MW00846707

Firestein & Kelley's Textbook of Rheumatology

Firestein & Kelley's Textbook of Rheumatology

ELEVENTH EDITION

Gary S. Firestein, MD

Distinguished Professor of Medicine
Dean and Associate Vice Chancellor
Clinical and Translational Research
University of California, San Diego School of Medicine
La Jolla, California

Ralph C. Budd, MD

University Distinguished Professor of Medicine and Microbiology and Molecular Genetics
Director
Vermont Center for Immunology and Infectious Diseases
The University of Vermont Larner College of Medicine
Burlington, Vermont

Sherine E. Gabriel, MD, MSc

President & The Robert C. and Naomi T. Borwell Presidential Professor
Rush University
Chief Academic Officer
Rush University System for Health
Chicago, Illinois

Gary A. Koretzky, MD, PhD

Professor of Medicine
Weill Cornell Medicine
Vice Provost for Academic Integration
Director, Cornell Center for Immunology
Cornell University
Ithaca, New York

Iain B. McInnes, CBE, PhD, FRCP, FRSE, FMedSci

Muirhead Professor of Medicine
Versus Arthritis Professor of Rheumatology
Director of Institute of Infection, Immunity, and Inflammation
College of Medical, Veterinary, and Life Sciences
University of Glasgow
Glasgow, United Kingdom

James R. O'Dell, MD, MACR, MACP

Stokes-Shackleford Professor and Vice Chair of Internal Medicine
University of Nebraska Medical Center
Chief of Rheumatology
Department of Medicine and Omaha Veterans Affairs
Omaha, Nebraska

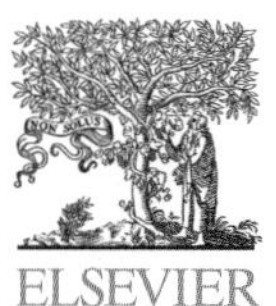

ELSEVIER

Elsevier
1600 John F. Kennedy Blvd.
Ste 1800
Philadelphia, PA 19103-2899

FIRESTEIN & KELLEY'S TEXTBOOK OF RHEUMATOLOGY, ELEVENTH EDITION ISBN: 978-0-323-63920-0

Volume 1 ISBN: 978-0-323-77639-4
Volume 2 ISBN: 978-0-323-77640-0

Notice

Practitioners and researchers must always rely on their own experience and knowledge in evaluating and using any information, methods, compounds or experiments described herein. Because of rapid advances in the medical sciences, in particular, independent verification of diagnoses and drug dosages should be made. To the fullest extent of the law, no responsibility is assumed by Elsevier, authors, editors or contributors for any injury and/or damage to persons or property as a matter of products liability, negligence or otherwise, or from any use or operation of any methods, products, instructions, or ideas contained in the material herein.

Previous editions copyrighted 2017, 2013, 2009, 2005, 2001, 1997, 1993, 1989, 1985, 1981.

Library of Congress Control Number: 2020939462

Senior Content Strategist: Nancy Anastasi Duffy
Senior Content Development Specialist: Anne Snyder
Publishing Services Manager: Catherine Jackson
Senior Project Manager: Daniel Fitzgerald
Designer: Margaret Reid

Printed in Canada

Last digit is the print number: 9 8 7 6 5 4 3 2 1

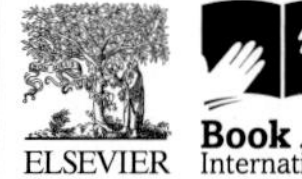
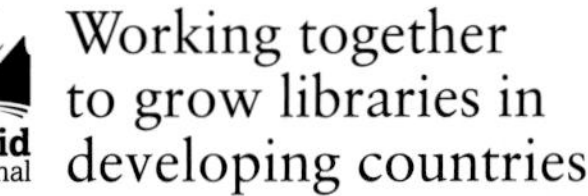

Sincerest thanks to my wonderful wife, Linda, and our children, David and Cathy, for their patience and support. Also, the editorial help of our two Cavalier King Charles dogs, Wrigley and Punkin, was invaluable.

Gary S. Firestein

Sincere thanks for the kind mentoring from Edward D. Harris, Jr., as well as for the support of my wife, Lenore, and my children, Graham and Laura.

Ralph C. Budd

To my three boys: my dear husband, Frank Cockerill, and our two wonderful sons, Richard and Matthew, for being my constant source of inspiration, love, and pride. And to my parents, Huda and Ezzat, for their love and tireless support.

Sherine E. Gabriel

My most sincere thanks to my many mentors, colleagues, and trainees who have taught me so much about medicine, rheumatology, and immunology. But none of my work would have been possible without the constant support of my wife, Kim, and daughter, Maya, who have always been at my side.

Gary A. Koretzky

To my wife, Karin, for her patience, understanding, and love, and to our wonderful girls, Megan and Rebecca, of whom I am so very proud and who continue to enlighten me.

Iain B. McInnes

Sincere thanks to my wife, Deb, for her patience and love, and to our wonderful children and grandchildren, who inspire me: Kim, Andy and Aiden, Jennie, Dan, Georgie and Niah, and Scott, Melissa, and Cecily. I also want to thank the members of my division, who continue to support me in all my efforts.

James R. O'Dell

The Textbook of Rheumatology *Editors also express gratitude and thanks to Linda Lyons Firestein, MD, who worked tirelessly to facilitate our organizational meetings and provided magnificent hospitality and sustenance throughout.*

Contributors

Steven B. Abramson, MD
Frederick H. King Professor of Internal Medicine
Chair
Department of Medicine
Professor of Medicine and Pathology
New York University Langone Medical Center
New York, New York
Pathogenesis of Osteoarthritis

Rohit Aggarwal, MD, MS
Associate Professor of Medicine
Division of Rheumatology and Clinical Immunology
University of Pittsburgh School of Medicine
Pittsburgh, Pennsylvania
Inflammatory Diseases of Muscle and Other Myopathies

Christine S. Ahn, MD, FAAD
Assistant Professor
Departments of Pathology and Dermatology
Wake Forest School of Medicine
Winston-Salem, North Carolina
Behçet's Disease

KaiNan An, PhD
Professor Emeritus
Department of Orthopedic Surgery
Mayo Clinic
Rochester, Minnesota
Biomechanics

Felipe Andrade, MD, PhD
Associate Professor of Medicine
Division of Rheumatology
The Johns Hopkins University School of Medicine
Baltimore, Maryland
Autoantibodies in Rheumatoid Arthritis

Stacy P. Ardoin, MD, MS
Associate Professor of Adult and Pediatric Rheumatology
Ohio State University
Nationwide Children's Hospital
Columbus, Ohio
Childhood-Onset Systemic Lupus Erythematosus, Drug-Induced Lupus in Children, and Neonatal Lupus

Abid Awisat, MD
Senior Physician
Rheumatology Unit
Bnai-Zion Medical Center
Haifa, Israel
Polyarteritis Nodosa and Related Disorders

Pedro Ming Azevedo, MD, PhD
Assistant Professor of Rheumatology
Evangelical University Hospital of Curitiba
Curitiba, Parana, Brazil
Rheumatic Fever and Post-streptococcal Arthritis

Fatima Barbar-Smiley, MD, MPH
Assistant Professor of Pediatrics
Pediatric Rheumatology
Nationwide Children's Hospital
Columbus, Ohio
Childhood-Onset Systemic Lupus Erythematosus, Drug-Induced Lupus in Children, and Neonatal Lupus

Medha Barbhaiya, MD, MPH
Assistant Attending Physician
Barbara Volcker Center for Women and Rheumatic Diseases
Hospital for Special Surgery
Assistant Professor of Medicine
Weill Cornell Medicine
New York, New York
Antiphospholipid Syndrome

Anne Barton, MBChB, MSc, PhD
Professor of Rheumatology
Centre for Musculoskeletal Research
The University of Manchester
Manchester, United Kingdom
Genetics of Rheumatic Diseases

Robert P. Baughman, MD
Professor of Medicine
Department of Internal Medicine
University of Cincinnati Medical Center
Cincinnati, Ohio
Sarcoidosis

Dorcas E. Beaton, BScOT, MSc, PhD
Senior Scientist
Institute for Work and Health
Affiliate Scientist
Li Ka Shing Knowledge Institute
St. Michael's Hospital
Associate Professor
Institute of Health Policy Management and Evaluation
University of Toronto
Toronto, Ontario, Canada
Assessment of Health Outcomes

Helen M. Beere, PhD
Department of Immunology
St. Jude Children's Research Hospital
Memphis, Tennessee
The Immunologic Repercussions of Cell Death

Edward M. Behrens, MD
Associate Professor
Pediatrics
Perelman School of Medicine at the University of Pennsylvania
Joseph Lee Hollander Chair of Pediatric Rheumatology
The Children's Hospital of Philadelphia
Philadelphia, Pennsylvania
Etiology and Pathogenesis of Juvenile Idiopathic Arthritis

Bonnie L. Bermas, MD
Professor of Medicine
Division of Rheumatology
University of Texas Southwestern Medical Center
Dallas, Texas
Pregnancy and Rheumatic Diseases

George Bertsias, MD, PhD
Assistant Professor in Rheumatology, Clinical Immunology, and Allergy
University of Crete Medical School
Iraklio, Greece
Treatment of Systemic Lupus Erythematosus

Meenakshi Bewtra, MD, MPH, PhD
Assistant Professor of Medicine and Epidemiology
Gastroenterology
Hospital of the University of Pennsylvania
Philadelphia, Pennsylvania
Inflammatory Bowel Disease–Associated Arthritis and Other Enteropathic Arthropathies

Nina Bhardwaj, MD, PhD
Director of Cancer Immunotherapy
Professor of Medicine
Ward-Coleman Chair in Cancer Research
The Tisch Cancer Institute
Icahn School of Medicine at Mount Sinai
New York, New York
Dendritic Cells

Clifton O. Bingham III, MD
Professor of Medicine
Division of Rheumatology
Johns Hopkins University School of Medicine
Baltimore, Maryland
Autoimmune Complications of Immune Checkpoint Inhibitors for Cancer

Linda K. Bockenstedt, MD
Harold W. Jockers Professor of Medicine
Internal Medicine/Rheumatology
Yale University School of Medicine
New Haven, Connecticut
Lyme Disease

Maarten Boers, MD, PhD, MSc
Professor of Clinical Epidemiology
Department of Epidemiology and Biostatistics
Amsterdam University Medical Centers, Vrije Universiteit
Staff Rheumatologist
Amsterdam Rheumatology and Immunology Center
Amsterdam University Medical Centers, Vrije Universiteit
Staff Rheumatologist
Reade Institute for Rehabilitation and Rheumatology
Amsterdam, Netherlands
Assessment of Health Outcomes

Eric Boilard, PhD
Full Professor
Immunity and Infectious Diseases
Universite Laval and CHU de Quebec
Quebec, Canada
Platelets and Megakaryocytes

Francesco Boin, MD
Professor of Medicine
Director
UCSF Scleroderma Center
University of California, San Francisco
San Francisco, California
Clinical Features and Treatment of Scleroderma

Dimitrios T. Boumpas, MD, FACP
Professor of Internal Medicine and Rheumatology
National and Kapodistrian University of Athens Medical School
"Attikon" University Hospital
Affiliated Investigator
Immunobiology
Biomedical Research Foundation of the Academy of Athens
Athens, Greece
Affiliated Investigator
Developmental and Functional Biology
Institute of Molecular Biology and Biotechnology—FORTH
Iraklio, Greece
Treatment of Systemic Lupus Erythematosus

Aline Bozec, PhD
Professor of Rheumatology and Immunology
Department of Internal Medicine 3
Friedrich Alexander Universität Erlangen-Nuremberg
Universitätsklinikum Erlangen
Erlangen, Germany
Biology, Physiology, and Morphology of Bone

Lori Broderick, MD, PhD
Assistant Professor
Pediatrics
University of California, San Diego
La Jolla, California
Pathogenesis of Inflammasome-Mediated Diseases

Matthew Brown, MBBS, MD, FRACP, FAHSM, FAA
Professor of Medicine
Director
Guy's and St Thomas' NHS Foundation Trust and King's College London NIHR Biomedical Research Centre
King's College London
London, United Kingdom
Ankylosing Spondylitis and Other Forms of Axial Spondyloarthritis

Christopher D. Buckley, MBBS, DPhil
Kennedy Professor of Translational Rheumatology
Rheumatology Research Group
Institute of Inflammation and Ageing
University of Birmingham
Birmingham, United Kingdom
Fibroblasts and Fibroblast-like Synoviocytes

Ralph C. Budd, MD
University Distinguished Professor of Medicine and Microbiology and Molecular Genetics
Director
Vermont Center for Immunology and Infectious Diseases
The University of Vermont Larner College of Medicine
Burlington, Vermont
T Lymphocytes

Nathalie Burg, MD
Assistant Professor
Division of Rheumatology
Weill Cornell Medicine
New York, New York
Neutrophils

Amy C. Cannella, MD, MS, RhMSUS
Associate Professor
Internal Medicine and Rheumatology
University of Nebraska Medical Center
Veterans Affairs Medical Center
Omaha, Nebraska
Ultrasound in Rheumatology
Traditional DMARDs: Methotrexate, Leflunomide, Sulfasalazine, Hydroxychloroquine, and Combination Therapies

Laura C. Cappelli, MD, MHS
Assistant Professor Medicine
Division of Rheumatology
Johns Hopkins School of Medicine
Baltimore, Maryland
Autoimmune Complications of Immune Checkpoint Inhibitors for Cancer

John D. Carter, MD
Professor of Medicine
Division of Rheumatology
University of South Florida Morsani School of Medicine
Tampa, Florida
Reactive Arthritis

Andrew C. Chan, MD, PhD
Genentech Research and Early Development
South San Francisco, California
Biomarkers in Rheumatology

Christopher Chang, MD, PhD, MBA
Clinical Professor of Medicine
Division of Rheumatology, Allergy and Clinical Immunology
University of California at Davis
Davis, California
Medical Director
Division of Pediatric Immunology and Allergy
Joe DiMaggio Children's Hospital
Hollywood, Florida
Osteonecrosis

Joseph S. Cheng, MD, MS
Frank H. Mayfield Professor and Chair
Department of Neurosurgery
University of Cincinnati College of Medicine
Cincinnati, Ohio
Neck Pain

Christopher P. Chiodo, MD
Chief
Foot and Ankle Division
Department of Orthopedic Surgery
Brigham and Women's Hospital
Boston, Massachusetts
Foot and Ankle Pain

Sharon A. Chung, MD, MAS
Associate Professor of Clinical Medicine
Division of Rheumatology
University of California, San Francisco
San Francisco, California
Anti-neutrophil Cytoplasmic Antibody–Associated Vasculitis

Leslie G. Cleland, MB BS, MD
Consultant Rheumatologist
Royal Adelaide Hospital
Clinical Professor
Department of Medicine
Adelaide University
Adelaide, South Australia, Australia
Nutrition and Rheumatic Diseases

Stanley Cohen, MD
Program Director
Rheumatology
Presbyterian Hospital
Clinical Professor
Internal Medicine
University of Texas Southwestern Medical School
Medical Director
Metroplex Clinical Research Center
Dallas, Texas
Intra-cellular Targeting Agents in Rheumatic Disease

Robert A. Colbert, MD, PhD
Senior Investigator
Clinical Director
National Institute of Arthritis, Musculoskeletal and Skin Diseases
National Institutes of Health
Bethesda, Maryland
Etiology and Pathogenesis of Spondyloarthritis

Paul P. Cook, MD, FACP, FIDSA
Professor of Medicine
Department of Medicine
Brody School of Medicine at East Carolina University
Greenville, North Carolina
Bacterial Arthritis

Joseph E. Craft, MD
Paul B. Beeson Professor of Medicine and Professor of Immunobiology, Internal Medicine and Immunobiology
Director
Investigative Medicine Program
Yale University School of Medicine
Attending in Rheumatology
Yale-New Haven Hospital
New Haven, Connecticut
Anti-nuclear Antibodies

Leslie J. Crofford, MD
Professor of Medicine
Director
Division of Rheumatology & Immunology
Vanderbilt University Medical Center
Nashville, Tennessee
Fibromyalgia
Therapeutic Targeting of Prostanoids

Bruce N. Cronstein, MD
Paul R. Esserman Professor of Medicine
Division of Rheumatology
New York University School of Medicine
New York, New York
Acute Phase Reactants

Mary K. Crow, MD
Physician-in-Chief
Chair
Department of Medicine
Benjamin M. Rosen Chair in Immunology and Inflammation Research
Hospital for Special Surgery
Chief
Division of Rheumatology
Joseph P. Routh Professor of Rheumatic Diseases in Medicine
Weill Cornell Medical College
New York, New York
Etiology and Pathogenesis of Systemic Lupus Erythematosus

Cynthia S. Crowson, PhD
Professor of Medicine and Biostatistics
Department of Health Sciences Research and Division of Rheumatology
Mayo Clinic
Rochester, Minnesota
Cardiovascular Risk in Inflammatory Rheumatic Disease

Sara J. Cuccurullo, MD
Clinical Professor and Chairman
Residency Program Director
Department of Physical Medicine and Rehabilitation
Hackensack Meridian School of Medicine at Seton Hall University
Rutgers Robert Wood Johnson Medical School
Vice President and Medical Director
JFK Johnson Rehabilitation Institute
Edison, New Jersey
Introduction to Physical Medicine and Rehabilitation

Gaye Cunnane, PhD, MB, FRCPI
Professor
Department of Medicine
Trinity College Dublin
Department of Rheumatology
St. James's Hospital
Dublin, Ireland
Relapsing Polychondritis
Hemochromatosis

Jeffrey R. Curtis, MD, MS, MPH
Harbert-Ball Professor of Medicine
Division of Clinical Immunology and Rheumatology
University of Alabama at Birmingham
Birmingham, Alabama
Clinical Research Methods in Rheumatic Disease

Nicola Dalbeth, MBChB, MD, FRACP
Professor and Rheumatologist
Department of Medicine
Faculty of Medical and Health Sciences
University of Auckland
Department of Rheumatology
Auckland District Health Board
Auckland, New Zealand
Clinical Features and Treatment of Gout

Maria Dall'Era, MD
Professor of Medicine
Medicine/Rheumatology
University of California San Francisco
San Francisco, California
Clinical Features of Systemic Lupus Erythematosus

Erika Darrah, PhD
Assistant Professor of Medicine
Division of Rheumatology
The Johns Hopkins University School of Medicine
Baltimore, Maryland
Autoantibodies in Rheumatoid Arthritis

Jonathan Dau, MD
Division of Rheumatology, Allergy, and Immunology
Massachusetts General Hospital
Boston, Massachusetts
Rheumatic Manifestations of HIV Infection

John M. Davis III, MD, MS
Associate Professor of Medicine
Division of Rheumatology
Mayo Clinic College of Medicine and Science
Rochester, Minnesota
History and Physical Examination of the Musculoskeletal System

Cosimo De Bari, MD, PhD, FRCP
Professor
Institute of Medical Sciences
University of Aberdeen
Aberdeen, United Kingdom
Regenerative Medicine and Tissue Engineering

Edward P. Debold, PhD
Associate Professor
Department of Kinesiology
University of Massachusetts
Amherst, Massachusetts
Muscle: Anatomy, Physiology, and Biochemistry

Francesco Dell'Accio, MD, PhD, FRCP
Professor
William Harvey Research Institute
Queen Mary, University of London
London, United Kingdom
Regenerative Medicine and Tissue Engineering

Paul J. DeMarco, MD, FACP, FACR, RhMSUS
Medical Director
The Center for Rheumatology and Bone Research
Arthritis and Rheumatism Associates PC
Wheaton, Maryland
Clinical Associate Professor of Medicine
Division of Rheumatology
Georgetown University School of Medicine
Washington, D.C.
Ultrasound in Rheumatology

Betty Diamond, MD
Professor
Center for Autoimmune, Musculoskeletal and Hematopoietic Diseases
Feinstein Institutes for Medical Research
Manhasset, New York
B Cells

Paul E. Di Cesare, MD
President
Di Cesare MD Consulting
Carlsbad, California
Pathogenesis of Osteoarthritis

Andrea di Matteo, MD
Rheumatology Unit
Department of Clinical and Molecular Sciences
Polytechnic University of Marche
Rheumatology Unit
Department of Clinical and Molecular Sciences
Ancona, Italy
Arthrocentesis and Injection of Joints and Soft Tissues

Rajiv Dixit, MD
Clinical Professor of Medicine
University of California, San Francisco
San Francisco, California
Director
Northern California Arthritis Center
Walnut Creek, California
Low Back Pain

Kenneth W. Donohue, MD
Assistant Professor
Department of Orthopaedic Surgery
Yale University
New Haven, Connecticut
Hand and Wrist Pain

Jeffrey Dvergsten, MD
Associate Professor of Pediatrics
Duke University School of Medicine
Durham, North Carolina
Juvenile Dermatomyositis, Scleroderma, Vasculitis, and Autoimmune Brain Disease

Hani S. El-Gabalawy, MD
Professor of Internal Medicine and Immunology
University of Manitoba
Winnipeg, Manitoba, Canada
Synovial Fluid Analyses, Synovial Biopsy, and Synovial Pathology

Bryant R. England, MD, PhD
Assistant Professor
Division of Rheumatology and Immunology
University of Nebraska Medical Center
Omaha, Nebraska
Clinical Features of Rheumatoid Arthritis

Doruk Erkan, MD
Associate Physician-Scientist
Barbara Volcker Center for Women and Rheumatic Diseases
Hospital for Special Surgery
Associate Professor of Medicine
Weill Cornell Medicine
New York, New York
Antiphospholipid Syndrome

Stephen Eyre, PhD
Professor
Centre for Musculoskeletal Research
The University of Manchester
Manchester, United Kingdom
Genetics of Rheumatic Diseases

Antonis Fanouriakis, MD
Rheumatology and Clinical Immunology
"Attikon" University Hospital
University of Athens
Athens, Greece
Treatment of Systemic Lupus Erythematosus

Ursula Fearon
Professor of Molecular Rheumatology
Trinity Biomedical Sciences Institute
Trinity College Dublin
The University of Dublin
Dublin, Ireland
Angiogenesis

Andrew Filer, MBChB, PhD
Reader in Translational Rheumatology
Institute of Inflammation and Ageing
The University of Birmingham
Honorary Consultant Rheumatologist
University Hospitals Birmingham NHS Foundation Trust
Birmingham, United Kingdom
Fibroblasts and Fibroblast-like Synoviocytes

David F. Fiorentino, MD, PhD
Professor
Department of Dermatology
Stanford University School of Medicine
Redwood City, California
Skin and Rheumatic Diseases

Gary S. Firestein, MD
Distinguished Professor of Medicine
Dean and Associate Vice Chancellor
Clinical and Translational Research
University of California, San Diego School of Medicine
La Jolla, California
Synovium
Etiology of Rheumatoid Arthritis
Pathogenesis of Rheumatoid Arthritis

Saloumeh K. Fischer, PhD
Department of BioAnalytical Sciences
Genentech Research and Early Development
South San Francisco, California
Biomarkers in Rheumatology

Felicity G. Fishman, MD
Assistant Professor
Department of Orthopaedic Surgery
Loyola University Medical Center
Maywood, Illinois
Hand and Wrist Pain

Oliver FitzGerald, MD, FRCPI, FRCP(UK)
Newman Clinical Research Professor
Rheumatology
St. Vincent's University Hospital and Conway Institute
University College Dublin
Dublin, Ireland
Psoriatic Arthritis

John P. Flaherty, MD
Professor of Medicine
Northwestern University Feinberg School of Medicine
Chicago, Illinois
Mycobacterial Infections of Bones and Joints
Fungal Infections of Bones and Joints

Cesar E. Fors Nieves, MD
Clinical Assistant Professor of Medicine
Division of Rheumatology
New York University School of Medicine
New York, New York
Acute Phase Reactants

Sherine E. Gabriel, MD, MSc
President & The Robert C. and Naomi T. Borwell Presidential Professor
Rush University
Chief Academic Officer
Rush University System for Health
Chicago, Illinois
Cardiovascular Risk in Inflammatory Rheumatic Disease

William Gallentine, MD
Professor
Pediatric Neurology and Epilepsy
Stanford University School of Medicine
Stanford, California
Juvenile Dermatomyositis, Scleroderma, Vasculitis, and Autoimmune Brain Disease

Philippe Gasque, PhD
Professor of Immunology
Immunology Laboratory Faculty of Medicine
University and CHU of La Réunion
St. Denis, Reunion Island, France
Viral Arthritis

Lianne S. Gensler, MD
Associate Professor of Medicine
Division of Rheumatology
University of California San Francisco
San Francisco, California
Ankylosing Spondylitis and Other Forms of Axial Spondyloarthritis

M. Eric Gershwin, MD
The Jack and Donald Chia Distinguished Professor of Medicine
Division of Rheumatology, Allergy and Clinical Immunology
University of California at Davis
Davis, California
Osteonecrosis

Mary B. Goldring, PhD
Senior Scientist
HSS Research Institute
Hospital for Special Surgery
Professor of Cell & Developmental Biology
Weill Cornell Graduate School of Medical Sciences
Weill Cornell Medical College
New York, New York
Cartilage and Chondrocytes

Steven R. Goldring, MD
Chief Scientific Officer Emeritus
Hospital for Special Surgery
Weill Cornell Medical College
New York, New York
Biology of the Normal Joint

Yvonne M. Golightly, PT, PhD
Assistant Professor of Epidemiology
University of North Carolina
Chapel Hill, North Carolina
Clinical Research Methods in Rheumatic Disease

Stuart Goodman, MD, PhD, FRCSC, FACS, FBSE, FICOR
Robert L. and Mary Ellenburg Professor of Surgery
Orthopaedic Surgery and (by courtesy) Bioengineering
Stanford University
Stanford, California
Hip and Knee Pain

Jonathan Graf, MD
Professor of Medicine
University of California San Francisco
Division of Rheumatology
Zuckerberg San Francisco General
San Francisco, California
Overlap Syndromes

Gerard Graham, PhD
Professor of Molecular and Structural Immunology
Institute of Infection, Immunity and Inflammation
University of Glasgow
Glasgow, Scotland, United Kingdom
Chemokines and Cellular Recruitment

Douglas R. Green, PhD
Peter C. Doherty Endowed Chair of Immunology
Department of Immunology
St. Jude Children's Research Hospital
Memphis, Tennessee
The Immunologic Repercussions of Cell Death

Adam Greenspan, MD, FACR
Professor of Radiology and Orthopedic Surgery
Section of Musculoskeletal Imaging
Department of Radiology
University of California Davis Health
Sacramento, California
Osteonecrosis

Christine Grimaldi, PhD
Director Biotherapeutic Bioanalysis
Drug Metabolism & Pharmacokinetics
Boehringer Ingelheim Pharmaceuticals, Inc.
Ridgefield, Connecticut
B Cells

Anika Grüneboom, PhD
Department of Internal Medicine 3—Rheumatology and Immunology
Friedrich Alexander Universität Erlangen-Nuremberg
Universitätsklinikum Erlangen
Erlangen, Germany
Biology, Physiology, and Morphology of Bone

Luiza Guilherme, PhD
Professor of Immunology
Heart Institute—InCor
University of São Paulo School of Medicine
Institute for Immunology Investigation
National Institute for Science and Technology
São Paulo, Brazil
Rheumatic Fever and Post-streptococcal Arthritis

Xavier Guillot, MD, PhD
Rheumatology Clinical Board
CHU of La Réunion
St. Denis, Reunion Island, France
Viral Arthritis

Rebecca Haberman, MD
Clinical Instructor of Medicine
Division of Rheumatology
New York University School of Medicine
New York, New York
Acute Phase Reactants

Rula A. Hajj-Ali, MD
Professor
Cleveland Clinic Lerner College of Medicine of Case Western Reserve University
Cleveland Clinic
Cleveland, Ohio
Primary Angiitis of the Central Nervous System

Dominik R. Haudenschild, PhD
Associate Professor
Department of Orthopaedic Surgery
University of California at Davis
Sacramento, California
Pathogenesis of Osteoarthritis

David B. Hellmann, MD
Vice Dean and Chairman
Department of Medicine
Johns Hopkins Bayview Medical Center
Baltimore, Maryland
Giant Cell Arteritis, Polymyalgia Rheumatica, and Takayasu's Arteritis

Hal M. Hoffman, MD
Professor
Pediatrics and Medicine
University of California, San Diego
La Jolla, California
Division Chief
Pediatric Allergy, Immunology, Rheumatology
Rady Children's Hospital San Diego
San Diego, California
Pathogenesis of Inflammasome-Mediated Diseases

V. Michael Holers, MD
Professor of Medicine and Immunology
Division of Rheumatology
University of Colorado School of Medicine
Aurora, Colorado
Complement System

Rikard Holmdahl, MD, PhD
Professor of Medical
Biochemistry and Biophysics
Karolinska Institute
Stockholm, Sweden
Experimental Models for Rheumatoid Arthritis

Joyce J. Hsu, MD, MS
Clinical Associate Professor
Pediatric Rheumatology
Stanford University School of Medicine
Stanford, California
Clinical Features and Treatment of Juvenile Idiopathic Arthritis

James I. Huddleston, III, MD
Associate Professor of Orthopaedic Surgery
Department of Orthopaedic Surgery
Stanford University Medical Center
Stanford, California
Hip and Knee Pain

Alan P. Hudson, PhD
Professor Emeritus
Immunology and Microbiology
Wayne State University School of Medicine
Detroit, Michigan
Reactive Arthritis

Gene G. Hunder, MS, MD
Professor of Medicine
Emeritus Staff Center
Mayo Clinic College of Medicine and Science
Rochester, Minnesota
History and Physical Examination of the Musculoskeletal System

Yoshifumi Itoh, PhD
Associate Professor
Kennedy Institute of Rheumatology
University of Oxford
Oxford, United Kingdom
Proteinases and Matrix Degradation

Johannes W.G. Jacobs, MD, PhD
Associate Professor of Rheumatology
Department of Rheumatology & Clinical Immunology
University Medical Center Utrecht
Utrecht, Netherlands
Glucocorticoid Therapy

Jacob L. Jaremko, MD, PhD, FRCPC
Associate Professor of Radiology
Department of Radiology and Diagnostic Imaging
University of Alberta
Alberta, Edmonton, Canada
Imaging in Rheumatic Diseases

Matlock A. Jeffries, MD
Assistant Professor
Department of Internal Medicine
Division of Rheumatology, Immunology, and Allergy
University of Oklahoma Health Sciences Center
Adjunct Assistant Member
Arthritis & Clinical Immunology Program
Oklahoma Medical Research Foundation
Oklahoma City, Oklahoma
Epigenetics of Rheumatic Diseases

Ho Jen, MD, FRCPC
Associate Clinical Professor of Radiology
Department of Radiology and Diagnostic Imaging
Division of Nuclear Medicine
University of Alberta
Alberta, Edmonton, Canada
Imaging in Rheumatic Diseases

Jaclyn Joki, MD
Attending Physician
Department of Physical Medicine and Rehabilitation
JFK Johnson Rehabilitation Institute
Clinical Assistant Professor
Rutgers Robert Wood Johnson Medical School
Assistant Professor
Hackensack Meridian School of Medicine at Seton Hall University
Edison, New Jersey
Introduction to Physical Medicine and Rehabilitation

Martha S. Jordan, PhD
Research Associate Professor
Pathology and Laboratory Medicine
Perelman School of Medicine
University of Pennsylvania
Philadelphia, Pennsylvania
Adaptive Immunity

Joseph L. Jorizzo, MD
Professor, Former and Founding Chair
Department of Dermatology
Wake Forest University School of Medicine
Winston-Salem, North Carolina
Professor of Clinical Dermatology
Weill Cornell Medical College
New York, New York
Behçet's Disease

Jorge Kalil, MD
Professor
Clinical Immunology and Allergy
Faculdade de Medicina Universidade de São Paulo
São Paulo, Brazil
Rheumatic Fever and Post-streptococcal Arthritis

Kenton R. Kaufman, PhD, PE
W. Hall Wendel, Jr., Musculoskeletal Research Professor
Director
Motion Analysis Laboratory
Professor of Biomedical Engineering
Mayo Clinic
Rochester, Minnesota
Biomechanics

Arthur Kavanaugh, MD
Professor of Medicine
Center for Innovative Therapy
Division of Rheumatology, Allergy, and Immunology
University of California, San Diego School of Medicine
La Jolla, California
Anti-cytokine Therapies

Robert T. Keenan
Associate Professor of Medicine
Vice Chief for Clinical Affairs
Division of Rheumatology
Duke University School of Medicine
Durham, North Carolina
Etiology and Pathogenesis of Hyperuricemia and Gout

Tony Kenna, PhD
Associate Professor
Queensland University of Technology
Institute of Health and Biomedical Innovation
Brisbane, Queensland, Australia
Ankylosing Spondylitis and Other Forms of Axial Spondyloarthritis

Darcy A. Kerr, MD
Assistant Professor of Pathology and Laboratory Medicine
Geisel School of Medicine at Dartmouth
Hanover, New Hampshire
Dartmouth-Hitchcock Medical Center
Lebanon, New Hampshire
Tumors and Tumor-like Lesions of Joints and Related Structures

Eugene Y. Kissin, MD, RhMSUS
Associate Professor of Medicine
Rheumatology
Boston University Medical Center
Boston, Massachusetts
Ultrasound in Rheumatology

Rob Knight, PhD
Professor
Departments of Pediatrics, Bioengineering, and Computer Science and Engineering
University of California, San Diego
La Jolla, California
The Microbiome in Health and Disease

Dwight H. Kono, MD
Professor of Immunology
Department of Immunology and Microbiology
The Scripps Research Institute
La Jolla, California
Autoimmunity and Tolerance

Gary A. Koretzky, MD, PhD
Professor of Medicine
Weill Cornell Medicine
Vice Provost for Academic Integration
Director, Cornell Center for Immunology
Cornell University
Ithaca, New York
Adaptive Immunity

Peter Korsten, MD
Rheumatologist
Department of Nephrology and Rheumatology
University Medical Center Göttingen
Göttingen, Germany
Sarcoidosis

Jennifer Kosty, MD
Assistant Professor
Department of Neurosurgery
Ochsner LSU Health Sciences Center
Shreveport, Louisiana
Neck Pain

Deborah Krakow, MD
Professor of Orthopaedic Surgery, Human Genetics, Pediatrics, and Obstetrics and Gynecology
David Geffen School of Medicine
University of California, Los Angeles
Los Angeles, California
Heritable Diseases of Connective Tissue

Deepak Kumar, PT, PHD
Assistant Professor
Physical Therapy and Athletic Training
Boston University
Assistant Professor
Boston University School of Medicine
Boston, Massachusetts
Treatment of Osteoarthritis

Helen J. Lachmann, MA, MBBChir, MD, FRCP, FRCPath
National Amyloidosis Centre
Royal Free Hospital London NHS Foundation Trust and University College Medical School
London, United Kingdom
Amyloidosis

Floris P.J.G. Lafeber, PhD
Professor
Department of Rheumatology & Clinical Immunology
University Medical Center Utrecht
Utrecht University
Utrecht, Netherlands
Hemophilic Arthropathy

Robert G.W. Lambert, MB, FRCR, FRCPC
Professor of Radiology
Department of Radiology and Diagnostic Imaging
University of Alberta
Alberta, Edmonton, Canada
Imaging in Rheumatic Diseases

Nancy E. Lane, MD
Distinguished Professor of Medicine, Rheumatology, Aging
Director of Center for Musculoskeletal Health
Department of Internal Medicine
UC Davis Health
UC Davis School of Medicine
Sacramento, California
Metabolic Bone Disease

Carol A. Langford, MD, MHS, FACP
Director
Center for Vasculitis Care and Research
Harold C. Schott Chair in Rheumatic and Immunologic Diseases
Cleveland Clinic
Associate Professor of Medicine
Cleveland Clinic Lerner College of Medicine of Case Western Reserve University
Cleveland, Ohio
Primary Angiitis of the Central Nervous System

Daniel M. Laskin, DDS, MS
Professor and Chairman Emeritus
Oral and Maxillofacial Surgery
Virginia Commonwealth University Schools of Dentistry and Medicine
Richmond, Virginia
Temporomandibular Joint Pain

Gregoire Lauvau, PhD
Professor
Department of Microbiology and Immunology
Albert Einstein College of Medicine
Bronx, New York
Innate Immunity

Tzielan C. Lee, MD
Clinical Associate Professor
Pediatric Rheumatology
Stanford University School of Medicine
Stanford, California
Clinical Features and Treatment of Juvenile Idiopathic Arthritis

David L. Leverenz, MD
Assistant Professor of Medicine
Division of Rheumatology and Immunology
Duke University Medical Center
Durham, North Carolina
Sjögren's Syndrome

Richard F. Loeser, MD
Herman and Louise Smith Distinguished Professor
Medicine
Division of Rheumatology, Allergy, and Immunology
Director
Thurston Arthritis Research Center
University of North Carolina
Chapel Hill, North Carolina
Cartilage and Chondrocytes

Carlos J. Lozada, MD
Professor of Clinical Medicine
Division of Rheumatology
University of Miami Miller School of Medicine
Miami, Florida
Rheumatic Manifestations of Hemoglobinopathies

Ofure Luke, MD
Attending Physician
Department of Physical Medicine and Rehabilitation
JFK Johnson Rehabilitation Institute
Assistant Professor
Hackensack Meridian School of Medicine at Seton Hall University
Edison, New Jersey
Introduction to Physical Medicine and Rehabilitation

Ingrid E. Lundberg, MD, PhD
Professor of Rheumatology
Division of Rheumatology
Department of Medicine, Solna, Karolinska Institutet
Stockholm, Sweden
Inflammatory Diseases of Muscle and Other Myopathies

Raashid Luqmani, BMedSci, BM, BS, DM, FRCP, FRCPE
Professor of Rheumatology
Nuffield Department of Orthopaedics, Rheumatology and Musculoskeletal Science
University of Oxford
Consultant Rheumatologist
Rheumatology Department
Nuffield Orthopaedic Centre
Oxford, United Kingdom
Polyarteritis Nodosa and Related Disorders

Frank P. Luyten, MD
Professor of Rheumatology
University Hospitals Leuven
Leuven, Belgium
Regenerative Medicine and Tissue Engineering

Reuven Mader, MD
Head
Rheumatic Diseases Unit
Ha'Emek Medical Center
Afula, Israel
Associate Clinical Professor, Emeritus
The B. Rappaport Faculty of Medicine
The Technion Institute of Technology
Haifa, Israel
Proliferative Bone Diseases

Conor Magee, MB BAO BCh
Rheumatology
St. Vincent's University Hospital and Conway Institute
University College Dublin
Dublin, Ireland
Psoriatic Arthritis

Walter P. Maksymowych, FRCP(C)
Professor of Medicine
Division of Rheumatology
University of Alberta
Edmonton, Alberta, Canada
Ankylosing Spondylitis and Other Forms of Axial Spondyloarthritis

Bernhard Manger, MD
Professor of Rheumatology and Immunology
Department of Internal Medicine 3
Friedrich-Alexander-Universität Erlangen-Nürnberg
Erlangen, Germany
Rheumatic Paraneoplastic Syndromes—Links Between Malignancy and Autoimmunity

Joseph A. Markenson, MD, MS
Professor of Clinical Medicine
Medicine/Rheumatology
Joan and Sanford Weill Medical College of Cornell University
Attending Physician
Rheumatology/Medicine
Hospital for Special Surgery
New York, New York
Arthritis Accompanying Endocrine and Metabolic Disorders

Scott David Martin, MD
Associate Professor of Orthopedics
Harvard Medical School
Director of Joint Preservation Service
Massachusetts General Hospital
Boston, Massachusetts
Shoulder Pain

Eric L. Matteson, MD, MPH
Professor of Medicine
Divisions of Rheumatology and Epidemiology
Mayo Clinic College of Medicine
Rochester, Minnesota
Cancer Risk in Rheumatic Diseases

Lara Maxwell, PhD, MSc
Managing Editor
Cochrane Musculoskeletal Group
University of Ottawa
Senior Methodologist
OMERACT, Ottawa
Ottawa, Ontario, Canada
Assessment of Health Outcomes

Katharine McCarthy, PharmD, BCACP
Clinical Pharmacist
University of Rochester Medical Center
Rochester, New York
Anti-cytokine Therapies

Iain B. McInnes, CBE, PhD, FRCP, FRSE, FMedSci
Muirhead Professor of Medicine
Versus Arthritis Professor of Rheumatology
Director of Institute of Infection, Immunity, and Inflammation
College of Medical, Veterinary, and Life Sciences
University of Glasgow
Glasgow, United Kingdom
Cytokines

Peter A. Merkel, MD, MPH
Chief of Rheumatology
Department of Medicine
Professor
Department of Medicine
Department of Biostatistics, Epidemiology, and Informatics
University of Pennsylvania
Philadelphia, Pennsylvania
Classification and Epidemiology of Systemic Vasculitis

Ted R. Mikuls, MD, MSPH
Umbach Professor of Rheumatology
Department of Internal Medicine
Division of Rheumatology and Immunology
University of Nebraska Medical Center
Omaha, Nebraska
Urate-Lowering Therapy
Clinical Features of Rheumatoid Arthritis

Mark S. Miller, PhD
Assistant Professor
Department of Kinesiology
University of Massachusetts
Amherst, Massachusetts
Muscle: Anatomy, Physiology, and Biochemistry

Devyani Misra, MD, MS
Divisions of Gerontology and Rheumatology
Beth Israel Deaconess Medical Center
Harvard Medical School
Boston, Massachusetts
Treatment of Osteoarthritis

Ali Mobasheri, BSc ARCS (Hons), MSc, DPhil (Oxon)
Professor of Musculoskeletal Biology
Research Unit of Medical Imaging, Physics and Technology
Faculty of Medicine
University of Oulu
Oulu, Finland
Senior Research Scientist
Department of Regenerative Medicine
State Research Institute Centre for Innovative Medicine
Vilnius, Lithuania
Centre for Sport, Exercise and Osteoarthritis Research Versus Arthritis
Queen's Medical Centre
Nottingham, United Kingdom
Cartilage and Chondrocytes

Kevin G. Moder, MD
Associate Professor of Medicine
Division of Rheumatology
Mayo Clinic College of Medicine and Science
Rochester, Minnesota
History and Physical Examination of the Musculoskeletal System

Paul A. Monach, MD, PhD
Lecturer
Division of Rheumatology, Inflammation, and Immunity
Brigham and Women's Hospital
Chief
Rheumatology Section
VA Boston Healthcare System
Boston, Massachusetts
Anti-neutrophil Cytoplasmic Antibody–Associated Vasculitis

Anna Montgomery, DPhil
Division of Rheumatology
Northwestern University Feinberg School of Medicine
Chicago, Illinois
Mononuclear Phagocytes

Vaishali R. Moulton, MD, PhD
Assistant Professor
Department of Medicine
Division of Rheumatology and Clinical Immunology
Beth Israel Deaconess Medical Center
Harvard Medical School
Boston, Massachusetts
Principles of Signaling

Catharina M. Mulders-Manders, MD
Department of Internal Medicine
Section Infectious Diseases
Radboud Expertise Centre for Immunodeficiency and Autoinflammation
Radboud University Medical Center
Nijmegen, Netherlands
Familial Autoinflammatory Syndromes

Luciana Ribeiro Muniz, PhD
Hematology and Oncology
Icahn School of Medicine at Mount Sinai
New York, New York
Dendritic Cells

Louise B. Murphy, PhD
Division of Population Health
Centers for Disease Control and Prevention
Atlanta, Georgia
Economic Impact of Arthritis and Rheumatic Conditions

Kanneboyina Nagaraju, DVM, PhD
Professor and Founding Chair
Pharmaceutical Sciences
School of Pharmacy and Pharmaceutical Sciences
Binghamton, New York
Inflammatory Diseases of Muscle and Other Myopathies

Rani Nasser, MD
Assistant Professor
Department of Neurosurgery
University of Cincinnati College of Medicine
Cincinnati, Ohio
Neck Pain

Amanda E. Nelson, MD, MSCR
Associate Professor of Medicine
Division of Rheumatology, Allergy, and Immunology
Thurston Arthritis Research Center
University of North Carolina at Chapel Hill
Chapel Hill, North Carolina
Clinical Features of Osteoarthritis

Tuhina Neogi, MD, PhD, FRCPC
Professor of Medicine
Rheumatology
Boston University School of Medicine
Professor of Epidemiology
Boston University School of Public Health
Boston, Massachusetts
Treatment of Osteoarthritis

Peter A. Nigrovic, MD
Associate Professor of Medicine
Harvard Medical School
Staff Pediatric Rheumatologist
Division of Immunology
Boston Children's Hospital
Director
Center for Adults with Pediatric Rheumatic Illness
Division of Rheumatology, Inflammation and Immunity, Brigham and Women's Hospital
Boston, Massachusetts
Mast Cells
Platelets and Megakaryocytes

James R. O'Dell, MD, MACR, MACP
Stokes-Shackleford Professor and Vice Chair of Internal Medicine
University of Nebraska Medical Center
Chief of Rheumatology
Department of Medicine and Omaha Veterans Affairs
Omaha, Nebraska
Traditional DMARDs: Methotrexate, Leflunomide, Sulfasalazine, Hydroxychloroquine, and Combination Therapies
Treatment of Rheumatoid Arthritis

Alexis Ogdie, MD, MSCE
Associate Professor of Medicine and Epidemiology
Rheumatology
Hospital of the University of Pennsylvania
Philadelphia, Pennsylvania
Inflammatory Bowel Disease–Associated Arthritis and Other Enteropathic Arthropathies

Mikkel Østergaard, MD, PhD
DMSc Professor of Rheumatology
Copenhagen Center for Arthritis Research
Center for Rheumatology and Spine Diseases
Rigshospitalet, Glostrup
Department of Clinical Medicine
University of Copenhagen
Copenhagen, Denmark
Imaging in Rheumatic Diseases

Michael A. Paley
Rheumatology Division
Department of Medicine
Washington University School of Medicine
St. Louis, Missouri
Innate Lymphoid Cells and Natural Killer Cells

Richard S. Panush, MD
Professor of Medicine
Division of Rheumatology
Keck School of Medicine
University of Southern California
Los Angeles, California
Occupational and Recreational Musculoskeletal Disorders

Stanford L. Peng, MD, PhD
Rheumatology
Swedish Community Specialty Clinic
Swedish Medical Center
Seattle, Washington
Anti-nuclear Antibodies

Harris Perlman, PhD
Chief of Rheumatology
Professor of Medicine
Mabel Greene Myers Professor of Medicine
Division of Rheumatology
Northwestern University Feinberg School of Medicine
Chicago, Illinois
Mononuclear Phagocytes

Shiv Pillai, MD, PhD
Professor of Medicine
Ragon Institute of MGH, MIT and Harvard
Harvard Medical School
Cambridge, Massachusetts
IgG_4-Related Disease

Michael H. Pillinger, MD
Professor of Medicine and Biochemistry and Molecular Pharmacology
Director
Rheumatology Training
Director
Masters of Science in Clinical Investigation Program
New York University School of Medicine
Section Chief
Rheumatology
New York Harbor Health Care System–NY Campus
Department of Veterans Affairs
New York, New York
Neutrophils
Etiology and Pathogenesis of Hyperuricemia and Gout

Gregory R. Polston, MD
Clinical Professor
Anesthesiology
University of California, San Diego
La Jolla, California
Analgesic Agents in Rheumatic Disease

Steven A. Porcelli, MD
Murray and Evelyne Weinstock Chair in Microbiology and Immunology
Department of Microbiology and Immunology
Albert Einstein College of Medicine
Bronx, New York
Innate Immunity

Mark D. Price, MD, PhD
Department of Orthopedic Surgery
Massachusetts General Hospital
Boston, Massachusetts
Foot and Ankle Pain

Astrid E. Pulles, MD
Department of Rheumatology & Clinical Immunology
Van Creveldkliniek
University Medical Center Utrecht
Utrecht University
Utrecht, Netherlands
Hemophilic Arthropathy

Karim Raza, FRCP, PhD
Professor of Rheumatology supported by Versus Arthritis
College of Medical and Dental Sciences
University of Birmingham
Honorary Consultant Rheumatologist
Sandwell and West Birmingham Hospitals NHS Trust
Birmingham, United Kingdom
Evaluation and Management of Early Undifferentiated Arthritis

Virginia Reddy, MD
Staff Physician
Division of Rheumatology
Texas Health Dallas
Dallas, Texas
Intra-cellular Targeting Agents in Rheumatic Disease

Ann M. Reed, MD
Professor and Chair
Department of Pediatrics
Duke University
Durham, North Carolina
Juvenile Dermatomyositis, Scleroderma, Vasculitis, and Autoimmune Brain Disease

John D. Reveille, MD
Professor
Division of Rheumatology
University of Texas Health Science Center at Houston
Houston, Texas
Rheumatic Manifestations of HIV Infection

Rennie L. Rhee, MD, MSCE
Assistant Professor of Medicine
Medicine/Rheumatology
University of Pennsylvania
Philadelphia, Pennsylvania
Classification and Epidemiology of Systemic Vasculitis

Christopher T. Ritchlin, MD, MPH
Professor of Medicine
Center for Musculoskeletal Research
University of Rochester Medical Center
Rochester, New York
Anti-cytokine Therapies

Angela B. Robinson, MD, MPH
Associate Professor
Pediatrics Institute
Cleveland Clinic Foundation
Cleveland, Ohio
Juvenile Dermatomyositis, Scleroderma, Vasculitis, and Autoimmune Brain Disease

Antony Rosen, MB, ChB, BSc (Hons)
Mary Betty Stevens Professor of Medicine
Professor of Pathology
Director
Division of Rheumatology
The Johns Hopkins University School of Medicine
Baltimore, Maryland
Autoantibodies in Rheumatoid Arthritis

James T. Rosenbaum, AB, MD
Professor of Ophthalmology, Medicine, and Cell Biology
Oregon Health and Science University
Chair of Ophthalmology Emeritus
Legacy Devers Eye Institute
Portland, Oregon
The Eye and Rheumatic Diseases

Andrew E. Rosenberg, MD
Vice Chair
Director of Bone and Soft Tissue Pathology
Department of Pathology
University of Miami Miller School of Medicine
Miami, Florida
Tumors and Tumor-like Lesions of Joints and Related Structures

Eric M. Ruderman, MD
Professor of Medicine/Rheumatology
Northwestern University Feinberg School of Medicine
Chicago, Illinois
Mycobacterial Infections of Bones and Joints
Fungal Infections of Bones and Joints

Kenneth G. Saag, MD, MSc
Jane Knight Lowe Professor of Medicine
Division of Clinical Immunology and Rheumatology
University of Alabama at Birmingham
Birmingham, Alabama
Clinical Research Methods in Rheumatic Disease
Bisphosphonates

Jane E. Salmon, MD
Collette Kean Research Chair
Medicine-Rheumatology
Hospital for Special Surgery
Professor of Medicine
Weill Cornell Medicine
New York, New York
Antiphospholipid Syndrome

Lisa R. Sammaritano, MD
Associate Professor of Clinical Medicine
Rheumatology
Hospital for Special Surgery
Weill Cornell Medicine
New York, New York
Pregnancy and Rheumatic Diseases

Jonathan Samuels, MD
Associate Professor of Medicine
Division of Rheumatology
NYU Langone Health
New York, New York
Pathogenesis of Osteoarthritis

Christy I. Sandborg, MD
Professor
Pediatric Rheumatology
Stanford University School of Medicine
Stanford, California
Clinical Features and Treatment of Juvenile Idiopathic Arthritis

Adam P. Sangeorzan, MD
Department of Orthopedic Surgery
Brigham and Women's Hospital
Boston, Massachusetts
Foot and Ankle Pain

Arthur C. Santora II, MD, PhD
Clinical Associate Professor
Division of Endocrinology, Metabolism and Nutrition
Rutgers Robert Wood Johnson School of Medicine
New Brunswick, New Jersey
Chief Medical Officer
Entera Bio Ltd.
Jerusalem, Israel
Bisphosphonates

Sebastian E. Sattui, MD
Hospital for Special Surgery
Weill-Cornell Medical School
New York, New York
Arthritis Accompanying Endocrine and Metabolic Disorders

Amr H. Sawalha, MD
Chief
Division of Pediatric Rheumatology
Director
Comprehensive Lupus Center of Excellence
University of Pittsburgh Children's Hospital of Pittsburgh
Pittsburgh, Pennsylvania
Epigenetics of Rheumatic Diseases

Amit Saxena, MD
Assistant Professor of Medicine
Division of Rheumatology
New York University School of Medicine
New York, New York
Acute Phase Reactants

Mansi Saxena, PhD
Associate Director
Vaccine and Cellular Therapy Laboratory
Hematology and Oncology
Icahn School of Medicine at Mount Sinai
New York, New York
Dendritic Cells

Carla R. Scanzello, MD, PhD
Section Chief
Rheumatology
Corporal Michael J. Crescenz VA Medical Center
Assistant Professor of Medicine
Medicine/Rheumatology
University of Pennsylvania
Philadelphia, Pennsylvania
Biology of the Normal Joint

Georg Schett, MD
Professor of Rheumatology and Immunology
Department of Internal Medicine 3
Friedrich Alexander Universität Erlangen-Nuremberg
Universitätsklinikum Erlangen
Erlangen, Germany
Biology, Physiology, and Morphology of Bone
Rheumatic Paraneoplastic Syndromes—Links Between Malignancy and Autoimmunity

Anne Grete Semb, MD, PhD
Consultant Cardiologist
Senior Researcher
Preventive Cardio-Rheuma Clinic
Department of Rheumatology
Diakonhjemmet Hospital
Oslo, Norway
Cardiovascular Risk in Inflammatory Rheumatic Disease

Ami A. Shah, MD, MHS
Associate Professor of Medicine
Division of Rheumatology
Johns Hopkins University School of Medicine
Baltimore, Maryland
Autoimmune Complications of Immune Checkpoint Inhibitors for Cancer

Binita Shah, MD, MS
Assistant Professor of Medicine
Division of Cardiology
New York University School of Medicine
New York, New York
Neutrophils

Faye A. Sharpley, MA, MSc, MBBChir, MRCP, FRCPATH
National Amyloidosis Centre
Royal Free Hospital London NHS Foundation Trust and University College Medical
School London, United Kingdom
Amyloidosis

Keith A. Sikora, MD
Assistant Clinical Investigator
National Institute of Arthritis, Musculoskeletal and Skin Diseases
National Institutes of Health
Bethesda, Maryland
Etiology and Pathogenesis of Spondyloarthritis

Anna Simon, MD, PhD
Associate Professor
Department of Internal Medicine
Section Infectious Diseases
Radboudumc Expertise Centre for Immunodeficiency and Autoinflammation
Radboud University Medical Center
Nijmegen, Netherlands
Familial Autoinflammatory Syndromes

Dawd S. Siraj, MD, MPH&TM, FIDSA, CTropMed
Professor of Medicine
Associate Program Director
Infectious Diseases Fellowship
Director
Global Health Pathway, Department of IM
Director
International Travel Clinic
Division of Infectious Diseases
University of Wisconsin-Madison
Madison, Wisconsin
Bacterial Arthritis

Linda S. Sorkin, PhD
Professor Emerita
Anesthesiology
University of California, San Diego
La Jolla, California
Neuronal Regulation of Pain and Inflammation

E. William St. Clair, MD
W. Lester Brooks, Jr. Professor of Medicine
Professor of Immunology
Chief
Division of Rheumatology and Immunology
Duke University Medical Center
Durham, North Carolina
Sjögren's Syndrome

Lisa K. Stamp, MBChB, FRACP, PhD
Professor
Department of Medicine
University of Otago, Christchurch
Christchurch, New Zealand
Nutrition and Rheumatic Diseases

John H. Stone, MD, MPH
Professor of Medicine
Harvard Medical School
Director
Clinical Rheumatology
Massachusetts General Hospital
Boston, Massachusetts
Immune Complex–Mediated Small Vessel Vasculitis
IgG_4-Related Disease

Lindsay C. Strowd, MD
Assistant Professor
Department of Dermatology
Wake Forest University School of Medicine
Winston-Salem, North Carolina
Behçet's Disease

Abel Suarez-Fueyo, PhD
Division of Rheumatology and Clinical Immunology
Department of Medicine
Beth Israel Deaconess Medical Center
Harvard Medical School
Boston, Massachusetts
Principles of Signaling

Camilla I. Svensson, MS, PhD
Professor
Physiology and Pharmacology
Karolinska Institutet
Stockholm, Sweden
Adjunct Associate Professor
Anesthesiology
University of California, San Diego
La Jolla, California
Neuronal Regulation of Pain and Inflammation

Nadera J. Sweiss, MD
Professor of Medicine
Division of Rheumatology
University of Illinois at Chicago
Chicago, Illinois
Sarcoidosis

Carrie R. Swigart, MD
Associated Professor of Orthopaedics and Rehabilitation
Yale University School of Medicine
New Haven, Connecticut
Hand and Wrist Pain

Zoltán Szekanecz, MD, PhD, DSc
Professor of Rheumatology, Immunology, and Medicine
University of Debrecen Faculty of Medicine,
Division of Rheumatology
Debrecen, Hungary
Angiogenesis

Stephen Tait, PhD
Cancer Research UK Beatson Institute
Institute of Cancer Sciences
University of Glasgow
Glasgow, United Kingdom
Metabolic Regulation of Immunity

Stacy Tanner, MD
Staff Clinician
Rheumatology
University of Manitoba
Winnipeg, Manitoba, Canada
Synovial Fluid Analyses, Synovial Biopsy, and Synovial Pathology

Peter C. Taylor, MA, PhD, FRCP
Professor of Musculoskeletal Sciences
Botnar Research Centre
Nuffield Department of Orthopaedics, Rheumatology and Musculoskeletal Sciences
University of Oxford
Oxford, United Kingdom
Cell-Targeted Biologics and Emerging Targets: Rituximab, Abatacept, and Other Biologics

William J. Taylor, MBChB, PhD, FRACP, FAFRM (RACP)
Associate Professor
Department of Medicine
University of Otago, Wellington
Wellington, New Zealand
Ankylosing Spondylitis and Other Forms of Axial Spondyloarthritis

Robert Terkeltaub, MD
Chief
Rheumatology Section
Veterans Affairs Healthcare System
Professor of Medicine
Division of Rheumatology, Allergy, and Immunology
University of California, San Diego
La Jolla, California
Calcium Crystal Disease: Calcium Pyrophosphate Dihydrate and Basic Calcium Phosphate

Argyrios N. Theofilopoulos, MD
Professor
Department of Immunology and Microbiology
The Scripps Research Institute
La Jolla, California
Autoimmunity and Tolerance

Thomas S. Thornhill, MD
Chairman Emeritus
Department of Orthopedic Surgery
Brigham and Women's Hospital
John B. and Buckminster Brown Professor of Orthopedic Surgery
Harvard Medical School
Boston, Massachusetts
Shoulder Pain

Michael Toprover, MD
Instructor
Division of Rheumatology
NYU Langone Health
New York, New York
Etiology and Pathogenesis of Hyperuricemia and Gout

Kathryn S. Torok, MD
Associate Professor
Pediatric Rheumatology
University of Pittsburgh School of Medicine
Pittsburgh, Pennsylvania
Juvenile Dermatomyositis, Scleroderma, Vasculitis, and Autoimmune Brain Disease

Michael J. Toth, PhD
Professor of Medicine
The University of Vermont College of Medicine
Burlington, Vermont
Muscle: Anatomy, Physiology, and Biochemistry

Michael J. Townsend, PhD
Department of Biomarker Discovery
Genentech Research and Early Development
South San Francisco, California
Biomarkers in Rheumatology

Elaine C. Tozman, MD
Associate Professor of Clinical Medicine
Rheumatology and Immunology
University of Miami Miller School of Medicine
Miami, Florida
Rheumatic Manifestations of Hemoglobinopathies

Leendert A. Trouw, PhD
Associate Professor
Department of Immunohematology and Bloodtransfusion
Leiden University Medical Center
Leiden, Netherlands
Complement System

George C. Tsokos, MD
Professor and Chief
Department of Medicine
Division of Rheumatology and Clinical Immunology
Beth Israel Deaconess Medical Center
Harvard Medical School
Boston, Massachusetts
Principles of Signaling

Peter Tugwell, MD
Professor of Medicine and Epidemiology and Community Medicine
University of Ottawa
Ottawa, Ontario, Canada
Assessment of Health Outcomes

Nicolas Vabret, PhD
Assistant Professor
Hematology and Oncology
Icahn School of Medicine at Mount Sinai
New York, New York
Dendritic Cells

Marlies C. van der Goes, MD, PhD
Department of Rheumatology
Meander Medical Center
Amersfoort, Netherlands
Glucocorticoid Therapy

Sjef van der Linden, MD, PhD
Professor of Rheumatology
Department of Internal Medicine
Division of Rheumatology
Maastricht University Medical Center
Maastricht, Netherlands, Department of Rheumatology, Immunology and Allergology
University of Bern, Inselspital
Bern, Switzerland
Ankylosing Spondylitis and Other Forms of Axial Spondyloarthritis

Jos W.M. van der Meer, MD, PhD
Professor of Medicine
Department of Internal Medicine
Radboud University Medical Center
Nijmegen, Netherlands
Familial Autoinflammatory Syndromes

Jacob M. van Laar, MD, PhD
Professor of Rheumatology
Rheumatology and Clinical Immunology
University Medical Center Utrecht
Utrecht, Netherlands
Immunosuppressive Drugs

Heather Van Mater, MD, MS
Associate Professor of Pediatrics
Duke University School of Medicine
Durham, North Carolina
Juvenile Dermatomyositis, Scleroderma, Vasculitis, and Autoimmune Brain Disease

Ronald F. van Vollenhoven, MD, PhD
Professor and Chair
Rheumatology and Clinical Immunology
Amsterdam University Medical Centers
Director
Amsterdam Rheumatology Center
Amsterdam, Netherlands
Evaluation of Monoarticular and Polyarticular Arthritis

Lize F. D. van Vulpen, MD, PhD
Internist-haematologist
Van Creveldkliniek
University Medical Center Utrecht
Utrecht University
Utrecht, Netherlands
Hemophilic Arthropathy

John Varga, MD
John and Nancy Hughes Professor
Department of Medicine
Northwestern University Feinberg School of Medicine
Chicago, Illinois
Etiology and Pathogenesis of Systemic Sclerosis

Raul A. Vasquez, MD
Director of Complex Spine Surgery
Baptist Health Neuroscience Center
Miami, Florida
Neck Pain

Douglas J. Veale, MD, FRCPI, FRCP (Lon)
Director of Translational Research Medicine
The Centre for Arthritis and Rheumatic Disease
St. Vincent's University Hospital
Professor of Medicine
University College Dublin
Fellow
Conway Institute of Biomolecular and Biomedical Medicine
Dublin, Ireland
Synovium
Angiogenesis

Richard J. Wakefield, BM, MD, FRCP
Leeds Institute of Rheumatic and Musculoskeletal Medicine
University of Leeds
Rheumatology
Leeds Teaching Hospitals Trust
Leeds, West Yorkshire, United Kingdom
Arthrocentesis and Injection of Joints and Soft Tissues

Mark S. Wallace, MD
Professor of Anesthesiology
University of California, San Diego
La Jolla, California
Analgesic Agents in Rheumatic Disease

Ruoning Wang, PhD
Principal Investigator
Center for Childhood Cancer and Blood Disease
The Research Institute at Nationwide Children's Hospital
Assistant Professor
Department of Pediatrics
The Ohio State University School of Medicine
Columbus, Ohio
Metabolic Regulation of Immunity

Tingting Wang, PhD
Center for Childhood Cancer and Blood Disease
The Research Institute at Nationwide Children's Hospital
Columbus, Ohio
Metabolic Regulation of Immunity

Victoria P. Werth, MD
Professor of Dermatology and Medicine
University of Pennsylvania
Chief
Dermatology
Corporal Michael J. Crescenz (Philadelphia) Veterans Administration Medical Center
Philadelphia, Pennsylvania
Skin and Rheumatic Diseases

Fredrick M. Wigley, MD
Martha McCrory Professor of Medicine
Division of Rheumatology
Johns Hopkins University School of Medicine
Baltimore, Maryland
Clinical Features and Treatment of Scleroderma

Deborah R. Winter, PhD
Assistant Professor of Medicine
Division of Rheumatology
Northwestern University Feinberg School of Medicine
Chicago, Illinois
Mononuclear Phagocytes

David Wofsy, MD
Professor
Medicine and Microbiology/Immunology
University of California San Francisco
San Francisco, California
Clinical Features of Systemic Lupus Erythematosus

Cyrus C. Wong, MD
Neurological Surgery
North Texas Neurosurgical and Spine Center
Fort Worth, Texas
Neck Pain

Wayne M. Yokoyama, MD
Sam J. and Audrey Loew Levin Professor of Arthritis Research
Rheumatology Division
Washington University School of Medicine
St. Louis, Missouri
Innate Lymphoid Cells and Natural Killer Cells

Richard Zamore, MD
Medicine/Rheumatology
University of Pennsylvania
Philadelphia, Pennsylvania
Inflammatory Bowel Disease–Associated Arthritis and Other Enteropathic Arthropathies

Ahmed S. Zayat, MRCP, MSc, MD
Leeds Institute of Rheumatic and Musculoskeletal Medicine
University of Leeds
Leeds, United Kingdom
Department of Rheumatology
Bradford Teaching Hospitals NHS Foundation Trust
Bradford, West Yorkshire, United Kingdom
Arthrocentesis and Injection of Joints and Soft Tissues

Yong-Rui Zou, PhD
Associate Professor
Center for Autoimmune, Musculoskeletal and Hematopoietic Diseases
Feinstein Institutes for Medical Research
Manhasset, New York
B Cells

Robert B. Zurier, MD
Professor of Medicine Chief of Rheumatology Emeritus
University of Massachusetts Medical School
Worcester, Massachusetts
Investigator
Autoimmunity and Musculoskeletal Disease Center
Feinstein Institute for Medical Research
Manhasset, New York
Prostaglandins, Leukotrienes, and Related Compounds

Preface

We are proud to present the 11th edition of the *Textbook of Rheumatology*. As with previous editions, we aim to provide a solid basic science framework, detailed pharmacology discussions of old and new anti-rheumatic agents, and an integrated approach to disease pathogenesis, clinical manifestations, and treatments. Before we begin each edition, the editors do some reality testing and examine the role of textbooks in an era of instant communication and easily accessible "quickie" medical review platforms that are sometimes part of electronic health record systems. We continue to believe that carefully moderated, integrated content like the *Textbook* remains a cornerstone of learning in medicine. This impression is supported by expanding *Textbook* access via the internet for institutions and individual learners. People speak with their "clicks," and it is clear that tomes like the *Textbook* continue to fill an important gap in education and training.

The theme of TOR11 is exemplified by our cover art, namely past, present, and future. The past is represented by a classic image of uric acid crystals in the ancient disease of gout. A photograph of a patient with active synovitis, still a common occurrence in our clinics, depicts the present. Finally, the future of rheumatology and actually science in general is exemplified by a hierarchical clustering of genomic data, which illustrates the power and importance of computational biology. We can expect new omics technologies and informatics to change the face of medicine and ultimately lead to an updated disease taxonomy that focuses less on phenotype and more on underlying mechanisms.

Our 11th edition also includes a new editor, Dr. Gary Koretzky, who brings a deep understanding of immunology in recognition that rheumatology is the exemplar of immunologic disease. Thus, the editors represent a broad swath of our specialty, from basic science to translational medicine to clinical care to population medicine. Of course, the true value of the book is derived from the effort and expertise of the many authors who spend countless hours writing and editing their sections. We are indebted to them and are confident that our readers will benefit greatly from their expertise.

The Editors

Contents

VOLUME I

Part 4: Broad Issues in the Approach to Rheumatic Disease

Part 5: Evaluation of Generalized and Localized Symptoms

Part 6: Differential Diagnosis of Regional and Diffuse Musculoskeletal Pain

Part 16: Rheumatic Diseases of Childhood

Part 17: Infection and Arthritis

Part 18: Arthritis Accompanying Systemic Disease

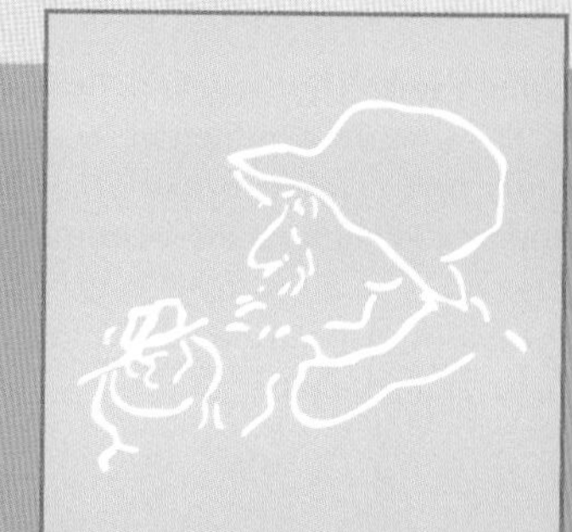

1 Biology of the Normal Joint

CARLA R. SCANZELLO AND STEVEN R. GOLDRING

KEY POINTS

Condensation of mesenchymal cells, which differentiate into chondrocytes, results in formation of the cartilage anlagen, which provides the template for the developing skeleton.

During development of the synovial joint, growth differentiation factor-5 regulates interzone formation, and interference with movement of the embryo during development impairs joint cavitation.

Members of the bone morphogenetic protein/transforming growth factor-β, fibroblast growth factor, and Wnt families and the parathyroid hormone–related peptide/Indian hedgehog axis are essential for joint development and growth plate formation.

The synovial lining of diarthrodial joints is a thin layer of cells lacking a basement membrane and consisting of two principal cell types—macrophages and fibroblasts.

The articular cartilage receives its nutritional requirements via diffusion from the synovial fluid, and interaction of the cartilage with components of the synovial fluid contributes to the unique low-friction surface properties of the articular cartilage.

Classification of Joints

Human joints, which provide the structures by which bones join with one another, may be classified according to the histologic features of the union and the range of joint motion. Three classes of joint design exist: (1) synovial or diarthrodial joints (Fig. 1.1), which articulate with free movement, have a synovial membrane lining the joint cavity, and contain synovial fluid; (2) amphiarthroses, in which adjacent bones are separated by articular cartilage or a fibrocartilage disk and are bound by firm ligaments, permitting limited motion (e.g., the pubic symphysis, intervertebral disks of vertebral bodies, distal tibiofibular articulation, and sacroiliac joint articulation with pelvic bones); and (3) synarthroses, which are found only in the skull (suture lines) where thin, fibrous tissue separates adjoining cranial plates that interlock to prevent detectable motion before the end of normal growth, yet permit growth in childhood and adolescence.

Joints also can be classified according to the connective tissues that join opposing bones. Symphyses have a fibrocartilaginous disk separating bone ends that are joined by firm ligaments (e.g., the symphysis pubis and intervertebral joints). In synchondroses, the bone ends are covered with articular cartilage, but no synovium or significant joint cavity is present (e.g., the sternomanubrial joint). In syndesmoses, the bones are joined directly by fibrous ligaments without a cartilaginous interface (the distal tibiofibular articulation is the only joint of this type outside the cranial vault).

Synovial joints are classified further according to their shapes, which include ball-and-socket (hip), hinge (interphalangeal), saddle (first carpometacarpal), and plane (patellofemoral) joints. These configurations reflect function, with the shapes and sizes of the opposing surfaces determining the direction and extent of motion. The various designs permit flexion, extension, abduction, adduction, or rotation. Certain joints can act in one (humeroulnar), two (wrist), or three (shoulder) axes of motion.

This chapter concentrates on the developmental biology and relationship between structure and function of a "prototypic," "normal" human diarthrodial joint—the joint in which arthritis is most likely to develop. Most of the research performed concerns the knee because of its accessibility, but other joints are described when appropriate.

Developmental Biology of the Diarthrodial Joint

Skeletal development is initiated by the differentiation of mesenchymal cells that arise from three embryonic sources: (1) neural crest cells of the neural ectoderm that give rise to craniofacial bones; (2) the sclerotome of the paraxial mesoderm, or somite compartment, which forms the axial skeleton; and (3) the somatopleure of the lateral plate mesoderm, which yields the skeleton of the limbs.[1] The appendicular skeleton develops in the human embryo from limb buds, which are first visible at approximately 4 weeks of gestation. Structures resembling adult joints are generated at approximately 4 to 7 weeks of gestation.[2] Many other crucial phases of musculoskeletal development follow, including vascularization of epiphyseal cartilage (8 to 12 weeks), appearance of villous folds in synovium (10 to 12 weeks), evolution of bursae (3 to 4 months), and the appearance of periarticular fat pads (4 to 5 months).

The upper limbs develop approximately 24 hours earlier than the analogous portions of the lower limbs. Proximal structures, such as the glenohumeral joint, develop before more distal ones, such as the wrist and hand. Consequently, insults to embryonic development during limb formation affect a more distal portion of the upper limb than of the lower limb. Long bones form as a result of replacement of the cartilage template by endochondral ossification. The stages of limb development are shown in Fig. 1.2.[2,3] The developmental sequence of the events occurring during synovial joint formation and some of the regulatory factors and extra-cellular matrix components involved are summarized in Fig. 1.3. The three main stages in joint development are interzone formation, cavitation, and morphogenesis, as described in detail in several reviews.[4-9]

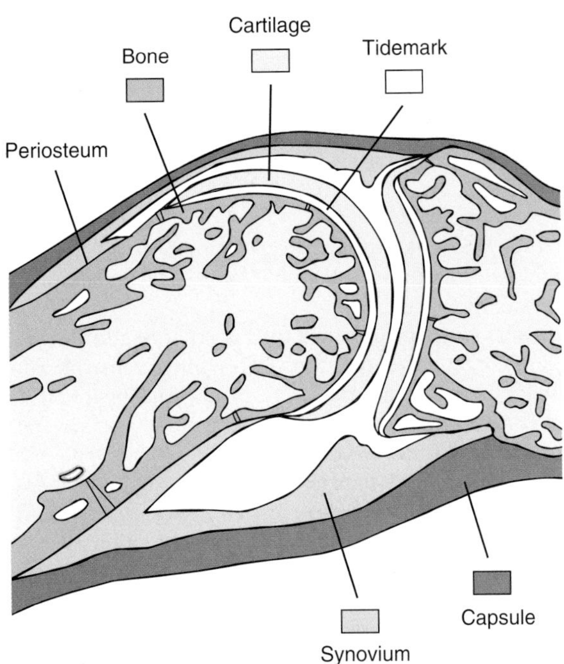

• **Fig. 1.1** A normal human interphalangeal joint, in sagittal section, as an example of a synovial, or diarthrodial, joint. The tidemark represents the calcified cartilage that bonds articular cartilage to the subchondral bone plate. (From Sokoloff L, Bland JH: *The musculoskeletal system.* Baltimore, Williams & Wilkins, 1975. Copyright 1975, the Williams & Wilkins Co, Baltimore.)

Interzone Formation and Joint Cavitation

The structure of the developing synovial joint and the process of joint cavitation have been described in many classic studies performed on the limbs of mammalian and avian embryos.[10] In the

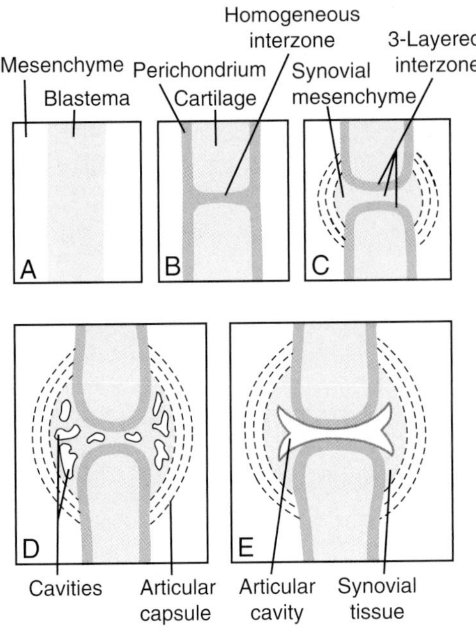

• **Fig. 1.2** The development of a synovial joint. (A) Condensation. Joints develop from the blastema, not the surrounding mesenchyme. (B) Chondrification and formation of the interzone. The interzone remains avascular and highly cellular. (C) Formation of synovial mesenchyme. Synovial mesenchyme forms from the periphery of the interzone and is invaded by blood vessels. (D) Cavitation. Cavities are formed in the central and peripheral interzone and merge to form the joint cavity. (E) The mature joint. (From O'Rahilly R, Gardner E: The embryology of movable joints. In Sokoloff L, editor: *The joints and synovial fluid,* vol 1, New York, Academic Press, 1978.)

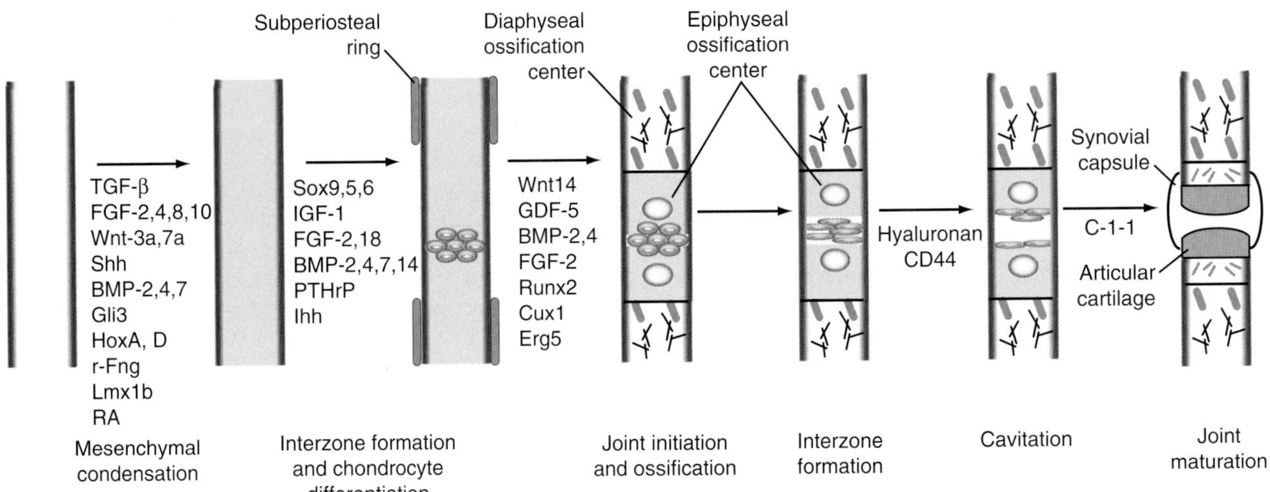

• **Fig. 1.3** Development of long bones and diathrodial joint formation from cartilage anlagen. *BMP,* Bone morphogenetic protein; *C-1-1,* Erg3 variant; *CD44,* cell determinant 44; *Cux,* cut-repeat homeobox protein; *Erg,* ETS-related gene 5; *FGF,* fibroblast growth factor; *GDF,* growth and differentiation factor; *Gli,* glioma-associated oncogene homolog; *Hox,* homeobox; *IGF,* insulin-like growth factor; *Ihh,* Indian hedgehog; *Lmx1b,* LIM homeodomain transcription factor 1b; *PTHrP,* parathyroid hormone–related protein; *RA,* retinoic acid; *r-Fng,* radical fringe; *Runx,* runt domain binding protein; *Shh,* Sonic hedgehog; *Sox,* SRY-related high mobility group-box protein; *TGF-β,* transforming growth factor-β; *Wnt,* wingless type.

human embryo, cartilage condensations can be detected at stage 17, when the embryo is small—approximately 11.7 mm long.[2,3] In the region of the future joint, after formation of the homogeneous chondrogenic interzone at 6 weeks (stages 18 and 19), a three-layered interzone is formed at approximately 7 weeks (stage 21), which consists of two chondrogenic, perichondrium-like layers that cover the opposing surfaces of the cartilage anlagen (embryonic pre-chondrogenic cell clusters) and are separated by a narrow band of densely packed cellular blastema that remains and forms the interzone. Cavitation begins in the central interzone at about 8 weeks (stage 23).

Although the cellular events associated with joint formation have been recognized for many years, only recently have the genes regulating these processes been elucidated.[6,7,9] These genes include growth differentiation factor (GDF)-5 (also known as cartilage-derived morphogenetic protein-1) and Wnt14 (also known as Wnt9a), which are involved in early joint development. Two major roles have been proposed for Wnt14. First, it acts at the onset of joint formation as a negative regulator of chondrogenesis. Second, it facilitates interzone formation and cavitation by inducing the expression of GDF-5; autotaxin; lysophosphatidic acid; the bone morphogenetic protein (BMP) antagonist, chordin; and the hyaluronan receptor, CD44.[4,11] Paradoxically, application of GDF-5 to developing joints in mouse embryo limbs in organ culture causes joint fusion,[12] suggesting that temporospatial interactions among distinct cell populations are important for the correct response. The current view is that GDF-5 is required at the early stages of condensations, where it stimulates recruitment and differentiation of chondrogenic cells, and later, when its expression is restricted to the interzone. Recent evidence from one study sheds light on the temporospatial sequence of events, and it suggests that there is a continuous recruitment of new GDF-5 expressing cells into the interzone during joint development that leads to lineage divergence at different stages. Early recruited GDF-5+ cells preferentially populate the developing epiphysis, and later recruited cells undergo chondrogenesis and contribute more to the developing articular surface.[13]

The distribution of collagen types and proteoglycans in developing avian and rodent joints is characterized histologically and by immunohistochemistry and in situ hybridization.[9,14,15] The matrix produced by mesenchymal cells in the interzone is rich in types I and III collagen, and during condensation, production switches to types II, IX, and XI collagens that typify the cartilaginous matrix. The messenger RNAs (mRNAs) encoding the small proteoglycans biglycan and decorin may be expressed at this time, but the proteins do not appear until after cavitation in the regions destined to become articular cartilage. The interzone regions are marked by the expression of genes encoding type IIA collagen by chondrocyte progenitors in the perichondrial layers, type IIB and XI collagens by differentiated chondrocytes in the cartilage anlagen, and type I collagen in the interzone and in the developing capsule and perichondrium (Fig. 1.4).[16]

The interzone region contains cells in two outer layers, where they are destined to differentiate into chondrocytes and become incorporated into the epiphyses, and in a thin intermediate zone where they are programmed to undergo joint cavitation and may remain as articular chondrocytes.[8] These early chondrocytes all arise from the same population of progenitors, but unlike the other chondrocytes of the anlagen, they do not activate matrilin-1 expression and are destined to form the articular surface.[17] As cavitation begins in this zone, fluid and macromolecules accumulate in this space and create a nascent synovial cavity. Blood vessels appear in the surrounding capsulosynovial blastemal mesenchyme before separation of the adjacent articulating surfaces. Although it was first assumed that these interzone cells undergo necrosis or programmed cell death (apoptosis), many investigators have found no evidence of DNA fragmentation preceding cavitation. In addition, no evidence exists that metalloproteinases are involved in loss of tissue strength in the region undergoing cavitation. Instead, the actual joint cavity seems to be formed by mechanospatial changes induced by the synthesis and secretion of hyaluronan via uridine diphosphoglucose dehydrogenase (UDPGD) and hyaluronan synthase. Interaction of hyaluronan and CD44 on the cell surface modulates cell migration, but the accumulation of hyaluronan and the associated mechanical influences force the cells apart and induce rupture of the intervening extra-cellular matrix by tensile forces. This mechanism accounts, partially, for observations that joint cavitation is incomplete in the absence of movement.[18-20] Equivalent data from human embryonic joints are difficult to obtain,[21] but in all large joints in humans, complete joint cavities are apparent at the beginning of the fetal period.

Cartilage Formation and Endochondral Ossification

The skeleton develops from the primitive, avascular, densely packed cellular mesenchyme, termed the *skeletal blastema.* Common precursor mesenchymal cells divide into chondrogenic, myogenic, and osteogenic lineages that determine the differentiation of cartilage centrally, muscle peripherally, and bone. The surrounding tissues, particularly epithelium, influence the differentiation of mesenchymal progenitor cells to chondrocytes in the cartilage anlagen. The cartilaginous nodules appear in the middle of the blastema, and simultaneously cells at the periphery become flattened and elongated to form the perichondrium. In the vertebral column, cartilage disks arise from portions of the somites surrounding the notochord, and nasal and auricular cartilage and the embryonic epiphysis form from the perichondrium. In the limb, the cartilage remains as a resting zone that later becomes the articular cartilage, or it undergoes terminal hypertrophic differentiation to become calcified (growth plate formation) and is replaced by bone (endochondral ossification). The latter process requires extra-cellular matrix remodeling and vascularization (angiogenesis). These events are controlled exquisitely by cellular interactions with the surrounding matrix, growth and differentiation factors, and other environmental factors that initiate or suppress cellular signaling pathways and transcription of specific genes in a temporospatial manner.

Condensation and Limb Bud Formation

Formation of the cartilage anlage occurs in four stages: (1) cell migration, (2) aggregation regulated by mesenchymal-epithelial cell interactions, (3) condensation, and (4) chondrocyte differentiation. Interactions with the epithelium determine mesenchymal cell recruitment and migration, proliferation, and condensation.[2,3,22] The aggregation of chondroprogenitor mesenchymal cells into precartilage condensations was first described by Fell[23] and depends on signals initiated by cell-cell and cell-matrix interactions, the formation of gap junctions, and changes in the cytoskeletal architecture. Before condensation, the prechondrocytic mesenchymal cells produce extra-cellular matrix that is rich in hyaluronan and type I collagen and type IIA collagen, which

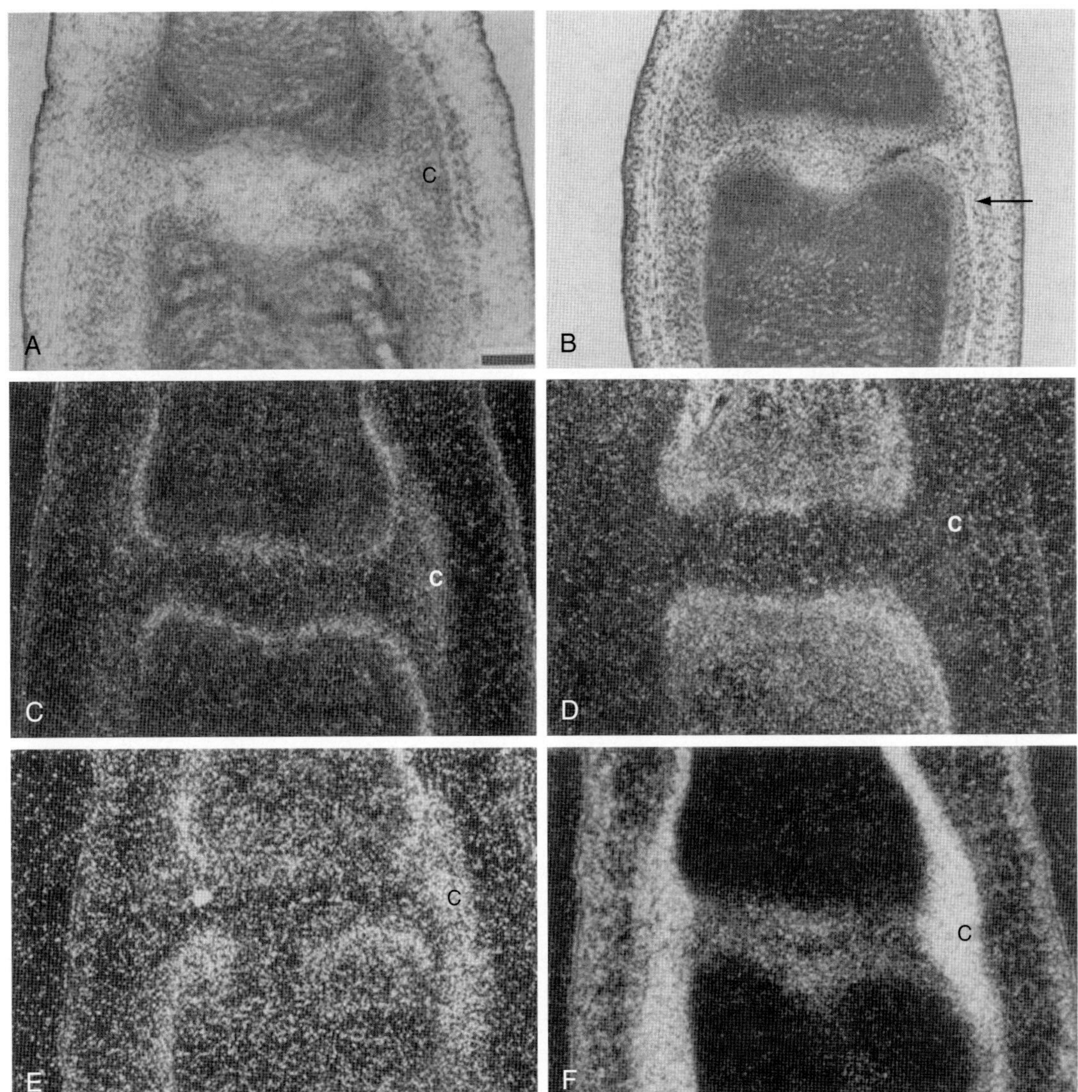

• **Fig. 1.4** In situ hybridization of a 13-day-old (stage 39) chicken embryo middle digit, proximal interphalangeal joint, midfrontal sections. (A) Bright-field image showing developing joint and capsule *(C)*. (B) Equivalent paraffin section of opposite limb of same animal, showing onset of cavitation laterally *(arrow)*. (C) Expression of type IIA collagen messenger RNA (mRNA) in articular surface cells, perichondrium, and capsule. (D) Type IIB collagen mRNA is expressed only in chondrocytes of the anlagen. (E) Type XI collagen mRNA is expressed in the surface cells, perichondrium, and capsule, with lower levels in chondrocytes. (F) Type I collagen mRNA is present in cells of the interzone and capsule. (C) through (F) images are dark field. Calibration bar = 1 μm. (From Nalin AM, Greenlee TK Jr, Sandell LJ: Collagen gene expression during development of avian synovial joints: transient expression of types II and XI collagen genes in the joint capsule. *Develop Dyn* 203:352–362, 1995.)

contains the exon-2–encoded aminopropeptide found in noncartilage collagens. The initiation of condensation is associated with increased hyaluronidase activity and the transient upregulation of versican, tenascin, syndecan, the cell adhesion molecules, neural cadherin (N-cadherin), and neural cell adhesion molecule (NCAM), which facilitate cell-cell interactions.[22,24]

Before chondrocyte differentiation, the cell-matrix interactions are facilitated by the binding of fibronectin to syndecan, thus downregulating NCAM and setting the condensation boundaries. Increased cell proliferation and extra-cellular matrix remodeling, with the disappearance of type I collagen, fibronectin, and N-cadherin, and the appearance of tenascins, matrilins, and thrombospondins, including cartilage oligomeric matrix protein (COMP), initiate the transition from chondroprogenitor cells to a fully committed chondrocyte.[1,24-26] N-cadherin and NCAM disappear in differentiating chondrocytes and are detectable later only in perichondrial cells. As discussed previously, recent evidence suggests that during joint development there is a continuous recruitment of new GDF-5–expressing cells into the interzone. These cells preferentially populate the developing epiphysis, and later, recruited cells undergo chondrogenesis and contribute to the developing articular surface.[13]

Much of the current understanding of limb bud development is based on early studies in chickens and recently in mice. The regulatory events are controlled by interacting patterning systems involving homeobox (Hox) transcription factors and fibroblast growth factor (FGF), hedgehog, transforming growth factor-β (TGF-β)/BMP, and Wnt pathways, each of which functions sequentially over time (see Fig. 1.3).[11,27-30] The HoxA and HoxD gene clusters are crucial for the early events of limb patterning in the undifferentiated mesenchyme, as they are required for the expression of FGF-8 and Sonic hedgehog (Shh),[31] which modulate the proliferation of cells within the condensations.[22] BMP-2, BMP-4, and BMP-7 coordinately regulate the patterning of limb elements within the condensations depending on the temporal and spatial expression of BMP receptors and BMP antagonists, such as noggin and chordin, as well as the availability of BMP- and TGF-β–induced SMADs (signaling mammalian homologues of *Drosophila* mothers against decapentaplegic).[32] BMP signaling is required for the formation of precartilaginous condensations and for the differentiation of precursors into chondrocytes,[33,34] acting, in part, by opposing FGF actions.[35] Growth of the condensation ceases when noggin inhibits BMP signaling and permits differentiation to chondrocytes. The cartilage formed serves as a template for formation of cartilaginous elements in the vertebra, sternum, and rib, and for limb elongation or endochondral bone formation.

Molecular Signals in Cartilage Morphogenesis and Growth Plate Development

The cartilage anlagen grow by cell division, deposition of extracellular matrix, and apposition of proliferating cells from the inner chondrogenic layer of the perichondrium. The nuclear transcription factor Sox9 is one of the earliest markers expressed in cells undergoing condensation and is required for the subsequent stage of chondrogenesis characterized by the deposition of matrix-containing collagens II, IX, and XI and aggrecan.[36] The expression of SOX proteins depends on BMP signaling via BMPR1A and BMPR1B, which are functionally redundant and active in chondrocyte condensations, but not in the perichondrium.[33] Sox5 and Sox6 are required for the expression of Col9a1, aggrecan, link protein, and Col2a1 during chondrocyte differentiation.[37] The runt-domain transcription factor, Runx2 (also known as core binding factor, Cbfa1), is expressed in all condensations including those that are destined to form bone.

Throughout chondrogenesis, the balance of signaling by BMPs and FGFs determines the rate of proliferation and the pace of the differentiation.[29,35,38] In the long bones, long after condensation, BMP-2, BMP-3, BMP-4, BMP-5, and BMP-7 are expressed primarily in the perichondrium, but only BMP-7 is expressed in the proliferating chondrocytes.[38] BMP-6 is found later, exclusively in hypertrophic chondrocytes along with BMP-2. More than 23 FGFs have been identified thus far.[39] The specific ligands that activate each FGF receptor (FGFR) during chondrogenesis in vivo have been difficult to identify because the signaling depends on the temporal and spatial location of not only the ligands but also the receptors.[40] FGFR2 is upregulated early in condensing mesenchyme and is present later in the periphery of the condensation along with FGFR1, which is expressed in surrounding loose mesenchyme. FGFR3 is associated with proliferation of chondrocytes in the central core of the mesenchymal condensation and overlaps with FGFR2. Proliferation of chondrocytes in the embryonic and postnatal growth plate is regulated by multiple mitogenic stimuli, including FGFs, which converge on cyclin D1.[41]

Early studies indicated that FGFR3 could serve as a master inhibitor of chondrocyte proliferation via Stat1 and the cell cycle inhibitor p21. FGFR3 activation downregulates AKT activity to decrease proliferation,[42] and MEK activation leads to decreased chondrocyte differentiation.[43] The physiologic FGFR3 ligands are not known, but FGF-9 and FGF-18 are good candidates because they bind FGFR3 in vitro and are expressed in the adjacent perichondrium and periosteum, forming a functional gradient.[29,44] FGF-18–deficient mice have an expanded zone of proliferating chondrocytes similar to that in FGFR3-deficient mice, and FGF-18 can inhibit Indian hedgehog (Ihh) expression. As the growth plate develops, FGFR3 disappears and FGFR1 is upregulated in the prehypertrophic and hypertrophic zones, where FGF-18 and FGF-9 regulate vascular invasion by inducing vascular endothelial growth factor (VEGF) and VEGFR1 and terminal differentiation.[39,45,46]

The proliferation of chondrocytes in the lower proliferative and prehypertrophic zones is under the control of a local negative feedback loop involving signaling by parathyroid hormone–related protein (PTHrP) and Ihh.[47] Ihh expression is restricted to the prehypertrophic zone, and the PTHrP receptor is expressed in the distal zone of periarticular chondrocytes. The adjacent, surrounding perichondrial cells express the Hedgehog receptor patched (Ptch), which, upon Ihh binding, similar to Shh in the mesenchymal condensations, activates Smo and induces Gli transcription factors, which can feedback regulate Ihh target genes in a positive (*Gli1* and *Gli2*) or negative *(Gli3)* manner.[48,49] Ihh induces expression of PTHrP in the perichondrium, and PTHrP signaling stimulates cell proliferation via its receptor expressed in the periarticular chondrocytes.[29,50] Recent evidence indicates that Ihh also acts independently of PTHrP on periarticular chondrocytes to stimulate differentiation of columnar chondrocytes in the proliferative zone, whereas PTHrP acts by preventing premature differentiation into prehypertrophic and hypertrophic chondrocytes, suppressing premature expression of Ihh.[51,52] Ihh and PTHrP, by transiently inducing proliferation markers and repressing differentiation markers, function in a temporospatial manner to determine the number of cells that remain in the chondrogenic lineage versus the number that enter the endochondral ossification pathway.[47] Components of the extra-cellular matrix also contribute to regulation of the different stages of growth plate development, including chondrogenesis and terminal differentiation, by interacting with signaling molecules and chondrocyte cell surface receptors.[53]

Endochondral Ossification

The development of long bones from the cartilage anlagen occurs by a process termed *endochondral ossification,* which involves terminal differentiation of chondrocytes to the hypertrophic phenotype, cartilage matrix calcification, vascular invasion, and ossification (see Fig. 1.3).[29,50,54] This process is initiated when the cells in the central region of the anlage begin to hypertrophy, increasing cellular fluid volume by almost 20 times. Ihh plays a pivotal role in regulating endochondral bone formation by synchronizing perichondrial maturation with chondrocyte hypertrophy, which, in turn, is essential for initiating the process of vascular invasion. Ihh is expressed in prehypertrophic chondrocytes as they exit the proliferative phase and enter the hypertrophic phase, at which time they begin to express hypertrophic chondrocyte markers type X collagen and alkaline phosphatase. These cells are responsible for laying down the cartilage matrix that subsequently undergoes mineralization. Wnt/β-catenin signaling promotes chondrocyte maturation by a BMP-2–mediated mechanism and induces chondrocyte hypertrophy partly by enhancing matrix metalloproteinase (MMP) expression and potentially by enhancing Ihh signaling and vascularization.[55]

Runx2 serves as an essential positive regulatory factor in chondrocyte maturation to hypertrophy. In Runx2-deficient mice, chondrocyte hypertrophy and terminal differentiation is blocked, and as a result endochondral ossification does not proceed. It is expressed in the adjacent perichondrium and in prehypertrophic chondrocytes and less in late hypertrophic chondrocytes, overlapping with Ihh, COL10A1, and BMP-6. IHH induces Gli transcription factors, which interact with Runx2 and BMP-induced SMADs to regulate transcription and expression of *COL10A1*.[56] A member of the myocyte enhancer factor (MEF) 2 family, MEF2C, stimulates hypertrophy partly by increasing Runx2 expression.[57] The class II histone deacetylase, HDAC4, prevents premature hypertrophy by directly suppressing the activities of Runx2 and MEF2C.[58] HDAC4 is in turn regulated by PTHrP and salt-inducible kinase 3 (SIK3).[59,60] Sox9,[61] FOXA2 and FoxA3,[62] Runx3,[63] Zfp521,[64] and peroxisome proliferator-activated receptor γ (PPARγ[65]) are also important transcriptional regulators of chondrocyte hypertrophy. MMP-13, a downstream target of Runx2, is expressed by terminal hypertrophic chondrocytes, and MMP-13 deficiency results in significant interstitial collagen accumulation, leading to the delay of endochondral ossification in the growth plate with increased length of the hypertrophic zone.[66,67]

Runx2 also is required for transcription activation of *COL10A1,* the gene encoding type X collagen, which is the major matrix component of the hypertrophic zone in the embryo and in the postnatal growth plate. Mutations in the *COL10A1* gene are associated with the dwarfism observed in human chondrodysplasias. These mutations affect regions of the growth plate that are under great mechanical stress, and the defect in skeletal growth may be due partly to alteration of the mechanical integrity of the pericellular matrix in the hypertrophic zone, although a role for defective vascularization also is proposed. The extra-cellular matrix remodeling that accompanies chondrocyte terminal differentiation is thought to induce an alteration in the environmental stress experienced by hypertrophic chondrocytes, which eventually undergo apoptosis.[68] Whether chondrocyte hypertrophy with cell death is the ultimate fate of hypertrophic chondrocytes or whether hypertrophy is a transient process that precedes osteogenesis is a subject of debate. However, recent genetic lineage tracing studies suggest that hypertrophic chondrocytes can survive at the chondro-osseous junction and become osteoblasts and osteocytes.[69,70]

Cartilage is an avascular tissue, and because the developing growth plate is relatively hypoxic, hypoxia inducible factor (HIF)-1α is important for survival as chondrocytes transition to hypertrophy. Under normoxia, the cell content of HIF-1α, -2α, and -3α is low because of oxygen-dependent hydroxylation by prolyl-hydroxylases, resulting in ubiquitination and degradation by the proteasome. In contrast, under hypoxia, prolyl-hydroxylase activity is reduced and the α subunits heterodimerize with the constitutive β-subunit members known as aryl hydrocarbon receptor nuclear translocators (ARNTs). HIFs are transcription factors that bind to hypoxia-responsive elements (HREs) in responsive genes. HIF-2α regulates endochondral ossification processes by directly targeting HREs within the promoters of the *COL10A1, MMP13,* and *VEGFA* genes.[71]

Vascular invasion of the hypertrophic zone is required for the replacement of calcified cartilage by bone. VEGF acts as an angiogenic factor to promote vascular invasion by specifically activating local receptors, including Flk1, which is expressed in endothelial cells in the perichondrium or surrounding soft tissues; neuropilin 1 (Npn1), which is expressed in late hypertrophic chondrocytes; or Npn2, which is expressed exclusively in the perichondrium. VEGF is expressed as three different isoforms: VEGF188, a matrix-bound form, is essential for metaphyseal vascularization, whereas the soluble form, VEGF120 (VEGFA), regulates chondrocyte survival and epiphyseal cartilage angiogenesis, and VEGF164 can be either soluble or matrix bound and may act directly on chondrocytes via Npn2. VEGF is released from the extra-cellular matrix by MMPs, including MMP-9, membrane-type (MT)1-MMP (MMP-14), and MMP-13. MMP-9 is expressed by endothelial cells that migrate into the central region of the hypertrophic cartilage.[72] MMP-14, which has a broader range of expression than MMP-9, is essential for chondrocyte proliferation and secondary ossification, whereas MMP-13 is found exclusively in late hypertrophic chondrocytes. Perlecan (Hspg2), a heparan sulfate proteoglycan in cartilage matrix, is required for vascularization in the growth plate through its binding to the VEGFR of endothelial cells, permitting osteoblast migration into the growth plate.[73]

A number of ADAM (a disintegrin and metalloproteinase) proteinases are also emerging as important regulators in growth plate development. For example, ADAM10 is a principle regulator of Notch signaling, which modulates endochondral ossification via RBPjk in chondrocytes[74] and promotes osteoclastogenesis at the chondro-osseous junction by regulating endothelial cell organization in the developing bone vasculature.[75] ADAM17 is the critical proteinase mediating cellular shedding of TNF but also the epidermal growth factor receptor (EGFR) ligands, including TGF-α. The EGFR signaling pathway induced by EGF and TGF-α plays a crucial role in the remodeling of the growth plate, where inactivation of EGFR results in the inability of hypertrophic chondrocytes to degrade the surrounding collagen matrix and to attract osteoclasts to invade and remodel the advancing growth plate under control of the osteoclast differentiation factor receptor activator of nuclear factor κB (NF-κB) ligand (RANKL).[76,77] Mice lacking ADAM17 in chondrocytes *(Adam17ΔCh)* show an expanded hypertrophic zone in the growth plate,[78] essentially phenocopying mice with defects in EGFR signaling in chondrocytes.[76] Tight regulation of EGFR signaling is important for cartilage and joint homeostasis, as shown in mice with cartilage-specific deletion of the mitogen-inducible gene 6 (MIG-6), a scaffold protein that binds EGFR and targets it for internalization and degradation.[79] These events of cartilage matrix remodeling and vascular invasion are required for the migration and differentiation of osteoclasts and osteoblasts, which remove the mineralized cartilage matrix and replace it with bone.

Development of Articular Cartilage

In the vertebrate skeleton, cartilage is the product of cells from three distinct embryonic lineages. Craniofacial cartilage is formed from cranial neural crest cells; the cartilage of the axial skeleton (intervertebral disks, ribs, and sternum) forms from paraxial mesoderm (somites); and the articular cartilage of the limbs is derived from the lateral plate mesoderm.[1] In the developing limb bud, mesenchymal cells form condensations in digital zones, followed by chondrocyte differentiation and maturation, whereas undifferentiated mesenchymal cells in the interdigital web zones undergo cell death. Embryonic cartilage is destined for one of several fates: it can remain as permanent cartilage (as on the articular surfaces of bones), or it can provide a template for the formation of bones by endochondral ossification. During development, cells in the cartilage anlage resembling the shape of the future bone undergo chondrocyte maturation expanding from the central site of the original condensation toward the ends of the forming bones. During joint cavitation, the peripheral interzone is absorbed into each adjacent cartilaginous zone, evolving into the articular surface. The articular surface is destined to become a specialized cartilaginous structure that does not normally undergo vascularization and ossification.[4,8,9]

Recent evidence indicates that postnatal maturation of the articular cartilage involves an appositional growth mechanism originating from progenitor cells at the articular surface rather than an interstitial mechanism. During formation of the mature articular cartilage, the differentiated articular chondrocytes synthesize the cartilage-specific matrix molecules, such as type II collagen and aggrecan (see Chapter 3). Through the processes described previously, the articular joint spaces are developed and lined on all surfaces either by cartilage or by synovial lining cells. These two different tissues merge at the enthesis, the region at the periphery of the joint where the cartilage melds into bone, and where ligaments and the capsule are attached. In the postnatal growth plate, the differentiation of the perichondrium also is linked to the differentiation of the chondrocytes in the epiphysis to form the different zones of the growth plate, contributing to longitudinal bone growth. Once the growth plate closes in the human joint, the adult articular cartilage must be maintained by the resident chondrocytes with low-turnover production of matrix proteins.[80,81]

Development of the Joint Capsule, Synovial Lining, Menisci, and Intracapsular Ligaments

The interzone and the contiguous perichondrial envelope, of which the interzone is a part, contain the mesenchymal cell precursors that give rise to other joint components, including the joint capsule, synovial lining, menisci, intracapsular ligaments, and tendons.[7-9] The external mesenchymal tissue condenses as a fibrous capsule. The peripheral mesenchyme becomes vascularized and is incorporated as the synovial mesenchyme, which differentiates into a pseudomembrane at about the same time as cavitation begins in the central interzone (stage 23, approximately 8 weeks). The menisci arise from the eccentric portions of the articular interzone. In common usage, the term *synovium* refers to the true synovial lining and the subjacent vascular and areolar tissue, up to—but excluding—the capsule. Synovial lining cells can be distinguished as soon as the multiple cavities within the interzone begin to coalesce. At first, these cells are exclusively fibroblast-like (type B) cells.

The synovial lining cells express the hyaluronan receptor CD44 and UDPGD, the levels of which remain elevated after cavitation. This increased activity likely contributes to the high concentration of hyaluronan in joint fluids. As the joint cavity increases in size, synovial-lining cell layers expand by proliferation of fibroblast-like cells and recruitment of macrophage-like (type A) cells from the circulation. In developing human temporomandibular joints, these type A cells can be detected by 12 weeks of gestation.[82] Further synovial expansion results in the appearance of synovial villi at the end of the second month, early in the fetal period, which greatly increases the surface area available for exchange between the joint cavity and the vascular space. Cadherin 11 is an additional molecule expressed by synovial lining cells.[83,84] It is essential for establishment of synovial lining architecture during development, where its expression correlates with cell migration and tissue outgrowth of the synovial lining.

The development and cellular composition of the synovium are discussed later.

The role of innervation in the developing joint is not well understood. A dense capillary network develops in the subsynovial tissue, with numerous capillary loops that penetrate into the true synovial lining layer. The human synovial microvasculature is already innervated by 8 weeks of gestation (stage 23), around the time of joint cavitation. Evidence of neurotransmitter function is not found until much later, however, with the appearance of the sensory neuropeptide substance P at 11 weeks. The putative sympathetic neurotransmitter, neuropeptide Y, appears at 13 weeks of gestation, along with the catecholamine-synthesizing enzyme tyrosine hydroxylase. The finding that the *Slit2* gene, which functions for the guidance of neuronal axons and neurons, is expressed in the mesenchyme and in peripheral mesenchyme of the limb bud (stages 23 to 28) suggests that innervation is an integral part of synovial joint development.[85]

Development of Nonarticular Joints

In contrast to articular joints, the temporomandibular joint develops slowly, with cavitation at a crown-rump length of 57 to 75 mm (i.e., well into the fetal stage). This slow development may occur because this joint develops in the absence of a continuous blastema and involves the insertion between bone ends of a fibrocartilaginous disk that arises from muscular and mesenchymal derivatives of the first pharyngeal arch. However, many of the same genes as those involved in articular joint development are involved in morphogenesis and growth of the temporomandibular joint.[86]

The development of other types of joints, such as synarthroses, is similar to that of diarthrodial joints except that cavitation does not occur, and synovial mesenchyme is not formed. In these respects, synarthroses and amphiarthroses resemble the "fused" peripheral joints induced by paralyzing chicken embryos, and they may develop as they do because relatively little motion is present during their formation.[87]

The intervertebral disk consists of a semiliquid nucleus pulposus (NP) in the center, surrounded by a multilayered fibrocartilaginous annulus fibrosus (AF), which is sandwiched between the cartilaginous end plates (EPs).[88] Between the EPs lies the vertebral body consisting of the growth plate, which later disappears, and the primary and secondary centers of ossification that fuse together. The cells in the NP arise from the embryonic notochord, and the notochord orchestrates somatogenesis, from which arises the ventral mesenchymal sclerotome that forms the AF of the intervertebral disk, as well as the vertebral bodies and ribs.[88] The NP acts as the center for controlling cell differentiation in the AF and EP through Shh signaling, which is regulated by Wnt signaling and, in turn, promotes growth and differentiation through downstream transcription factors, Brachyury and Sox9, and gene expression of extra-cellular matrix components.[89,90] The proteoglycans and collagens expressed during development of the intervertebral disk have been mapped and reflect the complex structure-function relationships that allow flexibility and resistance to compression in the spine.[91]

Organization and Physiology of the Mature Joint

The unique structural properties and biochemical components of diarthrodial joints make them extraordinarily durable load-bearing devices. The mature diarthrodial joint is a complex structure, influenced by its environment and mechanical demands (see Chapter 6). Joints have structural differences that are determined by their different functions. The shoulder joint, which demands an enormous range of motion, is stabilized primarily by muscles, whereas the hip, which requires motion and antigravity stability, has an intrinsically stable ball-and-socket configuration. The components of the "typical" synovial joint are the synovium, muscles, tendons, ligaments, bursae, menisci, articular cartilage, and subchondral bone. The anatomy and physiology of muscles are described in detail in Chapter 5.

Synovium

The synovium, which lines the joint cavity, is the site of production of synovial fluid that provides the nutrition for the articular cartilage and lubricates the cartilage surfaces. The synovium is a thin membrane between the fibrous joint capsule and the fluid-filled synovial cavity that attaches to skeletal tissues at the bone-cartilage interface and does not encroach on the surface of the articular cartilage. It is divided into functional compartments: the lining region (synovial intima), the subintimal stroma, and the neurovasculature (Fig. 1.5). The synovial intima, also termed *synovial lining,* is the superficial layer of the normal synovium that is in contact with the intra-articular cavity. The synovial lining is loosely attached to the subintima, which contains blood vessels, lymphatics, and nerves. Capillaries and arterioles generally are located directly underneath the synovial intima, whereas venules are located closer to the joint capsule.

A transition from loose to dense connective tissue occurs from the joint cavity to the capsule. Most cells in the normal subintimal stroma are fibroblasts and macrophages, although adipocytes and occasional mast cells are present.[92] These compartments are not circumscribed by basement membranes but nonetheless have distinct functions; they are separated from each other by chemical barriers, such as membrane peptidases, which limit the diffusion of regulatory factors between compartments. Synovial compartments are unevenly distributed within a single joint. Vascularity is high at the enthesis where synovium, ligament, and cartilage coalesce. Far from being a homogeneous tissue in continuity with the synovial cavity, synovium is highly heterogeneous, and synovial fluid may be poorly representative of the tissue-fluid composition of any synovial tissue compartment. In rheumatoid arthritis, the synovial lining of diarthrodial joints is the site of the initial inflammatory process. This lesion is characterized by proliferation of the synovial lining cells, increased vascularization, and infiltration of the tissue by inflammatory cells, including B and T lymphocytes, plasma cells, and activated macrophages (see Chapter 75).[93-96]

Synovial Lining

The synovial lining, a specialized condensation of mesenchymal cells and extra-cellular matrix, is located between the synovial cavity and stroma. In normal synovium, the lining layer is two to three cells deep, although intra-articular fat pads usually are covered by only a single layer of synovial cells, and ligaments and tendons are covered by synovial cells that are widely separated. At some sites, lining cells are absent, and the extra-cellular connective tissue constitutes the lining layer. Such "bare areas" become increasingly frequent with advancing age. Although the synovial lining is often referred to as the *synovial membrane,* the term *membrane* is more correctly reserved for endothelial and epithelial tissues that have basement membranes, tight intercellular junctions, and desmosomes. Instead, synovial lining cells lie loosely in a bed of hyaluronate interspersed with collagen fibrils; this is the macromolecular sieve that imparts the semipermeable nature of the synovium. The absence of any true basement membrane is a major determinant of joint physiology.

Early electron microscopic studies characterized lining cells as macrophage-derived type A and fibroblast-derived type B cells. High UDPGD activity and CD55 are used to distinguish type B synovial cells, whereas nonspecific esterase and CD68 typify type A cells. Normal synovium is lined predominantly by fibroblast-like synoviocytes, whereas macrophage-like synovial cells compose only 10% to 20% of lining cells (see Fig. 1.5).[94]

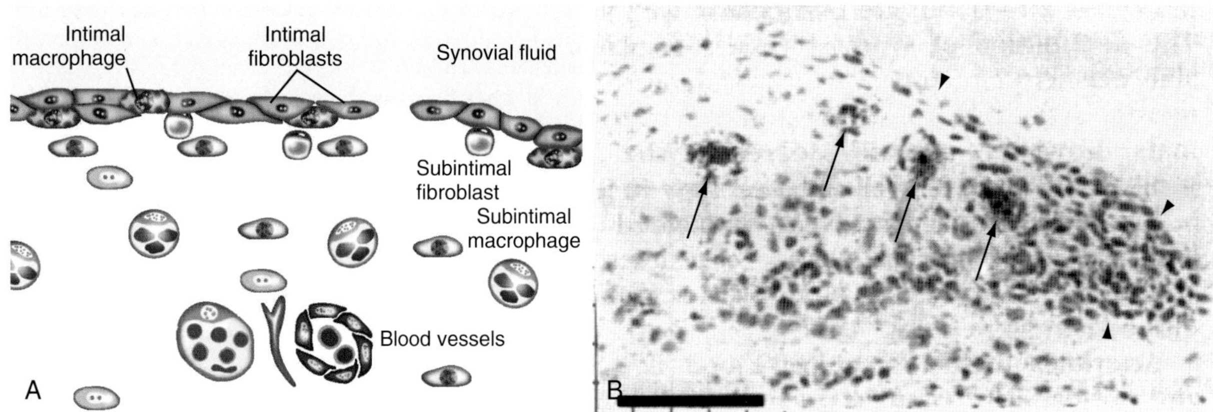

• **Fig. 1.5** (A) Schematic representation of normal human synovium. The intima contains specialized fibroblasts expressing vascular cell adhesion molecule-1 (VCAM-1), uridine diphosphoglucose (UDPG), and specialized macrophages expressing FcγRIIIa. The deeper subintima contains unspecialized counterparts. (B) Microvascular endothelium in human synovium contains receptors for the vasodilator/growth factor substance P. Silver grains represent specific binding of [^{191}I]Bolton Hunter–labeled substance P to synovial microvessels *(arrows). Arrowheads* indicate the synovial surface. Emulsion-dipped in vitro receptor autoradiography preparations with hematoxylin and eosin counterstain. Calibration bar = 1 μm. (A, from Edwards JCW: Fibroblast biology: development and differentiation of synovial fibroblasts in arthritis. *Arthritis Res* 2:344–347, 2000.)

Type A, macrophage-like synovial cells contain vacuoles, a prominent Golgi apparatus, and filopodia, but they have little rough endoplasmic reticulum. These cells express numerous cell surface markers of the monocyte-macrophage lineage, including CD16, CD45, CD11b/CD18, CD68, CD14, CD163, and the immunoglobulin (Ig)G Fc receptor, FcγRIIIa.[92,94] Synovial intimal macrophages are phagocytic and may provide a mechanism by which particulate matter can be cleared from the normal joint cavity. Similar to other tissue macrophages, these cells have little capacity to proliferate and are likely localized to the joint during development. The op/op osteopetrotic mouse that is deficient in macrophages because of an absence of macrophage colony-stimulating factor also lacks synovial macrophages, suggesting that type A synovial cells are of a common lineage with other tissue macrophages. Although they represent only a small percentage of the cells in the normal synovium, the macrophages are recruited from the circulation during synovial inflammation, potentially from subchondral bone marrow through vascular channels near the enthesis.

The type B, fibroblast-like synoviocytes contain fewer vacuoles and filopodia than type A cells and have abundant protein-synthetic organelles.[94] Similar to other fibroblasts, lining cells express genes encoding extra-cellular matrix components, including collagens, sulfated proteoglycans, fibronectin, fibrillin-1, and tenascin, and they express intra-cellular and cell surface molecules, such as vimentin and CD90 (Thy-1). They have the potential to proliferate, although proliferation markers are rarely seen in normal synovium. In contrast to stromal fibroblasts, synovial intimal fibroblasts express UDPGD and synthesize hyaluronan, an important constituent of synovial fluid.[92] They also synthesize lubricin, which, together with hyaluronan, is necessary for the low-friction interaction of cartilage surfaces in the diarthrodial joint. Synovial lining cells bear abundant membrane peptidases on their surface that are capable of degrading a wide range of regulatory peptides, such as substance P and angiotensin II.

Normal synovial lining cells also express a rich array of adhesion molecules, including CD44, the principal receptor for hyaluronan; vascular cell adhesion molecule (VCAM)-1; intercellular adhesion molecule (ICAM)-1; and CD55 (decay-accelerating factor).[94] They are essential for cellular attachment to specific matrix components in the synovial lining region, preventing loss into the synovial cavity of cells subjected to deformation and shear stresses during joint movement. Adhesion molecules such as VCAM-1 and ICAM-1 potentially are involved in the recruitment of inflammatory cells during the evolution of arthritis. Cadherins mediate cell-cell adhesion between adjacent cells of the same type. The identification of cadherin-11 as a key adhesion molecule that regulates the formation of the synovial lining during development and the synoviocyte function postnatally has provided the opportunity to examine its role in inflammatory joint disease.[83] Cadherin-11 is highly expressed in fibroblast-like cells at the pannus-cartilage interface in rheumatoid synovium, where it plays a role in the invasive properties of the synovial fibroblasts,[97] and treatment with a cadherin-11 antibody or a cadherin-11 fusion protein reduces synovial inflammation and cartilage erosion in an animal model of arthritis.[84]

Of interest, recent studies have highlighted the development and expansion of distinct synovial fibroblast populations in inflammatory arthritis, and data support a key role for these cells in the pathogenesis and maintenance of joint inflammation in rheumatoid arthritis.[98] The roles of synovitis and synovial angiogenesis are also of current interest in relation to the severity and progression of pain and joint damage in osteoarthritis (OA).[99-101]

Synovial Vasculature

The subintimal synovium contains blood vessels, providing the blood flow that is required for solute and gas exchange in the synovium itself and for the generation of synovial fluid.[102] The avascular articular cartilage also depends on nutrition in the synovial fluid, derived from the synovial vasculature. The vascularized synovium behaves similar to an endocrine organ, generating factors that regulate synoviocyte function and serving as a selective gateway that recruits cells from the circulation during stress and inflammation. Finally, synovial blood flow plays an important role in regulating intra-articular temperature.

The synovial vasculature can be divided on morphologic and functional grounds into arterioles, capillaries, and venules. In addition, lymphatics accompany arterioles and larger venules.[92] Arterial and venous networks of the joint are complex and are characterized by arteriovenous anastomoses that communicate freely with blood vessels in periosteum and periarticular bone. As large synovial arteries enter the deep layers of the synovium near the capsule, they give off branches, which bifurcate again to form "microvascular units" in the subsynovial layers. The synovial lining region, the surfaces of intra-articular ligaments, and the entheses (the angle of ligamentous insertions into bone) are particularly well vascularized.[103]

The distribution of synovial vessels, which were formed largely as a result of vasculogenesis during development of the joint, displays considerable plasticity. In inflammatory arthritis, the density of blood vessels decreases relative to the growing synovial mass, creating a hypoxic and acidotic environment.[104,105] Angiogenic factors such as VEGF, acting via VEGF receptors 1 and 2 (Flt1 and Flk2), and basic FGF promote proliferation and migration of endothelial cells, a process that is facilitated by matrix-degrading enzymes and adhesion molecules such as integrin αvβ3 and E-selectin, expressed by activated endothelial cells. Vessel maturation is facilitated by angiopoietin-1 acting via the Tie-2 receptor. The angiogenic molecules are restricted to the capillary epithelium in normal synovium, but their levels are elevated in inflamed synovium in perivascular sites and areas remote from vessels.[106,107]

Regulation of Synovial Blood Flow

Synovial blood flow is regulated by intrinsic (autocrine and paracrine) and extrinsic (neural and humoral) systems. Locally generated factors, such as the peptide vasoconstrictors angiotensin II and endothelin-1, act on adjacent arteriolar smooth muscle to regulate regional vascular tone.[103] Normal synovial arterioles are richly innervated by sympathetic nerves containing vasoconstrictors, such as norepinephrine and neuropeptide Y, and by "sensory" nerves that also play an efferent vasodilatory role by releasing neuropeptides, such as substance P and calcitonin gene–related peptide (CGRP). Arterioles regulate regional blood flow. Capillaries and postcapillary venules are sites of fluid and cellular exchange. Correspondingly, regulatory systems are differentially distributed along the vascular axis. Angiotensin-converting enzyme, which generates angiotensin II, is localized predominantly in arteriolar and capillary endothelia and decreases during inflammation. Specific receptors for angiotensin II and for substance P are abundant on synovial capillaries, with lower densities on adjacent arterioles. Dipeptidyl peptidase IV, a peptide-degrading enzyme, is specifically localized to the cell membranes of venular endothelium. The synovial vasculature is not only functionally compartmentalized from the surrounding stroma but also highly specialized along its arteriovenous axis. Other unique characteristics of the normal synovial vasculature include the presence of inducible nitric oxidase synthase–independent 3-nitrotyrosine, a reaction product of peroxynitrite, and the localization of the synoviocyte-derived CXCL12 chemokine on heparan sulfate receptors on endothelial cells, suggesting physiologic roles for these molecules in normal vascular function.

Joint Innervation

Dissection studies have shown that each joint has a dual nerve supply consisting of specific articular nerves that penetrate the capsule as independent branches of adjacent peripheral nerves and articular branches that arise from related muscle nerves. The definition of joint position and the detection of joint motion are monitored separately and by a combination of multiple inputs from different receptors in varied systems. Nerve endings in muscle and skin and in the joint capsule mediate sensation of joint position and movement. Normal joints have afferent (sensory) and efferent (motor) innervations consisting of both unmyelinated and sensory thick myelinated A fibers in ligaments, fibrous capsule, menisci, and adjacent periosteum, where they are thought to function primarily as sensors for pressure and movements. Sensory A and C fibers terminate as free nerve endings in the fibrous capsule, adipose tissue, ligaments, menisci, and the adjacent periosteum, where they are thought to act as nociceptors and contribute to the regulation of synovial microvascular function.

In normal synovium, a dense network of fine unmyelinated nerve fibers follows the courses of blood vessels and extends into the synovial lining layers. These nerve fibers are largely unmyelinated and are slow-conducting fibers; they may transmit diffuse, burning, or aching pain sensation. Sympathetic nerve fibers surround blood vessels, particularly in the deeper regions of synovium, and contain and release classic neurotransmitters, such as norepinephrine, and neuropeptides that are markers of sensory nerves including substance P, CGRP, neuropeptide Y, and vasoactive intestinal peptide.[102,108,109] Substance P and CGRP, in particular, have been implicated in modulating inflammation and the pain pathway in OA.[110] In addition, substance P is released from peripheral nerve terminals into the joint, and specific, G protein–coupled receptors for substance P are localized to microvascular endothelium in normal synovium. Abnormalities in neuropeptide release in arthritis may contribute to changes in vascular permeability and the failure of synovial inflammation to resolve.[111] The expression of substance P and CGRP are upregulated by nerve growth factor (NGF), which belongs to a family of neurotrophins that regulate neuronal growth during embryonic development. In addition to promoting nerve growth and mediating pain perception, NGF can act together with VEGF to promote blood vessel formation. Angiogenesis and nerve growth thus are linked by common pathways involving NGF, VEGF, and neuropeptides such as CGRP, neuropeptide Y, and semaphorins.[102,112,113]

Afferent nerve fibers from the joint play an important role in the reflex inhibition of muscle contraction. Trophic factors generated by motor neurons, such as the neuropeptide CGRP, are important in maintaining muscle bulk and a functional neuromuscular junction. Decreases in motor neuron trophic support during articular inflammation probably contribute to muscle wasting in arthritic conditions. Inflammation and excessive local neuropeptide release may result in the loss of nerve fibers, and synovial tissue proliferation without concomitant growth of new nerve fibers may lead to an apparent partial denervation of synovium in arthritis.[109] However, there is also evidence from humans and pre-clinical arthritis models of sprouting of sensory nerves in synovium, and ingrowth of neurovascular channels at the osteochondral junction.[102,114-116] Overall, aberrant innervation of synovium and other joint structures during arthritis development may contribute to changes in synovial joint homeostasis, motor neuron trophic support, and pain.

Mechanisms of joint pain have been reviewed in detail.[117-119] In a noninflamed joint, most sensory nerve fibers do not respond to movement within the normal range; these fibers are referred to as *silent nociceptors.* In an inflamed joint, however, these nerve fibers become sensitized by mediators such as bradykinin, neurokinin 1, NGF and prostaglandins, and the resulting peripheral sensitization leads to pain during normal joint movement, a characteristic symptom of arthritis.[110,120] Pain sensation is upregulated or downregulated further in the central nervous system, at the level of the spinal cord and in the brain, by central sensitization and "gating" of nociceptive input. A poor correlation often exists between the severity of apparent joint disease and perceived pain in people with chronic arthritis, and this may be a sign of sensitization either at the peripheral or central levels.

Synovial Fluid and Nutrition of Joint Structures

The volume and composition of synovial fluid are determined by the properties of the synovium and its vasculature. A normal joint contains a small quantity of fluid (2.5 mL in the knee), sufficient to coat the synovial and cartilage surfaces. Tendon sheath fluid and synovial fluid are biochemically similar. Both are essential for the nutrition and lubrication of adjacent avascular structures, including tendons and articular cartilage, and for limiting adhesion formation and maintaining movement. Characterization and measurement of synovial fluid constituents have proven useful for the identification of locally generated regulatory factors, markers of cartilage turnover, and the metabolic status of the joint, as well as for the assessment of the effects of therapy on cartilage homeostasis. However, interpretation of such data requires an understanding of the generation and clearance of synovial fluid and its various components.

Generation and Clearance of Synovial Fluid

Synovial fluid concentrations of a protein represent the net contributions of synovial blood flow, plasma concentration, microvascular permeability, and lymphatic removal and its production and consumption within the joint space. Synovial fluid is a mixture of a protein-rich ultrafiltrate of plasma and hyaluronan synthesized by synoviocytes.[93] Generation of this ultrafiltrate depends on the differences between intracapillary and intra-articular hydrostatic pressures and between colloid osmotic pressures of capillary plasma and synovial tissue fluid. Fenestrations (i.e., small pores covered by a thin membrane) in the synovial capillaries and the macromolecular sieve of hyaluronic acid facilitate rapid exchange of small molecules, such as glucose and lactate, assisted—in the case of glucose—by an active transport system. Proteins are present in synovial fluid at concentrations inversely proportional to molecular size, with synovial fluid albumin concentrations being about 45% of those in plasma. Concentrations of electrolytes and small molecules are equivalent to those in plasma.[121]

Synovial fluid is cleared through lymphatics in the synovium, assisted by joint movement. In contrast to ultrafiltration, lymphatic clearance of solutes is independent of molecular size. In addition, constituents of synovial fluid, such as regulatory peptides, may be degraded locally by enzymes, and low-molecular-weight metabolites may diffuse along concentration gradients into plasma. The kinetics of delivery and removal of a protein must be determined (e.g., using albumin as a reference solute) to assess the significance of its concentration in the joint.[122]

Hyaluronic acid is synthesized by fibroblast-like synovial lining cells, and it appears in high concentrations in synovial fluid at around 3 g/L, compared with a plasma concentration of 30 μg/L.[93] Lubricin, a glycoprotein that assists articular lubrication, is another constituent of synovial fluid that is generated by the lining cells.[123] It is now believed that hyaluronan functions in fluid-film lubrication, whereas lubricin is the true boundary lubricant in synovial fluid (see later discussion). Because the volume of synovial fluid is determined by the amount of hyaluronan, water retention seems to be the major function of this large molecule.

Despite the absence of a basement membrane, synovial fluid does not mix freely with extra-cellular synovial tissue fluid. Hyaluronan may trap molecules within the synovial cavity by acting as a filtration screen on the surface of the synovial lining, resisting the movement of synovial fluid out from the joint space. Synovial fluid proteins have a rapid turnover time (around 1 hour in normal knees), and equilibrium is not usually reached among all parts of the joint. However, the turnover time for hyaluronan in the normal joint (13 hours) is an order of magnitude slower than that of small solutes and proteins, so association with hyaluronan may result in trapping of solutes within synovial fluid. Tissue fluid around fenestrated endothelium reflects plasma ultrafiltrate most closely, with a low content of hyaluronate compared with synovial fluid. Locally generated or released peptides, such as endothelin and substance P, may attain much higher perivascular concentrations than those measured in synovial fluid.

In normal joints, intra-articular pressures are slightly subatmospheric at rest (0 to −5 mm Hg). During exercise, hydrostatic pressure in the normal joint may decrease further. Repeated abnormal mechanical stresses can interrupt synovial perfusion during joint movement, particularly in the presence of a synovial effusion. Resting intra-articular pressures in rheumatoid joints are around 20 mm Hg, whereas during isometric exercise, they may increase to greater than 100 mm Hg, well above capillary perfusion pressure and, at times, above arterial pressure.

Synovial Fluid as an Indicator of Joint Function

In the absence of a basement membrane separating synovium or cartilage from synovial fluid, measurements of synovial fluid may reflect the activity of these tissues. A wide range of regulatory factors and products of synoviocyte metabolism and cartilage breakdown may be generated locally within the joint, resulting in marked differences between the composition of synovial fluid and plasma ultrafiltrate. Because little capacity exists for the selective concentration of solutes in synovial fluid, solutes that are present at higher concentrations than in plasma are probably synthesized locally. It is necessary, however, to know the local clearance rate to determine whether the solutes present in synovial fluid at lower concentrations than in plasma are generated locally.[121,122] Because clearance rates from synovial fluid may be slower than those from plasma, synovial fluid levels of drugs or urate may remain elevated after plasma levels have declined.

Plasma proteins are less effectively filtered in inflamed synovium, perhaps because of increased size of endothelial cell fenestrations or because interstitial hyaluronate-protein complexes are fragmented by enzymes associated with the inflammatory process. Concentrations of proteins, such as α2 macroglobulin (the principal proteinase inhibitor of plasma), fibrinogen, and IgM, are elevated in synovial fluid from patients with arthritis (see Fig. 1.6), as are associated protein-bound cations. Membrane peptidases may limit the diffusion of regulatory peptides from their sites of release into synovial fluid. In inflammatory arthritis, fibrin deposits may additionally retard flow between the tissue and the liquid phase.

Investigators[124] analyzed synovial fluids and sera from a small series of patients with OA and rheumatoid arthritis using mass spectrometry and multiplex bead-based immunoassays. They identified more than a hundred proteins that were increased in the synovial fluid of patients with OA compared with healthy subjects. Of interest, they found that more than one-third of these were plasma proteins. They speculated that the elevation of these plasma proteins in the synovial fluid could be related to alterations in the endothelial barrier associated with local inflammation in the synovial tissue.

Synovial fluid alterations in joint disease may also reflect local aberrant production by cells within the joint. Investigators[125] utilized high-throughput proteomic analysis to define protein expression profiles of high abundance synovial fluid

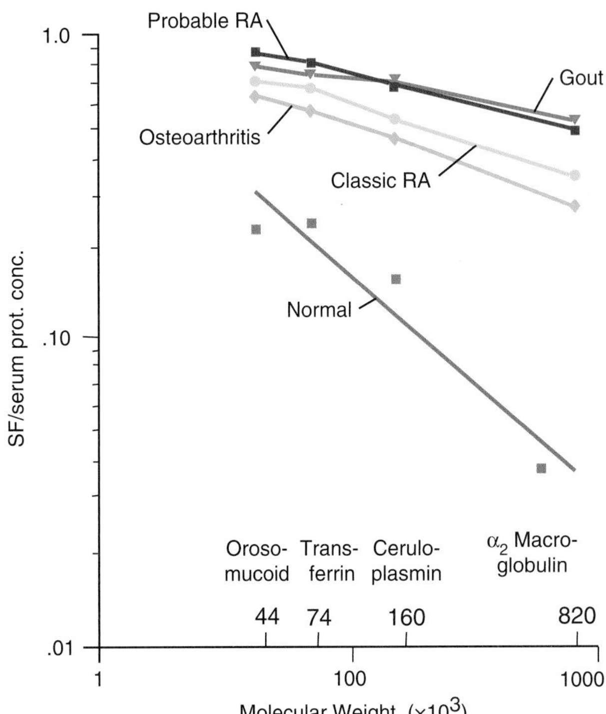

• **Fig. 1.6** Ratio of the concentration of proteins in synovial fluid to that found in serum, plotted as a function of molecular weight. Larger proteins are selectively excluded from normal synovial fluid, but this macromolecular sieve is less effective in diseased synovium. *Prot. conc.,* Protein concentration; *RA,* rheumatoid arthritis; *SF,* synovial fluid. (From Kushner I, Somerville JA: Permeability of human synovial membrane to plasma proteins. *Arthritis Rheum* 14:560, 1971. Reprinted with permission of the American College of Rheumatology.)

proteins in healthy subjects and in patients with early and late OA. They identified 18 proteins that were significantly differentially expressed between the osteoarthritic and control groups. Although all 18 were present in blood and could enter the joint through alterations in vascular permeability, these molecules were also products of synovial cells and chondrocytes. Investigators[126] further clarified that some of the OA proteome could result from local production, by comparing the synovial fluid protein composition with mRNA expression profiles of joint tissues. This analysis demonstrated that many of the proteins elevated in synovial fluid were derived from synovium or cartilage, providing direct evidence that cells within the joint were a source of the synovial fluid products. Proteins associated with oxidative damage and activation of mitogen-activated protein kinases were among the high-abundance molecules in the OA synovial fluids. They also identified members of the pro-inflammatory complement cascade. Of interest, these molecules have been implicated in the pathophysiology of both OA and rheumatoid arthritis.[127]

Lubrication and Nutrition of the Articular Cartilage

Lubrication

Synovial fluid serves as a lubricant for articular cartilage and a source of nutrition for the chondrocytes. Lubrication is essential for protecting cartilage and other joint structures from friction and shear stresses associated with movement under loading. There are two basic categories of joint lubrication. In fluid-film lubrication, cartilage surfaces are separated by an incompressible fluid film, and hyaluronan primarily provides this function. In boundary lubrication, specialized molecules attached to the cartilage surface permit surface-to-surface contact while decreasing the coefficient of friction. During loading, a noncompressible fluid film is trapped between opposing cartilage surfaces and prevents the surfaces from touching. Irregularities in the cartilage surface and its deformation during compression may augment this trapping of fluid. This stable film is approximately 0.1-μm thick in the normal human hip joint, but it can be much thinner in the presence of inflammatory synovial fluid or with increased cartilage porosity.[93]

Lubricin (also called superficial zone protein or proteoglycan 4) is the major boundary lubricant in the human joint.[123] Lubricin is a glycoprotein synthesized by synovial cells, superficial zone chondrocytes, meniscus, and tendon cells.[128,129] It has a molecular weight of 225,000, a length of 200 nm, and a diameter of 1 to 2 nm. Dipalmitoyl phosphatidylcholine, which constitutes 45% of the lipid in normal synovial fluid, acts together with lubricin as a boundary lubricant. In boundary lubrication, lubricin functions as a phospholipid carrier via a mechanism that is common to all tissues and protects the cartilage by reducing pathologic deposition of proteins at the cartilage surface.[130] It is enriched on the surface of articular cartilage, and although mechanisms that maintain its surface localization for boundary lubrication are unknown, recent work suggests that both noncovalent and covalent bonding with the COMP may be important.[131] People with loss-of-function mutations in the lubricin gene have the camptodactyly-arthopathy-coxa vara-pericarditis syndrome, which is associated with the development of severe premature OA.[132] Of interest, long-term overexpression of lubricin in animal models of OA protects against both age-related and post-traumatic OA through inhibition of transcriptional programs that promote cartilage catabolism and chondrocyte hypertrophy.[133]

Nutrition

As observed by Hunter in 1743,[134] normal adult articular cartilage contains no blood vessels, which is essential to maintain its mechanical properties. If vascularized, blood flow in cartilage would be repeatedly occluded during weight bearing and exercise, with reactive oxygen species generated during reperfusion resulting in repeated damage to cartilage matrix and chondrocytes. Chondrocytes synthesize specific inhibitors of angiogenesis that maintain articular cartilage as an avascular tissue.[135-138] As a result, chondrocytes normally live in a hypoxic and acidotic environment with extra-cellular fluid pH values around 7.1 to 7.2,[139] and use anaerobic glycolysis for energy production.[140,141] High lactate levels in normal synovial fluid, compared with paired plasma measurements, partially reflect this anaerobic metabolism.[141] The two sources of nutrients for articular cartilage are the synovial fluid and subchondral blood vessels.

The synovial fluid and, indirectly, the synovial lining, through which synovial fluid is generated, are the major sources of nutrients for articular cartilage. Nutrients may enter cartilage from synovial fluid either by diffusion or mass transport during compression-relaxation cycles.[142] Molecules as large as hemoglobin (65 kDa) can diffuse through normal articular cartilage,[143] and the solutes needed for cellular metabolism are much smaller. Diffusion of uncharged small solutes, such as glucose, is not impaired in matrices containing large amounts of glycosaminoglycans, and diffusivity of small molecules through hyaluronate is enhanced.[144,145]

Intermittent compression may serve as a pump mechanism for solute exchange in cartilage. The concept has arisen from observations that joint immobilization or dislocation leads to degenerative change, while exercise increases solute penetration into cartilage in experimental systems.[143] During weight bearing, fluid escapes from the load-bearing region by flow to other cartilage sites. When the load is removed, cartilage re-expands and draws back fluid, exchanging nutrients with waste materials.[146]

In a growing child, the deeper layers of cartilage are vascularized, such that blood vessels penetrate between columns of chondrocytes in the growth plate. It is likely that nutrients diffuse from these tiny end capillaries through the matrix to chondrocytes. Diffusion from subchondral blood vessels is not considered a major route for the nutrition of normal adult articular cartilage because of the barrier provided by its densely calcified lower layer. Nonetheless, partial defects may normally exist in this barrier,[147] and neovascularization of the deeper layers of articular cartilage in arthritis may contribute both to cartilage nutrition and to entry of inflammatory cells and cytokines.[148-150]

Mature Articular Cartilage

Articular cartilage is a specialized connective tissue that covers the weight-bearing surfaces of diarthrodial joints. The principal functions of cartilage layers covering bone ends are to permit low-friction, high-velocity movement between bones, to absorb the transmitted forces associated with locomotion, and to contribute to joint stability. Lubrication by synovial fluid provides frictionless movement of the articulating cartilage surfaces. Chondrocytes (see Chapter 3) are the single cellular component of adult hyaline articular cartilage and are responsible for synthesizing and maintaining the highly specialized cartilage matrix macromolecules. The cartilage extra-cellular matrix is composed of an extensive network of collagen fibrils, which confers tensile strength, and an interlocking mesh of proteoglycans, which provides compressive stiffness through the ability to absorb and extrude water. Numerous other noncollagenous proteins also contribute to the unique properties of cartilage (Table 1.1). Histologically, the tissue appears fairly homogeneous and clearly distinguished from the calcified cartilage and underlying subchondral bone (Fig. 1.7). However, significant topographical and regional differences exist in the molecular organization and composition of the articular cartilage, as described in Chapter 3.

Subchondral Bone

Subchondral bone is not a homogeneous tissue, and it consists of a layer of compact cortical bone and an underlying system of cancellous bone organized into a trabecular network.[151,152] The subchondral bone is separated from the overlying articular cartilage by a thin zone of calcified cartilage. This complex biocomposite of bone and calcified cartilage provides an optimal system for distributing loads that are transmitted from the weight-bearing surfaces lined by hyaline articular cartilage. The so-called tidemark defines the transition zone between the articular and calcified cartilage. Although the tidemark was originally believed to form a barrier to fluid flow, evidence shows that biologically active molecules can transit this zone, providing a mechanism by which products produced by chondrocytes and bone cells can influence the activity of the other cell type.[153,154] In addition, further communication is provided via products released from vascular elements in channels that penetrate the calcified cartilage from the adjacent marrow space.[148] Under physiologic conditions, the composition and structural organization of the subchondral bone and calcified cartilage are optimally adapted to transfer loads, but several conditions can lead to changes in structural and functional properties of these tissues.

The subchondral bone undergoes continuous structural reorganization throughout postnatal life. These alterations are mediated by the coordinated activity of bone-resorbing osteoclasts and bone-forming osteoblasts that remodel and adapt the bone in response to local biomechanical and biological signals.[155] Osteocytes are the bone cell type that regulates the bone remodeling process.[156,157] Osteocytes are distributed throughout the mineralized bone matrix, forming an interconnected network that is ideally positioned to sense and respond to local and systemic stimuli. These effects are mediated via both cell-cell interactions with osteoclasts and osteoblasts but also via signaling through the release of soluble mediators. These products include RANKL, the essential regulator of osteoclast differentiation and activity and its inhibitor osteoprotegerin (OPG),[158,159] as well as additional mediators, including prostanoids, nitric oxide, nucleotides, and a broad spectrum of growth factors and cytokines.[160] In addition to these factors, osteocytes also produce sclerostin and Dickkopf-related protein 1 (DKK-1), which are potent inhibitors of the Wnt/β-catenin pathway that regulates osteoblast-mediated bone formation.[161] The release of RANKL, OPG, and Wnt pathway regulators (DKK-1 and sclerostin) plays a major role in controlling the adaptation of the subchondral bone to alterations in mechanical loading in both physiologic and pathologic conditions.

The maintenance of the structural and functional integrity of articular cartilage and subchondral bone under physiologic loading is evidence of the unique and intimate interaction of these tissues, but controversy remains with regard to the relationship between them in the pathogenesis of OA.[162] Radin and Rose[163] proposed that the initiation of early alterations in articular cartilage is caused by an increase in subchondral bone stiffness that adversely affects the function of articular chondrocytes, leading

TABLE 1.1 Extra-cellular Matrix Components of Articular Cartilage[a]

Collagens
Type II
Type IX
Type XI
Type VI
Types XII, XIV
Type X (hypertrophic chondrocyte)
Proteoglycans
Aggrecan
Versican
Link protein
Biglycan (DS-PGI)
Decorin (DS-PGII)
Epiphycan (DS-PGIII)
Fibromodulin
Lumican
Proline/arginine-rich and leucine-rich repeat protein (PRELP)
Chondroadherin
Perlecan
Lubricin (SZP)
Other Noncollagenous Proteins (Structural)
Cartilage oligomeric matrix protein (COMP) or thrombospondin-5
Thrombospondin-1 and thrombospondin-3
Cartilage matrix protein (matrilin-1) and matrilin-3
Fibronectin
Tenascin-C
Cartilage intermediate layer protein (CILP)
Fibrillin
Elastin
Other Noncollagenous Proteins (Regulatory)
Glycoprotein (gp)-39, YKL-40
Matrix Gla protein (MGP)
Chondromodulin-I (SCGP) and chondromodulin-II
Cartilage-derived retinoic acid–sensitive protein (CD-RAP)
Growth factors
Cell Membrane–Associated Proteins
Integrins (α1β1, α2β1, α3β1, α5β1, α6β1, α10β1, αvβ3, αvβ5)
Anchorin CII (annexin V)
Cell determinant 44 (CD44)
Syndecan-1, 3, and 4
Discoidin domain receptor 2

[a]The collagens, proteoglycans, and other noncollagenous proteins in the cartilage matrix are synthesized by chondrocytes at different stages during development and growth of cartilage. In mature articular cartilage, proteoglycans and other noncollagen proteins are turned over slowly, whereas the collagen network is stable unless exposed to proteolytic cleavage. Proteins that are associated with chondrocyte cell membranes also are listed because they permit specific interactions with extra-cellular matrix proteins. The specific structure-function relationships are discussed in Chapter 3 and described in Table 3.1.

DS-PG, Dermatan sulfate proteoglycan; *SCGP,* small cartilage–derived glycoprotein; *SZP,* superficial zone protein; *YKL-40,* 40KD chitinase 3-like glycoprotein.

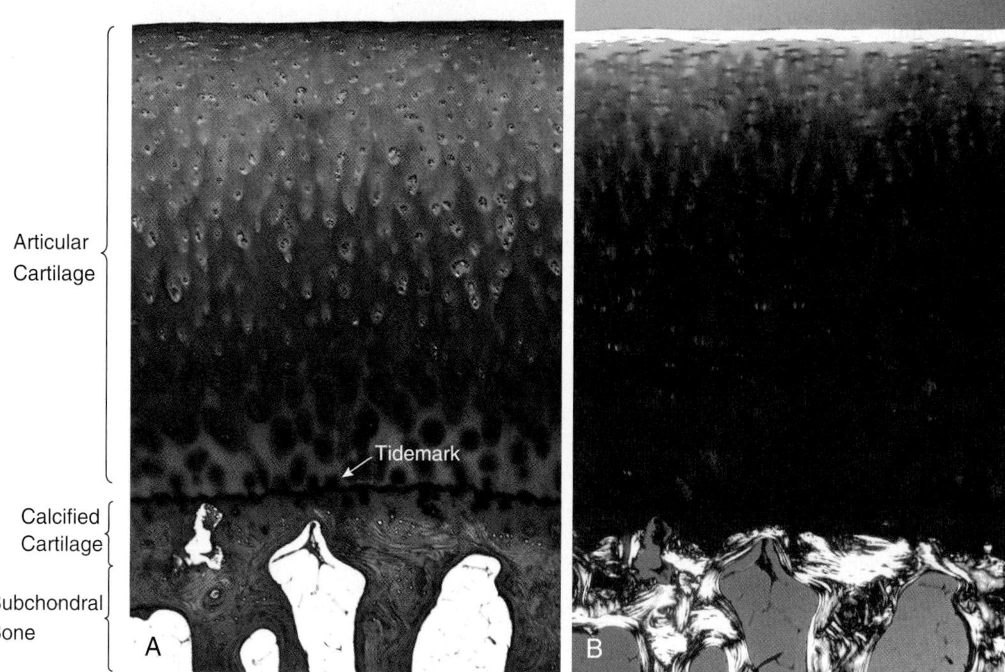

• **Fig. 1.7** Representative sections of normal human adult articular cartilage, showing nearly the same field in plain (A) and polarized (B) light. Note the clear demarcation of the articular cartilage from the calcified cartilage below the tidemark and the underlying subchondral bone. (Hematoxylin-eosin stain; original magnification ×60.) (Courtesy Edward F. DiCarlo, MD, Pathology Department, Hospital for Special Surgery, New York, N.Y.)

to deterioration in the properties of the articular cartilage and susceptibility to mechanical disruption. Alternatively, changes in subchondral bone stiffness may be a result of cartilage deterioration.[164-166] The alterations in subchondral bone and cartilage that accompany the osteoarthritic process are not restricted to these tissues but also affect the zone of calcified cartilage where there is evidence of vascular invasion, advancement of the calcified cartilage, and duplication of the tidemark that contributes to a decrease in articular cartilage thickness.[149,167] The penetration of the vascular channels from the subchondral bone and calcified cartilage into the deep zones of the articular cartilage permit exchange of fluids and soluble mediators between these tissues, providing an additional mechanism by which the subchondral bone and articular cartilage can affect the activity of cells within each of these tissues. These structural alterations in the articular cartilage and periarticular bone may also lead to modification of the contours of the adjacent articulating surfaces, further contributing to the adverse biomechanical environment.[163,168-170]

Tendons

Tendons are functional and anatomic bridges between muscle and bone.[171,172] Tendons focus the force of a large mass of muscle into a localized area on bone and, by splitting to form numerous insertions, may distribute the force of a single muscle to different bones. Tendons are formed of longitudinally arranged collagen fibrils embedded in an organized, hydrated proteoglycan matrix with blood vessels, lymphatics, and fibroblasts.[173] Cross-links between adjacent collagen chains or molecules contribute to the tensile strength of the tendon. Tendon collagen fibrillogenesis is initiated during early development by a highly ordered process of alignment involving the actin cytoskeleton and cadherin-11.[174,175] Many tendons, particularly those with a large range of motion, run through vascularized, discontinuous sheaths of collagen lined with mesenchymal cells resembling synovium (the tenosynovium). Gliding of tendons through their sheaths is enhanced by hyaluronic acid produced by the lining cells. Tendon movement is essential for the embryogenesis and maintenance of tendons and their sheaths.[176,177] Degenerative changes appear in tendons, and fibrous adhesions form between tendons and sheaths when inflammation or surgical incision is followed by long periods of immobilization.

At the myotendinous junction, recesses between muscle cell processes are filled with collagen fibrils, which blend into the tendon. At its other end, collagen fibers of the tendon typically blend into fibrocartilage, mineralize, and merge into bone through a fibrocartilaginous transition zone termed the *enthesis,* or insertion site.[178] In health, this graded, transitional structure allows for load transfer and minimization of stress at these attachments during movement. However, these attachment sites are susceptible to injury and degeneration, as well as inflammatory disease. Failure of the muscle-tendon apparatus is rare; when it does occur, it is the result of enormous, quickly generated forces across a joint and usually occurs at the enthesis where the tendon inserts into bone.[179] Factors that may predispose to tendon failure are aging processes, including loss of extra-cellular water and the increase in intermolecular cross-links of collagen; tendon ischemia; iatrogenic factors, including injection of glucocorticoids; and deposition of calcium hydroxyapatite crystals within the collagen bundles. Alterations in collagen fibril composition and structure are associated with tendon degeneration during aging and may predispose to enthesopathy and OA. Emerging studies are also shedding light on the importance of enthesial resident innate lymphoid cells, T lymphocytes, and the inflammatory cytokines IL-23, IL-17, TNF, and IL-22, which may drive enthesial inflammation in spondyloarthritis.[180]

Tendon fibroblasts synthesize and secrete collagens, proteoglycans, and other matrix components, such as fibronectin and tenascin C, as well as MMPs and their inhibitors, which can contribute to the breakdown and repair of tendon components.[173] Collagen fibrils in tendon are composed primarily of type I collagen with some type III collagen, but there are regional differences in the distribution of other matrix components. The compressed region contains the small proteoglycans, biglycan, decorin, fibromodulin, and lumican, as well as the large proteoglycan versican. The major components in the tensile region of the tendon are decorin, microfibrillar type VI collagen, fibromodulin, and the proline and arginine-rich end leucine-rich repeat protein (PRELP). The presence of COMP, aggrecan, biglycan, and collagen types II, IX, and XI is indicative of fibrocartilage. The collagen fiber orientation at the tendon-to-bone enthesis is important for maintaining microarchitecture by reducing the stress concentrations and shielding the outward splay of the insertion from the highest stresses.[181]

Understanding the structure and development of the enthesis has implications for tendon repair, because motion between a tendon graft and bone tunnel (i.e., in anterior cruciate ligament [ACL] repair) may impair early graft incorporation and lead to tunnel widening secondary to bone resorption.[182,183] Entheses develop during late fetal period but continue to mature during the early postnatal period. Clonal expansion of GDF5 progenitors promote the linear growth of the enthesis.[184] Recent work on Ihh signaling has demonstrated its importance in formation of the fibrocartilaginous zone, as Hedgehog responsive cells within this region mature from unmineralized to mineralized fibrochondrocytes.[184,185] The Ihh signaling pathway is reactivated during tendon-to-bone healing,[186] but this appears to be insufficient on its own to recapitulate the structure and strength of an enthesis attachment in pre-clinical models of tendon repair.[187] One potential reason may be the loss of Ihh responsive Gli1+ progenitor cells in the adult.[188] However, how Ihh signaling intersects with other mediators and developmental pathways (such as those involving Sox9, scleraxis, Mohawk, members of the TGF-β/BMP superfamily, and Wnt/β-catenin) in enthesis development needs further clarification to inform strategies for tendon repair in the future.[189-191]

Ligaments

Ligaments, which provide a stabilizing bridge between bones, permit a limited range of movement.[192] Ligaments often are recognized only as hypertrophied components of the fibrous joint capsule and are structurally similar to tendons.[193] Although the fibers are oriented parallel to the longitudinal axis of both tissues, the collagen fibrils in ligaments are nonparallel and arranged in fibers that are oriented roughly along the long axis in a wavy, undulating pattern, or "crimp," which can straighten in response to load. Some ligaments have a higher ratio of elastin to collagen (1 : 4) than do tendons (1 : 50), which permits a greater degree of stretch. Ligaments also have larger amounts of reducible cross-links, more type III collagen, slightly less total collagen, and more glycosaminoglycans compared with tendons. The cells in ligaments seem to be more metabolically active than the cells in tendons and have more plump cellular nuclei and higher DNA content.

During postnatal growth, the development of ligament attachment zones involves changes in the ratios and distribution of types I, III, and V collagen and in the synthesis of type II collagen and proteoglycans by fibrochondrocytes that develop from ligament cells at the attachment zone. Attachment zones are believed to permit gradual transmission of the tensile force between ligament and bone.

Ligaments play a major role in the passive stabilization of joints, aided by the capsule and, when present, menisci. In the knee, the collateral and cruciate ligaments provide stability when there is little or no load on the joint. As compressive load increases, there is an increasing contribution to stability from the joint surfaces themselves and the surrounding musculature. Injured ligaments generally heal well, and structural integrity is restored by contracture of the healing ligament so it can act again as a stabilizer of the joint.

Bursae

The many bursae in the human body facilitate gliding of one tissue over another, much as a tendon sheath facilitates movement of its tendon. Bursae are closed sacs usually located where muscles or tendons move over bony joints or prominences, lined sparsely with mesenchymal cells that are similar to synovial cells, but generally less well vascularized than synovium. Most bursae differentiate concurrently with synovial joints during embryogenesis. Throughout life, trauma or inflammation may lead to clinical bursitis, the development of new bursae, hypertrophy of previously existing ones, or communication between deep bursae and joints. In patients with rheumatoid arthritis, communications may exist between the subacromial bursae and the glenohumeral joint, between the gastrocnemius or semimembranosus bursae and the knee joint, and between the iliopsoas bursa and the hip joint. It is unusual, however, for subcutaneous bursae, such as the prepatellar bursa or olecranon bursa, to develop communication with the underlying joint.[194]

Menisci

The meniscus, a fibrocartilaginous, wedge-shaped structure, is best developed in the knee but also is found in the acromioclavicular and sternoclavicular joints, the ulnocarpal joint, and the temporomandibular joint. Until recently, menisci were thought to have little function and a quiescent metabolism with no capability of repair, although early observations indicated that removal of menisci from the knee could lead to premature arthritic changes in the joint. Evidence from arthroscopic studies of patients with ACL insufficiency indicates that disease of the medial meniscus correlates with that of the medial femoral cartilage. The meniscus is now considered to be an integral component of the knee joint that has important functions in joint stability, load distribution, shock absorption, and lubrication.[195,196]

The microanatomy of the knee meniscus is complex and age dependent.[197] The characteristic shapes of the lateral and the medial menisci are achieved early in prenatal development. At that time, the menisci are cellular and highly vascularized; with maturation, vascularity decreases progressively from the central margin to the peripheral margin. After skeletal maturity, the peripheral 10% to 30% of the meniscus remains highly vascularized by a circumferential capillary plexus and is well innervated. Tears in this vascularized peripheral zone may undergo repair and remodeling. The central portion of the mature meniscus is an avascular fibrocartilage, however, without nerves or lymphatics, consisting of cells surrounded by an abundant extra-cellular matrix of collagens, chondroitin sulfate, dermatan sulfate, and hyaluronic acid. Tears in this central zone heal poorly, if at all.

Collagen constitutes 60% to 70% of the dry weight of the meniscus and is mostly type I collagen, with lesser amounts of types III, V, and VI. A small quantity of cartilage-specific type II collagen is localized to the inner, avascular portion of the meniscus. Collagen fibers in the periphery are mostly circumferentially oriented, with radial fibers extending toward the central portion. Elastin content is around 0.6%, and proteoglycan content is around 2% to 3% dry weight. Aggrecan and decorin are the major proteoglycans in the adult meniscus. Decorin is the predominant proteoglycan synthesized in the meniscus from young people, whereas the relative proportion of aggrecan synthesis increases with age. Although the capacity of the meniscus to synthesize sulfated proteoglycans decreases after the teenage years, the age-related increases in expression of decorin and aggrecan mRNA suggest that the resident cells are able to respond quickly to alterations in the biomechanical environment.

The meniscus was defined originally as a fibrocartilage, based on the rounded or oval shape of most of the cells and the fibrous microscopic appearance of the extra-cellular matrix. Based on molecular and spatial criteria, three distinct populations of cells are recognized in the meniscus of the knee joint[198]:

1. The fibrochondrocyte is the most abundant cell in the middle and inner meniscus, synthesizing primarily type I collagen and relatively small amounts of type II and III collagens. It is round or oval in shape and has a pericellular filamentous matrix containing type VI collagen.
2. The fibroblast-like cells lack a pericellular matrix and are located in the outer portion of the meniscus. They are distinguished by long, thin, branching cytoplasmic projections that stain for vimentin. They make contact with other cells in different regions via connexin 43–containing gap junctions. The presence of two centrosomes, one associated with a primary cilium, suggests a sensory, rather than motile function that could enable the cells to respond to circumferential tensile loads rather than compressive loads.
3. The superficial zone cells have a characteristic fusiform shape with no cytoplasmic projections. The occasional staining of these cells in the uninjured meniscus with α-actin and their migration into surrounding wound sites suggest that they are specialized progenitor cells that may participate in a remodeling response in the meniscus and surrounding tissues.

Cell lineage tracing and gene profiling studies in mouse embryos have provided insight into the complexity of the meniscus and how it was formed.[199,200] Researchers have considerable interest in using this information to develop new strategies for meniscal repair and regeneration.

Conclusion

Normal human synovial joints are complex structures that comprise interacting connective tissue elements that permit constrained and low-friction movement of adjacent bones. The development of synovial joints in the embryo is a highly ordered process involving complex cell-cell and cell-matrix interactions that lead to the formation of the cartilage anlage, interzone, and joint cavitation. Understanding of the cellular interactions and molecular factors involved in cartilage morphogenesis and limb development has provided clues to understanding the functions of the synovium, articular cartilage, and associated structures in the mature joint.

The synovial joint is uniquely adapted to respond to environmental and mechanical demands. The synovial lining is composed of two to three cell layers, with no basement membrane separating the lining cells from the underlying connective tissue, which is innervated and vascularized. The synovium regulates molecular trafficking between the joint space and the vascular system, and it produces synovial fluid, which provides nutrition and lubrication to the avascular articular cartilage. Normal articular cartilage contains a single cell type, the articular chondrocyte, which is responsible for maintaining the integrity of the extra-cellular cartilage matrix. This matrix consists of a complex network of collagens, proteoglycans, and other noncollagenous proteins, which provide tensile strength and compressive resistance. Proper distribution and relative composition of these proteins is required for the maintenance and function of the articular cartilage during joint loading and motion. The subchondral bone and the overlying articular and calcified cartilage form a unique biocomposite that provides an optimal system for distributing loads during joint motion. The other tissue of the joint (tendons, ligaments, bursae) function to maintain stability and assist in joint motion.

Maintenance of the unique composition and organization of each joint tissue is crucial for normal joint function, which is compromised in response to inflammation, biomechanical injury, and aging. Knowledge of the normal structure-function relationships within joint tissues is essential for understanding the pathogenesis and consequences of joint diseases.

Full references for this chapter can be found on ExpertConsult.com.

Selected References

1. Olsen BR, Reginato AM, Wang W: Bone development, *Annu Rev Cell Dev Biol* 16:191–220, 2000.
2. O'Rahilly R, Gardner E: The timing and sequence of events in the development of the limbs in the human embryo, *Anat Embryol (Berl)* 148:1–23, 1975.
3. O'Rahilly R, Gardner E: The embryology of movable joints. In Sokoloff L, editor: *The joints and synovial fluid* (vol 1). New York, 1978, Academic Press, p 49.
4. Archer CW, Dowthwaite GP, Francis-West P: Development of synovial joints, *Birth Defects Res C Embryo Today* 69:144–155, 2003.
5. Zelzer E, Olsen BR: The genetic basis for skeletal diseases, *Nature* 423:343–348, 2003.
6. Goldring MB, Tsuchimochi K, Ijiri K: The control of chondrogenesis, *J Cell Biochem* 97:33–44, 2006.
7. Khan IM, Redman SN, Williams R, et al.: The development of synovial joints, *Curr Top Dev Biol* 79:1–36, 2007.
8. Pitsillides AA, Ashhurst DE: A critical evaluation of specific aspects of joint development, *Dev Dyn* 237:2284–2294, 2008.
9. Decker RS, Koyama E, Pacifici M: Genesis and morphogenesis of limb synovial joints and articular cartilage, *Matrix Biol* 39:5–10, 2014.
10. Pacifici M, Koyama E, Iwamoto M: Mechanisms of synovial joint and articular cartilage formation: recent advances, but many lingering mysteries, *Birth Defects Res C Embryo Today* 75:237–248, 2005.
11. Spater D, Hill TP, Gruber M, et al.: Role of canonical Wnt-signalling in joint formation, *Eur Cell Mater* 12:71–80, 2006.
12. Storm EE, Kingsley DM: GDF5 coordinates bone and joint formation during digit development, *Dev Biol* 209:11–27, 1999.
13. Shwartz Y, Viukov S, Krief S, et al.: Joint development involves a continuous influx of Gdf5-positive cells, *Cell Reports* 15:2577–2587, 2016.

14. Colnot CI, Helms JA: A molecular analysis of matrix remodeling and angiogenesis during long bone development, *Mech Dev* 100:245–250, 2001.
15. Colnot C, Lu C, Hu D, et al.: Distinguishing the contributions of the perichondrium, cartilage, and vascular endothelium to skeletal development, *Dev Biol* 269:55–69, 2004.
16. Nalin AM, Greenlee Jr TK, Sandell LJ: Collagen gene expression during development of avian synovial joints: transient expression of types II and XI collagen genes in the joint capsule, *Dev Dyn* 203:352–362, 1995.
17. Hyde G, Dover S, Aszodi A, et al.: Lineage tracing using matrilin-1 gene expression reveals that articular chondrocytes exist as the joint interzone forms, *Dev Biol* 304:825–833, 2007.
18. Pollard AS, McGonnell IM, Pitsillides AA: Mechanoadaptation of developing limbs: shaking a leg, *J Anat* 224:615–623, 2014.
19. Kahn J, Shwartz Y, Blitz E, et al.: Muscle contraction is necessary to maintain joint progenitor cell fate, *Dev Cell* 16:734–743, 2009.
20. Nowlan NC, Sharpe J, Roddy KA, et al.: Mechanobiology of embryonic skeletal development: insights from animal models, *Birth Defects Res C Embryo Today* 90:203–213, 2010.
21. Nowlan NC: Biomechanics of foetal movement, *Eur Cell Mater* 29:1–21, 2015, discussion 21.
22. Hall BK, Miyake T: All for one and one for all: condensations and the initiation of skeletal development, *Bioessays* 22:138–147, 2000.
23. Fell HB: The histogenesis of cartilage and bone in the long bones of the embryonic fowl, *J Morphol Physiol* 40:417–459, 1925.
24. DeLise AM, Fischer L, Tuan RS: Cellular interactions and signaling in cartilage development, *Osteoarthritis Cartilage* 8:309–334, 2000.
25. Eames BF, de la Fuente L, Helms JA: Molecular ontogeny of the skeleton, *Birth Defects Res C Embryo Today* 69:93–101, 2003.
26. Tuan RS: Biology of developmental and regenerative skeletogenesis, *Clin Orthop Relat Res* 427(Suppl):S105–S117, 2004.
27. Seo HS, Serra R: Deletion of Tgfbr2 in Prx1-cre expressing mesenchyme results in defects in development of the long bones and joints, *Dev Biol* 310:304–316, 2007.
28. Spagnoli A, O'Rear L, Chandler RL, et al.: TGF-beta signaling is essential for joint morphogenesis, *J Cell Biol* 177:1105–1117, 2007.
29. Long F, Ornitz DM: Development of the endochondral skeleton, *Cold Spring Harb Perspect Biol* 5:a008334, 2013.
30. Barna M, Niswander L: Visualization of cartilage formation: insight into cellular properties of skeletal progenitors and chondrodysplasia syndromes, *Dev Cell* 12:931–941, 2007.
31. Kmita M, Tarchini B, Zakany J, et al.: Early developmental arrest of mammalian limbs lacking HoxA/HoxD gene function, *Nature* 435:1113–1116, 2005.
32. Yoon BS, Lyons KM: Multiple functions of BMPs in chondrogenesis, *J Cell Biochem* 93:93–103, 2004.
33. Yoon BS, Ovchinnikov DA, Yoshii I, et al.: Bmpr1a and Bmpr1b have overlapping functions and are essential for chondrogenesis in vivo, *Proc Natl Acad Sci U S A* 102:5062–5067, 2005.
34. Retting KN, Song B, Yoon BS, et al.: BMP canonical Smad signaling through Smad1 and Smad5 is required for endochondral bone formation, *Development* 136:1093–1104, 2009.
35. Yoon BS, Pogue R, Ovchinnikov DA, et al.: BMPs regulate multiple aspects of growth-plate chondrogenesis through opposing actions on FGF pathways, *Development* 133:4667–4678, 2006.
36. Akiyama H, Chaboissier MC, Martin JF, et al.: The transcription factor Sox9 has essential roles in successive steps of the chondrocyte differentiation pathway and is required for expression of Sox5 and Sox6, *Genes Dev* 16:2813–2828, 2002.
37. Dy P, Smits P, Silvester A, et al.: Synovial joint morphogenesis requires the chondrogenic action of Sox5 and Sox6 in growth plate and articular cartilage, *Dev Biol* 341:346–359, 2010.
38. Minina E, Kreschel C, Naski MC, et al.: Interaction of FGF, Ihh/Pthlh, and BMP signaling integrates chondrocyte proliferation and hypertrophic differentiation, *Dev Cell* 3:439–449, 2002.
39. Itoh N, Ornitz DM: Functional evolutionary history of the mouse Fgf gene family, *Dev Dyn* 237:18–27, 2008.
40. Ornitz DM: FGF signaling in the developing endochondral skeleton, *Cytokine Growth Factor Rev* 16:205–213, 2005.
41. Beier F: Cell-cycle control and the cartilage growth plate, *J Cell Physiol* 202:1–8, 2005.
42. Priore R, Dailey L, Basilico C: Downregulation of Akt activity contributes to the growth arrest induced by FGF in chondrocytes, *J Cell Physiol* 207:800–808, 2006.
43. Murakami S, Balmes G, McKinney S, et al.: Constitutive activation of MEK1 in chondrocytes causes Stat1-independent achondroplasia-like dwarfism and rescues the Fgfr3-deficient mouse phenotype, *Genes Dev* 18:290–305, 2004.
44. Correa D, Somoza RA, Lin P, et al.: Sequential exposure to fibroblast growth factors (FGF) 2, 9 and 18 enhances hMSC chondrogenic differentiation, *Osteoarthritis Cartilage* 23:443–453, 2015.
45. Hung IH, Yu K, Lavine KJ, et al.: FGF9 regulates early hypertrophic chondrocyte differentiation and skeletal vascularization in the developing stylopod, *Dev Biol* 307:300–313, 2007.
46. Liu Z, Lavine KJ, Hung IH, et al.: FGF18 is required for early chondrocyte proliferation, hypertrophy and vascular invasion of the growth plate, *Dev Biol* 302:80–91, 2007.
47. Kronenberg HM: PTHrP and skeletal development, *Ann N Y Acad Sci* 1068:1–13, 2006.
48. Koziel L, Wuelling M, Schneider S, et al.: Gli3 acts as a repressor downstream of Ihh in regulating two distinct steps of chondrocyte differentiation, *Development* 132:5249–5260, 2005.
49. Hilton MJ, Tu X, Cook J, et al.: Ihh controls cartilage development by antagonizing Gli3, but requires additional effectors to regulate osteoblast and vascular development, *Development* 132:4339–4351, 2005.
50. Wuelling M, Vortkamp A: Transcriptional networks controlling chondrocyte proliferation and differentiation during endochondral ossification, *Pediatr Nephrol* 25:625–631, 2010.
51. Kobayashi T, Soegiarto DW, Yang Y, et al.: Indian hedgehog stimulates periarticular chondrocyte differentiation to regulate growth plate length independently of PTHrP, *J Clin Invest* 115:1734–1742, 2005.
52. Hilton MJ, Tu X, Long F: Tamoxifen-inducible gene deletion reveals a distinct cell type associated with trabecular bone, and direct regulation of PTHrP expression and chondrocyte morphology by Ihh in growth region cartilage, *Dev Biol* 308:93–105, 2007.
53. Tsang KY, Cheung MC, Chan D, et al.: The developmental roles of the extracellular matrix: beyond structure to regulation, *Cell Tissue Res* 339:93–110, 2010.
54. Sun MM, Beier F: Chondrocyte hypertrophy in skeletal development, growth, and disease, *Birth Defects Res C Embryo Today* 102:74–82, 2014.
55. Dao DY, Jonason JH, Zhang Y, et al.: Cartilage-specific beta-catenin signaling regulates chondrocyte maturation, generation of ossification centers, and perichondrial bone formation during skeletal development, *J Bone Miner Res* 27:1680–1694, 2012.
56. Amano K, Densmore M, Nishimura R, et al.: Indian hedgehog signaling regulates transcription and expression of collagen type X via Runx2/Smads interactions, *J Biol Chem* 289:24898–24910, 2014.
57. Arnold MA, Kim Y, Czubryt MP, et al.: MEF2C transcription factor controls chondrocyte hypertrophy and bone development, *Dev Cell* 12:377–389, 2007.
58. Bradley EW, McGee-Lawrence ME, Westendorf JJ: Hdac-mediated control of endochondral and intramembranous ossification, *Crit Rev Eukaryot Gene Expr* 21:101–113, 2011.
59. Sasagawa S, Takemori H, Uebi T, et al.: SIK3 is essential for chondrocyte hypertrophy during skeletal development in mice, *Development* 139:1153–1163, 2012.
60. Kozhemyakina E, Lassar AB, Zelzer E: A pathway to bone: signaling molecules and transcription factors involved in chondrocyte development and maturation, *Development* 142:817–831, 2015.

61. Dy P, Wang W, Bhattaram P, et al.: Sox9 directs hypertrophic maturation and blocks osteoblast differentiation of growth plate chondrocytes, *Dev Cell* 22:597–609, 2012.
62. Ionescu A, Kozhemyakina E, Nicolae C, et al.: FoxA family members are crucial regulators of the hypertrophic chondrocyte differentiation program, *Dev Cell* 22:927–939, 2012.
63. Kim EJ, Cho SW, Shin JO, et al.: Ihh and Runx2/Runx3 signaling interact to coordinate early chondrogenesis: a mouse model, *PLoS ONE* 8:e55296, 2013.
64. Correa D, Hesse E, Seriwatanachai D, et al.: Zfp521 is a target gene and key effector of parathyroid hormone-related peptide signaling in growth plate chondrocytes, *Dev Cell* 19:533–546, 2010.
65. Monemdjou R, Vasheghani F, Fahmi H, et al.: Association of cartilage-specific deletion of peroxisome proliferator-activated receptor gamma with abnormal endochondral ossification and impaired cartilage growth and development in a murine model, *Arthritis Rheum* 64:1551–1561, 2012.
66. Inada M, Wang Y, Byrne MH, et al.: Critical roles for collagenase-3 (Mmp13) in development of growth plate cartilage and in endochondral ossification, *Proc Natl Acad Sci U S A* 101:17192–17197, 2004.
67. Stickens D, Behonick DJ, Ortega N, et al.: Altered endochondral bone development in matrix metalloproteinase 13-deficient mice, *Development* 131:5883–5895, 2004.
68. Tsang KY, Chan D, Bateman JF, et al.: In vivo cellular adaptation to ER stress: survival strategies with double-edged consequences, *J Cell Sci* 123:2145–2154, 2010.
69. Tsang KY, Chan D, Cheah KS: Fate of growth plate hypertrophic chondrocytes: death or lineage extension? *Dev Growth Differ* 57:179–192, 2015.
70. Yang L, Tsang KY, Tang HC, et al.: Hypertrophic chondrocytes can become osteoblasts and osteocytes in endochondral bone formation, *Proc Natl Acad Sci U S A* 111:12097–12102, 2014.
71. Saito T, Fukai A, Mabuchi A, et al.: Transcriptional regulation of endochondral ossification by HIF-2alpha during skeletal growth and osteoarthritis development, *Nat Med* 16:678–686, 2010.
72. Ortega N, Wang K, Ferrara N, et al.: Complementary interplay between matrix metalloproteinase-9, vascular endothelial growth factor and osteoclast function drives endochondral bone formation, *Dis Models Mech* 3:224–235, 2010.
73. Ishijima M, Suzuki N, Hozumi K, et al.: Perlecan modulates VEGF signaling and is essential for vascularization in endochondral bone formation, *Matrix Biol* 31:234–245, 2012.
74. Hosaka Y, Saito T, Sugita S, et al.: Notch signaling in chondrocytes modulates endochondral ossification and osteoarthritis development, *Proc Natl Acad Sci U S A* 110:1875–1880, 2013.
75. Zhao R, Wang A, Hall KC, et al.: Lack of ADAM10 in endothelial cells affects osteoclasts at the chondro-osseus junction, *J Orthop Res* 32:224–230, 2014.
76. Zhang X, Siclari VA, Lan S, et al.: The critical role of the epidermal growth factor receptor in endochondral ossification, *J Bone Miner Res* 26:2622–2633, 2011.
77. Usmani SE, Pest MA, Kim G, et al.: Transforming growth factor alpha controls the transition from hypertrophic cartilage to bone during endochondral bone growth, *Bone* 51:131–141, 2012.
78. Hall KC, Hill D, Otero M, et al.: ADAM17 controls endochondral ossification by regulating terminal differentiation of chondrocytes, *Mol Cell Biol* 33:3077–3090, 2013.
79. Pest MA, Russell BA, Zhang YW, et al.: Disturbed cartilage and joint homeostasis resulting from a loss of mitogen-inducible gene 6 in a mouse model of joint dysfunction, *Arthritis Rheumatol* 66:2816–2827, 2014.
80. Bhattacharjee M, Coburn J, Centola M, et al.: Tissue engineering strategies to study cartilage development, degeneration and regeneration, *Adv Drug Deliv Rev* 84:107–122, 2015.
81. Hunziker EB, Lippuner K, Shintani N: How best to preserve and reveal the structural intricacies of cartilaginous tissue, *Matrix Biol* 39:33–43, 2014.
82. Carvalho de Moraes LO, Tedesco RC, Arraéz-Aybaret LA, et al.: Development of synovial membrane in the temporomandibular joint of the human fetus, *Eur J Histochem* 59:263–267, 2015.
83. Valencia X, Higgins JM, Kiener HP, et al.: Cadherin-11 provides specific cellular adhesion between fibroblast-like synoviocytes, *J Exp Med* 200:1673–1679, 2004.
84. Lee DM, Kiener HP, Agarwal SK, et al.: Cadherin-11 in synovial lining formation and pathology in arthritis, *Science* 315:1006–1010, 2007.
85. Holmes G, Niswander L: Expression of slit-2 and slit-3 during chick development, *Dev Dyn* 222:301–307, 2001.
86. Hinton RJ: Genes that regulate morphogenesis and growth of the temporomandibular joint: a review, *Dev Dyn* 243:864–874, 2014.
87. Nowlan NC, Prendergast PJ, Murphy P: Identification of mechanosensitive genes during embryonic bone formation, *PLoS Comput Biol* 4:e1000250, 2008.
88. Chan WC, Au TY, Tam V, et al.: Coming together is a beginning: the making of an intervertebral disc, *Birth Defects Res C Embryo Today* 102:83–100, 2014.
89. Winkler T, Mahoney EJ, Sinner D, et al.: Wnt signaling activates Shh signaling in early postnatal intervertebral discs, and re-activates Shh signaling in old discs in the mouse, *PLoS ONE* 9:e98444, 2014.
90. Dahia CL, Mahoney E, Wylie C: Shh signaling from the nucleus pulposus is required for the postnatal growth and differentiation of the mouse intervertebral disc, *PLoS ONE* 7:e35944, 2012.
91. Sivan SS, Hayes AJ, Wachtel E, et al.: Biochemical composition and turnover of the extracellular matrix of the normal and degenerate intervertebral disc, *Eur SpineJ* 23(Suppl 3):S344–S353, 2014.
92. Edwards JCW: Fibroblast biology. Development and differentiation of synovial fibroblasts in arthritis, *Arthritis Res* 2:344–347, 2000.
93. Hui AY, McCarty WJ, Masuda K, et al.: A systems biology approach to synovial joint lubrication in health, injury, and disease, *Wiley Interdiscip Rev Syst Biol Med* 4:15–37, 2012.
94. Bartok B, Firestein GS: Fibroblast-like synoviocytes: key effector cells in rheumatoid arthritis, *Immunol Rev* 233:233–255, 2010.
95. Bugatti S, Vitolo B, Caporali R, et al.: B cells in rheumatoid arthritis: from pathogenic players to disease biomarkers, *BioMed Res Int* 2014, 2014. 681-678.
96. Wechalekar MD, Smith MD: Utility of arthroscopic guided synovial biopsy in understanding synovial tissue pathology in health and disease states, *World J Orthop* 5:566–573, 2014.
97. Kiener HP, Niederreiter B, Lee DM, et al.: Cadherin 11 promotes invasive behavior of fibroblast-like synoviocytes, *Arthritis Rheum* 60:1305, 2009. –1310.
98. Mizoguchi F, Slowikowski K, Wei K, et al.: Functionally distinct disease-associated fibroblast subsets in rheumatoid arthritis, *Nat Commun* 9:789, 2018.
99. Scanzello CR, Albert AS, DiCarlo E, et al.: The influence of synovial inflammation and hyperplasia on symptomatic outcomes up to 2 years post-operatively in patients undergoing partial meniscectomy, *Osteoarthritis Cartilage* 21:1392–1399, 2013.
100. Henrotin Y, Pesesse L, Lambert C: Targeting the synovial angiogenesis as a novel treatment approach to osteoarthritis, *Ther Adv Musculoskelet Dis* 6:20–34, 2014.
101. Neogi T: Structural correlates of pain in osteoarthritis, *Clin Exp Rheumatol* 35(Suppl 107):S75–S78, 2017.
102. Mapp PI, Walsh DA: Mechanisms and targets of angiogenesis and nerve growth in osteoarthritis, *Nat Rev Rheumatol* 8:390–398, 2012.
103. Haywood L, Walsh DA: Vasculature of the normal and arthritic synovial joint, *Histol Histopathol* 16:277–284, 2001.
104. Szekanecz Z, Besenyei T, Szentpetery A, et al.: Angiogenesis and vasculogenesis in rheumatoid arthritis, *Curr Opin Rheumatol* 22:299–306, 2010.

105. Szekanecz Z, Besenyei T, Paragh G, et al.: New insights in synovial angiogenesis, *Joint Bone Spine* 77:13–19, 2010.
106. Uchida T, Nakashima M, Hirota Y, et al.: Immunohistochemical localisation of protein tyrosine kinase receptors Tie-1 and Tie-2 in synovial tissue of rheumatoid arthritis: correlation with angiogenesis and synovial proliferation, *Ann Rheum Dis* 59:607–614, 2000.
107. Gravallese EM, Pettit AR, Lee R, et al.: Angiopoietin-1 is expressed in the synovium of patients with rheumatoid arthritis and is induced by tumour necrosis factor alpha, *Ann Rheum Dis* 62:100–107, 2003.
108. McDougall JJ, Watkins L, Li Z: Vasoactive intestinal peptide (VIP) is a modulator of joint pain in a rat model of osteoarthritis, *Pain* 123:98–105, 2006.
109. Eitner A, Pester J, Nietzsche S, et al.: The innervation of synovium of human osteoarthritic joints in comparison with normal rat and sheep synovium, *Osteoarthr Cartil* 21:1383–1391, 2013.
110. Syx D, Tran PB, Miller RE, et al.: Peripheral mechanisms contributing to osteoarthritis pain, *Curr Rheum Reports* 20:9, 2018.
171. Benjamin M, Ralphs JR: The cell and developmental biology of tendons and ligaments, *Int Rev Cytol* 196:85–130, 2000.
172. Wang JH: Mechanobiology of tendon, *J Biomech* 39:1563–1582, 2006.
173. Vogel KG, Peters JA: Histochemistry defines a proteoglycan-rich layer in bovine flexor tendon subjected to bending, *J Musculoskelet Neuronal Interact* 5:64–69, 2005.
174. Canty EG, Starborg T, Lu Y, et al.: Actin filaments are required for fibripositor-mediated collagen fibril alignment in tendon, *J Biol Chem* 281:38592–38598, 2006.
175. Richardson SH, Starborg T, Lu Y, et al.: Tendon development requires regulation of cell condensation and cell shape via cadherin-11-mediated cell-cell junctions, *Mol Cell Biol* 27:6218–6228, 2007.
176. Nourissat G, Berenbaum F, Duprez D: Tendon injury: from biology to tendon repair, *Nat Rev Rheumatol* 11:223–233, 2015.
177. Sun HB, Schaniel C, Leong DJ, et al.: Biology and mechanoresponse of tendon cells: progress overview and perspectives, *J Orthop Res* 33:785–792, 2015.
178. Tan AL, Toumi H, Benjamin M, et al.: Combined high-resolution magnetic resonance imaging and histological examination to explore the role of ligaments and tendons in the phenotypic expression of early hand osteoarthritis, *Ann Rheum Dis* 65:1267–1272, 2006.
181. Thomopoulos S, Marquez JP, Weinberger B, et al.: Collagen fiber orientation at the tendon to bone insertion and its influence on stress concentrations, *J Biomech* 39:1842–1851, 2006.
182. Rodeo SA, Kawamura S, Kim HJ, et al.: Tendon healing in a bone tunnel differs at the tunnel entrance versus the tunnel exit: an effect of graft-tunnel motion? *Am J Sports Med* 34:1790–1800, 2006.

2 Synovium

DOUGLAS J. VEALE AND GARY S. FIRESTEIN

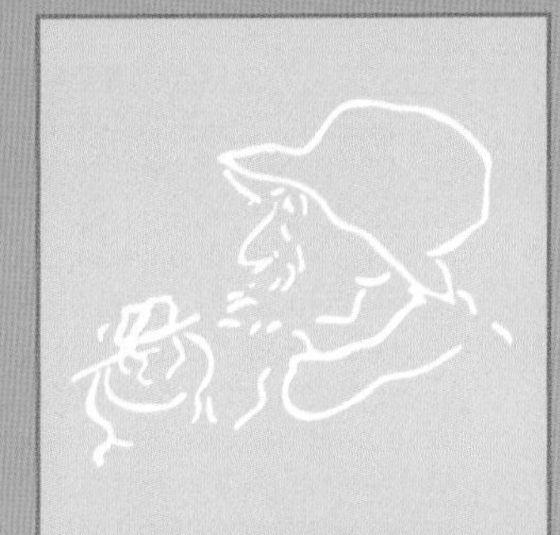

KEY POINTS

The synovium provides nutrients to cartilage and produces lubricants for the joint.

The intimal lining of the synovium includes macrophage-like and fibroblast-like synoviocytes.

The sublining in normal synovium contains scattered immune cells, fibroblasts, blood vessels, and fat cells.

Fibroblast-like synoviocytes in the intimal lining produce specialized enzymes that synthesize lubricants, such as hyaluronic acid.

Structure

The synovium is a membranous structure that extends from the margins of articular cartilage and lines the capsule of diarthrodial joints, including the temporomandibular joint[1] and the facet joints of vertebral bodies (Fig. 2.1).[2] The healthy synovium covers intra-articular tendons and ligaments, as well as fat pads, but not articular cartilage or meniscal tissue. Synovium also ensheaths tendons where they pass beneath ligamentous bands and bursae that cover areas of stress such as the patella and the olecranon. The synovial membrane is divided into two general regions: the intima, or synovial lining, and the subintima, otherwise referred to as the sublining. The intima represents the interface between the cavity containing synovial fluid and the subintimal layer. No well-formed basement membrane separates the intima from the subintima. In contrast to the pleura or pericardium, it is not a true lining because it generally lacks tight junctions, epithelial cells, and a well-formed basement membrane. The subintima is composed of fibrovascular connective tissue and merges with the densely collagenous fibrous joint capsule.

Synovial Lining Cells

The synovial intimal layer is composed of synovial lining cells (SLCs), which are arrayed on the luminal aspect of the joint cavity. SLCs, termed *synoviocytes,* are one to three cells deep, depending on the anatomic location, and extend 20 to 40 μm beneath the lining layer surface. The major and minor axes of SLCs measure 8 to 12 μm and 6 to 8 μm, respectively. The SLCs are not homogeneous and are conventionally divided into two major populations, namely, type A (macrophage-like) synoviocytes and type B (fibroblast-like) synoviocytes.[3]

Ultrastructure of Synovial Lining Cells

Transmission electron microscopic analysis shows that the intimal cells form a discontinuous layer, and thus the subintimal matrix can directly contact the synovial fluid (Fig. 2.2). The existence of two distinct cell types—type A and type B SLCs—was originally described by Barland and associates,[4] and several lines of evidence, including animal models, detailed ultrastructural studies, and immunohistochemical analyses, indicate that these cells represent macrophages (type A SLCs) and fibroblasts (type B SLCs). Studies of SLC populations in a variety of species, including humans, have found that macrophages make up anywhere from 20% and fibroblast-like cells approximately 80% of the lining cell.[5,6] The existence of the two cell types is substantiated by similar findings in a wide variety of species, including hamsters, cats, dogs, guinea pigs, rabbits, mice, rats, and horses.[6–14]

Distinguishing different cell populations that form the synovial lining requires immunohistochemistry or transmission light microscopy. At an ultrastructural level, type A cells are characterized by a conspicuous Golgi apparatus, large vacuoles, and small vesicles, and they contain little rough endoplasmic reticulum, giving them a macrophage-like phenotype (Fig. 2.3A and B). The plasma membrane of type A cells possesses numerous fine extensions, termed *filopodia,* that are characteristic of macrophages. Type A cells occasionally cluster at the tips of the synovial villi; this uneven distribution explains, at least in part, early reports that suggested that type A cells were the predominant intimal cell type.[4,8] However, the distribution is highly variable and can differ depending on the joint evaluated or even within an individual joint.

Type B SLCs have prominent cytoplasmic extensions that extend onto the surface of the synovial lining (Fig. 2.3C and D).[15] Frequent invaginations are seen along the plasma membrane, and a large indented nucleus relative to the area of the surrounding cytoplasm is also a feature. Type B cells have abundant rough endoplasmic reticulum widely distributed in the cytoplasm, and the Golgi apparatus, vacuoles, and vesicles are generally inconspicuous, although some cells have small numbers of prominent vacuoles at their apical aspect. Type B SLCs contain longitudinal bundles of different-sized filaments, which supports their classification as fibroblasts. Desmosomes and gap-like junctions have been described in rat, mouse, and rabbit synovium, but the existence of these structures in human SLCs has never been documented. Although occasional reports describe an intermediate synoviocyte phenotype, it is likely that these cells are functionally conventional type A or B cells.[16,17]

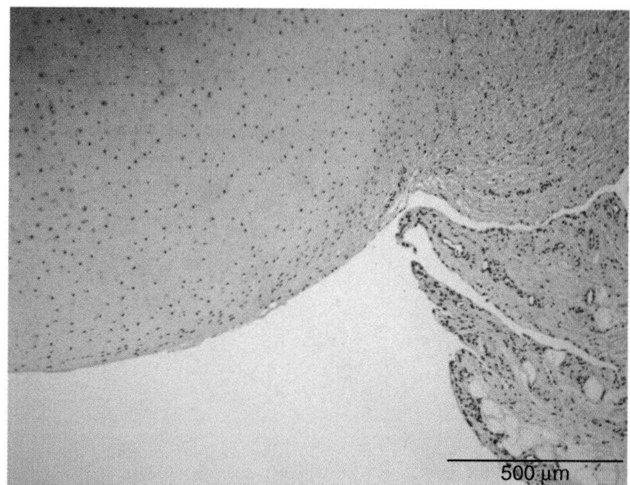

• **Fig. 2.1** The cartilage-synovium junction. Hyaline articular cartilage occupies the *left half* of this image, and fibrous capsule and synovial membrane occupies the *right half.* A sparse intimal lining layer with a fibrous subintima can be observed extending from the margin of the cartilage across the capsular surface to assume a more cellular intimal structure with areolar subintima.

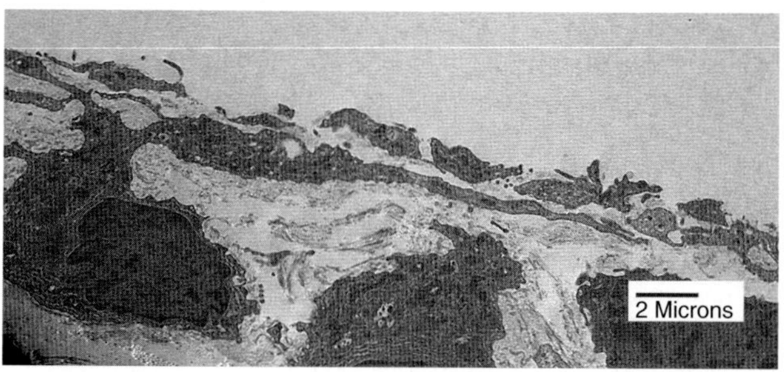

• **Fig. 2.2** Transmission electron photomicrograph of synovial intimal lining cells. The cell *on the left* exhibits the dendritic appearance of a synovial intimal fibroblast (type B cell). Other overlying fibroblast dendrites can be observed. Intercellular gaps allow the synovial fluid to be in direct contact with the synovial matrix.

Immunohistochemical Profile of Synovial Cells

Synovial Macrophages. Synovial macrophages and fibroblasts express lineage-specific molecules that can be detected by immunohistochemistry. Synovial macrophages express common hematopoietic antigen CD45 (Fig. 2.4A); monocyte/macrophage receptors CD163 and CD97; and lysosomal enzymes CD68 (Fig. 2.4B), neuron-specific esterase, and cathepsins B, L, and D. Cells expressing CD14, a molecule that acts as a co-receptor for the detection of bacterial lipopolysaccharide and is expressed by circulating monocytes and monocytes newly recruited to tissue, are rarely seen in the healthy intimal layer, but small numbers are found close to venules in the subintima.[18–24]

The Fcγ receptor, FcγRIII (CD16), which is expressed by Kupffer cells of the liver and type II alveolar macrophages of the lung, is expressed on a subpopulation of synovial macrophages.[25–27] The synovial macrophage population also expresses the class II major histocompatibility complex (MHC) molecule, which plays an important role in the immune response. More recently, the macrophages, which are responsible for the removal of debris, blood, and particulate material from the joint cavity and possess antigen-processing properties, have been found to express Z39Ig, a complement-related protein that is a cell surface receptor and immunoglobulin superfamily member involved in the induction of human leukocyte antigen, DR subregion (HLA-DR), and implicated in phagocytosis and antigen-mediated immune responses.[28–30]

Expression of the β2 integrin chains CD18, CD11a, CD11b, and CD11c varies; CD11a and CD11c may be absent or weakly expressed on a few lining cells.[31,32] Osteoclasts, which are tartrate resistant, acid phosphatase positive, and express the αVβ3 vitronectin and calcitonin receptors, do not appear in the normal synovium.

Synovial Intimal Fibroblasts. Synovial intimal and subintimal fibroblasts are indistinguishable by light microscopy. They generally are considered to be closely related in terms of cell lineage, but because of their different microenvironments, they do not always share the same phenotype. They possess prominent synthetic capacity and produce the essential joint lubricants hyaluronic acid (HA) and lubricin.[33] Intimal fibroblasts express uridine diphosphoglucose dehydrogenase (UDPGD), an enzyme involved in HA synthesis that is a relatively specific marker for this cell type. UDPGD converts UDP-glucose to UDP-glucuronate, one of the two substrates required by HA synthase for assembly of the HA polymer.[34] CD44, the nonintegrin receptor for HA, is expressed by all SLCs.[32,35,36] Recent studies in fibroblast-like synoviocytes from patients with rheumatoid arthritis (RA) have identified DNA methylation and transcriptome signatures that are joint-specific and may reflect distinct pathogenic processes.[37] Furthermore, epigenetic alterations discovered in the fibroblast-like synoviocytes may explain some of the nongenetic risk associated with RA.[38]

Synovial fibroblasts also synthesize normal matrix components, including fibronectin, laminin, collagens, proteoglycans, lubricin, and other identified and unidentified proteins. They have the capacity to produce large quantities of metalloproteinases, metalloproteinase inhibitors, prostaglandins, and cytokines. This capacity must provide essential biologic advantages, but the complex physiologic mechanisms relevant to normal function are incompletely delineated. Expression of selected adhesion molecules on synovial fibroblasts probably facilitates the trafficking of some cell populations, such as neutrophils, into the synovial fluid and the retention of others, such as mononuclear leukocytes, in the synovial tissue. Expression of metalloproteinases, cytokines, adhesion molecules, and other cell surface molecules is strikingly increased in inflammatory states. In a study comparing normal synovial tissue with that from subjects with seropositive arthralgia, osteoarthritis, early and established RA, the transcriptomic analysis revealed that expression of the immune checkpoint molecule, programmed death-1 (PD-1), was increased in early and established disease.[39] The ligands for PD-1, PD-L1, and PD-L2 are increased in synovial tissue on transcriptomic analysis; however, protein expression for the ligands is minimal even before the disease becomes clinically manifest, suggesting a homeostasis between PD-1 and its ligands in normal synovium that is lost in inflammation (Fig. 2.5). These data may explain why some patients receiving immune checkpoint inhibitors for treatment of cancer (e.g., nivolumab and pembrolizumab) may develop autoimmune inflammatory arthritis.

Specialized intimal fibroblasts express many other molecules that also might be expressed by the intimal macrophage population or by most subintimal fibroblasts, including decay-accelerating factor (CD55), vascular cell adhesion molecule–1,[33,40–43] and cadherin-11.[44,45] PGP.95, a neuronal marker, might be specific

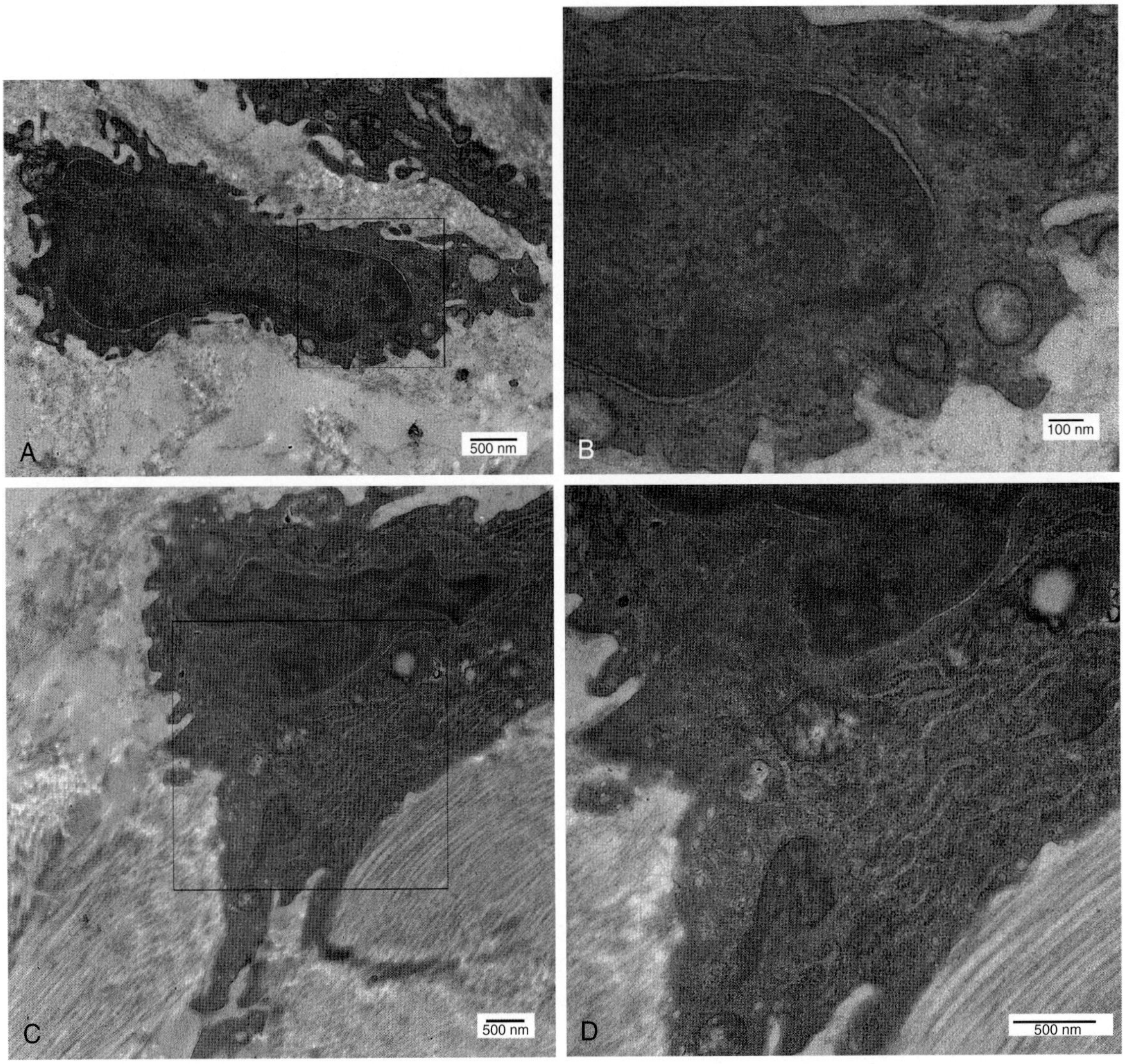

• **Fig. 2.3** Transmission electron photomicrographs of synovial intimal macrophages (type A cells) and fibroblasts (type B cells). (A) Low-powered magnification shows the surface fine filopodia, characteristic of macrophages, and a smooth-surfaced nucleus. (B) The *boxed area* in A is shown at a higher magnification, revealing numerous vesicles that are characteristic of macrophages. Absence of rough endoplasmic reticulum also is noted. (C) The convoluted nucleus along with the prominent rough endoplasmic reticulum *(boxed area)* is characteristic of a synovial intimal fibroblast (type B cell). (D) The rough endoplasmic reticulum is shown at greater magnification.

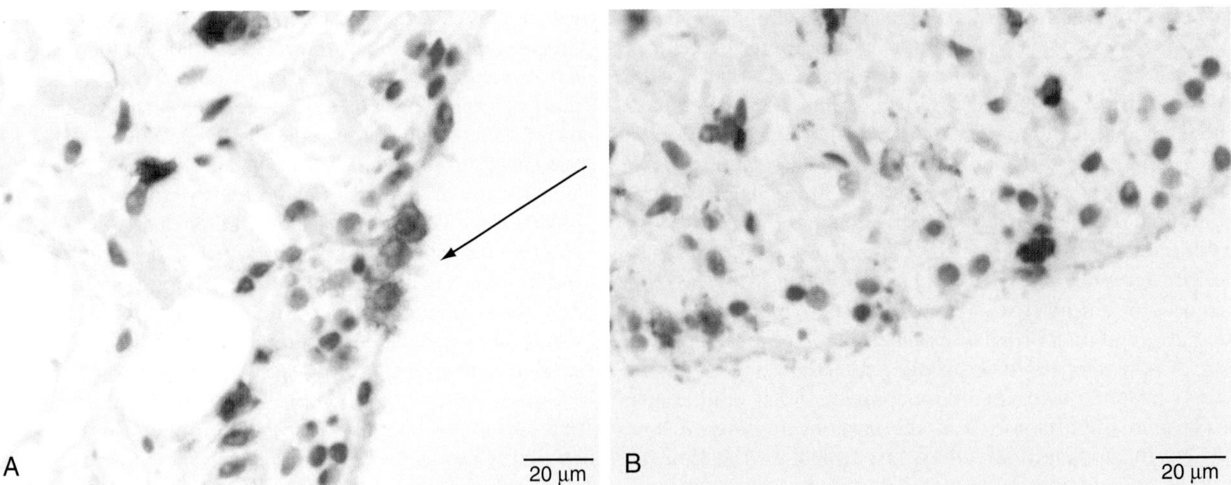

• **Fig. 2.4** Photomicrographs depicting synovial intimal macrophages by immunohistochemistry. Macrophages express CD45 (*arrow* in A) and CD68 (B), which are markers that identify hematopoietic cells (CD45) and macrophages (CD68).

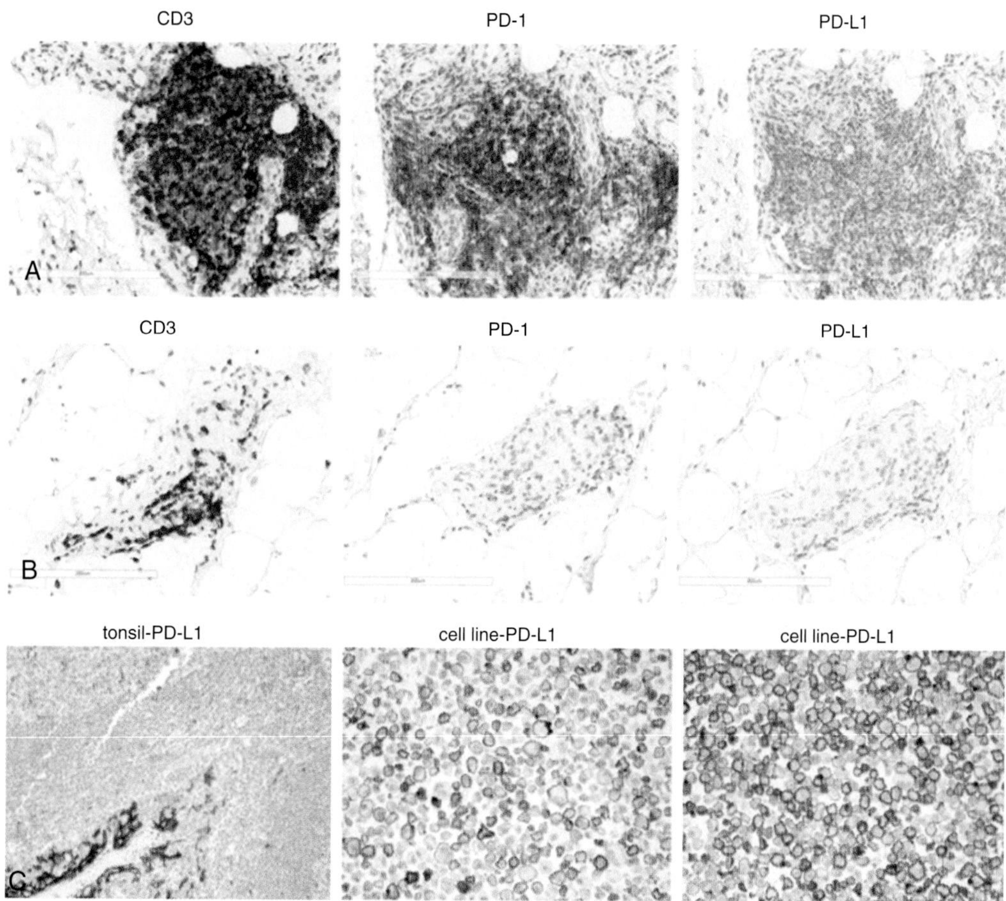

• **Fig. 2.5** Photomicrographs of synovial tissue and control tissue and cell line showing expression of CD3, PD-1, and PD-L1 in treatment-naïve early RA synovial biopsies. Immunohistochemistry analysis of (A) Synovium with abundant CD3, PD-1, and 5% PD-L1 staining. (B) Synovium with abundant CD3 and PD-1 staining, but less than 1% PD-L1 staining. (C) Positive PD-L1 staining control in human tonsil tissue *(left)* and positive PD-L1 staining control in cell line overexpressing PD-L1 at low *(middle)* and high density *(right)*, respectively. All images are shown at 20×.

for type B synoviocytes in some species.[46] Decay-accelerating factor, which is also expressed on many other cells (most notably erythrocytes), as well as bone marrow cells, interacts with CD97, a glycoprotein that is present on the surface of activated leukocytes, including intimal macrophages, and is thought to be involved in signaling processes early after leukocyte activation.[47,48] In contrast, FcγRIII is expressed by macrophages only when they are in close contact with decay-accelerating factor–positive fibroblasts or decay-accelerating factor–coated fibrillin-1 microfibrils in the extra-cellular matrix.[26]

Toll-like receptors (TLRs) are also expressed on intimal fibroblasts, including TLR2, which is activated by serum amyloid A (among other ligands), leading to angiogenesis and cell invasion that is mediated, at least in part, via the Tie2 signaling pathway.[49,50] Cadherins are a class of tissue-restricted transmembrane proteins that play important roles in homophilic intercellular adhesion and are involved in maintaining the integrity of tissue architecture. Cadherin-11, which was cloned from RA synovial tissue, is expressed in normal synovial intimal fibroblasts but not in intimal macrophages. Fibroblasts transfected with cadherin-11 form a lining-like structure in vitro, which implicates this molecule in the architectural organization of the synovial lining.[44,45,51] This suggestion is supported by the observation that cadherin-deficient mice have a hypoplastic synovial intimal lining and are resistant to inflammatory arthritis.[52] When fibroblasts expressing cadherin-11 are embedded in laminin microparticles, they migrate to the surface and form an intimal lining-like structure.[53] If macrophage lineage cells are included in the culture, they can co-localize with fibroblasts on the surface. Therefore, the organization of the synovial lining, including the distribution of type A and B cells, is orchestrated by fibroblast-like synoviocytes.

β1 and β3 integrins are present on all SLCs, forming receptors for laminin (CD49f and CD49b), types I and IV collagen (CD49b), vitronectin (CD51), CD54 (a member of the immunoglobulin superfamily), and fibronectin (CD49d and CD49e). CD31 (platelet–endothelial cell adhesion molecule), a member of the immunoglobulin superfamily expressed on endothelial cells, platelets, and monocytes, is weakly expressed on SLCs.[32]

Turnover of Synovial Lining Cells

Proliferation of SLCs in humans is low; normal human synovial explants have a labeling index of approximately 0.05% to 0.3%[54] when exposed to 3H thymidine.

This labeling index bears a striking contrast to labeling indices of approximately 50% for bowel crypt epithelium. Similar evidence of low proliferation is found in the synovium of rats and rabbits. The proportion of SLCs expressing the proliferation marker Ki67 is between 1 in 2800 and 1 in 30,000, confirming the relatively slow rate of in situ proliferation.[55] Proliferating cells are generally synovial fibroblasts,[22,56] a finding consistent with the concept that type A synovial cells are terminally differentiated macrophages. Mitotic activity of SLCs is low in inflammatory conditions, such as RA—a condition associated with SLC hyperplasia. Some investigators[57] have reported only rare mitotic figures in RA synovium samples.

Apart from the knowledge that synovial fibroblasts proliferate slowly, little is known about their natural life span, recruitment, or mode of death. Apoptosis is likely involved with maintaining synovial homeostasis, but cultured fibroblast-like synoviocytes tend to be resistant to apoptosis, and very few intimal lining cells display evidence of completed apoptosis by ultrastructural analysis or by labeling for fragmented DNA. The paucity of normal synovium samples for evaluation and the rapid clearance of apoptotic cells could confound the analysis.[58]

Origin of Synovial Lining Cells

There is little doubt that the type A SLC population is bone marrow–derived and represents cells of the mononuclear phagocyte system.[4] Studies in the Beige (bg) mouse, which harbors a homozygous mutation that confers the presence of giant lysosomes in macrophages, have confirmed the bone marrow origin of these cells.[59,60] Normal mice with bone marrow depleted through irradiation were rescued with bone marrow cells obtained from the bg mouse. Electron microscopic analysis of the synovium from recipient animals revealed that type A SLCs contained the giant lysosomes of the donor bg mouse and that these structures were never identified in type B cells. These findings provide powerful evidence that (1) type A SLCs represent macrophages, (2) they are recruited from the bone marrow, and (3) they are a distinct lineage from type B SLCs.

In addition to immunohistochemistry, several lines of evidence support the concept that type A SLCs are recruited from the bone marrow:

- The osteopetrotic (op/op) mouse, a spontaneously occurring mutant that fails to produce macrophage colony-stimulating factor because of a missense mutation in the *CSF1* gene,[61–63] has low numbers of circulating and resident macrophage colony-stimulating factor–dependent macrophages, including those in the synovium.
- Type A cells in rat synovium do not populate the joint until after the development of synovial blood vessels.[22]
- Type A SLCs are conspicuous around vessels in the synovium in neonatal mice.[6]
- When synovial explants are placed in culture, the reduction in type A SLCs is explained, in part, by their migration into the culture medium—an observation that reflects the process of migration of macrophages into the synovial fluid in vivo.[1,64]
- Macrophages constitute up to 80% of the cells found around venules in inflammatory conditions such as RA and are cleared rapidly (<48 hours) after successful treatment but will reaccumulate from the circulation if relapse occurs.[65]

Type B intimal cells represent a resident fibroblast population in the synovial lining, but little is known about the cells from which they derive and about how their recruitment is regulated. The existence of mesenchymal stem cells in the synovium suggests that these cells might differentiate into the synovial lining fibroblast. To date, a specific transcription factor directing mesenchymal stem cell differentiation into the synovial fibroblast, similar to factors required for commitment by this multipotential population into bone (CBFA-1), cartilage (SOX-9), and fat (peroxisome proliferator-activated receptor γ [PPARγ]), has not been identified.

Several important signaling pathways are activated in the inflamed synovium, including nuclear factor-κB (NF-κB), Janus kinase/signal transducer and activator of transcription (JAK/STAT), Notch, and hypoxia-inducible factor 1, α subunit (HIF-1α). NF-κB is a key transcriptional regulator in the inflamed synovium.[66] NF-κB signaling is complex and may be activated by cytokines, cell surface adhesion molecules, and hypoxia.[66,67] NF-κB activation could facilitate synovial hyperplasia by promoting proliferation and inhibiting apoptosis of RA fibroblast-like synoviocytes. One of the key roles of NF-κB is to protect RA fibroblast-like synoviocytes against apoptosis, possibly by countering the cytotoxicity of TNF and Fas ligand.[68]

JAK/STAT, Notch, and HIF-1α signaling pathways are also evident in inflamed synovium. STAT3 expression in the synovium correlates with synovitis and is activated by IL-6[69] but also indirectly by TNF. Notch signaling pathway components are predominantly localized to perivascular/vascular regions[70] and are regulated by vascular endothelial growth factor (VEGF) and ang2, which is consistent with the role of mediation of angiogenesis by Notch in inflammation and cancer.[70,71] Interestingly, hypoxia induces activation of phospho (p)-STAT3/p-STAT1, NF-κB, and Notch in synovial cells.[72] Furthermore, Notch/HIF-1α interactions in RA synoviocytes are in part mediated through STAT3 activation,[73] possibly through competition of STAT3 with von Hippel–Lindau tumor suppressor for binding to HIF-1α. Although no direct link between NF-κB and HIF-1α is demonstrated in the inflamed joint, preferential activation of the canonic NF-κB pathway occurs in RA synovial tissue obtained from patients with more hypoxic joints.[72]

Subintimal Layer

SLCs are not separated from the underlying subintima by a well-formed basement membrane composed of the typical trilaminar structure seen beneath epithelial mucosa. Nevertheless, most components of basement membrane are present in the extracellular matrix surrounding SLCs. These components include tenascin X, perlecan (a heparan sulfate proteoglycan), type IV collagen laminin, and fibrillin-1.[74,75] Of note is the absence of laminin-5 and integrin α3β3γ2, which are components of epithelial hemidesmosomes.[76]

The subintima is composed of loose connective tissue of variable thickness and variable proportions of fibrous/collagenous and adipose tissue, depending on the anatomic site. Under normal healthy conditions, inflammatory cells are virtually absent from the subintima, apart from a sprinkling of macrophages and scattered mast cells.[77] Human synovial tissue is a rich source of mesenchymal stem cells, and although it is unknown which compartment contains this cell population, some cells have the ability to self-renew and differentiate into bone, cartilage, and fat in vitro—a phenomenon that reflects the ability of the cell to regenerate in vivo.[78–80]

Three categories of subintima are well defined: areolar, fibrous, and fatty/adipose types. Under the light microscope, areolar-type subintima, the most commonly studied, generally is found in larger joints in which there is free movement. It is composed of fronds with a cellular intimal lining and loose connective tissue in the subintima, with little in the way of dense collagen fibers, and a rich vasculature. The fibrous subintima is composed of scant, dense, fibrous, poorly vascularized connective tissue, and it has an attenuated layer of SLCs. The adipose type, which contains abundant mature fat cells and has a single layer of SLCs, is seen more commonly with aging and in intra-articular fat pads.

The subintima contains types I, III, V, and VI collagen, glycosaminoglycans, proteoglycans, and extra-cellular matrices, including tenascin and laminins. Integrin receptors for collagens, laminin, and vitronectin are absent or at best weakly expressed by subintimal cells. In contrast, receptors for fibronectin (CD49d and CD49e) are detected, and CD44, the HA receptor, is strongly expressed in most subintimal cells. β2 integrins are largely limited to perivascular areas, particularly in the subintimal zone, as is CD54.[81]

Subintimal Vasculature

The vascular supply to the synovium is provided by many small vessels and is shared in part by the joint capsule, epiphyseal bone, and other perisynovial structures. Arteriovenous anastomoses communicate freely with the vascular supply to the periosteum and to periarticular bone. As large synovial arteries enter the deep layers of the synovium near the capsule, they branch to form microvascular units in the more superficial subsynovial layers. Precapillary arterioles probably play a major role in controlling circulation to the lining layer. The surface area of the synovial capillary bed is large, and because it runs only a few cell layers deep to the surface, it has a role in trans-synovial exchange of molecules. The intimal lining, however, is devoid of blood vessels. Although few in number, vessels in the normal synovium have an intact pericyte layer, suggesting vessel stability, in contrast to the inflamed joint, where a mix of mature and immature vessels were observed. Neural cell adhesion molecule (NCAM) deficiency and oxidative DNA damage suggest that vessels may remain in a plastic state even after pericyte recruitment.[82,83] After TNF blockade, synovial blood vessels become more stable and resemble normal synovium.

Numerous physical factors influence synovial blood flow. Heat promotes blood flow through synovial capillaries. Exercise enhances synovial blood flow to normal joints but may reduce the clearance rate of small molecules from the joint space. Immobilization reduces synovial blood flow, and pressure on the synovial membrane can act to tamponade the synovial blood supply.

Vascular endothelial lining cells express CD34 and CD31 (Fig. 2.6A). They also express receptors for the major components of basement membrane, including laminin and collagen IV, and the integrin receptors CD49a (laminin and collagen receptors), CD49d (fibronectin receptor), CD41, CD51 (vitronectin receptor), and CD61 (the β3 integrin subunit). Endothelial cells express CD44, the HA receptor, and CD62P (P-selectin), which acts as a receptor that supports binding of leukocytes to activated platelets and endothelium. They are only weakly positive in uninflamed synovium, however, for expression of CD54 (intercellular adhesion molecule-1), a receptor for β2 integrins expressed by many leukocytes. The endothelial cells of capillaries in the superficial zone of the subintima are strongly positive for HLA-DR expression by immunohistochemistry, whereas cells in the larger vessels in the deep aspect of the membrane are negative.[32,34]

Hypoxia is a key driver of endothelial cell activation and blood vessel formation in the inflamed joint. This theory was originally proposed in 1970,[84] when a synovial fluid electrode was used to demonstrate that a partial pressure of O_2 in a knee joint affected by RA was 26.5 mm Hg, which was significantly lower than that in joints affected by osteoarthritis (42.9 mm Hg) or traumatic effusions (63 mm Hg). This observation was supported by studies showing increased glycolytic metabolism in the joint suggestive of increased metabolic activity. Low pO_2 in the inflamed synovial membrane was confirmed with pO_2 probes, with mean levels approximately 3% compared with normal joints at 7%.[85] The degree of hypoxia in synovium affected by RA and normal synovium was inversely related to the number of blood vessels observed and their level of maturity. In patients responding to TNF blockade, the pO_2 increased, thus improving oxygenation to a level similar to that of normal joints.

Subintimal Lymphatics

Detailed analysis of the number and distribution of lymphatic vessels is made possible by the use of the antibody to the lymphatic vessel endothelial HA receptor (LYVE-1) (Fig. 2.6B).[86] This antibody is highly specific for lymphatic endothelial cells in lymphatic vessels and lymph node sinuses and does not react with endothelial cells of capillaries and other blood vessels that express CD34 and factor VIII–related antigen. Expression of LYVE-1 in lymphatic endothelial cells is used as a marker to show that lymphatic vessels are less common in the fibrous synovium compared with areolar and adipose variants of human subsynovial tissue. Detection of this molecule reveals that lymphatics are present in the superficial, intermediate, and deeper layers of synovial membrane in synovium from healthy people or patients with osteoarthritis and joints affected by RA, although the number in the superficial subintimal layer is low in normal synovium. Little difference in the distribution and number is noted between normal and osteoarthritis synovium, which is characterized by lack of villous hypertrophy. Lymphatic channels are plentiful, however, in the subintimal layer in the presence of villous edema hypertrophy and chronic inflammation.

Subintimal Nerve Supply

The synovium has a rich network of sympathetic and sensory nerves. The former, which are myelinated and detected with the antibody against S-100 protein, terminate close to blood vessels, where they regulate vascular tone (Fig. 2.6C through E). Sensory nerves respond to proprioception and pain via large myelinated nerve fibers and via small (<5 μm) unmyelinated or myelinated fibers with unmyelinated free nerve ends (nociceptors). The latter are immunoreactive in the synovium for neuropeptides, including substance P, calcitonin gene–related peptide, and vasoactive intestinal peptides.[87,88]

Function

Synthetic and protective functions of individual synovial cell populations are multiple and complex. The composite synovial structure, which includes cell populations and their products, vasculature, nerves, and the intercellular matrix, possesses several specialized functions that are essential for normal joint movement, synovial fluid formation, chondrocyte nutrition, and cartilage protection at multiple anatomic locations. These functions must be preserved over a lifetime to maintain maximal mobility and independence. Absence of essential constituents of synovial fluid or inadequate cartilage protection results in early articular malfunction, which may progress to local or generalized joint failure.

Joint Movement

Four characteristics of the synovium are essential for joint movement: deformability, porosity, nonadherence, and lubrication. In a healthy person, the synovium is a highly deformable structure

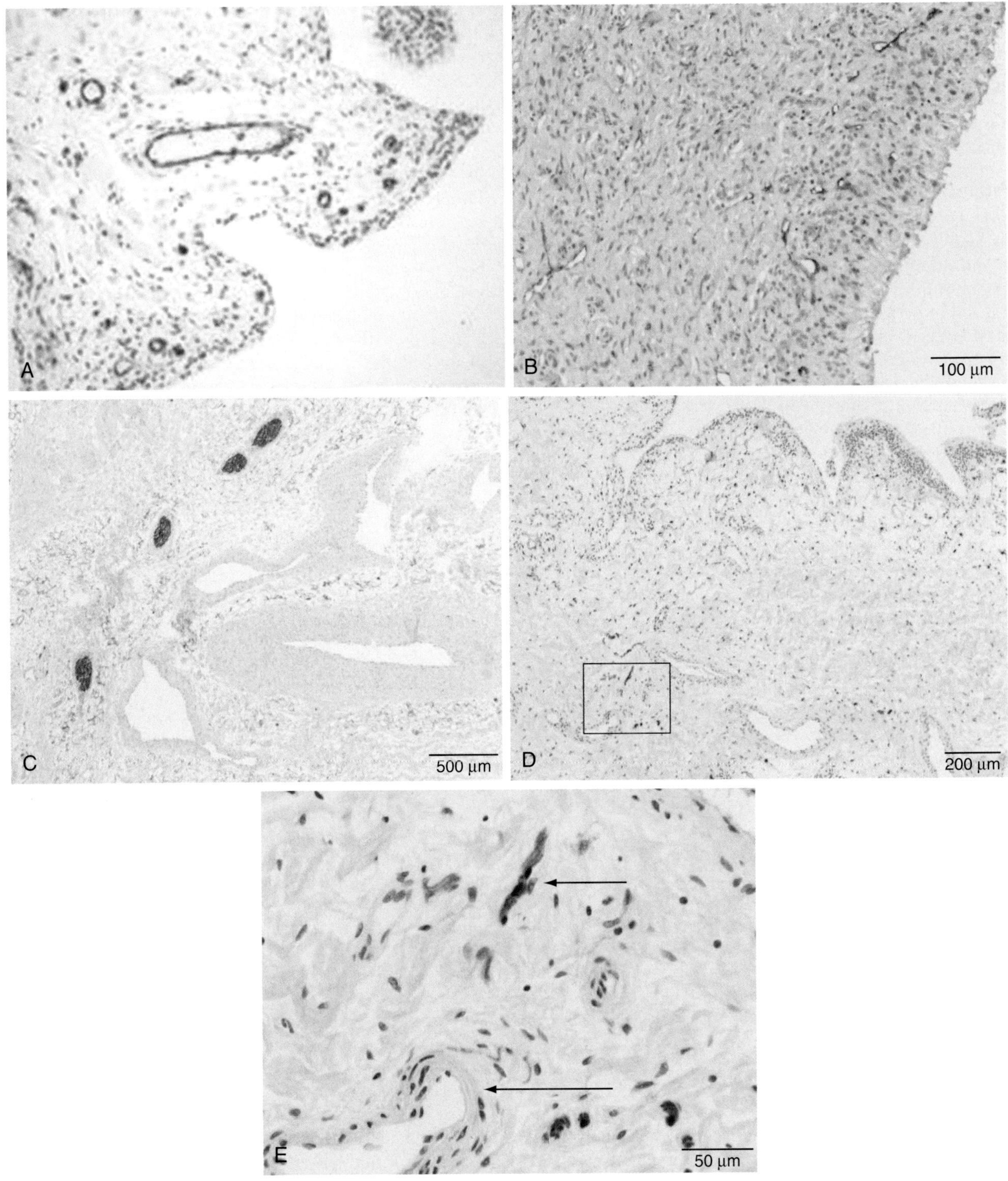

• **Fig. 2.6** Photomicrographs of synovium show lymphovascular and nervous structures by immunohistochemistry. (A) and (B) Areolar synovium featuring thin-walled vessels are highlighted with antibody to CD31 (A), and lymphatic vessels in an inflamed synovium are highlighted with antibody to lymphatic vessel endothelial HA receptor (LYVE-1) (B). (C) Deep in the synovial subintima, close to the joint capsule, medium-sized neurovascular bundles are present with nerves highlighted by antibody to S-100. (D) Within the more superficial synovium, small nerves decorated with S-100 are identified. (E) The *boxed area* in (D) is shown at a higher magnification. The *upper arrow* is directed at a nerve; the *lower arrow* is directed at a small vessel.

that facilitates movement between other adjacent, nondeformable structures within the joint. This unique facility of the synovium, to enable movement between tissues rather than within tissues, is emphasized[89] and can be attributed to the presence of a free surface that allows synovial tissue to remain separated from adjacent tissues. The ensuing space is maintained by the presence of synovial fluid.

Deformability

The deformability of normal synovium is considerable because it must accommodate the extreme positional range available to the joint and its adjacent tendons, ligaments, and capsule. When a finger is flexed, the palmar synovium of each interphalangeal joint contracts while the dorsal synovium expands; when the finger extends, the reverse mechanism occurs. This normal contraction and expansion of synovium seems to involve a folding and unfolding component and an elastic stretching and relaxation of the tissue. During repeated rapid movement, the synovial lining cannot be pinched between cartilage surfaces for it to successfully retain its integrity and the integrity of synovial blood vessels and lymphatics. Deformability also limits the extent of synovial ischemia-reperfusion injury during joint motion by maintaining a relatively low intra-articular pressure.

Porosity

The synovial microvasculature and the intimal lining must be porous to permit robust diffusion of nutrients to cartilage. The structure of the intimal lining is ideal for this requirement because of the relatively disorganized basement membrane and lack of tight junctions, although recent data suggest that macrophages in the lining form tight junctions that could be lost during inflammation.[89a] Plasma components freely diffuse into the intra-articular space, and most plasma components, including proteins, are present in synovial fluid at about one-third to one-half the plasma concentration.

Nonadherence

The third important characteristic of the synovium that facilitates joint movement is its nonadherence to opposing surfaces. Intimal cells on the synovial surface adhere to underlying cells and matrix but do not adhere to opposing synovial and cartilage surfaces. The mechanism that preserves this phenomenon of nonadherence is unknown and might involve the arrangement of cell surface and tissue matrix molecules, such as collagen, fibronectin, and HA. Alternatively, nonadherence may result, in part, from regular movement of the normal synovial lining.

Lubrication

The fourth characteristic of synovium that is essential for joint motion is an efficient lubrication mechanism to facilitate movement of cartilage on cartilage. The mechanisms of joint lubrication are complex and are an integral component of synovial physiology. In an articulating joint, cartilage is subjected to numerous compressive and frictional forces every day. Friction and wear can never be eliminated from a functioning joint. Adult chondrocytes do not normally divide in vivo, and damaged cartilage has limited capacity for self-repair. For a joint to maintain its function throughout a lifetime of use, protective biologic mechanisms, such as lubrication, help minimize wear and damage that result from normal daily activities. Synovial membrane may also contribute to concentration of lubricants in synovial fluid because it is a semi-permeable membrane. These functions have recently been replicated by a polytetrafluoroethylene membrane that can be used in a bioreactor system to modulate lubricant retention in bioengineered synovial fluid. Synoviocytes adherent to such membranes may serve as a source of lubricant and a barrier for lubricant transport.[90] Furthermore, cytokines can stimulate normal lubricant production 40-fold to 80-fold in such bioreactor systems (Fig. 2.7).[91]

The term *Boundary lubrication* refers to the protective effect of particular lubricating molecules adsorbing to a surface and repelling its opposing interface.[92] Bearing surfaces must generate a mutual repulsion to be lubricated in the boundary mode. Boundary lubricants exert their effects by changing the physicochemical characteristics of a surface, and they reduce articular friction and wear by providing a smooth and slippery coating. Friction is reduced by an interposed film of protective fluid that allows one surface to ride freely over another. The cartilage matrix is integral to this phenomenon because it is fluid filled and

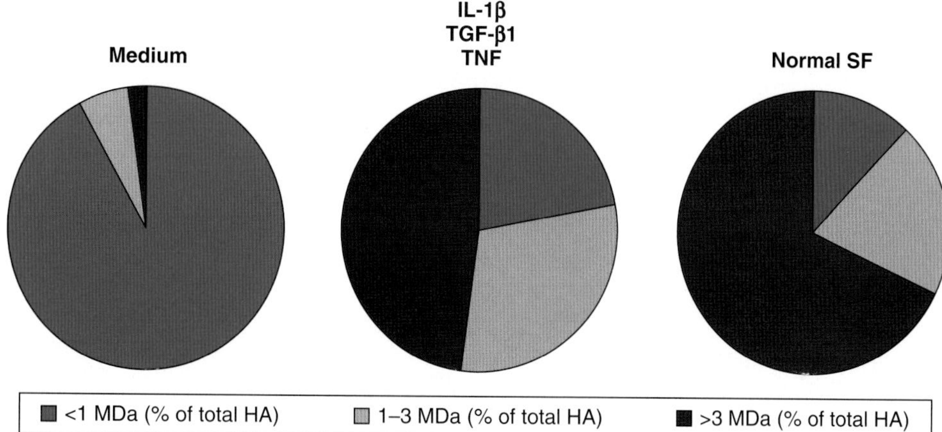

• **Fig. 2.7** The molecular size of synovial fluid hyaluronic acid (HA) (Normal SF), supernatants of cultured synoviocytes (Medium), and synoviocytes stimulated with a combination of IL-1β, TGF-β1 TNF. Note that cells stimulated with the cytokine cocktail closely approximate HA of normal SF compared with control cells, with high molecular weight species that promote a low friction environment. (Data from Blewis ME, Lao BJ, Schumacher BL, et al.: Interactive cytokine regulation of synoviocyte lubricant secretion. *Tissue Eng Part A* 16:1329–1337, 2010.)

compressible. Loaded cartilage extrudes lubricant fluid from its surface, and expressed fluid contributes to the separation of the two articulating surfaces. Scanning electron microscopy shows a continuous film of fluid that is only 100 nm thick; this film separates one surface from the other, preventing direct abrasive contact.[93] This ultrathin coating of lubricant resists distraction of the two articulating surfaces, enhancing joint stability. In healthy joints, another essential advantage of an intra-articular lubrication system is the effective prevention of pinching of adjacent, well-vascularized synovial membrane, a feature that is lost in the inflamed joint in which synovial membrane adheres to the cartilage surface.

Hyaluronic Acid. HA, a high-molecular-weight polysaccharide, is a major component of synovial fluid and cartilage.[94] It is produced in large amounts by mechanosensitive, fibroblast-like synoviocytes.[95,96] HA, which has three mammalian forms designated HAS1, HAS2, and HAS3,[97] is synthesized by HA synthase at the plasma membrane and is extruded directly into the extracellular compartment. HA synthase activity and HA secretion are stimulated by pro-inflammatory cytokines, including IL-1β and TGF-β.[95,98,99] Interestingly, although the levels of cytokines are increased in arthritic joints, the synovial fluid concentration of HA decreases.[100] HA is also synthesized by many other skeletal cells and is an important component of extra-cellular matrices. It is simultaneously a solid phase matrix element of cartilage and other tissues and a fluid phase element in the synovial space under normal and abnormal conditions.

HA has many biologic functions, which include effects on cell growth, migration, and adhesion. The regulatory role of HA is mediated through HA-binding proteins and receptors, including CD44, which are present on the cell surfaces of chondrocytes, lymphocytes, and other mononuclear cell populations. HA plays a crucial role in morphogenesis and in wound healing. HA also is a vital structural component of the synovial lining, and it has an essential role in the induction of joint cavitation during embryogenesis. HA, which is produced by synovium, was originally thought to be primarily a joint lubricant, and it is generally accepted that it plays a major physiologic role in maintaining synovial fluid viscosity. HA is important in normal joint function, not least through its capacity to provide effective shock absorption. HA might be a particularly important viscohydrodynamic lubricant at low-load interfaces, such as synovium-on-synovium and synovium-on-cartilage.[101] Synovial fluid HA, acting in combination with albumin, has a role in the attenuation of fluid loss from the joint cavity, particularly during periods of increased pressure, which can occur during sustained joint flexion.[102–104]

Lubricin. Compelling evidence suggests that lubricin, which was first described in the 1970s,[105] is the factor primarily responsible for boundary lubrication of diarthrodial joints.[106] Lubricin, a large secreted, mucin-like proteoglycan with an apparent molecular weight of 280 kDa, is a product of the gene proteoglycan 4 *(PRG4)*. It is a major component of synovial fluid and is present at the cartilage surface. The gene is highly expressed by human synovial fibroblasts and by superficial zone chondrocytes.[107] Lubricin is closely related to superficial zone protein, megakaryocyte-stimulating factor, and hemangiopoietin, which are encoded by the same gene but can differ in terms of post-translational modification. Superficial zone protein is expressed by SLCs and by superficial zone chondrocytes at the cartilage surface but not by intermediate or deep zone chondrocytes.[108] Some investigators suggest that lubricin may bind to the much longer hyaluronate polymers, distributing shear stress and stabilizing essential lubricant molecules.[109]

In an experimental model, lubricin seemed to have multiple functions in articulating joints and tendons, including protection of cartilage surfaces from protein deposition, cell adhesion, and inhibition of synovial cell overgrowth.[110] *Prg4*$^{-/-}$ mice, which were consistently normal at birth, showed progressive loss of superficial zone chondrocytes and increasing synovial cell hyperplasia (Fig. 2.8). The essential role of lubricin in maintaining joint integrity was shown by the identification of disease-causing mutations in patients with the autosomal-recessive disorder camptodactyly–arthropathy–coxa vara–pericarditis (CACP) syndrome.[111] CACP is a large joint arthropathy associated with the absence of lubricin from synovial fluid and ineffective boundary lubrication provided by the synovial fluid (Fig. 2.9).[109,112] In other studies of lubricin biology and joint integrity, experimental injury resulted in reduced synovial fluid lubricin concentrations, decreased boundary lubricating ability, and increased cartilage matrix degradation, each of which could be attributed to trauma-induced inflammatory processes.[107]

Other investigators argue against the importance of lubricin in joint lubrication; they propose that surface-active phospholipid, which is also secreted by intimal fibroblasts, is the essential boundary lubricant that reduces cartilage friction to remarkably low levels.[113] Lubricin could act as the carrier of surface-active phospholipid to articular cartilage, but that it is not the lubricant per se; they say the function of lubricin is similar to that of the well-characterized alveolar surfactant binding proteins in the lung.

Synovial Fluid Formation

In healthy people, a constant volume of synovial fluid is important during joint movement because it serves as a cushion for synovial tissue and as a reservoir of lubricant for cartilage. Many of the soluble components and proteins in synovial fluid exit the synovial microcirculation through pores or fenestrations in the vascular endothelium and then diffuse through the interstitium before entering the joint space. Synovial fluid is in part a filtrate of plasma to which additional components, including HA and lubricin, are added and removed by the SLCs (Fig. 2.10). As noted earlier, concentrations of electrolytes and small molecules in synovial fluid are similar to those in plasma. Synovial permeability to most small molecules is determined by a process of free diffusion through the double barrier of endothelium and interstitium, which is limited mainly by the intercellular space between SLCs. For most small molecules, synovial permeability is inversely related to the dimensions of the molecule.

Experimental evidence suggests that the exchange of small solutes is determined predominantly by the synovial interstitium and that permeability to proteins is mainly determined by the microvascular endothelium. The synovium should not be regarded as simply an inert membrane but as a complex regulatory tissue system. The small physiologic molecules that traverse the endothelium of synovial blood vessels and diffuse through intercellular spaces of the synovial lining before entering the synovial fluid include water, glucose, and many other essential nutrients and waste tissue metabolites. Evidence suggests that passage of some

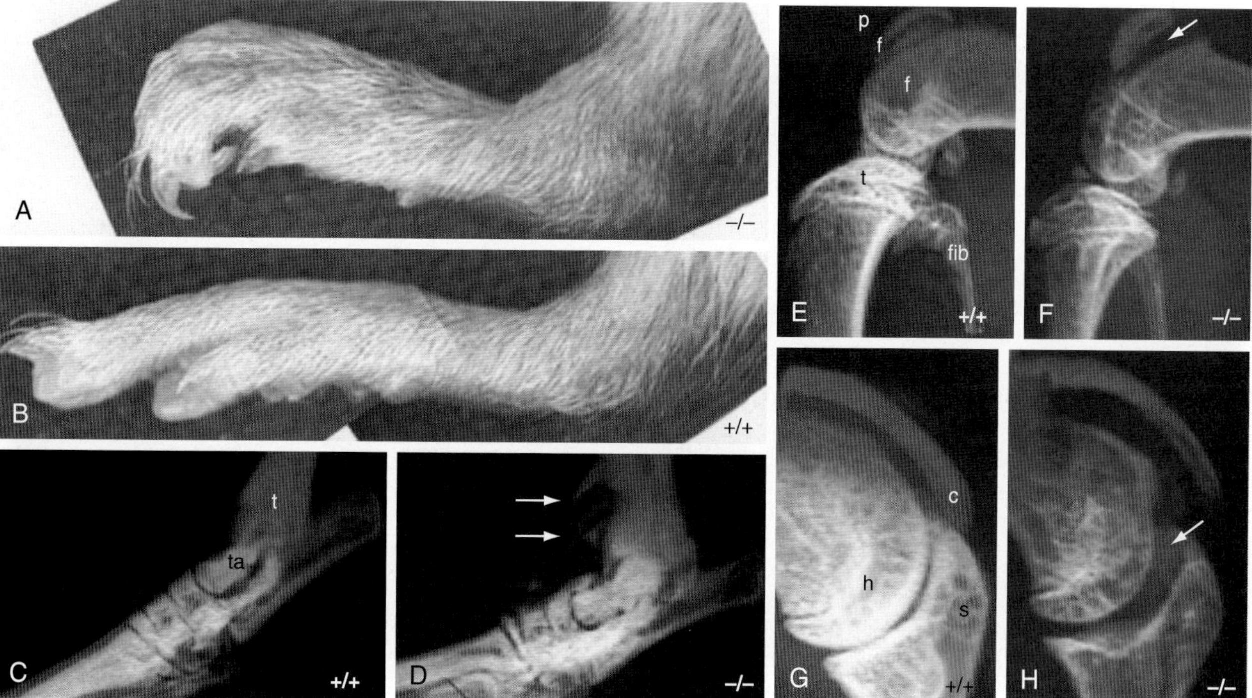

• **Fig. 2.8** Clinical appearance and radiographic changes in *Prg4*$^{-/-}$ mice. (A) and (B) Photographs of the hind paws of 6-month-old *Prg4*$^{-/-}$ (A) and wild-type (B) mice. Note the curved digits in the mutant mouse and swelling at the ankle joint. (C) and (D) Radiographs of the ankle joint of 9-month-old wild-type (C) and *Prg4*$^{-/-}$ mice (D). Structures corresponding to the tibia (t) and talus (ta) are indicated. Note the calcification of structures adjacent to the ankle (*arrows* in D). (E) Lateral knee radiograph of a 4-month-old wild-type mouse. Structures corresponding to the patella (p), femoral condyle (f), tibial plateau (t), and fibula (fib) are indicated. (F) Lateral knee radiograph of a 4-month-old *Prg4*$^{-/-}$ mouse. Note the increased joint space between the patella and femur *(arrow)* and osteopenia of the patella, femoral condyles, and tibial plateau. (G) Shoulder radiograph of a 4-month-old wild-type mouse. Structures corresponding to the humeral head (h), glenoid fossa of the scapula (s), and lateral portion of the clavicle (c) are indicated. (H) Shoulder radiograph of a 4-month-old *Prg4*$^{-/-}$ mouse. Note the increased joint space between the humerus and scapula *(arrow)* and osteopenia of the humeral head. (From Rhee DK, Marcelino J, Baker M, et al.: The secreted glycoprotein lubricin protects cartilage surfaces and inhibits synovial cell overgrowth. *J Clin Invest* 115:622–631, 2005.)

solutes across the synovium is facilitated by specific transport systems that possibly provide a "pump" mechanism capable of moving water out of the joint space.

Plasma proteins are able to cross the endothelium, traversing the synovial interstitium and entering the synovial fluid. The efficiency of this process is determined by the molecular size of the protein and the diameter of the endothelial pores. Smaller proteins, such as albumin, enter easily, whereas larger molecules, such as fibrinogen, gain access with greater difficulty. In contrast, the clearance or removal of proteins and other synovial fluid constituents is unrestricted and considerably more efficient through lymphatic drainage. The synovial fluid concentration of any protein reflects the dynamic balance between ingress and egress at a given time. Because egress is more efficient than ingress, joint space pressure is normally subatmospheric. Negative intra-articular pressure is thought to be important in maintaining joint stability. The synovial fluid-to-serum ratio of plasma proteins is inversely related to the molecular size of the protein. When the joint becomes inflamed, greater endothelial permeability permits more profuse ingress of all proteins, and the most obvious changes are noted in the concentrations of larger molecules. Increased synovial fluid volume also reduces the joint stability.

In contrast to hydrophilic molecules, fat-soluble molecules can diffuse through and between cell membranes, and their passage across the synovial surface is less restricted. The entire surface area of the synovium is available to lipophilic molecules that diffuse into and out of the joint space. Physiologically, the most important fat-soluble molecules are the respiratory gases, oxygen and carbon dioxide. When the joint is inflamed, synovial fluid may exhibit low partial pressure of oxygen, high partial pressure of carbon dioxide, decreased pH, and increased lactate production.[85] The resultant hypoxia and acidosis can have serious implications for the synovial microcirculation and chondrocyte metabolism.

Chondrocyte Nutrition

Another important function of synovium is to enhance the nutrition of chondrocytes, which reside in articular cartilage (see Chapter 3). Because articular cartilage is avascular, delivery of nutrients to chondrocytes and removal of metabolic breakdown products from the cartilage are believed to occur through synovial fluid and synovial tissue arterioles and venules, as well as through subchondral bone. Morphologic, physiologic, and pathologic studies have confirmed that solutes pass easily from the synovial fluid

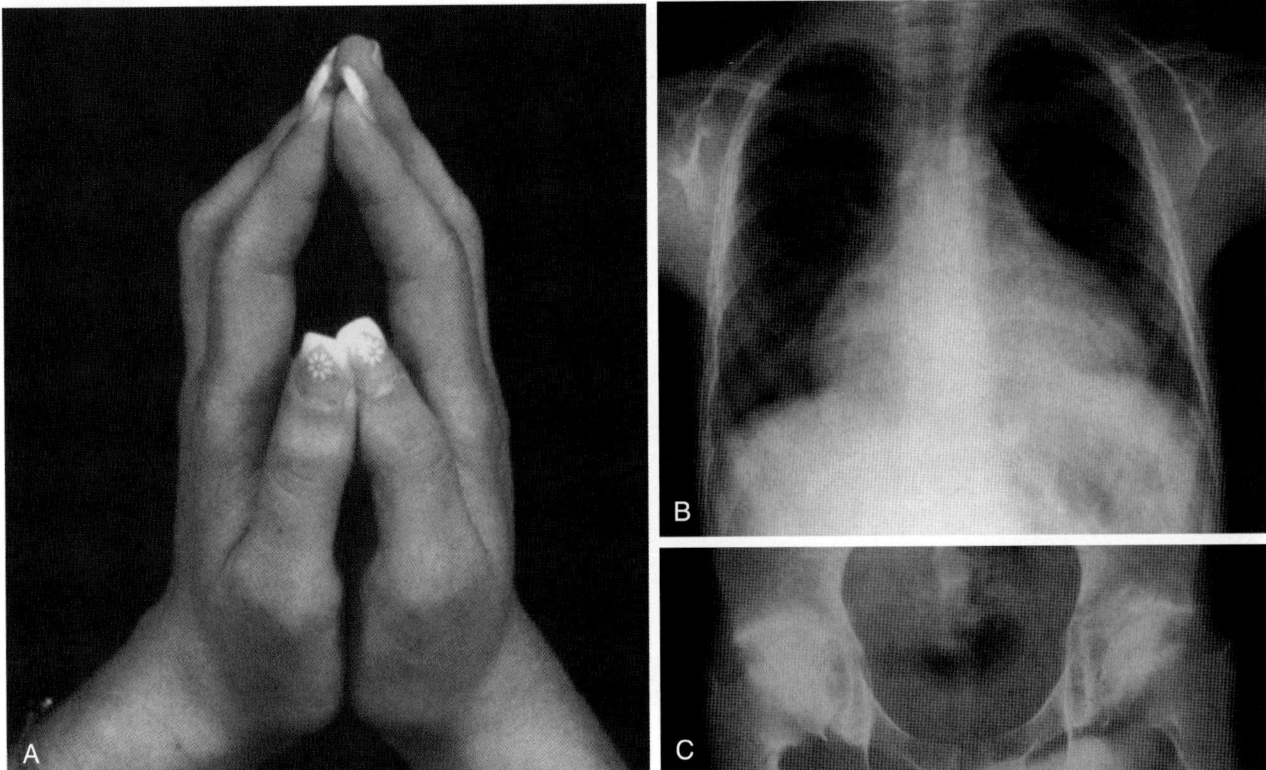

• **Fig. 2.9** Clinical features of camptodactyly–arthropathy–coxa vara–pericarditis (CACP) syndrome. (A) The characteristic deformity of the hands is shown. (B) A chest radiograph shows an enlarged cardiac outline caused by pericarditis. (C) Radiograph of the pelvis highlights coxa vara in a boy with CACP. (B and C, Courtesy Ronald Laxer, MD, Hospital for Sick Children, Toronto, Ontario, Canada.)

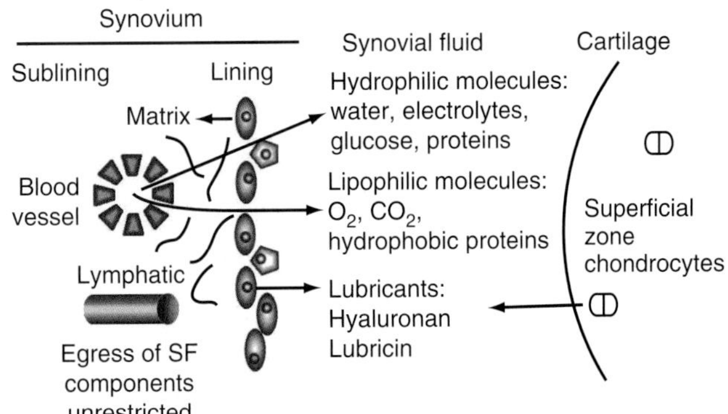

• **Fig. 2.10** Schematic representation of the formation of synovial fluid (SF). Many of the soluble components and proteins in SF exit the synovial subintimal microcirculation through pores or fenestrations in the vascular endothelium, then diffuse through the interstitium before entering the joint space. Synovial permeability to most small molecules is determined by a process of free diffusion through the double barrier of endothelium and interstitium, which is limited mainly by the intercellular space between synovial lining cells. Fat-soluble molecules can diffuse through and between cell membranes; their passage across the synovial surface is less restricted. Additional components, including hyaluronan and lubricin, are produced by synovial lining cells.

into cartilage, and that cartilage does not survive without synovial fluid contact in vivo. Within the cartilage matrix, three potential mechanisms for nutrient transfer have been proposed: diffusion, active transport by chondrocytes, and pumping by intermittent compression of cartilage matrix. A large proportion of hyaline cartilage lies within 50 μm of a synovial surface and its rich supply of blood vessels. Chondrocytes are well adapted to living in hypoxic conditions. Low oxygen tension promotes expression of the chondrocyte phenotype and cartilage-specific matrix formation. Reactive oxygen species also may play a crucial role in the regulation of some normal chondrocytic functions, such as cell activation, proliferation, and matrix remodeling.

Conclusion

The normal human synovial membrane is a highly specialized, multifunctional organ that is vital for mobility and survival. The intimal layer is composed of two distinct cell phenotypes with characteristics of macrophage and fibroblast lineages. Synovial macrophages express CD45, CD163, CD97, CD68, neuron-specific esterase, and cathepsins B, L, and D. Cells expressing CD14 are rarely seen in the healthy intimal layer. FcγRIII (CD16) is expressed by Kupffer cells of the liver and type II alveolar macrophages of the lung; CD16 is expressed on a subpopulation of synovial macrophages. Synovial macrophages also express the class II MHC molecule and play a central role in phagocytosis and in antigen-mediated immune responses.

Synovial intimal fibroblasts possess prominent synthetic capacity and produce the essential joint lubricants HA and lubricin. They also synthesize normal matrix components, including fibronectin, laminin, collagens, proteoglycans, lubricin, and other identified and unidentified proteins. In normal synovium, a delicate balance of checkpoint molecules appear to maintain homeostasis by way of epigenetic regulation, which is lost under inflammatory conditions when the tissue develops a capacity to produce large quantities of metalloproteinases, metalloproteinase inhibitors, prostaglandins, and cytokines. Expression of selected adhesion molecules on synovial fibroblasts probably facilitates the trafficking of some cell populations, such as polymorphs, into synovial fluid, and the retention of others, such as mononuclear leukocytes, within synovial tissue.

The subintimal layer is composed of a loose connective tissue matrix and contains branching blood and lymphatic vessels, a nerve supply, and a variety of resident cell populations, including infiltrating macrophages and fibroblasts. The nerve supply is important in regulating synovial blood flow. Lymphatic vessels allow egress of metabolic breakdown products from the synovium and synovial fluid. The structure of the subintimal layer varies according to the anatomic location and the local functional requirements.

Coordinated functions of the composite synovial membrane are essential for normal joint movement, formation of synovial fluid, nutrition of chondrocytes, and protection of cartilage. These functions must be preserved over a lifetime at multiple anatomic locations. Absence of essential constituents of synovial fluid, such as lubricin, or inadequate cartilage protection results in early articular malfunction, which may progress to variable degrees of joint failure. The characteristics of lubricin deficiency have been elegantly described in animal models and in humans. Additional studies may define novel clinical categories of degenerative polyarthritis that are associated with other specific disorders of synovial membrane function.

The references for this chapter can also be found on ExpertConsult.com.

References

1. Nozawa-Inoue K, Takagi R, Kobayashi T, et al.: Immunocytochemical demonstration of the synovial membrane in experimentally induced arthritis of the rat temporomandibular joint, *Arch Histol Cytol* 61:451–466, 1998.
2. Vandenabeele F, Lambrichts I, Lippens P, et al.: In vitro loading of human synovial membrane with 5-hydroxydopamine: evidence for dense core secretory granules in type B cells, *Arch Histol Cytol* 64:1–16, 2001.
3. Castor CW: The microscopic structure of normal human synovial tissue, *Arthritis Rheum* 3:140–151, 1960.
4. Barland P, Novikoff A, Novikoff AB, et al.: Electron microscopy of the human synovial membrane, *J Cell Biol* 14:207–220, 1962.
5. Krey PR, Cohen AS: Fine structural analysis of rabbit synovial cells in organ culture, *Arthritis Rheum* 16:324–340, 1973.
6. Okada Y, Nakanishi I, Kajikawa K: Ultrastructure of the mouse synovial membrane: development and organization of the extracellular matrix, *Arthritis Rheum* 24:835–843, 1981.
7. Groth HP: Cellular contacts in the synovial membrane of the cat and the rabbit: an ultrastructural study, *Cell Tissue Res* 164:525–541, 1975.
8. Roy S, Ghadially FN: Ultrastructure of normal rat synovial membrane, *Ann Rheum Dis* 26:26–38, 1967.
9. Wyllie JC, More RH, Haust MD: The fine structure of normal guinea pig synovium, *Lab Invest* 13:1254–1263, 1964.
10. Fell HB, Glauet AM, Barratt ME, et al.: The pig synovium. I. The intact synovium in vivo and in organ culture, *J Anat* 122:663–680, 1976.
11. Watanabe H, Spycher MA, Ruttner JR, et al.: Ultrastructural studies of rabbit synovitis induced by autologous IgG fragments. II. Infiltrating cells in the sublining layer, *Scand J Rheumatol Suppl* 15:15–22, 1976.
12. Linck G, Stoerkel ME, Petrovic A, et al.: Morphological evidence of a polypeptide-like secretory function of the B cells in the mouse synovial membrane, *Experientia* 33:1098–1099, 1977.
13. Johansson HE, Rejno S: Light and electron microscopic investigation of equine synovial membrane: a comparison between healthy joints and joints with intraarticular fractures and osteochondrosis dissecans, *Acta Vet Scand* 17:153–168, 1976.
14. Ghadially FN: *Fine structure of joints*, London, 1983, Butterworths.
15. Iwanaga T, Shikichi M, Kitamura H, et al.: Morphology and functional roles of synoviocytes in the joint, *Arch Histol Cytol* 63:17–31, 2000.
16. Graabaek PM: Ultrastructural evidence for two distinct types of synoviocytes in rat synovial membrane, *J Ultrastruct Res* 78:321–339, 1982.
17. Graabaek PM: Characteristics of the two types of synoviocytes in rat synovial membrane: an ultrastructural study, *Lab Invest* 50:690–702, 1984.
18. Edwards JCW: Fibroblast biology: development and differentiation of synovial fibroblasts in arthritis, *Arthritis Res* 2:344–347, 2000.
19. Athanasou NA: Synovial macrophages, *Ann Rheum Dis* 54:392–394, 1995.
20. Athanasou NA, Quinn J: Immunocytochemical analysis of human synovial lining cells: phenotypic relation to other marrow derived cells, *Ann Rheum Dis* 50:311–315, 1991.
21. Athanasou NA, Quinn J, Heryet A, et al.: The immunohistology of synovial lining cells in normal and inflamed synovium, *J Pathol* 155:133–142, 1988.
22. Izumi S, Takeya M, Takagi K, et al.: Ontogenetic development of synovial A cells in fetal and neonatal rat knee joints, *Cell Tissue Res* 262:1–8, 1990.
23. Edwards JC: The nature and origins of synovium: experimental approaches to the study of synoviocyte differentiation, *J Anat* 184:493–501, 1994.
24. Lau SK, Chu PG, Weiss LM: CD163: a specific marker of macrophages in paraffin-embedded tissue samples, *Am J Clin Pathol* 122:794–801, 2004.
25. Tuijnman WB, van Wichen DF, Schuurman HJ: Tissue distribution of human IgG Fc receptors CD16, CD32 and CD64: an immunohistochemical study, *APMIS* 101:319–329, 1993.
26. Edwards JCW, Blades S, Cambridge G: Restricted expression of Fc gammaRIII (CD16) in synovium and dermis: implications for tissue targeting in rheumatoid arthritis (RA), *Clin Exp Immunol* 108:401–406, 1997.
27. Bhatia A, Blades S, Cambridge G, et al.: Differential distribution of Fc gamma RIIIa in normal human tissues and co-localization with DAF and fibrillin-1: implications for immunological microenvironments, *Immunology* 94:56–63, 1998.
28. Walker MG: Z39Ig is co-expressed with activated macrophage genes, *Biochim Biophys Acta* 1574:387–390, 2002.
29. Kim JK, Choi EM, Shin HI, et al.: Characterization of monoclonal antibody specific to the Z39Ig protein, a member of immunoglobulin superfamily, *Immunol Lett* 99:153–161, 2005.
30. Lee MY, Kim WJ, Kang YJ, et al.: Z39Ig is expressed on macrophages and may mediate inflammatory reactions in arthritis and atherosclerosis, *J Leukoc Biol* 80:922–928, 2006.
31. el-Gabalawy H, Canvin J, Ma GM, et al.: Synovial distribution of alpha d/CD18, a novel leukointegrin: comparison with other integrins and their ligands, *Arthritis Rheum* 39:1913–1921, 1996.
32. Demaziere A, Athanasou NA: Adhesion receptors of intimal and subintimal cells of the normal synovial membrane, *J Pathol* 168:209–215, 1992.
33. Hui AY, McCarty WJ, Masuda K, et al.: A systems biology approach to synovial joint lubrication in health, injury, and disease, *Wiley Interdiscip Rev Syst Biol Med* 4:15–37, 2012.
34. Wilkinson LS, Pitsillides AA, Worrall JG, et al.: Light microscopic characterization of the fibroblast-like synovial intimal cell (synoviocyte), *Arthritis Rheum* 35:1179–1184, 1992.
35. Johnson BA, Haines GK, Haclous LA, et al.: Adhesion molecule expression in human synovial tissue, *Arthritis Rheum* 36:137–146, 1993.

36. Henderson KJ, Edwards JCW, Worrall JG: Expression of CD44 in normal and rheumatoid synovium and cultured fibroblasts, *Ann Rheum Dis* 53:729–734, 1994.
37. Ai R, Hammaker D, Boyle DL, et al.: Joint-specific DNA methylation and transcriptome signatures in rheumatoid arthritis identify distinct pathogenic processes, *Nat Commun* 7:118492016, 2016.
38. Whitaker JW, Shoemaker R, Boyle DL, et al.: An imprinted rheumatoid arthritis methylome signature reflects pathogenic phenotype, *Genome Med* 5:40, 2013.
39. Guo Y, Walsh AM, Canavan M, et al.: Immune checkpoint inhibitor PD-1 pathway is down-regulated in synovium at various stages of rheumatoid arthritis disease progression, *PLoS One* 13:e0192704, 2018.
40. Stevens CR, Mapp PI, Revell PA: A monoclonal antibody (Mab 67) marks type B synoviocytes, *Rheumatol Int* 10:103–106, 1990.
41. Pitsillides AA, Wilkinson LS, Mehdizadeh S, et al.: Uridine diphosphoglucose dehydrogenase activity in normal and rheumatoid synovium: the description of a specialized synovial lining cell, *Int J Exp Pathol* 74:27–34, 1993.
42. Wilkinson LS, Edwards JD, Paston RN, et al.: Expression of vascular cell adhesion molecule-1 in normal and inflamed synovium, *Lab Invest* 68:82–88, 1993.
43. Edwards JC, Wilkinson LS, Speight P, et al.: Vascular cell adhesion molecule 1 and alpha 4 and beta 1 integrins in lymphocyte aggregates in Sjögren's syndrome and rheumatoid arthritis, *Ann Rheum Dis* 52:806–811, 1993.
44. Valencia X, Higgins JM, Kiener HP, et al.: Cadherin-11 provides specific cellular adhesion between fibroblast-like synoviocytes, *J Exp Med* 200:1673–1679, 2004.
45. Kiener HP, Brenner MB: Building the synovium: cadherin-11 mediates fibroblast-like synoviocyte cell-to-cell adhesion, *Arthritis Res Ther* 7:49–54, 2005.
46. Kitamura HP, Yanase H, Kitamura H, et al.: Unique localization of protein gene product 9.5 in type B synoviocytes in the joints of the horse, *J Histochem Cytochem* 47:343–352, 1999.
47. Hamann J, Wishaupt JO, van Lier RA, et al.: Expression of the activation antigen CD97 and its ligand CD55 in rheumatoid synovial tissue, *Arthritis Rheum* 42:650–658, 1999.
48. Hamann J, Vogel B, van Schijadel GM, et al.: The seven-span transmembrane receptor CD97 has a cellular ligand (CD55, DAF), *J Exp Med* 184:1185–1189, 1996.
49. Ultaigh SN, Saber TP, McCormick J, et al.: Blockade of Toll-like receptor 2 prevents spontaneous cytokine release from rheumatoid arthritis ex vivo synovial explant cultures, *Arthritis Res Ther* 23(13), 2011.
50. Saber T, Veale DJ, Balogh E, et al.: Toll-like receptor 2 induced angiogenesis and invasion is mediated through the Tie2 signalling pathway in rheumatoid arthritis, *PLoS ONE* 6:e23540, 2011.
51. Kiener HP, Lee DM, Agarwal SK, et al.: Cadherin-11 induces rheumatoid arthritis fibroblast-like synoviocytes to form lining layers in vitro, *Am J Pathol* 168:1486–1499, 2006.
52. Lee DM, Kiener HP, Agarwal SK, et al.: Cadherin-11 in synovial lining formation and pathology in arthritis, *Science* 315:1006–1010, 2007.
53. Kiener HP, Watts GF, Cui Y, et al.: Synovial fibroblasts self-direct multicellular lining architecture and synthetic function in three-dimensional organ culture, *Arthritis Rheum* 62:742–752, 2010.
54. Mohr W, Beneke G, Mohing W: Proliferation of synovial lining cells and fibroblasts, *Ann Rheum Dis* 34:219–224, 1975.
55. Lalor PA, Garcia CH, O'Rourke LM, et al.: Proliferative activity of cells in the synovium as demonstrated by a monoclonal antibody, Ki67, *Rheumatol Int* 7:183–186, 1987.
56. Qu Z, Henderson B, Bitensky L, et al.: Local proliferation of fibroblast-like synoviocytes contributes to synovial hyperplasia: results of proliferating cell nuclear antigen/cyclin, c-myc, and nucleolar organizer region staining, *Arthritis Rheum* 37:212–220, 1994.
57. Coulton LA, Coates PJ, Ansari B, et al.: DNA synthesis in human rheumatoid and nonrheumatoid synovial lining, *Ann Rheum Dis* 39:241–247, 1980.
58. Hall PA, Edwards JC, Willoughby DA, et al.: Regulation of cell number in the mammalian gastrointestinal tract: the importance of apoptosis, *J Cell Sci* 107:3569–3577, 1994.
59. Edwards JC, Willoughby DA: Demonstration of bone marrow derived cells in synovial lining by means of giant intracellular granules as genetic markers, *Ann Rheum Dis* 41:177–182, 1982.
60. Edwards JC: The nature and origin of synovium: experimental approach to the study of synoviocyte differentiation, *J Anat* 184:493–501, 1994.
61. Yoshida H, Cecchini MG, Fleisch H, et al.: The murine mutation osteopetrosis is in the coding region of the macrophage colony stimulating factor gene, *Nature* 345:442–444, 1990.
62. Felix R, Cecchini MG, Fleisch H: Macrophage colony stimulating factor restores in vivo bone resorption in the op/op osteopetrotic mouse, *Endocrinology* 127:2592–2594, 1990.
63. Naito M, Palmer DG, Revell PA, et al.: Abnormal differentiation of tissue macrophage populations in "osteopetrosis" (op) mice defective in the production of macrophage colony-stimulating factor, *Am J Pathol* 139:657–667, 1991.
64. Hogg N, Palmer DG, Revell PA: Mononuclear phagocytes of normal and rheumatoid synovial membrane identified by monoclonal antibodies, *Immunology* 56:673–681, 1985.
65. Wijbrandts CA, Remans PH, Klarenbeek PL, et al.: Analysis of apoptosis in peripheral blood and synovial tissue very early after initiation of infliximab treatment in rheumatoid arthritis patients, *Arthritis Rheum* 58:3330–3339, 2008.
66. Müller-Ladner U, Gay RE, Gay S: Role of nuclear factor kappaB in synovial inflammation, *Curr Rheumatol Rep* 4:201–207, 2002.
67. Moynagh PN: The NF-κB pathway, *J Cell Sci* 118:4589–4592, 2005.
68. Miagkov AV, Kovalenko DV, Brown CE, et al.: NF-kappaB activation provides the potential link between inflammation and hyperplasia in the arthritic joint, *Proc Natl Acad Sci USA* 95:13859–13864, 1998.
69. Rosengren S, Corr M, Firestein GS, et al.: The JAK inhibitor CP-690,550 (tofacitinib) inhibits TNF-induced chemokine expression in fibroblast-like synoviocytes: autocrine role of type I interferon, *Ann Rheum Dis* 71:440–447, 2012.
70. Gao W, Sweeney C, Connolly M, et al.: Notch-1 mediates hypoxia-induced angiogenesis in rheumatoid arthritis, *Arthritis Rheum* 64:2104–2113, 2012.
71. De Bock K, Georgiadou M, Carmeliet P: Role of endothelial cell metabolism in vessel sprouting, *Cell Metab* 18:634–647, 2013.
72. Oliver KM, Garvey JF, Ng CT, et al.: Hypoxia activates NF-kappaB-dependent gene expression through the canonical signaling pathway, *Antioxid Redox Signal* 11:2057–2064, 2009.
73. Lee JH, Suk J, Park J, et al.: Notch signal activates hypoxia pathway through HES1-dependent SRC/signal transducers and activators of transcription 3 pathway, *Mol Cancer Res* 7:1663–1671, 2009.
74. Li TF, Boesler EW, Jimenez SA, et al.: Distribution of tenascin-X in different synovial samples and synovial membrane-like interface tissue from aseptic loosening of total hip replacement, *Rheumatol Int* 19:177–183, 2000.
75. Dodge GR, Boesler EW, Jimenez SA: Expression of the basement membrane heparan sulfate proteoglycan (perlecan) in human synovium and in cultured human synovial cells, *Lab Invest* 73:649–657, 1995.
76. Konttinen YT, Hoyland JA, Denton J, et al.: Expression of laminins and their integrin receptors in different conditions of synovial membrane and synovial membrane-like interface tissue, *Ann Rheum Dis* 58:683–690, 1999.
77. Dean G, Kruetner A, Ferguson AB, et al.: Mast cells in the synovium and synovial fluid in osteoarthritis, *Br J Rheumatol* 32:671–675, 1993.

78. Bentley G, Kreutner A, Ferguson AB: Synovial regeneration and articular cartilage changes after synovectomy in normal and steroid-treated rabbits, *J Bone Joint Surg Br* 57:454–462, 1975.
79. De Bari C, Sekiya I, Yagishita K, et al.: Multipotent mesenchymal stem cell from adult human synovial membrane, *Arthritis Rheum* 44:1928–1942, 2001.
80. Sakaguchi Y, Athanasou NA: Comparison of human stem cells derived from various mesenchymal tissues: superiority of synovium as a cell source, *Arthritis Rheum* 52:2521–2529, 2005.
81. Demaziere A, Athanasou NA: Adhesion receptors of intimal and subintimal cells of the normal synovial membrane, *J Pathol* 168:209–215, 1992.
82. Izquierdo E, Canete JD, Celis R, et al.: Immature blood vessels in rheumatoid synovium are selectively depleted in response to anti-TNF therapy, *PLoS ONE* 4:e8131, 2009.
83. Kennedy A, Ng CT, Biniecka M, et al.: Angiogenesis and blood vessel stability in inflammatory arthritis, *Arthritis Rheum* 62:711–721, 2010.
84. Lund-Olesen K: Oxygen tension in synovial fluids, *Arthritis Rheum* 13:769–776, 1970.
85. Ng CT, Biniecka M, Kennedy A, et al.: Synovial tissue hypoxia and inflammation in vivo, *Ann Rheum Dis* 69:1389–1395, 2010.
86. Xu H, Edwards J, Banerji S, et al.: Distribution of lymphatic vessels in normal and arthritic human synovial tissues, *Ann Rheum Dis* 62:1227–1229, 2003.
87. Bohnsack M: Distribution of substance-P nerves inside the infrapatellar fat pad and the adjacent synovial tissue: a neurohistological approach to anterior knee pain syndrome, *Arch Orthop Trauma Surg* 125:592–597, 2005.
88. McDougall JJ: Arthritis and pain: neurogenic origin of joint pain: a review, *Arthritis Res Ther* 10:220–230, 2006.
89. Henderson B, Edwards JCW: Functions of synovial lining. In Henderson B, Edwards JCW, editors: *The synovial lining in health and disease*, London, 1987, Chapman & Hall, pp 41–74.
89a. Culemann S, Gruneboom A, Nicolas-Avila JA, et al.: Locally renewing resident synovial macrophages provide a protective barrier for the joint, *Nature* 572:670–675, 2019.
90. Blewis ME, Lao BJ, Jadin KD, et al.: Semi-permeable membrane retention of synovial fluid lubricants hyaluronan and proteoglycan 4 for a biomimetic bioreactor, *Biotechnol Bioeng* 106:149–160, 2010.
91. Blewis ME, Lao BJ, Schumacher BL, et al.: Interactive cytokine regulation of synoviocyte lubricant secretion, *Tissue Eng Part A* 16:1329–1337, 2010.
92. Mazzucco D, Spector M: The role of joint fluid in the tribology of total joint arthroplasty, *Clin Orthop Relat Res* 429:17–32, 2004.
93. Clark JM, Norman AG, Kaab MJ, et al.: The surface contour of articular cartilage in an intact, loaded joint, *J Anat* 195:45–56, 1999.
94. Prehm P: Hyaluronan. In Steinbuchel A, editor: *Biopolymers*, Weinheim, Germany, 2002, Wiley-VCH-Verlag, pp 379–400.
95. Momberger TS, Levick JR, Mason RM: Hyaluronan synthesis by rabbit synoviocytes is mechanosensitive, *Matrix Biol* 24:510–519, 2005.
96. Momberger TS, Levick JR, Mason RM: Mechanosensitive synoviocytes: a Ca2+-PKCα-MAP kinase pathway contributes to stretch-induced hyaluronan synthesis in vitro, *Matrix Biol* 25:306–316, 2006.
97. Weigel PH, Hascall VC, Tammi M: Hyaluronan synthases, *J Biol Chem* 272:13997–14000, 1997.
98. Recklies AD, White C, Melching L, et al.: Differential regulation and expression of hyaluronan in human articular cartilage, synovial cells and osteosarcoma cells, *Biochem J* 354:17–24, 2001.
99. Tanimoto K, Itoh H, Sagawa N, et al.: Cyclic mechanical stretch regulates the gene expression of hyaluronic acid synthetase in cultured rabbit synovial cells, *Connect Tissue Res* 42:187–195, 2001.
100. Hui AY, McCarty WJ, Masuda K, et al.: A systems biology approach to synovial joint lubrication in health, injury, and disease, *Wiley Interdiscip Rev Syst Biol Med* 4:15–37, 2012.
101. Murakami T, Higaki H, Sawae Y, et al.: Adaptive multimode lubrication in natural synovial joints and artificial joints, *Proc Inst Mech Eng H* 212:23–35, 1998.
102. Levick JR: Fluid movement across synovium in healthy joints: role of synovial fluid macromolecules, *Ann Rheum Dis* 54:417–423, 1995.
103. Scott D, Coleman PJ, Mason RM, et al.: Molecular reflection by synovial lining is concentration dependent and reduced in dilute effusions in a rabbit model, *Arthritis Rheum* 43:1175–1182, 2000.
104. Sabaratnam S, Mason RM, Levick JR: Hyaluranon molecular reflection by synovial lining is concentration dependent and reduced in dilute effusions in a rabbit model, *Arthritis Rheum* 54:1673–1681, 2006.
105. Swann DA, Sotman S, Dixon M, et al.: The isolation and partial characterization of the major glycoprotein from the articular lubricating fraction from bovine synovial fluid, *Biochem J* 161:473–485, 1977.
106. Jay GD, Britt DE, Cha C-J: Lubricin is a product of megacaryocyte stimulating factor gene expression by human synovial fibroblasts, *J Rheumatol* 27:594–600, 2000.
107. Elsaid KA, Jay GD, Warman ML, et al.: Association of articular cartilage degradation and loss of boundary-lubricating ability of synovial fluid following injury and inflammatory arthritis, *Arthritis Rheum* 52:1746–1755, 2005.
108. Schumacher BL, Hughes CE, Kuettner KE, et al.: Immunodetection and partial cDNA sequence of the proteoglycan, superficial zone protein, synthesized by cells lining synovial joints, *J Orthop Res* 17:110–120, 1999.
109. Jay GD, Tantravahi U, Britt DE, et al.: Homology of lubricin and superficial zone protein (SZP): products of megakaryocyte stimulating factor (MSF) gene expression by human synovial fibroblasts and articular chondrocytes localized to chromosome 1q25, *J Orthop Res* 19:677–687, 2001.
110. Rhee DK, Marcelino J, Baker M, et al.: The secreted glycoprotein lubricin protects cartilage surfaces and inhibits synovial cell overgrowth, *J Clin Invest* 115:622–631, 2005.
111. Marcelino J, Carpten JD, Suwairi WM, et al.: CACP, encoding a secreted proteoglycan, is mutated in camptodactyly-arthropathy-coxa vara-pericarditis syndrome, *Nat Genet* 23:319–322, 1999.
112. Rhee DK, Marcelino J, Sulaiman A-M, et al.: Consequences of disease-causing mutations on lubricin protein synthesis, secretion, and post-translational processing, *J Biol Chem* 280:31325–31332, 2005.
113. Hills BA, Crawford RW: Normal and prosthetic synovial joints are lubricated by surface-active phospholipids: a hypothesis, *J Arthroplasty* 18:499–505, 2003.

3 Cartilage and Chondrocytes

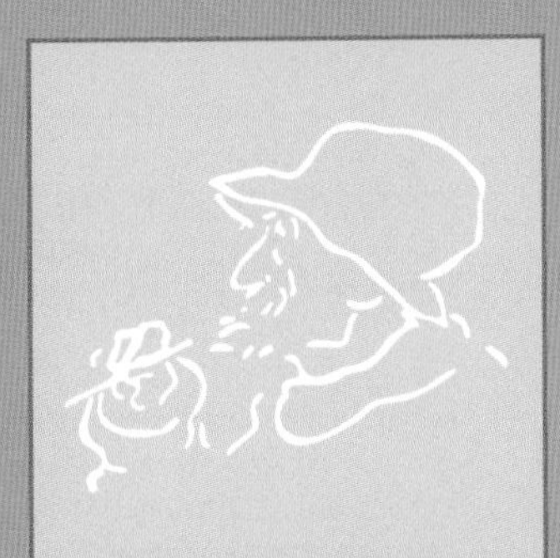

ALI MOBASHERI, MARY B. GOLDRING, AND RICHARD F. LOESER

KEY POINTS

Articular cartilage matrix is heterogeneous and contains a core matrisome of key extra-cellular matrix (ECM) proteins, of which the large aggregating proteoglycan aggrecan and collagen types II, IX, and XI are the major structural and functional constituents.

The collagen network of cartilage confers tensile strength, and large aggregating proteoglycans, such as aggrecan, provide resistance to compression.

Adult articular chondrocytes are nonmitotic cells that survive at low oxygen tension in an acidic and nutrient-challenged microenvironment in the absence of a vascular supply.

In response to trauma or inflammation, the metabolic activity of the chondrocyte is increased in response to catabolic and anabolic factors that regulate remodeling of the ECM.

Under physiologic conditions, the chondrocyte maintains low-turnover repair of proteoglycans, but the repair capacity, responses to anabolic factors, cell survival, and quality of the matrix decline with age.

Chondroprogenitor cells can be derived from multiple tissue sources, including bone marrow, synovium, and adipose tissue. There is emerging evidence for chondroprogenitors in adult articular cartilage, but their capacity for replacing chondrocytes or for repairing damaged matrix is not well established.

Introduction

Hyaline cartilage, including the articular cartilage of diarthrodial joints, consists of a single cellular component, the chondrocyte, which is embedded in a unique and complex matrix.[1] Adult articular chondrocytes are considered to be fully differentiated cells that maintain matrix constituents in a low-turnover state of equilibrium.[2] Chondrocytes serve diverse functions during development and postnatal life. In the embryo, chondrocytes arise from mesenchymal progenitors from diverse sources, including the cranial neural crest of the neural ectoderm, cephalic mesoderm, sclerotome of the paraxial mesoderm, and somatopleure of the lateral plate mesoderm, depending upon the ultimate location of the cartilage. The chondrocyte synthesizes the templates, or cartilage anlagen, through a process termed *chondrogenesis.*[3]

After mesenchymal condensation and chondroprogenitor cell (CPC) differentiation, chondrocytes undergo proliferation, terminal differentiation to chondrocyte hypertrophy, and apoptosis through a process termed *endochondral ossification,* whereby the hypertrophic cartilage is replaced by bone. A similar sequence of events occurs in the postnatal growth plate and leads to rapid growth of the skeleton. Processes that control the different stages of skeletal development are described in Chapter 1.

The permanent cartilage of articular surfaces, airways, ears, and nose persists throughout life.[4] In adults, the anatomic distribution of cartilage is restricted primarily to the joints, trachea, and nasal septum, where the major function is structural support. In joints, cartilage has the additional function of providing low-friction articulation. Adult articular cartilage comprises a specialized matrix of collagens, proteoglycans, and other cartilage-specific and nonspecific proteins. Adult articular chondrocytes, remnants of the resting or reserve chondrocytes that laid down the original cartilage matrix during chondrogenesis, are inactive metabolically, owing partially to the absence of a vascular supply and innervation in the tissue. However, there is accumulating evidence to suggest that chondrocytes undergo behavioral alterations and metabolic reprogramming in degenerative and inflammatory joint diseases. The clinical importance of the adult chondrocyte resides in its capacity to respond to mechanical stimuli, growth factors, and cytokines that may influence normal homeostasis in a positive or negative manner.[5–7]

Chondrocytes play important roles in the cellular taxonomy of arthritic diseases. In rheumatoid arthritis (RA), cartilage destruction occurs primarily in areas contiguous with the proliferating synovial pannus, although evidence indicates that the chondrocyte can respond to the inflammatory milieu and participate in degrading its own extra-cellular matrix (ECM). In osteoarthritis (OA), the chondrocyte plays a key role by reacting to structural changes in the surrounding cartilage matrix through the production of catabolic cytokines and anabolic factors, which act in an autocrine-paracrine manner.[8] The chondrocyte has limited capacity, which declines with age, to regenerate the normal cartilage architecture with zonal variations in the matrix network that was formed originally.[9] This chapter focuses on the structure and function of normal articular cartilage and the role of the chondrocyte in maintaining cartilage homeostasis and responding to adverse environmental insults that may modify cartilage integrity.

Cartilage Structure

Normal articular cartilage is a specialized tissue characterized macroscopically by its milky, shelled-almond (hyaline) appearance. It is an avascular tissue nourished by diffusion from the vasculature of the subchondral bone and from the synovial fluid. Articular cartilage is more than 70% water, and it is hypocellular compared with other tissues; chondrocytes constitute only 1% to 2% of its total volume.

Most of the dry weight of cartilage consists of two components: type II collagen and the large aggregating proteoglycan, aggrecan. Several "minor" collagens and small proteoglycans also contribute to the unique structural organization of the cartilage matrix.[10,11]

Among the organic constituents, collagen, primarily fibrillar type II, accounts for approximately 15% to 25% of the wet weight and about half of the dry weight except in the superficial zone, where it represents most of the dry weight. Proteoglycans, primarily aggrecan, account for 10% of the wet weight and about 25% of the dry weight. The highly cross-linked type II collagen–containing fibrils form a systematically oriented network that traps the highly negatively charged proteoglycan aggregates. Histochemical analysis of cartilage shows that proteoglycans can be stained reliably with Safranin O, Toluidine blue, or Alcian blue, although at low-substrate concentrations these methods are not stoichiometric.[12] Collagen also can be stained efficiently, but differentiation of collagen types requires immunostaining with specific antibodies. Less attention has been paid to less abundant and minor collagens, including types IV, VI, IX, X, XI, XII, XIII, and XIV.

Despite its thinness (≤7 mm) and apparent homogeneity, mature articular cartilage is a heterogeneous tissue with four distinct regions: (1) the superficial tangential (or gliding) zone, (2) the middle (or transitional) zone, (3) the deep (or radial) zone, and (4) the calcified cartilage zone, which is located immediately below the tidemark and above the subchondral bone (Fig. 3.1).[11] In the superficial zone, there are thin collagen fibrils in tangential array, and it contains a high concentration of the small proteoglycan decorin and a low concentration of aggrecan. The middle zone, comprising 40% to 60% of cartilage weight, consists of radial bundles of collagen fibrils that are thicker than in other zones. In the deep zone, the collagen fibrils become more perpendicular to the surface.

Cell density progressively decreases from the surface to the deep zone, where it is one-half to one-third the density of that in the superficial zone; chondrocytes in the deep and middle zones have cell volumes that are twice those of superficial chondrocytes. Cell morphology also changes across the different cartilage zones; cells in the superficial zone are relatively small, elongated in shape,

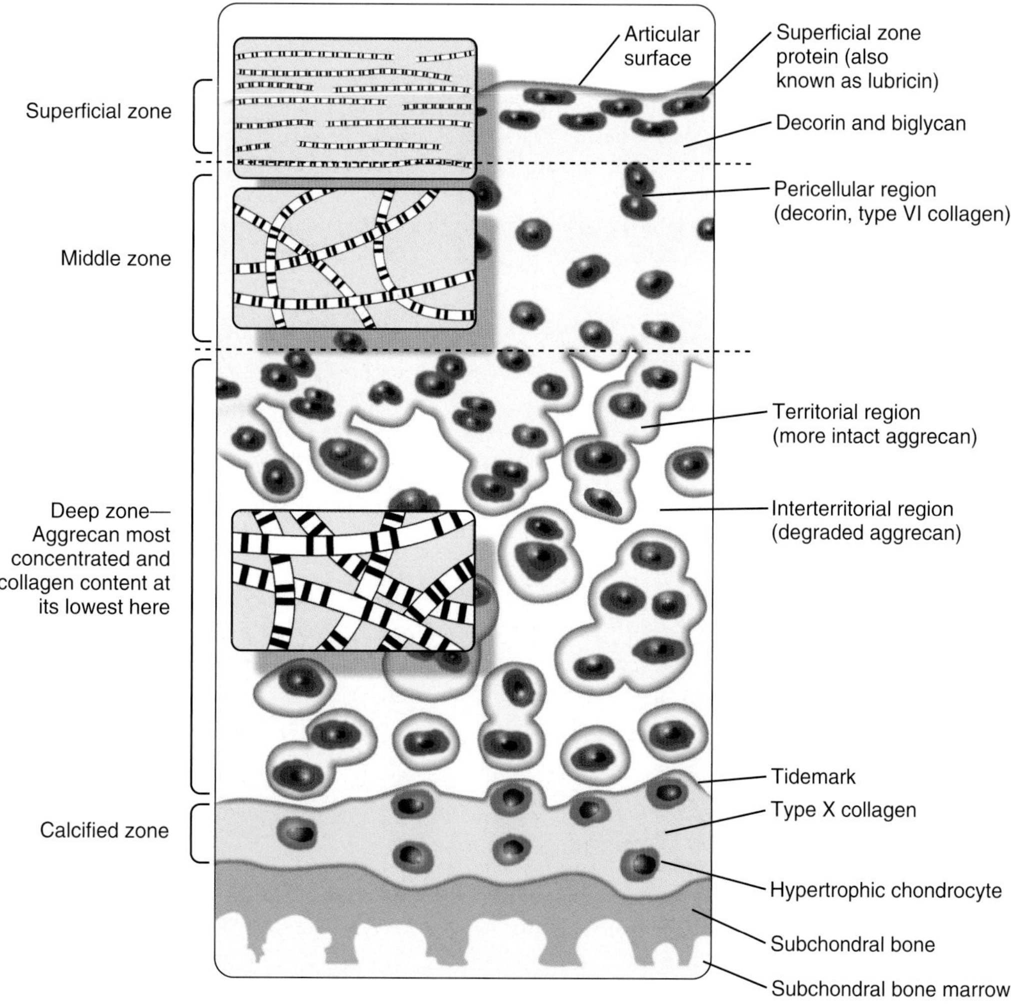

• **Fig. 3.1** The structure of human adult articular cartilage, showing zones of cellular distribution and the pericellular, territorial, and interterritorial regions of matrix organization. Insets show the relative diameters and orientations of collagen fibrils in the different zones. The positions of the tidemark and subchondral bone and other special features of matrix composition also are noted. (From Poole AR, Kojima T, Yasuda T, et al.: Composition and structure of articular cartilage: a template for tissue repair. *Clin Orthop Relat Res* [391S]:S26–S33, 2001. Copyright Lippincott Williams & Wilkins.)

aligned parallel to the surface, and lack an extensive pericellular matrix (PCM). Chondrocytes in the middle zone are spherical and do not exhibit an organized orientation relative to the surface. Cells in the deep zone exhibit extensive PCM deposition with chondrons in groups of three or more cells arranged in columns perpendicular to the articulating surface.[13]

Water is 75% to 80% of the wet weight in the superficial zone and progressively decreases to 65% to 70% with increasing depth. Compared with the middle and deep zones, greater amounts of collagen relative to proteoglycans are present in the superficial zone, and type I collagen may be present in addition to type II collagen. With increasing depth, the proportion of proteoglycan increases to 50% of the dry weight in the deep zone. The calcified zone is formed as a result of endochondral ossification and persists after growth plate closure with the histologically defined tidemark defining the boundary with the articular cartilage.[14,15] The calcified zone serves as an important mechanical buffer between uncalcified articular cartilage and subchondral bone (Fig. 3.2).

The physical properties of articular cartilage are determined by the unique fibrillar collagen network, which provides tensile strength, interspersed with proteoglycan aggregates that bestow compressive resilience.[16,17] Proteoglycans are associated with large quantities of water bound to the hydrophilic glycosaminoglycans (GAGs). This proteoglycan-rich ECM, with its tightly bound water, provides a high degree of resistance to deformation by compressive forces. The capacity to resist compressive forces is associated with the ability to extrude water as the cartilage compresses. When compression is released, the proteoglycans (now depleted of balancing counter ions that were removed with the water) contain sufficient fixed charge to reabsorb osmotically the water and small solutes into the matrix, which then rebounds to its original dimensions.

Structure-Function Relationships of Cartilage Matrix Components

ECM components synthesized by chondrocytes include highly cross-linked fibrils of triple-helical type II collagen molecules that interact with other collagens, aggrecan, small proteoglycans, and other cartilage-specific and nonspecific matrix proteins (Table 3.1).[10,11] The importance of these structural proteins may be observed in heritable disorders, such as chondrodysplasias, or in transgenic animals in which mutations or deficiencies in cartilage genes result in cartilage abnormalities. Deficiencies or disruptions in genes that encode the cartilage-specific collagens result, in some cases, in premature OA.[18] Knowledge of the composition of the cartilage matrix has permitted the development of methods for identifying molecular markers in serum and synovial fluid that can be used to monitor changes in cartilage metabolism and to assess cartilage damage in OA or RA.[19] Changes in the structural composition of cartilage can markedly affect its biomechanical properties.[7]

Cartilage Collagens

The major component of the collagen network in adult articular cartilage is the triple-helical type II collagen molecule, which is composed of three identical α chains ($(\alpha 1[II])_3$). These molecules are assembled in fibrils in a quarter-stagger array that can be observed by electron microscopy.[11,20] These fibrils are thinner than type I collagen–containing fibrils in skin because of the higher numbers of hydroxylysine residues that can form cross-links and the presence of other collagen and noncollagen components in the fibril. Type IIB collagen in articular cartilage is a product of alternative splicing

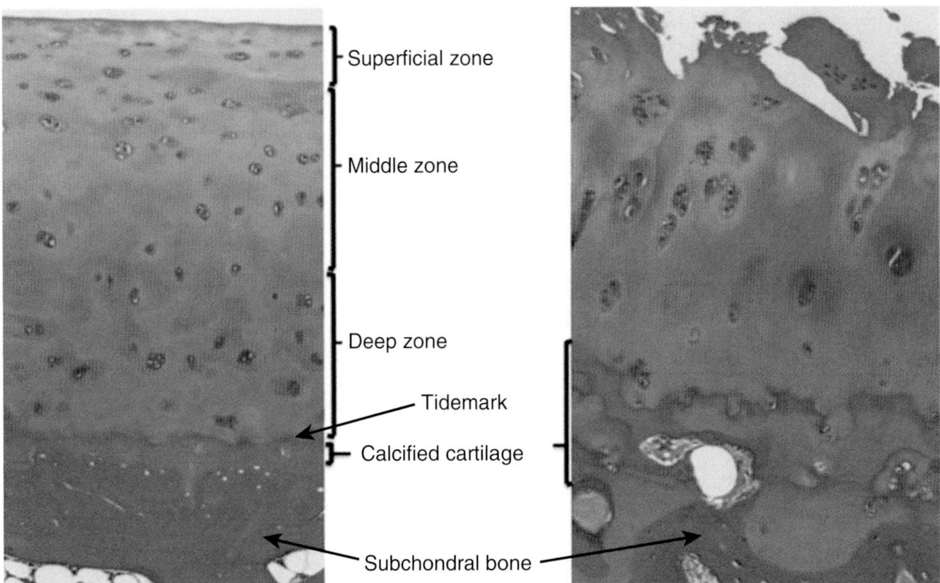

• **Fig. 3.2** The composition and cellular organization of healthy human adult articular cartilage *(left panel)* is more complex than it looks in this histological section showing chondrocytes distributed in matrix with homogeneous appearance and the clear demarcation *(tidemark)* between the articular cartilage and a thin zone of calcified cartilage next to the underlying subchondral bone. During the development of osteoarthritis, the normally quiescent chondrocytes become activated and undergo a phenotypic shift, resulting in surface fibrillation and degradation of cartilage matrix, the appearance of chondrocyte clusters, increased cartilage calcification associated with tidemark advancement or duplication, and vascular penetration from the subchondral bone *(right panel)*. Histology (Safranin O staining) provided by Cecilia Dragomir, Hospital for Special Surgery, New York, NY; 10× magnification. (Adapted from Goldring MB, Marcu KB: Epigenomic and microRNA-mediated regulation in cartilage development, homeostasis, and osteoarthritis. *Trends Mol Med* 18:109–118, 2012.)

TABLE 3.1 Extra-cellular Matrix Components of Cartilage

Molecule	Structure	Function and Location
Collagens		
Type II	$[\alpha 1(II)]_3$; fibril-forming	Tensile strength; major component of collagen fibrils
Type IX	$[\alpha 1(IX)\alpha 2(IX)\alpha 3(IX)]$; single CS or DS chain; $\alpha 1(II)$ gene encodes $\alpha 3(IX)$; FACIT	Tensile properties, interfibrillar connections; cross-links to surface of collagen fibril, NC4 domain projects into matrix
Type XI	$[\alpha 1(XI)\alpha 2(XI)\alpha 3(XI)]$; fibril-forming	Nucleation/control of fibril formation; within collagen fibril
Type VI	$[\alpha 1(VI)\alpha 2(VI)\alpha 3(VI)]$; microfibrils	Forms microfibrillar network, binds hyaluronan, biglycan, decorin; pericellular
Type X	$[\alpha 1(X)]_3$; hexagonal network	Support for endochondral ossification; hypertrophic zone and calcified cartilage
Type XII	$[\alpha 1(XII)]_3$; FACIT large cruciform NC3 domain	Associated with type I collagen fibrils in perichondrium and articular surface
Type XIV	$[\alpha 1(XIV)]_3$; FACIT	Associated with type I collagen; superficial zone
Type XVI	$[\alpha 1(XVI)]_3$; FACIT	Integrates with collagen II/XI fibrils
Type XXVII	*Col27a1* gene: 156 kb, 61 exons	Fibril-forming; developing cartilage
Proteoglycans		
Aggrecan	255 kDa core protein; CS/KS side chains; C-terminal EGF and lectin-like domains	Compressive stiffness through hydration of fixed charge density; binding through G1 domain to HA stabilized by link protein
Versican	265-370 kDa core protein; CS/DS side chains; C-terminal EGF, C-type lectin, and CRP-like domains	Low levels in articular cartilage throughout life; calcium-binding and selectin-like properties
Perlecan	400-467 kDa core protein; HS/CS side chains; no HA binding	Cell-matrix adhesion; pericellular
Biglycan	38 kDa; LRR core protein with two DS chains (76 kDa)	Binds collagen VI and TGF-β; pericellular
Decorin	36.5 kDa; LRR core protein with one CS or DS side chain (100 kDa)	Controls size/shape of collagen fibrils, binds collagen II and TGF-β; interterritorial
Asporin	40 kDa; LRR core protein; N-terminal extension of 15 aspartate residues	Binds collagen, modulates TGF-β function
Fibromodulin	42 kDa; containing KS chains in central LRR region and N-terminal tyrosine sulfate domains	Same as decorin
Lumican	38 kDa; structure similar to fibromodulin	Same as decorin
PRELP	44 kDa; LRR core protein; proline-rich and arginine-rich N-terminal binding domain for heparin and HS	Mediates cell binding through HS in syndecan
Chondroadherin	45 kDa; LRR core protein without N-terminal extension	Binding to cells via $\alpha 2\beta 1$ integrin
Other Molecules		
Hyaluronic acid (HA; hyaluronan)	1000-3000 kDa	Retention of aggrecan within matrix
Link protein	38.6 kDa	Stabilizes attachment of aggrecan G1 domain to HA
Cartilage oligomeric matrix protein (COMP)	550 kDa; five 110-kDa subunits; thrombospondin-like	Interterritorial in articular cartilage; stabilizes collagen network or promotes collagen fibril assembly; calcium binding
Cartilage matrix protein (CMP, or matrilin-1); matrilin-3	Three 50 kDa subunits with vWF and EGF domains	Tightly bound to aggrecan in immature cartilage
Cartilage intermediate-layer protein (CILP)	92 kDa; homology with nucleotide pyrophosphohydrolase without active site	Restricted to middle/deep zones of cartilage; increase in early and late osteoarthritis
Glycoprotein (gp)-39, YKL-40, or chitinase 3-like protein 1 (CH3L1)	39 kDa; chitinase homology	Marker of cartilage turnover; chondrocyte proliferation; superficial zone of cartilage

Continued

TABLE 3.1 **Extra-cellular Matrix Components of Cartilage—cont'd**

Molecule	Structure	Function and Location
Fibronectin	Dimer of 220 kDa subunits	Cell attachment and binding to collagen and proteoglycans; increased in osteoarthritis cartilage
Tenascin-C	Six 200-kDa subunits forming hexabrachion structure	Binds syndecan-3 during chondrogenesis; angiogenesis
Superficial zone protein (SZP), lubricin, or proteoglycan (PRG) 4	225 kDa, 200 nm length	Joint lubrication; superficial zone only
Membrane Proteins		
CD44	Integral membrane protein with extra-cellular HS/CS side chains	Cell-matrix interactions; binds HA
Syndecan-1, -3, -4	N-terminal HS attachment site; cytoplasmic tyrosine residues	Syndecan-3 is receptor for tenascin-C during cartilage development; cell-matrix interactions
Annexin V (anchorin CII)	34 kDa; homology to calcium-binding proteins calpactin and lipocortin	Cell surface attachment to type II collagen; calcium binding
Integrins (α1, α2, α3, α5, α6, α10; β1, β3, β5)	Two noncovalently linked transmembrane glycoproteins (α and β subunits)	Cell-matrix binding: α1β1/collagen I or VI, α2β1 or α3β1/collagen II, α5β1/fibronectin; intra-cellular signaling
Discoidin domain receptor 2	Receptor tyrosine kinase	Binds native type II collagen fibrils; Ras/ERK signaling
Transient receptor potential vanilloid 4 (TRPV4)	Ca^{2+} channel	Mechanosensor
Connexin 43	ATP release channel	Mechanosensor; primary cilia

CRP, Complement regulatory protein; *CS,* chondroitin sulfate; *DS,* dermatan sulfate; *EGF,* epidermal growth factor; *FACIT,* fibril-associated collagens with interrupted triple helices; *HA,* hyaluronic acid; *HS,* heparan sulfate; *KS,* keratan sulfate; *LRR,* leucine-rich repeat; *NC,* noncollagen; *PRELP,* proline-rich and arginine-rich end leucine-rich repeat protein; *TGF,* transforming growth factor; *vWF,* von Willebrand factor.

and lacks a 69 amino acid, cysteine-rich domain of the amino-terminal propeptide, which is encoded by exon 2 in the human type II collagen gene *(COL2A1).*[21] This domain is found in type IIA procollagen, which is expressed by CPCs during development, and in the amino propeptides of other interstitial collagen types, and may play a feedback-inhibitory role in collagen biosynthesis.[22] The reappearance of type IIA collagen in the midzone PCM and type X collagen, the hypertrophic chondrocyte marker, in the deep zone of OA cartilage suggests reversion to a developmental phenotype in an attempt to repair the damaged matrix.

Although collagens VI, IX, XI, XII, and XIV are quantitatively minor components, they may have important structural and functional properties and could represent a unique opportunity for the development of future biomarker tools for studying ECM repair and remodeling, especially in a regenerative context. Collagens IX and XI are relatively specific to cartilage, whereas collagens VI, XII, and XIV are widely distributed in other connective tissues. Collagen VI is present as microfibrils in the PCM and may play a role in cell attachment, and it interacts with other matrix proteins, such as hyaluronan, perlecan, biglycan, monomers or small aggregates of aggrecan, and type IX collagen, which are located there exclusively or at higher amounts than in the interterritorial matrix.[23] There are small amounts of collagen III in cartilage, and collagens VI and III may increase in OA cartilage.[10]

Type IX collagen is a proteoglycan and a collagen because it contains a chondroitin sulfate chain attachment site in one of the noncollagen domains. The helical domains of the type IX collagen molecule form covalent cross-links with type II collagen telopeptides and are attached to the fibrillar surface, as observed by electron microscopy. Type IX collagen may function as a structural intermediate between type II collagen fibrils and the proteoglycan aggregates, serving to enhance the mechanical stability of the fibril network and resist the swelling pressure of the trapped proteoglycans. Destruction of type IX collagen accelerates cartilage degradation and loss of function.

The α3 chain of type XI collagen has the same primary sequence as the α1(II) chain, and the heterotrimeric type XI collagen molecule is buried in the same fibril as type II collagen. Type XI collagen may have a role in regulating fibril diameter. The more recently discovered nonfibrillar fibril-associated collagens with interrupted triple helices (FACIT), XII and XIV, which are structurally related to type IX collagen, do not form fibrils by themselves but co-aggregate with fibril-forming collagens and modulate the packing of collagen fibers through domains projecting from their surfaces.

Cartilage Proteoglycans

The major proteoglycan in articular cartilage is the large aggregating proteoglycan aggrecan, which consists of a core protein of 225 to 250 kDa with covalently attached side chains of GAGs, including approximately 100 chondroitin sulfate chains, 30 keratan sulfate chains, and shorter *N*-linked and *O*-linked oligosaccharides.[10] Link protein, a small glycoprotein, stabilizes the noncovalent linkage between aggrecan and hyaluronic acid (also called *hyaluronan*) to form the proteoglycan aggregate that may contain 100 aggrecan monomers. The G1 and G2 N-terminal globular domains of aggrecan and its C-terminal G3 domain have distinct structural properties that function as integral parts of the aggrecan core protein and contribute cleavage products that accumulate with age or in OA. The G2 domain is separated from G1 by a linear interglobular domain and has two proteoglycan tandem repeats. The G3 domain contains sequence homologies to epidermal growth factor, lectin, and complement regulatory protein, and participates in growth regulation, cell recognition, intra-cellular trafficking, ECM assembly, and stabilization. About half of the aggrecan molecules in adult cartilage lack the G3 domain, probably as a result of proteolytic cleavage during matrix turnover. Small quantities of other large proteoglycans are found in cartilage, including versican, which forms aggregates with hyaluronic acid, and perlecan, which is nonaggregating; however, these proteoglycans function primarily during skeletal development, where versican is expressed in prechondrogenic condensations, and perlecan is expressed in the cartilage anlagen after expression of type II collagen and aggrecan.[24,25]

The nonaggregating small proteoglycans are not specific to cartilage, but in cartilage they serve specific roles in matrix structure and function, primarily by modulating collagen-fibril formation.[10,26] Of the more than 10 leucine-rich repeat (LRR) proteoglycans discovered so far, only osteoadherin is not present in cartilage. The 24-amino acid central LRR domain is conserved, but the N-terminal and C-terminal domains have patterns of cysteine residues involved in intrachain disulfide bonds that distinguish the four subfamilies: (1) biglycan, decorin, fibromodulin, and lumican; (2) keratocan and proline and arginine-rich end leucine-rich repeat protein (PRELP); (3) chondroadherin; and (4) epiphycan/PG-Lb and mimecan/osteoglycin. Biglycan may have two GAG chains—chondroitin sulfate or dermatan sulfate, or both—attached near the N-terminus through two closely spaced serine-glycine dipeptides. Decorin contains only one chondroitin sulfate or dermatan sulfate chain. Fibromodulin and lumican contain keratan sulfate chains linked to the central domain of the core protein and several sulfated tyrosine residues in the N-terminus. Negatively charged GAG side chains contribute to the fixed charge density of the matrix and, together with the highly anionic tyrosine-sulfation sites, permit multiple-site linkage between adjacent collagen fibrils, stabilizing the network. Decorin, the most extensively studied LRR proteoglycan, binds to collagens II, VI, XII, and XIV, and to fibronectin and thrombospondin. Biglycan, decorin, and fibromodulin bind transforming growth factor (TGF)-β and the epidermal growth factor receptor and may modulate growth, remodeling, and repair. PRELP and chondroadherin may regulate cell-matrix interactions through binding to syndecan and α2β1 integrin.

PRG4 (proteoglycan 4), also known as *lubricin* and *superficial zone proteoglycan (SZP),* is a large surface-active mucinous proteoglycan synthesized and secreted by chondrocytes located at the surface of articular cartilage and by some synovial lining cells.[27] PRG4 plays an important role in cartilage integrity in the synovial joint by providing boundary lubrication at the cartilage surface and contributing to the elastic absorption and energy dissipation of synovial fluid. Joint friction is elevated and accompanied by accelerated cartilage damage in humans and mice with a genetic deficiency of PRG4.[28,29] In healthy synovial joints, PRG4 molecules coat the cartilage surface, providing boundary lubrication and preventing cell and protein adhesion, inhibiting caspase-3 activation, thus preventing chondrocyte apoptosis.[30] The chondroprotective properties of PRG4 may be exploited to provide new therapeutic options for reducing friction in degenerative and inflammatory joint disorders.

Other Extra-cellular Matrix and Cell Surface Proteins

Several other noncollagenous matrix proteins may play important roles in determining cartilage matrix integrity.[31] Cartilage oligomeric protein (COMP), a member of the thrombospondin family, is a disulfide-bonded, pentameric, 550 kDa, calcium-binding protein that constitutes approximately 10% of the noncollagenous, nonproteoglycan protein in normal adult cartilage. COMP is located in the interterritorial matrix of adult articular cartilage, where it interacts with the COL3 and NC4 domains of type IX collagen that protrude from the fibril, stabilizing the collagen network. COMP is pericellular in the proliferating region of the growth plate, where it may have a role in cell-matrix interactions.[32] The cartilage matrix protein (or matrilin-1) and matrilin-3 are expressed in cartilage at certain stages of development. Matrilin-1 is present in the PCM of adult articular cartilage, and matrilin-1, -2, and -3 may be upregulated in articular cartilage during OA.[33]

Tenascin-C, a glycoprotein that is regulated in development, is characteristic of nonossifying cartilage. Similar to fibronectin, alternative splicing of tenascin-C mRNA gives rise to different protein products at different stages of chondrocyte differentiation. Both proteins are increased in OA cartilage and may serve specific functions in remodeling and repair.[34] The cartilage intermediate-layer protein (CILP) is expressed by chondrocytes in the middle to deep zones of articular cartilage as a precursor protein. When cleaved during secretion, CILP has structural similarities with nucleotide pyrophosphohydrolase, although it lacks the catalytic site, and it may play a role in pyrophosphate metabolism and calcification.[35] Asporin is related to decorin and biglycan and, similar to those other LRR proteins, may interact with and sequester growth factors such as TGF-β.[36] YKL-40/HC-gp39, also known as *chitinase 3-like protein 1,* is found only in the superficial zone of normal cartilage and stimulates proliferation of chondrocytes and synovial cells.[37] Chitinase 3-like protein 1 is induced by inflammatory cytokines and may function as a feedback regulator because it inhibits cytokine-induced cellular responses. Synthesis or release of these proteins or fragments is often increased in cartilage that is undergoing repair or remodeling, and they have been investigated as markers of cartilage damage in arthritis.

Morphology, Classification, and Normal Function of Chondrocytes

Morphology

The characteristic feature of the chondrocyte embedded in cartilage matrix is its rounded or polygonal morphology. The exception occurs at tissue boundaries, such as the articular surfaces of joints, where chondrocytes may be flattened or discoid. Intra-cellular features, including a rough endoplasmic reticulum (ER), a juxtanuclear Golgi apparatus, and deposition of glycogen, are characteristic of a synthetically active cell. The cell density of full-thickness, human, adult, femoral condyle cartilage is maintained at 14.5 (±3.0) × 10^3 cells/mm^2 from age 20 to 30 years. Although senescence of chondrocytes occurs with aging, mitotic figures are not observed in normal adult articular cartilage.

Chondrocytes possess mitochondria with varying degrees of structural and functional heterogeneity. Mitochondria are important for cartilage development and are primarily associated with cellular energetics and metabolism, but they are also important mediators of calcium accumulation needed for ECM calcification, especially in epiphyseal chondrocytes.[38] Chondrocyte mitochondrial impairment and dysfunction have been implicated in degenerative processes[39] and OA.[40] Mitochondrial degeneration can occur in response to oxidative damage, contributing to the age-related loss of chondrocyte function.[41]

Chondrocytes exhibit different behaviors depending on their position within the different cartilage layers, and these zonal differences in biosynthetic properties may persist in primary chondrocyte cultures. The primary cilia are important for spatial orientation of cells in developing growth plate and are sensory organelles in chondrocytes. Primary cilia are centers for Wnt and hedgehog signaling and contain mechanosensitive receptors, including the transient receptor potential vanilloid 4 (TRPV4), a Ca^{2+} permeable, nonselective cation channel, and connexin 43, an adenosine triphosphate (ATP) permeable gap junction channel involved in ATP release.[42,43]

Classification: Cell Origin and Differentiation

Chondrocytes arise in the embryo from mesenchymal origin during chondrogenesis, which is the earliest phase of skeletal development involving mesenchymal cell recruitment, migration, and condensation and differentiation of mesenchymal CPCs.[44,45] As described in detail in Chapter 1, chondrogenesis results in the formation of cartilage anlagen, or templates, at sites where skeletal elements form. This process is controlled by cell-cell and cell-matrix interactions and by growth and differentiation factors that initiate or suppress cellular signaling pathways and transcription of specific genes in a temporospatial manner (Fig. 3.3).[46]

Vertebrate limb development is controlled by interacting patterning systems involving fibroblast growth factor (FGF), hedgehog, bone morphogenetic protein (BMP), TGF-β, Wnt, and Notch pathways.[47–51] Wnt signaling, via the canonical β-catenin pathway and activation of TCF/Lef transcription factors, functions in a cell-autonomous manner to induce osteoblast differentiation and suppress chondrocyte differentiation in early

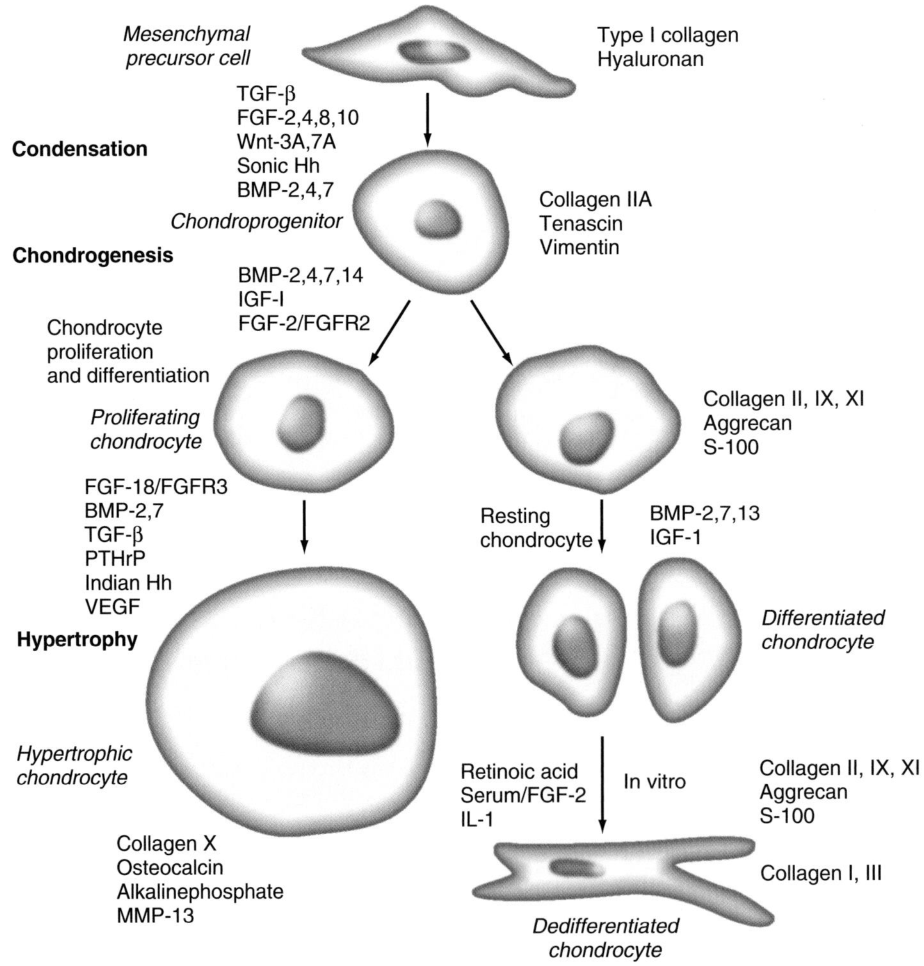

• **Fig. 3.3** Schematic representation of cellular phenotypes associated with developmental fates during condensation, chondrogenesis, chondrocyte proliferation, differentiation, and hypertrophy. Some of the regulatory factors active at different stages are listed to the left of the arrows. The major extra-cellular matrix genes are listed to the right of each cell type in which they are differentially expressed. *BMP,* Bone morphogenetic protein; *FGF,* fibroblast growth factor; *Hh,* hedgehog; *IGF,* insulin-like growth factor; *IL-1,* interleukin-1; *MMP,* matrix metalloproteinase; *PTHrP,* parathyroid hormone–related protein; *TGF-β,* transforming growth factor-β; *VEGF,* vascular endothelial growth factor; *Wnt,* wingless type.

chondroprogenitors. During chondrogenesis, Wnt/β-catenin acts at two stages: at low levels to promote chondroprogenitor differentiation and later at high levels to promote chondrocyte hypertrophic differentiation and subsequent endochondral ossification. The transcription factor, Sry-type high-mobility group box 9 (Sox9), is an early marker of the differentiating chondrocyte that is required for the onset of expression of type II collagen, aggrecan, and other cartilage-specific matrix proteins, such as type IX collagen.[48] Two other members of the SOX family, L-Sox5 and Sox6, are not present in early mesenchymal condensations but are required during overt chondrocyte differentiation, forming heterodimers that induce transcription more efficiently than Sox9 by itself. At different times during development, SOX proteins interact with SMADs (signaling through mammalian homologs of *Drosophila* mothers against decapentaplegic), which are functionally redundant and active in differentiating chondrocytes. Other transcription factors such as Gata4/5/6 and Nkx3.2 may interact directly or indirectly with Sox9 to upregulate the expression of *COL2A1* aggrecan *(ACAN),* and other cartilage-specific genes at early stages of chondrogenesis.[52]

In the embryonic or postnatal epiphyseal growth plates, molecules that promote matrix remodeling and angiogenesis facilitate endochondral ossification, whereby bone replaces the calcified cartilaginous matrix in the hypertrophic zone (see Chapter 1). Differentiated chondrocytes that remain in the reserve, or resting, zone become the cartilage elements in articular joints, or they can proliferate and undergo the complex process of terminal differentiation to hypertrophy marked by type X collagen. Indian hedgehog and parathyroid hormone–related protein (PTHrP) transiently induce proliferation and repress differentiation, determining the number of cells that enter the hypertrophic maturation pathway. The Runt domain transcription factor, Runx2 (also known as *core binding factor* or *Cbfa1*), serves as a positive regulatory factor in chondrocyte maturation to the hypertrophic phenotype and subsequent osteogenesis.[53] Runx2 is expressed in the adjacent perichondrium and in prehypertrophic chondrocytes, but less in late hypertrophic chondrocytes, and is required for expression of type X collagen and other markers of terminal differentiation.[44,52]

Numerous other transcription factors positively or negatively regulate chondrocyte terminal differentiation by controlling, in part, the expression or activity of Runx2.[52,53] BMP-induced Smad1 and interactions between Smad1 and Runx2 are required for the induction of chondrocyte hypertrophy. Histone deacetylase 4 (HDAC4), which is expressed later in prehypertrophic chondrocytes, prevents premature chondrocyte hypertrophy by interacting with Runx2 and inhibiting its activity.[54] The hypoxia-inducible factor (HIF)-1α contributes to chondrocyte survival during hypertrophic differentiation, owing partially to its regulation of vascular endothelial cell growth factor (VEGF) expression, and it prevents premature hypertrophy by directly suppressing Runx2 activity. The transcription factors involved in regulating gene expression during late-stage hypertrophy include Runx3, myocyte enhancer factor (MEF) 2C and 2D, Foxa2 and Foxa3, and Zfp521, in addition to Runx2.[44,52]

One major function of the chondrocyte is growth of the skeleton through increasing cell proliferation, production of ECM, and cell volume through hypertrophy. Lineage tracing studies indicate that Sox9-expressing cells are precursors for both articular and growth plate chondrocytes. Furthermore, cells expressing *Tgfbr2,* the gene encoding the TGF-β receptor (R) II in the interzone, can be traced to synovial lining, superficial meniscus, and ligaments and may persist as reserve progenitor cells that could later participate in regeneration. Finally, Gdf5, matrilin-1, and PTHrP appear to specify the eventual border between the articular cartilage surface and the joint space.[45] After cessation of growth, the resting chondrocyte remains as part of the supporting structures in articular, tracheal, and nasal cartilages, indicating that the fate of a chondrocyte depends on origin and location.[47]

Adult human articular cartilage contains CPCs that retain their expansion capacity with the potential of reproducing the structural and biomechanical properties of healthy articular cartilage. CPCs are stem/progenitor cells capable of chondrogenic differentiation and can be derived from multiple tissue sources including articular cartilage, synovium, and adipose tissue. CPCs reside not only in the superficial zone of articular cartilage but also in other zones of articular cartilage and in the neighboring tissues.[55] They have been classified as mesenchymal stem cells (MSCs) and have been postulated to play a role in responses to cartilage injury.[56] They can be identified by their colony forming ability, proliferative potential, telomere dynamics, multipotency, and expression of stem cell markers.[55] Therefore, they have potential applications in cartilage tissue engineering and may have clinical applications in cartilage repair.[57]

Normal Function of the Adult Articular Chondrocyte

The mature articular chondrocyte embedded in its ECM is a resting cell with no detectable mitotic activity and a low rate of synthetic activity, exemplified by long half-lives of the major ECM components. For example, the half-life of the aggrecan core protein is close to 25 years[58] whereas the half-life of type II collagen has been calculated to be 100 years.[59] Because articular cartilage is avascular, the chondrocyte must rely on diffusion from the articular surface or subchondral bone for exchange of nutrients and metabolites.[60] Chondrocytes maintain active membrane transport systems for exchange of cations, including Na^+, K^+, Ca^{2+}, and H^+, whose intra-cellular concentrations fluctuate with load and changes in the composition of the cartilage matrix.[61] The chondrocyte cytoskeleton is composed of actin, tubulin, and vimentin filaments, and the composition of these filament systems varies in the different cartilage zones.

Chondrocyte metabolism operates at low oxygen tension within the cartilage matrix, ranging from 10% at the surface to less than 1% in the deep zone. The consumption of oxygen by cartilage on a per-cell basis is only 2% to 5% of that in liver or kidney, although the amounts of lactate produced are comparable. Classical studies of oxygen consumption and glucose/lactate metabolism in cartilage suggest a shift in the major energy generating pathways as the oxygen environment is altered.[62,63]

Compared with highly metabolic cells such as neurons and cardiomyocytes, chondrocytes do not normally contain abundant mitochondria. Thus, energy metabolism depends strongly on glucose supply, and energy requirements may be modulated by mechanical stress. Glucose serves as the major energy source for chondrocytes and as an essential precursor for GAG synthesis. Facilitated glucose transport in chondrocytes is mediated by several distinct glucose transporter proteins (GLUTs) that may be constitutively expressed or induced by cytokines.[64] Chondrocytes express GLUT1, GLUT3, and several other glucose transporters.[64] GLUT1 is an abundant constitutively expressed GLUT that can be induced by hypoxia and pro-inflammatory cytokines. GLUT3 is responsive to hypoxia, growth factors, and cytokines. ATP-sensitive potassium [K(ATP)] channels can sense intra-cellular ATP/ADP (adenosine diphosphate) levels, being essential components of a glucose-sensing apparatus that couples glucose metabolism to ATP availability in chondrocytes. K(ATP) channels sense intra-cellular ATP and regulate the abundance of GLUT1 and GLUT3 according to functional demand.[65] Proteomic studies of chondrocytes have identified these and other intra-cellular proteins known to be involved in cell organization, energy protein fate, metabolism, and cell stress.[66] The relative expression of these proteins may determine the capacity of chondrocytes to survive in cartilage matrix and to modulate metabolic activity in response to environmental changes.

When cultured in a range of oxygen tensions between severe hypoxia (0.1% oxygen) and normoxia (21% oxygen), chondrocytes adapt to low oxygen tension by upregulating HIF-1α. Hypoxia via HIF-1α can stimulate chondrocytes to express GLUTs, angiogenic factors such as VEGF, and numerous genes associated with cartilage anabolism and chondrocyte differentiation.[67] In the growth plate, hypoxia and HIF-1α are associated with type II collagen production. HIF-1α is expressed in normal and OA articular cartilage, where it maintains tonic activity during physiologic hypoxia in the deeper layers associated with increased proteoglycan synthesis. In contrast to other tissues, however, HIF-1α is not completely degraded in cartilage when normoxic conditions are applied. Long-term systemic hypoxia (13%) may downregulate collagen and aggrecan gene expression in articular cartilage, whereas hyperoxia (55% oxygen) may increase the breakdown of cartilage collagens in articular cartilage in the presence of vascularized rheumatoid synovium. By modulating the intra-cellular expression of survival factors such as HIF-1α, chondrocytes have a high capacity to survive in the avascular cartilage matrix and to respond to environmental changes.[67]

The chondrocyte maintains a steady-state metabolism secondary to equilibrium between anabolic and catabolic processes, resulting in the normal turnover of matrix molecules. As mentioned earlier, normal adult articular cartilage exhibits low turnover of type II collagen and aggrecan core protein, whereas the GAGs on aggrecan are more readily replaced. Other cartilage ECM components, including biglycan, decorin, COMP, tenascins, and matrilins, incorporated previously into the matrix during development also may be synthesized by chondrocytes under low-turnover conditions. Regional differences in the remodeling activities of chondrocytes have been noted, however, and matrix turnover may be more rapid in the immediate pericellular zones. The metabolic potential of these cells is indicated by their capacity to proliferate in culture and to synthesize matrix proteins after enzymatic release from the cartilage of even elderly individuals. The complex composition of the articular cartilage matrix is more difficult for the chondrocyte to replicate if severe damage to the collagen network occurs.

Interactions of Chondrocytes With the Extracellular Matrix

Chondrocytes in vivo respond to structural changes in the cartilage ECM. The ECM not only provides a framework for chondrocytes suspended within it, but its constituents interact with cell surface receptors to provide signals that regulate many chondrocyte functions (Fig. 3.4).[8]

Integrins

The most prominent of the ECM receptors are the integrins, which are heterodimeric transmembrane receptors consisting of α and β subunits that link or "integrate" the ECM with the cytoskeleton. Integrins bind specifically to different cartilage matrix components and induce the formation of intra-cellular signaling complexes that regulate cell proliferation, differentiation, survival, and matrix remodeling. Integrins also may serve as mechanoreceptors that mediate responses to normal and abnormal loading of cartilage.[68] Chondrocytes express many different integrins that interact with cartilage ECM ligands, although most are not specific to this cell type. They include integrins that are receptors for collagen (α1β1, α2β1, α3β1, α10β1), fibronectin (α5β1, αvβ3, αvβ5), and laminin (α6β1). The integrin α1β1 has broader ligand specificity than the other collagen-binding integrins and mediates chondrocyte adhesion to pericellular type VI collagen and to the cartilage matrix protein, matrilin-1. The α2β1 integrin also binds to chondroadherin. The αv-containing integrins bind to vitronectin and osteopontin, in addition to serving as alternative fibronectin receptors. The α5β1 and αvβ3 integrins serve as receptors for different conformations of COMP.

Because α1β1, α2β1, and α10β1 are receptors for cartilage-specific type II collagen, there is great interest in determining whether they mediate differential responses of chondrocytes to changes in the ECM resulting from normal loading or pathologic changes. The α5β1 integrin is the prominent integrin in human adult articular cartilage. Depending on the method of analysis, adult chondrocytes also express α1β1 and αvβ5 integrins accompanied by weaker expression of α3β1 and αvβ3. Normal adult articular chondrocytes express little or no α2β1, whereas expression of α2β1 and α3β1 integrins is associated with a proliferative phenotype, as in fetal chondrocytes and in chondrosarcoma and chondrocyte cell lines. In growth plate chondrocytes, α5β1, αvβ5, and α10β1 are important for joint formation, chondrocyte proliferation, hypertrophy, and survival. Knockout of the β1 integrin subunit results in severe growth plate abnormalities and chondrodysplasias, whereas α1 integrin knockout mice develop spontaneous OA without growth plate abnormalities. In contrast, knockout of the α5 integrin subunit during joint development did not alter the synovial joints, but protected mice from surgically induced OA.[69] Importantly, α10β1 is the critical collagen receptor in skeletal development.[70]

Cellular binding to immobilized ECM proteins or integrin receptor aggregation with activating antibodies can promote numerous intra-cellular signaling events.[68] As in other cell types, integrin signaling is mediated by interaction with intra-cellular protein tyrosine kinases, such as pp125 focal adhesion kinase (FAK) and proline-rich tyrosine kinase 2 (Pyk2), which interact with the integrin cytoplasmic tail and induce a conformational change in the receptor subunits. Changes in organization of the cytoskeleton are associated with the formation of integrin-signaling complexes, which contain scaffolding proteins such as talin, paxillin, and α-actinin, in addition to FAK, Pyk2, and the integrin-linked kinase (ILK). Mice lacking ILK in cartilage display chondrodysplasia, a phenotype similar to that of cartilage-specific β1 integrin knockout mice. Developing chondrocytes express and secrete the protein integrin-β-like 1 (ITGBL1), which regulates integrin signaling to promote cartilage formation.[71] Decreased ITBGL1 is observed in arthritic cartilage, and its ectopic expression reduces the severity of surgically induced OA in mice.

Cooperative signaling among integrins and growth factors is a fundamental mechanism in the regulation of cellular functions.[68] Integrin aggregation and receptor occupancy enhance phosphorylation of growth factor receptors and activation of mitogen-activated protein kinases (MAPKs), notably extra-cellular signal-regulated kinase (ERK)-1 or ERK-2.[72] Integrins mediate the effects of mechanical forces through activation of cell signaling, a process termed *mechanotransduction*.[73]

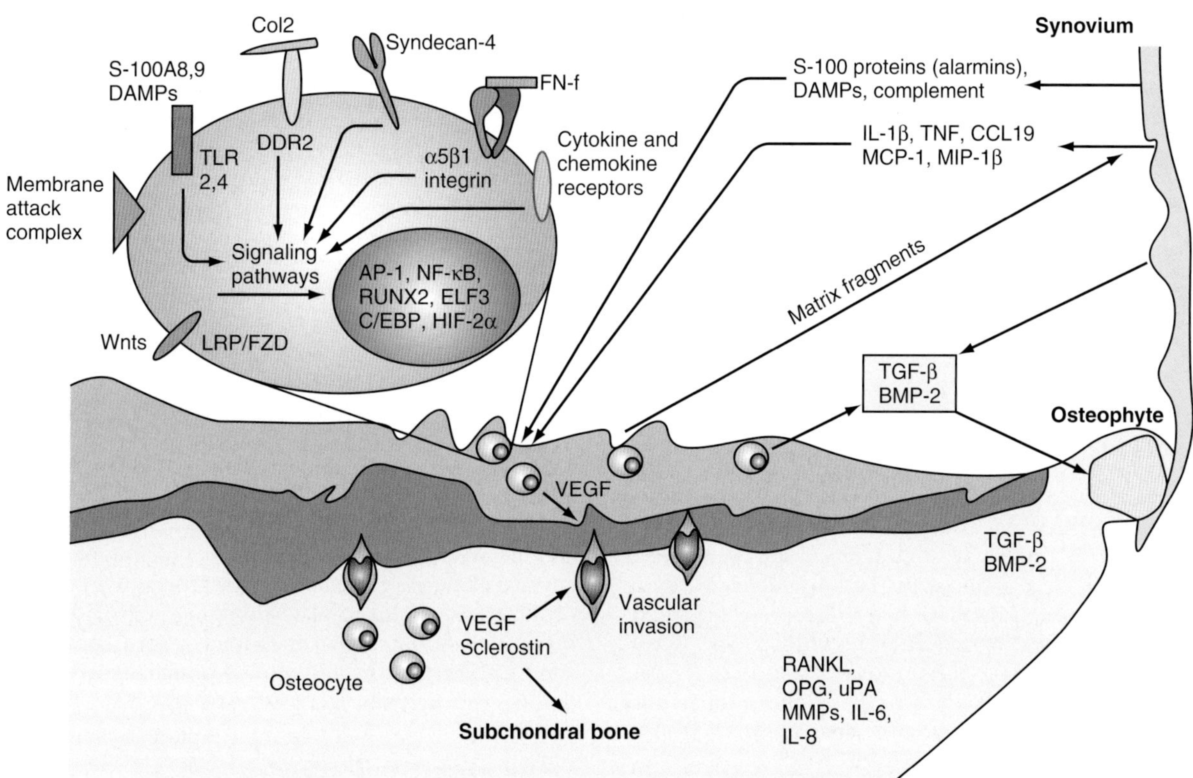

• **Fig. 3.4** Selected factors involved in the osteoarthritic process in the synovium, cartilage, and bone. Proteins including S100 proteins (alarmins) and damage-associated molecular pattern molecules (DAMPs), cytokines (interleukin (IL)-1β, tumor necrosis factor (TNF), IL-15, chemokines (C-C motif ligand 19 [CCL19]), monocyte chemotactic protein-1 (MCP-1), monocyte inflammatory protein (MIP-1β), and complement components released from the synovium can stimulate articular chondrocytes through activation of various cell surface receptors including Toll-like receptors (TLRs), cytokine and chemokine receptors, or by formation of the complement membrane attack complex. Other factors that activate cartilage matrix destruction include binding of native type II collagen to discoidin domain receptor 2 (DDR2), fibronectin fragments (FN-f) to the α5β1 integrin, Wnt proteins to LRP/frizzled (FZD) complexes, and extra-cellular ligands to the heparin sulfate proteoglycan syndecan-4. Syndecan-4 may also act by targeting a disintegrin and metalloproteinase with thrombospondin motifs-5 (ADAMTS-5) to the cell surface. Various signaling pathways lead to activation of a set of transcription factors that translocate to the nucleus and regulate expression of matrix degrading enzymes and inflammatory mediators. Matrix fragments released from the cartilage can stimulate further synovitis. Production of vascular endothelial growth factor (VEGF) in cartilage and bone stimulates vascular invasion from subchondral bone into the zone of calcified cartilage. VEGF, sclerostin, receptor activator of nuclear factor κ-B ligand (RANKL), osteoprotegerin (OPG), urokinase-type plasminogen activator (uPA), matrix metalloproteinase (MMP)s, IL-6, and IL-8 mediate bone remodeling and potentially diffuse to the cartilage to also promote cartilage matrix destruction. Transforming growth factor-β (TGF-β) and bone morphogenetic protein-2 (BMP-2) produced in the synovium, cartilage, and bone stimulate osteophyte formation. (Adapted from Loeser RF, Goldring SR, Scanzello CR, Goldring MB: Osteoarthritis: a disease of the joint as an organ. *Arthritis Rheum* 64:1697–1707, 2012.)

Normal chondrocytes use α5β1 as a mechanoreceptor. As the primary fibronectin receptor, α5β1 plays a role in cartilage degradation by binding to fibronectin fragments that upregulate matrix metalloproteinases (MMPs) such as MMP-3 and MMP-13. Chondrocyte binding to fibronectin fragments also increases the production of cytokines, chemokines, and other catabolic or inflammatory mediators through a mechanism requiring reactive oxygen species (ROS).[68]

Other Cell Surface Receptors on Chondrocytes

Other integral membrane proteins found in chondrocytes include cell determinant 44 (CD44), annexins, syndecans, and discoidin domain receptor 2 (DDR2). CD44 is a receptor for hyaluronan that in turn binds multiple aggrecan proteoglycan monomers to form a gel-like PCM. Through specific interactions with hyaluronan, CD44 has a role in assembly, organization, and maintenance of the chondrocyte PCM. CD44 expression is upregulated in chondrocytes in articular cartilage from RA patients and in experimental OA. Chondroprotective agents and anabolic factors may ameliorate cartilage matrix destruction by reducing CD44 fragmentation that disrupts hyaluronan-CD44 interactions and has adverse effects on the PCM.[74,75]

Annexin V, also known as *annexin CII,* is a 34 kDa integral membrane protein that binds type II collagen and shares extensive homology with the calcium-binding proteins calpactin and lipocortin. Annexins II, V, and VI have been detected in chondrocytes, where they likely play roles in physiologic mineralization of skeletal tissues and in pathologic mineralization of articular cartilage. Annexin V was first detected in chick cartilage and described as a type II collagen–binding protein that anchors chondrocytes to the ECM. In growth plate chondrocytes, annexins are required for calcium ion uptake and subsequent mineralization.[76] Annexin A6 is highly expressed in OA cartilage and plays a role in catabolic signaling.[77]

Syndecans have important roles during cartilage development and homeostasis. Syndecans link to the cell surface via glycosyl phosphatidylinositol and bind growth factors, proteinases and their inhibitors, and matrix molecules through heparan sulfate side chains on the extra-cellular domain.[78] Syndecan-1, syndecan-3, and syndecan-4 are upregulated in OA cartilage. Syndecan-4 is a positive effector of aggrecanase activity through controlling the synthesis of the stromelysin, MMP-3.

In contrast to integrins, which bind collagen fragments, DDR2 binds specifically to type II and X collagen fibrils, leading to activation of its integral receptor tyrosine kinase. DDR2 is upregulated in OA cartilage and induces specifically the expression of MMP-13 associated with cleavage of type II collagen. The serine proteinase, high temperature requirement A1 (HTRA1), which is induced by TGF-β and increased in OA articular cartilage, is responsible for disrupting the PCM, thereby exposing DDR2 to activation by fibrillar type II collagen.[79–84] Contributing to this process is connective tissue growth factor (CTGF), a latent TGF-β binding protein that controls the matrix sequestration and activation of TGF-β in mechanically injured cartilage.[80]

Angiogenic and Antiangiogenic Factors

Adult articular cartilage is among the few avascular tissues in mammalian organisms; its matrix composition and the presence of angiogenesis inhibitors make it resistant to vascular angiogenesis and invasion by inflammatory and neoplastic cells. Troponin I, MMP inhibitors, chondromodulin-I, and endostatin, a 20 kDa proteolytic fragment of type XVIII collagen, all function as endogenous angiogenic inhibitors in cartilage. In conditions in which extensive remodeling of ECM occurs, as in arthritis, the cartilage becomes susceptible to invasion by vascular endothelial and mesenchymal cells from the synovium and subchondral bone.[81] VEGF, which is an essential mediator of angiogenesis during endochondral ossification (see Chapter 1), is induced by inflammatory cytokines, hypoxia, and mechanical overload.[67,72] In OA, in which abnormal biomechanics and joint effusions cause severe hypoxia, chondrocytes produce VEGF, inducing angiogenesis at the chondro-osseous junction and contributing to expansion of the calcified cartilage, tidemark duplication, and cartilage thinning.[82] TGF-β-mediated angiogenesis in the subchondral bone may be among the earliest events driving OA,[83] where microcracks produced by mechanical stress and exacerbation of naturally occurring pores provide conduits for vascular invasion into the calcified cartilage and diffusion of small molecules.[15] In RA, ingrowth of blood vessels and synovial pannus into cartilage contributes to degradation of the cartilage matrix.

Gene expression profiling analyses comparing inflamed and noninflamed areas of synovium from the same OA patients identified STC1, encoding stanniocalcin-1, a molecule that plays roles in angiogenic sprouting via the VEGF/VEGF receptor 2 pathway, as the most highly upregulated gene in inflamed synovial membrane.[84] Articular cartilage is aneural, and the sensory nerve fibers observed in the vascular channels associated with osteochondral angiogenesis may constitute a potential source of symptomatic pain.[85] The clinical importance of these observations is supported by the report that VEGF blockade with bevacizumab inhibits post-traumatic OA in a rabbit model with pain relief associated with prevention of both synovitis and angiogenesis.[86]

Roles of Growth and Differentiation (Anabolic) Factors in Normal Cartilage Metabolism

Growth and differentiation factors generally are considered positive regulators of homeostasis in mature articular cartilage because of their capacity to stimulate chondrocyte anabolic activity and, in some cases, inhibit catabolic activity.[9,87] The best-characterized anabolic factors in the context of their production and action in articular cartilage include insulin-like growth factor I (IGF-I) and members of the FGF and TGF-β/BMP families. The PTHrP, Ihh, and the Wnt/β-catenin pathways have been implicated in maintenance of cartilage homeostasis or OA disease processes. Many of these factors also regulate chondrogenesis and endochondral ossification during skeletal development (see Chapter 1).[44,49,52] In adult cartilage, the expression and/or activity of growth factors declines with age, which is a risk factor for OA.[9]

Insulin-like Growth Factor

IGF-I was first described as *somatomedin C,* a serum factor controlling sulfate incorporation by articular cartilage in vitro, and it was later found to have the specific capacity to stimulate or maintain chondrocyte phenotype in vitro by promoting the synthesis of type II collagen and aggrecan. IGF-I is a competence factor for cell proliferation that is categorized more appropriately as a differentiation factor because its limited mitogenic activity seems to depend on the presence of other growth factors, such as FGF-2, a progression factor. IGF-I is considered an essential mediator of cartilage homeostasis through its capacity to stimulate proteoglycan synthesis, promote chondrocyte survival, and oppose the activities of catabolic cytokines in cooperation with other anabolic factors such as BMP-7. IGF-I and insulin can activate cell signaling via the IGF-I tyrosine kinase receptor or the type I insulin receptor at concentrations proportional to their binding affinities.[9] A study in rats showed that delivery of IGF-I to chondrocytes using unique nanocarriers reduces the severity of surgically induced OA.[88]

Specific IGF-binding proteins (IGFBPs) that do not recognize insulin also regulate IGF-I activity. Chondrocytes at different stages of differentiation express IGF-I and IGF receptors and different arrays of IGFBPs, providing a unique system by which IGF-I can exert different regulatory effects on these cells. IGFBP-2 and IGFBP-5 are positive regulators that increase proteoglycan synthesis in chondrocytes, whereas binding of IGFBP-3 to IGF-I negatively regulates the anabolic functions of IGF-I. IGFBP-3 may also directly inhibit chondrocyte proliferation in an IGF-independent manner.

In OA cartilage, the normal anabolic function of IGF-I may be disrupted because chondrocytes from animals with experimental arthritis and from patients with OA are hyporesponsive to IGF-I, despite normal or increased IGF-I receptor levels. This hyporesponsiveness has been attributed to excessive levels of reactive oxygen species seen in aged and OA cartilage, which alter the cell signaling response patterns to IGF-1.[89]

Fibroblast Growth Factor

Members of the FGF family, including FGF-2, FGF-4, FGF-8, FGF-9, FGF-10, and FGF-18, together with the FGF receptors, FGFR1, FGFR2, FGFR3, and FGFR4, coordinate patterning and cell proliferation during chondrogenesis and endochondral ossification in embryonic and postnatal growth plates.[49] The most extensively studied is FGF-2, or basic FGF, which is a potent mitogen for adult articular chondrocytes, but findings on its effects on the synthesis of cartilage matrix are contradictory, showing stimulation, inhibition, or no effect on proteoglycan synthesis.

The FGFs are generally considered homeostatic factors in joint tissues.[90,91] FGF-2 stored in the adult cartilage matrix is released with mechanical injury or with loading, suggesting a mechanism for modulating chondrocyte proliferation and anabolic activity. Different FGF receptors in cartilage may mediate opposing effects: FGF-2 promotes cartilage protection via FGFR3 and cartilage destruction via FGFR1.[92] Of the four receptors, FGFR1 and 3 are the most abundant, and the ratio of FGFR3 to FGFR1 is reduced in OA cartilage. Furthermore, cartilage-specific deletion of the *FGFR1* gene attenuates articular cartilage degeneration in mice.[93]

In cartilage development, FGF-18 negatively regulates chondrocyte proliferation and terminal differentiation in the growth plate via FGFR3. In articular cartilage, FGF-18 has a role in the maintenance of homeostasis via FGFR3 and protects against loading-induced damage in cartilage explants ex vivo.[94] In vivo, intra-articular administration of FGF-18 protects against cartilage damage in a rat model of injury-induced arthritis.[95] Thus, there is considerable interest in the potential of anabolic factors such as FGF-18 for enhancing cartilage regeneration with tissue engineering approaches.[96] A proof-of-concept trial with human recombinant FGF-18, sprifermin, showed statistically significant, dose-dependent improvement in prespecified secondary structural end points by magnetic resonance imaging (MRI), radiographic joint space narrowing, and Western Ontario and McMaster Universities Arthritis Index (WOMAC) pain scores.[97] Recent findings in pre-clinical models using sprifermin suggest clinical efficacy.[98]

Transforming Growth Factor-β/Bone Morphogenetic Protein Superfamily

Activities of the TGF-β/BMP superfamily in the skeleton were first discovered by Marshall Urist as constituents of demineralized bone that induced new bone formation when implanted into extraskeletal sites in rodents. These bioactive morphogens subsequently were extracted, purified, and cloned and were found to regulate the early commitment of mesenchymal cells to chondrogenic and osteogenic lineages during cartilage development and endochondral bone formation (Table 3.2). The TGF-β/BMP superfamily includes activins, inhibins, müllerian duct inhibitory substance, nodal, glial-derived neurotrophic factor, OP-1 (or BMP-7), and growth differentiation factors (GDFs), also called *cartilage-derived morphogenetic proteins* (CDMPs). In addition to regulating cartilage condensation and chondrocyte differentiation, members of this superfamily play key roles in site specification and cavitation of synovial joints (see Chapter 1) and in the development of other organ systems. Many of these factors, including BMP-2, BMP-6, BMP-7, BMP-9, TGF-β, and CDMP-1, can induce chondrogenic differentiation of mesenchymal progenitor cells in vitro. They also may have direct effects on mature articular chondrocytes in vivo and in vitro and are important for cartilage maintenance.[50]

TABLE 3.2 Bone Morphogenetic Protein Superfamily

Bone Morphogenetic Protein	Other Names	Potential Function
BMP-2	BMP-2A	Cartilage and bone morphogenesis
BMP-3	Osteogenin, GDF-10	Bone formation
BMP-4	BMP-2B	Cartilage and bone morphogenesis
BMP-5		Bone morphogenesis
BMP-6	Vegetal-related-1 (Vgr-1)	Cartilage hypertrophy
BMP-7	Osteogenic protein-1 (OP-1)	Cartilage and bone morphogenesis
BMP-8	Osteogenic protein-2 (OP-2)	Bone morphogenesis
BMP-9	GDF-2	Cartilage morphogenesis
BMP-10		Unknown
BMP-11	GDF-11	Unknown
BMP-12	GDF-7, CDMP-3	Cartilage morphogenesis
BMP-13	GDF-6, CDMP-2	Cartilage morphogenesis
BMP-14	GDF-5, CDMP-1	Cartilage morphogenesis

CDMP, Cartilage-derived morphogenetic protein; *GDF,* growth and differentiation factor.

Transforming Growth Factor-β

TGF-β was named on the basis of its discovery as a factor that could transform cells to grow in soft agar. TGF-β is not a potent inducer of chondrocyte proliferation; rather, it controls early mesenchymal cell condensation, as well as chondrocyte differentiation at early and late stages of chondrogenesis and endochondral ossification (see Chapter 1). Both inhibition and stimulation of the synthesis of aggrecan and type II collagen by TGF-β have been observed in vitro. Levels of TGF-β measured in synovial fluids of OA and RA patients may reflect anabolic processes in cartilage and other joint tissues. TGF-β may promote anabolism by inducing the expression of tissue inhibitors of MMP (TIMP).

TGF-β1, TGF-β2, and TGF-β3 generally are considered as potent stimulators of proteoglycan and type II collagen synthesis in primary chondrocytes and cartilage explants in vitro. However, TGF-β signaling can play both protective and deleterious roles in OA.[99] Although intra-articular injection of TGF-β stimulates proteoglycan synthesis and limits cartilage damage in inflammatory arthritis models, injection or adenovirus-mediated delivery of TGF-β1 may result in side effects in joint tissues, such as osteophyte formation, swelling, and synovial hyperplasia. Administration of agents that block TGF-β activity, such as the soluble form of TGF-βRII, inhibitory SMADs, or the physiologic antagonist, latency-associated peptide-1, increases proteoglycan loss and cartilage damage in experimental models of OA unless targeted specifically to bone.[83]

Aberrant TGF-β signaling in bone may be a key pathway in OA.[100] In the anterior cruciate ligament (ACL) transection model of OA, high doses of a TGF-β inhibitor administered systemically promote cartilage proteoglycan loss, whereas lower doses prevent the migration and/or localization of MSCs, osteoprogenitors, and osteoblasts in the subchondral bone of operated limbs and attenuate neovascularization and cartilage loss.[83] Transgenic expression of active TGF-β in osteoblasts induces the formation of nestin-positive MSCs in clusters, whereas knockout of *Tgfbr2* in nestin-positive MSCs prevents MSC migration to the subchondral bone and normalizes bone parameters, cartilage homeostasis, and limb function. Furthermore, implantation of a TGF-β-specific antibody in the subchondral bone attenuates the OA changes in both the cartilage and bone, suggesting that bone-targeted therapies may be useful in some forms of the disease.[83]

Bone Morphogenetic Proteins

BMPs constitute a large subclass of the TGF-β superfamily essential for normal appendicular skeletal and joint development.[101] The isolation and cloning of the first BMP family members from bone prompted a search for CDMPs—CDMP-1, CDMP-2, and CDMP-3—which are classified as GDF-5, GDF-6, and GDF-7. The BMPs may be divided into four distinct subfamilies based on the similarity of primary amino acid sequences: (1) BMP-2 and BMP-2B (BMP-4), which are 92% identical in the 7-cysteine region; (2) BMP-3 (osteogenin) and BMP-3B (GDF-10); (3) BMP-5, BMP-6, BMP-7 (OP-1), BMP-8 (OP-2), BMP-9 (GDF-2), BMP-10, and BMP-11 (GDF-11); and (4) BMP-12 (GDF-7 or CDMP-3), BMP-13 (GDF-6 or CDMP-2), BMP-14 (GDF-5 or CDMP-1), and BMP-15. BMP-1 is not a member of this family but is an astacin-related MMP that cleaves the BMP inhibitor chordin and acts as a procollagen C-proteinase.

Several BMPs, including BMP-2, BMP-7 (OP-1), and GDF-5/CDMP-1, can stimulate differentiation of mesenchymal precursors into chondrocytes and promote the differentiation of hypertrophic chondrocytes. BMP-2, BMP-4, BMP-6, BMP-7, BMP-9, and BMP-13 can enhance the synthesis of type II collagen and aggrecan by articular chondrocytes in vitro.[102] BMP-2 also is expressed in normal and OA articular cartilage, and it is a molecular marker, along with type II collagen and FGFR3, for the capacity of adult articular chondrocyte cultures to form stable cartilage in vivo. It is required for normal joint development, and loss of BMP-2 in mice results in spontaneous OA.[103] BMP-7 is expressed in mature articular cartilage and is possibly the strongest anabolic stimulus for adult chondrocytes in vitro because it increases aggrecan and type II collagen synthesis more strongly than IGF-I. In addition, BMP-7 reverses many of the catabolic responses induced by IL-1β, including induction of MMP-1 and MMP-13, downregulation of TIMP, and downregulation of proteoglycan synthesis in primary human articular chondrocytes. CDMP-2 is found in articular cartilage, skeletal muscle, placenta, and hypertrophic chondrocytes of the epiphyseal growth plate. CDMP-1 and CDMP-2 maintain the synthesis of type II collagen and aggrecan in mature articular chondrocytes, although they are less effective initiators of chondrogenesis than other BMPs in early progenitor cell populations in vitro.

BMPs have pleiotropic effects in vivo, however, acting in a concentration-dependent manner. While initiating chondrogenesis in the limb bud, they generally set the stage for bone morphogenesis (see Chapter 1). Several BMPs are true morphogens for other tissues, such as kidney, eye, heart, and skin.

Receptors, Signaling Molecules, and Antagonists That Mediate Chondrocyte Responses to Growth and Differentiation Factors

Major pathways activated by the growth and differentiation factors discussed earlier involve members of the ERK1/2, p38 MAPK, and phosphatidylinositol-3′-kinase (PI-3K)/v-akt murine thymoma viral oncogene homolog (AKT) pathways.[104] As in other cell types, FGF family members activate kinases of the ERK1/2 and p38 MAPK cascades in chondrocytes. Specific inhibitors of these pathways block FGF-2–induced and FGF-18–induced mitogenesis in chondrocytes and prevent FGF-2 induction of Sox9 in primary chondrocytes. The PI-3K pathway is required for the stimulation of proteoglycan synthesis by IGF-I in primary human articular chondrocytes, whereas the ERK1/2 pathway acts as a negative regulator.[9]

TGF-β and BMP family members transduce signals through the formation of heteromeric complexes of ligand-specific receptors, which have serine-threonine kinase activity. The specificity of subsequent signals is determined mainly by the type I receptors. Type I and type II receptors are required for signal transduction. Seven types of type I receptors, called *activin receptor–like kinases* (ALKs), have been identified in mammals and have similar structures. TGF-β interacts with TGFβRII, which recruits a TGF-β type I receptor (principally TGFβRI) to form a heterotrimeric receptor complex. The constitutively active TGFβRII kinase phosphorylates TGFβRI at serine and threonine residues. Three type I receptors, BMP type IA (BMPR-IA or ALK-3), BMPR-IB (ALK-6), and ALK-2, mediate BMP signaling. Although BMPR-1 receptors are able to bind ligand in the absence of type II BMP receptors, cooperativity has been shown in binding assays. On ligand binding, analogous to TGFβRI and TGFβRII, BMP type I receptors are phosphorylated by the BMP type II receptors, which include activin (Act) RII, ActRIIB, and T-ALK. Spatial and temporal differences in the distribution of these receptors in different tissues can govern the response patterns to different members of the TGF-β/BMP family.

The canonical SMAD pathway mediates TGF-β and BMP signaling through phosphorylation of receptor-activated SMADs (R-SMADs), which are related to the *Drosophila* mothers against decapentaplegic (MAD) and nematode SMADs signaling molecules. TGFβRI receptors (ALK 4, 5, and 7) phosphorylate Smad2 and 3 transcription factors. BMPs act primarily through ALK1, 2, 3, and 6 to activate Smad1, 5, and 8 and generally promote chondrocyte hypertrophic differentiation. The R-SMADs form complexes with the common Smad4 and translocate to the nucleus, where they bind to SMAD-specific DNA binding sites in the promoters of target genes.

The major route of TGF-β signaling in healthy articular cartilage is through canonical ALK5, which activates Smad2/3 to inhibit chondrocyte hypertrophy, but when TGF-β interacts with ALK1, it signals through Smad1/5/8 and induces MMP-13 and other degradative enzymes[99] and nerve growth factor (NGF).[105] Because the ALK1/ALK5 ratio is increased during aging,[99] this may account for the aberrant chondrocyte responses associated with the development of OA and off-target effects of TGF-β injections in joints that result in osteophyte formation and synovial fibrosis.

Further regulation is provided by inhibitory Smads, including Smad6 and Smurf1 and 2, which primarily inhibit Smad1/5/8 signaling by accelerating the proteosomal breakdown of phosphorylated Smads. The aberrant hypertrophic differentiation in Smad3-deficient mice can be rescued by restoring TGFβ-activated kinase 1 (TAK1) and activating transcription factor-2 (ATF2) signaling,[106] but inhibition of TAK1 or Janus kinase (JAK) can rescue impaired differentiation of MSCs in OA.[107]

BMP antagonists play important roles in spatial and temporal regulation of BMP activities during skeletal development. Originally discovered in *Xenopus,* they act as antagonists by determining the bioavailability of BMPs for binding to BMP receptors.[108] The roles of noggin and chordin seem to be crucial for determining boundaries during joint morphogenesis. They display different spatial and temporal patterns of expression, binding affinities, and susceptibility to proteinases that release BMP. BMPs bind to chordin and noggin via cysteine-rich domains that are similar to domains in the N-terminal propeptides of fibrillar procollagens I, II, III, and V, which also bind BMPs and are susceptible to cleavage by MMPs. BMP may be released from chordin by cleavage with MMPs or BMP-1/tolloid, whereas noggin binds BMP with high affinity and cannot be cleaved to release BMP.

Follistatin, gremlin, chordin, and chordin-like 2 are upregulated in OA cartilage. Follistatin, which has been linked to inflammatory processes; gremlin, which is associated with hypertrophic phenotype; and chordin appear at different stages of OA and with different topographic distribution. Because each antagonist binds preferentially to different BMPs, the differential expression may serve as a feedback mechanism to balance anabolic activities at different stages.

The Wnt/β-catenin pathway plays a role in both cartilage and bone development and pathology.[109] The cellular responses are governed by the availability of Wnt ligands in different tissues and their use of distinct, canonical versus noncanonical, pathways over the course of differentiation and during pathology.[109] The Wnt antagonists, including sclerostin (SOST), originally described as osteocyte-specific, dickkopf-related protein-1 (DKK-1), and secreted frizzled-related protein 1 (sFRP1), have been explored as regulators and biomarkers of articular cartilage homeostasis, because they may decrease hypertrophic conversion and expression of proteinases in vitro and, in some cases, in vivo.[110–113] Inhibition of Wnt signaling with small molecule inhibitors has emerged as a promising approach for disease modification in OA.[114,115]

Epigenetic Regulation of Cartilage Homeostasis

A host of epigenetic factors regulate chondrocyte gene expression and cartilage homeostasis including histone modifications such as acetylation and methylation, DNA methylation, and noncoding RNAs including microRNAs. Histone modification alters chromatin structure to regulate the accessibility of transcription factors and their associated proteins to specific locations in DNA and thereby regulate gene transcription. Histone modifications include acetylation, methylation, phosphorylation, ubiquitylation, and sumoylation. Perhaps the best studied in the context of chondrocyte biology is acetylation mediated by histone acetyl transferases and deacetylation mediated by the histone deacetylases. Histone acetylation and deacetylation can regulate both matrix gene expression and expression of matrix degrading enzymes depending on the specific histone site and cellular context.[116]

The sirtuins (Sirt) represent a family of NAD^+-dependent histone deacetylases. Chondrocytes express Sirt1, Sirt2, Sirt3, Sirt6, and Sirt7.[117] Loss of either Sirt1 or Sirt6 in mice results in a skeletal phenotype consistent with roles in cartilage development and homeostasis. Sirt1 is a positive regulator of cartilage matrix gene expression and chondrocyte survival, and the loss of Sirt1 in chondrocytes results in increased MMP-13 expression. Sirt6 is found primarily in the nucleus, where it protects from DNA damage and promotes chromatin stability. Mice haplodeficient in Sirt6 develop early onset OA.

DNA methylation of promoter sites most often inhibits gene transcription (gene silencing) while methylation at other sites can increase or decrease gene transcription. Genome-wide DNA methylation studies have found that thousands of genes in chondrocytes can undergo methylation, and methylation of specific genes can differ between normal cells and cells isolated from osteoarthritic joints.[118] Demethylation of the promoters of catabolic genes such as IL-1, MMP-13, and NF-κB could play a role in cartilage destruction in OA. Likewise, DNA hydroxymethylation of cytosines may also contribute to changes in gene expression seen in OA.[119]

MicroRNAs and long noncoding RNAs are additional epigenetic regulators that have been receiving increased attention. MicroRNAs negatively regulate the transcription of specific target genes. Hundreds of microRNAs have been discovered in normal and OA articular chondrocytes, but their function in cartilage has been determined for only a small number of these.[120,121] MicroRNAs are involved in skeletal development including chondrogenesis and in adult cartilage can promote either anabolic or catabolic activities, depending on the specific microRNA. For example, microRNA-675 upregulates type II collagen, microRNA-27b inhibits MMP-13, and microRNA-101 induces expression of cartilage degrading enzymes including *Adamts5*. Long noncoding RNAs, which are greater than 200 nucleotides in length, are also found in cartilage and can regulate gene transcription and translation, although currently their function is less well understood than the microRNAs.

Role of the Chondrocyte in Cartilage Pathology

The chondrocyte, the unique cell type in mature cartilage, maintains a stable equilibrium between the synthesis and the degradation of matrix components. During aging and joint diseases, such as RA and OA (see Chapters 75 and 104), this equilibrium is disrupted, and the rate of loss of collagens and proteoglycans from the matrix exceeds the rate of deposition of newly synthesized molecules. Cartilage destruction in OA is believed to be chondrocyte mediated in response to biomechanical insult and may occur directly or indirectly through the production of cytokines and cartilage matrix–degrading proteinases in cartilage and other joint tissues.[122] (Fig. 3.5).

During initial stages of OA, chondrocytes in vivo respond to abnormal biomechanical loading of the surrounding cartilage matrix by increasing cell proliferation and synthesis of matrix proteins, proteinases, and anabolic and catabolic factors. The earliest changes include the loss of negatively charged GAGs resulting in increased water content associated with swelling of the cartilage matrix. Macroscopic changes in the cartilage matrix composition are accompanied by the appearance of surface fibrillations or microscopic cracks in the superficial zone. As the disease progresses, fragmentation of the cartilage surface and fissures extending into the deeper cartilage layers lead to exposure of the underlying zones of calcified cartilage and subchondral bone. The aberrant behavior of OA chondrocytes is reflected in the formation of cell clusters and changes in quantity, distribution, or composition of matrix

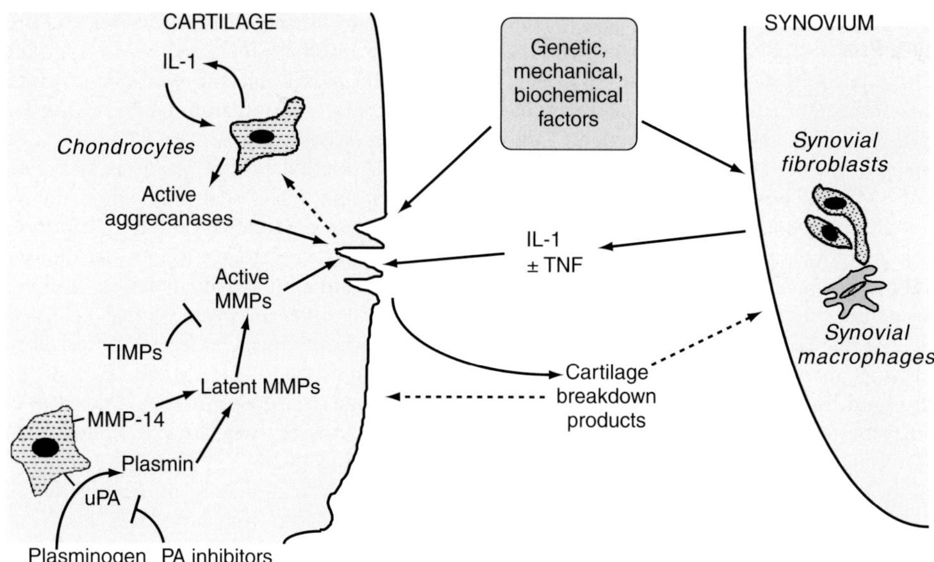

• **Fig. 3.5** The role of chondrocyte-derived proteinases in cartilage destruction in osteoarthritis. Although studies in vitro and in vivo have shown that the chondrocyte can respond directly to mechanical loading, to catabolic cytokines such as interleukin-1 (IL-1), to tumor necrosis factor (TNF), and to cartilage breakdown products, the initiating signals and their relative importance have not been defined clearly. *MMP,* Matrix metalloproteinase; *TIMP,* tissue inhibitor of metalloproteinase; *uPA,* urinary plasminogen activator. (Adapted from Goldring MB: Osteoarthritis and cartilage: the role of cytokines. *Curr Rheumatol Rep* 2:459–465, 2000.)

proteins. Genomic and proteomic analyses of global gene expression in cartilage have revealed increased anabolism reflected in increased levels of *COL2A1* and other cartilage-specific mRNAs in late OA, but also increased gene expression of noncartilage collagens and other matrix proteins. Evidence of phenotypic modulation is reflected in the increased gene expression of collagens I and III and the appearance of the hypertrophic chondrocyte marker, type X collagen, and other markers of terminal differentiation, suggesting recapitulation of a developmental program.[6,87] Prolonged oxidative stress, which occurs during aging and chronic inflammation, and metabolic stress due to diabetes and metabolic syndrome can induce biochemical changes, including glycation, carbonylation, lipoxidation, and nitrosylation, in cartilage structural proteins. These post-translational modifications induce aggregation and/or unfolding of cartilage matrix proteins, increasing their susceptibility to enzymatic cleavage and degradation.[123]

In contrast to OA, cartilage destruction in RA occurs primarily in areas contiguous with the proliferating synovial pannus as a result of the release and activation of proteinases from the synovial cells and, to some extent, at the cartilage surface exposed to matrix-degrading enzymes from polymorphonuclear leukocytes, or neutrophils, in the synovial fluids. In addition to the direct action of proteinases, RA synovial tissues contribute indirectly to cartilage loss by releasing cytokines and other mediators that act on the chondrocytes to produce dysregulation of chondrocyte function. Understanding of basic cellular mechanisms regulating chondrocyte responses to inflammatory cytokines has been inferred from numerous studies in vitro using cultures of cartilage fragments or isolated chondrocytes and is supported by studies in experimental models of inflammatory arthritis, such as collagen-induced arthritis and antigen-induced arthritis in mice.[124–126]

Direct analysis of cartilage or chondrocytes from OA patients undergoing joint replacement has yielded more information than is available from RA patients, where cartilage damage is extensive. These studies indicate that chondrocytes produce not only proinflammatory cytokines, but also inhibitory and anabolic cytokines that modulate responses. The impact of cytokines on chondrocyte function, particularly with respect to their various roles in cartilage destruction, has been reviewed extensively.[5,8,122] However, their role is unproven in OA initiation, where mechanotransduction events associated with activation of integrins, DDR-2, syndecans, and ion channels can be observed in chondrocytes due to abnormal biomechanics. Studies of cartilage degradation in genetically modified mouse strains that are resistant to or accelerate the development of OA spontaneously with aging or when subjected to excessive biomechanical injury have yielded information about the molecular effectors of the disease and potential targets for therapy.[124,127–129]

Cartilage Matrix–Degrading Proteinases

Chondrocytes synthesize and secrete MMPs in latent forms, which are activated outside the cells via activation cascades. An important cascade in cartilage is initiated by plasmin, the product of plasminogen activator activity, which may be produced by the chondrocyte; plasmin activates latent stromelysin (MMP-3), an activator of latent collagenases. In early studies, chondrocytes were among the first identified sources of TIMP-1, and they are now known to synthesize additional TIMPs, including TIMP-3, which is the major inhibitor of aggrecanase activities. TIMPs and MMPs detected in synovial fluids reflect the adaptive response to the local imbalance caused by increased production of active MMPs by chondrocytes and other joint tissues. Collagenases 1, 2, and 3 (MMP-1, MMP-8, and MMP-13); gelatinases (MMP-2 and MMP-9); stromelysin-1 (MMP-3); membrane type 1 MMP (MT1)-MMP (MMP-14); and the aggrecanases, ADAMTS-4 and ADAMTS-5, specifically degrade native collagens and proteoglycans in cartilage matrix (Table 3.3).[130,131]

TABLE 3.3 Chondrocyte Proteinases That Mediate Degradation of Cartilage Matrix

Proteinase Class	Cartilage Matrix Substrates	Activity
Matrix Metalloproteinases		
Collagenases (MMP-1, MMP-8, MMP-13)	Collagens I, II	Fibrillar domain, 3/4 from N-terminus N-telopeptide (MMP-13)
	Aggrecan core protein	Asn^{341}-Phe^{342} IGD
Stromelysins (MMP-3, MMP-10)	Aggrecan core protein Collagens IX, XI Link protein, fibronectin proMMPs, proTNF	Asn^{341}-Phe^{342} IGD Telopeptide region
Gelatinases (MMP-2, MMP-9)	Collagens II, XI Proteoglycans, link protein	Telopeptide or denatured collagen chains
Membrane-type MMPs MT-MMP-1 (MMP-14), MT-MMP-2, MT-MMP-3, MT-MMP-4 (MMP-15, MMP-16, MMP-17)	Collagen II Fibronectin, aggrecan ProMMP-2 ProMMP-13 ProTNF	Telopeptide
Matrilysin (MMP-7)	Link protein	
Enamelysin (MMP-20)	COMP, link protein	
Aggrecanases		
ADAMTS-1, ADAMTS-4, ADAMTS-5	Aggrecan core protein IGD	Glu^{373}-Ala^{374}, Glu^{1545}-Gly^{1546}, Glu^{1714}-Gly^{1715}, Glu^{1819}-Ala^{1820}, Glu^{1919}-Leu^{1920}
Serine		
Plasminogen activators (tPA, uPA)	Aggrecan, fibronectin, proMMPs	Activation of plasminogen gives rise to plasmin
Cathepsin G	Aggrecan, collagen II, proMMPs	
High temperature requirement A1 (HTRA1)	Matrilin 3, fibronectin, biglycan, fibromodulin, COMP, collagen VI	Degrades pericellular matrix
Cysteine		
Cathepsins B, K, L, S	Collagens IX, XI	Telopeptides (optimal pH 4.0-6.5)
	Link protein, aggrecan	
Aspartate		
Cathepsin D	Phagocytosed ECM components	In lysosomes (optimal pH 3.0-6.0)

ADAMTS, A disintegrin and metalloproteinase with thrombospondin-1 domains; *COMP,* cartilage oligomeric matrix protein; *ECM,* extra-cellular matrix; *IGD,* interglobular domain; *MMP,* matrix metalloproteinase; *MT-MMP,* membrane-type MMP; *proMMP,* proenzyme form of MMP; *TNF,* tumor necrosis factor; *tPA,* tissue-type plasminogen activator; *uPA,* urokinase-type plasminogen activator.

MMPs, aggrecanases, and the cleavage fragments generated by them are localized in regions of cartilage degradation and are detected in synovial fluids and cartilage from OA and RA patients.[5,6] Expression of MMP-13 in OA and RA cartilage and its ability to degrade type II collagen more effectively suggest a major role for this enzyme in cartilage degradation. Postnatal overexpression of constitutively active MMP-13 in cartilage in mice produces OA-like changes in knee joints, and knockout of the gene encoding MMP-13 protects cartilage against surgically induced OA.[132] Deficiency of DDR2, a collagen receptor whose activation is associated with upregulation of MMP-13, attenuates development of OA induced by DMM surgery.[133] Deficiencies of the Runx2 and HIF-2α transcription factors that are key regulators of MMP-13 also protect against OA development or progression.[134] Nuclear factor κB (NF-κB) signaling in response to upstream activating kinases can modulate the amplitude of MMP13 gene expression under inflammatory, mechanical, and oxidative stress.[135]

NF-κB is also required for activation of HIF-2α in articular cartilage.[134,136] HIF-2α directly targets hypoxia-responsive DNA elements in the promoter regions of MMP13, COL10A1, VEGFA, and other genes that are involved in chondrocyte dysfunction in OA.[137–139] In contrast, the upregulation of HIF-3α by PRG4 is associated with downregulation of HIF-1α and -2α target genes as part of a mechanism that protects against aging-related or post-traumatic OA development in mouse models.[140]

Although elevated levels of MMPs in RA synovial fluids likely originate from the synovium, intrinsic chondrocyte-derived chondrolytic activity is present at the cartilage-pannus junction and in deeper zones of cartilage matrix in some RA specimens. MMP-1 is expressed at lower levels than MMP-3 and MMP-13 in the RA synovial pannus but is also produced by chondrocytes. MMP-10, similar to MMP-3, activates procollagenases and is produced by the synovium and chondrocytes in response to inflammatory cytokines. MT1-MMP (MMP-14), produced principally by the synovial tissue, is important for synovial invasiveness and may also serve as an activator of other MMPs produced by chondrocytes.[141]

Several of the MMPs, including MMP-3, MMP-8, MMP-14, MMP-19, and MMP-20, are capable of degrading proteoglycans. Members of the reprolysin-related proteinases of the a disintegrin and metalloproteinase (ADAM) family, particularly ADAMTS-4 and ADAMTS-5, are now regarded as the principal mediators of aggrecan degradation.[142,143] The activities of MMPs and aggrecanases are complementary, however. Of the aggrecanases, ADAMTS-5 is associated with increased susceptibility to OA, as shown in *Adamts5*-deficient mice. TIMP-3, but not TIMP-1, TIMP-2, or TIMP-4, is a potent inhibitor of ADAMTS-4 and ADAMTS-5 in vitro, and TIMP-3 deficiency results in mild cartilage degradation similar to that seen in patients with OA.[144]

Cysteine proteinases, cathepsins B, K, S, and L, and the aspartic proteinase, cathepsin D, are lysosomal enzymes that may play a secondary role in cartilage degradation via intra-cellular digestion of products released by other proteinases.[145] Cathepsin B also may have a role in extra-cellular degradation of collagen telopeptides, collagens IX and XI, and aggrecan. Cathepsin K is expressed in synovial fibroblasts on the cartilage surface at the pannus-cartilage junction and is upregulated by inflammatory cytokines. Among the known cathepsins, cathepsin K is the only proteinase that is capable of hydrolyzing type I and type II collagens at multiple sites within the triple-helical regions, and its requirement for acidic pH may be provided by the microenvironment between the synovial pannus and the cartilage.[130]

Other MMPs, including MMP-16 and MMP-28, ADAM family members, including ADAM-17/TACE (TNF converting enzyme), ADAM-9, ADAM-10, and ADAM-12, and ADAMTS family members ADAMTS-2, ADAMTS-3, ADAMTS-7, ADAMTS-12, and ADAMTS-14 are expressed by chondrocytes, but their roles in adult cartilage have yet to be defined.[131,146,147] Identification of the precise roles of these proteinases and their endogenous inhibitors in chondrocyte-mediated cartilage degradation has provided the opportunity to develop targeted therapies that interfere with the activities of aggrecanases or MMPs without disrupting normal physiology.[148,149]

Balance of Cytokines in Cartilage Destruction

The roles of cytokines in cartilage metabolism must be considered in the context of the whole joint.[8] Sources of cytokines in the joint include the synovial macrophages and infiltrating mononuclear cells in the synovium, and the chondrocytes themselves.[122] Of the cytokines that affect cartilage metabolism, most are pleiotropic factors that were identified originally as immunomodulators but were found to regulate cellular functions in cells of mesenchymal origin. IL-1 and TNF not only stimulate chondrocytes to synthesize cartilage matrix–degrading proteinases, they also regulate matrix protein synthesis and cell proliferation. Considerable redundancy and overlap in biologic activities exist among the individual cytokines, and they do not act alone, but rather in synergy or partnership with or in opposition to other cytokines via cytokine networks. In addition to IL-1 and TNF, other catabolic cytokines have been characterized, as have inhibitory or anabolic cytokines produced by the chondrocytes themselves or by other cells in joint tissues (Table 3.4). Investigations in vitro and in vivo have begun to sort out the complexities of the cytokine networks and to determine how the balance in normal homeostasis can be restored when it is disrupted (Fig. 3.6). Studies of type II collagen–induced arthritis and other types of induced arthritis in transgenic animals with overexpressed or deleted genes encoding cytokines, their receptors, or activators have provided further insight into the roles of these factors in cartilage destruction.

TABLE 3.4 Cytokines That Regulate Cartilage Destruction

Catabolic	IL-1 Tumor necrosis factor IL-17 IL-18
Modulatory	IL-6 Leukemia inhibitory factor Oncostatin M IL-11
Inhibitory	IL-4 IL-10 IL-13 IL-1 receptor antagonist

IL, Interleukin.

Interleukin-1 and Tumor Necrosis Factor

Early work first identified IL-1 as a soluble factor, originally termed *catabolin,* in supernatants of normal, noninflamed porcine synovial fragment cultures that stimulated chondrocytes to degrade the surrounding cartilage matrix. Similar activities in culture supernatants from mononuclear cells and rheumatoid synovium were attributed to IL-1, and the catabolin isoforms were identified as IL-1α and IL-1β. Originally known as *cachectin,* TNF produces many effects on chondrocytes in vitro that are similar to those of IL-1β, including stimulation of the production of matrix-degrading proteinases and suppression of cartilage matrix synthesis. Although IL-1β is 100-fold to 1000-fold more potent on a molar basis than TNF, strong synergistic effects occur at low concentrations of the two cytokines together, eliciting more severe cartilage damage than injection of either cytokine alone.

The concept that TNF drives acute inflammation, whereas IL-1β has a pivotal role in sustaining inflammation and cartilage erosion, has been derived from work in animal models of RA using cytokine-specific neutralizing antibodies, soluble receptors, or receptor antagonists, and this has also been shown in transgenic or knockout mouse models. Since those early findings, numerous studies in vitro and in vivo indicate that IL-1 and TNF, originating primarily from the inflamed synovium, are catabolic cytokines involved in the destruction of articular cartilage in RA.[150] IL-1 receptor antagonist (IL-1Ra) is capable of blocking the actions of IL-1 if added at sufficiently high concentrations in vitro and was among the first agents to be developed for anti-cytokine therapy. However, anti-TNF therapy is more effective in RA than systemic IL-1Ra, and intra-articular IL-1Ra in OA joints requires delivery systems that maintain sufficiently high concentrations or stimulate local production.[151]

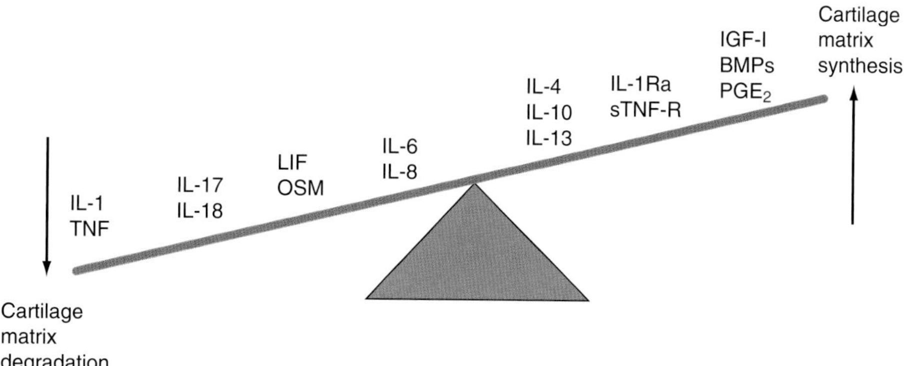

• **Fig. 3.6** The cytokine balance in cartilage metabolism. Soluble mediators toward the left of the balance promote the loss of cartilage matrix. Mediators on the right side prevent the synthesis or actions of catabolic cytokines and prevent loss of cartilage matrix. Anabolic factors, including insulin-like growth factor I (IGF-I) and bone morphogenetic proteins (BMPs), and prostaglandin E_2 (PGE_2) maintain or promote cartilage matrix synthesis. *IL-1,* Interleukin-1; *IL-1Ra,* IL-1 receptor antagonist; *LIF,* lymphocyte-activating factor; *OSM,* oncostatin M; *sTNF-R,* soluble TNF receptor; *TNF,* tumor necrosis factor. (Adapted from Goldring MB: Osteoarthritis and cartilage: the role of cytokines. *Curr Rheumatol Rep* 2:459–465, 2000.)

Major events in OA pathogenesis occur within the cartilage itself, and evidence suggests that chondrocytes participate in this destructive process not only by responding to cytokines released from other joint tissues but also by synthesizing them.[5,6] They may be exposed continuously to the autocrine and paracrine effects of IL-1 and other inflammatory mediators at high local concentrations. However, the role of IL-1 and TNF as key mediators of cartilage destruction in OA is being questioned due to their relatively low abundance in synovial fluid when compared with other cytokines and the failure of IL-1 or TNF inhibition to alter the symptoms or progression of OA.[152–154] The assumption has been that *IL1B* mRNA expressed in chondrocytes of OA cartilage could result in translation to pro-IL-1β and secretion of IL-1β. However, the inflammasome complex, consisting of nucleotide-binding domain, leucine rich repeat, and pyrin domain containing (NLRP)3, the adaptor protein ASC, and the IL-1β activator caspase-1, does not appear to be active in cartilage, thereby preventing secretion and autocrine activity of this cytokine. Furthermore, deficiency of genes encoding NLRP3 or IL-1β does not prevent catabolic responses induced by TNF, lipopolysaccharide (LPS), or mechanical load in cartilage explants from knockout mice.[155] These results suggest that locally produced IL-1β is not available to act in an autocrine or paracrine manner in cartilage, but rather this cytokine could be released from the synovium and other tissues to elicit chondrocyte responses.[155] Nevertheless, the low-grade inflammation associated with OA is subchronic, whereas systemic inflammation is defined as a two- to three-fold elevation of circulating inflammatory mediators, indicating that both cytokines will be much less abundant in OA compared with more inflammatory forms of joint disease.[122]

Cytokine Networks

The cytokine networks that affect chondrocytes must also be considered within the context of the whole joint (see Chapter 31).[5,6,8] IL-1β and TNF, as well as matrix fragments produced by cleavage by MMPs and other matrix-degrading enzymes, can induce chondrocytes to produce other pro-inflammatory cytokines, including IL-6, IL-7, leukemia inhibitory factor (LIF), IL-17, IL-18, IL-33, and chemokines. IL-6 seems to play a dual role by increasing expression of IL-1 receptor antagonist (IL-1Ra), soluble TNF receptor, and TIMPs, while also enhancing immune cell function and inflammation. The activity of IL-6 requires soluble IL-6 receptor to synergize with IL-1 to stimulate gene expression of MMPs and ADAMTS and to downregulate *COL2A1* and *ACAN* in cultured chondrocytes. IL-6 knockout mice are more susceptible to cartilage degeneration during aging, however, suggesting that this cytokine may play a protective role in normal physiology. Chondrocytes also produce macrophage migration inhibitory factor (MIF). MIF is increased in OA chondrocytes and, unlike IL-6, MIF knockout mice are protected from age-related OA but not surgically induced OA.[156]

Other members of the IL-6 family that act via receptors that heterodimerize with gp130 also may serve modulatory roles. IL-11 shares several actions of IL-6, including stimulation of TIMP production, without affecting MMP production by chondrocytes, and it may inhibit cartilage destruction. LIF participates in a positive feedback loop by increasing the production of IL-6 by chondrocytes. Oncostatin M (OSM), a product of macrophages and activated T cells, is a potent stimulator of chondrocyte production of MMPs and aggrecanases in synergism with IL-1β or TNF.

IL-17 and IL-18 are potent catabolic factors that stimulate the production of IL-1β, MMPs, and other pro-inflammatory and catabolic factors in human chondrocytes. IL-17 is produced by activated T helper type 1 (Th1), or $CD4^+$, lymphocytes and binds to a receptor that is not related to any known cytokine receptor family and can act in synergy with other cytokines. IL-17 can drive T cell–dependent erosive arthritis in TNF-deficient and IL-1Ra knockout mice, and treatment of mice with collagen-induced arthritis or antigen-induced arthritis with neutralizing IL-17 antibody effectively inhibits cartilage destruction in those models of RA. IL-18 is produced by macrophages, and its receptor shares homology with IL-1R1. IL-4, IL-10, IL-13, IL-37, and the naturally occurring IL-1Ra are classified as inhibitory cytokines because they decrease the production and activities of catabolic and pro-inflammatory cytokines in chondrocytes in vitro and suppress cartilage destruction in vivo (see Table 3.4). IL-4, IL-10, and IL-37 inhibit cartilage-degrading proteinases and reverse some effects of catabolic cytokines in vitro. IL-4 and IL-10 produce synergistic suppression of cartilage destruction in vivo. The efficacy of IL-4, IL-10, and IL-13 in retarding cartilage damage may be related in part to their stimulatory effects on IL-1Ra production, and their therapeutic application has been proposed as a means of restoring the cytokine balance in RA.

TABLE 3.5 Chemokines and Receptors in Chondrocytes[a]

Functional Name	Systematic Name	Chemokine Receptor
GROα	CXCL1	CXCR1, CXCR2
IL-8	CXCL8	CXCR1, CXCR2
MCP-1	CCL2	CCR2
MIP-1α	CCL3	CCR1, CCR5
MIP-1β	CCL4	CCR5
RANTES	CCL5	CCR1, CCR3, CCR5
SDF-1	CXCL12	CXCR4

[a]Chemokines are classified according to the positions of the first two cysteines (C) of the four conserved N-terminal cysteines: CC chemokine ligand (CCL), first two cysteines are adjacent; CXC chemokine ligand (CXCL), first two cysteines are separated by amino acid X other than cysteine; *CCR*, CC chemokine receptor; *CXCR*, CXC chemokine receptor; *GROα*, growth-related oncogene α; *IL-8*, interleukin-8; *MCP-1*, monocyte chemoattractant protein-1; *MIP-1*, macrophage inhibitory protein-1; *RANTES*, regulated on activation, normal T cell expressed and secreted; *SDF-1*, stromal-derived growth factor-1.

Other Mediators

Chondrocytes in OA cartilage, especially those in clonal clusters, also express the pattern recognition receptors (PRRs), including Toll-like receptors (TLRs) and the receptor for advanced glycation endproducts (RAGE). They are activated by ligands such as damage associated molecular patterns (DAMPs), also known as *alarmins*, including high mobility group box-1 (HMGB1), S100A8 (MRP8, calgranulin A) and S100A9 (MRP14, calgranulin B), serum amyloid A (SAA), collagen and proteoglycan constituents, and calcium pyrophosphate or hydroxyapatite crystals. DAMPs or other products released from damaged cartilage are evidence of adaptive immunity due to interactions of T cells,[125] but during established, chronic OA their role in innate immunity, in which they promote the initiation and perpetuation of the low-grade inflammation in OA joints, is of current interest.[157–159]

S100A8, S100A9, and S100A11 have critical roles in inflammatory arthritis and OA.[160,161] Activation of TLR or RAGE signaling drives inflammation-associated matrix catabolism through increased expression of inflammatory and catabolic genes, including MMP-3, MMP-13, and nitric oxide synthase (NOS)2, and increased ROS[158,162] matrix fragments, such as fibronectin fragments that are found in OA and RA cartilage and synovial fluid, can serve as biomarkers and also perform inflammatory and catabolic functions, stimulating the production of a host of pro-inflammatory factors and MMPs.[68]

Other candidates for innate effectors of the disease include the complement proteins, which are detected in synovial fluids of OA patients by proteomic analysis and can be activated by DAMPs.[163] The classical, mannose-binding lectin, and alternative complement pathways all converge on C3 to activate the membrane attack complex (MAC) formed from the complement effector C5b-C9. Knockout of the C5 and C6 components of MAC or pharmacological treatment with CR2-fH attenuates cartilage damage in the medial meniscectomy mouse OA model.[164]

The peroxisome proliferation-activated receptors (PPARs) are a family of transcription factors that play roles in a broad spectrum of physiological and pathological processes, including skeletal homeostasis. PPARγ is activated by the endogenous ligand 15-deoxy-$\Delta^{12,14}$ prostaglandin J_2 (PGJ_2). PPARγ activation opposes the induction of COX-2, iNOS, and MMPs and the suppression of aggrecan synthesis by IL-1. PPARα agonists may also protect chondrocytes against IL-1–induced responses by increasing the expression of IL-1Ra. In OA, the focus has been on the roles of PPARγ in obesity and inflammation and its capacity to decrease cartilage degradation in animal models of OA.[165–168]

Among the proteins that may be induced in chondrocytes in response to abnormal stimuli, the cytokine–induced suppressor of cytokine signaling 3 (SOCS3) acts as a feedback regulator to ameliorate adverse effects on chondrocyte functions.[169] Suppressors of cytokine signaling (SOCS) proteins are inhibitors of cytokines that signal via the JAK/STAT (signal transducer and activator of transcription) pathway in multiple cell types, including T cells, macrophages, chondrocytes, synoviocytes, osteoclasts, and osteoblasts. Investigators[170] examined the levels of SOCS proteins in cartilage specimens from a series of patients with OA and found that SOCS2 mRNA levels were markedly reduced in the OA chondrocytes compared to chondrocytes from normal cartilage.

Adipokines, including leptin, adiponectin, resistin, and visfatin, were identified originally as products of adipocytes and have roles in cartilage metabolism based on investigations in various experimental models.[171,172] Cytokines secreted by the white adipose tissue contribute to the low-grade inflammation in obesity-associated OA.[173] There is a balance between pro- and anticatabolic adipokines that are secreted by joint tissues, including the fat pad of the knee, suggesting complex interactions between systemic and local factors.[174]

Chemokines, which are small heparin-binding cytokines identified originally as chemotactic factors, are classified as C, CX3C, or CC molecules, indicating the presence of distinct N-terminal cysteine (C) residues. In addition to recruiting leukocytes to sites of inflammation in arthritic joints and mediating synovial fibroblast responses and actions, chemokines are capable of modulating chondrocyte functions that are associated with cartilage degradation. Chondrocytes, when activated by IL-1 and TNF, express several chemokines, including IL-8, monocyte chemoattractant protein (MCP)-1, MCP-4, macrophage inhibitory protein (MIP)-1α, MIP-1β, RANTES (regulated on activation normal T cell expressed and secreted), and growth-related oncogene (GRO)α; they also express the receptors that enable responses to some of these chemokines and that feedback-regulate synovial cell responses (Table 3.5).[175,176]

Normal and OA chondrocytes express the CC chemokines MCP-1, MIP-1α, MIP-1β, and RANTES. RANTES increases expression of its own receptor, CCR5. MCP-1 and RANTES increase MMP-3, iNOS, IL-6, and MMP-1 expression, inhibit proteoglycan synthesis, and enhance proteoglycan release from the chondrocytes. The growth factor TGFα, also produced by chondrocytes, can inhibit proteoglycan production and stimulate its degradation by upregulating MCP-1. Inhibition of the MCP-1 receptor CCR2 reduces the severity of cartilage degradation and pain in surgically induced arthritis in mice.[177] The RANTES receptors CCR3 and CCR5, but not CCR1, are expressed in normal cartilage, whereas all three receptors are expressed in OA cartilage or after stimulation of normal chondrocytes by IL-1β. Stromal cell–derived factor 1 (SDF-1) can be detected in OA and RA synovial fluids, and its receptor, CXCR4, is expressed by chondrocytes, but not by synovial fibroblasts, suggesting a direct influence of this chemokine on cartilage damage.[175]

Cytokine Signaling Pathways Involved in Cartilage Metabolism

Although the receptors for the various cytokines and associated adapter molecules are distinct, they share the capacity to activate some of the same signaling pathways (Fig. 3.7). The major pathways induced by catabolic cytokines involve signal transduction by the stress-activated protein kinases, JNKs and p38 kinases, and the NF-κB and PI-3K pathways.[5,6,104,178,179] The JAK/STAT pathway

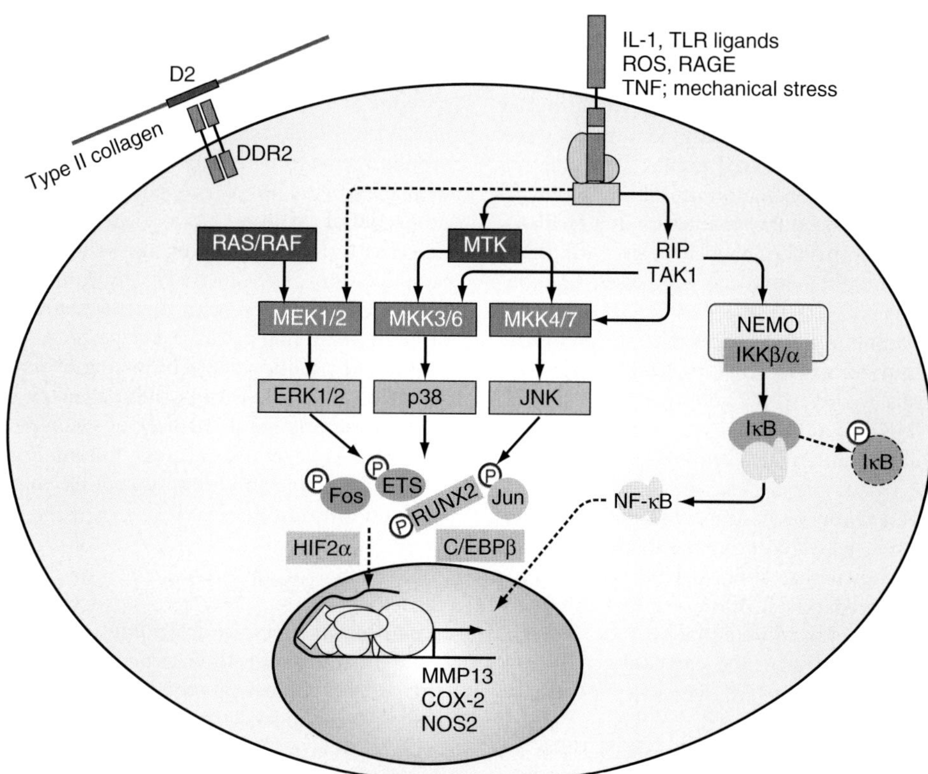

• **Fig. 3.7** Intra-cellular signaling pathways that regulate gene transcription in chondrocytes. Binding of the receptor tyrosine kinase, discoidin domain receptor (DDR) 2, to native type II collagen results in activation of RAS/RAF/MEK/ERK signaling in a manner independent of integrin- or cytokine-induced signaling. Interleukin (IL)-1, Toll-like receptor (TLR) ligand, reactive oxygen species (ROS), and advanced glycation endproducts (AGEs) interact with the cell through distinct receptors that transduce phosphorylation events and initiate various protein kinase cascades. Binding of IL-1 to the type I IL-1 receptor (IL-1R1) leads to recruitment of the IL-1R accessory protein (IL-1RAcP). Cytoplasmic Toll/IL-1 receptor (TIR) domains of the receptor recruit MyD88 via its TIR, and the MyD88 death domain (DD) recruits IL-1 receptor-associated kinases (IRAK and IRAK2) to the receptor complex before being rapidly phosphorylated and degraded. The IRAKs mediate tumor necrosis factor receptor-associated factor 6 (TRAF6) oligomerization, initiating various protein kinase cascades. The major pathways involve activation of (1) the stress-activated protein kinases, p38 mitogen-activated protein kinase (MAPK), and c-Jun N-terminal kinase (JNK), which lead to activation of activator protein-1 (AP-1) (cFos/cJun), activating transcription factor-2 (ATF-2), E26 transformation-specific (ETS) factors, HIF2α, Runx2, and C/EBPβ, among other transcription factors; and (2) inhibitor of κB (IκB) kinases α and β (IKK-α and IKK-β), which leads to activation of nuclear factor κB (NF-κB). TNF also stimulates these pathways, but mainly via TRAF2. Other signaling pathways may influence the target gene responses, such as growth factor-induced or chemokine-induced phosphatidylinositol 3-kinase (PI-3K) via the serine/threonine kinase, AKT/protein kinase B, and gp130 cytokine-induced Janus kinase (JAK)/signal transducer and activator of transcription (STAT) pathway. Responses of the target genes depend on the presence of DNA sequences within the respective promoters that bind to various transcription factors. (Adapted from Goldring MB: Chondrogenesis, chondrocyte differentiation, and articular cartilage metabolism in health and osteoarthritis. *Ther Adv Musculoskelet Dis* 4:269–285, 2012.)

is important for signaling by gp130 cytokines, including IL-6 and OSM.[180] Specific adapter molecules involved in the pathways induced by TNF receptors, which are members of the TNF receptor superfamily, are different from the adapter molecules used by IL-1 signaling pathways. The TNF receptor pathway uses TNF receptor–associated factor 2 (TRAF2), TRAF6, and the receptor interacting protein kinase, whereas the IL-1 receptor pathway uses TRAF6, IL-1 receptor–associated kinase (IRAK), and evolutionarily conserved signaling intermediate in Toll pathways (ECSIT) as adapter molecules. Signaling through TNF-RI associated with TNF receptor–associated death domain (TRADD) activates apoptosis, whereas TNF-RII signaling through TRAF2 activates JNK and NF-κB.

In contrast to ERK1 and ERK2, p38 and JNK signaling pathways are weakly activated by growth factors. Studies in chondrocytes in vitro have shown that the p38 and JNK cascades mediate the induction of proteinases and pro-inflammatory genes by IL-1 and TNF. These pathways also may be activated in chondrocytes by mechanical stress and cartilage matrix degradation products via integrins and other receptor-mediated events. Upregulation of IL-1 and TNF expression via mechanotransduction pathways suggests their involvement as secondary mediators in a feedback mechanism. At least four isoforms of p38 MAPK exist with different substrate specificities and differential effects on essential chondrocyte functions.

JNKs are serine threonine protein kinases that phosphorylate Jun family members, components of AP-1 transcription factors, and they exist in humans as three JNK isoforms: JNK1, JNK2, and JNK3. Activated JNK is detected in OA, but not in normal cartilage, and JNK inhibition attenuates cytokine-induced chondrocyte responses.

Members of the NF-κB family orchestrate mechanical, inflammatory, and oxidative stress–activated processes in chondrocytes. Numerous studies have shown that abnormal NF-κB signaling contributes to cartilage degradation in OA[181,182] and to phenotypic modulation and hypertrophic differentiation.[178,183] NF-κBs are released from inhibitory IκBs by the catalytic activities of the IKKα and IKKβ subunits of the IKK signalosome complex, permitting translocation of active NF-κB to the nucleus.[178] In response to a host of pro-inflammatory stimuli, IKKβ is the dominant IκBα kinase in vivo, whose activation is essential for the nuclear entry of canonical NF-κB heterodimers. NF-κB mediates the expression of cytokines and chemokines induced by fibronectin fragments, and inhibition of nuclear translocation or DNA-binding activity of NF-κB heterodimers of p65/p50 blocks pro-inflammatory and catabolic effects of IL-1 and TNF on chondrocytes. Chondrocyte phenotype appears to be subject to differential control by IKKβ-driven canonical NF-κB, which drives cartilage catabolism, and kinase independent IKKα, which promotes hypertrophic conversion.[184]

The IKKβ-driven, canonical NF-κB pathway signaling also has effects on downstream transcriptional regulators, including HIF-2α, β-catenin, Runx2, and the ETS factor, Elf3, thus linking inflammatory and oxidative stress responses with phenotypic and functional changes in chondrocytes.[134,136,185] In addition, NF-κB signaling plays a central role in disease progression and perpetuation, mediating a cascade of inflammatory responses triggered by advanced glycation end products, TLR ligands, or released ECM products, including fibronectin fragments, which lead to the continued expression of MMPs, aggrecanases, inflammatory cytokines, and chemokines, and to an abnormal differentiation status.

Aging of Articular Cartilage

It is important, but often difficult, to distinguish among the effects of aging itself and diseases such as OA that become more common with increasing age.[186,187] In both cases, biochemical alterations in matrix composition are reflected in changes in cartilage structure.[188] Age-related changes in the cartilage matrix and in chondrocyte function contribute to the development of OA but are distinct from OA (see Chapter 104 for a detailed discussion of the pathogenesis of OA). The thickness of articular cartilage, as shown by histology and magnetic resonance imaging, decreases with increasing age but remains intact in normal aged joints. Age-related changes in aggrecan size and the composition of the GAG chains result in decreased water content of cartilage, which may contribute to cartilage thinning and altered mechanical properties, including reduced resiliency during joint loading. Also contributing is the accumulation of unsubstituted proteoglycan core proteins of aggrecan and biglycan. Hyaluronan content increases in aged cartilage, but with reduced mean chain length, and link protein seems to be fragmented. Collagen fibrils become thinner with age and are less densely packed, which would alter the tensile properties of cartilage.

Perhaps the most striking age-related change in cartilage is the accumulation of advanced glycation end products, such as pentosidine, that form due to nonenzymatic glycation of long-lived proteins, including cartilage collagen and aggrecan. Advanced glycation end-products cause browning of tissues, and indeed cartilage from older adults can exhibit a yellow-brown hue in contrast to the glistening white cartilage of younger adults.[188] Pentosidine promotes collagen fiber cross-linking, making cartilage more "brittle" with age and more susceptible to damage from excessive mechanical loading.

Chondrocyte Aging

Chondrocyte function deteriorates with age such that catabolic activities and cell death become favored over anabolic activity.[186] This is due at least in part to the reduced production of pro-anabolic growth factors such as TGFβ and to the reduced responsiveness to growth factors such as IGF-1 and BMP-7. Because there is little to no cell proliferation in adult articular cartilage, the chondrocytes present in older adults are likely the same cells that were present in young adulthood. In contrast to other tissues such as epithelial tissue that have a continuous turnover of cells, the longevity of chondrocytes means that cellular damage, including DNA damage, can accumulate over many years leading to cell senescence. Chondrocyte senescence can also be promoted by increased levels of ROS due to age-related losses of antioxidant capacity and mitochondrial dysfunction, as well as the accumulated effects of excessive joint loading. Senescent cells lack the capacity to replicate while producing increased amounts of pro-inflammatory cytokines such as IL-6 and matrix degrading enzymes including the MMPs. This increased production of inflammatory mediators by senescent cells has been referred to as the senescence-associated secretory phenotype or SASP.[187] In fact, the SASP factors first identified in cultures of senescent fibroblasts are quite similar to the cytokines and MMPs found in OA cartilage, providing a direct link between chondrocyte senescence and OA.

Although senescent cells are more resistant to cell death than cells that maintain the capacity to proliferate, a decline in chondrocyte numbers in the articular cartilage occurs with age due to cell death and the lack of a supply of progenitor cells to replace lost cells. Although programmed cell death, or apoptosis, increases with age in adult rats and mice, this may be due to skeletal growth that occurs throughout life in these animals. In human adult cartilage, apoptotic cell removal does not seem to be common, however. Chondrocyte cell death in aged cartilage may be due to the reduction in autophagy.

Autophagy is an efficient housekeeping program used to maintain cellular function and homeostasis by removing damaged or malfunctioning cellular structures, eliminating exogenous cellular aggressors, and providing alternative sources of energy during ER stress, hypoxia, starvation, and other adverse events.[187,189] Reduced activity of 5′-AMP-activated kinase is associated with changes in energy metabolism and reduced autophagy. The loss of autophagy in articular cartilage during aging is associated with cell death and increasing OA severity because the chondrocyte is less resistant to mechanical or inflammatory stress.[190]

The age-related decline in chondrocyte autophagy could be related to decreased levels of forkhead-box class O (FOXO) transcription factors. FOXO1, FOXO3, and FOXO4 are found in articular chondrocytes, but with aging there is a reduction in FOXO1 and FOX3 levels associated with decreased autophagy.[191] FOXOs regulate the expression of autophagy genes, as well as antioxidants, including superoxide dismutase (SOD)-2 and catalase. Loss of FOXO activity results in reduced autophagy and increased susceptibility to oxidative stress, both of which would contribute to age-related OA.

Also compromised during aging is the unfolded protein response (UPR), which is a nonlysosomal pathway for ubiquitin/proteasome degradation of unfolded proteins eliminated from the ER.[162] The UPR enables chondrocyte survival in response to ER stress during growth plate development,[192] but also during inflammatory, mechanical, and oxidative stress in articular cartilage via C/EBP homologous protein (CHOP) and X-box protein 1 (XBP1).[162] Also related to autophagy are the classic cell survival signals, PI-3K and its downstream target, AKT, a serine-threonine kinase.[104] In addition, the impairment of chondrocyte mitochondrial function has emerged as a mechanism involved in impaired autophagy and deregulated bioenergetics during aging and OA development.[193]

Markers of Cartilage Matrix Degradation and Turnover

With increasing knowledge of the composition of the cartilage matrix, molecular markers in synovial fluid and body fluids such as urine, plasma, and serum have been identified for monitoring changes in cartilage metabolism and for assessing joint damage in arthritis.[194,195] Molecules originating from articular cartilage ECM, including aggrecan fragments containing chondroitin sulfate and keratan sulfate, type II collagen fragments, collagen pyridinoline cross-links, and COMP, usually are released as degradation products as a result of catabolic processes. Specific monoclonal antibodies have been developed for analyzing OA and RA body fluids for products of proteoglycan or collagen degradation (catabolic neoepitopes) or synthesis of newly synthesized matrix components (anabolic neoepitopes), which represent attempts to repair the damaged matrix. Different monoclonal antibodies can distinguish subtle biochemical differences in chondroitin sulfate or keratan sulfate chains that result from degraded versus newly synthesized proteoglycans. Such epitopes can be detected in the synovial fluids and sera of patients with OA and RA, and the synovial fluid-to-serum ratio has been suggested as a potential diagnostic indicator. The degradation of aggrecan in cartilage has been characterized using antibodies 846, 3B3(−), and 7D4, which detect chondroitin sulfate neoepitopes; 5D4, which detects keratan sulfate epitopes; and the VIDIPEN and NITEGE antibodies, which recognize aggrecanase and MMP cleavage sites within the interglobular G1 domain of aggrecan (see Chapter 8).[143,148]

Because collagens are the most abundant proteins in articular cartilage and type II collagen makes up approximately 50% of the cartilage ECM, many biomarker assays are designed to detect type II collagen breakdown products. It is possible to monitor the synthesis of type II collagen by measuring serum and synovial fluid levels of the carboxyl-terminal propeptide (CPII), and urinary excretion of hydroxylysyl pyridinoline cross-links or a cross-linked fragment of type II collagen (CTXII) may indicate collagen degradation. Specific antibodies that recognize epitopes on denatured type II collagen at the collagenase cleavage site are promising diagnostic reagents. These include the C12C antibody (previously known as *Col2-3/4C Long mono*) that has been used to detect specific cleavage of the triple helix of type II collagen in experimental models and in OA and RA cartilage. The ratios of these markers to the synthetic marker, CPII, are associated with a greater likelihood of radiologic progression in OA patients. These biomarker assays have been used as research tools and are currently being developed and validated as diagnostic tools for monitoring cartilage degradation or repair in OA and RA patient populations and for assessment of treatment efficacy.[194,195] Although a single marker may be insufficient, it could be possible eventually to identify a combination of biomarkers that discriminate between different stages of OA in different patient populations. There is potential for further development of biomarkers for use in future clinical trials.

Repair of Articular Cartilage

Articular cartilage has a poor capacity for regeneration, and pharmacologic enhancement of cartilage repair would have considerable potential in the treatment of arthritides and intra-articular fractures. The extent of intrinsic repair of a cartilage defect depends on the depth of the lesion and whether the defect penetrates the subchondral bone plate.[11] Owing to the avascularity of cartilage, it differs from most other tissues in its response to injury. The vascular-dependent inflammatory and reparative phases of the classic healing response are unavailable. Partial defects generally do not regenerate because resident chondrocytes cannot migrate into the defect, and there is no vascular access for progenitor cells. Deep cartilage defects with disruption of the subchondral bone plate initiate vascular responses, however, including bleeding, fibrin clot formation, and inflammation, which permit cell invasion from the blood or underlying bone marrow. These defects can be filled by fibrocartilage produced by progenitor cells found in the bone marrow including mesenchymal stem cells. Current procedures for cartilage repair include joint lavage, tissue debridement, microfracture of the subchondral bone, and transplantation of autologous or allogeneic osteochondral grafts, in addition to the ultimate therapy of total joint replacement.[11] These procedures may lead to the formation of fibrous tissue, chondrocyte death, and further cartilage degeneration, and they have variable success rates.

Transplantation of cultured autologous chondrocytes has been used successfully to repair small, full-thickness lesions in knee cartilage in young adults with sports injuries. Evidence of successful repair has been shown by turnover and remodeling of the initial fibrocartilaginous matrix formed by transplanted chondrocytes as the result of enzyme degradation and new synthesis of type II collagen. The donor site, although not load bearing, may undergo significant morbidity and osteoarthritic changes. Such procedures, however, show little difference in efficacy compared with microfracture of subchondral bone.[11]

Major challenges for cartilage repair include restoration of the three-dimensional collagen structure and integration of the newly synthesized matrix with resident tissue.[11] Novel approaches using autologous chondrocytes genetically engineered ex vivo to express anabolic factors have been explored to promote differentiation before implantation in the defect.[196] Because IGF-1 and TGF-β/BMP and FGF family members have roles in chondrogenesis and articular cartilage maintenance, they have been used as additive factors in tissue engineering strategies. The introduction of these factors into joints directly or by in vivo or ex vivo gene delivery or via injectable or implantable carriers has been investigated for the repair of small defects in animal models. Gene transfer of combinations of anabolic factors and inhibitory cytokines combined with cartilage engineering approaches may be a long-term goal for repair of extensive defects in RA or late OA patients and for prevention of further damage.

Recent investigations have focused on scaffolds with the mechanical and material properties of the osteochondral unit that will integrate with the host tissue and attract migration of chondrocytes or osteochondral progenitors from the subchondral bone.[197] Although these are promising strategies for the future based on in vitro and in vivo studies, many challenges remain, especially for cell-mediated cartilage repair. Among the cell sources are MSCs, which can be obtained from autologous adipose tissue, bone marrow, synovium, or muscle and expanded ex vivo in conditions that promote chondrogenesis, incorporated into scaffolds, and/or used as gene delivery vehicles to the site of cartilage damage.[196] Although adult articular chondrocytes have little intrinsic repair capacity, the potential of a small population of cartilage-derived stem or progenitor cells to be stimulated in situ is the subject of current investigations.[198]

Conclusion

As the single cellular component in adult articular cartilage, chondrocytes are responsible for maintaining the ECM components in a low-turnover state. The composition and organization of ECM macromolecules, unique to this tissue, are determined during chondrocyte differentiation in embryonic and postnatal development of cartilage. Adult chondrocytes are cytoplasmically isolated and exist in a hypoxic environment within articular cartilage. They exhibit low metabolic activity, partially as a result of the absence of blood vessels and nerves and display a rounded morphology that reflects their quiescent state, particularly in the middle and deep zones of cartilage. Chondrocytes interact with specific ECM components via cell surface receptors, including integrins, annexins, syndecans, DDR2, and CD44.

Studies in vitro and in vivo have shown that adult articular chondrocytes are capable of responding to biologic and mechanical stimuli that are anabolic or catabolic. Anabolic factors include members of the TGF-β/BMP and FGF families and IGF-I. Catabolic factors include pro-inflammatory cytokines, chemokines, DAMPs/alarmins, and adipokines, which stimulate the synthesis of matrix-degrading proteinases, such as MMPs and aggrecanases, in chondrocytes and increase intra-cellular events associated with inflammatory, mechanical, and oxidative stress processes. Many of the signaling pathways and transcription factors that mediate the responses of chondrocytes to these factors have been elucidated, but how they orchestrate specific chondrocyte functions is complex and is not fully understood. Under physiologic conditions, the adult articular chondrocyte maintains a stable equilibrium of low-turnover replacement of matrix components. Adult chondrocytes have a poor capacity for mediating effective repair of extensive cartilage lesions, and this capacity declines with age. Age-related changes in chondrocyte function decrease the ability of cells to maintain the tissue. There is decreased responsiveness to anabolic growth factors and increased production of pro-inflammatory factors due to cell senescence. Further understanding of how the adult articular chondrocyte functions within its unique environment and how this cell type undergoes metabolic reprogramming in a pro-inflammatory microenvironment would aid in the development of rational strategies for maintaining homeostasis and protecting against cartilage damage.

Full references for this chapter can be found on ExpertConsult.com.

Selected References

1. Archer CW, Francis-West P: The chondrocyte, *Int J Biochem Cell Biol* 35:401–404, 2003.
2. Archer CW, Morrison H, Pitsillides AA: Cellular aspects of the development of diarthrodial joints and articular cartilage, *J Anat* 184(Pt 3):447–456, 1994.
3. Hall BK: Chondrogenesis of the somitic mesoderm, *Adv Anat Embryol Cell Biol* 53:3–47, 1977.
4. Heinemeier KM, Schjerling P, Heinemeier J, et al.: Radiocarbon dating reveals minimal collagen turnover in both healthy and osteoarthritic human cartilage, *Sci Transl Med* 8:346ra390, 2016.
5. Goldring MB, Otero M: Inflammation in osteoarthritis, *Curr Opin Rheumatol* 23:471–478, 2011.
6. Goldring MB, Otero M, Plumb DA, et al.: Roles of inflammatory and anabolic cytokines in cartilage metabolism: signals and multiple effectors converge upon MMP-13 regulation in osteoarthritis, *Eur Cell Mater* 21:202–220, 2011.
7. Vincent TL, Wann AKT: Mechanoadaptation: articular cartilage through thick and thin, *J Physiol* 597:1271–1281, 2019.
8. Loeser RF, Goldring SR, Scanzello CR, et al.: Osteoarthritis: a disease of the joint as an organ, *Arthritis Rheum* 64:1697–1707, 2012.
9. Loeser RF, Gandhi U, Long DL, et al.: Aging and oxidative stress reduce the response of human articular chondrocytes to insulin-like growth factor 1 and osteogenic protein 1, *Arthritis Rheumatol* 66:2201–2209, 2014.
10. Heinegard D, Saxne T: The role of the cartilage matrix in osteoarthritis, *Nat Rev Rheumatol* 7:50–56, 2011.
11. Hunziker EB, Lippuner K, Shintani N: How best to preserve and reveal the structural intricacies of cartilaginous tissue, *Matrix Biol* 39:33–43, 2014.
12. Schmitz N, Laverty S, Kraus VB, et al.: Basic methods in histopathology of joint tissues, *Osteoarthritis Cartilage* 18(Suppl 3):S113–116, 2010.
13. Lotz MK, Otsuki S, Grogan SP, et al.: Cartilage cell clusters, *Arthritis Rheum* 62:2206–2218, 2010.
14. Lyons TJ, McClure SF, Stoddart RW, et al.: The normal human chondro-osseous junctional region: evidence for contact of uncalcified cartilage with subchondral bone and marrow spaces, *BMC Musculoskelet Disord* 7:52, 2006.
15. Burr DB, Gallant MA: Bone remodelling in osteoarthritis, *Nat Rev Rheumatol* 8:665–673, 2012.
16. Andriacchi TP, Favre J: The nature of in vivo mechanical signals that influence cartilage health and progression to knee osteoarthritis, *Curr Rheumatol Rep* 16:463, 2014.

17. Guo H, Maher SA, Torzilli PA: A biphasic finite element study on the role of the articular cartilage superficial zone in confined compression, *J Biomech* 48:166–170, 2015.
18. Sandell LJ: Etiology of osteoarthritis: genetics and synovial joint development, *Nat Rev Rheumatol* 8:77–89, 2012.
19. Hsueh MF, Onnerfjord P, Kraus VB: Biomarkers and proteomic analysis of osteoarthritis, *Matrix Biol* 39:56–66, 2014.
20. van Turnhout MC, Schipper H, Engel B, et al.: Postnatal development of collagen structure in ovine articular cartilage, *BMC Dev Biol* 10:62, 2010.
21. Patra D, DeLassus E, McAlinden A, et al.: Characterization of a murine type IIB procollagen-specific antibody, *Matrix Biol* 34:154–160, 2014.
22. McAlinden A, Traeger G, Hansen U, et al.: Molecular properties and fibril ultrastructure of types II and XI collagens in cartilage of mice expressing exclusively the alpha1(IIA) collagen isoform, *Matrix Biol* 34:105–113, 2014.
23. Wilusz RE, Sanchez-Adams J, Guilak F: The structure and function of the pericellular matrix of articular cartilage, *Matrix Biol* 39:25–32, 2014.
24. Wilusz RE, Defrate LE, Guilak F: A biomechanical role for perlecan in the pericellular matrix of articular cartilage, *Matrix Biol* 31:320–327, 2012.
25. Sgariglia F, Candela ME, Huegel J, et al.: Epiphyseal abnormalities, trabecular bone loss and articular chondrocyte hypertrophy develop in the long bones of postnatal Ext1-deficient mice, *Bone* 57:220–231, 2013.
26. Halper J: Proteoglycans and diseases of soft tissues, *Adv Exp Med Biol* 802:49–58, 2014.
27. Jay GD, Waller KA: The biology of lubricin: near frictionless joint motion, *Matrix Biol* 39:17–24, 2014.
28. Karamchedu NP, Tofte JN, Waller KA, et al.: Superficial zone cellularity is deficient in mice lacking lubricin: a stereoscopic analysis, *Arthritis Res Ther* 18:64, 2016.
29. Waller KA, Zhang LX, Elsaid KA, et al.: Role of lubricin and boundary lubrication in the prevention of chondrocyte apoptosis, *Proc Natl Acad Sci U S A* 110:5852–5857, 2013.
30. Larson KM, Zhang L, Badger GJ, et al.: Early genetic restoration of lubricin expression in transgenic mice mitigates chondrocyte peroxynitrite release and caspase-3 activation, *Osteoarthritis Cartilage* 25:1488–1495, 2017.
31. Onnerfjord P, Khabut A, Reinholt FP, et al.: Quantitative proteomic analysis of eight cartilaginous tissues reveals characteristic differences as well as similarities between subgroups, *J Biol Chem* 287:18913–18924, 2012.
32. Posey KL, Alcorn JL, Hecht JT: Pseudoachondroplasia/COMP—translating from the bench to the bedside, *Matrix Biol* 37:167–173, 2014.
33. Klatt AR, Becker AK, Neacsu CD, et al.: The matrilins: modulators of extracellular matrix assembly, *Int J Biochem Cell Biol* 43:320–330, 2011.
34. Halper J, Kjaer M: Basic components of connective tissues and extracellular matrix: elastin, fibrillin, fibulins, fibrinogen, fibronectin, laminin, tenascins and thrombospondins, *Adv Exp Med Biol* 802:31–47, 2014.
35. Bernardo BC, Belluoccio D, Rowley L, et al.: Cartilage intermediate layer protein 2 (CILP-2) is expressed in articular and meniscal cartilage and down-regulated in experimental osteoarthritis, *J Biol Chem* 286:37758–37767, 2011.
36. Xu L, Li Z, Liu SY, et al.: Asporin and osteoarthritis, *Osteoarthritis Cartilage*, 2015.
37. Ranok A, Wongsantichon J, Robinson RC, et al.: Structural and thermodynamic insights into chitooligosaccharide binding to human cartilage chitinase 3-like protein 2 (CHI3L2 or YKL-39), *J Biol Chem* 290:2617–2629, 2015.
38. Lee NH, Shapiro IM: Ca2+ transport by chondrocyte mitochondria of the epiphyseal growth plate, *J Membr Biol* 41:349–360, 1978.
39. Terkeltaub R, Johnson K, Murphy A, et al.: Invited review: the mitochondrion in osteoarthritis, *Mitochondrion* 1:301–319, 2002.
40. Loeser RF: Aging and osteoarthritis, *Curr Opin Rheumatol* 23:492–496, 2011.
41. Martin JA, Buckwalter JA: Aging, articular cartilage chondrocyte senescence and osteoarthritis, *Biogerontology* 3:257–264, 2002.
42. Wann AK, Zuo N, Haycraft CJ, et al.: Primary cilia mediate mechanotransduction through control of ATP-induced Ca2+ signaling in compressed chondrocytes, *FASEB J* 26:1663–1671, 2012.
43. Ruhlen R, Marberry K: The chondrocyte primary cilium, *Osteoarthritis Cartilage* 22:1071–1076, 2014.
44. Sun MM, Beier F: Chondrocyte hypertrophy in skeletal development, growth, and disease, *Birth Defects Res C Embryo Today* 102:74–82, 2014.
45. wwwwv
46. Tsang KY, Cheung MC, Chan D, et al.: The developmental roles of the extracellular matrix: beyond structure to regulation, *Cell Tissue Res* 339:93–110, 2010.
47. Wuelling M, Vortkamp A: Chondrocyte proliferation and differentiation, *Endocr Dev* 21:1–11, 2011.
48. Akiyama H, Lefebvre V: Unraveling the transcriptional regulatory machinery in chondrogenesis, *J Bone Miner Metab* 29:390–395, 2011.
49. Long F, Ornitz DM: Development of the endochondral skeleton, *Cold Spring Harb Perspect Biol* 5:a008334, 2013.
50. Wang W, Rigueur D, Lyons KM: TGFbeta signaling in cartilage development and maintenance, *Birth Defects Res C Embryo Today* 102:37–51, 2014.
51. Hosaka Y, Saito T, Sugita S, et al.: Notch signaling in chondrocytes modulates endochondral ossification and osteoarthritis development, *Proc Natl Acad Sci U S A* 110:1875–1880, 2013.
52. Kozhemyakina E, Lassar AB, Zelzer E: A pathway to bone: signaling molecules and transcription factors involved in chondrocyte development and maturation, *Development* 142:817–831, 2015.
53. Komori T: Signaling networks in RUNX2-dependent bone development, *J Cell Biochem* 112:750–755, 2011.
54. Bradley EW, McGee-Lawrence ME, Westendorf JJ: Hdac-mediated control of endochondral and intramembranous ossification, *Crit Rev Eukaryot Gene Expr* 21:101–113, 2011.
55. Candela ME, Yasuhara R, Iwamoto M, et al.: Resident mesenchymal progenitors of articular cartilage, *Matrix Biol* 39:44–49, 2014.
56. Vinod E, Boopalan P, Sathishkumar S: Reserve or resident progenitors in cartilage? Comparative analysis of chondrocytes versus chondroprogenitors and their role in cartilage repair, *Cartilage* 9:171–182, 2018.
57. Richardson SM, Kalamegam G, Pushparaj PN, et al.: Mesenchymal stem cells in regenerative medicine: focus on articular cartilage and intervertebral disc regeneration, *Methods* 99:69–80, 2016.
58. Maroudas A, Bayliss MT, Uchitel-Kaushansky N, et al.: Aggrecan turnover in human articular cartilage: use of aspartic acid racemization as a marker of molecular age, *Arch Biochem Biophys* 350:61–71, 1998.
59. Verzijl N, DeGroot J, Thorpe SR, et al.: Effect of collagen turnover on the accumulation of advanced glycation end products, *J Biol Chem* 275:39027–39031, 2000.
60. Goldring SR, Goldring MB: Changes in the osteochondral unit during osteoarthritis: structure, function and cartilage-bone crosstalk, *Nat Rev Rheumatol* 12:632–644, 2016.
61. Mobasheri A, Mobasheri R, Francis MJ, et al.: Ion transport in chondrocytes: membrane transporters involved in intracellular ion homeostasis and the regulation of cell volume, free [Ca2+] and pH, *Histol Histopathol* 13:893–910, 1998.
62. Lane JM, Brighton CT, Menkowitz BJ: Anaerobic and aerobic metabolism in articular cartilage, *J Rheumatol* 4:334–342, 1977.
63. Rajpurohit R, Koch CJ, Tao Z, et al.: Adaptation of chondrocytes to low oxygen tension: relationship between hypoxia and cellular metabolism, *J Cell Physiol* 168:424–432, 1996.
64. Mobasheri A, Bondy CA, Moley K, et al.: Facilitative glucose transporters in articular chondrocytes. Expression, distribution

and functional regulation of GLUT isoforms by hypoxia, hypoxia mimetics, growth factors and pro-inflammatory cytokines, *Adv Anat Embryol Cell Biol* 200:1, p following vi, 1–84.
65. Rufino AT, Rosa SC, Judas F, et al.: Expression and function of K(ATP) channels in normal and osteoarthritic human chondrocytes: possible role in glucose sensing, *J Cell Biochem* 114:1879–1889, 2013.
66. Ruiz-Romero C, Carreira V, Rego I, et al.: Proteomic analysis of human osteoarthritic chondrocytes reveals protein changes in stress and glycolysis, *Proteomics* 8:495–507, 2008.
67. Maes C, Carmeliet G, Schipani E: Hypoxia-driven pathways in bone development, regeneration and disease, *Nat Rev Rheumatol* 8:358–366, 2012.
68. Loeser RF: Integrins and chondrocyte-matrix interactions in articular cartilage, *Matrix Biol* 39:11–16, 2014.
69. Candela ME, Wang C, Gunawardena AT, et al.: Alpha 5 integrin mediates osteoarthritic changes in mouse knee joints, *PLoS One* 11:e0156783, 2016.
70. Lundgren-Akerlund E, Aszodi A: Integrin alpha10beta1: a collagen receptor critical in skeletal development, *Adv Exp Med Biol* 819:61–71, 2014.
71. Song EK, Jeon J, Jang DG, et al.: ITGBL1 modulates integrin activity to promote cartilage formation and protect against arthritis, *Sci Transl Med* 10, 2018.
72. Perera PM, Wypasek E, Madhavan S, et al.: Mechanical signals control SOX-9, VEGF, and c-Myc expression and cell proliferation during inflammation via integrin-linked kinase, B-Raf, and ERK1/2-dependent signaling in articular chondrocytes, *Arthritis Res Ther* 12:R106, 2010.
73. Roca-Cusachs P, Iskratsch T, Sheetz MP: Finding the weakest link: exploring integrin-mediated mechanical molecular pathways, *J Cell Sci* 125:3025–3038, 2012.
74. Ono Y, Ishizuka S, Knudson CB, et al.: Chondroprotective effect of kartogenin on CD44-mediated functions in articular cartilage and chondrocytes, *Cartilage* 5:172–180, 2014.
75. Luo N, Knudson W, Askew EB, et al.: CD44 and hyaluronan promote the bone morphogenetic protein 7 signaling response in murine chondrocytes, *Arthritis Rheumatol* 66:1547–1558, 2014.
76. Minashima T, Small W, Moss SE, et al.: Intracellular modulation of signaling pathways by annexin A6 regulates terminal differentiation of chondrocytes, *J Biol Chem* 287:14803–14815, 2012.
77. Minashima T, Kirsch T: Annexin A6 regulates catabolic events in articular chondrocytes via the modulation of NF-kappaB and Wnt/ss-catenin signaling, *PLoS One* 13:e0197690, 2018.
78. Pap T, Bertrand J: Syndecans in cartilage breakdown and synovial inflammation, *Nat Rev Rheumatol* 9:43–55, 2013.
79. Xu L, Golshirazian I, Asbury BJ, et al.: Induction of high temperature requirement A1, a serine protease, by TGF-beta1 in articular chondrocytes of mouse models of OA, *Histol Histopathol* 29:609–618, 2014.
80. Tang X, Muhammad H, McLean C, et al.: Connective tissue growth factor contributes to joint homeostasis and osteoarthritis severity by controlling the matrix sequestration and activation of latent TGFbeta, *Ann Rheum Dis* 77:1372–1380, 2018.
81. Suri S, Walsh DA: Osteochondral alterations in osteoarthritis, *Bone* 51:204–211, 2012.
82. Franses RE, McWilliams DF, Mapp PI, et al.: Osteochondral angiogenesis and increased protease inhibitor expression in OA, *Osteoarthritis Cartilage* 18:563–571, 2010.
83. Zhen G, Wen C, Jia X, et al.: Inhibition of TGF-[beta] signaling in mesenchymal stem cells of subchondral bone attenuates osteoarthritis, *Nat Med* 19:704–712, 2013.
84. Lambert C, Dubuc JE, Montell E, et al.: Gene expression pattern of cells from inflamed and normal areas of osteoarthritis synovial membrane, *Arthritis Rheumatol* 66:960–968, 2014.
85. Ashraf S, Mapp PI, Burston J, et al.: Augmented pain behavioural responses to intra-articular injection of nerve growth factor in two animal models of osteoarthritis, *Ann Rheum Dis* 73:1710–1718, 2014.
86. Nagai T, Sato M, Kobayashi M, et al.: Bevacizumab, an anti-vascular endothelial growth factor antibody, inhibits osteoarthritis, *Arthritis Res Ther* 16:427, 2014.
87. Mariani E, Pulsatelli L, Facchini A: Signaling pathways in cartilage repair, *Int J Mol Sci* 15:8667–8698, 2014.
88. Geiger BC, Wang S, Padera Jr RF, et al.: Cartilage-penetrating nanocarriers improve delivery and efficacy of growth factor treatment of osteoarthritis, *Sci Transl Med* 10, 2018.
89. Bolduc JA, Collins JA, Loeser RF: Reactive oxygen species, aging and articular cartilage homeostasis, *Free Radic Biol Med* 132:73–82, 2019.
90. Vincent TL: Fibroblast growth factor 2: good or bad guy in the joint? *Arthritis Res Ther* 13:127, 2011.
91. Vincent TL: Explaining the fibroblast growth factor paradox in osteoarthritis: lessons from conditional knockout mice, *Arthritis Rheum* 64:3835–3838, 2012.
92. Yan D, Chen D, Cool SM, et al.: Fibroblast growth factor receptor 1 is principally responsible for fibroblast growth factor 2-induced catabolic activities in human articular chondrocytes, *Arthritis Res Ther* 13:R130, 2011.
93. Weng T, Yi L, Huang J, et al.: Genetic inhibition of fibroblast growth factor receptor 1 in knee cartilage attenuates the degeneration of articular cartilage in adult mice, *Arthritis Rheum* 64:3982–3992, 2012.
94. Barr L, Getgood A, Guehring H, et al.: The effect of recombinant human fibroblast growth factor-18 on articular cartilage following single impact load, *J Orthop Res* 32:923–927, 2014.
95. Mori Y, Saito T, Chang SH, et al.: Identification of fibroblast growth factor-18 as a molecule to protect adult articular cartilage by gene expression profiling, *J Biol Chem* 289:10192–10200, 2014.
96. Ellman MB, Yan D, Ahmadinia K, et al.: Fibroblast growth factor control of cartilage homeostasis, *J Cell Biochem* 114:735–742, 2013.
97. Lohmander LS, Hellot S, Dreher D, et al.: Intraarticular sprifermin (recombinant human fibroblast growth factor 18) in knee osteoarthritis: a randomized, double-blind, placebo-controlled trial, *Arthritis Rheumatol* 66:1820–1831, 2014.
98. Sennett ML, Meloni GR, Farran AJE, et al.: Sprifermin treatment enhances cartilage integration in an in vitro repair model, *J Orthop Res* 36:2648–2656, 2018.
99. van der Kraan PM: The changing role of TGFβ in healthy, ageing and osteoarthritic joints, *Nat Rev Rheumatol* 13:155, 2017.
100. Bush JR, Beier F: TGF-[beta] and osteoarthritis–the good and the bad, *Nat Med* 19:667–669, 2013.
101. Nishimura R, Hata K, Matsubara T, et al.: Regulation of bone and cartilage development by network between BMP signalling and transcription factors, *J Biochem* 151:247–254, 2012.
102. Deng ZH, Li YS, Gao X, et al.: Bone morphogenetic proteins for articular cartilage regeneration, *Osteoarthritis Cartilage* 26:1153–1161, 2018.
103. Gamer LW, Pregizer S, Gamer J, et al.: The role of bmp2 in the maturation and maintenance of the murine knee joint, *J Bone Miner Res* 33:1708–1717, 2018.
104. Beier F, Loeser RF: Biology and pathology of Rho GTPase, PI-3 kinase-Akt, and MAP kinase signaling pathways in chondrocytes, *J Cell Biochem* 110:573–580, 2010.
105. Blaney Davidson EN, van Caam AP, Vitters EL, et al.: TGF-beta is a potent inducer of nerve growth factor in articular cartilage via the ALK5-Smad2/3 pathway. Potential role in OA related pain? *Osteoarthritis Cartilage*, 23:478–486, 2015.
106. Li TF, Gao L, Sheu TJ, et al.: Aberrant hypertrophy in Smad3-deficient murine chondrocytes is rescued by restoring transforming growth factor beta-activated kinase 1/activating transcription factor 2 signaling: a potential clinical implication for osteoarthritis, *Arthritis Rheum* 62:2359–2369, 2010.
107. van Beuningen HM, de Vries-van Melle ML, Vitters EL, et al.: Inhibition of TAK1 and/or JAK can rescue impaired chondrogenic

differentiation of human mesenchymal stem cells in osteoarthritis-like conditions, *Tissue Eng Part A*, 20:2243–2252, 2014.
108. Brazil DP, Church RH, Surae S, et al.: BMP signalling: agony and antagony in the family, *Trends Cell Biol*, 2015.
109. Lories RJ, Corr M, Lane NE: To Wnt or not to Wnt: the bone and joint health dilemma, *Nat Rev Rheumatol* 9:328–339, 2013.
110. van den Bosch MH, Blom AB, van Lent PL, et al.: Canonical Wnt signaling skews TGF-beta signaling in chondrocytes towards signaling via ALK1 and Smad 1/5/8, *Cell Signal* 26:951–958, 2014.
111. Lewiecki EM: Role of sclerostin in bone and cartilage and its potential as a therapeutic target in bone diseases, *Ther Adv Musculoskelet Dis* 6:48–57, 2014.
112. Bougault C, Priam S, Houard X, et al.: Protective role of frizzled-related protein B on matrix metalloproteinase induction in mouse chondrocytes, *Arthritis Res Ther* 16:R137, 2014.
113. Funck-Brentano T, Bouaziz W, Marty C, et al.: Dkk-1-mediated inhibition of Wnt signaling in bone ameliorates osteoarthritis in mice, *Arthritis Rheumatol* 66:3028–3039, 2014.
114. Lietman C, Wu B, Lechner S, et al.: Inhibition of Wnt/beta-catenin signaling ameliorates osteoarthritis in a murine model of experimental osteoarthritis, *JCI Insight* 3, 2018.
115. Deshmukh V, Hu H, Barroga C, et al.: A small-molecule inhibitor of the Wnt pathway (SM04690) as a potential disease modifying agent for the treatment of osteoarthritis of the knee, *Osteoarthritis Cartilage* 26:18–27, 2018.
116. Carpio LR, Westendorf JJ: Histone deacetylases in cartilage homeostasis and osteoarthritis, *Curr Rheumatol Rep* 18:52, 2016.
117. Dvir-Ginzberg M, Mobasheri A, Kumar A: The role of sirtuins in cartilage homeostasis and osteoarthritis, *Curr Rheumatol Rep* 18:43, 2016.
118. Rushton MD, Reynard LN, Barter MJ, et al.: Characterization of the cartilage DNA methylome in knee and hip osteoarthritis, *Arthritis Rheumatol* 66:2450–2460, 2014.
119. Taylor SE, Smeriglio P, Dhulipala L, et al.: A global increase in 5-hydroxymethylcytosine levels marks osteoarthritic chondrocytes, *Arthritis Rheumatol* 66:90–100, 2014.
120. Le LT, Swingler TE, Clark IM: Review: the role of microRNAs in osteoarthritis and chondrogenesis, *Arthritis Rheum* 65:1963–1974, 2013.

4

Biology, Physiology, and Morphology of Bone

ALINE BOZEC, ANIKA GRÜNEBOOM, AND GEORG SCHETT

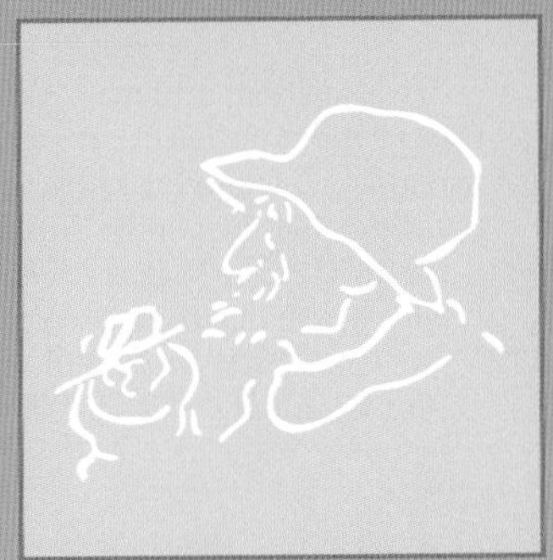

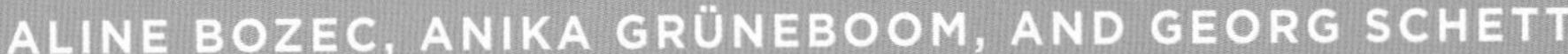

KEY POINTS

Intramembranous or endochondral ossification generates bone tissue.
Bones consist of a dense cortical shell and sponge-like trabecular network.
Bone formation depends on metabolically active osteoblasts synthesizing matrix proteins.
Bone marrow fat increases with age at the expense of osteoblasts.
Resorption of bone is mediated by multinucleated osteoclasts.
The most abundant cell type in bone is the osteocyte.
Bone is continuously rebuilt, a process known as ***bone remodeling.***
The immune system, in particular T lymphocytes, influences bone remodeling.
Neuroendocrine loops exert systemic control on bone remodeling.

Structure and Composition of Bone

Bone is a specialized connective tissue that assists in (1) locomotion, by providing the insertion site of the muscles; (2) protection of the internal organs and the bone marrow; and (3) metabolic function, such as storage and provision of calcium to the body. Bone consists of cells and the extra-cellular matrix, which is composed of type I collagen fibers and a number of noncollagenous proteins. The specific composition of the bone matrix allows its mineralization, which is a specific feature of bone.

The two major types of bones are flat bones, which are built by intramembranous ossification, and long bones, which emerge from endochondral ossification. Intramembranous bone formation is based on the condensation of mesenchymal stem cells, which directly differentiate into bone-forming osteoblasts. In contrast, during endochondral ossification of the long bones, the mesenchymal stem cells first differentiate into chondrocytes that will later be replaced by osteoblasts. Long bones consist of the following: (1) epiphyses, which are protrusions at the ends of the long bones; (2) diaphysis, constituting the bone's shaft; and (3) metaphyses, which are located between the epiphysis and the diaphysis (Fig. 4.1). The metaphysis is separated from the epiphysis by the growth plate, a proliferative cartilage layer that is essential for the longitudinal growth of bones. After the growth is completed, this cartilage layer is entirely remodeled into bone.

The external shape of bones is formed by a dense cortical shell (cortical or compact bone), which is particularly strong along the diaphysis, where the bone marrow is located. The cortical bone shell becomes progressively thinner toward the metaphyses and epiphyses, where most of the trabecular bone is located. Trabecular bone (also called *cancellous bone*) is a sponge-like network consisting of myriad highly interconnected bony trabeculae. The outer and the inner surfaces of cortical bone are covered by layers of osteogenic cells, termed the *periosteum* and the *endosteum,* which are involved in the growth of width by bone apposition at the periosteal sites and bone resorption at the endosteal sites.

Although cortical and trabecular bone is composed of the same cells and the same matrix components, there is a substantial difference between these two forms of skeletal tissue. Cortical bone almost exclusively consists of mineralized tissue (up to 90%), allowing it to fulfill its mechanical requirements. In contrast, only 20% of trabecular bone is mineralized tissue, with the bone marrow, blood vessels, and a network of mesenchymal stem cells constituting the remainder of the bone. As a consequence, trabecular bone shares a vast surface with the nonmineralized tissue, which is the basis for the metabolic function of bone, necessitating a high level of communication between the bone surface and the nonmineralized tissue.

Bone Vasculature

The metabolic function of the bone is dependent on being supplied with nutrients, oxygen, hormones, growth factors, and neurotransmitters. Bone marrow resident cells and mesenchymal stem cells respond to bone mediators but can also produce metabolic factors that are relevant for body homeostasis.[1,2] The exchange of such mediators into and out of the bone is mediated by a complex vascular system.

Oxygen is supplied by nutrient arteries; these enter the bone mainly at the metaphysis, run longitudinally along the bone shaft, and ramify towards the inner surface of the cortical bone, the endosteum. At this interface, the arteries form loops and interconnect with sinusoidal capillaries. This fenestrated venous vessel type allows a fast exchange of metabolites between the blood circulation and the bone marrow tissue. The sinusoids form a dense, irregular network that converges into a large central sinus in the middle of the bone marrow tissue. This central sinus exits the bone shaft and connects the bone marrow with the general blood circulation.[3–5]

In addition to the system of bone marrow vascularization, the mineralized bone also exhibits a dense vascular system, which is termed the *Haversian-Volkmann System.* This vascular network contains both arterial and venous vessels that ensure nutrient

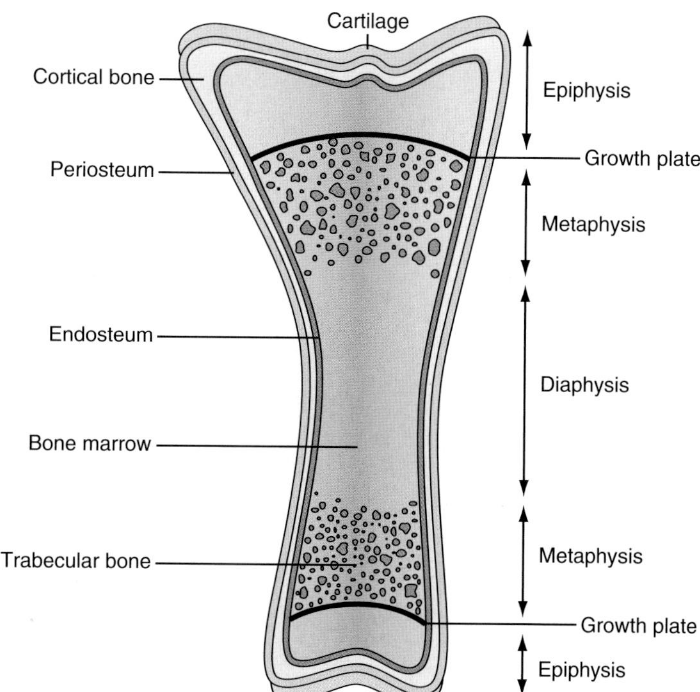

• **Fig. 4.1** Long bones consist of the epiphyses separated by growth plates from the metaphyses, which contain most of the trabecular bone. The outer lining of bone is the dense cortical bone, which is covered by the periosteum (outer surface) and the endosteum (inner surface). The latter connects bone to the bone marrow. The bony end plates are covered by the articular cartilage, consisting of a mineralized deep zone and a nonmineralized surface zone.

supply and metabolic exchange of the calcified bone tissue. Its structural organization is very complex because it can contain trans-cortical vessels (TCVs), which directly connect the bone marrow vascularization with the periosteum and the general circulation. Next to this, TCVs can show bifurcated or complex rope ladder–like morphologies (Fig. 4.2). Although their diameters are much smaller than those of nutrient arteries and central sinus exits, numbers of TCVs are drastically higher. Based on their multitude, they facilitate the major blood transport through the bone.[6,7]

At the endosteum, the vessels feed into the sinusoidal-arterial transition zones. These so-called *type H vessels* are also formed at the vascular transition zones of the metaphysis and exhibit specific metabolic profiles. Based on differences in tissue oxygenation and metabolic activity, they influence the growth potential and metabolism of hematopoietic stem cells as well as bone remodeling cells.[2,8,9] Thus, the vascular supply of nutrients and oxygen is not only relevant for bone marrow metabolism but also for the formation and destruction of the mineralized bone matrix.

Bone Matrix

The key protein component of bone is type I collagen. Collagen fibers follow specific directions, forming the basis for the lamellar structure of bone. This lamellar structure, which can be visualized when examining bone in the polarized light, allows dense packaging, resulting in optimal resistance to mechanical load. The lamellar collagen structures can be assembled in parallel (e.g., along the cortical bone surfaces and inside the bony trabeculae) or concentrically around blood vessels embedded in the Haversian channels of the cortical bone. Upon rapid deposition of new bone, such as during fracture healing, this lamellar structure is missing, and the bone is then called *woven bone.* Woven bone is consecutively remodeled into lamellar bone, which is also considered "mature" bone. The composition of the collagen backbone also assists in the deposition of spindle- or plate-shaped hydroxyapatite crystals, which contain calcium phosphate, thus allowing the calcification of the bone matrix.

In addition to type I collagen, other so-called noncollagenous proteins also exist in bone. Some of them, such as osteocalcin, osteopontin, and fetuin, are mineralization inhibitors, which serve to balance the degree of mineralization of the skeletal tissue. Aside from their intrinsic function in bone, noncollagenous proteins also exert important metabolic functions, such as the control of energy metabolism by osteocalcin.

Bone Cells: Osteoblasts

Osteoblasts are the bone-forming cells that derive from the mesenchymal stem cells of the bone marrow. Mesenchymal stem cells also form chondrocytes, myocytes, and adipocytes. Osteoblasts are cuboid-shaped cells that form clusters covering the bone surface. They are metabolically highly active, synthesizing the collagenous and noncollagenous bone matrix proteins that are excreted and then deposited between the osteoblasts and the bone surface. This newly built matrix, which is not yet calcified, is termed the *osteoid.* The lag phase between osteoid deposition and its mineralization is approximately 10 days. Osteoblast differentiation depends on the expression of two key transcription factors: runt domain transcription factor 2 (Runx2) and its target Osterix-1. The transcription factors confer the differentiation of mesenchymal cells into osteoblasts in response to external stimuli.[10] Prostaglandin E_2 (PGE_2), insulin-like growth factor (IGF)-1, parathyroid hormone (PTH), bone morphogenic proteins (BMPs), and Wingless and Int-1 (Wnt) proteins are key stimuli for osteoblast differentiation.[11,12] For instance, PGE_2 is an important anabolic factor for bone and induces the expression

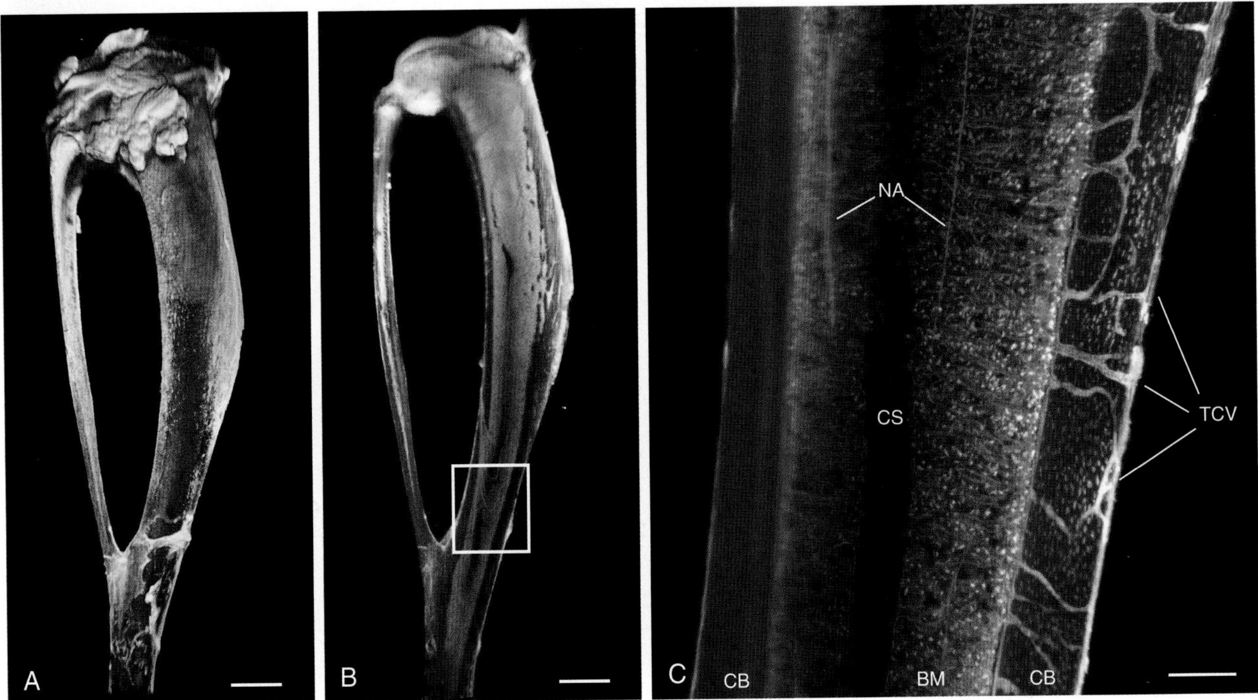

• **Fig. 4.2** Vascularization of long bones. (A) The three-dimensional rendering and (B) optical clipping of a light-sheet microscopy scanned murine tibia (autofluorescence, *gray*) shows the dense vascularization (CD31, *red*) of the bone marrow. Scale bars = 1000 μm. (C) Higher magnification scans of the indicated *white box* (B) emphasize the complex vascular organization of the bone tissue. Horizontally orientated sinusoids converge into the central sinus (CS), which runs longitudinally in the middle of the bone marrow shaft (BM) and is accompanied by nutrient arteries (NAs). In addition to the CS and NAs, the bone marrow vascularization is directly connected to the periosteum and the general circulation via trans-cortical vessels (TCVs), which pass the entire cortical bone (CB). Scale bar = 100 μm.

of bone sialoprotein and alkaline phosphatase in mesenchymal cells. BMPs and transforming growth factor (TGF)-β, which shares structural similarities with BMPs, foster osteoblast differentiation by activating intra-cellular Smad proteins. Finally, Wnt proteins, a family of highly conserved signaling molecules, are potent stimulators of osteoblast differentiation. Wnt proteins bind to surface receptors on mesenchymal cells, such as frizzled and LRP5, thereby eliciting activation and nuclear translocation of the transcription factor β-catenin, which induces the transcription of genes involved in osteoblast differentiation. Wnt proteins, thereby, act not only in close synergy with BMPs but also cross talk to the receptor activator of nuclear factor-κB ligand (RANKL)–osteoprotegerin (OPG) system, which is involved in the differentiation and function of bone-resorbing osteoclasts.

During aging, bone marrow adipocytes (BMAs) derived from bone marrow mesenchymal stem cells (BMSCs) accumulate, which correlates with osteoporosis. Activation of the nuclear receptor peroxisome proliferator-activated receptor gamma (PPAR-γ) promotes adipocyte differentiation.[13] However, activation of the Wnt/β-catenin signaling pathways stimulate BMSCs to differentiate into osteoblasts and inhibit adipogenesis.[14] BMAs are metabolically active cells that play an active role in energy storage, endocrine function, and bone metabolism.

Bone Cells: Osteocytes

Osteocytes are by far the most abundant cell type within bone. One cubic millimeter of bone contains up to 25,000 osteocytes that are well connected with each other and the bone surface by small tubes (canaliculi). This large and dense communication network inside the bone shares similarities to the nervous system. The surface of this network of lacunae contains the osteocytes and canaliculi, which consist of interconnecting filaments of the osteocytes. The network covers an area of 1000 to 4000 square meters. Osteocytes are derived from osteoblasts, which are subsequently entrapped in the bone matrix.[15] Osteocytes, however, also start to express genes that are specific for these cells and are not found in other cells, such as osteoblasts. One of the most interesting products of the osteocyte is sclerostin, a secreted molecule that binds lipoprotein receptor–related proteins (LRPs) and blocks Wnt-stimulated bone formation.[16] Consistent with its function as an inhibitor of bone formation, overexpression of sclerostin leads to low bone mass, whereas deletion of sclerostin leads to increased bone density and strength. This effect has recently been successfully used as a therapeutic strategy to increase bone mass by inhibiting sclerostin by a specific antibody.[17] Loss-of-function mutations in the human *SOST* gene that encodes sclerostin entail increased bone mass, a disease termed *sclerosteosis*.[18] Several local and systemic factors have been suggested as possible regulators of sclerostin expression by osteocytes. For instance, intermittent administration of PTH, which is associated with strong anabolic effects on the bone, potently inhibits sclerostin expression.

Recent genetic studies in mice have revealed that osteocytes provide the majority of the RANKL that controls osteoclast formation in cancellous bone.[19] Of note, osteocyte death is most strongly linked to the pathogenesis of osteonecrosis, a disease that occurs when excessive death of bone tissue and absence of bone regeneration result in the collapse of necrotic bone.[20]

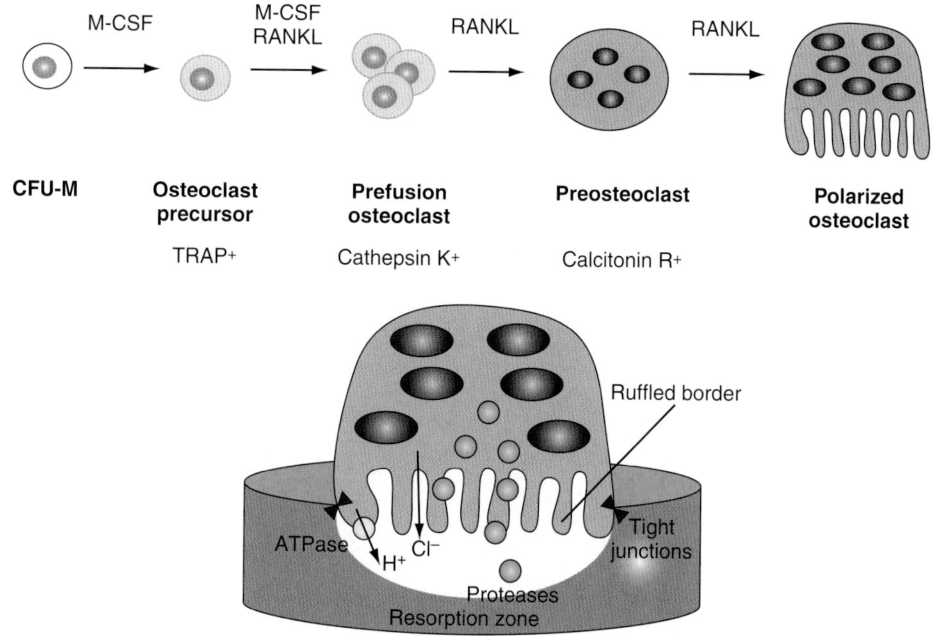

• **Fig. 4.3** Osteoclasts develop from mononuclear precursors (colony-forming unit macrophages [CFU-M]), which differentiate into mononuclear osteoclast precursors. These cells fuse and build a polykaryon, forming a preosteoclast. Final differentiation is characterized by cell polarization and acquisition of a ruffled border. *ATPase,* Adenosine triphosphatase; *M-CSF,* macrophage colony-stimulating factor; *RANKL,* receptor activator of nuclear factor-κB ligand; *TRAP,* tartrate-resistant acid phosphatase.

Bone Cells: Osteoclasts

Osteoclasts are multinucleated cells that contain up to 20 nuclei and are unique in their ability to resorb bone.[21,22] They are directly attached to the bone surface and build resorption lacunae (Howship lacunae). Apart from their multiple nuclei, another characteristic of the osteoclast is the *ruffled border,* a highly folded plasma membrane facing the bone matrix and designed to secrete and resorb proteins and ions into the space between the osteoclast and bone surface (Fig. 4.3). The space between this ruffled border and the bone surface is the place where bone resorption occurs. It is sealed by a ring of contractible proteins and tight junctions because it represents one of the few regions of the human body where a highly acidic milieu is found. Bone degradation by osteoclasts consists of two major steps: first, demineralization of inorganic bone components, and second, removal of organic bone matrix. To demineralize bone, osteoclasts secrete hydrochloric acid through proton pumps into the resorption lacunae. This proton pump requires energy that is provided by an adenosine triphosphatase (ATPase), allowing the enrichment of protons in the resorption compartment, which, in fact, represents an extracellular lysosome. In addition to protons and chloride, osteoclasts release matrix-degrading enzymes, including tartrate-resistant acid phosphatase (TRAP), lysosomal cathepsin K, and other cathepsins. Cathepsin K can effectively degrade collagens and other bone matrix proteins. Consequently, inhibitors of cathepsin K block osteoclast function and slow down bone resorption.

Osteoclasts originate from hematopoietic monocytic precursor cells and, upon the influence of specific signals, undergo a series of differentiation steps to become mature osteoclasts. Essential signals for osteoclast differentiation are macrophage colony-stimulating factor (M-CSF) and RANKL. During this differentiation and maturation process, osteoclasts acquire specific markers such as TRAP, fuse to multinucleated giant cells, and polarize on contact to bone. Osteoclastogenesis depends on an adequate microenvironment, which provides essential signals such as M-CSF and RANKL and certain cytokines such as TNF, which further enhance osteoclast differentiation. Mesenchymal cells such as preosteoblasts express M-CSF and RANKL and can induce osteoclast formation, highlighting the close interaction between bone formation and bone resorption.

RANKL, a TNF superfamily member, is a surface molecule expressed by osteocytes, preosteoblasts, and activated T cells.[23–25] Under steady-state conditions, its expression is induced in cells of the osteoblastic lineage in response to osteotrophic factors such as vitamin D, PTH, and prostaglandins, whereby the nuclear factor peroxisome proliferator-activated receptor–beta represents an essential checkpoint in the regulation of RANKL expression.[26] Moreover, inflammatory cytokines such as TNF, interleukin (IL)-1, and IL-17 can induce RANKL expression.[27–30] RANKL is essential for the final differentiation steps of osteoclasts, as well as for their bone-resorbing capacity, by engaging its receptor RANK on monocytic osteoclast-precursor cells. The interaction of RANKL with its receptor RANK is modulated by OPG, a secreted glycoprotein, which is identified as a soluble factor that strongly suppresses osteoclast differentiation both in vitro and in vivo. Interestingly, OPG expression is induced by estrogens, which explains the increase in osteoclast numbers and enhanced bone resorption during menopause. Accordingly, RANKL-deficient mice display severe osteopetrosis as a result of the lack of osteoclasts. With regard to the central role of the RANKL-RANK-OPG signaling system in bone resorption, researchers are increasingly interested in the therapeutic targeting of this system in human disease, and recent clinical trials involving post-menopausal osteoporosis have revealed the potent anti-resorptive effect of a neutralizing RANKL antibody (denosumab).[31] Beyond RANKL-RANK interactions, other important pro-osteoclastogenic signaling pathways are based on the triggering receptor expressed on myeloid cells (TREM) 2,

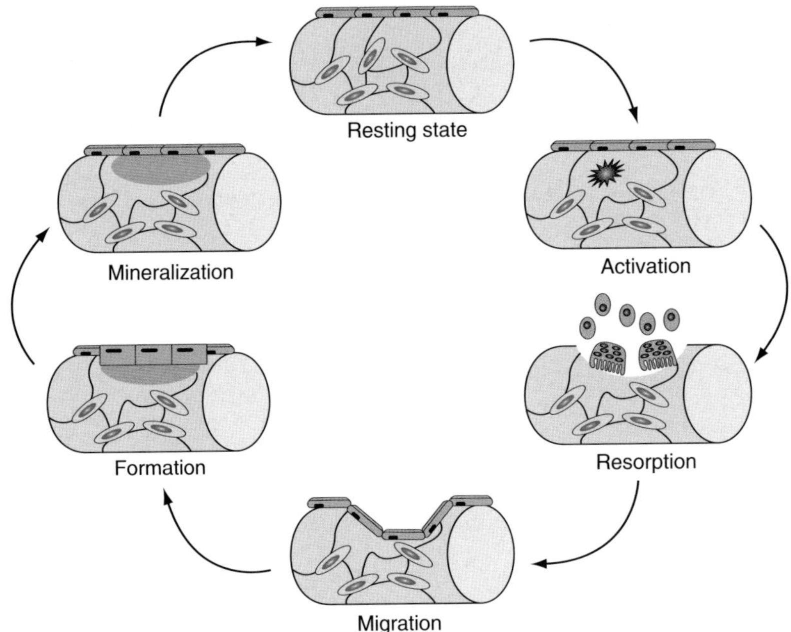

• **Fig. 4.4** Sequence of bone remodeling with *activation* characterized by sensing of damage by osteocytes, *resorption* by osteoclast differentiation and removal of bone matrix, *migration* of bone-lining mesenchymal cells into the lacuna, *formation* of new matrix by osteoblasts (cuboid cells), and *mineralization* of the newly synthesized matrix.

which interacts with the tyrosine kinase DAP12 and the osteoclast-associated immunoglobulin-like receptor (OSCAR). Both molecules are strong enhancers of osteoclastogenesis.[32]

Bone Remodeling Process

Developmental bone growth, postdevelopmental maintenance and repair of bone, and provision of calcium from the bone depend on a dynamic process called *bone remodeling* (Fig. 4.4). Factors yet unknown, which may likely be of mechanical nature and sensed by the osteocytes, initiate bone remodeling at a specific site. The death of osteocytes and the resulting metabolic changes leading to a lack of silencers for bone turnover, like sclerostin, may govern this activation process. It is followed by a resorptive phase dominated by osteoclast-mediated degradation of the bone matrix, resulting in a resorption lacuna. The naked bone surface inside this lacuna is subsequently populated by mesenchymal cells immigrating from the neighboring bone surface; the cells start differentiating into osteoblasts and produce the new bone matrix (also termed *osteoid*). This matrix then mineralizes, and the bone again returns to its resting state. This entire bone remodeling process takes about 3 to 6 months. Adults continuously remodel their skeleton, and this process occurs even faster during childhood and adolescence. In adults, the entire skeleton is remodeled in 7 to 10 years, which indicates that we fully replace our skeleton several times during our lifetime. Most of the bone remodeling happens in the trabecular bone, which promotes the building of an optimal inner microstructure adapted to the individual mechanical demands. Trabecular bone is the leading structure in the vertebral bodies (constituting up to two-thirds of the bone substance) and in long bones such as the femurs (constituting about 50% of the bone substance).

Normal physiologic circumstances ensure a balance between bone formation and bone resorption to maintain skeletal homeostasis. This bone remodeling process requires a tight mutual regulation of bone resorption by osteoclasts and bone formation by osteoblasts, a phenomenon called *coupling*. Coupling is regulated on at least three different levels: (1) by a direct interaction between osteoblasts and osteoclasts; (2) by local interactions between the immune system and bone cells; and (3) by neuroendocrine systemic control of bone metabolism.

Direct Interactions Between Osteoblasts and Osteoclasts

A proper coupling between bone formation and bone destruction is essential to maintain bone integrity (Fig. 4.5). This coupling process involves two main mechanisms; the first is the expression of the essential pro-osteoclastogenic cytokines by the osteoblast lineage, and the second involves the ephrin ligand/ephrin receptor bidirectional signaling.[33,34] Preosteoblasts are the main pro-osteoclastogenic cells in normal physiologic conditions and provide the first level of coupling between bone formation and bone resorption. In response to Wnt signaling, osteoblasts slowly lose their supportive activity for osteoclasts when they mature toward more mineralizing cells and then become the bone-embedded osteocytes. They then secrete antiosteoclastogenic molecules such as OPG and the Wnt inhibitors sclerostin, dickkopf-1 (DKK1), and secreted frizzled-related protein 1 (SFRP1), which either block osteoclast differentiation (OPG) or also inhibit the further differentiation of osteoblasts. A second level of coupling involves the expression of ephrin ligands on the surface of osteoclast progenitors that can bind to ephrin receptors and activate their tyrosine kinase activity. Two ephrin ligands regulate bone remodeling. The first, ephrin-B2, binds to the receptor EphB4 on osteoblast progenitors, increasing their differentiation and stimulating bone formation. The second, ephrin-A2, acts in an autocrine manner by binding to the EphA2 receptor on the osteoclasts, which promotes their differentiation in a paracrine manner on the osteoblasts, thus inhibiting their differentiation.

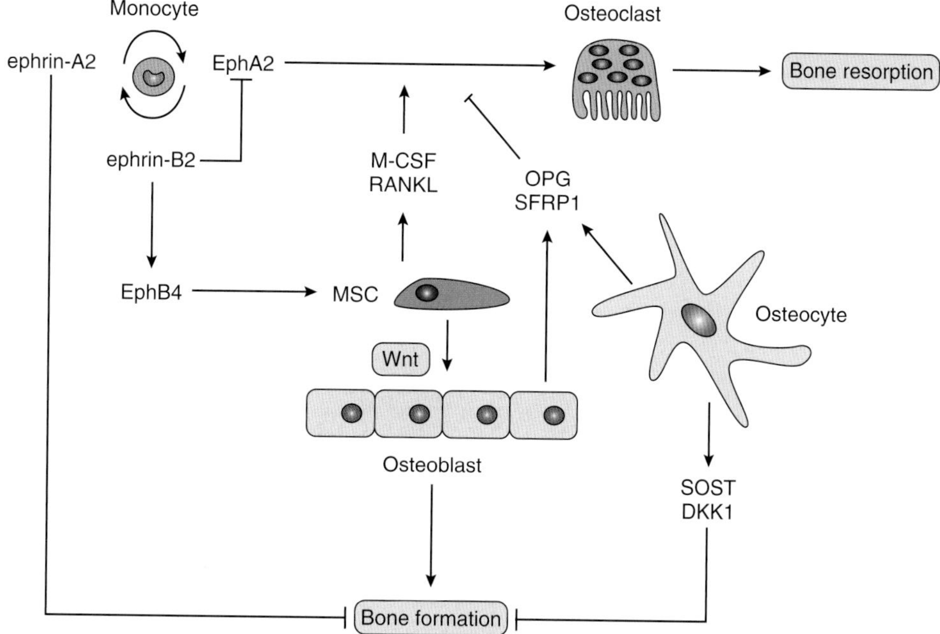

• **Fig. 4.5** Mesenchymal stem cells (MSCs) and preosteoblasts generated macrophage colony-stimulating factor (M-CSF) and receptor activator of nuclear factor-κB ligand (RANKL), supporting osteoclast differentiation. In contrast, mature osteoblasts suppress osteoclast differentiation by expression of osteoprotegerin (OPG) and secreted frizzled-related protein 1 (SFRP1). The ephrin-A2 system is an autocrine stimulator for osteoclasts and also blocks bone formation. In contrast, the binding of ephrin-B2 to its receptor ephrin-B4 stimulates osteoblast differentiation. Osteocyte-derived mediators such as sclerostin (SOST) and dickkopf-1 (DKK1) suppress bone formation by inhibiting the Wnt pathway.

Bone Remodeling by the Immune System

Aside from the reciprocal regulation of osteoblasts and osteoclasts, bone remodeling is also controlled by the immune system. Insights into the control of bone by the immune system have led to a new research field known as *osteoimmunology,* which has defined new pathways involved in immune regulation of post-menopausal osteoporosis and bone loss during inflammatory diseases.[35–37] Importantly, T cells influence the differentiation of osteoclasts, and hence activated T cells express RANKL, which not only stimulates osteoclastogenesis but also promotes the survival of dendritic cells.[38] RANKL expression has been found on various subsets of proliferative T cells (CD8 and CD4 and Th1 and Th2), as well as on FoxP3-expressing regulatory T cells (Tregs). Despite consistent expression of RANKL on various T cell lineages, individual T cells exert substantially different functions on the osteoclast, allowing a fine regulation of bone remodeling by the immune system. For instance, Th17 cells stimulate osteoclast differentiation via the production of IL-17.[30] Moreover, a subset of T cells expressing the IL-23 cytokine receptor is involved in bone remodeling, specifically at the insertion sites of the tendons.[39] In contrast, other T cell lineages express strong inhibitors of osteoclastogenesis, such as interferon (IFN)-γ in the case of Th1 cells, IL-4 in the case of Th2 cells, or cytotoxic T lymphocyte–associated antigen-4 (CTLA-4) in the case of regulatory T cells, and thereby provide protection from bone loss.[40–43]

Systemic Control of Bone Remodeling by Neuroendocrine Mechanisms

Bone remodeling is regulated not only locally but also by various systemic hormonal pathways, including the sex hormone and the growth hormone (GH)/IGF axes. In addition, two major systemic neuroendocrine regulators of bone homeostasis co-regulate bone, fat, and energy metabolism.[44,45] The two central players of this systemic loop seem to be osteocalcin and leptin. Osteocalcin is a hormone produced by mature osteoblasts and acts on the β cells of the pancreas to stimulate proliferation and thus insulin production in response to leptin.[45] In addition, osteocalcin can directly stimulate adipocytes to regulate insulin sensitivity. Leptin is a peptide hormone produced by adipocytes of the white adipose tissues. Leptin deficiency causes obesity and increased bone mass. Although the increased fat mass is certainly linked to the role of leptin in controlling appetite, the effect of leptin on bone and fat can be dissociated. Indeed, bone formation is negatively regulated by leptin through a hypothalamic pathway, the β-adrenergic sympathetic nervous system that mediates decreased osteoblast proliferation via the induction of clock genes in osteoblasts.[46,47] The question of how leptin regulates bone formation is debated. However, two potential hypothalamic relays have been identified. The first relay is the NPY peptide, a repressor of bone formation, which is silenced by leptin.[48] The second downstream modulator of leptin is neuromedin U, which inhibits clock gene expression and increases osteoblast proliferation.[49] These observations suggest that disturbance of the metabolic loops linking adipogenesis, osteogenesis, and insulin production have profound consequences on bone homeostasis.

Conclusion

Bone is continuously remodeled by bone-resorbing osteoclasts and bone-forming osteoblasts. This remodeling process allows the optimal adaptation of the bone architecture to individual demands and tight control of calcium homeostasis. Local factors control the bone remodeling process on the basis of osteoclast-osteoblast interactions, as well as by systemic immune and neuroendocrine factors controlling the bone-resorbing and bone-forming cells.

 The references for this chapter can also be found on ExpertConsult.com.

References

1. Filipowska J, Tomaszewski KA, Niedzwiedzki L, et al.: The role of vasculature in bone development, regeneration and proper systemic functioning, *Angiogenesis* 20:291–302, 2017.
2. Ramasamy SK, et al.: Blood flow controls bone vascular function and osteogenesis, *Nat Commun* 7:13601, 2016.
3. Ramasamy SK: Structure and functions of blood vessels and vascular niches in bone, *Stem Cells International* 2017:5046953, 2017.
4. Augustin HG, Koh GY: Organotypic vasculature: from descriptive heterogeneity to functional pathophysiology, *Science* 357, 2017.
5. Sivaraj KK, Adams RH: Blood vessel formation and function in bone, *Development* 143:2706–2715, 2016.
6. Grüneboom A, et al.: A network of trans-cortical capillaries as mainstay for blood circulation in long bones, *Nature Metabolism* 1:236–250, 2019.
7. Herisson F, et al.: Direct vascular channels connect skull bone marrow and the brain surface enabling myeloid cell migration, *Nat Neurosci* 21:1209–1217, 2018.
8. Kusumbe AP, Ramasamy SK, Adams RH: Coupling of angiogenesis and osteogenesis by a specific vessel subtype in bone, *Nature* 507:323–328, 2014.
9. Itkin T, et al.: Distinct bone marrow blood vessels differentially regulate haematopoiesis, *Nature* 532:323–328, 2016.
10. Hartmann C: Transcriptional networks controlling skeletal development, *Curr Opin Genet Dev* 19:437–443, 2009.
11. Karsenty G, Kronenberg HM, Settembre C: Genetic control of bone formation, *Ann Rev Cell Dev Biol* 25:629–648, 2009.
12. Takada I, Kouzmenko AP, Kato S: Wnt and PPARgamma signaling in osteoblastogenesis and adipogenesis, *Nat Rev Rheumatol* 5:442–447, 2009.
13. Battula VL, Chen Y, Cabreira Mda G, et al.: Connective tissue growth factor regulates adipocyte differentiation of mesenchymal stromal cells and facilitates leukemia bone marrow engraftment, *Blood* 122:357–366, 2013.
14. Day TF, Guo X, Garrett-Beal L, et al.: Wnt/beta-catenin signaling in mesenchymal progenitors controls osteoblast and chondrocyte differentiation during vertebrate skeletogenesis, *Dev Cell* 8:739–750, 2005.
15. Bonewald LF: The amazing osteocyte, *J Bone Miner Res* 26:229–238, 2011.
16. Van Bezooijen RL, Roelen BA, Visser A, et al.: Sclerostin is an osteocyte-expressed negative regulator of bone formation, but not a classical BMP antagonist, *J Exp Med* 199:805–814, 2004.
17. McClung MR, Grauer A, Boonen S, et al.: Romosozumab in postmenopausal women with low bone mineral density, *N Engl J Med* 370:412–420, 2014.
18. Balemans W, Ebeling M, Patel N, et al.: Increased bone density in sclerosteosis is due to the deficiency of a novel secreted protein (SOST), *Hum Mol Genet* 10:537–543, 2001.
19. Nakashima T, Hayashi M, Fukunaga T, et al.: Evidence for osteocyte regulation of bone homeostasis through RANKL expression, *Nat Med* 17:1231–1234, 2011.
20. Weinstein RS, Nicholas RW, Manolagas SC: Apoptosis of osteocytes in glucocorticoid-induced osteonecrosis of the hip, *J Clin Endocrinol Metab* 85(8):2907–2912, 2000.
21. Teitelbaum SL, Ross FP: Genetic regulation of osteoclast development and function, *Nat Rev Genet* 4:638–649, 2003.
22. Boyle WJ, Simonet WS, Lacey DL: Osteoclast differentiation and activation, *Nature* 423:337–342, 2003.
23. Wada T, Nakashima T, Hiroshi N, et al.: RANKL-RANK signaling in osteoclastogenesis and bone disease, *Trends Molec Med* 12:17–25, 2006.
24. Nakashima T, Hayashi M, Fukunaga T, et al.: Evidence for osteocyte regulation of bone homeostasis through RANKL expression, *Nat Med* 17:1231–1234, 2011.
25. Xiong J, Onal M, Jilka RL, et al.: Matrix-embedded cells control osteoclast formation, *Nat Med* 17:1235–1241, 2011.
26. Scholtysek C, Katzenbeisser J, Fu H, et al.: PPARβ/δ governs Wnt signaling and bone turnover, *Nat Med* 19:608–613, 2013.
27. McInnes IB, Schett G: Cytokines in the pathogenesis of rheumatoid arthritis, *Nat Rev Immunol* 7:429–442, 2007.
28. Lam J, Takeshita S, Barker JE, et al.: TNF-alpha induces osteoclastogenesis by direct stimulation of macrophages exposed to permissive levels of RANK ligand, *J Clin Invest* 106:1481–1488, 2000.
29. Zwerina J, Redlich K, Polzer K, et al.: TNF-induced structural joint damage is mediated by IL-1, *Proc Natl Acad Sci U S A* 104:11742–11747, 2007.
30. Sato K, Suematsu A, Okamoto K, et al.: Th17 functions as an osteoclastogenic helper T cell subset that links T cell activation and bone destruction, *J Exp Med* 203:2673–2682, 2006.
31. McClung MR, Lewiecki EM, Cohen SB, et al.: Denosumab in postmenopausal women with low bone mineral density, *N Engl J Med* 354:821–831, 2006.
32. Barrow AD, Raynal N, Andersen TL, et al.: OSCAR is a collagen receptor that costimulates osteoclastogenesis in DAP12-deficient humans and mice, *J Clin Invest* 121:3505–3516, 2011.
33. Matsuo K, Irie N: Osteoclast-osteoblast communication, *Arch Biochem Biophys* 473:201–209, 2008.
34. Zhao C, Irie N, Takada Y, et al.: Bidirectional ephrinB2-EphB4 signaling controls bone homeostasis, *Cell Metab* 4:111–121, 2006.
35. Lorenzo J, Horowitz M, Choi Y: Osteoimmunology: interactions of the bone and immune system, *Endocr Rev* 29:403–440, 2008.
36. David JP: Osteoimmunology: a view from the bone, *Adv Immunol* 95:149–165, 2007.
37. Takayanagi H: Osteoimmunology: shared mechanisms and crosstalk between the immune and bone systems, *Nat Rev Immunol* 7:292–304, 2007.
38. Wong BR, Josien R, Lee SY, et al.: TRANCE (tumor necrosis factor [TNF]-related activation-induced cytokine), a new TNF family member predominantly expressed in T cells, is a dendritic cell-specific survival factor, *J Exp Med* 186:2075–2080, 1997.
39. Sherlock JP, Joyce-Shaikh B, Turner SP, et al.: IL-23 induces spondyloarthropathy by acting on ROR-γt+ CD3+CD4-CD8- entheseal resident T cells, *Nat Med* 18:1069–1076, 2012.
40. Takayanagi H, Ogasawara K, Hida S, et al.: T-cell-mediated regulation of osteoclastogenesis by signalling cross-talk between RANKL and IFN-gamma, *Nature* 408:600–605, 2000.
41. Abu-Amer Y: IL-4 abrogates osteoclastogenesis through STAT6-dependent inhibition of NF-kappaB, *J Clin Invest* 107:1375–1385, 2001.
42. Zaiss MM, Axmann R, Zwerina J, et al.: Treg cells suppress osteoclast formation: a new link between the immune system and bone, *Arthritis Rheum* 56:4104–4112, 2007.
43. Bozec A, Zaiss MM, Kagwiria R, et al.: T cell costimulation molecules CD80/86 inhibit osteoclast differentiation by inducing the IDO/tryptophan pathway, *Sci Transl Med* 6:235ra60, 2014.
44. Rosen CJ: Bone remodeling, energy metabolism, and the molecular clock, *Cell Metab* 7:7–10, 2008.
45. Lee NK, Sowa H, Hinoi E, et al.: Endocrine regulation of energy metabolism by the skeleton, *Cell* 130:456–469, 2007.
46. Ducy P, Amling M, Takeda S, et al.: Leptin inhibits bone formation through a hypothalamic relay: a central control of bone mass, *Cell* 100:197–207, 2000.
47. Fu L, Patel MS, Bradley A, et al.: The molecular clock mediates leptin-regulated bone formation, *Cell* 122:803–815, 2005.
48. Baldock PA, Sainsbury A, Couzens M, et al.: Hypothalamic Y2 receptors regulate bone formation, *J Clin Invest* 109:915–921, 2002.
49. Sato S, Hanada R, Kimura A, et al.: Central control of bone remodeling by neuromedin U, *Nat Med* 13:1234–1240, 2007.

5

Muscle: Anatomy, Physiology, and Biochemistry

MARK S. MILLER, EDWARD P. DEBOLD, AND MICHAEL J. TOTH

KEY POINTS

- The structure and function of skeletal muscle and its neural recruitment pattern can change rapidly in response to activity level (i.e., plasticity).
- The smallest functional unit of muscle, the sarcomere, is composed of an almost crystalline array of filamentous proteins that convert metabolic energy into force and movement.
- Muscles are attached to the skeleton through collagenous tendons.
- Skeletal muscle contraction is controlled by the central nervous system through depolarization of specific efferent neurons called ***motor neurons.***
- Motor neurons innervate and depolarize muscle fibers through cholinergic synapses called ***neuromuscular junctions.***
- Afferent neurons provide the central nervous system with sensory information required for effective control of movement and posture.
- Force is transmitted to the exterior through two sets of protein cell adhesion complexes: integrins and dystroglycans.

Introduction

Approximately 660 skeletal muscles support and move the body under the control of the central nervous system (CNS). These muscles constitute up to 40% of adult human body mass. Most skeletal muscles are fastened by collagenous tendons across joints in the skeleton. The transduction of chemical energy into mechanical work by muscle cells leads to muscle shortening and consequent movement. A high degree of specialization in this tissue is evident from the intricate architecture and kinetics of intra-cellular membrane systems, the contractile proteins, and the molecular components that transmit force through the cell membrane to the extra-cellular matrix and tendons. Muscle cells normally exhibit wide variations in activity level and are able to adapt in size, isoenzyme composition, membrane organization, and energetics. In pathologic states, they often become deconditioned. These examples of plasticity can be surprisingly swift and extensive. This chapter outlines the structure and function of muscle and its relationship to associated connective tissue; this chapter will also introduce the basis for the highly adaptive response to altered functional demands and diseases.

Structure

Muscle Tissue

Parallel, aligned bundles of skeletal muscle fibers make up approximately 85% of the volume of muscle tissue and consist of a variety of signaling and contractile proteins (Table 5.1). Nerves, blood supply, and connective tissue structures that provide support, elasticity, and force transmission to the skeleton (see later discussion) constitute the remaining volume. Muscle fibers range in length from a few millimeters to 30 cm; in diameter, they range from 10 to 500 μm. Muscle fibers have a typical length of 3 cm and diameter of 100 μm. This elongated shape is determined by the organization of the contractile proteins that occupy most of the sarcoplasm. Each muscle has a limited range of shortening that is amplified into large motions by lever systems of the skeleton, usually operating at a mechanical disadvantage. Variations in geometric arrangements of the fibers—parallel, convergent (fan-shaped), pennate (feather-like), sphincter (circular), or fusiform (thick in the middle with tapered ends)—determine some of the mechanical properties. For example, a muscle with fibers aligned parallel to the force-generating axis will have more basic contractile units (i.e., sarcomeres, as discussed later) in series than a similarly sized pennate muscle, thus allowing the parallel muscle to contract more quickly, but with less force than the pennate muscle. Muscles designed for strength (e.g., gastrocnemius) are typically pennate, whereas those designed for speed (e.g., biceps) tend to have parallel fibers. Muscles are commonly arranged around joints as antagonistic pairs facilitating bidirectional motion. When one muscle (the agonist) contracts, another (its antagonist) is relaxed and passively extended. Their roles reverse to actively generate the opposite motion, unless the action occurs passively by the force of gravity.

An extensive network of areolar connective tissue, forming the endomysium, surrounds each muscle fiber. Fine nerve branches and small capillaries, which are necessary for the exchange of nutrients and metabolic waste products, penetrate this layer. The endomysium is continuous with the perimysium, a connective tissue network that ensheathes the *fasciculi* (or small parallel bundles of muscle fibers), *intrafusal fibers, larger nerves,* and *blood vessels.* The epimysium encompasses the entire muscle. All three layers of connective tissue contain mostly types I, III, IV, and V

TABLE 5.1 Signaling and Contractile Proteins of Skeletal Muscle

Protein	Molecular Weight (kDa)	Subunits (kDa)	Location	Function
Acetylcholine receptor	250	5 × 50	Postsynaptic membrane of neuromuscular junction	Neuromuscular signal transmission
Annexins	38	—	F-actin–binding protein	Membrane repair
Dihydropyridine receptor	380	1 × 160 1 × 130 1 × 60 1 × 30	T-tubule membrane	Voltage sensor
Dysferlin	230	—	Periphery of myofibers	Membrane repair
Ryanodine receptor	1800	4 × 450	Terminal cisternae of SR	SR Ca^{2+} release channel
Ca^{2+} ATPase	110	—	Longitudinal SR	Uptake of Ca^{2+} into the SR
Calsequestrin	63	—	Lumen of SR terminal cisternae	Binding and storage of Ca^{2+}
Troponin	70	1 × 18 1 × 21 1 × 31	Thin filament	Regulation of contraction
Tropomyosin	70	2 × 35	Thin filament	Regulation of contraction
Myosin	510	2 × 220 2 × 15 2 × 20	Thick filament	Chemomechanical energy transduction
Actin	42	—	Thin filament	Chemomechanical energy transduction
MM creatine phosphokinase	40	—	M line	ATP buffer, structural protein
α-Actinin	190	2 × 95	Z line	Structural protein
Titin	3000	—	From Z line to M line	Structural protein
Nebulin	600	—	Thin filaments, in the I band	Structural protein
Dystrophin	400	—	Sub-sarcolemma	Structural integrity of sarcolemma

ATP, Adenosine triphosphate; *ATPase*, adenosine triphosphatase; *SR*, sarcoplasmic reticulum.

collagen, with types IV and V predominating in the basement membranes surrounding each skeletal muscle fiber. The $\alpha 1_2 \alpha 2$-chain composition of the collagen IV isoform is the most prevalent and provides the mechanical stability and flexibility of the basil lamina.[1,2] The perimysium and endomysium merge at the junction between muscle fibers and tendons, aponeuroses, and fasciae. These layers give the attachment sites great tensile strength and distribute axial force into shear forces over a larger surface area.

Fiber Types

Muscles adapt to their specific functions. In any given muscle, part of this adaptation arises from its composition and organization of fiber types. Human skeletal muscle fibers can be classified according to their myosin heavy chain (MHC) isoform (I, IIA, or IIX). MHC molecules break down adenosine triphosphate (ATP) to produce the energy necessary for muscle contraction. The rate of ATP breakdown, or the adenosine triphosphatase (ATPase) rate, of the MHC isoforms is I < IIA < IIX, leading to contractions that are relatively slow in MHC I fibers, fast in MHC IIA fibers, and very fast in MHC IIX fibers. ATP synthesis primarily occurs through aerobic respiration (i.e., oxygen is required) in MHC I (slow oxidative) fibers. ATP synthesis is aided by the nature of MHC I fibers in that they have more mitochondria, an increased capillary blood supply, and more myoglobin compared with MHC IIX (fast glycolytic) fibers, which use anaerobic respiration (i.e., oxygen is not required) to restore their ATP levels. MHC I fibers produce less power than MHC IIX fibers but are more resistant to fatigue. MHC IIA (fast oxidative-glycolytic) fibers can use both aerobic and anaerobic respiration and fall in between MHC I and IIX fibers in terms of mitochondria, blood supply, myoglobin, power output, and fatigability. Although most human skeletal muscles contain a mixture of fiber types, MHC I and IIA fibers are most prevalent, with pure MHC IIX fibers being relatively rare. Notably, individual fibers can contain a mixture of MHC isoforms, leading to six different fiber types in humans ("pure": MHC I, IIA, and IIX; "mixed": MHC I/IIA, IIA/IIX, and I/IIA/IIX), which allows for a wide range of contractile properties. A list of various attributes of MHC isoforms can be found in Table 5.2.

TABLE 5.2 Classification of Muscle Fiber Types by Myosin Heavy Chain Isoform

General Features	MHC I	MHC IIA	MHC IIX
Mitochondria	Many	Intermediate	Few
Capillary blood supply	Extensive	Moderate	Moderate
SR membrane	Sparse	Extensive	Extensive
Z line	Wide	Moderate	Narrow
Protein Isoforms			
Myosin essential light chain	Slow and fast	Fast	Fast
Myosin regulatory light chain	Slow and fast	Fast	Fast
Myosin binding protein–C	Slow	Fast	Fast
Thin filament regulatory proteins	Slow	Fast	Fast
Mechanical Properties			
SR calcium ATPase rate	Slow	Fast	Fast
Actomyosin ATPase rate	Slow	Fast	Very fast
Contraction time	Slow	Fast	Very fast
Shortening velocity	Slow	Fast	Very fast
Power production	Low	Moderate	High
Resistance to fatigue	High	Moderate	Low
Metabolic Profile			
Oxidative capacity	High	Moderate	Low
Glycolytic capacity	Moderate	High	High
Glycogen	Low	High	High
Myoglobin	High	Moderate	Low

ATPase, Adenosine triphosphatase; *MHC*, myosin heavy chain; *SR*, sarcoplasmic reticulum.

During development, fiber-type specificity may be partially determined before innervation.[3] Although the biologic events and signals responsible for designating functional specialization in muscle fibers are not fully understood, classic cross-innervation experiments demonstrated that innervation can dynamically specify and modify the type of muscle fiber.[4] After cross-innervation, the functional and histologic properties listed in Table 5.2 shift toward the target fiber type over a few weeks' time, indicating the ability of muscles to adapt and remodel in accordance with the pattern of neuronal activity.

Events During Muscle Contraction

Neural Control

Voluntary control of muscle activation is a complex process. Afferent neurons emanating from sensory organs, such as cutaneous mechanoreceptors and thermoreceptors, pain receptors, joint receptors, and tendon organ and muscle spindles, provide the CNS with stimuli in the form of action potentials that, with or without additional stimuli from the brain, provide the necessary information for feedback control of effector organs via efferent neurons.[5] Efferent neurons are specifically called *motor neurons* if their axons innervate muscle. Many times, more afferent than efferent neurons afford effective feedback control of movement and posture. The afferent and efferent neurons are accompanied by Schwann cells, which are glial cells residing in the peripheral nervous system.[6] Neurons are termed *myelinated* if Schwann cells wrap around the axon at regularly spaced intervals. The points of bare axon between these Schwann cells are called *nodes of Ranvier*. Myelination enhances the velocity of action potential propagation by compelling a saltatory conduction of the action potential between neighboring nodes. Schwann cells may also fully, or nearly fully, cover the axon, thus rendering the neuron unmyelinated and relatively slow in action potential propagation. Three groups of myelinated motor neurons (α, β, and γ) are distinguished by diameter, propagation velocity, and target fiber type. Skeletal muscle fibers typically are innervated at several neuromuscular junctions along their length by branches of an α motoneuron (the largest and fastest) or a β motoneuron (Fig. 5.1). Muscle spindles are innervated by β or γ motoneurons, in addition to the afferent system, for sensing muscle length and force. A single motor neuron and the muscle fibers it innervates constitute a motor unit. When a motor neuron is excited, all fibers in the motor unit are triggered to contract simultaneously. A motor unit responsible for fine movement contains few muscle fibers, but motor units for gross movement generally contain many fibers. The level of muscle activation is controlled from the CNS by the number of motor units recruited and the stimulus rate.[7] Stimulus rate can be so infrequent as to elicit single muscle twitches, such as occur with the monosynaptic stretch reflex involving patellar tendon stretch and quadriceps activation. Conversely, the stimulus rate can be so frequent that individual twitches effectively fuse, causing nearly continuous activation of muscle force.[8]

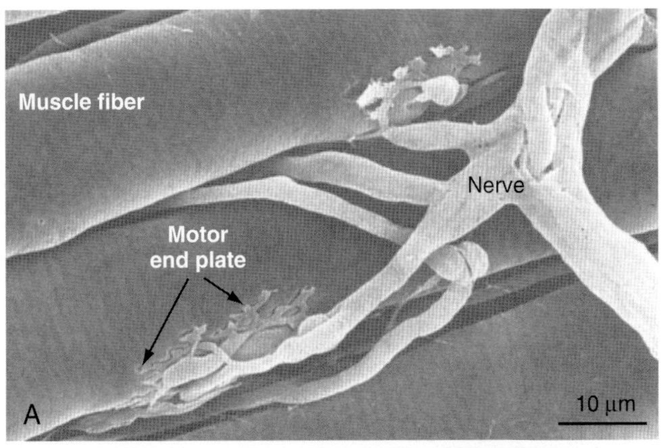

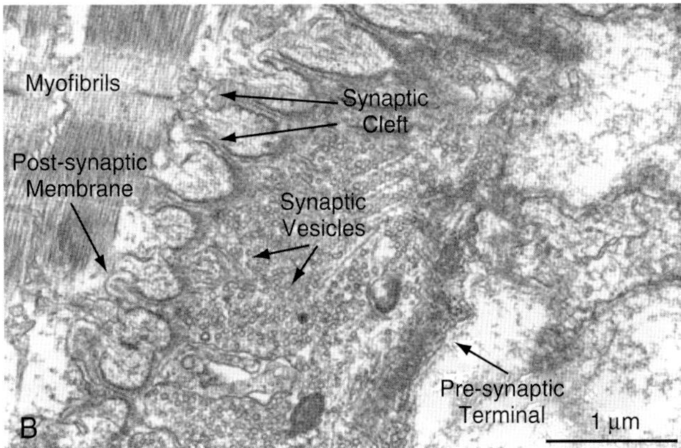

• **Fig. 5.1** Neuromuscular junction. (A) Scanning electron micrograph of an α motoneuron innervating several muscle fibers in its motor unit. Calibration bar = 10 μm. (B) Transmission electron micrograph. Calibration bar = 1 μm. (A, From Bloom W, Fawcett DW: *A textbook of histology*, ed 10. Philadelphia, WB Saunders, 1975. B, Courtesy Dr. Clara Franzini-Armstrong, University of Pennsylvania, Philadelphia.)

Neuromuscular Transmission

At the neuromuscular junction, the axon tapers, loses its myelin sheath, and ends as a pre-synaptic terminal crowded with vesicles that contain the neurotransmitter acetylcholine. The postsynaptic membrane of the muscle is indented into folds that increase its surface area and the number of nicotinic acetylcholine receptors bound therein (see Fig. 5.1). The junctional cleft is a 20 to 40 nm-wide space between the pre-synaptic and postsynaptic membranes.[9] When the motor neuron action potential reaches the pre-synaptic terminal, local voltage-gated Ca^{2+} channels open and extra-cellular Ca^{2+} streams into the terminal. Within milliseconds of Ca^{2+} influx, the acetylcholine-loaded vesicles fuse with the pre-neurosynaptic membrane.[10] Exocytosed acetylcholine rapidly diffuses across the junctional cleft and binds to the nicotinic acetylcholine receptors, which, in turn, open Na^+ and K^+ channels of the postneurosynaptic membrane. The membrane is locally depolarized, causing the initiation of an action potential which propagates along the muscle membrane (sarcolemma) at velocities up to 5 m/sec.

Excitation-Contraction Coupling

A network of tubules invaginate the sarcolemma and run deep into the muscle fiber. This transverse tubule network (T-tubules) pervades the fiber at regular intervals, coinciding with sarcomere boundaries along the length of the muscle, and surrounds the contractile apparatus with connected longitudinal and lateral segments (Fig. 5.2). The lumen of this network is open to the extracellular space and contains high Na^+ and low K^+ concentrations of interstitial fluid.[11] Action potentials at the surface membrane invade the entire T-tubular system. A specialized type of endoplasmic reticulum forms an entirely intra-cellular membrane system termed the *sarcoplasmic reticulum* (SR). Prevalent structures containing a T-tubule flanked by two terminal cisternae of the SR to form junctional complexes are termed *triads* (see Fig. 5.2). Terminal cisternae contain oligomers of the Ca^{2+}-binding protein calsequestrin that provide the fiber with an internal reservoir of calcium ions. Ca^{2+} channels, termed *dihydropyridine receptors* (DHPRs), are localized in the T-tubule membranes facing the cytoplasmic

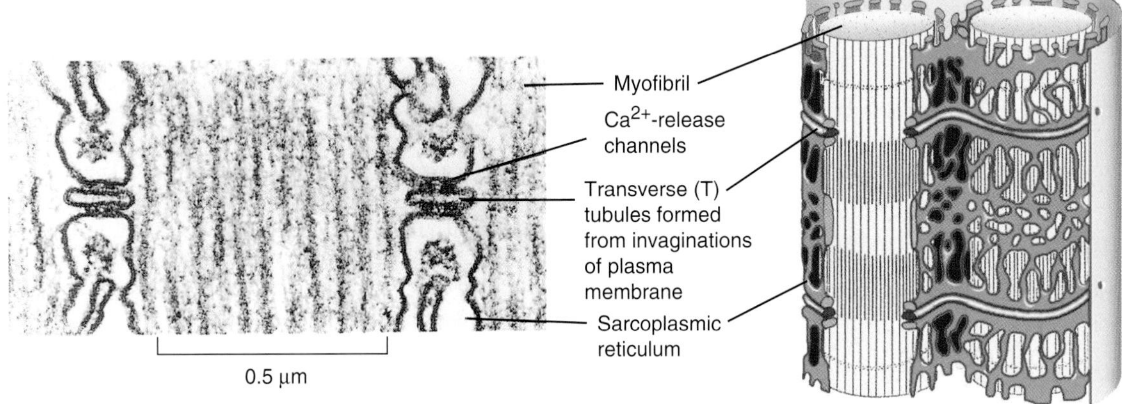

• **Fig. 5.2** Membrane systems that relay the excitation signal from the sarcolemma to the cell interior. In the electron micrograph, two T-tubules are cut in cross-section. Electron densities spanning the gap between T-tubules and sarcoplasmic reticulum membranes are the ryanodine receptors, which are channels that release calcium into the myoplasm. (From Alberts B, Bray D, Lewish J, et al.: *Molecular biology of the cell*, ed 2. New York, Garland Publishers, 1989. Micrograph courtesy Dr. Clara Franzini-Armstrong, University of Pennsylvania, Philadelphia.)

domain of SR Ca^{2+} release channels, also called *ryanodine receptors* (RyRs), in the terminal cisternae membranes.[12] These membrane proteins are further characterized in Table 5.1.

When an action potential depolarizes the T-tubular membrane, the DHPRs, primarily voltage sensors in skeletal muscle, transfer a signal from the T-tubules to the RyRs by direct interprotein coupling. Ca^{2+} is then released cooperatively through the RyRs from the SR into the myoplasm, where it activates the contractile machinery.[13] This sequence of events is termed *excitation-contraction coupling.*

Mutations in the α subunit of the DHPR in dysgenic mice lead to paralysis, because in these mutants, depolarization of the skeletal muscle membrane does not initiate release of Ca^{2+} from the SR. Excitation-contraction coupling can be restored in cultured cells from these mice by transfection with complementary DNA encoding for the DHPR,[14] and transfections using chimeric constructs[15] have pinpointed the domain within the DHPR that specifies skeletal- or cardiac-type excitation-contraction coupling.[16] Isoforms of the RyRs also help determine the characteristics of coupling between T-tubules and the SR.[17] Channelopathies in human skeletal and heart muscle have been linked to DHPR mutations.[18,19] Human malignant hyperthermia occurs in people with mutant RyRs that become trapped in the open state after exposure to halothane anesthetic agents.[20]

Contractile Apparatus

The specific locations and functions of the contractile proteins are listed in Table 5.1. Myofibrils (Fig. 5.3D) are long, 1 μm diameter cylindrical organelles that contain the contractile protein arrays responsible for work production, generation of force, and shortening. Each myofibril is a column of sarcomeres, the basic contractile units, that are approximately 2.5 μm in length and are delimited by Z lines (Fig. 5.3D and E) containing the densely packed structural protein α-actinin. The contractile and structural proteins within each sarcomere form a highly ordered, nearly crystalline lattice of interdigitating thick and thin myofilaments[21] (Fig. 5.3E, I, and J). Myofilaments are remarkably uniform in both length and lateral registration, even during contraction,[22] resulting in the cross-striated histologic appearance of skeletal and cardiac muscles. This highly periodic organization allows biophysical studies of muscle by sophisticated structural[21] and spectroscopic techniques.[23,24]

Thick filaments (1.6 μm long) that contain the motor protein myosin are located in the center of the sarcomere in the optically anisotropic A band (Fig. 5.3D). These thick filaments are organized into a hexagonal lattice stabilized by M protein[25] and muscle-specific creatine phosphokinase[26] in the M line (Fig. 5.3D and E). Myosin (Fig. 5.3K) is a highly asymmetric 470 kDa protein containing two 120 kDa globular NH_2-terminal heads, termed *cross-bridges* or *subfragment-1 (S1)* (Fig. 5.3L), and an α-helical coiled-coil rod that can be split enzymatically into two pieces, *subfragment-2* (S2) and light meromyosin (Fig. 5.3K). Two light chains, essential and regulatory, ranging from 15 to 22 kDa, are associated with the heavy chain in each S1 (Fig. 5.3L). The rod portions of approximately 300 myosin molecules polymerize in a three-stranded helix to form the backbone of each thick filament (Fig. 5.3J). The cross-bridges that protrude from these backbones contain ATPase and actin-binding sites responsible for the conversion of chemical energy into mechanical work. Besides their role in muscle contraction, at least 20 classes of nonmuscle myosins accomplish diverse tasks in cell motility such as chemotaxis, cytokinesis, pinocytosis, targeted vesicle transport, and signal transduction.[27] Thus, myosin is the target for mutations that lead to a number of inherited muscle and neurologic diseases.[28,29]

Thin filaments (Fig. 5.3I) are double-stranded helical polymers of actin that extend 1.1 μm from each side of the Z line and occupy the optically isotropic I band (Fig. 5.3D and E). A regulatory complex containing one tropomyosin molecule and three troponin subunits (TnC, TnT, and TnI) is associated with each successive group of seven actin monomers along the thin filament (Fig. 5.3I).[21] In the region where the thick and thin filaments overlap, the thin filaments are positioned within the hexagonal lattice equidistant from three thick filaments (Fig. 5.3F). Both sets of filaments are polarized. In an active muscle, an interaction between the two filaments causes a concerted translation of the thin filaments toward the M line that shortens the sarcomere; thus, the muscle fiber and the entire muscle shorten (Fig. 5.3A through D). Actin is ubiquitous in the cytoskeleton of eukaryotic cells and, like myosin, actin fulfills many roles in determining cell shapes and motions.[30,31] Control of the actin cytoskeleton and diseases due to mutations in actin-binding proteins are being intensively investigated.[32]

Two of the largest identified muscle proteins, titin and nebulin, function in assembly and maintenance of the sarcomeric structure. Individual titin molecules (~3000 kDa) are associated with the thick filament and extend from the M line to the Z line.[33] Titin contains repeating fibronectin-like immunoglobulin and unusual proline-rich domains that confer molecular elasticity on the resting sarcomere.[34] Nebulin (~800 kDa) is associated with the Z line and thin filaments.[33] Protein connections from the contractile apparatus through the sarcolemma to the extra-cellular matrix are described later in this chapter. The cytoskeleton of muscle fibers also contains cytoplasmic actin, microtubules, and intermediate filaments.[35]

Force Generation and Shortening

At rest, the thin filament regulatory proteins, troponin and tropomyosin, inhibit contraction by preventing myosin-actin strong-binding (Fig. 5.3I). During a twitch, Ca^{2+} released from the SR binds to TnC, relieving this inhibition and thus allowing cross-bridges to attach to actin. A contraction results from cyclic interaction between actin and myosin (the cross-bridge cycle) that produces a relative sliding force between thin and thick filaments,[36] which is ultimately powered by the energy derived from the hydrolysis of ATP to adenosine diphosphate (ADP) and inorganic phosphate (P_i).

A simplified model of the chemomechanical events in the cross-bridge cycle is illustrated in Fig. 5.4. Motor proteins, including myosin, can now be studied by single-molecule biophysical techniques, which provide unprecedented detail on their dynamics.[37] When Ca^{2+} is present, a complex of myosin, ADP, and P_i attaches to the thin filament (step a), and structural change within the myosin S1 initiates force production and the release of P_i (steps b and c).[38,39] The conformational change in the cross-bridge that leads to generation of force is a tilting motion of the light chain region.[40,41] Filament sliding that leads to shortening of the sarcomere occurs during a strain-dependent transition between two ADP states (step d). After ADP is released (step e), ATP binds to the active site and dissociates myosin from actin (step f). Myosin then hydrolyzes ATP (step g) to form the ternary myosin–ADP-P_i complex, which can reattach to actin for the next cycle.

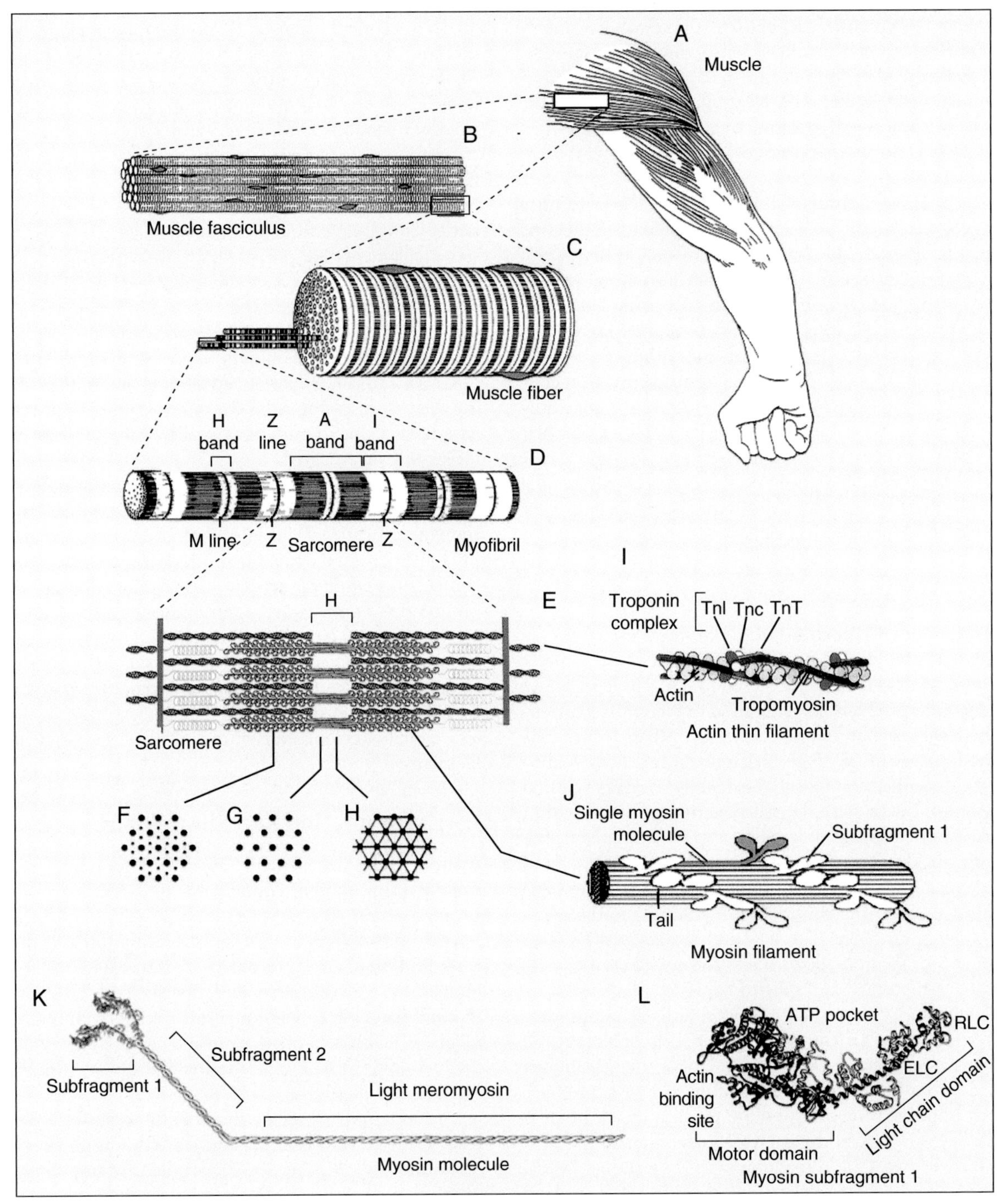

• **Fig. 5.3** Components of the contractile apparatus at successively increasing magnification from the whole muscle (A through C) to the molecular level (I through L). The myofibril (D) shows the banding pattern created by the lateral alignment of myofilaments (I and J) within the sarcomeres (D and E). Diagrams (F) through (H) show the cross-sectional structure of the filament lattice at various points within the sarcomere. Myosin is shown at the single two-headed molecule level (K), and the crystal structure of the globular motor domain is shown (L and subfragment 1) with the essential and regulatory light chains. *ATP,* Adenosine triphosphate; *ELC,* essential light chain; *RLC,* regulatory light chain. (A through K, Modified from Bloom W, Fawcett DW: *A textbook of histology*, ed 11. Philadelphia, WB Saunders, 1986; and L from Rayment I, Rypniewski WR, Schmidt-Base K, et al.: Three-dimensional structure of myosin subfragment-1: a molecular motor. *Science* 261:50–58, 1993.)

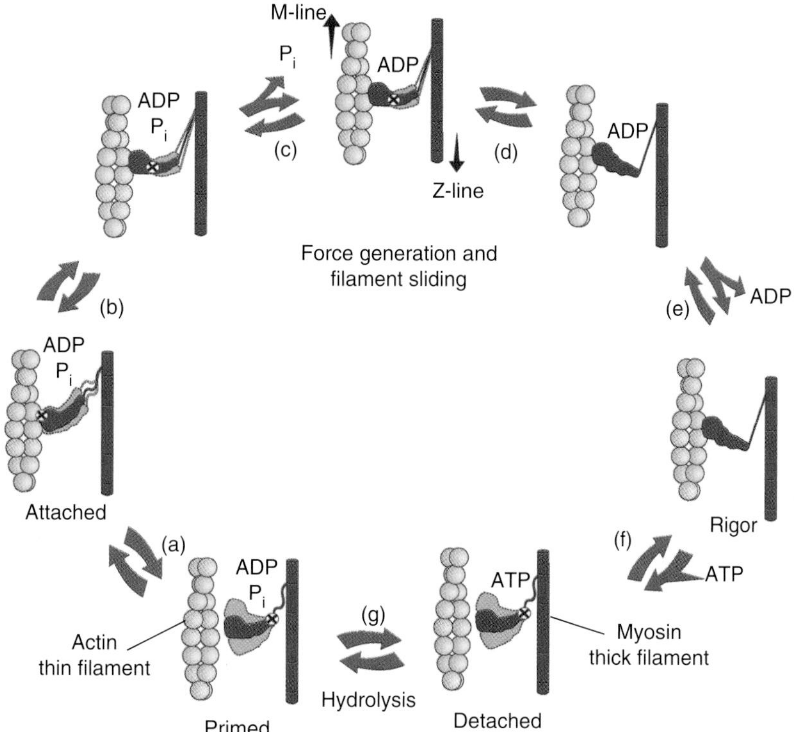

• **Fig. 5.4** The actomyosin cross-bridge cycle. Myosin molecules normally have two globular head regions (cross-bridges), but for clarity only one is shown. The ⊗ within the globular domain of myosin represents a hinge point with maximum flexibility. Each head binds with two actin monomers. The sequence of reactions consists of attachment (a); the force-generating transition (b); P_i release (c); force generation and filament sliding (d); ADP release (e); ATP binding and detachment (f); and ATP hydrolysis (g). The *lighter shaded* heads near detached and force-generating myosin heads indicate mobility of cross-bridges in these states. *ADP,* Adenosine diphosphate; *ATP,* adenosine triphosphate; *P_i,* inorganic phosphate.

If the mechanical load on the muscle is high, the contractile apparatus produces a force without changing length (an isometric contraction). If the load is moderate, the thin filaments slide actively toward the center of the sarcomere, resulting in shortening of the entire muscle. The width of the muscle increases during shortening, so the volume stays constant. Work production (concomitant force and sliding) is associated with an increase in the ATPase rate. Thermodynamic efficiency (mechanical power divided by energy liberated by ATPase activity) approaches 50%.[42] This is a remarkable figure given that manufactured combustion engines seldom achieve efficiencies greater than 20%.

Relaxation

The twitch is terminated by reversal of all steps in the activation. Ca^{2+} released from the SR is taken up again by Ca^{2+}-ATPase pumps located in longitudinal membranes of the SR. The myoplasmic Ca^{2+} concentration then decreases; then, Ca^{2+} dissociates from TnC, which deactivates the thin filament. When the number of attached cross-bridges declines below a certain threshold, tropomyosin inhibits further cross-bridge attachment, and tension declines to the resting level. Ca^{2+} diffuses within the longitudinal SR to calsequestrin sites in the terminal cisternae, ready to be released in the next twitch. Myosin continues to hydrolyze ATP at a low rate in relaxed muscle, which accounts for a sizable proportion of basal metabolism.

Transmission of Force to the Exterior

Cell-Matrix Adhesions

The muscle cell is connected to the basal lamina along its entire surface. Several transmembrane macromolecular complexes link the myofibrils and actin cytoskeleton to laminins and collagen in the extra-cellular matrix. Attachment complexes for muscle, analogous to the focal adhesions of motile and epithelial cells and to the adhesion plaques and intercalated disks in cardiac muscle, contain filamentous actin, vinculin, talin, and integrin (primarily the $\alpha7\beta1$ isoform), which is the transmembrane link to laminin (Fig. 5.5). In muscle, the main laminin isoforms are laminin-2 ($\alpha2\beta1\gamma1$) and laminin-4 ($\alpha2\beta2\gamma1$). In addition to providing mechanical coupling between the cytoskeleton and the extra-cellular matrix, the laminin-integrin system may provide a signaling pathway to regulate localized protein expression.[43] Defects in the expression of many of the cytoskeletal proteins lead to various forms of muscular dystrophy, as summarized in Table 5.3.[44]

A specialized linkage between the cytoskeleton and the basal lamina in muscle, complementary to the integrin focal adhesion system, is the dystrophin-glycoprotein complex (see Fig. 5.5). Dystrophin, a 427 kDa peripheral cytoskeletal protein, is postulated to function as a mechanical link between the cytoskeleton and the cell membrane or as a shock absorber, or to contribute mechanical strength to the membrane. Its absence or truncation causes Duchenne and Becker muscular dystrophies.[45]

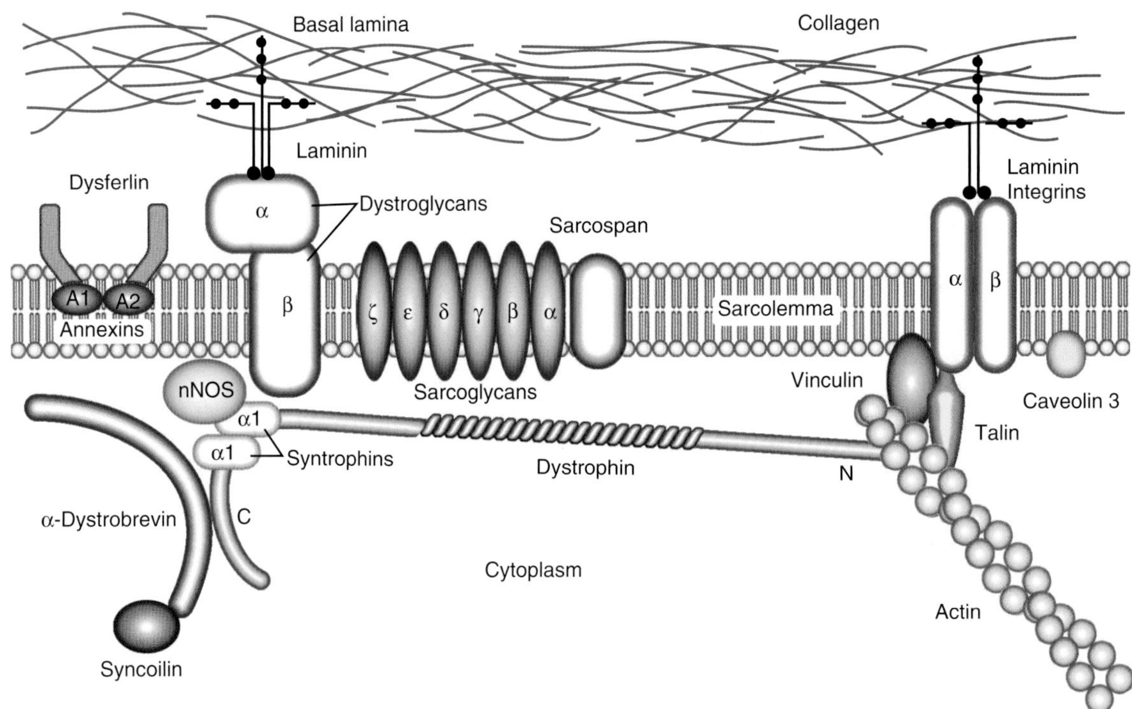

• **Fig. 5.5** Connections between the muscle cytoskeleton and the extra-cellular matrix. Actin is linked through integrins to the matrix, as in many cell types. Dystrophin forms an extra link through the dystroglycan-sarcoglycan complex of glycosylated proteins. The helical section of dystrophin is homologous to spectrin and may form homodimers or oligomers. Dystrophin links two intricate systems linking the sarcolemma to the basal lamina. The carboxy (COOH)-terminus of dystrophin is associated with the sarcoglycans, dystroglycans, dystrobrevin, syncoilin, neuronal nitric oxide synthase (nNOS), and the syntrophins. The NH_3-terminus links actin, vinculin, and the integrins with laminin and the basil lamina. These two adhesion systems provide a supportive substructure to maintain the integrity of the sarcolemma. The annexins and dysferlin have a role in muscle regeneration.

The N-terminus of dystrophin binds to actin via a region with sequence homology to the actin-binding domain of α-actinin. This end of the dystrophin molecule may be linked to the basal lamina via the same proteins described previously for focal adhesion-like complexes (see Fig. 5.5). The C-terminus binds to a transmembrane dystroglycan-sarcoglycan complex; in turn, this binds to the laminins. Muscular dystrophies of varied severity are associated with loss of these components (see Table 5.3).[46] Dystroglycans are also required for early embryonic development of muscle, possibly organizing laminin localization and assembly.[47,48] Utrophin, a smaller dystrophin-related protein (395 kDa), may also link the actin cytoskeleton to the dystroglycans, especially near the neuromuscular junction and in nonmuscle cells. Overexpression of this protein or truncated dystrophin constructs are promising avenues for gene therapy in people with Duchenne muscular dystrophy.[49] The unusual intricacy of cell-matrix connection systems in muscle may relate to the high forces generated during contraction.

Myotendinous Junction

The force of muscle contraction is transmitted to the skeleton via the tendons, which are composed of collagens type I and III, blood vessels, lymphatic ducts, and fibroblasts. At the ends of the muscle fibers, myofibrils are separated by invaginations of sarcolemma filled with long bundles of collagen arising from the tendon. These membrane folds increase the surface area for bearing the mechanical load by approximately 30-fold. Instead of terminating in the Z disks, actin filaments insert into a subsarcolemmal matrix containing α-actinin, vinculin, talin, and integrin. The force is transmitted through laminin to the collagen of the tendon.

Energetics

Metabolic pathways in muscle cells are specialized for the variable and at times extreme rates of ATP splitting by the contractile apparatus and membrane ionic pumps. Among the dozens of metabolic enzymes present, only the most important ones with regard to normal muscle function are mentioned here.

Buffering of Adenosine Triphosphate Concentration

The ATP content (~8 mM) is sufficient for only a few seconds of contraction, and thus rapid and effective buffering of ATP during contraction is essential for the maintenance of activity. ADP formed by the hydrolysis of ATP is rephosphorylated by transfer of a phosphate group from creatine phosphate (20 mM in a resting cell) by creatine phosphokinase located within the M line of the sarcomere (in the myoplasm) and between the inner and outer membranes of the mitochondria. Adenylate kinase, known in muscle as *myokinase,* catalyzes the transfer of a phosphate group between two ADP molecules, forming ATP and adenosine monophosphate (AMP). The by-products of the rapid enzymatic reactions that maintain ATP concentration are, therefore, creatine, P_i, and AMP. Some of the AMP is converted

TABLE 5.3 **Classification of Muscular Dystrophies**

Disease	Genetic Locus	Inheritance	Protein	Outcome
Duchenne/Becker		XR	Dystrophin	Lethal
Emery-Dreifuss		XR	Emerin, lamins A and C	40% lethality
Limb-Girdle Muscular Dystrophies				
LGMD 1A	5q31	AD	Myotilin	With LGMD, less-severe forms can emerge during the first three decades, leading to loss of ambulation after 30 yr of age; the most severe forms start at 3–5 yr of age and progress rapidly
LGMD 1B	1q11-q21	AD	Laminin A/C	
LGMD 1C	3p35	AD	Caveolin	
LGMD 1D	6q23	AD	—	
LGMD 1E	7q	AD	—	
LGMD 1F	7q32	AD	—	
LGMD 1G	4p21	AD	—	
LGMD 2A	15q15.1-q21.1	AR	Calpain 3	
LGMD 2B	2p13	AR	Dysferlin	
LGMD 2C	13q12	AR	γ-Sarcoglycan	
LGMD 2D	17q12-q21.33	AR	α-Sarcoglycan	
LGMD 2E	4q12	AR	β-Sarcoglycan	
LGMD 2F	5q33-q34	AR	δ-Sarcoglycan	
LGMD 2G	17q11-q12	AR	Telethonin	
LGMD 2H	9q31-q34.1	AR	E3-Ubiquitin ligase (TRIM32)	
LGMD 2I	19q13.3	AR	Fukutin-related protein	
LGMD 2J	2q24.3	AR	Titin	
LGMD 2K	9q34	AR	Protein O-mannosyltransferase	
CMDs With CNS Involvement				
Fukuyama CMD	9q31	AR	Fukutin	LE, 11–16 yr
Walker-Warburg CMD	1p32	AR	O-Mannosyltransferase	LE, <3 yr
Muscle-eye-brain CMD	1p32-34	AR	O-MNAGAT	LE, 10–30 yr
CMDs Without CNS Involvement				
Merosin-deficient classic type	6q2	AR	Merosin (laminin A_2)	Many patients never walk; others have an LGMD pattern
Merosin-positive classic type	4p16.3	AR	Selenoprotein N1, collagen VI α_2	Course stabilizes in late childhood; many continue to walk into adulthood
Integrin-deficient CMD	12q13	AR	Integrin α7	Presents early in infancy with hypotonia and delayed milestones
Other Dystrophies				
Facioscapulohumeral	4q35	AD	—	20% wheelchair bound
Oculopharyngeal	14q11.2-q13	AD/AR	Polyadenylate binding protein nuclear 1	Onset: ~48 yr, 100% symptomatic by age 70 yr
Myotonic dystrophy	19q13.3	AD	DMPK, CCHC-type zinc finger and CNBP	Onset: 50% show signs by age 20 yr; variable severity

AD, Autosomal dominant; *AR*, autosomal recessive; *CCHC*, cysteine and histidine amino acid sequence in this class of zinc finger; *CMD*, congenital muscular dystrophy; *CNBP*, cellular nucleic acid–binding protein; *CNS*, central nervous system; *DMPK*, dystrophia myotonica-protein kinase; *LE*, life expectancy; *LGMD*, limb-girdle muscular dystrophy; *O-MNAGAT*, O-mannose β-1,2-*N*-acetylglucosaminyl transferase; *XR*, X chromosome–related.

to inosine monophosphate by adenylate deaminase. Researchers have recently found that electrical conduction[50] drives the distribution of ATP throughout the highly connected mitochondria; this finding stands in contrast to the concept of facilitated diffusion as the driving force of ATP distribution.

Glycolysis

Muscles use some combination of glucose and fatty acids (and ketone bodies in some situations) as fuel, depending on their metabolic state (fasted vs. fed) and activity status (rested vs. exercise). The muscle compartment contains most of the body storage of glycogen, which is converted to glucose-6-phosphate for local use. Muscle fibers lack glucose-6-phosphatase and, thus, do not export glucose. During intense activity, especially in anaerobic conditions, the rate of glycolysis and the production of pyruvate exceed the rate of pyruvate consumption by the citric acid cycle. Excess pyruvate is reduced to lactate by lactate dehydrogenase, which has tissue-specific isoforms. The lactate-dehydrogenase reaction also produces nicotinamide adenine dinucleotide (NAD^+), which is necessary for glycolysis; however, lactate is not useful within the muscle. Lactate is freely permeable through the sarcolemma and can be transported through the blood to the liver, where it is converted back to pyruvate and then to glucose for use by other tissues. This sequence of steps, termed the *Cori cycle,* transfers some of the high metabolic load to the liver and "buys time" until oxidative metabolism is available.

Oxidative Phosphorylation

In aerobic conditions, pyruvate enters the mitochondria, where it is converted to acetyl-coenzyme A (CoA). Acetyl-CoA can enter the tricarboxylic acid cycle, where it is oxidized to carbon dioxide and water, generating reduced NAD (NADH). Fatty acids also contribute to the mitochondrial acetyl-CoA pool through the process of beta-oxidation. The reducing equivalents NADH and reduced form of flavin adenine dinucleotide ($FADH_2$) are subsequently oxidized by the electron transport chain, and an H^+ gradient is established across the mitochondrial membrane. This gradient is used to catalyze the phosphorylation of ADP to ATP by the mitochondrial ATP synthase. For example, when glycolysis and oxidative phosphorylation are combined, up to 38 ATP molecules can be generated by the oxidation of each molecule of glucose. This process is energetically much more favorable than the production of lactate, but it can occur only when molecular oxygen is available. Myoglobin is an iron-heme complex protein that facilitates oxygen transport within muscle cells. Tissue hydrostatic pressure in a contracting muscle often exceeds arterial perfusion pressure, so the strongest contractions are anaerobic. The content of oxidative enzymes, myoglobin, and mitochondria determines the predominant type of energy metabolism and varies in different muscle types, as was discussed previously (see Table 5.2).

Fatigue and Recovery

During intense or prolonged activity, muscle fatigue is caused by the accumulation of metabolites that suppress the generation of force at the contractile apparatus, during excitation-contraction coupling, or both.[51] Markedly increased myoplasmic P_i and H^+ concentrations and decreased creatine phosphate levels have been detected by magnetic resonance spectroscopy.[52] When the creatine phosphate level declines, maintained activity depends on glycogenolysis until glycogen stores are depleted. During prolonged intense activity, rate of energy production results in a greater number of metabolites (e.g., H^+ and P_i) than can be maintained in the cell, and force production declines well before the ATP concentration is compromised. Thus, fatigue of this nature results more from metabolite accumulation than ATP depletion.[53]

The chemomechanical link between P_i release and the generation of force (see Fig. 5.4) implies that increased myoplasmic P_i in fatigued muscle reduces the magnitude of force simply by mass action.[38] Decreased pH in the muscle, caused in part by accumulation of lactate and insufficient availability of acetylcholine at the neuromuscular junction, leads to failure of synaptic transmission and contributes to decreased work production. Because the respiratory and circulatory systems do not supply sufficient oxygen to support metabolism during intense activity, an oxygen debt is incurred. Blood flow and oxygen uptake continue at an enhanced level after the period of exercise to reclaim this energy. Rephosphorylation of creatine can take place within a few minutes, but glycogen resynthesis requires several hours. Recovery processes also involve restoration of ionic gradients across membrane-bound compartments and require consumption of further energy.

Plasticity

The size, strength, and endurance of a muscle are altered dramatically within weeks after changes in the demands for its use, mobility, or hormonal or metabolic environment. The effects of this adaptive response should be considered in any clinical situation that causes a substantial shift in these factors and with regard to the long-term quality of life of the patient.

Adaptation to Muscle Use/Disuse

Muscle is a use-dependent tissue, meaning that its functional characteristics are closely tied to the number and type of activity patterns that it experiences. Increased muscle use through physical exercise leads to adaptations in muscle fibers that include alterations in specific contractile, regulatory, structural, and metabolic proteins, as well as changes in neural recruitment patterns. The type (aerobic vs. resistance), frequency, intensity, and duration of a training stimulus and the external load influence the adaptive response.[54] Resistance training causes cross-sectional hypertrophy of primarily fast type II fibers (see Table 5.2) by increasing the size of existing fibers without inducing hyperplasia. This hypertrophy is driven primarily by increased myofilament protein, which occupies the vast majority of fiber volume (~80%), but other myocellular components (e.g., mitochondria) are also increased to maintain the relative volume fraction of each cellular component constant with hypertrophy. Aerobic training, on the other hand, enhances the oxidative capacity and volume density of mitochondria in oxidative type I and IIA fibers and generally does not induce hypertrophy. In this context, resistance training alters function by increasing the overall quantity of the muscle, whereas aerobic training alters the functional quality of the muscle to elicit greater endurance to repetitive contraction.

When physical activity is reduced—for instance, with bed rest during hospitalization—the cross-section of fibers decreases, which causes muscle weakness and reduced endurance. Of note, these changes are worsened by acute and chronic disease,[55] to the extent that up to 10% of muscle protein content can be lost per week.[56] After significant periods of muscle disuse, loss of muscle strength and endurance can progress to the point where patients are unable to accomplish simple activities of daily living. Although younger, healthier people tend to regain muscle size and function readily with exercise rehabilitation, the extent to which older people and those with chronic disease can recover from muscle disuse is impaired.[56a,56b]

Hormonal Control

Hormones acting in an endocrine or paracrine-autocrine fashion can alter muscle size, structure, and function. The most prominent hormonal controller of muscle is insulin, which regulates muscle anabolism in response to feeding by suppressing protein breakdown and facilitating protein synthesis via stimulation of amino acid uptake into muscle. In addition to insulin, insulin-like growth factor-I, which largely mediates the effects of growth hormone on muscle, stimulates the hypertrophy of existing muscle fibers by stimulating muscle protein synthesis and inhibiting protein breakdown, and it may contribute to muscle growth/regeneration through effects on muscle satellite cells.[57,58] In men, testosterone has anabolic effects on muscle, and conditions that reduce circulating testosterone levels lead to muscle atrophy and weakness.[58a] The role of testosterone in women is less certain. Estrogen in women may regulate muscle size and strength, although experimental evidence to support this contention in humans is limited,[58b] and the effects of estrogen on other metabolic processes in muscle appear to be relatively minor at concentrations observed during normal menstrual cycles and in the post-menopausal period.

In many acute and chronic illnesses, changes in the hormonal milieu can affect muscle; the predominant factors are cytokines and other inflammatory modulators,[59] although alterations in classic stress hormones, such as cortisol and glucagon,[60] likely also contribute. In most cases, the effect of these catabolic hormones is to direct amino acid substrates toward the liver to support the acute phase protein response. In addition, the type of persistent, low-grade inflammation that occurs with aging and in many chronic diseases may have similar detrimental effects on muscle when compounded over extended periods.

Aging

Sarcopenia, defined as loss of skeletal muscle mass and function with age, manifests as an inability to perform simple tasks of everyday life and contributes to disability, a greater risk for falls and fractures, an increase in all-cause mortality, and, in general, a poor quality of life. Healthy people exhibit approximately a 30% decrease in total muscle mass between the ages of 30 and 80 years. Although it is universally accepted that whole muscle force production is reduced with age,[61–64] disagreement exists about whether this effect is due solely to reduction in muscle mass or if loss of force production per unit muscle size is also a factor. Most single-fiber studies that have measured isometric force production per unit fiber cross-sectional area (i.e., accounting for age-related reductions in muscle size) show that aging decreases force-producing capabilities.[65–72] In addition, whole muscle[61,62,73–75] and single fiber[65,67–69,71,72,76] studies typically find decreases in contractile velocity with age, and this decrease leads to further reduction in the muscle performance of elderly people, especially for movements requiring high-velocity contractions. Altogether, these results suggest that aging slows portions of the fundamental contractile properties of skeletal muscle fibers, which decrease, at least in part, whole muscle performance.[77] Age-related changes in motor unit recruitment, activation of agonist and antagonist muscles, and fibrosis can exacerbate single fiber changes and further reduce whole muscle performance.

Conclusion

The complex functional capacity of muscle to produce finely tuned and coordinated movements is ultimately expressed as the transduction of chemical to mechanical energy by actomyosin. A twitch is initiated by the following mechanisms: an action potential propagated from the CNS along an α motoneuron, neuromuscular chemical transmission, direct protein–protein communication at the T-tubule–SR junction, Ca^{2+} diffusion in the myoplasm, and Ca^{2+} binding to thin filament regulatory proteins. Because the CNS controls activity through recruitment of motor units, gradation and coordination of movement depend critically on the pattern of connections between α motoneurons and muscle fibers and on variations of properties among motor units. Development, maintenance, and aging of the muscular system involve a complex series of genetic programs and cellular interactions that are beginning to be understood at the molecular level. Adaptation of motor unit properties is evident not only in training regimens but also in reduced activity caused by aging, disease, joint pain, and in compromised metabolic, hormonal, or nutritional conditions. Hence, the plasticity of muscle influences the clinical course of many diseases. In addition to its importance in pathophysiology, muscle serves as an excellent substrate for understanding the molecular basis of cell development, protein structure-function relationships, cell signaling, and energy transduction processes.

The references for this chapter can also be found on ExpertConsult.com.

References

1. Kuhn K: Basement membrane (type IV) collagen, *Matrix Biol* 14:439–445, 1995.
2. Hudson BG, Reeders ST, Tryggvason K: Type IV collagen: structure, gene organization, and role in human diseases. Molecular basis of Goodpasture and Alport syndromes and diffuse leiomyomatosis, *J Biol Chem* 268:26033–26036, 1993.
3. Miller JB, Stockdale FE: What muscle cells know that nerves don't tell them, *Trends Neurosci* 10:325–329, 1987.
4. Buller AJ, Eccles JC, Eccles RM: Differentiation of fast and slow muscles in the cat hind limb, *J Physiol* 150:399–416, 1960.
5. Hasan Z, Stuart DG: Animal solutions to problems of movement control: the role of proprioceptors, *Annu Rev Neurosci* 11:199–223, 1988.
6. Somjen G: Glial cells: functions. In Adelman G, editor: *Encyclopedia of neuroscience*, Boston, 1987, Birkhauser, pp 465–466.
7. Adrian ED, Bronk DW: The discharge of impulses in motor nerve fibres. Part II. The frequency of discharge in reflex and voluntary contractions, *J Physiol* 67:i3–i151, 1929.
8. Krarup C: Enhancement and diminution of mechanical tension evoked by staircase and by tetanus in rat muscle, *J Physiol* 311:355–372, 1981.
9. Kandel E, Schwartz J, Jessell T: *Principles of neural science*, ed 4, New York, 2000, McGraw-Hill.
10. Sudhof TC: The synaptic vesicle cycle: a cascade of protein-protein interactions, *Nature* 375:645–653, 1995.
11. Somlyo AV, Gonzalez-Serratos HG, Shuman H, et al.: Calcium release and ionic changes in the sarcoplasmic reticulum of tetanized muscle: an electron-probe study, *J Cell Biol* 90:577–594, 1981.

12. Franzini-Armstrong C, Protasi F: Ryanodine receptors of striated muscles: a complex channel capable of multiple interactions, *Physiol Rev* 77:699–729, 1997.
13. Rios E, Brum G: Involvement of dihydropyridine receptors in excitation-contraction coupling in skeletal muscle, *Nature* 325:717–720, 1987.
14. Tanabe T, Beam KG, Powell JA, et al.: Restoration of excitation-contraction coupling and slow calcium current in dysgenic muscle by dihydropyridine receptor complementary DNA, *Nature* 336:134–139, 1988.
15. Tanabe T, Beam KG, Adams BA, et al.: Regions of the skeletal muscle dihydropyridine receptor critical for excitation-contraction coupling, *Nature* 346:567–569, 1990.
16. Nakai J, Ogura T, Protasi F, et al.: Functional nonequality of the cardiac and skeletal ryanodine receptors, *Proc Natl Acad Sci U S A* 94:1019–1022, 1997.
17. Murayama T, Ogawa Y: Roles of two ryanodine receptor isoforms coexisting in skeletal muscle, *Trends Cardiovasc Med* 12:305–311, 2002.
18. Ptacek LJ: Channelopathies: ion channel disorders of muscle as a paradigm for paroxysmal disorders of the nervous system, *Neuromuscul Disord* 7:250–255, 1997.
19. Barchi RL: Ion channel mutations and diseases of skeletal muscle, *Neurobiol Dis* 4:254–264, 1997.
20. Gillard EF, Otsu K, Fujii J, et al.: A substitution of cysteine for arginine 614 in the ryanodine receptor is potentially causative of human malignant hyperthermia, *Genomics* 11:751–755, 1991.
21. Squire J: *The structural basis of muscular contraction*, New York, 1981, Plenum Press.
22. Sosa H, Popp D, Ouyang G, et al.: Ultrastructure of skeletal muscle fibers studied by a plunge quick freezing method: myofilament lengths, *Biophys J* 67:283–292, 1994.
23. Thomas DD: Spectroscopic probes of muscle cross-bridge rotation, *Annu Rev Physiol* 49:691–709, 1987.
24. Irving M, St Claire Allen T, Sabido-David C, et al.: Tilting of the light-chain region of myosin during step length changes and active force generation in skeletal muscle, *Nature* 375:688–691, 1995.
25. Chowrashi P, Pepe F: M-band proteins: evidence for more than one component. In Pepe F, Sanger J, Nachmias V, editors: *Motility in cell function*, New York, 1979, Academic Press.
26. Walliman T, Pelloni G, Turner D, et al.: Removal of the M-line by treatment with Fab′ fragments of antibodies against MM-creatine kinase. In Pepe F, Sanger J, Nachmias V, editors: *Motility in cell function*, New York, 1979, Academic Press.
27. Mermall V, Post PL, Mooseker MS: Unconventional myosins in cell movement, membrane traffic, and signal transduction, *Science* 279:527–533, 1998.
28. Hasson T: Unconventional myosins, the basis for deafness in mouse and man, *Am J Hum Genet* 61:801–805, 1997.
29. Redowicz MJ: Myosins and deafness, *J Muscle Res Cell Motil* 20:241–248, 1999.
30. Sheterline P, Clayton J, Sparrow J, editors: *Actin*, ed 4, New York, 1998, Oxford University Press.
31. Small JV, Rottner K, Kaverina I, et al.: Assembling an actin cytoskeleton for cell attachment and movement, *Biochim Biophys Acta* 1404:271–281, 1998.
32. Ramaekers FC, Bosman FT: The cytoskeleton and disease, *J Pathol* 204:351–354, 2004.
33. Wang K: Sarcomere-associated cytoskeletal lattices in striated muscle: review and hypothesis, *Cell Muscle Motil* 6:315–369, 1985.
34. Labeit S, Kolmerer B: Titins: giant proteins in charge of muscle ultrastructure and elasticity, *Science* 270:293–296, 1995.
35. Toyama Y, Forry-Schaudies S, Hoffman B, et al.: Effects of taxol and colcemid on myofibrillogenesis, *Proc Natl Acad Sci U S A* 79:6556–6560, 1982.
36. Goldman YE: Wag the tail: structural dynamics of actomyosin, *Cell* 93:1–4, 1998.
37. Leuba S, Zlatanova J, editors: *Biology at the single molecule level*, Oxford, United Kingdom, 2001, Pergamon Press.
38. Dantzig JA, Goldman YE, Millar NC, et al.: Reversal of the cross-bridge force-generating transition by photogeneration of phosphate in rabbit psoas muscle fibres, *J Physiol* 451:247–278, 1992.
39. Goldman YE: Kinetics of the actomyosin ATPase in muscle fibers, *Annu Rev Physiol* 49:637–654, 1987.
40. Forkey JN, Quinlan ME, Shaw MA, et al.: Three-dimensional structural dynamics of myosin V by single-molecule fluorescence polarization, *Nature* 422:399–404, 2003.
41. Dobbie I, Linari M, Piazzesi G, et al.: Elastic bending and active tilting of myosin heads during muscle contraction, *Nature* 396:383–387, 1998.
42. Huxley AF, Simmons RM: Proposed mechanism of force generation in striated muscle, *Nature* 233(5321):533–538, 1971.
43. Chicurel ME, Singer RH, Meyer CJ, et al.: Integrin binding and mechanical tension induce movement of mRNA and ribosomes to focal adhesions, *Nature* 392:730–733, 1998.
44. Kanagawa M, Toda T: The genetic and molecular basis of muscular dystrophy: roles of cell-matrix linkage in the pathogenesis, *J Hum Genet* 51:915–926, 2006.
45. Durbeej M, Campbell KP: Muscular dystrophies involving the dystrophin-glycoprotein complex: an overview of current mouse models, *Curr Opin Genet Dev* 12:349–361, 2002.
46. Matsumura K, Ohlendieck K, Ionasescu VV, et al.: The role of the dystrophin-glycoprotein complex in the molecular pathogenesis of muscular dystrophies, *Neuromuscul Disord* 3:533–535, 1993.
47. Campbell KP, Stull JT: Skeletal muscle basement membrane-sarcolemma-cytoskeleton interaction minireview series, *J Biol Chem* 278:12599–12600, 2003.
48. Henry MD, Campbell KP: A role for dystroglycan in basement membrane assembly, *Cell* 95:859–870, 1998.
49. Wells DJ, Wells KE: Gene transfer studies in animals: what do they really tell us about the prospects for gene therapy in DMD? *Neuromuscul Disord* 12(Suppl 1):S11–S22, 2002.
50. Glancy B, Hartnell LM, Malide D, et al.: Mitochondrial reticulum for cellular energy distribution in muscle, *Nature* 523(7562):617–620, 2015.
51. Fitts RH: Cellular mechanisms of muscle fatigue, *Physiol Rev* 74:49–94, 1994.
52. Meyer RA, Brown TR, Kushmerick MJ: Phosphorus nuclear magnetic resonance of fast- and slow-twitch muscle, *Am J Physiol* 248(3 Pt 1):C279–C287, 1985.
53. Debold EP: Recent insights into the molecular basis of muscular fatigue, *Med Sci Sports Exerc* 44(8):1440–1452, 2012.
54. Faulkner J, White T: Adaptations of skeletal muscle to physical activity. In Bouchard C, Shephard R, Stephens T, et al.: *Exercise, fitness, and health*, Champaign, Ill, 1990, Human Kinetics, pp 265–279.
55. Ferrando AA, Wolfe RR: Effects of bed rest with or without stress. In Kinney JM, Tucker HN, editors: *Physiology, stress and malnutrition: functional correlates, nutritional interventions*, New York, 1997, Lippincott-Raven, pp 413–429.
56. Gamrin L, Andersson K, Hultman E, et al.: Longitudinal changes of biochemical parameters in muscle during critical illness, *Metabolism* 46:756–762, 1997.
56a. Hvid L, Aagaard P, Justesen L, et al.: Effects of aging on muscle mechanical function and muscle fiber morphology during short-term immobilization and subsequent retraining, *J Appl Physiol* 109:1628–1634, 2010.
56b. Hvid LG, Suetta C, Nielsen JH, et al.: Aging impairs the recovery in mechanical muscle function following 4 days of disuse, *Exp Gerontol* 52:1–8, 2014.
57. Lamberts SW, van den Beld AW, van der Lely AJ: The endocrinology of aging, *Science* 278:419–424, 1997.
58. Florini JR, Ewton DZ, Coolican SA: Growth hormone and the insulin-like growth factor system in myogenesis, *Endocr Rev* 17:481–517, 1996.

58a. Mauras N, Hayes V, Welch S, et al.: Testosterone deficiency in young men: marked alterations in whole body protein kinetics, strength, and adiposity, *J Clin Endocr Metab* 83:1886–1892, 1998.
58b. Greising SM, Baltgalvis KA, Lowe DA, et al.: Hormone therapy and skeletal muscle strength: a meta-analysis, *J Gerontol A Biol Sci Med Sci* 64:1071–1081, 2009.
59. Lang CH, Frost RA, Vary TC: Regulation of muscle protein synthesis during sepsis and inflammation, *Am J Physiol Endocrinol Metab* 293:E453–E459, 2007.
60. Rooyackers OE, Nair KS: Hormonal regulation of human muscle protein metabolism, *Annu Rev Nutr* 17:457–485, 1997.
61. Thom JM, Morse CI, Birch KM, et al.: Triceps surae muscle power, volume, and quality in older versus younger healthy men, *J Gerontol A Biol Sci Med Sci* 60:1111–1117, 2005.
62. Petrella JK, Kim JS, Tuggle SC, et al.: Age differences in knee extension power, contractile velocity, and fatigability, *J Appl Physiol* 98:211–220, 2005.
63. Lanza IR, Towse TF, Caldwell GE, et al.: Effects of age on human muscle torque, velocity, and power in two muscle groups, *J Appl Physiol* 95:2361–2369, 2003.
64. Candow DG, Chilibeck PD: Differences in size, strength, and power of upper and lower body muscle groups in young and older men, *J Gerontol A Biol Sci Med Sci* 60:148–156, 2005.
65. Yu F, Hedstrom M, Cristea A, et al.: Effects of ageing and gender on contractile properties in human skeletal muscle and single fibres, *Acta Physiol (Oxford)* 190:229–241, 2007.
66. Trappe S, Gallagher P, Harber M, et al.: Single muscle fibre contractile properties in young and old men and women, *J Physiol* 552(Pt 1):47–58, 2003.
67. Ochala J, Dorer DJ, Frontera WR, et al.: Single skeletal muscle fiber behavior after a quick stretch in young and older men: a possible explanation of the relative preservation of eccentric force in old age, *Pflugers Arch* 452:464–470, 2006.
68. Ochala J, Frontera WR, Dorer DJ, et al.: Single skeletal muscle fiber elastic and contractile characteristics in young and older men, *J Gerontol A Biol Sci Med Sci* 62:375–381, 2007.
69. Larsson L, Li X, Frontera WR: Effects of aging on shortening velocity and myosin isoform composition in single human skeletal muscle cells, *Am J Physiol* 272(2 Pt 1):C638–C649, 1997.
70. Frontera WR, Suh D, Krivickas LS, et al.: Skeletal muscle fiber quality in older men and women, *Am J Physiol Cell Physiol* 279:C611–C618, 2000.
71. D'Antona G, Pellegrino MA, Adami R, et al.: The effect of ageing and immobilization on structure and function of human skeletal muscle fibres, *J Physiol* 552(Pt 2):499–511, 2003.
72. D'Antona G, Pellegrino MA, Carlizzi CN, et al.: Deterioration of contractile properties of muscle fibres in elderly subjects is modulated by the level of physical activity, *Eur J Appl Physiol* 100:603–611, 2007.
73. McNeil CJ, Vandervoort AA, Rice CL: Peripheral impairments cause a progressive age-related loss of strength and velocity-dependent power in the dorsiflexors, *J Appl Physiol* 102:1962–1968, 2007.
74. Valour D, Ochala J, Ballay Y, et al.: The influence of ageing on the force-velocity-power characteristics of human elbow flexor muscles, *Exp Gerontol* 38:387–395, 2003.
75. Kostka T: Quadriceps maximal power and optimal shortening velocity in 335 men aged 23-88 years, *Eur J Appl Physiol* 95:140–145, 2005.
76. Krivickas LS, Suh D, Wilkins J, et al.: Age- and gender-related differences in maximum shortening velocity of skeletal muscle fibers, *Am J Phys Med Rehabil* 80:447–455, 2001, quiz 456–457.
77. Miller MS, Bedrin NG, Callahan DM, et al.: Age-related slowing of myosin actin cross-bridge kinetics is sex specific and predicts decrements in whole skeletal muscle performance in humans, *J Appl Physiol* 115(7):1004–1014, 2013.

6 Biomechanics

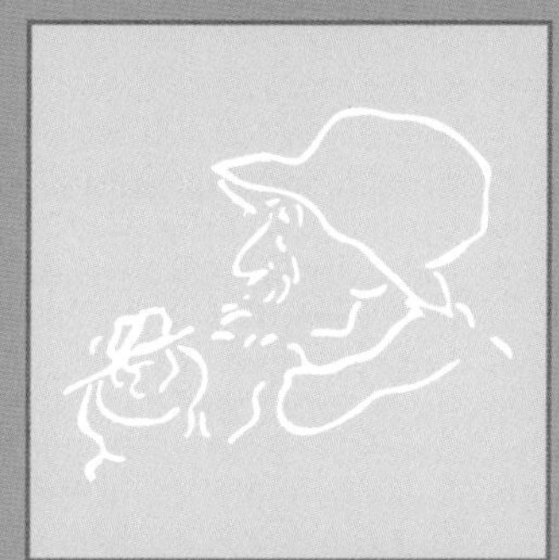

KENTON R. KAUFMAN AND KAINAN AN

KEY POINTS

- Kinematics is the study of the geometric and time-dependent aspects of motion without analyzing the forces causing the motion.
- Kinetics is the study of the forces that cause motion of a rigid body. These forces can be classified as either external forces or internal forces.
- The general unconstrained movement in three-dimensional space requires the description of three translations and three rotations to fully describe joint motion.
- External forces represent the action of objects contacting the body, gravitational forces, or force due to inertia of the body.
- Internal forces are the body's responses to external forces, which consist of muscle, ligament, and joint contact forces.
- Because of relatively smaller mechanical advantages, large muscle and tendon forces, and thus internal joint forces, are expected when performing any activities.
- The anatomic structure responsible for joint constraint can be divided into passive and active elements. Passive elements, consisting of the capsulo-ligamentous structures and bony articulating surfaces, provide the static constraints of the joint. The active elements include muscle-tendon units, which provide dynamic joint constraints.

Introduction

Biomechanics combines the field of engineering mechanics with the fields of biology and physiology. Biomechanics applies mechanical principles to the human body to understand the mechanical influences on bone and joint health. Forces that load the joints are generated by muscles and transmitted by tendons. Bones must withstand these forces. Developments in the field of biomechanics have improved our understanding of normal and pathologic gait, mechanics of neuromuscular control, and mechanics of growth and form. This knowledge contributed to the development of medical diagnostic and treatment procedures; it provided the basis for the design and manufacture of medical implants and orthotic devices and enhanced rehabilitation therapy practices. Biomechanics is also used to improve human performance in the workplace and in athletic competition.

Mechanics is a branch of physics that is concerned with the motion and deformation of bodies that are acted on by mechanical forces. Mechanics is one of the oldest physical sciences, dating back to Aristotle (384–322 BC), who conducted an organized analytical analysis of animal movement. Leonardo da Vinci (1452–1519) investigated the mechanics of the human body; his detailed anatomic sketches represent the birth of anatomy, as a discipline, and of mechanics as the science governing human motion. Although da Vinci wrote extensively on body mechanics, the man generally credited to be the father of modern biomechanics is Giovanni Alphonso Borelli (1608–1679). His book *De Motu Animalian* provided a quantitative graphical solution to a musculoskeletal biomechanics problem (Fig. 6.1).[1]

Engineering mechanics is the discipline devoted to the solution of mechanical problems through the integrated application of mathematical, scientific, and engineering principles. With roots in physics and mathematics, engineering mechanics is the basis of all engineering mechanical sciences. Engineering mechanics is an applied mechanics branch of the physical sciences. The broad field of applied mechanics can be further divided into three main parts: rigid body mechanics, deformable body mechanics, and fluid mechanics. In general, a material can be characterized as either a solid or fluid. Solid materials can be considered to be rigid or deformable. A rigid body is one that cannot be deformed. In reality, every object undergoes deformation to some extent when acted upon by external forces. However, this is a definition of convenience that is used to simplify complex problems. For example, during the study of movement in gait analysis, the bones are considered to be rigid bodies when compared with the soft tissues joining the bones. External loads applied to a rigid body result in internal loads, stresses, and deformations. The mechanics of deformable bodies deal with the relationships between externally applied loads and their internal effects. The mechanics of deformable bodies have strong ties with the field of materials science and are more complex when compared with the analyses required in rigid body mechanics. The purpose of this chapter is to introduce the reader to the field of biomechanics. We will focus on rigid body mechanics.

Basic biomechanics relies heavily on Newtonian mechanics. These laws were introduced by Sir Isaac Newton and form the basis for analyses in statics and dynamics. Statics analyzes the forces that occur in rigid bodies that are in static equilibrium. Dynamics is the study of bodies in motion. The general field of dynamics consists of two major areas: kinematics and kinetics. Ultimately, proper joint constraint and stability enables limb function in characteristic ways.

Kinematics

Kinematics is the study of the geometric and time-dependent aspects of motion without analyzing the forces causing the motion. Kinematic analysis is used to relate displacement, velocity, acceleration, and time. To study kinematics in an organized manner, it is common to classify the motion as translational, rotational, or general. Translational motion occurs when a straight line drawn between two points on the body remains in the same direction during the motion. Translational motion can be either

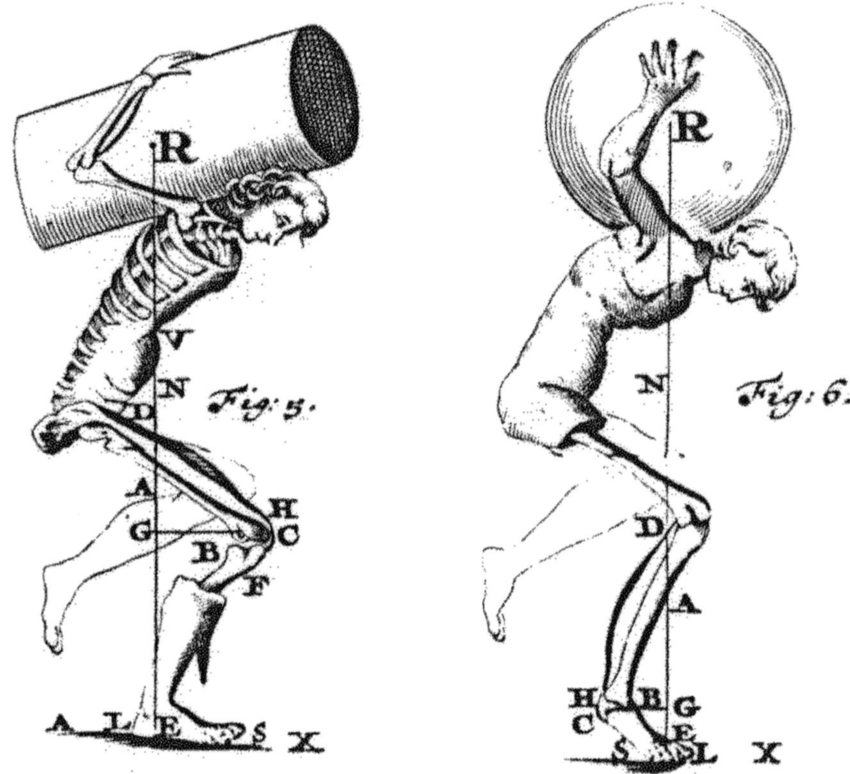

• **Fig. 6.1** Borelli's quantitative graphical solution to a musculoskeletal biomechanics problem. (From Borelli GA: *De motu anumalium*. Batavis, Lugduni, 1685.)

rectilinear motion (if the paths are straight lines) or curvilinear (if the paths are curved lines). Rotational motion occurs when the points on the body move in a circular path around an axis of rotation. The angular motion occurs about a central line known as the *axis of rotation*, which lies perpendicular to the plane of motion. The third class of motion is called *general motion* or *displacement*; this type of motion occurs if a body undergoes both translational and rotational motion simultaneously.

Kinematics can be analyzed in two-dimensional (2-D) or three-dimensional (3-D) space. When all points of a rigid body move parallel to a plane, the motion is referred to as *planar motion*, which can be thought of as 2-D motion. The more general type of rigid body motion is 3-D motion. Six independent parameters are required to describe 3-D motion. These parameters are called *degrees of freedom*, or the number of independent coordinates in a coordinate system that is required to completely specify the position of an object in space. A rigid body in space has a maximum of six degrees of freedom, consisting of three translations (expressed by linear coordinates) and three rotations (expressed by angular coordinates). The general movement of an object is defined by a vector quantity that is a combination of both linear and angular displacement. Velocity is the time-related change of displacement. Linear velocity is expressed in units of length per time (e.g., m/sec). Angular velocity is expressed in units of angular measure per time (e.g., rad/sec). Because velocities reflect vector quantities, both magnitude and direction must be specified. Acceleration is the time-rate of change of velocity. Linear acceleration is expressed in units of length per time squared (e.g., m/sec^2). Angular acceleration is the time rate of change in angular velocity (e.g., rad/sec^2). Accelerations are also vector quantities, and both magnitude and direction must be specified.

Kinematic techniques have been used to study body movements in both 2-D and 3-D space. The human body is typically modeled as a number of interconnected rigid body segments (Fig. 6.2). A coordinate system is affixed to each rigid body segment to establish an anatomic coordinate system. External markers are used to define orthogonal coordinate systems whose axes define the position of these body segments. Joint motion is then described as the relative motion of the distal body segment with respect to the proximal body segment. Limb segments are assumed to undergo angular displacement during human movement. However, more sophisticated analyses will also quantify the linear displacement that limb segments may undergo. These measures of relative segmental angles have been used to describe human walking and other activities of daily living.[2–7]

For example, knee motion in the sagittal plane can be characterized throughout the gait cycle (Fig. 6.3). At heel strike, the knee is nearly fully extended (with knee flexion of only five degrees). During midstance, the knee flexes to about 15 degrees, which occurs at 15% of the gait cycle. The knee joint is brought back into extension by midstance. At 50% of the gait cycle, opposite foot contact occurs. The weight is shifted to the opposite limb and the knee begins flexing. Toe-off occurs at 60% of the gait cycle. Peak knee flexion of 60 degrees occurs during the early portion of the swing phase. The knee motion can be described as two flexion waves, each starting in relative extension, progressing into flexion, and then returning again to extension. The first flexion wave, or stance phase knee flexion, acts as a shock absorber to aid weight acceptance. This curve peaks in early stance at opposite foot-off. The mechanical source for this shock absorber is the eccentrically contracting quadriceps muscles. The second flexion wave is necessary to clear the foot in

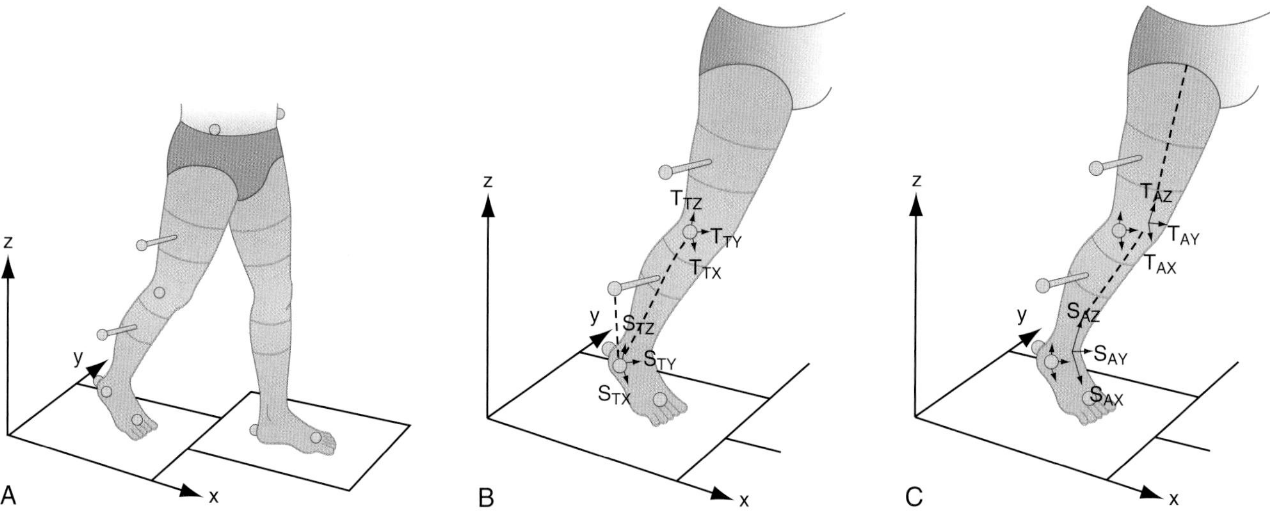

• **Fig. 6.2** The kinematic technique used to study body movement in three-dimensional space. Body-fixed reflective markers are used to establish anatomic coordinate systems. (A) Video camera measurement systems calculate the location of external markers placed on the body segments and are aligned with specific bony landmarks. (B) A body-fixed external coordinate system is then computed from three or more markers on each body segment. Body-fixed external coordinate systems are shown for the thigh (T_T) and shank (S_T). The coordinate system is shown for the three orthogonal directions (i.e., x, y, and z). The body-fixed thigh coordinate system is designated T_{Tx}, T_{Ty}, and T_{Tz}. (C) Using a subject-specific calibration relates the external coordinate system with an anatomic coordinate system through the identification of anatomic landmarks (e.g., the medial and lateral femoral condyles and medial lateral malleoli). The anatomic coordinate system for the thigh is then designated T_{Ax}, T_{Ay}, and T_{Az}. (From Kaufman KR: Objective assessment of posture and gait. In Bronstein AM, Brandt T, Marjorie H, editors: *Clinical disorders of balance, posture, and gait*. Oxford, England, A Hodder Arnold Publication, 2004.)

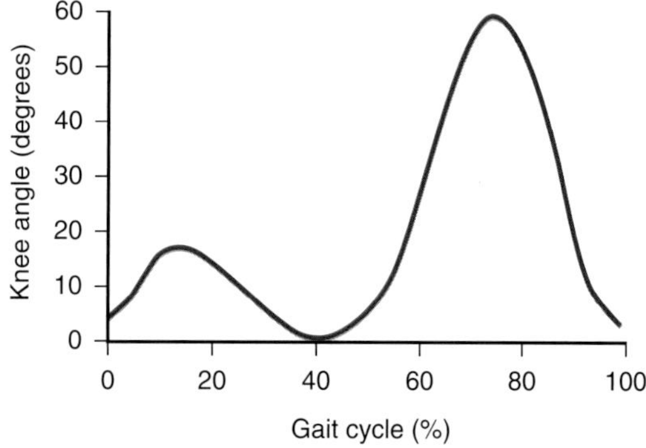

• **Fig. 6.3** Knee sagittal plane motion throughout the gait cycle. A positive value indicates knee flexion. For the first 60% of the gait cycle, the leg is in stance. The leg is in swing phase for the remainder of the gait cycle.

the early swing phase. The knee is rapidly flexed beginning just after heel rise to a maximum in the swing phase just as the swinging foot passes the opposite limb.

The complexity of kinematic analysis increases substantially when one moves from planar analysis to 3-D analysis. The complexity of the analysis arises from a technical difficulty—that is, large rigid body rotations cannot be treated as vectors and hence do not obey the vectorial principles of transformation, independence, and interchangeability of operations. For finite spatial rotation, the sequence of rotations is extremely important and must be specified for a unique description of joint motion.[8,9] For the same amount of rotation, different final orientations will result from different sequences of rotation (Fig. 6.4). However, with proper selection and definition of the axes of rotation between two bony segments, it is possible to make finite rotation sequence independent or communitive.[8,9]

Investigators in orthopedic biomechanics have adopted the concept of Eulerian angles to unify the definition of finite spatial rotation. In the selection of reference axes, one axis is fixed to the stationary segment and another axis is fixed to the moving segment (Fig. 6.5). In the knee joint, for example, the flexion/extension angle Φ occurs about a medial-laterally directed axis defined by a line connecting the medial and lateral femoral condyles. The axial rotation angle, Ψ, is measured about an axis defined by the line along the shaft of the tibia. The third axis, also defined as the *floating axis*, is orthogonal to the other two axes and defines abduction/adduction (Θ). These rotations match the Eulerian angle description and are thought to be performed in such a way as to bring the moving segment from the reference orientation into the current orientation. The advantage of using this system for description of the spatial rotation of anatomic joints is that the angular rotations do not have to be referred back to the neutral position of the joint because the rotation sequence can be independent, and thus, the measurement can be easily obtained and related to anatomic structures.

A complete analysis of total joint movement (i.e., six degrees of freedom) can be obtained using markers embedded in the bone[10,11] or dual fluoroscopic imaging techniques.[12,13] This general unconstrained movement in 3-D space requires the description of three translations and three rotations to fully describe joint motion. The most commonly used analytic method for description of six-degrees-of-freedom displacement of a rigid body is the screw displacement axis or helical axis.[14–16]

Kinetics

Kinetics is the study of the forces that cause motion of a rigid body. When unbalanced forces or moments are acting on a rigid body, it is under a nonequilibrium, or dynamic, condition, resulting

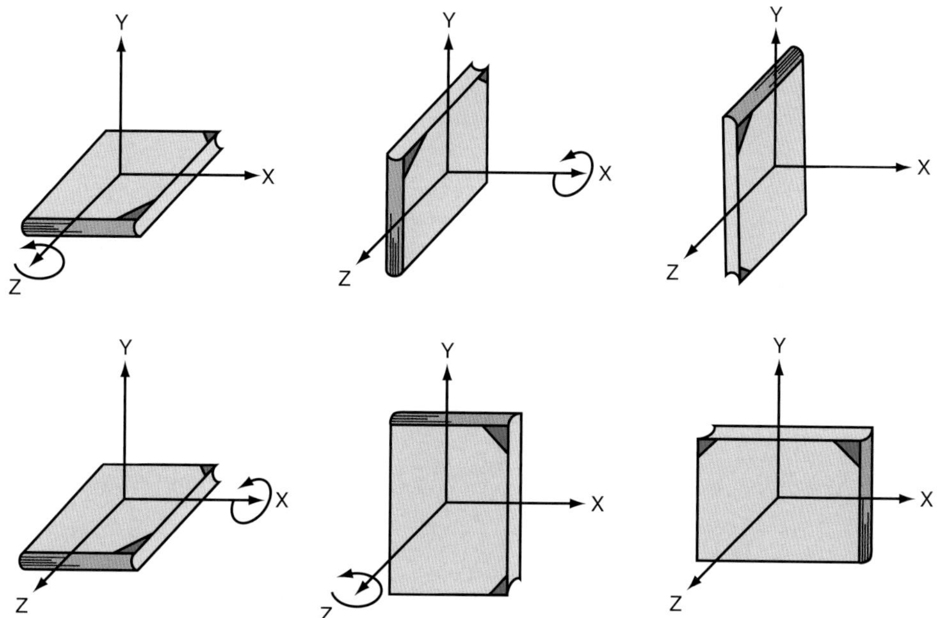

• **Fig. 6.4** Sequence dependence of rigid body motion. The object undergoes two rotations about the X-axis and Z-axis. The sequence of these rotations differs in the top and bottom rows. The result is that the final orientation of the object is different.

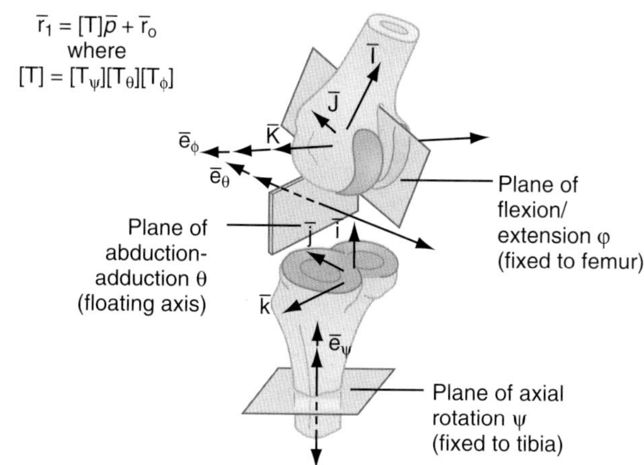

• **Fig. 6.5** Description of knee joint motion using the Eulerian angle system. An axis fixed to the distal femur defines flexion/extension motion, Φ. An axis, e_ψ, fixed to the proximal tibia along its anatomic axis defines internal external rotation, Ψ. A floating axis, e_θ, which is orthogonal to the other two axes, is used to measure abduction-adduction, θ. The rotation matrix [T] between the proximal and distal joint segment is then given by the multiplication of the three rotation matrices associated with the rotations around the three axes (i.e., $[T] = [T_\psi][T_\theta][T_\Phi]$). (From Chao EYS: Justification of triaxial goniometer for the measurement of joint rotation. *J Biomech* 13:989–1006, 1980.)

in motion. Understanding the kinetics of human movement provides a fundamental understanding of the musculoskeletal system. Before one can begin to analyze the forces during human movement, some basic definitions are necessary, and some basic assumptions must be made.

The key quantities in kinetics are *force, moment,* and *torque.* A force represents an interaction between two bodies. According to Newton's Second Law, force is any action that tends to change the state of rest or state of motion of a body to which it is applied. Forces can be contact forces (as when bodies touch each other) or field forces (as when bodies are separated by a distance, such as gravitational, electric, or magnetic forces). Forces are represented by *vectors*, which are composed of four components: magnitude, direction, sense, and position (also called *point of application*). The vector may be resolved into several component forces, usually along specified, mutually perpendicular coordinate axes. Conversely, forces can be summed using vectorial addition.

A moment represents the turning, twisting, or rotational effect of a force. A moment is a vector. A moment is defined as the product of the force and the perpendicular distance between the line of action of the force and the axis of rotation of the motion that the force produces (Fig. 6.6). Its magnitude is the force times the perpendicular distance to the axis of rotation. The direction of the moment is along the axis of rotation (or potential rotation) and, thus, perpendicular to the plane in which the twisting force is applied. The moment arm—that is, the distance used to calculate the moment—is the shortest distance from the force action line to the actual or potential pivot point of the system, regardless of the state of motion. Skeletal motions are the result of moments applied by muscles that cross the joints on which they act. The moment of a force about an axis measures the tendency of the force to impart to the body a motion of rotation about a fixed axis.

A torque is a special type of moment that results when a pair of forces that have equal magnitude, parallel lines of action, and opposite senses act on a body (Fig. 6.7). The magnitude of the torque is Fd, where *d* is the perpendicular distance between the two forces. The resultant force is zero because the two forces are equal and oppose each other.

Kinetics can be used to analyze forces affecting the musculoskeletal system. These forces can be classified as either external or internal. External forces represent the action of objects contacting the body, gravitational forces, or force due to inertia of the body. Internal forces are the body's responses to external forces. Internal forces consist of muscle, ligament, and joint

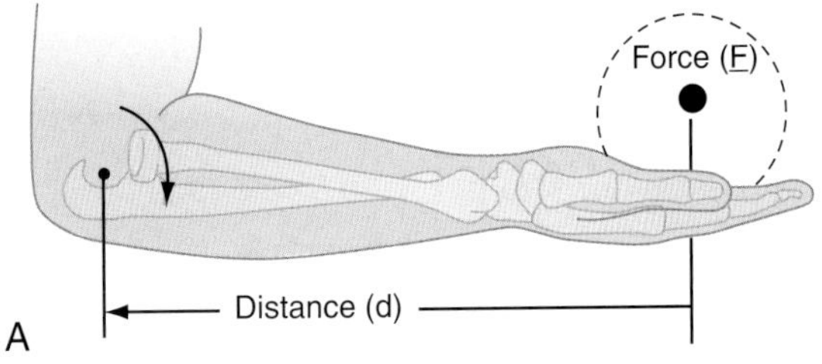

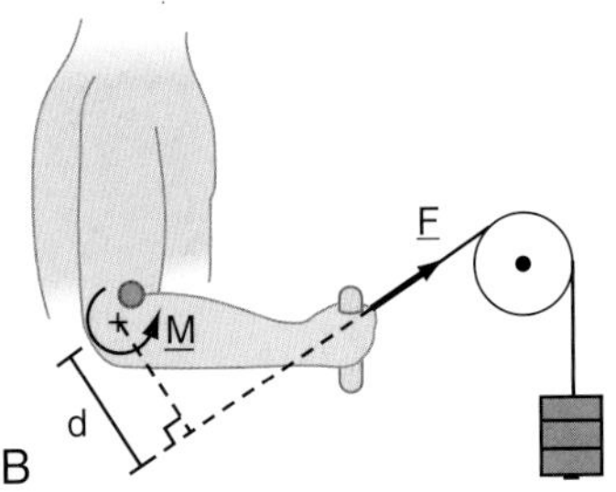

• **Fig. 6.6** The moment (M) of a force (F) about a point is equal to the force times the moment arm (d), which is the perpendicular distance between the point and the line of action of the force. The moment arm may be (A) or may not be (B) the distance along the limb segment to the axis of rotation. The moment arm is always the shortest distance between the line of force application and the axis of rotation.

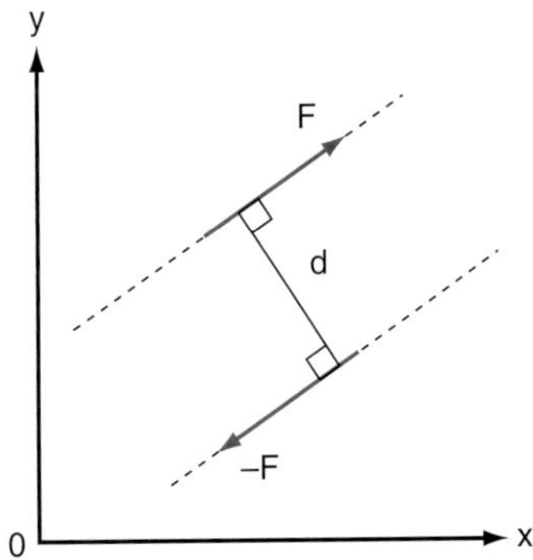

• **Fig. 6.7** A torque, or force couple, is created by two equal, noncollinear, and parallel but oppositely directed forces, F and –F. The magnitude of the torque is Fd, where *d* is the perpendicular distance between the two forces.

contact forces. In general, the limb segments are assumed to be rigid, which simplifies the analysis because it is assumed that the structure does not deform under load. Further, joints are assumed to be frictionless hinges.

Statics is the study of forces acting on a body at rest. When performing a force analysis, the body or part of a body at equilibrium may be isolated from the environment, and the environment is replaced by forces acting on the system, resulting in what is called a *free-body diagram.* Because both forces and moments are vectors, they must sum to zero in each of the three perpendicular directions (reference system). Consider a person standing quietly (Fig. 6.8). The person's weight (force of gravity) tends to pull the person toward the ground (Fig. 6.8A). The person does not move downward because the ground is pushing up with a total force equal in magnitude to the individual's weight (Newton's Third Law). If the person has his or her weight distributed symmetrically, then his or her weight is evenly shared by each lower extremity (Fig. 6.8A). The load under each foot can be represented by resultant ground reaction force (GRF) vectors, with one-half of the body weight supported by each foot. With one-half of body weight supported by each foot, the point of application of the resultant GRF passes approximately midway between the subject's two feet (Fig. 6.8B). No motion occurs because the external forces (i.e., body weight and the GRF) are balanced—they are equal and opposite in magnitude. When the person leans to one side (Fig. 6.8C), the GRF shifts in the direction that the person leans. Thus, overall body posture can affect the GRF location. If the person leans more, he or she will become unstable (i.e., the downward body weight vector will fall outside the base of support). To remain in static equilibrium, the subject requires additional support (Fig. 6.8D). The horizontal force applied to the upper body by the wall is balanced with an equal and opposite horizontal GRF component. Also, the two equal and opposite vertical forces are no longer aligned (i.e., collinear). They form a force couple that would tend to rotate the body in a counterclockwise direction. A second clockwise force couple formed by the two equal and opposite horizontal forces balances the counterclockwise force couple. As a result, the subject remains in both translational and rotational static equilibrium.

When unbalanced forces are present or no one is acting on a rigid body, it is under a nonequilibrium or dynamic condition, which results in motion. Newton's Second Law of Motion links the kinematics of a body to its kinetics. The Second Law states, "If the resultant force acting on a body is not zero, the body will have an acceleration proportional to the magnitude of the resultant and in the direction of this resultant force."[16a] Analysis of the motion of the limb segments requires a set of governing equations and assumptions. The equations assume that each limb segment is a rigid body moving in 3-D space. Therefore, six scalar equations of motion define the general 3-D forces and motion of each limb segment:

$$\Sigma F = ma$$

$$\Sigma M = I\alpha$$

where ΣF is the sum of forces in each of three orthogonal directions, ΣM is the sum of moments, I is the moment of inertia of the body, a is the linear acceleration of the body, m is the mass of the body, and α is the angular acceleration of the body. Newton's Second Law makes it possible to calculate the forces acting on the musculoskeletal systems from measurements of segment motion and mass. During normal ambulation, there is a medial and vertical GRF that balances the body weight and lateral inertial force. The vertical GRF component generally passes lateral to the body's center of mass during gait (Fig. 6.9A). The combined resultant GRF passes medial to the knee joint center, creating a load imbalance in the medial and lateral compartments of the knee. The medial and lateral compartments of the knee carry more load than the lateral compartment of the knee (Fig. 6.9B), and thus a higher degree of osteoarthritis (OA) typically develops in the medial compartment than in the lateral compartment. The resultant GRF vector creates a knee external adduction moment. Medial tibiofemoral OA is the most common form of OA, and it is apparent that medial knee OA is, at least partially, mechanically driven. Research scientists have implicated the peak external knee adduction moment in the progression of radiographic OA[17]; they identify this phenomenon as a marker of disease severity.[18,19]

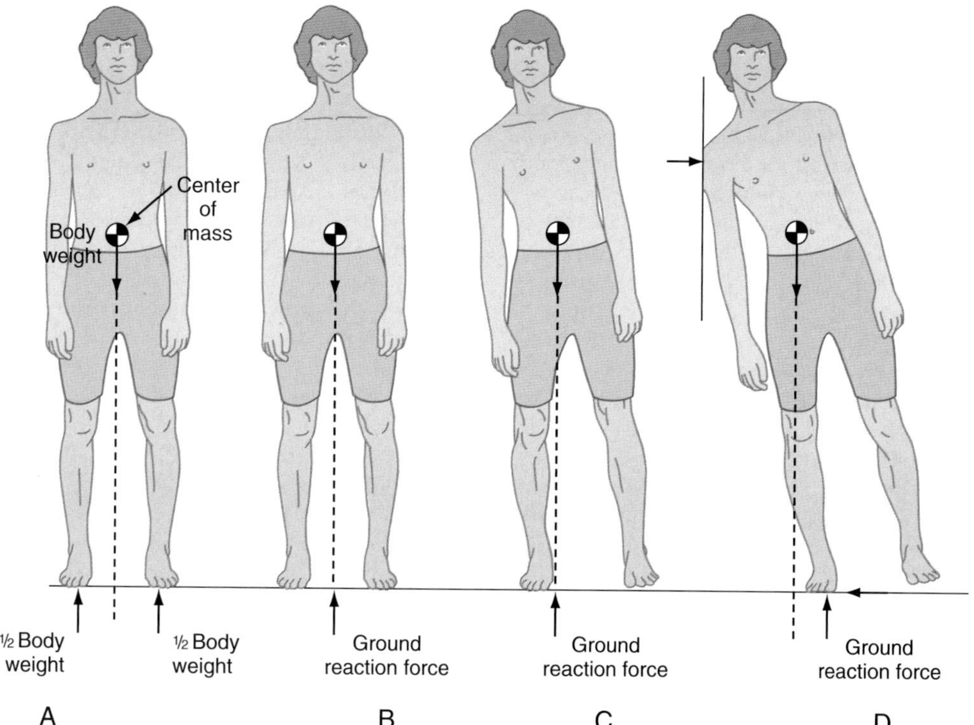

• **Fig. 6.8** Static force equilibrium. (A) When a person stands quietly with the body weight evenly distributed on both feet, that person can be considered to be in static equilibrium. (B) The loads under each foot can be combined into a single ground reaction force (GRF) equal to the sum of the forces under the two feet and located directly under the center of mass (COM), with a force equal to body weight. The GRF is located approximately midway between the two feet. (C) As body weight is shifted laterally, the GRF also shifts to remain under the COM. (D) When the body weight vector is shifted beyond the base of support (i.e., the lateral margin of the foot), an additional lateral force vector is required to maintain static equilibrium. (From Davis RB, Kaufman KR: Kinetics of normal walking. In Rose J, Gamble JG, editors: *Human walking*, ed 3. Philadelphia, Lippincott Williams & Wilkins, 2006.)

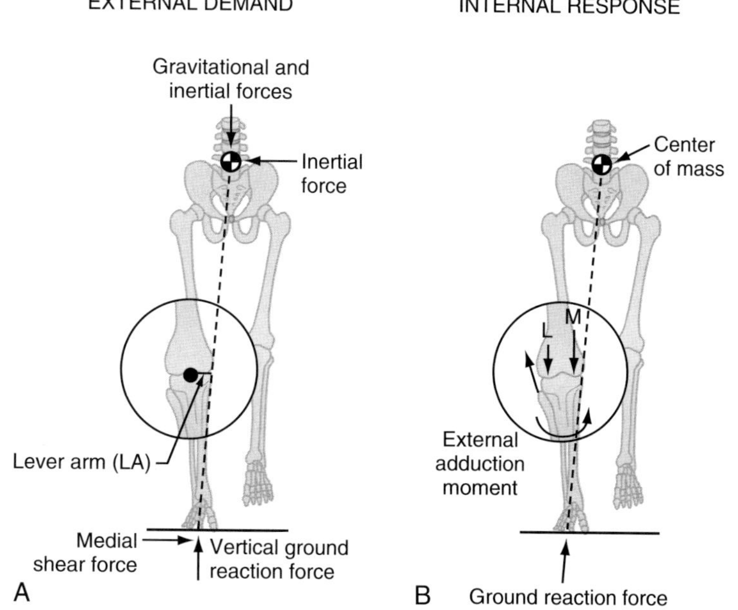

• **Fig. 6.9** Schematic of a person in single support during gait. (A) External demand. The body weight and vertical ground reaction force (GRF) force couple tend to rotate the body clockwise. The medial shear GRF and the corresponding lateral inertial force produce a force couple that tends to rotate the body counterclockwise. Thus, the body is in dynamic equilibrium. (B) Internal response. The resultant GRF passes medial to the knee joint, creating an external knee adduction moment. The external moment is balanced internally in the knee by creating a larger force on the medial tibial plateau (M) than on the lateral tibial plateau (L). Once again, the knee is in dynamic equilibrium.

Joint Biomechanics

Diarthrodial joints connect long bones to allow force transmission and joint rotation. The type of joint articulating motion depends on the shape of the joint surfaces. For example, the hip is a congruent ball and socket joint, the elbow is a congruent hinge joint, the knee and proximal interphalangeal joint are bicondylar joints, and the carpometacarpal joint of the thumb is a saddle joint. In general, the joint articulating motion can be described in terms of sliding, spinning, and rolling (Fig. 6.10). Sliding and spinning motions involve the relative translation of one surface against the other. Rolling has the least relative motion between articulating surfaces. The translational speeds range from 0.06 m/sec between the femoral head surface and acetabular surface during normal walking to 0.6 m/sec between the humeral head surface and glenoid surface during baseball pitching.[20]

Although diarthrodial joints experience an enormous amount of loading and motion, the cartilage surfaces undergo little wear and tear during normal conditions because of the special lubrication qualities of synovial fluid and the biphasic structure of the cartilage. Synovial fluid, which is secreted by the synovium into the joint space, contains mainly hyaluronate. Biomechanically, hyaluronate is a highly viscous liquid, with the shear stress depending on the rate of shear strain applied. As the shear rate increases, the viscosity of synovial fluid decreases. However, in the patient with rheumatoid arthritis, because of enzymatic degradation of the hyaluronate molecules, the viscosity of the rheumatoid synovial fluid does not have a normal shear rate dependency and is believed to be less effective in lubrication.[20]

Two lubrication mechanisms in the synovial joint provide minimal friction and cartilage wear: fluid film lubrication and boundary lubrication. During joint rotation, the sliding speed of the articulating surfaces and the viscosity of the synovial fluid create a thin film capable of supporting the load, which results in fluid film lubrication. When the joint is loaded, the two articulating surfaces approach each other, and a squeeze film is generated to support the load. The pressure developed in the lubricating fluid carries the load applied to the joint. The thin film of lubricant also produces a greater bearing surface. In addition, the cartilage is a biphasic porous medium. Water is bounded in the intrafibrillar space of the collagen matrix by proteoglycans. Intricate interaction of the mechanical stress, the electric charges, and the hydrodynamics result in a special fluid efflux pattern known as *elastohydrodynamic lubrication* (Fig. 6.11). The fluid exudation ahead of and imbibition behind the moving contact point of the articulating surface further facilitates the lubricant film.[20]

On occasion, heavy loading exceeds the capacity that the lubricant film can support. In this situation, the cartilage surfaces are in direct contact, and lubrication is provided by the mechanism of boundary lubrication.[20] Boundary lubrication is

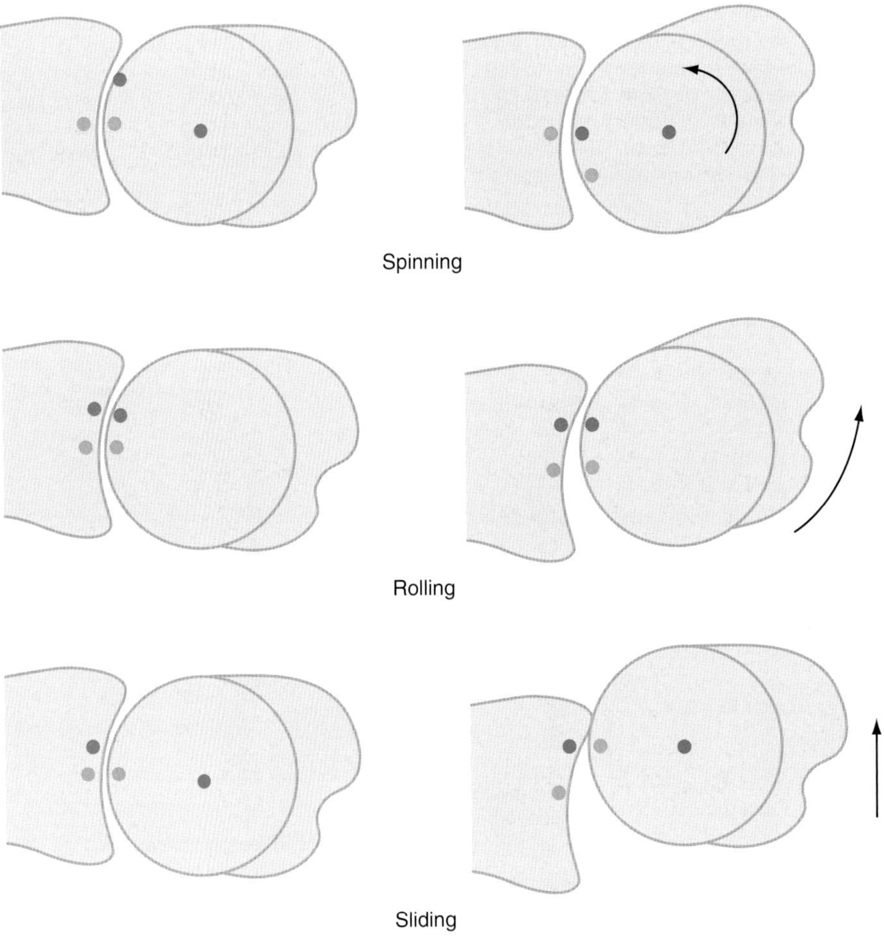

• **Fig. 6.10** The motions of joint articulation: spinning, rolling, and sliding. (From Morrey BF, Itoi E, An KN: Biomechanics of the shoulder. In Rockwood CA, Matsen, F, editors: *The shoulder*, ed 2, vol 1. Philadelphia, WB Saunders, pp 233–276, 1998.)

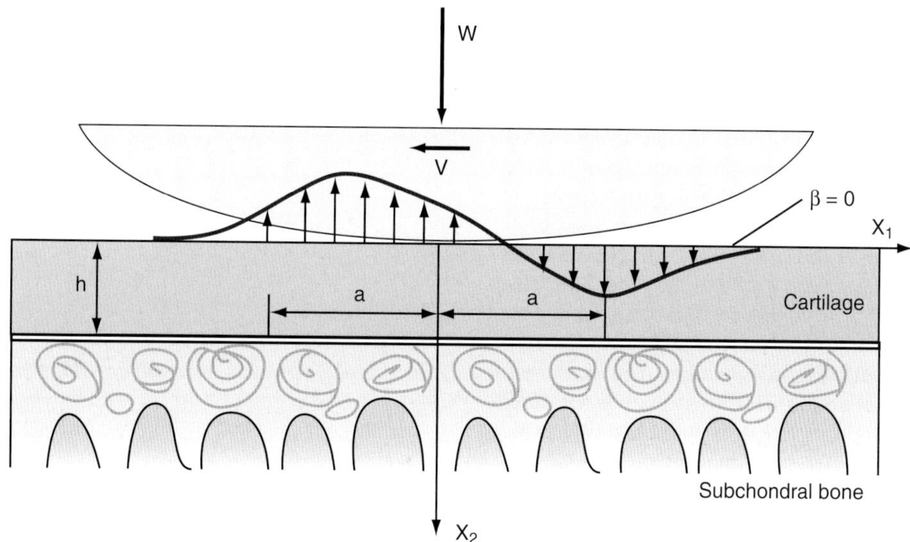

• **Fig. 6.11** Hydrodynamic lubrication. Surfaces moving relative to each other have an interposed viscous fluid that increases the pressure within the fluid to support the weight and keep the two surfaces separated. The pattern of predicted fluid exudation and imbibition over the articular surface (thickness = h) resulting from a frictionless, free-draining (β = 0) moving indenter is shown. *V* is the speed of the horizontal translation, and *W* is the resulting line load of a surface pressure distribution PA(×1) acting over a spread of |×1|<a. (From Mow VC, Soslowsky LJ: Friction, lubrication, and wear of diarthrodial joints. In Mow VC, Hayes WC, editors: *Basic orthopaedic biomechanics*, New York, Raven Press, pp 245–292, 1991.)

accomplished by a monolayer of glycoprotein called *lubricin*, a superficial zone protein. In the pathologic condition of OA, the structural properties of cartilage, such as porosity and permeability, are altered. The fluid efflux and the synovial fluid film are diminished, and boundary lubrication is the remaining mechanism of joint lubrication.

Joint Constraint and Stability

The human body is able to perform complex motions because the joints allow multiple degrees of freedom between articulating bones. Because of the variations in anatomic structures of the joints, various limbs have different movement characteristics and load transmissions. Adequate joint stability that balances motion and loads is necessary for a joint to function properly. Chronic disease or traumatic injury may cause damage to joint tissue, thus compromising the constraints and stability of the joint. To improve the diagnosis and treatment of such joint disorders, it is essential to understand the basic joint constraint mechanics which provides stability. The anatomic structure responsible for joint constraint can be divided into passive and active elements. Passive elements, consisting of the capsulo-ligamentous structures and bony articulating surfaces, provide static constraints of the joint. The active elements include muscle-tendon units, which provide dynamic constraints of the joint.

The contribution of capsulo-ligamentous structures to joint stability and constraint are determined by the change in length, the line of action, and the tissue material properties (Fig. 6.12). For a given loading and displacement of the joint, the greater the elongation of the soft tissue, the higher the passive tension generated by that tissue. However, the specific contribution of such passive tension to joint constraint further depends in turn on the relative line of action of the capsulo-ligament structures. Therefore, the relative locations of the origins and insertions of the ligaments may determine the contribution of the ligamentous tension in resisting joint displacement in three orthogonal directions. Surgical alternations of the soft tissue attachment to the bone would therefore change the joint constraints.

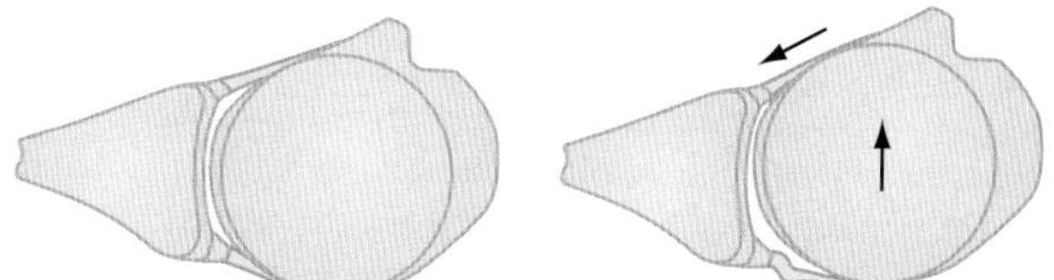

• **Fig. 6.12** When the joint is loaded or displaced, the capsulo-ligamentous tissues are stretched, and the passive tensions develop. The amount of tension developed depends on the amount of deformation and the material properties of the soft tissue. The location of the capsulo-ligamentous attachment on the bone and the direction of bony movement regulate not only the amount of deformation but also the direction of passive tension in stabilizing the joint.

Lengthening and shortening of the capsulo-ligament structures during joint loading and movement determine the tissue deformation. The tissue material properties, along with the amount of deformation, will determine the structure passive tension. For the same amount of deformation, the stiffer the tissue is, the higher the tension will be; likewise, the softer the tissue is, the lower the tension will be. Alterations of the material properties due to physiologic and pathologic conditions definitely alter the joint constraint and the articulation. For example, the tight posterior capsule of a baseball pitcher limits the range of physiologic motion. On the other hand, the softening of capsulo-ligamentous structures during pregnancy and in people with rheumatologic diseases could potentially lead to abnormal motion and contact stress on the joint surface. These alterations of soft tissue material properties must be considered as potentially critical factors in initiating early joint cartilage degeneration and may lead to the vicious cycle that perpetuates arthritis.

Experimentally, researchers assessed the significance of various passive anatomic structures to joint stability by using two methods: the stiffness test and the laxity test. The stiffness test is commonly used to determine the relative contributions of individual anatomic elements to joint constraint. The laxity test demonstrates the outcome of joint instability when one or more constraining units are compromised. In the stiffness test, the joint is displaced under controlled testing and the corresponding load is monitored. Based on the joint load–displacement curves, it is obvious that the load required to displace the joint is higher when all the ligaments are intact than when a ligament is lacerated. The difference in the constraining load between these two curves at the same joint displacement represents the contribution of that particular sectioned ligament to the joint constraint. Because the capsulo-ligamentous structures are passive tissues, as long as the joint displacement is controlled and experimentally reproduced, the relative contributions of individual tissues will not be dependent on the sectioning sequence of soft tissue. Contrary to the stiffness test, during which displacement is varied and load is measured, in the laxity test a specific load is applied to the joint and the extent of joint displacement is measured. Joint laxity is documented with changes in displacement as anatomic elements are removed. The joint laxity as observed and measured provides more of a clinical scenario of the joint instability experienced by a patient who has sustained a similar soft tissue injury.

In addition to soft tissue constraints, the joint articulating surface is an element that provides joint constraint and stability. Theoretically, its significance to joint stability is determined by both the geometric shapes of the joint surfaces and the amount of compressive force encountered between those two surfaces (Fig. 6.13A). When two curved surfaces articulate, a vertically applied force will induce either a transverse displacement or a transverse constraining force. The greater the congruency between the curved articulating surfaces, the greater the induced horizontal joint constraint force. This mechanism is sometimes referred to as *concavity-compression*. In the shoulder joint, for example, the relative translations between the glenoid and humeral head and the forces resisting translation were recorded. The stability ratio, defined as the peak translational force divided by the applied compressive force, was higher in the hanging-arm position than in glenohumeral abduction (Fig. 6.13B). The highest stability ratio was detected in the inferior and superior directions, and the anterior direction was associated with the lowest stability ratio. Resection of the glenoid labrum resulted in an average decrease in the stability ratio of 10%. In the treatment of traumatic recurrent anterior shoulder instability, patients with a large osseous glenoid defect are at risk for recurrent instability after arthroscopic Bankart repair. Bone grafting performed in shoulders with a large osseous glenoid defect to restore the articulating surface provides excellent clinical outcomes.[20a]

To benefit from the concavity-compression joint constraint, a compressive or oppositional force across the joint surface is required. This joint compressive force is usually generated by muscle contraction. The relative location and direction of the resultant joint force to the available articulating surfaces will determine the potential stability of the joint. For example, in the glenohumeral joint, if the resultant force is well located at the center of the glenoid articulating surface, the joint is considered stable. When the resultant force is directed outside the available joint surfaces, joint dislocation is most likely. However, when the resultant force is located within the joint surfaces but more toward the rim of the glenoid surface, the potential exists for joint subluxation. The interaction of muscle force resulting in a resultant joint constraint force is illustrated later.

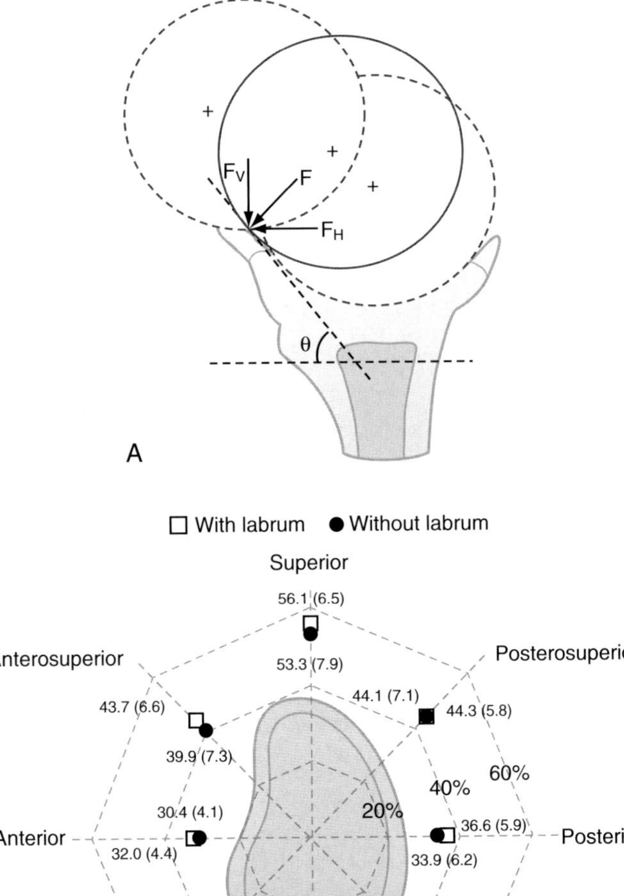

• **Fig. 6.13** Contributions of the articulating surface to joint stability. (A) Transverse displacement of bone in the curved joint requires elevation against the articulating surfaces. With compressive F_V applied, any transverse movement will encounter a resistance (F_H). If either the mating joint surface is flat (i.e., $\theta = 0$) or a compressive force, F_V is not available, there will be no transverse constraint ($F_H = 0$). (B) The stability ratio, defined as transverse constraint force F_H divided by the applied compressive force F_V, was measured in the glenohumeral joint with the labrum intact or absent. This measure indicates the stability through the joint-surface interaction, independent of the magnitude of the compressive force applied.

Intra-articular or intracapsular pressure is the other component of passive and static joint constraint (Fig. 6.14). The joint is usually surrounded by a capsule and sealed with synovial tissue. When the capsule is intact, any distraction force stretches and deforms the capsulo-ligamentous structure and will generate negative intra-articular pressure. This negative intra-articular pressure will counteract further displacement. When the joint capsule is vented, such negative pressure can no longer develop and cannot constrain the joint. Negative intracapsular pressure is, therefore, a constraint of all joints and is especially important for joints under gravitational distraction such as the shoulder joint.

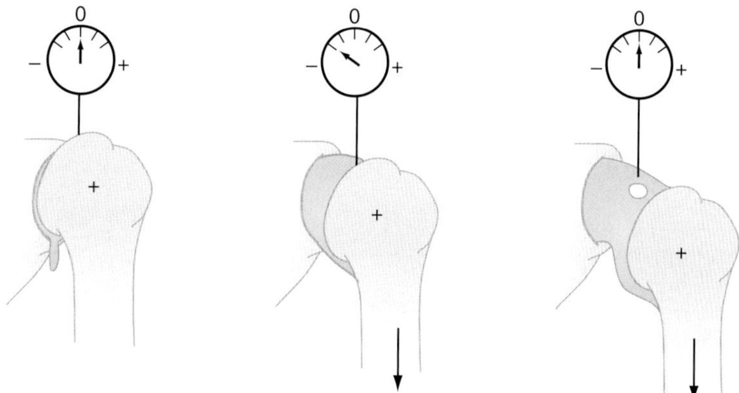

• **Fig. 6.14** Effect of negative intra-articular pressure on shoulder joint stability. In the normal situation, traction on the arm causes an increase in negative intra-articular pressure, and joint distraction is constrained. On the contrary, if the capsule is vented and air or fluid is introduced into the joint, traction on the arm no longer affects the intra-articular pressure; instead, the joint will be subluxed inferiorly.

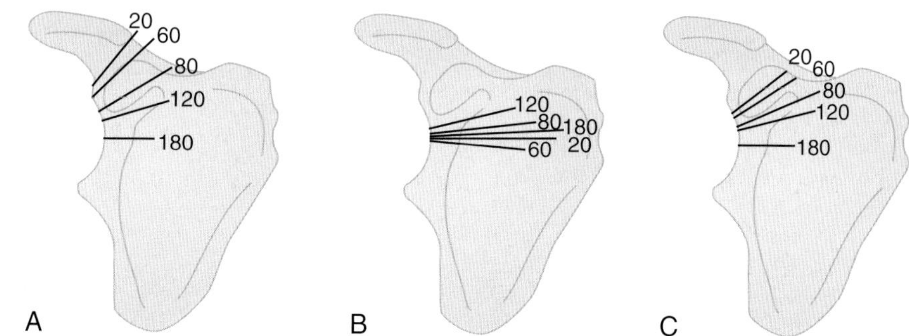

• **Fig. 6.15** Coordination of the muscle contractions to accomplish a given task is demonstrated by the situation when the deltoid and rotator cuff muscles work together to elevate the shoulder joint. (A) For patients with a rotator cuff tear, the shoulder elevation is accomplished by the deltoid muscle alone. The resultant joint force is directed superiorly because of the line of action of the deltoid muscle. In this situation, the joint is not stable and superior subluxation and migration results. (B) On the other hand, when elevating the shoulder with the rotator cuff muscle alone, the resultant joint force points toward the center of the glenoid surface, which makes the joint very stable. However, the magnitude of the joint resultant forces are relatively high, which may not be ideal for the cartilage tissue. (C) Ideally, shoulder elevation is accomplished with a combination of the deltoid muscles as the prime mover to provide strength and power, along with the rotator cuff muscles as the sterling in directing the joint resultant force to keep the joint in a more stable condition.

Active muscle contraction is also important for joint stability. Proper coordination of muscle contraction provides dynamic joint constraint. On the other hand, deficiency of muscle innervation or a tendon defect can result in unfavorable joint constraint and lead to joint instability. Importantly, muscle force can act as either a joint stabilizer or a joint dislocator. The contribution of muscles to joint constraint is similar to that of passive capsulo-ligamentous tension. It is determined by the line of action of the passive and active tension of the muscle. Based on the relative position of the bony structure and the direction of the joint displacement, the same muscle-tendon structure can contribute differently to joint constraint. When the joint is spanned by multiple muscles, the coordination of muscle contraction will ultimately determine the dynamic joint stability. For example, the contributions of muscle contractions to the articulating surfaces of the shoulder can be described in terms of the normal and shear directions (Fig. 6.15). The shear component has direct influence on the transverse translation of the bony element at the joint. In contrast, the normal force component of the muscle provides the compressive force to bring the surfaces together. A glenohumeral joint with a lax capsule and loose ligaments might be dynamically stabilized if the glenoid concavity is maintained and the functions of the external and internal rotators, which are efficient stabilizers, are enhanced. On the other hand, in a patient with a rotator cuff tear, the pull of the major movers, such as deltoids during arm elevation or forward rotation, will result in a resultant joint force in the superior and anterior directions; this results in superior impingement or anterior instability.

In general, muscle contraction will generate moments about all three axes of rotation of a given joint. However, when the constraints from other periarticular soft tissues are not available, the muscle will be primarily responsible for maintaining stability during the joint's rotation. If a muscle crosses multiple joints, the effect of muscle recruitment depends on the moment arms of all the joints it spans. The concept of biarticular muscle is of extreme clinical importance. For example, when considering rehabilitation after reconstructive surgery of the anterior cruciate ligament, the goal is to strengthen the muscles without excessive tension being placed on the ligament. Quadriceps loading, especially with the knee in a near extended position, would result in an anterior joint shear force and anterior displacement of the tibia with respect to the femur. This shear force would induce tension in the anterior cruciate ligament. To address this problem, investigators have employed closed kinetic-chain exercise. During closed-kinetic-chain–type exercises, such as the squat and the leg press, the foot is fixed, and knee motion is accompanied by motion at the hip and ankle joints. The GRF causes external flexion moments at both the knee and hip joints. The antagonistic muscle action of hamstrings at the knee joint is recruited to balance the hip flexion moment. Co-contraction of quadriceps and hamstrings at the knee joint reduces the anterior joint shear force and the tension in the anterior cruciate ligament.[21]

Mechanical Loading on Tendon

Tendons transmit the muscle contraction force to bone to cause limb movement. The force transmitted is primarily tensile force. In addition, specific portions of tendons also experience compression and shear force. Compression occurs when the tendon path is altered around a bony structure or pulley system. As a tendon is subjected to local compression, the mechanical loading does not distribute evenly within the tendon. The pressure decreases in deeper layers while the tension increases to the outer part. The overlapping of pressure and tension in the transition zone results in shear force inside the tendon. Furthermore, during tendon gliding against the surrounding tissues, shear force is generated on the contact surfaces of the tendon and surrounding tissues.

A tendon gliding through a pulley is analogous to a belt wrapped around a fixed mechanical pulley (Fig. 6.16). As the tendon moves proximally, the tensions in the tendon proximal and distal to the pulley (F_p and F_d) are related to the angle (θ) of the tendon segments wrapped around the pulley or arc of contact and the friction coefficient (μ).[22] Thus,

$$\text{Friction} = F_p - F_d = F_d\left(e^{\mu\theta} - 1\right)$$

This simple relationship clearly demonstrates the importance of the angle of contact and the friction coefficient. It explains why avoiding awkward joint postures is important ergonomically to reduce repetitive injury of soft tissue.

The three modes on mechanical loading (namely, tension, compression, and gliding) can be demonstrated by three scenarios at the shoulder joint (Fig. 6.17). The short head of the biceps brachii tendon is an example of the first scenario, in which the tendon mainly experiences tensile force alone. The second scenario, in which the tendon encounters tensile force and compression together, occurs internally at the bone insertion site of the supraspinatus tendon. The insertional area of the tendon encounters tensile force, as well as compression resulting from the transverse contact of the tendon with the attached bone. The third scenario occurs when the tendon is simultaneously subjected to tension, compression, and gliding. The long head of the biceps brachii tendon, where it passes through the bicipital groove, demonstrates an example of the third scenario. The supraspinatus tendon also fits the scenario, as well as the second scenario. Subacromial impingement of the supraspinatus tendon generates high compressive stress that varies along the supraspinatus tendon, depending on humeroscapular elevation. The mode of mechanical tendon loading is potentially correlated to the incidence of tendon degeneration. The tendons in the first scenario rarely experience degenerative tendinopathy. Tendons commonly affected with tendinopathy are represented in the other two scenarios, in which the affected areas normally sustain compression and shear force with or without gliding in addition to tensile force.

In conclusion, knowledge of biomechanical principles can help explain many commonly encountered situations in the musculoskeletal system, which contribute to musculoskeletal disease.

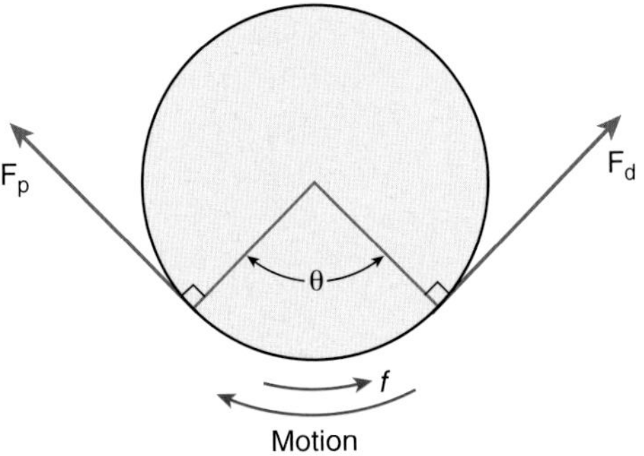

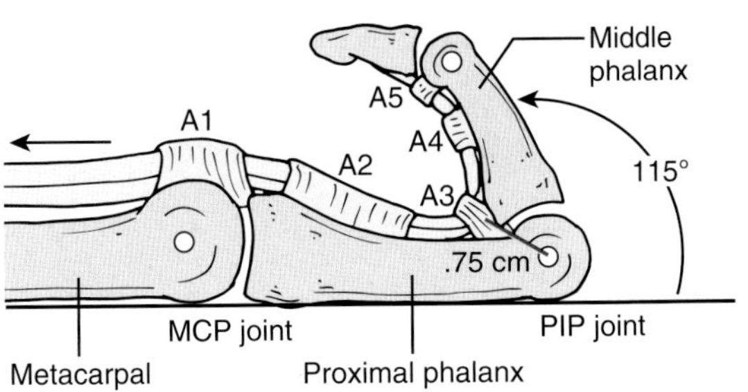

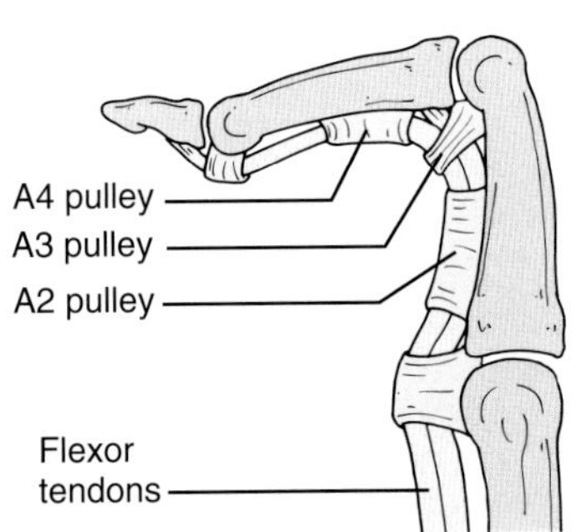

• **Fig. 6.16** To move the finger, the tendon glides through a pulley, which is analogous to a belt wrapped around a mechanical pulley. The tendon force must overcome the gliding resistance of the tendon and generate sufficient force to move the external load. The friction, *f*, of a tendon against the surrounding tissue is in the opposite direction of the tendon motion. The sliding resistance (friction) is the difference between the tension on the distal and proximal ends across the pulley (F_d and F_p respectively). *MCP,* Metacarpophalangeal; *PIP,* proximal interphalangeal.

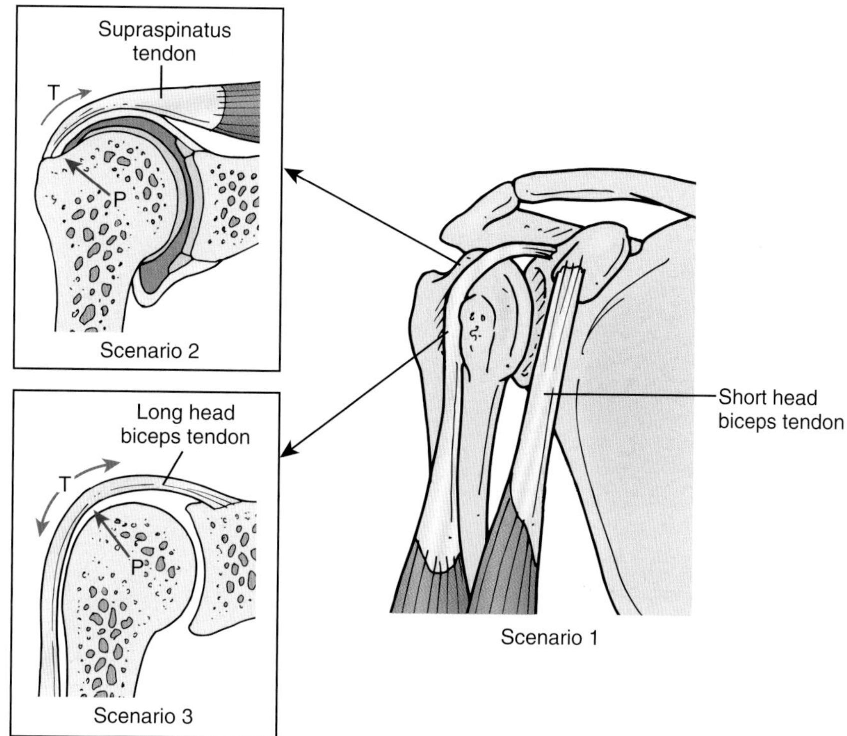

• **Fig. 6.17** Supraspinatus tendon and long head and short head biceps tendons. Scenario 1: tensile force only. Scenario 2: tensile force and compression. Scenario 3: tensile force and compression with gliding.

The references for this chapter can also be found on ExpertConsult.com.

References

1. Borelli GA: *De motu animalium*, Batavis, 1685, Lugduni.
2. Cappozzo A, Catani F, Croce UD, et al.: Position and orientation in space of bones during movement: anatomical frame definition and determination, *Clin Biomech* 10(4):171–178, 1995.
3. Inman V, Ralston H, Todd F: *Human walking*, Baltimore, 1981, Williams & Wilkins.
4. Kadaba M, Ramakrishnan H, Wootten M: Measurement of lower extremity kinematics during level walking, *J Orthop Res* 8(3):383–392, 1990.
5. Kaufman K, Hughes C, Morrey B, et al.: Gait characteristics of patients with knee osteoarthritis, *J Biomech* 34:907–915, 2001.
6. Perry J: *Gait analysis: normal and pathological function*, Thorofare, NJ, 1992, Slack.
7. Sutherland DH, Olshen R, Cooper L, et al.: The development of mature gait, *J Bone Joint Surg Am* 62(3):336–353, 1980.
8. Chao EYS: Justification of triaxial goniometer for the measurement of joint rotation, *J Biomech* 13:989–1006, 1980.
9. Grood E, Suntay W: A joint coordinate system for the clinical description of three-dimensional motions: applications to the knee, *J Biomech Eng* 105:136–143, 1983.
10. Selvik G: *A roentgen-stereophotogrammetric method for the study of the kinematics of the skeletal system*, Lund, Sweden, 1974, University of Lund.
11. Selvik G: A roentgen-stereophotogrammetric system. Construction, calibration and technical accuracy, *Acta Radiol Diagn (Stockh)* 24(4):343–352, 1983.
12. Li G, Wuerz TH, DeFrate LE: Feasibility of using orthogonal fluoroscopic images to measure in vivo joint kinematics, *J Biomech Eng* 126(2):314–318, 2004.
13. Tashman S, Anderst W: In-vivo measurement of dynamic joint motion using high speed biplane radiography and CT: application to canine ACL deficiency, *J Biomech Eng* 125(2):238–245, 2003.
14. Kinzel GL, Hall Jr AS, Hillberry BM: Measurement of the total motion between two body segments. I. Analytical development, *J Biomech* 5(1):93–105, 1972.
15. Spoor C, Veldpaus F: Rigid body motion calculated from spatial coordinates of markers, *J Biomech* 13:391–393, 1980.
16. Woltring HJ: On optimal smoothing and derivative estimation from noisy data in biomechanics, *Hum Mov Sci* 4(3):229–245, 1985.

16a. Newton I: *Philosophiæ Naturalis Principia Mathematica*, 5 July 1687.

17. Myazaki T, Wada M, Kawahara H, et al.: Dynamic load at baseline can predict radiographic disease progression in medial compartment knee osteoarthritis, *Ann Rheum Dis* 61:617–622, 2002.
18. Sharma L, Hurwitz DE, Thonar EJ, et al.: Knee adduction moment, serum hyaluronan level, and disease severity in medial tibiofemoral osteoarthritis, *Arthritis Rheum* 41(7):1233–1240, 1998.
19. Mundermann A, Dyrby CO, Andriacchi TP: Secondary gait changes in patients with medial compartment knee osteoarthritis: increased load at the ankle, knee, and hip during walking, *Arthritis Rheum* 52(9):2835–2844, 2005.
20. Mow VC, Flatow EL, Foster RJ: Biomechanics. In Simon SR, editor: *Orthopaedic basic science*, Rosemont, Ill, 1994, American Academy of Orthopaedic Surgeons, pp 397–446.

20a. Halder AM, Kuhl SG, Zobitz ME, et al.: Effects of the glenoid labrum and glenohumeral abduction on stability of the shoulder joint through concavity-compression: an in vitro study. *J Bone Joint Surg Am* 83:1062–1069, 2001.

21. Lutz GE, Palmitier RA, An KN, et al.: Comparison of tibiofemoral joint forces during open-kinetic-chain and closed-kinetic-chain exercises, *J Bone Joint Surg Am* 75A(5):732–739, 1993.
22. Uchiyama S, Coert JH, Berglund L, et al.: Method for the measurement of friction between tendon and pulley, *J Orthop Res* 13(1):83–89, 1995.

7 Regenerative Medicine and Tissue Engineering

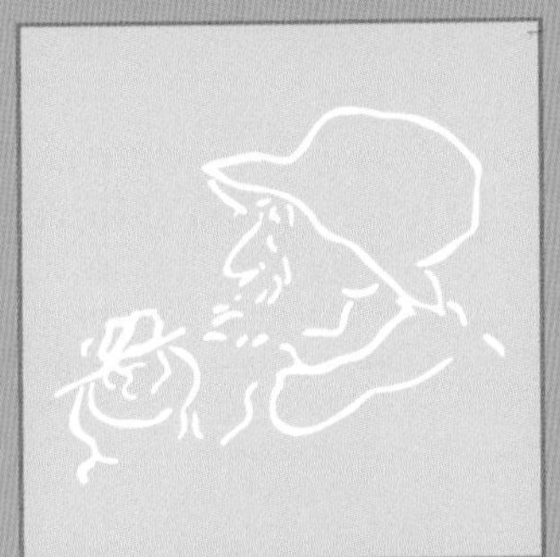

FRANK P. LUYTEN, COSIMO DE BARI, AND FRANCESCO DELL'ACCIO

KEY POINTS

Tissue repair and regeneration are partially determined by genetic factors.

Successful regeneration requires a balanced immune cell response.

The increased understanding of molecular signals governing native joint-resident stem cell function could lead to pharmacologic interventions that trigger intrinsic repair mechanisms to treat or prevent progression of damage.

Cell-based therapeutics and their combination products are complex regarding their mechanism of action and manufacturing and have evolved into advanced therapy medicinal products with a specific regulatory path.

Tissue engineering has adopted the concept of biomimetics of in vivo tissue development. *Developmental engineering* is the term used to describe a novel methodology for the rational and accurate design of robust, well-controlled manufacturing processes of "biologic spare parts."

Recent advances in regenerative medicine and tissue engineering relevant to rheumatology have entered clinical practice and include the biologic repair of joint surface defects and bone healing.

Introduction

Tissue destruction and joint failure are ultimately the disabling outcomes of most forms of inflammatory or degenerative arthritides.[1] The need for repair and regeneration of joints and joint-associated tissues is becoming more relevant as the dramatic advances of targeted treatments and improved disease management have allowed much more efficient control of inflammation and joint destruction.

In view of this, other aspects of joint biology require more attention—notably, and most importantly, the mechanisms driving tissue response and repair. Indeed, to restore the balance between tissue destruction and tissue repair (Fig. 7.1), we should be looking at the more complete picture, that is, the "systems biology" of the joint as an organ. Targeting tissue repair has entered our discipline, and investigating the potential to activate and enhance joint tissue repair mechanisms has become a prime goal. Introducing regenerative medicine approaches provides a significant opportunity to restore joint homeostasis and thus possibly provide a cure.

Regenerative medicine and tissue engineering (TE) seek to repair or regenerate damaged tissues and organs, regardless of the cause of the damage, ideally without scar tissue formation, thereby restoring both the structure and function of the damaged tissues/organs. Nature demonstrates that this goal is achievable, as successful wound healing and fracture repair are processes that happen routinely after birth. We also know, as demonstrated in fetal surgery, that scarless repair is partially dependent on age and context. Thus, it is attractive to envision that, with an in-depth understanding of the repair processes at the cellular and molecular level, we may be able to intervene quickly at the time of injury and guide the healing process more appropriately, thereby preventing scar formation. In view of this, there is increasing evidence that the role of the immune system is of importance in postnatal tissue regeneration, and that the further understanding of the crosstalk between the immune cells and the stem cells may be crucial for clinical success.[2]

Postnatal tissue healing mimics developmental processes of tissue formation. For example, it appears that the process of rebuilding an adult limb, such as seen in the axolotl, but also during fracture healing in higher species, has many similarities with how the limb forms in the embryo. Thus both limb formation and limb regeneration appear to use the same molecular pathways.[3] The remarkable advances in developmental biology during the past several decades have now provided the knowledge platform to advance into novel regenerative approaches in postnatal life. These advances not only include our understanding of the mechanisms of body axis formation and organogenesis but also impressive progress in stem cell biology, including the regulation of stemness, stem cell niches, lineage specification and cell differentiation, and the molecular pathways involved. Consequently, we have entered a new era in regenerative medicine and TE.[4,5] In this chapter we will review the approaches that seek to repair damaged and diseased synovial joints and skeletal structures.

When we aim to repair tissues, two mechanistic approaches are possible. The first approach consists of enhancing intrinsic repair mechanisms with stimulation of local cell proliferation, differentiation and tissue metabolic activity, and recruitment of endogenous progenitor populations into the damaged tissue. The second approach becomes necessary when intrinsic repair is insufficient and entails extrinsic repair, that is, TE approaches via manufacturing of cellular and/or combination products that can contribute mostly locally to tissue repair (Fig. 7.2).

Intrinsic Repair

In this section we will discuss the mechanism by which, in favorable conditions, joint tissues can repair after injury and how such mechanisms can be pharmacologically harnessed to prime and support repair in conditions in which spontaneous repair fails.

Genetic Basis of Tissue Repair

For many years it has been commonly accepted that "cartilage… when destroyed, is never recovered."[6] This statement probably still holds true for established defects (e.g., defects that have failed to heal and have become chronically symptomatic, and therefore come to the attention of the clinician); however, prospective imaging and arthroscopy studies have revealed that even in adult humans, acute cartilage defects are much more prevalent than suspected, even in asymptomatic subjects, and have some capacity for spontaneous healing.[7]

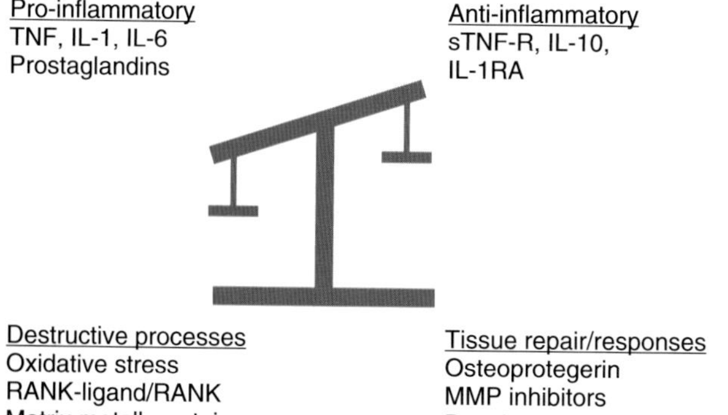

• **Fig. 7.1** The "systems biology" view of chronic arthritis. The severity and outcome of disease is determined by the balance between inflammation/destructive processes and anti-inflammatory signals with repair attempts. *BMP,* Bone morphogenetic protein; *ERK,* extra-cellular-signal regulated kinase; *FGF,* fibroblast growth factor; *IL,* interleukin; *MAPK,* mitogen-activated protein kinase; *MMP,* matrix metalloproteinase; *NF-κB,* nuclear factor-κB; *RANK,* receptor activator of nuclear factor-κB; *sTNFrec,* soluble tumor necrosis factor receptor; *TGF,* transforming growth factor; *TNF,* tumor necrosis factor.

Such studies showed that roughly half of adults without joint symptoms have chondral defects, and that about a third of such lesions improve spontaneously, a third remain stable, and the remainder worsen.[8,9]

In addition to comorbidities and environmental factors influencing the natural history of chondral defects (age, co-existing osteoarthritis [OA], high body mass, female sex, abnormal bone geometry, bone marrow lesions),[10,11] a prospective, magnetic resonance imaging (MRI)-based study in a sib-paired cohort[12] identified a very high (>80%) heritability of the rate of progression of chondral defects.

Nonetheless, in contrast with the remarkable progress in the identification of genetic markers predisposing to OA,[13,14] no quantitative trait linkage and association analysis study is available yet in humans with regard to the intrinsic capacity of repairing articular cartilage defects.

Although the evidence for the heritability of cartilage repair capacity in humans is still circumstantial, findings of animal studies are more convincing. Comparing the capacity of different inbred mouse strains to heal full-thickness cartilage defects, one group[15] demonstrated that different inbred mouse strains have a dramatically different capacity to heal cartilage defects and to avoid the onset of post-traumatic OA. This finding supports the concept that repair capacity has a genetic component. The development of such an animal model lends itself to genetic analysis. For instance, another group[16] took advantage of the different healing capacity of two strains of mice: LG/J, which can efficiently heal joint surface defects and experimental wounds to the cartilage of the pinna of the ear, and SM/J, which are poor healers. A set of recombinant inbred lines were obtained by crossing the

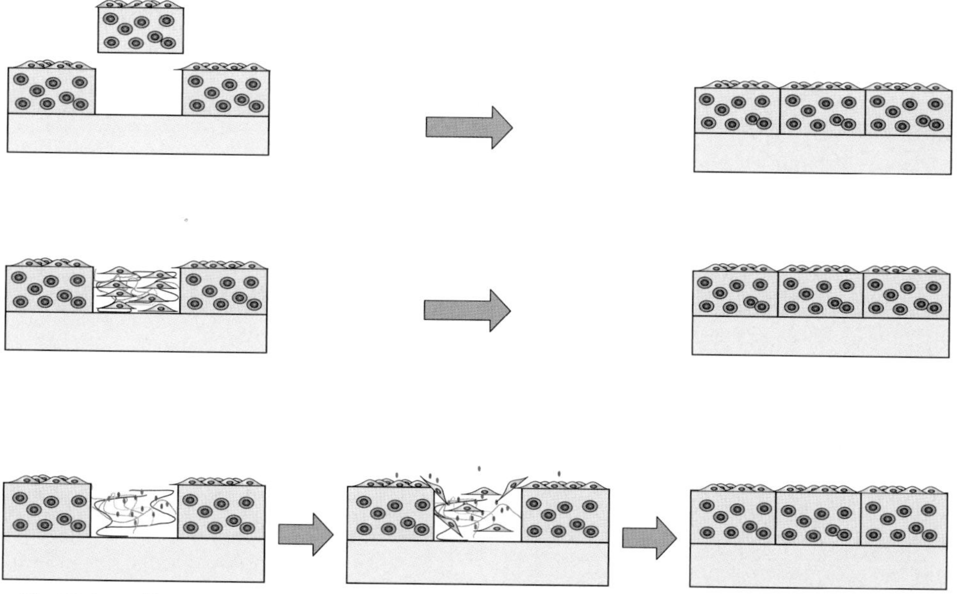

• **Fig. 7.2** In traditional tissue engineering *(top)*, the repair tissue is generated and matures in the laboratory and is inserted in the defect directly. No maturation is expected to happen in vivo. In cell-based approaches *(middle)*, nondifferentiated or partially differentiated in vitro expanded cells are implanted. Differentiation and remodeling are expected to happen in vivo. In cell-free approaches *(bottom)*, only biomaterials and bioactive molecules are implanted, which, in vivo, attract resident progenitor cells and induce their patterning and differentiation.

two strains. It was found that both the capacity of healing joint surface defects and the capacity to heal ear wounds were highly heritable and that they correlated with each other. This finding suggests that the capacity to heal cartilage is inheritable by itself, whether the cartilage is on the surface of a diarthrodial joint or in the pinna of the ear and is not just dependent on the resistance to develop OA or on factors extrinsic to cartilage such as bone shape/quality or synovitis. For example, the fact that homeostatic mechanisms affect the rate of OA progression suggests that the same genes associated with the predisposition to OA might affect also the capacity to repair; however, this assumption has never been rigorously tested experimentally. It must be remembered that other independent aspects come into play in the determination of OA progression, including joint shape,[17,18] body mass index, inflammation, and several other aspects that are also under genetic control.[19] Therefore, allelic variants that affect such parameters will also affect OA predisposition, independently from repair mechanisms intrinsic to the joint. Nevertheless, it is interesting that signaling molecules belonging to the same pathways have been associated with both OA and cartilage regeneration. For instance, loss of function alleles of the wingless type (Wnt) inhibitor FRZB are associated with OA predisposition,[20–22] and a single nucleotide polymorphism of the Wnt ligand WNT-3A has been associated with the heritability of cartilage repair capacity in mice.[23] Most of the genes identified in these screenings affect directly the behavior of joint resident stem cells or their interaction with joint tissues.

Signaling Pathways Orchestrating Joint Homeostasis and Surface Repair

Joint surface repair involves a number of events that are highly coordinated in space and time: when and for how long stem cells should proliferate; the path of their migration; the timing and extent of extra-cellular matrix production; and where and when, within the repair tissue, a stem cell should become an osteoblast or a chondrocyte are all processes regulated by soluble secreted molecular signals. Given the similarity between repair and embryonic joint morphogenesis, it is unsurprising that the major signaling molecules controlling these two processes are very similar: the transforming growth factor (TGF)-β superfamily, including the bone morphogenetic proteins (BMPs) and growth differentiation factors (GDFs), the Wnt family of proteins, the fibroblast growth factors (FGFs), the hedgehog proteins, parathyroid hormone (PTH)/PTH-related protein (PTHrP), and hedgehog and Notch signaling.[24] Next, we select a few examples of how these signaling pathways are involved in joint formation and their role in postnatal joint repair, with a specific focus on those that have led to advances in early clinical development in arthritic diseases.

PTHrP Signaling

PTHrP signaling during embryonic development of the skeletal elements contributes to the positional information and regulates the rate of differentiation of the chondrocytes through the epiphysis, preventing precocious or ectopic hypertrophic differentiation and endochondral bone formation.[25–28] In adulthood, the PTH/PTHrP receptor PPR is barely expressed in normal articular cartilage but is strongly upregulated in the intermediate layers of repair cartilage, just above the bottom layer of hypertrophic chondrocytes[29] and in osteoarthritic cartilage. Because hypertrophic differentiation of articular chondrocytes is not only a feature of OA but also drives cartilage breakdown[30,31] and PTH/PTHrP signaling is known to delay hypertrophy, investigators[32] tested whether a truncated form of human recombinant PTH currently used in the clinic for osteoporosis could improve the outcome of OA in mice. Indeed, human recombinant PTH could not only stop cartilage breakdown but also induced a regenerative effect. Unfortunately, the doses required to achieve this impressive effect in mice were very high and induced osteopetrosis. A restriction of the signaling domains to the tissue of interest is therefore required before this approach can be used in the clinic. Another caveat is that this study cannot discriminate between the effects on cartilage and those on the bone. In this context, it is noteworthy that strontium ranelate, another compound used as an anabolic agent in osteoporosis, was also able to reduce the rate of joint space narrowing and to improve symptoms in patients with OA.[33] Similar results were replicated in a rat and a dog model of instability-induced OA.[34,35]

Transforming Growth Factor-β/Bone Morphogenetic Protein Signaling

Recent data highlighted the relevance and critical role of members of the TGF-β superfamily (TGF-β, BMPs, and GDFs) in the biology of articular cartilage, bone, joints and joint-associated tissues, both during development and in postnatal tissue homeostasis, repair, and tissue response to injury and aging. TGF-β is involved in the maintenance and aging of articular cartilage and OA.[36] Despite the well-documented anabolic actions of TGF-β, excessive or sustained activation of this signaling pathway is detrimental to cartilage. In fact, overexpression of TGF-β[37] resulted in spontaneous osteoarthritis in mice and TGF-β or TGF-β receptor blockade protected cartilage integrity in models of osteoarthritis.[38–40]

BMPs have been reported to play major roles in articular cartilage metabolism, with BMP-7/osteogenic protein-1 (OP-1) being of particular interest.[41,42] In addition, modulation of TGF-β/BMP downstream receptor-Smad signaling plays an essential role in both the regulation of chondrocyte differentiation and the development and progression of OA.[43] Therefore, given overwhelming evidence of the regenerative potential of this family of growth and differentiation factors in pre-clinical models, it is not surprising that their therapeutic use is being explored in clinical studies and in indications such as long bone healing and OA. In addition, intense research is ongoing to identify modulators of the TGF-β/BMP receptor/Smad signaling pathways through peptide technology (peptidomimetics) or small molecule screens.[44] Because synovial joints allow for local treatment, it is expected that some newly identified compounds will first be tested as local applications, such as joint surface repair and monoarticular OA. BMP devices are already in the clinic for orthopedic applications such as spine fusion and the healing of nonunions.[45,46]

Fibroblast Growth Factor Signaling

Extensive investigations have identified fibroblast growth factor receptor (FGFR)3 signaling as a key regulator of chondrocyte and osteoblast function, both during development and postnatally. In particular, absence of signaling through FGFR3 in the joints of *Fgfr3*$^{-/-}$ mice leads to premature cartilage degeneration and early signs of OA.[47] One of the key ligands of FGFR3 signaling appears to be FGF18.[48] In the postnatal joint, FGF18 has significant anabolic effects on cartilage metabolism. Intra-articular injection of FGF18 induced a dose-dependent increase in cartilage formation and a reduction in cartilage degeneration scores in the medial tibial plateau of rats with OA.[49] Importantly, this effect was seen only in joints affected by OA, not in normal rat joints, suggesting a specific response to tissue injury. At the molecular level, this joint-protective effect may be due partially to its interaction with other signaling pathways such as BMP signaling by repressing noggin, a BMP antagonist.[50]

Wnt Signaling

Overwhelming evidence indicates a critical role for Wnt signaling in cartilage and bone biology, with a specific relevance to osteoporosis and OA (for a review, see ref. 51). Although Wnt signaling is essential for the development and homeostasis of synovial joints,[52–56] genetic studies in humans[20] and experimental data[22,57,58] demonstrate that excessive/uncontrolled activation of Wnt/β catenin signaling leads to reprogramming of articular chondrocytes toward catabolism or loss of their stable phenotype with subsequent loss of articular cartilage tissue structure and function. In particular, loss of function allelic variants of the Wnt inhibitor FRZB were associated with increased predisposition to develop OA.[20] Similarly, disruption of the *FRZB* gene in mice resulted in increased activity of the WNT signaling pathway and consequent increased bone stiffness and enhanced cartilage damage.[22] Importantly, upon induction of experimental OA, *Frzb*$^{-/-}$ mice showed greater cartilage loss than their wild-type counterparts.[59] Increased cartilage damage in *Frzb*$^{-/-}$ mice was associated with higher levels of β-catenin dependent Wnt signaling and with higher expression levels of matrix metalloproteinase (MMP)-3. Moreover, FRZB can directly inhibit MMP-3, probably through the netrin domain, indicating the potential complexity of the underlying mechanisms of observed phenomena.[60]

Tightly regulated Wnt signaling is critical for the homeostasis of synovial joints.[54,56,61,62] One study[63] demonstrated that in human and experimental murine arthritis, the inflammatory cytokine tumor necrosis factor drives the excessive production of the Wnt antagonist DKK1. The consequent excessive inhibition of the Wnt pathway was found to be responsible for bone resorption (erosions), typical of this arthritis model, as well as of rheumatoid arthritis (RA). Accordingly, blocking DKK1, and therefore de-repressing Wnt signaling, resulted in reversal of bone damage.[63] In the same model, direct activation of WNT signaling using the Wnt agonist R-Spondin 1 reversed not only the bone damage (also achieved with DKK1 blockade), but also the cartilage damage.[64] Therefore, both uncontrolled suppression and activation of the WNT signaling may lead to catabolism and cartilage loss. It appears that a tight control, both in terms of timing and magnitude, is essential not only to preserve homeostasis but even to induce tissue regeneration. For instance, controlled and temporary activation of β catenin signaling in adult mice led to an initial reduction of extra-cellular matrix (ECM), followed by chondrocyte proliferation and thickening of the articular cartilage.[62] Even more strikingly, although more remote from the context of joint disease, one study[65] demonstrated that although WNT signaling is essential for the capacity of some species (i.e., axolotl or *Xenopus* tadpoles) to regenerate entire limbs, it was sufficient to slightly modify the spatiotemporal distribution of WNT-β catenin activation to afford the chick embryo with the capacity to regenerate an entire limb.

In the clinical context of joint disease and regeneration, the complexity of Wnt signaling and its potential downstream effects may offer the opportunity to target catabolic effects while preserving the homeostatic ones. One group[66] demonstrated that WNT-3A drives chondrocyte proliferation through activation of the β catenin pathway and loss of differentiation through activation of CaMKII. Therefore, targeting CaMKII specifically allowed enhancement of differentiation without affecting proliferation.

Another opportunity concerns molecules that "buffer" Wnt signaling at homeostatic levels. For instance, WNT16 is a weak Wnt activator, which, however, prevents overactivation when more potent canonical Wnt molecules are present.[67] Genetic disruption of the *Wnt16* gene resulted in higher susceptibility to experimental osteoarthritis in mice and to a depletion of articular cartilage-residing progenitor cells.[67]

Better understanding of the downstream signaling mechanism and its regulation will be essential to target only the pathogenic effect of these pleiotropic signaling pathways in cartilage, bone, and the osteochondral junction.[68]

Growth Hormone/Insulin-like Growth Factor Axis

Other targets are activated by signaling molecules that play more prominent roles in postnatal skeletal growth. These proteins/pathways can be regarded as potential "anabolic" agents and could contribute to the restoration of joint homeostasis. In this regard, the growth hormone (GH)/insulin-like growth factor (IGF) axis is of interest. IGF-1 has been reported to be critical in the maintenance of the homeostasis of articular cartilage explants ex vivo.[69] Further evidence of its anabolic effect in in vivo models has led to the early clinical development of intra-articular treatments with IGF-1 in knee OA, although reports of clinical trials have not been published. Furthermore, it was reported that systemic administration of GH in horses may be beneficial to joint/articular cartilage biology because it increases IGF-1 levels in synovial fluid.[70] Improved formulations of GH have been explored to improve the duration and effect size in synovial joints.[71] Some evidence exists of a relationship between levels of IGF-1 and OA, further suggesting a potential benefit of targeting the GH/IGF-1 axis, particularly in OA. However, data thus far are inconclusive, and further systematic analysis of the hypothalamic-pituitary axis, including GH, IGF-1, and somatostatin, is required.[72]

As for all growth factor technologies, further studies are needed to address critical issues such as the relevant genetic background of the patients, stage of the disease process, and tissue specificity to restrict an effect to the targeted tissues, thereby avoiding systemic adverse effects.

Joint Resident Stem Cells

Stem cells persist in adult life to mediate tissue maintenance and regeneration. They have the capacity to self-renew (that is, to divide and produce more stem cells), thereby preserving a constant pool of stem cells, and to differentiate to replace the mature cells that are lost to physiologic turnover, injury, disease, or aging. Self-renewal and differentiation are regulated by stem cell intrinsic factors and signals from the surrounding microenvironment in which the stem cells reside, called the *stem cell niche*.

Stem cell niches have been described for a number of tissue types such as the hair follicle, intestine, and bone marrow.[73,74] In bone marrow the niches of hematopoietic stem cells (HSCs) have received considerable attention, and the understanding of HSCs has led to improvements of bone marrow transplantation outcomes in hematology. The HSC niches include the endosteal niche, where HSCs are in close contact with osteoblasts residing at the bone surface of the trabeculae, and the perivascular niche, where the HSCs are close to the sinusoids in the bone marrow.[60]

Mesenchymal stromal/stem cells (MSCs), which are derived from bone marrow and other connective tissues, including the synovium, have the ability to differentiate into chondrogenic and osteogenic lineage cells. Therefore, MSCs are of interest for their potential clinical use for joint tissue repair.

Evidence indicates that pericytes may be the native cells of the ex vivo MSCs.[75] Pericytes are located on the abluminal side of small blood vessels and are in close connection with the endothelial cells of the vessels. The proximity to vessels would allow MSCs to enter the bloodstream and migrate to sites of injury,[76] but it is not clear to what degree this happens and, importantly, if this phenomenon has clinical relevance. However, the notion that cells with MSC characteristics are derived from pericytes is challenged by the retrieval of MSC-like cells in articular cartilage,[77–79] notoriously an avascular tissue. Thus, pericytes are not the only source of MSCs, and such a relationship is likely to be tissue specific and context dependent.

The lack of an exclusive MSC marker in the joint has impeded studies of joint-resident MSCs.[80] One group[81] adopted a double-nucleoside-analog labeling method in a mouse model of joint surface injury to identify functional stem cells (i.e., long-term label-retaining cells that after injury undergo proliferation and differentiation).[81] This was based on the administration of two nucleoside analogs; iododeoxyuridine (IdU) was given before the injury followed by a washout period to identify label-retaining (slow-cycling) cells, and chlorodeoxyuridine (CldU) was given after the injury to label cells proliferating in response to the injury. In uninjured knees, IdU-label-retaining cells were detected in the synovium and were largely negative for CldU. Phenotypic analyses showed that these cells were nonhematopoietic and nonendothelial cells that expressed known MSC markers. After articular cartilage injury, there was marked accumulation of IdU and CldU double-positive cells, indicating that label-retaining cells proliferated to generate a pool of transit-amplifying cells. Furthermore, they formed ectopic cartilage, indicating that these cells can function as chondroprogenitors in their native environment.[81]

The label-retaining MSCs in the mouse synovium as identified by one group[81] were located in two niches, the lining niche and the sublining perivascular niche, the latter distinct from pericytes. In these two niches, MSCs could have distinct functions, but a hierarchy remains to be demonstrated (Fig. 7.3).

In recent years, lineage-tracing studies in mice have provided insights into the MSC populations that reside in the bone marrow, including the so-called *skeletal stem cells* (SSCs). In mouse bone marrow, perivascular MSCs are marked by Pdgfrα and Sca1,[82,83]

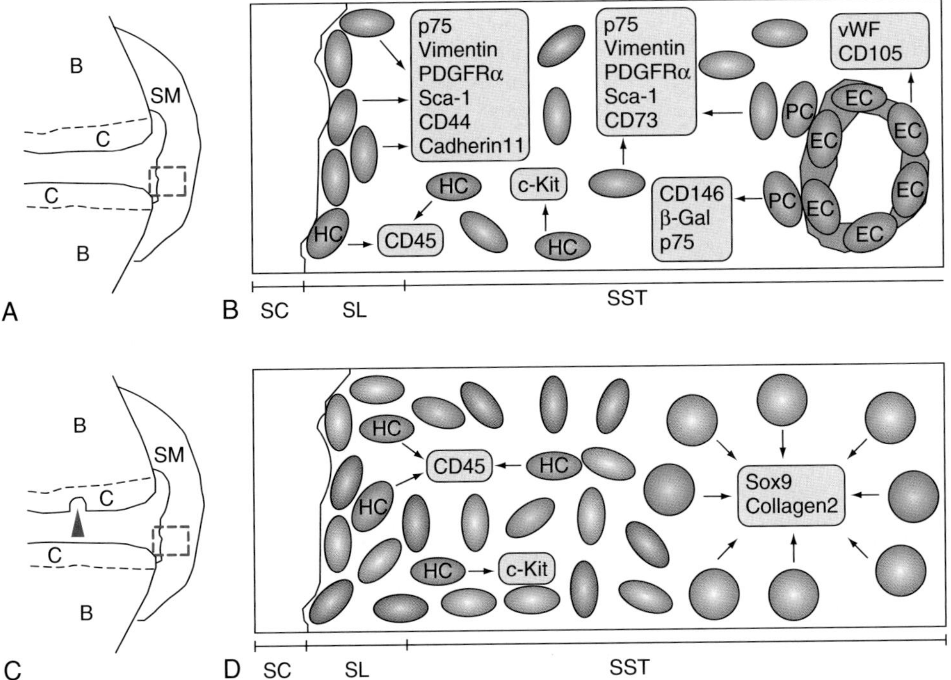

• **Fig. 7.3** Schematic representations of mesenchymal stem cells (MSCs) and their niches in synovium identified in mice using a double nucleoside analogue cell-labeling scheme.[123] (A) Schematic drawing of an uninjured control synovial joint. (B) Details of the dashed box in (A) showing cell populations in the synovium of uninjured joints. Iododeoxyuridine (IdU)-retaining cells *(green)* were located in both the synovial lining (SL) and the subsynovial tissue (SST). Subsets of IdU-positive cells displayed an MSC phenotype. IdU-negative cells *(blue)* included hematopoietic lineage cells (HC), endothelial cells (EC), pericytes (PC), and other cell types of unknown phenotype. (C) Schematic drawing of a synovial joint 12 days after articular cartilage injury in mice *(arrowhead)*. (D) Details of the dashed box in (C) showing cell populations in the synovium. Proliferating cells were detected in both the synovial lining and the subsynovial tissue and were either double positive for IdU and chlorodeoxyuridine (CldU; *orange*) or single positive for CldU *(red)*. Subsets of cells positive for IdU and CldU and cells positive only for IdU *(green)* expressed chondrocyte lineage markers. The boxed areas in (B) and (D) show cell phenotypes. *B,* Bone; *C,* cartilage; *p75,* low-affinity nerve growth factor receptor; *PDGFR,* platelet-derived growth factor receptor; *SC,* synovial cavity; *SM,* synovial membrane; *vWF,* von Willebrand factor. (From Kurth TB, Dell'Accio F, Crouch V, et al.: Functional mesenchymal stem cell niches in adult mouse knee joint synovium in vivo. *Arthritis Rheum* 63(5):1289–1300, 2011.)

Nestin (Nes)-GFP,[84,85] and Leptin-receptor (LepR),[86,87] with partial overlap between these cell populations. They support hematopoiesis and contribute to osteogenic and adipogenic lineages.[84,87] In addition, one study[88] identified a population of osteochondroreticular stem cells expressing Gremlin (Grem)1, distinct from Nes-GFP+ cells, which contribute to early postnatal growing bones and fracture repair in adult mice. Another study[89] proposed a model in mice whereby skeletogenesis would proceed through a hierarchy of lineage-restricted progenitors, and one primitive skeletal stem cell gives rise to all the cartilage, bone, and stromal lineages. The same team reported the identification in the human growth plate of a population of nonhematopoietic, nonendothelial cells enriched in SSCs able to self-renew and generate progenitors of bone, cartilage, and stroma, but not adipose tissue.[90]

Recently, by combining lineage tracing studies with single-cell RNA-sequencing analyses, investigators[91] identified a population of SSCs in mouse periosteum that is present in the long bones and calvarium, is distinct from other known SSCs, displays self-renewal ability, and forms bone via direct intramembranous ossification. These cells acquire the capacity to undergo endochondral bone formation during fracture healing after injury. A cell analogous to the mouse periosteal SSC appears to be present in the human periosteum.[91]

These studies provide evidence that growing bones, bone and bone marrow, and periosteum contain multiple pools of SSCs/MSCs, each with distinct functions.

Similarly, lineage tracing studies have provided important insights on the joint resident stem/progenitor cells and their involvement in joint development, maintenance, and repair. Synovial joint tissues, including articular cartilage and synovium, develop from progeny of cells of the embryonic joint interzone, a stripe of mesenchymal tissue that appears in the limb bud during development and is marked by the expression of growth and differentiation factor 5 (Gdf5).[56,92] The Gdf5-Cre mice developed by one group[92] contain a modified BAC that encompasses the *GDF5* gene inactivated by a knockin of Cre in the first exon, together with upstream regulatory elements driving Cre expression that are active in the knee joint interzone during development but not in adult knees.[93] These mice were used to show that Gdf5-lineage cells persisted in adult synovium as a subpopulation of the Pdgfrα-expressing MSCs, present predominantly in the synovial lining with a minor population in the sublining tissue.[94] They barely overlapped with SSC/MSC populations originally identified in bone marrow and also detected in the mouse synovium, marked by expression of Nestin[84] (Fig. 7.3), Leptin-receptor[87] or Grem-lin-1,[88] suggesting that they constitute a distinct lineage extending from embryonic development into adult life.[94]

After cartilage injury, Gdf5-lineage cells proliferated to underpin synovial lining hyperplasia, colonized the cartilage defect, and underwent chondrogenic differentiation in the repair tissue.[94] Conditional ablation of the transcriptional cofactor Yes-associated protein (YAP) in the Gdf5 lineage prevented the synovial lining hyperplasia and markedly reduced the contribution of Gdf5-lineage cells to cartilage repair.[94] After isolation and culture expansion, Gdf5-lineage cells retained ability to form cartilage and a synovial-lining-like layer. By comparison, other MSCs isolated from mouse knee joints (i.e., non-Gdf5-lineage) performed poorly in the chondrogenesis and synoviogenesis assays but showed osteogenic ability while the Gdf5-lineage MSCs were not osteogenic.[94] These findings demonstrated a functional heterogeneity of joint-resident MSCs, with Gdf5-lineage MSCs showing joint-relevant progenitor activity.

The Gdf5 lineage in adult life also includes articular cartilage cells, and there is evidence that progenitor cells are present in the cartilage. Archer reported the isolation of an MSC-like population from the superficial zone of the articular cartilage.[79] MSC properties in culture-expanded cells from articular cartilage were also described.[95] More recently, progenitor cells have been described in the articular cartilage in vivo. One group[96] generated mice carrying the tamoxifen-inducible CreERT2 knocked into the endogenous Prg4 locus (encoding proteoglycan 4 [Prg4], also known as *lubricin*), which is expressed by the superficial cells of the articular cartilage and cells in the lining layer of the synovium. Genetic lineage tracing showed that the progeny of Prg4+ cells differentiated into articular chondrocytes.[96] Prg4+ cells in the superficial layer of the cartilage divided slowly and express progenitor/stem cell markers.[97] Similar findings were observed using a different, BAC-based Prg4-CreERT2 model.[98] These studies demonstrated that postnatally the surface of the articular cartilage contains stem/progenitor cells.

In keeping with the study by one group,[94] another group[98] showed that after cartilage injury, the Prg4 lineage expanded in the synovial lining and contributed to the cartilage repair tissue. Because both Gdf5-lineage cells and Prg4-lineage cells are present in the synovium and in the superficial layer of articular cartilage, the tissue of origin of the chondroprogenitors that repair articular cartilage remains to be clarified. The lack of detectable proliferation of Gdf5-lineage and Prg4-lineage cells in the cartilage and their expansion in the synovium, contributing to synovial lining hyperplasia after injury,[94,98] suggest the prospect that the chondroprogenitors that repair cartilage originate from the synovium. The mechanisms are unclear and could include direct synovial attachment[98] and migration of synovial cells along the cartilage surface[99] or derived from the synovial fluid.[100–102] Indeed, studies have reported a raised number of MSCs in the synovial fluid[102] and bone marrow lesions of patients with OA.[103] An obvious question is why MSCs would fail to repair damaged cartilage in humans. It is possible that the MSC reparative function would be ineffective due to senescence[103,104] or adverse environmental conditions.

An understanding of the native MSCs and how signals at the niche sites are orchestrated toward joint homeostasis, remodeling, and repair will be essential to provide guidance regarding clinical applications that use cell-based approaches. The restoration of a functional niche will safeguard durable repair by ensuring lifelong replacement of mature cells. An exciting prospect is the pharmacologic targeting of MSCs and niche repair signals to promote joint surface repair and influence outcomes of joint disorders such as OA, with the ultimate goal of restoring joint homeostasis.

The Role of Inflammation and the Immune System

The immune system appears to play a critical role in the process of postnatal tissue regeneration after tissue damage. The immune system interferes in many ways including in debris clearance; in the regulation of local progenitor cell proliferation, cell specification and differentiation; and in the promotion of angiogenesis and tissue integration. Almost every cell type of the immune system is involved and includes the innate and adaptive immune system, depending on the phase of the regeneration process. The initial post-traumatic event activates the neutrophil defense system that triggers and modulates the post-traumatic inflammatory response (for a review, see ref. 105). Although neutrophils have always been considered as mediators of tissue damage, new data are revealing their role in activating post-traumatic homeostasis. For instance, Annexin 1-containing extra-cellular vesicles released by neutrophils in arthritis appear to protect cartilage from breakdown in models of inflammatory arthritis.[106]

Persistent and excessive inflammation is considered a pathogenic event that hampers repair; however, at the appropriate time and in the right amount, inflammation is essential to prime tissue repair. For instance,[107] TNF is expressed briefly at the site of bone fractures where it recruits neutrophils and monocytes through CC motif ligand 2 (CCL2). The local administration of low dose human recombinant TNF at the fracture site enhanced bone repair whereas inhibition of TNF or depletion of neutrophils impaired fracture repair. Crucially, systemic administration of TNF impaired fracture healing.[107]

Macrophages are key players in the early phase of the wound healing process, particularly M1 macrophages in debris clearance.[2,108] M1 macrophages, also known as pro-inflammatory macrophages, secrete inflammatory cytokines such as IL6, TNF, IL1β, and G-CSF, affecting the inflammatory response and initial cell proliferation, while M2 macrophages produce anti-inflammatory molecules such as IGF1 and TGFβ and are more involved in cell specification and differentiation. Although there is abundant evidence for the innate immune system being involved in tissue regeneration, the adaptive immune system has recently emerged as a key player. T-cells, in particular regulatory T-cells (T-reg), have been demonstrated to be involved in the repair and regeneration of various organs systems, including skeletal and heart muscle, skin, and long bones (for a review, see ref. 109). T-reg cells control the level of inflammation by promoting the M1 to M2 polarization. They activate tissue progenitors and tissue growth.

Conversely, adult stem cells interact with the immune system and can suppress and modulate the immune response to favor the repair response (for a review, see ref. 110).

Exploring the function of the immune system in regeneration has gained major attention, yet there is so much still to be investigated on how immunity controls the process. However, immune cells can also have a negative influence on regeneration, and a balanced immune response is key for a successful repair process.

Understanding how both the innate and adaptive immune system interact with the tissue resident progenitors and stem cells remains a key area of investigation (for a review, see ref. 111). This may in turn lead to fine tuning of the immune system to support regeneration and targeted therapeutic approaches with successful clinical outcomes.

Events Leading to Joint Surface Repair

In resting condition, articular cartilage has an extremely low rate of turnover. For instance, the half-life of type II collagen has been estimated as being around 117 years,[112] and articular chondrocytes are all essentially in the G0 of the cell cycle. After acute traumatic injury, however, chondrocytes deploy strong adaptive responses that ultimately result in a coordinated sequence of activation and chemotaxis of progenitors within the cartilage itself and in other joint tissues, along with cell proliferation and matrix turnover. In a number of cases, such adaptive responses are sufficient to repair damage and re-establish homeostasis.[32,113] However, if the injury exceeds the adaptive capacity or if the adaptive responses are hampered in some way, cartilage loss leads to OA and ultimately joint failure. In OA the "injury" (i.e., excessive mechanical load) is continuous, and no immediate loss of tissue occurs. In such a situation the homeostatic responses are more subtle and are heralded by the upregulation of the transcription factor SOX9 and its direct targets, type II collagen and aggrecan,[114–116] as well as a limited degree of chondrocyte proliferation. It is interesting to notice that such types of homeostatic responses persist even at late stages of OA.[117–121]

The sequence of events that leads to an adaptive response in cartilage is difficult to study in OA, which is a slow-progressing disease, but such study has been facilitated by the development of in vitro and in vivo models of acute injury. The first evidence of adaptive responses consisting of chondrocyte proliferation and new deposition of ECM dates back nearly one century (reviewed in Dell'accio and Vincent).[7] More accurate molecular analyses have identified several other components that are amenable for targeting. These components include an immediate molecular response, the activation and attraction of progenitors, breakdown of the residual mature ECM, the filling of the defect, tissue patterning, and, finally, tissue maturation—which, in humans, can take several years. In the entire joint, inflammation is an integral part of a natural response to injury, providing molecular signals and cascades that are likely to have distinct context and tissue-specific beneficial or detrimental effects. Studies aimed at teasing apart the "good" from the "bad" pathways will help modulate repair processes and restore/maintain joint homeostasis.

In therapeutic terms, therefore, it may be possible to target any of these phases, but it is likely that a stratified approach will be necessary to ensure efficacy and consistency. Such an approach will start with the understanding of which step of the homeostatic response has failed in groups of individual patients so that the approach will be targeted to the appropriate patients (Fig. 7.4).

Immediate Molecular Response

Scarification of the articular cartilage in vitro or in vivo induces a strong early molecular response dominated by the activation of signaling pathways known to play important roles in embryonic skeletogenesis.[15,122–127] Although this response is very rapid and transient, it primes a cascade of downstream steps. Probably the best known pathways involved in this phase are the WNT, FGF, and TGF-β/BMP pathways, which are discussed elsewhere in this chapter. It is important to say here, however, that although proof of concept for efficacy with each of these pathways has been provided in some way in different models, the disparate functions that these pleiotropic signaling molecules have in each different cell type remain a challenge. Tissue-targeted treatments will be of importance, including the use of novel smart delivery systems to confine the signaling domain of such powerful morphogens and avoid off-target effects.

Activation and Attraction of Mesenchymal Progenitors

There is increasing evidence that mesenchymal progenitors are implicated in the repair of joint surface defects. The understanding of the pathophysiologic mechanisms driving stem cell commitment and differentiation is paving the way to promising therapeutic interventions that exploit homeostatic mechanisms, as discussed previously. In 2012, one study[113] identified a small compound, kartogenin, which, by interacting with filamin A, regulates the activity of the CBFβ-RUNX1 transcriptional program in bone marrow–derived mesenchymal cells, inducing their chondrogenic differentiation. The delivery of kartogenin to mice subjected to instability-induced OA improved pain and resulted not only in the arrest of disease progression but even in regeneration of the cartilage tissue to some degree. Although kartogenin could induce

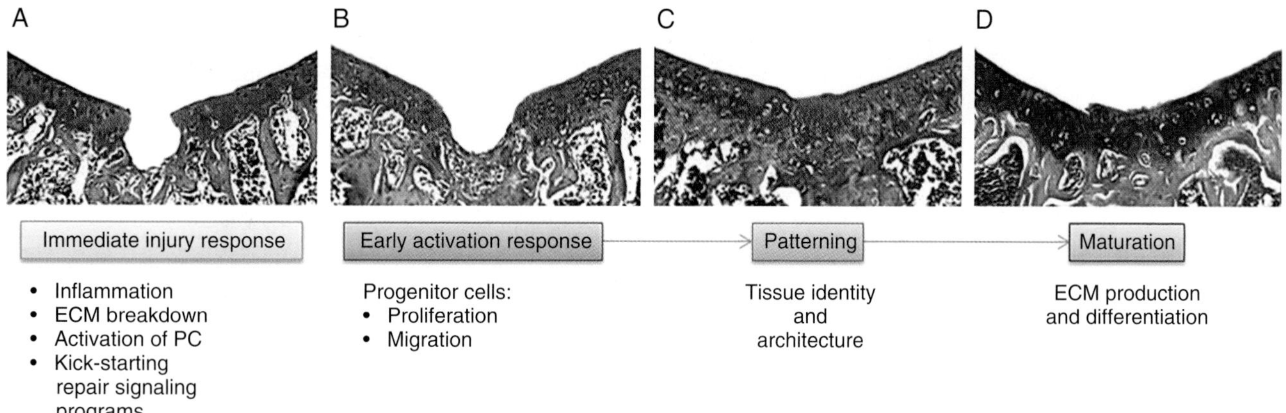

• **Fig. 7.4** Minutes after injury, tissues, including the articular cartilage, deploy a molecular response (A), which activates the migration of progenitor cells (B), the formation of a patterned repair tissues (C), and its maturation (D). *ECM,* Extra-cellular matrix; *PC,* progenitor cell.

chondrocytic differentiation of bone marrow stromal cells in vitro, it is not clear whether this effect on bone marrow stromal cells contributed to the chondroprotective effect of kartogenin in vivo. In fact, kartogenin could support harmonious skeletal growth, joint morphogenesis, and the resorption of the interdigital mesenchyme, which are otherwise stunted in ex vivo cultures of embryonic mouse limbs.[128] These effects were associated with the activation of several signaling pathways and particularly the TGF-β pathway. The effect of kartogenin is likely to be more complex than the simple capacity to induce chondrogenic differentiation of MSCs.

Patterning, Differentiation, Integration, and Remodeling

After the joint surface defect is filled with mesenchymal cells, the repair tissue needs patterning tissue maturation, integration, and remodeling to acquire the final architectural structure, with a properly layered cartilage and osteochondral junction. Interestingly, both morphologically and molecularly, the repair tissue in an osteochondral defect resembles the epiphysis of a developing skeletal element, with flat cells at the surface, then chondrocytes in different stages of maturation, and hypertrophic chondrocytes at the boundary with the bone front.[29] With time the bone front advances and, for successful repair, must arrest to leave a layer of permanent stable articular cartilage. Failure of this process results in failure of repair both in animal models[129,130] and also in humans, where excessive advancement of the bone front can lead to intra-articular osteophytes after surgical procedures such as bone marrow stimulation by microfracture.[131]

Emerging Clinical Applications Targeting Endogenous Repair

The successes in targeting homeostatic pathways to achieve cartilage repair in animal models stirred the interest of the pharmaceutical industry and led to the development of compounds currently in advanced states of clinical testing. Hereafter we summarize two of the most advanced examples of such a strategy.

Targeting FGF Signaling

FGF receptor 3–dependent signaling is essential for cartilage homeostasis and promotes cartilage anabolism. FGF-18 is a member of the FGF family of growth factors, which is highly specific for FGF receptor 3. The efficacy of intra-articular FGF-18 delivery was tested in a proof-of-concept placebo-controlled, double-blinded randomized clinical trial[132] in which safety and efficacy were assessed at 6 and 12 months. No safety issues were identified. The patients had moderate osteoarthritis (Kellgren-Lawrence score 2-3). Although no statistically significant difference was found in the primary efficacy endpoint (change in central medial femorotibial compartment cartilage thickness), the loss of cartilage thickness in the less severely affected lateral compartment was dose-dependently reduced.[132] Patients who received FGF-18 also had less pain. In addition to a possible underpowering of the study (for instance, the actual reduction of the cartilage thickness in the medial compartment in the placebo group was much smaller than expected from a cohort used for powering and an ambitious assumption of an expected 75% reduction in joint space narrowing compared with placebo), this study suggests that, at least with FGF-18, the best chances of success are with modest levels of cartilage loss, such as that present on the lateral condyle of the patients in this study. This raises the need for criteria to identify patients with early symptomatic knee OA who are at high risk of progression for inclusion in clinical trials and, ultimately, for treatment.[133]

Targeting Wnt Signaling

Excessive activation of Wnt signaling is a major driver of cartilage breakdown, but a physiologic level of Wnt activation is required to maintain joint stem cell populations and activate repair.[67] Therefore, inhibition of Wnt signaling has been pursued as a strategy. SB04690 is a small compound identified for its capacity to inhibit Wnt signaling in vitro.[134] The compound induced chondrogenesis in vitro and protected from cartilage loss in a severe model of osteoarthritis in rats.[134] In patients, a single intra-articular injection of SB04690 resulted in durable symptomatic relief and even radiologic evidence of thickening of the articular cartilage over 24 weeks. The remarkable long-term persistence of the compound within the tissue is possibly the reason for the long-term effect. These data need confirmation in an adequately powered phase III trial, and the precise mechanism of action needs to be clarified; nevertheless, such data, considered together with the success in pre-clinical models, may represent a major step forward towards pharmacologic cartilage regeneration.

SYMPTOMATIC FULL-THICKNESS JOINT SURFACE DEFECTS

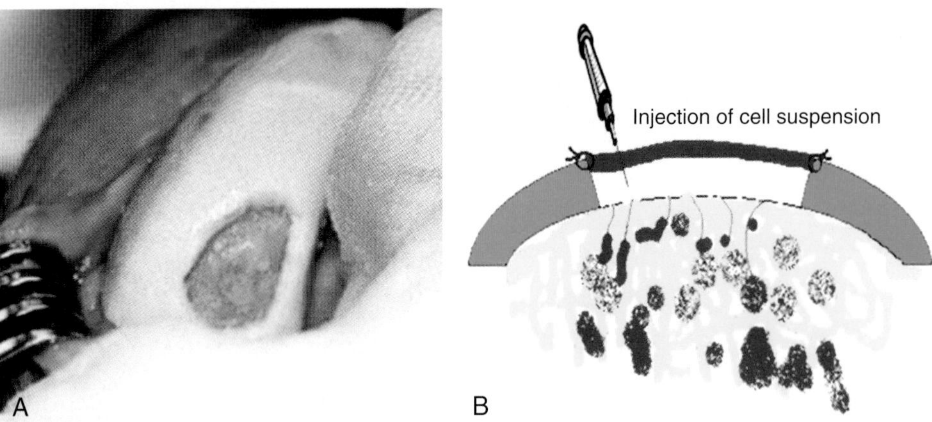

• **Fig. 7.5** (A) View at open knee surgery of a large full-thickness articular cartilage defect. Note the sharp borders of the lesion after surgical debridement. (B) A cell suspension, such as autologous chondrocytes, is injected beneath a periosteal flap or membrane sutured on the joint surface and sealed with fibrin glue to prevent leakage.

Extrinsic Repair: Current Therapeutic Interventions

Cell-based therapies and TE for joint surface repair using expanded articular chondrocytes have entered clinical practice with long-term follow-up data. At an earlier stage of clinical development are the use of adult stem cells (such as MSCs), which have shown promising pre-clinical and early clinical safety and efficacy data. The mechanisms whereby cellular therapies and combination products contribute to tissue repair are multiple and involve direct engraftment, proliferation, and differentiation to tissue-specific cell types but also include paracrine actions such as the secretion of growth and differentiation factors that enhance the local tissue response.[135] In addition, adult stem cells may have immunomodulatory properties, which have been clinically explored in graft-versus-host disease and autoimmune diseases.[136]

Joint Surface Defects

A variety of articular cartilage repair techniques have been developed, typically for the treatment of (sub)acute focal joint surface defects that are often associated with excessive joint loading, either as a result of high-impact trauma or cumulative low-impact repetitive overload. Joint surface lesions can extend to the subchondral bone (osteochondral defects) or be limited to the cartilage (chondral defects). Most chondral defects do not reach to the bone (partial thickness), and only about 5% are full thickness[137]; nevertheless, because most partial-thickness lesions are debrided at the time of surgery to full thickness, including the removal of the calcified layer (Fig. 7.5), repair strategies focus on the treatment of full-thickness defects. The best-established cell-based technology for the treatment of these lesions is autologous chondrocyte transplantation and variations thereof.

Autologous Chondrocyte Transplantation

Regeneration or repair of symptomatic articular cartilage defects has been at the forefront of regenerative medicine ever since 1994 when one group[138] reported a remarkably good clinical and structural outcome using a procedure called *autologous chondrocyte transplantation/implantation* (ACI). Briefly, cell populations were prepared by enzymatic release from a biopsy specimen of articular cartilage taken from an unloaded area in the symptomatic joint. The chondrocytes were subsequently expanded in vitro, and after six to eight population doublings, they were reimplanted in the joint surface defect under a periosteal flap taken from the tibia from the same patient. This procedure was then followed by a long rehabilitation period to reach its optimal outcome at 18 to 24 months. This high-profile publication attracted considerable interest and triggered a wave of basic, translational, and clinical research activities in the field. It also evolved quite quickly in 1997 in the marketing of Carticel, an autologous cell product for the repair of symptomatic condylar defects of the knee, by Genzyme Corporation (Cambridge, Mass.).

Progress has been made since then with studies aiming to improve and standardize the autologous chondrocyte preparation (the cell product), the development of other delivery systems for the chondrocytes and the replacement of the periosteal flap with a membrane of diverse composition, and a series of clinical studies. After a number of mostly open studies with diverse outcomes (for a review, see ref. 139), one study[140]—the first multicenter, prospective, randomized trial—failed to demonstrate that ACI was superior to microfracture, a technique mostly considered to be the standard of care for small (<2 to 3 cm^2) symptomatic joint surface defects. Microfracture is a bone marrow stimulation procedure and is based on the puncturing of the subchondral bone plate into the bone marrow, the generation of a blood clot containing precursor cell populations derived from the subchondral bone marrow, and the spontaneous transformation of the repair clot into a fibrocartilaginous repair tissue.[141] Microfracture is clearly associated with a clinical benefit and a filling of the joint surface defect with repair tissue, but it is generally accepted that this repair is not durable, resulting in a consistent decline in clinical outcome over the long term.[142,143] It is the aim of ACI to repair the cartilage defect with better quality tissue, mostly hyaline cartilage with tissue characteristics matching those of the neighboring tissue, thereby resulting in improved long-term outcomes (Fig. 7.6). Although one study[140] did not indicate clinical superiority of ACI over microfracture, there were some indications that good structural repair was associated with durable clinical outcome.[144]

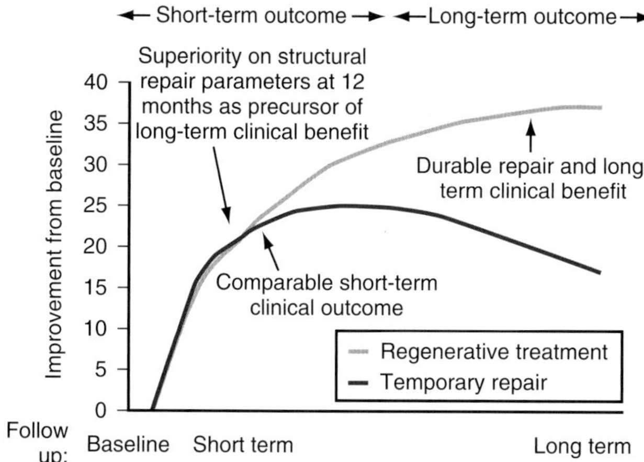

• **Fig. 7.6** The expected difference between repair of a joint surface lesion by a mechanism of scarring versus true tissue regeneration. Both treatment approaches (e.g., microfracture and autologous chondrocyte transplantation [ACI]) show clinically equal benefit at the short term, but repair tissue closer to the native tissue is seen with a regenerative approach (e.g., as seen in ACI). Long-term outcomes are more durable using regenerative approaches, in some cases leading to cure.

Subsequently, progress was made by improving the manufacturing process of the chondrocyte preparation. Indeed, in Europe, an autologous chondrocyte cell product called ChondroCelect (TiGenix, Leuven, Belgium) was developed and obtained the first cellular product central registration by the European Medicines Agency under the new advanced therapy medicinal product regulation. In a prospective randomized multicenter study, ChondroCelect, defined and characterized as a cell population capable of making stable cartilage in surrogate in vivo models and quality controlled through use of biomarkers, resulted in structurally superior repair tissue at 12 months after implantation compared with microfracture, with a superior clinical outcome at 3 years, but noninferiority in the overall population at 5 years.[145] The 5-year data demonstrated a clinically relevant superior outcome in the subpopulation of patients with relatively recent lesions (<3 years). This prospective, well-designed landmark clinical trial supports the concept that an improved understanding of the underlying biology and the consequent optimization of the manufacturing process lead to improved clinical outcome. In addition, stratification of patients will have a major impact on the potential for regenerative medicine approaches to move forward successfully to proper clinical use in daily practice.

The surgical delivery of these therapies is another important factor that requires standardization. In this regard, ACI is becoming a more easily controllable arthroscopic procedure. A recent study that used an arthroscopic approach reported a statistically better clinical outcome for matrix-applied autologous chondrocytes after 2 years when compared with microfracture.[146] Interestingly, in this case, structural repair as assessed by MRI and biopsy was not different from microfracture at 2 years.

Although still open for debate with respect to long-term clinical durability, there is a consensus that ACI, and variations thereof, can be considered a regenerative treatment with good structural and clinical outcome in the appropriate patients. Long-term clinical outcomes have been reported and indicate a good durability of the treatment in a substantial number of patients over periods exceeding 10 years.[147]

Importantly, the data indicate that the outcome is superior to standard care if the "proper" patients are treated. Positive predictors of good outcome include the age of the patient, the location of the defect, early intervention (<3 years after becoming symptomatic), good quality of chondrocytes, well-trained surgeons, adherence to rehabilitation protocols, and no signs of OA (as defined by the Kellgren II grading scale on standard radiographs).[148] Cost-effectiveness will certainly improve if the treatment also prevents the progression toward (early) OA, but these data are not yet available.

Other cell sources have been explored such as nasal chondrocytes. Chondrocytes derived from the nasal septum, with known capacity to generate hyaline-like cartilage, have been reported to be successful for knee cartilage defect repair in ten patients,[149] but large controlled trials are warranted to assess efficacy, and long-term follow-up is required.

Stem Cell–Based Approaches

The next wave of development is the use of progenitor cell populations, or the so-called *MSCs*, in particular via an allogeneic approach.

MSCs are easy to isolate, expandable in culture, and chondrogenic, and therefore they are attractive alternatives to chondrocytes in an ACI procedure. These properties of MSCs would allow upscaling and generation of large quality-controlled batches, thus circumventing the limitations and patient-to-patient variability of autologous cell protocols. For these reasons, the use of MSCs for joint surface repair is intensively sought[150–152] and has been explored in humans.[153] These studies have shown promising results, with cartilage formation and endochondral bone formation restoring the bone front. However, uplift of the bone front at the expense of the articular cartilage has been commonly observed[129] and has its clinical equivalent in intralesional osteophyte formation in patients after microfracture.[154] This "side effect" appears to be less frequent in patients treated with ACI,[155] suggesting that an imprinted memory of articular chondrocytes could preserve the normal thickness of the repair cartilage and limit the advancement of the bone front. This finding points to a need, when using MSCs, for strategies to enhance stable cartilage properties and reduce fibrous tissue and hypertrophic cartilage formation.

Another important area of investigation is the tissue source of MSCs. Adult bone marrow MSCs are leading candidates for use in the repair of cartilage defects and other skeletal tissues such as bone defects.[156] However, MSCs from bone marrow appear to have a high propensity to cartilage hypertrophy and bone formation[157,158] and may not be the ideal chondroprogenitors for the repair of articular cartilage. In this regard, superiority of MSCs from synovial membrane for cartilage formation in vitro when compared with MSCs from other tissue sources, including bone marrow and periosteum, has been reported.[159–161] Promising data using synovium-derived progenitors have been reported in vivo, but at this point the long-term outcome of these approaches is unclear.[162,163]

The differences in chondrogenic potency of MSC populations could find their origins in the distinctive molecular programs of embryonic formation of their native tissues, because lineage tracing studies in mice demonstrated a common developmental origin of articular cartilage and synovial membrane from the Gdf5-positive cells of the embryonic joint interzone.[56,92]

The solution to the challenge of stable-cartilage formation, displaying also the very specific articular cartilage characteristics, may come from the use of chondroprogenitors isolated from the articular cartilage itself, which display the ability to maintain chondrogenic potency upon extensive culture expansion.[164] A proof-of-principle pilot study in a goat model in vivo demonstrated the apparent noninferiority of these chondroprogenitors to form a cartilage-like repair tissue in a chondral defect when compared with full-depth chondrocytes.[165] Human long-term studies will be needed to demonstrate noninferiority of MSCs or any other stem/progenitor cell populations in clinical and structural outcomes when compared with the gold-standard articular cartilage–derived chondrocytes in ACI-like procedures.

The use of MSCs in joint resurfacing in animal models and humans reveals a variable structural outcome, ranging from hyaline-like cartilage to fibrous tissue. This finding has prompted interventions to support tissue maturation by using cartilage-promoting growth factors along with smart biomaterials.[166] However, the combination of cells, biomaterials, and morphogens would make the assessment of efficacy and toxicity more complex and the path from animal experimentation to clinical application arduous.

The use of allogeneic MSCs has shown an acceptable safety profile.[167] However, the pre-clinical data on the immunogenicity of MSCs are conflicting, and the acquired differentiated phenotype of the implanted stem cells may result in the loss of the immunologic privilege, with consequent rejection of the cells.[168,169]

Nonetheless, the use of allogeneic cells would allow manufacturing of large batches of cell products with specific clinical indications, off the shelf. Such an approach increases consistency and decreases costs of cell therapies, potentially accelerating the translational process toward routine clinical application.

Osteochondral Repair

Whereas regeneration strategies for chondral lesions have been tested in high-quality clinical trials, the management and repair of osteochondral defects, with damage to the articular cartilage and reaching deep into the subchondral bone, remains a significant problem (for a review, see Nukaravapu and Dorcemus[170]). Indeed, both the articular cartilage and subchondral bone need to be repaired with restoration of a new calcified layer and tidemark, fully integrated and aligned with the neighboring tissue. The major challenge lies in the development of biologically educated regenerative treatments for osteochondral defects without resorting to prostheses. Prosthetic joint resurfacing is irreversible and has, per definition, a limited life span, and revisions can be surgically challenging and are not ideal in younger patients with higher functional expectations.

The most common clinically used methods to treat osteochondral defects include debridement, bone marrow stimulation techniques such as microfracture, and the use of osteochondral allografts. Although they have shown some short-term positive results, the approaches taken are suboptimal and not curative and face serious drawbacks. Most of these treatments address only symptoms, and the use of allografts for larger osteochondral defects involves risks for immune rejection, disease transmission, and issues related to donor site morbidity and tissue availability. Currently, for osteochondral lesions bigger than 2.5 cm^2, the most commonly used clinical restorative method is ACI, using surgical variations with a so-called *sandwich approach*. However, the results are mixed and are neither robust nor predictable.

Several scaffold strategies have been developed and evaluated for osteochondral repair requiring bone, cartilage, and bone-cartilage interface regeneration. Indeed, one of the main aims in the development of repair strategies for osteochondral applications is to closely mimic the native osteochondral tissue gradient structure. The challenge is to create distinct but seamlessly integrated layers intended to repair articular cartilage, calcified cartilage, and bone.[171] Therefore, osteochondral TE research has been evolving from cell-based therapies to single-layer scaffold repair, followed by biphasic constructs, and ultimately to multiphasic constructs. Classically, biphasic materials entailing a cartilaginous layer and bone part have been described in several studies and have shown some success.[164,172] Among biphasic scaffolds, hybrids can be prepared by filling soft hydrogels into hard sponges. As an example of this approach, one group[173] successfully developed a composite construct consisting of a polylactide-co-glycolide (PLGA) sponge filled with fibrin gel, bone marrow MSCs, and TGF-β1 for full-thickness cartilage defect restoration in vivo. In vitro and in vivo studies in a rabbit model revealed that the PLGA/fibrin gel/MSCs/TGF-β1 constructs are an appealing candidate for osteochondral restoration.[173] This type of biphasic composite construct paved the way for the use of multilayered scaffolds for osteochondral defects.

After this progression, increasing interest is being devoted to gradient scaffolds with continuous interfaces to more faithfully mimic the natural hierarchic architecture. A clinical pilot study was performed in which a nanostructured, three-layered, collagen-hydroxyapatite construct was applied for the treatment of chondral and osteochondral lesions of the knee joint. This system was able to induce in situ regeneration via stem cells coming from the surrounding bone marrow in an innovative cell-free approach translatable to clinical practice.[174] In a sheep model, similar trilayered magnesium-hydroxyapatite-collagen type I composites were able to promote bone and cartilage tissue restoration by inducing the selective differentiation of resident progenitor cells, such as bone marrow–derived and/or synovium-derived cells, to osteogenic and chondrogenic lineages. Thus this approach indicates the potential of a suitable hybrid scaffold matrix that can direct and coordinate the process of bone and hyaline-like cartilage regeneration.[174] Other studies, also using biomimetic multilayered scaffolds, focused more on the development of a tidemark (intermediate layer). For example, hydroxyapatite/collagen bio-hybrid composites, prepared via a biologically inspired mineralization process, supported selective cell differentiation toward both osteogenic and chondrogenic lineages. Finally, continuous gradients in both material and bioactive signals take us one step further in scaffold complexity to achieve a high degree of mimicry. Continuous gradients can be added into hydrogels with incorporation of drug delivery systems (e.g., drug-loaded microspheres). As an elegant example of this approach, one group[173] incorporated recombinant human (rh) BMP-2 and rhIGF-1, microencapsulated in PLGA and silk microspheres, to form continuous concentration gradients in alginate gels and silk sponges. The combination of growth factors in different carrier systems enabled spatial control of the growth factors' distribution and temporal control of their release.

Although the use of tailored scaffolds associated with suitable factors and proper stem cell technology appears to be a more advanced TE strategy, the complexity intrinsic to such scaffolds presents a considerable set of technologic, regulatory, and financial challenges on the way to routine clinical application. Moreover, treatment approaches will have to be tailored to a number of variables including the size and location of the defect, the age of the patient, and the defined outcomes from symptomatic relief with limited loading to fully functional including sports activities.

Bone Regeneration

The most promising field to explore the full potential of regenerative medicine approaches in musculoskeletal medicine is bone regeneration. Bone already has a remarkable potential to heal postnatally, which indicates that all the necessary tools are available to obtain full tissue repair, without any tissue scarring, and thus also to obtain successful tissue integration and remodeling. We should thus try to fully understand how nature heals bone fractures postnatally and subsequently mimic these repair processes when bone healing goes wrong, such as in delayed healing and nonunions, for the repair of large bone defects such as avascular necrosis or after resection of bone tumors.

The standard of care in bone repair is the use of autologous bone grafts, which are typically obtained from the iliac crest. However, important developments have moved the boundaries in the field of bone engineering and include the development and improvement of biomaterials and new technologies in the design and production/manufacturing of these new biomaterials. It is not within the scope of this chapter, but suffice it to say that the spectrum of the smart biomaterials for bone engineering is vast, and recent progress has resulted in the production of resorbable and osteoconductive products, with some even displaying osteoinductive properties.[175] These latter characteristics have been obtained by coating biomaterials with bioactive factors, including growth factors such as the BMPs.[46] BMP devices have not only led to more robust and predictable outcomes in spine fusion but most importantly have demonstrated that recapitulation of embryonic tissue formation processes can lead to successful bone healing postnatally, as well as in long bone healing.

Despite all this progress, we still are not capable of healing large long bone defects in patients. In view of this, we and others believe that a combined implant incorporating smart and resorbable biomaterials, stem/progenitor cell populations, and growth factors will be required.[176] Failure of bone healing is typically associated with the lack of vascularization and the proper precursor cell populations not being available. Therefore, the generation of tissue-engineered viable implants will need to provide tools to enhance vascularization of the implant and promote cell survival to come to full fruition. Thus far, the results of the so-called *combination products* (scaffold and cells, eventually enriched with growth factors) have been somewhat disappointing. Lack of an underlying scientific basis for the design and manufacturing of these implants is probably responsible for a large part of this disappointment. Therefore, a bio-inspired model called *developmental engineering* was proposed and extensively described.[177,178] Recent publications indicate that this approach may be more successful than the traditional cells on the scaffold trial-and-error approach.[158]

Most importantly for the field are the need for good prospective multicenter clinical trials, and these are ongoing (see the World Health Organization International Clinical Trials Registry Platform and the European Union Drug Regulating Authorities Clinical Trials [EUDRACT] database) to better establish the clinical relevance of the different bone TE strategies. They include the direct percutaneous injection of expanded bone marrow MSCs in long bone nonunions, both autologous and allogenic, and the implantation of bone marrow–expanded MSCs with a bone substitute (hydroxy apatite/tricalcium phosphate carrier) in long bone nonunions. The development of some of the more complex TE techniques is raising further challenges, also with regard to the manufacturing of those products (for further review, see ref. 179).

Regeneration of Other Joint-Related Structures

Lesions of the articular cartilage are often associated with damage of other joint structures such as menisci, ligaments, and tendons, which need to be addressed to restore joint homeostasis. An attractive "holistic" approach to joint regeneration could be intra-articular delivery of MSCs. The injection of bone marrow MSCs in a hyaluronan suspension in a goat model of OA obtained by medial meniscectomy and anterior cruciate ligament resection resulted in a meniscus-like neo-tissue formation that provided protection from OA progression.[180] Similar data were obtained with intra-articular injection of synovial membrane–derived MSCs that promoted meniscus regeneration in a rat model.[181,182] Recently, a proof-of-concept phase I/II clinical trial assessed the safety and efficacy of intra-articular injection of autologous adipose-derived MSCs for knee OA. After a phase I study consisting of three dose-escalation cohorts with three patients each, phase II included nine patients receiving the high dose (1.0×10^8 MSCs). The primary outcomes were the safety and the Western Ontario and McMaster Universities Arthritis Index (WOMAC) at 6 months; secondary outcomes included clinical, radiologic, arthroscopic, and histologic evaluations. The intra-articular injection of MSCs into the osteoarthritic knee improved function and pain of the knee joint without causing adverse events and reduced cartilage defects by regeneration of hyaline-like articular cartilage.[183]

Systematic reviews of phase I/II clinical trials concluded that MSCs, obtained most commonly from bone marrow or adipose tissue and injected intra-articularly into the knee, are overall safe and well tolerated. MSCs can improve pain and function of the knee joint, with some histologic data suggesting formation of hyaline-like cartilage repair tissue.[184,185] A meta-analysis of 11 small trials of MSC therapy for knee OA, including a total of 582 knee OA patients, reported improvements across a range of clinical outcome measures.[186]

Most studies have used autologous cells, but allogeneic MSCs also appear to be safe.[187,188] Their use would allow upscaling of production of large batches of MSC preparations, thereby improving consistency of cell therapy. To reduce the costs and variability due to culture expansion, fresh bone marrow aspirate concentrate is being explored as a readily available source of autologous cells for intra-articular delivery, shown to be safe in 25 patients with knee OA.[189] Protocols for enrichment of clinical grade CD271+ MSCs from fresh bone marrow aspirate have been developed,[190] but clinical feasibility needs to be evaluated.

The mechanism of action of MSCs is not clear. Because the injected MSCs do not seem to contribute directly to joint tissue repair, they would instead mediate tissue repair largely via paracrine signals. In this regard, recent studies have reported that MSC-derived extra-cellular vesicles (small particles released from the cells and containing bioactive signaling molecules) can promote cartilage repair and protect against OA-induced cartilage degeneration.[108,191,192]

In summary, cell therapy appears to be safe. However, large, randomized, controlled studies are needed to demonstrate efficacy. Standardization of cell product manufacturing and delivery, as well as definition of target patient populations through stratification, will be needed for comparisons across clinical studies.[193]

Menisci

The menisci have a poor healing potential largely because their vascularity is restricted to the external third of the tissue.[194] A subtotal or total meniscectomy is now rarely performed in view of the high risk of OA development, but a partial meniscectomy can be necessary in symptomatic patients. The use of a cell-free biomaterial to replace part of the meniscus relies on repopulation of the scaffold by the host cells from the joint environment. The collagen meniscus implant (ReGen Biologics, Franklin Lakes, New Jersey) was the first regenerative method applied to meniscal tissue in clinical practice.[195–197] Noncontrolled case series have reported pain relief and functional improvement at 10-year follow-up.[198] Despite the wide clinical use, no randomized controlled trial supports the use of meniscal implants in routine clinical practice. The Actifit (Orteq Ltd, London) meniscus implant is a polyurethane-polycaprolactone–based synthetic meniscal substitute for partial meniscal defects,[199] but evidence about its safety and effectiveness is awaited.

Meniscal transplantation is a valid short-term option in selected patients with symptomatic, totally meniscectomized, aligned knees.[200] Limitations of this procedure include tissue availability, graft sizing, and risks of immune reaction and disease transmission. Fixation of the allograft also remains a significant challenge.

Regenerative medicine holds the potential for restoring anatomy and function of meniscal fibrocartilage. Several cell types have been assessed in meniscal TE, including meniscal cells from the meniscectomized meniscus itself; articular, costal, and nasal chondrocytes; MSCs; and embryonic stem cells (reviewed in ref. 201). They are seeded onto biomaterials, both natural and synthetic, which are anticipated to be biocompatible, biodegradable, bio-instructive (promoting cell differentiation and cell migration if cell free), biomimetic (mimicking architecture and biomechanics of the native meniscus), resistant to mechanical forces, porous (allowing diffusion of nutrients), and user friendly for the surgeon. Natural materials such as small intestine submucosa[202] and acellular porcine meniscal tissue[203] have high biocompatibility but do not allow varying structure geometry and adequate initial mechanical properties. Isolated tissue components such as collagens and proteoglycans allow generation of custom-made scaffolds with high biocompatibility.[204] However, these scaffolds usually have low biomechanical properties and are characterized by rapid biodegradation, and they are not sufficiently long to be completely replaced by the newly formed tissue.[201] Synthetic polymers (e.g., polyglycolic acid [PGA] and polylactic acid [PLA]) can be manufactured in custom-made shapes and with custom-made porosity and biomechanical properties, and the use of biopolymers such as silk fibrous protein has been explored to improve biocompatibility and biodegradability.[205] A possible solution is to couple the high biocompatibility of natural polymers with the superior mechanical strength and ease of being tailored of the synthetic polymers.[206]

A fascinating strategy entails the use of hydrogel materials,[207] because their semiliquid nature allows engineering anatomic geometries derived from medical imaging such as computed tomography.[208]

MSCs seeded onto a hyaluronan-collagen–based scaffold were used to repair a critical-size meniscal defect in an orthotopic rabbit model.[209] Although menisci repaired with the engineered tissue demonstrated a significantly better regeneration than did those repaired with the cell-free scaffold, the cell-loaded implants did not restore a normal meniscus.[209] Uncultured bone marrow cells in hyaluronan-collagen composite matrices stimulated the development of integrated meniscus-like repair tissue,[210] suggesting the feasibility of a one-step approach for partial meniscus TE.

Total meniscus TE offers an alternative to allografts to overcome the problems of availability, graft sizing, and immune reaction. The implantation of a PGA-PLGA scaffold seeded with allogeneic meniscal cells in a rabbit meniscectomy model resulted in a tissue histologically resembling normal meniscus.[211] Similar promising results were reported with a hyaluronic acid/polycaprolactone material seeded with expanded autologous articular chondrocytes in a sheep orthotopic model.[206] Investigators[205] reported the development of a TE meniscus based on a trilayered silk fibrous protein scaffold seeded with human culture-expanded fibroblasts in the outer part and chondrocytes in the inner part. The same authors reported the use of such trilayered scaffold seeded with human culture-expanded MSCs, showing native-like tissue structure and compressive properties in vitro.[212]

Despite the extensive pre-clinical and clinical investigations, none of the current strategies has demonstrated regeneration of a functional, durable meniscal tissue and full re-establishment of knee homeostasis. Advances in cell biology, biomaterial science, and bioengineering (e.g., bioreactors) have the potential to drive meniscus regeneration into more clinically relevant and feasible strategies.

Tendons

Common tendon injuries are tears of the rotator cuff, Achilles tendon, and flexor tendons of the hand. At present, they are treated with surgical repair and/or conservative approaches. Unfortunately, current treatment strategies fail to restore the functional, structural, and biochemical properties of the repaired tendons compared with native tendons. Tendon repair has been attempted with platelet-rich plasma, an autologous source of concentrated growth factors relevant to wound repair.[213] Numerous growth factors play a role in tendon healing, but the application of growth factors such as IGF-1, TGF-β, or GDF-5 (BMP-14) to clinical tendon repair remains challenging.[214]

In cases of severe tendon injury, surgical treatments may be used to repair or replace the damaged tendon with autografts, allografts, xenografts, or prosthetic devices. The unsatisfactory clinical outcomes with high failure rates[215] have prompted the development of TE strategies. With regard to the choice of cell types to use, the harvest of autologous tenocytes may cause secondary tendon defects, and thus dermal fibroblasts have been considered because they are easily accessible and do not cause major donor site morbidity.[216] In a recent clinical trial, an injection of dermal fibroblasts suspended in autologous plasma improved the healing of refractory patellar tendinopathy.[217] MSCs are another promising cell source for tendon TE. In a rabbit model, PGA sheets seeded with bone marrow MSCs enhanced mechanical strength when compared with a cell-free PGA scaffold.[218] Stem cells have also been identified in tendons.[219] Tendon-derived stem cells in fibrin glue, compared with fibrin glue alone, promoted superior tendon repair histologically and biomechanically.[220] Despite their potential advantages, the isolation of autologous cells would present the same donor site morbidities as tenocytes.

Three major categories of scaffolds are used in tendon TE: native tendon matrices, synthetic polymers, and derivatives of naturally occurring proteins. Cutting-edge processing protocols allow decellularized tendon scaffolds to maintain similar biomechanical properties compared with native tendon tissues.[221] Moreover, a number of ECM proteins and growth factors are preserved in acellular tendon,[222] suggesting potential biofunctionality of these scaffolds. Synthetic polymers such as PGA and poly-L-lactic acid have been used but have limitations, including the absence of biochemical motifs for cell attachment and the inability to regulate cell activity.[223] Scaffolds made from natural proteins and their derivatives may address these issues. Because tendon ECM is mainly composed of type I collagen, scaffolds based on collagen derivatives are highly biocompatible and exhibit superior biofunctionality by supporting cell adhesion and cell proliferation better than polyester materials.

A greater understanding of the molecular mechanisms underpinning tendon development and natural healing coupled with the advances in biomaterials and nanotechnology that allow a closer replication of the native tissues and delivery of growth factors with high spatiotemporal resolution and specificity[224] will allow tissue engineers to recapitulate tendon morphogenesis for repair. The insertion of tendons into bone remains a challenge.

The possibility of regeneration by triggering/enhancing the natural healing response is of interest. This goal could be achieved by using off-the-shelf biomaterials capable of delivering growth factors at specified times to recruit endogenous cells and direct repair to restore native tissue anatomy and function.[225] The application of biophysical modalities such as low-intensity pulsed ultrasound[226] is also promising for promotion of intrinsic healing and improving the mechanical properties of healing tendon-bone insertions.

Regenerative Medicine and Tissue Engineering in Arthritis

As we start to understand intrinsic tissue response mechanisms and attempts to counteract destructive processes by enhancing tissue repair, new therapeutic targets have been identified and targeted with "classic" pharmaceutical approaches such as the development of protein therapies and small molecules interfering with critical repair mechanisms. However, these approaches may still be far from sufficient and "too targeted," and therefore more comprehensive approaches may be needed. For this reason, cellular therapies and combination products have been explored. Indeed, cellular therapies will affect local processes in many ways as cell populations are manufactured so they deliver a vast array of secreted signals, also called their *secretome*, which is likely to influence local disease processes and enhance repair. Conversely, it becomes clear that the microenvironment will affect the cellular products and influence what they secrete and how they interact with the environment, including their engraftment, proliferation, differentiation, and tissue integration and remodeling.[227] Therefore, for regenerative medicine and cellular therapies to be successful, particularly in disease, we need to assess and quantify the microenvironment and mutual interactions between the cell-based product and the microenvironment, in particular also the immune system (see earlier). This approach points toward the importance of personalized medicine, and indeed, for regenerative medicine approaches to become cost-effective and successful, identifying the patients at risk and predicting responders to treatment will be of utmost importance.

Different cellular therapeutic approaches have been investigated in chronic inflammatory arthritis, with most data available on the use of adult MSCs. Proof-of-principle studies have been established for distinct indications. For inflammatory diseases such as RA and other autoimmune systemic diseases, the immune suppressive and immune modulatory effects of cellular therapies can contribute to the control of disease activity,[228] but this application is outside of the scope of this chapter.

Cellular therapies to enhance tissue repair have been explored quite extensively in pre-clinical animal models of post-traumatic OA.[180] The use of MSCs has been explored in patients with OA (see earlier).[153,229–233] The mechanisms through which they can influence the disease processes in OA appear diverse, as previously discussed, and include the so-called *trophic effects*, immune suppressive effects, and anti-inflammatory effects, as well as cell engraftment and contributing to the local de novo tissue formation, leading to meniscal and cartilage repair.[181,234] Because cellular products can potentially have all these effects, properly manufactured cell-based therapies might restore joint homeostasis thereby preventing disease progression in OA.

Conclusion

Regenerative medicine approaches are providing new and exciting opportunities in medicine in general and in the field of musculoskeletal disorders and diseases in particular. In orthopedics, cell-based tissue repair has entered the routine armamentarium and daily clinical practice. The development of injectable or arthroscopically implantable "regenerative biologics" will soon introduce regenerative medicine to the therapeutic options of rheumatologists. These options will include but are not limited to the repair of damaged joint surfaces, both chondral and osteochondral defects, the regeneration of difficult to heal fractured bones, the repair of damaged ligamentous structures, and the fabrication of a variety of "off the shelf" skeletal tissue structures, such as *viable* pieces of bones, ligaments, menisci, and other joint tissues. These regenerative treatments will not only be of use for post-traumatic damaged joints and skeletal tissues but also for (post)inflammatory and osteoarthritic joints.

Ultimately, the implantation of a *biologic* prosthesis with the potential of full tissue integration and remodeling is a dream target, and proof of principle exists that such a prosthesis may be within reach.[235,236] To achieve this goal in a more robust and predictable fashion, we need to change our strategy, using a bio-inspired engineering approach.[177,178] We proposed the term "developmental engineering" to describe a methodology for rational and accurate design of robust, well-controlled manufacturing processes. A close interaction between the efforts of biologists and engineers will speed up TE processes. Indeed, novel, enabling technologies such as bioreactors, biosensors, and three-dimensional (3-D) bioprinting will be required to achieve these goals.

The stage is set, and it is up to the biomedical TE community to break the boundaries toward the manufacturing of biologic spare parts of the body. It is anticipated that the musculoskeletal field, and thus patients with skeletal disorders and diseases, will benefit from this approach sooner rather than later.

Despite the advances in the field of tissue repair/regeneration in musculoskeletal conditions, these technologies are not yet in common use, and the National Health Services of several countries do not provide reimbursement. This situation is largely related to the high direct costs associated with such procedures, and cost-effectiveness remains a critical issue. A Swedish study has shown the health economic benefit of regenerative treatments when the reduction of disability, absenteeism, and other indirect costs are taken into account.[237] For those treatments to become affordable, however, a number of technologic gaps still need to be filled.

Furthermore, new emerging approaches are promising and include (1) the use of heterologous cell sources such as skeletal stem cells and induced pluripotent stem cells; (2) the harnessing of the intrinsic reparative mechanisms and homeostatic pathways through the use of bioactive molecules and/or acellular functionalized devices; and (3) the use of physical intervention to restore homeostasis, such as joint distraction,[238] which, by temporarily reducing the mechanical injury, would allow reparative mechanisms to take place.

At this stage we have obtained convincing evidence that regenerative musculoskeletal medicine has the potential for long-term, possibly lifelong efficacy in patients. The challenges have been identified and described. The growing knowledge in the molecular and cellular basis of the processes that drive tissue destruction and repair, disease progression, and homeostasis is paving the way by supplying an increasing number of targets for pharmacologic interventions, potential biomarkers, and a new generation of advanced therapeutic medicinal products. Finally, upscaling strategies and new enabling technologies such as 3-D bioprinting for tissue assembly provide a promising basis for the production of large living implants. While major milestones have been achieved, this is only the beginning of an exciting journey and the best is still to come!

 Full references for this chapter can be found on ExpertConsult.com.

Selected References

1. Luyten FR, Lories RJU, Verschueren P, et al.: Contemporary concepts of inflammation, damage and repair in rheumatic diseases, *Best Pract Res Cl Rh* 20(5):829–848, 2006.
2. Abnave P, Ghigo E: Role of the immune system in regeneration and its dynamic interplay with adult stem cells, *Semin Cell Dev Biol* 87:160–168, 2018.
3. Mariani FV: Proximal to distal patterning during limb development and regeneration: a review of converging disciplines, *Regen Med* 5(3):451–462, 2010.
4. Leucht P, Minear S, Ten Berge D, et al.: Translating insights from development into regenerative medicine: the function of Wnts in bone biology, *Seminars in Cell & Developmental Biology* 19(5):434–443, 2008.
5. Stoick-Cooper CL, Moon RT, Weidinger G: Advances in signaling in vertebrate regeneration as a prelude to regenerative medicine, *Gene Dev* 21(11):1292–1315, 2007.
6. Hunter W: Of the structure and disease of articulating cartilages (Reprinted from Philos-Trans-R-Soc-Lond, Vol 42, Pg 514-521, 1743), *Clin Orthop Relat R*(317)3–6, 1995.
7. Dell'accio F, Vincent TL: Joint surface defects: clinical course and cellular response in spontaneous and experimental lesions, *Eur Cells Mater* 20:210–217, 2010.
8. Ding CH, Cicuttini FM, Scott F, et al.: Natural history of knee cartilage defects and factors affecting change, *Arch Intern Med* 166(6):651–658, 2006.
9. Ding CH, Cicuttini FM, Scott F, et al.: The genetic contribution and relevance of knee cartilage defects: case-control and sib-pair studies, *Journal of Rheumatology* 32(10):1937–1942, 2005.
10. Davies-Tuck ML, Wluka A, Wang Y, et al.: The natural history of bone marrow lesions in community-based adults with no clinical knee osteoarthritis, *Annals of the Rheumatic Diseases* 68(6):904–908, 2009.
11. Wluka A, Wang Y, Davies-Tuck M, et al.: Bone marrow lesions predict progression of cartilage defects and loss of cartilage volume in healthy middle-aged adults without knee pain over 2 yrs, *Rheumatology* 47(9):1392–1396, 2008.
12. Zhai GJ, Ding CH, Stankovich J, et al.: The genetic contribution to longitudinal changes in knee structure and muscle strength—a sibpair study, *Arthritis Rheum-Us.* 52(9):2830–2834, 2005.
13. Reynard LN, Loughlin J: The genetics and functional analysis of primary osteoarthritis susceptibility, *Expert Rev Mol Med* 15, 2013.
14. Chapman K, Valdes AM: Genetic factors in OA pathogenesis, *Bone* 51(2):258–264, 2012.
15. Eltawil NM, De Bari C, Achan P, et al.: A novel in vivo murine model of cartilage regeneration. Age and strain-dependent outcome after joint surface injury, *Osteoarthr Cartilage* 17(6):695–704, 2009.
16. Rai MF, Hashimoto S, Johnson EE, et al.: Heritability of articular cartilage regeneration and its association with ear wound healing in mice, *Arthritis Rheum-Us.* 64(7):2300–2310, 2012.
17. Ding C, Cicuttini FM, Jones G: Tibial subchondral bone size and knee cartilage defects: relevance to knee osteoarthritis, *Osteoarthr Cartilage* 15(5):479–486, 2007.
18. Baker-LePain JC, Lane NE: Relationship between joint shape and the development of osteoarthritis, *Curr Opin Rheumatol* 22(5):538–543, 2010.
19. Buckwalter JA, Saltzman C, Brown T: The impact of osteoarthritis—implications for research, *Clin Orthop Relat R* 427:S6–S15, 2004.
20. Loughlin J, Dowling B, Chapman K, et al.: Functional variants within the secreted frizzled-related protein 3 gene are associated with hip osteoarthritis in females, *P Natl Acad Sci USA* 101(26):9757–9762, 2004.
21. Lories RJ, Boonen S, Peeters J, et al.: Evidence for a differential association of the Arg200Trp single-nucleotide polymorphism in FRZB with hip osteoarthritis and osteoporosis, *Rheumatology* 45(1):113–114, 2006.
22. Lories RJU, Peeters J, Bakker A, et al.: Articular cartilage and biomechanical properties of the long bones in Frzb-knockout mice, *Arthritis Rheum-Us.* 56(12):4095–4103, 2007.
23. Cheverud JM, Lawson HA, Bouckaert K, et al.: Fine-mapping quantitative trait loci affecting murine external ear tissue regeneration in the LG/J by SM/J advanced intercross line, *Heredity* 112(5):508–518, 2014.
24. Monteagudo S, Lories RJ: A notch in the joint that exacerbates osteoarthritis, *Nat Rev Rheumatol* 14(10):563–564, 2018.
25. Chung UI, Schipani E, McMahon AP, et al.: Indian hedgehog couples chondrogenesis to osteogenesis in endochondral bone development, *J Clin Invest* 107(3):295–304, 2001.
26. Guo J, Chung U, Kondo H, et al.: The PTH/PTHrP receptor can delay chondrocyte hypertrophy in vivo without activating phospholipase C, *Dev Cell* 3(2):183–194, 2002.
27. Kobayashi T, Chung UI, Schipani E, et al.: PTHrP and Indian hedgehog control differentiation of growth plate chondrocytes at multiple steps, *Development* 129(12):2977–2986, 2002.
28. Vortkamp A, Lee K, Lanske B, et al.: Regulation of rate of cartilage differentiation by Indian hedgehog and PTH-related protein, *Science* 273(5275):613–622, 1996.
29. Anraku Y, Mizuta H, Sei A, et al.: Analyses of early events during chondrogenic repair in rat full-thickness articular cartilage defects, *J Bone Miner Metab* 27(3):272–286, 2009.
30. Saito T, Fukai A, Mabuchi A, et al.: Transcriptional regulation of endochondral ossification by HIF-2 alpha during skeletal growth and osteoarthritis development, *Nat Med* 16(6):678–686, 2010.
31. Yang S, Kim J, Ryu JH, et al.: Hypoxia-inducible factor-2 alpha is a catabolic regulator of osteoarthritic cartilage destruction, *Nat Med* 16(6):687–693, 2010.
32. Sampson ER, Hilton MJ, Tian Y, et al.: Teriparatide as a chondroregenerative therapy for injury-induced osteoarthritis, *Sci Transl Med* 3(101), 2011.
33. Reginster JY, Badurski J, Bellamy N, et al.: Efficacy and safety of strontium ranelate in the treatment of knee osteoarthritis: results of a double-blind, randomised placebo-controlled trial, *Annals of the Rheumatic Diseases* 72(2):179–186, 2013.
34. Pelletier JP, Kapoor M, Fahmi H, et al.: Strontium ranelate reduces the progression of experimental dog osteoarthritis by inhibiting the expression of key proteases in cartilage and of IL-1 beta in the synovium, *Annals of the Rheumatic Diseases* 72(2):250–257, 2013.
35. Yu DG, Ding HF, Mao YQ, et al.: Strontium ranelate reduces cartilage degeneration and subchondral bone remodeling in rat osteoarthritis model, *Acta Pharmacol Sin* 34(3):393–402, 2013.
36. Davidson ENB, van der Kraan PM, van den Berg WB: TGF-beta and osteoarthritis, *Osteoarthr Cartilage* 15(6):597–604, 2007.
37. van Beuningen HM, Glansbeek HL, van der Kraan PM, et al.: Osteoarthritis-like changes in the murine knee joint resulting from

intra-articular transforming growth factor-beta injections, *Osteoarthritis Cartilage* 8(1):25–33, 2000.

38. Chen R, Mian M, Fu M, et al.: Attenuation of the progression of articular cartilage degeneration by inhibition of TGF-beta1 signaling in a mouse model of osteoarthritis, *Am J Pathol* 185(11):2875–2885, 2015.
39. Zhen G, Wen C, Jia X, et al.: Inhibition of TGF-beta signaling in mesenchymal stem cells of subchondral bone attenuates osteoarthritis, *Nat Med* 19(6):704–712, 2013.
40. Xie L, Tintani F, Wang X, et al.: Systemic neutralization of TGF-beta attenuates osteoarthritis, *Ann N Y Acad Sci* 1376(1):53–64, 2016.
41. Lories RJU, Derese I, Ceuppens JL, et al.: Bone morphogenetic proteins 2 and 6, expressed in arthritic synovium, are regulated by proinflammatory cytokines and differentially modulate fibroblast-like synoviocyte apoptosis, *Arthritis Rheum-Us.* 48(10):2807–2818, 2003.
42. Chubinskaya S, Hurtig M, Rueger DC: OP-1/BMP-7 in cartilage repair, *Int Orthop* 31(6):773–781, 2007.
43. van der Kraan PM, Davidson ENB, Blom A, et al.: TGF-beta signaling in chondrocyte terminal differentiation and osteoarthritis modulation and integration of signaling pathways through receptor-Smads, *Osteoarthr Cartilage* 17(12):1539–1545, 2009.
44. Hong CC, Yu PB: Applications of small molecule BMP inhibitors in physiology and disease, *Cytokine Growth F R* 20(5-6):409–418, 2009.
45. Garrison KR, Shemilt I, Donell S, et al.: Bone morphogenetic protein (BMP) for fracture healing in adults, *Cochrane Db Syst Rev* 6, 2010.
46. Giannoudis PV, Einhorn TA: Bone morphogenetic proteins in musculoskeletal medicine, *Injury* 40:1–3, 2009.
47. Valverde-Franco G, Binette JS, Li W, et al.: Defects in articular cartilage metabolism and early arthritis in fibroblast growth factor receptor 3 deficient mice, *Hum Mol Genet* 15(11):1783–1792, 2006.
48. Haque T, Amako M, Nakada S, et al.: An immunohistochemical analysis of the temporal and spatial expression of growth factors FGF 1, 2 and 18, IGF 1 and 2, and TGF beta 1 during distraction osteogenesis, *Histol Histopathol* 22(2):119–128, 2007.
49. Moore EE, Bendele AM, Thompson DL, et al.: Fibroblast growth factor-18 stimulates chondrogenesis and cartilage repair in a rat model of injury-induced osteoarthritis, *Osteoarthritis Cartilage* 13(7):623–631, 2005.
50. Reinhold MI, Abe M, Kapadia RM, et al.: FGF18 represses noggin expression and is induced by calcineurin, *J Biol Chem* 279(37):38209–38219, 2004.
51. Luyten FP, Tylzanowski P, Lories RJ: Wnt signaling and osteoarthritis, *Bone* 44(4):522–527, 2009.
52. Hartmann C, Tabin CJ: Wnt-14 plays a pivotal role in inducing synovial joint formation in the developing appendicular skeleton, *Cell* 104(3):341–351, 2001.
53. Guo X, Day TF, Jiang X, et al.: Wnt/beta-catenin signaling is sufficient and necessary for synovial joint formation, *Genes Dev* 18(19):2404–2417, 2004.
54. Yasuhara R, Ohta Y, Yuasa T, et al.: Roles of beta-catenin signaling in phenotypic expression and proliferation of articular cartilage superficial zone cells, *Lab Invest* 91(12):1739–1752, 2011.
55. Tamamura Y, Otani T, Kanatani N, et al.: Developmental regulation of Wnt/beta-catenin signals is required for growth plate assembly, cartilage integrity, and endochondral ossification, *J Biol Chem* 280(19):19185–19195, 2005.
56. Koyama E, Shibukawa Y, Nagayama M, et al.: A distinct cohort of progenitor cells participates in synovial joint and articular cartilage formation during mouse limb skeletogenesis, *Dev Biol* 316(1):62–73, 2008.
57. Zhu M, Tang DZ, Wu QQ, et al.: Activation of beta-catenin signaling in articular chondrocytes leads to osteoarthritis-like phenotype in adult beta-catenin conditional activation mice, *J Bone Miner Res* 24(1):12–21, 2009.
58. Enomoto-Iwamoto M, Kitagaki J, Koyama E, et al.: The Wnt antagonist Frzb-1 regulates chondrocyte maturation and long bone development during limb skeletogenesis, *Dev Biol* 251(1):142–156, 2002.
59. Lories RJ, Derese I, Luyten FP: Deletion of frizzled related protein (Frzb) reduces severity of ankylosis in a mouse model of spondyloarthritis, *Arthritis Rheum-Us.* 58(9):S347–S348, 2008.
60. Kiel MJ, Acar M, Radice GL, et al.: Hematopoietic stem cells do not depend on n-cadherin to regulate their maintenance, *Cell Stem Cell* 4(2):170–179, 2009.
61. Zhu M, Chen M, Zuscik M, et al.: Inhibition of beta-catenin signaling in articular chondrocytes results in articular cartilage destruction, *Arthritis Rheum-Us.* 58(7):2053–2064, 2008.
62. Yuasa T, Kondo N, Yasuhara R, et al.: Transient activation of Wnt/beta-catenin signaling induces abnormal growth plate closure and articular cartilage thickening in postnatal mice, *Am J Pathol* 175(5):1993–2003, 2009.
63. Diarra D, Stolina M, Polzer K, et al.: Dickkopf-1 is a master regulator of joint remodeling, *Nat Med* 13(2):156–163, 2007.
64. Kronke G, Uderhardt S, Kim KA, et al.: R-spondin 1 protects against inflammatory bone damage during murine arthritis by modulating the Wnt pathway, *Arthritis Rheum-Us.* 62(8):2303–2312, 2010.
65. Kawakami Y, Esteban CR, Raya M, et al.: Wnt/beta-catenin signaling regulates vertebrate limb regeneration, *Gene Dev* 20(23):3232–3237, 2006.
66. Nalesso G, Sherwood J, Bertrand J, et al.: WNT-3A modulates articular chondrocyte phenotype by activating both canonical and noncanonical pathways, *J Cell Biol* 193(3):551–564, 2011.
67. Nalesso G, Thomas BL, Sherwood JC, et al.: WNT16 antagonises excessive canonical WNT activation and protects cartilage in osteoarthritis, *Ann Rheum Dis* 76(1):218–226, 2017.
68. Monteagudo S, Lories RJ: Cushioning the cartilage: a canonical Wnt restricting matter, *Nat Rev Rheumatol* 13(11):670–681, 2017.
69. Luyten FP, Hascall VC, Nissley SP, et al.: Insulin-like growth-factors maintain steady-state metabolism of proteoglycans in bovine articular-cartilage explants, *Arch Biochem Biophys* 267(2):416–425, 1988.
70. Dart AJ, Little CB, Hughes CE, et al.: Recombinant equine growth hormone administration: effects on synovial fluid biomarkers and cartilage metabolism in horses, *Equine Vet J* 35(3):302–307, 2003.
71. Nemirovskiy O, Zheng YJ, Tung D, et al.: Pharmacokinetic/pharmacodynamic (PK/PD) differentiation of native and PEGylated recombinant human growth hormone (rhGH and PEG-rhGH) in the rat model of osteoarthritis, *Xenobiotica* 40(8):586–592, 2010.
72. Denko CW, Malemud CJ: Role of the growth hormone/insulin-like growth factor-1 paracrine axis in rheumatic diseases, *Semin Arthritis Rheu* 35(1):24–34, 2005.
73. Fuchs E, Tumbar T, Guasch G: Socializing with the neighbors: stem cells and their niche, *Cell* 116(6):769–778, 2004.
74. Augello A, Kurth TB, De Bari C: Mesenchymal stem cells: a perspective from in vitro cultures to in vivo migration and niches, *Eur Cells Mater* 20:121–133, 2010.
75. Crisan M, Yap S, Casteilla L, et al.: A perivascular origin for mesenchymal stem cells in multiple human organs, *Cell Stem Cell* 3(3):301–313, 2008.
76. Meirelles LD, Caplan AI, Nardi NB: In search of the in vivo identity of mesenchymal stem cells, *Stem Cells* 26(9):2287–2299, 2008.
77. Barbero A, Ploegert S, Heberer M, et al.: Plasticity of clonal populations of dedifferentiated adult human articular chondrocytes, *Arthritis Rheum-Us.* 48(5):1315–1325, 2003.
78. Dell'Accio F, De Bari C, Luyten FP: Microenvironment and phenotypic stability specify tissue formation by human articular cartilage-derived cells in vivo, *Exp Cell Res* 287(1):16–27, 2003.
79. Dowthwaite GP, Bishop JC, Redman SN, et al.: The surface of articular cartilage contains a progenitor cell population, *J Cell Sci* 117(6):889–897, 2004.
80. McGonagle D, Baboolal TG, Jones E: Native joint-resident mesenchymal stem cells for cartilage repair in osteoarthritis, *Nat Rev Rheumatol* 13(12):719–730, 2017.

81. Kurth TB, Dell'accio F, Crouch V, et al.: Functional mesenchymal stem cell niches in adult mouse knee joint synovium in vivo, *Arthritis Rheum* 63(5):1289–1300, 2011.
82. Morikawa S, Mabuchi Y, Kubota Y, et al.: Prospective identification, isolation, and systemic transplantation of multipotent mesenchymal stem cells in murine bone marrow, *J Exp Med* 206(11):2483–2496, 2009.
83. Park BW, Kang EJ, Byun JH, et al.: In vitro and in vivo osteogenesis of human mesenchymal stem cells derived from skin, bone marrow and dental follicle tissues, *Differentiation* 83(5):249–259, 2012.
84. Mendez-Ferrer S, Michurina TV, Ferraro F, et al.: Mesenchymal and haematopoietic stem cells form a unique bone marrow niche, *Nature* 466(7308):829–U59, 2010.
85. Isern J, Garcia-Garcia A, Martin AM, et al.: The neural crest is a source of mesenchymal stem cells with specialized hematopoietic stem-cell-niche function, *Elife* 3, 2014.
86. Ding L, Saunders TL, Enikolopov G, et al.: Endothelial and perivascular cells maintain haematopoietic stem cells, *Nature* 481(7382):457–462, 2012.
87. Zhou BO, Yue R, Murphy MM, et al.: Leptin-receptor-expressing mesenchymal stromal cells represent the main source of bone formed by adult bone marrow, *Cell Stem Cell* 15(2):154–168, 2014.
88. Worthley DL, Churchill M, Compton JT, et al.: Gremlin 1 identifies a skeletal stem cell with bone, cartilage, and reticular stromal potential, *Cell* 160(1-2):269–284, 2015.
89. Chan CK, Seo EY, Chen JY, et al.: Identification and specification of the mouse skeletal stem cell, *Cell* 160(1-2):285–298, 2015.
90. Chan CKF, Gulati GS, Sinha R, et al.: Identification of the human skeletal stem cell, *Cell* 175(1):43–56 e21, 2018.
91. Debnath S, Yallowitz AR, McCormick J, et al.: Discovery of a periosteal stem cell mediating intramembranous bone formation, *Nature* 562(7725):133–139, 2018.
92. Rountree RB, Schoor M, Chen H, et al.: BMP receptor signaling is required for postnatal maintenance of articular cartilage, *PLoS Biol* 2(11):e355, 2004.
93. Chen H, Capellini TD, Schoor M, et al.: Heads, shoulders, elbows, knees, and toes: modular Gdf5 enhancers control different joints in the vertebrate skeleton, *PLoS Genet* 12(11):e1006454, 2016.
94. Roelofs AJ, Zupan J, Riemen AHK, et al.: Joint morphogenetic cells in the adult mammalian synovium, *Nat Commun* 8, 2017.
95. Dell'Accio F, Vanlauwe J, Bellemans J, et al.: Expanded phenotypically stable chondrocytes persist in the repair tissue and contribute to cartilage matrix formation and structural integration in a goat model of autologous chondrocyte implantation (vol 21, pg 123, 2003), *J Orthop Res* 21(3):572, 2003.
96. Kozhemyakina E, Zhang M, Ionescu A, et al.: Identification of a Prg4-expressing articular cartilage progenitor cell population in mice, *Arthritis Rheumatol* 67(5):1261–1273, 2015.
97. Li L, Newton PT, Bouderlique T, et al.: Superficial cells are self-renewing chondrocyte progenitors, which form the articular cartilage in juvenile mice, *Faseb J* 31(3):1067–1084, 2017.
98. Decker RS, Um HB, Dyment NA, et al.: Cell origin, volume and arrangement are drivers of articular cartilage formation, morphogenesis and response to injury in mouse limbs, *Dev Biol* 426(1):56–68, 2017.
99. Hunziker EB, Rosenberg LC: Repair of partial-thickness defects in articular cartilage: cell recruitment from the synovial membrane, *J Bone Joint Surg Am* 78a(5):721–733, 1996.
100. Jones EA, English A, Henshaw K, et al.: Enumeration and phenotypic characterization of synovial fluid multipotential mesenchymal progenitor cells in inflammatory and degenerative arthritis, *Arthritis Rheum-Us.* 50(3):817–827, 2004.
101. Jones EA, Crawford A, English A, et al.: Synovial fluid mesenchymal stem cells in health and early osteoarthritis—detection and functional evaluation at the single-cell level, *Arthritis Rheum-Us.* 58(6):1731–1740, 2008.
102. Sekiya I, Ojima M, Suzuki S, et al.: Human mesenchymal stem cells in synovial fluid increase in the knee with degenerated cartilage and osteoarthritis, *J Orthop Res* 30(6):943–949, 2012.
103. Campbell TM, Churchman SM, Gomez A, et al.: Mesenchymal stem cell alterations in bone marrow lesions in patients with hip osteoarthritis, *Arthritis Rheumatol* 68(7):1648–1659, 2016.
104. Fellows CR, Williams R, Davies IR, et al.: Characterisation of a divergent progenitor cell sub-populations in human osteoarthritic cartilage: the role of telomere erosion and replicative senescence, *Sci Rep-Uk* 7, 2017.
105. Kovtun A, Messerer DAC, Scharffetter-Kochanek K, et al.: Neutrophils in tissue trauma of the skin, bone, and lung: two sides of the same coin, *J Immunol Res*, 2018.
106. Headland SE, Jones HR, Norling LV, et al.: Neutrophil-derived microvesicles enter cartilage and protect the joint in inflammatory arthritis, *Sci Transl Med* 7(315):315ra190, 2015.
107. Chan JK, Glass GE, Ersek A, et al.: Low-dose TNF augments fracture healing in normal and osteoporotic bone by up-regulating the innate immune response, *EMBO Mol Med* 7(5):547–561, 2015.
108. Zhang S, Chuah SJ, Lai RC, et al.: MSC exosomes mediate cartilage repair by enhancing proliferation, attenuating apoptosis and modulating immune reactivity, *Biomaterials* 156:16–27, 2018.
109. Li JT, Tan J, Martino MM, et al.: Regulatory t-cells: potential regulator of tissue repair and regeneration, *Front Immunol* 9:585, 2018.
110. Zachar L, Bacenkova D, Rosocha J: Activation, homing, and role of the mesenchymal stem cells in the inflammatory environment, *J Inflamm Res* 9:231–240, 2016.
111. Qi K, Li N, Zhang ZY, et al.: Tissue regeneration: the crosstalk between mesenchymal stem cells and immune response, *Cell Immunol* 326:86–93, 2018.
112. Verzijl N, DeGroot J, Thorpe SR, et al.: Effect of collagen turnover on the accumulation of advanced glycation end products, *J Biol Chem* 275(50):39027–39031, 2000.
113. Johnson K, Zhu ST, Tremblay MS, et al.: A stem cell-based approach to cartilage repair, *Science* 336(6082):717–721, 2012.
114. Bi WM, Deng JM, Zhang ZP, et al.: Sox9 is required for cartilage formation, *Nat Genet* 22(1):85–89, 1999.
115. Han Y, Lefebvre V: L-Sox5 and Sox6 drive expression of the aggrecan gene in cartilage by securing binding of Sox9 to a far-upstream enhancer, *Mol Cell Biol* 28(16):4999–5013, 2008.
116. Lefebvre V, Huang WD, Harley VR, et al.: SOX9 is a potent activator of the chondrocyte-specific enhancer of the pro alpha 1(II) collagen gene, *Mol Cell Biol* 17(4):2336–2346, 1997.
117. Aigner T, Zien A, Hanisch D, et al.: Gene expression in chondrocytes assessed with use of microarrays, *J Bone Joint Surg Am* 85a:117–123, 2003.
118. Appleton CTG, Pitelka V, Henry J, et al.: Global analyses of gene expression in early experimental osteoarthritis, *Arthritis Rheum-Us.* 56(6):1854–1868, 2007.
119. Karlsson C, Dehne T, Lindahl A, et al.: Genome-wide expression profiling reveals new candidate genes associated with osteoarthritis, *Osteoarthr Cartilage* 18(4):581–592, 2010.
120. Snelling S, Rout R, Davidson R, et al.: A gene expression study of normal and damaged cartilage in anteromedial gonarthrosis, a phenotype of osteoarthritis, *Osteoarthr Cartilage* 22(2):334–343, 2014.

8 Proteinases and Matrix Degradation

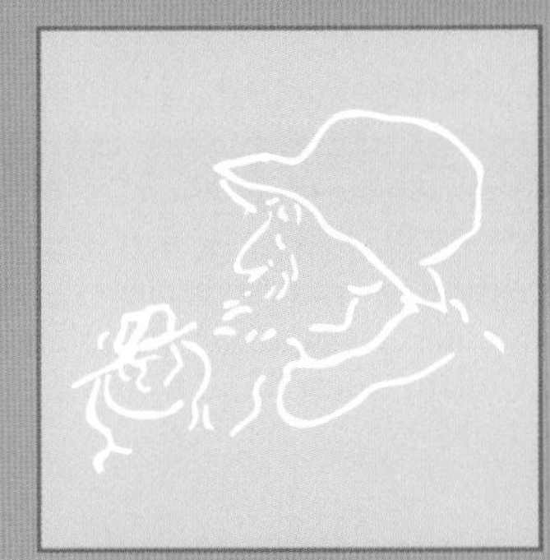

YOSHIFUMI ITOH

KEY POINTS

Proteinases are generally classified into aspartic proteinases, cysteine proteinases, serine proteinases, and metalloproteinases according to their catalytic mechanism.

Because of the optimal acidic pH and intra-cellular localization within lysosomes, most of the aspartic proteinases and cysteine proteinases are involved in intra-cellular degradation of extra-cellular matrix (ECM) components.

Serine proteinases and metalloproteinases are proteinases that act at neutral pH and play a central role in extra-cellular degradation of ECM macromolecules.

ECM-degrading metalloproteinases are composed mainly of the MMP (matrix metalloproteinase) and ADAMTS (a disintegrin and metalloproteinase with thrombospondin motifs) gene families.

Most endogenous proteinase inhibitors are proteinase class specific, whereas α2 macroglobulin inhibits the activities of all classes of proteinase.

The activities of ECM-degrading proteinases at the local tissues are regulated by the balance between the proteinases and their inhibitors, which may be determined by production rates of proteinases and inhibitors, their secretion, activation of proenzymes, and cell surface anchoring and recycling systems of the activated proteinases.

ProMMPs (precursors of MMPs) are activated via the extra-cellular, intra-cellular, and cell surface pathways depending on the enzymes.

Aggrecan and type II collagen, two major ECM components, may be degraded in articular cartilage by differential or complementary actions of the MMP and ADAMTS species in arthritides.

In rheumatoid arthritis, articular cartilage is destroyed by proteinases accumulated in synovial fluid, direct contact with proteolytic pannus, and proteinases derived from chondrocytes. Bone is resorbed by osteoclasts mainly by the action of cathepsin K and MMP-9 under acidic and hypercalcemic conditions in subosteoclastic compartments.

In osteoarthritis, chondrocyte-derived metalloproteinases, including the MMP and ADAMTS species, contribute primarily to the breakdown of articular cartilage.

Introduction

Extra-cellular matrix (ECM) is an important component of multicellular organisms, including humans. It provides the tissue architecture, fills the gaps between the cells, separates tissue components, acts as a scaffolding for migrating cells, acts as a growth factor pool, and sends the signals directly to the cells. While the cell-ECM interaction regulates various fundamental cellular functions, including growth, differentiation, apoptosis, and migration, upon tissue remodeling or cell migration in tissue, ECM becomes a physical barrier that needs to be degraded. ECM degradation is achieved by proteolytic enzymes, termed *endopeptidases* or *proteinases*. In normal healthy conditions, activity of ECM-degrading proteinases is under tight control, keeping tissue homeostasis. On the other hand, in pathologic conditions, activity of these proteinases are either elevated excessively for tissue destructive diseases or decreased for fibrotic diseases. Thus, regulatory mechanisms of ECM degradation are important to understand to reveal pathogenesis of these diseases. In rheumatoid arthritis and osteoarthritis, activity of ECM-degrading proteinases are elevated, causing destruction of joint tissue, including cartilage and bone. It is getting clearer that these unbalanced ECM metabolisms are due not only to upregulation of proteinase genes, but also to other factors. This chapter provides up-to-date information about ECM-degrading proteinases and their regulations in rheumatoid arthritis and osteoarthritis.

Extra-cellular Matrix-Degrading Proteinases

ECM is a meshwork of large macromolecules, and thus their degradation is caused by endopeptidases or proteinases that cleave internal peptide bonds of polypeptide chains. The impact of exopeptidases that cleave a few amino acids either from N- or C-terminus in ECM integrity is unlikely to be significant even if they exist. There are four different classes of proteinases that have been implicated in ECM degradation: aspartic proteinases, cysteine proteinases, serine proteinases, and metalloproteinases, which are classified according to their catalytic machinery.

Aspartic Proteinases

Most aspartic proteinases have two aspartic acid residues in their catalytic sites, where the nucleophile that attacks the scissile peptide bond is an activated water molecule. Mammalian aspartic proteinases include the digestive enzymes (pepsin and chymosin), the intra-cellular cathepsin D and cathepsin E, and rennin. Among the proteinases belonging to this group, cathepsin D is the major aspartic proteinase involved in ECM degradation. It exhibits proteolytic activity against most substrates such as aggrecan and collagen telopeptides with optimal pH between pH 3.5

and 5. Because of the acidic optimal pH and intra-cellular localization within lysosomes, cathepsin D is probably responsible for intra-cellular degradation of phagocytosed ECM fragments that previously were degraded in the extra-cellular spaces. However, a study on cartilage explant cultures using the aspartic proteinase inhibitor suggests the possibility that cathepsin D secreted extra-cellularly contributes to the degradation of aggrecan in articular cartilage.[1]

Cysteine Proteinases

Cysteine proteinases are endopeptidases in which the nucleophile of the catalytic site is the sulfhydryl group of a cysteine residue. The ECM-degrading cysteine proteinases include lysosomal cathepsins B, L, S, and K and the calpains (Table 8.1). Cathepsins B and L digest the telopeptide regions of fibrillar types I and II collagen, the nonhelical regions of types IX and XI collagen, and aggrecan at acidic pH. Cathepsin S has a similar spectrum of substrates within a broad range of pH values. Cathepsin K, also previously called *cathepsin O, O2,* or *X,* is a collagenolytic cathepsin that cleaves type I collagen at the triple helical regions at pH values between 4.5 and 6.6.[2] The proteinase also degrades gelatin and osteonectin. Cathepsin K is highly expressed in human osteoclasts,[3] and inactivating mutations or deletion of the gene result in an osteopetrotic phenotype in humans and animals; cathepsin K is thought to play a key role in osteoclast-dependent bone resorption (see later discussion). Because cathepsins B, L, S, and K are expressed in synovium or articular cartilage or both in rheumatoid arthritis and osteoarthritis, they may also be involved in the cartilage destruction through degradation of the ECM macromolecules when the local environment has shifted to acidic condition.[4]

Calpains are Ca^{2+}-dependent, papain-like cysteine proteinases that are ubiquitously distributed among mammalian cells. The best-characterized members of the calpain superfamily are μ-calpain and m-calpain, which also are called *conventional* (μ-calpain) and *classic* (m-calpain) *calpains.*[5] Calpains are involved in various pathologic conditions such as muscle dystrophy by acting intra-cellularly. They are present in the extra-cellular spaces and in osteoarthritic synovial fluid, and they can degrade aggrecan.

Serine Proteinases

Serine proteinases require the hydroxyl group of a serine residue acting as the nucleophile that attacks the peptide bond. Serine proteinases include the largest number of proteinases with around 40 family members. Most serine proteinases can degrade ECM macromolecules. The major ECM-degrading serine proteinases in joint tissues will be described below (see Table 8.1).

Neutrophil Elastase and Cathepsin G

Neutrophil elastase and cathepsin G are serine proteinases that are synthesized as precursors in promyelocytes in bone marrow and subsequently stored in the azurophil granules of polymorphonuclear leukocytes as active enzymes. Mature leukocytes do not synthesize elastase, but they mobilize azurophil granules to the cell surface and release the proteinases in response to various stimuli. Monocytes have low levels of elastase but lose the enzyme expression during the differentiation into macrophages. Neutrophil elastase and cathepsin G are basic glycoproteins with isoelectric points larger than 9 (neutrophil elastase) and about 12 (cathepsin G). They can be readily trapped in cartilage matrix that has a negative charge.

TABLE 8.1 Proteinases That May Be Involved in Degradation of Extra-cellular Matrix

Enzyme	Source	Inhibitor
Aspartic Proteinases		
Cathepsin D	Lysosome	Pepstatin
Cysteine Proteinases		
Cathepsin B	Lysosome	Cystatins
Cathepsin L	Lysosome	Cystatins
Cathepsin S	Lysosome	Cystatins
Cathepsin K	Lysosome	Cystatins
Calpain	Cytosol	Calpastatin
Serine Proteinases		
Neutrophil elastase	Neutrophils	α1 PI
Cathepsin G	Neutrophils	α1 Antichymotrypsin
Proteinase 3	Neutrophils	α1 PI, elafin
Plasmin	Plasma	Aprotinin
Plasma kallikrein	Plasma	Aprotinin
Tissue kallikrein	Glandular tissues	Aprotinin; kallistatin
tPA	Endothelial cells; chondrocytes	PAI-1; PAI-2
uPA	Fibroblasts; chondrocytes	PAI-1; PAI-2; PN-1
Tryptase	Mast cells	Trypstatin
Chymase	Mast cells	α1 PI
Metalloproteinases[a]		
MMPs	Tissue cells; inflammatory cells	TIMP-1, 2, 3, and 4; RECK for MMP-2, 7, 9, and 14
ADAMTSs	Tissue cells	TIMP-3
ADAMs	Tissue cells; inflammatory cells	TIMP-3; RECK for ADAM10

[a]For details of ADAMs, ADAMTSs, and MMPs, see Tables 8.2 and 8.3.

ADAMs, A disintegrin and metalloproteinases; *ADAMTSs,* a disintegrin and metalloproteinases with thrombospondin motifs; *MMPs,* matrix metalloproteinases; *PAI,* plasminogen activator inhibitor; *PI,* proteinase inhibitor, *PN,* proteinase nexin; *RECK,* reversion-inducing, cysteine-rich protein with Kazal motifs; *TIMP,* tissue inhibitor of metalloproteinases; *tPA,* tissue-type plasminogen activator; *uPA,* urokinase-type plasminogen activator.

Neutrophil elastase and cathepsin G cleave elastin; the telopeptide region of fibrillar collagen types I, II, and III; other collagen types IV, VI, VIII, IX, X, and XI; and other ECM components such as fibronectin, laminin, and aggrecan at neutral pH. These serine proteinases can also be involved indirectly in the breakdown of ECM by activating the zymogen of matrix metalloproteinases (proMMPs)[6] and by inactivating endogenous proteinase inhibitors such as α2 antiplasmin, α1 antichymotrypsin, and tissue inhibitors of metalloproteinases (TIMPs).

Mast Cell Chymase and Tryptase

Chymase and tryptase are packaged in secretory granules together with histamine and other mediators in mast cells, which are infiltrated in rheumatoid synovium. Chymase is a chymotrypsin-like proteinase with a broad spectrum of activity against ECM components such as type VI collagen[7] and aggrecan. It also activates proMMPs such as proMMP-1, 3, and 9.[6] Although prochymase is activated intra-cellularly and stored in the granules, the activity in the granules is limited at low pH and becomes fully active when released extra-cellularly. Tryptase is a trypsin-like proteinase that degrades type VI collagen and fibronectin; it also activates proMMP-3.[6]

Plasmin and Plasminogen Activators

Plasminogen is synthesized in the liver and secreted to plasma. It can bind to fibrin and to cells, and after activation by plasminogen activators, plasmin readily digests fibrin. Membrane-bound plasmin also degrades many ECM components, including proteoglycan, fibronectin, type IV collagen, and laminin. Other important functions of plasmin are to initiate the activation of proMMPs, activate latent cell-associated transforming growth factor (TGF)-β1, and act as proenzyme convertase. Plasmin is generated by activation of plasminogen by plasminogen activators, including tissue-type plasminogen activator (tPA) and urokinase-type plasminogen activator (uPA). The tPA is synthesized as a proenzyme of 70 kDa and is secreted into the circulating blood primarily by endothelial cells, fibroblasts, chondrocytes, and tumor cells.[8] The uPA was first purified from urine as a proenzyme of 54 kDa.[8] It is converted to the active form of two chains of 30 kDa and 24 kDa linked by a disulfide bond. Alternatively, a fully active form of 33 kDa can be generated by plasmin. The expression of uPA is found in various cells, including invasive cancer cells, migrating keratinocytes, and activated leukocytes in pathologic situations. Pro-uPA and two-chain uPA bind to a specific uPA receptor (uPAR), a glycosylphosphatidylinositol (GPI)–anchored glycoprotein expressed on the cell surface of fibroblasts, macrophages, and tumor cells. Receptor-bound uPA preferentially activates cell membrane–bound plasminogen into plasmin. Cell membrane–bound plasmin can activate receptor-bound pro-uPA. Despite the highly restricted substrate specificity of the plasminogen activators, uPA cleaves other proteins in vitro, including fibronectin, fibrinogen, diphtheria toxin, and possibly uPA itself.

Kallikreins

Two types of kallikreins, plasma and tissue kallikreins, have been identified. Plasma kallikrein, with two disulfide-linked chains (36 kDa and 52 kDa), is generated from prokallikrein of 88 kDa by coagulation factor XIIa or by kallikrein itself. It activates kininogens to bradykinin and activates proMMP-1 and proMMP-3.[6] Tissue kallikrein, which is synthesized in glandular tissues, releases Lys-bradykinin from kininogen and activates proMMP-8.[6]

Metalloproteinases

Similar to aspartic proteinases, metalloproteinases are endopeptidases in which the nucleophilic attack on a peptide bond is mediated by a water molecule. A divalent metal cation, usually zinc, activates the water molecule. Among the metalloproteinases, MMPs (matrix metalloproteinases), which are also designated as *matrixins* (a subfamily of the metzincin superfamily), are key ECM-degrading, zinc-dependent endopeptidases (Table 8.2). In addition, some members of the ADAMTS (a disintegrin and metalloproteinase with thrombospondin motifs) family, which is an MMP-related gene family within the metzincin family, are also responsible for the degradation of ECM, such as cartilage proteoglycan (Table 8.3). Only a few members of the ADAM (a disintegrin and metalloproteinase) family have limited activity to ECM components (Table 8.4).

Matrix Metalloproteinases

The human MMP family comprises 23 different members that have MMP designations (numbered according to a sequential numbering system) and common names coined by the authors of the published reports (see Table 8.2). On the basis of the biochemical properties provided by the domain structures and on their substrate specificity, these family members are classified into two major subgroups: secreted-type MMPs and membrane-anchored MMPs. MMP-4, 5, and 6 are excluded from the list because they are identical to other known MMPs (i.e., MMP-3 and 2). MMP-18 and 22 also are missing in Table 8.2 because they are assigned to *Xenopus* collagenase-4 and chicken MMP. Many of the secreted-type MMPs are composed of three basic domains—the prodomain, catalytic domain, and hemopexin-like domain—that are preceded by hydrophobic signal peptides (Fig. 8.1). The N-terminal prodomain has one unpaired cysteine in the conserved sequence of PRCGXPD. The cysteine residue in the sequence interacts with the catalytic zinc atom in the catalytic domain to maintain the proenzyme in an inactive state by preventing it from binding the water molecule to interact for the catalysis. The catalytic domain has the zinc-binding motif HEXGHXXGXXH, in which three histidines bind to and hold the catalytic zinc atom. The hemopexin-like domain, which is connected to the catalytic domain by the proline-rich hinge region, is considered as a molecular interaction interface and plays a role in determining the substrate specificity in some MMPs. In addition to these basic domains, gelatinases have additional insertions of three repeats of fibronectin type II domain in the catalytic domain (see Fig. 8.1), which provides them with collagen-binding properties. Matrilysins are the smallest MMP member, lacking the hemopexin-like domains. Furin-activated MMPs contain insertions of a basic amino acid motif of Arg-Xxx-Lys-Arg (RXKR) at the C-terminus of the prodomain that is recognized and cleaved by proprotein convertases, including furin (see Fig. 8.1). These enzymes are thus secreted to extra-cellular milieus as an active form. MMP-23 is synthesized as a type II transmembrane type MMP having type II transmembrane domain in the N-terminus of prodomain. It contains the RRRR sequence at the end of the prodomain that can be cleaved by proprotein convertases during secretion, which makes the enzyme a soluble enzyme. The domain structure of MMP-23 is also unique among MMP members as it has a cysteine array and an immunoglobulin-like domain instead of a hemopexin-like domain (see Fig. 8.1).

There are two types of membrane-type MMPs: type-I transmembrane type (MMP-14, -15, -16, and -24/MT1-, MT2-, MT3-, and MT5-MMPs) and GPI-anchored type (MMP-17 and -25/MT4- and MT6-MMPs).[7] Type I transmembrane-type MMPs have a stalk region, the transmembrane domain, and a short cytoplasmic tail downstream of the hemopexin domain in addition to the common domain composition (prodomain, catalytic domain, hinge, and hemopexin-like domain). GPI-anchored types are synthesized with hydrophobic GPI anchoring the signal peptide sequence following the stalk region at their C-terminus. This GPI-anchoring signal peptide is cleaved off and the ectodomain transferred to the de-novo synthesized GPI moiety by transamidase in endoplasmic reticulum (see Fig. 8.1).

TABLE 8.2 Substrates of Human Matrix Metalloproteinases

Enzymes	ECM Substrates	Non-ECM Substrates
Soluble MMPs		
Classic Collagenases		
MMP-1	Collagens I, II, III, VII, X; gelatins; aggrecan; link protein entactin; tenascin; perlecan	α2 Macroglobulin; IGF-BP-2, -3, and -5; (Interstitial Collagenase) α1 PI; α1 antichymotrypsin; pro-IL-1β; CTGF
MMP-8 (Neutrophil collagenase)	Collagens I, II, and III; gelatins; aggrecan; link protein	α1 PI
MMP-13 (Collagenase-3)	Collagens I, II, III, IV, IX, X, XIV; aggrecan; Fn; tenascin	CTGF; pro-TGF-β; α1 antichymotrypsin
Gelatinases		
MMP-2 (Gelatinase A)	Gelatins; collagens IV, V, VII, XI; Ln; Fn; elastin; aggrecan; link protein	Pro-TGF-β; FGF receptor I; MCP-3; IGFBP-5; pro-IL-1β; galectin-3; plasminogen
MMP-9 (Gelatinase B)	Gelatins; collagens III, IV, V; aggrecan; elastin; entactin; link protein	Pro-TGF-β; IL-2 receptor α; Kit-L; IGF-BP-3; pro-IL-1β; α1 PI; galectin-3; ICAM-1 plasminogen
Stromelysins		
MMP-3 (Stromelysin-1)	Aggrecan; decorin; gelatins; collagens III, IV, IX, X; Fn; Ln; tenascin; link protein; perlecan	IGF-BP-3; pro-IL-1β; HB-EGF; CTGF; E-cadherin; α1 antichymotrypsin; α1 PI; α2 macroglobulin; plasminogen; uPA; proMMP-1, 7, 8, 9, 13
MMP-10 (Stromelysin-2)	Aggrecan; Fn; Ln; collagens III, IV, V; link protein	ProMMP-1, 8, 10
Matrilysins		
MMP-7 (Matrilysin-1)	Aggrecan; gelatins; Fn; Ln; elastin; entactin; collagen IV; tenascin; link protein	Pro-α-defensin; Fas-L; β4 integrin; E-cadherin; pro-TNF; CTGF; HB-EGF; RANKL; IGF-BP-3; plasminogen
MMP-26 (Matrilysin-2)	Gelatin; collagen IV; Fn; fibrinogen	α1 PI; proMMP-9
Furin-Activated MMPs		
MMP-11 (Stromelysin-3)	Fn; Ln; aggrecan; gelatins	α1 PI; α2 macroglobulin; IGF-BP-1
MMP-21	Unknown	Unknown
MMP-28 (Epilysin)	Unknown	Casein
Other Secreted-Type MMPs		
MMP-12 (Metalloelastase)	Elastin; Fn; collagen V; osteonectin	Plasminogen; apolipoprotein A
MMP-19 (RASI-1)	Collagen IV; gelatin; Fn; tenascin; aggrecan; COMP; Ln; nidogen	IGF-BP-3
MMP-20 (Enamelysin)	Amelogenin; aggrecan; gelatin; COMP	Unknown
MMP-27	Unknown	Unknown
MMP-23	Gelatin	Unknown
Membrane-Type MMPs		
Type I Transmembrane-Type MMPs		
MMP-14 (MT1-MMP)	Collagens I, II, III; gelatins; aggrecan; Fn; Vn; Ln-1, -2, -4, -5; fibrin; perlecan;	ProMMP-2, -13; ADAM9; tTG; CD44; ICAM-1; LRP-1; syndecan 1; SLPI; CTGF; DR6, DJ-1; galectin-1, αV-integrin; C3b; EMMPRIN; ApoE; MICA; betaglycan; IL-8; Cyr61; dickkopf-1, KiSS-1, Dll1; peptidyl-prolyl cis-trans isomerase A
MMP-15 (MT2-MMP)	Fn; tenascin; nidogen; aggrecan; perlecan; Ln	ProMMP-2; tTG
MMP-16 (MT3-MMP)	Collagen III; Fn; gelatin	ProMMP-2; tTG
MMP-24 (MT5-MMP)	PG	ProMMP-2
GPI-Anchored-Type MMPs		
MMP-17 (MT4-MMP)	Gelatin; fibrinogen	Unknown
MMP-25 (MT6-MMP)	Gelatin; collagen IV; fibrin; Fn; Ln	ProMMP-2

ApoE, Apolipoprotein E; *C3b*, complement component 3; *COMP*, cartilage oligomeric matrix protein; *CTGF*, connective tissue growth factor; *Cyr61*, cysteine-rich angiogenic inducer 61; *Dll1*, delta-like1; *DR6*, death receptor-6; *ECM*, extra-cellular matrix; *FGF*, fibroblast growth factor; *Fn*, fibronectin; *GPI*, glycosylphosphatidylinositol; *HB-EGF*, heparin-binding epidermal growth factor; *ICAM-1*, intercellular adhesion molecule 1; *IGF-BP*, insulin-like growth factor binding protein; *IL*, interleukin; *KiSS-1*, kisspeptin; *Ln*, laminin; *LRP-1*, low density lipoprotein receptor-related protein 1; *MCP*, monocyte chemoattractant protein; *MICA*, MHC class I chain-related molecule A; *MMP*, matrix metalloproteinase; *PG*, proteoglycan; *PI*, proteinase inhibitor; *RANKL*, receptor activator for nuclear factor-κB ligand; *SLPI*, secretory leukocyte protease inhibitor; *TGF*, transforming growth factor; *TNF*, tumor necrosis factor; *tTG*, tissue transglutaminase; *uPA*, urokinase-type plasminogen activator.

TABLE 8.3 **Members of the ADAMTS Family**

ADAMTS	Other Names	Activity[a]	Functions	Tissue/Cell
ADAMTS	1C3-C5; METH1; KIAA1346	+	Digestion of aggrecan and versican; binding to heparin	Kidney; heart; cartilage
ADAMTS2	Procollagen N-proteinase	+	Processing of collagen I and II hPCPNI; PCINP N-propeptides	Skin; tendon
ADAMTS3	KIAA0366	+	Processing of collagen N-propeptides	Brain
ADAMTS4	KIAA0688; aggrecanase-1; ADMP-1	+	Degradation of aggrecan, brevican, and versican	Brain; heart; cartilage
ADAMTS5	ADAMTS11; aggrecanase-2; ADMP-2	+	Degradation of aggrecan	Uterus; placenta; cartilage
ADAMTS6	—	—	—	Placenta
ADAMTS7	—	—	—	Various tissues
ADAMTS8	METH-2	+	Degradation of aggrecan; inhibition of angiogenesis	Lung; heart
ADAMTS9	KIAA1312	+	Digestion of aggrecan	Cartilage
ADAMTS10	—	—	—	—
ADAMTS12	—	—	—	Lung (fetus)
ADAMTS13	VWFCP; C9orf8	+	Cleavage of von Willebrand factor	Liver; prostate; brain
ADAMTS14	—	+	Processing of collagen N-propeptides	Brain; uterus
ADAMTS15	—	+	Digestion of aggrecan	Liver (fetus); kidney (fetus)
ADAMTS16	—	+	Digestion of aggrecan	Prostate; brain; uterus
ADAMTS17	FLJ32769; LOC123271	—	—	Prostate; brain; liver
ADAMTS18	ADAMTS21; HGNC:16662	+	Digestion of aggrecan	Prostate; brain
ADAMTS19	—	—	—	Lung (fetus)
ADAMTS20	—	+	Digestion of versican (and aggrecan)	Brain; testis

[a] Proteinase activities are shown in 13 members of the ADAMTS family, but not in 6 other members.

ADAMTS, A disintegrin and metalloproteinases with thrombospondin motifs.

TABLE 8.4 **Members of the Human ADAM Family**

ADAM	Other Names	P/NP	Functions	Tissue/Cells
ADAM2	PH-30β; Fertilin-β α6β, and α9β	NP	Sperm/egg binding/fusion; binding to integrin αβ1	Sperm
ADAM7	EAP I; GP-83	NP	Binding to integrin α4β1, α4β7, and α9β1	Testis
ADAM8	MS2 (CD156)	P	Neutrophil infiltration; shedding of CD23	Macrophages; neutrophil
ADAM9	MDC9; MCMP; Meltrin-γ	P	Shedding of HB-EGF, TNF-p75 receptor, and APP; digestion of fibronectin and gelatin; binding to integrin α2β1, α6β1, α6β4, α9β1, and αVβ5	Various tissues
ADAM10	MDAM; Kuzbanian	P	Shedding of TNF, Delta, Delta-like 1, Jagged, N-cadherin, E-cadherin, VE-cadherin, Ephrin A2, Ephrin A5, Fas-l, IL-6R, APP, L1,CD44, and HB-EGF; digestion of collagen IV, gelatin, and myelin basic protein; presence of RRKR sequence	Kidney; brain; chondrocytes
ADAM11	MDC	NP	Tumor suppressor gene (?)	Brain

Continued

TABLE 8.4 Members of the Human ADAM Family—cont'd

ADAM	Other Names	P/NP	Functions	Tissue/Cells
ADAM12	Meltrin-α; MCMP; MLTN; MLTNA	P	Muscle formation; presence of RRKR sequence; binding to integrin α4β1 and α9β1; digestion of IGF-BP-3 and -5; shedding of HB-EGF and epiregulin; digestion of collagen IV, gelatin, and fibronectin	Osteoblasts; muscle cells; chondrocytes; placenta
ADAM15	Metargidin; MDC15; AD56; CR II-7	P	Expression in arteriosclerosis; binding to integrin αvβ3, α5β1, and α9β1; digestion of collagen IV and gelatin; shedding of CD23	Smooth muscle cells; chondrocytes; endothelial cells; osteoclasts
ADAM17	TACE; cSVP	P	Shedding of TNF, TGF-β, TNF-p75 receptor, RANKL, amphiregulin, epiregulin, HB-EGF, APP, L-selectin, and CD44; presence of RRKR sequence; binding to integrin α5β1	Macrophages; various tissues; carcinoma
ADAM18	tMDC III	NP	—	Testis
ADAM19	Meltrin-β; FKSG34	P	Formation of neuron; shedding of neuregulin, and RANKL; binding to integrin α4β1 and α5β1	Testis
ADAM20	—	P	Formation of sperm	Testis
ADAM21	—	P	—	Testis
ADAM22	MDC2	NP	—	Brain
ADAM23	MDC3	NP	Binding to integrin αvβ3	Brain; heart
ADAM28	e-MDC II; MDC-Lm; MDC-Ls	P	Digestion of VWF, IGF-BP-3, and CTGF; shedding of CD23; binding to integrin α4β1, α4β7, and α9β1	Epididymis; lung; stomach; pancreas
ADAM29	svph1	NP	—	Testis
ADAM30	svph4	P	—	Testis
ADAM32	AJ131563	NP	—	Testis
ADAM33	—	P	Mutation in bronchial asthma patients; shedding of APP and KL-1; digestion of insulin B chain; binding to integrin α4β1, α5β1, and α9β1	Lung (fibroblasts, smooth muscle cells)
ADAMDEC1	—	P	—	Lymphatic system; gastrointestinal system

ADAM, A disintegrin and metalloproteinase; *ADAMDEC1,* ADAM-like decysin 1; *APP,* amyloid precursor protein; *CTGF,* connective tissue growth factor; *HB-EGF,* heparin-binding epidermal growth factor; *IGF-BP,* insulin-like growth factor binding protein; *IL-6R,* interleukin-6 receptor; *KL-1,* kit ligand-1; *P/NP,* proteolytic/nonproteolytic; *RANKL,* receptor activator of nuclear factor-κB ligand; *TGF,* transforming growth factor; *TNF,* tumor necrosis factor; *VWF,* von Willebrand factor.

Collagenases (MMP-1, MMP-8, and MMP-13). The classic collagenases include MMP-1 (interstitial collagenase, collagenase-1), MMP-8 (neutrophil collagenase, collagenase-2), and MMP-13 (collagenase-3). These MMPs attack triple helical regions of interstitial collagen types I, II, and III at a specific single site after the Gly residue of the partial sequences Gly-(Ile or Leu)-(Ala or Leu), located about three-fourths of the distance from the N-terminus. This cleavage generates fragments approximately three-fourths and one-fourth of the size of the collagen molecules. A biochemical study has disclosed the molecular mechanism of the cleavage: MMP-1 unwinds the triple helical structure by interacting with the α2(I) chain of type I collagen and cleaves the three α chains in succession.[8] MMP-13 is unique in that it cleaves α chains of type II collagen at two sites of the Gly^{906}-Leu^{907} and Gly^{909}-Gln^{910} bonds.[9] All of these collagenases degrade the interstitial collagens, but their specific activities against the collagens are different; MMP-1, 8, and 13 relatively digest types III, I, and II collagen better than others, respectively. Although rodents such as mice were originally thought to have only two collagenases (*MMP-8* and *MMP-13*) and to lack the *MMP-1* gene, rodent homologues of the human *MMP-1* gene were cloned and named mouse collagenase A and B (*Mcol-A* and *Mcol-B*).[10] In addition to the interstitial fibrillar collagens, MMP-1, 8, and 13 degrade many other ECM macromolecules. MMP-1 digests entactin, collagen X, gelatins, perlecan, aggrecan, and cartilage link protein (see Table 8.2). MMP-8 digests aggrecan, gelatins, and cartilage link protein (see Table 8.2). MMP-13 hydrolyzes aggrecan; types IV, IX, X, and XIV collagens; fibronectin; and tenascin. Non-ECM substrates of MMP-1, 8, and 13 include α2 macroglobulin, α1 anti-proteinase inhibitor, α1 antichymotrypsin, insulin-like growth factor binding protein (IGF-BP)-2 and IGF-BP-3, connective tissue growth factor (CTGF), and pro-TGF-β (see Table 8.2).

Gelatinases (MMP-2 and MMP-9). MMP-2 (gelatinase A) and MMP-9 (gelatinase B) belong to the gelatinase subgroup. Both MMPs readily digest gelatins and cleave types IV and V collagen. Elastin, aggrecan, and cartilage link protein also are substrates of the gelatinases. Although MMP-2 and 9 share such substrates, they have different activities on several ECM macromolecules.

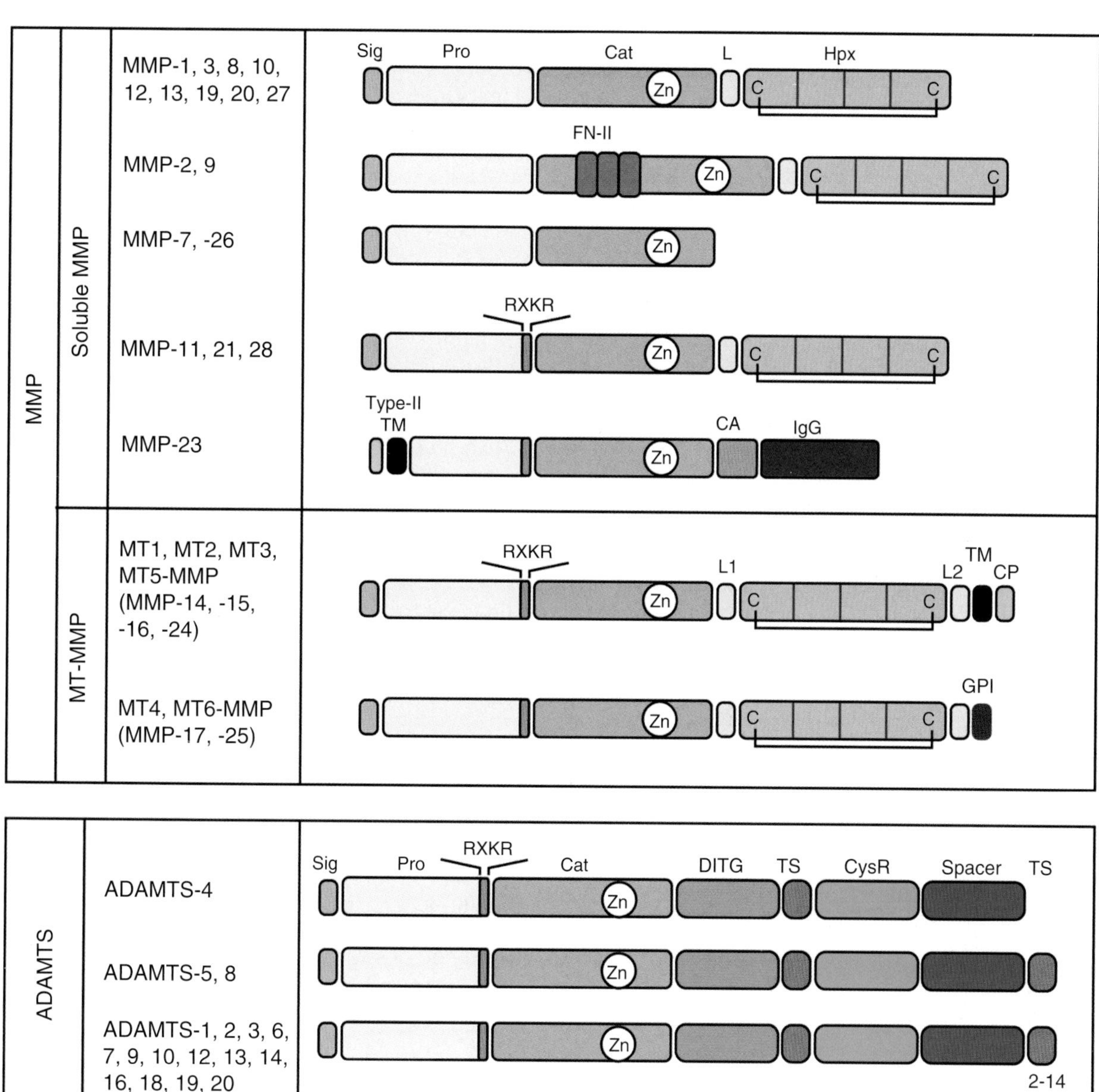

• **Fig. 8.1** Schematic representation of domain structure of metalloproteinases. MMP can be divided into two major groups: soluble MMPs and membrane-type MMPs, and they can be further classified into six subgroups in soluble MMPs and two subgroups in membrane-type MMPs according to their structures. MMP-11, 21, 28, and 23, and MT-MMPs have a basic motif of RXKR that is recognized and cleaved by proprotein convertases to activate the enzymes by removing their prodomain. ADAMTS enzymes also have a conserved domain structure and differ in the number of thrombospondin motifs (TS) at their C-terminus. ADAMTS-4 is the smallest, without a C-terminal TS, and ADAMTS-5 and 8 have two. Other members have 2 to 14 repeats. ADAM enzymes have a similarly conserved domain structure. ADAMTS and ADAM enzymes have an RXKR motif at the C-terminus of their propeptide from activation by proprotein convertases. *C,* Cysteine; *CA,* cysteine array; *Cat,* catalytic domain; *CP,* cytoplasmic domain; *CysR,* cysteine-rich domain; *DITG,* disintegrin-like domain; *EGF,* EGF-like domain; *FN-II,* fibronectin type II repeats; *GPI,* GPI-anchoring signal; *Hpx,* hemopexin domain; *IgG,* IgG-like domain; *L,* linker or hinge region; *L1,* linker 1 or hinge region; *L2,* linker 2 or stalk region; *Pro,* prodomain; *Sig,* signal peptide; *Spacer,* spacer domain; *TM,* transmembrane domain; *Type II TM,* type II transmembrane domain.

MMP-2, but not MMP-9, digests fibrillar type I and II collagens at the same site as collagenases, fibronectin, and laminin, and type III collagen and α2 chains of type I collagen are degraded only by MMP-9. The gelatinases also process directly TGF-β into an active ligand (see Table 8.2). MMP-2 and 9 cleave fibroblast growth factor receptor type I and interleukin (IL)-2 receptor type α (see Table 8.2). MMP-9 also releases soluble Kit-ligand. MMP-2 processes monocyte chemoattractant protein (MCP)-3 into an MCP-3 fragment deleting the N-terminal four amino acids, which can bind to CC-chemokine receptors and act as a general chemokine antagonist.

Stromelysins (MMP-3 and MMP-10). The subgroup of stromelysins consists of MMP-3 (stromelysin-1) and MMP-10 (stromelysin-2). They share 78% identity in amino acid sequence and have similar enzymatic properties. The enzymes hydrolyze numerous ECM macromolecules, including aggrecan, fibronectin, laminin, and collagen IV (see Table 8.2). Types III, IX, and X collagen and telopeptides of types I, II, and XI collagen also are digested by MMP-3. In addition to the ECM components, MMP-3 is active on IGF-BP-3, IL-1β, heparin-binding epidermal growth factor (HB-EGF), CTGF, E-cadherin, α1 antichymotrypsin, and α1 proteinase inhibitor (see Table 8.2). MMP-3 also activates many proMMPs. A similar activator function has been identified for MMP-10.

Matrilysins (MMP-7 and MMP-26). Matrilysins include MMP-7 (matrilysin-1) and MMP-26 (matrilysin-2), which are the smallest of the MMPs, having only the prodomain and catalytic domain. The substrate specificity of MMP-7 is similar to that of stromelysins, digesting numerous ECM components, including aggrecan; gelatins; fibronectin; laminin; elastin; entactin; types III, IV, V, IX, X, and XI collagen; fibrin/fibrinogen; vitronectin; tenascin; and link protein (see Table 8.2). Although these substrates overlap with the substrates of other MMPs, the specific activity of MMP-7 to most substrates is highest among the MMPs. Non-ECM molecules such as α-defensin, Fas ligand, β4 integrin, E-cadherin, plasminogen, TNF, and CTGF also are the substrates for MMP-7 (see Table 8.2). MMP-26 degrades gelatin, type IV collagen, fibronectin, fibrinogen, and α1 proteinase inhibitor, but information about other substrates is still limited.

Furin-Activated Matrix Metalloproteinases (MMP-11 and MMP-28). MMP-11 (stromelysin-3) and MMP-28 (epilysin) contain an RKRR sequence at the end of the prodomain, which is a unique motif for intra-cellular processing of proproteins to mature molecules by furin and other proprotein convertases. ProMMP-11 was activated during secretion by furin. MMP-11 shows only weak proteolytic activity against gelatin, laminin, fibronectin, and aggrecan, but it has respectable catalytic action in digesting α1 proteinase inhibitor, α2 macroglobulin, and IGF-BP-1 (see Table 8.2). MMP-28 can degrade casein, but its natural substrates are unknown.

Other Soluble MMP Enzymes (MMP-12, MMP-19, MMP-20, MMP-21, MMP-23, and MMP-27). MMP-12 (metalloelastase), MMP-19 (RASI-1), MMP-20 (enamelysin), MMP-21, and MMP-27 have structural characteristics similar to those of collagenases and stromelysins. These MMPs are not classified into the previously mentioned subgroups because their substrates and other biochemical characters are not fully examined at present. MMP-12, also called *metalloelastase*, digests elastin, fibronectin, collagen V, osteonectin, and plasminogen (see Table 8.2). MMP-19, which was originally reported as MMP-18 but renamed as MMP-19, cleaves type IV collagen, laminin, fibronectin, gelatin, tenascin, entactin, fibrin/fibrinogen, aggrecan, and cartilage oligomeric matrix protein (COMP; see Table 8.2). MMP-20 also degrades amelogenin, aggrecan, and COMP. Substrates of MMP-21 and 27 are unknown, however.

MMP-23 (cysteine array–MMP, MIFR) is unique among MMP enzymes as it is synthesized as a type II transmembrane-protein, but it becomes a soluble enzyme upon activation. MMP-23 is able to degrade gelatin, but no information about other substrates is available (see Table 8.2). A unique aspect of MMP-23 is that this MMP is expressed in only the reproductive organs of both males and females, such as the endometrium, ovary, testis, and prostate. However, its biologic functions are not understood.

Membrane-Type Matrix Metalloproteinases (MMP-14, MMP-15, MMP-16, MMP-17, MMP-24, and MMP-25, or MT1-MMP, MT2-MMP, MT3-MMP, MT4-MMP, MT5-MMP, and MT6-MMP). There are two types of MT-MMPs: type I transmembrane-type and GPI-anchored-type, and these MT-MMPs are unique in that they are expressed on the cell surface as an active form and function on the cell surface.[7] Type-I transmembrane type includes MMP-14 (MT1-MMP), MMP-15 (MT2-MMP), MMP-16 (MT3-MMP), and MMP-24 (MT5-MMP). All of these MT-MMPs can activate proMMP-2, but MT1-MMP is considered to be the major in vivo activator of proMMP-2 in various tissues (see later discussion). MT1-MMP also degrades a fibrillar collagen on the cell surface. Like other collagen-degrading MMP enzymes (MMP-1, -2, -8, and -13), it cleaves the triple helical part of collagen at ¾ from the N-terminus.[11] MT1-MMP also degrades other ECM components, including fibronectin, laminin, aggrecan, and gelatin (see Table 8.2).[11] MT2-MMP digests fibronectin, tenascin, nidogen, aggrecan, perlecan, and laminin.[12] MT3-MMP cleaves type III collagen, fibronectin, and gelatins.[13] MMP-17 (MT4-MMP) and MMP-25 (MT6-MMP) are GPI-anchored MMPs.[14,15] MT4-MMP and MT6-MMP can digest gelatin and fibrin/fibrinogen (see Table 8.2).

ADAM and ADAMTS Families

Two ADAM (a disintegrin and metalloproteinase) gene families exist: the enzymes with the transmembrane domain (ADAM) and secreted-type ADAM with thrombospondin motifs (ADAMTS; see Fig. 8.1). The active sites in the catalytic domains of most members of both gene families contain a common sequence of HEXGHXXGXXHD with the "Met-turn," which also is present in MMP members. The ADAMTS family includes 19 members. Although information about substrates and biologic functions is still limited, ADAMTS1-5, 8-9, 14-16, 18, and 20 are all ECM-degrading proteinases (see Table 8.3). ADAMTS1, 4, 5, 9, and 15 can preferentially cleave aggrecan at the five Glu-X bonds, including the Glu^{373}-Ala^{374} bond (the aggrecanase site). Because ADAMTS4 and ADAMTS5 are characterized as the first two aggrecanases, they are also named *aggrecanase-1* and *aggrecanase-2*, respectively[16,17]; versican is also digested by these proteinases,[18] and brevican is cleaved by ADAMTS4 (see Table 8.3).[19] The C-terminus–truncated ADAMTS4 also degrades fibromodulin and decorin.[20] ADAMTS16, 18, and 20 also appear to have weak aggrecanase activity. ADAMTS2 and 3 process the N-terminal prodomain of type I and II collagens and are named *procollagen N-proteinase*. Activity of procollagen N-proteinase also is known with ADAMTS14. ADAMTS13 is a von Willebrand factor–cleaving proteinase, and its mutation causes thrombotic thrombocytopenic purpura. Proteinase activities of other ADAMTS species are still unknown. The human genome contains 25 ADAM genes, including 4 pseudogenes, and thus the human ADAM family is composed of 21 members (see Table 8.4). Among the ADAMs, ADAM8-10, 12, 15, 17, 19-21, 28, 30, 33, and ADAM-like decysin 1 (ADAMDEC1) exhibit proteolytic activity (i.e., they are proteinase-type ADAMs; see Table 8.4). Although ADAM10, 12, and 15 degrade type IV collagen, the main substrates of these ADAMs are considered to be various membrane proteins, which include precursors of cytokines and growth factors such as TNF, HB-EGF, and neuregulin; IGF-BPs; receptors such as p75 TNF receptor; IL-1 receptor II; and other membrane proteins related to development such as Notch ligand and ephrin (see Table 8.4).[21–26] According to these data, a major function of the ADAMs is the membrane protein shedding. ADAM17 processes proTNF (type II transmembrane molecule) and releases the soluble TNF, and is thus called *TNF-converting enzyme* (TACE). ADAM17 is also involved in release of L-selectin, TGF-α, and p75 TNF receptor. ADAM9, 12, and 17 can shed HB-EGF from its precursor. ADAM12 and 28 cleave IGF-BP-3 and IGF-BP-5.[26,27] CD23 is shed by ADAM8, 15, and 28.[28] Other functions of ADAMs include binding to integrins, cell-cell interaction, cell migration, and signal transduction (see Table 8.4).[29]

Regulation of Proteinase Activity

The activities of ECM-degrading proteinases in tissues are regulated by different means, including their gene expression, activation of zymogen form, and inhibition by their endogenous inhibitors. Depending on the enzyme, some enzymes are also regulated by cell surface binding, endocytosis, and recycling.

Gene Expression

Matrix Metalloproteinases

Under physiologic conditions, cells express only limited levels of MMPs or TIMPs in tissues. However, under inflammatory conditions, expression of these genes are stimulated by cytokines and other factors. Neutrophils synthesize MMP-8 and MMP-9 during the differentiation and store them within the granules of the differentiated cells. Macrophages upon treatment with LPS or phorbormyristate acetate (12-O-tetradecanoylphorbol-13-acetate, PMA) express MMP-1, MMP-9, MT1-MMP and TIMP-1. Tumor cells express many MMPs such as MMP-1, 7, 9, 10, and MMP-14 (MT1-MMP), as well as TIMP-1, predominantly by oncogenic stimuli. The gene expression of *MMPs* and *TIMPs* in the tissue cell are regulated by numerous factors, including cytokines, growth factors, and chemical and physical stimuli. Much information is available for regulators of *MMP-1* and *MMP-3*, which are coordinately expressed in many cell types upon stimulation with cytokines and growth factors, factors acting at the cell surface, and chemical agents (Table 8.5). The upregulated production of MMP-1 and MMP-3 is suppressed by retinoic acid, TGF-β, and glucocorticoid. The gene expression of *MMP-7* and *MMP-9* is regulated by similar factors, but the regulation is stricter and fewer factors modulate the expression (see Table 8.5). *MMP-14* expression is upregulated by PMA, concanavalin A, fibrillar collagen, basic fibroblast growth factor, and TNF, and it is downregulated by glucocorticoids in various cells. TNF and IL-1α was reported to stimulate osteoarthritic chondrocytes to express the *MMP-14* gene. In contrast to these MMPs, MMP-2 and TIMP-2 are unique in that factors capable of enhancing the production of MMP-1, MMP-3, and TIMP-1 are inactive. *TIMP-1* expression is enhanced or suppressed in response to many factors, including cytokines, growth factors, and oncogenic transformation (see Table 8.5). Effects of these stimulatory factors are common to the gene expression of *MMPs*, but they are regulated independently. TGF-β, retinoic acid, progesterone, and estrogen enhance *TIMP-1* expression in fibroblasts, but they suppress the expression of *MMP-1* and *3*. Although information about stimulating and suppressive factors of *TIMP-1, 2*, and *3* is available (Table 8.5), factors controlling the gene expression of *TIMP-4* are not well known. Previous studies have identified the elements in the promoters of *MMPs* and *TIMPs*, which are related to or responsible for the stimulation or suppression of the gene expression with various factors. Regulation of the gene expression is generally explained by the structural characteristics of the promoters.

Serine Proteinases

Neutrophil elastase, cathepsin G, chymase, and tryptase are stored within the secretory granules and secreted into the extra-cellular milieu after activation of neutrophils and mast cells. The expression of these serine proteinases is controlled mainly by the cellular differentiation. Precursors of plasmin and plasma kallikrein are constitutively synthesized predominantly in the liver, circulate in the blood as zymogen forms (i.e., plasminogen and prekallikrein), and reach the inflamed tissues by being released from blood vessels. Plasminogen concentration in the plasma is roughly 200 μg/mL, and the activities in the tissues are controlled mainly through activation of the proenzymes by activators. The uPA and tPA molecules, activators of plasminogen, are synthesized by tissue cells, and their gene expression is regulated by many factors (see Table 8.6). The uPA synthesis is upregulated in many normal cell types and in transformed cells by agents that increase intra-cellular cyclic adenosine monophosphate (cAMP) levels (e.g., calcitonin, vasopressin, cholera toxin, and cAMP analogues); growth factors (e.g., EGF, platelet-derived growth factor, and vascular endothelial growth factor); cytokines (IL-1 and TNF); and phorbol esters, whereas glucocorticoid decreases the expression.[8] The expression of *tPA* is regulated by similar factors (see Table 8.6). In endothelial cells, proteinases are enhancers; thrombin and plasmin stimulate the production of tPA.[30] *PAI-1* and *2* also are regulated by common factors, many of which also enhance the production of uPA and tPA (see Table 8.6). Most serpins are constitutively produced in the liver and secreted to plasma.

Lysosomal Cysteine and Aspartic Proteinases

The expression of lysosomal cysteine proteinases, *cathepsins B, L,* and *K*, is generally constitutive, but cellular transformation is often associated with increased synthesis of cathepsins B and L. Cathepsin B transcription varies with cell type and the state of differentiation of tumor cells; it is increased in chondrocytes by IL-1. Malignant transformation, tumor promoters, and growth factors stimulate the synthesis of cathepsin L. *Cathepsin K* gene expression in monocyte-macrophage lineage depends on the cellular differentiation to osteoclasts, but all-*trans* retinoic acid upregulates the expression in rabbit osteoclasts. Lysosomal aspartic proteinase, *cathepsin D*, is constitutively expressed in almost all cells, although estradiol, calcitriol, and retinoic acid can regulate the expression.

Inhibition of Proteinases by Endogenous Inhibitors

Endogenous proteinase inhibitors control the activities of proteinases in vivo. The inhibitors are derived from plasma or cells in the local tissues. Plasma contains several proteinase inhibitors, and

TABLE 8.5 Factors That Modulate Synthesis of Matrix Metalloproteinases and Tissue Inhibitors of Metalloproteinases

Enzymes/TIMPs	Stimulating Factor[a]	Suppressive Factor
MMP-1	**Cytokines and growth factors:** IL-1; TNF; EGF; PDGF; bFGF; VEGF; NGF; TGF-α; IFN-α; IFN-β; IFN-γ; leukoregulin; relaxin **Factors acting at cell surface:** calcium ionophore A23187; cell fusion; collagen; concanavalin A; integrin receptor antibody; crystals of urate, hydroxyapatite, and calcium pyrophosphate; SPARC (osteonectin/BM 40); iron; extra-cellular matrix metalloproteinase inducer (EMMPRIN/CD147/basigin/M6 antigen); phagocytosis **Chemical agents:** cAMP; colchicine; cytochalasins B and D; LPS; pentoxifylline; TPA; calmodulin inhibitors; serotonin; 1,25-(OH)2 vitamin D3; platelet-activating factor; serum amyloid A; β-microglobulin **Physical factors:** heat shock; ultraviolet irradiation **Others:** viral transformation; oncogenes; autocrine agents; aging of fibroblasts	Retinoic acids; glucocorticoids; estrogen; progesterone; TGF-β; transmembrane neural cell adhesion and molecule; cAMP; IFN-γ; adenovirus E1A
MMP-2	TGF-β; concanavalin A; H-ras transformation; extra-cellular matrix metalloproteinase inducer (EMMPRIN/CD147/basigin/M6 antigen)	Adenovirus E1A
MMP-3	IL-1; TNF; EGF; concanavalin A; SPARC (osteonectin/BM 40); LPS; TPA; extra-cellular matrix metalloproteinase inducer (EMMPRIN/CD147/basigin/M6 antigen); viral transformation; oncogenes; integrin receptor antibody; heat shock; calcium ionophore A23187; cytochalasin B	Retinoic acids; glucocorticoids; estrogen; progesterone; TGF-β; adenovirus E1A
MMP-7	IL-1; TNF; EGF; TPA; LPS	Unknown
MMP-8	TNF; TPA; IL-1	Unknown
MMP-9	IL-1; TNF; EGF; TGF-β; TPA; H-ras; v-Src; SPARC (osteonectin/BM40)	Retinoic acids; adenovirus E1A
MMP-10	TPA; A23187; TGF-β; EGF	Unknown
MMP-11	Retinoic acids	bFGF
MMP-13	bFGF; TNF; TGF-β; fibrillar collagen	Unknown
MMP-14/MT1-MMP	Concanavalin A; TPA; bFGF; TNF; IL-1α; fibrillar collagen	Glucocorticoids
TIMP-1	IL-1; IL-6; IL-11; TPA; TGF-β; TNF; retinoic acids; LPS; progesterone; estrogen; oncogenic transformation; viral infection	Extra-cellular matrix; cytochalasins
TIMP-2	Progesterone	TGF-β; LPS
TIMP-3	EGF; TGF-β; TPA; TNF; glucocorticoids; oncostatin M	Unknown

[a]Factors regulating gene expression of other MMPs excluded from this table and TIMP-4 are unknown.

bFGF, Basic fibroblast growth factor; *cAMP,* cyclic adenosine monophosphate; *EGF,* epidermal growth factor; *IFN,* interferon; *IL,* interleukin; *LPS,* lipopolysaccharide; *MMP,* matrix metalloproteinase; *NGF,* nerve growth factor; *PDGF,* platelet-derived growth factor; *TGF,* transforming growth factor; *TIMP,* tissue inhibitor of metalloproteinases; *TNF,* tumor necrosis factor; *TPA,* 12-O-tetradecanoylphorbol-13-acetate; *VEGF,* vascular endothelial growth factor.

TABLE 8.6 Factors That Regulate Expression of Plasminogen Activators and Their Inhibitors

Enzyme/ Inhibitor	Stimulatory Factor	Suppressive Factor
uPA	TPA; IL-1; IFN-γ; EGF; PDGF; bFGF; VEGF; TGF-β; cholera toxin; cAMP; estrogen; calcitonin; vasopressin; disruption of E-cadherin–dependent cell-cell adhesion	Glucocorticoids; TGF-β
tPA	TPA; EGF; bFGF; VEGF; retinoic acids; glucocorticoids; cAMP; thrombin; plasmin; follicle-stimulating hormone; luteinizing hormone; gonadotropin-releasing hormone	TNF
PAI-1	IL-1; TNF; TGF-β; bFGF; VEGF; TPA; glucocorticoids	cAMP
PAI-2	TPA; LPS; TNF; colony-stimulating factor; cholera toxin; dengue virus	Glucocorticoids
PN-1	TPA; EGF; thrombin	Unknown

bFGF, Fibroblast growth factor; *cAMP,* cyclic adenosine monophosphate; *EGF,* epidermal growth factor; *IFN,* interferon; *IL,* interleukin; *LPS,* lipopolysaccharide; *PAI,* plasminogen activator inhibitor; *PDGF,* platelet-derived growth factor; *PN,* proteinase nexin; *TGF,* transforming growth factor; *TNF,* tumor necrosis factor; *TPA,* 12-O-tetradecanoylphorbol-13-acetate; *tPA,* tissue-type plasminogen activator; *uPA,* urokinase-type plasminogen activator; *VEGF,* vascular endothelial growth factor.

about 10% of all the plasma proteins are proteinase inhibitors. Many of them are proteinase class specific, but α2 macroglobulin inhibits the activities of proteinases from all classes. Major endogenous inhibitors of the ECM-degrading proteinases are listed in Table 8.7.

α2 Macroglobulin

The α2 macroglobulin (α2M) is a large glycoprotein of 725 kDa that consists of four identical subunits of 185 kDa that are linked in pairs by disulfide bonds. Almost all active proteinases, regardless of the proteinase classes, cleave a stretch within the molecule's so-called *bait region*, located near the center of the subunits. Upon cleaving the bait region, a conformational change of the α2M occurs and physically traps the proteinase within the molecular cage, resulting in a proteinase-α2M complex. Although the active site of the proteinase in the complex is free and remains active, the enzyme is trapped by the arms of the α2M and is prevented from interacting and degrading large macromolecules. Besides the function as a proteinase inhibitor, α2M may act as a carrier protein because it also binds to numerous growth factors and cytokines such as platelet-derived growth factor, basic fibroblast growth factor, TGF-β, insulin, and IL-1β. The α2M molecule is synthesized mainly in the liver but also locally by macrophages, fibroblasts, and adrenocortical cells. Concentration of the inhibitor in plasma is 250 mg/dL. Because of its large molecular weight, it is not present in non-inflammatory synovial fluid; however, during synovial inflammation, α2M penetrates into the joint cavity. Rheumatoid synovial fluid has about the same concentration of the inhibitor as plasma.

Inhibitors of Serine Proteinases

The primary inhibitors of serine proteinases include the members of the serpin (serine proteinase inhibitor) gene family, Kunitz-type inhibitors, and others (see Table 8.7). The serpins are glycoproteins of 50 to 100 kDa and share homology with human α1 proteinase inhibitor.[31] The major serpins involved in the regulation of ECM-degrading serine proteinases are α1 proteinase inhibitor, α1 antichymotrypsin, α2 antiplasmin, plasminogen activator inhibitors (PAI-1 and PAI-2), protein C inhibitor (PAI-3), C1-inhibitor, kallistatin, and proteinase nexin-1 (PN-1). The main proteinases inhibited by these molecules are listed in Table 8.7. Although PAI-1 and PAI-2 inhibit tPA and uPA, the inhibition by PAI-1 is more effective to tPA and that of PAI-2 is more efficient to uPA. Kunitz-type inhibitors include aprotinin, trypstatin, and PN-2, which is identical to a β-amyloid protein precursor. Secretory leukocyte proteinase inhibitor, which inhibits neutrophil elastase and cathepsin G, is present in many secretory and inflammatory fluids and in cartilage. Elafin is a serine proteinase inhibitor with 38% identity with the second domain of secretory leukocyte proteinase inhibitor; it inhibits neutrophil elastase and proteinase 3.

Inhibitors of Cysteine Proteinases

The members of the cystatin superfamily and calpastatin belong to the family of inhibitors of ECM-degrading cysteine proteinases (see Table 8.7). Cystatins that inhibit lysosomal cysteine proteinases consist of three groups. Subgroup 1 comprises stefins A and B. Each has a molecular mass of 11 kDa, and the stefins reside within cells. Subgroup 2 comprises cystatin C and S, each with a molecular mass of 13 kDa. They occur at relatively high concentrations in cerebrospinal fluid and saliva. Subgroup 3 comprises the kininogens. Kininogens that participate in blood coagulation and inflammation also are inhibitors of cysteine proteinases. Calpains are not inhibited by cystatins but are inhibited by calpastatin (120 kDa), which is a cytosolic specific inhibitor of calpain.

Tissue Inhibitors of Metalloproteinases

TIMPs are a gene family consisting of four different members with approximately 40% to 50% sequence identity (i.e., *TIMP-1, TIMP-2, TIMP-3,* and *TIMP-4*) that have molecular masses ranging from 21 to 28 kDa in humans. TIMPs inhibit the activities of MMPs by binding in a 1:1 molar ratio, forming tight, noncovalent complexes.[32] The exception is TIMP-1, which does not efficiently inhibit transmembrane-type MT-MMPs, including MT1-, MT2-, MT3-, and MT5-MMPs (MMP-14, 15, 16, and 24). TIMPs contain 12 highly conserved cysteine residues that form six intrachain disulfide bonds, which are essential for maintaining the correct structure of the molecule and stable inhibitory activity. TIMP molecules have two structurally distinct subdomains: an N-terminal subdomain that consists of loops 1 through 3 and a C-terminal subdomain that consists of loops 4 through 6. The N-terminal subdomain of each TIMP molecule contains the inhibitory activity for MMPs.[32] The crystal structures of the MMP/TIMP complexes show that the wedge-shaped TIMPs bind with their edge into the entire length of the active-site cleft of their cognate MMPs.[33] Efficient inhibitory activity of TIMP-2 to MMP-14 (MT1-MMP) are explained by the additional interaction between a quite long hairpin loop of TIMP-2 and a loop over the rim of the active-site cleft of MMP-14.[34] TIMP-1 and TIMP-2 are unique in that they make the complexes with proMMP-9 and proMMP-2 through their C-terminal subdomain and hemopexin domain of proMMP-9 and proMMP-2, respectively (i.e., the proMMP-9/TIMP-1 and proMMP-2/TIMP-2 complexes). Similar complex formation is also reported between TIMP-4 and proMMP-2. Because the MMP inhibitory sites of TIMPs in these complexes are not occupied, these proMMP/TIMP complexes are able to inhibit other MMPs. Interestingly, the proMMP-2/TIMP-2 complex is necessary for the efficient activation of proMMP-2 by MT1-MMP on the cell surface. MT1-MMP forms a homodimer on the cell surface through the hemopexin domain and the transmembrane domain. TIMP-2 binds to one of the MT1-MMP molecules in the dimer through the inhibitory domain and MMP-2 through C-terminal subdomain, forming a $(MT1\text{-}MMP)_2$-TIMP-2-ProMMP-2 complex on the cell surface (see later discussion). Thus TIMP-2 allow proMMP-2 to interact with MT1-MMP, which is essential for proMMP-2 activation.[7] In addition to MMP inhibition, TIMP-3 also inhibits ADAM10, 12, 17, 28, and 33, but not ADAM8, 9, and 19. TIMP-3 also inhibits ADAMTS4 and 5. The N-terminal inhibitory subdomain of TIMP-3 is critical for the inhibition of both MMPs and ADAM members, but the inhibitory mechanism seems to be slightly different.[35] The major interactions of TIMPs with the MMP involve two sections of polypeptide chain of the TIMP around the Cys^1 to Cys^{70} disulfide bond. Blocking the N-terminal α-amino group or the addition of an extra residue inactivates MMP inhibitory activity of TIMPs. However, such modification of TIMP-3 does not influence ADAM17 inhibition.[35] Besides inhibition of MMP/ADAM/ADAMTS enzymes, TIMPs also possess growth factor activity, antiangiogenic activity, and regulatory activity of apoptosis.[36] Another MMP inhibitor is *RECK* (reversion-inducing, cysteine-rich protein with Kazal

TABLE 8.7 Endogenous Inhibitors of Extra-cellular Matrix–Degrading Proteinases

Inhibitor	Size (kDa)	Source	Target Enzyme
α2 Macroglobulin	725	Plasma (liver); macrophages; fibroblasts	Most proteinases from all classes
Inhibitors of Serine Proteinase			
Serpins			
α1 Proteinase inhibitor	52	Plasma; macrophages	Neutrophil elastase, cathepsin G, proteinase 3
α1 Antichymotrypsin	58	Plasma	Cathepsin G; chymotrypsin; chymase; tissue kallikrein
α2 Antiplasmin	67	Plasma	Plasmin
Proteinase nexin-1	45	Fibroblasts	Thrombin; uPA; tPA; plasmin; trypsin; trypsin-like serine proteinase
PAI-1	45	Endothelial cells; fibroblasts; platelets; plasma	tPA; uPA
PAI-2	47	Plasma; macrophages	uPA; tPA
Protein C inhibitor	57	Plasma; urine	Active protein C; tPA; uPA; tissue kallikrein
C1-inhibitor	96	Plasma	Plasma kallikrein; C1 esterase
Kallistatin	92	Plasma; liver; stomach; kidney; pancreas	Tissue kallikrein
Kunins			
Aprotinin	7	Mast cells	Plasmin; kallikrein
Trypstatin	6	Mast cells	Tryptase
Proteinase nexin-2 (β-amyloid protein precursor)	100	Fibroblasts EGF binding protein; NGF-γ	Trypsin, chymotrypsin, factor XIa
Others			
SLPI	15	Bronchial secretions; seminal plasma; cartilage	Neutrophil elastase; cathepsin G; chymotrypsin; trypsin
Elafin	7	Horny layers of skin	Neutrophil elastase; proteinase 3
Inhibitors of Cysteine Proteinase			
Stefin A	11	Cytosol	Cysteine proteinases
Stefin B	11	Cytosol	Cysteine proteinases
Cystatin C	13	Body fluids	Cysteine proteinases
Cystatin S	13	Seminal plasma; tears; saliva	Cysteine proteinases
Kininogens	50-78/108-120	Plasma	Cysteine proteinases
Calpastatin	120	Cytosol	Calpains
Metalloproteinase Inhibitors			
TIMP-1	28	Connective tissue cells; macrophages	MMPs, ADAM10
TIMP-2	22	Connective tissue cells; macrophages	MMPs
TIMP-3	21/24[a]	Fibroblasts; synovial cells	MMPs; ADAMs; ADAMTS
TIMP-4	21	Heart; brain; testis	MMPs
RECK	110	Many tissue cells; fibroblasts	MMP-2; MMP-7; MMP-14 (MT1-MMP); ADAM10

ADAM, A disintegrin and metalloproteinase; *EGF*, epidermal growth factor; *MMP*, matrix metalloproteinase; *NGF*, nerve growth factor; *PA*, plasminogen activator; *PAI*, plasminogen activator inhibitor; *RECK*, reversion-inducing, cysteine-rich protein with Kazal motifs; *SLPI*, secretory leukocyte proteinase.

[a]Glycosylated form.

motifs).[37] RECK is a GPI-anchored glycoprotein harboring three inhibitor-like domains and inhibits at least MMP-2, 9, 14, and ADAM10.[38,39] Although this inhibitor seems to play a key role in the angiogenic processes in vivo,[37] the inhibitory mechanism of these enzymes and its functions in pathologic conditions such as arthritides remain to be further investigated.

Activation Mechanisms of the Zymogens of Matrix Metalloproteinases

All MMPs are synthesized as inactive zymogens (proMMPs), and activation of proMMPs is a prerequisite to express their activity. ProMMPs are kept inactive by their prodomain through an interaction between a cysteine-sulfhydryl group in the conserved sequence PRCGXPD and the zinc ion at the catalytic site, preventing the interaction of a water molecule with the catalytic zinc that is essential for the enzymatic reaction. Activation occurs by proteolytic removal of the prodomain that would expose the catalytic site. There are three pathways of proMMP activation dependent on the enzymes: extra-cellular activation, intra-cellular activation, and cell surface activation (Fig. 8.2).

Extra-cellular Activation

Many soluble MMPs (e.g., proMMP-1, 3, 7, 8-10, 12, and 13), are secreted as a zymogen form and need to be activated extra-cellularly. In vitro, the activation can be initiated by treatment with nonproteolytic agents that disturb interaction of the Cys within PRCGVPD motif in the prodomain with the catalytic zinc.[6,36] Such agents include thiol-modifying reagents, hypochlorous acid, sodium dodecyl sulfate, chaotropic agents, and physical factors (heat and acid exposure).[6] Among them, 4-aminophenylmercuric acetate (APMA) has been used for investigation of proMMP activation mechanism. Upon APMA treatment, APMA disturbs interaction of Cys in PRCGVPD motif and causes proMMP molecules to undergo autolytic processing at the upstream of PRCGVPD to remove a part of the prodomain.[6] Because the Cys no longer interacts with catalytic zinc, the intermediate form possesses a partial activity and intermolecularly removes the rest of the prodomain to generate the fully active form. This is called the *stepwise activation mechanism*. In the case of proMMP-9, APMA treatment only results in the cleavage of the Ala^{74}-Met^{75} bond upstream of the conserved sequence retaining the PRCGVPD sequence, but this intermediate form was found to be fully active. Concerning proMMP-9 activation in vivo during cerebral ischemia, nitric oxide is reported to activate proMMP-9 by S-nitrosylation.[40]

A major activation pathway in vivo is the proteolytic activation, and a similar stepwise activation can be applied to this mechanism. Different proteinases initially attack the stretch of the sequence within the prodomain's so-called bait region, which is upstream of the PRCGVPD motif of the domain. This partial removal of the prodomain disturbs interaction of Cys in PRCGVPD motif with catalytic zinc, generating a partially active intermediate form. This is followed by autolytic removal of the rest of the prodomain or by other MMPs.[6] The bait region can be attacked by different proteinases, which result in activation of particular MMPs. Potential activators of proMMPs are listed in Table 8.8. Plasmin may play a major role in the activation of proMMP-3 and proMMP-10 in vivo because treatment of these proMMPs with plasmin leads to full activation.[41] For proMMP-1 activation, plasmin alone results in only about 25% of the full MMP-1 activity, and full activation requires the subsequent cleavage of the Gln^{80}-Phe^{81} bond by MMP-3, 7, or 10.[6,42] MMP-3 and 10 can directly activate proMMP-7,[42] proMMP-8, proMMP-9,[43,44] and proMMP-13[45] into fully active forms. This intermolecular activation cascade of MMPs may be important for in vivo activation of soluble proMMPs.

Intra-cellular Activation

Some MMPs have a basic motif of RX(K/R)R sequence (X can be any amino acids) at the end of the prodomain that is recognized and cleaved by proprotein convertases (PCs) such as furin, a processing enzyme in the *trans*-Golgi apparatus. These MMPs are activated by PCs during secretion (see Fig. 8.2), which include proMMP-11, proMMP-23, proMMP-28, and proMT-MMPs. Intra-cellular activation of proMMP-11 and proMMP-14 (proMT1-MMP) by furin has been reported.[46,47] After the activation, active MMP-11 is secreted to extra-cellular milieu and active MMP-14 (MT1-MMP) is expressed on the cell surface. Because other proMT-MMPs, proMMP-23, and proMMP-28 also have the motif, PCs are responsible for the intra-cellular activation of these proMMPs. ADAM and ADAMTS family enzymes are also activated in this way because they have the same basic amino acid motif at the end of the prodomain.

Cell Surface Activation

ProMMP-2 is unique in that it is activated on the cell surface by MMP-14/MT1-MMP. The activation mechanism of proMMP-2 by MT1-MMP has been extensively investigated because it is considered to be a crucial step for cancer invasion and angiogenesis. Currently, the most accepted model for the activation of proMMP-2 by MT1-MMP is depicted in Fig. 8.2. MT1-MMP forms a homodimeric complex on the cell surface through the Hpx and the transmembrane domains.[48,49] Next, one of the MT1-MMP in this dimer complex is bound to and inhibited by TIMP-2. Because the C-terminal subdomain of TIMP-2, which has high affinity to the Hpx domain of proMMP-2, is available for interaction, the complex of $(MT1\text{-}MMP)_2$-TIMP-2 acts as a proMMP-2 activation receptor. Upon forming $(MT1\text{-}MMP)_2$-TIMP-2-proMMP-2 complex, the other MT1-MMP free from TIMP-2 in this complex cleaves a part of the proMMP-2 prodomain at Asn^{37}-Leu^{38} to generate an intermediate form of MMP-2, and autolytic action with another intermediate form of MMP-2 within the proximity removes a residual portion of the prodomain to generate a fully active enzyme.[50] Interestingly, activated MMP-2 can be released to extra-cellular milieu or functions on the cell surface by associating with TIMP-2 at the Hpx domain.[51] Other transmembrane type MT-MMPs, including MT2-MMP (MMP-15), MT3-MMP (MMP-16), and MT5-MMP (MMP-24), also activated proMMP-2,[52–55] but the in vivo role of proMMP-2 activation by these enzymes and the mechanism of activation are not clear. GPI-anchored MT4-MMP (MMP-17) does not activate proMMP-2. Another GPI-anchored MT6-MMP (MMP-25) initially activated proMMP-2, but later it was found that the full length enzyme is not able to activate proMMP-2 on the cell surface, although the isolated recombinant catalytic domain of MT6-MMP can activate proMMP-2 in a test tube. MT1-MMP (MMP-14) also activates proMMP-13 on the cell surface,[56] and this activation requires the hemopexin domain of MMP-13, but does not seem to require TIMP-2.[56,57] It was also reported that proMMP-7 is also activated on the cell surface, which was discovered through screening proMMP-7-binding molecules by a yeast two-hybrid screening.[58] ProMMP-7 is captured on the cell membrane by the interaction of the proMMP-7 prodomain with the C-terminal extra-cellular loop of CD151, a member of the transmembrane 4 superfamily, and is activated.[58] This cell surface activation of proMMP-7 requires a substrate of MMP-7. Because α chains of α3β1 and α6β4 integrins interact with CD151, these integrins may also be involved in the activation. Although the precise molecular mechanisms of this activation and the activator itself are still unclear, proMMP-7 and CD151 are overexpressed in osteoarthritic chondrocytes, and proMMP-7 is activated by the interaction with CD151 in articular cartilage of osteoarthritis.[59]

Endocytosis of ECM-Degrading Metalloproteinases

For MT-MMPs, endocytosis is a crucial regulatory mechanism. Some soluble enzymes are also known to be endocytosed via interaction with membrane proteins. In general, endocytosis is considered as a step of down regulation, but in some cases it is necessary for the enzyme to express their biologic function. It has been shown that MT1-MMP is endocytosed via both clathrin- and caveolae-dependent pathways.[60,61] The clathrin-dependent pathway is faster than the caveolae-dependent pathway, but it was also shown that clathrin-dependent endocytosis is required for MT1-MMP to promote cellular migration and invasion.[60] In the cytoplasmic domain of MT1-MMP, there is the LLY^{573} motif that is recognized by adaptor protein 2, a subunit of clathrin, and it is crucial for the enzyme to be endocytosed in this mechanism.[60] Just downstream of LLY^{573}, there is a Cys^{574}, which is post-translationally palmitoylated.[62] Interestingly, this palmitoylation was found to be crucial for the enzyme to be endocytosed via clathrin-dependent mechanism as well as for its cell migration promoting effect.[62] MT1-, MT3-, and MT5-MMP are endocytosed and recycled back to cell surface, and three amino acid motifs of DKV^{582} (MT1-MMP); EWV^{607} (MT3-MMP); and EWV^{645} (MT5-MMP) at their C-terminus were identified as recycling motifs.[63,64]

Endocytosis is the regulatory mechanism not only for MT-MMPs, but also for soluble enzymes. It was discovered that several ECM-degrading metalloproteinases and inhibitors are endocytosed via low-density lipoprotein receptor-related protein 1 (LRP1).

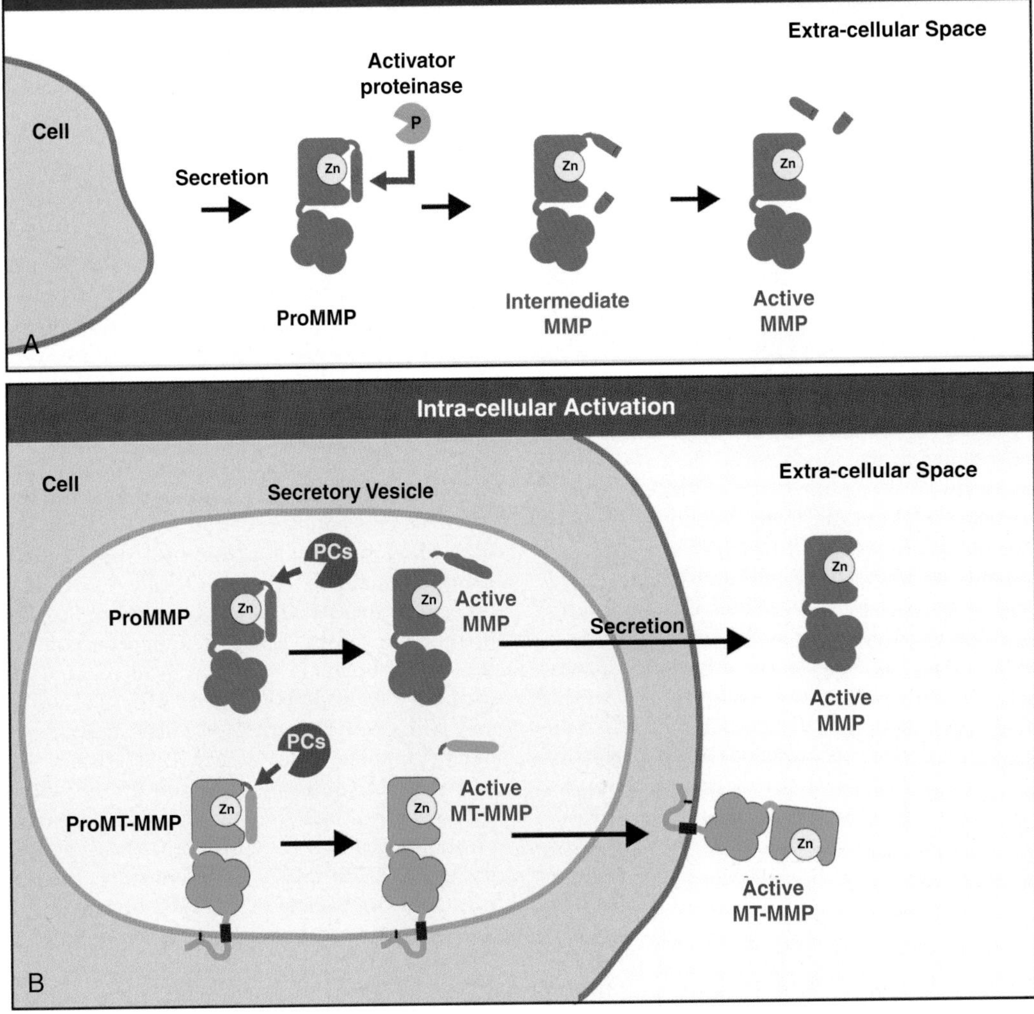

• **Fig. 8.2** Activation pathways of MMPs, ADAMs, and ADAMTSs. (A) Extra-cellular activation. Many proMMPs are secreted to extra-cellular space as an inactive form. Activator proteinases cleave a "bait region" within the prodomain *(highlighted in orange)* that results in an intermediate form of MMP. The intermediate enzyme possesses partial activity, and the inter molecular cleavage of intermediate MMPs removes the rest of prodomain, which converts the enzyme into a fully active MMP. (B) Intra-cellular activation. Some MMPs that contain four basic amino acids motif of RX(K/R)R at the end of the prodomain *(highlighted in orange)* are activated intra-cellularly during secretion by proprotein convertases (PCs). PCs recognize and directly cleave downstream of RX(K/R)R. These enzymes include MMP-11, -21, -28, -23, all MT-MMPs, ADAMTSs, and ADAM enzymes.

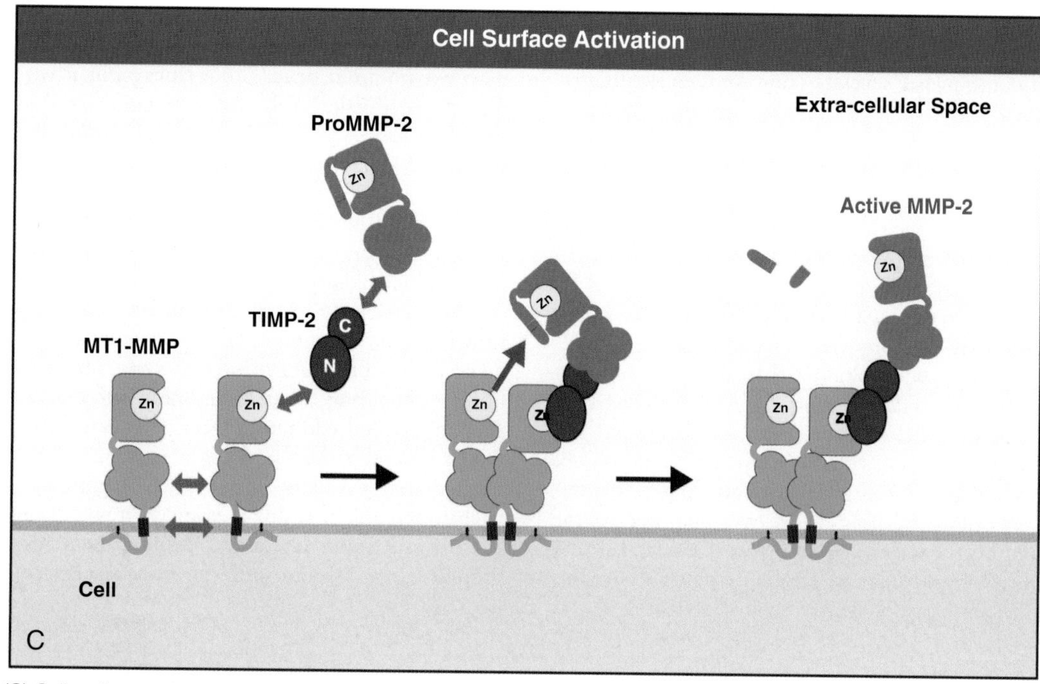

• Fig. 8.2, cont'd (C) Cell surface activation. The most accepted model of proMMP-2 by MT1-MMP on the cell surface is depicted. MT1-MMP expressed on the cell surface forms a homodimeric complex through its Hpx domain and the transmembrane domain. One of the MT1-MMP binds to TIMP-2 through an active site of the enzyme and inhibitory site of TIMP-2. The exposed C-terminal subdomain of TIMP-2 has high affinity to the Hpx domain of proMMP-2, resulting in formation of $(MT1\text{-}MMP)_2$-TIMP-2-proMMP-2 complex. MT1-MMP free from TIMP-2 within this complex then cleave the prodomain of proMMP-2 in the complex, resulting in an intermediate form of MMP-2. Proximal intermediate MMP-2 molecules then remove the rest of the prodomain to become fully active MMP-2. Activated MMP-2 can either stay on the cell surface or can be released to extra-cellular milieu.

TABLE 8.8 Activators of Pro-matrix Metalloproteinases

ProMMP	Activator
ProMMP-1	Trypsin (partial); plasmin (partial); plasma kallikrein (partial); chymase (partial); MMP-3; MMP-7; MMP-10; MMP-11
ProMMP-2	MT1-MMP; MT2-MMP; MT3-MMP; MT5-MMP
ProMMP-3	Plasmin; plasma kallikrein; trypsin; tryptase; chymase; cathepsin G; chymotrypsin; neutrophil elastase; thermolysin
ProMMP-7	MMP-3; MMP-10 (partial); trypsin; plasmin (partial); neutrophil elastase (partial)
ProMMP-8	MMP-3; MMP-10; tissue kallikrein; neutrophil elastase; cathepsin G; trypsin
ProMMP-9	MMP-3; MMP-2; MMP-7; MMP-10 (partial); MMP-13; trypsin; chymotrypsin; cathepsin G; tissue kallikrein
ProMMP-10	Plasmin; trypsin; chymotrypsin
ProMMP-11, 21, 28	Furin; PCs
ProMMP-13	MMP-2; MMP-3; MT1-MMP; plasmin
ProMT-MMPs	Furin; PCs

Pro-MMP, Pro-matrix metalloproteinase; *PCs,* proprotein convertases.

LRP-1 is synthesized as a 600 kDa precursor that is processed by proprotein convertases during secretion to the cell surface, resulting in a 515 kDa α chain and an 85 kDa β chain associated noncovalently. The α chain contains four extra-cellular binding regions for various molecules. It binds to extra-cellular molecules, rapidly endocytosed through clathrin-dependent mechanisms, and molecules bound to LRP-1 are degraded in lysosome. LRP-1 is widely expressed in different cell types and controls extra-cellular levels of numerous biologically active molecules to maintain tissue homeostasis.[65] Currently, more than 50 ligands have been characterized, including lipoproteins, ECM proteins, growth factors, cell surface receptors, proteinases, proteinase inhibitors, and secreted intra-cellular proteins.[65] In cartilage, it was shown that LRP-1 controls the Wnt/b-catenin signaling pathway by interacting with frizzled-1[66] and connective tissue growth factor (CCN2), and both regulate endochondral ossification and articular cartilage regeneration.[67] It has been shown that LRP-1 is also responsible for clearing extra-cellular MMP-2, MMP-9, MMP-13, ADAMTS5, TIMP-1, and TIMP-3.[68–71] LRP-1 was also reported to endocytose tPA, PAI-1, and uPA, and cathepsin D also binded to LRP-1 ectodomain.[69] Endocytic regulation of ECM-degrading enzymes in arthritic tissues is becoming an important area that directly influences disease progression, and further investigation is required.

Joint Tissue Destruction in Arthritis

Articular cartilage is the major organ that supports joint function by providing smooth joint movement and a shock-absorbing function. Cartilage is a unique tissue composed of a large volume of ECM and a small number of chondrocytes. The major cartilage ECM components are type II collagen and a large proteoglycan called aggrecan (about 45% each), and these components play crucial roles in cartilage function: aggrecan provides compressive resistance, and collagen provides cartilage architecture. Thus, degradation of these components severely compromises joint function. The major aggrecan-degrading enzymes are thought to be ADAMTSs, but MMPs also degrade it, while collagen degradation is carried out by collagen-degrading MMPs. In rheumatoid arthritis and osteoarthritis, these two subclasses of metalloproteinases are key in cartilage degradation. In rheumatoid arthritis, cartilage erosion is caused by invasion of inflamed synovial pannus tissue, by the enzymes present in the synovial fluid, and by chondrocytes-derived enzymes, while in osteoarthritis it is due to the enzymes produced by chondrocytes.

Upon disease onset, it is considered that aggrecan degradation proceeds before collagen degradation. Aggrecan is susceptible to degradation by many different proteinases, including MMPs, ADAMTSs, neutrophil elastase, cathepsin G, and cathepsin B. These enzymes are able to cleave peptide bonds between interglobular G1 and G2 domains. This cleavage effectively releases the major glycosaminoglycan-bearing aggrecan part (between G2 and G3 domain) from the hyaluronan attachment site (G1 domain) that provides a functional part of aggrecan within cartilage matrix (Fig. 8.3). The two major aggrecan fragments with the N-terminal sequences starting from Phe^{342} or Ala^{374} of the core protein are detected in joint synovial fluids from patients with various inflammatory arthritides and osteoarthritis. Many MMPs, including MMP-1, 2, 3, 7, 8, 9, 13, and MT1-MMP, preferentially cleave the Asn^{341}-Phe^{342} bond (the MMP site).[72] ADAMTS species, including ADAMTS1,[73] 4,[16] 5,[17] 8, 9, and 15, cleave the Glu^{373}-Ala^{374} bond (the aggrecanase site), in addition to other sites in the G2-G3 domains. Other minor components of cartilage are also degraded (see Fig. 8.3). Decorin, a leucine-rich repeat proteoglycan, is digested by MMP-2, 3, and 7,[74] as well as ADAMTS4.[20] Information is limited about the proteinases responsible for the degradation of other proteoglycans, including fibromodulin, lumican, biglycan, PRELP (arginine-rich end leucine-rich repeat protein), chondroadherin, and syndecan present in articular cartilage, although fibromodulin is cleaved by ADAMTS4.[20] Link protein that mediates interaction of aggrecan G1 domain and hyaluronan is susceptible to many proteinases such as MMP-1, 2, 3, 7-10, neutrophil elastase, and cathepsin G. Degradation of link protein may also contribute to releasing aggrecan from cartilage matrix.

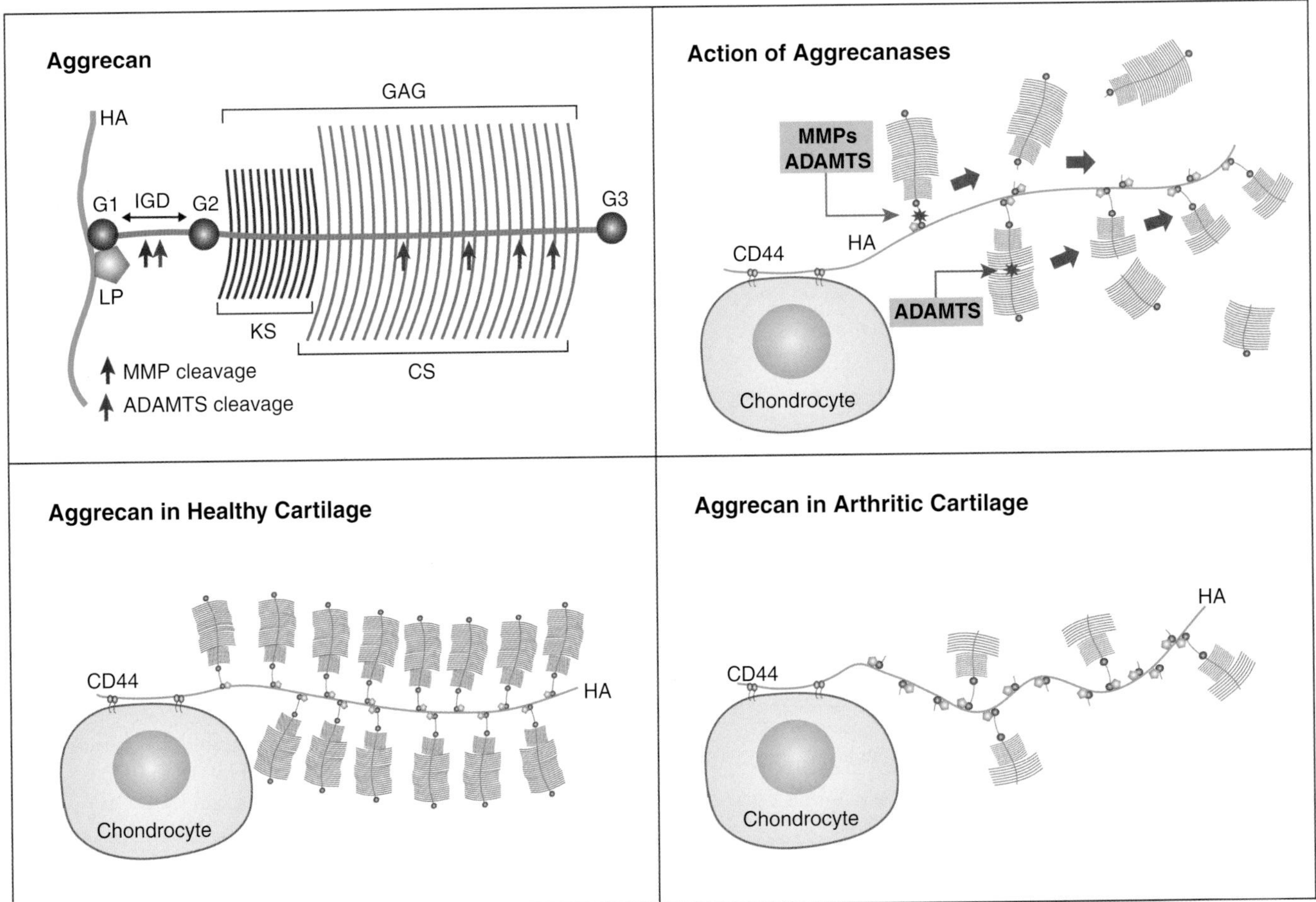

• **Fig. 8.3** Aggrecan degradation by MMPs and ADAMTS. Aggrecan is a large proteoglycan containing numerous chondroitin sulfate (CS) and keratan sulfate (KS) glycosaminoglycan (GAG) moieties, which are central to the function of the molecule as they draw water into the cartilage matrix, giving it the ability to withstand compression (normal cartilage). Aggrecan binds to hyaluronic acid (HA), which binds to chondrocytes through their HA receptors (such as CD44) through its globular domain 1 (G1) with the help of link protein (LP). Cleavage of aggrecan in the interglobular domain (IGD) between the N-terminal G1 and G2 globular domains by MMPs (Asn341 ~ Phe342 bond) and ADAMTSs (Glu373 ~ Ala374 bond) causes loss of the GAG species from the tissue and thus abrogates the function of the molecule (arthritic cartilage). ADAMTSs also cleave in the CS-chain attached region.

Fibrillar collagens (i.e., types I, II, and III collagens) are resistant to most proteinases at neutral pH because of their triple helical structures, except collagenases belonging to MMPs, including MMP-1, -2, -8, -13, and MT1-MMP. Among these fibrillar collagen types, Type III collagen can be degraded by noncollagenolytic enzymes, including MMP-3, -9, -16, and neutrophil elastase. Collagenases cleave the triple helical region of collagen molecules at ¾ from the N-terminus, and, upon this cleavage, the helical structures can be unwound at 37° C (i.e., body temperature) and become random peptides of gelatin. Once it becomes gelatin, it can be degraded into smaller peptides by gelatinases (MMP-2 and MMP-9) and many other proteinases. At both N- or C-terminus of fibrillar collagens, there are nonhelical telopeptide regions, and this part of collagens can be cleaved by various noncollagenolytic enzymes such as MMP-3, MMP-9, neutrophil elastase, cathepsin G, and cysteine proteinase cathepsins. Because collagen crosslinking occurs at the telopeptide region, this cleavage may contribute to depolymerizing the cross-linked collagens.

Fibronectin is degraded by many MMPs, including MMP-2, 3, 7, 10, 11, 13-16, 19, and other serine proteinases. COMP can be digested by MMP-19 and MMP-20. Proteinases capable of digesting cartilage matrix protein and cartilage intermediate layer protein are unknown, however.

Cartilage Destruction in Rheumatoid Arthritis

Rheumatoid arthritis is characterized by chronic proliferative synovitis, which shows hyperplasia of the synovial lining cells, inflammatory cell infiltration, and angiogenesis in the sublining cell layer (Fig. 8.4). Hyperplastic synovial lining cells are characterized to have an invasive character and overproduce MMP-1, 3, 9, 14, ADAMTS4, TIMP-1, and TIMP-3. Sublining fibroblasts produce MMP-2 and TIMP-2. Polymorphonuclear leukocytes infiltrated in the synovium and joint cavity keep MMP-8 in the specific granules and MMP-9 and neutrophil elastase, cathepsin G, and proteinase 3 in the azurophil granules. They are released from cells during phagocytosis of tissue debris and immune complexes. Other inflammatory cells in the synovium include macrophages, lymphocytes, and mast cells. Macrophages produce MMP-1, MMP-9, MT1-MMP, TIMP-1, and TIMP-2, and uPA, and cathepsins B, L, and D are also secreted from activated macrophages. T lymphocytes in the synovium synthesize MMP-9. Chymase and tryptase are degranulated from mast cells in response to

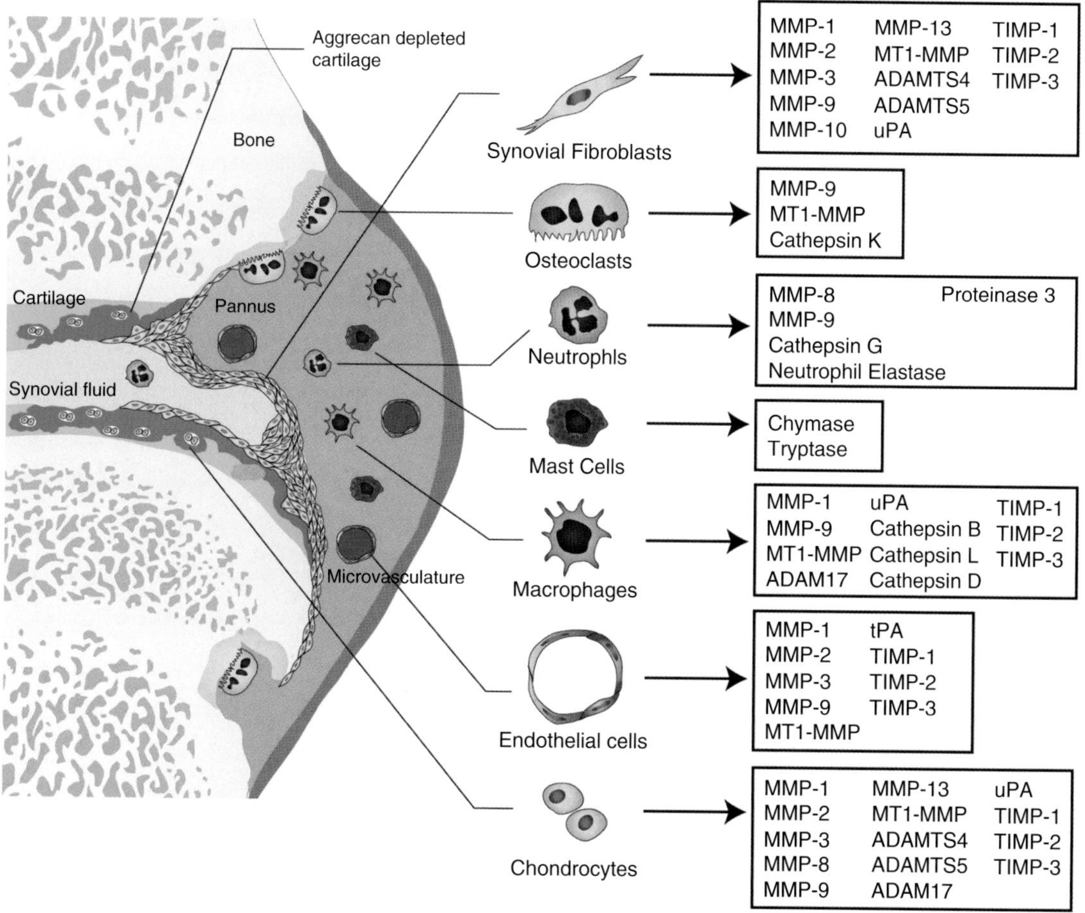

• **Fig. 8.4** Cells, proteinases, and their inhibitors that contribute to joint tissue destruction in rheumatoid arthritis. This illustration depicts a rheumatoid arthritic joint where the inflammed synovial pannus tissue invades and destroys cartilage and bone. Cartilage in *light blue* are intact while the ones in *dark blue* are aggrecan-depleted tissue. Synovial lining cells are activated, become hypertrophic, and invade into cartilage tissue. The bone matrix is degraded by osteoclasts. Polymorphonuclear neutrophils can be found in synovial fluid or synovial tissue. Macrophages and mast cells contribute not only to the inflammation, but also to cartilage degradation. Pannus tissue contains numerous microvasculatures that bring nutrients to the hypertrophic tissue. Chondrocytes in cartilage also contribute to the cartilage degradation.

activation by immune complexes. Endothelial cells express many MMPs, including MMP-1, 2, 3, 9, and MT1-MMP; tPA; and their inhibitors (see Fig. 8.4). However, these proteinases produced from endothelial cells may be involved in tissue remodeling during angiogenesis in the synovium rather than cartilage destruction. All of the soluble proteinases and inhibitors produced by synovial tissue cells and inflammatory cells are likely to be secreted into the synovial fluid and contribute to degradation of articular cartilage when active proteinases overwhelm inhibitors. MMP-1, 2, 3, 8, 9, ADAMTS4, TIMP-1, and TIMP-2 are detectable in rheumatoid synovial fluids, and the molar balance of MMPs to TIMPs in this compartment seems to tip to MMP activity as proteolytic activities are detectable in rheumatoid synovial fluids.[75] In the early stage of rheumatoid arthritis, the cartilage surface exposed to synovial fluid shows surface irregularity (fibrillation) and proteoglycan depletion without being covered by pannus tissue. This cartilage degradation may be caused by the action of the proteinases present in synovial fluid (Fig. 8.5). Among the MMPs detected in synovial fluids, MMP-3 has the highest concentration, and serum MMP-3 level can be used to monitor the activity of rheumatoid synovitis.[76–78] Articular cartilage in contact with synovial tissue is progressively degraded even in the early stage. This part of the synovial tissue becomes the pannus that further invades into and destructs cartilage tissue. This is a major pathway of cartilage erosion in rheumatoid arthritis, and it has been shown that MT1-MMP expressed in synovial fibroblasts is responsible for invasion of the pannus into the cartilage (see Fig. 8.5).[79,80] Analyses of rheumatoid arthritis joint specimens indicated that MT1-MMP is particularly overexpressed in the fibroblasts at the pannus-cartilage junction where they invade.[79] This unique expression pattern of MT1-MMP cannot be explained by inflammatory cytokines-driven gene expression, and it was reported that the upregulation of MT1-MMP is due to recognition of cartilage collagen by synovial fibroblasts through collagen receptor tyrosine kinase, discoidin domain receptor 2 (DDR2).[81] Collagen signaling through DDR2 upregulated *MT1-MMP* gene expression and function to degrade cartilage collagen matrix for invasion in synovial fibroblasts.[81] Interestingly, DDR2 cannot get activated by healthy intact cartilage but only by partially damaged, aggrecan-depleted cartilage, suggesting that aggrecan degradation needs to proceed before activation of the pannus invasion program.[81] Both MMPs and ADAMTSs are thought to play a role in aggrecan degradation, but ADAMTSs are thought to play a major role in the early stages of arthritis.[82] ADAMTS-1, -4, -5, -8, -9, -15, -16, and -18 can degrade aggrecan, but ADAMTS-5 is considered as a major aggrecanase because it possesses the strongest aggrecanase activity,[83,84] and ADAMTS-5 null mice are protected from cartilage degradation in antigen-induced arthritis.[85] Furthermore,

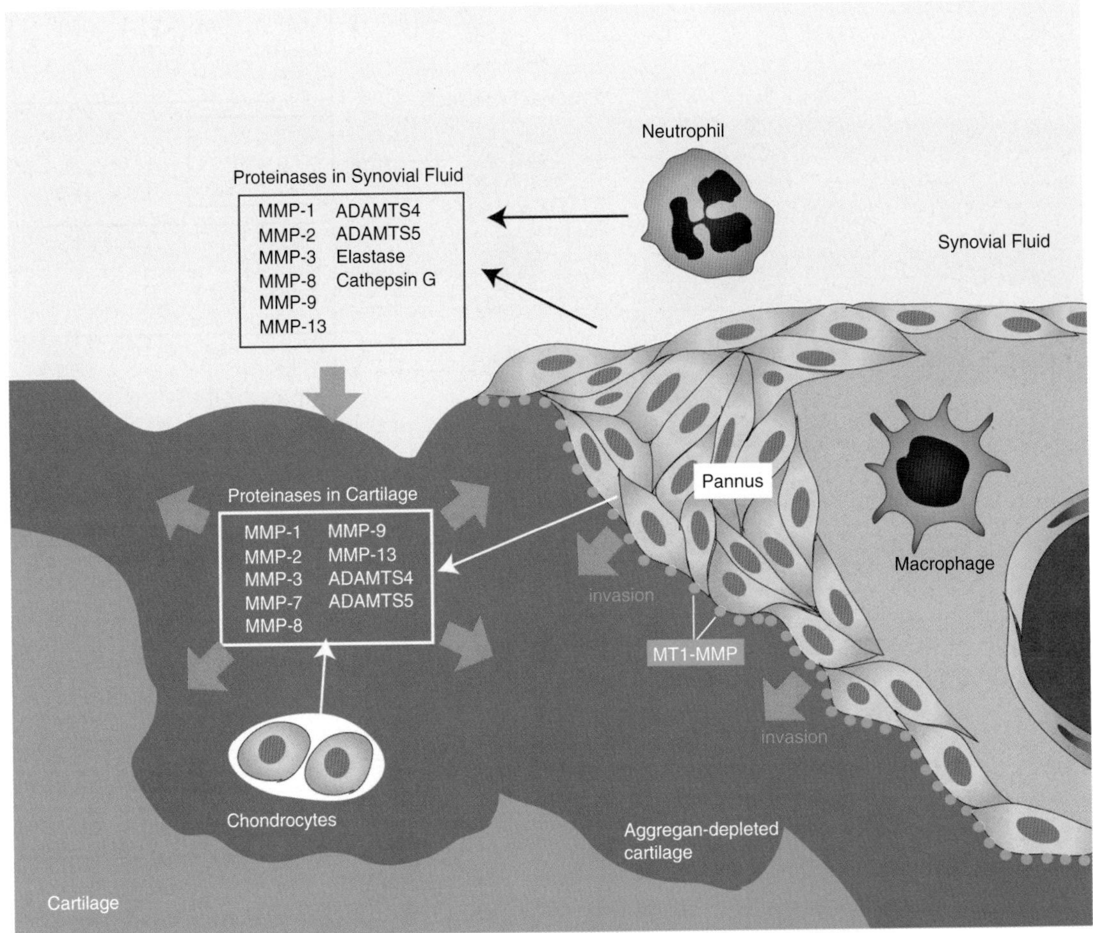

• **Fig. 8.5** Three pathways of cartilage matrix degradation. Cartilage matrix can be degraded in three pathways. Synovial tissue cells produce a large number of soluble proteinases and are considered to be secreted to synovial fluid. These enzymes attach to the cartilage surface. Chondrocytes in cartilage also produce proteinases. Together with proteinases secreted from synovial tissue into cartilage, they degrade cartilage from the inside. Finally, synovial fibroblasts express MT1-MMP at the cartilage pannus junction and degrade and invade the cartilage.

knockin mutant mice harboring a mutation in the ADAMTS cleavage site in the interglobular domain of aggrecan are also protected from cartilage degradation in the antigen-induced arthritis model.[86] These observations strongly suggest that aggrecan degradation is necessary for progression of cartilage degradation in inflammatory arthritis.

In addition to cells in inflamed synovial tissue, chondrocytes within cartilage tissue also produce cartilage-degrading proteinases upon pro-inflammatory stimulations (see Fig. 8.4). Various inflammatory cytokines stimulate chondrocytes to produce MMP-1, 2, 3, 7, 8, 9, 13, 14, 16, ADAM9, 10, 17, ADAMTS4, ADAMTS5, and other classes of proteinases. In rheumatoid arthritic cartilage, MMP-1, 2, 3, 7, 9, 13, and 14 are expressed in chondrocytes located in the proteoglycan-depleted zone. When large areas of the cartilage surface are ulcerated after degradation of cartilage ECM, death of chondrocytes occurs, leading to further progressive cartilage destruction.

Because MMPs play a central role in degradation of ECM molecules in rheumatoid arthritis and cancers, a number of MMP inhibitors were developed and subjected to clinical trials,[82,87–89] but all of them failed. MMP inhibitors for the treatment of patients with rheumatoid arthritis and osteoarthritis were withdrawn from the phase III trials, mainly because of a lack of efficacy.[88] In clinical trials for patients with cancer, most of the inhibitors had no definite benefit, and prolonged or high-dose treatment with broad-spectrum MMP inhibitors caused unexpected symptoms in the musculoskeletal system, such as inflammatory polyarthritis,[90] which are called musculoskeletal syndrome. The failure is considered to be due to the nature of active site-directed broad-spectrum inhibitors. In humans, there are 62 metalloproteinases, and many of these enzymes are important for normal tissue homeostasis. These small molecule inhibitors broadly inhibit the majority of these enzymes, causing unexpected side effects. Therefore, it is crucial to identify the responsible enzymes in the disease and inhibit them in a highly selective manner.

There are two potential MMPs that can be targeted in a selective manner and have shown an efficacy at least in animal models of arthritis. The first one is MMP-13, which is produced by rheumatoid synovial fibroblasts and chondrocytes upon stimulation with various inflammatory stimuli, including IL-1, TNF, IL-17, myeloid-related proteins (S100A8/S100A9), and oncostatin M.[91–94] High levels of MMP-13 are found in the synovial pannus at the cartilage junction.[95] There are small molecule inhibitors highly selective to MMP-13, and administration of this inhibitor inhibited development of arthritis in several inflammatory arthritis models, including the SCID mouse co-implantation model and collagen-induced arthritis model.[96] Another target is MT1-MMP (MMP-14). MT1-MMP is upregulated in rheumatoid synovial tissue[97–99] and is highly expressed in synovial fibroblasts at the pannus-cartilage junction.[79] Selective MT1-MMP inhibition by expressing a dominant negative form of MT1-MMP[79] or knocking down MT1-MMP[80] inhibited RASF invasion into cartilage in vitro. Also highly selective MT1-MMP inhibitory antibody DX2400 inhibited cartilage erosion in mice with collagen-induced arthritis.[100] These findings suggest that MT1-MMP is the enzyme that mediates synovial pannus invasion and cartilage erosion. As described earlier, selective MMP-13 inhibitor also inhibits cartilage erosion in animal models of arthritis.[96] Interestingly, silencing MMP-13 had no effect on RASF invasion into cartilage in vitro.[80] Therefore, both MMP-13 and MT1-MMP are involved in cartilage invasion, but their roles may be different: while MT1-MMP directly promotes RASF invasion by degrading cartilage collagen, the mechanism through which MMP-13 promotes invasion is unclear. MT1-MMP, as a cellular collagenase, also plays an essential role in angiogenesis[101] and monocyte endothelial transmigration[102,103] and thus may also promote disease through other mechanisms as well.

Bone Resorption in Rheumatoid Arthritis

Bone is composed of 40% organic component and 60% inorganic component, and the major organic component in mature bone is insoluble, highly cross-linked type I collagen (90% of all organic components), although type III and V collagens are also present. Other minor components in bone matrix are leucine-rich repeat proteoglycans (decorin and biglycan) and glycoproteins such as osteopontin, osteonectin (SPARC), osteocalcin (bone Gla-protein), and thrombospondin. Bone is resorbed by osteoclasts, and this is commonly observed at the bare zone, where pannus-like granulation tissue invades the bone marrow and destroys subchondral bone. Activated osteoclasts attach to only mineralized bone matrix, and this cell-matrix contact is carried out by αvβ3 integrin of osteoclasts attaching to Arg-Gly-Asp (RGD) sequence of osteopontin in the bone matrix. ECM degradation of the mineralized bone can occur only after demineralization of the bone matrix because proteinases cannot permeate the matrix components in the mineralized tissues. Matrix degradation by osteoclasts is performed in the subosteoclastic compartments, which have acidic (pH 4 to 5) and hypercalcemic (40 to 50 mM Ca^{2+}) conditions.[104] Under these conditions, a collagenolytic cysteine proteinase, cathepsin K, is thought to be responsible for bone resorption because of its collagenolytic activity with a broad pH optimum and selective expression in osteoclasts and giant cells of giant cell tumors. Mutations of human cathepsin K are responsible for pyknodysostosis, an autosomal recessive osteochondrodysplasia characterized by osteopetrosis and short stature.[105] *Cathepsin K*–deficient mice have a similar phenotype. Despite the importance of cathepsin K in bone resorption, osteoclastic bone resorption cannot be completely inhibited by cysteine proteinase inhibitors; it is inhibited to a similar degree by MMP inhibitors.[104] MMP-9 is highly expressed in osteoclasts in normal and rheumatoid bones[106] and giant cells of giant cell tumors. MMP-9 has telopeptidase activity against soluble and insoluble type I collagen and strong gelatinolytic activity.[43,106] ProMMP-9 can be activated by acid exposure, and when activated it is proteolytically active under acidic and hypercalcemic conditions.[106] *MMP-9*-deficient mice show a transient disturbance of growth plate development. Cathepsin K and MMP-9 may thus be involved in bone resorption in people with rheumatoid arthritis. Although MT1-MMP is also expressed in osteoclasts in rheumatoid arthritis,[98] evidence of the direct involvement in osteoclastic bone resorption is limited. MMP-7 may be involved in the solubilization of receptor activator of nuclear factor-κB ligand (RANKL) in a murine prostate cancer–induced osteolysis model,[107] but no data are available regarding the osteoclastic bone resorption in rheumatoid arthritis. For treatment of osteoporosis and/or destructive bone diseases, bisphosphonates that reduce bone turnover by inhibiting bone-resorbing activity of mature osteoclasts are commonly utilized. Denosumab, a human monoclonal antibody against RANKL, has been approved by the U.S. Food and Drug Administration and used for treatment of osteoporosis in people with rheumatoid arthritis. Cathepsin K inhibitors were considered to be promising drugs for treatment of post-menopausal osteoporosis because the reduction of osteoclast-stimulated bone formation is less compared with anti–bone resorptive drugs such as bisphosphonates.[108] These inhibitors were also expected to be useful for treatment of osteoporosis in people with rheumatoid arthritis. The drug went to phase III clinical trial, and it effectively increased bone densities. However, it also

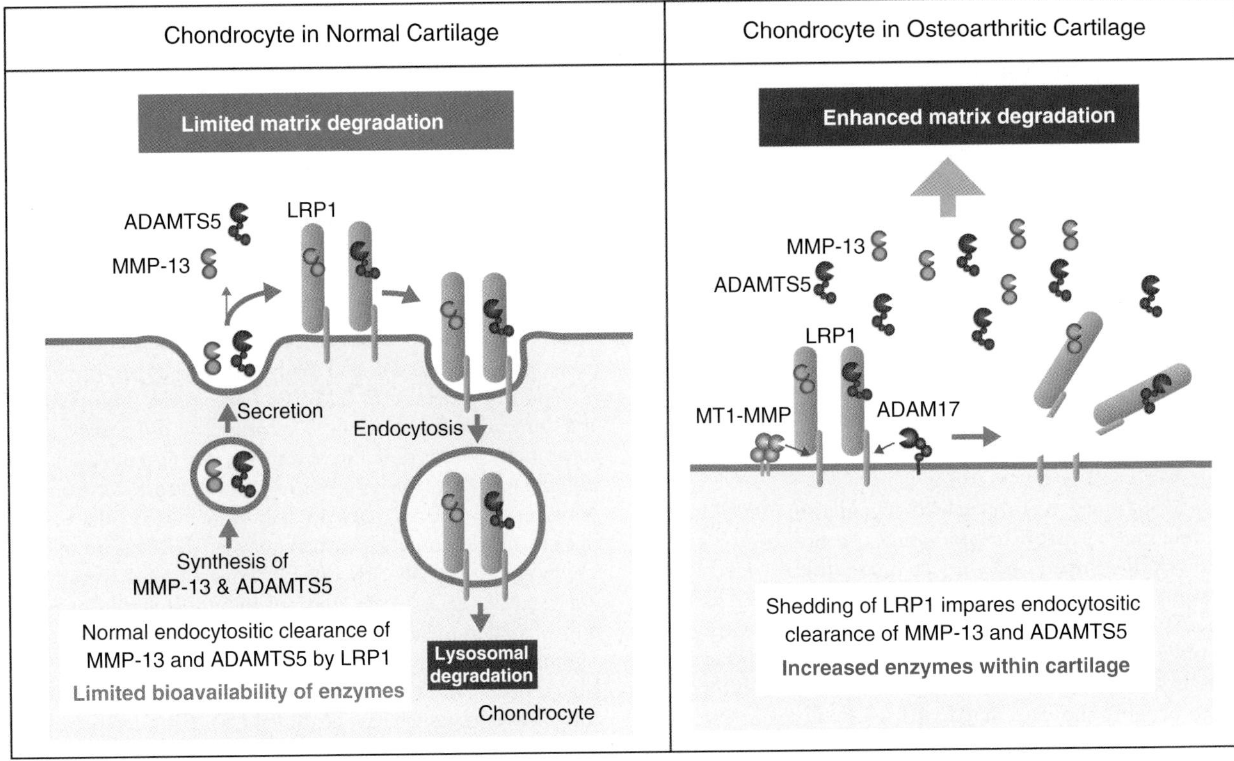

• **Fig. 8.6** Impaired endocytic regulation of proteinases in osteoarthritis. Chondrocytes in normal healthy cartilage spontaneously produce MMP-13 and ADAMTS5. However, LRP1-mediated endocytic clearance of these enzymes dominates and prevents matrix degradation. In osteoarthritis, chondrocytes overproduce MT1-MMP and ADAM17, and these enzymes shed ectodomain of LRP1, which impairs endocytic clearance of MMP-13 and ADAMTS5 and results in accumulation of these enzymes and cartilage matrix degradation. (Illustration was partially adapted from Yamamoto K, Santamaria S, Botkjaer KA, et al.: Inhibition of shedding of low-density lipoprotein receptor-related protein 1 reverses cartilage matrix degradation in osteoarthritis. *Arthritis Rheumatol* 69(6):1246–1256, 2017.)

increased the risk for stroke, which is something that needs to be prevented in this patient population, and development of the inhibitor was discontinued. Detailed mechanism of increased incidence of stroke upon cathepsin K inhibition has not been made clear, but it is likely to be due to other roles of cathepsin K.

Cartilage Degradation in Osteoarthritis

In osteoarthritis, the major cell type that produces cartilage degrading enzymes is chondrocyte. In early stages of the disease, aggrecan degradation proceeds before collagen degradation, and this step is considered to be crucial for the disease to further develop. A number of MMPs, including MMP-1,[109] -2,[110,111] -3,[112] -7,[113] -8,[109] -9,[111] -13,[9,109] and MT1-MMP,[110] are expressed in osteoarthritic cartilage. MMP-3, -7, and MT1-MMP are immunolocalized to chondrocytes in the proteoglycan-depleted zone of osteoarthritic cartilage, and the levels of their staining correlate directly with the histologic Mankin score.[110,112,113] Among the collagenolytic MMPs, MMP-13 is considered to be the key enzyme in degradation of cartilage collagen as no cartilage collagen degradation was observed in the mice lacking MMP-13 with the destabilization of the medial meniscus (DMM) surgery model.[114] Because MT1-MMP activates proMMP-13 on the cell surface,[56] MT1-MMP may play a key role in cartilage collagen degradation through activation of proMMP-13. The major aggrecan-degrading proteinases include MMPs and ADAMTSs, but ADAMTSs, especially ADAMTS5, are considered to play a key role. ADAMTS5 null mice, but not ADAMTS-4 null mice, were resistant from aggrecan degradation in the surgical DMM model of osteoarthritis.[115] Without ADAMTS5-dependent aggrecan degradation, cartilage tissue was completely protected. Thus, aggrecan degradation needs to occur before further cartilage destruction can occur, and ADAMTS5 is likely the key enzyme during the early stage of cartilage degradation in osteoarthritis. This is also supported by the biochemical property of ADAMTS5. Full-length ADAMTS5 possesses 33-fold more potent aggrecanase activity compared with full-length ADAMTS4 and 600-fold higher activity compared with truncated ADAMTS4.[83,84] In human osteoarthritic cartilage, ADAMTS4 can be induced by IL-1 and TNF, whereas ADAMTS5 expression is constitutive.[116] It has been found that constitutively expressed ADAMTS5, together with MMP-13, is constantly downregulated by low-density lipoprotein receptor–related protein 1 (LRP-1)-mediated endocytosis in normal cartilage, which explains why ADAMTS5 protein is difficult to detect in normal tissue (Fig. 8.6).[71] In human OA cartilage, LRP-1 is shed by MT1-MMP and ADAM17 that are highly upregulated in chondrocytes, causing a deficit in endocytic regulation of ADAMTS5 and MMP-13 (see Fig. 8.6).[117] Inhibition of LRP-1 shedding by highly selective inhibitors for MT1-MMP and ADAM17 in OA cartilage was found to reverse both aggrecan and cartilage degradation in the tissue,[117] suggesting that ADAMTS5-mediated aggrecan degradation is due to LRP-1 shedding, and local inhibition of MT1-MMP and ADAM17 may be an attractive potential therapeutic strategy.

The references for this chapter can also be found on ExpertConsult.com.

References

1. Handley CJ, Mok MT, Ilic MZ, et al.: Cathepsin D cleaves aggrecan at unique sites within the interglobular domain and chondroitin sulfate attachment regions that are also cleaved when cartilage is maintained at acid pH, *Matrix Biol* 20(8):543–553, 2001.
2. Bromme D, Okamoto K, Wang BB, et al.: Human cathepsin O2, a matrix protein-degrading cysteine protease expressed in osteoclasts. Functional expression of human cathepsin O2 in Spodoptera frugiperda and characterization of the enzyme, *J Biol Chem* 271(4):2126–2132, 1996.
3. Drake FH, Dodds RA, James IE, et al.: Cathepsin K, but not cathepsins B, L, or S, is abundantly expressed in human osteoclasts, *J Biol Chem* 271(21):12511–12516, 1996.
4. Salminen-Mankonen HJ, Morko J, Vuorio E: Role of cathepsin K in normal joints and in the development of arthritis, *Curr Drug Targets* 8(2):315–323, 2007.
5. Sorimachi H, Suzuki K: The structure of calpain, *Journal of biochemistry* 129(5):653–664, 2001.
6. Nagase H: Activation mechanisms of matrix metalloproteinases, *Biol Chem* 378(3-4):151–160, 1997.
7. Itoh Y: Membrane-type matrix metalloproteinases: their functions and regulations, *Matrix Biol*, 2015. 44-46207-223.
8. Chung L, Dinakarpandian D, Yoshida N, et al.: Collagenase unwinds triple-helical collagen prior to peptide bond hydrolysis, *EMBO J* 23(15):3020–3030, 2004.
9. Mitchell PG, Magna HA, Reeves LM, et al.: Cloning, expression, and type II collagenolytic activity of matrix metalloproteinase-13 from human osteoarthritic cartilage, *J Clin Invest* 97(3):761–768, 1996.
10. Balbin M, Fueyo A, Knauper V, et al.: Identification and enzymatic characterization of two diverging murine counterparts of human interstitial collagenase (MMP-1) expressed at sites of embryo implantation, *J Biol Chem* 276(13):10253–10262, 2001.
11. Ohuchi E, Imai K, Fujii Y, et al.: Membrane type 1 matrix metalloproteinase digests interstitial collagens and other extracellular matrix macromolecules, *J Biol Chem* 272(4):2446–2451, 1997.
12. d'Ortho MP, Will H, Atkinson S, et al.: Membrane-type matrix metalloproteinases 1 and 2 exhibit broad-spectrum proteolytic capacities comparable to many matrix metalloproteinases, *Eur J Biochem* 250(3):751–757, 1997.
13. Shimada T, Nakamura H, Ohuchi E, et al.: Characterization of a truncated recombinant form of human membrane type 3 matrix metalloproteinase, *Eur J Biochem* 262(3):907–914, 1999.
14. Itoh Y, Kajita M, Kinoh H, et al.: Membrane type 4 matrix metalloproteinase (MT4-MMP, MMP-17) is a glycosylphosphatidylinositol-anchored proteinase, *J Biol Chem* 274(48):34260–34266, 1999.
15. Kojima S, Itoh Y, Matsumoto S, et al.: Membrane-type 6 matrix metalloproteinase (MT6-MMP, MMP-25) is the second glycosylphosphatidyl inositol (GPI)-anchored MMP, *FEBS Lett* 480142–480146, 2000.
16. Tortorella MD, Burn TC, Pratta MA, et al.: Purification and cloning of aggrecanase-1: a member of the ADAMTS family of proteins, *Science* 284(5420):1664–1666, 1999.
17. Abbaszade I, Liu RQ, Yang F, et al.: Cloning and characterization of ADAMTS11, an aggrecanase from the ADAMTS family, *J Biol Chem* 274(33):23443–23450, 1999.
18. Sandy JD, Westling J, Kenagy RD, et al.: Versican V1 proteolysis in human aorta in vivo occurs at the Glu441-Ala442 bond, a site that is cleaved by recombinant ADAMTS-1 and ADAMTS-4, *J Biol Chem* 276(16):13372–13378, 2001.
19. Nakamura H, Fujii Y, Inoki I, et al.: Brevican is degraded by matrix metalloproteinases and aggrecanase-1 (ADAMTS4) at different sites, *J Biol Chem* 275(49):38885–38890, 2000.
20. Kashiwagi M, Enghild JJ, Gendron C, et al.: Altered proteolytic activities of ADAMTS-4 expressed by C-terminal processing, *J Biol Chem* 279(11):10109–10119, 2004.
21. Peschon JJ, Slack JL, Reddy P, et al.: An essential role for ectodomain shedding in mammalian development, *Science* 282(5392):1281–1284, 1998.
22. Sunnarborg SW, Hinkle CL, Stevenson M, et al.: Tumor necrosis factor-alpha converting enzyme (TACE) regulates epidermal growth factor receptor ligand availability, *J Biol Chem* 277(15):12838–12845, 2002.
23. Black RA: Tumor necrosis factor-alpha converting enzyme, *Int J Biochem Cell Biol* 34(1):1–5, 2002.
24. Yan Y, Shirakabe K, Werb Z: The metalloprotease Kuzbanian (ADAM10) mediates the transactivation of EGF receptor by G protein-coupled receptors, *J Cell Biol* 158(2):221–226, 2002.
25. Asakura M, Kitakaze M, Takashima S, et al.: Cardiac hypertrophy is inhibited by antagonism of ADAM12 processing of HB-EGF: metalloproteinase inhibitors as a new therapy, *Nat Med* 8(1):35–40, 2002.
26. Mochizuki S, Shimoda M, Shiomi T, et al.: ADAM28 is activated by MMP-7 (matrilysin-1) and cleaves insulin-like growth factor binding protein-3, *Biochem Biophys Res Commun* 315(1):79–84, 2004.
27. Loechel F, Fox JW, Murphy G, et al.: ADAM 12-S cleaves IGFBP-3 and IGFBP-5 and is inhibited by TIMP-3, *Biochem Biophys Res Commun* 278(3):511–515, 2000.
28. Fourie AM, Coles F, Moreno V, et al.: Catalytic activity of ADAM8, ADAM15, and MDC-L (ADAM28) on synthetic peptide substrates and in ectodomain cleavage of CD23, *J Biol Chem* 278(33):30469–30477, 2003.
29. Reiss K, Ludwig A, Saftig P: Breaking up the tie: disintegrin-like metalloproteinases as regulators of cell migration in inflammation and invasion, *Pharmacol Ther* 111(3):985–1006, 2006.
30. Saksela O, Rifkin DB: Cell-associated plasminogen activation: regulation and physiological functions, *Annu Rev Cell Biol*, 1988. 493–126.
31. Potempa J, Korzus E, Travis J: The serpin superfamily of proteinase inhibitors: structure, function, and regulation, *J Biol Chem* 269(23):15957–15960, 1994.
32. Murphy G, Willenbrock F: Tissue inhibitors of matrix metalloendopeptidases, *Methods in enzymology* 248496–248510, 1995.
33. Bode W, Fernandez-Catalan C, Tschesche H, et al.: Structural properties of matrix metalloproteinases, *Cell Mol Life Sci* 55(4):639–652, 1999.
34. Fernandez-Catalan C, Bode W, Huber R, et al.: Crystal structure of the complex formed by the membrane type 1-matrix metalloproteinase with the tissue inhibitor of metalloproteinases-2, the soluble progelatinase A receptor, *EMBO J* 17(17):5238–5248, 1998.
35. Wei S, Kashiwagi M, Kota S, et al.: Reactive site mutations in tissue inhibitor of metalloproteinase-3 disrupt inhibition of matrix metalloproteinases but not tumor necrosis factor-alpha-converting enzyme, *J Biol Chem* 280(38):32877–32882, 2005.
36. Visse R, Nagase H: Matrix metalloproteinases and tissue inhibitors of metalloproteinases: structure, function, and biochemistry, *Circ Res* 92(8):827–839, 2003.
37. Oh J, Takahashi R, Kondo S, et al.: The membrane-anchored MMP inhibitor RECK is a key regulator of extracellular matrix integrity and angiogenesis, *Cell* 107(6):789–800, 2001.
38. Noda M, Oh J, Takahashi R, et al.: RECK: a novel suppressor of malignancy linking oncogenic signaling to extracellular matrix remodeling, *Cancer Metastasis Rev* 22(2-3):167–175, 2003.
39. Muraguchi T, Takegami Y, Ohtsuka T, et al.: RECK modulates Notch signaling during cortical neurogenesis by regulating ADAM10 activity, *Nature neuroscience* 10(7):838–845, 2007.
40. Gu Z, Kaul M, Yan B, et al.: S-nitrosylation of matrix metalloproteinases: signaling pathway to neuronal cell death, *Science* 297(5584):1186–1190, 2002.

41. Nagase H: Human stromelysins 1 and 2, *Methods in Enzymology* 248449–248470, 1995.
42. Imai K, Yokohama Y, Nakanishi I, et al.: Matrix metalloproteinase 7 (matrilysin) from human rectal carcinoma cells. Activation of the precursor, interaction with other matrix metalloproteinases and enzymic properties, *J Biol Chem* 270(12):6691–6697, 1995.
43. Okada Y, Gonoji Y, Naka K, et al.: Matrix metalloproteinase 9 (92-kDa gelatinase/type IV collagenase) from HT-1080 human fibrosarcoma cells, *J Biol Chem* 26721712–26721719, 1992.
44. Ogata Y, Enghild JJ, Nagase H: Matrix metalloproteinase 3 (stromelysin) activates the precursor for the human matrix metalloproteinase 9, *J Biol Chem* 267(6):3581–3584, 1992.
45. Knäuper V, Lopez-Otin C, Smith B, et al.: Biochemical characterization of human collagenase-3, *J Biol Chem* 271(3):1544–1550, 1996.
46. Pei D, Weiss SJ: Furin-dependent intracellular activation of the human stromelysin-3 zymogen, *Nature* 375(6528):244–247, 1995.
47. Sato H, Kinoshita T, Takino T, et al.: Activation of a recombinant membrane type 1-matrix metalloproteinase (MT1-MMP) by furin and its interaction with tissue inhibitor of metalloproteinases (TIMP)-2, *FEBS Lett* 393(1):101–104, 1996.
48. Itoh Y, Takamura A, Ito N, et al.: Homophilic complex formation of MT1-MMP facilitates proMMP-2 activation on the cell surface and promotes tumor cell invasion, *EMBO J* 20(17):4782–4793, 2001.
49. Itoh Y, Ito N, Nagase H, et al.: The second dimer interface of MT1-MMP, the transmembrane domain, is essential for ProMMP-2 activation on the cell surface, *J Biol Chem* 283(19):13053–13062, 2008.
50. Will H, Atkinson SJ, Butler GS, et al.: The soluble catalytic domain of membrane type 1 matrix metalloproteinase cleaves the propeptide of progelatinase A and initiates autoproteolytic activation. Regulation by TIMP-2 and TIMP-3, *J Biol Chem* 271(29):17119–17123, 1996.
51. Itoh Y, Ito A, Iwata K, et al.: Plasma membrane-bound tissue inhibitor of metalloproteinases (TIMP)-2 specifically inhibits matrix metalloproteinase 2 (gelatinase A) activated on the cell surface, *J Biol Chem* 273(38):24360–24367, 1998.
52. Will H, Hinzmann B: cDNA sequence and mRNA tissue distribution of a novel human matrix metalloproteinase with a potential transmembrane segment, *Eur J Biochem* 231(3):602–608, 1995.
53. Takino T, Sato H, Shinagawa A, et al.: Identification of the second membrane-type matrix metalloproteinase (MT-MMP-2) gene from a human placenta cDNA library. MT-MMPs form a unique membrane-type subclass in the MMP family, *J Biol Chem* 270(39):23013–23020, 1995.
54. Pei D: Identification and characterization of the fifth membrane-type matrix metalloproteinase MT5-MMP, *J Biol Chem* 274(13):8925–8932, 1999.
55. Morrison CJ, Overall CM: TIMP independence of matrix metalloproteinase (MMP)-2 activation by membrane type 2 (MT2)-MMP is determined by contributions of both the MT2-MMP catalytic and hemopexin C domains, *J Biol Chem* 281(36):26528–26539, 2006.
56. Knäuper V, Will H, López-Otín C, et al.: Cellular mechanisms for human procollagenase 3 (MMP 13) activation: evidence that MT1 MMP (MMP 14) and gelatinase a (MMP 2) are able to generate active enzyme, *J Biol Chem* 271(29):17124–17131, 1996.
57. Knäuper V, Bailey L, Worley JR, et al.: Cellular activation of proMMP-13 by MT1-MMP depends on the C-terminal domain of MMP-13, *FEBS Lett* 532(1-2):127–130, 2002.
58. Shiomi T, Inoki I, Kataoka F, et al.: Pericellular activation of proMMP-7 (promatrilysin-1) through interaction with CD151, *Lab Invest* 85(12):1489–1506, 2005.
59. Fujita Y, Shiomi T, Yanagimoto S, et al.: Tetraspanin CD151 is expressed in osteoarthritic cartilage and is involved in pericellular activation of pro-matrix metalloproteinase 7 in osteoarthritic chondrocytes, *Arthritis Rheum* 54(10):3233–3243, 2006.
60. Uekita T, Itoh Y, Yana I, et al.: Cytoplasmic tail-dependent internalization of membrane-type 1 matrix metalloproteinase is important for its invasion-promoting activity, *J Cell Biol* 155(7):1345–1356, 2001.
61. Remacle A, Murphy G, Roghi C: Membrane type I-matrix metalloproteinase (MT1-MMP) is internalised by two different pathways and is recycled to the cell surface, *J Cell Sci* 116(Pt 19):3905–3916, 2003.
62. Anilkumar N, Uekita T, Couchman JR, et al.: Palmitoylation at Cys574 is essential for MT1-MMP to promote cell migration, *FASEB J* 19(10):1326–1328, 2005.
63. Wang X, Ma D, Keski-Oja J, et al.: Co-recycling of MT1-MMP and MT3-MMP through the trans-Golgi network. Identification of DKV582 as a recycling signal, *J Biol Chem* 279(10):9331–9336, 2004.
64. Wang P, Wang X, Pei D: Mint-3 regulates the retrieval of the internalized membrane-type matrix metalloproteinase, MT5-MMP, to the plasma membrane by binding to its carboxyl end motif EWV, *J Biol Chem* 279(19):20461–20470, 2004.
65. Lillis AP, Van Duyn LB, Murphy-Ullrich JE, et al.: LDL receptor-related protein 1: unique tissue-specific functions revealed by selective gene knockout studies, *Physiol Rev* 88(3):887–918, 2008.
66. Zilberberg A, Yaniv A, Gazit A: The low density lipoprotein receptor-1, LRP1, interacts with the human frizzled-1 (HFz1) and down-regulates the canonical Wnt signaling pathway, *J Biol Chem* 279(17):17535–17542, 2004.
67. Kawata K, Kubota S, Eguchi T, et al.: Role of LRP1 in transport of CCN2 protein in chondrocytes, *J Cell Sci* 125(Pt 12):2965–2972, 2012.
68. Troeberg L, Fushimi K, Khokha R, et al.: Calcium pentosan polysulfate is a multifaceted exosite inhibitor of aggrecanases, *FASEB J* 22(10):3515–3524, 2008.
69. Etique N, Verzeaux L, Dedieu S, et al.: LRP-1: a checkpoint for the extracellular matrix proteolysis, *Biomed Res Int* 2013:152163, 2013.
70. Yamamoto K, Murphy G, Troeberg L: Extracellular regulation of metalloproteinases, *Matrix Biol* 44-46:255-263, 2015 .
71. Yamamoto K, Okano H, Miyagawa W, et al.: MMP-13 is constitutively produced in human chondrocytes and co-endocytosed with ADAMTS-5 and TIMP-3 by the endocytic receptor LRP1, *Matrix Biol* 5657–5673, 2016.
72. Fosang AJ, Neame PJ, Last K, et al.: The interglobular domain of cartilage aggrecan is cleaved by PUMP, gelatinases, and cathepsin B, *J Biol Chem* 26719470–26719474, 1992.
73. Rodriguez-Manzaneque JC, Westling J, Thai SN, et al.: ADAMTS1 cleaves aggrecan at multiple sites and is differentially inhibited by metalloproteinase inhibitors, *Biochem Biophys Res Commun* 293(1):501–508, 2002.
74. Imai K, Hiramatsu A, Fukushima D, et al.: Degradation of decorin by matrix metalloproteinases: identification of the cleavage sites, kinetic analyses and transforming growth factor-beta1 release, *Biochem J* 322(Pt 3):809–814, 1997.
75. Yoshihara Y, Nakamura H, Obata K, et al.: Matrix metalloproteinases and tissue inhibitors of metalloproteinases in synovial fluids from patients with rheumatoid arthritis or osteoarthritis, *Ann Rheum Dis* 59(6):455–461, 2000.
76. Yamanaka H, Matsuda Y, Tanaka M, et al.: Serum matrix metalloproteinase 3 as a predictor of the degree of joint destruction during the six months after measurement, in patients with early rheumatoid arthritis, *Arthritis Rheum* 43(4):852–858, 2000.
77. Kobayashi A, Naito S, Enomoto H, et al.: Serum levels of matrix metalloproteinase 3 (stromelysin 1) for monitoring synovitis in rheumatoid arthritis, *Arch Pathol Lab Med* 131(4):563–570, 2007.
78. Catrina AI, Lampa J, Ernestam S, et al.: Anti-tumour necrosis factor (TNF)-alpha therapy (etanercept) down-regulates serum matrix metalloproteinase (MMP)-3 and MMP-1 in rheumatoid arthritis, *Rheumatology (Oxford)* 41(5):484–489, 2002.

79. Miller MC, Manning HB, Jain A, et al.: Membrane type 1 matrix metalloproteinase is a crucial promoter of synovial invasion in human rheumatoid arthritis, *Arthritis Rheum* 60(3):686–697, 2009.
80. Sabeh F, Fox D, Weiss SJ: Membrane-type I matrix metalloproteinase-dependent regulation of rheumatoid arthritis synoviocyte function, *J Immunol* 184(11):6396–6406, 2010.
81. Majkowska I, Shitomi Y, Ito N, et al.: Discoidin domain receptor 2 mediates collagen-induced activation of membrane-type 1 matrix metalloproteinase in human fibroblasts, *J Biol Chem* 292(16):6633–6643, 2017.
82. Murphy G, Nagase H: Reappraising metalloproteinases in rheumatoid arthritis and osteoarthritis: destruction or repair? *Nat Clin Pract Rheumatol* 4(3):128–135, 2008.
83. Fushimi K, Troeberg L, Nakamura H, et al.: Functional differences of the catalytic and non-catalytic domains in human ADAMTS-4 and ADAMTS-5 in aggrecanolytic activity, *J Biol Chem* 283(11):6706–6716, 2008.
84. Gendron C, Kashiwagi M, Lim NH, et al.: Proteolytic activities of human ADAMTS-5: comparative studies with ADAMTS-4, *J Biol Chem* 282(25):18294–18306, 2007.
85. Stanton H, Rogerson FM, East CJ, et al.: ADAMTS5 is the major aggrecanase in mouse cartilage in vivo and in vitro, *Nature* 434(7033):648–652, 2005.
86. Stracke JO, Hutton M, Stewart M, et al.: Biochemical characterization of the catalytic domain of human matrix metalloproteinase 19. Evidence for a role as a potent basement membrane degrading enzyme, *J Biol Chem* 275(20):14809–14816, 2000.
87. Overall CM, Lopez-Otin C: Strategies for MMP inhibition in cancer: innovations for the post-trial era, *Nat Rev Cancer* 2(9):657–672, 2002.
88. Catterall JB, Cawston TE: Drugs in development: bisphosphonates and metalloproteinase inhibitors, *Arthritis Res Ther* 5(1):12–24, 2003.
89. Turk B: Targeting proteases: successes, failures and future prospects. *Nature reviews, Drug discovery* 5(9):785–799, 2006.
90. Wojtowicz-Praga S, Torri J, Johnson M, et al.: Phase I trial of Marimastat, a novel matrix metalloproteinase inhibitor, administered orally to patients with advanced lung cancer, *J Clin Oncol* 16(6):2150–2156, 1998.
91. Koshy PJ, Lundy CJ, Rowan AD, et al.: The modulation of matrix metalloproteinase and ADAM gene expression in human chondrocytes by interleukin-1 and oncostatin M: a time-course study using real-time quantitative reverse transcription-polymerase chain reaction, *Arthritis Rheum* 46(4):961–967, 2002.
92. van Lent PL, Grevers L, Blom AB, et al.: Myeloid-related proteins S100A8/S100A9 regulate joint inflammation and cartilage destruction during antigen-induced arthritis, *Ann Rheum Dis* 67(12):1750–1758, 2008.
93. van Lent PL, Grevers LC, Blom AB, et al.: Stimulation of chondrocyte-mediated cartilage destruction by S100A8 in experimental murine arthritis, *Arthritis Rheum* 58(12):3776–3787, 2008.
94. Fearon U, Mullan R, Markham T, et al.: Oncostatin M induces angiogenesis and cartilage degradation in rheumatoid arthritis synovial tissue and human cartilage cocultures, *Arthritis Rheum* 54(10):3152–3162, 2006.
95. Konttinen YT, Salo T, Hanemaaijer R, et al.: Collagenase-3 (MMP-13) and its activators in rheumatoid arthritis: localization in the pannus-hard tissue junction and inhibition by alendronate, *Matrix Biol* 18(4):401–412, 1999.
96. Jüngel A, Ospelt C, Lesch M, et al.: Effect of the oral application of a highly selective MMP-13 inhibitor in three different animal models of rheumatoid arthritis, *Ann Rheum Dis* 69(5):898–902, 2010.
97. Konttinen YT, Ainola M, Valleala H, et al.: Analysis of 16 different matrix metalloproteinases (MMP-1 to MMP-20) in the synovial membrane: different profiles in trauma and rheumatoid arthritis, *Ann Rheum Dis* 58(11):691–697, 1999.
98. Pap T, Shigeyama Y, Kuchen S, et al.: Differential expression pattern of membrane-type matrix metalloproteinases in rheumatoid arthritis, *Arthritis Rheum* 43(6):1226–1232, 2000.
99. Konttinen YT, Ceponis A, Takagi M, et al.: New collagenolytic enzymes/cascade identified at the pannus-hard tissue junction in rheumatoid arthritis: destruction from above, *Matrix Biol* 17(8-9):585–601, 1998.
100. Kaneko K, Williams RO, Dransfield DT, et al.: Selective inhibition of membrane type 1 matrix metalloproteinase abrogates progression of experimental inflammatory arthritis: synergy with tumor necrosis factor blockade, *Arthritis Rheumatol* 68(2):521–531, 2016.
101. Zhou Z, Apte SS, Soininen R, et al.: Impaired endochondral ossification and angiogenesis in mice deficient in membrane-type matrix metalloproteinase I, *Proc Natl Acad Sci U S A* 97(8):4052–4057, 2000.
102. Matias-Roman S, Galvez BG, Genis L, et al.: Membrane type 1-matrix metalloproteinase is involved in migration of human monocytes and is regulated through their interaction with fibronectin or endothelium, *Blood* 105(10):3956–3964, 2005.
103. Sithu SD, English WR, Olson P, et al.: Membrane-type 1-matrix metalloproteinase regulates intracellular adhesion molecule-1 (ICAM-1)-mediated monocyte transmigration, *J Biol Chem* 282(34):25010–25019, 2007.
104. Delaisse J, Vaes G: Mechanism of mineral solubilization and matrix degradation in osteoclastic bone resorption. In Rifkin BRGC, editor: *Biology and physiology of the osteoclast*, Boca Raton, Fla, 1992, CRC Press, pp 289–314.
105. Gelb BD, Shi GP, Chapman HA, et al.: Pycnodysostosis, a lysosomal disease caused by cathepsin K deficiency, *Science* 273(5279):1236–1238, 1996.
106. Okada Y, Naka K, Kawamura K, et al.: Localization of matrix metalloproteinase 9 (92-kilodalton gelatinase/type IV collagenase = gelatinase B) in osteoclasts: implications for bone resorption, *Lab Invest* 72(3):311–322, 1995.
107. Lynch CC, Hikosaka A, Acuff HB, et al.: MMP-7 promotes prostate cancer-induced osteolysis via the solubilization of RANKL, *Cancer Cell* 7(5):485–496, 2005.
108. Boonen S, Rosenberg E, Claessens F, et al.: Inhibition of cathepsin K for treatment of osteoporosis, *Curr Osteoporos Rep* 10(1):73–79, 2012.
109. Shlopov BV, Lie WR, Mainardi CL, et al.: Osteoarthritic lesions: involvement of three different collagenases, *Arthritis Rheum* 40(11):2065–2074, 1997.
110. Imai K, Ohta S, Matsumoto T, et al.: Expression of membrane-type 1 matrix metalloproteinase and activation of progelatinase A in human osteoarthritic cartilage, *Am J Pathol* 151(1):245–256, 1997.
111. Mohtai M, Smith RL, Schurman DJ, et al.: Expression of 92-kD type IV collagenase/gelatinase (gelatinase B) in osteoarthritic cartilage and its induction in normal human articular cartilage by interleukin 1, *J Clin Invest* 92(1):179–185, 1993.
112. Okada Y, Shinmei M, Tanaka O, et al.: Localization of matrix metalloproteinase 3 (stromelysin) in osteoarthritic cartilage and synovium, *Lab Invest* 66(6):680–690, 1992.
113. Ohta S, Imai K, Yamashita K, et al.: Expression of matrix metalloproteinase 7 (matrilysin) in human osteoarthritic cartilage, *Lab Invest* 78(1):79–87, 1998.
114. Little CB, Barai A, Burkhardt D, et al.: Matrix metalloproteinase 13-deficient mice are resistant to osteoarthritic cartilage erosion but not chondrocyte hypertrophy or osteophyte development, *Arthritis Rheum* 60(12):3723–3733, 2009.
115. Glasson SS, Askew R, Sheppard B, et al.: Deletion of active ADAMTS5 prevents cartilage degradation in a murine model of osteoarthritis, *Nature* 434(7033):644–648, 2005.
116. NaitoS,ShiomiT,OkadaA,etal.:ExpressionofADAMTS4(aggrecanase-1) in human osteoarthritic cartilage, *Pathol Int* 57(11): 703–711, 2007.
117. Yamamoto K, Santamaria S, Botkjaer KA, et al.: Inhibition of shedding of low-density lipoprotein receptor-related protein 1 reverses cartilage matrix degradation in osteoarthritis, *Arthritis Rheumatol* 69(6):1246–1256, 2017.

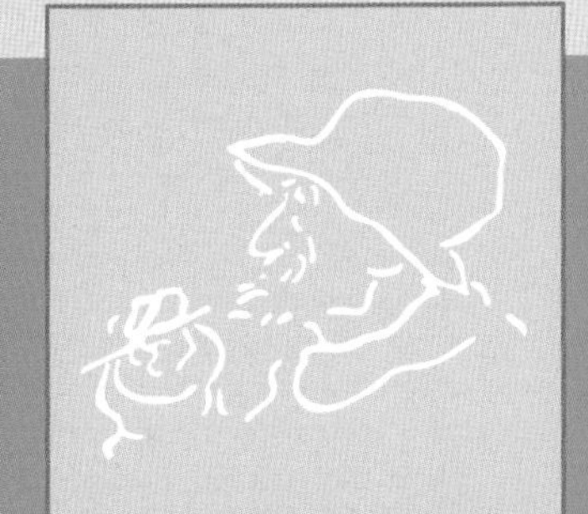

9 Dendritic Cells

MANSI SAXENA, NICOLAS VABRET, LUCIANA RIBEIRO MUNIZ, AND NINA BHARDWAJ

KEY POINTS

- Dendritic cells (DCs) together with monocytes and macrophages compose the mononuclear phagocyte system (MPS).
- DCs are professional antigen-presenting cells (APCs), abundant at body surfaces and within tissues, where they sense and sample the environment for self and non-self antigens.
- Three major subsets of DCs—plasmacytoid DCs (pDCs), conventional DCs (cDCs), and monocyte derived DCs (moDCs)—are characterized by distinct origins, receptors, and functions.
- Upon antigen capture, DCs undergo a process of "maturation" exemplified by enhanced antigen processing, induction of major histocompatibility complex (MHC) molecules, co-stimulatory molecules (CD80/86), and cytokine production. DCs migrate to primary and secondary lymphoid organs, where they present processed antigens to naïve T cells to induce immunity or tolerance.
- Mature DCs acquire the ability to differentiate naïve T cells into T helper (Th) 1, Th2, or Th17 cells, T follicular helper (Tfh), or regulatory T cells (Treg). Maturing DCs also express cytokines that enable the activation of B cells and natural killer (NK) cells and promote the recruitment of other innate immune effector cells.
- DCs are innate immune phagocytic cells, which sense the environment through membrane and cytosolic pattern recognition receptors (PRRs). DCs contribute to the maintenance of tolerance in the thymus and in the periphery, although their functions remain yet partially understood.
- There is a fine equilibrium in DC regulation between tolerogenic and inflammatory states, which can contribute to autoimmune diseases or to tolerance of tumors.
- DCs, as one of the main regulators of the immune response, can either be targeted or used as adjuvants to contain immunopathologies such as autoimmune diseases and cancers, respectively.

Introduction

In 1973 Ralph Steinman and Zanvil Cohn identified a new cell type in murine splenic cultures. They described these as adherent nucleated cells with multiple pseudopods. Owing to their unique morphology, they named them dendritic cells (DCs).[1] A decade later, in 1983, Steinman and Nussenzweig demonstrated that DC depletion completely ablated the stimulatory capacity in murine mixed lymphocyte reactions.[2] Further research revealed that DCs are specialized in acquiring and presenting antigens to T cells and have superior capacity over other antigen-presenting cells (APCs) in activating cytotoxic T lymphocytes (CTLs).[3,4] Moreover, a small number of DCs can directly or indirectly activate a large number of T cells, B cells, natural killer (NK) cells, and NK T cells, thus improving the efficiency of the immune response.[5–7] Furthermore, DCs express a plethora of activating and co-stimulatory receptors and ligands. As such it is no surprise that DCs are often referred to as "nature's adjuvants."

Under normal circumstances DCs exist in an immature form, populating practically every tissue in the body. DCs are activated upon encountering pathogen-associated molecular patterns (PAMPs) or danger-associated molecular patterns (DAMPs), which leads to a process of "maturation" that involves changes in the DC phenotype, antigen acquisition capacity, migration, and an ability to traffic to draining lymph nodes, where they prime cellular and humoral adaptive immune responses. Upon maturation, DCs process antigens (self and non-self) and then present them to antigen-specific adaptive immune cells (T cells and B cells) to induce immune responses to contain diseases such as cancer or infections, but also to maintain tolerance to self-antigens.[8] This chapter provides our current understanding of DC ontogeny and function as well as DCs' potential in clinical applications as immunotherapeutic agents.

Dendritic Cell Subsets and Development

DCs have been classified into subsets based on their location, function, and origin. It is currently believed that all DC subsets undergo four stages of development, namely hematopoietic precursors, DC precursors (pre-DC), immature DCs, and mature DCs. Pre-DCs are continuously produced at a steady rate in a pathogen-independent manner from CD34$^+$ hematopoietic stem cells (HSCs) within the bone marrow. Fms-like tyrosine kinase-3 ligand (Flt-3-L) and granulocyte-macrophage colony-stimulating factor (GM-CSF) represent key DC growth and differentiation factors.[9] The development of stromal cell culture systems, comprising of co-cultures of cord blood isolated CD34$^+$ HSCs and murine bone marrow stromal cells (OP9 cells) in the presence of factors such as stem cell factor (SCF), GM-CSF, and Flt3L have led to the identification of definitive pre-DCs that give rise to DC subsets found in the blood.[10] In humans, all DCs originate from granulocyte monocyte dendritic cell precursors (GMDP), which develop into monocyte dendritic cell precursors (MDP) within the bone marrow. MDPs subsequently give rise to two distinct lineages, the common dendritic cell progenitor (CDP) and the common myeloid progenitor (CMP). The CDPs differentiate

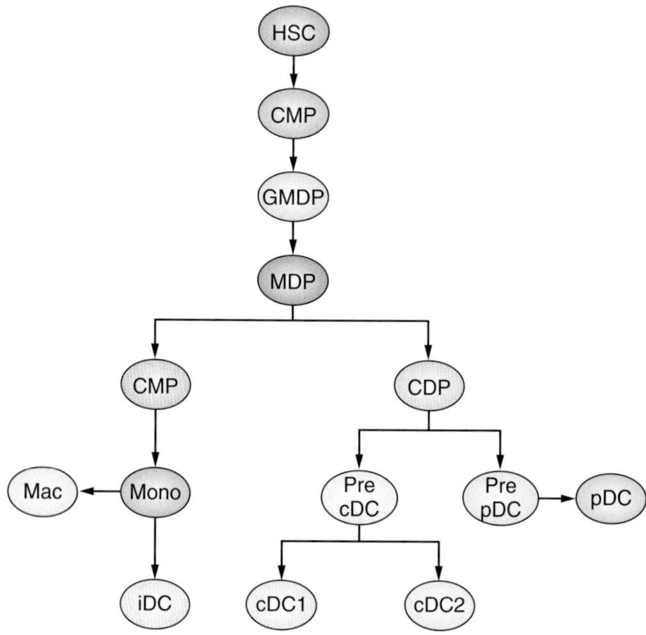

• **Fig. 9.1** Classical model of human dendritic cell (DC) Hematopoiesis. CD34+ hematopoietic stem cells (HSCs) differentiate into common myeloid progenitors (CMPs), which lead to granulocyte macrophage dendritic cell progenitor (GMDPs) and then macrophage dendritic cell progenitor (MDPs). MDPs bifurcate into either common myeloid progenitor (CMP) or common dendritic cell progenitor (CDP). CDPs eventually differentiate into pre-DCs and CMPs into monocytes. Monocytes give rise to macrophages and inflammatory DCs (iDCs) and pre-DCs ultimately give rise to cDC1, cDC2, and pDCs.

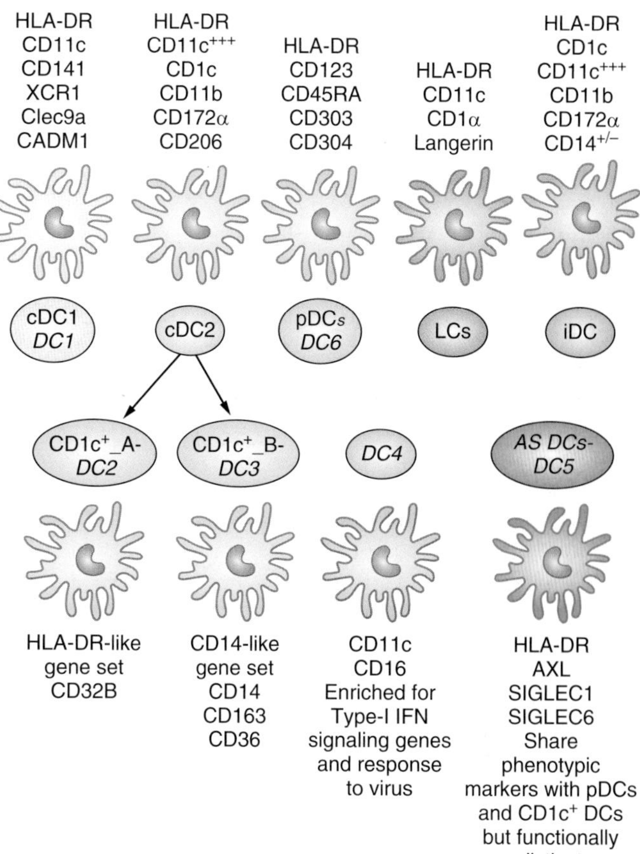

• **Fig. 9.2** Emerging human dendritic cell (DC) subset classification. Simplified depiction of common flow cytometry markers used to delineate different DC subsets, namely cDC1, cDC2, pDC, LCs, and iDCs. Recently, high throughput techniques and unbiased clustering of cells has shed new light on classical DC subset-phenotyping and identified additional two DC subsets within the cDC2 subset, CD1c_A and CD1c_B and one new subset under pDCs, the AS-DCs (Axl and Siglec6 positive DCs). The new subsets identified by investigators,[38] DC1-DC6, are marked by italics text. (Adapted from Saxena M, et al. Towards superior dendritic-cell vaccines for cancer therapy. *Nat Biomed Eng* 2[6]:341–346, 2018,[14] with permission.)

into pre-DCs that migrate out of the bone marrow and give rise to two classical DC subsets, the conventional DCs (cDCs) and plasmacytoid DCs (pDCs), whereas the CMPs differentiate into inflammatory DCs (iDCs), found in blood[11] (Fig. 9.1).

For ex vivo studies and phenotyping in humans, DCs are identified as cells lacking the expression of lineage markers CD3 (T cell marker), CD19, and CD20 (B cell markers), CD14 (monocytic marker), and CD56 (NK cell marker) and as being positive for HLA-DR.[12] Terminally differentiated DCs are broadly classified into four subsets, namely cDCs, pDCs, iDCs, and Langerhans cells (LCs). However, recent fate mapping studies have contested the classification of LCs as DCs, arguing that LCs fall into the tissue macrophage category.[13]

Conventional Dendritic Cells

cDCs comprise two subsets in humans and mice, cDC1 and cDC2 (see Fig. 9.1). In humans, cDC1s are commonly phenotyped by surface expression of Clec9a, CD141, low CD11c, XCR1, and CADM1 (Fig. 9.2) while murine cDC1s express CD8a and/or CD103. The cDC2 cells in humans are typically CD1c+, and they express high CD11c, CD11b, and CD172a (see Fig. 9.2). In mice they are CD4+ and CD11b+.[14–16] While both cDC1 and cDC2 can activate CD4+ and CD8+ T cells, several key differences distinguish cDC1s from cDC2s. For instance, cDC1s are considered more adept at antigen cross-presentation and at CD8+ T cell activation than any other APCs, including cDC2s. Cross-presentation is a unique antigen-presentation pathway that allows APCs to present exogenous antigens on class I MHC molecules; this pathway is described in detail later. Second, although cDC1 can be found in blood in small numbers, these cells are thought to primarily reside in the lymph node, while the cDC2s are migratory cells, outnumbering cDC1s in peripheral tissues by several fold.[15]

A key difference between DCs is the array of pattern recognition receptors (PRRs) expressed by each subset. PRRs are an important class of receptors that recognize pathogen-associated molecular patterns (PAMPs, expressed by microorganisms) or danger-associated molecular patterns (DAMPs, secreted by damaged cells). PRRs include secreted receptors such as MBL, CRP, SAP, LBP; cell-surface receptors like Toll-like receptors (TLRs1/2/4/5/6), CD14, MMR, MSR, MARCO,[17] and intra-cellular receptors such as TLRs3/7/8/9, RIG-I and MDA5, STING, DAI, AIM2, and NOD receptors. cDC1s primarily express TLR3 and TLR8 and in response to their stimulation secrete IL-12 as well as Type-III interferons. By contrast, cDC2s express and respond to a wider range of TLRs.[18]

The cDC1 and cDC2 cells exert distinct transcriptional programs.[10] cDC1s express interferon response element-8 (IRF8), Batf3, Bcl16, and Flt3, whereas the cDC2s express IRF4, Csl, and Klf4.[9,19] Notch signaling is a unique cell-to-cell signaling pathway that controls development of several immune cells including DCs. Stimulation of transmembrane Notch receptors by Delta-like ligands (DLL) 1, 3, and 4, or Jagged ligands (Jagged 1 and 2), leads to gamma-secretase driven Notch receptor cleavage. This event is followed by nuclear translocation of Notch intra-cellular domain and interaction with the transcription factor Csl (or RBPJ in mice). Overall, this pathway facilitates cellular development, maintenance, and differentiation programs.[20] The role of Notch signaling in DC differentiation has remained controversial with different research models yielding conflicting reports.[21] However, two independent groups recently confirmed the importance of Notch signaling in DC programming. Using the OP9 feeder culture system, Notch-2 signaling regulated pDC versus cDC differentiation from the precursor cells in both mice and humans.[10,22] Specifically, in the context of human cells, investigators demonstrated that expanding CD34⁺ cells (from either human cord blood or peripheral blood mononuclear cells [PBMCs]) with Flt3L, S-CSF, IL7, and thrombopoietin (TPO) for 7 days followed by co-culture with OP9 cells yielded a high number of pDCs but not many cDC1s. However, co-culturing CD34⁺ cells with a mixture of OP9 and OP9_DLL1 cells (OP9 cells expressing Notch ligand DLL1) remarkably increased the yield of cDC1s while moderately inhibiting the yield of pDCs.[10] These Notch-dependent cDC1 cells were functionally and transcriptionally similar to cDC1s found in blood, suggesting the significance of Notch signaling for cDC1 differentiation in vivo. Other studies in murine models have emphasized the role of Notch signaling in cDC2 development, particularly in context of T follicular cell activation and induction of B cell response during infection.[23]

Plasmacytoid Dendritic Cells

pDCs are distinguished by expression of CD123, CD303, CD304, and lack of CD11c (see Fig. 9.2). The geospatial distribution of pDCs is more restricted than cDCs. Although small numbers of pDCs can been found in blood and tissues such as nasal mucosa, pDCs primarily populate T cell areas of lymphoid tissues.[24] The production of extraordinarily high levels of Type-1 interferon is unique to this cell type and is important for initiating a strong antiviral innate response, promoting maturation of bystander CD11c⁺ cDCs and protecting cDCs from the cytopathic effect of viruses.[25] This response is primarily enabled by high expression of TLR7 and TLR9 on pDCs and their ability to rapidly present intra-cellular antigens, like those derived from viruses, to CD8⁺ T cells.[26,27]

Interestingly, upon activation, pDCs have been reported to differentiate into cells bearing similar characteristics to activated cDCs (such as high expression of class II MHC molecules and the capacity to prime naïve T cells) but express low levels of CD11c and lack the typical myeloid markers.[28,29] All these studies highlight the complexity and plasticity of DC development.

Inflammatory Dendritic Cells

iDCs arise from monocytic precursors during infection and inflammation in blood and migrate to the site of inflammation. iDCs are characterized by surface expression of CD1c, high expression of CD11c, CD11b, CD172a, and CD14 (see Fig. 9.2) and MCSFR and ZBTB46 as transcription factors.[30] iDCs can process and present antigens to both CD4⁺ and CD8⁺ T cells; however, their exact functional profile in vivo remains undetermined.[31] It is postulated that the monocyte-derived dendritic cells (moDCs) (Fig. 9.3), used in most DC-based cell therapy vaccines, closely resemble the in vivo iDCs. moDCs are generated from monocytes isolated from patient blood, and ex vivo differentiated into immature DCs under the influence of GM-CSF and IL4.[32]

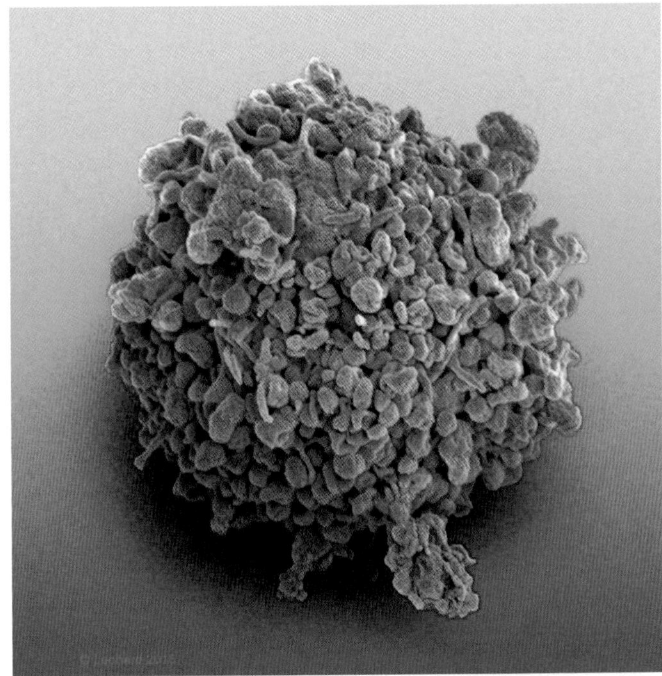

• **Fig. 9.3** Examples of monocyte-derived mature dendritic cell. The mononuclear cells were enriched by adherence, cultured with interleukin-4 (IL-4) and granulocyte-macrophage colony-stimulating factor (GM-CSF) for 6 days, and underwent maturation with PolyICLC for 24 hours. The cells were imaged by Transmission Electron Micrography. (Image provided by Andrew Paul Leonard, www. aplmicro.com.)

Langerhans Cells

LCs are self-renewing epidermal myeloid cells located in the epidermis, where they form a network between keratinocytes. LCs are also observed in squamous stratified epithelia, such as bronchiolar tissue, and in oral and genital mucous membranes. They can migrate and mature into DCs. LCs express shared common markers, such as CD11c, CD1a and the C-type lectin receptor (CLR) langerin (CD207) (see Fig. 9.2). A skin homing receptor, cutaneous lymphocyte-associated antigen (CLA), has been implicated in regulating the migratory potential of LCs.[33,34] Langerin, a common marker of LCs, delivers antigen through receptor-mediated endocytosis to Birbeck granules; these granules are structures connected to the endosomal network that are implicated in canonical and non-canonical antigen processing and presentation.[35] LCs were initially classified as DCs due to their function as APCs, their capacity for migrating to lymph nodes, and inducing T cell activation. However, recent developments in fate mapping studies suggest that LCs originate from the yolk sac progenitors and the fetal liver and differentiate into specialized tissue resident macrophages.[36,37]

New Developments in Dendritic Cell Classification

Using single-cell RNA sequencing, a recent study analyzed blood DCs with unbiased gene clustering and identified six DC subsets *(DC1-DC6)*. The new classification emerging from this study consists of (see Fig. 9.2):

- The *DC1* and *DC6* subsets corresponding to predefined cDC1 and pDC subsets.

- The *DC2* (CD1c+_A) and *DC3* (CD1c+_B) subsets were identified as two unique clusters under the cDC2 subset. Both *DC2* and *DC3* subsets express CD1c, CD11b, and CD11c but unlike *DC2*, the *DC3* subset was enriched for CD14 and acute and chronic inflammatory gene set.
- The *DC4* subset, negative for both CD141 and CD1c, was found enriched for CD16 and in genes involved in Type-I interferon secretion and response to virus.
- A novel but small subset, *DC5*, did not cluster with any other blood DC subset and can be identified by the expression of Axl and Siglec6, earning the name "AS-DCs." Despite sharing many markers with pDCs, AS-DCs are functionally, phenotypically, and morphologically distinct from pDCs.[38]

These results were corroborated by investigators, who employed flight mass cytometry (CyToF) to identify DC subsets in blood and tissue.[39] The authors also reported a conserved phenotype of cDC1 and cDC2 between blood and lymphoid organs while the skin DCs displayed tissue-specific phenotype with considerable inter-individual heterogeneity. However, the precise functionality of these newly discovered subsets remains to be determined.

In addition to subsets mentioned previously, other groups, over the years, have described atypical DC subsets that do not identify with any classical DC subset. These include a small pool of migratory precursor cells that originate from the CDPs in the bone marrow and can only differentiate into either CD1c$^+$ or CD141$^+$ cDCs.[40] A group of CD103$^+$ DCs in the intestinal LNs has been reported to induce expression of gut homing receptor, CCR9 on T cell and B cells through a retinoic acid receptor-dependent mechanism. Furthermore, intestinal CD103 DCs process dietary vitamin A into retinoic acid to support the differentiation of gut-homing FoxP3$^+$ regulatory T cells (Tregs).[41,42]

Dendritic Cell Maturation and Activation

DC maturation is a complex process that relies on key functional properties, such as activation by environmental sensing, antigen uptake, processing and presentation, migration, and T cell stimulation. The DC process of maturation is related to their environment and is therefore heterogeneous. It confers specific and distinctive functional properties to different DC subsets.[18]

DC maturation can be prompted by several activating cues such as pathogen or nonpathogen derived factors, cellular debris, stress signals, and receptor-ligand interaction, among others. In the steady state, cDCs are in a quiescent state that is characterized by a low surface expression of MHC molecules and co-stimulatory molecules, such as CD80, CD83, CD86, and CD40. Immunogenic conditioning of cDCs induces expression of class I and II MHC, T cell co-stimulatory molecules, such as CD80 and CD86, cytokines (e.g., TNF, IL-12, IL-18), and chemokines (e.g., RANTES, MIP-1α, IP-10). Additional changes include induction of CCR7, CCL19 and CCL21-dependent migration to follicular T cell–enriched zones in lymphoid organs and downregulation of receptors that serve to retain DCs at the site of activation (such as receptors for CCL3, CCL4 and CCL5). Upon antigen uptake the DCs are programmed to dampen antigen acquisition and processing and promote antigen presentation. DCs acquire the ability to induce clonal expansion and differentiation of antigen-specific naïve T cells into effector T cells.[43]

The activation and maturation event also polarizes the DCs toward a tolerogenic or immunogenic phenotype. Based on their environmental conditioning, DCs regulate the adaptation of T cell polarization to the specific nature of the stimuli. For example, activation of DCs in the absence of help from CD4$^+$ T cells, activation with suboptimal or prolonged innate stimuli, or maturation in response to stimuli like thymic stromal lymphopoietin (TSLP) which leads to induction of co-stimulatory molecules but does not induce an inflammatory cytokine response, can all lead to tolerogenic DCs. In the steady state, tolerogenic DCs are thought to present self-antigen and promote peripheral tolerance. However, in events of tumorigenesis or infection, tolerogenic DCs promote tumor evasion and inhibit pathogen clearance, respectively.[44–47] Indeed, tolerogenic DCs have often been observed in cases of chronic activation such as in cancer. Moreover, several pathogens have developed specific mechanisms of immune evasion via induction of tolerogenic DCs.[48]

Activation allows immature DCs to acquire a diverse array of antigens from pathogens, exosomes, apoptotic cells, etc.[49] Pathways of antigen acquisition include, micropinocytosis, macropinocytosis, receptor-mediated endocytosis, and phagocytosis. Activation and maturation via pattern recognition receptors (PRRs) is a key initial step in antigen acquisition, processing and presentation.

Pattern-Recognition Receptors and Dendritic Cell Maturation

DCs sense their environment through a broad panel of PRRs. PRRs are highly conserved innate immune receptors that detect PAMPs or endogenous DAMPs. PRRs are extremely diverse, detecting a wide range of molecular patterns, including proteins, lipids, carbohydrates, nucleic acids, and mineral crystals.[17] PRRs include the Toll Like Receptors (TLRs), the C-type lectin Receptors (CLRs), the Nod-like receptors (NLRs), the retinoic acid–inducible gene (RIG)-I–like receptors (RLRs), the scavenger receptors (SRs), the integrins, and others such as the Ig Fc receptors (FcRs). Triggering of PRRs such as TLRs or C-type lectins on DCs is thought to be critical for their functional maturation and the priming of T cell responses to infection, therefore coupling innate and adaptive immunity.

RLRs and Intra-cellular DNA Sensors. RIG-I and MDA5 RNA helicases are intra-cellularly expressed PRRs involved in the recognition of intra-cellular RNA upon viral infection[50] while cGAS and AIM2 receptors recognize intra-cellular DNA.[51]

TLRs. TLRs are a prominent class of PRRs that respond to PAMPs, such as peptidoglycan, lipopolysaccharide (LPS), and flagellin, and regulate DC functions. TLRs can be grouped into two subfamilies based on their subcellular localization: the TLRs expressed on the cell surface (in humans and mice, TLR1, TLR2, TLR5, and TLR6, and restricted to mice, TLR11, TLR12, and TLR13) and those localized to specialized endosomal compartments (TLR3, TLR7, TLR8, and TLR9). Finally, TLR4 can localize to both sites. Each DC subset expresses distinct panels of TLRs, which modulate their functional specialization. Human pDCs express high levels of nucleic acid-specific TLRs such as TLR7 and TLR9. TLR7 and TLR9 detect ssRNA and unmethylated cytosine-phosphatidyl-guanine (CpG) DNA, respectively, which are motifs usually found in both bacteria and viruses. TLR8 also recognizes bacterial ssRNA. Human CD1c$^+$ cDCs express mostly TLR1 through TLR8 and TLR10, whereas the CD141$^+$ cDCs express TLR3 and TLR7/8 and low levels of TLR1 and TLR2. Activation of DCs in response to binding of TLR agonists is controlled by signaling through the Toll/IL-1 receptor (TIR) domain present in the cytoplasmic domain of TLRs. TLR stimulation by self- and non-self-antigens can regulate cytokines such as TNF, IL-12, IL-6, IL-23, and IL-17, which have an important role in the polarization of T helper cell subsets during priming by DCs, and thus the functional consequences of DC activation.[52]

NLRs. Another important inflammatory signaling circuit governed by PRRs is the inflammasome pathway. The inflammasome is a multiprotein complex that can be activated through NLRs like NLRP3, NLRC4, or NLRP1 through PAMPs (such as pore-forming toxins, RNA and DNA, flagellin, β-glucans, and zymosan) or DAMPs (such as adenosine triphosphate [ATP], uric acid crystals, amyloid β, alum, silica and asbestos). Inflammasome activation induces the activation of key inflammatory cytokines, such as IL-1β and IL-18, and regulates an inflammatory cell death pathway known as pyroptosis.[53] Each NLR regulates a unique inflammasome activation cascade. NLRP3 inflammasome is activated in a two-step process.[54] The first step requires TLR2 or 4 driven upregulation of key inflammasome components, namely NLRP3, ASC, pro-IL-1β, and pro-IL18. The second step involves NLRP3 activation, assembly of the inflammasome complex, caspase1 cleavage and subsequent release of cytokines and possibly the induction of pyroptosis.[55]

CLRs. C-Type lectins are another family of PRRs that recognize sugar motifs in a calcium-dependent manner through their carbohydrate recognition functional domain. The repertoire of CLR expression varies among the different DC subsets and is tightly regulated by the interactions with the environment. CLRs are involved in endocytosis, phagocytosis, antigen processing, and presentation through regular class II MHC or by class I MHC cross-presentation. Several CLRs, such as DEC205, mannose receptor (MR), and DC immunoreceptor (DCIR), contribute to the cross-presentation of endocytosed antigens. DC-SIGN, a CLR expressed on many DCs is well known for interacting with pathogens like HIV-1 and 2, SIV etc. Some CLRs are mostly restricted to specific DC subsets such as langerin on LCs. BDCA-2 expressed by pDCs shares similar immunomodulatory properties as DEC-205 and has been targeted by recombinant antigens bound to antibodies in order to modulate DC function. This is accomplished by inducing antigen-specific tolerance or immune stimulation with the addition of a maturation signal. Finally, many CLRs recognize ligands expressed by apoptotic or necrotic cells and participate in the uptake of these dead cells by DCs, although most of the clearing process is mediated by neutrophils and macrophages. DNRG1 (CLEC9a) is expressed on CD141$^+$ DCs and recognizes F-actin, which is expressed at the surface of necrotic cells. This interaction induces immunogenic responses and promotes the cross-presentation of processed necrotic antigens on class I MHC. In the same way, macrophage-inducible C-type lectin (MINCLE), which is another CLR that recognizes necrotic cells, can induce inflammatory responses.[56]

Fc Receptors. FcRs, expressed by many immune cells, are important in regulation of immune responses to immune complexes composed of antigen bound to antibody and sometimes to components of the complement system. DCs express activating receptors FcγRI, FcγRIIA, FcγRIIIA, and inhibitory receptor FcγRIIB. Infected cells or pathogens coated with IgG activate FcγR-mediated clearance by antibody-dependent cell-mediated cytotoxicity (ADCC) or phagocytosis and/or indirectly through the release of cytokines.[17]

In addition to the receptors mentioned above, scavenger receptors (SRs) like CD36, CD-205, LOX-1, to name a few, promote DC activation and maturation. These receptors also regulate multiple cellular functions like pathogen clearance and apoptotic cell clearance. For example, CD36 on DCs detects phospholipid phoshatidylserine on apoptotic cells and facilitates apoptotic cell clearance. LOX-1 promotes DC activation by oxidized low density lipoprotein (LDL) and contributes to artherosclerosis.[57] Complement receptors on DCs regulate opsonization of pathogens and dying cells.[49] DCs also express receptors that specifically bind pathogens like CD4, CCR5 and CXCR4 that bind HIV. Other receptors aid in activating atypical immune cells. For example, the CD1 family of receptors allow DCs to present antigens such as sphingolipids, sulfatides and glycosphingolipids to activate γδT cells, and NK T cells. Hence, many distinct families of receptors, adorn and regulate DC function.[6,17,27]

Over the past decade it has become evident that DC activation, especially through TLRs, significantly influences not just antigen acquisition, but also the process of antigen presentation. TLR-induced DC activation induces an innate immune response conducive to micropinocytic antigen uptake, but only transiently, followed by a near cessation of antigen uptake.[58]

Antigen Processing and Presentation

DCs are specialized in antigen processing and can efficiently present endogenous and exogenous antigens in both class I and II MHC contexts. This activity is influenced by the maturation and activation status of the DC, which promotes phagolysosome maturation, peptide processing, peptide macropinocytosis, and DC metabolism to promote antigen processing and presentation of antigens by class I MHC and class II MHC, as well as lipid presentation by CD1 molecules.

Major Histocompatibility Complex Class I Antigen Presentation

DCs express class I MHC molecules on their cell surface bearing self or non-self peptides derived from the cytosol. These peptides are predominantly generated from ubiquitinated nascent, misfolded, and neosynthesized defective self-proteins, or defective ribosomal products (DRiPs). In the cytoplasm, the cytosolic proteasome, comprising of interferon regulated PA28 proteasome activator and leucine aminopeptidase, cleaves these proteins into peptides of appropriate length for presentation on class I MHC molecules.[59,60] Interestingly, DC maturation enhances antigen processing through upregulation of such immuneproteosomes. After being processed in the cytoplasm the trimmed peptides are translocated to the endoplasmic reticulum (ER) through the transporter associated with antigen processing (TAP) and further shortened to 8-9mer peptides, optimal length for loading onto class I MHC (Fig. 9.4). This shortening of peptides in the ER is performed by ER aminopeptidase-1 (ERAP-1). Once a stable class I MHC-antigen complex is formed, it is routed to the cell surface.

Cross-Presentation

DCs have the unique capacity to acquire antigens exogenously, internalize them, and process them for presentation on class I MHC molecules. This property is atypical because, in most cells, class I MHC molecules exclusively present endogenous proteins. Although the precise mechanism of cross-presentation remains controversial, it is well established that DCs use this process to activate CD8$^+$ T cells. DCs acquire antigens by endocytosis in the form of apoptotic cells, necrotic cells, antibody-opsonized cells, immune complexes, heat shock proteins, and exosomes, and even by nibbling of live cells.[61,62] Two main intra-cellular pathways, the

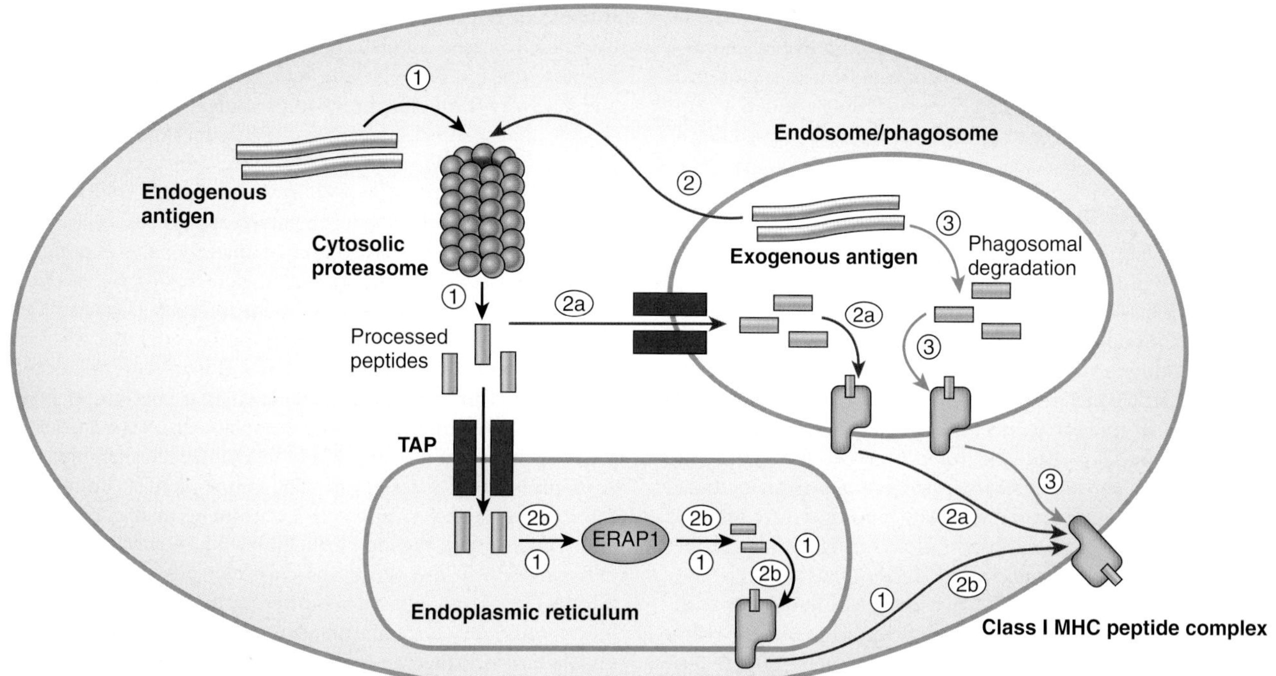

• **Fig. 9.4** Class I MHC antigen presentation by dendritic cells. DCs present endogenous antigens on class I MHC through the classical pathway *(1),* where endogenous antigens is degraded by the cytosolic proteasome. The degraded peptides are transported into the Endoplasmic Reticulum (ER) through TAP, further shortened through ERAP-1, loaded on to class I MHC and the class I MHC peptide complex is transported to the cell surface. *(2 and 3)* DCs also possess the unique capacity to process and present exogenous antigens on class I MHC, in a process called cross presentation through the cytosolic and the vacuolar pathways. *(2)* In the cytosolic pathway the exogenous antigen in the phagosomes or endosomes is transported into the cytosol and degraded by the cytosolic proteasome. Thereafter, either the peptides are transported back into the endosome *(2a)* for loading onto class I MHC or *(2b),* the peptides are transported into the ER and processed there for class I MHC loading. Finally, the class I MHC peptide complex is transported to the cell surface. *(3)* In the Vacuolar pathway, the exogenous antigen in the endosome or phagosome is processed within this compartment and loaded onto class I MHC. Class I MHC peptide complex is transported to the cell surface. *ERAP-1,* ER aminopeptidase-1; *TAP,* transporter associated with antigen processing.

cytosolic and the vacuolar pathways, traffic exogenous antigens from phagolysosomal compartments to the ER for cross-presentation (see Fig. 9.4).[63]

In the cytosolic pathway (also referred as *endosome-to-cytosol pathway*), antigens are transferred to the cytoplasm from the endosomal compartment and processed by the cytosolic proteasome. Thereafter the peptides are transported back into the endosome or to the ER where they are loaded onto class I MHC molecules. Class I MHC molecules, however, need to be present in the ER or the endosomes to be available for antigen loading. For this, either newly assembled class I MHC molecules are transported into the ER[64] or cell surface expressed class I MHC complexes are recycled back into the endosome for reloading[65] (see Fig. 9.4). This pathway is sensitive to proteasome inhibitors, suggesting that antigenic-proteins access the cytosol and are degraded by proteasomes. Yet, whether the peptide loading occurs via the classical class I MHC pathway described previously or in endocytic compartments remains to be fully determined.[66]

Antigen processing and loading through the vacuolar pathway is believed to occur in the endocytic compartments. This conclusion stems from the observations that inhibition of lysosomal proteolysis inhibits antigen presentation via this pathway, whereas inhibition of cytosolic proteasomes has no effect (see Fig. 9.4).[67] While some evidence suggests that cytosolic pathway maybe the predominant antigen processing mechanism here, there is no clear indication as to the relative contribution of cytosolic pathway over vacuolar pathway. Data from several groups indicate that DCs in general[68] and specific DC subsets such as the CD8α$^+$ DCs in mice and DC1s in humans are more specialized for cross-presentation than other APCs.[69,70] Recently, progress has been made in better understanding the cross-talk between the different cellular compartments that regulate the cross-presentation. Nair-Gupta and collaborators have identified an important role in DCs for communication between the endosomal recycling compartment (ERC), which is a key reservoir of class I MHC molecules, and the phagosome in cross-presentation. Trafficking from the ERC to phagosomes is controlled by the TLR-MyD88-IKK2 pathway, which stabilizes membrane interactions between the phagosome and the ERC, ensuring that ERC-deployed class I MHC are specifically routed to phagosomes engaged in TLR signaling. On the other hand, the class I MHC peptide loading complex (PLC) is recruited from another subcellular compartment, the ER and Golgi intermediate compartment (ERGIC), in a TLR-independent manner. The highly coordinated trafficking from ERC and ERGIC delivers essential components for cross-presentation to phagosomes during infection, and control of the ERC pathway by TLR signals favors phagosomes that contain microbial proteins for cross-presentation in the context of TLR-primed T cell co-stimulation.[65]

Interestingly, DCs have been documented to acquire complete functional class I MHC-antigen complex from a donor cell and decorate on their own (recipient) cell surface. This mode of antigen presentation has been coined "cross-dressing" and is postulated to boost a memory like response in previously primed CD8⁺ T cells.[71]

Major Histocompatibility Class II Antigen Presentation

While all nucleated cells express class I MHC, only APCs express class II MHC. Class II MHC presents short peptides to activate CD4⁺ T cells. Class II MHCα/β heterodimers rely on a specialized type II transmembrane chaperone protein, the invariant chain (Ii), for stable assembly in the ER. Assembled class II MHC molecules are transported and concentrated in multivesicular and multilamellar late endosomal compartments called class II MHC–containing compartments (MIICs). Antigens for class II MHC loading are acquired by APCs through macropinocytosis, receptor-mediated endocytosis, phagocytosis, and autophagy.[72] Antigens are retained within late endosome or phagosomes before fusing with lysosomes to form phagolysosomes. Concomitant TLR signals induce activation of the vacuolar proton pump that enhances lysosomal acidification and antigen proteolysis into antigenic peptides within phagolysosomes. Acidification of this compartment allows optimal activity of cathepsin S. Cathepsin S degrades the cytoplasmic tail of Ii, leaving a short peptide, the class II MHC–associated invariant-chain peptide (CLIP), bound to the peptide-binding groove and thus protected from proteases. CLIP is replaced by an antigenic peptide through the action of the catalyst-chaperone protein HLA-DM, which accelerates the rate of CLIP release, and the loaded class II MHC molecules are thought to be transported through cytoskeletal tubular structures that are directed toward the site of T cell interaction at the plasma membrane.[73–75]

DCs display several specializations in antigen processing/presentation mechanisms that distinguish them from other APCs. For instance, as opposed to macrophages that rapidly degrade internalized antigens, DCs process antigens slowly, thus allowing sufficient time for the DCs to mature and migrate to the lymphoid organs. Once mature, DCs increase proteolysis and quickly process antigens for MHC presentation for maximal T cell activation. TLR engagement regulates phagosome maturation,[74] enhances lysosomal acidification,[76] and increases antigen uptake transiently.[72] Class II MHC surface expression and turnover rates are regulated by cytoplasmic domain ubiquitination in DCs. This mechanism explains the expression of low levels of class II MHC molecules by immature DCs and their increase in half-life after maturation, sustaining antigen presentation after migration into secondary lymphoid organs.

T Cell Activation

T cells are primed and activated by DCs in the lymph nodes (see also Chapter 12). Lymph nodes are specialized immune organs situated at the confluence of lymphatic vessels and organized into the outermost cortex and inner medulla. The medulla contains macrophages and medullary cords, and plasma cells that secrete antibodies. The cortex is organized into two sections, the para-cortex region where T cells and APCs converge, and the outer-cortex where B cells form lymphoid follicles. The T cell-rich para-cortex is also referred to as the *T cell zone*.[77] Upon activation, immature cDCs migrate through afferent lymph from nonlymphoid tissues to the T cell zone in the lymph nodes. pDCs and naïve T cells migrate into T cell areas through the high endothelial venules (HEVs) of lymph nodes and marginal zone of the spleen, likely using CCR7 and CD62-L. Both activated blood cDCs and pDCs migrate in response to lymph node homing chemokines (CCL19 and CCL21) through expression of CCR7.[78]

An inflammatory gradient guides the movement of T cells and DCs around the lymph node. However, the exact composition of this gradient is uncertain. Similarly, while DC-T cell interaction is known to take place within the para-cortex, its exact location and kinetics are unknown. Furthermore, factors such as antigen burden (replicating infectious agent vs. non-replicative vaccine antigen) and the type of antigen (blood borne, cell free lymph borne, or carried by DCs) dictate the strength and kinetics of DC-T cell interaction.[77] Elegant intra-vital fluorescent microscopy in sophisticated murine models indicates that the lymph node-resident DCs and migratory DCs populate discrete sections of the para-cortex.[79] The murine models demonstrate that the resident cross-presenting cDCs (most likely equivalent to human cDC1 cells, though not yet validated) accumulate in the deep-cortex in close proximity to the incoming CD8⁺ T cells while the migratory cDCs remain in the peripheral cortex in proximity to the CD4⁺ T cells.[80,81] Thus, upon encountering antigens in the tissues or blood, migratory DCs mature, process, and present these antigens on MHCs and travel to the peripheral cortex of the lymph nodes where they activate the helper CD4⁺ T cells. Activated CD4⁺ T cells in turn facilitate activation of CD8⁺ T cells in deep-cortex by licensing the lymph node resident cross-presenting DCs.[82]

It is postulated that antigen-loaded DCs activate T cells over several hours and three dynamic phases requiring three distinct cell-to-cell signals.[83] First, incoming naïve T cells survey DCs in short bursts to find a matching antigen-MHC combination, aggregating each antigen specific signal. Second, once the activation signals reach a cumulative threshold, T cells initiate a sustained engagement with DCs, leading to their activation. Induction of memory T cells also takes place during this step. In the third phase, T cells start proliferating and break the prolonged DC engagement, reverting to transient contact.[83] Cell-free antigens that enter the lymph node though passive diffusion in the lymph are processed by a specialized DC subset residing within the lymphatic sinus epithelium. These DCs can rapidly activate T cells, bypassing the lengthy three phase process mentioned previously.[84] After clonal expansion, the activated antigen specific T cells exit the lymph node and go back in the circulation to locate their target cells.

During T cell activation, several factors influence generation of CD8⁺ memory T cells, such as the load of antigen on DCs and frequency of CD8⁺ T cell precursors.[85] Moreover, generation of effective CD8 memory T cells requires CD4⁺ T cell help in the form of secreted IL-2 and CD40L-CD40 interaction.[86] However, if the frequency of antigen specific CD8⁺ T cells is sufficiently high, the need for CD4⁺ T cell help may be dispensable for CD8⁺ T cell activation, but might still be required to establish memory responses, to protect primed CD8⁺ T cells from receptor mediated cell death and to avoid T cell exhaustion.[87]

Perhaps due to the army of co-stimulatory molecules involved in DC-T cell synapse, a small number of MHC-peptide complexes (<200) on the surface of mature DCs are sufficient to elicit a large T cell response, making DCs up to 1000 times more efficient at T cell activation than other APCs. The strength and duration of immunological synapse between T cells and DCs dictates the quality of T cell response based on three signals. Signal 1 is generated when the T cell receptor (TCR) engages a peptide–MHC complex on the APC. Signal 2 is generated when co-stimulatory molecules on APCs engage their ligands on T cells. This signal determines the qualitative and quantitative elements of T cell activation and differentiation, and is required for priming of naïve T cells. Co-stimulatory molecules include the CD80 and CD86 members of the B7 family, which ligate to CD28 on T cells, and members of the TNF family, such as CD40.[88] Other molecules play inhibitory roles upon encountering their receptors on T cells. For example, ICOS-L is present on both DC and B cells and engages ICOS on T cells to modulate T cell activity. Programmed death ligand 1 (PDL1) on DCs interacts with PD1 on T cells to downregulate T cell responses. It should be noted that many inhibitory TCRs like ICOS and PD1 are required to initiate T cell activation and in early stages of activation serve as markers of effector T cell functions. For example, mice lacking the expression of ICOS or ICOS-L failed to mount anti-tumor responses upon receiving anti-CTLA4 checkpoint therapy.[89] Moreover, emerging data indicate that CD80 on DCs interacts in cis with PDL1. Such CD80-PDL1 interaction on the DC cell surface inhibits binding of PDL1 with PD1 expressed on T cells, thus preventing T cell exhaustion.[90] Finally, signal 3 is derived from cytokines secreted by APCs. Cytokines such as IL-12 (for Th1) or IL-4 (for Th2) determine the skewing of the T cell response such that T cells may terminally differentiate toward either IFN-gamma producing Th1 cells (under the influence of IL-12), which eradicate intra-cellular pathogens (bacteria or viruses), or into IL-4, IL-5, and IL-13 producing Th2 cells (under the influence of IL-4), which promote elimination of extra-cellular infections. In addition, the signal 3 can also prompt differentiation into IL-10-secreting Treg cells that dampen Th1 response.[5]

Priming of naïve T cells by DCs into Th1 or Th2 cells is determined by multiple factors. DCs require expression of the transcription factor T bet for Th1 priming.[91] Activation of DCs with immunosuppressive stimuli like TSLP induces Th2 priming.[47] Prolonged and low level of DC activation exhausts the DCs inducingTh2 priming.[43] Low and high antigen dose induces Th2 and Th1 priming, respectively.[92]

In the past years, new $CD4^+$ T cell lineages have been discovered. These include Th9, Th22, and Th17. Of these, the Th17 lineage is best characterized.[93] Pro-inflammatory Th17 cells expressing IL-17 and the RAR-related orphan receptor γ (RORγt) transcription factor are aberrantly activated in multiple inflammatory disorders. Upon TLR stimulation, innate immune cells, including DCs, secrete IL-6, IL-23 and IL-1β. These cytokines, aided by TGF-β (secreted by other cells e.g., tumor cells) induce Th17 differentiation, subsequent production of IL-21, and expression of IL-23R. IL-21 amplifies Th17 differentiation and IL-23, which is produced by DCs, is needed for the maintenance of Th17 cells.[94] IL-1β and TGF-β are critical amplifiers of Th17 differentiation, especially in humans. IL-1β and IL-6 also promote the reprogramming of forkhead box $P3^+$ ($FoxP3^+$) Tregs to Th17. Hence, the pathological effect of Th17 is highly dependent upon the availability of other cytokines in the vicinity that could overtly amplify Th17-driven inflammation.[95]

Moreover, the signals received from priming DCs also impact the pathogenic potential of the T cells. Indeed, priming by immature DCs skews differentiation towards immunosuppressive Tregs.[96,97] However, even mature DCs have been reported to skew T cell differentiation to Tregs.[98]

Evidence is accumulating that pDCs, which were believed to play a role only in the innate immune response because of their ability to produce high levels of IFN-I, can present viral and tumor antigens to initiate both $CD4^+$ and $CD8^+$ T cell responses.[99] pDCs mature in response to viral infections (e.g., influenza and HIV), thereby providing an important link between innate and adaptive arms of the immune response. Studies using genetic depletion of pDCs in mice indicate that pDCs are primarily required to boost weak antiviral cytotoxic CD8+ T cell responses and may be dispensable against viral infections that elicit a robust CD8+ T cell response.[100]

B Cell Activation

B cells express both antigen-specific B cell receptors (BCRs) and various TLRs, thus allowing them to play a role in innate and adaptive immunity (see also Chapter 13). DCs present processed antigens to naïve T cells, while B cells recognize antigen in its unprocessed native state. DCs can activate B cells in an antigen-specific $CD4^+$ T cell–dependent manner. This action results in B cell activation and isotype switching to IgG, IgA, and IgE, as well as memory B cell generation in response to T-dependent antigens. DCs can also stimulate B cell proliferation by expression of B cell–activating factor (BAFF) and its closely related tumor necrosis family member APRIL (a proliferation-inducing ligand). Furthermore, inflammatory cytokines secreted by DCs can also affect B cell activation. IFN-α and IL-6, or ICAM-1, expressed by activated pDCs, regulate B cells to differentiate into plasma cells for T cell–independent antibody production. IFN-α can enhance antibody secretion in vivo and can induce cDCs to produce BAFF and APRIL, which trigger isotype switching independently of CD40 ligation.[101,102] In addition follicular DCs support B cell memory by continuously stimulating the B cells with antigen-antibody complexes in the germinal centers of the lymph nodes.[103]

Cross Talk Between Dendritic Cells and Innate Lymphoid Cells

Innate lymphoid cells (ILCs) are a recently described family of lymphoid cells that lack the ability to recognize antigens via rearranged receptors such as those expressed by T cells and B cells. ILCs can be classified into three different groups based on their immune function, the transcription factors they express, and the cytokines they produce upon activation.[104] ILCs are either cytotoxic, like the well-described NK cells, or "helper" ILCs, such as ILC1s, ILC2s, and ILC3s. ILC1s express T-bet and produce IFNγ to promote macrophage activation. The closely related ILC3s express RORγt, produce IL-22, and play a role in maintaining intestinal homeostasis. ILC2s are defined by their expression of IL-4, IL-5, IL-13 and their role during extra-cellular parasite infection and against allergens. The interactions between DCs and ILCs are complex and further define the importance of DCs as a critical link between innate and adaptive immunity.

DCs can promote ILC3 differentiation into ILC1s through IL-12 production.[105] However, this differentiation is reversible, and is notably controlled by the presence of IL-23, IL-1β, and retinoic acid produced by DCs in the inflamed gut.[105] DCs' ability to produce retinoic acid directly improves ILC3 activity by upregulating RORγt and IL-22 expression.[106,107] Finally, retinoic acid also controls ILCs tissue localization, by promoting a "switch" in ILCs expression of homing receptors, from lymphoid to gut.[108]

ILCs can also regulate DCs. ILC2-expression of IL-13 controlled the migration of activated lung DCs into draining lymph nodes, leading to the priming of naïve T cells and their differentiation into Th2 cells.[109] In the pancreas, IL-33-stimulated ILC2s produce IL-13 and GM-CSF, leading to retinoic acid production by DCs.[110] Finally, ILC3s activate DCs through the expression of membrane-bound lymphotoxin,[111,112] which allows them to modulate adaptive immune response through control of DC functions. It is interesting to observe that ILCs can promote T cell activation through DCs, and that DCs can in turn improve ILCs functions, providing theoretical basis for the establishment of positive feedback loops between ILCs, T cells, and DCs.

The interactions between NK cells and DCs are better characterized. Direct interactions between NK cells and mature DCs can result in NK cell activation as well as the potentiation of their cytolytic activity, and conversely, NK cells can induce further DC maturation. NK cells and DCs can form an immune synapse, probably helping directional and confined secretion of cytokines as well as facilitating receptor–ligand interactions. Activated NK cells induce DC activation through both cell-to-cell contact (involving NKp30) and TNF and IFN-γ secretion. In turn, activated DCs secrete IL-12/IL-18, IL-15, and IFN-α/β, which enhance IFN-γ secretion, proliferation, and cytotoxicity of NK cells. In some conditions, NK cells can lyse DCs through NKp30, although mature DCs are protected from cytolysis. This might represent a form of "cellular editing" whereby immature and tolerogenic DCs are cleared by NK cells in the course of an ongoing immune response.[113]

It is thus possible that DCs and NK cells play complementary roles in sensing pathogens, such that DCs could be the first to detect microbes through their expression of PRR (TLR, NOD proteins), whereas NK cells may get activated in the absence of overt inflammation but in the presence of ligands for activating NK-cell receptors, for example in tumors. Tumor cells frequently lose class I MHC expression or express NKG2D ligands, such as MIC-A/B. In both situations, either DCs or NK cells could create an inflammatory environment and induce the integrated activation of other cell types. Thus, in mice, infection by murine cytomegalovirus (CMV) induces pDCs to secrete high levels of IFN-α/β, but CD8α⁺ DC are the major producers of IL-12, and resistance to the virus is associated with expansion of Ly49H⁺ NK cells, driven by IL-12/IL-18. The interaction between NK cells and DCs likely takes place early during the course of an immune response. This allows DC to exploit the ability of NK cells to kill tumor- or virus- or parasite-infected cells and to cross-present this material to T cells.[114]

Activation of Other Elements of the Immune System

Apart from interactions with B cells, T cells and ILCs, DCs also regulate many other aspects of the immune system. For example, DCs boost anti-tumor responses by processing and presenting the synthetic ligand α-galactosyl ceramide on CD1 molecules to activate NK T cells.[115] Similarly, DCs engage CD1-restricted γδT cells to induce inflammatory response against pathogens such as, *Mycobacterium tuberculosis*. This interaction matures the DCs prompting secretion of IL-12, and induction of IFN-γ secretion by activated γδT cells.[116]

Overall, it is clear that DCs are integral regulators of immunity. Indeed, as mentioned above, DCs integrate immune responses from a myriad immune cells and influence many aspects of both innate and adaptive immune response (Fig. 9.5). Future studies will help determine the mechanism of how DCs can be best manipulated to harness the strongest immune response with least undesirable side effects.

Impairment of Dendritic Cell Biology in Disease

Dendritic Cells and Autoimmunity

While DCs promote tolerance via a variety of mechanisms, they can also promote autoimmunity through activation and differentiation of self-reactive T cells. At steady state, DCs participate in maintaining tolerance, but homeostatic balance can be altered by changes in DC number, phenotype, and function.[117] In pro-inflammatory settings, or when there is an absence of regulatory molecules, DCs can potentially present self-antigens to naïve T cells, thus promoting self-reactive T cell activation and contributing to autoimmunity.[118] DAMPs such as extra-cellular matrix breakdown products (heparan sulfate and hyaluronate), molecules released from necrotic cells (high-mobility group box 1 protein [HMGB1], uric acid, or even endogenous nucleic acids), fibronectin, and HSPs can all activate TLRs on cDCs and contribute to the generation of autoimmune responses.[119] Some of these conditions are discussed in more detail later.

One of the major models of systemic lupus erythematosus (SLE) proposes that DCs and other phagocytes in SLE patients have impaired abilities to clear apoptotic material from tissues, leading to disruption of peripheral mechanisms of tolerance against self-antigens.[120] Apoptotic blebs, containing clustered autoantigens, are formed at the surface of dying cells. If not cleared, the dying cell will shed these blebs and potentially activate other immune cells. DCs from SLE patients exhibit altered expression of CD40, CD86, Fcγ receptor,[121] and PD-L1, which can modulate T cell suppression.[122] Activated cDCs (possibly through immune complexes or cell derived microparticles) may promote lupus pathogenesis by presenting RNA-associated proteins and chromatin to self-reactive T cells.[123] In mouse models for SLE, activated DCs also enhance B cell proliferation, IL-6 and IFNγ secretion, and anti-nuclear antibodies production.[124,125] pDCs also play a central role in the development of SLE.[126–129] Notably, activation of the type I interferon pathway in SLE derives from chronic stimulation of TLR7, TLR9, and the STING pathway by persistent immune complexes containing endogenous nucleic acids, and in particular non-coding RNA and mitochondrial DNA.[130–134]

Aicardi-Goutieres syndrome (AGS) is an example of an autoimmune disease that results from excessive inflammation induced by the deregulation of Type I interferon immune response. It is hypothesized that mutations in genes involved in clearing apoptotic nucleic debris[135] or in negative regulation of interferon pathway (like SAMHD1)[136] are primarily responsible for AGS. Chronic and sustained production of type I IFNs has effects on both the innate and adaptive immune systems, leading to loss of tolerance and triggering of autoimmune disease. More specifically, it promotes differentiation of monocytes into activated iDCs, thus enhancing presentation of self-antigens, increasing the cytotoxicity of CD8⁺ T cells and NK cells, inducing plasma cell differentiation and subsequent generation of pathogenic autoantibodies.

Similar to SLE, moDC from patients with rheumatoid arthritis (RA) are more immunostimulatory than those from healthy individuals.[137,138] Additionally, synovial fluid in the joints of patients with RA has a high concentration of both myeloid and plasmacytoid DCs, and is enriched with pro-inflammatory cytokines and chemokines. Why RA synovial DCs are inflammatory and elevated in numbers remains unclear. However, it is strongly suggested than alterations of the synovial environment would

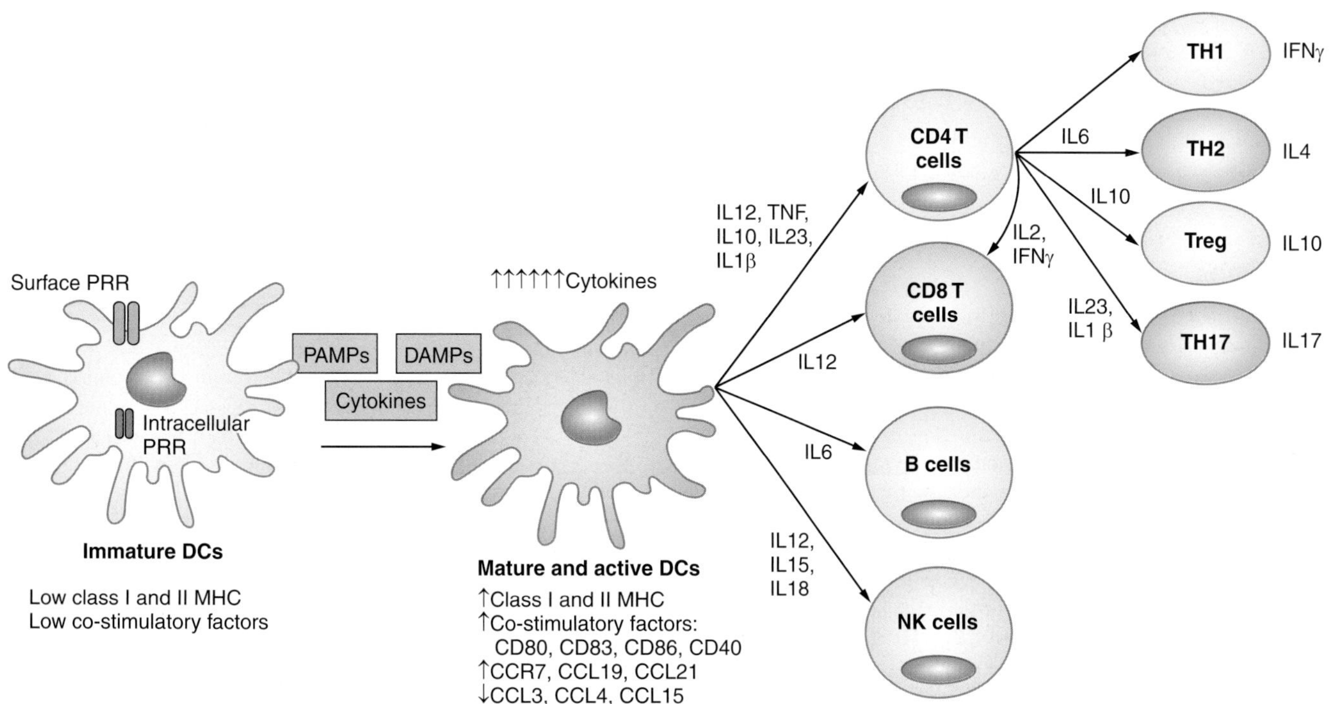

• **Fig. 9.5** Dendritic cells bridge the gap between innate and adaptive immunity. Dendritic cells (DCs) receive innate immune cues from the environment, in the form of microbe derived PAMPs, self-derived danger signals (DAMPs) or other factors like cytokines. These cues induce maturation and activation of DCs through the PRRs expressed either on DC surface or intra-cellularly. Depending upon the nature of stimuli the DCs, may be programmed to become activating or tolerogenic. DC maturation and activation is accompanied by antigen uptake, induction of class I and II MHC, increased expression of co-stimulatory factors like CD80, CD83, CD86 and CD40, induction of chemokine signaling (CCR7, CCL19, CCL21, etc) that guides the trafficking of DCs to the lymph nodes, decrease in chemokines like that restrict DC travel to lymphoid organs (CCL3, CCL4, CCL15, etc), an increase in innate cytokine secretion, etc. Cytokines secreted by activated and mature DCs drive differentiation of naïve immune cells into effector cells with distinct immunomodulatory properties. *DAMPs,* Danger associated molecular patterns; *PAMPS,* pathogen associated molecular patters; *PRR,* pattern recognition receptors.

stimulate DC-induced autoreactive effector T cell differentiation, causing RA development.

Multiple sclerosis (MS) is a chronic autoimmune inflammatory disease affecting the central nervous system (CNS). In the animal model of experimental autoimmune encephalomyelitis (EAE), several studies have shown improvement of disease severity through induction tolerogenic DCs.[139–143] However, EAE can also be induced in the absence of DCs, and the conditional depletion of DCs does not affect pathogenic Th priming in this model.[144,145] Thus, DCs altogether contribute and modulate the onset of EAE, but they are not strictly necessary for it and other APCs might promote harmful T cell differentiation.

Type 1 diabetes (T1D) is caused by dysregulated immune cell destruction of the insulin-generating pancreatic islet β-cells. In healthy individuals, DCs play a tolerogenic role in preventing T1D. However, activated DCs may also cross-present β-cell antigens to T cells initiating pathogenic T cell differentiation.[146,147] A distinct subset of AIRE+ DCs was described to express insulin antigen derived from β-cells, suggesting a role for tolerogenic DCs in controlling activation of insulin-reactive T cells.[148] Importantly, in T1D model of non-obese diabetic mouse, pDCs were required for initiating disease,[149] and were activated by self-DNA released from dying cells. In the same model, another study suggested that HMGB1, also released by dying pancreatic β-islet cells, was responsible for the activation of cDCs. Treatment of mice with antibody-mediated blockade of HMGB1 led to a reduction of incidence and disease onset, as well as decreased activation phenotype on DCs.[150]

Altogether, the major DC alterations that contribute to the break of tolerance during autoimmunity can be classified in four groups: changes in tissue DC concentration and distribution, inability to clear apoptotic cells, altered cytokines secretion, and impaired migration. When considering treatment approaches for autoimmune diseases, there is a need to correctly identify each of these parameters that control the balance between regulatory and pathogenic DC roles.

Dendritic Cells in Human Immunodeficiency

Recent studies of human immunodeficiencies have highlighted the transcription factors directing the development of DCs and emphasized their role in defense against microbial pathogens. Thus, in DC-monocyte-B cell-NK cell lymphoid deficiency (DCML), blood and interstitial DCs are absent along with monocytes and pDCs. The DCML is attributable to GATA-binding factor 2 (GATA2) mutations, a transcription factor involved in the homeostasis of HSCs. Patients with DCML deficiency have increased susceptibility to *Mycobacteria* spp., fungi, and viruses.[151] Another DC deficiency syndrome is caused by IRF8 mutations. The autosomal recessive K108E mutation leads to defects in peripheral cDCs, pDCs, and monocytes, with increased susceptibility to *Mycobacteria* spp., other intra-cellular bacteria and viruses, and is accompanied by a myeloproliferative syndrome. The dominant sporadic mutation T80A induces a specific loss of CD1c⁺ DCs, with increased susceptibility to mycobacterial infection but otherwise does not affect a normal life expectancy.[152]

Subversion of Dendritic Cell Function by Pathogens

Several pathogens have evolved mechanisms to inhibit DC functions, allowing them to persist in the host. Impairing DC functions leads to decreased T cell activation and efficacy, which promotes microbial immune escape.

A typical pathway targeted by pathogens is the antigen-presentation machinery, which is often actively downregulated in virus-infected cells. This is, for example, the case for human (HCMV), which induces downmodulation of class I or class II MHC molecules at the surface of infected cells.[153] Other chronic viruses well-known to perturb the immune responses also develop strategies to impair MHC expression through the specific activities of viral-encoded proteins. For example, HIV-1 protein Nef impairs both class I MHC and class II MHC surface expression.[154,155] Similarly Epstein-Barr virus proteins LMP2A and EBNA1 impair viral detection. LMP2A inhibits class II MHC expression[156] and EBNA1 contains a repeat sequence that prevents its processing by the proteasome and inhibits the production of DRiPS, overall leading to the disruption of peptide presentation on class I MHC.[157,158]

Another mechanism used by pathogens to impair DC functions consists in interfering with their ability to sense microbial ligands and produce interferons and other inflammatory cytokines. Almost all described viruses have developed multiple strategies to antagonize these pathways, and we will refer to another review that illustrates 10 different strategies developed by various viruses to antagonize interferon signaling.[159]

Further, in addition to inhibiting inflammatory cytokine production, pathogens also develop mechanisms to upregulate the production of immunosuppressive cytokines and negative immune regulators. Maybe the most evident example is once again HCMV, whose gene *UL111A* directly codes for a viral homolog of IL-10. Importantly, its production in infected cells in turn upregulates expression of endogenous IL-10 in monocytes.[160] High levels of the negative regulator PD-1 are measured at the surface of T cells during LCMV infection.[161] This is also the case for other viruses responsible for chronic infections, such as HIV[162] or hepatitis C virus (HCV).[163] The PD1/PD-L1 axis is not the only one perturbed by viral infection, and other negative regulators such as TIM-3 and LAG-3 were found upregulated, notably during HCV[164] and LCMV[165] infections, respectively.

Influenza virus (H1N1) induced a strong IFN-α response in pDCs at low titers of infectivity, but not at high titers, where they instead underwent apoptosis. It was proposed that this was a mechanism developed to protect the host from deleterious effects of virus-induced cytokine storm.[166] Another group reported that pDCs isolated from tonsils mounted a stronger interferon response to H3N2 influenza A infection compared with peripheral blood isolated pDCs. This study highlights the importance of taking into consideration the tissue adaptations when studying localized immune cell functions.[167]

Finally, DCs can be directly infected by viruses that use specific receptors to infect and replicate inside the cell. The measles virus uses DCs' expression of CD46, CD150, C-type lectin

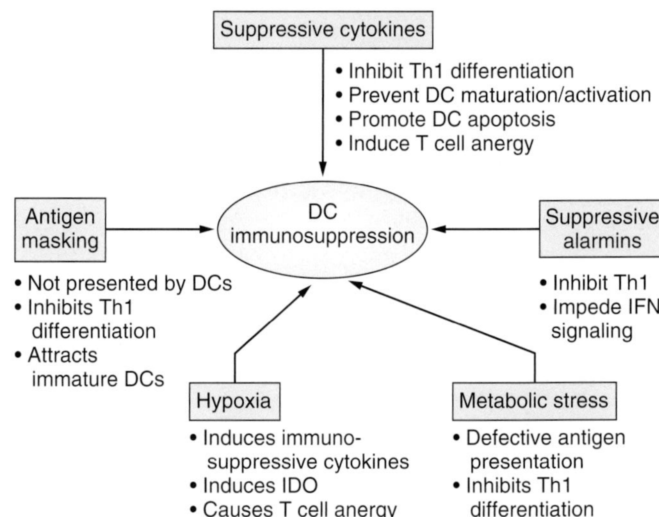

• **Fig. 9.6** Subversion of dendritic cell (DC) activity in cancer. The TME is enriched in immunosuppressive elements that serve to promote tumor growth by directly or indirectly inhibiting DC functions. These elements include suppressive cytokines, suppressive alarmins, hypoxia, metabolic stress, and evasive mechanisms such as antigen masking. Cumulatively these elements impair multiple aspects of DC function and result in absence of adequate Th1 differentiation in the tumor microenvironment. *IDO,* Indoleamine 2,3-dioxygenase; *IFN,* interferon; *Th1,* type 1 T helper cell. (From Saxena M, Bhardwaj N. Re-emergence of Dendritic Cell Vaccines for Cancer Treatment. *Trends Cancer* 4[2]:119–137, 2018,[48] with permission.)

DC-SIGN to enter DCs.[168] DC-SIGN is also notably used by Ebola[169] or Dengue virus.[170] In the case of HIV, DCs can mediate trans-infection of CD4⁺ T cells through the formation of an infectious synapse, carrying the virus with or without infection of the DCs themselves. DCs express the co-receptors CD4, CCR5, CXCR4, and again DC-SIGN, which are necessary for binding or entry of HIV.[171] Thus, HIV ultimately uses the migratory capacity of DCs and their repeated interaction with CD4⁺ T cells as a strategy to quickly propagate the infection through the host.

Dendritic Cell Dysfunction in Tumors

A straightforward model of DC-driven tumor immunity goes as such: (1) migratory DCs access tumor antigens in the TME. (2) DAMPs in the TME promote DC maturation and activation. (3) Tumor antigens are taken up by the DCs and either cross-presented on their class I MHC molecules[172] or migratory DCs carry the tumor antigen to the lymph nodes and transfer tumor antigen to lymph-node resident cross-presenting DCs.[173] (4) In the lymph nodes cross-presenting DCs activate T cells against the tumor antigens giving rise to anti-tumor CTLs. (5) Guided by the chemokine and inflammatory gradient the anti-tumor CTLs traffic back to the TME and proceed with tumor cell killing.[174] However, factors present in the TME actively suppress DC function, differentiation, and recruitment via multiple mechanisms (Fig. 9.6). Indeed, DCs in tumor biopsies have been reported to lack the functional capacity to activate and recruit T cells.[175,176] These observations are supported by murine studies that show that Batf3 knockout mice, deficient in cross-presenting DCs, experience aggravated tumorigenesis as compared to wild-type mice.[16]

Many tumors alter their antigen profile either through immune escape or antigen masking as a means of immune evasion. For example, tumor cells are known to alter their Muc1 antigen post-translationally through hypoglycosylation. DCs are unable to process the hypoglycosylated Muc1 and thus fail to activate T cells against this prominent tumor antigen.[177,178]

Immunosuppressive cytokines are expressed at high levels in the TME, and their levels are positively correlated with advanced cancer stages. Such cytokines include but are not limited to VEGF, TGF-β, IL10, granulocyte-colony stimulating factor (G-CSF), and IL-6. IL-6 drives chronic inflammation and induces downregulation of class II MHC, lymph-node homing receptor CCR7, and promotes differentiation towards immunosuppressive DCs.[179–181] IL-10 converts immunogenic DCs into tolerogenic DCs leading to the induction of anergic cytotoxic CD8$^+$ T cells.[182,183] Both IL-6 and IL-10 activate STAT3, a transcription factor aberrantly expressed in many tumors and associated with presence of immunosuppressive environment.[184]

Several studies indicate that in addition to promoting the growth of tumor vessels, VEGF secreted by tumors blocks the activation of transcriptional factor NF-κB and inhibits DC maturation.[185,186] Studies indicate that TGF-β in the TME plays a critical role in (a) altering the ability of DCs to respond to innate immune signaling,[187] (b) triggering DC differentiation towards an immature myeloid cell phenotype through transcriptional regulator ID1,[188] (c) inducing epigenetic modifications that impair DC differentiation and function,[189] (d) inhibiting DC egress thus trapping immature DCs in the TME, (e) suppressing the expression of IFN-γ, and (f) leading to a preferential recruitment of Tregs to the tumor.[190]

G-CSF produced by the cancer cells can inhibit the hematopoiesis of cDC1 in the bone marrow through downregulation of IRF8 transcription factor.[191] Migration of cDC1 is further reduced when lipid prostaglandin E2 expressed by tumor cells downregulates chemoattractant receptors XCR1, CCR1, and CCR5 on cDC1 surface[192] and when CCL4 expression is reduced upon activation of the WNT/β-catenin pathway.[193] Similarly, low concentration of FLT3L and other growth factors limit tumor cDC1 differentiation, expansion, and survival.[194]

The TME often exists in a persistent hypoxic state, thus fostering significant metabolic stress on the immune cells. Hypoxia modulates DCs to secrete factors (such as adenosine and indoleamine 2,3-dioxygenase) that promote T cell anergy and apoptosis.[195] Moreover the hypoxia in the TME induces an ER stress response in DCs that is mediated by the spliced transcription factor XBP1, and leads to abnormal accumulation of oxidized lipids rendering the DCs unable to process antigens and activate T cells.[196]

Yet another mechanism indeed used by the TME to evade immune detection is the modulation of DC functions to skew T cell differentiation. Overexpression of pro-tumorigenic alarmins such as matrix metalloproteinase-2 (MMP-2) conditions DCs to produce low levels of IL-12 and to express OX40-L, which biases anti-tumor CD4$^+$ T cells toward a suboptimal Th2 differentiation. This pathway involves the interaction of MMP-2 and TLR2 on DCs.[197,198] Similarly, Versican has been demonstrated to induce immune suppression in the TME.[199] Finally, a 2019 study identified a new pathway where regulatory T cells present in the TME inhibit cDC2's ability to drive anti-tumor conventional CD4$^+$ T cells differentiation. Importantly, the authors showed that the balance of human cDC2/Treg in the TME was predictive of anti-tumor responses and overall prognosis.[200]

Immunotherapeutic Strategies and Clinical Trials

In the era of immunotherapies, substantial progress has been made in understanding innate and adaptive immune responses and how they could be regulated and better targeted to contain immunopathologies. Various in vitro, in vivo and human studies indicate that optimal DC engagement is critical for eliciting an effective immune response by vaccines. Indeed, several early stage clinical trials have explored the effectiveness and safety of DC vaccines in raising an immune response against tumor antigens (e.g., non-Hodgkin's lymphoma, malignant melanoma, multiple myeloma, prostate cancer, renal cell carcinoma, breast cancer) or infectious disease pathogens (e.g., HIV). MoDCs are the most commonly used DCs for such purposes but some studies have used DCs generated from CD34$^+$ stem cells or DCs directly isolated from patient's blood (Fig. 9.7). Sipuleucel-T was the first cell based vaccine approved by the United States Food and Drug Association (FDA) for the treatment of castration-resistant prostate cancer. Sipuleucel-T, comprised of autologous, blood derived APCs, including monocytes and DCs, pulsed ex vivo with recombinant fusion protein of human prostatic acid phosphatase (PAP) and GM-CSF and re-infused in the patient. Unfortunately, despite inducing antigen specific T cell responses, the vaccine only yielded modest improvement in overall survival.[201] After the Sipuleucel-T disappointing clinical performance, it became apparent that a deeper understanding of DC biology, the DC subsets, methods for activating DCs, choosing the antigens and route of vaccine delivery, was required to harness these cells for vaccination purposes.[202]

Choosing the right set of antigens is a critical step for the success of DC-based therapy. moDC vaccines are traditionally loaded with shared tumor antigens or personalized, neo-antigens ex vivo and infused into the patients.[32] Investigators demonstrated that vaccinating patients with autologous moDCs loaded with personalized neoantigen peptides elicited a tumor specific CTL response.[203] Alternatively, DCs can be pulsed with a whole assortment of tumor antigens by loading with tumor lysates or upon phagocytosis of dying or opsonized autologous tumor cells.[204,205] In another approach DCs may be fused with tumor cells allowing the generation of hybrid cells with characteristic of DCs but expressing the whole set of tumor antigens.[206] Other innovative methods like RNA electroporation (Trimix DCs) and infection by recombinant viruses like lentivirus (SMART-DCs), poxvirus, herpes virus, and adeno-associated virus have been used to express antigens in DCs to improve cross-presentation and CTL activation.[207,208] In addition, DCs are being manipulated to express receptors specialized for internalizing antigen containing extra-cellular vesicles.[209]

The method for DC activation is a critical determinant of subsequent DC-induced immunity. Hence great care and thought needs to be taken when choosing to activate DCs using specific stimuli such as TLR ligands or modifying DCs to overexpress activating receptors. DCs may be activated by TLR ligands such as TLR-4 ligand, LPS, TLR3 ligand PolyICLC, TLR-7 ligand imiquimod/resiquimod or TLR-9 ligand unmethylated CpG oligonucleotides. Moreover, cytokines such as type I IFNs, IL-1β, IL-6, or TNF may be used to activate DCs ex vivo or in situ.[210] DCs can also be modified to express immunostimulatory molecules, such as transfection with RNA coding for CD40 ligand, CD70, and a constitutively active TLR-4 (Trimix DCs).[211] Moreover DCs may be manipulated using siRNA to silence the expression of inhibitory genes such as *PDL1* and *PDL2* (NCT02528682).[212]

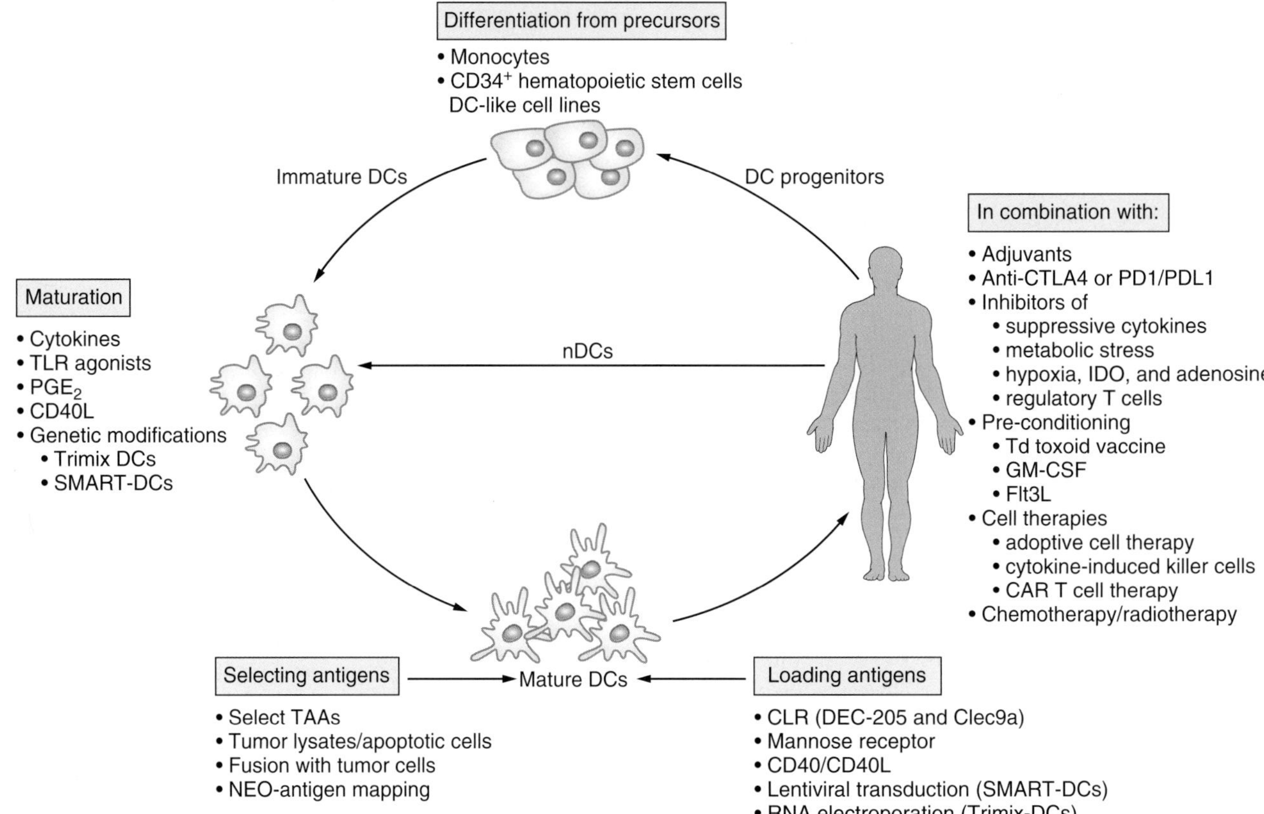

• **Fig. 9.7 Approaches for improving dendritic cell (DC) vaccines.** A summary of current approaches being tested in clinical trials to improve clinical efficacy of DC vaccines. (A) Differentiating immature DCs from precursors: patient-derived monocytes and CD34+ hematopoietic stem cells could be used to generate moDCs or XCR1+Clec9a+ DCs, or CD1d DCs or Langerhans cells, respectively. Natural/conventional DCs may also be directly isolated from patient blood. In the future, DC-like cell lines could be optimized to generate a universal immature DC line. (B) Maturing DCs: DCs can be matured using cytokines, TLR ligands, PGE2, CD40 ligand, or a combination of these. Maturation signals can be provided as exogenous stimuli or transfected/transduced into the immature DCs, as in the case of Trimix DCs and SMART DCs. (C) Selecting and loading antigens: whole tumor lysates or tumor cell fusion with DCs may be used. TAAs or neoantigens (personalized or shared) may be selected. Antigens are loaded on DCs in the form of short or long peptides through traditional DC priming, as DNA through lentiviral transduction, or in the form of RNA through electroporation. Antigens can be introduced with CLRs, mannose receptors, CD40L, or CD40-activating antibodies to improve cross-presentation. (D) Combinations: to maximize DC vaccine clinical efficacy the vaccine should be administered with the most suitable adjuvant in combination with (i) CTLA4 or PD1/PDL1 inhibitor, (ii) inhibitors of immune suppression, (iii) facilitators of DC mobilization such as Td toxoid vaccine, GM-CSF or Flt3L, (iv) other cell-based therapies such as CIKs, ACT, or CAR T cell therapy, and (v) in combination with standard chemotherapy and radiation therapy. *ACT,* Adoptive cell transfer therapy; *CAR,* chimeric antigen receptor; *CIKs,* cytokine-induced killer cells; *CLR,* C-type lectin receptor; *moDCs,* monocyte-derived DCs; *nDCs,* natural DCs; *PGE2,* prostaglandin E2; *TAAs,* tumor-associated antigens; *TLR,* Toll-like receptor. (From Saxena M, Bhardwaj N. Re-emergence of Dendritic Cell Vaccines for Cancer Treatment. *Trends Cancer* 4[2]:119–137, 2018,[48] with permission.)

Another strategy being tested is the targeting of DCs in situ. This strategy simplifies the vaccination pipeline because no ex vivo cell manipulation is required. Such approaches include using antibodies recognizing DC-specific surface molecules, such as Clec-9A, Clec12A, Mannose receptor, DEC-205, and CD40 as demonstrated in mouse models,[213] more recently in patients with cancer[214] and in clinical trials (NCT03358719, NCT02166905, NCT02376699, NCT02482168, NCT00648102, NCT00709462, and NCT01103635). Viral vectors, either in form of DC targeting viruses encoding tumor antigens or oncolytic virus armed for killing tumor cells, are being utilized to elicit and boost natural DC immunity in the TME.[215] Talimogene laherparepvec (TVEC), an attenuated GM-CSF-expressing herpes simplex virus, has been approved by the FDA for use as an intra-tumoral (IT) vaccine for the treatment of inoperable melanoma lesions.[216] TVEC improved the durable response rate in advanced unresectable melanoma (16.3% in the treated group vs. 2.1% in subjects receiving only GM-CSF; $P < .001$)[217] and is now being tested in combination with checkpoint inhibitors, ipilimumab or pembrolizumab. Early results of the TVEC and ipilimumab trial appear to be showing synergistic activity. Other strategies being tested for accessing DCs in vivo include use of nanoparticles,[218] modified RNA vaccines (NCT02410733), DNA vaccines, and vaccines containing manipulated autologous or non-autologous tumor cells (e.g., the GVAX platform using irradiated tumor cells modified to express GM-CSF).[18]

DCs can be activated in situ with IT injection of the TLR ligands. Indeed, TLR9 ligand CpG oligonucleotide (PF-3512676) was used to activate DCs in the TME of patients with low-grade B cell lymphoma and led to complete and partial clinical response with induction of tumor-specific $CD8^+$ T cell immunity.[219,220] Tumor regressions were observed in both injected and distant tumor sites. IT approaches are being tested with other immune modulators (e.g., Poly-IC, a TLR3 and MDA5 agonist, STING agonist),[221,222] and in combination with antibodies that target checkpoint molecules such as CTLA-4 and PD-1. To improve immunogenicity, investigators are preconditioning the vaccine site to stimulate local inflammation so as to enhance DC migration to the draining lymph nodes.[223] Flt3L is being used to enhance the frequency of pre-cDCs. Moreover, DC targeting vaccines such as DEC-205 monoclonal antibodies fused with tumor antigens are being tested in the clinic.[214] A recent study demonstrated that IT administration of Flt3L and PolyICLC in combination with radiation therapy could induce tumor regression in subjects with indolent non-Hodgkin's lymphoma. Importantly even the subjects that did not respond to this regimen became responsive to PD1 blockade therapy. Mechanistically this response was driven by Flt3L-mediated recruitment of cross-presenting DCs to the TME, where DCs were activated and matured by PolyICLC. The radiation therapy induced tumor cell death, releasing a multitude of tumor antigens and DAMPs that were acquired, processed, and presented by the DCs, leading to T cell activation against the tumor cells.[224] Other murine studies have also reported that treatment with Flt3L in combination with PolyICLC induces proliferation and activation of cross-presenting DCs and renders the tumor bearing host responsive to check point blockade.[225]

These studies support the use of in situ DC vaccines in synergy with chemotherapy and radiotherapy. Chemotherapy and radiotherapy trigger tumor cell death, which provides a source of tumor antigens to DCs while at the same time inducing exposure of immunogenic molecules on tumor cells.[226] Death of tumor cells from radiotherapy is also accompanied by release of DAMPS like HMGB1, which can trigger TLR4 and TLR2. Chemotherapy drugs, taxanes, induce release of cellular ATP, which potentiates inflammasome activation and IL-1β release. Finally, cyclophosphamide can cause secretion of type I IFN through release of tumor associated nucleic acids.[226]

Given the recent advances in the field it is apparent that no monotherapy can work as well as a combination therapy. DC immunotherapy will be most efficacious when co-administered with one or more additional interventions such as checkpoint inhibitors, drugs that inhibit immunosuppressive cells (temozolomide, cyclophosphamide or anti-CD25 antibodies that neutralize T regs or retinoic acid derivative all-trans-retinoic acid that prevents differentiation of myeloid suppressor cells), adoptive T cell transfer or radiation/chemotherapy.[227,228] The timing of vaccination is probably also crucial, and frequent immunizations may dramatically improve the clinical efficacy.[229] Ultimately, DCs may be more effective when given as immune prevention after tumor resection or in the neoadjuvant setting, where early studies suggest they may have impact.[230]

In the setting of HIV infection, a study in a small group of chronically infected individuals showed that vaccination with DCs loaded with chemically inactivated virus allowed stabilization and even suppression of viral load for an extended period of time without any other treatment.[231]

DCs are also key regulators of both central and peripheral tolerance. Indeed DCs act as both APCs and effector cells, producing pro-inflammatory molecules and regulating other effector cells. Hence, DCs may be targeted therapeutically to restore or induce tolerance in cases of autoimmunity or organ transplant, respectively. Some of the strategies to induce tolerized DCs include use of immune-suppressive cytokines like IL-10, TGF-β; use of checkpoint blockade proteins like fusion protein CTLA-4-Ig; inhibition of innate immune activation by using antagonists of TLRs and the use of pharmacological agents like corticosteroids, cyclosporine, rapamycin, mycophenolate mofetil, vitamin D_3, or prostaglandin E_2 and inhibitors of NF-κB.[232] Importantly, inhibitors of TNF, IL-1, and IL-6 are currently successfully being used to treat RA,[233] and their effect may, in part, be due to the ability of these cytokines to affect DC maturation. Further, a central role of synovial fluid GM-CSF in inducing a positive feedback loop activating DCs has recently been proposed.[234] DCs are also used in immunotherapy to induce tolerance in RA patients. DCs suppressed with a NF-κB inhibitor and loaded with citrullinated peptide antigens were reported to reduce antigen specific T cell response against citrullinated vimentin.[232] Another trial of tolerogenic DCs derived from $CD14^+$ monocytes and exposed to antigens in autologous synovial fluid demonstrated safety and feasibility.[235] Other similar trials are ongoing and demonstrate the important potential of DC–based immunotherapies to restore immune homeostasis and inhibit autoimmunity.

Future Directions

DCs are a heterogeneous population of bone marrow–derived mononuclear cells that are found in an immature state in almost all tissues in the body. As professional APCs, DCs are key effectors of innate immunity that stimulate naïve T cells, as well as B cells and NK cells, and initiate immune responses. In this way they contribute to protection against infections, maintenance of homeostasis, and also maintenance and regulation of tolerance. Their roles in tolerance regulation suggest that they might be key effectors in the development of autoimmune diseases and in graft tolerance and rejection. Several studies are under way to investigate and develop methodologies to specifically target the more relevant DCs subsets for use as cell based vaccines in the clinic.

Full references for this chapter can be found on ExpertConsult.com.

Selected References

1. Steinman RM, Cohn ZA: Identification of a novel cell type in peripheral lymphoid organs of mice. I. Morphology, quantitation, tissue distribution, *J Exp Med* 137:1142–1162, 1973.
2. Steinman RM, Gutchinov B, Witmer MD, et al.: Dendritic cells are the principal stimulators of the primary mixed leukocyte reaction in mice, *J Exp Med* 157:613–627, 1983.
3. Nussenzweig MC, Steinman RM, Gutchinov B, et al.: Dendritic cells are accessory cells for the development of anti-trinitrophenyl cytotoxic T lymphocytes, *J Exp Med* 152:1070–1084, 1980.
4. Steinman RM, Kaplan G, Witmer MD, et al.: Identification of a novel cell type in peripheral lymphoid organs of mice. V. Purification of spleen dendritic cells, new surface markers, and maintenance in vitro, *J Exp Med* 149:1–16, 1979.
5. Larsson M, et al.: Requirement of mature dendritic cells for efficient activation of influenza A-specific memory CD8+ T cells, *J Immunol* 165:1182–1190, 2000.
6. Nair S, Dhodapkar MV: Natural killer T cells in cancer immunotherapy, *Front Immunol* 8:1178, 2017.

7. Garcia-Marquez M, Shimabukuro-Vornhagen A, von Bergwelt-Baildon M: Complex interactions between B cells and dendritic cells, *Blood* 121:2367–2368, 2013.
8. Reis e Sousa C: Dendritic cells in a mature age, *Nat Rev Immunol* 6:476–483, 2006.
9. Collin M, Bigley V: Human dendritic cell subsets: an update, *Immunology* 154:3–20, 2018.
10. Balan S, et al.: Large-scale human dendritic cell differentiation revealing notch-dependent lineage bifurcation and heterogeneity, *Cell Reports* 24:1902–1915.e1906, 2018.
11. Breton G, Lee J, Liu K, et al.: Defining human dendritic cell progenitors by multiparametric flow cytometry, *Nat Protoc* 10:1407–1422, 2015.
12. See P, et al.: Mapping the human DC lineage through the integration of high-dimensional techniques, *Science* 356, 2017.
13. Sheng J, Ruedl C, Karjalainen K: Most tissue-resident macrophages except microglia are derived from fetal hematopoietic stem cells, *Immunity* 43:382–393, 2015.
14. Saxena M, Balan S, Roudko V, et al.: Towards superior dendritic-cell vaccines for cancer therapy, *Nat Biomed Eng* 2:341–346, 2018.
15. Granot T, et al.: Dendritic cells display subset and tissue-specific maturation dynamics over human life, *Immunity* 46:504–515, 2017.
16. Hildner K, et al.: Batf3 deficiency reveals a critical role for CD8alpha+ dendritic cells in cytotoxic T cell immunity, *Science* 322:1097–1100, 2008.
17. Woo SR, Corrales L, Gajewski TF: Innate immune recognition of cancer, *Annu Rev Immunol* 33:445–474, 2015.
18. Saxena M, Bhardwaj N: Turbocharging vaccines: emerging adjuvants for dendritic cell based therapeutic cancer vaccines, *Curr Opin Immunol* 47:35–43, 2017.
19. Murphy TL, et al.: Transcriptional control of dendritic cell development, *Annu Rev Immunol* 34:93–119, 2016.
20. Siebel C, Lendahl U: Notch signaling in development, tissue homeostasis, and disease, *Physiol Rev* 97:1235–1294, 2017.
21. Caton ML, Smith-Raska MR, Reizis B: Notch-RBP-J signaling controls the homeostasis of CD8- dendritic cells in the spleen, *J Exp Med* 204:1653–1664, 2007.
22. Kirkling ME, et al.: Notch signaling facilitates in vitro generation of cross-presenting classical dendritic cells, *Cell Reports* 23:3658–3672.e3656, 2018.
23. Briseno CG, et al.: Notch2-dependent DC2s mediate splenic germinal center responses, *Proc Natl Acad Sci USA* 115:10726–10731, 2018.
24. Salio M, et al.: Plasmacytoid dendritic cells prime IFN-gamma-secreting melanoma-specific CD8 lymphocytes and are found in primary melanoma lesions, *Eur J Immunol* 33:1052–1062, 2003.
25. McKenna K, Beignon AS, Bhardwaj N: Plasmacytoid dendritic cells: linking innate and adaptive immunity, *J Virol* 79:17–27, 2005.
26. Lui G, et al.: Plasmacytoid dendritic cells capture and cross-present viral antigens from influenza-virus exposed cells, *PLoS One* 4:e7111, 2009.
27. O'Brien M, et al.: CD4 receptor is a key determinant of divergent HIV-1 sensing by plasmacytoid dendritic cells, *PLoS Pathogens* 12:e1005553, 2016.
28. Grouard G, et al.: The enigmatic plasmacytoid T cells develop into dendritic cells with interleukin (IL)-3 and CD40-ligand, *J Exp Med* 185:1101–1111, 1997.
29. Rissoan MC, et al.: Reciprocal control of T helper cell and dendritic cell differentiation, *Science* 283:1183–1186, 1999.
30. Segura E, Amigorena S: Inflammatory dendritic cells in mice and humans, *Trends Immunol* 34:440–445, 2013.
31. Veglia F, Gabrilovich DI: Dendritic cells in cancer: the role revisited, *Curr Opin Immunol* 45:43–51, 2017.
32. O'Neill D, Bhardwaj N: Generation of autologous peptide- and protein-pulsed dendritic cells for patient-specific immunotherapy, *Methods Mol Med* 109:97–112, 2005.
33. Strunk D, Egger C, Leitner G, et al.: A skin homing molecule defines the langerhans cell progenitor in human peripheral blood, *J Exp Med* 185:1131–1136, 1997.
34. Ito T, et al.: A CD1a+/CD11c+ subset of human blood dendritic cells is a direct precursor of Langerhans cells, *J Immunol* 163:1409–1419, 1999.
35. Liu YJ: Dendritic cell subsets and lineages, and their functions in innate and adaptive immunity, *Cell* 106:259–262, 2001.
36. Otsuka M, Egawa G, Kabashima K: Uncovering the mysteries of langerhans cells, inflammatory dendritic epidermal cells, and monocyte-derived langerhans cell-like cells in the epidermis, *Front Immunol* 9:1768, 2018.
37. Doebel T, Voisin B, Nagao K: Langerhans cells—the macrophage in dendritic cell clothing, *Trends Immunol* 38:817–828, 2017.
38. Villani AC, et al.: Single-cell RNA-seq reveals new types of human blood dendritic cells, monocytes, and progenitors, *Science* 356, 2017.
39. Alcantara-Hernandez M, et al.: High-Dimensional phenotypic mapping of human dendritic cells reveals interindividual variation and tissue specialization, *Immunity* 47:1037–1050.e1036, 2017.
40. Breton G, et al.: Circulating precursors of human CD1c+ and CD141+ dendritic cells, *J Exp Med* 212:401–413, 2015.
41. Jaensson E, et al.: Small intestinal CD103+ dendritic cells display unique functional properties that are conserved between mice and humans, *J Exp Med* 205:2139–2149, 2008.
42. Agace WW, Persson EK: How vitamin A metabolizing dendritic cells are generated in the gut mucosa, *Trends Immunol* 33:42–48, 2012.
43. Langenkamp A, Messi M, Lanzavecchia A, et al.: Kinetics of dendritic cell activation: impact on priming of TH1, TH2 and nonpolarized T cells, *Nat Immunol* 1:311–316, 2000.
44. Albert ML, Jegathesan M, Darnell RB: Dendritic cell maturation is required for the cross-tolerization of CD8+ T cells, *Nat Immunol* 2:1010–1017, 2001.
45. Kurts C, et al.: CD4+ T cell help impairs CD8+ T cell deletion induced by cross-presentation of self-antigens and favors autoimmunity, *J Exp Med* 186:2057–2062, 1997.
46. Sporri R, Reis e Sousa C: Inflammatory mediators are insufficient for full dendritic cell activation and promote expansion of CD4+ T cell populations lacking helper function, *Nat Immunol* 6:163–170, 2005.
47. Soumelis V, et al.: Human epithelial cells trigger dendritic cell mediated allergic inflammation by producing TSLP, *Nat Immunol* 3:673–680, 2002.
48. Saxena M, Bhardwaj N: Re-emergence of dendritic cell vaccines for cancer treatment, *Trends in cancer* 4:119–137, 2018.
49. Skoberne M, Beignon AS, Larsson M, et al.: Apoptotic cells at the crossroads of tolerance and immunity, *Curr Top Microbiol Immunol* 289:259–292, 2005.
50. Chan YK, Gack MU: Viral evasion of intracellular DNA and RNA sensing, *Nat Rev Microbiol* 14:360–373, 2016.
51. Dhanwani R, Takahashi M, Sharma S: Cytosolic sensing of immuno-stimulatory DNA, the enemy within, *Curr Opin Immunol* 50:82–87, 2018.
52. Satoh T, Akira S: Toll-Like receptor signaling and its inducible proteins, *Microbiol Spectr* 4, 2016.
53. Saxena M, Yeretssian G: NOD-like receptors: master regulators of inflammation and cancer, *Front Immunol* 5:327, 2014.
54. Prochnicki T, Latz E: Inflammasomes on the crossroads of innate immune recognition and metabolic control. *Cell Metab* 26:71–79, 2017.
55. Fernandez MV, et al.: Ion efflux and influenza infection trigger NLRP3 inflammasome signaling in human dendritic cells, *J Leukoc Biol* 99:723–734, 2016.
56. Geijtenbeek TB, Gringhuis SI: C-type lectin receptors in the control of T helper cell differentiation, *Nat Rev Immunol* 16:433–448, 2016.
57. Wang D, et al.: Role of scavenger receptors in dendritic cell function, *Hum Immunol* 76:442–446, 2015.

58. Blander JM, Medzhitov R: On regulation of phagosome maturation and antigen presentation, *Nat Immunol* 7:1029–1035, 2006.
59. Comber JD, Philip R: MHC class I antigen presentation and implications for developing a new generation of therapeutic vaccines, *Ther Adv Vaccines* 2:77–89, 2014.
60. Macagno A, Kuehn L, de Giuli R, et al.: Pronounced up-regulation of the PA28alpha/beta proteasome regulator but little increase in the steady-state content of immunoproteasome during dendritic cell maturation, *Eur J Immunol* 31:3271–3280, 2001.
61. Leone DA, Rees AJ, Kain R: Dendritic cells and routing cargo into exosomes, *Immunol Cell Biol*, 2018.
62. Harshyne LA, Watkins SC, Gambotto A, et al.: Dendritic cells acquire antigens from live cells for cross-presentation to CTL, *J Immunol* 166:3717–3723, 2001.
63. Segura E, Amigorena S: Cross-Presentation in mouse and human dendritic cells, *Adv Immunol* 127:1–31, 2015.
64. Ackerman AL, Giodini A, Cresswell P: A role for the endoplasmic reticulum protein retrotranslocation machinery during crosspresentation by dendritic cells, *Immunity* 25:607–617, 2006.
65. Nair-Gupta P, et al.: TLR signals induce phagosomal MHC-I delivery from the endosomal recycling compartment to allow cross-presentation, *Cell* 158:506–521, 2014.
66. Embgenbroich M, Burgdorf S: Current concepts of antigen cross-presentation, *Front Immunol* 9:1643, 2018.
67. Gros M, Amigorena S: Regulation of antigen export to the cytosol during cross-presentation, *Front Immunol* 10:41, 2019.
68. Kamphorst AO, Guermonprez P, Dudziak D, et al.: Route of antigen uptake differentially impacts presentation by dendritic cells and activated monocytes, *J Immunol* 185:3426–3435, 2010.
69. Chiang MC, et al.: Differential uptake and cross-presentation of soluble and necrotic cell antigen by human DC subsets, *Eur J Immunol* 46:329–339, 2016.
70. Kretzer NM, et al.: RAB43 facilitates cross-presentation of cell-associated antigens by CD8alpha+ dendritic cells, *J Exp Med* 213:2871–2883, 2016.
71. Wakim LM, Bevan MJ: Cross-dressed dendritic cells drive memory CD8+ T-cell activation after viral infection, *Nature* 471:629–632, 2011.
72. Roche PA, Furuta K: The ins and outs of MHC class II-mediated antigen processing and presentation, *Nat Rev Immunol* 15:203–216, 2015.
73. Valladeau J, et al.: Langerin, a novel C-type lectin specific to langerhans cells, is an endocytic receptor that induces the formation of birbeck granules, *Immunity* 12:71–81, 2000.
74. Chow A, Toomre D, Garrett W, et al.: Dendritic cell maturation triggers retrograde MHC class II transport from lysosomes to the plasma membrane, *Nature* 418:988–994, 2002.
75. Boes M, et al.: T-cell engagement of dendritic cells rapidly rearranges MHC class II transport, *Nature* 418:983–988, 2002.
76. Savina A, et al.: NOX2 controls phagosomal pH to regulate antigen processing during crosspresentation by dendritic cells, *Cell* 126:205–218, 2006.
77. Groom JR: Moving to the suburbs: T-cell positioning within lymph nodes during activation and memory, *Immunol Cell Biol* 93:330–336, 2015.
78. Penna G, Vulcano M, Sozzani S, et al.: Differential migration behavior and chemokine production by myeloid and plasmacytoid dendritic cells, *Hum Immunol* 63:1164–1171, 2002.
79. Gerner MY, Kastenmuller W, Ifrim I, et al.: Histo-cytometry: a method for highly multiplex quantitative tissue imaging analysis applied to dendritic cell subset microanatomy in lymph nodes, *Immunity* 37:364–376, 2012.
80. Gerner MY, Casey KA, Kastenmuller W, et al.: Dendritic cell and antigen dispersal landscapes regulate T cell immunity, *J Exp Med* 214:3105–3122, 2017.
81. Kitano M, et al.: Imaging of the cross-presenting dendritic cell subsets in the skin-draining lymph node, *Proc Natl Acad Sci USA* 113:1044–1049, 2016.
82. Hor JL, et al.: Spatiotemporally distinct interactions with dendritic cell subsets facilitates CD4+ and CD8+ T cell activation to localized viral infection, *Immunity* 43:554–565, 2015.
83. Mempel TR, Henrickson SE, Von Andrian UH: T-cell priming by dendritic cells in lymph nodes occurs in three distinct phases, *Nature* 427:154–159, 2004.
84. Gerner MY, Torabi-Parizi P, Germain RN: Strategically localized dendritic cells promote rapid T cell responses to lymph-borne particulate antigens, *Immunity* 42:172–185, 2015.
85. Henrickson SE, et al.: Antigen availability determines CD8(+) T cell-dendritic cell interaction kinetics and memory fate decisions, *Immunity* 39:496–507, 2013.
86. Zhang S, Zhang H, Zhao J: The role of CD4 T cell help for CD8 CTL activation, *Biochem Biophys Res Commun* 384:405–408, 2009.
87. Williams MA, Bevan MJ: Immunology: exhausted T cells perk up, *Nature* 439:669–670, 2006.
88. Pardoll DM: Spinning molecular immunology into successful immunotherapy, *Nat Rev Immunol* 2:227–238, 2002.
89. Fan X, Quezada SA, Sepulveda MA, et al.: Engagement of the ICOS pathway markedly enhances efficacy of CTLA-4 blockade in cancer immunotherapy, *J Exp Med* 211:715–725, 2014.
90. Sugiura D, et al.: Restriction of PD-1 function by cis-PD-L1/CD80 interactions is required for optimal T cell responses, *Science* 2019.
91. Lugo-Villarino G, Maldonado-Lopez R, Possemato R, et al.: T-bet is required for optimal production of IFN-gamma and antigen-specific T cell activation by dendritic cells, *Proc Natl Acad Sci U S A* 100:7749–7754, 2003.
92. Kapsenberg ML: Dendritic-cell control of pathogen-driven T-cell polarization, *Nat Rev Immunol* 3:984–993, 2003.
93. Kara EE, et al.: Tailored immune responses: novel effector helper T cell subsets in protective immunity, *PLoS Pathogens* 10:e1003905, 2014.
94. Asadzadeh Z, et al.: The paradox of Th17 cell functions in tumor immunity, *Cell Immunol* 322:15–25, 2017.
95. Mangan PR, et al.: Transforming growth factor-beta induces development of the T(H)17 lineage, *Nature* 441:231–234, 2006.
96. Dhodapkar MV, Steinman RM: Antigen-bearing immature dendritic cells induce peptide-specific CD8(+) regulatory T cells in vivo in humans, *Blood* 100:174–177, 2002.
97. Steinman RM, et al.: Dendritic cell function in vivo during the steady state: a role in peripheral tolerance, *Ann N Y Acad Sci* 987:15–25, 2003.
98. Yamazaki S, et al.: Direct expansion of functional CD25+ CD4+ regulatory T cells by antigen-processing dendritic cells, *J Exp Med* 198:235–247, 2003.
99. Mitchell D, Chintala S, Dey M: Plasmacytoid dendritic cell in immunity and cancer, *J Neuroimmunol* 322:63–73, 2018.
100. Swiecki M, Colonna M: Unraveling the functions of plasmacytoid dendritic cells during viral infections, autoimmunity, and tolerance, *Immunol Rev* 234:142–162, 2010.
101. Fayette J, et al.: Human dendritic cells skew isotype switching of CD40-activated naive B cells towards IgA1 and IgA2, *J Exp Med* 185:1909–1918, 1997.
102. Bergtold A, Desai DD, Gavhane A, et al.: Cell surface recycling of internalized antigen permits dendritic cell priming of B cells, *Immunity* 23:503–514, 2005.
103. Kranich J, Krautler NJ: How follicular dendritic cells shape the B-cell antigenome, *Front Immunol* 7:225, 2016.
104. Vivier E, et al.: Innate lymphoid cells: 10 Years on, *Cell* 174:1054–1066, 2018.
105. Bernink JH, et al.: Interleukin-12 and -23 control plasticity of CD127(+) group 1 and group 3 innate lymphoid cells in the intestinal lamina propria, *Immunity* 43:146–160, 2015.
106. Mielke LA, et al.: Retinoic acid expression associates with enhanced IL-22 production by gammadelta T cells and innate lymphoid cells and attenuation of intestinal inflammation, *J Exp Med* 210:1117–1124, 2013.

107. van de Pavert SA, et al.: Maternal retinoids control type 3 innate lymphoid cells and set the offspring immunity, *Nature* 508:123–127, 2014.
108. Kim MH, Taparowsky EJ, Kim CH: Retinoic acid differentially regulates the migration of innate lymphoid cell subsets to the gut, *Immunity* 43:107–119, 2015.
109. Halim TY, et al.: Group 2 innate lymphoid cells are critical for the initiation of adaptive T helper 2 cell-mediated allergic lung inflammation, *Immunity* 40:425–435, 2014.
110. Dalmas E, et al.: Interleukin-33-Activated islet-resident innate lymphoid cells promote insulin secretion through myeloid cell retinoic acid production, *Immunity* 47:928–942.e7, 2017.
111. Tumanov AV, et al.: Lymphotoxin controls the IL-22 protection pathway in gut innate lymphoid cells during mucosal pathogen challenge, *Cell Host & Microbe* 10:44–53, 2011.
112. Kruglov AA, et al.: Nonredundant function of soluble LTalpha3 produced by innate lymphoid cells in intestinal homeostasis, *Science* 342:1243–1246, 2013.
113. Moretta A: The dialogue between human natural killer cells and dendritic cells, *Curr Opin Immunol* 17:306–311, 2005.
114. Iyoda T, et al.: The CD8+ dendritic cell subset selectively endocytoses dying cells in culture and in vivo, *J Exp Med* 195:1289–1302, 2002.
115. Fujii S, Shimizu K, Kronenberg M, et al.: Prolonged IFN-gamma-producing NKT response induced with alpha-galactosylceramide-loaded DCs, *Nat Immunol* 3:867–874, 2002.
116. Leslie DS, et al.: CD1-mediated gamma/delta T cell maturation of dendritic cells, *J Exp Med* 196:1575–1584, 2002.
117. Chung CY, Ysebaert D, Berneman ZN, et al.: Dendritic cells: cellular mediators for immunological tolerance, *Clin Dev Immunol* 2013:972865, 2013.
118. Liu J, Cao X: Regulatory dendritic cells in autoimmunity: a comprehensive review, *J Autoimmun* 63:1–12, 2015.
119. Marshak-Rothstein A: Toll-like receptors in systemic autoimmune disease, *Nat Rev Immunol* 6:823–835, 2006.
120. Biermann MH, et al.: The role of dead cell clearance in the etiology and pathogenesis of systemic lupus erythematosus: dendritic cells as potential targets, *Expert Rev Clin Immunol* 10:1151–1164, 2014.

10 Mononuclear Phagocytes

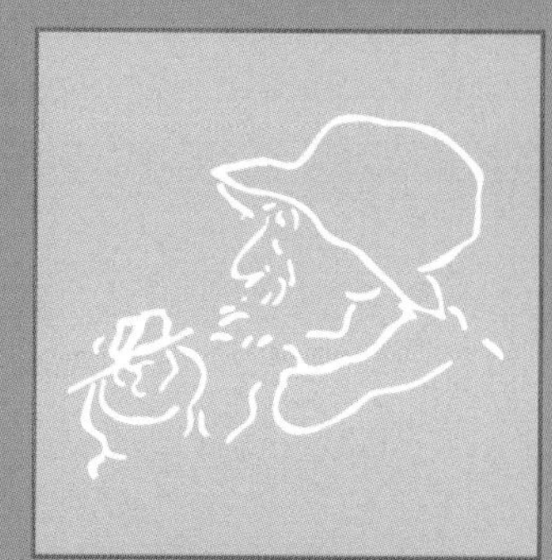

DEBORAH R. WINTER, ANNA MONTGOMERY, AND HARRIS PERLMAN

KEY POINTS

At least two populations of tissue macrophages exist: tissue-resident cells that are embryonically derived and a monocyte-derived population. Their functions may be discrete.

Macrophages are plastic and will change in response to environmental cues through pattern-recognition receptors and other sensors. These changes are regulated primarily at the epigenetic and transcriptional levels.

The M1/M2 paradigm does not fully characterize macrophage heterogeneity.

Synovial macrophages produce a variety of pro-inflammatory cytokines that contribute to synovitis and can be targeted with therapeutic agents.

Transcriptional profiling of synovial macrophages from patients with rheumatoid arthritis might provide insight into disease activity and response to therapy.

Introduction

Metchnikoff described macrophages in the early 1900s, but synovial macrophages were not identified until nearly 60 years later (Fig. 10.1). Three populations of synoviocytes were described based on electron microscopy and were termed type A, type B, and type C in the early 1960s.[1] It is now known that type A cells were synovial macrophages, type B were synovial fibroblasts, and type C were an undetermined population. Further studies in the 1980s and early 1990s refined the classification of synovial macrophages with the use of immunohistochemistry and known antibodies to antigen-presenting cells.[2] These studies were the first to suggest that the synovial macrophage population may be heterogeneous based on cell surface expression of proteins; location (lining vs. sublining); and production of cytokines, chemokines, and matrix metalloproteinases.[2] Additionally, the origin of synovial macrophages was linked to monocytes derived from the bone marrow, based on studies using radiation chimeras of beige mice.[3] Taken together, these fundamental studies provided the basis that the synovial macrophages were derived from hematopoietic progenitors and represented a heterogeneous population in both normal and inflamed synovium. The goal of this chapter is to provide an up-to-date review of macrophage biology and a revision of the current dogma of the mononuclear phagocyte system (MPS) as it relates to the pathogenesis of rheumatoid arthritis (RA).

Steady-State Development of Synovial Macrophages

Early studies in the 1960s and 1970s shaped our understanding of macrophage biology.[4,5] These studies determined that adult monocytes develop as precursors in the bone marrow and then enter the circulation to replenish macrophages in tissue through the use of radiolabeled monocyte progenitors. Nevertheless, more recent studies challenged these assumptions through the use of radiation chimeras, parabiotic mice, and lineage-tracing experiments. The current paradigm is that the vast majority of macrophages are "tissue-resident," developing during embryogenesis and self-renewing in most tissues in the absence of inflammatory stimuli or severe depletion.[6,7]

Initial studies suggested that, in adults, a common monocyte/dendritic cell (MDP) progenitor in the bone marrow leads to the development of monocytes, macrophages, and dendritic cells.[8] Recent studies, however, suggest that MDPs may also develop into other types of hematopoietic cells, such as lymphocytes.[9,10] The administration of nonlethal irradiation to induce death of hematopoietic cells and their precursors followed by administration of donor bone marrow (radiation chimeras) revealed populations of macrophages, including synovial macrophages, Langerhans cells, and microglia, that were resistant to irradiation and remained host origin, whereas the monocyte population was derived from donor hematopoietic cells. Moreover, parabiotic mice that share the same circulation showed that only a subset of macrophages such as heart, gut, and dermis exhibited a mixed population, whereas Langerhans cells, microglia, and alveolar macrophages were exclusively derived from the parent mouse. These studies were the first to provide support for an alternative hypothesis to the MPS regarding monocyte replacement and macrophage turnover in adult mice.[11]

Studies using radiation chimeras and parabiotic mice demonstrated that monocytes only populate tissue-resident macrophages in a few organs during steady-state conditions in adult mice. The origin of the adult tissue-resident macrophage, however, was unknown until the generation of fate-mapping and lineage-tracing mice. These mice express tamoxifen-induced Cre recombinase (Mer-cre-Mer) that enzymatically removes a stop codon flanked by *lox* sequences (floxed) on a reporter gene such as green fluorescent protein or yellow fluorescent protein, thus resulting in traceable fluorescence on the cells of interest. Runt-related transcription factor 1 (Runx1) is required for the development of erythro-myeloid precursors (EMP) and hematopoietic stem cells (HSC) from the hemogenic endothelium.[12] The YS-derived precursors are restricted to days E7.0 to 7.5, while expression at E8.5 is limited to the definitive hematopoiesis stage, which involves fetal monocyte differentiation into macrophages.[8] Runx1-Mer-cre-Mer mice, which have a tamoxifen-inducible cre recombinase flanked by two mutated estrogen receptors and a floxed neo into the Runx1 gene downstream of the proximal (P2) promoter were

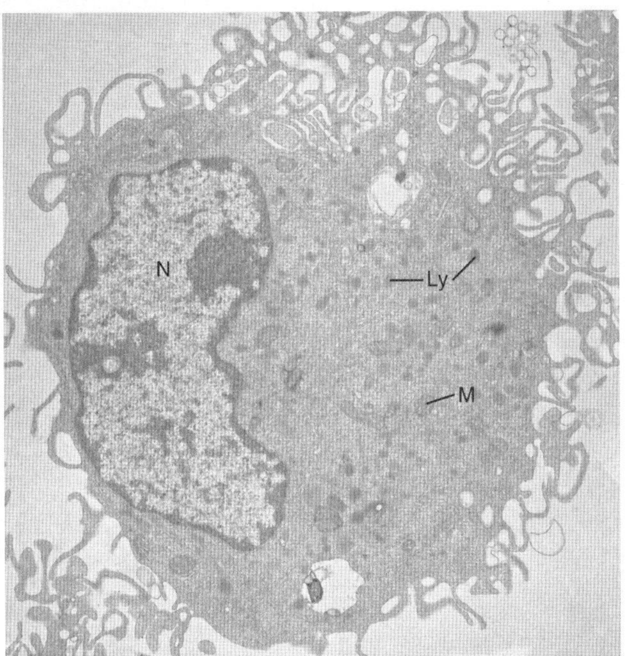

• **Fig. 10.1** Electron micrographs of type A and B cells in the synovium. Thin section of a bone marrow–derived mouse macrophage. Cells were cultured for 7 days and were fixed and processed for conventional electron microscopy. *Ly,* Lysosome; *M,* mitochondrion; *N,* nucleus. (Courtesy Chantal de Chastellier, Centre d'Immunologie de Marseille-Luminy, Marseille, France.)

crossed with fate mapping (reporter) mice and treated with tamoxifen to induce Cre recombination at day E7.0 versus E8.0.[11,13] These mice revealed that microglia were the predominant cell that fluorescently labeled at E7.5 and persisted throughout adulthood. In contrast, any macrophages that were positive at E7.5 lost their label during embryogenesis, which suggests that they were being replaced through nonlabeled precursors.[8,14,15] Consistent with this idea, the numbers of fluorescent positive monocytes and macrophages by the reporter gene increased progressively, whereas the numbers of positive microglia were negligible.[8,14,15]

Another study took advantage of embryos that lacked c-myb, a gene required for definitive hematopoiesis.[16] These mice were deficient for F4/80^{low}CD11b^{hi} myeloid cells but still retained the F4/80^{bright}CD11b^{low} macrophages, which were originally described as resident macrophages.[17,18] These data suggested that fetal macrophages arise from the c-myb-independent pathway in the yolk-sac (YS), whereas the majority of hematopoietic precursors require c-myb expressing progenitors.[16] In support of this idea, these investigators used Tie2-Mer-cre-Mer mice, because Tie2 is highly expressed in hemogenic endothelial progeny such as EMPs and fetal HSCs.[19,20] The addition of tamoxifen at E7.5, E8.5, or E9.0 revealed a differential labeling pattern of embryonic monocytes and macrophages in tamoxifen-treated Tie2-Mer-cre-Mer mice.[19,20] With induction at E7.5, adult tissue-resident macrophages were more labeled when compared with nonmacrophage leukocytes; at E8.5, the proportion of labeled tissue-resident macrophages and leukocytes were comparable; and at E9.5, the leukocytes were more labeled than the tissue-resident macrophages in the tamoxifen-treated Tie2-Mer-cre-Mer mice.[19,20] Taken together, these results suggest that the tissue-resident macrophage precursors are formed early in embryogenesis (i.e., E7.5) and resemble the EMPs. Moreover, the late EMPs or fetal HSCs require c-myb for the development of tissue-resident macrophages with the exception of microglia and some Langerhans cells. Further studies using c-kit-Mer-Cre-Mer mice supported the idea that embryonic HSC is crucial for the development of tissue-resident macrophages.[21] Nevertheless, it is possible that the loss of c-myb induces a redundant pathway that functions independent of c-myb.

More recent studies indicated that there are two decoupled waves of EMPs at days E7.5 (primitive hematopoiesis) and E8.5 (the transient definitive stage); the former is responsible for the development of the microglia, whereas the latter travels through the circulation and supports the development of fetal monocytes that traffic to the liver and then to the whole embryo through the circulation.[6,7,22,23] In this work, YS macrophages were depleted using an anti–colony stimulating factor (CSF) antibody injected at E6.5.[14] The fetal monocyte population was not affected, and the tissue-resident macrophage populations including the microglia were able to recover.[14] These data suggest that YS macrophages are not required for tissue-resident macrophage development and that there is another CSF-independent pathway. This concept is supported by the fact that YS macrophages were replaced in the embryo via fetal monocytes with the exception of microglial cells and a minor fraction of Langerhans cells over time, as observed through the injection of tamoxifen at early E8.5 or late E14.5 time points in Csf-Mer-cre-Mer and the Runx-Mer-cre-Mer mice or through the use of S100A4-cre mice, which labels myeloid cells after YS development when crossed with a reporter mouse.[14,15,19,20] Moreover, the fetal monocytes may be independent of HSC development because Flt3-cre/reporter mice, which label HSCs in adult mice, failed to label fetal HSCs sufficiently. Later stage EMPs, however, require c-myb to form the FL monocytes.[10,14,15,19,20]

Taken together, these data suggest that primitive hematopoiesis starts at E7 in YS and gives rise to EMPs that directly differentiate into microglia and a portion of Langerhans cells, bypassing the monocyte stage. Spatially and temporally regulated waves of hematopoiesis, including a transient definitive wave, also produce EMPs, which arise from YS at day E8 to E8.5; differentiate into fetal monocytes and progenitors for myeloid cells; and migrate via embryonic blood circulation to other tissues, including a fetal liver, to start the definitive hematopoietic stage. During this stage, almost all embryonic tissue macrophages are developed before the production of HSCs (Fig. 10.2).

It was well established in the late 1980s that human synovial macrophages are heterogeneous,[24] but the origin of these cells was unknown. Similar to other tissue macrophage populations in mice, murine synovial macrophages exist as monocyte-derived and YS-derived (tissue-resident) in a steady state[25] (Fig. 10.3). The monocyte-derived synovial macrophages are a minor population, have a high turnover rate, require M-CSF, are sensitive to irradiation, express class II major histocompatibility complex (MHC), and are poor phagocytes. In contrast, the YS-derived, tissue-resident macrophages self-populate, do not require M-CSF, are insensitive to irradiation, do not express class II MHC, and are phagocytic.[25] These studies document the origin of murine synovial macrophages, but it is still unknown whether human synovial macrophages develop in a similar manner to mice.

Transcriptional Regulation of Synovial Macrophages

Macrophage function is defined by the expression of genes that are influenced by ontogeny, stimuli, and environment[26] (Fig. 10.4).

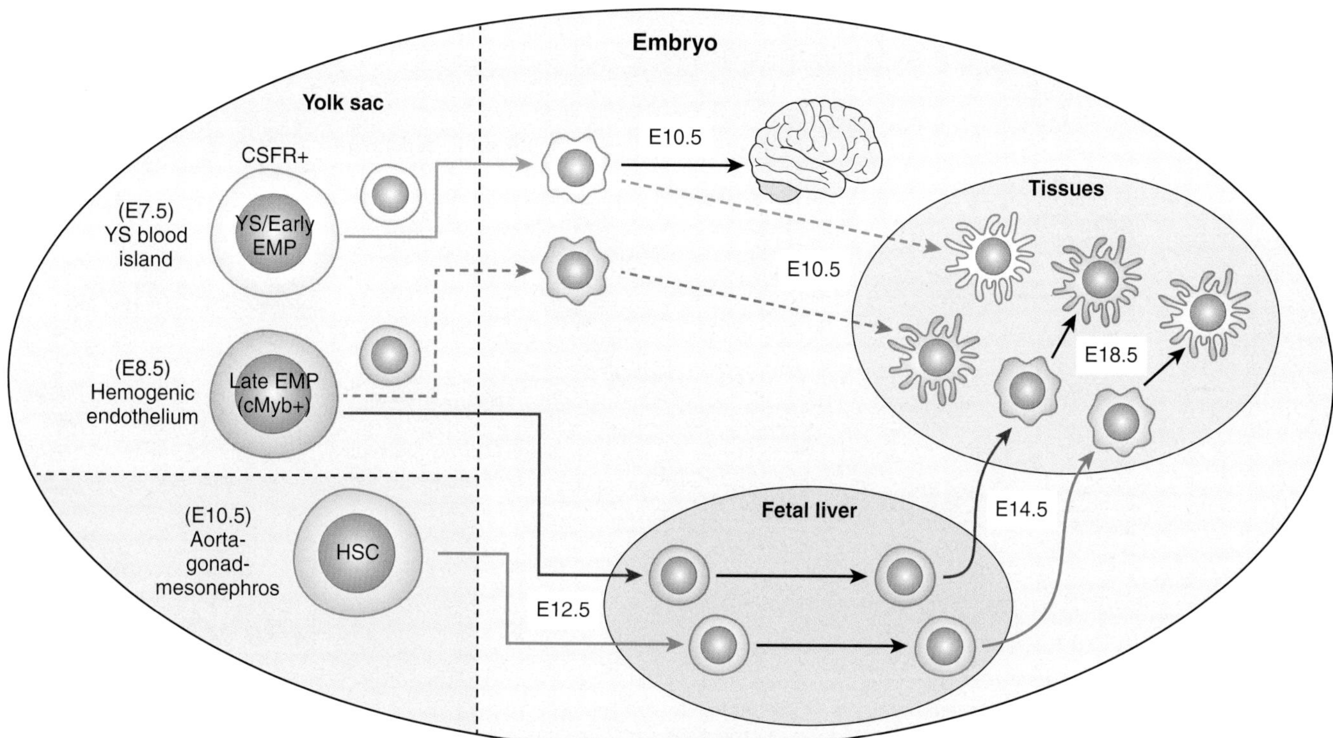

• **Fig. 10.2** Embryology of macrophages. There is a consensus that microglia are derived from the yolk sac. However, there are conflicting studies that suggest that they may also directly contribute to tissue macrophage bypassing the fetal liver stage. Starting at E12.5, late EMPs and HSCs migrate to the fetal liver and then become tissue macrophage around E14.5.

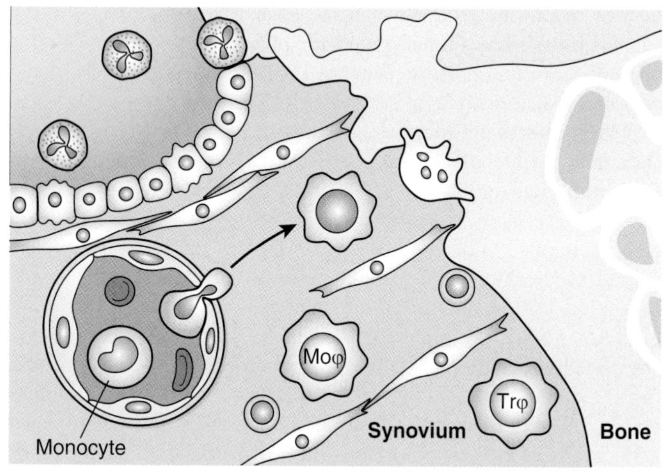

• **Fig. 10.3** Source of synovial macrophages. Synovial macrophages (Mφ) can be classified into 2 populations based on their origin. Tissue resident macrophages are derived from yolk sac progenitors during embryogenesis and persist into the adult where they are capable of self-renewal. Monocyte-derived macrophages undergo turnover from hematopoietic stem cells (HSCs) that differentiate into monocytes during postnatal development and throughout adulthood.

Macrophage genes are regulated by a complex network of transcription factors; proteins that recognize specific DNA sequences or motifs; and the cis-regulatory elements, such as enhancers, that they bind.[27] Multiple transcription factors have been proposed to specify macrophage fate based on the prevalence of their binding sites in macrophage-specific enhancers. Foremost among them is PU.1, which binds a large proportion of enhancers in macrophages[28–32] and will be further discussed later in this section. PU.1 binds enhancers in both peritoneal macrophages and splenic B cells, but only macrophages demonstrate co-binding with C/EBP and AP-1 factors.[30] C/EBPα and C/EBPβ have been implicated in macrophage development from HSCs.[30–34] C/EBPα is critical early on in hematopoiesis for commitment to the myeloid lineage, whereas C/EBPβ is expressed only upon differentiation from the macrophage progenitors.[35]

When compared with other myeloid cells, including monocytes and neutrophils, macrophages demonstrate increased binding of transcription factors in the MAF family.[32] Similarly, MAFB is important for microglia maturity: MAFB-null microglia fail to adapt the transcriptional profile associated with the adult brain.[36] MAF family transcription factors (TFs) may be necessary for terminal macrophage differentiation in tissues by regulating self-renewal.[37–39] In addition, the interferon regulatory factor (IRF) family motif, particularly as a composite with PU.1 (PU.1-IRF), is often found in macrophage enhancers.[28,29,40] The macrophage-specific factors described above do not bind in isolation; these TFs are often bound in combination with each other.

PU.1, a member of the ETS family, represents a special class of TFs known as *pioneers*.[41,42] Pioneers are master regulators that bind thousands of sites across the genome and are capable of increasing the chromatin accessibility of a region.[43–46] In this way, they establish enhancers at which other TFs can settle. PU.1 binding occurs in multiple hematopoietic cell types but is best known for its role in myeloid lineage specification.[47] The PU.1 motif is found in all macrophage progenitors from monocytes back through to HSCs.[31] PU.1 is necessary for the deposition and maintenance of macrophage enhancers and binds in combination with other macrophage-specific TFs.[48] Mutations between mouse

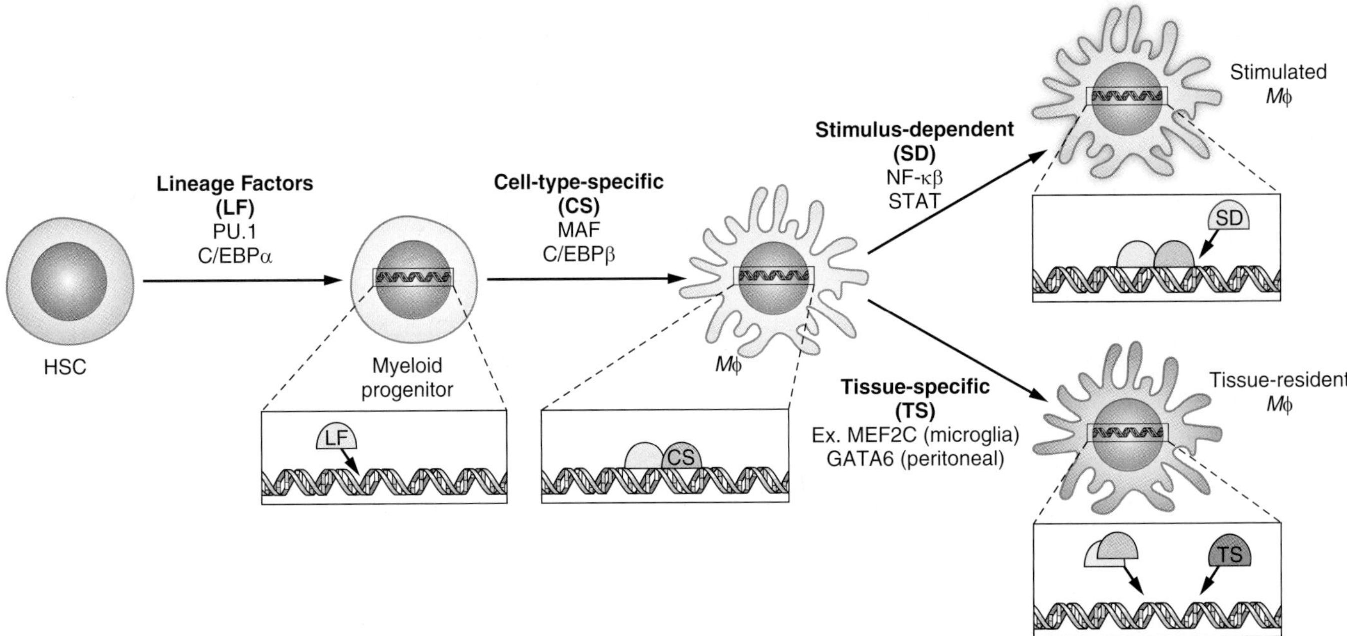

• **Fig. 10.4** Transcriptional regulation of macrophages (Mφ). Lineage transcription factors (TFs), such as PU.1 and C/EBPα, are necessary to specify the myeloid lineage from the HSC. Cell-type-specific TFs, such as MAF and C/EBPβ, distinguish macrophages from other myeloid cells. Stimulus-dependent TFs, such as NF-κβ and STAT, bind primarily to pre-established enhancers in stimulated Mφs. Tissue-specific enhancers, such as the MEF2C in microglia and GATA6 in the peritoneal Mφs, work in combination with cell-type-specific and lineage TFs to define the tissue-resident macrophage enhancer landscape.

strains that lead to the disruption of PU.1 motifs affect PU.1 binding, cofactor binding (such as CCAAT enhancer binding protein [C/EBP]α), and enhancer accessibility.[40,49] In normal hematopoiesis, the expression of PU.1 rather than GATA1 leads to commitment to the myeloid lineage over the erythroid lineage.[31,34] By upregulating myeloid genes and remodeling the enhancer landscape, PU.1, in combination with ectopic expression of C/EBPα or C/EBPβ, can force transdifferentiation of fibroblasts, B cells, and T cells into macrophage-like cells.[50–52] Not only are lineage-specifying TFs like PU.1 important for macrophage development, but they also determine response to stimuli.

Macrophages are adapted to turn on specific genes in response to stimuli. When bone marrow–derived macrophages (BMDMs) are treated with lipopolysaccharide (LPS), which is commonly used for macrophage stimulation, the majority of activated enhancers are previously primed.[28,53] Only a small subset of regions, known as *latent enhancers*, are opened de novo with stimulation.[54] Macrophages derived from human monocytes also demonstrate limited changes to the enhancer landscape when stimulated with LPS.[55] Similar results have been seen with other stimuli, such as Kdo2-lipid A (KLA) and TNF, where the stimulated enhancer landscape was largely composed of pre-existing enhancers.[30,56,57] Different sets of enhancers, however, are associated with different stimuli.[54] Primed enhancers are bound by lineage-specific TFs, such as PU.1 and C/EBPα.[30,54,56,57] With stimulation, stimulus-dependent TFs, such as NF-κβ and STAT, are recruited to a subset of these enhancers.[28,53,57,58] In this way, a macrophage-specific, stimulus-specific response is elicited. To investigate genome-wide binding in these experiments, high-throughput sequencing assays must be performed on macrophage populations. For this reason, much of these studies have been performed on macrophages cultured in vitro to obtain sufficient numbers and controlled conditions. Nevertheless, these macrophages may not fully reflect the function of macrophages in vivo in the local environment of the tissue. Although the underlying principles still apply, the in vitro response cannot capture the heterogeneity across macrophage populations.

Macrophages are often described as a plastic cell type because they are capable of adapting different functions depending on environmental signals. Since macrophages reside in almost every tissue of the body, they are exposed to a wide variety of local environments.[26] For example, macrophages in the peritoneum respond to retinoic acid in the environment, which leads to the induction of GATA6 for their characteristic gene expression.[59] GATA6 is a TF exclusively expressed in peritoneal macrophages compared with other tissue-resident macrophages, and the GATA motif is enriched at peritoneal-specific macrophage enhancers.[29,32] When macrophages are extracted from the peritoneum and grown in culture, they lose their distinctive enhancer landscape, but it is partially rescued by treatment with retinoic acid.[29] Similarly, microglia exhibit the highest expression of Mef2c, and microglia-specific enhancers are enriched for MEF2 motif.[29,32] Transforming growth factor (TGF)-β may be one of the key signals in the microglia environment, leading to the development of mature microglia and the establishment of the adult enhancer landscape.[29,36,60–62] Other tissue-specific TFs implicated by the macrophage enhancer landscape include peroxisome proliferator-activated receptor γ (PPARγ) in the lung; liver X receptor α (LXRα) in liver and spleen; retinoid X receptor (RXR) in lung and spleen; and runt-related transcription factors (RUNX) in intestinal macrophages.[32] These TFs bind in combination with general macrophage factors, such as PU.1, to regulate tissue-resident macrophage genes. A shared environmental signal across two macrophage populations, such as exposure to erythrocyte turnover in liver and spleen, may lead to a shared TF, but the collective binding of TFs in response to the assortment of signals in the unique environment leads to a distinct enhancer landscape regulating tissue-specific expression.

No study has compared the transcriptional landscape of synovial macrophages with other tissue-resident macrophage populations. One might predict, however, that synovial macrophage gene expression will be determined by a combination of cell-type-specific factors with tissue-specific factors that may overlap with those already seen or not, depending on the signals in the joint environment. Many of the studies listed in previous sections supporting macrophage-specific TFs were performed on mouse cells, but homologous proteins are likely to play a similar role in humans. Because it is difficult to obtain macrophage samples from human tissues, many of these factors have yet to be validated in humans.

Synovial Macrophage Production of Cytokines and Chemokines

Macrophages are plastic, which is not only governed by their origin (i.e., embryonic vs. monocyte-derived) but also by their microenvironment, especially during disease initiation, pathogenesis, and resolution.[32,63] The vast majority of our knowledge regarding synovial macrophages is attributed to studies that examined human synovial macrophages via dual immunohistochemistry or in situ hybridization of tissue sections from RA synovial tissue, synovial fluid macrophages in culture, and/or conversion of RA peripheral blood monocytes to macrophages in culture.[2,64,65] For most studies, synovial tissue was retrieved via joint replacement surgery of patients. Thus, these studies were unable to examine the synovium in early RA or in patients experiencing flares, although some groups were able to use percutaneous synovial biopsies or arthroscopic biopsies. Moreover, synovial tissue from osteoarthritis patients was commonly used as a comparison, which may not be ideal because osteoarthritis has an inflammatory component.[66] Nonetheless, the co-expression patterns of the synovial lining and sublining macrophages with transcription factors and cell signaling molecules such as nuclear factor-κB (NF-κB), activator protein-1 (AP-1), janus kinase/signal transducers and activators of transcription (JAK/STAT), C/EBP, c-Jun N-terminal kinase (JNK), extra-cellular regulating kinase (ERK), and p38, anti-apoptopic or proapoptotic proteins or cytokines/chemokines helped show pivotal and topographical roles for synovial macrophages during RA pathology.[2,64,65]

In culture, macrophages may be unstimulated or activated with pathogen-associated molecular patterns (PAMP) or damage-associated molecular patterns (DAMP), such as conventional and joint-specific agonists to the toll-like receptor pathways, the exogenous addition of TNF or IL-1β, and/or culture with macrophage (M)-CSF or granulocyte-macrophage (GM)-CSF on plastic dishes.[2,64,65] Through the studies, synovial macrophages were established to be one of the central producers of the cytokines TNF, IL-1, IL-6, IL-8, IL-10, IL-12, IL-18, IL-15, GM-CSF, and M-CSF, as well as chemokines such as CC motif ligand (CCL)3, CCL5, chemokine (CXC motif) ligand (CXCL)1, CXCL8, CCL2, and IL-8 in the joint.[2,64,65] Although collectively the cell culture experiments helped identify cell-specific production of individual cytokines and chemokines found in the synovium, they are fraught with potential issues that have only been recently identified due to technologic advances (i.e., bulk RNA sequencing and single-cell RNA sequencing). It has now become clear that macrophages express a different transcriptional profile in culture from those in tissue, due to the complex nature of the in vivo microenvironment. Synovial macrophages are continually in contact with other synovial cells and a milieu of cytokines and chemokines that could not be replicated in culture.[29,67] Moreover, culture conditions could never capture the heterogeneity of synovial macrophages, but would instead favor one or more of the individual population(s). The future of understanding synovial macrophages ex vivo will be through the development of organoid cultures and/or 3D micromass cultures that contain both synovial fibroblasts and macrophages under physiologic conditions, which develop a synovial lining-like structure.[68–72]

The M1 and M2 Paradigm Revisited

Over the past 30 years, macrophage biologists have created a paradigm that mimics the classical T helper (Th)1/Th2 mechanism for T-cells but can be applied to macrophages. Terms such as *activation* and *polarization* are commonly used to describe a particular state or phenotype of macrophage. One study described two phenotypes of macrophages: one activated by INFγ and called *classically activated* (M1), and one stimulated with IL-4 and referred to as *alternatively activated* (M2).[73] Cultured macrophages were classified into M1 and M2 phenotypes using mice that were biased towards Th1/Th2 readouts such as C57BL/6 and BALBc, respectively.[74] Typically, M1 (classically activated) macrophages treated with INFγ, LPS, GM-CSF, and TNF produce TNF, IL-1, IL-16, IL-23, IL-12, type I INF, inducible nitric oxide synthase (iNOS), and CXCL9, 10, and 11 and express class II MHC, CD80, CD86, CCR1, and CCR5 and promote Th1 responses.[75]

In contrast, M2 (alternatively activated) macrophages are induced by IL-4, IL-13, M-CSF, immune complexes, IL-10, and glucocorticoids, resulting in the expression of IL-4, IL-10, CCL16, 17, 18, 22 and 24, Chi3l3, arginase, Ym-1 and Relmα, CD163, CD206, and CCR3.[75] To work with the limited flexibility of the M1/M2 paradigm, others[76] established additional nomenclatures such as M2b (regulatory macrophages) and M2c (wound healing macrophages).[75] For example, immune complexes and Toll-like receptor (TLR) activation, apoptotic bodies, cyclic adenosine monophosphate (cAMP), prostaglandin E2, TGF-β, or IL-10 induce a remission/regulatory macrophage phenotype.[77]

There are many drawbacks to the M1/M2 nomenclature. The basis for this nomenclature was initially attributed to the generation of M-CSF or L929 treated bone marrow–derived macrophages or peritoneal cells in culture for 7 days, which does not parallel any in vivo macrophage population. In vivo, the local environment is flushed with stimulants affecting numerous transcriptional and translational programs that contain aspects of both classical and alternatively activated cells. Seminal studies by investigators showed that by adding one stimulant at a time, the transcriptional readouts were not able to fit into one single category.[78] Taken together, the M1/M2 macrophage paradigm is strictly a well-defined molecular event that is highly reproducible under controlled in vitro conditions but has little or no relevance in vivo.[75,78,79] Thus, in vivo macrophages may display characteristics or transcriptional profiles of pro-inflammatory as well as pro-fibrotic and/or proresolution signatures[75,79] and more likely exist within a spectrum of activation states.[76]

Macrophages in Murine Models of Inflammatory Arthritis

The hypertrophy of the synovial lining, as well as the increased cellularity of the synovial sublining, may be attributed to increased recruitment of immune cells (efflux of monocytes), reduced egress, local proliferation, or lack of death.[2] Animal models of RA-like disease that recapitulate various aspects of disease activity, which occur in RA patients (for a comprehensive review, please see reference 80), are effective to understand the mechanism behind the hyperplasia of the synovium (see Chapter 32). There are two main spontaneous models of arthritis (K/BxN and TNF-transgenic [Tg] mice). Previous studies have shown that mice expressing the KRN T-cell receptor (TCR) in the context of the class II MHC Allele H-2k (Ag7) develop a severe, spontaneous, symmetric, and erosive arthritis that resembles human RA.[81] K/BxAg7 (C57Bl/6 background) or K/BxN mice also develop noninfective endocarditis, another feature similar to humans with RA.[82] It was then determined that the Ag7 class II MHC allele presented endogenous glucose-6-phosphate isomerase (G6PI) peptides that were recognized as pathogenic by the KRN TCR. Importantly, 64% of patients with RA produce anti-G6PI antibodies, suggesting a similarity in the pathogenesis between the K/BxAg7 model and human disease.[83] The TNF transgenic model was generated through overexpression of the human TNF gene lacking post-transcriptional regulatory elements,[84] allowing for continued expression of TNF. The development and course of arthritis are dependent on the numbers of copies of the transgene but do not require lymphocytes as TNFTg RAG$^{-/-}$ mice still develop arthritis.

There are also inducible models of inflammatory arthritis.[84] Collagen-induced arthritis (CIA) is a chronic model of arthritis induced by immunization with collagen in complete Freund's adjuvant. This elicits a loss of tolerance to native collagen resulting in bone destruction and recruitment of immune cells.[80] Both K/BxN and CIA models recapitulate human disease with a chronic and destructive pathology involving the innate and adaptive immune system.[80,85] Further, K/BxN and CIA can be used as passive models through transfer of sera-containing anti-G6PI antibodies[86] or anti-collagen antibodies in the K/BxN serum transfer model (STIA) or collagen antibody induced model (CAIA), respectively. Both result in passive, resolving inflammatory arthritis in the recipient mice. The disease in STIA mice represents the effector phase of RA, is independent of lymphocytes,[87] and consists of an initiation, a developmental/propagation, and a resolution stage. Innate and adaptive immune components including B cells, T cells, neutrophils, mast cells, macrophages, complement factors, inflammatory cytokines (IL-1, TNF, IL-17), and Fc receptors contribute to the development of spontaneous arthritis and/or experimentally induced arthritis models.[88–90]

Monocyte and Macrophage Contribution to Synovial Hyperplasia

Monocytes are divided into at least two main populations: classical and nonclassical monocytes. Classical monocytes have a shorter life span and convert into nonclassical monocytes in bone marrow or the circulation. In mice, all monocytes are CD45$^+$CD11b$^+$CD115$^+$, but classical monocytes are further characterized as Ly6C$^+$CD62L$^+$CCR2$^+$CD43$^-$, whereas nonclassical monocytes are Ly6C$^-$CX3CR1$^+$CD62L$^-$CCR2$^-$CD43$^+$.[6] In humans, the classical monocyte population is considered CD45$^+$CD11b$^+$CD14^{++}CD16$^-$HLADR$^+$CCR2$^+$, while the nonclassical monocytes are CD45$^+$CD11b$^+$CD14$^+$CD16$^+$HLADR$^+$CX3CR1$^+$.[6] There are also intermediate populations that are in a state of conversion from a classical to nonclassical monocyte.[6] Although the exact roles for each population remain under investigation, it is clear that both populations of monocytes are involved in response to an insult. Nevertheless, the nonclassical monocytes may have an additional role as they are thought to patrol the vasculature to help maintain endothelial cells integrity and potentially limit the factors and cells which extravasate into tissues through the endothelium.[6]

Clodronate-loaded liposomes are commonly used to eliminate monocytes and tissue macrophages. When delivered systemically, clodronate-loaded liposomes deplete all bone marrow monocytes, circulating monocytes, splenic monocytes and macrophages, liver macrophages, and some kidney macrophages.[25] The synovium is spared, however, due to its low vascularity.[25] Systemic treatment of clodronate-loaded liposomes prevented STIA[25] and CIA because local delivery to the knee suppressed AIA and IL-1/mBSA induced arthritis.[91] Similarly, mice with a mutation in M-CSF (thus, deficient in monocytes and some tissue macrophages) or who lack GM-CSF fail to develop CIA and IL-1/mBSA induced arthritis.[25,92–94]

Treatment with an antagonistic M-CSF or GM-CSF antibody or an oral inhibitor of M-CSF also prevents CIA through the recruitment of monocytes.[92,95–97] Mice lacking CCR2, which have reduced numbers of classical monocytes, are still as equally susceptible to STIA as wild-type mice.[25,98] Further, antibody-mediated depletion of CCR2 does not affect the development of STIA,[25] and a CCR2-deficient model of TNFTg arthritis (CCR2$^{-/-}$TNFTg) displays an exacerbated form of arthritis.[99] Replacement of nonclassical monocytes restores the development of STIA following monocyte depletion with clodronate-loaded liposomes, whereas transfer of classical monocytes does not, and reduction in nonclassical monocytes via CX3CR1 depletion also leads to less STIA.[25,98] These findings suggest that nonclassical monocytes, not classical monocytes, are the critical population for development of inflammatory arthritis. Nevertheless, successful treatment of TNFTg arthritis with anti-TNF antibodies is associated with a reduced efflux of classical monocytes and enhanced classical monocyte apoptosis in the synovium of mice without impacting egress into the lymph node,[100] indicating that although classical monocytes may not be critical to disease initiation, they contribute significantly to pathology and progression of disease. Although monocytes may be essential for disease development, macrophages are critical for the remission phase as the deletion of both populations of synovial macrophages dramatically delays the spontaneous remission of inflammatory arthritis in mice. Taken together, these data demonstrate that individual cell populations have unique roles throughout the course of disease in inflammatory arthritis, which is influenced by the specific microenvironment created by the arthritis model.

Recently tissue-resident macrophages proliferated and maintained their niche. The increased numbers of macrophages were examined in bone marrow chimeric mice and following EDU treatment.[25] There was no change in the rate or numbers of proliferating monocytes or macrophages in the STIA model.[25] Moreover, mice lacking p21, a cell cycle inhibitor, led to increased STIA through hyperactivation of synovial macrophages.[101] Although these data do not rule out a contribution of monocyte and macrophage proliferation to arthritis development in other models of RA-like disease, the vast majority of studies indicate that the enhanced cellularity of the synovium is attributed to increased infiltration of leukocytes.[102]

A lack of apoptosis has also been suggested to contribute to the development and sustainment of inflammatory arthritis.[103] The apoptotic machinery has long been associated with determining and executing the fate of a cell. Cells undergo apoptosis via two

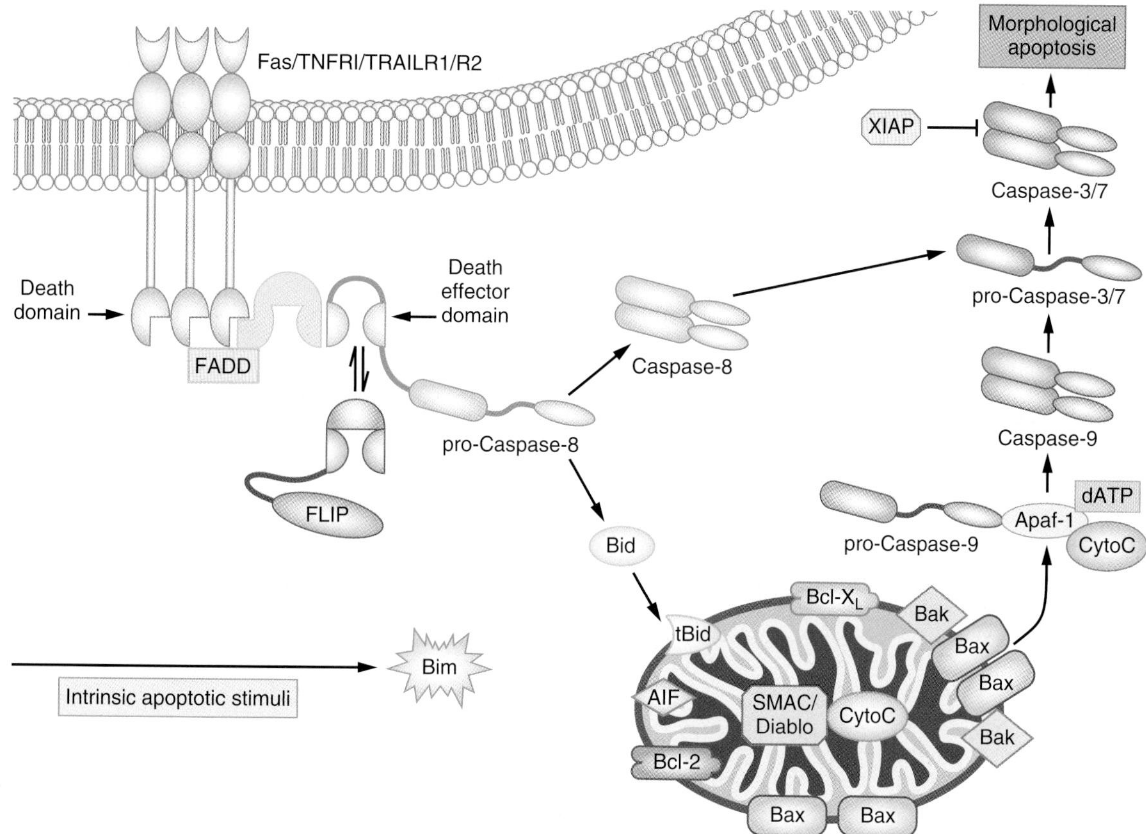

• **Fig. 10.5** Apoptotic pathways in macrophages. Schematic of extrinsic and intrinsic apoptotic pathways. The Fas apoptotic signaling pathways and the Bcl-2 family that controls the apoptotic signaling through the mitochondria are shown.

central but distinct pathways, an "extrinsic" pathway that requires binding of death ligands (Fas Ligand) to their cognate receptors (Fas) on the cell surface, and an "intrinsic" pathway in which mitochondria play a critical role (Fig. 10.5). The extrinsic pathway is suppressed by Flip, which binds to caspase 8, sequesters it, and prevents caspase 8 autocatalysis.[103] The intrinsic pathway is regulated by the Bcl-2 protein family, which is divided into antiapoptotic (Bcl-2, Bcl-xL, Mcl-1) and proapoptotic (Bax, Bak, Bim) members. While there are over 10 Bcl-2 homology (BH3)-only proteins (such as Bad, Bid, Bmf, Noxa, or Puma) or multi-BH domains (Bak and Bak), which are considered the inducers or executioners of mitochondrial apoptosis respectively, none of them result in spontaneous autoimmune-specific phenotype following deletion except Bim.[103] Increased expression of Flip, Mcl-1, and Bcl-2 and reduced expression of Bim have been reported in the human synovium.[104–109]

There are conflicting data regarding the development of inflammatory arthritis in mice lacking Fas that are dependent on the model of the disease. Fas-mutant mice did not develop CIA,[110] but they displayed accelerated STIA.[111] Nevertheless, mice lacking Fas specifically on myeloid cells exhibit less inflammatory arthritis, which may be due to reduced activation potential of the macrophage population.[112] Mice lacking Flip in myeloid cells, macrophages, and/or dendritic cells developed increased STIA or spontaneous arthritis.[113,114] Mice deficient for Bid or Bim also exhibit worse STIA than is associated with an increased number of synovial macrophages.[105,115] Systemic treatment with a BH3 mimetic that preferentially binds to macrophages is effective as a prophylactic and therapeutic for ameliorating STIA.[104]

Synovial Macrophages as a Possible Predictor of Disease Activity

Today, there are many options for therapy for patients with RA, yet there is little or no information that helps identify which therapy is best suited (i.e., a balance between efficacy and tolerance) for a particular patient (Fig. 10.6). Despite the many therapies for patients with RA, there is little information to guide the selection of the most effective treatment for an individual patient. Forty-sixty percent of patients with RA respond (defined by ACR50 response criteria) to conventional disease modifying anti-rheumatic drugs (cDMARDs)[116,117] or cDMARDs plus anti-TNF therapy.[118–126] Moreover, 20% to 40% of subjects in clinical trials never demonstrate even a minimal response (ACR20 response criteria) and are thus considered inadequate responders (cDMARD-IR).[122–128] There is a need to develop precision-based therapy for patients with RA, whereby clinical information such as novel biomarkers will enhance our ability to predict the therapeutic response and thereby limit ineffective therapy.

Biomarkers that indicate sensitivity or resistance to a particular therapy are sorely lacking in RA. For the most part, researchers have utilized peripheral blood, with minimal success.[129] Similarly, the results of genetic approaches have been disappointing.[108] More recent studies suggest the synovium, as the target organ in RA, may have greater potential in determining therapeutic response.[129] Early studies in the 1990s showed that the numbers of macrophages correlated with bone erosion in the joint, as well as being a common feature of early RA. The reduction of the numbers in subsynovial lining macrophages correlates with decreased

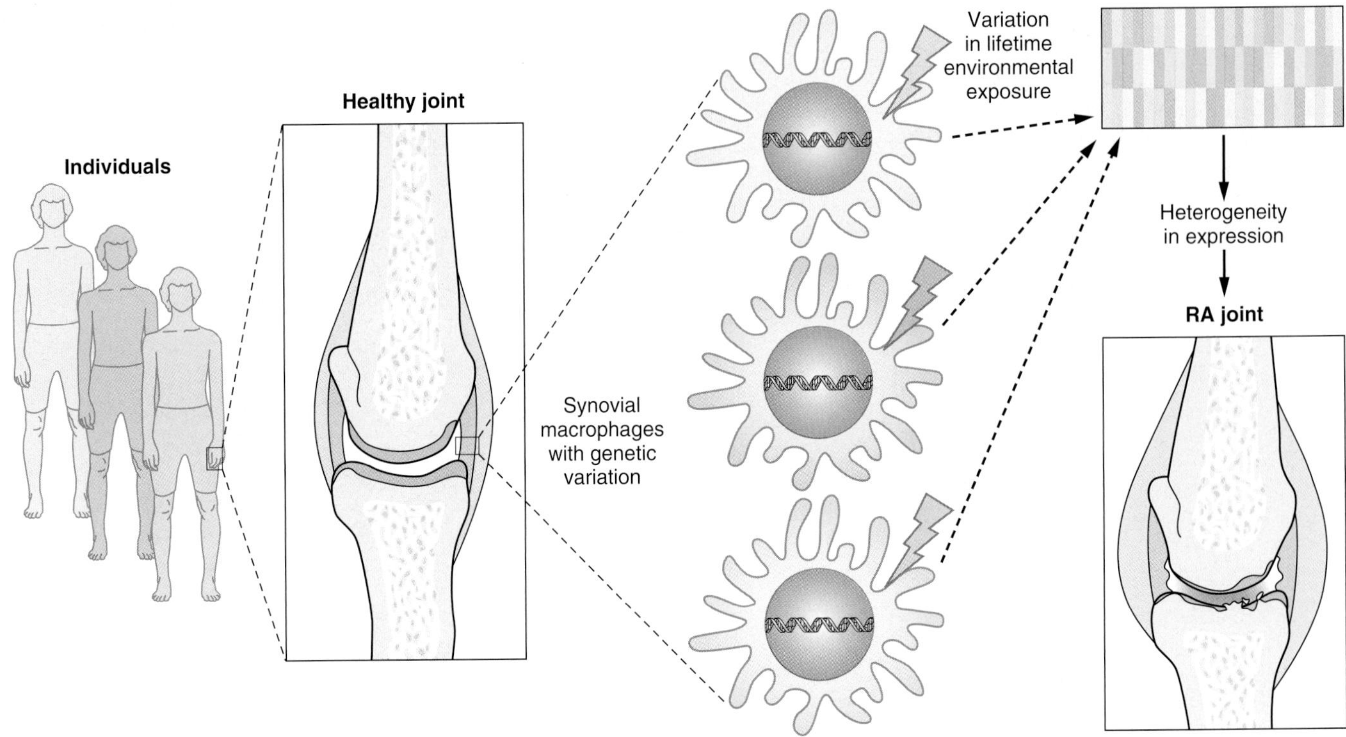

• **Fig. 10.6** Synovial macrophage heterogeneity in RA. Each individual has unique pattern synovial macrophages in their joints based on their genetic variation and lifetime environmental exposure. This combination of factors might lead to the development of inflammatory arthritis and accounts for the heterogeneity across patients.

DAS28 scores for some therapies but not for others (including rituximab, abatacept, and tofacitinib).[65] Nevertheless, previous studies demonstrated that the macrophages in the synovium are heterogeneous based on immunostaining and confirmed by FACS, Cy-ToF, and single-cell RNA sequencing.[130]

More recently, the transcriptional profile of synovial macrophages has altered our understanding of their function. Macrophages isolated from ultrasound-guided synovial tissue biopsies obtained from patients with RA identified transcriptional differences across patients based on RNA-seq studies.[131] Some patients cluster based on the similarity of their transcriptional profiles, which is associated with differences in disease activity.[131] Thus, some patients with controlled disease tend to share similar macrophage gene expression because their synovial macrophages are returning to normal function and beginning to resemble healthy cells. Six transcriptional modules of co-regulated genes from isolated synovial macrophages have been identified that might be associated with clinical disease status and cDMARD or biologic therapy (bDMARD).[131]

Some modules were negatively or positively correlated, respectively, with patients who are currently on biologics or have taken methotrexate in the past. Thus, it is possible that specific modules might help predict remission and include genes that directly relate to cytokines (TNF, IL-1β, and M-CSF), macrophage differentiation/survival (MAFB, C/EBPβ, C/EBPδ, SOD2, and Mcl-1), or activation (ICAM, PLAUR, and CD53). Other transcriptional modules were negatively and positively correlated with the degree of synovitis and may be better indicators of remission.[131] Other modules center on tissue-resident specific genes (Marco, CD14, and ApoE), immune response regulators (KLF2, XBP-1, TGFβ, and NF-κβ1a) and chemokines/MMP (CXCL3, CCL13, and TIMP1) or metabolic functions. Future studies will require an intensive understanding of the role that a particular biologic plays in macrophage activation and metabolism.

Recent studies have identified four populations of monocytes/macrophages using single-cell RNA-seq and confirmed by Cy-ToF (based on CCR2, CD11c, CD38).[132] One population was associated with IL-1β as well as genes affiliated with the LPS pathway in leukocyte-rich RA as compared to OA synovium. However, genes associated with NUPR separated monocytes/macrophages into another group that was associated with OA synovium.[132] Two other subsets of monocytes/macrophages contain genes associated with the phagocytosis and the interferon pathway, respectively. The IL-1β+ monocytes/macrophages comprised the bulk of myeloid cells in the RA synovium, while NUPR+ monocytes/macrophages were the largest myeloid cell subpopulation in the OA synovium.[132] Taken together, these data suggest that combining single-cell and bulk RNA-seq of isolated macrophages from synovial tissue may lead to the development of a precision medicine approach for RA.

Conclusion

RA is a chronic inflammatory and destructive arthropathy of unknown etiology. In patients with RA, there are increased numbers of monocytes, which normally exist as classical monocytes, intermediate monocytes, and nonclassical monocytes circulating in peripheral blood. Nonclassical monocytes are essential for murine models of disease, although whether these cells are also required in patients with RA is unknown. In the naïve mouse joint, there are at least two populations of ontologically distinct synovial macrophages, one from an embryonic origin (tissue-resident) and the other from circulating monocytes (monocyte-derived). Similar to mice, patients exhibit a heterogeneous population of synovial macrophages.

Monocytes differentiate into macrophages, leading to an elevation in their number, which is associated with articular destruction in the joints of patients with RA. Although extravasating monocytes can differentiate into both populations (tissue-resident and monocyte-derived) of synovial macrophages during the induction of inflammatory arthritis in mice, the role that each population plays in the perpetuation of inflammatory arthritis has not been defined. In RA, synovial macrophages are highly activated; express elevated levels of TLR 2, 4, and 7; and contribute directly and indirectly to synovial inflammation and destruction of cartilage and bone through the production of degradative enzymes, cytokines, and chemokines. TLR 2, 3, and 7 are also necessary for the development of inflammatory arthritis in mice. More importantly, macrophages are potent producers of IL-1β, IL-6, and TNF, three pro-inflammatory cytokines that contribute to RA pathogenesis. Further, reduced numbers of sublining macrophages are associated with successful response to therapy and better disease outcome in patients. Currently, approved therapeutics include monoclonal antibody inhibitors of TNF and IL-6, in addition to JAK inhibitors, CTLA4-Ig, and anti-CD20 antibodies, which all reduce macrophage numbers in synovial sublining, decrease synovial inflammation, and minimize bone destruction. Macrophages are also necessary for the remission phase, as deletion of both populations of synovial macrophages dramatically delays the spontaneous remission of inflammatory arthritis in mice. New studies using cutting edge technologies may potentially unlock a transcriptional profile in individual macrophage populations.

Full references for this chapter can be found on ExpertConsult.com.

Selected References

1. Barland P, Novikoff AB, Hamerman D: Electron microscopy of the human synovial membrane, *The Journal of Cell Biology* 14:207–220, 1962.
2. Hamilton JA, Tak PP: The dynamics of macrophage lineage populations in inflammatory and autoimmune diseases, *Arthritis and Rheumatism* 60:1210–1221, 2009.
3. Edwards JC, Willoughby DA: Demonstration of bone marrow derived cells in synovial lining by means of giant intracellular granules as genetic markers, *Annals of the Rheumatic Diseases* 41:177–182, 1982.
4. van Furth R, Cohn ZA: The origin and kinetics of mononuclear phagocytes, *The Journal of Experimental Medicine* 128:415–435, 1968.
5. van Furth R: Phagocytic cells: development and distribution of mononuclear phagocytes in normal steady state and inflammation. In Gallin JI, Goldstein IM, Snyderman R, editors: *Inflammation: Basic principles and clininal correlates*, New York, 1988, Raven Press, Ltd., pp 218–295.
6. Guilliams M, Mildner A, Yona S: Developmental and functional heterogeneity of monocytes, *Immunity* 49:595–613, 2018.
7. Bonnardel J, Guilliams M: Developmental control of macrophage function, *Curr Opin Immunol* 50:64–74, 2018.
8. Ginhoux F, Greter M, Leboeuf M, et al.: Fate mapping analysis reveals that adult microglia derive from primitive macrophages, *Science* 330:841–845, 2010.
9. Sathe P, Metcalf D, Vremec D, et al.: Lymphoid tissue and plasmacytoid dendritic cells and macrophages do not share a common macrophage-dendritic cell-restricted progenitor, *Immunity* 41:104–115, 2014.
10. Ginhoux F, Guilliams M: Tissue-resident macrophage ontogeny and homeostasis, *Immunity* 44:439–449, 2016.
11. Perdiguero EG, Geissmann F: The development and maintenance of resident macrophages, *Nature Immunology* 17:2–8, 2015.
12. Tober J, Yzaguirre AD, Piwarzyk E, et al.: Distinct temporal requirements for Runx1 in hematopoietic progenitors and stem cells, *Development* 140:3765–3776, 2013.
13. Samokhvalov IM, Samokhvalova NI, Nishikawa S: Cell tracing shows the contribution of the yolk sac to adult haematopoiesis, *Nature* 446:1056–1061, 2007.
14. Hoeffel G, Ginhoux F: Ontogeny of tissue-resident macrophages, *Frontiers in Immunology* 6:486, 2015.
15. Hoeffel G, Chen J, Lavin Y, et al.: C-Myb+ erythro-myeloid progenitor-derived fetal monocytes give rise to adult tissue-resident macrophages, *Immunity* 42:665–678, 2015.
16. Schulz C, Gomez Perdiguero E, Chorro L, et al.: A lineage of myeloid cells independent of Myb and hematopoietic stem cells, *Science* 336:86–90, 2012.
17. Hume DA, Irvine KM, Pridans C: The mononuclear phagocyte system: the relationship between monocytes and macrophages, *Trends Immunol* 40:98–112, 2019.
18. Gordon S, Plüddemann A: Tissue macrophages: heterogeneity and functions, *BMC Biol* 15:53, 2017.
19. Gomez Perdiguero E, Klapproth K, Schulz C, et al.: The origin of tissue-resident macrophages: when an erythro-myeloid progenitor is an erythro-myeloid progenitor, *Immunity* 43:1023–1024, 2015.
20. Gomez Perdiguero E, Klapproth K, Schulz C, et al.: Tissue-resident macrophages originate from yolk-sac-derived erythro-myeloid progenitors, *Nature* 518:547–551, 2015.
21. Sheng J, Ruedl C, Karjalainen K: Most tissue-resident macrophages except microglia are derived from fetal hematopoietic stem cells, *Immunity* 43:382–393, 2015.
22. T'Jonck W, Guilliams M, Bonnardel J: Niche signals and transcription factors involved in tissue-resident macrophage development, *Cell Immunol* 330:43–53, 2018.
23. Ginhoux F, Guilliams M: Tissue-resident macrophage ontogeny and homeostasis, *Immunity* 44:439–449, 2016.
24. Koch AE, Polverini PJ, Leibovich SJ: Functional heterogeneity of human rheumatoid synovial tissue macrophages, *J Rheumatol* 15:1058–1063, 1988.
25. Misharin AV, Cuda CM, Saber R, et al.: Nonclassical Ly6C(-) monocytes drive the development of inflammatory arthritis in mice, *Cell Reports* 9:591–604, 2014.
26. Amit I, Winter DR, Jung S: The role of the local environment and epigenetics in shaping macrophage identity and their effect on tissue homeostasis, *Nature Immunology* 17:18–25, 2016.
27. Winter DR, Amit I: The role of chromatin dynamics in immune cell development, *Immunological Reviews* 261:9–22, 2014.
28. Ghisletti S, Barozzi I, Mietton F, et al.: Identification and characterization of enhancers controlling the inflammatory gene expression program in macrophages, *Immunity* 32:317–328, 2010.
29. Gosselin D, Link VM, Romanoski CE, et al.: Environment drives selection and function of enhancers controlling tissue-specific macrophage identities, *Cell* 159:1327–1340, 2014.
30. Heinz S, Benner C, Spann N, et al.: Simple combinations of lineage-determining transcription factors prime cis-regulatory elements required for macrophage and B cell identities, *Molecular Cell* 38:576–589, 2010.
31. Lara-Astiaso D, Weiner A, Lorenzo-Vivas E, et al.: Chromatin state dynamics during blood formation, *Science* 345:943–949, 2014.
32. Lavin Y, Winter D, Blecher-Gonen R, et al.: Tissue-resident macrophage enhancer landscapes are shaped by the local microenvironment, *Cell* 159:1312–1326, 2014.
33. Ghisletti S, Natoli G: Deciphering cis-regulatory control in inflammatory cells, *Philosophical Transactions of the Royal Society of London Series B, Biological Sciences* 368:20120370, 2013.
34. Graf T, Enver T: Forcing cells to change lineages, *Nature* 462:587–594, 2009.

35. Iwasaki H, Akashi K: Myeloid lineage commitment from the hematopoietic stem cell, *Immunity* 26:726–740, 2007.
36. Matcovitch-Natan O, Winter DR, Giladi A, et al.: Microglia development follows a stepwise program to regulate brain homeostasis, *Science* 353:aad8670, 2016.
37. Aziz A, Soucie E, Sarrazin S, et al.: MafB/c-Maf deficiency enables self-renewal of differentiated functional macrophages, *Science* 326:867–871, 2009.
38. Kelly LM, Englmeier U, Lafon I, et al.: MafB is an inducer of monocytic differentiation, *Embo J* 19:1987–1997, 2000.
39. Soucie EL, Weng Z, Geirsdottir L, et al.: Lineage-specific enhancers activate self-renewal genes in macrophages and embryonic stem cells, *Science* 351:aad5510, 2016.
40. Heinz S, Romanoski C, Benner C, et al.: Effect of natural genetic variation on enhancer selection and function, *Nature* 503:487–492, 2013.
41. Winter DR, Jung S, Amit I: Making the case for chromatin profiling: a new tool to investigate the immune-regulatory landscape, *Nat Rev Immunol* 15:585–594, 2015.
42. Laslo P, Spooner C, Warmflash A, et al.: Multilineage transcriptional priming and determination of alternate hematopoietic cell fates, *Cell* 126:755–766, 2006.
43. Lupien M, Eeckhoute J, Meyer C, et al.: FoxA1 translates epigenetic signatures into enhancer-driven lineage-specific transcription, *Cell* 132:958–970, 2008.
44. Cirillo L, Lin F, Cuesta I, et al.: Opening of compacted chromatin by early developmental transcription factors HNF3 (FoxA) and GATA-4, *Molecular Cell* 9:279–289, 2002.
45. Cirillo L, Zaret K: An early developmental transcription factor complex that is more stable on nucleosome core particles than on free DNA, *Molecular Cell* 4:961–969, 1999.
46. Zaret KS, Carroll JS: Pioneer transcription factors: establishing competence for gene expression, *Genes & Development* 25:2227–2241, 2011.
47. Nutt S, Metcalf D, D'Amico A, et al.: Dynamic regulation of PU.1 expression in multipotent hematopoietic progenitors, *The Journal of Experimental Medicine* 201:221–231, 2005.
48. Laslo P, Spooner CJ, Warmflash A, et al.: Multilineage transcriptional priming and determination of alternate hematopoietic cell fates, *Cell* 126:755–766, 2006.
49. Link VM, Duttke SH, Chun HB, et al.: Analysis of genetically diverse macrophages reveals local and domain-wide mechanisms that control transcription factor binding and function, *Cell* 173, 2018. 1796-809.e17.
50. Xie H, Ye M, Feng R, et al.: Stepwise reprogramming of B cells into macrophages, *Cell* 117:663–676, 2004.
51. Feng R, Desbordes SC, Xie H, et al.: 1 and C/EBPalpha/beta convert fibroblasts into macrophage-like cells, *Proc Natl Acad Sci U S A* 105:6057–6062, 2008.
52. Laiosa CV, Stadtfeld M, Xie H, et al.: Reprogramming of committed T cell progenitors to macrophages and dendritic cells by C/EBP alpha and PU.1 transcription factors, *Immunity* 25:731–744, 2006.
53. Barish G, Yu R, Karunasiri M, et al.: Bcl-6 and NF-kappaB cistromes mediate opposing regulation of the innate immune response, *Genes & Development* 24:2760–2765, 2010.
54. Ostuni R, Piccolo V, Barozzi I, et al.: Latent enhancers activated by stimulation in differentiated cells, *Cell* 152:157–171, 2013.
55. Saeed S, Quintin J, Kerstens HH, et al.: Epigenetic programming of monocyte-to-macrophage differentiation and trained innate immunity, *Science* 345:1251086, 2014.
56. Escoubet-Lozach L, Benner C, Kaikkonen M, et al.: Mechanisms establishing TLR4-responsive activation states of inflammatory response genes, *PLoS Genetics* 7:e1002401, 2011.
57. Jin F, Li Y, Ren B, et al.: PU.1 and C/EBP(alpha) synergistically program distinct response to NF-kappaB activation through establishing monocyte specific enhancers, *Proceedings of the National Academy of Sciences of the United States of America* 108:5290–5295, 2011.
58. Kaikkonen M, Spann N, Heinz S, et al.: Remodeling of the enhancer landscape during macrophage activation is coupled to enhancer transcription, *Molecular Cell* 51:310–325, 2013.
59. Okabe Y, Medzhitov R: Tissue-specific signals control reversible program of localization and functional polarization of macrophages, *Cell* 157:832–844, 2014.
60. Gosselin D, Skola D, Coufal NG, et al.: An environment-dependent transcriptional network specifies human microglia identity, *Science* 356, 2017.
61. Butovsky O, Jedrychowski MP, Moore CS, et al.: Identification of a unique TGF-[beta]-dependent molecular and functional signature in microglia, *Nat Neurosci* 17:131–143, 2014.
62. Cohen M, Matcovitch O, David E, et al.: Chronic exposure to TGFβ1 regulates myeloid cell inflammatory response in an IRF7-dependent manner, *The EMBO Journal* 33:2906–2921, 2014.
63. Ginhoux F, Schultze JL, Murray PJ, et al.: New insights into the multidimensional concept of macrophage ontogeny, activation and function, *Nature Immunology* 17:34–40, 2016.
64. Kennedy A, Fearon U, Veale DJ, et al.: Macrophages in synovial inflammation, *Frontiers in Immunology* 2:52, 2011.
65. Udalova IA, Mantovani A, Feldmann M: Macrophage heterogeneity in the context of rheumatoid arthritis, *Nature Reviews Rheumatology* 12:472–485, 2016.
66. Conaghan PG, Cook AD, Hamilton JA, et al.: Therapeutic options for targeting inflammatory osteoarthritis pain, *Nat Rev Rheumatol* 15:355–363, 2019.
67. Helft J, Bottcher J, Chakravarty P, et al.: GM-CSF mouse bone marrow cultures comprise a heterogeneous population of CD11c(+)MHCII(+) macrophages and dendritic cells, *Immunity* 42:1197–1211, 2015.
68. Kiener HP, Watts GFM, Cui Y, et al.: Synovial fibroblasts self direct multiceullular lining architecture and synthetic function in three-dimensional organ culture, *Arthritis and Rheumatism*, 2009. In press.
69. Nozaki T, Takahashi K, Ishii O, et al.: Development of an ex vivo cellular model of rheumatoid arthritis: critical role of CD14-positive monocyte/macrophages in the development of pannus tissue, *Arthritis Rheum* 56:2875–2885, 2007.
70. Peck Y, Leom LT, Low PFP, et al.: Establishment of an in vitro three-dimensional model for cartilage damage in rheumatoid arthritis, *J Tissue Eng Regen Med* 12:e237–e249, 2018.
71. Sakuraba K, Fujimura K, Nakashima Y, et al.: Brief report: successful in vitro culture of rheumatoid arthritis synovial tissue explants at the air-liquid interface, *Arthritis Rheumatol* 67:887–892, 2015.
72. Solomon S, Masilamani M, Mohanty S, et al.: Generation of three-dimensional pannus-like tissues in vitro from single cell suspensions of synovial fluid cells from arthritis patients, *Rheumatol Int* 24:71–76, 2004.
73. Stein M, Keshav S, Harris N, et al.: Interleukin 4 potently enhances murine macrophage mannose receptor activity: a marker of alternative immunologic macrophage activation, *J Exp Med* 176:287–292, 1992.
74. Mills CD, Kincaid K, Alt JM, et al.: M-1/M-2 Macrophages and the Th1/Th2 paradigm, *J Immunol* 164:6166–6173, 2000.
75. Murray PJ, Allen JE, Biswas SK, et al.: Macrophage activation and polarization: nomenclature and experimental guidelines, *Immunity* 41:14–20, 2014.
76. Mosser DM, Edwards JP: Exploring the full spectrum of macrophage activation, *Nature Reviews Immunology* 8:958–969, 2008.
77. Fleming BD, Mosser DM: Regulatory macrophages: setting the threshold for therapy, *European Journal of Immunology* 41:2498–2502, 2011.
78. Xue J, Schmidt SV, Sander J, et al.: Transcriptome-based network analysis reveals a spectrum model of human macrophage activation, *Immunity* 40:274–288, 2014.

79. Martinez FO, Gordon S: The M1 and M2 paradigm of macrophage activation: time for reassessment, *F1000prime Reports* 6:13, 2014.
80. Bevaart L, Vervoordeldonk MJ, Tak PP: Evaluation of therapeutic targets in animal models of arthritis: how does it relate to rheumatoid arthritis? *Arthritis and Rheumatism* 62:2192–2205, 2010.
81. Matsumoto I, Staub A, Benoist C, et al.: Arthritis provoked by linked T and B cell recognition of a glycolytic enzyme, *Science* 286:1732–1735, 1999.
82. DeLong CE, Roldan CA: Noninfective endocarditis in rheumatoid arthritis, *Am J Med* 120:e1–2, 2007.
83. Schaller M, Burton DR, Ditzel HJ: Autoantibodies to GPI in rheumatoid arthritis: linkage between an animal model and human disease, *Nature Immunology* 2:746–753, 2001.
84. Li P, Schwarz EM: The TNF-alpha transgenic mouse model of inflammatory arthritis, *Springer Semin Immunopathol* 25:19–33, 2003.
85. Inglis JJ, Criado G, Medghalchi M, et al.: Collagen-induced arthritis in C57BL/6 mice is associated with a robust and sustained T-cell response to type II collagen, *Arthritis Research & Therapy* 9:R113, 2007.
86. Korganow AS, Ji H, Mangialaio S, et al.: From systemic T cell self-reactivity to organ-specific autoimmune disease via immunoglobulins, *Immunity* 10:451–461, 1999.
87. Monach PA, Mathis D, Benoist C: The K/BxN arthritis model, *Curr Protoc Immunol* Chapter 15:Unit 15.22, 2008.
88. Monach PA, Nigrovic PA, Chen M, et al.: Neutrophils in a mouse model of autoantibody-mediated arthritis: critical producers of Fc receptor gamma, the receptor for C5a, and lymphocyte function-associated antigen 1, *Arthritis and Rheumatism* 62:753–764, 2010.
89. Kyburz D, Corr M: The KRN mouse model of inflammatory arthritis, *Springer Semin Immunopathol* 25:79–90, 2003.
90. Ji H, Ohmura K, Mahmood U, et al.: Arthritis critically dependent on innate immune system players, *Immunity* 16:157–168, 2002.
91. van den Berg WB, van Lent PLEM: The role of macrophages in chronic arthritis, *Immunbiol* 195:614–623, 1996.
92. Campbell IK, Rich MJ, Bischof RJ, et al.: The colony-stimulating factors and collagen-induced arthritis: exacerbation of disease by M-CSF and G-CSF and requirement for endogenous M-CSF, *Journal of Leukocyte Biology* 68:144–150, 2000.
93. Yang YH, Hamilton JA: Dependence of interleukin-1-induced arthritis on granulocyte-macrophage colony-stimulating factor, *Arthritis and Rheumatism* 44:111–119, 2001.
94. Brodmerkel CM, Huber R, Covington M, et al.: Discovery and pharmacological characterization of a novel rodent-active CCR2 antagonist, INCB3344, *Journal of Immunology* 175:5370–5378, 2005.
95. Campbell IK, Hamilton JA, Wicks IP: Collagen-induced arthritis in C57BL/6 (H-2b) mice: new insights into an important disease model of rheumatoid arthritis, *European Journal of Immunology* 30:1568–1575, 2000.
96. Cook AD, Braine EL, Campbell IK, et al.: Blockade of collagen-induced arthritis post-onset by antibody to granulocyte-macrophage colony-stimulating factor (GM-CSF): requirement for GM-CSF in the effector phase of disease, *Arthritis Research* 3:293–298, 2001.
97. Ohno H, Uemura Y, Murooka H, et al.: The orally-active and selective c-Fms tyrosine kinase inhibitor Ki20227 inhibits disease progression in a collagen-induced arthritis mouse model, *Eur J Immunol* 38:283–291, 2008.
98. Jacobs JP, Ortiz-Lopez A, Campbell JJ, et al.: Deficiency of CXCR2, but not other chemokine receptors, attenuates autoantibody-mediated arthritis in a murine model, *Arthritis and Rheumatism* 62:1921–1932, 2010.
99. Puchner A, Saferding V, Bonelli M, et al.: Non-classical monocytes as mediators of tissue destruction in arthritis, *Ann Rheum Dis* 77:1490–1497, 2018.
100. Huang QQ, Birkett R, Doyle R, et al.: The role of macrophages in the response to TNF inhibition in experimental arthritis, *Journal of Immunology* 200:130–138, 2018.
101. Mavers M, Cuda CM, Misharin AV, et al.: Cyclin-dependent kinase inhibitor p21, via its C-terminal domain, is essential for resolution of murine inflammatory arthritis, *Arthritis and Rheumatism* 64:141–152, 2012.
102. Siouti E, Andreakos E: The many facets of macrophages in rheumatoid arthritis, *Biochem Pharmacol* 165:152–169, 2019.
103. Cuda CM, Pope RM, Perlman H: The inflammatory role of phagocyte apoptotic pathways in rheumatic diseases, *Nature Reviews Rheumatology* 12:543–558, 2016.
104. Scatizzi JC, Hutcheson J, Pope RM, et al.: Bim-Bcl-2 homology 3 mimetic therapy is effective at suppressing inflammatory arthritis through the activation of myeloid cell apoptosis, *Arthritis and Rheumatism* 62:441–451, 2010.
105. Scatizzi JC, Bickel E, Hutcheson J, et al.: Bim deficiency leads to exacerbation and prolongation of joint inflammation in experimental arthritis, *Arthritis and Rheumatism* 54:3182–3193, 2006.
106. Liu H, Eksarko P, Temkin V, et al.: Mcl-1 is essential for the survival of synovial fibroblasts in rheumatoid arthritis, *Journal of Immunology* 175:8337–8345, 2005.
107. Perlman H, Georganas C, Pagliari LJ, et al.: Bcl-2 expression in synovial fibroblasts is essential for maintaining mitochondrial homeostasis and cell viability, *Journal of Immunology* 164:5227–5235, 2000.
108. Sieberts SK, Zhu F, Garcia-Garcia J, et al.: Crowdsourced assessment of common genetic contribution to predicting anti-TNF treatment response in rheumatoid arthritis, *Nature Communications* 7:12460, 2016.
109. Perlman H, Pagliari LJ, Liu HT, et al.: Rheumatoid arthritis synovial macrophages express the Fas-associated death domain-like interleukin-1 beta-converting enzyme-inhibitory protein and are refractory to Fas-mediated apoptosis, *Arthritis and Rheumatism* 44:21–30, 2001.
110. Ma Y, Liu H, Tu-Rapp H, et al.: Fas ligation on macrophages enhances IL-1R1-Toll-like receptor 4 signaling and promotes chronic inflammation, *Nat Immunol* 5:380–387, 2004.
111. Brown NJ, Hutcheson J, Bickel E, et al.: Fas death receptor signaling represses monocyte numbers and macrophage activation in vivo, *Journal of Immunology* 173:7584–7593, 2004.
112. Huang QQ, Birkett R, Koessler RE, et al.: Fas signaling in macrophages promotes chronicity in K/BxN serum-induced arthritis, *Arthritis & Rheumatology* 66:68–77, 2014.
113. Huang QQ, Birkett R, Doyle RE, et al.: Association of increased F4/80high macrophages with suppression of serum-transfer arthritis in mice with reduced FLIP in myeloid cells, *Arthritis & Rheumatology* 69:1762–1771, 2017.
114. Huang QQ, Perlman H, Birkett R, et al.: CD11c-mediated deletion of Flip promotes autoreactivity and inflammatory arthritis, *Nature Communications* 6:7086, 2015.
115. Scatizzi JC, Hutcheson J, Bickel E, et al.: Pro-apoptotic Bid is required for the resolution of the effector phase of inflammatory arthritis, *Arthritis Research & Therapy* 9:R49, 2007.
116. O'Dell JR, Curtis JR, Mikuls TR, et al.: Validation of the methotrexate-first strategy in patients with early, poor-prognosis rheumatoid arthritis: results from a two-year randomized, double-blind trial, *Arthritis and Rheumatism* 65:1985–1994, 2013.
117. Saevarsdottir S, Wallin H, Seddighzadeh M, et al.: Predictors of response to methotrexate in early DMARD naive rheumatoid arthritis: results from the initial open-label phase of the SWEFOT trial, *Annals of the Rheumatic Diseases* 70:469–475, 2011.

118. Bathon JM, Martin RW, Fleischmann RM, et al.: A comparison of etanercept and methotrexate in patients with early rheumatoid arthritis, *The New England Journal of Medicine* 343:1586–1593, 2000.
119. Breedveld FC, Weisman MH, Kavanaugh AF, et al.: The PREMIER study: a multicenter, randomized, double-blind clinical trial of combination therapy with adalimumab plus methotrexate versus methotrexate alone or adalimumab alone in patients with early, aggressive rheumatoid arthritis who had not had previous methotrexate treatment, *Arthritis and Rheumatism* 54:26–37, 2006.
120. Emery P, Breedveld FC, Hall S, et al.: Comparison of methotrexate monotherapy with a combination of methotrexate and etanercept in active, early, moderate to severe rheumatoid arthritis (COMET): a randomised, double-blind, parallel treatment trial, *Lancet* 372:375–382, 2008.

11 Neutrophils

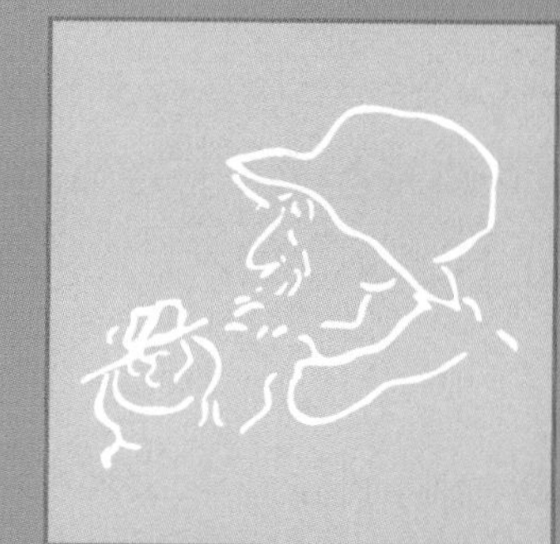

BINITA SHAH, NATHALIE BURG, AND MICHAEL H. PILLINGER

KEY POINTS

Neutrophils are myeloid-lineage cells characterized by the presence of granules containing enzymes and other potentially toxic agents involved in host defense.

Neutrophils are short-lived, terminally differentiated cells that exist primarily in the bloodstream, where they participate in host surveillance of foreign organisms.

Neutrophils function in acute inflammation and provide an essential defense against acute bacterial infections; abnormalities of neutrophil function are uncommon and impair ability to respond to life-threatening infections.

Key functions of neutrophils include phagocytosis and degradation of foreign particles, through activation of proteases and other antibiotic molecules, as well as generation of toxic oxygen radicals.

Neutrophil extra-cellular traps (NETs) are extruded neutrophil chromatin and granule enzymes that can trap and destroy bacteria, but also promote and resolve inflammation and may propagate autoimmunity.

Neutrophils play roles in many rheumatic conditions, both as effectors and as contributors to disease processes.

Overview

Neutrophils (polymorphonuclear neutrophils, PMNs) belong to the family of polymorphonuclear leukocytes, hematopoietically derived cells that share the features of a multilobed nucleus and highly developed intracytoplasmic granules (hence the alternative term *granulocytes* for this family of cells). On the basis of the cytochemical staining properties of their respective granules, three classes of polymorphonuclear leukocytes can be identified: neutrophils, eosinophils, and basophils. Whereas neutrophil granules stain with neutral dyes, eosinophil granules are most effectively stained with acidic dyes such as eosin, and basophil granules stain with basic dyes. In a standard polychromatic Wright stain of a peripheral blood smear, the cytoplasm of neutrophils, eosinophils, and basophils appears blue-pink, pink, and blue, respectively. These classes of polymorphonuclear leukocytes differ with respect to not only appearance, but also biochemistry and function. Polymorphonuclear leukocytes constitute an important part of the organism's system of innate immunity: their responses to foreign organisms, antigens, or both are preprogrammed and independent of prior exposure to the foreign particle.

Neutrophils are the body's first line of defense against foreign invaders and constitute a major cell type involved in acute and some forms of chronic inflammation. The importance of neutrophils in bacterial defense is illustrated by patients who have hereditary defects in neutrophil function and are prone to repeated and often life-threatening infections (discussed later in this chapter). Neutrophils are the most prevalent leukocytes in the bloodstream, typically constituting greater than 50% of all bloodstream leukocytes. During bacterial infection, the percentage of neutrophils may increase to 80% or more. In contrast, tissue concentrations of neutrophils during periods of homeostasis are thought to be low, but increase in response to infection or other triggers. Neutrophils may be considered to be surveillance cells, sweeping through the bloodstream, scanning for tissue infections or other inflammatory events. Unfortunately, the capacity of neutrophils to destroy foreign organisms is matched in some circumstances by a capacity for host tissue destruction. In this chapter, we review neutrophil development, structure, and function; the role of neutrophils in protecting against infection; and the role and impact of neutrophils in the pathogenesis and pathophysiology of immune deficiency and autoimmune and autoinflammatory diseases.

Neutrophil Development, Morphology, and Content

Neutrophil Myelopoiesis and Clearance

The neutrophil majority in the bloodstream is duplicated in the bone marrow, where 60% of hematopoietic capacity may be dedicated to neutrophil production. Daily, 10^{11} neutrophils are released into the bloodstream.[2] Neutrophil development in the marrow takes about 14 days, originating with the hematopoietic stem cell. Stem cells fated to become neutrophils first differentiate into myeloblasts, which retain the capacity to develop into eosinophils, basophils, and neutrophils. Subsequent differentiation leads to the neutrophilic promyelocyte, a dedicated precursor of the neutrophil, and proceeds through the stages of neutrophilic myelocyte, metamyelocyte, band cell, and mature neutrophil. At the metamyelocyte stage, neutrophil mitosis ceases, whereas neutrophil development and organization of granules continue. Only the mature neutrophil demonstrates the classic feature of a multilobed nucleus.[3] Neutrophils are terminally differentiated; they neither divide nor, as a general rule, alter their gross phenotype after their release from the marrow. However, in the setting of certain infections, such as helminths, some neutrophils may show a distinct profile of gene expression and a ring-form nucleus, in contrast to the typical multilobed cell seen in the peripheral blood.[4]

Given the origin of neutrophils from pluripotent stem cells, as well as the precise phases of their development, the mechanisms regulating neutrophil differentiation are of considerable interest.

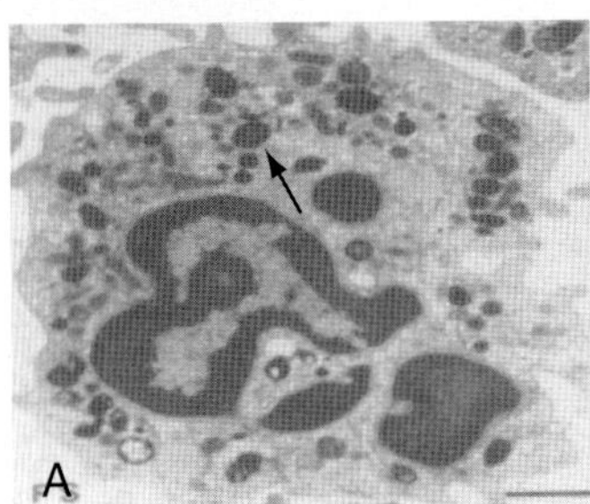

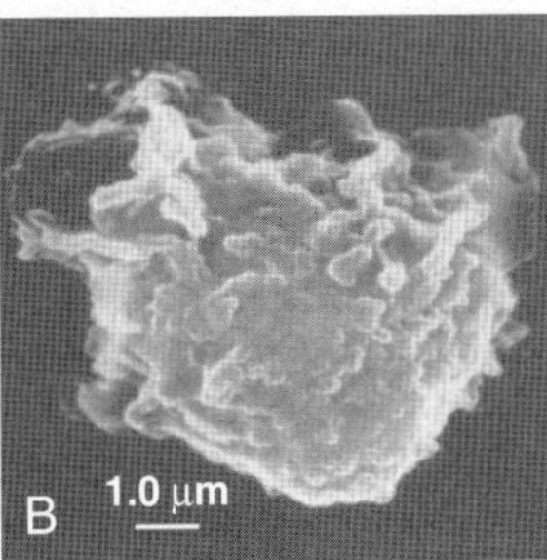

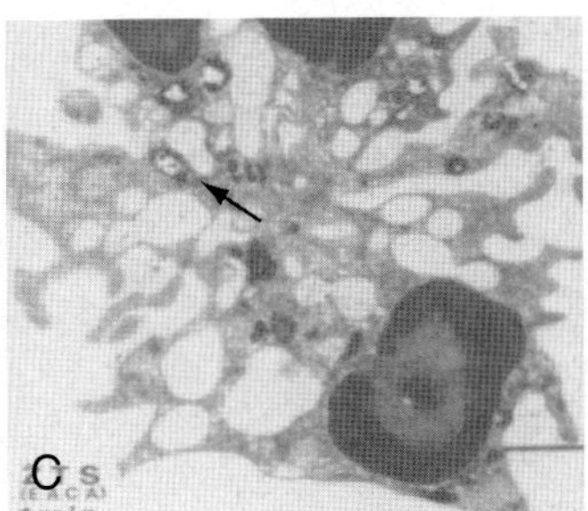

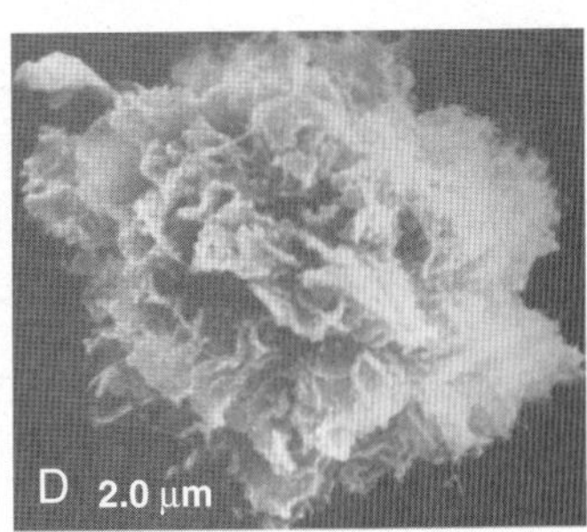

• **Fig. 11.1** Resting and stimulated neutrophil morphology. (A and B) Transmission (A) and scanning (B) electron micrographs of resting neutrophils. In (A) note the multilobed nucleus and the rich population of granules. At least two populations of granules may be discerned: The larger, darker granules represent the primary (azurophilic) granules, whereas the smaller, slightly paler granules are predominantly secondary (specific) granules and may include a population of gelatinase granules (*arrow* indicates primary granule). In (B) note the relatively smooth surface area with some membrane surface irregularities. (C and D) Transmission (C) and scanning (D) electron micrographs of neutrophils 1 minute after stimulation with zymosan. The cellular diameter is enlarged, and the overall surface (plasma) membrane area is greatly increased. Most of the membrane contributing to the increased surface area is supplied via the fusion of internal granule membranes with the plasma membrane. In (C) this fusion is apparent as the depletion of granules, leading to an appearance of empty vesicles (*arrow* indicates a partially depleted primary granule; clear circular areas represent fully depleted vesicles whose membranes are fused to the plasma membrane). In (D) this fusion is apparent as the increase in plasma surface membrane extensions, known as *lamellipodia*. (Courtesy G. Weissmann, NYU School of Medicine.)

Although this process remains incompletely understood, studies have emphasized the role of a particular complement of transcription factors and cytokines that seem to direct the early cells toward neutrophil development. Several myeloid factors are necessary for the transcriptional regulation of neutrophils including LEF-1, CCAAT enhancer binding proteins α, β, and ε (C/EBP-α, -β and -ε), and GFI-1. In contrast to other myeloid cells, lack of expression of the transcription factor GATA-1 also contributes to committed development of neutrophils.[5,6] Principal among the cytokines regulating granulopoiesis is granulocyte colony-stimulating factor (G-CSF). G-CSF effects include induction of myeloid differentiation, proliferation of granulocyte precursors, and release of mature neutrophils from the marrow.[7] Biologic effects of G-CSF are mediated through its receptor (G-CSFR or CD114), a member of the class I cytokine receptor family. Although other hematopoietic cytokines contribute to granulopoiesis in vivo (including granulocyte-macrophage colony-stimulating factor [GM-CSF], IL-6, and IL-3), their individual presence is not essential, as demonstrated by murine knockout experiments.

Once mature, neutrophils exit the bone marrow through the sinusoidal endothelium and enter the circulation, a process called *transcellular migration*.[8] Neutrophils released from the marrow have a bloodstream half-life of approximately 6 hours and a tissue half-life only marginally longer. Neutrophil life spans may be modulated by soluble signals; when exposed to stimuli such as TNF and Fas (CD95) ligand, neutrophils undergo apoptosis or programmed cell death.[9,10] The high output and short half-life of neutrophils imply that neutrophil clearance mechanisms must exist. Recently, the SDF-1/CXC chemokine receptor 4 (CXCR4) signaling system has been implicated in neutrophil clearance. CXCR4, a G-protein coupled receptor, is expressed at low levels in the mature neutrophil. As they age, neutrophils alter their phenotype and upregulate CXCR4. This change supports homing to the bone marrow via the chemoattractant stromal-derived factor 1 (SDF-1 or CXCL12). Once back in the marrow, senescent neutrophils are phagocytosed by stromal macrophages.[11] Senescent or apoptotic bloodstream neutrophils are also cleared by liver and spleen macrophages (reticuloendothelial system). Although little is known about the molecular mechanisms underlying neutrophil clearance in the liver and spleen, upregulation of the adhesion molecule P-selectin on Kupffer cells appears to be relevant. It remains a matter of speculation whether tissue neutrophils are cleared primarily via local macrophages or first passaged back through the lymphatic drainage system.

Neutrophil Morphology and Contents

Neutrophil nuclei tend to have more lobes than nuclei of other polymorphs, typically three to five (Figs. 11.1 and 11.2). In some circumstances, including vitamin B_{12} deficiency, neutrophil nuclei may become hypersegmented, with as many as seven lobes.[1] The multilobed nature of the neutrophil nucleus reflects a condensation of chromatin, suggesting that neutrophils might be incapable of transcription. It is now appreciated, however, that neutrophils retain the capacity for both constitutive and stimulated protein synthesis, albeit at a limited rate.[12]

Neutrophil granules identifiable by classic histochemical staining comprise two classes (Figs. 11.1 and 11.2). Two additional classes of granules require special techniques to recognize and identify them.

Primary Granules

Neutrophil primary granules form first (in myeloblasts and promyelocytes)[3] and, by virtue of their staining tendencies (affinity for the basic dye azure A), are also referred to as *azurophilic granules*.[13] These granules are oval or round and vary in size. They are similar, and functionally equivalent, to the lysosomes of other cells. Characteristic of azurophilic granules is the presence of myeloperoxidase (MPO), an enzyme that catalyzes the formation of hypochlorous acid from chloride in the presence of hydrogen peroxide (H_2O_2) (see *Respiratory Burst,* later). The presence of large amounts of this enzyme in azurophilic granules gives collections of neutrophils (pus) their typical greenish yellow color. Consistent with their functional role as lysosomes, azurophilic granules also contain a variety of proteases and other enzymes including elastase, lysozyme, acid phosphatase, cathepsins, and enzymes directed at nucleic acids and sugars (Table 11.1).[3] At the membrane level, however, they differ from true lysosomes in their lack of lysosome-associated membrane proteins I and II (LAMP-I and LAMP-II) and the mannose-6-phosphate receptor system.[14]

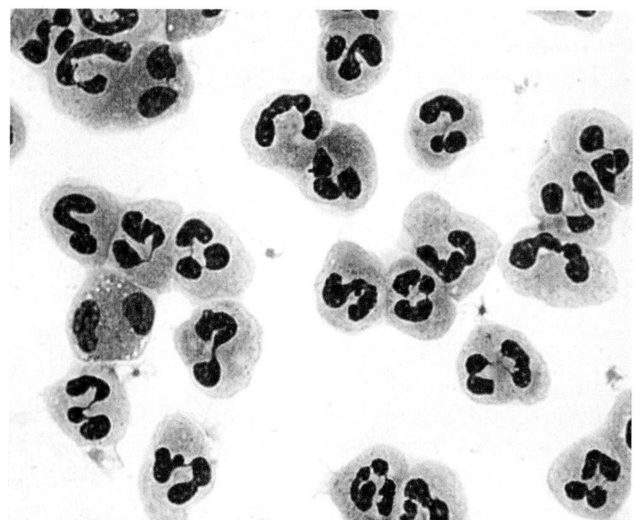

• **Fig. 11.2** Resting neutrophils and eosinophils under light microscopy. A blood smear stained with hematoxylin and eosin showing neutrophils and eosinophils; the three-lobulated nucleus (polymorphonuclear) cells are characteristic of neutrophil morphology. Two eosinophils are distinguished by their bilobed nuclei and pink-stained granules (eosin stains basic structures). (Courtesy K.A. Zarember, Laboratory of Host Defenses, National Institute of Allergy and Infectious Diseases, National Institutes of Health.)

Secondary Granules

In contrast to primary or azurophilic granules, neutrophil secondary granules constitute a population unique to neutrophils, a fact reflected in the alternatively employed nomenclature of specific granules. Specific granules possess an extensive array of membrane-associated proteins including cytochromes, signaling molecules, and receptors. Specific granules constitute a reservoir of proteins destined for topologically external surfaces of phagocytic vacuoles and the plasma membrane (see Table 11.1).[2,3] One particularly important family of proteinases found in neutrophil-specific granules are the matrix metalloproteinases (MMPs), including neutrophil collagenase-2 (MMP-8), gelatinase-B (MMP-9), stromelysin (MMP-3), and leukolysin (MMP-25). MMPs are stored as inactive proenzymes and undergo proteolytic activation after specific granule fusion with, and interaction with azurophilic granule contents in, the phagocytic vacuole.[3,15,16] MMP activation confers upon neutrophils the ability to alter and degrade integral membrane components of phagocytosed bacteria. Neutrophil MMP function is not limited to bacterial killing, however. For example, MMPs are also important for neutrophil extravasation and diapedesis (discussed in this chapter).[17]

Azurophilic and specific granules additionally contain antimicrobial proteins and peptides that are the cornerstone of innate immunity. A detailed description of the neutrophil's armamentarium against foreign invaders is beyond the scope of this chapter, but a few whose mechanisms of action have been elucidated warrant mention. Elastase, mentioned previously, aids in the killing of gram-negative bacteria via degradation of bacterial outer membrane protein A.[18] Elastase-deficient mice are more susceptible to infection with gram-negative (but not gram-positive) organisms than wild-type mice. The defensins, stored in azurophilic granules, accumulate in mg/mL concentrations in phagocytic vacuoles

TABLE 11.1 Partial Neutrophil Granule Contents

	Secretory Vesicles	Gelatinase Granules	Specific Granules	Azurophilic Granules
Relative size	Smallest	Intermediate	Intermediate	Largest
Soluble (matrix-associated) components	Plasma proteins	Gelatinase Acetyltransferase Arginase 1 Lysozyme Ficolin 1	Gelatinase MMP-3 MMP-8 MMP-9 Lactoferrin β_2-Microglobulin NGAL α_1-Anti-trypsin Lysozyme Haptoglobin hCAP-18	Myeloperoxidase Glucuronidase Elastase Lysozyme Proteinase 3 α_1-Anti-trypsin Defensins Cathepsin G BPI Azuricidin NSP4
Membrane-associated components	FMLP receptor SCAMP NRAMP2 VAMP2 CD11b/CD18 Cytochrome b_{558} Alkaline phosphatase Uroplasminogen activator CD10, CD13, CD16, CD45 CR1 Decay accelerating factor	FMLP receptor CD11b/CD18 Deacylating enzyme MMP-25 SCAMP CD177	CD11b/CD18 Cytochrome b_{558} CD66, CD67, CD177 Fibronectin receptor TNF receptor	CD63, CD68

BPI, Bactericidal/permeability-increasing protein; *FMLP*, formyl-methionyl-leucyl-phenylalanine; *MMP*, matrix metalloproteinase; *TNF*, tumor necrosis factor.

(discussed later) and render target (e.g., bacterial) cell membranes permeable. Based on their content, primary granules may be further subdivided into defensin-rich and defensin-poor granules, respectively.[19]

Bactericidal/permeability-inducing protein (BPI), also stored in azurophilic granules, acts in concert with the defensins; it potently neutralizes endotoxin and is cytotoxic to gram-negative bacteria.[20] BPI also enhances the activity of secretory phospholipase A_2, which has activity against gram-negative and gram-positive bacteria. Lactoferrin, found in specific granules, deprives microorganisms of iron and has antiviral and antibacterial effects. Other granule-associated proteins, such as cysteine-rich secretory protein 3 (CRISP3) and ficolin 1, have recently been described, although their functions are still unclear.

Gelatinase Granules and Secretory Vesicles

Special techniques have confirmed the existence of two additional classes of vesicles. Gelatinase granules are identical in size to specific granules and share some common proteins. As their name implies, however, gelatinase granules are distinguished by their high concentrations of gelatinase, a latent enzyme with the capacity for tissue destruction.[21] Secretory vesicles are smaller and lighter than the other classes and do not seem to contain proteolytic enzymes.[22] Rather, secretory vesicles are noteworthy for an extensive complement of membrane-associated proteins, including receptors otherwise identified with the plasma membrane. These and other data suggest that the secretory vesicle is a reservoir of neutrophil plasma membrane and other membrane proteins (see Table 11.1).

Neutrophil granule contents play important roles beyond their direct antimicrobial effects, including amplifying or dampening innate and adaptive immune responses. Lactoferrin released during phagocytosis inhibits proliferation of mixed lymphocyte cultures in vitro by decreasing release of IL-2, TNF, and IL-1β. On the other hand, proteinase 3 has been found to augment release of active TNF and IL-1β in monocyte/neutrophil co-cultures by releasing the membrane-bound forms of these cytokines.[23] Similarly, gelatinase B converts latent IL-1β into its active form, and potentiate IL-8 activity by truncating this chemoattractant and increasing its release, consequently amplifying neutrophilic influx.[24,25] Neutrophil elastase may also play a pro-inflammatory role by virtue of its ability to cleave and disrupt phosphatidyl serine receptors on macrophages. Apoptotic cells undergo membrane alterations that lead to expression of phosphatidyl serine on their outer membrane surface, and interaction of phosphatidyl serine with its receptor on macrophages leads to macrophage responses that downregulate inflammation through the generation of transforming growth factor (TGF)-β.[26] By disrupting these interactions, neutrophil elastase may permit inflammation to continue.

Neutrophil Activation and Signal Transduction

For bloodstream neutrophils to destroy foreign targets in the periphery, they must first sense the presence of such targets at a distance. They must then attach to the activated endothelium of blood vessels through multiple interactions involving adhesion molecules and their receptors (rolling and adhesion). After passing through the endothelium of postcapillary venules (diapedesis), neutrophils migrate to the source of the signal (chemotaxis). Finally, neutrophils must encounter a target, engulf it, and destroy it. Collectively, the processes that allow neutrophils to respond in these manners are referred to as *neutrophil activation.* Because of the potential for tissue destruction, neutrophil activation must be carefully regulated. The internal responses through which a cell translates an encounter with a stimulus into a particular phenotypic response are termed *signal transduction* (Fig. 11.3).[27]

Stimuli and Receptors

Classic neutrophil chemoattractants include lipid mediators (e.g., leukotriene B_4 [LTB_4], platelet-activating factor) and proteins/peptides (e.g., formylated peptides, the complement split product C5a, and the chemokine IL-8)[28] In vivo, chemoattractants are formed at sites of inflammation, either produced at the site by inflammatory cells (e.g., LTB_4 or IL-8) or liberated from presynthesized proteins, as in the case of C5a. The ability of formylated peptides such as *N*-formyl-methionyl-leucyl-phenylalanine to stimulate neutrophils probably represents a particularly ancient arm of the innate immune response because prokaryotic, but not eukaryotic (e.g., human), cells synthesize proteins whose first amino acid is a formylated methionine, allowing the more advanced organisms to recognize the more primitive ones. CXC chemokines are a group of chemoattractants characterized by the presence of two N-terminal cysteines *(C)* separated by any other amino acid *(X)* at the carboxy terminus. CXC chemokines that play a role in neutrophil recruitment include IL-8 (CXCL8), KC (CXCL1), and MIP-2 (CXCL2). In addition to their attractant activities, chemoattractants also stimulate most other aspects of neutrophil activation. Their individual potencies for particular responses differ, however, suggesting that they serve overlapping but distinct functions in neutrophil activation.[28,29]

Bloodstream activation of neutrophils depends on the presence of specific surface receptors. Most chemoattractant receptors belong to a class known as *seven-transmembrane-domain receptors* (also called *serpentine seven receptors* or *G protein-coupled receptors* [GPCRs]); these receptors are composed of a single protein chain whose hydrophobic domains snake across the plasma membrane a total of seven times.[30] Binding of chemoattractants to GPCRs occurs in a pocket on the extra-cellular face of the plasma membrane, at or below the level of the lipid hydrophobic head groups. Receptors for soluble ligands other than chemoattractants have also been identified on neutrophils, including receptors for growth factors, colony-stimulating factors, and cytokines. Growth factor receptors are members of the protein tyrosine kinase receptor family, in which ligand interaction with two identical or related receptors brings them into proximity, causing their cross-phosphorylation and activation. Receptors for a variety of inflammatory stimuli become highly expressed only in mature neutrophils.[31] These include CXC and CC chemokine receptors such as IL-8R-α and β; CXCR4 and CCR-1, 2, and 3; receptors for TNF and interferon (IFN)-α and -γ; and interleukin receptors IL1R, IL4R, IL6R, IL10R, and IL17R. Some nonchemoattractant ligands do not directly activate neutrophils but modulate their function. For example, pre-treatment of neutrophils with either insulin or GM-CSF results in amplification of subsequent neutrophil responses to chemoattractants, a process referred to as *priming.*[32]

Guanosine Triphosphate-Binding Proteins

Ligation of seven-transmembrane-domain receptors results in the activation of a class of intra-cellular effectors known as *heterotrimeric guanosine triphosphate (GTP)–binding proteins*, or G

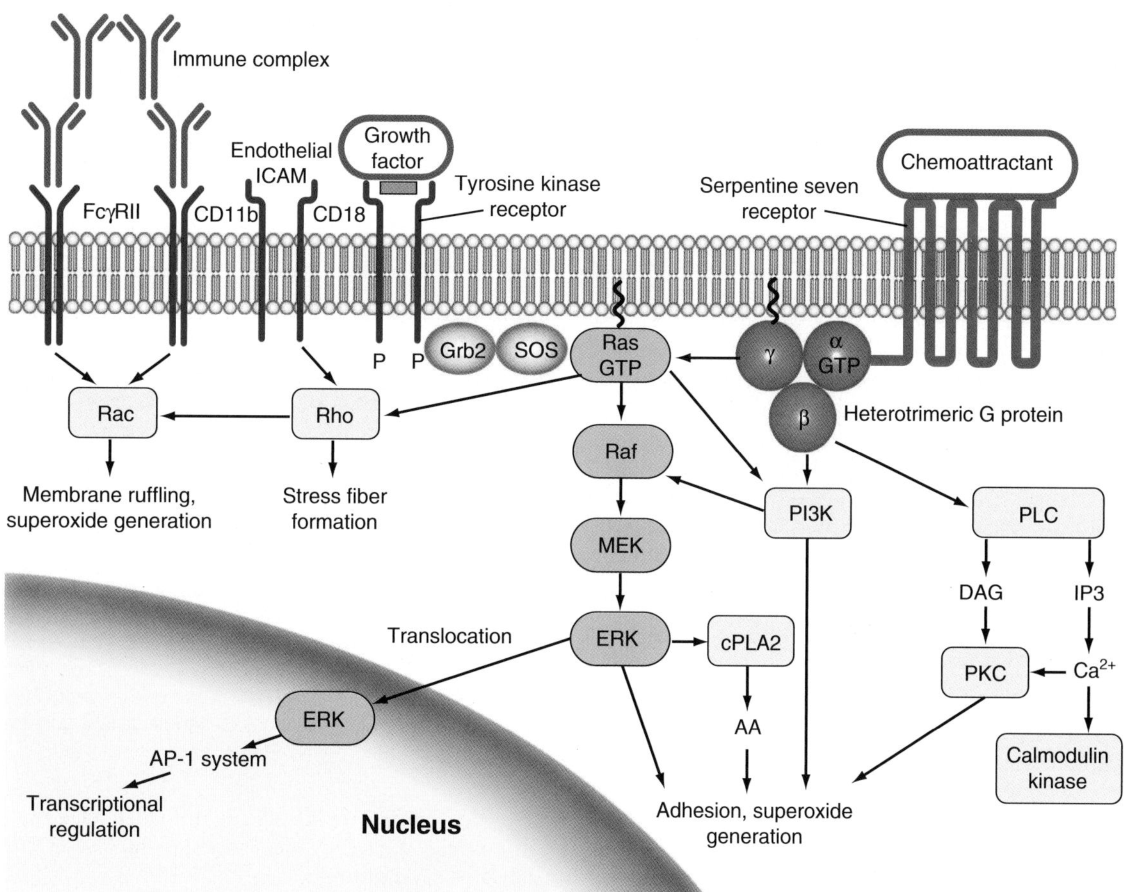

• **Fig. 11.3** Signaling pathways in neutrophil activation. Engagement of Fc, growth factor, and chemoattractant receptors and adhesion molecules initiate signaling pathways that result in pro-inflammatory neutrophil responses, including cytoskeletal and morphologic changes, activation of adhesion molecules and the superoxide generating system (NADPH oxidase), and regulation of transcription. Some of the well-established pathways participating in these responses are illustrated.

proteins. G proteins are composed of α, β, and γ subunits, and individual G protein types are distinguished by the particular α, β, and γ subunits they employ. In neutrophils, the predominant G proteins are of the G_i family. G protein γ subunits are modified by the addition of prenyl (polyisoprene) and carboxy-terminal methyl groups, which anchor them to the plasma membrane. All G proteins share the capacity, localized to their α subunits, to bind GTP and hydrolyze it to guanosine diphosphate (GDP). G proteins are active when GTP bound, but inactive in the GDP-bound form. Engagement of the appropriate serpentine-seven receptor promotes the binding of GTP on the α subunit. As a consequence of GTP binding, heterotrimeric G proteins dissociate into α and β/γ components, each with specific effector functions.[33]

A monomeric class of low-molecular weight (20 to 25 kDa) GTP-binding proteins (LMW-GBPs) is also important in neutrophil signal transduction. Because the first LMW-GBP described was the proto-oncogene Ras, these also are referred to as *Ras-related* or *Ras superfamily proteins,* or simply *small GTPases.* Small GTPases combine, in one molecule, the prenyl and methyl modifications of the G protein γ subunit with the GTP-binding capacity of the α subunit.[34] At least four families of small GTPases have been described: the Ras family, whose members play roles in activation as well as cell growth and division; the Rho family, which functions in cytoskeletal rearrangements; and the Rab and Arf families, crucial for vesicular and endomembrane trafficking.[35] All four classes of small GTPases are represented in neutrophils. The Rho family is thought to play the most direct role in neutrophil chemotaxis, with the Rho-family proteins Rac and Cdc42 regulating cytoskeletal rearrangements at the leading edge of neutrophil migration, and RhoA itself regulating arrangements at the uropod or trailing end.[36] (See also the section on chemotaxis.)

Second Messengers

Second messengers are small, diffusible molecules that are generated in response to stimuli and transmit signals from membrane receptors to downstream effector proteins. In the classic model of neutrophil activation, engagement of receptors results in the activation of phospholipase C, which cleaves phosphatidylinositol triphosphate (PIP_3) into diacylglycerol (DAG) and inositol 1,4,5-triphosphate (IP_3). DAG and IP_3 mediate the influx of cytosolic calcium and the activation of PKC, respectively. Other phospholipases present in the neutrophil include cytosolic phospholipase A_2 ($cPLA_2$), which cleaves phosphatidylcholine and/or ethanolamine from nuclear membrane lipids to generate arachidonic acid (AA), and phospholipase D, which cleaves phosphatidylcholine into phosphatidic acid and choline.[37] Although many second messengers are implicated in neutrophil activation, others may have inhibitory effects. For example, sphingosine and ceramide inhibit neutrophil phagocytosis.

In addition to lipids, other organic and inorganic second messenger molecules have been characterized. Intra-cellular concentrations of cyclic adenosine monophosphate (cAMP), a classic second messenger, increase rapidly in neutrophils exposed to both stimuli and inhibitors. cAMP in these settings is likely to provide a negative regulatory (off) signal because direct exposure to cAMP inhibits most neutrophil responses, primarily through the activation of protein kinase A (PKA).[29] (The anti-inflammatory effects of the phosphodiesterase 4 inhibitor apremilast are based on its ability to maintain cAMP levels and therefore sustain PKA activation.[38]) In contrast, increases in cyclic guanosine monophosphate (cGMP) have a modest enhancing effect on some neutrophil responses. Nitric oxide (NO), an important molecule in the regulation of host defense, is produced in neutrophils at low levels.[39] Studies have documented the capacity of NO to exert a variety of second messenger effects, including inhibition of reduced nicotinamide adenine dinucleotide phosphate (NADPH) oxidase, actin polymerization, and chemotaxis (discussed later). Conversely, excessive NO production has been implicated in many rheumatic diseases.[40]

Kinases and Kinase Cascades

Multiple kinases, proteins capable of enzymatically adding phosphate groups to target molecules, contribute to signaling in myeloid and nonmyeloid cells. PKC, now understood to be a family of kinases, was among the first kinases implicated in neutrophil activation in response to chemoattractants. The ability of phorbol myristate acetate (PMA), a synthetic activator of PKC, to stimulate neutrophil responses supports a role for PKC in neutrophil activation.[41] Conversely, inhibitors of PKC block stimulation of neutrophil functions.

The mitogen-activated protein kinases (MAPKs) are a family of serine threonine kinases, including the extra-cellular regulating kinase (ERK), p38, and c-Jun amino terminal kinase (JNK) families. In neutrophils, chemoattractants and other stimuli are capable of activating ERK, p38, and JNK, with time courses consistent with neutrophil activation. A role for ERK activation in signaling for both neutrophil O_2^- and neutrophil adhesion and phagocytosis has been demonstrated.[29,34,42] Phosphatidylinositol 3-kinase (PI3K) is a family of related enzymes that are found in abundance in neutrophils and primarily catalyze the phosphorylation, not of proteins, but of the three-position of phosphatidylinositol phospholipids. One of the main bioactive products of PI3K is PIP_3. Chemoattractants such as formyl-methionyl-leucyl-phenylalanine (FMLP) rapidly activate PI3K in neutrophils, where it participates in diverse neutrophil functions including O_2^- generation, adhesion, and degranulation.[43] PI3K also may regulate neutrophil survival and apoptosis.

Neutrophil Function

Adhesion

One of the earliest, crucial aspects of the inflammatory response is the ability of bloodstream neutrophils to adhere to vascular endothelium preparatory to movement into the tissues (Fig. 11.4). Stimulated neutrophils also possess the ability to adhere to each other (homotypic aggregation), which can bring bloodstream neutrophils into proximity with neutrophils already adherent to the vessel, or concentrate them at a site of inflammation. Several families of interacting adhesion molecules are displayed by neutrophils and endothelial cells, including selectins, integrins, intercellular adhesion molecules (ICAMs), and sialylated glycoproteins.

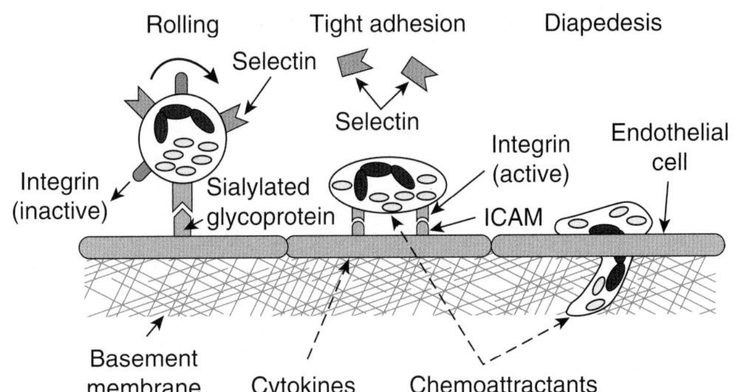

• **Fig. 11.4** Neutrophil adhesion to the vascular endothelium. *Left,* Rolling. An unstimulated neutrophil adheres with low affinity to the unstimulated endothelium of a postcapillary venule, a process mediated by the interaction of selectins (on neutrophil and endothelium) with sialylated glycoproteins and resulting in the rolling of neutrophils along the vessel wall. *Center,* Tight adhesion. Exposure of the neutrophil to chemoattractants results in activation of integrins (CD11a/CD18, CD11b/CD18); exposure of endothelium to cytokines results in the expression of intercellular adhesion molecules. These molecules interact, resulting in tight adhesion. Concurrently, selectins may be shed from the cell surfaces. *Right,* Diapedesis. A neutrophil undergoes diapedesis, passing across the endothelium and making its way through the basement membrane. Bloodstream neutrophils have the capacity to adhere to and move out of the vasculature in response to tissue signals for inflammation. *ICAM,* Intercellular adhesion molecule.

Selectins and Sialylated Glycoproteins

The selectin family includes three related molecules (L-selectin on leukocytes, E-selectin on endothelial cells, and P-selectin on activated platelets and endothelial cells). Selectins share a common structure of two or more complement regulatory domains, an epidermal growth factor–like domain and a lectin domain. Each selectin binds to a specific sialylated glycoprotein on the surface of its interacting cell: E-selectin binds to the sialyl Lewis^x antigen on neutrophils, P-selectin binds P-selectin glycoprotein-1 (PSGL-1) on neutrophils, and L-selectin binds PSGL-1 and GlyCAM-1 on the endothelium. Selectin/sialylated glycoprotein interactions are of low affinity and transient, and leukocytes therefore repetitively bind to, and release from, the endothelial surface. The result is a pool of bloodstream neutrophils that is, at any given time, loosely adherent to the vascular surface (i.e., marginated) and moving along it slowly in a rolling, tumbleweed-like motion. These neutrophils are therefore not sampled during routine clinical blood measurements. Exposure of neutrophils and endothelium to appropriate stimuli (e.g., adrenergic discharge, corticosteroids) leads to shedding of selectins and neutrophil release (demargination), with apparent increases in the measured peripheral neutrophil count.[44]

Integrins and Intercellular Adhesion Molecules

The integrins are a large family of heterodimeric molecules generated by various combinations of α and β chains. Like the selectins, integrins require divalent cations (Ca^{2+} or Mg^{2+} or both) to engage their ligands. Neutrophils express three β_2-type integrins, each constructed from a distinct α subcomponent (CD11a, CD11b, or CD11c) and a common β_2 chain (CD18). Integrins primarily use ICAMs as their counter-ligands. CD11b/CD18 (also called *Mac-1* or *CR3*) binds to fibrinogen, factor X, heparin, and the complement component iC3b in addition to ICAMs and is most strongly implicated in neutrophil/endothelial and neutrophil/neutrophil interactions. In contrast to the selectins, neutrophil CD11b/CD18 is constitutively expressed but inactive; stimulation of neutrophils results in changes in the CD11b/CD18 activation state and increases its affinity for ICAMs and other ligands.[45] Stimulation of endothelium with cytokines such as IL-1β results in increased expression of ICAM-1 and ICAM-2, providing a coordinate mechanism for the regulation of adhesion. In contrast to selectin-mediated adhesion, integrin/ICAM interactions are high-affinity and persistent. Stimulation of rolling neutrophils therefore results in their tight adhesion to vessel walls and constitutes the first committed step in the movement of neutrophils into tissues. Additionally, engagement of integrins by their counter-ligands sends signals into the cell ("outside in" signaling) that regulate selective cell responses such as cytoskeletal reorganization, oxidant production, and degranulation. Outside-in signaling through CD11b/CD18 also coordinates with signaling through Fc receptor FcγRIII (discussed later) to regulate a number of different functions, including phagocytosis of particles opsonized by IgG and the complement component iC3b and neutrophil-dependent adhesion in immune complex-mediated vascular inflammation.[46] Cross-talk between neutrophils and endothelial cells is a CD11b/CD18-dependent event: cross-linking of CD18 on neutrophils leads to increased endothelial permeability, probably through the release of neutrophil proteases.[47]

Data also strongly support that interactions between ICAMs and CD11a/CD18 (also known as *lymphocyte function-associated antigen-1*, or *LFA-1*) are necessary for neutrophil adhesion and emigration.[48] During neutrophil rolling on inflamed endothelium, neutrophil engagement by PSGL-1 leads to CD11a/CD18 activation, which in turn may contribute to neutrophil arrest.[49] Evidence suggests that CD11a/CD18 and CD11b/CD18 play slightly different roles, with CD11a/CD18 primarily regulating initial tight adhesion, and CD11b/CD18-ICAM mediating interactions allowing the cell to crawl over the endothelium to identify a possible location for transmigration (see below).[50] The function of CD11c/CD18 on neutrophils remains less clear.

Diapedesis and Chemotaxis

Diapedesis

The mechanism by which neutrophils pass through blood vessels (diapedesis) is not fully established. Although many experts consider that neutrophil diapedesis occurs between endothelial cells by disrupting cell-cell junctions,[44] some evidence suggests that neutrophils pass directly through pores generated within the endothelial cells themselves (Fig. 11.5).[51,52] Diapedesis requires homotypic interactions between adhesion molecules found on both neutrophils and endothelial cells which are known as *platelet-endothelial cell adhesion molecules* (PECAMs). PECAMs are concentrated at endothelial cell junctions, and antibodies that bind PECAMs inhibit transmigration in vitro by limiting neutrophils to the apical surface of the endothelium. Transmigrating neutrophils undergo upregulation of α6β1, an integrin that mediates binding to laminin (a key component of the perivascular basement membrane). Antibodies to α6β1 generally block neutrophil transmigration but fail to do so in a PECAM knockout mouse, implicating α6β1 and PECAM as both crucial to the passage of neutrophils out of the vasculature.[53] CD47, otherwise known as *integrin-associated protein,* and CD99, expressed on neutrophils and endothelial junctions, have also been implicated in neutrophil passage through the endothelium.

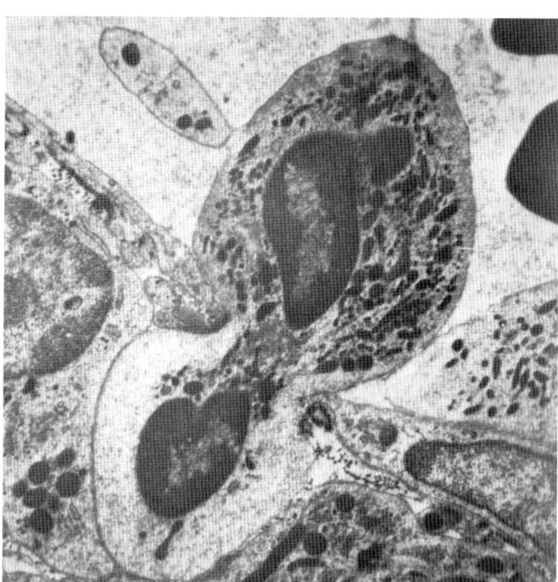

• **Fig. 11.5** Neutrophil diapedesis through the vascular endothelium. A neutrophil passaging between, or through, one or more endothelial cells is illustrated. The characteristic neutrophil multilobed nucleus and multiple granule types are visible. The leading edge of the neutrophil, passing through the endothelium, is relatively devoid of granule contents, suggesting that it represents the formation of a specialized structure for diapedesis, including the formation of F-actin cytoskeleton.

Once beyond the endothelium, neutrophils typically pause before traversing the basement membrane (basal lamina). Classic studies by Huber and Weiss[54] suggest that neutrophils pass through the basement membrane via transient disruption of its patency, without utilization of known proteases or oxygen radicals. The disruptions are rapidly reversed, through mechanisms likely involving endothelial tethering and release of the basement membrane. Speaking metaphorically, the endothelial cells may hold open the door of the tent (basement membrane) as the neutrophil enters, and then release it again after the neutrophil has passed through.

Chemotaxis

Chemotaxis in the direction of a molecular gradient is achieved by the extension of membrane ruffles (lamellipodia), followed by anchorage of the ruffles to the substrate and withdrawal of the trailing edge of the cell in the direction of movement. These changes are accomplished primarily through rearrangement of the actin cytoskeleton after sensing chemotactic gradients that signal through GPCRs and PI3K. Actin is a 41 kDa protein that exists as a soluble, globular monomeric form (G-actin) and as an insoluble linear polymer (F-actin). F-actin may be assembled (extended) at one end (barbed end) and disassembled at the other, under the control of regulatory molecules. During chemotaxis, F-actin formation and extension is concentrated at the leading edge of the neutrophil, permitting extension of the cell membrane (see Fig. 11.5). Chemoattractant receptors also concentrate at the leading edge, defining the cell's directional response to the gradient (headlight phenomenon). As the neutrophil moves along, receptors that were formerly at the leading edge are swept to the tail and internalized.[55]

Phagocytosis and Degranulation

Phagocytosis

Neutrophil phagocytosis of an encountered bacterium or other particle requires direct contact. Phagocytosis can be activated by direct neutrophil recognition of pathogen-associated molecular patterns (PAMPs), which are small molecule motifs found on or in bacteria or viruses (but not typically mammalian cells). PAMPs are recognized by Toll-like receptors (TLRs)[56] and other pattern recognition receptors (PRRs). Human neutrophils express all TLRs except for TLR3, and TLR activation stimulates human neutrophil phagocytosis by promoting structural and conformational changes.[57] However, neutrophils are generally poor at phagocytosing unmodified targets, particularly encapsulated bacteria. Phagocytosis is greatly enhanced by *opsonization* (from the Greek, "to prepare for the table"), the modification of a target via its decoration with immunoglobulin, complement components, or both (Fig. 11.6).

Neutrophils express two families of receptors for the Fc portion of complexed or aggregated IgG: low-affinity FcγRIIa and high-affinity FcγRIIIb.[58] During some infections, or after in vitro stimulation with interferon or G-CSF, neutrophils also express the high-affinity receptor FcγRI, which binds monomeric IgG.

FcγRIIa binds subclasses of IgG with varying efficiency depending on a polymorphism at amino acid position 131. FcγRIIIb polymorphisms of neutrophil antigens NA1 and NA2 also determine binding to IgG subclasses. Individuals homozygous for the NA2 allele have a lower capacity to mediate phagocytosis than individuals homozygous for the NA1 allele. These differences have important implications for rheumatic diseases in which immune complexes play an important role.

Phagocytosis is an active process involving simultaneous extension of the neutrophil membrane (filopodia and lamellipodia formation) around and invagination of the neutrophil at the locus of the target. Engagement of FcγR and complement receptors results in the activation of different signaling pathways that play distinct roles in phagocytosis.[59] Whereas engagement of CR3 (CD11b/CD18) results in actin stress fiber formation and invagination, engagement of FcγRII results primarily in extension of membranes out from, and around, the target. Signaling by these receptors depends on the activation of distinct members of the Rho family of LMW-GBPs.

Degranulation

Upon engaging a target, neutrophils degranulate, a term reflecting two possible and distinct events. Vesicles can fuse with the plasma membrane, spilling their contents into the extra-cellular space (see Fig. 11.1), or they can fuse with the phagocytic vacuole to form a phagolysosome. The former type of degranulation is regulated differentially from the latter and favors mobilization of lighter granules in response to stimuli (secretory vesicles > gelatinase granules > specific granules > azurophilic granules).[60] In the latter type of degranulation (phagolysosome formation), the preferential fusion of azurophilic granules with the phagocytic vacuole results in the delivery of proteolytic proenzymes, MPO, and antibacterial proteins to the site of an ingested bacterium.[61] Fusion of specific granules with the phagocytic vacuole then permits the delivery of collagenase, activation of azurophilic granule enzymes, and the appropriate localization of cytochrome b_{558}, a requisite for NADPH oxidase (discussed later). These regulated processes permit the maintenance of potentially toxic agents in inactive forms until they are required, at which point they are brought into proximity with each other and activated. Containment of the activated substances within the phagolysosome concentrates them near target bacteria, and minimizes host tissue damage and neutrophil autodestruction. However, control of granule content is imperfect, and toxic molecules may still spill into the extra-cellular milieu, particularly when the target is large (frustrated phagocytosis).

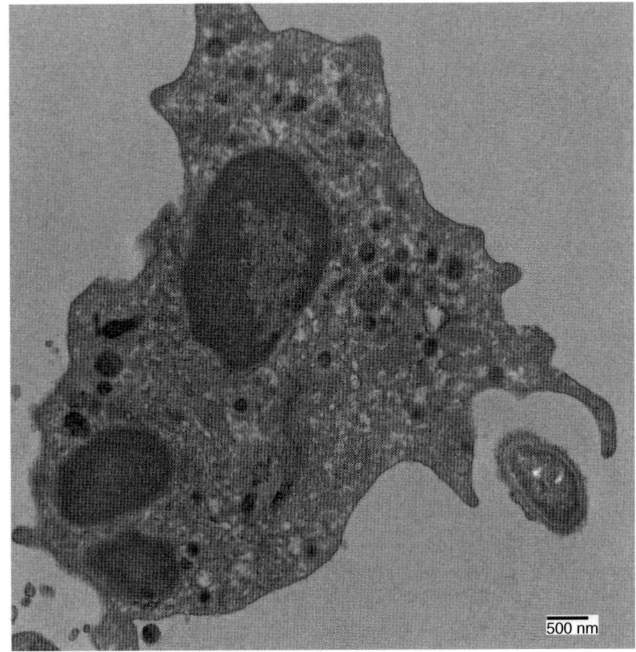

• **Fig. 11.6** Neutrophil engulfing bacteria. Neutrophils can internalize and kill many microbes, each phagocytic event resulting in the formation of a phagosome into which reactive oxygen species and hydrolytic enzymes are secreted. A transmission electron micrograph at the precise moment in which a bacterium is being phagocytosed by a neutrophil. (Courtesy K.A. Zarember, D.E. Greenberg, and K. Nagashima, Laboratory of Host Defenses, National Institute of Allergy and Infectious Diseases, National Institutes of Health.)

Respiratory Burst

In addition to the proteases and other antibacterial proteins contained in their granules, neutrophils have the capacity to kill bacteria through the generation of toxic oxygen metabolites such as NO, superoxide anion (O_2^-), and hydrogen peroxide (H_2O_2). This process, mediated by the NADPH oxidase system and frequently referred to as the *oxidative* or *respiratory burst,* is extremely potent and requires tight regulation to prevent neutrophil autodestruction.[62] The central component of NADPH oxidase is flavocytochrome b_{558}, which is localized to the membranes of specific granules and consists of two subunits: a 22-kDa component (gp22^{phox}, for *ph*agocyte *ox*idase) and a 91-kDa component (gp91^{phox}). This flavocytochrome lacks independent activity, however, and several cytosolic proteins are additionally required for oxidase activation, primarily a 47-kDa and a 67-kDa component (p47^{phox} and p67^{phox}).[63] On neutrophil stimulation, the p47^{phox} and p67^{phox} components translocate to the membranes to form an active complex with the flavocytochrome (Fig. 11.7). A fifth protein, p40^{phox}, associates with p47^{phox}/p67^{phox} and plays a less well-defined role in phagocytosis-induced superoxide production.[64,65] Finally, the small GTPase p21^{rac} also translocates to the complex in response to stimuli, and appears to contribute to oxidase activity in some way.[66,67]

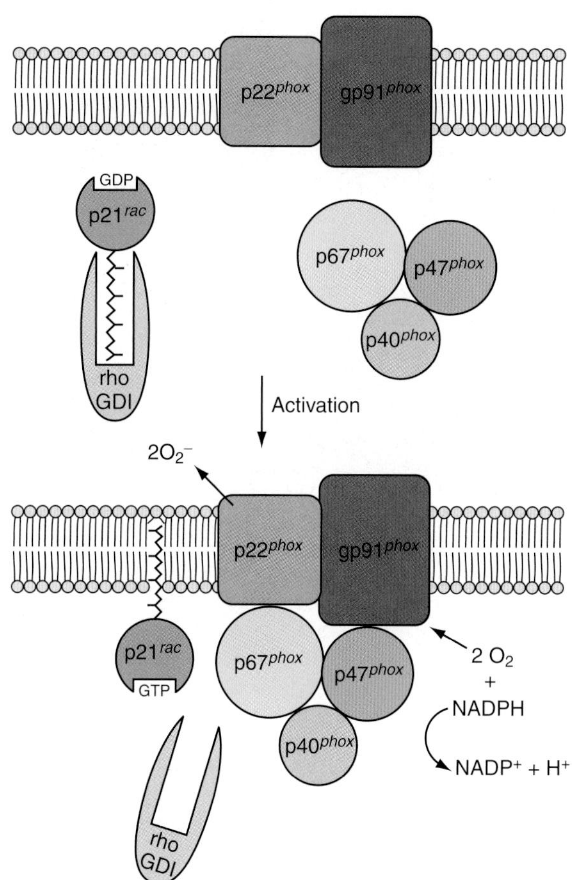

• **Fig. 11.7** Assembly of the neutrophil NADPH oxidase system. *Top,* Basic components of the NADPH oxidase as they are distributed in a resting state. The cytochrome b_{558}, composed of the two subunits $gp91^{phox}$ and $p22^{phox}$, are membrane associated, whereas $p47^{phox}$, $p67^{phox}$, and the more recently identified $p40^{phox}$ exist as a complex in the cytoplasm. $p21^{rac}$ in an inactive, GDP-bound form also resides in the cytoplasm, in association with a chaperone (Rho-GDI) that sheaths its hydrophobic tail to permit solubility. *Bottom,* Activation of the neutrophil leads to translocation of the cytosolic components of the oxidase to the neutrophil membrane, where they form an active complex with the cytochrome, resulting in the generation of oxygen. The potentially damaging oxidase system is carefully regulated through the segregation and assembly of its component parts.

When assembled and activated, the NADPH oxidase transfers electrons from NADPH to generate O_2^-:

$$2O_2 + NADPH \xrightarrow{\text{NADPH-Oxidase}} O_2^- + NADP^+ + H^+$$

A subsequent, spontaneous dismutase reaction rapidly produces hydrogen peroxide:

$$2O_2^- + H_2 \longrightarrow H_2O_2 + O_2$$

Although O_2^- and H_2O_2 can kill organisms in vitro, they are short lived and probably do not account for most of the bacterial killing capacity of the system under normal circumstances (indeed, many bacteria possess catalase, an enzyme that degrades H_2O_2). Instead, the production of H_2O_2 within the same space into which MPO has been released permits the generation of large quantities of hypochlorous acid (HOCL; chlorine bleach), a powerful oxidant with potent killing capacity. HOCL can also interact with proteins to form chloramines, less potent but longer-lived oxidants. Neutrophil oxidant production plays a key role in the body's defense against microorganisms. The view that oxidant production, via the production of HOCl by MPO, is the neutrophil's most powerful tool against microbes has been challenged, however. Mice lacking either NADPH oxidase or elastase and cathepsin G are susceptible to infection, implying that both arms of defense—oxidant production and protease-mediated microbial destruction—are equally crucial. Moreover, superoxide production in phagocytic vacuoles may indirectly promote protease function by causing the vacuolar pH to rise (secondary to the consumption of protons necessary to make H_2O_2), which, in turn, causes an influx of K^+. The resulting increase in ionicity liberates cationic proteases from the anionic proteoglycan matrix, freeing them to kill bacteria. In this newer model, oxidants are not primarily destructive to microbes, but rather are necessary to assist proteolytic damage.[68]

Neutrophil Production of Pro-inflammatory Mediators

Arachidonic Acid Metabolites

The capacity of stimulated neutrophils to liberate arachidonic acid (through the action of $cPLA_2$) from membranes has implications for acute inflammation. Although arachidonic acid has intrinsic chemoattractant and neutrophil-stimulatory properties, its metabolites are more crucial to its inflammatory effects.[42,69,70] Best recognized among these are the LTs. Neutrophils can produce LTB_4, a highly potent mediator for the chemoattraction of other neutrophils.[69] Intermediates of leukotriene production (e.g., 5-hydroxyeicosatetraenoic acid) also are produced by neutrophils and may have stimulatory properties.[42]

The cyclooxygenase (COX) (endoperoxide synthase) pathway is the other major pathway of arachidonic acid metabolism. Arachidonic acid metabolized by COX is converted into prostaglandin H, which undergoes further cell type-specific conversion to a variety of other prostaglandins.[71] The prostaglandin of most relevance to inflammation is PGE_2, whose numerous pro-inflammatory effects include increased vasodilation, vascular permeability, and pain. Interestingly, the direct effects of PGE_2 on neutrophils are largely inhibitory, probably through elevations of intra-cellular cAMP.[72] Although resting neutrophils exhibit little COX activity, persistent activation results in upregulation of COX-2, suggesting that neutrophils may contribute PGE_2 to both the inflammatory brew and the downregulation of their own activity.

Cytokine Production

Although the relative amount of cytokine production by neutrophils is small, the large numbers of neutrophils present in infected or inflammatory sites suggest that overall neutrophil cytokine production may play a role in recruiting additional neutrophils to the target area. Cytokines produced by neutrophils include chemokines such as IL-8, MIP-1α and MIP-1β (CCL3 and CCL4), and CXCL9 and -10, as well as growth-related oncogene-α (GRO-α), oncostatin M, and MCP-1. Neutrophils may also produce limited amounts of classical cytokines such as IL-1β, TNF, and IL-6, as well as anti-inflammatory cytokines such as IL-1ra.[12] Multiple lines of investigation suggest that neutrophils may also be a source for IL-17, a potent cytokine that can amplify neutrophil migration and recruitment.[73] The transcriptional program of terminally differentiated neutrophils requires a selective combination of stimulants for the production of specific chemokines. For example, in the presence of lipopolysaccharide, TNF drives neutrophil production of IL-8, GRO-α, and MIP-1, whereas IFN-γ drives CXCL9 and -10.[74]

Other neutrophil-derived molecules have been identified as bridging factors between innate and adaptive immunity. Activated neutrophils release both B-lymphocyte stimulator (BLyS)[75] and TNF-related apoptosis-inducing ligand (TRAIL).[76] While BLyS stimulates B cell proliferation (through the TNF receptors BAFF-R, TACI, and BCMA), TRAIL induces anti-tumor T cell effects and apoptosis.

TGF-β is a potent neutrophil chemoattractant at femtomolar concentrations, and its recruitment of neutrophils into an inflammatory space may lead to additional neutrophil cytokine production, including further production of TGF-β.[77] At higher concentrations, however, TGF-β has potent anti-inflammatory effects, and blocks neutrophil degranulation in response to LPS, FMLP, and TLR ligands.[26,78]

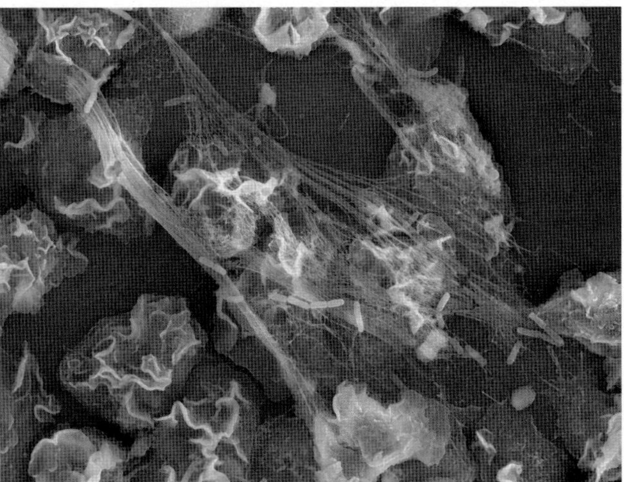

• **Fig. 11.8** Neutrophil extra-cellular traps (NETs). NETs are complex extracellular structures that are composed of chromatin, with specific proteins from the neutrophilic granules attached. NETs can trap gram-negative bacteria, gram-positive bacteria, and fungi. A scanning electron micrograph showing stimulated neutrophils forming NETs to trap *Shigella flexneri.* (Courtesy V. Brinkmann and A. Zychlinsky, Max Planck Institute for Infection.)

Neutrophil NETs and Microparticles

Recently discovered nonphagocytic mechanisms of neutrophil-mediated bacterial killing further augment host defense.

Neutrophil Extra-cellular Traps (NETs)

Neutrophil extra-cellular traps, or NETs, are extruded extracellular meshes composed of neutrophil-derived chromatin and granule proteins (Fig. 11.8).[79,80] The DNA that comprises the chromatin in NETs may originate from the neutrophil's nucleus (nDNA) and/or mitochondria (mtDNA).[81] Studies on these distinct types of NETosis have shown that while mtDNA extrusion can occur within 2 minutes, NETosis of nDNA typically takes more time (>2 hrs).

NETs may be formed and released in response to microbes as a mechanism of antimicrobial defense, or in response to sterile triggers such as cytokines, chemokines, immune complexes, or activated platelets present in inflammatory or autoimmune diseases.[82] NETs may be pro-inflammatory, anti-inflammatory, or both. While one study demonstrated aggregated NETs can create a physical barrier along large necrotic areas and thereby limit undesirable immune responses, NETs also contribute to the creation of the necrotic tissue.[83,84] As a part of their antimicrobial defense, NETs entrap bacteria while simultaneously providing a scaffold to promote high local concentrations of neutrophil antimicrobial components, thus killing microbes extra-cellularly.[79] In addition to killing microbes, NETs may simply inactivate microbes by cleaving virulence factors using highly concentrated adherent neutrophil proteins such as neutrophil elastase and cathepsin G. Furthermore, different neutrophil-derived granular proteins on the surface of NETs are associated with the elimination of different microbes (e.g., MPO for *Staphylococcus aureus,* calgranulin for fungi).[85,86] Several bacteria, however, degrade NETs via endonucleases.[87,88]

The release of NETs is typically associated with the suicide of neutrophils, characterized by chromatin decondensation, nuclear swelling, and membrane perforation (suicidal NETosis).[80] The process may be initiated by stimuli such as bacteria, viruses, and fungi that bind to receptors on the neutrophil surface such as Toll-like receptors or receptors for IgG-Fc or cytokines.[79] A subsequent release of calcium from the endoplasmic reticulum leads to the development of functional NADPH oxidase and generation of reactive oxygen species, which, in turn, trigger release of neutrophil elastase and MPO from azurophilic granules, neutrophil rupture, and release of the chromatin and granular proteins.[84] Interestingly, neutrophils in which oxidant production is blocked are unable to undergo NETosis, suggesting a role for oxidants in driving the NET process.[89–91] MPO binding of chromatin enhances nuclear decondensation, and may thereby also promote suicidal NETosis.[90] In addition, chromatin decondensation may also be driven by global transcriptional activation.[92] Once released from cells, chromatin decondensation appears to depend on histone hypercitrullination catalyzed by peptidylarginine deiminase 4 (an enzyme that also links to the assembly of NADPH oxidase),[93] as well as neutrophil elastase that digests nucleosomal histones or post-translational modification of core and linker histones.[89]

Not all NETosis leads to neutrophil destruction. In some situations neutrophils may alternatively undergo "vital NETosis," in which they eject their chromatin but remain otherwise structurally intact and retain the ability to chemotax and phagocytose microorganisms.[94] Vital NETosis occurs more quickly than suicidal NETosis, and is more likely to reflect release of mitochondrial rather than nuclear DNA, but like suicidal NETosis it depends on the generation of reactive oxygen species.[95–97] Vital NETosis occurs in response to *Staphylococcus aureus, Candida albicans,* and lipopolysaccharides on the surface of gram-negative bacteria, and in some cases involves Toll-like receptor 4 on platelets as a mediator.[98–100] Although the release of NETs may be mediated by multiple pathways, the mechanisms through which a neutrophil "decides" to undergo suicidal versus vital NETosis remain unclear.

Microparticles

Neutrophil-derived microparticles (microvesicles, exosomes) are emancipated, cytosol-entrapping vesicles derived from neutrophil plasma membrane. Like NETs, microparticles are previously unappreciated propagators of neutrophil-mediated outcomes (Fig. 11.9).[101] During activation, neutrophils release these heterogeneous vesicles,[102] which range in diameter between 100 and 1000 nm and express surface markers of their parent cells. Microparticles can bind to target cells (including endothelial cells) in a receptor-dependent manner and, in so doing, transfer parent

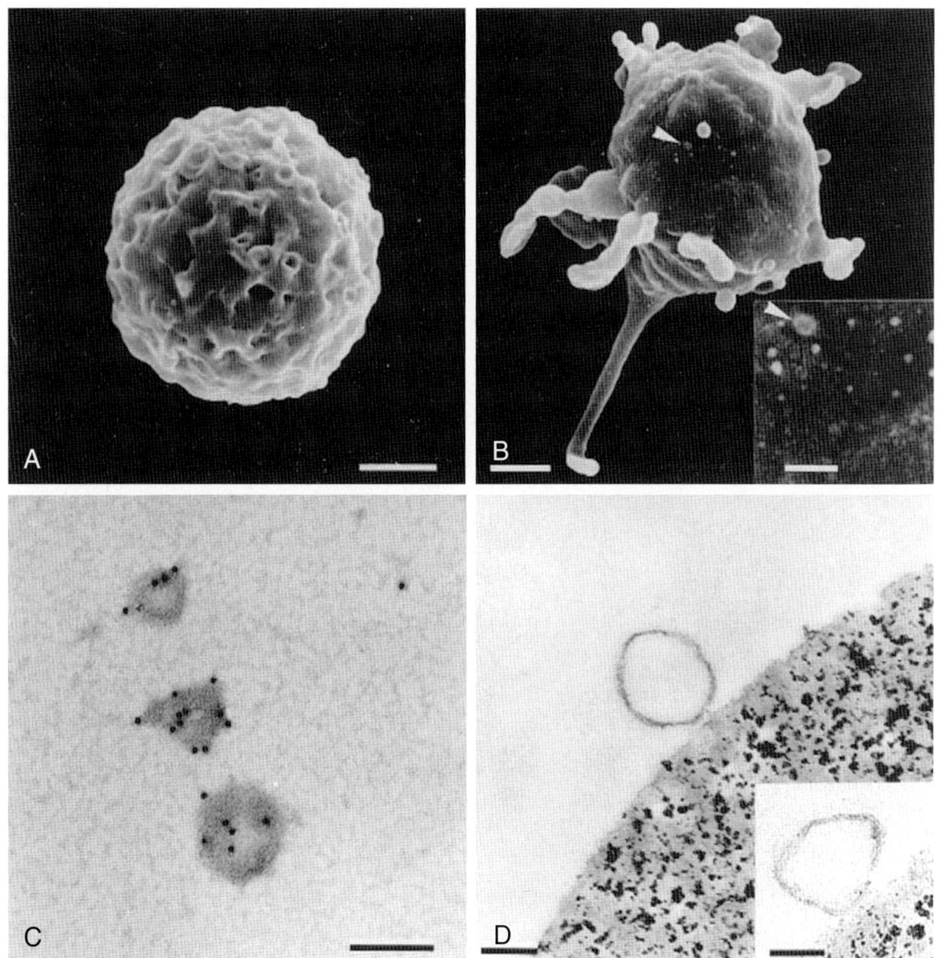

• **Fig. 11.9 Neutrophil microparticles.** (A) Scanning electron micrograph of a resting neutrophil (scale bar: 1.5 μm). (B) Scanning electron micrograph of a stimulated neutrophil in response to 0.1 μM FMLP. Note the large pseudopodia and budding of small vesicles (70–300 nm in size) from the neutrophil cell membrane (*arrowhead*; inset, higher magnification showing microparticle at arrowhead). (C) Transmission electron micrograph of immunogold-labeled microparticles, indicating the presence of antigens also found on the neutrophil cell surface (also seen in D) (scale bar: 150 nm). (D) Thin sections of microparticles precipitated with Dynabeads demonstrate bilamellar structure. (Copyright 1999. The American Association of Immunologists, Inc.)

cell mRNA and miRNA to drive transcellular responses. Neutrophil-derived microparticle numbers increase in sepsis as well as cardiovascular disease; they also appear to play a significant role in infection-mediated thrombosis (see also later).[102–105] Studies demonstrate that neutrophil-derived microparticles may promote both inflammatory effects via surface expression of L-selectin that allows adhesion of the microparticles to endothelial cells[106] and anti-inflammatory effects via increases in the release of TGF-β.[107]

NETs, Microparticles, and Thrombosis

Recent evidence indicates that neutrophils play a key role in the activation of platelets and thrombin, underlining the interaction between inflammation and thrombosis. Neutrophils that accumulate at sites of inflammation do so in concert with aggregating platelets, and further enhance platelet aggregation (Fig. 11.10); platelet-neutrophil complexes are elevated in patients with systemic lupus erythematosus and rheumatoid arthritis, likely due to neutrophil activation.[108] On the other hand, in the setting of vascular injury and endothelial damage, platelets activated in response to exposed collagen express P-selectin to promote neutrophil-platelet associations via neutrophil PSGL-1 counter-receptors. Subsequent activation of neutrophils leads to firmer bonds as a result of integrin CD11b/CD18 adhesion molecule activation.[109] Neutrophil-platelet interactions result in surface expression of tissue factor that can initiate the coagulation cascade.[110] More recent data suggest that in the setting of inflammation, neutrophils internalize platelet-derived microparticles via 12(S)-hydroxyeicosatetranoic acid, which in turn is produced by the interaction of inflammatory-induced secreted phospholipase A_2 IIA activity and 12-lipoxygenase expressed on the surface of platelet-derived microparticles.[111]

Neutrophil NETs have also been suggested to play roles in promoting clotting (including disseminated intravascular coagulation). In those cases, extruded neutrophil chromatin may directly increase thrombin generation and increase coagulation factor activity, as well as serve as a platform for the extra-cellular co-localization of neutrophil elastase and the anti-thrombotic tissue factor pathway inhibitor (TFPI).[112,113] Inactivation of TFPI

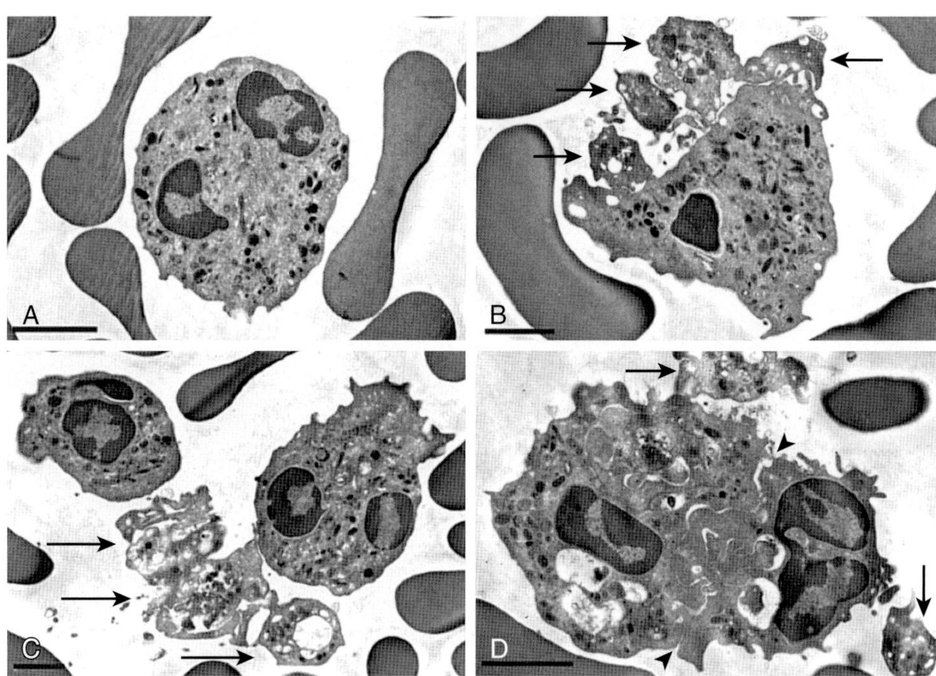

• **Fig. 11.10** Neutrophil-platelet interactions and neutrophil-neutrophil aggregation in blood specimens subjected to hydrodynamic shear, examined by transmission electron micrograph. (A) Single neutrophil with few to no adherent platelets appears round (unactivated). (B) Neutrophil bound to four platelets undergoes a shape change (i.e., activated by platelet contact). (C and D) Neutrophil aggregates observed with platelets forming bridges between neutrophils (C) and on the periphery of homotypically aggregating neutrophils (D). In (B and C) *arrows* mark platelets; in (D) *arrowheads* mark neutrophil-neutrophil contact region (scale bar in each panel: 2 μm). (Reproduced from Konstantopoulos K, Neelamegham S, Burns AR, et al. Venous levels of shear support neutrophil-platelet adhesion and neutrophil aggregation in blood via P-selectin and beta2-integrin. *Circulation* 1998; 98(9):873–882.)

by elastase then permits clotting to proceed.[114] NETs may also simply provide a scaffold for platelet adherence and subsequent aggregation.[115] In a flow restriction murine model of deep vein thrombosis, NETs were present in thrombi, and mice treated with DNAse or rendered neutropenic were protected against clot formation.[116]

Neutrophil-derived microparticles may also contribute to thrombosis. As microparticles contain many of the enzymes and surface proteins found on their parent neutrophil, thrombosis may be propagated via myeloperoxidase that leads to endothelial damage and via surface expression of the active form of β_2 integrins that activate platelets.[117,118]

Resolution of Neutrophil Inflammation

Inflammatory responses must eventually be resolved to avoid excessive tissue damage and initiate the healing process. Resolution of inflammation is an active and carefully regulated process. Pro-resolution signals include a number of lipid derivatives (resolvins, lipoxins, etc), annexin A1 and chemerin-derived peptides, and certain chemokines and cytokines.

Resolvins

Resolvins differ according to the lipid from which they derive. Resolvin E1 is derived from eicospentaenoic acid and inhibits monocytes, macrophages, and dendritic cells (DCs), as well as neutrophils.[119,120] Resolvin D derives from docosahexaenoic acid and is also a potent inhibitor of neutrophil diapedesis and migration.[121] Maresin 1 (macrophage mediator in resolving inflammation 1) has properties similar to the D-resolvins.[122] Some prostaglandins such as 15d-PGJ_2 also have anti-inflammatory properties.[123]

Lipoxins

Lipoxins are derived from arachidonic acid, but in contrast to leukotrienes and prostaglandins are potent anti-inflammatory molecules.[69] Lipoxin synthesis requires coordinated activity of neutrophil 5-lipoxygenase and a related enzyme (either 12-lipoxygenase or 15-lipoxygenase) from another cell type, either platelets or endothelial cells (Fig. 11.11).[124] Thus, in contrast to leukotrienes and prostaglandins, which are elevated early in inflammation, the requirement for a mixed population of inflammatory cells to accumulate to produce lipoxins may create a programmatic delay, permitting inflammation to reach an active stage before the anti-inflammatory processes kick in.[125] In some cases, apoptotic neutrophils at sites of inflammation are taken up by resident macrophages, promoting lipoxin A4 production.[126] Aspirin stimulates the generation of biologically active epilipoxins, suggesting a previously unappreciated mechanism for its anti-inflammatory action.[127]

Other Inflammation-Resolving Molecules

Following neutrophil activation, annexin A1 (lipocortin) is released in response to chemoattractants, downregulating transmigration and promoting neutrophil apoptosis and clearance.[128] Similar activities have been attributed to chemerin-derived peptides.[129] As noted earlier, activated neutrophils also produce IL-1 receptor antagonist (IL-1ra).[130] The efficacy of recombinant IL-1ra

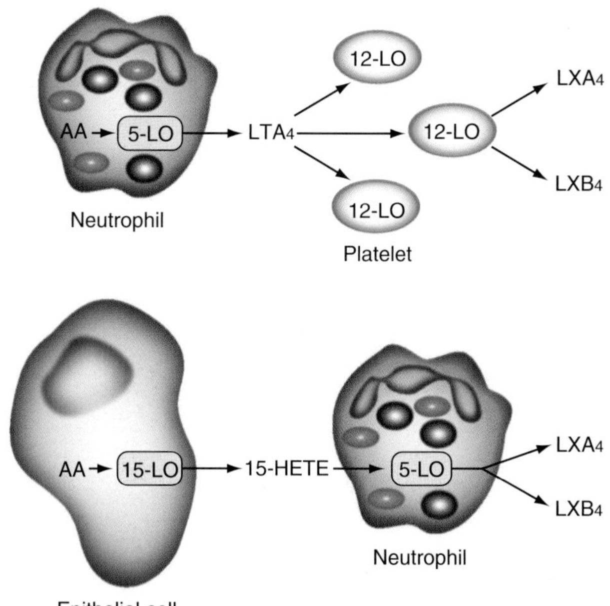

• **Fig. 11.11** Generation of the anti-inflammatory lipoxins A_4 and B_4 depends on the interaction between two different classes of inflammatory cells. Top, Lipoxin generation by neutrophils and platelets. Arachidonic acid (AA) generated by activated neutrophils is converted by neutrophil 5-lipoxygenase (5-LO) into leukotriene A_4 (LTA_4). LTA_4 may be converted by 12-LO in nearby platelets into lipoxin A_4 (LXA_4) and lipoxin B_4 (LXB_4). Bottom, Lipoxin generation by epithelial cells and neutrophils. AA generated by epithelial cells may be converted by 15-LO into 15-hydroxyeicosatetraenoic acid (15-HETE). In the setting of inflammation, 5-LO from adjacent neutrophils subsequently may convert 15-HETE into LXA_4 and LXB_4.

(anakinra) in treating rheumatoid arthritis and autoinflammatory diseases emphasizes its clinical importance in downregulating inflammation. An MMP-mediated mechanism of inflammatory resolution has also been identified. Macrophage-derived MMPs, such as MMP-1, MMP-3, and MMP-12, cleave CXC-chemokines to provoke the loss of their neutrophil-recruiting activity and dampen the influx of cells.[131]

Role of Apoptotic Neutrophils in Resolving Inflammation

Apoptotic neutrophils can inhibit live neutrophil chemotaxis and migration via release of lactoferrin and annexin A1.[132] Apoptotic neutrophils can also suppress granulopoiesis by inhibiting the proinflammatory consequences of IL-17/IL-23 axis activation. In this model, macrophages and DCs produce IL-23 at the site of insult, which in turn promotes IL-17 production by T cells (Th17, γ δ T cells, and natural killer [NK] T cells). As noted earlier, IL-17 is a powerful neutrophil chemoattractant. Recruited neutrophils undergo apoptosis and are phagocytosed by macrophages, resulting in a decrease of IL-23. This is followed by a reduction in IL-17 and G-CSF production, which downregulates granulopoiesis.[133]

An intriguing mechanism through which neutrophils might downregulate the action of protein inflammatory mediators has been defined. Apoptotic neutrophils (present during the resolving phase of inflammation) show increased expression of the chemokine receptor CCR5 on their surface (mediated by D and E resolvins), and this receptor can scavenge and reduce the soluble concentration of chemokines such as CCL3 and CCL5. These data emphasize again that neutrophils are not only inflammatory cells but may also play a direct role in the subsequent resolution of inflammation.[134]

Heritable Disorders of Neutrophil Function

A variety of acquired conditions result from neutrophil dysfunction and/or depletion, which can result from malignancies (myeloid leukemias), metabolic abnormalities (diabetes), and drugs (corticosteroids, chemotherapy). In addition, rare, congenital disorders of neutrophils have been identified (Table 11.2). In general, patients with congenitally impaired neutrophil function are prone to infection by bacteria (predominantly *Staphylococcus aureus, Pseudomonas* species, *Burkholderia*) and fungi *(Aspergillus, Candida),* less so by viruses and parasites. The major sites of infection include skin, mucous membranes, and lungs, but any site may be affected and spreading abscesses are common. Most of these diseases are potentially life threatening in the absence of available effective therapy.

Diseases of Diminished Neutrophil Number

Severe congenital neutropenia ([SCN], Kostmann's syndrome) results from marrow arrest of bone marrow myelopoiesis and leads to neutrophil counts persistently less than 0.5×10^9 cells/L. Monogenic autosomal dominant, autosomal recessive, sporadic, and polygenic subtypes have been identified, including mutations in the gene for neutrophil elastase and in HAX1, whose protein contributes to synthesis of G-CSF.[135–137] Patients are prone from early infancy to severe bacterial infections including omphalitis, pneumonia, otitis, gingivitis, and perirectal infections. Due to the lack of acute inflammation, infections tend to spread extensively before coming to attention, and rate of mortality is high. Therapy consists of antibiotics and long-term treatment with recombinant G-CSF, which may help maintain normal or near-normal neutrophil counts.

SCN patients are also at risk for acute myeloid leukemia (AML) and myelodysplastic syndrome, particularly those who respond poorly to G-CSF.[138] A milder form of neutropenia (benign congenital neutropenia) with higher neutrophil counts and fewer infections has also been observed. Another variant is cyclic neutropenia, which causes transient, recurrent neutropenia on a 21-day cycle. Studies suggest that defects in neutrophil elastase affect neutrophil survival in the marrow and may be responsible for severe congenital and cyclic neutropenia.[139] At least 52 different mutations in the *ELANE* gene, which encodes neutrophil elastase, have been described as the cause in around half of the patients.[140] Mutations in HAX-1 and glucose-6-phosphatase catalytic subunit 3 *(G6PC3)* genes account for a smaller proportion of SCN. Other, less frequent deficiencies include X-linked neutropenia, caused by constitutively active mutations of the *WASP* gene, and defects in several myeloid transcription factors.

Leukocyte Adhesion Deficiencies

Leukocyte adhesion disorders arise from defects in cell adhesion to extra-cellular matrix and vascular endothelium. Three distinct entities have been described in humans. Leukocyte adhesion deficiency type 1 (LAD-I) results from an autosomal recessive defect in ITGB2, which encodes the CD18 chain of β_2 integrins. Consequently, neutrophil β_2 integrins fail to form, and bloodstream neutrophils are unable to adhere firmly to vascular endothelium and transmigrate to sites of infection.[141,142] Phagocytosis is also impaired. The clinical picture is similar to that of the neutropenias, with recurrent life-threatening infections. Peripheral neutrophil counts are typically elevated, however, reflecting the intravascular

TABLE 11.2 Heritable Disorders of Neutrophil Function

Disorder	Defect	Inheritance	Presentation	Therapy	Typical Prognosis
Neutropenia					
Severe congenital neutropenia (Kostmann's syndrome)	Maturation arrest (<0.5 × 10^9 PMN/L)	AR (HAX1 mutations)	Bacterial infections (omphalitis, abscesses, gingivitis, UTIs)	RhG-CSF	Improved with treatment
Benign congenital neutropenia	Multiple etiologies (0.2-2 × 10^9 PMN/L)	Variable	Mild infections	None	Good
Cyclic neutropenia	Stem cell defect, elastase gene deficiency (nadir every 21 days)	AD (ELA2 mutations)	Infection during nadirs	RhG-CSF	Improved with treatment
Adhesion Deficiency					
Leukocyte adhesion deficiency type 1	Absent or abnormal CD18; deficiency in β_2-integrin chain of leukocyte adhesion molecules	AR	Leukocytosis; recurrent infections (skin mucous, membranes, gastrointestinal tract)	Marrow transplant	Fair-poor
Leukocyte adhesion deficiency type 2	Absent sialyl-Lewis^x	AR	Neutrophilia; infection; retardation, short stature		Poor
Leukocyte adhesion deficiency type 3	Impaired activation of Rap1 GTPase	AR	Leukocytosis; recurrent infections; bleeding tendency		Poor
Chemotaxis Deficiency					
Hyper-IgE syndrome	Chemotaxis defect	AD	Eczema; recurrent infections; elevated serum IgE levels	Skin care; antibiotics	Good
Granule Disorders					
Chédiak-Higashi syndrome	Defective lysosomal trafficking regulator gene	AR	Albinism; infection	Marrow transplant; antibiotics	Poor
Specific granule deficiency	Abnormal/reduced specific and azurophilic granules (lactoferrin deficiency)	AR?	Infection of skin, mucous membranes, lungs		Fair-good
Myeloperoxidase deficiency	Myeloperoxidase absent	Variable (mostly AR)	None	Transfusion of HLA identical leukocytes if severe	Excellent
p14 deficiency	Defective endosomal adapter protein gene	Recessive	Albinism; infection; short stature	None known to date	?
Oxidase Defects					
Chronic granulomatous disease (multiple types)	gp91^{phox} absent	X-linked 50%	Early childhood infections, especially skin and mucous membranes, abscesses	Interferon-γ	Improved with treatment
	p22^{phox} absent	AR 5%			
	p47^{phox} absent	AR 35%			
	p67^{phox} absent	AR 5%			
	p40^{phox} absent	AR 5%			

AR, Autosomal, recessive; *PMN*, polymorphonuclear neutrophil; *RhG-CSF*, recombinant human granulocyte colony-stimulating factor; *UTIs*, urinary tract infections.

accumulation of cells in the face of their inability to exit the vessels. Complete LAD-I manifests in infancy and is characterized by omphalitis, recurrent life-threatening bacterial and fungal infections, gingivitis, and delayed wound healing. Absence of pus at infection sites is a hallmark of LAD-I. Bone marrow transplantation is the only curative therapy.

LAD-II results from an autosomal recessive defect in the glycosylation of sialyl Lewis^x (SLex or CD15s), the neutrophil counter-ligand for endothelial selectins. Patients with LAD-II have neutrophils that are unable to roll along the endothelium and have symptoms similar to LAD-I but may also have mental retardation, short stature, distinctive facies, and the Bombay (hh) blood type.[143]

A third variant, LAD-III, has been described in which leukocytes have normal populations of surface integrins but lack the ability to signal these molecules into an active state.[143,144] Because integrin activation in this condition is also deficient in platelets, patients with LAD-III are at increased risk for infection and bleeding.

Granule Defects

Chédiak-Higashi syndrome is an autosomal recessive disorder in which granule subtypes—in neutrophils, lymphocytes, melanocytes, Schwann cells, and others—undergo disordered fusion, resulting in giant, dysfunctional granules. The cause seems to relate to a defect in the gene for lysosomal transport regulator (Lyst or CHS1).[145] Patients with Chédiak-Higashi syndrome present with partial oculocutaneous albinism, neutropenia, frequent infection, mild bleeding diathesis, and neurologic abnormalities. Most patients who survive childhood eventually enter a so-called "accelerated phase," a lymphoma-like infiltration of lymphocytes and histiocytes throughout the body, which is generally fatal.[146]

Other diseases of neutrophil granules have less ominous prognoses. A novel immunodeficiency syndrome relating to lack of the endosomal adapter protein p14 (encoded by the *ROBLD3* gene) has been described. Patients with this syndrome have congenital neutropenia with structurally abnormal neutrophil primary granules and abnormalities of B cells, cytotoxic T cells, and melanocytes. In addition to immunodeficiency, clinical findings include short stature and partial albinism.[147]

Oxidase Deficiencies—Chronic Granulomatous Disease

Chronic granulomatous disease (CGD) resembles other diseases of neutrophil dysfunction in that it results in severe, recurrent infections of the skin and mucous membranes. Osteomyelitis and intra-abdominal abscesses are common. Neutrophils from patients with CGD can adhere and migrate normally, but are unable to kill bacteria. Accordingly, they accumulate and persist at sites of infection and, rather than clear the target organism, tend towards granuloma formation. Cutaneous infections tend to show persistent drainage and scarring. The presence of even partially responsive neutrophils results in a lower frequency of sepsis in these patients relative to patients with absolute neutropenia. CGD is typically a disease of early childhood, although some milder cases may be recognized later in life.

CGD actually comprises a group of diseases. In each, a genetic defect in a different component of NADPH oxidase (gp91^{phox}, gp22^{phox}, p47^{phox}, or p67^{phox}) results in failure of neutrophils (and other phagocytes) to generate O_2^-, impairing both intra-cellular killing and the ability of neutrophils to generate NETs.[79,80,148] X-linked CGD affecting gp91^{phox} (*CYBB* gene) is the most common form and accounts for about 70% of cases, whereas the autosomal recessive forms are responsible for the rest.[149] Interestingly, patients with deficiencies of the fifth component of the NADPH oxidase (p40^{phox}) develop refractory inflammatory colitis.[65,150]

Treatment for CGD consists of aggressive antibiotic prophylaxis and therapy, along with long-term therapy with recombinant human IFN-γ to improve neutrophil function. Clinical trials of gene therapy for X-linked CGD have thus far yielded equivocal results.[151]

Defects of TLR Signaling

Defects in human TLR signaling, including IRAK-4 and MyD88 deficiencies, also lead to impaired neutrophil function and increased susceptibility to bacterial infections.[152,153]

Neutrophil Relevance to Rheumatic Disease

Neutrophil-Mediated Tissue Destruction

Despite sophisticated regulatory mechanisms, tissue destruction by neutrophils is common. In autoimmune diseases such as rheumatoid arthritis and systemic lupus erythematosus, neutrophils are activated by immune complexes via their Fc receptors, leading to release of proteolytic enzymes, chemokines, and the production of reactive oxygen species, all of which contribute to end-organ damage. Immune complexes activate the classical complement system leading to the production of C5a, a potent neutrophil chemoattactant, which in turn induces recruitment of neutrophils, with the potential to create a feed forward loop of inflammatory injury.[154] Immune complexes can also induce NETs,[155] which expose cytotoxic histones and other damage associated molecular patterns (DAMPs) and MMPs that cause endothelial cell damage.[156]

Neutrophils not only contribute to tissue damage, but may trigger the adaptive immune response by exposing nucleic acids, citrullinated proteins, and other known autoantigens[157–159] to plasmacytoid dendritic cells and monocytes,[160,161] leading to the production of IFN-α, an important mediator of some forms of autoimmunity.

Neutrophil Fc Receptor Polymorphisms and Rheumatic Disease

Given that polymorphisms of Fcγ R determine phagocytic capacity of IgG isotypes, it is not surprising that they determine susceptibility to diseases in which autoantibodies play a key role. Phagocytes from individuals with one Fcγ RIIa polymorphism (H131) are able to bind and phagocytose IgG_2; phagocytes from individuals with a different polymorphism (R131) cannot. In white European and African-American populations, patients with lupus nephritis have a higher frequency of the Fcγ RIIa-R131 allele than control groups; their relative inability to clear immune complexes may make them more susceptible to renal disease.[162] Platelets also express Fcγ RIIa, and it was recently shown that systemic lupus erythematosus (SLE) patients with the Fcγ RIIa-R131 allele have increased leukocyte-platelet aggregates and a higher incidence of carotid plaque compared with SLE patients with the control allele.[163] The significance of different Fc receptor polymorphisms may vary among rheumatologic diseases. One study found no association between Fcγ RIIa polymorphisms and likelihood of developing antineutrophil cytoplasmic antibody (ANCA)-associated vasculitides, but an overrepresentation of homozygosity for the Fcγ RIIIb NA1 allele among patients with anti-myeloperoxidase antibodies.[163a,163b] Recent studies have found no association between Fcγ RIIa, IIb, or IIIb haplotypes and rheumatoid arthritis susceptibility, but they did find a correlation between patients with extra-articular disease and the homozygous R/R 131 genotype. In contrast, Fcγ RIIIa receptor expression is increased in rheumatoid arthritis.[164]

Gout

Gout is the quintessential neutrophilic rheumatic disease. Although the initiation of an acute gouty attack involves the phagocytosis of urate crystals by synovial macrophages, and macrophage generation of cytokines such as IL-1β and IL-8, the hallmark of acute gout is the presence of enormous numbers of neutrophils (sometimes >100,000/mm^3) in the affected synovial fluid. Intra-articular urate crystals nonspecifically bind immunoglobulin and activate complement by the classic and alternative pathways. C5a liberated by this process attracts neutrophils to the joint space, where they phagocytose opsonized crystals via receptor-dependent mechanisms, resulting in further activation of the neutrophil and production of LTB_4, IL-8, and other mediators, promoting ingress of additional neutrophils. Naked urate crystals can also directly activate neutrophils. Neutrophils in the gouty joint may damage joint structures through discharge of contents directly into the joint fluid during crystal phagocytosis, or directly against cartilage during attempted phagocytosis of urate crystals embedded in or adherent to cartilage. Interaction of phagocytosed urate crystals with lysosomal membranes additionally results in the dissolution of the latter, spilling lysosomal proteases into the cytoplasm and, eventually, into the extra-cellular space.[165] Perhaps surprisingly, given their largely inflammatory role, recent studies implicate NETs as playing a role in the resolution, rather than the activation, of gouty inflammation. Monosodium urate (MSU) crystal arthritis is more severe and persists weeks longer in mice unable to make NETs, compared with controls. As increasing numbers of neutrophils are recruited to the synovial fluid, NETs aggregate and promote the degradation of key mediators such as IL-1β, thereby contributing to breaking the inflammatory cycle.[166] Interestingly, MSU-induced NETs have a much higher actin content than PMA-induced NETs. Because actin inhibits DNAse, MSU NETs may be less susceptible to DNase degradation, allowing their persistence in joints and tophi.[167] If gout-associated NETs serve to limit inflammation by degrading pro-inflammatory cytokines, their prolonged association with MSU crystals is consistent with the observation that tophi in chronic gout are frequently clinically quiescent.

Rheumatoid Arthritis

Rheumatoid arthritis (RA) may be conceptualized as a two-compartment inflammatory disease. In the synovium, lymphocytes, fibroblasts, and macrophages predominate, but the joint space contains mainly neutrophils. The classic model suggests that rheumatoid factor and/or anti-CCP-based immune complexes, produced in the pannus (inflamed synovium) and present in the joint space in high concentrations, can activate complement to recruit neutrophils into the joint space. The ability of rheumatoid synovial fibroblasts to secrete IL-1β, IL-8, and other cytokines indicates that pannus itself may play an important role in attracting neutrophils out of the bloodstream and into the joint.

Conversely, neutrophils in the RA joint may contribute to the propagation of pannus. RA neutrophils produce pro-inflammatory cytokines that may act on synovium, including oncostatin M, MIP-1α, and IL-8.[168] In animal models, injection of lysates of neutrophil granules into joints produces a synovitis histologically indistinguishable from rheumatoid synovitis, an effect that can be reproduced by injection with purified active or inactive myeloperoxidase.[169]

Neutrophil proteinase 3 may enhance the pro-inflammatory impact of synovial macrophages by cleaving and releasing active IL-1β and TNF from the surface of the latter. Neutrophil defensins enhance phagocytosis by macrophages and stimulate the activation and degranulation of mast cells, an interesting observation in light of a report that mice deficient in mast cells are resistant to the development of erosive arthritis.[170] Neutrophil proteases also enhance the adherence of rheumatoid synovial fibroblasts to articular cartilage, and neutrophils may regulate synovial vascularization through the production of vascular endothelial growth factor, leading to endothelial proliferation.

Studies by Lee and others confirm that neutrophils are necessary for the propagation of rheumatic disease in mouse models of RA. These studies implicate the ability of neutrophils to produce LTB_4, as well as the presence of FCγ RIIA and C5a receptors on the neutrophil surface as necessary for arthritis development.[171,172] Several studies have raised the unexpected possibility that, under certain conditions of stimulation, neutrophils can serve as antigen-presenting cells.[173] Neutrophils in RA synovial fluid synthesize and express large amounts of class II major histocompatibility complex.[174]

GWAS and epigenomic studies have shown that SNPs in the apoptosis-associated EnguLfment and Cell MOtility gene (ELMO) are linked to RA,[175] and the role of ELMO in arthritis pathogenesis has recently been linked to neutrophil transmigration. One study[176] compared severity of inflammation in myeloid-specific ELMO-knockout mice and controls using two mouse models of inflammatory arthritis. Their elegant studies demonstrated that ELMO expression in neutrophils is required for PMN transmigration into synovial tissues because it mediates an increase in PMN CD11b that is required for maximal inflammation in response to C5a and LTB_4. These data suggest that neutrophil ELMO is a potential target for therapies for RA.

Systemic Lupus Erythematosus

Until recently, the role of the neutrophil in lupus was considered to be limited to its function as an inflammatory effector. However, the discovery of NETs has led to a reconsideration of the neutrophil role in pathogenesis, not only via development of endothelial damage but also in the induction of autoimmunity. NETs express several autoantigens that are targets of lupus autoantibodies, particularly DNA.[177] While peptidylarginine deiminase facilitates NET formation, its inhibition is protective against organ damage in a model of murine lupus.[178] NETs can be dismantled by DNAse, and some patients with lupus cannot degrade NETs because of inhibitors of, or antibodies to, DNAse. In such patients the inability to degrade NETs has correlated with the presence of lupus nephritis,[179] and in a murine model DNAse-deficient mice rapidly develop antibodies to DNA and an SLE-like disease including nephritis.[180] Moreover, patients with low NET-degrading activity in their sera have higher levels of autoantibodies, and lower levels of C3 and C4, compared with patients with high NET-degrading activity.[181] Oxidized mtDNA from neutrophils had also recently been implicated in lupus pathogenesis, and specific inhibitors of mitochondrial reactive oxygen species decreased both the numbers of mtDNA NETs and the severity of lupus in MRL/lpr mice. Moreover, oxidized mtDNA induces type I IFNs in monocytes. The degree of DNA oxidation, rather than the identity of the DNA as mitochondrial, appeared to determine the capacity to induce type I IFNs.[182,183]

Despite the extensive data suggesting that NETs are implicated in the pathogenesis of SLE, it is noteworthy that lupus-prone MRL.Fas^{lpr} mice deficient in NAPDH oxidase (and therefore incapable of releasing at least some types of NETs) demonstrated higher levels of autoantibodies and exacerbated glomerulonephritis compared with controls, suggesting the possibility that at least some types of NETs are SLE-protective.[184]

Vasculitis

Neutrophils may be identified, to a greater or lesser degree, in the lesions of virtually all kinds of vasculitis. The mechanisms of neutrophil accumulation may vary, however, with different mechanisms predominating in different conditions. The early observation that infusions of allospecies serum produced acute inflammation in skin and joints (serum sickness), together with the appreciation that subcutaneous re-challenge with previously administered antigen leads to intense local inflammation (Arthus reaction), led to the development of a model in which immune complex deposition in blood vessels results in complement activation and an influx of neutrophils. Because immune complex formation is a hallmark of many small vessel vasculitides (e.g., essential mixed cryoglobulinemia, hypersensitivity vasculitis, Henoch-Schönlein purpura), it is likely that immune complex deposition is crucial to the genesis of these diseases. In several of these conditions, neutrophil disruption and fragmentation—*clasis*—is a prominent pathologic finding, leading to their designation under the rubric *leukocytoclastic vasculitis*. In some rheumatic diseases in which vasculitis is a secondary phenomenon, such as RA and systemic lupus erythematosus, the role of immune complex deposition is implicit. Patients with lupus experience transient accumulations of neutrophils (leukoaggregation) in small vessels of the lungs and other tissues, as a result of complement activation within these vessels or in the soluble phase.[185]

Induction of adhesion molecules on endothelial cells, neutrophils themselves, or both is an alternative mechanism through which neutrophil accumulation in vessels may be propagated. The Shwartzman phenomenon, in which reinjection of cellular material leads to vascular inflammation via a cytokine-dependent, immune complex–independent mechanism, is a model for this avenue to vasculitis. Adhesion molecule upregulation may be particularly relevant to vasculitides in which immune complex formation is not a hallmark. It is likely that many rheumatic diseases employ both immune complex–dependent and immune complex–independent mechanisms in the pathogenesis of neutrophil ingress into vascular structures. For example, one group has shown that endothelial cells demonstrate increased expression several adhesion molecules in skin biopsies from patients with systemic lupus erythematosus even in the absence of SLE-characteristic immune complexes.[186]

Several vasculitides are noteworthy for the presence, in the serum of affected patients, of antibodies directed at cytoplasmic components of neutrophils (ANCA). In these diseases, partial neutrophil degranulation, resulting in exposure of ANCA antigens (MPO, proteinase 3), appears to be critical for disease pathogenesis. ANCA-positive vasculitides are discussed in detail in Chapter 94.

Neutrophilic Dermatoses and Familial Mediterranean Fever

Sweet's syndrome is characterized by fever, neutrophilia, and painful erythematous papules, nodules, and plaques. The syndrome may be idiopathic, parainflammatory (e.g., associated with inflammatory bowel disease or infection), paraneoplastic (most commonly in the setting of leukemia), pregnancy related, or drug associated (usually after treatment with G-CSF). Clinically, Sweet's syndrome is a diagnosis of exclusion. Sweet's syndrome frequently appears after an upper respiratory tract infection and has a propensity to involve the face, neck, and upper extremities. When found on the legs, Sweet's syndrome lesions can be confused with erythema nodosum. Histopathology is characterized by dense neutrophilic infiltrate in the superficial dermis and edema of the dermal papillae and papillary dermis. Leukocytoclasia may suggest leukocytoclastic vasculitis, although vascular damage is absent. It is typically accompanied by peripheral neutrophilia. Treatment with systemic corticosteroids usually induces a dramatic resolution of the lesions and the systemic symptoms. Although the etiology of the disease is unclear, many authors believe that Sweet's syndrome may represent a hypersensitivity reaction to microbial or tumor antigens. Antibiotics do not influence the course of the disease in most patients.

Pyoderma gangrenosum is characterized by painful ulcerating cutaneous lesions over the lower extremities, usually in patients with an underlying inflammatory illness. Inflammatory bowel disease, RA, and seronegative arthritis are the most common associations, although an association with malignancy has also been reported. Fifteen percent of patients have a benign monoclonal gammopathy, usually IgA. Like Sweet's syndrome, pyoderma gangrenosum is a diagnosis of exclusion, is characterized on biopsy specimen by neutrophilic infiltrate, and usually remits with systemic corticosteroids, although topical and intralesional injections of corticosteroids may be beneficial as well. Other rare neutrophilic dermatoses include rheumatoid neutrophilic dermatitis, described as symmetric erythematous nodules on extensor surfaces of joints; bowel-associated dermatosis-arthritis syndrome occurring after bowel bypass surgery for obesity; and neutrophilic eccrine hidradenitis, sometimes linked to acute myelogenous leukemia.

In familial Mediterranean fever ([fMf], discussed in detail in Chapter 103), patients experience episodic inflammatory exacerbations, characterized by large influxes of neutrophils. A defect in the regulatory protein pyrin seems to permit the inappropriate development of inflammation, leading to the categorization of fMf as an autoinflammatory disease. Pyrin is expressed exclusively in myeloid cells including neutrophils and eosinophils.

Effects of Anti-rheumatic Agents on Neutrophil Functions

Many anti-rheumatic therapies currently in use have been documented to act at least partly at the level of the neutrophil.

Nonsteroidal Anti-inflammatory Drugs

By virtue of their ability to inhibit COX activity and prostaglandin production, moderate doses of nonsteroidal anti-inflammatory drugs (NSAIDs) have diverse effects on inflammation, including inhibition of vascular permeability and modulation of pain. At higher, clinically anti-inflammatory concentrations, NSAIDs inhibit chemoattractant-stimulated neutrophil CD11b/CD18-dependent adhesion and degranulation and NADPH oxidase activity.[195] It is unlikely, however, that these effects are due solely to COX inhibition because (1) as noted earlier, neutrophils exhibit little COX activity under normal circumstances, and (2) concentrations of NSAIDs required to inhibit neutrophil function exceed the concentrations required to inhibit COX. Salicylates may be unique as NSAIDs, both because of their ability to promote neutrophil-mediated, anti-inflammatory lipoxin A4 formation,[187] and because of their ability to inhibit neutrophil cell signaling at high concentrations.[196]

Glucocorticoids

Glucocorticoids exert potent effects on neutrophils, including inhibition of neutrophil phagocytic activity and adhesive function. The ability of steroids to increase peripheral blood neutrophil populations acutely—an effect known as *demargination*—is attributable to both a release of neutrophils from the bone marrow and the release (demargination) of neutrophils adherent to vessel walls. In addition, glucocorticoids lead to inhibition of phospholipase A_2, reducing leukotriene and prostaglandin production. Glucocorticoids may also downregulate the expression of COX-2 and stimulate the release of annexin A1, which inhibits arachidonate release from membranes. Effects of glucocorticoids on other cells may also reduce neutrophil responses indirectly through the suppression of cytokines at inflammatory sites.

Disease-Modifying Anti-rheumatic Drugs

Several disease-modifying anti-rheumatic drugs (DMARDs) have well-established effects on neutrophils. Methotrexate, widely used in RA, has no direct neutrophil effect but is capable of producing indirect effects, probably by virtue of its ability to stimulate the release of adenosine from surrounding cells. Some data suggest that methotrexate-induced adenosine release might inhibit phagocytosis, O_2^- production, and adhesion, and treatment of patients with methotrexate inhibits the capacity of neutrophils to generate LTB_4.[188,189] Sulfasalazine inhibits neutrophil chemotaxis, degranulation, and O_2^- generation; to decrease LTB_4 production; and to scavenge oxygen metabolites.[189]

Colchicine

Colchicine, a standard agent in the treatment of gout and fMf, inhibits microtubule formation and has pleiotropic effects on neutrophils, including inhibition of adhesion via decrements in selectin expression.[190] Additionally, colchicine has been observed to stimulate the expression of pyrin in neutrophils. Because pyrin is implicated in both fMf and gout, this observation suggests a previously unappreciated mechanism of action of colchicine in neutrophilic diseases.[191]

Biologic Agents

The current era of biologic therapies was first ushered in through the introduction of agents designed to block the effects of TNF or IL-1β. As noted earlier, IL-1β and TNF directly affect neutrophil function, including priming for stimulus-induced responses such as O_2^- production, cartilage destruction, and production of cytokines such as IL-8 and LTB_4. Nonetheless, studies examining the effects of anti-TNF treatment on neutrophil function measured ex vivo have not indicated extensive action. Treatment of patients with etanercept or adalimumab induced no effect on neutrophil ex vivo responses including chemotaxis, phagocytosis, and superoxide generation (although CD69 levels were reduced).[192,193] Reduction of neutrophil populations in RA joint effusions after anti-TNF therapy is more likely due to alteration of the inflammatory environment, rather than to direct effects on the neutrophils themselves. Similarly, recent studies indicate that anti-IL-6 therapy with tocilizumab may induce neutropenia in patients but has no direct effect on neutrophil function.[194] The role of IL-17 in neutrophil recruitment suggests that secukinumab, an anti-IL-17-directed agent, may function in part based on its ability to neutralize IL-17 stimulation of neutrophils.[197]

Conclusion

Without neutrophils, human life would be impossible. The complex machinery of neutrophil surveillance and response—the chemotactic, phagocytic, enzymatic, and oxidative defenses that enable neutrophils to sense and destroy foreign organisms—allows our bodies to abort many forms of infection, and to keep others at bay until more specific mechanisms can be roused. When improperly regulated, however, these same mechanisms become the basis of inflammatory and autoinflammatory disease, and potentially lead to tissue destruction. Moreover, it is increasingly appreciated that neutrophils play critical roles in bridging the gap between innate and acquired immunity. In several rheumatic diseases, the neutrophil therefore serves not merely as an effector cell, but as a direct participant in disease pathogenesis.

Full references for this chapter can be found on ExpertConsult.com.

Selected References

2. Borregaard N: Neutrophils, from marrow to microbes, *Immunity* 33(5):657–670, 2010.
3. Cowland JB, Borregaard N: Granulopoiesis and granules of human neutrophils, *Immunol Rev* 273(1):11–28, 2016.
6. Lawrence SM, Corriden R, Nizet V: The ontogeny of a neutrophil: mechanisms of granulopoiesis and homeostasis, *Microbiol Mol Biol Rev* 82(1):Epub, 2018.
11. Martin C, Burdon PC, Bridger G, et al.: Chemokines acting via CXCR2 and CXCR4 control the release of neutrophils from the bone marrow and their return following senescence, *Immunity* 19(4):583–593, 2003.
12. Tamassia N, Bianchetto-Aguilera F, Arruda-Silva F, et al.: Cytokine production by human neutrophils: revisiting the "dark side of the moon", *Eur J Clin Invest* 48(Suppl 2):e12952, 2018.
16. Murphy G, Bretz U, Baggiolini M, et al.: The latent collagenase and gelatinase of human polymorphonuclear neutrophil leukocytes, *Biochem J* 192:517–525, 1980.
17. Owen CA, Campbell EJ: The cell biology of leukocyte-mediated proteolysis, *J Leukoc Biol* 65(2):137–150, 1999.
18. Belaaouaj A, Kim KS, Shapiro SD: Degradation of outer membrane protein A in Escherichia coli killing by neutrophil elastase, *Science* 289(5482):1185–1188, 2000.
19. Rice WG, Ganz T, Kinkade JM, et al.: Defensin-rich dense granules of human neutrophils, *Blood* 70:757–765, 1987.
20. Schultz H, Weiss JP: The bactericidal/permeability-increasing protein (BPI) in infection and inflammatory disease, *Clin Chem Acta* 384:12–23, 2007.
21. Dewald B, Bretz U, Baggiolini M: Release of gelatinase from a novel secretory compartment of human neutrophils, *J Clin Invest* 70(3):518–525, 1982.
22. Borregaard N, Miller LJ, Springer TA: Chemoattractant-regulated mobilization of a novel intracellular compartment in human neutrophils, *Science* 237(4819):1204–1206, 1987.
25. Van den Steen PE, Proost P, Wuyts A, et al.: Neutrophil gelatinase B potentiates interleukin-8 tenfold by amino terminal processing, whereas it degrades CTAP-III, PF-4, and GRO-alpha and leaves RANTES and MCP-2 intact, *Blood* 96(8):2673–2681, 2000.
26. Huynh ML, Fadok VA, Henson PM: Phosphatidylserine-dependent ingestion of apoptotic cells promotes TGF-beta1 secretion and the resolution of inflammation, *J Clin Invest* 109(1):41–50, 2002.
28. Petri B, Sanz M-J: Neutrophil chemotaxis, *Cell and Tissue Res* 371:425–436, 2018.
29. Pillinger MH, Feoktistov AS, Capodici C, et al.: Mitogen-activated protein kinase in neutrophils and enucleate neutrophil cytoplasts: evidence for regulation of cell-cell adhesion, *J Biol Chem* 271(20):12049–12056, 1996.

30. Murdoch C, Finn A: Chemokine receptors and their role in inflammation and infectious diseases, *Blood* 95(10):3032–3043, 2000.
32. El-Benna J, Hurtado-Nedelec M, Marzaioli V, et al.: Priming of the neutrophil respiratory burst: role in host defense and inflammation, *Immunol Rev* 273(1):180–193, 2016.
33. Senarath K, Kankanamge D, Samaradivakara S, et al.: Regulation of G protein βγ signaling, *Int Rev Cell Mol Biol* 339:133–191, 2018.
41. Bertram A, Ley K: Protein kinase C isoforms in neutrophil adhesion and activation, *Arch Immunol Ther Exp* 59(2):79–87, 2011.
42. Capodici C, Pillinger MH, Han G, et al.: Integrin-dependent homotypic adhesion of neutrophils. Arachidonic acid activates Raf-1/Mek/Erk via a 5-lipoxygenase-dependent pathway, *J Clin Invest* 102(1):165–175, 1988.
44. Kolaczkowska E, Kubes P: Neutrophil recruitment and function in health and inflammation, *Nat Rev Immunol* 13(3):159–175, 2012.
47. Gautam N, Herwald H, Hedqvist Lindbom L: Signaling via beta(2) integrins triggers neutrophil-dependent alteration in endothelial barrier function, *J Exp Med* 191(11):1829–1839, 2000.
48. Ding ZM, Babensee JE, Simon SI, et al.: Relative contribution of LFA-1 and Mac-1 to neutrophil adhesion and migration, *J Immunol* 163(9):5029–5038, 1999.
49. Lefort CT, Ley K: Neutrophil arrest by LFA-1 activation, *Front Immunol* 3:157, 2012.
50. Schmidt S, Moser M, Sperandio M: The molecular basis of leukocyte recruitment and its deficiencies, *Mol Immunol* 55:49–58, 2013.
52. Cinamon G, Shinder V, Shamri R, et al.: Chemoattractant signals and β2 integrin occupancy at apical endothelial contacts combine with sheer stress signals to promote transendothelial neutrophil migration, *J Immunol* 173(12):7282–7291, 2004.
53. Dangerfield J, Larbi KY, Huang MT, et al.: PECAM-1 (CD31) homophilic interaction up-regulates α6β1 on transmigrated neutrophils in vivo and plays a functional role in the ability of α6 integrins to mediate leukocyte migration through the perivascular basement membrane, *J Exp Med* 196(9):1201–1211, 2002.
55. Petri B, Sanz MJ: Neutrophil chemotaxis, *Cell Tissue Res* 371(3):425–436, 2018.
57. Hayashi F, Means TK, Luster AD: Toll-like receptors stimulate human neutrophil function, *Blood* 102(7):2660–2669, 2003.
58. Futosi K, Fodor S, Mocsai A: Neutrophil cell surface receptors and their intracellular signal transduction pathways, *Int Immunopharmacol* 17(3):638–650, 2013.
60. Sengelov H, Follin P, Kjeldsen L, et al.: Mobilization of granules and secretory vesicles during in vivo exudation of human neutrophils, *J Immunol* 154:4157–4165, 1995.
64. Matute JD, Arias AA, Dinauer MC, et al.: p40phox: the last NADPH oxidase subunit, *Blood Cells Mol Dis* 35(2):291–302, 2005.
65. Nauseef WM, Borregaard N: Neutrophils at work, *Nat Immunol* 15(7):602–611, 2014.
68. Reeves EP, Lu H, Jacobs HL, et al.: Killing activity of neutrophils is mediated through activation of proteases by K+ flux, *Nature* 416(6878):291–297, 2002.
73. Li L, Huang L, Vergis AL, et al.: IL-17 produced by neutrophils regulates IFN-γ-mediated neutrophil migration in mouse kidney ischemia-reperfusion injury, *J Clin Invest* 120(1):331–342, 2010.
74. Theilgaard-Monch K, Jacobsen LC, Borup R, et al.: The transcriptional program of terminal granulocytic differentiation, *Blood* 105(4):1785–1796, 2005.
76. Cassatella MA: On the production of TNF-related apoptosis-inducing ligand (TRAIL/Apo-2L) by human neutrophils, *J Leukoc Biol* 79(6):1140–1149, 2006.
78. Shen L, Smith JM, Shen Z, et al.: Inhibition of human neutrophil degranulation by transforming growth factor-beta1, *Clin Exp Immunol* 149(1):155–161, 2007.
79. Brinkmann V, Reichard U, Goosmann C, et al.: Neutrophil extracellular traps kill bacteria, *Science* 303(5663):1532–1535, 2004.
80. Brinkmann V, Zychlinsky A: Beneficial suicide: why neutrophils die to make NETs, *Nat Rev Microbiol* 5(8):577–582, 2007.
81. Lood C, Blanco LP, Purmalek MM, et al.: Neutrophil extracellular traps enriched in oxidized mitochondrial DNA are interferogenic and contribute to lupus-like disease, *Nat Med* 22(2):146–153, 2016.
82. Delgado-Rizo V, Martinez-Guzman MA, Iniguez-Gutierrez L, et al.: Neutrophil extracellular traps and its implications in inflammation: an overview, *Front Immunol* 8:81–100, 2017.
83. Bilyy R, Fedorov V, Voyk V, et al.: Neutrophil extracellular traps form a barrier between necrotic and viable areas in acute abdominal inflammation, *Front Immunol* 7:424–430, 2016.
84. Wang J: Neutrophils in tissue injury and repair, *Cell Tissue Res* 371:531–539, 2018.
85. Parker H, Albrett AM, Kettle AJ, et al.: Myeloperoxidase associated with neutrophil extracellular traps is active and mediates bacterial killing in the presence of hydrogen peroxide, *J Leukoc Biol* 91(3):369–376, 2012.
86. Urban CF, Ermert D, Schmid M, et al.: Neutrophil extracellular traps contain calprotectin, a cytosolic protein complex involved in host defense against Candida albicans, *PLoS Pathog* 5(10), 2009:e1000639.
87. Berends ET, Horswill AR, Haste NM, et al.: Nuclease expression by Staphylococcus aureus facilitates escape from neutrophil extracellular traps, *J Innate Immun* 2(6):576–586, 2010.
88. Juneau RA, Stevens JS, Apicella MA, et al.: A thermonuclease of Neisseria gonorrhoeae enhances bacterial escape from killing by neutrophil extracellular traps, *J Infect Dis* 212(2):316–324, 2015.
89. Papayannopoulos V, Metzler KD, Hakkim A, et al.: Neutrophil elastase and myeloperoxidase regulate the formation of neutrophil extracellular traps, *J Cell Biol* 191(3):677–691, 2010.
90. Metzler KD, Fuchs TA, Nauseef WM, et al.: Myeloperoxidase is required for neutrophil extracellular trap formation: implications for innate immunity, *Blood* 117(3):953–959, 2011.
91. Akong-Moore K1, Chow OA, von Köckritz-Blickwede M, et al.: Influences of chloride and hypochlorite on neutrophil extracellular trap formation, *PLoS One* 7(8):e42984, 2012.
92. Khan MA, Palaniyar N: Transcriptional firing helps to drive NETosis, *Sci Rep* 7:41749–41764, 2017.
94. Yipp BG, Kubes P: NETosis. How vital is it, *Blood* 122(16):2784–2794, 2013.
96. Yousefi S, Mihalache C, Kozlowski E, et al.: Viable neutrophils release mitochondrial DNA to form neutrophil extracellular traps, *Cell Death Differ* 16(11):1438–1444, 2009.
98. Pilsczek FH, Salina D, Poon KK, et al.: A novel mechanism of rapid nuclear neutrophil extracellular trap formation in response to Staphylococcus aureus, *J Immunol* 185(12):7413–7425, 2010.
99. Byrd AS, O'Brien XM, Johnson CM, et al.: An extracellular matrix-based mechanism of rapid neutrophil extracellular trap formation in response to Candida albicans, *J Immunol* 190(8):4136–4148, 2013.
100. Clark SR, Ma AC, Tavener Sa, et al.: Platelet TLR4 activates neutropohil extracellular traps to ensnare bacteria in septic blood, *Nat Med* 13(4):463–469, 2007.
101. Johnson III BL, Kuethe JW, Caldwell CC: Neutrophil-derived microvesicles: emerging role of a key mediator to the immune response, *Endocr Metab Immune Disord Drug Targets* 14(3):210–217, 2014.
103. Watanabe J, Marathe GK, Neilsen PO, et al.: Endotoxins stimulate neutrophil adhesion followed by synthesis and release of platelet-activating factor in microparticles, *J Biol Chem* 278(35):33161–33168, 2003.
105. Nomura S, Ozaki Y, Ikeda Y: Function and role of microparticles in various clinical settings, *Thromb Res* 123(1):8–23, 2008.
106. Gasser O, Hess C, Miot S, et al.: Characterisation and properties of ectosomes released by human polymorphonuclear neutrophils, *Exp Cell Res* 285(2):243–257, 2003.

107. Gasser O, Schifferli JA: Activated polymorphonuclear neutrophils disseminate anti-inflammatory microparticles by exocytosis, *Blood* 104(8):2543–2548, 2004.
108. Joseph JE, Harrison P, Mackie IJ, et al.: Increased circulating platelet-leucocyte complexes and platelet activation in patients with antiphospholipid syndrome, systemic lupus erythematosus and rheumatoid arthritis, *Br J Haematol* 115(2):451–459, 2001.
111. Duchez AD, Boudreau LH, Naika GS, et al.: Platelet microparticles are internalized in neutrophils via the concerted activity of 12-lipoxygenase and secreted phospholipase A2-IIA, *Proc Natl Acad Sci USA* 112(27):E356–E373, 2015.
113. Kannemeir C, Shibamiya A, Nakazawa F, et al.: Extracellular RNA constitutes a natural procoagulant cofactor in blood coagulation, *Proc Natl Acad Sci USA* 104(15):6388–6393, 2007.
114. Massberg S, Grahl L, von Bruehl ML, et al.: Reciprocal coupling of coagulation and innate immunity via neutrophil serine proteases, *Nat Med* 16(8):887–896, 2010.
115. Fuchs TA, Brill A, Duerschmied D, et al.: Extracellular DNA traps promote thrombosis, *Proc Natl Acad Sci USA* 107(36):15880–15885, 2010.
116. von Brühl ML, Stark K, Steinhart A, et al.: Monocytes, neutrophils, and platelets cooperate to initiate and propagate venous thrombosis in mice in vivo, *J Exp Med* 209(4):819–835, 2012.
117. Pitanga TN, de Aragao Franca L, Rocha VC: Neutrophil-derived microparticles induce myeloperoxidase-mediated damage of vascular endothelial cells, *BMC Cell Biol* 14:21–30, 2014.
118. Pluskota E, Woody NM, Szpak D, et al.: Expression, activation, and function of integrin alphaMbeta2 (Mac-1) on neutrophil-derived microparticles, *Blood* 112(6):2327–2335, 2008.
120. Arita M, Ohira T, Sun YP, et al.: Resolvin E1 selectively interacts with leukotriene B4 receptor BLT1 and ChemR23 to regulate inflammation, *J Immunol* 178(6):3912–3917, 2007.
121. Serhan CN, Chiang N, Van Dyke TE: Resolving inflammation: dual anti-inflammatory and pro-resolution lipid mediators, *Nat Rev Immunol* 8(5):349–361, 2008.
122. Serhan CN, Yang R, Martinod K, et al.: Maresins: novel macrophage mediators with potent antiinflammatory and proresolving actions, *J Exp Med* 206(1):15–23, 2009.
123. Scher JU, Pillinger MH: 15d-PGJ2: the anti-inflammatory prostaglandin? *Clin Immunol* 114(2):100–109, 2005.
124. Chiang N, Arita M, Serhan CN: Anti-inflammatory circuitry: lipoxin, aspirin-triggered lipoxins and their receptor ALX, *Prostaglandins Leukot Essent Fatty Acids* 73(3-4):163–177, 2005.
125. Serhan CN: Lipoxins and aspirin-triggered 15-epi-lipoxins are the first lipid mediators of endogenous anti-inflammation and resolution, *Prostaglandins Leukot Essent Fatty Acids* 73(3-4):141–162, 2005.
126. Freire-de-Lima CG, Xiao YQ, Gardai SJ, et al.: Apoptotic cells, through transforming growth factor-beta, coordinately induce anti-inflammatory and suppress pro-inflammatory eicosanoid and NO synthesis in murine macrophages, *J Biol Chem* 281(50):38376–38384, 2006.
128. Perretti M, D'Acquisto F: Annexin A1 and glucocorticoids as effectors of the resolution of inflammation, *Nat Rev Immunol* 9(1):62–70, 2009. 2009.
130. McColl SR, Paquin R, Menard C, et al.: Human neutrophils produce high levels of the interleukin 1 receptor antagonist in response to granulocyte/macrophage colony-stimulating factor and tumor necrosis factor alpha, *J Exp Med* 176(2):593–598, 1992.
131. McQuibban GA, Gong JH, Tam EM, et al.: Inflammation dampened by gelatinase A cleavage of monocyte chemoattractant protein-3, *Science* 289(5482):1202–1206, 2000.
134. Ariel A, Fredman G, Sun YP, et al.: Apoptotic neutrophils and T cells sequester chemokines during immune response resolution through modulation of CCR5 expression, *Nat Immunol* 7(11):1209–1216, 2006.
135. Skokowa J, Germeshausen M, Zeidler C, et al.: Severe congenital neutropenia: inheritance and pathophysiology, *Curr Opin Hematol* 14(1):22–28, 2007.
137. Skokowa J, Dale DC, Touw IP, et al.: Severe congential neutropenias, *Nat Rev Dis Primers* 3:17032–17049, 2017.
139. Horwitz MS, Duan Z, Korkmaz B, et al.: Neutrophil elastase in cyclic and severe congenital neutropenia, *Blood* 109(5):1817–1824, 2007.
140. Zeidler C, Germeshausen M, Klein C, et al.: Clinical implications of ELA2-, HAX1-, and G-CSF-receptor (CSF3R) mutations in severe congenital neutropenia, *Br J Haematol* 144(4):459–467, 2009.
141. Anderson DC, Springer TA: Leukocyte adhesion deficiency: an inherited defect in the Mac-1, LFA-1, and p150,95 glycoproteins, *Annu Rev Med* 38:175–194, 1987.
142. Fagerholm SC, Guenther C, Llort Asens M, et al.: Beta2-integrins and interacting proteins in leukocyte trafficking, immune suppression, and immunodeficiency disease, *Front Immunol* 10:254, 2019.
145. Barbosa MD, Nguyen QA, Tcherneve VT, et al.: Identification of the homologous beige and Chediak-Higashi syndrome genes, *Nature* 382(6588):262–265, 1996.
146. Kaplan J, De Domenico I, Ward DM: Chediak-Higashi syndrome, *Curr Opin Hematol* 15(1):22–29, 2008.
148. Holland SM: Chronic granulomatous disease, *Hematol Oncol Clin North Am* 27(1):88–89, 2013.
149. van den Berg JM, van Koppen E, Ahlin A, et al.: Chronic granulomatous disease: the European experience, *PLoS One* 4(4):e5234, 2009.
150. Matute JD, Arias AA, Wright NA, et al.: A new genetic subgroup of chronic granulomatous disease with autosomal recessive mutations in p40 phox and selective defects in neutrophil NADPH oxidase activity, *Blood* 114(15):3309–3315, 2009.
151. Stein S, Ott MG, Schultz-Strasser S, et al.: Genomic instability and myelodysplasia with monosomy 7 consequent to EVI1 activation after gene therapy for chronic granulomatous disease, *Nat Med* 16(2):198–204, 2010.
152. Ku CL, von Bernuth H, Picard C, et al.: Selective predisposition to bacterial infections in IRAK-4-deficient children: IRAK-4-dependent TLRs are otherwise redundant in protective immunity, *J Exp Med* 204(10):2407–2422, 2007.
153. von Bernuth H, Picard C, Jin Z, et al.: Pyogenic bacterial infections in humans with MyD88 deficiency, *Science* 321(5889):691–696, 2008.
154. Mayadas TN, Cullere X, Lowell CA: The multifaceted functions of neutrophils, *Annu Rev Pathol* 9:181–218, 2014.
155. Chen K, Nishi H, Travers N, et al.: Endocytosis of soluble immune complexes leads to their clearance by FcgammaRIIIB but induces neutrophil extracellular traps via FcgammaRIIA in vivo, *Blood* 120(22):4421–4431, 2012.
156. Carmona-Rivera C, Zhao W, Yalavarthi S, et al.: Neutrophil extracellular traps induce endothelial dysfunction in systemic lupus erythematosus through the activation of matrix metalloproteinase-2, *Ann Rheum Dis* 74(7):1417–1424, 2015.
160. Garcia-Romo GS, Caielli S, Vega B, et al.: Netting neutrophils are major inducers of type I IFN production in pediatric lupus erythematosus, *Sci Transl Med* 3(73):73ra20, 2011.
162. Salmon JE, Millard S, Schacter LA, et al.: Fc gamma RIIA alleles are heritable risk factors for lupus nephritis in African Americans, *J Clin Invest* 97(5):1348–1354, 1996.
163. Barnard MR, Krueger LA, Freilinger 3rd AL, et al.: Whole blood analysis of leukocyte-platelet aggregates, *Curr Protoc Cytom* 2003; Ch 6:Unit 6.15.
164. Morgan AW, Barrett JH, Griffiths B, et al.: Analysis of Fcgamma receptor haplotypes in rheumatoid arthritis: FCGR3A remains a major susceptibility gene at this locus, with an additional contribution from FCGR3B, *Arthritis Res Ther* 8(1):R5, 2006.

166. Schauer C, Janko C, Munoz LE, et al.: Aggregated neutrophil extracellular traps limit inflammation by degrading cytokines and chemokines, *Nat Med* 20(5):511–517, 2014.
167. Chatfield SM, Grebe K, Whitehead LW, et al.: Monosodium urate crytals generate nuclease-resistant extracellular traps via a distinct molecular pathway, *J Immunol* 200(5):1802–1816, 2018.
171. Chen M, Lam BK, Kanaoka Y, et al.: Neutrophil-derived leukotriene B4 is required for inflammatory arthritis, *J Exp Med* 203(4):837–842, 2006.
172. Tsuboi N, Ernandez T, Li X, et al.: Human neutrophil FcγRIIA regulation by C5aR promotes inflammatory arthritis in mice, *Arthritis Rheum* 63(2):467–478, 2011.
173. Vono M, Lin A, Norrby-Teglund A, et al.: Neutrophils acquire the capacity for antigen presentation to memory CD4+ T cells in vitro and ex vivo, *Blood* 129(14):1991–2001, 2017.
174. Cross A, Bucknall RC, Cassatella MA: Synovial fluid neutrophils transcribe and express class II major histocompatibility complex molecules in rheumatoid arthritis, *Arthritis Rheumatol* 48(10):2796–2806, 2003.
175. Whitaker JW, Boyle DL, Bartok B, et al.: Integrative omics analysis of rheumatoid arthritis identifies non-obvious therapeutic targets, *PLoS One* 10(4):e0124254, 2015.
176. Arandjelovic S, Perry JSA, Lucas CD, et al.: A noncanonical role for the engulfment gene ELMO1 in neutrophils that promotes inflammatory arthritis, *Nat Immunol* 20(2):141–151, 2019.
177. Villanueva E, Yalavarthi S, Berthier CC, et al.: Netting neutrophils induce endothelial damage, infiltrate tissues, and expose immunostimulatory molecules in systemic lupus erythematosus, *J Immunol* 187(1):538–552, 2011.
179. Hakkim A, Fürnrohr BG, Amann K, et al.: Impairment of neutrophil extracellular trap degradation is associated with lupus nephritis, *Proc Natl Acad Sci USA* 107(21):9813–9818, 2010.
180. Sisirak V, Sally B, D'Agati V, et al.: Digestion of chromatin in apoptotoic cell microparticles prevents autoimmunity, *Cell* 166(1):88–101, 2016.
183. Lood C, Blanco LP, Purmalek MM, et al.: Neutrophil extracellular traps entriched in oxidized mitochondrial DNA are interferogenic and contribute to lupus-like disease, *Nat Med* 22(2):146–153, 2016.
190. Cronstein BN, Molad Y, Reibman J, et al.: Colchicine alters the quantitative and qualitative display of selectins on endothelial cells and neutrophils, *J Clin Invest* 96(2):994–1002, 1995.
191. Slobodnick A, Shah B, Pillinger MH, et al.: Colchicine: Old and new, *Am J Med* 128(5):461–470, 2015.
194. Wright HL, Cross AL, Edwards SW, et al.: Effects of IL-6 and IL-6 blockade on neutrophil function in vitro and in vivo, *Rheumatology* 53(7):1321–1331, 2014.
197. Isailovic N, Daigo K, Mantovani A, et al.: Interleukin-17 and innate immunity in infections and chronic inflammation, *J Autoimmun* 60:1–11, 2015.

12 T Lymphocytes

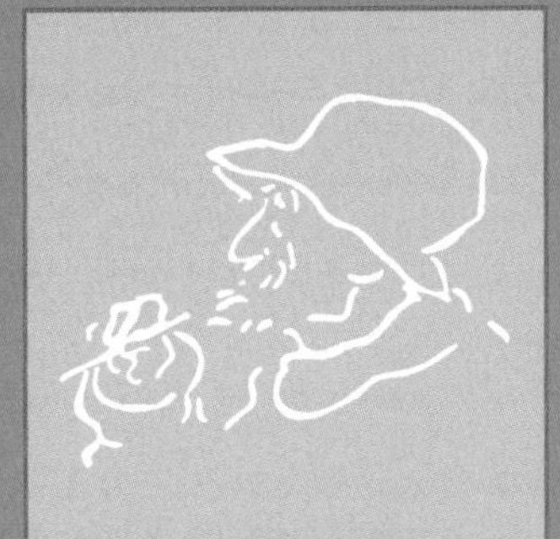

RALPH C. BUDD

KEY POINTS

T cells develop primarily in the thymus. The importance of the thymus is underscored by the absence of T cells in patients in whom the thymus has failed to develop (e.g., DiGeorge syndrome).

Thymic selection consists of a positive phase in which T cells must recognize self-major histocompatibility complex (MHC) molecules and a negative phase in which thymocytes bearing high-affinity T cell receptors for self-peptide MHC are deleted through apoptosis.

Only a small proportion of T cells emerge from the thymus as naïve T cells that are quiescent and produce relatively low levels of cytokines. After they acquire memory phenotype (CD45RO$^+$), they can produce high levels of cytokines.

Naïve T cells can undergo homeostatic proliferation to self-peptide/MHC in peripheral lymphoid tissues to generate a critical number of T cells. This process requires IL-7 and IL-15 and results in the upregulation of several cytolytic genes that can provoke inflammation. Lack of regulation of this process may contribute to various autoimmune disorders.

Th1 and Th17 cells accumulate at sites of inflammation such as rheumatoid synovium, whereas Th2 cells accumulate at sites of allergic responses such as asthma.

T cells undergo a tremendous change in metabolism as they transition from resting naïve T cells (oxidative phosphorylation) to proliferating effector T cells (glycolysis) to memory T cells (oxidative phosphorylation).

Introduction

The establishment and maintenance of immune responses, homeostasis, and memory depends to a large extent on T lymphocytes. T cells provide more than protection from infection and are involved in tumor surveillance as well as tissue homeostasis.[1] T cells thus confront the dilemma of generating a receptor that can recognize a broad array of antigens from foreign pathogens, tumors, and normal tissue without provoking an autoimmune response to the host. The price for generating an increasingly varied population of antigen receptors needed to recognize a wide spectrum of pathogens is the progressive risk of producing self-reactive lymphocytes. T lymphocytes are thus subjected to a rigorous selection process during development in the thymus to delete self-reactive T cells (i.e., central tolerance). In addition, premature activation of mature peripheral T cells is prevented by requiring two signals for activation (i.e., peripheral tolerance). Finally, the expansion of T cells that occurs during either homeostatic proliferation in the periphery or in response to an infection is resolved by the active induction of cell death. The consequences of inefficient lymphocyte removal at any one of these junctures could provoke an autoimmune diathesis. These issues are discussed in more detail in Chapter 19 on cell survival and death.

The activation of T lymphocytes yields a variety of effector functions that are pivotal to combating infections. Cytolytic T cells can kill infected cells through the release of granules containing perforin and granzymes that induce holes in cell membranes and cleave cellular substrates, respectively, or expression of ligands for death receptors such as Fas (CD95) or TNF receptor 1. Production of T cell cytokines such as interferon-γ (IFN-γ) by T helper (Th)1 cells (see below) can inhibit viral replication, whereas other cytokines such as interleukin (IL)-4, IL-5, and IL-21 by Th2 cells are critical for optimal B cell growth and immunoglobulin production.[2] However, this same armamentarium, if not tightly regulated, can also precipitate damage to host tissues and provoke autoimmune responses, such as in the synovium of inflammatory arthritides, pancreatic islets in type I diabetes, and the central nervous system in multiple sclerosis. Damage in these cases need not be directly the result of recognition of target tissues by the T cells. T cells may be activated elsewhere and then migrate to the tissue and damage innocent bystander cells. T cells may also promote autoimmunity through the augmentation of B cell responses. The following sections detail these events.

T Cell Development

T lymphocytes originate from bone marrow progenitors that migrate to the thymus for maturation, selection, and subsequent export to the periphery. T cells must traverse two stringent hurdles during their development. First, they must successfully rearrange the genes encoding the two chains of the T cell antigen receptor (TCR). Second, T cells must survive thymic selection during which T cells bearing a TCR th0at interacts strongly with self-major histocompatibility complex (MHC) molecules/peptides are eliminated (i.e., negative selection). This minimizes the chances of autoreactive T cells escaping to the periphery and is known as *central tolerance*. In addition, developing thymocytes must also make moderate interactions with self-MHC/peptides to survive (i.e., positive selection), as those T cells making no meaningful contact are also eliminated. The result of this "Goldilocks" concept of not too strong, not too weak TCR-MHC/peptide interactions is that less than 3% of developing thymocytes actually leave the thymus.

The TCR is an 80 to 90 kDa disulfide-linked heterodimer composed of a 48 to 54 kDa α chain and a 37 to 42 kDa β chain. An alternate TCR composed of γ and δ chains is expressed on 2% to 3% of peripheral blood T cells and is discussed below. The TCR has an extra-cellular ligand binding pocket for MHC/peptide and a short cytoplasmic tail that by itself cannot signal. Consequently, it is noncovalently associated with as many as five invariant chains of the CD3 complex, which relay information to the intra-cellular signaling machinery via immunoreceptor tyrosine activation motifs (ITAMs) (see later). The structure of the TCR gene locus is, not surprisingly, similar to immunoglobulin genes in B cells (see details in Chapter 13). To economically package up to 10^{15} TCR specificities within a genome of fewer than 30,000 genes, the process of gene rearrangement and splicing evolved using machinery similar to what already existed to promote gene translocations. The β- and δ-chain genes of the TCR contain 4 segments known as the V (variable), D (diversity), J (joining), and C (constant) regions. The α and γ chains are similar but lack the J component. Each of the segments has several family members (approximately 50 to 100 V, 15 D, 6 to 60 J, and 1 to 2 C members). An orderly process occurs during TCR gene rearrangement in which a D segment is spliced adjacent to a J segment, which is subsequently spliced to a V segment. Following transcription, the VDJ sequence is spliced to a C segment to produce a mature TCR messenger RNA. Arithmetically, this random rearrangement of a single chain of the TCR locus can give rise to minimally 50V × 15D × 6J × 2C or about 9000 possible combinations. At each of the splice sites, which must occur in-frame to be functional, additional nucleotides not encoded by the genome (so-called *N-region nucleotides*) can be incorporated, adding further diversity to the rearranging gene. The combinations from the two TCR chains, plus N-region diversity, yield at least 10 million theoretical possible combinations. The cutting, rearranging, and splicing are directed by specific enzymes. Mutations in the genes for these processes can result in an arrest in lymphocyte development. For example, mutation in the gene encoding a DNA-dependent protein kinase (DNA-PK) required for receptor gene recombination results in a severe combined immunodeficiency known as *scid*.

Because the developing T cell has two copies of each chromosome, there are two chances to successfully rearrange each of the two TCR chains. As soon as successful rearrangement occurs, further β-chain rearrangements on either the same or the other chromosome are suppressed, a process known as *allelic exclusion*. This limits the chance of dual TCR expression by an individual T cell. The high percentage of T cells that contain rearrangements of both β-chain genes attests to the inefficiency of this complex event. Rearrangement of the α chain occurs later in thymocyte development in a similar fashion, although without apparent allelic exclusion. This can result in dual TCR expression by a single T cell.

Development of T cells occurs within a microenvironment provided by the thymic epithelial stroma. The thymic anlage is formed from embryonic ectoderm and endoderm and is then colonized by hematopoietic cells, which give rise to dendritic cells, macrophages, and developing T cells. The hematopoietic and epithelial components combine to form two histologically defined compartments: the cortex, which contains immature thymocytes, and the medulla, which contains mature thymocytes (Fig. 12.1A). As few as 50 to 100 bone marrow–derived stem cells enter the thymus daily.

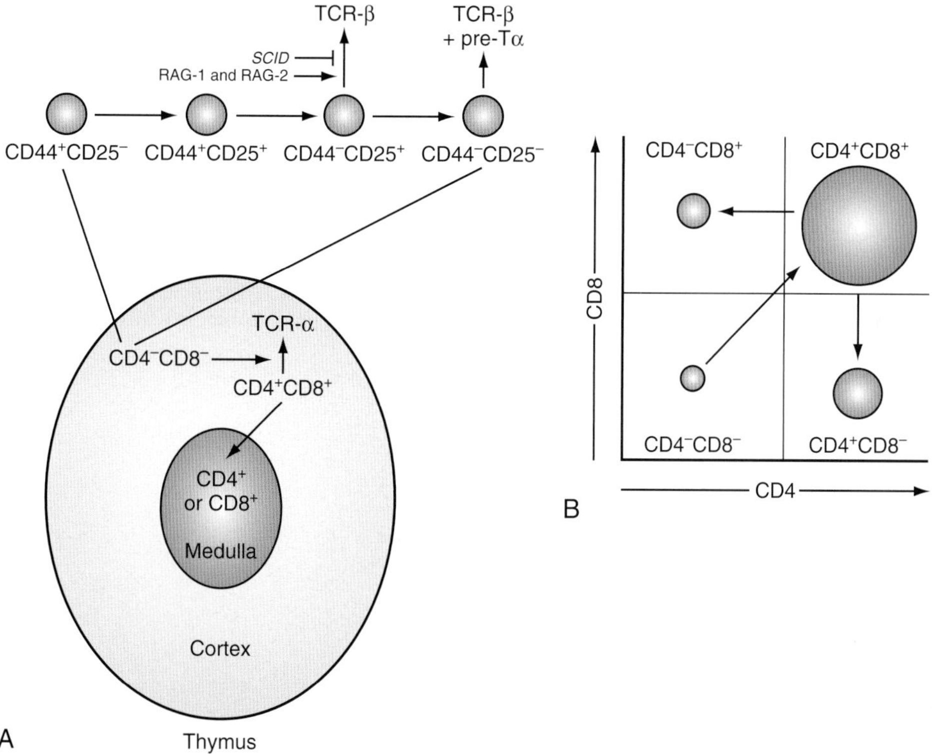

• **Fig. 12.1** Sequence of thymocyte development. (A) The earliest thymocyte precursors lack expression of CD4 and CD8 ($CD4^-CD8^-$). These can be further divided into four subpopulations based on the sequential expression of CD44 and CD25. It is at the $CD44^-CD25^+$ stage that the TCR-β chain rearranges. The *scid* mutation or deficiencies of the rearrangement enzymes Rag-1 and Rag-2 result in inability to rearrange the β chain and maturational arrest at this stage. Those thymocytes that successfully rearrange the β chain express it associated with a surrogate α chain known as pre-Tα. Concomitant with a proliferative burst, development can then progress to the $CD4^+CD8^+$ stage in the cortex where the TCR α chain rearranges and pairs with the β chain to express a mature TCR complex. These cells then undergo thymic positive and negative selection (as diagrammed in Figure 12.3B). Successful completion of this rigorous selection process results in mature $CD4^+$ or $CD8^+$ T cells in the medulla, which eventually emigrate to peripheral lymphoid sites. (B) Schematic two-color flow cytometry showing subpopulations of thymocytes defined by CD4 and CD8 expression in their relative proportions.

The stages of thymocyte development can be defined by the status of the TCR gene and the expression of CD4 and CD8, proceeding in an orderly fashion from $CD4^-8^- \rightarrow CD4^+8^+ \rightarrow CD4^+8^-$ or $CD4^-8^+$ (Fig. 12.1B). CD4 and CD8 define, respectively, the helper and cytolytic subsets of mature T cells.

$CD4^-8^-$ thymocytes can be further subdivided based on their expression of CD25 (the high affinity IL-2 receptor α chain) and CD44 (the hyaluronate receptor). Development proceeds in the following order: $CD25^-CD44^+ \rightarrow CD25^+CD44^+ \rightarrow CD25^+CD44^- \rightarrow CD25^-CD44^-$ (see Fig. 12.1). These subpopulations correspond to discrete stages of thymocyte differentiation. $CD25^-44^+$ cells contain TCR genes in germline configuration. These cells upregulate CD25 to give rise to $CD25^+CD44^+$ thymocytes, which now express surface CD2 and low levels of CD3ε. At the next stage ($CD25^+CD44^-$), there is a brief burst of proliferation followed by upregulation of the recombination-activating enzymes, RAG-1 and RAG-2, and the concomitant rearrangement of the genes of the TCR β chain. A small subpopulation of T cells rearranges and expresses a second pair of TCR genes known as γ and δ. Productive TCR β-chain rearrangement results in a second proliferative burst, yielding $CD25^-CD44^-$ thymocytes.

The TCR β chain cannot be stably expressed without an α chain. Because the TCR α chain has not yet rearranged, a surrogate invariant TCR pre-α chain is disulfide linked to the β chain. When associated with components of the CD3 complex, this allows a low-level surface expression of a pre-TCR and progression to the next developmental stage. Failure to successfully rearrange the TCR β chain results in a developmental arrest at the transition from CD25+CD44− to CD25-CD44−. This occurs in RAG-deficient mice as well as in *Scid* mice and humans.[3]

A number of transcription factors, receptors, and signaling molecules are required for early T cell development (Fig. 12.2). IKAROS encodes a transcription factor required for the development of cells of lymphoid origin. Notch-1, a molecule known to regulate cell fate decisions, is also required at the earliest stage of T cell lineage development.[4] Cytokines, including IL-7, promote the survival and expansion of the earliest thymocytes. In mice deficient for IL-7, its receptor components IL-7Rα or γ_c, or the cytokine receptor–associated signaling molecule Janus kinase (JAK)-3, thymocyte development is inhibited at the $CD25^-CD44^+$ stage. In humans, mutations in γ_c or JAK-3 result in the most frequent form of SCID.[5] Pre-TCR signaling is required for the $CD25^+CD44^- \rightarrow CD25^-CD44^-$ transition. Thus,

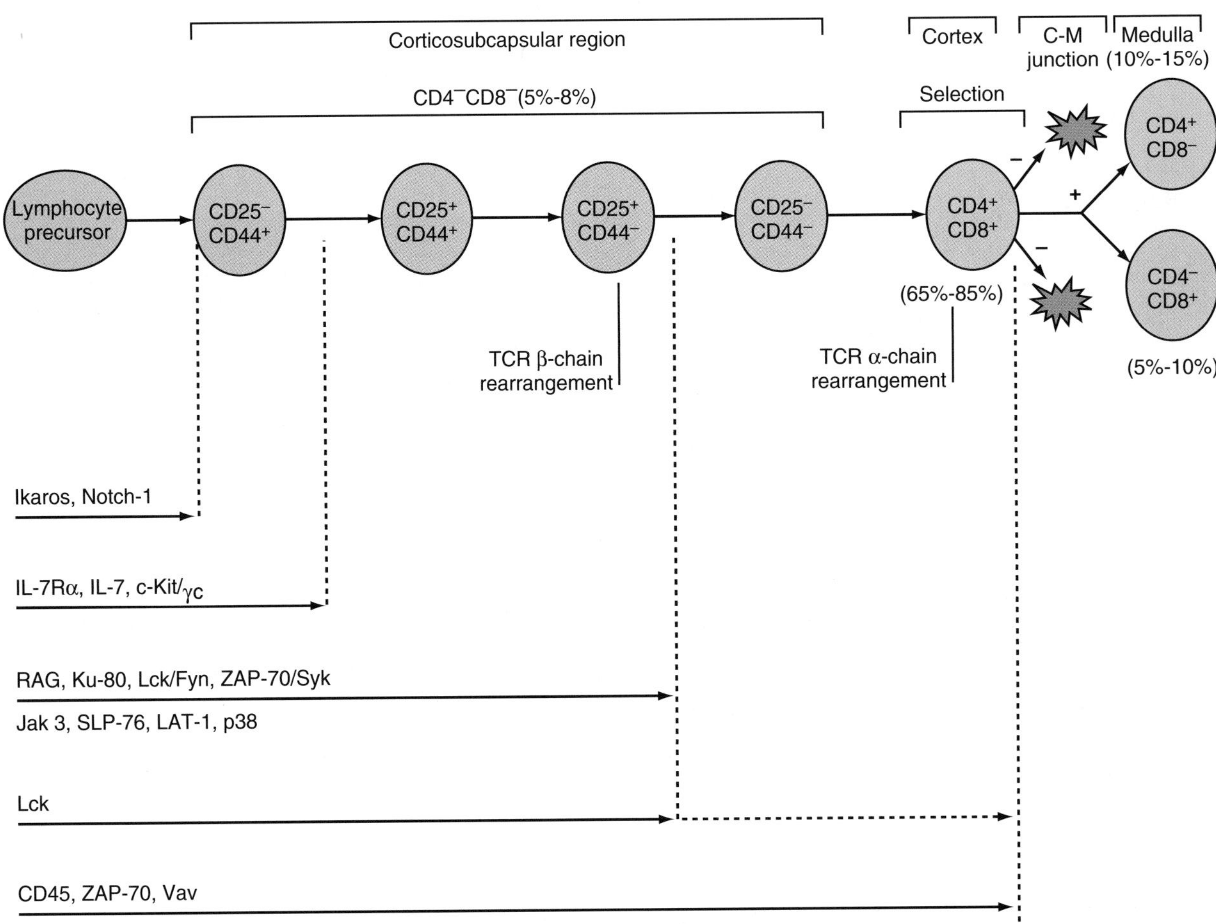

• **Fig. 12.2** Sequence of αβ T cell development in the thymus. The earliest thymocyte precursors lack expression of CD4 and CD8 ($CD4^-CD8^-$). These can be further divided into four subpopulations based on the sequential expression of CD25 and CD44. At the $CD25^+CD44^-$ stage, the TCR β chain rearranges and associates a surrogate α chain known as pre-Tα. Concomitant with a proliferative burst, thymocytes progress to the $CD4^+CD8^+$ stage, rearrange the TCR α chain, and express a mature TCR complex. These cells then undergo thymic positive and negative selection. Those thymocytes that survive this rigorous selection process differentiate into mature $CD4^+$ or $CD8^+$ T cells. Shown also are the various signaling molecules that are involved at specific stages of thymic development.

loss of TCR signaling components including Lck, SH2-domain–containing leukocyte protein-76 (SLP-76), and Linker for activation of T cells (LAT)-1 results in a block at this stage of T cell development. TCR signals are also required for differentiation of $CD4^+CD8^+$ to mature $CD4^+$ or $CD8^+$ cells. Humans deficient in ZAP-70 (see later) have $CD4^+$ but not $CD8^+$ T cells in the thymus and periphery.[6]

$CD25^-CD44^-$ cells upregulate expression of CD4 and CD8 to become $CD4^+8^+$, at which point the α chain of the TCR rearranges. Unlike the β chain, allelic exclusion of the α chain is not apparent. Rearrangement of the α chain can occur simultaneously on both chromosomes, and if one attempt is unsuccessful, repeat rearrangements to other Vα segments are possible. Reports exist of dual TCR expression by as many as 30% of mature T cells in which the same T cell expresses different α chains paired with the same β chain.[7] However, in most cases of dual TCR α chains, one is downregulated during positive selection by Lck and Cbl, through ubiquitination, endocytosis, and degradation.

Although the structure of immunoglobulin and TCR are quite similar, they recognize fundamentally different antigens. Immunoglobulins recognize intact antigens in isolation, either soluble or membrane bound, and are often sensitive to the tertiary structure. The TCRαβ recognizes linear stretches of antigen peptide fragments bound within the grooves of either class I or class II MHC molecules (Fig. 12.3A). Thymic selection molds the repertoire of emerging TCRs so that they recognize peptides within the groove of self-MHC molecules, ensuring the *self-MHC restriction* of T cell responses. The MHC structure is described in detail in Chapters 21 and 22. Pockets within the MHC groove bind particular residues along the peptide sequence of 7-9 amino acids for class I MHC and 9-15 amino acids for class II MHC molecules. As a result, certain amino acids make strong contact with the MHC groove while others are exposed to the TCR.

The contact between the TCR and MHC/peptide has been revealed by crystal structure to be remarkably flat, rather than a deep lock and key structure that one might imagine.[8] The TCR axis is tipped about 30 degrees to the long axis of the class I MHC molecule and is slightly more skewed for class II MHC. The affinity of the TCR for MHC/peptide is in the micromolar range. This is a lower affinity than many antibody-antigen affinities, and several logs less than many enzyme-substrate affinities. This has led to the notion that TCR interactions with MHC/peptide are brief, and successful activation of the T cell requires multiple interactions, resulting in a cumulative signal.

Once the T cell has successfully rearranged and expressed a TCR in association with the CD3 complex, it encounters the second major hurdle in T cell development, *thymic selection*. Selection has two phases, positive and negative, and the outcome is based largely upon the intensity of TCR signaling in response to interactions with self-MHC/peptides expressed on thymic epithelium and dendritic cells. TCR signals that are either too weak (death by neglect) or too intense *(negative selection)* result in elimination by apoptosis, whereas those with intermediate signaling intensity survive *(positive selection)* (Fig. 12.3B). Successful positive selection at the $CD4^+8^+$ stage is coincident with upregulation of surface TCR, the activation markers CD5 and CD69, and the survival factor Bcl-2. T cells bearing a TCR that recognizes class I MHC maintain CD8 expression, downregulate CD4, and become $CD4^-8^+$. T cells expressing a TCR that recognizes class II MHC become $CD4^+8^-$.

An enigma for thymic selection has been how to present the myriad self-proteins to developing thymocytes so that self-reactive thymocytes are effectively eliminated by negative selection. This

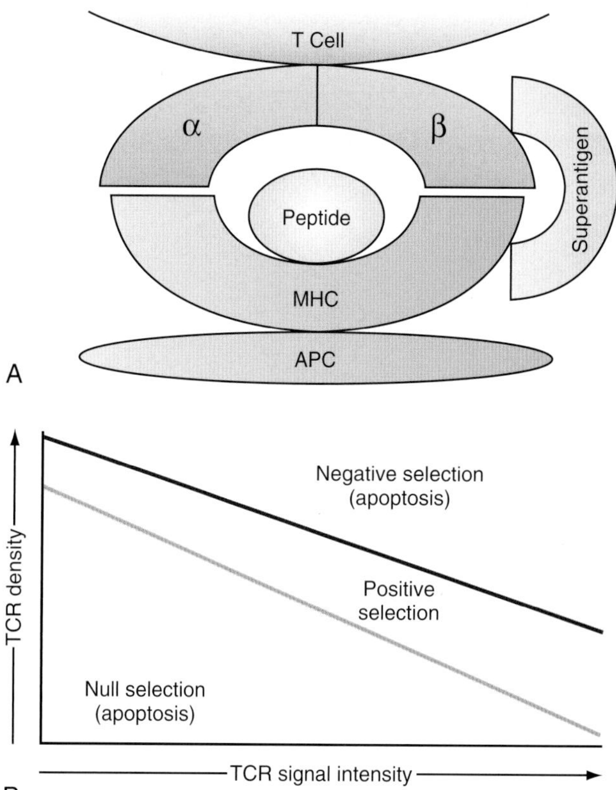

• **Fig. 12.3** TCR interaction with the MHC/peptide complex. (A) Polymorphic residues within the variable region of the α and β chains of the TCR contact determinants on the MHC molecule on an antigen presenting cell (APC) as well as with the peptide fragment that sits in the MHC binding groove. (B) A schematic diagram illustrating that during thymocyte development, those TCR conferring either a very low signal intensity (null selection) or high intensity (negative selection) each lead to apoptosis. Only those thymocytes whose TCR can engage MHC/peptides and confer moderate intensity survive by positive selection.

includes particularly those antigens with tissue or developmentally restricted expression. A solution was found with the discovery of the autoimmune regulator *(AIRE)* gene. AIRE is a transcription factor expressed by the medullary epithelium of the thymus that induces transcription of a wide array of organ-specific genes, such as insulin, that might otherwise be sequestered from developing thymocytes.[9] This effectively creates a self-transcriptome within the thymus against which autoreactive T cells can be deleted. Gene knockout mice of *AIRE*, and humans bearing *AIRE* mutations, manifest various autoimmune sequelae in a syndrome known as autoimmune polyendocrinopathy-candidiasis-ectodermal dystrophy (APECED).[10]

Not surprisingly, a variety of signaling molecules activated by TCR engagement are important to thymic selection. These include Lck, the Ras∏Raf-1∏MEK1∏ERK kinase cascade, the kinase ZAP-70, and the phosphatases CD45 and calcineurin, which are involved with positive selection. Among these, the Ras ∏ERK pathway is particularly important as dominant negative variants of these molecules can disrupt positive selection. Conversely, an activator of Ras known as *GRP1* assists with the positive selection of thymocytes expressing weakly selecting signals. These molecules are discussed in more detail in the section on TCR signaling. By contrast, although a number of molecules may promote negative selection, among them the mitogen-activated protein kinases (MAPKs) JNK and p38, there appears to be sufficient redundancy

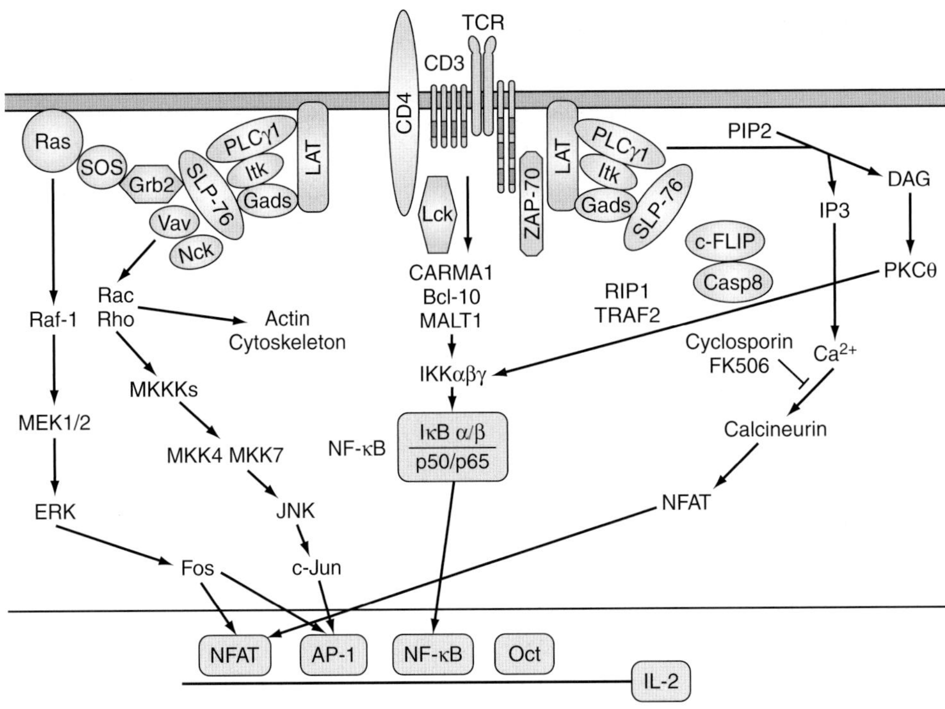

• **Fig. 12.4** TCR signal pathways. The schema shows the principle signal pathways resulting from TCR activation and how they impinge on the regulatory region of the *IL2* gene. See text for details.

so that only rarely does elimination of any one of these molecules alter the efficient deletion of thymocytes. The few exceptions include CD40, CD40L, CD30, or the proapoptotic Bcl-2 family member, Bim, where preservation of at least some thymocytes bearing self-reactive TCR could be observed in mice deficient in these molecules.[11]

The survivors of these stringent processes of TCR gene rearrangement and thymic selection represent less than 3% of total immature thymocytes. This is reflected by the presence of a high rate of cell death among developing thymocytes. This can be visualized by the measurement of DNA degradation, a hallmark of apoptosis, as shown in Fig. 12.4. The survivors become either CD4$^+$ helper or CD8$^+$ cytolytic T cells and reside in the thymic medulla for 12 to 14 days before emigrating to the periphery. The decision to become a CD4$^+$ versus CD8$^+$ T cell parallels the observation that long TCR interactions are required for CD4 progression, whereas shorter TCR engagement favors CD8 progression.[12]

Immunodeficiencies Resulting From Defects in T Cell Development

Given the vast number of events in T cell development, it is not surprising that multiple causes can underlie human T cell immunodeficiencies.[13] The influence of the thymic stroma on thymocyte ontogeny is underscored in the DiGeorge anomaly in which development of the pharyngeal pouches is disrupted and the thymic rudiment fails to form. This results in the failure of normal T cell development. Less severe T cell deficiencies are associated with a failure to express class I and/or class II MHC (the "bare lymphocyte syndrome"), which are directly involved with interactions required to induce the positive selection of, respectively, CD8$^+$ and CD4$^+$ mature T cells.

Metabolic disorders can affect thymocytes more directly. The absence of functional adenosine deaminase (ADA) and purine nucleoside phosphorylase (PNP) results in the buildup of metabolic byproducts that are toxic to developing T and B lymphocytes. This ultimately produces forms of severe combined immunodeficiency disorders (SCIDs).

Peripheral Migration and Homeostatic Proliferation of T Cells

In early life, the majority of T cells are newly emerged from the thymus and naïve. With age, memory T cells are generated from exposure to antigens, which plateaus in adulthood. This may parallel a shift in function toward tumor surveillance and tissue homeostasis. At this later stage, immunosenescence occurs with a decline in T cell function, which can result in immunodysregulation and inflammation.[1] The migration of naïve T cells to peripheral lymphoid structures or their infiltration into other tissues requires the coordinated regulation of an array of cell adhesion molecules. Entry from the circulation into tissues occurs via two main anatomic sites: the flat endothelium of the blood vessels and specialized postcapillary venules known as high endothelial venules (HEV). A three-step model has been described for lymphocyte migration: rolling, adhesion, and migration.[14] L-selectin expressed by naïve T cells binds via lectin domains to carbohydrate moieties of GlyCAM-1 and CD34 (collectively known as *peripheral node addressin*), which are expressed on endothelial cells, particularly high-endothelial venules (HEVs). The weak binding of CD62L to its ligand mediates a weak adhesion to the vessel wall which, combined with the force of blood flow, results in rolling of the T cell along the endothelium. The increased cell contact facilitates the interaction of a second adhesion molecule on lymphocytes, the integrin LFA-1 (CD11a/CD18), with its ligands, intercellular adhesion molecule (ICAM)-1 (CD54) and ICAM-2 (CD102). This results in the arrest of rolling and firm attachment. Migration into the extra-cellular matrix of tissues involves additional lymphocyte cell surface molecules such as the hyaluronate receptor (CD44) or the integrin α4β7 (CD49d/β7), which binds the mucosal addressin cell adhesion molecule-1 (MAdCAM-1) on endothelium of Peyer's patches and other endothelial cells.

Additional cytokines known as chemokines contribute to lymphocyte homing. Chemokines are structurally and functionally related to proteins bearing an affinity for heparan sulfate proteoglycan and promote migration of various cell types.[15] The chemokines RANTES, MIP-1α, MIP-1β, MCP-1, and IL-8 are produced by a number of cell types including endothelium, activated T cells, and monocytes and are present at inflammatory sites such as rheumatoid synovium (see Chapter 74).

Once mature T cells have reached the peripheral lymphoid tissues of lymph node and spleen, they undergo a slow rate of proliferation known as *homeostatic proliferation* in response to self-MHC/peptide complexes and the cytokines IL-7 and IL-15.[16] This serves to maintain the number of peripheral T cells and can become enhanced in response to lymphopenia, such as after chemotherapy or HIV infection.[17] Because homeostatic proliferation is driven by self-MHC/peptides and is thus inherently autoimmune, its acceleration could precipitate an autoimmune syndrome. In this regard, it is of interest that one of the standard murine models of autoimmunity is day 3 thymectomy, which results in lymphopenia and autoimmunity of various organs.[18] In addition, nonobese diabetic (NOD) mice have chronic lymphopenia that contributes to their diabetes,[19] and evidence of augmented homeostatic proliferation has been suggested to occur in rheumatoid arthritis (RA).[20] Homeostatic proliferation is also regulated by the death receptor Fas (CD95).[21] In the absence of Fas in mice or humans, T cells accumulate that express a gene profile that includes upregulation of pro-inflammatory molecules such as Fas ligand and Granzyme B, as well as the immunoinhibitory molecules programmed cell death 1 (PD-1) and LAG3.[22] This might serve to explain the clinical immunology paradox of sudden autoinflammatory features in immunodeficient individuals, such as the development of sudden psoriasis and psoriatic arthritis (PsA) in HIV-infected individuals.[23]

Activation of T Cells

Metabolic Switch

T cell activation initiates an intra-cellular signaling cascade that ultimately results in proliferation, effector function, or death, depending on the intensity of the TCR signal and associated signals. This requires a dramatic change in metabolism from largely oxidative phosphorylation to glycolysis to provide the synthetic machinery for proliferation and effector molecules.[24] This is detailed in Chapter 24. To guard against premature or excessive activation, T cells have a requirement of two independent signals for full activation. Signal 1 is an antigen-specific signal provided by the binding of the TCR to antigenic peptide complexed with MHC. Signal 2 is mediated by either cytokines or the engagement of co-stimulatory molecules such as B7.1 (CD80) and B7.2 (CD86) on the antigen-presenting cell (APC). Receiving only Signal 1 without co-stimulation results in T cell unresponsiveness or anergy, a process known as *peripheral tolerance.*

TCR Signal Regulation

TCR αβ and γδ have very short cytoplasmic domains and by themselves are unable to transduce signals. The molecules of the noncovalently associated CD3 complex couple the TCR to intra-cellular signaling machinery (see Fig. 12.4). The CD3 complex contains nonpolymorphic members known as CD3ε, CD3γ, CD3δ, as well as the ζ chain, which is a separate gene not genetically linked to the CD3 complex. Although the functional stoichiometry of the TCR complex is not completely defined, current data indicate that each TCR heterodimer is associated with 3 dimers: CD3εγ, CD3εδ, and ζζ or ζ. CD3ε, -γ, and -δ have an immunoglobulin-like extra-cellular domain, a transmembrane region, and a modest cytoplasmic domain, whereas ζ contains a longer cytoplasmic tail. The transmembrane domains of ζ and the CD3 chains contain a negatively charged residue that interacts with positively charged amino acids in the transmembrane domain of the TCR.

None of the proteins in the TCR/CD3 complex has intrinsic enzymatic activity. Instead, the cytoplasmic domains of the invariant CD3 chains contain conserved activation domains that are required for coupling the TCR to intra-cellular signaling molecules. These ITAMs contain a minimal functional consensus sequence of paired tyrosines (Y) and leucines (L): (D/E) XXYXXL$(X)_{6\text{-}8}$YXXL. ITAMs are substrates for cytoplasmic protein tyrosine kinases (PTKs), and upon phosphorylation they recruit additional molecules to the TCR complex.[25] Each ζ chain contains three ITAMs, whereas there is one in each of the CD3ε, -γ, and -δ chains. Thus, each TCR/CD3 complex can contain as many as 10 ITAMs.

Activation of PTKs is one of the earliest signaling events following TCR stimulation. Four families of PTKs are known to be involved in TCR signaling: Src, Csk, Tec, and Syk. The Src family members Lck and Fyn^T have a central role in TCR signaling and are expressed exclusively in lymphoid cells. Src PTKs contain multiple structural domains, including: (1) N-terminal myristylation and palmitoylation sites that allow association with the plasma membrane, (2) an Src homology (SH)3 domain that associates with proline-rich sequences, (3) an SH2 domain that binds phosphotyrosine-containing proteins, and (4) a carboxy-terminal negative regulatory site. Their catalytic activity is regulated by the balance between the actions of kinases and phosphatases. Activity is repressed by phosphorylation of a conserved carboxy-terminal tyrosine, and thus its dephosphorylation by the phosphatase CD45 is critical for the initiation of TCR-mediated signal transduction. In addition, autophosphorylation of other tyrosines within the kinase domain enhances catalytic activity. Lck is physically and functionally associated with CD4 and CD8. Fifty percent to 90% of total Lck molecules is associated with CD4 and 10% to 25% with CD8. CD4 and CD8 physically associate with the TCR/CD3 complex during antigen stimulation as a result of their interaction with class II and class I MHC molecules, respectively, and thus enhance TCR-mediated signals by recruiting Lck to the TCR complex. Lck phosphorylates the CD3 chains, TCRζ, ZAP-70, phospholipase C-γ1 (PLC-γ1), Vav, and Shc. Fyn binds TCRζ and CD3ε and, although its substrates are less well defined, T cells lacking Fyn have diminished response to TCR signals.[26] In addition, the SH2 and SH3 domains of Src PTKs can mediate their association with, respectively, phosphotyrosine- and proline-containing molecules.

Somewhat less is known about the Csk and Tec PTKs. Csk negatively regulates TCR signaling by phosphorylating the carboxy-terminal tyrosine of Lck and Fyn. Dephosphorylation of this negative regulatory tyrosine is mediated by the transmembrane tyrosine phosphatase CD45. CD45 activity is essential for TCR signaling as CD45-deficient T cells fail to activate by TCR stimulation. The Tec family member Itk is preferentially expressed in T cells and regulates PLC-γ.[27] T cells from Itk-deficient mice have diminished response to TCR stimulation.

Phosphorylation of the ITAM motifs on the CD3 complex recruits the Syk kinase family member ZAP-70 by its tandem SH2 domains. ZAP-70 is expressed exclusively in T cells and is required for TCR signaling. Following TCR stimulation, ZAP-70 is activated by phosphorylation of tyrosine 493 by Lck.[28] Loss-of-function hypomorphic alleles of ZAP-70 result in reduced TCR signaling and a propensity for autoimmune phenomena.[29]

Adaptor Proteins

Phosphorylation of tyrosine residues in ITAMs and PTKs following TCR stimulation creates docking sites for adaptor proteins. Adaptor proteins contain no known enzymatic or transcriptional activities but mediate protein-protein interactions or protein-lipid interactions. They function to bring proteins in proximity to their substrates and regulators, as well as sequester signaling molecules to specific subcellular locations. The protein complexes formed can function as either positive or negative regulators of TCR signaling, depending on the molecules they contain.

Two critical adaptor proteins for linking proximal and distal TCR signaling events are SLP-76 and LAT (see Fig. 12.4). Loss of these adaptor proteins has profound consequences for T cell development. Mice deficient for LAT or SLP-76 manifest a block in T cell development at the $CD4^-8^-$ $CD25^+CD44^+$ stage. LAT is constitutively localized to lipid rafts and, following TCR stimulation, is phosphorylated on tyrosine residues by ZAP-70. Phosphorylated LAT then recruits SH2-domain–containing proteins including PLCγ1, the p85 subunit of phosphoinositide-3 kinase, IL-2 inducible kinase (Itk), and the adaptors Grb2 and Gads. Because the SH3 domain of Gads is constitutively associated with SLP-76, this brings SLP-76 to the complex where it is phosphorylated by ZAP-70. SLP-76 contains three protein binding motifs: tyrosine phosphorylation sites, a proline-rich region, and an SH2 domain. The N-terminus of SLP-76 contains tyrosine residues that associate with the SH2 domains of Vav, the adaptor Nck, and Itk. Vav is a 95 kDa protein that acts as a guanine nucleotide exchange factor for the Rho/Rac/cdc42 family of small G proteins. The complex of LAT, SLP-76/Gads, PLCγ1, and associated molecules results in the full activation of PLCγ1 and activation of Ras/Rho guanosine triphosphatases (GTPases) and the actin cytoskeleton.

In addition to acting as positive regulators for TCR signaling, adaptors can also mediate negative regulation. As described previously, the activity of the Src family kinases is regulated by the interaction of kinases (Csk) and phosphatases (CD45) specific for inhibitory C-terminal phosphotyrosine, which is determined by the subcellular localization of these regulatory molecules. A second mechanism by which adaptor proteins can negatively regulate TCR stability is through regulation of protein stability. Proteins can be targeted for degradation by the conjugation of ubiquitin to lysine residues via a series of enzymatic reactions by E1, E2, and E3 ubiquitin ligases. Cbl-b, c-Cbl, ITCH, and GRAIL are E3 ligases, and mice lacking these proteins manifest T cell hyperproliferation and autoimmune phenotypes. For example, Cbl-b binds and ubiquitinates ZAP70, resulting in its degradation and reduced TCR signaling.[30]

Downstream TCR Signaling

The aforementioned signaling events couple TCR stimulation to downstream pathways that culminate in changes in gene transcription that are required for proliferation and effector function (see Fig. 12.4). One of the best-characterized genes induced following T cell activation is the T cell growth factor IL-2. Transcription of the *IL2* gene is regulated in part by the transcription factors AP-1, nuclear factor of activated T cells (NFAT), and nuclear factor (NF)-κB, all of which are activated following TCR stimulation. Proximal signaling events lead to the activation of Ras and PLCγ.[31] Ras initiates a cascade of kinases including Raf-1, MEK, and the MAPK ERK, which leads to the production of the transcription factor Fos. Ligation of the co-stimulatory molecule CD28 results in the activation of another member of the MAPK family, c-Jun N-terminal kinase (JNK), and phosphorylation of the transcription factor c-Jun. c-Jun and Fos associate to form AP-1. PLCγ hydrolyzes membrane inositol phospholipids to generate phosphoinositide second messengers including inositol 1,4,5-trisphosphate (IP_3) and diacylglycerol. IP_3 stimulates the mobilization of calcium from intra-cellular stores. Diacylglycerol activates protein kinase C (especially PCKθ in T cells) and, along with CARMA, connects with the NF-κB pathway.[31]

Increased intra-cellular calcium is central to many forms of cellular activation. Calcium activates the calcium/calmodulin-dependent serine phosphatase, calcineurin, which dephosphorylates NFAT.[33] Dephosphorylated NFAT translocates to the nucleus and, together with AP-1 and NF-κB, activates the *IL2* gene. The immunosuppressive agents Cyclosporin-A and FK-506 specifically inhibit the calcium-dependent activation of calcineurin, thereby blocking activation of NFAT and the transcription of NFAT-dependent cytokines such as IL-2, IL-3, IL-4, and granulocyte-macrophage colony-stimulating factor (GM-CSF). Recently it has been appreciated that differences in the amplitude and duration of calcium signals mediate different functional outcomes. Although high spikes of calcium are easily measured in lymphocytes during the first 10 minutes after antigen stimulation, sustained low-level calcium spikes over a few hours are necessary for full activation. These latter more subtle calcium fluxes are controlled by cyclic adenosine phosphate (ADP)-ribose and ryanodine receptors.[34] Selective inhibitors exist for these molecules, opening the potential for new specific blockers of T cell activation.

Co-stimulation

Signal 2 is mediated either by growth factor cytokines or through a co-stimulatory molecule, of which the prototype is CD28 on T cells interacting with CD80 (B7-1) or CD86 (B7-2) on APC. CD28 is a disulfide-linked homodimer constitutively expressed on the surface of T cells. Virtually all murine T cells express CD28, while in human T cells, nearly all $CD4^+$ and 50% of $CD8^+$ cells express CD28. The $CD28^-$ subset of T cells appears to represent a population that has undergone chronic activation and can manifest suppressive activity. Increased levels of $CD28^-$ T cells have been reported in several inflammatory and infectious conditions, including granulomatosis with polyangiitis, RA, and certain viral infections such as cytomegalovirus (CMV) and mononucleosis.[35–37] The cytoplasmic domain of CD28 has no known enzymatic activity but does contain two SH3 and one SH2 binding sites. CD28 interacts with PI_3 kinase and GRB2 and promotes JNK activation. CD28 ligation alone does not transmit a proliferative response to T cells, but in conjunction with TCR engagement augments the production of several cytokines, including IL-2, IL-4, IL-5, IL-13, IFN-γ, and TNF, as well as the chemokines IL-8 and RANTES at the level of both transcription and translation.

The ligands for CD28, CD80 (B7-1), and CD86 (B7-2) are expressed in a restricted distribution on B cells, dendritic cells, and monocytes. CD80 and CD86 have similar structures but share only 25% amino acid homology. They each contain rather short cytoplasmic tails that may signal directly and bind to CD28 with different avidities. Increased levels of soluble co-stimulatory molecules CTLA-4, CD28, CD80, and CD86 have been reported in systemic lupus erythematosus (SLE) patients and correlate with disease activity.[38]

The Immunologic Synapse

Antigen-specific interaction between the T cell and APC results in the formation of a specialized contact region called the *immunologic synapse* or *supramolecular activation cluster* (SMAC) (Fig. 12.5).[39] Synapse formation is an active, dynamic process that requires specific antigen and MHC. The synapse also overcomes the obstacles resulting from interactions of tall molecules (e.g., ICAM-1, LFA-1, and CD45) to promote T cell/APC contact that is mediated by short molecules (e.g., TCR, MHC, CD4, and CD8). Two stages of assembly have been described. During the nascent stage, cell adhesion molecules such as ICAM-1 on APC and LFA-1 on T cells make contact in a central zone, surrounded by an annulus of close contact between MHC and TCR.[39] Within minutes the engaged TCR migrates to the central area, resulting in a mature synapse in which the initial relationships are reversed; the central area (cSMAC) now contains TCR, CD2, CD28, and CD4 and is enriched for Lck, Fyn, and PKC-θ. Surrounding the central domain is a peripheral ring (pSMAC) that contains CD45, LFA-1, and associated talin. T cell activation also leads to compartmentalization of TCR signaling molecules to plasma membrane microdomains called *rafts*.[40] Rafts are composed primarily of glycosphingolipids and cholesterol and are enriched in signaling molecules, actin, and actin-binding proteins. Src family kinases, Ras-like G proteins, LAT, and phosphatidylinositol-anchored membrane proteins all localize to raft domains.

Full T cell activation requires engagement of a minimum of approximately 100 to 200 MHC/peptide molecules on an APC, which can serially stimulate 2000 to 8000 TCR. It has been estimated that naïve T cells also require a sustained signal for 15 to 20 hours to commit to proliferation.[27] T cells face a number of obstacles to achieving full activation, including the small physical size of the TCR and MHC molecules compared with other cell surface molecules, the low affinity of TCR for MHC/peptide complex, and the limited percentage of MHC molecules present on the APC that contain the antigenic peptide. The immunologic synapse helps provide a mechanism for overcoming these barriers and achieving the duration of TCR stimulation necessary to commit the cell to proliferation.[39] It has been shown that co-stimulatory signals may contribute to synapse formation by initiating the transport of membrane rafts containing the kinases and adaptor molecules required for TCR signaling to the site of contact.[41]

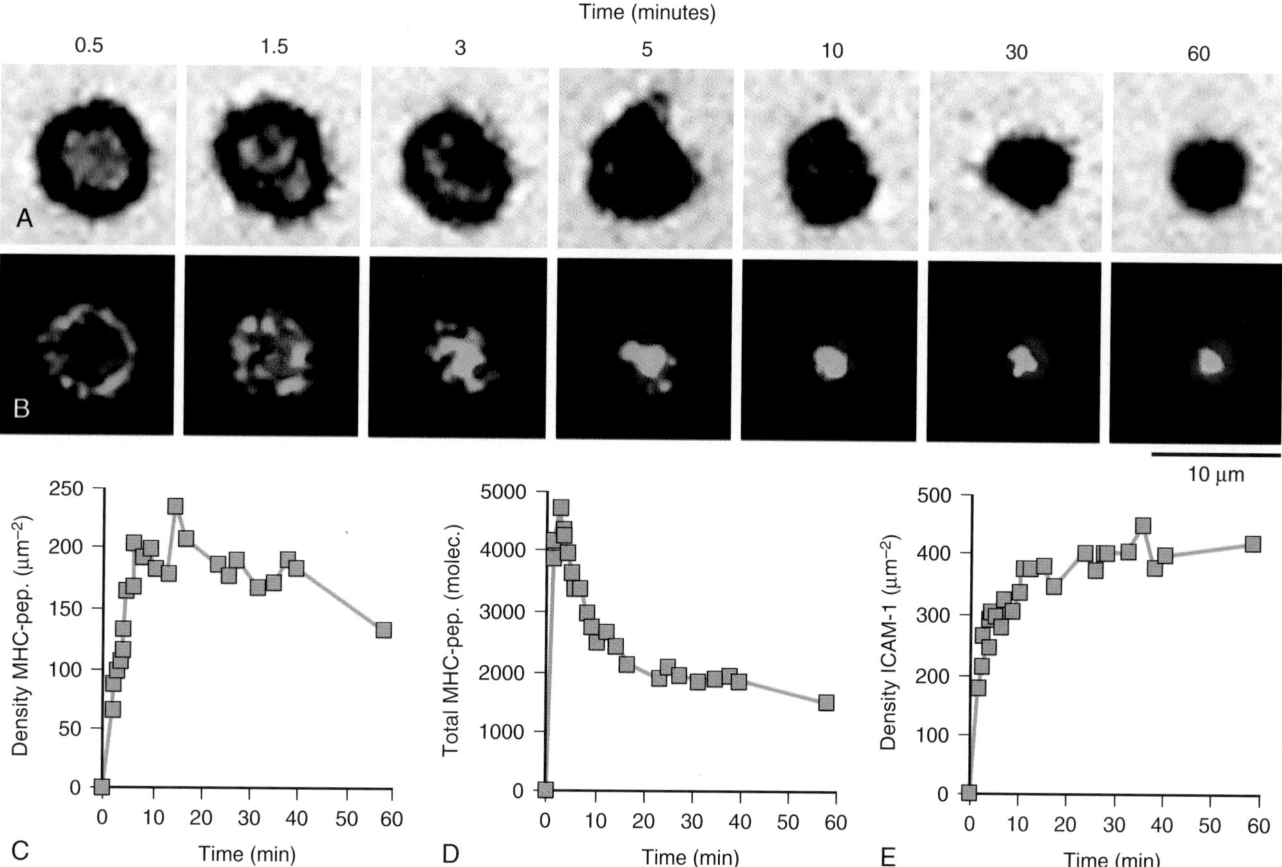

• **Fig. 12.5** Formation of the immunologic synapse. (A) Contact areas of T cells shown over the time points are indicated as dark gray against a light background. (B) Images containing Oregon green E^k-antigen (mouse cytochrome peptide 88-103) and Cy5 ICAM-1. (C) Density of accumulated E^k-MCC88-103. (D) Total accumulated E^k-MCC88-103. (E) Density of accumulated ICAM-1. (From Grakoui A, Bromley SK, Sumen C, et al.: The immunological synapse: a molecular machine controlling T cell activation. *Science* 285:221–227, 1999.)

Tolerance and Control of Autoreactive T Cells

The immune system is continually confronted by the dilemma of how to ensure that T cells are activated only under conditions in which there is a true need for a response to a foreign pathogen and not merely a self-component. As with many biologic filters, thymic negative selection is not 100% efficient, and not all self-reactive T cells are eliminated. Hence, a variety of fail-safe mechanisms are engaged to suppress the ability of these errant T cells to undergo premature clonal expansion. This is partly regulated by the requirement of two distinct signals from separate molecules (TCR and CD28) to be coordinately triggered for T cell activation and proliferation to proceed. If only one of the signals is received, the T cell will not proliferate and will actually enter a nonresponsive state known as *anergy*.

The anergy that results from the absence of a CD28 co-stimulatory signal manifests as a failure to fully couple the TCR signal to the Ras/MAPK pathway and consequent AP-1 transcriptional activity. An additional method of provoking an incomplete TCR signal and unresponsiveness is to make amino acid substitutions in the recognized peptide antigen. These so-called *altered peptide ligands* cause a suboptimal phosphorylation of TCRζ and consequent inefficient recruitment of ZAP-70.

Additional members of the CD28 family serve as inhibitory molecules, many of which have been targeted for therapeutic intervention of autoimmune disorders. Cytolytic T lymphocyte-associated protein 4 (CTLA-4) also binds to CD80 and CD86 with 20-fold higher affinity than CD28. Unlike CD28, CTLA-4 is expressed only transiently following T cell activation and confers an inhibitory signal for T cell proliferation.[42] In this capacity, CTLA-4 functions to limit T cell clonal expansion induced by CD28. The consequences of the loss of CTLA-4 negative regulation are striking. The genetic deletion of the *Ctla4* gene in mice results in enormous uncontrolled T cell expansion and an autoimmune syndrome.[43] *Ctla4* was also identified as a genetic risk factor in RA.[44] CTLA4-Ig (abatacept) is licensed for treatment of RA and PsA.

PD-1 is another member of the CD28 family that possesses an immunoreceptor tyrosine-based inhibitory motif (ITIM) within its cytoplasmic tail that associates with the tyrosine phosphatase SHP-2.[45] PD-1 does not bind the CD28/CTLA-4 ligands, CD80 or CD86, but rather binds to PD-L1 and PD-L2. PD-L1 is expressed by both lymphoid tissues (e.g., regulatory $CD4^+CD25^+$ T cells, inflammatory macrophages) as well as nonlymphoid tissues such as heart, placenta, lung, pancreas, and certain tumors. PD-L2 expression is more confined to macrophages and dendritic cells.[46] Ligation of PD-1 on T cells leads to cell cycle arrest. Treatment of mice with a blocking antibody to PD-L1 caused virus-specific $CD8^+$ T cells to undergo marked expansion.[45,46] The fact that many tumors also express PD-L1 enhances the interest in promoting anti-tumor responses with blocking antibodies to PD-1 or PD-L1. The fact that PD-1-deficient mice develop lupus-like arthritis and glomerulonephritis enhances interest in manipulating PD-1 for therapeutic purposes.[47] The use of anti-PD-1 and anti-PD-L1 immunotherapy for a variety of tumors is coupled with concern for potential autoimmune side effects (see Chapter 132).

Chronic exposure to certain inflammatory cytokines, most notably TNF, can also induce anergy. It has been appreciated for some time that T cells from rheumatoid synovium manifest profound deficiencies of proliferation and cytokine production,[48] and TNF is one of the major cytokines detectable in rheumatoid synovial fluid. Further studies demonstrated that chronic exposure of T cell clones to TNF for 10 to 12 days suppressed proliferative and cytokine responses to antigen by as much as 70%.[49] Furthermore, a single administration of anti-TNF receptor monoclonal antibody to patients with RA rapidly restored the response of peripheral T cells to mitogens and recall antigens.[49] Similar observations have been made in TCR transgenic mice following TNF exposure.[50]

An additional negative regulator for T cells is the B lymphocyte–induced maturation protein 1 (Blimp-1), which was initially identified in B lymphocytes. Blimp-1-deficient mice manifest augmented levels of peripheral effector T cells and develop severe colitis as early as 6 weeks of age.[51] Blimp-1 mRNA expression in T cells increases with TCR stimulation, and Blimp-1-deficient T cells manifested enhanced proliferation and produced more IL-2 and IFN-γ after activation.[51]

Regulatory T Cells

Another layer of cellular regulation occurs via a phenotypically defined subpopulation of $CD4^+CD25^+$ $FoxP3^+$ regulatory T cells (Tregs) that has the ability to inhibit antigen-induced proliferation.[52] This subset represents 5% to 15% of peripheral blood CD4 T cells and is at least partly thymic-dependent. The absence of regulatory T cells after day 3 thymectomy likely contributes to the development of autoimmune disease in these animals.[53] Diminished levels of $CD4^+CD25^+$ $FoxP3^+$ regulatory T cells have been observed in other autoimmune syndromes, and the transfer of Tregs to autoimmune mice has shown some alleviation of symptoms. The production of TGF-β and IL-10, and possibly expression of CTLA-4, appear to be critical to the suppressive activity of Tregs.[54] This is a very active area of research because of the potential therapeutic implications for autoimmune diseases and their possible role in generating IL-17–producing $CD4^+$ T cells (Th17; see below).[55] In this regard, studies to treat type I diabetes by increasing Treg number and function using anti-CD3 antibody or IL-2 are promising.[56] In addition, a genetic analysis of risk loci for RA identified the greatest enrichment of trimethylation of histone H3 at lysine 4 of RA risk factors in Tregs, out of 34 cell types studies, further supporting a role for Tregs in the pathogenesis of RA.[57]

Tregs also have important functions in tissue homeostasis, particularly in skin, fat, and muscle.[58] Whereas Tregs represent about 5% to 15% of $CD4^+$ T cells in peripheral blood, they account for 60% to 80% of $CD4^+$ T cells in adipose tissue, where they respond to IL-33 and are critical for adipocyte formation and insulin sensitivity.[58] In the skin, Tregs are located around hair follicles and are required for hair growth in a Notch-dependent manner.[59] They also accumulate in injured muscle and are important for the switch of infiltrating macrophages from inflammatory M1 phenotype to non-inflammatory M2 macrophages. Tregs also accumulate in muscular dystrophy.[60]

T Cell Subsets

$CD4^+$ Helper and $CD8^+$ Cytolytic T Cells

αβ T cells can be subdivided into two main subsets based on their recognition of peptides presented by class I or class II MHC molecules and their respective expression of CD8 or CD4. $CD4^+$ and $CD8^+$ T cells have different functions and recognize antigens derived from different cellular compartments. The peptides presented by class I MHC molecules are produced by the proteasome[61] and can be derived from either self-proteins or intracellular foreign proteins, as might occur during viral infection. Class II MHC-bound peptides are derived largely from extracellular infectious agents or self–cell surface proteins that have been engulfed and degraded in the lysosomal complex.

CD8$^+$ T cells, often referred to as *cytolytic T cells* (CTL), are very efficient killers of pathogen-infected cells. Given the ubiquitous expression of class I MHC molecules, mature CD8$^+$ CTL can recognize viral infections in a wide array of cells, in distinction to the more restricted distribution of class II molecules. CTL use three primary systems by which to kill target cells. The first is the release of two types of cytolytic granules, perforin and granzymes. Perforin, as the name implies, forms holes in the membrane of the target cell, similar to complement. This allows the granzymes contained in the granules to enter the target cell. Granzymes are serine proteases that cleave proteins within the target cell, ultimately leading to cell death. The cytolytic granules are released in the direction of the target cells to avoid collateral damage of bystander cells. The second pathway is secretion of IFN-γ, which has antimicrobial effects. The third pathway of CD8$^+$ CTL is by production of TNF and Fas-Ligand (FasL), which bind their respective receptors on target cells and induce apoptosis through activation of a caspase cascade. Similar to CD4, CD8 manifests an affinity for class I MHC molecules, enhances the signaling of CTL, and also binds Lck by its cytoplasmic tail.

CD4$^+$ T cells express a variety of cytokines and cell surface molecules that are important to B cell proliferation and immunoglobulin production, as well as to CD8$^+$ T cell function. Following antigen stimulation, CD4$^+$ T cells differentiate into different classes of effector T cells identified by their cytokine profiles, including T helper 1 (Th1), Th2, Th17, follicular helper T cells (Tfh; described below), and Treg cells (described above) (Fig. 12.6). The CD4 molecule is structurally related to immunoglobulins and has an affinity for nonpolymorphic residues on the class II MHC molecule. In this capacity CD4 presumably increases the efficiency with which CD4$^+$ T cells recognize antigen in the context of class II MHC molecules, whose expression is restricted to B cells, macrophages, dendritic cells, and a few other tissues during states of inflammation. In addition, the cytoplasmic tail of CD4 binds to Lck and promotes signaling by the TCR, as described earlier. However, ligation of CD4 prior to engagement of the TCR can render T cells susceptible to apoptosis upon subsequent engagement of the TCR.[62] This is clinically important in HIV infections in which the gp120 molecule of HIV binds to CD4 and primes the T cell to undergo cell death when later triggered by the TCR. Accelerated apoptosis of CD4$^+$ T cells has been demonstrated in AIDS patients.[63]

CD4 T Helper Subsets

CD4 T cells can be further subdivided based upon their cytokine profiles (see Fig. 12.6). Th1 cells produce IL-2, TNF, and IFN-γ and participate in cell-mediated inflammatory reactions and the

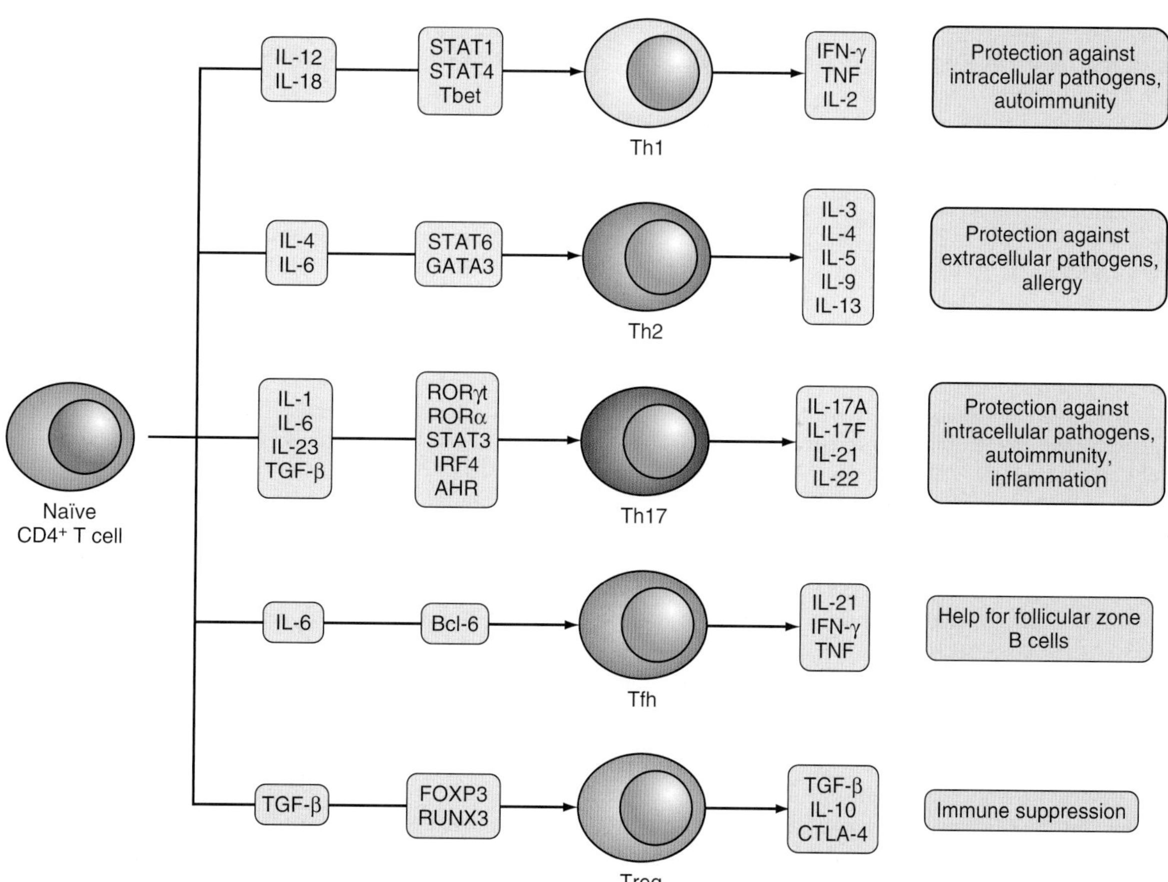

• **Fig. 12.6** T helper subsets. Naïve CD4 T cells can be polarized into producing particular patterns of cytokines depending upon the cytokine environment in which they develop and the expression of certain transcription factors. *AHR,* Aryl hydroxylase receptor.

activation of macrophages. Th2 cells, by contrast, produce IL-4, IL-5, IL-6, and IL-10. IL-4 and IL-5 are important B cell growth factors.[64] In addition, IL-4 promotes B cell secretion of immunoglobulin (Ig)G_1 and IgE, whereas IFN-γ drives IgG_{2a} production. A third group of cytokine-producing T cells are Th17 cells, which are important for driving many aspects of autoimmune inflammation. Both IFN-γ and the type 2 cytokine locus shared by *IL5, IL13*, and *IL4* are present only in vertebrates, whereas IL-17 is considerably more ancient in evolution, with orthologs in invertebrates; the sea urchin has 30 IL-17-like genes.[1]

These Th cytokine patterns have been best characterized during chronic infections. In general, a Th1 response helps eradicate intra-cellular microorganisms, such as *Leishmania major* and *Brucella abortus*,[65] whereas a Th2 cell response can better control extra-cellular pathogens, such as the helminth, *Nippostrongylus braciliensis*.[66] The cytokine profiles of Th1 and Th2 cells are mutually inhibitory, such that the Th1 cytokine IFN-γ, or IL-12 from APCs, suppresses Th2 responses and augments Th1 cytokine gene expression, whereas the Th2 cytokine IL-4, or IL-6 from APCs, promote the opposite pattern. Polarization of the cytokine environment also occurs at the sites of inflammation in many autoimmune syndromes. Th2 skewing has been observed in models of SLE where increased levels of immunoglobulins and autoantibodies are typical, as well as in chronic allergic conditions such as asthma.[67] In a variety of autoimmune disorders the infiltrating lymphocytes exhibit a bias toward Th1 cytokines. This occurs with brain-infiltrating lymphocytes in multiple sclerosis and its animal model experimental allergic encephalomyelitis (EAE),[68] β islet lymphocytes in diabetes,[69] and synovial lymphocytes in inflammatory arthritides.[70] Unlike the beneficial effects of Th1 responses during infections, these same cytokines can be quite deleterious in autoimmune disorders. Thus therapies based on inhibition of certain Th1 cytokines have been of considerable interest and often ameliorative, such as anti-TNF treatment of RA.[71] Several cytokines can have pleotropic effects, and predicting the effects of modulating their levels can be complex. For example, despite the tendency of IL-6 to promote a Th2 cytokine profile, nonetheless, blocking IL-6 is beneficial in RA.[72]

A subset of IL-17–producing CD4⁺ T cells (Th17) is critical for promoting a variety of autoimmune disorders. Th17 cells are regulated by the transcription factor RORγt and can be broadly divided into two groups: first, host protective cells that express both IL-17 and IL-10 and are activated by TGF-β and IL-6; and second, a highly inflammatory population that expresses IL-17, IL-22, and IFN-γ that are activated by IL-23 and IL-1β.[73,74] IL-22 has important functions at mucosal surfaces in host defense as well as in wound repair. It is produced primarily by Th17 CD4⁺ T helper cells and innate lymphocytes but acts only on nonhematopoietic stromal cells, particularly epithelial cells, keratinocytes, and hepatocytes.[74] In addition to strengthening epithelial barrier functions, excessive IL-22 can evoke pathology, such as psoriasis-like skin inflammation.[73] Injections of IL-23 into skin produced increased IL-17 in the epidermis and inflammatory lesions that resembled psoriasis.[75] Th17 CD4⁺ cells are increased in human psoriatic plaques,[75] in RA synovial fluid, and in multiple sclerosis.[76] Genome-wide association studies (GWAS) have linked genes involved with Th17 cells in RA and Crohn's disease.[74] Using a model of spontaneous autoimmune arthritis, synovial Th17 cells also produced CM-CSF, as well as stimulating fibroblast-like synoviocytes and synovial resident innate lymphocytes to make GM-CSF, which contributed to joint destruction.[77] In addition, anti-Th17 therapy is now approved for psoriasis, PsA, and ankylosing spondylitis.

An additional CD4 T helper subset is found in B cell follicles of secondary lymphoid organs due to their expression of the B cell follicle homing receptor CXCR5.[78] These Tfhs facilitate B cell activation and germinal center formation through expression of CD40L, IL-4, and IL-21. Dysregulation of Tfh function can result in autoantibody production and systemic autoimmunity.[79] Finally, CD4⁺FoxP3⁺ Tregs have been described earlier.

Naïve Versus Memory T Cells

CD4⁺ and CD8⁺ T cells emigrate from the thymus bearing a naïve phenotype. Naïve T cells produce IL-2 but only low levels of other cytokines and as such provide little B cell help. Naïve T cells express high levels of Bcl-2 and can survive for extended periods without antigen but require the presence of MHC molecules. Naïve T cells circulate from the blood to lymphoid tissues of the spleen and lymph nodes, where antigen, APC, T cells, and B cells are concentrated. Particularly important in this environment as APC are dendritic cells, which can migrate from other areas of the body such as the skin and are highly efficient at processing and presenting antigen to T cells (see Chapter 9). Dendritic cells express high and constitutive levels of class II MHC and co-stimulatory molecules CD80 (B7-1) and CD86 (B7-2) that are critical to promote proliferation of naïve T cells. In this capacity, dendritic cells are particularly adept at promoting clonal expansion of antigen-specific T cells. The development of MHC/peptide tetramer technology has allowed the direct quantitation of antigen-specific CD8 T cells using flow cytometry. Viral-specific CD8 T cells have a very robust ability to expand following infection, from levels that are undetectable to nearly 50% of the CD8 population, representing a nearly 1000-fold increase in only a few days.[80]

During the process of clonal expansion of naïve T cells, numerous genetic alterations occur in their differentiation into effector and eventually memory T cells. These are manifested primarily as increased expression of certain surface molecules involved with cell adhesion and migration (CD44, ICAM-1, LFA-1, α4β1 and α4β7 integrins, and the chemokine receptor CXCR3), activation (CD45 change from high molecular weight CD45RA to lower molecular weight CD45RO isotype), cytokine production (increased production of IFN-γ, IL-3, IL-4, and IL-5) and death receptors (e.g., Fas/CD95) (Table 12.1). More transiently induced are CD69, the survival factor Bcl-xL, and the high-affinity growth factor IL-2 receptor α chain (CD25). Survival of effector T cells to the memory stage is partly dependent upon the cytokines IL-7 and IL-15.[81]

The concept of immune memory has existed since the first successful vaccinations by Jenner for smallpox. A useful memory T cell marker in the murine system is CD44, the hyaluronate receptor. Surface CD44 is low on naïve T cells as they emerge from the thymus, but its expression is progressively upregulated concomitant with repeated rounds of T cell proliferation in response to foreign antigen or during homeostatic proliferation.[22] Expression of the IL-7 receptor identifies a subset of effector T cells that are destined to become memory T cells. The most notable phenotypic change for human memory T cells is from CD45RA to CD45RO (see Table 12.1). Using these markers, it has been possible to identify a variety of differences between naïve and memory T cells. Activation of memory T cells appears to be more efficient than that of naïve T cells and not to be absolutely dependent upon co-stimulation. Memory T cells are also able to migrate to nonlymphoid tissues such as lung, skin, liver, and joints.[82] Particularly interesting have been observations that the metabolic state of an

TABLE 12.1 **Surface Markers on Naïve and Memory T Cells**

Molecule	Other Designation	Molecular Weight (kDa)	Characteristic	EXPRESSION	
				Memory	Naïve
CD58	LFA-3	45-66	Ligand for CD2	++	+
CD2	T11	50	Alternative activation pathway	+++	++
CD11a/CD18	LFA-1	180-195	Receptor for ICAM-1, ICAM-2, ICAM-3	+++	++
CD29		130	β chain of β1 (VLA) integrins	++++	+
CD45RO		220	Isoform of CD45	++++	–
CD45RA		80-95	Isoform of CD45	–	++++
CD44	Pgp-1	90	Receptor for hyaluronic acid	+++	++
CD54	ICAM-1	120	Counterreceptor for LFA-1	+	–
CD26		40	Dipeptidyl peptidase IV	+	–
CD7		Multichain complex	T cell lineage marker	+/–	++
CD3		20-28	Part of TCR complex	+	+

CD, Cluster of differentiation; *ICAM,* intercellular adhesion molecule; *LFA,* leukocyte function–associated antigen; *TCR,* T cell antigen receptor; *VLA,* very late activation antigen.

effector T cell may profoundly affect which T cells survive to the memory state. Following their activation, T cells rapidly activate glycolysis, which provides many of the precursors needed for the synthesis of nucleic acids, amino acids, and lipids needed for proliferation and effector T cell function. However, the survival of T cells to the memory stage requires the return to a relatively nonglycolytic state of fatty acid metabolism and mitochondrial oxidative phosphorylation. Thus, improved survival of memory T cells has been conferred by agents such as rapamycin and metformin, which inhibit anabolic glycolytic metabolism and promote catabolic fatty acid metabolism.[83]

Nonconventional and Innate T Cells

In addition to the broad array of antigens recognized by conventional αβ T cells of the adaptive immune system, the immune system also contains subpopulations of innate-like T cells that express relatively invariant TCRs and may be specialized to recognize conserved structures that are either uniquely expressed by prokaryotic pathogens or on stressed host cells. These include γδ T cells, natural killer T (NKT) cells, and mucosal-associated invariant T (MAIT) cells.

γδ T Cells

γδ T cells are among the oddest of immunology's distinguished oddities.[84] They were identified after the serendipitous discovery of rearranged genes while searching for the TCR α–chain gene.[85] Structurally, the γ-chain locus contains at least 14 Vγ region genes (of which six are pseudogenes), each capable of rearranging to any of five Jγ regions and two Cγ regions. The δ-chain genes are nested within the α-chain gene locus. There are about six Vδ regions, two Dδ and two Jδ regions, and a single Cδ gene. Transcription of rearranged γ and δ genes begins prior to αβ genes and is apparent on days 15 to 17 of mouse thymus development, after which it declines in the adult thymus. In addition to the ordered appearance of TCR-γδ before TCR-αβ, there is also a highly ordered expression of γ and δ V-region genes during early thymic development. This results in successive waves of oligoclonal γδ T cells migrating to the periphery.

Evidence suggests that γδ T cells are beneficial in both infections and autoimmunity.[86–99] γδ T cells accumulate at inflammatory sites such as in RA,[100] celiac disease,[101] and sarcoidosis.[102] In addition, a role for γδ T cells in the immune response against tumors in humans is evident from a recent seminal study, which reported that "intratumor γδ T cells are the most favorable prognostic immune population across 39 cancer types in humans."[103]

γδ T cells are often highly lytic against transformed proliferative cells, infected cells, and infiltrating CD4+ T cells in inflammatory arthritis.[93,104,105] They can produce a variety of cytokines such as IFN-γ, TNF, and IL-17,[106] as well as insulin-like growth factor-1 (IGF1) and keratinocyte growth factor (KGF) that promote epithelial wound repair.[107] Studies from mice lacking γδ T cells have demonstrated that this T cell subset provides nonredundant protection against infections with bacteria, viruses, and protozoans and against tumors.[105,108,109]

These collective studies indicate that a principal function of γδ T cells is likely to respond to tissue injury of various causes. It is thus not surprising that γδ T cells are often suggested to be reactive to host components that are upregulated or exposed during cell injury.[110] Yet in the vast majority of cases, little if anything is known regarding the nature of these self-components or whether they actually engage the TCR-γδ. In contrast to αβ T cells, γδ T cells do not recognize peptide-MHC complexes but rather intact proteins. There is no evidence for antigen processing or for a presentation requirement by classic MHC.[106,111] Various ligands for γδ T cells have been proposed, although only a few have been confirmed to bind to TCR-γδ, and these lack any known unifying motif. Further understanding of TCR-γδ ligands is thus critical to understand their full function.

Human γδ T cell clones can be divided into two subsets based on expression of either Vδ1 or Vδ2. The predominant human γδ T cell subset in peripheral blood is Vδ2, which reacts to phosphorylated prenyl metabolites presented by butyrophilin.[112–117] These are products of microbes as well as self-antigens. However, the evidence is weak that these agents actually bind the TCR-γδ of Vδ2 T cells. Murine γδ T cells lack a homologous Vδ2 subset and do not respond to prenyl pyrophosphates.[107] Similarly, human Vδ1 γδ T cells, which also do not respond to prenyl pyrophosphates, reside in normal epithelial tissues of the skin and gastrointestinal tract. The epithelial layer of the gastrointestinal tract is also the most rapidly dividing tissue in adult mammals, with complete cellular renewal occurring every 4 to 5 days.[107] Thus, the Vδ1 subset is found in areas of rapid cell proliferation and cell death. These findings, coupled with observations that damaged murine keratinocytes express TCR-γδ ligands,[118] are consistent with a model in which Vδ1 T cells respond to potential ligands expressed by rapidly proliferating as well as by dying cells. The Vδ1 subset also accumulates in inflamed synovium in RA and Lyme arthritis.[93] Collectively, this suggests that γδ cells may recognize a class of antigens shared by a number of pathogens, as well as by damaged or transformed mammalian cells, and may provide insight into the role of γδ cells in infection and their accumulation at sites of inflammation.

Natural Killer T Cells

A minor subpopulation of T cells bearing the natural killer (NK) determinant manifests a highly restricted TCR repertoire. NKT cells are found within the $CD4^+$ and $CD4^-CD8^-$ T cell subsets and, in both mouse and human, express a very limited number of TCR-Vαβ-chains and an invariant α chain (Vα14 in mice, Vα24 in humans).[119] Furthermore, most NKT cells are restricted in their response to a nonpolymorphic class I MHC-like molecule, CD1d. Crystallographic analysis of CD1d has shown that it contains a deeper groove than traditional MHC molecules and is highly hydrophobic, conferring a preference for binding lipid moieties. Originally the sea sponge sphingolipid, α galactosylceramide, was the only known CD1d ligand. Now both endogenous and bacterial (*Sphingomonas* and *Borrelia burgdorferi*) sources of CD1d-binding sphingolipids have been identified.[120,121] This may represent another type of innate T cell response whereby bacterial lipids or lipopeptides may be presented to NKT cells to provoke a rapid early immune response.

The potential importance of NKT cells in autoimmune disease stems from their rapid production of high levels of certain cytokines, particularly IL-4 and IFNγ.[119] In this capacity, the IL-4 response may be important for modulating inflammatory responses dominated by Th1 infiltrates. This has been noted in the NOD mouse model of diabetes, which has reduced levels of NKT cells.[122] Adoptive transfer of NKT cells into NOD mice blocks the onset of diabetes.[123] A study extended this observation to human type I diabetes. The NKT cells of diabetic individuals produced more IFN-γ and less IL-4 than their unaffected siblings.[124] NKT cells have also been reported to be the predominant $CD4^+$ T cell in the airways of asthma patients.[125] Thus, this minor population of T cells may play a pivotal role in early innate responses to certain infections and also in the regulation of inflammatory sites.

MAIT Cells

Mucosal-associated invariant αβ T (MAIT) cells are a recently defined subpopulation that display a semi-invariant TCR and are restricted by the evolutionarily conserved MHC-related molecule MR1.[1] Human MAIT cells have been observed in blood, joints, lung, and liver and at various mucosa. They represent about 20% to 40% of T cells in the liver.[1] MAIT cells recognize small molecules created through the process of vitamin B2 *(riboflavin)* and B9 *(folic acid)* biosynthesis by bacteria and presented by MR1. This results in the release on innate pro-inflammatory cytokines and the ability to lyse bacterially infected cells. Similar to γδ T cells and NKT cells, MAIT cells have a memory-like phenotype *($CD44^+$, $CD45RO^+$, $CCR7^-$, $CD62L^{lo}$)* and can support adaptive immune responses. They also express high levels of CD161; IL-18 receptor; and chemokine receptors CCR5, CXCR6, and CCR6 on the cell surface. The presence of MAIT cells has been described in various autoimmune disorders, although their function is less clear. Again, similar to γδ T cells and NKT cells, MAIT cells may provoke inflammation nonspecifically through production of pro-inflammatory cytokines and cytolytic machinery.

Inflammation Mediated by T Cells

T cells can contribute to tissue inflammation by both antigen-specific and nonspecific mechanisms. The recognition of a foreign antigen, such as with viral infections, on a host cell can lead to T cell activation and the induction of host cell death by various cytolytic mechanisms, including perforin, granzymes, and Fas-Ligand. A similar process may occur when T cells react to self-antigens during augmented homeostatic proliferation and upregulation of the same cytolytic machinery. A third mechanism is the "innocent bystander" effect in which T cells activated by an antigen elsewhere and expressing Fas-Ligand migrate into various tissues and cause nonspecific organ injury to Fas-sensitive cells. This can be graphically demonstrated in mice transgenic for a specific foreign antigen. When the antigen is administered to the mice, responding T cells migrate to the liver and induce hepatocyte injury and inflammation in a Fas-Ligand-dependent manner.[126] This may represent a model of autoimmune hepatitis. In humans this is vividly apparent in toxic shock syndrome (TSS) in which a staphylococcal toxin TSST stimulates the expansion of a large subset of T cells resulting in injury to multiple organs.[127]

The concept of molecular mimicry, in which T cells responding to a foreign antigen might cross-react with a self-antigen, has long been a popular model for autoimmunity. This is best established for B cells in rheumatic heart disease where the antibody response to a Group A streptococcal wall component cross-reacts with cardiac myosin. A few similar reports have been noted for T cells. Investigators used the peptide sequence of myelin basic protein (MBP) recognized by specific T cell clones from patients with multiple sclerosis to search a database of infectious agents. Some of the candidate sequences obtained were able to stimulate the MBP-reactive T cell clones.[128] Another example is the outer surface proteins of *B. burgdorferi* known as OspA, which may trigger a cross-reactive T cell response to LFA-1.[129] The technology of MHC/peptide tetramers will enable investigators to determine the frequency of T cells bearing self-reactivity.

Modifications of self-proteins can also lead to new immunogenic determinants. An example is the response of certain $CD4^+$ T cells to citrullinated self-peptides,[130] which can be induced by autophagy, a reprocessing of organelles during cellular stress. In addition, class II HLA-DR4 molecules, a haplotype associated with RA, are very efficient at presenting citrullinated peptides to $CD4^+$ T cells.[130]

The cytokines produced by infiltrating T cells can also provoke inflammation. Tissue $CD4^+$ T cells in RA, type I diabetes, and multiple sclerosis share a similar Th1 cytokine pattern.[68–70] The importance of these cytokines in the inflammatory response was vividly illustrated in a murine study of type I diabetes. Islet-specific

CD4+ T cells were first incubated in vitro to develop into Th1 or Th2 cells. When adoptively transferred to naïve mice, although islet infiltrates developed in both groups of recipient mice, only those producing Th1 cytokines developed diabetes.[131] Evidence for the importance of these CD4+ cells derives from numerous studies showing the efficacy of CD4 depletion in animal models of these disorder.[132]

Termination of T Cell Responses

The rapid removal of the effector T cells after clearance of an infection is as important as the initial clonal expansion of responding T cells for the health of the organism. Failure to clear activated lymphocytes increases the risk of cross-reactivity with self-antigens and a sustained autoimmune reaction. To ensure that resolution of an immune response occurs rapidly, a number of processes promote active cell death of clonally expanded T cells. One means to control T cell proliferation is through limited availability of growth factors. Upon activation, T cells express receptors for various growth cytokines for approximately 7 to 10 days but only produce cytokines for a more limited period. This results in an unstable situation where T cells tend to outgrow the availability of growth cytokines. T cells expressing IL-2R, for example, in the absence of IL-2 will rapidly undergo programmed cell death. Another method is restimulation of TCR on actively dividing T cells, which triggers a death cascade known as activation-induced cell death (AICD).

The discovery of a family of death receptors expressed by T cells elucidated an additional regulatory process. These molecules are described more extensively in Chapter 19, The Immunologic Repercussions of Cell Death, and will thus be discussed here only as they relate to T cell function. The best described of these is Fas (CD95). Both Fas-deficient mice and humans bearing Fas mutations (Canele-Smith syndrome)[133] manifest a profound lymphadenopathy accompanied by an autoimmune syndrome. This underscores the importance of efficiently removing T cells after their activation. Nearly all cells have some level of surface Fas, whereas expression of its ligand (FasL) is restricted primarily to activated T cells and B cells. Consequently, regulation of Fas-mediated apoptosis is to a large extent under the governance of the immune system. FasL expression has also been reported for certain components of the eye, the Sertoli cells of the testis, and perhaps some tumors, providing "immune privileged" sites within which immune responses are difficult to initiate.[134] Expression of FasL by these nonlymphoid cells is thought to prevent immune responses at sites where such inflammation might cause tissue damage. During T cell activation, expression of FasL is rapidly induced, and these T cells readily kill Fas-sensitive target cells.

Proapoptotic members of the Bcl-2 family, Bim, Bad, and Bax, appear to regulate death in vivo from cytokine withdrawal or after acute foreign antigen stimulation, as with certain infections.[135] These molecules are related to the cell survival molecule Bcl-2 but are more truncated, containing only the BH3 domain of Bcl-2, hence their designation as the "BH3-only" family. They function as sentinels within the cell in that they are attached to various cytoskeletal proteins and organelles and sense cellular damage. If damage occurs they are released from these sequestered areas and migrate to the mitochondria to inhibit the survival function of Bcl-2.[135] By contrast, Fas serves to eliminate T cells following chronic TCR stimulation as occurs in homeostatic proliferation or chronic infections.[21,136]

Future Directions

As detailed more in Chapter 24, the metabolic state of T cells is now appreciated to greatly influence their function and survival. As mentioned earlier, resting naïve T cells and memory T cells manifest primarily mitochondrial oxidative phosphorylation and low levels of glycolysis, whereas effector T cells strongly upregulate glycolysis. This also leads to activation of caspase-3, which sensitizes the effector T cells to cell death.[137] The linking of glycolysis and proliferation to sensitization to cell death may provide a further fail-safe mechanism to guard against transitions to neoplasia or autoimmunity. Methods to manipulate T cell metabolism, particularly of highly proliferative glycolytic T cells (e.g., rapamycin) that may exist in autoimmune disorders, will likely receive considerable attention. Attention will also be focused on mitochondrial function of T cells; T cells in SLE patients, which have been reported to manifest enlarged mitochondria and reactive oxygen species[138] and so the reasons for these aberrations warrant explanation; and the possible therapeutic potential of mitochondrially targeted antioxidants.

An additional area of emerging interest in autoimmunity will be the possible contribution of dysregulated T cell homeostatic proliferation. Given that this process is driven by self-peptide/MHC complexes, and is thus inherently autoimmune, and also leads to upregulation of cytolytic machinery such as FasL and Granzyme B,[22] there is a need to further investigate its role in autoimmunity.

Full references for this chapter can be found on ExpertConsult.com.

Selected References

1. Kotas ME, Locksley RM: Why innate lymphoid cells? *Immunity* 48:1081–1090, 2018.
2. Pawson T, Scott JD: Signaling through scaffold, anchoring, and adaptor proteins, *Science* 278:2075–2080, 1997.
3. Mombaerts P, Iacomini J, Johnson RS, et al.: RAG-1-deficient mice have no mature B and T lymphocytes, *Cell* 68:869–877, 1992.
4. Radtke F, Wilson A, Stark G, et al.: Deficient T cell fate specification in mice with an induced inactivation of Notch1, *Immunity* 10:547–558, 1999.
5. Uribe L, Weinberg KI: X-linked SCID and other defects of cytokine pathways, *Semin Hematol* 35:299–309, 1998.
6. Elder ME, Lin D, Clever J, et al.: Human severe combined immunodeficiency due to a defect in ZAP-70, a T cell tyrosine kinase, *Science* 264:1596–1599, 1994.
7. Padovan E, Casorati G, Dellabona P, et al.: Expression of two T cell receptor a chains: dual receptor T cells, *Science* 262:422–424, 1993.
8. Garboczi DN, Ghosh P, Utz U, et al.: Structure of the complex between human T-cell receptor, viral peptide and HLA-A2, *Nature* 384:134–141, 1996.
9. Anderson MS, Venanzi ES, Klein L, et al.: Projection of an immunological self shadow within the thymus by the aire protein, *Science* 298:1395–1401, 2002.
10. Ramsey C, Winqvist O, Puhakka L, et al.: Aire deficient mice develop multiple features of APECED phenotype and show altered immune response, *Hum Mol Genet* 11:397–409, 2002.
11. Amakawa R, Hakem A, Kundig TM, et al.: Impaired negative selection of T cells in Hodgkin's disease antigen CD30-deficient mice, *Cell* 84:551–562, 1996.
12. Yasutomo K, Doyle C, Miele L, et al.: The duration of antigen receptor signalling determines CD4+ versus CD8+ T-cell lineage fate, *Nature* 404:506–510, 2000.

13. Buckley RH: Primary cellular immunodeficiencies, *J Allergy Clin Immunol* 109:747–757, 2002.
14. Butcher EC, Williams M, Youngman K, et al.: Lymphocyte trafficking and regional immunity, *Adv Immunol* 72:209–253, 1999.
15. Szekanecz Z, Kim J, Koch AE: Chemokines and chemokine receptors in rheumatoid arthritis, *Semin Immunol* 15:15–21, 2003.
16. Goldrath AW, Bogatzki LY, Bevan MJ: Naive T cells transiently acquire a memory-like phenotype during homeostasis-driven proliferation, *J Exp Med* 192:557–564, 2000.
17. Min B, McHugh R, Sempowski GD, et al.: Neonates support lymphopenia-induced proliferation, *Immunity* 18:131–140, 2003.
18. Yunis EJ, Hong R, Grewe MA, et al.: Postthymectomy wasting associated with autoimmune phenomena. I. Antiglobulin-positive anemia in A and C57BL-6 Ks mice, *J Exp Med* 125:947–966, 1967.
19. King C, Ilic A, Koelsch K, Sarvetnick N: Homeostatic expansion of T cells during immune insufficiency generates autoimmunity, *Cell* 117:265–277, 2004.
20. Koetz K, Bryl E, Spickschen K, et al.: T cell homeostasis in patients with rheumatoid arthritis, *Proc Natl Acad Sci U S A* 97:9203–9208, 2000.
21. Fortner KA, Budd RC: The death receptor Fas (CD95/APO-1) mediates the deletion of T lymphocytes undergoing homeostatic proliferation, *J Immuno* 175:4374–4382, 2005.
22. Fortner KA, Bond JP, Austin JW, et al.: The molecular signature of murine T cell homeostasis reveals both inflammatory and immune inhibition patterns, *J Autoimmun* 82:47–61, 2017.
23. Espinoza LR, Berman A, Vasey FB, et al.: Psoriatic arthritis and acquired immunodeficiency syndrome, *Arthritis Rheum* 31:1034–1040, 1988.
24. Frauwirth KA, Riley JL, Harris MH, et al.: The CD28 signaling pathway regulates glucose metabolism, *Immunity* 16:769–777, 2002.
25. Wange RL, Samelson LE: Complex complexes: signaling at the TCR, *Immunity* 5:197–205, 1996.
26. Appleby MW, Gross JA, Cooke MP, et al.: Defective T cell receptor signaling in mice lacking the thymic isoform of $p59^{fyn}$, *Cell* 70:751–763, 1992.
27. Gaud G, Lesourne R, Love PE: Regulatory mechanisms in T cell receptor signalling, *Nat Rev Immunol* 18:485–497, 2018.
28. van Oers NS, Killeen N, Weiss A: ZAP-70 is constitutively associated with tyrosine-phosphorylated TCR zeta in murine thymocytes and lymph node T cells, *Immunity* 1:675–685, 1994.
29. Hsu LY, Tan YX, Xiao Z, et al.: A hypomorphic allele of ZAP-70 reveals a distinct thymic threshold for autoimmune disease versus autoimmune reactivity, *J Exp Med* 206:2527–2541, 2009.
30. Naik E, Webster JD, DeVoss J, et al.: Regulation of proximal T cell receptor signaling and tolerance induction by deubiquitinase Usp9X, *J Exp Med.* 211:1947–1955, 2014.
31. Sun Z, Arendt CW, Ellmeier W, et al.: PKC-theta is required for TCR-induced NF-kappaB activation in mature but not immature T lymphocytes, *Nature* 404:402–407, 2000.
32. Deleted in review.
33. Crabtree GR, Olson EN: NFAT signaling: choreographing the social lives of cells, *Cell* 109(Suppl):S67–S79, 2002.
34. Guse AH, da Silva CP, Berg I, et al.: Regulation of calcium signalling in T lymphocytes by the second messenger cyclic ADP-ribose, *Nature* 398:70–73, 1999.
35. Lamprecht P, Moosig F, Csernok E, et al.: CD28 negative T cells are enriched in granulomatous lesions of the respiratory tract in Wegener's granulomatosis, *Thorax* 56:751–757, 2001.
36. Fletcher JM, Vukmanovic-Stejic M, Dunne PJ, et al.: Cytomegalovirus-specific CD4+ T cells in healthy carriers are continuously driven to replicative exhaustion, *J Immunol* 175:8218–8225, 2005.
37. Uda H, Mima T, Yamaguchi N, et al.: Expansion of a CD28-intermediate subset among CD8 T cells in patients with infectious mononucleosis, *J Virol* 76:6602–6608, 2002.
38. Wong CK, Lit LC, Tam LS, et al.: Aberrant production of soluble costimulatory molecules CTLA-4, CD28, CD80 and CD86 in patients with systemic lupus erythematosus, *Rheumatology* 44:989–994, 2005.
39. Grakoui A, Bromley SK, Sumen C, et al.: The immunological synapse: a molecular machine controlling T cell activation, *Science* 285:221–227, 1999.
40. Montixi C, Langlet C, Bernard A-M, et al.: Engagement of T cell receptor triggers its recruitment to low-density detergent-insoluble membrane domains, *EMBO J* 17:5334–5348, 1998.
41. Lee K-M, Chuang E, Griffen M, et al.: Molecular basis of T cell inactivation by CTLA-4, *Science* 282:2263–2266, 1998.
42. Krummel MF, Allison JP: CD28 and CTLA-4 have opposing effects on the response of T cells to stimulation, *J Exp Med* 182:459–465, 1995.
43. Tivol EA, Borriello F, Schweitzer AN, et al.: Loss of CTLA-4 leads to massive lymphoproliferation and fatal multiorgan tissue destruction, revealing a critical negative regulatory role of CTLA-4, *Immunity* 3:541–547, 1995.
44. Stahl EA, Raychaudhuri S, Remmers EF, et al.: Genome-wide association study meta-analysis identifies seven new rheumatoid arthritis risk loci, *Nat Genet* 42:508–514, 2010.
45. Ostrand-Rosenberg S, Horn LA, Haile ST: The programmed death-1 immune suppressive pathway: barrier to antitumor immunity, *J Immunol.* 193:3835–3841, 2014.
46. Khoury SJ, Sayegh MH: The roles of the new negative T cell costimulatory pathways in regulating autoimmunity, *Immunity* 20:529–538, 2004.
47. Nishimura H, Nose M, Hiai H, et al.: Development of lupus-like autoimmune diseases by disruption of the PD-1 gene encoding an ITIM motif-carrying immunoreceptor, *Immunity* 11:141–151, 1999.
48. Firestein GS, Zvaifler NJ: Peripheral blood and synovial fluid monocyte activation in inflammatory arthritis. I. A cytofluorographic study of monocyte differentiation antigens and class II antigens and their regulation by gamma-interferon, *Arthritis & Rheum* 30:857–863, 1987.
49. Cope AP, Londei M, Chu NR, et al.: Chronic exposure to tumor necrosis factor (TNF) in vitro impairs the activation of T cells through the T cell receptor/CD3 complex; reversal in vivo by anti-TNF antibodies in patients with rheumatoid arthritis, *J Clin Invest* 94:749–760, 1994.
50. Cope AP, Liblau RS, Yang XD, et al.: Chronic tumor necrosis factor alters T cell responses by attenuating T cell receptor signaling, *J Exp Med* 185:1573–1584, 1997.
51. Martins GA, Cimmino L, Shapiro-Shelef M, et al.: Transcriptional repressor Blimp-1 regulates T cell homeostasis and function, *Nat Immunol* 7:457–465, 2006.
52. Sakaguchi S, Sakaguchi N, Shimizu J, et al.: Immunologic tolerance maintained by CD25+ CD4+ regulatory T cells: their common role in controlling autoimmunity, tumor immunity, and transplantation tolerance, *Immunol Rev* 182:18–32, 2001.
53. Shevach EM, McHugh RS, Piccirillo CA, et al.: Control of T-cell activation by CD4+ CD25+ suppressor T cells, *Immunol Rev* 182:58–67, 2001.
54. Veldhoen M, Hocking RJ, Atkins CJ, et al.: TGFbeta in the context of an inflammatory cytokine milieu supports de novo differentiation of IL-17-producing T cells, *Immunity* 24:179–189, 2006.
55. Dong C: Diversification of T-helper-cell lineages: finding the family root of IL-17-producing cells, *Nat Rev Immunol* 6:329–333, 2006.
56. Nishio J, Feuerer M, Wong J, et al.: Anti-CD3 therapy permits regulatory T cells to surmount T cell receptor-specified peripheral niche constraints. *J Exp Med* 207: 1879-1889.
57. Okada Y, Wu D, Trynka G, et al.: Genetics of rheumatoid arthritis contributes to biology and drug discovery, *Nature* 506:376–381, 2014.

58. Li C, DiSpirito JR, Zemmour D, et al.: TCR transgenic mice reveal stepwise, multi-site acquisition of the distinctive fat-treg phenotype, *Cell* 174:285–299 e212, 2018.
59. Ali N, Zirak B, Rodriguez RS, et al.: Regulatory T cells in skin facilitate epithelial stem cell differentiation, *Cell* 169:1119–1129 e1111, 2017.
60. Villalta SA, Rosenthal W, Martinez L, et al.: Regulatory T cells suppress muscle inflammation and injury in muscular dystrophy, *Sci Transl Med* 6, 2014. 258ra142.
61. Pamer E, Cresswell P: Mechanisms of MHC class I—restricted antigen processing, *Annu Rev Immunol* 16:323–358, 1998.
62. Newell MK, Haughn LJ, Maroun CR, et al. Death of mature T cells by separate ligation of CD4 and the T-cell receptor for antigen, *Nature* 347:286–289, 1990.
63. Casella CR, Finkel TH: Mechanisms of lymphocyte killing by HIV, *Curr Opin Hematol* 4:24–31, 1997.
64. Schneider P, MacKay F, Steiner V, et al.: BAFF, a novel ligand of the tumor necrosis factor family, stimulates B cell growth, *J Exp Med* 189:1747–1756, 1999.
65. Street NE, Schumacher JH, Fong TA, et al.: Heterogeneity of mouse helper T cells. Evidence from bulk cultures and limiting dilution cloning for precursors of Th1 and Th2 cells, *J Immunol* 144:1629–1639, 1990.
66. Coffman RL, Seymour BW, Hudak S, et al.: Antibody to interleukin-5 inhibits helminth-induced eosinophilia in mice, *Science* 245:308–310, 1989.
67. Fuss IJ, Strober W, Dale JK, et al.: Characteristic T helper 2 T cell cytokine abnormalities in autoimmune lymphoproliferative syndrome, a syndrome marked by defective apoptosis and humoral autoimmunity, *J Immunol* 158:1912–1918, 1997.
68. Ruddle NH, Bergman CM, McGrath KM, et al.: An antibody to lymphotoxin and tumor necrosis factor prevents transfer of experimental allergic encephalomyelitis, *J Exp Med* 172:1193–1200, 1990.
69. Heath WR, Allison J, Hoffmann MW, et al.: Autoimmune diabetes as a consequence of locally produced interleukin-2, *Nature* 359:547–549, 1992.
70. Yssel H, Shanafelt MC, Soderberg C, et al.: Borrelia burgdorferi activates a T helper type 1-like T cell subset in Lyme arthritis, *J Exp Med* 174:593–601, 1991.
71. Elliott MJ, Maini RN, Feldmann M, et al.: Randomised double-blind comparison of chimeric monoclonal antibody to tumour necrosis factor alpha (cA2) versus placebo in rheumatoid arthritis, *Lancet* 344:1105–1110, 1994.
72. Choy EH, Isenberg DA, Garrood T, et al.: Therapeutic benefit of blocking interleukin-6 activity with an anti-interleukin-6 receptor monoclonal antibody in rheumatoid arthritis: a randomized, double-blind, placebo-controlled, dose-escalation trial, *Arthritis Rheum* 46:3143–3150, 2002.
73. Rutz S, Eidenschenk C, Ouyang W: IL-22, not simply a Th17 cytokine, *Immunol Rev* 252:116–132, 2013.
74. Gaffen S, Jain R, Garg AV, et al.: The IL-23-IL-17 immune axis: from mechanism to therapeutic testing, *Nat Rev Immunol.* 14:585–600, 2014.
75. Chan JR, Blumenschein W, Murphy E, et al.: IL-23 stimulates epidermal hyperplasia via TNF and IL-20R2-dependent mechanisms with implications for psoriasis pathogenesis, *J Exp Med* 203:2577–2587, 2006.
76. Steinman L: A brief history of T(H)17, the first major revision in the T(H)1/T(H)2 hypothesis of T cell-mediated tissue damage, *Nat Med* 13:139–145, 2007.
77. Hirota K, Hashimoto M, Ito Y, et al.: Autoimmune Th17 cells induced synovial stromal and innate lymphoid cell secretion of the cytokine GM-CSF to initiate and augment autoimmune arthritis, *Immunity* 48:1220–1232 e1225, 2018.
78. Fazilleau N, Mark L, McHeyzer-Williams LJ, et al.: Follicular helper T cells: lineage and location, *Immunity* 30:324–335, 2009.
79. Vinuesa CG, Cook MC, Angelucci C, et al.: A RING-type ubiquitin ligase family member required to repress follicular helper T cells and autoimmunity, *Nature* 435:452–458, 2005.
80. Doherty PC: The new numerology of immunity mediated by virus-specific CD8(+) T cells, *Curr Opin Microbiol* 1:419–422, 1998.
81. Purton JF, Tan JT, Rubinstein MP, et al.: Antiviral CD4+ memory T cells are IL-15 dependent, *J Exp Med* 204:951–961, 2007.
82. Masopust D, Vezys V, Marzo AL, et al.: Preferential localization of effector memory cells in nonlymphoid tissue, *Science* 291:2413–2417, 2001.
83. Pearce EL, Walsh MC, Cejas PJ, et al.: Enhancing CD8 T-cell memory by modulating fatty acid metabolism, *Nature* 460:103–107, 2009.
84. Saito H, Kranz DM, Takagaki Y, et al.: A third rearranged and expressed gene in a clone of cytotoxic T lymphocytes, *Nature* 312:36–40, 1984.
85. Saito H, Kranz DM, Takagaki Y, et al.: Complete primary structure of a heterodimeric T-cell receptor deduced from cDNA sequences, *Nature* 309:757–762, 1984.
86. Shi C, Sahay B, Russell JQ, et al.: Reduced immune response to Borrelia burgdorferi in the absence of γδ T cells, *Infect Immun* 79:3940–3946, 2011.
87. Hiromatsu K, Yoshikai Y, Matsuzaki G, et al.: A protective role of gamma/delta T cells in primary infection with Listeria monocytogenes in mice, *J Exp Med* 175:49–56, 1992.
88. Rosat JP, MacDonald HR, Louis JA: A role for gamma delta + T cells during experimental infection of mice with Leishmania major, *J Immunol* 150:550–555, 1993.
89. Kaufmann SH, Ladel CH: Role of T cell subsets in immunity against intracellular bacteria: experimental infections of knock-out mice with Listeria monocytogenes and Mycobacterium bovis BCG, *Immunobiology* 191:509–519, 1994.
90. Tsuji M, Mombaerts P, Lefrancois L, et al.: Gamma delta T cells contribute to immunity against the liver stages of malaria in alpha beta T-cell-deficient mice, *Proc Natl Acad Sci U S A* 91:345–349, 1994.
91. Mixter PF, Camerini V, Stone BJ, et al.: Mouse T lymphocytes that express a gamma delta T-cell antigen receptor contribute to resistance to Salmonella infection in vivo, *Infect Immun* 62:4618–4621, 1994.
92. Brennan FM, Londei M, Jackson AM, et al.: T cells expressing gamma delta chain receptors in rheumatoid arthritis, *J Autoimmun* 1:319–326, 1988.
93. Vincent M, Roessner K, Lynch D, et al.: Apoptosis of Fas high CD4+ synovial T cells by Borrelia reactive Fas ligand high gamma delta T cells in lyme arthritis, *J Exp Med.* 184:2109–2117, 1996.
94. Rust C, Kooy Y, Pena S, et al.: Phenotypical and functional characterization of small intestinal TcR gamma delta + T cells in coeliac disease, *Scand J Immunol* 35:459–468, 1992.
95. Balbi B, Moller DR, Kirby M, et al.: Increased numbers of T lymphocytes with gamma delta-positive antigen receptors in a subgroup of individuals with pulmonary sarcoidosis, *J Clin Invest* 85:1353–1361, 1990.
96. Peterman GM, Spencer C, Sperling AI, et al.: Role of gamma delta T cells in murine collagen-induced arthritis, *J Immunol* 151:6546–6558, 1993.
97. Pelegri C, Kuhnlein P, Buchner E, et al.: Depletion of gamma/delta T cells does not prevent or ameliorate, but rather aggravates, rat adjuvant arthritis, *Arthritis Rheum* 39:204–215, 1996.
98. Peng SL, Madaio MP, Hayday AC, et al.: Propagation and regulation of systemic autoimmunity by gamma delta T cells, *J Immunol* 157:5689–5698, 1996.
99. Mukasa A, Hiromatsu K, Matsuzaki G, et al.: Bacterial infection of the testis leading to autoaggressive immunity triggers apparently opposed responses of alpha beta and gamma delta T cells, *J Immunol* 155:2047–2056, 1995.
100. Brennan FM, Londei M, Jackson AM, et al.: T cells expressing gd chain receptors in rheumatoid arthritis, *J Autoimmun* 1:319–326, 1988.

101. Rust C, Kooy Y, Pena S, et al.: Phenotypical and functional characterization of small intestinal TcR gd+ T cells in coeliac disease, *Scand J Immunol* 35:459–468, 1992.
102. Balbi B, Moller DR, Kirby M, et al.: Increased numbers of T lymphocytes with gd+ antigen receptors in a subgroup of individuals with pulmonary sarcoidosis, *J Clin Invest* 85:1353–1361, 1990.
103. Gentles AJ, Newman AM, Liu CL, et al.: The prognostic landscape of genes and infiltrating immune cells across human cancers, *Nat Med* 21:938–945, 2015.
104. Wilhelm M, Kunzmann V, Eckstein S, et al.: Gammadelta T cells for immune therapy of patients with lymphoid malignancies, *Blood* 102:200–206, 2003.
105. Costa G, Loizon S, Guenot M, et al.: Control of Plasmodium falciparum erythrocytic cycle: gammadelta T cells target the red blood cell-invasive merozoites, *Blood* 118:6952–6962, 2011.
106. Zeng X, Wei Y-L, Huang J, et al.: Gamma delta T cells recognize a microbial encoded B cell antigen to initiate a rapid antigen-specific interleukin-17 response, *Immunity* 37:524–534, 2012.
107. Nielsen MM, Witherden DA, Havran WL: Gammadelta T cells in homeostasis and host defence of epithelial barrier tissues, *Nat Rev Immunol* 17:733–745, 2017.
108. Girardi M, Oppenheim DE, Steele CR, et al.: Regulation of cutaneous malignancy by gammadelta T cells, *Science* 294:605–609, 2001.
109. Born W, Cady C, Jones-Carson J, et al.: Immunoregulatory functions of gamma delta T cells, *Adv Immunol* 71:77–144, 1999.
110. Hirsh MI, Junger WG: Roles of heat shock proteins and gamma delta T cells in inflammation, *Am J Respir Cell Mol Biol* 39:509–513, 2008.
111. Chien YH, Konigshofer Y: Antigen recognition by gammadelta T cells, *Immunol Rev* 215:46–58, 2007.
112. Schoel B, Sprenger S, Kaufmann SH: Phosphate is essential for stimulation of V gamma 9V delta 2 T lymphocytes by mycobacterial low molecular weight ligand, *Eur J Immunol* 24:1886–1892, 1994.
113. Constant P, Davodeau F, Peyrat MA, et al.: Stimulation of human gamma delta T cells by nonpeptidic mycobacterial ligands, *Science* 264:267–270, 1994.
114. Tanaka Y, Sano S, Nieves E, et al.: Nonpeptide ligands for human gamma delta T cells, *Proc Natl Acad Sci U S A* 91:8175–8179, 1994.
115. Tanaka Y, Morita CT, Nieves E, et al.: Natural and synthetic nonpeptide antigens recognized by human gamma delta T cells, *Nature* 375:155–158, 1995.
116. Bukowski JF, Morita CT, Brenner MB: Human gamma delta T cells recognize alkylamines derived from microbes, edible plants, and tea: implications for innate immunity, *Immunity* 11:57–65, 1999.
117. Vavassori S, Kumar A, Wan GS, et al.: Butyrophilin 3A1 binds phosphorylated antigens and stimulates human gammadelta T cells, *Nat Immunol* 14:908–916, 2013.
118. Witherden DA, Ramirez K, Havran WL: Multiple receptor-ligand interactions direct tissue-resident gammadelta T cell activation, *Front Immunol* 5:602, 2014.
119. Bendelac A, Rivera MN, Park SH, et al.: Mouse CD1-specific NK1 T cells: development, specificity, and function, *Annu Rev Immunol* 15:535–562, 1997.
120. Kinjo Y, Wu D, Kim G, et al.: Recognition of bacterial glycosphingolipids by natural killer T cells, *Nature* 434:520–525, 2005.

13 B Cells

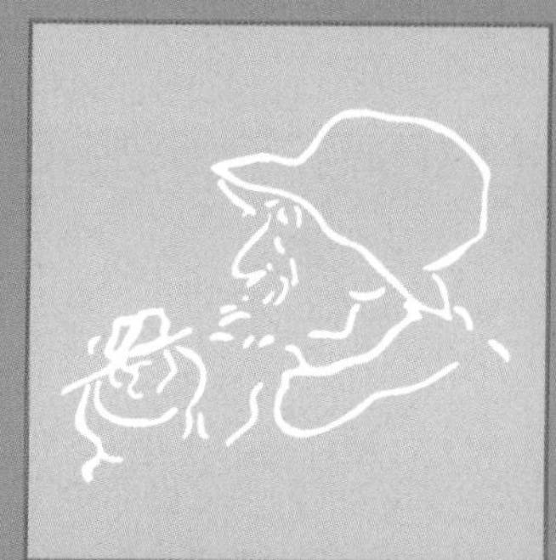

YONG-RUI ZOU, CHRISTINE GRIMALDI, AND BETTY DIAMOND

KEY POINTS

Immunoglobulins (Igs) are key to B cell function because they serve as both an antigen receptor and a major secreted product. The variable region binds antigen and is generated by random rearrangement of gene segments to give rise to numerous specificities. The constant region (Fc) defines the isotype and mediates effector functions.

Surface Ig is the major component of the B cell receptor complex, which regulates B cell selection, survival, and activation. Secreted Ig mediates antigen neutralization and opsonization with uptake by phagocytic cells, complement activation, and cellular activation or inhibition through engagement of receptors for the Fc region of Ig.

B cells are generated from hematopoietic precursors in the bone marrow and undergo several stages of maturation and selection before becoming immunocompetent, naïve B cells that reside in peripheral lymphoid organs. After antigen activation, B cells differentiate to memory cells and Ig-secreting plasma cells.

Follicular B cells respond to protein antigens in a T cell–dependent fashion and are the major source of B cell memory. B1 and marginal zone B cells are less dependent on T cell help and display limited heterogeneity of the B cell receptor.

Autoreactive B cells are generated in all individuals. Multiple checkpoints extinguish autoreactive B cells during early and later stages of B cell development. One or more of these checkpoints is breached in autoimmune-prone individuals, leading to the increased plasma cell differentiation from autoreactive B cells.

Introduction

The immune system is composed of numerous cells that are required to generate innate and adaptive immune responses. Adaptive responses are characterized by immunologic memory generated during the first exposure to an antigen, thereby permitting a rapid response to the antigen after subsequent exposure.

B cells are lymphocytes that recognize antigens through a molecule called the B cell receptor (BCR). The BCR is a surface immunoglobulin (Ig) molecule that recognizes the antigen and is associated with two additional proteins that transduce the signal. Upon encountering its antigen, a B cell begins a process of activation that leads to antibody secretion and memory formation regulated by interplay with antigen-activated T cells, dendritic cells (DCs), soluble factors, and in some cases follicular dendritic cells (FDCs). Both T and B lymphocytes can differentiate from naïve to memory cells, but only B cells have the capacity to fine-tune their antigen receptor structure to increase specificity and affinity, giving rise to more effective antibodies. Beyond immunoglobulin secretion, B cells regulate the immune response by cytokine secretion and antigen presentation to T cells in the context of class II major histocompatibility complex (MHC) molecules.

While much of the knowledge of B cell biology has been generated in mouse models, human B cell biology is described in this chapter whenever possible.

Immunoglobulins: Structure and Function

The hallmark of a B cell is the expression of the Ig molecules. There are two forms of Igs, membrane-bound Igs and secreted Igs, that are generated through alternative messenger RNA (mRNA) splicing. Cell surface Ig, also termed *BCR*, contributes to B cell maturation and survival and initiates an activation cascade after contact with antigens. Secreted Igs, referred to as *antibodies*, are produced by B cells after antigen activation to protect the host through neutralizing and eliminating the eliciting antigen.

Structurally, Igs are composed of four polypeptide chains: two identical light (L) chains with a molecular weight of approximately 25 kDa and two identical heavy (H) chains of 50 to 65 kDa. Each of the chains contains a folding motif that is highly conserved among proteins of the immune system, the *Ig domain*. These domains constitute the backbone of the Ig molecule and help permit pairing of the polypeptide chains (Fig. 13.1). The quaternary structure of an Ig molecule assumes a Y-shaped conformation that contains two functional moieties: two identical antigen-binding regions or variable regions, which are the arms of the "Y," and a constant region, which is the base of the "Y."[1]

This definition of functional moieties derives from early studies analyzing proteolytic fragments of Ig molecules. Cleavage with papain generates two identical fragments that retain antigen-binding capacity and hence are named *Fab*, as well as a distinct crystalizable fragment, the constant region (Fc), that mediates immune effector functions but is unable to interact with antigen.[2]

The antigen-binding regions are formed by pairing of the variable domain of the L chain (V_L) to the variable domain of the H chain (V_H). In contrast to the remainder of the molecule, great diversity exists in the amino acid sequence of the variable domains, which allows for a broad repertoire of Ig molecules that can recognize a wide array of antigens. Within the variable region of the Ig molecule are discrete regions, known as *complementary determining regions* (CDRs), that make direct contact with antigen. The amino acid sequences of the CDR are highly variable and are flanked by more conserved amino acid sequences called *framework regions*. The H- and L-chain molecules each contain three CDRs and four framework regions (see Fig. 13.1). The minimal antigenic determinant recognized by the variable regions of the H and L chains is known as an *epitope*, which

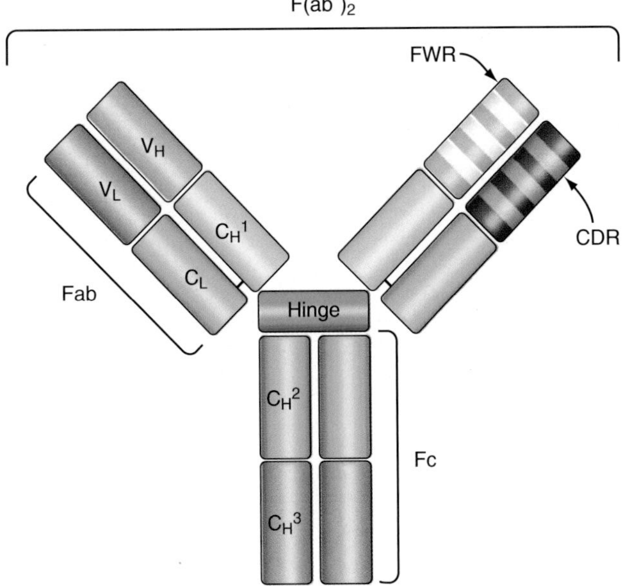

• **Fig. 13.1** Schematic of the antibody molecule. An antibody monomer consists of two heavy (H)-chain molecules covalently linked to two light (L)-chain molecules. The variable region is composed of the V_H and V_L domains of the H and L chains, respectively. Within the V_H and V_L domains are four framework regions (FWRs) and three complementary-determining regions (CDRs), which together make up the antigen-binding pocket. Papain digestion generates the Fab portion, which consists of V_H, C_H1, V_L, and C_L domains, and pepsin digestion generates two covalently linked Fabs, known as the F(ab′)$_2$. The Fc region of the H-chain constant region, which mediates immune effector functions, consists of the hinge domain (only in immunoglobulin [Ig]G, IgA, and IgD), which increases flexibility, and C_H2 and C_H3 domains.

may be a continuous or discontinuous region on a protein, carbohydrate, lipid, or nucleic acid. The presence of two identical variable regions in a single Ig molecule confers the capacity to interact with repetitive antigenic determinants present in multivalent antigens (i.e., polysaccharides) or enhances avidity by binding two separate antigen molecules containing the same antigenic determinant.[1]

The constant region directs the Ig effector functions that mediate the killing and removal of invading organisms and both the activation and homeostasis of the immune system. Strictly speaking, the constant region is formed by the constant domain of the L chain (C_L), which is paired to the first constant domain of the heavy chain (C_H1), and the remaining constant domains of the two heavy chains (C_H2, C_H3, and C_H4 in immunoglobulin M [IgM]), paired to each other. However, the functions associated with the constant region are mediated by the constant domains of the H chain.

Immunoglobulin Heavy Chain Constant Region

The specific binding interactions that occur between the Ig variable region and antigen may be sufficient to block microbial infectivity or neutralize toxins. However, the ability to eliminate pathogens is mediated by the Fc portion of the molecule. The Fc regions of antigen-antibody complexes are made accessible to serum factors that constitute the complement cascade or to cytotoxic and phagocytic cells that mediate the destruction and removal of pathogens. In mice and humans, there are five different types of H-chain constant regions, or isotypes, designated IgM (μ), IgD (δ), IgG (γ), IgA (α), and IgE (ε)[3]; each is encoded by a distinct constant region gene segment present in the H-chain locus of chromosome 4 in humans or chromosome 12 in mice. Each isotype is capable of specific effector functions, and each cellular receptor for Ig binds specific isotypes and initiates a distinct intra-cellular signaling cascade. The number of C_H domains, the presence of a hinge region to increase flexibility between Fab regions, the serum half-life, the ability to form polymers, complement activation, and Fc receptor binding vary among isotypes. Characteristics of the different Ig H-chain isotypes are presented in Table 13.1.[1,3,4] BCRs of different isotypes may also deliver different intra-cellular signals when activated by antigen. It should be noted that the interplay between antibodies and the cells that bear the Fc receptors extends beyond pathogen clearance and shapes the immune response by mediating activation or inhibition of specific cell types[5] and by mediating cell death.[6]

Immunoglobulin M

IgM is the first isotype expressed in developing B cells and the first antibody secreted during a primary immune response. It is found predominantly in serum but is also present in mucosal secretions and breast milk. Because the process that increases antibody affinity for a particular antigen (affinity maturation) has not yet been initiated during the early stages of a primary immune response, IgM antibodies usually exhibit low affinity. Their low affinity is balanced by the fact that much of the secreted IgM that exists is in pentameric form, generating multiple binding sites, providing high avidity for antigen and assisting with the binding of large, multimeric antigens. IgM also exists as a monomer and a hexamer, but only the pentameric form is linked by the polypeptide, called the *joining* (J) chain. The J chain allows the active transport of IgM to mucosal secretions.[7]

Many of the biologic functions of IgM are mediated by its ability to activate the classic complement pathway.[1] The complement cascade consists of a series of enzymes that, upon activation, mediate the removal and lysis of invading organisms. Deposition of antibody molecules or complement components on the surface of the antigen assists with phagocytosis. Proteins such as antibody and complement that enhance phagocytosis are called *opsonins.* Once the complement cascade has been activated, monocytes, macrophages, or neutrophils engulf opsonized particles through specific receptors present on phagocytic cells such as CD21, which recognizes fragments of the C3 complement component. Activation of the complement pathway also results in the generation of the membrane attack complex, which is composed of late complement components and directly lyses C3-opsonized pathogens. Because activation of the classic complement pathway requires exposed Fc regions to be spatially close, multimeric IgM is a potent activator of the classic complement pathway once it has bound its antigen. For example, hexameric IgM is between 20 and 100 times more potent as an inducer of complement activation than is monomeric IgM.[8] C1q is an early complement factor that binds to IgM, as well as IgG. Immune complexes containing C1q can downregulate immune responses because C1q binds LAIR-1, a negative regulator that is present on the cell surface of myeloid cells and lymphocytes. LAIR-1, when associated with C1q, can suppress inflammation by preventing DC maturation and activation induced by Toll-like receptors (TLRs).

Immunoglobulin G

IgG is the most common isotype found in serum, constituting about 70% of the circulating antibody. IgG antibodies are usually of higher affinity than IgM antibodies and predominate in a

TABLE 13.1 Properties of Human Immunoglobulin Isotypes

Characteristic	IgM	IgG	IgA	IgE	IgD
Structure	Pentamer, hexamer	Monomer	Dimer (IgA_2), monomer (IgA_1)	Monomer	Monomer
C_H domains	4	3	3	4	3
Serum values (mg/mL)	0.7-1.7	9.5-12.5	1.5-2.6	0.0003	0.04
Serum half-life (days)	5-10	7-24	11-14	1-5	2-8
Complement activation (classic)	Yes	Yes	No	No	No
FcR-mediated phagocytosis	No	Yes	Yes	No	No
Antibody-dependent cell mediated cytotoxicity	No	Yes	No	No	No
Placental transfer	No	Yes	No	No	No
Presence in mucosal secretions	Yes	No	Yes	No	No
Main biologic characteristic	Primary antibody response	Secondary antibody responses	Secreted immunoglobulin	Allergy and parasite reactivity	Marker for naïve B cells

C_H, Constant domain of the heavy chain; *FcR*, Fc receptor; *Ig*, immunoglobulin.

recall immune response. Four subclasses of IgG exist in humans: IgG1, IgG2, IgG3, and IgG4. IgG1 and IgG3 arise in response to viral and protein antigens. IgG2 is the main antibody present in response to polysaccharide antigens, and IgG4 participates in responses to nematodes and is observed in patients with IgG4-related systemic disease.[9]

All IgG subclasses exist as monomers and have a high structural similarity; however, minor differences result in distinct biologic effects. IgG3 and IgG1 are potent activators of the classic complement pathway, and IgG2 can initiate the alternative complement pathway.

All IgG subclasses engage specific Fcγ receptors (FcγRs) present on DCs, macrophages, neutrophils, and natural killer (NK) cells. The FcγRs on phagocytic cells, when cross-linked, mediate the removal of immune complexes from circulation and initiate antibody-dependent, cell-mediated cytotoxicity, resulting in the release of granules that contain perforin, a pore-forming protein, and enzymes known as *granzymes* that induce programmed cell death (apoptosis) of target cells.[10,11] FcγR engagement also allows the internalization and subsequent presentation of antigens in the context of class II MHC molecules.

Because IgG antibodies are the only ones that cross the placental barrier, they are critical for the survival of newborns. The transport of IgG from the maternal circulation into the fetal blood supply is mediated by the neonatal FcR (FcRn).[12] FcRn is also responsible for the long half-life of IgG in serum by blocking IgG catabolism.[13] FcRIIb is an important inhibitory receptor expressed on myeloid cells and B cells. Its function is discussed in more detail in the later Co-Receptors section.

Immunoglobulin A

Despite its relative low concentration in serum, more IgA is produced than all other isotypes combined. Most IgA exists as secretory IgA (SIgA) in mucosal cavities and in milk and colostrum, and only a small fraction is present in serum. Two subclasses of IgA exist in humans: IgA1 and IgA2. IgA1 is mainly produced as a monomer. In contrast, polymeric IgA2 is produced along mucosal surfaces.[14]

Polymeric IgA exists mainly as a dimer and includes a J chain (the same chain that links pentameric IgM). It is captured by the polymeric immunoglobulin receptor (pIgR) that is expressed on the basolateral surface of the epithelial cells and then transcytosed to the apical side. Release of IgA into mucosal secretions requires cleavage of the pIgR; a fragment known as the secretory component (SC) remains associated with SIgA and protects it from the action of proteases and increases its solubility in mucus, where it neutralizes toxins and inhibits the adherence of SIgA-coated micro-organisms to the mucosal surface.[15]

People with IgA deficiency are prone to respiratory tract and diarrheal infections, as well as an increased incidence of autoimmune disorders.[16] The presence of FcαR on the surface of neutrophils and macrophages has been suggested to play a regulatory role in the immune system; it is possible that autoimmune manifestations in IgA-deficient patients arise from the absence of immune regulation mediated by FcαR.[17]

Immunoglobulin E

IgE is involved in protection against parasitic infections but also triggers immune responses associated with allergic reactions. Only a small amount of IgE is detectable in serum, where it exists as a monomer.[18] Mast cells and basophils express a high-affinity IgE Fc receptor (FcεRI) that binds free IgE. Cross-linking of the FcεR by antigen-bound IgE induces degranulation and release of histamine, proteases, lipid mediators such as prostaglandin D_2, and leukotrienes, many of which are associated with anaphylaxis.

Immunoglobulin D

The role of IgD in the humoral response has been the subject of multiple speculations. IgD is found predominantly as cell surface Ig on mature naïve B cells. Soluble IgD is scarce in serum;

however, IgD-producing plasma cells are found in tonsils and tissue associated with the respiratory tract, where IgD binds to galectin-9 on basophils and mast cells to enhance protective humoral responses and inhibit IgE-induced allergic reactions.[19] High levels of secreted IgD can be found in patients with autoinflammatory syndrome.[20,21]

Light Chains

Two distinct L-chain polypeptides exist, designated κ and λ. L chains contain a variable and a single constant domain. Even though two L-chain isotypes exist, there is no known function associated with the L-chain constant region. The κ chain is used more often than the λ chain in human (65%) and mouse (95%) Ig molecules.[22]

Immunoglobulin Variable Region

The recognition of a virtually unlimited number of antigens requires a mechanism to generate Ig molecules with similarly broad specificities. The molecular basis of this process has been known for several years.[23] The Ig molecule is encoded by gene segments within distinct genetic loci residing on separate chromosomes (Fig. 13.2); the H-chain locus is on human chromosome 14,[24] the κ-chain locus is on chromosome 2, and the λ-chain locus is on chromosome 22.[25]

The H-chain variable region is encoded by a variable (V_H), diversity (D_H), and a joining (J_H) segment. The L chain is encoded by either Vκ and Jκ or V_λ and Jλ segments; it does not contain D segments. The human H-chain locus contains from 38 to 46 V_H, 23 D_H, and nine J_H functional genes (these numbers represent a typical haplotype but vary among individuals). The κ-chain locus contains approximately 31 to 35 V_κ genes and five J_κ functional genes; the λ-chain locus contains 29 to 32 Vλ genes and four or five Jλ functional genes.[26]

Generation of Immunoglobulin Diversity

In a developing B cell, different V_H, D_H, and J_H or V_L and J_L gene segments are randomly combined to generate a large number of different Ig molecules (see Fig. 13.2). This process, known as *V(D)J recombination,* occurs in the fetal liver or adult bone marrow, in the absence of antigen stimulation, and must be successful to continue with B cell maturation. Here, we present the molecular process, and later the functional and developmental consequences are discussed (see the B Cell Development section).

V(D)J recombination happens sequentially, beginning with the joining of one D_H segment to one J_H segment; then a V_H segment will be targeted to the rearranged D_HJ_H fragment. The absence of an in-frame recombination leads to recombination of the second allele. L-chain recombination also occurs in a stepwise manner. First, the κ locus is rearranged; in the absence of a productive κ-chain rearrangement, the λ locus undergoes recombination.[27]

The recombination machinery is composed of specific enzymes, including recombination-activating gene 1 and 2 (RAG-1 and RAG-2). The complex recognizes recombination signal sequences (RSS) that flank the V, D, and J gene segments. These highly conserved RSSs are composed of a palindromic heptamer (seven base pairs) followed by DNA spacers that are 12 or 23 base pairs in

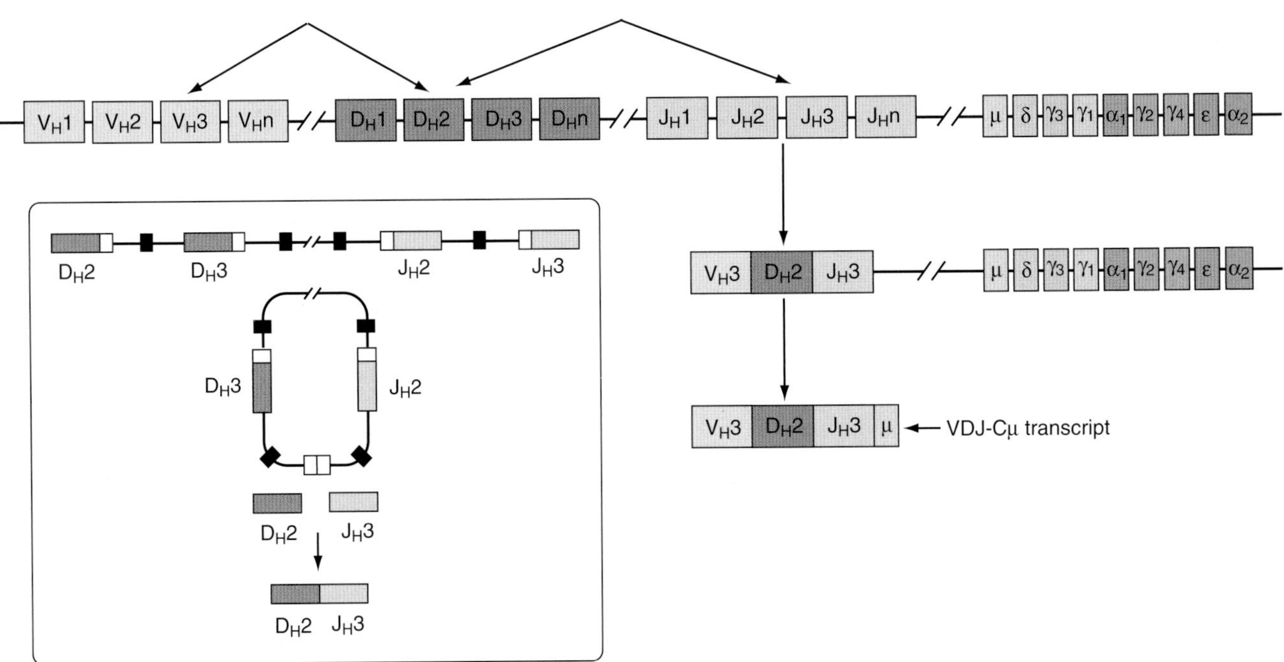

• **Fig. 13.2** V(D)J recombination at the immunoglobulin gene locus. V(D)J recombination at the heavy (H)-chain locus is depicted at the *top*. A single V_H gene segment randomly recombines with a D_H and J_H gene segment residing on the same chromosome. After $V_HD_HJ_H$ recombination, a transcript containing the immunoglobulin (Ig)M H-chain constant region gene (Cμ) is generated. The inset represents an example of V(D)J recombination occurring between a single D_H and J_H gene segment. The white squares represent the heptamer, and the black squares represent the nonamer recombination recognition sequences. After recognition and cleavage of these sequences, the coding junctions of the rearranged D_H and J_H gene segments are ligated. A V_H gene segment then recombines with the rearranged D_HJ_H segment. Light (L)-chain rearrangement is mediated by the same mechanism.

length and an adenosine/thymidine (AT)-rich nonamer.[28] Once the complex recognizes its target, it generates double-stranded DNA (dsDNA) breaks at the RSS sites. Next, the cellular DNA repair complex recognizes and joins the cleaved segments.

The random recombination that occurs among V, D, and J gene segments can generate a diverse Ig repertoire without the need for a large number of germline H- and L-chain genes. During H-chain recombination, nucleotides may be added at V_HD_H and D_HJ_H junctions by the enzyme terminal deoxynucleotidyl transferase (TdT). These non–germline-encoded sequences are known as *N additions.* As long as these nucleotide changes do not disrupt the reading frame or lead to the incorporation of premature stop codons, the random addition of N sequences increases the diversity of the amino acid sequence. Imprecise ligation at the coding junctions may result in the loss of nucleotides, thereby also enhancing diversity. Finally, random pairing of the H chains and L chains further diversifies the Ig repertoire.

B Cell Development

The final outcome of the maturation process is the generation of a pool of mature B cells with a diverse repertoire of Ig specificities that can recognize foreign and pathogenic antigens without compromising the integrity of the self. Therefore the process of generation of Ig diversity is coupled with the censoring of autospecificities.

B cells, as with all cells in the hematopoietic lineage, begin with the differentiation of noncommitted $CD34^+$ hematopoietic stem cells to lymphopoietic precursors with restricted lineage potential. These cells, known as *common lymphoid progenitors* (CLPs), have the potential to give rise to NK, T, and B cells. Early B cell progenitors begin to express genes for DNA rearrangement, as well as B cell program transcription factors. Multiple transcription factors act in concert, but Ikaros, E2A, EBF, and Pax5 appear to be the most important in B cell development.[29] Pax5 is considered the master transcriptional control for B cells because it is induced in early stages of B cell commitment and plays a dual role by repressing genes required for differentiation to the myelomonocytic lineage and activating B cell–specific genes such as Ig genes, CD19, and signaling molecules.[30]

Niches for Human B Lymphopoiesis

The development of hematopoietic stem cells ($CD34^+$) into mature B cells begins in the first weeks of uterine life. By the eighth gestational week, early B cell precursors can be identified in the fetal liver and omentum. From gestational week 34 and through adulthood, the bone marrow is the primary site of B lymphopoiesis.[31] It is unequivocally established that there are differences between the B cells that originate during fetal and adult lymphopoiesis in mice, and it is becoming clear that these differences extrapolate to human lymphopoiesis as well. B cell precursors are susceptible to estrogen, and the maturation of maternal B cells is arrested at the pro–B cell stage during pregnancy; in contrast, fetal B cell precursors lack estrogen receptors and consequently are unaffected by exposure to hormones.[32] B cells originating during prenatal life have a bias in the usage of D_H and J_H gene segments, and this, along with low expression of the enzyme TdT, leads to a more restricted Ig repertoire with shorter CDR3 sequences.[33]

Whether during fetal or adult lymphopoiesis, the maturation of B cells from CLP is contingent on the presence of stromal cells that provide both contact-dependent and soluble signals. Although the nature of the interactions provided by the stromal cells to create a lymphopoiesis-permissive environment is still largely unknown, they include both survival and proliferative signals. Interactions between chemokine CXCL12 and the integrin ligand vascular cell adhesion molecule-1 (VCAM-1) on the membrane of the stromal cells and CXCR4 and very late activation antigen-4 (VLA-4) on the early B cell progenitors are required for homing of the early B cell precursors to sites of lymphopoiesis and differentiation of B cells.[34] The molecules interleukin (IL)-7, IL-3, and the Fms-like tyrosine kinase-3 ligand (Flt-3L) promote B cell lymphopoiesis, although IL-7 appears to be dispensable for human B cell development. Matrix molecules in the microenvironment such as heparan sulfate proteoglycan are assumed to "trap" critical soluble factors.[35]

B Cell Ontogeny

The state of Ig gene rearrangement and the expression of intra-cellular and surface proteins define the stages of B cell lymphopoiesis into early B cell progenitors, pro-B, pre-B, immature, transitional, and mature naïve B cells (Table 13.2).[36] Once a CLP begins to express transcription factors required for B cell maturation, E2A and EBF, the cell becomes an early B cell progenitor. E2A and EBF enable transcription of the proteins involved in the recombination machinery (RAG-1/RAG-2). The beginning of D to J recombination on the IgH locus marks the progress to a pro-B stage.

Pro-B Cells

The pro-B cell stage is defined by the rearrangement of the IgH chain gene segments and synthesis of a μ-polypeptide. Pro-B cells are dependent on interactions with stromal cells. The VLA-4 integrin and CD44 both mediate adhesion to stromal cells, are highly expressed at this stage, and are believed to be important for continued development.[37] Pro-B cells also express high levels of B cell lymphoma 2 (Bcl-2), a molecule that protects cells from apoptosis. At the onset of the pro-B cell stage, the variable gene segments of both H- and L-chain loci are in the germline configuration but accessible to the recombination machinery. A D_H gene segment on one H-chain chromosome rearranges with a J_H gene segment residing on the same chromosome, often with the inclusion of nontemplate nucleotides at the junction of these two segments. Next, a V_H rearranges to the D_HJ_H gene segment. Completion of $V_HD_HJ_H$ gene rearrangement leads to the generation of an H-chain transcript that also contains the IgM constant region (C_μ), which is the constant region gene segment most proximal to the variable region gene segments on the chromosome (see Fig. 13.2).

The generation of a μ-polypeptide and its subsequent expression on the surface of the cell, together with a surrogate L chain formed by the λ5 and Vpre-B polypeptides, as well as the Igα/Igβ dimer—a complex known as the pre-B cell receptor (pre-BCR)—marks the end of this phase of gene recombination. This constitutes a critical developmental checkpoint and the entrance to the next developmental stage, known as the *pre-B cell.*[38] The requirement for a pre-BCR complex ensures that B cells without a productive H chain will die.

The pre-BCR stimulates pro-B cells with productive IgH rearrangement to proliferate. It also transduces a signal that the V(D)J rearrangement was successful and halts recombination of the second H-chain allele. This process, known as *allelic exclusion,* ensures that all Ig molecules generated within a single B cell are identical and have the same antigenic specificity. If no μ chain is generated, rearrangement is initiated on the other chromosome. If the second rearrangement also results in a nonproductive H-chain

TABLE 13.2 Human B Cell Maturation Markers During B Cell Development

Marker	HSC	Pro-B	Pre-B	Immature	Transitional 1	Transitional 2	Plasma
CD34	+	+	–	–	–	–	–
CD19	–	+	+	+	+	+	+
CD10	–	+	+	+	+	+	–
CD20	–	+	+	+	+	+	–
CD21	–	–	–	–	–	+	–
CD22	–	–	+	+	+	+	–
CD23	–	–	–	–	–	+	–
CD38	–	+	+	+	+	+	+
CD40	–	+	+	+	+	+	–
CD45	–	+	+	+	+	+	+
CD138	–	–	–	–	–	–	+
RAG-1	–	+	+	+/–	+/–	+/–	–
RAG-2	–	+	+	+/–	+/–	+/–	–
TdT	–	+	+	–	–	–	–
Igα	–	+	+	+	+	+	+
Igβ	–	+	+	+	+	+	+
Heavy chain	–	– (D_H–J_H)	+ (V_H–D_H-J_H)	+	+	+	+
Pre-BCR	–	–	+	–	–	–	–
Surface IgM	–	–	–	+	+	+	–
Surface IgD	–	–	–	–	–	+	–
Light chain	–	–	+ (V_κ-J_κ V_λ-J_λ)	+	+	+	+

BCR, B cell receptor; *CD*, cluster of differentiation; *HSC*, hematopoietic stem cell; *Ig*, immunoglobulin; *RAG*, recombination-activating gene; *Tdt*, terminal deoxynucleotidyl transferase.

molecule, the absence of a pre-BCR–mediated signal induces apoptosis. The odds of generating a productive rearrangement are one in three, and consequently, approximately 50% of the cells that begin recombination will be unable to proceed along a developmental pathway.

Pre-B Cells

The pre-B cell stage is characterized by L chain recombination. Initiation of this stage requires the presence of the pre-BCR and functional signal transduction machinery.

At the transitional stage from pro-B to pre-B cells, the expression of the pre-BCR induces a proliferative burst that generates daughter cells with the same H chain and potential for multiple specificities within daughter cells, each of which may produce a different L chain. Targeted disruption of genes encoding the pre-BCR complex such as the IgM transmembrane constant region domain, λ5, or the Igα and Igβ accessory molecules arrest B cell development. In addition, defects in the adapter molecule BLNK or the tyrosine kinase Btk lead to a serious impairment in pre-B cell maturation. It appears that the charged residues on pre-BCR induce self-aggregation, which activates constitutive internalization and signaling of the pre-BCR complex that leads to clonal expansion of B cell precursors with a fit pre-BCR.[39]

The expression of the pre-BCR is transient. After the proliferative burst, the μ H chain is present only in the cytoplasm as the pre-B cell rearranges an L chain. The general rearrangement process is similar to V(D)J rearrangement and is dependent on RAG-1/RAG-2 expression. Because TdT is not expressed at this stage, L chains do not usually contain N sequences at the V_LJ_L junction. At the end of this process, pairing of the newly minted L chain with the μ H chain leads to the surface expression of an IgM molecule, complexed with Igα and Igβ, to form the BCR complex. It is believed that surface expression of the BCR on immature B cells transduces signals that enforce allelic exclusion at the L-chain locus and downregulate expression of the RAG genes. This immature B cell has completed the gene rearrangement process and is now subject to repertoire selection.[40]

Immature B Cells

Once B cells express surface IgM in the bone marrow, they are subject to repertoire censoring. During this stage, cross-linking of the BCR by antigen leads to the activation of one of several tolerance mechanisms to diminish the fraction of autoreactive cells present in the mature repertoire. These mechanisms include deletion, receptor editing, and anergy (see later discussion on negative selection).

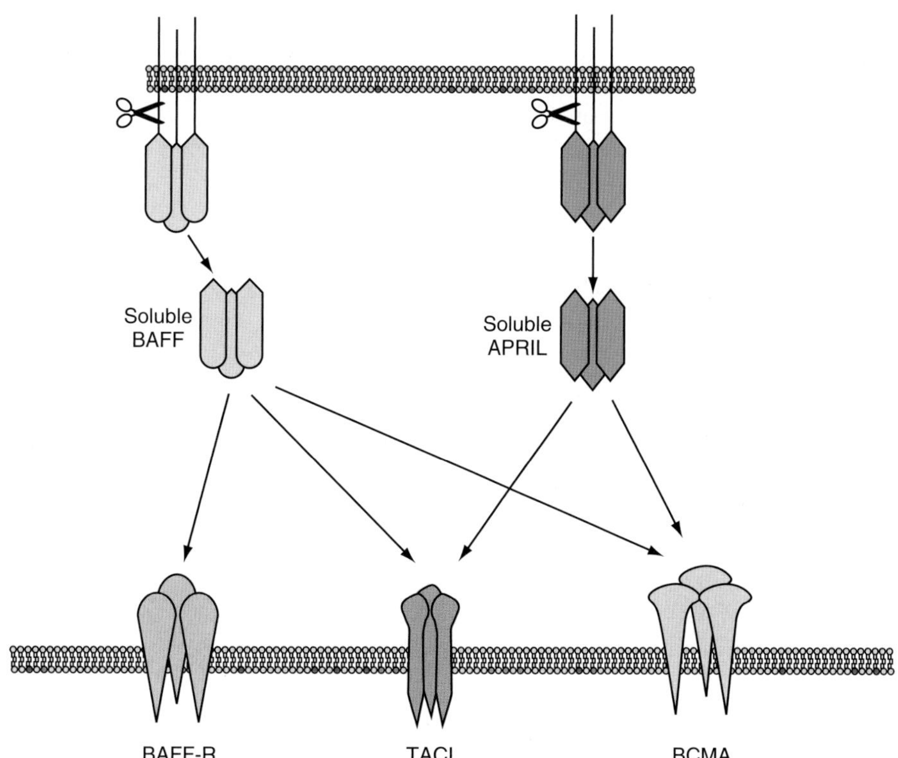

• **Fig. 13.3** The BAFF family of cytokines and their receptors. BAFF (also known as BLyS) and APRIL are expressed as membrane-bound proteins that can be cleaved by proteases to produce the soluble proteins. BAFF might bind the three known receptors: BAFF-R, TACI, and BCMA. APRIL only binds to BCMA and TACI.

During the maturation process in the bone marrow, the cells become less dependent on interactions with the stroma and move toward the sinusoidal lumen. Once they express IgM, they enter the blood, where they are called *transitional cells.*

Peripheral Naïve B Cell Subsets

As B cells mature and their dependence on stromal cells decreases, they leave the bone marrow and finish their maturation in the spleen before homing to other lymphoid tissue such as the lymph nodes, tonsils, and Peyer's patches of the intestine. It is in these secondary lymphoid organs where mature B cells interact with foreign antigen and specific humoral immune responses are activated.

The cytokine milieu surrounding the B cell is diverse and spatially and temporarily regulated. Two members of the TNF family, BAFF and APRIL, have emerged as key survival factors, particularly at two regulatory points in development and differentiation: the transition from an immature to a naïve B cell in the periphery and the survival of the newly produced plasma cells. BAFF (B cell–activating factor, BLyS) and APRIL (a proliferation-inducing ligand) are proteins produced by cells that take part in the innate response such as macrophages and DCs, as well as stromal cells, and are present as membrane-bound proteins or soluble trimers. They have three known receptors (BAFF-R, TACI, and BCMA) that are present on the membrane of B cells from the T2 stage to their final differentiation to plasma cells. BAFF binds the three receptors, whereas APRIL binds only TACI and BCMA. BAFF induces survival and activation of B cells when bound to BAFF-R, whereas BAFF signaling through TACI decreases the size of the B cell pool. APRIL does not participate in B cell homeostasis but seems to be critical to the survival of plasmablasts in the bone marrow.[41]

Enhanced survival and activation of autoreactive B cells have been demonstrated in mice that overexpress BAFF.[42] An increase in serum levels of BAFF has been observed in some patients with systemic lupus erythematosus (SLE), rheumatoid arthritis, and Sjögren's syndrome and is thought to contribute to pathogenesis because autoreactive B cells that would normally be censored can survive in the presence of excess BAFF (Fig. 13.3).[43]

Transitional B Cells

Once immature B cells egress from the bone marrow, they are called *transitional cells.* These cells are the earliest B cells found in the periphery in healthy subjects and move to the spleen to finish their maturation.

Transitional cells are the last B cell subpopulation that expresses the developmental marker CD24. At this stage B cells begin to express surface IgD, which harbors the same specificity as the IgM because the IgD H chain is encoded by the same VDJ fragments as IgM but expresses the C_δ instead of the C_μ domain. It is the expression of IgD that separates transitional cells into two different maturation stages. Transitional 1 (T1) B cells that do not express IgD are the recent bone marrow emigrants, and transitional 2 (T2) B cells that begin to express IgD represent the subsequent maturational stage.[44] The existence and functional characteristics of a third transitional stage (T3) are still debated.

Transitional cells constitute a stage subject to multiple regulatory processes. First, transitional cells must compete with naïve B cells already present in the periphery for a developmental niche. Transitional B cells are extremely dependent on BAFF. In its absence, B cell development does not progress beyond the T1 stage.[45] Second, T1 transitional cells are still highly susceptible to tolerance induction after BCR cross-linking. In T1 cells, cross-linking of the BCR ex vivo leads to cell death, whereas T2 cells respond to BCR cross-linking by proliferation and differentiation to the mature naïve B cell stage.

Mature B Cells

The final stages of maturation that occur in the spleen and give rise to the naïve B cell subset have not been fully elucidated, but the prevailing theory is that T2 B cells give rise to the circulating mature naïve cell population. In the mouse spleen, two populations of phenotypically and functionally different naïve B cells are recognized: follicular and marginal zone (MZ) B cells. Human naïve B cells constitute 60% to 70% of the circulating B cell repertoire and populate the spleen and lymph nodes. They include the equivalent of mouse follicular B cells and represent the circulating, nonantigen-exposed B cell subpopulation characterized by surface IgM and IgD expression, lack of CD27, and the presence of the membrane transporter ABC.[46] There is also a population in blood of IgM$^+$, CD27$^+$ B cells that have been likened to MZ B cells, which do not recirculate in the mouse.[47]

Marginal Zone B Cells

MZ B cells are a population of noncirculating mature B cells located in the MZ of the rodent spleen. In rodents, MZ B cells present clear phenotypic and functional differences from the cells present in the follicles, responding to blood-borne pathogens and to repetitive antigenic structures such as the ones present on polysaccharide antigens.

In the human spleen, the structural definition of the MZ does not correspond exactly to the area surrounding B cell follicles. However, there is a population with the functional characteristics of mouse MZ B cells: low activation thresholds, highly responsive to polysaccharide antigens, and with a clear surface phenotype. These cells, which are sometimes named *MZ-like* or *unswitched memory*, are not restricted to the human spleen but are found circulating in the peripheral blood, as well as in the lymph nodes, tonsils, and Peyer's patches.[47,48] They are defined as IgM^{high}, IgD^{low}, CD27$^+$, CD21$^+$, and CD1c$^+$.[48,49]

Given that these cells possess the "memory" marker CD27, it is suggested that they have experienced antigenic exposure; however, the presence of MZ-like B cells in subjects with X-linked agammaglobulinemia (a CD40L deficiency) suggests that even if antigen exposure has occurred, T cell help has not. Interestingly, MZ-like B cells, although already present at birth, do not seem to be fully functional at that time; infants up to age 2 years are particularly susceptible to infections by capsulated bacteria. This phenomenon might be due to the functional immaturity of the cells or to the lack of development of the antigen-trapping microstructure.

B1 Cells

In mice, B1 cells represent a minor population of B cells that reside predominantly in the pleural and peritoneal cavities. They are named *B1* because it is assumed that they are the first population of B cells to develop during intrauterine life. Functionally, B1 cells have been characterized as self-renewing cells that possess a limited BCR repertoire and respond with low affinity to a broad array of antigens, mainly phospholipids and carbohydrate structures in the bacterial cell wall. Despite their low numbers, these cells secrete most of the natural antibodies of the organism (antibodies that appear without evidence of previous immunization) and are assumed to be the precursors of most of the plasma cells that home to the intestinal lamina propria. Phenotypically, these cells are defined as IgM^{high} and IgD^{low}. About 70% of them express the marker CD5.

In humans, the definition of B1 cells is still unresolved. The CD5 marker has been used extensively as a surrogate marker for B1 cells with mixed success, given that activated human B cells also upregulate the expression of CD5.[50]

Sites of B Cell Homing and Activation

After the immature B cell stage, B cells home to secondary lymphoid organs, which contain the microenvironment and architecture necessary for the retention and activation of B cells. These organs include the spleen and lymph nodes, as well as lymphoid structures in mucosal tissue (e.g., Peyer's patches, appendix, and tonsils). The secondary lymphoid tissue is adapted to trap circulating antigen and expose the B cells to it and to provide interactions with T cells and other co-stimulatory cells. Peripheral lymphoid tissue contains specialized antigen-presenting cells known as *dendritic cells*. In the Peyer's patches of the intestines, foreign antigen is taken up in specialized epithelial cells known as *M cells*. Even though peripheral lymphoid tissues vary in structure and cellular organization, they all possess antigen-presenting cells and B cell–containing follicles surrounded by T cell–rich zones.[51] As explained in the following section, antigen, T cells, and DCs are required for B cell activation and differentiation into Ig-secreting plasma cells or memory B cells.

Circulation and Homing

B1 cells typically home to the peritoneal and pleural cavities and, to a lesser extent, the spleen. Naïve B cells enter the peripheral circulation by passing through the endothelial lining of the sinusoids of secondary lymphoid tissue and recirculating throughout the follicles of secondary lymphoid tissues. The entry, retention, and recirculation of B cells through secondary lymphoid organs depend on both adhesion molecules and chemokine receptors.[52,53] First, expression of LFA-1 and VLA-4 is required for entry into the lymphoid tissue, and then the chemokine receptors CXCR5 and CCR7 direct localization within the tissue. The CXCR5 molecule is expressed on all mature B cells and mediates B cell migration to follicles in response to the chemokine CXCL13, which is produced by follicular stromal cells. These cells, in turn, are regulated by lymphotoxin made by B cells. In the follicle, the B cells scan for antigen, making contact with potential antigen-bearing cells such as FDCs, subcapsular macrophages, and DCs. If the B cell does not encounter a cognate antigen, it will exit the lymphoid organ through the efferent lymphatics in response to the molecule sphingosine 1 phosphate (S1P). Neutralization of S1P leads to sequestration of B cells in lymphoid organs.[54]

Upon antigenic encounter, B cells are retained in the lymphoid organ because of the upregulation of CCR7. The ligands for CCR7 (CCL19 and CCL21) mediate the organization of the T cell zone and attract antigen-activated B cells to this border where cognate T cell–B cell interactions occur. In contrast, it is assumed that MZ-like B cells respond to antigen without the help of cognate T cells. In mice, MZ B cells are present exclusively in the spleen and do not recirculate; in humans they are found in the spleen and tonsils, as well as in blood. MZ B cells localize to the outer layers of the follicles, making them among the first cells to encounter blood-borne antigens. The adhesion molecules ICAM-1 and VCAM-1, as well as S1P and cannabinoid receptor 2, are responsible for sequestering MZ B cells within the marginal sinuses.

The interplay of chemokine expression and the induction of chemokine receptors play an important role in the germinal center (GC) response. The chemokine CXCL12 retains centroblasts in the dark zone during the process of somatic hypermutation and isotype class switching. CXCL13 regulates migration to the light zone, where survival and selection events are mediated by interactions with CXCR5-expressing T follicular helper (Tfh) cells and FDCs.[55] Later, CXCL12 promotes the migration of plasmablasts to the bone marrow, where they undergo further development into long-lived plasma cells.

Mucosa-Associated Compartments

Within the mucosal tissue, the sites of induction of immune responses are distinct from the site where the effector cells reside. There are two main sites for the induction of an immune response. The first is the mucosa-associated lymphoid tissue (MALT) that includes Peyer's patches, nasopharynx-associated tissue, and isolated lymphoid follicles, where exogenous antigen is displayed by specialized M cells that transport antigen to the follicle. The second site of induction includes mucosa-draining lymphoid nodes such as the mesenteric and cervical lymph nodes.

B cells reach these sites through the systemic circulation. Once they are stimulated by antigen and induced to differentiate, they home to the effector sites in the intestinal and respiratory lamina propria, where they differentiate into plasma cells and produce antibody mainly of the IgA isotype. An interesting characteristic of the plasma cells induced in the mucosal compartments is their selective homing to mucosal effector sites. Nasal activation leads to IgA-secreting cells with high levels of CCR10 and α4β1 integrin that home to the respiratory and genitourinary tracts in response to their ligands, CCL28 and VCAM-1. Migration to the intestinal lamina propria, in contrast, seems to be dependent on orally induced activation and subsequent expression on B cells of the chemokine receptor CCR9 and α4β7 integrin that bind to CCL25 and MADCAM1/VCAM-1, respectively.[56]

B Cell Activation and Differentiation

Upon encountering antigen, a B cell is triggered by the BCR signaling cascade to rapidly change its metabolic program from a quiescent to an activated state with an increase in glycolysis and upregulation of nutrient transporters.[57] Activated B cells, thus, amass energy and biomass needed for clonal expansion. The BCR signaling cascade ultimately initiates new gene expression that guides activated B cells to undergo either differentiation into memory B cells and plasma cells, or apoptosis. The end result of this process will depend on the characteristics of the antigen; the B cell subpopulation activated; the co-stimulatory signals provided by cytokines, growth factors, and T cells; and the microenvironment with its profile of nutrients and metabolites.

B Cell Receptor Signaling

The BCR complex is composed of surface Ig, noncovalently bound to a dimer formed by the molecules Igα and Igβ. The surface Ig on the naïve B cell includes both IgM and IgD. The role of surface Ig is to recognize foreign antigens; the Igα and Igβ molecules transduce the signal through their cytoplasmic tails that contain a particular amino acid sequence known as an *immunoreceptor tyrosine-based activation motif* (ITAM). This sequence contains two tyrosine residues that can be phosphorylated upon activation. After phosphorylation, the ITAM acts as a docking site for the Src homology-2 (SH2) domain to recruit tyrosine kinases and other signaling molecules.

BCRs on resting B cells are highly mobile within the plasma membrane, and they generate a ligand-independent tonic signal that is essential for B cell survival.[58,59] After cross-linking by antigen, BCRs aggregate and translocate to cholesterol- and sphingolipid-enriched membrane microdomains named *lipid rafts*.[60] The signal transduction events that occur after BCR cross-linking are mediated by the subsequent recruitment and activation of intracellular kinases including Lyn, Fyn, Btk, and Syk. The most proximal event after BCR cross-linking is the activation of Lyn, which results in the activation of the phosphatase CD45. CD45 removes the inhibitory phosphates on the ITAMs of Igα and Igβ, and the activation of Lyn leads to the activation of Syk and Btk.[58] There is evidence that ligation of CD19, an activating co-receptor of the BCR, leads to recruitment and activation of Vav, phosphatidylinositol 3-kinase (PI3K), Fyn, Lyn, and Lck.[61] Subsequently, the tyrosine kinases Syk and Btk are activated by tyrosine phosphorylation. The phosphorylation of Syk triggers the activation of phospholipase C (PLC), PI3K, and Ras pathways. The activation of Syk appears to be absolutely critical for BCR-mediated signal transduction because Syk-deficient cell lines exhibit a loss of BCR-induced signaling. Btk also appears to be required for the activation of second messenger pathways. In some patients with X-linked agammaglobulinemia, a mutation in the *Btk* gene results in impaired BCR signaling at the pre-B cell stage.[58] As a consequence, these patients have a greatly reduced number of mature B cells and generate poor antibody responses. In mice, however, a mutation in *Btk* leads to a disease known as *X-linked immunodeficiency.* B cell development is impaired at the transitional T2 stage, and B cells that do go on to maturity are unable to respond to certain T cell–independent antigens.

After recruitment and activation of the intra-cellular kinases, downstream pathways are initiated. Btk, Syk, and the adapter molecule BLNK are required for the activation of PLCγ. This leads to breakdown of phosphatidylinositol 4-phosphate to diacylglycerol (DAG) and inositol 1,4,5-triphosphate (IP_3) to trigger calcium release from intra-cellular stores and the subsequent translocation of nuclear factor of activated T cells (NFAT) to the nucleus. In addition, Btk activates Ras, which leads to nuclear translocation of the transcription factor activator protein-1 (AP-1). BCR cross-linking also activates mitogen-activated protein kinases (MAPKs) (Fig. 13.4).

Induction of these pathways ultimately transmits signals to the nucleus, where signals are integrated to regulate gene expression. One of the main transcriptional activators related to B cell activation is nuclear factor (NF)-κB, a family of transcriptional factors consisting of homodimers or heterodimers of different subunits. NF-κB regulates cellular processes leading to activation, differentiation into memory B cells and plasma cells, and apoptosis.

Co-receptors

Along with surface Ig, many molecules can modulate BCR signal transduction by either enhancing or diminishing the signal activated by antigen. These molecules include, but are not limited to, the B cell co-receptor complex (CD19/CD21/CD81/Leu-13), CD45, SHP1, SHP2, SH2 containing inositol 5-phosphatase

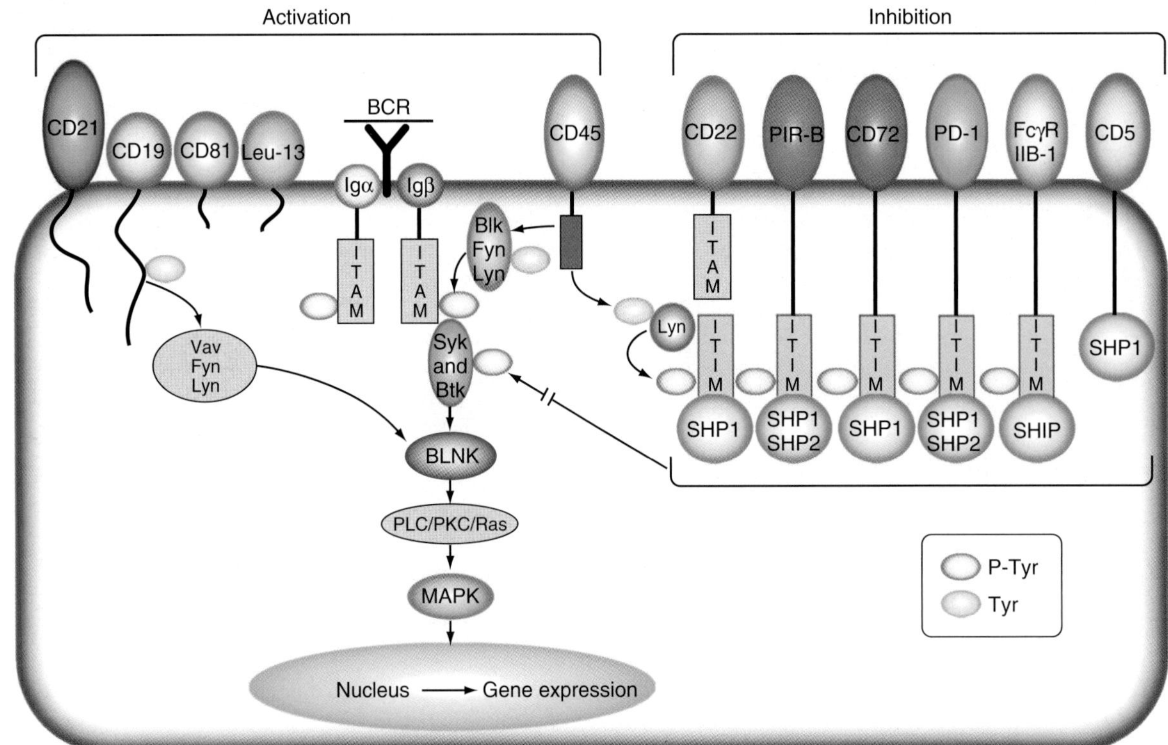

• **Fig. 13.4** Molecules that regulate the activation state of B cells. Co-ligation of surface immunoglobulin results in tyrosine phosphorylation at specific tyrosine residues present in the immunoreceptor tyrosine activation motif (ITAM) of Igα and Igβ cytoplasmic domains. This phosphorylation occurs after the removal of the inhibitory tyrosine residues of the B cell receptor (BCR)-associated cytoplasmic kinases such as Blk, Fyn, and Lyn, which is mediated by CD45. The phosphorylated ITAMs recruit and activate the Syk and Btk kinases, which in turn activate a series of second messenger pathways (PLC, PKC, and Ras) that result in the upregulation of genes required for B cell activation and survival. Co-ligation of the pre-BCR complex (CD19, CD21, CD81, and Leu-13) results in phosphorylation of tyrosine residues residing in the cytoplasmic domain of CD19. Cytoplasmic kinases including Vav, Fyn, and Lyn become activated and enhance the signaling mediated by the BCR. After the activation of distal mediators of BCR signaling such as PLC, PKC, and Ras, molecules of the mitogen-activated protein kinase (MAPK) pathway become activated and translocate to the nucleus to regulate gene expression. Signals mediated by CD22, PIR-B, CD72, PD-1, FcγRIIB1, and CD5 deliver negative signals that block the activation of distal molecules. After phosphorylation of the immunoreceptor tyrosine inhibition motif (ITIM), present in the cytoplasmic tail of these molecules, the phosphatases SHP1, SHP2, and SH2-containing inositol 5-phosphatase (SHIP) are recruited and activated.

(SHIP), CD22, FcγRIIB1, CD5, CD72, PIR-B, and PD-1 (see Fig. 13.4). The integration of all these signals sets the threshold for activation of the BCR signal.

The main positive regulator of B cell activation is the B cell co-receptor complex, composed of CD19, CD21, CD81, and an interferon-inducible molecule called *Leu-13*.[62] After antigen cross-linking of surface Ig, specific tyrosine residues contained within the CD19 cytoplasmic domain rapidly become phosphorylated. Although the natural ligand for CD19 is not known, in vitro studies have demonstrated that ligation of CD19 with anti-CD19 antibody lowers the threshold required for BCR-mediated B cell activation and enhances the proliferative effect of anti-IgM treatment on B cells.[63] A role for CD19 in B cell activation has been clearly defined in mice that either lack or overexpress CD19.[64] The CD19 molecule is required for T cell–independent and T cell–dependent B cell responses and for GC formation. The CD21 molecule serves as a receptor for cleavage fragments of the C3 component of complement. Cross-linking of the BCR and CD21 with complement-coated antigen has been proposed to trigger the activation of the cytoplasmic tail of CD19. Mice deficient in CD21 also have impaired responses to T cell–dependent and T cell–independent antigens and a defect in GC formation.[65] The functions of the remaining two components of the B cell co-receptor complex, CD81 and Leu-13, have not been characterized, although it is suggested that these molecules may mediate homotypic cell adhesion.

In contrast, CD22 that also associates with the BCR is primarily a negative regulator of BCR activation. Although CD22 contains an ITAM motif and is able to recruit Src tyrosine kinases to its cytoplasmic domain,[66] it also contains a specific motif known as the *immunoreceptor tyrosine-based inhibition motif* (ITIM). Similar to the ITAM, the ITIM contains a critical tyrosine residue. After activation of Lyn, it is believed that the ITIM of CD22 is phosphorylated by Lyn, leading to the recruitment and activation of phosphatases such as SHP1 that downregulate the activation cascade.[67]

FcγRIIB

Simultaneous ligation of both the BCR and FcγRIIB1 sends an inhibitory signal to diminish antigen activation of naïve and memory B cells. This inhibitory signal is activated by the presence of immune complexes and provides a negative feedback mechanism to attenuate an antigen-induced antibody response. After co-ligation of FcγRIIB1 and the BCR, Lyn phosphorylates FcγRIIB1.[68] The SHIP then associates with the FcγRIIB1 and mediates the dephosphorylation of phosphatidylinositol (3,4,5)-triphosphate (PIP_3), the major product of PI3K, thus inhibiting the recruitment and activation of Btk and Akt and attenuating BCR signaling.

CD5

The role of CD5 in B1a cell function is not well understood. After BCR cross-linking, CD5 is thought to mediate signals that induce apoptosis and block proliferation.[69] Cross-linking of CD5 with an anti-CD5 monoclonal antibody results in apoptosis. Some evidence indicates that CD5 recruits the inhibitory protein tyrosine phosphatase SHP1 to its cytoplasmic domain. However, unlike CD22 and FcγRIIB1, CD5 does not contain a consensus ITIM sequence and may recruit SHP1 indirectly.[70] The ligand-binding region of CD5 remains to be elucidated, but recent evidence suggests that CD5 may be a ligand for another negative regulator of BCR signaling, CD72.

CD72

CD72 is a transmembrane receptor that is expressed as a homodimer. The cytoplasmic tail of CD72 contains ITIMs. Mice with a targeted disruption of the CD72 gene reveal that CD72 plays a negative role in B cell activation, presumably through recruitment of SHP1. The B cell of CD72-deficient mice is similar to that of viable moth-eaten mice with expansion of B1 cells and B cells that are hyperresponsive to BCR cross-linking and are more resistant to BCR-mediated apoptosis.[71] There are several putative ligands for CD72, including CD5 and CD100.

Paired Ig-like Receptor

Paired Ig-like receptor (PIR)-A and PIR-B are expressed in a pairwise fashion, as the names imply. These receptors are believed to have opposing functions, with PIR-A inducing an activation signal and PIR-B inducing an inhibition signal. The ligands for PIR-A and PIR-B remain to be elucidated. Although little is known about the role of PIR-A in B cell activation, recent data demonstrate that PIR-B plays a role in downregulating B cell responses. The cytoplasmic tail of PIR-B possesses several ITIMs that recruit SHP1. Mice that harbor a targeted disruption of the PIR-B gene exhibit a phenotype similar to mice that are deficient in the other ITIM-bearing inhibitory receptors such as an expansion of B1 cells and B cell hyperresponsiveness.[72]

Programmed Cell Death Protein-1

Programmed cell death protein 1 (PD-1) is an inhibitory molecule expressed predominantly on activated B and T cells. The ligand-binding domain binds ligands PD-L1 and PD-L2, and the cytoplasmic tail of PD-1 contains ITIMs that recruit SHP2 to attenuate BCR signals. The B cells of PD-1–deficient mice are hyperresponsive to BCR signaling, and these mice display an augmented response to T cell–independent type II antigens. On certain genetic backgrounds, PD-1 deficiency leads to an autoimmune phenotype.[73]

Phosphatases

In general, intra-cellular signaling is regulated by a balance of phosphorylation and dephosphorylation. Protein tyrosine phosphatases (PTPs) play a major role in restraining the magnitude and duration of BCR signaling; among these, SHP1 is a potent negative regulator. SHP1 is found in association with transmembrane proteins such as CD22, FcγRIIB1, CD5, CD72, and PIR-B. SHP1 antagonizes BCR signaling by countering the action of protein tyrosine kinases.[70] The function of SHP1 has been extensively studied in mice that bear a naturally occurring mutation in the SHP1 gene. Mice with this genetic defect are known as *moth-eaten mice* because of the appearance of their fur. These mice have a decreased number of conventional B cells and an expansion of B1 cells, and they develop a fatal autoimmune and inflammatory disease.[74] The severe defect in B cell regulation underscores the importance of SHP1 in limiting the extent of BCR signaling. In contrast, the intracellular tyrosine phosphatase SHP2, although structurally similar to SHP1, seems to be a positive regulator of BCR signaling because it augments ERK responses.[75] The important role played by PTP in disease is also demonstrated by the discovery that a single mutation in the PTPN22, a protein that regulates Src family kinases, augments the risk of multiple autoimmune diseases.[76]

Another important regulator, SHIP, is an inositol phosphatase that inhibits B cell activation by removing the 5 phosphate from PIP_3, a critical component that recruits membrane association of pleckstrin homology (PH) domain containing signaling molecules, including PLCγ2, Btk, and Akt. Similar to SHP1 and SHP2, SHIP is recruited to an ITIM on FcγRIIB after BCR cross-linking. Mice deficient in SHIP display splenomegaly and elevated levels of serum antibody.[77]

Signal Transduction in Immature Versus Mature B Cells

An important event in BCR signaling is the recruitment of signaling components to lipid rafts, which are lipid-rich microdomains of the membrane that serve to bring together requisite signal molecules to facilitate integrated functions in three dimensions. After antigen engagement, the BCR translocates into lipid rafts and the BCR signaling cascade ensues because of the clustering of signaling components. In addition to activating signals, however, inhibitory components also localize to lipid rafts. As discussed later, BCR ligation mediates negative selection during the immature and transitional B cell stages and B cell activation during the mature B cell stage. The reason for these two distinct outcomes is not clear because the same signal components are present; however, differences in membrane cholesterol limit recruitment of the BCR to lipid rafts in immature B cells.[78] Evidence also indicates that the signal strength and duration and stage-specific expression patterns of signaling elements differ between immature and mature B cells.[79]

B Cell Activation

B cells develop without bias for a particular antigenic specificity, ensuring that a diverse repertoire of different Ig molecules is produced. After being stimulated by antigen and accessory cells such as DCs and T cells, antigen-activated B cells undergo clonal expansion; B cells that do not interact with antigen are destined to undergo programmed cell death in a matter of days or weeks. The B1 and B2 cell subsets are regulated by different activation mechanisms and are involved in different immune responses (Table 13.3).

TABLE 13.3 **Markers of Human Mature B Cell Subsets**

Characteristic	Naïve	Unswitched Memory	Switched Memory	B1
Surface IgM	High	High	Low	High
Surface IgD	Low	Low	High	Low
CD5	+	–	–	–/+
CD21	–	–	+	++
CD23	–	–	+	–
CD11b/CD18	+	+	–	–
Bone marrow progenitors	–	+	+	+
Self-renewal capacity	+	+	–	–
Response to T cell–independent antigens	+	+	+/–	+
Response to T cell–dependent antigens	+/–	+/–	+	+/–
Predominant isotype	IgM	IgM	IgG	IgM
Anatomic locations	Peritoneum, pleura, spleen	Peritoneum, pleura, spleen	Spleen, lymph nodes, Peyer's patches, tonsils, peripheral blood	Spleen, tonsils

CD, Cluster of differentiation; *Ig*, immunoglobulin.

B1 Cell Activation

B1 cells present in the pleural and peritoneal cavities respond to T cell–independent antigens. There are two classes of T cell–independent antigens: type I, which includes lipopolysaccharide, and type II, which includes large multivalent antigens with repetitive epitopes, often found on the surface of bacteria. T cell–independent antigens can directly activate B1 cells, resulting in the secretion of antibody. Soluble factors such as IL-5 and IL-10 also appear to be involved in the maintenance and activation of B1 cells.

B1 cells do not require interaction with antigen-specific T cells. However, activated T cells and macrophages may augment B1 cell activation, enhance Ig production, and influence isotype class switching such that B1 cells may also produce IgA and IgG.

Marginal Zone B Cell Activation

Marginal zone B (MZ B) cells are situated in the marginal sinuses, where specialized macrophages trap and remove antigen from the circulation. Like B1 cells, many MZ B cells express polyreactive BCRs that are specific for microbial antigens, including both protein and carbohydrate molecules. If micro-organisms reach the lymphoid organ from the blood, MZ B cells recognizing microbial carbohydrates elicit an innate-like T cell–independent response. MZ B cells can also mount a T cell–dependent response against microbial protein antigens. Soluble factors such as BAFF and T cell–derived cytokines are important for MZ B cell activation. MZ B cell activation can also be enhanced by CD40 ligand expressed on T cells, even though an antigen-specific (cognate) interaction with T cells is not necessary. Although the mechanism is not fully understood, MZ B cells are constitutively partially activated and differentiate rapidly into short-lived antibody-secreting plasma cells after activation by antigen. MZ B cells secrete predominantly IgM and, to a lesser extent, IgG antibodies without an affinity maturation process. Thus these antibodies display low to intermediate affinity.

Follicular B Cell Activation

Engagement of the BCR by antigen signals the B cells to engulf the antigen, process it intra-cellularly, and express peptide fragments bound to class II MHC molecules on its surface. After the expression of peptide fragments bound to class II MHC molecules, antigen-activated B cells present peptide to primed T helper (Th) cells. B cells and T cells interact through T cell receptor recognition of a peptide-MHC complex on the B cell and through engagement of co-stimulatory molecules B7 and CD40 on the B cell by CD28 and CD40L, respectively, on T cells (Fig. 13.5). Expression of the B7 molecule is upregulated on B cells after antigen stimulation. B cell activation during a T cell–dependent immune response also depends on engagement of the CD40 receptor expressed on B cells with the CD40 ligand (CD40L) expressed on T cells.[80] The importance of signal transduction events mediated by CD40-CD40L engagement is evident from studies of patients with X-linked hyper-IgM syndrome, an immunodeficiency disease resulting from a defect in CD40L. These individuals do not mount strong immune responses to T cell–dependent antigens; they have high concentrations of circulating IgM but only trace amounts of IgG and no affinity maturation of the antibody response. Th cells secrete cytokines such as IL-2, IL-3, IL-4, IL-5, IL-10, IL-17, IL-21, and IFN-γ and provide co-stimulatory signals that are important for B cell maturation and differentiation.[81]

Upon encountering antigen, a naïve B cell with high affinity for the antigen will activate and differentiate to a plasma cell that will secrete IgM or IgG antibodies without somatic mutations. If the activated B cell, however, harbors a receptor with low to intermediate affinity for antigen, the cell will migrate first to the border of the T cell zone and will begin the process of creating a GC.[82]

Germinal Centers

As B cells progress to form germinal centers (GCs), they interact with cognate T cells that are a specialized subpopulation of

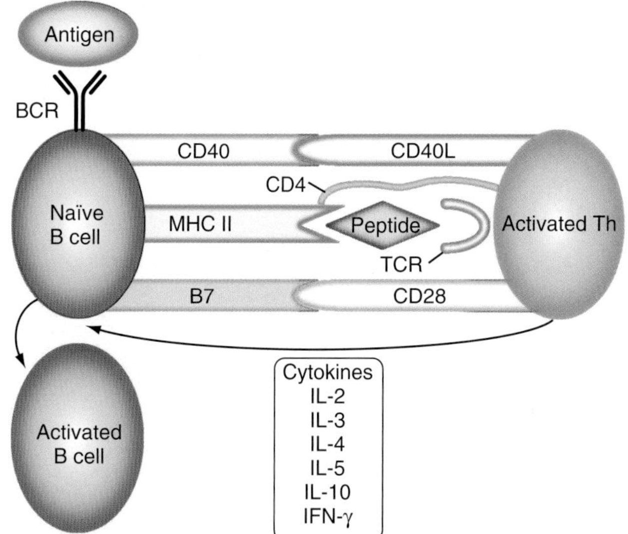

• **Fig. 13.5** B cells as antigen-presenting cells. Antigen bound to surface immunoglobulin on naïve B cells triggers endocytosis and intra-cellular processing of the antigen. B cells engage antigen-specific T helper (Th) cells through the recognition of foreign peptide by the T cell receptor (TCR) and through the binding of a conserved region of the class II major histocompatibility complex (MHC) molecule by CD4. Along with antigen binding, co-ligation of CD40 and B7 (expressed on B cells) with CD40L and CD28 (expressed on T cells) provides critical co-stimulatory signals and the secretion of cytokines required for B cell activation. *BCR,* B cell receptor; *IFN,* interferon; *IL,* interleukin.

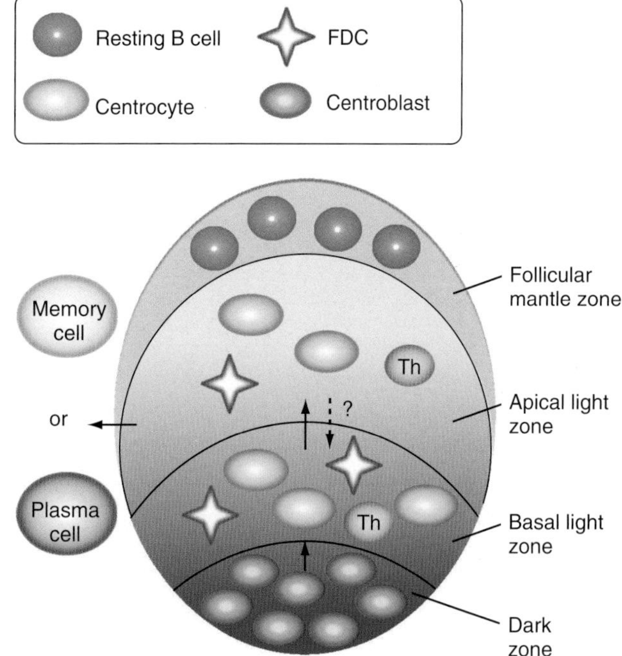

• **Fig. 13.6** B cell maturation in germinal centers. After exposure to antigen, B cells in the primary follicles form germinal centers or migrate to previously formed germinal centers. Centroblasts located in the dark zone undergo proliferation and acquire somatic mutations. A small number of proliferating centroblasts can give rise to a larger number of centrocytes present in the basal light zone. As these cells pass through a dense network of follicular dendritic cells (FDCs) and T helper (Th) cells, centrocytes bearing surface immunoglobulin receptors with high affinity for antigen undergo positive selection. Centrocytes in the apical light zone are nondividing cells that undergo differentiation into memory B cells or plasma cells. Centrocytes may return to the dark zone, where additional somatic mutations may be acquired. Resting B cells that are not activated by antigen are pushed aside to form the follicular mantle zone.

helper cells known as *Tfh cells.* The interaction between activated B cells and T cells through CD40 and CD40L induces expression of the transcription factor Bcl6 in both GC B cells and Tfh cells. Tfh cells express CXCR5 and S1P receptor 2 and therefore can migrate to and be retained in the B cell follicle, where, along with activated B cells, they form discrete structures known as *GCs.* It is in the GC that antigen-activated B cells undergo the process of class switch recombination (CSR) and affinity maturation through somatic hypermutation (SHM), and finally differentiate into memory B cells or long-lived plasma cells.

GCs can be subdivided into separate regions where the different stages of B cell differentiation take place (Fig. 13.6). The dark zone is the initial site of rapid proliferation, and B cells within the dark zone are called *centroblasts.* They are derived from a relatively small number of antigen-activated B cells (Table 13.4). Expression of the anti-apoptotic Bcl-2 protein is low in these cells, whereas expression of the proapoptotic Fas protein is upregulated. Low levels of Bcl-2 expression render developing B cells sensitive to apoptosis, but these cells can be rescued by antigen and CD40-CD40L interactions provided by antigen-specific Th cells. When these cells migrate to the light zone, they are termed *centrocytes* and encounter a dense network of FDCs and Tfhs (Fig. 13.7). B cells that express low affinity BCRs are outcompeted by B cells bearing higher affinity BCRs, whose enhanced antigen acquisition enables them to better interact with cognate Tfh, and thus they are selected to undergo more cell division.[83]

The process of SHM is activated during the centroblast stage. During this process, a nucleotide base-pair change is introduced in the DNA sequence of the variable region of Ig H- and L-chain genes, at approximately 10^{-3} per base pair per cell division. The mechanism for SHM is complex and requires the enzyme activation-induced cytidine deaminase (AICDA) to target to specific hotspot sequences.[84] The process of SHM is responsible for the affinity maturation of the antibody response. B cell clones that express surface Ig with an increased affinity for antigen are selectively expanded during the affinity maturation process, whereas B cells that express somatically mutated Igs with low affinity for antigen or novel binding to self-antigens are targeted for apoptosis or inactivation. The importance of somatic mutation and affinity maturation during an immune response is underscored by the fact that patients with mutations in the *AICDA* gene are immunocompromised.

AICDA is critical for not only somatic hypermutation but also for CSR. Although expression of IgM and IgD in B cells occurs through alternative splicing of a long transcript that contains coding regions for both the μ and δ chain, expression of any other Ig isotype requires the excision of all the H-chain genes between the recombined V(D)J region and the isotype to be expressed. Isotype switching requires preactivation of the particular H-chain locus to be involved in the recombination event, which is controlled by the cytokine milieu in which the cell is activated. AICDA induces the deamination of cytidine, creating dU:dG pairs (instead of dC:dG pairs) that activate the cellular DNA repair machinery and ultimately create circumstances that favor both CSR and SHM. For CSR, CD40-CD40L interactions and cytokines are also required.

TABLE 13.4 Markers of Antigen-Activated B Cells in Secondary Lymphoid Tissue

Marker	Naïve	Centroblast	Centrocyte	Memory	Plasma
Surface IgD	+	–	–	–	–
Surface IgM, IgG, IgA, or IgE	+	–	+	+	–
CD10	–	+	+	–	–
CD20	+	+	+	+	–
CD38	–	+	+	–	+
CD77	–	+	–	–	–
Presence of somatic mutation	–	+	+	+	+
Isotype class switch	–	–	+	+	+
Bcl-2	+	–	+/–[a]	+	+
Fas	+	+	+	+	–
AICDA	–	+	–	–	–
Blimp-1	–	–	–	?	+

[a]Bcl-2 is expressed in centrocytes only after interaction with follicular dendritic cells.

AICDA, Activation-induced cytidine deaminase; *Bcl-2*, B cell lymphoma 2; *Blimp-1*, B lymphocyte–induced maturation protein 1; *CD*, cluster of differentiation; *Ig*, immunoglobulin.

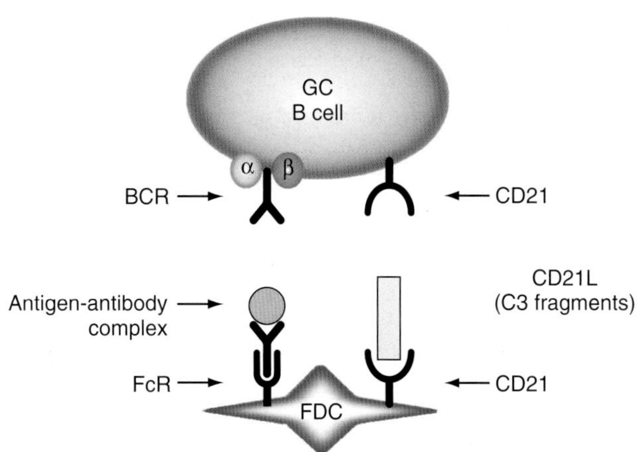

• **Fig. 13.7** Engagement of B cells with follicular dendritic cells (FDCs). Interaction between FDCs and B cells results in signals that mediate the positive selection of B cells in germinal centers (GCs). Antigen-antibody complexes trapped on the FDC surface deliver a signal to the B cell receptor (BCR). A second signal is delivered by the binding of CD21 on B cells to C3 complement components on the surface of FDCs. *FcR*, Fc receptor.

As centroblasts become centrocytes, they require survival signals from cognate Tfh cells to overcome their low level of Bcl-2 expression and high level of Fas expression. FDCs are stromal cells that trap antigen-antibody complexes by FcγR and complement receptors in bodies known as *iccosomes* (immune complex-coated bodies) on the cell surface. Iccosomes deliver an antigen-specific signal to B cells through the BCR (Fig. 13.8). Centrocytes with higher affinity BCR have a better chance to acquire antigen from FDCs and present antigen to cognate Tfh cells. These centrocytes receiving help signals from Tfh cells are saved from apoptosis by upregulation of the Bcl-2 molecule. Engagement of the complement receptors CR1 and CR2 (CD21 and CD35, respectively) on B cells by components of the C3 complement protein (iC3b, C3dg, and C3d) bound to FDCs may mediate a secondary co-stimulatory signal.[85] If centrocytes do not receive these positive selection signals, they rapidly die through a Fas-dependent pathway. Should they receive survival signals, they continue to differentiate into memory B cells or plasma cells.

Ectopic Lymphoid Structures

Despite being the prototypical structure for the induction of humoral immune responses, GCs are not found exclusively in lymphoid tissue. Ectopic lymphoid structures with GC-like characteristics are present in sites of chronic inflammation such as the synovium in people with rheumatoid arthritis, pancreatic islands in people with type 1 diabetes, and salivary glands of people with Sjögren's syndrome.[86]

These GC-like structures seem to develop as a consequence of chronic inflammation, which leads to the release of soluble mediators such as the chemokines CCL21 and CXCL12 that recruit lymphocytes.[87] These cells, once activated, secrete cytokines such as lymphotoxin that act in a paracrine manner and contribute to the organization of a GC-like structure that includes a dark and light zone with local induction of AICDA. In contrast to the GCs of the secondary lymphoid organs, these structures are not encapsulated. The B cells in these structures, therefore, are continuously exposed both to the local antigens that might be absent from the lymphoid organs[88] and to the inflammatory microenvironment that may facilitate bypass of the regulatory points in B cell differentiation, hence contributing to a potential autoimmune bias in these sites. Although no evidence exists that these structures are the underlying cause of any disease, in some diseases they may contribute to tissue pathology and augment the pool of

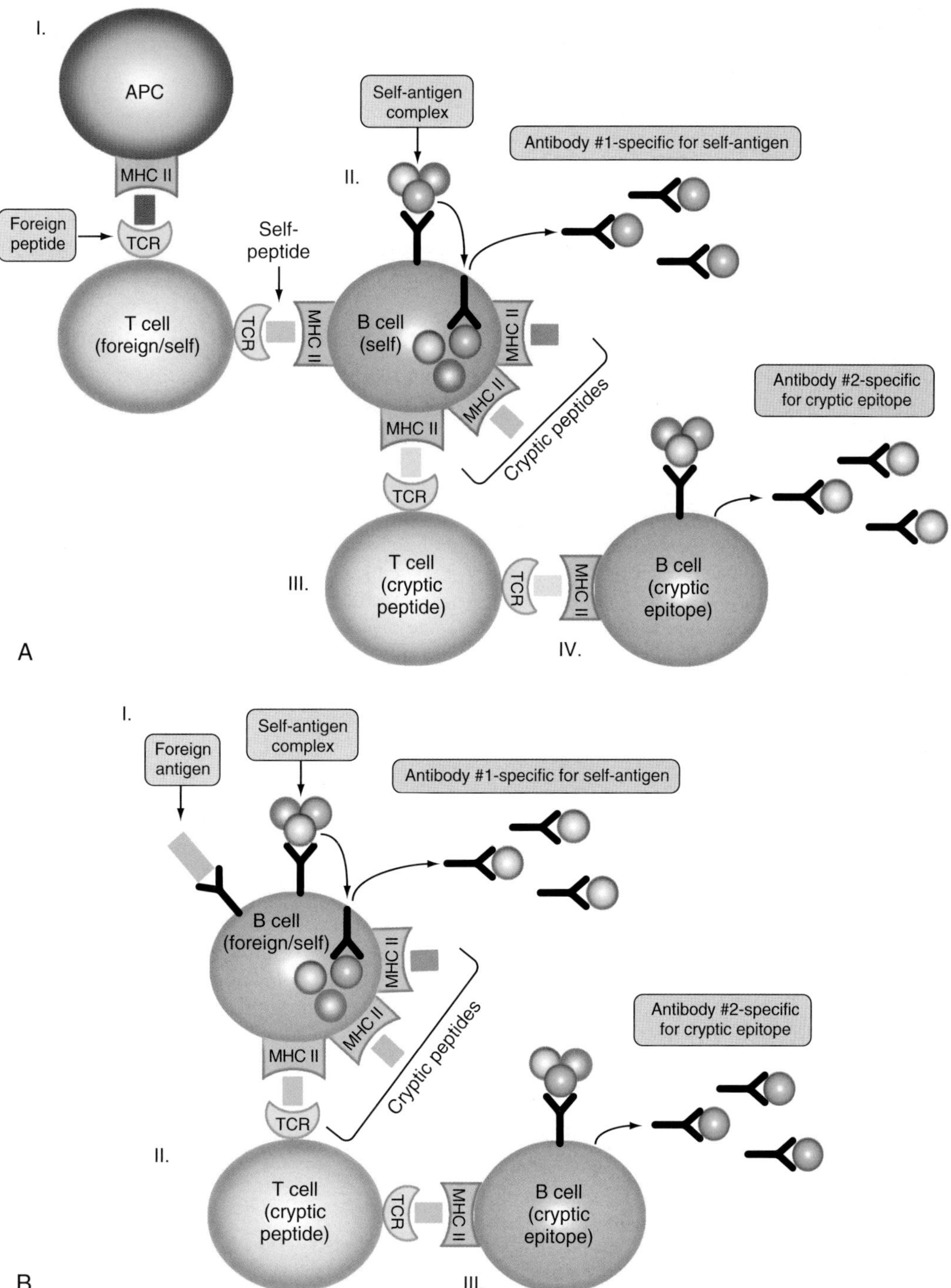

• **Fig. 13.8** Epitope spreading. (A) Epitope spreading by activation of cross-reactive T cells. *I,* After antigen presentation of a foreign peptide that is recognized by cross-reactive T cells, co-stimulatory signals are delivered to B cells with surface immunoglobulin receptors that recognize a self-antigen as part of a complex of self-molecules. *II,* The complex is engulfed by a self-reactive B cell, and antibodies specific for self-antigen are generated. *III,* Self-reactive B cells process the self-molecules and present cryptic peptide–class II major histocompatibility complex (MHC) complexes on the cell surface. *IV,* If these cryptic peptides are recognized by nontolerized autoreactive T cells, B cells specific for these cryptic peptides are activated, and the autoantibody response spreads to other components of the self-antigen complex. (B) Epitope spreading by activation of autoreactive B cells. *I,* A foreign antigen that mimics a self-molecule can mediate the endocytosis of a self-molecule that is included in a self-antigen complex. The self-molecules of the complex are processed and expressed on the cell surface of the B cell as cryptic peptide–class II MHC complexes. *II,* Cryptic peptides are recognized by nontolerized autoreactive T cells. *III,* These T cells provide co-stimulation to B cells that recognize cryptic peptides, resulting in the production of additional self-reactive antibodies. *APC,* Antigen-presenting cell; *TCR,* T cell receptor.

autoreactive plasma and memory cells. Not all ectopic lymphoid foci share characteristics with the GC. It is not known which structures are more damaging to tissue.

B Cell Differentiation

After antigen activation, B1 and MZ B cells rapidly differentiate into antibody-secreting plasma cells independent of T cell help. This innate-like humoral response generates mostly short-lived plasma cells that produce antibodies with low affinity, but it provides an early and fast protection against blood-borne microbes. It is antigen-activated follicular B cells that generate adaptive antibody responses through a GC reaction that give rise to long-lived memory B cells and plasma cells.

Memory B Cells

Postgerminal center memory B cells express Ig genes that have undergone CSR and SHM, and in humans they are distinguished by the presence of the marker CD27. The CD40-CD40L interaction contributes to directing GC B cells to mature into long-lived memory B cells. Like resting naïve B cells, memory B cells are in a metabolically quiescent state. Unlike naïve B cells, the survival of memory B cells does not depend on BAFF. The exact life span of memory B cells is unknown. It is postulated that these B cells either persist throughout the lifetime of the host[84] or are renewed constantly through either nonspecific stimulation[89] or antigen-specific stimulation.[90]

Quiescent memory B cells circulate throughout the body until specific antigen is re-encountered and triggers a potent secondary immune response. Memory B cells respond to antigen much faster, require lower amounts of antigen, and can even be induced in its absence by soluble mediators such as IL-2 or IL-15, in part because the BCR is already localized to lipid rafts. Subsequently, just like naïve B cells, memory B cells ingest antigen and express peptide–class II MHC fragments. After antigen presentation of peptide to Th cells, memory B cells undergo expansion and may differentiate to plasma cells.

Plasma Cells

The B cell differentiation cascade ends with the generation of a plasma cell. At the molecular level, the differentiation program is directed by the transcriptional repressor known as *B lymphocyte–induced maturation protein 1* (Blimp-1).[91] Blimp-1 induces a program in which plasma cells lose expression of several markers because they no longer express surface Ig, MHC molecules, or CD20. They initiate increased protein synthesis and secretion and consequently exhibit a large cytoplasm with a well-developed endoplasmic reticulum devoted to antibody production.

Blimp-1 also silences the expression of CXCR5, and thus B cells differentiating into plasma cells exit the lymphoid follicles and migrate to extrafollicular regions of secondary lymphoid tissue or to the bone marrow, where the final stage of plasma cell maturation occurs. B cells in the GC are induced to become plasma cells by IL-5, IL-6, and IL-21. Plasma cells have a variable life span that may be days for short-lived plasma cells that originate extrafollicular responses or years for long-lived plasma cells that arise from the GC response and home to the bone marrow.[92]

The longevity of plasma cells in the bone marrow depends on the presence of a niche that provides the survival factors CXCL12, IL-6, APRIL, and TNF. Cross-linking the FcγRIIb expressed by plasma cells induces apoptosis, a phenomenon that has been credited with pruning the plasma cell repertoire.[6]

Trafficking of Postimmune Cells

Plasma cells downregulate CXCR5 expression and elevate expression of EBI2, a chemotactic receptor that guides cells to outer follicle areas and extrafollicular regions. Both memory and plasma cells express CXCR4 that directs homing to the bone marrow but also allows localization in lymphoid tissues. Therefore CXCR4-expressing plasma cells can be found surrounding the GC or B cell follicles.[93] A subset of memory cells expresses CXCR3 and therefore migrates toward inflammatory chemokines such as CXCL9 and CXCL10.[94]

Nonconventional B Cell Activation

Although it is a central paradigm that B cells require cognate antigen for activation, infections induce an antibody response in which only a fraction of the responding B cells are specific for microbial antigen. This phenomenon, known as *polyclonal activation,* is induced by several mediators such as superantigen, cytokines, or noncognate T cell co-stimulation and leads to the production of self-reactive antibodies.

B cell superantigens include the *Staphylococcus aureus* protein A (SpA), the protein gp120 of HIV-1, and the erythrocyte membrane protein 1 of *Plasmodium falciparum.* These proteins share the ability to bypass the need to be recognized in the CDRs and bind instead to framework regions common to Ig gene families. They can therefore activate multiple clones; for example, SpA recognizes Igs of the V_H3 family that constitute up to 50% of the IgM repertoire.[95] Although the activation of multiple B cell clones by an organism might be seen as an advantage for the host, polyclonal activation leads to an extrafollicular response that, after a transient hyperglobulinemia, exhausts the B cell pool, leaving a vulnerable organism.

Noncognate activation of B cells clearly occurs in memory B cells that are easily activated by the presence of soluble mediators such as IL-2, IL-15, or CpG (see the Memory B Cells section).[89] In chronic infections, polyclonal activation seems to be a consequence of two nonmutually exclusive mechanisms. The simpler one is bystander activation of noncognate B cells by inflammatory cytokines. The second is $CD4^+$ T cell–mediated co-stimulation. Noncognate B cell activation carries the intrinsic risk of activating self-reactive B cells, as is observed in both experimental and natural infections.[96]

Mucosal T–Independent Class Switch Recombination

In the mucosa, IgA specific to commensal bacteria is induced through machinery that is T cell independent and occurs outside of organized lymphoid tissue.[97] Because this phenomenon is independent of T cells, other interactions must provide the required signals for CSR. One of the candidate molecules is BAFF, which is expressed by DCs in mucosal tissue. BAFF induces CSR in B cells in the presence of IL-10 or TGF-β, both of which are present in the mucosal microenvironment.[98]

Repertoire Selection

The ability to discriminate between foreign and self-antigens is as important as the capacity to mount a protective immune response. Any molecule derived from the intra-cellular or extra-cellular components of the host can be considered self-antigen; the censoring of the responses against these antigens occurs throughout B cell maturation and includes multiple mechanisms in the B cells themselves and in cells that cooperate in their activation and differentiation.

Tolerance

The random process of V(D)J recombination generates a diverse repertoire of BCRs that recognize virtually all antigens and thus, inevitably, also self-antigens. SHM during GC reactions also gives rise to B cells with autoreactive BCRs. These autoreactive B cells have to be purged by a process known as *tolerance*.

Tolerance is achieved through signals provided by the BCR, co-receptors, inflammatory mediators, and metabolic by-products that are integrated by the cell according to its developmental stage. BCR cross-linking during development or in the absence of co-stimulatory signals activates tolerance mechanisms in immature and transitional B cells. The same mechanisms that induce tolerance to self-antigen can induce tolerance to pathogens, and because some autoantigens are sequestered in sites of immune privilege, cells specific to them are not subject to tolerance mechanisms.

The tolerance mechanism depends on the developmental stage of the B cell and the strength of the BCR signal delivered by antigen. The strength of the signal depends on the degree of cross-linking of the BCR, which in turns depends on the concentration of self-antigen and the affinity of the antibody for self-antigen. With little receptor cross-linking, because of low antigen concentration or low affinity for antigen, there is no BCR signaling, and the autoreactive B cell is not tolerized. Three mechanisms mediate tolerance: receptor editing, anergy, and deletion. When mechanisms that regulate autoreactive B cells fail, the breakdown of self-tolerance can lead to the development of autoimmune disease.

During B cell development, autoreactive B cells are generated in the bone marrow after V(D)J rearrangement and expression of surface Ig on immature B cells. Because of the vast number of different antibody molecules that can be formed through the random recombination of H- and L-chain variable region genes and the random association of H- and L-chains, all individuals generate autoreactive B cells. The tolerance process that prevents the maturation of autoreactive B cells occurs with such efficiency that, despite the fact that more than 75% of immature B cells bear receptors with some degree of autoreactivity, about 30% of naïve B cells do so.[99]

Receptor Editing

A high degree of cross-linking of the BCR during development results in a process known as *receptor editing.* This process involves a secondary gene rearrangement of the H-chain or L-chain genes. Receptor editing requires reactivation of the recombination machinery and re-expression of RAG-1/RAG-2. When successful, receptor editing produces a BCR receptor with low or no affinity to the antigens present in its environment, and the cell is allowed to continue its development. RAG-1/RAG-2 can be seen in some cells in the GC or extrafollicular region as well, and some authors have interpreted this as evidence that receptor editing also occurs later in B cell development.

Deletion

Extensive BCR cross-linking also leads to apoptosis, thus deleting the autoreactive B cell. This was the first mechanism of tolerance described for B cells[100] and was long believed to be the main mechanism of central tolerance. However, deletion occurs only when cells are not able to decrease their autoreactivity by editing the BCR. Tolerance through deletion is mediated primarily through the activation of a series of endogenous proteases. In B cells the Fas pathway and the Bcl-2 pathway play important roles in regulating apoptosis.

Fas (also known as *CD95* or *Apo-1*), a member of the TNF receptor gene family, and Fas ligand are transmembrane proteins expressed on a variety of cell types. Clustering of Fas on the cell surface, which occurs when Fas molecules bind Fas ligand, activates apoptosis.[101] It appears that when B cells engage CD40L expressed on Th cells in the absence of BCR ligation, Fas signaling induces apoptosis.[102,103] Mutations in Fas *(lpr)* or Fas ligand *(gld)* in mice result in a SLE-like syndrome characterized by the production of pathogenic autoantibodies and lymphadenopathy. In humans, similar mutations lead to lymphadenopathy and anti-erythrocyte antibodies, but anti-DNA antibodies and glomerulonephritis are not found in these individuals.[104]

The Bcl-2 gene family is composed of molecules that either protect against or induce apoptosis in many cell types. Relative levels of these molecules dictate life and death of a cell. For example, excess Bcl-2 or Bcl-xL promotes cell survival, whereas excess Bax or Bim induces cell death.[105] Bcl-2 and Bcl-xL are upregulated at critical points during B cell development but can be easily counterbalanced on BCR cross-linking. The fact that certain mouse strains that overexpress Bcl-2 in B cells produce autoantibodies highlights the importance of apoptosis in tolerance.[106]

Anergy

Anergy is a hyporesponsive state considered to be induced in immature B cells when they undergo a modest degree of BCR cross-linking. Anergic B cells downregulate surface Ig receptors and display a desensitization of the BCR, blocking activation of downstream signaling. Anergic B cells are short lived. One group[107] performed classic studies on B cell tolerance induction in mice engineered to express an anti–hen egg lysozyme (HEL) antibody, along with soluble HEL, to act as a self-antigen. In the anti-HEL transgenic mouse model, B cells that encounter soluble, monovalent HEL are anergized. These B cells populate secondary lymphoid tissue but do not secrete anti-HEL antibody and are not recruited into B cell follicles. This phenomenon is known as *follicular exclusion.*[108]

Although anergy implies that the cells are not activated through BCR engagement, they *can* be activated by non–antigen-specific T cell co-stimulation, lipopolysaccharide, or IL-4. Exposure of anergic B cells in vivo to multivalent antigen in the presence of activated Th cells may also lead to their activation.[109] Consequently, it is suggested that anergic B cells may serve as a potential source of autoantibody and may be activated in inflammatory conditions.

B Cells as Immune Regulators

B cells produce cytokines in response to their environment. Several subsets of B cells have been reported to be able to suppress autoimmunity, including CD1d^{hi}CD5^{+} B cells and transitional B cells. All these B regulatory cells (Bregs) produce IL-10 to suppress immune responses.[110] The function of Bregs depends on stimulation through BCR and CD40. In healthy people, Bregs secrete IL-10 in response to CD40 engagement, whereas the equivalent population in patients with SLE fails to do so.[111] Bregs are also able to mediate immunosuppression through an IL-10–independent mechanism. Recent studies have identified IL-35 as an additional effector molecule for Breg function.[112,113] Some

IL-35–producing Bregs express CD138 and Blimp-1. Thus, activated B cells and plasma cells play an important role in regulating immune responses. These Bregs not only harness autoimmunity but also restrain immune responses against microbial infection.

Regulation by Small Molecules

Beyond the classic activators and regulators, the molecules described in the following sections play a particularly important role in the biology of B cells and are highlighted given their potential as biomarkers and therapeutic agents.

Vitamin D

Vitamin D is acquired from the diet or synthesized in the skin, followed by a conversion into a biologic product in the liver and kidney. The active metabolite, 1,25-dihydroxyvitamin D_3, decreases activation and proliferation of B cells, as well as differentiation to plasma cells. Circulating levels of vitamin D tend to be decreased in patients with autoimmune disease; whether this phenomenon contributes to the disease process is not known.

Estrogens

The role of estrogens in B cell–mediated autoimmune diseases has long been suggested by the female sex predominance within autoimmune diseases and may reflect a variety of effector mechanisms. However, estrogens modify the B cell repertoire, allowing survival of autoreactive B cells, and to alter the peripheral compartments in mice.[114]

Leptin

Although its first described role was as an endocrine hormone with a primary role in the control of metabolism, leptin later exhibited immune regulatory effects. For example, experimentally induced arthritis is attenuated in leptin receptor–deficient mice.[115] Leptin promotes B cell survival and proliferation through induction of Bcl-2 and cyclin D1.[116]

B Cell–Mediated Autoimmunity

B cell–mediated autoimmunity is the consequence of the production of self-reactive antibodies. We have detailed multiple mechanisms operating throughout B cell maturation and differentiation that are designed to avoid autoreactivity. The failure of only one tolerance checkpoint rarely leads to autoimmune disease[117]; it may, however, increase the level of circulating autoantibodies, without clinical disease.

The generation of a B cell–mediated autoimmune disease must involve (1) the generation of B cells bearing autoreactive BCRs; (2) failure of mechanisms that in the normal event will abrogate their maturation to short- or long-lived plasma cells; and (3) tissue malfunction induced by the autoantibody that leads to clinical symptoms.

Origin of Autoreactive B Cells

Theoretically, autoreactive cells can arise from any B cell subpopulation. In mice, B1 cells that bear BCRs with low affinities but high polyreactivity produce autoantibodies, but these autoantibodies help remove cellular debris and can protect the body from pathogenic autoreactivity. In addition, evidence indicates that MZ B cells secrete autoantibodies, which may also provide a physiologic rather than pathologic function.

A population of B cells, known as *autoimmunity-associated B cells (ABCs)*, has been found to expand in patients and mice with autoimmune diseases. ABCs display a unique phenotype, expressing the myeloid marker CD11c and the T-cell transcription factor T-bet. These cells seem to arise from antigen-experienced B cells driven by the T-bet transcriptional program. ABCs are not effectively activated by their BCR alone; however, when triggered with endosomal TLR ligands and IL-21 they rapidly switch from IgM to IgG2 production. ABCs from autoimmune animals and patients are reported to produce predominantly autoreactive IgG.[118,119]

Autoreactivity in the Preimmune B Cell Repertoire

Studies of the reactivity of human B cells have shown that in the healthy peripheral B cell compartment, about 30% of the naïve B cells bear some degree of autoreactivity; however, few of those can be considered potentially pathogenic given their low affinity for autoantigen.[99] In people with SLE, the frequency of autoreactive cells is as high as 50% in the naïve B cell population[120]; the frequency is greatest when disease is active and diminishes during periods of disease quiescence,[121] demonstrating that an inflammatory milieu may alter B cell selection.

Autoreactivity in the Postimmune B Cell Repertoire

Most of the autoantibodies in patients with autoimmune disease are generated through GC reaction because they have undergone CSR and display extensive somatic mutation. This observation suggests that the GC does not possess a fail-proof mechanism to effectively purge mutated autoreactive cells, although post-GC receptor editing and deletion of autoreactive B cells occurs. The understanding of the tolerance mechanisms that prevent the generation of autoreactive memory B cells and plasma cells is still incomplete.

Molecular Triggers of Autoimmunity

Several prevailing theories attempt to explain the activation and expansion of autoreactive B cells that should normally be silenced. Autoimmunity is thought to arise by a combination of environmental factors such as infectious agents that initiate an autoimmune response and genetic defects that alter B cell regulation. Proposed models for autoimmunity include (1) cross-reactivity of foreign antigen with self-antigen, (2) inappropriate co-stimulation, and (3) altered thresholds for BCR signaling.

Much of our understanding of the breakdown of self-tolerance and the progression of autoimmunity comes from the examination of mouse models. Autoimmune mouse models can be divided into two broad categories: induced autoimmunity and spontaneously occurring autoimmunity. Even though the progression of autoimmunity in humans is thought to be a highly complex process that involves multiple genetic and environmental factors, these animal models have provided much information about the molecular events that lead to a loss of self-tolerance.

Molecular Mimicry

One proposed model for the initiation of autoreactivity is that cross-reactive anti-self, anti-foreign B cells escape central tolerance because self-antigen is present at too low a concentration to trigger tolerance induction or because the affinity of the antibody for autoantigen is below the signaling threshold. These B cells become activated in the periphery by foreign pathogens resembling self-antigen and produce antibodies that bind both foreign and self-antigen. This cross-reactivity is known as *molecular mimicry*, and it is a popular model to explain the induction of many autoimmune disorders.[122] Once the pathogen is cleared, the autoantibody response is usually diminished because antigen-specific T cell help is no longer present, unless a high number of long-lived plasma cells have been generated. In the case of autoimmune-prone individuals, it is proposed that intrinsic B cell defects prevent the downregulation of autoantibody production, even after foreign antigen clearance. Several data support molecular mimicry as a trigger for B cell–mediated autoimmunity in some instances; for example, antibodies to infectious agents have been identified that cross-react with self-molecules associated with specific autoimmune diseases[123] (Table 13.5). Intriguing examples include the cross-reactivity observed between the M protein of group A *Streptococcus* and cardiac myosin in rheumatic heart disease and the cross-reactivity between *Campylobacter* and aquaporin.

Because both nonautoimmune and autoimmune-prone people have the capacity to generate autoantibodies, it is unlikely that cross-reactivity between foreign and self-antigens is solely responsible for breakdown of tolerance. A plausible explanation is that foreign antigen acts as a molecular trigger to initiate an immune response to self-molecules, and a defect in the mechanism that regulates B cell activation leads to the propagation of an autoimmune response.

In general, an initial immune response is generated against a dominant set of epitopes, followed by a later response to secondary or "cryptic" epitopes, a process known as *epitope spreading*.[124] Epitope spreading is an important aspect of a protective immune response because the ability to recognize multiple antigenic determinants increases the efficiency of the neutralization and removal of pathogens. When an autoimmune response has been triggered, epitope spreading can lead to the production of additional autoantibodies with specificity for multiple self-antigens. There are several proposed mechanisms by which epitope spreading triggers a cascade of T and B cell activation. For instance, antigen-presenting cells may present a foreign peptide that mimics a self-peptide to T cells (see Fig. 13.8A). Such cross-reactive T cells become activated and provide co-stimulation to autoreactive B cells that recognize self-antigen, which results in the production of autoantibodies specific for the antigen recognized by the T cell. After internalization of the self-antigen by the autoreactive B cells, the autoantigen is processed and new cryptic epitopes of the self-antigen are presented to T cells. A B cell binding to the self-antigen internalizes not only that self-antigen but also any complex of molecules that includes the self-antigen. The B cell may, therefore, present cryptic epitopes of many self-antigens and activate autoreactive T cells representing multiple autospecificities. In the periphery, T cells are present that have not been tolerized to these (cryptic) epitopes and thus are activated by self-peptide. These activated T cells in turn help provide co-stimulation and activate other autoreactive B cells.

Alternatively, cross-reactive B cells may be activated first after exposure to foreign antigen and T cell help (see Fig. 13.8B). These B cells internalize self-antigen and present cryptic peptides to T cells that have not been tolerized, leading to activation of autoreactive T cells and initiation of the cascade. Thus molecular mimicry and epitope spreading could lead to the activation of T cells and B cells specific for multiple autoantigens as long as the autoantigens form a complex in vivo.

TABLE 13.5 Evidence for Antibody Cross-Reactivity Between Foreign and Self-Antigens

Foreign Antigen	Self-Antigen
Yersinia, Klebsiella, Streptococcus[a]	DNA
Epstein-Barr virus nuclear antigen 1[a]	Ribonucleoprotein SmD
Streptococcus M protein[b]	Cardiac myosin
Coxsackie B3 capsid protein[c]	Cardiac myosin
Klebsiella nitrogenase[d]	Human leukocyte antigen B27
Yersinia lipoprotein[e]	Thyrotropin receptor
Mycobacteria heat shock protein[f]	Mitochondrial components
Escherichia, Klebsiella, Proteus[g]	Acetylcholine receptor
gpD derived from herpes simplex virus[g]	Acetylcholine receptor

Autoimmune disorders exhibiting cross-reactive antibodies: *a*, systemic lupus erythematosus; *b*, rheumatic fever; *c*, myocarditis; *d*, ankylosing spondylitis; *e*, Graves' disease; *f*, primary biliary cirrhosis; *g*, myasthenia gravis.

Supraoptimal B Cell Co-stimulation

It is evident that co-stimulatory signals provided by T cells play a critical role in B cell activation. Therefore inappropriate co-stimulation may lead to the propagation of an immune response directed against a self-antigen. The interaction between B7 on B cells and CD28 on T cells is crucial for the activation of antigen-specific T cells and B cells. When a genetically engineered protein that inhibits B7-CD28 interactions is administered to autoimmune mice, progression of disease is blocked.[125] Reciprocally, autoreactive B cells present in mice that constitutively overexpress B7 are not sensitive to Fas killing, and the mice display high serum autoantibody titers.[123] Overexpression of CD40 or CD40L may also activate autoreactivity. In vitro studies have demonstrated that CD40-CD40L ligation in the presence of IL-4 activates anergic cells. CD40L may be overexpressed in lymphoid cells of patients with SLE.[5,126]

Roquin-1/RC3H1, a putative ubiquitin E3 ligase, regulates differentiation of Tfh. Roquin-1 is an RNA binding protein that mediates mRNA degradation.[127] It represses the expression of multiple inflammatory cytokines, including ICOS, a co-stimulatory molecule that plays an important role in Tfh development and function. Tfh cells provide strong co-stimulation in the GC. Mice harboring a mutation in the gene encoding Roquin display high-affinity dsDNA antibodies as a result of increased numbers of Tfh and GC B cells.[128]

Interferon regulatory factor-4 binding protein (IBP) also regulates T cell co-stimulatory signals.[129] IBP is an activator of Rho guanosine triphosphatases (GTPases) and is recruited to the immunologic synapse after T cell receptor cross-linking to mediate the reorganization of the cytoskeleton. Mice deficient in IBP exhibit an autoimmune phenotype characterized by the production of dsDNA antibodies and glomerulonephritis. IBP plays an important role in the survival and effector function of memory T cells. In addition, IBP sequesters the transcription factor IRF4, thus preventing it from turning on expression of IL-17 and IL-21.[130]

TLRs belong to a family of pathogen recognition receptors that initiate innate immune responses to various components of pathogens. TLRs are expressed on the cell surface or are localized in the endosomes. Thus TLR4 on the plasma membrane binds bacterial lipopolysaccharides, and endosomal TLR7 and TLR9 recognize RNA and hypomethylated CpG-containing nucleic acid sequences, respectively, within B cells. Beside their role in DC maturation and T cell activation and differentiation, TLRs are directly involved in multiple steps of antibody responses. Some T cell–independent antigens, such as lipopolysaccharides (LPS), engage both BCRs and TLR signaling pathways that induce strong B cell activation. During a T cell–dependent response, co-stimulation of TLR enhances BCR-mediated uptake of antigen and boosts AICDA induction for CSR and GC reactions. TLR activation has also been linked with chronic inflammation and autoimmune diseases. Numerous studies suggest that engagement of the BCR and TLR with immune complexes containing nuclear antigens triggers the activation of anti-nuclear B cells, implying that TLR7 and TLR9 can function to enhance the activation of autoreactive B cells under some circumstances.[131–133]

B Cell Signaling Thresholds

The effects of altering the threshold for BCR signaling have been demonstrated in several mouse models. In transgenic mice that overexpress the BCR co-receptor complex component CD19, anergic B cells are activated and secrete autoantibody.[134] This result suggests that a decrease in the minimal requirement for antigen engagement of the BCR can lead to inappropriate activation of autoreactive B cells. Viable moth-eaten mice also develop an autoimmune syndrome due to a naturally occurring deficiency in the SHP1 phosphatase, a potent negative regulator of BCR signaling.[74] In these mice, B1 cells are responsible for the production of IgM anti-DNA antibodies. Transgenic mice deficient in other signaling molecules that alter threshold activation such as CD22[65] and Lyn[68] also produce autoantibodies. Thus, lowering thresholds for antigen-induced B cell activation can lead to the activation of autoreactive B cells.

It is now known that co-stimulation and the strength of T cell receptor signaling coordinate cellular metabolism and transcriptional programs to guide T cell differentiation into specialized effector subsets. It is not yet known whether parallel metabolic reprograming impacts B cell fates and functions. That anergic B cells are metabolically suppressed and that inhibiting glycolysis by 2-deoxy-glucose treatment in vivo seems to inhibit autoantibody production indicate that manipulations of immunometabolism can change the outcome of humoral responses.[135,136]

Conclusion

The generation of a diverse repertoire of antibody molecules provides an important line of defense against microbial infections. The immune system is exquisitely controlled at multiple levels to allow the maturation of B cells that produce protective antibodies while attempting to avoid the production of autoantibodies (Fig. 13.9). Only a small percentage of B cell precursors generated completes the

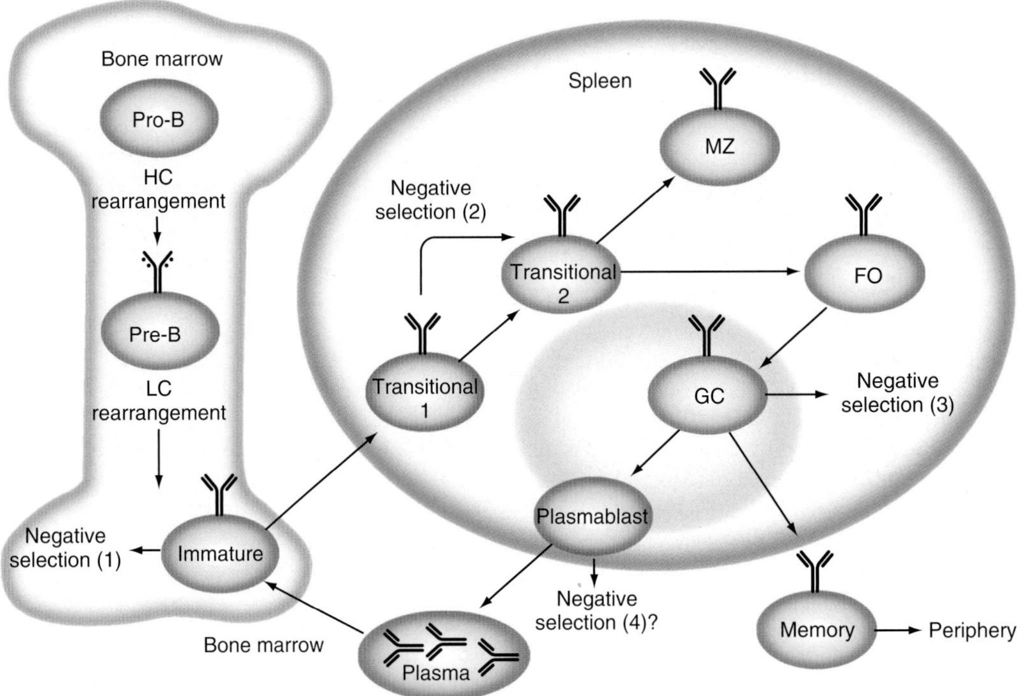

• **Fig. 13.9** Selection checkpoints during B cell maturation. Autoreactive B cells can be censored at multiple developmental checkpoints: *(1)* After surface expression of surface immunoglobulin, immature B cells that encounter autoantigen in the bone marrow are subject to negative selection. *(2)* B cells that are not eliminated in the bone marrow may undergo negative selection during the transitional B cell stage. Transitional B cells that emerge from this development stage give rise to follicular (FO) or marginal zone (MZ) B cells. Follicular B cells activated by antigen and the help of cognate T cells progress to the germinal center (GC) B cell stage. *(3)* Germinal center B cells that acquire high affinity for autoantigen by the process of somatic hypermutation may be eliminated in the germinal center to block their further maturation into long-lived plasma cells or memory cells. *(4)* There is evidence that autoreactive plasmablasts may also be subject to negative selection. Long-lived plasma cells that emerge from the selection process home primarily to the bone marrow, and memory B cells circulate throughout the periphery. *HC,* Heavy chain; *LC,* light chain.

maturation pathway. During the pro-B and pre-B cell stages of development, B cells with aberrantly rearranged H- or L-chain genes are eliminated. As the remaining precursor cells transit into the immature B cell stage, they are subject to negative selection; that is, immature B cells with autospecificity are either deleted or inactivated, whereas nonautoreactive B cells are released into the periphery. B cells that are stimulated by foreign antigen are selectively expanded and undergo further Ig gene diversification in peripheral lymphoid tissue. During this stage of development, B cells that express high-affinity BCRs undergo positive selection, whereas B cells with a diminished affinity or those that have acquired autoreactivity are eliminated. B cells that pass through these critical developmental checkpoints differentiate into long-lived memory B cells or plasma cells. The underlying causes of B cell–associated autoimmunity are not fully understood, but just as there are multiple checkpoints for the survival or activation of autoreactive B cells, it seems likely that multiple defects in the regulatory mechanisms that control B cell maturation and differentiation contribute to autoimmune disease.

Full references for this chapter can be found on ExpertConsult.com.

Selected References

1. Schroeder H, Wald D, Greenspan N: Immunoglobulins: structure and function. In Paul W, Editor: *Fundamental Immunology*, Philadelphia, Lippincott-Raven, 2008, pp 125–151.
2. Janeway C, Travers P, Walport M, et al.: The structure of a typical antibody molecule. In *Immunobiology*, New York, Garland, 2001, p 96.
3. Janeway C, Travers P, Walport M, et al.: Structural variation in immunoglobulin constant regions. In *Immunobiology*, New York, Garland, 2001, p 142.
4. Raghavan M, Bjorkman PJ: Fc receptors and their interactions with immunoglobulins, *Annu Rev Cell Dev Biol* 12:181–220, 1996.
5. Desai DD, Harbers SO, Flores M, et al.: Fc gamma receptor IIB on dendritic cells enforces peripheral tolerance by inhibiting effector T cell responses, *J Immunol* 178(10):6217–6226, 2007.
6. Xiang Z, Cutler AJ, Brownlie RJ, et al.: FcgammaRIIb controls bone marrow plasma cell persistence and apoptosis, *Nat Immunol* 8(4):419–429, 2007.
7. Johansen FE, Braathen R, Brandtzaeg P: Role of J chain in secretory immunoglobulin formation, *Scand J Immunol* 52(3):240–248, 2000.
8. Wiersma EJ, Collins C, Fazel S, et al.: Structural and functional analysis of J chain-deficient IgM, *J Immunol* 160(12):5979–5989, 1998.
9. Snapper C, Finkelman F: Immunoglobulin class switching. In Paul W, Editor. *Immunology*, Philadelphia Lippincott-Raven, 1999, p 831.
10. Froelich CJ, Hanna WL, Poirier GG, et al.: Granzyme B/perforin-mediated apoptosis of Jurkat cells results in cleavage of poly(ADP-ribose) polymerase to the 89-kDa apoptotic fragment and less abundant 64-kDa fragment, *Biochem Biophys Res Commun* 227(3):658–665, 1996.
11. Janssen EM, Lemmens EE, Gour N, et al.: Distinct roles of cytolytic effector molecules for antigen-restricted killing by CTL in vivo, *Immunol Cell Biol* 88(7):761–765, 2010.
12. Simister NE, Mostov KE: An Fc receptor structurally related to MHC class I antigens, *Nature* 337(6203):184–187, 1989.
13. Roopenian DC, Christianson GJ, Sproule TJ, et al.: The MHC class I-like IgG receptor controls perinatal IgG transport, IgG homeostasis, and fate of IgG-Fc-coupled drugs, *J Immunol* 170(7):3528–3533, 2003.
14. Macpherson AJ, McCoy KD, Johansen FE, et al.: The immune geography of IgA induction and function, *Mucosal Immunol* 1(1):11–22, 2008.
15. Woof JM, Kerr MA: The function of immunoglobulin A in immunity, *J Pathol* 208(2):270–282, 2006.
16. Yel L: Selective IgA deficiency, *J Clin Immunol* 30(1):10–16, 2010.
17. Pasquier B, Launay P, Kanamaru Y, et al.: Identification of FcalphaRI as an inhibitory receptor that controls inflammation: dual role of FcRgamma ITAM, *Immunity* 22(1):31–42, 2005.
18. Gould HJ, Sutton BJ: IgE in allergy and asthma today, *Nat Rev Immunol* 8(3):205–217, 2008.
19. Shan M, Carrillo J, Yeste A, et al.: Secreted IgD amplifies humoral T helper 2 cell responses by binding basophils via galectin-9 and CD44, *Immunity* 49(4):709–724 e8, 2018.
20. Chen K, Cerutti A: New insights into the enigma of immunoglobulin D, *Immunol Rev* 237(1):160–179, 2010.
21. Mulders-Manders CM, Simon A: Hyper-IgD syndrome/mevalonate kinase deficiency: what is new? *Semin Immunopathol* 37(4):371–376, 2015.
22. Gorman JR, Alt FW: Regulation of immunoglobulin light chain isotype expression, *Adv Immunol* 69:113–181, 1998.
23. Brack C, Hirama M, Lenhard-Schuller R, et al.: A complete immunoglobulin gene is created by somatic recombination, *Cell* 15(1):1–14, 1978.
24. Croce CM, Shander M, Martinis J, et al.: Chromosomal location of the genes for human immunoglobulin heavy chains, *Proc Natl Acad Sci U S A* 76(7):3416–3419, 1979.
25. McBride OW, Hieter PA, Hollis GF, et al.: Chromosomal location of human kappa and lambda immunoglobulin light chain constant region genes, *J Exp Med* 155(5):1480–1490, 1982.
26. Lefranc M: Nomenclature of the human immunoglobulin genes, *Curr Protoc Immmunol Appedix* 1, 2001. Appendix 1P.
27. Thomas LR, Cobb RM, Oltz EM: Dynamic regulation of antigen receptor gene assembly, *Adv Exp Med Biol* 650:103–115, 2009.
28. Akira S, Okazaki K, Sakano H: Two pairs of recombination signals are sufficient to cause immunoglobulin V-(D)-J joining, *Science* 238(4830):1134–1138, 1987.
29. Ramirez J, Lukin K, Hagman J: From hematopoietic progenitors to B cells: mechanisms of lineage restriction and commitment, *Curr Opin Immunol* 22(2):177–184, 2010.
30. Nutt SL, Heavey B, Rolink AG, et al.: Commitment to the B-lymphoid lineage depends on the transcription factor Pax5, *Nature* 401(6753):556–562, 1999.
31. Solvason N, Kearney JF: The human fetal omentum: a site of B cell generation, *J Exp Med* 175(2):397–404, 1992.
32. Igarashi H, Kouro T, Yokota T, et al.: Age and stage dependency of estrogen receptor expression by lymphocyte precursors, *Proc Natl Acad Sci U S A* 98(26):15131–15136, 2001.
33. Souto-Carneiro MM, Sims GP, Girschik H, et al.: Developmental changes in the human heavy chain CDR3, *J Immunol* 175(11):7425–7436, 2005.
34. Coulomb-L'Hermin A, Amara A, Schiff C, et al.: Stromal cell-derived factor 1 (SDF-1) and antenatal human B cell lymphopoiesis: expression of SDF-1 by mesothelial cells and biliary ductal plate epithelial cells, *Proc Natl Acad Sci U S A* 96(15):8585–8590, 1999.
35. Gupta P, McCarthy JB, Verfaillie CM: Stromal fibroblast heparan sulfate is required for cytokine-mediated ex vivo maintenance of human long-term culture-initiating cells, *Blood* 87(8):3229–3236, 1996.
36. Melchers F: Checkpoints that control B cell development, *J Clin Invest* 125(6):2203–2210, 2015.
37. Duchosal MA: B-cell development and differentiation, *Semin Hematol* 34(1 Suppl 1):2–12, 1997.
38. Herzog S, Reth M, Jumaa H: Regulation of B-cell proliferation and differentiation by pre-B-cell receptor signalling, *Nat Rev Immunol* 9(3):195–205, 2009.
39. Ohnishi K, Melchers F: The nonimmunoglobulin portion of lambda5 mediates cell-autonomous pre-B cell receptor signaling, *Nat Immunol* 4(9):849–856, 2003.

40. Lortan JE, Oldfield S, Roobottom CA, et al.: Migration of newly-produced virgin B cells from bone marrow to secondary lymphoid organs, *Adv Exp Med Biol* 237:87–92, 1988.
41. Mackay F, Schneider P: Cracking the BAFF code, *Nat Rev Immunol* 9(7):491–502, 2009.
42. Mackay F, Woodcock SA, Lawton P, et al.: Mice transgenic for BAFF develop lymphocytic disorders along with autoimmune manifestations, *J Exp Med* 190(11):1697–1710, 1999.
43. Moisini I, Davidson A: BAFF: a local and systemic target in autoimmune diseases, *Clin Exp Immunol* 158(2):155–163, 2009.
44. Carsetti R, Rosado MM, Wardmann H: Peripheral development of B cells in mouse and man, *Immunol Rev* 197:179–191, 2004.
45. Gross JA, Dillon SR, Mudri S, et al.: TACI-Ig neutralizes molecules critical for B cell development and autoimmune disease. Impaired B cell maturation in mice lacking BLyS, *Immunity* 15(2):289–302, 2001.
46. Wirths S, Lanzavecchia A: ABCB1 transporter discriminates human resting naive B cells from cycling transitional and memory B cells, *Eur J Immunol* 35(12):3433–3441, 2005.
47. Weller S, Braun MC, Tan BK, et al.: Human blood IgM "memory" B cells are circulating splenic marginal zone B cells harboring a prediversified immunoglobulin repertoire, *Blood* 104(12):3647–3654, 2004.
48. Kruetzmann S, Rosado MM, Weber H, et al.: Human immunoglobulin M memory B cells controlling Streptococcus pneumoniae infections are generated in the spleen, *J Exp Med* 197(7):939–945, 2003.
49. Weill JC, Weller S, Reynaud CA: Human marginal zone B cells, *Annu Rev Immunol* 27:267–285, 2009.
50. Griffin DO, Holodick NE, Rothstein TL: Human B1 cells in umbilical cord and adult peripheral blood express the novel phenotype CD20+ CD27+ CD43+ CD70, *J Exp Med* 208(1):67–80, 2011.
51. Manser T: Textbook germinal centers? *J Immunol* 172(6):3369–3375, 2004.
52. Kim CH: The greater chemotactic network for lymphocyte trafficking: chemokines and beyond, *Curr Opin Hematol* 12(4):298–304, 2005.
53. Muller G, Lipp M: Concerted action of the chemokine and lymphotoxin system in secondary lymphoid-organ development, *Curr Opin Immunol* 15(2):217–224, 2003.
54. Pereira JP, Kelly LM, Cyster JG: Finding the right niche: B-cell migration in the early phases of T-dependent antibody responses, *Int immunol* 22(6):413–419, 2010.
55. Allen CD, Ansel KM, Low C, et al.: Germinal center dark and light zone organization is mediated by CXCR4 and CXCR5, *Nat Immunol* 5(9):943–952, 2004.
56. Kiyono H, Fukuyama S: NALT- versus Peyer's-patch-mediated mucosal immunity, *Nat Rev Immunol* 4(9):699–710, 2004.
57. Boothby M, Rickert RC: Metabolic regulation of the immune humoral response, *Immunity* 46(5):743–755, 2017.
58. Kurosaki T: Molecular mechanisms in B cell antigen receptor signaling, *Curr Opin Immunol* 9(3):309–318, 1997.
59. Treanor B, Depoil D, Gonzalez-Granja A, et al.: The membrane skeleton controls diffusion dynamics and signaling through the B cell receptor, *Immunity* 32(2):187–199, 2010.
60. Cherukuri A, Dykstra M, Pierce SK: Floating the raft hypothesis: lipid rafts play a role in immune cell activation, *Immunity* 14(6):657–660, 2001.
61. Sato S, Jansen PJ, Tedder TF: CD19 and CD22 expression reciprocally regulates tyrosine phosphorylation of Vav protein during B lymphocyte signaling, *Proc Natl Acad Sci U S A* 94(24):13158–13162, 1997.
62. Bradbury LE, Kansas GS, Levy S, et al.: The CD19/CD21 signal transducing complex of human B lymphocytes includes the target of antiproliferative antibody-1 and Leu-13 molecules, *J Immunol* 149(9):2841–2850, 1992.
63. Carter RH, Fearon DT: CD19: lowering the threshold for antigen receptor stimulation of B lymphocytes, *Science* 256(5053):105–107, 1992.
64. Tedder TF, Inaoki M, Sato S: The CD19-CD21 complex regulates signal transduction thresholds governing humoral immunity and autoimmunity, *Immunity* 6(2):107–118, 1997.
65. Haas KM, Hasegawa M, Steeber DA, et al.: Complement receptors CD21/35 link innate and protective immunity during Streptococcus pneumoniae infection by regulating IgG3 antibody responses, *Immunity* 17(6):713–723, 2002.
66. Sato S, Miller AS, Inaoki M, et al.: CD22 is both a positive and negative regulator of B lymphocyte antigen receptor signal transduction: altered signaling in CD22-deficient mice, *Immunity* 5(6):551–562, 1996.
67. Muller J, Nitschke L: The role of CD22 and Siglec-G in B-cell tolerance and autoimmune disease, *Nat Rev Rheumatol* 10(7):422–428, 2014.
68. Chan VW, Meng F, Soriano P, et al.: Characterization of the B lymphocyte populations in Lyn-deficient mice and the role of Lyn in signal initiation and down-regulation, *Immunity* 7(1):69–81, 1997.
69. Bikah G, Carey J, Ciallella JR, et al.: CD5-mediated negative regulation of antigen receptor-induced growth signals in B-1 B cells, *Science* 274(5294):1906–1909, 1996.
70. Neel BG: Role of phosphatases in lymphocyte activation, *Curr Opin Immunol* 9(3):405–420, 1997.
71. Pan C, Baumgarth N, Parnes JR: CD72-deficient mice reveal non-redundant roles of CD72 in B cell development and activation, *Immunity* 11(4):495–506, 1999.
72. Ujike A, Takeda K, Nakamura A, et al.: Impaired dendritic cell maturation and increased T(H)2 responses in PIR-B(-/-) mice, *Nat Immunol* 3(6):542–548, 2002.
73. Nishimura H, Nose M, Hiai H, et al.: Development of lupus-like autoimmune diseases by disruption of the PD-1 gene encoding an ITIM motif-carrying immunoreceptor, *Immunity* 11(2):141–151, 1999.
74. Westhoff CM, Whittier A, Kathol S, et al.: DNA-binding antibodies from viable motheaten mutant mice: implications for B cell tolerance, *J Immunol* 159(6):3024–3033, 1997.
75. Qu CK, Yu WM, Azzarelli B, et al.: Biased suppression of hematopoiesis and multiple developmental defects in chimeric mice containing Shp-2 mutant cells, *Mol Cell Biol* 18(10):6075–6082, 1998.
76. Gregersen PK, Lee HS, Batliwalla F, et al.: PTPN22: setting thresholds for autoimmunity, *Semin Immunol* 18(4):214–223, 2006.
77. Helgason CD, Kalberer CP, Damen JE, et al.: A dual role for Src homology 2 domain-containing inositol-5-phosphatase (SHIP) in immunity: aberrant development and enhanced function of b lymphocytes in ship -/- mice, *J Exp Med* 191(5):781–794, 2000.
78. Karnell FG, Brezski RJ, King LB, et al.: Membrane cholesterol content accounts for developmental differences in surface B cell receptor compartmentalization and signaling, *J Biol Chem* 280(27):25621–25628, 2005.
79. Harnett MM, Katz E, Ford CA: Differential signalling during B-cell maturation, *Immunol Lett* 98(1):33–44, 2005.
80. van Kooten C, Banchereau J: Functional role of CD40 and its ligand, *Int Arch Allergy Immunol* 113(4):393–399, 1997.
81. Abbas AK, Murphy KM, Sher A: Functional diversity of helper T lymphocytes, *Nature* 383(6603):787–793, 1996.
82. Paus D, Phan TG, Chan TD, et al.: Antigen recognition strength regulates the choice between extrafollicular plasma cell and germinal center B cell differentiation, *J Exp Med* 203(4):1081–1091, 2006.
83. Gitlin AD, Shulman Z, Nussenzweig MC: Clonal selection in the germinal centre by regulated proliferation and hypermutation, *Nature* 509(7502):637–640, 2014.
84. Maruyama M, Lam KP, Rajewsky K: Memory B-cell persistence is independent of persisting immunizing antigen, *Nature* 407(6804):636–642, 2000.

85. Tew JG, Wu J, Qin D, et al.: Follicular dendritic cells and presentation of antigen and costimulatory signals to B cells, *Immunol Rev* 156:39–52, 1997.
86. Schroder AE, Greiner A, Seyfert C, et al.: Differentiation of B cells in the nonlymphoid tissue of the synovial membrane of patients with rheumatoid arthritis, *Proc Natl Acad Sci U S A* 93(1):221–225, 1996.
87. Gommerman JL, Browning JL: Lymphotoxin/light, lymphoid microenvironments and autoimmune disease, *Nat Rev Immunol* 3(8):642–655, 2003.
88. Aloisi F, Pujol-Borrell R: Lymphoid neogenesis in chronic inflammatory diseases, *Nat Rev Immunol* 6(3):205–217, 2006.
89. Bernasconi NL, Traggiai E, Lanzavecchia A: Maintenance of serological memory by polyclonal activation of human memory B cells, *Science* 298(5601):2199–2202, 2002.
90. Bachmann MF, Odermatt B, Hengartner H, et al.: Induction of long-lived germinal centers associated with persisting antigen after viral infection, *J Exp Med* 183(5):2259–2269, 1996.
91. Shaffer AL, Lin KI, Kuo TC, et al.: Blimp-1 orchestrates plasma cell differentiation by extinguishing the mature B cell gene expression program, *Immunity* 17(1):51–62, 2002.
92. Slifka MK, Ahmed R: Long-lived plasma cells: a mechanism for maintaining persistent antibody production, *Curr Opin Immunol* 10(3):252–258, 1998.
93. Kunkel EJ, Butcher EC: Plasma-cell homing, *Nat Rev Immunol* 3(10):822–829, 2003.
94. Muehlinghaus G, Cigliano L, Huehn S, et al.: Regulation of CXCR3 and CXCR4 expression during terminal differentiation of memory B cells into plasma cells, *Blood* 105(10):3965–3971, 2005.
95. Silverman GJ, Goodyear CS: Confounding B-cell defences: lessons from a staphylococcal superantigen, *Nat Rev Immunol* 6(6):465–475, 2006.
96. Hunziker L, Recher M, Macpherson AJ, et al.: Hypergammaglobulinemia and autoantibody induction mechanisms in viral infections, *Nat Immunol* 4(4):343–349, 2003.
97. Macpherson AJ, Gatto D, Sainsbury E, et al.: A primitive T cell-independent mechanism of intestinal mucosal IgA responses to commensal bacteria, *Science* 288(5474):2222–2226, 2000.
98. Litinskiy MB, Nardelli B, Hilbert DM, et al.: DCs induce CD40-independent immunoglobulin class switching through BLyS and APRIL, *Nat Immunol* 3(9):822–829, 2002.
99. Wardemann H, Yurasov S, Schaefer A, et al.: Predominant autoantibody production by early human B cell precursors, *Science* 301(5638):1374–1377, 2003.
100. Hartley SB, Goodnow CC: Censoring of self-reactive B cells with a range of receptor affinities in transgenic mice expressing heavy chains for a lysozyme-specific antibody, *Int Immunol* 6(9):1417–1425, 1994.
101. Ashkenazi A, Dixit VM: Death receptors: signaling and modulation, *Science* 281(5381):1305–1308, 1998.
102. Garrone P, Neidhardt EM, Garcia E, et al.: Fas ligation induces apoptosis of CD40-activated human B lymphocytes, *J Exp Med* 182(5):1265–1273, 1995.
103. Schattner EJ, Elkon KB, Yoo DH, et al.: CD40 ligation induces Apo-1/Fas expression on human B lymphocytes and facilitates apoptosis through the Apo-1/Fas pathway, *J Exp Med* 182(5):1557–1565, 1995.
104. Elkon KB, Marshak-Rothstein A: B cells in systemic autoimmune disease: recent insights from Fas-deficient mice and men, *Curr Opin Immunol* 8(6):852–859, 1996.
105. Knudson CM, Korsmeyer SJ: Bcl-2 and Bax function independently to regulate cell death, *Nat Genet* 16(4):358–363, 1997.
106. Strasser A, Whittingham S, Vaux DL, et al.: Enforced BCL2 expression in B-lymphoid cells prolongs antibody responses and elicits autoimmune disease, *Proc Natl Acad Sci U S A* 88(19):8661–8665, 1991.
107. Goodnow CC, Crosbie J, Adelstein S, et al.: Altered immunoglobulin expression and functional silencing of self-reactive B lymphocytes in transgenic mice, *Nature* 334(6184):676–682, 1988.
108. Cyster JG, Hartley SB, Goodnow CC: Competition for follicular niches excludes self-reactive cells from the recirculating B-cell repertoire, *Nature* 371(6496):389–395, 1994.
109. Cooke MP, Heath AW, Shokat KM, et al.: Immunoglobulin signal transduction guides the specificity of B cell-T cell interactions and is blocked in tolerant self-reactive B cells, *J Exp Med* 179(2):425–438, 1994.
110. Mauri C: Regulation of immunity and autoimmunity by B cells, *Curr Opin Immunol* 22(6):761–767, 2010.
111. Blair PA, Norena LY, Flores-Borja F, et al.: CD19(+)CD24(hi) CD38(hi) B cells exhibit regulatory capacity in healthy individuals but are functionally impaired in systemic lupus erythematosus patients, *Immunity* 32(1):129–140, 2010.
112. Shen P, Roch T, Lampropoulou V, et al.: IL-35-producing B cells are critical regulators of immunity during autoimmune and infectious diseases, *Nature* 507(7492):366–370, 2014.
113. Wang RX, Yu CR, Dambuza IM, et al.: Interleukin-35 induces regulatory B cells that suppress autoimmune disease, *Nat Med* 20(6):633–641, 2014.
114. Grimaldi CM, Cleary J, Dagtas AS, et al.: Estrogen alters thresholds for B cell apoptosis and activation, *J Clin Invest* 109(12):1625–1633, 2002.
115. Busso N, So A, Chobaz-Peclat V, et al.: Leptin signaling deficiency impairs humoral and cellular immune responses and attenuates experimental arthritis, *J Immunol* 168(2):875–882, 2002.
116. Lam QL, Wang S, Ko OK, et al.: Leptin signaling maintains B-cell homeostasis via induction of Bcl-2 and Cyclin D1, *Proc Natl Acad Sci U S A* 107(31):13812–13817, 2010.
117. Goodnow CC: Multistep pathogenesis of autoimmune disease, *Cell* 130(1):25–35, 2007.
118. Phalke S, Marrack P: Age (autoimmunity) associated B cells (ABCs) and their relatives, *Curr Opin Immunol* 55:75–80, 2018.
119. Rubtsova K, Rubtsov AV, Cancro MP, et al.: Age-associated B cells: A T-bet-dependent effector with roles in protective and pathogenic immunity, *J Immunol* 195(5):1933–1937, 2015.
120. Yurasov S, Wardemann H, Hammersen J, et al.: Defective B cell tolerance checkpoints in systemic lupus erythematosus, *J Exp Med* 201(5):703–711, 2005.

14 Fibroblasts and Fibroblast-like Synoviocytes

CHRISTOPHER D. BUCKLEY AND ANDREW FILER

KEY POINTS

- Fibroblasts are programmed epigenetically to determine the unique structure and function of different organs and tissues. These unique features might contribute to organ-specific disease.
- Tissue fibroblasts may be recruited from a number of sources and cell types including the bone marrow, blood, and local stromal cells and act as organ-specific innate immune sentinel cells.
- Under inflammatory conditions, fibroblasts become key immune system players by recruiting and modulating the behavior and survival of infiltrating immune cells.
- Fibroblasts can be programmed epigenetically through exposure to inflammatory and environmental stress such that they inappropriately prolong inflammation, which becomes persistent.
- Within the synovium, persistent abnormal behavior of fibroblasts in some diseases like rheumatoid arthritis results in continued damage to vital joint structures such as cartilage and bone, which, if untreated, will result in deformity and functional impairment.
- Recent advances in single cell transcriptomic analysis have demonstrated subpopulations of fibroblasts with discrete markers and functions within the synovium, with the potential to develop novel therapeutic approaches.

What Is a Fibroblast?

The architecture of organs and tissues is closely adapted to their function to provide microenvironments in which specialized functions may be carried out efficiently. The nature and character of such microenvironments are primarily defined by the stromal cells that reside within the tissues. The most abundant cell types of the stroma are fibroblasts, which are responsible for the synthesis and remodeling of extra-cellular matrix (ECM) components. In addition, their ability to produce and respond to growth factors and cytokines allows reciprocal interactions with adjacent epithelial and endothelial structures and with infiltrating leukocytes. Fibroblasts also integrate microenvironmental stimuli such as oxygen tension and pH. As a consequence, fibroblasts play a critical role during tissue development and homeostasis and are often described as having a "landscaping" function.

Fibroblast Identity and Microenvironments

Tissue-resident macrophages in the liver (Kupffer cells) and lung (alveolar macrophages) perform very different functions compared with macrophages in the brain (glial cells) or skin (Langerhans cells), yet they are all members of the monocyte/macrophage family. Until recently fibroblasts had been thought of as ubiquitous, generic cells with a common phenotype even within different tissues. However, we now know that fibroblasts from different organs are more like their macrophage counterparts, with unique morphologic features and repertoires of ECM proteins, cytokines, co-stimulatory molecules, and chemokines specialized to the different microenvironments in which they are found. This characterization also extends to their function as "immune sentinel" cells, expressing innate immune system pattern recognition receptors such as Toll-like receptors (TLRs), which trigger a pro-inflammatory response when ligated by bacterial or viral determinants.

Examination of fibroblast transcriptional profiles with use of microarray techniques reveals that fibroblasts retain a strong memory of their anatomic position and function in the body. Early studies demonstrated that fibroblast transcriptomes (i.e., the global picture of transcribed genes measured using microarrays) could be clustered into peripheral (synovial joint or skin fibroblasts) versus lymphoid (tonsil or lymph node) groups according to their organ of origin, with the potential to shift their transcriptional profiles upon exposure to inflammatory mediators such as TNF, IL-4, or interferon (IFN)-γ. More extensive analysis of expression profiles from primary human fibroblasts by one study[1] has shown large-scale differences related to three broad anatomic divisions: anterior-posterior, proximal-distal, and dermal-nondermal. Genes involved in pattern forming, cell signaling, and matrix remodeling were found to predominantly account for these divisions.[1] The gene expression profile of adult fibroblasts may therefore play a significant role in assigning positional identity within an organism.

More recently, it has become clear that these stable changes in gene transcription are brought about through epigenetic activation and silencing of the HOX family of landscaping genes.[2] Such epigenetic patterning, whereby covalent modifications are made to regulatory regions of DNA or to the histones around which the DNA is wrapped to control access of transcriptional complexes, is a prototype for the stable changes that are also seen in fibroblasts. Epigenetic modifications result in stable changes in gene expression that persist over cellular generations in the absence of mutation of the primary DNA sequence and therefore drive the persistence of disease, as is described in more detail in Chapter 26.

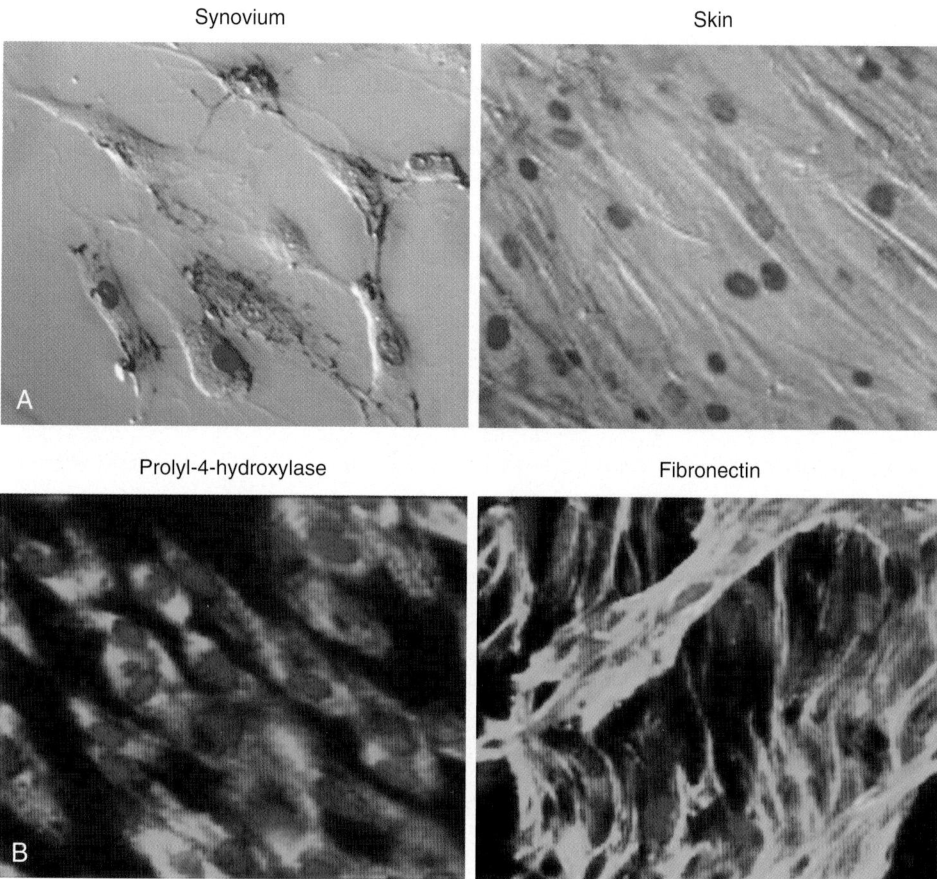

• **Fig. 14.1** Fibroblast phenotype. (A) Staining and differential interference contrast microscopy of live fibroblast cells in culture illustrating typical morphologic features and marked differences between synovial fibroblasts of the rheumatoid arthritis joint and skin fibroblasts. Red stain (fibronectin) demonstrates matrix production. Blue stain indicates nuclei. (B) Stromal cell status is confirmed by fluorescence microscopy of cells showing collagen synthetic enzymes (prolyl-4-hydroxylase) within and matrix production (fibronectin) on the surface of skin fibroblasts.

Embryologic Origins

The problem of distinguishing fibroblasts of differing origin or maturity has historically been difficult because of a lack of specific cell surface markers. Whereas cluster of differentiation (CD) markers have revolutionized the isolation and study of leukocyte subsets, relatively few, poor-quality discriminatory markers have been identified that allow the identification of fibroblast subpopulations. Therefore fibroblasts traditionally have been identified by their spindle-shaped structure (Fig. 14.1), elaboration of ECM, and lack of positive markers for endothelium, epithelial, and hemopoietic cells.

However, growing evidence indicates that fibroblasts are not a homogeneous population but exist as subsets of cells, much like tissue macrophages and dendritic cells (DCs). It is likely that connective tissue contains a mixture of distinct fibroblast lineages with mature fibroblasts existing side by side with more immature fibroblasts that are capable of differentiating into other connective tissue cells. Over the past 15 years studies have begun to identify novel markers that demarcate distinct subpopulations of stromal cells during development and have the potential to act as markers for different subpopulations of fibroblasts, each with different roles. Such markers include smooth muscle actin, which marks out a population of secretory, activated cells termed *myofibroblasts,* and more recently discovered markers such as CD248 and gp38 (podoplanin) (Table 14.1[3–14]; also see later discussion). More recently, the development of single cell transcriptomic techniques has enabled the discovery of discrete stromal and leukocyte clusters in tissues that allow correlation between protein-based markers and function among cells sorted from disaggregated tissue. This opens the door to new therapies that delete or promote differentiation of specific subpopulations within target tissues. Fibroblasts have been defined in terms of their embryologic origins and lineage relationships and are generally considered to be mesenchymal in origin. However, cell populations that appear to blur the distinction between hemopoietic and nonhemopoietic populations have now been identified. In addition, other unexpected shifts in lineage have been reported, including differentiation from neural stem cells into myeloid and lymphoid hemopoietic lineages. Classification by such lineages is therefore becoming increasingly untenable.

Origins of Fibroblasts in Tissue

Both inflammation and wound healing are characterized by the formation of new tissue. However, recent findings suggest that the new cells that form the remodeled tissues might not be derived from the proliferation of resident cells in the adjacent noninjured tissue, as was previously assumed. This finding is important because in both rheumatoid arthritis (RA) and fibrotic pathologic conditions, fibroblasts accumulate in excessive numbers despite apparently low proliferative rates. The principle

TABLE 14.1 Synovial Stromal Markers and Their Geographic and Functional Significance

Marker	Associated Cell Type	Synovial Location	Functional Significance
CD55	Fibroblast-like synoviocyte	Lining layer	Receptor/ligand for synovial macrophage CD97[3]
VCAM-1	Fibroblast-like synoviocyte	Lining layer	Activated lining layer fibroblasts; adhesion molecule[4]
α-SMA	Myofibroblast	Variable, minority subpopulation	Secretory, profibrotic fibroblast[5]
CD248/endosialin	Pericyte	Sublining fibroblasts, pericytes	Acute inflammation,[6] cancer and vasculogenesis[7]
gp38/podoplanin	Pericyte and lymphoid endothelium	Lining layer fibroblasts, pericytes, lymphoid endothelium	Structural, proangiogenic lymph node role[8]; promotes motility in cancer[9]
5B5/prolyl-4-hydroxylase	Broad fibroblast marker in vivo	Lining and sublining cells	Marks collagen synthetic machinery[10]
S-100A4/FSP-1/Mts-1	—	Lining and sublining cells, invasive regions	Cancer, invasiveness roles via motility and impaired apoptosis[11]
FAP	Associated with α-SMA$^+$ fibroblasts[12]	Lining layer	Role in cancer fibroblasts,[13] protective if ectoenzyme blocked in rheumatoid arthritis[14]

α-SMA, α-Smooth muscle actin; *FAP,* fibroblast activation protein; *VCAM-1,* vascular cell adhesion molecule-1.

origin for fibroblasts is from primary mesenchymal cells, and upon appropriate stimulation, fibroblasts can proliferate locally to generate new fibroblasts; however, although an increase in fibroblast numbers caused by local proliferation does occur, fibroblasts also may arise from other sources (Fig. 14.2). The first of these sources is local epithelial to mesenchymal transition (EMT). EMT is an essential, physiologically important developmental mechanism for diversifying cells in the formation of complex tissues. However, fibroblasts also appear to be derived by this process in adult tissue after epithelial stress such as inflammation or tissue injury. EMT both disaggregates epithelial cells and reshapes them for movement. The epithelium loses polarity as defined by the loss of adherens junctions, tight junctions, desmosomes, and cytokeratin intermediate filaments. Epithelial cells also rearrange their F-actin stress fibers and express filopodia and lamellipodia. A combination of cytokines and matrix metalloproteinases (MMPs) associated with digestion of the basement membrane is believed to be secreted and is important in the process. The transition of epithelial to mesenchymal cell populations occurs in cancer and in diseases of the lung and kidney, and the process has been implicated in fibrotic disease.[15] Early evidence suggests that a similar process may occur within the RA synovium.[16]

An alternative explanation for the accumulation of stromal cells in people with chronic inflammatory conditions such as RA lies in the possibility of blood-borne precursors. In the mid-1990s it was discovered that vascular precursors (angioblasts) circulate in the blood of healthy people and that they could be recruited to sites of vasculogenesis in a rabbit ischemic hind limb model.[17] This finding demonstrated that circulating mesenchymal precursors exist outside the hemopoietic system. Subsequent work has confirmed the presence of circulating cells of a mesenchymal phenotype in human subjects. These cells bear a remarkable resemblance to the synovial fibroblasts found in the joints of people with RA, which accumulate in large quantities in the joint lining despite little evidence of proliferation. Interestingly, one group[18] showed that an influx of such cells preceded inflammation in a mouse collagen-induced arthritis model, suggesting that a role may exist for blood-borne stromal cell precursors in the initiation of inflammatory diseases. Furthermore, synovial fibroblasts themselves may migrate in the bloodstream, at least between distant sections of human cartilage in severe combined immunodeficiency (SCID) mice,[19] raising an intriguing parallel to cancer and the radical concept of RA as a metastatic disease of the stroma.

Another circulating precursor cell that could account for the accumulation of fibroblasts in disease is the fibrocyte. Fibrocytes constitute 0.1% to 0.5% of nonerythrocytic cells in peripheral blood and rapidly enter sites of tissue injury and contribute to tissue remodeling in models of inflammatory lung disease.[20] Fibrocytes are adherent cells with a spindle-shaped structure. They express class II major histocompatibility complex (MHC) and type I collagen and arise from within the CD14$^+$ (monocyte) fraction of peripheral blood.[21] They are capable of matrix elaboration and differentiate along fibroblast lineages under the influence of cytokines, particularly transforming growth factor (TGF)-β. The mere fact that a cell type apparently arising from within the monocyte lineage may become a "mesenchymal" stromal cell such as a fibroblast implies a further degree of plasticity and blurring of the apparently clear dividing line that was previously thought to exist between hemopoietic and nonhemopoietic lineages.

Fibroblasts Versus Mesenchymal Progenitor Cells

The potential role of circulating mesenchymal cell precursors (variously termed *mesenchymal stem cells* [MSCs], *mesenchymal stromal cells,* or *mesenchymal progenitor cells* [MPCs]) as sources of tissue fibroblasts is highlighted by the remarkable capacity of these cells to differentiate into other members of the connective tissue family, including cartilage, bone, adipocyte, and smooth muscle cells. This ability was initially demonstrated in bone marrow stromal cells, RA synovial fibroblasts, and circulating mesenchymal cells. Therefore, a characteristic mesenchymal phenotype could be defined on the basis of the hypothesis that the rheumatoid synovium becomes

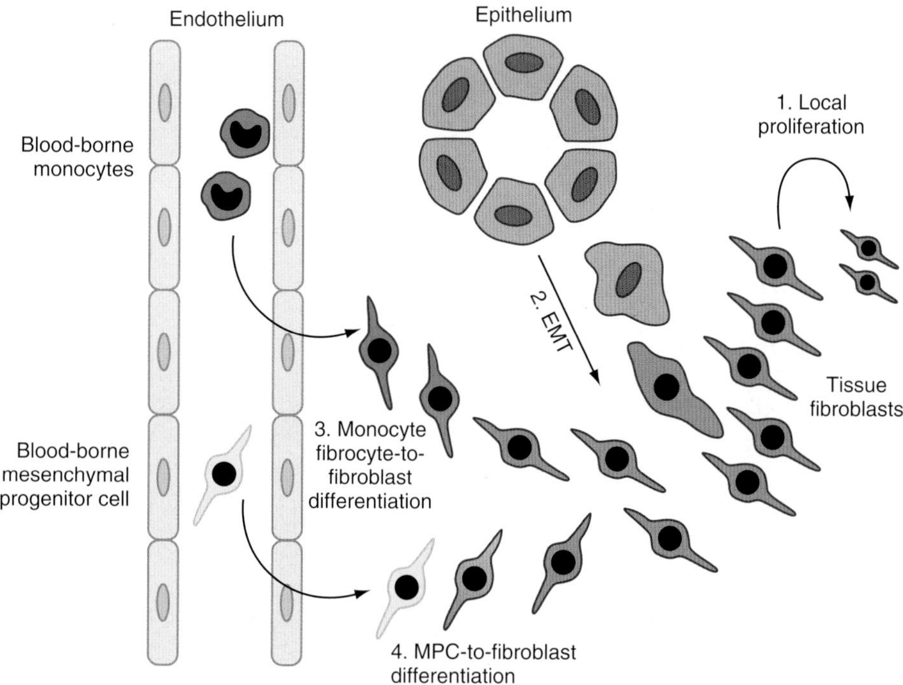

• **Fig. 14.2** Routes of differentiation to tissue fibroblasts. In response to wounding or inflammation, increased numbers of fibroblasts are produced within tissue. *1,* Fibroblasts can proliferate locally to generate new fibroblasts. *2,* The transition of epithelial to stromal cell populations occurs in cancer and diseases of the lung, kidney, and possibly the synovium. *3,* Fibrocytes arise from the monocyte population in blood and then differentiate toward fibroblasts in tissue. *4,* Blood-borne mesenchymal progenitor cells (MPC) may be recruited to tissues and undergo local differentiation to tissue fibroblasts. *EMT,* Epithelial to mesenchymal transition.

populated by a large proportion of circulating mesenchymal progenitor cells exported from the bone marrow. However, the property of trilineage differentiation ("pluripotentiality") is now a property of many adult tissue fibroblasts, although varying somewhat between fibroblasts from different tissues, implying a hitherto unsuspected degree of plasticity in the body's stromal cell populations.[22] The two previously separate fields of mesenchymal precursor cell biology and largely disease-centered fibroblast biology have therefore rapidly converged. However, the concept of bone marrow stromal precursors remains interesting; in chimeric murine models with bone marrow green fluorescent protein (GFP) expression, arthritic joints contained significantly more GFP^+ cells than did nonarthritic joints, supporting a bone marrow origin for expanded fibroblast populations.[23]

Physiologic Characteristics and Functions of Fibroblasts

Production of ECM Components

Ensuring ECM homeostasis is one of the primary functions of fibroblasts. To perform this function, fibroblasts must be able to produce and degrade ECM, as well as adhere to and interact with existing matrix components. Fibroblasts produce a number of ECM molecules—both fibrous proteins and polysaccharide gel components such as collagens, fibronectins, vitronectin, and proteoglycans—which are then assembled into a three-dimensional network. This mechanism provides a framework through which other cell types, which use varying strategies to navigate through the ECM, can move.[24] It also provides a substrate for the deposition of haptotactic (tissue rather than fluid-based) gradients of chemokines and stores of growth factors to direct cellular movement and behavior in a regional fashion.[25] The types of ECM molecules produced by individual populations of fibroblasts differ from tissue to tissue, reflecting the diversity of fibroblasts in different organs. For example, dermal fibroblasts produce significant amounts of type VII collagen, which adheres to the epidermal and dermal layers in the skin. Fibroblasts in other organs such as the lung and kidney produce mainly interstitial, fibrillar collagens (particularly types I and III).

In the synovial membrane, fibroblasts also have a barrier function, in that they provide the joint cavity and the adjacent cartilage with lubricating molecules such as hyaluronic acid, along with plasma-derived nutrients. Anatomically, the intimal synovial membrane is an unusual structure in that barrier function is maintained in the absence of a laminin-rich basement membrane, as occurs in epithelial structures. In addition to lacking a basement membrane, cellular contacts between the fibroblast-like synoviocytes also lack tight junctions and desmosomes. However, strong homophilic adhesion between synoviocytes is mediated by the adhesion molecule cadherin-11 (see later discussion), which is largely responsible for fibroblast organization into synovial tissue. In the presence of disease, fibroblasts must migrate to sites of tissue injury or remodeling and interact with ECM molecules through specific surface receptors. Through such receptors, fibroblasts must sense changes in both the structure and the cellular composition of connective tissues. They respond dynamically by adjusting the production of ECM components and cross-linking them into the appropriate matrix.

TABLE 14.2 **Fibroblast Cell Adhesion Molecules and Their Receptor/Ligand Molecules**

Family	CAM	Alternative Names	Ligands
Integrins	$\alpha_1\,\beta_1$	VLA-1	Laminin, collagen
	$\alpha_2\,\beta_1$	VLA-2	Laminin, collagen
	$\alpha_3\,\beta_1$	VLA-3	Laminin, collagen, fibronectin
	$\alpha_4\,\beta_1$	VLA-4, CD49d/CD29	VCAM-1, CS1 fibronectin
	$\alpha_5\,\beta_1$	VLA-5	Fibronectin
	$\alpha_6\,\beta_1$	VLA-6	Laminin
	$\alpha_L\,\beta_2$	LFA-1, CD11a/CD18	ICAM-1, ICAM-2, ICAM-3, JAM-A
	$\alpha_M\,\beta_2$	Mac-1, CR3, CD11b/CD18	ICAM-2, iC3b, fibrinogen, factor X
	$\alpha_X\,\beta_2$	P150, 95, CD11c/CD18	iC3b, fibrinogen
	$\alpha_E\,\beta_2$		E-cadherin
	$\alpha_4\,\beta_7$	CD49d	Fibronectin, VCAM-1, MAdCAM-1
	$\alpha_v\,\beta_3$	CD52/CD61, vitronectin receptor	Vitronectin, fibronectin, osteopontin, thrombospondin-1, tenascin
Ig superfamily	ICAM-1	CD54	LFA-1, Mac-1
	ICAM-2		LFA-1
	ICAM-3		LFA-1
	VCAM-1		$\alpha_4\,\beta_1$, $\alpha_4\,\beta_7$
	MAdCAM-1		$\alpha_4\,\beta_7$, L-selectin
Cadherins	E-cadherin	Cadherin-1	E-cadherin
	N-cadherin	Cadherin-2	N-cadherin
	Cadherin-11	OB-cadherin	Cadherin-11

ICAM, Intercellular adhesion molecule; *Ig*, immunoglobulin; *JAM*, junctional adhesion molecule; *LFA*, lymphocyte function–associated antigen; *Mac-1*, macrophage 1 antigen; *MAdCAM*, mucosal addressin cell adhesion molecule; *OB-cadherin*, osteoblast cadherin; *VCAM*, vascular cell adhesion molecule; *VLA*, very late antigen.

Attachment to and Interaction With Extra-cellular Matrix

Integrins

Integrins are key mediators of both cell-to-matrix and cell-to-cell adhesive interactions. They are expressed as transmembrane heterodimers containing one α- and one β-subunit, of which at least 25 αβ combinations are known (Table 14.2). The main adhesion molecules responsible for the attachment of fibroblasts to collagen are $\alpha_1\beta_1$ and $\alpha_2\beta$ integrins, whereas other β_1 integrins such as $\alpha_4\beta_1$ and $\alpha_5\beta_1$ mediate attachment of fibroblasts to fibronectin and its spliced variants. In addition, α_v integrins are responsible for attachment to vitronectin.

Syndecans

In addition to conventional integrin-to-ligand binding, additional accessory molecules allow for the integration of adhesive contacts and local growth factor signaling. Syndecans are a family of four single transmembrane domain proteins that carry three to five heparan sulfate and chondroitin sulfate chains, allowing for interaction with a large variety of ligands including fibroblast growth factors, vascular endothelial growth factor (VEGF), TGF-β, and ECM molecules such as fibronectin.[26] Syndecans are expressed on fibroblasts in a tissue-specific and development-dependent manner. Data from syndecan knockout mice indicate that syndecan-4 is involved in wound healing and that the response of syndecan-4–deficient fibroblasts to fibronectin attachment is significantly altered.[27]

Immunoglobulin Superfamily Receptors

The immunoglobulin (Ig) superfamily is a diverse group of transmembrane glycoproteins defined by the presence of one or more Ig-like repeats of 60 to 100 amino acids with a single disulfide bond.[28] Although it includes numerous adaptive immune system genes (e.g., Igs, T cell receptor, and MHC), adhesion proteins such as intercellular adhesion molecules (ICAMs) 1 to 3, vascular cell adhesion molecule-1 (VCAM-1), and mucosal addressin cell adhesion molecule (MAdCAM) mediate both cell-to-cell interactions and adhesive interactions with integrins (see Table 14.2).

Cadherins

Cadherins mediate homotypic, calcium-dependent adhesive interactions with the same cadherin species expressed by neighboring cells.[29] Classical cadherins possess five extra-cellular domains, a single-pass transmembrane domain, and a highly conserved cytoplasmic tail. The cytoplasmic tail interacts with β-catenin, which in turn binds α-catenin, forming a linkage between the cadherin-catenin complex and the actin cytoskeleton. Tightly regulated expression of cadherins is essential to embryogenesis but is also critical for tissue morphogenesis and tissue-specific cell differentiation. Cadherins also modulate cell proliferation and invasion through activation of intra-cellular signal transduction pathways, modulation of MMP production, and association with growth factor receptors.[30–32]

Adhesion Molecule-Mediated Signaling

Importantly, interaction with adhesion molecules not only regulates adhesion and motility but also directly influences activation status, apoptosis, and pro-inflammatory and anti-inflammatory responses in fibroblasts and other cells. The engagement of cell adhesion molecules such as integrin receptors on the surface of fibroblasts results in the formation of focal adhesion complexes, which activate intra-cellular signaling cascades that regulate cell proliferation and survival, the secretion of certain cytokines and chemokines, and matrix deposition and resorption. In particular, integrin-to-fibronectin engagement induces MMP expression, linking adhesion-to-matrix remodeling[33] (Fig. 14.3). Among the signaling molecules that transmit signals from the integrins to the cell interior, focal adhesion kinase (FAK) plays a central

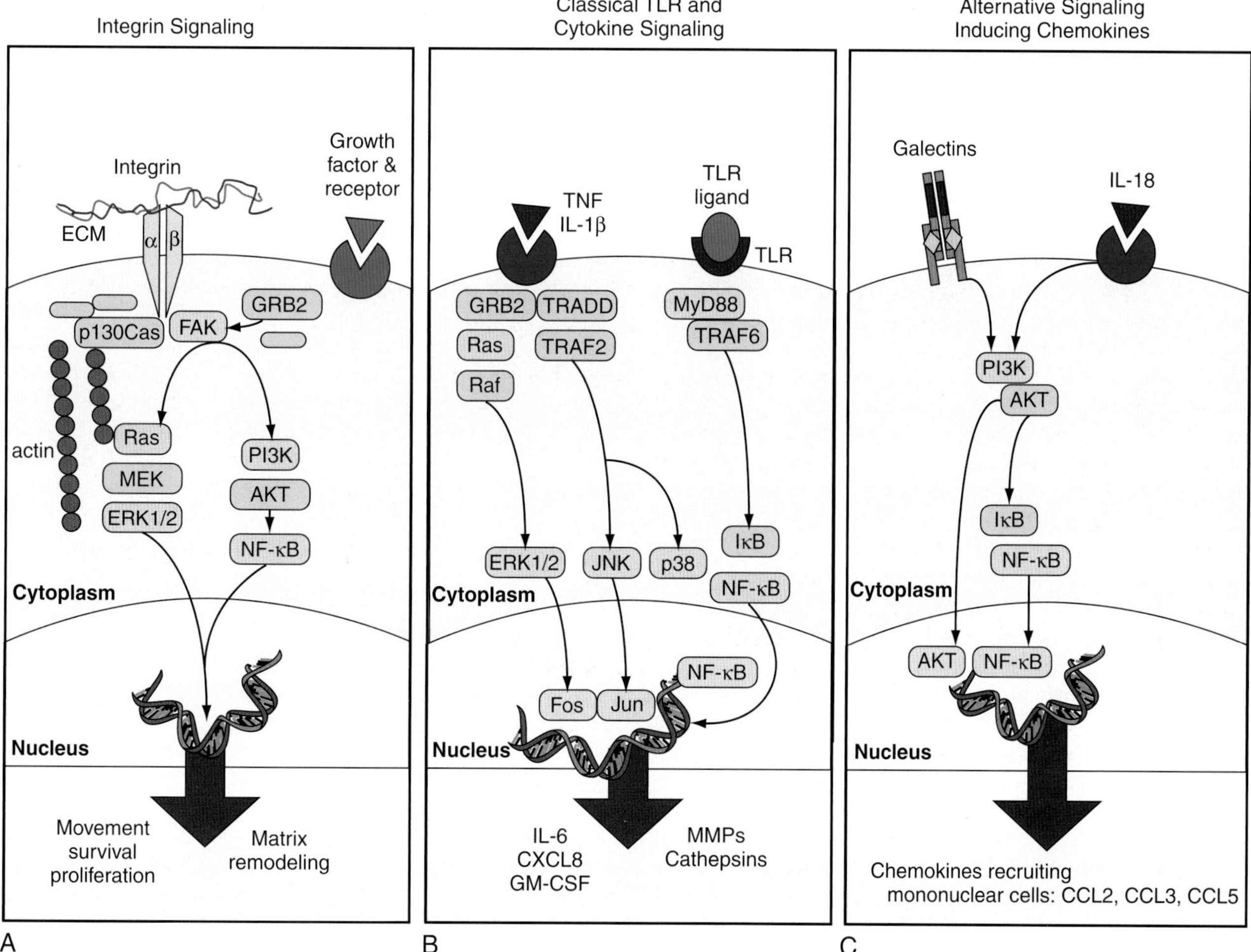

• **Fig. 14.3** Important signaling pathways in synovial fibroblasts. (A) Integrin signaling in fibroblasts. The engagement of integrins and extra-cellular matrix (ECM)–bound growth factors on the cell surface of fibroblasts results in the initiation of signaling cascades that result in changes in (1) cell motility through reorganization of the cytoskeleton, (2) cell survival (e.g., through activation of the Akt-NF-κB pathway), and (3) the production of matrix molecules, matrix-degrading enzymes, and soluble mediators through the activation of mitogen-activated protein kinases (MAPK). (B) The three MAPK pathways are also pivotal in pro-inflammatory cytokine activation of synovial fibroblasts, with tumor necrosis factor (TNF), interleukin (IL)-1β, and IL-6 all capable of activating the three main pathways. In particular, c-Jun N-terminal kinase (JNK) and p38 MAPK pathways are crucial to the production of matrix metalloproteinases (MMPs) such as the collagenases. Fos family members and Jun dimerize to form the activator protein-1 (AP-1) transcription factor for which binding sites are present on multiple pro-inflammatory genes, including the MMPs. (C) There is evidence for a discrete pro-inflammatory pathway for some ligands, which might bypass the classical MAPK and nuclear factor-κB (NF-κB)/AP-1 pathways, signaling via phosphatidylinositol 3-kinase (PI3K) to elicit secretion of chemokines. The chemokines specifically recruit the mononuclear cell population, which predominates in persistent inflammatory disease. *GM-CSF,* Granulocyte-macrophage colony-stimulating factor; *TLR,* Toll-like receptor.

role.[34] FAK, a tyrosine kinase, is recruited into newly established focal contacts and, in turn, recruits other adapter proteins such as p130Cas and Grb2. This process leads to phosphatidylinositide 3-kinase (PI3K) and Src-kinase activation and promotes the initiation of a variety of signaling cascades, culminating in phosphorylation of the extra-cellular regulating kinase (ERK) mitogen-activated protein kinases (MAPKs) and activation of transcription factors. Such pathways can also be activated through FAK-independent signaling events, such as through growth factor receptor ligation. The exact mechanisms by which different signals cooperate to mediate a specific response of fibroblasts and how this translates into distinct diseases are not yet fully defined.

Degradation of Extra-cellular Matrix by Fibroblasts

Remodeling of the ECM requires fibroblasts to express an extensive repertoire of matrix-degrading enzymes with varying specificity. Although these matrix-degrading enzymes are crucial to tissue maintenance and repair, inappropriate overexpression of such enzymes is a key factor in the joint damage, particularly to cartilage, that occurs in inflammatory disease. Such enzymes fall into a number of families, including MMPs, tissue inhibitors of metalloproteinases (TIMPs), cathepsins, and aggrecanases, which are covered in detail in Chapter 8.

With the exception of MMP-2 and the membrane-type (MT)-MMPs, which are constitutively expressed by fibroblasts, MMP expression is regulated by extra-cellular signals via transcriptional activation in fibroblasts. Three major groups of inducers can be differentiated: pro-inflammatory cytokines, growth factors, and matrix molecules. Among the cytokines, IL-1 is perhaps the most potent inducer of a variety of MMPs, including MMP-1, MMP-3, MMP-8, MMP-13, and MMP-14. Fibroblast growth factor (FGF) and platelet-derived growth factor (PDGF) are also known inducers of MMPs in fibroblasts because they potentiate the effect of IL-1 on MMP expression. All MMP promoter regions except MMP-2 contain activator protein-1 (AP-1) binding sites; however, there is good evidence that all MAPK families (ERK, c-Jun N-terminal kinase [JNK], and p38 pathways; see Fig. 14.3), in addition to activators of nuclear factor-κB (NF-κB), signal transducer and activator of transcription (STAT), and ETS transcription factors participate in MMP regulation.[35–39] Matrix proteins (i.e., collagen and fibronectin), and especially their degradation products, also activate MMP expression in fibroblasts, providing the possibility for site-specific MMP activation in regions of matrix breakdown.[40]

Fibroblasts as Innate Immune Sentinels

Classically, macrophages have been studied as sources of inflammatory cytokines and chemokines in response to innate immune stimuli and portrayed as immune sentinel cells accordingly. However, when activated by substances released during tissue injury or the products of invading microorganisms, fibroblasts are capable of elaborating a broad repertoire of inflammatory mediators, which fully justifies their classification as immune sentinel cells. Through expression of TLRs 2, 3, and 4, fibroblasts respond to bacterial products such as lipopolysaccharides (LPSs) by activating the classical NF-κB and AP-1 inflammatory pathways, generating chemokines capable of recruiting inflammatory cells, and generating metalloproteinases capable of degrading matrix.[41–43] However, TLR expression may be increased by pro-inflammatory cytokines TNF and IL-1β within the local microenvironment[44] and may also be activated by endogenous cellular debris such as necrotic cells in synovial fluid, leading to widespread fibroblast activation in disease.[45] As immune sentinels, fibroblasts are able to bridge the innate and adaptive immune responses through expression of the molecule CD40. This molecule was initially assumed to be restricted in its expression to antigen-presenting cells such as macrophages and DCs. However, it is widely expressed by fibroblasts within discrete tissues. CD40 engagement by its ligand CD40L expressed on a restricted population of immune cells, including activated T lymphocytes, is critical for the further induction of pro-inflammatory cytokines and chemokines during an immune response, as well as for antibody production by CD40-expressing B lymphocytes.

Fibroblasts also need to be able to respond to more generic danger signals. The intra-cellular apparatus for response to danger signals such as high levels of urate has recently been identified as the nucleotide-binding oligomerization domain (NOD)-like receptor family, which is made up of NOD and NALP (i.e., NACHT domain, leucine-rich repeat [LRR] domain, and pyrin domain [PYD]-containing protein) receptors. A high local level of urate released by dying cells triggers formation of the active NALP3 inflammasome complex, which results in release of IL-1.[46]

Expression of high levels of NOD-1, NOD-2, and NALP3 (cryopyrin) is seen in the RA synovium and can be induced in fibroblasts by TLR ligands and/or TNF. Furthermore, synergy between TLR and NOD stimulation, with increased IL-6 production in response to NOD-1, TLR2, and TLR4 ligands, has recently been demonstrated. The cytokine IL-17 also regulates multiple TLRs in RA synovial fibroblasts.

Role of Specialized Fibroblast Subsets Within Tissue Microenvironments

Combining surface markers with consistent function has been the key to decades of development in the field of leukocyte biology. By comparison, stromal cell biologists have had remarkably few such stable markers. However, this situation is now gradually changing, and certain areas of developmental biology have spearheaded identification of putative markers (such as CD248) through approaches such as immunization of animals with human fibroblasts and digesting and identifying stromal cell subpopulations in tractable organ systems. One example is the murine thymic stroma, in which subsets with both geographic and functional consistency have been identified. For instance, one study identified $CD45^-$, $gp38^+$ stromal cells in the thymus as T-zone fibroblastic reticular cells.[47] This population of cells, which is geographically restricted to the T zone, provides a limited pool of essential homeostatic survival factors, IL-7 and CCL19, for T lymphocytes, serving a key niche function for which adaptive immune cells must compete.[47] Also, gp38 marks populations of fibroblastic reticular cells within the lymph node that modulate trafficking of DCs.[48] Single cell based sequencing approaches to such cells have advanced our understanding of stromal diversity in the lymph node, revealing many stromal subpopulations within disaggregated lymph node tissue, with regional geography related to interactions with immune cells.[49]

A further subpopulation of specialized fibroblast-like cells of mesenchymal origin is the pericyte. These cells ensheath small blood vessels (i.e., arterioles, capillaries, and venules) and are involved in vasculogenesis, matrix stabilization, and immunologic defense. Pericytes have been hypothesized to represent the extralymphoid source of mesenchymal progenitor cells and express markers consistent with mesenchymal stem cells. Their further definition with newer stromal cell markers such as CD248 and CD146 will be able to establish a mesenchymal progenitor cell niche.[50]

Fibroblast-like Synoviocytes in the Normal Synovium

The normal synovium provides an excellent prototypic model of fibroblast subsets defined by known markers, some of which are responsive to disease. In healthy people the synovium is a delicate, thin, two-layer structure attaching bone and the joint capsule. One layer, a two- to three-cell-thick lining layer, is formed with roughly equal proportions of CD68$^+$, phagocytic type A macrophage-like synoviocytes, and type B mesenchymal, fibroblast-like synoviocytes (FLSs). This layer serves a barrier function, and FLS secretes lubricative substances, including hyaluronic acid and lubricin, along with secreting the lining layer matrix. The second layer is the sublining layer, which is composed of less densely packed fibroblasts and macrophages in a loose tissue matrix along with blood vessel networks. FLSs in the lining layer are associated with a number of cellular markers (see Table 14.1), including CD55 (decay accelerating factor [DAF]), VCAM-1 (which, outside of T cell–to-integrin interactions is generally only expressed by bone marrow fibroblasts providing support for the B cell developmental niche[51]), uridine diphosphoglucose dehydrogenase (UDPGD), reflecting the ability to synthesize hyaluronan, and the novel marker gp38.[52] Sublining FLSs are instead marked by the nonspecific cellular marker CD90 (Thy-1), which also recognizes endothelium, and by the recently discovered marker CD248, which marks both pericytes and stromal fibroblasts. Gp38 marks cells in the sublining region, including lymphatic endothelium (Fig. 14.4).

As mentioned earlier, the unique lining layer barrier function is not supported by a basement membrane and conventional tight junctions but instead by homotypic interactions between cadherin-11 molecules.[53] Randomly assorted cells expressing classical cadherins, such as cadherin-11, will sort themselves in a cadherin-specific manner, emphasizing their importance in the generation and maintenance of organ integrity. Cadherin-11 mediates selective association of mesenchymal rather than epithelial tissues, a function that is carried forward after embryogenesis in structures such as the joint, lung, and testis.[54] Cadherin-11 knockout mice exhibit a hypoplastic synovial lining that lacks the normal numbers of synovial lining cells and is deficient in ECM quantity.[55] Adhesion between type A and type B synoviocytes is maintained by ICAM-1:β_2 integrin and VCAM-1:$\alpha_4\beta_1$ integrin interactions.

By virtue of their role in defining the geography of specialized tissues, fibroblasts and other stromal cells exist in living organisms

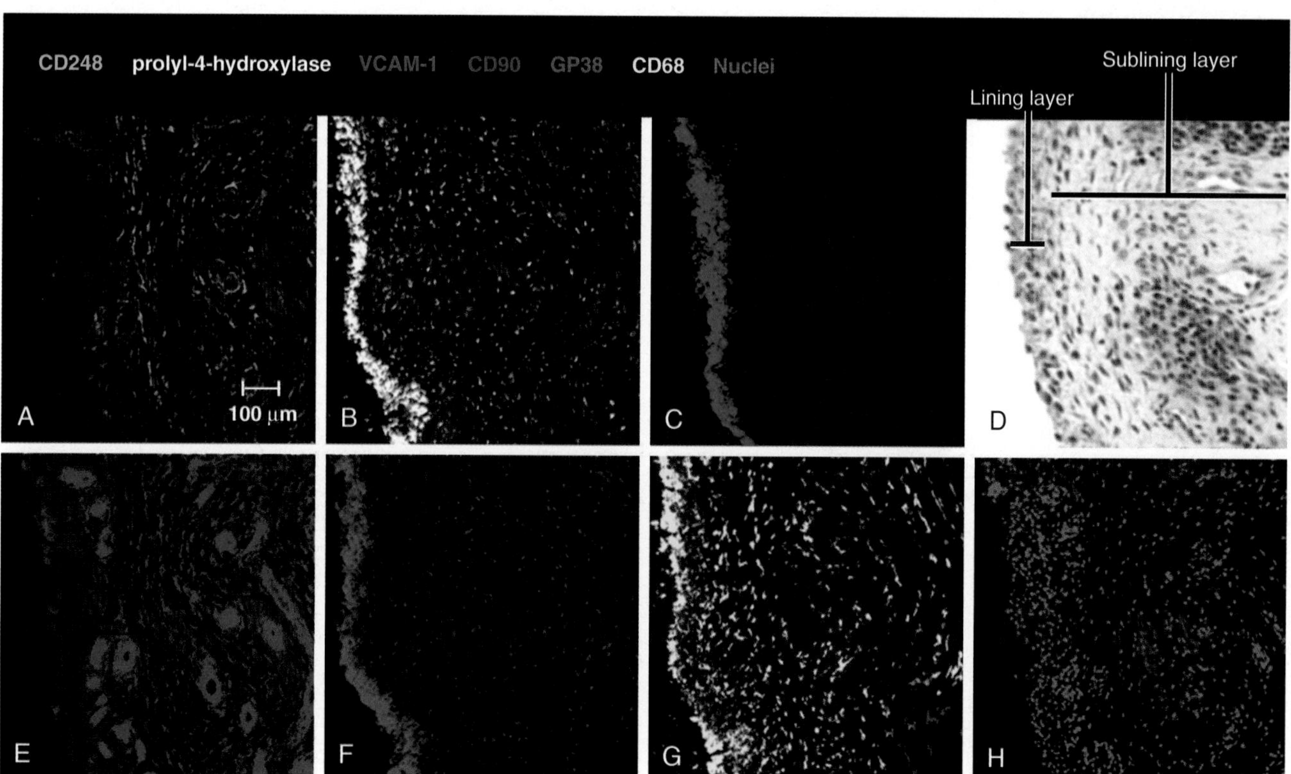

• **Fig. 14.4** Microscopic appearance of the synovium and stromal cell markers. The microscopic structure of hematoxylin and eosin–stained synovium is illustrated in (D), indicating lining and sublining layers. This geographic structure is reflected in serial frozen sections of rheumatoid arthritis synovium stained for stromal markers (A-C, E-G). For reference, a nuclear stain is shown in H. (A) CD248 stains only sublining fibroblasts. (B) Prolyl-4-hydroxylase stains most populations of synovial fibroblasts. (C) Vascular cell adhesion molecule-1 (VCAM-1) (CD106) characteristically stains only the lining layer. (E) CD90 (Thy-1) stains predominantly sublining layers but also strongly stains endothelial cells, outlining synovial vasculature. (F) gp38 marks lining layer cells and a proportion of sublining cells. (G) CD68 highlights macrophage-like synovial cells in the lining layer and resident tissue macrophages in the sublining layer.

within three-dimensional environments, whereas the vast majority of experiments performed using fibroblasts in the laboratory are still conducted within two-dimensional environments. Furthermore, fibroblasts are frequently grown in nonphysiologic stimuli such as serum, to which fibroblasts would not normally be exposed unless tissue damage were to occur. Behavior is significantly different when cells are cultured in artificial three-dimensional environments.[56] It is therefore all the more remarkable that fibroblasts cultured using conventional two-dimensional techniques retain characteristics such as positional memory and unique cytokine profiles.

Recent work has addressed the issue of three-dimensional synovial models. In so-called *micromass cultures,* FLS, but not dermal fibroblasts, within laminin-containing spheres reproduced a lining layer structure with production of lubricin, support for co-cultured monocytic cells, and expansion of the membrane upon stimulation with pro-inflammatory stimuli such as TNF. Some cells also remained in a "sublining" zone of low density.[57] FLSs therefore have the ability to self-organize in a tissue organoid, which recapitulates some of the key features of the synovium. This finding is further evidence of the robustness of epigenetic programming, which determines site and organ specialization.

Fibroblasts in Rheumatic Diseases

Role of Fibroblasts in Persistent Inflammation

Inflammatory reactions proceed against the backdrop of specialized stromal microenvironments. The response to tissue damage involves a carefully choreographed series of interactions among diverse cellular, humoral, and connective tissue elements. For an inflammatory lesion to resolve, dead or redundant cells that were recruited and expanded during the active phases of the response must be removed. In addition, resident fibroblasts attempt to repair damaged tissue.

It is becoming increasingly clear that fibroblasts are not only passive players in immune responses but also actively determine the switches that govern progression from acute to chronic inflammation, as well as those governing resolution or the progression to chronic, persistent inflammation. The "switch to resolution" is an important signal that permits tissue repair to take place and enables immune cells to return to draining lymphoid tissues (lymph nodes) for immunologic memory to become established. However, in chronic immune-mediated inflammatory diseases such as RA, fibroblasts contribute to the inappropriate recruitment and retention of leukocytes in a site- or organ-dependent manner, leading to tissue- and site-specific initiation and subsequent relapse of chronic persistent inflammatory disease, effectively a "switch to persistence."[58]

It is now recognized that fibroblasts themselves may undergo fundamental changes while responding to such environmental stimuli. It is known that during wound healing and under profibrotic conditions, some fibroblast-like cells are transformed into myofibroblasts, which are distinct from tissue fibroblasts in terms of both their phenotype and their behavior.[59] The mechanisms underlying such persistent phenotypic change, which is maintained through cellular generations, are highly likely to involve epigenetic modifications of gene promoters and their closely related histones (see Chapter 26). This has been shown recently in both human and murine renal fibrotic disease, where hypermethylation of the promoter region of a ras oncogene inhibitor led to gene silencing, ras pathway activation, and hence persistent fibrogenesis.[60] Such fibrotic transformation of fibroblasts is also characteristic of systemic sclerosis, a generalized fibrotic disorder that affects the skin and various internal organs such as the lungs, heart, and gastrointestinal tract (see Chapter 88). The overproduction of ECM components, particularly type I, III, VI, and VII collagen, by skin fibroblasts is a hallmark of this disease and is closely linked to the disease-specific activation of these fibroblasts. This pattern of activation includes not only a distinct profile of ECM overproduction but also altered responses to both inflammatory mediators and immune cells.[61] Although the phenotype of fibroblasts in RA is not fundamentally profibrotic in this sense, the hallmark of these cells, both in vitro and in vivo, is also a persistently imprinted phenotype that is maintained even in the absence of continuous stimulation by inflammatory triggers or leukocytes.

Fibroblast-like Synoviocytes in Rheumatoid Arthritis

In inflammatory arthritis such as RA, the two compartments of the synovium undergo radical change. The lining layer undergoes dramatic hyperplasia, sometimes reaching 10 to 20 cells in depth, with both type A and type B cell populations expanded and becoming merged with the sublining. At the articular borders of the synovium, the thickened synovial lining layer may become a mass of "pannus" tissue rich in FLS and osteoclasts, which aggressively invade the adjacent articular cartilage and subchondral bone, respectively. The sublining layer also undergoes expansion, with sometimes huge infiltrates of inflammatory cells including macrophages, mast cells, T cells, B cells, and plasma cells in addition to DCs. T and B lineage cells may remain in diffuse infiltrates or may coalesce into aggregates of cells varying from simple perivascular "cuffs" a few cells in diameter to structures resembling B cell follicles in up to 20% of samples.[62] This increased activity is supported by further ECM production and neoangiogenesis, although the inflamed synovium remains in a state of relative hypoxia.[63]

As mentioned previously, cadherin-11 serves a vital role in preserving the integrity of the synovial lining layer, and cadherin-11 knockout mice display a hypoplastic lining layer. However, when cadherin-11 knockout mice are evaluated in the K/BxN serum transfer model, invasiveness is reduced with a 50% reduction in inflammation. Similarly, cultured fibroblasts with mutant cadherin-11 constructs also demonstrate impaired invasiveness into cartilage.[55,64] Cadherin-11 expression is also much higher in RA than in osteoarthritis (OA) or normal synovium. This unique structural molecule may therefore emerge as a therapeutic target[55]; because of shared roles in invasive disease, targeting of this molecule in breast cancer is currently in development.[65]

Persistent Activated Fibroblast Phenotype in the Rheumatoid Arthritis Synovium

Increased expression of cadherin-11 is but one facet of the persistent, activated phenotype of rheumatoid FLS, which remains stable even after culturing in vitro for many months. These cells play a direct role in tissue damage through secretion of multiple MMPs and cathepsins, which degrade cartilage and bone tissues in the joint. In vitro functional assays such as the laminin invasion assay produce intriguing results, in which the degree of invasion with a given in vitro cultured fibroblast sample correlates with the degree of radiographic progression seen in the joints of the patient from whose samples the fibroblasts were initially cultured.[66] The most compelling evidence for a persistent phenotype is the attachment to and invasion of fibronectin-rich matrix such as human cartilage in the absence of functioning leukocyte immune cells in the SCID mouse model of arthritis.[67] Here, fibroblasts in a tissue construct with human cartilage are implanted under the kidney capsule or skin of immune-incompetent SCID or $Rag^{-/-}$ mice. Multiple-passage cultured rheumatoid FLSs, but not OA or normal FLSs, invade and destroy the co-implanted human cartilage. This model has been used to explore the in vivo mechanisms governing invasiveness. For example, targeting MMP-1 and cathepsin L using ribozymes inhibits cartilage destruction.[68,69] The effectiveness of glucocorticoids and the relative efficacy of different formulations of methotrexate in preventing erosions have also been examined.[70,71]

Unbiased approaches to determining the key regulators of fibroblast invasiveness have made rapid recent progress. Transcriptomic approaches linking gene expression in RA fibroblasts and macrophages have revealed invasiveness pathways within fibroblasts regulated by complementary macrophage inflammatory pathways that are strongly driven by IL-1β stimulation. Key genes include periostin osteoblast-specific factor (POSTN) and twist basic helix–loop–helix transcription factor 1 (TWIST1).[72,73] The impact of TNF and IL-17 stimulation on the transcriptome of RA fibroblasts has been examined, revealing critical hypoxia regulated genes linked to invasiveness, including MMP-2 and the chemokine receptor CXCR4, which is already implicated in disease persistence.[74]

An alternative unbiased approach to dissecting function involves the parallel study of cellular enzymes mediating tyrosine phosphorylation of key signaling molecules (protein tyrosine phosphatases [PTPs]). Investigation of the PTPome of synovial fibroblasts in RA compared with OA revealed a dual role for SH2 domain–containing phosphatase 2 (SHP2); knockdown of this enzyme reduced both invasiveness and survival of RA FLSs, suggesting a pivotal signaling molecule.[73]

Fibroblasts implanted with cartilage migrate to a contralateral cell-free implant, and subcutaneous, intraperitoneal, and intravenously injected fibroblasts will also migrate to sections of human cartilage, suggesting a tropism to damaged cartilage tissue. This important finding raises the question of which cell populations are grown from the synovium when tissue is digested and adherent cells are cultured in vitro: lining layer cells, sublining cells, or a mixture of both? From a methodologic perspective, answering this question is a challenge. However, we do know from transcriptomic approaches that the phenotype remains more stable in tissue culture than might be expected, with little transcriptional divergence over the first two to four passages and the level of differentially expressed genes between parallel cultures rising to greater than 10% only after passage 7.[75]

These models demonstrate the remarkably stable and disease-specific phenotype of cultured RA synovial fibroblasts, which includes high basal and stimulated expression of signature cytokines such as IL-6 and chemokines (discussed later).[76] RA synovial fibroblasts also express characteristic adhesion and immune-modulating molecules such as VCAM-1, galectin-3, and a specific repertoire of TLRs, which initiate innate immune cellular responses. A satisfactory molecular explanation for the stable phenotype of RA synovial fibroblasts has until recently evaded the field. However, epigenetic changes including DNA methylation; histone modifications such as acetylation, methylation, and citrullination; and altered micro RNA (miRNA) expression have now been suggested to underlie the observed persistent changes in fibroblast gene transcription and post-transcriptional repression (see Chapter 26). Further characteristic aspects of the RA FLS phenotypes and their biology are discussed extensively in Chapter 75.

Interactions of Fibroblasts With Leukocytes

Recruitment of Inflammatory Infiltrates Into the Joint

Stromal elements such as synovial fibroblasts are subject to a pro-inflammatory cytokine network within the inflamed synovium. Direct-contact interactions with other infiltrating cells such as T lymphocytes lead to high levels of expression of many inflammatory chemokines (see Fig. 14.3). Neutrophil-attracting chemokines are expressed at high levels by stimulated fibroblasts and include CXCL8 (IL-8), CXCL5 (ENA-78), and CXCL1 (GRO-α).[77–79] Monocytes and T cells are recruited by a range of chemokines found at high levels in the synovium; CXCL10 (IP-10) and CXCL9 (Mig) are highly expressed in synovial tissue and fluid.[80] CXCL16 is also highly expressed in the RA synovium and acts as a potent chemoattractant for T cells.[81] CCL2 (MCP-1) is found in synovial fluid and is known to be produced by synovial fibroblasts; it is considered to be a pivotal chemokine for the recruitment of monocytes.[82] CCL3 (MIP-1α), CCL4 (MIP-1β), and CCL5 (RANTES) are chemotactic for monocytes and lymphocytes and are known products of synovial fibroblasts.[80,83] CCL20 (MIP-3α) is also overexpressed in the synovium and has a similar chemoattractant profile via its specific receptor, CCR6.[84] CX3CL1 (fractalkine) is also widely expressed in the rheumatoid synovium. A number of chemokine receptors differs between peripheral blood and synovial leukocytes, suggesting that they are enriched in the synovium either though their selective recruitment by endothelial-expressed chemokines or after upregulation by the microenvironment after their recruitment.

Fibroblast Support for Leukocyte Survival

Stromal cell support for the survival of leukocyte populations fulfills a physiologic role in certain organs within the body. The selective recruitment and support of hemopoietic subsets is an essential physiologic function of stromal cells in specific microenvironments. For instance, immature B lymphocytes are completely dependent on factors such as IL-6 produced by bone marrow stromal cells. Although the bone marrow niche plays a critical role in the early development of all hemopoietic leukocyte populations, it also acts as an active reservoir for terminally differentiated leukocyte subpopulations, including CD4 and CD8 T cells and neutrophils. The bone marrow stromal microenvironment therefore maintains not only the selective survival, differentiation, and proliferation of all lineages of immature hemopoietic cells but also, in some cases, the survival of their mature counterparts. The stromal microenvironment plays a crucial role in the maintenance of such survival niches, which are not generic but are highly specific to certain organs and tissues, resulting in site-specific differences in the ability of different stromal cells to support the differential accumulation of leukocyte subsets.

In the case of an inflammatory response, successful resolution requires the removal of the vast majority of immune cells that were recruited and expanded during the active phase of the inflammation. A number of studies have shown that during the resolution phase of viral infections, the initial increase in T cell numbers in peripheral blood that is seen within the first few days is followed by a wave of apoptosis occurring in the activated T cells. This situation is mirrored within tissues, where apoptosis induced by the molecule Fas occurs at the peak of the inflammatory response and may be responsible for limiting the extent of the immune response. In contrast, the resolution phase appears to be principally triggered by cytokine-deprivation–induced apoptosis, during which leukocytes compete for a shrinking pool of survival factors provided by the microenvironment, leading to programmed death of those cells, which are surplus to requirements.

In RA the resolution phase of inflammation becomes disordered. Recent studies have shown that a failure of synovial T cells to undergo apoptosis contributes to the persistence of the inflammatory infiltrate. The T cell survival pathway shares all the essential hallmarks of a stromal cell, cytokine-mediated mechanism (high B cell lymphoma [Bcl]-X_L, low Bcl-2, and lack of cell proliferation). Type I IFNs (IFN-α and -β), which are produced by synovial fibroblasts and macrophages, have been identified as one of the principal factors responsible for prolonged T cell survival in the rheumatoid joint (Fig. 14.5).[58] Interestingly, although type I IFN is beneficial in multiple sclerosis (a disease in which tissue scarring and low levels of T cell infiltrates are observed), these results suggest that type I IFN is not likely to be a successful therapy for people with RA, a prediction that has been borne out in clinical trials.[85] It is likely that this mechanism of stromal cell–induced leukocyte survival occurs in many chronic inflammatory conditions in which T cells accumulate.

Not surprisingly, other leukocyte subpopulations derive support from stromal cells. Although fibroblast support for T cell and B cell survival exhibits site-specific properties, neutrophil survival is dependent on prior cytokine activation of fibroblasts and shows no differences between fibroblasts taken from different anatomic sites.[76] Plasma cells are, of course, rescued from apoptosis within the bone marrow stem cell niche,[86] but mast cells of the gut are rescued by intestinal fibroblasts,[87] whereas dermal fibroblasts maintain Langerhans-like cells in the skin.[88] Fibroblast modulation of inflammatory and differentiation pathways in monocyte lineage cells has become a recent focus as the role of differentially polarized macrophage populations becomes more prominent. Recent transcriptomic analyses of co-cultured RA FLSs and macrophages demonstrated not only that shared inflammatory pathways are present in both cell types but that co-cultured RA FLSs modulate up to a third of TNF-regulated pathways in macrophages.[89]

Fibroblast-Mediated Retention of Leukocytes in Tissue

Although inhibition of T cell death by stromal cells at sites of chronic inflammation contributes to T cell accumulation, it is unlikely to be the only mechanism because lymphocytes should be able to leave the inflamed tissue during the resolution of inflammation, even if their death is inhibited. A number of studies have recently reported that the synovial microenvironment contributes directly to the inappropriate retention of T cells within the joint by an active chemokine-dependent process. The presence of high levels of inflammatory chemokines, produced by stromal cells, is a characteristic of environments such as the rheumatoid synovium. However, recent data suggest that, paradoxically, constitutive chemokines, which are involved in the recruitment of lymphocytes to secondary lymphoid tissues, are ectopically expressed in immune-mediated inflammatory diseases. The constitutive chemokine CXCL12 (SDF-1) and its receptor CXCR4 emerged as unexpected but crucial players in the accumulation of T lymphocytes within the rheumatoid synovial microenvironment. This chemokine-receptor pair plays an important role, both in the constitutive traffic of lymphocytes and in the recruitment and retention of hemopoietic cells within the bone marrow. Unexpectedly, CD45RO$^+$ T lymphocytes in the rheumatoid synovium were found to express CXCR4 receptors at high levels in the rheumatoid synovium. The CXCR4 ligand CXCL12 was highly expressed on endothelial cells at the sites of T cell accumulation.[90,91] In addition, stromal cell–derived TGF-β is responsible for upregulation of CXCR4 receptors on T cells in the synovium.[90] Evidence also suggests that the stability of lymphocyte infiltrates is reinforced by a positive feedback loop whereby tissue CXCL12 promotes CD40 ligand expression on T cells, which in turn stimulates further CXCL12 production by CD40-expressing synovial fibroblasts. Furthermore, levels of CXCL12 secreted by synovial fibroblasts are controlled in part by T cell–derived IL-17.[92]

Therefore, clear evidence supports the hypothesis that aberrant ectopic constitutive expression of chemokines such as CXCL12, CCL19, and CCL21 by synovial stromal cells contributes to the retention of T cells within the RA synovium.

Other cell constituents of the rheumatoid inflammatory infiltrate may be affected by the CXCL12/CXCR4 axis. One study[93] has shown increased expression of CXCL12/CXCR4 by monocyte/macrophage cells in RA compared with OA. In addition, using implanted human synovial tissue in SCID mice, they demonstrated that monocytes are recruited into transplanted synovial tissue by CXCL12.[93] Contact-mediated B cell survival induced by synovial fibroblasts also depends on CXCL12, B cell activating factor (BAFF)/BLyS, and CD106 (VCAM-1)–dependent mechanisms that are independent of TNF.[51,94] Overexpression of CXCL12 has also been identified as a distinct feature of RA, as opposed to OA synovia, using complementary DNA arrays. Data validating these findings in vivo have come from a collagen-induced arthritis model of RA in DBA/1 IFN-γ receptor-deficient mice, where administration of the specific CXCR4 antagonist AMD3100 significantly ameliorated disease severity.[95] In another murine collagen-induced arthritis model, the small molecule CXCR4 antagonist 4F-benzoyl-TN14003 ameliorated clinical severity and suppressed delayed-type hypersensitivity (DTH) responses.[96] The CXCL12/CXCR4 constitutive chemokine pair therefore seems to play an important role in lymphocyte retention in RA.

These experiments demonstrate that understanding the behavior of fibroblasts and leukocytes within microenvironments necessarily requires that we model the interactions of all the cellular populations concerned. An elegant example of this approach in vitro is the work of one group, who developed a flow-based model of cellular recruitment to the rheumatoid synovium.[97] Co-culturing fibroblasts from skin and RA synovial membrane with endothelial cells showed that IL-6 released from synovial (but not skin) fibroblasts was able to induce production of chemokines and adhesion molecules, resulting in greater neutrophil recruitment by synovial fibroblasts. Subsequent work interrogating the system using low-density gene arrays demonstrated that the effect of neutrophil-attracting chemokines such as CXCL5 released from synovial fibroblasts was dependent on the function of the chemokine transporter molecule DARC (Duffy antigen receptor for chemokines), which was also induced by fibroblast-to-endothelial cell co-culture.[97]

Constitutive Chemokines and Lymphoid Neogenesis

RA is one of a number of inflammatory diseases in which the organization of the inflammatory infiltrate shares characteristics of lymphoid tissue. Follicular hyperplasia with germinal center formation can occur in autoimmune

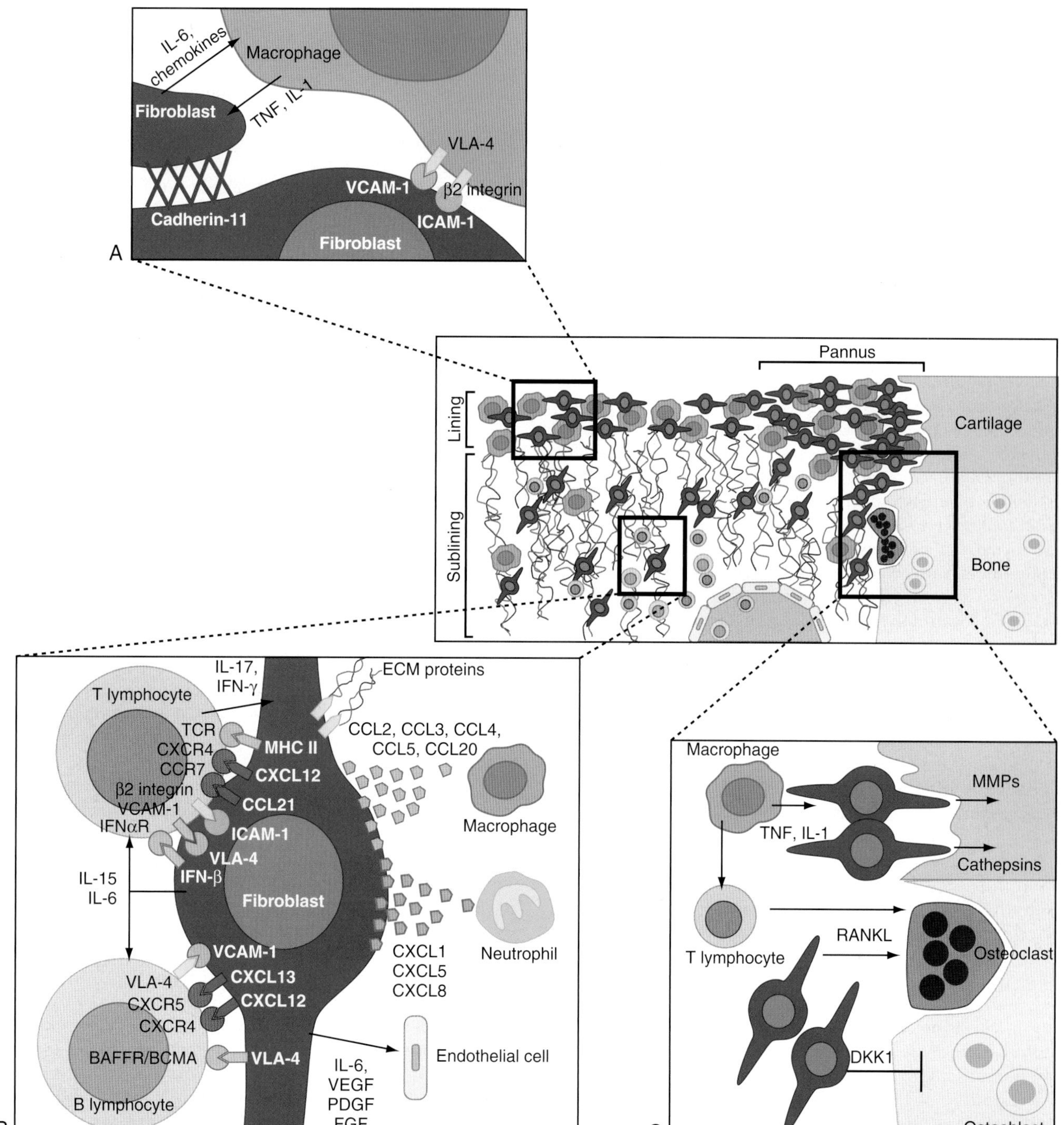

• **Fig. 14.5** Cell-cell interactions in the synovium. Synovial fibroblasts interact with multiple cell types in the rheumatoid arthritis (RA) synovium to maintain persistence of inflammation and continued joint destruction. (A) Fibroblast-like synoviocytes in the RA synovial lining interact with macrophage-like synoviocytes through both secretion of soluble factors and cell surface receptor interactions to maintain lining layer structure and promote the activation of both cell types. Key soluble interactions include production of interleukin (IL)-1 and tumor necrosis factor (TNF) by macrophages and IL-6 by fibroblasts. Adhesive interactions consist of integrin-receptor interactions as described in the text and the critical presence of homotypic interaction through cadherin-11. (B) Sublining synovial fibroblasts interact with numerous cell types including mast cells and plasma cells (not shown), T cells, B cells, interstitial macrophages, and endothelial cells, leading to their recruitment, retention, activation, and differentiation. Both cell surface receptor interactions and secreted mediators are important in this process. T cell–fibroblast interactions include T cell recruitment and retention by fibroblast-secreted chemokines such as CXCL12, CCL5, and CX3CL1 (fractalkine). In addition, fibroblasts may activate T cells through antigen presentation, co-stimulatory receptors (e.g., CD40 and intercellular adhesion molecule-1 [ICAM-1]), and cytokine secretion. Fibroblast cytokines such as IL-6 and IL-15 may be particularly important for differentiation of the Th17 T cell subset, and secretion of interferon (IFN)-β supports T cell survival. Fibroblasts, in turn, are activated by these cell surface interactions and by T cell cytokines, including IL-17 and IFN-γ. B cells are similarly recruited and retained through fibroblast secretion of chemokines such as CXCL12 and CXCL13 and through cell surface adhesion interactions (e.g., very late activation antigen-4 [VLA-4] and vascular cell adhesion molecule-1 [VCAM-1]). Critical survival and differentiation signals are maintained through fibroblast secretion of BAFF (BLyS) and APRIL. Neutrophils and monocyte/macrophage lineage cells are also recruited by fibroblast chemokine production. Macrophages, in turn, help activate synovial sublining fibroblasts through the production of cytokines such as IL-1 and TNF. Finally, synovial sublining fibroblasts promote angiogenesis through the production of proangiogenic factors such as vascular endothelial growth factor (VEGF) and platelet-derived growth factor (PDGF) and may help direct endothelial recruitment of inflammatory cells through secretion of cytokines such as IL-6. (C) Pannus tissue, an extension of the hyperplastic synovial lining consisting of both activated macrophage-like synoviocyte (MLS) and fibroblast-like synoviocyte (FLS), actively degrades both cartilage and bone through production of matrix degrading enzymes such as matrix metalloproteinases (MMPs) and cathepsins. In addition, fibroblasts and T cells secrete receptor activator of nuclear factor-κB ligand (RANKL), which promotes osteoclast differentiation and activation, leading to bone erosions. Furthermore, production of dickkopf-1 (DKK1) inhibits wnt signaling pathways, which normally promote anabolic osteoblast activity, preventing repair of bone erosions. *CD40L,* CD40 ligand; *ECM,* extra-cellular matrix; *FGF,* fibroblast growth factor; *IFNαR,* interferon-α/β receptor; *MHC II,* class II major histocompatibility complex; *TCR,* T cell receptor.

thyroid disease, myasthenia gravis, Sjögren's syndrome, and RA and may occur during infection with *Helicobacter pylori* and *Borrelia burgdorferi*. The lymphoid infiltrates in the rheumatoid synovium can be divided into at least three distinct histologic groupings, varying from diffuse lymphocyte infiltrates through organized lymphoid aggregates to clear germinal center reactions. Moreover, there is conflicting evidence that such distinct histologic types correlate with other serum indicators of disease activity. This form of inflammatory lymphoid neogenesis relies on inappropriate but highly organized temporal and spatial expression by fibroblasts of the constitutive chemokines, particularly CXCL13 and CCL21, which are required for physiologic lymphoid organogenesis.

The elegant choreography of lymphocyte-stromal interactions within lymph nodes is organized by expression of adhesive and chemotactic cues in overlapping and combinatorial fashions. Once they have encountered new antigen, DCs specialized in the presentation of antigen to lymphocytes undergo a process of maturation under the local influence of inflammatory cytokines and bacterial and viral products. As a result, inflammatory chemokine receptors are downregulated, and upregulation of the constitutive receptors CCR4, CCR7, and CXCR4 occurs, causing DCs to migrate into local draining lymphatics and thereby into peripheral lymph nodes. Trafficking of B and T cells is regulated by CXCL13 (BCA-1), its receptor CXCR5, and CCL21 and CCL19 (ELC), which are both CCR7 agonists. Within the lymph node, CXCR5-bearing B cells are attracted to follicular areas, whereas T cells and DCs are maintained within parafollicular zones by local expression of CCL21 and CCL19. Some T cells that have been successfully presented with their cognate antigen by DCs then upregulate CXCR5, allowing them to migrate toward and interact with B cells.[98–100]

The genesis of lymphoid follicular structures in diseases such as diabetes and RA appears to rely on expression of such constitutive chemokines, in association with the lymphotoxins α and β (LT-α and LT-β) and TNF.[101] In this context it is important to note that transgenic animals overexpressing the TNF gene display increased formation of focal lymphoid aggregates and develop a chronic arthritis similar to RA.[102] Clearly, one of the many mechanisms of action of TNF inhibitor therapy may be the dissolution of such aggregates. In transgenic mouse models, expression of CXCL13 in the pancreatic islets was sufficient for the development of T and B cell clusters, but because they lacked follicular dendritic cells, it was not sufficient for true germinal center formation.[103] CCL21 does appear to be sufficient in some cases for lymph node formation; murine pancreatic islet models have demonstrated formation of lymph node–like structures in the presence of CCL21 and lymphoid infiltrates in response to CCL19 expression. The degree of lymphoid organization seen in the rheumatoid synovium correlates with expression of the chemokines CCL21 and CXCL13, although these chemokines are also associated with less organized lymphoid aggregates.[104] Expression of CCL21 is restricted to a population of perivascular fibroblastic reticular cells with common phenotype and function in secondary lymphoid and inflammatory aggregate tissues.[105] CXCR5 is overexpressed in the rheumatoid synovium, consistent with a role in recruitment and positioning of B and T lymphocytes within lymphoid aggregates of the RA synovium. It therefore seems likely that expression of lymphoid-constitutive chemokines contributes significantly to the entry, local organization, and exit of lymphocytes in the RA synovium. It also seems that the ectopic expression of chemokines is a general characteristic of a number of chronic rheumatic conditions because another B cell–attracting chemokine, CXCL13 (BCA-1), is inappropriately expressed by fibroblasts in the salivary glands of patients with Sjögren's syndrome.[106]

Interestingly, the ectopic lymphoid structures seen in RA are capable of appropriate secondary lymphoid tissue functions, including the production of class-switched high-affinity antibody production, as evidenced by the expression of activation-induced cytidine deaminase (AID), the enzyme required for somatic hypermutation and class switch recombination (CSR) of Ig genes.[107] CXCR3-expressing plasma cells are also present in the rheumatoid synovium, and their recruitment is once more supported by ectopic production of the CXCR3 ligand CXCL9 by fibroblasts, particularly in the sublining region where aggregates are located.[108]

Role of Fibroblast Subsets in Disease

It has long been hypothesized that expanded populations of synovial fibroblasts discussed earlier may correspond with functionally diverse fibroblast lineages and subpopulations. Based on microarray analysis, the transcriptional profile of RA synovial fibroblasts clustered into two broad groups representing "high" (myofibroblastic) and "low" (growth factor producing) populations.[5] These clusters were representative of the heterogeneity and the degree of inflammation in the tissue of origin, suggesting that transcriptionally and functionally distinct populations of fibroblasts exist in joints. For example, some CD248$^+$ cells may correspond with a pluripotential, stem cell–like population of pericytic cells lying in close apposition to endothelial cells, which provide a supply of new stromal cells during inflammation.[109] Interestingly, deletion or removal of the intra-cellular portion of CD248 can reduce stromal cell accumulation and ameliorate models of arthritis such as murine collagen antibody-induced arthritis (CAIA).[110] Furthermore, the prevailing conditions of hypoxia within the rheumatoid synovium may enhance expression of CD248, which is regulated by hypoxia-inducible factor-2 (HIF-2) binding to a hypoxia response element, and which in turn participates in angiogenesis.[111]

Whether such markers remain associated with functionally distinct subpopulations or simply contribute to a larger local pool of multipotential mesenchymal precursors is as yet unknown, but the discovery of markers apparently linked to function has provided the tools with which such questions can be answered. The surface marker gp38 (podoplanin) is a potential therapeutic target that marks populations of fibroblasts (fibroblastic reticular cells) that modulate trafficking of immune cells such as dendritic cells within the lymph node.[48] The surface marker gp38 is highly expressed in lining layer fibroblasts in RA, and its synovial expression is reduced during TNF blockade. In vitro data support a relationship with inflammation, because gp38 expression is induced by pro-inflammatory cytokines, whereas silencing reduces IL-6 and IL-8 production.[112,113]

Just as in the field of lymph node stromal biology, disaggregation of synovial tissue followed by single cell transcriptomic analyses is beginning to demonstrate the diversity of fibroblast clusters based on shared transcriptional profiles. Disaggregated tissue can be sorted to refine smaller subpopulations for transcriptomic analysis after single cell RNA sequencing, and it can also be subjected to antibody-based mass cytometry techniques that allow up to 40 multiplexed markers to be analyzed in parallel. This approach was used to isolate and study fibroblasts in the OA and RA synovium based on a sorting strategy for gp38-positive cells that excluded leukocytes and endothelial cells.[114] Stromal diversity was observed using single cell sequencing of populations from disaggregated synovium, identifying key surface determinants of fibroblast subpopulations as CD90, gp38, and CD34, with a lesser contribution from cadherin 11. The three discrete clusters of cells demonstrated distinct functions in tissue culture, including proliferation, invasiveness, support for osteoclast differentiation, and cytokine secretion.[115] This work identifies lining and sublining populations as having distinct functional roles, with greater diversity in the sublining compartment. An unbiased single cell approach to identifying synovial populations in disaggregated tissue also confirmed the presence of up to 13 synovial cellular populations, containing at least three fibroblast subpopulations.[116] Additional studies are required to determine if the subsets represent terminal differentiation of cell types or a continuum of cell phenotype.

Epigenetic Regulation of Fibroblast Gene Expression in Rheumatic Disease

Epigenetic regulation implies heritable alterations in regulation of gene transcription in the absence of genetic mutation. The epigenetic code, itself regulated by dedicated enzyme complexes, consists of two main groups of covalent modifications: first, methylation and hydroxymethylation of CpG dinucleotides in DNA gene promotor regions, and second, multiple modifications of the histone proteins around which DNA is packaged in chromatin, including acetylation, methylation, and citrullination.[117] These modifications control the access of transcription complexes to chromatin. Global changes in DNA methylation have been recorded in RA FLS, paralleling those seen in human tumors; using demethylating agents to induce global DNA demethylation in "normal" synovial fibroblasts induces genes suggestive of change toward an RA FLS-like phenotype.[118] Similarly, global changes in histone acetylation and levels of the histone acetyltransferase (HAT) and histone deacetylase (HDAC) complexes that are responsible for their control have been demonstrated in RA FLS.[119,120] HDAC inhibitors have also been suggested to show beneficial effects in vitro and in ex vivo models using synovial tissue.[121,122]

Transcriptomics has been used to identify genes overexpressed in RA FLS, which has identified promoter hypomethylation in the critical T-box transcription factor 5 *(TBX5)* gene and specific local histone modifications such as histone 4 lysine 4 trimethylation that correspond with open chromatin structure and active transcription. TBX5 emerges as a target of cytokine (IL-1β) and TLR stimulation and a driver of multiple pathways, including chemokine expression, thus identifying a key element in the epigenetic regulation of established RA FLS.[123] Other genes recently identified as subject to epigenetic regulation in RA FLS include the cytokine IL-6[124] and the chemokine CXCL12.[125] Cytokine stimulation can regulate promoter DNA methylation, demonstrating a reversible, short-term hypomethylation of candidate genes in response to IL-1β in OA and RA fibroblasts mediated via changes in DNA methyltransferase activity. However, although this suggests that pro-inflammatory cytokines can drive epigenetic regulation, the repertoire of promoters modified by IL-1β exposure was limited, suggesting that additional factors influence the persistent changes seen in long-standing disease.[126] Whole methylome comparative analysis of RA FLS and OA FLS reveals epigenetic change in key genes, including the key signaling component STAT3, and MAP3K5 (ASK1), a key component of TLR-induced inflammatory pathways and apoptosis in response to cellular stress.[127,128] Recent work has documented the epigenetic landscape of RA and OA FLS, systematically linking DNA to histone modifications and identifying characteristic signatures of disease and function such as invasiveness.[129] Intriguingly, studies of fibroblasts from patients with very early disease suggest that epigenetic changes are present in the earliest stages of clinically apparent RA, and that disease-specific epigenetic changes in synovial fibroblasts are not simply the product of prolonged exposure to high levels of inflammation.[130]

Rapid advances helped define the altered, profibrotic phenotype of fibroblasts in systemic sclerosis. Once again initial studies have focused on genome-wide regulation; blockade in dermal fibroblasts of histone 3 lysine 27 trimethylation, a well-characterized histone modification associated with gene silencing, led to dramatic increases in collagen release in vitro and in animal models of fibrosis.[131] Focused work on proteins interacting with Wnt pathways that regulate both bone turnover and fibrotic processes revealed hypermethylation of the promoters of DKK1 and SFRP1. Use of the whole genome demethylating agent 5-azacytidine reversed this modification and ameliorated experimental fibrosis.[132] Although this represents a nonspecific approach to modifying regulation of individual genes, 5-aza-cytidine is already in use in the treatment of multiple myeloma, and such drugs are the precursors of newer agents that will target regulation of specific groups of genes via blockade of regulatory subunits of the chromatin-modifying complexes that generate and remove epigenetic modifications.[133]

Proof of the concept that epigenetic regulation determines disease phenotype comes from a recent genome-wide DNA methylation study comparing fibroblasts from scleroderma patients with diffuse disease, patients with limited disease, and control subjects. Not only were differentially methylated DNA sites found between the groups, but these sites were also frequently related to key genes in fibrotic pathways, including the metalloprotease ADAM12, collagen genes, and transcription factors of the RUNX family that are known to drive collagen synthesis. Multiple additional candidates identified by this study will further elucidate the roles and interactions of fibroblasts in scleroderma.[134]

Targeting global epigenetic change, although a potential therapeutic in the context of a hematologic malignancy such as myeloma, is unlikely to be acceptable in the treatment of chronic inflammatory disease, as reflected in the high levels of adverse events seen in early phase trials in people with juvenile idiopathic arthritis (JIA).[135] Our ability to target specific epigenetic modification complexes and thus influence individual genes or groups of genes is currently limited[136] but will rapidly expand over the coming years.

MicroRNAs and Fibroblast-like Synoviocytes

MiRNAs are small, approximately 22-nucleotide-long RNAs that regulate the expression of multiple genes through interactions with both the 3′ untranslated region (UTR) of gene transcripts and RNA-induced silencing complexes.[137] This in turn interferes with translation of messenger RNA (mRNA) into protein or induces mRNA degradation. Currently around 1900 miRNAs have been identified in humans, although many of the target genes of miRNAs are yet to be described.

MiRNAs are frequently grouped alongside epigenetic modifications as key controllers of altered gene expression in disease. Underlying this association is the high degree of epigenetic regulation of miRNA genes. This phenomenon has been demonstrated at the level of individual genes, as in the case of miR-203, which is overexpressed in RA FLS under the control of DNA methylation, leading to enhanced expression of MMPs and IL-6.[138] A similar regulatory relationship has also been demonstrated at a whole genome level: Comparing RA FLS and OA FLS, a range of differentially expressed miRNAs were identified and in close proximity to differentially methylated CpG rich regions of DNA, suggesting that differences in miRNA profiles are closely related to DNA methylation. These differential CpG region methylation and miRNA expression data sets have been further combined in silico to predict networks of miRNA targets that may be modified in the aggressive RA FLS phenotype.[139]

Two miRNAs, miR-146a and miR-155, are vital for immune function, are overexpressed in RA FLS compared with OA FLS, and are subject to induction by cytokines and TLR ligands. The miRNA miR-155 drives changes in MMP repertoire,[140] although in vitro studies suggest a regulatory role leading to overall repression of MMP production.[141] The importance of miR-146a in anti-inflammatory regulatory networks has been highlighted through work with the arthritogenic Chikungunya virus. Chikungunya virus–infected synovial fibroblasts upregulate miR-146a, which in turn downregulates pro-inflammatory signaling factors such as TRAF6, IRAK1, and IRAK2, resulting in a corresponding decrease in NF-κB phosphorylation. This finding highlights the critical involvement of this miRNA in the regulation of inflammation.[142]

Increased RA FLS survival is linked to miRNAs; the miR-34 promoter becomes hypermethylated in RA FLS, leading to reduced responsiveness to FasL and TNF-related apoptosis-inducing ligand (TRAIL)-mediated apoptosis.[143] More recently, mutations in p53 in RA have been linked to miRNA-regulated proliferation of RA FLS; mutated forms of p53 are not capable of driving the expression of miR-22, which represses the pro-proliferation protein Cry61. This finding fits with observations of decreased miR-22 expression in RA compared with OA synovial tissue, providing a potential explanation for increased RA FLS numbers in the synovium.[144] MiR-20 has also been implicated in regulation of cell survival and inflammation; overexpression of MiR-20 in RA FLS reduced ASK1 mRNA stability and inhibited LPS-induced IL-6 and CXCL10 expression.[145] This finding adds to the increasing data demonstrating a role for miRNAs in regulation of TLR-induced responses; for example, previous work has shown that miR-19a/b regulates TLR2 expression in RA FLS.[146] More recently, the fundamental embryonic epigenetic patterning and epigenetic marks of fibroblasts from different joints in the body has been undertaken, revealing not only the important role played by noncoding RNA species such as miRNAs, but also that such patterning plays a role in differential function at different sites. For instance, epigenetic regulation provides an explanation for a greater tendency towards cartilage degradation in the joints of the hand compared with shoulder or knee joints.[147,148]

Modulation of miRNA expression has significant therapeutic potential as a means of regulating networks of related genes rather than current approaches targeting single cytokines or cell types. Multiple approaches are being taken to develop miRNA therapeutics, including administering exogenous miRNAs and treatment with compounds that either stimulate or inhibit the expression of endogenous miRNAs. For instance, the compound denbinobin upregulates the expression of miR-146a, which in turn ablates the responsiveness of OA FLS to IL-1β.[149]

Lessons Learned From Cancer

Alongside the field of inflammation, oncology has also been experiencing a surge in interest in the biology of fibroblasts and stromal cells, as well as the mechanisms by which they interact with primary transformed tumor cells.[150] A number of important cytokines that contribute to cancerous transformation of healthy cells by so-called cancer-associated fibroblasts has been described, including hepatocyte growth factor (HGF) and TGF-β. Crucially, tumor-associated fibroblasts appear able to transform normal cells, in addition to premalignant cells.[150] The importance of tumor-associated fibroblasts, termed *cancer-associated fibroblasts (CAFs),* has been demonstrated in breast cancer: human breast cancer implants were unable to grow successfully when implanted into mice without their co-administration with human tumor–derived fibroblasts.[151] Intriguingly, similar molecular signals have been implicated in the predilection for cancer cells to metastasize to certain sites. In particular, the ectopic expression and function of the CXCL12/CXCR4 ligand-receptor pair, in a manner reminiscent of RA, have been implicated in the persistence and tissue tropism of metastatic cells in breast cancer. Tumor-associated fibroblasts secrete CXCL12, resulting in increased promotion of carcinoma cell proliferation, migration, and invasion compared with control fibroblasts but also leading to recruitment of endothelial cell precursors.[152,153]

Furthermore, molecules that mark fibroblast subpopulations in the joint are associated with active, invasive cancer. These molecules include the expression of tumor-associated stromal markers such as fibroblast activation protein (FAP),[12,13] galectin-3,[154,155] and S-100A4.[156] Interestingly, galectin-3 subjects to epigenetic regulation.[155,157] Both gp38 and CD248 are also heavily implicated in tumor progression.[9,158]

These similarities between RA synovial fibroblasts and CAFs overlap with observations that the persistent phenotype of RA synovial fibroblasts itself includes elements normally associated with "transformed" cells. These elements include loss of density and anchorage limitation for growth, which usually curtails in vitro fibroblast culture, firm adherence to ECM components of cartilage, and the invasiveness that is most aptly demonstrated in the chimeric SCID mouse model. Another defining characteristic of RA synovial fibroblasts that helps explain their phenotype is dysregulation of proto-oncogenes and tumor suppressor genes. Once again, epigenetic regulation is likely to underlie this phenotype. However, the precise mechanisms maintaining the persistent phenotype at a whole genome level are yet to be elucidated.

Furthermore, RA is a systemic disease involving multiple joints; therefore, whether the fibroblast phenotype results from a global change in fibroblast gene expression or whether the phenotype is locally imprinted by exposure to a characteristic cytokine, matrix, and cellular milieu is yet to be established. Recent data now appear to confirm that human RA synovial fibroblasts within the SCID mouse model may travel systemically through lymphatics and the bloodstream to unpopulated samples of cartilage and then invade.[19] Therefore, at least one possibility is that locally imprinted, "activated" fibroblasts may export destructive arthritis to joints where mild injury or immune response has occurred over time. In the cancer field, the concept of tumor stroma "normalization" has now become an accepted aspect of new oncology therapies. Clinical studies of angiogenesis inhibitors and antibodies against ECM components such as tenascin have been favorable, whereas inhibitors of MMPs, overexpression of TIMPs, and blockade of integrin signaling have all shown promise in pre-clinical trials.[159] Results of studies examining the interactions between endothelial cells and their associated pericytes underlie the importance of targeting the stroma as a whole.

One study[160] has shown that endothelial cells release PDGF, which induces VEGF production from pericytes, leading to bidirectional conversations between the two cell types. Interrupting these conversations by using PDGF inhibitors has proven to be more effective therapy than using VEGF inhibitors alone. Interestingly, although VEGF inhibitors lost their inhibitory effect in later stage tumors, targeting of the pericytes helped even late-stage tumors regress.[160] The authors have subsequently shown that pericyte precursors are partly recruited from the bone marrow to tumor perivascular sites.[161]

The cyclin-dependent kinases (CDKs) are a family of enzymes that maintain cellular proliferation and survival under tight control, balanced by specific inhibitors (CDKis). CDK dysregulation has been demonstrated in many tumors, and their manipulation has consequently been exploited to develop anticancer drugs including the CDKi roscovitine.[162] RA fibroblasts express low levels of the CDKi p21,[163] and adenovirus-mediated p21 gene transfer into RA fibroblasts both induces cell cycle arrest and downregulates expression of cytokines, MMPs, and cathepsins,[164] suggesting a novel therapy targeting a disease-specific phenotype in RA FLS. Inhibition of TNF pathways and CDK inhibition recently synergize in ameliorating murine collagen-induced arthritis without increasing immune suppression. This approach, currently in early phase trials in RA, may therefore have significant benefits.[165]

Conclusion

Fibroblasts are structural mesenchymal cells that form the cellular infrastructure for most internal organs, as well as for bordering membranes such as the synovial membrane. They are prominently involved in the deposition and resorption of the ECM and thus are responsible for maintaining tissue homeostasis. However, fibroblasts are far more than structural, passively responding cells that build the "backbone" for organ-specific function. Rather, they are sensitive to environmental changes. They react in a specific manner to a variety of stimuli and are capable of actively influencing not only the composition of the ECM but also the cellular composition of tissues and barrier membranes. Under inflammatory disease conditions, fibroblasts act as organ-specific, innate immune system sentinel cells and are involved in the progression of organ damage, as well as in the switch from acute resolving to chronic persisting inflammation. We now know that functionally distinct fibroblast subsets exist and can be identified with new markers to understand better mechanisms of developmental patterning, wound healing, and persistent inflammatory responses, which appear to depend in large part on epigenetic modifications. This notion is particularly true for fibroblast-like synoviocytes, which play a critical role in the pathogenesis of RA and possess a characteristic, invasive, and activated phenotype. In addition to contributing to the recruitment of inflammatory cells to the joint, they modulate the survival and behavior of these cells and are, in turn, regulated by the newly recruited cells. More importantly, fibroblast-like synoviocytes are crucial components in the hyperplastic lining layer and in cartilage destruction. New data raise the possibility of epigenetically programmed aggressive cells exporting arthritis from inflamed to uninflamed joints in the early stages of arthritis, but at the same time offering the possibility of specifically targeting stromal subpopulations of choice.

Full references for this chapter can be found on ExpertConsult.com.

Selected References

1. Rinn JL, et al.: Anatomic demarcation by positional variation in fibroblast gene expression programs, *PLoS Genet* 2(7):e119, 2006.
2. Rinn JL, et al.: Functional demarcation of active and silent chromatin domains in human HOX loci by noncoding RNAs, *Cell* 129(7):1311–1323, 2007.
3. Hamann J, et al.: Expression of the activation antigen CD97 and its ligand CD55 in rheumatoid synovial tissue, *Arthritis Rheum* 42(4):650–658, 1999.
4. Wilkinson LS, et al.: Expression of vascular cell adhesion molecule-1 in normal and inflamed synovium, *Lab Invest* 68(1):82–88, 1993.
5. Kasperkovitz PV, et al.: Fibroblast-like synoviocytes derived from patients with rheumatoid arthritis show the imprint of synovial tissue heterogeneity: evidence of a link between an increased myofibroblast-like phenotype and high-inflammation synovitis, *Arthritis Rheum* 52(2):430–441, 2005.
6. Lax S, et al.: CD248/Endosialin is dynamically expressed on a subset of stromal cells during lymphoid tissue development, splenic remodeling and repair, *FEBS Lett* 581(18):3550–3556, 2007.
7. Tomkowicz B, et al.: Interaction of endosialin/TEM1 with extracellular matrix proteins mediates cell adhesion and migration, *Proc Natl Acad Sci U S A* 104(46):17965–17970, 2007.
8. Katakai T, et al.: Lymph node fibroblastic reticular cells construct the stromal reticulum via contact with lymphocytes, *J Exp Med* 200(6):783–795, 2004.
9. Wicki A, et al.: Tumor invasion in the absence of epithelial-mesenchymal transition: podoplanin-mediated remodeling of the actin cytoskeleton, *Cancer Cell* 9(4):261–272, 2006.
10. Smith SC, et al.: An immunocytochemical study of the distribution of proline-4-hydroxylase in normal, osteoarthritic and rheumatoid arthritic synovium at both the light and electron microscopic level, *Br J Rheumatol* 37(3):287–291, 1998.
11. Senolt L, et al.: S100A4 is expressed at site of invasion in rheumatoid arthritis synovium and modulates production of matrix metalloproteinases, *Ann Rheum Dis* 65(12):1645–1648, 2006.
12. Bauer S, et al.: Fibroblast activation protein is expressed by rheumatoid myofibroblast-like synoviocytes, *Arthritis Res Ther* 8(6):R171, 2006.
13. Henry LR, et al.: Clinical implications of fibroblast activation protein in patients with colon cancer, *Clin Cancer Res* 13(6):1736–1741, 2007.
14. Ospelt C, et al.: Inhibition of fibroblast activation protein and dipeptidylpeptidase 4 increases cartilage invasion by rheumatoid arthritis synovial fibroblasts, *Arthritis Rheum* 62(5):1224–1235, 2010.
15. Kalluri R, Neilson EG: Epithelial-mesenchymal transition and its implications for fibrosis, *J Clin Invest* 112(12):1776–1784, 2003.
16. Steenvoorden MM, et al.: Transition of healthy to diseased synovial tissue in rheumatoid arthritis is associated with gain of mesenchymal/fibrotic characteristics, *Arthritis Res Ther* 8(6):R165, 2006.
17. Asahara T, et al.: Isolation of putative progenitor endothelial cells for angiogenesis, *Science* 275(5302):964–967, 1997.
18. Marinova-Mutafchieva L, et al.: Inflammation is preceded by tumor necrosis factor-dependent infiltration of mesenchymal cells in experimental arthritis, *Arthritis Rheum* 46(2):507–513, 2002.
19. Lefevre S, et al.: Synovial fibroblasts spread rheumatoid arthritis to unaffected joints, *Nat Med* 15(12):1414–1420, 2009.
20. Phillips RJ, et al.: Circulating fibrocytes traffic to the lungs in response to CXCL12 and mediate fibrosis, *J Clin Invest* 114(3):438–446, 2004.
21. Abe R, et al.: Peripheral blood fibrocytes: differentiation pathway and migration to wound sites, *J Immunol* 166(12):7556–7562, 2001.

22. Haniffa MA, et al.: Adult human fibroblasts are potent immunoregulatory cells and functionally equivalent to mesenchymal stem cells, *J Immunol* 179(3):1595–1604, 2007.
23. Li X, Makarov SS: An essential role of NF-kappaB in the "tumor-like" phenotype of arthritic synoviocytes, *Proc Natl Acad Sci U S A* 103:17432–17437, 2006.
24. Friedl P, Zanker KS, Brocker EB: Cell migration strategies in 3-D extracellular matrix: differences in morphology, cell matrix interactions, and integrin function, *Microsc Res Tech* 43(5):369–378, 1998.
25. Kuschert GS, et al.: Glycosaminoglycans interact selectively with chemokines and modulate receptor binding and cellular responses, *Biochemistry* 38(39):12959–12968, 1999.
26. Echtermeyer F, et al.: Syndecan-4 core protein is sufficient for the assembly of focal adhesions and actin stress fibers, *J Cell Sci* 112(Pt 20):3433–3441, 1999.
27. Echtermeyer F, et al.: Delayed wound repair and impaired angiogenesis in mice lacking syndecan-4, *J Clin Invest* 107(2):R9–R14, 2001.
28. Petruzzelli L, Takami M, Humes HD: Structure and function of cell adhesion molecules, *Am J Med* 106(4):467–476, 1999.
29. Wheelock MJ, Johnson KR: Cadherins as modulators of cellular phenotype, *Annu Rev Cell Dev Biol* 19:207–235, 2003.
30. Tran NL, et al.: Signal transduction from N-cadherin increases Bcl-2. Regulation of the phosphatidylinositol 3-kinase/Akt pathway by homophilic adhesion and actin cytoskeletal organization, *J Biol Chem* 277(36):32905–32914, 2002.
31. Kim JB, et al.: N-Cadherin extracellular repeat 4 mediates epithelial to mesenchymal transition and increased motility, *J Cell Biol* 151(6):1193–1206, 2000.
32. Hazan RB, et al.: Exogenous expression of N-cadherin in breast cancer cells induces cell migration, invasion, and metastasis, *J Cell Biol* 148(4):779–790, 2000.
33. Werb Z, et al.: Signal transduction through the fibronectin receptor induces collagenase and stromelysin gene expression, *J Cell Biol* 109(2):877–889, 1989.
34. Mitra SK, Hanson DA, Schlaepfer DD: Focal adhesion kinase: in command and control of cell motility, *Nat Rev Mol Cell Biol* 6(1):56–68, 2005.
35. Westermarck J, Seth A, Kahari VM: Differential regulation of interstitial collagenase (MMP-1) gene expression by ETS transcription factors, *Oncogene* 14(22):2651–2660, 1997.
36. Li WQ, Dehnade F, Zafarullah M: Oncostatin M-induced matrix metalloproteinase and tissue inhibitor of metalloproteinase-3 genes expression in chondrocytes requires Janus kinase/STAT signaling pathway, *J Immunol* 166(5):3491–3498, 2001.
37. Mengshol JA, et al.: Interleukin-1 induction of collagenase 3 (matrix metalloproteinase 13) gene expression in chondrocytes requires p38, c-Jun N-terminal kinase, and nuclear factor kappaB: differential regulation of collagenase 1 and collagenase 3, *Arthritis Rheum* 43(4):801–811, 2000.
38. Barchowsky A, Frleta D, Vincenti MP: Integration of the NF-kappaB and mitogen-activated protein kinase/AP-1 pathways at the collagenase-1 promoter: divergence of IL-1 and TNF-dependent signal transduction in rabbit primary synovial fibroblasts, *Cytokine* 12(10):1469–1479, 2000.
39. Brauchle M, et al.: Independent role of p38 and ERK1/2 mitogen-activated kinases in the upregulation of matrix metalloproteinase-1, *Exp Cell Res* 258(1):135–144, 2000.
40. Loeser RF, et al.: Fibronectin fragment activation of proline-rich tyrosine kinase PYK2 mediates integrin signals regulating collagenase-3 expression by human chondrocytes through a protein kinase C-dependent pathway, *J Biol Chem* 278(27):24577–24585, 2003.
41. Pierer M, et al.: Chemokine secretion of rheumatoid arthritis synovial fibroblasts stimulated by toll-like receptor 2 ligands, *J Immunol* 172(2):1256–1265, 2004.
42. Ospelt C, et al.: Overexpression of toll-like receptors 3 and 4 in synovial tissue from patients with early rheumatoid arthritis: toll-like receptor expression in early and longstanding arthritis, *Arthritis Rheum* 58(12):3684–3692, 2008.
43. Brentano F, et al.: Pre-B cell colony-enhancing factor/visfatin, a new marker of inflammation in rheumatoid arthritis with pro-inflammatory and matrix-degrading activities, *Arthritis Rheum* 56(9):2829–2839, 2007.
44. Seibl R, et al.: Expression and regulation of Toll-like receptor 2 in rheumatoid arthritis synovium, *Am J Pathol* 162(4):1221–1227, 2003.
45. Brentano F, et al.: RNA released from necrotic synovial fluid cells activates rheumatoid arthritis synovial fibroblasts via Toll-like receptor 3, *Arthritis Rheum* 52(9):2656–2665, 2005.
46. Martinon F, et al.: Gout-associated uric acid crystals activate the NALP3 inflammasome, *Nature* 440(7081):237–241, 2006.
47. Link A, et al.: Fibroblastic reticular cells in lymph nodes regulate the homeostasis of naive T cells, *Nat Immunol* 8(11):1255–1265, 2007.
48. Acton SE, et al.: Podoplanin-rich stromal networks induce dendritic cell motility via activation of the C-type lectin receptor CLEC-2, *Immunity* 37(2):276–289, 2012.
49. Rodda LB, et al.: Single-cell RNA sequencing of lymph node stromal cells reveals niche-associated heterogeneity, *Immunity* 48:1014–1028 e1016, 2018.
50. Augello A, Kurth TB, De Bari BC: Mesenchymal stem cells: a perspective from in vitro cultures to in vivo migration and niches, *Eur Cell Mater* 20:121–133, 2010.
51. Burger JA, et al.: Fibroblast-like synoviocytes support B-cell pseudoemperipolesis via a stromal cell-derived factor-1- and CD106 (VCAM-1)-dependent mechanism, *J Clin Invest* 107(3):305–315, 2001.
52. Boland JM, et al.: Clusterin is expressed in normal synoviocytes and in tenosynovial giant cell tumors of localized and diffuse types: diagnostic and histogenetic implications, *Am J Surg Pathol* 33(8):1225–1229, 2009.
53. Valencia X, et al.: Cadherin-11 provides specific cellular adhesion between fibroblast-like synoviocytes, *J Exp Med* 200(12):1673–1679, 2004.
54. Kimura Y, et al.: Cadherin-11 expressed in association with mesenchymal morphogenesis in the head, somite, and limb bud of early mouse embryos, *Dev Biol* 169(1):347–358, 1995.
55. Chang SK, Gu Z, Brenner MB: Fibroblast-like synoviocytes in inflammatory arthritis pathology: the emerging role of cadherin-11, *Immunol Rev* 233(1):256–266, 2010.
56. Friedl P, et al.: CD4+ T lymphocytes migrating in three-dimensional collagen lattices lack focal adhesions and utilize beta1 integrin-independent strategies for polarization, interaction with collagen fibers and locomotion, *Eur J Immunol* 28(8):2331–2343, 1998.
57. Kiener HP, et al.: Synovial fibroblasts self-direct multicellular lining architecture and synthetic function in three-dimensional organ culture, *Arthritis Rheum* 62(3):742–752, 2010.
58. Buckley CD, et al.: Fibroblasts regulate the switch from acute resolving to chronic persistent inflammation, *Trends Immunol* 22(4):199–204, 2001.
59. Kissin EY, Merkel PA, Lafyatis R: Myofibroblasts and hyalinized collagen as markers of skin disease in systemic sclerosis, *Arthritis Rheum* 54(11):3655–3660, 2006.
60. Bechtel W, et al.: Methylation determines fibroblast activation and fibrogenesis in the kidney, *Nat Med* 16(5):544–550, 2010.
61. Distler O, et al.: Overexpression of monocyte chemoattractant protein 1 in systemic sclerosis: role of platelet-derived growth factor and effects on monocyte chemotaxis and collagen synthesis, *Arthritis Rheum* 44(11):2665–2678, 2001.
62. Takemura S, et al.: Lymphoid neogenesis in rheumatoid synovitis, *J Immunol* 167(2):1072–1080, 2001.

63. Taylor PC, Sivakumar B: Hypoxia and angiogenesis in rheumatoid arthritis, *Curr Opin Rheumatol* 17(3):293–298, 2005.
64. Kiener HP, et al.: Cadherin 11 promotes invasive behavior of fibroblast-like synoviocytes, *Arthritis Rheum* 60(5):1305–1310, 2009.
65. Assefnia S, et al.: Cadherin-11 in poor prognosis malignancies and rheumatoid arthritis: common target, common therapies, *Oncotarget* 5(6):1458–1474, 2014.
66. Tolboom TC, et al.: Invasiveness of fibroblast-like synoviocytes is an individual patient characteristic associated with the rate of joint destruction in patients with rheumatoid arthritis, *Arthritis Rheum* 52(7):1999–2002, 2005.
67. Muller-Ladner U, et al.: Synovial fibroblasts of patients with rheumatoid arthritis attach to and invade normal human cartilage when engrafted into SCID mice, *Am J Pathol* 149(5):1607–1615, 1996.
68. Rutkauskaite E, et al.: Ribozymes that inhibit the production of matrix metalloproteinase 1 reduce the invasiveness of rheumatoid arthritis synovial fibroblasts, *Arthritis Rheum* 50(5):1448–1456, 2004.
69. Schedel J, et al.: Targeting cathepsin L (CL) by specific ribozymes decreases CL protein synthesis and cartilage destruction in rheumatoid arthritis, *Gene Ther* 11(13):1040–1047, 2004.
70. Lowin T, et al.: Glucocorticoids increase alpha5 integrin expression and adhesion of synovial fibroblasts but inhibit ERK signaling, migration, and cartilage invasion, *Arthritis Rheum* 60(12):3623–3632, 2009.
71. Fiehn C, et al.: Methotrexate (MTX) and albumin coupled with MTX (MTX-HSA) suppress synovial fibroblast invasion and cartilage degradation in vivo, *Ann Rheum Dis* 63(7):884–886, 2004.
72. You S, et al.: Identification of key regulators for the migration and invasion of rheumatoid synoviocytes through a systems approach, *Proc Natl Acad Sci U S A* 111(1):550–555, 2014.
73. Stanford SM, et al.: Protein tyrosine phosphatase expression profile of rheumatoid arthritis fibroblast-like synoviocytes: a novel role of SH2 domain-containing phosphatase 2 as a modulator of invasion and survival, *Arthritis Rheum* 65(5):1171–1180, 2013.
74. Hot A, et al.: IL-17 and tumour necrosis factor alpha combination induces a HIF-1alpha-dependent invasive phenotype in synoviocytes, *Ann Rheum Dis* 71(8):1393–1401, 2012.
75. Neumann E, et al.: Cell culture and passaging alters gene expression pattern and proliferation rate in rheumatoid arthritis synovial fibroblasts, *Arthritis Res Ther* 12(3):R83, 2010.
76. Filer A, et al.: Differential survival of leukocyte subsets mediated by synovial, bone marrow, and skin fibroblasts: Site-specific versus activation-dependent survival of T cells and neutrophils, *Arthritis Rheum* 54(7):2096–2108, 2006.
77. Koch AE, et al.: Epithelial neutrophil activating peptide-78: a novel chemotactic cytokine for neutrophils in arthritis, *J Clin Invest* 94(3):1012–1018, 1994.
78. Koch AE, et al.: Growth-related gene product alpha. A chemotactic cytokine for neutrophils in rheumatoid arthritis, *J Immunol* 155(7):3660–3666, 1995.
79. Koch AE, et al.: Synovial tissue macrophage as a source of the chemotactic cytokine IL-8, *J Immunol* 147(7):2187–2195, 1991.
80. Patel DD, Zachariah JP, Whichard LP: CXCR3 and CCR5 ligands in rheumatoid arthritis synovium, *Clin Immunol* 98(1):39–45, 2001.
81. Nanki T, et al.: Pathogenic role of the CXCL16-CXCR6 pathway in rheumatoid arthritis, *Arthritis Rheum* 52(10):3004–3014, 2005.
82. Villiger PM, Terkeltaub R, Lotz M: Production of monocyte chemoattractant protein-1 by inflamed synovial tissue and cultured synoviocytes, *J Immunol* 149(2):722–727, 1992.
83. Hosaka S, et al.: Expression of the chemokine superfamily in rheumatoid arthritis, *Clin Exp Immunol* 97(3):451–457, 1994.
84. Matsui T, et al.: Selective recruitment of CCR6-expressing cells by increased production of MIP-3 alpha in rheumatoid arthritis, *Clin Exp Immunol* 125(1):155–161, 2001.
85. van HJ, et al.: A multicentre, randomised, double blind, placebo controlled phase II study of subcutaneous interferon beta-1a in the treatment of patients with active rheumatoid arthritis, *Ann Rheum Dis* 64(1):64–69, 2005.
86. Merville P, et al.: Bcl-2+ tonsillar plasma cells are rescued from apoptosis by bone marrow fibroblasts, *J Exp Med* 183(1):227–236, 1996.
87. Sellge G, et al.: Human intestinal fibroblasts prevent apoptosis in human intestinal mast cells by a mechanism independent of stem cell factor, IL-3, IL-4, and nerve growth factor, *J Immunol* 172(1):260–267, 2004.
88. Takashima A, et al.: Colony-stimulating factor-1 secreted by fibroblasts promotes the growth of dendritic cell lines (XS series) derived from murine epidermis, *J Immunol* 154(10):5128–5135, 1995.
89. Donlin LT, et al.: Modulation of TNF-induced macrophage polarization by synovial fibroblasts, *J Immunol* 193(5):2373–2383, 2014.
90. Buckley CD, et al.: Persistent induction of the chemokine receptor CXCR4 by TGF-beta 1 on synovial T cells contributes to their accumulation within the rheumatoid synovium, *J Immunol* 165(6):3423–3429, 2000.
91. Nanki T, et al.: Stromal cell-derived factor-1-CXC chemokine receptor 4 interactions play a central role in CD4+ T cell accumulation in rheumatoid arthritis synovium, *J Immunol* 165(11):6590–6598, 2000.
92. Kim KW, et al.: Up-regulation of stromal cell-derived factor 1 (CXCL12) production in rheumatoid synovial fibroblasts through interactions with T lymphocytes: role of interleukin-17 and CD40L-CD40 interaction, *Arthritis Rheum* 56(4):1076–1086, 2007.
93. Blades MC, et al.: Stromal cell-derived factor 1 (CXCL12) induces monocyte migration into human synovium transplanted onto SCID mice, *Arthritis Rheum* 46(3):824–836, 2002.
94. Ohata J, et al.: Fibroblast-like synoviocytes of mesenchymal origin express functional B cell-activating factor of the TNF family in response to proinflammatory cytokines, *J Immunol* 174(2):864–870, 2005.
95. Matthys P, et al.: AMD3100, a potent and specific antagonist of the stromal cell-derived factor-1 chemokine receptor CXCR4, inhibits autoimmune joint inflammation in IFN-gamma receptor-deficient mice, *J Immunol* 167(8):4686–4692, 2001.
96. Tamamura H, et al.: Identification of a CXCR4 antagonist, a T140 analog, as an anti-rheumatoid arthritis agent, *FEBS Lett* 569(1–3):99–104, 2004.
97. Lally F, et al.: A novel mechanism of neutrophil recruitment in a coculture model of the rheumatoid synovium, *Arthritis Rheum* 52(11):3460–3469, 2005.
98. Luther SA, et al.: Differing activities of homeostatic chemokines CCL19, CCL21, and CXCL12 in lymphocyte and dendritic cell recruitment and lymphoid neogenesis, *J Immunol* 169(1):424–433, 2002.
99. Cyster JG: Chemokines and cell migration in secondary lymphoid organs, *Science* 286(5447):2098–2102, 1999.
100. Ebisuno Y, et al.: Cutting edge: the B cell chemokine CXC chemokine ligand 13/B lymphocyte chemoattractant is expressed in the high endothelial venules of lymph nodes and Peyer's patches and affects B cell trafficking across high endothelial venules, *J Immunol* 171(4):1642–1646, 2003.
101. Hjelmstrom P, et al.: Lymphoid tissue homing chemokines are expressed in chronic inflammation, *Am J Pathol* 156(4):1133–1138, 2000.
102. Keffer J, et al.: Transgenic mice expressing human tumour necrosis factor: a predictive genetic model of arthritis, *EMBO J* 10(13):4025–4031, 1991.
103. Luther SA, et al.: BLC expression in pancreatic islets causes B cell recruitment and lymphotoxin-dependent lymphoid neogenesis, *Immunity* 12(5):471–481, 2000.

104. Manzo A, et al.: Systematic microanatomical analysis of CXCL13 and CCL21 in situ production and progressive lymphoid organization in rheumatoid synovitis, *Eur J Immunol* 35(5):1347–1359, 2005.
105. Manzo A, et al.: CCL21 expression pattern of human secondary lymphoid organ stroma is conserved in inflammatory lesions with lymphoid neogenesis, *Am J Pathol* 171(5):1549–1562, 2007.
106. Amft N, et al.: Ectopic expression of the B cell-attracting chemokine BCA-1 (CXCL13) on endothelial cells and within lymphoid follicles contributes to the establishment of germinal center-like structures in Sjögren's syndrome, *Arthritis Rheum* 44(11):2633–2641, 2001.
107. Humby F, et al.: Ectopic lymphoid structures support ongoing production of class-switched autoantibodies in rheumatoid synovium, *PLoS Med* 6(1):e1, 2009.
108. Tsubaki T, et al.: Accumulation of plasma cells expressing CXCR3 in the synovial sublining regions of early rheumatoid arthritis in association with production of Mig/CXCL9 by synovial fibroblasts, *Clin Exp Immunol* 141(2):363–371, 2005.
109. Crisan M, et al.: A perivascular origin for mesenchymal stem cells in multiple human organs, *Cell Stem Cell* 3(3):301–313, 2008.
110. Maia M, et al.: CD248 and its cytoplasmic domain: a therapeutic target for arthritis, *Arthritis Rheum* 62(12):3595–3606, 2010.
111. Ohradanova A, et al.: Hypoxia upregulates expression of human endosialin gene via hypoxia-inducible factor 2, *Br J Cancer* 99(8):1348–1356, 2008.
112. Ekwall AK, et al.: The tumour-associated glycoprotein podoplanin is expressed in fibroblast-like synoviocytes of the hyperplastic synovial lining layer in rheumatoid arthritis, *Arthritis Res Ther* 13(2):R40, 2011.
113. Del Rey MJ, et al.: Clinicopathological correlations of podoplanin (gp38) expression in rheumatoid synovium and its potential contribution to fibroblast platelet crosstalk, *PLoS ONE* 9(6):e99607, 2014.
114. Donlin LT, et al.: Methods for high-dimensonal analysis of cells dissociated from cyropreserved synovial tissue, *Arthritis Res Ther* 20:139, 2018.
115. Mizoguchi F, et al.: Functionally distinct disease-associated fibroblast subsets in rheumatoid arthritis, *Nat Commun* 9:789, 2018.
116. Stephenson W, et al.: Single-cell RNA-seq of rheumatoid arthritis synovial tissue using low-cost microfluidic instrumentation, *Nat Commun* 9:791, 2018.
117. Tarakhovsky A: Tools and landscapes of epigenetics, *Nat Immunol* 11(7):565–568, 2010.
118. Karouzakis E, et al.: DNA hypomethylation in rheumatoid arthritis synovial fibroblasts, *Arthritis Rheum* 60(12):3613–3622, 2009.
119. Huber LC, et al.: Histone deacetylase/acetylase activity in total synovial tissue derived from rheumatoid arthritis and osteoarthritis patients, *Arthritis Rheum* 56(4):1087–1093, 2007.
120. Kawabata T, et al.: Increased activity and expression of histone deacetylase 1 in relation to tumor necrosis factor-alpha in synovial tissue of rheumatoid arthritis, *Arthritis Res Ther* 12(4):R133, 2010.
129. Ai R, et al.: Comprehensive epigenetic landscape of rheumatoid arthritis fibroblast-like synoviocytes, *Nature Communications* 9:1921, 2018.
147. Frank-Bertoncelj M, et al.: Epigenetically-driven anatomical diversity of synovial fibroblasts guides joint-specific fibroblast functions, *Nat Commun* 8:14852, 2017.
148. Ai R, Hammaker D, Boyle DL, et al.: Joint-specific DNA methylation and transcriptome signatures in rheumatoid arthritis identify distinct pathogenic processes, *Nat Commun* 7:11849, 2016.

15 Mast Cells

PETER A. NIGROVIC

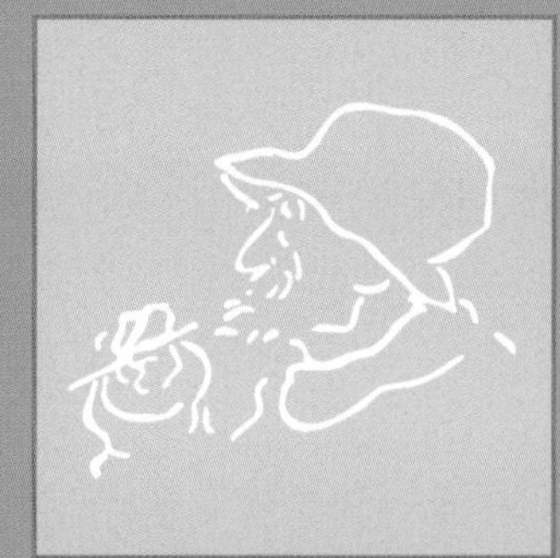

KEY POINTS

Mast cells arise in the bone marrow, circulate as immature precursors, and develop into functional mast cells after entering peripheral tissues.

The phenotype of mast cells is diverse, plastic, and governed by signals from lymphocytes, fibroblasts, and other elements of the microenvironment.

In healthy tissues, mast cells serve as immunologic sentinels and participate in innate and adaptive immune responses to bacteria and parasites.

Mast cells accumulate in injured and inflamed tissue, where they may amplify or suppress inflammation.

Mast cells have been implicated in multiple immune-mediated diseases, including inflammatory arthritis, although their role as a therapeutic target remains uncertain.

Introduction

Although mast cells are best known for their role in allergy and anaphylaxis, the immune function of this bone marrow–derived lineage far outstrips its participation in immunoglobulin (Ig)E-driven disease. Mast cells are resident broadly in vascularized tissues but cluster near interfaces with the external world in skin and mucosa, as well as in the linings of vulnerable body cavities and near blood vessels and nerves. In these locations, mast cells serve as immune sentinels, equipped with an array of pathogen receptors and an armamentarium of mediators capable of rapidly recruiting immune effector cells. Mast cells also accumulate in sites of tissue injury and chronic inflammation, although their role in such locations remains uncertain. Other functions for this lineage, conserved by evolution for more than 500 million years, continue to be defined.

Circumstantial and experimental evidence implicates mast cells in the pathogenesis of rheumatic diseases. Mast cells reside constitutively in the normal synovium and are found in large numbers in inflamed synovial tissue, whereas mast cell mediators are identified in inflammatory joint fluid. Moreover, models have indicated that mast cells can contribute importantly to the pathogenesis of experimental arthritis. Mast cells have also been implicated in other autoimmune conditions, including multiple sclerosis, bullous pemphigoid, and systemic sclerosis.

Basic Biology of Mast Cells

Development and Tissue Distribution

Mast cells are distinctive in appearance. Ranging in size from 10 to 60 μm and with a centrally located round or oval nucleus, their abundant cytoplasm is filled with multiple small granules. They were named *Mastzellen* in 1878 by the German pathologist Paul Ehrlich, who believed that they were overfed connective tissue cells (*mästen*, in German, means to feed or fatten an animal). Electron microscopy reveals that the plasma membrane of the mast cells exhibits multiple thin cytoplasmic extensions, providing a broad interface with the surrounding tissue (Fig. 15.1A). The tissue distribution of mast cells is extensive; within tissue, mast cells tend to cluster around blood vessels and nerves and near epithelial and mucosal surfaces. They are also found in the lining of vulnerable body cavities such as the peritoneum and the diarthrodial joint. Given this localization, mast cells are among the first immune cells to encounter pathogens invading into tissue from the external world or via the bloodstream, consistent with their role as immune sentinel cells.

Mast cells are of hematopoietic origin, arising in the bone marrow and depositing in tissues after migrating through the bloodstream (Fig. 15.2). Unlike other myeloid cells, such as monocytes and neutrophils, mast cells do not terminally differentiate in the bone marrow but rather circulate as rare progenitors (0.005% of leukocytes), bearing the surface signature $CD34^+$/c-Kit^+/$Fc\varepsilon RI^+$.[1] Further developmental details have been worked out most extensively in the mouse. A burst of circulating progenitors late in gestation suggests the possibility that mast cells may populate the tissues primarily during early development, with later recruitment restricted to the inflammatory context, as appears to be the case for certain populations of murine tissue macrophages. After entering the tissues, murine mast cells may mature into classic granulated cells or remain as ungranulated progenitors, awaiting local signals to differentiate fully. Comparison of murine lung and intestine has demonstrated that these tissues use distinct pathways to regulate the constitutive and inducible recruitment of mast cell progenitors, illustrating that mast cell homing is a precisely controlled process.[2,3]

Once resident in tissues, mast cells may live for many months. Mature mast cells remain capable of mitotic division, although recruitment of circulating progenitors appears to greatly exceed local replication as a pathway to expand the number of tissue mast cells. Mechanisms of reducing mast cell numbers include apoptosis, as demonstrated in tissue mast cells deprived of the cytokine stem cell factor (SCF), a critical survival signal for mast cells. Under certain conditions, mast cells can also emigrate via the lymphatics, appearing in draining lymph nodes much in the manner of dendritic cells.[4] The pathways that license mast cell accumulation in inflamed tissues are incompletely defined but include tissue production of factors such as IL-4 and IL-33 that attenuate mast cell apoptosis.[5,6]

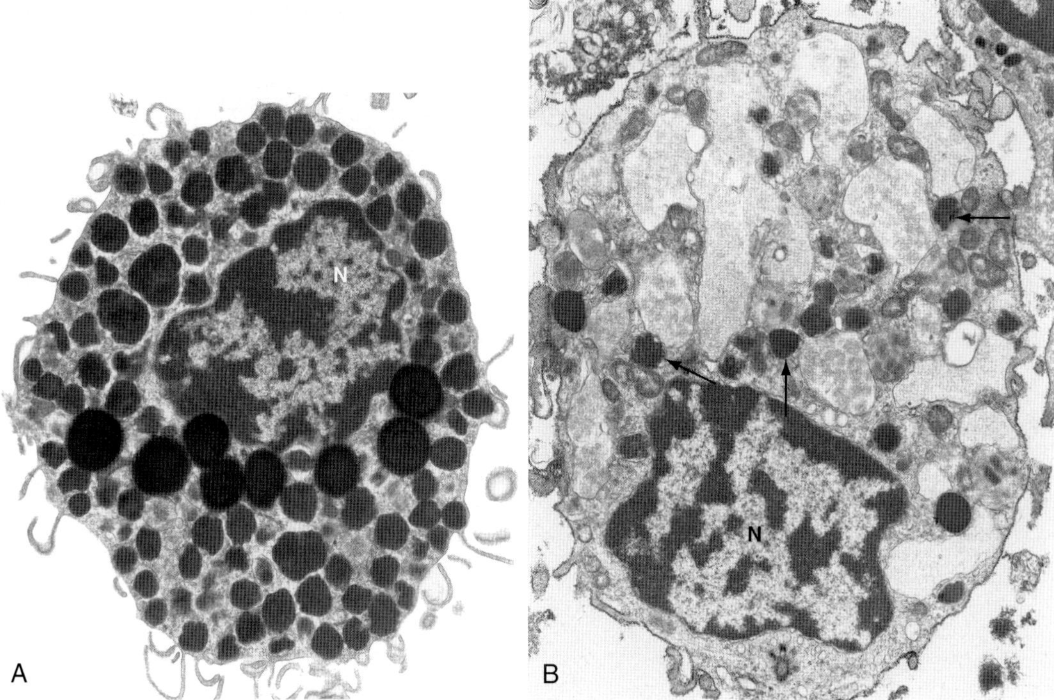

• **Fig. 15.1** Mast cell morphology. (A) Intact mast cell. (B) Mast cell that has undergone anaphylactic degranulation; note how fusion of intra-cellular granules has resulted in formation of a labyrinth of interconnected channels by which granule contents may be expelled from the cell. *Arrows* indicate remaining granules. *N,* Nucleus. (Images courtesy of Dr. A. Dvorak, Beth Israel Deaconess Medical Center, Boston, MA. From Dvorak AM, Schleimer RP, Lichtenstein LM: Morphologic mast cell cycles. *Cell Immunol* 105: 199-204, 1987; and Galli SJ, Dvorak AM, Dvorak HF: Basophils and mast cells: morphologic insights into their biology, secretory patterns, and function. In Ishizaka K, editor: *Progress in Allergy: Mast Cell Activation and Mediator Release*, Basel, 1984, S Karger, pp 1-141.)[146,147]

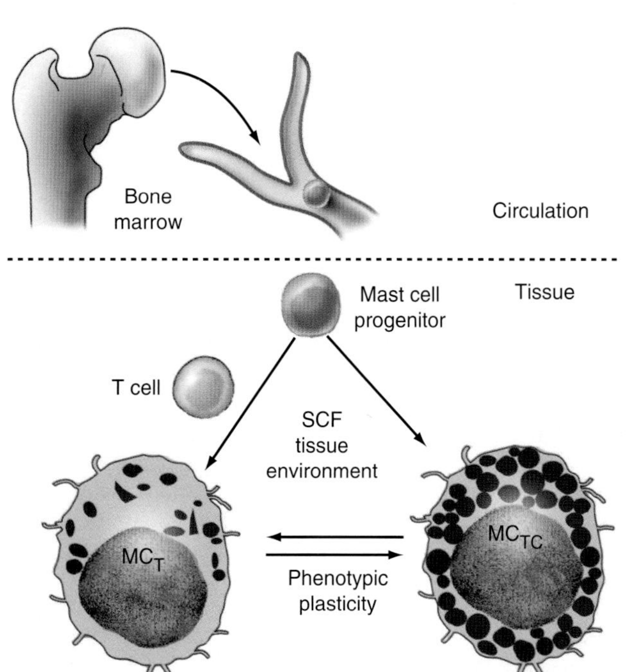

• **Fig. 15.2** Mast cell origin and differentiation. Mast cells arise in the bone marrow, circulate as committed progenitors, and differentiate into mature mast cells upon entering tissue. Human mast cells may be classified on the basis of granule proteases into tryptase+ mast cells (MC$_{TC}$) and tryptase+/chymase+ mast cells (MC$_{TC}$), with characteristic tissue localization and mediator production.

Mast Cell Heterogeneity: Common Progenitor, Multiple Subsets, Phenotypic Plasticity

Whereas all types of mast cells derive from a common progenitor lineage, the phenotype of fully differentiated tissue mast cells is heterogeneous. Human mast cells are conventionally divided into two broad classes on the basis of the protease contents of their granules (see Fig. 15.2). MC$_{TC}$ display rounded granules containing the enzymes tryptase and chymase, whereas the smaller and more irregularly shaped granules of MC$_T$ contain tryptase but not chymase. MC$_{TC}$ also express other proteases, including carboxypeptidase and cathepsin G. These subtypes differ in tissue distribution. MC$_{TC}$ tend to be found in connective tissue, such as in normal skin, muscle, the intestinal submucosa, and the normal synovium, whereas MC$_T$ predominate in mucosal sites, including the lining of the gut and respiratory tract, although in fact both are present in many locations. Beyond the protease signature, other differences between these subsets include their profile of cytokine elaboration, as well as cell surface receptor expression; however, tissue-specific phenotypic differences are noted within each type as well (i.e., neither MC$_{TC}$ nor MC$_T$ are homogenous cellular subsets).

The relationship between MC$_{TC}$ and MC$_T$ mast cells is controversial. Are they committed subsets, akin to CD4 and CD8 lymphocytes, or functional states that mast cells assume under the influence of the microenvironment? In mice, where an analogous distinction exists between connective tissue mast cells (CTMCs) and mucosal mast cells (MMCs), evidence for phenotypic plasticity is strong. Both in culture and in vivo, single CTMCs may differentiate into (or give rise to) MMCs and vice versa. Mast cells with intermediate protease expression are found, and serial observations suggest that exposure to an inflammatory stimulus can induce progressive change from one class to another, although whether this occurs at a single-cell level has not been definitively established. Similarly, in murine and human mastocytosis, clonally expanded mast cells display divergent phenotypes depending on the tissue of residence. Immunoreceptors such as FcγRIIb are expressed by human mast cells in some tissues but not others.[7] In mice, gene expression signatures differ between mast cells harvested from different locations, although broad patterns remain similar, distinguishing these cells clearly from other lineages (including basophils).[8] In aggregate, these data favor the hypothesis that mast cells assume their phenotype under the control of local signals but can change their phenotype in accordance with local conditions.

Stem Cell Factor

One of the most important signals from tissue to local mast cells is SCF. The receptor for SCF, c-Kit, is expressed widely on hematopoietic lineages early in differentiation, but among mature lineages only mast cells express c-Kit at a high level. Stimulation of mast cells by SCF promotes maturation and phenotypic differentiation, blocks apoptosis, and induces chemotaxis. It may also activate mast cells directly to release mediators. In both mice and humans, SCF remains an irreplaceable survival signal for tissue mast cells. Accordingly, mice with defects in SCF or c-Kit are strikingly deficient in mature tissue mast cells (examples include W/W^v, Sl/Sl^d, and W^{sh} strains). Similarly, clonal mast cells obtained from patients with systemic mastocytosis commonly exhibit activating mutations in *KIT*.

SCF occurs in two alternate forms resulting from differential mRNA splicing: soluble and membrane bound. The importance of this latter form is clear from Sl/Sl^d mice, which lack only the membrane-bound isoform yet exhibit very few tissue mast cells. SCF is synthesized by multiple lineages, including mast cells themselves. Expression by fibroblasts is especially important, given the intimate physical contacts observed between fibroblasts and mast cells in situ. The SCF/c-Kit axis mediates cell-cell adhesion between mast cells and fibroblasts independent of the kinase activity of the receptor. Rodent mast cells co-cultured with fibroblasts demonstrate enhanced survival, connective-tissue phenotypic differentiation, and heightened capacity to elaborate pro-inflammatory eicosanoids, effects mediated at least in part by direct contact, including interactions between SCF and c-Kit. The extent of similar regulation in human mast cells is uncertain. Expression of SCF has also been documented on other lineages including macrophages, vascular endothelium, and airway epithelium and is likely a critical pathway by which tissues modulate the local mast cell population.

T Lymphocytes and Other Cells

T lymphocytes exert a profound effect on mast cell phenotype. Severe combined immunodeficiency (SCID) mice that lack T cells fail to develop mucosal mast cells, a defect that can be corrected by T cell engraftment.[9] An analogous observation has been made in humans deficient in T cells due to congenital or acquired immunodeficiency. Intestinal biopsy in these patients shows that MMCs (MC_T) are strikingly reduced, whereas CTMCs (MC_{TC}) are present in normal numbers.[10] The pathways by which T cells exert this striking effect are not defined, although T cell cytokines such as IL-3, IL-4, IL-6, IL-9, and transforming growth factor (TGF)-β may have profound effects on the phenotype of mast cells matured in culture. By contrast, interferon (IFN)-γ inhibits mast cell proliferation and may induce apoptosis. These observations imply that cells recruited to an inflamed tissue may impact the phenotype of local mast cells. The rheumatoid synovium may well exemplify this phenomenon; normally populated by MC_{TC} mast cells, large numbers of MC_T mast cells are identified in the inflamed synovium, typically in regions rich in infiltrating leukocytes, whereas MC_{TC} mast cells reside in deeper, more fibrotic areas of the joint.[11] Interestingly, regulatory T cells (Tregs) can also directly impact mast cell function, including recruitment, receptor expression, degranulation, and cytokine production.[12–15]

Other cells aside from T cells can interact with mast cells in the tissues. Fibroblasts and mast cells commonly demonstrate close physical interactions. Beyond SCF, fibroblasts elaborate cytokines such as the IL-1 family member IL-33, which can exert effects on mast cell protease expression, effector phenotype, and survival.[6,16,17] Dendritic cells have also been implicated in the recruitment of mast cells into inflamed tissues.[18]

Different Functions for MC_T and MC_{TC} Mast Cells

The preservation of distinct types of mast cells in multiple species implies distinct roles for these subtypes. However, the understanding of functional differences between MC_T and MC_{TC} remains limited. One hypothesis is that MC_T play a pro-inflammatory role and MC_{TC} specialize in matrix remodeling. This hypothesis makes sense of (1) the promotion of MC_T development by T cells patrolling the tissues; (2) the partition of MC_T and MC_{TC} mast cells to inflamed and fibrotic areas, respectively; and (3) the preferential expression of the pro-inflammatory mediators IL-5 and IL-6 by MC_T and the profibrotic IL-4 by MC_{TC}.[19] Not all observations fit comfortably into this dichotomy, however. For example, the potently pro-inflammatory anaphylatoxin receptor C5aR (CD88) is expressed on MC_{TC} but not on MC_T.[20] Ultimately, too little is known about the actual functional importance of these subsets to permit firm conclusions.

Mast Cell Activation

Immunoglobulin E

The canonical pathway to mast cell activation is via IgE and its receptor FcεRI. With a K_a of 10^{10} L/M, this receptor is essentially constantly saturated with IgE at typical serum concentrations, to which perivascular mast cells are exposed through direct sampling of the luminal contents.[21] Such binding not only sensitizes mast cells to the target antigen but also helps promote mast cell survival and cytokine production. Crosslinking FcεRI-bound IgE by multivalent antigen, and in some circumstances even by monovalent antigen, induces a brisk and vigorous response.[22] Within minutes, granules within the mast cell fuse together and with the surface membrane, creating a set of labyrinthine channels that allow rapid release of granule contents (see Fig. 15.1B). This compound exocytosis event, termed *anaphylactic degranulation*, is followed within minutes by the elaboration of eicosanoids newly synthesized from arachidonic acid cleaved from internal membrane lipids. Alternately, for cell-bound antigen opsonized by IgE, mast cells can disgorge their granules directly upon the targeted cell in a structure termed an *antibody-dependent degranulatory synapse*.[23] Signals transduced via FcεRI also induce the transcription of new genes and elaboration of a wide range of chemokines and cytokines (Fig. 15.3). Both degranulation and mediator production exhibit partial dependence on a rapid switch of mast cell metabolism in favor of glycolysis.[24] Upon termination of the stimulation event, the surface membrane closes over the granule-formed channels, which

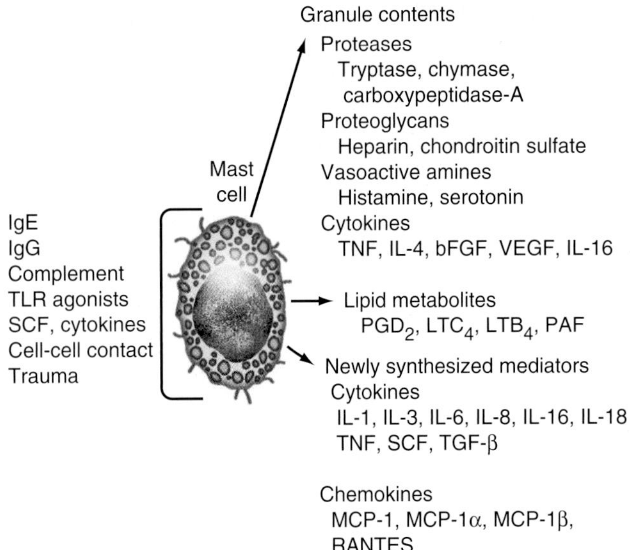

• **Fig. 15.3** Mediator production by human mast cells (partial list). The set of mediators liberated upon activation will vary depending on the state of differentiation of the mast cell and the nature of the stimulus. See Reference 148 for a complete mediator list and references. *bFGF,* Basic fibroblast growth factor; *LTB_4,* leukotriene B_4; *LTC_4,* leukotriene C_4; *MCP-1,* monocyte chemoattractant protein-1; *MIP,* macrophage inflammatory protein; *PAF,* platelet activating factor; *PDGF,* platelet-derived growth factor; *PGD_2,* prostaglandin D_2; *RANTES,* released upon activation, normal T-cell expressed and secreted; *TGF-β,* transforming growth factor-β; *TNF,* tumor necrosis factor; *VEGF,* vascular endothelial growth factor.

subsequently bud off within the cytoplasm, re-creating discrete granules using the original membranes. These granules are then recharged with mediators in a process that occurs gradually over days to weeks.

Immunoglobulin G and Immune Complexes

IgE is only one among many pathways of mast cell activation. One key trigger for mast cell activation in both humans and mice is IgG, acting via receptors for the Fc portion of IgG (FcγR). The importance of this pathway was demonstrated first in mice rendered genetically deficient in IgE. Contrary to expectations, these animals remain susceptible to anaphylaxis mediated through IgG and the low-affinity IgG receptor FcγRIII.[25] The human counterpart of this receptor, FcγRIIa, is equally capable of inducing activation of human mast cells.[26,27] Human mast cells can also be induced to express the high-affinity IgG receptor FcγRI, rendering them susceptible to IgG-mediated activation.[28]

IgG receptors contribute to involvement of mast cells in antibody-driven diseases. Thus, in the mouse, mast cells participate in IgG-mediated immune complex peritonitis, the cutaneous Arthus reaction, and experimental murine bullous pemphigoid. Activation via Fc receptors also mediates mast cell participation in antibody-mediated murine arthritis.[29]

Soluble Mediators and Cell-Cell Contact

Mast cells coordinate with immune and nonimmune lineages via mechanisms beyond antibody response, including soluble mediators and surface receptors. Examples of such signals include the cytokine TNF and the neurogenic peptide substance P, which can induce mast cell degranulation. Peptide secretagogues (including substance P) and many pharmaceutical compounds that elicit pseudo-allergic reactions (e.g., morphine) activate mast cells via the G-protein-coupled receptor MRGPRX2.[30] Mast cells can be activated by complement, including the anaphylatoxin C5a.[27] Physical contact with other cells can also induce mast cell activation. For example, CD30 on lymphocytes can interact with CD30L on mast cells to induce production of a range of chemokines.[31] Interestingly, ligation of CD30L does not induce release of granule contents or lipid mediators, illustrating the selectivity of response of which mast cells are capable.

Danger and Injury

Mast cells are equipped to recognize danger in the absence of guidance from other lineages via a range of pathogen receptors, including multiple Toll-like receptors (TLRs) and CD48, a surface protein recognizing the fimbrial antigen FimH. These receptors are implicated in the response of mast cells to pathogens and could potentially contribute to mast cell engagement in diseases such as atopic dermatitis, in which skin becomes abnormally colonized with bacteria. Mast cells can also be activated by the complement-derived anaphylatoxins C3a and C5a.[27,32] Mast cells can respond directly to physical stimuli including trauma, temperature, and osmotic stress. Finally, mast cells can be triggered by danger signals released by injured bystander cells, such as IL-33 and uric acid crystals.[33,34] Together, these receptors enable mast cell involvement in a broad range of immune and nonimmune processes.

Inhibitory Signals for Mast Cells

As with other immune lineages, mast cells are subject to both negative and positive regulation. Cytokines that inhibit aspects of mast cell function include TGF-β and IL-10. Inhibitory receptors on the mast cell surface include the IgG receptor FcγRIIb and the phosphatidyl serine receptor CD300A. The importance of these receptors is demonstrated in genetically deficient animals. Mice lacking FcγRIIb demonstrate a striking propensity to activation via both IgG and IgE (which binds with low affinity to both FcγRIIb and FcεRI).[35,36] Ligation of FcγRIIb via IgG directed against allergens may blunt IgE-mediated mast cell activation, accounting in part for the efficacy of immunotherapy in allergic disease.[37,38] CD300A mediates suppression of mast cell activation by apoptotic debris.[39] Modulating the surface expression of inhibitory receptors is a potentially important regulator of the activation threshold for mast cells in tissues.

Mast Cell Mediators

Granule Contents: Proteases, Amines, Proteoglycans, and Cytokines

Mature mast cells package a range of mediators in their granules that are ready for immediate release through fusion with the surface membrane. The most abundant of these are the neutral proteases, named for their enzymatic activity at neutral pH, but vasoactive amines, proteoglycans such as heparin, and pre-formed cytokines play distinct roles in the biologic consequences of mast cell degranulation. The release of these mediators is not all or none. In addition to anaphylactic degranulation, mast cells may release only a few granules at a time in a process termed *piecemeal degranulation.* Mast cells can release one type of granule but not another. Alternately, mast cells may be induced to elaborate cytokines and chemokines without any release of granule contents, as illustrated by activation via CD30L, and may release their proteases packaged in microvesicles budded from the cell surface.[31,40] Thus, although the mast cell is well equipped to release large volumes of pre-formed mediators, it is equally capable of responses tailored to the activating stimulus.

Tryptase. Named for its enzymatic similarity to pancreatic trypsin, tryptase is the most abundant granule protein in human mast cells. It is also a specific marker for mast cells, synthesized in scant amounts by basophils but by no other lineage. The enzyme found in granules is the β isomer, which is the product of two distinct genes and is enzymatically active upon formation of a homotetramer that relies on the scaffolding function of the proteoglycan heparin. Mast cells also synthesize α tryptase, a protein incapable of forming homotetramers and thus enzymatically inactive. Unlike β tryptase, the α isomer is not stored in granules but is constitutively released into circulation, where its function is unknown. The distinction between tryptase isomers is important for diagnostic reasons: as a marker of degranulation, systemic levels of β tryptase constitute a marker of recent anaphylaxis.[41] By contrast, α trypsin levels reflect total body mast cell load and serve as a useful biomarker in systemic mastocytosis.[42]

Tryptase cleaves structural proteins such as fibronectin and type IV collagen and enzymatically activates stromelysin, an enzyme responsible for activating collagenase. Fibrinogen is another substrate, potentially implicating mast cells in prevention of fibrin deposition and blood coagulation in the tissues.[43] Tryptase also promotes hyperplasia and activation of fibroblasts, airway smooth muscle cells, and epithelium. Cleavage of protease-activated receptors such as PAR2 may contribute to some of these activities, although other studies document PAR2-independent tryptase activation of mesenchymal cells. In aggregate, these effects suggest an important role for tryptase in matrix remodeling. A further contribution to the inflammatory milieu is suggested by the capacity of tryptase to promote neutrophil and eosinophil recruitment and to cleave C3, C4, and C5 to generate anaphylatoxins. Interestingly, tryptase can potentially suppress inflammation by cleaving IgE and IL-6.[44,45]

Chymase. This chymotrypsin-like neutral protease is found in the MC_{TC} subset of human mast cells, packaged within the same granules as tryptase. Like tryptase, chymase can cleave matrix components and activate stromelysin, although it can also activate collagenase directly, suggesting a role in matrix remodeling. Chymase can activate angiotensin I, leading to angiotensin converting enzyme (ACE)-independent activation of the potent vasoconstrictor angiotensin II. Chymase also affects cytokine function, cleaving pro-IL-1β to generate active cytokine and inactivate proinflammatory cytokines such as IL-6 and TNF, as well as "alarmins," including heat shock protein 70 and IL-33.[46]

β-Hexosaminidase. This enzyme is found in lysosomes from many cell types. In mast cells it is abundant in secretory granules, where it is released into the surrounding environment during degranulation. Recent studies have found that this enzyme is capable of degrading bacterial cell peptidoglycan, and release by mast cells plays an important role in the defense against experimental staphylococcal infection in mice.[47]

Vasoactive Amines. Human mast cells are capable of synthesizing and storing the biogenic amines histamine and serotonin, which are implicated in vascular leak. Histamine, by far the more abundant, is a vasoactive amine found in both MC_T and MC_{TC}, as well as other lineages. Histamine is involved in the wheal-and-flare response to cutaneous allergen challenge via augmented vascular permeability, transendothelial vesicular transport, and neurogenic vasodilation. These effects are mediated principally via the H1 receptor. Three other histamine surface receptors, H2, H3, and H4, are distributed widely on immune and nonimmune lineages, with effects as diverse as gastric acid secretion, Langerhans cell migration, and B cell proliferation. Another important mechanism underlying mast cell-induced vascular leak is heparin-mediated bradykinin production (as discussed in the following section).

Heparin and Chondroitin Sulfate E. These large proteoglycans enable the ordered packing of mediators within human mast cell granules. Negatively charged carbohydrate side chains complex tightly with positively charged proteins, enabling the accumulation of very high concentrations of β tryptase and other proteases. Heparin, produced exclusively by mast cells, facilitates the activity of tryptase by making possible proteolytic self-activation within the granule and stabilizing the active tetrameric form of this enzyme. Heparin also has a wide range of effects beyond the mast cell. It is potently angiogenic. Heparin binding activates antithrombin III, providing the basis for use as an anticoagulant, while inhibiting chemokines and both classic and alternative pathways of complement activation, as well as the function of Treg cells. The physiologic role of these extra-cellular activities is uncertain. Of more evident in vivo relevance is that the negatively charged surface of heparin enables activation of factor XII. This zymogen then activates kallikrein, an enzyme that in turn cleaves high-molecular-weight kininogen to generate bradykinin, a potent mediator of vascular leak. This mechanism contributes to the antihistamine-resistant edema observed in patients with hereditary angioedema from lack of C1 esterase inhibitor, an inhibitor of activated factor XII and kallikrein.[48]

Pre-formed Cytokines and Chemokines. Mast cells store certain mediators in their granules for rapid release. The first of these to be documented was TNF.[49] In the mouse, this pool of TNF is implicated in the rapid recruitment of neutrophils to the peritoneum during peritonitis.[50,51] Exocytosed granules appear to release TNF gradually into the environment, enhancing the immunostimulatory effect of the cytokine as TNF-containing granules reach draining lymph nodes, helping promote development of the mature immune response.[52–54] Other cytokines that may be stored in granules include IL-4, IL-16, IL-17A, basic fibroblast growth factor (bFGF), and vascular endothelial growth factor (VEGF). Stored chemokines include the neutrophil chemoattractants CXCL1 and CXCL2.[55]

Newly Synthesized Mediators: Lipid Mediators, Cytokines, Chemokines and Growth Factors

Beyond pre-formed mediators, activated mast cells generate a range of mediators de novo. These mediators are released minutes to hours after stimulation, broadening and extending the impact of activated mast cells on surrounding tissues.

Lipid Mediators. Within minutes of activation, mast cells begin to release metabolites of membrane phospholipids. This process is rapid because the relevant enzymes, beginning with phospholipase A2, which is responsible for harvesting phospholipids from the outer leaflet of the nuclear membrane, are already present in the cytoplasm and need only to be activated through signals mediated by calcium flux and the phosphorylation of intra-cellular messengers. The hallmark prostaglandin of human mast cells is prostaglandin D_2 (PGD_2), which induces bronchoconstriction, vascular leak, and neutrophil recruitment. Smaller amounts of other prostaglandins, as well as thromboxane, are also made. Mast cell-derived leukotrienes (LTs) have similar but generally more potent activity. LTC_4 is the major leukotriene species generated by human mast cells, and, together with its metabolites LTD_4 and LTE_4, serves as a potent inducer of vascular leak. Smaller amounts of the chemotaxins LTB_4 and platelet-activating factor (PAF) are also generated. The profile of lipid mediators produced by mast cells changes with local environmental signals and the resulting state of differentiation. Thus mast cells from skin generate PGD_2 in excess of LTC_4, whereas both species are elaborated in roughly equal proportion by mast cells isolated from lung and osteoarthritic synovium.

Cytokines, Chemokines, and Growth Factors. Within hours of activation, mast cells begin to elaborate newly synthesized mediators as the end result of induced gene transcription and translation. The range of such mediators is broad (see Fig. 15.3). They include the canonical pro-inflammatory mediators TNF, IL-1, and IL-6; the Th2 cytokines IL-4, IL-5, IL-10, and IL-13; the "alarmin" IL-33; chemotactic factors including IL-8, macrophage inflammatory protein (MIP)-1α, CXCR1, CXCR2, and RANTES (regulation upon activation normal T cell expressed and presumably excreted); and growth factors for fibroblasts, blood vessels, and other cells such as bFGF, VEGF, and platelet-derived growth factor (PDGF). IL-17 is detected in tissue mast cells and can be generated by mast cells stimulated in culture.[56,57] As noted earlier, some of these cytokines may also be stored pre-formed in granules for rapid release. The panel of mediators generated depends on the state of differentiation, as well as the activating signal, and may occur in the absence of degranulation.

TABLE 15.1 Participation of Mast Cells in Murine Models of Disease (Partial List)

Beneficial to Host	Harmful to Host
Angiogenesis	Anaphylaxis*
Anxiety control	Arthritis*
Bacterial cystitis	Aortic aneurysm*
Bacterial peritonitis*	Asthma*
Bladder epithelium exfoliation*	Atherosclerosis*
Bone remodeling	Atopic dermatitis
Brain trauma	Atrial fibrillation
Dengue fever	Autoinflammatory disease
Dermatitis*	Bacterial cystitis
Envenomation*	Burn
Glomerulonephritis*	Bullous pemphigoid*
Graft tolerance*	Cardiac fibrosis
Intestinal epithelial barrier*	Cardiomyopathy
Lung infection, bacterial*	Chronic obstructive pulmonary disease
Lung infection, viral*	Colitis
Parasites, intestine*	Colon polyps
Parasites, muscle	Cystic fibrosis
Parasites, skin	Dermatitis, irritant*
Peptic ulcer disease	Dermatitis, sunburn
Thromboembolism	Gastritis
Tumor suppression*	Glomerulonephritis*
Wound healing*	Gout
	Immune complex peritonitis*
	Ischemia-reperfusion injury
	Kidney injury*
	Lung fibrosis
	Malaria
	Multiple sclerosis*
	Myocardial infarct size
	Myositis*
	Neurogenic inflammation*
	Obesity*
	Peritonitis, irritant*
	Peritoneal adhesions
	Pneumonitis
	Renal fibrosis*
	Renal ischemia-reperfusion
	Retinopathy*
	Scleroderma
	Sepsis*
	Tumor angiogenesis

Mast cells are implicated in these processes by virtue of phenotypic abnormalities in mast cell–deficient mice or in mice lacking mast cell–specific mediators. The asterisk (*) indicates that the phenotype is reversible by engraftment with cultured mast cells, providing direct evidence for a role for this lineage.

Role of Mast Cells in Health and Disease

The understanding of the role of mast cells in health and disease has been aided greatly by the availability of mice that lack mast cells entirely or are deficient in mast cell–specific products such as heparin or granule proteases. These mice are viable, excluding an obligate role for mast cells in the structure and function of most tissues. Yet when they are under physiologic stress, such as that imposed by experimental models of disease, multiple differences from wild-type mice become evident. In many cases, these abnormalities may be corrected by engraftment with cultured mast cells, directly implicating mast cells in a remarkably broad range of disease processes (Table 15.1). The extrapolation of such experiments to human disease is limited by multiple factors. Most evidently, mice are not humans, and the experimental systems employed typically model at best only certain aspects of the corresponding human condition. Further, many of these mice exhibit "off-target" phenotypes outside of the mast cell lineage, complicating interpretation of the data, especially when results in one mast cell–deficient mouse strain diverge from those observed in another. These discrepancies have occasioned considerable controversy in the mast cell literature. However, together with in vitro experiments using human mast cells, and careful study of individuals in different states of health and disease, animal experiments have contributed greatly to the understanding of mast cell physiology and pathophysiology.

Mast Cells in Allergy: Anaphylaxis, Allergic Disease, and Asthma

Mast cells are the primary mediator of IgE-mediated systemic anaphylaxis. This is demonstrated in mast cell–deficient mice, where resistance to anaphylaxis may be restored by engraftment with mast cells.[58] In humans, participation of mast cells in anaphylaxis has been documented through the detection of elevated serum levels of β tryptase, a specific marker of mast cell degranulation.[41] Mast cells can be triggered upon contacting antigen directly or, in some cases, after blood-borne antigen is passed to mast cells by perivascular dendritic cells.[59] Of note, anaphylaxis may also be mediated by IgG, a context in which mast cells play only a partial role, while neutrophils assume primacy.[60] Mast cells accumulate in atopic mucosal tissues where they degranulate upon exposure to antigen and contribute prominently to tissue edema and the overproduction of mucous. Mast cells accumulate in the asthmatic airway, including within the smooth muscle lining the airways, and have been implicated by human and animal data in airway hyper-reactivity and mucosal changes.

Mast Cells in Nonallergic Inflammation

Pathogen Defense: Mast Cells as Sentinels of Innate Immunity

The involvement of mast cells in atopic disease is clear but does not explain their remarkable evolutionary conservation. Rather, mast cells must somehow contribute to the survival of the organism. The most probable mechanism by which mast cells convey a survival advantage is in the defense against infection. This role is reflected in the localization of mast cells near epithelial surfaces, around blood vessels, and in other locations of potential invasion by pathogens.

Mast cells are competent defensive cells against bacteria. They express TLRs and other receptors against bacterial antigens, and upon activation are able to phagocytose bacteria and generate anti-microbial molecules such as cathelicidin. However, given their relatively small numbers, the most important function of mast cells in immune defense is likely as sentinels, monitoring for early traces of infection and rapidly mobilizing neutrophils and other inflammatory cells when needed. Such a role has been clearly demonstrated in murine bacterial peritonitis, where mast cell–deficient animals exhibit a high mortality. This susceptibility correlates with delayed recruitment of neutrophils via TNF and leukotrienes; both neutrophil influx and survival may be restored by correction of the mast cell deficit, although in the case of severe infection, mast cell TNF may actually contribute to mortality.[51,61,62] Clearance of bacteria from the lungs is delayed in mast cell–deficient mice and can be similarly restored by exogenous mast cells.[51] Analogous observations have been made in other models of bacterial infection. Thus, mast cells likely play an important role in the defense of the host against bacterial infection.

Mast cells are also implicated in the defense against parasites. Mast cell–deficient animals exhibit abnormal clearance of multiple parasites from gut and skin. The mechanism of this defense remains uncertain but may include direct attack upon pathogens, recruitment of inflammatory lineages such as neutrophils and eosinophils, lysis of tight junctions in the mucosal lining to facilitate the expulsion of helminths, and expansion of protective innate ILC2 lymphocytes.[63–65]

More limited data implicate mast cells in the defense against viruses, including dengue, vaccinia, and cytomegalovirus. The role of mast cells in this setting includes recruitment of CD8 T cells and other cytotoxic lineages, as well as production of type I IFNs to help neighboring cells resist infection.

Mast Cells and the Adaptive Immune Response

In addition to recruiting innate effector cells, mast cells mobilize T and B lymphocytes, the adaptive arm of the immune system. Mast cells may express class II major histocompatibility complex (MHC), as well as co-stimulatory molecules such as CD80, rendering them effective antigen-presenting cells for CD4 T cells.[66] Mast cells can also mobilize and potentiate CD8 T cell responses.[67,68] They can migrate from peripheral tissues to lymph nodes carrying antigen and contribute to the recruitment of T cells to lymph nodes via mediators including MIP-1β and TNF.[4,52] Indeed, infection-induced lymph node hyperplasia is abrogated in the absence of mast cells. Further, mast cells can recruit CD4 and CD8 effector T cells to peripheral tissues via LTB_4, among other mediators.[69] Finally, mast cells contribute to the migration of cutaneous Langerhans cells and other dendritic cells to lymph nodes via mediators including histamine and mast cell granules.[70,71] By means of the inducible expression of CD40L and cytokines, mast cells stimulate B cells and induce class switching to IgA or IgE.[72,73] The physiologic importance of these effects vary with circumstances. For example, under some conditions, delayed-type hypersensitivity responses in skin are mast cell dependent, whereas under others, mast cells play no role. The potential importance of the mast cell in adaptive immunity is highlighted by the demonstration that mast cell activators are effective vaccine adjuvants.[53]

Neurogenic Inflammation

In addition to their perivascular localization, mast cells cluster near and sometimes within peripheral nerves. A discrete function for them in these locations has not yet been defined, although the potential for bidirectional neuroimmune interaction is clear. Mast cell mediators such as histamine can directly activate neurons, whereas mast cells residing near stimulated neurons can be induced to degranulate. Indeed, vascular leak and neutrophil infiltration arising from infiltration of skin with the neurogenic mediator substance P are mediated by mast cells.[74,75] Thus neurons likely recruit mast cells as local effectors of neurogenic inflammation.

Autoimmune Disease

Reconstitution experiments in mast cell–deficient mice have implicated mast cells in a variety of pathologic conditions (see Table 15.1). These include murine models of autoimmune diseases such as bullous pemphigoid, multiple sclerosis, scleroderma, and inflammatory arthritis. In mice with pemphigoid, mast cells that are triggered via IgG antibodies against a hemidesmosomal antigen recruit neutrophils, which are responsible for blister formation.[76] The role of mast cells in murine experimental autoimmune encephalomyelitis (EAE) is more complex. Although the resistance of mast cell–deficient W/W^v mice to EAE corrects with mast cell engraftment, these cells fail to repopulate the brain and spinal cord, indicating that mast cells are not obligate local effector cells in this model.[77,78] One mechanism for this activity appears to be the promotion of the adaptive immune response, because mast cell engraftment into W/W^v animals improves T cell responses to immunization with the inciting myelin antigen.[79,80] The contribution of mast cells to human scleroderma remains unknown, although they express TGF-β in sclerodermatous skin and interact closely with local lymphocytes and fibroblasts, even forming gap junctions that enable cytoplasmic continuity with the latter cells.[81,82] Humans with polymyositis, but not dermatomyositis, exhibit increased density of mast cells in inflamed muscle; a similar phenotype is noted in dermatomyositis skin.[83,84] Murine studies suggest that these cells may play a role in disease pathogenesis, because experimental myositis is attenuated in mast cell–deficient animals, a defect that corrects partially with mast cell engraftment.[84] The participation of mast cells in arthritis is discussed in detail in a later section.

Mast Cells as Anti-inflammatory Cells

Within the past decade, it has become evident that mast cells may also help moderate the immune response. One mechanism for this effect is degradation of pro-inflammatory mediators. Mast cell proteases may cleave and inactivate the cytokines IL-5, IL-6, IL-13, IL-33, and TNF, as well as endothelin-1 and the anaphylatoxin C3a. Proteases degrade tissue-derived danger signals, including heat shock protein 70. The importance of this anti-inflammatory activity has been demonstrated in a murine sepsis model, where mast cells reduced mortality by restraining excess inflammation in a protease-dependent manner.[85]

More broadly, mast cells produce mediators such as IL-10 that have immunosuppressive activity, and even otherwise pro-inflammatory mediators such as TNF and granulocyte-macrophage colony-stimulating factor (GM-CSF) can be immunosuppressive under appropriate circumstances.[86,87] Mast cells promote immunologic tolerance to skin grafts and limit tissue inflammation related to ultraviolet light injury.[45,86,88,89] Data suggest a role for mast cell–produced IL-2 in the promotion of Treg responses that limit experimental dermatitis and development of IL-10–producing regulatory B cells while promoting development of regulatory T cells.[90–92] Mast cells may play a permissive role in the immunosuppressive activity of murine myeloid-derived suppressor cells, an activity that may be beneficial or harmful to the host.[93,94]

Mast Cells and Connective Tissue

Wound Healing and Tissue Fibrosis

Mast cells have long been noted to accumulate at the borders of healing wounds. In healthy human subjects undergoing experimental wounding and recurrent biopsies, mast cell numbers increase sixfold by day 10 after the initial incision. These mast cells localize preferentially to fibrotic areas of the wound and strongly express IL-4, a cytokine capable of inducing fibroblast proliferation and collagen synthesis.[95] In vitro studies confirm the stimulatory effects of mast cells on fibroblast growth; candidate fibroblast mitogens in addition to IL-4 include tryptase, histamine, LTC_4, and bFGF. Indeed, W/W^v animals exhibit delayed contracture and healing of skin wounds in a manner reparable by local engraftment with cultured mast cells, though other mast cell–deficient mice exhibit no defect in wound healing.[96,97]

Mast cells accumulate in sites of pathologic fibrosis, including the skin and lungs of patients with scleroderma. Because experimental skin fibrosis proceeds in mast cell–deficient mice with few if any differences in intensity or kinetics, it is unlikely that mast cells are an obligate effector lineage in human scleroderma, although they may contribute to disease progression.[98]

Bone

Mast cells are also implicated in the remodeling of bone. Mast cells accumulate in sites of healing fracture and may contribute to normal bone turnover.[99,100] Mast cells accumulate in osteoporotic bone, and systemic osteoporosis is a known complication of systemic mastocytosis.[101,102] Heparin can directly promote differentiation and activation of osteoclasts. Mast cell products such as IL-1, TNF, and MIP-1α have similar activity.

Angiogenesis

Another potentially important activity of mast cells on the stroma is angiogenesis. Mast cells are not required for the development of the normal vasculature, as is evident in the viability of mast cell–deficient mice. However, mast cells cluster at sites of early blood vessel growth in tumors and contribute appreciably to physiologic angiogenesis under certain experimental conditions. Heparin was the first proangiogenic mast cell mediator identified; bFGF and VEGF are other potent stimulators of endothelial migration and proliferation.

Mast Cells in Arthritis

The normal synovium is populated by a limited number of mast cells. These cells are not found in the immediate lining layer but rather reside in the synovial sublining near blood vessels and nerves, constituting almost 3% of cells within 70 μM of the synovial lumen.[103] In both mice and humans, their phenotype is principally MC_{TC}, similar to mast cells found in most other connective tissue sites.[11,104] The several-fold increased density of mast cells in the immediate vicinity of the synovial lining, compared with more distant connective tissue, supports the hypothesis that mast cells contribute to immune surveillance of the articular cavity.[11] Extrapolating from the activity of mast cells near other vulnerable body cavities, such as the peritoneum, it is likely that synovial mast cells monitor the joint for early evidence of infection.

Under inflammatory arthritis, the population of synovial mast cells expands remarkably (Fig. 15.4). More than two-thirds of synovial specimens from patients with rheumatoid arthritis (RA) exhibit abnormal numbers of mast cells, averaging in excess of tenfold above normal.[105] Consistent with these histologic findings, synovial fluid from rheumatoid joints contains appreciable quantities of histamine and tryptase.[106,107] Unlike the normal joint, in the RA joint both subtypes of mast cells are present in roughly equal numbers, with MC_T cells located nearer to the pannus and infiltrating leukocytes while MC_{TC} cells cluster in deeper, more fibrotic areas of the synovium.[11] Mast cells can appear near the junction of pannus and cartilage.[108] Rare mast cells are also identified in synovial fluid.[109] The absence of mitotic figures and of staining for the proliferation antigen Ki-67 suggests that they arise not from local replication but rather by recruitment of circulating progenitors.[110] Although the signals driving this recruitment are unknown, inflammatory cytokines such as TNF enhance expression of the mast cell chemotactic and survival factor SCF on synovial fibroblasts, suggesting one mechanism.[111] Indeed, degree of inflammation is the best predictor of the number of mast cells within the joint.[105,112,113] Incompletely identified factors in RA synovial fluid can potently promote mast cell differentiation and growth.[114]

Hyperplasia of the mast cell population is observed in a wide range of inflammatory joint disorders (Table 15.2). Synovial mast cells expressing IL-17A have been observed in spondyloarthropathy, raising the possibility that they may be an important local source of this cytokine.[115] Expansion is also noted in osteoarthritis

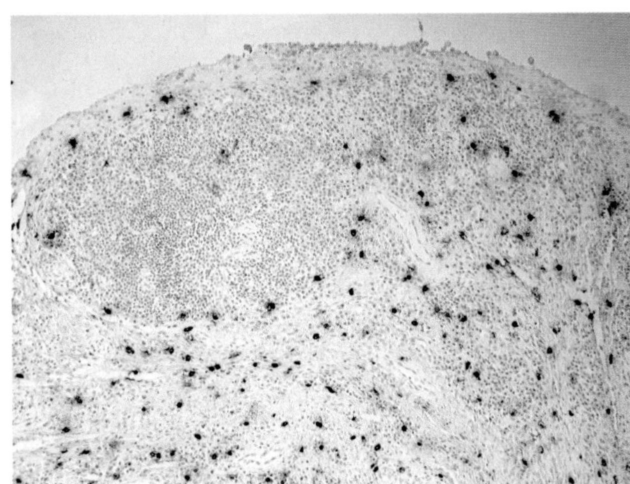

• **Fig. 15.4** Mast cells in the rheumatoid synovium. Stained red by an antibody against tryptase, mast cells are abundant in this synovial biopsy from a patient with chronic rheumatoid arthritis. Note the proliferation of mast cells in the synovial sublining. (Reproduced with permission from reference 116. From Nigrovic PA, Lee DM: Synovial mast cells: role in acute and chronic arthritis. *Immunol Rev* 217: 19-37, 2007.)

(OA), often to densities observed in RA.[116] The levels of histamine and tryptase in OA synovial fluid are also comparable. Interestingly, unlike in RA, the expansion in OA results from an increase in numbers of MC_T mast cells, the subtype generally associated with T cells and inflammation.[11,117] The role of these cells in OA biology remains to be defined.

Studies of human synovial mast cells confirm that they can be activated via pathways relevant to arthritis biology, including complement, Fc receptors, and TLR ligands.[28,118,119] Mast cells are also a potential source of citrullinated autoantigens implicated in RA, although their relative importance in this context is unknown.[120]

TABLE 15.2 Joint Diseases With Documented Synovial Mastocytosis

Chronic infection
Gout
Juvenile idiopathic arthritis
Osteoarthritis
Psoriatic arthritis
Rheumatoid arthritis
Rheumatic fever
Traumatic arthritis
Tuberculosis

See Reference 116 for supporting references.

Mast Cells in Acute Arthritis: Insights From Animal Models

Experimental work in mice has shed light on the role of mast cells in inflammatory arthritis. Several mast cell–deficient strains demonstrate resistance to arthritis induced by IgG autoantibodies, a defect that may be repaired by engraftment with cultured mast cells expressing receptors for IgG and C5a.[27,29,121–123] A number of mechanisms contribute to this arthritogenic activity. First, mast cells induce vascular permeability, facilitating entry of autoantibodies into the joint.[124,125] Second, mast cells release pro-inflammatory mediators including IL-1 that help establish inflammation, presumably via effects on endothelium and other local populations such as macrophages and fibroblasts.[29,123] These actions appear to be most critical at the initiation of disease, constituting a "jump start" for acute inflammation within the joint.[29] This function is in line with the activity of mast cells in other models of IgG-mediated disease, such as IgG-mediated immune complex peritonitis, murine bullous pemphigoid, and anaphylaxis. In each of these models, mast cells resident in tissue for immune defense become co-opted by autoantibodies to initiate inflammatory pathology (Fig. 15.5, *top*). Mast cells have also been

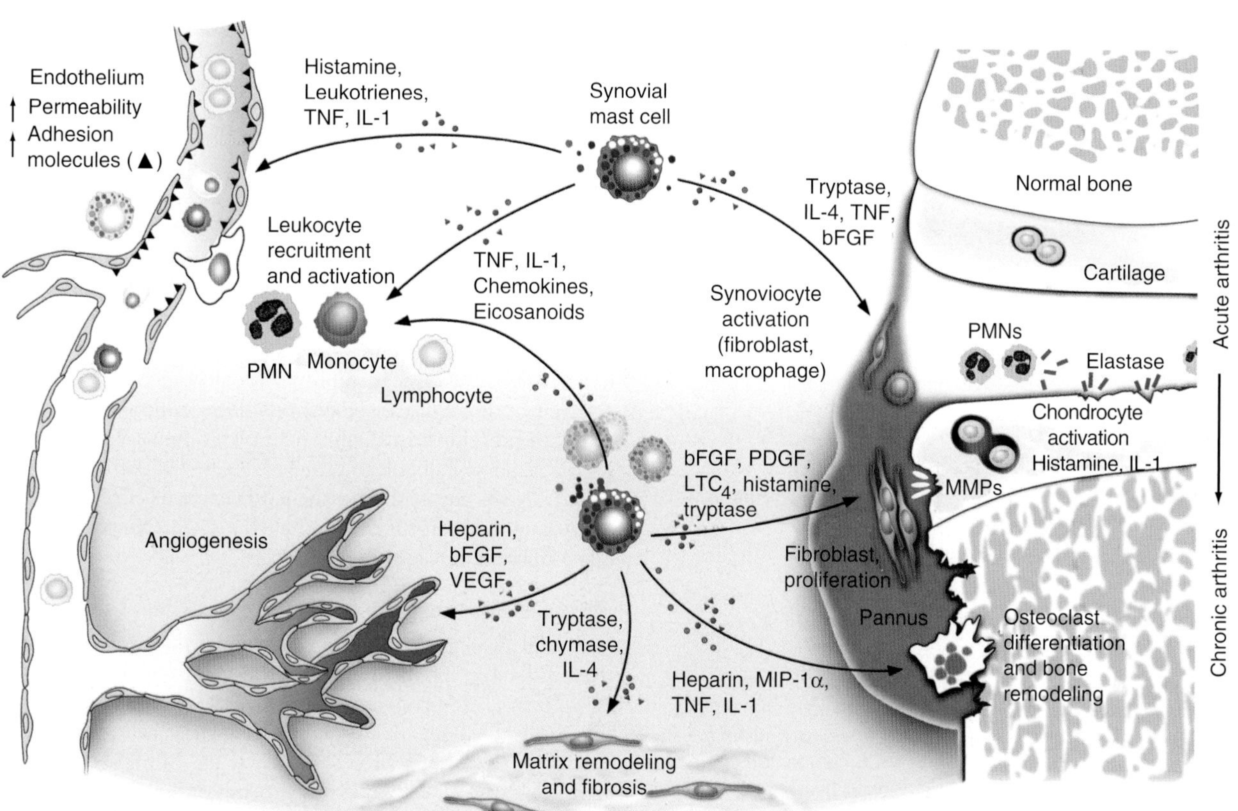

• **Fig. 15.5** Potential roles of mast cells in acute and chronic arthritis. In the acute phase of joint inflammation, mast cells may contribute to initiation of arthritis by inducing vascular permeability, recruiting and activating circulating leukocytes, and stimulating local fibroblasts and macrophages. In established arthritis, these activities may be joined by effects on the stroma, including the promotion of pannus formation, angiogenesis, fibrosis, and injury to cartilage and bone. Potential anti-inflammatory effects of mast cells are not depicted. The mediators listed are representative and do not represent a complete list. (From Nigrovic PA, Lee DM: Synovial mast cells: role in acute and chronic arthritis. *Immunol Rev* 217: 19-37, 2007.)

implicated in uric acid crystal sensing and cytokine production in experimental gout.[34]

Of note, not all mice lacking mast cells are resistant to experimental arthritis (Fig. 15.6).[29,126–128] This discordance reflects factors including intensity of the arthritogenic stimulus, arthritis susceptibility of the nonhematopoietic background, and accompanying abnormalities in other immune lineages.[129] Correspondingly, mice lacking specific mast cell proteases exhibit partial protection from arthritis.[130–132] Thus mast cells represent a potential contributor to joint inflammation but their importance varies with context.

Mast Cells in Chronic Arthritis

In contrast to acute joint inflammation, the role of mast cells in chronic arthritis is poorly understood. The sheer numbers of these cells in arthritic synovium implies a substantial role. Taking into account the spectrum of mast cell activity elsewhere, it is likely that mast cells participate both in the inflammatory process and in the mesenchymal response (see Fig. 15.5, *bottom*).[116]

An ongoing contribution of mast cells to inflammatory arthritis is suggested by several observations. First, as noted, prominent among infiltrating synovial mast cells are MC_T cells, typically associated elsewhere with the elaboration of cytokines such as IL-6 with documented pathogenic activity in RA. Immunofluorescence staining has identified TNF and IL-17 in mast cells from inflamed synovium,[57,133,134] and the elaboration of other pro-inflammatory mediators is probable. Second, mast cells from RA but not OA synovium express the receptor for the anaphylatoxin C5a, a mediator readily documented in synovial fluid.[118] Immune complexes within RA joints represent a likely pathway to activation of synovial mast cells. Indeed, ultrastructural data support ongoing degranulation of mast cells in the RA synovium.[117] Finally, studies of c-Kit inhibitors in murine

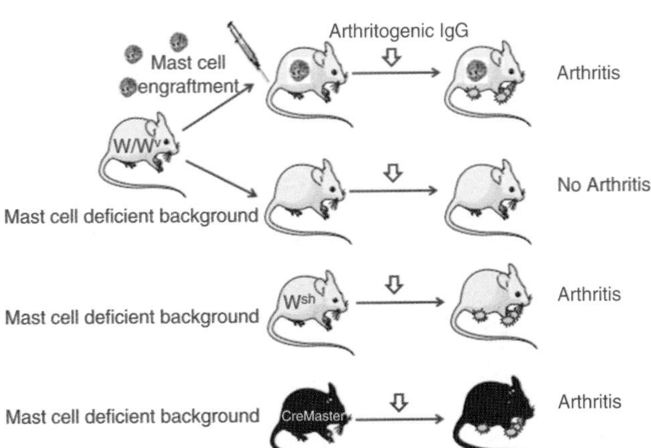

• **Fig. 15.6** Murine studies exploring the role of mast cells in arthritis. W/W^v mice, lacking mast cells through compound heterozygous mutation at the *W* locus encoding c-Kit, are normally resistant to joint inflammation mediated by arthritogenic IgG, and this resistance can be overcome by selective engraftment with cultured mast cells *(top)*. However, this genetic defect carries other hematopoietic implications, including a reduction in neutrophils and megakaryocytes, and occurs on a stromal background that is also generally resistant to disease. By contrast, mast cells are not required in certain other mice that also lack cells, including W^{sh} and CreMaster, where the hematopoietic and stromal context are more favorable for development of disease. These studies demonstrate that mast cells can play a key role in the development of arthritis but can also be "bypassed" by other host factors in the context of a strong proarthritis signal and a favorable genetic background.[129]

and human arthritis suggest efficacy, although it remains unclear whether these agents functionally antagonize tissue mast cells and whether such antagonism explains their efficacy, because these agents impact multiple kinases and affect a broad range of lineages.[135,136]

The effect of mast cells on the established inflammatory synovial infiltrate is difficult to predict. Depletion of mast cells in established murine collagen–induced arthritis was not associated with a change in clinical indices, although methodological limitations render this finding difficult to interpret.[137] Activated mast cells may promote the recruitment and activation of leukocytes. Alternately, protease cleavage of inflammatory mediators and the elaboration of cytokines such as IL-10 and TGF-β could downmodulate inflammation, potentially by promoting Treg function, as has been observed in tolerance of skin grafts in mice.[88]

Mast cells likely modulate the stromal response to inflammation. Expansion and activation of synovial fibroblasts is a key pathogenic process within RA, and the capacity of mast cells to promote such changes is well established. Through interaction with osteoclasts, mast cells could promote both focal erosions and periarticular osteopenia. Mast cell tryptase not only promotes inflammation but also can contribute directly to joint injury by activating synovial fibroblasts to produce chemokines and by cleaving substrates such as cartilage aggrecan, both directly and through proteolytic activation of matrix metalloproteinases.[130,131,138–140] Finally, by producing proangiogenic mediators, mast cells may enable growth of the vascular supply required for the profound expansion of the thin synovial layer into thick pannus. Confirmation of these roles awaits further experimental data.

Therapeutic Potential of Mast Cell Antagonism in Rheumatic Disease

The broad involvement of mast cells in health and disease suggests that targeting this lineage could have potential therapeutic value. Multiple strategies for blocking mast cell activity are under active consideration. In the context of atopic disease, targeting IgE and its receptor FcεRI offers the appealing prospect of antagonizing a pathway of direct disease relevance while retaining most protective mast cell functions. In rheumatic diseases, however, such specificity will be more difficult to achieve because the pathways by which mast cells are engaged, and their downstream effector responses, are typically relevant for immune defense and shared by multiple hematopoietic lineages.

Mast Cell Protease Inhibition

Mast cell proteases make up the bulk of the protein content of these cells and are in many cases largely or entirely specific to this lineage, as previously described. Targeting these proteins therefore offers a pathway to selective mast cell antagonism, in particular because mast cell proteases are implicated directly in arthritis pathogenesis, both as pro-inflammatory factors and as mediators of tissue injury.[130,131,140] Protease inhibitors have been generated but are not currently in active clinical development for arthritis.

SCF/c-Kit Antagonism

Given the critical importance of the SCF/c-Kit axis for the development and survival of mast cells, attention has focused on the potential of kinase inhibitors as mast cell antagonists. Although no inhibitors are fully specific to c-Kit, the tyrosine kinase inhibitors imatinib and mastinib and the downstream protein kinase C inhibitor midostaurine exhibit relative selectivity for c-Kit and have clinical utility in some cases of systemic mastocytosis.[141] These treatments may be complicated by neutropenia and thrombocytopenia, reflecting the importance of c-Kit in other hematopoietic lineages. Imatinib has proven effective in severe refractory human asthma.[142] Imatinib is effective in murine arthritis, in doses that affect in vitro mast cell activation; similarly, treatment of human synovial cultures induces apoptosis of mast cells and limits cytokine production.[57,133,135] However, the action of this agent on multiple lineages obscures the role of mast cell targeting in these results, even in vitro.[135] Interestingly, imatinib is less effective at antagonizing c-Kit stimulation from immobilized SCF, as between tissue-resident mast cells and their adjacent fibroblasts.[143] Further, in vitro and in vivo data suggest that c-Kit signaling can be at least partially replaced by other survival signals from the inflamed environment, such as IL-33. Together, these results suggest that c-Kit blockade is unlikely to represent a mast cell–specific therapeutic approach, although effects on mast cells may certainly contribute to the clinical improvement suggested by series of patients with rheumatic diseases, including RA, treated with kinase inhibitors.

Signaling Pathways

Mast cells share pathways of intra-cellular signaling with other cells, but disproportionate use of individual pathways could offer the potential for pharmacologic specificity. Examples of such pathways include the delta isoform of phosphoinositide 3 kinase (PI3Kδ) and Ras guanine nucleotide-releasing protein-4 (RasGRP4). PI3Kδ is involved in intra-cellular signaling in mast cells, including downstream of c-Kit, and mice lacking this receptor exhibit a partial deficiency of mast cells in some tissues and a striking reduction of IgE-mediated signaling and anaphylaxis. Mice lacking RasGRP4, a guanine nuclear exchange factor expressed principally in mast cells, exhibit impaired mediator production by this lineage and impaired inflammation in models of colitis and arthritis.[144,145] Antagonism of targets such as these could limit the contribution of mast cells to human disease, although the clinical efficacy and side effect profile of such blockade will depend greatly on the availability of redundant pathways within human mast cells and the expression of these targets in other lineages.

Conclusions

Mast cells are potent immune cells characterized by phenotypic diversity and an extremely broad range of functions in health and disease. In addition to mediating atopic disease, mast cells represent important sentinels against pathogen invasion. Under certain conditions it is likely that they also participate in the control of the immune response and the remodeling of tissue matrix. Aberrant activation of mast cells by autoantibodies and potentially other signals has been identified in a range of inflammatory diseases, including arthritis. Such activation may represent a key pathologic step in the development of tissue inflammation and injury and could present an interesting target for the development of anti-inflammatory therapies.

Full references for this chapter can be found on ExpertConsult.com.

Selected References

1. Dahlin JS, et al.: Lin- CD34hi CD117int/hi FcεRI+ cells in human blood constitute a rare population of mast cell progenitors, *Blood* 127:383–391, 2016.
4. Wang HW, Tedla N, Lloyd AR, et al.: Mast cell activation and migration to lymph nodes during induction of an immune response in mice, *J Clin Invest* 102:1617–1626, 1998.
5. Burton OT, et al.: Direct effects of IL-4 on mast cells drive their intestinal expansion and increase susceptibility to anaphylaxis in a murine model of food allergy, *Mucosal Immunol* 6:740–750, 2013.
6. Wang JX, et al.: IL-33/ST2 axis promotes mast cell survival via BCLXL, *Proc Natl Acad Sci U S A* 111:10281–10286, 2014.
7. Burton OT, et al.: Tissue-specific expression of the low-affinity igg receptor, FCγRIIb, on human mast cells, *Front Immunol* 9:1244, 2018.
8. Dwyer DF, Barrett NA, Austen KF, Immunological Genome Project Consortium: Expression profiling of constitutive mast cells reveals a unique identity within the immune system, *Nat Immunol* 17:878–887, 2016.
11. Gotis-Graham I, McNeil HP: Mast cell responses in rheumatoid synovium. Association of the MCTC subset with matrix turnover and clinical progression, *Arthritis Rheum* 40:479–489, 1997.
16. Kaieda S, et al.: Interleukin-33 primes mast cells for activation by IgG immune complexes, *PLoS One* 7:e47252, 2012.
17. Kaieda S, et al.: Synovial fibroblasts promote the expression and granule accumulation of tryptase via interleukin-33 and its receptor ST-2 (IL1RL1), *J Biol Chem* 285:21478–21486, 2010.
21. Cheng LE, Hartmann K, Roers A, et al.: Perivascular mast cells dynamically probe cutaneous blood vessels to capture immunoglobulin E, *Immunity* 38:166–175, 2013.
22. Felce JH, et al.: CD45 exclusion- and cross-linking-based receptor signaling together broaden FcεRI reactivity, *Sci Signal* 11, 2018.
23. Joulia R, et al.: Mast cells form antibody-dependent degranulatory synapse for dedicated secretion and defence, *Nat Commun* 6:6174, 2015.
24. Phong B, Avery L, Menk AV, et al.: Cutting edge: murine mast cells rapidly modulate metabolic pathways essential for distinct effector functions, *J Immunol* 198:640–644, 2017.
25. Oettgen HC, et al.: Active anaphylaxis in IgE-deficient mice, *Nature* 370:367–370, 1994.
26. Zhao W, et al.: Fc gamma RIIa, not Fc gamma RIIb, is constitutively and functionally expressed on skin-derived human mast cells, *J Immunol* 177:694–701, 2006.
27. Nigrovic PA, et al.: C5a receptor enables participation of mast cells in immune complex arthritis independently of Fcγ receptor modulation, *Arthritis Rheum* 62:3322–3333, 2010.
28. Lee H, et al.: Activation of human synovial mast cells from rheumatoid arthritis or osteoarthritis patients in response to aggregated IgG through Fcγ receptor I and Fcγ receptor II, *Arthritis Rheum* 65:109–119, 2013.
29. Nigrovic PA, et al.: Mast cells contribute to initiation of autoantibody-mediated arthritis via IL-1, *Proc Natl Acad Sci U S A* 104:2325–2330, 2007.
30. McNeil BD, et al.: Identification of a mast-cell-specific receptor crucial for pseudo-allergic drug reactions, *Nature* 519:237–241, 2015.
34. Reber LL, et al.: Contribution of mast cell-derived interleukin-1β to uric acid crystal-induced acute arthritis in mice, *Arthritis Rheumatol* 66:2881–2891, 2014.
35. Takai T, Ono M, Hikida M, et al.: Augmented humoral and anaphylactic responses in Fc gamma RII-deficient mice, *Nature* 379:346–349, 1996.
36. Ujike A, et al.: Modulation of immunoglobulin (Ig)E-mediated systemic anaphylaxis by low-affinity Fc receptors for IgG, *J Exp Med* 189:1573–1579, 1999.

37. Burton OT, et al.: Oral immunotherapy induces IgG antibodies that act through FcγRIIb to suppress IgE-mediated hypersensitivity, *J Allergy Clin Immunol* 134:1310-1317 e6, 2014.
38. Burton OT, Tamayo JM, Stranks AJ, et al.: Allergen-specific IgG antibody signaling through FcγRIIb promotes food tolerance, *J Allergy Clin Immunol* 141:189-201 e3, 2018.
41. Schwartz LB, Metcalfe DD, Miller JS, et al.: Tryptase levels as an indicator of mast-cell activation in systemic anaphylaxis and mastocytosis, *N Engl J Med* 316:1622–1626, 1987.
42. Schwartz LB, et al.: The alpha form of human tryptase is the predominant type present in blood at baseline in normal subjects and is elevated in those with systemic mastocytosis, *J Clin Invest* 96:2702–2710, 1995.
48. Oschatz C, et al.: Mast cells increase vascular permeability by heparin-initiated bradykinin formation in vivo, *Immunity* 34:258–268, 2011.
49. Gordon JR, Galli SJ: Mast cells as a source of both preformed and immunologically inducible TNF-alpha/cachectin, *Nature* 346:274–276, 1990.
50. Zhang Y, Ramos BF, Jakschik BA: Neutrophil recruitment by tumor necrosis factor from mast cells in immune complex peritonitis, *Science* 258:1957–1959, 1992.
51. Malaviya R, Ikeda T, Ross E, et al.: Mast cell modulation of neutrophil influx and bacterial clearance at sites of infection through TNF-alpha, *Nature* 381:77–80, 1996.
52. McLachlan JB, et al.: Mast cell-derived tumor necrosis factor induces hypertrophy of draining lymph nodes during infection, *Nat Immunol* 4:1199–1205, 2003.
53. McLachlan JB, et al.: Mast cell activators: a new class of highly effective vaccine adjuvants, *Nat Med* 14:536–541, 2008.
55. De Filippo K, et al.: Mast cell and macrophage chemokines CXCL1/CXCL2 control the early stage of neutrophil recruitment during tissue inflammation, *Blood* 121:4930–4937, 2013.
57. Noordenbos T, et al.: Interleukin-17-positive mast cells contribute to synovial inflammation in spondylarthritis, *Arthritis Rheum* 64:99–109, 2012.
58. Martin TR, Galli SJ, Katona IM, et al.: Role of mast cells in anaphylaxis. Evidence for the importance of mast cells in the cardiopulmonary alterations and death induced by anti-IgE in mice, *J Clin Invest* 83:1375–1383, 1989.
59. Choi HW, et al.: Perivascular dendritic cells elicit anaphylaxis by relaying allergens to mast cells via microvesicles, *Science* 362, 2018.
60. Jonsson F, et al.: Mouse and human neutrophils induce anaphylaxis, *J Clin Invest* 121:1484–1496, 2011.
61. Echtenacher B, Mannel DN, Hultner L: Critical protective role of mast cells in a model of acute septic peritonitis, *Nature* 381:75–77, 1996.
62. Piliponsky AM, et al.: Mast cell-derived TNF can exacerbate mortality during severe bacterial infections in C57BL/6-KitW-sh/W-sh mice, *Am J Pathol* 176:926–938, 2010.
64. Shin K, et al.: Mouse mast cell tryptase mmcp-6 is a critical link between adaptive and innate immunity in the chronic phase of trichinella spiralis infection, *J Immunol* 180:4885–4891, 2008.
66. Lotfi-Emran S, et al.: Human mast cells present antigen to autologous CD4(+) T cells, *J Allergy Clin Immunol* 141:311–321 e10, 2018.
67. Stelekati E, et al.: Mast cell-mediated antigen presentation regulates CD8+ T cell effector functions, *Immunity* 31:665–676, 2009.
69. Ott VL, Cambier JC, Kappler J, et al.: Mast cell-dependent migration of effector CD8+ T cells through production of leukotriene B4, *Nat Immunol* 4:974–981, 2003.
71. Dudeck J, et al.: Engulfment of mast cell secretory granules on skin inflammation boosts dendritic cell migration and priming efficiency, *J Allergy Clin Immunol*, 2018.
72. Gauchat JF, et al.: Induction of human IgE synthesis in B cells by mast cells and basophils, *Nature* 365:340–343, 1993.
73. Merluzzi, S. et al. Mast cells enhance proliferation of B lymphocytes and drive their differentiation toward IgA-secreting plasma cells. *Blood* 115, 2810-2817.
76. Chen R, et al.: Mast cells play a key role in neutrophil recruitment in experimental bullous pemphigoid, *J Clin Invest* 108:1151–1158, 2001.
81. Hugle T, Hogan V, White KE, et al.: Mast cells are a source of transforming growth factor beta in systemic sclerosis, *Arthritis Rheum* 63:795–799, 2011.
82. Hugle T, White K, van Laar JM: Cell-to-cell contact of activated mast cells with fibroblasts and lymphocytes in systemic sclerosis, *Ann Rheum Dis* 71:1582, 2012.
83. Shrestha S, et al.: Lesional and nonlesional skin from patients with untreated juvenile dermatomyositis displays increased numbers of mast cells and mature plasmacytoid dendritic cells, *Arthritis Rheum* 62:2813–2822, 2010.
84. Yokota M, et al.: Roles of mast cells in the pathogenesis of inflammatory myopathy, *Arthritis Res Ther* 16:R72, 2014.
85. Maurer M, et al.: Mast cells promote homeostasis by limiting endothelin-1-induced toxicity, *Nature* 432:512–516, 2004.
86. de Vries VC, et al.: Mast cells condition dendritic cells to mediate allograft tolerance, *Immunity* 35:550–561, 2011.
87. Rivellese F, et al.: Ability of interleukin-33- and immune complex-triggered activation of human mast cells to down-regulate monocyte-mediated immune responses, *Arthritis Rheumatol* 67:2343–2353, 2015.
88. Lu LF, et al.: Mast cells are essential intermediaries in regulatory T-cell tolerance, *Nature* 442:997–1002, 2006.
90. Hershko AY, et al.: Mast cell interleukin-2 production contributes to suppression of chronic allergic dermatitis, *Immunity* 35:562–571, 2011.
92. Morita H, et al.: An interleukin-33-mast cell-interleukin-2 axis suppresses papain-induced allergic inflammation by promoting regulatory T cell numbers, *Immunity* 43:175–186, 2015.
98. Bradding P, Pejler G: The controversial role of mast cells in fibrosis, *Immunol Rev* 282:198–231, 2018.
99. Severson AR: Mast cells in areas of experimental bone resorption and remodelling, *Br J Exp Pathol* 50:17–21, 1969.
100. Silberstein R, Melnick M, Greenberg G, et al.: Bone remodeling in W/Wv mast cell deficient mice, *Bone* 12:227–236, 1991.
101. Frame B, Nixon RK: Bone-marrow mast cells in osteoporosis of aging, *N Engl J Med* 279:626–630, 1968.
102. Fallon MD, Whyte MP, Teitelbaum SL: Systemic mastocytosis associated with generalized osteopenia. Histopathological characterization of the skeletal lesion using undecalcified bone from two patients, *Hum Pathol* 12:813–820, 1981.
103. Castor W: The microscopic structure of normal human synovial tissue, *Arthritis Rheum* 3:140–151, 1960.
104. Shin K, et al.: Lymphocyte-independent connective tissue mast cells populate murine synovium, *Arthritis Rheum* 54:2863–2871, 2006.
105. Crisp AJ, Chapman CM, Kirkham SE, et al.: Articular mastocytosis in rheumatoid arthritis, *Arthritis Rheum* 27:845–851, 1984.
106. Frewin DB, Cleland LG, Jonsson JR, et al.: Histamine levels in human synovial fluid, *J Rheumatol* 13:13–14, 1986.
107. Buckley MG, et al.: Mast cell activation in arthritis: detection of alpha- and beta-tryptase, histamine and eosinophil cationic protein in synovial fluid, *Clin Sci (Lond)* 93:363–370, 1997.
108. Bromley M, Fisher WD, Woolley DE: Mast cells at sites of cartilage erosion in the rheumatoid joint, *Ann Rheum Dis* 43:76–79, 1984.
109. Malone DG, Irani AM, Schwartz LB, et al.: Mast cell numbers and histamine levels in synovial fluids from patients with diverse arthritides, *Arthritis Rheum* 29:956–963, 1986.
110. Ceponis A, et al.: Expression of stem cell factor (SCF) and SCF receptor (c-kit) in synovial membrane in arthritis: correlation with synovial mast cell hyperplasia and inflammation, *J Rheumatol* 25:2304–2314, 1998.

111. Kiener HP, et al.: Tumor necrosis factor alpha promotes the expression of stem cell factor in synovial fibroblasts and their capacity to induce mast cell chemotaxis, *Arthritis Rheum* 43:164–174, 2000.
112. Malone DG, Wilder RL, Saavedra-Delgado AM, et al.: Mast cell numbers in rheumatoid synovial tissues. Correlations with quantitative measures of lymphocytic infiltration and modulation by antiinflammatory therapy, *Arthritis Rheum* 30:130–137, 1987.
113. Gotis-Graham I, Smith MD, Parker A, et al.: Synovial mast cell responses during clinical improvement in early rheumatoid arthritis, *Ann Rheum Dis* 57:664–671, 1998.
114. Firestein GS, et al.: Cytokines in chronic inflammatory arthritis. I. Failure to detect T cell lymphokines (interleukin 2 and interleukin 3) and presence of macrophage colony-stimulating factor (CSF-1) and a novel mast cell growth factor in rheumatoid synovitis, *J Exp Med* 168:1573–1586, 1988.
115. Chen S, et al.: Histologic evidence that mast cells contribute to local tissue inflammation in peripheral spondyloarthritis by regulating interleukin-17A content, *Rheumatology (Oxford)*, 2018.
116. Nigrovic PA, Lee DM: Synovial mast cells: role in acute and chronic arthritis, *Immunol Rev* 217:19–37, 2007.
117. Buckley MG, Gallagher PJ, Walls AF: Mast cell subpopulations in the synovial tissue of patients with osteoarthritis: selective increase in numbers of tryptase-positive, chymase-negative mast cells, *J Pathol* 186:67–74, 1998.
118. Kiener HP, et al.: Expression of the C5a receptor (CD88) on synovial mast cells in patients with rheumatoid arthritis, *Arthritis Rheum* 41:233–245, 1998.
119. Suurmond J, et al.: Toll-like receptor triggering augments activation of human mast cells by anti-citrullinated protein antibodies, *Ann Rheum Dis* 74:1915–1923, 2015.
120. Arandjelovic S, McKenney KR, Leming SS, et al.: ATP induces protein arginine deiminase 2-dependent citrullination in mast cells through the P2X7 purinergic receptor, *J Immunol* 189:4112–4122, 2012.
121. Lee DM, et al.: Mast cells: a cellular link between autoantibodies and inflammatory arthritis, *Science* 297:1689–1692, 2002.
122. Corr M, Crain B: The role of FcgammaR signaling in the K/B x N serum transfer model of arthritis, *J Immunol* 169:6604–6609, 2002.
123. Guma M, et al.: JNK1 controls mast cell degranulation and IL-1{beta} production in inflammatory arthritis, *Proc Natl Acad Sci U S A* 107:22122–22127, 2010.
124. Wipke BT, Wang Z, Nagengast W, et al.: Staging the initiation of autoantibody-induced arthritis: a critical role for immune complexes, *J Immunol* 172:7694–7702, 2004.
125. Binstadt BA, et al.: Particularities of the vasculature can promote the organ specificity of autoimmune attack, *Nat Immunol* 7:284–292, 2006.
126. Zhou JS, Xing W, Friend DS, et al.: Mast cell deficiency in Kit(W-sh) mice does not impair antibody-mediated arthritis, *J Exp Med* 204:2797–2802, 2007.
127. Feyerabend TB, et al.: Cre-mediated cell ablation contests mast cell contribution in models of antibody- and T cell-mediated autoimmunity, *Immunity* 35:832–844, 2011.
128. Schubert N, et al.: Mast cell promotion of T cell-driven antigen-induced arthritis despite being dispensable for antibody-induced arthritis in which T cells are bypassed, *Arthritis Rheumatol* 67:903–913, 2015.
129. Cunin P, et al.: Megakaryocytes compensate for Kit insufficiency in murine arthritis, *J Clin Invest* 127:1714–1724, 2017.
130. McNeil HP, et al.: The mouse mast cell-restricted tetramer-forming tryptases mouse mast cell protease 6 and mouse mast cell protease 7 are critical mediators in inflammatory arthritis, *Arthritis Rheum* 58:2338–2346, 2008.
131. Shin K, et al.: Mast cells contribute to autoimmune inflammatory arthritis via their tryptase/heparin complexes, *J Immunol* 182:647–656, 2009.
132. Stevens RL, et al.: Experimental arthritis is dependent on mouse mast cell protease-5, *J Biol Chem* 292:5392–5404, 2017.
133. Juurikivi A, et al.: Inhibition of c-kit tyrosine kinase by imatinib mesylate induces apoptosis in mast cells in rheumatoid synovia: a potential approach to the treatment of arthritis, *Ann Rheum Dis* 64:1126–1131, 2005.
134. Hueber AJ, et al.: Mast cells express IL-17A in rheumatoid arthritis synovium, *J Immunol* 184:3336–3340, 2010.
135. Paniagua RT, et al.: Selective tyrosine kinase inhibition by imatinib mesylate for the treatment of autoimmune arthritis, *J Clin Invest* 116:2633–2642, 2006.
136. Tebib J, et al.: Masitinib in the treatment of active rheumatoid arthritis: results of a multicentre, open-label, dose-ranging, phase 2a study, *Arthritis Res Ther* 11:R95, 2009.
137. van der Velden D, et al.: Mast cell depletion in the preclinical phase of collagen-induced arthritis reduces clinical outcome by lowering the inflammatory cytokine profile, *Arthritis Res Ther* 18:138, 2016.
138. Palmer HS, et al.: Protease-activated receptor 2 mediates the proinflammatory effects of synovial mast cells, *Arthritis Rheum* 56:3532–3540, 2007.
139. Sawamukai N, et al. Mast cell-derived tryptase inhibits apoptosis of human rheumatoid synovial fibroblasts via rho-mediated signaling. *Arthritis Rheum* 62, 952-959.
140. Magarinos NJ, et al.: Mast cell-restricted, tetramer-forming tryptases induce aggrecanolysis in articular cartilage by activating matrix met alloproteinase-3 and -13 zymogens, *J Immunol* 191:1404–1412, 2013.
141. Ustun C, DeRemer DL, Akin C: Tyrosine kinase inhibitors in the treatment of systemic mastocytosis, *Leuk Res* 35:1143–1152, 2011.
142. Cahill KN, et al.: KIT inhibition by imatinib in patients with severe refractory asthma, *N Engl J Med* 376:1911–1920, 2017.
143. Tabone-Eglinger S, et al.: Niche anchorage and signaling through membrane-bound Kit-ligand/c-kit receptor are kinase independent and imatinib insensitive, *FASEB J* 28:4441–4456, 2014.
144. Adachi R, et al.: Ras guanine nucleotide-releasing protein-4 (Ras-GRP4) involvement in experimental arthritis and colitis, *J Biol Chem* 287:20047–20055, 2012.
145. Zhu M, Fuller DM, Zhang W: The role of Ras guanine nucleotide releasing protein 4 in Fcγ epsilonRI-mediated signaling, mast cell function, and T cell development, *J Biol Chem* 287:8135–8143, 2012.

16

Innate Lymphoid Cells and Natural Killer Cells

MICHAEL A. PALEY AND WAYNE M. YOKOYAMA

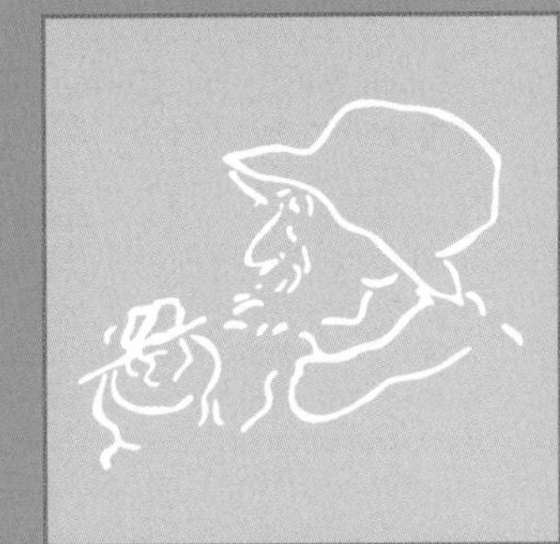

KEY POINTS

- Innate lymphoid cells (ILCs) and natural killer (NK) cells are components of the innate immune system that protect against invading pathogens.
- ILCs and NK cells contribute to immune responses by amplifying inflammation or facilitating wound healing via the production of cytokines.
- By functioning in an antigen-independent manner, these cells augment the early immune response, limit pathogen replication, and "buy time" for the adaptive immune response of B and T cells to develop and control offending agents.
- Emerging data implicate ILCs and NK cells in rheumatologic conditions.

Introduction

As constituents of innate immunity, innate lymphoid cells (ILCs) and natural killer (NK) cells can provide early host responses against a variety of pathogens, including viruses, bacteria, fungi, and parasites.[1,2] The diversity of ILC and NK cell responses parallels the biology of T cells (Fig. 16.1).[3,4] Therefore, much of the current understanding of ILC biology is built upon the scaffold of T cell differentiation.

ILCs are divided into three types based on development and function, such as cytokine production. Type 1 ILCs (ILC1s) produce interferon-γ (IFN-γ) and require the T-box transcription factor T-bet for their development, paralleling Th1 cells. ILC2s produce the type 2 cytokines IL-5 and IL-13, and are programmed by the transcription factors GATA3 and RORα,[2] resembling Th2 cells. ILC3s includes two members, distinguished by expression of a natural cytotoxicity receptor (NCR) (i.e., NCR^+ ILC3s and NCR^- ILC3s), require the transcription factor RORγt, and produce IL-17 and/or IL-22, akin to Th17 cells.

Two additional subsets, NK cells, studied for more than 40 years, and lymphoid tissue-inducer (LTi) cells are also considered innate lymphocytes and have been previously classified as belonging to ILC1s and ILC3s, respectively, but are now recognized as distinct cell lineages. While NK cells share a primary feature of ILC1s, such as the production of IFN-γ, several properties of NK cells clearly distinguish them from other ILCs. For example, under homeostatic conditions, NK cells actively circulate between the blood and multiple organs,[5] while ILCs predominantly remain in extra-lymphoid tissues and rarely circulate.[6] In addition, NK cells are primed to rapidly kill virally infected or transformed malignant cells, whereas ILC1s have reduced cytotoxic capacity.[7] Furthermore, ILC1s and NK cells arise from distinct developmental pathways (discussed in the next section). As a result, NK cells likely play a distinct role in human pathophysiology compared with ILC populations.

LTi cells share many features with ILC3s, such as the transcription factors RORγt, Tox, AHR, TCF1, and Notch as well as the production of cytokines IL-17, IL-22, and lymphotoxin.[2,8] However, unlike ILC3s, LTi cells are essential during embryonic development to form secondary lymphoid tissue, such as lymph nodes and Peyer's patches.[9–11] This is a distinctive function of LTi cells. Similarly, LTi cells can also contribute to the development of tertiary lymphoid structures within organs subjected to chronic inflammation. In contrast to secondary lymphoid tissue, however, this is not a unique capacity of LTi cells as other cell types, such as T or NK cells, are able to initiate tertiary lymphoid tissue development.[12] LTi cells can also be distinguished from ILC3s by the chemokine receptor CCR6[13] and a distinct developmental pathway (discussed in the next section). As a result, LTi cells are now considered a subset on their own.

Distinguishing Human ILCs and NK Cells

ILCs and NK cells are defined as lymphoid cells that do not require antigen receptor rearrangement for their development, unlike T and B cells, and can now be clearly distinguished from other leukocytes. For example, ILCs and NK cells lack proteins expressed on specific cell types, such as CD3 and CD5 (T cells), CD19 and CD20 (B cells), and CD13 and CD14 (myelomonocytes).[5]

Discriminating between ILCs and NK cells has become important as cells formerly thought to be immature NK cells were subsequently identified as ILCs. For example, most ILCs are dependent on the cytokine IL-7 and therefore can be identified by the expression of the IL-7 receptor (CD127), whereas NK cells utilize IL-15 for survival and have high expression of the IL-2/IL-15 receptor β chain (CD122).[2] In addition, NK cells can be identified based on the expression of the transcription factor Eomesodermin (EOMES), the cytolytic molecules granzyme and perforin, their MHC-binding receptors, and CD16, an Fc receptor responsible for antibody-dependent cellular cytotoxicity (ADCC).[5] Despite these acknowledged differences, there is significant overlap between ILCs and NK cells, which still contributes to challenges in cell identification.

T-cell	Effector molecules		Innate cell	Activating cytokines
Th1	IFN-γ, TNF, IL-2	IFN-γ	ILC1	IL-12, IL-18
Th2	IL-4, IL-5, IL-13, L-25, AREG	IL-4, IL-5, IL-13, IL-9, AREG	ILC2	IL-25, IL-33, TSLP
Th17	IL-17, IL-21, IL-22	IL-17, IL-22, GM-CSF, lymphotoxin	ILC3	IL-1β, IL-23
CD8 T cell	Perforin granzymes IFN-γ, TNF	Perforin granzymes IFN-γ, TNF	NK cell	IL-2, IL-12, IL-18

• **Fig. 16.1** Lineage of innate lymphoid cells and corresponding T cells. Each type of innate lymphoid cell is illustrated alongside the cytokines that trigger its activation (i.e., "activating cytokines") as well as the cytokines that the innate cells release to potentiate an immune response (i.e., "effector molecules"). For each innate cell type, the corresponding T cell population is presented with its own effector molecules to illustrate the overlap between T cell and innate cell functions. *AREG,* Amphiregulin; *GM-CSF,* granulocyte-macrophage colony-stimulating factor; *IFN,* interferon; *IL,* interleukin; *TNF,* tumor necrosis factor; *TSLP,* thymic stromal lymphopoietin.

Target Recognition by NK Cells and Killer Immunoglobulin-like Receptors (KIRs)

One of the main functions of NK cells is direct killing of infected or transformed target cells with the help of germline-encoded NK cell receptors. The major family of these receptors is the killer immunoglobulin-like receptors (KIRs), consisting of both activation and inhibitory receptors.[14] There are several KIR isoforms with two or three Ig-like domains (2D or 3D). Inhibitory receptors are designated as having long cytoplasmic tails, such as KIR2DL1, with intra-cellular immunoreceptor tyrosine-based inhibitory motifs (ITIMs). Those with short cytoplasmic domains, such as KIR2DS1, are activation receptors because they couple to signaling chains with immunoreceptor tyrosine-based activation motifs (ITAMs), similar to those in the T or B cell antigen receptor complexes. NK cells integrate the positive and negative signals from these respective receptors to determine whether to kill a target cell and release pro-inflammatory cytokines or to remain quiescent (Fig. 16.2).

In addition to providing the first line of defense against virally infected or transformed cells, NK cells can cooperate with adaptive immunity to accelerate pathogen elimination. For example, NK cells are central mediators of ADCC, where (1) antibodies bind antigens on the surface of an infected or malignant cell, (2) NK cells use their low affinity Fc receptor for IgG (CD16) to recognize the cell-bound antibodies, and (3) subsequent CD16 crosslinking results in degranulation and lysis of the target cell.[15] This antibody-mediated destruction of target cells by NK cells appears to be operative in a variety of clinical settings, including B cell depletion with the monoclonal anti-CD20 antibody rituximab for rheumatoid arthritis and vasculitis.[15–17]

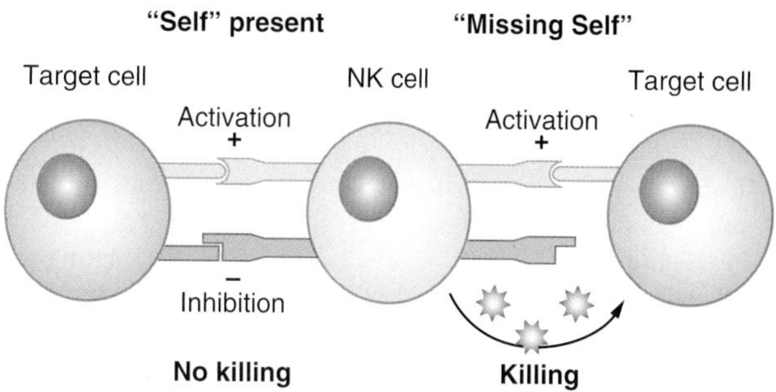

• **Fig. 16.2** Regulation of natural killer (NK) cell killing based on "missing self." NK cells integrate activation and inhibitory signals to determine target cell killing. For target cells that express self-class I MHC molecules *(left)*, the signals for NK cell activation *(green)* and inhibition *(red)* are appropriately balanced, which prevents NK cell killing. In contrast, virally infected or transformed target cells that decrease self-class I MHC expression *(right)* remove ligands for inhibitory NK cell receptors. This tips the overall signaling towards NK cell activation, which leads to NK cell-mediated killing. The process of specifically killing cells that have lost self-MHC molecules is termed "missing self," since class I MHC is nearly ubiquitously expressed.

Due to this ability to elicit effector functions, CD16 is considered among the activation receptors on NK cells, which also include the natural cytotoxicity receptors (NKp46, NKp44, NKp30), NKG2C, NKG2D, and several KIRs (KIR2DS1, KIR2DS2, KIR2DS4).[18] The ligands for these activation receptors have not all been identified, but they include alleles of the human leukocyte antigen (HLA) locus, including HLA-C (for KIR2DS1), HLA-E (NKG2C), and HLA-G (KIR2DL4).[18]

Ligands for NKG2D include MICA, MICB, and ULBP1-4, which are generally not expressed well under normal conditions but can be upregulated during periods of cell stress, such as during infection or malignancy. The corresponding activation receptor (NKG2D) can then trigger NK cell killing, thereby limiting the spread of infection or cancer.

Activation receptors trigger effector functions through their association with type I transmembrane-anchored proteins that contain a cytoplasmic ITAM: FcR γ, CD3 ζ, and DAP12.[18,19] Upon ligation of the activating receptor, tyrosine residues in the ITAMs are phosphorylated through Src family kinases (e.g., Lck, Lyn, Fyn, Src, Yes, and Fgr).[18] These phosphorylation events lead to activation of the Syk family tyrosine kinases that trigger additional downstream signaling events involving phospholipase C-γ (PLC-γ) and Vav, which subsequently lead to actin reorganization, degranulation, and activation of the transcription factors NFAT, NF-κB, ERK, and AKT with associated transcriptional changes.[18] While some activation receptors are able to elicit effector functions in isolation, other receptors only mediate activity in combination with other co-receptors.[19]

In contrast to activation receptors, NK cell inhibitory receptors contain a cytoplasmic ITIM. Members of the inhibitory receptor group include 2B4, KLRG1, NKG2A, KLRB1, LAIR1, LILRB1, and several KIRs (KIR2DL1, KIR2DL2, KIR2DL3, KIR3DL1, KIR3DL2).[18] When the inhibitory receptor is crosslinked, the ITIM is tyrosine-phosphorylated, which can recruit the tyrosine phosphatases SHP-1 or SHP-2, or the SH2 domain-containing inositol 5′phosphatase-1 (SHIP-1).[19] Positioning SHP-1 and SHP-2 at the immunologic synapse by ITIMs leads to dephosphorylation of adapter signaling molecules, such as VAV, which abrogates ITAM-mediated signaling.[20] Similarly, recruitment of SHIP leads to degradation of the signaling molecules $PI(3,4,5)P_3$ and IP_3, which inhibits parallel signaling pathways downstream of ITAM signaling.[20] Inhibitory receptor signaling is able to counteract activation receptors, protecting potential target cells from NK cell killing.

The ligands for the inhibitory receptors are frequently class I MHC alleles, such as HLA-A3/A11 (for KIR3DL2), HLA-C (KIR2DL1, KIR2DL2, and KIR2DL3), HLA-E (NKG2A), or any HLA class I (LILRB1).[18] Notably, HLA-C alleles can be grouped into two broad categories based on amino acid residue 80, which dictates recognition by certain KIR isotypes (i.e., KIR2DL1 is specific for HLA-C [Lys80] while KIR2DL2 and KIR2DL3 are specific for HLA-C [Asn80]), indicating stringent specificity of KIRs for their HLA ligands, similar to the exquisite specificity of TCRs.

Biology of ILCs and NK Cells

ILCs and NK cells both originate from hematopoietic stem cells (HSCs) in the bone marrow. HSCs give rise to the common lymphoid precursor (CLP), which is the progenitor for B cells, T cells, NK cells, and ILCs. CLPs subsequently differentiate into the common innate lymphoid progenitor (CILP), the branch-point for ILC and NK cell commitment (Fig. 16.3).

ILC Development

CILPs generate common helper innate lymphoid progenitors (CHILPs) under the influence of the transcription factors GATA3, TCF-1, and ID2.[2,21] In addition to the ILC1, ILC2, and ILC3 lineages, CHILPs are also precursors to LTi cells. The transcription factor PLZF, however, directs CHILPs to differentiate into the innate lymphoid cell precursor (ILCP), preventing formation of LTi cells. ILCPs are the direct precursor to ILC1s, ILC2s, and ILC3s.

The differentiation of ILCPs into ILC1s, ILC2s, and ILC3s is heavily influenced by environmental cytokines. For example, the cytokines IL-12, IL-15, and IL-18 lead ILCPs to differentiate into ILC1s and produce IFN-γ.[22,23] In contrast, IL-7, IL-25, and IL-33 promote the formation of ILC2s, while IL-7, IL-23, and retinoic acid drive ILC3 differentiation.[21] Once formed, however, these ILC lineages are malleable and demonstrate plasticity. For example, ILC1s can convert to ILC2s, while ILC2s can be induced to produce the ILC1-defining cytokine IFN-γ.[24–26] Similarly, there may also be conversion between ILC1s and ILC3s.[3,27,28] Thus, ILCs can facilitate multiple pro-inflammatory processes, a feature currently under intense investigation.

NK Cell Development

Under the direction of several transcription factors (TOX, NFIL3, ID2, PU.1, Runx3, and ETS1), CILPs develop into NK cell precursors (NKPs),[2] which are characterized by expression of CD122 without NK cell lineage markers.[29] The expression of CD122 and other components of the IL15R are critical for NK cell development, as NKPs and their mature progeny are dependent on IL-15 for survival. NKPs further develop into immature then finally mature NK cells under the coordination of Gata-3, IRF-2, CEBP-γ, MEF, MITF, and two T-box transcription factors (T-BET and EOMES).[2,30,31] Unlike mice where NK development largely takes place in the bone marrow, human NK cell development may also occur in secondary lymphoid tissues, such as the lymph node or spleen.[5] This process of maturation is characterized by the acquisition of several surface receptors (CD16, KIRs, NKp30, NKp46, 2B4, NKG2A, NKG2C, NKG2D), effector molecules (perforin), and glycoproteins (CD56, CD57).[32]

The glycoprotein CD56 distinguishes two populations of mature human NK cells ($CD56^{bright}$ and $CD56^{dim}$).[33,34] These two populations differ in terms of phenotype and functional capacity, with $CD56^{bright}$ NK cells having robust proliferation and production of IFN-γ in response to IL-2, IL-12, IL-15, and IL-18, whereas $CD56^{dim}$ NK cells express CD16, are highly cytotoxic, and produce IFN-γ in the context of target cell recognition.[32] These two subsets of NK cells also differ in terms of anatomic prevalence; while $CD56^{dim}$ NK cells comprise 90% of circulating NK found in the blood, the majority of NK cells found in secondary lymphoid organs are $CD56^{bright}$.[32]

$CD56^{bright}$ and $CD56^{dim}$ NK cells have been hypothesized to be developmentally related, with the $CD56^{bright}$ NK cells giving rise to $CD56^{dim}$ NK cells.[35] This is supported by observations that $CD56^{bright}$ NK cells contain longer telomeres, have more robust proliferation after stimulation, and can generate $CD56^{dim}$ NK cells after an in vitro culture.[32] This model of linear differentiation has been suggested to occur during development and homeostasis. Data from nonhuman primates suggest, however, that these two populations undergo little transition during homeostasis.[36] Instead, $CD56^{bright}$ NK cells may only give rise to $CD56^{dim}$ NK cells in substantial numbers during generation or replenishment of the NK cell pool, such as during development, after bone marrow transplantation, or after targeted NK cell ablation via IL-15 deprivation.[36]

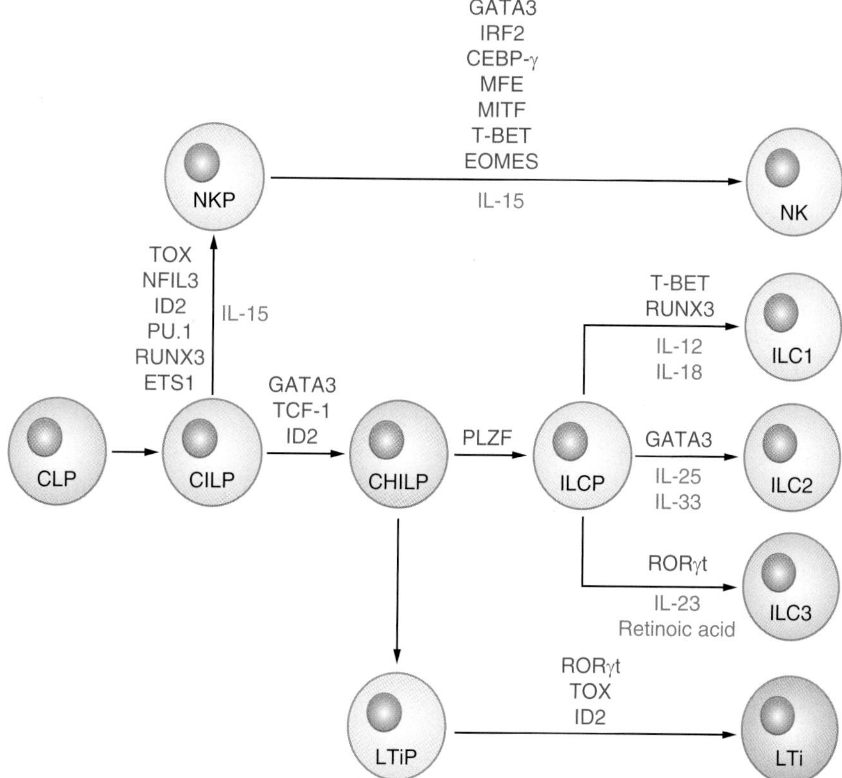

• **Fig. 16.3** ILC and NK cell development. Development is illustrated from left to right. Transcription factors regulating each step of development are shown in *red*. Specific cytokines that support each developmental step are shown in *blue*. *CHILP,* Common helper innate lymphoid progenitors; *CILP,* common innate lymphoid progenitor; *CLP,* common lymphoid precursor; *ILC,* innate lymphoid cell; *ILCP,* innate lymphoid cell precursor; *LTI,* lymphoid tissue inducer cell; *LTiP,* lymphoid tissue inducer precursor; *NK,* natural killer; *NKP,* natural killer cell precursor.

NK Cell Function

The two well-defined features of NK cells are their ability to lyse target cells and produce inflammatory cytokines. In contrast with T and B cells from the adaptive immune response, NK cell function does not require prior exposure to the offending tumor or viral pathogen, but instead is present on the initial encounter.[37] NK cell activity is, however, finely tuned based on the process of licensing and the state of NK cell activation (discussed in the next section).

The importance of NK cells in combating viral infection has been established from humans with NK cell deficiencies. A patient with complete and relatively selective NK cell deficiency suffered two life-threatening herpesvirus infections: disseminated varicella zoster virus and cytomegalovirus pneumonitis at ages 13 and 17, respectively.[38] In addition to NK cell deficiency, impaired NK cell function also leads to increased vulnerability to herpesviruses. Small case series of siblings have demonstrated that NK functional defects may lead to severe infections from EBV[39] and HSV.[40] Thus, NK cells play a critical role in human immunity to viral pathogens.

NK cells have other functions in addition to elimination of target cells. For example, NK cells accumulate at the maternal-fetal interface in the placenta and have been suggested to play a supportive role in pregnancy by preventing trophoblast invasion and the development of pre-eclampsia.[41,42] These uterine NK cells have a distinct transcriptional program compared to traditional NK cells, possibly due to the non-inflammatory requirements of fetal-placental development.[43] As a result, NK cell function can be heavily influenced by its surrounding environment.

Regulation of NK Cell Activation, Licensing, and Missing Self

While mature NK cells are functional at a basal resting state, activation of NK cells through inflammatory cytokines and cell-cell contact greatly enhances NK cell activity. Several cytokines activate NK cells, such as IFN-α, IFN-β, IL-12, IL-15, and IL-18.[44] Upon activation, NK cells produce pro-inflammatory cytokines such as IFN-γ, TNF, and granulocyte-macrophage colony-stimulating factor (GM-CSF).[45–48] These inflammatory cytokines are important to augment anti-viral and anti-tumor responses. In addition, NK cells can release chemokines to recruit additional immune cells to initial sites of inflammation.

Most ligands for the KIRs on NK cells belong to the HLA region, a locus with high genomic variability. Moreover, the KIRs themselves are highly polymorphic. As a result, inherited KIR ligands and KIRs show profound variability from one individual to the next, risking the possibility of autoreactivity in individuals who do not inherit the right combination of cognate ligands for their inhibitory receptors. Consequently, the NK cell population must finely tailor its potential for activation, a process termed licensing.

Licensing is an education process for NK cells that depends on exposure to host class I MHC. Experiments in mice have demonstrated that genetic lesions affecting normal expression of all class I MHC proteins do not affect NK cell number but lead to severe NK cell defects, such as dysfunctional NK killing and cytokine production, contrary to what would be otherwise expected by the missing-self hypothesis, as discussed in the next section. Reintroduction of a selected class I MHC gene allows NK cells with receptors that specifically recognize that class I MHC protein to become fully functional.[49] This process has also been observed in humans for specific pairings of inhibitory receptors and their corresponding HLA allele.[50,51] As a result, NK cells are only "licensed" (or educated) when they recognize self-class I MHC proteins.

As mentioned previously, several ligands for NK inhibitory receptors are class I MHC proteins, HLA-A, -B, and -C. The function of these class I MHC proteins is to present intra-cellular antigens to cytotoxic CD8 T cells. This allows CD8 T cells to identify virally infected cells due to the presentation of viral antigens. Consequently, to evade CD8 T cell responses, multiple viruses decrease or remove class I MHC genes from the surface of the infected cell. Class I MHC downregulation, however, enables NK cell killing, providing a critical role for NK cells in eliminating viruses that utilize this immune-evasion strategy.[37]

This function of NK cells is described by the "missing self" hypothesis since class I MHC is nearly ubiquitously expressed and normally prevents NK cells from killing target cells due to inhibitory receptors that bind class I MHC. When the target cell reduces the expression of class I MHC (such as during viral infection) (i.e., missing self), the NK cell receives less inhibitory signals, tipping the balance towards NK cell activation and target cell killing. Thus, the "missing self" hypothesis is a major guiding principle of NK cell function,[37] but current hypotheses suggest that missing self reactivity requires licensed NK cells that were educated by self-class I MHC molecules.

The Evolution of Missing Self

"Missing self" appears to have developed in parallel in separate mammalian species, a prime example of convergent evolution. For example, while human NK cells utilize an assortment of KIRs, mice do not have KIRs and instead independently evolved a collection of structurally distinct receptors, termed the Ly49 family, that are not present in humans but serve the same purpose.[44] While the mammalian strategy to detect "missing self" is young in evolutionary terms, cytotoxic cells themselves are phylogenetically old.[52] Indeed, cell-mediated cytotoxicity may have even evolved prior to the evolution of adaptive immunity and the development of recombination-activating gene (RAG) in jawed fish. In support of this, cell-mediated cytotoxicity occurs not only in multiple non-mammalian vertebrates,[52] but also in invertebrates, protecting the host from invasive cells from another individual of the same species, presumably by discriminating "self" from "non-self."[53] Thus, in contrast to the self- versus nonself-discrimination present in both vertebrate and invertebrate species, class I MHC-dependent "missing self" likely evolved more recently under species-specific, selective pressures.

ILC Functions

As mentioned previously, ILCs broadly function in parallel to their CD4 Th cell counterparts. However, there are several notable differences between ILCs and Th cells. In contrast to T cells, ILCs do not express unique rearranged antigen receptors (i.e., the T cell receptor). Instead, similar to NK cells, ILCs can respond quickly to inflammatory cytokines to potentiate an immune response. While T cells and B cells must undergo several days of proliferation and differentiation to acquire effector functions, due to clonal selection, cytokine-induced activation allows ILCs (and NK cells) to respond rapidly in the early phases of an immune response. An additional feature that accelerates the ILC response over T cells is that ILCs are resident in the tissues, already present at the site of initial inflammation, while T cells generally circulate and must home to inflammatory foci.

Role of NK Cells in Health and Disease

NK Cell Correlates With Rheumatologic Diseases

NK cells have been examined in multiple rheumatologic conditions. Multiple autoimmune diseases are associated with fewer circulating NK cells and/or reduced NK cell functionality.[54] Whether this is an initial risk factor or secondary to the development of a systemic inflammatory disorder remains unclear. Moreover, reduced NK cell cytotoxicity appears to be a common feature of rheumatologic disorders, but this finding should be interpreted with caution. Disorders with excess production of NK cells, such as chronic NK cell lymphocytosis, are associated with increased production of immature NK cells that have not yet acquired full effector functions.[55,56] As a result, autoimmune diseases that accelerate NK cell development could be associated with reduced NK cell killing, regardless of whether diminished cytotoxicity was a factor in developing the rheumatic disorder. Nevertheless, these correlations raise the possibility that NK cells participate in rheumatologic diseases.

Rheumatoid Arthritis and NK Cells

Similar to other autoimmune conditions, features of NK cells are altered in the setting of rheumatoid arthritis (RA). For example, the frequency and cytotoxicity of circulating NK cells in the blood are reduced while the ability for NK cells to produce IFN is not impaired.[57] In contrast, examination of the inflamed joints of RA patients has revealed an expansion of $CD56^{bright}$ NK cells, a lineage with enhanced cytokine production but reduced cytotoxicity.[58,59] Thus, decreased circulating NK cells may be the result of trafficking to the inflamed tissue, but it is possible the diminished cytotoxicity may be a risk factor for the development of RA.

Systemic Lupus Erythematosus and NK Cells

Studies in systemic lupus erythematosus (SLE) have reported low numbers of circulating NK cells and reduced NK cell killing. While improvement in SLE disease activity led to normalization of NK cell numbers, the defect in NK cell killing remained.[60–62] Thus, NK cell cytotoxicity appears permanently altered in the setting of SLE and may be a contributing risk factor for the development of disease, though considerations mentioned previously for RA may apply.

Juvenile Idiopathic Arthritis and NK Cells

Patients with juvenile idiopathic arthritis (JIA) have also been reported to have diminished levels of peripheral blood NK cells.

This observation was most extreme in patients with the systemic form of JIA.[63] NK cells in JIA patients were also less effective killers, expressing lower levels of the cytotoxic molecule perforin.[64]

Macrophage Activation Syndrome/Hemophagocytic Lymphohistiocytosis and NK Cells

Macrophage activation syndrome (MAS) is a rare robust inflammatory disorder associated with rheumatologic diseases. MAS shares a strong clinical overlap with hemophagocytic lymphohistiocytosis (HLH). Unlike some rheumatologic conditions, MAS/HLH has a robust mouse model. NK cells and cytotoxic CD8 T cells from mice deficient in the cytotoxic molecule perforin are unable to kill virally infected cells. Infection of these mice with specific viruses leads to a robust inflammatory response that resembles HLH and is eventually fatal.[65,66] This is thought to be due to a persistent viral stimulus of the immune system because the cytotoxic cells are unable to clear the virus. In support of this, persistent stimulation of innate immunity through Toll-like receptor 9 (TLR9) leads to macrophage activation syndrome-like disease in mice.[67]

Consistent with the mouse models, NK cell defects likely underlie a large subset of human cases of MAS and HLH. For example, mutations in the cytotoxic molecule perforin that lead to loss of expression and absent NK cell killing have been identified in inherited forms of HLH.[68,69] Furthermore, NK cell defects have been found in sufficient frequency in these diseases that they were included as part of a proposed diagnostic criteria for HLH and MAS.[70,71]

KIR/HLA and Their Association With Autoimmune Disease

Through genetic studies, several rheumatologic conditions have been associated with specific HLA and KIR alleles. For example, a meta-analysis has suggested KIR2DL3, KIR2DL5, KIR3DL3, and KIR2DS5 decrease the risk of developing RA.[72] In contrast, a genome-wide association study associated the LILRB3 locus, which encodes an NK inhibitory receptor, as a risk allele for developing Takayasu's arteritis.[73] By comparison, inheritance of the activating receptor KIR2DS2 in the absence of the inhibitory KIR2DL2 is associated with scleroderma.[74] Thus, the relative risk or benefit of specific KIR alleles varies by rheumatologic condition.

While genetic HLA associations with disease risk are generally thought to be due to the role of HLA in antigen presentation to T cells, it remains possible that the risk association may also be related to the binding of HLA alleles to NK cell activation or inhibitory receptors. For instance, a specific HLA-C allele (HLA-C*06:02) is associated with the development of psoriasis and psoriatic arthritis.[75–77] One notable feature of HLA-C*06:02 is that it does not bind the inhibitory KIR, KIR2DL1.[77] As a result, NK cells may be predisposed towards activation without such inhibitory signaling. Consistent with this hypothesis, patients who inherit the activating receptors KIR2DS1 and KIR2DS2 with HLA-C*06:02 homozygosity have increased risk of developing psoriatic arthritis.[77]

The genetic association between KIR and autoimmune diseases implicates NK cells in playing a pathogenic role in these disorders. However, this interpretation warrants caution. While KIRs were first identified on NK cells, KIRs are now known to be expressed by other immune cells. For example, RA patients with vasculitis were more likely to have inherited the activating receptor KIR2DS2 compared with RA patients without vasculitis or healthy controls.[78] However, in that study, CD4 T cells were demonstrated to have higher expression of KIR2DS2 in RA vasculitis cases compared with healthy controls, raising the possibility that the risk for RA vasculitis from KIR2DS2 may be mediated by CD4 T cells instead of, or in addition to, NK cells. Similarly, patients with HLA-B27-associated spondyloarthropathy have higher expression of the inhibitory receptor KIR3DL2 on NK cells and CD4 T cells,[79,80] and KIR3DL2-expressing CD4 T cells are enriched in the synovial fluid of patients with spondyloarthritis.[80] In addition, the interaction between HLA-B27 and KIR3DL2 appears to increase the survival of this particular CD4 T cell population.[80] Thus, some of the pathogenesis associated with HLA-KIR interactions may be mediated by non-NK cells, particularly T cells.

ILCs and Potential Contributions to Rheumatologic Disease

ILC populations have been reported to be altered in the setting of autoimmune disease. In psoriatic arthritis, synovial fluid contains elevated numbers of both ILC1s and NKp44$^+$ ILC3s. The synovial ILC3s produce the inflammatory cytokine IL-17, a pathogenic cytokine in psoriatic arthritis that is currently targeted by biologic therapy.[81] Similarly in ankylosing spondylitis, specific subpopulations of ILC3s are increased in the gut, blood, synovial fluid, and bone marrow. These ILC3s produce IL-17, which is also a target in ankylosing spondylitis.[81] Thus, targeted therapy for different forms of spondyloarthritis may work through successfully mitigating ILC function.

It is difficult to discern the relative contribution of ILCs to the development of rheumatologic conditions after the disease has been established. However, certain single-nucleotide polymorphisms (SNPs) associated with inflammatory bowel disease or RA are located in regulatory regions of the genome called *super-enhancers* that are specifically used by ILCs compared with T cells.[82] This work suggests that genomic variations that influence ILC behaviors may increase the risk of developing autoimmune disease.

In addition, recent work has highlighted ILC alterations in individuals at risk for rheumatologic disorders before the development of full-fledged disease. Specifically, a study examined lymph node biopsies from subjects with early RA, subjects with pre-clinical RA due to the presence of autoantibodies, and healthy controls. Compared to healthy controls, subjects with early RA or pre-clinical RA demonstrated increased ILC1s.[83] These disturbances in ILC populations that occur during the earliest detectable phases of disease support the possibility that ILCs participate in the development of rheumatologic disorders.

Summary

ILCs and NK cells provide important innate immune functions in antipathogen and anti-tumor immunity, both before and in concert with the adaptive immune response. In addition, there is emerging evidence that ILCs and NK cells may participate in inappropriate autoimmune responses and contribute to rheumatologic disease. However, whether specifically detecting or manipulating ILCs and NK cells will have diagnostic or therapeutic benefit in patients with autoimmune disorders remains to be determined.

The references for this chapter can also be found on ExpertConsult.com.

References

1. Paul WE: *Fundamental immunology*, ed 7, Wolters Kluwer Health/ Lippincott Williams & Wilkins, 2013.
2. Vivier E, et al.: Innate lymphoid cells: 10 years on, *Cell* 174:1054–1066, 2018.
3. Vonarbourg C, et al.: Regulated expression of nuclear receptor RORgammat confers distinct functional fates to NK cell receptor-expressing RORgammat(+) innate lymphocytes, *Immunity* 33:736–751, 2010.
4. Bernink JH, et al.: Human type 1 innate lymphoid cells accumulate in inflamed mucosal tissues, *Nat Immunol* 14:221–229, 2013.
5. Freud AG, Mundy-Bosse BL, Yu J, et al.: The broad spectrum of human natural killer cell diversity, *Immunity* 47:820–833, 2017.
6. Gasteiger G, Fan X, Dikiy S, et al.: Tissue residency of innate lymphoid cells in lymphoid and nonlymphoid organs, *Science* 350:981–985, 2015.
7. Klose CSN, et al.: Differentiation of type 1 ILCs from a common progenitor to all helper-like innate lymphoid cell lineages, *Cell* 157:340–356, 2014.
8. Melo-Gonzalez F, Hepworth MR: Functional and phenotypic heterogeneity of group 3 innate lymphoid cells, *Immunology* 150:265–275, 2017.
9. Eberl G, et al.: An essential function for the nuclear receptor RORgamma(t) in the generation of fetal lymphoid tissue inducer cells, *Nat Immunol* 5:64–73, 2004.
10. Strober W: The LTi cell, an immunologic chameleon, *Immunity* 33:650–652, 2010.
11. Cherrier M, Eberl G: The development of LTi cells, *Curr Opin Immunol* 24:178–183, 2012.
12. Jones GW, Hill DG, Jones SA: Understanding immune cells in tertiary lymphoid organ development: it is all starting to come together, *Front Immunol* 7:401, 2016.
13. Zhong C, Zheng M, Zhu J: Lymphoid tissue inducer-A divergent member of the ILC family, *Cytokine Growth Factor Rev* 42:5–12, 2018.
14. Campbell KS, Purdy AK: Structure/function of human killer cell immunoglobulin-like receptors: lessons from polymorphisms, evolution, crystal structures and mutations, *Immunology* 132:315–325, 2011.
15. Seidel UJ, Schlegel P, Lang P: Natural killer cell mediated antibody-dependent cellular cytotoxicity in tumor immunotherapy with therapeutic antibodies, *Front Immunol* 4:76, 2013.
16. Stone JH, et al.: Rituximab versus cyclophosphamide for ANCA-associated vasculitis, *N Engl J Med* 363:221–232, 2010.
17. Edwards JC, et al.: Efficacy of B-cell-targeted therapy with rituximab in patients with rheumatoid arthritis, *N Engl J Med* 350:2572–2581, 2004.
18. Lanier LL: Up on the tightrope: natural killer cell activation and inhibition, *Nat Immunol* 9:495–502, 2008.
19. Long EO, Kim HS, Liu D, et al.: Controlling natural killer cell responses: integration of signals for activation and inhibition, *Annu Rev Immunol* 31:227–258, 2013.
20. Vivier E, Nunes JA, Vely F: Natural killer cell signaling pathways, *Science* 306:1517–1519, 2004.
21. Cherrier DE, Serafini N, Di Santo JP: Innate lymphoid cell development: A T cell perspective, *Immunity* 48:1091–1103, 2018.
22. Bernink JH, et al.: Interleukin-12 and -23 Control plasticity of CD127(+) group 1 and group 3 innate lymphoid cells in the intestinal lamina propria, *Immunity* 43:146–160, 2015.
23. Fuchs A, et al.: Intraepithelial type 1 innate lymphoid cells are a unique subset of IL-12- and IL-15-responsive IFN-gamma-producing cells, *Immunity* 38:769–781, 2013.
24. Ohne Y, et al.: IL-1 is a critical regulator of group 2 innate lymphoid cell function and plasticity, *Nat Immunol* 17:646–655, 2016.
25. Bal SM, et al.: IL-1beta, IL-4 and IL-12 control the fate of group 2 innate lymphoid cells in human airway inflammation in the lungs, *Nat Immunol* 17:636–645, 2016.
26. Silver JS, et al.: Inflammatory triggers associated with exacerbations of COPD orchestrate plasticity of group 2 innate lymphoid cells in the lungs, *Nat Immunol* 17:626–635, 2016.
27. Cella M, Otero K, Colonna M: Expansion of human NK-22 cells with IL-7, IL-2, and IL-1beta reveals intrinsic functional plasticity, *Proc Natl Acad Sci U S A* 107:10961–10966, 2010.
28. Klose CS, et al.: A T-bet gradient controls the fate and function of CCR6-RORgammat+ innate lymphoid cells, *Nature* 494:261–265, 2013.
29. Geiger TL, Sun JC: Development and maturation of natural killer cells, *Curr Opin Immunol* 39:82–89, 2016.
30. Gordon SM, et al.: The transcription factors T-bet and Eomes control key checkpoints of natural killer cell maturation, *Immunity* 36:55–67, 2012.
31. Leong JW, Wagner JA, Ireland AR, et al.: Transcriptional and post-transcriptional regulation of NK cell development and function, *Clin Immunol* 177:60–69, 2017.
32. Luetke-Eversloh M, Killig M, Romagnani C: Signatures of human NK cell development and terminal differentiation, *Front Immunol* 4:499, 2013.
33. Lanier LL, Le AM, Civin CI, et al.: The relationship of CD16 (Leu-11) and Leu-19 (NKH-1) antigen expression on human peripheral blood NK cells and cytotoxic T lymphocytes, *J Immunol* 136:4480–4486, 1986.
34. Cooper MA, et al.: Human natural killer cells: a unique innate immunoregulatory role for the CD56(bright) subset, *Blood* 97:3146–3151, 2001.
35. Moretta L: Dissecting CD56dim human NK cells, *Blood* 116:3689–3691, 2010.
36. Wu C, et al.: Clonal expansion and compartmentalized maintenance of rhesus macaque NK cell subsets, *Sci Immunol* 3, 2018.
37. Yokoyama WM, Kim S: How do natural killer cells find self to achieve tolerance? *Immunity* 24:249–257, 2006.
38. Biron CA, Byron KS, Sullivan JL: Severe herpesvirus infections in an adolescent without natural killer cells, *N Engl J Med* 320:1731–1735, 1989.
39. Fleisher G, et al.: A non-x-linked syndrome with susceptibility to severe Epstein-Barr virus infections, *J Pediatr* 100:727–730, 1982.
40. Lopez C, et al.: Correlation between low natural killing of fibroblasts infected with herpes simplex virus type 1 and susceptibility to herpesvirus infections, *J Infect Dis* 147:1030–1035, 1983.
41. Moffett-King A: Natural killer cells and pregnancy, *Nat Rev Immunol* 2:656–663, 2002.
42. Hiby SE, et al.: Combinations of maternal KIR and fetal HLA-C genes influence the risk of preeclampsia and reproductive success, *J Exp Med* 200:957–965, 2004.
43. Koopman LA, et al.: Human decidual natural killer cells are a unique NK cell subset with immunomodulatory potential, *J Exp Med* 198:1201–1212, 2003.
44. Yokoyama WM, Kim S, French AR: The dynamic life of natural killer cells, *Annu Rev Immunol* 22:405–429, 2004.
45. Fehniger TA, Carson WE, Caligiuri MA: Costimulation of human natural killer cells is required for interferon gamma production, *Transplant Proc* 31:1476–1478, 1999.
46. Fehniger TA, et al.: Differential cytokine and chemokine gene expression by human NK cells following activation with IL-18 or IL-15 in combination with IL-12: implications for the innate immune response, *J Immunol* 162:4511–4520, 1999.
47. Cooper MA, et al.: Interleukin-1beta costimulates interferon-gamma production by human natural killer cells, *Eur J Immunol* 31:792–801, 2001.
48. Lauwerys BR, Renauld JC, Houssiau FA: Synergistic proliferation and activation of natural killer cells by interleukin 12 and interleukin 18, *Cytokine* 11:822–830, 1999.
49. Yokoyama WM, Kim S: Licensing of natural killer cells by self-major histocompatibility complex class I, *Immunol Rev* 214:143–154, 2006.
50. Anfossi N, et al.: Human NK cell education by inhibitory receptors for MHC class I, *Immunity* 25:331–342, 2006.

51. Kim S, et al.: HLA alleles determine differences in human natural killer cell responsiveness and potency, *Proc Natl Acad Sci U S A* 105:3053–3058, 2008.
52. Yoder JA, Litman GW: The phylogenetic origins of natural killer receptors and recognition: relationships, possibilities, and realities, *Immunogenetics* 63:123–141, 2011.
53. Khalturin K, Becker M, Rinkevich B, et al.: Urochordates and the origin of natural killer cells: identification of a CD94/NKR-P1-related receptor in blood cells of Botryllus, *Proc Natl Acad Sci U S A* 100:622–627, 2003.
54. French AR, Yokoyama WM: Natural killer cells and autoimmunity, *Arthritis Res Ther* 6:8–14, 2004.
55. Orange JS, Chehimi J, Ghavimi D, et al.: Decreased natural killer (NK) cell function in chronic NK cell lymphocytosis associated with decreased surface expression of CD11b, *Clin Immunol* 99:53–64, 2001.
56. French AR, et al.: Chronic lymphocytosis of functionally immature natural killer cells, *J Allergy Clin Immunol* 120:924–931, 2007.
57. Grunebaum E, Malatzky-Goshen E, Shoenfeld Y: Natural killer cells and autoimmunity, *Immunol Res* 8:292–304, 1989.
58. Dalbeth N, Callan MF: A subset of natural killer cells is greatly expanded within inflamed joints, *Arthritis Rheum* 46:1763–1772, 2002.
59. Pridgeon C, et al.: Natural killer cells in the synovial fluid of rheumatoid arthritis patients exhibit a CD56bright,CD94bright,CD158 negative phenotype, *Rheumatology (Oxford)* 42:870–878, 2003.
60. Yabuhara A, et al.: A killing defect of natural killer cells as an underlying immunologic abnormality in childhood systemic lupus erythematosus, *J Rheumatol* 23:171–177, 1996.
61. Sibbitt Jr WL, Mathews PM, Bankhurst AD: Natural killer cell in systemic lupus erythematosus. Defects in effector lytic activity and response to interferon and interferon inducers, *J Clin Invest* 71:1230–1239, 1983.
62. Henriques A, et al.: NK cells dysfunction in systemic lupus erythematosus: relation to disease activity, *Clin Rheumatol* 32:805–813, 2013.
63. Villanueva J, et al.: Natural killer cell dysfunction is a distinguishing feature of systemic onset juvenile rheumatoid arthritis and macrophage activation syndrome, *Arthritis Res Ther* 7:R30–37, 2005.
64. Fogel LA, Yokoyama WM, French AR: Natural killer cells in human autoimmune disorders, *Arthritis Res Ther* 15:216, 2013.
65. Matullo CM, O'Regan KJ, Hensley H, et al.: Lymphocytic choriomeningitis virus-induced mortality in mice is triggered by edema and brain herniation, *J Virol* 84:312–320, 2010.
66. Storm P, Bartholdy C, Sorensen MR, et al.: Perforin-deficient CD8+ T cells mediate fatal lymphocytic choriomeningitis despite impaired cytokine production, *J Virol* 80:1222–1230, 2006.
67. Behrens EM, et al.: Repeated TLR9 stimulation results in macrophage activation syndrome-like disease in mice, *J Clin Invest* 121:2264–2277, 2011.
68. Stepp SE, et al.: Perforin gene defects in familial hemophagocytic lymphohistiocytosis, *Science* 286:1957–1959, 1999.
69. Kogawa K, et al.: Perforin expression in cytotoxic lymphocytes from patients with hemophagocytic lymphohistiocytosis and their family members, *Blood* 99:61–66, 2002.
70. Henter JI, et al.: HLH-2004: diagnostic and therapeutic guidelines for hemophagocytic lymphohistiocytosis, *Pediatr Blood Cancer* 48:124–131, 2007.
71. Kumar B, Aleem S, Saleh H, et al.: A personalized diagnostic and treatment approach for macrophage activation syndrome and secondary hemophagocytic lymphohistiocytosis in adults, *J Clin Immunol* 37:638–643, 2017.
72. Aghaei H, Mostafaei S, Aslani S, et al.: Association study between KIR polymorphisms and rheumatoid arthritis disease: an updated meta-analysis, *BMC Med Genet* 20:24, 2019.
73. Renauer PA, et al.: Identification of susceptibility loci in IL6, RPS9/LILRB3, and an intergenic locus on chromosome 21q22 in takayasu arteritis in a genome-wide association study, *Arthritis Rheumatol* 67:1361–1368, 2015.
74. Momot T, et al.: Association of killer cell immunoglobulin-like receptors with scleroderma, *Arthritis Rheum* 50:1561–1565, 2004.
75. Okada Y, et al.: Fine mapping major histocompatibility complex associations in psoriasis and its clinical subtypes, *Am J Hum Genet* 95:162–172, 2014.
76. Gladman DD, Cheung C, Ng CM, et al.: HLA-C locus alleles in patients with psoriatic arthritis (PsA), *Hum Immunol* 60:259–261, 1999.
77. Nelson GW, et al.: Cutting edge: heterozygote advantage in autoimmune disease: hierarchy of protection/susceptibility conferred by HLA and killer Ig-like receptor combinations in psoriatic arthritis, *J Immunol* 173:4273–4276, 2004.
78. Yen JH, et al.: Major histocompatibility complex class I-recognizing receptors are disease risk genes in rheumatoid arthritis, *J Exp Med* 193:1159–1167, 2001.
79. Chan AT, Kollnberger SD, Wedderburn LR, et al.: Expansion and enhanced survival of natural killer cells expressing the killer immunoglobulin-like receptor KIR3DL2 in spondylarthritis, *Arthritis Rheum* 52:3586–3595, 2005.
80. Ridley A, et al.: Activation-induced killer cell immunoglobulin-like receptor 3DL2 binding to HLA-B27 licenses pathogenic T cell differentiation in spondyloarthritis, *Arthritis Rheumatol* 68:901–914, 2016.
81. Wenink MH, Leijten EFA, Cupedo T, et al.: Review: innate lymphoid cells: sparking inflammatory rheumatic disease? *Arthritis Rheumatol* 69:885–897, 2017.
82. Koues OI, et al.: Distinct gene regulatory pathways for human innate versus adaptive lymphoid cells, *Cell* 165:1134–1146, 2016.
83. Rodriguez-Carrio J, et al.: Brief report: altered innate lymphoid cell subsets in human lymph node biopsy specimens obtained during the at-risk and earliest phases of rheumatoid arthritis, *Arthritis Rheumatol* 69:70–76, 2017.

17 Platelets and Megakaryocytes

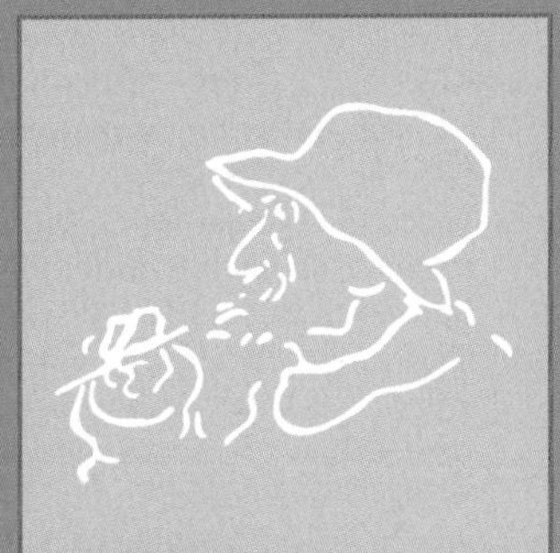

ERIC BOILARD AND PETER A. NIGROVIC

KEY POINTS

- Platelets are small subcellular fragments that circulate in blood, where they promote hemostasis.
- Platelets express receptors and a multitude of mediators recognized as being active in inflammation.
- Inhibition of platelet functions generally involves blockade of G protein–coupled receptor soluble agonists (e.g., thromboxane, thrombin, and adenosine diphosphate). However, platelet immunoreceptor tyrosine-based activation motif signaling at the site of inflammation is also implicated.
- Platelets likely contribute to inflammation in rheumatic diseases, including rheumatoid arthritis and systemic lupus erythematosus.
- Megakaryocytes can act as pro-inflammatory cells independently of platelets and have been implicated in arthritis through animal models.
- Blockade of platelet pro-inflammatory functions could represent an approach to treatment of the rheumatic diseases and their associated cardiovascular risks.

Introduction

Platelets patrol the vasculature to promote hemostasis. In blood, platelets represent the second most abundant cellular lineage after the red blood cell, outnumbering leukocytes by several orders of magnitude. When damage to the vasculature occurs, platelets quickly respond to prevent blood loss. In addition to their recognized role in thrombosis, platelets are emerging as important participants in the separation of blood and lymphatic systems, in maintenance of vasculature integrity in inflammation, and in immune responses. Accumulating evidence suggests that platelets and their bioactive mediators are important contributors to the pathogenesis of rheumatic diseases. The source cell for platelets, the megakaryocyte, also has immune sensing and effector capacity and has itself been implicated experimentally in systemic inflammatory disease

Platelet Structure

Platelets are small subcellular fragments that circulate in blood. In humans, normal platelet counts range between 150 × 10^6/mL and 450 × 10^6/mL, making them the second most abundant cell lineage present in blood after erythrocytes. Structurally, resting platelets resemble irregular discs that are 2 to 5 μm in diameter and 0.5 μm thick, with a volume of 6 to 10 femtoliters. In comparison, lymphocytes and neutrophils have a volume of 218 and 330 femtoliters, respectively.[1,2] Because of their small size and discoid shape, platelets are continuously pushed by the blood flow toward the edge of blood vessels, positioning them optimally to recognize endothelial injury. Thus because of their structure and abundance in the blood, platelets are positioned to fulfill their hemostatic function: the maintenance of vascular integrity.[3]

The cytoskeleton maintains the platelet's discoid shape.[4] A spectrin-based cytoskeleton is associated with the cytoplasmic side of the plasma membrane, microtubule coils form along the circumference of the cell, and 2000 to 5000 linear polymers of actin, the most abundant protein expressed by platelets, fill the cytoplasm.[5–7] These cytoskeletal components maintain the platelet's structure in the setting of high fluid shear forces and also enable conformational changes with activation to form finger-like filopodia and pseudopods.[8] Under these conditions, the platelet structure is remodeled dramatically, changing from a disk to spiny sphere.

The resting platelet plasma membrane is composed of phospholipids that appear smooth on electron microscopy, with a fine corrugated surface.[9,10] The surface membrane contains channels and sinuous invaginations called the *open canicular system (OCS)*.[11] The OCS increases the platelet surface area in direct contact with the extra-cellular milieu. Plasma components such as serotonin and fibrinogen are imported into platelets through this system, and the OCS serves as a conduit for the release of mediators stored within the platelet.[12,13] The channels that constitute the OCS are also a source of membrane necessary for the profound morphologic changes, such as the formation of filopodia and spreading that occur rapidly when platelets are activated, increasing their exposed surface by 420%.[14] Adherent platelets trail long (250 μm) tendrils into the blood vessel lumen, further increasing their contact surface and helping them interact with circulating leukocytes.[15]

The platelet cytoplasm includes numerous small organelles with three main types of secretory granules: α-granules, dense bodies (δ-granules), and lysosomes (Table 17.1). The α-granules are the most abundant organelle in platelets (40 to 80 per platelet).[16,17] They are round or oval, have a diameter of 200 to 500 nm, and contain proteins in their lumens or membrane, including von Willebrand factor (vWF), P-selectin, coagulation factor V, thrombospondin, fibrinogen, platelet factor-4 (also known as CXCL4), and growth factors such as platelet-derived growth factor (PDGF) and transforming growth factor-β (TGF-β).[18] Dense

TABLE 17.1 Platelet Components Implicated in the Inflammatory Response

	Platelet Component	Actions
Surface molecules	P-selectin (CD62P), PECAM (CD31), GPIbα	Adhesive targets for leukocytes
	PAF, ROS	Neutrophil activation
	CD154 (CD40 ligand)	Agonist for endothelial cells
Soluble factors	Serotonin, histamine	Regulators of vascular permeability
	β-Thromboglobulin, PF4	Chemotaxis
	Acid hydrolases, ROS	Tissue destruction
	PDGF, TGF-β	Cellular mitogens, chemoattractant
End products of platelet procoagulant activity	Thrombin, fibrin	Promote leukocyte accumulation

GPI, Glycosyl phosphatidylinositol; *PAF*, platelet-activating factor; *PDGF*, platelet-derived growth factor; *PECAM*, platelet–endothelial cell adhesion molecule; *PF4*, platelet factor-4; *ROS*, reactive oxygen species; *TGF*, transforming growth factor.

bodies are smaller than α-granules, are fewer in number (4 to 8 per platelet), and are rich in calcium, magnesium, adenosine diphosphate (ADP), adenosine triphosphate (ATP), serotonin, and histamine.[19,20] Calcium and serotonin are responsible for the opacity of dense bodies on electron microscopy. Platelets also usually bear approximately one lysosome (sometimes none and never more than three). These lysosomes may serve as an endosomal digestion compartment, but the importance of this function in hemostasis is unknown. Proteolysis can also take place in platelet proteasomes.[21] The proteasome is necessary for platelet function, because its pharmacological blockade by the proteasome inhibitor bortezomib (given to patients with multiple myeloma) inhibits platelet thrombotic activities and platelet production.[22,23] Platelets express residual fragments of Golgi complexes and functional mitochondria (4 to 7 per platelet), which are implicated in the production of energy and platelet activation.[21,24]

Platelet Production

The great majority of the platelets will never be involved in any hemostatic process and will be eliminated at senescence through the reticuloendothelial system in the liver and spleen. Because of their relatively short life span in circulation (10 days), approximately 100 billion platelets must be produced every day in the human body. Platelets are not cells per se; they are fragments derived from megakaryocytes and, consequently, they are without a nucleus.[25,26] The megakaryocyte arises from a master stem cell in the bone marrow under the control of thrombopoietin, a hormone produced in the liver and kidneys that promotes megakaryocyte maturation, number, and size and forestalls megakaryocyte apoptosis.[27,28] Thrombopoietin is a soluble, 80 to 90 kDa protein that acts through binding to its receptor, c-Mpl, which is expressed by megakaryocytes and platelets. The binding of thrombopoietin to platelets induces its catabolism. More thrombopoietin is thus available in people with lower platelet counts, thereby driving megakaryocyte activity. However, serum thrombopoietin levels remain normal in severely thrombocytopenic mice, and mice deficient in apoptosis-regulatory molecules (e.g., Bax and Bak) exhibit high levels of thrombopoietin despite the increased platelet counts, thus suggesting that thrombopoietin metabolism by platelets is not the only determinant of platelet biogenesis. This mechanism may involve glycoprotein Ibα (GPIbα), a receptor expressed by platelets, as its ablation in mice or its absence in humans is associated with reduced levels of hepatic thrombopoietin.[29] Further, aging platelets directly induce thrombopoietin expression in hepatocytes because they are cleared through an interaction between desialyated platelet surface glycans and the hepatic asialyloglycoprotein receptor.[30]

Cytokines such as IL-1, IL-3, IL-6, IL-11, stem cell factor (also called Kit ligand), and granulocyte-macrophage colony-stimulating factor (GM-CSF) amplify megakaryocyte production.[31–33] Enhanced platelet production can be assessed by measurement of the mean platelet volume, a measure that is often part of a complete blood cell count. A larger average platelet size is seen when platelet production by megakaryocytes is increased, generally reflecting compensation for accelerated platelet destruction as seen in immune thrombocytopenic purpura (ITP), myeloproliferative diseases, and Bernard-Soulier syndrome.[34]

The mature megakaryocyte is a giant cell (50 to 100 μm in diameter) resulting from repeated cycles of endomitosis, which means that it undergoes repeated cycles of DNA replication without cell division, leading to polyploidy, typically up to 16N (128N can be observed).[35] This amplification of DNA results in gene amplification and increases protein production, which is necessary for the generation of up to 5000 platelets per megakaryocyte. During platelet formation, long (millimeters in length) cytoplasmic extensions emanate from the megakaryocyte and protrude out of the bone marrow in the interior of vascular sinusoids. These extensions, called *proplatelet processes*, elongate through the action of microtubules, which also serve as a track for the transportation of membranes, organelles, and granules from the mother megakaryocyte distally into nascent proplatelets. Actin filaments participate in proplatelet branching. Cytoplasmic continuity between the mother megakaryocyte and nascent proplatelets also enables platelets to bear functional microRNA and messenger RNA, as well as the molecular machinery required to translate the latter efficiently into protein.[36,37]

Fragments from proplatelet processes are next released into the blood as either globular pre-platelets or as barbell-shaped proplatelets (Fig. 17.1). These interconvertible forms generate platelets upon fission. Furthermore, individual human platelets can divide.[38] Thus platelet maturation likely continues in the circulation. Interestingly, megakaryocytes can migrate into the bloodstream, and evidence suggests that an appreciable proportion of

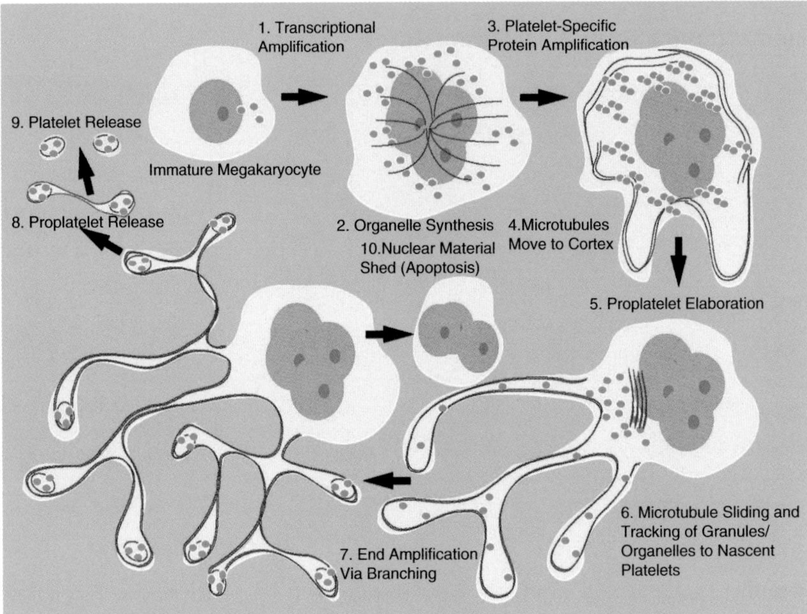

• **Fig. 17.1** Platelet biogenesis according to the proplatelet model. (From Italiano JE Jr, Hartwig J: Megakaryocyte development and platelet formation. In Michelson AD, editor: *Platelets*, ed 3, Amsterdam, 2013, Elsevier, pp 27–50.)

platelets is generated by the megakaryocytes that have taken up residence in the lungs.[25,39,40]

Platelets and Hemostasis

The sum of the processes by which the loss of blood is prevented is called *hemostasis*. Intravital microscopic analyses, performed as early as 1882 by the Italian scientist Bizzozero, demonstrated that platelets could recognize a damaged blood vessel and form a plug.[1] Since then, the molecular participants in the promotion of hemostasis have been described. The intact endothelium produces molecules, such as prostacyclin (PGI_2), nitric oxide, and thrombomodulin, which, conjointly with cell-associated ecto-adenophosphatase (ADPase; CD39),[41] inhibit platelet activation. Endothelial injury triggers vasoconstriction, which reduces blood flow and exposes the subendothelial matrix. At this stage, the main platelet glycoprotein (GP) receptors implicated are the members of the GP Ib-IX-V complex (25,000 copies/platelet), and the integrin αIIbβ3 (GPIIb-IIIa complex; 80,000 copies/platelet).[42,43]

Under high shear, the GPIb-IX-V complex attaches to vWF, which is itself bound to the wound rich in collagen fibers, mediating transient adhesion (also referred to as tethering).[44] Glycoprotein VI (GPVI), which is expressed as a complex with the homodimeric Fc receptor γ chain,[45,46] and the integrin α2β1 stabilize the association by binding collagen directly. Although GPIIb-IIIa is a receptor for several ligands (fibronectin, fibrinogen, vWF, thrombospondin, and vitronectin), only its activated form binds fibrinogen. Platelet activation through GPIb-IX and GPVI thus promotes inside-out signaling, leading to GPIIb-IIIa activation and the binding of the latter to fibrinogen, thereby bridging platelets together and recruiting additional platelets onto adhered spread platelets.[42–44,47,48] Deficiency of components of the GPIb-IX-V complex and the GPIIb-IIIa complex leads to the congenital bleeding disorders Bernard-Soulier disease and Glanzmann's thrombasthenia, respectively.[49,50] vWF catabolism is mediated by the metalloprotease ADAMTS-13, which is expressed in plasma and acts as a natural anti-thrombotic agent. Mutations of ADAMTS-13 or depletion by autoantibodies cause familial and acquired thrombocytopenic purpura, respectively.

Platelet activation engages intra-cellular signaling. The actin cytoskeleton pushes the granules toward the platelet membrane. Granule fusion with the plasma membrane is mediated by soluble N-ethylmaleimide-sensitive factor attachment protein (SNAP) receptor (SNARE) complexes, leading to release of granule content through the OCS route.[51] The release of ADP further activates platelets through P2Y12 receptors. Because phospholipids serve as a reservoir of fatty acid, such as arachidonic acid (AA), the cleavage of phospholipids by phospholipase A2 generates lysophospholipids, which can be metabolized into platelet activating factor (PAF) and AA. AA is the substrate of cyclo-oxygenase 1 (COX-1) present in platelets, leading to generation of thromboxane A_2.[52] Thromboxane A_2 is highly potent at inducing platelet aggregation and vasoconstriction, acting via the thromboxane A_2 receptor. As a result, growth of the platelet plug occurs and the blood coagulation cascade is initiated, leading to thrombin generation and fibrin clot formation. In line with the significance of these activation pathways, the inhibition of ADP activity using antagonists of P2Y12 receptors (such as clopidogrel) and of the biosynthesis of thromboxane A_2 using COX-1 inhibitors (such as acetylsalicylic acid) is frequently applied in people at risk of myocardial infarction and thrombotic stroke.

Platelets also respond to activation and shear stress through the release of small extra-cellular vesicles called *microparticles* or microvesicles. Microparticles, originally termed "platelet dust,"[53] are produced by cytoplasmic blebbing and fission. They measure approximately 100 to 1000 nm in diameter and are distinct from the exosomes that are smaller (50 to 100 nm in diameter) and originate from multivesicular bodies and α-granules through exocytosis.[54] Megakaryocytes can also elaborate microparticles directly, independent of platelet synthesis.[55] Platelets and megakaryocytes are the most abundant source of microparticles in circulating blood, as identified by expression of GPIIb (CD41).[56]

During microparticle release, loss of membrane asymmetry generally occurs, leading to exposure of phosphatidylserine (PS) on the microparticle surface.[57] Exposed PS can support blood coagulation.[58] Platelet microparticles are implicated in the pathogenesis of several inflammatory pathologies, including rheumatic diseases (see below).

Beyond their role in the defense of injured blood vessels, platelets appear to play an incompletely understood role in the maintenance of endothelial integrity. Patients with severe thrombocytopenia have been noted to develop abnormalities of the endothelium such as thinning, fenestrations, and enhanced vascular permeability.[59,60] Accordingly, animals with profound experimental thrombocytopenia experience bleeding at the site of inflammation in skin, lung, or brain.[59–62]

Signaling Pathways in Platelet Activation

ADP, thromboxane A_2, and thrombin, the latter through its binding to protease-activating receptors (PARs), share signaling via G protein–coupled receptors (GPCRs).[62,63] However, GPCR signaling is dispensable for the prohemostatic role of platelets in inflammation, pointing to the existence of other significant activation signaling pathways in platelets.

Immunoreceptor tyrosine-based activation motif (ITAM) signaling can play such a role. Platelets express three receptors that belong to the family of ITAM receptors: Fc receptor γIIA (a low affinity receptor for IgG immune complexes),[64] Fc receptor γ chain, which is noncovalently associated with GPVI and is necessary for GPVI function,[45,46] and the C-type lectin 2 (CLEC2), a receptor for podoplanin.[65]

Fc receptor γIIA (FcγRIIA) is expressed on human platelets but is absent in mice,[64,66] and its activation is critical in the pathogenesis of immune-mediated thrombocytopenia, bacterial sepsis–associated thrombocytopenia, disseminated intravascular coagulation, and various thrombotic manifestations of antiphospholipid antibody syndrome.[62,67] Importantly, FcγRIIA also amplifies platelet aggregation and thrombus formation by contributing to integrin outside-in signaling.[62,63]

To determine how platelets prevent hemorrhage during inflammation, transgenic mice expressing a chimeric human IL-4 receptor α/GPIbα (hIL-4Rα/GPIbα) protein instead of GPIbα on the platelet surface were used to induce thrombocytopenia. By infusion of antibodies against hIL-4Rα, profound thrombocytopenia was generated and hemorrhages were detected in the skin after inducing an Arthus reaction. Because wild-type (WT) platelets are insensitive to platelet depletion by anti-IL4Rα (they don't express the chimeric α/GPIbα [hIL-4Rα/GPIbα] protein), WT platelets were transfused in thrombocytopenic mice and could rescue mice from bleeding at the site of inflammation.[61] Importantly, transfused platelets lacking the expression of GPVI and CLEC2 failed to prevent bleeding in skin during an Arthus reaction, demonstrating the key role of GPVI and CLEC2 signaling in the maintenance of endothelial integrity by platelets.[61]

Another prohemostatic role of platelet ITAMs is the separation of blood and lymphatic vessels.[68] Mouse embryos deficient for CLEC2 display blood-filled lymph sacs and die shortly after birth, reminiscent of lethality seen in mice lacking spleen tyrosine kinase (Syk) and SLP-76, two kinases downstream of CLEC2 signaling.[69–72] Blood-filled lymphatic vessels also develop in lethally irradiated mature mice transplanted with bone marrow lacking CLEC2, Syk, or SLP-76, and they die of lymphatic dysfunction, demonstrating that CLEC2 and its signaling are implicated in the separation of blood and lymph in the adult.[62,73] It is not known whether drugs intended to target Syk in the treatment of chronic inflammatory conditions might have an impact on blood-lymphatic vessel separation.

Similarly to most hematopoietic cells, platelets also express immunoreceptor tyrosine-based inhibition motif (ITIM)-containing receptors. Although ITIM receptors, such as PECAM-1 and G6b-B, are best known for their role in the attenuation of ITAM-mediated platelet activation, studies show that they may also contribute to platelet reactivity or production.[74]

Together, these observations illustrate that not all functions of platelets can be blocked simply through "classic" anti-platelet drugs such as antagonists of ADP, acetylsalicylic acid, and thrombin (Fig. 17.2).

The Platelet as an Inflammatory Cell

Nucleated thrombocytes, called *hemocytes*, participate both in hemostasis and in immune defense in lower vertebrates (amphibians, birds, fish, and reptiles).[75] It is generally accepted that these more primitive multifunctional cells slowly evolved to the more specialized role of the mammalian platelets. The platelet nevertheless maintains a broad repertoire of inflammatory mediators, and growing evidence points to an active role of the platelet in innate and adaptive immunity.

Inflammation occurs during innate and adaptive immune responses and in tissue repair and can sometime contribute critically to human disease. A central event in inflammation is the recruitment of leukocytes. When a blood vessel is damaged, not only do platelets rapidly seal the vascular leak, but they also recruit leukocytes that serve to combat potential infection at the injured site. Because of their abundance in blood and their adhesive receptors, platelets are perfectly positioned to have an impact on immune cell extravasation. Platelet P-selectin interacts with leukocyte P-selectin glycoprotein ligand-1 (PSGL-1), allowing leukocytes to roll on adherent activated platelets. Firm adhesion of leukocytes follows through the interaction between leukocyte integrin αMβ2 (CD11b/CD18, Mac-1) and platelet GPIb.[76,77]

CD40L (CD154) is a transmembrane protein and is part of the TNF receptor family that is expressed by both T cells and platelets. Its counterligand CD40 is expressed by macrophages, dendritic cells, B cells, platelets themselves, and other lineages, including endothelial cells. Platelet-derived CD40L can support B cell differentiation and immunoglobulin class switching and induces the expression of intercellular adhesion molecule-1 (ICAM-1), vascular cell adhesion molecule-1 (VCAM-1), and release of chemokine (CC motif) ligand 2 (CCL2) by endothelial cells, promoting leukocyte adhesion and extravasation.[75] Because platelets are the largest reservoir of soluble CD40L in the human body, plasma levels of CD40L correlate with platelet activation.

Platelets also express Toll-like receptors (TLRs), which are members of a family of pattern recognition receptors that recognize well-conserved molecular motifs common among pathogens. Platelets express TLRs 1 through 9, and platelet TLR stimulation provokes thrombocytopenia and engages TNF production in vivo.[78–81] When platelet TLR4 is activated by bacterial lipopolysaccharide (LPS), it promotes the interaction of platelets with neutrophils, helping trigger neutrophil degranulation and release of neutrophil extra-cellular traps (NETs) that stretch downstream of the platelet-neutrophil aggregate in blood.[82] NETs are readily observed in RA, systemic lupus erythematosus (SLE), and gout. Whether platelet-induced NETosis is beneficial or detrimental is unclear, but recent

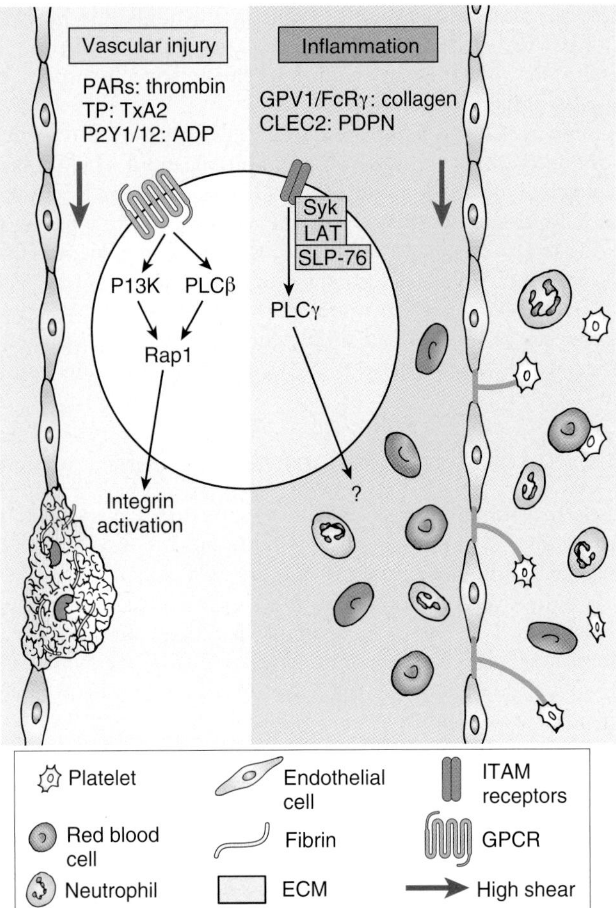

• **Fig. 17.2** Platelet-dependent hemostasis after vascular injury and at sites of inflammation. Schematic representation of important molecular mechanisms regulating platelet-dependent hemostasis. At sites of vascular injury, platelet activation and adhesion is strongly dependent on soluble agonists and their respective G protein–coupled receptors (GPCRs) expressed on the platelet surface. Engagement of GPCRs leads to the rapid activation of phospholipase Cβ2 (PLCβ2) and phosphatidylinositol 3-kinase (PI3K), events that are critical for the activation of the small guanosine triphosphatase Rap1, affinity regulation in platelet integrins, and platelet aggregate formation. The contribution of immunoreceptor tyrosine-based activation motif (ITAM)–coupled receptors to platelet activation at sites of vascular injury is weak when compared with GPCRs. In contrast, hemostasis at sites of inflammation depends primarily on platelet ITAM signaling and is independent of major platelet adhesion receptors. In these inflammatory conditions, platelets can also contribute to neutrophil extravasation and formation of neutrophil extra-cellular traps. These findings suggest a model in which platelets get activated under low-flow/no-flow conditions in the extravascular space, leading to the release of soluble factors that secure vascular integrity. Both the signaling response downstream of PLCγ2 and the platelet-derived mediator(s) critical for vascular integrity in inflammation are currently unknown. *CLEC2,* C-type lectin 2; *ECM,* extra-cellular matrix; *FcRγ,* Fc receptor γ chain; *GPVI,* glycoprotein VI; *LAT,* linker for activation of T cells; *PAR,* protease activated receptor; *PDPN,* podoplanin; *SLP-76,* SH2 containing leukocyte protein of 76 kDa; *TP,* TxA2 receptor; *TxA2,* thromboxane A_2. (Modified from Boulaftali Y, Hess PR, Kahn ML, Bergmeier W: Platelet immunoreceptor tyrosine-based activation motif [ITAM] signaling and vascular integrity. *Circ Res* 114:1174–1184, 2014. Reprinted with permission from the American Heart Association.)

observations in gout suggest that NETs may form aggregates that trap cytokines and thereby limit inflammation.[83–86]

Apart from their surface receptors, platelet-derived soluble molecules also contribute to inflammation via mediators including growth factors, cytokines, chemokines, and lipid mediators (see Table 17.1). Activated platelets release PDGF and TGF-β, which are responsible for the fibroproliferative response in chronic inflammation. PDGF is chemotactic for smooth muscle cells, fibroblasts, and macrophages and is central in wound healing.[87] Platelets represent a major pool of TGF-β in humans (milligrams of TGF-β/kilogram) and regulate its blood levels.[75] TGF-β is also chemoattractant for leukocytes, and its main function appears to be the inhibition of inflammation, because its systemic administration can reduce the development of inflammatory arthritis in rats,[88] and TGF-β is also necessary for the development of $CD4^+CD25^+FoxP3^+$ regulatory T (Treg) cells.[75] However, fine control of its expression is important because TGF-β overexpression is potentially profibrotic.[89]

Other members of the platelet secretome implicated in the intertwined prohemostatic and pro-inflammatory reactions are the CXC chemokine PF4 and the CC chemokine RANTES (regulated upon activation, normal T cell expressed and secreted), stored in α-granules. Because patients who have gray platelet syndrome (and thus are deficient in platelet α-granules) do not experience recurrent infections, platelet pro-inflammatory activity may reside in other storage compartments or may reflect newly synthesized mediators. Indeed, activated platelets can rapidly synthesize and release IL-1β.[36,90] In sum, platelets are versatile players in inflammation. The fact that platelets express inflammatory mediators, which appear to be mostly dispensable for their hemostatic functions, supports the idea that they might contribute to inflammatory conditions, such as rheumatic diseases.

The Megakaryocyte as an Inflammatory Cell

Compared with platelets, evidence for a role for megakaryocytes in systemic inflammation is more limited.[91] Like platelets, megakaryocytes can express several members of the TLR family, including TLRs 1, 2, 3, 4, and 6.[92–97] TLR5 mRNA transcripts are expressed in murine lung megakaryocytes.[2] The functional consequences of activation via these receptors are poorly understood but might include acceleration of megakaryocyte maturation and platelet production.[96,98,99] Human megakaryocytes, like human platelets, can express the low-affinity IgG receptor FcγRIIA.[100,101] Murine studies suggest that stimulation via Fc receptors might enhance release of megakaryocyte microparticles, an observation that reflects stimulation of the high-affinity receptor FcγRI by noncanonical ligands such as C-reactive protein.[102] The IgE receptor FcεRI is also expressed but serves primarily to pass this receptor to platelets, because human platelets but not megakaryocytes express this receptor at the cell surface.[103] The role of these receptors in megakaryocyte function in vivo has not been explored.

Megakaryocytes might also contribute to adaptive immunity. Like platelets, megakaryocytes express CD40L.[104] In the marrow environment, megakaryocytes promote plasma cell survival, potentially via IL-6 and a proliferation-inducing ligand (APRIL).[105] Megakaryocytes can take up exogenous antigen and cross-present this in the context of class I major histocompatibility complex (MHC), enabling immune thrombocytopenia in a murine experimental model.[106]

Megakaryocytes can elaborate a range of distinct cytokines, chemokines, and other mediators.[91] The bone marrow niche is characterized by high concentrations of PF4 and TGF-β of megakaryocyte origin that participate in the regulation of hematopoietic stem cells.[107–109] Expression of the neutrophil chemoattractants CXCL1 and CXCL2 (corresponding to human IL-8) enable megakaryocytes to regulate neutrophil egress from bone marrow. In fact, granulocyte colony-stimulating factor (G-CSF)–mediated release of murine marrow neutrophils is mediated by megakaryocytes that release CXCL1/2 in response to thrombopoietin generated by G-CSF–sensing cells in the marrow stroma; correspondingly, administration of thrombopoietin can cause an increase in circulating neutrophil count.[110]

Megakaryocytes are also able to produce IL-1α and IL-1β as free cytokine or packaged within microparticles.[40,102,111–114] Correspondingly, engraftment of WT but not IL-1–deficient megakaryocytes restores the susceptibility of certain disease-resistant mice to arthritis, even independent of their platelets, establishing a potential role for megakaryocytes in IL-1–driven systemic inflammatory disease.[102]

A final, intriguing interaction of megakaryocytes in immunity is termed *emperipolesis*. This term, derived from the Greek *em* "inside," *peri* "around," and *polesis* "wandering," refers to the observation that leukocytes can be seen moving about within megakaryocytes in fresh marrow specimens.[115] Marrow histologic sections show active emperipolesis in 2% to 5% of megakaryocytes in bone marrow sections, both human and murine, with neutrophils represented disproportionately.[116] Emperipolesis increases markedly under pathologic conditions, including hematologic malignancy and myelofibrosis.[117–119] Recent development of an in vitro model of emperipolesis, together with ultrastructural imaging and in vivo murine experiments, have established that emperipolesis represents a novel pathway for the exchange of membrane and other material between megakaryocytes and neutrophils, which emerge viable from the interaction.[120] The effect of this exchange on the function of megakaryocytes, platelets, and neutrophils remains to be established (Fig. 17.3).

Platelets, Megakaryocytes, and Rheumatic Diseases

Rheumatoid Arthritis

Variations in platelet number and signs of platelet activation are seen in people with RA. Thrombocytosis (increased platelet number) is frequent in people with active RA[121,122] and correlates with disease severity and relapses, suggesting that their production might be induced by inflammatory cytokines such as IL-1, IL-6, or TNF.[32,123] By contrast, thrombocytopenia in RA may result from treatments such as gold, cyclophosphamide, methotrexate, and azathioprine that can suppress megakaryocyte development. More rare is drug-induced immune thrombocytopenia, in which immunoglobulin G (IgG)-coated platelets are eliminated in the spleen, a feature seen in 1% to 3% of patients injected intramuscularly with gold salts.[124] In Felty's syndrome, a rare but severe complication in people with seropositive RA, splenomegaly results in enhanced platelet clearance, but hemorrhage is rare because platelets generally remain above 50,000 platelets per microliter.[125]

In RA, the hallmarks of platelet activation are apparent in both blood and synovial fluid. Platelet-leukocyte aggregates, platelet microparticles, soluble P-selectin, and soluble CD40L are increased in the blood of people with RA compared with healthy people. Although microparticles released from megakaryocytes maintain the expression of both GPVI and CLEC-2, those released by platelets lose the expression of GPVI. In RA patients, platelet microparticles harboring CLEC-2, but not GPVI, are found increased in blood, thus suggesting that platelets actively contribute to the generation of microparticles in RA.[126] Platelets isolated from the blood of people with RA are hyperresponsive to stimuli in vitro, suggesting that they might be primed in vivo.[127–135] Platelets and platelet-derived proteins have been identified in the inflamed synovial cavity,[122,136–138] and platelet CLEC2 is detected in synovium in conjunction with platelet thrombi and fibrin deposition in synovial vessels.[139–141] Platelet microparticles, identified through expression of GPIIb (CD41), have been detected in the synovial fluid of people with

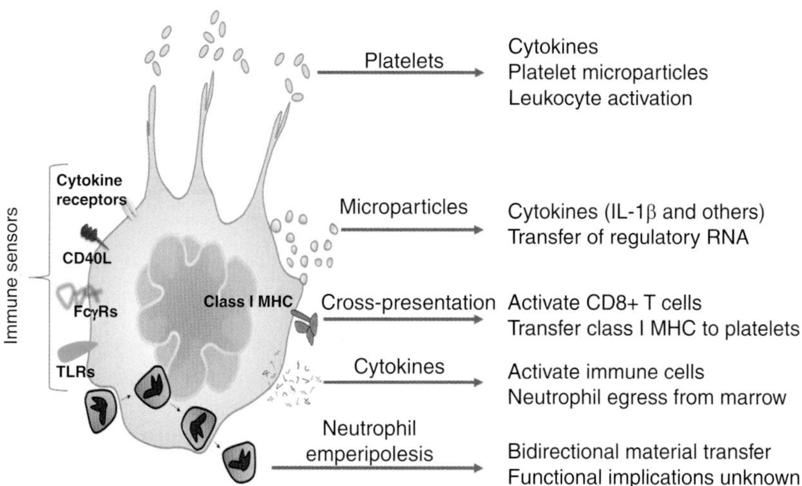

• **Fig. 17.3** Megakaryocytes as immune cells. Megakaryocytes possess the capacity to mediate systemic immune impact via distinct pathways, including platelet production; megakaryocyte microparticle release; antigen uptake; and presentation on class I major histocompatibility complex (MHC) proteins, cytokines, and uptake and release of neutrophils and potentially other lineages in a cell-in-cell reaction termed emperipolesis. (Figure modified from Cunin and Nigrovic, *J Leuk Biol* 2019 in press.)

RA.[142–145] Platelet microparticles are much more abundant in RA synovial fluid than in osteoarthritis fluid, but they are also detected at significant levels in joint fluid from active psoriatic arthritis, juvenile idiopathic arthritis, and gout. In RA, platelet microparticles express autoantigens such as citrullinated fibrinogen and vimentin and are coated with autoantibodies and complement in synovial fluid, but not in the blood of people with RA or in psoriatic arthritis synovial fluid.[143,146] Platelet microparticles therefore could represent an important source of autoantigens in people with RA. Further, platelet microparticles likely represent an important nucleating factor for the immune complexes that are abundant in seropositive, but not seronegative, people with RA.[147,148]

Whereas platelet adherence to migrating leukocytes represents one potential route for the accumulation of platelet-derived components in the synovial fluid, a permeable vasculature will also permit direct entry of platelet microparticles. Under inflammatory conditions, platelets can mediate the vascular permeability, leading to extravasation of fluid and tissue edema.[149] Injection of platelet extracts into the skin of human volunteers induces swelling, tenderness, and redness, and platelets injected in the skin of animals triggers neutrophil accumulation and edema.[150]

Because the synovial vasculature is more permeable in RA,[139,140,151,152] the role of platelets in vascular permeability was evaluated in arthritic mice using intravital imaging.[139] Gaps in the blood vessels of the inflamed joint allowed fluorescent microbeads that had been intravenously injected in the tail vein to accumulate inside the synovial tissue, outside the vasculature. Notably, these gaps were absent in healthy mice, and no microbeads could reach nondiseased joints. The gaps were created by platelet-derived serotonin. Serotonin is stored in dense granules after its import through the serotonin transporter, the same serotonin reuptake receptor that is a target of anti-depressant agents, and fluoxetine could reduce the vascular permeability in the arthritic joint.[139] Thus, at least in mice, platelets play a key role in the ongoing maintenance of enhanced vascular permeability in the inflamed synovium.

Platelet depletion in mice reduces joint inflammation in the K/BxN mouse model of arthritis (Fig. 17.4).[139,142,153] Using this model, activation of platelets triggered microparticle production through GPVI and occurred independently of P2Y12, GPIb, and thromboxane A_2. GPVI-induced microparticles contain both IL-1α and IL-1β and thereby activate fibroblast-like synoviocytes to produce inflammatory cytokines.[142] These results point to GPVI and its ITAM signaling cascade as possible targets for the treatment of arthritis (Fig. 17.5).

Finally, megakaryocytes have been implicated as mediators of inflammatory arthritis even independent of their platelets. For example, mice bearing mutations affecting the SCF receptor Kit, instrumental in megakaryocyte development, have multiple hematopoietic aberrancies. A relative deficiency of megakaryocytes was implicated by the ability to restore susceptibility to IgG-mediated arthritis by engraftment of megakaryocytes but not neutrophils or platelets.[102] This effect was mediated through megakaryocyte-derived IL-1, potentially transferred to synovial tissues via IL-1-rich microparticles released by megakaryocytes entrapped in the pulmonary vascular bed. These observations, still to be tested in humans, suggest that pulmonary megakaryocytes could act as an "in-line sensor" with the potential to sense and respond to diverse triggers and thereby contribute to systemic inflammation.[91]

Systemic Lupus Erythematosus

Elevated levels of thromboxane,[154] soluble and surface P-selectin,[155–157] platelet-monocyte aggregates,[158] platelet microparticles,[54,132,159] and platelet ultrastructural changes such as blebbing[160] are evident in the blood of patients with SLE. Complement C4d and IgG antibodies against GPIIbIIIa and GPVI[161–163] are reported on the platelet surface in people with SLE, and anti-DNA antibodies abundant in SLE may cross-react with GPIIbIIIa.[161]

Platelets may also bind immune complexes through FcγRIIA, a receptor implicated genetically in the pathogenesis of SLE.[164,165] Indeed, the sera of people with SLE, but not of healthy volunteers, trigger expression of the platelet activation marker P-selectin via FcγRIIA.[166,167] Upon activation through FcγRIIA, platelets trigger production of IFN-α by myeloid and plasmacytoid dendritic cells, promoting generation of autoantibodies by B cells.[166] Using SLE-prone mouse models, platelets actively promote the disease, because platelet depletion and inhibition of platelet function (using P2Y12 blockers) both significantly ameliorate proliferative nephritis[166,168,169] (Fig. 17.6).

Patients with SLE are at higher risk of thrombosis, potentially correlating with elevated levels of platelet-derived microparticles.[170] The elevated levels of circulating soluble CD40L in SLE are mainly due to the release of CD40L from activated platelets, correlating with disease activity.[166] The impact of the blockade of CD40L in SLE has been evaluated in two distinct clinical trials. Although inhibition of CD40L in patients with active proliferative lupus nephritis efficiently reduced proteinuria, the trial

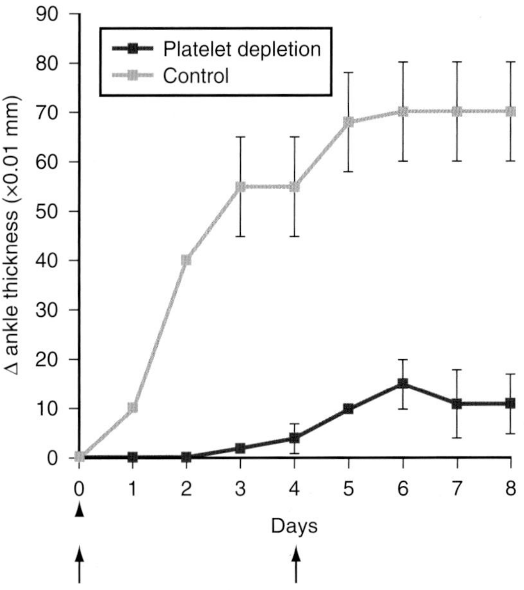

• **Fig. 17.4** Platelets can be involved in the development of arthritis. The passive K/BxN model of arthritis is induced by administration of arthritogenic serum containing antibodies to glucose-6-phosphate isomerase (GPI). The graph shows arthritis severity after K/BxN serum transfer in mice administered a platelet-depleting antibody *(red squares)* or isotype control antibody *(blue squares)*. Data show the mean ± standard error of the mean (SEM).[44] *Arrows* indicate parenteral administration of platelet-depleting antibody; *arrowhead,* K/BxN serum administration. These findings suggest that platelets are required for arthritis development in vivo in this model. (From Boilard E, Nigrovic PA, Larabee K, et al: Platelets amplify inflammation in arthritis via collagen-dependent microparticle production. *Science* 327:580–583, 2010.)

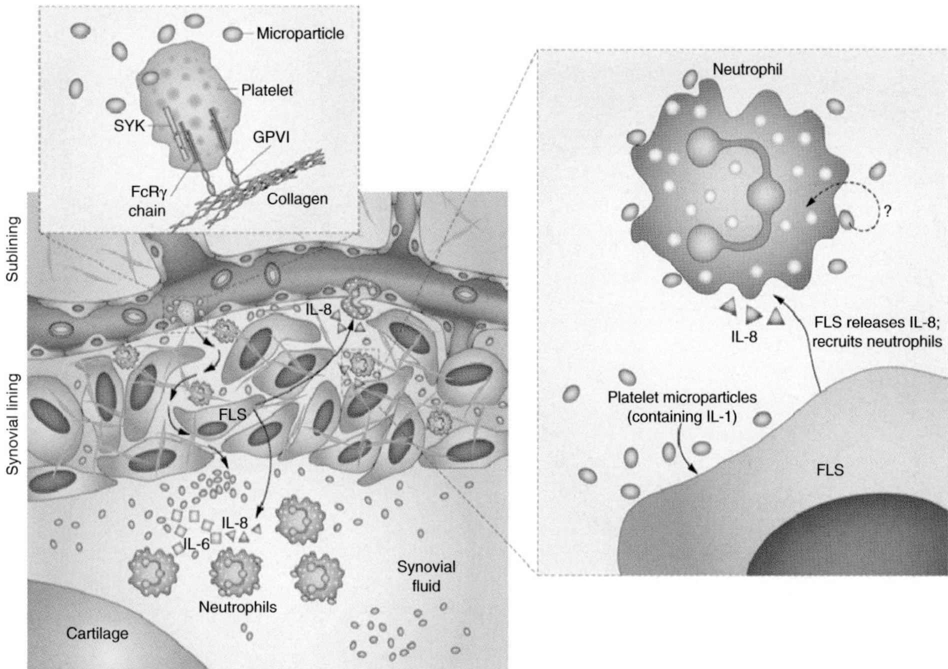

• **Fig. 17.5** Mechanism by which platelets can enhance inflammation in rheumatoid arthritis (RA). Glycoprotein (GP)VI-expressing platelets activated by GPVI ligands (collagen or laminin) produce IL-1-rich microparticles *(main panel* and *insets)*. The precise anatomic location of platelet activation and the route by which microparticles enter the joint remain speculative but may implicate transportation by leukocytes and the presence of gaps between the endothelial cells in the joint vasculature and created by platelet-derived serotonin. GPVI stimulation mediates platelet activation via Src kinases and is dependent on SYK activity *(top inset)*. Platelet microparticles (~100 to 1000 nm in diameter), detectable at high levels in inflammatory synovial fluid, interact with tissue cells including fibroblast-like synoviocytes (FLS) and synovial fluid leukocytes *(right inset),* eliciting further inflammatory effector functions from target cells and thereby amplifying synovitis. In the case of FLS, platelet microparticles promote production of IL-6, IL-8, and other mediators capable of leukocyte chemoattraction to the joint *(right inset)*. Platelet microparticles attached to neutrophils, as found in diseased synovial fluid, may also stimulate neutrophil effector functions. (From Boilard E, Blanco P, Nigrovic PA: Platelets: active players in the pathogenesis of arthritis and SLE. *Nat Rev Rheumatol* 8:534–542, 2012. Reprinted with permission from Nature Publishing Group.)

was terminated prematurely because of thromboembolic events in patients treated with the drug.[171] Correspondingly, thrombosis was induced in FcγRIIA transgenic mice intravenously injected with complexes composed of anti-CD40 and soluble CD40L, activating platelets through its unique Fc receptor.[172] In a second study, the inhibition of CD40L failed to have an impact on SLE features, and no adverse events were observed.[171,173]

Other Rheumatic Diseases

Platelets most likely participate in other rheumatic disorders. Activated platelets, platelet aggregates, soluble P-selectin, and platelet-derived microparticles have been observed in people with antiphospholipid syndrome, systemic sclerosis, ankylosing spondylitis, Arthus reaction, and Raynaud's phenomenon.[158,174–183] Although the treatment of Raynaud's phenomenon by anti-depressants targeting serotonin uptake appears to be effective,[184] pointing to a potential role for platelet-derived serotonin, the actual role of platelets in Raynaud's remains to be established.

Conclusion

A key role of platelets and megakaryocytes in the prevention of hemorrhage is well known. Platelets also have less generally appreciated roles in the maintenance of endothelial integrity, in the regulation of vascular permeability, in separating blood vessels from lymphatics, and in modulating the severity and course of inflammation. Megakaryocytes also appear to have a range of immune functions independent of their platelets. Growing recognition of these nonhemostatic functions has led to a new appreciation of the potential role of platelets and megakaryocytes in the rheumatic diseases, including RA and lupus. Whereas multiple pathways can contribute to platelet activation, traditional anti-thrombotic agents are unlikely to be sufficient to intervene therapeutically in the immune biology of the platelet. Further research is required to advance our comprehension of the diverse roles of platelets and megakaryocytes in host defense and in inflammatory disease, with the ultimate goal of developing ways to interfere selectively with their roles in disease while maintaining their contribution to vascular integrity.

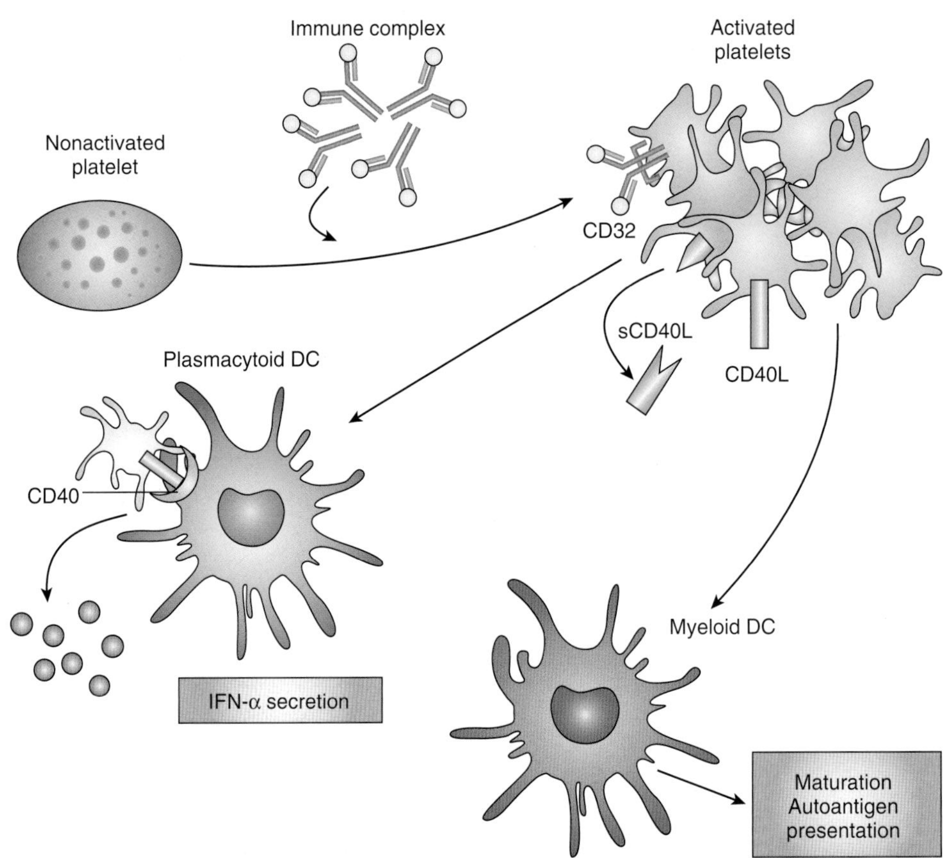

• **Fig. 17.6** Platelet activation processes involved in systemic lupus erythematosus (SLE). Platelets activated by circulating immune complexes express surface CD40 ligand (CD40L), which promote platelet aggregation, binding to myeloid dendritic cells (DCs) to induce their maturation, and binding to plasmacytoid DCs to promote interferon (IFN)-α secretion. *sCD40L,* Soluble CD40 ligand; *SLE,* systemic lupus erythematosus. (From Boilard E, Blanco P, Nigrovic PA: Platelets: active players in the pathogenesis of arthritis and SLE. *Nat Rev Rheumatol* 8:534–542, 2012. Reprinted with permission from Nature Publishing Group.)

Full references for this chapter can be found on ExpertConsult.com.

Selected References

3. White JG: Platelet structure. In Michelson AD, editor: *Platelets*, ed 3, Amsterdam, 2013, Elsevier, pp 117–144.
4. Hartwig JH: The platelet cytoskeleton. In Michelson AD, editor: *Platelets*, ed 3, Amsterdam, 2013, Elsevier, pp 145–168.
5. Fox JE, Boyles JK, Berndt MC, et al.: Identification of a membrane skeleton in platelets, *J Cell Biol* 106:1525–1538, 1988.
14. Escolar G, Leistikow E, White JG: The fate of the open canalicular system in surface and suspension-activated platelets, *Blood* 74:1983–1988, 1989.
15. Tersteeg C, Heijnen HF, Eckly A, et al.: FLow-induced PRotrusions (FLIPRs): a platelet-derived platform for the retrieval of microparticles by monocytes and neutrophils, *Circ Res* 114:780–791, 2014.
16. King SM, Reed GL: Development of platelet secretory granules, *Semin Cell Dev Biol* 13:293–302, 2002.
18. Maynard DM, Heijnen HF, Horne MK, et al.: Proteomic analysis of platelet alpha-granules using mass spectrometry, *J Thromb Haemost* 5:1945–1955, 2007.
22. Shi DS, Smith MC, Campbell RA, et al.: Proteasome function is required for platelet production, *J Clin Invest* 124:3757–3766, 2014.
23. Gupta N, Li W, Willard B, et al.: Proteasome proteolysis supports stimulated platelet function and thrombosis, *Arterioscler Thromb Vasc Biol* 34:160–168, 2014.
24. Choo HJ, Saafir TB, Mkumba L, et al.: Mitochondrial calcium and reactive oxygen species regulate agonist-initiated platelet phosphatidylserine exposure, *Arterioscler Thromb Vasc Biol* 32:2946–2955, 2012.
25. Hartwig J, Italiano Jr J: The birth of the platelet, *J Thromb Haemost* 1:1580–1586, 2003.
26. Josefsson EC, Dowling MR, Lebois M, et al.: The regulation of platelet life span. In Michelson AD, editor: *Platelets*, ed 3, Amsterdam, 2013, Elsevier, pp 51–66.
27. Kaushansky K, Broudy VC, Lin N, et al.: Thrombopoietin, the Mp1 ligand, is essential for full megakaryocyte development, *Proc Natl Acad Sci U S A* 92:3234–3238, 1995.
28. Akkerman JW: Thrombopoietin and platelet function, *Semin Thromb Hemost* 32:295–304, 2006.
30. Grozovsky R, Begonja AJ, Liu K, et al.: The Ashwell-Morell receptor regulates hepatic thrombopoietin production via JAK2-STAT3 signaling, *Nat Med* 21:47–54, 2015.
36. Denis MM, Tolley ND, Bunting M, et al.: Escaping the nuclear confines: signal-dependent pre-mRNA splicing in anucleate platelets, *Cell* 122:379–391, 2005.
37. Landry P, Plante I, Ouellet DL, et al.: Existence of a microRNA pathway in anucleate platelets, *Nat Struct Mol Biol* 16:961–966, 2009.
38. Schwertz H, Koster S, Kahr WH, et al.: Anucleate platelets generate progeny, *Blood* 115:3801–3809, 2010.
39. Italiano JE, Jr, Hartwig J: Megakaryocyte development and platelet formation. In Michelson AD, editor: *Platelets*, ed 3, Amsterdam, 2013, Elsevier, pp 27–50.

42. George JN: Platelets. *Lancet* 355:1531–1539, 2000.
43. Nieswandt B, Varga-Szabo D, Elvers M: Integrins in platelet activation, *J Thromb Haemost* 7(Suppl 1):206–209, 2009.
44. Clemetson KJ: Platelets and primary haemostasis, *Thromb Res* 129(3):220–224, 2012.
45. Jandrot-Perrus M, Busfield S, Lagrue AH, et al.: Cloning, characterization, and functional studies of human and mouse glycoprotein VI: a platelet-specific collagen receptor from the immunoglobulin superfamily, *Blood* 96:1798–1807, 2000.
46. Clemetson JM, Polgar J, Magnenat E, et al.: The platelet collagen receptor glycoprotein VI is a member of the immunoglobulin superfamily closely related to FcalphaR and the natural killer receptors, *J Biol Chem* 274:29019–29024, 1999.
48. Zaffran Y, Meyer SC, Negrescu E, et al.: Signaling across the platelet adhesion receptor glycoprotein Ib-IX induces alpha IIbbeta 3 activation both in platelets and a transfected Chinese hamster ovary cell system, *J Biol Chem* 275:16779–16787, 2000.
50. Nurden AT: Platelet membrane glycoproteins: a historical review, *Semin Thromb Hemost* 40:577–584, 2014.
51. Koseoglu S, Flaumenhaft R: Advances in platelet granule biology, *Curr Opin Hematol* 20:464–471, 2013.
52. Nieswandt B, Pleines I, Bender M: Platelet adhesion and activation mechanisms in arterial thrombosis and ischaemic stroke, *J Thromb Haemost* 9(Suppl 1):92–104, 2011.
54. Buzas EI, Gyorgy B, Nagy G, et al.: Emerging role of extracellular vesicles in inflammatory diseases, *Nat Rev Rheumatol* 10:356–364, 2014.
55. Flaumenhaft R, Dilks JR, Richardson J, et al.: Megakaryocyte-derived microparticles: direct visualization and distinction from platelet-derived microparticles, *Blood* 113:1112–1121, 2009.
56. Arraud N, Linares R, Tan S, et al.: Extracellular vesicles from blood plasma: determination of their morphology, size, phenotype and concentration, *J Thromb Haemost* 12:614–627, 2014.
57. Morel O, Jesel L, Freyssinet JM, et al.: Cellular mechanisms underlying the formation of circulating microparticles, *Arterioscler Thromb Vasc Biol* 31:15–26, 2011.
58. Owens 3rd AP, Mackman N: Microparticles in hemostasis and thrombosis, *Circ Res* 108:1284–1297, 2011.
59. Goerge T, Ho-Tin-Noe B, Carbo C, et al.: Inflammation induces hemorrhage in thrombocytopenia, *Blood* 111:4958–4964, 2008.
60. Ho-Tin-Noe B, Demers M, Wagner DD: How platelets safeguard vascular integrity, *J Thromb Haemost* 9(Suppl 1):56–65, 2011.
61. Boulaftali Y, Hess PR, Getz TM, et al.: Platelet ITAM signaling is critical for vascular integrity in inflammation, *J Clin Invest* 123:908–916, 2013.
62. Boulaftali Y, Hess PR, Kahn ML, et al.: Platelet immunoreceptor tyrosine-based activation motif (ITAM) signaling and vascular integrity, *Circ Res* 114:1174–1184, 2014.
63. Stegner D, Haining EJ, Nieswandt B: Targeting glycoprotein VI and the immunoreceptor tyrosine-based activation motif signaling pathway, *Arterioscler Thromb Vasc Biol* 34:1615–1620, 2014.
65. Suzuki-Inoue K, Fuller GL, Garcia A, et al.: A novel Syk-dependent mechanism of platelet activation by the C-type lectin receptor CLEC-2, *Blood* 107:542–549, 2006.
66. McKenzie SE, Taylor SM, Malladi P, et al.: The role of the human Fc receptor Fc gamma RIIA in the immune clearance of platelets: a transgenic mouse model, *J Immunol* 162:4311–4318, 1999.
68. Osada M, Inoue O, Ding G, et al.: Platelet activation receptor CLEC-2 regulates blood/lymphatic vessel separation by inhibiting proliferation, migration, and tube formation of lymphatic endothelial cells, *J Biol Chem* 287:22241–22252, 2012.
69. Clements JL, Lee JR, Gross B, et al.: Fetal hemorrhage and platelet dysfunction in SLP-76-deficient mice, *J Clin Invest* 103:19–25, 1999.
70. Abtahian F, Guerriero A, Sebzda E, et al.: Regulation of blood and lymphatic vascular separation by signaling proteins SLP-76 and Syk, *Science* 299:247–251, 2003.
71. Ichise H, Ichise T, Ohtani O, et al.: Phospholipase Cgamma2 is necessary for separation of blood and lymphatic vasculature in mice, *Development* 136:191–195, 2009.
72. Finney BA, Schweighoffer E, Navarro-Nunez L, et al.: CLEC-2 and Syk in the megakaryocytic/platelet lineage are essential for development, *Blood* 119:1747–1756, 2012.
73. Hess PR, Rawnsley DR, Jakus Z, et al.: Platelets mediate lymphovenous hemostasis to maintain blood-lymphatic separation throughout life, *J Clin Invest* 124:273–284, 2014.
75. Semple JW, Italiano JE, Freedman J: Platelets and the immune continuum, *Nat Rev Immunol* 11:264–274, 2011.
76. Ehlers R, Ustinov V, Chen Z, et al.: Targeting platelet-leukocyte interactions: identification of the integrin Mac-1 binding site for the platelet counter receptor glycoprotein Ibalpha, *J Exp Med* 198:1077–1088, 2003.
77. Furie B, Furie BC: The molecular basis of platelet and endothelial cell interaction with neutrophils and monocytes: role of P-selectin and the P-selectin ligand, PSGL-1, *Thromb Haemost* 74:224–227, 1995.
78. Andonegui G, Kerfoot SM, McNagny K, et al.: Platelets express functional Toll-like receptor-4, *Blood* 106:2417–2423, 2005.
79. Cognasse F, Hamzeh H, Chavarin P, et al.: Evidence of Toll-like receptor molecules on human platelets, *Immunol Cell Biol* 83:196–198, 2005.
80. Aslam R, Speck ER, Kim M, et al.: Platelet Toll-like receptor expression modulates lipopolysaccharide-induced thrombocytopenia and tumor necrosis factor-alpha production in vivo, *Blood* 107:637–641, 2006.
81. Semple JW, Aslam R, Kim M, et al.: Platelet-bound lipopolysaccharide enhances Fc receptor-mediated phagocytosis of IgG-opsonized platelets, *Blood* 109:4803–4805, 2007.
82. Brinkmann V, Reichard U, Goosmann C, et al.: Neutrophil extracellular traps kill bacteria, *Science* 303:1532–1535, 2004.
83. Schauer C, Janko C, Munoz LE, et al.: Aggregated neutrophil extracellular traps limit inflammation by degrading cytokines and chemokines, *Nat Med* 20:511–517, 2014.
84. Khandpur R, Carmona-Rivera C, Vivekanandan-Giri A, et al.: NETs are a source of citrullinated autoantigens and stimulate inflammatory responses in rheumatoid arthritis, *Sci Transl Med* 5, 2013. 178ra40.
85. Garcia-Romo GS, Caielli S, Vega B, et al.: Netting neutrophils are major inducers of type I IFN production in pediatric systemic lupus erythematosus, *Sci Transl Med* 3:73ra20, 2011.
86. Hakkim A, Furnrohr BG, Amann K, et al.: Impairment of neutrophil extracellular trap degradation is associated with lupus nephritis, *Proc Natl Acad Sci U S A* 107:9813–9818, 2010.
87. Ross R, Raines EW, Bowen-Pope DF: The biology of platelet-derived growth factor, *Cell* 46:155–169, 1986.
89. Denton CP, Abraham DJ: Transforming growth factor-beta and connective tissue growth factor: key cytokines in scleroderma pathogenesis, *Curr Opin Rheumatol* 13:505–511, 2001.
90. Lindemann S, Tolley ND, Dixon DA, et al.: Activated platelets mediate inflammatory signaling by regulated interleukin 1beta synthesis, *J Cell Biol* 154:485–490, 2001.
121. Selroos O: Thrombocytosis in rheumatoid arthritis, *Scand J Rheumatol* 1:136–140, 1972.
123. Ertenli I, Kiraz S, Ozturk MA, et al.: Pathologic thrombopoiesis of rheumatoid arthritis, *Rheumatol Int* 23:49–60, 2003.
125. Bowman SJ: Hematological manifestations of rheumatoid arthritis, *Scand J Rheumatol* 31:251–259, 2002.
127. Wang F, Wang NS, Yan CG, et al.: The significance of platelet activation in rheumatoid arthritis, *Clin Rheumatol* 26:768–771, 2007.
129. Mac Mullan PA, Peace AJ, Madigan AM, et al.: Platelet hyper-reactivity in active inflammatory arthritis is unique to the adenosine diphosphate pathway: a novel finding and potential therapeutic target, *Rheumatology (Oxford)* 49:240–245, 2010.
130. Knijff-Dutmer EA, Koerts J, Nieuwland R, et al.: Elevated levels of platelet microparticles are associated with disease activity in rheumatoid arthritis, *Arthritis Rheum* 46:1498–1503, 2002.
131. Bunescu A, Seideman P, Lenkei R, et al.: Enhanced Fcgamma receptor I, alphaMbeta2 integrin receptor expression by monocytes and neutrophils in rheumatoid arthritis: interaction with platelets, *J Rheumatol* 31:2347–2355, 2004.

132. Sellam J, Proulle V, Jungel A, et al.: Increased levels of circulating microparticles in primary Sjögren's syndrome, systemic lupus erythematosus and rheumatoid arthritis and relation with disease activity, *Arthritis Res Ther* 11:R156, 2009.
133. Goules A, Tzioufas AG, Manousakis MN, et al.: Elevated levels of soluble CD40 ligand (sCD40L) in serum of patients with systemic autoimmune diseases, *J Autoimmun* 26:165–171, 2006.
134. Pamuk GE, Vural O, Turgut B, et al.: Increased platelet activation markers in rheumatoid arthritis: are they related with subclinical atherosclerosis? *Platelets* 19:146–154, 2008.
135. Gitz E, Pollitt AY, Gitz-Francois JJ, et al.: CLEC-2 expression is maintained on activated platelets and on platelet microparticles, *Blood* 124:2262–2270, 2014.
136. Ginsberg MH, Breth G, Skosey JL: Platelets in the synovial space, *Arthritis Rheum* 21:994–995, 1978.
137. Yaron M, Djaldetti M: Platelets in synovial fluid, *Arthritis Rheum* 21:607–608, 1978.
138. Endresen GK: Investigation of blood platelets in synovial fluid from patients with rheumatoid arthritis, *Scand J Rheumatol* 10:204–208, 1981.
139. Cloutier N, Pare A, Farndale RW, et al.: Platelets can enhance vascular permeability, *Blood* 120:1334–1343, 2012.
141. Del Rey MJ, Fare R, Izquierdo E, et al.: Clinicopathological correlations of podoplanin (gp38) expression in rheumatoid synovium and its potential contribution to fibroblast platelet crosstalk, *PLoS ONE* 9:e99607, 2014.
142. Boilard E, Nigrovic PA, Larabee K, et al.: Platelets amplify inflammation in arthritis via collagen-dependent microparticle production, *Science* 327:580–583, 2010.
143. Cloutier N, Tan S, Boudreau LH, et al.: The exposure of autoantigens by microparticles underlies the formation of potent inflammatory components: the microparticle-associated immune complexes, *EMBO Mol Med* 5:235–249, 2013.
144. Gyorgy B, Szabo TG, Turiak L, et al.: Improved flow cytometric assessment reveals distinct microvesicle (cell-derived microparticle) signatures in joint diseases, *PLoS ONE* 7:e49726, 2012.
145. Boudreau LH, Duchez AC, Cloutier N, et al.: Platelets release mitochondria serving as substrate for bactericidal group IIA secreted phospholipase A2 to promote inflammation, *Blood* 124:2173–2183, 2014.
146. Biro E, Nieuwland R, Tak PP, et al.: Activated complement components and complement activator molecules on the surface of cell-derived microparticles in patients with rheumatoid arthritis and healthy individuals, *Ann Rheum Dis* 66:1085–1092, 2007.
149. Bozza FA, Shah AM, Weyrich AS, et al.: Amicus or adversary: platelets in lung biology, acute injury, and inflammation, *Am J Respir Cell Mol Biol* 40:123–134, 2009.
150. Vieira de Abreu A, Rondina MT, Weyrich AS, et al.: Michelson AD, editor: *Platelets,* ed 3, Amsterdam, 2013, Elsevier, pp 733–767.
153. Mott PJ, Lazarus AH: CD44 antibodies and immune thrombocytopenia in the amelioration of murine inflammatory arthritis, *PLoS ONE* 8:e65805, 2013.
155. Nagahama M, Nomura S, Ozaki Y, et al.: Platelet activation markers and soluble adhesion molecules in patients with systemic lupus erythematosus, *Autoimmunity* 33:85–94, 2001.
156. Tam LS, Fan B, Li EK, et al.: Patients with systemic lupus erythematosus show increased platelet activation and endothelial dysfunction induced by acute hyperhomocysteinemia, *J Rheumatol* 30:1479–1484, 2003.
157. Ekdahl KN, Bengtsson AA, Andersson J, et al.: Thrombotic disease in systemic lupus erythematosus is associated with a maintained systemic platelet activation, *Br J Haematol* 125:74–78, 2004.
158. Joseph JE, Harrison P, Mackie IJ, et al.: Increased circulating platelet-leucocyte complexes and platelet activation in patients with antiphospholipid syndrome, systemic lupus erythematosus and rheumatoid arthritis, *Br J Haematol* 115:451–459, 2001.
160. Pretorius E, du Plooy J, Soma P, et al.: An ultrastructural analysis of platelets, erythrocytes, white blood cells, and fibrin network in systemic lupus erythematosus, *Rheumatol Int* 34:1005–1009, 2014.
161. Zhang W, Dang S, Wang J, et al.: Specific cross-reaction of anti-dsDNA antibody with platelet integrin GPIIIa49-66, *Autoimmunity* 43:682–689, 2010.
163. Takahashi H, Moroi M: Antibody against platelet membrane glycoprotein VI in a patient with systemic lupus erythematosus, *Am J Hematol* 67:262–267, 2001.
164. Reveille JD: The genetic basis of autoantibody production, *Autoimmun Rev* 5:389–398, 2006.
165. Balada E, Villarreal-Tolchinsky J, Ordi-Ros J, et al.: Multiplex family-based study in systemic lupus erythematosus: association between the R620W polymorphism of PTPN22 and the FcgammaRIIa (CD32A) R131 allele, *Tissue Antigens* 68:432–438, 2006.
166. Duffau P, Seneschal J, Nicco C, et al.: Platelet CD154 potentiates interferon-alpha secretion by plasmacytoid dendritic cells in systemic lupus erythematosus, *Sci Transl Med* 2:47ra63, 2010.
167. Berlacher MD, Vieth JA, Heflin BC, et al.: FcgammaRIIa ligation induces platelet hypersensitivity to thrombotic stimuli, *Am J Pathol* 182:244–254, 2013.
170. Pereira J, Alfaro G, Goycoolea M, et al.: Circulating platelet-derived microparticles in systemic lupus erythematosus. Association with increased thrombin generation and procoagulant state, *Thromb Haemost* 95:94–99, 2006.
171. Boumpas DT, Furie R, Manzi S, et al.: A short course of BG9588 (anti-CD40 ligand antibody) improves serologic activity and decreases hematuria in patients with proliferative lupus glomerulonephritis, *Arthritis Rheum* 48:719–727, 2003.
172. Robles-Carrillo L, Meyer T, Hatfield M, et al.: Anti-CD40L immune complexes potently activate platelets in vitro and cause thrombosis in FCGR2A transgenic mice, *J Immunol* 185:1577–1583, 2010.
173. Kalunian KC, Davis Jr JC, Merrill JT, et al.: Treatment of systemic lupus erythematosus by inhibition of T cell costimulation with anti-CD154: a randomized, double-blind, placebo-controlled trial, *Arthritis Rheum* 46:3251–3258, 2002.
174. Postlethwaite AE, Chiang TM: Platelet contributions to the pathogenesis of systemic sclerosis, *Curr Opin Rheumatol* 19:574–579, 2007.
175. Silveri F, De Angelis R, Poggi A, et al.: Relative roles of endothelial cell damage and platelet activation in primary Raynaud's phenomenon (RP) and RP secondary to systemic sclerosis, *Scand J Rheumatol* 30:290–296, 2001.
176. Chiang TM, Takayama H, Postlethwaite AE: Increase in platelet non-integrin type I collagen receptor in patients with systemic sclerosis, *Thromb Res* 117:299–306, 2006.
177. Wang F, Yan CG, Xiang HY, et al.: The significance of platelet activation in ankylosing spondylitis, *Clin Rheumatol* 27:767–769, 2008.
178. Hara T, Shimizu K, Ogawa F, et al.: Platelets control leukocyte recruitment in a murine model of cutaneous Arthus reaction, *Am J Pathol* 176:259–269, 2010.
179. Pauling JD, O'Donnell VB, McHugh NJ: The contribution of platelets to the pathogenesis of Raynaud's phenomenon and systemic sclerosis, *Platelets* 24:503–515, 2013.
180. Iversen LV, Ostergaard O, Ullman S, et al.: Circulating microparticles and plasma levels of soluble E- and P-selectins in patients with systemic sclerosis, *Scand J Rheumatol* 42:473–482, 2013.
181. Guiducci S, Distler JH, Jungel A, et al.: The relationship between plasma microparticles and disease manifestations in patients with systemic sclerosis, *Arthritis Rheum* 58:2845–2853, 2008.
182. Oyabu C, Morinobu A, Sugiyama D, et al.: Plasma platelet-derived microparticles in patients with connective tissue diseases, *J Rheumatol* 38:680–684, 2011.
183. Pamuk GE, Turgut B, Pamuk ON, et al.: Increased circulating platelet-leucocyte complexes in patients with primary Raynaud's phenomenon and Raynaud's phenomenon secondary to systemic sclerosis: a comparative study, *Blood Coagul Fibrinolysis* 18:297–302, 2007.
184. Coleiro B, Marshall SE, Denton CP, et al.: Treatment of Raynaud's phenomenon with the selective serotonin reuptake inhibitor fluoxetine, *Rheumatology (Oxford)* 40:1038–1043, 2001.

18 Principles of Signaling

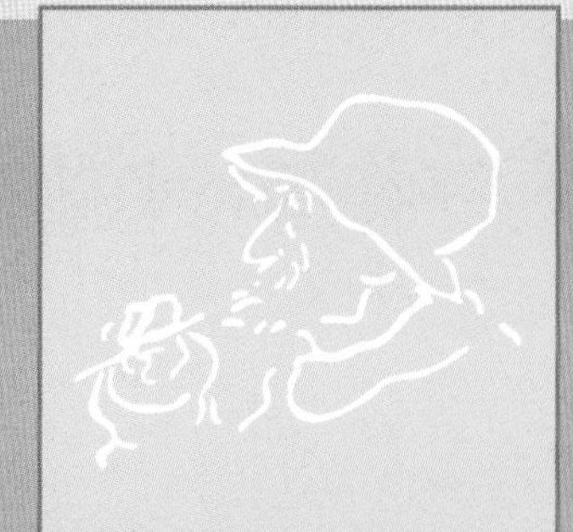

ABEL SUAREZ-FUEYO, VAISHALI R. MOULTON, AND GEORGE C. TSOKOS

KEY POINTS

Cells of the immune system sense environmental stimuli via receptors, which may be expressed on the cell surface or may be intra-cellular.

Interaction of ligands with receptors initiates signaling cascades, which relay the extra-cellular stimuli within the cell and alter cellular function.

Signaling pathways typically involve phosphorylation (by kinases) and dephosphorylation (by phosphatases) of molecules.

Signaling eventually leads to cellular responses such as changes in growth, activation, proliferation, and differentiation.

Introduction

Immune cells respond to a vast variety of stimuli to carry out their role in maintaining the immune system. Physiologic and innocuous and foreign or dangerous signals must be recognized and communicated within the cell, where they culminate into cellular responses such as changes in shape, motility, growth, activation, differentiation, or production of effector molecules. Distinct cascades of interacting molecules connect the perceived stimuli and relay information into the cytosol and/or nucleus to initiate these effector functions either directly or through initiation of gene transcription and protein translation programs. Signaling pathways can be categorized based on the mechanisms by which environmental stimuli are sensed, such as cell surface receptor-mediated interactions or intra-cellular detection of lipid-soluble molecules. Receptor-mediated signaling can further be classified by the presence or absence of enzymatic activity. This chapter focuses on fundamental concepts of signaling based on these groups of receptors and their intra-cellular signaling pathways.

Receptors With Enzymatic Activity

Many ligands are water soluble and therefore impermeable through the lipid bilayer of the plasma membrane; they interact with cognate receptors on the cell surface. These ligands include antigens, immune complexes, chemokines, cytokines, and microbial components. Interactions of ligands with their receptors initiate downstream catalytic activity and recruitment of similar signaling molecules or adaptor molecules. Receptors with enzymatic activity comprise extra-cellular ligand-binding domains, membrane-spanning domains, and intra-cellular signaling domains. Intrinsic enzymatic activity within the receptor includes kinase, phosphatase, or guanylate cyclase activity.

The receptor tyrosine kinase (RTK) family is a common class of these receptors. The human RTK family consists of 20 subfamilies that detect ligands such as stem cell factor (SCF), insulin, epidermal growth factor (EGF), vascular endothelial growth factor (VEGF), platelet-derived growth factor (PDGF), colony-stimulating factor (CSF), and fibroblast growth factor (FGF).[1] These receptors are generally inactive until bound by their ligands, which induce clustering and dimerization of the receptors and autophosphorylation of their kinase domains (Fig. 18.1A). Upon activation, other kinases or cytoplasmic molecules are recruited for activation and transmission of signals downstream. In addition to receptor binding, ligands, along with accessory molecules, may also mediate receptor dimerization. FGF, for example, partners with heparan sulfate proteoglycans to cross-link and dimerize FGF receptors (FGFR).[2] Some receptors may dimerize even in the absence of ligands, such as the disulfide-linked insulin receptor and the insulin-like growth factor (IGF)-1 receptors. Ligand binding induces structural changes to activate these receptors and signaling by diverse mechanisms.[1]

Phosphorylation occurs at tyrosine, serine, or threonine residues. The phosphotyrosine residue is recognized by proteins containing Src homology (SH)2 and phosphotyrosine-binding (PTB) domains. These proteins may be kinases or phosphatases or lack enzymatic activity and act as intermediates known as *adaptor proteins*. SH2 domain proteins include phospholipase Cγ (PLCγ), phosphatidyl inositol-3-OH kinase (PI3K), and SHP phosphatases. Grb-2 and IRS are examples of adaptor proteins, of which Grb-2 recruits the guanine nucleotide exchange factor (GEF) SOS. SOS activates the small G protein Ras to activate the mitogen-activated protein kinase (MAPK) pathway.

Transforming growth factor (TGF)-β is an anti-inflammatory cytokine, which binds to receptors similar to the RTK family and regulates a variety of cellular processes.[3] The TGF-β ligand superfamily includes bone morphogenetic proteins, growth and differentiation factors (GDFs), activin, and TGF-β1, 2, and 3. TGF-β binding to a type II receptor that bears a serine threonine kinase mediates phosphorylation of a type I receptor to form a heterotrimeric complex with the ligand. This complex recruits and phosphorylates the intra-cellular SMAD proteins. The SMAD proteins include the receptor-activated (r)-Smads 1, 2, 3, 5, and 9. Once phosphorylated, the r-Smads 2 and 3 oligomerize with a common mediator, Smad4, and translocate to the nucleus to regulate gene transcription (see Fig. 18.1B).[4]

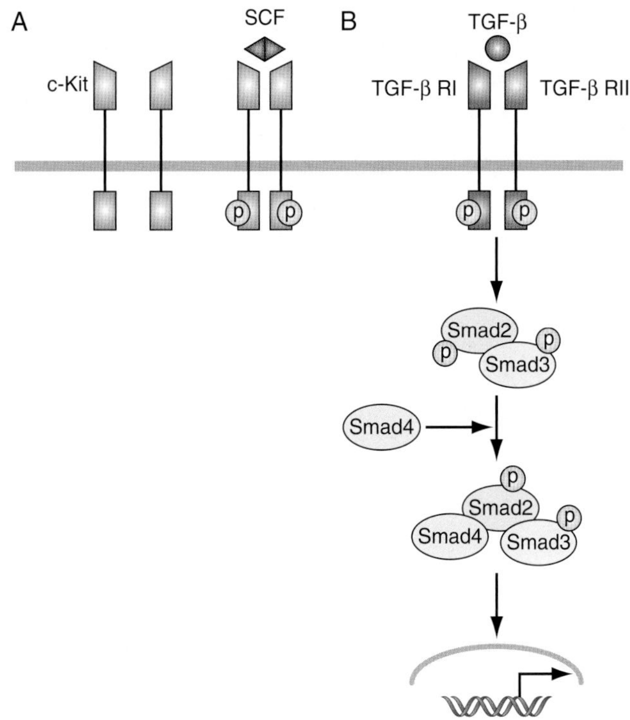

• **Fig. 18.1** (A) Receptor tyrosine kinase c-kit, the receptor for stem cell factor (SCF) is depicted in the inactive form as monomers *(left)*. Upon binding to its ligand, the receptor dimerizes, and the kinase domains phosphorylate each other *(right)*. (B) Schematic depicting the transforming growth factor (TGF)-β–TGFβR signaling pathway. *P,* Phosphate.

Some receptors have phosphatase activity and are known as *protein tyrosine phosphatases* (PTP). For example, the Src family kinases contain an activating and an inhibitory tyrosine residue. C-terminal Src kinase (Csk) phosphorylates the inhibitory tyrosine, whereas the transmembrane tyrosine phosphatase CD45 removes this phosphate, which is required for initiation of signaling in lymphocytes.

Receptors That Recruit Molecules With Enzymatic Activity

Immunoreceptors: T Cell Receptor, B Cell Receptor, and FcRs

Immune cells express antigen recognition receptors that are generated and selected for in a complex fashion.[5,6] T cells and NKT cells express T cell receptor (TCR) and recognize peptides or lipids associated with the major histocompatibility complex (MHC), or CD1d, respectively. B cells, through the B cell receptor (BCR), recognize soluble antigens. Lymphoid and myeloid cells, such as NK cells and macrophages, express receptors of the FcR family, which cause activation upon detection of antibodies in complex with antigen. These receptors are heteromultimeric complexes, with a subunit of one or two chains that recognize the ligand, co-receptors (CD4, CD8, or CD19), and associated or adaptor molecules that contain from one to six immunoreceptor tyrosine-based activation motif (ITAM) domains (Fig. 18.2).

Antigen recognition by the immune receptor and co-receptor triggers the recruitment and activation of membrane proximal early kinases, including Src, Syk, and Tec, which phosphorylate tyrosines of the ITAM domains in the chains associated with the immune receptors. The Src family phosphotyrosine kinases (PTK) comprise eight kinases (Fgr, Fyn, Src, Yes, Blk, Hck, Lck, Lyn), which are recruited through their SH2 domain. The Tec family consists of five different kinases (Bmx, Btk, Itk, Tec, and Txk/Rlk), which translocate to the cell membrane through their pleckstrin homology (PH) domain to bind PIP_3. Alternatively, they are recruited via their SH2 domains, which recognize ITAM motifs on adaptor proteins (e.g., BLNK in B cells, or SLP-76 and LAT in T cells). The principal downstream target of Tec kinases is PLCγ.[7,8] Their function is regulated by the kinase Csk and the protein tyrosine phosphatase CD45.

ITAM phosphorylation leads to recruitment and activation of Syk family kinases recruited through SH2 domains. BCRs recruit Syk, whereas ZAP-70 binds to phospho-ITAMs of CD3ζ within the TCR. Both kinases are implicated in the signaling of Fc receptors because Syk associates with their common gamma chain, although some incorporate CD3ζ to recruit ZAP-70. These then undergo autophosphorylation to create sites for interaction with SH2 proteins.[7]

Co-stimulatory Receptors

T cell activation requires two signals, one mediated through the T cell receptor and a second signal called *co-stimulation*. This signal is provided by a family of receptor-ligand molecules that mediate interactions between T cells and antigen-presenting cells. The B7/CD28 is one of the most well-studied pathways of co-stimulation. B7-1 and B7-2 are expressed by APCs and bind CD28 on T cells. This interaction triggers downstream signaling to amplify the primary signal and initiate effector responses. CD28 is phosphorylated by Lck and activates the PLCγ and PI3K/Akt pathways. An important consequence of this signaling pathway is to enhance mRNA stability of IL-2, which is responsible for the dramatic increase in IL-2 secretion. Cytotoxic T lymphocyte antigen (CTLA)4 is closely related to CD28 in structure, can bind to B7 molecules but with much higher avidity, and curbs the activation and proliferation of T cells.[9] In addition to the B7-CD28 pairing, other co-stimulatory molecules include the inducible co-stimulator (ICOS), which is induced on activated T cells and interacts with B7-H2/ICOSL on activated dendritic cells, monocytes, and B cells. Another class of co-stimulatory molecules is the signaling lymphocyte activation molecule (SLAM) family, a subtype of the immunoglobulin superfamily consisting of nine transmembrane proteins. SLAMs are important for multiple cell types, including T, B, and NK cells, and mediate their effects via homophilic and heterophilic interactions. The SLAM proteins bear a tyrosine-based switch motif through which they bind SH2-bearing proteins SLAM-associated protein (SAP) and EAT2 with high affinity.[10]

Once activated, T cells express other co-stimulatory molecules, such as CD40L and the programmed cell death (PD)1 receptor. CD40L interacts with CD40 on APCs, and this induces signals, which play an important role in effector functions, such as activation of B cells, to produce antibodies. A co-stimulatory inhibitory pathway involves PD1 on T cells binding to B7-H1/PDL1 and B7-DC/PDL2 expressed on APCs.[11] PD1 belongs to the immunoglobulin superfamily, and its intra-cellular domain bears an immunoreceptor tyrosine-based inhibitory motif (ITIM) and an immunoreceptor tyrosine-based switch motif (ITSM). The tyrosine in the ITSM binds to the phosphatases SHP1 and SHP2,

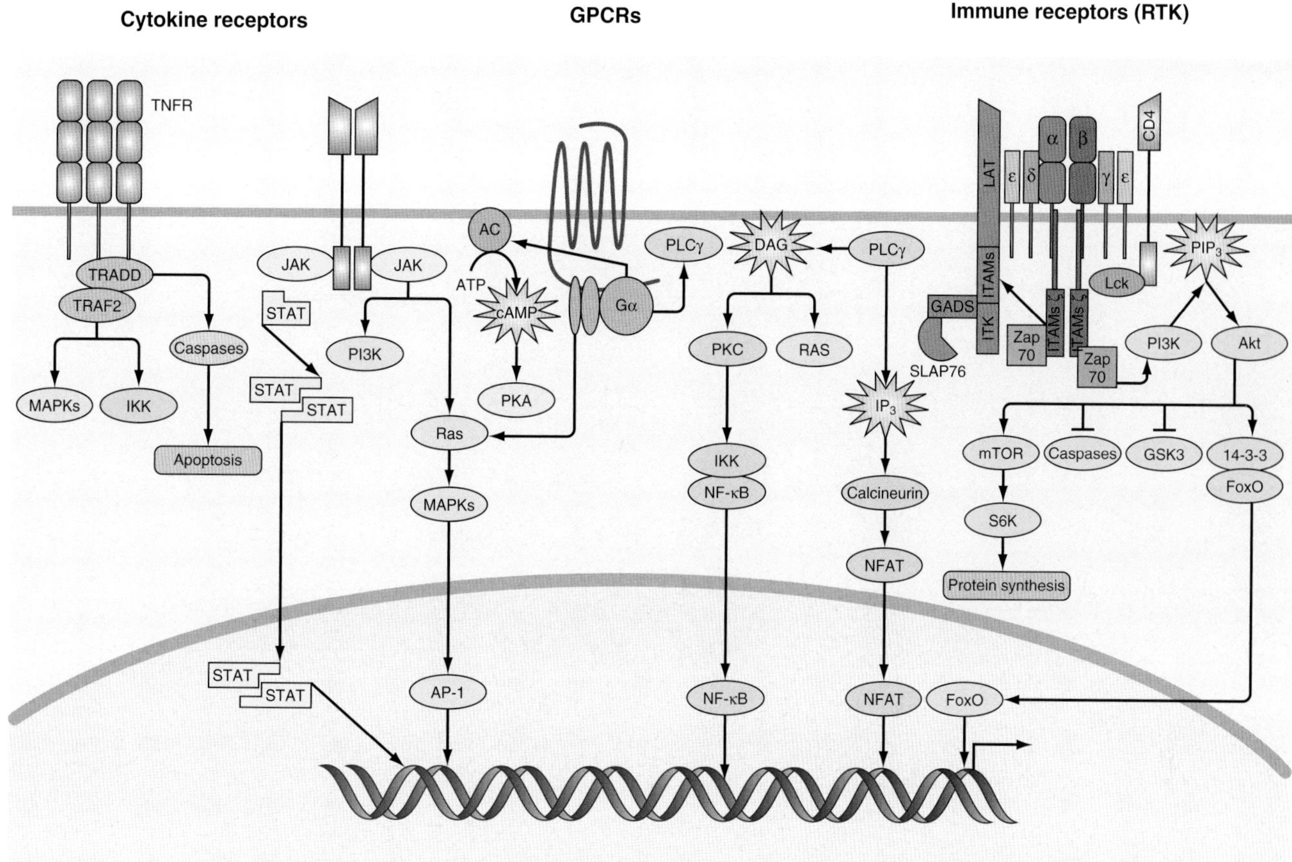

• **Fig. 18.2** Schematic depicting signaling pathways through cytokine receptors, G protein–coupled receptors (GPCRs), and immune receptors. *AC,* Adenyl cyclase; *AP-1,* activator protein-1; *GADS,* growth factor receptor-bound protein-2-related adaptor protein-2; *ITAM,* immunoreceptor tyrosine activation motif; *JAK,* Janus kinase; *LAT,* linker for activation of T cells; *MAPK,* mitogen-activated protein kinase; *NFAT,* nuclear factor of activated T cells; *PI3K,* phosphatidyl inositol-3-OH kinase; *PIP_3,* phosphatidylinositol-3,4,5-triphosphate; *PKA,* protein kinase A; *PLC,* phospholipase C; *SLAP,* Src-like adaptor protein; *STAT,* signal transducer and activator of transcription; *TNFR,* tumor necrosis factor receptor; *TRAF,* TNFR-associated factor; *TRADD,* TNFR-associated death domain.

which act to inhibit the PI3K/Akt pathway. PD1 signaling inhibits induction of the antiapoptotic molecule BcL-xL and transcription factors such as T-bet, GATA-3, and Eomes, which are important for T cell differentiation.

Thus, co-stimulatory signals not only activate cells to promote proliferation and effector functions required in the immune response but also are inhibitory to curb excessive activation and are important for tolerance induction.

Cytokine Receptors

Cytokines are soluble peptide regulators with profound effects on immune homeostasis and autoinflammatory disease.[12] Cytokine receptors are organized into four classes on the basis of their domain and structure:

1. Class I receptors are characterized by a WSXWS motif and can be subdivided on the basis of structural homology or the use of shared signaling subunits. Examples include receptors for IL-2, IL-6, IL-7, IL-15, and for hormones such as erythropoietin and prolactin.[13]
2. Class II receptors include those for type I and II interferon (IFN), IL-10, IL-20, IL-22, IL-26, IL-28, and IL-29.[14] IFNs are glycoproteins commonly generated as a downstream effect of pathogen detection. They are divided into three classes on the basis of the receptors that they activate. Type I IFNs bind the IFNA receptor (IFNAR); this group includes IFN-α, IFN-β, IFN-ε, IFN-κ, and IFN-ω. IFN-γ is the sole member of type II in humans, and it binds IFNGR. Type III IFNs activate a receptor complex consisting of IL-10R2 and IFNLR1; this group includes IL-29, IL-28A, and IL-28B. Activation stimulates the Janus kinase (JAK)/signal transducer and activator of transcription (STAT) signal cascades and transcriptional changes made in cooperation with interferon regulatory factor (IRF) proteins. The expression of so-called *interferon signature genes* (ISG) promotes anti-viral activities, increased MHC presentation, and apoptosis.
3. TNF receptors share structures with some noncytokine receptors, such as CD95.[15] The TNF superfamily consists of 19 ligands and 29 receptors, which play varied roles in inflammation, apoptosis, and proliferation.[16] TNF and lymphotoxin-α (also known as TNFβ) were the first two members identified and share approximately 50% homology in their protein sequence. Other members of this superfamily include lymphotoxin-β, CD40L, FasL, CD30L, 4-1BBL, CD27L, OX40L, TNF-related apoptosis-inducing ligand (TRAIL), lymphotoxin-like ligand

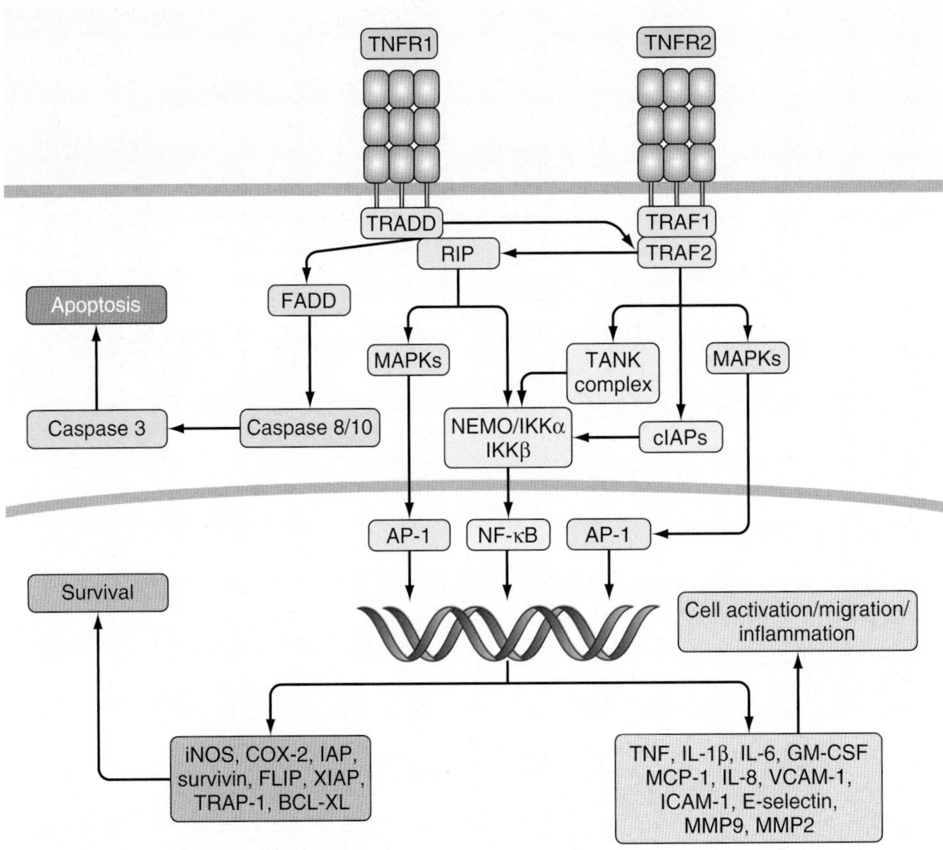

• **Fig. 18.3** Tumor necrosis factor receptor 1 (TNFR1) and TNFR2 signaling pathways. *AP,* Activator protein; *BCL,* B cell lymphoma; *cIAPs,* cellular inhibitors of apoptosis; *COX,* cyclooxygenase; *FADD,* Fas-associated protein with death domain; *FLIP,* FLICE-like inhibitory protein; *GM-CSF,* granulocyte-macrophage colony-stimulating factor; *IAP,* inhibitor of apoptosis; *ICAM,* intercellular adhesion molecule; *IKK,* IκB (inhibitor of κB) kinase; *iNOS,* inducible nitric oxide synthetase; *MAPK,* mitogen-activated protein kinases; *MCP,* monocyte chemotactic protein; *MMP,* matrix metalloproteinase; *NEMO,* NF-κB essential modulator; *NF-κB,* nuclear factor-κB; *RIP,* receptor-interacting serine/threonine-protein kinase 1; *TANK,* TRAF family member-associated NF-κB activator; *TRADD,* tumor necrosis factor receptor type 1–associated death domain; *TRAP,* TNF receptor-associated protein; *VCAM,* vascular cell adhesion protein; *XIAP,* X-linked inhibitor of apoptosis protein.

competitive with gD-1 HSV for HVEM expressed on T cells (LIGHT), receptor activator of NF-κB ligand (RANKL), TNF-related weak inducer of apoptosis (TWEAK), a proliferation-inducing ligand (APRIL), B cell–activating factor (BAFF), vascular endothelial cell-growth inhibitor (VEGI), ectodysplasin A (EDA)-A1, EDA-A2, and glucocorticoid-induced TNF receptor (TNFR) family ligand (GITRL). TNF binds to two distinct receptors: TNFR1 and TNFR2 (Fig. 18.3). Receptors of the TNF superfamily can be categorized based on the presence or absence of an intra-cellular death domain (DD), of which the D-containing receptors are ubiquitous in expression. TNFR1 contains a DD and is expressed in virtually all cell types, whereas TNFR2 is expressed mainly on immune cells, endothelial cells, and nerve cells. TNF is expressed both in soluble form and as a transmembrane protein on the cell surface, whereas lymphotoxin-α is only expressed as soluble protein. TNF signaling induces several signaling pathways, including activation of NF-κB, MAPK, and apoptosis.

4. IL-1 receptors can be considered analogous to Toll-like receptors (TLRs).[17]

These receptor complexes present two or more single-pass transmembrane subunits that include domains that recruit signaling proteins upon activation and subunits with extra-cellular binding domains. Whereas class I and II cytokine receptors use the JAK-STAT signaling pathway, TNFRs use adaptor molecules called *TNFR-associated factors* (TRAFs) to recruit complexes with different functions.

Adhesion Molecules

A variety of cellular functions, including lymphocyte activation, migration, and cell-cell interaction, involve adhesion molecules. These include selectins, integrins, and immunoglobulin superfamily molecules. L-selectin (CD62L) is important for lymphocyte homing to lymphoid tissues. Activated lymphocytes downregulate L-selectin and upregulate other adhesion/migratory molecules, such as CD44, a transmembrane protein, which recognizes hyaluronic acid and is critical for migration into peripheral sites of inflammation. CD44 lacks intrinsic kinase activity, but the cytoplasmic domain associates with Src family kinases Lck and Fyn. In addition, the cytoplasmic tail binds to the phosphorylated ezrin/radixin/moesin (pERM) proteins, which cross-link actin cytoskeleton proteins to CD44.[18] CD44 signaling also activates PI3K/Akt cell survival pathways.[19]

Integrins are heterodimeric cell surface proteins that provide interactions with other cells and the extra-cellular matrix, allowing for migration to effector sites. Various chemokines can activate integrins to mediate migration into lymphoid or nonlymphoid tissues. T lymphocyte integrins include leukocyte function–associated antigen (LFA)-1, LPAM-1, and very late activation antigen (VLA)-4, which bind immunoglobulin superfamily members ICAM-1, MAdCAM-1, and VCAM-1, respectively. Integrin activation results in inside-out signaling, which regulates the affinity of the integrin receptor to the extra-cellular ligands. Elements of this signaling pathway include the small GTPase RAP1 and its GEFs talin and kindlin3.[20–22]

Seven-Transmembrane Domain Receptors

G Protein–Coupled Receptors

G protein–coupled receptors (GPCRs) are a large family of approximately 350 members that bind a variety of ligands, including hormones, lipids, chemokines, and leukotrienes. They are seven-transmembrane domain-bearing proteins that associate with an intra-cellular trimeric G protein (α, β, or γ) and are organized into five families: rhodopsin, secretin, glutamate, adhesion, and Frizzled/Taste2 (Table 18.1). Ligand binding promotes the exchange of guanine diphosphate (GDP) for guanine triphosphate (GTP) and dissociation of the Gα and β subunits from the receptor subunit.

Based on their α-subunits, G proteins are divided into four subfamilies: Gαs, Gαi/o, Gαq/11, and Gα12/13. Each Gα has specific targets: Gαs and Gαi/o activate or repress adenyl cyclase (AC), regulating cyclic adenosine monophosphate (cAMP) levels to impact several ion channels and the activation of protein kinase A (PKA), whereas Gαq/11 activates phospholipase C (PLC)-β to generate IP_3 and diacylglycerol (DAG) from PIP_2, ultimately leading to Ca^{2+} and protein kinase C (PKC) pathway activation. The targets for Gα12/13 are three RhoGEFs that activate the small GTPase Rho, critical for cytoskeleton regulation via the stress-activated MAPK pathway. Alternatively, the Gβγ-complexes regulate several ion channels, specific isoforms of AC, PLC, and PI3K (see Fig. 18.2).[23] Gβγ dimers activate the Rho family G proteins to regulate actin filament reorganization and therefore induce cytoskeletal changes and impact cellular trafficking. These changes are important in response to chemokines, anaphylatoxins, or histamine. Sphingosine-1-phosphate (S1P) is a lipid-signaling molecule present in blood and lymph. Its receptor is abundantly expressed on endothelial cells and is important for lymphocytes exiting from the thymus and lymph nodes.

TABLE 18.1 Examples of G Protein–Coupled Receptors (GPCR) and Their Ligands

GPCR Superfamily	GPCR Family	GPCR	Ligands
Rhodopsin	Adenosine receptor	$A_{2A}R$	Adenosine
	Chemokine receptor	CXCR4	SDF1
		CCR2	CCL2
		CCR3	CCL5 CCL7 CCL11 CCL13 CCL26
		CCR4	CCL2 CCL4 CCL5 CCL17 CCL22
		CCR5	CCL3 CCL4 CCL5
	Bradykinin receptor	B_2R	Bradykinin
	Anaphylatoxin receptor	C5aR	C5a
	S1P receptor	S1P1	S1P
	Protease-activated receptor	PAR-1	Thrombin
		PAR-2	Trypsin
	Prostaglandin receptor	EP_2/EP_4	Prostaglandin E2
Adhesion		CD97	CD55
Secretin		GCG-R	Glucagon
Glutamate		Kainate GluR	Glutamate
Frizzled/Taste2		FZ5	Wnt5a

Wingless Type Signaling Pathways

The wingless type (Wnt) signaling pathway is a complex signaling pathway[24] that, depending on the nature of the ligands and downstream events, can be divided into two classes: the canonical and the noncanonical pathways. The canonical pathway includes Wnt1 class ligands (Wnt2, Wnt3, Wnt3a, and Wnt8a), which bind to Frizzled (Frz) receptors and their co-receptors, LRP5 and LRP6. When activated, Frz and LRP recruit and inhibit the cytoplasmic APC/Axin destruction complex, integrated by protein kinases such as casein kinase (CK)-1 and glycogen synthase kinase (GSK)-3b, the tumor suppressor adenomatous polyposis coli (APC) protein, and the scaffolding protein Axin, to stabilize β-catenin.[25] The canonical Wnt pathway is mainly involved in cell proliferation and differentiation.[26]

Noncanonical Wnt signaling is initiated by the Wnt5a types (Wnt4, Wnt5a, Wnt5b, Wnt6, Wnt7a, and Wnt11), which bind to Frz receptors, activate Dishevelled (Dvl), and, depending on the phenotypic response, are classified as Wnt/planar cell polarity (PCP) or Wnt/Ca^{2+} pathways.[27,28] The Wnt/Ca^{2+} pathway activates the Phospholipase C (PLC) pathway, which leads to the release of calcium and the activation of protein kinase C, CaMKII, and calcineurin, as well as the transcription factor nuclear factor associated with T cells (NFAT), to regulate cytoskeletal rearrangements, cell adhesion, and migration.[29] In the PCP pathway, Wnt ligands are recognized by Frz/retinoic acid-related orphan receptor (ROR)/RTK complexes.[30] This pathway activates Rho and Rac,[31] leading to cytoskeletal rearrangements and cell motility through the activation of Rho–associated kinase (ROCK)[32] and the c–Jun N–terminal kinase (JNK) signaling pathway.[31]

Innate Receptor Signaling

TLRs and nucleotide-binding oligomerization-like receptors (NLRs) constitute the major pathogen sensors of innate immunity and work in a cell autonomous fashion to initiate anti-microbial responses, including inflammation and apoptosis (Fig. 18.4). The major downstream effect of the cascades initiated by pathogen-associated molecular pattern (PAMP) recognition is IRF transcriptional activation of IFN genes that mediate inflammation and tissue repair. PAMPs are detected in endosomes and on the surface of cells by a variety of TLRs. These receptors have leucine-rich repeat domains to detect ligands, a single-pass membrane domain, and an intra-cellular Toll–interleukin-1 receptor (TIR) motif for downstream signaling. Their activities are most relevant in macrophages, monocytes, and dendritic cells.

TLR1, 2, 4, and 6 recognize varieties of endotoxin lipopolysaccharides from gram-negative bacteria, whereas TLR3, 7, 8, and 9 respond to nucleic acids that may also derive from viruses. TLR11 detects profilin protein, and the ligand for TLR10 remains uncharacterized. Response to ligand binding includes dimerization of receptors, which promotes docking of a variety of adaptor proteins, including myeloid differentiation factor (MyD)88, TIR-domain–containing adaptor protein-inducing IFN-β (TRIF), TIR-associated protein (TIRAP), and TRIF-related adaptor molecule (TRAM). A common downstream target of these cascades is NF-κB, which stimulates the transcription of inflammatory cytokines and IFN.

NLRs detect cytosolic PAMPs and endogenous inflammatory signals. Common motifs in these receptors include the nucleotide-binding oligomerization domain (NOD) and leucine-rich repeat (LRR). There are more than 20 versions of these receptors in mammals. The best-characterized is NOD1/CARD4 and NOD2/CARD15. NOD1 senses meso-diaminopimelic acid, found in gram-negative strains, whereas the NOD2 ligand is muramyl dipeptide, present in all bacteria.

C-type lectin receptors (CLRs) recognize carbohydrate structures and have an important role in inducing pro- and anti-inflammatory responses. Some CLRs, like Dectin-1, dendritic cell, and natural killer cell lectin group receptor 1 (DNGR1), have integral ITAMs in their cytoplasmatic tails. Others, like Dectin-2, macrophage C-type lectin (MCL), and macrophage-inducible C-type lectin (MINCLE), use the signaling adaptor Fc receptor γ-chain (FcRγ), whereas NKG2D, CLEC5A, and liver and lymph node sinusoidal endothelial cell C-type lectin (LSECtin) associate with DAP10. These receptors recruit SYK kinase, which activates the complex caspase-recruitment domain protein 9 (CARD9)–B cell lymphoma/leukemia 10 (BCL-10)–mucosa-associated lymphoid tissue lymphoma translocation protein 1 (MALT1) to induce NF-κB-dependent pro-inflammatory responses. DC-SIGN associates with the adaptor lymphocyte-specific protein 1 (LSP1) and can recruit the serine/threonine-protein kinase RAF1 signalosome, leading to phosphorylation and acetylation of p65 and therefore increasing pro-inflammatory responses. Phosphorylated p65 may also interact with transcription factor RELB to form a transcriptionally inactive dimer during Dectin 1-triggered noncanonical NF-κB signaling. DAP10 recruits the p85 subunit of PI3K and a growth factor receptor-bound protein 2 (GRB2)–VAV1 signaling, which leads to the activation of extra-cellular signal-regulated kinase 1 (ERK1) and ERK2. Other CLRs, like myeloid inhibitory C-type lectin (MICL), negatively regulate the signaling pathways induced by other receptors through recruiting tyrosine and inositol phosphatases, including SHIP1 and SHP1, and they are generally thought to suppress the inflammatory pathways. Some other CLRs (including CD93, L-selectin, layilin, and thrombomodulin) activate the ezrin, radixin, and moesin (ERM) complex proteins, reorganizing the actin cytoskeleton. Polycystic kidney disease 1 (PKD1) forms part of a Ca^{2+} channel and may function as an atypical G protein-coupled receptor, regulating several intra-cellular signaling pathways, including mammalian

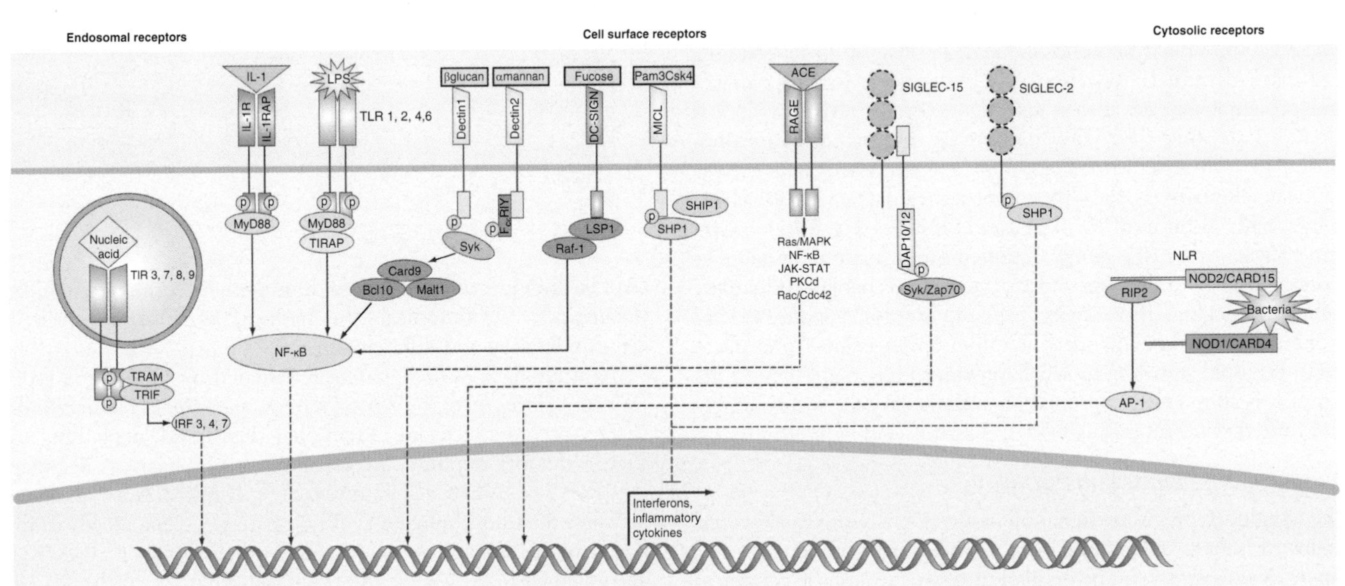

• **Fig. 18.4** Schematic depicting signaling through endosomal receptors, cell surface Toll-like receptors (TLRs), C-type lectin receptors (CLRs), receptor for advanced glycation end-products (RAGE), sialic acid-binding immunoglobulin-type lectins (Siglecs), and cytosolic nucleotide binding oligomerization domain (NOD)-like receptors (NLRs). *AP-1,* Activator protein-1; *CARD,* caspase recruitment domain; *1RAP,* IL-1 receptor accessory protein; *IRF,* interferon regulatory factor; *LPS,* lipopolysaccharide; *MyD88,* myeloid differentiation factor 88; *NF-κB,* nuclear factor-κB; *TIRAP,* Tir-domain–containing adaptor protein; *TRAM,* TRIF-related adaptor molecule; *TRIF,* Tir-domain–containing adaptor-inducing interferon-β.

target of rapamycin (mTOR) complex 1 (mTORC1) and WNT–β-catenin signaling.[33] RAGE (receptor for advanced glycation end products) is a member of the superfamily of Ig molecules and is able to bind a large variety of ligands, including advanced glycation end-products (AGEs) and damage-associated molecular patterns (DAMPs) such as HMGB1. LPS and LPA are also RAGE ligands, as are Mac-1 and complement factor 1q. Depending on the presence of different adaptor molecules and the existence of co-receptors, RAGE signaling is cell specific, involving molecules like AKT, Egr–1, the extra-cellular signal-regulated kinases (ERK1/2), GSK3β, mDia1, MEK, NF-κB, p38, p–c–Src, PI3K, PKC, Rac, Ras, ROS, or STAT3.[34]

Sialic acid-binding immunoglobulin-type lectins (Siglecs) recognize different sialylated glycoconjugates, which can lead to the activation or inhibition of the immune response. These receptors are divided into two subgroups based on sequence homology: CD33-related Siglecs, which show low gene conservation but a high degree of sequence identity, and the CD33-nonrelated, which consists of Siglec-1 (Sialoadhesin), Siglec-2 (CD22), Siglec-4 (myelin-associated glycoprotein, MAG), and Siglec-15. At a functional level, the Siglec receptors can be subdivided into those associated with DAP (DAP12 and DAP10), of which Siglec-15 is the most studied, and those with ITIMs in their cytosolic tail. While DAP-associated Siglecs can activate Zap70 and Syk pathways, leading to activation, the ITIM-bearing Siglecs recruit SHP1 and SHP2 inhibiting kinase dependent pathways.[35]

Intra-cellular Receptor Signaling

Steroid hormones synthesized from cholesterol in the adrenals and gonads, and vitamin D from dietary sources or produced by photochemistry in the skin, exert direct effects on gene expression via interaction with nuclear receptors. Because they are lipid soluble, these hormones can diffuse through plasma membranes to the nucleus to interact with receptors that directly modulate transcription, making them potent and common drug targets. In addition to endogenous molecules, many xenobiotics, such as endocrine disruptors, modulate these receptors. Almost half of the roughly 50 mammalian nuclear receptors have poorly characterized or multiple low-affinity ligands and are therefore known as *orphan receptors.*

Nuclear hormone receptors are broadly divided into two classes. Type I are retained in the cytoplasm until ligand binding drives a conformational change that releases binding partners, such as heat shock proteins, after which they translocate to the nucleus. Examples include the glucocorticoid, androgen, and estrogen receptors. Glucocorticoid agonists, such as dexamethasone and prednisolone, are important immunosuppressants. Activation not only drives gene expression changes following nuclear translocation but also transrepression of pro-inflammatory transcriptional complexes, such as AP-1 and NF-κB.

Another type I nuclear receptor of importance in immune signaling is the RAR-related orphan receptor γ (RORγ). Derived from the *RORC* gene, mRNA for this protein is detectable in a variety of tissues, but its physiologic role is largely restricted to the RORγt isoform, critical for the development and maintenance of Th17 cells. This T helper is the primary source of pro-inflammatory IL-17, which makes RORγt a target for novel drug antagonists.[36]

Type II nuclear receptors generally reside on deoxyribonucleic acid and are inhibited by co-repressor proteins until ligand detection. Examples include thyroid hormone receptor (TR), retinoic acid receptor (RAR), and vitamin D receptor (VDR). They act as heterodimers in conjunction with co-receptors, the most common of which is the retinoid X receptor (RXR). Although its major action is to regulate calcium absorption in the intestine and bone remodeling, vitamin D has increasingly been recognized as an immune modulator. Macrophages within granulomas convert vitamin D into its active form as part of an innate immune regulatory cascade.[37] Activated monocytes also generate this metabolite, and its effects are potentiated by IFN-γ. In contrast, IL-4 generated by Th2 attenuates vitamin D effects, perhaps by stimulating its degradation.

Adaptor Molecules

Adaptor proteins are noncatalytic and act as docking sites for other proteins via different motifs. These proteins help receptors recruit signaling proteins and activate different pathways.

Transmembrane Adaptor Proteins

CD3 complex, CD79, and FceR1 are molecules that associate to TCR, BCR, or other receptors, respectively, and consist of one to six chains that contain ITAM domains, which undergo phosphorylation and recruit other proteins through their SH2 domain (see Fig. 18.2).

DAP10 and DAP12 signaling subunits are highly conserved in evolution and are expressed in a wide variety of cells but especially in those of the innate immune system. DAP12 bears a single ITAM, which, after tyrosine phosphorylation, recruits and activates Syk in myeloid cells and Syk and ZAP70 in NK cells. DAP10 has a YINM sequence in its cytoplasmatic tail, which, after tyrosine phosphorylation, allows the binding of phosphatidylinositol-3 kinase (PI3K) and a Grb2–Vav1–SOS1 complex.

Linker for activation of T cells (LAT) is a transmembrane protein, whereas SH2-domain–containing leukocyte protein-76 (SLP-76) and BLNK are cytoplasmic. In their absence, activation of Src and Syk kinases fail to stimulate the pathway and calcium flux induced by PLCγ.[38]

Grb2 Family

Grb2, a member of the Grb2 family of proteins together with GADS and GRAP, is an adaptor protein required for signaling by nearly all RTKs. Grb2 associates with the guanine nucleotide exchange factor (GEF) SOS or Vav using its SH3 domains and becomes recruited to phosphorylated RTKs through its SH2 domain. This event translocates SOS and Vav close to Ras and Rac, allowing them to catalyze the exchange of GDP to GTP.

Other molecules with similar function and structure are Crk and CrkL, which play an important role in B cells, among other cells.

Tumor Necrosis Factor Receptor Signaling Adaptor Molecules

Upon TNF binding to the TNFR1, the DD recruits the TNFR-associated DD (TRADD) protein, an adaptor protein which subsequently recruits the Fas-associated protein with DD (FADD). This triggers activation of caspase 8 and caspase 3, leading to apoptosis. TNF may also activate apoptosis through the mitochondrial pathway, cytochrome C release, and activation of caspase 9 and caspase 3.

On the other hand, TNF can activate NF-κB, leading to cell survival and proliferation. This pathway involves TNF binding to TNFR1 and recruitment of TRADD, followed by TNFR-associated factor 2 (TRAF2/TRAF5), receptor-interacting protein (RIP), TAK1, and IκB kinase (IKK). TNF–TNFR1 signaling regulates proliferation through TRAF2 to activate MEKK1, MKK7, and JNK. p38 MAPK is activated through TRAF2 and MKK3.[39,40]

TNFR2 can bind TRAF2 directly and indirectly recruit TRAF1, TRAF-associated NF-κB activator (TANK), and cellular inhibitors of apoptosis (cIAPs), thereby activating the NF-κB pathway. In addition, TNFR2 signaling can also activate the MAPK pathways efficiently. Despite the general belief that TNFR1 signaling induces apoptosis and the TNFR2 pathway is prosurvival, cross-talk exists between the two pathways, and TNFR2 signaling may also lead to apoptosis in some cells.[41]

Myeloid Differentiation Primary Response Gene 88 and IL-1R Associated Kinase

Interaction of TLRs with components of bacterial and viral pathogens, or the activation of the receptors for IL-1, IL-18 or IL-33, leads to the recruitment of the adaptor molecule myeloid differentiation primary response gene 88 (MyD88), followed by the recruitment and interaction of different subunits of the IL-1R–associated kinase (IRAK) family to form a complex known as the Myddosome, which switches on pro-inflammatory pathways.[16,42]

TRIF

Production of type I IFNs depends on TRIF signaling. TRIF recruits TRAF3, RIP1, and RIP3 and is also implicated in the activation of IRAK1 and IRAK2.

TRAM and TIRAP

These adaptor molecules act as bridging adaptors for MyD88 and TRIF in the context of specific TLRs. In this way, TIRAP binds MyD88 to TLR2 and TLR4, whereas TRAM couples TRIF to TLR4.

Second Messengers

Some of the proteins recruited and activated after the binding of the ligand generate second messengers, which include small, nonprotein molecules such as phospholipids and calcium. Two enzymes that have a major role in the generation of lipid second messengers are PLC and PI3K.

Phospholipase C Signaling: Calcium Flux and Protein Kinase C Activation

Activated PLC leads to the generation of IP_3 and DAG from PIP_2. IP_3 is a soluble second messenger, which leads to the release of stored Ca^{2+} into the cytoplasm. This second messenger activates calmodulin and other Ca^{2+}-binding proteins. Calmodulin activates Ras/MAPK via indirect activation of Ras or directly through activation of Raf-1.[43] In addition, calmodulin activates the serine/threonine phosphatase calcineurin, which dephosphorylates NFAT. This exposes a nuclear localization signal (NLS), which leads to nuclear import and transcription regulation.[44] On the other hand, DAG acts as a second messenger to stimulate PKC. These proteins are also related to the control of NF-κB (via phosphorylation of IKK) and activator protein (AP)-1 transcription factors.[45]

PI3K/Akt Pathway

The PI3K family is divided into three classes on the basis of structure, regulation, and lipid substrate specificity. The focus of this discussion will be on class I because it controls the Akt/mTOR pathway, which is involved in proliferation, differentiation, motility, and intra-cellular trafficking (see Fig. 18.2).[46] Class I PI3Ks are composed of four heterodimeric proteins, including a catalytic (p110) and a regulatory (p85) subunit, and generate PIP_3 upon activation. The group is further divided into subclasses on the basis of the regulatory subunit they bind. Class IA is composed of p110 α, β, and δ catalytic subunits, which bind isoforms of p85 and are activated by tyrosine kinase–associated receptors. Phosphorylation of different ITAMs causes recruitment of PI3K through the SH2 domain and, eventually, generation of PIP_3 from PIP_2.[47] Akt is a serine/threonine kinase that is recruited to the plasma membrane through its PH domain and binds PIP_3. Akt is activated by phosphorylation by phosphoinositide-dependent kinase 1 (PDK-1) and mTOR complex 2. Active Akt phosphorylates a number of targets such as FOXO1, 3A and 4, GSK3α/β, RAF1, TSC2, and PRAS40 (both of which are then inhibited, allowing mTOR 1 function), IKKα (leading to activation of NF-κB), p21CIP1, BAD, or caspase 9.

Signaling Pathways

The binding of a ligand to its receptor triggers several events that lead to the activation of different and specific signaling pathways. These pathways lead to the modification of cell behavior at different levels, including cytoskeleton and metabolic changes and activation of transcription factors.

JAK/STAT Pathway

The mammalian JAK family includes four tyrosine kinases: JAK1, JAK2, JAK3, and tyrosine kinase 2 (Tyk2) (Fig. 18.5). All four proteins have a conserved kinase domain and a related pseudokinase regulatory domain. JAK1 and JAK2 are involved in a wide range of cellular functions in growth and development, hematopoiesis, and inflammation, whereas JAK3 and Tyk2 are primarily important in the immune response. JAKs are controlled predominantly by post-translational mechanisms. More than 30 class I cytokine receptors and approximately 12 class II cytokine receptors activate the JAK family members. JAK structure is distinct from other tyrosine kinases. The N-terminal of these proteins contains two domains: an SH2 domain and a band 4.1 ezrin radixin moesin (FERM) domain. Interestingly, however, the SH2 domains do not function as phosphotyrosine residues but instead act as scaffolds. Upon cytokine-receptor binding, JAKs are reciprocally activated by phosphorylation and phosphorylate receptor cytoplasmic tail regions. This leads to recruitment and activation of the SH2 domain-containing proteins known as the *STATs* (STAT1, 2, 3, 4, 5A, 5B, and 6). The STAT proteins share a high homology in their SH2 domain: a DNA-binding domain and a transactivation domain. STATs bind to the phosphorylated receptor through their SH2 domain and are activated in response to phosphorylation by JAKs. Upon phosphorylation, STATs undergo conformational changes, detach from the receptor, and dimerize with another STAT molecule. Dimers may be homo- or heterodimers, which subsequently translocate to the nucleus to regulate gene expression.[48,49]

Different STATs are important for the signaling of distinct cytokines and/or growth factors/hormones (see Fig. 18.5). In addition to the STAT proteins, JAK activation also leads to recruitment of SHP2 and Shc, p85, and suppressor of cytokine signaling (SOCS)-3, which leads to regulation of Ras/MAPK and PI3K cascades. STAT proteins continually traffic between the cytoplasm and nucleus to mediate their function as transcription factors.[50] However, not all STATs travel in the same manner. STAT1 and STAT4 entry into the nucleus depends on their tyrosine phosphorylation and, importantly, dimerization, which creates a nuclear localization signal. Unphosphorylated STAT2 is constantly imported into the nucleus in complex with IRF-9, but is shuttled back into the cytoplasm because of its dominant nuclear export signal. After phosphorylation, it can dimerize with STAT1 to import the complex into the nucleus. STAT3, 5, and 6 are continually imported to the nucleus regardless of their tyrosine phosphorylation state.

Cytokine responses and the JAK-STAT pathway are under tight control of molecules, including PTPs, protein inhibitor of activated STATs (PIAS), and SOCS proteins.[51] PTPs include SH2-containing PTP1 (SHP1), SHP2, CD45, and T cell PTP (TCPTP). The PTP and PIAS proteins, although not exclusive regulators of the JAK-STAT pathway, also regulate other cellular functions. PIAS inhibit the STATs by interfering with their DNA binding function and also, likely, by recruiting histone deacetylases. The SOCS family consists of eight members: SOCS 1-7 and cytokine-induced STAT inhibitors (CISs), which block STAT activation. SOCS3 acts mainly by binding to the JAK and the cytokine receptor, which leads to inhibition of STAT3 activation. Besides STAT3, SOCS3 can also regulate signaling through other STATs. SOCS3 can either inhibit JAK activation or lead to ubiquitin-proteasome–mediated degradation of the receptor.

Mammalian/Mechanistic Target of Rapamycin (mTOR) Pathway

Mammalian/mechanistic target of rapamycin (mTOR) is a central integrator of growth signals and cellular metabolism with an important role in both innate and adaptive immune responses. mTOR exists in two structurally distinct complexes: mTOR complex 1 (mTORC1), which associates with the adaptor Raptor, and mTORC2, which associates with Rictor.[52,53] Activation of mTORC1 by the PI3K/AKT pathway leads to the phosphorylation of ribosomal protein S6 kinase (S6K), eukaryotic translation initiation factor 4E (eIF4E), and 4E binding proteins (4E-BPs) to promote the translation of metabolic enzymes required for proliferation,[54] and the synthesis of transcription factors such as Myc and HIF-1α critical for metabolic reprogramming.[55] mTORC1 is also involved in the regulation of pyrimidine biosynthesis, mitochondrial tetrahydrofolate (mTHF) cycle, and stimulation of lipid and sterol biosynthesis through activation of S6K, ATF4, and sterol regulatory binding element proteins (SREBPs).[56]

Activation of AKT through phosphorylation at Ser473 residue by mTORC2 can lead to the enhancement of glycolytic metabolism through the induction of the enzyme glucokinase (GCK).[57] In addition, mTORC2-dependent acetylation and phosphorylation of FoxO1 acts as a switch toward pro-growth metabolism.[58]

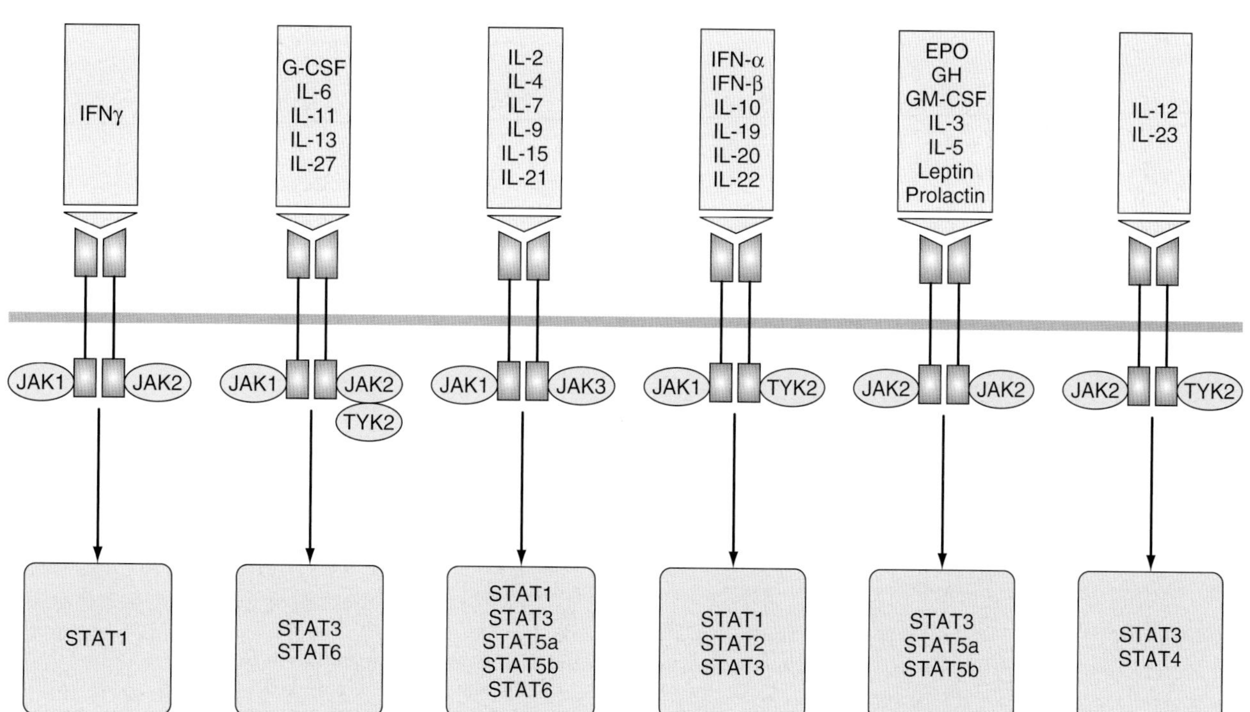

• **Fig. 18.5** Janus kinase (JAK)/signal transducer and activator of transcription (STAT) pathway. Activation of different JAK/STAT combinations by major cytokines. Cytokine receptors recruit and activate specific pairs of JAK kinases, which induce STAT phosphorylation and dimerization. STAT dimers translocate into the nucleus, where they act as transcription factors. *EPO,* Erythropoietin; *G-CSF,* granulocyte-colony stimulating factor; *GH,* growth hormone; *GM-CSF,* granulocyte-macrophage colony-stimulating factor; *IFN,* interferon.

MAPK Pathway

A wide range of extra-cellular signals, including cytokines, stress, and growth factors, can activate a series of MAPKs to ultimately regulate gene expression and diverse cellular processes, including growth, proliferation, survival, and inflammatory immune responses. The MAPK signal cascades involve three tiers of activation (Fig. 18.6). The first level of activation is the MAPK kinase kinase (MAPKKK or MAP3K), which includes activated Raf, apoptosis signal-regulating kinase (ASK)1, MEKK1-4, MLK, and TGF-β–associated kinase (TAK)1. MAPKKK phosphorylates and activates the next tier MAPKK, examples of which include MEK1/2 and the MKKs. MAPKK then phosphorylates the third tier of MAPK molecules, which includes three families, namely, ERK1/2, JNK, and p38 (α, β, γ, and δ), the latter two of which are stress-activated MAPKs. Finally, ERK, JNK, and p38 activate transcription factors, which include Ets, Elk-1, c-Myc activating transcription factor (ATF)2, p53, cAMP response element binding protein (CREB), NF-κB, and AP-1. Activation of transcription factors may occur through direct phosphorylation or via modulation of ribosomal S6 kinase activity in the case of CREB and via IKK in the case of NF-κB. JNK also regulates activity of nontranscription factors, such as the apoptosis-related Bcl-2 molecules.

Distinct signals activate the three families of MAPKs (although there can be considerable cross-talk): ERK1/2, p38, and JNK. ERK1 and 2 are serine/threonine kinases that are components of the Ras-Raf-MEK-ERK cascade of the MAPK pathways.[59] Whereas Raf and MEK kinases have limited substrate specificity, ERK1/2 phosphorylate and activate a vast number of cellular targets, including a large number of transcription factors. ERK1/2 are activated by a variety of cellular stimuli, including bradykinin, epidermal growth factor, FGF, insulin IGF1, PDGF, cytokines, and osmotic stress. Activation of this pathway regulates cell adhesion, migration, survival, proliferation, and differentiation. The p38 α and β isoforms are ubiquitous in their distribution; the γ isoform is mainly expressed in skeletal muscle; and the δ isoform is expressed in the testes, pancreas, and the small intestine. p38 MAPK is activated via pro-inflammatory cytokines and lipopolysaccharide (LPS). The p38 MAPK is critically important for the production of IL-1, TNF, and IL-6 pro-inflammatory cytokines. The JNK proteins are encoded by JNK1, JNK2, and JNK3 genes, and alternative splicing results in additional isoforms and complexity. JNK1 and JNK2 are ubiquitous in their tissue distribution, whereas JNK3 is expressed mostly in the brain, heart, and testis. Pro-inflammatory cytokines, such as IL-1 and TNF, and UV radiation lead to JNK phosphorylation. The JNKs are involved in modulation of the extra-cellular matrix by regulating production of metalloproteinases.[60] A specific subgroup of protein tyrosine phosphatases that inactivate the MAPKs are called MAPK phosphatases (MKPs) and include MKP1, 3, 5, and 7, which can inactivate JNK and provide a means to regulate MAPK activity.

Therefore the MAPKs integrate signals from different receptors to regulate transcription factors to control a variety of overlapping genes and to ultimately regulate cellular survival, proliferation, and differentiation under physiologic and pathologic conditions.[61–63]

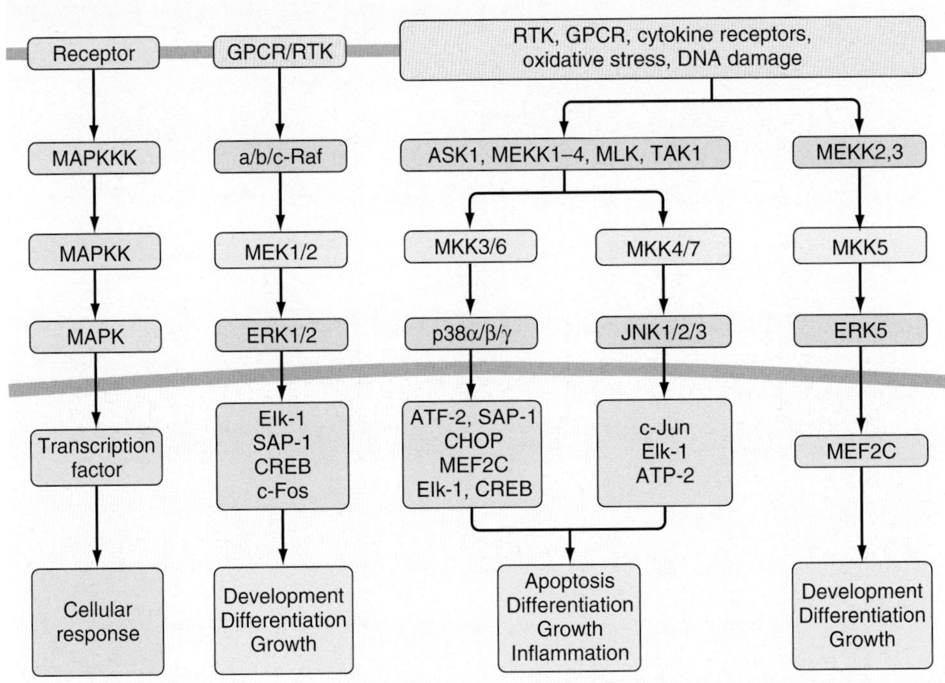

• **Fig. 18.6** Mitogen-activated protein kinase pathway (MAPK). A general schematic of the MAPK signaling pathway is shown on the *left*. On the *right* are specific receptors and three tiers in the MAPK cascades. Transcription factors and cellular responses activated by the different pathways are indicated. *ASK,* Apoptosis signal-regulating kinase; *ATF2,* activating transcription factor 2; *C/EBP,* CCAAT enhancer binding protein; *CHOP,* C/EBP homologous protein; *CREB,* cyclic adenosine monophosphate (AMP) response element–binding protein; *ERK,* extra-cellular signal-regulated kinase; *GPCR,* G protein–coupled receptor; *JNK,* c-Jun N-terminal kinase; *MEF2C,* myocyte-enhancer factor 2C; *MLK,* mixed lineage kinases; *RTK,* receptor tyrosine kinase; *SAPK,* stress-activated protein kinase; *TAK,* TGF-β–associated kinase.

IRAK

Interleukin-1 receptor-associated kinase (IRAK) is a family of kinases implicated in the signal transduction of the TLR/IL-1R family. Four members have been identified.

IRAK4 is the first member recruited by MyD88, and it has an important role for the MyD88-dependent activation of NF-κB and MAPKs and production of inflammatory mediators. Interaction with other members of IRAK family leads to differential signaling.[64–66] Recruitment of IRAK1 has a critical function in plasmacytoid dendritic cells for the production of IFN-γ and is also involved in the activation of the NLRP3 inflammasome, which leads to IL-18 production.[67,68] IRAK2, which is, with IRAK4, part of the Myddosome, has a role in the activation of nuclear factor (NF)-kB[41] and can interact with the TLR3 signaling adaptor Mal/TIRAP. Along with IRAK1, IRAK2 is important in the formation of polyubiquitin chains associated with TNFR-associated factor 6 (TRAF6) signaling. Unlike the other IRAK family members, IRAK3 is only expressed in monocytes and macrophages and is a negative regulator of TLR signaling.[69]

Transcription Factors

One of the important effects of the different cell signaling pathways is the activation of transcription factors. These proteins eventually activate or repress the expression of specific genes through the binding to specific regions within their promoters.

Nuclear Factor (NF)-κB

NF-κB transcription factors can act both as activators or repressors for gene expression. There are five members in mammalians: RelA (p65), RelB, c-Rel, p50/p105 (NF-κB1), and p52/p100 (NF-κB2), which form different complexes by combinations that can be homo- and heterodimers. NF-κB complexes are retained in the cytoplasm by a family of inhibitory proteins known as *inhibitors of NF-κB* (IκBs). IKK, which is the activator of NF-κB, is composed of two catalytic subunits and one regulatory subunit known as the *NF-κB essential modulator* (NEMO). Activation of NF-κB typically involves the phosphorylation of IκB by the IκB kinase (IKK) complex, which results in IκB degradation and translocation of NF-κB to the nucleus, where it drives the transcription of pro-inflammatory cytokines, such as IL-6, IL-18, chemokines, cyclooxygenase 2 (COX-2), and 5-lipoxygenase (5-LOX), controlling programmed cell death (apoptosis), cell adhesion, and proliferation, among other pathways.[70]

Activator Protein (AP)-1

The AP-1 family in humans is composed of homo- and heterodimer members of the ATF (ATF2, ATF3/LRF1, B-ATF, JDP1, and JDP2), Fos (c-Fos, FosB, Fra-1, and Fra-2), Jun (c-Jun, JunB, and JunD), and MAF (c-Maf, MafB, MafA, MafG/F/K, and Nrl) protein families. The AP-1 complex binds to the promoters of specific genes and transactivates or represses them.[71]

NFAT

There are four NFAT proteins in mammalian cells, NFAT1-4, which are expressed in different cell types from the immune system. NFAT-family proteins are activated by calcium signaling downstream of various receptors, including TCR, BCR, FcR, and receptors coupled to certain heterotrimeric G proteins. NFAT is involved in regulation of cytokines like IL-2 and different surface receptors.[44]

CREB/CREM

The cyclic AMP responsive element-binding protein (CREB) and the cAMP responsive element modulator (CREM) are two transcription factors involved, among others, in the regulation of IL-2. They compete for binding to the promoter of IL-2 where CREB exerts a positive effect on transcription and CREM is a negative regulator.[72,73]

Conclusion

Discovery of these signaling pathways has provided valuable insights into immune pathogenesis of autoimmune and immunodeficiency diseases. Many receptors and/or signaling pathways are potential therapeutic targets for immune-mediated diseases. Because many of the signaling pathways and molecules are widely expressed, carefully balancing the risk and benefit of perturbing them will be a critical component of a drug development program.

The references for this chapter can also be found on ExpertConsult.com.

References

1. Lemmon MA, Schlessinger J: Cell signaling by receptor tyrosine kinases, *Cell* 141(7):1117–1134, 2010.
2. Schlessinger J: Receptor tyrosine kinases: legacy of th first two decades, *Cold Spring Harb Perspect Biol* 6(3), 2014.
3. Massagué J: TGFβ signalling in context, *Nat Rev Mol Cell Biol* 13(10):616–630, 2012.
4. Morikawa M, Koinuma D, Miyazono K, et al.: Genome-wide mechanisms of Smad binding, *Oncogene* 32(13):1609–1615, 2013.
5. Hertz M, Kouskoff V, Nakamura T, et al.: V(D)J recombinase induction in splenic B lymphocytes is inhibited by antigen-receptor signalling, *Nature* 394(6690):292–295, 1998.
6. Love PE, Bhandoola A: Signal integration and crosstalk during thymocyte migration and emigration, *Nat Rev Immunol* 11(7):469–477, 2011.
7. Bradshaw JM: The Src, Syk, and Tec family kinases: distinct types of molecular switches, *Cell Signal* 22(8):1175–1184, 2010.
8. Mano H: Tec family of protein-tyrosine kinases: an overview of their structure and function, *Cytokine Growth Factor Rev* 10(3–4):267–280, 1999.
9. Chen L, Flies DB: Molecular mechanisms of T cell co-stimulation and co-inhibition, *Nat Rev Immunol* 13(4):227–242, 2013.
10. Detre C, Keszei M, Romero X, et al.: SLAM family receptors and the SLAM-associated protein (SAP) modulate T cell functions, *Semin Immunopathol* 32(2):157–171, 2010.
11. Francisco LM, Sage PT, Sharpe AH: The PD-1 pathway in tolerance and autoimmunity, *Immunol Rev* 236:219–242, 2010.
12. Shachar I, Karin N: The dual roles of inflammatory cytokines and chemokines in the regulation of autoimmune diseases and their clinical implications, *J Leukoc Biol* 93(1):51–61, 2013.
13. Wang X, Lupardus P, Laporte SL, et al.: Structural biology of shared cytokine receptors, *Annu Rev Immunol* 27:29–60, 2009.
14. Renauld J-C: Class II cytokine receptors and their ligands: key antiviral and inflammatory modulators, *Nat Rev Immunol* 3(8):667–676, 2003.

15. Locksley RM, Killeen N, Lenardo MJ: The TNF and TNF receptor superfamilies: integrating mammalian biology, *Cell* 104(4):487–501, 2001.
16. Kawai T, Akira S: TLR signaling, *Cell Death Differ* 13(5):816–825, 2006.
17. Dunne A, O'Neill LAJ: The interleukin-1 receptor/Toll-like receptor superfamily: signal transduction during inflammation and host defense, *Sci STKE Signal Transduct Knowl Environ* 2003(171):re3, 2003.
18. Ponta H, Sherman L, Herrlich PA: CD44: from adhesion molecules to signalling regulators, *Nat Rev Mol Cell Biol* 4(1):33–45, 2003.
19. Baaten BJ, Li C-R, Bradley LM: Multifaceted regulation of T cells by CD44, *Commun Integr Biol* 3(6):508–512, 2010.
20. Hogg N, Patzak I, Willenbrock F: The insider's guide to leukocyte integrin signalling and function, *Nat Rev Immunol* 11(6):416–426, 2011.
21. Shattil SJ, Kim C, Ginsberg MH: The final steps of integrin activation: the end game, *Nat Rev Mol Cell Biol* 11(4):288–300, 2010.
22. Springer TA, Dustin ML: Integrin inside-out signaling and the immunological synapse, *Curr Opin Cell Biol* 24(1):107–115, 2012.
23. Wettschureck N, Offermanns S: Mammalian G proteins and their cell type specific functions, *Physiol Rev* 85(4):1159–1204, 2005.
24. Nusse R, Lim X: *The Wnt homepage* (website). http://web.stanford.edu/group/nusselab/cgi-bin/wnt/. Accessed January 30, 2019.
25. Nusse R, Clevers H: Wnt/β-Catenin signaling, disease, and emerging therapeutic modalities, *Cell* 169(6):985–999, 2017.
26. Niehrs C, Acebron SP: Mitotic and mitogenic Wnt signalling, *EMBO J* 31(12):2705–2713, 2012.
27. Kühl M: Non-canonical Wnt signaling in Xenopus: regulation of axis formation and gastrulation, *Semin Cell Dev Biol* 13(3):243–249, 2002.
28. Pandur P, Maurus D, Kühl M: Increasingly complex: new players enter the Wnt signaling network, *Bio Essays News Rev Mol Cell Dev Biol* 24(10):881–884, 2002.
29. Kohn AD, Moon RT: Wnt and calcium signaling: beta-catenin-independent pathways, *Cell Calcium* 38(3–4):439–446, 2005.
30. Famili F, Perez LG, Naber BA, et al.: The non-canonical Wnt receptor Ryk regulates hematopoietic stem cell repopulation in part by controlling proliferation and apoptosis, *Cell Death Dis* 7(11):e2479, 2016.
31. Habas R, Dawid IB, He X: Coactivation of Rac and Rho by Wnt/Frizzled signaling is required for vertebrate gastrulation, *Genes Dev* 17(2):295–309, 2003.
32. Marlow F, Topczewski J, Sepich D, et al.: Zebrafish Rho kinase 2 acts downstream of Wnt11 to mediate cell polarity and effective convergence and extension movements, *Curr Biol CB* 12(11):876–884, 2002.
33. Brown GD, Willment JA, Whitehead L: C-type lectins in immunity and homeostasis, *Nat Rev Immunol* 18(6):374–389, 2018.
34. Kierdorf K, Fritz G: RAGE regulation and signaling in inflammation and beyond, *J Leukoc Biol* 94(1):55–68, 2013.
35. Bornhöfft KF, Goldammer T, Rebl A, et al.: Siglecs: a journey through the evolution of sialic acid-binding immunoglobulin-type lectins, *Dev Comp Immunol* 86:219–231, 2018.
36. Kojetin DJ, Burris TP: REV-ERB and ROR nuclear receptors as drug targets, *Nat Rev Drug Discov* 13(3):197–216, 2014.
37. Lagishetty V, Liu NQ, Hewison M: Vitamin D metabolism and innate immunity, *Mol Cell Endocrinol* 347(1–2):97–105, 2011.
38. Yablonski D, Weiss A: Mechanisms of signaling by the hematopoietic-specific adaptor proteins, SLP-76 and LAT and their B cell counterpart, BLNK/SLP-65, *Adv Immunol* 79:93–128, 2001.
39. Aggarwal BB, Gupta SC, Kim JH: Historical perspectives on tumor necrosis factor and its superfamily: 25 years later, a golden journey, *Blood* 119(3):651–665, 2012.
40. Bradley JR, Pober JS: Tumor necrosis factor receptor-associated factors (TRAFs), *Oncogene* 20(44):6482–6491, 2001.
41. Naudé PJW, den Boer JA, Luiten PGM, et al.: Tumor necrosis factor receptor cross-talk, *FEBS J* 278(6):888–898, 2011.
42. Lin S-C, Lo Y-C, Wu H: Helical assembly in the MyD88-IRAK4-IRAK2 complex in TLR/IL-1R signalling, *Nature* 465(7300):885–890, 2010.
43. Agell N, Bachs O, Rocamora N, et al.: Modulation of the Ras/Raf/MEK/ERK pathway by Ca (2+), and calmodulin, *Cell Signal* 14(8):649–654, 2002.
44. Macian F: NFAT proteins: key regulators of T-cell development and function, *Nat Rev Immunol* 5(6):472–484, 2005.
45. Tan S-L, Parker PJ: Emerging and diverse roles of protein kinase C in immune cell signalling, *Biochem J* 376(Pt 3):545–552, 2003.
46. Manning BD, Cantley LC: AKT/PKB signaling: navigating downstream, *Cell* 129(7):1261–1274, 2007.
47. Deane JA, Fruman DA: Phosphoinositide 3-kinase: diverse roles in immune cell activation, *Annu Rev Immunol* 22:563–598, 2004.
48. O'Shea JJ, Holland SM, Staudt LM: JAKs and STATs in immunity, immunodeficiency, and cancer, *N Engl J Med* 368(2):161–170, 2013.
49. Rawlings JS, Rosler KM, Harrison DA: The JAK/STAT signaling pathway, *J Cell Sci* 117(Pt 8):1281–1283, 2004.
50. Reich NC: STATs get their move on, *JAK-STAT* 2(4):e27080, 2013.
51. Carow B, Rottenberg ME: SOCS3, a major regulator of infection and inflammation, *Front Immunol* 5:58, 2014.
52. Kim D-H, Sarbassov DD, Ali SM, et al.: mTOR interacts with raptor to form a nutrient-sensitive complex that signals to the cell growth machinery, *Cell* 110(2):163–175, 2002.
53. Sarbassov DD, Guertin DA, Ali SM, et al.: Phosphorylation and regulation of Akt/PKB by the rictor-mTOR complex, *Science* 307(5712):1098–1101, 2005.
54. Morita M, Gravel S-P, Chénard V, et al.: mTORC1 controls mitochondrial activity and biogenesis through 4E-BP-dependent translational regulation, *Cell Metab* 18(5):698–711, 2013.
55. Barnhart BC, Lam JC, Young RM, et al.: Effects of 4E-BP1 expression on hypoxic cell cycle inhibition and tumor cell proliferation and survival, *Cancer Biol Ther* 7(9):1441–1449, 2008.
56. Ben-Sahra I, Hoxhaj G, Ricoult SJH, et al.: mTORC1 induces purine synthesis through control of the mitochondrial tetrahydrofolate cycle, *Science* 351(6274):728–733, 2016.
57. Kishore M, Cheung KCP, Fu H, et al.: Regulatory T cell migration is dependent on glucokinase-mediated glycolysis, *Immunity* 47(5):875–889.e10, 2017.
58. Masui K, Tanaka K, Akhavan D, etal.: mTOR complex 2 controls glycolytic metabolism in glioblastoma through FoxO acetylation and upregulation of c-Myc, *Cell Metab* 18(5):726–739, 2013.
59. Roskoski R: ERK1/2 MAP kinases: structure, function, and regulation, *Pharmacol Res* 66(2):105–143, 2012.
60. Sweeney SE, Firestein GS: Mitogen activated protein kinase inhibitors: where are we now and where are we going? *Ann Rheum Dis* 65(Suppl 3):iii83–iii88, 2006.
61. Dong C, Davis RJ, Flavell RA: MAP kinases in the immune response, *Annu Rev Immunol* 20:55–72, 2002.
62. Huang G, Shi LZ, Chi H: Regulation of JNK and p38 MAPK in the immune system: signal integration, propagation and termination, *Cytokine* 48(3):161–169, 2009.
63. Guma M, Firestein GS: c-Jun N-terminal kinase in inflammation and rheumatic diseases, *Open Rheumatol J* 6:220–231, 2012.
64. Kawagoe T, Sato S, Jung A, et al.: Essential role of IRAK-4 protein and its kinase activity in Toll-like receptor-mediated immune responses but not in TCR signaling, *J Exp Med* 204(5):1013–1024, 2007.
65. Kawagoe T, Sato S, Matsushita K, et al.: Sequential control of Toll-like receptor-dependent responses by IRAK1 and IRAK2, *Nat Immunol* 9(6):684–691, 2008.
66. Koziczak-Holbro M, Glück A, Tschopp C, et al.: IRAK-4 kinase activity-dependent and -independent regulation of lipopolysaccharide-inducible genes, *Eur J Immunol* 38(3):788–796, 2008.

67. Fernandes-Alnemri T, Kang S, Anderson C, et al.: Cutting edge: TLR signaling licenses IRAK1 for rapid activation of the NLRP3 inflammasome, *J Immunol Baltim Md 1950* 191(8):3995–3999, 2013.
68. Lin K-M, Hu W, Troutman TD, et al.: IRAK-1 bypasses priming and directly links TLRs to rapid NLRP3 inflammasome activation, *Proc Natl Acad Sci U S A* 111(2):775–780, 2014.
69. Kobayashi K, Hernandez LD, Galán JE, et al.: IRAK-M is a negative regulator of Toll-like receptor signaling, *Cell* 110(2):191–202, 2002.
70. Perkins ND: Integrating cell-signalling pathways with NF-κB and IKK function, *Nat Rev Mol Cell Biol* 8(1):49–62, 2007.
71. Karin M, Liu Z g, Zandi E: AP-1 function and regulation, *Curr Opin Cell Biol* 9(2):240–246, 1997.
72. Elliott MR, Tolnay M, Tsokos GC, et al.: Protein kinase a regulatory subunit type IIβ directly interacts with and suppresses CREB transcriptional activity in activated T cells, *J Immunol* 171(7):3636–3644, 2003.
73. Liao W, Lin J-X, Leonard WJ: Interleukin-2 at the crossroads of effector responses, tolerance, and immunotherapy, *Immunity* 38(1):13–25, 2013.

19

The Immunologic Repercussions of Cell Death

HELEN M. BEERE AND DOUGLAS R. GREEN

KEY POINTS

- Apoptosis is a discrete form of cell death induced by multiple stimuli and mediated by a group of cysteine proteases known as caspases. This type of cell death is characterized by the degradation of nuclear DNA and is generally non-inflammatory.
- Apoptosis and caspase activation can be triggered extra-cellularly by engagement of death receptors, or intrinsically by mitochondrial damage and release of cytochrome-c and Smac/DIABLO, which function to activate caspases at the apoptosome.
- The Bcl-2 family includes both pro- and anti-apoptotic proteins that control cell death by regulating the mitochondrial outer membrane potential (MOMP).
- Necrosis and necroptosis are both death processes that involve swelling of cells and rupture of the plasma membrane, resulting in inflammation.
- Necroptosis is a specialized form of necrosis that is initiated by death ligands and regulated by signaling pathways that are also important for the regulation of apoptosis.
- Nod-like receptor (NLR) molecules act as cell stress sensors to trigger inflammasome assembly and activation of caspase-1 to mediate the processing of the pro-inflammatory cytokines IL-1β and IL-18 and the cleavage of Gasdermin-D to trigger formation of a membrane pore, through which active IL-1β and IL-18 are released and pyroptosis is induced.
- Autophagy is a normal cellular response to nutrient deprivation that is characterized by the degradation and recycling of cellular components.

Introduction

Cell death can proceed by one of several distinct pathways in response to signals arising from intra- and extra-cellular stresses such as DNA damage, metabolic disruption, or infection. The removal of damaged or redundant cells is critical for development, tissue turnover, and restoration of homeostasis following tissue damage or disease—but once destined to die, why does it matter how the cell engages this death?

It turns out that not all cell deaths are created equal, at least in the context of immune function. A dead or dying cell can modulate the immune response via multiple mechanisms, including the release of cytokines and chemokines. Furthermore, it is the specific type of cell death engaged that determines the nature of those signals and whether or not that cell death process is non-inflammatory or pro-inflammatory—or even, in some cases, actively suppresses inflammation. In this review, we will introduce several different types of cell death and discuss the defining features of each. The impact of these cell death pathways on immune function will be discussed in the context of disease pathologies associated with aberrant immune regulation and defects in cell death pathways.

Types of Cell Death

Apoptosis

Perhaps the best characterized of the cell death pathways is apoptosis (type I cell death), characterized by key phenotypic characteristics including perturbation and blebbing of the plasma membrane from which small membrane bound vesicles, so-called "apoptotic bodies," are released. The plasma membrane maintains its integrity but undergoes lipid reorganization to externalize phospholipids on the cell surface. This particular event is critical with regard to how apoptotic cells are detected by the immune system. Within a cell dying by apoptosis, chromatin condenses and internucleosomal DNA cleavage proceeds, before which the dying cell then begins to shrink and, if adherent, detaches from neighboring cells and surrounding stroma and matrix.

These changes are mediated by the induced enzymatic activity of a family of cysteine proteases, the caspases that mediate the apoptotic demise of the cell and, as such, caspase activation represents one of the most universal and informative descriptive biochemical features of apoptotic cell death. There are several different caspases, each activated and regulated by different signaling pathways so that apoptotic cell death can be engaged in response to multiple types of damage or stress.

Once caspases have cleaved their target substrates, the now apoptotic cell is rapidly removed from the body via phagocytosis. Therefore, in contrast to other types of cell death, apoptosis generally, but not always, fails to evoke an inflammatory response. Even so, the term "immunologically silent," often used to describe apoptosis, is somewhat misleading. Following their engulfment by phagocytes, apoptotic cells can remain a source of signals able to regulate components of immune function.

Necrosis—Classic or Noncanonical?

Necrosis (type III cell death) is likely familiar to most as a nonprogrammed, disordered type of death, characterized by swelling of both the cell and its intra-cellular organelles, rupture of the plasma membrane, and release of intra-cellular contents. Such death can be triggered by stresses such as altered tonicity, heat, or physical trauma, and by intra-cellular events such as Ca^{2+} efflux or a rapid decrease in adenosine triphosphate (ATP) levels. "Programmed necrosis" or necroptosis is similarly characterized by rupture of the plasma membrane but is fundamentally distinct from "classic" necrosis, in that it is mediated by specific signaling pathways. Nonetheless, cellular rupture, irrespective of associated signaling events, releases numerous immune activators or danger-associated molecule patterns (DAMPs) to generate a potent inflammatory response.

Features typically associated with apoptosis can be detected in cells undergoing necroptotic death, including the externalization of inner membrane phosphatidyl-serine, partial chromatin condensation, and phagocytic uptake. The requirement for caspase activity is generally used to discriminate apoptosis from necrosis (but see pyroptosis, discussed in the following section). However, caspase activity, critical for apoptosis, is not only dispensable for necroptotic cell death but in some cases actually requires the active inhibition of one specific caspase for programmed necrosis to proceed (discussed later).

Necroptosis can be induced by death receptors of the TNF superfamily, members of the immune sensing Toll-like receptors (TLRs), and as part of the interferon response. Accordingly, a close, and in some cases overlapping, functional relationship, between signaling components of the immune system and those of necroptosis has emerged. Several components of the upstream death receptor signaling machinery are common to both apoptosis and necroptosis but, downstream, specialized death pathway-specific adapters ensure the appropriate engagement of each form of cell death. For example, in the case of necroptosis, the critical effector molecules are the receptor interacting protein kinase 3 (RIPK3) and its substrate, mixed lineage kinase domain-like (MLKL).

Pyroptosis

Pyroptosis, also a form of regulated necrosis, is mediated by the catalytic activity of the "inflammatory caspases," which include caspase-1 and, under some circumstances, caspase-4 and caspase-5 (caspase-11 in rodents).[1,2] Pyroptosis is mediated by one caspase substrate, which causes cellular lysis that is preceded by a marked increase in cell size, attributed to a caspase-dependent formation of membrane pores, which is thought to provoke a consequent disruption of ionic gradients across the cell membrane and an increase in osmotic pressure that causes water influx, cell swelling, and membrane rupture. There is, however, evidence that additional steps are required for full cell lysis.[3] The resulting release of intra-cellular contents provides a localized pool of potential pro-inflammatory molecules that include both direct activators of immune cells as well as so-called "danger signals" that trigger the production of inflammatory molecules from other cells. Because caspase-1 (but not caspase-4, -5, or -11) can also cleave and activate executioner caspases (e.g., caspase-3 and caspase-7, see later), caspase-1 activation can induce apoptosis when the substrate responsible for pyroptosis is absent.

Autophagy

Autophagy is a catabolic process in which cellular components are enclosed within a double membrane bound vesicle or autophagosome, before being targeted to lysosomes for degradation. Autophagy plays a role in cell survival by providing energy and metabolites during times of starvation and for the removal of damaged organelles and long-lived proteins. It may also engage cell death (type II cell death), particularly under conditions in which autophagy is enforced. However, the lack of stringent experimental discrimination between autophagy-induced cell death and autophagy arising as a consequence of cell death has proven a rich source of controversy. Consequently, the term "autophagic cell death" must only be applied from a functional perspective and only to scenarios in which cell death can be inhibited by the suppression of key regulators of autophagy. This excludes most examples in mammalian systems, and our understanding of autophagic cell death is limited, with very little insight into the physiologic conditions under which it is engaged. While autophagy regulates cell death pathways as well as immune responses, we do not consider it further herein.

Molecular Mechanisms of Caspase Activation

Caspases and Apoptosis

Apoptotic cell death is executed by one or more caspases, a family of cysteine proteases with selectivity for aspartate (Asp/D) residues that cleave their target substrates after tetrapeptide sequences containing aspartic acid at the P1 position, for example, DEVD.[4] All caspases are synthesized as inactive monomeric zymogens with an N-terminal prodomain and a C-terminal protease domain, consisting of a large and a small subunit and the catalytic cysteine residue, require dimerization, in addition to other events for catalytic competence.

Caspases are categorized according to their general function. The executioner caspases, caspases-3, -6, and -7, are responsible for the cleavage of substrates to effect cellular destruction and clearance of the dead cell. In contrast, the initiator caspases, including caspases-8 and -9 (and caspase-10 in humans) provide the molecular "ignition" to trigger the proteolytic cascade and facilitate executioner function. The inflammatory caspase, caspase-1, can also trigger apical events; although its role is largely in immune regulation, it can participate in apoptosis under some circumstances (noted previously).

Caspase Substrates of Note

The initiator caspases are responsible for two critical cleavage events: (1) autocleavage to induce stabilization of the active dimer (caspases-8 and -10) or destabilization (caspases-9 and -1); and (2) the cleavage and activation of the executioner caspases-3 and -7 that can, in turn, cleave and activate another executioner caspase, caspase-6. It is therefore important to note that while proper cleavage of an executioner caspase is evidence of its activation, cleavage of an initiator caspase is not necessarily evidence of its activation.

Once active, executioner caspases cleave numerous target substrates, including inhibitor of caspase-activated DNase (ICAD), which inhibits active CAD, the caspase-activated DNase responsible for DNA fragmentation,[5,6] poly-ADP-ribosyltransferase (PARP), a DNA repair enzyme,[7] components of the cytoskeleton and matrix, and targets responsible for phosphatidylserine externalization, critical for phagocytic uptake and removal of dead cells.

The inflammatory caspase, caspase-1, cleaves two pro-inflammatory cytokines, IL-1β and IL-18, to generate bioactive cytokines that are released upon pyroptosis. Unlike caspase-1, the other inflammatory caspases-4, -5, and -11 do not cleave the proforms of these cytokines. Additional caspase-1 substrates include components of the actin cytoskeleton, the cellular inhibitor of apoptosis proteins (cIAPs), and metabolic enzymes, although the relevance of these cleavage events to caspase-1-dependent cell death remains poorly characterized. Gasdermin-D (GsdmD) is cleaved by all of these inflammatory caspases (but not executioner caspases), and upon cleavage forms pores in the plasma membrane responsible for pyroptosis.[8–13]

Another caspase substrate effectively blurs the distinction between apoptosis and necrosis. Like GsdmD, another member of this family, GsdmE, is capable of forming destructive plasma membrane pores upon its cleavage. However, GsdmE is cleaved by caspase-3 and caspase-7 (and not inflammatory caspases) and, therefore, cells that express GsdmE, upon induction of apoptosis, have features of both forms of cell death (this has been called "secondary necrosis").[14,15]

Caspase Regulation: Activation and Inhibition

Initiator and executioner caspases require different mechanisms of activation. Initiator or apical caspases have long prodomains and exist as inactive monomers that must be dimerized to generate and stabilize the catalytic site. This is mediated by the formation of oligomeric signaling complexes, comprising the apical caspase, specialized adapter proteins, and additional regulatory proteins. In contrast, the executioner caspases exist as preformed inactive dimers with minimal prodomains that are rendered active by enzymatic cleavage of a DEVD site within the linker region between the large and small subunits. In this way, dimerization of an apical caspase, enforced by recruitment to its specific activation complex, generates an active enzyme that, in turn, cleaves and activates downstream executioner caspases to mediate proteolysis of specific target substrates and cellular destruction.

Caspase Inhibitors (IAPs)

Inhibitor of apoptosis proteins (IAPs), characterized by one or more copies of a motif called the baculovirus IAP repeat (BIR), can bind to and suppress active caspases.[16] First identified in viruses, IAPs ensure viral replication by inhibiting caspase activity in the host cell to sustain cell survival.[17–19] Subsequently, BIR-containing proteins were identified in vertebrates that included XIAP,[20] c-IAP1, c-IAP2,[21] NAIP,[22,23] and survivin.[24]

It is only XIAP that directly blocks apoptosis by interacting with and inhibiting active caspases.[20] XIAP is characterized by three BIR domains, with BIR3 and adjacent RING domain mediating the inhibition of caspase-9 and BIR2 and adjoining linker region suppressing the executioner caspases-3 and -7.[25] XIAP, as well as c-IAP1 and c-IAP2, can function as E3-ligases to promote ubiquitination and proteasomal degradation of their target protein substrates.[26] In this way, XIAP can also halt caspase activity by inducing protein degradation. Although XIAP-deficient mice have no obvious developmental defects,[27] there are certain circumstances in which XIAP may be a critical determinant of cellular sensitivity to certain apoptotic pathways (discussed in more detail later).

Playing CARDS (and DEDs)—Activation Platforms of the Initiator Caspases

The recruitment of apical caspases to large protein complexes is determined by the specialized adapter molecules within these complexes and the reciprocal binding domain within the caspase itself. The prodomain of the initiator caspases contains one of two specialized binding domains, the CARD (caspase recruitment domain), present in caspases-1, -2, -4, -5 -9, -11, and -12, and the DED domain, found in caspases-8 and -10. The DED and CARD domains display no sequence homology, although structurally they are similar in that they form so-called "death folds." The death domain (DD) and pyrin (PyD) domains, although not a structural feature of caspases themselves, are found in other proteins that participate in caspase activation.

The Inflammasome—Activation Platform for Procaspase-1

Caspase-1 is the prototypical human inflammatory caspase and exists as an inactive monomer that is activated by its CARD-dependent recruitment to a multiprotein complex, the "inflammasome." Caspase-1 is essential for the processing of the inactive proforms of IL-1β and IL-18 to generate active cytokines, the release of which occurs via a noncanonical secretory pathway that also requires caspase-1 function. Initiation of caspase-1-dependent IL-1β/IL-18 release is most often associated with components of pathogenic organisms, collectively termed pathogen-associated molecular patterns (PAMPs), which function by engaging members of the Nod-like receptor (NLR) family in the cytosol (discussed in the following section).

The DISC—Activation Platform for Procaspase-8

Activation of caspase-8 and caspase-10 (found in humans and not rodents) is triggered via death receptors, a subset of the TNF receptor family when ligated by their cognate death ligand, also TNF-like molecules. Depending upon which accessory protein is recruited to the signaling complex, procaspase-8 cleavage and/or activation can participate in one of several biologic pathways.

Constitutively trimerized death receptor is activated by trimers of death ligand to form homotypic DD-DD interactions with one of several adapter molecules including FADD, to reveal the DED domain and recruitment of procaspase-8 or procaspase-10 via one of their two DED domains. Enforced dimerization and activation of these procaspases promotes the cleavage and activation of the effector caspases-3 and-7. That is, unless procaspase-8 forms heterodimers with a catalytically inert homolog, c-FLIP$_L$ (herein, FLIP$_L$), a negative regulator of procaspase-8 activity. FLIP-procaspase-8 heterodimers, although lacking the ability to promote apoptosis, retain sufficient catalytic activity to inhibit an alternative form of cell death, necroptosis, which is discussed in more detail later.

The Apoptosome—Activation Platform for Procaspase-9

Procaspase-9 activation is mediated via its recruitment to a large protein complex called the apoptosome, comprising procaspase-9, APAF-1 (apoptotic protease activating factor-1), and additional regulatory proteins.[28,29] APAF-1 is a specialized adapter protein containing an N-terminal CARD domain and a C-terminal protein-binding domain consisting of multiple WD repeats. APAF-1 is a cytosolic molecule, triggered to undergo self-oligomerization by the binding of cytochrome-*c* following its release from the mitochondrial intermembrane space.[29] Association with cytochrome-*c*, together with the binding of deoxynucleotides (dATP), unmasks

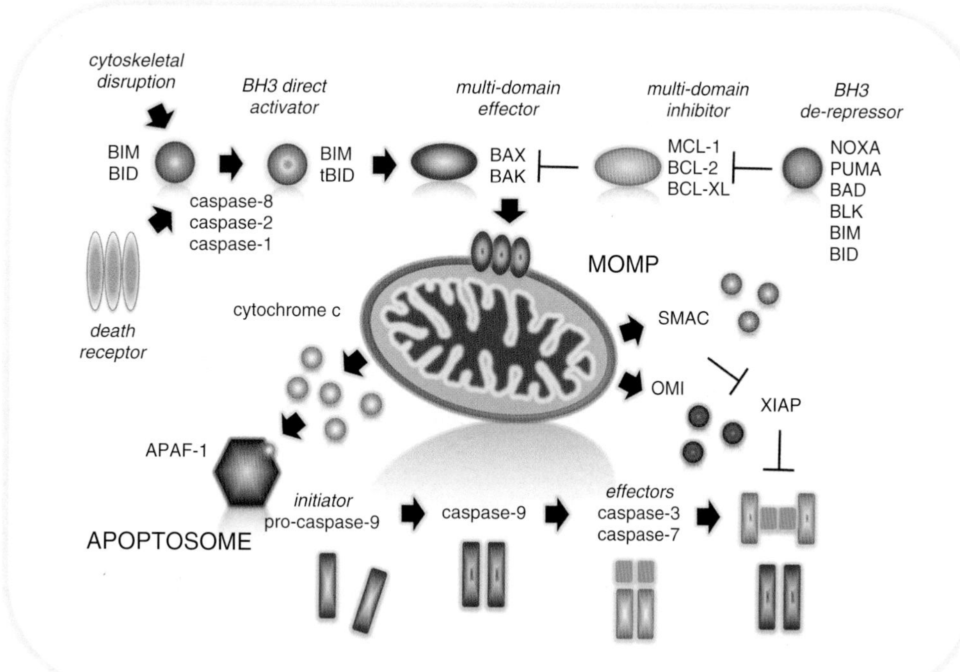

• **Fig. 19.1** Bcl-2 protein-regulated mitochondrial outer membrane permeabilization (MOMP) is a critical event in the intrinsic apoptosis pathway. Bcl-2 proteins regulate MOMP in response to a multitude of signals to engage the intrinsic apoptotic pathway. The multidomain proapoptotic effector molecules BAX and BAK undergo several modifications including conformational change and oligomerization to induce MOMP. The multidomain anti-apoptotic Bcl-2 proteins including Bcl-2, Bcl-XL, and MCL-1 inhibit BAX/BAK-induced MOMP. The proapoptotic BH3 only effector proteins activate BAX and BAK either by direct activation (direct BH3 activators include BIM and BID) or indirectly by displacement of inhibitory anti-apoptotic Bcl-2 proteins (de-repressor BH3 proteins include NOXA, PUMA, and BAD). BH3 proteins act as sensors to different types of stress and can be modified by several mechanisms. For example, BID is cleaved and activated by caspase-8 in response to death receptor-mediated signaling events while BIM activation can be mediated by disruption of the cytoskeleton. MOMP permits the release of several intermembrane space proteins including cytochrome-*c*, SMAC, and OMI, all of which regulate the apoptotic pathway. Cytochrome-*c* binds to the adapter protein APAF-1 to trigger the recruitment of inactive procaspase-9 monomers and assembly of the apoptosome complex. This results in the self-cleavage of procaspase-9 to generate catalytically active caspase-9 dimers, which then cleave and activate the executioner caspases-3 and -7. XIAP, an E3 ligase, negatively regulates the activity of caspases-9, -7, and -3 either by blocking of the catalytic site or by promoting their ubiquitin-dependent degradation. SMAC and OMI bind to or cleave XIAP, respectively, to inhibit its activity and promote apoptosis.

the C-terminal CARD domain of APAF-1, allowing it to interact with the CARD domain of procaspase-9.[30] Once activated, caspase-9 then cleaves to activate the executioner caspases-3 and -7.

Mitochondria and Apoptosis—INTRINSIC Apoptosis

Caspase-dependent apoptosis is broadly defined as two pathways that, for the most part, proceed independently of one another—the mitochondria-dependent "intrinsic" pathway and the "extrinsic" pathway that is mediated by death receptor/death ligand interaction. The former, dependent upon the initiator caspase-9, is characterized by mitochondrial outer membrane permeabilization (MOMP) to release cytochrome-*c*, an intermembrane component of the electron transport chain, into the cytosolic space.[31–33] Once released, cytochrome-*c* binds to APAF-1 to facilitate assembly of the apoptosome and activation of procaspase-9 (see previous). Several additional proteins are also released that include SMAC (second mitochondrial-derived activator of caspase), also known as DIABLO, OMI/Htr2A, and AIF.[34–36] SMAC and OMI participate indirectly in caspase activation through binding and antagonism of XIAP (discussed in more detail later).

Regulation of Mitochondrial Outer Membrane Permeabilization (MOMP)

MOMP is one of the primary features of the intrinsic apoptotic pathway and is positively and negatively regulated by the Bcl-2 (B cell lymphoma-2) family of proteins (Fig. 19.1) (reviewed in refs. 37, 38). Bcl-2 proteins are grouped into those that promote and those that suppress cell death by directly or indirectly regulating MOMP according to specific structural features.[39]

The proapoptotic multidomain effector proteins, BAX and BAK, directly permeabilize the outer mitochondrial membrane while the anti-apoptotic family members including Bcl-2 itself, Bcl-X_L, A1, Bcl-B, Bcl-W, and Mcl-1 function primarily to prevent MOMP. The proapoptotic BH3 only proteins, including BID, BIM, PUMA, NOXA, HRK, BIK, BMF, and BAD, also promote MOMP, but do so indirectly, either by activating the effectors, BAX and BAK, or inhibiting the anti-apoptotic Bcl-2 proteins.[40]

Monomeric BAX is found in the cytosol, while BAK resides on the outer mitochondrial membrane, anchored by its carboxy-terminal region. Conversion to their active state requires transient interaction with one or more of the BH3-only proteins to induce a change in their conformation, multimerization into large homo-oligomers and, in the case of BAX, translocation to the outer mitochondrial membrane. The subsequent release of intermembrane space proteins requires membrane permeabilization, but whether BAX and BAK oligomers achieve this directly by membrane insertion and forming pores themselves, or indirectly, by triggering the formation of lipid pores, has yet to be resolved. Nonetheless, following permeabilization, cytochrome-*c*, SMAC (DIABLO), and OMI (Htr2A) are released from the mitochondrial intermembrane space into the cytosol to activate caspases and mediate apoptotic cell death.

A third Bcl-2 family member, BOK, can similarly induce cell death via MOMP. BOK protein is inherently unstable and under constitutive conditions is degraded via the endoplasmic reticulum (ER)–associated degradation pathway (ERAD).[41] Inhibition of the proteasome or various forms of ER stress leads to the stabilization and accumulation of BOK protein to promote MOMP and trigger apoptotic cell death. However, the precise role of BOK remains somewhat of a mystery—neither the ablation of BOK expression nor its co-deletion with BAX or BAK revealed any overt developmental phenotype.[42] Interestingly, however, BOK, unlike either BAX or BAK, is frequently deleted in cancers.[43]

Insertion of BAX or BAK into the outer mitochondrial membrane exposes the BH3 domain, allowing self-oligomerization to induce MOMP or, alternatively, interaction with an anti-apoptotic Bcl-2 protein to inhibit it. In contrast, the sequestration and neutralization of the anti-apoptotic Bcl-2 proteins by the BH3-only proteins increases the likelihood of BAX and BAK activation to induce MOMP. Specific members of the BH3 protein family, BID, BIM, and PUMA, so-called "direct activators," are able to trigger the conversion of BAX and BAK from their constitutively inert state into active oligomers capable of inducing MOMP.

The engagement of cell death in the context of caspase inhibition can promote a type of cell death that is also characterized by MOMP and Bcl-2 protein function—so-called caspase-independent cell death (CICD). This type of cell death is perhaps most commonly observed during development and particularly under conditions in which certain pathways of caspase activation are inactivated, such as in the APAF-1 deficient model. In this case, cells die due to a bioenergetic catastrophe, as mitochondrial function is lost upon MOMP.

Post-translational Regulation of Bcl-2 Protein Function

Bcl-2 proteins are regulated at the transcriptional level, and can also be regulated by several post-translational modifications including phosphorylation, ubiquitin-mediated degradation, protease-mediated cleavage, myristiolyation, and neddylation. Although the precise functional consequences of these modifications are not clear in many cases, there are a few exceptions.

Kinase-mediated phosphorylation of the BH3-only proteins BIM and BAD is critical for the integration of upstream signaling events associated with growth factor withdrawal and activation of downstream apoptotic effectors. Phosphorylation of BIM at serine-69 by the mitogen-activated protein kinase (MAPK) extra-cellular-regulating kinase (ERK) induces the proteasomal degradation of BIM.[44] In contrast, the phosphorylation of BIM by the MAPK, c-Jun N-terminal kinase (JNK), stabilizes the protein to facilitate BAX-dependent cell death.[45] AKT-dependent phosphorylation of BAD at residues Ser-112 and Ser-136 promotes the association of BAD with 14-3-3,[46] while the dephosphorylation of BAD in response to nutrient deprivation neutralizes its proapoptotic activity by triggering its interaction with Bcl-X_L or Bcl-2.[47–49]

Multiple phosphorylation and ubiquitylation events also contribute to the regulation of MCL-1 stability.[50] Disruption of AKT activity under conditions of nutrient withdrawal relieves the inhibition of the kinase, GSK3, which phosphorylates MCL-1 to promote its degradation.[51] Interaction between MCL-1 and MULE, an E3 ligase, when disrupted by a proapoptotic BH3-only protein such as NOXA, allows the ubiquitlylation and degradation of MCL-1.[52] Other proteins that control the stability of MCL-1 include FBW-7,[53] a tumor suppressor frequently deleted in cancers, and the deubiquitinase USP9X,[54] expressed in many tumor types. The turnover of the anti-apoptotic proteins Bcl-2 and Bcl-XL are similarly subject to regulation by post-translational modification.[55,56] For example, ERK1/2-mediated modification of a serine residue (Ser-70) within the flexible loop between the BH3 and BH4 domains[57] or on serine-87 of Bcl-2 both exacerbate its anti-apoptotic activity, at least in part, by maintaining protein stability.[58] Dephosphorylation by PPA2 opposes this activity and neutralizes the anti-apoptotic activity of Bcl-2.[59] In contrast, the anti-apoptotic activity of Bcl-x_L is disrupted by the deamidation of two asparagine residues in the unstructured loop between BH4 and BH1.[60]

Specific cleavage events can also contribute to the function of certain Bcl-2 proteins. The BH3-only protein BID is unique among its BH3 relatives in that in its native state, its BH3 domain is buried within the tertiary structure of the molecule, rendering it inactive. However, cleavage of a flexible linker within BID by one of several proteases, including caspases-8[61] and -2,[62] granzyme B,[63] lysosomal proteases (cathepsins),[64] and the calcium-activated protease, calpain,[65] generates an active cleavage product, tBID, rendering it able to associate with anti-apoptotic proteins or function as a direct activator of BAX and BAK. In this way, upstream cytosolic events leading to the activation of these proteases can engage mitochondria-dependent apoptosis by the direct cleavage and activation of the BH3 protein, BID. Calpain-mediated cleavage of BAX to enhance its proapoptotic activity has also been described,[66] although the physiologic significance of this event has yet to be fully delineated.

Multiple transcription factors have been implicated in the regulation of both pro- and anti-apoptotic Bcl-2 gene expression, including p53, nuclear factor κB (NF-κB), and FOXO3a. Several micro RNAs (miRNAs), including MiR-17-92, Mir-15, and Mir-16, specifically reduce the levels of BIM and Bcl-2 RNAs. Several of the Bcl-2 proteins exist as multiple splice variants, including Bcl-XL, BAX, and PUMA, although their specific roles are poorly defined. However BIM, found as multiple isoforms, including BIM-S, BIM-L, and BIM-EL, appear to harbor differing pro-apoptotic potencies as a consequence of the presence or absence of a dynein light chain-binding region. Anoikis, apoptotic cell death arising from perturbation of the cytoskeleton and detachment of cells from the basement membrane, is mediated by BIM and another BH3 protein, BMF. BIM is anchored to the microtubule complex, while BMF is sequestered by the actin cytoskeleton, each by their respective dynein light chain binding regions. Disruption of the cytoskeleton induces the release of BIM and BMF to promote MOMP and engage apoptosis.

Alternative/Additional Roles of Bcl-2 Proteins

Our discussion of Bcl-2 function has focused on their role in cell death in the context of MOMP regulation. Although a critically important role, it is becoming apparent that the collective activity of Bcl-2 proteins is not restricted to the regulation of cell death, but that it likely has significant impact in several additional signaling pathways including the regulation of mitochondrial dynamics,[67] the response to DNA damage,[68,69] metabolic bioenergetics,[70–72] Ca^{2+} homeostasis,[73] ER function, and autophagy.[74]

Death Receptor–Associated Signaling Events—EXTRINSIC Apoptosis

The death ligands and their receptors exist as preformed trimers and represent subsets of the TNF and TNF receptor (TNFR) superfamilies, respectively. The receptors include TNF-R1, CD95 (also known as Fas or Apo-1), DR3 (death receptor 3), the TRAIL (TNF-related apoptosis ligand) receptors, TRAIL receptor-1 (or DR4), TRAIL receptor-2 (also known as DR5 in humans), and death receptor 6 (DR6). Their corresponding activating ligands are TNF itself, CD95-ligand (or FasL), and TRAIL, all of which engage apoptosis. Neither DR3 nor DR6 promote apoptosis. Interaction between a death receptor and its appropriate ligand induces a conformational change to expose the DD, a specialized protein-association domain in the receptor, making it available for interaction with one of several DD-containing adapter proteins.

Interaction between FasL (CD95 ligand) and its receptor Fas (CD95) triggers the recruitment of the DD-containing adapter protein FADD. This is accompanied by a conformational change in FADD to reveal a second specialized binding domain, the DED. Assembly of the mature signaling complex or CD95 death inducing complex (DISC) is completed by the recruitment of procaspase-8 via interaction between one of two DEDs in its prodomain and the DED of FADD. The consequent dimerization of procaspase-8 permits self-cleavage and stabilization of the active caspase, leading in turn to the proteolysis and activation of the effector caspases-3 and -7. DISC formation is negatively regulated by the dimerization of caspase-8 with its catalytically inactive homolog, FLIP. Although this interaction prevents the dimerization and cleavage of caspase-8, it does not completely inhibit its catalytic activity. This results in the cleavage of FLIP but, importantly, not the induction of apoptosis. Recently, studies have further characterized the complexity of binding among FADD, FLIP, and caspase-8, demonstrating it to be an important determinant of the type of cell death that proceeds, apoptosis or necroptosis (discussed in detail in the following section).

The signaling events elicited by activation of the TNFR1 are complex, subject to a variety of regulatory mechanisms, and leading to cellular survival, apoptosis, or programmed necrosis, depending upon the specific identity of the proteins recruited to the TNFR1 receptor-signaling complex, termed Complex I, IIa, and IIb (details are described in Fig. 19.2). TNFR1 activation can be mediated by one of two ligands, TNF itself or lymphotoxin, both of which trigger conformational changes within the intra-cellular domain of the receptor to expose the DD as well as an additional binding site for an E3-ligase, TNF-receptor associated factor-2 (TRAF2). Subsequent recruitment of TRADD to TNFR1 via their respective DD domains serves to both stabilize the TRAF2-TNFR1 interaction and recruit RIPK1. RIPK1 is a functionally versatile molecule, able to contribute to the activity of several TNRR1 signaling complexes, some of which require its kinase activity and others that do not. In Complex I, RIPK1 acts to recruit additional signaling components to the TNFR1 complex in a kinase-independent manner once modified by TRAF2-mediated lysine 63-linked polyubiquitylation. One of these is NEMO (NF-κB essential modulator), a component of the IKK (IκB kinase) complex that stimulates the phosphorylation, ubiquitylation, and degradation of IκBα to reveal the transcriptional activity of NF-κB. It is important to note that, under these conditions, cell death does not proceed, but instead NF-κB induces the transcription of genes that contribute to cellular survival, including cIAP1, cIAP2, and $FLIP_L$, and others that participate in inflammatory responses.

Under some conditions, the TRADD-TRAF-2-RIPK1 signaling complex is released from TNFR1, where the DD domain of TRADD, available after detachment from the TNFR1, now recruits FADD. This scenario is compatible with the formation of one of two signaling complexes, termed Complex IIa and IIb. Recruitment of $FLIP_L$ to form heterodimers with caspase-8 prevents the assembly of catalytically active caspase-8 homodimers to inhibit apoptosis but in a manner that retains the ability of caspase-8 to cleave and inactivate RIPK1 and RIPK3. However, in the absence of $FLIP_L$, the catalytic activity of caspase-8 is unrestrained and therefore able to promote apoptosis. In contrast, inhibition of caspase-8, or its requisite adapter, FADD, promotes assembly of Complex IIb, also termed the necrosome, by allowing the recruitment and stabilization of RIPK1 and RIPK3 to instead trigger necroptosis. In this way, $FLIP_L$ provides a critical point at which TNFR1 signaling events are integrated to determine the mode of cell death engaged.

Molecular Interaction With the Mitochondrial Pathway—Caspase-8 and BID

For the most part, the apical signaling events of the intrinsic and extrinsic apoptotic pathways proceed independently of one another, converging only at the terminal executioner phase of caspase-3 activation. However, MOMP, typically associated with the intrinsic death pathway, can also participate in death receptor-mediated apoptosis by virtue of caspase-8-mediated cleavage and activation of the BH3 protein, BID. XIAP appears to be the critical determinant of the relative involvement of BID-mediated MOMP in the extrinsic apoptosis pathway.[75]

XIAP binds to and blocks the proteolytic activities of caspase-9, -3, and -7 but not caspase-8, unless displaced by SMAC and OMI, both of which are released from the mitochondria upon MOMP. Thus, when XIAP is expressed, the activation of BID and promotion of MOMP are required for death receptor-induced apoptosis, via the derepression of XIAP by SMAC and OMI.

Caspases and Pyroptosis

Assembly and activation of the inflammasome complex to initiate the production of the pro-inflammatory cytokines, IL-1β and IL-18, represents a critical component of the host innate immune system to protect against infection and sterile insults. The initiating event for inflammasome assembly is the detection of a "stressor" by one of several sensor molecules or nucleotide-binding domains, leucine-rich repeat-containing (NBD-LRR) or NLRs. Activators of NLRs, collectively termed DAMPS, can be of endogenous, exogenous, self, or foreign origin although most are commonly associated with components of infectious agents or PAMPS.

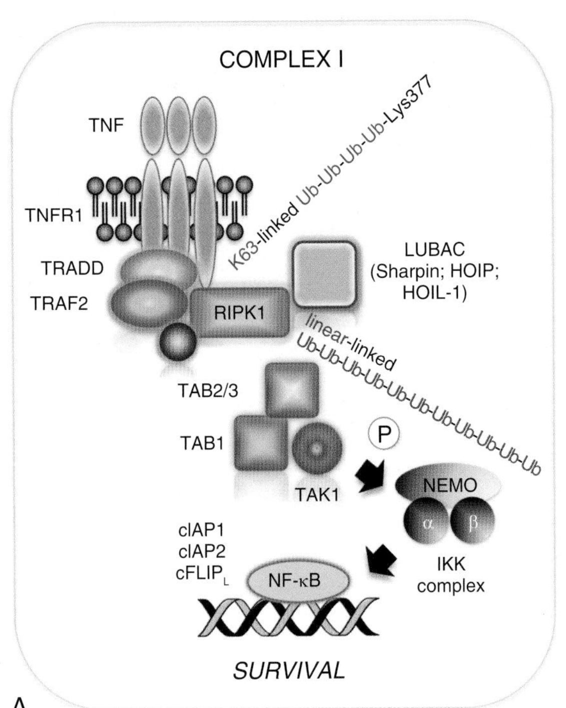

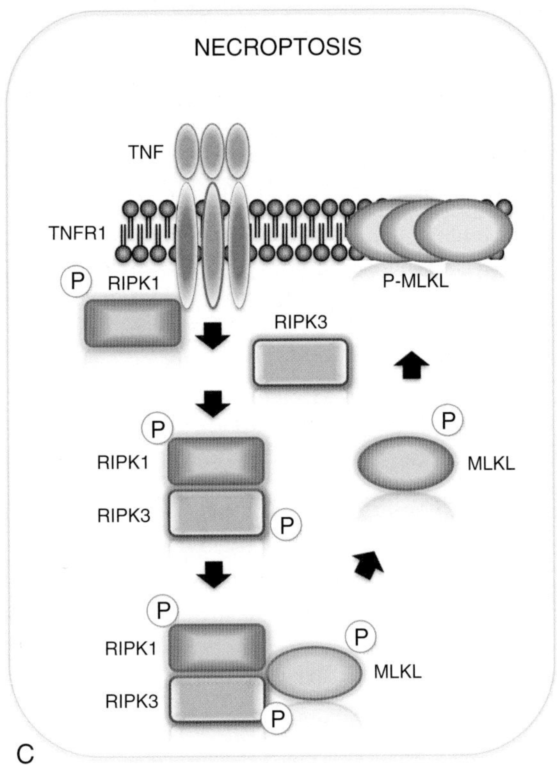

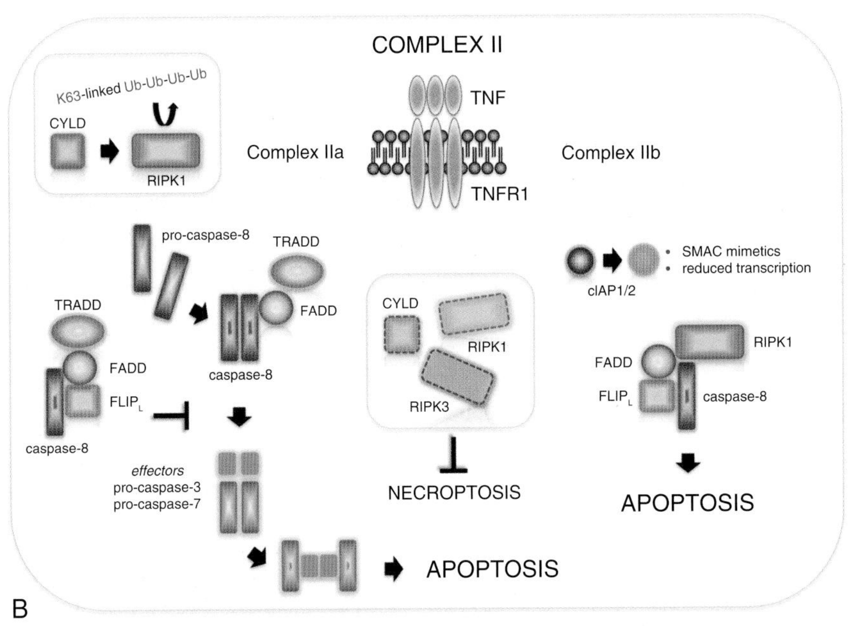

• **Fig. 19.2** Multiple TNF-TNFR1 complexes can be formed, each leading to a different biologic outcome. (A) COMPLEX I: Binding of TNF to its trimeric receptor TNFR1 triggers assembly of Complex I that comprises TRADD, RIPK1, and the E3 ubiquitinases, cIAP1, cIAP2, TRAF2, and HOIL-1 of the LUBAC complex. cIAP1/2 mediates the K63-linked polyubiquitylation of RIPK1 on lysine 377 to promote RIPK1-dependent stabilization of complex I and recruitment of the (i) TAB-TAK complexes and (ii) NF-κB activation IKK complex to the ubiquitin chain. The E3 ligase activity of the LUBAC Complex further contributes to RIPK1 ubiquitylation, complex stability, and NF-κB activation. NF-κB-dependent transcription of cFLIP$_L$ and cIAP1/2 contribute to cellular survival by the stabilization of Complex I and inhibition of proapoptotic Complex II assembly. (B) COMPLEX IIa: The formation of Complex IIa is triggered by TNF-TNFR1 interaction and occurs in the cytosolic compartment under conditions in which Complex I is destabilized. One way this can occur is via the activity of CYLD, a deubiquitylase that removes K63-linked polyubiquitin from RIPK1 to promote the destabilization of Complex I and dissociation of RIPK1 to participate in alternative TNF-induced signaling complexes. Complex IIa assembly involves the indirect recruitment of FADD to TNFR1 via TRADD. This promotes the association of procaspase-8 monomers to form catalytically active caspase-8 dimers. Active caspase-8 can then cleave and activate the downstream executioner caspases-3 and -7 to mediate apoptotic cell death. FLIP$_L$ can also bind to FADD and/or procaspase-8. Under these conditions, caspase-8 in dimerization with FLIP$_L$ is catalytically active but not fully processed, displays altered substrate specificity, and cannot engage apoptosis. COMPLEX IIb (ripoptosome): Under conditions in which cIAPs are reduced or inhibited, stable RIPK1-dependent Complex I formation is less favored and an alternative Complex IIb can assemble. This cytosolic complex is TRADD-independent and comprises RIPK1, FADD, and FLIP$_L$-caspase-8 heterodimers. Under these conditions the proapoptotic RIPK1 function is favored. FLIP$_L$ can also bind to FADD and acts as a competitive inhibitor of caspase-8-FADD association to prevent apoptosis. Changes in the levels of RIPK3, MLKL, and caspase-8 activation can alternatively lead to necroptosis. (C) TNF-induced necroptosis: Induction of necroptosis in response to TNF-TNFR1 ligation. Oligomerization of RIPK1 and RIPK3 induces the autophosphorylation of RIPK3 to recruit and phosphorylate MLKL in a RIPK3 dependent manner. How MLKL then induces rupture of the plasma membrane remains unclear, but suggested mechanisms include direct permeabilization by MLKL itself or MLKL-dependent recruitment of $Ca2^+$ and/or K^+ ion channels to effect changes in ion homeostasis, cellular swelling, and eventual rupture of the plasma membrane.

NLRs are among the so-called pattern-recognition receptors (PPRs) that encompass TLRs, C-type lectin receptors (CLRs), the absent in melanoma 2 (AIM2)–like receptor (ALR) families, and retinoic acid inducible gene (RIG)–I-like receptors (RLRs). NLR members include NLRP1 (NOD-, LRR-, and pyrin-containing domain 1), NLRP3, NLRP6, NLRP7, NLRP12, and NLRC4 (also named IPAF), and are characterized by three distinct domains. The N terminal region that confers the functional classification of the NLR contains a pyrin, caspase recruitment domain (CARD) or baculovirus inhibitory domain, the central domain, NBD or NACHT domain (nucleotide-binding domain) that mediates dNTP hydrolysis and multimerization, and the C-terminal leucine rich repeat (LRR) domain. It is the LRR domain, ascribed autoinhibitory function in several inflammasome complexes, that promotes structural stability and a variety of protein-protein interactions.

The inflammasome, although structurally analogous to the caspase-8 activating DISC and the caspase-9 activating apoptosome in general terms, differs from these caspase-activation complexes in one significant way. The inflammasome complex can vary in its molecular composition by virtue of different adapter molecules that are themselves, characterized by one of several different protein binding domains (Fig. 19.3). Despite the compositional variations of inflammasome complexes, their primary role is to induce caspase activity via direct or indirect interaction with the CARD domain of caspase-1. One of the most common adapter molecules required for inflammasome assembly is ASC (apoptotic speck-forming CARD), which mediates IL-1 and IL-18 processing via homomultimeric interactions between its CARD domain and that of caspase-1. ASC also contains a pyrin domain (PyD), a death domain (DD) that mediates interaction between the PyD domain of several members of the NLR family including NLRP1, NLRP3, NLRP 6, NLRP7, NLRP12, and NLRC4 to promote inflammasome assembly. Activating ligands are derived from multiple sources and include endogenous ligands such as glucose and amyloid-β, environmental stressors including asbestos and ultraviolet (UV) irradiation and those derived from infectious agents of bacterial, viral, fungal, and protozoan origin.

The NLRP3 Inflammasome

Assembly of an active NLRP3-containing inflammasome requires, in most cases, two independent signaling events—the first primes the cells and arises from NF-κB activation mediated by TLR or TNF-R1 to induce expression of NLRP3 and other inflammasome components,[76] while the second event is mediated by activation of NLRP3 via one of several DAMPS or PAMPs that include asbestos,[77] amyloid-β,[78] uric acid,[79] muramyl-dipeptide,[80] and calcium pyrophosphate dihydrate (CPPD)[81] as well as bacterial RNAs[82] and viral components derived from multiple pathogens (Fig. 19.3A). In response to these triggers, NLRP3, via its PYD domain, associates with the PYD-containing adapter ASC. The CARD domain of ASC then interacts with that of caspase-1 to promote inflammasome formation, the processing of IL-1β and IL-18, and activation of Gasdermin-D to induce pyroptosis.

The promiscuous nature of NLRP3 activation is likely to represent a common activation mechanism rather than multiple factors directly interacting with NLRP3 to promote inflammasome assembly. However, despite this assertion, a unifying mechanism has yet to emerge, although many potential triggers have been proposed (see Fig. 19.2A). These include several mitochondrially localized events such as reactive oxygen species (ROS) production,[83] oxidation of mitochondrial DNA,[84] translocation of cardiolipin,[85] and direct association between K63 ubiquitinated NLRP3[86] and mitochondrial anti-viral signaling (MAVS) proteins[87] or mitofusin 2.[88] Molecules that physically interact with NLRP3 to promote inflammasome assembly include double-stranded RNA-dependent protein kinase (PKR)[89] and guanylate binding protein (GBP).[90] Several additional regulatory factors include K^+ efflux,[91,92] Ca^{2+} influx,[93,94] ATP-triggered puraminergic signaling events,[95] and interaction with chaperone proteins including HSP90 and SGT1 via the LRR domain of NLRP3 to maintain a stable but inactive complex.[96]

Multiple inherited and de novo mutations in the NLRP3 gene have been identified, many clustered within the NBD domain, rendering a genetic predisposition to increased formation of the NALP3-containing inflammasome. Increased IL-1β production contributes to the pathophysiology of a family of cryopryinopathies or cryopyrin-associated periodic fever syndromes (CAPS) including familiar cold-induced autoinflmammatory syndrome (FCAS), Muckle-Wells syndrome (MWS), and neonatal onset multisystem inflammatory disorder or chronic infantile neurologic cutaneous and articular syndrome (NOMID/CINCA).[97] Genetic characterization of a contributory role for NLRP3 in CAPS was identified using murine knock-in models harboring specific NLRP3 mutations associated with MWS and FCAS.[98] These NLRP3 mutations, when introduced into cells of the hematopoietic compartment, manifested in several clinical features of the human syndromes, including neutrophil infiltration into the skin, periodic bouts of fever, and elevated Th17-associated cytokines. These symptoms were largely alleviated by anti-IL-1 treatment, suggesting that the underlying pathophysiology can be attributed to increased IL-1β secretion as a consequence of the enhanced formation of NLRP3-containing inflammasomes.

Several other pathophysiologies associated with exuberant production of pro-inflammatory cytokines, including IL-1β, have also implicated NLRP3 function. NLRP3-dependent inflammasome formation can be triggered by the mislocalization of endogenous molecules including those typically associated with gout, an inflammatory disease arising from deposition of monosodium urate (MSU) crystals in the joints, cholesterol deposits in atherosclerotic plaques, and insoluble aggregates of β-amyloid, a feature of Alzheimer's disease. Tissue damage arising from ischemic-reperfusion injury or that associated with excessive inflammation in the lung during pulmonary fibrosis or asthma is characterized by the release of multiple DAMPS including extra-cellular ATP, uric acid, the purinergic receptor P2X7, and hyaloronan, a component of the extra-cellular matrix—all of which can directly induce the formation of an NLRP3-dependent inflammasome. Furthermore, lung inflammation arising from environmental factors such as asbestos and silica may well be attributable to the reported NLRP3-dependent production of IL-1β and IL-18 triggered by these agents. Although a direct role for NLRP3 in all of these aberrant inflammatory scenarios remains to be fully tested, a contributory role in the associated pathophysiologies seems likely.

The NLRP3-containing inflammasome is an essential component of the host immune response to numerous bacterial, fungal, and viral pathogens. Examples include *Staphylococcus aureus,*

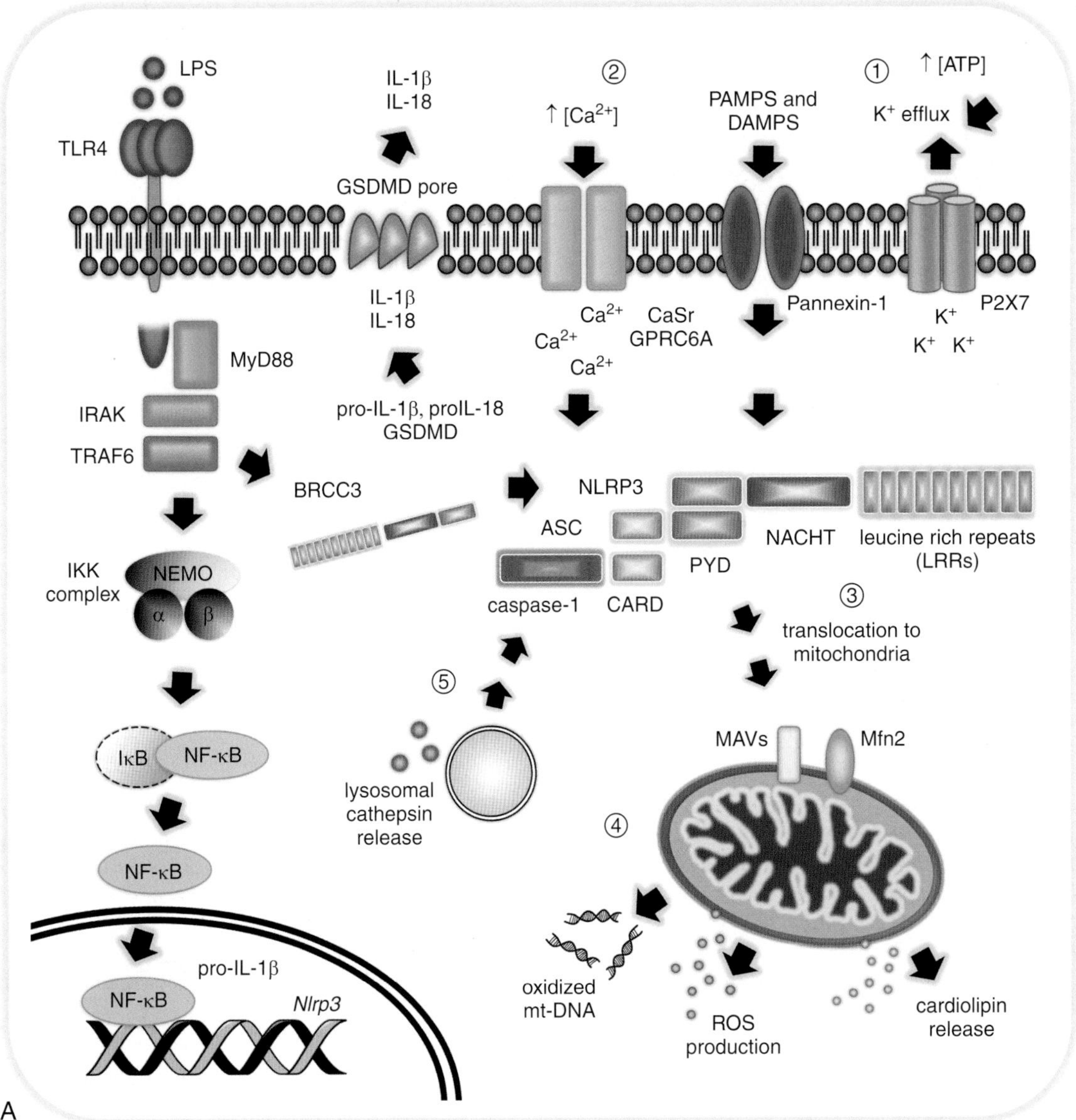

• **Fig. 19.3** The inflammasome is the activation platform for caspase-1 and is represented by different complexes according to the identity of the specific NLR and adapter proteins. (A) NLRP3 (NALP3) canonical inflammasome. NLRP3 inflammasome assembly is induced by viral and bacterial PAMPS and DAMPS arising from environmental and self-derived origins. Examples include pore forming toxins, amyloid aggregates, extra-cellular ATP, hyaluronan, monosodium urate (MSU) crystals, asbestos, silica, alum, and ultraviolet irradiation. NLRP3 inflammasome assembly is mediated by interaction between the PYD domains of NLRP3 and ASC and a CARD-CARD interaction between ASC and caspase-1. This results in the activation of caspase-1, cleavage of Gasdermin-D (GSDMD), pro-IL-1β, and pro-IL-18 and their subsequent release as bioactive molecules via the gasdermin pore. How NLRP3 is activated in response to all these different stimuli is unclear, although several mechanisms have been proposed: *1.* Elevation in extra-cellular [ATP] triggers K^+ efflux via the ATP-gated K^+ channel, P2X7, and assembly of pannexin-1 pores, through which PAMPS and DAMPs may enter the cytosol; *2.* Increased availability of Ca2+ ions from endogenous stores and extra-cellular sources also activates NLRP3 inflammasome assembly. Several mechanisms have been proposed including entry of extra-cellular calcium via the G protein coupled calcium-sensing receptors (CaSRs). Mitochondria may function as a source of several activating stimuli; *3.* Interaction of NLRP3 with MAVS (mitochondrial anti-viral signaling) proteins or mitofusin 2 (Mfn2); *4.* In response to the mitochondrial release of cardiolipin, ROS, or oxidized DNA; *5.* Lysosomal rupture and release of cathepsins. In addition to one or more of these activating stimuli, an NF-κB priming signal, triggered via TLRS or TNFR1 (LPS-mediated TLR4 activation is shown), induces the transcription of NLRP3 and pro-IL-1β. De-ubiquitination of NLRP3 via BRCC3 is also required to permit assembly of the NLRP3 inflammasome. (B) NLRC4 inflammasome. Flagellin and components of the type III and type IV bacterial secretion machinery trigger NLRC4 inflammasome assembly via the NACHT domain of the NAIP proteins. NAIP1 acts as the upstream sensor of needle proteins, those of NAIP2 sense rod proteins and NAIP5/6 BIRS are triggered by flagellin. Interaction between the NIAPs and NLRC4 may then trigger oligomerization of NLRC4, and direct interaction between the CARD domains of NLRC4 and caspase-1 then complete assembly of the inflammasome. Active caspase-1 converts pro-IL-1β/IL-18 to their active form and cleaves GSDMD to trigger assembly of a gasdermin pore. Pyroptosis and associated cell lysis releases active IL-1β/IL-18. Under some circumstances, ASC can also play a role. (C) NLRP1b inflammasome. Activators include ATP, bacterial peptidoglycan dipeptide (MDP), and lethal toxin from *Bacillus anthracis*. Caspase-1 CARD can directly interact with NLRP1b CARD to form the inflammasome. ASC may stabilize this interaction and potentiate inflammasome activity. Cleavage of the FIIND domain of NLRP1b may be required for its activity. (D) AIM2 inflammasome. Activators of the AIM2 inflammasome include DNA from intra-cellular bacteria and viruses as well as self-derived DS DNA. Cytosolic DNA binds to the HIN200 domain of AIM2 to trigger its interaction with ASC via their respective PYD domains. Caspase-1 is then recruited via its CARD domain to bind with the CARD domain of ASC. Once activated, caspase-1 cleaves pro-IL-1β and pro-IL-18 to generate the mature proteins, which exit the cell via the Gasdermin-D pore in the plasma membrane.

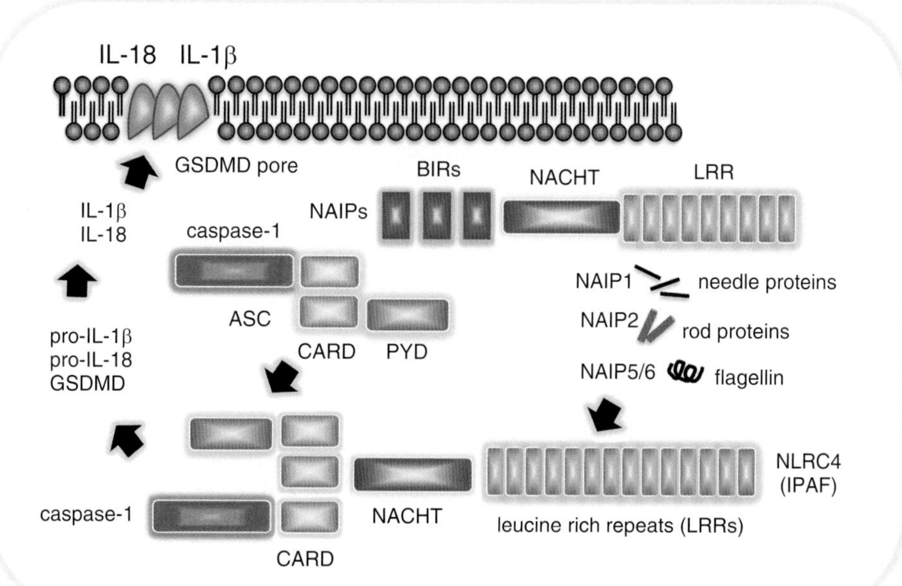

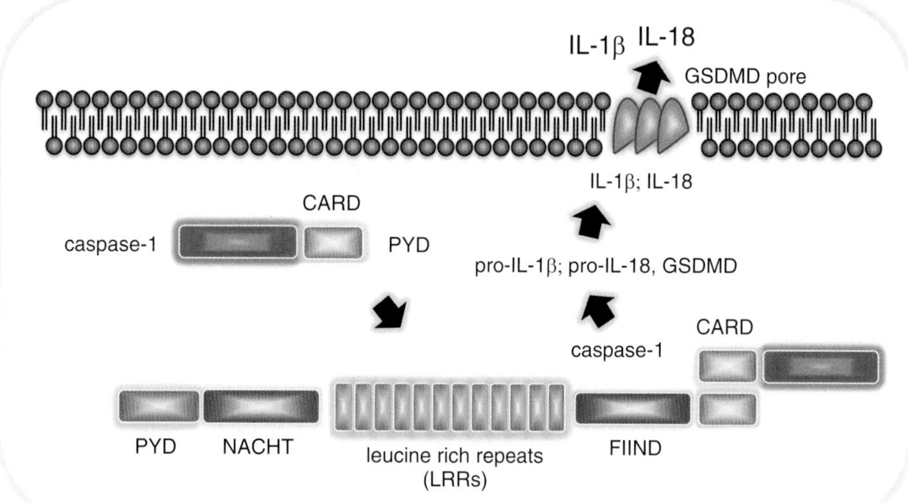

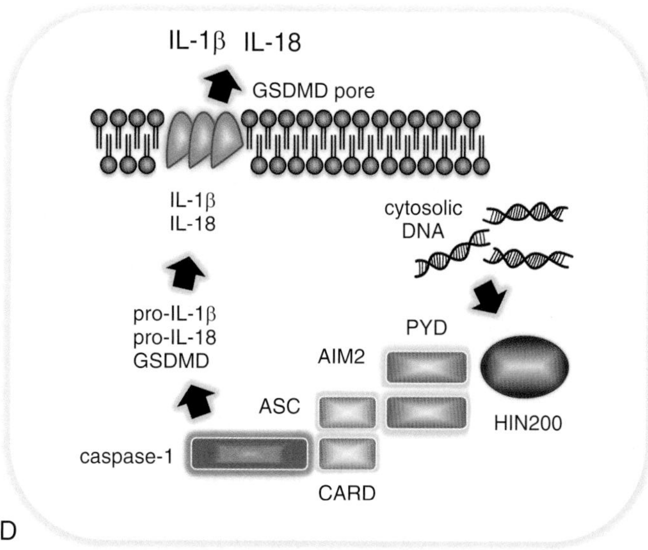

• **Fig. 19.3, cont'd**

Listeria monocytogenes, Escherichia coli, Klebsiella pneumonia, Shigella flexneri, Candida albicans, and *Saccharomyces cerevisiae.*[99] Several of these organisms express pore-forming toxins that induce membrane rupture and NLRP3-dependent inflammasome activation and/or pyroptosis. These include Toxins A and B from *Clostridium difficile,*[100] pneumolysin from *Streptococcus pneumonia,*[101] nigericin from various strains of *Streptomyces,*[102] α-, β-, and γ-hemolysins, the virulence factors from *Staphylococcus aureus,*[103] and listeriolysin from *Listeria monocytogenes.*[104]

Host-mediated immunity against some DNA viruses including influenza,[105,106] herpes,[107,108] and Sendai[109] may also involve activation of the NLRP3 inflammasome.[110] However, identification of AIM2 as the primary sensor of nucleic acids to trigger ASC-dependent inflammasome activation[111] may limit the general role of NLRP3 under some conditions. Nevertheless, clearly NLRP3 is a critical component of effective host defense against multiple bacterial pathogens and DAMPS of self-derived origin.

The NLRC4 Inflammasome

NLRC4 itself contains a CARD domain, capable of direct interaction with the CARD of caspase-1, thereby negating the requirement for an adapter such as ASC to promote caspase-1 activation and release of IL-1β and IL-18 (Fig. 19.3B).[112–114] Cytosolic assembly of the NLRC4 inflammasome is triggered by components of the Type III or Type IV secretion systems or by flagellate bacteria including *Shigella flexneri, Pseudomonas aeruginosa,* and *Salmonella typhirium.* NLRC4 is a unique member of the NLR family in that the mechanism mediating its response to pathogens is known. Members of the NLR-apoptosis inhibitory protein (NAIP) family, 6 paralogs in mice, function as the upstream sensors to then directly engage NLRC4 inflammasome assembly and IL-1β maturation.[115]

Two independent NLRC4 gain-of function point mutations were recently described, both of which rendered the NLRC4 inflammasome constitutively active and were associated with periodic bouts of fever.[116–118] Functional analyses revealed aberrant IL-1β/IL-18 production and an increased susceptibility to pyroptosis within macrophage populations isolated from patients.

The NLRP1b Inflammasome (Fig. 19.3C)

NLRP1, the first NLR to be identified as an inflammasome mediator,[119] is encoded by a single gene in humans but by three orthologs in the mouse, denoted Nlrp1a, Nlrp1b, and Nlrp1c.[120] Unlike human NLRP1, which contains a pyrin domain, the murine paralogs do not and are composed of a nucleotide binding domain, an LRR region, a FIIND ("function to find" domain), and a C terminal CARD. Muramyl dipeptide (MDP), a minimal bioactive peptidoglycan peptide common to both positive and negative bacteria, was initially identified as a ligand for Nlrp1b-mediated inflammasome formation. However, whether Nlrp1b-mediated inflammasome formation and caspase-1 processing requires pyrin domain-dependent association with ASC or instead occurs via a direct interaction between NLRP1 and caspase-1 via their respective CARD domains remains unclear.[121]

Lethal toxin (LT), the major virulence factor of *Bacillus anthracis,* is a potent ligand for Nlrp1b-dependent inflammasome formation and triggers IL-1β and IL-18 processing and extensive pyroptosis of macrophages. LT promotes the cleavage of Nlrpb1,[122,123] an event that is reportedly both necessary and sufficient[124] for inflammasome assembly.

Interestingly, an activating mutation of NLRP1 and consequent predisposition to inflammasome formation, although associated with lethal systemic inflammation via IL-1β, also led to caspase-1 activity and extensive pyroptosis in the hematopoietic compartment independently of IL-1β production. Nlrp1a-mediated inflammasome formation and pyroptosis may therefore have additional roles independently of that of IL-1β-mediated inflammation.

The NLRP6 Inflammasome

NLRP6 is expressed predominantly in gut epithelial cells and can mediate ASC-dependent assembly of the inflammasome, caspase-1 processing, and enhanced secretion of IL-1β and IL-18. Mice lacking Nlrp6, ASC, or caspase-1 exhibited a marked exacerbation in colitis and an enhanced susceptibility to damage-associated gut tumorigenesis[125–128] that was attributed to the disruption of epithelial cell turnover and indicates that localized inflammation is critical for tissue repair. In contrast, the amelioration of colitis in mice lacking Nlrp6 and IL-1β production aligns instead with the destructive consequences of the inflammatory response.[129] One intriguing reconciliation of these opposing findings may lie in the observation that NLRP6, by promoting ASC-dependent inflammasome assembly and IL-18 secretion, regulates the gut flora to maintain integrity of the epithelial barrier and reduce the incidence of colitis.[130,131] Therefore NLRP6 deficiency negatively regulates inflammasome assembly, promotes aberrant colonization of the gut by damage-inducing microbiota, and leads to a localized inflammatory response.

In contrast to what we believe to be the primary pro-inflammatory role of the other NLRs, NLRP6 instead may negatively regulate inflammatory signaling to retard pathogen clearance. Accordingly, mice lacking Nlrp6 are highly resistant to *Listeria monocytogenes, Salmonella typhimurium,* and *E. coli* that is attributed to NLRP6-mediated suppression of TLR-generated MAPK and NF-κB signaling events.[132] Whether this finding is representative of a subclass of NLRs that function as critical immune suppressors remains to be determined. It does, however, provide tantalizing evidence of regulatory crosstalk between the NLRs and members of the TLR family.

The AIM2 Inflammasome

AIM2, although not an NLR, is a pyrin-containing protein, responsive to cytosolic DNA[133] of either pathogen or host origin and able to mediate inflammasome formation (Fig. 19.3D).[134,135] AIM2, via its HIN-200 domain,[136] directly associates with its trigger, DNA, to recruit the adapter ASC in a PyD-dependent manner to promote caspase-1 activation.[137,138]

AIM2, by regulating the levels of IL-1β and IL-18, plays a critical role in antipathogen immunity to several cytosol-replicating bacteria such as *Francisella tularenis*[111,139,140] and *Listeria monocytogenes* and the DNA viruses, vaccinia and cytomegalovirus.[111] The mechanism(s) via which AIM2 can sense cytosolic DNA has yet to be fully elucidated, although type I interferon signaling events can contribute to the response to bacterial DNA although not to that of viral origin.[140,141]

The ability of AIM2 to recognize and respond to cytosolic DNA of host origin is thought to mediate the pathophysiology of self-driven inflammatory responses including systemic lupus erythematosus[142] and psoriasis.[143]

Noncanonical Inflammasomes

The family of inflammatory caspases, in addition to caspase-1, includes murine caspase-11, and human caspases-4 and -5. Caspase-11 can induce pyroptosis in a manner that is independent of any known inflammasome. Several pathogenic bacteria, including *E. coli, Vibrio cholera, Salmonella typhimurium,* and *Legionella pneumophila,* induce the activation of procaspase-4, -5, -11. Expression of caspase-11 is induced by several proinflammatory stimuli including TLR4-TRIF activation via LPS, interferons IFNγ and IFNβ that is at least partially dependent on NF-κB and STAT signaling. Lipid A, a core structural moiety of lipopolysaccharide (LPS), was identified as the requisite trigger for caspase-4, caspase-5, and caspase-11 activation and pyroptosis following challenge with gram-negative bacteria. The activation of these caspases appears to occur by a direct interaction between LPS and the CARD of the caspase itself.[144] The initiation of a process by the very same molecule responsible for its execution introduces an unexpected twist in our understanding of caspase biology and to the fundamental regulation of innate immunity. Whether this observation is only the first to define caspases as a novel class of receptors for pathogen-derived PAMPs remains to be seen.

Not all pyroptosis and IL-1β production is mediated by activation of caspase-1. In several studies, caspase-8, perhaps in a complex with MALT-1 and ASC, can mediate the processing of IL-1β and activation of Gasdermin-D to effect pyroptosis.[145–147] It remains to be determined if this noncanonical caspase-8 inflammasome can be engaged in response to other extra-cellular pathogens, or, indeed, if the activity of other apical caspases can be similarly co-opted for host immune defense.

Molecular Pathways of Regulated Necrosis

Necrosis and Secondary Necrosis

Necrosis can be induced either directly by stimuli such as ATP depletion, nutrient withdrawal, and excessive ROS or, alternatively, as a consequence of apoptosis and is termed "secondary necrosis." Cells undergoing secondary necrosis are characterized by chromatin condensation, a feature typically associated with apoptosis, and plasma membrane permeabilization, one of the hallmarks of necrosis. As noted previously, secondary necrosis can occur as a consequence of the cleavage of Gasdermin-E by executioner caspases, causing the formation of plasma membrane pores.

Necrosis and the Mitochondrial Permeability Transition

MOMP, most often a feature of apoptotic cell death, can also be associated with necrotic cell death arising from ischemia-reperfusion injury. Under these conditions, the loss of outer mitochondrial membrane integrity is attributed to activation of the permeability transition pore (PTP), a channel in the inner mitochondrial membrane, resulting in dissipation of the transmembrane potential, or mitochondrial permeability transition (MPT), swelling of the mitochondrial matrix, and, ultimately, rupture of the outer mitochondrial membrane and release of its contents into the cytosol. Importantly, however, there is no strong evidence to indicate that this activates apoptotic signaling, as would be the case if MOMP were mediated in a Bax/Bak-dependent manner.

PARP and Necrosis (Parthanatos)

The generation of ATP to provide the necessary energy to sustain normal cellular function is mediated by the collective activities of glycolysis, the Kreb's cycle, and oxidative phosphorylation. Disruption of these pathways or an enhanced demand for intracellular energy consumption can lead to bioenergetic failure and engagement of necrosis. PARP is an essential enzyme for DNA repair, an energy-costly process that utilizes large amounts of nicotinamide adenine dinucleotide (NAD^+), thereby limiting mitochondrial ATP generation. As a consequence, cellular damage that demands excessive PARP-dependent DNA repair can disrupt oxidative phosphorylation, leading to necrotic cell death, also known as parthanatos (Thanatos—personification of death).

Ferroptosis

Ferroptosis or iron-dependent cell death is distinct from other forms of death by morphologic and metabolic criteria. Cells undergoing ferroptosis are characterized by mitochondria that are smaller in size but with an increase in the density of their membranes.[148] The identification of several genes required for ferroptosis including citrate synthase, an acyl Co-A synthase family member (ACSF2) and an enzyme required for synthesis of poly-unsaturated fatty acids (ACSL4), both of which are involved in mitochondrial fatty acid metabolism, suggesting that lipid synthesis could represent one pathway through which ferroptosis may be regulated.[149–151] Indeed, ferroptosis depends on the presence of poly-unsaturated fatty acids.[152] Further characterization indicates that ferroptosis is induced by iron-dependent production of lipid peroxides via the Fenton reaction, dependent upon hydrogen peroxide (which in turn may depend on mitochondrial metabolism).[153]

Peroxidized lipids are extremely toxic, as they promote a feed-forward peroxidation in the presence of oxygen, destabilizing cellular membranes. The only lipid peroxidase in the cell, GPX4, is a seleno-protein required for the prevention of ferroptosis. GPX4 must be "recharged" by glutathione (GSH) to sustain its peroxidase activity. Therefore, inhibitors of GPX4 or treatments (or conditions) that deplete GSH (inhibition of cystine import via the System Xc^- transporter, cysteine/cystine deprivation) promote ferroptosis.[152]

Not all cells are sensitive to the induction of ferroptosis by GPX4 inhibition or GSH depletion. Remarkably, a wide variety of cancer cell lines that are relatively resistant to ferroptosis attain a dependence on GPX4 following treatment with a range of chemotherapeutic agents that kill a majority of the cells. Those that persist in the face of such treatment ("persister cells") become highly susceptible to GPX4 inhibition.[154,155]

Necroptosis

Until relatively recently, our understanding of necrosis was somewhat limited, fueled largely by the presumed absence of any underlying molecular mechanism. However, the identification of a form of regulated or programmed necrosis, necroptosis, has invigorated research efforts into determining the molecular basis for this type of death, how it contributes to host biology, and whether its regulatory pathways may be exploited for clinical benefit.[156,157]

Although several stimuli can induce programmed necrosis, TNF and activation of its death receptor, TNFR1, has provided most insight into the molecular basis of this type of necrotic cell death (see Fig. 19.2C). As we have already discussed, TNFR1 signaling is complex, with TNFR1-induced NF-κB activation promoting cellular survival and death receptor induced caspase-8 activation critical for the induction of apoptosis. However, long before we had defined its molecular basis or had a name for it, an alternative form of death receptor-induced death was described that proceeded independently of caspase activation and required RIPK1 activity.[158–160] Recent genetic studies have characterized this form of TNF-induced caspase-independent cell death as necroptosis and defined key components of death receptor signaling, including caspase-8, $FLIP_L$, and FADD as essential regulators.

An Unanticipated Finding of a Caspase Needed for Cell Survival

Tantalizing suggestions of an unidentified death pathway involving caspase-8, FADD, and FLIP arose from apparent contradictory findings that were not easily reconciled with their known role in apoptosis. These included the unexpected embryonic lethality associated with the deletion of caspase-8 or FADD, two proteins that prior to these studies were exclusively associated with promoting apoptotic cell death and therefore predicted to phenocopy the cellular accumulation observed in embryos lacking Apaf-1 or caspase-9.[161–163] These findings were reconciled by the genetic rescue of the early lethality of caspase-8 or FADD deficiencies by the co-deletion of either of two related kinases, receptor-interacting serine/threonine-protein kinases (RIPK) 1 and 3.[164–166] Programmed necrosis, or necroptosis, is therefore a death pathway that is mediated by RIPK1/3 but only in the absence of caspase-8 activity.

The overlapping requirement for several of the signaling components required for both TNF-induced apoptosis and TNF-induced necroptosis begs the question as to how the activity of caspase-8 is regulated under physiologic conditions to engage cell death via apoptosis or necroptosis, and even, under some circumstances, to sustain cellular survival.

Molecular Regulation of Programmed Necrosis

The realization that RIPK3 was required for TNF-induced RIPK1-dependent necrosis provided a critical piece of a mechanistic puzzle[167–169] that was completed by the subsequent identification of MLKL as the target of RIPK3 and terminal effector of necroptosis.[170,171] Interaction between catalytically active RIPK1 and RIPK3 is mediated by their respective receptor interacting protein (RIP) homotypic interaction motifs (RHIM).[167,168,172] Neither the homodimerization of the N termini of RIPK1 lacking a RHIM domain ($RIPK1^{ΔRHIM}$) nor heterodimerization of $RIPK1^{ΔRHIM}$ and $RIPK3^{ΔRHIM}$ is able to trigger necroptosis. However, enforced dimerization of either the N termini of RIPK1 or $RIPK1^{ΔRHIM}$ and RIPK3 are both able to do so, as are homo-oligomers, but not dimers of the C termini of $RIPK3^{ΔRHIM}$ as well as dimers of the N termini of $RIPK3^{ΔRHIM}$.[173]

RHIM-dependent interaction between RIP1 and RIP3 kinases triggers self-propagation of large hetero-oligomeric RIPK complexes that are essential for both kinase activity and execution of necroptosis.[167,168,172] Characterization of these high order RIPK1/3 oligomers revealed strikingly similar characteristics to amyloid aggregates and an underlying mechanism by which kinase activation and necrosome assembly mutually reinforce each other.[174] Amyloid-like structures can be toxic in and of themselves. However, acquisition of kinase activity as a consequence of RIPK1/3 complex assembly is more compatible with the requirement for specific RIPK substrates to mediate necroptosis, rather than the complexes themselves causing toxicity. Recently identified is the RIPK-dependent phosphorylation of the pseudokinase, MLKL, to induce its activation, oligomerization, and translocation to the plasma membrane.[170,171,175] The swelling and loss of membrane permeability in cells dying by necroptosis is attributed to the ability of MLKL to disrupt ion homeostasis. Whether this occurs by the direct binding of MLKL to phospholipid components of the plasma membrane or by its association with Ca^{2+} or sodium channels remains to be determined.[176–179]

RIPK1—Apoptosis, Necroptosis, or Survival

While the activity of RIPK1 is critical for TNFR1-mediated activation of RIPK3 and execution of necroptosis, it is now apparent that its ability to regulate cell death mechanisms also encompasses roles in TNF-induced apoptosis under certain conditions as well as suppressing the aberrant inflammation associated with RIPK3 and caspase-8 activities. RIPK1 therefore clearly represents a critical signaling nexus within several pathways including those induced by TNF, TLRs, DNA-sensing pathways, and interferons. The diverse consequences of its regulatory activities are evidenced by its impact on multiple downstream signaling pathways and their biologic consequences.[180]

Deletion of RIPK1 is associated with perinatal lethality characterized by multiorgan inflammation and widespread cell death.[181] However, mice harboring one of several homozygous point mutations that eliminate RIPK1 kinase activity are viable.[182–184] Recent genetic studies have begun to elucidate not only the molecular basis for the postnatal lethality associated with RIPK1 deletion but also the identity of signaling pathways regulated by RIPK1 and the mechanisms mediating its effects. While the individual deletion of FADD, RIPK3, or caspase-8 all fails to impact the lethal phenotype observed in $RIPK1^{-/-}$ mice, the ablation of both RIPK3 and caspase-8 or RIPK3 and FADD in the context of $RIPK1^{-/-}$ completely rescues postnatal lethality.[185–187] Development also proceeds normally in mice lacking both RIPK1 and RIPK3 and the requisite adapter molecule for caspase-8 activation, FADD.[185] The unambiguous conclusion from these studies is that RIPK1 is an inhibitor of two independent pathways associated with embryonic lethality—one that is mediated by FADD/caspase-8 and the other, a lethal RIPK3-mediated pathway. This is consistent with roles for RIPK1 in the inhibition of both apoptosis and necroptosis. But have we not just discussed the requirement for RIPK1 in promoting cell death? In fact, this assertion too is supported by unambiguous genetic data—specifically that the embryonic lethality associated with ablation of caspase-8 or FADD is completely rescued by the co-deletion of RIPK3 or RIPK1.[165,166] The simple conclusion, then, is that RIPK1 must drive or mediate the lethal signal resulting from the ablation of caspase-8 or FADD. Must we therefore reach the "not so simple" conclusion, then, that RIPK1 can both promote and inhibit cell death? As we will now discuss, that indeed is the case.

Homodimerization and activation of caspase-8 can be triggered by the ligation of TNFR1 via the adapter proteins TRADD and FADD to promote apoptosis.[162,188,189] NF-κB, also activated by TNFR1 ligation, can inhibit caspase-8-dependent cell death by inducing transcription of FLIP, a catalytically inactive form of caspase-8. FLIP, by forming heterodimers with caspase-8, prevents the homodimerization of caspase-8 to inhibit apoptosis. RIP1K, by acting as a scaffold protein within this signaling complex, may provide a critical activation signal for NF-κB[190] or facilitate amplification of NF-κB-mediated transcription.[191–193] Either way, RIPK1 activity can contribute to cellular survival under conditions of TNFR1 ligation. Murine embryonic fibroblasts (MEFs) deficient for RIPK1, but not those expressing a kinase-dead version of RIPK1, are more sensitive to TNF-induced apoptosis.[191] Furthermore, intestine-specific ablation of RIP1K in adult mice is associated with a postnatal lethality, characterized by extensive apoptosis of the gut epithelium and generalized inflammation. This RIPK1 null phenotype can be rescued by the tissue specific co-deletion of caspase-8 or FADD but not by the introduction of catalytically inactive RIPK1.[194,195] The observed accumulation of cIAP1 and TRAF2 in tissues lacking RIPK1 is consistent with a model in which the alleviation of cIAP1/TRAF2 mediated stabilization of NIK leads to increased NF-κB activity that promotes TNF transcription to induce apoptosis. This is supported by the rescue, albeit partial, of the excessive apoptosis associated with gut-specific ablation of RIPK1 as well as $ripk1^{-/-}/ripk3^{-/-}$-induced lethality, by the co-deletion of TNFR1.

RIPK1 can also mediate FADD-dependent caspase-8 activation to promote apoptosis in response to several stimuli including depletion of cIAPs, TNF, and TLR activation.[196–198] Homotypic interaction between the DDs of FADD and RIPK1 to recruit and activate procaspase-8 constitutes the so-called "ripoptosome." TLR-induced ripoptosome formation is mediated by interaction of the respective RHIM domains of TRIF and RIPK1.[199–201] This prodeath role of RIPK1 is substantiated by several genetic studies in which the absence of RIPK1 (or caspase-8) can rescue the embryonic lethality associated with catalytically inactive $RIPK3^{D161N}$.[183] In a similar manner, ablation of MLKL, the target of RIPK3 and required for necroptosis, instead can promote apoptosis via a RIPK3/RIPK1/caspase-8-dependent pathway.[202]

The death-inducing role of RIPK1 is also evident in RIPK3/MLKL-dependent necroptosis, but only under circumstances in which caspase-8 activity is disrupted. RHIM-mediated interaction between the RIPK1 and RIPK3 is essential for RIP3K activity and the induction of necroptosis by ligation of TNFR1. For this, RIP1K absolutely requires its kinase activity, although the precise reason remains unclear, as RIPK1-mediated phosphorylation of itself, but not RIPK3 can be detected. Potentially, therefore, autophosphorylation and a consequent conformational change of RIPK1 may mediate its interaction with RIPK3, or alternatively, additional RIPK1 substrates that participate in the activation of RIPK3 to promote necroptosis remain to be identified.

RIPK1-Independent Necroptosis

While the ubiquitous activity of RIPK1 can be utilized for cellular survival, apoptosis, or programmed necrosis, RIPK3/MLKL-dependent necroptosis can also proceed in the absence of RIPK1[203] (Fig. 19.4A). TRIF, the signaling adapter associated with activation of TLRs 3 or 4, can directly bind and activate RIPK3 to promote necroptosis in the absence of RIPK1.[204] TRIF-independent TLR signaling can also induce necroptosis by autocrine- or paracrine-mediated TNF activities.[205] The DNA sensor, DAI, is activated by viral infection and contains an RHIM domain that can also directly engage RIPK3 function to promote necroptosis in the absence of RIPK1.[206–208] Type I (α/β) and II (γ) interferons can also engage necroptosis under conditions in which either caspase-8 or FADD is inactivated. Although interferon-induced necroptosis is mediated via a RIPK1-RIPK3 complex, the kinase activity of RIPK1 is not required. Instead, the RNA-responsive kinase (PKR) interacts with RIPK1 to induce the formation of RIPK1-RIPK3 heterodimers and necroptosis.[203–209] If RIPK1 is present under any of these circumstances, necroptosis can only proceed if the proapoptotic FADD-caspase-8-FLIP axis is disrupted.

These observations are consistent with RIPK1-dependent inhibition of RIPK3/MLKL-mediated necroptosis. RIPK1 can suppress RIPK3-mediated necroptosis via two known pathways. The first requires its association with FADD to assemble the FADD-caspase-8-FLIP complex to facilitate the formation of FLIP-caspase-8 heterodimers (see Fig. 19.4B). These heterodimers, while unable to cleave and activate caspase-8 to promote apoptosis,[210–212] are sufficiently active to cleave components of the necrosome and its regulators,[166,213] including both RIPK1 and RIPK3, and suppress MLKL-mediated necroptosis.[214–216] In an alternative scenario, necroptosis initiated by caspase inhibition and TLR ligation or interferon treatment is inhibited by the disruption of RIPK1 activity with necrostatin[204,205,217] (see Fig. 19.4C). Furthermore, a catalytically inactive RIPK1 mutant, or RIPK1-bound to necrostatin, can still associate with RIPK3 when triggered by TLR signaling and caspase inhibition but does so in a manner that precludes interaction between RIPK3 and MLKL.[185]

Pro-inflammatory Effects of Programmed Necrosis

Murine models in which the expression and/or function of RIPK3 or MLKL are disrupted have provided at least some insight into the in vivo role of necroptosis in inflammation. Deletion of RIPK3 prevents the spontaneous inflammation associated with tissue specific deletion of FADD in the intestinal epithelial compartment[218] and skin keratinocytes,[219] consistent with a pro-inflammatory role of necroptosis. Similarly, the inflammatory consequences of tissue-specific deletion of caspase-8 in either the gut or the skin are abrogated by the co-deletion of RIPK3.[220] Deletion of RIPK3 or MLKL also ameliorated necroptosis of keratinocytes and immune infiltration into skin deficient for epidermal RIPK1.[194] The RIPK1 inhibitor, necrostatin, has also been a useful tool with which to interrogate the significance of necroptotic signaling events under a variety of physiologic conditions and to determine if the inhibition of necroptosis may be therapeutically advantageous.[221] The realization, however, that RIPK1 function is dispensable for RIPK3-MLKL-dependent necroptosis under certain conditions should be factored into any conclusion that relies solely on the use of necrostatin. Nonetheless, in several models that mimic a variety of pathophysiologic conditions including ischemic brain injury, myocardial infarction, and kidney ischemia-reperfusion injury, necrostatin provided significant protection against tissue damage and, in some cases, offset detrimental immune cell infiltration.[222]

The mechanism(s) by which necroptosis triggers inflammation have yet to be fully defined but likely involve the associated release of DAMPS to trigger a myriad of inflammatory signaling events[223] or indirectly by compromising the integrity of epithelial barriers in tissues such as the skin or gut.[224] Perhaps more intriguingly, however, is the delineation of RIPK-3-dependent pro-inflammatory

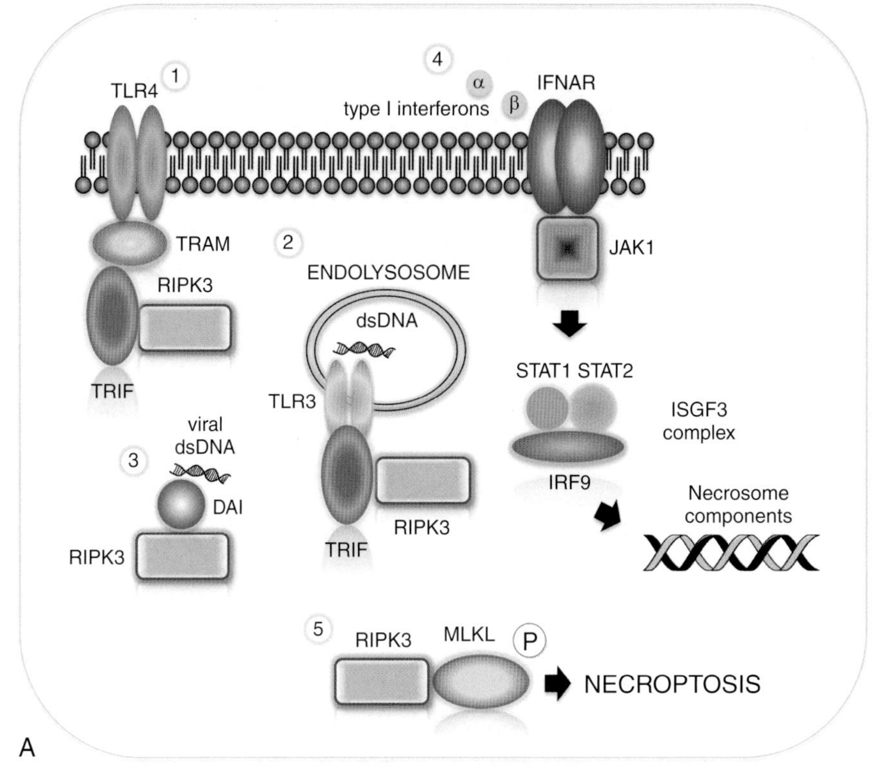

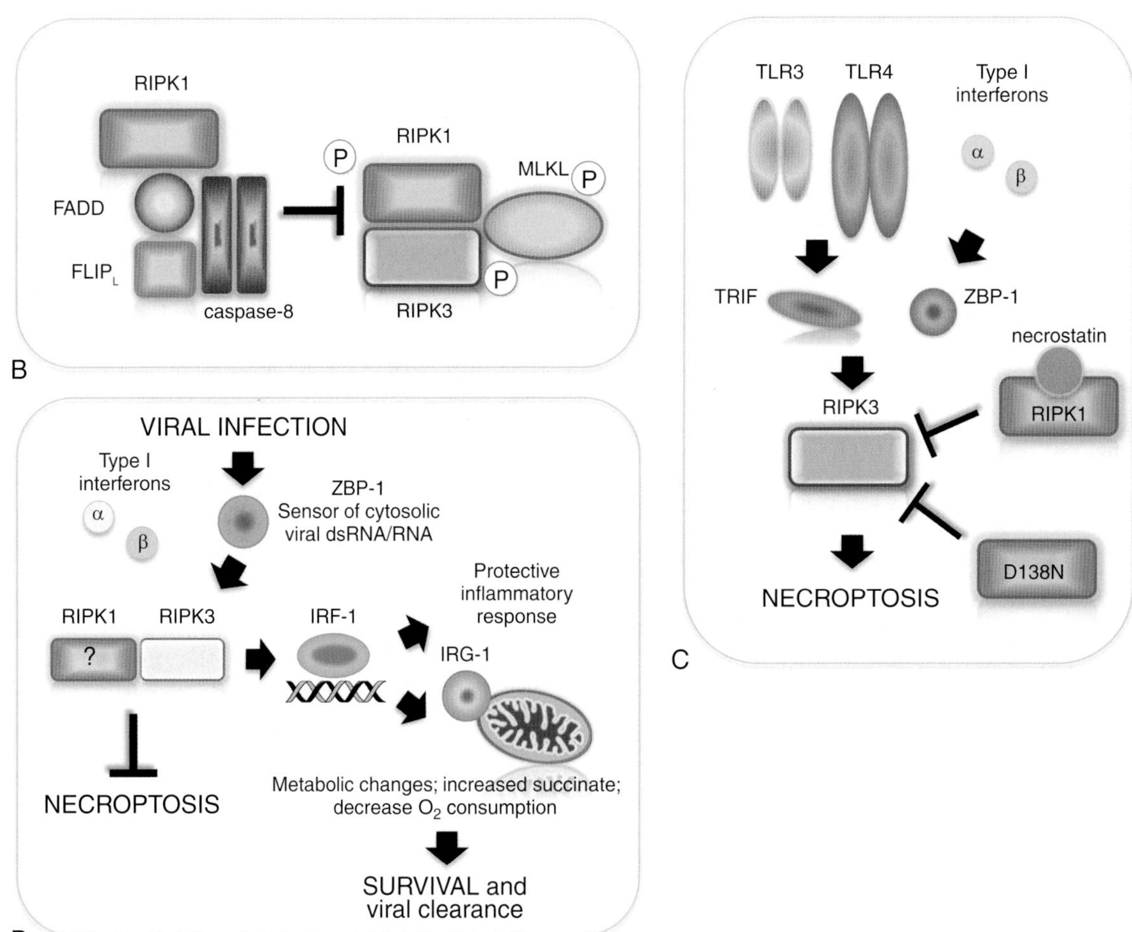

• **Fig. 19.4** "Signal 2"-dependent necroptosis. (A) Necroptosis can be engaged in a RIPK1-independent manner in response to TLR4 *(1)*, TLR3 *(2)*, DAI *(3)*, and type I interferons *(4)*. Each of these pathways results in RIPK3-dependent recruitment and activation of MLKL to promote necroptosis *(5)*. RIPK1 can actively suppress RIPK3 via two pathways. (B) RIPK1-DD interacts with FADD-DD to recruit FLIP$_L$ and caspase-8, resulting in the inhibition of caspase-8 induced apoptosis but retention of sufficient caspase-8 activity to cleave and inactivate RIPK1 and RIPK3 to disrupt the MLKL activating complex. (C) TLR activation or type I interferons activate RIPK3 via the adapters TRIF or ZBP-1, respectively, to induce necroptosis. Kinase inactive RIPK1 or its inhibition by necrostatin can suppress necroptosis. Therefore kinase inactive RIPK1 can block RIPK3-MLKL-dependent necroptosis. (D) RIPK3-mediated inflammation independent of necroptosis is triggered by its interaction with ZBP-1, a sensor of cytosolic viral dsRNA/DNA. Increased transcription of inflammatory genes and IRF-1 mediated changes in mitochondrial metabolism contribute to the anti-viral immune response. The role of RIPK1 in this context remains unclear.

pathways that proceed in the absence of necroptosis. The role of RIPK1 in this context remains unclear[225–233] (see Fig. 19.4D).

Cell Death and Immunity

"Like All Successful Relationships, It's Complex"

Key components of inflammatory responses, such as TNF, can induce cell death and, in a reciprocal manner, dead or dying cells can significantly impact immune function. Cell death plays critical roles in development of the immune system, maintenance of normal homeostasis, and in regulating immune function in response to pathogenic invasion.

Upon engulfment of dying cells by macrophages and dendritic cells, the mode by which the cell died influences the biology of the engulfing cell. With respect to macrophages, engulfment of a necrotic cell promotes inflammatory cytokine production, while uptake of an apoptotic cell promotes transition to a state, referred to as M2, which is anti-inflammatory (reviewed in ref. 234) and involved in tissue repair.[235,236] This may account for the presence of immunosuppressive macrophages in the tumor microenvironment, and manipulation of the processes involved in digestion of the corpse can promote inflammation[237] and anti-tumor immunity.[238]

Upon engulfment of dying cells, dendritic cells can present peptides derived from the corpse on class I major histocompatibility complex (MHC) molecules to promote $CD8^+$ T cell responses, a process refered to as "cross-presentation." Here, again, the mode of cell death appears to be important. While uptake of apoptotic cells promotes some cross-presentation, this is dramatically increased when cells that have died by necroptosis are engulfed.[239] This is likely to have implications for tumor immunotherapy.

The simple dichotomy that suggests that apoptosis is anti-inflammatory while necrosis promotes inflammation does not appear to extend to the activation of adaptive T cell responses. Extensive evidence exists that apoptotic cells can be immunogenic or non-immunogenic, depending on the treatment that induced the cell death. This has led to the concept of "immunogenic cell death" and the search for treatments that promote it.[240] Indeed, treatments that promote immunogenic cell death represent effective cancer therapies that rely on an intact immune system for optimal benefit. What makes a cell death immunogenic has been correlated with several events associated with the dying cell, including the cell surface exposure of the ER protein calreticulin. Whether the effects are on dendritic cell cross-presentation or other aspects of the initiation of the adaptive immune response are not clear.

Caspase-1 is at the epicenter of inflammatory responses and host immune defense by virtue of its ability to cleave and activate pro-IL-18 and pro-IL-1β. Pathogens express multiple virulence factors able to disrupt inflammasome assembly and/or its downstream pro-inflammatory effects (reviewed in refs. 241 to 243). A few examples are given in the following section.

Strategies to Inhibit Cell Death Pathways

Poxvirus family members express one of several so-called "serpins," including cowpox virus protein cytokine response modifier A (CRMA), SPI-1, and SPI-2, which directly inhibit the enzymatic activity of caspase-1 and caspase-8.[244–246] CRMA acts as a pseudosubstrate for caspase-1, forming a covalent bond with the active site cysteine in caspase-1 to render it catalytically inert.[247,248] Additional mechanisms through which virulence factors can disrupt the pro-inflammatory activity of inflammasomes include the secretion of soluble scavenger proteins that neutralize host-derived cytokines such as an IL-1β receptor able to bind to and inactivate host-derived IL-1β[249] and soluble IL-18 inhibitory binding proteins to neutralize host derived IL-18.[250] Several virulence factors can also directly disrupt inflammasome formation, primarily by the expression of decoy proteins. Examples include the herpes virus–derived protein, ORF63, an NLRP1 homolog that lacks both the CARD and pyrin interaction motifs that, by associating with host NLRP1 or NLRP3, prevents caspase-1 recruitment and activation.[251] Virally derived pyrin-only proteins (POPs) also act as decoys to sequester PYD-containing host proteins involved in inflammasome assembly, including the adapter protein ASC.[252,253] Bacterial factors that function to dysregulate the inflammasome-IL-1β/IL-18 axis include the Yersinia Yop proteins, negative regulators of Rho GTPases that inhibit caspase-1 activation[254] and mask recognition by the NLRs, NLRP3 and NLRC4, to prevent inflammasome assembly.[255]

As we have already discussed, mammalian cells express their own caspase inhibitor, XIAP. But so too do pathogens—in fact the first IAP to be identified was isolated from baculoviruses and provided the basis for their subsequent identification in vertebrates based on BIR domain homology. CRMA, expressed by pox viruses and a potent inhibitor of caspase-1 function, can also inhibit the catalytic activity of caspase-8 function. Baculovirus also expresses p35 protein which, once cleaved and processed, functions as a pseudosubstrate for caspases, thereby binding to and inhibiting the catalytically active cysteine and preventing proteolysis of target substrates.

Herpes viruses, including murine cytomegalovirus (MCMV), can circumvent death of the infected host cell by expressing the viral inhibitor of caspase-8 processing (vICA). Clearly, while this activity may effectively suppress caspase-8-dependent apoptosis and limit viral replication, it coincidentally triggers necroptosis—an alternative cell death pathway also with a critical role in anti-viral immunity. However, cells infected by MCMV neither succumb to apoptosis nor necroptosis as it also expresses the RHIM-like domain containing protein, vIRA, product of the M45 gene that prevents interaction between RIPK3 and DNA activator of interferon (DAI), a sensor of viral infection. The viral protease, NS3/4a, binds to mitochondria, where it cleaves an important signaling adapter, MAVS, thus preventing viral clearance by endogenous interferon production. Viral infection also triggers TNF production as part of the host defense mechanism to induce necroptosis. Both $Ripk1^{-/-}$ and $Ripk3^{-/-}$ cells are refractive to TNF-induced programmed necrosis as evidenced by abrogation of necrosis and inflammation in mice deficient for RIPK3. However, the failure to induce necroptosis manifests as uncontrolled viral replication, an inability to clear infection and, ultimately, death of the host. Thus, it is possible that necroptosis may act as a form of defense against viral infection.

Bacteria have also evolved multiple mechanisms to regulate cell death and inflammatory pathways, both of which can be detrimental to their survival (reviewed in refs. 242, 243). TNF-induced signaling is frequently targeted by components of pathogenic bacteria, both to prevent bacterial elimination by the inflammatory response and cell death, which, as a rich source of PAMPs, can also trigger inflammation and limit bacterial replication. NF-κB, a component of TNF-induced signaling, is a critical regulator of inflammation via the transcriptional induction of several cytokines. NLEB and various homologs, expressed by *Salmonella* and other pathogenic *E. coli* strains, are potent inhibitors of TNF-induced NF-κB activation via multiple mechanisms (reviewed elsewhere).

Conclusion and Clinical Potential

Several pharmacologic regulators of cell death are currently under development and/or in the clinic for their potential application to a range of pathologies including those characterized by aberrant cell death and immune dysfunction.

Caspase Inhibitors

Several pharmacologic inhibitors used experimentally include the peptide-based inhibitors z-VAD-fmk Z-Val-Ala-DL-Asp-FMK (fluoromethylketone) and qVD-oph Quinoline-Val-Asp Difluorophenoxymethylketone and Emricasan (IDN-6556), a small molecule pan caspase inhibitor. In all cases, the specificity of caspase inhibitors must be treated with caution, as they frequently inhibit other proteases, including calpains and cathepsins. Inhibitors that are putatively specific for individual caspases must be similarly questioned, as these specificities are, at best, confined to narrow dose ranges. Likely due, at least in part, to these caveats, clinical evaluation of several caspases inhibitors has revealed toxicity and poor efficacy and the trials have failed to progress. Currently, the IDN-6556 Emricasan remains the only caspase-inhibitor under clinical evaluation for the treatment of non-alcoholic steatohepatitis cirrhosis.

Necroptosis Inhibitors

The role of the RIP kinases in necroptosis has prompted the search for inhibitors of these kinases. The RIPK1 inhibitor Necrostatin-1, widely used experimentally, also inhibits the enzyme IDO (indoleamine 2,3-dioxygenase), which has immunologic consequences. Another RIPK1 inhibitor, Necrostatin-1s, however, does not have this cross reactivity. RIPK3 inhibitors are also described, including GSK2399872B. Necroptosis can also be inhibited by targeting MLKL. Necrosulfonamide inhibits human but not rodent MLKL, and the latter can be inhibited by GW806742X. Currently, no inhibitors of necroptosis are approved for human use.

Pyroptosis Inhibitors

With the delineation of a role for gasdermins in mediating pyroptotic cell death, a Gasdermin-D inhibitor N-acetyl-Phe-Leu-Thr-Asp-chloromethylketone (Ac-FLTD-CMK) has recently been described[8] that is able to suppress cleavage of Gasdermin-D by the inflammatory caspases and inhibit pyroptosis and IL-1β release. Several NLRP3 inhibitors have also been described, including the small molecule MCC-950 that inhibits both canonical and noncanonical NLRP3 inflammasome activation, CY-09 and OLT1177, which block the ATPase activity of NLRP3, and Tranilast, a drug used for the treatment of a variety of inflammatory disorders that was recently described to suppress NLRP3 oligomerization.[256,257] It remains to be seen whether additional inflammasome inhibitors will emerge as clinically viable options for the treatment of IL-1β–associated inflammatory disorders.

BH3 Mimetics

Several inhibitors of anti-apoptotic Bcl-2 proteins are described, including Obatoclax (inhibitor of Bcl-2 proteins), Gossypol (AT-101) (inhibitor of anti-apoptotic Bcl-2 proteins), and Sabutoclax (inhibitor of Bcl-2 proteins), although none of these have specificity for their targets. Of much more utility are the BH3 mimetic compounds, which include the experimental compounds ABT-737 (inhibitor of Bcl-X_L, Bcl-2, and Bcl-W), WEHI-539 (Bcl-XL selective inhibitor) and UMI-77 (MCL1 selective inhibitor), and the drugs Navitoclax (inhibitor of Bcl-XL, Bcl-2, and Bcl-W), Venetoclax (Bcl-2 selective inhibitor), A-1155463 (Bcl-X_L selective inhibitor), and several MCL-1 selective inhibitors (S63845, AZD5991, AMG176). The BH3 mimetics show exquisite specificity for the anti-apoptotic Bcl-2 proteins and are in clinical trials for a number of human malignancies. The Bcl-2 selective inhibitor Venetoclax has been approved for use in patients with chronic lymphocytic leukemia and acute myeloid leukemia.

IAP Inhibitors

As we discussed previously, ubiquitination is a powerful modulator of multiple pathways including the TNFR1 signaling complex to regulate the selective engagement of cellular survival or the death pathways, apoptosis and necroptosis. The use of SMAC (second mitochondrial-derived activator of caspases) mimetics (SMs), which function as antagonists of IAP function and promote the autoubiquitination and degradation of IAPs, can overcome cellular survival and increase the sensitivity of cells to RIP kinase-mediated necrosis. This approach could be of clinical importance by circumventing the commonly observed resistance of cancer cells to apoptotic death and instead evoking death in a RIPK dependent manner. As we begin to understand how RIPK-mediated death may intersect with immune function, it may also be possible to utilize SMAC mimetics to prime immune function against tumor-derived antigens.

As we reach some level of understanding of the molecular pathways of cell death and develop therapeutic agents to manipulate these pathways, the beginnings of an era of cell death therapy has arrived. While the treatment of cancer represents first steps in the emergence of this era, we can foresee applications in inflammatory and immune-mediated diseases as well. To reach this goal, however, we must continue to explore and dissect the complex interactions between the processes of cell death and the regulation of the immune response.

Full references for this chapter can be found on ExpertConsult.com.

Selected References

1. Bergsbaken T, Fink SL, Cookson BT: Pyroptosis: host cell death and inflammation, *Nat Rev Microbiol* 7(2):99–109, 2009.
2. Shi J, Gao W, Shao F: Pyroptosis: gasdermin-mediated programmed necrotic cell death, *Trends Biochem Sci* 42(4):245–254, 2017.
3. Davis MA, et al.: Calpain drives pyroptotic vimentin cleavage, intermediate filament loss, and cell rupture that mediates immunostimulation, *Proc Natl Acad Sci U S A* 116(11):5061–5070, 2019.
4. Alnemri ES: Mammalian cell death proteases: a family of highly conserved aspartate specific cysteine proteases, *J Cell Biochem* 64(1):33–42, 1997.
5. Sakahira H, Enari M, Nagata S: Cleavage of CAD inhibitor in CAD activation and DNA degradation during apoptosis, *Nature* 391(6662):96–99, 1998.
6. Enari M, et al.: A caspase-activated DNase that degrades DNA during apoptosis, and its inhibitor ICAD, *Nature* 391(6662):43–50, 1998.
7. Lazebnik YA, et al.: Cleavage of poly(ADP-ribose) polymerase by a proteinase with properties like ICE, *Nature* 371(6495):346–347, 1994.

8. Yang J, et al.: Mechanism of gasdermin D recognition by inflammatory caspases and their inhibition by a gasdermin D-derived peptide inhibitor, *Proc Natl Acad Sci U S A* 115(26):6792–6797, 2018.
9. Shi J, et al.: Cleavage of GSDMD by inflammatory caspases determines pyroptotic cell death, *Nature* 526(7575):660–665, 2015.
10. Ding J, et al.: Pore-forming activity and structural autoinhibition of the gasdermin family, *Nature* 535(7610):111–116, 2016.
11. Kayagaki N, et al.: Caspase-11 cleaves gasdermin D for non-canonical inflammasome signalling, *Nature* 526(7575):666–671, 2015.
12. Liu X, et al.: Inflammasome-activated gasdermin D causes pyroptosis by forming membrane pores, *Nature* 535(7610):153–158, 2016.
13. Ruan J, et al.: Cryo-EM structure of the gasdermin A3 membrane pore, *Nature* 557(7703):62–67, 2018.
14. Wang Y, et al.: Chemotherapy drugs induce pyroptosis through caspase-3 cleavage of a gasdermin, *Nature* 547(7661):99–103, 2017.
15. Rogers C, et al.: Cleavage of DFNA5 by caspase-3 during apoptosis mediates progression to secondary necrotic/pyroptotic cell death, *Nat Commun* 8:14128, 2017.
16. Hawkins CJ, et al.: Anti-apoptotic potential of insect cellular and viral IAPs in mammalian cells, *Cell Death Differ* 5(7):569–576, 1998.
17. Bump NJ, et al.: Inhibition of ICE family proteases by baculovirus antiapoptotic protein p35, *Science* 269(5232):1885–1888, 1995.
18. Xue D, Horvitz HR: Inhibition of the Caenorhabditis elegans cell-death protease CED-3 by a CED-3 cleavage site in baculovirus p35 protein, *Nature* 377(6546):248–251, 1995.
19. Clem RJ, Fechheimer M, Miller LK: Prevention of apoptosis by a baculovirus gene during infection of insect cells, *Science* 254(5036):1388–1390, 1991.
20. Deveraux QL, et al.: X-linked IAP is a direct inhibitor of cell-death proteases, *Nature* 388(6639):300–304, 1997.
21. Duckett CS, et al.: A conserved family of cellular genes related to the baculovirus iap gene and encoding apoptosis inhibitors, *EMBO J* 15(11):2685–2694, 1996.
22. Liston P, et al.: Suppression of apoptosis in mammalian cells by NAIP and a related family of IAP genes, *Nature* 379(6563):349–353, 1996.
23. Roy N, et al.: The gene for neuronal apoptosis inhibitory protein is partially deleted in individuals with spinal muscular atrophy, *Cell* 80(1):167–178, 1995.
24. Ambrosini G, Adida C, Altieri DC: A novel anti-apoptosis gene, survivin, expressed in cancer and lymphoma, *Nat Med* 3(8):917–921, 1997.
25. Sun C, et al.: NMR structure and mutagenesis of the inhibitor-of-apoptosis protein XIAP, *Nature* 401(6755):818–822, 1999.
26. Vaux DL, Silke J: IAPs, RINGs and ubiquitylation, *Nat Rev Mol Cell Biol* 6(4):287–297, 2005.
27. Harlin H, et al.: Characterization of XIAP-deficient mice, *Mol Cell Biol* 21(10):3604–3608, 2001.
28. Zou H, et al.: Apaf-1, a human protein homologous to C. elegans CED-4, participates in cytochrome c-dependent activation of caspase-3, *Cell* 90(3):405–413, 1997.
29. Li P, et al.: Cytochrome c and dATP-dependent formation of Apaf-1/caspase-9 complex initiates an apoptotic protease cascade, *Cell* 91(4):479–489, 1997.
30. Qin H, et al.: Structural basis of procaspase-9 recruitment by the apoptotic protease-activating factor 1, *Nature* 399(6736):549–557, 1999.
31. Liu X, et al.: Induction of apoptotic program in cell-free extracts: requirement for dATP and cytochrome c, *Cell* 86(1):147–157, 1996.
32. Kluck RM, et al.: The release of cytochrome c from mitochondria: a primary site for Bcl-2 regulation of apoptosis, *Science* 275(5303):1132–1136, 1997.
33. Yang J, et al.: Prevention of apoptosis by Bcl-2: release of cytochrome c from mitochondria blocked, *Science* 275(5303):1129–1132, 1997.
34. Du C, et al.: Smac, a mitochondrial protein that promotes cytochrome c-dependent caspase activation by eliminating IAP inhibition, *Cell* 102(1):33–42, 2000.
35. Suzuki Y, et al.: A serine protease, HtrA2, is released from the mitochondria and interacts with XIAP, inducing cell death, *Mol Cell* 8(3):613–621, 2001.
36. Susin SA, et al.: Bcl-2 inhibits the mitochondrial release of an apoptogenic protease, *J Exp Med* 184(4):1331–1341, 1996.
37. Volkmann N, et al.: The rheostat in the membrane: BCL-2 family proteins and apoptosis, *Cell Death Differ* 21(2):206–215, 2014.
38. Tait SW, Green DR: Mitochondrial regulation of cell death, *Cold Spring Harb Perspect Biol* 5(9), 2013.
39. Moldoveanu T, et al.: Many players in BCL-2 family affairs, *Trends Biochem Sci* 39(3):101–111, 2014.
40. Bender T, Martinou JC: Where killers meet—permeabilization of the outer mitochondrial membrane during apoptosis, *Cold Spring Harb Perspect Biol* 5(1):a011106, 2013.
41. Llambi F, et al.: BOK is a non-canonical BCL-2 family effector of apoptosis regulated by ER-associated degradation, *Cell* 165(2):421–433, 2016.
42. Ke F, et al.: Consequences of the combined loss of BOK and BAK or BOK and BAX, *Cell Death Dis* 4, 2013:e650.
43. Beroukhim R, et al.: The landscape of somatic copy-number alteration across human cancers, *Nature* 463(7283):899–905, 2010.
44. Luciano F, et al.: Phosphorylation of Bim-EL by Erk1/2 on serine 69 promotes its degradation via the proteasome pathway and regulates its proapoptotic function, *Oncogene* 22(43):6785–6793, 2003.
45. Lei K, Davis RJ: JNK phosphorylation of Bim-related members of the Bcl2 family induces Bax-dependent apoptosis, *Proc Natl Acad Sci U S A* 100(5):2432–2437, 2003.
46. Datta SR, et al.: 14-3-3 proteins and survival kinases cooperate to inactivate BAD by BH3 domain phosphorylation, *Mol Cell* 6(1):41–51, 2000.
47. Yang E, et al.: Bad, a heterodimeric partner for Bcl-XL and Bcl-2, displaces Bax and promotes cell death, *Cell* 80(2):285–291, 1995.
48. Zha J, et al.: Serine phosphorylation of death agonist BAD in response to survival factor results in binding to 14-3-3 not BCL-X(L), *Cell* 87(4):619–628, 1996.
49. Datta SR, et al.: Akt phosphorylation of BAD couples survival signals to the cell-intrinsic death machinery, *Cell* 91(2):231–241, 1997.
50. Perciavalle RM, Opferman JT: Delving deeper: MCL-1's contributions to normal and cancer biology, *Trends Cell Biol* 23(1):22–29, 2013.
51. Maurer U, et al.: Glycogen synthase kinase-3 regulates mitochondrial outer membrane permeabilization and apoptosis by destabilization of MCL-1, *Mol Cell* 21(6):749–760, 2006.
52. Zhong Q, et al.: Mule/ARF-BP1, a BH3-only E3 ubiquitin ligase, catalyzes the polyubiquitination of Mcl-1 and regulates apoptosis, *Cell* 121(7):1085–1095, 2005.
53. Inuzuka H, et al.: SCF(FBW7) regulates cellular apoptosis by targeting MCL1 for ubiquitylation and destruction, *Nature* 471(7336):104–109, 2011.
54. Schwickart M, et al.: Deubiquitinase USP9X stabilizes MCL1 and promotes tumour cell survival, *Nature* 463(7277):103–107, 2010.
55. Ito T, et al.: Bcl-2 phosphorylation required for anti-apoptosis function, *J Biol Chem* 272(18):11671–11673, 1997.
56. Kutuk O, Letai A: Regulation of Bcl-2 family proteins by post-translational modifications, *Curr Mol Med* 8(2):102–118, 2008.
57. Deng X, et al.: Survival function of ERK1/2 as IL-3-activated, staurosporine-resistant Bcl2 kinases, *Proc Natl Acad Sci U S A* 97(4):1578–1583, 2000.
58. Deng X, et al.: Mono- and multisite phosphorylation enhances Bcl2's antiapoptotic function and inhibition of cell cycle entry functions, *Proc Natl Acad Sci U S A* 101(1):153–158, 2004.
59. Deng X, Gao F, May WS: Protein phosphatase 2A inactivates Bcl2's antiapoptotic function by dephosphorylation and up-regulation of Bcl2-p53 binding, *Blood* 113(2):422–428, 2009.

60. Deverman BE, et al.: Bcl-xL deamidation is a critical switch in the regulation of the response to DNA damage, *Cell* 111(1):51–62, 2002.
61. Li H, et al.: Cleavage of BID by caspase 8 mediates the mitochondrial damage in the Fas pathway of apoptosis, *Cell* 94(4):491–501, 1998.
62. Bonzon C, et al.: Caspase-2-induced apoptosis requires bid cleavage: a physiological role for bid in heat shock-induced death, *Mol Biol Cell* 17(5):2150–2157, 2006.
63. Barry M, et al.: Granzyme B short-circuits the need for caspase 8 activity during granule-mediated cytotoxic T-lymphocyte killing by directly cleaving Bid, *Mol Cell Biol* 20(11):3781–3794, 2000.
64. Stoka V, et al.: Lysosomal protease pathways to apoptosis. Cleavage of bid, not pro-caspases, is the most likely route, *J Biol Chem* 276(5):3149–3157, 2001.
65. Chen M, et al.: Bid is cleaved by calpain to an active fragment in vitro and during myocardial ischemia/reperfusion, *J Biol Chem* 276(33):30724–30728, 2001.
66. Wood DE, et al.: Bax cleavage is mediated by calpain during drug-induced apoptosis, *Oncogene* 17(9):1069–1078, 1998.
67. Karbowski M, et al.: Role of Bax and Bak in mitochondrial morphogenesis, *Nature* 443(7112):658–662, 2006.
68. Zinkel SS, et al.: A role for proapoptotic BID in the DNA-damage response, *Cell* 122(4):579–591, 2005.
69. Kamer I, et al.: Proapoptotic BID is an ATM effector in the DNA-damage response, *Cell* 122(4):593–603, 2005.
70. Danial NN, et al.: BAD and glucokinase reside in a mitochondrial complex that integrates glycolysis and apoptosis, *Nature* 424(6951):952–956, 2003.
71. Gimenez-Cassina A, Danial NN: Regulation of mitochondrial nutrient and energy metabolism by BCL-2 family proteins, *Trends Endocrinol Metab* 26(4):165–175, 2015.
72. Perciavalle RM, et al.: Anti-apoptotic MCL-1 localizes to the mitochondrial matrix and couples mitochondrial fusion to respiration, *Nat Cell Biol* 14(6):575–583, 2012.
73. Pinton P, Rizzuto R: Bcl-2 and Ca2+ homeostasis in the endoplasmic reticulum, *Cell Death Differ* 13(8):1409–1418, 2006.
74. Levine B, Sinha S, Kroemer G: Bcl-2 family members: dual regulators of apoptosis and autophagy, *Autophagy* 4(5):600–606, 2008.
75. Jost PJ, Grabow S, Gray D, et al.: XIAP discriminates between type I and type II FAS-induced apoptosis, *Nature* 460(7258):1035–1039, 2009. Epub 2009 Jul 22.
76. Bauernfeind FG, et al.: Cutting edge: NF-kappaB activating pattern recognition and cytokine receptors license NLRP3 inflammasome activation by regulating NLRP3 expression, *J Immunol* 183(2):787–791, 2009.
77. Dostert C, et al.: Innate immune activation through Nalp3 inflammasome sensing of asbestos and silica, *Science* 320(5876):674–677, 2008.
78. Halle A, et al.: The NALP3 inflammasome is involved in the innate immune response to amyloid-beta, *Nat Immunol* 9(8):857–865, 2008.
79. Martinon F, et al.: Gout-associated uric acid crystals activate the NALP3 inflammasome, *Nature* 440(7081):237–241, 2006.
80. Martinon F, et al.: Identification of bacterial muramyl dipeptide as activator of the NALP3/cryopyrin inflammasome, *Curr Biol* 14(21):1929–1934, 2004.
81. Pazar B, et al.: Basic calcium phosphate crystals induce monocyte/macrophage IL-1beta secretion through the NLRP3 inflammasome in vitro, *J Immunol* 186(4):2495–2502, 2011.
82. Kanneganti TD, et al.: Bacterial RNA and small antiviral compounds activate caspase-1 through cryopyrin/Nalp3, *Nature* 440(7081):233–236, 2006.
83. Zhou R, et al.: A role for mitochondria in NLRP3 inflammasome activation, *Nature* 469(7329):221–225, 2011.
84. Shimada K, et al.: Oxidized mitochondrial DNA activates the NLRP3 inflammasome during apoptosis, *Immunity* 36(3):401–414, 2012.
85. Iyer SS, et al.: Mitochondrial cardiolipin is required for Nlrp3 inflammasome activation, *Immunity* 39(2):311–323, 2013.
86. Guan K, et al.: MAVS promotes inflammasome activation by targeting ASC for K63-linked ubiquitination via the E3 ligase TRAF3, *J Immunol*, 2015.
87. Subramanian N, et al.: The adaptor MAVS promotes NLRP3 mitochondrial localization and inflammasome activation, *Cell* 153(2):348–361, 2013.
88. Ichinohe T, et al.: Mitochondrial protein mitofusin 2 is required for NLRP3 inflammasome activation after RNA virus infection, *Proc Natl Acad Sci U S A* 110(44):17963–17968, 2013.
89. Lu B, et al.: Novel role of PKR in inflammasome activation and HMGB1 release, *Nature* 488(7413):670–674, 2012.
90. Shenoy AR, et al.: GBP5 promotes NLRP3 inflammasome assembly and immunity in mammals, *Science* 336(6080):481–485, 2012.
91. Petrilli V, et al.: Activation of the NALP3 inflammasome is triggered by low intracellular potassium concentration, *Cell Death Differ* 14(9):1583–1589, 2007.
92. Munoz-Planillo R, et al.: K(+) efflux is the common trigger of NLRP3 inflammasome activation by bacterial toxins and particulate matter, *Immunity* 38(6):1142–1153, 2013.
93. Murakami T, et al.: Critical role for calcium mobilization in activation of the NLRP3 inflammasome, *Proc Natl Acad Sci U S A* 109(28):11282–11287, 2012.
94. Lee GS, et al.: The calcium-sensing receptor regulates the NLRP3 inflammasome through Ca2+ and cAMP, *Nature* 492(7427):123–127, 2012.
95. Riteau N, et al.: ATP release and purinergic signaling: a common pathway for particle-mediated inflammasome activation, *Cell Death Dis* 3:e403, 2012.
96. Mayor A, et al.: A crucial function of SGT1 and HSP90 in inflammasome activity links mammalian and plant innate immune responses, *Nat Immunol* 8(5):497–503, 2007.
97. Broderick L, et al.: The inflammasomes and autoinflammatory syndromes, *Annu Rev Pathol* 10:395–424, 2015.
98. Brydges SD, et al.: Inflammasome-mediated disease animal models reveal roles for innate but not adaptive immunity, *Immunity* 30(6):875–887, 2009.
99. Cassel SL, Joly S, Sutterwala FS: The NLRP3 inflammasome: a sensor of immune danger signals, *Semin Immunol* 21(4):194–198, 2009.
100. Ng J, et al.: Clostridium difficile toxin-induced inflammation and intestinal injury are mediated by the inflammasome, *Gastroenterology* 139(2):542–552, 552 e1-3, 2010.
101. Witzenrath M, et al.: The NLRP3 inflammasome is differentially activated by pneumolysin variants and contributes to host defense in pneumococcal pneumonia, *J Immunol* 187(1):434–440, 2011.
102. Mariathasan S, et al.: Cryopyrin activates the inflammasome in response to toxins and ATP, *Nature* 440(7081):228–232, 2006.
103. Munoz-Planillo R, et al.: A critical role for hemolysins and bacterial lipoproteins in Staphylococcus aureus-induced activation of the Nlrp3 inflammasome, *J Immunol* 183(6):3942–3948, 2009.
104. Meixenberger K, et al.: Listeria monocytogenes-infected human peripheral blood mononuclear cells produce IL-1beta, depending on listeriolysin O and NLRP3, *J Immunol* 184(2):922–930, 2010.
105. Ichinohe T, et al.: Inflammasome recognition of influenza virus is essential for adaptive immune responses, *J Exp Med* 206(1):79–87, 2009.
106. Ichinohe T, Pang IK, Iwasaki A: Influenza virus activates inflammasomes via its intracellular M2 ion channel, *Nat Immunol* 11(5):404–410, 2010.
107. Nour AM, et al.: Varicella-zoster virus infection triggers formation of an interleukin-1beta (IL-1beta)-processing inflammasome complex, *J Biol Chem* 286(20):17921–17933, 2011.
108. Johnson KE, Chikoti L, Chandran B: Herpes simplex virus 1 infection induces activation and subsequent inhibition of the IFI16 and NLRP3 inflammasomes, *J Virol* 87(9):5005–5018, 2013.

109. Park S, et al.: The mitochondrial antiviral protein MAVS associates with NLRP3 and regulates its inflammasome activity, *J Immunol* 191(8):4358–4366, 2013.
110. Xiao TS: The nucleic acid-sensing inflammasomes, *Immunol Rev* 265(1):103–111, 2015.
111. Rathinam VA, et al.: The AIM2 inflammasome is essential for host defense against cytosolic bacteria and DNA viruses, *Nat Immunol* 11(5):395–402, 2010.
112. Duncan JA, Canna SW: The NLRC4 inflammasome, *Immunol Rev* 281(1):115–123, 2018.
113. Hu Z, et al.: Structural and biochemical basis for induced self-propagation of NLRC4, *Science* 350(6259):399–404, 2015.
114. Li Y, et al.: Cryo-EM structures of ASC and NLRC4 CARD filaments reveal a unified mechanism of nucleation and activation of caspase-1, *Proc Natl Acad Sci U S A* 115(43):10845–10852, 2018.
115. Tenthorey JL, et al.: The structural basis of flagellin detection by NAIP5: A strategy to limit pathogen immune evasion, *Science* 358(6365):888–893, 2017.
116. Canna SW, et al.: An activating NLRC4 inflammasome mutation causes autoinflammation with recurrent macrophage activation syndrome, *Nat Genet* 46(10):1140–1146, 2014.
117. Kitamura A, et al.: An inherited mutation in NLRC4 causes autoinflammation in human and mice, *J Exp Med* 211(12):2385–2396, 2014.
118. Romberg N, et al.: Mutation of NLRC4 causes a syndrome of enterocolitis and autoinflammation, *Nat Genet* 46(10):1135–1139, 2014.
119. Martinon F, Burns K, Tschopp J: The inflammasome: a molecular platform triggering activation of inflammatory caspases and processing of proIL-beta, *Mol Cell* 10(2):417–426, 2002.
120. Boyden ED, Dietrich WF: Nalp1b controls mouse macrophage susceptibility to anthrax lethal toxin, *Nat Genet* 38(2):240–244, 2006.

20 Innate Immunity

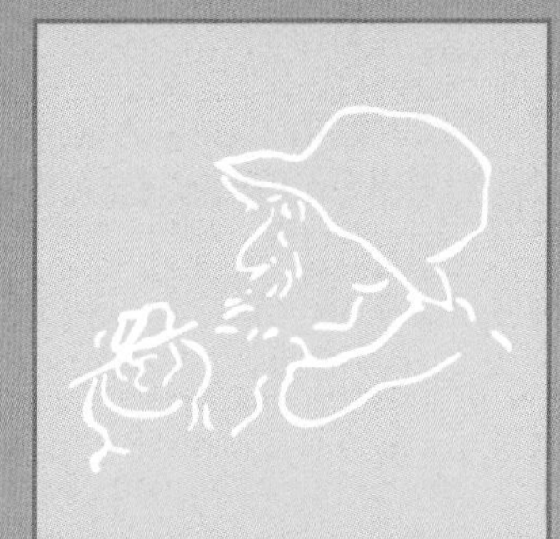

GREGOIRE LAUVAU AND STEVEN A. PORCELLI

KEY POINTS

- Innate immunity depends on recognition of conserved molecular patterns found in many microorganisms.
- Several families of pattern recognition receptors are responsible for triggering innate immune responses.
- Toll-like receptors and other pattern recognition receptors with leucine-rich repeat domains play a key role in innate immune recognition.
- Anti-microbial peptides are important effectors of innate immunity.
- Phagocytic cells and several types of innate-like lymphocytes are key cell types in mediating innate immunity.
- Innate immune responses have a strong impact on the development of adaptive immunity.
- Some defects in the innate immune system are associated with a predisposition to infection or to autoimmune disease.

Introduction

It has become common practice in immunology to divide the mechanisms involved in host defense into adaptive and innate components. This approach provides a useful framework for classifying the numerous cells, receptors, and effector molecules that combine to make up the vertebrate immune system (Table 20.1). A specific immune response, such as the production of antibodies or T cells against a particular pathogen, is referred to as *adaptive immunity* because it represents an adaptation that occurs during the lifetime of an individual as a result of exposure to that pathogen. Adaptive immune responses involve the clonal expansion of T and B lymphocytes bearing a large repertoire of somatically generated receptors that can be selected to recognize virtually any pathogen. The adaptive immune system of any given person is profoundly molded by the immunologic challenges encountered by that person during the course of a lifetime. A hallmark of adaptive immune responses is that they are highly specific for the triggering agent, and they provide the basis for immunologic memory. This property of memory endows the adaptive immune response with its "anticipatory" property, which provides increased resistance against future infection with the same pathogen and also allows vaccination against future infectious threats.

Adaptive immunity is essential for the survival of all mammals and most other vertebrates, but a wide variety of other mechanisms that do not involve antigen-specific lymphocyte responses are also involved in successful immune protection. These diverse mechanisms are collectively known as *innate immunity* because they are not dependent on prior exposure to specific pathogens for their amplification. Such responses are controlled by the products of germline genes that are inherited and similarly expressed by all healthy people. Innate immune mechanisms involve both constitutive and inducible components and use a wide variety of recognition and effector mechanisms. It has become clear in recent years that innate immune responses have a profound influence on the generation and outcome of adaptive immune responses. This ability of the innate immune system to instruct the responses of the adaptive immune system suggests many ways in which innate immunity can influence the development of both long-term specific immunity and autoimmune disease.

Evolutionary Origins of Innate Immunity

In spite of its obvious importance for most vertebrate organisms, the adaptive immune system is a relatively recent evolutionary development (Fig. 20.1). In the great majority of present-day vertebrate species, the adaptive immune system is based on the ability to generate large families of variable lymphocyte receptors with immunoglobulin-like structures. This ability has been conserved as a result of the acquisition of a specialized recombination system that mediates the assembly of gene segments in the T cell and B cell receptor families, which most likely occurred through invasion of the genome of a primitive vertebrate by a transposable element or virus carrying this machinery.[1,2] This critical step in the evolution of the immune system can be traced back to the emergence of the ancestors of present-day jawed fish, which represent the most primitive extant species known to have adaptive immune systems based on the generation of large families of specific immunoglobulin-type receptors.[3] Recently, other systems of variable lymphocyte receptors that are unrelated to immunoglobulins but also provide the basis for an adaptive immune response have been discovered in primitive jawless fish such as lampreys and hagfish.[4,5] This finding shows that at least two different strategies for the creation of an adaptive immune system emerged at the dawn of vertebrate evolution about 500 million years ago, and it emphasizes the importance of adaptive immunity for survival and further evolution of the vertebrate lineages.

Given this key role of adaptive immunity in the evolution and survival of vertebrates, it is surprising that all invertebrate animals appear to lack the ability to generate lymphocyte populations bearing large families of clonally diverse antigen receptors.[6,7] In these animals, protection against pathogen invasion depends entirely on innate immunity, elements of which appear to exist in all animals and plants and must have evolved with the earliest multicellular forms of life. In many cases, components of the innate immune system are significantly conserved in structure and function in animals from the lowliest invertebrates to the most complex vertebrates. This preservation of innate immune mechanisms, with

TABLE 20.1 Contrasting Features of Innate and Adaptive Immune Systems

Property	Innate Immune System	Adaptive Immune System
Receptors	Relatively few (several hundred?)	Many (potentially 10^{14} or more)
	Fixed in genome	Encoded in gene segments
	Gene rearrangement not required	Gene rearrangement required
Distribution	Nonclonal	Clonal
	All cells of a class identical	All cells of a class distinct
Targets	Conserved molecular patterns	Details of molecular structure
	Lipopolysaccharides	Proteins
	Lipoteichoic acids	Peptides
	Glycans and peptidoglycans	Carbohydrates
	Others	
Self–non–self-discrimination	Perfect: selected over evolutionary time	Imperfect: selected in individual somatic cells
Action time	Immediate or rapid (seconds to hours)	Delayed (days to weeks)
Response	Microbicidal effector molecules	Clonal expansion or anergy of specific T and B lymphocytes
	Anti-microbial peptides	Cytokines (IL-2, IL-4, IFN-γ, others)
	Superoxide	Specific antibody production
	Nitric oxide	Specific cytolytic T cell generation
	Cytokines (IL-1, IL-6, others)	
	Chemokines (IL-8, others)	

IFN, Interferon; *IL*, interleukin.

Modified from Medzhitov R, Janeway CA Jr: Innate immune recognition. *Annu Rev Immunol* 20:197, 2002.

their functions largely intact, over such vast evolutionary distances is a clear indication of their importance, even in animals that have developed sophisticated adaptive immune responses.

Pathogen Recognition by the Innate Immune System

Some mechanisms of innate immunity are constitutive, meaning that they are continuously expressed and are not significantly modulated by the presence or absence of infection. Examples include the barrier functions provided by epithelial surfaces continuously exposed to microbial flora, such as those of the skin and intestinal and genital tracts. In contrast, the inducible mechanisms of innate immunity involve increased production of mediators and upregulation of effector functions that eliminate microorganisms. Induction occurs as a result of exposure to a wide variety of microbes and represents a less specific form of immune recognition than that associated with the specific antibodies and T cells that mediate adaptive immunity. The basic principle underlying this form of response is a process known as *pattern recognition.* This recognition strategy is based on the detection of commonly occurring and conserved molecular patterns that are essential products or structural components of microbes.

PAMPs and DAMPs: Patterns for Innate Immune Recognition

Pathogen-Associated Molecular Patterns

The general name given to the targets of innate immune recognition in microbes is *pathogen-associated molecular patterns* (PAMPs). These structural features or components distinctive for microorganisms are not normally found in the animal host. The best-known example of a PAMP is bacterial lipopolysaccharide (LPS), a ubiquitous glycolipid constituent of the outer membranes of gram-negative bacteria. Another important example is the peptidoglycan structure present as the basic cell wall component in nearly all bacteria. These structures may vary partially from one bacterium to another, but the basic elements are conserved, thus providing the possibility of recognizing a broad array of pathogens by sensing a single or a relatively small number of PAMPs. Many PAMPs that serve as targets of recognition for the innate immune response are now known to be associated with bacteria, fungi, and viruses.

In addition to allowing direct recognition of molecules produced by various microorganisms, the innate immune system is able to respond to the patterns of host-derived molecules released by cells undergoing necrotic death. The molecules recognized are generally referred to as *damage-associated* or *danger-associated molecular patterns* (DAMPs) and include multiple different families of proteins, as well as nonproteinaceous substances such as uric acid microcrystals.[8–10] Thus the response to DAMPs can be an indirect response to microbial invasion, or it can be triggered by other types of tissue damage such as ischemia to result in sterile inflammation.

Pattern Recognition Receptors

Recognition of PAMPs and DAMPs is mediated by a collection of germline-encoded molecules known collectively as *pattern recognition receptors* (PRRs) (Table 20.2). These receptors are host proteins that have evolved, through many millions of years of natural selection, to possess precisely defined specificities for particular PAMPs or DAMPs expressed by microorganisms. The total number of PRRs present in complex vertebrates such as humans is estimated to be several hundred—a number limited by the size of the genome of any animal and the number of genes it can dedicate to immune protection. The human genome, for example, is estimated to contain approximately 19,000 to 20,000 protein-coding genes, most of which are not related directly to the immune system. This example demonstrates one of the strong points of contrast between the innate and adaptive immune systems, because the latter can possess in the range of 10^{14} different somatically generated receptors for foreign antigens in the form of antibodies

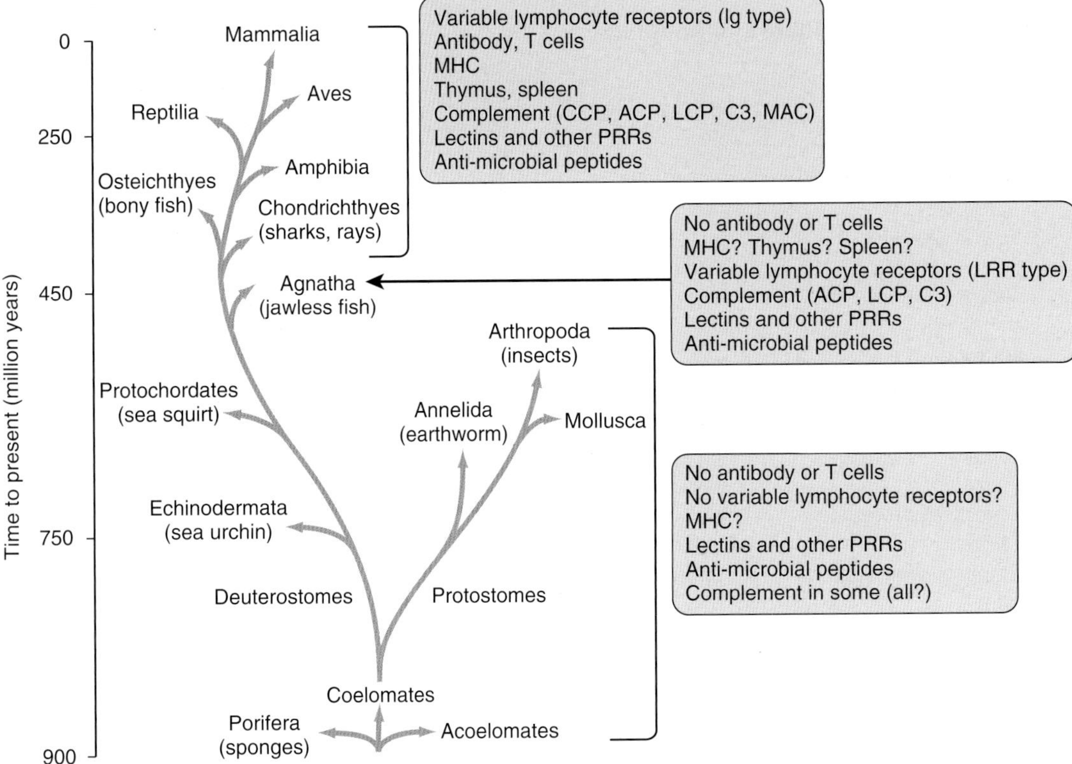

• **Fig. 20.1** Ancient evolutionary origin of the innate immune system. Studies of the immune systems of a wide range of vertebrates and invertebrates have revealed that even the most primitive invertebrates possess many components of innate immunity (e.g., pattern recognition receptors of the lectin and Toll-like families, anti-microbial peptides, and complement proteins). The innate immune system is thus extremely ancient, having arisen early in the evolution of multicellular life. In contrast, the adaptive immune system is a much more recent development that did not appear until emergence of the ancestors of present-day sharks and rays, approximately 400 million years ago. The first species to acquire an adaptive immune system based on immunoglobulin (Ig)-type receptors must have arisen after the appearance of the direct ancestors of present-day jawless fish (lampreys and hagfish), which are the most highly evolved living species that lack the ability to generate large families of variable Ig-type lymphocyte receptors *(arrow). ACP,* Alternative complement pathway; *CCP,* classic complement pathway; *LCP,* lectin-activated complement pathway; *LRR,* leucine-rich repeat domain; *MAC,* membrane attack complex; *MHC,* major histocompatibility complex; *PRR,* pattern recognition receptor. (Modified from Sunyer JO, Zarkadis IK, Lambris JD: Complement diversity: a mechanism for generating immune diversity? *Immunol Today* 19:519, 1998.)

and T cell receptors. With its much more limited array of receptors, the innate immune system uses the strategy of targeting highly conserved PAMPs that are shared broadly by large classes of microorganisms. Because most pathogens contain PAMPs, this strategy allows the generation of at least partial immunity against most infections.

PRRs are expressed by many cell types; some are specialized effector cells of the immune system (e.g., neutrophils, macrophages, dendritic cells, and lymphocytes), and others are not generally regarded as part of the immune system (e.g., epithelial and endothelial cells). Unlike the T and B cell receptors used for adaptive immune recognition, expression of PRRs is not clonal, which means that all receptors displayed by a given cell type (e.g., macrophages) have identical structure and specificity. When PRRs are engaged by recognition of their associated PAMPs or DAMPs, effector cells bearing the PRRs are triggered to perform their immune effector functions immediately, rather than after undergoing proliferation and expansion, as in the case of adaptive immune responses. This mechanism accounts for the much more rapid onset of innate immune responses.

Considerable progress has been made toward identifying many of the important PRRs involved in the induction of innate immunity. These receptors can be classified into three functional classes: secreted, endocytic, and signaling PRRs (see Table 20.2). In addition, many of the known PRRs can be classified into structurally defined families on the basis of a few characteristic protein domains. Among these, the best known include proteins with calcium-dependent lectin domains, scavenger receptor domains, and leucine-rich repeat domains (LRRs).

Pattern Recognition Receptors of the Lectin Family

Calcium-dependent lectin domains are common modules of secreted and membrane-bound proteins involved in the binding of carbohydrate structures. A well-characterized PRR belonging to this class is the *mannan-binding lectin* (MBL), also known as *soluble mannose-binding protein,* which represents a secreted PRR that functions in initiation of the complement cascade (Fig. 20.2).[11–14] This protein is synthesized primarily in the liver on a constitutive basis, although its production can be increased as an acute phase reactant after many types of infection. MBL binds to carbohydrates on the

TABLE 20.2 Pattern Recognition Receptors

Receptor Class	Examples	Prominent Sites of Expression	Major Ligands	Function
Secreted PRRs	Collectins Mannan-binding lectin Ficolins Surfactant proteins (SP-A, SP-B) Pentraxins Short pentraxins (CRP, SAP) Long pentraxins	Plasma	Carbohydrate arrays typical of bacterial capsules, fungi, and other microbes Apoptotic cells and cellular debris, including chromatin	Complement activation Opsonization
Endocytic PRRs	Lectin-family receptors Macrophage mannose receptor DEC-205 Dectin-1 Scavenger receptor A MARCO Complement receptors CD11b/CD18 (CR3) CD21/35 (CR2/1)	Macrophages, dendritic cells, some endothelia, epithelia, and smooth muscle cells	Cell wall polysaccharides (mannans and glucans), LPS, LTA, and opsonized cells and particles	Pathogen uptake by phagocytes Delivery of ligands to antigen-processing compartments Clearance of cellular and extracellular debris
Signaling PRRs	Toll-like receptors Nod-like receptors Pyrin domain proteins PYHIN proteins RIG-I-like receptors	Macrophages, dendritic cells, epithelia	Multiple conserved pathogen-associated molecular patterns (LPS, LTA, dsRNA, lipoproteins, flagellin, viral or bacterial DNA, others)	Activation of inducible innate immunity (anti-microbial peptides, cytokines, reactive oxygen or nitrogen intermediates) Instruction of adaptive immune response

CARD, Caspase activation and recruitment domain; *CR,* complement receptor; *CRP,* C-reactive protein; *DEC-205,* dendritic and epithelial cells, 205 kDa; *dsRNA,* double-stranded RNA; *LPS,* lipopolysaccharide; *LTA,* lipoteichoic acid; *MARCO,* macrophage receptor with collagenous structure; *NOD,* nucleotide-binding oligomerization domain; *PRR,* pattern recognition receptor; *PYHIN,* pyrin and HIN-200 domain containing proteins; *RIG-I,* retinoic acid inducible gene-I; *SAP,* serum amyloid P protein; *SP,* surfactant protein.

outer membranes and capsules of many bacteria, as well as fungi, some viruses, and parasites. Although mannose and fructose sugars bound by MBL can also be found on the surfaces of normal mammalian cells, they are present at too low a density or in the wrong orientation to efficiently engage the lectin domains of MBL. In contrast, the coats of many microorganisms contain an array of these sugars, which allows strong binding of MBL. Thus, in this case, the spacing and orientation of specific carbohydrate residues constitute the PAMP that triggers the activation of innate immunity by MBL. MBL functions as one of a small number of secreted PRRs that can initiate the lectin pathway of complement activation. At least two other soluble proteins with lectin activity in human plasma, known as *ficolins* (ficolin/P35 and H-ficolin), can also activate this pathway after their interaction with bacterial polysaccharides.[14,15]

Several of the soluble lectin-type PRRs also play an important role in the opsonization of microbes by binding to their surfaces and directing them to receptors on phagocytic cells. Among these are two pulmonary surfactant proteins, SP-A and SP-D, which similarly recognize and bind to the surface sugar codes of microbes in the respiratory tract.[16] These molecules are similar in structure to MBL, having both collagen-like and lectin domains, and together they constitute a family of soluble PRRs known as *collectins.*[14] Another family of soluble PRRs that performs a similar function in plasma is the pentraxins, so called because they are formed by the association of five identical protein subunits.[17,18] This family includes the acute-phase reactants C-reactive protein (CRP) and serum amyloid P protein (SAP), along with a number of so-called *long pentraxins,* which have an extended polypeptide structure with homology to the classic short pentraxins (i.e., CRP and SAP) only at their carboxy-terminal domains. Long pentraxins are expressed in a variety of different tissues and cells, and their specific functions are mostly unknown. However, the long pentraxin PTX3 plays an important, nonredundant role in resistance to fungal infection in mice, and recent studies indicate that PTX3 is essentially a functional ancestor of antibodies that recognizes microbes and promotes their clearance through complement activation and phagocytosis.[18,19]

In addition to these soluble proteins, a large number of membrane-bound glycoproteins with lectin domains are known to exist; some of them participate in innate immunity by serving as endocytic PRRs for the uptake of microbes or microbial products[20,21] (see Fig. 20.2). One of the most extensively studied of these is the macrophage mannose receptor (MMR).[22] Although originally identified on alveolar macrophages and known to be expressed on macrophage subsets throughout the body, this receptor is also expressed on a variety of other cell types, including certain endothelia, epithelia, and smooth muscle cells. The MMR is a membrane-anchored, multilectin domain–containing protein that mediates the binding of a broad range of pathogens, leading to their internalization via endocytosis and phagocytosis. Although the major function of the MMR appears to be directing the uptake of its ligands, evidence suggests that this receptor may be capable of signaling to modify macrophage functions after receptor engagement.[23] Another member of this receptor family, the β-glucan binding cell-surface lectin known as *dectin-1,* has a role in the modulation of inflammation in a mouse model of infection-induced arthritis.[24]

Pattern Recognition Receptors of the Scavenger Receptor Family

The scavenger receptor family contains a broad range of structurally diverse cell surface proteins that are expressed most prominently on macrophages, dendritic cells, and endothelial cells[25,26] (see Fig. 20.2). Although they were originally defined by their ability to bind and take up modified serum lipoproteins, they also bind a wide range of other ligands, including bacteria and some of their associated products. Multiple members of this family have been implicated as PRRs for innate immunity, including the scavenger receptor A (SR-A) and a related molecule called the *macrophage receptor with collagenous structure* (MARCO).[27] Both of these molecules contain a scavenger receptor cysteine-rich domain in the distal ends of their membranes and a collagen-like stalk with a triple-helical structure. Both are known to bind bacteria, and SR-A also binds well-known PAMPs such as lipoteichoic acids and LPS.[28,29] Mice that have been made deficient in SR-A by targeted gene disruption show increased susceptibility to infections caused by a variety of bacteria, thus providing strong evidence of the role of scavenger receptors in protective immunity, most likely through the activation of innate immune mechanisms.[30,31] Members of the class B scavenger receptor family, including CD36 and SR-BI/CLA-1, have also been found to recognize a variety of pathogen-derived molecules.[25] Although these members of the scavenger receptor family clearly function as endocytic PRRs in the uptake of microbes, their potential to serve as signaling receptors has not yet been established. However, several scavenger receptors play a co-receptor role in the signal transduction process mediated by members of the Toll-like receptor (TLR) family (discussed in a later section), most likely by capturing specific ligands and transferring them to adjacent TLRs.[25]

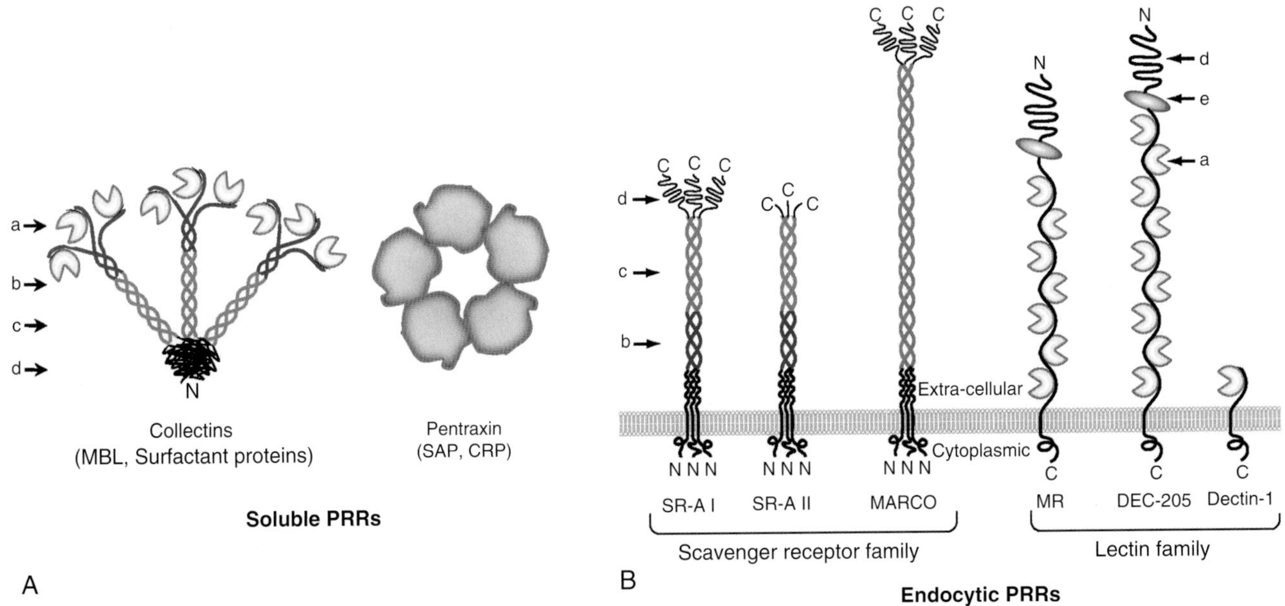

• **Fig. 20.2** Structure of representative soluble and endocytic pattern recognition receptors. (A) General structure of members of the collectin family is illustrated on the *left*, including mannan-binding lectin (MBL) and pulmonary surfactant proteins. MBL is a multimer protein structure with multiple carbohydrate-binding lectin domains. Three identical 32 kDa polypeptides associate to form a subunit, which then oligomerizes to form functional complexes (the trimeric form consisting of three subunits is illustrated, which is one of several different oligomer sizes that has been observed for MBL). Each polypeptide in the subunit contains (a) multiple calcium-dependent (C-type) lectin domains that bind various carbohydrate ligands, (b) the α-helical coiled-coil domain, (c) the collagen-like domain, which is implicated in the binding of polyanionic ligands, and (d) an N-terminal cysteine-rich domain. In contrast, the general structure of pentraxin family proteins is represented on the *right*, consisting of a ring of five identical globular subunits. These include the serum amyloid P protein (SAP) and C-reactive protein (CRP), which bind lipoprotein ligands and bacterial cell wall phosphocholine respectively in a calcium-dependent manner to activate the classical complement pathway. (B) Endocytic pattern recognition receptors of the scavenger receptor and lectin families. *Left,* Illustrations of three members of the scavenger receptor family. These trimeric complexes of type II transmembrane polypeptides have their N-terminals positioned in the cytoplasm and their C-terminals in the extra-cellular space. Three distinct extra-cellular structural domains are indicated: (b) the α-helical coiled-coil domain (absent in macrophage receptor with collagenous structure [MARCO]), which is believed to assist in receptor trimerization; (c) the collagen-like domain, which is implicated in the binding of polyanionic ligands; and (d) the scavenger receptor cysteine-rich (SRCR) domain (absent in SR-A II), which has no currently known function. *Right,* Three examples of lectin domain endocytic pattern recognition receptors: macrophage mannose receptor (MR), DEC-205 and Dectin-1. Distinct extra-cellular domains in these receptors include (d) a cysteine-rich N-terminal domain, (e) a fibronectin-like domain, and (a) single or multiple calcium-dependent (C-type) lectin domains that bind various carbohydrate ligands. N indicates N-terminus, and C indicates C-terminus of polypeptide chains.

Pattern Recognition Receptors With Leucine-rich Repeat Domains

LRRs are structural modules found in many proteins, including PRRs involved in signaling the activation of innate immunity. Molecules in this class include, most notably, the family of mammalian TLRs, which are membrane-bound signal-transducing molecules that play a central role in the recognition of extra-cellular and vacuolar pathogens.[32] Two families of cytoplasmic LRR-containing receptors have also been identified; they play a prominent role in the innate immune recognition of PAMPs expressed by intracellular pathogens. These include the families of caspase activation and recruitment domain (CARD) proteins and of pyrin domain proteins.[33] These molecules are closely related in structure and function to proteins found in invertebrates and plants involved in pathogen resistance, highlighting the ancient origin of these pathways for host defense; they appear to have been recognizably conserved throughout approximately 1 billion years of evolution.

Toll-like Receptors. The first member of the Toll family to be discovered was the *Drosophila* Toll protein, which was identified as a component of a signaling pathway that controls dorsoventral polarity during development of the fly embryo.[34] The sequence of Toll showed it to be a transmembrane protein with a large extra-cellular domain containing multiple tandemly repeated LRRs at the N-terminal end, followed by a cysteine-rich domain and an intracellular signaling domain (Fig. 20.3). A role for Toll in immune responses was suggested by the observation that its intra-cellular domain shows homology to the mammalian IL-1R cytoplasmic domain.[35] This association was later confirmed in studies showing that Toll was critical for the antifungal response in the fly, linking this pathway for the first time to innate immunity.[36] Identification of *Drosophila* Toll eventually led to a search for similar proteins in mammals; this effort has been richly rewarded, yielding a family of 10 TLRs in humans and 12 in mice.[37,38] Among these, TLR1 through TLR9 are conserved between mice and humans, TLR10 is present only in humans, and TLR11 through TLR13 are expressed only in mice.[37,38] All these molecules contain large extra-cellular domains with multiple LRRs, as well as intra-cellular signaling domains known as Toll/IL-1R, or TIR, domains.[39] Many of these TLRs have been linked to innate immune responses against various PAMPs of different microorganisms.[40]

Toll-like Receptor 4 and the Response to Lipopolysaccharide. The first human TLR to be identified was the molecule now designated TLR4, which is a major component in the response to one of the most common of all PAMPs: bacterial LPS.[41] Earlier studies on the response to LPS had identified two proteins, CD14 and LPS-binding protein, as molecules involved in the binding of LPS to the surface of LPS-responsive cells. However, these molecules did not possess any potential for transducing signals into the cell, so it was unclear how LPS binding would lead to the activation of cellular responses associated with gram-negative bacterial infection. The answer was provided by positional cloning studies of the gene responsible for the phenotype in the LPS-hyporesponsive C3H/HeJ mouse.[42] This study revealed a single amino acid substitution in the signaling domain of TLR4. Specific deletion of

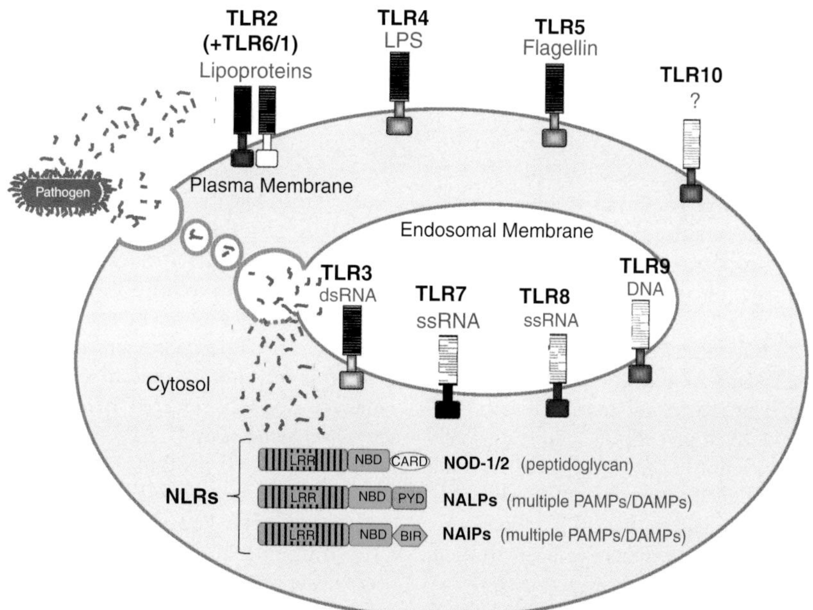

• **Fig. 20.3** Membrane Toll-like receptors (TLRs) and cytoplasmic nod-like receptors (NLRs). Schematic illustration of human TLR and NLR families. The ten human TLRs are transmembrane proteins either inserted in the plasma membrane or in the membranes delimiting endosomal compartments. The leucine-rich repeat (LRR) domains face either the extra-cellular environment or the luminal space of the endosomes. Together, these receptors detect a wide array of different microbial PAMPs, both in the extra-cellular and intra-cellular environment. Major known ligands for each TLR are shown *in red font*. Note that TLR2 is known to form heterodimers with TLR6 and TLR1, whereas the other TLRs appear to function as monomers or ligand-induced homodimers. Also shown are the general structures of the major cytosolic NLRs, which are divided into three major subfamilies. These detect a range of PAMPs and DAMPs in the cytosol through their LRR domains, which induces oligomerization through the nucleotide binding domain (NBD). The resulting molecular complexes (termed *inflammasomes* in some cases) transmit signals to activate inflammatory pathways via signaling domains. These include the CARD (caspase activation and recruitment domain), PYD (pyrin domain), and BIR (Baculovirus inhibitor of apoptosis repeat) domains.

the *TLR4* gene by targeted gene disruption in mice subsequently confirmed the essential role of this molecule in the response to LPS, because TLR4 knockout mice have almost no response to LPS and are highly resistant to endotoxic shock.[43,44] Biochemical studies provide further support for TLR4 as a component of the LPS receptor; they show that LPS bound to the surface of cells is in close contact with both CD14 and TLR4, as well as another protein called *MD-2,* which appears to perform an accessory function in the binding of LPS to the receptor complex.[45] Additional studies have elucidated many of the downstream elements in the signaling pathways that connect TLR4 to the activation of genes associated with inducible innate immunity.[46,47] Studies of Toll signaling pathways in *Drosophila* have identified the transcription factor nuclear factor-κB (NF-κB) as one of the key effectors of gene activation after the engagement of Toll. This basic pathway in the fly appears to be largely conserved in TLR signaling in higher animals, including mammals.[48,49]

Other Pathogen-Associated Molecular Patterns Recognized by Toll-like Receptors. The search for ligands that lead to signaling through various TLRs has demonstrated that this family of PRRs is collectively responsible for innate immune responses to an extraordinary array of PAMPs. In addition to its central role in the signaling of responses to LPS, TLR4 is involved in responses to multiple different self-ligands and non–self-ligands.[40] The antimitotic agent and cancer chemotherapy drug paclitaxel (Taxol) mimics LPS-induced signaling in mouse cells through a pathway that requires both TLR4 and MD-2.[50] Other foreign ligands of TLR4 include the fusion protein (F protein) of respiratory syncytial virus[51] and the heat shock protein 60 (HSP60) of chlamydia.[52] TLR4 can signal in response to mammalian HSP60, a protein expressed at increased levels and most likely released by stressed or damaged cells.[53] This represents a variation of the pattern recognition principle in which the pattern is an endogenous molecule released by damaged host cells that serves as a DAMP, rather than a PAMP produced directly by a pathogen. Other examples of recognition of DAMPs by TLR4 include responses to oligosaccharide breakdown products of tissue hyaluronans and responses to the extra-domain A region of fibronectin produced by alternative RNA splicing in response to tissue injury or inflammation.[40,54]

The range of PAMPs recognized through TLR2 is probably even greater than for TLR4. TLR2 is known to be involved in signaling in response to multiple PAMPs of gram-negative and gram-positive bacteria, including such structures as bacterial glycolipids, bacterial lipoproteins, parasite-derived glycolipids, and fungal cell wall polysaccharides.[40] TLR2 does not function independently in responding to these PAMPs; rather, it forms heterodimers with TLR1 or TLR6. This ability to pair with other TLRs appears to be unique to TLR2, because other TLRs that have been studied carefully (e.g., TLR4 and TLR5) most likely function only as monomers or homodimers. Other TLRs with currently defined ligands are TLR5 (involved in the response to bacterial flagellin), TLR3 (double-stranded RNA), TLR7 (single-stranded RNA), and TLR9 (unmethylated bacterial DNA).[40] Most, if not all, microbes contain multiple PAMPs that are recognized by different TLRs. For example, a typical bacterium expressing LPS also contains unmethylated DNA and thus generates signals not only through TLR4 but potentially through TLR9 as well. Because different TLRs are capable of activating distinct signaling cascades, the ability of a single cell to detect several different features of a pathogen simultaneously with multiple TLRs may help the innate immune response to be more finely tuned to respond to a particular challenge.[55]

NLR, STING, and RLR Proteins. There are a large number of cytosolic proteins that have structural similarities to membrane-bound TLRs and that function as sensors for PAMPs of intra-cellular pathogens and as regulators of innate immune responses (see Fig. 20.3). Many of these proteins contain LRR domains and have been classified on the basis of their incorporation of a CARD or pyrin domain. The nomenclature and classification schemes for this growing family of innate immune sensors and regulators are still evolving, although the most recent literature shows a trend toward referring to this group of proteins as the *NLR family,* an acronym that stands for either "nucleotide-binding domain, leucine-rich repeat proteins"[56,57] or "Nod-like receptors."[37] The first intra-cellular microbial sensors in this family to be described were the Nod1 and Nod2 proteins, which contain LRR domains linked to a central nucleotide binding domain (NBD, also designated as *NOD* or *NACHT domains*) and an N-terminal CARD domain.[58] As in the case of TLRs, the LRR domains of these proteins appear to be involved in the direct recognition of pathogen-derived molecules and a variety of host components that function as DAMPs, and their CARD domains are linked to downstream signaling for the activation of innate immunity. Although originally implicated in the response to bacterial LPS, it is now well accepted that both Nod1 and Nod2 are primarily involved in the recognition of muropeptide monomers released from bacterial cell wall peptidoglycans.[33] Signals resulting from the recognition of peptidoglycan components by Nod1 and Nod2 lead to activation of the NF-κB pathway, as in the case of TLR signaling. However, other signaling pathways also appear to be engaged, such as activation of procaspase-1 and caspase-9 by CARD domain interactions, leading to increased production of IL-1β and cell death through a process referred to as *pyroptosis.*[56]

The pyrin domain–containing proteins represent a major subgroup of NLRs that are believed to signal in response to microbial invasion or cellular stress. The prototype member of this family is pyrin, which is the product of the gene that is mutated in people with familial Mediterranean fever.[59] Although pyrin itself lacks an LRR domain, numerous other members of this family contain an LRR linked to a central NOD domain and an N-terminal pyrin domain. These family members include cryopyrin (also known as *NLRP3* or *NALP3*), which is mutated in patients with a range of hereditary inflammatory diseases referred to collectively as *cryopyrin-associated periodic syndromes* (CAPS).[56] Cryopyrin, together with these multiple related proteins, constitutes a large set of related proteins known as the NLRP (NLR-PYRIN domain) or NALP (NACHT-LRR-PYRIN domain–containing proteins) family.[33] The human genome contains 14 genes encoding NLRP proteins, the precise functions of which are still largely unknown.[37] However, several NLRP proteins, particularly NLRP3 and NLRP1, and also the closely related NAIP protein, have been identified as key components in the formation of intra-cellular complexes known as *inflammasomes.*[10] These cytosolic protein complexes serve as activating platforms that are involved in the activation of caspases—that is, intra-cellular proteases required for the processing of inflammatory cytokines such as IL-1β and IL-18.[56,60] Direct recognition of specific PAMPs by NLRP proteins remains to be established, although initial studies implicate these proteins as direct or indirect sensors of various stimuli, including constituents of bacteria (peptidoglycan, bacterial RNA, and exotoxins), viruses (double-stranded RNA), and uric acid crystals.[37,56,61–64]

In addition to the likely role of NLRP proteins in sensing foreign nucleic acids as PAMPs, recent studies have characterized a complex array of other proteins that serve as sensors for intra-cellular DNA or RNA and are likely to play major roles in anti-viral innate immunity. One prominent example is the family of PYHIN proteins, which are cytosolic or nuclear proteins containing PYRIN domains linked to a DNA-binding domain known as HIN-200.[65] Some of these proteins, such as the absent in melanoma-2 (AIM2) protein, have been clearly established to act as sensors for intra-cellular viral DNA that can trigger a range of innate immune responses. A range of other candidate intra-cellular proteins have been identified that make important contributions to the innate response to DNA, particularly those that act through signaling pathways mediated by the adaptor protein called stimulator of interferon genes (STING).[66,67] STING is a transmembrane dimeric protein in the endoplasmic reticulum membrane that weakly recognizes double-stranded (ds) DNA but is strongly activated by cyclic dinucleotides, which can either be directly produced by intra-cellular bacteria as PAMPs or generated as DAMPs by the cyclic guanosine monophosphate–adenosine monophosphate (GMP-AMP) synthase cGAS when it is activated by binding cytosolic dsDNA. In addition to these cytosolic DNA sensors, there is a growing list of cytosolic RNA sensing proteins; the most well studied at present are the RIG-I-like receptors (RLRs). The RLRs include the retinoic acid–inducible gene-I (RIG-I), melanoma differentiation factor 5 (MDA5), and laboratory of genetics and physiology 2 (LGP2) proteins.[68] These proteins are expressed in the cytosol of most cells and respond to structural motifs present in many viral RNA molecules to induce type I interferon (IFN) and other anti-viral effectors. Together, these multiple sensors of cytosolic nucleic acids serve to trigger inflammatory responses against a large spectrum of microbial pathogens, including DNA and RNA viruses, and to make potentially important contributions to autoimmune and inflammatory diseases.[69]

Effector Mechanisms of Innate Immune Responses

The ability to recognize pathogens through PRRs allows activation of numerous anti-microbial effector mechanisms by the innate immune response. These responses lead to the killing of pathogens through production of effector molecules with direct microbicidal activities, including the membrane attack complex of complement, a variety of anti-microbial peptides, and the caustic reactive oxygen and reactive nitrogen intermediates generated within phagocytic cells. In invertebrates, these mechanisms represent virtually the entire protective response against microbial invaders. However, in most vertebrates, including mammals, innate immune recognition also has profound effects on triggering and programming the adaptive immune response that follows somewhat later. This ability of the innate immune system to instruct the adaptive response has major implications for the development of long-term protective immunity to infection and may play a critical role in mechanisms leading to autoimmunity.

Cell Types Mediating Innate Immunity

Many types of cells have the ability to mount at least a limited response to PAMPs, but the most effective cell types in this regard are the specialized phagocytes, such as macrophages, neutrophils, and dendritic cells. Upon recognition of microbial stimuli, these cells have the ability to upregulate nicotinamide adenine dinucleotide phosphate (NADPH) oxidase by assembling the components of this enzyme complex on phagosomal membranes, leading to an oxidative burst that produces microbicidal superoxide ions.[70] Many phagocytic cells also increase their expression of inducible nitric oxide synthase (iNOS, or NOS2) upon contact with various PAMPs.[71] This increased expression leads to the production of reactive nitrogen intermediates, including nitric oxide and peroxynitrite, which have potent direct antimicrobicidal activities. These responses are synergistic because the anti-microbial activity of the phagocyte oxidase system is frequently enhanced by the expression of reactive nitrogen intermediates.

Innate-like Lymphocytes

A number of distinct lymphocyte subsets also play important roles in innate immune responses. Among these subsets are a complex mixture of lymphocytes that lack markers of the T and B cell lineages and are collectively referred to as *innate lymphoid cells* (ILCs). The complexity of ILC populations is currently still being unraveled. Recent classifications recognize three distinct lineages designated ILC1, ILC2, and ILC3 cells that are distinguished by phenotypic markers and by secretion of different cytokines.[72] The cytokine secretion profiles of these ILC subsets and some aspects of their functions in immunity parallel closely those of conventional T helper cell subsets (i.e., Th1, Th2, and Th17 cells).[73] The ILC1 subset is composed of IFN-γ–secreting populations, which include natural killer (NK) cells. These lymphocytes do not express receptors generated by somatic recombination and thus depend on germline-encoded receptors for signaling their responses against pathogen-infected cells.[72] NK cells participate in the early innate response against virally, and probably bacterially, infected cells through expression of cytotoxic activity and secretion of cytokines.[74]

Several other subsets of lymphocytes belonging to the T and B cell lineages have been identified as participants in the rapid response against pathogens to which the host has not previously been exposed. Although these cells express clonally variable, somatically rearranged antigen receptors (T cell antigen receptors or membrane immunoglobulins) and thus could be classified as components of the adaptive immune system, their manner of functioning is much more characteristic of innate than adaptive immunity. These innate-like lymphocytes (ILLs) may represent remnants of the earliest primitive adaptive immune system, and they appear to have been conserved to varying degrees because they continue to make specialized contributions to host immunity.[75]

Among the currently recognized ILLs are two B cell populations, known as the *B1* and *marginal zone B cell subsets*.[76,77] These B cell populations are involved in the spontaneous production of natural antibodies, which are largely germline-encoded immunoglobulins that are reactive to commonly expressed microbial determinants. In addition, both of these B cell populations generate rapid T cell–independent responses after bacterial challenges and thus contribute to the first line of immune defense that precedes the onset of adaptive immunity. A subset of B1 cells is the Innate Response Activator (IRA) B cells; this unique subset originates from serosal sites and co-secretes substantial amounts of granulocyte-macrophage colony-stimulating growth factor (GM-CSF) and IL-3 upon bacterial LPS recognition in the spleen and the lung. While IRA B cell-derived GM-CSF protects against bacterial sepsis by promoting protective IgM production and increased phagocyte clearance, it can also drive pathologic changes such as atherosclerosis by enhancing splenic extramedullary hematopoiesis and pro-inflammatory phagocyte production.[78]

Among the T cells, three populations of ILLs have been identified and characterized in detail: γδ T cells, NK T cells, and mucosal-associated invariant T (MAIT) cells. The γδ T cells express somatically rearranging receptors that use a limited number of variable region genes and are thought to recognize a narrow spectrum of foreign or self-ligands.[79] In humans, the specificities of two subsets of γδ T cells have been at least partially defined. One of these subsets, the major circulating population expressing the Vδ2 gene product, responds rapidly and without prior immunization to a variety of small alkyl phosphate and alkyl amine compounds that are produced by many bacteria.[80] Another subset, characterized by its expression of the Vδ1 gene product, responds to class I major histocompatibility complex (MHC)–related self-molecules of the class I MHC chain–related A and B (MICA/B) and CD1 families.[79] These molecules may serve as markers of cellular stress and are upregulated on cells in the context of infection or inflammation, leading to the activation of Vδ1-bearing γδ T cells.

A similar principle appears to be involved in the functioning of NK T cells, which are so named because of their co-expression of an αβ T cell antigen receptor and a variety of receptor molecules that are typically associated with NK cells.[81,82] Similar to γδ T cells, NK T cells have somatically rearranged antigen receptors that use a limited array of V genes and most likely recognize a narrow range of foreign or self-antigens. A major population of NK T cells is reactive with the class I MHC–like CD1d molecule, and these ILLs are activated by recognition of a variety of lipid or glycolipid ligands that can be presented by CD1d. Several bacterial glycolipids have been identified as specific antigens that stimulate NK T cells, suggesting that these cells may be rapid responders that contribute to innate antibacterial immunity.[81] A wide variety of mouse disease models have shown that NK T cells also make significant contributions to the development of adaptive immune responses and may play a particularly important role in immunoregulation to prevent autoimmunity.[81] Similarly, MAIT cells are a separate population of innate-like T cells that have recently been shown to use their αβ T cell antigen receptors to recognize common vitamin B metabolites that are produced and secreted by a wide range of bacteria.[83]

Anti-microbial Peptides

Anti-microbial peptides are the key effector molecules of inducible innate immunity in many invertebrates and are being increasingly recognized as important elements of innate immunity in higher animal species, including mammals.[84] They are evolutionarily ancient components of host defense that are widely distributed throughout all multicellular organisms in the animal and plant kingdoms. More than 1000 such peptides have been identified, and their diversity is so great that it is difficult to categorize them. However, at a structural and mechanistic level, most of these peptides share several basic features. They generally are composed of amino acids arranged to create an amphipathic structure with hydrophobic and cationic regions. The cationic regions target a fundamental difference in membrane design between microbes and multicellular animals, which is the abundance of negatively charged phospholipid head groups on the outer leaflet of the lipid bilayer. The preferential association of anti-microbial peptides with microbial membranes leads to membrane-disrupting activity, most likely involving the interaction of the hydrophobic regions of the peptide with membrane lipids.[85]

Anti-microbial peptides produced in response to engagement of various PRRs account for most of the inducible immunity against microbes noted in many invertebrate animals and plants. Although these peptides are probably less central to host immunity in most vertebrates, evidence indicates that they make important contributions to immunity in more highly evolved animals, including mammals.[86] In humans, active anti-microbial peptides, such as the α- and β-defensins, are constitutively or inducibly produced in skin and epithelia of the gastrointestinal and respiratory tracts.[87] These molecules most likely act as natural preservatives of epithelia that are colonized or frequently exposed to microbial flora. Because the acquisition of resistance against these agents by sensitive microbial strains is extremely unusual, anti-microbial peptides are of great interest as templates for the development of new anti-microbial pharmaceuticals.[87–89]

Influence of Innate Mechanisms on Adaptive Immunity

In addition to functioning as a first line of defense against invading pathogens, a critical feature of the innate immune system in higher animals such as mammals is its effect on activating the adaptive immune system. In fact, it is now clear that in most situations, the adaptive immune system mounts a response to a pathogen only after the pathogen has generated signals via PRRs of the innate immune system. This principle serves as the basis for the adjuvant effect, which is the observation that antibody and T cell responses are efficiently generated against protein antigens only if these are introduced together with a nonspecific activator of the immune system, which is generically known as an *adjuvant.* Most adjuvants are in fact extracts or products of bacteria, and it is clear that in most or all cases, adjuvant effects result from activation of the innate immune response.[90]

Innate immune responses can prime or potentiate the adaptive immune response in many ways (Fig. 20.4). In the case of T cell responses, one extremely important and well-recognized mechanism involves the upregulation of co-stimulatory molecules. T cells require at least two signals to become activated from a naïve resting state. One signal is provided through the T cell antigen receptor by its binding to a specific peptide ligand presented by a class I or II MHC molecule. The second signal is provided by one of several co-stimulatory ligands that are expressed by specialized antigen-presenting cells such as dendritic cells. The best studied of these are the molecules of the B7 family, B7-1 (CD80) and B7-2 (CD86), which engage the activating receptor CD28 on the surface of the T cell. Expression of B7 family co-stimulatory molecules on the surface of antigen-presenting cells is controlled by the innate immune system, such that these molecules are induced to appear at functional levels only after PRRs, such as members of the TLR family, have been activated by recognition of their cognate PAMPs or DAMPs.[41]

Innate immune signaling through TLRs has a major impact on the responses of phagocytic antigen-presenting cells; it also provides an important second signal for immunoglobulin production by B cells. In the case of phagocytic cells, uptake of microbes by phagocytosis and subsequent maturation of the phagosome are stimulated by concurrent TLR signaling.[91] In dendritic cells, which are the predominant antigen-presenting cells for the priming of T cell responses, TLR signaling has a major impact on whether antigens from phagocytosed microbes are effectively presented on class II MHC molecules.[92] For B cells responding to foreign antigens, it

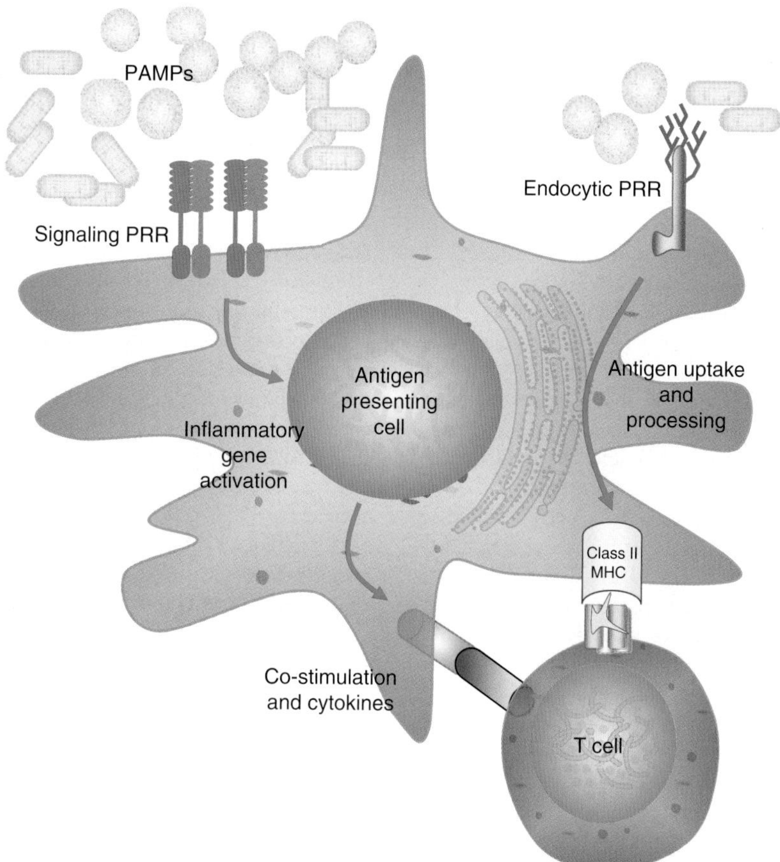

• **Fig. 20.4** Instruction on the adaptive immune response by the innate immune system. When an antigen-presenting cell (APC) comes into contact with pathogen-bearing pathogen-associated molecular patterns (PAMPs), responses are triggered via innate immune mechanisms that dramatically alter the ability of the APC to stimulate an adaptive (T cell–mediated) immune response. For example, signals generated by contact with PAMPs such as lipopolysaccharide (LPS) with Toll-like receptor 4 (TLR4) lead to the activation of transcription factor nuclear factor-κB (NF-κB), which enters the nucleus of the APC and assists in switching on genes for cytokines (e.g., IL-1, -6, and -12 and a variety of chemokines) and co-stimulatory molecules (e.g., the B7 family members CD80 and CD86). In addition, binding of the pathogen to endocytic pattern recognition receptors (PRRs) such as the mannose receptor (MR), leads to delivery of the pathogen to endosomes (Endo) and lysosomes (Lys). There, the protein antigens of the pathogen are partially degraded to generate antigenic peptides that can be presented by class II major histocompatibility complex (MHC) molecules for recognition by the T cell antigen receptors (TCRs) of specific T cells. These effects of pattern recognition by the innate immune system lead to expression of the signals required for activation of quiescent antigen-specific T cells and the subsequent generation of specific antibodies.

has been demonstrated that concurrent signaling through TLRs is necessary for the efficient stimulation of T cell–dependent differentiation into plasma cells and subsequent antibody secretion.[93] This concept is also relevant for T cell responses to autoantigens, including several prominent nuclear antigens that are targets of autoantibodies in rheumatic disease.[94–96]

Innate immune responses also trigger the production of many cytokines and chemokines, which enhance the development of adaptive immune responses and change the nature of the adaptive response generated. For example, contact between dendritic cells and PAMPs such as LPS or bacterial lipoproteins leads to the production of IL-12 as a result of signaling through TLRs.[90,97] This cytokine acts on antigen-specific T cells to promote their differentiation into T helper type 1 cells, which are associated with the production of IFN-γ and other effector mechanisms that favor the clearance of bacterial pathogens.[98] In the case of myeloid lineage dendritic cells, signaling through TLRs (and potentially other PRRs) induces a process known as *maturation,* which is associated with increased expression of antigen-presenting and co-stimulatory molecules that enables the efficient priming of naïve antigen-specific T cells.[99]

This requirement for the innate immune response to "switch on" the expression of molecules required for the priming and differentiation of T cell responses helps ensure that pro-inflammatory adaptive immune responses occur mainly in the setting of a relevant infectious challenge. After activation, helper T cells control other components of adaptive immunity, such as the activation of cytotoxic T cells, B cells, and macrophages. Innate immune recognition, therefore, appears to control all major aspects of the adaptive immune response through the initial recognition of infectious microbes by PRRs. The discovery of self-molecules that act as DAMPs further extends this paradigm to include immune responses that are triggered by tissue damage. This more extended view, sometimes referred to as the "danger model," helps explain why certain self-ligands produced or released in the setting of infection or tissue damage can function in essentially the same manner as the PAMPs associated with microorganisms.[100,101]

Trained Immunity: Blurring the Distinction Between Innate and Adaptive Responses

While conventional T cells are one of the central components of adaptive immunity, recent work has called attention to the innate-like properties of a population of CD8+ T cells with memory phenotype, also known as *virtual memory CD8+ T cells*. Similar innate-like properties have also been shown to be acquired in some cases by conventional vaccine-induced memory CD8+ T cells. These properties include functional attributes similar to classic NK cells, such as rapid cytokine secretion and cytolytic function, in response to a specific set of inflammatory signals and independently of cognate antigen stimulation.[102] Conversely, in recent years, NK cells and monocytes, which represent characteristic cells of the innate immune system, have been found to exhibit a form of immunologic memory that is now referred to as "trained immunity."[103] The most compelling evidence for this is derived from studies of NK cell responses to murine cytomegalovirus infection or hapten immunization. These studies reveal that following such exposures, NK cells can expand and differentiate into long-lived progeny that show improved effector functions upon secondary encounters with the original or related stimuli. Similar findings have been reported for monocytes, from which improved effector responses are observed upon secondary encounters with particular pathogens or PAMPs.[103] Such training, which amplifies subsequent encounters with various stimuli, largely occurs though epigenetic reprogramming and the alterations of chromatin accessibility in these cells and their progenitors. This trained immunity remains distinct from classical immunologic memory since it relies on recognition by germline encoded nonpolymorphic receptors, but it demonstrates the ability of some classic innate immune effector cells to possess a form of memory, thus blurring in some situations the traditional demarcation between innate and adaptive immunity.

Disease Associations Involving Innate Immunity

Given the obvious role of the innate immune response in virtually all types of infectious disease, one might expect that gross defects in the mechanisms of innate immunity occur relatively rarely and in association with clinical immunodeficiency. In fact, increasing evidence indicates that mutations that inactivate various innate immune pathways can lead to increased pathogen sensitivity in both laboratory mice and humans.[11,30,86,104,105] Because many of the pathways leading to innate immunity are amplified during recurrent or prolonged activation of the immune system, they must also participate in mediating tissue damage in chronic inflammatory disease. In addition, certain self-molecules that are produced or released at increased levels as a result of inflammation, including heat shock proteins, nucleic acids, and microcrystals of monosodium urate or calcium pyrophosphate, may act as DAMPs.[52,94,95,106,107] These self-molecules may signal through TLRs or other PRRs to stimulate adjuvant-like effects that increase the potential for autoreactive lymphocytes to be activated. Along these lines, gain of function mutations in the cytosolic dsDNA sensors STING and cGAS are associated with systemic lupus erythematosus (SLE), Aicardi-Goutieres syndrome (AGS), and STING-associated vasculopathy with onset in infancy (SAVI).[69]

Perhaps a more surprising finding has been that some defects in innate immunity are associated with a markedly increased predisposition to autoimmune disease. Several different mechanisms have been proposed to explain this paradoxical association. Mechanisms of the innate immune response play an important role in the clearance of self-antigens released from necrotic or apoptotic cells, resulting in a non-inflammatory clearance of self-antigens that tends to favor tolerance rather than the stimulation of immune responses.[108] Failure of such clearance may lead to excessive exposure to self-antigens, triggering normally silent autoreactive lymphocyte clones to expand and differentiate into effector cells. This mechanism may account for the development of lupus-like autoimmunity in mice with targeted deletion of the gene for the short pentraxin SAP, which, along with other components of the innate immune system, appears to play a significant role in the clearance of DNA-chromatin complexes.[109] Reduced levels of serum mannose-binding lectin in humans also appear to be a risk factor for the development of SLE, possibly because of the role of this soluble PRR in facilitating the clearance of apoptotic cells.[110]

Deficiencies of early components of the classic pathway of complement activation have been strongly associated with lupus-like autoimmunity in both humans and mouse models.[111–115] This association may be the result of alterations in the clearance of apoptotic cells or other sources of self-antigens, resulting in increased stimulation of normally silent autoreactive lymphocytes.[116,117] An alternative, but nonexclusive, mechanism relates to involvement of the complement system, particularly the early components C1 and C4, in facilitating the induction of self-tolerance by the adaptive immune system by increasing the localization of autoantigens such as double-stranded DNA and nucleoproteins within the primary lymphoid compartment.[111,118,119] Thus, a deficiency of C1 or C4 appears to result in the failure to delete or functionally inactivate autoreactive B cell clones as they arise during lymphopoiesis in the bone marrow.[118,120] Studies carried out in mouse models suggest that this tolerance-inducing mechanism is partially disrupted in animals that are deficient in a variety of other components of innate immunity, including SAP and the complement receptors CD21/CD35.[109,118]

Multiple examples of links between defects in signaling receptors of the innate immune system and chronic inflammatory diseases have emerged from studies of the CARD and pyrin families of cytosolic PRRs.[37,56] The first association of this type was provided by genetic mapping studies that identified the Nod2 protein as the product of the inflammatory bowel disease 1 (IBD1) locus, which contributes to disease susceptibility in a subset of patients with Crohn's disease.[121–124] This soluble PRR of the CARD family normally functions by inducing cytokine production in response to bacterial peptidoglycan, but mutant alleles associated with increased risk of Crohn's disease are defective in this function.[121] In this case, it may be failure of innate immunity to adequately control bacterial colonization or infection in the intestine that leads to the final expression of disease. Consistent with this view, a recent study has demonstrated diminished expression of a class of anti-microbial peptides (β-defensins known as *cryptdins*) in Paneth cells from the ileum of patients with Crohn's disease and *Nod2* mutations.[125] Other findings suggest that defective signaling by mutant variants of *Nod2* can result in reduced production of immunoregulatory cytokines such as IL-10, perhaps resulting in uncontrolled inflammation in the intestine.[126] Other studies have established links between various members of the pyrin family and specific chronic inflammatory disorders. These links include the causative association of mutations in pyrin with familial Mediterranean fever and of cryopyrin with cryopyrin-associated periodic syndromes.[56,59] These diseases and other chronic inflammatory or autoimmune disorders associated with specific deficiencies in innate immune mechanisms are frequently considered together as autoinflammatory diseases.[127] Recognition that these diseases are frequently associated with dysregulation of inflammatory cytokine production, in particular IL-1β, has led to some striking therapeutic advances in the treatment of selected patients using systemic administration of the IL-1 receptor antagonist anakinra.[128–130]

Deficiencies in at least two populations of ILLs, NK cells and NK T cells, have been associated with multiple autoimmune syndromes in both humans and mice.[81,131–133] This finding is believed to reflect a significant role for these ILLs in regulating adaptive immune responses, although the precise mechanisms by which they act still are not fully understood. Given the complex interplay between innate immunity and adaptive immunity, it is extremely likely that associations between alterations in innate immunity and autoimmune diseases will continue to emerge. As for some of the examples cited here, a fuller understanding of these associations is likely to lead to new and successful therapies for autoimmune and autoinflammatory diseases.

Future Directions

In the past two decades of research in immunology, we have seen a great emphasis on the fundamental role played by innate immune mechanisms in all immune responses. The innate immune system in humans represents the accumulation of many stages of evolution and natural selection that began with the most primitive organisms. Because of the ancient origins of the innate immune system, some of the most important discoveries in the field of innate immunity have come from studies of relatively simple animals such as flies and worms. Now that many of the pieces of this elaborate system have been discovered and categorized, continued research efforts are turning increasingly toward exploring the roles of various components of innate immunity in the human immune system. These efforts are very likely to yield insights into many currently unexplained diseases and may provide targets for new therapeutics.

Connection to the Clinic

- Innate immune responses serve as the foundation of all immunity; they participate at some level in all infectious, inflammatory, and autoimmune diseases.
- Drugs targeting specific innate immune effectors are beginning to emerge as useful therapeutic agents.
- Innate immune receptors are responsible for triggering the clinical syndromes associated with uric acid crystals and potentially other types of crystal-induced arthritis.
- Primary defects in specific innate immune molecules have been identified as the cause of a range of uncommon disorders known as *autoinflammatory diseases.*
- Many systemic autoimmune diseases are associated with genetic polymorphisms of molecules involved in innate immune responses.
- Research into innate immunity has provided important new insight into potential mechanisms for common autoimmune diseases such as Crohn's disease and SLE.

Full references for this chapter can be found on ExpertConsult.com.

Selected References

1. Schatz DG: Transposition mediated by RAG1 and RAG2 and the evolution of the adaptive immune system, *Immunol Res* 19:169–182, 1999.
2. Flajnik MF: A cold-blooded view of adaptive immunity, *Nat Rev Immunol* 18:438, 2018.
3. Pancer Z, Cooper MD: The evolution of adaptive immunity, *Annu Rev Immunol* 24:497, 2006.
4. Boehm TL, McCurley N, Sutoh Y, et al.: VLR-based adaptive immunity, *Annu Rev Immunol* 30:203, 2012.
5. Boehm T, Hirano M, Holland SJ, et al.: Evolution of alternative adaptive immune systems in vertebrates, *Annu Rev Immunol* 36:19, 2018.
6. Hoffmann JA, Reichhart JM: Drosophila innate immunity: an evolutionary perspective, *Nat Immunol* 3:121, 2002.
7. Kingsolver MB, Huang Z, Hardy RW: Insect antiviral innate immunity: pathways, effectors, and connections, *J Mol Biol* 425:4921, 2013.
8. Castiglioni A, Canti V, Rovere-Querini P, et al.: High-mobility group box 1 (HMGB1) as a master regulator of innate immunity, *Cell Tissue Res* 343:189, 2011.
9. Kataoka H, Kono H, Patel Z, et al.: Evaluation of the contribution of multiple DAMPs and DAMP receptors in cell death-induced sterile inflammatory responses, *PLoS ONE* 9:e104741, 2014.
10. Hayward JA, Mathur A, Ngo C, et al.: Cytosolic recognition of microbes and pathogens: inflammasomes in action, *Microbiol Mol Biol Rev* 82, 2018.
11. Jack DL, Klein NJ, Turner MW: Mannose-binding lectin: targeting the microbial world for complement attack and opsonophagocytosis, *Immunol Rev* 180(86), 2001.
12. Eisen DP: Mannose-binding lectin deficiency and respiratory tract infection, *J Innate Immun* 2:114, 2010.
13. Garred P, Genster N, Pilely K, et al.: A journey through the lectin pathway of complement-MBL and beyond, *Immunol Rev* 274:74, 2016.
14. Howard M, Farrar CA, Sacks SH: Structural and functional diversity of collectins and ficolins and their relationship to disease, *Semin Immunopathol* 40:75, 2018.
15. Matsushita M: Ficolins: complement-activating lectins involved in innate immunity, *J Innate Immun* 2:24, 2010.
16. Seaton BA, Crouch EC, McCormack FX, et al.: Structural determinants of pattern recognition by lung collectins, *Innate Immun* 16:143, 2010.
17. Cieślik P, Hrycek A: Long pentraxin 3 (PTX3) in the light of its structure, mechanism of action and clinical implications, *Autoimmunity* 45:119, 2012.
18. Daigo K, Inforzato A, Barajon I, et al.: Pentraxins in the activation and regulation of innate immunity, *Immunol Rev* 274:202, 2016.
19. Bottazzi B, Garlanda C, Cotena A, et al.: The long pentraxin PTX3 as a prototypic humoral pattern recognition receptor: interplay with cellular innate immunity, *Immunol Rev* 227(9), 2009.
20. Taylor PR, Martinez-Pomares L, Stacey M, et al.: Macrophage receptors and immune recognition, *Annu Rev Immunol* 23:901, 2005.
21. Graham LM, Brown GD: The dectin-2 family of C-type lectins in immunity and homeostasis, *Cytokine* 48:148, 2009.
22. Martinez-Pomares L: The mannose receptor, *J Leukoc Biol* 92:1177, 2012.
23. Nigou J, Zelle-Rieser C, Gilleron M, et al.: Mannosylated lipoarabinomannans inhibit IL-12 production by human dendritic cells: evidence for a negative signal delivered through the mannose receptor, *J Immunol* 166:7477, 2001.
24. Rosenzweig HL, Clowers JS, Nunez G, et al.: Dectin-1 and NOD2 mediate cathepsin activation in zymosan-induced arthritis in mice, *Inflamm Res* 60:705, 2011.

25. Canton J, Neculai D, Grinstein S: Scavenger receptors in homeostasis and immunity, *Nat Rev Immunol* 13:621, 2013.
26. PrabhuDas MR, Baldwin CL, Bollyky PL, et al.: A consensus definitive classification of scavenger receptors and their roles in health and disease, *J Immunol* 198:3775, 2017.
27. Jing J, Yang IV, Hui L, et al.: Role of macrophage receptor with collagenous structure in innate immune tolerance, *J Immunol* 190:6360, 2013.
28. Hampton RY, Golenbock DT, Penman M, et al.: Recognition and plasma clearance of endotoxin by scavenger receptors, *Nature* 352:342, 1991.
29. Dunne DW, Resnick D, Greenberg J, et al.: The type I macrophage scavenger receptor binds to gram-positive bacteria and recognizes lipoteichoic acid, *Proc Natl Acad Sci U S A* 91:1863, 1994.
30. Thomas CA, Li Y, Kodama T, et al.: Protection from lethal gram-positive infection by macrophage scavenger receptor-dependent phagocytosis, *J Exp Med* 191(147), 2000.
31. Haworth R, Platt N, Keshav S, et al.: The macrophage scavenger receptor type A is expressed by activated macrophages and protects the host against lethal endotoxic shock, *J Exp Med* 186:1431, 1997.
32. Kawai T, Akira S: The role of pattern-recognition receptors in innate immunity: update on Toll-like receptors, *Nat Immunol* 11:373–384, 2010.
33. Werts C, Girardin SE, Philpott DJ: TIR, CARD and PYRIN: three domains for an antimicrobial triad, *Cell Death Differ* 13:798, 2006.
34. Hashimoto C, Hudson KL, Anderson KV: The Toll gene of Drosophila, required for dorsal-ventral embryonic polarity, appears to encode a transmembrane protein, *Cell* 52:269, 1988.
35. Gay NJ, Keith FJ: Drosophila Toll and IL-1 receptor, *Nature* 351:355, 1991.
36. Lemaitre B, Nicolas E, Michaut L, et al.: The dorsoventral regulatory gene cassette spatzle/Toll/cactus controls the potent antifungal response in Drosophila adults, *Cell* 86:973, 1996.
37. Fukata M, Vamadevan AS, Abreu MT: Toll-like receptors (TLRs) and Nod-like receptors (NLRs) in inflammatory disorders, *Semin Immunol* 21:242, 2009.
38. Takeda K, Akira S: Toll-like receptors, *Curr Protoc Immunol* 109:11, 2015.
39. Gay NJ, Symmons MF, Gangloff M, et al.: Assembly and localization of Toll-like receptor signalling complexes, *Nat Rev Immunol* 14:546, 2014.
40. Sasai M, Yamamoto M: Pathogen recognition receptors: ligands and signaling pathways by Toll-like receptors, *Int Rev Immunol* 32:116–133, 2013.
41. Medzhitov R, Preston-Hurlburt P, Janeway Jr CA: A human homologue of the Drosophila Toll protein signals activation of adaptive immunity, *Nature* 388:394, 1997.
42. Poltorak A, He X, Smirnova I, et al.: Defective LPS signaling in C3H/HeJ and C57BL/10ScCr mice: mutations in TLR4 gene, *Science* 282:2085, 1998.
43. Hoshino K, Takeuchi O, Kawai T, et al.: Cutting edge: Toll-like receptor 4 (TLR4)-deficient mice are hyporesponsive to lipopolysaccharide: evidence for TLR4 as the LPS gene product, *J Immunol* 162:3749, 1999.
44. Takeuchi O, Hoshino K, Kawai T, et al.: Differential roles of TLR2 and TLR4 in recognition of gram-negative and gram-positive bacterial cell wall components, *Immunity* 11:443, 1999.
45. da Silva CJ, Soldau K, Christen U, et al.: Lipopolysaccharide is in close proximity to each of the proteins in its membrane receptor complex transfer from CD14 to TLR4 and MD-2, *J Biol Chem* 276:21129, 2001.
46. Kawai T, Akira S: TLR signaling, *Cell Death Differ* 13:816, 2006.
47. Balka KR, De Nardo D: Understanding early TLR signaling through the Myddosome, *J Leukoc Biol*, 2018.
48. Belvin MP, Anderson KV: A conserved signaling pathway: the Drosophila Toll-dorsal pathway, *Annu Rev Cell Dev Biol* 12:393, 1996.
49. Brennan JJ, Gilmore TD: Evolutionary origins of Toll-like receptor signaling, *Mol Biol Evol* 35:1576, 2018.
50. Kawasaki K, Gomi K, Nishijima M: Cutting edge: Gln22 of mouse MD-2 is essential for species-specific lipopolysaccharide mimetic action of taxol, *J Immunol* 166:11, 2001.
51. Haynes LM, Moore DD, Kurt-Jones EA, et al.: Involvement of Toll-like receptor 4 in innate immunity to respiratory syncytial virus, *J Virol* 75:10730, 2001.
52. Vabulas RM, Ahmad-Nejad P, da Costa C, et al.: Endocytosed HSP60s use Toll-like receptor 2 (TLR2) and TLR4 to activate the Toll/interleukin-1 receptor signaling pathway in innate immune cells, *J Biol Chem* 276:31332, 2001.
53. Ohashi K, Burkart V, Flohe S, et al.: Cutting edge: heat shock protein 60 is a putative endogenous ligand of the Toll-like receptor-4 complex, *J Immunol* 164:558, 2000.
54. Okamura Y, Watari M, Jerud ES, et al.: The extra domain A of fibronectin activates Toll-like receptor 4, *J Biol Chem* 276:10229, 2001.
55. Underhill DM, Ozinsky A: Toll-like receptors: key mediators of microbe detection, *Curr Opin Immunol* 14:103, 2002.
56. Jha S, Ting JP-Y: Inflammasome-associated nucleotide-binding domain, leucine-rich repeat proteins and inflammatory diseases, *J Immunol* 183:7623, 2009.
57. Jones JD, Vance RE, Dangl JL: Intracellular innate immune surveillance devices in plants and animals, *Science* 354, 2016.
58. Kufer TA, Banks DJ, Philpott DJ: Innate immune sensing of microbes by Nod proteins, *Ann N Y Acad Sci* 1072:19, 2006.
59. Ting JP, Kastner DL, Hoffman HM: CATERPILLERs, pyrin and hereditary immunological disorders, *Nat Rev Immunol* 6:183, 2006.
60. Zambetti LP, Laudisi F, Licandro G, et al.: The rhapsody of NLRPs: master players of inflammation ... and a lot more, *Immunol Res* 53:78, 2012.
61. Martinon F, Petrilli V, Mayor A, et al.: Gout-associated uric acid crystals activate the NALP3 inflammasome, *Nature* 440:237, 2006.
62. Kanneganti TD, Ozoren N, Body-Malapel M, et al.: Bacterial RNA and small antiviral compounds activate caspase-1 through cryopyrin/Nalp3, *Nature* 440:233, 2006.
63. Kanneganti TD, Body-Malapel M, Amer A, et al.: Critical role for cryopyrin/Nalp3 in activation of caspase-1 in response to viral infection and double-stranded RNA, *J Biol Chem* 281:36560, 2006.
64. Boyden ED, Dietrich WF: Nalp1b controls mouse macrophage susceptibility to anthrax lethal toxin, *Nat Genet* 38:240, 2006.
65. Schattgen SA, Fitzgerald KA: The PYHIN protein family as mediators of host defenses, *Immunol Rev* 243:109, 2011.
66. Paludan SR, Bowie AG: Immune sensing of DNA, *Immunity* 38:870, 2013.
67. Chen Q, Sun L, Chen ZJ: Regulation and function of the cGAS-STING pathway of cytosolic DNA sensing, *Nat Immunol* 17:1142, 2016.
68. Vabret N, Blander JM: Sensing microbial RNA in the cytosol, *Front Immunol* 4:468, 2013.
69. Li Y, Wilson HL, Kiss-Toth E: Regulating STING in health and disease, *J Inflamm (Lond)* 14(11), 2017.
70. Nauseef WM, Borregaard N: Neutrophils at work, *Nat Immunol* 15:602, 2014.
71. Fang FC: Antimicrobial reactive oxygen and nitrogen species: concepts and controversies, *Nature Rev Microbiol* 2:820, 2004.
72. Walker JA, Barlow JL, McKenzie ANJ: Innate lymphoid cells—how did we miss them? *Nat Rev Immunol* 13:75, 2013.
73. McKenzie ANJ, Spits H, Eberl G: Innate lymphoid cells in inflammation and immunity, *Immunity* 41:366, 2014.
74. Lee SH, Biron CA: Here today—not gone tomorrow: roles for activating receptors in sustaining NK cells during viral infections, *Eur J Immunol* 40:923, 2010.

75. Bendelac A, Bonneville M, Kearney JF: Autoreactivity by design: innate B and T lymphocytes, *Nat Rev Immunol* 1:177, 2001.
76. Zhang X: Regulatory functions of innate-like B cells, *Cell Mol Immunol* 10(113), 2013.
77. Cerutti A, Cols M, Puga I: Marginal zone B cells: virtues of innate-like antibody-producing lymphocytes, *Nat Rev Immunol* 13:118, 2013.
78. Chousterman BG, Swirski FK: Innate response activator B cells: origins and functions, *Int Immunol* 27:537, 2015.
79. Bonneville M, O'Brien RL, Born WK: Gamma delta T cell effector functions: a blend of innate programming and acquired plasticity, *Nat Rev Immunol* 10:467, 2010.
80. Adams EJ, Gu S, Luoma AM: Human gamma delta T cells: Evolution and ligand recognition, *Cell Immunol* 296:31, 2015.
81. Cerundolo V, Kronenberg M: The role of invariant NKT cells at the interface of innate and adaptive immunity, *Semin Immunol* 22:59, 2010.
82. Crosby CM, Kronenberg M: Tissue-specific functions of invariant natural killer T cells, *Nat Rev Immunol* 18:559, 2018.
83. Kjer-Nielsen L, Patel O, Corbett AJ, et al.: MR1 presents microbial vitamin B metabolites to MAIT cells, *Nature* 491:717, 2012.
84. Zasloff M: Antimicrobial peptides of multicellular organisms, *Nature* 415:389, 2002.
85. Steinstraesser L, Kraneburg U, Jacobsen F, et al.: Host defense peptides and their antimicrobial-immunomodulatory duality, *Immunobiology* 216:322, 2011.
86. Mansour SC, Pena OM, Hancock R: Host defense peptides: front-line immunomodulators, *Trends Immunol* 35:443, 2014.
87. Hazlett L, Wu M: Defensins in innate immunity, *Cell Tissue Res* 343:175, 2011.
88. Shai Y: From innate immunity to de-novo designed antimicrobial peptides, *Curr Pharm Des* 8:715, 2002.
89. Kang HK, Kim C, Seo CH, et al.: The therapeutic applications of antimicrobial peptides (AMPs): a patent review, *J Microbiol* 55(1), 2017.
90. Maisonneuve C, Bertholet S, Philpott DJ, et al.: Unleashing the potential of NOD- and Toll-like agonists as vaccine adjuvants, *Proc Nat Acad Sci U S A* 111:12294, 2014.
91. Blander JM, Medzhitov R: Regulation of phagosome maturation by signals from Toll-like receptors, *Science* 304:1014, 2004.
92. Blander JM, Medzhitov R: Toll-dependent selection of microbial antigens for presentation by dendritic cells, *Nature* 440:808, 2006.
93. Pasare C, Medzhitov R: Control of B-cell responses by Toll-like receptors, *Nature* 438:364, 2005.
94. Leadbetter EA, Rifkin IR, Hohlbaum AM, et al.: Chromatin-IgG complexes activate B cells by dual engagement of IgM and Toll-like receptors, *Nature* 416:603, 2002.
95. Lau CM, Broughton C, Tabor AS, et al.: RNA-associated autoantigens activate B cells by combined B cell antigen receptor/Toll-like receptor 7 engagement, *J Exp Med* 202:1171, 2005.
96. Suthers AN, Sarantopoulos S: TLR7/TLR9- and B cell receptor-signaling crosstalk: promotion of potentially dangerous B cells, *Front Immunol* 8:775, 2017.
97. Barton GM, Medzhitov R: Control of adaptive immune responses by Toll-like receptors, *Curr Opin Immunol* 14:380, 2002.
98. Murphy KM, Stockinger B: Effector T cell plasticity: flexibility in the face of changing circumstances, *Nat Immunol* 11:674, 2010.
99. Palucka K, Banchereau J, Mellman I: Designing vaccines based on biology of human dendritic cell subsets, *Immunity* 33:464, 2010.
100. Seong SY, Matzinger P: Hydrophobicity: an ancient damage-associated molecular pattern that initiates innate immune responses, *Nat Rev Immunol* 4:469, 2004.
101. Shi Y, Evans JE, Rock KL: Molecular identification of a danger signal that alerts the immune system to dying cells, *Nature* 425:516, 2003.
102. Lauvau G, Goriely S: Memory CD8+ T cells: orchestrators and key players of innate immunity? *PLoS Pathog* 12:e1005722, 2016.
103. Netea MG, Joosten LA, Latz E, et al.: Trained immunity: a program of innate immune memory in health and disease, *Science* 352:aaf1098, 2016.
104. Casanova JL, Abel L, Quintana-Murci L: Human TLRs and IL-1Rs in host defense: natural insights from evolutionary, epidemiological, and clinical genetics, *Annu Rev Immunol* 29:447, 2011.
105. Corr SC, O'Neill LA: Genetic variation in Toll-like receptor signalling and the risk of inflammatory and immune diseases, *J Innate Immun* 1:350, 2009.
106. Liu-Bryan R, Scott P, Sydlaske A, et al.: Innate immunity conferred by Toll-like receptors 2 and 4 and myeloid differentiation factor 88 expression is pivotal to monosodium urate monohydrate crystal-induced inflammation, *Arthritis Rheum* 52:2936, 2005.
107. Liu-Bryan R, Pritzker K, Firestein GS, et al.: TLR2 signaling in chondrocytes drives calcium pyrophosphate dihydrate and monosodium urate crystal-induced nitric oxide generation, *J Immunol* 174:5016, 2005.
108. Gershov D, Kim S, Brot N, et al.: C-reactive protein binds to apoptotic cells, protects the cells from assembly of the terminal complement components, and sustains an antiinflammatory innate immune response: implications for systemic autoimmunity, *J Exp Med* 192:1353, 2000.
109. Kravitz MS, Pitashny M, Shoenfeld Y: Protective molecules—C-reactive protein (CRP), serum amyloid P (SAP), pentraxin3 (PTX3), mannose-binding lectin (MBL), and apolipoprotein A1 (Apo A1), and their autoantibodies: prevalence and clinical significance in autoimmunity, *J Clin Immunol* 25:582, 2005.
110. Tsutsumi A, Takahashi R, Sumida T: Mannose binding lectin: genetics and autoimmune disease, *Autoimmun Rev* 4:364, 2005.
111. Leffler J, Bengtsson AA, Blom AM: The complement system in systemic lupus erythematosus: an update, *Ann Rheum Dis* 73:1601, 2014.
112. Einav S, Pozdnyakova OO, Ma M, et al.: Complement C4 is protective for lupus disease independent of C3, *J Immunol* 168:1036, 2002.
113. Paul E, Pozdnyakova OO, Mitchell E, et al.: Anti-DNA autoreactivity in C4-deficient mice, *Eur J Immunol* 32:2672, 2002.
114. Mitchell DA, Pickering MC, Warren J, et al.: C1q deficiency and autoimmunity: the effects of genetic background on disease expression, *J Immunol* 168:2538, 2002.
115. Chen Z, Koralov SB, Kelsoe G: Complement C4 inhibits systemic autoimmunity through a mechanism independent of complement receptors CR1 and CR2, *J Exp Med* 192:1339, 2000.
116. Munoz LE, Lauber K, Schiller M, et al.: The role of defective clearance of apoptotic cells in systemic autoimmunity, *Nat Rev Rheumatol* 6:280, 2010.
117. Mevorach D: Clearance of dying cells and systemic lupus erythematosus: the role of C1q and the complement system, *Apoptosis* 15:1114, 2010.
118. Prodeus AP, Goerg S, Shen LM, et al.: A critical role for complement in maintenance of self-tolerance, *Immunity* 9:721, 1998.
119. Paul E, Carroll MC: SAP-less chromatin triggers systemic lupus erythematosus, *Nat Med* 5:607, 1999.
120. Goodnow CC, Cyster JG, Hartley SB, et al.: Self-tolerance checkpoints in B lymphocyte development, *Adv Immunol* 59:279, 1995.

21 Adaptive Immunity

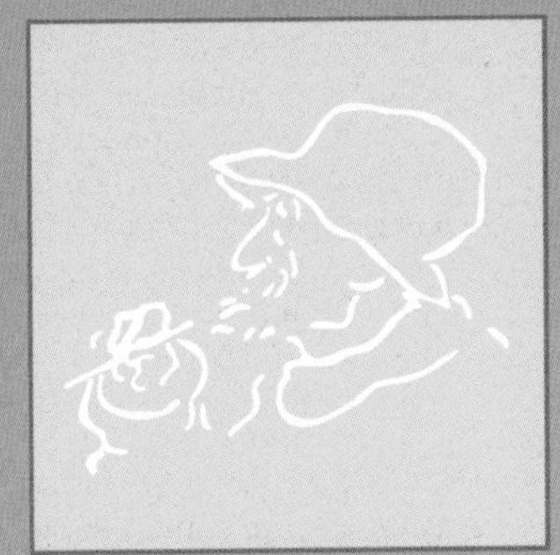

MARTHA S. JORDAN AND GARY A. KORETZKY

KEY POINTS

There are two arms of the adaptive immune system: B cells that provide humoral immunity and T cells that confer cell-based immunity.

B and T lymphocytes rearrange genomic DNA to create a vast array of antigen-specific receptors.

Characteristics of the adaptive immune system include exquisite sensitivity to antigen, tolerance to self, rapid expansion and then elimination of antigen-specific cells responding to a challenge, and memory for a more robust response when a pathogen is reencountered.

Adaptive immune cells develop in primary lymphoid organs, migrate through the body, become activated in secondary lymphoid structures, then home to tissues to exert their effector functions.

Activation of the adaptive immune system involves finely orchestrated interactions with cells of the innate immune system.

Adaptive immune cells take on a variety of effector functions determined by the inciting antigen, the innate immune cells present during activation, and the cytokine environment present at the time of activation.

Impaired adaptive immune cell development and function as well as overexuberant responses can lead to severe pathology.

Introduction

There are many interwoven components that collectively make up the vertebrate immune system. These individual parts can be grouped into two major arms: the innate and adaptive immune systems. The innate arm, as more fully described in Chapter 20, consists of cells with receptors designed to identify and respond to "danger" signals in the environment. The response is rapid and stereotypic in that the same response is elicited every time with the same kinetics and same effector response. This quick and robust response is complemented by the slower and more "fine-tuned" activation and execution of effector functions exhibited by adaptive immune cells. However, coordination of these nonredundant immune cell groups is key for maximal protection against invading pathogens as well as surveillance and elimination of host cells that have been altered, such as those that have undergone malignant transformation.

This chapter is a general introduction to adaptive immune cells, how they develop, function, and interact with cells of the innate immune system as well as the tissues in which they reside. We will discuss how the adaptive immune system, and thus the development and function of its constituents, are shaped by several cardinal features including specificity/diversity, tolerance, expansion/contraction, and memory. A brief discussion of the phylogenetic development of the adaptive immune system is included as well as a review of the tissues in the body where lymphocyte activation occurs. Adaptive immune cells do not function in isolation, and a brief description of how innate and adaptive immune system cells interact with each other then follows. The chapter concludes with a brief discussion of the disease consequences of dysfunction of adaptive immune lineages, presaging material that is presented in the more disease-focused chapters of the text that detail the role of the adaptive immune cells in the pathogenesis of rheumatic diseases.

Phylogenetic Appearance of the Adaptive Immune System

Understanding how the immune system evolved phylogenetically can provide insights into the mechanisms of mammalian immune system-mediated protection, the etiologies of immune system-mediated disorders, and potentially provide clues into novel means to modulate immune system function for therapeutic purposes.[1–3] Innate immune functions, relying on germ line encoded cell surface receptors that distinguish nonself from self by recognizing discreet molecular patterns, are found at the earliest stages of phylogeny in the animal kingdom and throughout the plant world.[4,5] The various effector cell lineages of the innate immune system evolved over time, acquiring different capabilities, presumably responding to challenges by pathogens. Approximately 500 million years ago the first evidence for receptor recombination, and hence the ability to generate a diverse universe of antigen receptors not encoded directly by the genome, was seen with the evolution of chordates.[1] This allowed for finer discrimination between self-proteins and foreign antigens. It is in organisms that developed at this time that the earliest T cells (responsible for cell-mediated immunity; see Chapter 12) and B cells (responsible for antibody production; see Chapter 13) are found.

The key evolutionary advances required for adaptive immune cell development were the appearance of elements in the genome that could recombine to create novel receptors, the enzymatic machinery to allow for this recombination to occur,[6] and molecules present on cells that could bind to and present antigen to adaptive immune cells.[7] Importantly, because rearrangement of the genome has inherent risks (mutation that may result in unrestrained cell growth or imminent cell death), it was essential for recombination leading to antigen receptor production to be restricted in space (specific genomic loci) and in time (those periods during cellular maturation when receptor development occurs). While there has been evolution of all of these components, the basic rules for antigen receptor creation date to the earliest adaptive immune cells. Exactly how the different components of antigen receptor rearrangement and expression evolved from precursor genetic elements remains an area of investigation.

One of the most intriguing findings that emerged from studies of the evolution of the adaptive immune system is that this process occurred twice, both times with a similar solution in principle, but with two different mechanisms.[8] Specifically, although the two branches of vertebrates, the jawed vertebrates and the jawless fish (lamprey and hagfish), both evolved adaptive immune systems, these evolutionary branches employed different molecular approaches to achieve this goal. The jawed vertebrates evolved the genomic organization allowing for receptor diversity, the enzymes required for receptor gene recombination to occur along with key target recognition sites near the antigen receptor genes for these enzymes to act, and forerunners of the major histocompatibility complex critical for function of cell-mediated immunity (see section on T cells later). In contrast, while the jawless vertebrates also evolved adaptive immune cell function, the solution to receptor diversity differed. These organisms possess three sets of leucine-rich variable lymphocyte receptors (VLRs) that emerged through gene conversion.[9] Two of these receptor families function in cells similar to T lineages of jawed vertebrates and the third is operative in cells with similarity to B cells. Intriguingly, the VLRs of the jawless fish bear little resemblance to the antigen-specific receptors of their cousins, yet the two systems seem to function similarly. This example of convergent evolution speaks to the enormous pressure (and presumably selective advantage) to having immune cells that can detect subtle antigenic variability.

Cardinal Features of the Adaptive Immune System

Specificity/Diversity

As discussed in Chapter 20 and throughout this text as it applies to rheumatologic disease processes, the innate immune system consists of cells with receptors designed to identify and respond to "danger" signals in the environment. This is accomplished by "hard-wired" expression of receptors that detect molecular patterns existing in pathogens, but largely absent from host cells. For example, lipopolysaccharide (LPS) is a component of the cell wall of microorganisms that are often pathogenic but is not produced by eukaryotic host cells.[10] Receptors for LPS[11,12] are present on innate immune cells that may encounter an infectious agent at the earliest stage of invasion and signal the presence of danger to these cells. These innate immune cells, in turn, produce mediators and adopt effector functions to rid the host of the pathogen. Unlike the innate immune system, which is triggered by molecular patterns that generally exist in pathogens and are for the most part absent in host cells, the adaptive immune system can be triggered by antigens that are nearly identical to self-molecules (Table 21.1). Indeed, there are only minute differences between a self-protein and a molecule with a similar function but which arises from a potential pathogen and can be identified as foreign by antigen-specific T or B cells. Importantly, each T or B cell expresses a single variety of an antigen receptor; hence a large number of cells, all with different antigen specificity, is generated to ensure protection of the host. Given the enormity of potential antigens to which the adaptive immune system must respond, it is impossible to "pre-wire" T and B cells to express sufficient number of receptors to capture all of the potential antigens to which a response is needed. Even if this was possible, mutation within microorganisms would quickly make them resistant to the receptors encoded by the mammalian genome. Hence, a system was required to both expand the potential reactivity of adaptive immune cells beyond the specificities that could be encoded in the genome and to enable a system that was not restricted to the antigens that exist today. The elegant solution to this problem of generating diversity in the antigen receptor repertoire involves a complex process of receptor gene rearrangement, a process that is the sine qua non of the adaptive immune system.[13,14] As noted previously, this occurred with the development of chordates and has evolved into an increasingly robust system for host protection.

Tolerance

One unavoidable consequence of random reassortment of genetic elements to create a diverse repertoire of antigen receptors is the risk of expressing receptors that are reactive to self-tissues. The host must therefore employ mechanisms to protect itself against these B and T cells which, if left unchecked, could do irreparable damage to tissues. These protective measures are collectively known as *immune tolerance.*

Immunologists distinguish two main types of tolerance, that which occurs in the primary lymphoid organs where B and T cells are generated (central tolerance) and that which occurs in the periphery after lymphocyte development is complete (peripheral tolerance).[15] For B cells, central tolerance therefore occurs primarily in the bone marrow,[16] and for T cells this occurs in the thymus.[17] The main mechanism of central tolerance is accomplished by deletion of potentially self-reactive lymphocytes. Cells are tested at various checkpoints during their development for autoreactivity and, if the degree of such reactivity is excessive, as manifested by robust production of key second messengers when either the antigen receptor for B cells (B cell receptor; BCR) or T cells (T cell receptor; TCR) is triggered during development, cellular maturity ceases and the developing lymphocytes undergo apoptosis. Other, nondeletional forms of tolerance are operational during lymphocyte development. For example, in some B cells the BCR is "edited" through further mutation.[16] In other cases, T cells with autoreactive receptors are allowed to develop, but the T cells that develop (regulatory T cells) adopt inhibitory function that quells immune responses in the periphery.[18,19]

Although central tolerance is an effective process, there are cells that emerge from the lymphocyte generative organs that still have the potential for autoreactivity. Hence, mechanisms must be in place to guard against destruction of self-tissues after T and B cellular maturation is complete. The means that are employed are known collectively as *peripheral tolerance* and involve myriad mechanisms.[20] These include the requirement for multiple signals to be delivered for a productive adaptive immune response to occur. The best example of this is that stimulation of the TCR alone on naïve T cells fails to elicit a T cell effector response, but instead induces a state of T cell nonresponsiveness.[21] For a T cell to become activated in the periphery, it is necessary for there to be a signal delivered by the TCR and by other activating co-receptors. This "brake" on T cell responses prevents effectors from doing damage to the host if conditions are not appropriate for the effectors to exert their functions. In addition to this requirement for "co-stimulation," the environment of the secondary lymphoid organs includes cells from various lineages whose role is to actively inhibit the function of effector T cells, either through products

TABLE 21.1 Cardinal Features of the Adaptive Immune Response

Features of Adaptive Immunity		Mechanism
Specificity and diversity	Each lymphocyte expresses a unique antigen receptor. Enormous diversity.	Lymphocytes utilize somatic gene recombination to generate unique antigen receptors capable of responding to a precise epitope or peptide from a foreign antigen. The process of antigen receptor rearrangement allows for diversity.
Tolerance	Lymphocytes that express autoreactive receptors with the potential to injure self-tissues are eliminated during development (central tolerance) or are inhibited in the periphery (peripheral tolerance) to protect the host.	Tolerance is achieved through "negative selection" as developing lymphocytes with autoreactive receptors receive strong signals that result in apoptosis. Cells with autoreactive receptors that escape deletion can be inhibited in the periphery through failed co-stimulation, an immunosuppressive cytokine environment, or by the action of regulatory cells.
Expansion and contraction	Activation through the antigen receptor triggers clonal expansion of individual lymphocytes. These clonally expanded lymphocytes maintain their antigen specify. Once a pathogen is cleared, the vast majority of activated cells undergo apoptosis.	Lymphocytes undergo metabolic remodeling to support massive proliferation and expansion. Lymphocyte intrinsic and extrinsic mechanisms are thought to regulate clonal contraction following elimination of an invading organism.
Memory	Lymphocytes activated previously by a pathogen can respond rapidly upon subsequent infection with the same pathogen, resulting in faster clearance. The memory response can often prevent symptoms of infection.	During an immune response, a subset of cells differentiates into memory cells. Memory cells are long-lived cells, capable of quickly responding to the same antigen that activated them initially.

they elaborate or through signals they deliver via cell-cell contacts. Some of these mechanisms have been co-opted by tumor cells as they develop in the host, inhibiting the adaptive immune response that has the potential to eliminate that tumor.[22,23] Understanding the variety of signals that modulate a peripheral immune response is therefore critical for us to learn how to maximally manipulate the immune system to either enhance or diminish responses as needed for therapeutic purposes.

Expansion/Contraction

Given the universe of potential antigens against which the adaptive immune system must be primed to react, it stands to reason that the number of cells bearing receptors for a particular antigen prior to exposure to that antigen (the so-called *precursor frequency*) must be relatively small.[24] However, to combat a replicative pathogen a large number of effector cells is required. Hence, once stimulated by antigen under the appropriate activating conditions, B and T cells undergo massive expansion in number.[25] This generally takes a number of days, emphasizing the importance of the innate immune system to keep the pathogen in check until B and T cell numbers increase sufficiently to mount a successful effector response. The lymphocyte expansion begins in the secondary lymphoid organs (SLOs); however, effector cells continue to increase in number as B and T cells migrate to the tissues and the site of the antigenic challenge.

Once a pathogen has been cleared, it is essential for the expanded population of effector cells to be reduced in number. Thus, effector B and T cells are programmed to die after a period of time to ensure a return to homeostasis. This is accomplished by activation-induced expression of receptors on these cells, such as Fas and Fas-ligand, which induce apoptosis when engaged.[26] Failure of this to occur results in accumulation of activated cells, and in the case of a number of human syndromes, massive lymphadenopathy and the accumulation of autoreactive cells that drive destruction of various self-tissues.[27]

Memory

One of the most important attributes of the adaptive immune system is its ability to respond more robustly when a pathogen is encountered subsequent to the host's first exposure. This property, known as immunologic memory, is present in both the B and T cell compartments and is manifested by a speedier and more efficacious response to the pathogenic challenge.[28,29] The memory property of the immune system has been exploited by the developers of vaccinations, where the initial inciting antigenic challenge is delivered through an attenuated pathogen or an isolated immunodominant determinant of that pathogen that by itself is not deleterious. This results in elicitation of an immune response without an initial illness, but one that primes the vaccine recipient for a robust memory response should the intact pathogen be encountered at a later time. Exploiting this adaptive immune system property has made vaccines one of the most successful public health innovations in the history of medicine.

Although it is clear that immunologic memory does exist, the molecular underpinnings of this process are still incompletely understood. Additionally, recent data indicate clearly that there are subsets of memory B and T cells that differ in location in the body, longevity of the cells themselves, and the means by which these cells respond to rechallenge.[30–32] Different types of memory cells can be identified by markers they bear, making it possible to study these cells in isolation, and, as experimental techniques improve, in vivo during an immune response. Controversy also remains regarding whether cells are destined to become memory early on in an immune response or if the memory compartment develops

TABLE 21.2 Properties of BCR and TCR

	BCR	TCR
Structure	IgG, V, C	TCR, β (γ), α (δ), V, C
Proteins	Two heavy chains + two light chains Membrane bound or secreted	α and β chains or γ and δ chains Membrane bound
Antigen Recognition	Macromolecules - Proteins - Lipids - Polysaccharides Small chemicals	Peptide:MHC complexes (α / β T cells) Lipids or Lipid:MHC complexes (alternative lineages)
Antigen Presentation	Native protein, linear, or conformational recognition	13-25 amino acid linear peptides presented by class I MHC 8-10 amino acid linear peptides presented by class II MHC
Alterations after Maturation	Isotype switching Somatic mutation	None

stochastically during the contraction phase that follows immune cell expansion.[33,34] Data also indicate, particularly in studies of T cells, that there are inherent metabolic differences between effector and memory cells, indicating a difference in energy requirements.[35–37] Furthermore, naïve, effector, and memory cells have different transcriptional profiles associated with different epigenetic marks.[38,39] As work in this area continues to develop, it will likely be possible to pharmacologically manipulate B and T cells to favor or disfavor survival and function of effector versus memory cells.

Cells of the Adaptive Immune System

B and T cells comprise the cells of the adaptive immune system. While both cell types adhere to the cardinal features described previously, they have very different and distinct roles in providing protection to the host. Importantly, however, dysregulation of either lineage may result in significant, even life-threatening pathology. General features of these cell types are discussed below and described in greater depth in Chapters 12 and 13.

B Cells and Humoral Immunity

B cells are named for their generative organ in chickens, the Bursa of Fabricius, a model system for some of the earliest studies done to define this lineage of cells.[40,41] In mammals, B cells originate and develop in the bone marrow before they are exported to the circulation to populate SLOs and the tissues.[42]

Mature B cells are responsible for humoral immunity, the arm of the adaptive immune system that relies on the production of antibodies for protection of the host. Antibodies are simply the soluble form of the BCR that is expressed on the B cells and is responsible for binding antigens.[43] Antibodies may coat (opsonize) pathogens, targeting them for engulfment by cells of the reticuloendothelial system, or they may bind to inactive surface receptors on pathogens or toxins that may have been produced. Antibodies consist of two proteins, designated the *light* and *heavy chains* (Table 21.2). Each of these proteins has a variable region and a constant region. The former arises from recombined gene segments (and hence is unique to a particular antibody) and is responsible for binding to antigen; the latter is the product of an invariant gene segment. Adding further diversity to B cell biology are the different classes of antibodies, designated IgM, IgG, IgA, IgD, and IgE, each with different effector functions. Naïve B cells (those that have not encountered a stimulatory antigen) express IgM and IgD, but may "class switch" following activation, by linking their variable regions to a different constant region gene.[44] What class of antibody will eventually be secreted is a function of many factors including the type of antigen that elicited the immune response, the location of the B cell that was stimulated, and the local environment when the stimulation event occurred.

After maturation in the bone marrow, B cells leave this organ and travel through the circulation to secondary lymphoid organs throughout the body. B cells express cell surface molecules that direct them to substructures within the SLOs to maximize their potential to encounter antigen through their BCR. Using their BCR, B cells can detect either soluble or membrane-bound antigen. Following ligation of the BCR, and under the appropriate activating conditions (e.g. a permissive cytokine environment and "help" from T cells), antigen-specific B cells expand in number and mature into antibody secreting plasma cells.[45] Instead of expressing membrane-bound BCRs, plasma cells produce large quantities of antibodies that are secreted into the circulation. Importantly, because this switch to production of secreted antibodies does not alter the antibody specificity, the antigen that elicited the initial B cell response will be recognized by circulating antibody. However, as the B cell response to antigen progresses, B cells may alter their variable regions through a process known as somatic hypermutation.[46] The goal of this process is to generate antibodies with increasing affinity for antigen, improving opportunities for pathogen clearance.

Beyond manufacturing and secreting antibody, B cells serve other immune system functions. Through cell surface receptors and ligands, B cells make contacts with other immune cells and influence their behaviors. The importance of B cells and the intricate roles they play in immune function have become increasingly evident with the advent of therapies that deplete B cells (e.g., rituximab) and that have effects that cannot be explained solely by loss of antibody production. The full panoply of B cell functions remains to be defined and, with further elucidation, will suggest new therapeutic modalities for adaptive immune system modulation.

Contrasting the BCR With the TCR

Although T and B cells share many similarities, there are key features that distinguish these lineages from each other. Many of these features stem from inherent differences between the antigen receptors these cells express and how BCRs and TCRs are activated. As noted previously, there are two forms of the BCR, a cell surface variant that is expressed on the B cell making it sensitive to antigens in the environment, and a circulating variant that is secreted as antibody to exert humoral immune effector functions. In contrast, the TCR is only found as a cell surface structure and is not secreted. Hence, the TCR is not itself an effector molecule but only serves as a surface-bound detector for foreign antigens. Another significant difference between the BCR and TCR is that following antigen receptor gene rearrangement, the nucleotides that encode the TCR are fixed; there is no opportunity for the TCR to undergo mutations as B cells do during somatic hypermutation or class switching. Thus, once expressed on a T cell, the TCR is not altered throughout the lifetime of the cell. Perhaps the most biologically important distinction between the TCR and BCR relates to the types of antigen to which these receptors respond. B cells respond to native antigen, recognizing large molecular conformations that fit snugly into the antigen combining site of the BCR. In contrast, the TCR recognizes short peptide fragments that are embedded in proteins of the major histocompatibility complex (MHC) present on the cell surface of other cells. These peptides (generally 8 to 10 or 13 to 25 amino acids long depending on binding, respectively, to class I or class II MHC molecules) arise from degradation of proteins that have been engulfed by an antigen presenting cells (APCs) or by sampling proteins made by the APCs themselves.[47] The term *MHC restriction* refers to the requirement of the TCR to recognize peptides in the context of self-MHC complexes. The biological underpinning for MHC restriction comes from the fact that the TCR has reactivity not only against the short peptide within the MHC-binding pocket, but also for amino acids found in the MHC molecules themselves. Hence, T cells must have some degree of self-reactivity (through recognition of the host's own MHC) to become activated.[48]

T-Cell Mediated Immunity

There are two major types of T cells: CD4+ and CD8+. These T cells mediate very different types of effector functions once they leave the thymus. Briefly, CD4+ cells function mainly by producing cytokines and expressing surface proteins that interact with other cells of the innate and adaptive immune systems.[49] These mediators may promote effector functions of other cells by enhancing their potency and, in the case of B cells, support class switching and secretion of antibody. Importantly, CD4+ T cells are not a uniform lineage. Indeed, multiple CD4+ T cell subsets have been identified, characterized by signature transcription factors and the specific cytokines they elaborate. Some CD4+ T cells (T regulatory cells) can even suppress immune responses, either by the products they produce or the cell-cell interactions they mediate.[19] Dysregulation or imbalanced function of these subsets tracks with clinical manifestations of a number of important immune-mediated diseases, including many with rheumatologic manifestations. Similar to CD4+ T cells, CD8+ T cells also produce a number of cytokines that help coordinate the activity of innate immune cells. However, the classic functional property of CD8+ T cells is their cytotoxicity directed against cells that stimulate their TCR.[50] When infected cells present pathogen-derived peptides on their class I MHC molecules, CD8+ cells, whose TCRs recognize that specific peptide-MHC combination, lyse these infected cells, thereby contributing to clearance of pathogens that reside within cells.

Development of Adaptive Immune Cells

Primary Lymphoid Organs

The sites of development of the adaptive immune cell lineages are designated *primary lymphoid organs.* For T cells, this is the thymus; and for B cells, the bone marrow. It is in these primary lymphoid structures where antigen receptor gene rearrangement occurs and where initial selection events take place ensuring that the antigen receptor that has been generated has appropriate antigen reactivity for development to proceed.

B Cell Development in the Bone Marrow

B cells begin their developmental program in the bone marrow as precursor cells mature from common lymphoid progenitors (CLPs). These B cell precursors, marked by expression of the B220 isoform of the cell surface protein CD45, advance through multiple stages of development that are defined by expression of numerous other cell surface as well as intra-cellular proteins.[51] The earliest committed B lineage cells, the pro-B cells, are marked by rearrangement of their immunoglobulin heavy chain locus, followed by progression to the pre-B cell stage where the heavy chain is expressed with an invariant (surrogate) light chain (Fig. 21.1A). Successful rearrangement of this "pre-B cell receptor" triggers proliferation of developing B cells followed by quiescence and subsequent rearrangement of the light chain locus. B cells with

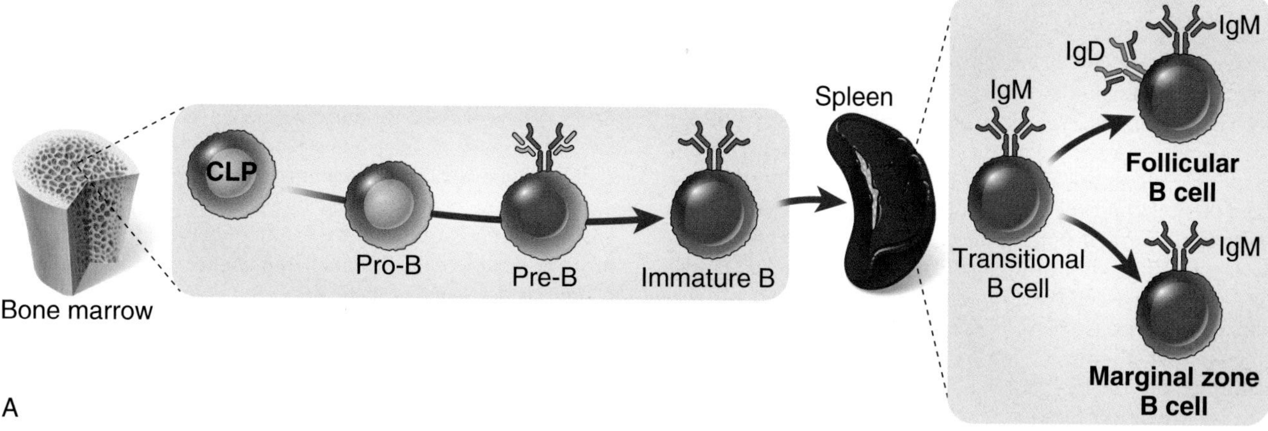

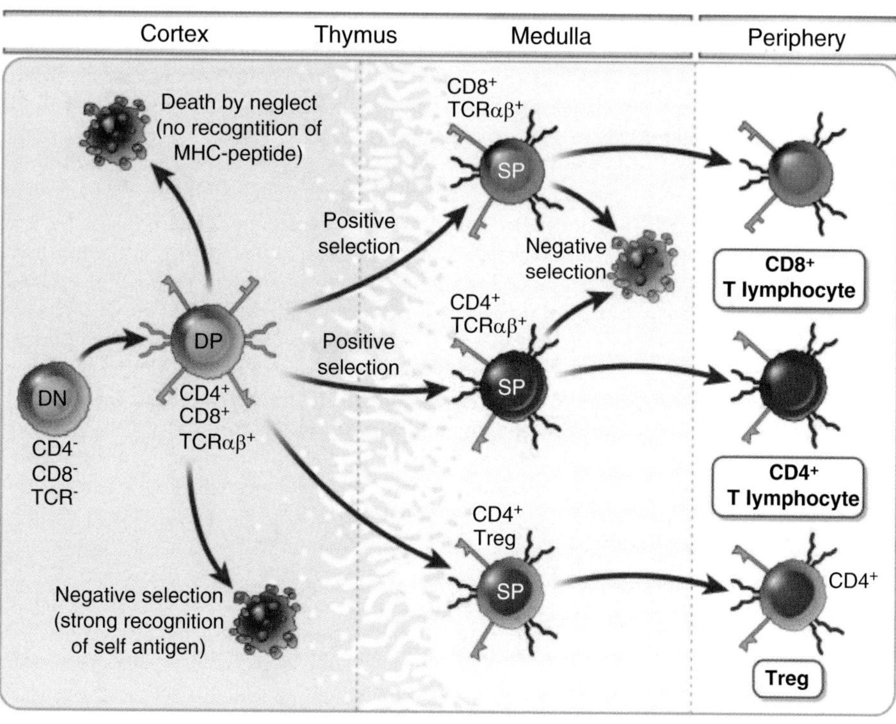

• **Fig. 21.1** Schematic of adaptive immune cell development. (A) B cells begin their maturation in the bone marrow differentiating from the common lymphoid progenitor (CLP). They progress from the pro-B to pre-B stage, where they express the pre-B cell receptor, then develop into immature B cells that express a mature IgM-BCR. In the spleen, B cells finish their maturation, becoming follicular B cells that express IgM and IgD, or marginal zone B cells. (B) DN thymocytes rearrange their TCR genes and upregulate expression of CD4 and CD8, at which time these early thymocytes are subjected to positive and negative selection events. Traditional α/β CD4 and CD8 T cells emerge from the thymus and enter the peripheral lymphatic system. The thymus also generates other types of T cells, including T regulatory cells as well as alternative lineages such as γ/δ T and NKT cells. (Adapted from Abbas, *Cellular and Molecular Immunology*, 9e, Figure 8.15.)

successful immunoglobulin light chain pairing with the heavy chain develop further into immature B cells that express surface-bound IgM.[52]

Expression of surface IgM marks a critical stage for developing B cells, for it is at this time these cells are subjected to selection.[16] Active forms of B cell tolerance include deletion of B cells expressing receptors with high affinity to self-proteins or induction of anergy, a state in which B cells do not die, yet cannot be activated. A third mechanism by which autoreactive B cell receptors can be limited is through a process termed *receptor editing*. This process allows for further rearrangement of the light chain in B cells that generated a deletional signal upon first encounter with self-proteins. If the newly rearranged light chain no longer transmits a strong signal (indicating that autoreactivity has diminished), the immature B cell can be rescued from deletion. Not all autoreactive B cells are purged from the B cell repertoire. Some B cells with specificity for self-proteins are simply "ignorant" in that under normal conditions, the interaction affinity with their cognate antigen is quite low or they simply do not come in contact with it. However, these cells have the potential to become activated in certain circumstances, including inflammatory settings, with the potential to cause or exacerbate autoimmune disorders.

T Cell Development in the Thymus

The thymus, consisting of paired lobes, is located just beneath the sternum in the anterior mediastinum. Each thymic lobe contains a central medullary region and peripheral cortex. The cell types that make up the thymus include the stroma, intrinsic to the thymus itself, and a number of hematopoietic lineages that seed the thymus from the circulation and stay as resident cells or are present in the thymus on a transient basis.[53] The relative size of the thymus is greatest in the neonatal period, coincident with a robust period of T cell development. Like most organs, the thymus increases in size as the host grows, but after puberty gradually becomes smaller, although some T cell development continues to occur throughout the lifespan.

T cells derive from precursor cells that originate in the bone marrow, but complete their development in the thymus.[54] The earliest T cell precursors enter the thymus at the corticomedullary junction then migrate to the cortex (see Fig. 21.1B). These early T cells are defined as *triple-negative* as they lack surface molecules that are the hallmarks of mature T cells, the TCR (and its associated proteins designated *CD3*) and either CD4 or CD8. Like the BCR, the TCR consists of two proteins, in this case the α and β chains (see Table 21.2). Each has unique variable regions that arise from rearranging genes, and constant elements that are the same among TCR. The first stage in T cell development is rearrangement of the genes encoding the β chain of the antigen receptor. At this point, developing T cells must pass a checkpoint known as β-selection. Because gene rearrangement of the TCR chains is a random event, it is possible for recombination to result in encoding a β-chain that is incapable of being expressed (for example, due to insertion of a stop codon). β-selection tests the ability of the β-chain to pair with an invariant, non-rearranging pre-TCR α-chain and to signal to key downstream molecules, marking rearrangements that have resulted in a functional protein.[55] Cells that pass β-selection, rearrange their TCR α-chain, begin to express both CD4 and CD8 (becoming double-positive [DP] thymocytes), and become subject to positive selection. Positive selection of DP thymocytes is mediated by cortical medullary epithelial cells that express both class I and class II MHC.[56] If the successful selection steps involve antigen presented by class I MHC, the DP cells downregulate CD4 and complete their maturation as CD8 single positive cells, whereas if selection involves antigen presented by class II, CD8 is silenced and the resulting mature T cell is CD4+. However, the vast majority of thymocytes fail positive selection and die by apoptosis because they demonstrate insufficient reactivity to self-MHC (recall, T cells respond to both peptide antigen and self-MHC molecules). Some thymocytes also undergo negative selection at this stage due to too strong of an interaction with peptide-MHC complexes. Those that do survive migrate to the medulla where they encounter APCs that express low levels of many of the peripheral proteins a T cell might encounter in the periphery.[57] If there is substantial reactivity with the TCR, this interaction is interpreted as autoreactivity, and these cells fail negative selection and die by apoptosis. These sequential steps shape the TCR repertoire of the pool of cells that ultimately reach the circulation and the SLOs.

In addition to T cells that express highly variable α- and β-chain antigen receptors, there are other subpopulations of T cells that develop in the thymus and migrate to the periphery. These include cells that express a receptor composed of two other proteins (designated γ and δ) that bear similarity to α- and β-chains and also arise from rearranged genes to create diverse antigen receptors.[58] Another population, labelled natural killer T (NKT) cells, also develops in the thymus. These cells have characteristics of both T cells and NK cells. NKT cells utilize α- and β-chains for their antigen receptors; however, NKT cells make use of a limited repertoire of the genes for these proteins and hence have much less potential for recognition of diverse antigens.[59] The γ/δ T cells and NKT cells are responsive to different types of antigens than classical α/β T cells and are not restricted by classical MHC molecules. Our emerging understanding of the role of these cell lineages in host protection and their potential importance in immune-mediated diseases is described in more detail in Chapter 12.

Anatomic Organization of the Peripheral Adaptive Immune System

Secondary Lymphoid Organs

SLOs include the spleen, regional lymph nodes, and mucosal-associated lymphoid tissues. The immunologic purpose of the SLOs is to concentrate antigens in a permissive environment, making it possible for circulating lymphocytes to find and respond to their antigenic triggers. The spleen is the major site for concentration of blood-borne antigens, while lymph nodes and mucosal-associated lymphoid tissues are essential for capturing antigens that have been picked up in the tissues by resident APCs. The architecture of the SLOs and how cells are directed into these organs juxtaposes T cells and B cells with key stromal elements and other cells of the immune system to maximize their potential for activation when appropriate conditions are met. Cell-cell interactions and the production of inhibitory cytokines in the SLOs are also critical for promoting peripheral tolerance to prevent autoreactive lymphocytes from exerting damaging effects on self-tissues.

Spleen

The spleen is a multifunctional organ that rests in the left upper quadrant of the abdominal cavity and generally weighs between 150 and 200 grams in a normal-sized adult. Phagocytes in the red pulp are key for removing aged red blood cells and for engulfing and destroying antibody-coated bacteria and other particles from the circulation. The importance of the spleen in protection from pathogenic encapsulated bacteria is demonstrated by the increased morbidity of such infections in patients following splenectomy or functional asplenia from disorders such as sickle cell disease.[60]

The spleen is also the major site for the initiation of an immune response against bloodstream antigens and as such receives approximately 5% of the cardiac output. Blood enters the splenic hilum via the splenic artery, which then branches into a series of trabecular arteries. As the vessels travel deeper into the splenic parenchyma, they progressively branch into a series of central arterioles that empty into a network of sinuses, which bathe the lymphocyte-rich white pulp (Fig. 21.2A–C). The interface between the red and white pulp, known as the marginal zone, is where circulating antigens encounter B cells and/or are captured by innate immune cells to be processed for presentation to T cells that also enter the spleen via its circulation. Segregation of lineages of lymphocytes into particular regions of the spleen increases the efficiency of immune cell activation as these regions are preferentially rich in the innate immune cells most critical for communication with B versus T cells. B cells congregate in the spleen into regions known as follicles[61] whereas T cells reside within the T cell zone.

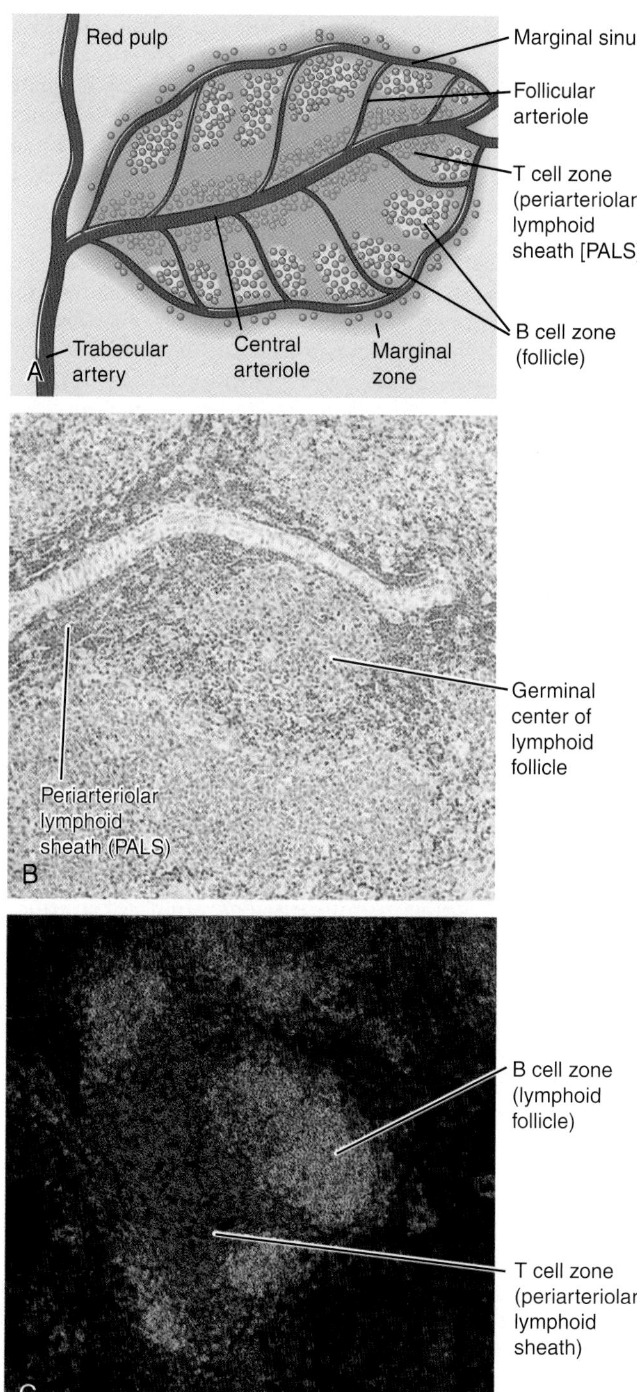

• **Fig. 21.2** Morphology of the spleen. (A) Schematic diagram of the spleen. (B) Photomicrograph of a section of human spleen. Shown is the trabecular artery surrounded by the adjacent periarteriolar lymphoid sheath and adjacent to a lymphoid follicle containing a germinal center. Bordering these areas is the red pulp. (C) Immunohistochemical staining of a spleen section identifies T cells *(red)* and B cells *(green)* in the spleen. These stains demarcate the T and B cell zones, respectively. (Courtesy of Drs. Kathryn Pape and Jennifer Walter, University of Minnesota School of Medicine, Minneapolis. Adapted from Abbas, *Cellular and Molecular Immunology*, 9e, Figure 2.17.)

Resident within the follicle are cells of mesenchymal origin known as follicular dendritic cells (FDCs) that capture antigens that are able to activate the BCR on naïve B cells.[62] Upon antigen recognition, B cells internalize and process the antigen and present it to CD4+ T cells at the interface of the T cell and B cell zones. Once provided T cell help, proliferating B cells within the follicles may form germinal centers,[63] specialized collections of B cells where antibody class switching and affinity maturation occurs. Germinal centers are also the site where differentiation into memory B cells or plasma cells capable of producing large quantities of antibody occurs.

Each lymphocyte subset is attracted to their respective regions by specific soluble mediators known as *chemokines.* Chemokines are a class of low molecular weight chemotactic cytokines, which function as attractants for leukocytes bearing receptors for that specific chemokine. Chemokines are essential for normal homeostasis of the immune system by ensuring that lymphocyte progenitors migrate to appropriate regions within primary lymphoid organs and that mature, naïve cells populate their correct niche within SLOs.[54,64–66] Following activation in SLOs, chemokines also play a key role in directing effector cells to the appropriate tissues where they can exert their protective functions. There are four subfamilies of chemokines grouped as CXC, CC, CX3C, and XC based upon structural similarities within each category.[66] The different receptors respond to their cognate chemokines and activate signaling pathways that direct migration of target cells, and in some circumstances activate the target cells. One example of coordinated lymphocyte movements directed by chemokine:receptor pairs is that of CCR7 and CXCR5. High CCR7 expression on naïve T cells (and activated APCs) directs these cells to the T cell zone where their ligand is present,[67] whereas cells in the splenic B cell zone elaborate chemokines that bind CXCR5 expressed by naïve B cells, resulting in their migration to the follicle.[68] Once activated, B cells downregulate CXCR5 and upregulate CCR7, thus allowing for their transient movement to the T:B interphase where they can be further activated. Conversely, a small population of T cells upregulate CXCR5 and downregulate CCR7, which causes them to move into the B cell follicle where they support B cell responses.

B and T cells that find their cognate antigen and are activated in the spleen leave the organ via the portal circulation. As part of their activation program, their chemokine receptors and adhesion molecules (see later) are altered, ultimately directing the cells to the tissues. Those B and T cells that fail to be activated in the spleen also re-enter the circulation, but instead of homing to tissues, remain in the circulation where they can re-enter other SLOs in search of an antigenic signal.

Lymphatics

Lymphocytes are unique cells in the body because they circulate through two parallel circulations, the blood and lymphatic vessels. Lymphatics are an open vascular network that serves to drain tissue spaces, as well as the SLOs, and carry lymphocytes and fluids (known collectively as *lymph*) to the heart where the lymph is admixed with blood. One important function of the lymphatic system is to ensure that fluids leaving the blood stream capillaries to bathe the tissues are returned to the circulation. It is estimated that approximately 3 liters of such fluid is generated each day. Failure of the lymphatics to maintain fluid homeostasis results in lymphedema, a condition that can become a debilitating disorder.[69] Lymphatics draining the tissues also play a critical role in delivering activated APCs (with the antigens they present) to regional lymph nodes, thereby concentrating antigen in sites accessible to patrolling T cells. Lymphatics are also key to direct lymphocytes from SLOs back into the circulation, as the network of lymphatic vessels end in the thoracic duct, which itself empties into the superior vena cava and subsequently the heart. Using the combined blood and lymphatic circulatory networks allows for continued migration of lymphocytes into the SLOs where antigen encounters occur, but also allows for activated lymphocytes to leave the lymphoid system and home to the tissues where their effector functions may be needed. How lymphatics develop is an area of considerable investigation, with a number of recent discoveries describing their formation and maintenance. This work will certainly provide additional insights into the regulation of lymphocyte circulation as well as clues for new approaches for the treatment of lymphatic disruption.

Lymph Nodes and Mucosal Lymphoid Tissue

Lymph nodes are the SLOs found at the intersection of blood and lymphatic vessels.[70,71] "True" lymph nodes are encapsulated organs, strategically located throughout the body to drain the various tissues. Mucosal lymphoid tissues do not have a capsule, but in virtually all other regards they are similar to lymph nodes and hence are grouped together in this description.

The lymph node capsule covers the cortex, which in turn surrounds the paracortex and then the medulla. Lymph nodes are vascularized by lymphatics originating in the tissues that deliver APCs that have been activated in the periphery (typically by "danger signals" associated with pathogen encounters) and are able to present antigen to arriving T cells. Afferent lymphatics enter the lymph node through the capsule and empty into the marginal sinus (Fig. 21.3A). Lymph bathes the node allowing APCs to find their niche, largely through chemokine/chemokine receptor interactions. Lymph then collects in the efferent lymphatics, which leaves the lymph node and eventually makes its way to the thoracic duct, the heart, and the blood vessel circulation. Lymphocytes enter the lymph node through the blood circulation, flowing into the lymph node stroma via post capillary venules designated *high endothelial venules.* Similar to the spleen, the lymph node architecture allows for spatial discrimination between T cell (parafollicular cortex) and B cell (follicular and germinal center) zones that are populated with the appropriate stromal elements, APCs, and support cells for the distinct lymphocyte populations (see Figs. 21.3B and C). Lymphocytes dwell in the lymph node long enough to survey the environment for cognate antigen, then leave the lymph node via the efferent lymphatics to re-enter the blood circulation. As in the spleen, should a productive encounter with antigen occur, cells emigrating from the lymph node alter expression of key receptors that will ultimately direct them to the tissues. Nonactivated cells maintain their naïve phenotype and recirculate from the blood stream back to SLOs.

As every clinician knows well, lymph nodes are the location for expansion of the adaptive immune cell population responsive to an antigenic challenge. The extensive cell division is manifest as clinical lymphadenopathy. Under normal circumstances, following removal of the pathogen that incited the expanded immune response, lymph nodes are also the site of the subsequent contraction phase eliminating the vast majority of the activated cells. Failure of this contraction to occur may result in persistent lymphadenopathy and survival of autoreactive cells, a hallmark of a number of rheumatic diseases.

The largest collections of lymphoid tissues in the body are found associated with mucosal surfaces. This makes a great deal of immunological sense as these surfaces represent the barrier between the host and the outside world replete with potential pathogens. Hence, there are significant collections of B and T cells in the tonsils, adenoids, and along the respiratory mucosa, throughout the gut, and surrounding the urogenital tracts. These lymphoid collections are not encapsulated and are not considered by some investigators as true SLOs. However, they function in many of the same ways, have a similar architecture, and support B and T cell recirculation, activation, and tolerance induction as do encapsulated lymph nodes. Although there are many anatomical and functional similarities, mucosal-associated lymphoid structures also have unique properties related to the types of antigenic challenges that predominate in their particular locations.[72] For example, Peyer's patches in the gut express specialized chemokines to attract particular classes of lymphocytes and are the most important site of IgA production. Similarly, intestinal and respiratory collections of lymphoid tissue are important locations for cytokine production that drive a particular subset of CD4+ T cells, known as *Th2*[73] cells, that are responsive to helminth infections, given the importance of these barrier surfaces to protect against ingested or inhaled parasites.

Tertiary Lymphoid Structures

Tertiary lymphoid structures, also known as *ectopic lymphoid follicles,* are organized collections of lymphocytes and stromal elements that occur outside of the normal SLOs.[74] While these structures resemble SLOs in many ways, they are distinguished from SLOs by the fact that they occur in organs not typically associated with lymphoid development or where a primary adaptive immune response (stimulation of naïve cells to become effectors) takes place. The distinction between tertiary lymphoid structures and SLOs is debated where some investigators consider mucosal-associated lymphoid structures as part of the normal SLO network, while others consider all lymphocyte collections that lack a defined capsule as being part of the tertiary lymphoid structures system. Tertiary lymphoid structures often appear in response to chronic inflammatory conditions and are a hallmark of a number of autoimmune disorders. Such examples include collections of organized lymphoid collections in the synovium of patients with rheumatoid arthritis[75] or in salivary glands of individuals with Sjögren's syndrome.[76,77] It is thought that immune activation in these sites potentiates disease through continued stimulation of potentially self-reactive lymphocytes.

Trafficking of Adaptive Immune Cells

Egress From the Thymus and Lymph Nodes

For lymphocytes to exert their functions, they must enter and leave the circulation at various times. For example, maturing thymocytes remain resident in the thymus throughout their development, but then leave to begin their surveillance in the SLOs. Similar to residency time in the thymus, T cells must remain in the SLOs long enough to encounter representative APCs to allow for activation to occur. However, the likelihood that such an encounter will occur at any point in time is low, so there must be a mechanism for T cells to leave any particular lymph node to re-enter the circulation and then to enter another lymph node where an APC with the appropriate antigen can be found. Recent work has shown that control of lymphocyte egress from primary and secondary lymphoid organs relies on the dynamic expression of a subclass of receptors for sphinogosine 1 phosphate (S1P1).[78–80] Binding of S1P1 receptor type 1 by S1P1 is critical for exit of lymphocytes into the circulation and travel to the next set of SLOs for sampling of antigens or to tissues in the case of T cells that have been activated in the SLOs. Understanding the biology of lymphocyte egress has been exploited for therapeutic benefit

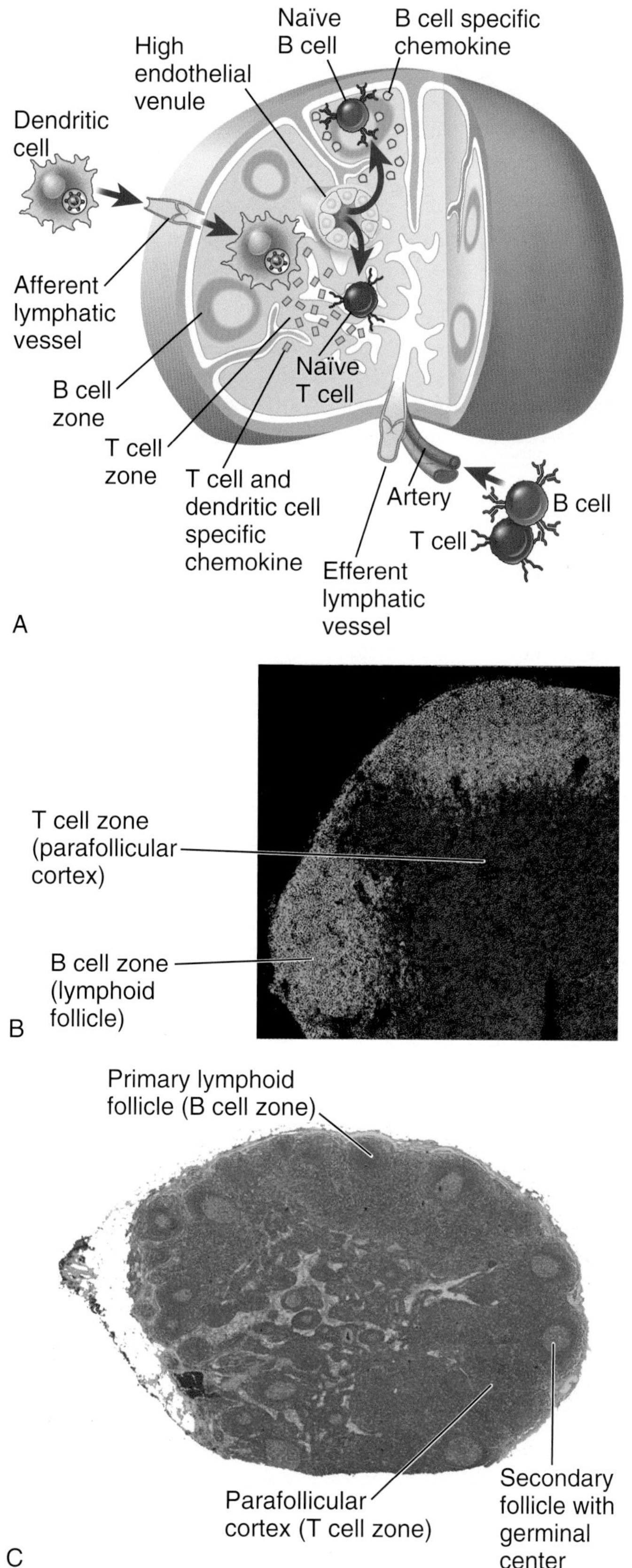

• **Fig. 21.3** Morphology of the lymph node. (A) Schematic diagram of cell migration in the lymph node. Lymphocytes enter the lymph node through high endothelial venules, then are directed by chemokine gradients to specific T or B cell zones. These cells leave the lymph node through the efferent lymphatic vessel. Dendritic cells enter via the afferent lymphatic vessel, then migrate to the T cell zone for antigen presentation. (B) Immunohistochemical staining of a lymph node section is shown. T cells clustered in the T cell zone are stained red and B cells in the lymphoid follicle or B cell zone are stained in green. (C) Light micrograph of a lymph node in which the T cell zone and B cell zone can be appreciated, as well as follicles containing germinal centers. (B, Courtesy of Drs. Kathryn Pape and Jennifer Walter, University of Minnesota School of Medicine, Minneapolis; C, Courtesy of Dr. James Gulizia, Department of Pathology, Brigham and Women's Hospital, Boston, Massachusetts; A–C were adapted from Abbas, *Cellular and Molecular Immunology*, 9e, Figures 2.14 and 2.15.)

with the introduction of FTY720, an agent that, when modified in the body, acts to internalize the S1P1 receptor, preventing T cell egress from both the thymus and lymph nodes. Use of FTY720 to sequester potentially autoreactive T cells and prevent their migration to peripheral organs has proven an effective strategy for multiple sclerosis.[81] Studies are ongoing to determine use of this agent in other immune-mediated disorders.[82–84]

Lymphocyte Migration and Circulation to SLOs and Peripheral Tissues

There are multiple mechanisms that govern the appropriate migration of progenitor T and B cells into their generative organs, then for mature cells to travel through the circulation, transit through SLOs, and eventually reach their target tissues.[54,85] These mostly rely on cell surface receptors expressed on the lymphocytes that drive directional chemotaxis of these cells (chemokine receptors) and other receptors on their surfaces that promote adhesion when the cells traffic to the appropriate location (integrins). T cells and B cells express different family members of these receptors that direct homing to appropriate locations in the body. Of note, expression of chemokine receptors is not static, but instead changes as cells undergo developmental progression and activation. Hence, for example, naïve cells express a suite of chemokine receptors that direct these cells to SLOs and their appropriate APCs. Once activated, however, a different set of such receptors is expressed to direct the effector lymphocytes away from the SLOs and, instead, to the peripheral tissues. Beyond this, sublineages of lymphocytes also express characteristic chemokine receptors that are, in turn, responsive to tissue-specific ligands that are often expressed preferentially after contact with particular classes of antigens. This helps ensure the trafficking of the appropriate effector cells to the areas of greatest need.

In addition to chemokines and their receptors, integrins and their ligands are critical for lymphocyte trafficking. Unlike chemokines, which are soluble mediators that initiate leukocyte chemotaxis, integrin ligands are found on cell surfaces. The interaction between integrins and their ligands is important at a number of steps during lymphocyte circulation, as they enter and then migrate to appropriate regions within SLOs, as they leave these organs, and then as they extravasate into tissues and travel through the endothelial layers and parenchmya.[86] Elegant studies have unraveled the multistep process by which integrins function to facilitate leukocyte migration through the bloodstream and then into tissues.[87] A key first step for T and B cells to leave the high-flow, turbulent circulation is for these cells to be captured by the vascular endothelium at the entry point into the SLOs or tissues. This is accomplished by interactions between integrins on the adaptive immune cells and their ligands. For naïve T cells, the integrin/receptor pair that is most critical is L-selectin (CD62L) on the lymphocyte that interacts with one of the members of the peripheral node addressin (PNAd) family, GlycCAM-1 or CD34 on lymph node high endothelial venules, or MadCAM-1 in Peyer's patches. These interactions are not high affinity, and the lymphocytes arrest for only a short period of time. However, other signals, for example those delivered by chemokines, alter the integrins themselves on the T cells, increasing the affinity of the interactions between the integrins and their ligands. This process, known as *inside-out signaling*, where second messengers activated by other receptors signal to integrins and change their characteristics,[88] allows naïve T cells to arrest firmly on the endothelial surface, then crawl between endothelial cell junctions into the lymph node parenchyma. From there, the lymphocytes follow chemokine gradients and populate their appropriate niche.

Productive interactions between naïve lymphocytes and their antigens in the SLOs stimulate a number of intra-cellular signals. One consequence of these activation events is increased expression of integrins and increased integrin affinity for ligand. This allows for more efficient arrest of the activated lymphocytes on endothelial surfaces in the region of inflamed tissues, once the activated lymphocytes leave the SLOs and survey the tissues through the bloodstream.[89] For example, activated T cells express high levels of CD44, VLA-4, and VLA-5, molecules that bind tissue matrix components (such as hyaluronic acid, fibrin, and fibronectin) that increase with inflammation. Hence, as activated T cells pass near such regions, their integrins will bind avidly to their cognate ligands, arrest along the endothelium, and facilitate entry of the cells into the tissues. Collectively, the response to chemokines and increased function of integrins brings activated lymphocytes to the regions where they are most needed, areas of tissue damage and active inflammation (Fig. 21.4).

Cell-to-Cell Interactions That Support Development of an Immune Response

T cells and B cells do not function in isolation but are highly dependent on cooperation with cells of the innate immune system for their function (Fig. 21.5). The most obvious example of this is that naïve T cells only become activated after encountering APCs with the appropriate peptide antigen displayed by the correct (for that TCR) MHC molecules. Importantly, however, APCs provide other cell surface structures that are critical for activating and shaping the adaptive immune response. One of the most important discoveries related to T cell biology stemmed from the observation that stimulation of T cells via a peptide:MHC combination on APCs (known as signal 1) is not sufficient to elicit a T cell response, and, in fact, stimulating T cells solely through this mechanism results in T cells becoming either temporarily or permanently unresponsive (anergic). Hence, activation of T cells requires stimulation of the TCR in combination with engagement of other T cell surface receptors by ligands present on APCs. These other receptors are known collectively as co-stimulatory receptors, and the signal delivered by their engagement has been designated signal 2. The chance that this required second signal will be delivered is augmented through stabilizing the interaction between T cells and APCs. This is accomplished in part by inside-out signaling from the TCR which, like signals from chemokines, increases affinity of integrins, such as lymphocyte function associate antigen-1 (LFA-1) on T cells that then bind more tightly to their ligands, intercellular adhesion molecule-1 (ICAM-1) on the APC.[90]

The most potent and best studied signal 2 is delivered by the co-stimulatory receptor CD28. In addition to CD28,[91] however, there are a number of other co-stimulatory receptors that serve to reinforce or prolong T cell activation, including adhesion proteins that stabilize the interaction of T cells and the APC, other members of the CD28 superfamily[92] such as inducible T cell co-stimulator (ICOS), as well as several members of the TNF and TNF receptor family of co-stimulatory proteins such as OX40 and 4-1BB. Much work is being done to understand better the biology of these receptors and their ligands, which are often upregulated on activated cells of the innate immune system.

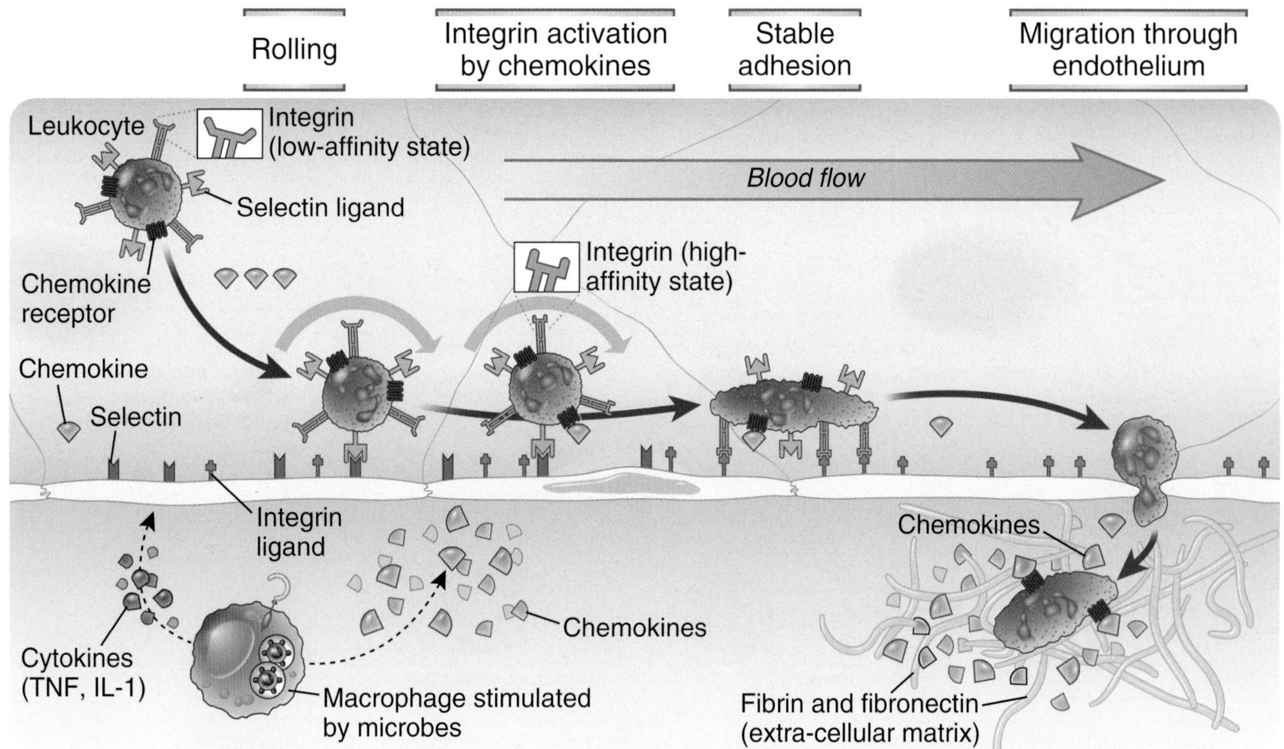

• **Fig. 21.4** Lymphocyte migration into tissues. At sites of infection, activated macrophages secrete cytokines that induce expression of selectins, integrin ligands, and chemokines on the tissue endothelium. Leukocytes are first tethered to the tissue endothelium through weak interactions with selectins and integrin ligands. These interactions mediate rolling of leukocytes on the tissue surface under sheer force of blood flow. Chemokine signals induce leukocyte integrins to adopt a high-affinity binding state, resulting in firm adhesion of leukocytes to the endothelium and ultimately migration into the infected tissue. (Adapted from Abbas, *Cellular and Molecular Immunology*, 9e, Figure 3.3.)

Of equal importance to those signals that co-stimulate T cells are those that function to dampen their responses.[93] Inhibitory receptors, such as programmed cell death 1 (PD-1) and cytotoxic T-lymphocyte associated protein 4 (CTLA-4) begin to be expressed on activated T cells as a way to regulate the magnitude of their response. Signaling through these receptors can directly interfere with the positive signal provided by co-stimulatory receptors. Additionally, because CTLA-4 binds to the same ligands (B7.1 and B7.2) as CD28, CTLA-4 can directly interfere with CD28 engagement. Given the powerful impact of both co-stimulatory and inhibitory signals on T cell homeostasis, it is no surprise that enhancing or limiting engagement of these types of receptors is actively being pursued as means to treat immune-mediated disorders and modulate the immune response to malignancy.[94,95]

In addition to signals delivered through direct cell-cell contact, innate immune cells elaborate a large number of cytokines, such as IL-12, and other soluble mediators that bind to receptors on T cells.[96] These cytokines, often described as *signal 3,* have a profound influence on the magnitude as well as the type of T cell effector response that will be manifest. As with the co-stimulatory versus inhibitory signals described previously, cytokines from innate immune cells do not always promote immune responses. There are many inhibitory cytokines, IL-10[97] and TGF-β[98] being classic among this group, that suppress the activation of adaptive immune cells. Moreover, just as the cytokine microenvironment generated by innate cells directs the differentiation of T cells, T cell derived cytokines can impact innate cell function. One example is macrophage differentiation into inflammatory versus suppressive subtypes. This process is dependent in part on the cytokine environment generated by the T cells in the vicinity.[99] Despite the complex nature of cytokines and their cellular functions, many have become attractive pharmacologic targets, with inhibition of TNF or its receptors being the most successful to date for the treatment of immune-mediated rheumatologic conditions.[100]

T cells are the major source of "help" for B cells, providing both cell-to-cell interactions and soluble factors required for B cell activation. B cells that have taken up antigen via their BCR can process that antigen and present it as peptide:class II MHC complexes to CD4+ T cells. In turn, CD4+ helper T cells provide stimulatory signals, of which CD40 ligand (CD40L) is perhaps the best-described.[101] Ligation of CD40 on B cells induces a host of B cell functions, including proliferation, immunoglobulin class-switching, and somatic hypermutation within the variable regions of the BCR to increase antibody affinity within germinal centers.[63] CD40L expression is also accompanied by secretion of one of a number of T cell derived cytokines (including IL-4, a potent B cell proliferation factor), which direct B cells to class-switch their immunoglobulins to specific isotypes best suited to combat the infection at hand. In addition to providing stimulation for B cells, CD40 ligation on innate immune cells is also critical for generating a robust immune response. Macrophages require CD40 ligation for full activation and upregulation of their anti-microbial activity, and ligation of CD40 on dendritic cells is a potent signal for their final maturation.

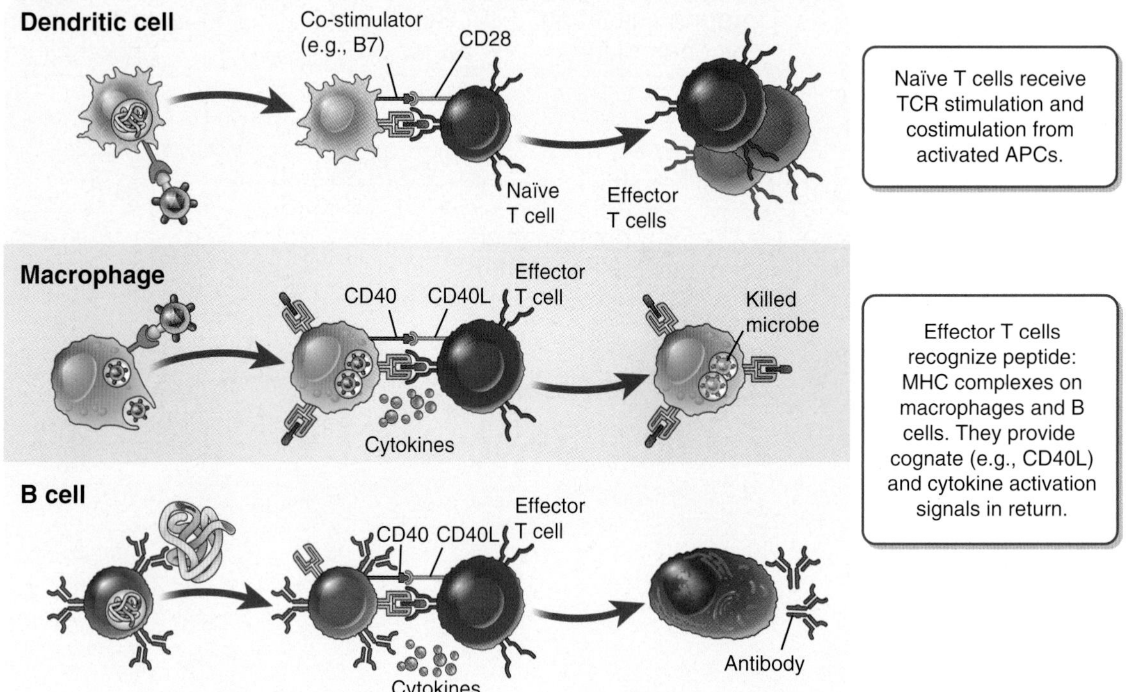

• **Fig. 21.5** Cell-to-cell interactions are required for immune responses. Cell contact dependent- and independent-interactions between immune cells are required for optimal immune cell activation and the subsequent development of a productive immune response. Three such interactions are illustrated here. Dendritic cells serve as potent antigen-presenting cells to naïve T cells, providing not only peptide:MHC complexes but co-stimulation that is required for T cell activation. Activated T cells upregulate surface expression of CD40L that binds to CD40 on the macrophage and mediates activation of these cells. In turn, the activated macrophages secrete cytokines that help direct T cell differentiation. Interactions between B cells and T cells include presentation of peptide:MHC complexes by B cells to T cells, and the provision of both cognate (CD40:CD40L) as well as soluble cytokines from T cells to direct B cell antibody production. (Adapted from Abbas, *Cellular and Molecular Immunology*, 9e, Figure 6.2.)

Innate immune cells also modulate the B cell response through altering the cytokine microenvironment. For example, innate cell production of type I interferons can render B cells more sensitive to BCR stimulation,[102] thus enhancing their activation, a property that may significantly impact severity of a number of rheumatologic disorders. As another example, within the bone marrow, eosinophils provide plasma cells with critical cytokines (APRIL and IL-6) to sustain their long-term survival and thus support "immunological memory."[103]

Consequences of Failed Development or Activation of the Adaptive Immune System

Defects in the development or function of adaptive immune cells have serious consequences for the host. This has been shown in both experimental animal models and strikingly in patients with genetic or acquired abnormalities of the B and/or T cell compartments. Understanding the molecular underpinnings of these disorders has provided important insights into the fundamental biology of the immune system and disease pathogenesis, and has also given rise to potential targets for pharmaceutical agents that have proven extremely effective in a number of rheumatic (and other) disease states.

B Cell Deficiency and Hyperactivity

X-linked (Bruton's) agammaglobulinemia was described in 1952 as an immunodeficiency affecting young boys.[104] This disorder, the first immunodeficiency identified in human patients, is characterized by the lack of circulating antibody resulting in frequent, severe bacterial infections that may be life threatening. Subsequent studies revealed that the lack of antibody is due to the absence of mature B lymphocytes in these patients. Since the description of this disease, decades of investigation have provided insights into the molecular events critical for B cell development and subsequent B cell activation. Among these discoveries was the identification of key enzymes that coordinate B cell function following engagement of the BCR by antigen. One of these enzymes is a protein tyrosine kinase essential for a B cell activation signal to occur. This kinase, now known as Bruton's tyrosine kinase (BTK), functions to couple engagement of the stimulated BCR to the downstream biochemical events critical for B cell maturation and division. The absence of BTK in patients with Bruton's agammaglobulinemia abrogates the ability of the BCR to "signal," hence arresting B cell development at an early stage in the bone marrow.[105,106]

While it was long known that the absence of circulating antibody in patients with Bruton's agammaglobulinemia could be remedied by regular infusions of intravenous gamma globulin, identification of the molecular basis for this disease provides new opportunities not only for treatment of this particular disease, but also more widely for therapeutic interventions. In the case of Bruton's agammaglobulinemia, understanding the molecular underpinnings of this disorder sets the stage for eventual cure by gene replacement therapy. Although this is not currently an approved mode of therapy, it is likely that advances in the field will result in ex vivo correction of the gene in patient-derived stem cells with subsequent infusion into patients for reconstitution of corrected, autologous hematopoietic progenitor cells.[107] Beyond this, however, the discovery of BTK and its essential role in B cell proliferation has already provided a new avenue for treatment of patients with B cell leukemias and lymphomas.[108–110] Drugs that interfere with BTK function, in clinical use since 2013, are now firmly established as an effective immunotherapy and have dramatically altered the course of disease in a subset of patients. Numerous studies are in progress evaluating the use of BTK inhibition in rheumatic diseases, in particular rheumatoid arthritis, with results expected to be forthcoming.

For many years, B cell biologists sought discovery of cell surface markers that would uniquely identify B cells for their studies. The cell surface antigen, CD20, emerged as one such marker and the development of reagents directed against this protein added greatly to the fundamental study of B cell function. Given the importance of B cells and antibodies in disease pathogenesis, investigators quickly realized that anti-CD20 antibodies had the potential not only to identify B cells for study, but to target B cells for immune destruction and therapeutic advantage. It has now been more than 20 years that anti-CD20 antibodies have been available for the elimination of B cells in the setting of B cell malignancies.[111] Since that time, indications for the use of anti-CD20 antibodies have expanded to include immune-mediated diseases that are triggered or perpetuated by over-exuberant B cell function, including rheumatoid arthritis, microscopic polyangiitis, and granulomatosis with polyangiitis.[112] Interestingly, one adverse effect that may occur with anti-CD20 therapy is hypogammaglobulinemia, the condition that in many ways heralded our understanding of the role of B cells as a critically important immune lineage.

T Cell Deficiency and Hyperactivity

That the thymus and thymus-derived T cells play an essential, nonredundant role in host defense was not appreciated until the 1960s. Studies in mice by Jacques Miller in 1961 showed that neonatal thymectomy resulted in loss of T cells and coincident immune deficiency.[113] These findings were extended to human patients in the mid-1960s with the identification of DiGeorge syndrome, a disorder that includes among its manifestations the congenital lack of the thymus with consequent absence of circulating T cells. DiGeorge patients suffer from serious infections, particularly due to intra-cellular pathogens.[114] These findings were extended in "nude" mice, an important animal model of thymic deficiency. Experiments in murine model systems and further evaluation of patients with T cell defects established that the thymus is not a vestigial organ, but instead plays a critical role in host defense as the generative organ for T cells.

As an appreciation developed for the central role played by T cells in host defense, patients with T cell defects were described. Some of these individuals had abnormalities restricted to the T cell compartment, while others manifested dysfunction in multiple immune lineages.[115] This underscored both some of the common features of immune cell development as well as the functional interdependence of cells of the immune system. For example, loss of T cells precludes T cells from providing "help" to B cells and is manifested by diminished antibody production and near absence of class-switched antibodies. As our understanding of T cell biology became more sophisticated, an understanding of different T cell effector subsets grew. This work both led and was enhanced by the discovery of patients with selective defects in T cell compartments. A key example of such discoveries includes the identification of patients harboring mutations in *FOXP3*, a gene required for the development of regulatory T cells, a T cells subset that functions to inhibit responses of other effector T cells.[116] Loss of regulatory T cells was found to be causal for the wide range of devastating autoimmunity afflicting patients with immunodysregulation polyendocrinopathy enteropathy x-linked (IPEX) syndrome.[117]

Discoveries related to the biology of T cells and the unique properties of T cell activation have led to numerous approaches to either augment or diminish T cell function in vivo to ameliorate disease. For example, understanding the requirement of co-stimulation for activation of T cells led to reagents that block the interaction between CD28 on T cells and its ligand on APCs. This blockade diminishes T cell reactivity and has become an established treatment for rheumatoid arthritis.[118] Recent years have also seen remarkable success in treating cancer with so-called *checkpoint blockade reagents.* Instead of preventing stimulation of activating co-receptors, these drugs interfere with the "break" on T cell activation by blocking engagement of inhibitory T cell receptors by their ligands on APCs.[119] As would be expected, one of the adverse events seen with immunotherapeutic checkpoint blockade is the emergence of autoimmunity, underscoring the precarious balance the immune system must maintain to eliminate dangers from the host, while ensuring the health of self-tissues.[120]

Conclusion

Adaptive immunity is an essential component of the finely orchestrated immune system network that provides for defense of the host. T and B cells play nonredundant roles that function collaboratively with the phylogenetically more ancient cells of the innate immune system and collectively protect individuals from a range of challenges, from external pathogens to mutation and damage of one's own cells. While the innate immune system is pre-wired to detect molecular patterns that signal danger, the adaptive immune system evolved to be highly specific and able to detect minute changes signaling "foreignness." Beyond its specificity and diversity, the adaptive immune system possesses memory so that subsequent encounters with pathogens are dealt with more quickly and efficiently. The flip side of the potential of the adaptive immune system to recognize foreign antigens is the risk for autoimmunity, requiring multiple mechanisms to achieve and maintain tolerance to self.

Understanding the fundamental biology of adaptive immune cells has led to a greater appreciation for how these processes may go awry, leading to immune-mediated tissue destruction, a hallmark of many rheumatic disorders. New knowledge that we have gained about adaptive immune cell function has also given important insights into novel approaches to pharmacologically modulate immune function. This has led to remarkable therapeutic advances for important diseases and has put us on the threshold of continued progress in designing new therapies and personalizing those that are now available to the best advantage of our patients. However, understanding the "on-target" and the less well explained adverse effects of many of these novel agents will require further investigation into the fundamental biology of cells of the adaptive immune system.

The references for this chapter can also be found on ExpertConsult.com.

References

1. Flajnik MF, Kasahara M: Origin and evolution of the adaptive immune system: genetic events and selective pressures, *Nat Rev Genet* 11(1):47–59, 2010.
2. Parra D, Takizawa F, Sunyer JO: Evolution of B cell immunity, *Annu Rev Anim Biosci* 1:65–97, 2013.
3. Cooper MD, Herrin BR: How did our complex immune system evolve? *Nat Rev Immunol* 10(1):2–3, 2010.
4. Muthamilarasan M, Prasad M: Plant innate immunity: an updated insight into defense mechanism, *J Biosci* 38(2):433–449, 2013.
5. Buchmann K: Evolution of innate immunity: clues from invertebrates via fish to mammals, *Front Immunol* 5:459, 2014.
6. Carmona LM, Schatz DG: New insights into the evolutionary origins of the recombination-activating gene proteins and V(D)J recombination, *FEBS J* 284(11):1590–1605, 2017.
7. Kaufman J: Unfinished business: evolution of the MHC and the adaptive immune system of jawed vertebrates, *Annu Rev Immunol* 36:383–409, 2018.
8. Boehm T: Design principles of adaptive immune systems, *Nat Rev Immunol* 11(5):307–317, 2011.
9. Saha NR, Smith J, Amemiya CT: Evolution of adaptive immune recognition in jawless vertebrates, *Semin Immunol* 22(1):25–33, 2010.
10. Alexander C, Rietschel ET: Bacterial lipopolysaccharides and innate immunity, *J Endotoxin Res* 7(3):167–202, 2001.
11. Hoshino K, Takeuchi O, Kawai T, et al.: Cutting edge: toll-like receptor 4 (TLR4)-deficient mice are hyporesponsive to lipopolysaccharide: evidence for TLR4 as the Lps gene product, *J Immunol* 162(7):3749–3752, 1999.
12. Shi J, Zhao Y, Wang Y, et al.: Inflammatory caspases are innate immune receptors for intracellular LPS, *Nature* 514(7521):187–192, 2014.
13. Jung D, Giallourakis C, Mostoslavsky R, et al.: Mechanism and control of V(D)J recombination at the immunoglobulin heavy chain locus, *Annu Rev Immunol* 24:541–570, 2006.
14. Schatz DG, Spanopoulou E: Biochemistry of V(D)J recombination, *Curr Top Microbiol Immunol* 290:49–85, 2005.
15. Xing Y, Hogquist KA: T-cell tolerance: central and peripheral, *Cold Spring Harb Perspect Biol* 4(6), 2012.
16. Nemazee D: Mechanisms of central tolerance for B cells, *Nat Rev Immunol* 17(5):281–294, 2017.
17. Gascoigne NR, Rybakin V, Acuto O, et al.: TCR signal strength and T cell development, *Annu Rev Cell Dev Biol* 32:327–348, 2016.
18. Jordan MS, Boesteanu A, Reed AJ, et al.: Thymic selection of CD4+CD25+ regulatory T cells induced by an agonist self-peptide, *Nat Immunol* 2(4):301–306, 2001.
19. Josefowicz SZ, Lu LF, Rudensky AY: Regulatory T cells: mechanisms of differentiation and function, *Annu Rev Immunol* 30:531–564, 2012.
20. Walker LS, Abbas AK: The enemy within: keeping self-reactive T cells at bay in the periphery, *Nat Rev Immunol* 2(1):11–19, 2002.
21. Schwartz RH: T cell anergy, *Annu Rev Immunol* 21:305–334, 2003.
22. Gajewski TF, Meng Y, Harlin H: Immune suppression in the tumor microenvironment, *J Immunother* 29(3):233–240, 2006.
23. Riaz N, Havel JJ, Makarov V, et al.: Tumor and microenvironment evolution during immunotherapy with nivolumab, *Cell* 171(4), 2017. 934-949.e916.
24. Jenkins MK, Moon JJ: The role of naive T cell precursor frequency and recruitment in dictating immune response magnitude, *J Immunol* 188(9):4135–4140, 2012.
25. Heinzel S, Marchingo JM, Horton MB, et al.: The regulation of lymphocyte activation and proliferation, *Curr Opin Immunol* 51:32–38, 2018.
26. Green DR, Droin N, Pinkoski M: Activation-induced cell death in T cells, *Immunol Rev* 193:70–81, 2003.
27. Zheng L, Li J, Lenardo M: Restimulation-induced cell death: new medical and research perspectives, *Immunol Rev* 277(1):44–60, 2017.
28. Chang JT, Wherry EJ, Goldrath AW: Molecular regulation of effector and memory T cell differentiation, *Nat Immunol* 15(12):1104–1115, 2014.
29. Inoue T, Moran I, Shinnakasu R, et al.: Generation of memory B cells and their reactivation, *Immunol Rev* 283(1):138–149, 2018.
30. Weisel F, Shlomchik M: Memory B cells of mice and humans, *Annu Rev Immunol* 35:255–284, 2017.
31. Becattini S, Latorre D, Mele F, et al.: T cell immunity. Functional heterogeneity of human memory $CD4^+$T cell clones primed by pathogens or vaccines, *Science* 347(6220):400–406, 2015.
32. Hale JS, Youngblood B, Latner DR, et al.: Distinct memory CD4+ T cells with commitment to T follicular helper- and T helper 1-cell lineages are generated after acute viral infection, *Immunity* 38(4):805–817, 2013.
33. Youngblood B, Hale JS, Kissick HT, et al.: Effector CD8 T cells dedifferentiate into long-lived memory cells, *Nature* 552(7685):404–409, 2017.
34. Barnett BE, Ciocca ML, Goenka R, et al.: Asymmetric B cell division in the germinal center reaction, *Science* 335(6066):342–344, 2012.
35. O'Neill LA, Kishton RJ, Rathmell J: A guide to immunometabolism for immunologists, *Nat Rev Immunol* 16(9):553–565, 2016.
36. Patel CH, Powell JD: Targeting T cell metabolism to regulate T cell activation, differentiation and function in disease, *Curr Opin Immunol* 46:82–88, 2017.
37. Klein Geltink RI, O'Sullivan D, Corrado M, et al.: Mitochondrial priming by CD28, *Cell* 171(2);385-397.e311 2017.
38. Böttcher J, Knolle PA: Global transcriptional characterization of CD8+ T cell memory, *Semin Immunol* 27(1):4–9, 2015.
39. Wherry EJ: T cell exhaustion, *Nat Immunol* 12(6):492–499, 2011.
40. Cooper MD, Peterson RD, Good RA: Delineation of the thymic and bursal lymphoid systems in the chicken, *Nature* 205:143–146, 1965.
41. Cooper MD, Raymond DA, Peterson RD, et al.: The functions of the thymus system and the bursa system in the chicken, *J Exp Med* 123(1):75–102, 1966.
42. LeBien TW, Tedder TF: B lymphocytes: how they develop and function, *Blood* 112(5):1570–1580, 2008.
43. Reth M: Antigen receptors on B lymphocytes, *Annu Rev Immunol* 10:97–121, 1992.
44. Stavnezer J, Guikema JE, Schrader CE: Mechanism and regulation of class switch recombination, *Annu Rev Immunol* 26:261–292, 2008.
45. Yoshida T, Mei H, Dörner T, et al.: Memory B and memory plasma cells, *Immunol Rev* 237(1):117–139, 2010.
46. Methot SP, Di Noia JM: Molecular mechanisms of somatic hypermutation and class switch recombination, *Adv Immunol* 133:37–87, 2017.
47. Amigorena S: Antigen presentation: from cell biology to physiology, *Immunol Rev* 272(1):5–7, 2016.
48. La Gruta NL, Gras S, Daley SR, et al.: Understanding the drivers of MHC restriction of T cell receptors, *Nat Rev Immunol* 18(7):467–478, 2018.
49. Luckheeram RV, Zhou R, Verma AD, et al.: $CD4^+$T cells: differentiation and functions, *Clin Dev Immunol* 2012:925135, 2012.
50. Mittrücker HW, Visekruna A, Huber M: Heterogeneity in the differentiation and function of $CD8^+$T cells, *Arch Immunol Ther Exp (Warsz)* 62(6):449–458, 2014.

51. Hardy RR, Hayakawa K: B cell development pathways, *Annu Rev Immunol* 19:595–621, 2001.
52. Reth M, Nielsen P: Signaling circuits in early B-cell development, *Adv Immunol* 122:129–175, 2014.
53. Rodewald HR: Thymus organogenesis, *Annu Rev Immunol* 26:355–388, 2008.
54. Love PE, Bhandoola A: Signal integration and crosstalk during thymocyte migration and emigration, *Nat Rev Immunol* 11(7):469–477, 2011.
55. Kreslavsky T, Gleimer M, Miyazaki M, et al.: β-Selection-induced proliferation is required for αβ T cell differentiation, *Immunity* 37(5):840–853, 2012.
56. Klein L, Kyewski B, Allen PM, et al.: Positive and negative selection of the T cell repertoire: what thymocytes see (and don't see), *Nat Rev Immunol* 14(6):377–391, 2014.
57. Anderson MS, Su MA: AIRE expands: new roles in immune tolerance and beyond, *Nat Rev Immunol* 16(4):247–258, 2016.
58. Nielsen MM, Witherden DA, Havran WL: γδ T cells in homeostasis and host defence of epithelial barrier tissues, *Nat Rev Immunol* 17(12):733–745, 2017.
59. Crosby CM, Kronenberg M: Tissue-specific functions of invariant natural killer T cells, *Nat Rev Immunol* 18(9):559–574, 2018.
60. Pearson HA, Spencer RP, Cornelius EA: Functional asplenia in sickle-cell anemia, *N Engl J Med* 281(17):923–926, 1969.
61. Cyster JG: B cell follicles and antigen encounters of the third kind, *Nat Immunol* 11(11):989–996, 2010.
62. Heesters BA, Myers RC, Carroll MC: Follicular dendritic cells: dynamic antigen libraries, *Nat Rev Immunol* 14(7):495–504, 2014.
63. Victora GD, Nussenzweig MC: Germinal centers, *Annu Rev Immunol* 30:429–457, 2012.
64. Schulz O, Hammerschmidt SI, Moschovakis GL, et al.: Chemokines and chemokine receptors in lymphoid tissue dynamics, *Annu Rev Immunol* 34:203–242, 2016.
65. Zhiming W, Luman W, Tingting Q, et al.: Chemokines and receptors in intestinal B lymphocytes, *J Leukoc Biol* 103(5):807–819, 2018.
66. Griffith JW, Sokol CL, Luster AD: Chemokines and chemokine receptors: positioning cells for host defense and immunity, *Annu Rev Immunol* 32:659–702, 2014.
67. Förster R, Davalos-Misslitz AC, Rot A: CCR7 and its ligands: balancing immunity and tolerance, *Nat Rev Immunol* 8(5):362–371, 2008.
68. Vinuesa CG, Linterman MA, Yu D, et al.: Follicular helper T cells, *Annu Rev Immunol* 34:335–368, 2016.
69. Grada AA, Phillips TJ: Lymphedema: Pathophysiology and clinical manifestations, *J Am Acad Dermatol* 77(6):1009–1020, 2017.
70. Fu YX, Chaplin DD: Development and maturation of secondary lymphoid tissues, *Annu Rev Immunol* 17:399–433, 1999.
71. Gasteiger G, Ataide M, Kastenmüller W: Lymph node—an organ for T-cell activation and pathogen defense, *Immunol Rev* 271(1):200–220, 2016.
72. Lefrançois L, Puddington L: Intestinal and pulmonary mucosal T cells: local heroes fight to maintain the status quo, *Annu Rev Immunol* 24:681–704, 2006.
73. Kubo M: Innate and adaptive type 2 immunity in lung allergic inflammation, *Immunol Rev* 278(1):162–172, 2017.
74. Jones GW, Jones SA: Ectopic lymphoid follicles: inducible centres for generating antigen-specific immune responses within tissues, *Immunology* 147(2):141–151, 2016.
75. Corsiero E, Nerviani A, Bombardieri M, et al.: Ectopic lymphoid structures: powerhouse of autoimmunity, *Front Immunol* 7:430, 2016.
76. Bird AK, Meednu N, Anolik JH: New insights into B cell biology in systemic lupus erythematosus and Sjögren's syndrome, *Curr Opin Rheumatol* 27(5):461–467, 2015.
77. Espitia-Thibault A, Masseau A, Néel A, et al.: Sjögren's syndrome-associated myositis with germinal centre-like structures, *Autoimmun Rev* 16(2):154–158, 2017.
78. Cyster JG, Schwab SR: Sphingosine-1-phosphate and lymphocyte egress from lymphoid organs, *Annu Rev Immunol* 30:69–94, 2012.
79. Pereira JP, Xu Y, Cyster JG: A role for S1P and S1P1 in immature-B cell egress from mouse bone marrow, *PLoS One* 5(2):e9277, 2010.
80. Proia RL, Hla T: Emerging biology of sphingosine-1-phosphate: its role in pathogenesis and therapy, *J Clin Invest* 125(4):1379–1387, 2015.
81. Brinkmann V, Billich A, Baumruker T, et al.: Fingolimod (FTY720): discovery and development of an oral drug to treat multiple sclerosis, *Nat Rev Drug Discov* 9(11):883–897, 2010.
82. Han Y, Li X, Zhou Q, et al.: FTY720 abrogates collagen-induced arthritis by hindering dendritic cell migration to local lymph nodes, *J Immunol* 195(9):4126–4135, 2015.
83. Huang J, Zhang T, Wang H, et al.: Treatment of experimental autoimmune myasthenia gravis rats with FTY720 and its effect on Th1/Th2 cells, *Mol Med Rep* 17(5):7409–7414, 2018.
84. Tsai HC, Han MH: Sphingosine-1-Phosphate (S1P) and S1P signaling pathway: therapeutic targets in autoimmunity and inflammation, *Drugs* 76(11):1067–1079, 2016.
85. Cyster JG: Chemokines, sphingosine-1-phosphate, and cell migration in secondary lymphoid organs, *Annu Rev Immunol* 23:127–159, 2005.
86. Vestweber D: How leukocytes cross the vascular endothelium, *Nat Rev Immunol* 15(11):692–704, 2015.
87. Luo BH, Carman CV, Springer TA: Structural basis of integrin regulation and signaling, *Annu Rev Immunol* 25:619–647, 2007.
88. Ginsberg MH, Partridge A, Shattil SJ: Integrin regulation, *Curr Opin Cell Biol* 17(5):509–516, 2005.
89. Rose DM, Alon R, Ginsberg MH: Integrin modulation and signaling in leukocyte adhesion and migration, *Immunol Rev* 218:126–134, 2007.
90. Smith-Garvin JE, Koretzky GA, Jordan MS: T cell activation, *Annu Rev Immunol* 27:591–619, 2009.
91. Esensten JH, Helou YA, Chopra G, et al.: CD28 Costimulation: From mechanism to therapy, *Immunity* 44(5):973–988, 2016.
92. Chen L, Flies DB: Molecular mechanisms of T cell co-stimulation and co-inhibition, *Nat Rev Immunol* 13(4):227–242, 2013.
93. Schildberg FA, Klein SR, Freeman GJ, et al.: Coinhibitory pathways in the B7-CD28 ligand-receptor family, *Immunity* 44(5):955–972, 2016.
94. Topalian SL, Drake CG, Pardoll DM: Immune checkpoint blockade: a common denominator approach to cancer therapy, *Cancer Cell* 27(4):450–461, 2015.
95. Baumeister SH, Freeman GJ, Dranoff G, et al.: Coinhibitory pathways in immunotherapy for cancer, *Annu Rev Immunol* 34:539–573, 2016.
96. Lin JX, Leonard WJ: Fine-tuning cytokine signals, *Annu Rev Immunol*, 2019.
97. Saraiva M, O'Garra A: The regulation of IL-10 production by immune cells, *Nat Rev Immunol* 10(3):170–181, 2010.
98. Chen W, Ten Dijke P: Immunoregulation by members of the TGFβ superfamily, *Nat Rev Immunol* 16(12):723–740, 2016.
99. Geissmann F, Gordon S, Hume DA, et al.: Unravelling mononuclear phagocyte heterogeneity, *Nat Rev Immunol* 10(6):453–460, 2010.
100. Croft M, Siegel RM: Beyond TNF: TNF superfamily cytokines as targets for the treatment of rheumatic diseases, *Nat Rev Rheumatol* 13(4):217–233, 2017.
101. Quezada SA, Jarvinen LZ, Lind EF, et al.: CD40/CD154 interactions at the interface of tolerance and immunity, *Annu Rev Immunol* 22:307–328, 2004.
102. Domeier PP, Chodisetti SB, Schell SL, et al.: B-cell-intrinsic type 1 interferon signaling is crucial for loss of tolerance and the development of autoreactive B cells, *Cell Rep* 24(2):406–418, 2018.
103. Chu VT, Fröhlich A, Steinhauser G, et al.: Eosinophils are required for the maintenance of plasma cells in the bone marrow, *Nat Immunol* 12(2):151–159, 2011.

104. Bruton OC: Agammaglobulinemia, *Pediatrics.* 9(6):722–728, 1952.
105. Vetrie D, Vorechovský I, Sideras P, et al.: The gene involved in X-linked agammaglobulinaemia is a member of the src family of protein-tyrosine kinases, *Nature* 361(6409):226–233, 1993.
106. Tsukada S, Saffran DC, Rawlings DJ, et al.: Deficient expression of a B cell cytoplasmic tyrosine kinase in human X-linked agammaglobulinemia, *Cell* 72(2):279–290, 1993.
107. Shillitoe B, Gennery A: X-linked agammaglobulinaemia: Outcomes in the modern era, *Clin Immunol* 183:54–62, 2017.
108. Ponader S, Burger JA: Bruton's tyrosine kinase: from X-linked agammaglobulinemia toward targeted therapy for B-cell malignancies, *J Clin Oncol* 32(17):1830–1839, 2014.
109. Byrd JC, Furman RR, Coutre SE, et al.: Targeting BTK with ibrutinib in relapsed chronic lymphocytic leukemia, *N Engl J Med* 369(1):32–42, 2013.
110. Wang ML, Rule S, Martin P, et al.: Targeting BTK with ibrutinib in relapsed or refractory mantle-cell lymphoma, *N Engl J Med* 369(6):507–516, 2013.
111. Pierpont TM, Limper CB, Richards KL: Past, present, and future of rituximab-the world's first oncology monoclonal antibody therapy, *Front Oncol* 8:163, 2018.
112. Schioppo T, Ingegnoli F: Current perspective on rituximab in rheumatic diseases, *Drug Des Devel Ther* 11:2891–2904, 2017.
113. Miller JF: Immunological function of the thymus, *Lancet* 2(7205):748–749, 1961.
114. Sullivan KE: Chromosome 22q11.2 deletion syndrome and DiGeorge syndrome, *Immunol Rev* 287(1):186–201, 2019.
115. Buckley RH: Molecular defects in human severe combined immunodeficiency and approaches to immune reconstitution, *Annu Rev Immunol* 22:625–655, 2004.
116. Hori S, Nomura T, Sakaguchi S: Control of regulatory T cell development by the transcription factor Foxp3, *Science* 299(5609):1057–1061, 2003.
117. Bennett CL, Christie J, Ramsdell F, et al.: The immune dysregulation, polyendocrinopathy, enteropathy, X-linked syndrome (IPEX) is caused by mutations of FOXP3, *Nat Genet* 27(1):20–21, 2001.
118. Kremer JM, Westhovens R, Leon M, et al.: Treatment of rheumatoid arthritis by selective inhibition of T-cell activation with fusion protein CTLA4Ig, *N Engl J Med* 349(20):1907–1915, 2003.
119. Sharma P, Allison JP: The future of immune checkpoint therapy, *Science* 348(6230):56–61, 2015.
120. van der Vlist M, Kuball J, Radstake TR, et al.: Immune checkpoints and rheumatic diseases: what can cancer immunotherapy teach us? *Nat Rev Rheumatol* 12(10):593–604, 2016.

22

Autoimmunity and Tolerance

DWIGHT H. KONO AND ARGYRIOS N. THEOFILOPOULOS

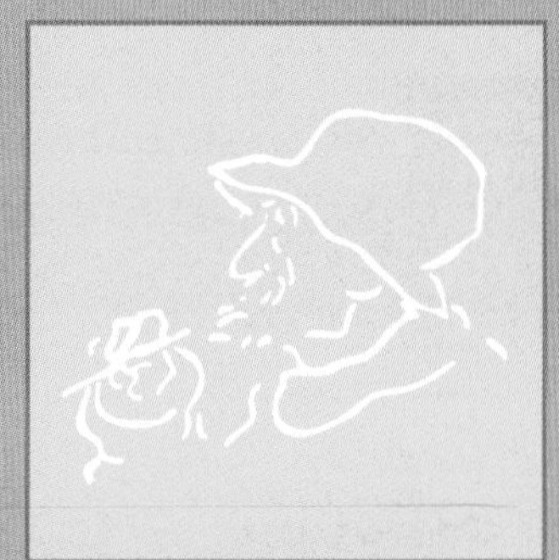

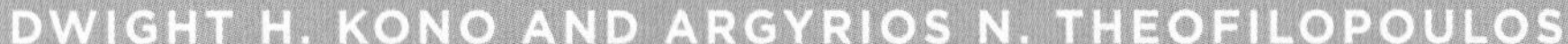

KEY POINTS

Autoimmunity ranges from physiologic levels of autoreactivity to overt autoimmune disease, in part reflecting the complexity of the immune system, the presence of multiple layers of tolerance mechanisms, and genetic heterogeneity.

Autoimmune diseases can be classified by the extent of organ involvement (organ-specific to systemic), innate immune system requirements, and effector mechanisms. However, each type of autoimmune disease has unique pathophysiologic characteristics.

Advances in defining the mechanisms underlying autoimmune diseases have been greatly facilitated by delineation of the innate and adaptive immune systems.

Susceptibility to autoimmune disease is multifactorial and involves genetic, environmental, sex, and other factors, with genetic predisposition usually playing a central role. The contributions of these factors are typically heterogeneous, partial, and additive, and can increase or decrease susceptibility.

Animal models of autoimmunity contribute to fundamental insights into genetic, mechanistic, and pathologic processes. Spontaneous animal models do not exist for most autoimmune diseases.

Progress delineating pathways has identified key genes and molecules in autoimmune diseases that are already targeted in clinical practice or hold therapeutic promise.

Introduction

Autoimmune diseases represent a significant health burden for 3% to 9% of the general population, and rheumatology, perhaps more than any medical subspecialty, encompasses a broad array of such diseases that affect a wide range of organ systems (Table 22.1).[1–4] Consequently, rheumatologists have a great interest in defining the causes and pathophysiology of autoimmunity and in applying this information in the clinic.

The immune system must effectively defend against a diverse universe of pathogens while simultaneously maintaining tolerance to self-antigens. Recent advances have begun to clarify how this equilibrium is established and sustained and, importantly, have identified many critical factors and processes involved in the pathogenesis of autoimmune diseases. This chapter provides a general overview of autoimmunity, covering the definition of the term, general tolerance mechanisms for T and B lymphocytes, theories of how tolerance can be breached, and ways in which genetic and environmental factors have been implicated in breaking tolerance and producing disease. Emphasis is placed on manifestations and mechanisms related to rheumatologic diseases.

Definition and Classification of Pathogenic Autoimmunity

Autoimmunity—that is, the immune response against self—evokes the specter of "horror autotoxicus," a term coined by Paul Ehrlich at the turn of the 20th century to depict the perceived disastrous consequences of this condition.[5] In fact, autoreactivity is more nuanced, ranging from a low "physiologic" level of self-reactivity essential for lymphocyte selection and maintenance of normal immune system homeostasis, to an intermediate level of autoimmunity that manifests as circulating autoantibodies and tissue infiltrates that are not associated with clinical consequences, to pathogenic autoimmunity associated with immune-mediated dysfunction or injury.[6] From the clinical perspective, it is the transformation to pathogenic autoimmunity that demarcates significant from insignificant self-reactivity.

The diagnosis of an autoimmune disease is generally based on the presence of adaptive immune system–mediated disease caused by self-reactive antibodies, T cells, or both. For many common autoimmune diseases, more definitive evidence for an autoimmune cause has come from studies showing transfer of disease by autoantibodies or self-reactive T cells and from animal models exhibiting congruent characteristics. However, no universally accepted criteria exist, and some less well-characterized diseases that are currently considered to be autoimmune may turn out to have other causes.

An example of disorders that exhibit some characteristics of autoimmunity but are distinct in their pathogenesis are the autoinflammatory diseases.[7–15] These diseases are predominantly rare monogenic disorders typified by intermittent bouts of fever, rash, serositis, and arthritis caused by a widening spectrum of defects in the control of basic inflammatory pathways. Included in this category are familial Mediterranean fever, the cryopyrinopathies, hyperimmunoglobulinemia D with recurrent fever, familial cold urticaria, Blau syndrome, and others. These syndromes could be considered part of a broader definition of autoreactivity in which the autoinflammatory diseases mediated entirely through the innate arm of the immune system comprise one end of the spectrum, while at the other end are the autoimmune diseases that require both the innate and adaptive responses. Indeed, the possibility of a less stringent demarcation has been suggested by disorders such as Behçet's disease, systemic juvenile rheumatoid arthritis,

TABLE 22.1 Rheumatologic Autoimmune Diseases

Rheumatoid arthritis
Juvenile rheumatoid arthritis
Systemic lupus erythematosus
Neonatal lupus
Systemic sclerosis CREST syndrome
Overlap syndromes
Antiphospholipid syndrome
Vasculitis Giant cell arteritis/polymyalgia rheumatica Takayasu's arteritis Granulomatosis with polyangiitis Churg-Strauss syndrome Polyarteritis nodosa Microscopic polyangiitis
Polymyositis/dermatomyositis
Relapsing polychondritis
Sjögren's syndrome
Behçet's disease
Kawasaki's disease
Sarcoidosis

CREST, Calcinosis, Raynaud's phenomenon, esophageal dysmotility, sclerodactyly, and telangiectasia.

and Crohn's disease, which appear to manifest various degrees of both autoinflammatory and autoimmune features. Similarly, the interferonopathies, a subset of the autoinflammatory diseases caused by mutations that alter the processing or sensing of cytoplasmic nucleic acids, are associated with high levels of type I interferons, interferon-associated pathology, and lupus-like manifestations.[16,17]

Autoimmune diseases can be classified as systemic or organ-specific depending on the extent of their clinicopathology (Table 22.2). The systemic category includes systemic lupus erythematosus (SLE), rheumatoid arthritis (RA), scleroderma, antiphospholipid syndrome (aPL), primary Sjögren's syndrome, dermatomyositis, and systemic vasculitides. In systemic disease, autoimmunity targets ubiquitously expressed self-antigens, and end-organ injury is typically mediated by autoantibodies and, less commonly, T cells. In contrast, in organ-specific diseases, the self-antigens are typically cell- or tissue-specific in location or accessibility, and end-organ damage or dysfunction can be mediated by antibodies and/or T cells. Some of the more notable examples in this group, which span virtually all organ systems, include Hashimoto's thyroiditis, Graves' disease, multiple sclerosis (MS), neuromyelitis optica, type 1 diabetes mellitus (T1DM), pemphigus vulgaris, autoimmune hemolytic anemia, idiopathic thrombocytopenic purpura, and myasthenia gravis. It should be emphasized, however, that although the distinction of systemic and organ-specific disorders provides a conceptual framework, the individual pathophysiologies are more diverse than is implied by this simple classification. Autoimmune diseases are also classified by hypersensitivity reaction type based on the mechanism of adaptive immune system–mediated injury,[18] a topic that will be discussed later in the chapter.

Animal Models of Autoimmunity

Much of what is known about the immune system and autoimmunity has been derived from studies in animals, particularly the mouse, which has an immune system and genome composition similar to that of humans. Many well-characterized autoimmune models exist in which investigators can manipulate genomes and immune systems, test interventions, and modify environments. Animal models of autoimmune disease can be divided into three main types based on their derivation: (1) spontaneous, (2) genetically modified, and (3) induced. Some of the more common or notable models are listed in Table 22.3.

Within the spontaneous group are models of SLE, RA, and T1DM. The lupus-prone strains commonly develop anti-DNA and immune-complex-mediated kidney damage, but they also possess unique phenotypic characteristics and differ in the genes underpinning susceptibility.[19] The SKG arthritis model is a spontaneous, inflammatory, and erosive arthritis caused by a ZAP70 mutation that, similar to RA, is associated with rheumatoid factor (RF) and antibodies to citrullinated proteins.[20] T1DM develops in nonobese (NOD) mice and biobreeding (BB) rats as a result of T cell-mediated destruction of β-islet cells.[21]

The genetically modified group, encompassing transgenic, site-directed genetic replacement (gene knockout or knockin), and *N*-ethyl *N*-nitrosourea (ENU)-mutagenized mice, is by far the largest, with more than 100 different models of lupus and many models of organ-specific diseases, particularly T1DM and MS.[19,21,22] The lupus models, primarily single gene knockout or transgenic mice, have provided a wealth of information related to immune tolerance and disease pathogenesis. Some examples are: (1) confirmation of human SLE gene associations and elucidation of mechanisms, such as C1q and Fc gamma receptor IIb (FcγRIIb) knockout mice; (2) discovery of novel mechanisms such as altered messenger RNA (mRNA) regulation in San Roque and miR-17-92 transgenic mice; and (3) identification of new pathways relevant to therapy, such as B cell-activating factor of tumor necrosis factor family (BAFF) transgenic.

An example of an arthritis model created by genetic modification is the K/BxN mouse, a B6xNOD hybrid expressing a transgenic T cell receptor, named KRN, that recognizes a bovine ribonuclease peptide on H-2K.[23] An acute severe inflammatory arthritis develops in these mice that is caused by antibodies to glucose-6-phosphate isomerase (GPI), an antigen that, although intra-cellularly and ubiquitously expressed, is mainly accessible to antibodies in joints.[24] Although there is no evidence that antibodies to GPI cause RA or other arthritides, the model has nevertheless been useful for investigating inflammatory mechanisms in arthritis.[25]

Other genetically modified models of spontaneous arthritis include the human T-lymphotropic virus (HTLV)-1 tax transgenic, the TNF transgenic, the IL-1 receptor antagonist (IL-1ra) transgenic, and a gain-of-function knockin mutant of CD130, the signaling component of receptors for several cytokines including IL-6, IL-11, IL-27, and leukemia inhibitory factor (LIF).[26] Several genetically modified models of T cell-mediated organ-specific disease have been developed that consist of T cell receptor (TCR) transgenic T cells that recognize tissue-specific antigens in organs such as the brain and pancreatic islets or employ a slightly modified version in which mice are double transgenic for both an antigen expressed in a tissue of interest and the corresponding TCR.[27–30] By allowing analysis of single autoreactive T cell clones, these models have yielded considerable insights into tolerance mechanisms and disease pathophysiology. Similarly, autoreactive B cell receptor transgenics or knockin models have been developed that have been crucial for defining B cell tolerance mechanisms.[31–37]

TABLE 22.2 Classification, Mechanisms, and Models of Autoimmune Diseases

Syndrome	AutoAg	Consequence	Hypersensitivity Type[a]	Animal Model (Example)
Systemic				
aPL syndrome	β2-GP1 (apoH)	Vascular thrombosis, recurrent miscarriages	II	(NZW x BXSB)F1
Microscopic angiitis	p-ANCA (MPO)	Glomerulonephritis, leukocytoclastic vasculitis, mononeuritis multiplex, lung inflammation	III	Anti-MPO
Granulomatosis with polyangiitis	c-ANCA (PR3)	Vasculitis of kidney, upper airway, and lungs	III	None
Cryoglobulinemia	Unknown	Cutaneous vasculitis, glomerulonephritis	III	MRL-*Fas^lpr*
SLE	Nuclear antigens plus others	Glomerulonephritis, skin lesions, arthritis, CNS lupus, and others	III	MRL-*Fas^lpr*, BWF1, BXSB, NZM2410
Systemic sclerosis	Unknown	Fibrosis of multiple organs	III	Tsk/+ mice, bleomycin-induced
RA[b]	RF IgG immune complexes; citrullinated proteins; other joint antigens	Arthritis and associated manifestations rheumatoid nodules, rheumatoid lung, Felty's syndrome	III	CIA, PGIA, AA, SKG, K/BxN, BxD2, citrullinated-protein-immunized DR4-IE transgenic
Organ-Specific				
Grave's disease	TSH receptor	Stimulation of receptor; hyperthyroidism	II	EAT
Myasthenia gravis	ACh receptor	Receptor blockade/modulation; neuromuscular paralysis	II	EAMG
Autoimmune hemolytic anemia	RBC surface Ag	C′ and FcgR-mediated cell destruction; anemia	II	NZB
Idiopathic thrombocytopenic purpura	Platelet integrin GpIIb:IIIa	Thrombocytopenia; purpura, bleeding	II	(NZW x BXSB)F1
Goodpasture's syndrome	Type IV collagen[a] and other basement membrane Ags	Pulmonary hemorrhage, glomerulonephritis	II	Anti-CIV, anti-laminin
Pemphigus vulgaris	Epidermal cadherin (Dsg3)	Bullous skin lesions	II	Anti-Dsg3
Neonatal lupus	Ro/La	Cutaneous LE, heart block	II	Anti-Ro52[316]
T1DM	Pancreatic β-cell antigens	Pancreatic islet inflammation, diabetes	IV	NOD, BB
Multiple sclerosis	CNS antigens; MBP, PLP, MOG in animal models	Progressive CNS inflammation and paralysis	IV	EAE, Theiler's virus infection

[a]Most likely hypersensitivity type.

[b]Both systemic and organ-specific.

AA, Adjuvant arthritis; *ACh,* acetylcholine; *ANCA,* anti-neutrophil cytoplasmic antibody; *anti-CIV,* anti-type IV collagen; *anti-Dsg3,* anti-desmoglein 3; *β2-GP1,* β2-glycoprotein 1; *CIA,* collagen-induced arthritis; *EAE,* experimental autoimmune encephalomyelitis; *EAMG,* experimental autoimmune myasthenia gravis; *EAT,* experimental autoimmune thyroiditis; *MBP,* myelin basic protein; *MOG,* myelin oligodendrocyte glycoprotein; *MPO,* myeloperoxidase; *PGIA,* proteoglycan-induced arthritis; *PLP,* proteolipid protein; *PR3,* proteinase 3; *RF,* rheumatoid factor; *TSH,* thyroid stimulating hormone. Other abbreviations are mouse strains.

The induced models encompass a wide variety of both systemic and organ-specific diseases. More commonly studied models of systemic disease include tetramethylpentadecane (TMPD, also called pristane)-induced autoimmunity, mercury-induced autoimmunity, and chronic graft-versus-host disease.[38–41] All models bear similarities to human SLE in producing anti-nuclear antibodies and immune complex deposits, but they differ in pathophysiology and strain susceptibility. For the induced models of organ-specific diseases, a common approach is to immunize rodents with a self-antigen or closely related peptide or foreign antigen, plus a strong adjuvant, usually complete Freund's. This approach makes it possible to induce autoimmunity in virtually all organ systems and to produce diseases mediated by cellular as well as humoral mechanisms. Some of the more commonly studied organ-specific models developed by this approach include collagen-induced arthritis (CIA), proteoglycan-induced arthritis (PGIA), and experimental autoimmune encephalomyelitis (EAE), but many others exist that are directed to the thyroid, eye, gonad, nerves, neuromuscular junction (acetylcholine receptor), muscle, heart, adrenal gland, bladder, stomach, liver, inner ear, kidney, and

TABLE 22.3 Partial List of Autoimmune Disease Models

Model	Autoimmune Disease	Species	Notable Characteristics
Spontaneous Variant			
MRL-Fas^{lpr}	SLE	Mouse	Fas mutation, defective apoptosis, lymphoproliferation, human counterpart ALPS
(NZBxNZW)F1	SLE	Mouse	Female predominance
NZB	SLE, AIHA	Mouse	Anti-RBC
BXSB	SLE	Mouse	Yaa mutation (duplication of X-chrom. containing TLR7 gene on Y-chrom.)
(NZWxBXSB)F1	SLE, APS, ITP	Mouse	Anti-cardiolipin, anti-platelet
BXD2	SLE, RA	Mouse	Lupus and inflammatory arthritis
SKG	RA	Mouse	ZAP-70 mutation
NOD	T1DM	Mouse	MHC (H-2^{g7}) similar to T1DM-predisposing HLA
BB	T1DM	Rat	Lymphopenia
Genetically Modified			
C1q ko	SLE	Mouse	Defective clearance of apoptotic cells
FcgRIIb ko	SLE	Mouse	Impair regulation of B cell and APCs
BAFF Tg	SLE	Mouse	Enhanced survival of B cells
TLR7 Tg	SLE	Mouse	Enhanced survival and activation of B cells and DCs
Sanroque mice (*roquin* gene)	SLE	Mouse	*Rc3h1* M199R mutation increases ICOS expression and T_{FH} cell expansion
miR-17-92 Tg	SLE	Mouse	miRNA induced autoimmunity
K/BxN, TCR Tg	RA	Mouse	Arthritis mediated by anti-GPI
MBP-specific TCR Tg mice	MS	Mouse	Spontaneous autoimmune encephalomyelitis
Double Tg: anti-GP TCR and insulin promoter-GP (GP = LCMV glycoprotein)	T1DM	Mouse	Ignorant Tg T cells are activated by infection with LCMV causing insulitis and diabetes
Induced			
TMPD (pristane)-induced autoimmunity	SLE	Mouse	IFN-α- and TLR7-dependent
Hg-induced autoimmunity	SLE	Mouse, rat	IFN-γ dependent
Chronic graft-versus-host disease	SLE	Mouse	Parent CD4 T cells into F1
Collagen-induced arthritis	RA	Mouse, rat	Autoimmunity to type II collagen
PG-induced arthritis	RA	Mouse	Autoimmunity to proteoglycan
Adjuvant arthritis	RA	Rat	Inflammatory arthritis induced by complete Freund's adjuvant or mineral oil
Citrullinated-protein-immunized DR4-IE transgenic	RA	Mouse	Autoimmunity to citrullinated-fibrinogen or enolase (human and bacterial)
EAE	MS	Mouse, rat	Autoimmunity to MBP, MOG, or PLP depending on MHC haplotype
EAT	Thyroiditis	Mouse, rat	Autoimmunity to thyroglobulin
EAMG	MG	Rat	Autoimmunity to acetylcholine receptor

AIHA, Autoimmune hemolytic anemia; *ALPS,* autoimmune proliferative syndrome; *APS,* antiphospholipid syndrome; *EAE,* experimental autoimmune encephalomyelitis; *GPI,* glucose-6-phosphate isomerase; *ko,* gene knockout; *ITP,* idiopathic thrombocytopenic purpura; *MBP,* myelin basic protein; *MOG,* myelin oligodendrocyte glycoprotein; *MS,* multiple sclerosis; *PLP,* proteolipid protein; *T1DM,* type 1 diabetes mellitus; *Tg,* transgenic; *TMPD,* 2,6,10,14-tetramethylpentadecane.

prostate tissues. In certain susceptible strains of rats, a progressive inflammatory erosive arthritis called *adjuvant arthritis* can also be induced by intradermal injection of complete Freund's adjuvant, or by mineral oil components of Freund's adjuvant such as TMPD. Other induced models of arthritis include streptococcal cell wall and antigen-induced arthritis.[26] Arthritis characterized by synovial hyperplasia and ankylosis was reported in human leukocyte antigen (HLA)-DR4-IE transgenic mice immunized with human citrullinated fibrinogen or enolase.[42,43]

Tolerance Mechanisms

Increasing insights into mechanisms of self-nonself discrimination have emerged during the past few decades, in parallel with growing knowledge of the immune system. In 1960, the Nobel Prize in Physiology and Medicine was awarded to Burnet and Medawar for advancing the critical concept that tolerance was imposed by clonal deletion of self-reactive lymphocytes during early development, that is, central tolerance.[44,45] The subsequent discovery that mature B cells undergo somatic hypermutation in the periphery led to the hypothesis by Bretscher and Cohn that the production of autoantibodies might be impeded by the need for both B and T cell compartments to breach tolerance.[46] In 1975, while studying allogeneic responses, Lafferty and Cunningham posited that activation of T cells involved the passing of a second signal that need not be antigen-related, thereby implicating co-stimulation from antigen-presenting cells (APCs) as a critical factor in lymphocyte activation.[47] In 1987, the nature of the co-stimulation, or two-signal, requirement was further defined when Jenkins and Schwartz showed that engagement of antigen receptor alone without a second signal resulted in functional inactivation of T cells.[48] An elegant mechanism for self-nonself discrimination was then advanced by Janeway in 1989 when he hypothesized that APCs remain quiescent unless activated by the engagement of pattern recognition receptors (PRRs) by microbial products.[49] This concept was further extended by Matzinger in 1994 to a "danger model" that includes activation of the immune system by both foreign and endogenous factors associated with tissue stress and damage.[50] These models laid the foundation for the current, more complex view of self-nonself

TABLE 22.4 Multiple Tiers of Tolerance

Type	Cell Type	Site	Mechanism
Central Compartment			
Central tolerance	T cells	Thymus	Primarily deletion, anergy, possibly editing
	B cells	Bone marrow	Editing, anergy, deletion
Peripheral Compartment			
Immature B cell tolerance	Transitional 1 (T1) B cells	Periphery	Deletion, anergy upon activation
Peripheral anergy	T and B cells	Secondary lymphoid organs and peripheral tissue	Inadequate signal induces cell inactivation
Ignorance	T cells; maybe B cells	Peripheral and secondary lymphoid organs	Insufficient self-antigen or co-stimulation
Inaccessible self-antigen	T and B cells	Peripheral organs	Sequestration, crypticity
Regulation	T and B cells	Secondary lymphoid organs and site of inflammation	Suppression by regulatory cells via intercellular signals and cytokines
Clonal deletion following activation	T and B cells	Site of inflammation and secondary lymphoid organs	Apoptosis caused by a decline in survival factors
Cytokine deviation	T cells	Site of inflammation and secondary lymphoid organs	Differentiation toward less pathogenic Th subsets
Postsomatic hypermutation	B cells	Germinal center	Insufficient CD4 T cell help, deletion (via *Fas*)
Tissue resistance	B and T cells	Peripheral tissues	Inhibitory intercellular signals and cytokines
Innate Mechanisms			
PRR engagement required for activation	Innate cells	Site of inflammation	Simple mechanism for self-nonself discrimination
Suppression of adaptive immune responses	Immature and mature DC	Site of inflammation and secondary lymphoid organs	Delivery of inhibitory signals and activation of Treg
Clearance of apoptotic cells	Complement, phagocytes	Peripheral tissues	Removal of potential pro-inflammatory material and self-antigens
Complement-mediated effects on adaptive responses	Lymphocytes, innate cells	Secondary lymphoid organs and peripheral tissue	Modulation of activation

PRR, Pattern recognition receptor; *Treg,* regulatory T cell.

discrimination, in which tolerance is imposed by both innate and adaptive immune systems through layers of mechanisms occurring at various stages, called "self-tolerance checkpoints," throughout lymphocyte development and activation (Table 22.4).

Clone-Specific Self-Nonself Recognition

In contrast to innate immune cells, which are activated primarily by hardwired microbial PRRs, lymphocytes have broad specificity and therefore self-nonself discrimination must be implemented at the clonal level. To achieve this objective, T and B cells utilize several mechanisms that can be grouped into three general strategies. First, the type of response is controlled by developmental stage. For example, immature lymphocytes respond to strong antigen receptor stimulation by cell death, whereas a similar signal in mature cells leads to activation. Through this mechanism, self-reactive clones are eliminated from the nascent lymphocyte repertoire before they can cause injury. Second, activation of mature lymphocytes requires, in addition to antigen receptor engagement, a second co-stimulatory signal, the absence of which results in anergy or cell death. For the most part, this requirement limits reactivity to self because co-stimulatory signals are largely provided by cells of the innate immune system. Third, lymphocytes are fine-tuned in various ways by a fairly extensive list of modulating factors necessary for controlling self-reactive clones.[51–53] In B cells, but not T cells, this includes an inverse correlation of antigen receptor (membrane immunoglobulin [Ig]M) expression and ability to flux calcium with the degree of self-reactivity.[54]

Examples of defects affecting a broad range of other surface receptors on lymphocytes include those with prosurvival (IL-7R, BAFF receptor [BAFFR], and IL-2R), proapoptotic (TNF receptors [TNFRs], Fas ligand [FasL], and TNF-related apoptosis-inducing ligand [TRAIL]), co-stimulatory (CD28, CD40, and Toll-like receptors [TLRs]), differentiating (IL-12R, IL-4R, interferon-γ receptor [IFNγR], IL-23R, retinoic acid receptor, transforming growth factor-β receptors [TGF-βRs], signaling lymphocyte activation molecule [SLAM]/SLAM-associated protein [SAP] family members, OX40, and inducible co-stimulator [ICOS]/ICOS ligand [ICOSL]), inhibitory (FcγRIIb, CD22, cytotoxic T lymphocyte-associated antigen-4 [CTLA4], and programmed cell death protein 1 [PD-1]), antigen receptor signal modulating (CD19 and CD45), and activating (SAP/SLAM family members) functions, and they influence the development of autoimmunity.[19] Collectively, these self-nonself recognition mechanisms provide the basic cellular means by which the innate and adaptive immune systems render T and B cell clonotypes tolerant to self-antigens and resistant to autoimmune disease.

The Innate System and Tolerance

Given its vital role in initiating and modulating adaptive immune responses, it is not surprising that the innate immune system strongly influences both tolerance and autoimmunity. Indeed, although its contributions have yet to be fully delineated, several ways in which self-tolerance is influenced by the innate arm have been defined.

First, activation of the innate immune system under normal circumstances typically requires engagement of microbial PRRs, which endows the immune system with a direct and simple way to distinguish foreign-antigens from self-antigens.[55] PRRs recognize common structures on pathogens and also a few self-molecules, such as certain damage-associated molecular patterns (DAMPs)—for example, heat shock proteins[56]—which are released during cellular stress, injury or death. PRRs can be classified by their location into the following types: secreted (e.g., collectins, pentraxins, and ficolins), plasma transmembrane (e.g., TLRs, certain C-type lectin receptors, and N-formyl methionine receptors), endosomal (e.g., TLRs), and cytosolic (e.g., retinoic acid inducible gene I [RIG-I]-like receptors, NOD-like receptors, and DNA receptors: IFI16, AIM2, and the cyclic guanosine monophosphate–adenosine monophosphate synthase [cGAS]–stimulator of interferon genes [STING] pathway).[57–59] The importance of this mechanism is illustrated by the finding that overexpression of TLR7 by spontaneous gene duplication or transgenic approaches promotes systemic autoimmunity.[60] This outcome occurs because certain PRRs, such as TLR7 and TLR9, which equally sense both foreign and self-nucleic acids, avoid significant exposure to endogenous nucleic acids by virtue of their location in subcellular compartments.[61] However, in the case of TLR7, overexpression allows for normally substimulatory amounts of self RNA to activate immune cells, thereby bypassing the usual requirement for RNA from microbial exposure.

Second, some cells of the innate immune system actively suppress adaptive immune system activation under certain conditions. For example, both immature and mature dendritic cells (DCs) promote tolerance by inducing CD4 T regulatory (Treg) cells and other mechanisms.[62,63]

Third, failure of the rapid non-inflammatory clearance of apoptotic cells, another critical function of the innate immune system,[64,65] can result in an increased supply of self-antigenic material including nucleic acids, secondary necrosis, and release of pro-inflammatory factors, leading to systemic autoimmunity.[66] Accordingly, deficiencies in several key apoptotic cell clearance molecules are associated with autoimmunity, including: (1) the Tyro3-Axl-Mer receptors on phagocytes that bind, through Gas6 or protein S, the exposed phosphatidylserine (PS) on apoptotic cells,[67] (2) the milk fat globule-epidermal growth factor 8 (MFG-E8) protein that bridges the αvβ3 integrin on phagocytes and PS on apoptotic cells,[68,69] (3) Tim4 expressed on the surface of resident macrophages that bind PS,[70] (4) the 12/15 lipoxygenase that controls which macrophage subpopulations phagocytize apoptotic cells,[71] and (5) natural IgM, C1q, or C1q receptor (SCARF1) that binds to, and enhances clearance of, apoptotic cells.[72–75]

Fourth, several complement components have been directly implicated in autoimmunity. For example, SLE is associated with deficiencies of proximal components of the classical pathway, including C1q, C4, and C2. Although the mechanism for this association is uncertain, defective clearance of apoptotic material/immune complexes and a shift in the activation threshold of lymphocytes have been suggested.[76] In the chronic graft-versus-host disease model of lupus, C1q also restrains autoimmunity by interacting with the mitochondrial cell-surface protein p32/gC1qR to alter cell metabolism and dampen CD8 T cell responses to self-antigens.[77] Another example is that deficiency of CD55 (or decay-accelerating factor), a cell surface protein that restricts complement activation, is associated with enhanced T cell responses and exacerbation of neuroinflammation and lupus in animal models.[78,79]

Fifth, the innate system could be a major source of self-antigenic material. For example, neutrophil extra-cellular traps (NETs), the nuclear material-containing web-like structure extruded by neutrophils to combat bacterial infection, contain a compelling collection of modified autoantigens, but thus far their role in patients remains to be firmly established.[80] Thus, at many levels, the innate immune system plays a critical role in maintaining tolerance and controlling autoimmunity.

T Cell Tolerance

T cells are critical players in not only achieving, but also fine tuning, tolerance to a high degree of specificity. Several mechanisms have been identified that can be divided into three main areas: central tolerance wherein T cells first acquire their antigen receptor, peripheral tolerance where T cells encounter self-antigens not present in the thymus, and postactivation regulation wherein activated and expanded T cell clones undergo apoptosis or are returned to their preactivation state. Central tolerance, as alluded to earlier, is imposed on T cells with self-reactive specificities during thymocyte development by mechanisms utilizing primarily deletion, to a lesser extent anergy, and possibly receptor editing of the TCR α-chain.[81,82] This process, although highly effective, is not completely efficient, and T cells with autoreactivity—primarily those with intermediate to low affinity to self or those that recognize self-antigens poorly expressed in the thymus—emigrate to the periphery in significant numbers. This leakiness is probably necessary to generate a broad repertoire, but then creates vulnerability to autoimmunity and necessitates peripheral tolerance mechanisms.

In the periphery, multiple mechanisms for avoiding autoreactivity have been identified. Among these, a common explanation is that most self-antigens are not accessible to trigger a response, a situation that can be caused by low abundance, specific characteristics of the self-antigen, or location. This mechanism is supported experimentally by the finding that T cells expressing a transgenic TCR to certain tissue-specific antigens are not deleted or activated, nor do they cause autoimmune disease. Yet, these so-called "ignorant" T cells are fully functional and respond to self-antigen when presented in a conventional context.[30,83] For a few self-antigens, such as those expressed in the anterior chamber of the eye, central nervous system (CNS), or other so-called *immune privileged sites*—as originally defined by their ability to accept allograft transplants—resistance to self-reactivity is also partly from anatomic sequestration caused by limited access of blood-borne cells and the absence of conventional lymphatic drainage,[84] although the latter is not universally accepted.[85,86] Nevertheless, other anatomic structures that enable separation of immune cells from the brain such as endothelial, epithelial, and glial cell barriers that establish compartments within the CNS, have been identified with higher resolution imaging.[85] Sequestration is important because T cells are typically first activated in secondary lymphoid organs and subsequently migrate to target organs where reactivation by local APCs and the production of pro-inflammatory factors lead to tissue damage.[87] Anatomic sequestration alone, however, is not sufficient for tissues to support immunologic privilege, and, as will be discussed later, such sites employ a host of additional local mechanisms.[88,89]

Another peripheral mechanism is the aforementioned two-signal paradigm in which T cell activation requires both TCR engagement and a co-stimulatory signal usually provided by CD28. Because the two ligands for CD28, CD80, and CD86 are primarily expressed at high levels on activated professional APCs, presentation of self-antigen by quiescent APCs would lead to tolerance. Indeed, immature DCs promote tolerance in this manner by constitutively presenting low doses of self-antigen on major histocompatibility complexes (MHCs), resulting in cell death or anergy of the corresponding T cells.[90]

Peripheral tolerance is also maintained by active suppression via immunoregulatory cells of the immune system, among which $CD4^+$ regulatory T cells (Tregs) are the best characterized.[91–96] They constitute a distinct αβ-T cell subset generated in the thymus (thymus [tTreg] or also called *natural Treg [nTreg]*) or are differentiated in the periphery from naïve or mature CD4 T cells exposed to TGF-beta (peripheral [pTreg] and induced [iTreg] subsets). Tregs are developmentally induced by the forkhead boxP3 (FOXP3) transcription factor. They typically express high levels of CTLA-4 and the IL-2 receptor component, IL-2Rα (CD25), and require IL-2 for survival. Tregs participate in every adaptive immune response, are critical for maintaining the proper level of immune response, and are activated at the same time as conventional T cells. Suppression is thought to be mediated in large part by initial downregulation of DC function through CTLA-4 engaging and reducing CD86/80 expression and then inhibition of T cell activation by competition for IL-2, production of immunosuppressive cytokines (such as TGF-β, IL-10, and IL-35), and expression of inhibitory surface molecules (CD39, CD73, lymphocyte activating 3 [LAG3], and T cell immunoreceptor with Ig and ITIM domains [TIGIT]).[95–97] These actions globally suppress immune and inflammatory cells that are in proximity to Tregs and regardless of lymphocyte specificity.[98] Treg cells also exhibit functional adaptability that includes differentiation into subsets (Th1, Th2, Th17, Tfr),[99] similar to conventional effector CD4 T cells; although Tregs are a highly stable lineage, under certain conditions lineage instability with conversion to conventional CD4 T cells has been described.[100–102] Tissue-resident subsets of Tregs, in addition to their immunosuppressive function, express tissue-specific transcription factors and elaborate mediators that promote homeostasis and healing in many organ system components including adipose tissue, muscle, lung, gut, and skin.[99,103] Other T cells with regulatory activity in autoimmunity, including Tr1, $CD8^+$ Treg, Qa-1/HLA-E-restricted CD8 T cells, and γδ T cells, have been described but are less well characterized.[104–108] Because of the ability of Tregs to target specific organs or cell types, including antigen-specific lymphocytes, there is considerable interest in applying various types of regulatory T cell strategies to treat autoimmune diseases.[109–111]

Tissues themselves also employ mechanisms that suppress self-reactivity and contribute to the establishment of immune privilege.[88,112–114] These tissues can be considered to comprise four general categories: First, certain tissues are decorated with cell surface inhibitory molecules, such as the proapoptotic FasL and TRAIL, lymphocyte inhibitory and Treg promoting PD-L2, and complement regulatory proteins, CD55 and CD46, which can potentially eliminate or impede the activation of autoreactive T cells. Second, soluble inhibitors of inflammation and immune activation are secreted by particular tissues. Notably, in the aqueous humor of the eye, there is a broad spectrum of such factors that include TGF-β, α-melanocyte-stimulating hormone, vasointestinal peptide, calcitonin gene-related protein, somatostatin, macrophage inhibitory factor, and complement inhibitors. Third, lymph node resident stromal cells induce tolerance of CD8 T cells that recognize peripheral tissue-restricted self-antigens.[115,116] Thus, it has been proposed that stromal cells in lymph node and tissues may serve to provide a means to eliminate T cells that bind to tissue-restricted antigens not expressed in the thymus. Fourth, the anterior chamber of the eye elicits a unique type of altered immune response through a complex multistep process termed *anterior chamber–associated immune deviation* (ACAID), which leads to a dampened, less tissue-destructive, response.[88,114,117] Although ACAID was long thought to be important for tolerance, it has recently been argued that its primary function may be to modulate the immune response so the eye can respond to infection without damaging its integrity.[118]

Another possible peripheral mechanism is immune deviation, wherein polarization away from a predisposing cytokine pattern—such as from a Th1 to a Th2 profile—by administering or blocking specific cytokines, suppresses the development of autoimmune disease.[119] Similarly, activation of natural killer (NK) T cells with α-GalCer, which induces IFN-γ production, is associated with dampening of the adaptive Th1 and Th17 effector responses and protection from experimental autoimmune uveitis.[120] In these models, autoreactive T cells are activated but do not produce the pro-inflammatory factors necessary for tissue damage.

In addition to central and peripheral tolerance, the immune system must also avert autoimmunity by suppressing or eliminating T cells after their activation or expansion. This regulation is mediated by several processes, including upregulation of inhibitory receptors such as CTLA4 and PD-1,[121] expression of proapoptotic receptors such as Fas, synthesis of metabolic enzymes such as indoleamine-2,3-dioxygenase (IDO),[122] and release of intra-cellular proapoptotic factors such as Bim. Deficiencies of such mediators that control the magnitude of T cell responses are associated with severe expansion of lymphocyte populations and with varying degrees of autoimmunity. This has been clearly documented by the frequent development of autoimmune disease in cancer patients treated with "checkpoint blockade" such as inhibitors of CTLA4 and PD-1.[123]

B Cell Tolerance

B cells are not only required for antibody production, but serve as potent APCs for T cells and follicular DCs and can also act in regulation.[124,125] Moreover, depletion of B cells with rituximab has shown promise even in autoimmune diseases considered to be mediated by T cells such as T1DM[126] and MS.[127] Therefore, substantial interest exists for defining both mechanisms of B cell tolerance and the specific role of B cell tolerance in autoimmune disease.[128]

Before discussing specific tolerance mechanisms, however, it should be emphasized that the fate of B cells after engagement of their antigen receptors (BCRs) is highly dependent on developmental stage, context and strength of signal, and the nature of the antigen, probably more so than for T cells because B cells are subjected to less stringent selection during central tolerance. Several checkpoints considered important for controlling autoreactive B cells and maintaining self-tolerance have been identified and include many central and peripheral mechanisms similar to those described for T cells, as well as a few additional ones.

Central tolerance of B cells takes place in the bone marrow during pre-B to immature B cell transition as they express rearranged immunoglobulin (Ig) genes on their surface.[129] It appears that the dominant mechanism for B cells with high affinity to membrane-bound self-antigen is receptor editing (replacement of light [L] chain) and, to a lesser extent, deletion, whereas soluble self-antigens induce both receptor editing and anergy.[130,131] Anergic B cells are detectable in the periphery as an $IgD^{+}IgM^{-}$ population[132] or in mice as splenic transitional 3 (T3) B cells.[133] They are short lived at least in part because they downregulate the BAFFR, which is required for their survival, putting them at a competitive disadvantage with other immature B cells, and they are less able to enter B cell follicles.

In the periphery, the earliest tolerance checkpoint occurs at the transitional 1 (T1) B stage over a 2-day interval before maturation to T2 and later naive B cell subsets.[129,134–136] T1 B cells are the immediate bone marrow emigrant population, retain an immature phenotype, and are dependent on BAFF for survival. Importantly, they undergo apoptosis and not activation when stimulated, which results in deletion of B cells that recognize peripheral self-antigens not expressed in the bone marrow compartment. Thus, this mechanism, which is unique to B cells, essentially represents an extension of central tolerance to the periphery. Self-reactive B cells can also downmodulate their surface IgM,[54] which allows them to escape deletion and affords the host a broader repertoire despite the risk of autoimmunity.

Other peripheral tolerance mechanisms are achieved in much the same way as those previously described for T cells, but they differ qualitatively as a result of distinct differentiation pathways and differences in antigen recognition by B cells and T cells—that is, BCRs can bind to virtually all tertiary structures, whereas TCRs are restricted to recognizing self-MHC/peptide complexes on host cell surfaces. Accordingly, B cells can be ignorant of their corresponding self-antigen because of insufficient quantity or access[31] or can undergo anergy and ultimately cell death if engagement of the BCR occurs without co-stimulation, that is, two signals.[137]

Another notable checkpoint occurs during T-dependent immune responses, as B cells undergo affinity maturation in germinal centers (GCs) and acquire new specificities that may include self-reactivity. Evidence suggests that tolerance at this juncture is often defective in autoimmune diseases, because most autoantibodies have acquired autoreactivity through somatic hypermutation and are class switched,[138–140] both of which are indicative of GC maturation. Although studies have provided significant insights into GC processes involved in the selection of B cell clones with high affinity to foreign antigens, the manner in which tolerance of class-switched autoreactive B cells is achieved remains less well defined. Nevertheless, the strongest evidence suggests that (1) autoreactive B cells compete poorly for the cognate T cell help essential for GC B cell survival because the autoreactive BCR would bind less well to the original antigen, resulting in less internalization of antigen for processing and presentation to T cells,[141–143] and (2) B cells that acquire BCRs with reactivity to high density membrane self-antigens are deleted by a Fas-dependent mechanism.[144,145]

Theories of Autoimmunity

Development of autoimmune diseases is influenced by genetic and, to varying degrees, environmental, sex, and other factors, with current evidence supporting a model in which genetic predisposition is required (Fig. 22.1). Therefore, theories of autoimmunity

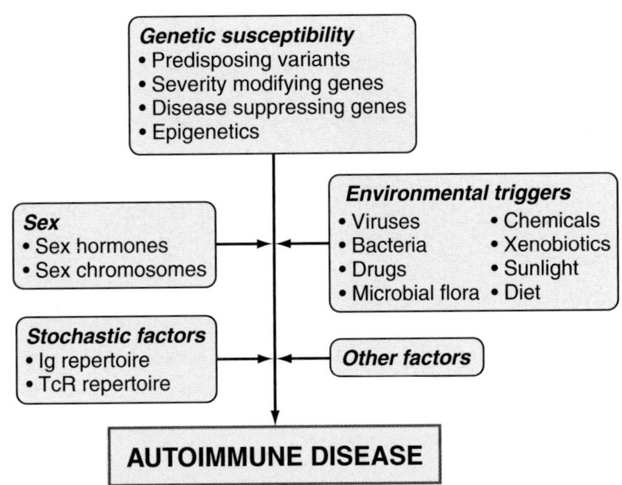

• **Fig. 22.1** Etiology of autoimmune diseases. Autoimmune diseases are usually caused by the additive effects of autoimmunity-promoting environmental, sex, and other factors superimposed on significant underlying genetic predisposition.

and loss of tolerance are closely intertwined with genetic influences. In addition, such theories must also explain how tolerance is breached when autoimmunity is induced in otherwise healthy animals. Upon taking both these factors into account and applying a reductionist perspective, theories of autoimmune disease can be consolidated into two main mechanisms representing separate ends of a continuum, with most diseases having some elements of both. On one end, loss of tolerance and consequent autoimmune disease is caused by genetically imposed defects in central and/or peripheral tolerance mechanisms, whereas on the other end, autoimmunity arises from the conventional immune response to self-antigens for which tolerance is normally incompletely established (Table 22.5). In general, most systemic autoimmune diseases are caused by tolerance defects, whereas organ-specific diseases can be mediated by either mechanism.

Defective Tolerance

Although it can be inferred that loss of tolerance underlies autoimmunity, the specific tolerance defects causing common autoimmune diseases have been difficult to delineate, presumably because of modest defects at multiple checkpoints. Nevertheless, studies of monogenic human autoimmune diseases and animal models have identified a wide range of defects in the various layers of central and peripheral tolerance. Such defects are caused by diverse genetic abnormalities and are mediated by a variety of lymphoid and nonlymphoid cell types. A few representative examples will be discussed.

Central tolerance is essential for eliminating nascent self-reactive lymphocytes, so it is not surprising that autoimmunity can develop from a breakdown in this process. Nevertheless, this mechanism was only firmly established after the discovery that mutations in the transcription factor, autoimmune regulator (AIRE), were the cause of autoimmune polyglandular syndrome 1 (APS-1, also called autoimmune polyendocrinopathy-candidiasis-ectodermal dystrophy [APECED]), a rare inherited disease associated with T cell-mediated autoimmune destruction of multiple endocrine organs.[146–148] *Aire*-deficient mice developed a similar syndrome caused by the reduced expression of thousands of mostly peripheral tissue genes in the thymic medullary epithelium and consequent failure to eliminate T cells recognizing those

TABLE 22.5 Mechanisms of Autoimmunity

Examples	Disease	Mechanism
Defective Tolerance		
Central Defects		
AIRE deficiency	APECED syndrome	Failure to delete autoreactive T cells because of reduced expression of peripheral antigens in thymus
ZAP-70 deficiency	Inflammatory erosive arthritis (mice)	Defective T cell activation and thymic selection
Peripheral Defects		
FAS/FASLG deficiency	Autoimmune lymphoproliferative syndrome (ALPS)	Defective apoptosis
Rc3h1 (M199R) mutation	Lupus (mice)	Increased ICOS on T_{FH} cells promotes their expansion
TREX1 (DNase II) deficiency	Aicardi-Goutières syndrome, chilblain lupus	Accumulation of intra-cellular DNA induces IFN-α production
FOXP3 deficiency	IPEX syndrome	Absence of Treg cells
PD-1 deficiency	Lupus, myocarditis (mice)	Defective peripheral tolerance of T cells
Activation of Nontolerant Lymphocytes		
Penetrating injury	Sympathetic ophthalmia	Release of self-antigen in an inflammatory milieu
Coxsackie B virus infection	T1DM (mice)	Infection mediated release of self-antigen in an inflammatory milieu
Immunization with self-antigen and strong adjuvant	EAE (mice)	Activation of ignorant T cells
Protein citrullination	RA	Generation of neo self-antigens
Altered structure of collagen IV caused by sulfilimine bonds	Goodpasture's syndrome	Formation of conformational neo self-antigens
Cross-reactivity of Group A streptococcal and cardiac antigens	Rheumatic fever	Molecular mimicry
Lymphopenia caused by disease-associated IL-21 production	T1DM (NOD mice)	Lymphopenia-induced homeostatic proliferation

AIRE, Autoimmune regulator; *ALPS,* autoimmune lymphoproliferative syndrome; *APECED,* autoimmune polyendocrinopathy candidiasis ectodermal dystrophy; *DNA,* deoxyribonucleic acid; *DNase,* deoxyribonuclease; *EAE,* experimental autoimmune encephalomyelitis; *ICOS,* inducible co-stimulator; *IFN,* interferon; *IL,* interleukin; *IPEX,* immune dysregulation, polyendocrinopathy, enteropathy X-linked; *NOD,* nonobese diabetic; *PD-1,* programmed cell death protein 1; *RA,* rheumatoid arthritis; *T1DM,* type 1 diabetes mellitus; *Tfh,* follicular helper T cell; *Treg,* regulatory T cell.

gene products. Evidence suggests AIRE achieves this selectivity by binding to certain repressive transcription complexes, such as MBD1-ATF7ip, that target specific methylated cytosine-phosphatidyl-guanine (CpG) dinucleotides in genetic regions encoding tissue-specific antigens. AIRE also promotes, through positive selection, the perinatal thymic generation of CD4$^+$ Foxp3$^+$ regulatory T cells (Tregs) that express peripheral antigen specificities[149] (Tregs, discussed later) and exhibits sex hormone-biased thymic expression, with females showing lower expression of peripheral tissue-specific genes, consistent with their higher prevalence of autoimmune disease.[150] More recently, additional transcription factors, FEZF2 and PRDM1, also regulated expression of peripheral tissue-specific antigens in thymic medullary cells and prevent autoimmune disease in mice.[151,152]

Another example of altered thymic selection leading to autoimmunity, in this instance caused by an intrinsic defect in the T cells, is the aforementioned ZAP70 arthritis model.[153] Here, a function-impairing mutation in the C-terminal SH2 domain of ZAP70, a Syk family tyrosine kinase activated by the TCR complex ζ-chain, reduces TCR signaling, causes defective conventional T cell and nTreg development in the thymus, and seemingly enhances positive selection of autoreactive T cells.[154] Interestingly, using several ZAP70 mutants, it was shown that susceptibility to arthritis and other autoimmune diseases was altered by only slight differences in ZAP70-mediated signaling strength, the strain background, and the type of microbial PRR exposure.[154,155]

For B cells, major defects in central tolerance leading to autoimmunity have been more difficult to prove and no AIRE-like equivalent has been discovered, presumably because immature B cells continue the selection process for a couple of days after egress from the bone marrow, allowing direct exposure to peripheral antigens. Nevertheless, defective central tolerance of B cells in autoimmunity has been suggested by the finding of a higher frequency of naive mature B cells with self-reactivity in patients with SLE and RA.[156–158]

In the periphery, FAS deficiency provides an example of defective peripheral tolerance promoting autoimmunity.[159] FAS is a proapoptotic surface receptor that plays a critical role in maintaining immune homeostasis by eliminating undesired cells. Defects in FAS cause autoimmune lymphoproliferative syndrome (ALPS, also called *Canale-Smith syndrome*) and, in mice, lymphoproliferative (lpr) disease, both of which exhibit massive enlargement of secondary lymphoid organs caused mainly by the accumulation of a normally rare, so-called *double negative* subset of T cells lacking both CD4 and CD8 co-receptors, along with a variety of autoimmune manifestations. *Lpr* mice are defective in eliminating B cells that acquire self-reactivity in the periphery, a process that typically occurs in the GC during somatic hypermutation.[144] Similar abnormalities are found in humans and mice with defects in the ligand for FAS (FASLG).[160]

Peripheral tolerance is also breached by overexpression of the co-stimulatory molecule ICOS on T follicular helper (Tfh) cells in *San Roque* mice. These mice have a point mutation in the *Rc3h1* gene, a RING-type ubiquitin ligase that impairs its ability to degrade ICOS mRNA.[161] Increased expression of ICOS promotes the expansion of Tfh cells and GCs, production of IL-21, and autoimmunity.[162]

An example of a lymphocyte-extrinsic cause for loss of tolerance and autoimmunity is deficiency in the 3′ repair exonuclease 1 (TREX1, deoxyribonuclease [DNase] III). Loss-of-function mutations in TREX1 have been implicated in Aicardi-Goutières syndrome, a rare progressive encephalopathy associated with elevated interferon-α levels in the cerebral spinal fluid, and chilblain lupus, a rare form of SLE characterized by painful bluish-red inflammatory skin lesions typically affecting areas exposed to cold temperatures.[163,164] Autoimmunity is thought to be caused by the intra-cellular accumulation of single-stranded DNA (ssDNA) reportedly derived from endogenous retro-elements normally degraded by TREX1, resulting in the activation of the intra-cellular DNA sensor STING and consequent overproduction of IFN-α.[165–167] Intriguingly, oxidized DNA, which is abundant in NETs and in ultraviolet-induced skin lesions, is resistant to TREX1 degradation and can promote STING activation and type I IFN production,[168] suggesting that the TREX1 pathway may play a more general role in SLE pathogenesis. The importance of DNA disposal in lupus has been further illustrated by the association of DNASE I and DNASE1L3 deficiencies with development of lupus in humans and mice.[169–172]

Defective regulation can also result in loss of tolerance and autoimmune disease, as illustrated by the absence of Tregs.[173,174] In humans, monogenic deficiency of the *FOXP3* gene, which is required for Treg development, is associated with the immune dysregulation, polyendocrinopathy, enteropathy X-linked (IPEX) syndrome, a severe systemic autoimmune disease associated with diarrhea, eczematous dermatitis, and endocrinopathy, which is usually fatal within the first year. T1DM, autoimmune cytopenias, and nephritis are among other, less common, autoimmune manifestations of this syndrome. Similar findings are observed in *scurfy* mice, which have a spontaneous function-impairing mutation of *Foxp3*.

Autoimmunity Caused by Activation of Non- or Partially Tolerant T Cells

The other main theory is that autoimmunity develops through the conventional activation of self-reactive T cells that have not been deleted in the thymus and remain oblivious to the corresponding self-antigen after emigration. Such ignorant T cells, commonly found in the periphery of both healthy humans and animals, can be activated by antigen presented by professional APCs in the context of an innate inflammatory milieu. Once activated, T cells are able to gain access to virtually all tissues and, when activated again locally, can elaborate pro-inflammatory factors, causing tissue damage.[87] Breach of tolerance by this mechanism is most often associated with organ-specific diseases, presumably because tissue-specific antigens are less likely to be expressed in the thymus. This theory is supported by the finding that type 1 diabetes is prevented in BB rats and NOD mice by intrathymic transplantation of pancreatic islets,[175,176] or inhibited in NOD mice by intrathymic administration of glutamic acid decarboxylase (GAD), a major β-islet autoantigen in this model.[177,178] Similarly, EAE can be prevented by intrathymic administration of either the immunizing antigen, myelin basic protein, or its major encephalitogenic epitope,[179] and autoantibody production can be delayed in lupus-prone mice following intrathymic injections of polynucleosomes.[180] Taken together, these data support the concept that autoimmunity can be caused by the activation of lymphocytes to self-antigens that had incomplete central tolerance. This mechanism is similar to the mechanism underlying the APECED syndrome caused by AIRE deficiency, but in this instance central tolerance is not known to be defective.

Breach of tolerance by ignorant lymphocytes depends on many factors, including the (1) nature of the self-antigen, (2) extent of exposure to antigen, (3) antigen receptor affinity, (4) frequency of autoreactive lymphocytes, (5) types and levels of co-stimulatory molecule expression, (6) cytokine and chemokine profiles, and (7) presence of inflammation.[30,181–187] It should also be emphasized that despite the presence of lymphocytes that recognize self-antigen, under normal conditions peripheral tolerance mechanisms are difficult to overcome. Consequently, although the experimental autoimmune models are highly reproducible, they require supraphysiologic amounts of self-antigen, strong adjuvant, specific MHC haplotypes, and a susceptible background to break tolerance. These findings are consistent with the fact that autoimmunity does not develop in most individuals and speaks to the robustness of the tolerance process that must be overcome. Although it is difficult to prove which of these mechanisms are applicable in patients, they provide frameworks for understanding how autoimmunity can develop, along with guidance in devising interventions.

Similar to immune responses in general, key factors for the initiation of autoimmunity are innate inflammatory and co-stimulatory factors that promote the initial activation and expansion of naive autoreactive lymphocytes. This mechanism is thought to contribute to the autoimmune response by the release of self-antigens after cell damage or death, increased MHC/peptide expression, upregulation of co-stimulatory factors, and activation of professional APCs.[182,183,188] Indeed, moderate to severe tissue necrosis is often associated with some evidence of autoreactivity, although this condition rarely progresses to autoimmune disease.[189,190] In autoimmune diseases, chronic cell and tissue injury and the continual release of self-antigens under conditions favorable for antigen presentation and co-stimulation promote epitope spreading and the activation of an expanding repertoire of lymphocytes that recognize autoantigens beyond the initiating autoantigen.[191,192] This process is thought to at least partially account for the often progressive course of autoimmunity. Overall, these and other findings support the theory that, under certain conditions such as infection or trauma, self-antigens are released and, in the presence of inflammatory factors and an activated innate immune system, there is triggering and expansion of previously ignorant self-antigen-recognizing lymphocytes that can lead to autoimmune disease.

In addition to the release of sequestered self-antigens, the initial activation of non-tolerant lymphocytes has been postulated to occur in several other ways. Some investigators have suggested that the initial response may be directed toward certain determinants[193,194] based on the concept of "crypticity," essentially the presence of a hierarchy of dominant and cryptic epitopes on a protein because of differences in binding affinity to the MHC, protein processing, preference for presentation by different APCs, and the repertoire of epitope-specific T cells.[192,195] It is therefore posited that during thymic selection, T cells that engage the few dominant epitopes are eliminated, whereas those recognizing the less antigenic, but more abundant, cryptic epitopes are spared. The latter T cells then emigrate to the periphery, where they can be activated by the corresponding cryptic epitope under certain inflammatory conditions.

Another mechanism by which self-antigens can activate nontolerant lymphocytes is through the production of neo self-antigens after post-translational or chemical modifications. A prominent example of this mechanism is the formation of citrullinated proteins caused by the deimination of arginine residues by peptidyl-arginine deiminase (PADI) enzymes. Several citrullinated proteins are not only major targets of autoantibodies in a subset of RA, but are thought to play a significant role in disease pathogenesis.[196–198] Deficiency of L-isoaspartate O-methyltransferase (PIMT), which catalyzes the repair of isoAsp proteins formed by the spontaneous conversion of aspartic acid to its isoaspartyl derivative, also results in accumulation of isoAsp proteins and development of lupus in a mouse model.[199] Furthermore, in the PL/J model of EAE, acetylation of the encephalitogenic Ac1-11 peptide of myelin basic protein (MBP) is required for T cell activation even though unmodified peptide binds to MHC.[200] These and other studies suggest that protein modifications can generate new epitopes either directly by creating new structures such as citrulline, or indirectly by altering MHC binding or modifying sites of peptide processing to produce new and/or cryptic self-peptides.[201]

Neo self-antigens can also arise from changes in overall structure, for example, by the formation of immunogenic IgG-containing immune complexes from nonantigenic soluble monomeric IgG, which can induce rheumatoid factors, antibodies to the Fc portion of complexed IgG.[202,203] Likewise, in Goodpasture's disease, a configuration change in type IV collagen due to sulfilimine bonds produces a neotarget for pathogenic autoantibodies, a mechanism coined *conformeropathy*.[204]

Another potential mechanism for triggering autoimmunity in susceptible people is lymphopenia-induced homeostatic expansion of T cells.[205,206] Expansion occurs because of greater availability of survival-promoting cytokines (IL-7, IL-15) that, when combined with low-affinity engagement of the TCR to self-peptide/MHC, induces low-grade proliferation without full activation. It was therefore hypothesized that the requirement for self-reactivity could, after repeated rounds of lymphopenia, result in the preferential expansion of autoreactive T cells and, consequently, autoimmunity.[205] This hypothesis is supported by the presence of lymphopenia in people with certain autoimmune diseases, such as SLE and RA, autoimmune manifestations in some primary immunodeficiencies with lymphopenia, and several experimental autoimmune models.

In addition to self-antigens, foreign antigens with sufficient sequence or structural similarity can cross-activate nontolerant self-recognizing T (and B) lymphocytes, a mechanism termed *molecular mimicry*.[207] For T cells, several findings support this possibility: (1) cross-reactivity requires only short peptide lengths of 8 to 15 amino acids, (2) T cell recognition is highly degenerate depending on only a few key amino acid residues, and it is possible to have mimotopes with no identical amino acids at any position,[208,209] (3) the estimation that a single T cell, despite requiring anchor residues to bind the HLA, can react with 10^4 to more than 10^8 different peptides,[210] (4) MBP-specific T cells cloned from patients with MS can be stimulated by diverse microbial peptides,[211,212] and (5) infection with a modified Theiler's virus expressing a foreign cross-reactive peptide (*Haemophilus influenzae* protease IV protein that shares only 6/13 amino acids) induced T cells against a myelin protein, proteolipid protein (PLP), resulting in autoimmune CNS disease.[213] To date, however, there is no compelling evidence to connect a specific microbial T cell mimotope to any autoimmune disease.[214,215]

In contrast, fairly good evidence indicates that molecular mimicry affects self-reactive B cells in a few autoimmune diseases. The best examples include cross-reactivity of (1) bacterial adhesin FimH with lysosomal membrane protein 2 (LAMP2) in anti-neutrophil cytoplasmic antibody (ANCA)-positive pauci-immune focal necrotizing glomerulonephritis,[216] (2) group A streptococcal carbohydrate epitope, N-acetyl glucosamine, and M protein with cardiac myosin in rheumatic fever,[217] and (3) *Campylobacter jejuni* lipo-oligosaccharide with ganglioside GM1 on peripheral nerves in the acute motor axonal neuropathy subtype of Guillain-Barré syndrome because of an identical determinant, Gal β1–3 GalNAc β1–4 (NeuAc α2-3) Galβ.[218,219] Overall, however, although molecular mimicry is an attractive hypothesis, supportive evidence for most autoimmune diseases is lacking. Whether this situation is because of technical issues that impede detection, such as multiple mimotopes from diverse sources, diverse HLA haplotypes, and the considerable plasticity of the T cell receptor, or whether mimicry is an uncommon cause of autoimmune disease remains an open question.

Immunologic Mechanisms of Tissue Inflammation and Dysfunction

The same effector mechanisms used by the immune system to neutralize pathogens are exploited in autoimmunity to inflict a wide range of deleterious effects on self-molecules, cells, and tissues. These mechanisms have been broadly grouped into hypersensitivity types II to IV, which encompass antibody-, immune complex-, and T cell-mediated processes, respectively (see Table 22.2).

In type II reactions, pathologic autoantibodies bind to self-antigens primarily located on cell-surfaces or in tissues and mediate autoimmune disease by three general mechanisms: (1) altering the function of the target antigen, (2) promoting cell injury or death, and (3) inducing inflammation. Blocking or enhancing self-molecule function represents a special kind of type II hypersensitivity response in which autoantibodies alone are sufficient to effect autoimmune manifestations. Examples include the agonist anti–thyroid-stimulating hormone (TSH) receptor antibodies in Graves' disease that stimulate thyrocyte growth and production of thyroid hormone, the anti–acetylcholine receptor antibodies that block neuromuscular transmission in myasthenia gravis, and anti–β2-glycoprotein I antibodies in antiphospholipid syndrome that alter the regulation of anticoagulant activity.[220] Direct cell injury or death is mediated by the binding of IgM or IgG to surface antigens, leading to cell lysis directly by complement activation or to phagocytosis via interaction of deposited C3 fragments with CR1 and CR3 receptors. Bound IgG also promotes phagocytosis through its interaction with Fc receptors. Examples include autoimmune hemolytic anemia, idiopathic thrombocytopenia, and autoimmune neutropenia. Finally, antibodies bound to tissue antigens promote inflammation by activating complement, which generates the chemoattractant C5a and leukocyte-activating C3 fragments, and by FcγR binding, which activates immigrating leukocytes such as neutrophils and macrophages, as well as tissue resident mast cells and basophils. These cells produce pro-inflammatory factors that further expand the inflammatory response by recruiting and then activating additional circulating leukocytes.

Type III responses are caused by abnormal deposition of immune complexes of IgG antibody and soluble antigen in tissues. Such complexes, which also contain bound C3 complement fragments, are normally cleared from the circulation by complement receptors on red blood cells (RBCs) and by complement receptors and FcγRs on mononuclear phagocytes and platelets. However, this clearance can be overwhelmed under certain conditions such as overabundant production or immune complexes composed of excess antigen, wherein less antibody coverage reduces complement deposition and aggregation of Fc regions, leading to less efficient clearance. Once deposited in tissues, immune complexes initiate, through complement activation and FcγR binding, the same inflammatory cascades as type II responses. SLE and RA are autoimmune diseases mediated by this mechanism.

Type IV hypersensitivity encompasses cell and tissue injury mediated by activated T cells through their cytolytic activity in the case of CD8 T cells or the production of pro-inflammatory factors primarily by the CD4 subset. Apart from direct evidence of this mechanism in animal models using approaches that are not feasible in human studies, indirect evidence supporting this mechanism includes a higher frequency of autoreactive T cells with effector function in patients with autoimmune diseases, immunopathologic findings similar to T cell-mediated autoimmune models, and inhibition with T cell-blocking agents such as cyclosporin A.[221] T1DM and MS are examples of type IV reactions.

It should be mentioned that these classifications are general, and for some diseases the underlying effector mechanism may be more complex. In RA, for example, the mechanism responsible for injury or dysfunction probably involves more than one hypersensitivity type,[222,223] whereas in others, such as SLE, different clinical manifestations are mediated by different mechanisms; for example, anti-neuronal antibody-mediated CNS disease is a type II process whereas glomerulonephritis is type III.[224–227] Finally, for diseases such as dermatomyositis and systemic sclerosis, the type of mechanism mediating tissue injury remains to be defined.

Pathophysiology of Autoimmune Rheumatic Diseases

Although the general principles underlying loss of tolerance and autoimmunity provide a useful conceptual foundation, the actual pathophysiologies suggested by the few better-defined autoimmune diseases are likely to also employ specific and unique mechanisms. Two notable examples of this phenomenon are the pathophysiology of anti-nuclear antibody production in SLE and the development of arthritis in RA. These examples will be briefly discussed in the context of their broader significance to autoimmune diseases.

Recent findings suggest a model of SLE pathophysiology that provides a mechanism explaining why anti-nuclear antibodies are virtually always present in lupus despite substantial genetic and clinical heterogeneity.[60,228] First, autoreactive B cells are activated when self-reactive BCRs bind to nucleic acid–containing antigens (nucleosomes, oxidized mitochondrial DNA,[229] or ribonucleoprotein [RNP]) and internalize them into the endolysosome compartment, where the released nucleic acids engage TLR7 and TLR9, and provide a second signal. Such activated B cells act as potent APCs for T lymphocytes and after class-switch recombination produce IgG autoantibodies. Next, plasmacytoid DCs (pDCs) and DCs are activated by a similar mechanism following uptake of autoantibody nucleic acid–containing complexes by FcγRIIA (FcγRIII in mice). Elaboration of lupus-promoting cytokines such as type I IFN and BAFF by pDCs and DCs, as well as enhanced antigen presentation, are thought to further drive loss of tolerance, activation of autoreactive B cells, and autoantibody production, thereby resulting in an amplification loop. Thus, in people susceptible to lupus, confinement of nucleic acid–binding TLRs to endolysomes is not enough of a barrier to block their activation by normally innocuous amounts of self-nucleic acids. This mechanism provides an explanation for the high prevalence of autoantibodies in SLE that bind to nucleic acids such as DNA as well as to antigens physically associated with nucleic acids such as histones, RNPs, myeloperoxidase (ANCA), and surface molecules on many cell types including platelets, lymphocytes, neutrophils, and even RBCs. Autoantibodies to cell surface targets are likely induced by apoptotic bodies containing nucleic acids.[230] Importantly, this explanation suggests the possibility that other autoimmune diseases might also be mediated by specific PRRs.[231,232]

The pathophysiology of RA also involves common and specific pathways that together promote inflammatory synovitis in roughly three phases,[233–238] which is best described in the HLA-DR1*401 (DR4) anti-citrullinated protein antibody (ACPA) subset of patients who have greater disease severity. The initial pre-clinical phase that can occur years before onset of arthritis is postulated to involve the activation of T cells and B cells at extra-articular inflammatory sites where cyclic citrullinated proteins (CCPs) are produced, in part, by the release of peptidylarginine deiminase from apoptosing granulocytes and monocytes. The HLA-DRB1 shared epitope, which specifically binds and presents citrullinated self-peptides, is thought to predispose to this type of response. Targets for ACPA include fibrinogen, vimentin, α-enolase, and others, and these antibodies are thought to play a major role in disease pathogenesis, although the mechanism remains uncertain. The specific triggers of ACPA response are also not firmly established, but evidence strongly suggests that inflammation at mucosal sites, caused by environmental factors such as smoking, silicosis, periodontal disease, and the gut microbiome, is responsible for initiating a limited ACPA response that expands in scope and consistency with clinical progression.

The next early "clinically evident" arthritis phase is characterized by localization of the immune response and inflammation in joints. The resulting immune complexes and activated T cells lead to further stimulation of macrophages, synovial fibroblasts, endothelial cells, mast cells, osteoclasts, and platelets,[239] concurrent with the eventual production of pro-inflammatory factors such as TNF, IL-1, IFN-γ, IL-17A, IL-23, chemokines, matrix metalloproteinases, osteopontin, and many others that contribute to synovitis, pannus formation, bone erosion, and cartilage destruction. Indeed, unique populations of PD-1^{hi}CXCR5^{-} CD4 T cells in RA synovium and peripheral blood have been identified that express factors promoting B cell help and likely contribute to this process.[240] This activity leads to the third chronic "established" RA phase, predominantly inflammatory and tissue-damaging, which is mediated largely by activated fibroblast-like synoviocytes, which produce a wide array of pro-inflammatory mediators that promote recruitment and activation of circulating and resident immune cells.[241] It has also been suggested that the spread of arthritis to unaffected joints could, in fact, be mediated by transmigration of these activated fibroblast-like synovial cells.[242] The pathophysiology of the ACPA subset of RA provides another example of the collaboration of the innate and adaptive arms of the immune system in autoimmune disease, but it also has two unique features. First, the major autoantigen, citrullinated protein, is a neoantigen specifically targeted in this disease, and second, tissue damage is to a large extent mediated by fibroblast-like synoviocytes.

Genetics of Autoimmune Diseases

During the past three decades, substantial insight into the genetic landscape responsible for autoimmune disease susceptibility has emerged from both human and animal studies. This progress was greatly facilitated by the availability of genomic sequences, improved definition of genetic variations and haplotypes among human populations, consortia with collections of patients and control subjects in the thousands, and numerous major technical and analytical advances.[243,244] In particular, genetic studies have progressed from testing a few specific candidate polymorphisms to genome-wide family analyses of hundreds of cases, and even larger scale genome-wide association studies (GWASs) involving thousands,[245,246] making it possible to not only verify known genetic associations, but to also capture common disease-predisposing variants with modest effects. Combined, these approaches have identified more than 100 candidate genes or loci in SLE and RA and in other rheumatologic diseases such as systemic sclerosis, Kawasaki's disease, Behçet's disease, spondylitis, and ANCA-associated vasculitis (reviewed in references 247-260; http://www.genome.gov/gwastudies). These candidates span the gamut of innate and adaptive immune systems, but they also include some loci with genes of unknown immunologic function. For example, in SLE—one of the best defined at the genetic level of any rheumatic disease—candidate genes are involved in antigen presentation (HLA-DR3), B and T cell receptor signaling (*PTPN22, BANK1,* and *BLK*), CD4 T helper cell regulation (OX40L, *TNFSF4*, and *CTLA4*), T cell-mediated regulation *(PDCD1)*, cytokine signaling *(STAT4)*, interferon and TLR7/9 signaling (*IRF5, TNFAIP3, IRAK1, IRF7,* and *TYK2*), Fc receptor function (one of which, *FCGR2A*, has been implicated in the transport of nucleic acid–containing immune complexes to TLR7/9-containing endosomes), neutrophil function *(ITGAM)*, clearance of self-antigens (*C1Q, C2,* and *C4*), clearance of intracytoplasmic DNA *(TREX1)*, and also several loci-containing genes with no known connection to the immune system or lupus. Together, these candidates provide clues to specific pathways involved in SLE, which indeed has dovetailed well with genetic studies in mice.[19]

From GWAS and other studies, including those in animal models, several general conclusions can be made about genetic susceptibility in the more common autoimmune diseases. First, autoimmune diseases are associated with a large number of susceptibility genes that have an impact on a wide range of immunologic, cellular, and end-organ functions in ways that enhance, modify, or even suppress relevant pathophysiologic processes.

Second, considerable genetic heterogeneity exists at both the individual and population levels regardless of whether the phenotype is relatively uniform, as in RA, or diverse, as in SLE. Thus, although there are a large number of predisposing genes, having only a subset of these genes is generally sufficient for disease development. Whether this heterogeneity is caused by variants affecting a few common pathways or numerous unique pathways remains unclear.

Third, the vast majority of candidate genes or loci have only modest effect sizes, with most odds ratios less than 1.5, although in some diseases, notably SLE, a few rare variants, such as *C1Q*-deficiency associated with a greater than 90% incidence of SLE and *TREX1* mutations leading to chilblain lupus, have been identified that are highly penetrant. Although rare and often exhibiting clinical presentations not typical of SLE, monogenic lupus-like diseases have nonetheless provided valuable insights into the complexity of genetic variation-phenotype associations and related pathologic mechanisms.[261] Another salient finding derived from GWAS analysis is that, for most autoimmune diseases, HLA alleles consistently have the highest or among the highest effect sizes. This finding accords well with the central role of antigen presentation and T cells in directing the adaptive immune response to specific antigens. Overall, however, for most candidate variations, defining the mechanism and proving a role in autoimmune disease will be hampered by their low effect sizes.

Fourth, some of the variant genes and loci are shared among autoimmune diseases, suggesting common underlying mechanisms.[262] Noteworthy examples are the association of *PTPN22* with a wide range of autoimmune diseases, including T1DM, RA, SLE, juvenile idiopathic arthritis (JIA), Graves' disease, systemic sclerosis, myasthenia gravis, generalized vitiligo, and granulomatosis with polyangiitis, but not MS,[263] and the association of *STAT4* with RA, SLE, systemic sclerosis, and Sjögren's syndrome.[264,265] This finding supports a role for such broadly predisposing genetic factors in the known occurrence of multiple different autoimmune diseases in some families.

Fifth, common single nucleotide polymorphism-defined variants account for only a portion of overall heritability in autoimmune diseases, that is approximately 20% to 60%[243,244,266] of which the HLA region typically accounts for a substantial part. Several reasons for the missing heritability have been suggested: (1) failed detection because of inadequate single-nucleotide polymorphism (SNP) coverage or the presence of disease-promoting non-SNP genomic variations such as copy number variants, (2) a large number of common variants with modest to marginal effects (odds ratio <1.1 to 1.2) that are undetectable despite large study sizes given that the statistical power is reduced by both smaller effect size and lower variant frequency in the population, and (3) uncommon variants (1% to 5%) or rare disease-associated risk alleles (<1% frequency). Illustrating the hurdles that must be overcome to identify these rare variants on a genome wide scale, it was estimated that 25,000 cases plus a replication set would be required for a well-powered study.[267] Notably, for many traits, common single-nucleotide variations with small effect sizes below that detectable by GWAS with large effect sizes have been suggested to account for a majority of missing heritability.[268] Such a situation would present significant challenges to further defining genetic susceptibility and to incorporate gene variant-specific programs in patient care.[269]

Sixth, most common SNP variants associated with diseases do not affect coding regions, making it difficult to determine if the SNP variant is the actual change associated with disease. Nonetheless, some of these have been identified within the regulatory regions of disease-related genes and include a subset of enhancers, called *superenhancers* or *stretch enhancers*, which can function as lineage-determining master transcription factors that regulate cell identity.[270] An example is the association of SNPs in the super-enhancer region of BACH2, a regulator of T cell activation, with several autoimmune diseases including RA, Crohn's disease, MS, and T1DM.[270] Furthermore, the Janus kinase (JAK) inhibitor tofacitinib approved for the treatment of RA altered the expression of RA risk genes within predicted superenhancer regulatory nodes. Thus, finer characterization of the noncoding enhancer and superenhancer regions for different immune cell types and other autoimmune diseases could yield new insights into pathways central to pathogenesis and with therapeutic potential.

Seventh, the application of transcriptomics, the high-throughput profiling of virtually all RNAs, for cells or tissues from patients is a powerful approach that has led to the identification of therapeutic targets such as type I IFN, IL-1, and IL-17 for autoimmune diseases.[271,272] This technology, by defining the broad gene expression patterns associated with various disease states, has the potential for advancing both understanding of basic pathogenesis and many areas of clinical practice including diagnosis, patient stratification, and monitoring.[271]

Finally, information gleaned from genetic studies to date has not been useful for identifying people at risk, and it is thought that this situation will remain so because of the small effect sizes and relatively high frequency of known risk alleles combined with incomplete coverage of heritability.[244] Nevertheless, these data and newer technology-driven approaches have helped define disease-relevant pathways, and within that context have provided clues and support for developing therapeutic strategies.

Sex and Autoimmunity

A significant female sex bias in autoimmunity was identified early on and was considered an important clue to disease pathogenesis.[273] The strength of this predilection, however, varies among autoimmune disorders, with female prevalence in the 80% to 95% range for thyroiditis, SLE, Sjögren's syndrome, and antiphospholipid syndrome; in the 60% to 75% range for RA, scleroderma, myasthenia gravis, and MS; and close to 50% for T1DM and autoimmune myocarditis.[274] Why some autoimmune diseases are affected more by sex than others is not known, but the lack of common or distinguishing characteristics in those diseases with higher female predominance suggests the possibility of multiple mechanisms.

Indeed, to differing extents depending on the disease, both sex hormones and sex chromosomes have been implicated in this dichotomy.[275–279] In terms of sex hormones, substantial evidence from in vitro, animal, and clinical studies supports a role for both female and male sex steroids in modifying the incidence and severity of autoimmunity. For example, in people with SLE, both estrogens and prolactin exacerbate disease. In animal studies, they promote loss of tolerance and expansion of B cell populations, which, for estrogens, was also associated with enhanced survival and greater expression of B cell lymphoma 2 (Bcl-2).[280] Importantly, studies of lupus-prone mice involving combinations of castration and hormone replacement convincingly demonstrated a disease-promoting effect of female hormones on spontaneous systemic autoimmunity.[281]

Evidence also supports a role for sex chromosomes in autoimmune disease susceptibility. People with Klinefelter's syndrome (XXY) have a higher than expected incidence of SLE, whereas there is contrastingly suggestive under-representation in Turner's syndrome (XO).[282,283] Furthermore, using genetic and gonad manipulation in mice that allowed direct comparison of the effects of one or two X chromosomes on autoimmunity, susceptibility to both EAE in SJL mice and TMPD-induced lupus was more severe in mice with XX.[284,285] Another potential contributing factor is the biallelic expression of the aforementioned TLR7 lupus-risk gene in some B cells, monocytes, and pDCs due to incomplete X-chromosome inactivation at the single cell level in females.[286] Biallelic expression in B cells correlated with more TLR7 protein, greater response to TLR7 ligand, and a propensity to class switch, findings that support an increased predisposition to lupus.

The influence of sex on the immune response to the microbiome and other environmental factors has also been implicated in autoimmune disease susceptibility.[277,287] Thus, the additive contribution of several sex hormones, the number or extent of inactivation of X-chromosomes, and types of interaction with the environment, rather than a single factor, modulate the overall sex differences in predisposition.

Microbial and Other Environmental Triggers

As alluded to previously, considerable evidence indicates that environmental factors can exert varying degrees of influence on the development of autoimmune diseases. A clear causal effect has been documented for a few disorders, whereas the low concordance rate (20% to 50%) among monozygotic twins in common autoimmune diseases supports the presence of a significant environmental component. Nevertheless, the specific environmental factors and the extent to which they contribute to disease induction and exacerbation remain largely unknown for the majority of autoimmune disorders. The reasons for this lack of knowledge are likely manifold and, depending on the disease, may include unsuspected or unknown environmental culprits, multiple independent factors, additive factors contributing to cumulatively small portions of the overall environmental effect, a highly variable or prolonged interval between exposure and disease onset, and a low incidence of autoimmune disease after exposure. Moreover, another general impediment is the difficulty of proving causation with epidemiologic data. Because of these difficulties, animal studies have been invaluable in allowing controlled experimentation, and much of what we understand mechanistically has come through this approach.

Despite the aforementioned limitations, a broad range of environmental factors have been implicated, albeit with varying levels of confidence.[288] Notably, the most prominent are infection and exposure to microbial products, which epidemiologic and animal models suggest can either enhance or inhibit autoimmunity depending on the type of exposure and disease.[289,290] Rheumatologic examples include reactive arthritis after certain enteric infections, chronic Lyme arthritis resulting from *Borrelia burgdorferi*, and the association of oral *Porphyromonas gingivalis* (which expresses a peptidylarginine deiminase that can citrullinate proteins) with RA. Several mechanisms by which microbes are postulated to induce or exacerbate autoimmunity include: (1) molecular mimicry,[217] (2) bystander activation of autoreactive T cells by pathogen-activated APCs,[291,292] (3) inflammation of the target tissue and the release of immunologically hidden self-antigens,[293] (4) production of disease-promoting cytokines, such as IFN-α,[60,294] (5) expansion of pathogenic immune cells including Th17 T cells and plasmacytoid DCs,[292,295–297] and (6) release of metabolites that affect the frequencies of autoreactive and regulatory T cells or inflammation.[298,299]

Inhibition of autoimmune diseases by pathogens was initially suggested by epidemiologic evidence in people with T1DM and MS, consistent with the "hygiene hypothesis"—that is, a lower incidence of infectious burden is responsible for an increasing incidence of allergic and autoimmune diseases in Western countries.[300,301] This concept has since been supported by additional epidemiologic and experimental data, although the microbial pathogens, type of exposure, and mechanisms remain largely uncertain. Studies of T1DM in NOD mice, which gets worse in clean conditions and better with exposure to microbial products, showed that alterations in gut microbiota, which can interact with and modulate the host immune and inflammatory apparatus, could account for a significant portion of the environmental effects and even influenced the female sex bias.[302–305] Many of these mechanisms do not require a specific pathogen but can be mediated by a wide spectrum of organisms. Additionally, in some animal models, autoimmune disease develops under germ-free conditions, thereby excluding an absolute requirement for microbial environment or infection. In this case, one would infer that the trigger is provided by self, most likely cell damage–derived products. Examples include T1DM in NOD mice and BB rats, APECED in Aire-deficient mice, IPEX in the presence of Foxp3 deficiency, and lupus in MRL-lpr mice.[306–310] Interestingly, however, in MRL-*lpr* mice, the addition of a filtered diet containing fewer pathogen-associated molecular patterns (PAMPs) reduces disease severity. This finding suggests that microbial products at least partially affect disease susceptibility in this model and points to the difficulty of completely excluding a role for microbial organisms.

Finally, studies are increasingly uncovering striking relationships between the microbiome (the collective genomes of microbes living inside and on the body), altered immune system homeostasis, and autoimmune diseases.[311,312] In addition to the previous examples, studies have found associations of gut dysbiosis in SLE. The gut pathobiont *Enterococcus gallinarum* was implicated in promoting leakiness of the gut mucosal barrier, colonization of extra-intestinal organs, and lupus in both SLE patients and a mouse model.[292] Impressively, lupus was prevented in mice by treatment with antibiotics or vaccination against *E. gallinarum*. In another study, a fivefold greater representation of *Ruminococcus gnavus* was detected in two independent cohorts of SLE, and its presence correlated with reduced taxonomic complexity of the microbiome, antibodies to *R. gnavus*, increased disease activity, and greater severity.[313]

In terms of the other nonmicrobial environmental factors, some of the general types that have been implicated include: (1) drugs, such as procainamide, gold salts, and interferons, which typically cause mild autoimmunity that resolves after discontinuation; (2) trauma, exemplified by sympathetic ophthalmia caused by penetrating injury to the eye globe; and (3) diverse environmental agents such as adulterated oil (which causes toxic oil syndrome), ultraviolet radiation (which exacerbates systemic autoimmunity), iodine (which causes autoimmune thyroiditis), silica (which is associated with RA, SLE, and systemic sclerosis), and tobacco smoke (which is associated with ACPA and HLA-DR4$^+$ RA).[198,288]

Conclusion

Since 1904, when Donath and Landsteiner reported the first evidence of self-reactivity in paroxysmal hemoglobinuria,[314] the field of autoimmunity has progressed tremendously at both the clinical and basic science levels. Notably, substantial progress has been made since the previous edition of this book in genetic susceptibility, environmental factors (particularly the microbiome), and pathophysiology, notably with the continued refinement of the many pathways that connect cause with immunopathology. Advances have continued to better inform how the innate response plays key roles in both initiating autoimmunity and determining the type of adaptive autoimmune response and autoimmune disease. Genetic studies have advanced to larger GWAS projects and with larger focus on identifying and characterizing causative variants underlying mechanisms. Advances in the understanding of disease pathogenesis, primarily in more common rheumatologic diseases, have further solidified and extended existing frameworks, which researchers can build on to identify critical pathways and molecules. Of importance to patient care has been the successful bench-to-bedside translation approach that has resulted in the introduction of new therapies to the clinic. Despite this progress, there are many important facets of autoimmunity that remain unresolved, and patient care remains suboptimal. Importantly, the highly sought-after objective of specifically re-establishing tolerance in patients has remained elusive despite considerable effort,[315] and currently more broadly immunosuppressing therapies are only partially effective and are associated with significant side effects. Consequently, there continues to be a critical need to investigate the basic processes that underpin the rheumatologic autoimmune diseases and to leverage this to develop effective and safe therapies.

Full references for this chapter can be found on ExpertConsult.com.

Selected References

1. Shapira Y, Agmon-Levin N, Shoenfeld Y: Geoepidemiology of autoimmune rheumatic diseases, *Nat Rev Rheumatol* 6:468–476, 2010.
2. Cooper GS, Bynum ML, Somers EC: Recent insights in the epidemiology of autoimmune diseases: improved prevalence estimates and understanding of clustering of diseases, *J Autoimmun* 33:197–207, 2009.
3. Jacobson DL, Gange SJ, Rose NR, et al.: Epidemiology and estimated population burden of selected autoimmune diseases in the United States, *Clin Immunol Immunopathol* 84:223–243, 1997.
4. NIH progress in autoimmune diseases research, National Institutes of Health Publication No. 05-514 2005.
5. Silverstein AM: *A history of immunology*, ed 2, London, 2009, Elsevier Inc.
6. Olsen NJ, Karp DR: Autoantibodies and SLE: the threshold for disease, *Nat Rev Rheumatol* 10:181–186, 2014.
7. Masters SL, Simon A, Aksentijevich I, et al.: Horror autoinflammaticus: the molecular pathophysiology of autoinflammatory disease (*), *Annu Rev Immunol* 27:621–668, 2009.
8. Ombrello MJ, Kastner DL: Autoinflammation in 2010: expanding clinical spectrum and broadening therapeutic horizons, *Nat Rev Rheumatol* 7:82–84, 2011.
9. Schroder K, Tschopp J: The inflammasomes, *Cell* 140:821–832, 2010.
10. Martinon F, Aksentijevich I: New players driving inflammation in monogenic autoinflammatory diseases, *Nat Rev Rheumatol* 11:11–20, 2015.
11. van Kempen TS, Wenink MH, Leijten EF, et al.: Perception of self: distinguishing autoimmunity from autoinflammation, *Nat Rev Rheumatol* 11:483–492, 2015.
12. Stoffels M, Kastner DL: Old dogs, new tricks: monogenic autoinflammatory disease unleashed, *Annu Rev Genomics Hum Genet* 17:245–272, 2016.
13. Van Gorp H, Van Opdenbosch N, Lamkanfi M: Inflammasome-dependent cytokines at the crossroads of health and autoinflammatory disease, *Cold Spring Harb Perspect Biol* 11, 2019.
14. Manthiram K, Zhou Q, Aksentijevich I, et al.: The monogenic autoinflammatory diseases define new pathways in human innate immunity and inflammation, *Nat Immunol* 18:832–842, 2017.
15. Martinez-Quiles N, Goldbach-Mansky R: Updates on autoinflammatory diseases, *Curr Opin Immunol* 55:97–105, 2018.
16. Uggenti C, Lepelley A, Crow YJ: Self-awareness: nucleic acid-driven inflammation and the type I interferonopathies, *Annu Rev Immunol*, 2019.
17. Lee-Kirsch MA: The type I interferonopathies, *Annu Rev Med* 68:297–315, 2017.
18. Gell PGH Coombs RRA: *Clinical aspects of immunology*, ed 1, Oxford, 1963, Blackwell.
19. Kono DH Theofilopoulos AN. Genetics of lupus in mice, in *Systemic Lupus Erythematosus*, eds. R. G. Lahita, Academic Press, San Diego, 2011, 63-105.
20. Sakaguchi N, Takahashi T, Hata H, et al.: Altered thymic T-cell selection due to a mutation of the ZAP-70 gene causes autoimmune arthritis in mice, *Nature* 426:454–460, 2003.
21. Yang Y, Santamaria P: Lessons on autoimmune diabetes from animal models, *Clin Sci (Lond)* 110:627–639, 2006.
22. Benson RA, McInnes IB, Garside P, et al.: Model answers: rational application of murine models in arthritis research, *Eur J Immunol* 48:32–38, 2018.
23. Kouskoff V, Korganow AS, Duchatelle V, et al.: Organ-specific disease provoked by systemic autoimmunity, *Cell* 87:811–822, 1996.
24. Wipke BT, Wang Z, Kim J, et al.: Dynamic visualization of a joint-specific autoimmune response through positron emission tomography, *Nat Immunol* 3:366–372, 2002.
25. Matsumoto I, Lee DM, Goldbach-Mansky R, et al.: Low prevalence of antibodies to glucose-6-phosphate isomerase in patients with rheumatoid arthritis and a spectrum of other chronic autoimmune disorders, *Arthritis Rheum* 48:944–954, 2003.
26. van den Berg WB: Lessons from animal models of arthritis over the past decade, *Arthritis Res Ther* 11:250, 2009.
27. Goverman J, Woods A, Larson L, et al.: Transgenic mice that express a myelin basic protein-specific T cell receptor develop spontaneous autoimmunity, *Cell* 72:551–560, 1993.
28. Lafaille JJ, Nagashima K, Katsuki M, et al.: High incidence of spontaneous autoimmune encephalomyelitis in immunodeficient anti-myelin basic protein T cell receptor transgenic mice, *Cell* 78:399–408, 1994.
29. Katz JD, Wang B, Haskins K, et al.: Following a diabetogenic T cell from genesis through pathogenesis, *Cell* 74:1089–1100, 1993.
30. von Herrath MG, Evans CF, Horwitz MS, et al.: Using transgenic mouse models to dissect the pathogenesis of virus-induced autoimmune disorders of the islets of Langerhans and the central nervous system, *Immunol Rev* 152:111–143, 1996.
31. Akkaraju S, Canaan K, Goodnow CC: Self-reactive B cells are not eliminated or inactivated by autoantigen expressed on thyroid epithelial cells, *J Exp Med* 186:2005–2012, 1997.
32. Rathmell JC, Cooke MP, Ho WY, et al.: CD95 (Fas)-dependent elimination of self-reactive B cells upon interaction with CD4+ T cells, *Nature* 376:181–183, 1995.
33. Li Y, Li H, Ni D, et al.: Anti-DNA B cells in MRL/lpr mice show altered differentiation and editing pattern, *J Exp Med* 196:1543–1552, 2002.
34. Heltemes-Harris L, Liu X, Manser T: Progressive surface B cell antigen receptor down-regulation accompanies efficient development of antinuclear antigen B cells to mature, follicular phenotype, *J Immunol* 172:823–833, 2004.
35. Clarke SH: Anti-Sm B cell tolerance and tolerance loss in systemic lupus erythematosus, *Immunol Res* 41:203–216, 2008.
36. Murakami M, Honjo T: Anti-red blood cell autoantibody transgenic mice: murine model of autoimmune hemolytic anemia. [Review] [43 refs], *Semin Immunol* 8:3–9, 1996.
37. Kim-Saijo M, Akamizu T, Ikuta K, et al.: Generation of a transgenic animal model of hyperthyroid Graves' disease, *Eur J Immunol* 33:2531–2538, 2003.
38. Reeves WH, Lee PY, Weinstein JS, et al.: Induction of autoimmunity by pristane and other naturally occurring hydrocarbons, *Trends Immunol* 30:455–464, 2009.
39. Pollard KM, Hultman P, Kono DH: Immunology and genetics of induced systemic autoimmunity, *Autoimmun Rev* 4:282–288, 2005.
40. Via CS: Advances in lupus stemming from the parent-into-F1 model, *Trends Immunol* 31:236–245, 2010.
41. Yu X, Petersen F: A methodological review of induced animal models of autoimmune diseases, *Autoimmun Rev* 17:473–479, 2018.
42. Hill JA, Bell DA, Brintnell W, et al.: Arthritis induced by post-translationally modified (citrullinated) fibrinogen in DR4-IE transgenic mice, *J Exp Med* 205:967–979, 2008.
43. Kinloch AJ, Alzabin S, Brintnell W, et al.: Immunization with Porphyromonas gingivalis enolase induces autoimmunity to mammalian alpha-enolase and arthritis in DR4-IE-transgenic mice, *Arthritis Rheum* 63:3818–3823, 2011.
44. Burnet FM: Immunological recognition of self, *Science* 133:307–311, 1961.
45. Billingham RE, Brent L, Medawar PB: Actively acquired tolerance of foreign cells, *Nature* 172:603–606, 1953.
46. Bretscher P, Cohn M: A theory of self-nonself discrimination, *Science* 169:1042–1049, 1970.
47. Lafferty KJ, Cunningham AJ: A new analysis of allogeneic interactions, *Aust J Exp Biol Med Sci* 53:27–42, 1975.
48. Jenkins MK, Schwartz RH: Antigen presentation by chemically modified splenocytes induces antigen-specific T cell unresponsiveness in vitro and in vivo, *J Exp Med* 165:302–319, 1987.
49. Janeway Jr CA: Approaching the asymptote? Evolution and revolution in immunology, *Cold Spring Harb Symp Quant Biol* 54(Pt 1):1–13, 1989.
50. Matzinger P: Tolerance, danger, and the extended family, *Annu Rev Immunol* 12:991–1045, 1994.

51. Ohashi PS, DeFranco AL: Making and breaking tolerance, *Curr Opin Immunol* 14:744–759, 2002.
52. Goodnow CC, Vinuesa CG, Randall KL, et al.: Control systems and decision making for antibody production, *Nat Immunol* 11:681–688, 2010.
53. Goodnow CC: Multistep pathogenesis of autoimmune disease, *Cell* 130:25–35, 2007.
54. Zikherman J, Parameswaran R, Weiss A: Endogenous antigen tunes the responsiveness of naive B cells but not T cells, *Nature* 489:160–164, 2012.
55. Janeway Jr CA, Medzhitov R: Innate immune recognition, *Annu Rev Immunol* 20:197–216, 2002.
56. Piccinini AM, Midwood KS: DAMPening inflammation by modulating TLR signalling, *Mediators Inflamm* 2010, 2010.
57. Iwasaki A, Medzhitov R: Regulation of adaptive immunity by the innate immune system, *Science* 327:291–295, 2010.
58. Wu J, Chen ZJ: Innate immune sensing and signaling of cytosolic nucleic acids, *Annu Rev Immunol* 32:461–488, 2014.
59. Brubaker SW, Bonham KS, Zanoni I, et al.: Innate immune pattern recognition: a cell biological perspective, *Annu Rev Immunol* 33:257–290, 2015.
60. Theofilopoulos AN, Gonzalez-Quintial R, Lawson BR, et al.: Sensors of the innate immune system: their link to rheumatic diseases, *Nat Rev Rheumatol* 6:146–156, 2010.
61. Wagner H: The sweetness of the DNA backbone drives Toll-like receptor 9, *Curr Opin Immunol* 20:396–400, 2008.
62. Maldonado RA, von Andrian UH: How tolerogenic dendritic cells induce regulatory T cells, *Adv Immunol* 108:111–165, 2010.
63. Mayer CT, Berod L, Sparwasser T: Layers of dendritic cell-mediated T cell tolerance, their regulation and the prevention of autoimmunity, *Front Immunol* 3:183, 2012.
64. Ravichandran KS: Find-me and eat-me signals in apoptotic cell clearance: progress and conundrums, *J Exp Med* 207:1807–1817, 2010.
65. Colonna L, Lood C, Elkon KB: Beyond apoptosis in lupus, *Curr Opin Rheumatol* 26:459–466, 2014.
66. Nagata S, Hanayama R, Kawane K: Autoimmunity and the clearance of dead cells, *Cell* 140:619–630, 2010.
67. Rothlin CV, Lemke G: TAM receptor signaling and autoimmune disease, *Curr Opin Immunol* 22:740–746, 2010.
68. Hanayama R, Tanaka M, Miyasaka K, et al.: Autoimmune disease and impaired uptake of apoptotic cells in MFG-E8-deficient mice, *Science* 304:1147–1150, 2004.
69. Peng Y, Elkon KB: Autoimmunity in MFG-E8-deficient mice is associated with altered trafficking and enhanced cross-presentation of apoptotic cell antigens, *J Clin Invest* 121:2221–2241, 2011.
70. Miyanishi M, Segawa K, Nagata S: Synergistic effect of Tim4 and MFG-E8 null mutations on the development of autoimmunity, *Int Immunol* 24:551–559, 2012.
71. Uderhardt S, Herrmann M, Oskolkova OV, et al.: 12/15-lipoxygenase orchestrates the clearance of apoptotic cells and maintains immunologic tolerance, *Immunity* 36:834–846, 2012.
72. Botto M: Links between complement deficiency and apoptosis, *Arthritis Res* 3:207–210, 2001.
73. Chen Y, Khanna S, Goodyear CS, et al.: Regulation of dendritic cells and macrophages by an anti-apoptotic cell natural antibody that suppresses TLR responses and inhibits inflammatory arthritis, *J Immunol* 183:1346–1359, 2009.
74. Ehrenstein MR, Notley CA: The importance of natural IgM: scavenger, protector and regulator, *Nat Rev Immunol* 10:778–786, 2010.
75. Ramirez-Ortiz ZG, Pendergraft 3rd WF, Prasad A, et al.: The scavenger receptor SCARF1 mediates the clearance of apoptotic cells and prevents autoimmunity, *Nat Immunol* 14:917–926, 2013.
76. Cook HT, Botto M: Mechanisms of disease: the complement system and the pathogenesis of systemic lupus erythematosus, *Nat Clin Pract Rheumatol* 2:330–337, 2006.
77. Ling GS, Crawford G, Buang N, et al.: C1q restrains autoimmunity and viral infection by regulating CD8(+) T cell metabolism, *Science* 360:558–563, 2018.
78. Liu J, Miwa T, Hilliard B, et al.: The complement inhibitory protein DAF (CD55) suppresses T cell immunity in vivo, *J Exp Med* 201:567–577, 2005.
79. Miwa T, Maldonado MA, Zhou L, et al.: Deletion of decay-accelerating factor (CD55) exacerbates autoimmune disease development in MRL/lpr mice, *Am J Pathol* 161:1077–1086, 2002.
80. Knight JS, Kaplan MJ: Lupus neutrophils: 'NET' gain in understanding lupus pathogenesis, *Curr Opin Rheumatol* 24:441–450, 2012.
81. McCaughtry TM, Hogquist KA: Central tolerance: what have we learned from mice? *Semin Immunopathol* 30:399–409, 2008.
82. Jenkins MK, Chu HH, McLachlan JB, et al.: On the composition of the preimmune repertoire of T cells specific for peptide-major histocompatibility complex ligands, *Annu Rev Immunol* 28:275–294, 2010.
83. Zinkernagel RM, Pircher HP, Ohashi P, et al.: T and B cell tolerance and responses to viral antigens in transgenic mice: implications for the pathogenesis of autoimmune versus immunopathological disease, *Immunological reviews* 122:133–171, 1991.
84. Weller RO, Galea I, Carare RO, et al.: Pathophysiology of the lymphatic drainage of the central nervous system: Implications for pathogenesis and therapy of multiple sclerosis, *Pathophysiology* 17:295–306, 2010.
85. Engelhardt B, Vajkoczy P, Weller RO: The movers and shapers in immune privilege of the CNS, *Nat Immunol* 18:123–131, 2017.
86. Louveau A, Harris TH, Kipnis J: Revisiting the mechanisms of CNS immune privilege, *Trends Immunol* 36:569–577, 2015.
87. Kawakami N, Flugel A: Knocking at the brain's door: intravital two-photon imaging of autoreactive T cell interactions with CNS structures, *Semin Immunopathol* 32:275–287, 2010.
88. Niederkorn JY: See no evil, hear no evil, do no evil: the lessons of immune privilege, *Nat Immunol* 7:354–359, 2006.
89. Caspi RR: A look at autoimmunity and inflammation in the eye, *J Clin Invest* 120:3073–3083, 2010.
90. Steinman RM, Hawiger D, Nussenzweig MC: Tolerogenic dendritic cells, *Annu Rev Immunol* 21:685–711, 2003.
91. Smigiel KS, Srivastava S, Stolley JM, et al.: Regulatory T-cell homeostasis: steady-state maintenance and modulation during inflammation, *Immunol Rev* 259:40–59, 2014.
92. Grant CR, Liberal R, Mieli-Vergani G, et al.: Regulatory T-cells in autoimmune diseases: Challenges, controversies and-yet-unanswered questions, *Autoimmun Rev* 14:105–116, 2015.
93. Ohkura N, Kitagawa Y, Sakaguchi S: Development and maintenance of regulatory T cells, *Immunity* 38:414–423, 2013.
94. Liston A, Gray DH: Homeostatic control of regulatory T cell diversity, *Nat Rev Immunol* 14:154–165, 2014.
95. Dominguez-Villar M, Hafler DA: Regulatory T cells in autoimmune disease, *Nat Immunol* 19:665–673, 2018.
96. Wing JB, Tanaka A, Sakaguchi S: Human FOXP3(+) regulatory T cell heterogeneity and function in autoimmunity and cancer, *Immunity* 50:302–316, 2019.
97. Sakaguchi S, Yamaguchi T, Nomura T, et al.: Regulatory T cells and immune tolerance, *Cell* 133:775–787, 2008.
98. Tarbell KV, Yamazaki S, Olson K, et al.: CD25+ CD4+ T cells, expanded with dendritic cells presenting a single autoantigenic peptide, suppress autoimmune diabetes, *J Exp Med* 199:1467–1477, 2004.
99. Wing JB, Tekguc M, Sakaguchi S: Control of germinal center responses by T-follicular regulatory cells, *Front Immunol* 9:1910, 2018.
100. Zhou L, Chong MM, Littman DR: Plasticity of CD4+ T cell lineage differentiation, *Immunity* 30:646–655, 2009.
101. Komatsu N, Okamoto K, Sawa S, et al.: Pathogenic conversion of Foxp3+ T cells into TH17 cells in autoimmune arthritis, *Nat Med* 20:62–68, 2014.
102. Levine AG, Mendoza A, Hemmers S, et al.: Stability and function of regulatory T cells expressing the transcription factor T-bet, *Nature* 546:421–425, 2017.

103. Panduro M, Benoist C, Mathis D: Tissue Tregs, *Annu Rev Immunol* 34:609–633, 2016.
104. Apetoh L, Quintana FJ, Pot C, et al.: The aryl hydrocarbon receptor interacts with c-Maf to promote the differentiation of type 1 regulatory T cells induced by IL-27, *Nat Immunol* 11:854–861, 2010.
105. Blink SE, Miller SD: The contribution of gammadelta T cells to the pathogenesis of EAE and MS, *Curr Mol Med* 9:15–22, 2009.
106. Dinesh RK, Skaggs BJ, La Cava A, et al.: CD8+ Tregs in lupus, autoimmunity, and beyond, *Autoimmun Rev* 9:560–568, 2010.
107. Jiang H, Chess L: Qa-1/HLA-E-restricted regulatory CD8+ T cells and self-nonself discrimination: an essay on peripheral T-cell regulation, *Hum Immunol* 69:721–727, 2008.
108. Fujio K, Okamura T, Yamamoto K: The family of IL-10-secreting CD4+ T cells, *Adv Immunol* 105:99–130, 2010.
109. Bluestone JA, Buckner JH, Fitch M, et al.: Type 1 diabetes immunotherapy using polyclonal regulatory T cells, *Sci Transl Med* 7:315ra189, 2015.
110. Marek-Trzonkowska N, Mysliwiec M, Iwaszkiewicz-Grzes D, et al.: Factors affecting long-term efficacy of T regulatory cell-based therapy in type 1 diabetes, *J Transl Med* 14:332, 2016.
111. Clemente-Casares X, Blanco J, Ambalavanan P, et al.: Expanding antigen-specific regulatory networks to treat autoimmunity, *Nature* 530:434–440, 2016.
112. Wing K, Sakaguchi S: Regulatory T cells exert checks and balances on self tolerance and autoimmunity, *Nat Immunol* 11:7–13, 2010.
113. Francisco LM, Sage PT, Sharpe AH: The PD-1 pathway in tolerance and autoimmunity, *Immunol Rev* 236:219–242, 2010.
114. Caspi RR: Ocular autoimmunity: the price of privilege? *Immunol Rev* 213:23–35, 2006.
115. Fletcher AL, Malhotra D, Turley SJ: Lymph node stroma broaden the peripheral tolerance paradigm, *Trends Immunol* 32:12–18, 2011.
116. Turley SJ, Fletcher AL, Elpek KG: The stromal and haematopoietic antigen-presenting cells that reside in secondary lymphoid organs, *Nat Rev Immunol* 10:813–825, 2010.
117. Streilein JW: Ocular immune privilege: therapeutic opportunities from an experiment of nature, *Nat Rev Immunol* 3:879–889, 2003.
118. Matzinger P, Kamala T: Tissue-based class control: the other side of tolerance, *Nat Rev Immunol* 11:221–230, 2011.
119. Finkelman FD: Relationships among antigen presentation, cytokines, immune deviation, and autoimmune disease, *J Exp Med* 182:279–282, 1995.
120. Grajewski RS, Hansen AM, Agarwal RK, et al.: Activation of invariant NKT cells ameliorates experimental ocular autoimmunity by a mechanism involving innate IFN-gamma production and dampening of the adaptive Th1 and Th17 responses, *J Immunol* 181:4791–4797, 2008.

23 The Microbiome in Health and Disease

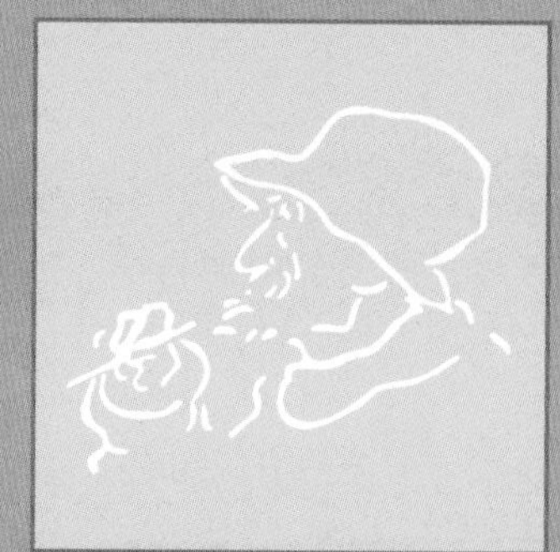

ROB KNIGHT

KEY POINTS

The human microbiome is a complex ecosystem that contains more cells than the human body and at least as many as 100 times the number of genes as the human genome.

Different parts of the body have different microbiomes with almost no overlap in species among them; however, the gut microbiome, in particular, can produce chemical and immunologic effects throughout the body.

Unlike the human genome, which is almost identical between different people, the human microbiome is almost completely different between different people; however, within a single person, it is relatively stable over time.

Sources of variation in the microbiome include age, long-term diet, geography, medications (including those other than antibiotics), and disease; however, human genetics has a surprisingly modest impact.

Many diseases throughout the body, including inflammatory bowel disease, cardiovascular disease, rheumatoid arthritis, multiple sclerosis, Parkinson's disease, and autism, have been associated with the gut microbiome in humans and have been studied in depth in animal models to determine mechanism.

Study of the human microbiome is highly interdisciplinary; it combines ideas from microbiology, biochemistry, molecular biology, ecology, statistics, and computer science.

The links between inflammatory arthritis and the gut and oral microbiomes in rodents and humans were some of the first examples of long-range interactions that drove the field; further mechanisms, which link the microbiome to specific biochemical and immunologic pathways in the host, point the way to applying these principles to rheumatic diseases, generally.

The Human Microbiome

The view that each human is a single physiologic unit specified by the human genome is giving way to the view that each of us is an ecosystem, and the human body is host to trillions of microbes. Many gene functions, which we require for health, are encoded not in our own genome but in these microbial genomes (the microbiome); therefore, the extensive variation in the microbiome may be more closely associated with diseases, especially those linked to the immune system, than variation in the human genome. Furthermore, unlike the human genome, which is fixed at conception, the human microbiome changes during development and can be further modified through diet, medications, and lifestyle factors, which provides new avenues for therapy.

Fifteen years ago, little was known about the human microbiome, and it was widely assumed that the differences in colonization between different individuals could be of little importance for health. This view was exacerbated by the difficulty of growing most kinds of microbes associated with the human body, under standard culture conditions, and by the difficulty of distinguishing microbes by microscopy. However, the rise of culture-independent methods (so-called *next-generation sequencing* techniques that reduced the cost of obtaining DNA sequences by orders of magnitude) and advances in computational tools led to an explosion of association studies linking the human microbiome to a wide range of different diseases; these approaches were complemented with laboratory studies, including the powerful gnotobiotic mouse model, that allowed key mechanisms linking the microbiome to diseases throughout the body to be deduced.[1,2] Among the first diseases outside the gut to be linked to the gut microbiome using these techniques was rheumatoid arthritis (RA)[3]; although progress linking the gut microbiome has been more rapid in other areas of medicine. This chapter describes what the microbiome is, principles of host-microbe interactions, experimental and computational techniques for assessing microbiome changes, what is known about the microbiome's effects throughout the body, and how these techniques will likely be applicable in the future to understanding, diagnosing, and treating rheumatic diseases.

What Is the Microbiome?

Each of our bodies is host to ~39 trillion microbial cells, outnumbering the ~30 trillion human cells that we think of as "us."[4] These microbial cells constitute what is known as the *microbiota*; their genes, the microbiome.[5] However, in colloquial use, the "microbiome" is often used to describe the organisms as well. Astonishing as the idea is that we are only 43% human at the cell level, the disparity is even more profound when we consider unique genes. At latest count, the human genome contains 21,306 protein-coding genes,[6] but estimates of the size of the gene catalog of the human microbiome obtained by different methods have consistently ranged from 2 million to 20 million,[5,7–10] which is orders of magnitude larger. Although billions of dollars have been spent linking the human genome to disease, the much larger number of unique genes in the microbiome, with their antigens and biochemical activities that are absent from the human genome, have received far less attention, although recent evidence suggests that they are at least as closely linked to many clinically relevant traits, such

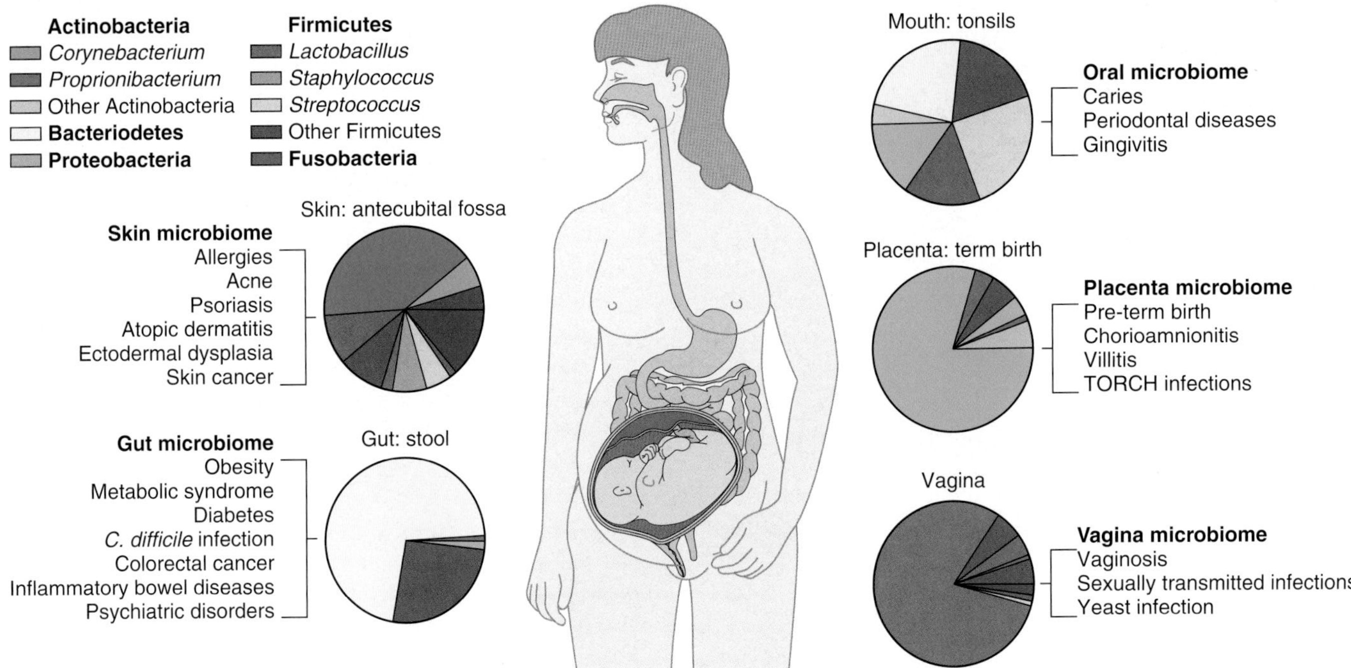

• **Fig. 23.1** Distribution of microbes across the body, and links to human diseases. Many microbiomes, most notably the gut microbiome, have effects at distal sites. (From José E. Belizário and Mauro Napolitano: Human microbiomes and their roles in dysbiosis, common diseases, and novel therapeutic approaches. Front. Microbiol., 06 October 2015.)

as high-density lipoprotein (HDL) cholesterol, lactose consumption, waist and hip circumference, and body mass index (BMI), as they are human genes.[11] Furthermore, each individual's human genes are fixed at conception (barring a few mutations), but one's microbial genes change profoundly throughout the first 3 years of life and continue to be plastic throughout the lifespan. Therefore, the potential for fundamentally new therapeutic approaches is tremendous, although the potential for non–evidence-based false hope is also considerable.

Microbes in the human body (Fig. 23.1) have a wide range of physiologic effects and come from all three domains of cellular life—the bacteria, the archaea, and the eukaryotes—plus viruses. Most attention has focused on the causative agents of infectious disease, such as the bacterium enteropathogenic *Escherichia coli* (EPEC), the fungus *Candida albicans*, or viruses, such as herpes simplex virus 1 (HSV-1). However, the vast majority of the cells in the microbiota, and the vast majority of unique strains and species, are harmless or beneficial.

Two important myths about the microbiome were dispelled by the high-throughput molecular techniques described later in the chapter. First, it was once assumed that each person had "a microbiome," given the ability of microbes to transfer across the body. Second, it was assumed that we all share a "core microbiome" that consists of a sizeable fraction of the total number of species, decorated with relatively unimportant variations. For example, at the planning meeting for the National Institutes of Health (NIH)-funded Human Microbiome Project at the Banbury Center at Cold Spring Harbor in 2008, much of the discussion focused on the idea that a human microbiome project would be like a human genome project, in which one individual is sequenced deeply, and then a population study is performed to identify the variants against this background. Both concepts turned out to be completely wrong. Even in the NIH-funded Human Microbiome Project, the number of shared genera declined precipitously as the number of subjects examined increased, and the different sites on the body separated radically from one another,[8] such that the difference in microbial ecology between the mouth and gut of the same person were as different from one another as the microbes in the water from a coral reef versus the microbes in the soil of a prairie[12] (Fig. 23.2). Attempts to find correlations among different microbiome sites in healthy people have largely failed, despite substantial effort. However, clinical observations of different microbiomes as biomarkers for clinical disease at distal sites, including RA,[3] suggest that such connections may exist in diseased states (see Fig. 23.1).

Principles of Host-Microbiome Interaction

Intriguingly, although the range of taxonomic composition of the microbiome at a given body site varies dramatically, the range of functions encoded by their gene products is much more consistent. In the Human Microbiome Project data, two samples from the gut that are completely different in terms of the families of microbes they contain have a consistent repertoire of gene functions, which differentiates them from the mouth or from the vagina.[8] Just as in other ecological systems, completely different species assemblages can converge on the same functional result. For example, grasslands or rainforests in South America and Africa can look remarkably similar across continents, even though no species are shared between the grasslands or between the rainforests in the two continents. Because of the complexity of understanding the interactions of the many genes in the microbiome, and because most of their functions are either not known or known only at very high levels (for example, "transporter protein"), most work to date has focused on associating particular categories of gene functions with the phenotypic state of the host, or on studies of the functions of individual genes in individual species of bacteria (mostly pathogens). Consequently, there is still much to discover

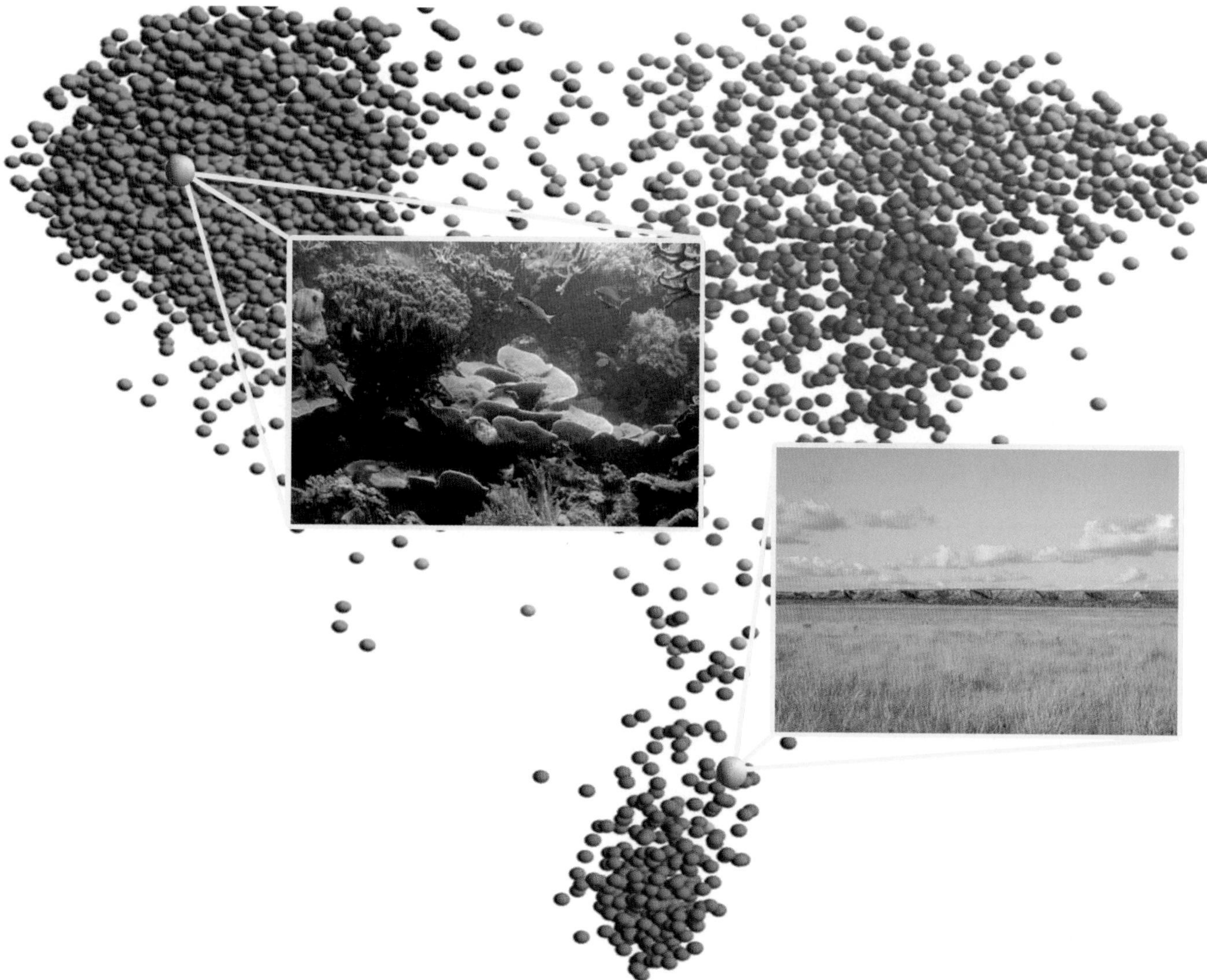

• **Fig. 23.2** Differences in microbial ecology in different parts of the same individual's body are vastly different to one another, and indeed comparable to the differences between different physical environments. This Principal Coordinates Analysis plot, which is based on UniFrac distances, integrates the Human Microbiome Project data with the Earth Microbiome Project data. Different colors represent different human body habitats. The layout algorithm calculates distances between each pair of samples using a phylogenetic tree relating the bacteria in those samples *(UniFrac)*; two points are closer if they share more similar microbes, and farther apart if their microbes are more dissimilar. The figure highlights the idea that the microbial community distance between the oral and fecal microbiome of one subject *(yellow points)* is comparable to the microbial community distance between microbes in the water of a coral reef and microbes in the soil of a prairie, as measured by UniFrac.

about these functional relationships and mechanisms that associate specific microbial genes and their molecular products with disease. However, progress can be made despite this complexity. One analogy is to nutrition: although running a sample of your morning cup of coffee through a mass spectrometer will result in thousands of mass peaks, mostly representing molecules that have never been characterized, we know that caffeine is an active ingredient that explains many of its physiologic effects. Similarly, individual microbes within microbiomes can have large effects, as in the case of *Prevotella copri* in inducting RA,[3] or *Christensenella* spp. in reducing adiposity.[13] In both cases, microbial strains of large effect were identified in population studies, then isolated and transferred into rodent models to demonstrate activity that explained the effects.

Because microbial genes are both more numerous and more diverse than human genes, they provide many molecular functions that are not provided by proteins encoded in the human genome. For example, they can synthesize vitamins and branched-chain amino acids (although not in amounts sufficient for health), antibiotics, secondary bile acids, and many other compounds. Individual species such as *Clostridium sporogenes* metabolize aromatic amino acids into compounds that accumulate in plasma, such as indole-propionic acid[14]; other classes of enzyme, such as trimethylamine lyase (TMA lyase) are more broadly distributed in different groups of bacteria and process dietary carnitine and choline into trimethylamine, which is then processed into trimethylamine-N-oxide (TMAO) in the liver and contributes to atherosclerosis through an inflammatory process.[15] It has even been estimated that ~10% of metabolites circulating in mammalian blood are derived from microbes.[16] Microbially derived metabolites can explain complex interactions among diet, the microbiome, and susceptibility to both chronic and infectious disease. For example, desaminotyrosine, a compound produced from dietary flavonoids by particular strains of bacteria, reduces mortality of mice exposed to influenza from 95% to 25% by priming the amplification loop of Type I interferon signaling, but both the microbes and the dietary precursors of the molecule are required to achieve this effect.[17] Because this result was both unexpected and recent, it is likely that further work in humans will uncover unexpected links among diet, the microbiome, the immune system, and disease susceptibility.

What Affects the Microbiome?

The microbiome within a body site is affected by many factors, and different studies are beginning to agree on which of these factors have the largest effect size. Despite intense interest in the question of whether host genetics shape the human microbiome, the effects of human genes on microbiome composition have been remarkably modest, explaining less than 2% of the variation in the gut microbiome overall in multiple studies, including twin studies and studies that assess the human genotype directly[11,13,18,19]; host genetic effects on the oral microbiome have similarly been minimal.[20,21] The most profound impact on the microbiome is the age of the subject; newborns have largely undifferentiated microbiomes that depend primarily on delivery mode, with the microbiomes in all body habitats of newborns delivered vaginally resembling the microbiome of their mother's vagina, whereas those delivered by C-section instead resemble adult skin.[22] The gut microbiome then develops to resemble the adult state over the first 3 years of life (Fig. 23.3),[19,23] with the development of other microbiomes not yet studied at the same level of temporal resolution.

Within adults, the largest single driving effect on microbiomes across the body is lifestyle. Hunter-gatherers, such as the Yanomami in the Amazon basin and the Hadza in Africa's Great Rift Valley, have markedly different microbiomes across the body, including entire phyla that are not found in populations that have taken up farming, let alone those that inhabit air-conditioned dwellings in urbanized environments.[24–29] For example, spirochetes appear to have been lost from the gut in most human populations, except those living the most remote lifestyles; in contrast, Verrucomicrobia (primarily *Akkermansia muciniphila*) and *Bacteroides spp.* are far more common in more industrialized populations.[29]

The second strongest effect in the gut, which has been better studied than other habitats, is diet, with the ratio of proteins to carbohydrates in particular having a large influence of the ratio of two major taxa, *Bacteroides* and *Prevotella*[30]; and the number of different species of plants and the frequency of consumption of salty and sugary snacks also has notable effects.[31] However, long-term diet seems to have the most important effect; studies attempting to shift the microbiome using even extreme short-term dietary interventions have had surprisingly modest effect sizes, with changes typically being small compared with the differences among individuals and often with the same intervention driving the microbiome in different directions in different individuals.[30,32]

Medications, including antibiotics and proton pump inhibitors, have large effects on the microbiome in large cohort studies,[31,33,34] although concordance in the ranks of these effect sizes has generally been poor. However, in vitro studies demonstrate that many medications not previously thought of as anti-microbial have large effects on the growth and survival of individual human gut microbes, including antipsychotics.[35] Age among adults consistently has a large impact on the gut microbiome[19,23,31,33,34]; it is not as dramatic as during the first 3 years of life, but it likely acts as an important confounding factor in many studies seeking links between the human microbiome and disease phenotypes. Household has a surprisingly large effect, with co-habiting adults typically converging in terms of their microbiome at multiple sites on the body including the gut, mouth, and skin.[11,36] Indeed, dog owners and their dogs come to resemble one another in terms of their microbiome. This observation is consistent with the observation that cage effects on the microbiome in mice are large and that therefore

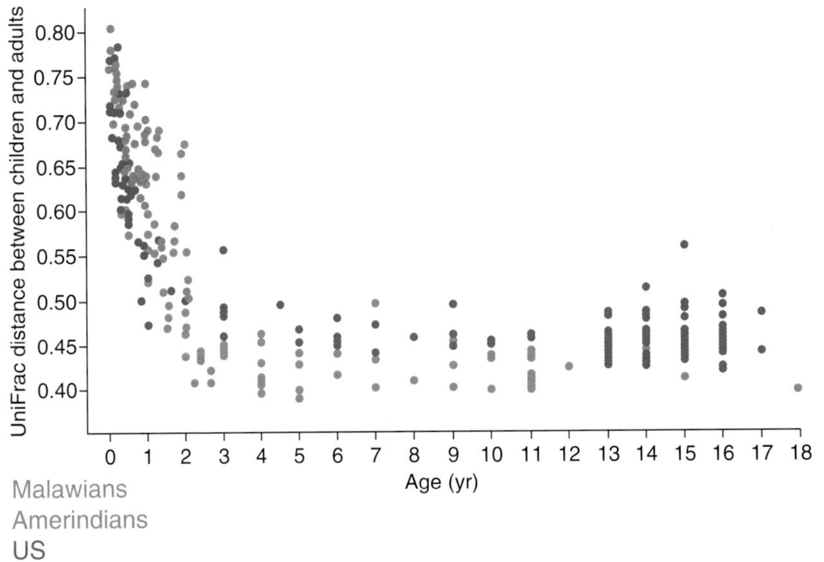

• **Fig. 23.3** Approach of the developing infant gut microbiome to the adult state during the first 3 years of life. UniFrac distances between children and adults decrease with increasing age of children in each population. Each point indicates the average distance between a child and all adults who are from the same country but are, otherwise, unrelated; the vast majority of the convergence to the adult state completes by 3 years of age. Results derive from bacterial V4 16S rRNA gene amplicon data. (From Yatsunenko T, Rey FE, Manary MJ, et al.: Human gut microbiome viewed across age and geography. *Nature* 486(7402):222–227, 2012.)

experiments linking specific factors, such as single-gene knockouts, to the microbiome must be repeated in many cages to be reliable[37] (although coprophagy rates are presumably lower among humans, the fecal-oral route is still important in our species for spreading pathogenic microbes, and may also spread nonpathogens). Intriguingly, according to one case study, surgery dramatically affected the human gut microbiome; in 1 day, an 8-inch resection of the sigmoid colon achieved a difference within the patient comparable to the largest differences among individuals.[31] Similarly, effects of bariatric surgery on the gut microbiome have been reported to be very large.[38] Intriguingly, in bariatric surgery, the change in the microbiome is remarkably fast and is linked to metabolic changes in weight loss before reduced caloric intake could have an effect; however, the mechanisms of these changes—and whether the metabolic switch can trigger without surgery—are still active areas of research as of this writing. A general theory of large versus small effects on the microbiome, and how to reshape the microbiome in specific directions, has yet to develop.

How Is the Microbiome Determined From a Sample?

The current state of microbiome science is that there are many association studies in humans, and causal mechanistic work primarily in mouse models, but little in the way of commercially available and medically validated microbiome-based diagnostics or therapeutics. However, the potential for such therapeutics is high given the advanced state of animal model work.

There are several different approaches to reading out the microbiome, and each way has specific strengths and weaknesses (Fig. 23.4).[2,39,40] Traditional microbiologic work relies on culturing organisms, typically in liquid culture or on a petri dish, but is limited to the minority of organisms that can be cultured. However, culture-based assays are still the gold standard for infectious disease diagnosis. Culture-independent approaches, which rely on direct molecular analysis of the sample, are able to reveal more of the microbial community including those organisms that are difficult or impossible to culture, but are typically not yet as sensitive as culture-based assays, which in some cases can detect a single cell of a pathogen.

One of the most important culture-independent approaches is 16S rRNA gene amplicon sequencing, which relies on the universal nature of the 16S rRNA gene (the product of which forms the backbone of the small subunit of the ribosome) and the presence of both conserved regions that act as anchors for polymerase chain reaction (PCR) primers and variable regions, which can be used as nametags for identification of particular organisms. In this approach, a specific region of the 16S rRNA gene is amplified and sequenced, providing a readout of what kinds of organisms are in a specific sample. However, 16S rRNA analysis is limited because different species can be identical along the length of the amplified fragment, or even along the length of the entire 16S rRNA. Alternative markers, such as the internally transcribed spacer (ITS) region, can provide more specific identifications at the expense of generality because this region evolves so rapidly in bacteria that different PCR primers must be designed for each genus. However, fungal ITS sequencing is widely used for fungal taxonomic identification, in part because the 18S rRNA is identical for entire families of fungi and therefore cannot be used for specific identifications. Designing good PCR primers is difficult, and using well-established primer pairs, such as the 515-806 pair (relative to the *E. coli* 16S rRNA) used by the Earth Microbiome Project,[12,41] is a better plan than designing new primers from scratch.

Other forms of culture-independent nucleic acid sequence analysis that are widely used are shotgun metagenomics (analysis of the total DNA in a sample), and shotgun metatranscriptomics (analysis of total RNA). Shotgun metagenomics, in principle, provides access to all of the organisms in a sample, including viruses and fungi (which cannot be seen with 16S rRNA gene amplicon sequencing because they do not have 16S rRNA genes) with resolution down to single nucleotide variants. However, this increased resolution comes at much greater expense (traditionally, 100 to 1000 times the sequencing cost) and much greater computational difficulty. There are two general strategies to analyzing metagenomic or metatranscriptomic data. The first, reference-based, relies on mapping sequences to a reference database using tools, such as Kraken[42] or Centrifuge.[43] However, sequences that are not in the reference database are missed, which is problematic especially for types of body habitats or human populations that have not been extensively studied, and the rate of off-target matches is high enough that careful filtering is required to avoid false positive detection of pathogens (or even of species that are definitely not in the sample, such as the duck-billed platypus[44]). The second is known as *assembly-based*, and it relies on putting together an incredibly complex puzzle of tens of millions to billions of short (typically, 150 to 250 base pairs) DNA fragments into complete genomes, or, more typically, *contigs*, which represent fragments of genomes with algorithms, such as MetaSPAdes.[45] These longer assemblies can be assigned to particular taxonomic groups more reliably than short-read DNA sequences, but the assembly procedure is extremely computationally expensive and cannot be performed on an ordinary laptop or desktop computer.

Technologies that offer longer DNA sequence reads than Illumina sequencing (e.g., PacBio or Oxford Nanopore), synthetic long-read technologies (e.g., Illumina TSLR [now discontinued]), or 10X offer considerable promise because long sequences are much easier to assemble than short ones. However, these techniques are expensive and more error prone than Illumina sequencing, which limits current applicability. Once the sequences, assembled or unassembled, have been obtained, the next step is to assign functions to each gene, typically by matching them against reference databases of genes with known functions.[46] An intriguing recent approach is using shallow-coverage (1 million sequences per sample) short-read DNA sequencing with statistical corrections to perform taxonomic characterization on a sample; the cost can be comparable to 16S rRNA amplicon profiling, but accuracy is not affected by PCR primers.[47] Considerations with RNA analysis are similar to those with DNA analysis, except that transcripts cannot be assembled into complete genomes. In principle, transcripts yield useful information about gene expression that cannot be obtained at the DNA level, but RNA degrades very rapidly (the median half-life of an mRNA in *E. coli* is 2 to 5 minutes depending on growth rate),[48] so samples must be preserved very rapidly to prevent degradation artifacts. The interpretation of metatranscriptomic data in biospecimens (e.g., stool) is unclear.

Beyond nucleic acid analysis, metaproteomics (analysis of the proteins in a complex sample by multidimensional liquid chromatography followed by tandem mass spectrometry) and metabolomics (analysis of the small molecules, typically by gas chromatography or liquid chromatography followed by tandem mass spectrometry) hold considerable promise for microbiome analysis, but these are still very much emerging techniques.

Broad view					Narrow view
Metabolomics (non-protein small molecules)	**Metaproteomics** (protein) **Metatranscriptomics** (RNA)	**Shotgun sequencing** (complete genomes, "Metagenomics")	**Amplicon sequencing** (partial genomes)	**PCR panels** (qPCR, RT-PCR)	**Culture** (traditional method for bacteria; also some archaea and viruses)
All small molecules made by all organisms present Targeted: better for known metabolites (i.e., bile acids) Non-targeted: better for novel compounds, discovery Good for looking at functional changes No link to specific organisms	All protein or RNA made by all organisms present Good for looking at functional changes No link to specific organisms	Every organism present will have most of the genomes sequenced: all bacteria fungi, viruses, etc. This includes the host/patient, discuss if using biopsy samples All organisms present No functional changes	Most selected organisms present, depending on method used (no viruses) Most selected organisms present — uses 16S, 18S or ITS as "barcode"	Can include a single type or a select combination of organisms Generally up to around 24 per sample Limited in scope to known specific organisms in selected panel	A small number of known organisms that will grow on specific media under aerobic conditions Anaerobes can be isolated and grown, but many difficulties are present Limited in scope to known organisms under specific conditions
All organisms (including host)	RNA viruses and all organisms (including host)	All organisms (including host)	Bacteria and some archaea for 16S Eukaryotes only for 18S Fungi only for ITS	Viruses and other selected organisms (depends on panel used)	Bacteria, fungi, archaea, and viruses (depends on media used)
High throughput 96 samples per run ~48 hours $$$	High throughput 96-384 samples per run ~48 hours $$$$	High throughput 384 samples per run ~48 hours $$$	High throughput 384 samples per run ~48 hours $$	Low throughput Max 30 pooled samples per run 1 to 5 hours $$	Low throughput 1 sample per media used 24 to 48 hours $

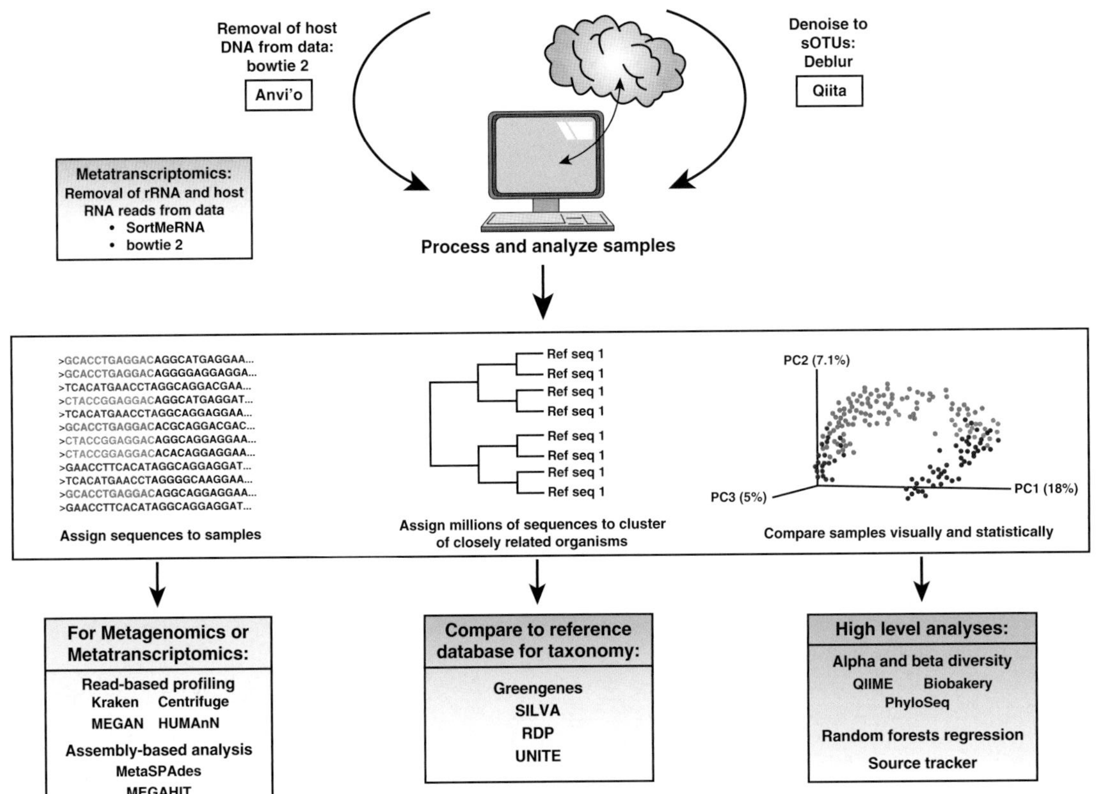

• **Fig. 23.4** Once samples are collected, the samples can be put through molecular preparations and DNA sequencing to generate microbiome data. Two common types of protocols are amplicon sequencing and shotgun sequencing. In amplicon sequencing, the polymerase chain reaction (PCR) primers are used to target a specific region of a specific gene, focusing sequencing effort on just those fragments. One of the most widely used protocols targets the V4 region of the 16S rRNA gene. In shotgun sequencing, the DNA in the sample is randomly sheared and sequenced, generating data from many different parts of the genome. The specifics of the molecular protocol used before shotgun sequencing are important for what type of data are being examined, and this type of sequencing can be used, for example, for metagenomics and metatranscriptomics. The initial processing performed on the data after sequencing depends on the type of sequencing performed. For amplicon studies, one common strategy is to upload the data into Qiita and to use Deblur to resolve sequence data into single-sequence variants called sub-operational taxonomic units (sOTUs). Taxonomic assignments, generally, are performed using naive Bayes classifiers, such as the Ribosomal Database Project (RDP) classifier, as implemented in the q2-feature-classifier against reference databases, such as Greengenes, SILVA, RDP, or UNITE (fungal internal transcribed spacer [ITS]) depending on the amplicon target. Shotgun sequencing of host-associated samples first requires preprocessing to remove either host DNA before analysis. Typically, the shotgun data then are summarized using tools, such as Kraken, MEtaGenome ANalyzer (MEGAN), or HUMAnN2 to generate taxonomic or functional profiles, or are assembled with tools, such as metaSPAdes and MEGAHIT. For both sequencing methods, higher-level analyses (e.g., α and β diversity, taxonomic profiling, and machine learning) subsequently are used to assay patterns of microbiome variation in the context of the study design. Metagenomic assemblies also can be analyzed through platforms, such as Anvi'o.SourceTracker, a Bayesian estimator of the sources that make up each unknown community, which is useful for classifying microbial samples according to the environment of origin. Citizen Science platforms, such as the American Gut Project, standardize the molecular work and bioinformatic processing to generate a basic summary report of the content of an individual's sample. In the case of the American Gut Project, the samples also are placed into the context of a few other popular microbiome studies through data integration. (From Allaband C, McDonald D, Vazquez-Baeza Y, et al.: Microbiome 101: Studying, analyzing, and interpreting gut microbiome data for clinicians. *Clin Gastroenterol Hepatol* 17(2):218–230, 2019.)

However, metabolomics is well established for analysis of urine or plasma samples and linking the resulting metabolites, including microbially produced metabolites, to human phenotypes.

How Are Microbiome Data Interpreted?

Once the molecular analysis has been performed, the next step is to link the features (microbial taxa, genes, transcripts, proteins, or metabolites) to host phenotypes of interest. This general strategy resulted in many of the known links between the human gut microbiome and phenotypes, which range from the obvious (inflammatory bowel disease [IBD], irritable bowel syndrome), to the more surprising (obesity, RA, cardiovascular disease), to phenotypes completely unsuspected a decade ago (autism, Parkinson's disease, multiple sclerosis) (see Fig. 23.1). This is typically done by analysis of a *feature table*, which is a matrix showing the count or proportion of each feature in each sample. There are considerable statistical challenges in doing so because the data are sparse (i.e., many of the entries in the table are zero because most microbes are not found in most samples), compositional (relative rather than absolute abundance data), and highly multivariate. As a result, standard statistical approaches to association or correlation fail either because too many different comparisons are applied to achieve statistical significance after correction for multiple comparisons or because the statistical models underlying tests, such as the familiar t test or Pearson correlation coefficient, are not appropriate and yield high false discovery rates.[48a]

Approaches that are useful for microbiome data analysis typically come from ecology, where techniques for analyzing complex communities have a long history. Some of the important concepts are alpha diversity, beta diversity, and taxonomy. Alpha diversity is, essentially, the complexity within a single sample, typically with components of richness (the number of kinds of organisms, genes, molecules, etc.) and evenness (whether all the entities are about equal in abundance, or if they differ). Beta diversity is the dissimilarity between two different samples, which can be combined across many samples to understand gradients, timeseries data, or population structure at the whole-community level. Taxonomy is aggregating the exact DNA sequences into higher levels, such as species, genera, phyla, etc. Some of the most useful approaches in dealing with these kinds of data include the following: statistical tests for association between particular microbes and microbial groups with phenotype, which use specialized approaches, such as ALDEx2 (analysis of variance [ANOVA]-like differential expression[49]; analysis of compositions (ANCOMs)[50]; phylogenetic isometric log ratio (PhILR)[51]; principal balances,[52] in which principal coordinates analysis and non-metric multidimensional scaling produce plots of a reduced dimensionality representation of the whole data set, which can then be tested for association with phenotype using permutational multivariate analysis of variance (PERMANOVA),[53] and inference of correlation networks among microbes using correlation techniques, such as SparCC (sparse correlations for compositional data)[54] or CoNet.[55] Machine learning techniques, notably Random Forests classifiers, have proven extremely useful for a wide range of classification and regression tasks in the microbiome, and can both provide models for separating cases from controls as well as identify optimized lists of microbes or genes to provide such classification,[56] sometimes reducing thousands of features to a model with only a couple of dozen, which could then be used to design a targeted assay. Many of these tools are wrapped into pipelines, such as Quantitative Insights Into Microbial Ecology (QIIME),[57] which take the raw sequence data or count tables and perform these types of statistical analyses. Database resources, such as Qiita,[58] facilitate application of these tools to existing data sets, which span hundreds of thousands of biologic specimens from thousands of studies, including newly collected data (Fig. 23.5).

What Can the Microbiome Be Used for Today?

In the context of individual studies, these approaches have been highly successful in linking different aspects of the microbiome (the overall pattern of taxa or genes, or individual taxa or genes) to a wide range of human phenotypes. Both the gut microbiome and the oral microbiome have been implicated in RA[3] and in systemic lupus erythematous.[59,60] The gut microbiome has also been implicated in differential response (efficacy and/or toxicity) to many drugs used for RA and lupus, including methotrexate,[61] TNF inhibitors,[62,63] steroids,[64] nonsteroidal anti-inflammatory drugs (NSAIDs),[65,66] and analgesics.[67] Although, in turn, many of these drugs appear to influence the microbiome, so causal relationships are typically unclear at this point. Because microbes also metabolize many drugs, which makes them more or less active, future efficacy and toxicity studies will also need to take the microbiome into consideration. Further, most of these drugs have been studied in nonrheumatologic contexts, so applicability of the results to rheumatology remains to be determined because the same drug may have different effects or may be metabolized differently in a disease-affected microbiome. However, generalizing the results across cohorts to produce a clinically valid test based on the microbiome, either for diagnosis of disease or as a companion diagnostic, has been elusive to date. Meta-analyses and combined analyses of microbiome studies have been challenging because technical differences among studies (for example, in DNA extraction methods, choice of PCR primers or other "library construction methods" to prepare DNA for sequencing on modern instruments, and in bioinformatics) often have much larger effect sizes than the biologic differences between cases and controls.[68,69] Even in cohort studies where technical approaches have been kept constant, microbiome markers that separate cases from controls in one city may not generalize to another city because the same microbes that differentiate cases from controls in one city may also differentiate controls in that city from controls in another city, which may lead to incorrect classifications.[70] Although progress has been made in identifying microbial features of other autoimmune diseases, notably IBD, across different populations extending even from the United States to China,[71] the limits of applicability of these approaches are not yet known.

Right now, microbiome studies are primarily useful for gaining insight into potential, new disease mechanisms and interactions among microbes, drugs, and the immune system. Human case-control studies demonstrate the differences between cases and controls. This suggests that there is a microbiome difference of interest. These then translate into mouse studies to determine mechanism. For example, researchers can transplant either a whole human microbiome or defined communities of microbial strains of interest into germ-free mice raised without any microbes; then, the researchers can study the resulting "gnotobiotic mice" in depth (e.g., performing genetic knockouts on either the host or microbial side to test specific mechanisms). The results can then be applied to designing human intervention trials that test the applicability of these mechanisms in clinical

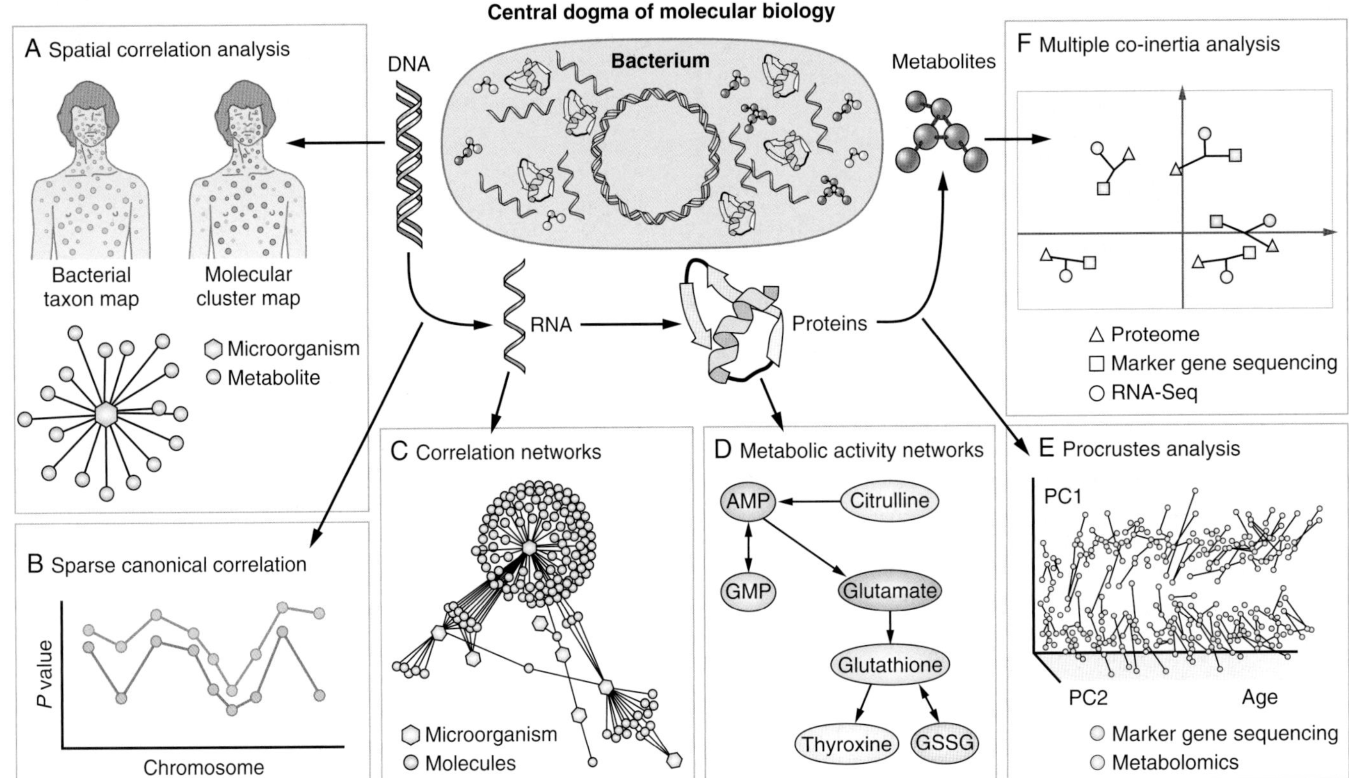

• **Fig. 23.5** The central dogma of molecular biology, which concerns the progression from genes to downstream metabolic products, is reflected by the compendia of corresponding "omes," which co-occur within the cell. Linking the knowledge from different omics studies constitutes a multi-omics analysis. Panels around the cell represent some integration examples of various omics data with marker gene sequencing. (A) Three-dimensional visualization of mapped molecular and microbial (or any other) features aids our understanding of spatial correlation thereof. (B) Sparse canonical correlation analysis identifies linear combinations of the two sets of variables that are highly correlated with each other. (C) Correlation network analysis shows clustering of a particular microorganism with metabolites that are potentially produced and/or processed by it. (D) Metabolic activity networks help to predict microbial community structure and function by mathematical modelling of the molecular mechanisms of particular organisms. (E) Procrustes analysis enables the direct comparison of different omics data sets with the same internal structure on a single principal coordinates (PC) analysis plot to reveal trends in the data. (F) Multiple co-inertia analysis (MCIA) enables multidimensional comparisons through graphic representation so that the similarity of different omics data can be more easily understood. *GSSG*, Oxidized glutathione; *RNA-Seq*, RNA sequencing. (From Knight R, Vrbanac A, Taylor BC, et al.: Best practices for analysing microbiomes. *Nat Rev Microbiol* 16(7):410–422, 2018.)

settings. Although studies of other conditions, such as IBD or obesity, are far along this path, with microbiome-directed stratification of interventions already working in research settings (although not yet clinical ones), these approaches have not yet been tried in RA, systemic lupus erythematosus (SLE), or other diseases of interest to rheumatology; however, the pathway is clear from other studies (Fig. 23.6).

What Microbiome Principles From Other Areas of Medicine or Biology Can Be Applied to Rheumatology?

Microbiome studies directly relevant to rheumatology are still in their infancies because researchers discovered the associations between the microbiome and RA 5 years after the discovery of the associations between the microbiome and obesity and IBD; however, mechanistic studies of the microbiome in RA and subsequent transfer of aspects of phenotype from humans to germ-free animals via the microbiome were among the first studies of this kind, and they served as a paradigm for the field. However, these types of studies receive lower funding than other areas of research. However, studies of other aspects of microbiome science that are further ahead, notably metabolic disease, cancer, and other types of molecular assays clearly point to directions that could benefit many aspects of rheumatology practice.

First, most current studies of RA, SLE, ankylosing spondylitis (AS), Sjögren's syndrome, and other diseases of interest to rheumatologists are small sample numbers. Because the human microbiome is highly individualized and multivariate, studies in the dozens of patients often lead to inconsistent results, especially when different methods are used to perform the studies. Large systematic studies using the same methods on hundreds to thousands of treatment-naïve subjects will be required for robust results because they have been in other diseases, such as Crohn's disease.[72] Choice of controls may also be important. For example, given the convergence in the microbiome state of individuals living together,[11,36] household controls who are discordant for disease may be especially useful for highlighting disease association in matched-pairs study designs.

Second, most current studies use a case-control paradigm, which examines a single disease versus healthy controls. This approach often reveals general signals of inflammation, such as increased *Enterobacteriaceae* and *Prevotella*, rather than specific markers of individual disease. Because, as noted earlier, meta-analyses across

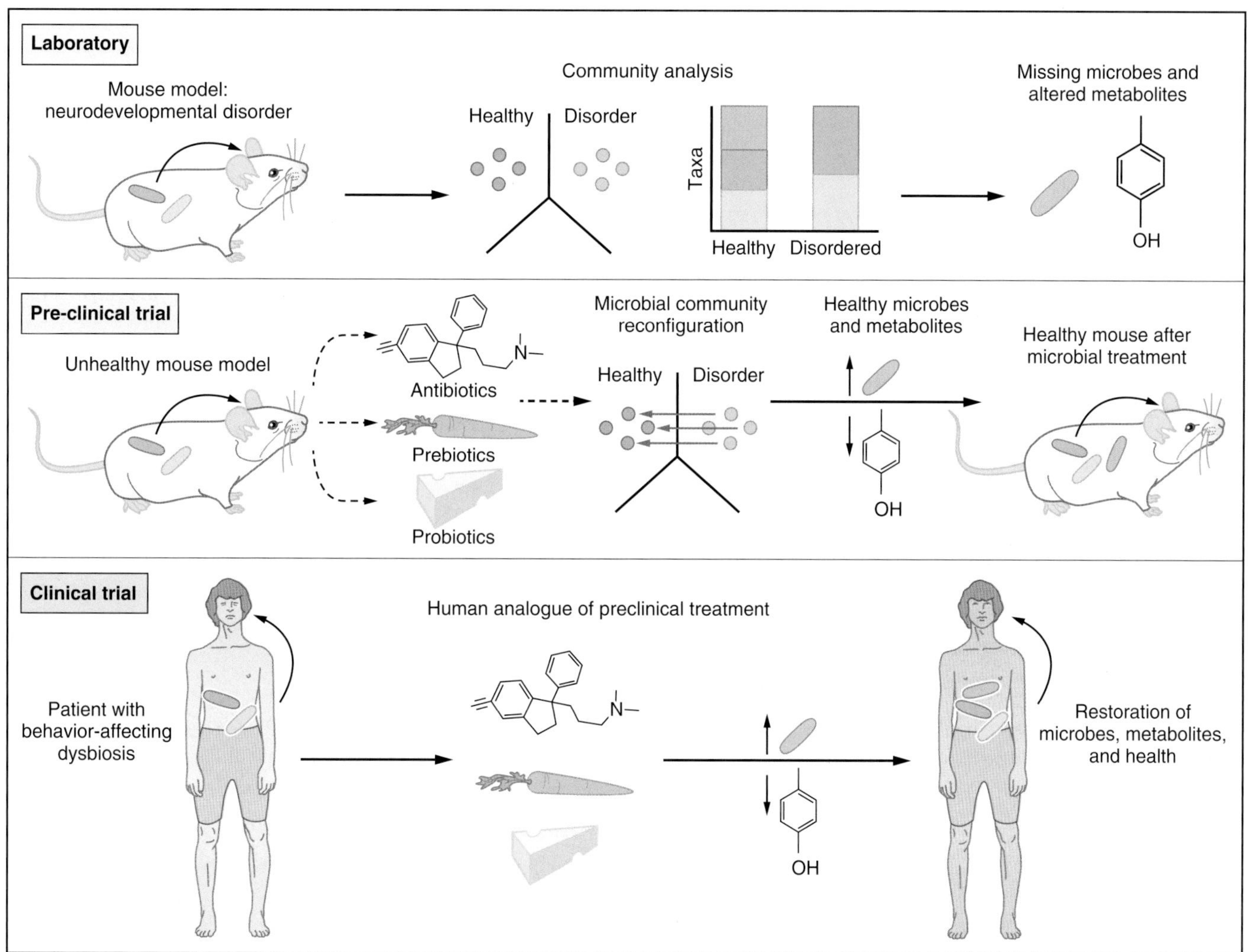

• **Fig. 23.6** Evolution of a pipeline for therapeutic strategies for neurodevelopmental disorders based on microbiome and metabolite profiling. *(Top),* Experiments using mouse models (for example, an MIA mouse with symptoms of autism spectrum disorder (ASD) and potentially other behavioral disorders) and subsequent community profiling can provide a mechanistic understanding of the importance of specific gut microbes and their metabolites in triggering the illness process, especially when lead compounds or microbes are applied to germ-free mice. *(Middle),* Potential treatments to restore the healthy state of the mouse model (replacements of the identified missing microbes and/or the differences in metabolites they cause) can be tested and validated in pre-clinical trials, including different strategies for altering the microbial community and/or metabolite profile. For example, introducing a beneficial microbe, such as the probiotic strains of *Bacteroides fragilis* used by Hsaio et al., may decrease a harmful metabolite rather than increase a beneficial one. *(Bottom),* Formulation and application of analogous treatments in human trials may lead to new ways to treat the behavioral and physiologic problems associated with human neurodevelopmental disorders. Careful clinical trials will be needed in humans because the effects of a given microbe and metabolite may differ in different species. (From Gilbert JA et al.: Toward effective probiotics for autism and other neurodevelopmental disorders. *Cell* 55(7):1446–1448, 2013.)

different studies is challenging,[68] although easier with new tools,[58] understanding which microbial genes are shared across diseases and which are unique to specific diseases will be as important as understanding which human risk alleles are specific to individual autoimmune conditions, versus which are shared between many autoimmune conditions. For example, although many risk alleles have been identified within the human genome for RA,[73] many are shared with other autoimmune diseases ranging from type 1 diabetes to celiac disease.[74]

Third, case-control studies using a single timepoint are at a severe disadvantage relative to studies that examine autoimmune disease over a longer period, tracking microbiome associations with cycles of flare and remission. It is increasingly apparent from longitudinal studies of IBD that dynamics are important, and taking into account the dynamics of disease from multiple samples can both provide insight into the disease process itself and provide improved microbial biomarkers relative to a single timepoint.[75,76] Applying these concepts to rheumatology could be of tremendous value, given the similarities in disease dynamics.

Fourth, large differences in the microbiome among healthy populations pose important challenges in generalizing results of studies that examine one population, because the same microbes that distinguish cases and controls in one population may yield diagnostic models that fail in other populations.[70] Consequently, multicenter studies that span different geographic regions, different levels of urbanization, and different diets, along with careful characterization of these parameters as well as other covariates now known to have large effects on the microbiome, including medications for other disorders, will be essential for scaling up research-quality differences among populations into robust diagnostics that can guide clinical practice. These multicenter studies must use the same technical methods.[69] Premature application of lessons from small individual studies into commercial microbiome-based tests, which are ineffective in other areas, provides an important cautionary example. For example, early studies in mice[77] and humans[7,78] suggested that the ratio of two phyla (i.e., Firmicutes and Bacteroidetes) was important for obesity. Although this result has been consistent in mice, results in human cohorts have been inconsistent.[79,80] However, these mixed results have not dissuaded companies from selling tests to reveal "microbiome-based obesity," which relies on this ratio.

Fifth, studies of the microbiome are starting to move from reading out current state to predicting future state. For example, subjects with gingivitis are prone to relapse into a microbiome state that resembles their specific initial state if their gingivitis is treated but allowed to relapse.[81] Similarly, early-life microbiome differences within the first 2 years of life are associated with BMI at age 12.[82] The potential to use large prospective stool collection studies, such as the FINRISK 2002 collection from more than 7500 subjects in Finland, to define microbes and their metabolites, which predict future health outcomes, is considerable; stool collections that are being performed now will be similarly useful in the future provided that the same subjects can be tracked over time.

Sixth, studies need to move from observational to interventional, as they have in other fields. The first step, already performed for RA, is to demonstrate that traits can be transferred from human subjects into mouse models by transferring the microbiome.[3] Identifying heritable components of the microbiome, which are associated with disease, can be useful for narrowing down these results from the whole microbiome to individual microbes of large effect.[13] Likewise, so can the use of personalized culture collections, which demonstrate that strains of bacteria grown in culture can recapitulate the results from transferring a whole stool sample[83]; both of these approaches have been useful in the study of metabolic syndrome. Sampling the microbiome, before a clinical intervention, and then testing whether patients can be stratified for response based on the microbiome, and/or whether mice to which the microbiome of individual patients has been transferred also respond the same way to that intervention, has been an extraordinarily fruitful approach, especially for cancer immunotherapy.[84–86] However, it should be noted that the actual microbiome biomarkers of immunotherapy efficacy differed among three very similar studies. Studies of insulin response and metabolic syndrome fared better; researchers predicted subject-specific postprandial glucose responses via a machine learning model, which they trained on one set of subjects and validated on another independent set.[87] This study was recently replicated by independent investigators using a cohort on another continent,[88] pointing the way towards how similar studies could be done for rheumatic disease. One important distinction is that postprandial glucose response can be measured in minutes using continuous glucose monitoring, which allows for very detailed assessment of the effects of different intervention; developing a comparable, continuous monitoring system for inflammation, although beyond current technical capability, should be a high priority for future development as a major enabling technology for these kinds of studies.

Finally, detailed mechanistic understanding of the interplay among the microbiome, metabolism, immune system, and other aspects of host gene expression and function will enable much less empirical and more hypothesis-driven research into microbiome mechanisms. These studies will parallel work on autism, wherein the maternal immune activation mouse model, an altered microbiome in the pups, produces a specific metabolite called 4-ethylphenylsulfate (4-EPS) that leads to compulsive behavior, communications deficits, cognitive deficits, and gut barrier dysfunction; many of these effects can be suppressed by introduction of a beneficial microbe (i.e., *Bacteroides fragilis*) from the human gut microbiome, which suppresses 4-EPS production[89] and subsequently demonstrates the involvement of specific populations of T helper 17 (Th17) cells in the fetal brain.[90] This demonstration of plausibility of mechanism linking the microbiome to a complex disease at a distal site led to further research, which investigated whether fecal microbiota transplant (i.e., transplant of gut microbes from a healthy donor to a patient) improved both gastrointestinal and cognitive symptoms associated with autism in a small, open-label clinical trial,[91] and it led to a double-blind placebo-controlled trial of a prebiotic intervention using galactooligosaccharide, a sugar that can only be metabolized by bacteria, which also improved both gastrointestinal and behavioral symptoms of autism.[92] Although these findings need to be replicated in additional studies, the concept that a disorder as complex as autism might be traced to the gut microbiome and alleviated by microbiome-directed therapies holds hope that other complex immune-linked disorders might benefit from similar approaches. Microbes can also be thought of as occupying specific ecological niches, so colonization with beneficial microbes may prevent pathogens that trigger inflammatory processes from gaining a foothold later. For example, *Clostridium difficile* is repelled by healthy microbiomes and primarily colonizes individuals whose gut ecosystems have been depleted by clindamycin.

How Will the Microbiome Be Useful to Rheumatologists in the Future?

Taken together, these principles from other areas of microbiome research suggest that it is plausible, although by no means certain, that the microbiome could be applied to rheumatology in the following ways, ordered from nearest- to longest-term:

- In animal models of rheumatic disease, the microbiome may explain and reconcile differences in results in animals obtained from or housed in different facilities with different microbiome backgrounds.
- Rheumatic diseases not yet linked to the microbiome may be associated in case-control studies with different microbiome features.
- Patients may be stratified for treatment with different drugs based on their microbiomes before treatment. This stratification may account for the ability of microbes in the gut (or, more speculatively, elsewhere in the body) to degrade a specific drug, modify it into a more or less toxic form, or stimulate or dampen aspects of host immune response.
- Diagnostic models may be developed where, from a stool sample (or, more speculatively, other microbiome sample) or a readout of the microbiome, or its products fed into a machine learning system, which is trained on healthy subjects and subjects with a range of different indications; this allows for a specific form of rheumatic disease to be identified rapidly. However, the need for large and diverse populations, ideally across multiple countries, as training data currently limits this type of application.
- The microbiome or its products may be tracked longitudinally to assess whether a therapy is working or to predict flare or remission. An exciting possibility here is that microbiome adaptation to therapy may explain loss of efficacy. However, the

per-assay cost of microbiome research and the cost and difficulty of returning serial samples collected at home, in a way that preserves specimens, currently limits this type of application.

- In cases where a test indicates that a patient is unlikely to respond well to treatment because of their microbiome state, or in a case where the microbiome is contributing to disease, the microbiome might be modified by probiotics (adding microbes), prebiotics (adding fertilizer for particular kinds of microbes), synbiotics (the combination of probiotics and prebiotics), targeted antibiotics, fecal microbiota transplant, drugs that target microbial enzymes rather than human enzymes, or other microbiome-directed therapies. However, our knowledge of how to modify the microbiome in a specific way is still in its infancy; considerable research both on empirical strategies to change the microbiome and into the biologic mechanisms that underpin these changes remains to be done. Additionally, substantial regulatory barriers slow progress in fecal microbiota transplant and in the use of novel microbes isolated from the human body; the U.S. Food and Drug Administration (FDA) regulates these methods as drugs and subjects them to the full sequence of clinical trials.

Overall, the microbiome holds considerable promise for improved conceptual understanding, diagnosis, and treatment of rheumatic disease; researchers have proven the microbiome to be useful for modifying RA in animal models.[3,93,94] Although these specific results may not translate to humans, the roadmap for a concerted research program that leverages progress in other areas of microbiome research is clear and has an excellent chance of rapidly delivering benefits in some areas of patient care (e.g., especially those areas related to treatment stratification).

The references for this chapter can also be found on ExpertConsult.com.

References

1. Gilbert JA, Blaser MJ, Caporaso JG, et al.: Current understanding of the human microbiome, *Nat Med* 24(4):392–400, 2018.
2. Knight R, Callewaert C, Marotz C, et al.: The microbiome and human biology, *Annu Rev Genomics Hum Genet* 18:65–86, 2017.
3. Scher JU, Sczesnak A, Longman RS, et al.: Expansion of intestinal Prevotella copri correlates with enhanced susceptibility to arthritis, *Elife* 2:e01202, 2013.
4. Sender R, Fuchs S, Milo R: Are we really vastly outnumbered? Revisiting the ratio of bacterial to host cells in humans, *Cell* 164(3):337–340, 2016.
5. Turnbaugh PJ, Ley RE, Hamady M, et al.: The human microbiome project, *Nature* 449(7164):804–810, 2007.
6. Pertea M, Shumate A, Pertea G, et al.: Thousands of large-scale RNA sequencing experiments yield a comprehensive new human gene list and reveal extensive transcriptional noise, *bioRxiv* 332825, 2018.
7. Gill SR, Pop M, Deboy RT, et al.: Metagenomic analysis of the human distal gut microbiome, *Science* 312(5778):1355–1359, 2006.
8. Human Microbiome Project C: Structure, function and diversity of the healthy human microbiome, *Nature* 486(7402):207–214, 2012.
9. Lloyd-Price J, Mahurkar A, Rahnavard G, et al.: Strains, functions and dynamics in the expanded Human Microbiome Project, *Nature* 550(7674):61–66, 2017.
10. Qin J, Li R, Raes J, et al.: A human gut microbial gene catalogue established by metagenomic sequencing, *Nature* 464(7285):59–65, 2010.
11. Rothschild D, Weissbrod O, Barkan E, et al.: Environment dominates over host genetics in shaping human gut microbiota, *Nature* 555(7695):210–215, 2018.
12. Thompson LR, Sanders JG, McDonald D, et al.: A communal catalogue reveals Earth's multiscale microbial diversity, *Nature* 551(7681):457–463, 2017.
13. Goodrich JK, Waters JL, Poole AC, et al.: Human genetics shape the gut microbiome, *Cell* 159(4):789–799, 2014.
14. Dodd D, Spitzer MH, Van Treuren W, et al.: A gut bacterial pathway metabolizes aromatic amino acids into nine circulating metabolites, *Nature* 551(7682):648–652, 2017.
15. Wang Z, Klipfell E, Bennett BJ, et al.: Gut flora metabolism of phosphatidylcholine promotes cardiovascular disease, *Nature* 472(7341):57–63, 2011.
16. Wikoff WR, Anfora AT, Liu J, et al.: Metabolomics analysis reveals large effects of gut microflora on mammalian blood metabolites, *Proc Natl Acad Sci U S A* 106(10):3698–3703, 2009.
17. Steed AL, Christophi GP, Kaiko GE, et al.: The microbial metabolite desaminotyrosine protects from influenza through type I interferon, *Science* 357(6350):498–502, 2017.
18. Turnbaugh PJ, Hamady M, Yatsunenko T, et al.: A core gut microbiome in obese and lean twins, *Nature* 457(7228):480–484, 2009.
19. Yatsunenko T, Rey FE, Manary MJ, et al.: Human gut microbiome viewed across age and geography, *Nature* 486(7402):222–227, 2012.
20. Demmitt BA, Corley RP, Huibregtse BM: Genetic influences on the human oral microbiome, *BMC Genomics* 18(1):659, 2017.
21. Stahringer SS, Clemente JC, Corley RP, et al.: Nurture trumps nature in a longitudinal survey of salivary bacterial communities in twins from early adolescence to early adulthood, *Genome Res* 22(11):2146–2152, 2012.
22. Dominguez-Bello MG, Costello EK, Contreras M, et al.: Delivery mode shapes the acquisition and structure of the initial microbiota across multiple body habitats in newborns, *Proc Natl Acad Sci U S A* 107(26):11971–11975, 2010.
23. Koenig JE, Spor A, Scalfone N, et al.: Succession of microbial consortia in the developing infant gut microbiome, *Proc Natl Acad Sci U S A* 108(Suppl 1):4578–4585, 2011.
24. Blaser MJ, Dominguez-Bello MG, Contreras M, et al.: Distinct cutaneous bacterial assemblages in a sampling of South American Amerindians and US residents, *ISME J* 7(1):85–95, 2013.
25. Clemente JC, Pehrsson EC, Blaser MJ, et al.: The microbiome of uncontacted Amerindians, *Sci Adv* 1(3), 2015.
26. Contreras M, Costello EK, Hidalgo G, et al.: The bacterial microbiota in the oral mucosa of rural Amerindians, *Microbiology* 156(Pt 11):3282–3287, 2010.
27. Fragiadakis GK, Smits SA, Sonnenburg ED, et al.: Links between environment, diet, and the hunter-gatherer microbiome, *Gut Microbes*1–12, 2018.
28. Obregon-Tito AJ, Tito RY, Metcalf J, et al.: Subsistence strategies in traditional societies distinguish gut microbiomes, *Nat Commun* 6:6505, 2015.
29. Smits SA, Leach J, Sonnenburg ED, et al.: Seasonal cycling in the gut microbiome of the Hadza hunter-gatherers of Tanzania, *Science* 357(6353):802–806, 2017.
30. Wu GD, Chen J, Hoffmann C, et al.: Linking long-term dietary patterns with gut microbial enterotypes, *Science* 334(6052):105–108, 2011.
31. McDonald D, Hyde E, Debelius JW, et al.: American gut: an open platform for citizen science microbiome research, *mSystems* 3(3), 2018.
32. David LA, Maurice CF, Carmody RN, et al.: Diet rapidly and reproducibly alters the human gut microbiome, *Nature* 505(7484):559–563, 2014.
33. Falony G, Joossens M, Vieira-Silva S, et al.: Population-level analysis of gut microbiome variation, *Science* 352(6285):560–564, 2016.

34. Zhernakova A, Kurilshikov A, Bonder MJ, et al.: Population-based metagenomics analysis reveals markers for gut microbiome composition and diversity, *Science* 352(6285):565–569, 2016.
35. Maier L, Pruteanu M, Kuhn M, et al.: Extensive impact of non-antibiotic drugs on human gut bacteria, *Nature* 555(7698):623–628, 2018.
36. Song SJ, Lauber C, Costello EK, et al.: Cohabiting family members share microbiota with one another and with their dogs, *Elife* 2:e00458, 2013.
37. Goodrich JK, Di Rienzi SC, Poole AC, et al.: Conducting a microbiome study, *Cell* 158(2):250–262, 2014.
38. Zhang H, DiBaise JK, Zuccolo A, et al.: Human gut microbiota in obesity and after gastric bypass, *Proc Natl Acad Sci U S A* 106(7):2365–2370, 2009.
39. Allaband C, McDonald D, Vazquez-Baeza Y, et al.: Microbiome 101: studying, analyzing, and interpreting gut microbiome data for clinicians, *Clin Gastroenterol Hepatol* 17(2):218–230, 2019.
40. Knight R, Vrbanac A, Taylor BC, et al.: Best practices for analysing microbiomes, *Nat Rev Microbiol* 16(7):410–422, 2018.
41. Caporaso JG, Lauber CL, Walters WA, et al.: Ultra-high-throughput microbial community analysis on the Illumina HiSeq and MiSeq platforms, *ISME J* 6(8):1621–1624, 2012.
42. Wood DE, Salzberg SL: Kraken: ultrafast metagenomic sequence classification using exact alignments, *Genome Biol* 15(3):R46, 2014.
43. Kim D, Song L, Breitwieser FP, et al.: Centrifuge: rapid and sensitive classification of metagenomic sequences, *Genome Res* 26(12):1721–1729, 2016.
44. Gonzalez A, Vazquez-Baeza Y, Pettengill JB, et al.: Avoiding pandemic fears in the subway and conquering the platypus, *mSystems* 1(3), 2016.
45. Nurk S, Meleshko D, Korobeynikov A, et al.: metaSPAdes: a new versatile metagenomic assembler, *Genome Res* 27(5):824–834, 2017.
46. Franzosa EA, McIver LJ, Rahnavard G, et al.: Species-level functional profiling of metagenomes and metatranscriptomes, *Nat Methods* 15(11):962–968, 2018.
47. Hillmann B, Al-Ghalith GA, Shields-Cutler RR, et al.: Evaluating the information content of shallow shotgun metagenomics, *mSystems* 3(6), 2018.
48. Esquerre T, Laguerre S, Turlan C, et al.: Dual role of transcription and transcript stability in the regulation of gene expression in Escherichia coli cells cultured on glucose at different growth rates, *Nucleic Acids Res* 42(4):2460–2472, 2014.
48a. Gloor GB, Wu JR, Pawlowsky-Glahn V, et al.: It's all relative: analyzing microbiome data as compositions, *Ann Epidemiol* 26(5):322–329, 2016.
49. Fernandes AD, Reid JN, Macklaim JM, et al.: Unifying the analysis of high-throughput sequencing datasets: characterizing RNA-seq, 16S rRNA gene sequencing and selective growth experiments by compositional data analysis, *Microbiome* 2:15, 2014.
50. Mandal S, Van Treuren W, White RA, et al.: Analysis of composition of microbiomes: a novel method for studying microbial composition, *Microb Ecol Health Dis* 26:27663, 2015.
51. Silverman JD, Washburne AD, Mukherjee S, et al.: A phylogenetic transform enhances analysis of compositional microbiota data, *Elife* 6, 2017.
52. Morton JT, Sanders J, Quinn RA, et al.: Balance trees reveal microbial niche differentiation, *mSystems* 2(1), 2017.
53. Anderson M: A new method for non-parametric multivariate analysis of variance, *Austral Ecology* 26(1):32–46, 2001.
54. Friedman J, Alm EJ: Inferring correlation networks from genomic survey data, *PLoS Comput Biol* 8(9):e1002687, 2012.
55. Faust K, Raes J: CoNet app: inference of biological association networks using Cytoscape, *F1000Res* 5:1519, 2016.
56. Knights D, Parfrey LW, Zaneveld J, et al.: Human-associated microbial signatures: examining their predictive value, *Cell Host Microbe* 10(4):292–296, 2011.
57. Caporaso JG, Kuczynski J, Stombaugh J, et al.: QIIME allows analysis of high-throughput community sequencing data, *Nat Methods* 7(5):335–336, 2010.
58. Gonzalez A, Navas-Molina JA, Kosciolek T, et al.: Qiita: rapid, web-enabled microbiome meta-analysis, *Nat Methods* 15(10):796–798, 2018.
59. Li Y, Wang H, Li X, et al.: Disordered intestinal microbes are associated with the activity of systemic lupus erythematosus, *Clin Sci (Lond)* 133:821–838, 2019.
60. van der Meulen TA, Harmsen HJM, Vila AV, et al.: Shared gut, but distinct oral microbiota composition in primary Sjogren's syndrome and systemic lupus erythematosus, *J Autoimmun* 97:77–87, 2019.
61. Zhou B, Xia X, Wang P, et al.: Induction and amelioration of methotrexate-induced gastrointestinal toxicity are related to immune response and gut microbiota, *EBioMedicine* 33:122–133, 2018.
62. Bazin T, Hooks KB, Barnetche T, et al.: Microbiota composition may predict anti-Tnf alpha response in spondyloarthritis patients: an exploratory study, *Sci Rep* 8(1):5446, 2018.
63. Picchianti-Diamanti A, Panebianco C, et al.: Analysis of gut microbiota in rheumatoid arthritis patients: disease-related dysbiosis and modifications induced by etanercept, *Int J Mol Sci* 19(10), 2018.
64. Jain R, Hoggard M, Zoing M, et al.: The effect of medical treatments on the bacterial microbiome in patients with chronic rhinosinusitis: a pilot study, *Int Forum Allergy Rhinol*, 2018.
65. Edogawa S, Peters SA, Jenkins GD, et al.: Sex differences in NSAID-induced perturbation of human intestinal barrier function and microbiota, *FASEB J* fj201800560R, 2018.
66. Maseda D, Zackular JP, Trindade B, et al.: Nonsteroidal anti-inflammatory drugs alter the microbiota and exacerbate clostridium difficile colitis while dysregulating the inflammatory response, *MBio* 10(1), 2019.
67. Clayton TA, Baker D, Lindon JC, et al.: Pharmacometabonomic identification of a significant host-microbiome metabolic interaction affecting human drug metabolism, *Proc Natl Acad Sci U S A* 106(34):14728–14733, 2009.
68. Lozupone CA, Stombaugh J, Gonzalez A, et al.: Meta-analyses of studies of the human microbiota, *Genome Res* 23(10):1704–1714, 2013.
69. Sinha R, Abu-Ali G, Vogtmann E, et al.: Microbiome Quality Control Project C et al: Assessment of variation in microbial community amplicon sequencing by the Microbiome Quality Control (MBQC) project consortium, *Nat Biotechnol* 35(11):1077–1086, 2017.
70. He Y, Wu W, Zheng HM, et al.: Regional variation limits applications of healthy gut microbiome reference ranges and disease models, *Nat Med* 24(10):1532–1535, 2018.
71. Zhou Y, Xu ZZ, He Y, et al.: Gut microbiota offers universal biomarkers across ethnicity in inflammatory bowel disease diagnosis and infliximab response prediction, *mSystems* 3(1), 2018.
72. Gevers D, Kugathasan S, Denson LA, et al.: The treatment-naive microbiome in new-onset Crohn's disease, *Cell Host Microbe* 15(3):382–392, 2014.
73. Yarwood A, Huizinga TW, Worthington J: The genetics of rheumatoid arthritis: risk and protection in different stages of the evolution of RA, *Rheumatology (Oxford)* 55(2):199–209, 2016.
74. Zhernakova A, van Diemen CC, Wijmenga C: Detecting shared pathogenesis from the shared genetics of immune-related diseases, *Nat Rev Genet* 10(1):43–55, 2009.
75. Halfvarson J, Brislawn CJ, Lamendella R, et al.: Dynamics of the human gut microbiome in inflammatory bowel disease, *Nat Microbiol* 2:17004, 2017.
76. Vazquez-Baeza Y, Gonzalez A, Xu ZZ, et al.: Guiding longitudinal sampling in IBD cohorts, *Gut* 67(9):1743–1745, 2018.
77. Ley RE, Backhed F, Turnbaugh P, et al.: Obesity alters gut microbial ecology, *Proc Natl Acad Sci U S A* 102(31):11070–11075, 2005.

78. Ley RE, Turnbaugh PJ, Klein S, et al.: Microbial ecology: human gut microbes associated with obesity, *Nature* 444(7122):1022–1023, 2006.
79. Walters WA, Xu Z, Knight R: Meta-analyses of human gut microbes associated with obesity and IBD, *FEBS Lett* 588(22):4223–4233, 2014.
80. Sze MA, Schloss PD: Looking for a signal in the noise: Revisiting obesity and the microbiome, *MBio* 7(4), 2016.
81. Huang S, Li R, Zeng X, et al.: Predictive modeling of gingivitis severity and susceptibility via oral microbiota, *ISME J* 8(9):1768–1780, 2014.
82. Stanislawski MA, Dabelea D, Wagner BD, et al.: Gut microbiota in the first 2 years of life and the association with body mass index at age 12 in a Norwegian birth cohort, *MBio* 9(5), 2018.
83. Ridaura VK, Faith JJ, Rey FE, et al.: Gut microbiota from twins discordant for obesity modulate metabolism in mice, *Science* 341(6150):1241214, 2013.
84. Gopalakrishnan V, Spencer CN, Nezi L, et al.: Gut microbiome modulates response to anti-PD-1 immunotherapy in melanoma patients, *Science* 359(6371):97–103, 2018.
85. Matson V, Fessler J, Bao R, et al.: The commensal microbiome is associated with anti-PD-1 efficacy in metastatic melanoma patients, *Science* 359(6371):104–108, 2018.
86. Routy B, Le Chatelier E, Derosa L, et al.: Gut microbiome influences efficacy of PD-1-based immunotherapy against epithelial tumors, *Science* 359(6371):91–97, 2018.
87. Zeevi D, Korem T, Zmora N, et al.: Personalized nutrition by prediction of glycemic responses, *Cell* 163(5):1079–1094, 2015.
88. Mendes-Soares H, Raveh-Sadka T, Azulay S, et al.: Assessment of a personalized approach to predicting postprandial glycemic responses to food among individuals without diabetes, *JAMA Netw Open* 2(2):e188102, 2019.
89. Hsiao EY, McBride SW, Hsien S, et al.: Microbiota modulate behavioral and physiological abnormalities associated with neurodevelopmental disorders, *Cell* 155(7):1451–1463, 2013.
90. Choi GB, Yim YS, Wong H, et al.: The maternal interleukin-17a pathway in mice promotes autism-like phenotypes in offspring, *Science* 351(6276):933–939, 2016.
91. Kang DW, Adams JB, Gregory AC, et al.: Microbiota transfer therapy alters gut ecosystem and improves gastrointestinal and autism symptoms: an open-label study, *Microbiome* 5(1):10, 2017.
92. Grimaldi R, Gibson GR, Vulevic J, et al.: A prebiotic intervention study in children with autism spectrum disorders (ASDs), *Microbiome* 6(1):133, 2018.
93. Evans-Marin H, Rogier R, Koralov SB, et al.: Microbiota-dependent involvement of Th17 cells in murine models of inflammatory arthritis, *Arthritis Rheumatol* 70(12):1971–1983, 2018.
94. Rogier R, Evans-Marin H, Manasson J, et al.: Alteration of the intestinal microbiome characterizes preclinical inflammatory arthritis in mice and its modulation attenuates established arthritis, *Sci Rep* 7(1):15613, 2017.

24 Metabolic Regulation of Immunity

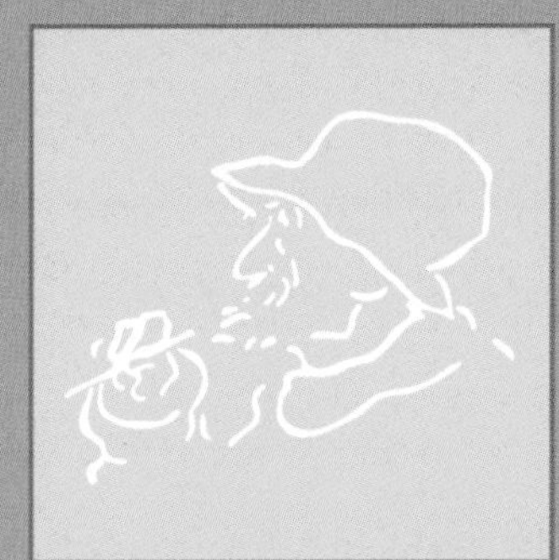

RUONING WANG, TINGTING WANG, AND STEPHEN TAIT

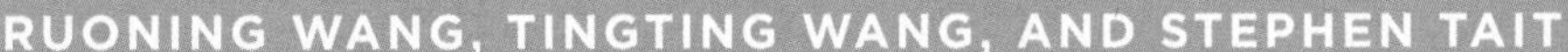

KEY POINTS

- Immune signaling drives metabolic reprogramming in both innate and adaptive immune cells.
- The metabolic shift renders immune cells highly dependent on certain metabolic pathways.
- Mitochondria serve as signaling hubs for directing innate and adaptive immune responses.
- The availability of extra-cellular metabolites mediates the intercellular metabolic cross-talk that affects the immune response.

Introduction

The evolution of vertebrate immunity has culminated in an effective and complex chain reaction that is composed of a rapid activation of specialized innate immune cells—primarily neutrophils, macrophages, and dendritic cells (DCs)—followed by the proliferative burst and functional polarization of adaptive B and T cells. Because the invading pathogens of vertebrates often rapidly reproduce and spread in their host, an effective host-mediated immune response must be fast and energy intensive. An immune signaling–driven metabolic reprogramming in both innate and adaptive immune cells is essential for their activation, proliferation, and polarization and for the subsequent functional events elicited by these cells (Figs. 24.1 and 24.2).

Metabolic Rewiring in Innate Immunity

Macrophage Metabolism

Macrophages, together with DCs, are considered first-line effectors of innate immunity. Based on their specific functional activities after pathogen or cytokine stimulation, macrophages can be largely defined as two different subtypes: the classically activated macrophage subset (M1) and the alternatively activated macrophage phenotype (M2). The classical activation of macrophages is often induced by a combination of bacterial product lipopolysaccharide (LPS) and cytokines such as interferon-γ (IFN-γ), whereas the polarization of macrophages via the alternative activation program is triggered by exposure to the cytokines interleukin (IL)-4 or IL-13.[1] M1 macrophages produce nitric oxide (NO), a product of inducible nitric oxide synthase (iNOS)–mediated breakdown of arginine, reactive oxygen species (ROS), and pro-inflammatory cytokines, including TNF, IL-1β, IL-6, and IL-12, thus mounting a rapid, effective response against highly proliferative intra-cellular pathogens. In contrast, M2 phenotype macrophages produce high levels of IL-10 and IL-1 receptor antagonist (IL-1ra), meanwhile shifting arginine catabolism from iNOS-mediated production of NO to an arginase I (Arg I)–mediated breakdown of arginine into urea and ornithine, thus functioning in anti-parasitic responses, promoting tissue healing, and, in general, dampening inflammation.[2–4] Therefore, M1 macrophages promote inflammation, whereas M2 macrophages suppress inflammation and promote tissue repair. In addition to the differential engagement of an iNOS-dependent or Arg I–dependent arginine catabolic program, the differences of M1 and M2 macrophages are also reflected in their other metabolic profiles. Whereas the inflammatory M1 macrophages predominantly engage glycolysis and the pentose phosphate shunt (PPP), the anti-inflammatory M2 macrophages actively engage lipid oxidation.[1,5]

Heightened glycolysis is required for adenosine triphosphate (ATP) generation in M1 macrophages and also provides many glycolytic intermediate metabolites, which are direct precursors for lipid and amino acid biosynthesis. Whereas newly synthesized lipids are involved in the dramatic intra-cellular membrane reorganization after pathogen invasion, both lipids and amino acids are required for the production and secretion of pro-inflammatory cytokines.[6–9] Meanwhile, the PPP pathway provides nicotinamide adenine dinucleotide phosphate (NADPH), which functions in maintaining reduced glutathione and limiting oxidative stress in M1 macrophages.[10–12] Enhanced glycolysis and PPP in M1 macrophages also results in glucose depletion and an acidified microenvironment, resulting in a hostile environment that may suppress pathogen proliferation.[13] It has been demonstrated that the metabolic reprogramming in M1 macrophages is tightly coordinated by transcriptional and post-translational regulation of metabolic enzymes. LPS stimulation in M1 macrophages leads to a transcriptional induction of glycolytic enzymes such as phosphoglycerate kinase (PGK), the glucose transporter-1 (GLUT-1), and ubiquitous 6-phosphofructo-2-kinase/fructose-2, 6-bisphosphatase (uPFK2) to promote glycolysis, meanwhile suppressing the expression of mitochondrial enzymes.[14,15] In addition, LPS stimulation results in a robust NO production, which not only plays an indispensable role in destroying invading microorganisms but also results in a suppression of mitochondrial oxidative phosphorylation, likely via S-nitrosylation of mitochondrial metabolic enzymes.[16,17] The transcriptional factor hypoxia-inducible

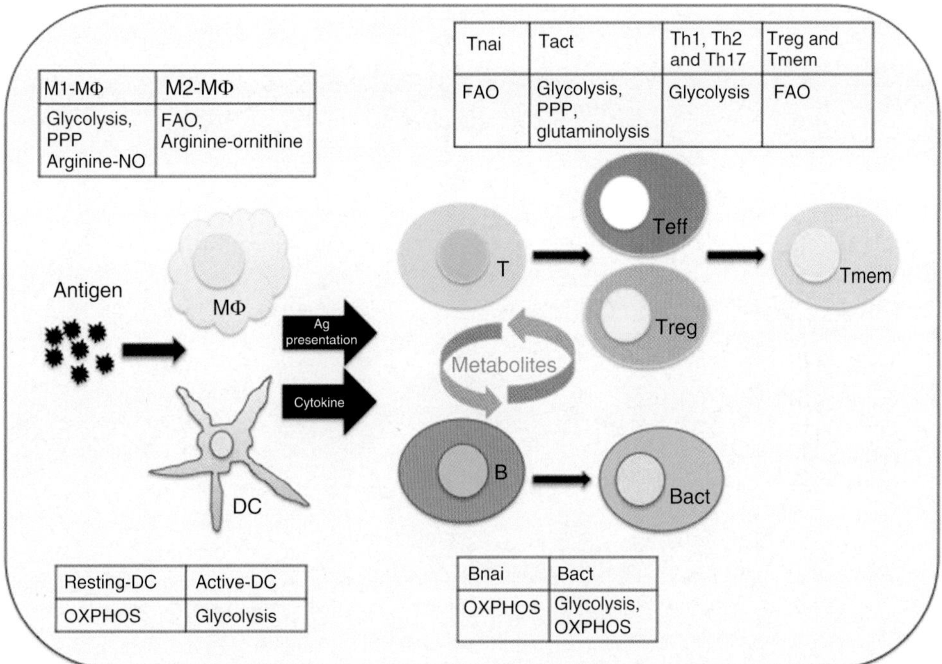

• **Fig. 24.1** Metabolic reprogramming and interplay in immunity. Resting dendritic cells (DCs) mainly rely on the mitochondrial oxidative phosphorylation (OXPHOS) metabolic pathway, whereas active DCs rapidly switch from OXPHOS to glycolysis after activation. M1 macrophages (MΦ) engage glycolysis, pentose phosphate shunt (PPP), and inducible nitric oxide synthase (iNOS)–mediated arginine catabolism that generates nitric oxide (NO), whereas M2 MΦ predominantly rely on fatty acid oxidation (FAO) and convert arginine to ornithine and urea. Upon antigen and cytokine stimulation, naïve T (Tnai) cells become active and undergo a metabolic reprogramming from FAO to glycolysis, PPP, and glutaminolysis. Active T (Tact) cells then differentiate into effector T (Teff) cells with heightened glycolysis, as well as regulatory T (Treg) and memory T (Tmem) cells that depend on FAO. Unlike T cells, naïve B (Bnai) cells rely on OXPHOS, whereas active B (Bact) cells display a balanced increase in glycolysis and OXPHOS. Beyond this, the different immune populations may interplay with each other through competing nutrients or formation of metabolic symbiosis.

factor-1α (HIF-1α) has also been implicated in the regulation of glycolysis, in addition to its role in promoting the transcription of proangiogenic factors and pro-inflammatory cytokines in macrophages.[14,18] In response to LPS stimulation, succinate and itaconate are generated through the TCA cycle and serve as important signaling metabolites in macrophages to modulate innate immune response.[19] Succinate enhances the expression of pro-inflammatory cytokine IL-1β via stabilizing HIF-1α, while itaconate acts as anti-inflammatory metabolite.[20–22]

On the other hand, a rapid downregulation of carbohydrate kinase–like protein (CARKL) after LPS stimulation is required for shunting glucose catabolism into the oxidative arm of the PPP pathway in M1 macrophages. CARKL possesses the same catalytic activity as the sedoheptulose kinase, which promotes metabolic flux through a nonoxidative arm and consequentially reduces metabolic flux through the oxidative arm of the PPP. The nonoxidative arm of the PPP is designed to generate ribose-5-phosphate (R5P), whereas the oxidative arm of the PPP produces NADPH, thus modulating redox balance. Intriguingly, M2 macrophages display higher CARKL expression than do M1 macrophages, implicating CARKL as a rheostat for coordinating macrophage metabolic routes and functional polarizations.[23] Beyond this, IL-4, an M2 macrophage stimulator, dramatically induces the signal transducer and activator of transcription 6 (STAT6), which promotes the transcription of Arg1, thus shifting arginine catabolism from iNOS-mediated production of NO to the production of urea and ornithine.[24] STAT6 also cooperates with peroxisome proliferator-activated receptor γ (PPARγ)-coactivator-1β (PGC-1β) to induce the expression of genes involved in fatty acid oxidation (FAO) and mitochondrial biogenesis in M2 macrophages.[25]

Dendritic Cell Metabolism

DCs, which are key players in immunity and tolerance, play a crucial role in driving T cell activation and differentiation via antigen presentation and production of cytokines. DCs can be divided into several subsets, including conventional DCs (cDCs), inflammatory DCs (infDCs), and plasmacytoid DCs (pDCs).[26–28] Resting DCs, which are largely immature and poorly immunogenic, mainly rely on the mitochondrial oxidative phosphorylation (OXPHOS) metabolic pathway. While resting DCs are able to consume glucose to fuel subsequent OXPHOS, DCs also possess glycogen store, which plays a key role in maintaining nutrient homeostatic and regulating optimal immune function of DCs.[29,30] Upon the stimulation of pathogen-derived Toll-like receptor (TLR) ligands, DCs become active and immunogenic and undergo a rapid metabolic switch from OXPHOS to glycolysis to fulfill their bioenergetic needs.[31–33] In addition, many intermediate metabolites of the glycolytic pathway provide a carbon source for amino acid biosynthesis and de novo fatty acid synthesis, the latter of which is required for the synthesis of endoplasmic reticulum (ER) and Golgi membranes to promote the

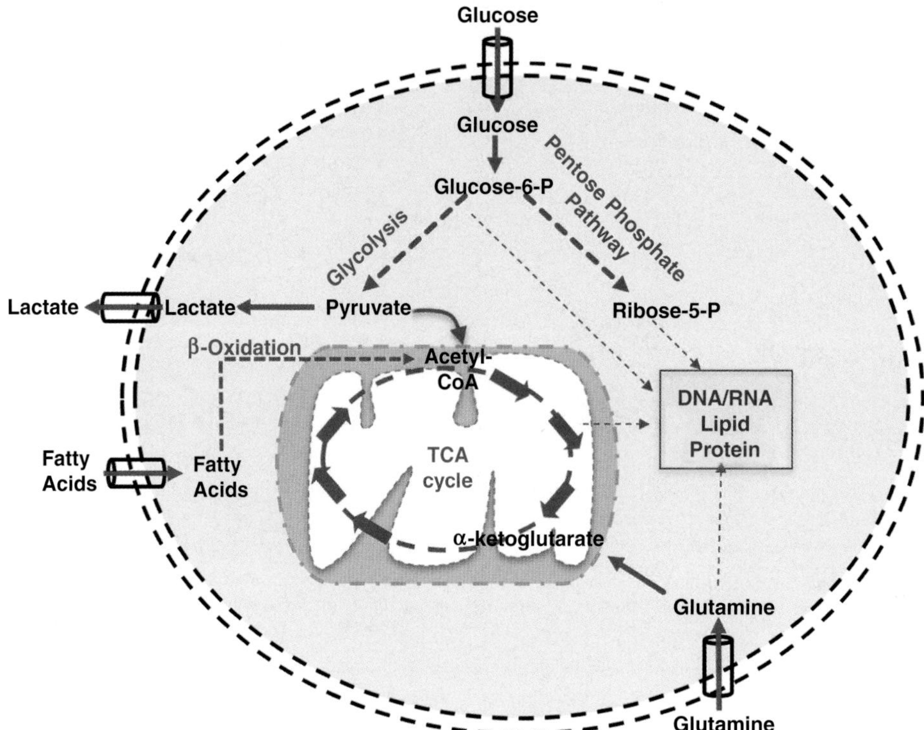

• **Fig. 24.2** Schematic view of central carbon metabolism. Central carbon metabolic pathways are branched pathways that interconnect with each other, enabling the production of the target metabolic products from various sources. The pentose phosphate pathway branches away from glycolysis to produce nicotinamide adenine dinucleotide phosphate (NADPH) and ribose at glucose-6-phosphate. The carbons of glucose are further funneled toward lactate production (aerobic glycolysis) or acetyl-CoA (the TCA cycle) at pyruvate. Fatty acid beta-oxidation generates acetyl-CoA that enters the TCA cycle. In addition to acetyl-CoA, the TCA cycle in mitochondria is fueled by anapleurotic substrates including α-ketoglutarate (α-KG), derived from glutamine. Collectively, the catabolic pathway of glucose, glutamine, and free fatty acids are coordinated to support cell proliferation and function by generating energy, maintaining redox homeostasis, and providing biosynthetic building blocks of macromolecules.

synthesis, transportation, and secretion of proteins associated with DC activation and maturation.[31,34] Mechanistically, the engagement of TLR ligands leads to the activation of phosphatidylinositol 3-kinase (PI3K)/protein kinase B (Akt) pathway, which may directly promote GLUT membrane translocation and enhance glucose uptake in DCs.[31,35,36] As an essential downstream signaling node of the PI3K/Akt signaling pathway, the mammalian target of rapamycin (mTOR) has also been implicated in modulating metabolic programs in both cDCs and infDCs.[31,36,37] The activation of mTOR results in the expression and stabilization of transcription factor HIF-1α, which regulates the expression of genes involved in glycolysis. The transcription factor sterol-regulatory element binding protein (SREBP) is another downstream target of mTOR and is responsible for controlling genes relevant in lipid synthesis.[38–40] Similar to M1 macrophages, an iNOS-derived NO may play a critical role in suppressing mitochondrial OXPHOS, thus promoting the metabolic shift from mitochondrial-dependent metabolism to glycolysis in DCs. Other reports also suggested that the autocrine production of type 1 IFN is required for the metabolic switch in cDCs.[32,33,41] Whereas the engagement of glycolysis is required for TLR-induced DC activation and immunogenicity, mitochondrial OXPHOS is likely involved in DC-mediated immune tolerance. Consistent with findings in other immune cells, recent studies indicated that adenosine monophosphate (AMP)–activated protein kinase (AMPK) and peroxisome proliferator-activated receptor-γ coactivator (PGC)-1α form a signaling axis to coordinately regulate mitochondrial biogenesis, OXPHOS, and other catabolic metabolisms in DCs, thus favoring the acquisition of tolerogenic DCs.[31,42–45]

Metabolic Rewiring in Adaptive Immunity

T Cell Metabolism

As an essential component of adaptive immunity, T cells can recognize foreign antigen and rapidly transit from a quiescent to an active state that is concomitant with cell growth (increase of cell size) and proliferation. Subsequently, activated and proliferating T cells can differentiate into various functional subsets, which are determined by the nature of antigen stimulation and the surrounding cytokine milieu. Subsequent to the peak of T cell expansion and antigen clearance, the vast majority of T cells will die by programmed cell death (apoptosis) during a phase of contraction. The remaining population returns to a quiescent state and gives rise to the memory subset, which responds more quickly and effectively upon encountering the same pathogen. To fulfill their bioenergetic and biosynthetic demands coupled with various functional stages, T cells actively engage distinct signaling pathways and transcriptional modulators to alter their metabolic programs accordingly.

T Cell Activation

Upon the engagement of antigen and co-stimulatory molecules, resting T cells undergo a rapid growth and proliferation process. Concomitant with this process, and as a result of activation signaling, T cells reprogram their metabolic profile, shifting from FAO to robust aerobic glycolysis, PPP, and glutaminolysis. Naïve T cells rely on OXPHOS, generating energy to meet the basic needs for cell function and survival. Heightened aerobic glycolysis and glutaminolysis in activated T cells not only support ATP generation but also provide biosynthetic intermediates as building blocks of amino acids, nucleotides, and lipids to fulfill the biosynthetic demands of rapid cell growth and proliferation. In addition, glutaminolysis and glycolysis in active T cells provide carbon and nitrogen for other growth and proliferation-associated biosynthetic pathways, such as hexosamine and polyamine biosynthesis. Shunting of glucose into the PPP pathway results in the production of R5P and NADPH. Whereas R5P is a precursor for ribonucleotide biosynthesis, NADPH determines cellular redox balance and coordinates to FFA and cholesterol biosynthesis through the provision of reducing equivalents.[46–49]

The rewiring of metabolic pathways upon T cell activation is coordinately regulated by several signaling pathways, including mitogen-activated protein kinase (MAPK)/extra-cellular signal-regulated kinase (ERK) and PI3K/Akt/mTOR cascades.[46,50] The activation of Akt signaling promotes the expression and cell surface trafficking of GLUT-1 to the cell surface, facilitating glucose uptake.[51,52] On the other hand, ERK signaling promotes glutamine uptake via modulation of sodium-dependent neutral amino acid transporter-2 (SNAT2) expression and cell membrane trafficking.[53] Beyond the regulation of glucose and glutamine uptake, T cell activation signaling drives a global metabolo-transcriptome, including most of the key metabolic enzymes involved in the aforementioned catabolic and biosynthetic pathways. Interrogation of the promoters of these genes and subsequent genetic modulation of candidate transcriptional factors in T cells revealed that the proto-oncogene Myc is required in T cell activation–driven glucose and glutamine catabolism.[46,50] Meanwhile, metabolic genes involved in lipid metabolism and de novo cholesterol biosynthesis and transport are under the dynamic regulation of transcriptional factors, nuclear receptor liver X receptor (LXR), and the orphan steroid receptor estrogen receptor-related α (ERRα).[54–56]

T Cell Differentiation

After a rapid initial growth phase, T cells enter a proliferation phase and subsequently differentiate into various phenotypic and functional subtypes. In response to the distinct antigen challenge and extra-cellular cytokine signal, activated $CD4^+$ T cells differentiate into immune suppressive regulatory T cells (Tregs) or inflammatory T effector cells, such as T helper (Th)1, Th2, and Th17 (see Chapter 12). Th1 cells mediate responses to intracellular pathogens. Th2 cells control responses to extra-cellular bacteria and helminths. Th17 cells are important in anti-fungal defense and inflammation.[57–59] Despite their distinct functions in immunity, Th1, Th2, and Th17 cells all sustain heightened glycolysis, whereas Treg cells show decreased glycolysis.[55,60] Although the regulatory mechanism of elevated glycolysis in Th1 and Th2 cells remains unclear, HIF-1α is indispensable for driving Th17 differentiation and sustaining elevated glycolysis during Th17 differentiation.[55,60] Consistent with the crucial role of mTOR in regulating T effector development,[61,62] the expression of HIF-1α is dependent on the function of mTOR during Th17 differentiation. Whereas heightened glycolysis is necessary for Th17 differentiation and function,[60] HIF-1α appears to also directly regulate Th17 differentiation, at least in part through direct transcriptional activation of the Th17 master transcription factor, RAR-related orphan receptor γ (RORγt), thereby enhancing Th17 differentiation.[63] On the other hand, HIF-1α suppresses Treg differentiation, partially by antagonizing forkhead box protein 3 (Foxp3), a master transcriptional factor for Treg differentiation.[63] Treg cells act as immunologic suppressors by dampening T cell activation and inflammatory response. In contrast to other Th cells that actively engage glycolytic programs, Treg cells exhibit a reliance on mitochondrial-dependent oxidation of lipids for energy production.[55] Consistent with this mechanism, exogenous fatty acid supplementation inhibits Th1, Th2, and Th17 differentiation while modestly enhancing Treg differentiation.[55] In addition, butyrate, a commensal microbe-derived short-chain fatty acid, preferentially induces Treg differentiation. However, this effect may be due to the inhibition of histone deacetylase activity by butyrate.[64,65] Similar to CD4 T cells, activated CD8 T cells also switch from FAO to aerobic glycolysis and sustain elevated glycolysis and anabolic metabolism for CD8 T cell growth and differentiation into cytotoxic T cells.[66] After the peak of cell proliferation and differentiation, the metabolic profile of T cells shifts from glycolysis back to FAO, partially as a result of decreased mTOR signaling.[67–69] Intriguingly, a significant portion of substrates of FAO are de novo synthesized in CD8 memory T cells.[70] The metabolic switch is postulated to be required for the generation of memory CD8 T cells. Taken together, T cell activation and differentiation are tightly coupled with metabolic reprogramming.

B Cell Metabolism

B cells, which produce antibodies against pathogens, represent another critical component in adaptive immunity. Whereas T cells rapidly engage robust glycolytic programs upon antigen stimulation, B cells display a balanced increase in aerobic glycolysis and mitochondrial glucose oxidation after the engagement of the B cell antigen receptor (BCR) or LPS-mediated activation of TLR signaling. This balanced increase is likely because of a proportionally upregulated GLUT and mitochondrial mass.[71,72] Accumulating evidence has indicated that the engagement of glycolysis is tightly regulated by intra-cellular signal transduction pathways after B cell activation and is required for B cell proliferation and antibody production. It has been reported that the PI3K/Akt pathway is indispensable for glucose uptake and utilization, because the activation of Akt is sufficient to increase glucose metabolism in B cells.[73–75] Differentiation of B cells into immunoglobulin-secreting plasma cells is accompanied by the expansion of the intra-cellular membrane network, where immunoglobulin is produced and secreted. Such endomembrane network expansion requires the engagement of de novo lipogenesis. The PI3K/Akt signaling pathway is required to activate ATP-citrate lyase (ACLY), a key enzyme that channels the carbon of glucose to lipids through conversion of citrate to cytosolic acetyl-coenzyme A (CoA).[76,77] In addition, IL-4 promotes B cell survival by regulating glucose metabolism via the Janus kinase 1/3 (JAK1/3)-STAT6 signaling pathway.[71] Poly (adenosine diphosphate [ADP]-ribose) polymerase 14 (PARP14), an ADP ribosyltransferase, may represent another important downstream effector of IL-4 signaling, interplaying with STAT6 and modulating glycolysis in B cells.[78] Although HIF-1α is required for regulating glycolysis in B cell development in bone marrow,[79] it is dispensable for driving glycolysis in active B cells. Rather, an Myc-dependent upregulation of GLUT1 and likely other glycolytic genes are required for engaging glycolysis after B cell activation.[72]

Mitochondria and Immunity

Mitochondria play multiple, key roles in immunity. In addition to their critical biosynthetic function, mitochondria are intimately involved in immunity, where they serve as both initiators and transducers of various signaling cascades. Immunity can be divided into innate, pre-existing, or acquired, such that it develops after pathogenic challenge. Direct signaling roles for mitochondria have been best described in the context of innate immunity. Innate immune cells including macrophages or DCs detect infectious pathogens or damaged cells through pathogen recognition receptors (PRRs).[80] PRRs recognize conserved molecular patterns shared by microorganisms (pathogen-associated molecular patterns [PAMPs]) and damaged cells (damage-associated molecular patterns [DAMPs]). PRR pathway activation leads to the production of various pro-inflammatory and anti-microbial cytokines, including type 1 IFNs and IL-1. Through their action, these cytokines simultaneously create an anti-microbial environment and stimulate the development of adaptive immunity against the invading pathogen. As we will now discuss, mitochondria regulate multiple aspects of innate immune signaling, where they serve as both initiators and effectors of PRR signaling. We will review the roles of mitochondria in transducing signals elicited by three separate PRR families: retinoic acid inducible gene (RIG-I)–like receptors (RLRs), TLRs, and nuclear oligomerization domain (NOD)–like receptors (NLRs).

Mitochondria and NOD-like Receptor Signaling

Many PAMPs and DAMPs activate cytoplasmic complexes called *inflammasomes* (see Chapter 99).[81] After activation, inflammasomes activate the protease caspase-1, which, in turn, cleaves various pro-inflammatory cytokines, leading to their maturation and cellular release. The best-described cytoplasmic NLR is NLRP3. NLRP3 inflammasomes recruit and activate caspase-1 via the adaptor protein ASC. Various roles for mitochondria in promoting NLRP3-activation have been proposed; for example, recent data implicate the mitochondrial protein MAVS in NLRP3 inflammasome activation. MAVS is a key player in antiviral immunity engaged by RLR; however, it also interacts with NLRP3, leading to NLRP3 mitochondrial recruitment, thus promoting NLRP3-inflammasome assembly and activation.[82,83] Nevertheless, although it facilitates NLRP3 activation, MAVS is not essential because MAVS-deficient cells retain NRLP3 activity.[84]

In a separate study, microtubule-dependent transport of mitochondria to the endoplasmic reticulum (ER) promotes NLRP3-inflammasome activation by bringing together the key inflammasome-adaptor molecule, ASC (present on mitochondria) with NLRP3 (present on the ER).[85] Supporting this model, previous work has shown that active NLRP3 inflammasomes reside at mitochondrial-ER contacts.[86] Interestingly, mitochondrial transport depends upon acetylated tubulin, suggesting that mitochondrial metabolism (producing the acetyl-CoA required for acetylation) may also regulate inflammasome activity. Why would recruitment of NLRP3 to the mitochondria, either via MAVS or ASC, facilitate inflammasome activation? Potentially, mitochondria simply act as a physical scaffold that promotes inflammasome assembly. Alternatively, mitochondria may actively participate in inflammasome activation. Along these lines, different studies have shown that mitochondrial ROS promote NLRP3 activity.[86,87] Various DAMPs and PAMPs trigger mitochondrial ROS, and blocking ROS production (using ROS scavengers) can effectively block NLRP3-inflammasome activation.[86] It is not clear how ROS promotes NLRP3-inflammasome activation; similarly, it is not known how such diverse stimuli give rise to ROS. Besides mitochondrial ROS, other mitochondrial molecules such as cardiolipin and mitochondrial DNA (mtDNA) have been proposed to facilitate NLRP3 activation.[87,88] As we have discussed, there are numerous means by which mitochondria may promote NLRP3 activity; nevertheless, these means remain controversial. Whether mitochondria are required for NLRP3 activation is a question that may be readily addressed using a recently described method to generate mitochondria-deficient cells.[89]

Mitochondria and RIG-I-like Signaling

RLRs are the primary means by which cytoplasmic viral double-stranded RNA (dsRNA) is detected. RLR signaling ultimately leads to the production of type 1 IFN and pro-inflammatory cytokines, thereby inhibiting viral replication and promoting acquired immunity. In simplistic terms, binding of viral dsRNA to RIG-I or melanoma differentiation–associated protein 5 (MDA5) triggers its binding to MAVS, which is located on the mitochondrial outer membrane. MAVS then undergoes oligomerization, permitting it to bind adaptor molecules TRAF3 and TRAF6; these molecules subsequently activate interferon regulatory factor (IRF) and nuclear factor-κB (NF-κB) transcription factors, leading to antiviral interferon and pro-inflammatory cytokine production.[90] MAVS is a resident mitochondrial outer membrane protein, and various reports highlight an active role for mitochondrial dynamics in regulating RLR- and MAVS-dependent signaling (Fig. 24.3).

Mitochondria are constantly undergoing rounds of fission and fusion with one another, thereby promoting mitochondrial homeostasis. Interestingly, RLR signaling via MAVS requires mitochondrial fusion because cells deficient in mitofusins (MFN) 1 and 2 or optic atrophy type 1 (OPA-1)—all proteins that are required for mitochondrial fusion—are defective in MAVS signaling.[91,92] Similarly, Ψ disruption of mitochondrial membrane potential (Ψ_m), leading to mitochondrial fragmentation, also inhibits MAVS-dependent signaling.[93] It remains unclear why an intact mitochondrial network supports MAVS signaling, although in research that potentially addresses this question, MAVS activation occurs in a prion-like manner, whereby one activated MAVS molecule activates another.[94,95] Potentially, a continuous, fused mitochondrial network facilitates sufficient MAVS oligomerization to support downstream signaling. It is important to note that because of its pleiotropic effects, disruption of mitochondrial membrane potential may affect MAVS signaling by additional means beyond disrupting mitochondrial fusion. Similarly, MFN2 has additional fusion-independent functions, for example, in mitochondrial-ER tethering.[96]

Mitochondria and Toll-like Receptor Signaling

TLRs are localized at both the plasma membrane and various intra-cellular organelles that include lysosomes and endosomes. This nine-membered family responds to various PAMPs derived from bacteria, viruses, fungi, and parasites, transducing signals that ultimately lead to the production of pro-inflammatory cytokines.

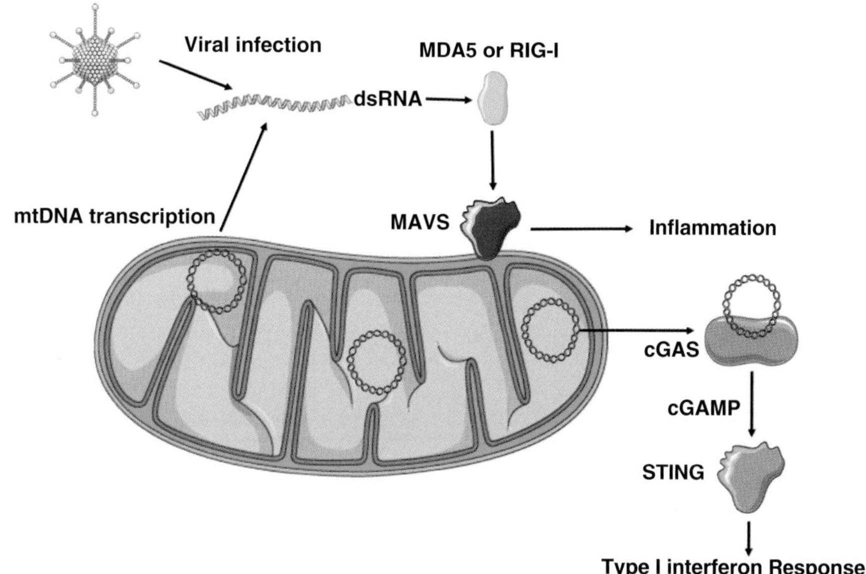

• **Fig. 24.3** Mechanisms of mitochondrial activation of innate immunity. Specific viral infections and transcription of circular mtDNA give rise to dsRNA. dsRNA is detected by cytoplasmic innate immune receptors, MDA5 and RIG-I. Upon binding dsRNA, MDA-5 and RIG-I bind mitochondrial localized MAVS leading to downstream inflammatory signaling. mtDNA can also drive inflammatory signaling directly. Following mitochondrial release, mtDNA is detected by the DNA sensor cGAS, leading to generation of the secondary messenger cGAMP. cGAMP activates STING, leading to a type 1 interferon response.

A key facet of innate immunity is the destruction of intra-cellular bacteria. After phagocytosis, ROS are induced, leading to the killing of intra-cellular bacteria. Most ROS produced during this process originate from NADPH oxidases; however, recent evidence also demonstrates an important role for TLR-driven mitochondrial ROS.[97] Triggering of specific TLRs triggers translocation of the TLR-adaptor molecule, TRAF6, to the mitochondria. At the mitochondria, TRAF6 ubiquitylates evolutionarily conserved signaling intermediate in Toll pathways (ECSIT), a protein implicated in complex I assembly.[98] Through means that are unclear, ubiquitinated ECSIT triggers mitochondrial ROS production and pathogen clearance. Beyond these effects, TLR engagement effects mitochondrial metabolism in other ways. For example, LPS increases the mitochondrial Krebs cycle intermediate metabolite, succinate, which induces pro-inflammatory IL-1β expression.[18]

Mitochondria as a Source of Danger Signals

Thus far we have discussed mitochondria as key signaling platforms in a variety of innate signaling cascades. Likely stemming from their bacterial ancestry, mitochondria also represent a rich source of DAMPs. Chief among these is mtDNA, which contains hypomethylated cytosine-phosphatidyl-guanine (CpG) motifs similar to bacterial DNA. In line with a pro-inflammatory function, direct injection of mtDNA, but not nuclear DNA, leads to inflammation.[99] Moreover, systemic release of mtDNA after trauma has been proposed to underlie systemic inflammatory response syndrome, a form of septic shock.[100] mtDNA released during apoptotic cell death is a potent activator of cyclic GMP-AMP synthase (cGAS)–stimulator of interferon genes (STING) signaling leading to a pro-inflammatory type I interferon response.[101,102] Recognition of mtDNA by the cytosolic DNA sensing enzyme cGAS leads to production of the secondary messenger cGAMP, which activates STING; during cell death, mitochondrial inner membrane permeabilization enables mtDNA release into the cytosol whereupon it activates cGAS-STING[103,104] (see Fig. 24.3). mtDNA dependent activation of cGAS-STING signaling also serves as an important anti-viral innate immune mechanism.[105] Besides mtDNA, other mitochondrial molecules may also serve as DAMPs. Recent studies also found that nuclear DNA damage can generate ssDNA in the cytoplasm, leading to the activation of cGAS-cGAMP-STING pathway that determines the immunologic outcomes of DNA damage,[106] and mitochondrial double-stranded RNA can activate anti-viral signaling pathway that triggers IFN-I response.[107] Again, similar to bacteria, mitochondria also use *N*-formyl-methionine as the translation initiating residue. Both can stimulate cytokine production after binding of formyl peptide receptors (FPRs).[100] Finally, due to bidirectional transcription of their circular DNA genome, mitochondria are an endogenous source of dsRNA.[108] dsRNA can activate various innate immune signaling pathways. Accordingly, under conditions where mitochondria dsRNA degradation is inhibited, it can activate MDA5-dependent anti-viral signaling (see Fig. 24.3).

Metabolic Interplay in the Immune Microenvironment

Aerobic glycolysis, glutaminolysis, and other amino acid catabolism are dominant metabolic routes for many pathogen-encountered immune cells. Thus, those heightened catabolic pathways cause local depletion of nutrients (e.g., glucose and glutamine) and local accumulation of metabolic end- or by-products (e.g., lactate, proton, and NO) in infection and inflammatory sites. The similarity of metabolic programs among some immune cells may lead to a potential metabolic antagonism for limited nutrient sources. On the contrary, some immune cells may preferentially utilize metabolic products of others to form a potential metabolic symbiosis (see Fig. 24.1).

Metabolic Antagonism in Immunity

The metabolic competition among active T cells, B cells, and DCs may lead to a rapid, albeit transient, nutrient depletion after immune activation. The restriction of glucose and glutamine results in metabolic stress and, consequentially, elicits signaling responses through AMPK and mTOR to modulate immune responses.[47,62,109] In addition, the depletion of extra-cellular tryptophan or arginine by DCs and macrophages that express amino acid catabolic enzymes such as indolamine 2,3-dioxygenase (IDO), tryptophan-2,3-dioxygenase (TDO), and arginase I (Arg I) often results in the depletion of local amino acids, and consequentially the activation of the protein kinase general control nonrepressed 2 (GCN2) in T cells.[110–113] Therefore Th17 differentiation is suppressed, whereas Treg development and T cell anergy are enhanced.[111,114]

The secreted metabolic products may dramatically change the local metabolic environment and may form additional metabolic antagonism to shape immune cell functions. The lactate and carbon dioxide produced from glycolysis and glutaminolysis lead to microenvironment acidification, which suppresses T cell proliferation, impairs NK cell and T cell cytokine production, and has a profound impact on monocyte differentiation.[115–118] Beyond this, the cross-membrane transport of sodium ions is intimately coupled with proton and amino acids transport and has a profound impact on immune function.[119,120] Recent studies showed that high-sodium chloride conditions induce the development of pathogenic Th17 cells with elevated release of pro-inflammatory cytokines (granulocyte-macrophage colony-stimulating factor [GM-CSF], TNF, and IL-2) and thus promote tissue inflammation.[121,122] Also, iNOS-mediated breakdown of arginine into NO affects both the intra-cellular and extra-cellular redox balance and consequentially elicits immune modulatory effects.[123,124]

Metabolic Symbiosis in Immunity

Lactate mediates a form of metabolic symbiosis in muscle, brain, and certain tumors.[125–127] Although it has not been demonstrated, the preference of mitochondrial-dependent oxidative metabolism of Treg cells indicates the possibility that Treg cells may utilize lactate and form a metabolic symbiosis with other lactate-producing immune cells. The concentration of lactate in vertebrate plasma ranges from 1 to 30 mM under physiologic and pathologic conditions.[128] Early studies have shown that lactate enhances Treg differentiation through the stimulation of IL-2 production and, in another case, promotes the development of myeloid-derived suppressor cells (MDSCs).[118,129,130] In addition, lactate and acidic environments have a profound impact on tumor-associated macrophages (TAMs), promoting tumor angiogenesis.[116,131–133] Beyond this, the breakdown of tryptophan to kynurenine and potentially other intermediate metabolites in antigen-presenting cells results in the accumulation of nature ligands of aryl hydrocarbon receptor (AHR) in the local microenvironment, which plays a broad role in modulating immunity.[134,135] As such, extra-cellular accumulation of kynurenine elicits an AHR-mediated response to reciprocally enhance function of Tregs and suppress the function of effector T (Teff) cells and immunogenicity of DCs.[136–138] Thus kynurenine may mediate another form of metabolic symbiosis in immunity.

Conclusion

In this chapter, we illustrate the relevant metabolic aspects of immune cells that have recently been revealed. In addition, we discuss the potential regulatory mechanism of metabolic reprogramming and the consequences of metabolic intervention on specific metabolic pathways in the immune response. The metabolic shift in immune cells during the transition between rest and activation is often associated with dramatically increased bioenergetic and biosynthetic demands. This may also lead active immune cells to become "addicted" to certain metabolic pathways in ways that resting cells are not. Thus, the modulation of such addiction, in terms of the biologic effects of enhancement or inhibition of specific pathways in immune cells, may offer novel therapeutic regimes to improve immunologic unresponsiveness or to suppress excessive immune responses, respectively. In addition to other known soluble protein factors, such as cytokines and chemokines, the availability of specific metabolites in the infection/inflammation microenvironment may be part of a pro-inflammatory or anti-inflammatory signaling circuit that affects the immune response. This is independent of their roles of bioenergetic fuels and may represent a general feature of the intercellular metabolic cross-talk mediated by metabolites. The revived interest in cell metabolism has revealed many fundamental biologic insights and will likely generate new therapeutic strategies for immunologic diseases in the near future.

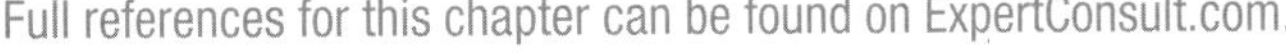
Full references for this chapter can be found on ExpertConsult.com.

Selected References

1. Martinez J, Verbist K, Wang R, et al.: The relationship between metabolism and the autophagy machinery during the innate immune response, *Cell Metab* 17:895–900, 2013.
2. Gordon S: Alternative activation of macrophages, *Nat Rev Immunol* 3:23–35, 2003.
3. Thompson RW, Pesce JT, Ramalingam T, et al.: Cationic amino acid transporter-2 regulates immunity by modulating arginase activity, *PLoS Pathog* 4:e1000023, 2008.
4. Qualls JE, Subramanian C, Rafi W, et al.: Sustained generation of nitric oxide and control of mycobacterial infection requires argininosuccinate synthase 1, *Cell Host Microbe* 12:313–323, 2012.
5. Mills E, O'Neill LA: Succinate: a metabolic signal in inflammation, *Trends Cell Biol* 24:313–320, 2014.
6. Stubbs M, Kuhner AV, Glass EA, et al.: Metabolic and functional studies on activated mouse macrophages, *J Exp Med* 137:537–542, 1973.
7. Shapiro H, Lutaty A, Ariel A: Macrophages, meta-inflammation, and immuno-metabolism, *Scientific World Journal* 11:2509–2529, 2011.
8. Bordbar A, Mo ML, Nakayasu ES, et al.: Model-driven multi-omic data analysis elucidates metabolic immunomodulators of macrophage activation, *Mol Syst Biol* 8:558, 2012.
9. Galvan-Pena S, O'Neill LA: Metabolic reprograming in macrophage polarization, *Front Immunol* 5:420, 2014.
10. Newsholme P, Costa Rosa LF, Newsholme EA, et al.: The importance of fuel metabolism to macrophage function, *Cell Biochem Funct* 14:1–10, 1996.
11. Maeng O, Kim YC, Shin HJ, et al.: Cytosolic NADP(+)-dependent isocitrate dehydrogenase protects macrophages from LPS-induced nitric oxide and reactive oxygen species, *Biochem Biophys Res Commun* 317:558–564, 2004.

12. Pollak N, Dolle C, Ziegler M: The power to reduce: pyridine nucleotides—small molecules with a multitude of functions, *Biochem J* 402:205–218, 2007.
13. Bellocq A, Suberville S, Philippe C, et al.: Low environmental pH is responsible for the induction of nitric-oxide synthase in macrophages. Evidence for involvement of nuclear factor-kappaB activation, *J Biol Chem* 273:5086–5092, 1998.
14. Cramer T, Yamanishi Y, Clausen BE, et al.: HIF-1alpha is essential for myeloid cell-mediated inflammation, *Cell* 112:645–657, 2003.
15. Rodriguez-Prados JC, Traves PG, Cuenca J, et al.: Substrate fate in activated macrophages: a comparison between innate, classic, and alternative activation, *J Immunol* 185:605–614, 2010.
16. Moncada S, Erusalimsky JD: Does nitric oxide modulate mitochondrial energy generation and apoptosis? *Nat Rev Mol Cell Biol* 3:214–220, 2002.
17. Doulias PT, Tenopoulou M, Greene JL, et al.: Nitric oxide regulates mitochondrial fatty acid metabolism through reversible protein S-nitrosylation, *Sci Signal* 6:rs1, 2013.
18. Tannahill GM, Curtis AM, Adamik J, et al.: Succinate is an inflammatory signal that induces IL-1beta through HIF-1alpha, *Nature* 496:238–242, 2013.
19. Murphy MP, O'Neill LAJ: Krebs cycle reimagined: the emerging roles of succinate and itaconate as signal transducers, *Cell* 174:780–784, 2018.
20. Mills EL, Kelly B, Logan A, et al.: Succinate dehydrogenase supports metabolic repurposing of mitochondria to drive inflammatory macrophages, *Cell* 167:457–470.e13, 2016.
21. Bambouskova M, Gorvel L, Lampropoulou V, et al.: Electrophilic properties of itaconate and derivatives regulate the IkappaBzeta-ATF3 inflammatory axis, *Nature* 556:501–504, 2018.
22. Mills EL, Ryan DG, Prag HA, et al.: Itaconate is an anti-inflammatory metabolite that activates Nrf2 via alkylation of KEAP1, *Nature* 556:113–117, 2018.
23. Haschemi A, Kosma P, Gille L, et al.: The sedoheptulose kinase CARKL directs macrophage polarization through control of glucose metabolism, *Cell Metab* 15:813–826, 2012.
24. Sinha P, Clements VK, Miller S, et al.: Tumor immunity: a balancing act between T cell activation, macrophage activation and tumor-induced immune suppression, cancer immunology, immunotherapy, *CII* 54:1137–1142, 2005.
25. Vats D, Mukundan L, Odegaard JI, et al.: Oxidative metabolism and PGC-1beta attenuate macrophage-mediated inflammation, *Cell Metab* 4:13–24, 2006.
26. Collin M, McGovern N, Haniffa M: Human dendritic cell subsets, *Immunology* 140:22–30, 2013.
27. Merad M, Sathe P, Helft J, et al.: The dendritic cell lineage: ontogeny and function of dendritic cells and their subsets in the steady state and the inflamed setting, *Annu Rev Immunol* 31:563–604, 2013.
28. Mildner A, Jung S: Development and function of dendritic cell subsets, *Immunity* 40:642–656, 2014.
29. Pearce EJ, Everts B: Dendritic cell metabolism, *Nat Rev Immunol* 15:18–29, 2015.
30. Thwe PM, Pelgrom L, Cooper R, et al.: Cell-intrinsic glycogen metabolism supports early glycolytic reprogramming required for dendritic cell immune responses, *Cell Metab* 26:558–567.e5, 2017.
31. Krawczyk CM, Holowka T, Sun J, et al.: Toll-like receptor-induced changes in glycolytic metabolism regulate dendritic cell activation, *Blood* 115:4742–4749, 2010.
32. Everts B, Amiel E, van der Windt GJ, et al.: Commitment to glycolysis sustains survival of NO-producing inflammatory dendritic cells, *Blood* 120:1422–1431, 2012.
33. Pantel A, Teixeira A, Haddad E, et al.: Direct type I IFN but not MDA5/TLR3 activation of dendritic cells is required for maturation and metabolic shift to glycolysis after poly IC stimulation, *PLoS Biol* 12:e1001759, 2014.
34. Everts B, Pearce EJ: Metabolic control of dendritic cell activation and function: recent advances and clinical implications, *Front Immunol* 5:203, 2014.
35. Weichhart T, Saemann MD: The PI3K/Akt/mTOR pathway in innate immune cells: emerging therapeutic applications, *Ann Rheum Dis* 67(Suppl 3):iii70–74, 2008.
36. Amiel E, Everts B, Freitas TC, et al.: Inhibition of mechanistic target of rapamycin promotes dendritic cell activation and enhances therapeutic autologous vaccination in mice, *J Immunol* 189:2151–2158, 2012.
37. Wang Y, Huang G, Zeng H, et al.: Tuberous sclerosis 1 (Tsc1)-dependent metabolic checkpoint controls development of dendritic cells, *Proc Natl Acad Sci U S A* 110:E4894–4903, 2013.
38. Land SC, Tee AR: Hypoxia-inducible factor 1alpha is regulated by the mammalian target of rapamycin (mTOR) via an mTOR signaling motif, *J Biol Chem* 282:20534–20543, 2007.
39. Jantsch J, Chakravortty D, Turza N, et al.: Hypoxia and hypoxia-inducible factor-1 alpha modulate lipopolysaccharide-induced dendritic cell activation and function, *J Immunol* 180:4697–4705, 2008.
40. Wobben R, Husecken Y, Lodewick C, et al.: Role of hypoxia inducible factor-1alpha for interferon synthesis in mouse dendritic cells, *Biol Chem* 394:495–505, 2013.
41. Cleeter MW, Cooper JM, Darley-Usmar VM, et al.: Reversible inhibition of cytochrome c oxidase, the terminal enzyme of the mitochondrial respiratory chain, by nitric oxide. Implications for neurodegenerative diseases, *FEBS Lett* 345:50–54, 1994.
42. Lagouge M, Argmann C, Gerhart-Hines Z, et al.: Resveratrol improves mitochondrial function and protects against metabolic disease by activating SIRT1 and PGC-1alpha, *Cell* 127:1109–1122, 2006.
43. Rangasamy T, Williams MA, Bauer S, et al.: Nuclear erythroid 2 p45-related factor 2 inhibits the maturation of murine dendritic cells by ragweed extract, *Am J Respir Cell Mol Biol* 43:276–285, 2010.
44. Svajger U, Obermajer N, Jeras M: Dendritic cells treated with resveratrol during differentiation from monocytes gain substantial tolerogenic properties upon activation, *Immunology* 129:525–535, 2010.
45. Carroll KC, Viollet B, Suttles J: AMPKalpha1 deficiency amplifies proinflammatory myeloid APC activity and CD40 signaling, *J Leukoc Biol* 94:1113–1121, 2013.
46. Wang R, Dillon CP, Shi LZ, et al.: The transcription factor Myc controls metabolic reprogramming upon T lymphocyte activation, *Immunity* 35:871–882, 2011.
47. Wang R, Green DR: Metabolic checkpoints in activated T cells, *Nat Immunol* 13:907–915, 2012.
48. Wang R, Green DR: Metabolic reprogramming and metabolic dependency in T cells, *Immunol Rev* 249:14–26, 2012.
49. Wang R, Green DR: The immune diet: meeting the metabolic demands of lymphocyte activation, *F1000 Biol Rep* 4:9, 2012.
50. Grumont R, Lock P, Mollinari M, et al.: The mitogen-induced increase in T cell size involves PKC and NFAT activation of Rel/NF-kappaB-dependent c-myc expression, *Immunity* 21:19–30, 2004.
51. Frauwirth KA, Riley JL, Harris MH, et al.: The CD28 signaling pathway regulates glucose metabolism, *Immunity* 16:769–777, 2002.
52. Jacobs SR, Herman CE, Maciver NJ, et al.: Glucose uptake is limiting in T cell activation and requires CD28-mediated Akt-dependent and independent pathways, *J Immunol* 180:4476–4486, 2008.
53. Carr EL, Kelman A, Wu GS, et al.: Glutamine uptake and metabolism are coordinately regulated by ERK/MAPK during T lymphocyte activation, *J Immunol* 185:1037–1044, 2010.
54. Bensinger SJ, Bradley MN, Joseph SB, et al.: LXR signaling couples sterol metabolism to proliferation in the acquired immune response, *Cell* 134:97–111, 2008.

55. Michalek RD, Gerriets VA, Jacobs SR, et al.: Cutting edge: Distinct glycolytic and lipid oxidative metabolic programs are essential for effector and regulatory CD4+ T cell subsets, *J Immunol* 186:3299–3303, 2011.
56. Kidani Y, Elsaesser H, Hock MB, et al.: Sterol regulatory element-binding proteins are essential for the metabolic programming of effector T cells and adaptive immunity, *Nat Immunol* 14:489–499, 2013.
57. Romagnani S: Type 1 T helper and type 2 T helper cells: functions, regulation and role in protection and disease, *Int J Clin Lab Res* 21:152–158, 1991.
58. Korn T, Bettelli E, Oukka M, et al.: IL-17 and Th17 cells, *Annu Rev Immunol* 27:485–517, 2009.
59. Luckheeram RV, Zhou R, Verma AD, et al.: CD4(+)T cells: differentiation and functions, *Clin Dev Immunol* 2012:925135, 2012.
60. Shi LZ, Wang R, Huang G, et al.: HIF1alpha-dependent glycolytic pathway orchestrates a metabolic checkpoint for the differentiation of TH17 and Treg cells, *J Exp Med* 208:1367–1376, 2011.
61. Peter C, Waldmann H, Cobbold SP: mTOR signalling and metabolic regulation of T cell differentiation, *Curr Opin Immunol* 22:655–661, 2010.
62. Chi H: Regulation and function of mTOR signalling in T cell fate decisions, *Nat Rev Immunol* 12:325–338, 2012.
63. Dang EV, Barbi J, Yang HY, et al.: Control of T(H)17/T(reg) balance by hypoxia-inducible factor 1, *Cell* 146:772–784, 2011.
64. Arpaia N, Campbell C, Fan X, et al.: Metabolites produced by commensal bacteria promote peripheral regulatory T-cell generation, *Nature* 504:451–455, 2013.
65. Furusawa Y, Obata Y, Fukuda S, et al.: Commensal microbe-derived butyrate induces the differentiation of colonic regulatory T cells, *Nature* 504:446–450, 2013.
66. Finlay D, Cantrell DA: Metabolism, migration and memory in cytotoxic T cells, *Nat Rev Immunol* 11:109–117, 2011.
67. Araki K, Turner AP, Shaffer VO, et al.: mTOR regulates memory CD8 T-cell differentiation, *Nature* 460:108–112, 2009.
68. Pearce EL, Walsh MC, Cejas PJ, et al.: Enhancing CD8 T-cell memory by modulating fatty acid metabolism, *Nature* 460:103–107, 2009.
69. van der Windt GJ, Everts B, Chang CH, et al.: Mitochondrial respiratory capacity is a critical regulator of CD8+ T cell memory development, *Immunity* 36:68–78, 2012.
70. O'Sullivan D, van der Windt GJ, Huang SC, et al.: Memory CD8(+) T cells use cell-intrinsic lipolysis to support the metabolic programming necessary for development, *Immunity* 41:75–88, 2014.
71. Dufort FJ, Bleiman BF, Gumina MR, et al.: Cutting edge: IL-4-mediated protection of primary B lymphocytes from apoptosis via Stat6-dependent regulation of glycolytic metabolism, *J Immunol* 179:4953–4957, 2007.
72. Caro-Maldonado A, Wang R, Nichols AG, et al.: Metabolic reprogramming is required for antibody production that is suppressed in anergic but exaggerated in chronically BAFF-exposed B cells, *J Immunol* 192:3626–3636, 2014.
73. Donahue AC, Fruman DA: Proliferation and survival of activated B cells requires sustained antigen receptor engagement and phosphoinositide 3-kinase activation, *J Immunol* 170:5851–5860, 2003.
74. Doughty CA, Bleiman BF, Wagner DJ, et al.: Antigen receptor-mediated changes in glucose metabolism in B lymphocytes: role of phosphatidylinositol 3-kinase signaling in the glycolytic control of growth, *Blood* 107:4458–4465, 2006.
75. Woodland RT, Fox CJ, Schmidt MR, et al.: Multiple signaling pathways promote B lymphocyte stimulator dependent B-cell growth and survival, *Blood* 111:750–760, 2008.
76. Bauer DE, Hatzivassiliou G, Zhao F, et al.: ATP citrate lyase is an important component of cell growth and transformation, *Oncogene* 24:6314–6322, 2005.
77. Dufort FJ, Gumina MR, Ta NL, et al.: Glucose-dependent de novo lipogenesis in B lymphocytes: a requirement for atp-citrate lyase in lipopolysaccharide-induced differentiation, *J Biol Chem* 289:7011–7024, 2014.
78. Cho SH, Ahn AK, Bhargava P, et al.: Glycolytic rate and lymphomagenesis depend on PARP14, an ADP ribosyltransferase of the B aggressive lymphoma (BAL) family, *Proc Natl Acad Sci U S A* 108:15972–15977, 2011.
79. Kojima H, Kobayashi A, Sakurai D, et al.: Differentiation stage-specific requirement in hypoxia-inducible factor-1alpha-regulated glycolytic pathway during murine B cell development in bone marrow, *J Immunol* 184:154–163, 2010.
80. Janeway Jr CA, Medzhitov R: Innate immune recognition, *Annu Rev Immunol* 20:197–216, 2002.
81. Strowig T, Henao-Mejia J, Elinav E, et al.: Inflammasomes in health and disease, *Nature* 481:278–286, 2012.
82. Park S, Juliana C, Hong S, et al.: The mitochondrial antiviral protein MAVS associates with NLRP3 and regulates its inflammasome activity, *J Immunol* 191:4358–4366, 2013.
83. Subramanian N, Natarajan K, Clatworthy MR, et al.: The adaptor MAVS promotes NLRP3 mitochondrial localization and inflammasome activation, *Cell* 153:348–361, 2013.
84. Allam R, Lawlor KE, Yu EC, et al.: Mitochondrial apoptosis is dispensable for NLRP3 inflammasome activation but non-apoptotic caspase-8 is required for inflammasome priming, *EMBO Rep* 15:982–990, 2014.
85. Misawa T, Takahama M, Kozaki T, et al.: Microtubule-driven spatial arrangement of mitochondria promotes activation of the NLRP3 inflammasome, *Nat Immunol* 14:454–460, 2013.
86. Zhou R, Yazdi AS, Menu P, et al.: A role for mitochondria in NLRP3 inflammasome activation, *Nature* 469:221–225, 2011.
87. Nakahira K, Haspel JA, Rathinam VA, et al.: Autophagy proteins regulate innate immune responses by inhibiting the release of mitochondrial DNA mediated by the NALP3 inflammasome, *Nat Immunol* 12:222–230, 2011.
88. Iyer SS, He Q, Janczy JR, et al.: Mitochondrial cardiolipin is required for Nlrp3 inflammasome activation, *Immunity* 39:311–323, 2013.
89. Tait SW, Oberst A, Quarato G, et al.: Widespread mitochondrial depletion via mitophagy does not compromise necroptosis, *Cell Rep* 5:878–885, 2013.
90. Dixit E, Kagan JC: Intracellular pathogen detection by RIG-I-like receptors, *Advances in immunology* 117:99–125, 2013.
91. Castanier C, Garcin D, Vazquez A, et al.: Mitochondrial dynamics regulate the RIG-I-like receptor antiviral pathway, *EMBO Rep* 11:133–138, 2010.
92. Pourcelot M, Arnoult D: Mitochondrial dynamics and the innate antiviral immune response, *FEBS J* 281:3791–3802, 2014.
93. Koshiba T, Yasukawa K, Yanagi Y, et al.: Mitochondrial membrane potential is required for MAVS-mediated antiviral signaling, *Sci Signal* 4:ra7, 2011.
94. Hou F, Sun L, Zheng H, et al.: MAVS forms functional prion-like aggregates to activate and propagate antiviral innate immune response, *Cell* 146:448–461, 2011.
95. Cai X, Chen J, Xu H, et al.: Prion-like polymerization underlies signal transduction in antiviral immune defense and inflammasome activation, *Cell* 156:1207–1222, 2014.
96. de Brito OM, Scorrano L: Mitofusin 2 tethers endoplasmic reticulum to mitochondria, *Nature* 456:605–610, 2008.
97. West AP, Brodsky IE, Rahner C, et al.: TLR signalling augments macrophage bactericidal activity through mitochondrial ROS, *Nature* 472:476–480, 2011.
98. Vogel RO, Janssen RJ, van den Brand MA, et al.: Cytosolic signaling protein Ecsit also localizes to mitochondria where it interacts with chaperone NDUFAF1 and functions in complex I assembly, *Genes Dev* 21:615–624, 2007.

99. Collins LV, Hajizadeh S, Holme E, et al.: Endogenously oxidized mitochondrial DNA induces in vivo and in vitro inflammatory responses, *J Leukoc Biol* 75:995–1000, 2004.
100. Zhang Q, Raoof M, Chen Y, et al.: Circulating mitochondrial DAMPs cause inflammatory responses to injury, *Nature* 464:104–107, 2010.
101. Rongvaux A, Jackson R, Harman CC, et al.: Apoptotic caspases prevent the induction of type I interferons by mitochondrial DNA, *Cell* 159:1563–1577, 2014.
102. White MJ, McArthur K, Metcalf D, et al.: Apoptotic caspases suppress mtDNA-induced STING-mediated type I IFN production, *Cell* 159:1549–1562, 2014.
103. McArthur K, Whitehead LW, Heddleston JM, et al.: BAK/BAX macropores facilitate mitochondrial herniation and mtDNA efflux during apoptosis, *Science* 359, 2018.
104. Riley JS, Quarato G, Cloix C, et al.: Mitochondrial inner membrane permeabilisation enables mtDNA release during apoptosis, *EMBO J* 37, 2018.
105. West AP, Khoury-Hanold W, Staron M, et al.: Mitochondrial DNA stress primes the antiviral innate immune response, *Nature* 520:553–557, 2015.
106. Li T, Chen ZJ: The cGAS-cGAMP-STING pathway connects DNA damage to inflammation, senescence, and cancer, *J Exp Med* 215:1287–1299, 2018.
107. Dhir A, Dhir S, Borowski LS, et al.: Mitochondrial double-stranded RNA triggers antiviral signalling in humans, *Nature* 560:238–242, 2018.
108. Young PG, Attardi G: Characterization of double-stranded RNA from HeLa cell mitochondria, *Biochem Biophys Res Commun* 65:1201–1207, 1975.
109. Waickman AT, Powell JD: mTOR, metabolism, and the regulation of T-cell differentiation and function, *Immunol Rev* 249:43–58, 2012.
110. Nicholson LB, Raveney BJ, Munder M: Monocyte dependent regulation of autoimmune inflammation, *Curr Mol Med* 9:23–29, 2009.
111. Sundrud MS, Koralov SB, Feuerer M, et al.: Halofuginone inhibits TH17 cell differentiation by activating the amino acid starvation response, *Science* 324:1334–1338, 2009.
112. Bunpo P, Cundiff JK, Reinert RB, et al.: The eIF2 kinase GCN2 is essential for the murine immune system to adapt to amino acid deprivation by asparaginase, *J Nutr* 140:2020–2027, 2010.
113. Huang L, Baban B, Johnson 3rd BA, et al.: Dendritic cells, indoleamine 2,3 dioxygenase and acquired immune privilege, *Int Rev Immunol* 29:133–155, 2010.
114. Munn DH, Sharma MD, Baban B, et al.: GCN2 kinase in T cells mediates proliferative arrest and anergy induction in response to indoleamine 2,3-dioxygenase, *Immunity* 22:633–642, 2005.
115. Fischer K, Hoffmann P, Voelkl S, et al.: Inhibitory effect of tumor cell-derived lactic acid on human T cells, *Blood* 109:3812–3819, 2007.
116. Samuvel DJ, Sundararaj KP, Nareika A, et al.: Lactate boosts TLR4 signaling and NF-kappaB pathway-mediated gene transcription in macrophages via monocarboxylate transporters and MD-2 up-regulation, *J Immunol* 182:2476–2484, 2009.
117. Dietl K, Renner K, Dettmer K, et al.: Lactic acid and acidification inhibit TNF secretion and glycolysis of human monocytes, *J Immunol* 184:1200–1209, 2010.
118. Husain Z, Huang Y, Seth P, et al.: Tumor-derived lactate modifies antitumor immune response: effect on myeloid-derived suppressor cells and NK cells, *J Immunol* 191:1486–1495, 2013.
119. Estrella V, Chen T, Lloyd M, et al.: Acidity generated by the tumor microenvironment drives local invasion, *Cancer Res* 73:1524–1535, 2013.
120. Reshkin SJ, Cardone RA, Harguindey S: Na+-H+ exchanger, pH regulation and cancer, *Recent Patents Anticancer Drug Discov* 8:85–99, 2013.

25 Genetics of Rheumatic Diseases

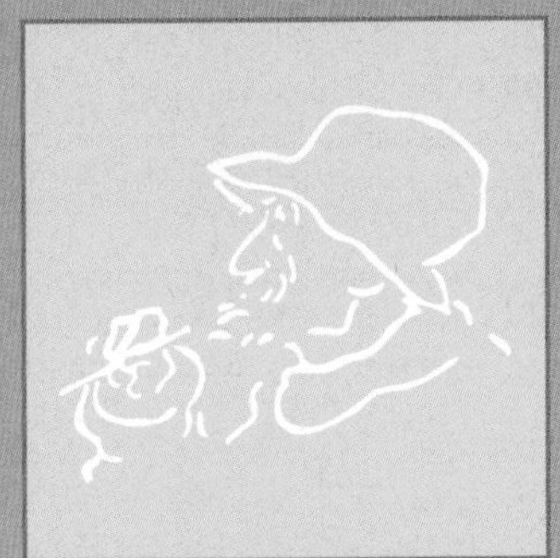

STEPHEN EYRE AND ANNE BARTON

KEY POINTS

- New genomic techniques have led to the discovery of genetic polymorphisms, which can contribute to the rheumatic diseases.
- In many cases, the genes and variants associated with disease have not yet been defined, although a locus of association has been identified.
- Exploiting genetic data provides insights into important key risk pathways, the cell types responsible for disease, and potential targets for novel drug development.
- Genetic testing has not translated into the clinical setting for most diseases—more work is required to identify signatures of drug response and prognosis.

Introduction

Many of the musculoskeletal diseases seen by rheumatologists in routine clinics are thought to arise as a result of an environmental insult that triggers disease in a genetically susceptible individual. As such, they are called *complex diseases* because both genes and environment contribute to the risk of disease development. Genetic risk factors are easier to study than environmental risk factors because genetic variants are present from conception (and therefore, must have been present before disease onset and could contribute to disease susceptibility and severity), are stable throughout life, and are easily measured. This contrasts with environmental risk factors where information is often collected after the patient has developed disease but the exposure could have occurred many years before disease onset, thereby introducing recall bias; or the exposure is measured after initial symptom onset, making it difficult to separate cause from effect. Furthermore, environmental risk factors often cannot be reliably or consistently measured. Thus, while research has identified a few environmental factors that predispose to disease, there has been an explosion of knowledge about the genetic contribution to many rheumatic diseases.

Evidence for a Genetic Component to Rheumatic Diseases

To justify investigating the genetic basis of any disease, it is first necessary to have some evidence that genes play a role. This evidence comes from twin or family studies most commonly, although adoption and migration studies can also support a genetic component. Classical twin studies compare the incidence of disease concordance in monozygotic (MZ) and dizygotic (DZ) twin pairs. Higher disease concordance in MZ twins provides support for a genetic etiology and can be used to estimate the heritability of disease. The percentage concordance of disease in MZ twins at one point in time will underestimate the genetic contribution to risk in diseases of late age at onset, like many musculoskeletal disorders. This is because, as time progresses, the concordance rate in MZ twins is likely to increase as their age increases. Thus, the concordance rate from one twin study in the UK found a rate of 15% in MZ twins and 4% in DZ twins, equating to a 60% heritability.[1]

For less common rheumatic diseases, it may be impossible to collect enough data on twin pairs to interpret the data reliably. However, family studies can also indicate a genetic contribution to disease. The sibling recurrence risk ratio is defined as:

$$\lambda_s = \frac{\text{Risk of recurrence in a sibling of affected individuals}}{\text{General population risk}}$$

Diseases that show an increased prevalence in family members are likely to have a genetic component. Obtaining a reliable value of λs depends on having accurate estimates of disease prevalence in the two comparison groups. This is not a trivial matter. A firm diagnosis of rheumatic disease is difficult to make in large population surveys, with errors in both directions possible. Underestimation may occur because of the lack of reporting of disease that is no longer active. Overestimation may result from inadequate distinction between different forms of rheumatic disease. Table 25.1 shows the heritability estimates (where available) and sibling recurrence risk ratios for some of the rheumatic diseases.

If genome-wide genotype data are available, it is now also possible to estimate heritability from the data itself using statistical methods that assume that patients with a disease are more genetically similar overall than controls and several such methods are available.[2] However, in some cases, the genetic data can suggest lower heritability than the original twin/family estimates; for example, an estimation of "callous-unemotional" behavior based on twin study methodology yielded a heritability estimate of 64%, as compared to a GCTA that yielded a heritability estimate of 7%.[3]

TABLE 25.1 Sibling Recurrence Risks and Heritability Estimates for Some Common Rheumatic Diseases

Rheumatic Disease	Sibling Recurrence Risk	Heritability
Rheumatoid arthritis	3-19	60
Juvenile idiopathic arthritis	15-20	
Psoriatic arthritis	40	
Ankylosing spondylitis	54	>90
Systemic lupus erythematosus	20-40	66
Osteoarthritis		
Hip	2-4	60%
Knee	2-5	40%
Hand	4	60%

TABLE 25.2 Glossary of Terms

Allele	Alternative form, or variant, of a gene at a particular locus
Alloantisera	Antisera that detect antigenic differences between individuals in the population; the term is most often used to refer to sera that detect antigenic (i.e., structural) differences among human leukocyte antigen molecules carried by different individuals
Haplotype	A group of alleles at adjacent or closely linked loci on the same chromosome that are usually inherited together as a unit
Heterozygote	An individual who inherits two different alleles at a given locus on two homologous chromosomes
Heterozygosity	A measure at a particular locus of the frequency with which heterozygotes occur in the population
Linkage	The tendency toward the co-inheritance within a family of two genes that lie near each other on the genome; complete linkage occurs when parents who are heterozygous at each locus are unable to produce recombinant gametes
Linkage disequilibrium	The preferential association in a population of two alleles or mutations that occurs more frequently than predicted by chance; linkage disequilibrium is detected statistically and, except in unusual circumstances, it implies that the two alleles lie near each other on the genome
Polymorphism	The degree of allelic variation at a locus within a population; specific criteria differ, but a locus is said to be polymorphic if the most frequent allele does not occur in >98% of the population; occasionally, polymorphism can be used in the same way as allele to refer to a particular genetic variant
Penetrance	The conditional probability of disease (or phenotype) given the presence of a risk genotype

Study Design

There are a number of important considerations when designing a study to identify genetic variants contributing to disease. These include the use of linkage versus (Table 25.2) association approaches, case-control versus family based studies, the choice of marker to be tested and candidate gene versus whole genome methods. The choice may be driven by cost considerations, power, and/or the availability of samples. The differing approaches have been outlined in more detail in the following sections.

Linkage Studies

Linkage methods depend on the ability to track polymorphic markers in families and to show that these genetic markers cosegregate with the disease phenotype in families where there are multiple members affected. Thus multiplex families are required for linkage analysis. The details of the statistical methods are complex but are generally based on examining the likelihood of a particular pattern of co-inheritance of marker and disease (linkage), compared with the likelihood that there is no linkage (the null hypothesis). A measure of this likelihood is referred to as the *LOD* (log of the odds) score, with an LOD score greater than 3 generally interpreted to indicate significant evidence of linkage when markers across the entire genome are examined.[4]

Linkage analysis has been applied with great success to the analysis of rheumatic diseases that exhibit a clear Mendelian pattern of inheritance (e.g., dominant or recessive). For example, in 1992, familial Mediterranean fever was mapped to chromosome 16,[5] and this led to the identification of mutations in the *MEFV* gene as being causal in this disease.[6] The *MEFV* gene encodes a protein known as *pyrin*, thought to be important in regulation of the innate immune response, particularly in response to interferon gamma stimulation. In addition, an entirely new class of familial periodic fever syndromes has been localized to mutations in the TNF receptor 1 gene on chromosome 12.[7] Thus for highly penetrant Mendelian disorders with a clear pattern of inheritance, classical linkage analysis is a powerful means of identifying the underlying molecular basis of disease. However, for complex diseases alternative approaches based on the affected sibling pair (ASP) method are required.[8] This method is based on a simple question: When two siblings are both affected with a disease, do they share alleles at particular genetic markers more frequently than would be expected by chance? Fig. 25.1 illustrates this basic approach. In this family, two siblings are affected and the first-born sibling (sib 1) has inherited alleles 1 and 3 at a marker locus, X. By the laws of Mendelian inheritance, sibling 2 has a 25% chance of inheriting the same two alleles; a 25% chance of inheriting neither of these alleles (i.e., sib 2 inherits 2,4 and shares nothing with sib 1 at locus X) and a 50% chance of inheriting one. This 25:50:25 distribution of sharing is expected if there is no linkage between the disease and the marker locus. However, if a gene that lies near the marker locus is involved in disease risk, a significant deviation toward increased sharing among affected siblings will be observed. The closer the marker is to the disease locus, the greater the deviation will be from

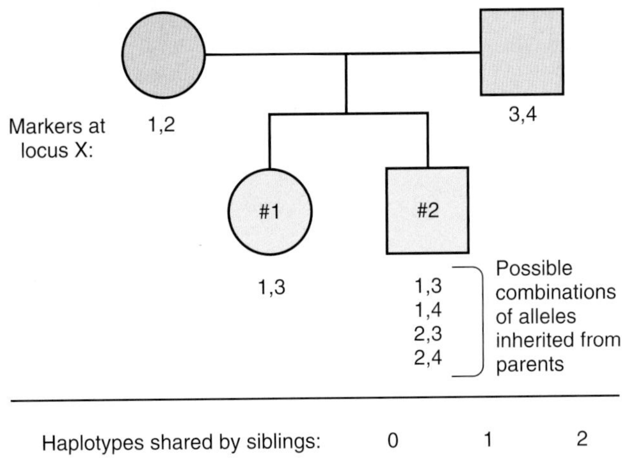

• **Fig. 25.1** A nuclear family with two affected children (affected sibling pair). The possible distribution of alleles at an autosomal locus, X, is shown for sib 2, along with the predicted frequency of shared haplotypes among the sibs. In these families researchers can detect linkage using affected sibling pair analysis (see text).

a 25:50:25 distribution. By examining large numbers of affected sibling pairs in this manner, the investigator can develop statistical evidence that this is the case. ASP analysis has a number of distinct advantages and disadvantages. Only affected individuals are used, and the problem of falsely assigning a family member as "unaffected" is eliminated. This is a major issue for many musculoskeletal diseases where the disease may not express itself until later in life. ASP analysis can be done without assuming a specific model of inheritance (i.e., recessive or dominant). As with linkage in general, the ASP methods suffer from having relatively low power to detect genes that confer only modest risk. This means that large numbers (hundreds or thousands) of families with affected siblings are required to obtain statistically significant results.

ASP linkage analysis has resulted in a few successes, most notably the identification of the *NOD2* gene as a major risk factor for Crohn's disease.[9,10] Furthermore, the presence of a linkage peak (LOD score > 3.5) on chromosome 2q in RA ASPs[11] led to the identification of the *STAT4* gene as a risk gene for RA, as well as systemic lupus erythematosus (SLE).[12] Thus, although challenging to carry out, linkage can occasionally be applied successfully to complex diseases.

Population-Association Studies

The most common way to establish whether a genetic variant (allele) confers risk for a disease is by performing a case-control study. In this type of study, subjects are initially identified according to whether they have the disease, and individuals without the disease are the controls. The risk of disease in those carrying a particular variant is described using the odds ratio (OR). An OR of 1 indicates that the genetic factor confers no risk for the disease. An OR less than 1 suggests that the genetic factor under study is negatively associated with the disease (i.e., it is protective). Traditionally, ORs are reported with respect to the less common genetic variant (minor allele), so an OR of less than 1 indicates that the major allele confers risk. Sometimes, however, the OR with respect to the risk variant (whether the major or minor allele) is reported and, in that case, the ORs are always greater than 1 if the result is statistically significant.

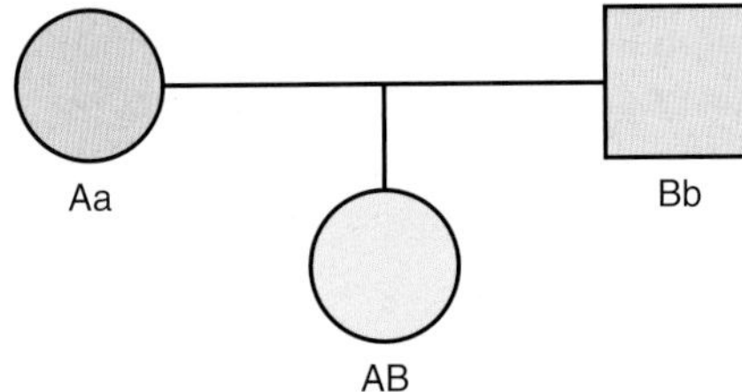

• **Fig. 25.2** Illustration of the trio family used for transmission disequilibrium test analysis.

One of the potential drawbacks of case-control association studies is that spurious association can occur if the cases and controls are not sampled from the same population (population stratification). An example would be if all disease cases were samples from a Scottish population and all controls from a Spanish population. The gene variant conferring red hair color is more prevalent in the Scottish population with or without disease. Therefore, the red hair color gene would be associated with disease in such a study but the association would be a false positive. In reality, if information is available on a large number of genetic variants across the genome or for variants known to differ across populations of different ancestry, methods exist to correct for population stratification in the analysis but the best solution is to consider this potential confounder in the study design. While family-based association designs, such as the transmission disequilibrium test (TDT)[13] (which calculates any deviation from the 50:50 random chance of passing a specific allele from a parent to an affected child [Fig. 25.2]), use parental control genotypes to eliminate the risk of population stratification, it is generally more expensive to collect and genotype trio families, so most studies use a case-control approach.

Choice of Genetic Marker to Test

There has been an explosion in new genetic knowledge over the past few years and this is likely to continue for some time. A number of initiatives have sequenced individuals of various ancestries to create a reference catalogue of the common sequence variation across the human genome (e.g., www.uk10k.org). The most common form of variation across the genome is where a single base change occurs, for example, from adenine (A) to guanine (G) in the DNA sequence. Such changes are called single nucleotide polymorphisms (SNPs) and there are now more than 30 million SNPs referenced for *Homo sapiens* in dbSNP, an online SNP reference database (www.ncbi.nlm.nih.gov/SNP/). In addition to SNPs, there are tens of thousands of variable numbers of tandem repeats (VNTRs) variants and insertions and deletions[14] providing other sources of genetic variation that can be associated with human disease. For example, Huntington's disease is caused by variable number of repeats of a CAG triplet within the Huntingtin gene. Smaller insertions and deletions are also frequent and the number of these genetic variants will grow substantially as more human genomes are fully sequenced.

Candidate Gene Versus Genome-wide Association Studies

The first wave of genetic studies of complex diseases focused on candidate gene studies. The candidate genes investigated were selected based on biological plausibility, because they were associated with another disease or based on animal model studies.

However, the prior probability of detecting association to one gene among the at least 30,000 known protein-coding genes is very low, especially when only one or a few markers were tested at the genomic locus, as was generally the case in such candidate gene studies. Furthermore, few studies tested large sample sizes of cases and controls and so were underpowered to generate robust findings. Nonetheless, several genes of large effect sizes were consistently detected, notably the *HLA* and *PTPN22* genetic associations observed with many complex diseases.

The acceleration in the knowledge of genetic variation across the genome, coupled with sweeping technologic advances, has meant that it is now possible to test SNP markers spanning the genome for evidence of association, so-called genome-wide association studies (GWAS). The era of SNP-based GWAS began in earnest in 2005, when the complement regulatory protein Factor H was identified as a significant risk factor for age-related macular degeneration.[15] A major advance was made in 2007 with the realization that for most complex diseases, effect sizes of individual variants on disease would be modest, hence large sample sizes would be required to robustly detect association. This was heralded by the pioneering Wellcome Trust Case Control Consortium (WTCCC) study.[16] The WTCCC study was the first to utilize a respectably powered study design, including 2000 cases from seven diseases and 3000 common controls; association was tested to 500,000 SNP markers spanning the genome and robust statistical thresholds were applied to claim confirmed significance. Novel loci were identified, and subsequent, better powered studies in larger independent sample sizes identified further loci. In the intervening 10 years, GWAS studies have proven to be particularly fruitful when applied to autoimmune disorders. Together, there are now nearly 200 distinct chromosomal regions that have been identified as containing risk loci for major autoimmune diseases (http://www.genome.gov/multimedia/illustrations/GWAS). As large datasets are assembled for some of the rarer or less studied autoimmune disorders, GWAS will continue to play a major role in dissecting the genetic contribution to musculoskeletal diseases.

Genome-wide Association Studies

Compared with linkage analysis, association methods have much greater statistical power to detect genetic effects.[17] However, in contrast to the relatively modest numbers of markers used for linkage studies, hundreds of thousands or even millions of genetic markers are currently utilized to carry out GWAS. The issue of testing so many markers raises the possibility of detecting association by chance alone. Hence, the genetics community has implemented thresholds for claims of confirmed association, based on the fact that there are estimated to be 1 million independent (noncorrelated) SNPs across the genome; applying a Bonferroni correction for 1 million markers equates to exceeding a statistical threshold of $P < 5 \times 10^{-8}$ to report confirmed association. In turn, this has implications for study power, which is related to the effect size of the locus, the statistical threshold, and the frequency of the risk allele, which all impact the sample size required to detect association. Thus, the smaller the effect size expected, the lower the *P* value threshold used, and the lower the frequency of the minor allele, the larger the sample size required to have power to detect association. The effect size reflects the contribution of a particular locus to disease susceptibility and is measured by the OR. ORs are often overestimated in the first study in which a locus is reported to be associated with a disease because of the phenomenon of "winner's curse"[18]: as most studies are underpowered to detect all susceptibility loci, if association is detected, it is likely that, by chance, the risk allele is enriched in the population tested. In independent populations, the true frequency of the risk allele will be lower so a larger sample size is required to replicate the association.

The success of whole genome association studies is critically dependent on taking advantage of the underlying haplotype structure of the genome, which in turn reflects the ubiquitous presence of linkage disequilibrium (LD) across the genome. LD refers to the fact that genetic variants at adjacent loci often tend to be found together more frequently than expected by chance. LD over long distances is a particularly prominent feature of the human leukocyte antigen (HLA) region.

Linkage Disequilibrium

The concept of LD is central to understanding the significance of any genetic association with disease. LD exists when the frequency of two alleles occurring together on the same haplotype exceeds that predicted by chance. For example, a common major histocompatibility complex (MHC) haplotype that exhibits LD in the white population carries a certain combination of alleles, A*0101-B*0801-DRB1*03011, commonly referred to as the A1-B8-DR3 haplotype (also known as the "8.1" haplotype).[19] This haplotype is present in about 9% of the Danish population, a typical white Northern European group. To understand why this reflects the presence of LD, consider the fact that the A1 allele is present in 17% of Danes and the B8 allele is present in 12.7% of Danes. They could be expected to be found together only 12.7% × 17% = 2.1% of the time, much less than observed (9%).

Detailed maps of LD are widely available online for the entire human genome, with easy-to-use visualization tools (see http://www.haplotype-reference-consortium.org/). The lower portion of Fig. 25.3 shows a visualization of LD using the D′ measure for a region around the *PTPN22* gene on chromosome 1. The D′ value between any two markers is reflected by the heat map (red D′ = 1; white D′ = 0). In this case, LD extends well beyond *PTPN22* itself. Indeed, as indicated in the figure, the SNP marker rs6679677 was used by the WTCCC[16] to detect the underlying association of rheumatoid arthritis (RA) with *PTPN22* even though this marker is 100 kb distant from the causative SNP at rs2476601, which lies within the *PTPN22* gene.

To understand how LD occurs, it is useful to remember that, during meiosis, recombination occurs resulting in a shuffling of the genome. An analogy is shuffling a pack of cards. Three likely explanations for LD exist. First, the population may have originated from a mixture of two populations, one of which had a high frequency of a particular haplotype. If this happened recently, there would not have been time (i.e., a sufficient number of generations) to randomize alleles at closely linked loci by recombination at meiosis; this is known as *population admixture.* In the analogy of the playing cards, consider the situation of two suits of cards (diamonds and spades, for example) that have been shuffled together less than 10 times to mix them. When the cards are dealt, there will be large runs of sequential cards of the same suit. Inasmuch as human history is marked by large population migrations, it is probable that population admixture explains many examples of LD. A second explanation, related to the first, rests on the observation that certain regions of the genome tend to exhibit relatively low levels of meiotic recombination (in the card analogy, for some reason, some cards are never separated by shuffling; they are stuck together) for reasons related to the underlying genomic structure. Thus genetic variants within these regions tend to stay together on the same haplotype over many generations, even if haplotypes were introduced into a population in the distant past. A third explanation for LD posits that the alleles in LD may be maintained together because of a selective advantage. For example, going back to the A1-B8-DR3 haplotype mentioned earlier, one could postulate an advantage for immune defense when alleles on this haplotype are maintained and regulated together in the same individual. Thus individuals with this haplotype may have had a survival advantage in times when infection in childhood was the greatest cause of death. The haplotype would become more common in the population but now that people are surviving into older age, the same haplotype may predispose to autoimmune disease as a result of a heightened immune response. Although plausible, this hypothesis is difficult to prove for any particular haplotype.

LD is useful for mapping associated variants because, as Fig. 25.3 shows, for the region around the *PTPN22* gene on chromosome 1, common variation in large segments of most genetic regions can be interrogated using just a few markers that "tag" the common haplotypes (see Fig. 25.3).

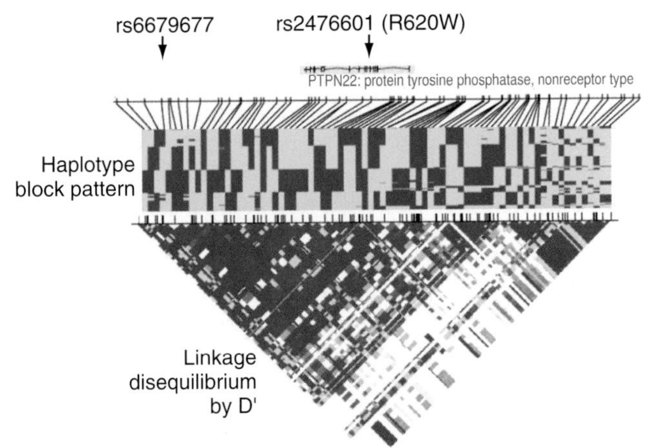

• **Fig. 25.3** Map of the region around the *PTPN22* locus on chromosome 1p13 covering approximately 200,000 base pairs. The blue and yellow haplotype pattern in the central part of the figure was generated by looking at combinations of single nucleotide polymorphism (SNP) alleles in 90 white subjects from the HapMap Project. Note that despite the large number of SNPs, a limited number of haplotype patterns are observed, generating a kind of bar code for each subject. The lower portion of the figure shows a heat map in which the intensity of red color reflects the degree of correlation (linkage disequilibrium [LD] measured by D′) among SNPs across the region (indicated by *tick marks*). Note that widely separated SNPs are highly correlated. Two markers associated with type 1 diabetes (and other autoimmune diseases) are shown at the top. Marker rs2476601 is likely to be the causative variant in this region and results in an amino acid change at codon 620. Note that another marker (rs6679677) nearly a distance of 100 kb also strongly associates with diabetes, emphasizing that it is difficult to assign the causative locus on the basis of associations alone when extensive linkage disequilibrium exists in a region.

Common Versus Rare Variants

There remains debate about the overall genetic "architecture" of human disease.[20] Until recently, there has been an assumption that common allelic variants are likely to account for a large portion of the genetic risk for common diseases in the population. This is based on the common disease, common variant hypothesis that assumes that common diseases will be caused by variants in the population that do not individually have a large effect on disease risk, do not affect reproductive fitness, and so persist and are common in the population.[21] If a variant had a large effect on disease risk, it would be likely to reduce reproductive fitness and therefore would not survive over generations, so disease frequency would be rare. By common variants, we generally mean variants that are present in the population at frequencies of 5% or more, and certainly not less than 1%. Findings from many complex diseases provide partial support for this theory; for example, the HLA alleles and the *PTPN22* gene variant that are associated with many rheumatic diseases are examples where the risk variants occur at reasonable frequency in the population. However, the common variants identified, to date, do not explain all of the genetic contribution to disease and there is no a priori reason to reject the hypothesis that many rare variants actually account for a significant fraction of the genetic burden of disease. The main reason that common variants have been a focus of research is because the current technologies are particularly well suited to investigating them, meaning that the common disease common variant hypothesis is a self-fulfilling prophecy. However, the advent of new technologies now permits sequencing of the whole genome although few studies have applied this to common diseases to date and those that have yielded disappointing results; for example, one large study of inflammatory bowel disease compared whole-genome sequencing of more than 4000 cases with 3600 controls but did not identify any low frequency variants (frequency ~1%) that had not already been identified using standard approaches.[22]

Interpreting Statistical Association From Case-Control Studies

Almost all of the studies of complex diseases in recent years have reported statistical associations that are detected by means of retrospective case-control studies. It is essential to understand the strengths and weaknesses of this approach to genetic analysis to judge the significance of these associations. In general, there are three possible reasons for detecting an association between a particular allele and a disease, once acceptable statistical criteria are met (see earlier section). First, the allele under investigation may be directly involved in the pathogenesis of the disease. A second reason that must be considered is the possibility that the result is an artifact of population stratification of patients and controls. Methods for correcting for underlying population genetic substructure are now widely accepted and indeed are often required for publication in leading genetics journals, so this should be less of an issue. Finally, a third (and common) reason for observing a genetic association is that the causative gene is actually in LD with the marker allele being tested. Therefore, once an association signal is detected, further fine-mapping is required to locate the markers with the greatest evidence of statistical association and explore whether these variants could be functional and, therefore, causal.

Rheumatoid Arthritis Susceptibility Genes

Before the GWAS era, there were only two loci that could be confidently assigned as having a role in susceptibility risk to RA. These are still the largest genetic risk factors known to date for RA: the *HLA-DRB1* and *PTPN22* genes. In common with the vast majority of autoimmune diseases, the HLA region confers, by far, the largest genetic risk for RA—accounting for approximately 60% of the genetic load.

Human Leukocyte Antigen Class I and Class II Isotypes: Functional Correlates

HLA class II molecules have a restricted tissue distribution, generally limited to antigen-presenting cells of the immune system such as B cells, macrophages, dendritic cells, and some subsets of T cells. This reflects the fact that HLA class II molecules are primarily involved in presenting foreign antigens to $CD4^+$ T cells during the initiation and propagation of the immune response. However, the expression of HLA class II molecules can also be induced on a variety of other cell types by inflammatory cytokines such as interferon-γ, enabling these cells to engage in antigen presentation to $CD4^+$ T cells. In contrast, HLA class I molecules are widely distributed on all somatic cells, with the exception of red blood cells. This distribution reflects their predominant role in presenting antigen to $CD8^+$ effector or cytotoxic T cells. Another major functional difference between class I and class II molecules is related to the source of peptide antigens that are found in the antigen-binding cleft. In general, class I molecules present peptide antigens derived from proteins that are actively synthesized within the endoplasmic reticulum, whereas HLA class II molecules present antigens that are taken up from outside of the cell by endocytosis. These differences are reflected in the antigen processing machinery and the different trafficking patterns of class I and class II molecules inside the cell. Chapters 10 and 19 discuss this complex process in detail.

Rheumatoid Arthritis: HLA-DRB1 Associations and the "Shared Epitope"

Stastny reported the first associations of RA with HLA class II alleles in the 1970s.[23] This was done using cellular and antibody reagents that are no longer routinely used for HLA typing; however, the nomenclature for HLA alleles still derives from these early typing methods. The DRB1*0401 allele (corresponding to the "Dw4 " type in Stastny's original report) was the first HLA polymorphism to be associated with RA. Numerous studies have generally confirmed that this allele is the most strongly associated with RA, at least in white populations. However, several other HLA-DRB1 alleles have also been associated with RA, although the strength of these associations varies. In some ethnic groups, RA is not associated with HLA-DR4 alleles, but rather with HLA-DR1[24] or HLA-DR10.[25] Experts now widely accept that the following alleles are the major contributors to RA risk at the DRB1 locus: DRB1*0401, *0404, *0405, *0101, and *1001. In addition, minor variants of these alleles and others (e.g., DRB1*1402) may also contribute to susceptibility, and DRB1*0901 is a susceptibility allele in Asians, where this allele is common. Most of these risk alleles share a common sequence: Q or K-R-R-A-A, which has been termed the *shared epitope* (SE).[26] This structural feature is located on the α-helical portion of the DR β chain in a position where it may influence both peptide binding and T cell receptor interactions with the DRB1 molecule. In the case of the DRB1*1001 risk allele, one amino acid varies from this consensus by a conservative change, with an R at position 70, as does DRB1*0901.

A number of different hypotheses have been advanced to explain the SE association with RA. Given that this region of the genome codes for amino acids that sit within and inform the shape of the groove of the DRB1 protein responsible for binding and presenting peptide antigens to the immune system, an obvious possibility is that a specific RA, probably auto, antigen is being presented to the immune system in such a way as to illicit an erroneously controlled immune response, leading ultimately to the inflammatory destruction of joint tissue. Many years of investigations have failed to demonstrate convincingly the RA autoantigen presented by the shared epitope, although many antigens have been suggested as possibilities. In view of the strong association of the SE alleles with anti-citrullinated peptide antibodies (ACPA), it is of interest that citrullinated peptides may have a particular affinity for DRB1*0401 alleles.[27] A second major hypothesis posits that these risk alleles regulate the formation of the peripheral T cell repertoire, by acting to select for particular T cell receptors (TCRs) during thymic selection. There is elegant experimental evidence in humans to support a role for DR4 alleles in shaping the peripheral T cell repertoire.[28] However, it is unclear whether this effect on the TCR repertoire is really related to disease susceptibility. Researchers have proposed a number of other interesting hypotheses, involving molecular mimicry,[29,30] allele specific differences in intra-cellular trafficking,[31] and regulation of nitric oxide production,[32] but these require further experimental confirmation.

The SE hypothesis has come under scrutiny, in recent years, because it is quite clear that it is not a complete explanation for the *HLA* associations with RA. This is evident from the fact that not all SE-positive alleles carry the same degree of genetic risk and the strength of the association varies in different populations. In general, *DRB1*0101* alleles carry lower levels of risk for RA than the *DRB1*0401* and **0404* alleles,[33] and yet *DRB1*0101* is the major risk allele in some ethnic groups. The SE itself does not appear to associate strongly with RA in African-American and some Hispanic populations.[34,35] Furthermore, certain combinations of *DRB1* alleles carry especially high risk.[36] Thus the combination of *DRB1*0401* with **0404* carries an OR of higher than 30 in Caucasian populations.[33] This compares with OR values in the range of 4 or 5 for either allele alone. Table 25.3 summarizes some of these relationships.

The idea of the SE involvement in RA, first suggested in 1987, is still largely correct but has been modified slightly in recent years. Using massively high throughput genetic technologies, coupled with powerful bioinformatic and statistical analysis, the association to RA in the *HLA-DRB1* gene has been refined to three amino acids, independently associated with susceptibility to RA, two of these amino acids being located within the SE region.[37] Current understanding of the RA associations within the HLA region suggests an amino acid at position 11 or 13 (the two positions are in high LD) of *HLA-DRB1*—still within the peptide binding groove but not within the classical SE motif—is most associated with disease susceptibility, followed by two further associations at amino acids 71 and 74—within the SE. In

TABLE 25.3 Genotype Relative Risks of DRB1 Genotypes for Rheumatoid Arthritis

DRB1 Genotype	Relative Risk	*P* Value
0101/DRX	2.3	10^{-3}
0401/DRX	4.7	10^{-11}
0404/DRX	5	10^{-9}
0101/0401	6.4	10^{-4}
0401/0404	31.3	10^{-32}

addition, amino acids in *HLA-B* (at position 9) and *HLA-DPB1* (at position 9) also show robust association with RA, even after correcting for the association with HLA-DRB1 amino acids. Together, these five amino acids explain almost all of the association observed at the MHC genomic region in ACPA positive European RA subjects.

The other gene robustly associated with RA susceptibility in the premodern genetics era is *PTPN22*. In 2004, an association between the intra-cellular phosphatase, *PTPN22*, was reported for a number of autoimmune diseases, including type 1 diabetes (T1D),[38] RA,[39] SLE,[40] and autoimmune thyroid disease.[41] With ORs consistently in the range of 1.5 to 2, this was the first compelling demonstration that a specific common allelic variant outside of *HLA* gene region can confer risk for multiple different autoimmune phenotypes and the finding has been consistently replicated.[42] In this case, a nonsynonymous change in one of several SH3 binding sites in PTPN22 (a tryptophan substitution for arginine at codon 620) disrupted the normal association of PTPN22 with cytosolic src kinase (CsK), an intra-cellular tyrosine kinase.[38,39] Multiple lines of evidence support the notion that csk is an important negative regulator of T cell function. One of csk's key substrates is a tyrosine present in lck, an enzyme essential for T cell activation. When csk acts on lck, lck no longer is able to support signalling via the T cell antigen receptor. Given its role in regulating csk, it was not surprising to find that knockout of *PTPN22* in rodents leads to dramatic overactivity of T cells, but the exact functional consequence of the human risk allele remains controversial. However, there is little doubt that PTPN22 is involved in setting thresholds for TCR signaling through Lck,[43,44] as well as B cell receptor signaling.[45] PTPN22 is also found in many other hematopoietic cells and its function in these cells is largely unknown.

The *PTPN22* RA risk allele is actually protective for Crohn's disease and has no role in risk for multiple sclerosis, emphasizing the likely presence of distinct mechanisms of pathogenesis in these disorders.[46] This offers a fascinating insight into disease mechanism, and obviously has implications in areas such as drug development, where an agonist may well be effective for RA, and other autoimmune diseases, but exacerbate Crohn's disease. Thus *PTPN22* is a prime example of how the discovery of new disease associations with relatively modest effect can redirect hypothesis-driven research into new pathways.

The Genome-wide Association Studies Era of Rheumatoid Arthritis Genetics

The step change in the discovery of RA susceptibility genes was achieved in 2007 with the WTCCC[16] and followed from the huge advances in the knowledge of the genetic architecture of the human genome and the enormous advancements in genotyping technology, enabling the design of chip arrays capable of analyzing more than 500,000 variants in a single experiment at a cost-effective price. It also coincided with the realization, by the genetics community, that large sample sizes of both cases and controls would be required to achieve adequate power and that new, robust statistical methodologies would have to be developed to analyze the resulting data. GWAS approaches have been improved over time, with ever greater numbers of genetic variants being analyzed in ever-increasing sample sizes, such that the latest RA genetic study incorporated 29,880 RA cases and 73,758 controls, and brought the total of confirmed genetic loci involved in susceptibility to 101.[47]

Even though there is still much to uncover in the genetic data, there is much we can learn from the 101 loci currently known for RA:

- *There are probably more genetic loci associated with RA left to discover.* It is notoriously difficult to estimate the true size of the genetic component to a complex disease, like RA. The twin studies used to estimate the heritability of RA have been relatively small and led to quite disparate estimates but, even using the lower estimates, the current confirmed genetic findings only account for around 60% of the genetic component to RA susceptibility. Many theories have been suggested for this "missing" genetic heritability.[48] This includes the role of epistasis, a multiplicative interaction between genes or between genes and environmental factors, conferring greater risks than simple additive carriage alone. Other theories include the involvement of genetic variations, which have not been well investigated yet, such as copy number variants and rare variants; these types of variants are generally not well captured using current genotyping technologies. Epigenetics, non–sequence-related changes to the DNA, may also play a role. It appears likely, though, that a combination of overestimating the genetic component of RA and the existence of many more genetic loci that contribute to the susceptibility of RA with ever-decreasing effect sizes are likely to play the major role. There is a large number of genetic variants that are strongly associated with disease susceptibility, but at a significance level where findings cannot be claimed as confirmed ($P < 10^{-5}$ but $> 10^{-8}$). Studies in other diseases and traits (e.g., height, inflammatory bowel disease) have illustrated that the more samples that are tested, the more confirmed loci are obtained—a story found, and likely to be continued, in RA.[49,50]
- *Not all risk variants are required in every patient.* The genetic variants that are being discovered to be associated with disease are generally quite common—present in over 5% of the population. As such many people without disease have a "genetic risk score" and carry risk variants. Similarly all patients will have a genetic risk score, which is generally higher than controls, but which is based on carriage of a subset of risk variants, never all. Determining which specific variants are important in subsets of patients has the potential to stratify patients into a more homogeneous subgroup, potentially with benefits for treatment therapy and outcome predictions. Statistical modeling has indicated those patients who carry a subset of risk variants (*HLA, PTPN22,* and *STAT4*) can have an OR of developing RA of over 15 compared with those who do not have these variants.[51] This work, and other continuing efforts, will provide insights into the highest risk groups and their eventual outcome and response to different therapies.
- *HLA associations are different in the serotypes of RA and, although by far the strongest genetic association, are neither necessary nor sufficient to cause disease.* The long established association of RA with the *HLA* locus gives us a great wealth of information about the disease. The vastly increased frequency of a distinct set of amino acids of the *DRB1* locus in *HLA* suggests the presentation of a common antigen is important in most, but not all, RA patients. This is clearly distinct from other autoimmune diseases, which may be strongly associated with the *HLA* locus, but with different genes or alleles. Furthermore, there is clear evidence that anti-cyclic citrullinated peptide (CCP) seropositive and seronegative patients show association to different amino acids within the *HLA-DRB1*.[52] Similar to the landscape in seropositive disease, seronegative disease has independent

genetic associations with both class II *(HLA-DRB1)* and class I *(HLA-B)* HLA genes. Again the independent associations are seen at position 11 in *HLA-DRB1* and at position 9 in *HLA-B*, both within the peptide binding grooves. These amino acid positions therefore have an association to both forms of disease, but importantly the risk of seropositive and seronegative disease is to distinct amino acid residues, suggesting separate antigens may be important in the different forms of RA. For example, serine, at position 11, is protective for ACPA+ disease, but confers risk for ACPA– disease.[52]

Along with other evidence that the genetic loci associated with the disease serotypes are different, in both strength and effect,[53] the HLA locus gives compelling evidence that the two forms of disease are indeed genetically distinct. Within the seropositive subgroup, there is a hierarchy of risk dependent on the amino acid present at each of the five most important sites within the HLA locus and this hierarchy of risk also correlates with disease severity.[37,54]

- *There are overlaps and also clear differences between the genetic risk factors for RA in different populations and ethnicities.* The latest large-scale meta-analysis, bringing the confirmed number of genes associated with RA to 101, was an international study using large cohorts of Asian and Caucasian samples.[47] The study showed that many RA loci are shared among these groups. These included key immune genes, such as *IL6R, STAT4, TNFAIP3,* and *IRF5.* Although these loci are shared among RA patients from different ethnic backgrounds, it is still to be established whether the same genetic variant is causal in both populations. Association with different causal genetic variants mapping to the same gene is observed in different autoimmune diseases; for example, different genetic variants within and around the *TNFAIP3* gene are associated with both RA and SLE, but it is not clear whether this is true of RA in different populations.[55,56] If different causal variants were identified in different populations of the same disease, it would indicate that the gene is fundamental to disease susceptibility, but that the genetic mutation arose on different ancestral backgrounds. Some genetic loci are shared between the two ethnicities, but as yet with no obvious candidate gene as the likely causal target. For example, strong associations with RA can be found to the promoter region of *AFF3,* a transcription factor with an unknown function in immune disease, in both the Asian and Caucasian populations.[47] There are also associated loci that are population-specific, offering a fascinating insight into the different pathways, different evolutionary constraints, and the different gene/environment interactions that may play a role in disease onset. These genes, surprisingly, include the *REL* gene, a subunit of NF-κB, a key driver of the immune response and a pathway strongly implicated in the majority of autoimmune diseases. The association at *REL* is only found in European populations, and is absent in Asian cohorts. Other, European only, susceptibility loci include *IL2RA, PRKCQ, CD5, CD28,* and *INGR2.* Loci restricted to Asian populations include *PRKCH, CD83,* and *IL3,* perhaps indicating disparate immune pathways that ultimately lead to RA in the different populations.
- Overlap exists between autoimmune diseases. One of the remarkable findings in the modern genetic GWAS era has been the unexpected and significant overlap in genetic risk factors between different diseases, particularly among autoimmune diseases. In fact, this led to the instigation of a successful study to design a custom Illumina genotyping array—"immunochip"—that densely mapped the shared genetic loci in a wide range of autoimmune diseases, including RA, T1D, inflammatory bowel disease, and celiac disease.[57,58] That study is the starting point for in-depth investigations as to the extent of genetic sharing between diseases, whether that be the same variant associated with groups of diseases or shared loci but with different causal variants. Some of the most interesting insights may be gained by understanding which loci are associated uniquely with a particular disease. Already, the analysis has offered a fascinating insight into cross-disease genetic risk. For example, although the majority of autoimmune diseases, including RA, share a risk variant within the *PTPN22* gene, the same variant is protective for Crohn's disease. Similarly, at the *IL6R* gene, a genetic variant protective for RA and cardiovascular disease confers risk for asthma. Interestingly this variant is highly correlated with soluble IL6R levels and functions by increasing the cleaving of IL6R from the membrane bound to the soluble form. This increase in soluble IL6R mimics the action of the therapeutic agent, tocilizumab, a soluble IL6R agent used in the treatment of RA, but there is no published evidence to suggest that the drugs exacerbate existing asthma or precipitate new cases. For RA, the greatest overlap with disease currently appears to be with T1D, although this may be due to the larger sample sizes tested in these diseases, yielding larger numbers of confirmed associations. Perhaps the more interesting aspect of the genetic overlap between diseases is the genes that are unique to a disease. For RA there appears to be only two genes out of the 101 identified, to date, which are unique to disease susceptibility. The first is the *PADI4* gene, which encodes a protein responsible for the citrullination of proteins, and may be expected to be RA specific, given the specificity of ACPA autoantibodies in disease. More surprisingly the gene encoding a general cytokine, *CCL21,* also seems to be uniquely associated with RA. This chemokine, responsible for the formation of lymph nodes, including tertiary, ectopic nodes, T cell migration across lymph nodes, and which has also been implicated in angiogenesis, may well explain the pannus formation and nodule formation characteristic of RA.
- *Most genetic variants associated with musculoskeletal diseases are not located within genes.* In contrast to what was expected before the GWAS era, in the 101 loci that have been associated with RA, only 14 are within protein coding regions. These include genes such as *PTPN22, IL6R, TYK2,* and *IRAK1,* known to be pivotal in T cell immunity. A protein coding variant associated with RA is also in the *PAD14* gene, important in the citrullination of peptides, with obvious links to ACPA positive disease. In the remaining RA loci the associated variants are outside protein coding genes, but around 13 have been linked to probable causal genes through correlation of expression. These genes include *TRAF1, CD28, CD40,* and *IRF5,* again all strongly implicated in T cell immunity.

The fact that over 80% of disease associated variants lie outside protein coding regions of the genome means that the genetic changes that increase the risk of developing disease are likely to regulate gene expression rather than fundamentally altering protein structure or function. We also know that these regulatory regions can act over long distances, often "skipping" the closest gene, so it is not always obvious which genes are being targeted by the associated genetic variants[59]; therefore a major task in interpreting the GWAS findings is to assign a gene and mechanism to the associated variants. Major advances in genetic engineering have occurred since the discovery of bacterial products that can alter or regulate the DNA sequence, called CRISPR/Cas9, and which can be targeted to specific areas of DNA by using guide RNAs; this is revolutionizing the study of how genetic variants affect gene function (Fig. 25.4). By perturbing the implicated regulatory regions it is now possible to determine the genes, mechanism, and cell types likely to be involved in disease.[60] This is obviously pivotal to the understanding of disease and a full translation of GWAS results.

- *Genetics can provide clues as to how disease is initiated and maintained, including the cell type that is the most important in disease initiation.* Both T and B cells have been implicated as the key drivers of RA. By studying the epigenetic marks that show regions of the DNA genome that are active in each cell type, it has been reported that there is an enrichment of RA genetic associations in regions of active DNA in CD+ T cells, implicating this cell type in susceptibility.[61] Further genomic work, utilizing single cell mass cytometry (CyTOF), has demonstrated how a particular PD-1 high subset of CD4+ T cells is enriched in synovium tissue from RA patients, supporting the genetic evidence for the key role of T cells in disease.[62] Interpretation of the GWAS signals is complicated.

Juvenile Idiopathic Arthritis

JIA is perhaps the most heterogeneous of complex rheumatic disorders. It is classified into several subgroups, incorporating number and chronicity of joint involvement, as well as comorbidity and autoantibody status. Although the subgrouping of JIA into classes may be contentious, clear delineation exists between the major classes. Subgroups exist that also have psoriasis, spine involvement, a systemic disease, and both antibody positive and antibody negative disease. It may be speculated that these are early forms of PsA, AS, SLE, RA, and "true" JIA—indeed genetics has a clear role in gaining insight into the overlap between these forms of disease.

The major genetic locus in the susceptibility to JIA is the *HLA* region, conferring up to 13% of the total genetic risk to disease.[63] When detailed analysis of that region was applied, it was shown that each JIA category potentially has an adult counterpart; for example, the RF-positive polyarthritis association at HLA-DRB1 amino acid at position 11/13 mirrors the association in adult seropositive RA, while the combined oligoarthritis and RF-negative polyarthritis dataset shared the same association with adult seronegative RA.[64] The finding of genetic similarity in adult RA- and RF-positive JIA also extends beyond just the MHC region.[65] This could potentially inform treatment selection in JIA and extend the choice of therapies based on disease in adults.

Genetic studies have also confirmed that systemic-onset JIA is distinct from other subsets,[66] and this reflects the clinical picture where treatment for systemic-onset JIA responds to blockade of the IL1 pathway, unlike other forms of JIA.

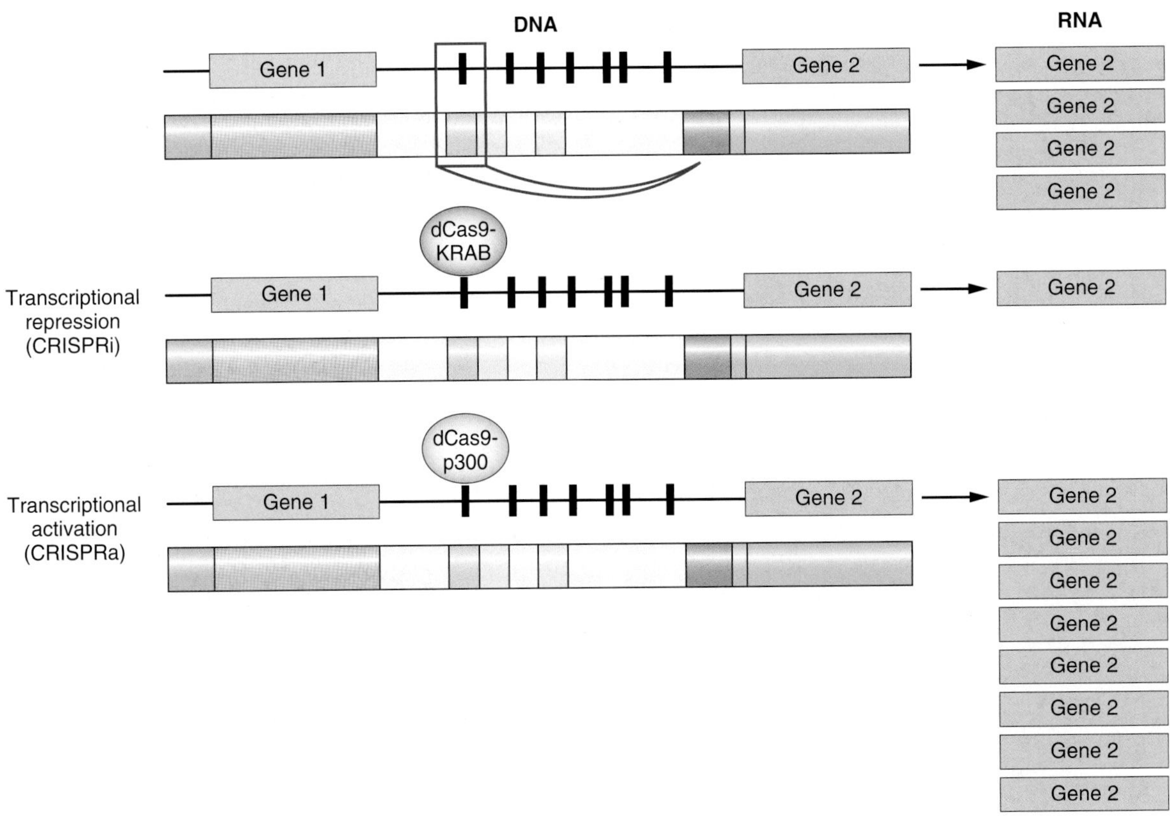

• **Fig. 25.4** dCas9-mediated transcriptional modulation. Schematic shows how CRISPR/Cas9 can be used to investigate regulatory regions containing disease associated SNPs. Here it is hypothesized that the regulatory region containing an associated variant *(orange region)* interacts with the promoter of gene 2 *(red region)* to affect transcription. This hypothesis can be tested by using CRISPR, with dCas9-KRAB to repress the target region, or dCas9-p300 to activate the region. The result on gene expression is measured via qPCR, or RNA-seq, which measure the number of gene transcripts produced following the perturbation (number of boxes of gene 2) to provide empiric evidence as to the action of the disease associated regulatory region.

Outside the HLA region, GWAS and Immunochip studies have led to identification of 17 genes robustly confirmed to be associated with JIA susceptibility.[63] Knowledge of these genes has already provided insights into the pathogenesis of disease. For example, although JIA shares many loci with the adult form of RA, the IL2 pathway appears to be more prevalent in the juvenile form of disease, with IL2 and IL2RA conferring larger effect sizes than in RA, and other genes in the pathway also being associated, including *PTPN2* and *RUNX1*. The IL2 pathway is enriched in T1D, a disease that appears to share more genetic loci with JIA than it does with RA.

Psoriatic Arthritis

Genealogical and family studies suggest that the genetic contribution to psoriatic arthritis (PsA) is greater than that to psoriasis alone. Family studies have estimated the sibling recurrence risk to be in the region of 40, yet many of the susceptibility loci identified are shared with psoriasis. This is hardly surprising as most patients with PsA will have psoriasis and GWAS studies have, so far, been performed using only modest sample sizes of PsA patients. Early GWAS studies identified the *TRAF3IP2* gene as associated with PsA, with an effect size larger than psoriasis.[67] However, association at this locus was also observed in samples from patients with psoriasis, some of whom may also have had PsA, illustrating the difficulty of proving the existence of PsA-specific loci. In a follow-up study investigating 17 loci that did not reach genome-wide levels of significance in the original GWAS, association with the *RUNX3* gene was confirmed in both PsA and psoriasis.[68] The largest genetic study, to date, used the Immunochip array to test nearly 2000 PsA patients and 9000 controls.[69] Eight loci showed confirmed evidence for association at genome-wide significance levels, seven of which have previously been reported to be associated with psoriasis *(MHC, TRAF3IP2, IL12B, IL23R, IL23A-STAT2, TNIP1, TYK2)*. However, the SNPs predisposing to disease appear to be different between psoriasis and PsA for at least one locus, *IL23R*. That finding was subsequently replicated in independent data sets.[70] Furthermore, two PsA-specific loci were identified: one at chromosome 5q31 and the other in the MHC *(HLA-B27)*. The association with the MHC is complex with three major associations detected with PsA: the classical psoriasis-associated *HLA-C*0602*; *HLA-B27*; and *HLA-A*02*.[71] However, when age at psoriasis onset is accounted for in the analysis, it was shown that HLA*0602 is associated with skin disease (psoriasis) but not joint disease (PsA).[72] Furthermore, amino acid at position 97 (on the HLA B27 risk allele) differentiates PsA from cutaneous psoriasis. This is the same position that confers risk for AS but different amino acids at the same position have different effects: asparagine is associated with both but a serine increases risk of PsA but not AS. It is likely that as sample sizes improve for PsA, further loci will be identified and it will be possible to dissect the shared and distinct loci for these overlapping diseases. This is important because it would potentially pave the way for screening patients with psoriasis for the risk of developing PsA.

Ankylosing Spondylitis

Family studies indicate that there is a substantial genetic component to AS, with a sibling recurrence risk of 9.2% compared with 0.1% to 0.4% in the general population.[73] Based on these figures, the heritability has been estimated to exceed 95%.

The strongest genetic susceptibility factor for ankylosing spondylitis (AS) is carriage of the *HLA-B27* allele. In white populations, more than 90% of patients with AS carry *HLA-B27*, in contrast to approximately 8% of unaffected individuals, giving estimated relative risk (RR) values of 50 to 100 or higher.[74] However, only 2% of people who are *HLA-B27* positive will go on to develop AS, indicating the presence of other genetic, environmental, and stochastic risks. The consistency of the association with AS across most ethnic groups lends support to the contention that the *HLA-B27* alleles are directly involved in disease pathogenesis.[75,77] *HLA-B27* is also associated with reactive arthritis and with the arthritis seen in the context of inflammatory bowel disease. The serologic specificity of HLA-B27 actually encompasses many distinct HLA class I alleles. These alleles differ from one another at a number of amino acid positions, most of which involve amino acid substitutions in and around the peptide binding pocket. This fact leads naturally to the question of whether there are differences among these B27 alleles in terms of disease association. Most data indicate that this is not the case, although there may be some exceptions in some populations.[75] These exceptions may provide clues to the role of the HLA-B27 molecule in pathogenesis. Overall, however, it appears that most of the structural differences among the *B27* alleles do not affect disease risk.

Outside the HLA gene region, genetic studies have identified a further 48 risk loci, to date.[76,77] These findings have highlighted several important insights into underlying disease pathways and mechanisms. First, the association of several aminopeptidase genes (*ERAP1*, *ERAP2*, *LNPEP*, and *NPEPPS*) has reinforced the importance of antigen presentation in AS pathogenesis because these genes encode proteins that trim peptides to be presented to HLA molecules. Interestingly, the *ERAP1* association is only found in *HLA-B27* positive individuals and was one of the first examples of genetic epistasis (i.e., the presence of both *HLA-B27* and *ERAP1* risk variant increased disease risk multiplicatively).[78] By contrast, *ERAP2* is also associated with *HLA-B27* negative AS. Studies in mice implicate *ERAP1* in viral peptide generation and presentation, specifically. Second, there is enrichment of genes involved in the *IL-23* pathway, including *IL23R, IL-12B*, and *IL27*. The pathway drives the differentiation of CD4+ Th17 cells, which produce IL-17. Encouragingly, phase 3 clinical trials of biologic drugs targeting the IL23 and IL-17 signaling pathways have shown promising results in AS patients.[79] Third, pathways involving T cell differentiation (*EOMES, IL7R, RUNX3, ZMIZI, BACH2*, and *SH2B3*) and G-protein coupled receptors (*GPR35, GPR37, GPR65*, and *GPR25*) have also been identified. Although the *IL1* gene cluster has been implicated in some studies, findings have been inconsistent and trials of an anti-IL1 biologic drug, anakinra, were not successful for the treatment of AS.[80,81] Finally, there appears to be considerable overlap in the genes predisposing to AS and Crohn's disease. Given that up to 60% of AS patients have been reported to show histopathologic evidence of gut inflammation and that a pathway comprising genes involved in the defense against pathogens has been identified in Crohn's disease, there is now considerable interest in the role of the gut microbiome in predisposing to AS.[82]

Systemic Lupus Erythematosus—Identification of the Interferon Pathway

In 2005 researchers showed that interferon regulatory factor 5 *(IRF5)* was associated with susceptibility to systemic lupus,[83] and they replicated this finding shortly thereafter.[84] This was a satisfying observation because activation of interferon pathways is clearly central to the pathogenesis of lupus and related disorders.[85] Since these original observations, it is now apparent that multiple genes in interferon pathways are involved in lupus susceptibility.[86] Interferon has emerged as a potential drug target, and there is renewed appreciation and interest in the role of interferon regulation in the immune response generally.[87] The involvement of multiple genes in interferon pathways as risk factors for autoimmune diseases provides important support for continuing biologic studies in this field, as well as the potential for new insights into the details of how this pathway is regulated.

Researchers into the genetic contribution to SLE have pioneered the way in determining critical biologic pathways that lead to disease. These breakthroughs have arisen from the usual GWAS and Immunochip routes, but have also incorporated robust findings from family and single gene studies and transethnic studies. Monogenetic disorders, such as Aicardi-Goutières syndrome, share many of the phenotypes of the complex genetic form of SLE.[88] Using family linkage approaches, key genes and biologic pathways have been uncovered in these studies, including *TREX1*, important in IFN-α production, complement deficiency, and FasL implicated in apoptosis.

Putting these discoveries with the data generated from case-control association studies has led to the provisional identification of four key pathways involved in SLE susceptibility. These are the type 1 interferon pathway, as exemplified by the association of *IRF5, IFIH, TYK2*; the NfKB pathway *(TNFAIP3, IRAK1)*; B and T cell signaling *(PTPN22, BLK)* pathways; and apoptosis *(ITGAM, FCGR2A)* (reviewed in reference 89). These groundbreaking findings are the first steps toward a stratified medicine approach, implicating as they do that SLE is not a single disease and revealing the key pathways that can be used to designate subtypes of disease. In clinic SLE patients with a B cell signal-driven disease, for example, could be grouped together and may well respond better to a specific therapeutic approach.

Osteoarthritis

Osteoarthritis (OA) is the most common musculoskeletal disorder, yet, as a result of its high prevalence in so-called "healthy control populations," identifying genes underlying disease has been very challenging as large numbers of "controls" will go on to develop OA in the future. Furthermore, different patterns of clinical joint involvement are apparent and were described before the era of genetics. Genetic studies have confirmed that different genes could contribute to these phenotypic subgroups. GWAS have now confirmed association to 30 genomic intervals at genome-wide thresholds[90] and although some loci associate with OA in a specific joint, the latest GWAS study has indicated a high degree of genetic sharing between knee and hip OA.[91]

It should be noted that, as in other GWAS, it is often a chromosomal region that is associated rather than being able to pinpoint a single gene. The locus is often named according to the gene closest to the strongest association signal or the most likely candidate based on existing knowledge. However, in most cases, the gene conferring risk has not yet been conclusively identified. The best investigated locus, to date, is the *GDF5* locus mapping to chromosome 20. Interestingly, this is one of two regions (*GDF5* and *DOT1L*) that are also inversely associated with height (i.e., the risk allele for OA is associated with being smaller).[92] *GDF5* codes for a growth factor protein, important in chondrogenesis and bone growth. Indeed, a number of OA susceptibility genes, such as *RUNX2, SMAD3*, and *PTHLH*, are important in skeletal and bone development, highlighting the importance of bone morphology in disease, but genes involved in inflammation have not been identified. The largest OA GWAS to date utilized the UK Biobank GWAS data from more than 300,000 individuals. Not only did the study add nine novel associations to the list of OA loci, it demonstrated a causative affect, through Mendelian randomization, of body mass index in increasing the risk of developing OA.

Clinical Translation

GWAS is only a starting point in understanding the genetic basis of musculoskeletal diseases. As described previously, the technique often identifies a region of interest but, ultimately, experimental verification and functional studies are required to identify the important variants and the gene it is regulating. Only once the causal genes have been defined can reliable pathway analysis be undertaken. At the time of writing, in only a few cases has the causal gene within an associated locus been unequivocally identified.[57] However, genetic studies could potentially be used to inform clinical practice in other ways, as outlined.

Identification of Drug Targets—Lessons From Genetics

Three of the genes identified in RA GWAS are the targets for drugs that are highly effective in the management of disease activity: abatacept is an analogue of the molecule encoded by the *CTLA-4* gene; tocilizumab is a biologic drug that perfectly mimics the action of the RA-associated variant within the *IL6R* gene, while tofacitinib acts on the JAK/STAT pathway in which the RA associated gene, *TYK2*, is crucially involved. Indeed, drug targets have been reported to be enriched in the largest analysis of RA genetic studies, which identified more than 100 RA susceptibility genes.[47] Therefore, genetic studies can highlight novel targets or pathways for drug development. Supported by genetic data, several drugs targeting the IL17 and IL23 pathways in PsA and AS are licensed or are in early phase trials, including drugs targeting the interferon pathway in SLE. In JIA, the variants in the *IL1RN* gene has been reported to be associated with systemic-onset JIA and IL1 is the target of anakinra, which is used to treat systemic-onset JIA.[93] Indeed, high expression alleles correlated with nonresponse to anakinra and, if replicated, could be used to inform treatment selection in the future.

Prognosis

It is recognized that huge variability exists in the course of musculoskeletal diseases but few reliable predictors of outcome have yet been identified. In RA, the presence of ACPA as measured by anti-CCP antibody status is more predictive of the development of erosions than the presence of rheumatoid factor at baseline but does not completely explain the variance in outcome.[94] However, it is expected that disease severity will be genetically determined and a family study in early RA has provided support for this.[95]

A number of other non-HLA genes or genetic loci have been investigated in terms of whether they can predict severity. The most consistent evidence for association with severity is for *HLA-DRB1* SE alleles. The *TRAF1/C5* locus has also been associated with joint erosions in multiple populations[96–99] but was not replicated in a subsequent study.[100] Two studies have reported association of the IL4R with outcome.[101,102] A further two studies have reported association of the IL2RA gene with erosions.[103,104] However, findings for many have not been replicated in all studies and none of the variants provide sufficient discrimination to be of clinical utility alone.

Treatment Response

There are several biologic therapies available, particularly for RA, which target specific pathways. However, for each drug or drug class, less than half of the patients treated achieve remission. Currently, drugs are used on a trial and error basis, often in the order they came to market rather than on any scientific rationale. It would be tempting to speculate that remission rates would be improved if the initial biologic used was selected to target the major pathway mediating inflammation in individual patients. This is the concept of precision medicine. The prerequisite is to define the pathways involved in individuals. Currently this is limited because, at most associated loci, the gene responsible is not known. As explained previously, gene names are often assigned to a locus based on biologic plausibility or because they are the closest gene to the most associated variant in a region. However, there are numerous examples where this assumption has been proven wrong. For example, the SNP rs12740374, strongly associated with cholesterol levels, is found within the gene *CELSR2* but convincingly confers its functional effect on cholesterol levels by changing the expression of *SORT1* in the liver, a gene separated from *CELSR2* on the chromosome by two other genes (*PSRC1* and *MYBPHL*).[105] If the wrong gene is assigned to a locus, then downstream pathway analysis to define subgroups of patients by the predominant pathway involved may be catastrophically compromised and treatment response rates, based on such groupings, are unlikely to be improved. Therefore, precision medicine, using genetic biomarkers, is only likely to become a reality once the genes responsible for the association signal in a region are identified.

In the meantime, efforts are ongoing to assign patients to strata according to their known treatment response to drugs, stratified medicine. In several countries, longitudinal cohort studies are underway in which genetic data are being generated from patients who have received a drug, usually a biologic drug, and whose response to therapy has been recorded using standardized definitions of response. In Europe and, increasingly in the United States, the outcome measure used is usually the change in disease activity score across 28 joints (DAS28) or EULAR response criteria, which are based on the DAS28.[106,107] Studies to identify genetic predictors of response lag behind those of studies of susceptibility for several reasons. First, the difference between responders to a drug and nonresponders is more subtle than between patients with a disease and control individuals without. Issues about how moderate responders are classified can complicate the phenotype definition, for example. Furthermore, the outcome measure itself is a composite score comprising both subjective (tender joint count, patient global health score) and objective measures (swollen joint count, erythrocyte sedimentation rate, or C-reactive protein). However, several studies have shown that the subjective components have low heritability estimates and so will have weak genetic associations at best, yet the tender joint count receives double the weighting of the swollen joint count in calculating the DAS28.[108] Second, the genetic studies performed so far have been in modest sample sizes. For example, one of the first GWAS of tumor necrosis factor inhibitor (TNFi) response was performed in 566 patient samples, encompassing good, bad, and moderate responders, so study power has been a major limitation.[109] Third, biologics acting on the same pathway have been grouped, as in the study described, but there is evidence that etanercept has different properties to monoclonal TNFi drugs. Therefore, progress in stratified medicine has been slow but international collaboration led to the first moderately sized GWAS, which identified the *CD84* gene as approaching genome-wide significance levels for association with response to etanercept.[110] Independent studies from Denmark and Spain have replicated association to the *PDE3A-SLCO1C1*. In a combined analysis, the association statistic exceeded genome-wide thresholds,[111] but a subsequent UK study did not replicate the findings.[112] A systematic review has identified six loci with replicated evidence for association but, even combined, these only had moderate power to predict response/nonresponse to TNFi.[113] Efforts are continuing, but we can already conclude that there is no major genetic determinant of TNFi response of an effect size similar to that of the *HLA* region with RA. Instead, response is likely to be mediated by a large number of genes, each with a small individual effect, and that signatures of response might be more realistic.

Identification of High-Risk Groups

Given the low prevalence of many rheumatic diseases (with the exception of OA) and the low effect sizes for most of the risk loci identified, it is unlikely that population screening to identify groups at risk of disease will ever be feasible. Even for age-related macular degeneration, where large effect sizes at a modest number of genes have been found, the sensitivity and specificity of the testing means that population screening will probably not be cost-effective. However, genetic testing may be of more use in an already high-risk group; for example, in RA, those with a family history of disease or who are ACPA positive. It may be more feasible for PsA where patients with psoriasis are already at higher risk for developing PsA than the general population. This could pave the way for preventative therapies for high-risk individuals in the future and several cohort studies are underway to identify other factors which may increase risk further.

This is now a tremendously exciting time to be involved in the genetics of rheumatic disease. Years of investment and collaboration between leading international consortia have had a tangible impact in determining changes to genomic regions that increase the risk of developing disease. The next phase in rheumatic genetic research is to develop ways to translate these findings into clinical benefit. Large collections of biologically relevant samples, coupled with advances in methodologies, including single cell techniques, proteomics and metabolomics, have the potential to link these risk genetic changes to a clinically meaningful phenotypic outcome. In addition, the genes and genetic pathways, which are important in disease, are high priority targets for both novel and repositioned therapeutics. Advances in genetic engineering and genome therapy, already impacting single gene disorders and in cancer, have the potential to influence the therapeutic choices and outcome in patients. Finally, by better understanding the genetic mechanism underpinning disease, with novel molecular and nuclear DNA techniques, it will be possible to better stratify patients into more homogeneous disease types, potentially improving diagnosis and disease outcome.

The references for this chapter can also be found on ExpertConsult.com.

References

1. MacGregor AJ, Snieder H, Rigby AS, et al.: Characterizing the quantitative genetic contribution to rheumatoid arthritis using data from twins, *Arthritis Rheum* 43(1):30–37, 2000.
2. Evans LM, Tahmasbi R, Vrieze SI, et al.: Comparison of methods that use whole genome data to estimate the heritability and genetic architecture of complex traits, *Nat Genet* 50(5):737–745, 2018.
3. Viding E, Price TS, Jaffee SR, et al.: Genetics of callous-unemotional behavior in children, *PLoS One* 8(7):e65789, 2013.
4. Ott J, Bhat A: Linkage analysis in heterogeneous and complex traits, *Eur Child Adolesc Psychiatry* 8(Suppl 3):43–46, 1999.
5. Pras E, Aksentijevich I, Gruberg L, et al.: Mapping of a gene causing familial Mediterranean fever to the short arm of chromosome 16, *N Engl J Med* 326(23):1509–1513, 1992.
6. Ancient missense mutations in a new member of the RoRet gene family are likely to cause familial Mediterranean fever. The International FMF Consortium. *Cell* 1997; 90(4):797–807, 1997.
7. Hull KM, Drewe E, Aksentijevich I, et al.: The TNF receptor-associated periodic syndrome (TRAPS): emerging concepts of an autoinflammatory disorder, *Medicine (Baltimore)* 81(5):349–368, 2002.
8. Risch NJ: Searching for genetic determinants in the new millennium, *Nature* 405(6788):847–856, 2000.
9. Hugot JP, Chamaillard M, Zouali H, et al.: Association of NOD2 leucine-rich repeat variants with susceptibility to Crohn's disease, *Nature* 411(6837):599–603, 2001.
10. Ogura Y, Bonen DK, Inohara N, et al.: A frameshift mutation in NOD2 associated with susceptibility to Crohn's disease, *Nature* 411(6837):603–606, 2001.
11. Amos CI, Chen WV, Lee A, et al.: High-density SNP analysis of 642 Caucasian families with rheumatoid arthritis identifies two new linkage regions on 11p12 and 2q33, *Genes Immun* 7(4):277–286, 2006.
12. Lee HS, Remmers EF, Le JM, et al.: Association of STAT4 with rheumatoid arthritis in the Korean population, *Mol Med* 13(9-10):455–460, 2007.
13. Spielman RS, McGinnis RE, Ewens WJ: Transmission test for linkage disequilibrium: the insulin gene region and insulin-dependent diabetes mellitus (IDDM), *Am J Hum Genet* 52(3):506–516, 1993.
14. Sebat J, Lakshmi B, Malhotra D, et al.: Strong association of de novo copy number mutations with autism, *Science* 316(5823):445–449, 2007.
15. Klein RJ, Zeiss C, Chew EY, et al.: Complement factor H polymorphism in age-related macular degeneration, *Science* 308(5720):385–389, 2005.
16. Genome-wide association study of 14,000 cases of seven common diseases and 3,000 shared controls, *Nature* 447(7145):661–678, 2007.
17. Palmer LJ, Cardon LR: Shaking the tree: mapping complex disease genes with linkage disequilibrium, *Lancet* 366(9492):1223–1234, 2005.
18. Zollner S, Pritchard JK: Overcoming the winner's curse: estimating penetrance parameters from case-control data, *Am J Hum Genet* 80(4):605–615, 2007.
19. Price P, Witt C, Allcock R, et al.: The genetic basis for the association of the 8.1 ancestral haplotype (A1, B8, DR3) with multiple immunopathological diseases, *Immunol Rev* 167:257–274, 1999.
20. Pritchard JK, Cox NJ: The allelic architecture of human disease genes: common disease-common variant…or not? *Hum Mol Genet* 11(20):2417–2423, 2002.
21. Peng B, Kimmel M: Simulations provide support for the common disease-common variant hypothesis, *Genetics* 175(2):763–776, 2007.
22. Luo Y, de Lange KM, Jostins L, et al.: Exploring the genetic architecture of inflammatory bowel disease by whole-genome sequencing identifies association at ADCY7, *Nat Genet* 49(2):186–192, 2017.
23. Stastny P: Association of the B-cell alloantigen DRw4 with rheumatoid arthritis, *N Engl J Med* 298(16):869–871, 1978.
24. Nichol FE, Woodrow JC: HLA DR antigens in Indian patients with rheumatoid arthritis, *Lancet* 1(8213):220–221, 1981.
25. Sanchez B, Moreno I, Magarino R, et al.: HLA-DRw10 confers the highest susceptibility to rheumatoid arthritis in a Spanish population, *Tissue Antigens* 36(4):174–176, 1990.
26. Gregersen PK, Silver J, Winchester RJ: The shared epitope hypothesis. An approach to understanding the molecular genetics of susceptibility to rheumatoid arthritis, *Arthritis Rheum* 30(11):1205–1213, 1987.
27. Hill JA, Southwood S, Sette A, et al.: Cutting edge: the conversion of arginine to citrulline allows for a high-affinity peptide interaction with the rheumatoid arthritis-associated HLA-DRB1*0401 MHC class II molecule, *J Immunol* 171(2):538–541, 2003.
28. Walser-Kuntz DR, Weyand CM, Weaver AJ, et al.: Mechanisms underlying the formation of the T cell receptor repertoire in rheumatoid arthritis, *Immunity* 2(6):597–605, 1995.
29. Roudier J, Petersen J, Rhodes GH, et al.: Susceptibility to rheumatoid arthritis maps to a T-cell epitope shared by the HLA-Dw4 DR beta-1 chain and the Epstein-Barr virus glycoprotein gp110, *Proc Natl Acad Sci U S A* 86(13):5104–5108, 1989.
30. Albani S, Keystone EC, Nelson JL, et al.: Positive selection in autoimmunity: abnormal immune responses to a bacterial dnaJ antigenic determinant in patients with early rheumatoid arthritis, *Nat Med* 1(5):448–452, 1995.
31. Auger I, Toussirot E, Roudier J: HLA-DRB1 motifs and heat shock proteins in rheumatoid arthritis, *Int Rev Immunol* 17(5-6):263–271, 1998.
32. Ling S, Li Z, Borschukova O, et al.: The rheumatoid arthritis shared epitope increases cellular susceptibility to oxidative stress by antagonizing an adenosine-mediated anti-oxidative pathway, *Arthritis Res Ther* 9(1):R5, 2007.
33. Hall FC, Weeks DE, Camilleri JP, et al.: Influence of the HLA-DRB1 locus on susceptibility and severity in rheumatoid arthritis, *QJM* 89(11):821–829, 1996.
34. McDaniel DO, Alarcon GS, Pratt PW, et al.: Most African-American patients with rheumatoid arthritis do not have the rheumatoid antigenic determinant (epitope), *Ann Intern Med* 123(3):181–187, 1995.
35. Teller K, Budhai L, Zhang M, et al.: HLA-DRB1 and DQB typing of Hispanic American patients with rheumatoid arthritis: the "shared epitope" hypothesis may not apply, *J Rheumatol* 23(8):1363–1368, 1996.
36. Nepom BS, Nepom GT, Mickelson E, et al.: Specific HLA-DR4-associated histocompatibility molecules characterize patients with seropositive juvenile rheumatoid arthritis, *J Clin Invest* 74(1):287–291, 1984.
37. Raychaudhuri S, Sandor C, Stahl EA, et al.: Five amino acids in three HLA proteins explain most of the association between MHC and seropositive rheumatoid arthritis, *Nat Genet* 44(3):291–296, 2012.
38. Bottini N, Musumeci L, Alonso A, et al.: A functional variant of lymphoid tyrosine phosphatase is associated with type I diabetes, *Nat Genet* 36(4):337–338, 2004.
39. Begovich AB, Carlton VE, Honigberg LA, et al.: A missense single-nucleotide polymorphism in a gene encoding a protein tyrosine phosphatase (PTPN22) is associated with rheumatoid arthritis, *Am J Hum Genet* 75(2):330–337, 2004.
40. Kyogoku C, Langefeld CD, Ortmann WA, et al.: Genetic association of the R620W polymorphism of protein tyrosine phosphatase PTPN22 with human SLE, *Am J Hum Genet* 75(3):504–507, 2004.
41. Criswell LA, Pfeiffer KA, Lum RF, et al.: Analysis of families in the multiple autoimmune disease genetics consortium (MADGC) collection: the PTPN22 620W allele associates with multiple autoimmune phenotypes, *Am J Hum Genet* 76(4):561–571, 2005.

42. Gregersen PK, Lee HS, Batliwalla F, et al.: PTPN22: setting thresholds for autoimmunity, *Semin Immunol* 18(4):214–223, 2006.
43. Vang T, Congia M, Macis MD, et al.: Autoimmune-associated lymphoid tyrosine phosphatase is a gain-of-function variant, *Nat Genet* 37(12):1317–1319, 2005.
44. Rieck M, Arechiga A, Onengut-Gumuscu S, et al.: Genetic variation in PTPN22 corresponds to altered function of T and B lymphocytes, *J Immunol* 179(7):4704–4710, 2007.
45. Arechiga AF, Habib T, He Y, et al.: Cutting edge: the PTPN22 allelic variant associated with autoimmunity impairs B cell signaling, *J Immunol* 182(6):3343–3347, 2009.
46. De Jager PL, Sawcer S, Waliszewska A, et al.: Evaluating the role of the 620W allele of protein tyrosine phosphatase PTPN22 in Crohn's disease and multiple sclerosis, *Eur J Hum Genet* 14(3):317–321, 2006.
47. Okada Y, Wu D, Trynka G, et al.: Genetics of rheumatoid arthritis contributes to biology and drug discovery, *Nature* 506(7488):376–381, 2014.
48. Eichler EE, Flint J, Gibson G, et al.: Missing heritability and strategies for finding the underlying causes of complex disease, *Nat Rev Genet* 11(6):446–450, 2010.
49. Yang J, Benyamin B, McEvoy BP, et al.: Common SNPs explain a large proportion of the heritability for human height, *Nat Genet* 42(7):565–569, 2010.
50. Jostins L, Ripke S, Weersma RK, et al.: Host-microbe interactions have shaped the genetic architecture of inflammatory bowel disease, *Nature* 491(7422):119–124, 2012.
51. McClure A, Lunt M, Eyre S, et al.: Investigating the viability of genetic screening/testing for RA susceptibility using combinations of five confirmed risk loci, *Rheumatology (Oxford)* 48(11):1369–1374, 2009.
52. Han B, Diogo D, Eyre S, et al.: Fine mapping seronegative and seropositive rheumatoid arthritis to shared and distinct HLA alleles by adjusting for the effects of heterogeneity, *Am J Hum Genet* 94(4):522–532, 2014.
53. Viatte S, Plant D, Bowes J, et al.: Genetic markers of rheumatoid arthritis susceptibility in anti-citrullinated peptide antibody negative patients, *Ann Rheum Dis* 71(12):1984–1990, 2012.
54. Han B, Pouget JG, Slowikowski K, et al.: A method to decipher pleiotropy by detecting underlying heterogeneity driven by hidden subgroups applied to autoimmune and neuropsychiatric diseases, *Nat Genet* 48(7):803–810, 2016.
55. Thomson W, Barton A, Ke X, et al.: Rheumatoid arthritis association at 6q23, *Nat Genet* 39(12):1431–1433, 2007.
56. Graham RR, Cotsapas C, Davies L, et al.: Genetic variants near TNFAIP3 on 6q23 are associated with systemic lupus erythematosus, *Nat Genet* 40(9):1059–1061, 2008.
57. Eyre S, Bowes J, Diogo D, Lee A, et al.: High-density genetic mapping identifies new susceptibility loci for rheumatoid arthritis, *Nat Genet* 44(12):1336–1340, 2012.
58. Cortes A, Brown MA: Promise and pitfalls of the immunochip, *Arthritis Res Ther* 13(1):101, 2011.
59. Martin P, McGovern A, Orozco G, et al.: Capture Hi-C reveals novel candidate genes and complex long-range interactions with related autoimmune risk loci, *Nat Commun* 6:10069, 2015.
60. Simeonov DR, Gowen BG, Boontanrart M, et al.: Discovery of stimulation-responsive immune enhancers with CRISPR activation, *Nature* 549(7670):111–115, 2017.
61. Trynka G, Sandor C, Han B, et al.: Chromatin marks identify critical cell types for fine mapping complex trait variants, *Nat Genet* 45(2):124–130, 2013.
62. Rao DA, Gurish MF, Marshall JL, et al.: Pathologically expanded peripheral T helper cell subset drives B cells in rheumatoid arthritis, *Nature* 542(7639):110–114, 2017.
63. Hinks A, Cobb J, Marion MC, et al.: Dense genotyping of immune-related disease regions identifies 14 new susceptibility loci for juvenile idiopathic arthritis, *Nat Genet* 45(6):664–669, 2013.
64. Hinks A, Bowes J, Cobb J, et al.: Fine-mapping the MHC locus in juvenile idiopathic arthritis (JIA) reveals genetic heterogeneity corresponding to distinct adult inflammatory arthritic diseases, *Ann Rheum Dis* 76(4):765–772, 2017.
65. Hinks A, Marion MC, Cobb J, et al.: Brief report: the genetic profile of rheumatoid factor-positive polyarticular juvenile idiopathic arthritis resembles that of adult rheumatoid arthritis, *Arthritis Rheumatol* 70(6):957–962, 2018.
66. Ombrello MJ, Arthur VL, Remmers EF, et al.: Genetic architecture distinguishes systemic juvenile idiopathic arthritis from other forms of juvenile idiopathic arthritis: clinical and therapeutic implications, *Ann Rheum Dis* 76(5):906–913, 2017.
67. Huffmeier U, Uebe S, Ekici AB, et al.: Common variants at TRAF3IP2 are associated with susceptibility to psoriatic arthritis and psoriasis, *Nat Genet* 42(11):996–999, 2010.
68. Apel M, Uebe S, Bowes J, et al.: Variants in RUNX3 contribute to susceptibility to psoriatic arthritis, exhibiting further common ground with ankylosing spondylitis, *Arthritis Rheum* 65(5):1224–1231, 2013.
69. Bowes J, Budu-Aggrey A, Huffmeier U, et al.: Dense genotyping of immune-related susceptibility loci reveals new insights into the genetics of psoriatic arthritis, *Nat Commun* 6:6046, 2015.
70. Budu-Aggrey A, Bowes J, Loehr S, et al.: Replication of a distinct psoriatic arthritis risk variant at the IL23R locus, *Ann Rheum Dis* 75(7):1417–1418, 2016.
71. Okada Y, Han B, Tsoi LC, et al.: Fine mapping major histocompatibility complex associations in psoriasis and its clinical subtypes, *Am J Hum Genet* 95(2):162–172, 2014.
72. Bowes J, Ashcroft J, Dand N, et al.: Cross-phenotype association mapping of the MHC identifies genetic variants that differentiate psoriatic arthritis from psoriasis, *Ann Rheum Dis* 76(10):1774–1779, 2017.
73. Tsui FW, Tsui HW, Akram A, et al.: The genetic basis of ankylosing spondylitis: new insights into disease pathogenesis, *Appl Clin Genet* 7:105–115, 2014.
74. Brewerton DA, Hart FD, Nicholls A, et al.: Ankylosing spondylitis and HL-A 27, *Lancet* 1(7809):904–907, 1973.
75. Reveille JD, Ball EJ, Khan MA: HLA-B27 and genetic predisposing factors in spondyloarthropathies, *Curr Opin Rheumatol* 13(4):265–272, 2001.
76. Ellinghaus D, Jostins L, Spain SL, et al.: Analysis of five chronic inflammatory diseases identifies 27 new associations and highlights disease-specific patterns at shared loci, *Nat Genet* 48(5):510–518, 2016.
77. Cortes A, Hadler J, Pointon JP, et al.: Identification of multiple risk variants for ankylosing spondylitis through high-density genotyping of immune-related loci, *Nat Genet* 45(7):730–738, 2013.
78. Reveille JD, Sims AM, Danoy P, et al.: Genome-wide association study of ankylosing spondylitis identifies non-MHC susceptibility loci, *Nat Genet* 42(2):123–127, 2010.
79. Braun J, Baraliakos X, Deodhar A, et al.: Effect of secukinumab on clinical and radiographic outcomes in ankylosing spondylitis: 2-year results from the randomised phase III MEASURE 1 study, *Ann Rheum Dis* 76(6):1070–1077, 2017.
80. Haibel H, Rudwaleit M, Listing J, et al.: Open label trial of anakinra in active ankylosing spondylitis over 24 weeks, *Ann Rheum Dis* 64(2):296–298, 2005.
81. Sims AM, Timms AE, Bruges-Armas J, et al.: Prospective meta-analysis of interleukin 1 gene complex polymorphisms confirms associations with ankylosing spondylitis, *Ann Rheum Dis* 67(9):1305–1309, 2008.
82. Van PL, Van den Bosch FE, Jacques P, et al.: Microscopic gut inflammation in axial spondyloarthritis: a multiparametric predictive model, *Ann Rheum Dis* 72(3):414–417, 2013.
83. Sigurdsson S, Nordmark G, Goring HH, et al.: Polymorphisms in the tyrosine kinase 2 and interferon regulatory factor 5 genes are associated with systemic lupus erythematosus, *Am J Hum Genet* 76(3):528–537, 2005.

84. Graham RR, Kozyrev SV, Baechler EC, et al.: A common haplotype of interferon regulatory factor 5 (IRF5) regulates splicing and expression and is associated with increased risk of systemic lupus erythematosus, *Nat Genet* 38(5):550–555, 2006.
85. Crow MK: Interferon pathway activation in systemic lupus erythematosus, *Curr Rheumatol Rep* 7(6):463–468, 2005.
86. Flesher DL, Sun X, Behrens TW, et al.: Recent advances in the genetics of systemic lupus erythematosus, *Expert Rev Clin Immunol* 6(3):461–479, 2010.
87. Crow MK: Interferon-alpha: a therapeutic target in systemic lupus erythematosus, *Rheum Dis Clin North Am* 36(1):173–186, x, 2010.
88. Rice GI, Kasher PR, Forte GM, et al.: Mutations in ADAR1 cause Aicardi-Goutieres syndrome associated with a type I interferon signature, *Nat Genet* 44(11):1243–1248, 2012.
89. Liu Z, Davidson A: Taming lupus-a new understanding of pathogenesis is leading to clinical advances, *Nat Med* 18(6):871–882, 2012.
90. Gonzalez A: Osteoarthritis year 2013 in review: genetics and genomics, *Osteoarthritis Cartilage* 21(10):1443–1451, 2013.
91. Zengini E, Hatzikotoulas K, Tachmazidou I, et al.: Genome-wide analyses using UK Biobank data provide insights into the genetic architecture of osteoarthritis, *Nat Genet* 50(4):549–558, 2018.
92. Sanna S, Jackson AU, Nagaraja R, et al.: Common variants in the GDF5-UQCC region are associated with variation in human height, *Nat Genet* 40(2):198–203, 2008.
93. Arthur VL, Shuldiner E, Remmers EF, et al.: IL1RN variation influences both disease susceptibility and response to recombinant human interleukin-1 receptor antagonist therapy in systemic juvenile idiopathic arthritis, *Arthritis Rheumatol* 70(8):1319–1330, 2018.
94. Bukhari M, Thomson W, Naseem H, et al.: The performance of anti-cyclic citrullinated peptide antibodies in predicting the severity of radiologic damage in inflammatory polyarthritis: results from the Norfolk Arthritis Register, *Arthritis Rheum* 56(9):2929–2935, 2007.
95. Knevel R, Grondal G, Huizinga TW, et al.: Genetic predisposition of the severity of joint destruction in rheumatoid arthritis: a population-based study, *Ann Rheum Dis* 71(5):707–709, 2012.
96. Kurreeman FA, Padyukov L, Marques RB, et al.: A candidate gene approach identifies the TRAF1/C5 region as a risk factor for rheumatoid arthritis, *PLoS Med* 4(9):e278, 2007.
97. Plant D, Thomson W, Lunt M, et al.: The role of rheumatoid arthritis genetic susceptibility markers in the prediction of erosive disease in patients with early inflammatory polyarthritis: results from the Norfolk Arthritis Register, *Rheumatology (Oxford)* 50(1):78–84, 2011.
98. Viatte S, Plant D, Lunt M, et al.: Investigation of rheumatoid arthritis genetic susceptibility markers in the early rheumatoid arthritis study further replicates the TRAF1 association with radiological damage, *J Rheumatol* 40(2):144–156, 2013.
99. Mohamed RH, Pasha HF, El-Shahawy EE: Influence of TRAF1/C5 and STAT4 genes polymorphisms on susceptibility and severity of rheumatoid arthritis in Egyptian population, *Cell Immunol* 273(1):67–72, 2012.
100. Knevel R, de Rooy DP, Gregersen PK, et al.: Studying associations between variants in TRAF1-C5 and TNFAIP3-OLIG3 and the progression of joint destruction in rheumatoid arthritis in multiple cohorts, *Ann Rheum Dis* 71(10):1753–1755, 2012.
101. Krabben A, Wilson AG, de Rooy DP, et al.: Association of genetic variants in the IL4 and IL4R genes with the severity of joint damage in rheumatoid arthritis: a study in seven cohorts, *Arthritis Rheum* 65(12):3051–3057, 2013.
102. Leipe J, Schramm MA, Prots I, et al.: Increased Th17 cell frequency and poor clinical outcome in rheumatoid arthritis are associated with a genetic variant in the IL4R gene, rs1805010, *Arthritis Rheumatol* 66(5):1165–1175, 2014.
103. Knevel R, de Rooy DP, Zhernakova A, et al.: Association of variants in IL2RA with progression of joint destruction in rheumatoid arthritis, *Arthritis Rheum* 65(7):1684–1693, 2013.
104. Ruyssen-Witrand A, Lukas C, Nigon D, et al.: Association of IL-2RA and IL-2RB genes with erosive status in early rheumatoid arthritis patients (ESPOIR and RMP cohorts), *Joint Bone Spine* 81(3):228–234, 2014.
105. Musunuru K, Strong A, Frank-Kamenetsky M, et al.: From noncoding variant to phenotype via SORT1 at the 1p13 cholesterol locus, *Nature* 466(7307):714–719, 2010.
106. van Gestel AM, Prevoo ML, van't Hof MA, et al.: Development and validation of the European League Against Rheumatism response criteria for rheumatoid arthritis. Comparison with the preliminary American College of Rheumatology and the World Health Organization/International League Against Rheumatism Criteria, *Arthritis Rheum* 39(1):34–40, 1996.
107. Prevoo ML, van't Hof MA, Kuper HH, et al.: Modified disease activity scores that include twenty-eight-joint counts. Development and validation in a prospective longitudinal study of patients with rheumatoid arthritis, *Arthritis Rheum* 38(1):44–48, 1995.
108. Massey J, Plant D, Hyrich K, et al.: Genome-wide association study of response to tumour necrosis factor inhibitor therapy in rheumatoid arthritis, *Pharmacogenomics J*, 18:657–664, 2018.
109. Plant D, Bowes J, Potter C, et al.: Genome-wide association study of genetic predictors of anti-tumor necrosis factor treatment efficacy in rheumatoid arthritis identifies associations with polymorphisms at seven loci, *Arthritis Rheum* 63(3):645–653, 2011.
110. Cui J, Stahl EA, Saevarsdottir S, et al.: Genome-wide association study and gene expression analysis identifies CD84 as a predictor of response to etanercept therapy in rheumatoid arthritis, *PLoS Genet* 9(3), 2013:e1003394.
111. Acosta-Colman I, Palau N, Tornero J, et al.: GWAS replication study confirms the association of PDE3A-SLCO1C1 with anti-TNF therapy response in rheumatoid arthritis, *Pharmacogenomics* 14(7):727–734, 2013.
112. Smith SL, Plant D, Lee XH, et al.: Previously reported PDE3A-SLCO1C1 genetic variant does not correlate with anti-TNF response in a large UK rheumatoid arthritis cohort, *Pharmacogenomics* 17(7):715–720, 2016.
113. Bek S, Bojesen AB, Nielsen JV, et al.: Systematic review and meta-analysis: pharmacogenetics of anti-TNF treatment response in rheumatoid arthritis, *Pharmacogenomics J* 17(5):403–411, 2017.

26 Epigenetics of Rheumatic Diseases

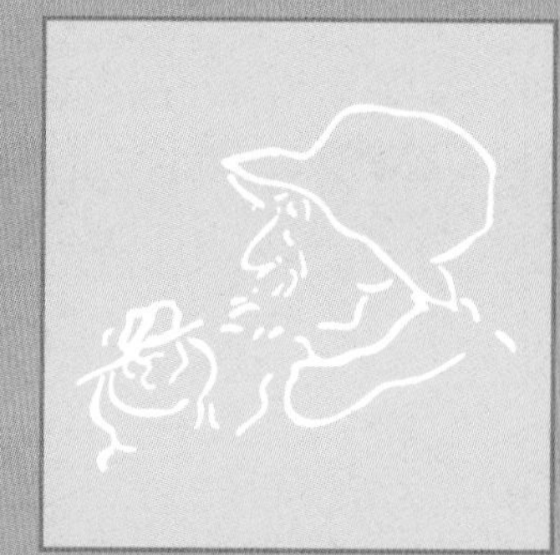

AMR H. SAWALHA AND MATLOCK A. JEFFRIES

KEY POINTS

Epigenetic mechanisms include DNA methylation, histone modifications, and noncoding RNA regulation. Collectively, these mechanisms determine chromatin architecture, accessibility of genetic loci to transcriptional machinery, and gene expression levels.

Epigenetic changes are cell-type specific, and epigenetic mechanisms play an important role in regulating the normal immune response, such as T cell differentiation.

Alterations in the epigenetic landscape are increasingly recognized as playing an important role in the pathogenesis of rheumatic diseases.

Epigenome-wide studies in rheumatology have focused primarily on DNA methylation changes, and this identified novel target genes and pathogenic mechanisms in immune-mediated diseases.

The epigenome is dynamic, allowing for the development of novel biomarkers for disease activity, specific disease manifestations, and response to treatment.

Some epigenetic changes reflect the effect of environmental triggers that cause disease in a genetically susceptible host. An integrated "omics" approach would help to better understand disease pathogenesis in rheumatology.

The developing field of epigenetic editing has the potential to both prove "causality" of epigenetic changes associated with rheumatic conditions and to potentially reverse epigenetic modifications associated with these diseases. Cell-type specific epigenetic editing approaches promise potential therapeutic value in the future.

Introduction

Epigenetics refers to changes in gene regulation without changes in the DNA sequence. These changes are often described as "heritable," indicating a relative stability of epigenetic changes during cell division. Three main epigenetic mechanisms are thought to operate in concert to regulate chromatin architecture, and thereby the accessibility of regulatory regions within the genome to transcriptional machinery. Therefore, epigenetic changes are often described as "silencing" or "activating," indicating the net effect of a given epigenetic change on gene expression (transcription). DNA methylation, histone modifications, and regulatory RNAs (such as microRNAs) have evolved in mammalian systems to provide a complex array of epigenetic changes that determine specific chromatin architecture in any given genetic locus to regulate gene expression. These epigenetic mechanisms are essential during development and tissue differentiation, as well as in dictating the repertoire of genes expressed by the various cell types and tissues. Every nucleated cell contains the same repertoire of the human genome, yet each cell type maintains a specific assortment of expressed genes that is necessary for its function, while the rest of the genome is silenced. This silencing is achieved by epigenetic changes and the relative presence or absence of transcription factors. Indeed, two factors have to co-exist for any gene to be expressed in any cell type: chromatin accessibility and appropriate transcription factors. If either of the two is absent in a particular gene locus, that gene cannot be expressed.

Epigenetic Regulation

The genetic material (DNA) that carries the genetic code within nucleotide bases is tightly packed within the nucleus with histone proteins to form the chromatin. The chromatin basic units are known as *nucleosomes*, which consist of ~147 bp of DNA wrapped twice around a core protein octamer consisting of two each of H2A, H2B, H3, and H4 histone proteins.[1] This architectural arrangement serves two main purposes. First, it allows for the genomic material to be compacted in such a way that it fits within the tight space of the nucleus, and second, it provides an avenue for regulating gene expression through epigenetic modifications, as will be described in more detail.

DNA methylation is the most studied epigenetic mechanism and is considered the cornerstone of epigenetic regulation. *DNA methylation* refers to the addition of a methyl group (–CH3) to the fifth carbon of cytosine rings.[2] This reaction is mediated by a group of enzymes called *DNA methyltransferases* (DNMTs). DNMT3A and DNMT3B are considered de novo DNMTs as they determine and establish DNA methylation patterns in utero[3] and do not rely on copying pre-existing DNA methylation patterns. DNMT3 ligand (DNMT3L) is a recently discovered catalytically inactive member of the DNMT family that works in concert with DNMT3A and DNMT3B to establish genomic methylation patterns.[4] DNMT1 is the "maintenance" DNMT as it maintains DNA methylation patterns throughout cell division ex utero.[5–7] Of course, though this is a general rule there are exceptions, and some redundancies within the DNMTs as a group in specific situations and cell types have been described. The methyl group in DNA methylation reactions is derived from *S*-adenosylmethionine, which gets converted to *S*-adenosyl-homocysteine after donating a methyl group (Fig. 26.1). Therefore, dietary

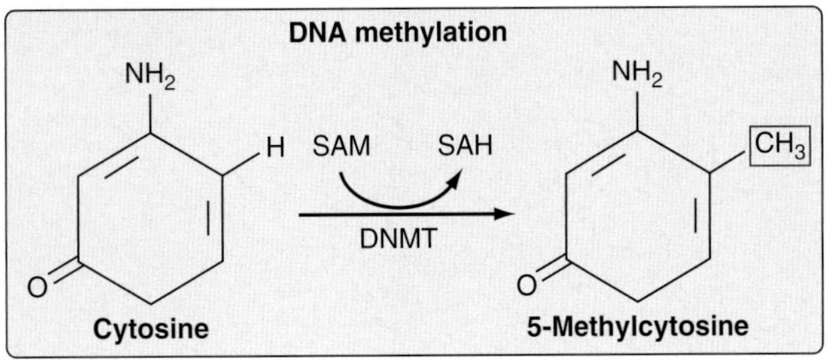

DNA methylation

NH2 — H — SAM — SAH — DNMT — NH2 — CH3

Cytosine — 5-Methylcytosine

• **Fig. 26.1** *DNA methylation* refers to the addition of a methyl group to the fifth carbon in cytosine rings. Most DNA methylation occurs in cytosine residues within cytosine-guanosine (CG) dinucleotides, although non-CG cytosine methylation has also been recently described. DNA methylation is mediated by DNA methyltransferase enzymes (DNMT) that use *S*-adenosyl-methionine as the methyl group donor. *SAH,* *S*-adenosyl-homocysteine; *SAM,* *S*-adenosyl-methionine.

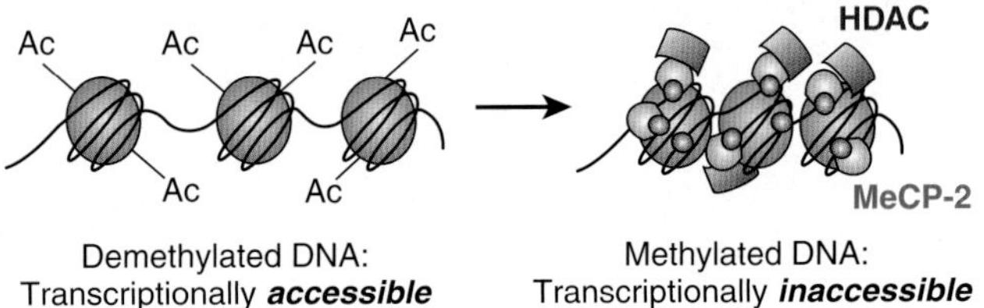

• **Fig. 26.2** DNA methylation represses gene expression. Transcriptionally accessible regions in the genome are generally characterized by DNA demethylated and histone tail acetylation. When DNA gets methylated *(red circles)*, it recruits methyl-binding domain, including proteins such as MeCP-2 *(green)*, which in turn recruits histone deacetylase (HDAC) 1 and 2. HDACs cleave off the acetyl group from histone tails, increasing the charge attraction between DNA and histone cores and thereby increasing chromatin compaction and reducing accessibility to transcription factors. The presence of methyl-binding proteins and HDACs also physically hinders transcription factor binding.

changes that affect micronutrient levels in *S*-adenosyl-methionine metabolism can potentially alter DNA methylation and provide a link between metabolism and gene expression patterns.[8] DNA methylation most often occurs in cytosine residues within cytosine-guanosine dinucleotides (CG). However, non-CG methylation, which is very frequent in plants, has been also been described in mammalian cells. This typically occurs in cytosines within CA or CT dinucleotides and is generally restricted to embryonic stem cells and developing brain tissue.[9,10]

DNA methylation in promoter or regulatory sequences within the genome generally silences gene expression. Demethylation or hypomethylation, on the other hand, is associated with active transcription. DNA methylation inhibits gene expression by several mechanisms. One important mechanism is by interacting with and inducing histone deacetylation (Fig. 26.2). Methylated DNA recruits methyl-binding domain-containing proteins such as methyl-CpG-binding protein 2 (MeCP-2). MeCP-2 recruits and binds histone deacetylases (HDAC1 and HDAC2), and the latter cleave off the acetyl groups from acetylated histone tails, thereby increasing the charge attraction between the histone core and DNA strands and inducing a compact chromatin architecture that becomes inaccessible to the transcriptional machinery, resulting in gene silencing.[11,12]

Conversely, the removal of DNA methylation marks results in gene activation and occurs via both active and passive mechanisms.[13] Passive demethylation occurs with a failure of the normal copying of the DNA methylation pattern (via DNMT1) to newly synthesized DNA strands during cellular division. Active DNA demethylation also occurs and involves a conversion of 5′-methylcytosine to 5′-hydroxymethylcytosine mediated by 10-11-10 gene family members (TETs). Following this first critical and rate-limiting step, hydroxymethylcytosine is then converted to subsequent chemical intermediates, finally undergoing base-excision repair (BER) to produce unmethylated cytosine.[14,15]

There are a number of histone tail modifications that play a role in epigenetic regulation. As mentioned, histone acetylation (primarily of histones H3 and H4) is associated with transcriptional accessibility and active gene expression. Deacetylation of H3 and H4 silences gene expression. Other histone tail modifications have variable effects on gene expression, depending on the specific modification and the specific location of these modifications within histone proteins. The details of these histone changes are beyond the scope of this chapter, but generally they include acetylation, methylation, phosphorylation, ubiquitination, and others.[16] The complexity of the effects of histone changes on chromatin architecture has been increasingly recognized. Mapping chromatin modifications across the genome and in multiple cell types and tissues has resulted in a better understanding of chromatin regulation and architecture, as has been demonstrated by the ENCODE project.[17]

The importance of gene regulation by noncoding (nc) RNA (such as microRNAs) was recognized with a Nobel Prize in Medicine and Physiology awarded in 2006. MicroRNAs are small RNA molecules generally between 19 and 25 nucleotides that regulate the expression of target genes by binding to regulatory elements within their specific target genes such as the 3′ untranslated regions (3′-UTR).[18] For example, X chromosome inactivation is partially directed by coating of the chromosome in a short noncoding RNA known as the *X-inactive specific transcript* (X-ist).[19] Long noncoding RNAs (lncRNAs) are intricately linked with paternal imprinting (the process by which the redundant copies of each gene, either maternal or paternal in origin, are inactivated).[20,21] Several novel functions of miRNAs have been proposed, and several new classes of larger noncoding RNA with important transcriptional significance have been recently described, including Piwi-interacting RNAs (piRNAs), small nucleolar RNAs (snoRNAs), circular RNAs (circRNAs), and others. Our knowledge of the different types of regulatory RNAs, their biology and regulatory potential and function, and the specific target regions and genes they regulate is constantly evolving. In this chapter, we will focus on microRNAs as the most studied regulatory RNA in the context of autoimmune and rheumatic conditions. A timeline for some of the major epigenetic discoveries and progress is outlined in Fig. 26.3.

Epigenetics and the Immune Response

Epigenetic mechanisms are critically involved in the regulation of multiple aspects of the normal immune response.[22] We will only discuss a few examples herein, to demonstrate two important points to the reader of this textbook: the importance of epigenetic changes in the normal functions of immune cells that are thought to be key in the development of autoimmune and inflammatory diseases, and the utmost importance of examining specific cell types (not a mixture of cells) in epigenetic studies in immune-mediated diseases.

T cell activation is associated with rapid production of IL-2, resulting in a feedback loop of further expression of the high affinity IL-2 receptor alpha (IL-2Rα or CD25) and more IL-2

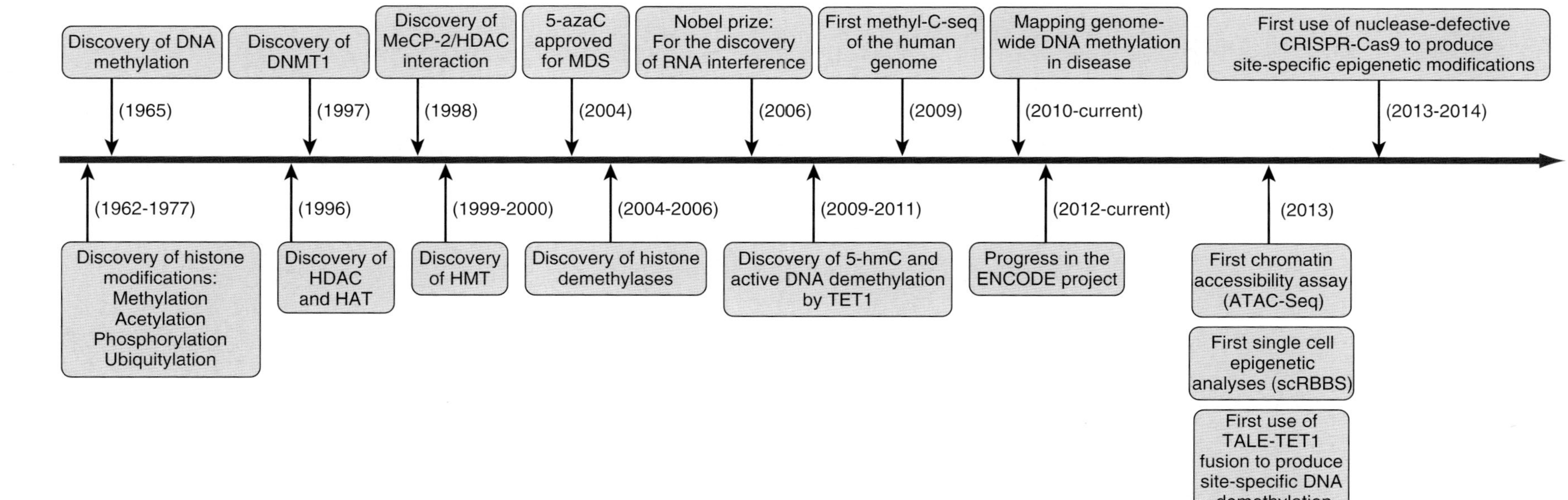

• **Fig. 26.3** The timeline for key discoveries and progress in epigenetics. *DNMT1,* DNA methyltransferase 1; *ENCODE,* Encyclopedia of DNA Elements; *HAT,* histone acetyltransferase; *HDAC,* histone deacetylase; *HMT,* histone methyltransferase; *MDS,* myelodysplastic syndrome; *TET1,* 10-11 translocation methylcytosine dioxygenase 1.

production (autocrine mechanism). This rapid and efficient IL-2 production is associated with a robust and rapid demethylation of the *IL2* promoter sequence. Indeed, this demethylation starts within minutes after T cell stimulation, and therefore is clearly independent of cell cycle or cell division.[23,24] This was a strong argument for the presence of an active DNA demethylation process, discussed in the previous section.[14,15]

The differentiation of naïve CD4+ T cells to Th1 and Th2 effector cells is accompanied by essential- and locus-specific epigenetic changes.[22] In naïve CD4+ T cells, the Th1 locus *(IFNG)* and the Th2 locus (*IL4*, *IL5*, and *IL13* common locus control region) are inaccessible for transcription as the DNA is methylated and histone tails in these two loci are deacetylated, resulting in compact chromatin that is transcriptionally repressive. Upon Th1 differentiation the Th1 locus *(IFNG)* gets demethylated and histone tails become acetylated, leading to a locus-specific chromatin accessibility and the production of the key Th1 cytokine IFN-γ. At the same time, the Th2 locus control region becomes even more methylated compared with naïve CD4+ T cells, to ensure no production of Th2 cytokines.[25,26] The exact opposite happens in the Th2 locus control region and the Th1 *IFNG* locus upon naïve CD4+ T cell differentiation into Th2 effector cells.[27–29] Importantly, these locus-specific methylation changes are maintained upon memory Th1 and Th2 cell generation, to ensure a rapid clonal T cell response upon re-exposure to the same pathogen. Indeed, the 2 to 3 days it generally takes for an initial Th1 or Th2 immune response is largely the time needed for the aforementioned locus-specific methylation changes to happen, and this explains why a second-exposure response from memory T cells is much faster.[30] The development of IL-17 producing Th17 cells is similarly accompanied by chromatin remodeling in the *IL17A* and *IL17F* loci.[31]

Regulatory T cells (Treg) demethylate the *FOXP3* genetic locus, resulting in the ability to produce FOXP3, a key transcription factor in the immune-regulatory function of these cells.[32] Specifically, the initiation and maintenance of *FOXP3* expression are highly driven by demethylation of conserved noncoding sequences (or CNSs), which include a number of transcription factor binding sites, within the first exon. Demethylation of these CNS regions is found in Treg cell precursors even before *Foxp3* expression is initiated, demonstrating the concept of epigenetic "poising." Demethylation of these regions is critical for stable, long-term expression of *FOXP3* and a suppressive Treg phenotype.[33] Therefore, locus-specific epigenetic changes play a critical role in the differentiation of T cells into specific subsets with a specific cellular function and cytokine-producing capacity.

Challenges Faced in Translational Epigenetics Research

Epigenetic control mechanisms are fundamental to setting and maintaining gene expression patterns in humans. This breadth can make it somewhat difficult to design epigenetic research experiments in a way that strong conclusions may be drawn. For example, differentiating "real" epigenetic changes within a specific individual cell population from "artifactual" variations in epigenetic patterns caused by changes in composition of subpopulations within a sample of interest has been a substantial hurdle to epigenetic research. Indeed, computational approaches to the estimation of cell subpopulations within, for example, whole blood specimens, have been widely adopted.[34–36] This potential confounding of epigenetic patterns by compositional differences leads thoughtful researchers to carefully select their tissue of interest for epigenome-wide analyses to select the most specific subpopulation possible. Although the importance of narrowly defining cell types to be studied has been recognized as critical in epigenetic phenotyping for some time, it has only been recently that technological advances and scientific knowledge have advanced enough to make this a reality. This potential confounding may also be applied to the patient phenotypes being analyzed, as most studies are (to this day) conducted on an admixture of patient phenotypes that have been defined as a single entity of rheumatic disease. As an example, patients with systemic lupus erythematosus with mainly mucocutaneous or arthritic complaints are likely to represent a distinct phenotype when compared to lupus patients who present with hematologic disease and nephritis and will likely have substantial variations in epigenetic patterns of diseased tissues. Similarly, newly described endophenotypes (that is, patient groups defined by molecular characteristics, i.e., the lupus "interferon-high" patient) would also be expected to be epigenetically distinct from one another. In fact, epigenetic variation clustering is sometimes used to define new endophenotypes de novo, as in the "inflammatory signature" chondrocyte subtype of osteoarthritis discussed later. Although this phenomenon can be a shortcoming of epigenetic studies aimed at linking epigenetic changes with pathophysiology, it can actually be viewed as a benefit in studies leveraging epigenetic changes of readily accessible tissues for biomarker research, as discussed later. The astute reader will note that the majority of studies we will discuss were performed on more general cellular populations. A detailed methodological discussion of each study is beyond our scope; suffice it to say that studies wherein more attention was paid to carefully phenotyping both patients and the tissues of interest should instill a higher level of confidence than more general, less well-defined study populations.

Epigenetics in Rheumatic Diseases

Systemic Lupus Erythematosus

The etiology of systemic lupus erythematosus (hereafter, lupus) is incompletely understood. There is a strong and growing body of literature that supports a role for epigenetic changes in the pathogenesis of lupus.[37–39] Most of these studies are focused on T cells, as demethylated T cells have been shown sufficient to induce lupus in animal models. Initial studies in the epigenetics of lupus, and in rheumatology in general, originated from Dr. Bruce Richardson's work at the University of Michigan. As a result of this work, and subsequent work by others, epigenetics is now in the center of the current paradigm of lupus pathogenesis. Indeed, epigenetics provides a link between environmental triggers and genetic susceptibility in autoimmune diseases.

DNA Methylation Regulation and Candidate Gene Studies in Lupus T Cells

Initial studies demonstrated that procainamide and hydralazine cause drug-induced lupus by demethylating T cells, thereby resulting in T cell autoreactivity. Both inhibit the activity of the maintenance DNA methyltransferase DNMT1. Procainamide directly inhibits DNMT1 in T cells, while hydralazine inhibits MEK/ERK signaling, which regulates and mediates DNMT1 expression.[40,41] CD4+ T cells treated with procainamide or hydralazine, the DNA methylation inhibitor 5-azacytidine, or MEK/ERK pathway inhibitors, overexpress mRNA and proteins encoded by methylation-sensitive genes (such as CD11a, CD70, perforin, CD40L, and killer cell immunoglobulin-like receptor [KIR] family) and become autoreactive and capable of killing autologous macrophages and stimulating B cell immunoglobulin production in vitro.[37] In vivo experiments, using adoptive transfer of similarly treated and demethylated T cells into syngeneic mice, cause autoantibody production and a lupus-like disease.[37] T cells isolated from lupus patients demonstrate reduced MEK/ERK signaling, reduced DNMT1 expression and activity, and demethylation of the promoter sequences, resulting in overexpression of CD11a, CD70, perforin, CD40L, and KIRs, similar to 5-azaC treated T cells.[37] Therefore, T cells from lupus patients resemble normal T cells treated with MEK/ERK pathway inhibitors or DNA methylation inhibitors. The extent of MEK/ERK signaling defect and reduction in DNMT1 expression in lupus T cells is proportional to disease activity, with T cells isolated from active lupus patients showing more extensive demethylation compared to patients with inactive disease.[42]

To further provide a proof of principle that reduced MEK/ERK signaling in T cells can result in T cell demethylation and lupus, rather than the alternative possibility that the observed MEK/ERK signaling defect in lupus is the result of and not causal to the disease, a transgenic mouse model with induced T cell MEK/ERK signaling defect was generated.[43] These mice demonstrated that inducing a defect in the MEK/ERK signaling pathway results in reduced DNMT1 expression, demethylation of methylation sensitive genes, and overexpression of these same genes, similar to T cells isolated from lupus patients.[43,44] Further, this mouse model developed anti-dsDNA antibodies and a T cell interferon expression signature, reminiscent of the interferon signature in lupus patients.[43] On a genetic background permissive to autoimmunity, these mice also develop clinical lupus-like disease such as glomerulonephritis.[44] Taken together, inducing a DNA methylation defect in T cells is sufficient to cause autoimmunity in an autoimmune-resistant genetic background, and clinical lupus-like phenotype in the presence of a genetic background that is permissive to autoimmunity. This resembles the observation in humans taking hydralazine (which is a MEK/ERK inhibitor), with the majority of patients developing autoantibodies and only a small fraction, presumably those with genetic background for lupus, developing a clinical lupus-like disease. Furthermore, investigations have demonstrated that the lupus-prone mouse strain MRL/*lpr* possesses CD70 demethylation in CD4+ T cells that is similar to human lupus patients.[45] These observations provide a basis for genetic–epigenetic interaction in the pathogenesis of lupus, other evidence for which is discussed later.

Subsequent studies mapped the origin of the MEK/ERK signaling defect in lupus T cells, causing the observed DNA methylation defect, to an upstream signaling defect in PKCδ.[46] Interestingly, oxidative stress such as oxygen-free radical species can induce a defect in PKCδ signaling similar to that observed in lupus T cells, resulting in T cell DNA demethylation.[47,48] These data provide a link between environmental triggers of oxidative stress, such as infections, and autoimmunity in the susceptible host. Infections are known to induce flares in lupus patients, and this might be mediated at least partly by increased oxidative stress resulting in T cell demethylation. In fact, mitochondrial dysfunction resulting in increased production of reactive oxygen species and reduced levels of the antioxidant glutathione has been reported in lupus T cells.[49] Increased oxidative stress in lupus T cells also results in activation of the mTOR signaling pathway, which also inhibits DNMT1.[49] Treatment of lupus patients with the antioxidant and glutathione precursor *N*-acetylcysteine blocked mTOR in T cells and improved disease activity.[50]

Recent data have also provided evidence for additional mechanisms that play a role in inducing DNA methylation defect in lupus T cells. For example, protein phosphatase 2A (PP2A), which is involved in multiple cellular processes including proliferation and activation, is overexpressed in lupus T cells. Increased PP2A expression and activity have been linked to reduced IL-2 production, which is characteristic of lupus T cells.[51] Recent evidence suggests that increased PP2A might induce a DNA methylation defect in lupus T cells by causing a MEK/ERK signaling defect, thereby reducing DNMT1 expression. Indeed, suppressing PP2A in lupus T cells enhanced MEK/ERK signaling, increased *DNMT1* mRNA expression, and reduced the expression of methylation sensitive genes such as *CD70*.[52] Further, increased PP2A induces epigenetic changes in the *IL17* locus, enhancing IL-17 production from lupus T cells. PP2A catalytic subunit (PP2Ac) transgenic mice develop an IL-17 dependent glomerulonephritis.[53]

The growth arrest and DNA damage-induced 45α (GADD45α), which is involved in DNA repair and DNA demethylation, is overexpressed at the mRNA and protein levels in lupus CD4+ T cells.[54] Inhibiting GADD45 α in lupus CD4+ T cells using siRNA resulted in increased methylation of *ITGAL* (encoding CD11a) and *TNFSF7* (encoding CD70) promoter regions and reduced *ITGAL* and *TNFSF7* mRNA expression, reduced T cell proliferation, and reduced T cell autoreactivity as measured by B cell co-stimulation.[54]

Other contributing factors to the DNA methylation defect and overexpression of methylation-sensitive genes in lupus CD4+ T cells include downregulation of regulatory factor X1 (RFX1). RFX1 recruits DNMT1 and HDAC1 and suppresses CD11a and CD70 expression, and underexpression of RFX1 is associated with demethylation and increased expression in CD11a and CD70 in lupus CD4+ T cells.[55]

Genome-wide DNA Methylation Studies in Systemic Lupus Erythematosus

A number of genome-wide methylation studies have been recently performed in lupus. These studies provide an unbiased view of the DNA methylome, and have identified a number of novel differentially methylated genetic loci that might be important in the pathogenesis of this disease. Using a group of twins discordant for lupus, one group investigated lupus-associated DNA methylation changes in ~1500 CpG sites in peripheral blood leukocytes.[56] This first genome-wide study of DNA methylation in lupus was shortly followed by another study examining ~27,000 CpG sites in CD4+ T cells from lupus patients compared to healthy age-, sex-, and ethnicity-matched controls.[57] Several differentially methylated regions were identified in CD4+ T cells, including hypomethylation of *CD9* (T cell co-stimulatory molecule), *MMP9* (matrix metalloproteinase involved in autoimmunity), *PDGFRA* (platelet-derived growth factor receptor alpha precursor), *CASP1* (caspase 1), and interferon-regulated genes such as *IFI44L* and *BST2*.[57] Subsequent work by investigators[58] identified genome-wide DNA methylation changes across more than 485,000 methylation sites in naïve CD4+ T cells in lupus. This study included a discovery and a replication cohort, to robustly identify and replicate DNA methylation changes, coupled with gene expression profiling in a subset of the same samples. This study demonstrated for the first time a robust and consistent hypomethylation in interferon signature genes in lupus, which proceeds gene expression. Therefore, it appears that naïve CD4+ T cells in lupus patients are poised at the epigenetic level to produce type-I interferon-regulated genes even before T cell activation (Fig. 26.4). These data provided a

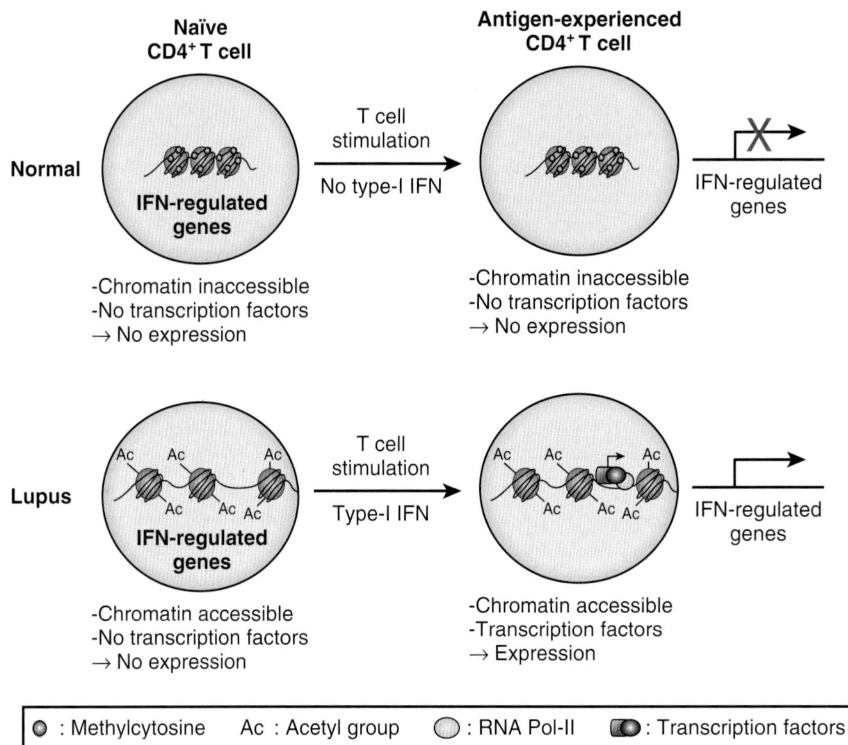

• **Fig. 26.4** Interferon-regulated genes are epigenetically "poised" in naïve CD4+ T cells in lupus, as abnormal DNA methylation exists in lupus T cells before activation. A model whereby interferon-regulated genes are epigenetically poised to respond to type-I interferon upon T cell activation in lupus is proposed. These data provide evidence for an epigenetic architecture favoring, and providing an explanation for, type-I interferon hyper-responsiveness in lupus T cells.

mechanistic explanation for the previously reported increased type-I interferon sensitivity in lupus PBMCs and adds yet an additional pathogenic role for abnormal DNA methylation in the pathogenesis of lupus.[58] In 2014, one group[59] conducted a genome-wide DNA methylation study coupled with transcriptome and microRNome analysis in lupus CD4+ T cells and identified additional DNA methylation changes in lupus, such as the differential methylation and overexpression of novel target genes including *NLRP2* (inflammasome component gene), *CD300LB* (a pro-inflammatory nonclassical activating receptor of the immunoglobulin superfamily), and *S1PR3* (a pro-inflammatory G protein-coupled receptor). Further, this study localized some methylation changes that are specific to clinical disease subsets in lupus, such as kidney and skin disease.[59]

Recent analyses have investigated genome-wide DNA methylation patterns in additional inflammatory cell subsets in lupus patients. A study examining methylation patterns in CD4+ T cells, CD19+ B cells, and CD14+ monocytes in systemic lupus erythematosus (SLE) confirmed the previous observations described in naïve CD4+ T cells, replicated a widespread and substantial type-I interferon hypomethylation signature in each of these cell types, and identified a DNA methylation shift in genes related to MAPK signaling (within the aforementioned MEK/ERK pathway).[60] Several lines of evidence have recently implicated a potential role for abnormal, pro-inflammatory neutrophils in lupus pathology, including a subset known as *low-density granulocytes* (or LDGs). LDGs in particular are suggested to induce end-organ tissue damage in lupus, including skin disease, glomerulonephritis, and endothelial damage.[61] In 2015, one study[62] evaluated differential DNA methylation patterns within neutrophils from lupus patients, and again encountered a robust and widespread DNA demethylation signature within both neutrophils and autologous LDGs; indeed, the hypomethylation pattern was nearly identical within the two cell subsets, with the exception of hypomethylation within a cytoskeleton-regulating gene *(RAC1)* in LDGs. LDGs are more prone to produce neutrophil extra-cellular traps (NETs) composed of extruded chromatin material,[61] which can in turn stimulate a variety of inflammatory cytokine signals, including interferon alpha production from plasmacytoid dendritic cells.[63] One group hypothesized that this interferon production from extra-cellular NETs may be enhanced in SLE owing to increased stimulation via TLR9 induced by this substantially hypomethylated DNA of lupus NETs.

Another lupus-related cell subset gaining substantial attention recently is the CD4+CD28+KIR+CD11a^{hi+} cells. The relative abundance of this cell subtype correlates with lupus disease activity, and the expression of *KIR* in CD4+CD28+CD11a^{hi+} cells can be induced via treatment with a demethylating agent.[64] This cell subtype expresses a variety of genes known to be hypomethylated in CD4+ T cells from lupus patients, including *CD70* and *CD40L*. In 2018, one study[65] comprehensively examined the epigenome and transcriptome of this cell subtype and again demonstrated global DNA hypomethylation, along with specific demethylation of 235 genes, including a variety of pro-inflammatory cytokines, adhesion molecules, Toll-like receptor genes, and matrix metalloproteinases.

Genetic–Epigenetic Interaction in Lupus

MeCP-2 (encoded by *MECP2*) is a key transcriptional regulator that is intimately involved in DNA methylation-mediated transcriptional repression. Numerous studies have identified and replicated the genetic association between *MECP2* and lupus, suggesting that genetic variants within *MECP2* are associated with increased risk for lupus.[66–68] This was the first link suggesting a potential role for genetic–epigenetic interaction in the pathogenesis of lupus. Subsequent studies indicated that the lupus-risk variant in *MECP2* is associated with increased mRNA expression of one *MECP2* transcript variant in stimulated but not unstimulated T cells, and that mice overexpressing human MeCP-2 develop anti-nuclear antibodies and a gene expression profile characterized by an interferon signature in activated CD4⁺ T cells.[69] Importantly, the DNA methylome of stimulated T cells from healthy individuals carrying the lupus-risk variant in *MECP2* reveals hypomethylation of several interferon-regulated genes.[69]

Genetic–epigenetic interaction plays a role in flare severity in lupus patients. There is a positive correlation between genetic risk to T cell DNA methylation ratio and lupus disease activity in lupus patients.[70] Moreover, male lupus patients require a higher genetic risk and/or lower T cell DNA methylation to achieve a lupus flare of equal severity to women.[70] Genetic risk alone or T cell DNA methylation alone could not explain the difference between men and women in lupus flare severity. These data provide further evidence for genetic–epigenetic interaction in lupus, and suggest that while genetic risk is relatively stable over time, dynamic changes in T cell DNA methylation might play an important role in lupus flares, in interaction with the genetic susceptibility for lupus.

Recent advances in genome-wide DNA methylation methodologies have made possible more detailed analyses of the interactions between epigenetic modifications and underlying genetic risk for autoimmune and rheumatic conditions. These associations, specifically between DNA methylation changes and genetic susceptibility loci, are known as *methylation quantitative trait loci* (meQTLs). Imgenberg-Kreuz[71] in 2017 published a large meQTL analysis performed on 548 SLE patients and 587 healthy controls using a mixed whole blood tissue sample. Like previous genome-wide DNA methylation studies, they again saw a pattern of DNA hypomethylation of interferon-regulated genes. They also identified seven meQTLs, located within the genes encoding CD45, *class III MHC, HRF1BP1, IRF5, IRF7, IKZF3,* and *UBE2L3.* This study strongly suggests that lupus risk alleles may exert their pathogenic influence at least in part by colluding with local epigenetic patterns.

Histone Modifications in Systemic Lupus Erythematosus

Histone acetylation status is a product of the balance between histone acetyltransferases and histone deacetylases. As the name implies, the former increases histone acetylation while the latter leads to its reduction. As discussed, histone acetylation/deacetylation determines chromatin accessibility, and is influenced by the DNA methylation status (see Fig. 26.2). One of the earliest reports related to histone changes in lupus suggested that histone deacetylase inhibitors can abrogate lupus-like disease in murine models. Histone deacetylase inhibitors downregulated the production of several cytokines including IFNγ, IL-12, IL-10, and IL-6 in MRL/*lpr* mice. Further, mice treated with histone deacetylase inhibitors showed global increase in histone H3 and H4 acetylation as expected, and, more importantly, demonstrated significant improvement in renal diseases.[72] Similarly, NZB/W lupus-prone mice treated with a histone deacetylase inhibitor also showed improvement of renal disease, reduction in Th17 cells, and increased Tregs and acetylation of the Treg key transcription factor *FoxP3.* Therefore, histone deacetylase inhibitors might provide therapeutic effect in lupus by altering T cell subsets and reducing pathogenic Th17 cells while increasing Tregs.[73]

Gene-specific studies in human disease demonstrated the importance of histone changes in suppressing IL-2 and inducing IL-17 production in lupus T cells.[74] In lupus monocytes, *TNF* (encoding TNF) locus is more acetylated compared with normal control monocytes, and this hyperacetylation is associated with increased *TNF* mRNA expression.[75] At a genome-wide level, and while histone changes in lupus have not been as extensively studied as DNA methylation, CD4⁺ T cells from lupus patients demonstrate reduced global H3 and H4 acetylation.[76] This is consistent with the beneficial effect of HDAC inhibitors in lupus mice discussed previously. Mapping histone H4 acetylation in lupus monocytes suggested that the majority of hyperacetylated loci are potentially regulated by type-1 interferons.[77]

A rising area of SLE epigenetic research, and potential therapy, involves the transcription regulator enhancer of zeste homolog 2 (EZH2). EZH2 is a histone lysine methyltransferase and part of the polycomb repressor complex PRC2, which functions by trimethylating lysine 27 of histone H3, resulting in repression of gene expression. A study in 2016 demonstrated an enrichment of EZH2 binding sites among differentially methylated genomic locations correlated with lupus disease activity.[78] Interestingly enough, EZH2 expression is at least partially regulated by another level of epigenetic control, microRNAs miR-26a and miR-101, in response to glucose restriction.[79] MiR-26a expression was indeed positively correlated with lupus disease activity scores.[78] In a follow-up study in 2017, researchers both confirmed overexpression of EZH2 and reduced expression of miR-26a and miR-101 in lupus.[80] Furthermore, they examined the epigenetic consequences of EZH2 overexpression in CD4⁺ T cells, and found substantial differential methylation, particularly in cell adhesion and leukocyte migration-related genes. Linking these epigenetic findings to cellular phenotype, they then demonstrated increased capacity of EZH2-overexpressing T cells to adhere to endothelial cells, suggesting a potential future therapeutic avenue for SLE treatment.[80]

MicroRNAs and the Pathogenesis of Lupus

Differential expression of microRNAs has been reported in multiple cell types in lupus patients.[18,81] As microRNA expression is involved in the regulation of multiple aspects of the normal immune response, it is not surprising that changes in the microRNA milieu can be associated with autoimmunity. Some of the dysregulated microRNAs in lupus tie in specific and credible pathogenic aspects of the disease, and therefore can be targeted as novel therapeutic targets in the future. Overexpression of several microRNAs in lupus CD4⁺ T cells contributes to the DNA methylation defect described previously. The expression of microRNAs miR-126 and miR-148a is increased in lupus CD4⁺ T cells and directly target and inhibit *DNMT1.*[82,83] MiR-21, which is also upregulated in lupus CD4⁺ T cells, inhibits DNA methylation by targeting *RASGRP1,* an upstream component in the MEK/ERK signaling pathway that regulates *DNMT1* expression.[83] These data demonstrate the interaction between two distinct epigenetic mechanisms in lupus: DNA methylation and microRNA regulation.

An example of downregulated microRNAs in lupus is miR-31. Downregulation of miR-31, which directly targets and represses RhoA, contributes to impaired IL-2 production in lupus T cells.[84] Another downregulated microRNA in lupus is miR-146a, which targets several interferon-related genes, such as *IRAK1, TRAF6, IRF5,* and *STAT1.*[85,86] Downregulation of miR146a results in increased activation of type I interferon, a characteristic pathogenic feature of lupus.[86] Of interest, a genetic association between the *miR146a* locus and lupus has been described and the risk variant in this locus is associated with downregulation of miR146a.[87] This is another example of genetic–epigenetic interaction in lupus, whereby a genetic variant might contribute to lupus pathogenesis by affecting the expression of an epigenetic affecter molecule. Another such example is the genetic polymorphism in the 3′UTR region in *TLR7* in lupus patients, which is located in a binding site for miR-3148, suggesting that this genetic variant in *TLR7* might induce pathogenicity by altering the epigenetic regulation of *TLR7*. Indeed, the lupus-associated variant in this locus is associated with increased TLR7 mRNA and protein expression, and the mRNA expression levels of *TLR7* in lupus and normal PBMCs was inversely correlated with miR-3148 expression.[88]

LncRNAs have also been explored in the context of SLE. In one experiment, investigators demonstrated differential expression of nearly 2000 lncRNAs in CD3$^+$ T cells of lupus patients.[89] Two in particular, uc001ykl.1 and ENST00000448942, were strongly correlated with various clinical parameters in these patients, including the presence of anti-Smith antibodies, erythrocyte sedimentation rate (ESR), and c-reactive protein (CRP). Differential expression of lncRNA-mRNA matched pairs has also been noted in peripheral blood mononuclear cells of lupus patients.[90] The expression of lncRNAs in monocyte-derived dendritic cells has also been correlated with disease activity scores (SLEDAI) in lupus patients.[91]

Rheumatoid Arthritis

Fibroblast-like synoviocytes (FLS) are thought to play an important role in rheumatoid arthritis (RA). They are activated and produce a number of pro-inflammatory cytokines in joints of RA patients. Further, this pro-inflammatory phenotype is associated with increased production of specific matrix metalloproteinases in the synovial fluid, leading to joint destruction. Earlier studies showed that FLS in RA patients are characterized by global DNA hypomethylation and as a result express L1 retrotransposable elements, and this global hypomethylation is presumably due to decreased expression of DNMT1.[92] Treating normal FLS with DNA methylation inhibitors results in phenotypic changes resembling activated FLS from RA patients, and in overexpression of several genes, including *miR-203*, which is increased in RA FLS and correlates with levels of IL-6 production.[93] Multiple other microRNAs are also overexpressed in RA FLS, such as miR-155 which is similarly upregulated in RA PBMCs and synovial macrophages.[94,95] MiR-155 is a pro-inflammatory microRNA, as miR-155 deficient mice are resistant to collagen-induced arthritis.[95] MiR-223 is overexpressed in the synovium, peripheral blood naïve CD4$^+$ T cells, and the serum in RA patients, and its expression levels in the serum correlate with disease activity in treatment-naïve early RA.[96–98] The overall role of miR-223 as a therapeutic target in RA remains controversial. Overexpression of miR-223 suppresses osteoclastogenesis in vitro, suggesting a potential beneficial therapeutic effect of miR-223 overexpression[97]; however, suppressing miR-223 in vivo ameliorates arthritis, bone erosions, and osteoclastogenesis in mice with collagen-induced arthritis,[99] suggesting a pathogenic effect of this same microRNA molecule. Of interest, miR-146a is downregulated in lupus peripheral blood leukocytes but is overexpressed in PBMCs and FLS from RA patients,[94,100] although the exact role of miR-146a in RA has not been clearly elucidated.

Global reductions in T cell DNA methylation levels and DNA methyltransferase activity has been described in RA patients, but to a lesser extent than what has been observed in active lupus.[101] Further, a genome-wide DNA methylation study in peripheral blood leukocytes from twin pairs discordant for RA failed to show DNA methylation differences, contrary to lupus in the same study.[56] A demethylated "senescent" CD4$^+$ T cell subset (CD4$^+$CD28$^-$ T cells) is expanded in RA, and overexpresses a number of proteins encoded by methylation-sensitive genes such as CD70, perforin, and KIRs.[102] How much of a role and what causal role this T cell subset plays in RA is currently not clear, but is unlikely to be specific for RA as this T cell subset is expanded in multiple chronic inflammatory diseases. It is interesting, however, that this CD4$^+$CD28$^-$ T cell subset is found in atherosclerotic lesions and is implicated in plaque development and rupture[103,104] given that RA is an independent risk factor for atherosclerotic cardiovascular disease.

Genome-wide DNA methylation studies in RA have focused on elucidating DNA methylation differences between FLS from patients compared with osteoarthritis controls. In one study examining genomic DNA isolated from FLS of six RA patients and five osteoarthritis controls, a number of differentially methylated genes that could play a role in RA were revealed. These include hypomethylation of *CASP1*, *STAT3*, *MMP20*, *TRAF2*, and *MEFV*, among others.[105] Hypomethylation was enriched in pathways related to cell migration, adhesion, and extra-cellular matrix interactions. Interestingly, several CG sites in TNF encoding gene *(TNF)* were hypermethylated in RA FLS.[105] A recent study added to these data, demonstrating differences in DNA methylation and gene transcription signatures in RA versus osteoarthritis control FLS, but also showing substantial differences in epigenetic and transcriptomic patterns in knee joints compared to hip joints.[106] These differences between knee and hip joints were concentrated in inflammatory gene pathways, including IL-6 signaling and the JAK-STAT pathway, IL-17A signaling, and TGF-beta signaling. These data suggest that joint-specific differences in natural history and drug response seen in RA patients may, at least in part, be due to epigenetic variation in joint tissues. Another study examined and integrated changes in the DNA methylome with microRNA expression and gene expression analysis in FLS from six RA and six OA patients.[107] This study identified differential methylation in novel genes in RA including hypomethylation in *IL6R*, *CD74*, *TNFAIP8*, and *CAPN8*, and hypermethylation in *DPP4*, *CCR6*, and *HOXC4*, among others. These data also demonstrated inverse correlation between DNA methylation levels and gene expression in over 200 genes in RA. Importantly, several novel dysregulated microRNAs were revealed in this study, such as miR-503, miR-551b, miR-550, and miR-625*.[107]

A number of genome-wide DNA methylation studies of RA patients' peripheral blood cells have also been performed. In 2014, one study determined DNA methylation patterns in CD3$^+$ T cells and CD19$^+$ B cells from RA patients, using Illumina 450k array technology.[108] Unlike findings in primary Sjögren's syndrome (discussed later), they found evidence for more differential methylation within RA patient T cells compared to B cells, and identified a set of 32 genes with concordant differential methylation in both cell types.[108] The same group published a follow-up study in 2016, in which they examined T and B cells from early (treatment-naïve) RA patients.[109] They demonstrated a distinct methylation signature in each cell type, again showed more differential methylation in T cells than B cells, and identified a methylation "signature" consisting of 150 CpG sites in T lymphocytes and 113 CpG sites in B lymphocytes that accurately clustered all RA patients separately from controls.[109] In 2017, one group[110] examined CD4$^+$ T cells from a Han Chinese RA patient cohort, and described significant differential DNA methylation of the human leukocyte antigen (HLA) region. Interestingly, the global reductions in DNA methylation in RA peripheral blood cell subpopulations appear to be reversible by disease-modifying treatment. In a 2015 study, another group[111] examined global DNA methylation levels of five major blood cell subpopulations (T, B, NK, monocyte, and polymorphonuclear leukocytes) from early RA patients before and 1 month after treatment with the first-line RA disease modifying drug methotrexate. Following drug therapy, global DNA methylation significantly increased in T cells and monocytes, to levels indistinguishable from controls; this change was accompanied by increases in the de novo and maintenance DNA methyltransferases DNMT1 and DNMT3A, respectively.

Advances in sequencing technology over the past few years have led to ever-expanding epigenetic maps of cells involved in RA pathogenesis. For example, a 2017 study identified distinct transcriptomes and epigenomes among *HOX* genes in FLS from different joints, translating into joint-specific synovial fibroblast phenotypes producing a unique microenvironment in each joint.[111a] A comprehensive analysis of the epigenetic landscape of RA FLS was published in 2018.[111b] This study leveraged cutting-edge techniques, including whole-genome DNA methylation and RNA transcription analysis, histone modifications, and open chromatin analysis via Assay for Transposase-Accessible Chromatin using Sequencing (ATAC-Seq), along with a novel method for integration and interrogation of the multidimensional relationships of these various levels of epigenetic regulation. Although they identified a number of epigenetically conserved, RA-associated regions, particularly among enhancers and promoters, there were several unexpected pathways found. These included the Huntington's Disease Signaling pathway, with the Huntington-interaction protein-1 suggested as a mediator of FLS matrix invasion.

Genetic–epigenetic interactions have also been demonstrated in RA. In one large study including genetic and epigenetic data from several hundred RA cases and matched controls, DNA methylation levels in two clusters within the major histocompatibility complex (MHC) region were found to be strongly correlated with both RA and with the underlying genetic sequence in peripheral blood lymphocytes.[112] In 2015, one group[113] published a large-scale integrative-omics study to identify genetic–epigenetic interactions in RA. They considered genomic locations that met three criteria for pathogenic significance: genetic risk (based on genome-wide association studies [GWASs]), differential gene expression in RA FLS, and epigenetic risk via differential DNA methylation in RA FLS. They identified several candidate genes not previously linked to RA pathogenesis, including *AIRE, CASP8, CSF2, ELMO1, ETS1, HLA-DQA1,* and *LBH.*[113] In 2016, this same group expanded their analysis to include differentially methylated CpG sites located outside of "traditional" promoter regulatory regions; specifically, they included enhancer regions in a new analysis.[114] In their new analysis, they identified a novel enhancer associated with the *LBH* gene, which demonstrated hypomethylation in RA FLS, and was enriched in activating histone H3K4me1 marks. Furthermore, they demonstrated a meQTL at this location, wherein the underlying RA-associated genetic risk allele conspired with RA-associated DNA demethylation to substantially increase gene expression beyond what was seen in non–risk-allele control patients. These data strongly suggest that DNA methylation may act as an intermediary of genetic risk in RA, similar to the risk-enhancing effects of meQTLs in SLE and OA, discussed elsewhere in this chapter.

Primary Sjögren's Syndrome

Primary Sjögren's syndrome (pSS) is a systemic autoimmune disease characterized by lymphocytic infiltration of exocrine glands and primarily salivary and lacrimal glands, resulting in dryness of the eyes and mouth. Global DNA methylation levels in labial salivary gland epithelial cells from patients with pSS are decreased, and this reduction correlates with lower DNMT1 levels and increased expression of the demethylating co-factor GADD45α.[111] The presence and extent of the DNA methylation defect in salivary gland epithelial cells in pSS correlate with the presence of B cell infiltrates, which was confirmed in vitro using salivary gland epithelial cell/B cell co-culture.[115] However, no global reduction in peripheral blood B cell or T cell methylation levels was detected.[115] Gene-specific DNA methylation studies in peripheral blood $CD4^+$ T cells in pSS revealed demethylation and overexpression of the co-stimulatory molecule CD70, similar to what had been previously observed in lupus patients.[116] In contrast, *FOXP3* is hypermethylated and transcriptionally repressed in $CD4^+$ T cells from pSS, which is consistent with the Treg functional defect reported in pSS.[117]

The first genome-wide DNA methylation study of pSS, performed in 2014, examined DNA methylation differences in more than 485,000 methylation sites in naïve $CD4^+$ T cells compared to age-, sex-, and ethnicity-matched controls.[118] This study identified 753 differentially methylated sites, with the majority being hypomethylated in pSS compared with controls. Several hypomethylated genes of interest in pSS include *CD247, TNFRSF25, PTPRC, GSTM1*, and *PDCD1*. Several interferon-regulated genes were also hypomethylated, consistent with an interferon signature in pSS.[118] *LTA*, which encodes lymphotoxin alpha (LTα, or TNFβ) and promotes interferon production, was also hypomethylated in naïve $CD4^+$ T cells in pSS. LTα is overexpressed in the serum and salivary gland from patients with pSS, and a clinical trial to block the lymphotoxin pathway as a therapeutic option in pSS is underway. An interesting group of solute carrier protein genes was also differentially methylated in naïve $CD4^+$ T cells from pSS.[118]

Subsequent genome-wide DNA methylation studies have been conducted in pSS in other cell subtypes. In 2014, one study[119] determined changes in DNA methylation patterns using the same 450k technology as Altorok in $CD4^+$ T cells and $CD19^+$ B cells from pSS patients, and demonstrated an increased frequency of epigenetic alterations in B cells, such as genes found to be differentially methylated clustered in signaling pathways related to cytokines (IL4 and IL8), as well as chemokine signaling (CXCR4), and B cell receptor signaling. In 2016, Imgenberg-Kreuz[120] examined $CD19^+$ B cells and identified, similar to SLE patients, a hypomethylation signature in interferon-regulated genes, including *MX1, IFI44L,* and *PARP9*, and demonstrated increased gene expression of several interferon-regulated genes associated with gene DNA hypomethylation. Interestingly, they went on to show similar DNA methylation differences in cells obtained from minor salivary gland biopsies, and identified a meQTL within the human leukocyte antigen (HLA) region as well as two pSS-associated susceptibility alleles located within interferon regulatory factor 5 *(IRF5)*. Also in 2016, one group[121] determined that reductions in DNA methylation of the Sjögren's syndrome B (SSB) gene promoter P1 in minor salivary gland tissue was associated with both lymphocyte infiltration into salivary glands and with increasing titers of anti-SSB (also known as *anti-La*) autoantibodies in pSS patients. Further adding to evidence for altered DNA methylation in salivary gland tissues, another group[122] in 2016 showed persistent alterations in DNA methylation patterns in long-term cultures of salivary gland epithelial cells from pSS patients, again mostly in interferon-regulated genes. Taken together, these studies strongly suggest, similar to SLE, a role for epigenetic dysregulation of interferon-regulated genes in the pathogenesis of pSS. Importantly, these alterations extend to the target tissues of pSS pathophysiology, namely, the salivary glands.

Systemic Sclerosis

Systemic sclerosis (scleroderma) is an autoimmune disease characterized by immune activation, vasculopathy including microvascular endothelial cell dysfunction, and excessive collagen production and fibrosis of the skin and internal organs. Epigenetic studies in scleroderma have therefore focused on fibroblasts, microvascular endothelial cells, and CD4⁺ T cells.[123,124]

Fibroblasts from scleroderma patients underexpress FLi-1, a negative regulator of collagen synthesis,[125] which is hypermethylated in fibroblasts from scleroderma patients compared with controls.[126] Further, H3 and H4 acetylation levels are reduced in the *FLI1* promoter region, probably contributing to its transcriptional repression. Treating scleroderma fibroblasts with DNA methylation inhibitors combined with histone deacetylase inhibitors increases *FLI1* expression and restores collagen production to levels comparable with normal fibroblasts.[126] These data suggest that hypermethylation and hypoacetylation of *FLI1* in scleroderma fibroblasts might play a role in the pathogenesis of this profibrotic disease. Indeed, DNMT1 protein levels and the protein levels of the histone deacetylases HDAC1 and HDAC6 were elevated in scleroderma fibroblasts,[126] which could explain the hypermethylated and hypoacetylated repressive status of *FLI1*. Recent data suggest that the Wnt pathway signaling antagonist genes *DKK1* and *SFRP1* are underexpressed and silenced by hypermethylation in scleroderma fibroblasts.[127] Importantly, inhibiting DNMT1 reduced canonical Wnt pathway signaling in scleroderma fibroblasts and reduced bleomycin-induced fibrosis in mice.[127] Multiple microRNAs are dysregulated in scleroderma fibroblasts compared with controls, with several targeting components in TGFβ signaling. For example, miR-21 and miR-146 are overexpressed, putatively targeting SMAD4 and SMAD7, respectively.[124]

A recent genome-wide DNA methylation study in skin fibroblasts from diffuse and limited scleroderma patients identified a large number of differentially methylated genes between patients and age-, sex-, and ethnicity-matched healthy controls.[128] It is interesting that despite previous reports showing increased DNMT1 expression in scleroderma fibroblasts, most DNA methylation changes observed using this genome-wide unbiased approach were hypomethylation changes in patients compared with healthy controls. This report revealed methylation changes that are common between diffuse and limited disease, and also subset-specific DNA methylation changes. Hypomethylated genes in both diffuse and limited scleroderma included collagen genes such as *COL4A2* and *COL23A1*, *PAX9*, *TNXB*, *ITGA9*, *ADAM12*, and the RUNX transcription family members *RUNX1*, *RUNX2*, and *RUNX3*. Increased mRNA expression levels in multiples of these hypomethylated genes were also demonstrated in the same study.[128]

Studies in microvascular endothelial cells in scleroderma demonstrated increased methylation in *BMPRII*-encoding bone morphogenic protein receptor II, which plays a role in endothelial cell resistance to apoptosis. BMPRII is underexpressed in microvascular endothelial cells from scleroderma patients, and in vitro treatment with DNA methylation/histone deacetylase inhibitors restores expression levels of BMPRII to levels similar to healthy controls.[129] CD4⁺ T cells in scleroderma patients express less DNMT1 compared with normal controls,[130] and overexpress proteins encoded by methylation sensitive genes such as *CD70* and *CD40L*, and the promoter sequences of these genes are hypomethylated.[131,132] This is very similar to what has been previously observed in lupus CD4⁺ T cells. At least one genome-wide DNA methylation analysis of circulating inflammatory cells has also been conducted in the context of systemic sclerosis. One group[133] in 2018 published an analysis of CD4⁺ and CD8⁺ T cells from scleroderma patients. Similar to what has been seen in other systemic autoimmune diseases, they identified substantial epigenetic dysregulation of the type-I interferon signaling pathway in both CD4⁺ and CD8⁺ T cells. Additionally, they determined significant elevations of both type I interferon-alpha and -beta proteins in the sera of scleroderma patients.[133]

A few studies have also recently demonstrated associations between histone post-translational modification changes and scleroderma pathology. Histone deacetylase 5 (HDAC5) is an enzymatic effector of histone post-translational modifications, and is linked to angiogenesis; specifically, HDAC5 expression is inversely correlated with angiogenic activity in endothelial cells.[134,135] In a 2016 study, one group[136] examined the role of HDAC5 in impaired angiogenesis in endothelial cells from scleroderma patients. They first demonstrated increases in *HDAC5* expression in dermal endothelial cells isolated from scleroderma patients, then went on to show that knockdown of *HDAC5* by short interfering RNA (siRNA) restores normal angiogenesis in scleroderma endothelial cells in vitro. Finally, they demonstrated that knockdown of *HDAC5* resulted in widespread epigenetic changes, as measured by increases in open chromatin regions identified through transposase–accessible chromatin using sequencing (ATAC–seq). Remarkably, gene ontology analysis of locations "opened up" following *HDAC5* knockdown revealed 16 genes known to be involved in angiogenesis and 3 involved in fibrosis, 8 of which were differentially expressed following *HDAC5* knockdown. This study offers a good example of the types of epigenetic-cellular phenotype analyses that are critical to link epigenetic associations with disease pathophysiology.

Behçet's Disease

Behçet's disease is an immune-mediated inflammatory disease characterized by recurrent oral-genital ulcers, inflammatory eye disease, skin involvement, CNS involvement, and recurrent thrombosis. The etiology of Behçet's disease is incompletely understood, but, unsurprisingly, genetic and environmental factors play a role in the pathogenesis of the disease. A recent genome-wide DNA methylation study of Behçet's disease shed light on the epigenetic architecture of CD4⁺ T cells and monocytes in Behçet's disease patients with active untreated disease compared to healthy age-, sex-, and ethnicity-matched controls.[137] The study identified key differentially methylated loci and pathways across the genome in Behçet's disease that can be targeted for the development of novel therapeutic interventions in the future. Several regulatory and structural cytoskeletal components showed consistent DNA methylation change in both CD4⁺ T cells and in monocytes in this disease. Differentially methylated genes in Behçet's disease include *RAC1*, *RSG14*, *FSCN2*, among others. Moreover, these epigenetic changes were dynamic, as the study showed clear evidence for reversibility of DNA methylation changes when the same patients were examined at a subsequent time point after disease remission.[137] Therefore, this study of Behçet's disease provides evidence that DNA methylation does change throughout the course of the disease, and that some of these epigenetically altered loci can be explored as novel disease biomarkers and therapeutic targets.

Differential DNA methylation of other cell types has also been associated with Behçet's disease. For example, interferon regulatory factor 8 *(IRF8)* is hypermethylated in dendritic cells of ocular Behçet's patients, and is associated with decreased gene expression; correction of this hypermethylation with 5-aza-2′-deoxycytidine increased *IRF8* expression and downregulated the expression of a variety of co-stimulatory molecules and interleukins, suggesting a potential epigenetic therapy for Behçet's.[138]

Osteoarthritis

Several recent genome-wide DNA methylation studies in articular cartilage tissue have been reported and suggest that epigenetic profiling can identify novel candidate genes and disease aspects, therapeutic targets, disease subsets, and epigenetic biomarkers for disease severity in osteoarthritis (OA).[139,140] In a study examining DNA methylation in ~27,000 CG methylation sites in cartilage tissue from knee OA patients compared with cadaveric controls, 91 differentially methylated CG sites were identified between the two groups. Importantly, genome-wide methylation data and gene expression profiling identified a cluster of OA patients with substantial differential methylation within inflammatory genes.[139] These data suggested that epigenetic and transcriptional profiling can identify disease endophenotypes in OA, which could help target specific therapeutic options in a more individualized manner in the future. Another study examined DNA methylation changes in hip joint OA across more than 485,000 methylation sites using a unique approach comparing eroded with noneroded cartilage tissue from the same joint.[140] This eliminates any confounding effect from genetic variation across the groups. Remarkably, ~40% of genetic risk variants previously reported in OA showed evidence of differential methylation in this study, suggesting that genetic–epigenetic interaction might play a role in the pathogenesis of OA and that genetic or epigenetic alteration in these same genes is associated with OA risk. The study identified a total of 550 differentially methylated genes in OA, with over two-thirds of them hypomethylated. Bioinformatic analysis to identify common regulating factors among these differentially methylated genes identified TGF-β1 and several microRNAs such as miR-128, miR-27a, and miR-9. Importantly, this study showed correlation between DNA methylation in 20 CG sites and histological severity scores in OA.[140] Subsequent studies have confirmed these previous findings across several cohorts. A consistent pattern has emerged, including the aforementioned inflammatory subset as well as substantial differences in DNA methylation between knee and hip OA samples.[141]

Like SLE and RA, researchers have also examined the interaction of epigenetic variation and genetic susceptibility in OA. One study identified 31 genes for which changes in DNA methylation were affected by local genetic variation, and 26 genes for which changes in gene expression were affected by both local epigenetic patterns and genetic variation.[142] A second study published in 2015 performed a methylation quantitative trait loci (meQTL) analysis in knee and hip OA cartilage samples, focusing on 16 previously identified European OA genetic susceptibility loci.[143] Four meQTLs were identified, consisting of nine CpG sites in which genetic variation was associated with changes in local DNA methylation patterns. Interestingly, the effects of these variations on gene transcription patterns were seen both in diseased and disease-free tissue. A later study confirmed a meQTL within the *SUPT3H/RUNX2* region and demonstrated that alterations in gene expression produced by changes in DNA methylation within this region are amplified by the presence of an underlying OA genetic risk allele.[144] Similar effects have also been noted in the iodothyronine deiodinase 2 gene *(DIO2)*, where DNA methylation levels mediate the OA susceptibility effect of the SNP locus *rs225014*.[145]

There has also been interest in epigenetic changes within noncartilage joint tissue, specifically subchondral bone. The first study in this regard characterized the methylome of subchondral bone underlying eroded and intact cartilage sections of end-stage OA hip patient joints.[146] It identified an order of magnitude more differentially methylated CpG sites in subchondral bone than the matched overlying cartilage, with 44% of differentially methylated genes in cartilage also being differentially methylated in subchondral bone. Gene ontology suggested differential methylation of TGF-beta-related genes and various cytokines. A second study in 2016 divided subchondral bone into three distinct regions of the tibial plateau, corresponding to early, intermediate, and late disease, and the corresponding overlying cartilage.[147] Interestingly, they were able to determine that DNA methylation changes occurring both in subchondral bone and cartilage appear first in the subchondral bone compartment. Gene ontology analysis demonstrated differential methylation of genes involved in both stem cell development and differentiation and a cluster of homeobox family *(HOX)* genes, as well as a TGF-beta signature.

Epigenetic Modifications as Biomarkers of Rheumatic Disease

Beyond contributions to disease pathogenesis, epigenetic changes may also offer easily accessible biomarkers to diagnose, predict severity of, or predict response to therapy for many rheumatic diseases. In SLE, a study in 2015 examined peripheral blood mononuclear cell DNA methylation patterns from lupus patients, healthy controls, and non-lupus autoimmune rheumatoid arthritis and Sjögren's syndrome patients for potential disease-associated biomarkers.[148] They identified differentially methylated locations within the *IFI44L* gene as highly associated with SLE, confirming two specific CpG sites within this region in a much larger group of patients as part of a discovery cohort using a high-throughput bisulfite pyrosequencing method. They confirmed the utility of DNA methylation of these two CpG sites in multiple validation cohorts, including among the same ethnic group (Chinese) and among a different ethnic group (Europeans). Among Chinese patients, this assay performed with a sensitivity in the 90% range, whereas in Europeans it performed in the 70% to 80% range. A subsequent study in 2016[149] identified a differential methylation in naive T cells of a single CpG within the *CHST12* gene from lupus patients as highly associated with the presence of lupus nephritis with a sensitivity of 86% and specificity of 71%. Other studies have similarly noted strong associations between DNA methylation alterations and disease activity in SLE. These include *IL10* and *IL12* correlation with lupus disease activity,[150] and *IL6* methylation correlations with lupus disease activity, flare, and serum complement levels.[151,152] *FOXP3* DNA methylation has also been associated with lupus disease activity,[153] and retroviral element *HERV-E* and *HERV-K* methylation has been associated with both disease activity and several autoantibody specificities.[154,155]

Future Directions

Epigenetic dysregulation has been increasingly recognized as a major factor involved in the pathogenesis of rheumatic diseases. The past many years have witnessed a growing interest in studying epigenetic differences between patients with various autoimmune, inflammatory, and non-inflammatory rheumatic conditions and normal healthy controls. The availability of unbiased genome-wide approaches has broadened our knowledge and allowed for the identification of novel epigenetically altered genetic loci that can help to better understand disease pathogenesis and identify novel targets for therapy.

With this plethora of epigenetic and epigenomic studies in rheumatology, several issues need to be carefully kept in mind. Epigenetic changes are cell-type specific, and therefore, moving forward, it is of utmost importance that very specific cell subsets should be examined to accurately capture epigenetic differences between patients and controls, which represent genuine disease-associated differences, rather than effect of differences in cellular constituents or cell activation status between patients and controls. Adequately powered studies to address the clinical heterogeneity of the disease of interest, careful phenotyping of patients, and careful selection of matched healthy controls should be emphasized. New technologies have recently emerged allowing ever-more-detailed phenotyping of cellular subsets, including the ultimate in subphenotyping: single cell analyses,[156] which may become the standard form of epigenetic analysis in the future. This careful attention to adequate phenotyping of both patients and tissues of interest must become the rule rather than the exception if we are to draw well-reasoned conclusions regarding epigenetic associations with disease.

As discussed in the previous section, the dynamic nature of epigenetic changes may allow for the development of novel disease biomarkers. Indeed, there is paucity in rheumatology of reliable biomarkers. Future studies would focus and expand on disease subset specific epigenetic changes. We hope to answer questions such as what specific DNA methylation changes could predict nephritis in a lupus patient, what specific epigenetic changes could predict the development of lymphoma in a Sjögren's syndrome patient or severe lung involvement in a scleroderma patient, what epigenetic changes may predict rapid disease progression in OA patients, and so on. Some of the epigenetic changes that we need to discover and validate in future studies can also help assess disease activity, predict disease flares, or determine what treatment option to use in an increasingly personalized medicine approach. One way to achieve this is to conduct longitudinal epigenetic studies in rheumatology, following the same group of patients over time, rather than the more commonly used cross-sectional approach. A longitudinal approach would also help address the question of "cause" versus "effect" in epigenomic changes we associate with the various diseases. Ideally, a longitudinal approach following and collecting biological samples from a group of individuals before they develop disease would be most informative in dissecting the issue of causality.

Another, and potentially quite powerful, technique to examine the causality of epigenetic changes is the emerging field of epigenetic editing. Spurred by the development of novel DNA localization and binding technologies, most notably nuclease-defective Cas9 proteins (dCas9, part of the clustered regularly interspersed short palindromic repeats, or CRISPR, system), epigenetic editing approaches have now been demonstrated in several cell types. A sequence-specific epigenetic editing system generally consists of at least three parts: a DNA binding module, a flexible linker, and a catalytically active epigenetic modification module (Fig. 26.5). To date, epigenetic editing has been demonstrated using a variety of enzymatic effectors, including DNA "demethylation" via conversion of 5-methylcytosine to 5-hydroxymethylcytosine with aforementioned TET proteins,[157] DNA methylation via the mammalian DNA methyltransferase DNMT3a[158,159] or bacterial methyltransferase m.SssI,[160] histone acetylases including p300[161] and CBP,[162] and histone lysine demethylase LSD1.[162] Two studies directly demonstrating epigenetic editing in rheumatic diseases have been published. The first used dCas9-TET1 and dCas9-p300 constructs targeted to the T cell–specific demethylated region (TSDR) of mouse *Foxp3* in a mouse T cell line in vitro, where they demonstrated that both DNA demethylation and histone acetylation of this *Foxp3* region increased and stabilized expression of this key regulatory gene and partially prevented a loss of *Foxp3* expression after an inflammatory stimulus, and enhanced epigenetically edited cells' ability to suppress effector T cell expansion in vitro.[163] The second study implemented a refined version of a dCas9-TET1 DNA demethylation system known as *Suntag*, which allows multiple TET1 effectors to be tethered to a single dCas9 molecule (first demonstrated by one study).[164] This study targeted several regions in the human *FOXP3* gene, including the TSDR, proximal promoter, and CNS1 region in the Jurkat T cell line.[165] They demonstrated substantial reductions in DNA methylation upon epigenetic editing, associated with overexpression of *FOXP3* when targeting each of the three regions. Furthermore, they demonstrated suppression of $CD4^+$ $CD25^-$ effector T cell expansion upon co-culture with epigenetically edited T cells.

A second critical study in the field of epigenetic editing was published by one group in 2018.[166] In this paper, the investigators delivered the DNA methylation inhibitor 5-azacytidine, known to cause lupus in mice when given systemically, specifically to $CD4^+$ and $CD8^+$ T cells via a cutting-edge nanolipogel technique. Contrary to expectations, they found that delivery to either cell subtype suppressed lupus disease activity in lupus-susceptible MRL*lpr* mice; specifically, targeted therapy reduced proteinuria, reduced multiple serum pro-inflammatory cytokine levels, and reduced skin manifestations. The authors went on to show that targeting 5-azacytidine to $CD4^+$ T cells results in increases in regulatory T cell number, likely by demethylating *Foxp3*. Targeting this drug to $CD8^+$ T cells resulted in a significant decrease in the autoreactive so-called "double negative" T cell pool in mice, representing a population of $CD4^-$ $CD8^-$ cells thought to be pathogenic in murine lupus, likely by reducing stimulation-dependent *Cd8* downregulation in $CD8^+$ cells.[166] Although still in its infancy, the field of epigenetic editing, through both specific genomic targeting and delivery to particular cell subtypes, holds great promise for correcting many of the epigenetic aberrancies that have been demonstrated associated with autoimmune diseases.

Future studies in epigenomics in rheumatology should also address more comprehensively genetic–epigenetic interaction, and the interaction between environmental triggers of disease, epigenomic changes, and the disease genetic background. Studies have already been initiated to examine allele-specific epigenetic changes to understand how some genetic variants that are associated with diseases induce risk. These efforts will need

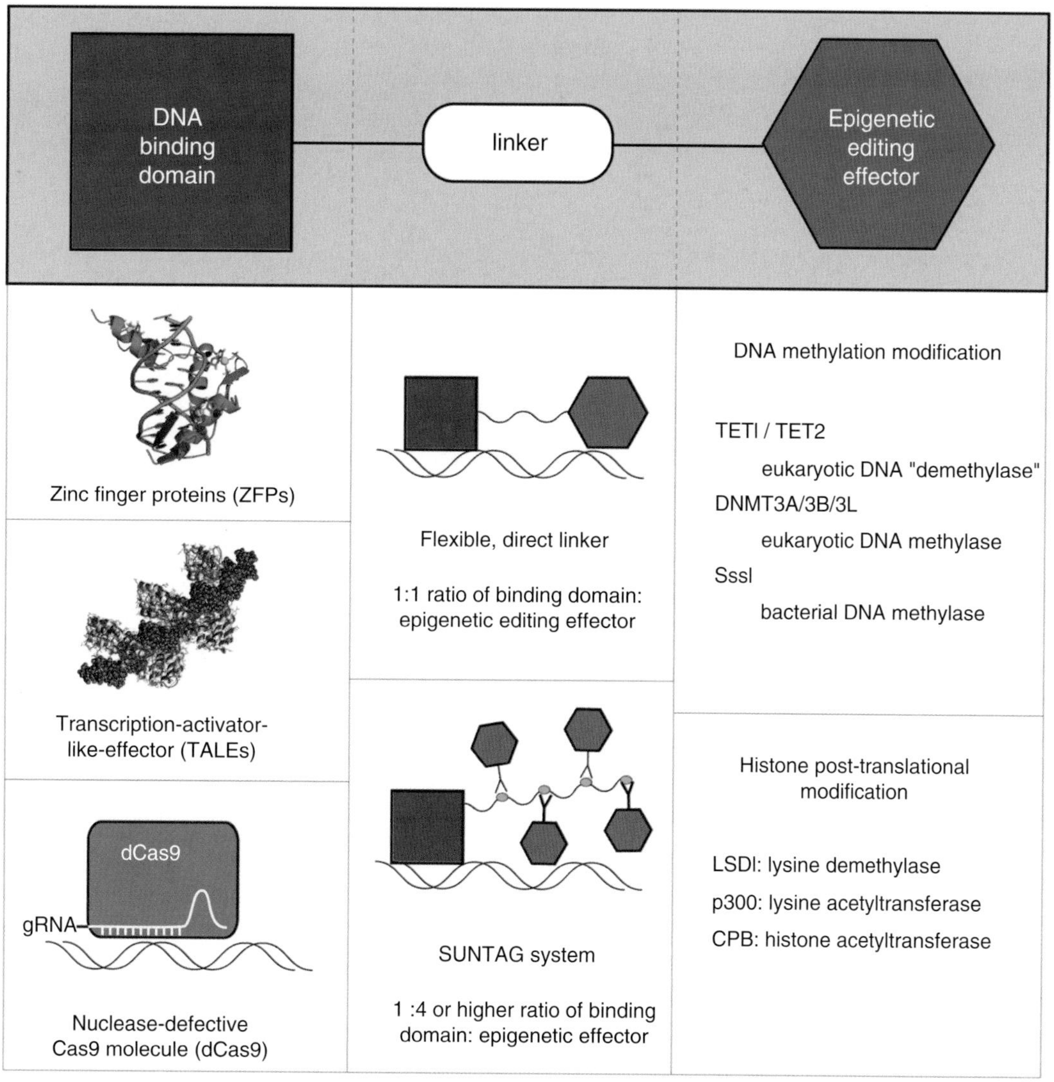

DNA binding domain

linker

Epigenetic editing effector

Zinc finger proteins (ZFPs)

Transcription-activator-like-effector (TALEs)

dCas9

gRNA

Nuclease-defective Cas9 molecule (dCas9)

Flexible, direct linker

1:1 ratio of binding domain: epigenetic editing effector

SUNTAG system

1 :4 or higher ratio of binding domain: epigenetic effector

DNA methylation modification

TETI / TET2

eukaryotic DNA "demethylase"

DNMT3A/3B/3L

eukaryotic DNA methylase

SssI

bacterial DNA methylase

Histone post-translational modification

LSDI: lysine demethylase

p300: lysine acetyltransferase

CPB: histone acetyltransferase

• **Fig. 26.5** Epigenetic editing techniques rely on targeting of epigenetic "effectors" to specific genomic locations. These systems universally have three components: a DNA binding domain, a linker region, and an epigenetic editing effector. Recent refinements have included the introduction of nuclease-defective dCas9 as a DNA binding domain and the Suntag system as a linker, allowing multiple epigenetic effector domains to be tethered to each DNA binding domain, increasing both specificity and efficiency of induced epigenetic modifications.

to be expanded to a genome-wide level. An integrated "-omics" approach that includes the genome, epigenome, transcriptome, and exposome (environmental exposures) would be very informative to comprehensively understand and better treat rheumatic diseases in the very near future.

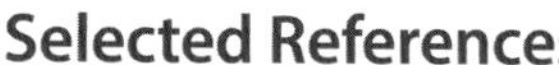
Full references for this chapter can be found on ExpertConsult.com.

Selected References

1. Luger K, Mäder AW, Richmond RK, et al.: Crystal structure of the nucleosome core particle at 2.8 A resolution, *Nature* 389:251–260, 1997.
2. Razin A, Riggs AD: DNA methylation and gene function, *Science* 210:604–610, 1980.
3. Okano M, Bell DW, Haber DA, et al.: DNA methyltransferases Dnmt3a and Dnmt3b are essential for de novo methylation and mammalian development, *Cell* 99:247–257, 1999.
4. Jurkowska RZ, Rajavelu A, Anspach N, et al.: Oligomerization and binding of the Dnmt3a DNA methyltransferase to parallel DNA molecules: heterochromatic localization and role of Dnmt3L, *J Biol Chem* 286:24200–24207, 2011.
5. Riggs AD: X inactivation, differentiation, and DNA methylation, *Cytogenet Cell Genet* 14:9–25, 1975.
6. Bird AP, Southern EM: Use of restriction enzymes to study eukaryotic DNA methylation: I. The methylation pattern in ribosomal DNA from Xenopus laevis, *J Mol Biol* 118:27–47, 1978.
7. Holliday R, Pugh JE: DNA modification mechanisms and gene activity during development, *Science* 187:226–232, 1975.
8. Oaks Z, Perl A: Metabolic control of the epigenome in systemic lupus erythematosus, *Autoimmunity* 47:256–264, 2014.
9. Lister R, Pelizzola M, Dowen RH, et al.: Human DNA methylomes at base resolution show widespread epigenomic differences, *Nature* 462:315–322, 2009.
10. Lister R, Mukamel EA, Nery JR, et al.: Global epigenomic reconfiguration during mammalian brain development, *Science* 341:1237905, 2013.

11. Nan X, Ng HH, Johnson CA, et al.: Transcriptional repression by the methyl-CpG-binding protein MeCP2 involves a histone deacetylase complex, *Nature* 393:386–389, 1998.
12. Jones PL, Veenstra GJ, Wade PA, et al.: Methylated DNA and MeCP2 recruit histone deacetylase to repress transcription, *Nat Genet* 19:187–191, 1998.
13. Wu H, Zhang Y: Reversing DNA methylation: mechanisms, genomics, and biological functions, *Cell* 156:45–68, 2014.
14. Ito S, Shen L, Dai Q, et al.: Tet proteins can convert 5-methylcytosine to 5-formylcytosine and 5-carboxylcytosine, *Science* 333:1300–1303, 2011.
15. He Y-F, Li B-Z, Li Z, et al.: Tet-mediated formation of 5-carboxylcytosine and its excision by TDG in mammalian DNA, *Science* 333:1303–1307, 2011.
16. Xu Y-M, Du J-Y, Lau ATY: Posttranslational modifications of human histone H3: an update, *Proteomics* 14:2047–2060, 2014.
17. ENCODE Project Consortium: An integrated encyclopedia of DNA elements in the human genome, *Nature* 489:57–74, 2012.
18. Shen N, Liang D, Tang Y, et al.: MicroRNAs—novel regulators of systemic lupus erythematosus pathogenesis, *Nat Rev Rheumatol* 8:701–709, 2012.
19. Beard C, Li E, Jaenisch R: Loss of methylation activates Xist in somatic but not in embryonic cells, *Genes Dev* 9:2325–2334, 1995.
20. Sleutels F, Zwart R, Barlow DP: The non-coding Air RNA is required for silencing autosomal imprinted genes, *Nature* 415:810–813, 2002.
21. Thakur N, Tiwari VK, Thomassin H, et al.: An antisense RNA regulates the bidirectional silencing property of the Kcnq1 imprinting control region, *Mol Cell Biol* 24:7855–7862, 2004.
22. Sawalha AH: Epigenetics and T-cell immunity, *Autoimmunity* 41:245–252, 2008.
23. Bruniquel D, Schwartz RH: Selective, stable demethylation of the interleukin-2 gene enhances transcription by an active process, *Nat Immunol* 4:235–240, 2003.
24. Bird A: Il2 transcription unleashed by active DNA demethylation, *Nat Immunol* 4:208–209, 2003.
25. Mullen AC, Hutchins AS, High FA, et al.: Hlx is induced by and genetically interacts with T-bet to promote heritable T(H)1 gene induction, *Nat Immunol* 3:652–658, 2002.
26. Agarwal S, Rao A: Modulation of chromatin structure regulates cytokine gene expression during T cell differentiation, *Immunity* 9:765–775, 1998.
27. Lee DU, Agarwal S, Rao A: Th2 lineage commitment and efficient IL-4 production involves extended demethylation of the IL-4 gene, *Immunity* 16:649–660, 2002.
28. Santangelo S, Cousins DJ, Winkelmann NEE, et al.: DNA methylation changes at human Th2 cytokine genes coincide with DNase I hypersensitive site formation during CD4(+) T cell differentiation, *J Immunol* 169:1893–1903, 2002.
29. Young HA, Ghosh P, Ye J, et al.: Differentiation of the T helper phenotypes by analysis of the methylation state of the IFN-gamma gene, *J Immunol* 153:3603–3610, 1994.
30. Cuddapah S, Barski A, Zhao K: Epigenomics of T cell activation, differentiation, and memory, *Curr Opin Immunol* 22:341–347, 2010.
31. Akimzhanov AM, Yang XO, Dong C: Chromatin remodeling of interleukin-17 (IL-17)-IL-17F cytokine gene locus during inflammatory helper T cell differentiation, *J Biol Chem* 282:5969–5972, 2007.
32. Kim H-P, Leonard WJ: CREB/ATF-dependent T cell receptor–induced FoxP3 gene expression: a role for DNA methylation, *J Exp Med* 204:1543–1551, 2007. Rockefeller University Press.
33. Janson PCJ, Winerdal ME, Marits P, et al.: FOXP3 promoter demethylation reveals the committed Treg population in humans, *PLoS One* 3:e1612, 2008.
34. Jaffe AE, Irizarry RA: Accounting for cellular heterogeneity is critical in epigenome-wide association studies, *Genome Biol* 15:R31, 2014.
35. Houseman EA, Accomando WP, Koestler DC, et al.: DNA methylation arrays as surrogate measures of cell mixture distribution, *BMC Bioinformatics* 13:86, 2012.
36. Bakulski KM, Feinberg JI, Andrews SV, et al.: DNA methylation of cord blood cell types: Applications for mixed cell birth studies, *Epigenetics* 11:354–362, 2016.
37. Altorok N, Sawalha AH: Epigenetics in the pathogenesis of systemic lupus erythematosus, *Curr Opin Rheumatol* 25:569–576, 2013.
38. Guo Y, Sawalha AH, Lu Q: Epigenetics in the treatment of systemic lupus erythematosus: potential clinical application, *Clin Immunol* 155:79–90, 2014.
39. Richardson BC, Patel DR: Epigenetics in 2013. DNA methylation and miRNA: key roles in systemic autoimmunity, *Nat Rev Rheumatol* 10:72–74, 2014.
40. Scheinbart LS, Johnson MA, Gross LA, et al.: Procainamide inhibits DNA methyltransferase in a human T cell line, *J Rheumatol* 18:530–534, 1991.
41. Deng C, Lu Q, Zhang Z, et al.: Hydralazine may induce autoimmunity by inhibiting extracellular signal–regulated kinase pathway signaling, *Arthritis and Rheum* 48:746–756, 2003. Wiley Subscription Services, Inc., A Wiley Company.
42. Zhang Y, Zhao M, Sawalha AH, et al.: Impaired DNA methylation and its mechanisms in CD4+ T cells of systemic lupus erythematosus, *J Autoimmun* 41:92–99, 2013. Elsevier.
43. Sawalha AH, Jeffries M, Webb R, et al.: Defective T-cell ERK signaling induces interferon-regulated gene expression and overexpression of methylation-sensitive genes similar to lupus patients, *Genes Immun* 9:368–378, 2008.
44. Strickland FM, Hewagama A, Lu Q, et al.: Environmental exposure, estrogen and two X chromosomes are required for disease development in an epigenetic model of lupus, *J Autoimmun* 38:J135–J143, 2012.
45. Sawalha AH, Jeffries M. Defective DNA methylation and CD70 overexpression in CD4+ T cells in MRL/lpr lupus–prone mice. Eur J Immunol. Wiley Online Library; 2007. Available: https://onlinelibrary.wiley.com/doi/abs/10.1002/eji.200636872.
46. Gorelik G, Fang JY, Wu A, et al.: Impaired T cell protein kinase Cδ activation decreases ERK pathway signaling in idiopathic and hydralazine-induced lupus, *J Immunol Am Assoc Immunol* 179:5553–5563, 2007.
47. Gorelik GJ, Yarlagadda S, Patel DR, et al.: Protein kinase Cδ oxidation contributes to ERK inactivation in lupus T cells, *Arthritis Rheum* 64:2964–2974, 2012.
48. Li Y, Gorelik G, Strickland FM, et al.: Oxidative stress, T cell DNA methylation, and lupus, *Arthritis Rheumatol* 66:1574–1582, 2014.
49. Perl A: Oxidative stress in the pathology and treatment of systemic lupus erythematosus, *Nat Rev Rheumatol* 9:674–686, 2013.
50. Lai Z-W, Hanczko R, Bonilla E, et al.: N-acetylcysteine reduces disease activity by blocking mammalian target of rapamycin in T cells from systemic lupus erythematosus patients: a randomized, double-blind, placebo-controlled trial, *Arthritis and Rheum* 64:2937–2946, 2012. Wiley Online Library.
51. Katsiari CG, Kyttaris VC, Juang Y-T, et al.: Protein phosphatase 2A is a negative regulator of IL-2 production in patients with systemic lupus erythematosus, *J Clin Invest* 115:3193–3204, 2005.
52. Sunahori K, Nagpal K, Hedrich CM, et al.: The catalytic subunit of protein phosphatase 2A (PP2Ac) promotes DNA hypomethylation by suppressing the phosphorylated mitogen-activated protein kinase/extracellular signal-regulated kinase (ERK) kinase (MEK)/phosphorylated ERK/DNMT1 protein pathway in T-cells from controls and systemic lupus erythematosus patients, *J Biol Chem ASBMB* 288:21936–21944, 2013.
53. Apostolidis SA, Rauen T, Hedrich CM. Protein phosphatase 2A enables expression of IL-17 through chromatin remodeling. *J Biol Chem* 288:26775–26784, 2013. Available: http://www.jbc.org/content/early/2013/08/05/jbc.M113.483743.short.
54. Li Y, Zhao M, Yin H, et al.: Overexpression of the growth arrest and DNA damage—induced 45α gene contributes to autoimmunity by promoting DNA demethylation in lupus T cells, *Arthritis and Rheum* 62:1438–1447, 2010. Wiley Online Library.

55. Zhao M, Sun Y, Gao F, et al.: Epigenetics and SLE: RFX1 downregulation causes CD11a and CD70 overexpression by altering epigenetic modifications in lupus CD4+ T cells, *J Autoimmun* 35:58–69, 2010.
56. Javierre BM, Fernandez AF, Richter J, et al.: Changes in the pattern of DNA methylation associate with twin discordance in systemic lupus erythematosus, *Genome Res* 20:170–179, 2010.
57. Jeffries MA, Dozmorov M, Tang Y, et al.: Genome-wide DNA methylation patterns in CD4+ T cells from patients with systemic lupus erythematosus, *Epigenetics* 6:593–601, 2011.
58. Coit P, Jeffries M, Altorok N, et al.: Genome-wide DNA methylation study suggests epigenetic accessibility and transcriptional poising of interferon-regulated genes in naive CD4+ T cells from lupus patients. *J Autoimmun* 43:78–84, 2013. Available: https://www.sciencedirect.com/science/article/pii/S0896841113000504.
59. Zhao M, Liu S, Luo S, et al.: DNA methylation and mRNA and microRNA expression of SLE CD4+ T cells correlate with disease phenotype, *J Autoimmun* 54:127–136, 2014.
60. Absher DM, Li X, Waite LL, et al.: Genome-wide DNA methylation analysis of systemic lupus erythematosus reveals persistent hypomethylation of interferon genes and compositional changes to CD4+ T-cell populations, *PLoS Genet* 9:e1003678, 2013.
61. Villanueva E, Yalavarthi S, Berthier CC, et al.: Netting neutrophils induce endothelial damage, infiltrate tissues, and expose immunostimulatory molecules in systemic lupus erythematosus, *J Immunol* 187:538–552, 2011.
62. Coit P, Yalavarthi S, Ognenovski M, et al.: Epigenome profiling reveals significant DNA demethylation of interferon signature genes in lupus neutrophils, *J Autoimmun* 58:59–66, 2015.
63. Knight JS, Kaplan MJ: Lupus neutrophils: "NET" gain in understanding lupus pathogenesis, *Curr Opin Rheumatol* 24:441–450, 2012.
64. Strickland FM, Patel D, Khanna D, et al.: Characterisation of an epigenetically altered CD4(+) CD28(+) Kir(+) T cell subset in autoimmune rheumatic diseases by multiparameter flow cytometry, *Lupus Sci Med* 3:e000147, 2016.
65. Gensterblum E, Renauer P, Coit P, et al.: CD4+CD28+KIR+CD11ahi T cells correlate with disease activity and are characterized by a pro-inflammatory epigenetic and transcriptional profile in lupus patients, *J Autoimmun* 86:19–28, 2018.
66. Sawalha AH, Webb R, Han S, et al.: Common variants within MECP2 confer risk of systemic lupus erythematosus, *PLoS One* 3:e1727, 2008.
67. Webb R, Wren JD, Jeffries M, et al.: Variants within MECP2, a key transcription regulator, are associated with increased susceptibility to lupus and differential gene expression in patients with systemic lupus erythematosus, *Arthritis Rheum* 60:1076–1084, 2009.
68. Kaufman KM, Zhao J, Kelly JA, et al.: Fine mapping of Xq28: both MECP2 and IRAK1 contribute to risk for systemic lupus erythematosus in multiple ancestral groups, *Ann Rheum Dis* 72:437–444, 2013.
69. Koelsch KA, Webb R, Jeffries M, et al.: Functional characterization of the MECP2/IRAK1 lupus risk haplotype in human T cells and a human MECP2 transgenic mouse, *J Autoimmun* 41:168–174, 2013.
70. Sawalha AH, Wang L, Nadig A, Michigan Lupus Cohort, et al.: Sex-specific differences in the relationship between genetic susceptibility, T cell DNA demethylation and lupus flare severity, *J Autoimmun* 38:J216–J222, 2012.
71. Imgenberg-Kreuz J, Carlsson Almlöf J, Leonard D, et al.: DNA methylation mapping identifies gene regulatory effects in patients with systemic lupus erythematosus, *Ann Rheum Dis* 77:736–743, 2018.
72. Mishra N, Reilly CM, Brown DR, et al.: Histone deacetylase inhibitors modulate renal disease in the MRL-lpr/lpr mouse, *J Clin Invest* 111:539–552, 2003.
73. Regna NL, Chafin CB, Hammond SE, et al.: Class I and II histone deacetylase inhibition by ITF2357 reduces SLE pathogenesis in vivo, *Clin Immunol* 151:29–42, 2014.
74. Rauen T, Hedrich CM, Tenbrock K, et al.: cAMP responsive element modulator: a critical regulator of cytokine production, *Trends Mol Med* 19:262–269, 2013.
75. Sullivan KE, Suriano A, Dietzmann K, et al.: The TNFα locus is altered in monocytes from patients with systemic lupus erythematosus, *Clin Immunol* 123:74–81, 2007.
76. Hu N, Qiu X, Luo Y, et al.: Abnormal histone modification patterns in lupus CD4+ T cells, *J Rheumatol* 35:804–810, 2008.
77. Zhang Z, Song L, Maurer K, et al.: Global H4 acetylation analysis by ChIP-chip in systemic lupus erythematosus monocytes, *Genes Immun* 11:124–133, 2010.
78. Coit P, Dozmorov MG, Merrill JT, et al.: Epigenetic reprogramming in naive CD4+ T cells favoring T cell activation and non-Th1 effector T cell immune response as an early event in lupus flares, *Arthritis Rheumatol* 68:2200–2209, 2016.
79. Zhao E, Maj T, Kryczek I, et al.: Cancer mediates effector T cell dysfunction by targeting microRNAs and EZH2 via glycolysis restriction, *Nat Immunol* 17:95–103, 2016.
80. Tsou P-S, Coit P, Kilian NC, et al.: EZH2 modulates the DNA methylome and controls T cell adhesion through junctional adhesion molecule-A in lupus patients, *Arthritis Rheumatol*, 2017.
81. Zan H, Tat C, Casali P: MicroRNAs in lupus, *Autoimmunity* 47:272–285, 2014.
82. Zhao S, Wang Y, Liang Y, et al.: MicroRNA-126 regulates DNA methylation in CD4+ T cells and contributes to systemic lupus erythematosus by targeting DNA methyltransferase 1, *Arthritis and Rheum* 63:1376–1386, 2011. Wiley Online Library.
83. Pan W, Zhu S, Yuan M, et al.: MicroRNA-21 and microRNA-148a contribute to DNA hypomethylation in lupus CD4+ T cells by directly and indirectly targeting DNA methyltransferase 1, *J Immunol* 184:6773–6781, 2010.
84. Fan W, Liang D, Tang Y, et al.: Identification of microRNA-31 as a novel regulator contributing to impaired interleukin-2 production in T cells from patients with systemic lupus erythematosus, *Arthritis and Rheum* 64:3715–3725, 2012. Wiley Online Library.
85. Taganov KD, Boldin MP, Chang K-J, et al.: NF-κB-dependent induction of microRNA miR-146, an inhibitor targeted to signaling proteins of innate immune responses, *Proc Natl Acad Sci U S A* 103:12481–12486, 2006.
86. Tang Y, Luo X, Cui H, et al.: MicroRNA-146a contributes to abnormal activation of the type I interferon pathway in human lupus by targeting the key signaling proteins, *Arthritis and Rheum* 60:1065–1075, 2009. Wiley Online Library.
87. Luo X, Yang W, Ye D-Q, et al.: A functional variant in microRNA-146a promoter modulates its expression and confers disease risk for systemic lupus erythematosus, *PLoS Genet* 7:e1002128, 2011.
88. Deng Y, Zhao J, Sakurai D, et al.: MicroRNA-3148 modulates allelic expression of toll-like receptor 7 variant associated with systemic lupus erythematosus, *PLoS Genet* 9:e1003336, 2013.
89. Li L-J, Zhao W, Tao S-S, et al.: Comprehensive long non-coding RNA expression profiling reveals their potential roles in systemic lupus erythematosus, *Cell Immunol* 319:17–27, 2017.
90. Luo Q, Li X, Xu C, et al.: Integrative analysis of long non-coding RNAs and messenger RNA expression profiles in systemic lupus erythematosus, *Mol Med Rep* 17:3489–3496, 2018.
91. Wang Y, Chen S, Chen S, et al.: Long noncoding RNA expression profile and association with SLEDAI score in monocyte-derived dendritic cells from patients with systematic lupus erythematosus, *Arthritis Res Ther* 20:138, 2018.
92. Karouzakis E, Gay RE, Michel BA, et al.: DNA hypomethylation in rheumatoid arthritis synovial fibroblasts, *Arthritis Rheum* 60:3613–3622, 2009.
93. Stanczyk J, Ospelt C, Karouzakis E, et al.: Altered expression of microRNA-203 in rheumatoid arthritis synovial fibroblasts and its role in fibroblast activation, *Arthritis and Rheum* 63:373–381, 2011. Wiley Online Library.
94. Pauley KM, Satoh M, Chan AL, et al.: Upregulated miR-146a expression in peripheral blood mononuclear cells from rheumatoid arthritis patients, *Arthritis Res Ther* 10:R101, 2008.
95. Kurowska-Stolarska M, Alivernini S, Ballantine LE, et al.: MicroRNA-155 as a proinflammatory regulator in clinical and

experimental arthritis, *Proc Natl Acad Sci U S A* 108:11193–11198, 2011.
96. Fulci V, Scappucci G, Sebastiani GD, et al.: miR-223 is overexpressed in T-lymphocytes of patients affected by rheumatoid arthritis, *Hum Immunol* 71:206–211, 2010.
97. Shibuya H, Nakasa T, Adachi N, et al.: Overexpression of microRNA-223 in rheumatoid arthritis synovium controls osteoclast differentiation, *Mod Rheumatol* 23:674–685, 2013.
98. Filková M, Aradi B, Senolt L, et al.: Association of circulating miR-223 and miR-16 with disease activity in patients with early rheumatoid arthritis, *Ann Rheum Dis* 73:1898–1904, 2014.
99. Li Y-T, Chen S-Y, Wang C-R, et al.: Brief report: amelioration of collagen-induced arthritis in mice by lentivirus-mediated silencing of microRNA-223, *Arthritis Rheum* 64:3240–3245, 2012.
100. Stanczyk J, Pedrioli DML, Brentano F, et al.: Altered expression of MicroRNA in synovial fibroblasts and synovial tissue in rheumatoid arthritis, *Arthritis Rheum* 58:1001–1009, 2008.
101. Richardson B, Scheinbart L, Strahler J, et al.: Evidence for impaired T cell DNA methylation in systemic lupus erythematosus and rheumatoid arthritis, *Arthritis Rheum* 33:1665–1673, 1990.
102. Liu Y, Chen Y, Richardson B: Decreased DNA methyltransferase levels contribute to abnormal gene expression in "senescent" CD4+ CD28- T cells, *Clin Immunol* 132:257–265, 2009. Elsevier.
103. Liuzzo G, Goronzy JJ, Yang H, et al.: Monoclonal T-cell proliferation and plaque instability in acute coronary syndromes, *Circulation* 101:2883–2888, 2000.
104. Gerli R, Schillaci G, Giordano A, et al.: CD4+CD28- T lymphocytes contribute to early atherosclerotic damage in rheumatoid arthritis patients, *Circulation* 109:2744–2748, 2004.
105. Nakano K, Whitaker JW, Boyle DL, et al.: DNA methylome signature in rheumatoid arthritis, *Ann Rheum Dis* 72:110–117, 2013.
106. Ai R, Hammaker D, Boyle DL, et al.: Joint-specific DNA methylation and transcriptome signatures in rheumatoid arthritis identify distinct pathogenic processes, *Nat Commun* 7:11849, 2016.
107. de la Rica L, Urquiza JM, Gómez-Cabrero D, et al.: Identification of novel markers in rheumatoid arthritis through integrated analysis of DNA methylation and microRNA expression, *J Autoimmun* 41:6–16, 2013.
108. Glossop JR, Emes RD, Nixon NB, et al.: Genome-wide DNA methylation profiling in rheumatoid arthritis identifies disease-associated methylation changes that are distinct to individual T- and B-lymphocyte populations, *Epigenetics* 9:1228–1237, 2014.
109. Glossop JR, Emes RD, Nixon NB, et al.: Genome-wide profiling in treatment-naive early rheumatoid arthritis reveals DNA methylome changes in T and B lymphocytes, *Epigenomics* 8:209–224, 2016.
110. Guo S, Zhu Q, Jiang T, et al.: Genome-wide DNA methylation patterns in CD4+ T cells from Chinese Han patients with rheumatoid arthritis, *Mod Rheumatol* 27:441–447, 2017.
111. de Andres MC, Perez-Pampin E, Calaza M, et al.: Assessment of global DNA methylation in peripheral blood cell subpopulations of early rheumatoid arthritis before and after methotrexate, *Arthritis Res Ther* 17:233, 2015.
112. Liu Y, Aryee MJ, Padyukov L, et al.: Epigenome-wide association data implicate DNA methylation as an intermediary of genetic risk in rheumatoid arthritis, *Nat Biotechnol* 31:142–147, 2013.
113. Whitaker JW, Boyle DL, Bartok B, et al.: Integrative omics analysis of rheumatoid arthritis identifies non-obvious therapeutic targets, *PLoS One* 10:e0124254, 2015.
114. Hammaker D, Whitaker JW, Maeshima K, et al.: LBH gene transcription regulation by the interplay of an enhancer risk allele and DNA methylation in rheumatoid arthritis: genomic regulation of LBH in rheumatoid arthritis, *Arthritis and Rheumatol* 68:2637–2645, 2016.
115. Thabet Y, Le Dantec C, Ghedira I, et al.: Epigenetic dysregulation in salivary glands from patients with primary Sjögren's syndrome may be ascribed to infiltrating B cells, *J Autoimmun* 41:175–181, 2013.
116. Yin H, Zhao M, Wu X, et al.: Hypomethylation and overexpression of CD70 (TNFSF7) in CD4+ T cells of patients with primary Sjögren's syndrome, *J Dermatol Sci* 59:198–203, 2010.
117. Yu X, Liang G, Yin H, et al.: DNA hypermethylation leads to lower FOXP3 expression in CD4+ T cells of patients with primary Sjögren's syndrome, *Clin Immunol* 148:254–257, 2013.
118. Altorok N, Coit P, Hughes T, et al.: Genome-wide DNA methylation patterns in naive CD4+ T cells from patients with primary Sjögren's syndrome: DNA methylation in naive CD4+ T cells in primary SS, *Arthritis and Rheumatol* 66:731–739, 2014.
119. Miceli-Richard C, Wang-Renault S-F, Boudaoud S, et al.: Overlap between differentially methylated DNA regions in blood B lymphocytes and genetic at-risk loci in primary Sjögren's syndrome, *Ann Rheum Dis* 75:933–940, 2016.
120. Imgenberg-Kreuz J, Sandling JK, Almlöf JC, et al.: Genome-wide DNA methylation analysis in multiple tissues in primary Sjögren's syndrome reveals regulatory effects at interferon-induced genes, *Ann Rheum Dis* 75:2029–2036, 2016.

27 Complement System

V. MICHAEL HOLERS AND LEENDERT A. TROUW

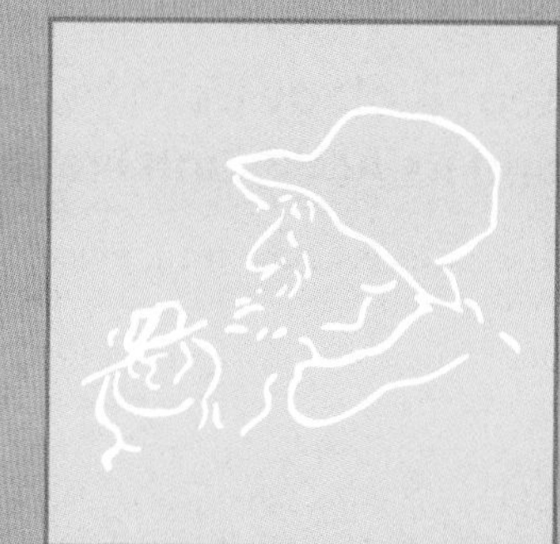

KEY POINTS

The complement system is a delicately balanced protein activation cascade that includes many activators as well as a series of regulators that prevent unwanted and disproportional complement activation under physiologic conditions.

In several forms of arthritis as well as vasculitis and other rheumatic and autoimmune diseases, complement is activated in damaged tissues.

Deposition of autoantibodies represents an important trigger for complement activation.

Measuring complement levels and activation fragments is useful in the diagnosis and follow-up of patients who have systemic lupus erythematosus, but it is not validated in many other rheumatic conditions.

Complement proteins may play additional roles outside the traditional complement activation cascades, including removal of debris as well as promotion of intra-cellular processes important in pathogen clearance, cytokine polarization, and the regulation of cellular metabolism.

Introduction

The time when complement was mainly considered an anti-bacterial defense mechanism via the pore-forming membrane attack complex is long gone. In addition to great progress in understanding the molecular functioning of complement proteins, substantial changes have occurred in the possibilities of modulating complement activation therapeutically in patients, and more are on the near horizon. Therefore, the goal of this chapter is to provide rheumatologists with an updated review of the physiologic and pathologic roles played by the complement system in the context of rheumatic and autoimmune diseases. Furthermore, large numbers of functional and quantitative tests have been developed and are currently available to monitor complement levels and complement activation, but the interpretation of these results is not always straightforward. This chapter will provide guidance in the interpretation of complement activation and laboratory test results in the context of the several rheumatic conditions.

Functions of the Complement System

The complement system was discovered more than a century ago and until relatively recently was considered to be a mechanism only involved in the defense against infections. In the experiments that led to the identification of complement, scientists learned that a substance with the capacity to kill bacteria was present in the cell-free fraction of blood. The substance was heat labile, unstable, and present in all individuals, whereas antibodies were heat stabile and required prior exposure to or immunization with, for example, certain bacteria. Sets of mixing experiments finally revealed that for the observed cytotoxic and lytic effects, both antibodies and this substance were required. Because this substance was considered to "complement" the action of the antibodies to mediate lysis and host protection, the name *complement* was coined.[1]

Given that the identification of complement was based on pathogen lysis and killing experiments and that for many years the laboratory readouts for complement activity were based on red blood cell lysis assays, an important role for this lytic process as an effector mechanism of complement was assumed. Today it is understood, though, that although complement-mediated lysis does take place in vivo and may contribute to tissue damage, defense against infections and self-tissue damage is not dependent on this mechanism. Thus, complement has several other effector mechanisms that may overall have more impact than the simple insertion of lytic pores. Opsonization and generalized immune activation via anaphylatoxins, opsonization, and possibly intracellular complement effects represent more important mechanisms used by the system to mediate host protection in concert with the remainder of the innate and adaptive immune system.[1,2]

In addition to mediation of innate immune defense and instruction of adaptive immune responses, complement is important in clearance of waste, such as apoptotic and necrotic cells, as well as immune complexes, prions, and amyloid-β aggregates. Complement is also involved in other cascades and processes such as coagulation, tissue repair, angiogenesis, placentation, and tumor cell survival.[3] These multifactorial activities mean that unraveling the contribution of complement activation to a clinical condition is often difficult, because a similar deposition of C3b could either contribute to tissue damage and/or stimulate other protective activities such as regeneration. For example, the molecule C1q can contribute to immune complex–mediated damage in people with systemic lupus erythematosus (SLE), whereas deficiency of C1q is the strongest genetic risk factor for the development of SLE through activities that may be independent of downstream complement activation.[4] Collectively, these examples illustrate that the interpretation of laboratory results, including the activity levels of the pathways, the presence of circulating activation fragments, or tissue depositions, is not always straightforward. Although our understanding of the overall role of complement in rheumatic diseases is far from complete, this chapter provides an overview of current insights.

Terminology Used to Describe Complement and Its Activation Fragments

The nomenclature used to describe the different complement factors, especially the convertases and the activation products, may appear confusing. However, some logic can be found in the nomenclature.[5] Complement proteins are mostly indicated by a capital letter followed by a number and a lowercase letter suffix (e.g., C5a and C5b). The molecular part designated with the letter *a* indicates the smaller molecular fragment, whereas the designation *b* indicates the larger fragment. The only exception to this rule is C2, for which the large cleavage fragment is indicated by the letter *a* and the small part by the letter *b.* Although this particular point remains under review, in this chapter the larger fragment of C2 is referred to in the original manner as *C2a.*[5]

The three activation pathways of complement—that is, the classical pathway, the lectin pathway, and the alternative pathway—converge to cleave and activate the central component C3 (Fig. 27.1). After cleavage of C3, all three pathways use the same terminal pathway that generates the membrane attack complex (MAC; see Fig. 27.1).

The nine proteins of the first pathway to be discovered, the classical pathway, are designated with an uppercase letter *C,* followed by a number (e.g., C2). Although most of these numbers are in a logical numeric order, one exception exists—C4—which is cleaved in sequence with C2 and before C3. The components of the lectin pathway are largely similar to those of the classical pathway, but the proteins unique to the lectin pathway do not have a similar logical nomenclature. For the alternative pathway, however, most of the proteins involved are indicated by the word *factor* followed by an uppercase letter (e.g., factor B). Enzymatically active component or protein complexes are often indicated by a bar above the name (e.g., $\overline{\text{C3Bb}}$). After inactivation by complement inhibitors, several complement proteins can no longer participate in further complement activation and are indicated with a lowercase prefix *i,* indicating "inactivated" (e.g., iC3b). However, these factors can demonstrate additional activities, such as iC3b interacting with specific receptors such as complement receptor 3 (CR3).

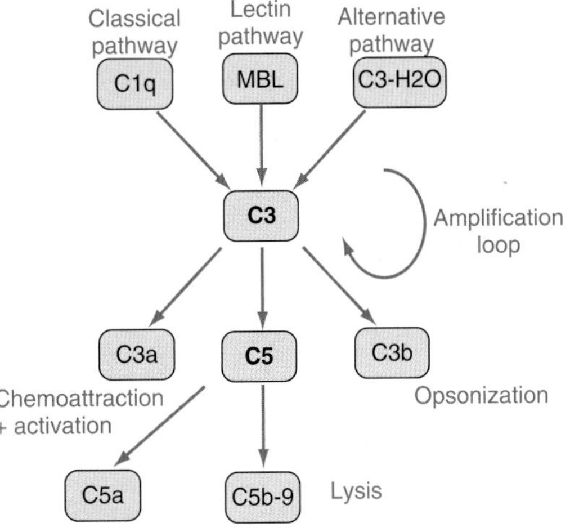

• **Fig. 27.1** Schematic overview of the complement activation pathways. Key initial target recognition molecules for each of the pathways are highlighted, as well as the components and activation products.

Activation Pathways

Traditionally, three different pathways of complement activation are distinguished: the classical pathway, the lectin pathway, and the alternative pathway (see Fig. 27.1). In addition to these three pathways, several "shortcuts" collectively referred to as *extrinsic complement activation* also have been described and will be discussed only briefly.

The classical pathway becomes activated when its recognition molecule C1q binds to one of its ligands. Whereas initially mainly surface-bound immunoglobulin (Ig)M and complexed IgG were thought to be the main ligands for C1q, the list of relevant ligands has now been expanded and includes, among others, C-reactive protein (CRP), DNA, microbial components, and apoptotic and necrotic cells.[4,6] C1q is initially part of the C1 complex, which also comprises two C1r and two C1s molecules. After the binding of C1q to its ligands, a consecutive activation of C1r and C1s takes place.[7] The activated form of C1s now has the capacity to cleave C4 to C4a and C4b, exposing a hidden thioether residue that leads to the immediate covalent attachment of C4b on surfaces close to the place where C1q was binding to its ligands. This quick and covalent binding ensures that opsonization takes place at the right place as directed by its target-bound ligands.

Next, activated C1s also cleaves C4b-bound C2, generating C2a and C2b. The result of this cleavage is the formation of the classical pathway C3-convertase C4b2a. As the name implies, the C3 convertase is an enzymatic protein complex that has the capacity to cleave C3 into its active fragments C3a (an anaphylatoxin) and C3b (an opsonin), which, like C4b, bind instantly and covalently to nearby surfaces. C3 is considered to be the central component of complement activation because it is at this point that the three activation pathways converge to follow the same terminal pathway of complement activation, leading to the formation of the MAC (see Fig. 27.1).

The lectin pathway is similar to the classical pathway, except for the fact that it uses different recognition molecules (mannan-binding lectin [MBL], ficolins, and collectins) and different serine proteases (the MBL-associated serine proteases [MASPs] (see Fig. 27.1).[8] Most importantly, the ligands that are recognized by the lectin pathway are different and mainly comprise patterns of modified carbohydrates. After binding of MBL, MASP-2 will cleave both C4 and C2, generating exactly the same C3 convertase as in the classical pathway. MASP-1 will cleave MASP-2, and MASP-3 plays an important role by cleaving profactor D into an active molecule.[9]

The alternative pathway is different from the other two pathways and serves two purposes. It is an important activation pathway in its own right, using a tick-over mechanism, and its constituents also serve as an amplification loop for the classical and alternative pathways. The tick-over mediated activation of the alternative pathway refers to the fact that a small fraction of the circulating C3 is hydrolyzed to C3(H_2O). This hydrolyzed form of C3 exposes a binding site for factor B. After binding, factor B is cleaved by factor D, generating a fluid-phase C3-convertase C3(H_2O) Bb that cleaves native C3 into C3a and C3b. Similar to C4b, this C3b also binds covalently to a surface and serves as the starting point for the generation of a new C3 convertase, C3bBb. However, on host cells this initial binding of C3b is quickly neutralized by the action of several complement inhibitors, especially factor H, whereas insufficient inhibition of this alternative pathway initiation exists on the surface of foreign cells, resulting in strong deposition of C3b and C3 convertases, thereby making the difference between self and non-self.

Properdin is a molecule that stabilizes the alternative pathway C3 convertase by forming a complex, C3bBbP, which allows a longer half-life. However, on certain target surfaces properdin can also serve as a pattern recognition molecule that can localize complement activation to surfaces of pathogens or dead cells by attracting C3b, allowing the formation of the alternative pathway C3 convertase.[10] The amplification function of the alternative pathway is often neglected, but as much as 80% of the C3 deposited during complement activation via the classical or lectin pathway, or the alternative pathway initiation itself, may be the result of the amplification loop.[11] This loop is activated simply by the deposition of C3b, which, independent of the pathway by which it was generated, serves as the starting point for more alternative pathway activation as the alternative pathway C3 convertase is built upon this bound C3b. Notably, a series of structure-function studies have recently illuminated the molecular mechanisms by which these proteins interact and are regulated.[12]

The terminal pathway of complement activation represents the common final pathway used by all three routes of complement activation. As more and more C3b fragments are generated by way of either the classical, lectin, or alternative pathway or its amplification loop, the C3 convertases also start to acquire additional C3b molecules, C4b2aC3b and C3bBbC3b. These complexes gain a unique property: they now can serve as C5 convertases that cleave C5 into C5a, a very potent anaphylatoxin, and C5b. C5b interacts with C6 and C7, and this complex becomes attached to the cell surface, followed by interaction with C8. However, it is not until several C9 molecules are inserted into the complex that a pore is actually formed in the cell membrane. This final complex is referred to as the *membrane attack complex (MAC)* or *C5b-9*. Insertion of many copies of the MAC can lead to cellular activation, apoptosis, or lysis, depending on the dosage and the cell type involved.[13]

As previously mentioned, other processes have been described that lead to complement activation via mechanisms that differ from the traditional complement pathways. *Extrinsic complement activation* refers to situations in which complement proteins can be cleaved, and hence activated, via noncomplement proteins such as plasmin, thrombin, elastase, and plasma kallikrein.[14,15] For example, cleavage of C5 by these proteases can yield bioactive C5a.[14,15]

Regulation of Complement Activation

Because the complement system is very aggressive and has the potential to be highly damaging, it is not surprising that the human body is equipped with a large array of complement regulators and inhibitors (Table 27.1). These proteins ensure that complement activation is limited in time and in place to ensure maximal effectiveness in fighting infections and clearing debris while minimizing the collateral damage to healthy host tissue.[16] One other important aspect of efficient regulation is the importance of maintaining sufficient levels of complement fragments so they are available to fight infections. In case of deficiencies of fluid-phase complement inhibitors factor I and factor H, the complement system becomes activated via the alternative pathway and does not stop until all complement is consumed, resulting in a secondary C3 deficiency. Both fluid-phase and membrane-bound complement inhibitors function primarily via a similar mechanism of putting a break on unwanted complement activation at several levels of the complement cascades: initiation, formation of C3 convertases, and MAC insertion.

Fluid-phase regulators circulate together with all the other complement proteins and prevent complement activation under physiologic conditions (Fig. 27.2). C1 esterase (C1-INH) inhibits several enzymes of the classical and lectin pathways: C1r, C1s, and MASPs, as well as proteins from the contact system that generate vasoactive compounds. One of the main fluid-phase inhibitors is factor H, which can serve both as a decay-accelerator (decreasing the half-life of C3 convertases) and as a cofactor for the enzymatic degradation of C3b by factor I.[17] The cell surface regulatory activities of factor H are counteracted by a series of factor H related proteins, which exhibit many types of functions but one of the most important being blocking of the binding of factor H to target surfaces where it would regulate the convertases.[18] The degrading enzyme factor I is present in the circulation without a known inhibitor but only works to degrade C3b in the presence of a cofactor.[19] Once C3b is bound by, for example, factor H, then factor I comes into action and cleaves C3b to iC3b. The iC3b—that is, inactivated C3b—now can no longer serve as a starting point for the formation of a new C3 convertase, but it can still be recognized by complement receptors. Whereas factor H is the main fluid-phase regulator for the alternative pathway, C4b binding protein (C4BP) serves a similar role, mainly for the classical and lectin pathways.[20] Vitronectin and clusterin are fluid-phase regulators of the insertion of the MAC. Finally, carboxypeptidase-N quickly converts the potent anaphylatoxins C3a and C5a into less active, des-arginated forms.

Membrane-bound regulators provide important protection against excessive complement attack on host cells (see Fig. 27.2). Most membrane-bound inhibitors work at the level of the C3 and C5 convertases, with the exception of CD59, which inhibits the insertion of the MAC into the cell membranes. Decay-accelerating factor (DAF; CD55) and complement receptor 1 (CR1; CD35) inhibit the action of C3 convertases by reducing their half-life. Membrane-cofactor protein (MCP; CD46) and CR1 serve as cofactors for the action of factor I.

Receptors for Complement Fragments

Even though complement may be best known for its capacity to induce lysis via the MAC, its capacity to activate (immune) cells via complement receptors may actually be much more important in health and disease. Complement receptors (Table 27.2) are present on a large array of immune cells and stromal cells, and the integrated signals lead to a wide variety of biologic processes such as cellular activation, differentiation, and apoptosis. Three types of receptors can be distinguished depending on the type of ligands; C1q, anaphylatoxins C3a and C5a, and C3 and C4 degradation products.

Several receptors for C1q have been proposed over the years, and most of these molecules actually do bind C1q, but whether they are essential C1q signaling molecules is sometimes debated. It is clear that C1q can have effects on cells, inducing migration and phagocytosis as well as promoting anti-inflammatory clearance mechanisms, but the nature or combinations of receptors and binding proteins remain the subject of further studies.

Biologic effects of the anaphylatoxin C3a are mediated via the C3a receptor (C3aR), which is present on mast cells, smooth

TABLE 27.1 Established Complement Regulators

Negative Regulators	Alternate Names	Function
C1-INH	SERPIN1	Inhibits C1r/s and MASPs
sMAP	MAP19	Binds to MBL, competes with MASPs
MAP-1	MAP44	Binds to MBL/ficolins/collectins; inhibits C4 deposition
C4BP	C4b-binding protein	Accelerates decay of LP/CP convertases; cofactor for fI
Factor H	CFH	Recognizes self-surfaces; blocks convertase assembly; accelerates convertase decay; cofactor for fI
FHL-1	Reconectin, CFHL1	Accelerates convertase decay; cofactor for fI
MCP	CD46	Membrane bound cofactor for fI
DAF	CD55	Membrane bound accelerator of decay of convertases
CD59	Protectin	Membrane bound protein; binds to C8 and C9; prevents assembly of TCC
CFHR-1	FHR-1	Recognizes self-surfaces and C5; inhibits C5 cleavage and TCC formation
Vitronectin	S-protein	Binds to C5b-9; prevents assembly of TCC
Clusterin	Apolipoprotein J; SP-40,40	Binds to C7-C9; prevents assembly of TCC
Carboxypeptidase-N		Degrades C3a and C5a to des-Arg forms
Positive Regulators/Modulators		
Properdin	Factor P	Stabilization of AP C3 and C5 convertases; surface ligand recognition (some settings)
CFHRs (complement factor H-related proteins)	FHRs	Competition with Factor H; several other inter-related functions

CFHR-1, Complement factor H–related protein; *DAF*, decay-accelerating factor; *FHL-1*, factor H-like protein 1; *fI*, factor I; *MAP-1*, MBL/ficolin associated protein-1; *MASP*, MBL-associated serine protease; *MBL*, mannan-binding lectin; *MCP*, membrane cofactor protein; *sMAP*, small mannose-binding lectin–associated protein; *TCC*, terminal complement complex.

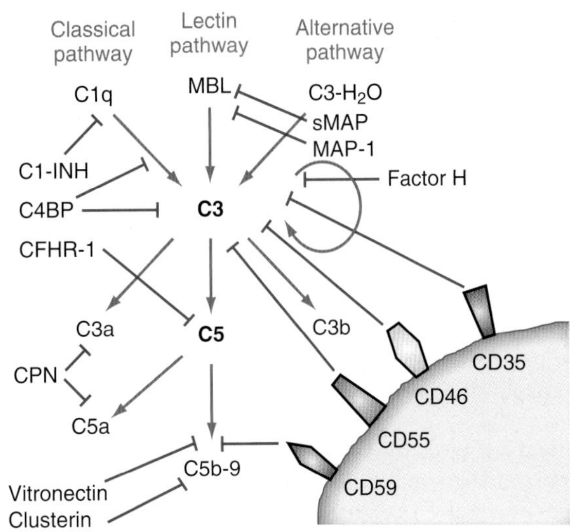

• **Fig. 27.2** Schematic overview of the different complement inhibitors acting on the complement cascade. Well-characterized complement inhibitors are highlighted, together with the parts of the complement cascade that they primarily inhibit. Note that Factor I is not indicated; Factor I is the enzyme that, together with some of the inhibitors highlighted in the scheme, cleaves and inactivates C3b and C4b.

muscle cells, epithelial and endothelial cells, and cells of the myeloid lineage. Triggering of this receptor can lead to cellular activation, degranulation, and chemotaxis. Signaling via the C3aR may be either pro-inflammatory or anti-inflammatory depending on the context. Detection of anaphylatoxin C5a is mediated via the C5a receptor, C5aR1 (CD88). The C5a receptor is also present on a wide array of immune and nonimmune cells. Triggering results in strong chemotaxis, cellular activation, degranulation, and general immune activation. An alternative C5a receptor also exists, C5aR2 (also known as C5L2), which binds C5a strongly and $C5a_{desarg}$ weakly, and may also interact with C3a/$C3a_{desarg}$. C5aR2 also demonstrates context-dependent pro- or anti-inflammatory activities. Recently, protease activated receptors 1 and 4 have been identified as receptors for the C4a fragment.[21]

Cellular recognition of C3 and C4 fragments is mediated via the complement receptors CR1, CR2, CR3, and CR4. Despite their similar names, they have different structures, ligands, expression profiles, and functions. CR1 (CD35), which is expressed on several immune cells and on erythrocytes, both enhances phagocytosis by binding to C3b and C4b and serves as a complement regulator that, via factor I, degrades its ligands.[22] CR1 is the only cofactor that allows a second cleavage of iC3b by factor I, generating C3dg. CR1 also serves an important role in transporting

TABLE 27.2 Schematic Overview of the Main Complement Receptors

Receptors	Alternative Names	Function
CR1	CD35; C3b/C4b receptor	Binds C3b/iC3b; induces phagocytosis; accelerates decay of convertases; cofactor for fI; immune complex clearance
CR2	CD21; C3d receptor	Binds iC3b/C3dg/C3d; lowers threshold for B cell activation with CD19 complex; primary Epstein-Barr virus receptor
CR3	CD11b/CD18; Mac-1; integrin αMβ2	Induces phagocytosis through interaction with iC3b; modulates IL-12 family in APCs
CR4	CD11c/CD18; integrin αXβ2	Induces phagocytosis through interaction with iC3b
C3aR		Binds C3a; triggers pro/anti-inflammatory signaling
C5aR1	CD88	Binds C5a; triggers pro-inflammatory and immunomodulatory signaling
C5aR2	C5L2, GPR77	Binds C5a (strongly) and C5adesArg (weakly); might bind C3a/C3adesArg; function not fully defined
PAR1/PAR4	Protease activated receptors 1 and 4	Binds C4a and increases endothelial cell activation and permeability
CRIg	Z93Ig, VSIG4	Induces phagocytosis through interaction with iC3b/C3c; regulatory effect on C5 convertases
cC1qR	Calreticulin	Recognizes bound C1q; induces phagocytic signaling through CD91
gC1qR	C1q-binding protein	Recognizes C1q; potential role in phagocytosis and signaling; modulates IL-12 on APCs
C1qRp	CD93 + unknown protein	Part of receptor complex that binds C1q and mediates phagocytosis

APC, Antigen-presenting cell; *fI*, factor I.

Modified from Ricklin D, Hajishengallis G, Yang K, Lambris JD: Complement: a key system for immune surveillance and homeostasis. *Nat Immunol* 11:785–797, 2010.

complement-opsonized immune complexes via erythrocytes to the reticuloendothelial system for clearance. The C3b/C4b-opsonized immune complexes bind via CR1 to the erythrocytes (immune adherence), which deliver the immune complexes to the liver and spleen, where macrophage-like cells remove the immune complexes. These macrophages do not cleave the immune complexes but, rather, cleave CR1 to release the immune complexes from the erythrocytes.[23] The erythrocytes that re-enter the circulation therefore express less residual CR1 on their surface, a phenomenon observed in patients with active lupus, in whom this immune complex transport and clearance is an important process, and often disrupted in a manner that promotes inappropriate deposition of complexes in tissues such as the lung. CR1 on granulocytes and monocytes will induce internalization and degradation of complement-opsonized immune complexes, whereas CR1 on follicular dendritic cells will result in the extra-cellular trapping and presentation of the immune complexes and antigens they contain.

CR2 (CD21) is expressed on B cells and follicular dendritic cells. On the B cells it serves as a co-receptor for signaling through the B cell receptor. The presence of C3d/C3dg on antigens reduces the threshold for B cell activation significantly, resulting in amplified B cell activation and differentiation.[24]

CR3 (CD11b-CD18) and CR4 (CD11c-CD18) are integrin receptors expressed on myeloid cells that both bind iC3b.[25] Both receptors strongly enhance phagocytosis, and CR3 is also involved in shaping the cytokine responses and immune activation in general.

Functions of the Complement System

Innate Immune Responses

As was previously alluded to, complement plays an important role in the innate defense against invading microorganisms. Whereas the MAC is responsible for complement-mediated lysis of myriad targets, deficiencies of proteins within the MAC from C5-C8 are only associated with infections with *Neisseria*. In contrast, deficiency for C3 is associated with a large array of recurrent infections. Together these findings indicate that the killing of microorganisms does not rely on the MAC, with the exception of *Neisseria*. Apparently, for all other types of infectious organisms, the innate immune defense uses mechanisms in addition to complement-mediated lysis to actually kill the microbes. This process is mediated largely via opsonization with C3b and cellular uptake via complement receptors and in parallel the activation of immune cells via C3a and C5a. Complement also interacts with other systems of innate immune defense, such as the cellular Toll-like receptors (TLRs).[26] A clear bidirectional interaction takes place between those systems; for example, triggering via the C3aR or C5aR/C5L2 may affect the cellular response to lipopolysaccharide (LPS) via TLR4.

Several proteins of the complement system also interact with the cascade of coagulation, collectively enhancing local clotting reactions to prevent the spread of possible pathogens. This bidirectional interaction involves, for example, C5a, which enhances the expression of tissue factor (TF)[27] and stimulates coagulation, whereas in the other direction thrombin cleaves C5 and generates C5a.[14]

Clearing Immune Complexes and Apoptotic Material

The important contribution of complement toward clearance of immune complexes and dead cells became apparent from studies of complement-deficient people. Deficiency of the early components of the classical pathway is associated with development of SLE, with greater risk associated with early components of the complement cascade (C1q–/– > C4–/– > C2–/–). When accumulation of apoptotic cells was also noted in C1q-deficient mice, the waste disposal hypothesis was put forward.[28] C1q can bind to apoptotic and necrotic cells and both directly lead to clearance through C1q receptors as well as induce classical pathway activation.[29,30] In the absence of the early classical pathway components, apoptotic cells are not cleared efficiently.[31] Importantly, whereas early complement components bind to apoptotic cells to enhance opsonization and phagocytosis, the binding of fluid-phase inhibitors provides protection against excessive complement attack and lysis.[32]

Clearance of immune complexes is influenced by complement via two mechanisms. The first is the clearance of immune complexes to prevent their tissue precipitation,[33] a process mainly mediated via the classical pathway and transport via erythrocytes through interactions with the surface-bound complement receptor type 1(CR1) that interacts with C3b/C4b-bound targets. The second mechanism involves solubilization of already existing immune complexes, which is mainly mediated via the alternative pathway. In addition to apoptotic material and immune complexes, many other forms of debris are cleared in ways that involve complement activation, such as amyloid-β deposits, urate crystals, cholesterol crystals, oxidized lipids, and extra-cellular DNA.

Regulating Adaptive Immune Responses

The complement system plays an important role in shaping the adaptive immune response. Whereas initially the focus was mainly on B cells and antibody responses, the focus has shifted to the T cell–dendritic cell interface, and now even toward the intra-cellular environment of T cells. C3dg, a degradation product of C3b, serves as a natural adjuvant by providing co-stimulatory signals to B cells via binding to CR2 in the B cell co-receptor complex, co-associating the B cell receptor with CR2/CD19 complexes.[34] In addition to activating B cells, CR2 is also involved in the capture and prolonged presentation of complement-opsonized antigens on follicular dendritic cells.[24] Complement also has an impact on the effector arm of antibodies, not just via the classical pathway, but also by influencing the expression levels and activities of cellular Fcγ receptors. C5aR triggering alters the expression levels of activating and inhibiting Fcγ receptors in such a way that cells are more prone to respond to antibody triggering.[35] Interestingly, Fcγ receptor signaling can enhance synthesis of C5,[36] reinforcing the C5a-Fcγ receptor cross-talk.[35,36]

Direct effects of complement on T cell immunity were concluded from experiments with complement-deficient animals, for example, in the context of transplant rejection.[37] The local production of the anaphylatoxins C3a and C5a in the T cell–dendritic cell synapse highly determines the outcome of these cognate interactions.[38] Expression levels of complement inhibitory molecules such as DAF (CD55) have an impact on the degree of complement activation and hence the degree of dendritic cell and T cell activation. In addition, specific triggering of membrane-bound complement inhibitory molecules such as CD59 and DAF can limit their activation or even skew toward a regulatory T cell phenotype.[39,40]

Noncanonical Functions of Complement

Recently, important roles for intra-cellular complement factors have been identified that appear to expand the impact of this system outside of its long-appreciated roles. These include promoting human T helper 1 (Th1) responses as well as regulating cell processes through fundamental mechanisms such as directing metabolic pathways and regulating autophagy.[2] Understanding these "non-canonical" activities of complement should provide additional insights into how one can modulate the pathway in a manner that is beneficial to patients.

Measuring Complement Activation

Many different assays are available to monitor the activity and activation of complement and the antigenic levels of complement proteins.[41] Depending on the clinical question, various substrates and assays, or different combinations of assays, are used. Deposition of activated complement fragments in target organs—for example, the renal glomeruli—along with evidence of systemic depletion of C3 and C4 provides important clinical information regarding the occurrence of active lupus nephritis.

The most commonly used assays to determine the functional activity of complement are based on hemolytic assays for classical pathway and alternative pathway activity (CH50 and AP50, respectively). The CH50 quantitates the ability of serum to lyse sheep erythrocytes that have been opsonized by antibodies. The assay for the alternative pathway, AP50, records the ability to lyse 50% of rabbit erythrocytes in a buffer that does not allow the classical pathway to be active. The CH50 and AP50 determine the dilution of serum required to achieve this 50% lysis, and, as such, these assays provide quantitation of overall activity from the initiation of the pathway to the insertion of the MAC. These assays can be used to screen for deficiencies but can also be used for the evaluation of disease activity and consumption of complement, as, for example, in the context of a flare in patients with SLE. More modern tests now provide plate-bound variants so that the classical, alternative, and lectin pathways can all be individually screened for activity.[42] These assays are much easier to perform; however, they typically provide less quantitative insight but only a more qualitative answer, and hence these assays are more suited to identify deficiencies than to monitor disease activity.

The presence of ongoing activation of complement in patients can be concluded from the measurement of complement activation products—for example, C3a, C5a, C4d, C3d, iC3b, and C5b-9. Monitoring of the levels of these markers over time allows evaluation of the underlying disease activity. However, in daily practice they are less often used because of the price, lack of availability in routine laboratories, and difficulty of interpretation. As is the case with complement assays in general, the quality of the sample and the capability of the testing laboratory highly determine the reliability of the test. Complement is a heat-sensitive system in which some enzymes will relatively quickly lose their activity, and complement activation fragments may be generated during inappropriate handling of samples.

The antigenic screening for complement proteins C3 and C4 is regularly carried out in most laboratories around the world that perform routine tests, mostly based on nephelometric or turbidimetric assays. These robust assays are often used for the diagnosis and follow-up of patients with SLE in particular.

Several autoantibodies that react with complement proteins have been described.[43] In rheumatology, several autoantibodies such as anti–C1-INH, anti-CR1, and anti–Factor H have been described, but many laboratories that perform routine diagnostic tests offer only the detection of anti-C1q autoantibodies. These anti-C1q autoantibodies are especially relevant in the context of lupus nephritis.[44]

Complement Deficiency

Primary Complement Deficiency

Primary deficiencies have been described for nearly all complement proteins. The most common deficiencies are depicted in Table 27.3. Most deficiencies are inherited as autosomal recessive traits, except for the X-linked genes properdin and factor D, which display an autosomal dominant pattern, and the acquired X-linked somatic mutations of the glycophosphatidylinositol (GPI) anchor that result in DAF and CD59 deficiency.[45] Almost all of the circulating factor deficiencies are associated with increased risk for bacterial infections, although for some deficiencies this association only becomes apparent in otherwise immunocompromised hosts. At the time of their discovery, it came as a surprise that for the early classical pathway components—C1q, C4, and C2—their deficiency was highly associated with the development of clinical autoimmunity presenting as SLE-like syndromes.[46] Interestingly, this phenomenon is restricted to SLE, because these deficiencies have not manifested as Sjögren's syndrome, rheumatoid arthritis (RA), or vasculitis. Although SLE develops in a large portion of people deficient for the early components of the classical pathway, only a very small fraction of all patients with SLE are genetically deficient for one of these early classical pathway components. During flares of their disease, many patients with SLE can display very low levels of these classical pathway components, but this phenomenon is primarily related to immune complex–mediated activation and depletion and is hence a secondary deficiency, as outlined in the next section. C1q deficiency is most strongly associated with SLE (90%), followed by C4 (70%) and C2 (15%) deficiencies. C1q deficiency is rare, with approximately 70 cases currently known,[47] and C1r and C1s deficiency is also rare.[48] Next to increased risk for infections, these patients display a greater than 90% frequency of SLE.

The genes encoding C4 are polymorphic and have undergone ancestral duplication and mutation, giving rise to two genes designated *C4A* (encoding the acidic C4A) and *C4B* (encoding the basic C4B), which are not to be mistaken for the cleavage products C4a and C4b. It has been suggested that functional differences between *C4A* and *C4B* affect the risk for development of SLE, as well as the severity of disease. Homozygous deficiency of C4A, the form of C4 that can interact best with immune complexes, is a susceptibility factor for SLE.[49] In addition to complete genetic deficiency, low copy number variation also has been associated with increased risk for SLE,[50] but this association has not yet been well established.

C2 deficiency is relatively more common, with an estimated frequency of 1:20,000 in white populations.[51] The frequency of SLE in C2-deficient people is approximately 15%, and the clinical presentation is suggested to be different from the SLE associated with C1q or C4 deficiency.[51]

Deficiencies of other complement factors such as C3, factor B, factor D, and properdin are particularly associated with severe infections.[52] Deficiencies of other factors such as MBL, with an estimated frequency of 1:10 in Caucasians, are associated with infections mainly in otherwise immunocompromised people.[52] The question of whether MBL deficiency is associated with increased risk for SLE and RA remains controversial, but if any effect exists, it is most likely small. Interestingly, deficiencies of components of the MAC do not lead to highly increased risk of infections in general but only to infections with *Neisseria*.[52]

TABLE 27.3 Schematic Overview of the Main Genetically Driven Complement Deficiencies

Protein	Frequency[a]	Disease Association
C1q	Rare; <100 cases	SLE; glomerulonephritis; infections
C1r or C1s	Rare; <50 cases	SLE; glomerulonephritis
C2	1:20,000	SLE; infections
C4	Rare; <50 cases	SLE; glomerulonephritis; infections
C3	Rare; <50 cases	Recurrent infections; SLE; glomerulonephritis
MBL	Common; 1:10	Susceptibility to infections
Factor D	Rare; <20 cases	*Neisseria* infections
Properdin	Rare; <100 cases	Meningococcal disease
C5/6/7/8	Rare; <100 cases	Usually healthy; some *Neisseria* infections
C9	1:1000 in Japan	Usually healthy; some *Neisseria* infections
C1-INH	1:50,000	Hereditary angioedema
FHR-1/3	Varies by population	AMD/IgANeph/SLE risk

[a]Estimated frequency in the Caucasian population (with the exception of protein C9).

MBL, Mannan-binding lectin; *SLE*, systemic lupus erythematosus.

Modified from Sturfelt G, Truedsson L: Complement in the immunopathogenesis of rheumatic disease. *Nat Rev Rheumatol* 8:458–468, 2012.

Secondary Complement Deficiency

Secondary, or acquired, complement deficiency is mainly the result of increased consumption via activation rather than decreased production. Secondary deficiency may occur as a consequence of lack of inhibition, such as in the absence of factor I or factor H, resulting in deregulated activation and depletion of the alternative pathway components, thus leading to a secondary C3 deficiency with an increased risk of infections.[53] However, by far most cases of (partial) secondary deficiency occur because complement activation is consuming more complement proteins than the liver and other tissues can synthesize. Especially in SLE, decreased levels of CH50 and AP50 are detected, which are proportional to decreased circulating levels of C1q, C3, and C4.[54] Hypocomplementemia is a poor prognostic sign in people with SLE because it is related to complement consumption via activation on affected tissues such as the kidneys.[54] Decreased levels of classical pathway proteins are also observed in subsets of patients who have disorders such as mixed cryoglobulinemia and Sjögren's syndrome. In the latter condition, decreased levels of C3 and C4 have been repeatedly identified as markers of unfavorable outcomes, such as lymphoma, severe disease manifestations, and premature death.[55]

Targeted Complement Therapeutics

For rheumatic diseases, therapeutic intervention focused on complement is aimed either at (1) restoring normal complement function by replenishing deficient components or (2) inhibiting complement activation.

Reconstituting the primary deficiency is a method that has been used for many years. Either purified complement proteins such as MBL and C1-INH or fresh frozen plasma is infused to correct the missing factor. Many complement factors are produced by the liver, and it is worth noting that liver transplantation can reverse certain deficiency states, such as for MBL,[56] although obviously this is not a therapeutic option. However, for C1q, which is mainly produced by cells of hematopoietic origin such as macrophages and dendritic cells,[57] it is possible to reverse the deficiency phenotype completely through hematologic stem cell transplantation. This procedure has been successfully applied, resulting in restoration of circulating C1q levels and diminishment of lupus symptoms.[58]

Despite the important scientific insight that is provided by the association between complement deficiency and rheumatic diseases, it must be noted that this association represents a minute fraction of the patients who have these diseases. In line with what was called the *lupus paradox*, missing complement leads to SLE, but in most patients with SLE, complement contributes to tissue damage, and therefore complement inhibition might be the more appropriate type of intervention. Several clinically approved interventions currently exist (reviewed in detail elsewhere).[59] One example is soluble CR1 (sCR1). CR1, which is mainly expressed on erythrocytes, mediates complement inhibition by serving as a cofactor for factor I–mediated inactivation of C3b and C4b and as an accelerator of the decay of C3 convertases.[22] Interestingly, the soluble version of CR1 also retains these activities, and modified forms of sCR1 have been suggested to be effective for the treatment of myocardial infarction and other indications.[60] Another main target of intervention is C5—either the C5 molecule itself or the interaction of C5a with the C5a receptor using blocking antibodies or peptides. A humanized antibody to C5 was developed and has been used successfully in the treatment of paroxysmal nocturnal hemoglobinuria (PNH), atypical hemolytic uremic syndrome (aHUS), neuromyelitis optica, and myasthenia gravis, and it is currently being tested for several other conditions.[59] Currently, inhibitors of the C5a receptor are being tested in clinical trials, and have demonstrated beneficial outcomes in ANCA-associated vasculitis.[61]

Complement in Rheumatic Diseases

Systemic Lupus Erythematosus

The involvement of complement activation in SLE is easily appreciated; not only are affected tissues decorated by activated complement fragments, but serum levels of several key complement components are decreased because of consumption.[54] As mentioned earlier, the lupus paradox makes it difficult to establish if complement plays an essential role in human SLE. On the basis of the tissue deposition of C1q and the heavily decreased levels of circulating C1q during a flare, one would assume that C1q would play an essential role by binding to deposited immune complexes and activating the classical pathway. However, C1q-deficient patients are not protected from lupus. On the contrary, they have a very high chance of developing SLE-like disease, which likely indicates that C1q is involved in two different processes. One process relates to the onset/development of SLE, and the other process relates to the final pathways of tissue destruction that are known to involve, but not totally depend on, complement classical pathway activation.

SLE is mainly characterized by a breakdown of tolerance against nuclear components, such as double-stranded DNA. Immune complexes are formed between these anti-nuclear antibodies and their antigens, which are released from dead cells. These immune complexes deposit in tissues, where complement activation contributes to tissue damage by the formation of the MAC and the release of pro-inflammatory mediators such as C5a. In addition, the immune complexes stimulate plasmacytoid dendritic cells (pDCs) to produce type I interferons, further stimulating the disease process.[62] The interaction of ligands with CR2 on follicular dendritic cells may also promote interferon release in lupus patients.[63] Lupus nephritis is a complicated process that is reviewed in detail elsewhere.[64] Substantial clinical information is available for lupus nephritis with regard to the relationship with tissue deposition of complement, decreased circulating levels, and clinical flares of the nephritis.

Circulating levels of C3 and C4 are included in the disease activity index SLEDAI.[65] Measuring cell-bound complement activation fragments, rather than decreased circulating levels of complement, is suggested as possibly being a more sensitive way to analyze complement activation in SLE,[54] but thus far this method has not replaced established assays in laboratories around the world that perform routine testing.

Anti-C1q autoantibodies can be detected in SLE, and their presence is associated with lupus nephritis.[66] In particular, the absence of anti-C1q autoantibodies is strongly associated with lack of renal involvement.[67] Because anti-C1q autoantibodies can also occur in healthy people who do not have any renal problems, for many years it was unclear how anti-C1q autoantibodies could contribute to renal disease in people with lupus.[44] However, mouse studies have revealed that anti-C1q autoantibodies only contribute to renal damage if sufficient immune complexes containing C1q are present in the glomeruli.[68]

Because complement seems to play such a prominent role in lupus nephritis, clinical trials have been conducted to study whether blocking complement would be beneficial.[69] However, the first small study on this topic that targeted C5 did not reveal an effect during a relatively short follow-up period.[69]

Rheumatoid Arthritis

A contribution of complement to the pathogenesis of RA can be concluded from the observed complement tissue deposition,[70] decreased levels of complement components in synovial fluid,[71] and the presence of complement activation fragments,[72,73] as previously reviewed.[74] However, the pronounced systemic hypocomplementemia that is observed during flares in SLE is not observed in people with RA. In addition, the complement deficiencies of the classical pathway that are associated with SLE may involve some arthritis but do not predispose to RA. Whereas over the years different views have existed regarding the contribution of autoantibodies, B cells, T cells, and other immune players, currently an emphasis has been placed on B cells and the autoantibodies they produce.[75] In addition to the well-known rheumatoid factor (RF), anti-citrullinated protein antibodies (ACPAs)[76] and the recently identified antibodies against carbamylated proteins (anti-CarP autoantibodies)[77] are thought to be involved in the disease process.

Interestingly, these antibodies can already be detected in serum many years before the diagnosis of RA is made.[78,79] In addition, tissue-specific autoantibodies such as anti–type II collagen may be involved in a subset of patients.[80] A contribution of these autoantibodies is inferred from the clinical associations between the presence of the antibodies and more severe joint damage.[77,80,81] In addition, experimental evidence in animal models suggests a directly pathogenic role for these autoantibodies.[82,83]

In vitro, ACPAs are able to trigger complement activation.[84] Interestingly, this action was mediated not just via the expected classical pathway but also via the alternative pathway of complement activation.[84] In mouse models for arthritis, it actually seems that only the alternative and perhaps the lectin pathways are absolutely required for antibody-mediated arthritis to develop, without any essential contribution of the classical pathway activation proteins.[85]

Complement activation fragments can be detected in people with RA, but the concentrations are much higher in synovial fluid compared with serum.[72,73,86–88] These data indicate that complement is activated not systemically but mainly locally in the affected joints. The cause of this local complement activation is not known but likely involves several sources that are not mutually exclusive. Immune complexes formed by autoantibodies binding to joint specific antigens, dead cells that accumulate during chronic inflammatory reactions in the joint, or matrix components released from damaged cartilage may all contribute to the observed complement activation.[80,84,89,90] Release of C3a and C5a, as well as sublytic insertion of the MAC, may activate immune cells, along with synoviocytes. In addition, insertion of the MAC may be involved in the generation of citrullinated antigens in the joint,[91] possibly providing antigen for ACPAs to bind to and subsequently form immune complexes.

From animal models of arthritis it may be concluded that complement plays an essential role in the development of full-blown arthritis.[74] However, at present it is not known if complement activation plays an essential role in arthritis in humans. Several clinical intervention studies aimed at blocking complement activation or inhibiting the signaling via complement receptors have been performed or are currently under way. Inhibition of C5a–C5a receptor signaling has thus far been unsuccessful.[92] Humanized monoclonal antibodies targeting C5 have been proven to be well tolerated in a phase I study and additionally showed modest beneficial effects in a phase II study.[69] However, thus far this biologic agent has not reached clinical use, most likely for economic reasons. Many experimental treatments that rely on different modes of action are being tested in pre-clinical models and include locally produced blocking minibodies[93] or targeted inhibition using constructs consisting of CR2 to bind to activated complement fragments, as well as use of factor H domains to inhibit complement.[94,95]

For other forms of inflammatory arthritis, the body of evidence supporting a role for complement in the disease processes is small.[96] For example, in psoriatic arthritis, increased levels of C3 were reported with no signs of activation, likely as a result of the acute-phase response.[97] Authors of several studies reported that complement activation in osteoarthritis (OA) and spondyloarthritis either did not exist or was limited, with only low levels of complement activation in reactive arthritis.[70,97,98] More recently, though, presence of complement activation in human synovial fluid and a necessary role for complement activation in an experimental model of OA have been demonstrated.[99] However, overall it seems that determination of the relative contribution of complement activation to the disease processes underlying these conditions would benefit from additional studies, especially in patients.

Other Systemic Rheumatic Conditions

In many and perhaps all systemic rheumatic conditions, a role for complement can be concluded on the basis of either changed serum levels or tissue deposition of activated complement components.[96] In several conditions hypocomplementemia—that is, low C3 and/or C4—has been included in criteria and disease activity scores.[46] However, the mechanism responsible for the observed effects on complement and how this contributes to the overall disease process in these systemic rheumatic conditions remain to be established. With the large number of complement therapeutic programs underway, with inhibitors of all major components of the complement system included, it is likely that the next decade will reveal what complement activation contributes to the pathogenesis of many rheumatic diseases through the pre-clinical to clinical disease course.

Conclusion

In this chapter an overview of the current understanding of the role played by the complement system in health and in rheumatic conditions is provided. For many years the role of complement in rheumatic diseases was largely limited to measuring complement consumption as biomarkers of disease activity. Now, as the first drugs that target complement activation are becoming available in the clinic, a new era has begun as we begin to understand the extent to which complement activation plays an essential role in disease processes. Because of all the positive effects of complement in the body, it will need to be established whether long-term complement inhibition in rheumatic diseases will ever become standard treatment or whether it will be limited to specific clinical conditions, such as a flare of lupus nephritis. In addition, the complement biomarker field is developing rapidly, and choosing the right biomarker for a specific clinical problem is an interesting future challenge.

The references for this chapter can also be found on ExpertConsult.com.

References

1. Ricklin D, Hajishengallis G, Yang K, et al.: Complement: a key system for immune surveillance and homeostasis, *Nat Immunol* 11:785–797, 2010.
2. Kolev M, Le Friec G, Kemper C: Complement—tapping into new sites and effector systems, *Nat Rev Immunol* 14:811–820, 2014.
3. Holers VM: Complement and its receptors: new insights into human disease, *Ann Rev Immunol* 32:433–459, 2014.
4. Lu J, Kishore U: C1 complex: an adaptable proteolytic module for complement and non-complement functions, *Front Immunol* 8:592, 2017.
5. Kemper C, Pangburn MK, Fishelson Z: Complement nomenclature 2014, *Mol Immunol* 61:56–58, 2014.
6. Nayak A, Pednekar L, Reid KB, et al.: Complement and non-complement activating functions of C1q: a prototypical innate immune molecule, *Innate Immun* 18:350–363, 2012.
7. Gaboriaud C, Thielens NM, Gregory LA, et al.: Structure and activation of the C1 complex of complement: unraveling the puzzle, *Trends Immunol* 25:368–373, 2004.
8. Garred P, Genster N, Pilely K, et al.: A journey through the lectin pathway of complement-MBL and beyond, *Immunol Rev* 274:74–97, 2016.
9. Takahashi M, Ishida Y, Iwaki D, et al.: Essential role of mannose-binding lectin-associated serine protease-1 in activation of the complement factor D, *J Exp Med* 207:29–37, 2010.

10. Spitzer D, Mitchell LM, Atkinson JP, et al.: Properdin can initiate complement activation by binding specific target surfaces and providing a platform for de novo convertase assembly, *J Immunol* 179:2600–2608, 2007.
11. Harboe M, Mollnes TE: The alternative complement pathway revisited, *J Cell Mol Med* 12:1074–1084, 2008.
12. Ricklin D, Reis ES, Mastellos DC, et al.: Complement component C3—The "Swiss Army Knife" of innate immunity and host defense, *Immunol Rev* 274:33–58, 2016.
13. Cole DS, Morgan BP: Beyond lysis: how complement influences cell fate, *Clinical Science* 104:455–466, 2003.
14. Huber-Lang M, Sarma JV, Zetoune FS, et al.: Generation of C5a in the absence of C3: a new complement activation pathway, *Nat Med* 12:682–687, 2006.
15. Markiewski MM, Nilsson B, Ekdahl KN, et al.: Complement and coagulation: strangers or partners in crime? *Trends Immunol* 28:184–192, 2007.
16. Sjoberg AP, Trouw LA, Blom AM: Complement activation and inhibition: a delicate balance, *Trends Immunol* 30:83–90, 2009.
17. Zipfel PF, Skerka C: Complement regulators and inhibitory proteins, *Nat Rev Immunol* 9:729–740, 2009.
18. Medjeral-Thomas N, Pickering MC: The complement factor H–related proteins, *Immunol Rev* 274:191–201, 2016.
19. Nilsson SC, Sim RB, Lea SM, et al.: Complement factor I in health and disease, *Mol Immunol* 48:1611–1620, 2011.
20. Blom AM, Villoutreix BO, Dahlback B: Complement inhibitor C4b-binding protein-friend or foe in the innate immune system? *Mol Immunol* 40:1333–1346, 2004.
21. Wang H, Ricklin D, Lambris JD: Complement-activation fragment C4a mediates effector functions by binding as untethered agonist to protease-activated receptors 1 and 4, *PNAS* 114:10948–10953, 2017.
22. Krych-Goldberg M, Atkinson JP: Structure-function relationships of complement receptor type 1, *Immunol Rev* 180:112–122, 2001.
23. Craig ML, Bankovich AJ, Taylor RP: Visualization of the transfer reaction: tracking immune complexes from erythrocyte complement receptor 1 to macrophages, *Clin Immunol* 105:36–47, 2002.
24. Roozendaal R, Carroll MC: Complement receptors CD21 and CD35 in humoral immunity, *Immunol Rev* 219:157–166, 2007.
25. Dustin ML: Complement receptors in myeloid cell adhesion and phagocytosis, *Microbiol Spec*, 2016. 10.1128/microbiolspec. MCHD-0034-2016.
26. Hajishengallis G, Lambris JD: Crosstalk pathways between Toll-like receptors and the complement system, *Trends Immunol* 31:154–163, 2010.
27. Ritis K, Doumas M, Mastellos D, et al.: A novel C5a receptor-tissue factor cross-talk in neutrophils links innate immunity to coagulation pathways, *J Immunol* 177:4794–4802, 2006.
28. Manderson AP, Botto M, Walport MJ: The role of complement in the development of systemic lupus erythematosus, *Annu Rev Immunol* 22:431–456, 2004.
29. Nauta AJ, Trouw LA, Daha MR, et al.: Direct binding of C1q to apoptotic cells and cell blebs induces complement activation, *Eur J Immunol* 32:1726–1736, 2002.
30. Navratil JS, Watkins SC, Wisnieski JJ, et al.: The globular heads of C1q specifically recognize surface blebs of apoptotic vascular endothelial cells, *J Immunol* 166:3231–3239, 2001.
31. Gullstrand B, Martensson U, Sturfelt G, et al.: Complement classical pathway components are all important in clearance of apoptotic and secondary necrotic cells, *Clin Exp Immunol* 156:303–311, 2009.
32. Trouw LA, Bengtsson AA, Gelderman KA, et al.: C4b-binding protein and factor H compensate for the loss of membrane bound complement inhibitors to protect apoptotic cells against excessive complement attack, *J Biol Chem* 282:28540–28548, 2007.
33. Arason GJ, Steinsson K, Kolka R, et al.: Patients with systemic lupus erythematosus are deficient in complement-dependent prevention of immune precipitation, *Rheumatology (Oxford)* 43:783–789, 2004.
34. Dempsey PW, Allison ME, Akkaraju S, et al.: C3d of complement as a molecular adjuvant: bridging innate and acquired immunity, *Science* 271:348–350, 1996.
35. Shushakova N, Skokowa J, Schulman J, et al.: C5a anaphylatoxin is a major regulator of activating versus inhibitory FcgammaRs in immune complex-induced lung disease, *J Clin Invest* 110:1823–1830, 2002.
36. Kumar V, Ali SR, Konrad S, et al.: Cell-derived anaphylatoxins as key mediators of antibody-dependent type II autoimmunity in mice, *J Clin Invest* 116:512–520, 2006.
37. Pratt JR, Basheer SA, Sacks SH: Local synthesis of complement component C3 regulates acute renal transplant rejection, *Nat Med* 8:582–587, 2002.
38. Strainic MG, Liu J, Huang D, et al.: Locally produced complement fragments C5a and C3a provide both costimulatory and survival signals to naive CD4+ T cells, *Immunity* 28:425–435, 2008.
39. Kemper C, Chan AC, Green JM, et al.: Activation of human CD4+ cells with CD3 and CD46 induces a T-regulatory cell 1 phenotype, *Nature* 421:388–392, 2003.
40. Longhi MP, Sivasankar B, Omidvar N, et al.: Cutting edge: murine CD59a modulates antiviral CD4+ T cell activity in a complement-independent manner, *J Immunol* 175:7098–7102, 2005.
41. Mollnes TE, Jokiranta TS, Truedsson L, et al.: Complement analysis in the 21st century, *Mol Immunol* 44:3838–3849, 2007.
42. Seelen MA, Roos A, Wieslander J, et al.: Functional analysis of the classical, alternative, and MBL pathways of the complement system: standardization and validation of a simple ELISA, *J Immunol Methods* 296:187–198, 2005.
43. Dragon-Durey MA, Blanc C, Marinozzi MC, et al.: Autoantibodies against complement components and functional consequences, *Mol Immunol* 56:213–221, 2013.
44. Mahler M, van Schaarenburg RA, Trouw LA: Anti-C1q autoantibodies, novel tests, and clinical consequences, *Front Immunol* 4:117, 2013.
45. Risitano AM: Paroxysmal nocturnal hemoglobinuria and other complement-mediated hematological disorders, *Immunobiology* 217:1080–1087, 2012.
46. Sturfelt G, Truedsson L: Complement in the immunopathogenesis of rheumatic disease, *Nat Rev Rheumatol* 8:458–468, 2012.
47. Schejbel L, Skattum L, Hagelberg S, et al.: Molecular basis of hereditary C1q deficiency—revisited: identification of several novel disease-causing mutations, *Genes Immun* 12:626–634, 2011.
48. Wu YL, Brookshire BP, Verani RR, et al.: Clinical presentations and molecular basis of complement C1r deficiency in a male African-American patient with systemic lupus erythematosus, *Lupus* 20:1126–1134, 2011.
49. Sturfelt G, Truedsson L, Johansen P, et al.: Homozygous C4A deficiency in systemic lupus erythematosus: analysis of patients from a defined population, *Clin Genet* 38:427–433, 1990.
50. Yang Y, Chung EK, Wu YL, et al.: Gene copy-number variation and associated polymorphisms of complement component C4 in human systemic lupus erythematosus (SLE): low copy number is a risk factor for and high copy number is a protective factor against SLE susceptibility in European Americans, *Am J Hum Genet* 80:1037–1054, 2007.
51. Pickering MC, Botto M, Taylor PR, et al.: Systemic lupus erythematosus, complement deficiency, and apoptosis, *Adv Immunol* 76:227–324, 2000.
52. Skattum L, van DM, van der Poll T, et al.: Complement deficiency states and associated infections, *Mol Immunol* 48:1643–1655, 2011.
53. Nilsson SC, Trouw LA, Renault N, et al.: Genetic, molecular and functional analyses of complement factor I deficiency, *Eur J Immunol* 39:310–323, 2009.
54. Leffler J, Bengtsson AA, Blom AM: The complement system in systemic lupus erythematosus: an update, *Ann Rheum Dis* 73:1601–1606, 2014.
55. Theander E, Manthorpe R, Jacobsson LT: Mortality and causes of death in primary Sjogren's syndrome: a prospective cohort study, *Arthritis Rheum* 50:1262–1269, 2004.
56. Bouwman LH, Roos A, Terpstra OT, et al.: Mannose binding lectin gene polymorphisms confer a major risk for severe infections after liver transplantation, *Gastroenterology* 129:408–414, 2005.

57. Castellano G, Woltman AM, Nauta AJ, et al.: Maturation of dendritic cells abrogates C1q production in vivo and in vitro, *Blood* 103:3813–3820, 2004.
58. Arkwright PD, Riley P, Hughes SM, et al.: Successful cure of C1q deficiency in human subjects treated with hematopoietic stem cell transplantation, *J Allergy Clin Immunol* 133:265–267, 2014.
59. Ricklin D, Lambris JD: Complement in immune and inflammatory disorders: therapeutic interventions, *J Immunol* 190:3839–3847, 2013.
60. Rioux P: TP-10 (AVANT Immunotherapeutics), *Curr Opin Investig Drugs* 2:364–371, 2001.
61. Thurman JM, Frazer-Abel A, Holers VM: The evolving landscape for complement therapeutics in rheumatic and autoimmune diseases, *Arth Rheum* 69:2102–2113, 2017.
62. Lovgren T, Eloranta ML, Bave U, et al.: Induction of interferon-alpha production in plasmacytoid dendritic cells by immune complexes containing nucleic acid released by necrotic or late apoptotic cells and lupus IgG, *Arthritis Rheum* 50:1861–1872, 2004.
63. Das A, Heesters BA, Bialas A, et al.: Follicular dendritic cell activation by TLR ligands promotes autoreactive B cell responses, *Immunity* 46:106–119, 2017.
64. Lech M, Anders HJ: The pathogenesis of lupus nephritis, *J Am Soc Nephrol* 24:1357–1366, 2013.
65. Bombardier C, Gladman DD, Urowitz MB, et al.: Derivation of the SLEDAI. A disease activity index for lupus patients. The Committee on Prognosis Studies in SLE, *Arthritis Rheum* 35:630–640, 1992.
66. Siegert C, Daha M, Westedt ML, et al.: IgG autoantibodies against C1q are correlated with nephritis, hypocomplementemia, and dsDNA antibodies in systemic lupus erythematosus, *J Rheumatol* 18:230–234, 1991.
67. Trendelenburg M, Marfurt J, Gerber I, et al.: Lack of occurrence of severe lupus nephritis among anti-C1q autoantibody-negative patients, *Arthritis Rheum* 42:187–188, 1999.
68. Trouw LA, Groeneveld TW, Seelen MA, et al.: Anti-C1q autoantibodies deposit in glomeruli but are only pathogenic in combination with glomerular C1q-containing immune complexes, *J Clin Invest* 114:679–688, 2004.
69. Barilla-Labarca ML, Toder K, Furie R: Targeting the complement system in systemic lupus erythematosus and other diseases, *Clin Immunol* 148:313–321, 2013.
70. Konttinen YT, Ceponis A, Meri S, et al.: Complement in acute and chronic arthritides: assessment of C3c, C9, and protectin (CD59) in synovial membrane, *Ann Rheum Dis* 55:888–894, 1996.
71. Swaak AJ, van RA, Planten O, et al.: An analysis of the levels of complement components in the synovial fluid in rheumatic diseases, *Clin Rheumatol* 6:350–357, 1987.
72. Jose PJ, Moss IK, Maini RN, et al.: Measurement of the chemotactic complement fragment C5a in rheumatoid synovial fluids by radioimmunoassay: role of C5a in the acute inflammatory phase, *Ann Rheum Dis* 49:747–752, 1990.
73. Moxley G, Ruddy S: Elevated C3 anaphylatoxin levels in synovial fluids from patients with rheumatoid arthritis, *Arthritis Rheum* 28:1089–1095, 1985.
74. Okroj M, Heinegard D, Holmdahl R, et al.: Rheumatoid arthritis and the complement system, *Ann Med* 39:517–530, 2007.
75. Scott DL, Wolfe F, Huizinga TW: Rheumatoid arthritis, *Lancet* 376:1094–1108, 2010.
76. Schellekens GA, de Jong BA, van den Hoogen FH, et al.: Citrulline is an essential constituent of antigenic determinants recognized by rheumatoid arthritis-specific autoantibodies, *J Clin Invest* 101:273–281, 1998.
77. Shi J, Knevel R, Suwannalai P, et al.: Autoantibodies recognizing carbamylated proteins are present in sera of patients with rheumatoid arthritis and predict joint damage, *Proc Natl Acad Sci U S A* 108:17372–17377, 2011.
78. Nielen MM, van SD, Reesink HW, et al.: Specific autoantibodies precede the symptoms of rheumatoid arthritis: a study of serial measurements in blood donors, *Arthritis Rheum* 50:380–386, 2004.
79. Shi J, van de Stadt LA, Levarht EW, et al.: Anti-carbamylated protein (anti-CarP) antibodies precede the onset of rheumatoid arthritis, *Ann Rheum Dis* 73:780–783, 2014.
80. Mullazehi M, Wick MC, Klareskog L, et al.: Anti-type II collagen antibodies are associated with early radiographic destruction in rheumatoid arthritis, *Arthritis Res Ther* 14:R100, 2012.
81. Huizinga TW, Amos CI, AH vdH-vM, et al.: Refining the complex rheumatoid arthritis phenotype based on specificity of the HLA-DRB1 shared epitope for antibodies to citrullinated proteins, *Arthritis Rheum* 52:3433–3438, 2005.
82. Kuhn KA, Kulik L, Tomooka B, et al.: Antibodies to citrullinated proteins enhance tissue injury in experimental arthritis, *J Clin Invest* 116:961–973, 2006.
83. Sokolove J, Johnson DS, Lahey LJ, et al.: Rheumatoid factor as a potentiator of anti-citrullinated protein antibody mediated inflammation in rheumatoid arthritis, *Arth Rheum* 66:813–821, 2015.
84. Trouw LA, Haisma EM, Levarht EW, et al.: Anti-cyclic citrullinated peptide antibodies from rheumatoid arthritis patients activate complement via both the classical and alternative pathways, *Arthritis Rheum* 60:1923–1931, 2009.
85. Ji H, Ohmura K, Mahmood U, et al.: Arthritis critically dependent on innate immune system players, *Immunity* 16:157–168, 2002.
86. Brodeur JP, Ruddy S, Schwartz LB, et al.: Synovial fluid levels of complement SC5b-9 and fragment Bb are elevated in patients with rheumatoid arthritis, *Arthritis Rheum* 34:1531–1537, 1991.
87. Mollnes TE, Paus A: Complement activation in synovial fluid and tissue from patients with juvenile rheumatoid arthritis, *Arthritis Rheum* 29:1359–1364, 1986.
88. Morgan BP, Daniels RH, Williams BD: Measurement of terminal complement complexes in rheumatoid arthritis, *Clin Exp Immunol* 73:473–478, 1988.
89. Happonen KE, Heinegard D, Saxne T, et al.: Interactions of the complement system with molecules of extracellular matrix: relevance for joint diseases, *Immunobiology* 217:1088–1096, 2012.
90. Trouw LA, Blom AM, Gasque P: Role of complement and complement regulators in the removal of apoptotic cells, *Mol Immunol* 45:1199–1207, 2008.
91. Romero V, Fert-Bober J, Nigrovic PA, et al.: Immune-mediated pore-forming pathways induce cellular hypercitrullination and generate citrullinated autoantigens in rheumatoid arthritis, *Sci Transl Med* 5:209ra150, 2013.
92. Vergunst CE, Gerlag DM, Dinant H, et al.: Blocking the receptor for C5a in patients with rheumatoid arthritis does not reduce synovial inflammation, *Rheumatology (Oxford)* 46:1773–1778, 2007.
93. Durigutto P, Macor P, Ziller F, et al.: Prevention of arthritis by locally synthesized recombinant antibody neutralizing complement component C5, *PLoS ONE* 8, 2013. e58696.
94. Banda NK, Levitt B, Glogowska MJ, et al.: Targeted inhibition of the complement alternative pathway with complement receptor 2 and factor H attenuates collagen antibody-induced arthritis in mice, *J Immunol* 183:5928–5937, 2009.
95. Holers VM, Rohrer B, Tomlinson S: CR2-mediated targeting of complement inhibitors: bench-to-bedside using a novel strategy for site-specific complement modulation, *Adv Exp Med Biol* 735:137–154, 2013.
96. Ballanti E, Perricone C, Greco E, et al.: Complement and autoimmunity, *Immunol Res* 56:477–491, 2013.
97. Chimenti MS, Perricone C, Graceffa D, et al.: Complement system in psoriatic arthritis: a useful marker in response prediction and monitoring of anti-TNF treatment, *Clin Exp Rheumatol* 30:23–30, 2012.
98. Sjoholm AG, Berglund K, Johnson U, et al.: C1 activation, with C1q in excess of functional C1 in synovial fluid from patients with rheumatoid arthritis, *Int Arch Allergy Appl Immunol* 79:113–119, 1986.
99. Wang Q, Rozelle AL, Lepus CM, et al.: Identification of a central role for complement in osteoarthritis, *Nat Med* 17:1674–1679, 2011.

28 Prostaglandins, Leukotrienes, and Related Compounds

ROBERT B. ZURIER

KEY POINTS

Eicosanoid biosynthesis is catalyzed by cyclooxygenases and lipoxygenases.

Conversion of the endoperoxide intermediate prostaglandin H_2 requires activity of specific terminal synthases.

Eicosanoids and their receptors regulate inflammatory and immune responses.

Synthesis of eicosanoids is modified by the administration of precursor fatty acids.

Introduction

The addition of oxygen to arachidonic acid and other polyunsaturated fatty acids that are not bound to membrane phospholipids in nearly all human cell types results in the formation of several classes of bioactive products termed *eicosanoids*. Eicosanoids include prostaglandins (PGs), prostacyclin (PGI), thromboxanes (TXs), leukotrienes (LTs), and lipoxins (LXs). All of these compounds are crucial to the regulation of immunity and inflammation, among other physiologic and pathologic processes. Although eicosanoids are derived from C20 polyunsaturated fatty acids (eicosa = 20), only a small percentage of these polyenoic acids form the eicosanoids: dihomo-γ-linolenic acid (DGLA), which is 8,11,14-eicosatrienoic acid; arachidonic acid (AA), which is 5,8,11,14-eicosatetraenoic acid; and eicosapentaenoic acid (EPA), which is 5,8,11,14,17-EPA (Fig. 28.1).

Two groups of fatty acids are essential to the body: the omega-6 series derived from linoleic acid (18 : 2 n-6) and the omega-3 series derived from α-linolenic acid (18 : 3 n-3). The *n* refers to the number of carbon atoms from the methyl (omega) end of the fatty acid chain to the first double bond (i.e., omega-3 and omega-6 designations). Using this notation, *18* refers to the number of carbon atoms in the fatty acid. The degree of unsaturation (the number of double carbon-carbon bonds) follows the number of carbon atoms. Fatty acids are metabolized by an alternating sequence of desaturation (removal of two hydrogen atoms) and elongation (addition of two carbon atoms). Membrane phospholipids are the main storage site for polyunsaturated fatty acids and are particularly rich in eicosanoid precursors, which are located at the sn-2 position (Fig. 28.2). Because mammalian cells cannot interconvert n-3 and n-6 fatty acids, the composition of membrane phospholipids is determined by exogenous sources of fatty acids.

Biosynthesis of Eicosanoids

Phospholipases

The presence of phospholipase A_2 (PLA_2) in lysosomes or bound to cell membranes catalyzes the breaking of the sn-2 bond, facilitating the release of AA or other polyunsaturated fatty acids (see Fig. 28.2). The enzyme is crucial to regulation of eicosanoid synthesis because it is in the nonesterified state that the polyunsaturated precursors enter into the cascades that lead to eicosanoid formation. Only a scant amount of oxidation at carbon 15 of AA occurs catalytically when the fatty acid is still covalently bound as part of a phospholipid.[1]

A large number of PLA_2 isoforms have been characterized and grouped based on primary structure, localization, and Ca^{2+} requirements.[2] Cytosolic PLA_2 ($cPLA_2$) group IV is the major catalyst of arachidonate release that leads to PG and LT production. The structure of $cPLA_2$ reveals a monomeric cytosolic protein with a molecular size of 85 kDa. Lysophospholipids "left over" after the action of PLA_2 are direct precursors of platelet-activating factor (PAF), a potent mediator of inflammation, which is generated by acylation (i.e., the addition of fatty acid) in the open sn-2 position of the lysophospholipid.

Four distinct types of PLA_2 activities hydrolyze fatty acids esterified at the sn-2 position. Secretory PLA_2 ($sPLA_2$) has small disulfide cross-linked proteins that require Ca^{2+} in millimolar concentrations for optimal activity. $cPLA_2$ has larger proteins that require Ca^{2+} in micromolar concentrations, which are AA selective and can deacylate diacylphospholipids completely, preventing accumulation of potentially toxic lysophospholipids. Ca^{2+}-independent PLA_2 ($iPLA_2$) exhibits specificity for plasmalogen substrates. Finally, PAF acetylhydrolase (PAF-PLA_2) has a series of isozymes specific for short chains.[3,4]

Under basal conditions, AA is liberated by $iPLA_2$ and then reincorporated into cell membranes (reacylated). It is unavailable for appreciable eicosanoid biosynthesis. The acylase enzymes competitively inhibit the cyclooxygenase (COX) isoenzymes. After receptor activation and cell stimulation, intra-cellular Ca^{2+} levels increase and the Ca^{2+}-dependent $cPLA_2$ liberates arachidonate at a rate that

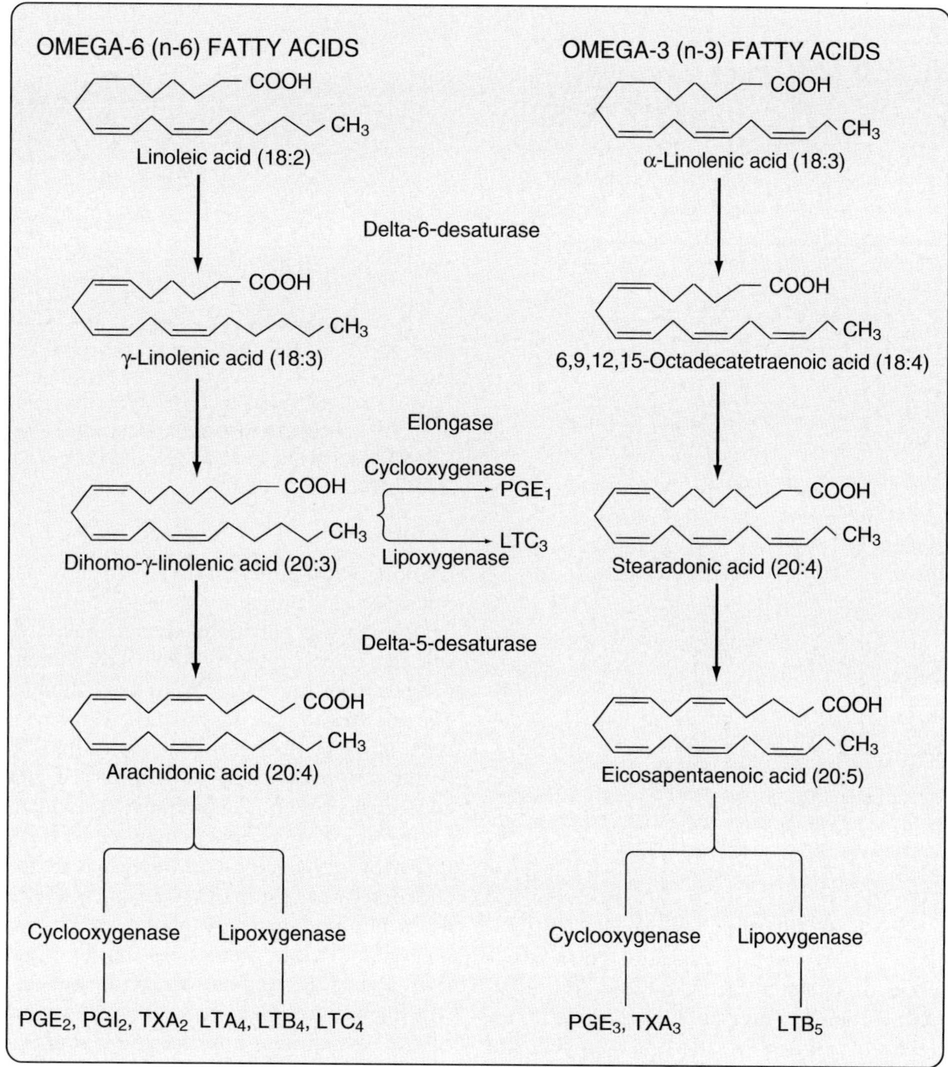

• **Fig. 28.1** Metabolic pathways of essential fatty acids. The pathways involve progressive desaturation alternating with elongation. Eicosanoid precursors include dihomo-γ-linolenic acid, arachidonic acid, and eicosapentaenoic acid. *LT,* Leukotriene; *PG,* prostaglandin; *TX,* thromboxane.

exceeds the rate of reacylation, leading to arachidonate metabolism by COX isoenzymes and by lipoxygenases (LOXs). Initial formation of prostaglandin (PG)E_2 seems to be due to preferential coupling among $cPLA_2$, COX-1, and cytosolic PGH-PGE isomerase. More intense inflammation leads to the participation of secreted $sPLA_2$ and amplification of PGE_2 biosynthesis by inducible COX-2. Thus, it is an oversimplification to regard the availability of AA as the sole rate-limiting step in cellular eicosanoid biosynthesis.

Phospholipase C (PLC) hydrolyzes the polar head group (e.g., inositol and choline) from phospholipids to yield diacylglycerol (DAG) and the polar head group. Direct protein isolation and molecular cloning studies have revealed multiple PLC isozymes in mammalian tissues. Phosphatidylinositol-PLC occurs in cytosolic (cPLC) and secreted (sPLC) forms and can be divided into three major classes (PLC-β, PLC-γ, and PLC-δ) based on substrate specificity. PLC with specificity for phosphatidylinositol and phosphorylated phosphatidylinositol is a key component of phosphatidylinositol-mediated signaling pathways. DAG is an activator of protein kinase C (PKC), and rapid production of this lipid by phosphatidylinositol-PLC hydrolysis of the phosphorylated phosphatidylinositol pool is a primary step in signaling. Further AA is made available by the sequential actions of diglyceride lipase and monoglyceride lipase.[5] PLC with activity on phosphatidylcholine has also been identified. Peripheral blood monocytes from patients with rheumatoid arthritis (RA) exhibit greater PLA_2 and PLC activity than do cells from healthy volunteers. PLA_2 concentrations did not correlate with disease activity, but the greatest increases in PLC enzyme activity were seen in cells from patients with the most severe, persistent, proliferative disease, not in cells from patients with the most active disease at the time the cells were studied.[6] In accord with the need for balance in regulation of the inflammatory response, $sPLA_2$, numbering nine members in humans, has both inflammatory and anti-inflammatory actions. Thus group V $sPLA_2$ counters the inflammatory activity of group IIA $sPLA_2$ by regulating cysteinyl LT synthesis and promoting immune complex clearance in a murine model of autoimmune erosive inflammatory arthritis. It is of interest that concentrations of IIA $sPLA_2$ are far greater than those of V $sPLA_2$ in synovial fluid from patients with RA.[7] In keeping with the fact that nothing in biology and the pathogenesis of disease is simple is the observation that treatment of patients who have RA with $sPLA(_2)$-IIA inhibitors has only transient benefit, and that $sPLA(_2)$-IIA has activity (induction of COX-2) independent of its enzyme activity.[8]

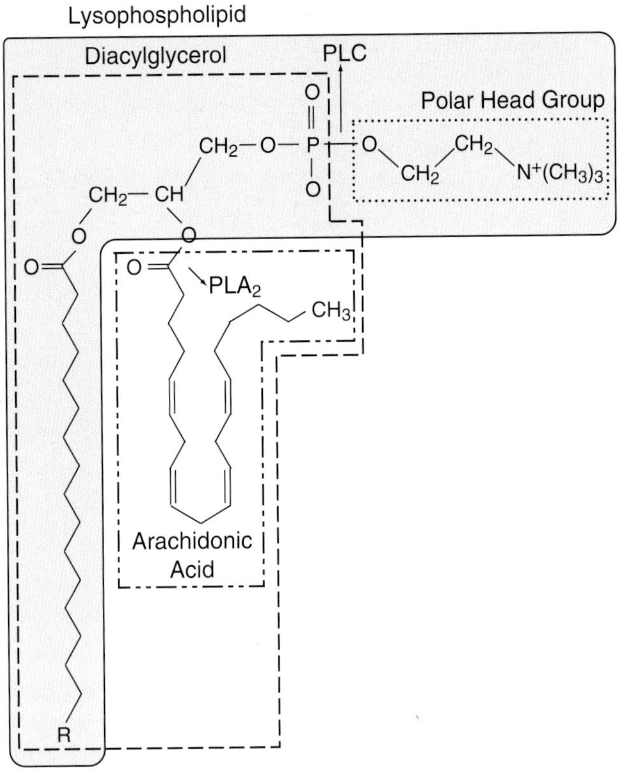

• **Fig. 28.2** Arachidonic acid release from phospholipid. Phosphatidylcholine, the major membrane storage site for polyunsaturated fatty acids, is depicted. *PLA_2*, Phospholipase A_2; *PLC*, phospholipase C.

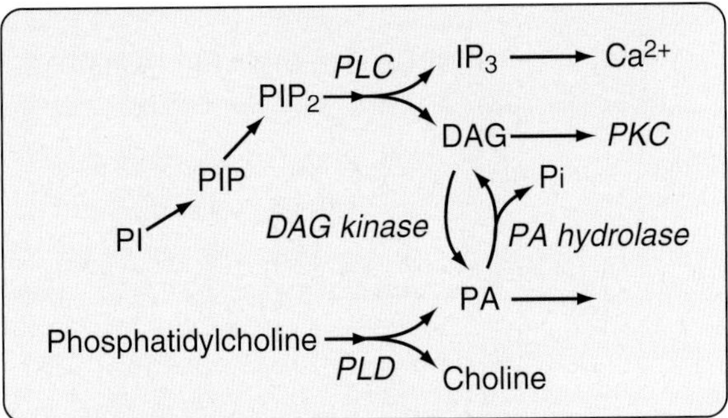

• **Fig. 28.3** Reactions catalyzed by phospholipases C and D, illustrating interconversion of diacylglycerol (DAG) and phosphatidic acid (PA). *IP_3*, Inositol-1,4,5-triphosphate; *Pi*, inorganic phosphate; *PI*, phosphatidylinositol; *PIP*, phosphatidylinositol phosphate; *PIP_2*, phosphatidylinositol-4,5-bisphosphonate; *PKC*, protein kinase C; *PLC*, phospholipase C; *PLD*, phospholipase D.

Hydrolysis of phospholipids by phospholipase D (PLD) produces phosphatidic acid (PA) and the respective polar head groups. The capacity of cells to interconvert PA and DAG through the action of specific cellular phosphatases and kinases (Fig. 28.3) suggests that AA release from DAG and a variety of intra-cellular signaling and protein-trafficking events may be regulated by PLD activity. The targets of phosphorylation within the PLD_2 molecule that are key to its regulation have been mapped. PLD may be activated after or independent of PLC activation.[9]

The tetraenoic precursor (AA) is the most abundant of the three eicosanoid precursor fatty acids in the cells of people who eat usual Western-style diets. Metabolites of AA constitute the "2" series (dienoic) PGs (two double bonds in the molecule), and the metabolic pathway has acquired the familiar name "arachidonic acid (AA) cascade." Diets enriched in eicosapentaenoic or γ-linolenic acid, the other eicosanoid precursors, lead to formation of different eicosanoids. Fig. 28.4 illustrates the COX and 5-lipoxygenase (5-LOX) pathways of the cascade.

Because phospholipases are involved in cell signaling and acute inflammation, which sometimes escapes regulation and resolution, inhibitors of $sPLA_2$, $cPLA_2$, and PLD are being developed. It will be important to improve the selectability of these inhibitors.[10]

Cyclooxygenase Pathway

The first step in the biosynthesis of "prostanoids" (e.g., PGs, TXs, and PGI) is catalyzed by the bifunctional PG endoperoxide synthase 1 isozyme (also known as *prostaglandin G/H synthase 1* [PGHS-1] and *COX-1*) and PGHS-2 (COX-2). COX is a homodimeric enzyme that integrates into only a single leaflet of the lipid bilayer of the cell membrane. The COX active site is a long hydrophobic channel. Aspirin and most other nonsteroidal anti-inflammatory drugs (NSAIDs) exclude arachidonate from the upper portion of the channel.[11] To form the characteristic five-carbon ring structure (TXs contain a six-member ring), the precursor fatty acids must have double bonds at carbons 8, 11, and 14 (numbering from the carboxyl group). When a molecule of oxygen is inserted across carbons 9 and 11, ring closure occurs enzymatically across C8 and C12, creating the unstable PG endoperoxide PGG. Subsequent peroxidation yields PGH with formation of the cyclopentane ring. PGH serves as the common precursor for PGs, PGI, and TXs that are formed under the influence of terminal synthases (see Fig. 28.4). In addition to the activity of phospholipases, regulation of PG synthesis also occurs at the level of PGHS gene expression. PGHS levels are increased by IL-1, platelet-derived growth factor, and epidermal growth factor, which are compounds that increase PG synthesis.

Cell membranes constitute the source of substrate AA and the site of action of eicosanoid-forming enzymes. PG synthesis can also occur in lipid bodies, which are non–membrane-bound, lipid-rich cytoplasmic inclusions that develop in cells associated with inflammation. Lipid bodies isolated from human monocytes express PGHS activity, are reservoirs of arachidonyl phospholipids, and can function as domains of PG synthesis during an inflammatory reaction.[12]

PGHS, the well-known target of NSAIDs, exists in two isoforms. These isoforms are similar in terms of amino acid identities (about 60%), catalytic properties, and substrate specificity, but they differ in their genomic regulation.[13]

Regulation of Cyclooxygenase-1 Expression

The gene encoding COX-1 *(PTGS1)* is preferentially expressed constitutively at high levels in some cell lineages, including endothelium, monocytes, platelets, renal collecting tubules, and seminal vesicles. Because the expression level of the enzyme does not vary greatly, it has been difficult to study its transcriptional regulation. The gene has a TATA-less promoter that contains multiple start sites for transcription. The Sp1/Cis regulatory elements in the promoter bond the Sp1 transcription factor to induce COX-1 gene expression. In addition, COX-1 and COX-2 splice variants may function in tissue-specific normal and pathologic processes and may represent new targets for therapy.[14] The localization of COX-1 in nearly all tissues under basal conditions suggests that its major function is to provide eicosanoids for physiologic

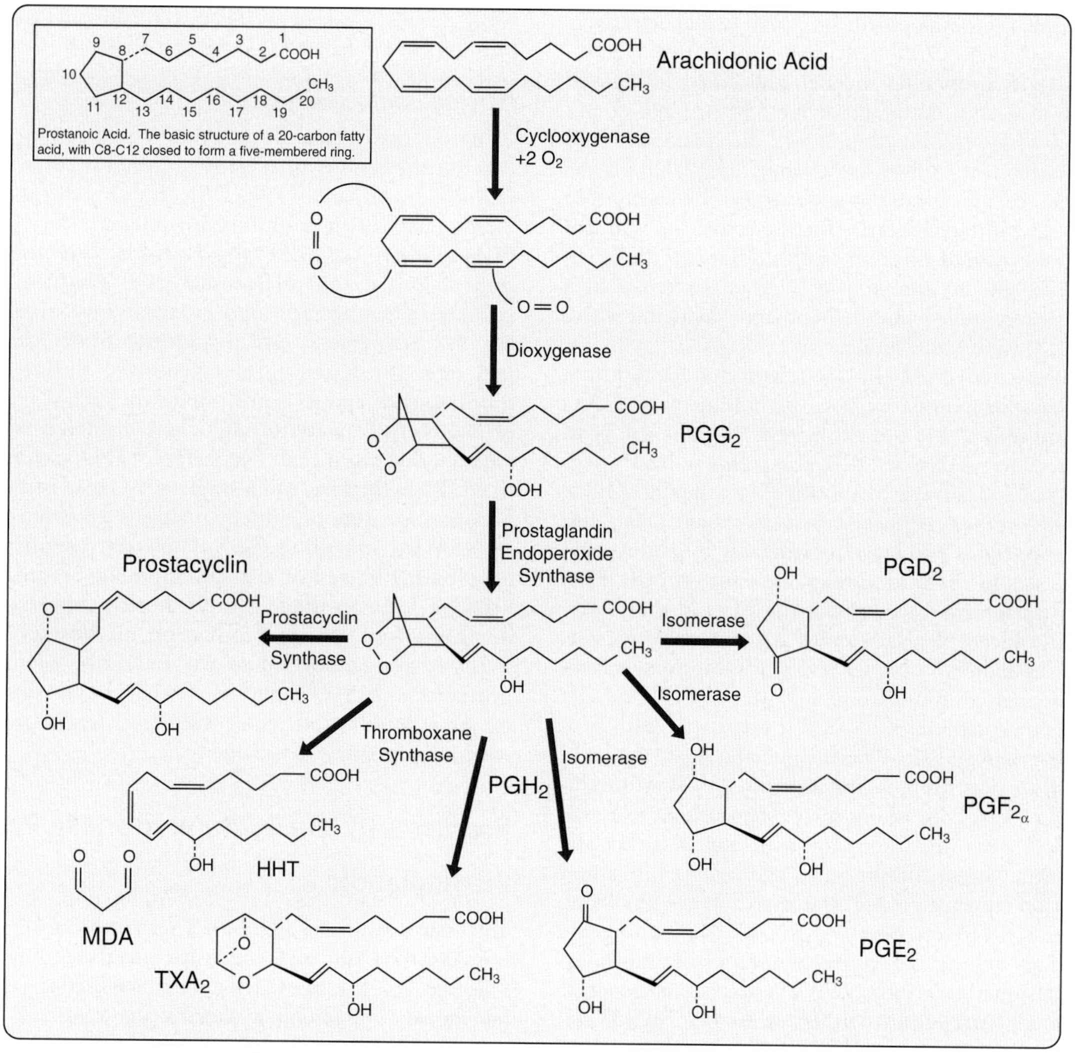

• **Fig. 28.4** Cyclooxygenase pathway of arachidonic acid metabolism. *HHT,* Hydroxyheptadeca-trienoic acid; *MDA,* malondialdehyde; *PG,* prostaglandin; *TX,* thromboxane.

regulation, which is seen clearly in platelets that do not have nuclei and cannot produce an inducible enzyme on activation. Rather, TXs are produced constitutively so that platelet aggregation can be completed.

Regulation of Cyclooxygenase-2 Expression

The regulated formation of eicosanoids implies that cells have an ability to amplify the rate and amount of eicosanoid synthesis. Several processes contribute to that regulation, including the silencing of $sPLA_2$ expression by COX-2 and autoinactivation ("suicide inactivation") of COX-2 and other oxygenases and synthases. In addition, the COX-2 transcript contains at least 12 copies of the AUUUA RNA motif, which makes it unstable and subject to rapid degradation. Factors that regulate COX-2 expression are specific for the physiologic processes involved. Expression of COX-2 in the macula densa in the kidney depends on luminal salt concentrations. Transcriptional activation of the COX-2 gene by mediators of inflammation such as IL-1β and TNF is likely regulated by the transcription factors nuclear factor-κB (NF-κB) and CCAAT/enhancer binding protein (C/EBP). Perhaps the most crucial of the several demonstrated regulatory sequences in the 5′ flanking regions of the gene for COX-2 is the activating transcription factor/cyclic adenosine monophosphate (cAMP) response element (ATF/CRE), a site that is activated by the transcriptional activator protein-1 (AP-1) and the cAMP regulatory binding protein. Now that quantitative polymerase chain reaction analysis is used routinely to examine gene expression, it is clear that COX-2 is constitutively expressed under basal conditions at levels too low to be detected by Northern blot analysis.[15] Depending on cell and tissue specificity, several signaling pathways (kinases, Rho, cyclic guanosine monophosphate, and Wnt) and transcription factors (NF-κB, AP-1, and NF of activated T cells [NFAT]) are involved in COX-2 expression.[16]

COX-1 and COX-2 affect a balance in several physiologic and pathologic situations. Of particular interest are their actions in the kidney and stomach. During times of low blood volume, the kidney releases angiotensin and other factors to maintain blood pressure by systemic vasoconstriction. Angiotensin also provokes PG synthesis in the kidney. COX-1, expressed in vessels, glomeruli, and collecting ducts, produces vasodilating PGs, which maintain renal plasma flow and glomerular filtration during conditions of systemic vasoconstriction. In the antrum of the stomach, COX-1 leads to production of PGs, which increase gastric blood flow and mucus secretion. Inhibition of COX-1 by NSAIDs prevents these protective mechanisms and results in renal ischemia and damage, and gastric ulcers (mainly antral) in susceptible people. These observations led to the development of NSAIDs that selectively inhibit COX-2 and spare COX-1. AA gains access to the active site of COX via a hydrophobic channel, and access is blocked by insertion of an acetyl residue on serine 530 in COX-1 and serine 516 in COX-2. The irreversibility of the interaction and the unique expression of COX-2 in the anucleate platelet is the reason for the clinical efficacy of low-dose aspirin. Nonacetylated NSAIDs compete with arachidonate for the active site and can interfere with the sustained effects of aspirin. Although the structures of COX isozymes are similar, COX-2 is characterized by a side-pocket extension to the hydrophobic channel, which is where the selective COX-2 inhibitors localize.[13]

The major adverse effects of NSAIDs, gastroduodenal injury, and impaired renal function are caused by inhibition of COX-1, whereas promotion of MI and stroke rests on their ability to inhibit COX-2. Nevertheless, COX-2 also seems to have a regulating role in renal, brain, gastrointestinal, ovarian, and bone function. COX-2 is also expressed in endothelial cells, and its inhibition suppresses prostacyclin synthesis by endothelial cells.[17] COX-2 acts in the initiation and resolution of inflammation. Its expression increases transiently early in the course of carrageenan-induced pleurisy in rats. Later in the response, COX-2 is expressed at even higher levels, leading to synthesis of PGD_2 and its dehydration product 15-deoxy-δ12,14-PGJ_2 (15δPGJ_2). Early expression of COX-2 is associated with production of inflammatory PGs, whereas the later peak results in production of PGs that suppress inflammation.[18] That inflammation occurs in COX-2 knockout mice[19] reminds us, as Lewis Thomas stated,[20] that "inflammation will take place at any cost." Nonetheless, the search for more selective and localized COX-2 inhibition continues. One strategy is achieved by using the mechanism of RNA interference (RNAi). Nonpathogenic *Escherichia coli* are engineered to invade tumor cells (and perhaps could be designed to invade synovial cells) and to generate anti–COX-2 small interfering (si)RNA molecules (siCOX-2), thereby silencing overexpressed COX-2. The involvement of micro (mi)RNAs in COX-2 post-transcriptional regulation suggests a possible endogenous silencing mechanism to reduce COX-2 expression.[21]

Cyclooxygenase-3 and Other Variants

Acetaminophen, similar to NSAIDs, suppresses pain and fever. Acetaminophen, however, is not an anti-inflammatory agent and, despite its extensive use, its mechanism of action has not been apparent. The finding that acetaminophen inhibits COX activity more in canine brain homogenates than in spleen homogenates gave rise to the concept that variants of the COX enzyme exist that are differentially sensitive to acetaminophen. COX-3 is a splice variant of COX-1 that retains the intron-1 gene sequence at the messenger (m)RNA level, which encodes a 30 amino acid sequence inserted into the N-terminal hydrophobic signal peptide of the enzyme protein. COX-3 protein and mRNA transcripts have been identified in human tissues, as well as in rats. They have been found most abundantly in the cerebral cortex and heart, although the mechanism for conversion of COX-3 mRNA to active enzyme is not clear.[11,22] These findings led to a search for other COX variants. A COX-2 variant induced by 0.5 mM diclofenac via stimulation of the nuclear receptor peroxisome proliferator-activated receptor γ (PPARγ) (the receptor for the pro-resolving 15-deoxy-δ12,14 PGJ_2) has been discovered. Whereas induction of COX-2 by lipopolysaccharide (LPS) results in release of the inflammatory cytokines IL-6 and TNF, diclofenac-induced COX-2 leads to release of the anti-inflammatory cytokines transforming growth factor (TGF)-β and IL-10.

Prostaglandin Synthases

Conversion of the endoperoxide intermediate PGH_2 to PGs requires the activity of specific terminal synthases. Hematopoietic PGD synthase (H-PGDS) catalyzes the isomerization of PGH_2 to PGD_2 in immune and inflammatory cells. Cytosolic PGE synthase (cPGES) is responsible for constitutive expression of PGE_2, and microsomal PGE synthase 1 (mPGES-1) induces PGE in response to inflammatory stimuli. At least 10 enzymes convert PG precursors into biologically active PGs, and reactive oxygen species generated during an inflammatory response lead to expression of mPGES-1.[23,24] Suppression of PG synthase activity might be considered as an alternative strategy that would fall between global blockade by inhibition of COX and blockade of a single eicosanoid receptor. Increased fibrosis may now be added to the well-known adverse effects of NSAIDs, including COX-2 selective agents.[25] Thus efforts have been directed at the development of drugs that inhibit mPGES-1, rather than COX-2, thereby suppressing PGE_2 production while sparing production of prostacyclin.[26] Because PGE_2 is also important to the induction of matrix metalloproteinases (MMP)-3 and MMP-13, suppression of mPGES-1 might counteract articular cartilage degradation in patients with inflammatory arthritis.[27]

Products of the Cyclooxygenase Pathway

Prostaglandins

The basic structure of all PGs is a "prostanoic acid" skeleton, which is a 20-carbon fatty acid with a five-membered ring at C8 through C12 (see Fig. 28.4, *inset*). The term *prostaglandins* is employed widely but should be used only to describe the oxygenation products that contain the five-membered carbon ring. A family of acidic lipids found first in human seminal fluid, PGs were misnamed because it was thought that they were produced in the prostate gland rather than in the seminal vesicles.[28–30] The alphabetic PG nomenclature (e.g., PGE, PGF, and PGD) is related to the chemical architecture of the cyclopentane ring. PGE and PGF differ only in the presence of a ketone or hydroxyl function at C9 (see Fig. 28.4). These compounds are made by different enzymes (e.g., PGE_2 and PGD_2 are made by isomerases, and $PGF_{2\alpha}$ is made by a reductase). In the nomenclature, a subscript numeral after the letters indicates the degree of unsaturation in the alkyl and carboxylic acid side chains. The numeral *1* indicates the presence of a double bond at C13-C14 (PGE_1), *2* marks the presence of an additional double bond at C5-C6 (PGE_2), and *3* denotes a third double bond at C17-C18 (PGE_3).

PGs are produced on demand and generally exert their effects on the cell of origin or nearby structures. They are not stored in cells and are degraded rapidly in vivo by 15-hydroxyprostaglandin dehydrogenase (PGDH) during one passage through the lungs. Abundant experimental evidence supports the view that PGs participate in the development of the inflammatory response. PGE_2 is a central component of the inflammasome-dependent induction of the eicosanoids that leads to loss of intravascular fluid.[31] PGs are probably better, however, at potentiating the effects of other mediators of inflammation than they are at inducing inflammation directly. PGE compounds and intermediate hydroperoxides of AA increase pain sensitivity to bradykinin and histamine. The effects of PGE are cumulative, depending on concentration and time. Even small amounts of PGs, if allowed to persist at the site of injury, may in time cause pain.

PGE_2 stimulates bone resorption,[32] and its 13,14-dihydro derivative is nearly as potent, which is of interest because derivatives of the biologically active PGs are usually assumed to be of no functional significance. Addition of serum to the culture medium stimulates bone resorption, a process that is complement dependent and PG mediated. The mechanism may help explain bone erosion in joints of patients with RA, in which complement is activated and PGE_2 concentrations are high. The observation that PGE_1 can stimulate bone formation[33] suggests that PGs physiologically participate in the coordination of bone formation and resorption. For example, primary idiopathic hypertrophic osteoarthropathy, a familial disorder, is associated with mutations in PGDH and subsequent impairment of PG degradation. These patients have chronically elevated levels of PGE and exhibit digital clubbing and evidence of both increased bone formation and resorption in their phalanges.[34] Many effects of IL-1 and TNF on cells are associated with stimulation of PG production and inflammation. Cartilage explants from patients with osteoarthritis (OA) express COX-2 (but not COX-1) and release 50 times more PGE_2 in culture than does cartilage from healthy subjects and 18 times more PGE_2 than does normal cartilage stimulated with cytokines plus LPS. Explants from patients with OA release IL-1β, whereas normal cartilage does not express mRNA for pro-IL-1β or release IL-1β spontaneously. It seems that in OA—and probably in RA—upregulation of cartilage IL-1β and subsequent production of PGE_2 leads to cartilage degradation.[35,36]

Mast cells, sometimes overlooked as important in inflammatory responses, are seen in large numbers in synovium from patients early in the course of RA.[37] PGD_2, the major PG formed by mast cells, is also produced by eosinophils and type 2 (T helper [Th]2) lymphocytes. PGD_2 induces chemotaxis of Th2 cells via activation of the chemoattractant receptor-homologous molecule (CRTH2) expressed on Th2 cells, and CRTH2 antagonists block that action and reduce allergen-induced inflammation. PGJ_2, formed from the dehydration of PGD_2, functions as a brake on the inflammatory response. It reduces macrophage activation, reduces nitric oxide production from stimulated cells, and induces apoptosis in tumor cell lines. PGJ_2 is metabolized to 15-deoxy-δ12,14 PGJ_2 and δ12 PGJ_2, which are also biologically active.[38] The biologic activity of PGA, formed from loss of water from the cyclopentane ring, is not completely clear. In vitro, however, PGA_2 induces apoptosis in HL-60 cells and acts through a nuclear receptor to increase insulin sensitivity.[39]

Prostacyclin

PGI, discovered in 1976,[40] has been purified, and the complementary (c)DNA for PGI synthase has been cloned. In addition to a cyclopentane ring, a second ring is formed by an oxygen bridge between carbons 6 and 9. PGI is generated from PGH_2 by a distinct prostacyclin synthase, a 56 kDa member of the cytochrome P-450 superfamily of enzymes found predominantly in endothelial and vascular smooth muscle cells.[15] Production of PGI can be stimulated by thrombin or generated by transfer of PGH_2 from platelets (the endoperoxide steal), or it can be stimulated by contact with activated leukocytes or by stretching of the arterial wall. PGI is a powerful vasodilator that inhibits platelet aggregation through activation of adenylate cyclase, which leads to an increase in intra-cellular cAMP. It is metabolized rapidly (the half-life in plasma is less than one circulation time) to the more stable, less biologically active 6-keto-$PGF_{1\alpha}$. The enzymatic products of its conversion—2,3-dinor-6-keto $PGF_{1\alpha}$ and 6,15-di-keto-2,3-dinor $PGF_{1\alpha}$—are also chemically stable and have little biologic activity. They are the major metabolites of prostacyclin excreted in urine, in which they can be assayed as indicators of PGI generation.

PGI generated in the vessel wall has anti-platelet and vasodilator actions, whereas TXA_2 generated by platelets from the same precursors induces platelet aggregation and vasoconstriction. These two eicosanoids represent biologically opposite poles of a mechanism for regulating the interaction between platelets and the vessel wall and of formation of hemostatic plugs and intra-arterial thrombi. Given the central role of platelets in inflammatory reactions, an appropriate PGI-TX balance is important to regulation of inflammation. The balance may be altered in patients with antiphospholipid antibody syndrome, in patients treated with cyclosporine, and in patients treated with NSAIDs, especially patients treated with selective COX-2 inhibitors. Although COX-2 inhibitors reduce recurrence of colorectal adenomas, they increase the risk for cardiovascular events, such as myocardial infarction and stroke.[41]

Intravascular infusion of PGI also reduces some of the clinical changes associated with pulmonary embolism. The instability of PGI makes it cumbersome to administer therapeutically. Nonetheless, it has been used with limited success to treat peripheral vascular disease, including Raynaud's phenomenon. New therapeutics for treatment of pulmonary hypertension, including patients with sarcoidosis and systemic sclerosis, are PGI analogues and PGI receptor antagonists.[42,43] Inhaled PGI analogues may help overcome some of the adverse events that result from intravenous administration of these drugs.[44]

Thromboxanes

The endoperoxide PGH_2 can be converted into TXs after the action of the enzyme TX synthase, a microsomal 60 kDa member of the cytochrome P-450 family, which is quite active in the platelet. The gene that encodes the enzyme has been cloned. TXs contain a six-member oxane ring instead of the cyclopentane ring of the PGs. TX synthase converts PGH_2 into equal amounts of TXA_2 and 12L-hydroxy-5,8,10-heptadecatrienoic acid. TXA_2 stimulates platelet activation, contributes to intravascular aggregation of platelets, and contracts arteriolar and bronchiolar smooth muscles. It is hydrolyzed rapidly (the half-life is 30 seconds) to the inactive, stable, measurable product, TXB_2, and its actions are limited to the microenvironment of its release.

The extraordinary rapidity with which platelets adhere to damaged tissue, aggregate, and release potent biologically active materials suggests that the platelet is well suited to be a cellular trigger for the inflammatory process. Efforts directed at suppression of TX synthesis and platelet aggregation may result in limitation of inflammatory responses, especially in coronary arteries. Inhibition of platelet aggregation may be important to the anti-inflammatory effects of aspirin and other NSAIDs. Long-term administration of low doses of aspirin (40 mg/day—the lowest dose predicted to cause total inhibition of TX formation in serum, according to mathematic modeling) has inhibitory effects on platelet function ex vivo that are indistinguishable from the effects caused by giving 325 mg/day of aspirin.[45] Aspirin acetylation of COX in platelets occurs in the portal vein, where the aspirin concentration is high before it is metabolized in the liver, which explains why the 81-mg dose of aspirin is effective in prevention of heart attacks and strokes. Platelets lose their ability to aggregate until new platelets are formed in about a week.[11] Nonetheless, the response to aspirin can vary among individuals. Biomarker testing for TX production and assessment of aspirin efficacy—which is not done as routinely as necessary—can reduce the risks associated with aspirin therapy.[46] High platelet turnover in some patients with chronic inflammation may diminish the efficacy of aspirin, a phenomenon called *aspirin resistance*.[47]

Selective inhibition of TX synthase represents an approach that may be used to suppress TXA_2 synthesis without depressing prostacyclin formation. The endoperoxide steal seems to function in vivo after administration of a TX synthase inhibitor. Antagonists of the receptors shared by endoperoxide and TXA_2 have been developed, and these agents inhibit platelet aggregation in patients who are recalcitrant to TX synthase inhibition. Novel agents targeting TX receptors and TX synthase have improved treatment of vasculitis and cardiovascular and renal diseases.[48] More specific inhibition of TX action may become possible now that TX receptors have been cloned and characterized.[49]

Lipoxygenase Pathways

In contrast to the COX pathway, in which stable products have three atoms of oxygen covalently attached to AA from 2 moles of molecular oxygen, LOXs insert a single oxygen atom into the molecular structure of AA. Separate LOXs exist in certain cells and have strict structural requirements for their substrates. Three major mammalian LOXs insert their oxygen atoms into the 5, 12, or 15 position of AA, with formation of a new double bond and hydroperoxy group. The hydroperoxy fatty acids (hydroxyperoxyeicosatetraenoic acid [HPETE]) can be reduced by peroxidases in the cell to yield the corresponding hydroxy fatty acids (hydroxyeicosatetraenoic acid [HETE]). The exclusive LOX product of the human platelet is 12-HPETE, which, upon reduction of the hydroperoxy group, yields 12-HETE. In contrast, the human neutrophil makes predominantly 5-HPETE, but when high concentrations of AA are added, cells exhibit 15-LOX. LOXs that act on AA are found in the cytosol fraction of cells.

The human 5-LOX gene has been isolated and characterized[50,51] and produces a 78 kDa enzyme. In myeloid cells the 5-LOX pathway leads to formation of the biologically active LTs (Fig. 28.5) that were originally found in leukocytes and that contain three conjugated double bonds (trienes). Cell activation leads to translocation of 5-LOX from cytosol to the nuclear membrane, where it encounters the 18 kDa, 5-LOX–activating protein (FLAP). AA is also translocated to FLAP for presentation to 5-LOX. In addition, upon cell stimulation, $cPLA_2$ is activated and also associates with the nuclear membrane, close to FLAP. Thus FLAP inhibition represents an approach to suppression of inflammation.[52] The ability of macrophages and dendritic cells to respond appropriately during innate immune responses is likely regulated by 5-LOX and 12-LOX.[53] The unstable HPETE is the initial metabolite of each LOX pathway. HPETE is reduced to the more stable HETE or is converted by 5-LOX to LTA_4. LTA_4 can be converted to LTB_4 (in neutrophils and macrophages) or conjugated with reduced glutathione to form LTC_4 (in eosinophils, mast cells, endothelial cells, and macrophages). In contrast to LOX, which is mainly distributed in myeloid cells, LTA_4 hydrolase (5,12-dihydroxyeicosatetraenoic acid), a zinc-requiring enzyme that converts LTA_4 to LTB_4, is widely distributed. From the DNA sequence, it was suggested that mRNA for LTA_4 has a short half-life, which accounts for the properties of extremely rapid production and shutdown of LTB_4 and other eicosanoid biosynthesis.

LTA_4 can be exported from the cell of origin and converted in other cells by LTA_4 hydrolase to LTB_4. This variation on the endoperoxide steal—perhaps better called *transcellular metabolism*—also applies to conversion of LTA_4 to LTC_4 by LTC_4 synthase, a glutathione-*S*-transferase.[54] Although human endothelial cells do not produce terminal products of the 5-LOX system, they do generate LTC_4 from LTA_4 provided by neutrophils. LTC_4 and its products, LTD_4 and LTE_4, constitute the biologic mixture previously known as slow-reacting substance of anaphylaxis. LTD_4 and LTE_4 arise from LTC_4 after sequential removal of γ-glutamic acid and glycine from LTC_4. The enzyme γ-glutamyl transpeptidase is present in many cells as part of a complex enzymatic system involved in glutathione biosynthesis and amino acid transport. In many systems the major sulfidopeptide LT has been reported to be LTD_4, rather than the precursor LTC_4. Removal of glycine from LTD_4 results in LTE_4, with concomitant loss of a significant amount of biologic activity. The principal route of inactivation of LTB_4 is by omega oxidation.

Products of the Lipoxygenase Pathways

The biologic effects of compounds produced in the LOX pathway indicate their importance in inflammatory diseases.[55] They are the major mediators of inflammation formed by the oxygenation of AA and are implicated as key mediators in several diseases, including inflammatory bowel disease, systemic sclerosis, psoriasis, and RA.

5-HETE and 5-HPETE stimulate the generation of superoxide in human neutrophils. These compounds also augment intracellular calcium levels, facilitating PKC-dependent activation of a superoxide-generating system of neutrophils. LTB_4 increases adherence of leukocytes to endothelial cells, a response that is augmented by exposure of the endothelial cells to TNF. LTB_4 does not seem to have a direct vascular contractile action because it is inactive in the hamster cheek pouch preparation and several other microvasculature systems. In rabbit skin, administration of LTB_4 with a vasodilator PG induces plasma exudation, which suggests that LTB_4 may enhance vascular permeability. Increased venule permeability does occur in response to LTC_4, LTD_4, and LTE_4. LTB_4 is a potent chemotactic factor for neutrophils and is weakly chemotactic for eosinophils. LTB_4 and, to a lesser extent, 5-HETE enhance migration of T lymphocytes in vitro. Synovial cells produce 5-HETE but do not produce significant amounts of LTB_4. Nevertheless, macrophages that invade the synovium in patients with RA generate substantial quantities of 5-lipoxygenation and 15-lipoxygenation products, including LTB_4. In addition to local signs of inflammation induced by products of the LOX pathway, these compounds may contribute to the pain, tenderness, and aching common in patients with RA. LTB_4 also seems to serve an immunoregulatory function. It stimulates differentiation of competent $CD8^+$ T lymphocytes from precursors lacking the CD8 marker. LTB_4 also stimulates interferon (IFN)-γ and IL-2 production by T cells, and biosynthesis of IL-1 by monocytes.[56]

Synovial cell proliferation and endothelial cell proliferation are central to propagation of the rheumatoid joint lesion. LTB_4 and the cysteinyl LTs act as growth or differentiation factors for several cell types in vitro. These compounds also increase proliferation of fibroblasts when PG synthesis is inhibited.[57] These findings emphasize the importance of interactions between the COX and LOX pathways and limit efficacy of NSAID therapy in patients with RA.

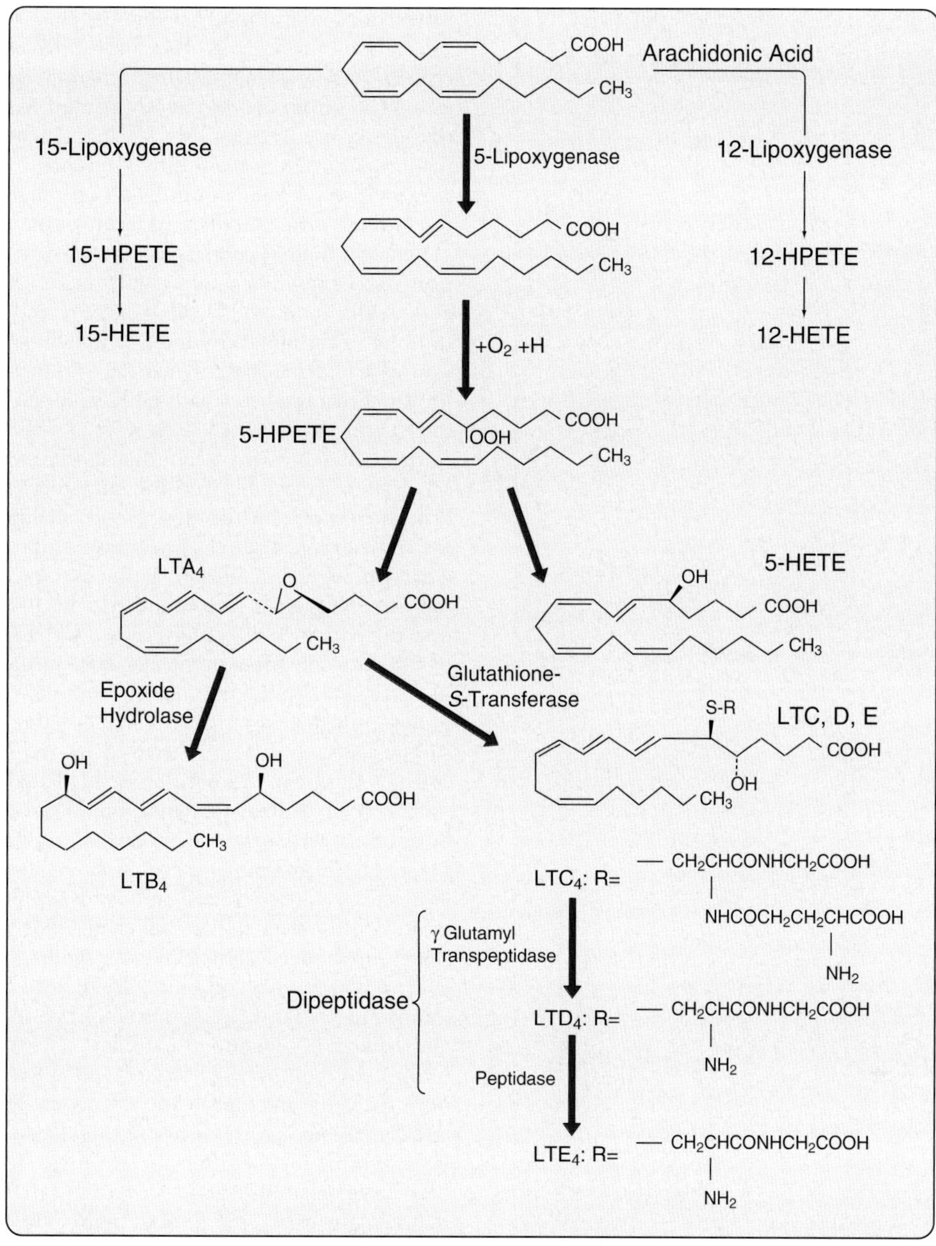

• **Fig. 28.5** 5-Lipoxygenase pathway of arachidonic acid metabolism. *HETE,* Hydroxyeicosatetraenoic acid; *HPETE,* hydroxyperoxyeicosatetraenoic acid; *LT,* leukotriene.

Strategies for inhibiting production or antagonizing the actions of LTs include the development of selective LT receptor antagonists and inhibition of the production of LT by blocking the action of 5-LOX. Inhibition of enzymes distal in the LT cascade, such as LTA_4 hydrolase,[58] is also a promising strategy for the development of anti-inflammatory drugs. A compound that inhibits binding of 5-LOX to FLAP exhibits anti-inflammatory effects in animal models. Although LOX inhibitors have not been very useful for treatment of patients with inflammatory diseases, development of new compounds, based on a better understanding of the molecular aspects of inhibitory activities, seems more promising.[59] In addition, the existing agents may be aiming at the wrong target. Fibroblasts such as synovial cells do not make much LTB_4, but they do make 12-HETE, a growth factor, through a cytochrome P-450 pathway.[60] Cytochrome P-450 inhibitors may be more to the therapeutic point.[61]

LOX activities do not lead solely to production of mediators of inflammation. DGLA is converted by 15-LOX into 15-HETE, which is incorporated into DAG and exerts anti-inflammatory effects partly by interfering with PKC-β activity. A LOX product of linoleic acid, 13-hydroxyoctadecadienoic acid, also suppresses inflammation and cell proliferation by a similar mechanism.[62] EPA is converted by LOX into 15-hydroxyeicosapentaenoic acid, which also exhibits anti-inflammatory properties.[63]

Lipoxins and Resolution of Inflammation

Another large family of AA metabolites arises from the sequential action of 5-LOXs and 15-LOXs. The addition of 15-HPETE and 15-HETE to human leukocytes results in the formation of a pair of oxygenated products containing a unique conjugated tetraene. One compound (LXA_4) was identified as

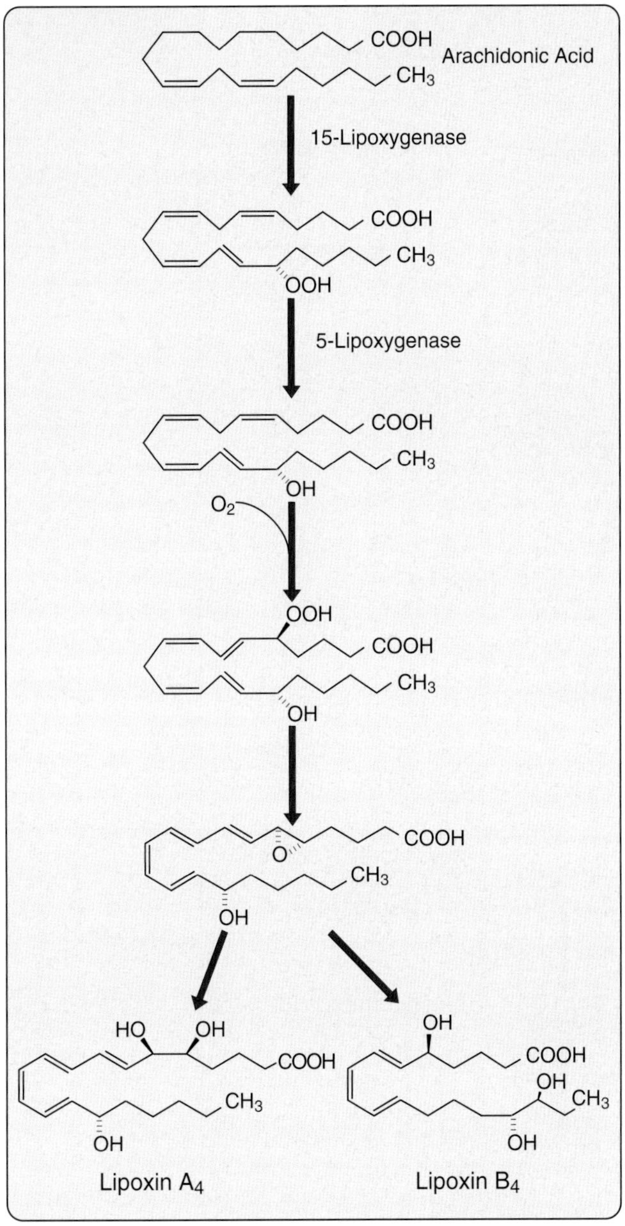

• **Fig. 28.6** Lipoxin biosynthesis. The lipoxins result from the sequential action of 15-lipoxygenase and 5-lipoxygenase on arachidonic acid.

5,6,15L-trihydroxy-7,9,11,13-eicosatetraenoic acid, and the other proven to be its positional isomer (LXB_4), 5D-14,15-trihydroxy-6,8,10,12-eicosatetraenoic acid (Fig. 28.6). Because both of these compounds can arise through an interaction between LOX pathways, the trivial name *lipoxins* (i.e., lipoxygenase interaction products) was introduced. Platelet 12-LOX can transform neutrophil LTA_4 to LXs. The complete stereochemistry and multiple routes of biosynthesis for biologically active LXA_4 and LXB_4 have been determined.[64]

The fact that macrophages of rainbow trout generate LXs rather than LTs or PGs as their major products of AA metabolism indicates that LXs have a long evolutionary history. LTs and LXs can be generated in parallel in fish. In humans, the process has diverged to a two-cell system. Biosynthesis of eicosanoids by transcellular and cell-cell interactions is recognized as an important way to generate and amplify lipid-derived mediators. LXs can be generated within the vascular lumen during platelet-leukocyte interactions and at mucosal surfaces via leukocyte–epithelial cell interactions. In humans, LXs are formed in vivo during multicellular responses such as inflammation, atherosclerosis, and in asthma. These tetraene-containing products serve as stop signals in that they prevent leukocyte-mediated tissue injury. Acute inflammation is a primitive protective response,[65] and chronic inflammation involves failure of mechanisms designed to stop the acute response. A major problem in joints of patients with RA, and of patients with other conditions associated with chronic inflammation and tissue injury, is that inflammation fails to resolve. LXs and aspirin-induced 15-epilipoxins are endogenous components of events governing resolution of inflammation. Aspirin acetylation of COX-2 in endothelial cells suppresses PG synthesis but leads to generation of 15R-HETE from AA, which is transformed to 15-epilipoxin by leukocytes in a transcellular biosynthetic route involving vascular endothelial cells or epithelial cells. These 15-epilipoxins exhibit anti-inflammatory and anti-proliferative actions in vitro and in vivo. Stable analogues of LXA_4 and of aspirin-triggered LX (ATL) have also suppressed inflammation in animal models. In addition, acting as antagonists at the receptor CysLT1, ATL analogues counteract the inflammatory actions of cysteinyl LTs.[66] These observations may lead to the development of new anti-inflammatory drugs. For example, induction by IFN of particular genes is important to the pathogenesis of systemic lupus erythematosus (SLE). A stable synthetic analogue of LXA_4 suppressed several IFN-induced genes and reduced kidney damage in a murine model of immune-mediated nephritis.[67]

LXs block human polymorphonuclear leukocyte chemotaxis but stimulate monocyte chemotaxis and adherence. Monocytes do not release mediators of inflammation in response to LXs, however, and LXs are converted rapidly by monocytes to inactive compounds. This selective effect on chemotaxis suggests that LXs play a role in wound healing. LXA_4 antagonizes LTD_4-induced vasoconstriction in vivo and blocks binding of LTD_4 to its receptors on mesangial cells. LXA_4 suppresses LTB_4-induced plasma leakage and leukocyte migration, and blocks LTB_4-induced neutrophil inositol triphosphate generation and calcium mobilization, but not superoxide anion generation. Conversely, LXA_4 activates PKC and is more potent in this regard than DAG and AA. LXA_4 seems to be specific for the γ subspecies of PKC. These results indicate that LXs regulate the actions of vasoconstrictor LTs and suggest that LXA_4 may be an important modulator of intra-cellular signal transduction.

It was long thought that resolution of inflammation was a passive process. Contrary to this belief, the inflammatory response does not dissipate but is mediated actively by products of COX and LOX, and acetylation of these enzymes.[68] The discovery that omega-6 and omega-3 polyunsaturated fatty acids are also substrates for enzymatic oxygenation reactions that produce lipid mediators with potent anti-inflammatory and proresolution actions has advanced our understanding of the inflammatory response. In addition to LXs, entire spectra of specialized pro-resolving mediators (SPM) have been uncovered. These SPMs include resolvins, protectins, and maresins.[69] Like LXs, resolvins are formed via specific transcellular biosynthetic pathways from both n-6 and n-3 fatty acids. EPA-derived (E series) cellular interaction products formed in resolving exudates have been termed *resolvins* (RvE1, RvE2, and RvE3). The omega-3 docosahexaenoic acid (DHA) can be catalyzed via the 15-LOX pathway to dihydroxy products (D series resolvins D1-D5) that also stimulate resolution of inflammation and enhance innate host defense mechanisms. LXs and resolvins act as endogenous

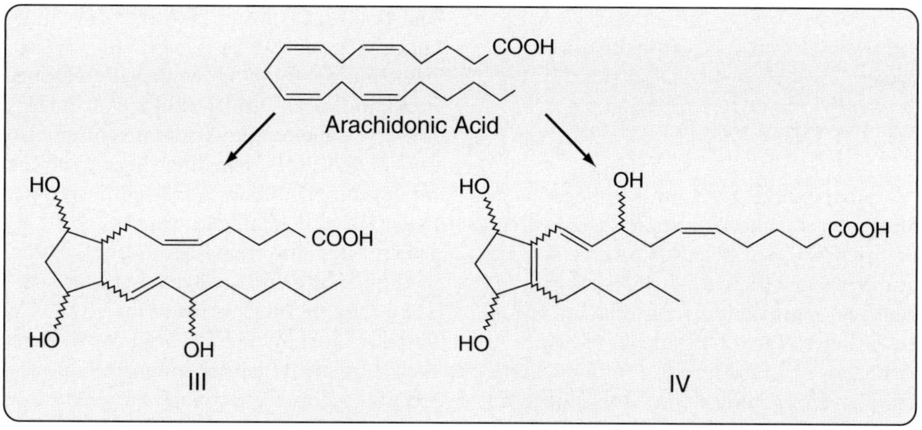

• **Fig. 28.7** Isoprostane $F_{2\alpha}$ structures. *Jagged lines* indicate that stereochemistry is uncertain.

receptor agonists at low concentrations (pM to nM) and at specific G protein–coupled membrane spanning receptors to actively downregulate inflammatory events and to stimulate resolution of an inflammatory exudate. A single cell type can also form oxygenated lipid mediators with counter-regulatory actions. DHA can also be catalyzed via the 15-LOX pathway to a dihydroxy product termed *protectin D1* (PD1), which can protect against tissue damage and activate resolution of inflammation. In a second single oxygenation route, a lipid mediator termed *maresin* (macrophage mediators in resolving inflammation) is formed via the action of human 12-LOX. The maresin biosynthetic pathway is activated in macrophages during phagocytosis. Maresin 1 (MaR1) reduces neutrophil migration and increases macrophage phagocytosis of apoptotic cells, thereby exhibiting the hallmarks of SPM. It now seems clear that the failure of resolution programs contributes to progression of diseases characterized by chronic inflammation.[70]

Isoeicosanoids

Isoeicosanoids, which are isomers of enzymatically derived eicosanoids, are derived from the free radical–mediated peroxidation auto-oxidation of both omega-6 and omega-3 fatty acids.[71] Isoeicosanoids include members of the F, D, and E isoprostanes, isothromboxanes, and isoleukotrienes. Analysis of the isoprostanes indicates that they reflect lipid peroxidation in vivo and are therefore used as markers of oxidative stress. One F-type isoprostane, isoprostane $F_{2\alpha}$ III (formerly 8-isoprostaglandin $F_{2\alpha}$), has been studied in detail because of its biologic activity in vitro. Isoprostane $F_{2\alpha}$ III (Fig. 28.7) is a potent vasoconstrictor and may function as a mitogen, with actions that are blocked by TX receptor antagonists. Although isoprostanes may act as ligands at TX or PG receptors (e.g., 8,12-isoprostane $F_{2\alpha}$ III activates the $PGF_{2\alpha}$ receptor), they also activate specific isoprostane receptors.

Isoprostanes

What all isoprostanes have in common, and what distinguishes them from the PGs, is the fact that the top (α) and the bottom (ω) side chains are always syn—that is, crowded together on the same face of the cyclopentane ring. The minimal requirement for generation of an isoprostane is a polyunsaturated fatty acid with three contiguous methylene-interrupted double bonds, a requirement met by dozens of naturally occurring polyunsaturated fatty acids. Brain tissue contains particularly high levels of fatty acids formed from DHA (C22:6 n-3). By the same peroxidation process undergone by AA, DHA in nerve cell membranes is converted to several neuroprostanes. Of these, F4-neuroprostane is a biomarker for several neurodegenerative diseases. A similar mechanism in plants yields phytoprostanes from α-linolenic acid. In contrast to conventional, enzymatically derived PGs that are formed intra-cellularly and released immediately, isoprostanes are formed in the cell membrane, cleaved by phospholipases, circulate in plasma, and are excreted in urine. As stable end products of lipid peroxidation, endogenously formed isoprostanes are useful markers of oxidative stress and independent risk markers for coronary artery disease. They are increased in several diseases, including acute respiratory distress syndrome, in which polymorphonuclear leukocytes generate reactive oxygen species that damage pulmonary epithelium. The immune cells in inflamed tissues are exposed to reactive oxygen intermediates produced by neutrophils and other phagocytic cells. Oxidants are also generated as mediators in intra-cellular signaling pathways by cytokines such as IL-1β and TNF. Isoprostanes are important to and are biomarkers for inflammatory conditions such as vasculitis and RA, and they are assayed in biologic fluids and tissues. Because isoprostanes are released pre-formed, their production is not blocked by NSAIDs, which suppress metabolism of free AA. It is possible that inflammation that is unresponsive to NSAIDs may yield to inhibition of isoprostanes. In keeping with the notion of eicosanoids as regulators, however, some isoprostanes suppress release of mediators of inflammation from macrophages, and a phytoprostane (E1-phytoprostane) signals through PPARγ and NF-κB to suppress IL-12 production by activated dendritic cells and to reduce cytokine production by Th1 and Th2 cells.[72,73]

Endocannabinoids

Groups of naturally occurring members of the eicosanoid superfamily that can activate cannabinoid receptors and are derivatives of long-chain fatty acids have been referred to as *endocannabinoids*. They are not stored in cells. Rather, they are synthesized rapidly in the manner of PGs and LTs from lipid precursors, and are released from—among other cells—cells of the immune system during immune/inflammatory responses. They can then activate cannabinoid receptors on the same or adjacent cells and are metabolized rapidly by the specific serine hydrolase, fatty acid amide hydrolase (FAAH), or by monoglyceride lipase or *N*-acetylethanolamine. Thus inhibition of FAAH offers a strategy for treatment of chronic inflammatory pain.[74] One of the most important endocannabinoids is anandamide (from the Sanskrit word for "bliss"), the amide conjugate of AA and ethanolamine (arachidonoyl

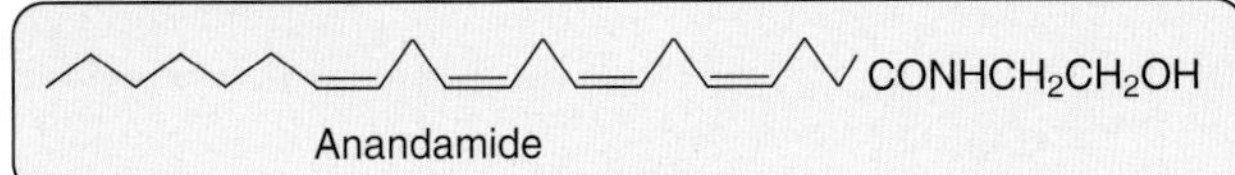

• **Fig. 28.8** Chemical structure of anandamide (arachidonoyl ethanolamide).

ethanolamide; Fig. 28.8). Anandamides and other endocannabinoids, such as 2-arachidonylglycerol and virodamine, are involved in a wide range of regulatory functions, including pain perception and modulation of immune responses, actions mediated via cannabinoid 1 (CB1) and CB2 receptor subtypes, resulting in activation of G proteins of the G(i/o) family. Of particular relevance to joint tissue injury is the capacity of anandamide to suppress TNF-induced NF-κB activation by direct inhibition of IκB kinase, an action that is independent of CB1 or CB2 activation.

Acid congeners of anandamides are lipoamino acids (elmiric acids) that exist as endogenous substances, regulate tissue levels of anandamide, and exhibit anti-inflammatory effects and the capacity to assist resolution of inflammation. One such compound, *N*-arachidonylglycine (NAGly), is found in many tissues at higher concentrations than anandamide. It has analgesic actions similar to those reported for anandamide but does not exhibit psychotropic action. A library of elmiric acids (n-3 and n-6) has been synthesized. Several of these compounds exhibit anti-inflammatory activity, likely in part by increasing production of PGJ_2, and they also modulate immune responses.[75–77]

Discovery of naturally occurring and synthetic analogues and metabolites of anandamide suggest that a family of such biologically active substances exists. The polyunsaturated amides dihomo-γ-linolenoyl (20:3 n-6) and adrenoyl (22:4 n-6) ethanolamides have been found in the mammalian brain.[78] N-3 fatty acid ethanolamides also exist in mammalian tissues. That anandamide can enhance its own synthesis in macrophages suggests the presence of a rapid response to counter excessive inflammatory or immune responses. Anandamide is converted by COX-2 (but not by COX-1) into PGE_2 or $PGF_{2\alpha}$ ethanolamide directly, without going through free AA.[78] These novel PGs ("prostamides") are pharmacologically active.[79] Because anandamide is a substrate for COX-2, inhibitors of COX-2 may reduce anandamide metabolism, with a subsequent increase in concentration of the anandamide. A combination of anandamide with NSAIDs reduces gastric damage and produces synergistic analgesia in experimental models.[80] NAgly, a naturally occurring lipoamino acid, is also a substrate for COX-2, giving rise to amino acid conjugates of the PGs.[81]

Eicosanoid Receptors

For many years, it was thought that the lipophilic eicosanoids—in contrast to the peptide molecules for which receptors were characterized routinely—simply "diffused" into cell membranes or were carried in by a binding protein. The isolation and cloning of eicosanoid receptors changed that thinking.[82]

Prostaglandin Receptors

PGs exert most of their actions through G protein–coupled receptors (GPCRs). Receptors for the COX products are designated P receptors, depending on the prostanoid that has the most affinity for them. These receptors include the PGD receptors (DP); four subtypes of the PGE receptor (EP1 through EP4); the PGF receptor (FP); the PGI_2 receptor (IP); and the TX receptor (TP). The IP, DP, EP2, and EP4 receptors mediate increases in cellular cAMP, whereas the TP, FP, and EP1 receptors induce calcium mobilization. EP2, EP4, and IP regulate macrophage cytokine production in a similar manner. As might be expected, signaling through these receptors is more complicated. Studies designed to understand PGE_2 signaling suggest the involvement of phosphatidylinositol-3-kinase (PI3K), mitogen-activated protein kinase (MAPK), and Wnt pathways in EP2R/EP4R regulation of cell growth, migration, and apoptosis.[34] PGE_2 is the most abundant of the major eicosanoids in the joint space of patients with RA. The molecular mechanisms whereby PGE_2 actions are mediated by each EP subtype have been explained using mice deficient in each subtype.[83] Identification of PGD_2 as the ligand for the DP2 receptor led to the development of DP2 receptor antagonists for treatment of asthma and airway inflammation.[84]

The modification of immune cell and surrounding cell functions by prostanoids during immune or inflammatory responses is influenced by the different repertoire of PG receptors expressed on these cells. Mice deficient in each EP receptor subtype have been generated, and highly selective agonists for these receptors have been developed. As noted, PGE can suppress or induce bone formation.[34] EP2 and EP4 knockout mice exhibit inflammation-induced bone resorption and impaired osteoclastogenesis. The receptor mediating PGE-induced bone formation is unknown, although it has been proposed that EP2R and EP4R mediate the anabolic effects of PGE_2 on bone. In animal models, acute inflammation and pain are completely absent in IP-deficient mice. The profile of PG formation changes as the inflammatory response evolves to a more chronic state, so other receptors are probably involved. It is unlikely that blockade of one receptor will completely block an inflammatory response. More encouraging is the fact that PGs participate in allodynia, a pain response to a usually nonpainful stimulus. Knowing the contribution of P receptors to allodynia should lead to better treatment of neuropathic pain and myofascial pain syndromes such as fibromyalgia.

Stimulation of TX/endoperoxide receptors (TP) elicits platelet aggregation and contraction of vascular smooth muscle and promotes expression of adhesion molecules with subsequent movement of monocytes/macrophages from the circulation to tissue. Thus TP antagonists reduce vascular inflammation, are antithrombotic, and maintain vasodilation, actions that mark them as potential agents for treatment of conditions characterized by chronic inflammation.[85]

The availability of cloned P receptors should assist in the development of more effective receptor-active compounds. The PGI_2 analogue iloprost is useful for treatment of peripheral vascular disease and pulmonary hypertension. Although iloprost binds to IP with high affinity, it also binds to EP1 and EP3. It may be that targeting activation, blockade, or both of a single P receptor or a specific set of P receptors will provide advantages compared with compounds that work "upstream," such as the COX-2 inhibitors or traditional NSAIDs. For example, it is clear that E prostaglandins are the most important of the endogenous eicosanoids for modulation of the function and mucosal integrity of the gastrointestinal tract. Protection by PGE_2 against acid reflux esophagitis and against ethanol- and indomethacin-induced gastric mucosa injury is mimicked by EP1 agonists and attenuated by an EP1 antagonist, whereas EP4 antagonism does not affect the integrity of gastrointestinal mucosa. In addition, PGE_2 does not exhibit gastric cytoprotection in EP1 knockout mice. In the small intestine, the protective effect of PGE_2 on indomethacin-induced damage is mimicked by both EP3 and EP4 agonists.

Further evidence of the importance of eicosanoids in immune cell function and regulation of immune responses derives from experiments with mice deficient in PG receptors, which indicate that PGE_2 assists and amplifies IL-12–mediated Th1 cell differentiation and IL-23–mediated Th17 cell expansion. These PGE_2 actions and those of PGD_2 and PGI_2—also discovered using receptor-deficient mice—contribute to the development of immune diseases.[86] Mice lacking the $PGF_{2\alpha}$ receptor are protected against bleomycin-induced pulmonary fibrosis,[87] a finding with implications for treatment of systemic sclerosis.

The implications for therapy derived from this new knowledge are clear and exciting, but prostanoid analogues with selective binding properties need to be developed. Some progress has been made, and it seems that deletion of P receptors, with the exception of EP4, is not associated with serious problems of fetal development or physiologic function in animals.

Leukotriene Receptors

Surface receptors for LTB_4, denoted BLT1 and BLT2 (LTB_4 R-1 and LTB_4 R-2), and for the cysteinyl (cys) LTs, produced by cells of the innate immune system, including Th2 lymphocytes, also exert their actions through transmembrane-spanning GPCRs. High-affinity LTB_4 receptors transduce chemotaxis and adhesion responses, whereas low-affinity receptors are responsible for the secretion of granule contents and superoxide generation. Recognition that cysLTs are important to the pathogenesis of diseases characterized by acute and chronic inflammation prompted the development of selective cysLT receptor antagonists.[88,89] BLT2 knockout mice express normal levels of BLT1 but are protected from development of disease in the K/BxN model of inflammatory arthritis.[90] The COX-1–derived ligand 12(S)-hydroxyheptadeca-5Z,8E,10E-trienoic acid (12-HHT), which is produced during thromboxane synthesis, is an endogenous high-affinity ligand for BLT2 (now called BLT2/HHTR), another example of a connection between the LOX and COX pathways. LTB_4 in particular among the LTs is involved in the development of atherosclerosis, which has emerged as a major concern for patients with inflammatory arthritis and lupus. The receptor for cysLTs includes two subtypes: $CysLT_1$ and $CysLT_2$. The molecular structure of $CysLT_2$ has been constructed. $CysLT_1$ contains 336 amino acid residues, and the gene encoding the receptor is located on the X chromosome. $CysLT_2$ contains 345 amino acids with 40% sequence identity to $CysLT_1$. $CysLT_1$ mediates calcium mobilization and inhibition of adenylate cyclase, whereas $CysLT_2$ mediates calcium mobilization and increased cAMP concentrations. The preferred ligands for $CysLT_1$ are $LTD_4 > LTC_4 > LTE_4$. $CysLT_2$ binds LTC_4 and LTD_4 equally, whereas LTE_4 exhibits low affinity for the receptor. Both receptors have wide tissue and cellular distribution, including a presence in cells that participate in immune responses.[3] Most actions of the cysLTs are mediated by $CysLT_1$. More than a dozen chemically distinct, specific, and selective antagonist drugs that block the binding of LT to $CysLT_1$ have been identified. Clinically, these compounds have been used mainly in the treatment of asthma. Development of selective LTB_4 receptor antagonists, which are useful in pre-clinical models, may lead to their use in inflammatory disease.[91] A challenge to the design of "anti-receptor therapy" is the genetic variation in GPCRs that can be associated with disease.[92] Adding to the complexity is the fact that variants may result in altered predisposition to disease, rather than manifestation of the disease. Each variant provides an opportunity to understand receptor function such as recycling or desensitization, thus enhancing the potential for the development of therapy.

Lipoxin Receptors

LXs can act at their own specific receptors for LXA_4 and LXB_4, and LXA_4 can interact with a subtype of LTD_4 receptors. LXs can also act at intra-cellular targets within their cell of origin or after uptake by another cell. The seven-transmembrane-spanning, G protein–coupled LXA_4 receptor named ALX/FPR2 (Kd ~ 0.7 nM) has been cloned and characterized. Signaling involves a novel polyisoprenyl-phosphate pathway that regulates phospholipase D.[93] LX actions are cell type specific. The monocyte and neutrophil LXA_4 receptors are identical at the DNA sequence level, but they evoke different responses, and the LXA_4 receptor on endothelial cells seems to be a structurally distinct form. LXA_4 also binds to the human orphan receptor GPR32, a member of the chemoattractant receptor family. Like LXA_4, 15-epi-LXA_4 is an anti-inflammatory SPM that binds and activates ALX/FPR2 (Kd ~ 2 nM). Lipoxin B_4 (LXB_4) and aspirin-triggered 15-epi LXB_4 also have anti-inflammatory actions by oral administration and topical application. Stereoselective actions of these compounds indicate they have their own yet-to-be-identified receptors. The resolvins, derived from omega-3 fatty acids, activate the receptors GPR32 and ChemR23.

Nuclear Receptors

Nuclear receptors are a superfamily of ligand-regulated transcription factors that interact with other transcription factors and with co-regulators that either enhance (co-activators) or inhibit (co-repressors) transcription. The major nuclear receptors involved in regulation of inflammation are the glucocorticoid receptors (GRs), peroxisome proliferator-activated receptors, liver X receptors (LXRs), and the orphan receptor nuclear receptor–related 1 protein (Nurr1). Other members of the nuclear receptor family that contribute to regulation of inflammation include estrogen receptors, vitamin D receptors, and retinoic acid receptors. The clinical efficacy of glucocorticoids is well known, but knowledge of their mechanisms of action has been slow to emerge. The ability of GRs to repress inflammatory responses is due in part to interference with other signal-dependent transcription factors and disruption of activator/co-activator complexes. PPARs are members of the nuclear receptor family of transcription factors, a large and diverse group of proteins that mediate ligand-dependent transcriptional activation and repression. PPARs were first cloned as nuclear receptors that mediate the effects on gene transcription of synthetic compounds called *peroxisome proliferators.* Several mechanisms account for the anti-inflammatory action of PPARγ, including inhibition of NF-κB; inhibition of transcription of genes encoding for IL-1β, IL-12, MMP-9, and chemokines; and promotion of expression of anti-inflammatory mediators, including IL-10 and LXR. PPARγ can be modulated by post-translational modifications (PTMs). Thus regulation of PTMs may be a better approach to disease therapy than the existing PPARγ activators.[94] Interest in PPARs increased dramatically when they were activated by medically relevant compounds, including NSAIDs and PGD_2 and its metabolite 15-deoxy-δ12,14 PGJ_2.[95] Most information available on the potential role of PPARs in inflammation relates to PPARγ. One PPARα agonist, palmitoyl ethanolamide, shows promise for relief of chronic pain.[96] PPARα is expressed mainly in tissues that have a high fatty acid catabolism, including liver and the immune system. LTB_4 is an activator and natural ligand of PPARα. Activation of PPARα results in induction of genes involved in fatty acid oxidation pathways that degrade fatty acids and derivatives, including LTB_4. Thus a feedback mechanism that controls inflammation is established. Mechanisms for the anti-inflammatory actions of PPARβ/δ include induction of an anti-inflammatory co-repressor protein, inhibition of NF-κB, and induction of anti-inflammatory mediators. Experiments with PPAR knockout mice indicate that PPARα suppresses LTB_4-induced inflammation. PPAR agonists that target PPAR action more selectively are being developed.[97] Overexpression of Nurr receptors reduces inflammatory cytokine expression, and mutations in the Nurr1 gene are associated with diminished counter-regulation of inflammation.[98]

Several kinases that facilitate co-repressor turnover have been identified. These kinases represent important pharmacologic targets because their inhibition should block gene expression of inflammatory mediators while bypassing the clinically significant adverse events associated with direct targeting of the nuclear receptors. For example, cartilage matrix degradation is prevented by inhibition of a cyclin-dependent kinase.[98]

Platelet-Activating Factor

PAF (1-0-alkyl-2-acetyl-sn-glycero-3-phosphocholine) is a potent mediator of inflammation that causes neutrophil activation, increased vascular permeability, vasodilation, and bronchoconstriction, in addition to platelet activation. PAF is formed by a smaller number of cell types than the eicosanoids, mainly leukocytes, platelets, and endothelial cells. Because of the extensive distribution of these cells, however, the actions of PAF can manifest in virtually every organ system. In contrast to the two long-chain acyl groups present in phosphatidylcholine, PAF contains a long-chain alkyl group joined to the glycerol backbone in an ether linkage at position 1 and an acetyl group at position 2 (Fig. 28.9). PAF represents a family of phospholipids (PAF-like lipids: PAF-LL) because the alkyl group at position 1 can vary in length from 12 to 18 carbons. PAF, similar to the eicosanoids, is not stored in cells. Rather, it is synthesized when cells are stimulated, at which time the composition of the alkyl group may change. The immediate effects of PAF are mediated through a cell surface GPCR, PAFR. PAFR is coupled to Gi, Gq, and G12/13. Activation of PAFR results in inhibition of cAMP, mobilization of calcium, and activation of MAPKs, whereas long-term responses depend on intra-cellular receptor activation.[99]

Despite the potent inflammatory effects of PAF, its inhibition in animal models does not lead to marked suppression of inflammatory responses. PAF acetylhydrolase (PAF-AH) circulates in blood in association with lipoproteins, is found in atherosclerotic lesions, and hydrolyzes PAF, and was thus considered to have anti-inflammatory properties and to be a marker for cardiovascular disease. At the same time, however, PAF-AH also generates compounds that have pro-inflammatory activity, which likely explains why, in three clinical trials, a PAF-AH inhibitor failed to influence C-reactive protein levels, coronary atherosclerosis, or time to cardiovascular death.[100,101] Nonetheless, targeting PAF metabolism, signaling, and the PAF receptor, as monotherapy or with other agents, is a promising approach to suppression of inflammation and carcinogenesis.[102]

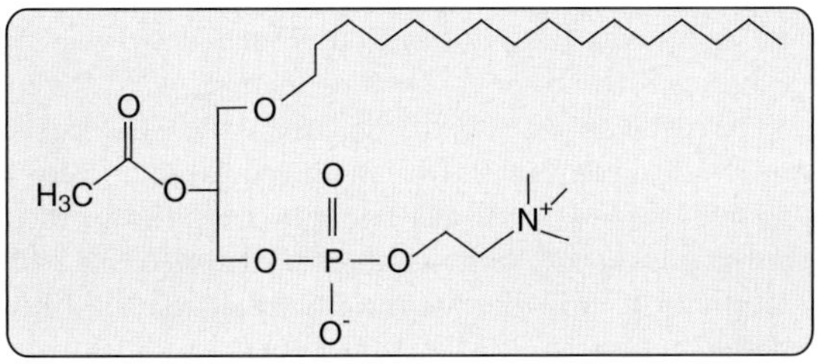

• **Fig. 28.9** Chemical structure of platelet-activating factor.

Eicosanoids as Regulators of Inflammation and Immune Responses

In addition to their well-known actions as mediators of inflammation, the stable PGs PGE_1 and PGI_2 have anti-inflammatory, inflammatory, and immunomodulatory actions.[103,104] As noted,[68–70] PGJ, LXs, and an array of eicosanoids act as brakes to protect against runaway inflammatory responses. Even LTB_4 is capable of modulating inflammation and immune responses.[56] The observations that PGE_1 inhibits platelet aggregation and that it suppresses acute and chronic inflammation and joint tissue injury in animal models[105] led to the notion that COX products of AA metabolism might have anti-inflammatory activity. As it became more clear that NSAIDs have anti-inflammatory effects other than interference with COX production and subsequent PG inhibition,[106] consideration was given to the potential protective effects of PGs.

PGE_1 has remained an orphan among the eicosanoids, mainly because of a long-held notion that not enough of it is made by human cells to be of use and that its biologic effects are no different from the effects of PGE_2 and PGI_2. Contrary to popular belief, PGE_1 is found in physiologically important amounts in humans. Lost in the vast literature on the "AA cascade" are the early observations of Bygdeman and Samuelsson,[107] who found (using bioassay) that the concentration of PGE_1 in human seminal plasma (16 μg/mL) was higher than that of PGE_2 (13 μg/mL), PGE_3 (3 μg/mL), $PGF_{1\alpha}$ (2 μg/mL), and $PGF_{2\alpha}$ (12 μg/mL). One group[108] found PGE_1 to be the sole PGE in human thymus. PG immunoassays usually do not distinguish between PGE_1 and PGE_2. To identify PGE_1, it must first be separated from PGE_2 by thin-layer or high-performance liquid chromatography. When such methods have been used, PGE_1 has been identified consistently in platelets, leukocytes, macrophages, vas deferens, oviducts, uterus, heart, and skin.[109] Evidence from in vitro and in vivo experiments indicates that PGs, notably PGE compounds, can suppress diverse effector systems of inflammation. PGE can enhance and diminish cellular and humoral immune responses, observations that reinforce a view of these compounds as regulators of cell function. These actions of eicosanoids depend on the stimulus to inflammation, the predominant eicosanoid produced at a particular time in the host response, and the profile of eicosanoid-receptor expression.[110,111]

The "2" series prostaglandins (i.e., E2, D2, and I2) also regulate T cell function and immune responses. PGE_2 reduces production of several inflammatory cytokines, including TNF, IFN-γ, and IL-12, and reduces IFN-α production by plasmacytoid dendritic cells (PDCs) from patients with SLE. PGE_2-treated PDCs from patients with SLE also induce $CD4^+$ T cell proliferation and skew cytokine production toward a Th2 profile.[112] Another example of an endogenous link between the COX and LOX pathways is provided by the observation that PGE_2 preserves resolution of inflammation in the murine collagen–induced arthritis model by increasing production of the pro-resolving LXA_4.[113]

Modulation of Eicosanoid Synthesis by Administration of Precursor Fatty Acids

The relationship between essential fatty acids and PGs was discovered simultaneously and independently by two groups.[114,115] Both groups reported that AA was converted to PGE_2, and shortly thereafter they showed that PGE_1 is formed from DGLA.[116] Attempts to modify eicosanoid production have been directed at providing fatty acids other than AA as substrates for oxygenation enzymes in an effort to generate a unique eicosanoid profile with immunosuppressive and anti-inflammatory effects.[63,117] The fatty acids themselves, by virtue of their incorporation into signal-transduction elements, also have effects independent of the eicosanoid effects on cells involved in inflammation and immune responses.[118]

Experiments directed at suppression of TX synthesis, enhancement of PGI production, and inhibition of platelet aggregation have been done in an effort to limit inflammatory responses. EPA is not found in appreciable amounts in cells from people who eat a Western-style diet. Fish oil lipids, which are rich in EPA (20:5 n-3), inhibit formation of COX products (e.g., TXA_2 and PGE_2) derived from AA, and the newly formed TXA_3 has much less ability than TXA_2 to constrict vessels and aggregate platelets. Production of PGI_2 (prostacyclin) by endothelial cells is not reduced appreciably by increased EPA content, and the physiologic activity of newly synthesized PGI_3 is added to that of PGI_2. Administration of fish oil to humans leads to reduced production of LTB_4 by means of 5-LOX in stimulated neutrophils and monocytes and induces EPA-derived LTB_5, which is far less biologically active than LTB_4. Fish oil also reduces production of IL-1β, TNF, and PAF by activated blood monocytes. In randomized controlled trials of administration of fish oil to patients with RA, tender joint counts and duration of morning stiffness were reduced, and use of NSAIDs decreased. Fish oil treatment of patients with early RA (<12 months) reduces the triple therapy conventional disease-modifying anti-rheumatic drug (DMARD) failure rate and increases the American College of Rheumatology (ACR) remission rate.[119] Because NSAIDs confer an increased risk for cardiovascular disease and increased mortality from cardiovascular disease occurs in patients with RA, an added benefit of fish oil for patients with RA may be reduced risk of cardiovascular disease directly and by virtue of less use of NSAIDs.[120] Another potential benefit of an increase in dietary omega-3 fatty acids might be greater formation, from EPA and DHA, of resolvins, protectins, and maresins, all of which participate in resolution of inflammation.[66,68–70]

The other "alternative" eicosanoid precursor fatty acid, DGLA (20:3 n-6), is also increased by administration of certain plant seed oils, notably oils extracted from the seeds of *Oenothera biennis* (evening primrose) and *Boragio officinalis* (borage), which contain relatively large amounts of GLA. GLA is converted to DGLA, the immediate precursor of PGE_1, an eicosanoid with known anti-inflammatory and immunoregulating properties.[103] Administration of GLA to volunteers and patients with RA results in increased production of PGE_1 and reduced production of the inflammatory eicosanoids PGE_2, LTB_4, and LTC_4 by stimulated peripheral blood monocytes. In addition to competing with AA for oxidative enzymes, DGLA cannot be converted to inflammatory LTs. Rather, it is converted by means of 15-LOX to a 15-hydroxy-DGLA, which has the capacity to inhibit 5-LOX and 12-LOX activities. DGLA should have anti-inflammatory actions because of its capacity to reduce synthesis of oxygenation products of AA through the COX and LOX pathways.[117,121]

In addition to their roles as precursors of eicosanoids, essential fatty acids are important for the maintenance of cell membrane structure and function, and they protect the gastric mucosa from NSAID-induced injury. DGLA can also modulate immune responses in an eicosanoid-independent manner. DGLA suppresses IL-2 production by human peripheral blood monocytes in vitro, suppresses proliferation of IL-2–dependent human peripheral blood and synovial tissue T lymphocytes, and reduces expression of activation markers on T lymphocytes directly in a manner that is independent of its conversion to eicosanoids. Oral administration of oils enriched in GLA, but not administration of oils enriched in linoleic acid (the parent n-6 fatty acid) or α-linolenic acid (the parent n-3 fatty acid), reduces proliferation of human lymphocytes activated through the T cell receptor complex.[122]

The addition of GLA to peripheral blood mononuclear cells in vitro or oral administration of GLA to volunteers reduces production of IL-1β and TNF from stimulated cells and reduces autoinduction of IL-1β, preserving the protective effects of IL-1β, while suppressing excessive production of the cytokine.[123] GLA has suppressed acute and chronic inflammation, including arthritis, in several animal models; and randomized, double-blind, placebo-controlled trials of GLA in patients with RA and active synovitis indicated that GLA treatment results in statistically significant and clinically relevant reduction in signs and symptoms of disease activity compared with baseline and placebo. GLA also reduces the need for NSAID and corticosteroid therapy.[124,125]

EPA suppresses conversion of DGLA to AA, and a combination of EPA-enriched and GLA-enriched oils exhibited synergy in its capacity to reduce the induction of synovitis in animal models.[126] In addition, administration of black currant seed oil, which contains the n-3 fatty acid α-linolenic acid (which is converted to EPA) and the n-6 GLA, suppresses active synovitis in patients with RA.[127] The synergy observed in the animal models was not reprised in an 18-month double-blind trial of a combination of fish oil and borage oil in patients with RA. Nevertheless, treatment with each oil alone and with the combination resulted in meaningful clinical responses equivalent to treatment with methotrexate, including a reduction in drug therapy greater than that seen in matched patients from an RA registry. In addition, all three treatment groups exhibited significantly reduced total and low-density lipoprotein cholesterol and triglycerides, increased high-density lipoprotein cholesterol, and an improved plasma atherogenic index.[128,129] Much larger amounts of the polyunsaturated fatty acids (GLA, EPA, and DHA) can be delivered in far smaller capsules than are needed to accommodate the natural oils, a strategy that should be adopted to improve compliance.

Full references for this chapter can be found on ExpertConsult.com.

Selected References

1. Brash AR: Specific lipoxygenase attack on arachidonic acid and linoleate esterified in phosphatidylcholine: precedent for an alternative mechanism in activation of eicosanoid biosynthesis, *Adv Prostaglandin Thromboxane Leukot Res* 15:197–199, 1985.

2. Dennis EA, Cao J, Hsu YH, et al.: Phospholipase A2 enzymes: physical structure, biological function, disease implication, chemical inhibition, and therapeutic intervention, *Chem Rev* 111:6130, 2011.
3. Krizaj J: Roles of secreted phospholipases A2 in the mammalian immune system, *Protein Pept Lett* 21:1201–1208, 2014.
4. Sun GY, Chuang DY, Zong Y, et al.: Role of cytosolic phospholipase A2 in oxidative and inflammatory signaling pathways in different cell types in the central nervous system, *Mol Neurobiol* 50:6–14, 2014.
5. Hasham SN, Pillarisetti S: Vascular lipases, inflammation, and atherosclerosis, *Clin Chim Acta* 372:179, 2006.
6. Bomalaski JS, Clark MA, Zurier RB: Enhanced phospholipase activity in peripheral blood monocytes from patients with rheumatoid arthritis, *Arthritis Rheum* 29:312, 1986.
7. Boillard E, Lai Y, Larabee K, et al.: A novel anti-inflammatory role for phospholipase A2 in immune complex-mediated arthritis, *EMBO Mol Med* 2:172, 2010.
8. Bryant KJ, Bidgood MJ, Lei PW: A bifunctional role for group IIA secreted phospholipase A2 in human rheumatoid fibroblast-like synoviocyte arachidonic acid metabolism, *J Biol Chem* 286:2492, 2011.
9. Gomez-Cambronero J: New concepts in phospholipase D signaling in inflammation and cancer, *Sci World J* 10:1356, 2010.
10. Budd DC, Qian Y: Development of lysophosphatidic acid pathway modulators as therapies for fibrosis, *Future Med Chem* 5:2013, 1935.
11. Botting RM: Vane's discovery of the mechanism of action of aspirin changed our understanding of its clinical pharmacology, *Pharmacol Rep* 62:518, 2010.
12. Bozza PT, Yu W, Penrose JF, et al.: Eosinophil lipid bodies: specific, inducible intracellular sites for enhanced eicosanoid formation, *J Exp Med* 186:909, 1997.
13. Smith WL, DeWitt DL, Garavito RM: Cyclooxygenases: structural, cellular, and molecular biology, *Annu Rev Biochem* 69:145, 2000.
14. Roos KL, Simmons DL: Cyclooxygenase variants: the role of alternative splicing, *Biochem Biophys Res Commun* 338:62, 2005.
15. Rouzer CA, Marnett LJ: Cyclooxygenases: structural and functional insights, *J Lipid Res* 50:S29, 2009.
16. Telliez A, Furman C, Pommery N, et al.: Mechanisms leading to COX-2 expression and COX-2 induced tumorigenesis: topical therapeutic strategies targeting COX-2 expression and activity, *Anticancer Agents Med Chem* 6:187, 2006.
17. Debey S, Meyer-Kirchrath J, Schror K: Regulation of cyclooxygenase-2 expression in iloprost in human vascular smooth muscle cells: role of transcription factors CREB and ICER, *Biochem Pharmacol* 65:979, 2003.
18. Morris T, Stables M, Gilroy DW: New perspectives on aspirin and the endogenous control of acute inflammatory resolution, *Sci World J* 6:1048, 2006.
19. Dinchuk JE, Car BD, Focht RJ, et al.: Renal abnormalities and an altered inflammatory response in mice lacking cyclooxygenase II, *Nature* 378:406, 1995.
20. Lewis T: *The lives of a cell*, New York, 1995, Penguin.
21. Cornett AL, Lutz CS: Regulation of COX-2 expression by miR-146a in lung cancer cells, *RNA* 20:1419–1430, 2014.
22. Snipes JA: Cloning and characterization of cyclooxygenase-1b (putative Cox-3) in rat, *J Pharm Exp Ther* 313:668, 2005.
23. Wu KK, Liou JY: Cellular and molecular biology of prostacyclin synthase, *Biochem Biophys Res Commun* 338:45, 2005.
24. Korbecki J, Baranowska-Bosiacka I, Gutowska I, et al.: The effect of reactive oxygen species on the synthesis of prostanoids from arachidonic acid, *J Physiol Pharmacol* 64:409, 2013.
25. Liu F, Mih JD, Shea BS, et al.: Feedback amplification of fibrosis through matrix stiffening and COX-2 suppression, *J Cell Biol* 190:693, 2010.
26. Koeberle A, Werz O: Inhibitors of the microsomal prostaglandin E(2) synthase-1 as alternative to non steroidal anti-inflammatory drugs (NSAIDs)—a critical review, *Curr Med Chem* 16:4274, 2009.
27. Gosset M, Pigenet A, Salvat C, et al.: Inhibition of matrix metalloproteinase-3 and -13 synthesis induced by IL-1β in chondrocytes from mice lacking microsomal prostaglandin E synthase-1, *J Immunol* 185:6244, 2010.
28. Kurzrock R, Lieb CC: Biochemical studies of human semen, II: the action of semen on the human uterus, *Proc Soc Exp Biol Med* 28:268, 1930.
29. von Euler US: On the specific vasodilating and plain muscle stimulating substances from accessory genital glands in man and certain animals (prostaglandin and vesiglandin), *J Physiol (Lond)* 88:213, 1936.
30. Bergstrom S, Ryhage R, Samuelsson B: The structure of prostaglandins E_1, F_1, and F_2, *Acta Chem Scand* 16:501, 1962.
31. Rodriguez M, Domingo E, Municio C, et al.: Polarization of the innate immune response by prostaglandin E2: a puzzle of receptors and signals, *Mol Pharmacol* 85:187, 2014.
32. Raisz LG: Pathogenesis of osteoporosis: concepts, conflicts, and prospects, *J Clin Invest* 115:3318, 2005.
33. Marks SC, Miller SC: Prostaglandins and the skeleton: the legacy and challenges of two decades of research, *Endocr J* 1:337, 1993.
34. Blackwell CA, Raisz LG, Pilbeam CC: Prostaglandins in bone: bad cop, good cop? *Trends Endocrinol Metab* 21:294, 2010.
35. Abramson SB, Yazici Y: Biologics in development for rheumatoid arthritis: relevance to osteoarthritis, *Adv Drug Deliv Rev* 58:212, 2006.
36. Abramson SB: Developments in the scientific understanding of osteoarthritis, *Arthritis Res Ther* 11:227, 2009.
37. Hueber AJ, Asquith DL, Miller AM, et al.: Mast cells express IL-17A in rheumatoid arthritis synovium, *J Immunol* 184:3336, 2010.
38. Scher JU, Pillinger MH: The anti-inflammatory effects of prostaglandins, *J Investig Med* 57:703, 2009.
39. Zhu X, Walton RG, Tian L, et al.: Prostaglandin A2 enhances cellular insulin sensitivity via a mechanism that involves the orphan nuclear receptor NR4A3, *Horm Metab Res* 45:213, 2013.
40. Moncada S, Gryglewski R, Bunting S, et al.: An enzyme isolated from arteries transforms prostaglandin endoperoxides to an unstable substance that inhibits platelet aggregation, *Nature* 263:633, 1976.
41. Bertagnolli MM, Eagle CJ, Zauber AG, et al.: Celecoxib for the prevention of sporadic colorectal adenomas, *N Engl J Med* 355:873, 2006.
42. Zamanian RT, Kudelko KT, Sung YK, et al.: Current clinical management of pulmonary arterial hypertension, *Circ Res* 115:131–147, 2014.
43. Sharma M, Pinnamaneni S, Aronow WS, et al.: Existing drugs and drugs under investigation for pulmonary arterial hypertension, *Cardiol Rev* 22:297–305, 2014.
44. Vorhies EE, Caruthers RL, Rosenberg H, et al.: Use of inhaled iloprost for the management of postoperative pulmonary hypertension in congenital heart surgery patients: review of a transition protocol, *Pediatr Cardiol* 35:1337–1343, 2014.
45. Remuzzi G, Fitzgerald GA, Patrono C: Thromboxane synthesis and action within the kidney, *Kidney Int* 41:1483, 1992.
46. Neath SX, Jefferies JL, Berger JS, et al.: The current and future landscape of urinary thromboxane testing to evaluate atherothrombotic risk, *Rev Cardiovasc Med* 15:119, 2014.
47. Floyd CN, Ferro A: Mechanisms of aspirin resistance, *Pharmacol Ther* 141(69), 2014.
48. Sakariassen KS, Alberts P, Fontana P, et al.: Effect of pharmaceutical interventions targeting thromboxane receptors and thromboxane synthase in cardiovascular and renal diseases, *Future Cardiol* 5:479, 2009.

49. Shankar H, Kahner B, Kunapuli SP: G-protein dependent platelet signaling: perspectives for therapy, *Curr Drug Targets* 7:1253, 2006.
50. Osher E, Weisinger G, Limor R, et al.: The 5 lipoxygenase system in the vasculature: emerging role in health and disease, *Mol Cell Endocrinol* 252:201, 2006.
51. Chang WC, Chen BK: Transcription factor Sp1 functions as an anchor protein in gene transcription of human 12(S)-lipoxygenase, *Biochem Biophys Res Commun* 338:117, 2005.
52. Corser-Jensen CE, Goodell DJ, Freund RK, et al.: Blocking leukotriene synthesis attenuates the pathophysiology of traumatic brain injury and associated cognitive deficits, *Exp Neurol* 256:7–16, 2014.
53. Rådmark O, Werz O, Steinhilber D, et al.: 5-Lipoxygenase, a key enzyme for leukotriene biosynthesis in health and disease, *Biochim Biophys Acta* 1851:331, 2015.
54. Folco G, Murphy RC: Eicosanoid transcellular biosynthesis: from cell-cell interactions to in vivo tissue responses, *Pharmacol Rev* 58:375, 2006.
55. Korotkova M, Lundberg IE: The skeletal muscle arachidonic acid cascade in health and inflammatory disease, *Nat Rev Rheumatol* 10:295, 2014.
56. Le Bel M, Brunet A, Gosselin J: Leukotriene B4, an endogenous stimulator of the innate immune response against pathogens, *J Innate Immun* 6:159, 2014.
57. Kanaoka Y, Boyce JA: Cysteinyl leukotrienes and their receptors; emerging concepts, *Allergy Asthma Immunol Res* 6:288, 2014.
58. Caliskan B, Banoglu E: Overview of recent drug discovery approaches for new generation leukotriene A4 hydrolase inhibitors, *Expert Opin Drug Discov* 8(49), 2013.
59. Bukhari SN, Lauro G, Jantan I, et al.: Pharmacological evaluation and docking studies of alpha,beta-unsaturated carbonyl based synthetic compounds as inhibitors of secretory phospholipase A2, cyclooxygenases, lipoxygenase and proinflammatory cytokines, *Bioorg Med Chem* 22:4151, 2014.
60. Nieves D, Moreno JJ: Hydroxyeicosatetraenoic acids released through cytochrome P450 pathway regulate 3T6 fibroblast growth, *J Lipid Res* 47:2681–2689, 2006.
61. Meirer K, Steinhilber D, Proschak E: Inhibitors of the arachidonic acid cascade: interfering with multiple pathways, *Basic Clin Pharmacol Toxicol* 114:83, 2014.
62. Mani I, Iversen L, Ziboh VA: Upregulation of nuclear PKC and MAP-kinase during hyperproliferation of guinea pig epidermis: modulation by 13-(s) hydroxyoctadecadienoic acid (13-HODE), *Cell Signal* 10(143), 1998.
63. Calder PC: Marine omega-3 fatty acids and inflammatory processes: Effects, mechanisms, and clinical relevance, *Biochim Biophys Acta* 1851:469–484, 2014.
64. Serhan CN, Cish CB, Brannon J, et al.: Anti-microinflammatory lipid signals generated from dietary N-3 fatty acids via cyclooxygenase-2 and transcellular processing: a novel mechanism for NSAID and N-3 PUFA therapeutic actions, *J Physiol Pharmacol* 51:643, 2000.
65. Ryan GB, Majno G: Acute inflammation. A review, *Am J Pathol* 86:185, 1977.
66. Serhan CN, Chiang N: Resolution phase mediators of inflammation: agonists of resolution, *Curr Opin Pharmacol* 13(1), 2013.
67. Ohse T, Ota T, Godson C, et al.: Modulation of interferon induced genes by lipoxin analogue in anti-glomerular basement membrane nephritis, *J Am Soc Nephrol* 15:919, 2004.
68. Buckley CD, Gilroy DW, Serhan CN: Proresolving lipid mediators and mechanisms in the resolution of acute inflammation, *Immunity* 40:315, 2014.
69. Serhan CN, Levy: Pro-resolving lipid mediators are leads for resolution physiology, *Nature* 510(92), 2014.
70. Spite M, Claria J, Serhan CN: Resolvins, specialized pro-resolving lipid mediators, and their potential roles in metabolic diseases, *Cell Metab* 19:21, 2014.
71. Vigor C, Bertrand-Michel J, Pinot E, et al.: Nonenzymatic lipid oxidation products in biological systems: assessment of the metabolites from polyunsaturated fatty acids, *J Chromatogr B Analyt Technol Biomed Life Sci* 964:65–78, 2014.
72. Leung KS, Galano JM, Durand T, et al.: Current development in non-enzymatic lipid peroxidation products, isoprostanoids, and isofuranoids in novel biological samples, *Free Radic Res* 49:816–826, 2014.
73. Bauerova K, Acquaviva A, Ponist S, et al.: Markers of inflammation and oxidative stress studied in adjuvant induced arthritis in the rat on systemic and local level affected by pinosylvin and methotrexate and their combination, *Autoimmunity* 48:46–56, 2014.
74. Pertwee RG: Elevating endocannabinoid levels: pharmacological strategies and potential therapeutic applications, *Proc Nutr Soc* 73:96, 2014.
75. Burstein S: The elmiric acids: biologically active anandamide analogs, *Neuropharmacology* 55:1259, 2008.
76. Sido JM, Nagarkatti PS, Nagarkatti M: Role of endocannabinoid activation of peripheral CB1 receptors in the regulation of autoimmune diseases, *Int Rev Immunol* 34:403–414, 2014.
77. Witkampf R, Meijerink J: The endocannabinoid system: an emerging key player in inflammation, *Curr Opin Clin Nutr Metab Care* 17:130, 2014.
78. Alhouayek M, Muccioli GG: COX-2 derived endocannabinoid metabolites as novel inflammatory mediators, *Trends Pharmacol Sci* 35:284, 2014.
79. Davis MP: Cannabinoids in pain management: CB1, CB2 and non-classic receptor ligands, *Expert Opin Investig Drugs* 23:1123, 2014.
80. Cipriano M, Bjorklund E, Wilson AA, et al.: Inhibition of fatty acid amide hydrolase and cyclooxygenase by the N-(3-methylpyridin-2-yl)amide derivatives of flurbiprofen and naproxen, *Eur J Pharmacol* 720:383, 2013.
81. Kohno M, Hasegawa H, Inoue A, et al.: Identification of N-arachidonylglycine as the endogenous ligand for the orphan G-protein-coupled receptor GPR18, *Biochem Biophys Res Commun* 347:827, 2006.
82. Hata AN, Breyer RM: Pharmacology and signaling of prostaglandin receptors: multiple roles in inflammation and immune modulation, *Pharmacol Ther* 103:147, 2006.
83. Clark P, Rowland S, Denis D: MF498[N-{[4-(5,9-diethoxy-6-oxo-6,8-dihydro-7H-pyrrolo[3,4-g]quinolin-7-yl)-3-methylbenzyl] sulfonyl}-2-(2-methoxyphenyl)acetamide], a selective prostanoid receptor 4 antagonist, relieves joint inflammation and pain in rodent models of rheumatoid and osteoarthritis, *J Pharmacol Exp Ther* 325:425, 2008.
84. Norman P: Update on the status of DP2 receptor antagonists: from proof of concept through clinical failures to promising new drugs, *Expert Opin Investig Drugs* 23(55), 2014.
85. Capra V, Back M, Angiolillo DJ, et al.: Impact of vascular thromboxane prostanoid receptor activation on hemostasis, thrombosis, oxidative stress, and inflammation, *J Thromb Haemost* 12:126, 2014.
86. Sakata D, Yao C, Narumiya S: Emerging roles of prostanoids in T cell-mediated immunity, *IUBMB Life* 62:591, 2010.
87. Oga T, Matsuoka T, Yao C, et al.: Prostaglandin F(2alpha) receptor signaling facilitates bleomycin-induced pulmonary fibrosis independently of transforming growth factor-beta, *Nat Med* 15:1426, 2009.
88. Kanaoka Y, Boyce JA: Cysteinyl leukotrienes and their receptors; emerging concepts, *Allergy Asthma Immunol Res* 6:288, 2014.
89. Theron AJ, Steel HC, Tintiger GR, et al.: Cysteinyl leukotriene receptor-1 antagonists as modulators of innate immune cell function, *J Immunol Res* 2014:608930, 2014.
90. Mathis SP, Jala VR, Lee D, et al.: Nonredundant roles for leukotriene receptors BLT1 and BLT2 in inflammatory arthritis, *J Immunol* 185:3049, 2010.
91. Di Gennaro A, Haeggstrom JZ: Targeting leukotriene B4 in inflammation, *Expert Opin Ther Targets* 18:79, 2014.

92. Thompson MD, Hendy GN, Percy ME, et al.: G protein-coupled receptor mutations in human genetic disease, *Methods Mol Biol* 1175:153, 2014.
93. Back M, Powell WS, Dahlen S-E, et al.: Update on leukotriene, lipoxin and oxoeicosanoid receptors: IUPHAR Review 7, *Br J Pharmacol* 171:3551, 2014.
94. Choi SS, Park J, Choi JH: Revisiting PPARγ as a target for treatment of metabolic disorders, *BMB Rep* 47:599–608, 2014.
95. Ricote M, Li AC, Willson TM, et al.: The peroxisome-proliferator-activated receptor-gamma is a negative regulator of macrophage activation, *Nature* 391(79), 1998.
96. Freitag CM, Miller RJ: Peroxisome proliferator-activated receptor agonists modulate neuropathic pain: a link to chemokines? *Front Cell Neurosci* 8:238, 2014.
97. Wright MB, Bortolini M, Tadayyon M, et al.: Minireview: Challenges and opportunities in development of PPAR agonists, *Mol Endocrinol* 28:1756–1768, 2014.
98. Yik JH, Hu Z, Kumari R, et al.: Cyclin-dependent kinase 9 inhibition protects cartilage from the catabolic effects of proinflammatory cytokines, *Arthritis Rheumatol* 66:1537, 2014.
99. Xu H, Valenzuela N, Fai S, et al.: Targeted lipidomics—advances in profiling lysophosphocholine and platelet-activating factor second messengers, *FEBS J* 280:5652, 2013.
100. Marathe GK, Pandit CL, Lakshmikanth VH, et al.: To hydrolyse or not to hydrolyse: the dilemma of platelet activating factor acetyl hydrolase (PAF-AH), *J Lipid Res* 55:1847, 2014.
101. Stafforini DM, Zimmerman GA: Unraveling the PAF-AH/Lp-PLA2 controversy, *J Lipid Res* 55:1811, 2014.
102. Yu Y, Zhang M, Cai Q, et al.: Synergistic effects of combined platelet-activating factor receptor and epidermal growth factor receptor targeting in ovarian cancer cells, *J Hematol Oncol* 7:39, 2014.
103. Zurier RB: Prostaglandins: then, now, and next, *Semin Arth Rheum* 33:137, 2003.
104. Manferdini C, Maumus M, Gabusi E, et al.: Adipose-derived mesenchymal stem cells exert anti-inflammatory effects on chondrocytes and synoviocytes from osteoarthritic patients through prostaglandin E2, *Arthritis Rheum* 65:1271, 2013.
105. Zurier RB, Hoffstein S, Weissmann G: Suppression of acute and chronic inflammation in adrenalectomized rats by pharmacologic amounts of prostaglandins, *Arthritis Rheum* 16:606, 1973.
106. Weissmann G, Montesinos MC, Pillinger M, et al.: Non-prostaglandin effects of aspirin III and salicylate: inhibition of integrin-dependent human neutrophil aggregation and inflammation in COX2 and NF kappa B (P105)-knockout mice, *Adv Exp Med Biol* 507:571, 2002.
107. Bygdeman M, Samuelsson B: Quantitative determination of prostaglandins in human semen, *Clin Chim Acta* 10:566, 1964.
108. Karim SMM, Soindler M, Williams ED: Distribution of prostaglandins in human tissues, *Br J Pharmacol Chemother* 31:340, 1967.
109. Horrobin DF: The roles of essential fatty acids in the development of diabetic neuropathy and other complications of diabetes mellitus, *Prostaglandins Leukot Essent Fatty Acids* 31:181, 1988.
110. Ricciotti E, Fitzgerald GA: Prostaglandins and inflammation, *Arterioscler Thromb Vasc Biol* 31:986, 2011.
111. Torres R, Herrerias A, Sera-Pages M, et al.: Locally administered prostaglandin E_2 prevents aeroallergen-induced airway sensitization in mice through immunomodulatory mechanisms, *Pharmacol Res* 70(50), 2013.
112. Fabricus D, Neubauer M, Mandel B, et al.: Prostaglandin E2 inhibits IFN-α secretion and Th1 costimulation by human plasmacytoid dendritic cells via E-prostanoid 2 and E-prostanoid 4 receptor engagement, *J Immunol* 184:677, 2010.
113. Chan MM, Moore AR: Resolution of inflammation in murine autoimmune arthritis is disrupted by cyclooxygenase-2 inhibition and restored by prostaglandin E2-mediated lipoxin A4 production, *J Immunol* 184:6418, 2010.
114. van Dorp DA, Beer Thuis RK, Nugteren DH: The biosynthesis of prostaglandins, *Biochim Biophys Acta* 90:204, 1964.
115. Bergstrom S, Daniellson H, Samuelsson B: The enzymatic formation of prostaglandin E2 from arachidonic acid, *Biochim Biophys Acta* 90:207, 1964.
116. Bergstrom S, Daniellson H, Klenberg D, et al.: The enzymatic conversion of essential fatty acids into prostaglandins, *J Biol Chem* 239:4006, 1964.
117. Yates CM, Calder PC, Rainger GE: Pharmacology and therapeutics of omega-3 polyunsaturated fatty acids in chronic inflammatory disease, *Pharmacol Ther* 141:272, 2014.
118. Legrand-Poels S, Esser N, L'homme L, et al.: Free fatty acids as modulators of the NLRP3 inflammasome in obesity/type 2 diabetes, *Biochem Pharmacol* 92:131–141, 2014.
119. Proudman SM, James MJ, Spargo LD, et al.: Fish oil in recent onset rheumatoid arthritis: a randomized, double blind controlled trial within algorithm-based drug use, *Ann Rheum Dis* 74(89–95), 2015.
120. Kremer JM: Effects of modulation of inflammatory and immune parameters in patients with rheumatic and inflammatory disease receiving dietary supplementation of n-3 and n-6 fatty acids, *Lipids* 31:S253, 1996.

29 Chemokines and Cellular Recruitment

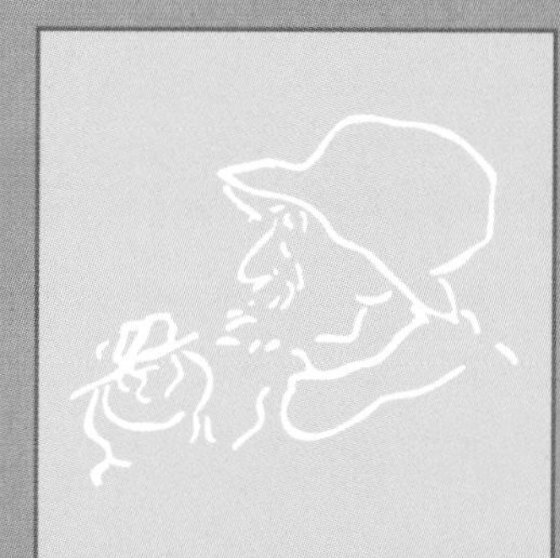

GERARD GRAHAM

KEY POINTS

- Chemokines are the primary regulators of in vivo leukocyte migration and are defined on the basis of the presence of a conserved cysteine motif in their mature sequences.
- Chemokines bind to receptors belonging to the G-protein coupled receptor family, as well as to atypical chemokine receptors.
- These chemoattractant proteins regulate the recruitment of leukocytes from the vasculature, as well as their intratissue migration dynamics.
- Chemokines are central players in a range of key pathologies, including immune and inflammatory diseases, HIV, and cancer.

Introduction

Chemokines are central regulators of leukocyte migration in vivo. In this chapter, I review the chemokine family, describing its evolutionary origin and in vivo functions, and then go on to summarize the understanding of the roles for chemokines in disease. Throughout this chapter, I have also highlighted certain complexities associated with chemokine biology in terms of an understanding, and targeting, of their roles in pathology.

Defining Membership of the Chemokine Family

The word *chemokine* is an amalgamation of two words: chemotactic and cytokine. Chemokines are therefore cytokine-like molecules that control directed cellular migration (chemotaxis) in vitro and in vivo. Importantly, not all cytokines that exhibit chemotactic behavior are members of the chemokine family. Thus, for example, IL-2,[1] IL-18,[2] and transforming growth factor (TGF)-β[3] can display chemotactic activity, but they are not chemokines. In fact, membership of the chemokine family is strictly defined on the basis of a conserved cysteine motif in the mature secreted protein.[4] As shown in Fig. 29.1, the large chemokine family is divided into four subfamilies according to the specific nature of this motif. A cytokine that is chemotactic but which lacks one of these variations on the cysteine motif is not a member of the chemokine family. Equally, a protein bearing one of these cysteine motifs but which displays no chemotactic activity will still be biochemically identified as a chemokine. The chemokine family is therefore strictly defined on the basis of biochemistry and not function.

The largest of the four subfamilies is the CC, or beta, chemokine subfamily, so-called because the first two cysteines are juxtaposed. The cysteines are essential for disulfide bond formation and form disulfide bonds between cysteines 1 and 3 and cysteines 2 and 4.[5] These are essential for proper folding of the mature chemokine protein and are indispensable for function.[6] There are currently 28 known members of the CC chemokine subfamily. The second largest subfamily is the CXC, or alpha, chemokine subfamily. This family differs from the CC chemokine family on the basis of the presence of a variable amino acid (designated X) between the first two cysteines. Again, disulfide bonding occurs between cysteines 1 and 3 and cysteines 2 and 4. Currently, we have identified 17 members of the CXC chemokine subfamily. In addition to the CC and CXC chemokines, there are two much smaller subfamilies, namely the XC subfamily, which has only two of the conserved cysteine residues and comprises only two related chemokines, and the CX3C subfamily, which has three amino acids between the first two cysteines and comprises only a single member.

Chemokines are classic secreted proteins that bear signal peptides on the amino-terminus, which are then cleaved off during secretion. There are two major variations on this basic processing model. CX3CL1[7] and CXCL16[8] are produced with a carboxy-terminal mucin stalk, which embeds them in the cellular membrane. These chemokines can be produced in a membrane-anchored form, as well as in a soluble form after cleavage from the mucin stalk, using tumor necrosis factor converting enzyme (TACE)-like enzymes.[9] In addition, there exists a murine-specific variant of the chemokine CCL27, which lacks a signal peptide and is targeted for nuclear translocation.[10,11] The role of this variant in the murine immune response is still unclear.

Ultimately the chemokine family is strictly defined on the basis of a conserved cysteine motif and is divided into four subfamilies according to the specific nature of this motif.

The Chemokine Nomenclature System

Chemokine nomenclature has been a source of complexity and confusion, both for people new to the chemokine field and for those who have worked with chemokines for many years. Historically, one of the problems was that some chemokines were identified by numerous different labs within a short time of each other and given separate trivial names in key publications. This was particularly problematic during the 1990s when "data-mining" allowed for the rapid identification of novel members of structurally defined families such as chemokines. Thus, for example, SLC, 6-CKine, TCA4, and Ckb9 are all names for the same chemokine,

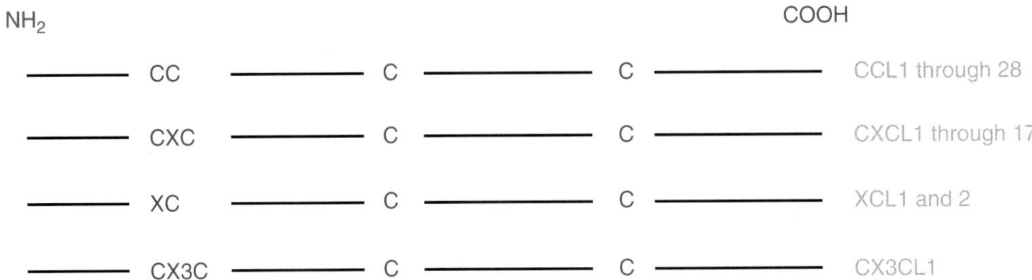

• **Fig. 29.1** A diagram showing the relative distribution of cysteine residues in the four chemokine subfamilies. In addition, the diagram summarizes the chemokine nomenclature, with CC chemokines being labeled CCL, CXC chemokines labeled CXCL, and the XC and CX3C chemokines labeled XCL and CX3CL, respectively. Note that the *black line* depicted on either side of the cysteine residues represents the remaining amino acid sequences of the intact protein.

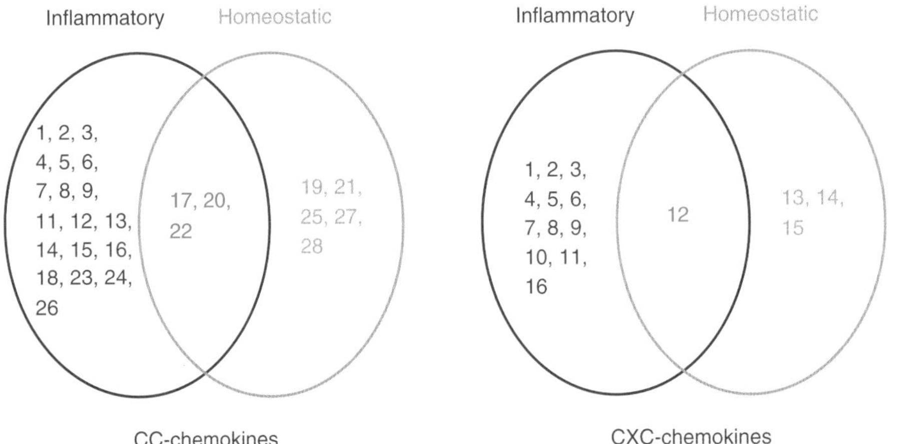

• **Fig. 29.2** A Venn diagram representation of the division of CC and CXCL chemokines into inflammatory and homeostatic subsets, along with an indication of those that display biology intermediate between these two subsets. The numbers in the ovals represent the numbered chemokine (e.g., CCL1, CCL19).

and there are many other examples of such nominative complexity. Moreover, in an example of another confusing aspect of chemokine nomenclature, IL-8 is not an interleukin at all but rather a chemokine (which is now known as CXCL8).

For these reasons, at the turn of the century, the chemokine community decided on a systematic nomenclature system for the molecules.[12] The nomenclature system defines the chemokines as ligands. Thus CC chemokines are referred to as CC ligands or CCLs, CXC ligands are CXCLs, and XC and CX3C ligands are XCLs and CX3CLs. The numbering system simply refers to the order in which the cDNA sequences for the chemokines were deposited in the genomic databases. In other words, CCL1 was the first CC chemokine identified and CCL28 was the most recent—and probably last—of the CC chemokines. According to this nomenclature, the chemokine that was previously known by such names as SLC and 6-Ckine is now referred to as CCL21. The nomenclature system has been universally adopted by chemokine biologists, immunologists, and others working with these molecules.

The Inflammatory and Homeostatic Chemokine Model

Chemokines play diverse and complex roles in regulating in vivo leukocyte migration (Fig. 29.2). To simplify chemokine biology, they are typically referred to as being either inflammatory or homeostatic, according to the contexts in which they function.[12,13] Inflammatory chemokines are not expressed in resting tissues but can be induced to extremely high expression levels after infection, wounding, or insult to any tissue in the body. In fact, it is likely that inflammatory chemokines can be expressed by any cell type undergoing stress, infection, or damage. Inflammatory chemokines direct recruitment of inflammatory leukocytes to the damaged or infected site and then are transcriptionally silenced as a prelude to the resolution of the inflammatory response. The ability of inflammatory chemokines to be made at any body site experiencing trauma allows for an immediate and directed recruitment of inflammatory leukocytes to the specific site of damage.

In contrast, homeostatic chemokines are not typically regarded as being inducible but are expressed at low and steady levels by specific cells within individual tissues. Homeostatic chemokines are involved in more precise tissue navigation processes. For example, the skin expresses the chemokine CCL27, which, through its receptor CCR10, ensures the homing of T-cells specifically to the skin.[14] In the gut, CCL25 is expressed and interacts with the chemokine receptor CCR9 on gut-homing T cells.[15] Hematopoietic stem cells express the chemokine receptor CXCR4, which binds the chemokine CXCL12 (which is expressed by bone marrow stromal cells) and allows for the precise recruitment of stem cells to bone marrow niches.[16–18]

The inflammatory-homeostatic distinction is not completely clean, and a number of chemokines perform both inflammatory and homeostatic roles. Nevertheless, it remains a useful description of the extremes of chemokine biology and provides a context in which to interpret chemokine and chemokine receptor function.

The Chemokine Receptor Family

Despite occasional reports to the contrary, chemokine receptors appear to exclusively belong to the family of 7-transmembrane-spanning, G-protein-coupled receptors.[19] To date, 19 signaling chemokine receptors have been identified. Importantly, unlike the ligands, it is not possible to exhaustively screen for chemokine-specific receptors in genomic databases. As a result, it remains possible that there are other chemokine receptors amongst the existing pool of "orphan" GPCRs. Again, there is a systematic nomenclature for chemokine receptors. Fortunately the receptors typically only bind chemokines from one or other of the ligand families. Thus we can define CC chemokine receptors (CCRs), CXC chemokine receptors (CXCRs), XCRs, and CX3CRs. As with the ligands, the numbering of receptors reflects the order in which the cDNAs were deposited in the genomic databases; CCR1 is the first CC-chemokine receptor identified and CCR10 the most recent. To date, 10 receptors for CC chemokines, 7 receptors for CXC chemokines, and single receptors for the XC and CX3C chemokines have been identified. As with the ligands, chemokine receptors can be classified as being either inflammatory or homeostatic, according to the cell types in which they are expressed. Inflammatory chemokine receptors, such as CCR1 and CXCR2, are typically expressed on inflammatory leukocytes and support the recruitment of innate immune cells to sites of tissue injury or infection. In contrast, homeostatic receptors, such as CCR9 and CCR10, are expressed on lymphocyte subsets and confer on them specific tissue tropisms.

Despite being specific for one or other of the ligand subfamilies, interactions between chemokines and their receptors are extraordinarily complex.[20,21] As shown in Table 29.1, although some chemokine receptors bind relatively few ligands, a number of them (particularly those involved in inflammation, as described in the previous section) are capable of binding numerous ligands and displaying extensive promiscuity. To complicate things further, a number of the ligands display unfaithfulness to individual receptors. For example, CCL3 does not just bind to CCR1; it also binds to CCR3 and CCR5. The promiscuity and unfaithfulness of receptor-ligand interactions has led to much confusion in terms of understanding chemokine and receptor function in the context of inflammation. In fact, it has been one of the confounding factors that has hampered the generation of a clear model of chemokine function in inflammatory disease. What is not clear, and is the subject of some controversy in the field, is whether the promiscuous interaction of ligands with the receptors is evidence of fundamental and extensive redundancy in the chemokine system.[22–24] This issue has not yet been resolved, but recent clear demonstration of biased signaling[25] through G-protein coupled receptors (i.e., different signaling downstream of individual ligand interactions with the same receptor) suggests that there is scope for interpreting the promiscuity as being a basis for exquisite subtlety rather than simply redundancy.

Atypical Chemokine Receptors

In addition to the classic signaling chemokine receptors, there exists a small subfamily of receptors that display alternative signaling responses to ligands and are typically expressed on stromal cell types.[26–28] These are the atypical chemokine receptors (ACKRs) and, to date, four atypical chemokine receptors have been identified. These are detailed in Table 29.2, along with their ligand-binding profiles.

ACKR1 is something of an outlier in this family in that it is located in a genomic region that is remote from the other classic chemokine receptors and atypical chemokine receptors and there is little primary structural identity with the other chemokine receptors. It is unique amongst chemokine receptors in its ability to bind chemokines from more than one subfamily and is able to comprehensively bind inflammatory chemokines from both the CC and CXC chemokine subfamilies. Data suggest an important role for ACKR1 in the carriage of chemokines across vascular endothelial cells,[29] as well as in malarial pathogenesis[30] and hematopoietic stem cell development and differentiation.[31]

TABLE 29.1 Known Chemokine Receptors and Their Identified Chemokine Ligands

Receptor	Ligands
CCR1	CCL3, 5, 7, 8, 13, 14, 15, 16, 23
CCR2	CCL2, 7, 8, 13, 15
CCR3	CCL3, 4, 5, 7, 11, 13, 15, 24, 26, 28
CCR4	CCL17,22
CCR5	CCL,3,4,5,7 14, 16
CCR6	CCL20
CCR7	CCL19, 21
CCR8	CCL1, CCL18
CCR9	CCL25
CCR10	CCL27, 28
CXCR1	CXCL5, 6, 8
CXCR2	CXCL1, 2, 3, 5, 6, 7, 8
CXCR3	CXCL9, 10, 11
CXCR4	CXCL12
CXCR5	CXCL13
CXCR6	CXCL16
CXCR8	CXCL17
XCR1	XCL1, 2
CX3CR1	CX3CL1

TABLE 29.2 Known Atypical Chemokine Receptors and Their Identified Chemokine Ligands

Receptor	Ligands
ACKR1	CCL2, 3, 4, 5, 7, 11, 13, 14, 17, CXCL5, 6, 8, 11
ACKR2	CCL2, 3, 4, 5, 7, 11, 13, 14, 17, 22
ACKR3	CXCL11, 12
ACKR4	CCL19, 21, 25

ACKR2, 3, and 4 are clearly related to the other chemokine receptors and sit within the major chemokine receptor chromosomal loci.[32] These receptors are able to act as chemokine-scavenging receptors[33–37] and play an important role in fine-tuning chemokine activity in a variety of contexts. ACKR2 exclusively binds inflammatory CC chemokines and plays a crucial role in resolving inflammatory responses,[38–41] placental function,[42,43] and branching morphogenesis in development.[44,45] ACKR3 binds CXCL11 and CXCL12[46] and plays essential developmental roles, as evidenced by elegant studies in zebrafish[47] and by the perinatal lethality of the homozygous knockout mice.[48] Finally, ACKR4 binds the homeostatic CC chemokines CCL19, CCL21, and CCL25.[49] It plays an important role in establishing gradients to support the regulation of dendritic cell migration into the lymph node parenchyma.[50] It is also highly expressed in the thymus, although its role in this tissue remains obscure.[51]

Chemokines in an Evolutionary Context

Chemokines and their receptors are vertebrate-specific molecules; pre-vertebrate species such as Drosophila do not possess chemokines. Chemokines and their receptors first appeared in evolution approximately 600 million years ago in jawless fish,[52,53] and the primordial role for the first chemokines was almost certainly to regulate stem cell migration during development.[54] One of the most ancient, and highly conserved, chemokines that we know of is CXCL12. In mammalian embryogenesis, this molecule is essential for the migration of primordial germ cells to the genital ridge,[55,56] the movement of hematopoietic stem cells from fetal liver to the bone marrow,[57,58] and the migration of vascular and neural progenitor cells.[57,59,60] Mice deficient in CXCL12 die at birth as a result of severe bone marrow failure.[57,58] Studies on zebrafish have also indicated that interference with CXCL12 results in infertility in adult fish as a result of compromised primordial germ cell migration.[55,61] CXCL12 is also crucial for the migration of a population of cells along the lateral line of the developing zebrafish.[62,63] Thus the ancient, and highly conserved, role for chemokines was to regulate stem cell migration during embryogenesis.

From CXCL12, and through a process of gene duplication, the chemokine system has expanded to the point that mammals have approximately 45 different chemokines, which involve themselves in exquisitely subtle ways in regulating in vivo leukocyte migration. Nevertheless, we retain the essential dependence on CXCL12 for successful embryologic development. In terms of receptors, the most ancient are almost certainly the CXCL12 receptor CXCR4, which is expressed on stem cell populations and required for their migration within the embryo, and ACKR3, which fine tunes CXCL12 expression and presentation to finesse the developmental process.

How Chemokines Attract Cells to Particular In Vivo Destinations

Presented chemokines have to perform two distinct functions in terms of supporting leukocyte migration to specific tissues. First, they have to inform cells in the circulation that they are at the right place to leave and enter the tissue under either inflammatory or homeostatic conditions. Second, they need to facilitate the movement of extravasated cells within the sublumenal tissue. These will be dealt with separately.

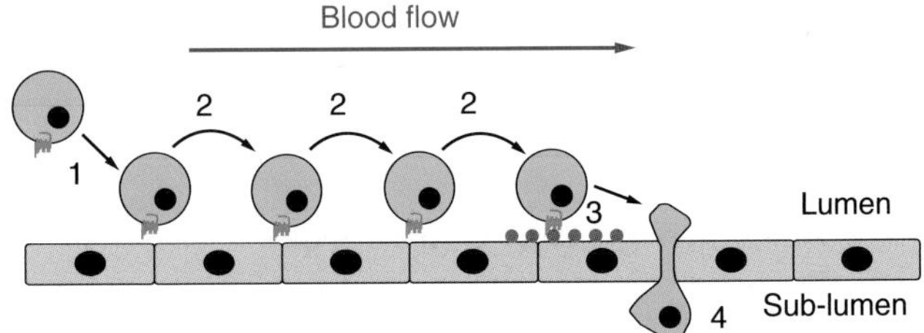

• **Fig. 29.3** A diagrammatic representation of the leukocyte adhesion cascade. This diagram shows *(1)* the initial weak interactions of leukocytes *(green cells)* with the lumenal face of the endothelium *(yellow cells)* under shear-flow; *(2)* selectin-dependent rolling of leukocytes along the endothelial surface; *(3)* chemokine receptor signaling induced integrin-dependent tight binding to the endothelial surface; and *(4)* transendothelial migration.

Chemokines in the Leukocyte Adhesion Cascade

Leukocytes use combinations of molecules to determine, in time and space, where to exit the vasculature and enter the tissues.[64,65] As summarized in Fig. 29.3, the leukocytes initially roll on the lumenal endothelial surface via "stuttering" interactions with selectins. When the rolling leukocyte encounters the chemokine for which it has the appropriate receptor, the chemokine induces "inside-out" signaling, which activates cell surface integrins and mediates firm adhesion to the vascular lumen.[66,67] This is then followed by transendothelial migration, which is when leukocytes traverse the endothelial layer and enter the sublumenal tissue. Much has been written about the relevance of chemokine gradients in attracting cells in vivo. Nevertheless, in the context of the leukocyte adhesion cascade and the regulation of the exit of leukocytes from the vasculature, it is clear that chemokine gradients cannot be supported within a living circulatory system. In fact, most analyses indicate that chemokines are presented to rolling leukocytes bound to glycosaminoglycan molecules[68,69] within the hydrated glycocalyx layer[70] of the endothelial cells. Precisely how the chemokines are presented has not been worked out, but numerous studies using enzymes that deplete glycosaminoglycan components of the glycocalyx[71] have shown a clearly important role for proteoglycan presentation of chemokines in mediating extravasation of leukocytes into sublumenal tissues.

Chemokine Functions Within a Tissue

Although the role of chemokines in recruiting cells from the vasculature is fairly well understood, our knowledge of the involvement of chemokines in intratissue migration is not as well developed. It is clear that numerous chemokine ligands are expressed within tissues and therefore are likely to contribute to the movement of extravasated cells in the tissue compartment. In addition, chemokines are involved in the exit of dendritic cells from peripheral tissues to enable them to migrate through the lymphatic system to lymph nodes and engage in antigen presentation.[72,73] In this regard, it has been demonstrated that gradients of the chemokine CCL21 emanate from lymphatic endothelial surfaces and serve to recruit dendritic cells into the lymphatic circulation.[34]

Interestingly, it may not simply be intratissue migration that is regulated by the chemokines; there is evidence that chemokines also increase the speed of cell movement within tissues.[74] In the lymph node, this is seen as being advantageous in terms of enhancing antigen presentation.

Considerable work still needs to be done to fully understand the role of chemokines in tissues. This issue is fraught with complexity as, in inflamed tissues, multiple chemokines binding to the same receptors are simultaneously present. How leukocytes integrate this information to facilitate specific kinetic and dynamic responses is not yet understood.

Chemokines and Their Receptors in Disease

Chemokines and their receptors play pivotal roles in three main classes of pathologies: (1) immune and inflammatory diseases, (2) HIV pathogenesis, and (3) cancer.

Immune and Inflammatory Diseases

Essentially all pathologies, whether inflammatory, autoimmune, or allergic, that involve leukocytes are centrally dependent on chemokines.[21,75] For example, for inflammatory cells to migrate to rheumatoid joints,[76–78] psoriatic plaques,[79,80] or destructive lesions in multiple sclerosis (MS),[81,82] local chemokine production is required and pathologic inflammatory sites are rich sources of a diverse array of inflammatory chemokines. Especially in inflamed conditions, as leukocytes enter the sites, the sites typically respond by producing more inflammatory chemokines, thereby amplifying the inflammatory response. In addition, in autoimmune diseases, chemokines are indispensable for dendritic cell (DC) and T cell migration to secondary lymphoid organs and for overall antigen presentation.[83] In allergic diseases such as asthma, specific chemokines have been associated with the recruitment of T helper (Th)2 cells, as well as mast cells and eosinophils.[84,85] A strong association between chemokines and chemokine receptors and the development of atherosclerotic plaques has also been demonstrated in pre-clinical and clinical studies.[86,87] Indeed, numerous polymorphisms in key inflammatory chemokine receptors such as CCR2 and CX3CR1 display strong links with the pathogenesis of atherosclerosis. The clear association of inflammatory chemokines with destructive inflammatory pathologies has highlighted chemokines and their receptors as being important therapeutic targets. In essence, all inflammatory, allergic, and autoimmune diseases have a fundamental reliance on chemokines and their receptors.

HIV Pathogenesis

Although not related to inflammatory or immune dysfunction, chemokine receptors are now known to be essential in HIV pathogenesis.[88] Specifically, the chemokine receptor CCR5 acts as the principal co-receptor (along with CD4) for initial infection with M-tropic HIV strains.[89] Allied to this discovery is the observation that individuals with T cells overproducing ligands for this receptor have historically displayed a longer time for conversion from HIV infection to full-blown AIDS.[90] This is now known to be a direct result of these chemokines competing with HIV for binding to CCR5. In addition, individuals homozygous for a polymorphism in CCR5 known as Δ32 are essentially refractory to HIV infection.[91] This polymorphism results in the deletion of 32 base pairs from the CCR5 genomic locus, yielding an inactive truncated receptor. The polymorphism arose among Northern Europeans; among people of northern European descent today, it is present at a frequency of 15% heterozygosity and 1% homozygosity.[92] Some confusion exists around the precise in vivo role for CCR5 because homozygous null individuals do not display overt immunologic or inflammatory deficiencies. Indeed, sporadic reports suggest that they display reduced inflammatory responses in a range of diseases, including rheumatoid arthritis (RA)[93] and MS.[94]

What is known, however, is that people who are homozygous null for CCR5 have an increased chance of developing lethal encephalitis in response to West Nile virus infection.[95–97] It is likely therefore that CCR5 has very specific roles to play at least in the context of encephalitic viral infections.

Importantly, and in contrast to inflammatory diseases, pharmacologic targeting of CCR5 has been highly successful, and a high-quality pharmacologic blocker known as Maraviroc[98] is licensed for use as an anti-HIV medication. In addition to CCR5, another prominent HIV co-receptor, CXCR4, plays roles later in the in vivo evolution of the disease.[99] As the virus evolves in vivo it develops the ability to interact with both CCR5 and CXCR4 and ultimately exclusively with CXCR4. It is the switch to CXCR4 use that triggers the development of full-blown AIDS.[100,101] Why individuals cannot be directly infected with CXCR4-dependent virus is not known, and CCR5 remains almost exclusively the receptor required for initial viral entry.

Cancer

Chemokines are also major contributors to tumorigenesis.[102,103] This contribution starts at the very initial points of the tumorigenic process, and a number of studies have demonstrated that oncogenic genomic events are strong inducers of chemokine expression.[104,105] This is likely to be a by-product of the cells responding to the stress of the oncogenic event by sending out "rescue" signals. These chemokines are pathologically important as they recruit leukocyte subtypes, such as macrophages, which contribute directly to tumor promotion.[106] To date, numerous chemokines have been implicated in cancer development. In metastasis, there are now significant data indicating that a number of cancers use chemokine receptors to migrate to their metastatic destinations.[107–109]

Overall, chemokines and their receptors are potentially important therapeutic targets in cancer.

Conclusion

In summary, chemokines are key regulators of in vivo leukocyte migration. They comprise a vertebrate-specific and biochemically defined family and play essential roles in biology and pathology. They are therefore important therapeutic targets, particularly in the context of inflammatory disease.

The references for this chapter can also be found on ExpertConsult.com.

References

1. Wilkinson PC, Newman I: Chemoattractant activity of IL-2 for human lymphocytes: a requirement for the IL-2 receptor beta-chain, *Immunology* 82(1):134–139, 1994.
2. Komai-Koma M, Gracie JA, Wei X-q, et al.: Chemoattraction of human T cells by IL-18, *J Immunol* 170(2):1084–1090, 2003.
3. Wahl SM, Hunt DA, Wakefield LM, et al.: Transforming growth factor type beta induces monocyte chemotaxis and growth factor production, *P Natl Acad Sci USA* 84(16):5788–5792, 1987.
4. Rot A, von Andrian UH: Chemokines in innate and adaptive host defense: basic chemokinese grammar for immune cells, *Annu Rev Immunol* 22:891–928, 2004.

5. Rajarathnam K, Sykes BD, Dewald B, et al.: Disulfide bridges in interleukin-8 probed using non-natural disulfide analogues: dissociation of roles in structure from function, *Biochemistry* 38(24):7653–7658, 1999. Epub 1999/07/01.
6. Fernandez EJ, Lolis E: Structure, function, and inhibition of chemokines, *Annu Rev Pharmacol Toxicol* 42(1):469–499, 2002.
7. Bazan JF, Bacon KB, Hardiman G, et al.: A new class of membrane-bound chemokine with a CX3C motif, *Nature* 385(6617):640–644, 1997. Epub 1997/02/13.
8. Matloubian M, David A, Engel S, et al.: A transmembrane CXC chemokine is a ligand for HIV-coreceptor Bonzo, *Nat Immunol* 1(4):298–304, 2000. Epub 2001/03/23.
9. Garton KJ, Gough PJ, Blobel CP, et al.: Tumor necrosis factor-alpha-converting enzyme (ADAM17) mediates the cleavage and shedding of fractalkine (CX3CL1), *J Biol Chem* 276(41):37993–38001, 2001. Epub 2001/08/10.
10. Baird JW, Nibbs RJ, Komai-Koma M, et al.: ESkine, a novel beta-chemokine, is differentially spliced to produce secretable and nuclear targeted isoforms, *J Biol Chem* 274(47):33496–33503, 1999.
11. Nibbs RJ, Graham GJ: CCL27/PESKY: a novel paradigm for chemokine function, *Expert Opin Biol Ther* 3(1):15–22, 2003.
12. Zlotnik A, Yoshie O: Chemokines: a new classification system and their role in immunity, *Immunity* 12(2):121–127, 2000.
13. Mantovani A: The chemokine system: redundancy for robust outputs, *Immunol Today* 20(6):254–257, 1999.
14. Homey B, Alenius H, Muller A, et al.: CCL27-CCR10 interactions regulate T cell-mediated skin inflammation, *Nat Med* 8(2):157–165, 2002. Epub 2002/02/01.
15. Kunkel EJ, Campbell JJ, Haraldsen G, et al.: Lymphocyte CC chemokine receptor 9 and epithelial thymus-expressed chemokine (TECK) expression distinguish the small intestinal immune compartment: epithelial expression of tissue-specific chemokines as an organizing principle in regional immunity, *J Exp Med* 192(5):761–768, 2000. Epub 2000/09/07.
16. Lapidot T, Dar A, Kollet O: How do stem cells find their way home? *Blood* 106(6):1901–1910, 2005.
17. Lapidot T, Petit I: Current understanding of stem cell mobilization: the roles of chemokines, proteolytic enzymes, adhesion molecules, cytokines, and stromal cells, *Exp Hematol* 30(9):973–981, 2002.
18. Wright DE, Bowman EP, Wagers AJ, et al.: Hematopoietic stem cells are uniquely selective in their migratory response to chemokines, *J Exp Med* 195(9):1145–1154, 2002.
19. Bachelerie F, Ben-Baruch A, Burkhardt AM, et al.: International union of pharmacology. LXXXIX. Update on the extended family of chemokine receptors and introducing a new nomenclature for atypical chemokine receptors, *Pharmacol Rev* 66(1):1–79, 2014.
20. Schall TJ, Proudfoot AE. Overcoming hurdles in developing successful drugs targeting chemokine receptors. *Nat Rev Immunol.* 11(5):355–363.
21. Viola A, Luster AD: Chemokines and their receptors: drug targets in immunity and inflammation, *Annu Rev Pharmacol Toxicol* 48:171–197, 2008.
22. Schall TJ, Proudfoot AEI: Overcoming hurdles in developing successful drugs targeting chemokine receptors, *Nat Rev Immunol* 11(5):355–363, 2011.
23. Steen A, Larsen O, Thiele S, et al.: Biased and G protein-independent signaling of chemokine receptors, *Front Immunol* 5:277, 2014.
24. Dyer DP, Medina-Ruiz L, Bartolini R, et al.: Chemokine receptor redundancy and specificity are context dependent, *Immunity* 50(2):378–389e5, 2019.
25. Jorgensen AS, Rosenkilde MM, Hjorto GM: Biased signaling of G protein-coupled receptors—from a chemokine receptor CCR7 perspective, *Gen Comp Endocrinol* 258:4–14, 2018. Epub 2017/07/12.
26. Bachelerie F, Graham GJ, Locati M, et al.: New nomenclature for atypical chemokine receptors, *Nat Immunol* 15(3):207–208, 2014.
27. Bachelerie F, Graham GJ, Locati M, et al.: An atypical addition to the chemokine receptor nomenclature: IUPHAR Review 15, *Br J Pharmacol* 172(16):3945–3949, 2015. Epub 2015/05/12.
28. Nibbs RJB, Graham GJ: Immune regulation by atypical chemokine receptors, *Nat Rev Immunol* 13(11):815–829, 2013.
29. Middleton J, Neil S, Wintle J, et al.: Transcytosis and surface presentation of IL-8 by venular endothelial cells, *Cell* 91(3):385–395, 1997.
30. Rot A: Contribution of Duffy antigen to chemokine function, *Cytokine Growth Factor Rev* 16(6):687–694, 2005.
31. Duchene J, Novitzky-Basso I, Thiriot A, et al.: Atypical chemokine receptor 1 on nucleated erythroid cells regulates hematopoiesis, *Nat Immunol* 18(7):753–761, 2017.
32. Nomiyama H, Osada N, Yoshie O: A family tree of vertebrate chemokine receptors for a unified nomenclature, *Dev Comp Immunol* 35(7):705–715, 2011.
33. Fra AM, Locati M, Otero K, et al.: Cutting edge: scavenging of inflammatory CC chemokines by the promiscuous putatively silent chemokine receptor D6, *J Immunol* 170(5):2279–2282, 2003.
34. Weber M, Blair E, Simpson CV, et al.: The chemokine receptor D6 constitutively traffics to and from the cell surface to internalize and degrade chemokines, *Mol Biol Cell* 15(5):2492–2508, 2004.
35. Hoffmann F, Mueller W, Schuetz D, et al.: Rapid uptake and degradation of CXCL12 depend on CXCR7 carboxyl-terminal serine/threonine residues, *J Biol Chem* 287(34):28362–28377, 2012.
36. Naumann U, Cameroni E, Pruenster M, et al. CXCR7 functions as a scavenger for CXCL12 and CXCL11, *PloS One* 5(2):e9175.
37. Bryce SA, Wilson RA, Tiplady EM, et al.: ACKR4 on stromal cells Scavenges CCL19 to enable CCR7-dependent trafficking of APCs from inflamed skin to lymph nodes, *J Immunol* 196(8):3341–3353, 2016. Epub 2016/03/16.
38. Graham GJ: D6 and the atypical chemokine receptor family: novel regulators of immune and inflammatory processes, *Eur J Immunol* 39(2):342–351, 2009.
39. Martinez de la Torre Y, Locati M, Buracchi C, et al.: Increased inflammation in mice deficient for the chemokine decoy receptor D6, *Eur J Immunol* 35(5):1342–1346, 2005.
40. Graham GJ: D6/ACKR2, *Front Immunol* 6:280, 2015. Epub 2015/06/23.
41. Jamieson T, Cook DN, Nibbs RJ, et al.: The chemokine receptor D6 limits the inflammatory response in vivo, *Nat Immunol* 6(4):403–411, 2005.
42. Madigan J, Freeman DJ, Menzies F, et al.: Chemokine scavenger D6 is expressed by trophoblasts and aids the survival of mouse embryos transferred into allogeneic recipients, *J Immunol* 184(6):3202–3212, 2010.
43. Martinez de la Torre Y, Buracchi C, Borroni EM, et al.: Protection against inflammation- and autoantibody-caused fetal loss by the chemokine decoy receptor D6, *Proc Natl Acad Sci U S A* 104(7):2319–2324, 2007.
44. Lee KM, Danuser R, Stein JV: The chemokine receptors ACKR2 and CCR2 reciprocally regulate lymphatic vessel density, *Embo J* 33(21):2564–2580, 2014. Epub 2014/10/02.
45. Wilson GJ, Hewit KD, Pallas KJ, et al.: Atypical chemokine receptor ACKR2 controls branching morphogenesis in the developing mammary gland, *Development* 144(1):74–82, 2017. Epub 2016/11/27.
46. Burns JM, Summers BC, Wang Y, et al.: A novel chemokine receptor for SDF-1 and I-TAC involved in cell survival, cell adhesion, and tumor development, *J Exp Med* 203(9):2201–2213, 2006.
47. Boidajipour B, Mahabaleshwar H, Kardash E, et al.: Control of chemokine-guided cell migration by ligand sequestration, *Cell* 132(3):463–473, 2008.
48. Sierro F, Biben C, Martinez-Munoz L, et al.: Disrupted cardiac development but normal hematopoiesis in mice deficient in the

second CXCL12/SDF-1 receptor, CXCR7, *Proc Natl Acad Sci U S A* 104(37):14759–14764, 2007.
49. Townson JR, Nibbs RJ: Characterization of mouse CCX-CKR, a receptor for the lymphocyte-attracting chemokines TECK/mCCL25, SLC/mCCL21 and MIP-3beta/mCCL19: comparison to human CCX-CKR, *Eur J Immunol* 32(5):1230–1241, 2002.
50. Ulvmar MH, Werth K, Braun A, et al.: The atypical chemokine receptor CCRL1 shapes functional CCL21 gradients in lymph nodes, *Nat Immunol* 15(7):623–630, 2014.
51. Lucas B, White AJ, Ulvmar MH, et al.: CCRL1/ACKR4 is expressed in key thymic microenvironments but is dispensable for T lymphopoiesis at steady state in adult mice, *Eur J Immunol* 45(2):574–583, 2015. Epub 2014/12/19.
52. Bajoghli B: Evolution and function of chemokine receptors in the immune system of lower vertebrates, *Eur J Immunol* 43(7):1686–1692, 2013.
53. Bird S, Tafalla C: Teleost chemokines and their receptors, *Biology* 4(4):756–784, 2015.
54. DeVries ME, Kelvin AA, Xu L, et al.: Defining the origins and evolution of the chemokine/chemokine receptor system, *J Immunol* 176(1):401–415, 2006. Epub 2005/12/21.
55. Doitsidou M, Reichman-Fried M, Stebler J, et al.: Guidance of primordial germ cell migration by the chemokine SDF-1, *Cell* 111(5):647–659, 2002.
56. Ara T, Nakamura Y, Egawa T, et al.: Impaired colonization of the gonads by primordial germ cells in mice lacking a chemokine, stromal cell-derived factor-1 (SDF-1), *Proc Natl Acad Sci U S A* 100(9):5319–5323, 2003.
57. Zou YR, Kottmann AH, Kuroda M, et al.: Function of the chemokine receptor CXCR4 in haematopoiesis and in cerebellar development, *Nature* 393(6685):595–599, 1998.
58. Ma Q, Jones D, Borghesani PR, et al.: Impaired B-lymphopoiesis, myelopoiesis, and derailed cerebellar neuron migration in CXCR4- and SDF-1-deficient mice, *P Natl Acad Sci USA* 95(16):9448–9453, 1998.
59. Killian ECO, Birkholz DA, Artinger KB: A role for chemokine signaling in neural crest cell migration and craniofacial development, *Dev Biol* 333(1):161–172, 2009.
60. Tachibana K, Hirota S, Iizasa H, et al.: The chemokine receptor CXCR4 is essential for vascularization of the gastrointestinal tract, *Nature* 393(6685):591–594, 1998.
61. Molyneaux KA, Zinszner H, Kunwar PS, et al.: The chemokine SDF1/CXCL12 and its receptor CXCR4 regulate mouse germ cell migration and survival, *Development* 130(18):4279–4286, 2003.
62. Valentin G, Haas P, Gilmour D: The chemokine SDF1a coordinates tissue migration through the spatially restricted activation of Cxcr7 and Cxcr4b, *Curr Biol* 17(12):1026–1031, 2007.
63. Valentin G, Haas P, Gilmour D: The chemokine SDF1a coordinates tissue migration through the spatially restricted activation of Cxcr7 and Cxcr4b, *Current Biology* 17(12):1026–1031, 2007.
64. Nourshargh S, Alon R: Leukocyte migration into inflamed tissues, *Immunity* 41(5):694–707, 2014.
65. Ley K, Laudanna C, Cybulsky MI, et al.: Getting to the site of inflammation: the leukocyte adhesion cascade updated, *Nat Rev Immunol* 7:678, 2007.
66. Alon R, Ley K: Cells on the run: shear-regulated integrin activation in leukocyte rolling and arrest on endothelial cells, *Curr Opin Cell Biol* 20(5):525–532, 2008.
67. Montresor A, Toffali L, Constantin G, et al.: Chemokines and the signaling modules regulating integrin affinity, *Front Immunol* 3:127, 2012.
68. Handel TM, Johnson Z, Crown SE, et al.: Regulation of protein function by glycosaminoglycans—as exemplified by chemokines, *Annu Rev Biochem* 74(1):385–410, 2005.
69. Proudfoot AEI: Chemokines and glycosaminoglycans, *Front Immunol* 6:246, 2015.
70. Weinbaum S, Tarbell JM, Damiano ER: The structure and function of the endothelial glycocalyx layer, *Annu Rev Biomed Eng* 9(1):121–167, 2007.
71. Bao X, Moseman EA, Saito H, et al.: Endothelial heparan sulfate controls chemokine presentation in recruitment of lymphocytes and dendritic cells to lymph nodes, *Immunity* 33(5):817–829, 2010.
72. Forster R, Braun A, Worbs T: Lymph node homing of T cells and dendritic cells via afferent lymphatics, *Trends in Immunology* 33(6):271–280, 2012.
73. Forster R, Schubel A, Breitfeld D, et al.: CCR7 coordinates the primary immune response by establishing functional microenvironments in secondary lymphoid organs, *Cell* 99(1):23–33, 1999.
74. Worbs T, Mempel TR, Bolter J, et al.: CCR7 ligands stimulate the intranodal motility of T lymphocytes in vivo, *J Exp Med* 204(3):489–495, 2007.
75. Gerard C, Rollins BJ: Chemokines and disease, *Nat Immunol* 2(2):108–115, 2001.
76. Haringman JJ, Ludikhuize J, Tak PP: Chemokines in joint disease: the key to inflammation? *Ann Rheum Dis* 63(10):1186–1194, 2004.
77. Koch AE: Chemokines and their receptors in rheumatoid arthritis: future targets? *Arthritis Rheum* 52(3):710–721, 2005.
78. Robinson E, Keystone EC, Schall TJ, et al.: Chemokine expression in rheumatoid arthritis (RA): evidence of RANTES and macrophage inflammatory protein (MIP)-1 beta production by synovial T cells, *Clin Exp Immunol* 101(3):398–407, 1995.
79. Homey B: Chemokines and chemokine receptors as targets in the therapy of psoriasis, *Curr Drug Targets Inflamm Allergy* 3(2):169–174, 2004.
80. Nickoloff BJ, Xin H, Nestle FO, et al.: The cytokine and chemokine network in psoriasis, *Clin Dermatol* 25(6):568–573, 2007.
81. Godiska R, Chantry D, Dietsch GN, et al.: Chemokine expression in murine experimental allergic encephalomyelitis, *J Neuroimmunol* 58(2):167–176, 1995.
82. Zhang GX, Baker CM, Kolson DL, et al.: Chemokines and chemokine receptors in the pathogenesis of multiple sclerosis, *Mult Scler* 6(1):3–13, 2000.
83. Forster R, Davalos-Misslitz AC, Rot A: CCR7 and its ligands: balancing immunity and tolerance, *Nat Rev Immunol* 8(5):362–371, 2008.
84. Chantry D, Burgess LE: Chemokines in allergy, *Curr Drug Targets Inflamm Allergy* 1(1):109–116, 2002.
85. Schuh JM, Blease K, Kunkel SL, et al.: Chemokines and cytokines: axis and allies in asthma and allergy, *Cytokine Growth Factor Rev* 14(6):503–510, 2003.
86. Barlic J, Murphy PM: Chemokine regulation of atherosclerosis, *J Leukoc Biol* 82(2):226–236, 2007.
87. Braunersreuther V, Mach F, Steffens S: The specific role of chemokines in atherosclerosis, *Thromb Haemost* 97(5):714–721, 2007.
88. Broder CC, Collman RG: Chemokine receptors and HIV, *J Leukoc Biol* 62(1):20–29, 1997.
89. Dragic T, Litwin V, Allaway GP, et al.: HIV-1 entry into CD4+ cells is mediated by the chemokine receptor CC-CKR-5, *Nature* 381(6584):667–673, 1996.
90. Cocchi F, DeVico AL, Garzino-Demo A, et al.: Identification of RANTES, MIP-1α, and MIP-1β as the major HIV-suppressive factors produced by CD8+ T cells, *Science* 270(5243):1811–1815, 1995.
91. Samson M, Libert F, Doranz BJ, et al.: Resistance to HIV-1 infection in caucasian individuals bearing mutant alleles of the CCR-5 chemokine receptor gene, *Nature* 382(6593):722–725, 1996.
92. Novembre J, Galvani AP, Slatkin M: The geographic spread of the CCR5 Δ32 HIV-resistance allele, *PLOS Biol* 3(11):e339, 2005.
93. Prahalad S: Negative association between the chemokine receptor CCR5-Delta32 polymorphism and rheumatoid arthritis: a meta-analysis, *Genes Immun* 7(3):264–268, 2006. Epub 2006/03/17.

94. Song GG, Lee YH: A Meta-analysis of the relation between chemokine receptor 5 delta32 polymorphism and multiple sclerosis susceptibility, *Immunol Invest* 43(4):299–311, 2014.
95. Glass W, Lim J, Cholera R, et al.: Chemokine receptor CCR5 promotes leukocyte trafficking to the brain and survival in West Nile virus infection, *J Exp Med* 202:1087–1098, 2005.
96. Glass WG, McDermott DH, Lim JK, et al.: CCR5 deficiency increases risk of symptomatic West Nile virus infection, *J Exp Med* 203(1):35–40, 2006.
97. Suthar MS, Diamond MS, Gale Jr M: West Nile virus infection and immunity, *Nat Rev Microbiol* 11(2):115–128, 2013.
98. Meanwell NA, Kadow JF: Drug evaluation: Maraviroc, a chemokine CCR5 receptor antagonist for the treatment of HIV infection and AIDS, *Curr Opin Investig Drugs* 8(8):669–681, 2007.
99. Oberlin E, Amara A, Bachelerie F, et al.: The CXC chemokine SDF-1 is the ligand for LESTR/fusin and prevents infection by T-cell-line-adapted HIV-1, *Nature* 382(6594):833–835, 1996.
100. Kalinkovich A, Weisman Z, Bentwich Z: Chemokines and chemokine receptors: role in HIV infection, *Immunol Lett* 68(2–3):281–287, 1999.
101. Rowland-Jones S: The role of chemokine receptors in HIV infection, *Sex Transm Infect* 75(3):148–151, 1999.
102. Balkwill F: Cancer and the chemokine network, *Nat Rev Cancer* 4(7):540–550, 2004.
103. Balkwill FR: The chemokine system and cancer, *J Pathol* 226(2):148–157, 2012.
104. Sparmann A, Bar-Sagi D: Ras-induced interleukin-8 expression plays a critical role in tumor growth and angiogenesis, *Cancer Cell* 6(5):447–458, 2004. Epub 2004/11/16.
105. Yi F, Jaffe R, Prochownik EV: The CCL6 chemokine is differentially regulated by c-Myc and L-Myc, and promotes tumorigenesis and metastasis, *Cancer Res* 63(11):2923–2932, 2003. Epub 2003/06/05.
106. Noy R, Pollard JW: Tumor-associated macrophages: from mechanisms to therapy, *Immunity* 41(1):49–61, 2014. Epub 2014/07/19.
107. Ben-Baruch A: Organ selectivity in metastasis: regulation by chemokines and their receptors, *Clin Exp Metastasis* 25(4):345–356, 2008.
108. Muller A, Homey B, Soto H, et al.: Involvement of chemokine receptors in breast cancer metastasis, *Nature* 410(6824):50–56, 2001.
109. Zlotnik A: Chemokines and cancer, *Int J Cancer* 119(9):2026–2029, 2006.

30 Angiogenesis

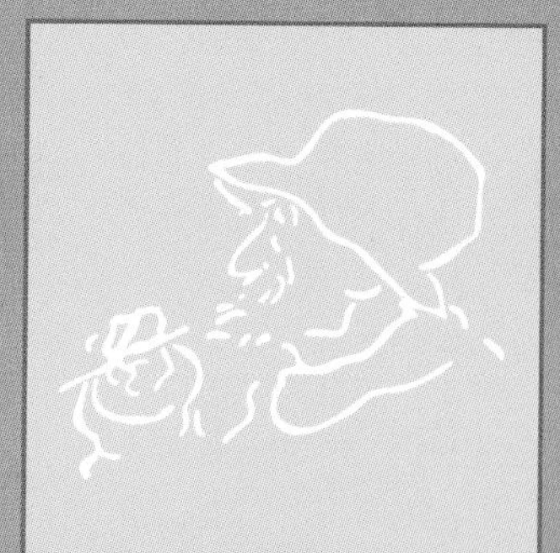

URSULA FEARON, ZOLTÁN SZEKANECZ, AND DOUGLAS J. VEALE

KEY POINTS

Angiogenesis is the sprouting of new vessels from pre-existing vessels.
Synovial angiogenesis facilitates leukocyte extravasation into the joint.
Angiogenic blood vessel growth and migration relies on tip-stalk cell communication.
Angiogenesis is tightly controlled by pro- and anti-angiogenic mediators, including growth factors, chemokines, cytokines, and matrix remodelling proteins.
Metabolic changes in EC dictates their phenotypic fate.

Introduction

Angiogenesis is a dynamic multistep process that contributes to normal physiologic processes, but is also a key mechanism in a number of pathologic conditions including inflammatory arthritis (IA).[1–4] Angiogenesis is the formation of new blood vessels whereby new capillaries sprout from existing blood vessels. The early development of a rich vascular network facilitates leukocyte extravasation into the joint, in addition to supplying the nutrients required for the expansion of resident cells. Angiogenesis is tightly controlled by both pro- and anti-angiogenic factors and is driven by numerous growth factors and pro-inflammatory cytokines in the inflamed joint. Activation of endothelial cells (EC) by proangiogenic stimuli results in the secretion of degradative enzymes that dissolve the EC basement membrane and the extracellular matrix (ECM) components. Migration of ECs through the connective tissue matrix results in the formation of primary capillary sprouts. This is followed by EC proliferation, migration, tip-stalk cell selection, sprout elongation, synthesis of basement membrane, and lumen formation.

Endothelial Cells

Endothelial Permeability

EC line the lumina of blood vessels, thus they separate and connect the blood and the ECM of the vessel wall. The main function of ECs is to contain and distribute blood, facilitate gas and fluid exchange, regulate coagulation cascades, interact with circulating leukocytes to facilitate inflammation, and interact with SMC/pericytes to regulate vascular tone. The endothelium is involved in numerous homeostatic mechanisms, as well as in pathologic states.[1–4] In inflammatory states, such as arthritis, ECs interact with other cell types including leukocytes, fibroblasts, and pericytes. ECs express numerous cell adhesion molecules (CAMs), adhere to ECM components, and secrete a number of inflammatory mediators, such as cytokines, nitric oxide (NO), prostaglandins, endothelin 1 (ET-1), and proteases, and thus they regulate inflammation in the surrounding tissue. ECs are also active responders to external stimuli as they may become targets of inflammatory mediators produced by leukocytes.[1–10]

Vascular endothelium undergoes morphologic changes during the inflammatory response including vasodilatation and increased permeability (leakage), which result from several mechanisms including EC contraction and retraction, leukocyte- or anti-EC antibody (AECA)-mediated vascular injury and regeneration.[1,6,11,12] ECs release vasodilatory mediators including prostacyclin (PGI_2), NO, and platelet-activating factor (PAF).[1,2,7,13] Factors triggering endothelial leakage include, among others, histamine, serotonin, complement factors, bradykinin, leukotrienes, PAF, and AECA. EC adhesion accompanied by cytoskeletal reorganization occurs upon EC activation by pro-inflammatory cytokines such as IL-1, TNF, or interferon-γ (IFN-γ).[1–3,13–15]

Endothelial Injury and Regeneration

In inflammation, endothelial injury is caused by inflammatory cells, as well as soluble mediators.[3,16–18] Various mediators produced by ECs themselves and other cells lead to endothelial injury. ECs synthesize NO, prostaglandins, ET-1, and other substances.[1–3,10,18–20] During inflammation, ECs and leukocytes produce high amounts of NO,[3,21] which interacts with ROI.[13,19,20] EC injury also involves ROI and matrix metalloproteinase (MMP) enzymes produced by inflammatory leukocytes.[18,19,22–25] Asymmetric dimethylarginine (ADMA) is a naturally produced amino acid that circulates in the plasma. Increased ADMA production is associated with vascular injury, as well as inflammatory rheumatic diseases.[3,22,23] ET-1, a vasoconstrictor peptide, activates leukocyte adhesion and is involved in ECM remodeling and vascular injury.[13,24]

Angiogenesis

Synovial angiogenesis is a cascade of tightly regulated steps, which includes enzymatic degradation of capillary basement membrane, EC activation and proliferation, tip cell selection, directed

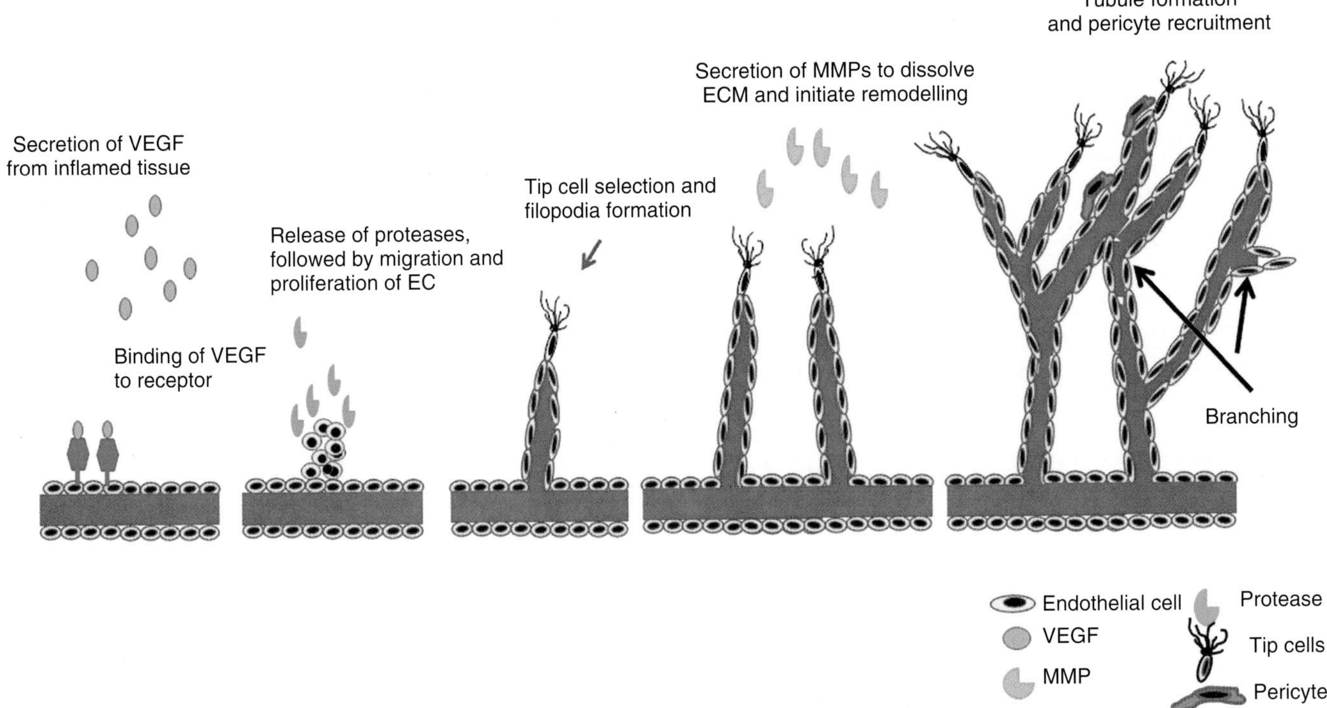

• **Fig. 30.1** Sprouting angiogenesis. VEFG is produced and secreted from inflamed tissue. VEGF binds to and activates receptors expressed on endothelial cells present on the pre-existing synovial blood vessels. Activation of endothelial cells results in the release of enzymes called *proteases* that degrade the basement membrane to allow endothelial cells to escape from the original (parent) vessel walls. Based on the VEGF gradient tip cell, selection occurs and ECs then proliferate towards the angiogenic stimulus into the surrounding microenvironment, forming solid sprouts that connect to their neighboring vessels. To further support this process ECs secrete MMP enzymes that degrade extra-cellular matrix in front of the sprouting vessel, thus further accommodating the growth of the new vessels within the pre-existing architecture. As the vessel extends, the sprouts form loops to become a fully formed vessel lumen. Pericytes are then recruited to form the outer layer of the blood vessel.

migration of ECs, tubulogenesis, vessel fusion, and pericyte stabilization.[25–28] While there are many different forms of angiogenesis including (1) sprouting, (2) intussusceptive, (3) vessel co-option, and (4) vessel mimicry, the most well described in inflammatory conditions is "sprouting" angiogenesis.

Sprouting Angiogenesis

Inflamed tissues produce and release proangiogenic growth factors (described later), which bind to receptors expressed on the EC of the nearby pre-existing blood vessels (Fig. 30.1).[29–30] Once activated, ECs release enzymes known as *proteases* that degrade the surrounding basement membrane, facilitating the detachment and escape of ECs from their parent vessel wall. ECs then proliferate towards the angiogenic stimulus into the surrounding microenvironment, forming solid sprouts that connect to their neighboring vessels. To further support this process ECs secrete MMP enzymes that degrade ECM in front of the sprouting vessel, thus further accommodating the growth of the new vessels within the pre-existing architecture. As the vessel extends the sprouts form loops to become a fully formed vessel lumen. Pericytes are then recruited to form the outer layer of the blood vessel. Finally, tight interjunctional complexes are formed through increased expression of adhesion molecules, followed by basement membrane deposition.

Endothelial Subtypes

Blood vessels are composed of developmentally related but functionally distinct ECs (Fig. 30.2). There are three EC subsets, tip cells, stalk cells, and phalanx cells, which have distinct cellular fates and functions (migration, proliferation, and quiescence).[29–33] Their specialized function is key to the development of a proper functioning vessel, which is defined by their spatial organization within the inflamed microenvironment and is dependent on the signals they sense. Thus a coordinated response by ECs is critical to this process, and all three EC cell types must "know" the phenotypic profile of their neighboring cells, which in turn will dictate their function. In order for a proper functioning sprout, some ECs will migrate (tip cells), other ECs will divide and form the lagging cells (stalk cells), while other ECs remain quiescent (phalanx).

Sprouting initiation requires one EC to respond to a stimulus, which senses higher concentrations of the stimulus compared to their neighboring EC.[34] This EC cell becomes the tip cell at the forefront of vessel branching and is highly polarized and migratory. Tip cells have a specific molecular signature characterized by Delta-like ligand-4 (Dll4), a Notch ligand, the surface adhesion glycoprotein CD34, the axon guidance receptor Unc5B, neuropilin-1, CXCR4, and VEGFR-2/-3,[35,36] expression of which is increased in the vascular regions of the inflamed synovium.[37–40] Essential for the tip cell phenotype is lamellipodial and filopodial formation. Lamellipodia are short cytoskeletal actin projections on the leading edge of the tip cell, whereas filopodia consist of long spiky protrusions that extend beyond the leading edge of the cell. Lamellipodia and filopodia probe the environment, detect gradients of navigatory cues, and interpret combinatorial

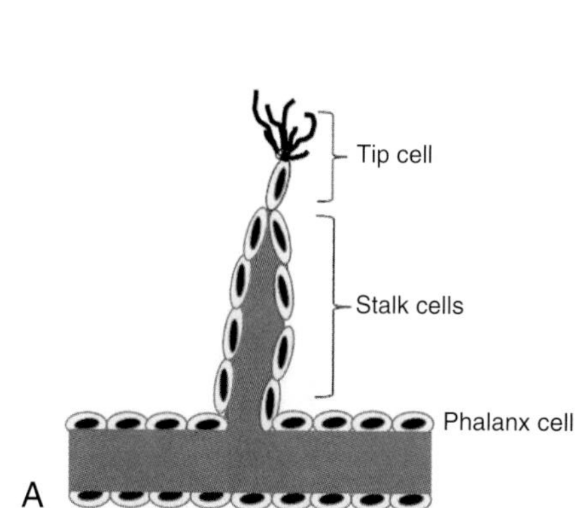

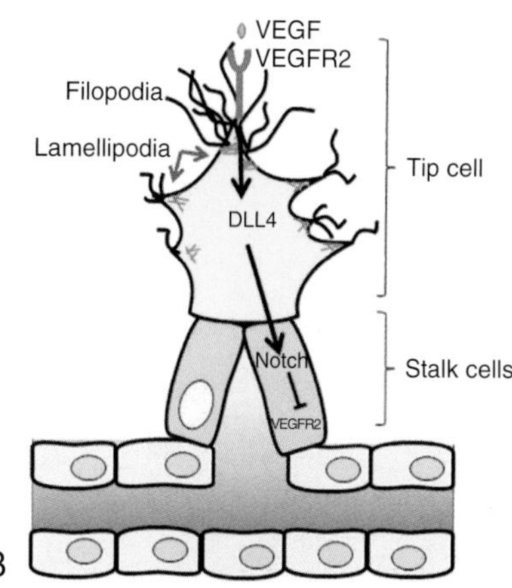

• **Fig. 30.2** Endothelial cell subtypes and lateral inhibition. (A) Blood vessels are composed of developmentally related but functionally distinct endothelial cells (ECs). There are three EC subsets, tip cells, stalk cells, and phalanx cells, which have distinct cellular fates and functions (migration, proliferation, and quiescence, respectively). (B) Lateral inhibition. The tip cell is selected based on the fact that it senses the highest concentration of VEGF. Binding of VEGF to the VEGFR on the tip cell induces expression of DLL-4 in the tip cell, which in turn, binds to Notch on the neighboring EC. Notch activation inhibits VEGFR signaling, making this cell less sensitive to VEGF stimulation and thus limiting its ability to activate DLL-4 in the neighboring cell. This inhibits tip cell formation and promotes the stalk cell phenotype in this cell. Once selected, migratory tip cells form lamellipodia and filopodial extensions that sprout towards the VEGF gradient, further strengthening their position as the tip cell. The adjacent stalk cell now follows the guiding tip cell and proliferates to support sprout elongation.

molecular codes that dictate the directional migration of tip cells. This involves actin cytoskeletal rearrangement and activation of the Rho-family of GTPases, which include Cdc42, Rac1, and RhoA.[41–46] In response to a positive stimulus, Cdc42 induces filopodial formation and cell polarization via microtubule organization, Rac1 regulates lamellipodial formation, whereas RhoA induces stress fiber formation via the Rho-associated serine threorine protein kinase (ROCK), promoting forward movement of the tip cell.[41–46] Lamellipodia and filopodia also form focal adhesion points, through activation of focal adhesion kinase (FAK), which connect the cytoskeleton to ECM, leading to stress fiber rearrangement of actin/myosin filaments that pulls the cell forward, thus inducing migration. Pro-inflammatory mediators including TNF, IL-17A, and TLR-agonists alter cytoskeletal dynamics and induce integrin expression (β1 and αvβv3), with subsequent activation of Cdc42 and Rac1 in vitro,[47–50] consistent with the observed increased expression of specific integrins and FAKs in RA synovial vascular regions.[47–50] Once the tip cell is selected, the neighboring ECs are prevented from becoming tip cells and become stalk cells. Stalk cells proliferate in order to increase mass and surface area of the growing blood vessel, and in contrast to tip cells, do not display filopodial extensions.[51,52] Once the lumen is fully formed and blood flow is established, the migratory activity and proliferation of the tip and stalk EC stop and they revert back to the quiescent EC phenotype, the phalanx cells.[53–55]

Tip-Stalk Cell Lateral Inhibition

How ECs are directed to become tip, stalk, and phalanx cells relies on tip-stalk cell communication, a process dependent on the Notch signaling pathway (see Fig. 30.2), which plays a pivotal role in vascular development and cell-cell communication.[56–59] The Notch receptors and ligands are transmembrane proteins, thus Notch signals require cell-cell contact. Four Notch receptors have been described in mammals with ligands encoded by Jagged-1, 2 and Delta-like 1, 3, 4 (DLL-1, DLL-3, DLL-4) genes.[60–67] Cleavage of Notch receptors releases Notch intra-cellular domain, which translocates into the nucleus,[66–67] regulating downstream target genes Hrt (Hes-related transcriptional repressors) and Hes (Hairy/Enhancer of Split).[57,67]

Vascular endothelial growth factor (VEGF) receptor signaling is the primary stimulator of tip cell formation. The tip cell is selected based on the fact that it senses the highest concentration of VEGF. Binding of VEGF to the VEGFR on the tip cell induces expression of DLL-4 in the tip cell[68,69] (see Fig. 30.2). In turn, DLL-4 binds to Notch on the neighboring EC and inhibits VEGFR signaling, making this cell less sensitive to VEGF stimulation and thus limiting its ability to activate DLL-4 in the neighboring cell. This inhibits tip cell formation and promotes the stalk cell phenotype, thus creating a feedback loop that allows the leading tip cell to maintain its position.[70] Once selected, migratory tip cells form filopodial extensions and sprout towards the VEGF gradient,[71,72] further strengthening their position as the "tip cell." The adjacent stalk cell now follows the guiding tip cell and proliferates to support sprout elongation.[72] Expression of Notch 1IC, its ligand DLL4, and downstream components is increased in the inflamed synovium,[37,69,73] localized to synovial blood vessels, and regulated by hypoxia and the complimentary action of VEGF/Ang2.[37,69,73] Moreover, Notch signaling is thought to promote integrin/FAK-mediated pathways,[74–76] known to be overexpressed in inflamed synovium.[47–50,76]

Vessel Stabilization and Maturity

Pericytes are critical players in the microcirculation, and the maturation and stability of the blood vessel depends on their presence and interaction with ECs. Pericytes reside within the basement membrane, align themselves along the vessel wall, and interact with EC through direct interdigitations.[77] Functionally, pericytes are involved in the regulation of blood vessel diameter, vessel permeability, EC proliferation, angiogenesis, and leukocyte recruitment.[78–81] Initiation of new blood vessels occurs in the presence of high levels of VEGF and angiopoietin 2 (Ang2), which interact to induce angiogenesis,[69] both of which are significantly expressed

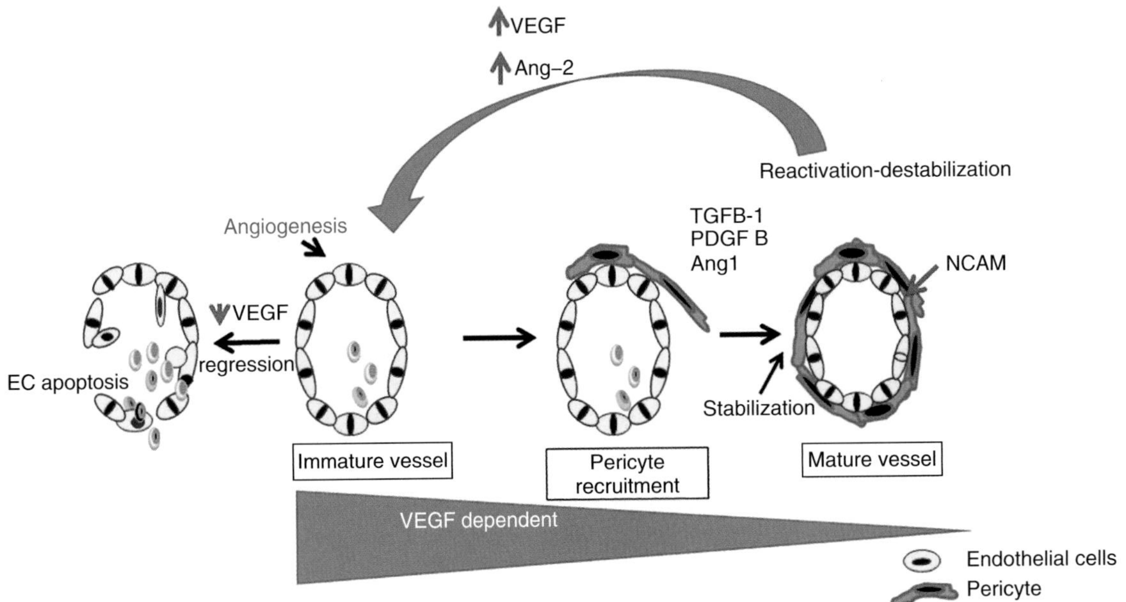

• **Fig. 30.3** Blood vessel maturation and stabilization. Initiation of new blood vessels occurs in the presence of high levels of VEGF and angiopoietin 2 (Ang2) which interact to induce angiogenesis. At this early stage, the immature vessel is vulnerable (no pericyte coverage), and if VEGF and Ang2 are withdrawn the vessel will regress and undergo EC apoptosis. As the vessel matures, it becomes less dependent on VEGF and other factors become important, including platelet derived growth factor-B, (PDGF-B/PDGFR-β), Ang1, and transforming growth factor-β (TGF-β), which recruit supporting pericytes around the EC wall. Close alignment of EC and pericytes is also mediated by neural cell adhesion molecule (NCAM). If the EC/pericyte interactions are not fully intact the vessel can be re-exposed to high levels of VEGF and Ang2, which can reactivate and destabilize the vessel once again, further exacerbating disease.

in the inflamed synovium early in disease[82–85] (Fig. 30.3). At this early stage, the immature vessel is vulnerable (no pericyte coverage), and if VEGF and Ang2 are withdrawn the vessel will regress through EC apoptosis. As the vessel matures, it becomes less dependent on VEGF, and other factors become important, including the prominent signaling pathways, platelet derived growth factor-B, (PDGF-B/PDGFR-β), Ang1, and transforming growth factor-β (TGF-β),[86–89] which recruit supporting pericytes around the EC wall. In the context of IA, a significant number of immature vessels are present in the inflamed synovium,[79,80] where incomplete EC/pericyte interactions have been observed and are associated with hypoxia and increased oxidative damage.[79,90] Close alignment of ECs and pericytes is also mediated by neural cell adhesion molecule (NCAM),[91] lack of which has also been observed in the IA joint.[79] If the EC/pericyte interactions are not fully intact the vessel can be re-exposed to high levels of VEGF and Ang2, which can reactivate and destabilize the vessel once again, further exacerbating disease. Pericytes will also influence the local ECM to guide endothelial migration by modulating deposition of basement membrane proteins.[92,93] Furthermore, EC–pericyte cell interactions alter the expression of ECM-binding integrins by both cell types, which are required for the newly formed matrix.[94] Once vascular tubes are formed, pericyte-derived tissue inhibitor of metalloproteinase-3 (TIMP-3) inhibits proteolysis of matrix proteins.[95]

Regulators of Angiogenesis

Several inflammatory mediators including growth factors (GF), cytokines, chemokines and their receptors, certain CAMs, as well as other mediators can modulate neovascularization in RA (Table 30.1) (reviewed in references 26, 96–99).

Growth Factors

Hypoxia is a major pathogenic factor in arthritis-associated angiogenesis.[79] VEGF is induced by hypoxia and hypoxia-inducible factors (HIF-1α and HIF-2α) in RA. Interactions between VEGF and Ang1/Ang2 have been implicated in the regulation of blood vessel maturation.[100] Ang1 plays a critical role in pericyte recruitment and vessel stabilization. On the other hand, Ang2 exerts an antagonizing effect leading to vessel regression, however, in the presence of VEGF it promotes capillary sprouting.[98–100] VEGF, HIF-1α, HIF-2α, Ang1, and Tie2 have all been detected in the RA synovium already in the very early phase of the disease.[26,69,82,96] Expression of Ang1, Ang2, and their receptor Tie2 correlates with progression of disease in collagen induced arthritis (CIA) models, with blockade of Tie2 ameliorating bone destruction.[101,102] Studies have shown that Tie2 mediates Toll-like receptor 2 (TLR-2)-induced angiogenesis in RA.[103] Other angiogenic mediators, such as pro-inflammatory cytokines (e.g., IL-6, IL-17, IL-18), monocyte/macrophage migration inhibitory factor (MIF), endothelin 1, and others may also stimulate angiogenesis via VEGF-dependent mechanisms.[96,104] More recently, the role of the GATA4 transcription factor has been implicated in VEGF-dependent angiogenesis underlying arthritis and pannus formation.[105]

Other GFs implicated in synovial angiogenesis include fibroblast GF (FGF-1 and -2), epidermal GF (EGF), hepatocyte GF (HGF), keratinocyte GF (KGF), insulin-like GF I (IGF-I), connective tissue GF (CTGF), placenta GF (PlGF) platelet-derived GF (PDGF), as well as transforming GF β (TGF-β). All of these GFs have been implicated in synovial angiogenesis either through VEGF-dependent or -independent mechanisms. Moreover, many of these growth factors are bound to heparin and heparan sulfate proteoglycans in the synovial ECM and they are mobilized by proteases during synovial neovascularization.[26,96,99,104,105,106]

TABLE 30.1 Some Angiogenic and Angiostatic Factors in Rheumatoid Arthritis

	Mediators	Inhibitors
Chemokines	CXCL1, CXCL5, CXCL7, CXCL8, CXCL12, CCL2, CCL21, CCL23, CX3CL1	CXCL4, CXCL9, CXCL10, CCL21
Matrix molecules	Type I collagen, fibronectin, laminin, heparin, heparan sulphate	Thrombospondin, RGD sequence
Cell adhesion molecules	β_1 and β_3 integrins, E-selectin, P-selectin, CD34, VCAM-1, endoglin, PECAM-1, VE-cadherin, Le^y/H, MUC18, galectin 9	RGD sequence (integrin ligand)
Growth factors	VEGF, bFGF, aFGF, PDGF, EGF, IGF-I, HIF-1, TGF-β[a]	TGF-β[a]
Cytokines	TNF, IL-15, IL-18, CCN1	IL-4, IL-35, IFN-α, IFN-γ
Proteases	MMPs, plasminogen activators	TIMPs, plasminogen activator inhibitors
Others	Angiogenin, substance P, prolactin	DMARDs, infliximab, etanercept, angiostatin, endostatin

[a]Mediators with both pro- and anti-angiogenic effects

aFGF, Acidic fibroblast growth factor; *bFGF,* basic fibroblast growth factor; *CCN1,* cysteine-rich 61; *DMARDs,* disease-modifying anti-rheumatic drug; *EGF,* endothelial growth factor; *HIF-1,* hypoxia-inducible factor-1; *IFN,* interferon; *IGF,* insulin-like growth factor; *MMPs,* matrix metalloproteinases; *MUC18,* mucin-like protein 18; *PDGF,* platelet-derived growth factor; *PECAM,* platelet-endothelial adhesion molecule; *RGD,* arginine-glycineaspartate; *TGF,* transforming growth factor; *TIMPs,* tissue inhibitors of metalloproteinase; *TNF,* tumor necrosis factor; *VCAM,* vascular cell adhesion molecule; *VEGF,* vascular endothelial growth factor.

Cytokines and Chemokines

Pro-inflammatory cytokines may exert direct angiogenic activity or may act indirectly via VEGF-dependent pathways. Among these mediators, TNF, IL-1α and β, IL-6, IL-8, IL-15, IL-17, IL-18, oncostatin M, MIF, granulocyte (G-CSF), granulocyte-macrophage colony-stimulating factors (GM-CSF), and cysteine-rich 61 (CCN1) have been implicated in synovial angiogenesis.[26,48,96,107,108] For example, TNF induces VEGF production by various cell types such as macrophages and ECs.[109,110] These inflammatory molecules also increase the expression of other angiogenic mediators including chemokines, CAMs, and MMPs and may also influence the Ang1/Tie2 axis.[26,48,96,107,108] For example, IL-17A induces angiogenesis, cell migration, and cell invasion in RA, mechanisms that are mediated in part through chemokine- and cytoskeleton-dependent pathways.[48] Recently, CCN1, an important pro-inflammatory cytokine, promoted VEGF production by osteoblasts and increased angiogenesis in arthritis.[108] On the other hand, some cytokines, such as IFNα, IFNγ, IL-4, IL-12, and leukemia inhibitory factor (LIF) suppress angiogenesis, mostly by inhibiting VEGF-dependent pathways.[96] More recently, IL-35 inhibits synovial angiogenesis by blocking VEGF as well as STAT1 signaling.[111]

A number of chemokines and chemokine receptors have been implicated in angiogenesis underlying RA.[96,112,113] The angiogenic nature of most CXC chemokines has been associated with the glutamyl-leucyl-arginyl (ELR) amino acid sequence. The most relevant ELR-containing, angiogenic CXC chemokines include CXCL1, CXCL5, CXCL7, and CXCL8.[96,112–114] In contrast, most ELR-lacking CXC chemokines (CXCL4, CXCL9, CXCL10) inhibit angiogenesis.[112] However, as one exception to the rule, CXCL12 is an angiogenic chemokine that lacks the ELR motif.[26,112] The CXCL12/CXCR4 axis is fundamentally important in vasculogenesis as it attracts endothelial progenitor cells (EPCs) to line the newly formed blood vessels.[26] Among CC chemokines, CCL2 induces EC chemotaxis in vitro and angiogenesis in vivo. CCL23 has been implicated in the migration of vascular ECs and MMP production. CX_3CL1 (fractalkine) is involved in both angiogenesis and atherosclerosis underlying RA.[96,113] Among chemokine receptors, CXCR2 may be the most relevant one to ELR-containing angiogenic CXC chemokines such as CXCL1, CXCL5, and CXCL8 on ECs. The importance of the CXCL12/CXCR4 axis in vasculogenesis was highlighted previously. CCR2-CCL2 and CCR7-CCL21 interactions are also involved in synovial neovascularization.[96,112] Chemokines may also act indirectly to support angiogenesis through the attraction of leukocytes to the inflamed synovium, further inducing neovascularization. For example, CCL2 is a major chemoattractant of monocytes/macrophages, which are a major source of angiogenic mediators. CX3CL1 (fractalkine) also recruits leukocytes and promotes angiogenesis independently.[112,113]

Matrix Remodeling: The Role of Adhesion Molecules

Remodeling of the ECM involves several ECM components, CAMs, and proteases, which have also been implicated in inflammatory angiogenesis.[96,97,115,116] For example, type I collagen, fibronectin, laminin, vitronectin, tenascin, and proteoglycans mediate, while thrombospondin 1 (TSP-1) inhibits EC adhesion and neovascularization.[96,115] As described earlier, some GFs bind to proteoglycans during angiogenesis.[97,115] Among CAMs, most β_1 and β_3 integrins, E-selectin, the L-selectin ligand CD34, selectin-related glycoconjugates including Lewis^y/H and MUC18, vascular cell adhesion molecule 1 (VCAM-1), platelet-endothelial CAM 1 (PECAM-1), endoglin, and junction-adhesion molecules (JAMs) are expressed on the EC surface and promote angiogenesis.[26,96,97,116–118]

Recent evidence suggests mammalian lectins, such as galectin 9, have been implicated in arthritis-associated angiogenesis.[119] MMPs, ADAM, and ADAMTS proteases digest the ECM, release GFs and other angiogenic mediators, and thus promote synovial angiogenesis.[96,97,115]

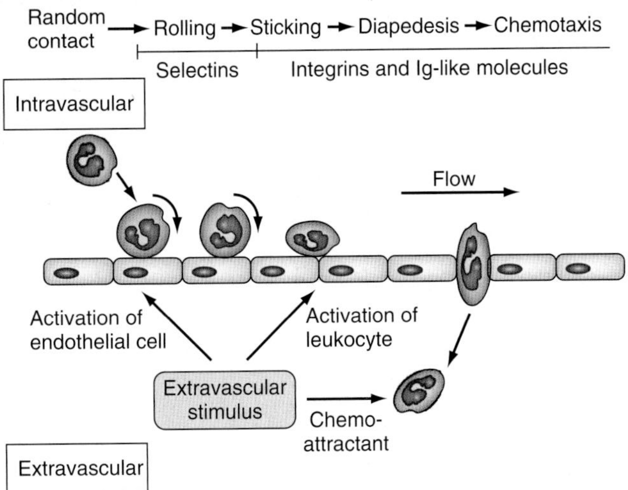

• **Fig. 30.4** The process of leukocyte extravasation in inflammation. During leukocyte adhesion and transendothelial migration, an early, weak adhesion termed *rolling* occurs first. This step involves mainly selectins and their ligands and leads to leukocyte activation. Firm adhesion involves mostly integrin-CAM dependent interactions, as well as the secretion of numerous chemokines. Chemokines preferentially attract endothelium-bound leukocytes. Leukocytes migrate through the endothelial bed via a process known as *diapedesis*.

Remodeling of the ECM is a critical step during the angiogenic process. Among the players involved in synovial neovascularization described earlier, the TSP-1-TGF-β-CTGF axis is a good example for GF-ECM crosstalk during angiogenesis.[120] Among CAMs, integrins and their ligands and E-selectin have been implicated in cell-ECM interactions during ECM remodeling demonstrated to be of significant importance in angiogenesis.[26,50,96] Among integrins, the αvβ3 integrin, as well as the *ITGAV* gene play a critical role in angiogenesis. This integrin has become a major target for specific therapy.[26,47,96,121] FAKs are involved in αvβ3 integrin signaling underlying synovial inflammation and angiogenesis.[47,50] Moreover, MMPs and other proteases that digest ECM components play a crucial role in the process of remodeling.[96,122,123]

Transendothelial Leukocyte Recruitment During Angiogenesis

Leukocyte Extravasation in Inflammation

Adhesion of peripheral blood leukocytes to endothelium leads to the process of leukocyte transendothelial migration into the inflamed joint (Fig. 30.4).[116,123] During leukocyte adhesion and transendothelial migration, an early, weak adhesion termed *rolling* occurs first. This step involves mainly selectins and their ligands and leads to leukocyte activation. Firm adhesion involves mostly integrin-dependent interactions, primarily ICAM-1 and VCAM-1, as well as the secretion of numerous chemokines. Chemokines preferentially attract endothelium-bound leukocytes. Transendothelial migration may be the point of no return in inflammation.[116,124]

Regulation of Leukocyte Migration by Chemokines During Angiogenesis

Chemokines may induce CAM expression and thus promote cell adhesion and angiogenesis. For example, CCL2 regulates β_3 integrin expression through the Ets-1 transcription factor.[125] Stimulation of CXCR1- and CXCR2-dependent pathways in arthritis models resulted in increased neutrophil adhesion to endothelium.[126] Thus, various chemokines and chemokine receptors are involved in driving leukocyte transendothelial migration.

As described earlier, numerous ELR-containing CXC chemokines, CC chemokines, CX_3CL1 (fractalkine), and their receptors have been implicated in angiogenesis underlying RA.[96,112] Chemokine-induced neovascularization may involve CAMs. For example, CCL2-induced angiogenesis may occur via β_3 integrins.[126]

Hypoxia, Cell Metabolism, and Angiogenesis

Hypoxia

The hypothesis that the inflamed joint is hypoxic was originally proposed based on studies demonstrating increased surrogate markers of hypoxia in the synovial cavity or synovial fluid (SF) of patients with RA.[127,128] This was confirmed in subsequent studies using specific oxygen probes, which demonstrated that the inflamed synovium was profoundly hypoxic, with low pO_2 levels associated with increased synovial vascularity, growth factor expression, and oxidative damage, paralleled by a lack of NCAM expression.[79,129,130] Studies have shown that hypoxia induces the expression of VEGF, its receptor VEGFR, angiopoietins, MCP-1, IL-8, and MMPs, from synovial cells/explants under hypoxia conditions.[129] In addition, hypoxia can potentiate the effects of IL-17A, IL-1β and TNF on angiogenic and invasive mechanisms in RA through HIF-1α and NF-κB activation.[131–133] Activation of HIF-1α through transient silencing of prolyl hydroxylases (PHD) in synovial fibroblasts induces the expression of many proangiogenic/inflammatory mediators.[134] Furthermore, synovial expression of Notch signaling components is associated with low synovial pO_2 levels,[37] and is induced by hypoxia and VEGF/Ang2 in vitro.[27,69] Interestingly, Notch−1 silencing inhibits hypoxia−induced HIF−1α expression, angiogenesis, EC migration/invasion, and activity of MMP−2 and MMP−9, thus creating complex bidirectional signaling interactions that regulate synovial angiogenesis.[37]

Cell Metabolism

Evidence for a key role of metabolism in the regulation of synovial inflammation has emerged, where proliferation and rapid activation of immune and stromal cells require a switch in their cell metabolism from oxidative phosphorylation to glycolysis.[135,136] While in the context of synovial EC very little is known, tumor studies have demonstrated that the three EC subsets (tip, stalk, and phalanx cells) differ in their energy, biomass, and redox requirements.[137–138] It is now apparent that metabolic changes in EC dictate their phenotypic differentiation into tip, stalk, or phalanx cells, with tip and stalk cells showing increased glycolytic rates compared to phalanx EC.[139] In IA, synovial blood vessels display enhanced expression of the glucose transporter GLUT1, glycolytic enzymes, metabolic intermediate receptors, and components of the mitochondrial electron transport chain, NADPH oxidase (NOX).[140–143] In particular, two glycolytic rate-limiting enzymes, 6-phosphofructo-2-kinase/fructose-2,6-bisphosphatase 3 (PFKFB3) and Hexokinase 2 (HK2), which regulate EC angiogenesis, are significantly increased in synovial vascular regions and mediate VEGF induced-sprout formation.[141,142] Indeed, cancer studies have shown that these glycolytic enzymes are compartmentalized to the tip cell, with high localized expression in the sensing filopodia, thus generating rapid ATP for tip cell migration.[137,139] Blockade of PFKFB3 inhibits angiogenic tube formation, secretion of proangiogenic mediators, and key signaling pathways in RAFLS and EC.[140] Consistent with these studies, PFKFB3 and/or HK2 inhibition reduces disease severity in disease models driven by pathogenic angiogenesis including RA, psoriasis, and IBD.[137,141,142] Enriched synovial vascular expression of another metabolic enzyme, glucose-6-phosphate isomerase (G6PI), which plays a crucial role in glycolysis and gluconeogenesis, has also recently been shown, with in vitro G6PI loss-of-function assays demonstrating the requirement of G6PI in mediating hypoxia-induced angiogenesis in RA.[143] Finally, in animal models of arthritis the metabolic intermediate succinate induced synovial angiogenesis through VEGF-dependent HIF-1α pathways.[144]

Targeting Angiogenesis

Currently, disease-modifying anti-rheumatic agents (DMARDs) such as rofecoxib, dexamethasone, chloroquine, sulfasalazine, methotrexate, azathioprine, cyclophosphamide, leflunomide, thalidomide, tacrolimus, minocycline, and anti-TNF therapies nonspecifically suppress angiogenesis.[145–147] The anti–IL-6 receptor antibody tocilizumab reduced serum levels of VEGF[148] and synovial microvessel density in RA.[149] Another cytokine that both directly and indirectly induces synovial angiogenesis is IL-18, blockade of which reduces secretion of proangiogenic mediators from synovial cells, and inhibits disease progression in a CIA model of arthritis.[150] While phase 1 clinical trials of humanized neutralizing antibodies against IL-18pb showed a dose-dependent pharmacokinetics with no adverse events in moderate to severe RA, further trials have not been performed.[151] Studies have also shown that tofacitinib (JAK-STAT inhibitor), which is widely approved for treatment of RA, reduces the secretion of proangiogenic mediators in vitro and in vivo.[152,153] Furthermore, JAK-STAT signaling pathways also interact with both HIF-1α and Notch signaling,[154] in addition to specific glycolytic enzymes.[152]

Several studies have examined blocking angiogenic pathways such as VEGF, its receptors, or the angiopoietins in models of arthritis, both in vitro and in vivo.[101,155,156] Bevacizumab, an anti-VEGF monoclonal antibody,[157] is approved for colon, kidney, and lung cancer, however, efficacy has not been observed in RA. A soluble Tie2 receptor transcript delivered via an adenoviral vector attenuated the incidence and severity in CIA models.[101] A double anti-angiogenic protein (DAAP; a dimeric decoy receptor) that strongly binds to Ang1, Ang2, and VEGF, had better protective effects than VEGF-Trap or Tie2-Fc on both inflammation and bone destruction in the CIA models of arthritis.[158] This study also showed that DAAP had beneficial combination effects with TNFi, suggesting that coordinated blocking of angiogenic activities by DAAP with TNFi might represent a promising therapeutic approach to RA.

Inhibitors against tyrosine kinases, NF-κB signaling, MAPK-PI3K signaling, and FAK signaling have all been developed.[26] Sunitinib, a multitargeted receptor tyrosine kinase (RTK) inhibitor that is FDA approved for treatment of specific cancers, inhibits synovial neoangiogenesis and joint destruction in CIA models. Other tyrosine kinase inhibitors approved for cancer include Pazopanib and PD166866, however, they have not been tested in inflammatory diseases.[26] Recent studies have examined noncanonical NF-κB pathways, with studies showing that mice deficient in NF-κB-inducing kinase (NIK) have a reduction in synovial blood vessels, paralleled by significantly less inflammation in the adjuvant-induced arthritis model.[159] MAPK inhibitors, including tacrolimus, the ERK inhibitor-FR180204, and a p38 inhibitor reduce EC proliferation and migration, secretion of growth factors, and inhibit radiographic damage in animal models of arthritis.[26] Despite this data, many of these inhibitors failed in RA clinical trials due to lack of efficacy or toxic effects.

Given the role of Notch signaling in tip cell selection and filopodial protrusion, studies have also examined targeting Notch signaling in addition to integrin-FAK mediated pathways. Inhibition of Notch signaling with γ-secretase inhibitors and nanoparticle delivery significantly reduced cytokine/chemokine and growth factor expression, in addition to attenuation of disease severity in RA animal models.[160,161] Several in vitro studies have shown that FAK inhibitors (Pf-573,228 and FAK inhibitor-14) decrease VEGF-induced EC migration and angiogenic tube formation. Several FAK inhibitors including defactinib, TAE226, PF-562,271, and GSK225-6098 have been developed,[26] however these peptides have yet to be tested in clinical trials. Vitaxin (MEDI-522), a humanized monoclonal IgG1 antibody that specifically binds to the αvβ3 integrin that is expressed on synovial blood vessels at an early stage of disease, inhibits synovial angiogenesis and disease severity in animal models of arthritis.[162] These pre-clinical studies led to a phase II clinical trial in RA; however, its efficacy was limited.[163]

As highlighted earlier, chemokines play a key role in proangiogenic mechanisms in IA, with many studies focusing on the CXCL12–CXCR4/CXCR7 signaling axis. Monoclonal antibodies or antagonists against CXCL12, CXCR4, or CXCR7 have demonstrated significant reduction in blood vessel numbers, T-cell infiltration, and joint inflammation in various animal models of arthritis.[26,99] Neutralization of MIF suppresses synovial vascularization and joint swelling in experimental arthritis.[164] Milatuzumab (an anti-CD74 monoclonal antibody), which targets CD74, a part of the MIF receptor, is currently in phase I clinical trials for the treatment of systemic lupus erythematosus (SLE) (clinicaltrials.gov). While several pharmacologic inhibitors of this axis are in phase I-II clinical trials for different cancers, they have not yet been tested in RA.

Finally, metabolic pathways have been implicated in disease pathogenesis. In particular, PFKFB3 and HK2 inhibition reduced angiogenic mediators in synovial cells in vitro/ex vivo, in addition to reducing severity of disease in animal models of arthritis.[141–143] Furthermore, targeting metabolic intermediates such as succinate is also a promising therapeutic avenue, where their cellular accumulation regulates synovial angiogenesis and synovial fibroblast invasiveness.[141]

In summary, angiogenesis is one of the primary events in synovial pathogenesis, activation of which facilitates leukocyte infiltration, leading to pannus expansion and joint invasion. Many therapeutic approaches have successfully resolved arthritic joint vascularization in pre-clinical models, however, this has not translated successfully to the clinic. It is likely that novel strategies that target multiple pathways or combining anti-angiogenic therapies with current treatments may be utilized in future IA therapies.

Full references for this chapter can be found on ExpertConsult.com.

Selected References

1. Szekanecz Z, Koch AE: Vascular endothelium and immune responses: implications for inflammation and angiogenesis, *Rheum Dis Clin North Am* 30(1):97–114, 2004.
2. Szekanecz Z, Koch AE: Endothelial cells in inflammation and angiogenesis, *Curr Drug Targets Inflamm Allergy* 4(3):319–323, 2005.
3. Tesfamariam B, DeFelice AF: Endothelial injury in the initiation and progression of vascular disorders, *Vascul Pharmacol* 46(4):229–237, 2007.

4. Szekanecz Z, Koch AE: Cell-cell interactions in synovitis. Endothelial cells and immune cell migration, *Arthritis Res* 2(5):368–373, 2000.
5. Lum H, Roebuck KA: Oxidant stress and endothelial cell dysfunction, *Am J Physiol Cell Physiol* 280(4):C719–C741, 2001.
6. Savage CO: Vascular biology and vasculitis, *APMIS Suppl* (127)37–40, 2009.
7. Pober JS, Cotran RS: Cytokines and endothelial cell biology, *Physiol Rev* 70(2):427–451, 1990.
8. Widlansky ME, Gokce N, Keaney Jr JF, et al.: The clinical implications of endothelial dysfunction, *J Am Coll Cardiol* 42(7):1149–1160, 2003.
9. Blann AD, Woywodt A, Bertolini F, et al.: Circulating endothelial cells. Biomarker of vascular disease, *Thromb Haemost* 93(2):228–235, 2005.
10. Giannotti G, Landmesser U: Endothelial dysfunction as an early sign of atherosclerosis, *Herz* 32(7):568–572, 2007.
11. Buckley CD, Rainger GE, Nash GB, et al.: Endothelial cells, fibroblasts and vasculitis, *Rheumatology (Oxford)* 44(7):860–863, 2005.
12. Zhang C: The role of inflammatory cytokines in endothelial dysfunction, *Basic Res Cardiol* 103(5):398–406, 2008.
13. Brenner BM, Troy JL, Ballermann BJ: Endothelium-dependent vascular responses. Mediators and mechanisms, *J Clin Invest* 84(5):1373–1378, 1989.
14. Joris I, Majno G, Corey EJ, et al.: The mechanism of vascular leakage induced by leukotriene E4. Endothelial contraction, *Am J Pathol* 126(1):19–24, 1987.
15. Bodolay E, Csipo I, Gal I, et al.: Anti-endothelial cell antibodies in mixed connective tissue disease: frequency and association with clinical symptoms, *Clin Exp Rheumatol* 22(4):409–415, 2004.
16. Gonzalez-Gay MA, Gonzalez-Juanatey C, Martin J: Inflammation and endothelial dysfunction in rheumatoid arthritis, *Clin Exp Rheumatol* 24(2):115–117, 2006.
17. Szekanecz Z, Kerekes G, Der H, et al.: Accelerated atherosclerosis in rheumatoid arthritis, *Ann N Y Acad Sci* 1108:349–358, 2007.
18. Varani J, Ginsburg I, Schuger L, et al.: Endothelial cell killing by neutrophils. Synergistic interaction of oxygen products and proteases, *Am J Pathol* 135(3):435–438, 1989.
19. Kvietys PR, Granger DN: Role of reactive oxygen and nitrogen species in the vascular responses to inflammation, *Free Radic Biol Med* 52(3):556–592, 2012.
20. Feletou M, Kohler R, Vanhoutte PM: Endothelium-derived vasoactive factors and hypertension: possible roles in pathogenesis and as treatment targets, *Curr Hypertens Rep* 12(4):267–275, 2010.
21. Gunnett CA, Lund DD, McDowell AK, et al.: Mechanisms of inducible nitric oxide synthase-mediated vascular dysfunction, *Arterioscler Thromb Vasc Biol* 25(8):1617–1622, 2005.
22. Kemeny-Beke A, Gesztelyi R, Bodnar N, et al.: Increased production of asymmetric dimethylarginine (ADMA) in ankylosing spondylitis: association with other clinical and laboratory parameters, *Joint Bone Spine* 78(2):184–187, 2011.
23. Zsuga J: [Asymmetric dimethil-arginine (ADMA) as a link between insulin resistance and atherosclerosis], *Ideggyogy Sz* 61(5-6):183–192, 2008.
24. Zouki C, Baron C, Fournier A, et al.: Endothelin-1 enhances neutrophil adhesion to human coronary artery endothelial cells: role of ET(A) receptors and platelet-activating factor, *Br J Pharmacol* 127(4):969–979, 1999.
25. Folkman J, Watson K, Ingber D, et al.: Induction of angiogenesis during the transition from hyperplasia to neoplasia, *Nature* 339(6219):58–61, 1989.
26. Tas SW, Maracle CX, Balogh E, et al.: Targeting of proangiogenic signalling pathways in chronic inflammation, *Nat Rev Rheumatol* 12(2):111–122, 2016.
27. Szekanecz Z, Besenyei T, Paragh G, et al.: New insights in synovial angiogenesis, *Joint Bone Spine* 77(1):13–19, 2010.
28. Leblond A, Allanore Y, Avouac J: Targeting synovial neoangiogenesis in rheumatoid arthritis, *Autoimmun Rev* 16(6):594–601, 2017.
29. Gerhardt H, Golding M, Fruttiger M, et al.: VEGF guides angiogenic sprouting utilizing endothelial tip cell filopodia, *J Cell Biol* 161(6):1163–1177, 2003.
30. Eelen G, Cruys B, Welti J, et al.: Control of vessel sprouting by genetic and metabolic determinants, *Trends Endocrinol Metab* 24(12):589–596, 2013.
31. Carmeliet P, De Smet F, Loges S, et al.: Branching morphogenesis and antiangiogenesis candidates: tip cells lead the way, *Nat Rev Clin Oncol* 6(6):315–326, 2009.
32. Gerhardt H, Betsholtz C: How do endothelial cells orientate? *EXS* (94)3–15, 2005.
33. Dorrell MI, Aguilar E, Friedlander M: Retinal vascular development is mediated by endothelial filopodia, a preexisting astrocytic template and specific R-cadherin adhesion, *Invest Ophthalmol Vis Sci* 43(11):3500–3510, 2002.
34. Ruhrberg C, Gerhardt H, Golding M, et al.: Spatially restricted patterning cues provided by heparin-binding VEGF-A control blood vessel branching morphogenesis, *Genes Dev* 16(20):2684–2698, 2002.
35. del Toro R, Prahst C, Mathivet T, et al.: Identification and functional analysis of endothelial tip cell-enriched genes, *Blood* 116(19):4025–4033, 2010.
36. Strasser GA, Kaminker JS, Tessier-Lavigne M: Microarray analysis of retinal endothelial tip cells identifies CXCR4 as a mediator of tip cell morphology and branching, *Blood* 115(24):5102–5110, 2010.
37. Gao W, Sweeney C, Connolly M, et al.: Notch-1 mediates hypoxia-induced angiogenesis in rheumatoid arthritis, *Arthritis Rheum* 64(7):2104–2113, 2012.
38. Schubert T, Denk A, Mägdefrau U, et al.: Role of the netrin system of repellent factors on synovial fibroblasts in rheumatoid arthritis and osteoarthritis, *Int J Immunopathol Pharmacol* 22(3):715–722, 2009.
39. Ikeda M, Hosoda Y, Hirose S, et al.: Expression of vascular endothelial growth factor isoforms and their receptors Flt-1, KDR, and neuropilin-1 in synovial tissues of RA, *J Pathol* 191(4):426–433, 2000.
40. Paavonen K, Mandelin J, Partanen T, et al.: Vascular endothelial growth factors C and D and their VEGFR-2 and 3 receptors in blood and lymphatic vessels in healthy and arthritic synovium, *J Rheumatol* 29(1):39–45, 2002.
41. Tan W, Palmby TR, Gavard J, et al.: An essential role for Rac1 in endothelial cell function and vascular development, *FASEB J* 22(6):1829–1838, 2008.
42. Connolly JO, Simpson N, Hewlett L, et al.: Rac regulates endothelial morphogenesis and capillary assembly, *Mol Biol Cell.* 13(7):2474–2485, 2002.
43. Caron C, DeGeer J, Fournier P, et al.: CdGAP/ARHGAP31, a Cdc42/Rac1 GTPase regulator, is critical for vascular development and VEGF-mediated angiogenesis, *Sci Rep* 7(6):27485, 2016.
44. Philippova M, Ivanov D, Allenspach R, et al.: RhoA and Rac mediate endothelial cell polarization and detachment induced by T-cadherin, *FASEB J* 19(6):588–590, 2005.
45. Davis GE, Bayless KJ: An integrin and Rho GTPase-dependent pinocytic vacuole mechanism controls capillary lumen formation in collagen and fibrin matrices, *Microcirculation* 10(1):27–44, 2003.
46. Hoang MV, Whelan MC, Senger DR: Rho activity critically and selectively regulates endothelial cell organization during angiogenesis, *Proc Natl Acad Sci USA* 101(7):874–947, 2004.
47. Connolly M, Veale DJ, Fearon U: Acute serum amyloid A regulates cytoskeletal rearrangement, cell matrix interactions and promotes cell migration in rheumatoid arthritis, *Ann Rheum Dis* 70(7):1296–1303, 2011.
48. Moran EM, Connolly M, Gao W, et al.: Interleukin-17A induction of angiogenesis, cell migration, and cytoskeletal rearrangement, *Arthritis Rheum* 63(11):3263–3273, 2011.
49. McGarry T, Veale DJ, Gao W, et al.: Toll-like receptor 2 (TLR2) induces migration and invasive mechanisms in rheumatoid arthritis, *Arthritis Res Ther* 17:153, 2015.

50. Shahrara S, Castro-Rueda HP, Haines GK, et al.: Differential expression of the FAK family kinases in rheumatoid arthritis and osteoarthritis synovial tissues, *Arthritis Res Ther* 9(5):R112, 2007.
51. Fantin A, Lampropoulou A, Gestri G, et al.: NRP1 Regulates CDC42 activation to promote filopodia formation in endothelial tip cells, *Cell Rep* 11(10):1577–1590, 2015.
52. Bussmann J, Wolfe SA, Siekmann AF: Arterial-venous network formation during brain vascularization involves hemodynamic regulation of chemokine signaling, *Development* 138(9):1717–1726, 2011.
53. Eichmann A, Le Noble F, Autiero M, et al.: Guidance of vascular and neural network formation, *Curr Opin Neurobiol* 15(1):108–115, 2005.
54. Iruela-Arispe ML, Davis GE: Cellular and molecular mechanisms of vascular lumen formation, *Dev Cell* 16(2):222–231, 2009.
55. Stratman AN, Davis GE: Endothelial cell-pericyte interactions stimulate basement membrane matrix assembly: influence on vascular tube remodeling, maturation, and stabilization, *Microsc Microanal* 18(1):68–80, 2012.
56. Milner LA, Bigas A: Notch as a mediator of cell fate determination in hematopoiesis: evidence and speculation, *Blood* 93(8):2431–2448, 1999.
57. Artavanis-Tsakonas S, Rand MD, Lake RJ: Notch signaling: cell fate control and signal integration in development, *Science* 284(5415):770–776, 1999.
58. Gridley T: Notch signaling in vascular development and physiology, *Development* 134(15):2709–2718, 2007.
59. Iso T, Hamamori Y, Kedes L: Notch signaling in vascular development, *Arterioscler Thromb Vasc Biol* 23(4):543–553, 2003.
60. Armulik A, Abramsson A, Betsholtz C: Endothelial/pericyte interactions, *Circ Res* 97(6):512–523, 2005.
61. Li L, Huang GM, Banta AB, et al.: Cloning, characterization, and the complete 56.8-kilobase DNA sequence of the human NOTCH4 gene, *Genomics* 51(1):45–58, 1998.
62. Uyttendaele H, Marazzi G, Wu G, et al.: Notch4/int-3, a mammary proto-oncogene, is an endothelial cell-specific mammalian Notch gene, *Development* 122(7):2251–2259, 1996.
63. Knust E, Dietrich U, Tepass U, et al.: EGF homologous sequences encoded in the genome of Drosophila melanogaster, and their relation to neurogenic genes, *EMBO J* 6(3):761–766, 1987.
64. Fleming RJ, Scottgale TN, Diederich RJ, et al.: The gene Serrate encodes a putative EGF-like transmembrane protein essential for proper ectodermal development in Drosophila melanogaster, *Genes Dev* 4(12A):2188–2201, 1990.
65. Lindsell CE, Shawber CJ, Boulter J, et al.: Jagged: a mammalian ligand that activates Notch1, *Cell* 80(6):909–917, 1995.
66. Weinmaster G: Notch signaling: direct or what? *Curr Opin Genet Dev* 8(4):436–442, 1998.
67. Mumm JS, Kopan R: Notch signaling: from the outside in, *Dev Biol* 228(2):151–165, 2000.
68. Roca C, Adams RH: Regulation of vascular morphogenesis by Notch signaling, *Genes Dev* 21(20):2511–2524, 2007.
69. Gao W, Sweeney C, Walsh C, et al.: Notch signalling pathways mediate synovial angiogenesis in response to vascular endothelial growth factor and angiopoietin 2, *Ann Rheum Dis* 72(6):1080–1088, 2013.
70. Hellström M, Phng LK, Hofmann JJ, et al.: Dll4 signalling through Notch1 regulates formation of tip cells during angiogenesis, *Nature* 445(7129):776–780, 2007.
71. Lamalice L, Houle F, Jourdan G, et al.: Phosphorylation of tyrosine 1214 on VEGFR2 is required for VEGF-induced activation of Cdc42 upstream of SAPK2/p38, *Oncogene* 23(2), 2004. 434-4.
72. Hoang MV, Whelan MC, Senger DR: Rho activity critically and selectively regulates endothelial cell organization during angiogenesis, *Proc Natl Acad Sci U S A* 101(7):1874–1879, 2004.
73. Choe JY, Hun Kim J, Park KY, et al.: Activation of dickkopf-1 and focal adhesion kinase pathway by tumour necrosis factor α induces enhanced migration of fibroblast-like synoviocytes in rheumatoid arthritis, *Rheumatology (Oxford)* 55(5):928–938, 2016.
74. D'Souza B, Miyamoto A, Weinmaster G: The many facets of Notch ligands, *Oncogene* 27(38):5148–5167, 2008.
75. Redmond L, Ghosh A: The role of Notch and Rho GTPase signaling in the control of dendritic development, *Curr Opin Neurobiol* 11(1):111–117, 2001.
76. Nam EJ, Sa KH, You DW, et al.: Up-regulated transforming growth factor beta-inducible gene h3 in rheumatoid arthritis mediates adhesion and migration of synoviocytes through alpha v beta3 integrin: regulation by cytokines, *Arthritis Rheum* 54(9):2734–2744, 2006.
77. Tilton RG, Kilo C, Williamson JR: Pericyte-endothelial relationships in cardiac and skeletal muscle capillaries, *Microvasc Res* 18(3):325–335, 1979.
78. Hirschi KK, D'Amore PA: Pericytes in the microvasculature, *Cardiovasc Res* 32(4):687–698, 1996.
79. Kennedy A, Ng CT, Biniecka M, et al.: Angiogenesis and blood vessel stability in inflammatory arthritis, *Arthritis Rheum* 62(3):711–721, 2010.
80. Izquierdo E, Cañete JD, Celis R, et al.: Immature blood vessels in rheumatoid synovium are selectively depleted in response to anti-TNF therapy, *PLoS One* 4(12):e8131, 2009.
81. Ayres-Sander CE, Lauridsen H, Maier CL, et al.: Transendothelial migration enables subsequent transmigration of neutrophils through underlying pericytes, *PLoS One* 8(3):e60025, 2013.
82. Fearon U, Griosios K, Fraser A, et al.: Angiopoietins, growth factors, and vascular morphology in early arthritis, *J Rheumatol* 30(2):260–268, 2003.
83. Fraser A, Fearon U, Reece R, et al.: Matrix metalloproteinase 9, apoptosis, and vascular morphology in early arthritis, *Arthritis Rheum* 44(9):2024–2028, 2001.
84. van de Sande MG, de Launay D, de Hair MJ, et al.: Local synovial engagement of angiogenic TIE-2 is associated with the development of persistent erosive rheumatoid arthritis in patients with early arthritis, *Arthritis Rheum* 65(12):3073–3083, 2013.
85. Salvador G, Sanmartí R, Gil-Torregrosa B, et al.: Synovial vascular patterns and angiogenic factors expression in synovial tissue and serum of patients with rheumatoid arthritis, *Rheumatology (Oxford)* 45(8):966–971, 2006.
86. Li LY, Barlow KD, Metheny-Barlow LJ: Angiopoietins and Tie2 in health and disease, *Pediatr Endocrinol Rev* 2(3), 2005. 399-40.
87. Biel NM, Siemann DW: Targeting the Angiopoietin-2/Tie-2 axis in conjunction with VEGF signal interference, *Cancer Lett* 380(2):525–533, 2016.
88. Folkman J, D'Amore PA: Blood vessel formation: what is its molecular basis? *Cell* 87(7):1153–1155, 1996.
89. Potente M, Gerhardt H, Carmeliet P: Basic and therapeutic aspects of angiogenesis, *Cell* 146(6):873–887, 2011.
90. Balogh E, Veale DJ, McGarry T, et al.: Oxidative stress impairs energy metabolism in primary cells and synovial tissue of patients with rheumatoid arthritis, *Arthritis Res Ther* 20(1):95, 2018.
91. Xian X, Håkansson J, Ståhlberg A, et al.: Pericytes limit tumor cell metastasis, *J Clin Invest* 116(3):642–651, 2006.
92. Davis GE: Angiogenesis and proteinases: influence on vascular morphogenesis, stabilization and regression, *Drug Discov Today Dis Models* 8(1):13–20, 2011.
93. Stratman AN, Malotte KM, Mahan RD, et al.: Pericyte recruitment during vasculogenic tube assembly stimulates endothelial basement membrane matrix formation, *Blood* 114(24):5091–5101, 2009.
94. Davis GE, Norden PR, Bowers SL: Molecular control of capillary morphogenesis and maturation by recognition and remodeling of the extracellular matrix: functional roles of endothelial cells and pericytes in health and disease, *Connect Tissue Res* 56(5):392–402, 2015.
95. Saunders WB, Bohnsack BL, Faske JB, et al.: Coregulation of vascular tube stabilization by endothelial cell TIMP-2 and pericyte TIMP-3, *J Cell Biol* 175(1):179–191, 2006.

96. Szekanecz Z, Koch AE: Mechanisms of Disease: angiogenesis in inflammatory diseases, *Nat Clin Pract Rheumatol* 3(11):635–643, 2007.
97. Folkman J: Angiogenesis in cancer, vascular, rheumatoid and other disease, *Nat Med* 1(1):27–31, 1995.
98. Veale DJ, Fearon U: Inhibition of angiogenic pathways in rheumatoid arthritis: potential for therapeutic targeting, *Best Pract Res Clin Rheumatol* 20(5):941–947, 2006.
99. Maracle CX, Tas SW: Inhibitors of angiogenesis: ready for prime time? *Best Pract Res Clin Rheumatol* 28(4):637–649, 2014.
100. Asahara T, Chen D, Takahashi T, et al.: Tie2 receptor ligands, angiopoietin-1 and angiopoietin-2, modulate VEGF-induced postnatal neovascularization, *Circ Res* 83(3):233–240, 1998.
101. Chen Y, Donnelly E, Kobayashi H, et al.: Gene therapy targeting the Tie2 function ameliorates collagen-induced arthritis and protects against bone destruction, *Arthritis Rheum* 52(5):1585–1594, 2005.
102. Malik NM, Jin P, Raatz Y, et al.: Regulation of the angiopoietin-Tie ligand-receptor system with a novel splice variant of Tie1 reduces the severity of murine arthritis, *Rheumatology (Oxford)* 49(10):1828–1839, 2010.
103. Saber T, Veale DJ, Balogh E, et al.: Toll-like receptor 2 induced angiogenesis and invasion is mediated through the Tie2 signalling pathway in rheumatoid arthritis, *PLoS One* 6(8):e23540, 2011.
104. Shibuya M: Vascular endothelial growth factor-dependent and -independent regulation of angiogenesis, *BMB Rep* 41(4):278–286, 2008.
105. Jia W, Wu W, Yang D, et al.: GATA4 regulates angiogenesis and persistence of inflammation in rheumatoid arthritis, *Cell Death Dis* 9(5):503, 2018.
106. Colville-Nash PR, Willoughby DA: Growth factors in angiogenesis: current interest and therapeutic potential, *Mol Med Today* 3(1):14–23, 1997.
107. Marrelli A, Cipriani P, Liakouli V, et al.: Angiogenesis in rheumatoid arthritis: a disease specific process or a common response to chronic inflammation? *Autoimmun Rev* 10(10):595–598, 2011.
108. Chen CY, Su CM, Hsu CJ, et al.: CCN1 promotes VEGF production in osteoblasts and induces endothelial progenitor cell angiogenesis by inhibiting mir-126 expression in rheumatoid arthritis, *J Bone Miner Res* 32(1):34–45, 2017.
109. Yoshida S, Ono M, Shono T, et al.: Involvement of interleukin-8, vascular endothelial growth factor, and basic fibroblast growth factor in tumor necrosis factor alpha-dependent angiogenesis, *Mol Cell Biol* 17(7):4015–4023, 1997.
110. Leibovich SJ, Polverini PJ, Shepard HM, et al.: Macrophage-induced angiogenesis is mediated by tumour necrosis factor-alpha, *Nature* 329(6140):630–632, 1987.
111. Wu S, Li Y, Yao L, et al.: Interleukin-35 inhibits angiogenesis through STAT1 signalling in rheumatoid synoviocytes, *Clin Exp Rheumatol* 36(2):223–227, 2018.
112. Szekanecz Z, Koch AE: Chemokines and angiogenesis, *Curr Opin Rheumatol* 13(3):202–208, 2001.
113. Szekanecz Z, Koch AE: Successes and failures of chemokine-pathway targeting in rheumatoid arthritis, *Nat Rev Rheumatol* 12(1):5–13, 2016.
114. Koch AE, Volin MV, Woods JM, et al.: Regulation of angiogenesis by the C-X-C chemokines interleukin-8 and epithelial neutrophil activating peptide 78 in the rheumatoid joint, *Arthritis Rheum* 44(1):31–40, 2001.
115. Madri JA, Pratt BM: Endothelial cell-matrix interactions: in vitro models of angiogenesis, *J Histochem Cytochem* 34(1):85–91, 1986.
116. Agarwal SK, Brenner MB: Role of adhesion molecules in synovial inflammation, *Curr Opin Rheumatol* 18(3):268–276, 2006.
117. Isozaki T, Amin MA, Ruth JH, et al.: Fucosyltransferase 1 mediates angiogenesis in rheumatoid arthritis, *Arthritis Rheumatol* 66(8):2047–2058, 2014.
118. Naik TU, Naik MU, Naik UP: Junctional adhesion molecules in angiogenesis, *Front Biosci* 13:258–262, 2008.
119. O'Brien MJ, Shu Q, Stinson WA, et al.: A unique role for galectin-9 in angiogenesis and inflammatory arthritis, *Arthritis Res Ther* 20(1):31, 2018.
120. Rico MC, Rough JJ, Del Carpio-Cano FE, et al.: The axis of thrombospondin-1, transforming growth factor beta and connective tissue growth factor: an emerging therapeutic target in rheumatoid arthritis, *Curr Vasc Pharmacol* 8(3):338–343, 2009.

31 Cytokines

IAIN B. MCINNES

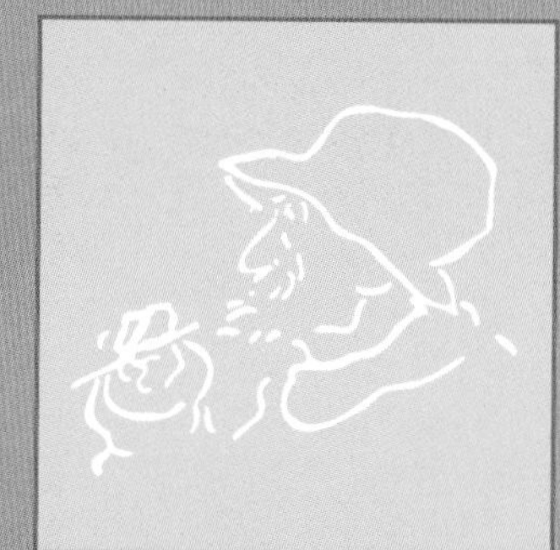

KEY POINTS

Cytokines are peptides that have a fundamental role in communication within the immune system and in allowing the immune system and host tissue cells to exchange information.

Cytokines act via binding to a receptor that in turn sends a signal to the recipient cell, leading to a change in function or phenotype. Such signal cascades are complex and integrate a variety of environmental factors.

Cytokines exist in broad families that are structurally related but exhibit diverse function (e.g., the TNF/TNF receptor superfamily, IL-1 superfamily, and IL-6 superfamily).

Cytokines may contain shared subunits such that therapeutic targeting of one subunit can inhibit the activity of two discrete cytokines (e.g., IL-12 [p35/p40], IL-23 [p19, p40]).

Cytokine targeting has proven effective in many rheumatic diseases, particularly therapeutics that inhibit TNF or IL-6. Many more cytokines are currently under investigation as therapeutic targets or as therapeutic agents.

Introduction

Immune function depends on the biologic activities of numerous small glycoprotein messengers termed *cytokines*. Originally discovered and defined on the basis of their functional activities, cytokines are now designated primarily by structure. Typically, cytokines exhibit broad functional activities that not only mediate effector and regulatory immune function but also have wider effects across a range of tissues and biologic systems. Additional features are the capacity to work in synergy one with another and to utilize shared signaling components.[1] As such, cytokines play a role not only in host defense but also in a variety of normal physiologic and metabolic processes. By this means they integrate de facto host defense and host metabolic function. The Human Genome Project has assisted with the discovery of numerous cytokines, facing considerable challenges in resolving their respective and synergistic functions in complex tissues in health and disease. However, such understanding is essential with the increasing application of cytokine-targeted therapies in the clinic. This chapter reviews general features of cytokine biology and the cellular and molecular networks within which cytokines operate; the focus is on the effector functions of cytokines that are important in chronic inflammation and in rheumatic diseases.

Classification of Cytokines

In the absence of a unified classification system, cytokines are variously identified by numeric order of discovery (currently IL-1 through IL-41)[2]; by a given functional activity (e.g., TNF and granulocyte colony-stimulating factor [G-CSF]); by kinetic or functional role in inflammatory responses (e.g., early or late, innate or adaptive, and pro-inflammatory or anti-inflammatory); by primary cell of origin (e.g., monokine = monocyte derivation and lymphokine = lymphocyte derivation); and, more recently, by structural homologies shared with related molecules. Superfamilies of cytokines share sequence similarity and exhibit homology and some promiscuity in their reciprocal receptor systems (Fig. 31.1). They do not necessarily exhibit functional similarity. Cytokine superfamilies also contain important regulatory cell membrane receptor-ligand pairs, reflecting evolutionary pressures that use common structural motifs in diverse immune functions in higher mammals. The TNF/TNF receptor superfamily[3] contains immunoregulatory cytokines including TNF, lymphotoxins, and cellular ligands such as CD40L, which mediates B cell and T cell activation, and FasL (CD95), which promotes apoptosis. Similarly, the IL-1/IL-1 receptor superfamily[4] contains cytokines including IL-1β, IL-1α, IL-18, IL-33, and IL-36 (α, β, γ); receptor antagonists including IL-1RA, IL-36 receptor antagonist, and IL-38; and an anti-inflammatory cytokine, namely IL-37, which mediates physiologic and host-defense function, but this family also includes the Toll-like receptors (TLRs), a series of mammalian pattern-recognition molecules with a crucial role in recognition of microbial species early in innate responses.

Assessing Cytokine Function In Vitro and In Vivo

Although they were originally identified by bioactivity and quantified by bioassay, most cytokines are now identified via homologous receptor binding or sequence homology in gene databases. They are quantified in biologic solutions by enzyme-linked immunosorbent assay, multiplex technology, or meso platform techniques, with the latter allowing many cytokines (25 to 360) to be measured in single, small sample volumes (~20 μL). Cytokines are also assessed in experimental systems at the messenger RNA (mRNA) level, often using quantitative polymerase chain reaction (PCR) or Taqman low-density array (TLDA)-based approaches; the latter allows many cytokines to be identified in small samples simultaneously. RNA sequencing also detects cytokines commonly in complex tissue biopsy analyses. Post-transcriptional regulation of cytokines is common, however, suggesting cautious interpretation of mRNA data alone. Function is thereafter assessed by identification of the cellular source of cytokine, determination of native stimuli, characterization of receptor distribution, and determination of function in target cells. Experimental in vivo models use

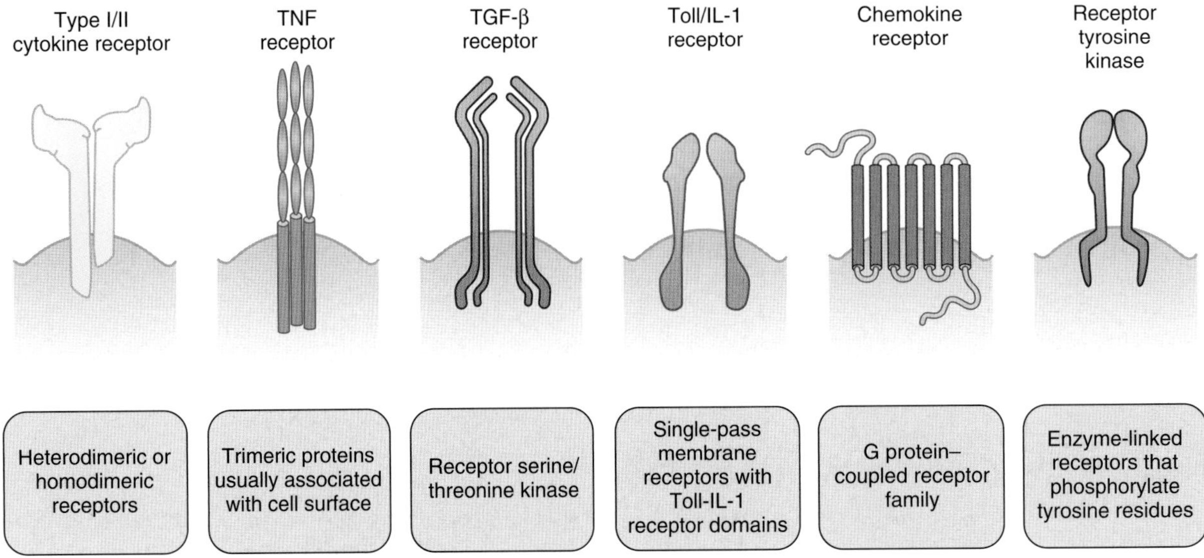

• **Fig. 31.1** Cytokine receptors. Cytokines, chemokines, and growth factors bind to many different types of surface receptors in the cell membrane. The figure shows several distinct families and representative ligands that are critical. Each receptor type is associated with distinct signaling mechanisms that orchestrate and integrate the cellular response after ligand binding. *TGF-β,* Transforming growth factor-β; *TNF,* tumor necrosis factor.

the addition of neutralizing cytokine-specific antibodies or soluble receptors (often as fragment crystallizable fusion or pegylated proteins to enhance half-life and modulate functional interaction with leukocytes) to modulate cytokine function. Genetically modified knockout and knockin mice (cytokine or receptor modified by embryonic stem cell technology) or transgenic mice (tissue/cell lineage–specific overexpression) have proven particularly useful. Conditional gene-targeting approaches (e.g., using the Cre system) facilitate circumvention of embryonic lethal deficiencies or allow kinetic evaluation of the relative contribution of a cytokine throughout a response. Moreover, recent multiphoton microscopic techniques have allowed the additional evaluation of cytokine contributions in three-dimensional tissue orientation and in real time in vivo. Cytokine function is normally assessed in vitro in primary or transformed cell lines stimulated in the presence or absence of recombinant cytokine or specific anti-cytokine antibody or soluble receptor. Gene knock-down approaches with use of small interfering (si)RNA or antisense oligonucleotides are also increasingly employed. Recently CRISPR (clustered regularly interspaced short palindromic repeats) and TALEN (transcription activator-like effector nucleases)-based technologies have facilitated highly specific cytokine and cytokine receptor knock-down cell work.

This general approach has been crucial in rheumatic disease research. Studies in which cytokine addition and neutralization occur in synovial tissue explants or disaggregated cell populations, chondrocyte explants, bone culture models, skin, and renal tissue explants and cell lines have been informative. Ex vivo methodologies now include intra-cellular fluorescence activated cell sorter methods, confocal and laser scanning microscopy, and quantitative histologic evaluation using automated image analysis. Such modalities, particularly when used in human therapeutic cytokine neutralization studies in which inflammatory tissues are obtained throughout therapeutic interventions, advance the understanding of basic and pathogenetic cytokine function. Analysis of synovial biopsy specimens obtained before and after TNF inhibitor, abatacept, rituximab, tocilizumab, IL-1RA, IL-10, interferon (IFN)-β, and JAK inhibitor administration in people with rheumatoid arthritis (RA) provides the strongest evidence for the success of this approach.[5–7]

Cytokine Receptors

Cytokine receptors exist in structurally related superfamilies and comprise high-affinity molecular signaling complexes that assist in cytokine-mediated communication (see Fig. 31.1). Such complexes often include heterodimeric or heterotrimeric structures that use unique, cytokine-specific recognition receptors together with common receptor chains shared across a cytokine superfamily. Examples include the use of the common γ chain receptor by IL-2, IL-4, IL-7, IL-9, IL-15, and IL-21, and glycoprotein (gp)130 by members of the IL-6 family.[8,9] Alternatively, distinct receptors may use shared signaling domains. Homologous death domains are found in many TNF-receptor family members. Similarly, the IL-1 signaling domain is common to not only IL-1R but also other IL-1R superfamily members, including IL-18R, IL-33R, and the TLRs.[4] Unrelated cytokine receptor systems exhibit close cross-communication on the cell membrane, allowing a cell to integrate a variety of external stimuli to optimize signaling pathways and the cellular response in real time in a changing environment. Although best elucidated in the epidermal growth factor receptor system, this mechanism also has been identified for members of the common γ chain signaling family. Signaling pathways that subserve these responses are discussed in detail elsewhere (see Chapter 18—they have become of particular relevance with the advent of Janus kinase [JAK] inhibitors across rheumatology).

Cytokine receptors can operate via several mechanisms. Membrane receptors, with intra-cellular signaling domains intact, can transmit signals to the target cell nucleus after soluble cytokine binding and promote effector function (Fig. 31.2). Membrane receptors may bind cell membrane cytokines assisting cross-talk between adjacent cells. Membrane-bound and soluble cytokines may promote distinct receptor function. Useful exemplars exist relevant to the rheumatic diseases. Thus TNF binds TNF-RI and

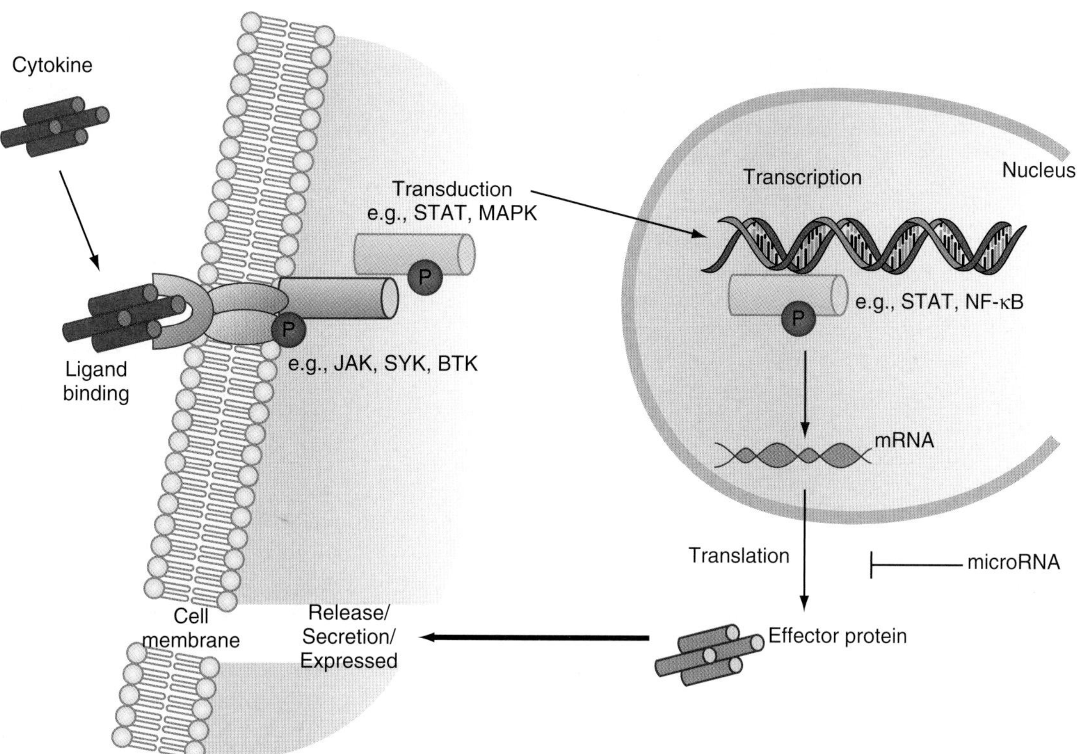

• **Fig. 31.2** Cytokine signaling and regulation. After ligand binding, cytokine receptors activate a series of signaling molecules that are associated with the cytoplasmic portion of the receptor or the plasma membrane. In this figure, Janus kinase (JAK) or spleen tyrosine kinase (SYK) is activated, which in turn phosphorylates additional cytoplasmic molecules (signal transducer and activator of transcription [STAT] and mitogen-activated protein kinase [MAPK]) that then can migrate to the nucleus and either directly or through additional intermediaries activate gene transcription. Messenger RNA (mRNA) levels can also be regulated after transcription by microRNAs. Ultimately, the translated proteins can be processed and released by the cell into the microenvironment or presented on the plasma membrane to other cells. *BTK,* Bruton's tyrosine kinase; *NF-κB,* nuclear factor-κB.

TNF-RII with similar affinity, but it has a slower rate of dissociation from TNF-RI. Soluble TNF may dissociate rapidly from TNF-RII to bind TNF-RI, promoting preferential signaling by the latter (ligand passing).[3] In contrast, during cell-cell contact, stable TNF/TNF-RI and TNF/TNF-RII complexes form, allowing for differential signaling contribution by TNF-RI and TNF-RII.

Cytokine receptor/cytokine complexes also may operate in trans, whereby component parts of the ligand-receptor complex are derived from adjacent cells. IL-15/IL-15Rα complexed on one cell may bind IL-15Rβ/γ on another.[10] Receptors also exist in soluble form, derived either from alternative mRNA processing to generate receptor-lacking transmembrane or intra-cellular domains or from enzymatic cleavage of receptor from the cell surface (e.g., soluble TNF-R [sTNF-R] and soluble IL-1R1 [sIL-1R1]). Soluble receptors may act to antagonize cytokine function, thus regulating responses. Soluble receptors also may pre-form complexes with cytokine to promote subsequent ligand-receptor assembly on the target cell membrane and enhance function. Soluble receptors can deliver cytokine to the cell membrane via ligand passing. IL-6 provides a particularly important example given its core role in a range of rheumatic disorders. IL-6 binds to a heterodimeric receptor (IL-6R and gp130) and provokes cell activation via conventional signal pathways that involve signal transducer and activator of transcription (STAT)-3. Thus IL-6 may activate a cell expressing the combination of IL-6R and gp130 by conventional (cis) signaling. In addition, however, circulating soluble IL-6R may form functional gp130/IL-6R effector complexes on any cell expressing membrane gp130 and by this means confer on circulating IL-6 the ability to exert broad functional effects (trans signaling). Finally, it is now recognized that some cytokines with the capacity to be retained in the membrane may themselves function as signaling molecules (reverse signaling).

Regulation of Cytokine Expression

Cytokines are synthesized in the Golgi apparatus and may traffic through the endoplasmic reticulum to be released as soluble mediators, remain membrane bound, or be processed into cytosolic forms that can traffic intra-cellularly, even returning to the nucleus, where they can act as transcriptional regulators. Cytokines mediate autocrine function either through release or membrane expression and immediate receptor ligation on the source cell or intra-cellularly within the source cell. Alternatively, cytokines operate in a paracrine manner, allowing cellular communication beyond that assisted by local cell-cell contact. The distance and kinetics for effective function may be limited,[11] however, by numerous factors, including physicochemical considerations of the peptide structure itself, extra-cellular matrix binding (e.g., to heparan sulfate), enzymatic degradation, or the presence of soluble receptors or novel cytokine-binding proteins in the inflammatory milieu.

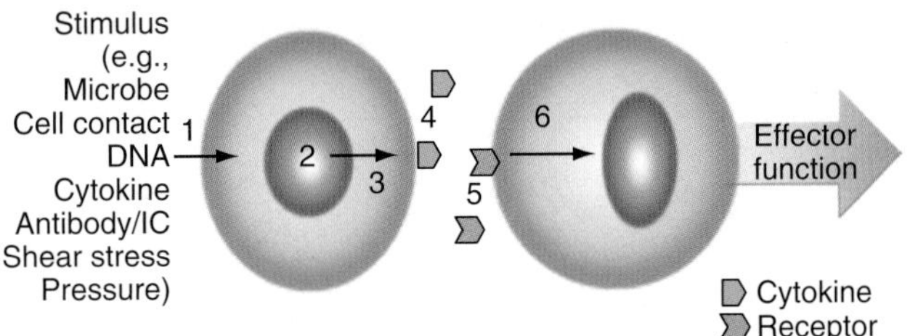

• **Fig. 31.3** Overview of cytokine regulatory function. Numerous and diverse stimuli *(1)* promote cytokine expression arising either from novel gene expression *(2)* or from activation of pre-formed cytokine *(3)*. Cytokine proteins are thereafter expressed in the cytosol, on the cell membrane, or in soluble form in the extra-cellular environment *(4)*. Cytokines bind to reciprocal receptors that reside either on the membrane of a target cell or in the soluble phase *(5)*. Membrane receptors, on cytokine ligation, signal to the recipient cell nucleus *(6)* and drive novel gene expression to promote effector function. Each phase of cytokine function offers rich therapeutic potential. *IC,* Immune complexes.

Numerous factors promote cytokine expression in vivo (Fig. 31.3), including cell-cell contact, immune complexes/autoantibodies, local complement activation, microbial species and their soluble products (particularly via TLRs and nucleotide oligomerization domain [NOD]-like receptors [NLRs]), molecular markers of tissue damage (DAMPs), reactive oxygen and nitrogen intermediates, trauma, shear stress, ischemia, radiation, ultraviolet light, extra-cellular matrix components, DNA (mammalian or microbial), heat shock proteins, electrolytes (e.g., K^+ via P_2X7 receptors), and cytokines themselves operating in autocrine loops. Commonly used in vitro stimuli include many of these factors and chemical entities including phorbol esters, calcium ionophores, lectins (e.g., phytohemagglutinin), and receptor-specific antibodies, such as anti-CD3 and anti-CD28 for T cell activation or anti-immunoglobulin and anti-CD40 for B cells.

Cytokine regulation within the cell can be usefully considered at several levels (see Fig. 31.2). Transcriptional regulation depends on the recruitment of discrete transcription factors to the cytokine promoter region. Transcription factor binding allows for numerous signal pathways to regulate cytokine expression across a range of stimuli. Several transcription factors (e.g., nuclear factor-κB [NF-κB], activator protein [AP]-1, and nuclear factor of activated T cell) are crucial in cytokine production. Sequence polymorphism within cytokine promoters offers potential for differential cytokine expression between individuals that could confer selective advantage against infection but could also increase susceptibility to, or progression of, autoimmunity. In general, the net effect of haplotypes may be more important at the functional level or only play a role in the context of networks where multiple minor polymorphisms can synergize, particularly when their relevance to disease entities is considered. Finally, a number of microRNAs have been identified that regulate cytokine release in the context of rheumatic diseases.[12]

Post-transcriptional regulation is important in determining longevity of cytokine expression. This regulation may operate by promoting translational initiation, mRNA stability, and polyadenylation. AU-rich elements (AREs) within the 52 or 32 untranslated regions (UTRs) of cytokine mRNA are crucial for stability.[13] For TNF, regulatory proteins bind AREs to mediate such effects. HuR and AUF1 exert opposing effects, stabilizing and destabilizing ARE-containing transcripts.[14] TIA-1 and TIAR have been identified as RNA recognition motif family members[15] that function as translational silencers. Macrophages from TIA-1–deficient macrophages produce excess TNF, whereas TIA-1–deficient lymphocytes exhibit normal TNF release, suggesting distinctions in mRNA regulation in discrete cell types.[16] Alternatively, cytokines may generate stable mRNA a priori to assist with subsequent rapid response in tissues. The IL-15 mRNA 52 UTR contains 12 AUG triplets that significantly reduce the efficiency of IL-15 translation. Deletion of this sequence permits IL-15 secretion.[17]

Post-translational regulation also modulates cytokine expression via several mechanisms. Patterns of glycosylation are important for cytokine function and may regulate intra-cellular trafficking.[17] Modified leader sequences can alter intra-cellular trafficking of cytokines. Some cytokines are translated without functional leader sequences. Their secretion depends on nonconventional secretory pathways that are poorly understood. IL-1β employs, among other pathways, a purine receptor–dependent pathway (P_2X_7) for cellular release.[18] Enzymatic activation of cytokines is common, whereby nonfunctional promolecules are cleaved to generate functional subunits. Examples include the cleavage by caspase 1 of pro-IL-1β to generate active IL-1β and, similarly, of pro-IL-18 to generate an active 18 kDa species.[19] This organized process occurs both sequentially (in time) and by orientation within the cell (in space). IL-1 processing occurs in a protein complex within the cytosol termed the *inflammasome.* The latter has attracted considerable interest as a therapeutic target in conditions such as crystal-induced arthritis and in diseases that arise from mutations in certain inflammasome genes (e.g., cryopyrin; see Chapters 11 and 18).

Alternative processing pathways for cytokines include the serine proteases, proteinase 3 and elastase, and adamalysin family members. Enzyme cleavage pathways operate within and outside cells, providing for extra-cellular cytokine activation. Similarly, cell membrane enzymes serve to cleave membrane-expressed cytokine. Members of the adamalysin family regulate TNF release; a TNF-converting enzyme cleaves and mediates the release of TNF and its receptors.[20] Extensive molecular machinery exists to regulate tightly not only the production and stability of cytokine mRNA but also its translation and cellular expression and distribution. At each level, opportunities exist for intervention and therapeutic cytokine modulation; thus far, however, no successful medicines have emerged from this approach.

Effector Function of Cytokines

Cytokines possess pleiotropic and potent effector function in acute and chronic inflammatory responses. The identity, receptor specificity, and key effects of cytokines understood to have particular importance in the pathogenesis of human autoimmunity and chronic inflammation are summarized in Tables 31.1 through 31.8.

Cytokines operate at every stage in the crucial early events that promote acute inflammation. Cells that make up the innate immune response, including neutrophils, natural killer (NK) cells, macrophages, mast cells, and eosinophils, all produce and respond to cytokines generated within seconds of tissue insult. Cytokines prime leukocytes for response to microbial and chemical stimuli, upregulate adhesion molecule expression on migrating leukocytes and endothelial cells, and amplify the release of reactive oxygen intermediates, nitric oxide, vasoactive amines, and neuropeptides, as well as the activation of kinins and arachidonic acid derivatives, prostaglandins, and leukotrienes, which regulate cytokine

TABLE 31.1 **IL-1 Superfamily Cytokines With Roles in Rheumatic Disease**

Cytokine	Size (kDa)[a]	Receptors	Major Cell Sources	Key Functions
IL-1β	35 (pro)	IL-1RI	Monocytes; B cells; fibroblasts; chondrocytes; keratinocytes	Fibroblast cytokine, chemokine, MMP, iNOS, PG release ↑
	17 (active)	IL-1RAcP IL-1RII (decoy)		Monocyte cytokine, ROI, PG ↑ Osteoclast activation Chondrocyte GAG synthesis ↓; iNOS, MMP, and aggrecanase ↑ Endothelial adhesion-molecule expression
IL-1α	35 (pro)[b]	IL-1RI	Monocytes; B cells; PMNs; epithelial cells; keratinocytes	Similar to IL-1β
	17 (active)	IL-1RAcP IL-1RII (decoy)		Autocrine growth factor (e.g., keratinocytes)
IL-1Ra	22	IL-1RI	Monocytes	Antagonize effects of IL-1β and IL-1α
		IL-1RAcP IL-1RII		
IL-18	23 (pro)	IL-18R	Monocytes; PMNs; dendritic cells; platelets; endothelial cells	T cell effector polarization (Th1 with IL-12/ Th2 with IL-4)
	18 (active)	IL-18Rβα		Chondrocyte GAG synthesis ↓; iNOS expression NK activation; cytokine release; cytotoxicity Monocyte cytokine release; adhesion molecule expression PMN activation; cytokine release; migration Endothelial cells—proangiogenic
IL-36 (αβγ)	35	IL-1Rrp2	Macrophages, DC, lymphocytes, epithelial cells (skin, bronchial), FLS	Innate immune cell activation, cytokine production
		IL-1RAcP		Keratinocyte proliferation
IL-37	35	IL-18Rα	Ill-defined	General anti-inflammatory function: transgenic mice protected from colitis, ischemia reperfusion injury
IL-33	30 (pro)	ST2L	Epithelial cells; monocytes; smooth muscle cells; keratinocytes	Promote Th2 cell activation, mast cell activation, and cytokine production
	18 (active)	IL-1RAcP		

[a]Pro forms cleaved to active moieties by proteases including caspase-1, calpain, elastase, and cathepsin G.

[b]Pro-IL-1α retains bioactivity before cleavage.

DC, Dendritic cell; *FLS*, fibroblast-like synoviocyte; *GAG*, glycosaminoglycan; *iNOS*, inducible nitric oxide synthase; *MMP*, matrix metalloproteinase; *NK*, natural killer; *PG*, peptidoglycan; *PMN*, polymorphonuclear neutrophil; *ROI*, reactive oxygen intermediates; *Th*, T helper.

release. Similarly, cytokines regulate the expression of complement processing and membrane defense molecules, scavenger receptors, NLRs, and TLRs. Cytokines, particularly IL-1, TNF, and IL-6, are crucial in driving the acute-phase response. Some moieties are designated “alarmins” on the basis of their very rapid induction or prior expression and critical early role in initiating inflammation (e.g., IL-33 and high mobility group box 1 [HMGB1]). Tables 31.1 through 31.8 provide descriptions of the function of cytokines expressed within the acute inflammatory response.

Cytokines critically modulate the cellular interactions that characterize chronic inflammation. Studies using real-time image analytic techniques such as two-photon microscopy and confocal scanning suggest continuous cellular motility during inflammation. Inflammatory lesions might properly be considered fluid states in which individual cells under cytokine control transiently contribute to organized functional subunits—such as the ectopic germinal center, synovial lining layer, or renal interstitial nephritis—yet remain competent to migrate thereafter under the influence of chemokines on the extra-cellular matrix (see Chapter 29). Cytokines also may promote cell death (apoptosis) either by withdrawal (e.g., IL-2, IL-7, IL-15, and type I IFNs) or by binding cytokine receptors containing death

TABLE 31.2 Tumor Necrosis Factor Superfamily Cytokines[a] With Potential Role in Rheumatic Disease

Cytokine	Size (kDa)	Receptors	Major Cell Sources	Selected Functions
TNF	26 (pro)	TNF-RI (p55)	Monocytes; T, B, NK cells; PMNs; eosinophils; mast cells; fibroblasts; keratinocytes; glial cells; osteoblasts; smooth muscle	Monocyte activation, cytokine, and PG ↑ PMN priming, apoptosis, oxidative burst ↑ Endothelial cell adhesion molecule, cytokine release ↑; fibroblast proliferation and collagen synthesis ↓
		TNF-RII (p75)		MMP and cytokine ↑ T cell apoptosis; clonal (auto)regulation; TCR dysfunction Adipocyte FFA release ↑ Endocrine effects—ACTH, prolactin ↑; TSH, FSH, GH ↓
LTα	22-26	TNF-RI	T cells; monocytes; fibroblasts; astrocytes; myeloma; endothelial cells; epithelial cells	Peripheral lymphoid development
		TNF-RII		Otherwise similar bioactivities to TNF
RANK ligand	35	RANK	Stromal cells; osteoblasts; T cells	Stimulates bone resorption via osteoclast maturation and activation Modulation of T cell–DC interaction
OPG	55	RANKL	Stromal cells, osteoblasts	Soluble decoy receptor for RANKL
BLyS[b]	18-32	TACI BCMA	Monocytes; T cells; DCs	B cell proliferation, Ig secretion, isotype switching, survival
		BLyS-R		T cell co-stimulation
APRIL	–	TACI	Monocytes; T cells; tumor cells	B cell proliferation
		BCMA		Tumor proliferation

[a]Additional members of importance include TRAIL, TWEAK, CD70, FasL, and CD40L. At least 18 members of the family are now described.

[b]Also called *B cell activating factor*, belonging to the TNF family (BAFF).

ACTH, Adrenocorticotropic hormone; *APRIL*, a proliferation inducing ligand; *BCMA*, B cell maturation protein; *BLyS*, B lymphocyte stimulator protein; *DC*, dendritic cell; *FFA*, free fatty acid; *FSH*, follicle-stimulating hormone; *GH*, growth hormone; *Ig*, immunoglobulin; *LT*, lymphotoxin; *MMP*, matrix metalloproteinase; *NK*, natural killer; *OPG*, osteoprotegerin; *PG*, peptidoglycan; *PMN*, polymorphonuclear neutrophil; *RANKL*, receptor activator of NF-κB ligand; *TACI*, transmembrane activator and calcium modulator and cyclophilin ligand; *TCR*, T cell receptor; *TNF*, tumor necrosis factor; *TRAIL*, TNF-related apoptosis-inducing ligand; *TSH*, thyroid-stimulating hormone; *TWEAK*, TNF-like weak inducer of apoptosis.

domains (e.g., TNF-R1). Cytokines contribute at every stage of inflammatory lesion development in a dynamic equilibrium, rather than in a static, linear manner. Chronic inflammation in rheumatic disease usually contains cytokine activities reminiscent of innate and acquired immune responses. For convenience, cytokines can be considered by their effect on cell subsets and cellular interactions (see Fig. 31.2, which describes the role of cytokine activity in a developing and chronic lesion). It is critical to recall that cytokines can contribute both pro- and anti-inflammatory effects depending on the time and context of their expression.

T cells depend on cytokine function at every developmental stage from bone marrow stem cell maturation, through thymic education, to functional determination and maturation after primary or secondary antigen exposure. The latter is of prime importance because re-education of phenotypic T cell responses may be achieved through alteration of the ambient cytokine milieu. T cell receptor–peptide–major histocompatibility complex (MHC) interactions during T cell–dendritic cell interaction rely on co-stimulatory molecule and local cytokine expression to determine the functional outcome (see Tables 31.3 and 31.4). IL-12, in the presence of IL-18, promotes type 1 phenotypic development, characterized ultimately by IFN-γ producing T helper (Th) type 1 effector cells.[21] IFN-γ drives macrophage priming and activation and adhesion molecule expression and promotes granuloma formation and microbial killing. IFN-γ has a complex role in tissue destruction, however, with contradictory data obtained in inflammation models in IFN-γ-deficient and IFN-γ receptor–deficient mice. IFN-γ ultimately may retard tissue destruction, perhaps by suppressing osteoclast activation.[22]

T cell subsets that secrete IL-17A predominantly (Th17 effector cells), together with IL-22 and TNF, are critical in a number of autoimmune diseases. Type 17 cells (either $CD4^+$ or $CD8^+$) are generated in the presence of IL-6 and transforming growth factor (TGF)-β, expanded by IL-1β and IL-23, and antagonized by IL-25 (IL-17E), IL-10, and IFN-γ. Type 17 cell differentiation has proven rather dynamic and plastic in terms of pathologic potential. IL-17A provides a direct and rapid route to tissue damage via such means as neutrophil recruitment and activation, chondrocyte

TABLE 31.3 Cytokines Associated Predominantly With Effector Function for T Cells[a]

Cytokine	Size (kDa)	Receptors	Major Cell Sources	Key Functions
Type II Interferon				
IFN-γ	20-25	IFNγR	Th/c1 cells; NK cells; γδT cells; B cells; macrophage/DCs	Macrophage activation, DC APC function ↑
				Endothelial adhesion molecule ↑
				Class II MHC expression ↑
				T cell growth ↓; opposes Th2 responses
				Bone resorption ↓; fibroblast collagen synthesis
4α-Helix Family				
IL-2	15	IL-2Rα	Th/c cells; NK cells	T cell division; maturation; cytokine release; cytotoxicity
		IL-2/15Rβ γ chain		NK cell cytokine release; cytotoxicity; monocyte activation
				Lymphocyte apoptosis ↓
IL-4	20	IL-4Rα/γ chain	Th/c cells (Th2); NK cells	Th2 differentiation, maturation, apoptosis ↓
		IL-4Rα/IL-13R1		B cell maturation; isotype switch (IgE)
				Eosinophil migration, apoptosis ↓ Endothelial activation; adhesion molecule expression
IL-5	25 monomer	IL-5Rα	Th/c2 cells; NK cells; mast cells; epithelial cells	B cell differentiation; immunoglobulin production (IgA)
	50 homodimer	IL-5Rβ		Eosinophil differentiation and activation
				Th/c maturation
IL-17 Family[b]				
IL-17A/F	20-30	IL-17R	T cells (Th17); fibroblasts	Chemokine release, fibroblast cytokine release, MMP release ↑ Osteoclastogenesis; hematopoiesis Chondrocyte GAG synthesis ↓ Leukocyte cytokine production ↑
IL-25 (IL-17E)	20-30	IL-17R	Th2 cells	Th2 cytokine release; B cell IgA and IgE synthesis; eosinophilia; epithelial cell hyperplasia

[a]Additional T cell–derived cytokines of potential interest include IL-13 from Th2 and NK2 cells.

[b]IL-17 family also contains IL-17B and IL-17C, the distinct functions of which are currently unclear.

APC, Antigen presenting cell; *DC,* dendritic cell; *GAG,* glycosaminoglycan; *IFN,* interferon; *Ig,* immunoglobulin; *IL,* interleukin; *MHC,* major histocompatibility complex; *MMP,* matrix metalloproteinase; *NK,* natural killer; *Th/c,* T helper/cytotoxic.

activation, keratinocyte activation, osteoclast activation, and fibroblast-like synoviocyte (FLS) activation.[23] Other lineages, such as innate lymphoid cells, likely also contribute to pathogenesis via IL-17 expression. Clinical trials that target IL-17A have been successful in a variety of rheumatic diseases and clearly demonstrate a pivotal role in psoriasis, psoriatic arthritis, and spondyloarthritis. The role for IL-17A in RA is much less clear because selective inhibitors have limited benefit in that disease, although perhaps there will be a role in pre-RA.

IL-4 dominance during T cell–dendritic cell interactions in the presence of IL-33 leads to type 2 responses, which promote humoral immunity driven by Th2 cells synthesizing primarily IL-4, IL-5, IL-10, and IL-13. Resulting pathogenesis more likely may be B cell mediated. Cytokines that predispose to regulatory T cell development are unclear, although high levels of IL-10 or TGF-β have been suggested in this context.[24] Effector T cells can operate via secretion of cytokines to patterns determined by their prior activatory conditions.

In the context of disease, it is likely that T cells are activated by interactions with diverse moieties, including extra-cellular matrix components and, in some disease states, autoantigens. In

TABLE 31.4 Cytokines Described Initially With Primary Role in Regulation of T Cells[a]

Cytokine	Size	Receptors	Major Cell Sources	Key Functions
IL-12	IL-12/23p40	IL-12Rα	Macrophages; DCs	Th1 cell proliferation, maturation
	IL-12p35	IL-12Rβ1		T cell cytotoxicity
		IL-12Rβ2		B cell activation
IL-15	15 kDa	IL-15Rα	Monocytes; fibroblast; mast cells; B cells; PMNs; DCs	T cell chemokinesis, activation, memory maintenance
		IL-2/15Rβ γ chain		NK cell maturation, activation, cytotoxicity Macrophage activation, suppression (dose dependent) PMN activation, adhesion molecule, oxidative burst Fibroblast activation B cell differentiation and isotype switching
IL-21	15 kDa	IL-21R γ chain	Activated T cells; others (?)	B cell activation
IL-23	59 kDa	IL-23R	Macrophages; DCs	Th17 cell expansion and activation; IL-17 release

[a]Cytokines included in this table are now understood to exhibit considerable functional heterogeneity as shown. Other T cell regulatory cytokines have been described, including IL-27, the functions of which are currently under investigation.

DC, Dendritic cells; *NK,* natural killer; *PMN,* polymorphonuclear neutrophil; *Th,* T helper.

TABLE 31.5 IL-10 Superfamily Cytokines[a]

Cytokine	Receptors	Cellular Sources	Key Functions
IL-10	IL-10R1	Monocytes; T cells; B cells; DCs; epithelial cells; keratinocytes	Macrophage cytokine release, iNOS, ROI ↓; soluble receptor ↑
	IL-10R2		T cell cytokine release, MHC expression ↓; anergy induction Treg cell maturation; effector function (?) DC activation, cytokine release ↓ Fibroblast MMP, collagen release ↓; no effect on TIMP B cell isotype switching enhanced
IL-19	IL-20R1/IL-20R2	Monocytes; others (?)	Monocyte cytokine and ROI release; monocyte apoptosis
IL-20	IL-22R/IL-20R2 IL-20R1/IL-20R2	Keratinocytes; others (?)	Autocrine keratinocyte growth regulation
IL-22	IL-22R/IL-10R2	Th17 cells; CD8 T cells; γδ T cells; NK cells	Acute-phase response, keratinocyte activation proliferation ↑
IL-24	IL-22R/IL-20R2 IL-20R1/IL-20R2	Monocytes; T cells	Tumor apoptosis; Th1 cytokine release by PBMC

[a]Additional members include IL-26, IL-28, and IL-28A. Many functions of the IL-10 superfamily are as yet poorly understood, but they likely reside beyond the immune system.

DC, Dendritic cell; *iNOS,* inducible nitric oxide synthase; *MMP,* matrix metalloproteinase; *NK,* natural killer; *PBMC,* peripheral blood mononuclear cells; *ROI,* reactive oxygen intermediates; *Th,* T helper; *TIMP,* tissue inhibitor of metalloproteinase; *Treg,* regulatory T cell.

addition, T cells can be activated by cell-contact with adjacent macrophages and potentially stromal cells[25–32] via cytokine driven autocrine loops. By this means, cytokines can promote chronicity by activating T cells to promote inflammation regardless of local (auto) antigen recognition; this mechanism has enormous therapeutic potential.

Agonist/Antagonist Cytokine Activities in Chronic Inflammation

Complex regulatory interactions exist to suppress ongoing inflammatory responses. This suppression is often achieved via parallel secretion of antagonistic cytokines and soluble receptors to regulate cytokine effector pathways. Th1 responses are suppressed

TABLE 31.6 IL-6 Superfamily Cytokines[a]

Cytokine	Size (kDa)	Receptors	Major Cell Sources	Key Functions
IL-6	21-28	IL-6R[b] gp130	Monocytes; fibroblasts; B cells; T cells	B cell proliferation; immunoglobulin production Hematopoiesis, thrombopoiesis T cell proliferation, differentiation, cytotoxicity Hepatic acute-phase response Hypothalamic-pituitary-adrenal axis Variable effects on cytokine release by monocytes
Oncostatin M	28	OMR gp130	Monocytes; activated T cells	Megakaryocyte differentiation Fibroblast, TIMP, and cytokine release Acute-phase reactants, fibroblast protease inhibitors ↑ Monocyte TNF release ↓; IL-1 effector function ↓ Hypothalamic-pituitary axis ↑; corticosteroid release Modulatory effect on osteoblast (?) Pro-inflammatory effects in some models (?)
Leukemia inhibitory factor	58	LIFR gp130	Fibroblasts; monocytes; lymphocytes; mesangial cells; smooth muscle cells; epithelial cells; mast cells	Acute-phase reactants ↑ Hematopoiesis, thrombopoiesis Role in neural development, neural effector function, implantation Bone metabolism; extra-cellular matrix regulation Leukocyte adhesion molecule expression Eosinophil priming Mixed pro-inflammatory versus anti-inflammatory effects in models

[a]Additional members of potential importance include IL-11, cardiotropin-1, and ciliary neurotrophic factor. Note overlapping effects within family.

[b]Membrane or soluble form can dimerize gp130 to promote signaling, which promotes signal transduction.

gp130, Glycoprotein 130; *LIFR,* leukemia inhibitory factor receptor; *OMR,* oncostatin M receptor; *TIMP,* tissue inhibitor of metalloproteinase; *TNF,* tumor necrosis factor.

partly by cytokines of the Th2 type (e.g., IL-4 and IL-10), and, consequently, exaggerated Th1 responses arise in models in which the Th2 response is deficient.[21] Th1 and Th2 cells similarly limit Th17 cell expansion.[23] Similar regulatory loops operate for other leukocytes, exemplified by the yin-yang effects of TNF and IL-10 on macrophage cytokine release and effector function.[33]

Inhibitory cytokine activities are usually defined with respect to a pro-inflammatory cytokine, and in other contexts they may have quite distinct functions, rendering prediction of their net contribution to an inflammatory response difficult. IL-10 and IL-35 oppose many of the pro-inflammatory effects of TNF and IL-1β (e.g., it reduces adhesion molecule expression, MHC expression, and MMP release, and activates Tregs, respectively), but IL-10 can potently activate B cell activation and immunoglobulin secretion.[33] Similarly, TNF may have an important role in regulating T cell function because T cells removed from sites of chronic inflammation exhibit a suppressed capacity to signal via their T cell receptor, which recovers on TNF neutralization.[34] Such regulation is complicated further by the precise ratio of cytokine to soluble receptor, such as TNF to sTNF-R or IL-10 to sIL-10R within the local environment. Commensurate with this, administration of anti-inflammatory cytokines such as IL-4, IL-10, and IL-11 has generally proven disappointing in the context of clinical inflammatory diseases. An important caveat is the potential requirement of combinations of cytokines to suppress inflammation optimally (e.g., combinations including IL-4, IL-10, and IL-11). Further functional antagonism is exemplified in the antagonistic activities of IL-1β and IL-1Ra and of IL-18 and IL-18 binding protein in regulating macrophage activation.

B Cells and Cytokine Release in Chronic Inflammation

Cytokines are crucial to B cell maturation, proliferation, activation, isotype switching, and survival. They are comprehensively discussed in Chapter 13 and also highlighted in Tables 31.1 through 31.8.

Innate Cell Lineages in Chronic Inflammation

Cytokines potently activate innate response cells that contribute to the chronic inflammatory lesion of a variety of rheumatic diseases. Tables 31.1 through 31.8 document relevant examples in which neutrophils, NK cells, eosinophils, and mast cells may be recruited and activated by the presence of appropriate cytokine combinations.

Growth Factors in Chronic Inflammation

Many data document the importance of growth factor families in chronic inflammation. TGF-β superfamily members, including TGF-β isoforms and bone morphogenetic protein

TABLE 31.7 Growth Factors Relevant to Rheumatic Diseases

Cytokine	Receptors	Cellular Sources	Key Functions
TGF-β[a]	Type I TGFβR	Broad—including fibroblasts, monocytes, T cells, platelets	Wound repair, matrix maintenance, and fibrosis
Isoforms 1-3[b]	Type II TGFβR		Initial activation then suppression of inflammatory responses
	Others		T cell (Treg and Th17) and NK cell proliferation and effector function ↓ Early-phase leukocyte chemoattractant, gelatinase, and integrin expression ↑ Early macrophage activation then suppression, reduced iNOS expression
BMP family (BMP2-15)	BMPRI	Varied (e.g., epithelial and mesenchymal embryonic tissues); bone-derived cell lineages	Regulate critical chemotaxis, mitosis, and differentiation processes during chondrogenesis and osteogenesis, tissue morphogenesis (e.g., heart, skin, eye)
	BMPRII		
PDGF	PDGFRα	Platelets; macrophages; endothelial cells; fibroblasts; glial cells; astrocytes; myoblasts; smooth muscle cells	Local paracrine or autocrine growth factor for variety of lineages
	PDGFRβ		Wound healing
FGF family	FGFR (various) Basic FGF Acidic FGF	Widespread	Growth and differentiation of mesenchymal, epithelial, and neuroectodermal cells

[a]Members of TGF-β superfamily include BMP, growth and differentiation factor, inhibinA, inhibinB, müllerian inhibitory substance, glial-derived neurotrophic factor, and macrophage inhibitory cytokine.

[b]Bound to latency-associated peptide to form small latency complex and to latent TGF-β binding protein to form large latent complex; activated by proteolytic and nonproteolytic pathways.

BMP, Bone morphogenetic protein; *FGF,* fibroblast growth factor; *iNOS,* inducible nitric oxide synthase; *NK,* natural killer; *PDGF,* platelet-derived growth factor; *TGF,* transforming growth factor; *Th,* T helper; *Treg,* regulatory T cell.

family members, warrant particular reference. TGF-β is critically involved in processes of cell proliferation, differentiation, inflammation, and wound healing.[35] Bone morphogenetic proteins, in addition to regulating inflammatory responses, are paramount in determining cartilage and bone tissue development and remodeling.[36] As such, they are of increasing interest in the pathogenesis of several rheumatic diseases.

Cytokine Effects Beyond Immune Regulation

A striking feature of the cytokine field concerns the broad functional pleiotropy exemplified in the effects of cytokines in normal physiologic and adaptive processes. Cytokine activities are found in muscle, adipose tissue, central nervous system, and liver, mediating normal regulation of metabolic pathways and modulation imposed by altered tissue conditions. Examples are found not only in the release of adipokines that regulate adipose metabolic pathways but also in the release of conventional cytokines by fat pads in inflammatory synovitis. Because cytokines thereby likely mediate normal and pathophysiologic activities in many tissues, they may underlie the co-morbidity that is observed in vascular, central nervous system, and bone tissues in several rheumatic diseases. Thus, cytokines or their receptors arising from the primary target tissues (e.g., joint and kidney) may "leak" into the circulation and promote additional pathology in other tissues. Commensurate with this targeting, such cytokines may modulate this co-morbid risk, which is now exemplified in the reduction of vascular morbidity in patients receiving TNF inhibitors. However, paradoxical effects occur—for example, tocilizumab inhibits IL-6R, and in so doing it elevates total and low-density lipoprotein cholesterol. The long-term implications of this effect for vascular risk are not yet clear but provide abundant evidence for complex interactions between cytokine and metabolic processing.

Conclusion

Cytokines represent a diverse family of glycoproteins that are active across a broad range of tissues. Their pleiotropic functions and propensity for synergistic interactions and functional redundancy render them intriguing therapeutic targets. Thus far, single cytokine targeting has proven useful in several rheumatic disease states. Further elucidation of the biology and functional interactions within this expanding family of bioactive moieties is likely to prove informative in resolving pathogenesis and in generating novel therapeutic options. In particular, biologic agents that target cytokines will increasingly unravel a novel molecular taxonomy for the rheumatic diseases.[37–39]

TABLE 31.8 Miscellaneous Cytokines With Potential Roles in Rheumatic Diseases

Cytokine	Size (kDa)	Receptors	Cellular Sources	Key Functions
MIF	12	Unclear	Macrophages; activated T cells; fibroblasts (synoviocytes)	Macrophage cytokine release, phagocytosis, NO release ↑
				T cell activation; DTH
				Fibroblast proliferation; COX expression; PLA_2 expression
				Intrinsic oxidoreductase activity ("cytozyme")
HMGB1	30	RAGE, dsDNA	Widespread expression; necrotic cells; macrophages; pituicytes	DNA-binding transcription factor
		Others (?)		Necrosis-induced inflammation
				Macrophage activation—delayed pro-inflammatory cytokine
				Smooth muscle chemotaxis
				Disrupts epithelial barrier function
				Bactericidal (direct)
GM-CSF	14-35	GM-CSFRα	T cells; macrophages; endothelial cells; fibroblasts	Granulocyte and monocyte maturation; hemopoietic effects
		GM-CSFRβ		Leukocyte PG release; DC maturation
				Pulmonary surfactant turnover
G-CSF	19	G-CSFR	Monocytes; PMNs; endothelial cells; fibroblasts; various tumor cells; stromal cells	Granulocyte maturation; promotes PMN function
M-CSF	28-44	M-CSFR	Monocytes; fibroblasts; endothelial cells	Monocyte activation, maturation
IL-32α-δ	Unknown	Unknown	Monocytes; T cells; NK cells; epithelial cells	Promotes pro-inflammatory cytokine release from variety of cells
Type I interferons IFN-α/β family	Various	IFNαβR	Widespread	Anti-viral response
				Broad immunomodulatory effects (promotes MHC expression)
				Macrophage activation; lymphocyte activation and survival
				Anti-proliferative, cytoskeletal alteration, differentiation ↑

COX, Cyclooxygenase; *DC*, dendritic cell; *dsDNA*, double-stranded DNA; *DTH*, delayed-type hypersensitivity; *G-CSF*, granulocyte colony-stimulating factor; *GM-CSF*, granulocyte-macrophage colony-stimulating factor; *HMGB*, high mobility group box chromosomal protein; *IFN*, interferon; *M-CSF*, macrophage colony-stimulating factor; *MHC*, major histocompatibility complex; *MIF*, macrophage inhibitory factor; *NO*, nitric oxide; *PG*, prostaglandin; *PLA*, phospholipase A; *PMN*, polymorphonuclear neutrophil; *RAGE*, receptor for advanced glycation end products.

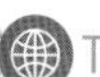 The references for this chapter can also be found on ExpertConsult.com.

References

1. McInnes IB, Buckley CD, Isaacs JD: Cytokines in rheumatoid arthritis—shaping the immunological landscape, *Nat Rev Rheumatol* 12(1):63–68, 2016.
2. Catalan-Dibene J, McIntyre LL, Zlotnik A: Interleukin 30 to Interleukin 40, *J Interferon Cytokine Res* 38(10):423–439, 2018.
3. Locksley RM, Killeen N, Lenardo MJ: The TNF and TNF receptor superfamilies: integrating mammalian biology, *Cell* 104:487, 2001.
4. Garlanda C, Dinarello C, Mantovani A: The interleukin-1 family: back to the future, *Immunity* 39:1003, 2013.
5. Bresnihan B, Baeten D, Firestein GS, et al.: OMERACT 7 Special Interest Group: synovial tissue analysis in clinical trials, *J Rheumatol* 32:2481, 2005.
6. Haringman JJ, Gerlag DM, Zwinderman AH, et al.: Synovial tissue macrophages: a sensitive biomarker for response to treatment in patients with rheumatoid arthritis, *Ann Rheum Dis* 64:834, 2005.
7. Boyle DL, Soma K, Hodge J, et al.: The JAK inhibitor tofacitinib suppresses synovial JAK1-STAT signalling in rheumatoid arthritis, *Ann Rheum Dis* 74(6):1311–1316, 2015.
8. Gadina M, Hilton D, Johnston JA, et al.: Signaling by type I and II cytokine receptors: ten years after, *Curr Opin Immunol* 13:363, 2001.
9. Bravo J, Heath JK: Receptor recognition by gp130 cytokines, *EMBO J* 19:2399, 2000.
10. Dubois S, Mariner J, Waldmann TA, et al.: IL-15Ralpha recycles and presents IL-15 in trans to neighboring cells, *Immunity* 17:537, 2002.
11. Francis K, Palsson BO: Effective intercellular communication distances are determined by the relative time constants for cyto/chemokine secretion and diffusion, *Proc Natl Acad Sci U S A* 94:12258, 1997.
12. Alivernini S, Gremese E, McSharry C, et al.: MicroRNA-155-at the critical interface of innate and adaptive immunity in arthritis, *Front Immunol* 8:1932, 2018.
13. Kontoyiannis D, Pasparakis M, Pizarro TT, et al.: Impaired on/off regulation of TNF biosynthesis in mice lacking TNF AU-rich elements: implications for joint and gut-associated immunopathologies, *Immunity* 10(387), 1999.

14. Anderson P: Post-transcriptional regulation of tumour necrosis factor alpha production, *Ann Rheum Dis* 59(3), 2000.
15. Gueydan C, Droogmans L, Chalon P, et al.: Identification of TIAR as a protein binding to the translational regulatory AU-rich element of tumor necrosis factor alpha mRNA, *J Biol Chem* 274:2322, 1999.
16. Saito K, Chen S, Piecyk M, et al.: TIA-1 regulates the production of tumor necrosis factor in macrophages, but not in lymphocytes, *Arthritis Rheum* 44:2879, 2001.
17. Budagian V, Bulanova E, Paus R, et al.: IL-15/IL-15 receptor biology: a guided tour through an expanding universe, *Cytokine Growth Factor Rev* 17:259, 2006.
18. Ferrari D, Chiozzi P, Falzoni S, et al.: Extracellular ATP triggers IL-1 beta release by activating the purinergic P2Z receptor of human macrophages, *J Immunol* 159:1451, 1997.
19. Fantuzzi G, Dinarello CA: Interleukin-18 and interleukin-1 beta: two cytokine substrates for ICE (caspase-1), *J Clin Immunol* 19(1), 1999.
20. Wallach D, Varfolomeev EE, Malinin NL, et al.: Tumor necrosis factor receptor and Fas signaling mechanisms, *Annu Rev Immunol* 17:331, 1999.
21. Liew FY: T(H)1 and T(H)2 cells: a historical perspective, *Nat Rev Immunol* 2(55), 2002.
22. Takayanagi H, Kim S, Taniguchi T: Signaling crosstalk between RANKL and interferons in osteoclast differentiation, *Arthritis Res* 4(Suppl 3):S227, 2002.
23. Weaver CT, Harrington LE, Mangan PR, et al.: Th17: an effector CD4 T cell lineage with regulatory T cell ties, *Immunity* 24:677, 2006.
24. Shevach EM, DiPaolo RA, Andersson J, et al.: The lifestyle of naturally occurring CD4+ CD25+ Foxp3+ regulatory T cells, *Immunol Rev* 212:60, 2006.
25. Yamamura Y, Gupta R, Morita Y, et al.: Effector function of resting T cells: activation of synovial fibroblasts, *J Immunol* 166:2270, 2001.
26. Unutmaz D, Pileri P, Abrignani S: Antigen-independent activation of naive and memory resting T cells by a cytokine combination, *J Exp Med* 180(1159), 1994.
27. McInnes IB, Leung BP, Liew FY: Cell-cell interactions in synovitis: interactions between T lymphocytes and synovial cells, *Arthritis Res* 2(374), 2000.
28. Sebbag M, Parry SL, Brennan FM, et al.: Cytokine stimulation of T lymphocytes regulates their capacity to induce monocyte production of tumor necrosis factor-alpha, but not interleukin-10: possible relevance to pathophysiology of rheumatoid arthritis, *Eur J Immunol* 27:624, 1997.
29. Dayer JM, Burger D: Cytokines and direct cell contact in synovitis: relevance to therapeutic intervention, *Arthritis Res* 1(17), 1999.
30. Ribbens C, Dayer JM, Chizzolini C: CD40-CD40 ligand (CD154) engagement is required but may not be sufficient for human T helper 1 cell induction of interleukin-2- or interleukin-15-driven, contact-dependent, interleukin-1beta production by monocytes, *Immunology* 99:279, 2000.
31. Hayes AL, Smith C, Foxwell BM, et al.: CD45-induced tumor necrosis factor alpha production in monocytes is phosphatidylinositol 3-kinase-dependent and nuclear factor-kappaB-independent, *J Biol Chem* 274:33455, 1999.
32. Foey A, Green P, Foxwell B, et al.: Cytokine-stimulated T cells induce macrophage IL-10 production dependent on phosphatidylinositol 3-kinase and p70S6K: implications for rheumatoid arthritis, *Arthritis Res* 4(64), 2002.
33. Fickenscher H, Hor S, Kupers H, et al.: The interleukin-10 family of cytokines, *Trends Immunol* 23:89, 2002.
34. Cope AP: Studies of T-cell activation in chronic inflammation, *Arthritis Res* 4(Suppl 3):S197, 2002.
35. Chen W, Wahl SM: TGF-beta: receptors, signaling pathways and autoimmunity, *Curr Dir Autoimmun* 5:62, 2002.
36. Abe E: Function of BMPs and BMP antagonists in adult bone, *Ann N Y Acad Sci* 1068:41, 2006.
37. Schett G, Elewaut D, McInnes IB, et al.: How cytokine networks fuel inflammation: toward a cytokine-based disease taxonomy, *Nat Med* 19:822, 2013.
38. McInnes IB, Schett G: The pathogenesis of rheumatoid arthritis, *N Engl J Med* 365:2205, 2011.
39. McInnes IB, Schett G: Cytokines in the pathogenesis of rheumatoid arthritis, *Nat Rev Immunol* 7:429, 2007.

32 Experimental Models for Rheumatoid Arthritis

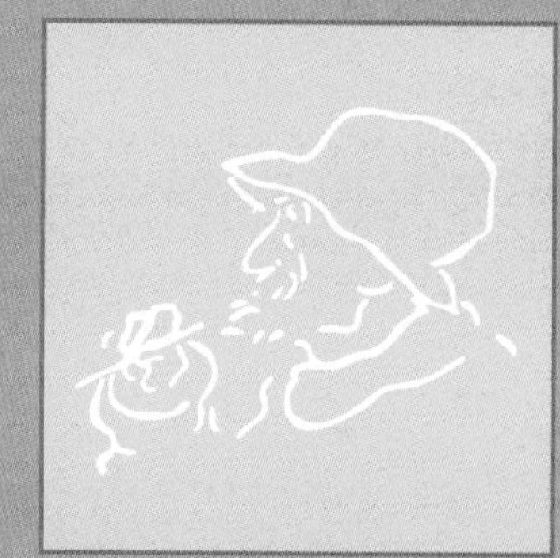

RIKARD HOLMDAHL

KEY POINTS

Animal models are tools to understand the basic mechanisms believed to cause or perpetuate rheumatoid arthritis (RA).

There are many different pre-clinical models for RA, some of which are standard, such as the collagen-induced arthritis (CIA) model, collagen antibody-induced arthritis (CAIA) model, and adjuvant (pristane)-induced arthritis model.

Arthritis can be induced in animals by immunization with cartilage components, adjuvants, bacterial or viral components, or genetic modification.

Pre-clinical models have a defined disease course and are useful for analysis of the discrete phases of biology mediating RA: priming, disease onset, and chronicity.

Animal models allow for controlled experiments with specific variations of environment and genetics.

Experimental models provide direction for novel approaches to treatment, such as cytokine inhibition and tolerance induction.

Introduction

For a deeper understanding of the complexity of the pathogenesis of rheumatoid arthritis (RA), the use of animal models is a necessity. Obviously a disease identical to RA in humans cannot develop in animals because they are of different species with different genetics and environments.

The three main advantages of using animal models are as follows:

1. Inbred animal strains can be genetically altered and environmentally controlled.
2. Manipulative experiments can be made. The genome of inbred strains can be changed by mutations, insertions, and deletions. The environment can also be changed in a controlled way; they can be immunized or infected, which may lead to arthritis. Controlled experiments can be performed.
3. It is more ethical to use animals instead of humans.

To evaluate and select proper animal models for RA, it is of value to be able to reproduce some of the basic features of the disease. The following are hallmarks of RA pathogenesis (see also Chapter 75):

- *The pathogenesis of disease usually starts before the clinical diagnosis is evident.* An autoimmune and inflammatory process precedes the clinical onset by up to several years.
- *Tissue-specificity.* The clinical onset is due to a tissue-specific inflammatory attack affecting diarthrodial, peripheral, and cartilaginous joints. Although systemic immune responses as well as manifestations are usually present, the inflammation is mainly directed towards peripheral joints.
- *Chronicity.* The inflammation fails to be downregulated and continues to occur in tissues in which no causative infectious pathogens have so far been demonstrated. Acute joint involvement is a common manifestation in both physiological responses to infections and in connection with other inflammatory disorders, but in RA, chronicity is an essential characteristic. The disease course may proceed with identifiable relapses, but there is usually a steady progression of joint destruction.
- *Autoantibodies.* The development of RA is preceded and associated with elevated levels of autoantibodies in serum. Anti-citrullinated protein antibodies (ACPA) have the highest specificity and sensitivity followed by antibodies to immunoglobulin (rheumatoid factors), but antibodies to other antigens do also occur in subsets of patients, like antibodies to collagen type II (CII), hnRNP-A2, and other post-translationally modified entities such as carbamylation and acetylation (see also Chapter 74).
- *Class II major histocompatibility complex (MHC) association.* The genetic influence is significant but complex. By far, the largest genetic contribution comes from class II genes in the major histocompatibility complex. In particular, certain structures in the peptide-binding pocket of human leukocyte antigen (HLA)-DR4 molecules are highly associated with RA. Several other loci confirm involvement of adaptive immunity (e.g., loci containing *PTPN22, CTLA4, IL21*), which strengthens the view that RA is an autoimmune disease.

Accumulating data suggest that RA develops in three discrete stages: priming, onset, and chronicity (Table 32.1). The disease priming process starts several years before clinical onset with enhanced levels of autoantibodies (ACPA and rheumatoid factor [RF]) and a higher level of inflammation markers. It is likely that the etiologic factors are operating at this early time.[1] Smoking and various chronic infections, such as periodontitis, may be associated with the early disease process.[2] This process, however, is not joint specific and a further spreading of the autoimmune reactivity towards joint structures is likely to occur before the clinical onset of arthritis. Because a classification of RA requires the chronic development of arthritis and the involvement of several joints, the diagnosis is normally made months or years after the inflammatory attacks on the joints begin. Thus only the chronic stage has so far been classified and studied in patient cohorts. Animal models, in contrast, are mainly used for studies of the initial stages and are not normally used to describe the established chronic stage (see Table 32.1).

TABLE 32.1 **Three Stages of Rheumatoid Arthritis Development in Human and Animal Models**

Disease Stage	Studies in Humans	Studies in Animal Models	Stage-Suitable Models
Pre-RA	Limited number of studies	Many studies but not mimicking pre-RA	No models mimicking pre-classic RA with both class II MHC association and ACPA response. The most promising models involve induction of autoimmunity by various adjuvant components.
Clinical onset	Limited number of studies	Many studies	Most models useful. Each model may involve specific pathways leading to subtypes of arthritis.
Chronic arthritis	Almost all studies	Limited number of studies and only a few models	DA rat or C57Bl mouse strains may show chronic relapsing models with adjuvant (pristane)- or cartilage/antigen-induced arthritis. Several spontaneous arthritis models show chronic progressive arthritis.

RA develops in three discrete steps, but the focus on the different stages has been different in human RA and animal models.
ACPA, Anti-citrullinated protein antibody; *MHC*, major histocompatibility complex; *RA*, rheumatoid arthritis.

In all three phases, an infectious agent may play a critical role but with different mechanisms. The first priming phase is thought to be dependent on chronic inflammation within mucosal tissues, leading to uncontrolled exposure of post-translational modified proteins, such as citrullinated proteins, to T and B cells. In genetically susceptible individuals, an autoimmune response may be allowed to develop. Alternatively, the inflammatory targeting to the joints, and the chronic relapsing pattern, could also be explained by a breakdown of tolerance to joint localized antigens.

It is likely that the adaptive immune system is critical for the initiation and onset of disease, especially because these stages seem to be strongly associated with class II MHC and lymphocyte activation genes. Nevertheless, there is no strong evidence that the chronic relapsing stage is driven by the adaptive immune system as chronically activated fibroblast and macrophages could also potentially drive the disease.

Thus the cause and driving forces are not yet clarified and are likely to operate differently in different individuals, leading to the syndrome we call *rheumatoid arthritis*.

Animal models are excellent tools for understanding the basic mechanisms of the immune system and how they may cause and regulate disease development and progression. Disease models allow for the analysis of distinct pathways and are likely to reflect distinct subsets of the human disease. The recent advancement of different animal models that mimic different aspects of human diseases as well as the improvement in genetic techniques has dramatically increased their usefulness. The present overview will not only include models for RA, but will also briefly add models with related disease pathways, such as psoriatic arthritis, reactive arthritis, axial spondyloarthritis (AxSpA), Lyme disease, and septic arthritis (summarized in Table 32.2). Nevertheless, there is a focus on the classic models for RA, which are commonly used in both industry and academia: the adjuvant arthritis (AA) model in the rat, the collagen-induced arthritis (CIA) model, and the collagen antibody-induced arthritis (CAIA) model.

Arthritis Caused by Infectious Agents

Several infectious agents may invade joints where they persist and cause arthritis. As with most persisting infectious agents, a balance between the parasite and the host is usually achieved. Thus inflammatory consequences may not only be caused directly by the parasite but also by an aberrant inflammatory response of the host. When microorganisms are present in the target tissue, chronic autoimmunity could be maintained by different mechanisms, such as superantigen-mediated T cell activation, a cross-reactive immune response, or the presence of adjuvant material enhancing autoantigen presentation. Several such arthritogenic agents have been described in experimental animals, and some of these mimic a corresponding infectious disease in humans.

Mycoplasma Arthritides

Arthritis associated with mycoplasma infection is endemic among farm animals. It is also possible to induce arthritis in rodents after inoculation with *Mycoplasma arthritidis*. Nevertheless, *Mycoplasma* bacteria are not found in joints with RA, although it may cause arthritis in individuals with severe B cell deficiency. Inoculation of mice induces a mild chronic arthritis in conjunction with the persistence of the microorganism, but this is driven by immune activation by a mycoplasma-derived superantigen.[3] In accordance with observations in humans, B cell–deleted mice are more susceptible to *Mycoplasma*-induced arthritis.

Lyme Arthritis

Borrelia is a spirochete that may persist in joints and cause arthritis. The clinical picture is chronic and resembles RA—it, too, is genetically associated with class II-DR4 MHC. Live bacteria persist in the joints, but in many patients it has been difficult to identify the spirochete in the arthritic joints. Mice infected with *Borrelia* develop arthritis similar to the human version of the disease. Similar to humans, MHC controls the susceptibility to arthritis, and the immune response associated with human class II MHC expressed in mice is directed to *Borrelia*-derived antigens.[4] The persistence of the spirochete seems to be a requirement for the development of arthritis, although some mouse strains do not develop arthritis despite high levels of bacteria in the joints.

Staphylococcal Arthritis

Septic arthritis is most commonly caused by a persistent infection of *Staphylococcus aureus*. The bacteria tend to be encapsulated in tissues such as joint synovia and persist for years. Inoculation

TABLE 32.2 **Overview of Animal Arthritis Models**

Model	Species	Genetics	Disease Characteristics	References
Arthritis Caused by Infection				
Mycoplasma-induced arthritis	Rats and mice	More pronounced in B cell-deficient mice	Mild chronic arthritis	3
Borrelia-induced arthritis	Mice	Major histocompatibility complex (MHC)	Severe and erosive arthritis with spirochetes in the joints	79
Staphylococcus-induced arthritis	Rats and mice	MHC	Severe arthritis	5
Yersinia-induced arthritis	Rats and mice	Lewis (LEW) and spontaneous hypertensive (SHR) rats but not dark agouti (DA) and Brown Norway (BN) rats	Severe arthritis with bacteria in the joints	80
Arthritis Caused by Bacterial Fragments				
Mycobacterium-induced arthritis (adjuvant arthritis [AA])	Rats	MHC, non-MHC genes (LEW>F344)	Acute and generalized inflammatory disease including erosive arthritis	8
Streptococcal cell wall–induced arthritis	Mice and rats	Non-MHC genes (LEW>F344), (DBA/1=Balb/c>B10)	Severe and erosive arthritis	81
Arthritis Induced by Adjuvant				
Avridine-induced arthritis (AvIA)	Rats	MHC (f)	Very severe, erosive, and chronic arthritis	82
Oil (mineral oil)-induced arthritis (OIA)	DA rats	non-MHC loci on chromosomes 4, 10	Acute and self-limited inflammation of peripheral joints	12
Pristane-induced arthritis (PIA)	Rats	MHC, non-MHC loci on chromosomes 1, 4, 6, 12, 14	Chronic and erosive arthritis in peripheral joints Can be passively transferred with T cells	13, 20, 83
PIA	Mice	MHC (q, d)?, *Ncf1* Balb/c, DBA, and C3H gene backgrounds	Chronic and generalized lupus-type of inflammatory disease also affecting joints	22
Mannan induce psoriasis and psoriatic arthritis (MIP)	Mice	B10.Q, B10.RIII. Arthritis enhanced by mutation in *Ncf1*	Psoriasis and psoriasis arthritis developing a few days after injection of mannan. Macrophage, gd T cell, and neutrophil dependent	27
Arthritis Induced by Cartilage Protein Immunization				
CII (heterologous or homologous CII in mineral oil)-induced arthritis (CIA)	Rats	MHC (a, l, f, and u), non-MHC loci on chromosomes 1, 4, 7, 10	Erosive and chronic arthritis in peripheral joints	33
CII (heterologous or homologous CII in CFA)-induced arthritis (CIA)	Mice	MHC (q and r), non-MHC loci on chromosomes 1, 2, 3, 6, 7, 8, 10, 15	Erosive and chronic arthritis in peripheral joints	37
CXI (rat CXI in IFA)-induced arthritis	Rats	MHC (f, u)	Severe and chronic arthritis	31
Human proteoglycan (in complete Freund's adjuvant)–induced arthritis	BALB/c mice	MHC (d), several non-MHC loci	Chronic arthritis	30
Cartilage oligomeric matrix protein (COMP) (in mineral oil)–induced arthritis	Rats, mice	MHC (RT1u, H2q)	Acute and chronic arthritis	32, 59
Glucose-6-phosphate isomerase (G6PI)–induced arthritis	Mice	MHC (H2q)	Self-limited arthritis	62

Continued

TABLE 32.2 **Overview of Animal Arthritis Models—cont'd**

Model	Species	Genetics	Disease Characteristics	References
Antibody-Induced Arthritis Models				
Collagen antibody-induced arthritis (CAIA)	Mice	Balb/c>DBA/1>C57Bl Ncf1	Anti-CII antibodies induce a mild arthritis within 2 days. If subsequently injected with lipopolysaccharide (LPS), a more severe, self-limited arthritis develops. If injected with mannan, a severe chronic relapsing arthritis develops, in particular in Ncf1-deficient mice	38, 84
KxB/N serum-induced arthritis (SIA)	Mice		Serum from transgenic KxB/N induces arthritis within 2 days, which will heal after a few weeks	85
"Spontaneous" Arthritis Models				
HLA-B27 transgenic animals	Rat	B27 heavy chain transgene	Ankylosing spondylitis, colitis, balanitis, arthritis	6
The MRL/lpr mouse (mutation in the *Fas* gene controlling apoptosis)	Mice	Lpr	Generalized inflammation as a part of lupus disease, which also affects the joints	68
Stress-induced arthritis	DBA/1 mice	Non-MHC genes	Enthesopathic response with no evidence for immune involvement. A model for psoriasis arthritis	67, 86
Tumor necrosis factor (TNF) transgenic mice (overpro-duction of TNF)	Mice	TNF transgene	Erosive arthritis as well as generalized tissue inflammation	69
IL-1R antagonist deficient mouse	Balb/c mice	IL-1Ra deficiency	Arthritis	72
Gp130 IL-6R mutated mouse	C57 Black mice	IL-6R mutation	Arthritis	73
K/BxN	K/BxN mice	TCR transgenic specific for a G6PI-derived peptide	Severe arthritis with autoreactivity to G6PI	74
Zap70 mutation	Balb/c mice	Spontaneous mutation in *Zap70*	Severe arthritis with autoreactivity	25
Severe combined immunodefi-ciency (SCID) mouse	Mice	Local injection of fibroblasts into immunodeficient SCID mouse	Sustained destructive arthritis	75

with certain *Staphylococcus aureus* strains induces septic arthritis in many mouse and rat strains.[5] Severe and prolonged arthritis develops in infected joints, mimicking the human situation. Interestingly, protection of the host is critically dependent on the innate defense, such as neutrophils and complement, whereas the adapted immune response is not effective. Instead, the apparently aberrant adapted immune response promotes arthritis.

Arthritis and Ankylosing Spondylitis Induced by Intra-cellular Bacteria

Some bacteria with the capacity to invade cells upon infection (e.g., *Yersinia*) are known to be related to postinfectious arthritides, such as reactive arthritis and ankylosing spondylitis. These diseases are genetically associated with HLA-B27, a class I MHC allele of the B locus. It has been possible to reproduce the human disease to a large extent in HLA-B27 transgenic mice and rats.[6,7] In B27-transgenic rats, ankylosing spondylitis, balanitis, colitis, dermatitis, and arthritis occur spontaneously. If the rats are made germ-free, however, the joint manifestations are no longer present. This phenomenon indicates the importance of a so far unknown infectious agent. Importantly the development of arthritis is most likely related to the triggering of inflammation by adjuvant fragments from the pathogen.

Arthritis Caused by Bacterial Fragments

Postinfectious arthritis may develop after bacterial infections. The occurrence of arthritis can be dependent on several different bacteria-derived compounds, such as cell wall fragments, DNA, and heat shock proteins. Bacterial cell wall fragments are difficult for macrophages to degrade and may cause prolonged activation of synovial macrophages. The first animal model for RA to be described was the so-called *adjuvant arthritis* (AA) induced in rats after injection of mycobacterium cell walls suspended in mineral oil (i.e., complete Freund's adjuvant [CFA]).[8] Only rats (and not mice or primates) develop arthritis after mycobacterium challenge, although joint-related granuloma formation may occur also in humans treated with mycobacterium-containing vaccine. CFA is a potent adjuvant that activates a multitude of pattern recognition

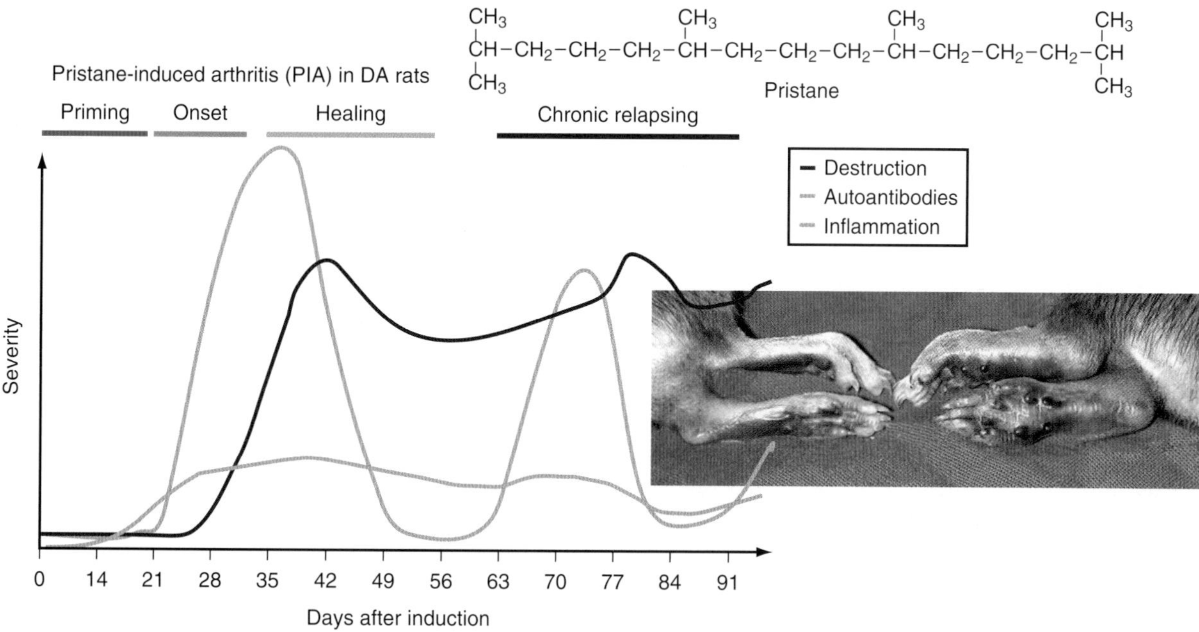

• **Fig. 32.1** Pristane-induced arthritis in dark agouti rats. Induced with pristane subcutaneously. Development of severe and chronic relapsing arthritis starting 10 to 14 days after injection

receptors, activating antigen-presenting cells and enhancing T cell immunity. Subcutaneous injection of CFA in rats leads to granulomatous inflammation in many organs, such as the spleen, liver, bone marrow, skin, and eyes, and causes profound inflammation in peripheral joints. AA is severe but self-limited, and the inflammation subsides after 5 to 7 weeks. The mycobacterium cell wall fragments are most likely disseminated throughout the body and engulfed by tissue macrophages, which have difficulties in degrading the bacterial cell wall structures and are therefore transformed into an activated state, which can trigger inflammation.

AA can be abrogated by elimination of the classic αβ type of T cells, and spleen-derived T cells can transfer the disease. The specificity of such T cells has not been reproducibly demonstrated, although some possibilities have been suggested, including bacterial structures and cross-reactive self-components. Although a role for heat shock proteins as T cell antigens has not been confirmed, they play a regulatory role for the development of arthritis. A minimal arthritogenic structure in the mycobacteria cell wall is the peptidoglycan component muramyl dipeptide. Interestingly, T cells do not recognize this structure, but it has potent adjuvant capacity as it activates the inflammasome by stimulating innate immune receptors (NOD2) and antigen-presenting cells. In addition, the unmethylated DNA of bacteria independently trigger arthritis in mice and contribute to the arthritic severity of AA in rats. The bacterial DNA trigger Toll-like receptors on both antigen-presenting cells and inflammatory macrophages and will, therefore, interact with both T cell–dependent and inflammatory pathways. Another T cell–dependent arthritogenic pathway is triggered by the mineral oil in which the mycobacteria is suspended, as is discussed later in more detail. Thus, this classic adjuvant-induced arthritis (AIA) is mediated by different and interacting pathways, dependent on both different mycobacterium cell components as peptidoglycans, DNA, and heat shock proteins but also dependent on adjuvant activity mediated by the oil used to suspend the mycobacteria.

Postinfectious arthritis has also been observed to occur after streptococcal infections. A rapidly developing form of arthritis has been observed after systemic inoculation of streptococcal cell wall fragments in rats and mice but not in primates.[9] Parenterally injected peptidoglycans rapidly disseminate throughout the body, including the joints. These structures are difficult for the macrophages to degrade and, consequently, synovial macrophages are persistently activated. T cells are necessary for the initiation and perpetuation of the arthritis.

Chronic parodontitis, caused by *Porphyromonas gingivalis,* has been suggested to be involved in the initiation of RA,[10] but so far no arthritis has been induced in animal models by using live bacteria or immunization with *P. gingivalis*–derived components.

Adjuvant-Induced Arthritis

The induction of arthritis in rats was found to be dependent not only on the mycobacteria but also on the oil into which the mycobacterium fragments were suspended (reviewed in ref. 11). Interestingly, some oils were found to support the induction of arthritis, whereas others did not. Many years later, it was noted that the mineral oils that supported the induction of arthritis were in fact arthritogenic by themselves.[12] It was also found that subcutaneous administration of nonbacterial adjuvant compounds, such as pristane, hexadecane, and squalene, were highly effective in inducing arthritis.[13–15] In most cases, these adjuvant compounds produce inflammation confined to the joints and offer more appropriate experimental models for RA than the earlier commonly used AA (i.e., mycobacterium in oil induced arthritis) model.

Mineral oil–induced arthritis (OIA), avridine-induced arthritis (AvIA), pristane-induced arthritis (PIA), hexadecane-induced arthritis, and squalene-induced arthritis in the rat share many common features but differ by the degree of chronic development (Fig. 32.1). They are induced with adjuvant compounds that lack immunogenic capacity (i.e., no specific immune responses are elicited). Instead, they are rapidly spread throughout the body after a single subcutaneous injection, penetrate through cell membranes into cells, and interact with yet unknown cell surface receptors and intra-cellular proteins. One or two weeks after injection, arthritis suddenly develops. The arthritis appears in the peripheral joints, with a similar distribution as seen in RA. Occasionally, other joints are involved, but systemic manifestations in other tissues have so far not been reported. In certain rat strains, especially in the PIA model, the arthritis proceeds as a chronic relapsing disease. Interestingly a systemic immune response occurs that leads to production of antibodies to RA33 and RF but not ACPA, whereas an immune response to cartilage proteins appear in the more chronic development of the disease.[16] A role for cartilage proteins in regulation of disease activity is seen because the disease can be prevented and, in fact, therapeutically ameliorated by nasal vaccination with various cartilage proteins. Interestingly the first acute phase of the disease is class II MHC–dependent and αβ T cells play a critical role in all stages of the disease. T cell transfer of the disease seems to be oligoclonal rather than monoclonal and so far antigen-specific T cells have not been identified.[17] A role for environmental infectious agents is not likely because no difference in disease susceptibility could be seen in germ-free rats, although only conventional rats respond to heat shock proteins.[18] So far, there is no evidence for recognition by lymphocyte receptors or receptors involved in the innate immune system.

Surprisingly, some of the arthritogenic adjuvants are components already present in the body before injection. For example, pristane is a component of chlorophyll and is normally ingested by all mammals, including laboratory rats. Pristane is taken up through the intestine and spread throughout the body. Nevertheless, they all share the capacity to penetrate into cells where they can change membrane fluidity and modulate transcriptional regulation and in higher doses induce apoptosis. The injection route and dose is critical (i.e., it is decisive for which cell is first activated and to what extent).

The PIA model has been subjected to genetic analysis showing that the disease is polygenic,[19] and the identified loci control distinct phases of the disease, such as arthritis onset, clinical severity, joint erosion, and chronicity. Some of the underlying genes have been identified. The strongest effect is mediated through a polymorphism of the *Ncf1* gene of both inbred and wild rat populations.[20] The *Ncf1* gene codes for the p47phox component of the NOX2 complex and controls the oxidative burst. Surprisingly a lower oxidative burst capacity was associated with more severe arthritis. The effect was found to operate before T cell activation, and therefore it also controls the degree of autoimmunity, linking innate and adaptive immunity. Importantly, several other genes including class II MHC genes, which control the adaptive T cell response, and a C-type lectin gene cluster (APLEC), which is likely to have importance in the uptake of antigen to antigen-presenting cells, also control PIA (reviewed in ref. 21).

AA is not easily inducible in species other than rats. Of the above mentioned AIA models, only PIA has been described in mice.[22] Nevertheless, the induction of PIA in mice requires repeated intraperitoneal injections of pristane, which triggers a widespread inflammatory disease with a late and insidious onset. The induced disease mimics systemic lupus erythematosus (SLE) rather than RA[23] and is known as *pristane-induced lupus* (PIL). The disease is clearly different from PIA in the rat; the same inducing protocol does not induce disease in the rat and the disease course and characteristics are different. Another adjuvant-related model is the induction of mild arthritis after intra-articular injection of agents that activate macrophages, such as unmethylated DNA.[24] It has recently been found that several mouse models earlier believed to be spontaneous are critically dependent on adjuvants and should therefore be classified as AIA.

From the observation that a BALB/c substrain in Japan spontaneously developed arthritis, a causative amino acid–replacing mutation in the *ZAP70* gene was identified.[25] The mutation *(W163C)* caused a weaker T cell receptor (TCR)–mediated signalling and a disturbed T cell selection in thymus. It resulted in the activation of autoreactive IL-17 secreting T cells, stimulating synovial fibroblasts to secrete granulocyte-macrophage colony-stimulating factor (GM-CSF) and thereby initiating arthritis.[26] The arthritis, however, did not develop in specific pathogen-free conditions and it could be shown that injection of beta-glycan or mannan induced the arthritis. Thus this model seems to be an AIA in mice. The resulting arthritis, however, may differ depending on the inducing agent and the genetic background. For example, injection of mannan in certain mouse strains with a deficiency in reactive oxygen species production results in a disease that mimics psoriatic arthritis rather than the classic RA.[27]

Some other spontaneous arthritis models, such as the KxB/N model or the IL-1R deficient mouse, are likely mediated by an adjuvant component because arthritis either does not develop or is dramatically attenuated under germ-free conditions.[28,29] The causative arthritogenic effect is mediated by intestinal bacteria, segmented filamentous bacteria (SFB),[28] and lactobacillus,[29] respectively.

Taken together, there is today a set of useful adjuvant type of arthritis models in both mice and rats.

Cartilage Protein-Induced Arthritis

Arthritis is inducible with several different cartilage proteins, such as aggrecan,[30] collagen type XI (CXI),[31] cartilage oligomeric matrix protein (COMP),[32] and CII.[33] These various models have different characteristics and genetics. Collagen-induced arthritis (CIA), induced with CII, is the most commonly used model for RA today and was first demonstrated in the rat[33] and later reported in other species, such as mice[34] and primates.[35]

CII-Induced Arthritis

Immunization with the major collagen in cartilage, CII, leads to an autoimmune response and, as a consequence, sudden onset of severe arthritis. It is usually necessary to emulsify the CII in adjuvant, such as mineral oil in the rat and CFA in the mouse, but the disease can be distinguished from the various forms of AA. The susceptibility of the CIA model varies considerably depending on the experimental animal strain, the adjuvant used, and whether the CII used is of self (homologous CII) or nonself (heterologous CII) origin.

In both rats and mice immunized with heterologous CII, a severe, erosive polyarthritis develops 2 to 3 weeks after immunization but usually subsides within 3 to 4 weeks (Fig. 32.2). The most commonly used DBA/1 strain thus develops a severe but only an acute disease. Nevertheless, a genetic influence is obvious because mice on the less susceptible C57Bl backgrounds develop a milder arthritis, which may later develop into a more chronic relapsing disease course (Fig. 32.3). In all of the models, the erosive inflammatory phase is followed by a healing phase, with pronounced formation of new cartilage and bone that can be difficult to distinguish clinically from active inflammation. The disease is critically dependent on both a T and a B cell response to CII, and pathogenic antibodies play a role in the inflammatory attack on the joints.[36] Importantly, isolation of monoclonal antibodies specific to CII can induce arthritis,[37] which has developed into a useful new animal model called the *collagen antibody-induced*

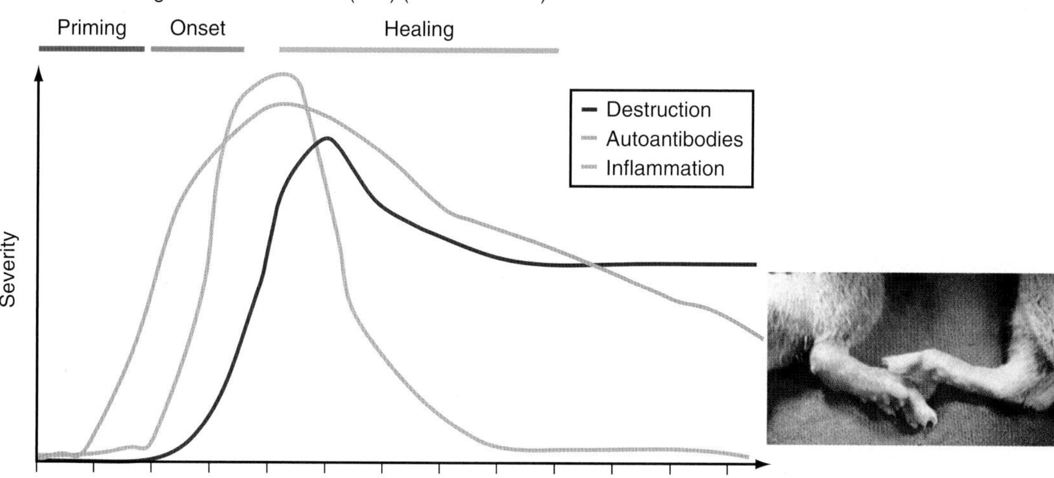

• **Fig. 32.2** Collagen-induced arthritis in DBA/1 mice. Induced after immunization with heterologous (bovine, chicken, rat) collagen type II emulsified in complete Freund's adjuvant. Severe arthritis starts 3 to 4 weeks after immunization. Although the arthritis is severe and gives dramatic erosions and bone remodeling, there is no chronic relapsing inflammatory disease course.

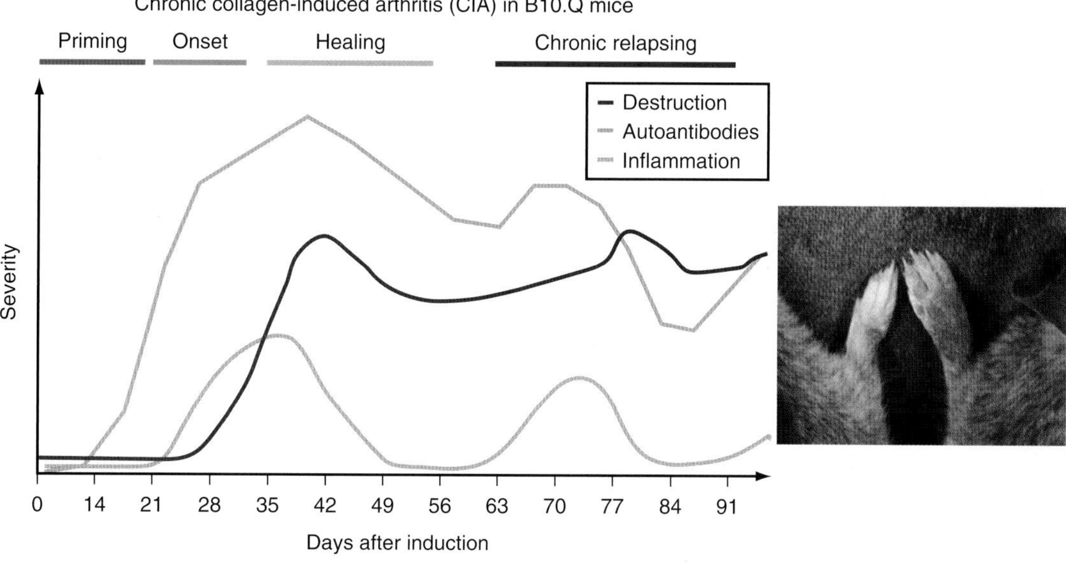

• **Fig. 32.3** Collagen-induced arthritis in B10.Q mice. Induced after immunization with rat collagen type II emulsified in complete Freund's adjuvant. Mild arthritis starts 3 to 5 weeks after immunization. The arthritis is mild but causes inflammatory joint erosions and bone remodeling. It is, however, often followed by a chronic disease with inflammatory relapses.

arthritis (CAIA) model[38] (Fig. 32.4). These CII-specific antibodies bind to the cartilage and destabilize the cartilage matrix. The formation of local immune complexes activates neurons, inducing pain-like effects.[39,40] Subsequently the inflammatory response is triggered with fixation of complement attraction of neutrophilic granulocytes, and activation of FcR expressing inflammatory cells in a process independent of the adaptive immune system.[41] Interestingly the epitopes recognized on CII predominantly contain arginines that can be citrullinated.[42] The major CII epitopes are citrullinated and cross-reactive anti-citrullinated monoclonal antibodies induce arthritis, indicating an important link to RA.[43] Nevertheless, the antibody response to citrullinated proteins in CIA is of a much lower titer and lacks important qualities seen in the human ACPA response, such as citrulline peptide promiscuity and N-glycosylation in the antigen-binding domain.[44]

The disease provoked after immunization with homologous CII in both rats and mice is not as easily inducible, but once started it is severe and tends to be more chronic than the disease induced with heterologous CII. The pathogenic events in the chronic disease phase are largely unknown but are most likely dependent on both autoreactive B and T cell activity. Nevertheless, the CIA model is the most extensively investigated model for RA and has provided valuable insights into the genetic control of the arthritic process and of the autoimmune interactions with cartilage. It has also been useful for the development of new therapeutic approaches and for drug screening.

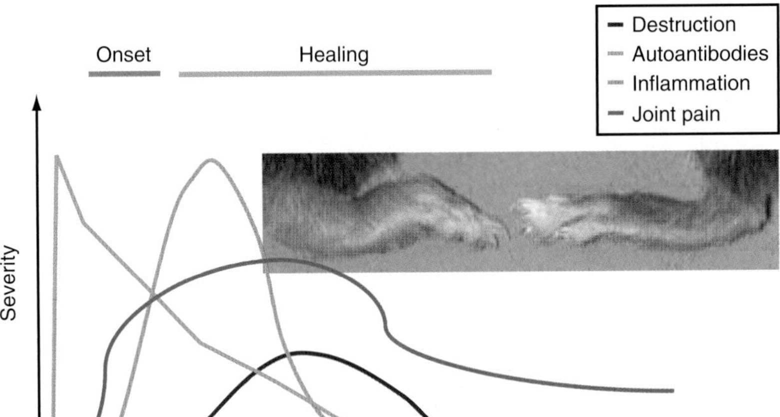

• **Fig. 32.4** Collagen antibody-induced arthritis (CAIA) in DBA/1 mice. Induced after intravenous injection of a defined set of monoclonal antibodies to collagen type II. The mice change behavior due to pain in the joints around 24 hours, mild arthritis starts 48 hours after injection, and severe arthritis starts after an additional boost with injection of lipopolysaccharide (LPS) intraperitoneally. The arthritis is acute with mild joint erosions but with no bone remodeling. The disease is acute and resolves within a few weeks.

Genetic Basis of Collagen-Induced Arthritis

Susceptibility to CIA varies dramatically between different inbred strains. CIA is a complex, polygenic disease, in similarity with the AA models described above. In the CIA model the autoimmune process is already determined by induction through immunization with a defined antigen. Not surprisingly, the class II MHC polymorphism is important for determining susceptibility, but there is also a major influence by a large number of genes outside the MHC region. The major gene regions have been identified through genetic segregation experiments in both mice and rats, which have given an overall picture of the genetic inheritance of the susceptibility.[45] As in other complex diseases, these genes operate in concert and can only be identified through isolation in a controlled genetic and environmental context. Some of the major genes have, however, been positioned in both rats and mice, including class II MHC genes, *Ncf1,* and complement C5. The *Ncf1* gene was defined through analysis of PIA and CIA in rats.[20] A spontaneous mutation in the mouse *Ncf1* gene, when combined with the CIA-susceptible class II MHC allele Aq in the C57Bl/10 mouse, causes a chronic relapsing form of CIA.[46] In addition, these mice tend to develop a severe form of chronic arthritis in the postpartum period, with the spontaneous development of autoimmunity to CII. Subsequent studies have identified *Ncf1* as a major genetic factor in both RA and SLE.[47–49]

Another genetic polymorphism of importance is the complement C5, which is deficient in many mouse strains. The deficiency leads to a relative resistance to CIA, suggesting a role for complement pathways in arthritis, which in fact is the opposite of its role in mycoplasma-induced arthritis. A role for alternative complement pathways, as well as Fc receptor–mediated pathways, has been demonstrated using both the CIA and CAIA models.[50,51] The rapid progress of genome-wide association analysis of large human cohorts today gives direct information on involved genes and gene clusters in common diseases, such as RA. Nevertheless, the animal models are needed to understand their functional relevance, and for this, the genes controlling the corresponding disease in the animals need to be identified.

Autoimmunity Associated With the Major Histocompatibility Complex in Collagen-Induced Arthritis

Early observations using the CIA model in both mice and rats indicated a role for the MHC region. In the mouse, CIA induced with either heterologous or homologous CII is most strongly associated with the $H2^q$ and $H2^r$ haplotypes, whereas most other haplotypes, such as b, s, d and p, are relatively resistant.[52] The major underlying gene within the $H2^q$ haplotype has been identified as the A^q beta gene.[53] Moreover, the immunodominant peptide derived from the CII molecule bound to the arthritis-associated q variant of the A (A^q) molecule has been found to be located between positions 259 and 271 of CII.[54] This peptide can be glycosylated on the central lysine side chain and is recognized by most of the CII-reactive T cells. Interestingly the peptide is also bound by DR4 (DRB1*0401/DRA) and DR1 molecules, (i.e., the shared epitope, which is associated with RA). Mice that transgenically express DR4 or DR1 are susceptible to CIA, respond to CII259-271 peptide and CII-reactive T cells from RA patients, and seem to predominantly recognize the glycosylated forms of the CII259-271 peptide.[55] Importantly, CII is normally expressed in the thymus but not the glycosylated modification, leading to an escape of central tolerance.[56] These findings suggest a model for studies of RA that not only mimic some basic pathogenic events but might also share some critical structural similarities.

Arthritis is also inducible in mouse strains that do not express q or r. A commonly used model is to induce arthritis with high doses of chicken or bovine CII emulsified in *Mycobacterium tuberculosis*-containing CFA, but this is not a CIA model because the arthritis is dependent on various contaminants in the CII preparation, such as another matrix protein or the pepsin used for the preparation.[57] Such T cell reactivity could help B cells produce antibodies to CII because these contaminants aggregate with CII, which could explain the development of arthritis. Thus, if strain restrictions exist for a given experimental protocol, it is preferable to instead use the CAIA model.

It is important to emphasize that the identified structural interaction between class II MHC+ peptide complexes and T cells does not give us the answer to the pathogenesis of CIA (or RA), but rather, a better tool for further analysis. An important question is how the immune system interacts with the peripheral joints (i.e., how autoreactive T and B cells are normally tolerized and what happens in the pathologic situation after their activation by CII immunization). Many of the T cells reactive with the rat CII259-271 peptide do not cross-react with the corresponding peptide from mouse CII. The difference between the heterologous and the homologous peptide is position 266, in which the rat has a glutamic acid (E) and the mouse an aspartic acid (D), which leads to a weaker binding of the mouse peptide to A^q. The importance of this minor difference was demonstrated in transgenic mice expressing CII mutated to express a glutamic acid at this position.[58] When mutated CII was expressed in cartilage, the T cell response to CII was partially but not completely tolerized. The mice were susceptible to arthritis, but the incidence was low, similar to what is seen in mice immunized with homologous CII. This finding shows that a normal interaction between cartilage and T cells leads to the activation of T cells but with less capacity to induce arthritis or with regulatory properties. These CII autoreactive T cells may, under extreme circumstances (such as CII immunization), be pathogenic. In contrast, B cells reactive with CII are not tolerized, and as soon as the T cells are activated, even in a partially tolerized state, they may help B cells to produce autoreactive and pathogenic antibodies.

Induction of Arthritis With Other Cartilage and Joint-Related Proteins

CXI-Induced Arthritis

CXI is structurally similar to CII and is, to a large extent, co-localized. CXI is a heterotrimer with three different α chains where one is shared with CII (the a3 chain). Both heterologous and homologous CXI induce arthritis in rat strains.[31] Interestingly the induction with homologous CXI gives a chronic relapsing disease, which is distinctly different from the heterologous CXI-induced disease and CII-induced CIA.

Cartilage Oligomeric Matrix Protein-Induced Arthritis

Another cartilage protein is cartilage oligomeric matrix protein (COMP). Homologous COMP induces arthritis in both rats and mice.[32,59]

Proteoglycan (Aggrecan)-Induced Arthritis

Other major components of joint cartilage are proteoglycans, of which the largest is aggrecan. Immunization of Balb/c mice with fetal human aggrecan induces chronic arthritis.[30] Both B and T cells are involved in the pathogenesis. Autoreactive T cells have been isolated and respond to the G1-domain of aggrecan, in which neoepitopes are created.[60] T cell receptor transgenic mice spontaneously develop arthritis at old age. The disease has been genetically mapped and shares many gene regions in common with CIA.

TABLE 32.3 Some Environmental Effects on Arthritis Models

Environmental Effect	Effect on Arthritis	Reference
Cage Grouping	+	67
Noise Stress	++	87
Predator Stress	–	88
Pregnancy	–	89
Postpartum	+	90
Estrogen	–	91
Darkness	+	92
Infections	–/+	18, 28, 93, 94

–, Decreased arthritis; +, increased arthritis.

Antigen-Induced Arthritis

Antigen-induced arthritis is a classic model of RA that is induced by immunizing animals with a foreign antigen, usually bovine serum albumin, and subsequently injecting the same antigen into a joint. A pronounced T cell–dependent, immune complex-mediated, and destructive arthritis develops in the injected joint as a result. The model is very well controlled and has been used to understand the effector phase of joint inflammation and cartilage destruction.[61]

Glucose-6-Phosphate Isomerase–Induced Arthritis

The successful induction of arthritis after immunization with recombinant glucose-6-phosphate isomerase (GPI) in adjuvant[62] stems from the identification of the K/BxN model in which transgenic T cells specific for GPI leads to spontaneous arthritis in nonobese diabetic (NOD) mice.[63] GPI-induced arthritis is MHC dependent and associated with the $H2^q$ haplotype (as CIA), and GPI peptides with an Aq-binding capacity can induce arthritis.[64,65] GPI has a unique affinity for cartilage because it binds with high affinity to cartilage proteoglycans,[65] and spontaneous immune activation in the K/BxN mouse seems to primarily arise in lymph nodes draining joints.[66]

Spontaneous Arthritis

Many of the classic inbred mouse and rat strains tend to spontaneously develop arthritis, especially under certain environmental influences (Table 32.3). In some strains, such as DBA/1, the grouping of males easily induces intermale aggressiveness; such stress seems to be associated with the development of severe arthritis.[67] This stress-induced arthritis is very different from inflammatory arthritis models like CIA and has less inflammatory synovial infiltrate, but with enthesopathy and new cartilage and bone formation; in many ways, it is more similar to psoriasis arthritis than RA. There are also a number of genetic mutations that strongly enhance arthritis development. One such mutation occurs in the *Fas* gene, which is of critical importance for apoptosis. In the MRL mouse background, arthritis develops along with a severe lupus disease.[68] Other examples are the previously mentioned mutations in the *Ncf1*[46] or *ZAP70*[25] genes.

Spontaneous Arthritis in Genetically Modified Strains

Importantly, models that develop spontaneous arthritis can be created by genetically modifying mouse strains. The prime example of this is the demonstration that overexpression of TNF leads to severe arthritis.[69] This model has been extremely useful in delineating the role of TNF in mediating arthritis. Other genetic mutations leading to overexpression of TNF also lead to the spontaneous development of severe arthritis, such as deletion of an upstream regulatory element controlling TNF secretion in fibroblast[70] or the deletion of DNasII,[71] which leads to aberrant secretion of TNF by chronically stimulated macrophages. Mice overproducing TNF can develop arthritis despite a functional immune system and are thus operating entirely through innate inflammatory mechanisms. Another important lesson from the TNF-overproducing mice is that it primarily leads to the development of arthritis, although in some situations colitis and encephalomyelitis may also develop.

Subsequently, several other genetically modified mouse strains developing arthritis have been reported. A mouse deficient for the IL-1 receptor antagonist[72] developed arthritis that not only affected the downstream effector functions but was also dependent on T cell activation.

A mutation in the gp130 IL-6 receptor was observed to lead to arthritis in elderly mice.[73] Interestingly the mutation led to an accumulation of polyclonal autoreactive CD4$^+$ T cells that secreted inflammatory cytokines, indicating a regulatory role of the IL-6 receptor of the adaptive immune system.

Another type of spontaneous arthritis was observed in a T cell receptor transgenic mouse in which the TCR recognized a peptide derived from the ubiquitously occurring protein glucose-6-phosphate isomerase (G6PI) bound to the class II MHC protein Ag7 in the K/BxN mouse.[74] Nevertheless, as discussed in a preceding section, the arthritis requires SFB bacteria in the intestinal flora, which indicates that this disease is not strictly spontaneous but rather induced by a bacterial adjuvant stimulation. The pathogenic effector pathway in this model is dependent on antibodies reactive with G6PI. This serum-induced arthritis (SIA) can be transferred with sera from K/BxN mice and the antibodies bind to precipitated GPI on the cartilage surface, mimicking the pathogenesis of anti-CII antibodies in the CAIA model. The use of the G6PI antibody-induced arthritis has been instrumental in finding early inflammatory steps in the joint attack, which involves complement activation through the alternative pathway, and neutrophil infiltration. The joints are specifically targeted in the disease and it remains to be determined how T cells and antibodies recognize this systemically expressed autoantigen in a joint-specific context.

Another type of model is induction arthritis after transplantation of human synovial fibroblasts into severe combined immunodeficiency (SCID) mice.[75,76] The same type of arthritis develops after transfer of murine fibroblast cell lines.[77] This model is likely to reflect inherent properties of fibroblast-mediated mechanisms, showing different features as compared with other arthritis models such as CIA and PIA.

These models most likely represent various aspects of the processes leading to arthritis, which will be determined by the transgene or defective gene, or due to transplantation of specific cells.

Use of Animal Models

Increasing the Knowledge of Disease Pathways

An ideal model for human RA should mimic the complexity of the human disease in being polygenic and dependent on environmental factors. The animal models have the advantage that both genetics and environment can be better controlled. There are many forms of arthritis, and the different clinical varieties are likely to continue to be subdivided just as has happened with ACPA$^+$ RA and seronegative RA, whereas the animal models from the beginning represent very divergent pathways and diseases that lead to arthritis.

Ideally, animal models should mimic the various subtypes of RA. With increasing knowledge of RA, such as the identification of ACPA as a predictive biomarker, and the identification of new genes associated with RA, there will be new demands on the animal models. Thus there is not yet an animal model that reflects the production of ACPA[78] nor has a properly humanized mouse strain been developed that pathophysiologically mimics the genetic polymorphism identified in humans. To introduce new genes (e.g., human class II MHC) or environmental factors (e.g., smoking), a proper and well-controlled genetic and environmental context is critical. For example, the introduction of the human class II MHC as transgenes in the mouse has led to a number of artifacts, some of them related to the nonphysiologic interactions between human and mouse genes. Nevertheless, as long as the mouse models have been studied with a well-controlled genetic and environmental context, they have and will contribute detailed information on the molecular pathogenesis that leads to arthritis. For this work, the possibilities to genetically modify both mice and rats is a powerful tool, and the possibility to make controlled experiments is a critical advantage.

Developing New Therapeutic Strategies

To test new drugs and therapies, it will be necessary to select from the different models available. Obviously, there is no optimal model for RA and there will never be one. The models described, however, are useful because they represent different aspects of RA pathogenesis. Thus, depending on the questions to be asked or symptoms to be treated, different models may be used. The most common model used today for testing new therapeutic approaches is the CIA model, which should be included as a reference model. The usefulness of this model has been confirmed with the anti-TNF treatment, which was subsequently introduced in RA.

Recapitulating the three stages through which RA develops—priming, onset, and chronicity—reasonable criteria are that the animal models should be useful for studies of specific pathways of importance in these stages. A common mistake is to only use acute models and to only use disease prevention and not established chronic disease as a readout. It is also of critical importance to be aware of the specific environmental influences on arthritis development in rodent. Of particular importance are stress effects, which are easily produced by mixing mice from different litters in the same cage which will lead to cage-dependent effects. Other important factors are sex hormones and, most likely, neurohormones, which play an important role modulating disease activity—seen as effects by estrous cycling, pregnancy, and light effects. Not only do environmental effects need to be controlled but genetic effects do, too. The control of genetics is usually achieved by testing standardized inbred strains. The problem is that these vary considerably between different colonies, mainly because of genetic contamination. In spite of these problems, there is no question that both environment and genetics can be better controlled in experimental animal models than in studies directly involving the human population.

Ethical Considerations

One important drawback of using experimental models for RA is the suffering of animals. Nevertheless, in the light of various human activities that use animals, the use of them in research seems to be the easiest to defend. In fact, it would be unethical not to use them for research because it would prohibit further understanding of human diseases, thereby letting humans suffer from something that may be possible to cure or prevent. It should also be emphasized that the recent development of animal models for RA has refined them to be of more specific use, which has decreased animal suffering. For example, the historically most commonly used model for RA, the mycobacterium-induced AA, is a systemic and severe inflammatory disease, whereas PIA and CIA are more specific diseases of the joints.

Conclusion

Experimental animal models are essential tools not only for investigating the basic mechanisms leading to RA but also for the development of new therapies. Many models have been described, and each represents different aspects of the disease; it is therefore important to use different models. It has been emphasized that the models used should reflect essential clinical hallmarks of RA, and they should reflect the fact that RA is a polygenic disease triggered by unknown and multifactorial environmental factors.

The references for this chapter can also be found on ExpertConsult.com.

References

1. Aho K, Palosuo T, Raunio V, et al.: When does rheumatoid disease start? *Arthritis Rheum* 28:485–489, 1985.
2. Klareskog L, Lundberg K, Malmstrom V: Autoimmunity in rheumatoid arthritis: citrulline immunity and beyond, *Adv Immunol* 118:129–158, 2013.
3. Cole BC, Knudtson KL, Oliphant A, et al.: The sequence of the Mycoplasma arthritidis superantigen, MAM: identification of functional domains and comparison with microbial superantigens and plant lectin mitogens, *J Exp Med* 183(3):1105–1110, 1996.
4. Iliopoulou BP, Guerau-de-Arellano M, Huber BT: HLA-DR alleles determine responsiveness to Borrelia burgdorferi antigens in a mouse model of self-perpetuating arthritis, *Arthritis Rheum* 60(12):3831–3840, 2009.
5. Bremell T, Lange S, Yacoub A, et al.: Experimental *Staphylococcus aureus* arthritis in mice, *Infect Immun* 59:2615–2623, 1991.
6. Hammer RE, Maika SD, Richardson JA, et al.: Spontaneous inflammatory disease in transgenic rats expressing HLA-B27 and human beta2m: An animal model of HLA-B27-associated human disorders, *Cell* 63:1099–1112, 1990.
7. Taurog JD, Richardson JA, Croft JT, et al.: The germfree state prevents development of gut and joint inflammatory disease in HLA-B27 transgenic rats, *J Exp Med* 180(6):2359–2364, 1994.
8. Pearson CM, Wood FD: Studies of polyarthritis and other lesions induced in rats by injection of mycobacterial adjuvant. I. General clinical and pathologic characteristics and some modifying factors, *Arthritis Rheum* 2:440–459, 1959.
9. Koga T, Kakimoto K, Hirofuji T, et al.: Acute joint inflammation in mice after systemic injection of the cell wall, its peptidoglycan, and chemically defined peptidoglycan subunits from various bacteria, *Infection Immun* 50:27–34, 1985.
10. Lundberg K, Kinloch A, Fisher BA, et al.: Antibodies to citrullinated alpha-enolase peptide 1 are specific for rheumatoid arthritis and cross-react with bacterial enolase, *Arthritis Rheum* 58(10):3009–3019, 2008.
11. Holmdahl R, Lorentzen JC, Lu S, et al.: Arthritis induced in rats with non-immunogenic adjuvants as models for rheumatoid arthritis, *Immunol Rev* 184:184–202, 2001.
12. Holmdahl R, Goldschmidt TJ, Kleinau S, et al.: Arthritis induced in rats with adjuvant oil is a genetically restricted, alpha beta T-cell dependent autoimmune disease, *Immunology* 76(2):197–202, 1992.
13. Vingsbo C, Sahlstrand P, Brun JG, et al.: Pristane-induced arthritis in rats: a new model for rheumatoid arthritis with a chronic disease course influenced by both major histocompatibility complex and non-major histocompatibility complex genes, *Am J Pathol* 149:1675–1683, 1996.
14. Carlson BC, Jansson AM, Larsson A, et al.: The endogenous adjuvant squalene can induce a chronic T-cell-mediated arthritis in rats, *Am J Pathol* 156(6):2057–2065, 2000.
15. Hultqvist M, Olofsson P, Gelderman KA, et al.: A new arthritis therapy with oxidative burst inducers, *PLoS Med* 3(9):e348, 2006.
16. Tuncel J, Haag S, Carlsen S, et al.: Class II major histocompatibility complex-associated response to type XI collagen regulates the development of chronic arthritis in rats, *Arthritis Rheum* 64(8):2537–2547, 2012.
17. Holmberg J, Tuncel J, Yamada H, et al.: Pristane, a non-antigenic adjuvant, induces MHC class II-restricted, arthritogenic T cells in the rat, *J Immunol* 176(2):1172–1179, 2006.
18. Björk J, Kleinau S, Midtvedt T, et al.: Role of the bowel flora for development of immunity to hsp 65 and arthritis in three experimental models, *Scand J Immunol* 40:648–652, 1994.
19. Vingsbo-Lundberg C, Nordquist N, Olofsson P, et al.: Genetic control of arthritis onset, severity and chronicity in a model for rheumatoid arthritis in rats, *Nat Genet* 20(4):401–404, 1998.
20. Olofsson P, Holmberg J, Tordsson J, et al.: Positional identification of Ncf1 as a gene that regulates arthritis severity in rats, *Nat Genet* 33(1):25–32, 2003.
21. Yau AC, Holmdahl R: Rheumatoid arthritis: identifying and characterising polymorphisms using rat models, *Dis Model Mech* 9(10):1111–1123, 2016.
22. Wooley PH, Seibold JR, Whalen JD, et al.: Pristane-induced arthritis. The immunologic and genetic features of an experimental murine model of autoimmune disease, *Arthritis Rheum* 32:1022–1030, 1989.
23. Satoh M, Reeves WH: Induction of lupus-associated autoantibodies in BALB/c mice by intraperitoneal injection of pristane, *J Exp Med* 180(6):2341–2346, 1994.
24. Deng GM, Nilsson IM, Verdrengh M, et al.: Intra-articularly localized bacterial DNA containing CpG motifs induces arthritis, *Nat Med* 5(6):702–705, 1999.
25. Sakaguchi N, Takahashi T, Hata H, et al.: Altered thymic T-cell selection due to a mutation of the ZAP-70 gene causes autoimmune arthritis in mice, *Nature* 426(6965):454–460, 2003.
26. Hirota K, Hashimoto M, Ito Y, et al.: Autoimmune th17 cells induced synovial stromal and innate lymphoid cell secretion of the cytokine GM-CSF to initiate and augment autoimmune arthritis, *Immunity* 48(6):1220–1232 e5, 2018.
27. Khmaladze I, Kelkka T, Guerard S, et al.: Mannan induces ROS-regulated, IL-17A-dependent psoriasis arthritis-like disease in mice, *Proc Natl Acad Sci U S A* 111(35):E3669–E3678, 2014.
28. Wu HJ, Ivanov II , Darce J, et al.: Gut-residing segmented filamentous bacteria drive autoimmune arthritis via T helper 17 cells, *Immunity* 32(6):815–827, 2010.

29. Abdollahi-Roodsaz S, Koenders MI, Walgreen B, et al.: Toll-like receptor 2 controls acute immune complex-driven arthritis in mice by regulating the inhibitory Fcgamma receptor IIB, *Arthritis Rheum* 65(10):2583–2593, 2013.
30. Zhang Y, Guerassimov A, Leroux JY, et al.: Arthritis induced by proteoglycan aggrecan G1 domain in BALB/c mice. Evidence for T cell involvement and the immunosuppressive influence of keratan sulfate on recognition of T and B cell epitopes, *J Clin Invest* 101(8):1678–1686, 1998.
31. Cremer MA, Ye XJ, Terato K, et al.: Type XI collagen-induced arthritis in the Lewis rat. Characterization of cellular and humoral immune responses to native types XI, V, and II collagen and constituent alpha-chains, *J Immunol* 153(2):824–832, 1994.
32. Carlsen S, Nandakumar KS, Backlund J, et al.: Cartilage oligomeric matrix protein induction of chronic arthritis in mice, *Arthritis Rheum* 58(7):2000–2011, 2008.
33. Trentham DE, Townes AS, Kang AH: Autoimmunity to type II collagen: an experimental model of arthritis, *J Exp Med* 146:857–868, 1977.
34. Courtenay JS, Dallman MJ, Dayan AD, et al.: Immunization against heterologous type II collagen induces arthritis in mice, *Nature* 283:666–667, 1980.
35. Yoo TJ, Kim SY, Stuart JM, et al.: Induction of arthritis in monkeys by immunization with type II collagen, *J Exp Med* 168:777–782, 1988.
36. Stuart JM, Dixon FJ: Serum transfer of collagen induced arthritis in mice, *J Exp Med* 158:378–392, 1983.
37. Holmdahl R, Rubin K, Klareskog L, et al.: Characterization of the antibody response in mice with type II collagen-induced arthritis, using monoclonal anti-type II collagen antibodies, *Arthritis Rheum* 29:400–410, 1986.
38. Nandakumar KS, Svensson L, Holmdahl R: Collagen type II-specific monoclonal antibody-induced arthritis in mice: description of the disease and the influence of age, sex, and genes, *Am J Pathol* 163(5):1827–1837, 2003.
39. Nandakumar KS, Bajtner E, Hill L, et al.: Arthritogenic antibodies specific for a major type II collagen triple-helical epitope bind and destabilize cartilage independent of inflammation, *Arthritis Rheum* 58(1):184–196, 2008.
40. Bas DB, Su J, Sandor K, et al.: Collagen antibody-induced arthritis evokes persistent pain with spinal glial involvement and transient prostaglandin dependency, *Arthritis Rheum* 64(12):3886–3896, 2012.
41. Rowley MJ, Nandakumar KS, Holmdahl R: The role of collagen antibodies in mediating arthritis, *Mod Rheumatol* 18(5):429–441, 2008.
42. Haag S, Schneider N, Mason DE, et al.: Identification of new citrulline-specific autoantibodies, which bind to human arthritic cartilage, by mass spectrometric analysis of citrullinated type II collagen, *Arthritis Rheumatol* 66(6):1440–1449, 2014.
43. Uysal H, Bockermann R, Nandakumar KS, et al.: Structure and pathogenicity of antibodies specific for citrullinated collagen type II in experimental arthritis, *J Exp Med* 206(2):449–462, 2009.
44. Ge C, Xu B, Liang B, et al.: Structural basis of cross-reactivity of anti-citrullinated protein antibodies, *Arthritis Rheumatol*, 2018.
45. Ahlqvist E, Ekman D, Lindvall T, et al.: High-resolution mapping of a complex disease, a model for rheumatoid arthritis, using heterogeneous stock mice, *Hum Mol Genet* 20(15):3031–3041, 2011.
46. Hultqvist M, Olofsson P, Holmberg J, et al.: Enhanced autoimmunity, arthritis, and encephalomyelitis in mice with a reduced oxidative burst due to a mutation in the Ncf1 gene, *Proc Natl Acad Sci U S A* 101(34):12646–12651, 2004.
47. Olsson LM, Nerstedt A, Lindqvist AK, et al.: Copy number variation of the gene NCF1 is associated with rheumatoid arthritis, *Antioxid Redox Signal*, 2011.
48. Zhao J, Ma J, Deng Y, et al.: A missense variant in NCF1 is associated with susceptibility to multiple autoimmune diseases, *Nat Genet* 49(3):433–437, 2017.
49. Olsson LM, Johansson AC, Gullstrand B, et al.: A single nucleotide polymorphism in the NCF1 gene leading to reduced oxidative burst is associated with systemic lupus erythematosus, *Ann Rheum Dis* 76(9):1607–1613, 2017.
50. Kleinau S, Martinsson P, Heyman B: Induction and suppression of collagen-induced arthritis is dependent on distinct fcgamma receptors, *J Exp Med* 191(9):1611–1616, 2000.
51. Banda NK, Takahashi K, Wood AK, et al.: Pathogenic complement activation in collagen antibody-induced arthritis in mice requires amplification by the alternative pathway, *J Immunol* 179(6):4101–4109, 2007.
52. Wooley PH, Luthra HS, Stuart JM, et al.: Type II collagen induced arthritis in mice. I. Major histocompatibility complex (I-region) linkage and antibody correlates, *J Exp Med* 154:688–700, 1981.
53. Brunsberg U, Gustafsson K, Jansson L, et al.: Expression of a transgenic class II Ab gene confers susceptibility to collagen-induced arthritis, *Eur J Immunol* 24(7):1698–1702, 1994.
54. Michaëlsson E, Andersson M, Engström A, et al.: Identification of an immunodominant type-II collagen peptide recognized by T cells in H-2q mice: self tolerance at the level of determinant selection, *Eur J Immunol* 22(7):1819–1825, 1992.
55. Bäcklund J, Carlsen S, Höger T, et al.: Predominant selection of T cells specific for glycosylated collagen type II peptide (263-270) in humanized transgenic mice and in rheumatoid arthritis, *Proc Natl Acad Sci U S A* 99(15):9960–9965, 2002.
56. Raposo B, Merky P, Lundqvist C, et al.: T cells specific for post-translational modifications escape intrathymic tolerance induction, *Nat Commun* 9(1):353, 2018.
57. Bäcklund J, Li C, Jansson E, et al.: C57BL/6 mice need MHC class II Aq to develop collagen-induced arthritis dependent on autoreactive T cells, *Ann Rheum Dis* 72(7):1225–1232, 2013.
58. Malmström V, Michaëlsson E, Burkhardt H, et al.: Systemic versus cartilage-specific expression of a type II collagen-specific T-cell epitope determines the level of tolerance and susceptibility to arthritis, *Proc Natl Acad Sci U S A* 93(9):4480–4485, 1996.
59. Carlsén S, Hansson AS, Olsson H, et al.: Cartilage oligomeric matrix protein (COMP)-induced arthritis in rats, *Clin Exp Immunol* 114(3):477–484, 1998.
60. Boldizsar F, Kis-Toth K, Tarjanyi O, et al.: Impaired activation-induced cell death promotes spontaneous arthritis in antigen (cartilage proteoglycan)-specific T cell receptor-transgenic mice, *Arthritis Rheum* 62(10):2984–2994, 2010.
61. van Lent PL, Hofkens W, Blom AB, et al.: Scavenger receptor class A type I/II determines matrix metalloproteinase-mediated cartilage destruction and chondrocyte death in antigen-induced arthritis, *Arthritis Rheum* 60(10):2954–2965, 2009.
62. Schubert D, Maier B, Morawietz L, et al.: Immunization with glucose-6-phosphate isomerase induces T cell-dependent peripheral polyarthritis in genetically unaltered mice, *J Immunol* 172(7):4503–4509, 2004.
63. Matsumoto I, Staub A, Benoist C, et al.: Arthritis provoked by linked T and B cell recognition of a glycolytic enzyme, *Science* 286(5445):1732–1735, 1999.
64. Iwanami K, Matsumoto I, Tanaka Y, et al.: Arthritogenic T cell epitope in glucose-6-phosphate isomerase-induced arthritis, *Arthritis Res Ther* 10(6):R130, 2008.
65. Studelska DR, Mandik-Nayak L, Zhou X, et al.: High affinity glycosaminoglycan and autoantigen interaction explains joint specificity in a mouse model of rheumatoid arthritis, *J Biol Chem* 284(4):2354–2362, 2009.
66. Mandik-Nayak L, Wipke BT, Shih FF, et al.: Despite ubiquitous autoantigen expression, arthritogenic autoantibody response initiates in the local lymph node, *Proc Natl Acad Sci U S A* 99(22):14368–14373, 2002.
67. Holmdahl R, Jansson L, Andersson M, et al.: Genetic, hormonal and behavioural influence on spontaneously developing arthritis in normal mice, *Clin Exp Immunol* 88(3):467–472, 1992.

68. Hang L, Theofilopoulos AN, Dixon FJ: A spontaneous rheumatoid arthritis-like disease in MRL/l mice, *J Exp Med* 155:1690–1701, 1982.
69. Keffer J, Probert L, Cazlaris H, et al.: Transgenic mice expressing human tumour necrosis factor: a predicitive genetic model of arthritis, *EMBO J* 10:4025–4031, 1991.
70. Kontoyiannis D, Pasparakis M, Pizarro TT, et al.: Impaired on/off regulation of TNF biosynthesis in mice lacking TNF AU-rich elements: implications for joint and gut-associated immunopathologies, *Immunity* 10(3):387–398, 1999.
71. Kawane K, Ohtani M, Miwa K, et al.: Chronic polyarthritis caused by mammalian DNA that escapes from degradation in macrophages, *Nature* 443(7114):998–1002, 2006.
72. Horai R, Saijo S, Tanioka H, et al.: Development of chronic inflammatory arthropathy resembling rheumatoid arthritis in interleukin 1 receptor antagonist-deficient mice, *J Exp Med* 191(2):313–320, 2000.
73. Sawa S, Kamimura D, Jin GH, et al.: Autoimmune arthritis associated with mutated interleukin (IL)-6 receptor gp130 is driven by STAT3/IL-7-dependent homeostatic proliferation of CD4+ T cells, *J Exp Med* 203(6):1459–1470, 2006.
74. Kouskoff V, Korganow AS, Duchatelle V, et al.: Organ-specific disease provoked by systemic autoimmunity, *Cell* 87(5):811–822, 1996.
75. Geiler T, Kriegsmann J, Keyszer GM, et al.: A new model for rheumatoid arthritis generated by engraftment of rheumatoid synovial tissue and normal human cartilage into SCID mice, *Arthritis Rheum* 37(11):1664–1671, 1994.
76. Lefevre S, Knedla A, Tennie C, et al.: Synovial fibroblasts spread rheumatoid arthritis to unaffected joints, *Nat Med* 15(12):1414–1420, 2009.
77. Lange F, Bajtner E, Rintisch C, et al.: Methotrexate ameliorates T cell dependent autoimmune arthritis and encephalomyelitis but not antibody or fibroblast induced arthritis, *Ann Rheum Dis* 64(4):599–605, 2005.
78. Vossenaar ER, Nijenhuis S, Helsen MM, et al.: Citrullination of synovial proteins in murine models of rheumatoid arthritis, *Arthritis Rheum* 48(9):2489–2500, 2003.
79. Schaible UE, Kramer MD, Wallich R, et al.: Experimental Borrelia burgdorferi infection in inbred mouse strains: antibody response and association of H-2 genes with resistance and susceptibility to development of arthritis, *Eur J Immunol* 21(10):2397–2405, 1991.
80. Hill JL, Yu DT: Development of an experimental animal model for reactive arthritis induced by Yersinia enterocolitica infection, *Infect Immun* 55(3):721–726, 1987.
81. Dalldorf FG, Cromartie WJ, Anderle SK, et al.: The relation of experimental arthritis to the distribution of streptococcal cell wall fragments, *Am J Pathol* 100:383–402, 1980.
82. Vingsbo C, Jonsson R, Holmdahl R: Avridine-induced arthritis in rats; a T cell-dependent chronic disease influenced both by MHC genes and by non-MHC genes, *Clin Exp Immunol* 99(3):359–363, 1995.
83. Tuncel J, Haag S, Hoffmann MH, et al.: Animal Models of rheumatoid arthritis (i): pristane-induced arthritis in the rat, *PLoS One* 11(5):e0155936, 2016.
84. Hagert C, Sareila O, Kelkka T, et al.: chronic active arthritis driven by macrophages without involvement of t cells: a novel experimental model of rheumatoid arthritis, *Arthritis Rheumatol* 70(8):1343–1353, 2018.
85. Korganow AS, Ji H, Mangialaio S, et al.: From systemic T cell self-reactivity to organ-specific autoimmune disease via immunoglobulins, *Immunity* 10(4):451–461, 1999.
86. Corthay A, Hansson AS, Holmdahl R: T lymphocytes are not required for the spontaneous development of entheseal ossification leading to marginal ankylosis in the DBA/1 mouse, *Arthritis Rheum* 43(4):844–851, 2000.
87. Rogers MP, Trentham DE, Dynesius-Trentham R, et al.: Exacerbation of collagen arthritis by noise stress, *J Rheumatol* 10:651–654, 1983.
88. Rogers MP, Trentham DE, McCune WJ, et al.: Effect of psychological stress on the induction of arthritis in rats, *Arthritis Rheum* 23:1337–1341, 1980.
89. Waites GT, Whyte A: Effect of pregnancy on collagen-induced arthritis in mice, *Clin Exp Immunol* 67:467–476, 1987.
90. Mattsson R, Mattsson A, Holmdahl R, et al.: Maintained pregnancy levels of oestrogen afford complete protection from post-partum exacerbation of collagen-induced arthritis, *Clin Exp Immunol* 85(1):41–47, 1991.
91. Jansson L, Mattsson A, Mattsson R, et al.: Estrogen induced suppression of collagen arthritis. V: physiological level of estrogen in DBA/1 mice is therapeutic on established arthritis, suppresses anti-type II collagen T-cell dependent immunity and stimulates polyclonal B-cell activity, *J Autoimmunity* 3:257–270, 1990.
92. Hansson I, Holmdahl R, Mattsson R: Constant darkness enhances autoimmunity to type II collagen and exaggerates development of collagen-induced arthritis in DBA/1 mice, *J Neuroimmunol* 27(1):79–84, 1990.
93. Wing K, Klocke K, Samuelsson A, et al.: Germ-free mice deficient of reactive oxygen species have increased arthritis susceptibility, *Eur J Immunol* 45(5):1348–1353, 2015.
94. Kohashi O, Kohashi Y, Takahashi T, et al.: Suppressive effect of Escherichia Coli on adjuvant-induced arthritis in germ-free rats, *Arthritis Rheum* 29(4):547–553, 1986.

33 Neuronal Regulation of Pain and Inflammation

CAMILLA I. SVENSSON AND LINDA S. SORKIN

KEY POINTS

Pain signaling is amplified by inflammation.

Peripheral sensory neurons have efferent functions that contribute to inflammation, including axon and dorsal root reflexes.

Neurogenic inflammation results in flare, edema, and increased pain.

Subclinical inflammation and other non-inflammatory mechanisms can induce and sustain pain prior to, and subsequent to, clinical inflammation.

The sympathetic nervous system modulates many immune cell functions and peripheral somatic nerve terminals via adrenergic receptors.

Vagal nerve stimulation attenuates disease activity in many models of inflammatory arthritis.

Neural control of inflammation involves multiple feedback loops involving somatic, sympathetic, and parasympathetic nervous systems and the hypothalamic-pituitary-adrenal axis.

Introduction

Historically, pain was viewed as a symptom of inflammation and not as an actively contributing factor to the inflammatory process. Nonetheless, in the early 1900s, researchers noted that stimulation of dorsal roots and dorsal root ganglia (DRG) neurons resulted in peripheral vasodilation,[1] suggesting that sensory neurons not only conduct information to the spinal cord but also have an efferent function. Thus, the foundation was laid for future investigators to show that the four cardinal signs of inflammation—erythema, warmth, swelling, and hypersensitivity—all can result from neural activation, today referred to as *neurogenic inflammation*. Hence, nervous system activation by inflammatory mediators leads to increased excitability of peripheral nociceptive sensory fibers, causing inflammatory pain. Conversely, the nervous system feeds back on the peripheral inflammatory process. This effect is achieved by output systems at multiple levels, including primary afferent fibers (axonal reflex), spinal cord (dorsal root reflexes), and the brain (neuroendocrine functions and autonomic activation). Thus, a bidirectional relationship exists between the inflammatory process and sensory neuron activation.

A 1903 report concluded that the sympathetic nerve influenced the course of inflammation by nervous functions other than vasoconstriction and vasodilatation.[2] Since then, several interactions between the sympathetic nervous system and the immune system have been identified. Multiple neuromediators, including norepinephrine, neuropeptide Y (NPY), and adenosine triphosphate (ATP) are released from sympathetic terminals; however, the majority of research has focused on norepinephrine. Most immune cells express functional adrenergic and NPY receptors, which translate neuronal signals into immune cell signals.[3] A role for the parasympathetic nervous system, in particular the vagus nerve, in immune regulation has also been demonstrated,[4] although the efferent linkage is a matter of heated debate.[3,5,6]

Primary Afferent Fibers

Nociceptors—that is, peripheral receptors that signal pain—are classically thought to transmit information regarding real or impending tissue damage from external sources. Nociceptors are typically divided into groups based on the type of stimulus that activate them. Accordingly, thermal nociceptors respond to heat or cold and chemical nociceptors to exogenous agents, such as chemical irritants, or endogenous ligands, such as ATP or protons. Mechanical nociceptors respond to noxious pressure and tissue distortion. Nociceptors that respond to multiple modalities (e.g., both mechanical and thermal stimuli) are classified as polymodal nociceptors. Evidence is accumulating that, in addition to sensing changes in the interface with the outside environment, many nociceptive fibers signal variations in acidity, temperature, carbon dioxide, and the metabolic state of the internal environment from a predetermined set point. Thus nociceptors can also be thought of as homeostatic sensors and are elements of a feedback loop.[7,8] During chronic inflammation and pathologic pain states, these feedback mechanisms frequently go awry and become players in the pathology.

Nociceptors are called *free nerve endings* because they are not encapsulated or associated with traditional receptor structures, although they are frequently in close contact with small distal blood vessels, lymphatic vessels, and tissue-resident immune cells.[9] Nociceptors detect noxious stimuli and transduce them into action potentials (APs) that move toward the central nervous system (CNS). In addition, some receptors are found along the length of the axon and, when activated by specific agonists, also generate APs and cause the release of other neurotransmitters.[10,11] Nociceptors are primarily associated with two major axonal types: Aδ fiber (finely myelinated) and C fiber (unmyelinated) axons. A different nomenclature is sometimes employed for afferent fibers from joint and muscle; type III is roughly equivalent to Aδ fibers and type IV is similar to C fibers. All primary afferents are glutamatergic and many contain one or more peptide neurotransmitters, including substance P (SP), calcitonin gene–related peptide (CGRP), somatostatin, and galanin. Over the last decades, scientists have characterized and sorted sensory neurons into different categories based on (1) marker expression, such as tropomyosin receptor kinase A (TrkA)-positive versus TrkA-negative isolectin B4 (IB4)-positive nerve fibers,[12] (2) functionality (as described in the previous section), or (3) single cell transcriptome clustering.[13–15]

Skin

The skin is highly innervated with sensory nerve fibers, which can respond to pain, temperature, and touch. Finely myelinated Aδ and unmyelinated C fibers comprise the majority of the dermal and epidermal innervation and can be activated by noxious mechanical, thermal, or chemical stimulus. Many of these fibers are polymodal nociceptors and can respond to all three stimuli.[16–19] Sympathetic efferent fibers are also present, although they represent a minority of the cutaneous nerve fibers. These autonomic nerve fibers are confined to the dermis, where they innervate blood vessels, lymphatic vessels, hair follicles, and apocrine and eccrine glands.[19,20]

Joint Afferents

Although most joint structures are innervated, importantly, they do not have equivalent innervation density. Nociceptors innervate the synovium, fibrous capsules, ligaments, infrapatellar fat pad, and bone, but are not found in adult cartilage and innervate only the outer third of the menisci. Only 20% of fibers in articular nerves are myelinated, with the preponderance being nociceptive finely myelinated Aδ (group III) fibers. Unmyelinated fibers are distributed between sympathetic efferent (discussed in a later section) and C (group IV) nociceptors, with the latter comprising almost half of the total population.[21,22] Nociceptors in the joint can be activated by noxious levels of pressure and joint hyperrotation. During inflammation and after tissue damage, these fibers may become sensitized due to the presence of inflammatory mediators such as cytokines and prostaglandin E2, whereupon they fire APs in response to previously subthreshold stimuli.[23,24] Sensitization results in movements within the normal range being perceived as painful. Certain C fibers do not respond to any mechanical stimuli unless they have first been subjected to an inflammatory environment; these fibers are referred to as *silent nociceptors* (see later discussion). Sympathetic fibers regulate blood flow and articular vessel permeability in the joint.[25]

Bone

Bone is innervated by Aδ, C, and sympathetic efferent fibers, but not by Aβ fibers.[26,27] These fibers are distributed in the periosteum, mineralized bone, and bone marrow.[28–32] In contrast to skin, which has a lower percentage of TrkA-expressing sensory fibers, the TrkA receptor is expressed by the majority of myelinated and unmyelinated sensory nerve fibers that innervate the periosteum, bone marrow, and mineralized bone.[33,34] Most nerve fibers in the bone are associated with blood vessels.[32,35] In the periosteum, nerve fibers are arranged into a fishnet-like network, possibly to detect mechanical injury and protect the underlying structure.[36] Thus Aδ and C fibers innervate different layers of the bone and likely contribute to pain. Sympathetic fibers have been implicated in the regulation of bone destruction and formation[37,38] and may contribute to pain via alteration of bone metabolism.[39]

Fascia

Fascia is innervated by Aδ and C fibers. Although innervation is readily detectable in the outer layers next to the skin, the middle layer containing the thick collagen fiber bundles does not appear to be innervated by nociceptors and the reported innervation of the inner layer overlying the muscle differs among different reports.[40–44] In fascia, the Aδ fibers are exclusively mechanoreceptors, whereas the C fibers include a large percentage of polymodal nociceptors. In experiments on human volunteers, noxious stimulation of the lumbar fascia evokes pain.[45] There is a higher density of nociceptors in the fascia than are found in the underlying muscle. Consequently, injections of pain-producing agents into the fascia are more painful than the same injections into skin or muscle.[43] Complete Freund's adjuvant (CFA)–induced inflammation causes an increase in the density of CGRP- and SP-positive fibers in the inner and outer layer of the thoracolumbar fascia.[46] Thus fascia may be a source of pain in fasciitis and nonspecific low back pain.

Muscle and Tendon

Skeletal muscle and tendons are innervated by Aδ and C fibers. The nerve fiber density in the connective tissue around tendons, at least of the rat calcaneal tendon, is several times higher than in the gastrocnemius soleus muscle.[47] In contrast, collagen fiber bundles of the tendon are almost devoid of free nerve endings. The high fiber density in the peritendineum may explain the prevalence of tenderness or pain in the tissue around the tendon and the insertion site.[48]

Sensitization

Sensitization is defined as a reduced threshold to activation and increased responsiveness, and it occurs at all levels of the neuraxis. It can occur instantaneously or have longer latency and duration. Short-term sensitization can result from receptor phosphorylation or dephosphorylation or trafficking of receptors and channels into or out of the plasma membrane. Longer-lasting sensitization can occur after increased synthesis of receptors and ion channels.[49]

Factors such as pro-inflammatory eicosanoids, cytokines, growth factors,[50–53] glutamate,[54,55] and protons (acidity)[56] that are released during inflammation and tissue damage can sensitize sensory neurons. Thus inflammation can lead to an increased and prolonged activation of peripherally located neurons in response to both noxious and innocuous stimuli, a process known as *peripheral sensitization*.

Under normal circumstances, the free nerve endings of nociceptors have high thresholds to mechanical and thermal stimuli.[57] Hyperalgesic priming is another form of sensitization. An initial injury elicits nociceptor sensitization and hyperalgesia and then resolves. However, if priming has occurred a second injury will cause a prolonged sensitization and nociception in response to what originally were subthreshold stimuli.[58,59]

Finally, there is a population of C fibers present in the joint, colon, bladder, and skin that is normally unresponsive to mechanical stimulation.[60–65] These nociceptors are known as *mechanically insensitive afferents* or silent nociceptors and are thought not to be involved in mechanical pain signaling in healthy individuals. During inflammation and after tissue damage, however, the silent nociceptors can be "un-silenced" and start to respond to innocuous stimuli like light touch and normal joint movement, as well as noxious stimuli. Although the molecular mechanism that mediates the un-silencing of silent nociceptors is still under investigation, endogenous inflammatory mediators such as nerve growth factor (NGF) appear to drive this process.[66,67] Peripheral sensitization increases the magnitude and duration of signal transmission to the CNS, which often leads to central sensitization. If this occurs the pain sensation may be magnified and prolonged.

Release of inflammatory mediators within the CNS contributes to central sensitization, pathological pain, and illness behavior.[68] Sensitization of the spinal cord occurs via a number of processes, including increased hyperexcitability of spinal cord neurons through N-methyl-D aspartate (NMDA) receptor activation,[69] reduced activation of inhibitory interneurons,[70] expansion of the neuronal receptive fields,[71] and glial cell activation in the spinal cord, which can lead to an increased production and release of inflammatory and growth-associated mediators such as TNF, IL-1β, IL-18, prostaglandins, and brain-derived growth factor (BDNF). These factors can contribute to the fine tuning of both excitatory and inhibitory synaptic integration, which ultimately enhances pain signal transmission to the brain.[52,72] Chronic afferent activity from the spinal cord can subsequently lead to a reorganization of the cortex and increased amygdala activation, facilitated by a decreased inhibitory control through the pain-related deactivation medial prefrontal cortex.[73–75]

Pain Prior to Clinical Inflammation

Arthralgia (joint pain without clinical evidence of inflammation) is often experienced before the onset of joint pathology in conditions such as rheumatoid arthritis (RA) and can develop without signs of synovitis.[76–78] Although the symptoms in the pre-arthritis phase of arthralgia can be considerable and lead to functional limitations,[79] the origin of symptoms in this phase is insufficiently known. The “pre-RA” patients with arthralgia can be positive for anti-citrullinated protein antibodies (ACPA) or rheumatoid factor (RF),[80] but may also remain seronegative for these autoantibodies. In ACPA-positive pre-RA individuals, bone marrow edema correlates with joint tenderness, and subclinical synovitis correlates with tenderness in ACPA-negative pre-RA individuals,[81] suggesting different pathways for pain in these two subcategories of patients. Interestingly, transfer of ACPA purified from RA patient blood and synovial fluid to mice induces long-lasting pain-like behavior without generating visual or histologic signs of inflammation,[82] and injection of anti–type II collagen antibodies or immunization against collagen type II generates pain-like behavior in mice prior to signs of joint inflammation. Furthermore, pre-clinical studies show that the immune complex can exert direct actions on nociceptors via neuronally expressed Fcγ receptors prior to establishment of joint inflammation.[83–85] Thus accumulating data suggests that subclinical inflammation and/or associated processes in the joint leads to the release of factors that sensitize joint nociceptors.

Persistent Pain Despite Suppression of Inflammation

While there is a close and bidirectional relationship between inflammation and pain, there is evidence that other processes also contribute to pain chronicity in conditions like RA. Although initiation, change, or increase in disease-modifying anti-rheumatic drug (DMARD) therapy can lead to reductions in pain that are both statistically and clinically significant, pain still remains troublesome for a substantial percentage of patients, despite the lack of residual inflammation, assessed as no swollen joints and normal erythrocyte sedimentation rate (ESR) levels.[86,87] Thus pain may not solely be sustained by inflammatory processes even when the condition is considered mainly of inflammatory character. In osteoarthritis (OA) and RA, regions distal or remote from the affected joints can also display increased pain sensitivity,[88–90] indicating pain augmentation by the CNS and/or a blunting of normal anti-nociceptive modulation. A systematic review concluded that central sensitization is present in people with RA.[91] Pathology of the peripheral or central nervous systems can directly cause neuropathic pain in the absence of nociceptive input and peripheral tissue damage. Recent studies using the painDETECT questionnaire show that a subpopulation of RA patients may have a neuropathic component[92–94] and direct measurements revealed that 33% of people with RA who reported neuropathic symptoms displayed clinical evidence of neuropathology.[95] Pre-clinical models of arthritis also suggest that pain-like behavior outlasts joint inflammation[96,97] and that certain types of joint inflammation and joint pathologies may drive specific changes in the sensory nervous system that are also initiated by nerve injury.[61,98,99]

Efferent Functions of Primary Afferent Fibers

Neurogenic Inflammation

In the absence of actual tissue injury, activation of peripheral nerves or their terminals results in peripheral release of the same neurotransmitters as are released from their central (spinal) terminals. Action potentials in nociceptors going toward the spinal cord (orthodromic) elicit pain sensations. APs traveling away from the spinal cord (antidromic) lead to a peripheral release of neurotransmitters throughout all branches of that fiber, a process called the “axon reflex” (Fig. 33.1). Peripheral release of the neuropeptides SP and CGRP induces increased blood flow and vascular permeability, respectively, and gives rise to neurogenic inflammation.[100–103] This “injury free” inflammation manifests as low levels of redness (flare) from increased blood flow and vasodilation, edema secondary to increased plasma extravasation, and nociception/pain after activation of additional nociceptive terminals.

Peptidergic C fibers and sympathetic efferents in synovium have trophic effects on mast cell density, providing one specific avenue by which the CNS could influence neurogenic inflammation and other inflammatory states. Interestingly, primary afferent peptides activate resident keratinocytes and induce upregulation of pro-inflammatory cytokines and nerve growth factor.[104] This may play a role in some chronic inflammatory diseases such as psoriasis.

Capsaicin activates the vanilloid receptor subtype 1 (TRPV1), expressed on peptide containing C fibers; this elicits a sensation of burning pain and causes neurogenic inflammation. Cutting the dorsal root eliminates sensory traffic between the spinal cord and periphery while maintaining the integrity of the sympathetic nervous system and the peripheral terminal (Fig. 33.2). Significantly, cutting the lumbar sensory roots reduces intradermal capsaicin-induced increases in blood flow and edema, indicating that there is an active spinal cord contribution to neurogenic inflammation. Similar prevention of capsaicin-induced increases of blood flow and paw edema are

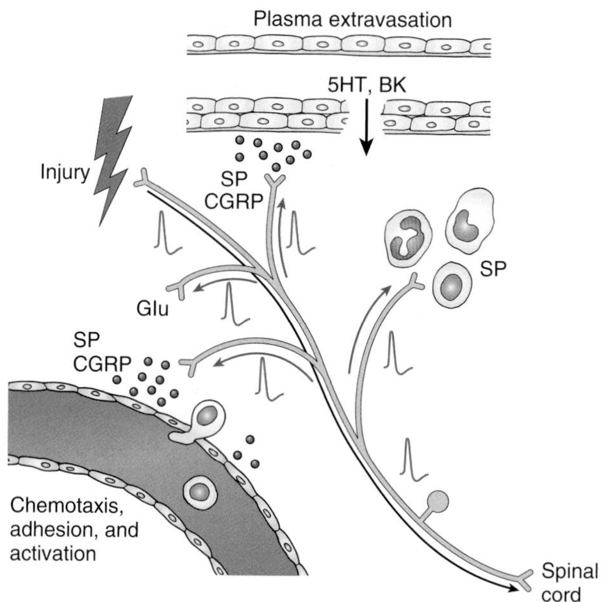

• **Fig. 33.1** The axon reflex is initiated by nociceptor activation in peripheral tissue by injury and inflammation. When noxious stimuli activate primary afferent fibers, action potentials (APs) are conveyed toward the spinal cord *(black arrows)*. When terminal branches or axon collaterals merge, APs travel down every branch, including anterogradely *(red arrows)*. Thus antidromic axon reflexes are generated and induce peripheral release of glutamate and neuropeptides. Neurotransmitter release signals to vascular endothelial cells to increase blood flow and induces plasma extravasation (leakage of vascular proteins, 5-hydroxytryptamine [5HT] and bradykinin [BK], and edema), which degranulates mast cells and activates other nerve fibers. Although the axon reflex by itself is not sufficient to recruit immune cells, in a primed system it facilitates recruitment of inflammatory leukocytes. Taken together, these actions produce the flare around an injury site. *CGRP,* Calcitonin gene–related peptide; *Glu,* glutamate; *SP,* substance P.

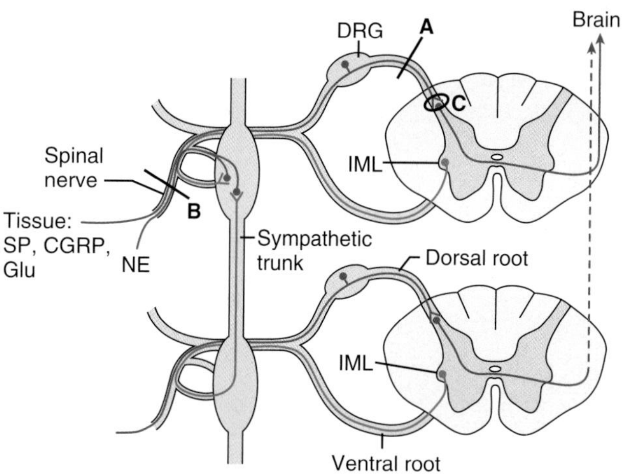

• **Fig. 33.2** Wiring diagrams of lesions used to assess pathways of neural control of inflammation. Cross-sections of two sequential segments of thoracic spinal cord are illustrated. At each level, a sensory neuron *(purple)*, sympathetic preganglionic neuron (*blue*, located in the intermediolateral cell column [IML]) and a sympathetic postganglionic fiber *(red,* only shown in one segment) are illustrated. Preganglionic fibers synapse in sympathetic ganglia at their entry level and also send collaterals to other sympathetic ganglia along the chain. Dorsal rhizotomy (lesion A) severs only the sensory afferent fibers. Spinal nerve transection (lesion B) severs the sensory fibers and the efferent sympathetic postganglionic axons, including those innervating the vasculature. Intrathecal capsaicin destroys (bilaterally) the central terminals of the peptidergic C fiber (lesion C); importantly, the cell bodies in the dorsal root ganglia (DRG) and peripheral terminals are left intact. If capsaicin is given neonatally, all of the peptidergic fibers are lost. *CGRP,* Calcitonin gene–related peptide; *Glu,* glutamate; *n.,* nerve; *NE,* norepinephrine; *SP,* substance P.

observed after chemically-induced loss of peptidergic C fibers, depletion of their neurotransmitters, and administration of SP-receptor antagonists, manipulations which reduce sensory trafficking from the periphery to the spinal cord.[100,105–108]

Neurogenic Anti-inflammation

Efferent activity in the peripheral nerve also has anti-inflammatory influences. Under conditions of bacterial infection, CFA-induced inflammation, and in the serum transfer-induced arthritis (passive K/BxN mouse model), nociceptors release neuropeptides (somatostatin, galanin, and CGRP) that modulate draining lymph nodes and can reduce pro-inflammatory cytokine release by infiltrating macrophages. Somotostatin and galanin also directly inhibit peripheral release of sensory neuropeptides from peptidergic terminals and thus inhibit plasma extravasation.[109,110] Not surprisingly, animals with a genetic alteration that reduces nociceptor activity or animals with a loss of peptidergic C fibers have reduced pain behavior. Unexpectedly, under the inflammatory conditions (e.g., bacterial infection) previously noted, these animals display increased edema and immune cell infiltration.[111–113] This change in sign may be due to decreased release of anti-inflammatory neuropeptides from the deleted or altered nociceptors. Certainly, an anti-inflammatory role for somatostatin is a reasonable supposition as treatment with a long-lasting somatostatin analogue elicits improvement in patients with refractory RA.[114] Interestingly, patients with greatly elevated plasma somatostatin levels demonstrate a rapidly developing RA upon resolution of the endocrine abnormality.[115] In keeping with a prominent role for efferently released somatostatin, topical therapy with a capsaicin cream in patients with degenerative spine diseases elicits a prominent increase in plasma somatostatin, along with pain relief.[116] Factors controlling the final pro- and anti-inflammatory balance of neurogenically released primary afferent neurotransmitters remain undefined.

Dorsal Root Reflex

The dorsal root reflex (DRR) is a strictly somatic positive feedback mechanism that engages neurogenic inflammation after intense peripheral activation of nociceptive afferent fibers (Fig. 33.3). Orthodromic APs in Aδ and C fibers activate ascending spinal nociceptive pathways and γ-aminobutyric acid (GABA)–containing inhibitory neurons within the spinal cord via glutamatergic linkages. The inhibitory (GABA) neurons have collaterals synapsing on $GABA_A$ receptors on the central terminals of the Aδ and C fibers.[117–120] Low-frequency firing in this system elicits pre-synaptic inhibition of the afferent fibers via primary afferent depolarization (PAD) and decreases spinal neurotransmitter release, resulting in an inhibited signal.[121] In marked contrast, substantial tissue inflammation or injury leads to excessive firing of the primary afferent fibers and greatly enhances spinal release of GABA.[122,123] This results in enough PAD to trigger APs in the afferent fibers that travel anterograde from the spinal cord to the injured tissue. Neurogenic inflammation, triggered

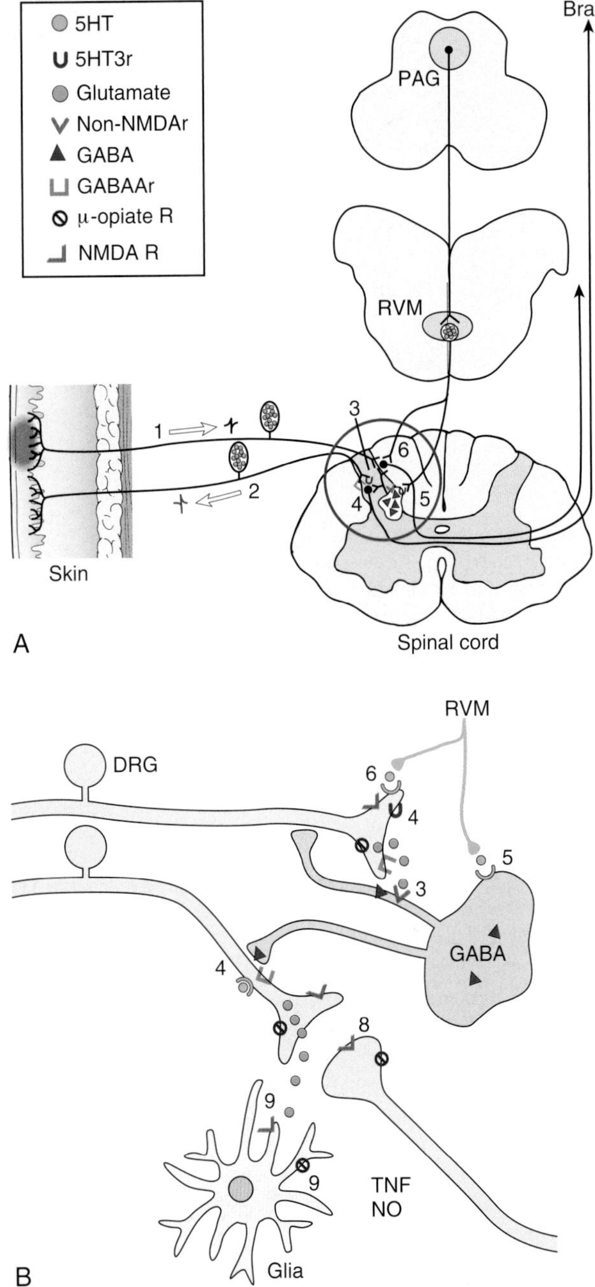

• **Fig. 33.3** (A) The dorsal root reflex (DRR). (B) Enlargement of inset in (A). A DRR is induced when *(1)* action potentials (APs) reach the spinal cord and then *(2)* anterograde propagation back to the tissue occurs. It is dependent on the central terminals of the afferent fibers being stimulated at an intensity that causes primary afferent depolarization (PAD) at a level that exceeds action potential (AP) threshold. As pictured, the afferent action potential activates *(3)* a non–N-methyl-D-aspartate (NMDA) linkage on a γ-aminobutyric acid (GABA) ergic neuron. *(4)* Excess GABA acts on a $GABA_A$ receptor on the central terminal to elicit PAD. Antagonism of GABA and/or non-NMDA receptors blocks DRR. *(5)* The system may also be triggered via 5-hydroxytryptamine (5HT) release from the raphe-spinal system acting on 5HT-3 receptors on the inhibitory interneuron or *(6)* on the terminal endings. Activation of spinal opiate receptors and NMDA receptor antagonism is also effective in some longer-lasting models. These agents may work by *(7)* blocking pre-synaptic release of neurotransmitters, either by direct inhibition or removal of glutamatergic positive feedback. Alternatively, they can *(8)* act postsynaptically on pain transmission neurons or *(9)* by blocking glial activation and the resultant central release of pro-inflammatory agents such as nitric oxide (NO) and tumor necrosis factor (TNF). *DRG,* Dorsal root ganglia; *PAG,* periaqueductal gray; *RVM,* rostral ventromedial medulla.

by peripheral release of neurotransmitters, including glutamate, SP, and CGRP, then occurs.

Significantly, DRRs have been recorded in nerves contralateral to the initiating tissue insult.[124–126] This occurrence is consistent with the concept that inflammation in one limb results in inflammation in the mirror-image contralateral limb.[126–128] This appears to be a neuronal polysynaptic pathway.[128] Importantly, experimental monoarthritis can produce a cellular infiltrate and increased temperature that is specific to the mirror-image contralateral joint.[129] These studies postulate a role for sympathetic efferent fibers on the noninjured side.

Pain Transmission in the Dorsal Horn

The nociceptive sensory primary afferent fibers traverse from the peripheral tissue to the spinal dorsal horn, regardless of their innervated structure. Not surprisingly, spinal nociceptive projection neurons reflect the termination pattern of the primary afferents. Aδ and C fibers project to the superficial dorsal horn (Laminae I-II),[130–133] the area with the largest concentration of nociceptive-specific neurons. These neurons are subdivided into those having predominant input from Aδ or C fibers and convey information regarding sharp or burning pain, respectively.[134] The neurons in the lateral deep dorsal horn (Lamina V) receive nociceptive input from cutaneous and articular Aδ nociceptive afferents[130] and also have low-threshold Aβ input.

Projection neurons receiving information concerning pain and inflammation convey this information to a wide variety of supraspinal structures. These neurons contribute to sensory discriminative, homeostatic, and affective components of pain, as well as to the autonomic responses to nociceptive stimuli. The classic spinothalamic tract (STT) projects to the contralateral ventral posterior thalamus (VPL) and on to somatosensory cortex. This pathway plays a prominent role in the discrimination of nociceptive stimuli.[135] A second STT tract (arising exclusively from lamina I neurons) projects to contralateral thalamus and then to the anterior cingulate, which contributes to the affective but not the sensory component of pain. A third STT pathway to the medial thalamus also receives an exclusive lamina I projection and projects to the contralateral posterior insula, as well as to cortical area 3a. This area is thought to be the cortical processing area for homeostatic input, describing the extra-cellular milieu of the chemodetecting nociceptive C fibers and inflammatory pain, respectively. Both play as yet undefined roles in sensory discrimination and affect.

The spinomesencephalic and spinoreticular tracts project throughout the brain stem reticular formation and midbrain. Importantly the spinoreticular pathway has bilateral projections. The parabrachial region in the midbrain has numerous two-way interconnections with autonomic control centers throughout the brain stem[136] and projects to limbic structures, including the amygdala. There is also a lamina I dorsal horn projection to medullary noradrenergic nuclei that integrates autonomic input and projects back down to the preganglionic neurons of the intermediate horn, and thus participates in important sympathetic spino-bulbo-spinal feedback loops. The vagal nucleus solitarius is also a termination site for lamina I neurons, thus involving the parasympathetic nervous system (Fig. 33.4A).

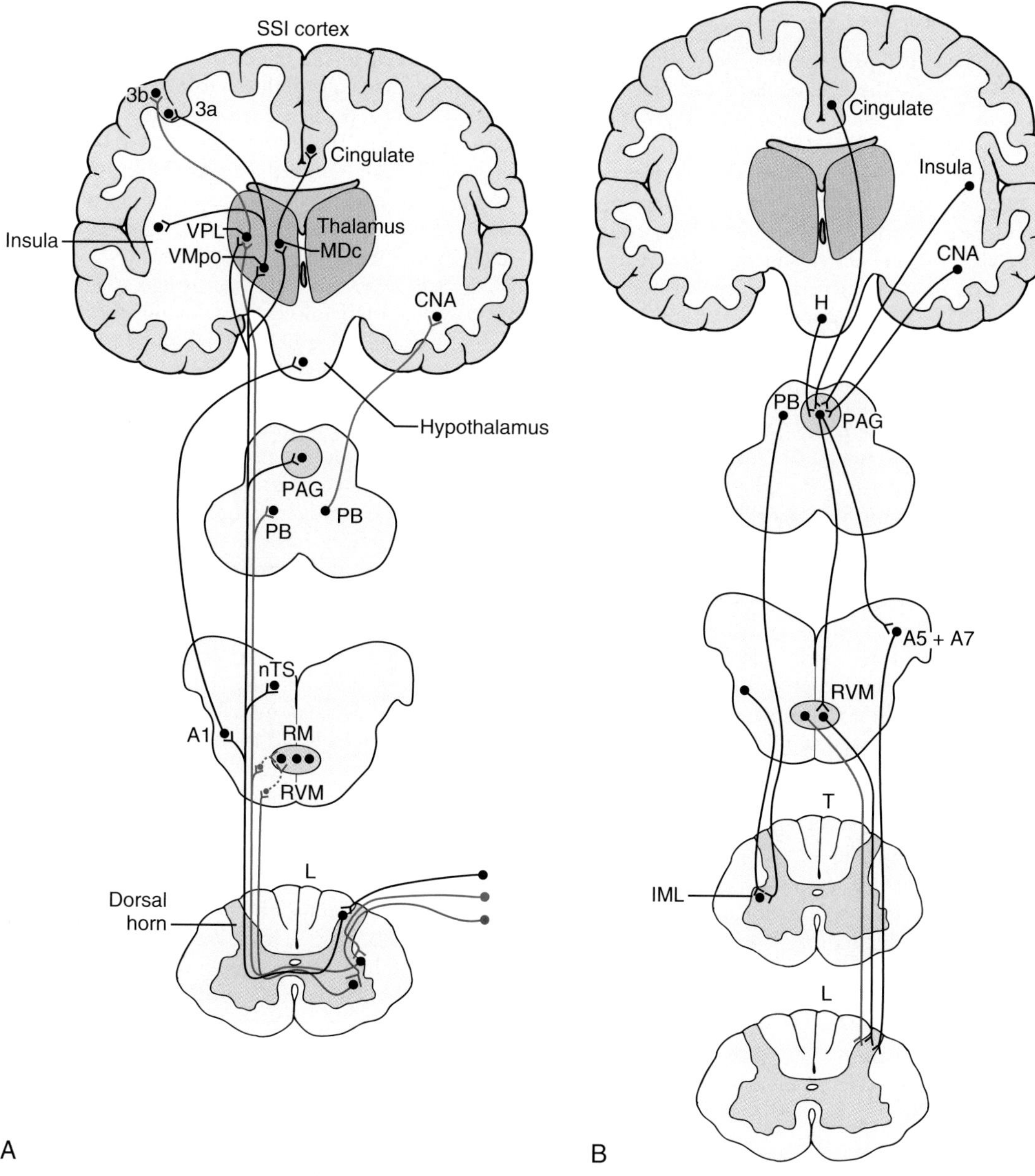

• **Fig. 33.4** (A) Ascending pain pathways. Nociceptive afferent fibers enter the spinal cord through the dorsal root and activate neurons in laminae I *(black),* V *(blue)* and VII-VIII *(red)*. Lamina I neurons have strong monosynaptic C fiber input (slow, burning pain) and project directly to the vagal nuclei (nTS), periaqueductal gray (PAG), parabrachial nucleus (PB) and thalamic nuclei, mediodorsal thalamic nucleus (MDc), and posterior ventral medial nucleus (VMpo), with a weaker projection to the ventral posterior thalamus (VPL). Importantly, the spinovagal connection is triggered by visceral but not cutaneous nociceptive stimulation. Lateral PAG projects onto the amygdala (CNA), whereas the VMpo projects further to the insula cortex and area 3a in the deep primary somatosensory cortex (SSI). Thus area 3a has predominantly C fiber input, perhaps accounting for its association with burning pain and inflammation. The MDc projects onto the cingulate gyrus (area 24c). There is also a lamina I projection to several of the catecholamine cell groups in the ventrolateral medulla, including the nucleus of solitary tract (nTS), and A1, a relay to the hypothalamus, which participates in nociceptive stimulation-induced release of adrenocorticotrophic hormone (ACTH). Lamina V-VIII neurons also project to the brain stem reticular formation and PAG and onto the VPL thalamus. Whereas all of the other spinal projections are primarily contralateral, the spinoreticular tract is bilateral (not illustrated). *Dotted lines* indicate indirect connections. (B) Descending modulatory pathways. Several cortical areas project to the ventrolateral PAG, including the insula, cingulate, frontal lobe, and amygdala. There is also a prominent connection from the hypothalamus. PAG, in turn, projects to several of the noradrenergic brain stem nuclei (including A5 and A7) and to nuclei of the rostral ventromedial medulla (RVM). Importantly, these RVM neurons contain substance P and other neurotransmitters, as well as serotonin, and wield bidirectional (excitatory and inhibitory) control over ascending pain impulses. Descending control over preganglionic neurons in the intermediolateral cell column (IML) come from the lateral PB and ventrolateral medulla. *CNA,* Central nucleus of the amygdala; *H,* hypothalamus; *L,* lumbar; *T,* thoracic.

Descending Modulation

Early literature suggested that pain-selective descending modulation was all inhibitory.[137] The backbone of the best-studied descending system includes a linkage from ascending projection neurons to the periaqueductal gray (PAG). An indirect descending linkage from PAG to the spinal cord by way of the raphe nuclei, or via the brain stem noradrenergic nuclei (Fig. 33.4B), completes the negative feedback loop. Parts of this loop have been examined after joint inflammation where activity in the afferent primary afferents and the descending leg increase in parallel, resulting in inhibition of the nociceptive projection neurons and amelioration of the ascending nociceptive activity.[138] The PAG processes indirect input from ascending pain pathways, the limbic system, and cortical pain-processing centers. Stimulation of ventrolateral PAG is strongly analgesic.[139] The raphe nuclei have a prominent serotonergic projection to the superficial dorsal horn. Serotonin (5-hydroxytryptamine [5HT]) released in the spinal cord can be anti-nociceptive (1) if it acts on 5HT-1 or 5HT-2 receptors on pain projection neurons, or (2) if low levels of 5HT bind to the excitatory 5HT-3 receptor found on GABAergic inhibitory interneurons in the superficial dorsal horn.

Nevertheless, under other conditions, ascending activity in the projection neurons results in a positive feedback loop, which enhances nociception.[140] Serotonin acting on 5HT-3 receptors is proalgesic because (1) in the presence of inflammation, additional high-level 5HT-3 receptor activation of the inhibitory neuron acts just like excessive GABA and results in DRR generation, enhanced inflammation, and pain[126] and (2) some nociceptive projection neurons also have 5HT-3 receptors.[141] Enhanced pain associated with joint and tissue inflammation, but not with surgical incision, is subject to facilitatory influences from the raphe region.[142–144] The parallel PAG-spinal noradrenergic pathway has similar facilitatory and inhibitory feedback components. Inflammation in hairy, but not glabrous, skin is subject to an α2-adrenergic–mediated descending inhibition via this pathway.[145] Clinically, intrathecal administration of α2-adrenergic agonists produces analgesia. Much like the receptor dichotomy seen for the serotonergic system, however, α1-adrenergic antagonists produce pain facilitation.

Neuronal Regulation of Inflammation in Acute Inflammatory Models

Acute inflammation can be induced by injection of kaolin and carrageenan into the knee joint. In this model, DRRs were recorded from Aβ, Aδ, and C fibers (group II, III, and IV), indicating that they are generated in the large myelinated fibers as well as the finely myelinated and unmyelinated nociceptive afferents.[146] If acute inflammation has a DRR component, then spinal blockade of either the glutamate receptor (non-NMDA) on the spinal inhibitory interneuron or antagonism of the pre-synaptic $GABA_A$ receptor located on the central terminal of the nociceptive afferent fiber should reduce DRR reflexes and peripheral signs of inflammation.

Pre-treatment with either of these two classes of agents is effective not only in blocking the anterogradely transmitting DRRs[147] but also in reducing the edema and temperature increase in the inflamed joint or tissue and pain behavior.[148–150] NMDA or $GABA_B$ receptor antagonists are without effect in this simple acute model. These data are consistent with involvement of the DRR originating in the articular afferents, as previously outlined. These data argue against a requirement for spinal glia, whose activation is more closely linked to NMDA receptor–mediated spinal sensitization, playing a prominent role in this reflexive activity. Unexpectedly, spinal post-treatment with the non-NMDA and $GABA_A$ antagonists partially reversed already established knee joint swelling but did not reduce the elevated joint temperature,[151] indicating perhaps that different aspects of the inflammation are under separate controls and that, even in acute models, these paradigms change after initiation of inflammation.

Experiments were repeated using capsaicin injection into the skin rather than injection of kaolin and carrageenan into the joint. Intradermal capsaicin also induced anterograde DRRs in Aδ and C fibers but, unlike the joint afferents, not in the larger Aβ fibers.[152,153] Pre-treatment and post-treatment with spinal $GABA_A$ and non-NMDA glutamate receptor antagonists were effective in this model, but, in contrast to the previous paradigm, spinal NMDA receptor antagonists also blocked the enhanced DRRs, as well as reducing the surrounding flare and edema.[152]

The anatomical substrate of the DRR theory requires involvement of sensory fibers running through the dorsal root for both the afferent and efferent legs of the reflex in addition to spinal inhibitory interneurons. Theoretically, it does not require the autonomic nervous system, supraspinal centers, or the adrenohypothalamic axis. Neither DRRs nor edema in the acute inflammatory phase of the kaolin/carrageenan model are blocked by surgical sympathectomy or high spinal cord transection, but functional separation of primary afferents from the CNS by dorsal root section, lidocaine application to the peripheral nerve, or nerve crush prevent their development.[148,154] Nevertheless, reduction in peripheral inflammation due to the functional loss of primary afferent fibers does not indicate whether the nerve fibers are a necessary part of the afferent, the efferent, or both legs of the reflex. A corollary to the need for GABA release from the inhibitory interneuron for DRRs is that anything that hyperactivates the interneuron will increase neurogenic inflammation, and factors that inhibit the inhibitory interneuron decrease the peripheral effect. As previously stated, serotonin, acting on postsynaptic 5HT-3 receptors on the interneuron, facilitates GABA release.[155] Thus, although supraspinal circuitry is not necessary for DRR-induced neurogenic inflammation, activation of either the PAG or the raphe nuclei can enhance the phenomena.[126,156]

Results were somewhat different when zymosan was injected into the knee joints of mice. Peripheral inflammation and pain behavior in this model were enhanced by spinal $GABA_B$ receptor agonists, which, presumably acting on sympathetic preganglionic neurons via a p38 linkage, activated the sympathetic efferent fibers to elicit neutrophil infiltration of the joint, as well as to increase local levels of TNF and IL-1β but not IL-10.[157] Administration of spinal $GABA_B$ or p38 antagonists, sympathectomy, or peripheral adrenergic antagonism blocked the enhanced responses to spinal GABA.

Another model of acute knee inflammation, which is induced by injection of lipopolysaccharide (LPS) into a knee joint previously primed with carrageenan, generates a reactive monoarthritis with leukocyte infiltration into synovial fluid, synthesis of pro-inflammatory cytokines, and joint swelling as indices of inflammation. This model is fundamentally different from the previous kaolin/carrageenan one in that spinal administration of glial inhibitors prevented signs of inflammation.[158] This outcome is consistent with the observed dependence of joint damage and inflammation in this model on NMDA receptor activation.[159]

Pre-treatment with spinal TNF inhibitors or neutralizing antibody also reduced vascular leakage into the knee and infiltration of polymorphonuclear leukocytes into the synovial fluid.[158,160] A spinal PAD inhibitor, which acts by blocking DRRs, also successfully blocked signs of peripheral inflammation in this model.[158] Co-administration of PAD and glial inhibitors did not produce an additive effect, indicating, perhaps, that they are in series within a common pathway. Thus, in this third intermediate duration model, DRRs are linked to spinal modulation of peripheral inflammation in tandem with a requirement for glial activation. These results were unaffected by corticosteroid synthesis inhibitors indicating a lack of participation of the hypothalamic-pituitary-adrenal (HPA) axis.

Spinal administration of morphine also prevented knee swelling and preserved joint integrity in the monoarthritis model.[159] The spinal opiate could be acting via (1) pre-synaptic inhibition of the nociceptive afferent signal, reduction of afferent transmitter release, and blockade of GABAergic interneuron activation, GABA release, and the DRR (i.e., blocking the afferent leg of the reflex) or (2) by postsynaptic inhibition of glia or neurons along the nociceptive transmission pathway. As activated glia release TNF and nitric oxide (NO), which contribute to spinal sensitization, activation of ascending pathways, and potential involvement of sympathetic pathways, their inhibition would inhibit CNS outflow systems (Fig. 33.3).

In a fourth type of model, cutaneous acute inflammation was induced by intradermal or subcutaneous injection of paw carrageenan. Intrathecal pre-treatment with a nonsteroidal anti-inflammatory drug (NSAID), morphine, or agents that inhibit the NO/cyclic guanosine (cGMP) pathway all blocked edema without reducing neutrophil infiltration.[161,162] Mechanistically, these agents collectively reduce neurotransmitter release from the spinal end of excited nociceptors. In similar experiments, spinal pre-treatment with either 5HT-1 receptor agonists or 5HT-2 receptor antagonists reduced paw swelling.[162,163] This outcome would fit with a blockade of DRRs, but not of other elements, that elicit immune cell chemotaxis.

In marked contrast, spinal administration of adenosine A1-specific (A1) but not adenosine A2-specific (A2) agonists inhibited neutrophil accumulation due to intradermal carrageenan.[164,165] The adenosine effect was mimicked by a spinal NMDA antagonist and reversed by spinal NMDA agonists. This latter experiment demonstrated that the NMDA linkage is downstream of the adenosine effect.[166] Inhibition of cellular infiltrates highlight that the spinal A1 protective effect goes beyond merely blocking the DRRs through direct inhibition of the spinal terminals. Interestingly, paw carrageenan elicits a massive reduction in peripheral adenosine, which is time linked to neutrophil infiltration. Adenosine loss, as well as the increase in neutrophil accumulation, is blocked by spinal pre-treatment with an NMDA antagonist.

Peripheral adenosine acting on A2 receptors inhibits peripheral neutrophil infiltration,[167,168] and thus maintenance of peripheral adenosine is thought to be the basis of the antiallodynic activity of both the spinal adenosine A1 agonists and NMDA receptor antagonists.[164] Spinal adenosine A1–mediated modulation of inflammation is also dependent on an intact dorsal root (sensory fibers) but is not dependent on the sympathetic efferent fibers.[165] Unlike the other cutaneous models, intradermal carrageenan-induced inflammation was not affected by spinal inhibition of non-NMDA glutamatergic receptors or by functional elimination of capsaicin-sensitive C fibers.

The several different acute models mentioned above differ with regard to source (skin vs joint) and peripheral stimulus (pure nociceptive, e.g., capsaicin, vs an irritant or an inflammation-causing agent), as well as stimulus intensity and consistency of examined elements. Despite the complexity of comparing these diverse paradigms, some conclusions can be made. Pain behavior co-varied with signs of inflammation, edema, and macrophage infiltration. All models, except for the mouse knee zymosan and paw carrageenan studies where DRRs were not examined, were dependent on dorsal root reflexes. By definition, this requires intact afferent and efferent nociceptive sensory fibers and increased activation of inhibitory interneurons via $GABA_A$ or serotonergic receptors. Although all the models required spinal glutamate receptor activation, there were distinct differences among the models. The kaolin/carrageenan knee and paw capsaicin injections were both dependent on spinal non-NMDA receptor activation. Because the first glutamatergic synapse from the primary afferent is thought to be via non-NMDA receptors, this is consistent. Models that require NMDA receptor activation are more likely to engage glial activation and perhaps central sensitization. NMDA receptor dependence does not seem to correlate to the site of inflammation or the injected substance.

Neuronal Regulation of Inflammation in Chronic Models of Inflammation

Animal models with joint inflammation that lasts for weeks or more are used to study spinal cord control of peripheral inflammation in RA and include adjuvant-induced arthritis (AIA) in rats, antigen-induced arthritis (AA) in mice, and collagen-induced arthritis (CIA) in mice. As with the acute inflammatory models, section of major lumbar nerve trunks greatly diminished development of these symptoms in the denervated limb.[169,170]

Capsaicin administered in different conditions is a frequently used tool to examine the mechanism in these models. Upon first contact with locally injected capsaicin, afferent C fibers emit APs, which in turn evoke burning pain. Higher doses or repeated application of capsaicin desensitizes sensory neurons, and eventually nerve conduction through the treated segment is selectively blocked in capsaicin-sensitive (a subpopulation of peptidergic C) fibers. Intrathecal injection of high dose capsaicin leads to destruction of axon terminals in the primary afferent terminal regions of the spinal cord (see Fig. 33.2). Systemic capsaicin administration to neonatal rats destroys subpopulations of DRG cells, including both central and peripheral processes, reflected by loss of SP and CGRP immunoreactivity and sensory deficits. When intrathecal or systemic neonatal capsaicin pre-treatment was used to eliminate only the central peptidergic sensory fibers, or both their central and peripheral terminals, respectively, severity of the inflammation in the AIA model was consistently ameliorated, indicating that this subpopulation of sensory afferent fibers and some element that they activate in the spinal cord contributes to the inflammation.[128,171–173] Interestingly, capsaicin pre-treatment at doses sufficient to reduce sensory activity also reduced AIA-induced T cell infiltration into the synovium.[173]

The commonality among the three lesions is loss of the peptidergic afferent fiber connection and preservation of the sympathetic efferent fibers.[174] Additionally, motor function is preserved after rhizotomy and capsaicin (see Fig. 33.2). In a combined lesion study in which animals were pre-treated as neonates with systemic capsaicin to produce a bilateral loss of the peptidergic afferent fibers, in conjunction with a unilateral rhizotomy, joint injury was reduced on the capsaicin-only side, whereas the lesion-plus-capsaicin side displayed increased disease severity.[128] These results show that the effect of peripheral denervation on the severity of joint inflammation in the rat is not dependent only on loss of a particular subset of neurons but rather reflects changes in the activity of both afferent and efferent peripheral neurons. In addition to the complexity of the wiring, it is necessary to involve additional autonomic and endocrine feedback loops to explain the system.

In accordance with the effect of spinal A1 adenosine receptor agonists on dermal neutrophil infiltration in an acute inflammation model, continuous spinal administration of an adenosine A1 receptor agonist greatly ameliorated all of the clinical AIA symptoms. Spinal treatment was beneficial even if it was started as late as 8 days after immunization when animals first presented with clinical signs, but there was a much smaller, nonsignificant effect on paw swelling when the course of treatment began after clinical signs were well established (day 14).[175] Noxious stimulation of afferent fibers resulted in an increase in c-Fos expression in the nuclei of nociceptive neurons in the spinal dorsal horn, which is thought to reflect increased activity levels.[176]

Despite the more than 80% decrease in AIA-induced presentation of clinical symptoms observed with intrathecal adenosine A1 agonist treatment, simultaneous reduction of the AIA-induced c-Fos expression in the superficial dorsal horn was only 22%.[175] Reduction of c-Fos expression in deeper spinal laminae was not affected by the A1 agonist. Taken together, this implies that pain is only marginally reduced by the spinal adenosine agonist and illustrates the dichotomy between successful alleviation of clinical signs of arthritis and only modest reduction in pain. As in the acute intradermal carrageenan model, anti-inflammatory and anti-nociceptor results were observed with either intrathecal administration of a TNF-neutralizing antibody or a p38 mitogen activated protein kinase (MAPK) inhibitor.[177] In addition, these agents also suppressed synovial infiltration of immune cells and expression of the pro-inflammatory cytokines IL-1β, IL-6, and TNF and matrix metalloproteinase (MMP)-3.[159,177] Interestingly, spinal expression of TNF and interferon (IFN)-β and late stage pain behavior varies between male and female mice in the K/BxN serum transfer model of arthritis, as does the efficacy of various spinally administered therapeutics.[178]

Arthritis induces a relative increase in sympathetic tone compared to that of the parasympathetic nervous system; this change in autonomic output ratio is also prevented by blocking the effects of spinal TNF.[179] Continuous spinal administration of morphine or the NMDA antagonist ketamine throughout a 3-week course of AIA caused a major decrease in joint swelling and synovial infiltration of inflammatory cells.[159] This is likely the result of a loss of DRRs due to pre-synaptic actions on μ-opioid and NMDA receptors, respectively. Nevertheless, as both manipulations block the ascending pain signal, they could have also altered autonomic outflow. The opioid-associated reduction in swelling was maintained over the entire period, and tolerance did not develop.

Sympathetic Effects on Peripheral Inflammation Are Time Dependent

When activated, most sympathetic postganglionic neurons release norepinephrine, which activates adrenergic receptors expressed on the peripheral target tissue. There are two adrenergic receptor types (α and β) that have several receptor subtypes (α1, α2, α3, β1, and β2). Cells of the innate immune system appear to express α1, α2, and β2 receptors, whereas those of the adaptive immune system primarily express the β2 subtype.[3] Importantly, stimulation of individual receptor subtypes can elicit different functional effects. For example, macrophages can be activated via α2-receptor stimulation, whereas β2-receptor stimulation has a suppressive effect.[3] Thus, the role of the sympathetic nervous system in immune cell functioning is complex, and directed pharmacologic studies show mixed results in animal models of arthritis, both ameliorating and exacerbating disease severity. It has been suggested that during the early phase of inflammation, there is "a shift in the autonomic balance toward a sympathetically dominated state."[179] This relationship may be bidirectional as patients with chronic RA display an increased sympathetic tone,[180] whereas patients with chronic hypertension exhibit a higher inflammatory index.[181] Puzzlingly, some inflammatory states seem to evoke a systemic-wide sympathetic response, whereas in others the response is relatively local and confined to the area of the inciting inflammation.

A better explained discrepancy between models is due to a potential functional loss of sympathetic innervation of the inflamed tissue over time; this loss has been observed in patients with RA and in animal models of RA.[182–184] Indeed, an inverse relationship has been demonstrated between numbers of tyrosine hydroxylase (TH)–positive nerve fibers (a catecholaminergic marker of sympathetic neurons) and both the inflammation index and levels of released IL-6 in synovial tissue of patients with RA.[185] This reduction in adrenergic nerve endings is specific and may be due to increased secretion of mediators of sympathetic axon repulsion, such as semaphorin 3c, which does not affect peptidergic sensory nerve fibers.[186]

In marked contrast to the previous anatomical findings, 4 weeks after CFA injection into the tibial-tarsal joint of the male rat, there in a marked increase in both sympathetic and peptidergic innervation of the ankle synovium. This is accompanied by sympathetic fiber ingrowth into the upper dermal layer over the joint, an area normally devoid of sympathetic innervation.[187] Late post-treatment with guanethidine to block sympathetic outflow successfully blocked or attenuated pain behavior induced by cutaneous stimulation in this model. Similarly, CFA injection into the knee of female, aged mice induces both sensory and sympathetic sprouting along with pronounced pain behavior and robust $CD68^+$ macrophage infiltration into the joint.[188] Thus, although the clinical data appear to consistently support the loss of innervation,[25] especially sympathetic, in arthritic joints, the pre-clinical data allow for some differences that have yet to be established.

Agents released from the sympathetic terminals contribute to increases in joint and tissue swelling in the early phases of arthritis. Mechanisms can vary from increases in blood flow to redistribution, migration, and chemotaxis of leukocytes toward the site of inflammation and β2-mediated release of interleukins and other algesic agents from resident keratinocytes.[189] Sympathectomy prior to or at induction of AIA, CIA, and AA, with a loss of the sympathetic terminals in the inflamed joint, results in amelioration of bone damage and a delay in onset of the clinical symptoms.[128,190,191] In contrast, when the sympathetic nervous system is interrupted after the early phases of inflammation, it either does not alter joint swelling and histopathologic scores or exacerbates the disease. These studies suggest that the sympathetic nervous system has time-dependent, immunomodulating effects in arthritis models. Prior to the immunization phase or at the early stage of inflammation, it has pro-inflammatory effects, and after the onset, it may have anti-inflammatory effects.

The biphasic nature of the sympathetic system is most prominent in the pre-clinical polyarthritis models where swelling and inflammatory signs are present throughout the full duration of the experiment, usually about 2 months. In the acute monoarthritis model mentioned previously, joint swelling presents on day 1 and resolves in 7 to 10 days.[192] As in the polyarthritis model, chemical sympathectomy prior to symptom presentation in the monoarthritis model ameliorated the disease and post-treatment had no effect. Nevertheless, if a second flare is induced by a second injection of the antigen into the joint after the first flare has resolved, preinjection sympathectomy is once again effective. This outcome implies that in this model and, perhaps, in clinical RA, the sympathetic terminals return and become functional between flares.

Examination of adrenergic receptor subtypes in more detail suggests a prominent role for β2-adrenergic receptors in the sympathetic nervous system's time-dependent, immunomodulating effect. Rats with continuous administration of a catecholamine reuptake inhibitor or a β2-adrenergic receptor antagonist that began prior to disease induction showed a delayed presentation of clinical signs and less severe joint damage than did control subjects.[193] Smaller protective effects of these agents on joint injury were obtained when treatment was confined to the period either before or after presentation of clinical disease, indicating that reduction of endogenous catecholamines was beneficial throughout the entire 28-day time course.

Subsequent studies from other groups confirmed the role of early systemic β2-receptor activation as contributory to joint damage and report that administration of β2 agonists at or shortly after disease onset increased the severity of the disease. In vivo studies on the function of α-adrenergic receptor subtypes in experimental arthritis have shown that administration of a nonselective α1/2 antagonist before immunization had no effect, whereas administration at the time of immunization increased severity and at the time of disease onset reduced severity. Thus, taken together, the significance of different adrenergic receptor subtypes at different times is unclear, although it seems that both α- and β-adrenergic receptors contribute to inflammation.

Beyond these adrenergic-dependent mechanisms, there are adrenergic-independent components of the inflammation. Local production of inflammatory agents such as bradykinin act directly on sympathetic terminal varicosities to release prostaglandins and adenosine.[194] This process still occurs after surgical sympathectomy at the sympathetic trunk, which leaves the postganglionic fibers and terminals intact, but is deleted by chemical sympathectomies (see Fig. 33.2). Many of the complexities concerning sympathetic effects arise from the fact that both adenosine and norepinephrine have concentration-dependent preferences for different receptor subtypes. Different outcomes (pro-inflammatory or anti-inflammatory) result from the subtypes activated.

Vagal nerve and parietal cortex stimulation of awake rats can activate the locus coeruleus and PAG, areas that are known to modulate the autonomic nervous system and pain behavior. Recent work indicates that this stimulation can also reduce zymosan-induced neutrophil infiltration into the knee joint, edema, and local synovial levels of TNF, IL-1β, and IL-6. This amelioration was dependent on the physical integrity of the sympathetic nervous system and was prevented by peripheral administration of adrenergic antagonists.[195,196]

Parasympathetic Effects on Peripheral Inflammation

The vagus nerve (VN) plays a key role as a parasympathetic interface between the brain and body. Over the past two decades, there has been a dramatic advancement in our understanding of the neuroanatomical, cellular, and molecular mechanisms by which VN activity contributes to modulation of immune function and suppression of inflammation. The afferent vagal fibers originate from internal organs and project to the nucleus tractus solitarius (NTS) in the medulla of the brain stem, with the cell bodies of the vagal sensory neurons located in the nodose ganglia. The efferent fibers of the VN originate in the dorsal motor nucleus in the medulla and innervate the digestive tract. Part of the gut, including the rectum, are innervated through the sacral parasympathetic nucleus.[197] The afferent VN is sensitive to inflammatory mediators such as IL-1, prostaglandin E2 (PGE2), and pathogen-associated molecular pattern molecules (PAMPs) and thus transfer important information regarding the inflammatory status to supraspinal sites. Increased activity in afferent VN projections to NTS is conveyed to corticotropin-releasing factor (CRF)–containing neurons, with subsequent release of adrenocorticotropic hormone from the pituitary gland, which stimulates the adrenal glands to release glucocorticoids. Thus, afferent VN signaling leads to activation of the HPA and consequently decreased peripheral inflammation through the action of glucocorticoids (Fig. 33.5A).

In addition to activation of the HPA axis, VN signaling can reduce inflammation via a vagovagal reflex where activation of vagal afferents, in response to peripheral inflammation, activate vagal efferent fibers leading to suppression of the inflammatory process. This connection was first postulated by one group based on their finding that stimulation of vagal efferents (by electrical stimulation of the distal end of a cut VN) prevented LPS-induced septic shock.[198] Since then, it has been demonstrated that electrical and pharmacologic stimulation of the VN controls inflammation and improves survival in a number of different experimental models of infectious and inflammatory disorders.[199] This reflex is referred to as the *cholinergic anti-inflammatory pathway* because it culminates in the peripheral release of acetylcholine (ACh).

The anti-inflammatory action of released ACh involves its binding to nicotinic ACh receptor subunit 7 (α7nAChR) on macrophages, which reduces the release of cytokines such as TNF.[4,200,201] The exact anatomical interaction in the cholinergic anti-inflammatory pathway, however, is still a matter of debate. The VN does not directly interact with resident macrophages in the spleen or gut, and several possibilities have been proposed. In the gut, the vagal modulation of intestinal resident macrophages appears to occur indirectly through activation of enteric neurons located within the gut muscularis. The nerve endings of these cholinergic myenteric neurons receiving vagal input are located in close proximity to resident macrophage-like cells[202,203] (Fig. 33.5B).

A likely explanation defines vagal modulation of macrophages in the spleen as a multistep indirect process. First, activity in the efferent VN signals to the celiac-mesenteric ganglion where it activates the splenic sympathetic nerve. This leads to the release of norepinephrine from splenic nerve endings that terminate in close proximity to immune cells in the spleen. NE binds β2-adrenergic receptors on splenic T lymphocytes and stimulates

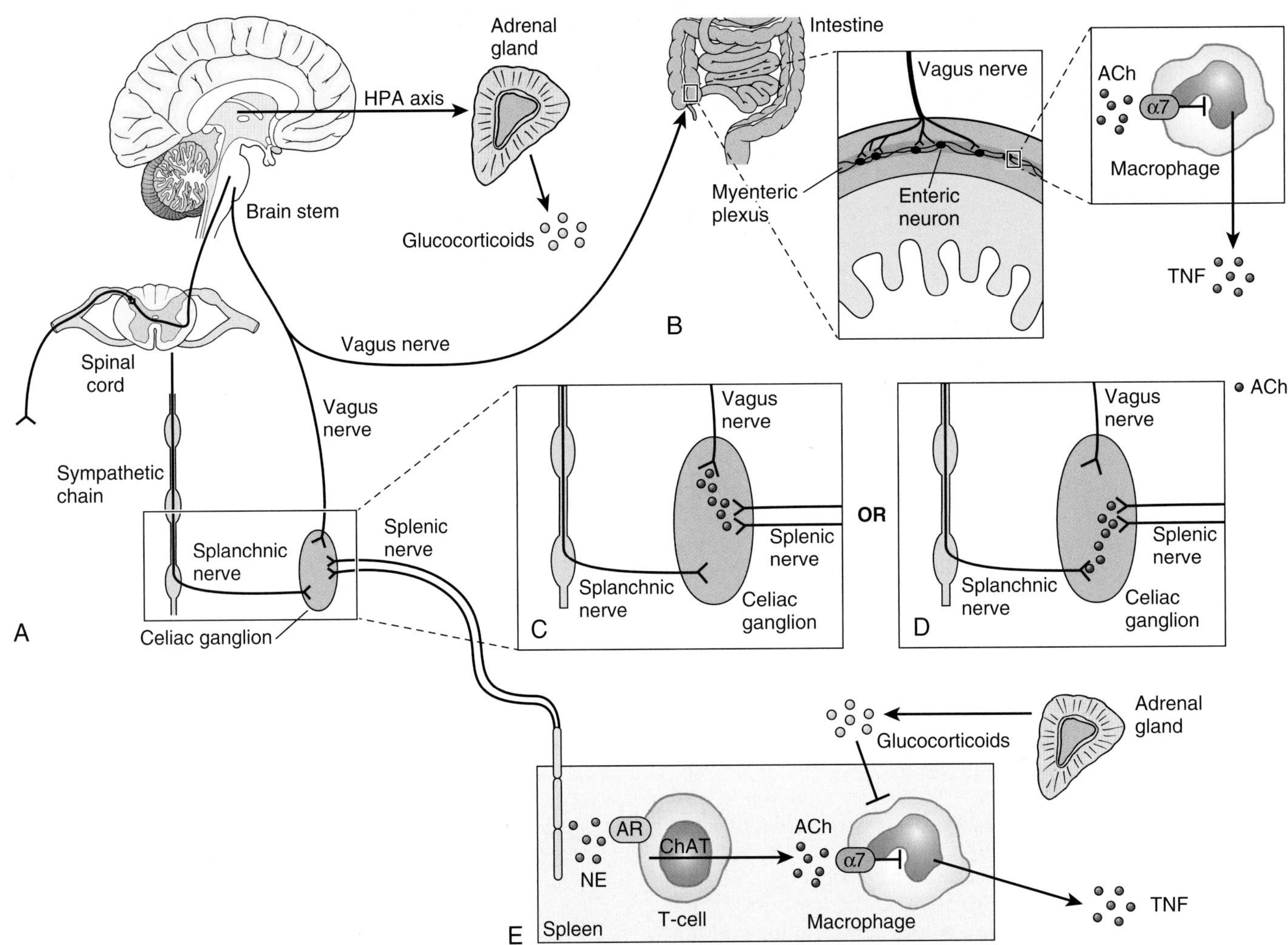

• **Fig. 33.5** The inflammatory reflex. (A) The HPA axis. After sensory input to the brain stem, signals are also relayed to the nuclei controlling the function of the hypothalamic-pituitary-adrenal (HPA) axis. This results in an increased release of glucocorticoids from the adrenal gland and subsequent suppression of cytokine release and inflammation, connecting the neuronal network to humoral anti-inflammatory mechanisms. (B) Vagal anti-inflammatory pathway to the gut. The efferent vagus nerve projects to cholinergic myenteric neurons in the enteric ganglia, which release ACh that stimulates α7nAChRs on resident macrophages in the muscle layers of the gut. (C) The cholinergic anti-inflammatory reflex. The illustrations depict the classic vagal theory of the inflammatory reflex, where stimulation of the efferent arm of the vagus nerve emerging from the dorsal motor nucleus signals to the celiac ganglion, where the splenic nerve is activated by acetylcholine (ACh) released from the vagus nerve. ACh activates nAChRa7 receptors in splenic neurons, which leads to release of norepinephrine (NE) from the splenic nerve into the spleen. NE activates β2-adrenergic receptors of choline acetyltransferase (ChAT)-expressing T cells. These T cells then produce and release ACh, which acts on α7nACh receptors (α7) on macrophages and other immune cells and suppresses release of cytokines like TNF. These cells are stimulated to produce and secrete ACh that activates nAChRa7 on macrophages, inhibiting TNF release. It is possible that NE acts on β-adrenergic receptors on macrophages and suppresses their production of TNF. (D) In another hypothesis, increased activity across synapses between splanchnic and splenic neurons in the celiac ganglion drive norepinephrine release into the spleen (E). In this hypothesis, splanchnic sympathetic nerves are the efferent arm in the inflammatory reflex, not the vagus nerve.

choline acetyl transferase (ChAT)-mediated ACh release, which in turn activates α7nAChR on macrophages and thereby suppresses the release of pro-inflammatory cytokines and inflammation (Fig. 33.5C). It has been suggested that enhanced vagal tone and α7nAChR activation increases the levels of the anti-inflammatory cytokine IL-10 and concomitantly may induce the macrophage switch from pro-inflammatory M1 macrophages to anti-inflammatory M2 macrophages.[198,204–207] At the molecular level, activation of α7nAChR on macrophages can downregulate cytokine production via inhibiting the nuclear factor (NF)-κB and janus kinase (JAK)/signal transducer and activator of transcription (STAT) pathways.[208,209]

Electrical and pharmacologic activation of the VN has shown promising results as a means to reduce the inflammatory response in experimental animal models (e.g., of endotoxemia, burn injuries, colitis, pancreatitis, and arthritis).[199] For example, reducing afferent VN activity by bilateral cervical vagotomy or systemic atropine and increasing efferent VN activity by electrical stimulation reduced the expected edema induced by carrageenan.[198,210] Similar benefits were observed with vagal stimulation and systemic treatment with nicotine or an α7nAChR-specific agonist in the CIA model (decreased edema, pannus formation, and bone erosion).[211–213] In addition, α7-deficient mice showed a marked increase in synovial inflammation compared with wild-type littermates.[214]

The cytokine induction in response to LPS stimulation in whole blood cultures established from healthy human volunteers subjected to noninvasive VNS or sham stimulation was examined. LPS-induced levels of TNF, IL-1β, IL-8, and MCP-1 were lower and IL-10 levels higher in blood cultures from VNS than sham-stimulated individuals.[215] The same group showed that noninvasive VNS blocks noxious thermal stimulation-induced activity throughout the nociceptive matrix, including somatosensory, insular, and cingulate cortices,[216] suggesting that VNS reduces the physiologic response to noxious thermal stimuli and impacts neural circuits important for pain processing and autonomic output.

Recent work shows reduced vagal tone in RA patients[217] and in patients at risk of developing RA,[218] suggesting the possibility that altered vagal function precedes development of the disease. The first patient studies to examine the effect of vagus nerve stimulation (VNS) on clinical parameters in RA have been completed. An implanted device was used for 6 weeks of VNS in two cohorts of RA patients refractory to either methotrexate or multiple DMARDs. Clinical improvement was observed and correlated with reduction in TNF levels, although the study was open label and needs to be confirmed in a double-blind prospective trial.[201,218]

There are conflicting findings regarding the involvement of cholinergic and noradrenergic nerves targeting the spleen. In some studies, vagotomy has not resulted in modulation of LPS-induced TNF release and, in the same setting, splanchnic nerve section generated an increase in TNF levels.[219,220] Furthermore, it has been questioned whether vagal efferents have functional connections to the splenic nerve in the celiac ganglion.[221] Thus it has been proposed that rather than direct vagal efferent projections to the celiac ganglion, noradrenergic input to the spleen is controlled by traditional preganglionic sympathetic input from the spinal cord (Fig. 33.5D and E).[6] This concept is in line with reflex activation of the sympathetic nervous system during inflammation, where the efferent arm is the splanchnic nerve that inhibits the excessive release of inflammatory cytokines in the spleen and other organs innervated by postganglionic sympathetic neurons. It does not, however, provide an explanation for the wealth of experimental data showing anti-inflammatory responses to selective stimulation of vagal efferent nerve fibers. Hence, additional studies are needed to determine the exact neuronal component of the inflammatory reflex.

Role of Pain in Inflammatory Disease

The impact of CNS activation in regulation of inflammation may not be inherently obvious. In addition to generating pain sensations, activation of nociceptors leads to local axon reflexes that cause the release of neurotransmitters from peripheral sensory nerve terminals. This mechanism regulates not only small blood vessels but also chemotaxis and activation of immune cells, mainly in a pro-inflammatory fashion, and importantly, it is spatially confined. Activation of nociceptors can also generate dorsal root reflexes, which, in addition to driving neurogenic inflammation at the site of peripheral stimulation, can cause similar responses on the mirror-image body site.

In contrast, autonomic stimulation has both localized and systemic effects on inflammation. Sympathetic outflow might affect the inflammatory process in specific sympathetically innervated tissues or immune organs such as lymph nodes and spleen or have a more general impact by driving systemic release of catecholamines from adrenal medulla and thus affect immune cells. Although linkages delineating the vagal anti-inflammatory pathway are still being defined, evidence for a parasympathetic influence on the immune system is strong. Somatosensory and autonomic neuroimmune interactions are much more intricate than previously thought. Furthermore, it is quite likely that it is not individual neural processes and molecules but rather specific combinations of activating and suppressing neuronal signaling that influence different stages and types of immune responses.

Preventing or reducing sensory nervous system activity is a therapeutic target, primarily focused on controlling pain. Because activation of nociceptors drives the neuronal release of factors that trigger neurogenic inflammation, however, treatment of immune disorders may need to include targeting of nociceptors as well as immune cells. Thus an increased understanding of the molecular interplay between the sensory nervous system and the immune system and the ability to regulate excitability of sensory neurons may have important therapeutic consequences in a number of diseases, including (but not limited to) migraine, arthritis, asthma, and inflammatory bowel disease.

The role of the autonomic nervous system in immunoregulation has led to the proposal of new anti-inflammatory therapeutic approaches for chronic inflammatory conditions. Based on the animal models previously discussed, it can be envisioned that regulating the activity in the sympathetic or parasympathetic nervous system can control inflammation. No clinical study of adrenergic agents as a treatment strategy for patients with chronic inflammatory joint disease has been published. Because data targeting adrenergic receptors obtained from animal models are somewhat variable, additional research is needed to fully understand how catecholamines influence the functional state of specific immune cell populations; without that information, it is difficult to draw definitive conclusions as to which treatment would be beneficial for which patient groups.

With regard to the parasympathetic nervous system and treatment, the two major options are pharmacologic activation of the α7nAChR or vagal stimulation. Nicotine is a potent α7nAChR agonist, but the therapeutic value of nicotine is limited because of its lack of specificity and toxicity. More specific α7nAChR agonists are well tolerated in healthy volunteers and in patients with schizophrenia.[222,223] Nevertheless, the LPS-induced innate immune response (release of TNF, IL-6, IL-10, and IL-1 receptor antagonist) in humans was not reduced by the highest tolerable dose of GTS-21, an α7nAChR agonist, compared with placebo.[224] Vagal stimulation is already in use clinically for treatment of refractory epilepsy and depression.[225,226] Intriguingly, long-term vagal stimulation in patients with epilepsy caused a normalization of plasma cytokines and cortisol levels compared with the control group.[227] VNS in RA patients appears to inhibit cytokine production and improved the clinical score. The local and systemic targets of vagal signals, however, may be more complex than anticipated, as may be the interaction between the sympathetic and parasympathetic system in the context of anti-inflammatory actions. Thus further pre-clinical and clinical studies exploring the potential and safety of using vagal stimulation as therapy for patients with inflammatory disorders are warranted.

 Full references for this chapter can be found on ExpertConsult.com.

Selected References

3. Bellinger DL, Lorton D: Autonomic regulation of cellular immune function, *Auton Neurosci* 182:15–41, 2014.
4. Chavan SS, Tracey KJ: Essential Neuroscience in Immunology, *J Immunol* 198:3389–3397, 2017.
6. Martelli D, Farmer DGS, Yao ST: The splanchnic anti-inflammatory pathway: could it be the efferent arm of the inflammatory reflex? *Exp Physiol* 101:1245–1252, 2016.
8. Craig AD: Interoception: the sense of the physiological condition of the body, *Curr Opin Neurobiol* 13:500–505, 2003.
9. Heppelmann B, Messlinger K, Neiss WF, et al.: Fine sensory innervation of the knee joint capsule by group III and group IV nerve fibers in the cat, *J Comp Neurol* 351:415–428, 1995.
10. Sorkin LS, Xiao WH, Wagner R, et al.: Tumour necrosis factor-alpha induces ectopic activity in nociceptive primary afferent fibres, *Neuroscience* 81:255–262, 1997.
11. Bernardini N, Neuhuber W, Reeh PW, et al.: Morphological evidence for functional capsaicin receptor expression and calcitonin gene-related peptide exocytosis in isolated peripheral nerve axons of the mouse, *Neuroscience* 126:585–590, 2004.
15. Zeisel A, Hochgerner H, Lönnerberg P, et al.: Molecular architecture of the mouse nervous system, *Cell* 174:999–1014, 2018. e22.
16. Treede RD, Meyer RA, Campbell JN: Myelinated mechanically insensitive afferents from monkey hairy skin: heat-response properties, *J Neurophysiol* 80:1082–1093, 1998.
18. Dubin AE, Patapoutian A: Nociceptors: the sensors of the pain pathway, *J Clin Invest* 120:3760–3772, 2010.
19. Roosterman D, Goerge T, Schneider SW, et al.: Neuronal control of skin function: the skin as a neuroimmunoendocrine organ, *Physiol Rev* 86:1309–1379, 2006.
23. Schaible HG, Schmidt RF: Excitation and sensitization of fine articular afferents from cat's knee joint by prostaglandin E2, *J Physiol* 403:91–104, 1988.
24. Schaible H-G, Richter F, Ebersberger A, et al.: Joint pain, *Exp Brain Res* 196:153–162, 2009.
25. Schaible H-G, Straub RH: Function of the sympathetic supply in acute and chronic experimental joint inflammation, *Auton Neurosci* 182:55–64, 2014.
29. Chartier SR, Mitchell SAT, Majuta A, et al.: The changing sensory and sympathetic innervation of the young, adult and aging mouse femur, *Neuroscience* 387:178–190, 2018.
33. Castañeda-Corral G, Jimenez-Andrade JM, Bloom AP, et al.: The majority of myelinated and unmyelinated sensory nerve fibers that innervate bone express the tropomyosin receptor kinase A, *Neuroscience* 178:196–207, 2011.
34. Jimenez-Andrade JM, Mantyh WG, Bloom AP, et al.: A phenotypically restricted set of primary afferent nerve fibers innervate the bone versus skin: therapeutic opportunity for treating skeletal pain, *Bone* 46:306–313, 2010.
41. Tesarz J, Hoheisel U, Wiedenhöfer B, et al.: Sensory innervation of the thoracolumbar fascia in rats and humans, *Neuroscience* 194:302–308, 2011.
45. Schilder A, Hoheisel U, Magerl W, et al.: Sensory findings after stimulation of the thoracolumbar fascia with hypertonic saline suggest its contribution to low back pain, *Pain* 155:222–231, 2014.
46. Mense S, Hoheisel U: Evidence for the existence of nociceptors in rat thoracolumbar fascia, *J Bodyw Mov Ther* 20:623–628, 2016.
49. Hucho T, Levine JD: Signaling pathways in sensitization: toward a nociceptor cell biology, *Neuron* 55:365–376, 2007.
52. Ji R-R, Chamessian A, Zhang Y-Q: Pain regulation by non-neuronal cells and inflammation, *Science* 354:572–577, 2016.
53. Pinho-Ribeiro FA, Verri WA, Chiu IM: Nociceptor sensory neuron–immune interactions in pain and inflammation, *Trends Immunol* 38:5–19, 2017.
54. Carlton SM, Zhou S, Coggeshall RE: Evidence for the interaction of glutamate and NK1 receptors in the periphery, *Brain Res* 790:160–169, 1998.
55. Du J, Koltzenburg M, Carlton SM: Glutamate-induced excitation and sensitization of nociceptors in rat glabrous skin, *Pain* 89:187–198, 2001.
56. Steen KH, Reeh PW, Anton F, et al.: Protons selectively induce lasting excitation and sensitization to mechanical stimulation of nociceptors in rat skin, in vitro, *J Neurosci* 12:86–95, 1992.
57. Basbaum AI, Bautista DM, Scherrer G, et al.: Cellular and molecular mechanisms of pain, *Cell* 139:267–284, 2009.
58. Reichling DB, Levine JD: Critical role of nociceptor plasticity in chronic pain, *Trends Neurosci* 32:611–618, 2009.
59. Kandasamy R, Price TJ: The pharmacology of nociceptor priming. In *Handbook of experimental pharmacology* (vol 227). 2015, pp 15–37.
63. Schmidt R, Schmelz M, Forster C, et al.: Novel classes of responsive and unresponsive C nociceptors in human skin, *J Neurosci* 15:333–341, 1995.
65. Gold MS, Gebhart GF: Nociceptor sensitization in pain pathogenesis, *Nat Med* 16:1248–1257, 2010.
66. Prato V, Taberner FJ, Hockley JRF, et al.: Functional and molecular characterization of mechanoinsensitive "silent" nociceptors, *Cell Rep* 21:3102–3115, 2017.
67. Weinkauf B, Schultz C, Obreja O, et al.: Nerve growth factor induces sensitization of nociceptors without evidence for increased intraepidermal nerve fiber density, *Pain* 154:2500–2511, 2013.
68. Watkins LR, Maier SF: Beyond neurons: evidence that immune and glial cells contribute to pathological pain states, *Physiol Rev* 82:981–1011, 2002.
69. Latremoliere A, Woolf CJ: Central sensitization: a generator of pain hypersensitivity by central neural plasticity, *J Pain* 10:895–926, 2009.
70. Todd AJ: Plasticity of inhibition in the spinal cord, *Handb Exp Pharmacol* 227:171–190, 2015.
71. Cervero F: Spinal cord hyperexcitability and its role in pain and hyperalgesia, *Exp Brain Res* 196:129–137, 2009.
72. Old EA, Clark AK, Malcangio M: The role of glia in the spinal cord in neuropathic and inflammatory pain. In *Handbook of experimental pharmacology* (vol 227). 2015, pp 145–170.
73. Bushnell MC, Ceko M, Low LA: Cognitive and emotional control of pain and its disruption in chronic pain, *Nat Rev Neurosci* 14:502–511, 2013.
75. Thompson JM, Neugebauer V: Amygdala plasticity and pain, *Pain Res Manag* 2017:1–12, 2017.
78. Molendijk M, Hazes JMW, Lubberts E: From patients with arthralgia, pre-RA and recently diagnosed RA: what is the current status of understanding RA pathogenesis ? *RMD Open* 1–11, 2018.
79. Brinck RM ten, Steenbergen HW van, Mangnus L, et al.: Functional limitations in the phase of clinically suspect arthralgia are as serious as in early clinical arthritis; a longitudinal study, *RMD Open* 3:e000419, 2017.
80. Rantapää-Dahlqvist S, Jong BAW De, Berglin E, et al.: Antibodies against cyclic citrullinated peptide and iga rheumatoid factor predict the development of rheumatoid arthritis, *Arthritis Rheum* 48:2741–2749, 2003.
82. Wigerblad G, Bas DB, Fernades-Cerqueira C, et al.: Autoantibodies to citrullinated proteins induce joint pain independent of inflammation via a chemokine-dependent mechanism, *Ann Rheum Dis* 75:730–7398, 2016.
84. Qu L, Zhang P, LaMotte RH, et al.: Neuronal Fc-gamma receptor I mediated excitatory effects of IgG immune complex on rat dorsal root ganglion neurons, *Brain Behav Immun* 25:1399–1407, 2011.
85. Bersellini Farinotti A, Wigerblad G, Nascimeto D, et al.: Cartilage bining antibodies induce pain through immune complex mediated stimulation of neurons, *J Exp Med* 216:1904–1924, 2019.

86. Altawil R, Saevarsdottir S, Wedrén S, et al.: Remaining pain in early rheumatoid arthritis patients treated with methotrexate, *Arthritis Care Res (Hoboken)* 68:1061–1068, 2016.
87. McWilliams DF, Walsh DA: Factors predicting pain and early discontinuation of tumour necrosis factor-α-inhibitors in people with rheumatoid arthritis: results from the British society for rheumatology biologics register, *BMC Musculoskelet Disord* 17:337, 2016.
89. Fridén C, Thoors U, Glenmark B, et al.: Higher pain sensitivity and lower muscle strength in postmenonpausal women with early rheumatoid arthritis compared with age-matched healthy women—a pilot study, *Disabil Rehabil* 35:1350–1356, 2013.
90. Leffler A-S, Kosek E, Lerndal T, et al.: Somatosensory perception and function of diffuse noxious inhibitory controls (DNIC) in patients suffering from rheumatoid arthritis, *Eur J Pain* 6:161–176, 2002.
92. Ahmed S, Magan T, Vargas M, et al.: Use of the painDETECT tool in rheumatoid arthritis suggests neuropathic and sensitization components in pain reporting, *J Pain Res* 7:579–588, 2014.
94. McWilliams DF, Walsh DA: Pain mechanisms in rheumatoid arthritis, *Clin Exp Rheumatol* 35:S94–S101, 2017.
96. Bas DB, Su J, Sandor K, et al.: Collagen antibody-induced arthritis evokes persistent pain with spinal glial involvement and transient prostaglandin dependency, *Arthritis Rheum* 64:3886–3896, 2012.
97. Christianson CA, Corr M, Firestein GS, et al.: Characterization of the acute and persistent pain state present in K/BxN serum transfer arthritis, *Pain* 151:394–403, 2010.
106. Lembeck F, Holzer P: Substance P as neurogenic mediator of antidromic vasodilation and neurogenic plasma extravasation, *Naunyn Schmiedebergs Arch Pharmacol* 310:175–183, 1979.
108. Willis W: Dorsal root potentials and dorsal root reflexes: a double-edged sword, *Exp Brain Res* 124:395–421, 1999.
111. Chiu IM, Heesters BA, Ghasemlou N, et al.: Bacteria activate sensory neurons that modulate pain and inflammation, *Nature* 501:52–57, 2013.
112. É Borbély, Botz B, Bölcskei K, et al.: Capsaicin-sensitive sensory nerves exert complex regulatory functions in the serum-transfer mouse model of autoimmune arthritis, *Brain Behav Immun* 45:50–59, 2015.
113. Helyes Z, Szabó A, Németh J, et al.: Antiinflammatory and analgesic effects of somatostatin released from capsaicin-sensitive sensory nerve terminals in a Freund's adjuvant-induced chronic arthritis model in the rat, *Arthritis Rheum* 50:1677–1685, 2004.
116. Horváth K, Boros M, Bagoly T, et al.: Analgesic topical capsaicinoid therapy increases somatostatin-like immunoreactivity in the human plasma, *Neuropeptides* 48:371–378, 2014.
119. Bernardi PS, Valtschanoff JG, Weinberg RJ, et al.: Synaptic interactions between primary afferent terminals and GABA and nitric oxide-synthesizing neurons in superficial laminae of the rat spinal cord, *J Neurosci* 15:1363–1371, 1995.
122. Castro-Lopes JM, Tavares I, Tölle TR, et al.: Carrageenan-induced inflammation of the hind foot provokes a rise of GABA-immunoreactive cells in the rat spinal cord that is prevented by peripheral neurectomy or neonatal capsaicin treatment, *Pain* 56:193–201, 1994.
125. Bagust J, Kerkut GA, Rakkah NI: The dorsal root reflex in isolated mammalian spinal cord, *Comp Biochem Physiol A Comp Physiol* 93:151–160, 1989.
126. Peng YB, Wu J, Willis WD, et al.: GABA(A) and 5-HT(3) receptors are involved in dorsal root reflexes: possible role in periaqueductal gray descending inhibition, *J Neurophysiol* 86:49–58, 2001.
129. Kidd BL, Mapp PI, Gibson SJ, et al.: A neurogenic mechanism for symmetrical arthritis, *Lancet* 2:1128–1130, 1989.
132. Schaible HG, Grubb BD: Afferent and spinal mechanisms of joint pain, *Pain* 55:5–54, 1993.
133. Schaible HG, Schmidt RF, Willis WD: Responses of spinal cord neurones to stimulation of articular afferent fibres in the cat, *J Physiol* 372:575–593, 1986.
135. Vierck CJ, Whitsel BL, Favorov OV, et al.: Role of primary somatosensory cortex in the coding of pain, *Pain* 154:334–344, 2013.
138. Cervero F, Schaible HG, Schmidt RF: Tonic descending inhibition of spinal cord neurones driven by joint afferents in normal cats and in cats with an inflamed knee joint, *Exp Brain Res* 83:675–678, 1991.
140. Kovelowski CJ, Ossipov MH, Sun H, et al.: Supraspinal cholecystokinin may drive tonic descending facilitation mechanisms to maintain neuropathic pain in the rat, *Pain* 87:265–273, 2000.
141. Suzuki R, Morcuende S, Webber M, et al.: Superficial NK1-expressing neurons control spinal excitability through activation of descending pathways, *Nat Neurosci* 5:1319–1326, 2002.
144. Pogatzki EM, Urban MO, Brennan TJ, et al.: Role of the rostral medial medulla in the development of primary and secondary hyperalgesia after incision in the rat, *Anesthesiology* 96:1153–1160, 2002.
146. Sluka KA, Rees H, Westlund KN, et al.: Fiber types contributing to dorsal root reflexes induced by joint inflammation in cats and monkeys, *J Neurophysiol* 74:981–989, 1995.
148. Sluka KA, Lawand NB, Westlund KN: Joint inflammation is reduced by dorsal rhizotomy and not by sympathectomy or spinal cord transection, *Ann Rheum Dis* 53:309–314, 1994.
149. Sluka KA, Westlund KN: Centrally administered non-NMDA but not NMDA receptor antagonists block peripheral knee joint inflammation, *Pain* 55:217–225, 1993.
150. Sluka K, Willis W, Westlund K: Joint inflammation and hyperalgesia are reduced by spinal bicuculline, *Neuroreport* 5:109–112, 1993.
152. Lin Q, Wu J, Willis WD: Dorsal root reflexes and cutaneous neurogenic inflammation after intradermal injection of capsaicin in rats, *J Neurophysiol* 82:2602–2611, 1999.
157. Bassi GS, Malvar D do C, Cunha TM, et al.: Spinal GABA-B receptor modulates neutrophil recruitment to the knee joint in zymosan-induced arthritis, *Naunyn Schmiedebergs Arch Pharmacol* 389:851–861, 2016.
159. Boettger MK, Weber K, Gajda M, et al.: Spinally applied ketamine or morphine attenuate peripheral inflammation and hyperalgesia in acute and chronic phases of experimental arthritis, *Brain Behav Immun* 24:474–485, 2010.
161. Brock SC, Tonussi CR: Intrathecally injected morphine inhibits inflammatory paw edema: the involvement of nitric oxide and cyclic-guanosine monophosphate, *Anesth Analg* 106:965–971, 2008.
164. Bong GW, Rosengren S, Firestein GS: Spinal cord adenosine receptor stimulation in rats inhibits peripheral neutrophil accumulation. The role of N-methyl-D-aspartate receptors, *J Clin Invest* 98:2779–2785, 1996.
165. Sorkin LS, Moore J, Boyle DL, et al.: Regulation of peripheral inflammation by spinal adenosine: role of somatic afferent fibers, *Exp Neurol* 184:162–168, 2003.
167. Cronstein BN, Levin RI, Philips M, et al.: Neutrophil adherence to endothelium is enhanced via adenosine A1 receptors and inhibited via adenosine A2 receptors, *J Immunol* 148:2201–2206, 1992.
170. Kane D, Lockhart JC, Balint PV, et al.: Protective effect of sensory denervation in inflammatory arthritis (evidence of regulatory neuroimmune pathways in the arthritic joint), *Ann Rheum Dis* 64:325–327, 2005.
174. Holzer P: Capsaicin: cellular targets, mechanisms of action, and selectivity for thin sensory neurons, *Pharmacol Rev* 43:143–201, 1991.
175. Boyle DL, Moore J, Yang L, et al.: Spinal adenosine receptor activation inhibits inflammation and joint destruction in rat adjuvant-induced arthritis, *Arthritis Rheum* 46:3076–3082, 2002.
177. Boyle DL, Jones TL, Hammaker D, et al.: Regulation of peripheral inflammation by spinal p38 MAP kinase in rats, *PLoS Med* 3:e338, 2006.
179. Boettger MK, Weber K, Grossmann D, et al.: Spinal tumor necrosis factor alpha neutralization reduces peripheral inflammation and hyperalgesia and suppresses autonomic responses in experimental arthritis: a role for spinal tumor necrosis factor alpha during

induction and maintenance of peripheral inflammation, *Arthritis Rheum* 62:1308–1318, 2010.

180. Pongratz G, Straub RH: Role of peripheral nerve fibres in acute and chronic inflammation in arthritis, *Nat Rev Rheumatol* 9:117–126, 2013.
183. Mapp PI, Kidd BL, Gibson SJ, et al.: Substance P-, calcitonin gene-related peptide- and C-flanking peptide of neuropeptide Y-immunoreactive fibres are present in normal synovium but depleted in patients with rheumatoid arthritis, *Neuroscience* 37:143–153, 1990.
184. Straub RH, Härle P: Sympathetic neurotransmitters in joint inflammation, *Rheum Dis Clin North Am* 31:43–59, 2005.
185. Miller LE, Jüsten HP, Schölmerich J, et al.: The loss of sympathetic nerve fibers in the synovial tissue of patients with rheumatoid arthritis is accompanied by increased norepinephrine release from synovial macrophages, *FASEB J* 14:2097–2107, 2000.
186. Miller LE, Weidler C, Falk W, et al.: Increased prevalence of semaphorin 3C, a repellent of sympathetic nerve fibers, in the synovial tissue of patients with rheumatoid arthritis, *Arthritis Rheum* 50:1156–1163, 2004.
187. Longo G, Osikowicz M, Ribeiro-da-Silva A: Sympathetic fiber sprouting in inflamed joints and adjacent skin contributes to pain-related behavior in arthritis, *J Neurosci* 33:10066–10074, 2013.
188. Jimenez-Andrade JM, Mantyh PW: Sensory and sympathetic nerve fibers undergo sprouting and neuroma formation in the painful arthritic joint of geriatric mice, *Arthritis Res Ther* 14:R101, 2012.
190. Härle P, Pongratz G, Albrecht J, et al.: An early sympathetic nervous system influence exacerbates collagen-induced arthritis via CD4+CD25+ cells, *Arthritis Rheum* 58:2347–2355, 2008.
192. Ebbinghaus M, Gajda M, Boettger MK, et al.: The anti-inflammatory effects of sympathectomy in murine antigen-induced arthritis are associated with a reduction of Th1 and Th17 responses, *Ann Rheum Dis* 71:253–261, 2012.
194. Green PG, Miao FJ, Strausbaugh H, et al.: Endocrine and vagal controls of sympathetically dependent neurogenic inflammation, *Ann N Y Acad Sci* 840:282–288, 1998.
195. Bassi GS, Dias DPM, Franchin M, et al.: Modulation of experimental arthritis by vagal sensory and central brain stimulation, *Brain Behav Immun* 64:330–343, 2017.
198. Borovikova LV, Ivanova S, Zhang M, et al.: Vagus nerve stimulation attenuates the systemic inflammatory response to endotoxin, *Nature* 405:458–462, 2000.
199. Hoover DB: Cholinergic modulation of the immune system presents new approaches for treating inflammation, *Pharmacol Ther*, 2017.
200. Wang H, Yu M, Ochani M, et al.: Nicotinic acetylcholine receptor alpha7 subunit is an essential regulator of inflammation, *Nature* 421:384–388, 2003.
201. Levine YA, Grazio S, Miljko S, et al.: Vagus nerve stimulation inhibits cytokine production and attenuates disease severity in rheumatoid arthritis, *Proc Natl Acad Sci*, 2016.
202. Matteoli G, Gomez-Pinilla PJ, Nemethova A, et al.: A distinct vagal anti-inflammatory pathway modulates intestinal muscularis resident macrophages independent of the spleen, *Gut* 63:938–948, 2014.
204. Rasmussen SE, Pfeiffer-Jensen M, Drewes AM, et al.: Vagal influences in rheumatoid arthritis, *Scand J Rheumatol* 47:1–11, 2018.
206. Zhang Q, Lu Y, Bian H, et al.: Activation of the α7 nicotinic receptor promotes lipopolysaccharide-induced conversion of M1 microglia to M2, *Am J Transl Res* 9:971–985, 2017.
210. Borovikova LV, Ivanova S, Nardi D, et al.: Role of vagus nerve signaling in CNI-1493-mediated suppression of acute inflammation, *Auton Neurosci* 85:141–147, 2000.
211. Levine YA, Koopman FA, Faltys M, et al.: Neurostimulation of the cholinergic anti-inflammatory pathway ameliorates disease in rat collagen-induced arthritis, *PLoS One* 9:e104530, 2014.
212. Maanen MA van, Lebre MC, Poll T van der, et al.: Stimulation of nicotinic acetylcholine receptors attenuates collagen-induced arthritis in mice, *Arthritis Rheum* 60:114–122, 2009.
214. Maanen MA van, Stoof SP, Larosa GJ, et al.: Role of the cholinergic nervous system in rheumatoid arthritis: aggravation of arthritis in nicotinic acetylcholine receptor α7 subunit gene knockout mice, *Ann Rheum Dis* 69:1717–1723, 2010.
215. Lerman I, Hauger R, Sorkin L, et al.: Noninvasive transcutaneous vagus nerve stimulation decreases whole blood culture-derived cytokines and chemokines: a randomized, blinded, healthy control pilot trial, *Neuromodulation* 19:283–290, 2016.
216. Lerman I, Davis B, Huang M, et al.: Noninvasive vagus nerve stimulation alters neural response and physiological autonomic tone to noxious thermal challenge, *PLoS One* 14:e0201212, 2019.
217. Kosek E, Altawil R, Kadetoff D, et al.: Evidence of different mediators of central inflammation in dysfunctional and inflammatory pain—Interleukin-8 in fibromyalgia and interleukin-1 β in rheumatoid arthritis, *J Neuroimmunol* 280:49–55, 2015.
218. Koopman FA, Maanen MA van, Vervoordeldonk MJ, et al.: Balancing the autonomic nervous system to reduce inflammation in rheumatoid arthritis, *J Intern Med* 282:64–75, 2017.
219. Martelli D, Yao ST, McKinley MJ, et al.: Reflex control of inflammation by sympathetic nerves, not the vagus, *J Physiol* 592:1677–1686, 2014.
221. Bratton BO, Martelli D, McKinley MJ, et al.: Neural regulation of inflammation: no neural connection from the vagus to splenic sympathetic neurons, *Exp Physiol* 97:1180–1185, 2012.
225. Mohr P, Rodriguez M, Slavíčková A, et al.: The application of vagus nerve stimulation and deep brain stimulation in depression, *Neuropsychobiology* 64:170–181, 2011.

34 Clinical Research Methods in Rheumatic Disease

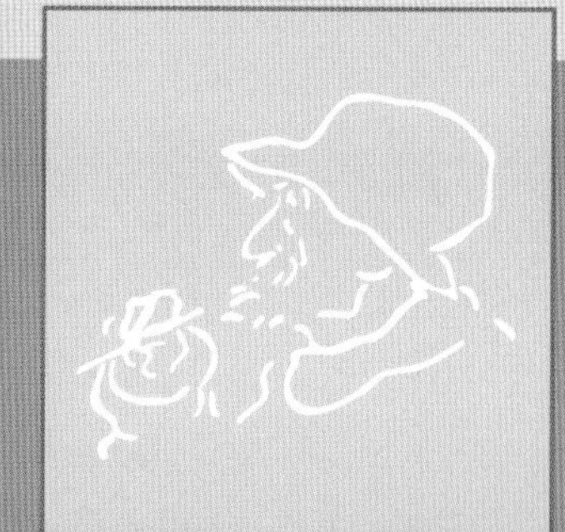

JEFFREY R. CURTIS, YVONNE M. GOLIGHTLY, AND KENNETH G. SAAG

KEY POINTS

Epidemiology is the study of the distribution of disease and its determinants in populations. Epidemiologic methods can be used to describe the frequency or development of disease and to determine underlying risk factors.

Prevalence is the frequency of disease in the population at a given time, including both existing and new cases. Incidence measures the development of disease over a specified period of time in an initially disease-free population.

The odds ratio (OR) compares the odds of disease in an exposed population with those in a population without the exposure or risk factor under study. The relative risk (RR) is the risk of development of disease during a specific time period in an exposed population compared with an unexposed population.

Threats to the validity of a study include chance, systematic bias, and confounding. Confounding occurs when an extraneous factor, associated with both the exposure of interest and the disease, but which is not part of the causal pathway between exposure and disease, is superimposed on the true risk factor-disease relationship.

Case-control studies examine exposures in a population that already has the disease, and compares them with exposures in otherwise comparable but disease-free individuals derived from the same source population. This study design may be subject to recall bias, in which individuals with disease are more likely to recall exposure to risk factors than those without the disease, but it may be the design of choice for rare diseases.

Cohort studies follow groups of individuals with and without an exposure of interest to measure the development of disease with time. Because the exposure assessment precedes the disease, time can help determine causation.

Randomized controlled trials most closely resemble formal experiments in which the exposure and the response are compared between groups that receive the active intervention and those that receive a placebo or other comparator.

A pragmatic clinical trial provides evidence of real world effectiveness, and an adaptive clinical trial allows for planned changes to the intervention at interim time points based on specific response targets.

Introduction

Epidemiology is the study of the distribution of disease and its determinants in populations.[1] Its purpose is to describe the frequency of disease and to determine risk factors and causes responsible for variation in disease occurrence. Comparison of the relative strengths of risk factors and assessment of their generalizability can allow truth to be inferred to a broader population. Causality is often difficult to discern in observational investigations, particularly based on the results from a single study. The criteria proposed to assess the likelihood of a cause-effect relationship include consideration of the strength of the association, biologic credibility, consistency with other investigations, the temporal sequence, and a dose-response relationship.[2] This chapter will explain basic epidemiologic concepts and definitions; describe major epidemiologic study designs, their strengths and weaknesses, and their usefulness in inferring causality; and demonstrate specific applications of these principles to the study of rheumatic diseases. The term *disease* will be used to represent a disease, death, or other health outcome of interest, and the term *exposure* will be used to represent a risk or protective factor examined for its association with disease.

Measures of Disease Occurrence

The frequency of a disease in a population at any given time is referred to as its *prevalence*. Measured at one point in time, prevalence is the proportion of individuals with a disease of the total population under study. Importantly, the numerator makes no distinction between new and established cases of disease. Multiple estimates of disease prevalence estimated over time are commonly used to determine trends in disease occurrence or the need for health services. The following factors affect prevalence: whether the disease results in premature mortality, and the number of new cases arising in the population (i.e., incidence).

Incidence

To determine the likelihood that disease will develop with time, repeated observations of the same people are required to determine

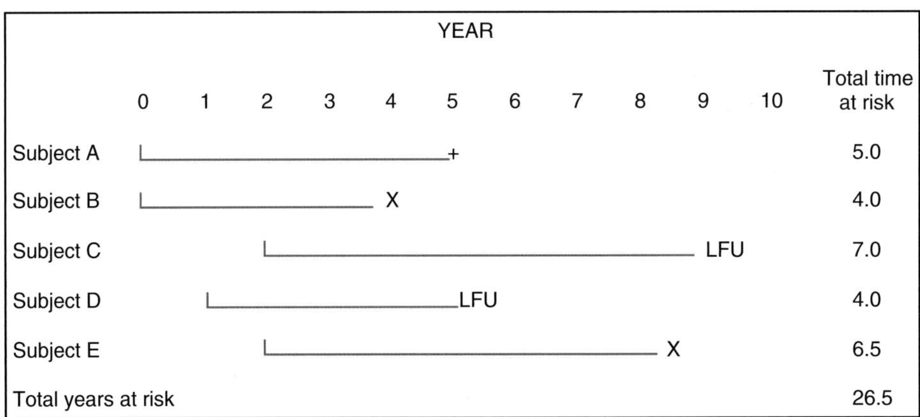

• **Fig. 34.1** Hypothetical calculation of person-time at risk for study of incidence of systemic lupus erythematosus for 10 years. |, Beginning of observation period; +, died; *LFU,* lost-to-follow-up; *X,* developed disease.

in whom disease develops and in whom it does not. Incidence proportion, or risk, is the frequency of new cases during a specified time, out of those at risk for, but without, the disease at baseline. During the observation period, a person may manifest the disease in question, die from competing risks (e.g., another health condition), or be lost to follow up. All of these situations result in that person no longer contributing time at risk to the denominator. The concept of person-time includes the actual time at risk contributed by each individual. For example, consider the hypothetical example of incidence of systemic lupus erythematosus (SLE) during a 10-year period (Fig. 34.1). The disease may not develop in Person A during the observation period, but he or she may die at year 5 of a competing cause; this person contributes 5 person years to the denominator. SLE might develop in Person B 4 years after the study begins, when he or she is thus no longer at risk; this person contributes 4 person years of time at risk to the denominator. Person C joins the study at year 2 and is lost to follow-up at year 9, contributing 7 years of time at risk. Person D joins the study at year 1 and is lost to follow-up at year 5, for a total of 4 years of person time at risk. Person E joins the study at year 2 and manifests SLE halfway between year 8 and year 9, contributing 6.5 person years at risk. Incidence rate is defined by the following[2]:

$$\text{Incidence Rate} = \frac{\text{New cases developing during time period of observation}}{\text{Total person} - \text{time at risk for each individual without the disease at study entry}}$$

In the example, two new cases of SLE are observed and the total person time from people A through E at risk equals 5.0 + 4.0 + 7.0 + 4.0 + 6.5 = 26.5 person years. Thus, the incidence rate is 2 cases per 26.5 person years, or 1 case per 13.25 person years. This may be expressed as 0.0754 cases per person year or 7.54 cases per 100 person years. Estimating an incidence rate generally assumes that the rate is constant over the observation period. If needed, stratification can be performed on key factors (e.g., age, birth cohort) relating to the circumstance where the incidence rate may be changing over time.

Measures of Effect

The association between the disease and exposures or risk factors may be even more important than the description of the frequency of disease or its development. One way to examine the association between a risk factor and an outcome is to compare the prevalence or incidence of disease in groups with a given exposure to those without that exposure. To assess the potential exposure/disease association, it is critical that the exposed and unexposed groups are comparable. Measures to delineate this relationship between disease occurrence and exposure vary according to study design. Cross-sectional surveys and case-control studies utilize the odds ratio (OR), which is a measure of the odds (prevalence odds = prevalence/1-prevalence; incidence odds = incidence/1-incidence) of disease in the exposed group compared with the unexposed group. Longitudinal designs can calculate a ratio of risks (RR) of the incidence of disease or an outcome event in the exposed compared with the unexposed groups. If the amount of follow-up time in which the disease or event can occur is the same in all groups (e.g., all patients have follow-up of exactly one year), then risk is simply defined as the probability of the disease or outcome occurring in that period of time. The RR, or *relative risk*, between exposed and unexposed individuals describes the relative likelihood of the event occurring in the exposed group versus the unexposed group. If patients contribute unequal amounts of follow-up time, an incidence rate, or risk per unit time, is more appropriate to calculate. If one wishes to compare the incidence rates between exposed and unexposed individuals, an incidence rate ratio can be computed. Some statistical techniques, such as a Cox Proportional Hazard analysis, estimate a hazard ratio, which is a close approximation of the incidence rate ratio.

Data Sources for Research in Rheumatology

An increasing variety of data sources exist for rheumatology research (Table 34.1).

Traditionally, disease-specific registries have served this purpose, which might be located at a single academic medical center or span multiple sites.[3,4] Although traditional registries can address a broad range of clinical effectiveness and safety questions, they are usually labor-intensive to create and maintain, expensive, and challenged to enroll adequate numbers of patients to address rare but serious safety questions. Traditional registries also may be subject to selection bias both in who participates (e.g., healthy volunteers) and who remains in the registry (e.g., patients with a severe illness who may be more likely to drop out over time).

In part, for these reasons, administrative claims data obtained from large health plans and insurers have been used to study safety and effectiveness questions. Although these typically lack

TABLE 34.1 Comparison of Data Types Relevant to Rheumatology Research

Type of Data	Examples	Clinical Outcomes	Safety	Health Care Utilization, Economics	Potential Limitations
Traditional registry/ cohort	Corrona	Excellent	Excellent	Fair	Operational cost to create and maintain; size; potential concern for selection bias (generalizability)
Administrative Health Plan Claims	Medicare, commercial health plans (e.g., Optum, HealthCore, Marketscan)	Generally infeasible	Excellent[a]	Excellent	Lack of information on disease severity, activity
Single-specialty EHR (retrospective[b])	ACR RISE registry (rheumatology) THIN database (U.K. primary care)	Good (for metrics routinely measured by clinicians)	Generally infeasible	Fair	Lack of information from any other providers (e.g., hospitalization)
Multi-specialty EHR	PCORnet	Fair	Good	Good (usually not comprehensive)	Feasibility to access if data is held by multiple stakeholders; lack of comprehensiveness for the study of safety questions
Patient registries	ArthritisPower FORWARD	Good (for patient-centric metrics)	Fair	Generally infeasible	Without linkages to external data, information is largely patient-reported with potential concerns re: validity for some data elements
Linked data sources between >1 different data types above	Generally infeasible	Excellent	Excellent	Excellent	More clarity

ACR, American College of Rheumatology; *EHR*, electronic health record.

[a]For certain outcomes where high quality validation studies are available.

[b]Where prospective data collection is possible, clinical outcomes can be captured with whatever detail that participating physicians are willing to provide.

information on disease activity and severity, their comprehensive nature and complete follow-up may well suit the study of safety questions, health service utilization, and health economic questions. More recently, large-scale electronic medical record data sources have been used to create large cohorts.[5] Perhaps the most well-known example of a large scale electronic health record (EHR)-based registry in rheumatology is the American College of Rheumatology's Rheumatology Informatics System for Effectiveness (RISE) registry, which extracts data elements from the EHRs of rheumatologists. RISE currently captures data from more than 1000 rheumatology providers and encompasses the data of more than 1 million rheumatology patients. The limitation to this type of single-specialty EHR-based cohort is the inherent problem that rheumatologists may not record the complete set of comorbidities relevant to a patient, especially if those conditions are managed by other specialists (e.g., uveitis, co-managed by ophthalmology). Moreover, a single-specialty EHR-based cohort will typically miss out-of-office care (e.g., hospitalization, emergency department visits), making it difficult to study safety comprehensively. As a partial solution, a multi-specialty, multi-site EHR-based infrastructure called *National Patient-Centered Clinical Research Network (PCORnet)* was created in the U.S., funded by the Affordable Care Act, and includes data from multiple health systems and primary care and specialty providers.[6] Currently encompassing EHR data for more than 100 million people, PCORnet continues to grow and provides opportunity to study a variety of outcomes relevant to spondyloarthritis (SpA). Importantly, however, as much as 80% of the information in EHR records may be represented as unstructured data (i.e., free text), and methods to convert this text into structured data elements suitable for analysis are time-consuming and resource-intensive to apply.

Common strengths and limitations of each of the above data sources are summarized in Table 34.1. Recognizing that all data sources have potential gaps, the opportunity to link across data sources and overcome the limitations in one data source with the strengths of another is now a possibility. A variety of methods can be used to link data, varying two important features including (1) whether unique identifiers are available (e.g., social security numbers, medical record number, health plan ID); and (2) whether or not personal identifying information can be exchanged between the parties directly.[7,8] Regardless, a variety of methods exist to link data, irrespective of limitations in whether unique identifiers are available or the extent of shareable information is limited. In fact, even in circumstances where no data can be directly exchanged, combining results across data sources in a distributed data network is possible.[9]

Clinical Research Study Designs

Clinical research study designs include ecological studies, cross-sectional surveys, case-control studies, case-cohort studies, cohort studies, self-controlled study designs, quasi-experimental designs, and randomized controlled clinical trials. The latter is frequently considered the most rigorous study design and the one most closely representing a formal experiment. Each study design has its own inherent strengths and weaknesses (Table 34.2), and the choice of study design depends upon the research question, the rarity of the disease under study, the availability of appropriate study and comparable control populations, resources available to conduct the study, and logistics.[10,11]

Observational Studies

In observational studies, the exposure is not randomly distributed in a population. The investigator observes the exposure rather than selects (i.e., via randomization) the exposure status of an individual.[12] Types of observational studies include ecological, cross-sectional, case-control, and cohort.

Ecological Studies

In this study design, the unit of observation is a group rather than an individual.[13] Aggregate data on rates of disease and risk factors are compared to examine associations between disease frequencies and exposures. The ecological study is frequently a design of expediency and can generate hypotheses for more rigorous testing in studies by using individual-level data.[11] One of its chief drawbacks is its high susceptibility to confounding. This occurs when an extraneous factor, not on the causal pathway, masks the true relationship between exposure and disease by virtue of its association with both.[14] Further, associations in the aggregate may not necessarily hold true for the individual.[11] This concept is termed the *ecological fallacy*. As a hypothetical example, rates of specific kinds of cancers may be high in countries in which cigarette sales are also high. Whether the individuals who are buying and presumably smoking the cigarettes are the same individuals in whom cancer develops is not known from this study design. A variant on this type of study design is called a *trend-in-trend analysis*, which is a study design that requires a strong time in exposure but may allow for adjusting for some types of bias.[15]

Cross-Sectional Surveys

The goal of this study design is usually descriptive, including all individuals, with and without the disease under study, in the population, or a representative sample of them, at one point in time with no follow-up period. In a population-based cohort or registry, surveys can estimate prevalence of a particular disease in the population and determine need for health services and resource allocation.[11] Typically, information about risk factors is obtained simultaneously. Such risk factor data may or may not represent the most relevant time of exposure, nor can it be determined whether the exposure preceded or resulted from the disease.[10]

An example of a cross-sectional survey, conducted approximately once per decade in the United States, is the National Health and Nutrition Examination Survey (NHANES). This survey samples a proportion of the residents in the contiguous 48 states and measures various health outcomes and habits, such as blood pressure, serum lipids, height, weight, smoking, and dietary intake. These surveys have been used in rheumatology to determine the prevalence of radiographic knee and hip osteoarthritis (OA), as well the prevalence of spondyloarthritis according to defined classification criteria, in various age, sex, and race/ethnicity subgroups.[16]

Case-Control Studies

Much maligned by the uninitiated because of its susceptibility to bias, the case-control study can be the study design of choice—or sometimes the *only* appropriate study design—in certain situations, particularly when the disease under study is rare. This type of study usually includes fewer individuals and is much less costly and more efficient than cohort studies. These advantages stem from the fact that it is composed of individuals who already have the disease under study, compared with the cohort study in which researchers must wait for the disease to develop in a small proportion of a large cohort with time. Most important in the design of a case-control study are: (1) the choice of the control group, which must be comparable to the cases; and (2) recognition of potential biases that may threaten validity. In general, a case-control study is a proxy for the cohort study that is not considered feasible to conduct.

Strictly defined, the case-control study compares a group of individuals with the disease under study with a control population without the disease. Both groups are drawn from the same source population.[1,14] The source population may be the residents of a particular geographic area or a hospital's referral base. The control group serves as an estimate of the distribution of the exposure in the source population, and consequently, the control group must be sampled independently of exposure status.[1,14] For example, if researchers are interested in examining the possible association between smoking and progressive systemic sclerosis (PSS), the controls must be from the same source population that generated the cases of patients with PSS, if this can be determined, and must be sampled without regard to their smoking status.

Selection of Controls for Case-Control Study

If the source of the cases is a well-defined population, the controls can be sampled directly from that population. If the source population is too large to allow a complete enumeration, controls may be matched to each case by their residence in the same neighborhood. In the past, random-digit dialing had been used to select controls, but this labor-intensive method omits those without land line telephones or those who cannot be reached; random digit dialing became somewhat impractical in later years.[1] If the cases are drawn from a particular hospital or clinic, then the source population should represent people who would be treated in that hospital or clinic if they developed the disease under study, but frequently, this source population can be difficult to identify and is influenced by referral practices.[1] Hospital or clinic controls can be used, but this method can have particular pitfalls because the controls might not be selected independently of the exposure in the source population. For instance, in a hospital-based study of smoking in SLE, individuals hospitalized for other diseases, such as myocardial infarction or pneumonia, might have exposures different from the source population in general, especially if the exposure, in this case smoking, causes or prevents the "control" disease selected. One way to avoid this is to exclude diseases known to be associated with the exposure under study, but this may create other biases. Another tactic could be to select hospital controls with diseases thought to be unrelated to the disease or exposures

TABLE 34.2 Common Epidemiologic Study Designs and Their Strengths and Weaknesses

Study Design	Definition	Measure of Effect	Strengths	Weaknesses
Ecological	Aggregate data on exposures and disease; unit of analysis is a group, not an individual	Odds ratio	Inexpensive Short duration Hypothesis-generating	Susceptibility to confounding Ecological fallacy
Cross-sectional survey	Data on exposures and disease obtained at one time from all individuals in an area (or a sample thereof) with and without disease	Prevalence Odds ratio	Can study several outcomes Short duration Can generate population prevalence estimates of disease and risk factor distributions	May not be able to determine whether disease preceded exposure Not practical for rare diseases Cannot produce incidence or relative risk estimates
Case-control	Study of exposure/disease relationship in cases with a disease and controls without that disease, who are selected from source population from which the cases arose	Odds ratio	Best for studying rare conditions or those with long latency Short duration Small sample[a] Inexpensive[a] Odds Ratio can approximate Relative Risk	Inefficient for rare exposures Potential bias from sampling cases and controls separately May not be able to determine whether exposure preceded disease Potential recall bias Potential survivor bias Cannot produce prevalence or incidence estimates
Cohort	Individuals without disease are followed during a period of time to determine which characteristics predict who will get the disease and who will not	Incidence Relative risk	Can determine sequence of events Less susceptibility to survivor bias and bias in measuring predictors Can study multiple outcomes Can generate population incidence, relative risk	Frequently requires large samples Not feasible for rare outcomes More expensive Long duration
Prospective	Study sample selected by investigator and followed forward in time for development of disease	Incidence Relative risk	Investigator control over selection of participants and measures	Increased expense Long duration
Retrospective	Study sample and measurement of exposures and disease during a period of time have already occurred	Incidence Relative risk	Less expensive Short duration	Less control over selection of participants and measures
Nested case-control and case-cohort	Case-control study within the context of a prospective or retrospective cohort	Incidence Relative risk	Underlying cohort design Relatively inexpensive, compared to measurement on entire cohort	May require bank of samples that can be assayed at later date until or after outcomes occur
Randomized clinical trial	Exposure (pharmaceutical, nonpharmacologic device, educational intervention) manipulated by investigator	Relative risk Hazard ratio	Most closely emulates an experiment Strongest design to produce evidence for cause and effect Random assignment of intervention minimizes confounding May be faster and cheaper for some study questions than observational studies	Costly in time and money Some research questions not suitable because of rare disease or ethical barriers May not be generalizable if highly controlled environment does not reflect "real world" common practice May have narrow scope and study question
Pragmatic clinical trial	Effectiveness of interventions evaluated in usual clinical practice conditions	Relative risk Hazard ratio	Tests whether intervention works in real-life practice setting Participants more likely to represent most individuals with the condition of interest Results may be more generalizable to clinical care and more relevant to patients than efficacy trial	Participants and providers may be unblinded, so it is important that assessors are blinded to group assignment

[a]Relative to cohort study design.

Modified from Hennekens CH and Buring JE: Epidemiology in medicine, Little Brown and Company, 1987; and Hulley SB, Cummings SR: Designing clinical research: an epidemiologic approach, Williams & Wilkins, 1988.

under study, such as traumatic leg fractures,[1] or to use several control groups selected by different methods.[11] For instance, sample controls might be chosen from hospitalized patients with diseases other than that under study, nonhospitalized patients in the same medical care system, or nonhospitalized individuals in the general population, comparing each control group separately with the diseased group.

Weaknesses of the Case-Control Design

It is not possible to derive incidence or prevalence estimates from a case-control study. The greatest threat to validity is the inherent susceptibility to bias that can exist in this study design because the cases and controls are sampled separately, and the assessment of exposure variables is retrospective.[11] Matching the cases and controls on factors, such as age, sex, or race/ethnicity, can help ensure comparability of cases and controls to a degree. As mentioned earlier, more than one control group, selected in different ways, can be used to see whether findings are consistent across control groups with different sampling biases. A nested case-control design (described later), in which a case-control study is performed within a larger cohort study, has the advantage of minimizing sampling bias because the cases and the controls would have been previously sampled in identical fashion into the parent cohort study.[11]

The other chief source of bias in the case-control study is recall bias, which occurs when exposures predating the disease are differentially reported by the controls and the cases, the latter of whom may have incentive to remember and report exposures. This can be partially prevented by using exposure data measured before the disease occurred, if available, and by blinding the observer and the participant to the exposure under investigation, or if possible, blinding them even to the specific disease under study and therefore, to case or control status. For example, in a case-control study examining racial/ethnic variation as the exposure variable of interest in SLE, race/ethnicity is immutable and thus not subject to recall bias. In contrast, if study participants know or suspect that prior exposure to hair dye, for instance, is the exposure of interest in the same case-control study, those with disease may be more prone to "remember" their exposure than those without disease. Investigators can obtain information about multiple potential exposures or even include several "dummy" exposures to mask the real hypothesis to try to minimize this type of bias, although this likely would only detect the occurrence of such bias, and not necessarily correct for it.[17]

Cohort Studies

Cohort studies follow groups of individuals without the disease in question during a period of time to describe the development or incidence of disease and to compare the incidence of the disease itself, or disease- or exposure-related outcomes between groups with different risk factors or exposures. Cohorts can be prospective or retrospective.[1,11]

Prospective Cohort Study

Prospective cohorts are characterized by the selection of the cohort and measurement of risk factors or exposures before the outcome has occurred, thereby establishing time sequence or temporality, an important factor in determining causality. This design provides a distinct advantage versus the case-control study, in which exposure and disease are assessed simultaneously.

The primary disadvantage to the prospective cohort study is its expense. It requires large numbers of individuals to be followed up, potentially for long periods of time. Biases can creep in, particularly if there is significant loss to follow up. This study design is highly inefficient and inappropriate for study of rare diseases, but its efficiency increases while the frequency of the disease in the population increases.[11] For example, a prospective cohort study would be inappropriate to study PSS because of its rarity but excellent to study a common condition, such as OA.[18,19] A prospective cohort may better allow for the potential that risk factors for disease onset (e.g., incident cases) may differ from risk factors for disease progression among those with prevalent disease. Carefully considering the expected temporal and causal relationships between risk factors, disease onset, and subsequent outcomes is also critical.

Retrospective Cohort Study

In a retrospective cohort study, individuals are followed during a period of time, but the cohort selection and collection of data have already occurred, sometimes for a different purpose than the current disease under study. For example, a cohort of individuals with small vessel vasculitis seen at a particular hospital between 1990 and 1992 could be identified, and data abstracted regarding baseline serologies, physical examination findings, and biopsy results when the patients were first evaluated. Then, examination of outcomes, such as stroke or development of dialysis-dependent renal disease, could be ascertained in 2000, by medical record review or by re-contact with the individuals so identified. Because exposure or risk factor assessment precedes assessment of outcome, this study design can establish temporality, as in a prospective cohort, and is less subject to recall bias that can hinder case-control studies. By selecting the cases and controls from the same source population, this study design also avoids some of the selection biases of case-control studies, in which the cases and controls are sampled separately. The retrospective cohort design is cheaper and more efficient than a prospective cohort, but because the data collection has already occurred, inferences from such a study are highly dependent upon the quality, completeness, and appropriateness of the original risk factor assessments to study their association with the disease in question.[11]

Nested Case-Control, Case-Cohort, and Case-Cohort Studies

These studies are case-noncase studies that occur within the context of a prospective or retrospective cohort, and are particularly useful to assess risk factor variables that would be too expensive to measure among all members of the cohort, such as biologic or genetic measurements.[11] In these designs, all members of a cohort who have experienced a particular outcome during the observation period (cases) are selected and compared with a subset of individuals within that same cohort. Full exposure or risk factor information is then collected. Sampling of these noncases differs between the nested case-control and case-cohort designs. In nested case-control studies, controls are sampled from individuals at risk for the outcome (i.e., they do not yet have the outcome but might have it in the future) at the same time that cases are identified. Controls may be selected to match cases on potential confounding variables (see "Confounding" section later), forming matched sets of cases and controls. In the nested case-control sample (i.e., cases and sampled controls for each case), exposure variables and covariates are then observed. In case-cohort studies, controls are derived from a subcohort sampled from the baseline cohort.[20]

This subcohort is a random sample of the entire cohort, which means that selection of this subcohort is independent of whether or not an individual becomes a case; the subcohort may contain cases by chance. Data on exposures and covariates from the cases and subcohort sample are then collected and observed. Although the analysis is slightly more complicated, a potential benefit of a case-cohort study design is that the same comparison cohort can be used repeatedly to study a variety of outcomes rather than have to select multiple sets of controls (i.e., noncases) unique to each outcome.

Self-Controlled Study Designs

A family of study designs with growing popularity for the study of intermittent exposures are self-controlled methods. These encompass a variety of options, including the case crossover self-controlled case series, case time control studies, and several variants.[21–23] All of these allow a given person to serve as her/his own control, where the question being asked as part of the study hypothesis is not, "why did the event occur in this patient?" but rather, "why did the event occur NOW in this patient?" Various control periods in remote time blocks prior to an exposure or outcome are used to measure risk factor(s) of interest, comparing the occurrence of the risk factor in an at-risk period versus one or more control periods. The principal advantage to these methods is that they effectively control for within-person confounding for time-invariant factors, because individuals are compared only to themselves at a different point in time (earlier or later). A number of assumptions are built in which helpfully are often different than for other study designs such as a cohort study. Importantly, a critical requirement for self-controlled study designs is that exposure must be intermittent, have minimal carryover effect, and ideally, have a short and well-defined latency period between exposure and outcome. For example, the association between acute hypersensitivity events and biologic exposure has been evaluated in rheumatoid arthritis (RA) patients using a case crossover design. This study design was felt to be most suitable given that hypersensitivity reactions were expected to occur within 24 hours of intravenous administration. Rituximab and infliximab were found to have significant higher risks for hypersensitivity reactions compared to IV abatacept.[24]

Clinical Trials

General Principles of Clinical Trial Design

The study designs described previously in this chapter are all observational designs that include no experimental manipulation of the exposure or outcome. Experimental study designs or interventions include clinical trials, field trials, pragmatic trials, and community intervention trials.[13] Inferences from such trials of treatments assigned randomly to a large enough sample are much less likely to suffer from biases and other threats to validity than observational designs. In theory, randomization should eliminate most confounding, although some variation in risk factors between the intervention and control groups may occur by chance. This is more likely if the study size is small, and this possibility should always be ascertained and addressed in the analysis if necessary. The validity of conclusions from a randomized controlled trial (RCT) depends, in part, upon the avoidance of loss to follow up or participant dropout.

RCTs can be conducted for pharmacologic or nonpharmacologic interventions, such as dietary, physical activity, assistive devices, or educational interventions. Trials can include single or multiple dosages of the study intervention; placebo controls; active comparator controls, in which the intervention of interest is compared to another agent where its efficacy is known; and combinations of interventions. For example, the Glucosamine/Chondroitin Arthritis Intervention Trial (GAIT) compared glucosamine hydrochloride alone, chondroitin sulfate alone, the combination of glucosamine and chondroitin with placebo, an active comparator (i.e., celecoxib), for their effects on symptoms of OA of the knee.[25–28] The Intensive Diet and Exercise for Arthritis (IDEA) trial was a nonpharmacologic, rigorous, weight loss intervention in which intensive dietary restriction, exercise, and the combination of diet and exercise were compared.[29] Such nonpharmacologic trials may include an "attention-control," in which the control group does not get the specific intervention of interest, but does get at least a minimal amount of attention from the investigator because it is known that even minimal contact with the participants in a study can improve outcomes.[30] An attention control will also help facilitate subgroup analyses of patients who are more engaged with the intervention and the control arm, albeit who will no longer benefit from randomization. Optimally, to minimize bias, the study should be double-blind, in which the assignment of treatment is unknown to the participant and to the data collector evaluating the participant's response. A cross-over design is a within-patient design which allows each participant to be his/her own control and receive either the active intervention and a subsequent "washout" period, in which no active or inactive treatment is given, and then the control treatment, or vice-versa. This design has some advantages, particularly in sample size requirements, but can be biased if there is a significant carry-over effect of the active treatment into the "control" observation period.[13] Response to treatment may also differ depending upon whether the active treatment is received before or after the placebo or other comparator.[31,32] In circumstances where there is relatively rapid washout of an effect, an n-of-1 trial design might be performed,[33] where patients are randomized to various sequences of treatments over time. This study design has been used successfully in prior studies of nonsteroidal anti-inflammatory drugs (NSAIDs) and paracetamol effectiveness in OA.[34]

Other important considerations in RCTs are the selection and means of assessment of primary and secondary outcomes, which must be pre-specified. Outcomes can include measures of disease modification, symptom modification, and frequency of side-effects or other poor outcomes. Increasingly, both regulatory agencies and consumers of such studies want to see patient-reported outcomes (PROs) (see later). Symptom modification trials are frequently of short duration and less expensive than disease modification trials, which generally are interested in longer-term outcomes. In RCTs of biologics for RA, for instance, effects on symptoms can frequently be measured in weeks to months, whereas effects on prevention or healing of radiographic erosions may require longer follow-up times.[35] Disease modification trials in OA that use radiographs generally require large numbers of individuals followed up for at least 2 years; this is predominantly because responsiveness to change in minimal joint space width is improved in studies of 2 years duration.[36,37] Outcomes based on magnetic resonance imaging exhibit moderate evidence for construct and predictive validity and good evidence for reliability and responsiveness; this likely allows for smaller sample sizes and shorter observation periods to demonstrate an effective response.[38] The Osteoarthritis Research Society International made recommendations to the Federal Drug Administration about study design, imaging modalities of choice, and other issues regarding structure modification in OA in 2011.[38]

Other trial designs can apply interventions to entire communities or to health care workers with measurement of outcome in their patients. An example of the latter would be the Patient and Provider Interventions for Managing Osteoarthritis in Primary Care study,[39] in which patient-specific treatment recommendations for behavioral and clinical treatment of knee and hip OA (e.g., weight management, physical activity) are given to providers at the time of care. The physicians receive the intervention; whether a particular intervention is prescribed, and whether it improves patient symptoms, is measured by assessing the patient. Behavioral interventions often take the form of "quality improvement" studies. Their status as research has in the past been somewhat uncertain, but helpfully, changes to the federal common rule in 2019 allow for simpler informed consent mechanisms for these minimal risk studies.[40]

Although RCTs represent the "ultimate" study design closest to a controlled experiment, there are significant potential threats to its validity. Importantly, not all conditions can be subject to randomization. For example, in studying the association between cigarette smoking and RA, it would be unethical to randomly assign participants to smoking; thus, only observational studies are possible. Another example might be to assess the impact of adherence to a therapy. It is not feasible to randomize patients to be adherent to therapy, and a number of unmeasured factors may co-occur with adherence behaviors.[41] Another challenge of RCTs is that they generally are too short in duration to adequately assess therapeutic safety for many drugs and devices for which longer term outcomes are of public health interest. One of the most important biases can occur when there is large loss to follow-up. To minimize this type of bias, every effort should be made to continue to obtain outcome information on all participants, even those who otherwise discontinue study assignment to therapy. Because all predictors of dropout cannot be known, and because dropouts may differ from individuals who remain in a study in ways that cannot be controlled, conventional analyses of treatment status are likely confounded.[13] Data may be analyzed in an intention-to-treat fashion, in which all randomly assigned participants are analyzed as a member of the group to which they were initially randomized, regardless of whether they actually adhered to the group assignment, but this analytical method can be biased by noncompliance leading to a misclassification of treatment status.[13] One method for dealing with treatment noncompliance, suggested by Mark and Robins,[42] includes making the assigned treatment a fixed covariate and received treatment a time-dependent exposure in a structural failure-time model. Completer, or "according to protocol," analyses are often also performed, in which only those who adhered to their assigned group treatment are included in the analysis. Per protocol analyses are generally not the primary analysis for efficacy in therapeutic trials, but they may be the most important analysis to examine for safety outcomes. Pre-randomization screening and run-in periods before randomization can help to avoid randomly assigning those unlikely to adhere to or complete the protocol, thereby minimizing expense and dilution of effects.[43,44] Other issues to consider in the interpretation of results of RCTs are generalizability and the difference between efficacy in a controlled environment and effectiveness in the real world of everyday practice (see section on pragmatic clinical trials). Post-marketing observations can often reveal side-effects or unintended consequences of interventions that may not be apparent within the context of relatively small, highly regulated trials.

Noninferiority Trials

The most common type of RCT is the superiority trial, in which investigators determine whether a new treatment is more effective than placebo, no treatment, a lower dose of the test treatment, or an established treatment that is widely used or has known effectiveness. Noninferiority trials, on the other hand, are used to determine whether the effect of a new treatment is no worse than a reference treatment.[45–47] This differs from an equivalence trial, which aims to demonstrate that the effect of a new treatment is similar to the effect of the reference treatment.[46]

Designing and interpreting noninferiority trials can be challenging because of several weaknesses of this study compared with superiority trials. Intention-to-treat analysis (a commonly used approach in superiority trials, in which not all participants may have completed the treatment protocol) is not possible in noninferiority trials. Intention-to-treat tends to bias results towards the null (treatment equivalence), which, in a noninferiority trial, would result in an inferior treatment being incorrectly labeled as *noninferior*.[45,46] Thus, a per protocol analysis should generally accompany a more traditional intention-to-treat analysis. Additionally, an inferiority margin must be predetermined, and this margin may be subjectively based on the expectation of a minimally important effect or, more objectively, on the effect of the reference treatment in prior studies.[45,47] For the latter, the assumption is that the effect of the reference treatment in the noninferiority trial is similar to its effect in prior trials, which may not be true if the current and prior trials differ based on critical factors (i.e., study population).[45,46] Several recent examples of noninferiority trials have been recently published in rheumatology, where the noninferiority margin has been specified as the half-width of the difference between an active treatment (e.g., a biologic therapy) and placebo.[48] Another disadvantage of noninferiority trials is that they are often much larger and more expensive than a superiority trial, depending on the noninferiority margin chosen.

Pragmatic and Adaptive Design Clinical Trials

Pragmatic trials evaluate the effectiveness of interventions in usual clinical practice conditions.[49] This study design differs from efficacy trials (Fig. 34.2), which test interventions in ideal conditions among participants meeting strict inclusion and exclusion criteria. A continuum exists between pragmatic and efficacy trial designs,[50] and a purely pragmatic trial design is rare. Efficacy trials examine whether the intervention works among patients with specific demographic and clinical characteristics under certain conditions, whereas pragmatic trials examine whether the intervention works in real-life practice settings in a way that is relevant to the patients and generalizable in routine conditions. Thus, pragmatic trials offer higher external validity, whereas efficacy trials offer higher internal validity. Because exclusion criteria are intentionally less rigorous (e.g., only excluding individuals for whom there are significant safety concerns that preclude study participation), participants selected for pragmatic trials are likely to represent most individuals with the condition or disease of interest. For example, in the Benefits of Effective Exercise for Knee Pain (BEEP) study,[51] the investigators purposely chose to not use radiographic diagnosis of knee OA as a criterion for study inclusion because they wanted study participants to represent patients typically seen in primary care.

Adaptive trial designs can make clinical trials more efficient and less costly by permitting planned changes (established a priori) to the study approach after its initiation.[52] These trial designs were developed for oncology but have expanded to other disease areas,

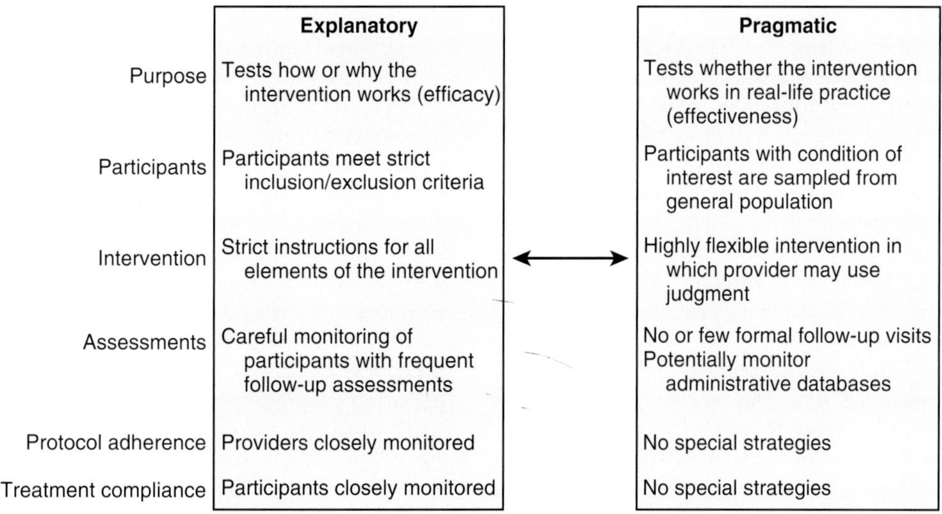

• **Fig. 34.2** Clinical trials: explanatory to pragmatic continuum.

including cardiovascular disease and rheumatology. Often with these designs, the objectives are to reduce sample size, required resources, and costs while maintaining study validity and reliability. Prior to study commencement, the adaptive clinical trial design requires a protocol that describes a series of decision rules for the intervention, including if and when the intervention may be implemented, how to deliver the intervention, and what modifications or adaptations can be made to the intervention (e.g., type, intensity) for a specified participant. These changes may be applied if a participant does not meet a certain response target at an interim time point.[53] Based on interim analyses, ineffective treatments or doses may be promptly discontinued and proportions of participants in treatment arms can be altered. One type of adaptation intervention is Sequential Multiple Assignment Randomized Trial (SMART), which includes multiple stages at which participants are randomized to different treatment components.[54] For example, researchers conducted a two-stage SMART design in a trial of 99 participants with knee OA and subsyndromal depression to compare different sequences of cognitive behavioral therapy (CBT) and physical therapy for prevention of new episodes of depression or anxiety.[55] Stage 1 determined the relative effectiveness of CBT (8 sessions), physical therapy (8 sessions), and usual care. Participants who did not respond to the Stage 1 intervention were randomized to another intervention or were provided with four additional sessions of the intervention they received in Stage 1.

Cluster (Group)-Randomized Implementation Trials

A cluster-randomized implementation trial does not randomly assign at the individual-level, but rather by group (e.g., clinical practices or hospital sites). This type of trial design is especially useful in comparative effectiveness and implementation studies, particularly if the intervention is implemented at the cluster level,[56] such as among teams of health care providers or at a physician level. Also, the cluster-randomized design may help prevent treatment group contamination by separating groups by location or time.[56] For example, a cluster-randomized trial of a behavioral intervention for a treat-to-target approach was conducted in RA patients, and the cluster-randomization was chosen in order to minimize the influence of the intervention on clinician behaviors.[57] However, contamination can occur in cluster-randomized trials if there is spillover of the exposure to treatment and control conditions between the clusters. For example, an educational intervention might be administered at the patient level that aims to "activate" patients in an effort to influence the patient-to-physician communication about effective osteoporosis treatment prescription. Because prescribing occurs by doctors, random assignment is performed at the doctor level and patients are nested within clusters of doctors. If a doctor is randomly assigned to the control cluster, but some of her patients are inadvertently exposed to the educational intervention, this contamination could affect her management of her other patients in the control arm of the study and adversely impact the internal validity of the study findings. To reduce the risk of recruitment bias, participants or recruiters of participants should be blinded to cluster assignment at time of enrollment,[58] or random assignment of clusters can occur after enrollment of groups. Standard approaches to calculating sample size would provide an underestimate. To account for the lack of independence among individuals within the same cluster, the average cluster size and degree of correlation within clusters must be considered and the "design effect" (inflation factor) should be included in sample size calculations, and more patients will be required in such a design.[49] Power is more influenced by the number of clusters rather than the size of the cluster.[59] Furthermore, analytic approaches should account for the unit of analysis (the cluster),[59] such as mixed linear models, hierarchical linear modeling, and generalized estimating equations.

Comparative Effectiveness Research and Patient-Centered Outcomes Research

Although all of the previously mentioned study designs have a role in fostering medical research, their ultimate goals are as follows: to generate new evidence of the efficacy and/or effectiveness of treatments in informing medical decisions to be made by multiple parties (i.e., by clinicians, patients, and caregivers), to reduce health care costs, and to improve outcomes. Comparative effectiveness research (CER) generates evidence on the real-world effectiveness and safety of treatments with the goal of determining which treatment is best for particular groups of people with certain conditions to improve the quality of treatments and outcomes.[60] Systematic reviews and meta-analyses may be conducted in which all results from existing studies are compiled and the benefits and risks of the treatments are evaluated across different populations. Alternatively, new studies may be conducted to examine the effectiveness of treatments, including their benefits, side effects, and costs compared to other available treatments for a given outcome in a specified population. The Institute of Medicine (IOM) Committee on Comparative Effectiveness Research Prioritization selected 100 health topics requiring CER, including OA (musculoskeletal disorders), and rheumatoid and psoriatic arthritis (immune system, connective tissue, and joint disorders), based on the input of public and private stakeholders.[60] For additional information on the national priorities of CER, the IOM's Initial National Priorities on Comparative Effectiveness Research is available at the National Academies Press website (www.nap.edu).

A newer variant of CER is patient-centered outcomes research (PCOR), which was enhanced in the U.S. in 2010 by the creation of the Patient-Centered Outcomes Research Institute (PCORI). PCOR emphasizes the relevance of research questions to patients and encourages their engagement as an active part of the research process, not merely as research participants. One of the prominent goals of PCORI is to harness the power of regional and national electronic health record data systems, along with patient-facing data within 20 patient registries, via the creation of a nationwide CER infrastructure, PCORnet.[61]

Patient-Reported Outcomes

Central to PCOR is measuring the outcomes that matter most to patients. International efforts that are supported and endorsed by organizations, such as United Kingdom's National Institute for Health, and Care Excellence (NICE) and the German Institute for Quality and Efficiency in Health Care (IQWiG),[62] are advancing the promotion of patient engagement to define and improve quality of care criteria for specific conditions, and great strides have occurred in rheumatology around PROs; these are discussed in Chapter 33. Both older PROs, such as the Health Assessment Questionnaire (HAQ) and somewhat newer ones such as Routine Assessment of Patient Index Data (RAPID 3) are critical to the study of many of our disease states. For even newer PROs, the field is moving toward computer adaptive testing (CAT), which uses item response theory (IRT).[63] The principle of this newer form of PROs is to use the response of an initial question to guide the next PRO question. For example, a patient who can run a mile is not asked about their ability to walk two blocks, but is next given survey items selected based on their performance level noted. Population normative data are growing for these approaches, and one initiative called the Patient-Reported Outcomes Information System (PROMIS)[64] and has gained international recognition as a newer state-of-the-art PRO measure. The PROMIS system has been supported by the NIH and evaluated and refined by numerous researchers and is disease agnostic, allowing for cross-comparisons across health conditions. PROMIS encompasses multiple comprehensive health domains that are impacted by chronic illness (e.g., pain and its effect on activity, fatigue, participation in social roles), and scores have been normalized and benchmarked to the general population. Performance of many PROMIS instruments has been tested and has good validity in rheumatic disease populations[65,66] and can be time-saving compared to legacy PRO measures.[67]

Biosensors in Clinical Research

Advances in technology have made way for patient outcomes to now feature biologic data captured using "wearables." Devices popularized by consumer device companies (e.g., Fitbit, Apple) have gained considerable stature in medical research and have also found a foothold in studies of patients with rheumatologic illness where regular measure of physical function, such as step counts and other measures of mobility, energy expenditure, activity, and sleep measurements at night, can provide valuable surrogates of function. The ability to not only passively track activity without the need for patients to repeatedly answer questionnaires over time but also to correlate with clinical measures (e.g., arthritis flare)[68–70] and perhaps even to predict future health events, provides unprecedented opportunities to support medical research and improve care. The data streams available from these devices are often available at a precision of one minute resolution, or even more frequently. Limitations to these devices include the following: a need for typical linkage to portable computing platforms (e.g., smartphone apps, especially third-party apps); the proprietary nature of the device algorithms (e.g., mathematical formulas analyzing activities [e.g., sleep, etc.]; challenges inherent in motivating patients to continue to wear these devices as part of a research study or registry[71]; and interpreting the data streams to derive clinical meaning from them. These issues make the area of wearables and biosensors a promising yet challenging new domain for research methods.

Biases in Study Design

Error in a study may be random (chance) or systematic (bias). Bias can result from errors in the selection of participants, errors in measurement of a variable, or in confounding. Bias may produce an incorrect conclusion about the association between an exposure and disease.

Selection Bias

The procedures used to select participants for a study or factors related to study participation may result in a different exposure-disease association between participants and nonparticipants. Selection bias may occur in any study design but most notably in retrospective or case-control studies where the exposure and outcome both occur before selection of participants. Differential participation may arise in cohort studies or clinical trials with loss to follow-up particularly if participants leave the study for reasons related to the exposure or the disease.

Information and Recall Bias

Errors in the measurement or collection of information may occur. If a variable is measured categorically, information about a participant may be placed in the wrong category, or misclassified. Nondifferential misclassification of an exposure occurs when misclassification is not related to the presence of disease.[1] Misclassification is differential if exposure differs by disease status.[1] Similarly, misclassification of a disease is nondifferential if it does not differ by exposure status; it is differential if it varies by exposure status. Nondifferential misclassification biases an association between exposure and disease towards the null except if the association is the null. Differential misclassification may bias the association in either direction.

In case-control studies, those who are cases may have a different recall of their exposure history than those who are noncases. This difference in recall can introduce a bias that inflates the estimate of an association between exposure and disease. Recall bias is differential misclassification because the exposure is misclassified differently among cases and controls.[1] For example, women who deliver a child with a birth defect may have a much different likelihood to recall medications taken during pregnancy and other potentially harmful exposure. Methods for reducing recall bias include structuring questions to improve recall for both groups, selecting a control group that would be more likely to have good recall of exposure history, or use of information other than contemporary interviews, such as medical records.[1]

Collider Stratification Bias

A variable is considered to be a collider when it is causally associated with two other variables. In causal diagrams, the arrows from the two variables both point towards the collider variable, which differs from a confounder where both arrows point away from the confounding variable. Thus, spurious associations can be created by inappropriately conditioning on a collider during statistical analysis, with stratification, or with selection of a sample. A notable example is conditioning on pre-existing baseline radiographic OA in an observational study of the association of obesity and progression of radiographic OA. In this example, there is a genetic factor that increases the risk of both incident and progressive radiographic OA, but it is not a confounder because it is not associated with obesity prior to development of radiographic OA.[72] Pre-existing baseline radiographic OA likely results from both obesity and the genetic factor; consequently, it is a collider variable. Restricting the study population to individuals with pre-existing baseline radiographic OA (index event) introduces index event bias and leads to an erroneous path between obesity and the genetic factor, although obesity and the genetic factor are not related. This results in a biased estimate of obesity and progression of radiographic OA potentially towards the null. Another example is the false inverse association of smoking and RA progression that results when the study population is restricted to individuals with baseline RA (index event bias).[73] Unknown or unmeasured risk factors (URFs) are not associated with smoking before incident RA; therefore, they are not confounders. However, limiting analyses to only individuals with RA creates a spurious path between smoking and URFs. If smoking appears to be inversely linked with URFs in analyses, the estimate of the association between smoking and RA progression will be towards the null or negative (Fig. 34.3). Strategies to reduce bias include careful consideration through causal diagrams of the time sequence of all variables related to a specified research question, use of incident rather than prevalent exposures, and examination of worsening disease in the full sample rather than progression in a sample restricted to baseline disease.[72,73]

Confounding

Confounding occurs when there is a "mixing of effects" between the exposure, outcome, and a third factor.[74] Specifically, a confounding variable is a risk factor for the disease or outcome; it associates with the main exposure and is not an intermediate step on the casual pathway from exposure to disease.[13] For example, when examining leg length inequality as a risk factor for lower extremity OA in a cohort study, a likely confounding variable would be injury to the lower limb. Injury is a risk factor for OA; it associates with leg length inequality (i.e., a severe injury to a lower limb can result in a shortening of that limb), and it precedes both OA and leg length inequality. Methods used to control confounding include stratifying data by the confounding variable or including the variable as a covariate in multivariable statistical models. Matching may reduce confounding in case-control studies. In experimental studies, random assignment is a strategy to reduce confounding and would be expected to achieve balance in the confounding factor in large samples.

The amount of confounding is an important consideration in determining whether one should control for it in analyses.[13] If the estimate of an association minimally changes after adjusting for a potential confounding variable (e.g., unadjusted OR = 2.62, adjusted OR = 2.58), the inclusion of the variable as a covariate in a multivariable model may not be necessary. However, if the estimate changes profoundly (e.g. >10%, unadjusted OR = 2.62, adjusted OR = 1.05), then methods to control confounding should be used to reduce bias in the association. However, the observation that adjusting for a covariate produces a meaningful difference in an effect estimate like an OR does not necessarily assure that the factor is a confounder; subject matter expertise typically is required to inform this conclusion.

Confounding by Indication and Channeling in Observational Studies of Therapeutics

In observational studies of therapeutics, delivery of treatment is not randomized, and the reason for treatment may be based on risk for the outcome.[75,76] Because risk profiles between treated and comparison groups may differ, results may be biased. Channeling occurs in observational studies when drugs are prescribed (i.e., *channeled*) to patients differently based on prognostic characteristics (e.g., disease activity) or disease severity.[77] Channeling can make study outcomes related to a drug appear better or worse than they truly are, which can incorrectly attribute health benefits or adverse events to the drug. Confounding by indication is a type of channeling bias that occurs when the indication for which a drug is prescribed (drug exposure) is an independent risk factor for the outcome.[75,76] There has been considerable controversy in

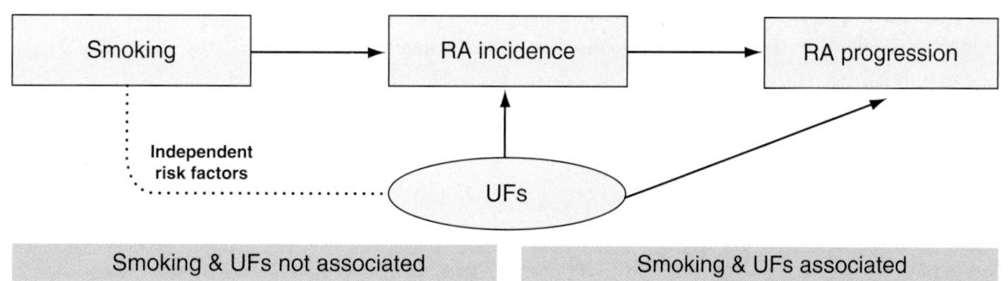

• **Fig. 34.3** Temporal and causal relationship diagram between smoking and unmeasured factors on RA. *RA,* Rheumatoid arthritis; *UFs,* unmeasured factors. (Adapted by permission from Springer Nature: Nature Reviews Rheumatology. Choi, H. et al: *Nat Rev Rheumatol* 10[7]:403–412, 2014.)

RA, for example, about the role of low-dose glucocorticoids and their association with adverse outcomes, such as infections and cardiovascular disease. It is clear that considerable confounding is present by indication or severity around glucocorticoid use, whereby patients with more active/severe RA are more likely to be prescribed glucocorticoids. These same patients, in turn, are also the group most likely to experience an adverse outcome that may or may not be fully attributable to the low-dose glucocorticoid, but instead to their underlying disease state.[78]

Analytic Methods to Address Confounding by Indication

Methods available for accounting for confounding by indication in observational studies include propensity scores, instrumental variables (IVs), and marginal structural models (MSMs). By way of contrast with traditional multivariable models, where covariates are modeled to adjust for their influence on an outcome, a propensity score is the probability that a participant received a treatment (exposure).[79] In a randomized controlled study, the propensity score for each participant should be 0.5 if assignment was determined by a coin toss. In observational studies, the propensity score is unknown and is estimated based on participant characteristics, typically measured at baseline and using prior information. Information collected after the treatment is initiated is generally not used, given that these "downstream" effects are likely to have been influenced by the treatment, so it would be inappropriate to adjust for them because they lie on the causal pathway. The propensity score can be used analytically in different ways to assist with balancing comparison groups to make them analogous. Methods to use propensity scores to control for bias include matching (either 1:1, or variable ratio 1:n matching), weighting (e.g. inverse probability of treatment weighting), or stratification (e.g., typically quintiles, or deciles). In considering propensity score strata, the observational study becomes similar to a randomized block study, in which each block represents a group of participants with the same likelihood of treatment. However, despite common and increasing use of propensity scores in the medical literature over time, propensity scores on expectation balance only measure confounders. Unlike randomization, propensity scores provide no guarantee that unmeasured confounders will be balanced. The suggestion has been proffered, with empiric support, that a set of "high dimensional" data, such as might be found in large administrative health plan claims data sources or electronic health record data, might serve as a proxy for unmeasured confounders and control for confounding better than would be obtained by selecting covariates based on subject matter expertise alone.[80] Both simulations and empiric evidence suggest that high dimensional propensity scores may achieve better control for confounding than traditional propensity scores in certain settings; although, this is not always uniformly the case.[81]

The use of IVs is another approach to control for confounding by indication. The overall goal is to select a factor or instrument that strongly associates with the treatment but has no other independent association with the outcome or possible confounders (co-variates). A variety of instruments in the medical literature have been used, including driving distance to a needed resource, the availability of a particular type of medical service in a community, or physician predilection to prefer certain types of treatments, independent of patient characteristics. Using this instrument to "substitute" for the main exposure variable may achieve better control for confounding and result in less bias. An example in rheumatology is an observational study of the association of cyclo-oxygenase (COX)-2 selective NSAIDs (also known as *coxibs*) with gastrointestinal (GI) bleeding.[82] In this study, the most recent NSAID prescription written by a given physician (to either a traditional nonselective or a coxib) for a prior patient was used as an instrument to adjust for confounding by indication associated with the preferential choice of coxibs for patients at higher risk of GI bleeding. Because instrumental variable methods use a two-stage approach for estimation, the precision of the estimate (i.e., confidence interval widths) are generally wider than using traditional methods. Thus, IV analyses are generally not used for the primary analysis but rather as a secondary or confirmatory approach. Last, an even newer method involves MSMs with inverse probability weighting, which affords a sophisticated analytic approach and partially addresses the issues of time-varying confounding. Although MSM has been used in past studies to evaluate the effects of biologic and glucocorticoid exposure on mortality and other outcomes, the more complicated statistical programming required and challenges in interpreting the results may hinder use of this method for routine analysis.[83,84]

Effect Measure Modification

Two factors are considered to be independent if the combination of their effects is equal to their joint effects. If the effect of one factor depends on the effect of another, effect measure modification exists. This concept is also known as *statistical interaction*. Examining effect measure modification allows researchers to investigate whether the association between exposure and disease differs across subgroups. For example, one study[85] reported a strong association between past history of smoking and RA in men (OR, 2.0; 95% CI, 1.2 to 3.2), but not women (OR, 0.9; 95% CI, 0.6 to 1.3). Upon further exploration, this association was only seen among men with rheumatoid factor-positive RA. If effect measure modification is not considered, results could be biased, or important groups for targeting interventions could be missed.

Screening

Screening is an important public health strategy in reducing morbidity and mortality.[74] Screening tests classify a person who is asymptomatic as likely or unlikely to have the disease. This differs from diagnostic tests, which determine whether a person with signs or symptoms of a disease truly has the disease. If a screening test suggests a high likelihood of disease, then further diagnostic evaluation may occur to confirm disease presence. Although not applicable in all diseases, the early detection of disease when a person is asymptomatic is felt to result in more effective treatment than if disease detection occurs later when symptoms develop with advanced disease.[74] To determine the validity of a screening or diagnostic test, one must establish the sensitivity or specificity of the test. Often, a new test may be compared with a "gold standard" of the definition of a disease, although this standard may not encompass all signs and symptoms of that disease.

Sensitivity

Sensitivity is the probability that a test will correctly classify a case among those who have the disease. This is expressed as a proportion of the number of cases identified by the test as being positive out of the total number of individuals with the disease. In screening, sensitivity is the probability of correctly classifying an

TABLE 34.3 Hypothetical Distribution of Patients by Disease and Test Result

	Disease	No Disease	Total
Positive Test	37	4	41
Negative Test	6	62	68
Total	43	66	109

individual as a detectable, pre-clinical case. For example, if a test correctly provides a positive test result for 37 out of 43 people with disease, the sensitivity of the test is 86% (Table 34.3).

Specificity

Specificity is the probability that a test will correctly classify a noncase. This is expressed as a proportion of the number of individuals without disease identified by the test as being negative out of the total number of individuals without disease. If a test correctly provides a negative test result for 62 out of 66 people without disease, the specificity of the test is 94% (see Table 34.3).

Predictive Value

Predictive values are used to interpret the results of a test by examining the correct classification of individuals according to the test result. This measure is valuable because whether a person is truly a case or noncase may be difficult to know (for determining sensitivity or specificity), but a positive or negative result of a test is known. The positive predictive value is a proportion of the number of true cases identified among all individuals with positive test results. For example, if 37 people truly have disease out of 41 with a positive test result, the positive predictive value is 90% (see Table 34.3). A negative predictive value is a proportion of individuals who are noncases identified among all those with negative test results. If 62 people truly do not have disease out of 68 with a negative test result, the negative predictive value is 94% (see Table 34.3). Unlike the sensitivity and specificity of a test, which generally is considered invariant to the prevalence of the disease in the population, the positive and negative predictive values of a screening test is dependent on the population prevalence. A low prevalence condition will make even a highly specific test have a low positive predictive value. For example, if the prevalence of undiagnosed ankylosing spondylitis (AS) in a population is 0.5% (5 per 1000), then even a reasonably sensitive and specific test such as HLA B27+ (positive in 90% of AS patients and negative in approximately 93% of patients who do not have AS) would result in a positive predictive value of only about 6%.

Conclusion

Epidemiologic methods can be used to measure frequency or development of disease or outcomes and evaluate risk or protective factors in disease occurrence. Choice of study design depends on multiple factors, including the research question, disease under study, availability of appropriate study populations, and resources available. Each study design has its own set of advantages and disadvantages, with the clinical trial considered the most rigorous.

The references for this chapter can also be found on ExpertConsult.com.

References

1. Rothman K: *Epidemiology: an introduction*, New York, 2002, Oxford University Press, Inc.
2. Bradford Hill A: The environment and disease: association or causation ? *Proc R Soc Med* 58:295–300, 1965.
3. Mease PJ, Karki C, Palmer JB, et al.: Clinical characteristics, disease activity, and patient-reported outcomes in psoriatic arthritis patients with dactylitis or enthesitis: results from the corrona psoriatic arthritis/spondyloarthritis registry, *Arthritis Care Res (Hoboken)* 69:1692–1699, 2017.
4. Mease PJ, Karki C, Palmer JB, et al.: Clinical and patient-reported outcomes in patients with psoriatic arthritis (PSA) by body surface area affected by psoriasis: results from the Corrona PsA/Spondyloarthritis Registry, *J Rheumatol* 44:1151–1158, 2017.
5. Papp K, Gottlieb AB, Naldi L, et al.: Safety surveillance for ustekinumab and other psoriasis treatments from the Psoriasis Longitudinal Assessment and Registry (PSOLAR), *J Drugs Dermatol* 14:706–714, 2015.
6. Yazdany J, Bansback N, Clowse M, et al.: Rheumatology informatics system for effectiveness: a national informatics-enabled registry for quality improvement, *Arthritis Care Res (Hoboken)* 68:1866–1873, 2016.
7. Agiro A, Chen X, Eshete B, et al.: Data linkages between patient-powered research networks and health plans: a foundation for collaborative research, *J Am Med Inform Assoc*, 2019.
8. Curtis JR, Chen L, Bharat A, et al.: Linkage of a de-identified United States rheumatoid arthritis registry with administrative data to facilitate comparative effectiveness research, *Arthritis Care Res (Hoboken)* 66:1790–1798, 2014.
9. Li X, Fireman BH, Curtis JR, et al.: Validity of privacy-protecting analytical methods that use only aggregate-level information to conduct multivariable-adjusted analysis in distributed data networks, *Am J Epidemiol* 188:709–723, 2019.
10. Hennekens CH, Buring JE: *Epidemiology in medicine*, Boston-Toronto, 1987, Little Brown and Company.
11. Hulley S, Cummings S: *Designing clinical research*, Philadelphia, 1988, Lippincott Williams & Wilkins.
12. Koepsell T, Weiss N: *Epidemiologic methods: studying the occurrence of illness*, New York, 2003, Oxford University Press.
13. Rothman K, Greenland S: *Modern epidemiology*, Philadelphia, 1998, Lippincott Williams & Wilkins.
14. Rothman K: *Modern epidemiology*, Boston/Toronto, 1986, Little Brown and Company.
15. Ji X, Small DS, Leonard CE, et al.: The Trend-in-trend research design for causal inference, *Epidemiology (Cambridge, Mass)* 28:529–536, 2017.
16. Dillon CF, Rasch EK, Gu Q, et al.: Prevalence of knee osteoarthritis in the United States: arthritis data from the Third National Health and Nutrition Examination Survey 1991-94, *J Rheumatol* 33:2271–2279, 2006.
17. Cooper GS, Dooley MA, Treadwell EL, et al.: Smoking and use of hair treatments in relation to risk of developing systemic lupus erythematosus, *J Rheumatol* 28:2653–2656, 2001.
18. Felson DT, Zhang Y, Hannan MT, et al.: Risk factors for incident radiographic knee osteoarthritis in the elderly: the Framingham Study, *Arthritis Rheum* 40:728–733, 1997.
19. Jordan JM, Helmick CG, Renner JB, et al.: Prevalence of knee symptoms and radiographic and symptomatic knee osteoarthritis in African Americans and Caucasians: the Johnston County Osteoarthritis Project, *J Rheumatol* 34:172–180, 2007.
20. Ganna A, Reilly M, de Faire U, et al.: Risk prediction measures for case-cohort and nested case-control designs: an application to cardiovascular disease, *Am J Epidemiol* 175:715–724, 2012.

21. Consiglio GP, Burden AM, Maclure M, et al.: Case-crossover study design in pharmacoepidemiology: systematic review and recommendations, *Pharmacoepidemiol Drug Saf* 22:1146–1153, 2013.
22. Petersen I, Douglas I, Whitaker H: Self controlled case series methods: an alternative to standard epidemiological study designs, *BMJ* 354:i4515, 2016.
23. Suissa S: The case-time-control design: further assumptions and conditions, *Epidemiology* 9:441–445, 1998.
24. Yun H, Xie F, Beyl RN, et al.: Risk of hypersensitivity to biologic agents among medicare patients with rheumatoid arthritis, *Arthritis Care Res (Hoboken)* 69:1526–1534, 2017.
25. Sawitzke AD, Shi H, Finco MF, et al.: The effect of glucosamine and/or chondroitin sulfate on the progression of knee osteoarthritis: a report from the glucosamine/chondroitin arthritis intervention trial, *Arthritis Rheum* 58:3183–3191, 2008.
26. Clegg DO, Reda DJ, Harris CL, et al.: Glucosamine, chondroitin sulfate, and the two in combination for painful knee osteoarthritis, *N Engl J Med* 354:795–808, 2006.
27. Sawitzke AD, Shi H, Finco MF, et al.: Clinical efficacy and safety of glucosamine, chondroitin sulphate, their combination, celecoxib or placebo taken to treat osteoarthritis of the knee: 2-year results from GAIT, *Ann Rheum Dis* 69:1459–1464, 2010.
28. The NIH Glucosamine/Chondroitin Arthritis Intervention Trial (GAIT), *J Pain Palliat Care Pharmacother* 22:39–43, 2008.
29. Messier SP, Legault C, Mihalko S, et al.: The Intensive Diet and Exercise for Arthritis (IDEA) trial: design and rationale, *BMC Musculoskelet Disord* 10:93, 2009.
30. Rene J, Weinberger M, Mazzuca SA, et al.: Reduction of joint pain in patients with knee osteoarthritis who have received monthly telephone calls from lay personnel and whose medical treatment regimens have remained stable, *Arthritis Rheum* 35:511–515, 1992.
31. Schiff MH, Jaffe JS, Freundlich B: Head-to-head, randomised, crossover study of oral versus subcutaneous methotrexate in patients with rheumatoid arthritis: drug-exposure limitations of oral methotrexate at doses >/=15 mg may be overcome with subcutaneous administration, *Ann Rheum Dis* 73:1549–1551, 2014.
32. Trudeau J, Van Inwegen R, Eaton T, et al.: Assessment of pain and activity using an electronic pain diary and actigraphy device in a randomized, placebo-controlled crossover trial of celecoxib in osteoarthritis of the knee, *Pain Pract* 15:247–255, 2015.
33. Gabler NB, Duan N, Vohra S, et al.: N-of-1 trials in the medical literature: a systematic review, *Med Care* 49:761–768, 2011.
34. Wegman ACM, van der Windt DAWM, de Haan M, et al.: Switching from NSAIDs to paracetamol: a series of n of 1 trials for individual patients with osteoarthritis, *Ann Rheum Dis* 62:1156–1161, 2003.
35. van der Heijde D, Klareskog L, Rodriguez-Valverde V, et al.: Comparison of etanercept and methotrexate, alone and combined, in the treatment of rheumatoid arthritis: two-year clinical and radiographic results from the TEMPO study, a double-blind, randomized trial, *Arthritis Rheum* 54:1063–1074, 2006.
36. Reichmann WM, Maillefert JF, Hunter DJ, et al.: Responsiveness to change and reliability of measurement of radiographic joint space width in osteoarthritis of the knee: a systematic review, *Osteoarthritis Cartilage* 19:550–556, 2011.
37. Brandt KD, Mazzuca SA, Conrozier T, et al.: Which is the best radiographic protocol for a clinical trial of a structure modifying drug in patients with knee osteoarthritis? *J Rheumatol* 29:1308–1320, 2002.
38. Conaghan PG, Hunter DJ, Maillefert JF, et al.: Summary and recommendations of the OARSI FDA osteoarthritis Assessment of Structural Change Working Group, *Osteoarthritis Cartilage* 19:606–610, 2011.
39. Allen KD, Bosworth HB, Chatterjee R, et al.: Clinic variation in recruitment metrics, patient characteristics and treatment use in a randomized clinical trial of osteoarthritis management, *BMC Musculoskelet Disord* 15:413, 2014.
40. U.S. Department of Health and Human Services (HHS): Federal policy for the protection of human subjects: six month delay of the general compliance date of revisions while allowing the use of three burden-reducing provisions during the delay period, *Federal Register* 83(118):28497–28520, 2018.
41. Curtis JR, Larson JC, Delzell E, et al.: Placebo adherence, clinical outcomes, and mortality in the Women's Health initiative randomized hormone therapy trials, *Medical Care* 49:427–435, 2011.
42. Mark SD, Robins JM: A method for the analysis of randomized trials with compliance information: an application to the Multiple Risk Factor Intervention Trial, *Control Clin Trials* 14:79–97, 1993.
43. Brandt KD, Mazzuca SA: Lessons learned from nine clinical trials of disease-modifying osteoarthritis drugs, *Arthritis Rheum* 52:3349–3359, 2005.
44. Brandt KD, Mazzuca SA, Katz BP, et al.: Effects of doxycycline on progression of osteoarthritis: results of a randomized, placebo-controlled, double-blind trial, *Arthritis Rheum* 52:2015–2025, 2005.
45. Piaggio G, Elbourne DR, Altman DG, et al.: Reporting of noninferiority and equivalence randomized trials: an extension of the CONSORT statement, *JAMA* 295:1152–1160, 2006.
46. Snapinn SM: Noninferiority trials, *Curr Control Trials Cardiovasc Med* 1:19–21, 2000.
47. D'Agostino Sr RB, Massaro JM, Sullivan LM: Non-inferiority trials: design concepts and issues—the encounters of academic consultants in statistics, *Stat Med* 22:169–186, 2003.
48. Weinblatt ME, Schiff M, Valente R, et al.: Head-to-head comparison of subcutaneous abatacept versus adalimumab for rheumatoid arthritis: findings of a phase IIIb, multinational, prospective, randomized study, *Arthritis Rheum* 65:28–38, 2013.
49. Friedman L, Furberg C: *Fundamentals of clinical trials*, New York, 2010, Springer.
50. Thorpe KE, Zwarenstein M, Oxman AD, et al.: A pragmatic-explanatory continuum indicator summary (PRECIS): a tool to help trial designers, *J Clin Epidemiol* 62:464–475, 2009.
51. Foster NE, Healey EL, Holden MA, et al.: A multicentre, pragmatic, parallel group, randomised controlled trial to compare the clinical and cost-effectiveness of three physiotherapy-led exercise interventions for knee osteoarthritis in older adults: the BEEP trial protocol (ISRCTN: 93634563), *BMC Musculoskelet Disord* 15:254, 2014.
52. Kairalla JA, Coffey CS, Thomann MA, et al.: Adaptive trial designs: a review of barriers and opportunities, *Trials* 13:145, 2012.
53. Lei H, Nahum-Shani I, Lynch K, et al.: A "SMART" design for building individualized treatment sequences, *Annu Rev Clin Psychol* 8:21–48, 2012.
54. Collins LM, Murphy SA, Strecher V: The multiphase optimization strategy (MOST) and the sequential multiple assignment randomized trial (SMART): new methods for more potent eHealth interventions, *Am J Prev Med* 32:S112–S118, 2007.
55. Karp JF, Dew MA, Wahed AS, et al.: Challenges and solutions for depression prevention research: methodology for a depression prevention trial for older adults with knee arthritis and emotional distress, *Am J Geriatr Psychiatry* 24:433–443, 2016.
56. Hutton JL: Are distinctive ethical principles required for cluster randomized controlled trials? *Stat Med* 20:473–488, 2001.
57. Harrold LR, Reed GW, John A, et al.: Cluster-randomized trial of a behavioral intervention to incorporate a treat-to-target approach to care of us patients with rheumatoid arthritis, *Arthritis Care Res (Hoboken)* 70:379–387, 2018.
58. Allen KD, Bosworth HB, Brock DS, et al.: Patient and provider interventions for managing osteoarthritis in primary care: protocols for two randomized controlled trials, *BMC Musculoskelet Disord* 13:60, 2012.
59. Campbell MK, Piaggio G, Elbourne DR, et al.: Consort 2010 statement: extension to cluster randomised trials, *BMJ* 345:e5661, 2012.
60. Medicine Io: *Initial national priorities for comparative effectiveness research*, Washington, DC, 2009, The National Academies Press.

61. Collins FS, Hudson KL, Briggs JP, et al.: PCORnet: turning a dream into reality, *J Am Med Inform Assoc* 21:576–577, 2014.
62. Doward LC, Gnanasakthy A, Baker MG: Patient reported outcomes: looking beyond the label claim, *Health Qual Life Outcomes* 8:89, 2010.
63. Jette AM, McDonough CM, Ni P, et al.: A functional difficulty and functional pain instrument for hip and knee osteoarthritis, *Arthritis Res Ther* 11:R107-R, 2009.
64. Cella D, Riley W, Stone A, et al.: The Patient-Reported Outcomes Measurement Information System (PROMIS) developed and tested its first wave of adult self-reported health outcome item banks: 2005-2008, *J Clin Epidemiol* 63:1179–1194, 2010.
65. Bingham Iii CO, Gutierrez AK, Butanis A, et al.: PROMIS Fatigue short forms are reliable and valid in adults with rheumatoid arthritis, *J Patient Rep Outcomes* 3:14, 2019.
66. Katz P, Pedro S, Michaud K: Performance of the patient-reported outcomes measurement information system 29-item profile in rheumatoid arthritis, osteoarthritis, fibromyalgia, and systemic lupus erythematosus, *Arthritis Care Res (Hoboken)* 69:1312–1321, 2017.
67. Yun H, Nowell WB, Curtis D, et al: Assessing RA Disease Activity with PROMIS Measures using Digital Technology. *Arthritis Care Res*; 0.
68. Jacquemin C, Molto A, Servy H, et al.: Flares assessed weekly in patients with rheumatoid arthritis or axial spondyloarthritis and relationship with physical activity measured using a connected activity tracker: a 3-month study, *RMD Open* 3:e000434, 2017.
69. Jacquemin C, Servy H, Molto A, et al.: Physical activity assessment using an activity tracker in patients with rheumatoid arthritis and axial spondyloarthritis: prospective observational study, *JMIR Mhealth Uhealth* 6:e1, 2018.
70. Gossec L, Guyard F, Leroy D, et al.: Detection of flares by decrease in physical activity, collected using wearable activity trackers, in rheumatoid arthritis or axial spondyloarthritis: an application of Machine-Learning analyses in rheumatology, *Arthritis Care Res (Hoboken)*, 2018.
71. Nowell WB, Curtis D, Thai M, et al.: Digital interventions to build a patient registry for rheumatology research, *Rheum Dis Clin North Am* 45:173–186, 2019.
72. Zhang Y, Niu J, Felson DT, et al.: Methodologic challenges in studying risk factors for progression of knee osteoarthritis, *Arthritis Care Res* 62:1527–1532, 2010.
73. Choi HK, Nguyen US, Niu J, et al.: Selection bias in rheumatic disease research, *Nat Rev Rheumatol* 10:403–412, 2014.
74. Aschengrau III A: *GRS: essentials of epidemiology in public health*, Sudbury, MA, 2008, Jones and Bartlett Publishers.
75. Signorello LB, McLaughlin JK, Lipworth L, et al.: Confounding by indication in epidemiologic studies of commonly used analgesics, *Am J Ther* 9:199–205, 2002.
76. Salas M, Hotman A, Stricker BH: Confounding by indication: an example of variation in the use of epidemiologic terminology, *Am J Epidemiol* 149:981–983, 1999.
77. Blais L, Ernst P, Suissa S: Confounding by indication and channeling over time: the risks of beta 2-agonists, *Am J Epidemiol* 144:1161–1169, 1996.
78. van Sijl AM, Boers M, Voskuyl AE, et al.: Confounding by indication probably distorts the relationship between steroid use and cardiovascular disease in rheumatoid arthritis: results from a prospective cohort study, *PloS One* 9:e87965-e, 2014.
79. Austin PC: An Introduction to propensity score methods for reducing the effects of confounding in observational studies, *Multivariate Behav Res* 46:399–424, 2011.
80. Schneeweiss S, Rassen JA, Glynn RJ, et al.: High-dimensional propensity score adjustment in studies of treatment effects using health care claims data, *Epidemiology* 20:512–522, 2009.
81. Guertin JR, Rahme E, Dormuth CR, et al.: Head to head comparison of the propensity score and the high-dimensional propensity score matching methods, *BMC Med Res Methodol* 16:22, 2016.
82. Brookhart MA, Wang PS, Solomon DH, et al.: Evaluating short-term drug effects using a physician-specific prescribing preference as an instrumental variable, *Epidemiology* 17:268–275, 2006.
83. Lewis JD, Scott FI, Brensinger CM, et al.: Increased mortality rates with prolonged corticosteroid therapy when compared with antitumor necrosis factor-alpha-directed therapy for inflammatory bowel disease, *Am J Gastroenterol* 113:405–417, 2018.
84. Robins JM, Hernan MA, Brumback B: Marginal structural models and causal inference in epidemiology, *Epidemiology* 11:550–560, 2000.
85. Krishnan E, Sokka T, Hannonen P: Smoking-gender interaction and risk for rheumatoid arthritis, *Arthritis Res Ther* 5:R158–R162, 2003.

35 Economic Impact of Arthritis and Rheumatic Conditions

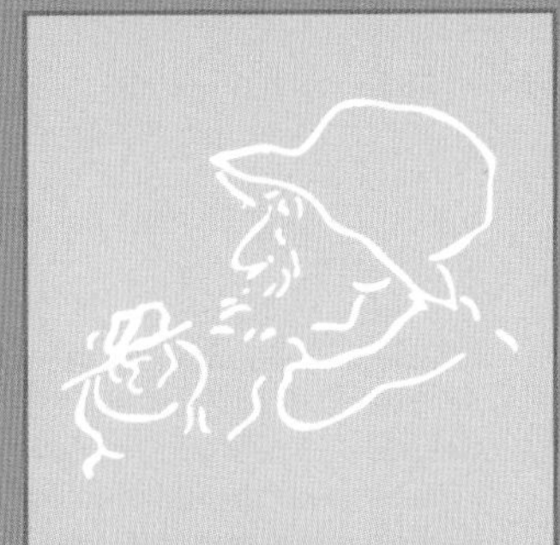

LOUISE B. MURPHY

KEY POINTS

- For conditions with lower mortality rates, such as arthritis and rheumatic conditions, cost-of-illness (COI) estimates can provide evidence on the impact on quality of life.
- COI is reported as direct and indirect costs where direct costs are medical expenditures and indirect costs are lost earnings and other measures of lost productivity.
- In the past two decades, several events have influenced medical costs and earnings losses including introduction of the biologics, increasing utilization of joint replacement surgeries, aging of the population (and corresponding increase in the number of adults with arthritis and other rheumatic conditions).
- The increasing use of biologic agents for rheumatoid arthritis (RA) has led to a rapid increase in the direct costs associated with this condition; costs of these agents alone exceed the total direct and indirect costs of rheumatoid arthritis during the prebiologics era.
- In 2013, total U.S. national direct and indirect all-cause costs for arthritis were $609.8 billion, which was equivalent to almost 4% of the 2013 U.S. Gross Domestic Product, and represented half of the $1.2 trillion national medical expenditures in Medical Expenditure Panel Survey (MEPS).
- In 2013, total arthritis-attributable costs were $304 billion ($140 billion in medical expenditures and $164 billion in earnings losses).
- Comorbidities, which are very common among adults with arthritis and rheumatic conditions, represent a substantial percentage of all-cause costs, especially direct costs.
- Out-of-pocket costs are increasing for adults with arthritis, which could ultimately offset some of the advancements in patient outcomes.

Introduction

Cost-of-illness (COI) studies are conducted to describe the economic impact of medical conditions. Estimates from these studies are used to convey the personal and societal impact of disease. COI is reported as direct and indirect costs where direct costs are medical expenditures and indirect costs are lost earnings and other measures of lost productivity. For conditions with lower mortality rates, such as arthritis and rheumatic conditions, COI estimates can provide evidence on the impact of quality of life.

The COI literature began to grow in the 1960s with the emergence of a new discipline, health economics. Today there is substantial literature on arthritis and rheumatic conditions including specific conditions such as osteoarthritis (OA), rheumatoid arthritis (RA), and systemic lupus erythematosus (SLE). These studies come from various settings and different sources including clinics, described in this chapter, and health systems, administrative records such as billing information, registries, and population-health surveys; the majority of these studies are based on clinic data, and many of these are from tertiary care centers. The convergence of multiple events in the past two decades has influenced direct and indirect costs including introduction of the biologics, increasing utilization of joint replacement surgeries, aging of the population and a corresponding increase in the number of adults with arthritis and other rheumatic conditions, and the Great Recession of 2008-09 and sequelae, where individuals with arthritis were more likely to stop work and less likely to start working than those without arthritis.[1] The evolution in costs of RA because of biologics is particularly striking because current medical total costs are considerably higher than combined medical costs and wage losses during the prebiologic era.[2] While studies of direct costs represent a larger percentage of the COI literature than indirect costs, the latter are an essential component because arthritis and other rheumatic conditions can be highly disabling, leading to premature departure from the workforce and ultimately resulting in substantial annual and lifetime earnings losses.[2]

Health economics integrates the principles and methods of economics with disciplines that measure and improve health such as medicine, social and behavioral science, health policy, and epidemiology. Health economists strive to identify the most efficient, cost-effective, and equitable use of health resources. Theoretically, health care spending ensures that health care resources are allocated equitably and used efficiently.[3] This means that people with similar health status have relatively equal access to evidence-based health care services and that these resources are used efficiently to produce these desired health outcomes. Efficient use of health care resources may increase the likelihood that resources are available to a larger number of individuals.

Equitable access to health resources in the United States is an ongoing focus of health care providers, researchers, and policy

The findings and conclusions in this report are those of the authors and do not necessarily represent the official position of the Centers for Disease Control and Prevention.

makers[4] and has been the impetus for health care reform.[5] In recent years, there has been growing attention to altering cost sharing policies (that is, shifting to consumers paying a greater percentage of health care costs)[6] and resulting effects on access to medical treatments and potential adverse effects.[6] For those with arthritis, there has been attention on interest into access to medications like the biologics, which can be costly.[7] Access to other specialty care, such as joint replacements,[8] and physical or occupational therapy[9] are also of concern.

Estimating COI can be an important step for health economists' deliberations to identify individuals and groups whose health status and outcomes have the greatest personal and societal economic impact and therefore a high need for interventions that are efficient, accessible, and improve their health and wellbeing (Table 35.1). For example, in the United States, federal, state, and local governments provide public health insurance, such as Medicare,[10] which is generally available to all U.S. citizens and permanent residents age ≥ 65 years, and COI estimates specific to payer types may be particularly relevant.[11] High medical expenditures do not necessarily indicate inefficiencies and/or compromised access to care. The underlying assumption of health economists is that health is a good, that is, something that satisfies human wants and provides utility. Analyses such as cost-effectiveness studies examine whether the investment in health through medical expenditures yields evidence-based benefits at a cost that is acceptable to payers, individuals, and society. For example, although medical costs for joint replacements are relatively high, researchers conducting cost effectiveness studies conclude that the economic and quality of life benefits (for example, reduced disability) of this procedure justify this sizeable investment (Table 35.2).[12]

COI estimates from population-based data represent the costs for all individuals in the population. This chapter focuses on population-based estimates (i.e., estimates derived from a nationally representative data source, or from a study representing a defined geographic area such as, for example, estimates from the Rochester Epidemiology Project, which represents all residents in Olmstead County, Minnesota). This chapter describes the economic impact of arthritis and the rheumatic conditions and includes studies from all settings. As demonstrated in this chapter, there are a limited number of population-based studies and considerably more information from other data sources that provide complementary details in interpreting the population-based estimates.

Methods used to generate population-based COI estimates have advanced in recent decades; two important reasons are the increased availability of individual-level data and the development and refinement of statistical methods. One early approach to estimating medical costs, which is still used today, is multiplying disease prevalence by cost estimates from medical records, such as hospital admissions and ambulatory care, for groups of individuals. A corresponding approach for indirect estimates is applying the estimated prevalence of those not working to wages. While there are methodological concerns about this approach, including the potential for double counting of costs,[13] this may be the only option when individual level data are unavailable for estimating economic impact.[14] As Finkelstein and Corso[14] acknowledge: "Even with these shortcomings, carefully documented COI studies are certainly more valuable than the alternative of providing no information on the economic burden associated with particular illnesses and injuries."

Recognizing the limitations in interpreting estimates from group level data, in 1997, the U.S. government began an annual and ongoing survey, the Medical Expenditure Panel Survey (MEPS), which collects extensive individual-level information on a range of

TABLE 35.1 Principal Methods to Assess Costs of Illness

There are two principal methods to assess the costs of illness:
(1) The human capital approach, developed by Dorothy Rice when she was at the U.S. Social Security Administration and later the National Center for Health Statistics,[122,124] and
(2) The willingness-to-pay approach.[125]

The two methods do not differ in the way that they assess the direct costs of medical care. For the indirect costs associated with loss of function and the intangible impacts of disease, the human capital approach uses the market value of the labor to reduce the impacts (e.g., by hiring a replacement worker).

In a variant of the human capital approach called the "friction method,"[126] the losses are estimated from the perspective of the employer and only last until the replacement worker is hired and then achieves the same productivity as the worker who left as a result of disease.

At that point, an employer would be said to incur no additional costs from the onset of the prior incumbent's disease. The willingness-to-pay approach values the loss of function as the amount the affected individual would pay to restore the function, which may be more, the same, or less than the amount it would take to replace the worker in the labor market.

The human capital approach is no doubt more reliable in estimating the economic impact of the lost productivity of affected individuals because the cost of labor is well established in all advanced societies and, therefore, easy to estimate.

The human capital approach, however, usually only enumerates the intangible impacts of disease (e.g., the burden associated with the experience of intense pain), but does not translate them into economic terms. The willingness-to-pay approach is theoretically capable of incorporating all of the costs of disease in those terms, although as a practical matter there are problems associated with attempting to do so.[127]

From Yelin E: Economic burden of rheumatic diseases. In Firestein GS, et al, editors: *Kelley and Firestein's textbook of rheumatology*. Philadelphia, 2017, Elsevier.

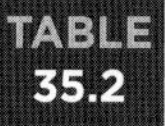

TABLE 35.2 Economic Methods to Assess the Value of Health Interventions

A concise review has been published of the methods to estimate the relationship between health care expenditures and the returns of these expenditures in terms of health-related quality of life, including one of its domains, employment.[128]

When one cannot show that alternative levels of health expenditures will result in improved outcomes, one merely attempts to reduce the wastage of health expenditures, the subject of "cost-minimization studies."

When alternative treatments for a condition are available, one uses "cost-effectiveness analysis," which shows the relative returns from these alternatives in a common natural metric (e.g., longevity).

When one is comparing alternative investments across conditions, one needs an outcome metric that applies to all conditions equally; often the easiest outcome to measure in common terms is the dollar value of lost wages, the subject of "cost-benefit analysis." However, there are inherent problems in translating outcomes into dollar terms.

Accordingly, economists have developed such common metrics as the quality-adjusted life year, which takes into account the value individuals in society place on achieving a common outcome (economists use the term *utility* for these evaluations and the term *cost-utility analysis* for assessing the returns on alternative health expenditures).

Modified from Yelin E: Economic burden of rheumatic diseases. In Firestein GS, et al, editors: *Kelley and Firestein's textbook of rheumatology*. Philadelphia, 2017, Elsevier.

topics including socio-demographic and health status characteristics, all types of health care utilization, measures of access to care, and employment history.[15,16] MEPS allows researchers to generate standardized COI direct and indirect cost estimates for specific conditions at a national and individual level and has become the most frequently used data source for generating population-based direct and indirect cost estimates in the United States. MEPS data are collected systemically from the U.S. population and statistical techniques are used to make estimates representative of the U.S. civilian noninstitutionalized population. The ongoing nature of MEPS allows the calculation of estimates for fairly rare conditions such as RA, because the uniformity of data collected across several years at a time permits analysts to combine multiple years of data to provide sufficient sample size for reliable estimates.[17] Additionally, for some self-reported data such as medications, diagnoses, and insurance coverage, MEPS validates information for at least a subset of respondents, comparing self-reported information with medical and pharmacy records and billing information. Most cost studies, including those based on MEPS, provide estimates of actual costs or expenditures rather than charges; the former is money that was exchanged for a service whereas charges indicate the amount asked for by a health care provider.

The one facet of COI that cannot be examined using MEPS is indirect costs because of premature mortality. For conditions such as inflammatory rheumatic conditions where increased mortality is high,[18–21] describing COI without estimating lost earnings among those who die prematurely may lead to underestimation of costs. However, this underestimation may not occur when considering costs for the overall disease groups of both arthritis and rheumatic condition and musculoskeletal conditions; results from a Canadian study that included estimates of premature mortality in indirect costs found that premature mortality represented only 4% of indirect costs with the remaining costs being long term disability.[22]

COI estimates have been generated from MEPS for arthritis and rheumatic diseases overall and specific conditions such as RA and musculoskeletal conditions.[17,23–26] The focus of this chapter is on arthritis and other rheumatic conditions overall and for specific arthritis types with additional discussion of the economic impact of musculoskeletal conditions.

Cost-of-Illness Studies of Arthritis and the Rheumatic Conditions

Arthritis and Rheumatic Conditions

A series of recent MEPS-based studies of arthritis and rheumatic conditions (also referred to as arthritis) over the past 20 years demonstrate the persistently high direct and indirect costs of arthritis. Of note is that these population-based cost studies, discussed later, used variants of a definition of arthritis and rheumatic diseases that capture individuals with a range of conditions considered arthritis and/or treated by a rheumatologist including OA, RA, SLE, gout, and fibromyalgia.[27] This definition, which appears on many population-health surveys in the United States and internationally, is part of the public health approach to arthritis,[28,29] which strives to complement and extend the benefits of clinical care. That is, individuals identified by this definition could benefit from evidence-based interventions that reduce the adverse effects (such as pain and reduced physical function and mental health) that are common among all types of arthritis; the population health interventions proven to benefit individuals with arthritis are described later in this section.

Direct Costs

In 2013, total national direct all-cause arthritis costs were $609.8 billion, which was equivalent to almost 4% of the 2013 U.S. Gross National Product, and represented half of the $1.2 trillion national medical expenditures in MEPS.[30] In this MEPS study, all-cause costs are the sum of all costs for individuals with a medical condition; for adults with arthritis, they represent total medical costs incurred for all their health care utilization, regardless of cause. Separate from all-cause estimates are "condition-attributable," which for adults with arthritis, represent the specific costs attributable to arthritis and are interpreted as the dollar amount that could be averted if the condition was prevented. In 2013, approximately a fifth of direct costs incurred by adults with arthritis ($139.8 billion) was attributable to arthritis. Three in four U.S. adults with arthritis also report 1 or more other chronic conditions, and a substantial portion of the remaining all-cause costs is attributable to comorbidities.[30]

Total national all-cause costs for adults with arthritis increased by approximately 10% from 2008 to 2014 whereas total national arthritis-attributable costs rose but then dropped to 2008 levels.[31] The rise in the number of adults with arthritis from 56.1 million in 2008 to 65.1 million in 2014 largely accounts for increases; in 2014, there were 9 million more people with arthritis in the general population whereas both average per person total all-cause and arthritis-attributable costs fell by 5% and 36%, respectively, in the same period. The important role of the increasing number of adults with arthritis and costs observed in this study is consistent with two earlier studies comparing trends in costs among adults with arthritis.[32,33]

Across time and studies, the largest portion of both all-cause and arthritis-attributable medical expenditures across health care utilization categories is for ambulatory care services, representing from a third to a half of medical expenditures.[27,31–34] Since 2002, medication costs have risen to the second-most expensive arthritis-attributable costs, where average per person costs are $500[30,31]; in 1997, before the 1998 commercial release of the first biologic etanercept, medications accounted for the smallest portion of arthritis-attributable expenditures.[34] In both 2013 and 2014, arthritis-attributable inpatient costs were third-most expensive, followed by costs for other services (emergency room visits, home health care, vision and dental care, and medical devices).

Attributable estimates can also be generated for the underlying reasons for the costs, such as pain or functional limitations. For example, an analysis of direct costs among adults with arthritis or joint pain in the 2011 MEPS found that functional limitations accounted for almost a quarter of medical costs of average per person costs ($1,638 of $6,773), suggesting that preventing functional limitations would reduce medical costs.[35] Preventing and reducing functional limitations are fundamental objectives of health care providers when treating arthritis and other rheumatic conditions and also for arthritis public health investigators who, based on the public health approach to arthritis, recommend low-cost and evidence-based public health interventions such as weight loss/control, regular physical activity, and participation in self-management education programs.[28,29] Benefits of these interventions, which have been evaluated among adults with several types of arthritis and rheumatic conditions including those in the definition, include reduced pain and improved physical function and mental health.[36–40] These evidence-based self-management interventions, developed for individuals with a range of chronic conditions, improve outcomes for other chronic conditions (for example, reduced shortness of breath among individuals with asthma and chronic obstructive pulmonary disease).[39] Nevertheless, despite evidence that these programs result in substantial improvements in quality of life, to date, there is no evidence that they result in reduced direct and indirect costs.

Cost Sharing

Both payers and adults with arthritis bear the medical costs of adults with arthritis: In 2014, on average, each person with arthritis paid $1,099 in out-of-pocket medical expenses, which was almost double that for those without arthritis ($531).[31] Cost-sharing can have unintended consequences. A Canadian study, comprising poor and elderly adults, examined health outcomes before and after the implementation of a medication cost sharing policy.[9] Rates of serious adverse event and emergency room visits increased as out-of-pocket expenses. These adverse outcomes were associated with self-rationing of medications (for example, took them less frequently than prescribed or bought only the medications they could afford, which were not necessarily their essential medications). The reduced access that may come with cost-sharing has been recognized by professional organizations such as the American College of Rheumatology, which, in its Position Statement on Patient Access to Biologics, advocates against excessive coinsurance to ensure equitable access to these medications.[41] In the United States (2009-2011), among all U.S. adults with arthritis, one in seven reported that they were unable to afford prescription medications because of costs.[42]

Indirect Costs

In 2013, arthritis-attributable earnings losses averaged $4,040 per person and $163.7 billion nationally; an estimated 9.4 million adults with arthritis age 18 to 64 years were not working. Total national indirect arthritis-attributable costs now represent a higher percentage of total national arthritis-attributable costs compared with previous estimates; in 2013, they represented 54% of total national arthritis-attributable costs compared with 41% and 42% in 1997 and 2003, respectively.[30,33,34] The difference in the percentage of adults with arthritis working in 1997 compared with 2013 increased (in 1997 and 2003, the difference was 11 and 14 percentage points, respectively).[30,34] Some of this increase may be attributable to the lingering effects of the 2008-09 Great Recession. That is, compared with those without arthritis, adults with arthritis were less likely to return to work as the economy began bouncing back after this recession[1]; following the recession, it took several years for employment rates in the general population to rebound,[44] and return to work may have been even slower for adults with arthritis who can be susceptible to the phenomenon of "last hired and first fired."[45] Early intervention, such as job accommodations, which are legally required in the United States under the Americans with Disabilities Act, and improved job management (for example, reduced pace, reducing hours worked) may be a promising strategy for keeping individuals with arthritis in the workforce.[46]

Musculoskeletal Conditions

The disease grouping musculoskeletal conditions includes osteoporosis, spine disorders, injuries, and arthritis and other rheumatic diseases. The growing economic impact of musculoskeletal conditions in the United States and throughout the world, especially in mid- to low-income nations, is well documented.[25,47] The Global Burden of Disease study estimated that worldwide, in 2016, 1.3 billion individuals had a musculoskeletal condition, and these conditions were the leading cause of disability worldwide and annually, account for 138 billion years disability-adjusted life years.[48] In 2012 to 2014, direct and indirect costs for musculoskeletal conditions represented 5.8% (2014 dollars) of the U.S. Gross Domestic Product (GDP), which was an increase of approximately two percentage points from the mid- to late-1990s, when it represented 3.4% of the GDP (1996-1998).[25] Nonarthritis musculoskeletal conditions are costly and very common among adults with arthritis.[49–51]

In the 2012 to 2014 MEPS, each year, an estimated 108 million U.S. adults reported a musculoskeletal condition. Annual average per person all-cause medical expenditures were $8,206 for a national total of $882.5 billion.[25] Medical costs attributable to musculoskeletal conditions represented 18%, or $162.4 billion, of all-cause costs. Both national all-cause and MSK-attributable medical costs have been rising steadily and, like arthritis, this reflects a growing number of individuals with these conditions. For example, whereas average per person MSK-attributable medical costs have decreased over time ($2,243 in 2008-2010 compared with $1,510 in 2012-2014), the number of adults age 18 years and older with MSK conditions rose by 6.4 million in this time period from 101.1 million in 2008-2010 to 107.5 million in 2012-2014. Interestingly, the slight decrease in all-cause musculoskeletal medical costs among adults with arthritis in this time period was the biggest reason why all-cause per person medical costs declined in this time period, and these decreases offset increases in cost for the other four condition groups (osteoporosis, spine disorders, injuries, and other MSK conditions). Across these condition groups, in 2012 to 2014, annual average costs per person were highest for osteoporosis (~$13,000) and lowest for those with injuries (~$8,000).

Similar to arthritis, across the four health care utilization categories examined, ambulatory care accounted for the largest percentage of both all-cause and MSK-attributable medical costs; in 2012 to 2014, it represented 34% and 50% of total all-cause and MSK-attributable national direct costs, respectively.[25] For MSK conditions, the second-most expensive category was inpatient care, accounting for 27% of costs. Prescriptions were third (24%), followed by other costs (15%), which includes emergency room visits, dental and vision care, and home health care. For MSK-attributable costs, national costs for each of the non-ambulatory care groups represented a similar portion of costs (15% to 29%).

All-cause indirect costs for musculoskeletal conditions represented only 10% ($97.5 billion) of total all-cause direct and indirect costs ($980 billion). Unlike other conditions reported in this chapter, average per person earnings losses attributable to MSK conditions were higher than the all-cause earnings losses ($2,432 and $1,490). One group[25] notes that "persons with musculoskeletal conditions experience a greater loss of wages than would be expected based on their characteristics other than work history."

International Estimates of Musculoskeletal Conditions, Including Arthritis and Rheumatic Conditions

Studies on the economic impact of arthritis and other musculoskeletal conditions have been conducted in several nations including Australia,[52] Canada,[22,53] the Netherlands,[54] the United Kingdom,[13] and Sweden.[55] The methods for these population-based studies differ from those used in the MEPS analyses described above, and these studies' findings complement knowledge about economic impact gained from U.S. studies.

One challenge in comparing costs for arthritis with other chronic conditions is that methods used to estimate costs can differ substantially, rendering studies incomparable. However, a study in the Netherlands used similar methods across disease groups and found that musculoskeletal conditions ranked second among all major diagnostic groups in medical costs, exceeding coronary and other circulatory conditions and only being eclipsed by "mental retardation."[54]

Whereas many indirect cost studies present estimates of lost wages, two Canadian and a United Kingdom study demonstrate the importance of estimating costs of long-term disability and lost productivity. In the first Canadian study, using 2000 data (in 2008 Canadian dollars), all-cause direct and indirect costs for arthritis were $7.7 billion dollars, which represented 29% of total all-cause costs for musculoskeletal disease ($22.3 billion); the latter represented approximately 2.9% of Canada's Gross National Product ($748,998 million) in 2000.[22,22a] For arthritis all-cause costs, indirect costs—represented by long-term disability ($4,969 billion) and premature mortality ($213.6 million)—were considerably greater than the direct costs for arthritis, suggesting that not including the costs of long-term disability and premature death can lead to underestimated population-level costs. The second Canadian study estimated that the productivity losses arising from unemployment, reduced performance, and occupational changes at work were, on average, $11,553 (Canadian dollars for year 2000) for each person with arthritis.[56] The United Kingdom study examining annual arthritis costs (reported in 2008) found that total all-cause arthritis costs (i.e., OA and RA combined) were £30.7 billion; direct costs represented 20% (6.1 billion); indirect costs were £14.8 billion (including costs of being unable to work, absenteeism, reduced productivity, and informal caretakers); and quality of life costs (that is, the value of healthy life lost) were £9.8 billion and represented 32%.[13] It is noted in an earlier section of this chapter that health spending in the United States is considerably higher than that in other nations, which may account for some of the much lower ratio of indirect to direct estimates in the United States compared with these international analyses; nevertheless, including additional measures of indirect costs that reflect disability, lost productivity, and costs of informal caretakers in future population-based U.S. studies will provide additional insights on the high impact of arthritis and other musculoskeletal conditions on society.

The demographic structure of developed nations represented in these studies is similar; many developed countries have projected a pandemic of arthritis and other musculoskeletal disease, and evidence from epidemiologic studies in the United States and Canada suggests that these projections are being realized.[57,57a,58,58a] Projections have been used to estimate future costs; for example, a recent Australian study projected a 38% increase in health care costs from 2015 to 2030 corresponding with the projected increase in the number of adults with arthritis in this period ($5.5 billion in 2015 and estimated to rise to $7.6 billion by 2030).[52]

Rising prevalence of physical inactivity may have a role in increased costs of arthritis and other musculoskeletal conditions. For example, obesity is a risk factor for several types of arthritis and other musculoskeletal conditions and may increase the number of individuals with these conditions.[59,60] It is also a risk factor for joint replacements, which are costly,[61] and it, as well as physical inactivity, increase risk of costly comorbidities such as diabetes, heart disease, and cancer.[62] To the author's knowledge, there are no conclusive studies linking costs to increases in these risk factors, to date.

Cost of Specific Arthritis Types

Across specific types of arthritis and rheumatic conditions, the first COI studies were conducted for RA, and this condition continues to be studied extensively especially with the introduction of the biologics. However, there is sizable literature on the economic impact of SLE and OA, and at least a few studies on the costs associated with ankylosing spondylitis, psoriatic arthritis (PsA), gout, and fibromyalgia.

Rheumatoid Arthritis

The literature on costs of RA is substantial, reflecting costs from a range of perspectives (individual with the condition, the share of total costs paid out-of-pocket; payer, share paid by health insurance plans or national health insurance; and society, focusing on total resources devoted to health care for the condition, independent of who pays for those resources, as well as productivity losses), time since diagnosis (that is, prevalent or incident cases), and the effects of specific treatments including the biologic agents.[63–70]

In studies prior to introduction of biologics, which typically included prevalent cases (mostly those with longstanding disease), average direct costs in most studies ranged from $5,000 to $7,000 per year; indirect costs were, on average, two and three times more. Although, hospital admissions among those with RA were uncommon (<10%), approximately two-thirds of direct costs were for hospital admissions; surgical interventions, mostly joint replacements, were the primary reason for these costs.

In the prebiologic era, medical costs were generally low among those with RA who were not hospitalized. In 1995, one study found the average cost for most people was $5,919 per year and the median costs was $2,715; however, a small percentage of individuals in this study incurred considerable expenses (90th and 95th percentiles were >$8,000 and >$30,000, respectively).[71]

Indirect costs were considerably higher than direct costs with the high frequency of work disability (prevalence ranging from 34% to 59% across studies) being a driver of this.[72] Studies across several countries show that work disability can occur soon after symptom onset: 20% to 70% of individuals with RA were work disabled within 5 to 10 years of symptom onset (50% of individuals become work disabled after 4.5 to 22 years).[73] Individuals with RA may be at risk for living in poverty. One study of individuals with RA age 55 to 64 years found that compared with those still in the workforce, the median household incomes of those who had retired prematurely was $20,000 less ($50,000 and $30,000) and that early retirees were more likely than their working peers to have household incomes below the poverty line (11% and 2%).[74]

Whereas historically, indirect costs were higher than direct costs, now medical care expenditures for RA for biologic agents alone are greater than the total direct and indirect costs reported in prebiologic studies. MEPS provides important population-based estimates to complement knowledge from clinic-based studies. A recent population-based study of current medical expenditures and earnings losses associated with arthritis demonstrates the direct to indirect cost ratio.[17] In the 2008 to 2012 MEPS, annual national all-cause direct and indirect medical expenditures were $46 billion; of this, $32.6 billion were medical expenditures and $13.1 billion were lost earnings.[17] This ratio, albeit smaller, persisted for the RA-attributable direct to indirect costs ($13.8 and $7.9 billion, respectively).

In this MEPS study, where annual per person all-cause direct costs $19,040, the most notable gradient in average per person all-cause direct costs among adults with RA was for educational attainment where expenditures rose with increasing education levels; there was a $9,000 difference between those with less than a high school education ($16,527) and with a college degree ($25,526).[17]

Employment differences remain an important concern for adults with arthritis; among adults with RA of working age (18 to 64 years), there was an approximately 30 percentage point difference in annual working prevalence: 56.1% and 87.9% among those with and without RA, respectively.[17] Each year, those with RA earned, on average, approximately $15,000 less than those without RA.

An advantage of this population-based study is that it included individuals with RA across a range of disease severity whereas studies of individuals from tertiary care centers or health plans may not include those with less severe rheumatoid arthritis. Of note is that even for extremely large population-based studies such as MEPS (for example, in 2016, data were collected from more than 33,000 children and adults), it is typically not possible to generate accurate and reliable estimates for some conditions because there is an insufficient number of people with the condition. However, because MEPS is an ongoing survey with consistent data collection methods for the past decade, the study authors were able to generate annual estimates using 2008 to 2012 MEPS data. An important consideration for interpreting many RA costs studies is how individuals with RA are identified; for conditions such as RA, when clinical diagnostic information is unavailable (such as self-report surveys and administrative data), typically analysts use an algorithm to identify those who are most likely to have the condition. In contrast, in the MEPS study described immediately above, survey respondents meeting the following criteria were classified as having RA: self-reported ever having RA and at least five prescriptions or ambulatory care visits associated with RA.

These MEPS-based estimates illustrate the substantial economic impact of this rare disease but with the limited population-based estimates available, other data sources help to deconstruct these estimates. In the early 2000s, in some RA patient groups, nearly a half received[75]; considering annual initiation rates of biologics among adults with RA covered by public and private insurers, it has been suggested that current prevalence of use may be currently at least this high.[76] Several studies have described the costs for, or costs that are attributable to, biologics; one study reported annual per person costs of biologics (i.e., etanercept, adalimumab, and infliximab) of $26,000, although other studies have presented lower costs.[77] A recent meta-analysis examining total direct medical costs reported that total medical costs for RA patients taking biologics were almost three times those of all RA patients ($36,053 and $12,509),[67] a pattern that was reported very soon after the introduction of biologic use.[78] A relatively early study in the biologic era projected the potential impact of the biologics on the Danish health care service would raise national medical costs by 50% to 500%.[79] Currently, biologics represent 38% of U.S. prescription spending, and account for 70% of drug spending growth from 2010 to 2015.[80]

The lower costs of biosimilars are projected to slow the increase in medication costs and reduce biologic spending by $54 billion from 2017 to 2026.[80,81] Findings from an analysis of 2017 Medicare Part D data suggest that for biosimilars may not produce costs savings for Medicare Part D beneficiaries, given the structure and cost-sharing elements of these plans.[82] This study compared total and out-of-pocket costs of a biologic and biosimilar treatment for RA (infliximab and infliximab-dyyb, respectively), based on a standard 2017 Part D benefit. In that year, Medicare Part D beneficiaries had a deductible ($400), after which they transitioned to a phase where they had coverage to $3,700 (they were responsible for 25% of costs). Once individuals reached the upper limit of this coverage, they moved into a gap phase where they assumed a higher level of cost sharing; whereas biosimilars were less expensive than biologics, the percentage of costs that individuals had to cover was less for the biologics than for biosimilars (40% and 51%). Additionally, the manufacturer's coupon (50%) could not be applied to biosimilars, unlike biologics. Ultimately individuals assumed higher levels of out-of-pocket expenses for biosimilars than biologics. This analysis suggests that without the benefits of gap discounts, projected annual out-of-pocket cost for one biosimilar (infliximab-dyyb) is higher than infliximab ($5,118 and $3,432, respectively).

Although medical management of RA has changed dramatically in the past two decades, work issues are still common and start soon after disease onset, leading to corresponding high indirect costs. In addition to lost earnings, costs of absenteeism are high.[83] There is equivocal evidence that increased use of biologics corresponds with reduced work disability, absenteeism (missed days from work), especially for those with early RA, and presenteeism (ill health at work), but many of the previous employment patterns, reported before and in the early days of the biologics, are still applicable.[46,83,84] For example, a 2001 study showed that indirect costs for absenteeism were highest in the first 3 years of disease and then declined, but ultimately indirect costs, because of work disability, offset some of the reduced costs from absenteeism.[84]

The high costs of medical care associated with RA have implications for patient level treatment decisions and for payers. Studies, including those examining the cost-effectiveness of biologics demonstrate that individuals taking biologics have reduced disability and improved quality of life.[85,85a] It is plausible that biologic initiation for all who need them can reduce costs, by decreasing the need for other costly utilizations such as medical costs for joint replacements, and indirect costs from lost wages. To date, there is inconclusive evidence whether increases in biologic use have led to decreases in joint replacements for RA and work disability. For work disability, it is unclear whether this change is an artifact of the simultaneous increase in biologics and recovery from the 2008 Great Recession.[1] The cost-effectiveness literature has grown, and across cost-effectiveness studies, conclusions are mixed about biologics. A recent systematic review of cost-effectiveness studies highlights an important issue when interpreting these cost-effectiveness studies[85]: The criteria used to determine cost-effectiveness, incremental cost-effectiveness ratio (ICER), differs across countries and jurisdictions or may not be used (for example, the U.S. Patient Protection and Affordable Care Act does not permit use of ICERs because of concerns that they lead to government rationing of high health care costs.[5,86] One group[85] concludes that whether biologics are cost-effective is ultimately determined by the threshold of the ICER being used.

Systemic Lupus Erythematosus

Whereas the first studies examining the costs of RA emerged in the mid-1970s, studies examining costs of SLE appeared two decades later. Now, there is substantial literature spanning multiple continents extending the literature beyond studies of undifferentiated SLE to the impact of levels of disease activity[87] and organ manifestations[88–90] on direct and indirect costs. For medical costs, organ involvement, especially renal failure, and neuropsychiatric impairment, lead to high direct costs because of hospitalization.[91]

Before the introduction of biologics for the treatment of RA, direct costs for SLE were slightly higher than for RA, but those with SLE incurred less inpatient costs.[88–91] For those with SLE, average medical care costs were about $7,000 per year with a range from slightly more than $4,000 to just under $14,000. On average, hospitalizations accounted for considerably less than half of direct costs, despite high inpatient costs for the small percentage who were admitted, whereas medications accounted for about a quarter. Costs of ambulatory care and medications were of the same magnitude.

An international study conducted two decades ago, which remains instructive, examined patterns in costs for three countries, the United States, the United Kingdom, and Canada.[92] To ensure that prices for services did not affect their estimates, the authors used the same unit prices for each country. Costs of SLE in Canada and the United Kingdom were of similar magnitude, but both were about 10% to 15% less than in the United States. This extra level of expenditure in the United States did not result in better outcomes.

Across studies examining how specific levels of disease activity and specific organ manifestations affect direct and indirect costs, it is evident that lupus nephritis is highly influential. Other factors associated with higher costs include renal damage, neuropsychiatric manifestations including memory impairment, and global measures of disease activity and severity and disease flare. For example, in one study, SLE patients experiencing flares incurred twice the total costs of SLE as those without flares; those with renal or neuropsychiatric flares had the highest levels of costs.[91] In another, higher severity was associated with increased utilization and costs for many aspects of clinical care, such as greater medication use (specifically, corticosteroids, immunosuppressants, and antihypertensives) and more frequent specialist and emergency room visits and hospitalizations.[93] Effective treatment to prevent damage accrual to specific organs or to reduce the frequency and severity of flares may result in a substantial reduction in the costs of SLE. SLE direct costs may rise in coming years because of biologics, although the effectiveness of the biologics for treating SLE is challenged by the clinical heterogeneity of this condition.[94,95] Currently, existing biologics are also being used to treat SLE; with the exception of one, belimumab, these biologics are being used off-label.[96,97] Additional biologics targeted to SLE are in development.

Indirect costs have been measured using more heterogeneous methods than for direct costs, but for studies with similar methods, indirect costs exceed direct costs by an average of about 2:1.[98] Indirect costs are high in SLE due to high rates of employment loss; among those employed at disease onset, an estimated 15% may be unemployed within the first 5 years of diagnosis, 40% within the first decade, and 63% within the first two decades.[99] These rates of work loss are worthy of concern; an additional contributor to poor labor outcomes for people with SLE is that the presence of fatigue, pain, and neurocognitive deficits may mask detection of other diseases with similar symptoms.[100]

Work loss costs can be substantial for individuals with SLE because the age of SLE onset is, on average, 10 years younger for SLE compared with RA and there are high levels of temporary or permanent work loss among those with SLE.[100,101] Similar to direct costs, indirect costs rise with severity of disease manifestations.[101] Flares are an important predictor of both increased frequency and duration in absence from work. The unpredictability of the disease can influence ability to return to work and poor mental health outcomes are more common among those who aren't working. Because lupus can strike at such a young age, it can limit educational attainment and in turn, lifelong employment and income trajectories, ultimately diminishing ability to acquire assets for retirement.[101] To date, the economic impact from recent gains in survival has not been examined.

Connective Tissue Disease (Including Systemic Lupus Erythematosus)

Recent United States all-cause direct estimates for connective tissue disease, from the 2008 to 2014 MEPS, were $15.8 billion (average cost per person was $19,702).[24] Across all those with connective tissue disease, ambulatory care represented a third of these costs, followed by inpatient care (28%), prescriptions (25%), and other costs (15%) including emergency room visits, home health care, and vision and dental. Access to care is a substantial issue for SLE and delays can have critical implications for disease outcomes; in this study, groups with the lowest average costs per person were those with no health insurance ($5,631) and non-Hispanic blacks ($14,564). In previous studies, the uninsured and non-Hispanic blacks with SLE received poorer quality of care and had higher rates of poor outcomes such as pregnancy failures, organ failure, and premature mortality.[102–105]

In the MEPS based study described above, the authors examined individuals with connective tissue disease (ICD-9-CM 710) because the condition is so rare, and even after combining 7 years of data for those with SLE (ICD-9-CM 710.0), there was an insufficient sample size to generate statistically reliable estimates; in fact, they were unable to generate earnings loss estimates for connective tissue disease because of the small sample size when restricted to working age adults.[24]

Osteoarthritis

There are limited population-based studies of the economic impact of OA. Nevertheless it is evident that with increased joint replacement utilization, for which OA is the most common indication, that each year, OA accounts for an increasingly larger portion of overall health care utilization and costs in the United States and internationally. In the United States, hospitalizations for joint replacements rose almost fourfold from 1993 (323,804 discharges) to 2016 (1,205,651 discharges), and in 2013, OA was the second-most expensive condition treated in U.S. hospitals (hospitalization costs were $16.5 billion).[106,107] These hospitalizations were costly for both private and public payers as it was the most expensive source of hospitalization costs for private insurers and the second-most for Medicare.[106,107] In the 1990s, most joint replacement costs were borne by Medicare because older adults (≥65 years) accounted for almost all joint replacement utilization, but the increased utilization among middle age adults (45 to 64 years) has resulted in increased costs for private payers.[108]

While joint replacements are an important component of OA costs, pain and comorbidities are strongly associated with both direct and indirect OA costs.[51,109] In the United States, annual all-cause medical expenditures and earnings losses were $486.4 billion among the estimated 32.5 million United States adults with OA in 2008 to 2014.[26] At $136.8 billion, total national direct and indirect costs attributable to OA were approximately a quarter of all-cause costs.

Direct costs ($373.2 billion), calculated for all adults age 18 years and older, represented three-quarters (77%) of the all-cause direct and indirect costs among adults with OA ($486.4 billion).[26] Average direct costs for each adult with OA were $11,502 with a strong age gradient in average per person costs ($7,988 among younger adults [ages 18 to 44 years] to $12,714 among older adults [ages ≥65 years]). Across all age groups, average per person medical costs were highest among those with any limitation in work, school, or housework ($17,136).

For OA-attributable costs, total indirect national costs ($71.3 billion; average per person = $4,274) were slightly higher than total direct national costs ($65.5 billion; average per person = $2,018). Furthermore, whereas total national OA-attributable direct costs represented approximately 18% of all-cause costs, total national OA-attributable indirect costs comprised 63% of all-cause indirect costs. The substantial difference in all-cause and attributable direct costs overall is largely because of statistical adjustment for the costs of comorbidities; the smaller difference between all-cause and OA-attributable indirect costs, which were calculated among working age adults, is because they likely have fewer comorbidities. The national indirect all-cause costs for OA ($113.2 billion), calculated for adults age 18 to 64 years, were considerably lower because only half of all adults with OA are of the traditional working age.

A notable problem when using self-reported diagnostic information in surveys such as MEPS can be inaccuracy of self-reported diagnosis; self-reported OA is one such example because multiple studies, including those using MEPS data, show that accuracy of self-reported OA is low. For example, in one MEPS study, only 10% of people who had been diagnosed with OA (ICD-9-CM 715) reported having it.[109a] For this reason, individuals with OA in the MEPS study immediately above were identified with an algorithm that accounted for potential errors in self-reporting. One component of this algorithm was exclusion of individuals who reported that they had ever been diagnosed with RA because frequently, individuals with OA erroneously self-report RA instead of OA. For this reason, COI studies using only self-reported OA status to ascertain individuals with OA may be biased towards underreporting and have limited generalizability to the general population.[110]

Gout

An analysis of 2008 to 2012 MEPS data found that in the United States, annual all-cause costs among individuals with gout were $26 billion.[111] Total direct costs were $36.6 billion with average costs of $11,936 per person; most of all-cause costs are likely for treatment of comorbidities such as obesity, hypertension, type II diabetes, and heart disease which are very common among those with gout.[111a] As described below, total costs were lower than total direct costs because individuals with gout earned $10 billion more than those without gout. Hospitalizations and long-term care likely account for a meaningful percentage of costs because in 2013, a diagnosis of gout was associated with 2.9% of hospital visits for any diagnosis and 3.3% of all hospital charges billed. Individuals with uncontrolled gout, and frequent flares, have the highest costs.[112,113] In contrast, gout accounted for only 0.5% of ambulatory care visits for any diagnosis. From 1993 to 2011, hospitalizations with a diagnosis of gout increased, which is believed to be because of the rise of obesity and hypertension.[114]

The annual prevalence of working in 2008 to 2012 was only slightly higher for those without gout (with and without gout were 85% and 88% respectively).[111] Because each individual with gout earned, on average, $6,810 more than those without gout, adults with gout earned $10 billion more than those without.

Back Conditions

MEPS data are suitable for estimating the economic impact associated with back problems because they do not require a specific health care provider diagnosis and can be reported by an individual experiencing a back problem. Using MEPS, Yelin[2] estimated that the number of people with self-reported back problems increased by 19%, or 6 million more people from 1996-1998 (27.4 million) to 2002-2004 (32.9 million). Prevalence rose by 12% during this time, to 11.3%.

Total direct costs for each person with back problems increased by about 25% across this time period, from $4,756 to $5,923 (2004 U.S. dollars); this increase was largely because of an 88% increase in the cost of medicine prescribed for back problems.[2] From 1996 to 1998 to 2002 to 2004, direct costs for back problems increased from the equivalent of 1.2% to 1.7% of GDP because of both the increase in the direct costs per person and the increase in prevalence. Average earnings losses with back problems were low, averaging $1,871 for each of the 24.3 million among working age adults (18 to 64 years) with back problems; in total, earnings losses for back problems equaled 0.4% of the 2004 U.S. GDP. Although back problems are a common cause of work loss, earnings losses are relatively low because the majority of people with back problems experience temporary disability rather than permanent work loss.

Ankylosing Spondylitis

Similar to the other inflammatory conditions described above, direct and indirect costs among those with ankylosing spondylitis are high. A 2005 review of costs reported that the total costs associated with ankylosing spondylitis including direct costs ranged between $7,243 and $11,840, amounts comparable with the cost of RA in the prebiologic era.[115] Similar to the transition to the biologic era with RA, direct costs are expected to rise with the increasing use of biologics for management of ankylosing spondylitis (estimates of TNF inhibitor utilization range from 0% [Hong Kong, Chile, and Uruguay] to 55% [United States] across 15 countries).[115,116] Individuals with ankylosing spondylitis have a particularly high need for assistive devices and caretakers are a meaningful contributor to direct costs.[117]

Across countries, the distribution among cost categories differs. Individuals with ankylosing spondylitis in the United States may have unmet needs for care because insurance coverage for physical therapy and hospital admissions varies; as a result, a larger proportion of total costs of the condition are attributable to wage losses than in other nations.

Fibromyalgia

Although published a decade ago, the summary of the literature by one study[118] is the most comprehensive discussion of the economic impacts of fibromyalgia. Fibromyalgia is a chronic widespread pain syndrome whose symptoms include sleep disturbance and depression. Fibromyalgia disproportionately affects women.[119] Because fibromyalgia studies have not accounted for loss of caretaking and household management, direct medical care costs, averaging between $5,000 and $6,000 in the studies reviewed by one group, are much higher than indirect costs from earnings losses (averaged between $2,000 and $3,000). This occurs although a relatively high percentage of those who are employed at onset either stop working, reduce their hours, or are short-term disability recipients. Of note is that those with fibromyalgia frequently use job management strategies (change job tasks or switch jobs to accommodate the symptoms) to stay in the workforce. The studies reviewed report that direct costs associated with fibromyalgia are higher before diagnosis because of the costs of the workup; following diagnosis, ambulatory care and medications for management of symptoms (such as pain and depression) account for most direct cost spending.

To date, there are no published U.S. population-based cost estimates of fibromyalgia. A MEPS-based study examining sensitivity of the ICD-9-CM code for self-reported fibromyalgia, where the gold standard was health care provider record of diagnosis, found a low sensitivity (≤0.34) (Miriam Cisternas, personal communications, 2014). This indicated that estimating fibromyalgia was not feasible in MEPS but may be with the change to ICD-10-CM because of the more specific diagnostic codes for fibromyalgia (Miriam Cisternas, personal communications, 2014).

Psoriatic Arthritis

The limited number of international studies examining direct and indirect costs of PsA indicate that costs for this condition are even higher than those for other inflammatory conditions because individuals are typically managing two complex conditions simultaneously, psoriasis and PsA itself and are more likely to have additional comorbidities.[120] While both direct and indirect costs reported for this condition have been consistently high, the relatively recent introduction of biologics for treatment of psoriatic arthritis has, similarly to RA, changed the distribution of total costs among individuals with PsA, with direct costs now exceeding indirect costs. It has been concluded that the improvements in productivity realized through use of the biologics has offset some of the biologics' costs.

Summary

Overall, COI studies convey the impact of direct and indirect costs associated with, and attributable to, arthritis and the rheumatic conditions for individuals, health systems, and society overall. Costs are projected to rise with the growing number of individuals with these conditions and increasing use of costly medications (e.g., biologics) and medical procedures (e.g., joint replacements).[52] Increases in out-of-pocket expenses and the costs of medications, such as biologics, can create barriers to access to care among adults with arthritis and rheumatic conditions. For example, a 2018 systematic review found that increases in out-of-pocket expenses were associated with reductions in medication adherence among individuals with rheumatoid arthritis[121]; individuals who are not working and experiencing earnings losses may be even more vulnerable. Medical treatments like the biologics and joint replacements can improve quality of life and may extend workforce participation. Increased access to these treatments may enable additional adults with arthritis and rheumatic conditions can experience these benefits.

 Full references for this chapter can be found on ExpertConsult.com.

Selected References

1. Theis KA, Roblin D, Helmick CG, et al.: Employment exit and entry among U.S. adults with and without arthritis during the great recession. A longitudinal study: 2007-2009, NHIS/MEPS, *Work* 60(2):303–318, 2018.
2. Yelin E: Economic burden of rheumatic diseasess. In Firestein GS, Gabriel SE, Mcinnes IB, et al.: *Kelley and Firestein's textbook of rheumatology*, Philadephia, 2017, Elsevier.
3. Gold MR, Spiegel JE, Russell LB, et al.: *Cost-effectiveness in health and medicine*, New York, 1996, Oxford University Press.
4. National Prevention Council, *National Prevention Strategy.* 2011, U.S. Department of Health and Human Services, Office of the Surgeon General: Washington, D.C. p. 125. https://www.hhs.gov/sites/default/files/disease-prevention-wellness-report.pdf.
5. 11th US Congress (2009-2010) H.R. 3590 Patient Protection and Affordable Care Act.
6. Crowley R, Daniel H, Cooney TG, Health and Public Policy Committee of the American College of Physicians, et al.: Envisioning a better U.S. health care system for all: coverage and cost of care, *Ann Intern Med* 172(supp 2):S7–S32, 2020.
7. Putrik P, Ramiro S, Kvien TK, et al.: Inequities in access to biologic and synthetic DMARDs across 46 European countries, *Ann Rheum Dis* 73(1):198–206, 2014.
8. Hausmann LRM, Brandt CA, Carroll CM, et al.: Racial and ethnic differences in total knee arthroplasty in the Veterans Affairs Healthcare System (2001-2013), *Arthritis Care Res (Hoboken)* 69:1171–1178, 2017.
9. Kolasinski SL, Neogi T, Hochberg MC, et al.: 2019 American College of Rheumatology/Arthritis Foundation guideline for the management of osteoarthritis of the hand, hip, and knee, *Arthritis Care Res (Hoboken)* 72(2):149–162, 2020.
10. Centers for Medicaid and Medicare Services: Original Medicare (Part A and B) eligibility and enrollment. Available from: https://cms.gov/Medicare/Eligibility-and-Enrollment/OrigMedicarePartABEligEnrol, 2020.
11. Putrik P, Ramiro S, Kvien TK, et al.: Inequities in access to biologic and synthetic DMARDs across 46 European countries, *Ann Rheum Dis* 73(1):198–206, 2014.
12. Kamaruzaman H, Kinghorn P, Oppong R: Cost-effectiveness of surgical interventions for the management of osteoarthritis: a systematic review of the literature, *BMC Musculoskelet Disord* 18(1):183, 2017.
13. Oxford Economics: The economic costs of arthritis for the US economy 2010. Available from https://www.oxfordeconomics.com/publication/download/222531.
14. Finkelstein E, Corso P: Cost-of-illness analyses for policy making: a cautionary tale of use and misuse, *Expert Rev Pharmacoecon Outcomes Res* 3(4):367–369, 2003.
15. Cohen JW, Cohen SB, Banthin JS: The medical expenditure panel survey: a national information resource to support healthcare cost research and inform policy and practice, *Med Care* 47(7 Suppl 1):S44–50, 2009.
16. Agency for Healthcare Research and Quality. Medical Expenditure Panel Survey 2019. Available from: https://meps.ahrq.gov/mepsweb/.
17. Hochberg MC, Cisternas MG, Watkins-Castillo SI. Rheumatoid arthritis. 2018. In The Burden of Musculoskeletal Diseases in the United States [Internet]. 4th. Available from: https://www.boneandjointburden.org/fourth-edition/iiib21/rheumatoid-arthritis.
18. Widdifield J, Paterson JM, Huang A, et al.: Causes of Death in rheumatoid arthritis: how do they compare to the general population? *Arthritis Care Res* 70(12):1748–1755, 2018.
19. Widdifield J, Bernatsky S, Paterson JM, et al.: Trends in excess mortality among patients with rheumatoid arthritis in Ontario, Canada, *Arthritis Care Res* 67(8):1047–1053, 2015.
20. Humphreys JH, Warner A, Chipping J, et al.: Mortality trends in patients with early rheumatoid arthritis over 20 years: results from the Norfolk Arthritis Register, *Arthritis Care Res* 66(9):1296–1301, 2014.
21. Jorge AM, Lu N, Zhang Y, et al.: Unchanging premature mortality trends in systemic lupus erythematosus: a general population-based study (1999-2014), *Rheumatology (Oxford, England)* 57(2):337–344, 2018.
22. O'Donnell S, Lagacé C, Diener A, Roberge H, Tanguay S. Life with arthritis in Canada: a personal and public health challenge. 2011. Public Health Agency of Canada. Available from: https://www.canada.ca/content/dam/phac-aspc/migration/phac-aspc/cd-mc/arthritis-arthrite/lwaic-vaaac-10/pdf/arthritis-2010-eng.pdf.

23. Yelin E, Cisternas MG, Watkins-Castillo SI. Impact of Musculoskeletal Diseases on the US Economy: US Bone and Joint Initiative; 2014 [cited 2019]. Available from: https://www.boneandjointburden.org/2013-report/impact-musculoskeletal-diseases-us-economy/x5.
24. Hochberg MC, Cisternas MG, Watkins-Castillo SI. Connective Tissue Disorders. 2018. In: The Burden of Musculoskeletal Diseases in the United States [Internet]. 4th. Available from: https://www.boneandjointburden.org/fourth-edition/iiib23/connective-tissue-disorders.
25. Yelin E, Cisternas MG, Watkins-Castillo SI. Burden from Musculoskeletal Conditions in the US Economy. 2018. In: The Burden of Musculoskeletal Diseases in the United States [Internet]. 4th. Available from: https://www.boneandjointburden.org/2014-report/xd0/musculoskeletal-medical-care-expenditures.
26. Hochberg MC, Cisternas MG, Watkins-Castillo SI. Osteoarthritis. 2018 2018. In: The Burden of Musculoskeletal Diseases in the United States [Internet]. 4th. Available from: https://www.boneandjointburden.org/fourth-edition/iiib10/osteoarthritis.
27. Murphy LB, Cisternas MG, Greenlund KJ, et al.: Defining arthritis for public health surveillance: methods and estimates in four US population health surveys, *Arthritis Care Res* 69(3):356–367, 2017.
28. Ellis BM, Conaghan PG: Reducing arthritis pain through physical activity: a new public health, tiered approach, *Br J Gen Pract* 67(663):438–439, 2017.
29. Hootman JM, Helmick CG, Brady TJ: A public health approach to addressing arthritis in older adults: the most common cause of disability, *Am J Public Health* 102(3):426–433, 2012.
30. Murphy LB, Cisternas MG, Pasta DJ, et al.: Medical expenditures and earnings losses among US adults with arthritis in 2013, *Arthritis Care Res* 70(6):869–876, 2018.
31. Raval AD, Vyas A: Trends in healthcare expenditures among individuals with arthritis in the United States from 2008 to 2014, *J Rheumatol* 45(5):705–716, 2018.
32. Cisternas MG, Murphy LB, Yelin EH, et al.: Trends in medical care expenditures of US adults with arthritis and other rheumatic conditions 1997 to 2005, *J Rheumatol* 36(11):2531–2538, 2009.
33. Yelin E, Murphy L, Cisternas MG, et al.: Medical care expenditures and earnings losses among persons with arthritis and other rheumatic conditions in 2003, and comparisons with 1997, *Arthritis Rheum* 56(5):1397–1407, 2007.
34. Yelin E, Cisternas MG, Pasta DJ, et al.: Medical care expenditures and earnings losses of persons with arthritis and other rheumatic conditions in the United States in 1997: total and incremental estimates, *Arthritis Rheum* 50(7):2317–2326, 2004.
35. Williams EM, Walker RJ, Faith T, et al.: The impact of arthritis and joint pain on individual healthcare expenditures: findings from the Medical Expenditure Panel Survey (MEPS), 2011, *Arthritis Care Res* 19(1):38, 2017.
36. Kelley GA, Kelley KS, Hootman JM: Effects of exercise on depression in adults with arthritis: a systematic review with meta-analysis of randomized controlled trials, *Arthritis Care Res* 17:21, 2015.
37. Kelley GA, Kelley KS, Callahan LF: Community-deliverable exercise and anxiety in adults with arthritis and other rheumatic diseases: a systematic review with meta-analysis of randomised controlled trials, *BMJ Open* 8(2):e019138, 2018.
38. Kelley GA, Kelley KS, Hootman JM, et al.: Effects of community-deliverable exercise on pain and physical function in adults with arthritis and other rheumatic diseases: a meta-analysis, *Arthritis Care Res* 63(1):79–93, 2011.
39. Brady TJ, Murphy L, O'Colmain BJ, et al.: A meta-analysis of health status, health behaviors, and health care utilization outcomes of the chronic disease self-management program, *Prev Chronic Dis* 10:120112, 2013.
40. Atukorala I, Makovey J, Lawler L, et al.: Is there a dose-response relationship between weight loss and symptom improvement in persons with knee osteoarthritis? *Arthritis Care Res* 68(8):1106–1114, 2016.
41. American College of Rheumatology: Position Statement: patient Access to BIologics. Available from: https://www.rheumatology.org/Portals/0/Files/Patient%20Access%20to%20Biologics%20aka%20Model%20Biologics.pdf, 2017.
42. Murphy LB, Yelin E, Theis KA: Compromised access to prescriptions and medical care because of cost among US adults with arthritis, *Best Pract Res Clin Rheumatol.* 26(5):677–694, 2012.
43. Deleted in review.
44. Center on Budget and Policy Priorities. Chart Book: The Legacy of the Great Recession 2019. Available from: https://www.cbpp.org/research/economy/chart-book-the-legacy-of-the-great-recession.
45. Kaye HS. The Impact of the 2007-2009 Recession on Workers with Disabilities. 2019. Available from: http://www.tilrc.org/assests/news/publications/recession_impact_on_workers_with_disabilities_10-2011.pdf.
46. Verstappen SM, Boonen A, Bijlsma JW, et al.: Working status among Dutch patients with rheumatoid arthritis: work disability and working conditions, *Rheumatology (Oxford, England)* 44(2):202–206, 2005.
47. Briggs AM, Woolf AD, Dreinhofer K, et al.: Reducing the global burden of musculoskeletal conditions, *Bull World Health Organ* 96(5):366–368, 2018.
48. Global Burden of Disease 2016 Disease and Injury Incidence and Prevalence Collaborators: Global, regional, and national incidence, prevalence, and years lived with disability for 328 diseases and injuries for 195 countries, 1990-2016: a systematic analysis for the Global Burden of Disease Study 2016, *Lancet (London, England)* 390(10100):1211–1259, 2017.
49. Strine TW, Hootman JM: US national prevalence and correlates of low back and neck pain among adults, *Arthritis Rheum* 57(4):656–665, 2007.
50. Ma VY, Chan L, Carruthers KJ: Incidence, prevalence, costs, and impact on disability of common conditions requiring rehabilitation in the United States: stroke, spinal cord injury, traumatic brain injury, multiple sclerosis, osteoarthritis, rheumatoid arthritis, limb loss, and back pain, *Arch Phys Med Rehabil* 95(5):986–995.e1, 2014.
51. Gabriel SE, Crowson CS, Campion ME, et al.: Direct medical costs unique to people with arthritis, *J Rheumatol* 24(4):719–725, 1997.
52. Ackerman IN, Bohensky MA, Pratt C, et al.: Counting the Costs. Part 1: Healthcare costs. The current and future burden of arthritis. 2016. Melbourne EPi Center at the University of Melbourne. Available from: https://arthritisaustralia.com.au/wordpress/wp-content/uploads/2017/09/Final-Counting-the-Costs_Part1_MAY2016.pdf.
53. Badley EM: The economic burden of musculoskeletal disorders in Canada is similar to that for cancer, and may be higher, *J Rheumatol* 22(2):204–206, 1995.
54. Meerding WJ, Bonneux L, Polder JJ, et al.: Demographic and epidemiological determinants of healthcare costs in Netherlands: cost of illness study, *BMJ* 317(7151):111–115, 1998.
55. Jonsson D, Husberg M: Socioeconomic costs of rheumatic diseases. Implications for technology assessment, *Int J Technol Assess Health Care* 16(4):1193–1200, 2000.
56. Li X, Gignac MA, Anis AH: The indirect costs of arthritis resulting from unemployment, reduced performance, and occupational changes while at work, *Med Care* 44(4):304–310, 2006.
57. Barbour KE, Helmick CG, Boring M, et al.: Vital Signs: prevalence of Doctor-diagnosed arthritis and arthritis-Attributable Activity Limitation—United States, 2013-2015, *MMWR Morb Mortal Wkly Rep* 66(9):246–253, 2017.
57a. Hootman JM, Helmick CG: Projections of US prevalence of arthritis and associated activity limitations, *Arthritis Rheum* 54(1):226–229, 2006.
59. Hussain SM, Urquhart DM, Wang Y, et al.: Fat mass and fat distribution are associated with low back pain intensity and disability: results from a cohort study, *Arthritis Res Ther* 19(1):26, 2017.

60. Deshpande BR, Katz JN, Solomon DH, et al.: Number of persons with Symptomatic knee osteoarthritis in the US: impact of race and ethnicity, age, sex, and obesity, *Arthritis Care Res* 68(12):1743–1750, 2016.
61. George J, Klika AK, Navale SM, et al.: Obesity epidemic: is its impact on total joint arthroplasty underestimated? An analysis of national trends, *Clin Orthop Relat Res* 475(7):1798–1806, 2017.
62. Guh DP, Zhang W, Bansback N, et al.: The incidence of co-morbidities related to obesity and overweight: a systematic review and meta-analysis, *BMC Public Health* 9:88, 2009.
63. Cooper NJ: Economic burden of rheumatoid arthritis: a systematic review, *Rheumatology (Oxford, England)* 39(1):28–33, 2000.
64. Pugner KM, Scott DI, Holmes JW, et al.: The costs of rheumatoid arthritis: an international long-term view, *Semin Arthritis Rheum* 29(5):305–320, 2000.
65. Chevat C, Pena BM, Al MJ, et al.: Healthcare resource utilisation and costs of treating NSAID-associated gastrointestinal toxicity. A multinational perspective, *PharmacoEconomics* 19(Suppl 1):17–32, 2001.
66. Lubeck DP: A review of the direct costs of rheumatoid arthritis: managed care versus fee-for-service settings, *PharmacoEconomics* 19(8):811–818, 2001.
67. Hresko A, Lin TC, Solomon DH: Medical care costs associated with rheumatoid arthritis in the US: a systematic literature review and meta-analysis, *Arthritis Care Res* 70(10):1431–1438, 2018.
68. Hunsche E, Chancellor JV, Bruce N: The burden of arthritis and nonsteroidal anti-inflammatory treatment. A European literature review, *PharmacoEconomics* 19(Suppl 1):1–15, 2001.
69. Rat AC, Boissier MC: Rheumatoid arthritis: direct and indirect costs, *Joint Bone Spine* 71(6):518–524, 2004.
70. Bansback N, Ara R, Karnon J, et al.: Economic evaluations in rheumatoid arthritis: a critical review of measures used to define health States, *PharmacoEconomics* 26(5):395–408, 2008.
71. Yelin E, Wanke LA: An assessment of the annual and long-term direct costs of rheumatoid arthritis: the impact of poor function and functional decline, *Arthritis Rheum* 42(6):1209–1218, 1999.
72. Felts W, Yelin E: The economic impact of the rheumatic diseases in the United States, *J Rheumatol* 16(7):867–884, 1989.
73. Verstappen SM: Rheumatoid arthritis and work: the impact of rheumatoid arthritis on absenteeism and presenteeism, *Best Pract Res Clin Rheumatol* 29(3):495–511, 2015.
74. Allaire S, Wolfe F, Niu J, et al.: Work disability and its economic effect on 55-64-year-old adults with rheumatoid arthritis, *Arthritis Rheum* 53(4):603–608, 2005.
75. Wolfe F, Michaud K: Biologic treatment of rheumatoid arthritis and the risk of malignancy: analyses from a large US observational study, *Arthritis Rheum* 56(9):2886–2895, 2007.
76. Desai RJ, Solomon DH, Jin Y, et al.: Temporal trends in use of biologic DMARDs for rheumatoid arthritis in the United States: a cohort study of publicly and privately insured patients, *J Manag Care Spec Pharm* 23(8):809–814, 2017.
77. Gu T, Shah N, Deshpande G, et al.: Comparing biologic cost per treated patient across indications among adult US managed care patients: a retrospective cohort study, *Drugs Real World Outcomes* 3(4):369–381, 2016.
78. Michaud K, Messer J, Choi HK, et al.: Direct medical costs and their predictors in patients with rheumatoid arthritis: a three-year study of 7,527 patients, *Arthritis Rheum* 48(10):2750–2762, 2003.
79. Sorensen J, Andersen LS: The case of tumour necrosis factor-alpha inhibitors in the treatment of rheumatoid arthritis: a budget impact analysis, *PharmacoEconomics* 23(3):289–298, 2005.
80. Mulcahy AW, Hlavka JP, Case SR: Biosimilar cost savings in the United States: initial experience and future potential, *Rand Health Q* 7(4):3, 2018.
81. Dorner T, Strand V, Cornes P, et al.: The changing landscape of biosimilars in rheumatology, *Ann Rheum Dis* 75(6):974–982, 2016.
82. Yazdany J, Dudley RA, Lin GA, et al.: Out-of-Pocket costs for infliximab and its biosimilar for rheumatoid arthritis under Medicare Part D, *Jama* 320(9):931–933, 2018.
83. Hallert E, Husberg M, Jonsson D, et al.: Rheumatoid arthritis is already expensive during the first year of the disease (the Swedish TIRA project), *Rheumatology (Oxford, England)* 43(11):1374–1382, 2004.
84. Merkesdal S, Ruof J, Schoffski O, et al.: Indirect medical costs in early rheumatoid arthritis: composition of and changes in indirect costs within the first three years of disease, *Arthritis Rheum* 44(3):528–534, 2001.
85. Joensuu JT, Huoponen S, Aaltonen KJ, et al.: The cost-effectiveness of biologics for the treatment of rheumatoid arthritis: a systematic review, *PloS One* 10(3):e0119683, 2015.
86. Neumann PJ, Ganiats TG, Russell LB, et al.: *Cost effectiveness in health and medicine*, ed 3, New York, 2017, Oxford.
87. Lacaille D, Clarke AE, Bloch DA, et al.: The impact of disease activity, treatment and disease severity on short-term costs of systemic lupus erythematosus, *J Rheumatol* 21(3):448–453, 1994.
88. Carls G, Li T, Panopalis P, et al.: Direct and indirect costs to employers of patients with systemic lupus erythematosus with and without nephritis, *J Occup Environ Med* 51(1):66–79, 2009.
89. Clarke AE, Panopalis P, Petri M, et al.: SLE patients with renal damage incur higher health care costs, *Rheumatology (Oxford, England)* 47(3):329–333, 2008.
90. Pelletier EM, Ogale S, Yu E, et al.: Economic outcomes in patients diagnosed with systemic lupus erythematosus with versus without nephritis: results from an analysis of data from a US claims database, *Clin Ther* 31(11):2653–2664, 2009.
91. Zhu TY, Tam LS, Lee VW, et al.: The impact of flare on disease costs of patients with systemic lupus erythematosus, *Arthritis Rheum* 61(9):1159–1167, 2009.
92. Clarke AE, Petri MA, Manzi S, et al.: An international perspective on the well being and health care costs for patients with systemic lupus erythematosus. Tri-Nation Study Group, *J Rheumatol* 26(7):1500–1511, 1999.
93. Clarke AE, Urowitz MB, Monga N, et al.: Costs associated with severe and nonsevere systemic lupus erythematosus in Canada, *Arthritis Care Res* 67(3):431–436, 2015.
94. Aytan J, Bukhari MA: Use of biologics in SLE: a review of the evidence from a clinical perspective, *Rheumatology (Oxford, England)* 55(5):775–779, 2016.
95. He J, Li Z: An era of biological treatment in systemic lupus erythematosus, *Clin Rheumatol* 37(1):1–3, 2018.
96. Gatto M, Kiss E, Naparstek Y, et al.: In-/off-label use of biologic therapy in systemic lupus erythematosus, *BMC Med* 12:30, 2014.
97. Ryden-Aulin M, Boumpas D, Bultink I, et al.: Off-label use of rituximab for systemic lupus erythematosus in Europe, *Lupus Sci Med* 3(1):e000163, 2016.
98. Sutcliffe N, Clarke AE, Taylor R, et al.: Total costs and predictors of costs in patients with systemic lupus erythematosus, *Rheumatology (Oxford)* 40(1):37–47, 2001.
99. Yelin E, Trupin L, Katz P, et al.: Work dynamics among persons with systemic lupus erythematosus, *Arthritis Rheum* 57(1):56–63, 2007.
100. Scofield L, Reinlib L, Alarcon GS, et al.: Employment and disability issues in systemic lupus erythematosus: a review, *Arthritis Rheum* 59(10):1475–1479, 2008.
101. Agarwal N, Kumar V: Burden of lupus on work: issues in the employment of individuals with lupus, *Work* 55(2):429–439, 2016.
102. Krishnan E, Hubert HB: Ethnicity and mortality from systemic lupus erythematosus in the US, *Ann Rheum Dis* 65(11):1500–1505, 2006.
103. Yazdany J, Feldman CH, Liu J, et al.: Quality of care for incident lupus nephritis among Medicaid beneficiaries in the United States, *Arthritis Care Res* 66(4):617–624, 2014.
104. Barber MRW, Clarke AE: Socioeconomic consequences of systemic lupus erythematosus, *Curr Opin Rheumatol* 29(5):480–485, 2017.
105. Mendoza-Pinto C, Mendez-Martinez S, Soto-Santillan P, et al.: Socioeconomic status and organ damage in Mexican systemic lupus erythematosus women, *Lupus* 24(11):1227–1232, 2015.

106. Torio CM, Moore BJ: *National Inpatient Hospital Costs: the Most Expensive Conditions by Payer, 2013: Statistical Brief #204. Healthcare Cost and Utilization Project (HCUP) Statistical Briefs*, Rockville, MD, 2016, Agency for Healthcare Research and Quality (US).
107. Agency for Healthcare Research and Quality. HCUPnet. Healthcare Cost and Utilization Project (HCUP), 1993 to 2016. 2019. Available from: https://www.hcup-us.ahrq.gov/reports/statbriefs/sb204-Most-Expensive-Hospital-Conditions.jsp.
108. Losina E, Thornhill TS, Rome BN, et al.: The dramatic increase in total knee replacement utilization rates in the United States cannot be fully explained by growth in population size and the obesity epidemic, *J Bone Joint Surg Am* 94(3):201–207, 2012.
109. Gabriel SE, Crowson CS, Campion ME, et al.: Indirect and nonmedical costs among people with rheumatoid arthritis and osteoarthritis compared with nonarthritic controls, *J Rheumatol* 24(1):43–48, 1997.
110. Kotlarz H, Gunnarsson CL, Fang H, et al.: Insurer and out-of-pocket costs of osteoarthritis in the US: evidence from national survey data, *Arthritis Rheum* 60(12):3546–3553, 2009.
111. Hochberg MC, Cisternas MG, Watkins-Castillo SI. Gout. 2018. In: The Burden of Musculoskeletal Diseases in the United States [Internet]. 4th. Available from: https://www.boneandjointburden.org/fourth-edition/iiib30/gout.
112. Lee YY, Kuo LN, Chen JH, et al.: Prescribing patterns and healthcare costs of gout, *Curr Med Res Opin* 1–18, 2018.
113. Flores NM, Nuevo J, Klein AB, et al.: The economic burden of uncontrolled gout: how controlling gout reduces cost, *J Med Economics* 22(1):1–6, 2019.
114. Lim SY, Lu N, Oza A, et al.: Trends in gout and rheumatoid arthritis hospitalizations in the United States, 1993-2011, *JAMA* 315(21):2345–2347, 2016.
115. Boonen A, van der Heijde D: Review of the costs of illness of ankylosing spondylitis and methodologic notes, *Expert Rev Pharmacoecon Outcomes Res* 5(2):163–181, 2005.
116. Reveille JD, Ximenes A, Ward MM: Economic considerations of the treatment of ankylosing spondylitis, *Am J Med Sci* 343(5):371–374, 2012.
117. Woolf AD: Economic burden of rheumatic diseasess. In Firestein GS, Gabriel SE, Mcinnes IB, et al.: *Kelley and Firestein's textbook of rheumatology*, ed 8, Philadephia, 2009, Saunders-Elsevier.
118. Annemans L, Le Lay K, Taieb C: Societal and patient burden of fibromyalgia syndrome, *PharmacoEconomics* 27(7):547–559, 2009.
119. Clauw DJ: Fibromyalgia: a clinical review, *JAMA* 311(15):1547–1555, 2014.
120. D'Angiolella LS, Cortesi PA, Lafranconi A, et al.: Cost and cost effectiveness of treatments for psoriatic arthritis: a systematic literature review, *PharmacoEconomics* 36(5):567–589, 2018.

36 Assessment of Health Outcomes

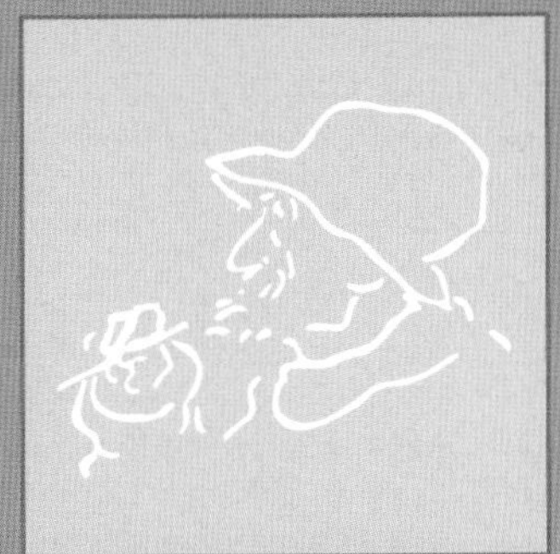

DORCAS E. BEATON, MAARTEN BOERS, PETER TUGWELL, AND LARA MAXWELL

KEY POINTS

The decision of what to measure as a health outcome and how to measure it is a choice that will define what you are able to see in terms of the impact of a disease and the benefits and harms of interventions.

Choosing the right instrument involves accumulating enough evidence to suggest it can be used in your intended setting. Both practical evidence of its feasibility and content and mathematical evidence of its measurement properties should be taken into account. Methods have been developed to guide this decision making.

Core outcome sets define a small set of important outcomes that are recommended for use. They provide a good starting point for deciding on outcomes and outcome measures.

Introduction

Health outcomes, those outcomes that reflect both the expected and unexpected impacts of a disease or its treatment,[1] and their accurate measurements are increasingly important in an era of accountability, patient-centered orientation, and quality in our health care system.[2] Although outcomes themselves are not new, there has been a distinct shift toward ensuring we capture what has often been missing—that is, what matters to patients.[3–6] Each outcome is like a window, offering a particular view of the impact of a disease, so the choice of outcomes inevitably influences the information available to patients, researchers, clinicians, guideline committees, and policy makers when it comes to answers to their most pressing questions. The goal of health outcome assessment is to have windows facing in the right direction to get the full view of the outcomes of our care and a good-quality, clear glass in that window to do the job well. Health outcome assessment is about putting important views in front of key decision makers in a way that they can use.[3,4,7] This chapter will provide practical advice on how to choose what should be measured and how to measure it, drawing on information from organizations engaged in making sure the right outcomes are available for decision making.

We will draw on the experience in rheumatology through OMERACT (Outcome Measures in Rheumatology),[8–10] an international consensus-based group established in 1992 that works within the arthritis communities (i.e., clinicians, researchers, patients, payors, regulators, industry) to define domains and instruments of importance in different rheumatologic conditions. We will also touch on the work of other international groups, which focus closely on outcomes and often work collaboratively with OMERACT in advancing methods for the development of core outcome sets. Core sets or core outcome sets will be mentioned throughout the chapter and refer to an agreed upon set of outcomes that will be used in all research or clinical practices, providing a small set of windows that we know we will have in each study. Other outcomes can also be chosen for a specific need, but these core outcomes will be there to allow comparisons across studies. The essential components of health outcome assessment are similar across all these organizations.

Health Outcome Assessments

Although the latter part of the 20th century saw the proliferation of instruments to capture outcomes such as functioning and health-related quality of life, the last 10 to 15 years has seen advances in working toward agreements on what outcomes and instruments should be used in research or clinical practice so that results can be compared to inform decision making. Perhaps the strongest force in the last decade is the recognition of patient perspective and patient-reported outcomes by the patient-centered care initiatives internationally.

There are many different guidelines and guidance statements associated with the selection of any outcome and especially with patient-reported outcomes.[11] Some standards, such as the U.S. Food and Drug Administration (FDA) guidance statement (currently under revision)[12,13] and the OMERACT Filter renewal,[9,14–16] define what evidence is needed to be confident in an instrument to perform certain measurements.[17] Other standards, such as the Core Outcome Measurement in Effectiveness Trials (COMET), focus on determining the outcome domains of importance in a core set by advancing consensus-based approaches to doing so.[18,19] Many focus on the appraisal and synthesis of studies on the performance of instruments, in efforts led by groups such as the Evaluation of the Measurement of Patient-Reported Outcomes (EMPRO)[20] and the Consensus-Based Standards for the Selection of Health Status Measurement Instruments (COSMIN),[21,22] which outline methods for systematic reviews (search, appraisal, and synthesis) of studies of measurement properties (www.cosmin.nl). PRO Measurement Information System (PROMIS), a federally funded initiative in the United States (www.healthmeasures.net), has created a large item bank calibrated to the general population that can be applied through computer adaptive testing (CAT). It provides shorter assessments, avoiding items that can be predictably answered (e.g., if you can run a mile, you can likely walk around the block, so that question is not asked). These can also be used across different conditions. This system is now gathering evidence of its performance in different clinical and research settings and its comparability and calibration to many legacy or well-used instruments.[23] Paper versions or short forms of the item banks are available to give comparable results. Finally, there are organizations trying to pull all this information on outcomes and instruments together for people through the creation of what they consider suitable sets of outcomes: both what should be measured and how it should be measured. Two organizations are particularly relevant in rheumatology: OMERACT, which examines core outcome sets for research, and the International Consortium for Health Outcome Measurement (ICHOM), which looks at core outcomes for clinical practice and quality improvement. Both work on defining a small set of prioritized outcome domains and matching high-quality instruments that should be used across outcome assessments. These two organizations will be mentioned again in a later section. These and other organizations were formed to deal with a growing number of instruments, a growing body of literature on measurement properties, and a number of studies and trials that could not be compared because they did not measure the same outcomes or used different tools. Agreement on a core outcome set means that at least that core of outcomes will be the same across our work, allowing more of the high-quality and often costly research being conducted to be included in systematic reviews, guideline development, and comparative effectiveness research.

The overlap and collaboration across these organizations is welcome, with specific strengths coming from each and more convergence happening across groups, especially evident in recent years.[15,22,24]

What Needs to Be Measured: Defining Measurement Needs

The process of deciding on the outcomes to include in either research or clinical settings begins by defining the specific need.[15,17,25] There are three parts to this: Who, Why, and What?

The Target Population

The target population is critical to define and keep in mind throughout the health outcome assessment process. Although clinicians "know" this in their understanding of the disease, it is often overlooked when deciding on a health outcome assessment and the relevance of a domain or instrument. A given instrument may, for example, work very well in severe osteoarthritis of the hip but not be sensitive to the early symptoms of the disease. Patients in those two states may also have different ideas of what is important in terms of outcomes. It is equally important to consider whether you want an instrument to assess individual patients (e.g., in care) or to describe one or more groups of patients (e.g., to describe group mean change in a clinical trial). The former demands much higher levels of things like reliability and precision.[26]

Defining the Reason for Measuring

Clarity about how you intend to use the scores from an instrument/index, or your purpose for measuring, is important for defining which attributes need to be prioritized in your decision making. Kirshner and Guyatt describe three purposes: descriptive (measurement of a domain to get a snapshot of it at one point in time only), predictive (using an outcome instrument to provide information about another future outcome, such as the Health Assessment Questionnaire [HAQ]'s ability to predict mortality in arthritis), and evaluative (measure change during time, such as the benefit or harm from treatment), where the focus is on the amount of change, rather than what the absolute score is on the scale at any point in time.[27] In this chapter, we focus on two of the purposes most relevant to the way health outcome assessments are used to capture the effect of interventions in research and practice: descriptively (the level of health outcome state at one point in time) and evaluatively (changes in health outcome).[27] Predictive uses are equally valid, but less likely to be described as an outcome in health outcome assessment. A predictive use might be to measure the domain at an initial visit to predict the likely course and make a decision on how to treat the patient. Each purpose, descriptive, evaluative, and predictive, requires slightly different types of evidence to support an argument that an instrument will work well in that setting. Evaluative purposes, for example, place a lot more emphasis on the elements around change, such as responsiveness to clinical changes and test-retest reliability. These are not as important for descriptive applications where change is not the focus. Knowing your purpose ahead of time will guide you to the right kind of evidence in thinking about the quality of an instrument.

What Do You Want to Measure?

Perhaps the most important step at this stage is to define the concept you want/need to measure (the "what"). Health outcome assessment has tended to focus on things that are meaningful and relevant to the clinician or researcher. Over the past two decades, international organizations, regulators, and clinical practice groups have begun to focus on patient experience as key to identifying what to measure in health outcome assessments.[3,4,28] Hearing patients and their experiences has created a new understanding of concepts such as fatigue[29] or rheumatoid arthritis (RA) flares.[30] It has also helped us to define novel domains such as cognitive dysfunction in many inflammatory disease groups or a patient's sense of recovery.[31] New instruments have arisen to address a new understanding of the co-occurrence of intermittent and constant pain associated with osteoarthritis (OA) pain.[32] Hearing what is important to patients means actively listening. Patient experience is often captured through rigorous qualitative methods aimed at understanding the lived experience of the disease or the domain or interest. A series of individual interviews or focus groups are used to hear that collective voice and tease out the specific ways that patients talk about things like pain or function. Engaging patients in this process of deciding on outcomes is the best way to ensure the outcomes you are considering accurately capture their experience. The more effectively domains and instruments can capture our patients' experiences, the closer we will be to having the right set of tools in our outcome assessment in research or clinical practice.

Generating ideas of what should be measured can also be facilitated by using a conceptual framework. These frameworks not only

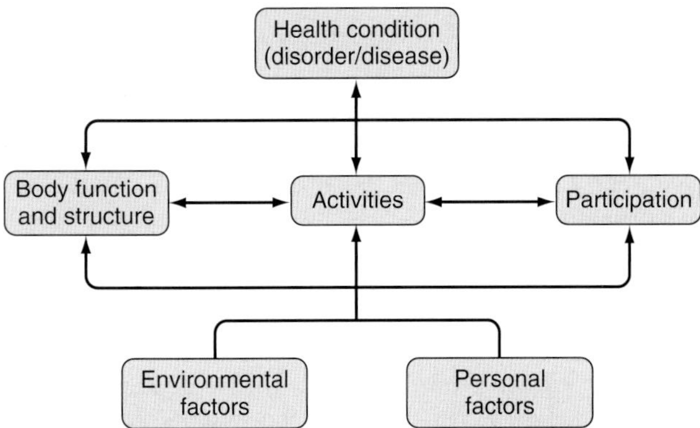

• **Fig. 36.1** The International Classification of Functioning (ICF) conceptual framework showing the hypothesized relationships between domains of impairment, activity limitations, and participation restrictions and the direct influence of environmental and personal factors on these domains.

define the breadth of areas that can be measured to gain a good understanding of a health condition's impact but also hypothesize the relationship between those areas of health and what other factors might be influencing them. The advantage of a framework is that it usually covers a wide range of manifestations of the impact of a disease and can draw you to broader windows or view on outcomes.[33] One framework, the International Classification of Functioning, Disability, and Health (ICF), was endorsed by the World Health Organization in 2001[34,35] and describes three main concepts (Fig. 36.1): (1) impairments (symptoms, structural limitations), (2) activity limitations (difficulties while performing tasks), and (3) participation restrictions (difficulties in social role participation like parenting or working). Several domains or outcomes could be imagined within each, such as pain and range of motion, physical functioning, and work role functioning. Around these main areas, the ICF adds the importance of environmental factors (job demands, environmental barriers, weather) and personal factors (predispositions, coping strategies). OMERACT made use of the ICF's concepts when formulating its framework for core domain set development; it defined four core areas for outcome assessment: pathophysiologic manifestations, life impact (including activity limitations and participation restrictions), resource utilization, and adverse events (including death).[9] Similar to the ICF, the OMERACT model requires the consideration of important contextual factors, both environmental and personal.[9] The OMERACT framework was recently adopted by the COMET group in their taxonomy of potential outcomes.[23] In the development of the core domain set, OMERACT requires groups to include at least one domain for each of the three core areas, with resource use still considered optional. This ensures a minimum content validity of the core domain sets, which means that the full breadth of outcomes will be carefully considered.[8,9,16]

A good starting point for identifying outcomes is to search the current literature for domains that have been used, such as all the clinical trials in a condition of interest.[36] This approach, however, reinforces current practices and might well miss that important patient perspective or a core area from a framework.[8,28] Reviews of current practices are therefore best supplemented with qualitative, inductive approaches.

Having generated a number of domains, it would be impractical to measure all of them. Groups must figure out ways to agree on the most critical outcomes for research or practice. Consensus methods, such as a Delphi survey, are used often to rate the outcomes that are critical for all outcome assessments.[37] OMERACT uses consensus methods, including this survey, but when interpreting results we separate the patients' perspectives from the clinicians'. A study of flare in RA, for example, demonstrated that patients and clinicians do not always see importance in the same way and that the patients' perspectives were what was missing in the outcome batteries.[30] Ensuring you can see where patients agree or disagree with other parties is critical as their numbers in decision-making groups are often fewer than those of researchers/clinicians and their input might easily get lost. Involving patients as research partners in the entire domain selection process can offer tremendous insight into the lived experiences of people with the disease at every step of the decision-making process.[16,38] When patients are considered equal voices in deciding what should be included in a core set, the results will likely be more patient-centered and comprehensive.

Domain selection does not stop at the label. Detailed definitions and descriptions of the lived experience are needed. Quotes from qualitative work are one way to ensure future users will understand its scope (the breadth and depth of the outcome domain and what experiencing a high level of it would feel like, as well as experiencing a low or moderate level). This type of detail becomes the standard for assessing the match of a future instrument with that concept and content.[16]

At this point, the measurement need should be defined: who do you want to measure this in, why are you measuring (are you describing a health state at one point in time, a change in state in a randomized trial setting, or a change of state in a clinical practice), and what are you going to measure? Thinking about these questions carefully and explicitly should precede the selection of an instrument so that the instrument meets the need and not the reverse.

Outcome Measures in Arthritis

Arthritis has the advantage of being ahead of the field in terms of measuring patient-centered outcomes with some of the early disability and pain scales. They have also been involved in the organization of core sets for a number of decades through OMERACT. Well-designed core outcome sets should be able to capture key areas of health from the perspective of patients, clinicians, researchers, industry leaders, and policy makers. At OMERACT, several core sets have been developed and many are currently being reviewed. Table 36.1A and Table 36.1B list the core domain sets (what should be measured in each trial) for several rheumatologic diseases, many of which were revisited and endorsed at the 2018 OMERACT meeting.[39–57]

The first column shares the core areas and domains nominated in at least one core set within each. The core areas are the broad headings suggested by the most recent OMERACT Filter 2.1, used to ensure full consideration is given across the impact of the disease.[8,9] OMERACT tries to ensure that at least one outcome domain is covered in each core area (life impact, pathophysiologic manifestations, adverse effects, death, and, optionally, resource utilization). The remaining columns show selections for core sets in different rheumatic disease, at present. There are many things in common. For example, most sets contain or recommend inclusion of pain, physical function, some form of overall appraisal of disease impact, and markers of inflammation. Many also include the need to measure disease activity or damage to structures themselves. Some core sets contain domains reflecting the unique aspects of the disease (e.g., spinal mobility in ankylosing spondylitis)[48] or the unique target of the study (e.g., tophi in measuring response in gout)[57] (see Tables 36.1A and 36.1B).

Deciding on an Instrument for a Health Outcome Assessment

Armed with a well-articulated need (already knowing who you want to measure this in, why you want to measure it, and what exactly you want to be able to capture), the selection of "how" to measure that outcome (instrument selection) is a step-by-step process. At OMERACT, people are asked to make sure their chosen instrument has satisfactorily met the requirements of the Filter 2.1. This means that there is sufficient, quality evidence that it meets the three pillars of the original OMERACT Filter. In other words, it is truthful, discriminating (able to detect differences between trial arms), and feasible to use (in terms of burden and time).[10] In developing the Filter 2.1, OMERACT reorganized these pillars into a set of four signaling questions, which are ordered in increasing difficulty to reflect an increased investment of time and effort. The first two steps are deciding if the instrument is a match for the target concept and then if it is feasible to use it in the intended setting. The other two questions are more oriented to measurement properties. In total, there are three pillars, four signaling questions, and seven measurement properties to get to one answer. What we will describe here is a decision-making process that can be used to assess whether a given instrument fits with the articulated measurement need. This process, depicted in Fig. 36.2, builds on the work of Law,[58] Lohr,[59] Kirshner,[60] Mokkink,[20] FDA Guidance,[12] and Reeve,[11] as well as years of experience at OMERACT, and is the heart of the OMERACT Filter 2.1 for instrument selection.[10,15] More detail can be found in the OMERACT handbook, including a fillable workbook (https://omeract.org/handbook/), to move you through the process.

The instrument selection algorithm (see Fig. 36.2) has three key features that deserve attention. First, it always starts with a firm statement of the measurement need (Who, Why, and What, as described in the previous section). Second, a lot of the initial work must be done through the group (clinicians, researchers, and the patient partner), who offer guided reflections on what they think of the instrument itself, the practical issues of using it, and whether it looks like it is covering enough content before looking at more statistical evidence of reliability and correlational validity (i.e., correlations and effect-size statistics).[61,62] This leads to the third point, which is that the inability to confirm either of the first two signaling questions indicates an irreconcilable mismatch (triggering a "no" in the instrument selection algorithm) and suggests that you are better off finding another candidate instrument. Conversely, if you have made it past this prestatistical appraisal with either a solid "yes" (marked as green, go) or a "maybe" (some concerns, but still go ahead; marked with an amber or cautionary rating), you are likely holding a good instrument worthy of investment in reviewing or creating evidence of its ability to perform in this situation. With these overarching points in mind, let us look at the process.

Signaling Question 1: Is It a Good Match With the Target Domain?

Think about your concept or domain and then decide, based on the description of the candidate instrument, the nature of the items/elements assessed, and the response categories or scales used, whether there is a match between the instrument's concept and the measurement need (concept, population, purpose).[25] At this stage, input from patients is critical. They can review content, see if their experience is fully captured by this outcome instrument, and note whether the score seems to make sense. Patients may provide different levels of input, depending on whether the instrument is a questionnaire, a performance-based instrument, an observer-based assessment of physical signs, or a biomarker (soluble, tissue, or imaging). For questionnaires, cognitive interviews can be useful to help elicit some understanding of how patients formulate their responses and understand an item. Similar procedures can be brought into play for other types of instruments. Gathering a set of responses to the instrument in a group of patients/respondents can highlight items with high missing values (perhaps a sensitive topic) or floor/ceiling effects, suggesting an instrument will not be able to go further in this direction.[12,59] If the instrument is not a good match, start with another candidate instrument.[63]

Signaling Question 2: Is It Feasible to Use?

Feasibility covers the practical aspects of using the instrument in its intended setting.[10,58,59] Does it take too much time? Are the licensing costs too high? Does it require special equipment? Is it too burdensome for your patients (e.g., language, literacy, acceptability of questions, time of procedure, physical discomfort) or observers (training)? For both patient- and clinician-observed outcomes, consideration of the format and the response categories are important. For example, are procedural and calibration instructions clear for an imaging outcome? Are the results of the score easily interpretable? A negative response to any of these questions could direct you to another, more feasible instrument. Feasibility, or the practicalities of using the instrument, can often make or break a decision about a candidate instrument.[10,59,61,62] Many of these questions can be answered with a thorough review of the actual instrument and information on its administration by a clinical or research team with patient input. Patient partners are invaluable at this time, particularly in their opinion of the meaning of an item, the clarity of the wording, and the comprehensiveness of the instrument's content.[38]

Signaling Question 3: Do the Numeric Scores Make Sense?

Having convinced yourself of the content and practical feasibility of the scale, the next step begins the more data-intensive evaluation. Instruments are tested to see if there is enough evidence to support their use in your intended application (your measurement need).[15,64,65] Evidence should come from similar enough settings to your own (patients, severity, culture).

Checking Whether the Items Fit Onto the Intended Scale

Instruments that are questionnaires or a set of items combined into one final score are often checked for their *structural validity*. That is, they are checked to confirm the structure of the items/components onto their scales, as per the developer's intention. Structural validity is assessed through approaches such as factor analysis if the instrument was designed to have multiple items of a trait that are summed together or item response theory (IRT)[66,67] to assess whether the items designed to capture consecutive levels of the trait along the continuum are doing a satisfactory job. The choice is dependent on the approach that is being used for scoring the instrument. For example, IRT-scored scales, where each item is weighted based on the level it represents of the attribute, are often linked to a CAT platform to make assessments shorter and equally efficient. PROMIS is an excellent example of this (www.healthmeasures.net). Further details on how to conduct factor analysis or IRT analyses are beyond the scope of this chapter, but

TABLE 36.1A Domains Endorsed for Inclusion in OMERACT Core Outcome Sets of Joint Health Conditions, Organized by Core Areas (Manifestations, Life Impact, Societal/Resource Use, and Life Span/Death)

Core Areas and Domains[8,9,39]	Rheumatoid Arthritis[30,40–42]	Psoriatic Arthritis[43]	GOUT		OSTEOARTHRITIS		Ankylosing Spondylitis[47]	Polymyalgia Rheumatica[48]	Shoulder[49]	Juvenile Idiopathic Arthritis[50]
			Acute[44]	Chronic[44]	Hip and Knee[45]	Hand[46]				
Manifestations/Abnormalities										
Symptoms										
Pain										
Fatigue										
Sleep										
Musculoskeletal Signs										
Tenderness/Pain										
Swelling										
Combined										
Stiffness										
Performance										
Signs at Other Sites										
Skin/Subcutis										
Other/Multiple										
Global Assessment (Disease Activity)										
Patient										
Physician										
Biomarkers										
Imaging										
Soluble										
Life Impact										
Health-related QoL										
Physical Function/Disability										
Emotional Well-Being										
Psychosocial Impact										
Role Participation										
Societal/Resource Use										
Costs/HCU										
Work Disability as Cost										
Life Span/Death										
Number of Deaths										

(Dark shading) Mandatory domain; measure in all clinical trials or in specific, defined circumstances.
(Light shading) Important but optional domain.

Note: The clinical conditions included in this table are placed here as a way of separating the conditions into two tables and do not imply a formal definition of "joint health conditions."
More detail on domain sets is available in references 30, 39–50.
HCU, Health care utilization; *QoL*, quality of life.

readers should be aware of their value in verifying that the items can confidently be put into the score as recommended.[66,67]

Evidence Supporting the Validity of the Numeric Score in Setting

An instrument is built by understanding a concept and then identifying the items, response, and scoring systems that seem to capture it well. From that point forward, you can use the score to directly quantify the concept. When selecting an instrument, you want to make sure that there is enough evidence that such use is valid (i.e., that a score is a good representation of that domain of interest in your patients and setting). Evidence for this comes from placing the instrument in different scenarios and seeing if the scores perform the way an excellent measure of the domain should.[17,65,68]

One approach is to make comparisons with similar scales or related constructs (e.g., high and low levels of pain might be compared to a measure of pain impact and estimates of synovitis might come from different imaging approaches) and is often called *construct validity*. Logical arguments or scenarios are established before analysis, the direction and magnitude of the expected relationship is declared, and then the relationship is tested.[15,25,59,64] Ideally, you should test in situations where the comparisons with highly related comparators (high correlations), as well as those where no

TABLE 36.1B Domains Endorsed in OMERACT Core Outcome Sets of Diseases Manifesting in Systemic Involvement, Organized by Core Areas (Manifestations, Life Impact, Societal/Resource Use, and Life Span/Death)

Core Areas and Domains[8,9,39]	Systemic Lupus Erythematosus[51]	Vasculitis ANCA-Associated[52]	Fibromyalgia Syndrome[53]	Osteoporosis[54]	CTD-ILD[55]	Myositis[56]	Behçets[57]
Manifestations/Abnormalities							
Symptoms							
Pain							
Fatigue							
Sleep							
Other							
Musculoskeletal Signs							
Tenderness/Pain							
Deformity							
Signs at Other Sites							
Skin/Subcutis							
Other/Multiple							
Global Assessment (Disease Activity)							
Patient							
Biomarkers							
Imaging							
Soluble							
Other/Multiple							
Life Impact							
Health-Related QoL							
Physical Function/Disability							
Depression							
Dyscognition							
Societal/Resource Use							
Costs/HCU							
Life Span/Death							
Number of Deaths							
	Mandatory domain; measure in all clinical trials or in specific, defined circumstances.						
	Important but optional domain.						

Note: The clinical conditions included in this table are placed here as a way of separating the conditions into two tables and do not imply a formal definition of "systemic rheumatologic health conditions." More detail on domain sets is available in references 51–57.

CTD-ILD, Connective tissue disease-interstitial lung disease; *HCU,* health care utilization; *QoL,* quality of life.

relationship is expected (low, no correlation), will provide more confidence in what this tool is capable of measuring. Comparisons should also be made among groups known to differ by the target domain (people working or unable to work, for example, might be expected to have different physical functioning), a comparison called *known groups*. Again, a logical argument is proposed (e.g., disease activity indices should have higher scores in a person in a flare vs people in remission), and then the score is checked to see if it matches the theory. If there is not enough evidence that matches your type of need or patient group, you can either look for another instrument (because you have not been able to build an argument supporting its validity) or you can conduct a study to create that evidence and then continue to advance your understanding of the instrument and how you can use it.

It is important to understand the precision of measurement as well. In multi-item questionnaires, we might look at the consistency of responses across items (e.g., internal consistency using Cronbach's alpha coefficients, which range from 0 to 1, with [higher being the preference until 0.95]). For imaging techniques, we need to look for calibration of the machine(s) and, if there is more than one person doing the testing or making the observation, inter-rater reliability.

Inter-rater reliability is especially important for clinician-observed outcomes, such as range of motion or grip strength, or imaging outcomes where different raters might be interpreting something like joint space from an image. In these situations, the rater is a source of important variability in the score, and any error between raters needs to be estimated. The preferred statistic is one

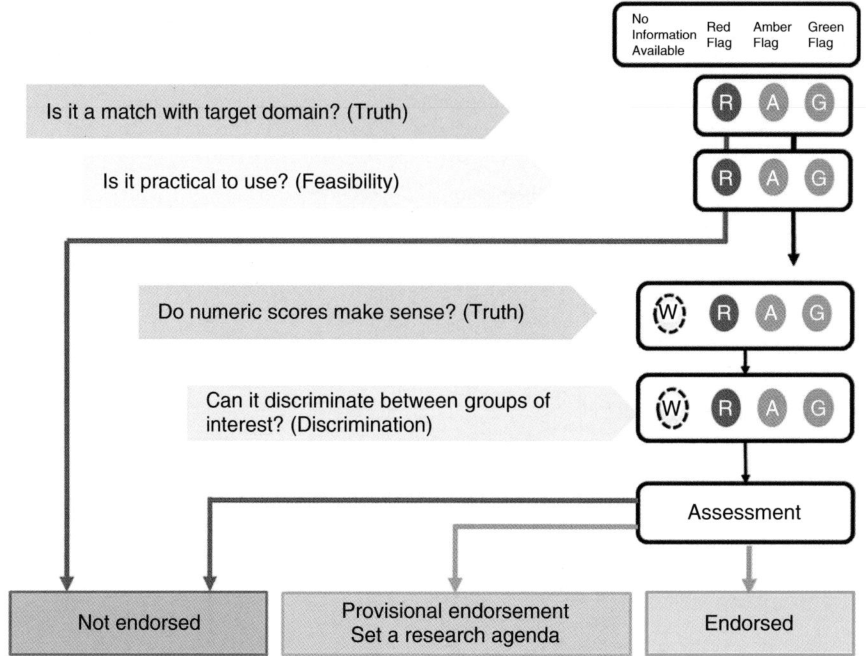

• **Fig. 36.2** Instrument selection algorithm showing the decision-making process for the fit of a candidate measure with your target measurement need, according to the OMERACT Filter 2.1. The first two signaling questions can be completed by appraisal of the instrument itself with input from patients. The last two require data from the literature. Many instruments are discarded as a poor fit in questions 1 and 2. Instruments that make it past that level often do well and groups are encouraged to create the evidence if it is missing in the literature. (@2018 OMERACT Handbook; www.omeract.org.)

that looks for the exact same number/score/rating coming from the different sources (raters, devices). The Intraclass Correlation Coefficient (ICC) and weighted kappa are well suited to look for exact agreement rather than just the trend captured by a correlation coefficient alone.[69]

Signaling Question 4: Can It Discriminate Between Groups of Interest?

After getting a general sense of the evidence supporting the cross-sectional validity and reliability of the instrument, we sometimes wish to know whether this outcome is able to measure change during a period of time. This is only important if you are going to measure and make statements about a change in score (e.g., if a change of 20 points was observed). If your goal is to describe an outcome state at one point in time, such as the level of pain after a treatment or the presence of a finding, you do not need to answer signaling question 4. When looking at change is the focus of our use of the instrument's scores, however, there are additional pieces of evidence that we need. We are looking for a few different things: (1) Do we have evidence that the scores will remain the same when the target concept has not changed during a period of time (test-retest reliability)? (2) When the concept changes, does the score on the instrument change as well (responsiveness and sensitivity to the target construct of change)? And (3) Do we have evidence to support how to use change scores as thresholds of meaning? We will now review each of these questions.

Test-Retest Reliability

Test-retest reliability requires two administrations of the instrument during a period of time when no change in the target concept has occurred. As a reader of reliability studies, you should feel convinced that no change in the target domain (e.g., pain, function, or disease activity) could have occurred in these patients between testing times.[59,60] In such a situation, we would like to see no change in the instrument's scores. Often, people conducting studies of test-retest reliability will establish a clinical situation in which no change should have occurred, or they will use an external anchor (e.g., a question about whether the patient's pain is the same as last time) to identify patients who have not changed. The responses from only those who are stable are used for test-retest reliability. Similar to interobserver reliability, the ICC is the preferred statistic for continuous scores, and weighted kappa, its equivalent, is the preferred statistic for categorical scores.[69] The cutoffs are the same, and a coefficient can be converted into a "minimal detectable change"[70] = $1.96 \times s(2[1\text{-}r])^{1/2}$, where s = standard deviation and r = test-retest reliability (ICC).[26,70] Ninety-five percent of people who are stable will have change scores less than this value, hence a change greater than this is not likely to occur in a stable patient. This becomes a possible lower boundary of meaningful change for an individual. It could be that individuals assess smaller changes to be meaningful, but our instrument is not sensitive enough to detect such changes reliably. Anything below that boundary could also be random error.

Responsiveness

Responsiveness is perhaps best thought of as longitudinal construct validity. It is defined as the ability to detect change when it has occurred and involves setting up a situation of change and then testing the ability of an instrument to capture it. Similar to construct validity, it depends on an a priori situation, allowing you to identify patients/respondents who have changed (e.g., natural course of disease, treatment of known efficacy, or change as indicated on an external anchor). Several situations where change is expected are woven into a study, and hopefully are close in direction and magnitude to what you want to be able to capture when using the instrument. Statistics that capture the signal (change score) over background noise (some estimate of variability in scores, such as a standard deviation) are used to summarize responsiveness. It is easy to focus on the amount of change recorded and be impressed by a large effect size; however, it is critical to match the change in the instrument's scores with the type or amount of change that was actually expected in that testing situation. A large change is not useful if we were expecting a small one; it only suggests excessive signal and noise. The amount of change expected in a study of responsiveness should be carefully described in the publication for the readers. Users of the literature should then make sure it is similar enough to their own needs to be useful as evidence.[71]

As mentioned, responsiveness is often summarized with statistics of signal (change) over noise (error), such as the standardized response mean (mean change/standard deviation of change), *t* statistic (mean change/standard error), or effect size (mean change over standard deviation of baseline).[69,72] Deyo and Centor also describe the correlational approach (correlate change and another indicator of change) as a direct parallel to cross-sectional construct validity correlated change scores with an external marker (another credible estimate of change).[72] They also suggest a receiver-operator characteristic curve approach (various change scores against an external marker [criterion in ROC] that the person changed). This offers information on the sensitivity and specificity of different change scores for application to individuals, as well as an overall summary for the entire score's ability to discriminate between changed and unchanged groups.[72] All of these approaches are dependent on the external anchor, which is a question or a way of knowing that a change has occurred. Deciding on this anchor is an important part of the study. As a reader of the literature, you should be convinced that the anchor for change that was used is credible and that it and the whole situation of change are close enough to your intended application for you to be able to make use of the evidence.

Discrimination Between Treatment Arms in a Trial/Cohort

One important type of change at OMERACT is the ability to detect change in a clinical trial, similar to the trials we are preparing a core outcome set for. This adds a layer to responsiveness, making it important not only to pick up change but also to do it well enough to detect the relative difference in that change between a treatment and control arm. Placebo-controlled trials are rarely used once a therapy is accepted in a field. Trials will use the established therapy as a comparator (called *comparative effectiveness research*) in a noninferiority design, so the responsiveness of an instrument will need to be sensitive in a comparison of one active treatment versus another or to show that the new treatment is equivalent to another. This could be done in a series of comparisons in large cohorts. For example, cohorts of people on two different treatments or people within a cohort who could be subdivided into those who were somewhat better and those who were dramatically improved could be used. Relative change between these subgroups would then be compared. Several such tests might be needed to build confidence in the performance of the instrument. The summary statistics, effect-size statistics, can be adapted for a direct comparison of change in two groups, as illustrated by Buchbinder[73] or Verhoeven[74] by adjusting the numerator to be relative change and the denominator to be a pooled standard deviation.

Thresholds of Meaning

The final step for this signaling question, which is often deemed the most elusive, is determining thresholds that are meaningful from the score. Responder analyses that quantify outcome as the proportion who have improved, recovered, or responded to therapy are dependent on having established thresholds of meaning. Care must therefore be taken to make sure these are accurate thresholds so that we can avoid misclassifying someone as being better or worse off than they are. The two most common thresholds of meaning involve determining meaningful levels or benchmarks in a state (level of pain, function) that has meaning and determining meaningful thresholds of change (a small but important change, for example). We will discuss the key features of each of these.

Thresholds Related to a Certain State. Clinicians want to know if pain is at a tolerable level or if a patient is in a low disease state, which requires us to be able to understand and benchmark scores. Some work has been done in this area, particularly in rheumatology. Both patient acceptable symptom states (PASS),[75,76] for what patients deem to be tolerable levels of symptoms (i.e., pain <2/10), and estimates of states reflecting low disease activity scores (LDAS)[77,78] are examples of this type of threshold. Patients often frame an important response to treatment in the form of meeting these types of thresholds. As one group describes, benchmarking allows us to ask if someone is feeling good, rather than if they are feeling better.[79]

Thresholds in Meaning Around Changes in State. Thresholds are often set to help people interpret changes in state. Sometimes, this is based on experience, reflections on observed trends in data, case studies, or consensus. The idea is to get an understanding of when a change in score is indicating an improvement or deterioration worthy of attention. The focus is on the amount of change.

The American College of Rheumatology (ACR) took the core set measures and determined that if one observed a 20% change in joint count, swollen joint count, and in at least three of the following: (1) erythrocyte sedimentation rate (ESR) or C-reactive protein (CRP); (2) physician global, patient global, pain, or (3) physical disability, then one had a clinical response, and the individual would be classified as a responder. Subsequently, research has also used thresholds of 50% and 70%. The ACR20 is widely used, defining responses across a wide variety of domains and discriminating well in clinical trials.[74]

Another important threshold is the minimal important difference (MID) in score (improvement or deterioration). There are many different ways to determine this but recently clinicians, researchers, and regulators place more value on approaches that use an external anchor to first determine who has had a small but important change.[13] The anchor might be a patient-reported rating of change, patient and clinician agreement about change, or a change in another closely related marker. A certain level on the anchor is carefully chosen to reflect when the important change has occurred. This then becomes the standard for determining the MID. Like so much of measurement testing, the quality of the resultant MID is dependent on the quality of the anchor. To improve the quality, one can use multiple anchors and triangulate the results to build confidence in the MID value. When the instrument relates to life impact, symptoms, or role functioning, patients can be welcome experts in the development or choice of these anchors and the thresholds on them that should indicate a small but important change. Many options are available to compare the result of the standard with that of the candidate instruments but one predominates: treating a number of change score like a diagnostic test and looking at the sensitivity (true positive rate) and specificity (true negative rate) of each in comparison with the chosen anchor. Receiver operator characteristic (ROC) curves can help determine the change score on the instrument that best represents that of the anchor (i.e., the one with the best sensitivity and specificity for the purpose).

MID values will vary depending on the anchor used or the approach chosen, the baseline state of the patients, and for improvements versus deterioration.[80–85] Being transparent about this variability is important. Farrar[86] advocates plotting the distribution of change scores (cumulative distribution ideal) and then visually showing the location of the change scores that reflect the calculated MIDs. The impact is to immediately show the differences in the proportion that would be described as improved across different MID values. It could also be used to show the comparison of the treatment arms in a trial showing any shifts in the description of the differences between the groups. Triangulating across the MIDs helps build confidence in the results of a trial.[84,86]

Similar graphs can be stratified by the groups defined on the anchor (i.e., improved, no change, worse). If we have a trustworthy anchor, we should see nonoverlapping distributions. If they overlap, it would suggest that the anchor is not leading to a clean separation of change scores. If it is misclassifying people as being improved or not, another anchor might be able to create a clearer threshold MID.[13] Readers are encourage to explore this reference for this emerging method.

Both of these plotting techniques promote showing the data in a way that it can be easily interpreted and limitations in the interpretation can be seen.[86]

Combined Approaches: Change and State. An attractive, but often overlooked, option is to combine the last two approaches. For example, in 1996, the European League Against Rheumatism (EULAR) defined clinical response as a change in the Disease Activity Score (DAS)-28 of more than 1.2 (change) plus a final DAS28 score of less than 2.4 (final state).[87] In doing so, this suggested both the need to change and the need to end at a very low disease activity level before being classified as a clinical response. Jacobson did the same in defining an individual's response to psychotherapy where change alone was not good enough to claim success; one needed to induce a change that could get a person to a good (i.e., non-depressed, non-anxious) state. Jacobson operationalized using change greater than day-to-day variability in score to indicate the change induced by the psychotherapy (change > error [minimal detectable change from reliability analyses]), and the person's final score had to be normal.[88] Studies on how patients themselves often define being "better" echo this combination of change and final health state.[31,79]

Is the Instrument Good Enough?

There is an element of judgment involved in each of the signaling questions above, and perfect evidence across all of the signaling questions is very unlikely.

In OMERACT decision making, green, amber, and red synthesis readings are used. Green means confidently supportive, red means against, and amber suggests that there are some questions and caution about the performance of the instrument for each signaling question (see Fig. 36.2).[15] In the end, an overall judgment is made as to whether the instrument has enough evidence to support it in OMERACT core sets or in monitoring programs and value in care as suggested by groups like ICHOM.[89]

Examples of Arthritis Instruments

Rheumatology research studies have used a wide variety of instruments. Although only a few of them have been evaluated fully according to the processes described above, they give a wide range of evidence that users could consider, and they serve as solid examples of types of instruments that might be used in the field. We will briefly review some of the more commonly encountered instruments used for arthritis, as organized by the four core areas described previously.

Indicators of Pathophysiologic Manifestations of the Disease

Disease activity is one of the most frequently encountered indicators of pathophysiologic manifestations of rheumatologic diseases. Two of the most commonly used indicators of disease activity (indicators of the inflammatory activity) are the DAS[87] and DAS28[90] in rheumatoid arthritis, in which a set of the core outcomes (i.e., acute-phase reactants, joint counts, and global ratings) are combined to form a weighted score that provides a score of 2 to 10 (DAS) or 0 to 9 (DAS28). Based on these scores, cutoffs were established to define high, moderate, and low disease states. In 2010, new criteria for remission in RA have been proposed. These new criteria recognize that disease activity is not always sensitive enough to perform at extremely low levels of functioning, leading others to refine scales or develop new ones to improve reach.[91] Other examples of disease activity indices (DAIs) include the Bath Ankylosing Spondylitis Disease Activity Index (BASDAI).[92] When more than one is available, it is helpful to seek direct comparisons of instruments. Groups are also working on worsening and moving out of remission as a key threshold of meaning for disease activity indices.[30,93]

Damage indices are indicators of structural damage to joints, typically shown by joint space narrowing, erosions, subchondral cysts, or osteophytes. In RA, particular attention has been paid to this by Van der Heijde, who reviews three approaches (Sharp, Larsen/Scott, and Van der Heijde), which are used to assess joint damage and progression in joint damage by using change greater than the smallest detectable change around error.[47]

Symptoms

Another pathophysiologic manifestation of the disease would be the intensity of symptoms like pain. Pain is usually measured by using a 10-cm visual analog scale or a 0 to 10 numeric rating scale of the intensity of the pain.[94] This simple instrument has been well tested and is easily understood by patients. Hawker led an initiative to better understand pain in hip arthritis and found patients describing qualitative visual analog differences in their intermittent and constant pain. This resulted in a new instrument to be considered for pain.[32,95] Fatigue is another important symptom, which many patients feel is quite distinct from being "tired."[29,96,97] In the area of sleep, work done through OMERACT on the measurement of the problem provides a recent strong example of moving through the concept of impairment of sleep, defining it, and then focusing on the available scales that capture that concept and definition.[98,99]

Life Impact of the Disease

General Health Status

Generic health outcomes provide information on an aspect of health across many conditions. Thus, theoretically, comparisons can be made of the impact of low back pain with that of arthritis or diabetes. This depends on how well an instrument captures the impact in each disease group. In addition to this comparability, generic instruments have the advantage of covering a broader range of health issues that may otherwise be overlooked (e.g., mental health or role functioning). Nevertheless, generic instruments, because of their breadth, tend not to delve into the depth of experience in any one disease. As a result, they are often weaker in their ability to detect specific impacts and their sensitivity to different levels of impact or change in impact should be checked. Popular examples of a generic instrument include the Short Form (SF)-36 and Euroqol (EQ-5D).[100] Although many instruments show evidence of validity in rheumatologic populations,[100] different studies' results may not be comparable if each used a different health status scale.[101,102]

Utilities: Value of Health State

Where health status scales describe someone's state of health, utility scales try to capture the value of that health state, setting death at zero and full health at one.[103] The emphasis is not upon describing the state alone, but on assigning a value, worth, or preference to that state.[103,104] Utilities play a key role in determining quality-adjusted life-years (QALY) and cost per QALY estimates. Several different approaches can be used to measure utilities, from direct estimation of value of current life (standard gamble, time trade-off) to indirect weights that are applied to multi-item/attribute scales, such as the EQ-5D, SF-36 subset of items, and the Health Utility Index (HUI).[103–105] This challenging outcome is a current area of activity at OMERACT.[105]

Physical Functioning Scales

Physical functioning is an outcome of importance for many patients with arthritis, who are focused on the ability to do many of the demands of daily life. Often, it is measured by using the HAQ Disability Index (HAQ-DI),[100] which covers 20 items that examine different domains of daily functioning. Patients score each item on a 0 to 3 scale, in which 3 represents the greatest disability. Scores are obtained for each domain and then combined for a total score expressed on the same 0 to 3 scale. Scores are adjusted to a worse health state (a 2/3) if a support is used to complete a task. More details on the HAQ-DI are widely available in print and on the Internet.

PROMIS/Health Measures offer a physical functioning instrument both on their direct entry CAT platform and as a paper form (www.healthmeasures.net) that has been tested in musculoskeletal disorders and compared to several of the arthritis scales, like the HAQ-DI.[21] There are other scales or subscales that assess physical function that have been described by one group.[106]

Self-Efficacy/Effective Consumer

Self-management is becoming a part of programs for individuals with multiple chronic conditions.[107] For patients with arthritis, these programs improve levels of self-efficacy: the confidence one has in the ability to manage pain and disease effectively. Lorig's Self-Efficacy Scale is one of the most commonly used outcomes for this type of study.[108] Tugwell's group has developed a complementary "effective consumer scale," which captures the degree to which the patient is effectively managing his or her own health care decisions, interactions with the health care team, and disease monitoring.[109] It is an instrument with demonstrated reliability, validity, and responsiveness in arthritis, and consumers with arthritis support it.[110]

Social Role Functioning

With the shift toward more effective management of earlier rheumatic disease, more people with arthritis are able to stay at work or in other life roles. Outcomes must shift to match the disease's lived experience, and in thinking about work outcomes as an example, less focus is now needed on absenteeism or withdrawal from the workforce and more attention can be paid to capturing how people function while at work.[40,96,111] Similarly, focus is needed on how people balance their multiple roles at and outside of work (work-life balance) or function in valued life activities outside of work (leisure, volunteer work). Social role functioning outcomes are particularly challenging because they come with a number of contextual factors that need to be considered. For example, is it part-time or full-time work? Does the valued leisure activity involve high levels of physical functioning or is it more sedentary? These factors can impact how a person functions in their leisure or work roles and may reduce comparability of the numeric scores from a global scale of leisure or productivity if they are not considered. These concepts will need to be considered carefully and outcome instruments reflecting this tested or developed in the future.

Patient-Specific Indices

Patient-specific scales allow the patient to nominate his or her own items, in effect creating their own customized outcome scale. Most researchers encourage three to five items to be nominated, often those that are most challenging for the person. A surprising number of these scales have been developed and reviewed by investigators.[112] Each taps into very relevant content for patients, and because of this, they can be responsive to change.[73] The challenge is in the mathematics and how to analyze the numeric score that has been created by different sets of items for each person. Analysis that focuses on individual-level quantification is likely best (e.g., the percentage of people who reach their goal or improve in their selected activities). Another challenge is that over time, certain items might become less important and there often is no way to substitute in other items. It is increasingly recognized that life span should enter our outcome frameworks.

Resource Utilization and Costs

Costs of the ingredients associated with treatment (drugs, equipment, and physician visits) are all important when considering the benefit of one treatment versus another. Thus OMERACT Filter 2.1 includes resource utilization as an important but optional area to consider in developing core outcome sets.[9] This could include direct costs, as well as indirect costs (e.g., lost productivity and caregiving). Harmonization is important to get a comparable estimates of cost across studies.

Toxicity/Adverse Events

Medical and nonmedical management of many rheumatic conditions carries a risk of adverse events,[113] many of them unexpected. Because patients, clinicians, and policy makers need to balance benefits versus harms when considering intervention, a comprehensive documentation of a range of adverse events is important in outcomes assessments separate from the treatment benefits.[8,9,12] Rheumatologic conditions are associated with increased mortality, and because mortality is a mandatory reporting condition in any clinical trial, it should be tracked in health outcome assessments in arthritis.

Areas of Growth in Health Outcome Assessment

Systematic Reviews of Measurement Properties

With the growth in the number of articles published on measurement properties for a given tool, we are seeing the growth in the number of reviews and, more recently, systematic reviews of the measurement properties in the literature (*n* >1000, www.cosmin.nl). By systematic, we mean standardized methods for searching the literature, selection of articles as relevant, critical appraisal for risk of bias, and synthesis. There are several approaches recommended for the critical appraisal step in these reviews; however, COSMIN is the most frequently used resource both for search strategies and for a scored critical appraisal instrument (recently focusing more on risk of bias).[114]

Similar to a systematic review of effectiveness studies, a lot of work is involved in systematically reviewing the articles and coming to a decision. For an instrument, one is effectively doing a mini review for each property. The results are brought together to give an overall appraisal of the instrument's ability to capture and represent the target domain in the planned application. Currently, many different approaches are being used, which could lead to different conclusions. Nevertheless, we are optimistic that the groups will be able to work together on essential elements and come to the same conclusions about the quality of an instrument.

Adaptation to an Ongoing Disease

In this chapter, we focused on the measurement of health states and also on their improvement or deterioration over time. Nevertheless, people with chronic diseases may successfully adapt to ongoing disease using behavioral strategies or by cognitively reshaping their idea of what "good health" means.[115,116] These adaptations may alter the way a person responds to a survey and an outcome might capture successful coping rather than response to a treatment. In some circles, this is called *adjustment*, in others a *response shift*.[115,116] Ongoing work is underway to capture this adaptation and decide how it should be integrated into our understanding of a patient's outcome.

Conclusion

Patient-centered care initiatives have brought a lot of attention to the topics raised in this chapter. A commitment to outcomes that matter, and increased rigor in the standards these measures must achieve to be used in clinical care or labeling means that the coming years will see even more advances and choices in health outcomes measurement. Core outcome sets are developed to ensure studies field a minimum set of outcome domains with proper instruments to improve systematic reviews and guideline development. Such core sets are not meant to restrict a researcher's choice of outcome, but rather to increase comparability across studies, interventions, and patient experiences. Our experiences in RA, where the core set was widely endorsed, have been very positive with over 70% of trials now fielding the core set of outcomes and allowing more comparability between these studies.[117]

In the future, more and more outcomes will be captured using electronic formats. The capacity to do so is present, affording a greater opportunity for more streamlined assessments using IRT with applications of CAT platforms such as for the PROMIS tools (www.healthmeasures.net). The ability to link these electronic outcome scores to health records or administrative databases increases the likelihood of having PROMs and other important clinical outcome assessments as a voice in decisions about the programs of care, policy making, or clinical decision making. They will become part of what is available in "big data." Such efforts, however, require collaboration and cooperation across measurement efforts, heeding Cano's call for international consensus on measurement and metrology.[6] There are still many challenges to face together, one of the greatest being the interpretability of the scores. When is a pain score low enough to be considered acceptable or tolerable? When is a flare starting? When should we consider an improvement in health a success or a justification for new resources?

Health outcome assessment is well advanced in arthritis care, and we acknowledge the years of work and commitment of many professional and patient/consumer groups. Advances will continue in the use of technology, the breadth and depth of our outcomes, and the quality of measurement methods. The voice of our key stakeholders from patients to investigators, payers, policy makers, and researchers should continue to advance and refresh what we measure in outcome assessments because measuring what matters is the key to advancing the meaningfulness of our research and our care.

The references for this chapter can also be found on ExpertConsult.com.

References

1. Last JM: *A dictionary of epidemiology*, ed 4, Toronto, 2001, Oxford University Press.
2. Orszag PR, Emanuel EJ: Health care reform and cost control, *N Engl J Med* 363(7):601–603, 2010.
3. Frank L, Basch E, Selby JV: The PCORI perspective on patient-centered outcomes research, *JAMA* 312(15):1513–1514, 2014.
4. Gabriel SE, Normand SL: Getting the methods right–the foundation of patient-centered outcomes research, *N Engl J Med* 367(9):787–790, 2012.
5. Coulter A: Measuring what matters, *BMJ* 356:j816, 2017.
6. Cano SJ, Pendrill LR, Barbic SP, et al.: Patient-centred outcome metrology for healthcare decision-making, *J Phys* 1044, 2018, Epublication.
7. Methodology Committee of the Patient-Centered Outcomes Research Institute (PCORI): Methodological standards and patient-centeredness in comparative effectiveness research: the PCORI perspective, *JAMA* 307(15):1636–1640, 2012.
8. Boers M, Kirwan JR, Wells G, et al.: Developing core outcome measurement sets for clinical trials: OMERACT filter 2.0, *J Clin Epidemiol* 67(7):745–753, 2014.
9. Boers M, Beaton D, Shea BJ, et al.: OMERACT Filter 2.1: elaboration of the conceptual framework for outcome measurement in health intervention studies, *J Rheumatol* 46(8):1021–1027, 2019.
10. Boers M, Brooks P, Strand V, et al.: The OMERACT Filter for outcome measures in rheumatology, *J Rheumatol* 25(2):198–199, 1998.
11. Reeve BB, Wyrwich KW, Wu AW, et al.: ISOQOL recommends minimum standards for patient-reported outcome measures used in patient-centered outcomes and comparative effectiveness research, *Qual Life Res* 22(8):1889–1905, 2013.
12. U.S. Department of Health and Human Services Food and Drug Administration Center for Drug Evaluation and Research (CDER): Guidance for industry: patient-reported outcome measures: use in medical product development to support labeling claims. http://www fdagov/cder/gdlns/prolbl.htm, 2009.

13. United States Food and Drug Administration. Discussion Document for Patient-Focused Drug Development Public Workshop on Guidance 3: Select, develop or modify fit for purpose clinical outcome assessments. Workshop October 15-16 2018. https://www.fda.gov/downloads/Drugs/NewsEvents/UCM620708.pdf. Accessed 12/31/2018.
14. Tugwell P, Boers M, D'Agostino MA, et al.: Updating the OMERACT filter: implications of filter 2.0 to select outcome instruments through assessment of "truth": content, face, and construct validity, *J Rheumatol* 41(5):1000–1004, 2014.
15. Beaton DE, Maxwell L, Shea B et al. Instrument selection using the OMERACT Filter 2.1: The OMERACT Methodology. *J Rheumatology* 46(8):1028–1035, 2019.
16. Maxwell LJ, Beaton DE, Shea BJ, et al.: Core domain set selection according to OMERACT Filter 2.1: The 'OMERACT Methodology', *J Rheumatol* 46(8):1014–1020, 2019.
17. Kane MT: Validating the interpretations and uses of test scores, *J Educ Meas* 50(1):1–73, 2013.
18. Williamson PR, Altman DG, Blazeby JM, et al.: Developing core outcome sets for clinical trials: issues to consider, *Trials* 213(132), 2012.
19. Kirkham JJ, Davis K, Altman DG, et al.: CoreOutcome Set-STAndards for Development: the COS-STAD recommendations, *PLoS Med* 14(11):e1002447, 2017a.
20. Valderas JM, Ferrer M, Mendivil J, et al.: Development of EMPRO: a tool for the standardized assessment of patient-reported outcome measures, *Value Health* 11(4):700–708, 2008.
21. Mokkink LB, Terwee CB, Patrick DL, et al.: The COSMIN checklist for assessing the methodological quality of studies on measurement properties of health status measurement instruments: an international Delphi study, *Qual Life Res* 19(4):539–549, 2010.
22. Prinsen CA, Vohra S, Rose MR, et al.: How to select outcome measurement instruments for outcomes included in a "Core Outcome Set"—a practical guide, *Trials* 17(1):449, 2016.
23. Witter JP: Introduction: PROMIS a first look across diseases, *J Clin Epidem* 73:87–88, 2016.
24. Dodd S, Clarke M, Becker L, et al.: A taxonomy has been developed for outcomes in medical research to help improve knowledge discovery, *J Clin Epidem* 96:84–92, 2018.
25. Kane MT: Validation as a pragmatic, scientific activity, *J Educ Meas* 50(1):115–122, 2013.
26. McHorney CA, Tarlov AR: Individual patient monitoring in clinical practice: are available health status surveys adequate? *Qual Life Res* 4:293, 1995.
27. Kirshner B, Guyatt GH: A methodological framework for assessing health indices, *J Chronic Dis* 38(1):27–36, 1985.
28. El Miedany Y, El Gaafary M, El Aroussy N, et al.: Patient centricity: Can PROM's fill the gap between the physician perspective and the dynamtic pattern of atient perceived remission in rheumatoid arthritis, *J Rheumatol Arthritic Dis* 3(2):1–7, 2018.
29. Hewlett S, Choy E, Kirwan J: Furthering our understanding of fatigue in rheumatoid arthritis, *J Rheumatol* 39(9):1775–1777, 2012.
30. Bykerk VP, Lie E, Bartlett SJ, et al.: Establishing a Core Domain Set to measure rheumatoid arthritis flares: report of the OMERACT 11 RA Flare Workshop, *J Rheumatol* 41(4):799–809, 2014.
31. Beaton DE, Tarasuk V, Katz JN, et al.: Are you better? A qualitative study of the meaning of being better, *Arthritis Care Res* 7(3):313–320, 2001.
32. Hawker GA, Davis AM, French MR, et al.: Development and preliminary psychometric testing of a new OA pain measure–an OARSI/OMERACT initiative, *Osteoarthritis Cartilage* 16(4):409–414, 2008.
33. Mayo NE, Figueiredo S, Ahmed S, et al.: Montreal Accord on Patient-reported outcomes (PROs) use series—Paper 2: terminology proposed to measure what matters in health, *J Clin Epidemiol* 89:119–124, 2017.
34. World Health Organization: *International Classification of functioning, disabilty and health*, Geneva, 2001, World Health Organization.
35. Stucki G, Boonen A, Tugwell P, et al.: The World Health Organisation International Classification of Functioning, Disability and Health (ICF): a conceptual model and interface for the OMERACT process, *J Rheumatol* 34:600–606, 2007.
36. Page MJ, McKenzie JE, Green SE, et al.: Core domain and outcome measurement sets for shoulder pain trials are needed: systematic review of physical therapy trials, *J Clin Epidemiol* 68(11):1270–1281, 2015.
37. Sinha IP, Smyth RL, Williamson PR: Using the delphi technique to determine which outcomes to measure in clinical trials: recommendations for the future based on a systematic review of existing studies, *PLoS Med* 8(1):e1000393, 2011.
38. de Wit M, Kirwan JR, Tugwell P. et al.: Successful stepwise development of patient research partnership: 14 years' experience of actions and consequences in outcome measures in rheumatology (OMERACT) Patient (2017), 10:141–152.
39. Wolfe F, Lassere M, van der Heijde D, et al.: Preliminary core set of domains and reporting requirements for longitudinal observational studies in rheumatology, *J Rheumatol* 26:484–489, 1999.
40. Boers M, Tugwell P, Felson DT, et al.: World Health Organization and International League of Associations for Rheumatology core endpoints for symptom modifying antirheumatic drugs in rheumatoid arthritis clinical trials, *J Rheumatol* 21(Suppl 41):86–89, 1994.
41. Felson DT, Anderson JJ, Boers M, et al.: The American College of Rheumatology preliminary core set of disease activity measures for rheumatoid arthritis clinical trials, The Committee on Outcome Measures in Rheumatoid Arthritis Clinical Trials, *Arthritis Rheum* 36(6):729–740, 1993.
42. Kirwan J, Minnock P, Abebajo A, et al.: Patient perspective: fatigue as a recommended patient-cetnred outcome measure in rheumatoid arthritis, *J Rheum* 34(5):1174–1177, 2007.
43. Orbai AM, Mease PJ, deWit M, et al.: Report of the GRAPPA-OMERACT Psoriatic Arthritis Working Group from the GRAPPA 2015 Annual Meeting, *J Rheumatol* 43(5):965–969, 2016.
44. Schumacher HR, Taylor W, Edwards L, et al.: Outcome domains for studies of acute and chronic gout, *J Rheumatol* 36:2342–2345, 2009.
45. Smith TO, Hawker GA, Hunter DJ, et al.: The OMERACT-OARSI core domain set for measurement in clinical trials of hip and/or knee osteoarthritis, *J Rheumatol* 46(8):981–989, 2019.
46. Kloppenburg M, Boyesen P, Visser AW, et al.: Report from the OMERACT Hand Osteoarthritis Working Group: set of core domains and preliminary set of instruments for use in clinical trials and observational studies, *J Rheumatol* 42, 2015. 2190–7.
47. van der Heijde D, van der Linden S, Dougados M, et al.: Ankylosing spondylitis: plenary discussion and results of voting on selection of domains and some specific instruments, *J Rheumatol* 26:1003–1005, 1999.
48. Mackie SL, Twohig H, Neill LM, et al.: The OMERACT Core domain set for outcome measures for clinical trials in polymyalgia rheumatica, *J Rheumatol* 44:1515–1521, 2017.
49. Ramiro S, Page M, Whittle S, et al.: The OMERACT core domain set for clinical trials of shoulder disorders, *J Rheumatol* 46(8):969–975, 2019.
50. Morgan E, Munro J, Horonjeff J, et al.: Establishing an updated core domain set for studies in juvenile idiopathic arthritis: a report from the OMERACT 2018 JIA Workshop, *J Rheumatol* 46(8):1006–1013, 2019.
51. Smolen JS, Strand V, Cardiel M, et al.: Randomized clinical trials and longitudinal observational studies in systemic lupus erythematosus: consensus on a preliminary core set of outcome domains, *J Rheumatol* 26(2):504–507, 1999.
52. Merkel PA, Aydin SZ, Boers M, et al.: The OMERACT core set of outcome measures for use in clinical trials of ANCA-Associated Vasculitis, *J Rheumatol* 38:1480–1486, 2011.

53. Mease P, Arnold LM, Choy EH, et al.: Fibromyalgia syndrome module at OMERACT 9: domain construct, *J Rheumatol* 36(10):2318–2329, 2009.
54. Sambrook PN, Cummings SR, Eisman JA, et al.: Guidelines of osteoporosis trials, *J Rheumatol* 24:1234–1236, 1997.
55. Khanna D, Mitto S, Aggarwal R, et al.: Connective tissue disease-associated interstitial lung diseases–report from OMERACT CTD-ILD working group, *J Rheumatol* 42:2168–2171, 2015.
56. Regardt M, Mecoli C, Park JK, et al.: OMERACT 2018 modified patient-reported outcome domain core set in the life impact area for adult idiopathic inflammatory myopathies, *J Rheumatol* 46(10):1351–1354, 2019.
57. Hatemi G. Personal communication (domains endorsed at OMERACT2018 but manuscript not yet published)
58. Law M: Measurement in occupational therapy: scientific criteria for evaluation, *CJOT* 54(3):133–138, 1987.
59. Lohr KN, Aaronson NK, Alonso J, et al.: Evaluating quality-of-life and health status instruments: development of scientific review criteria, *Clin Ther* 18(5):979–992, 1996.
60. Kirshner B, Guyatt G: A methodological framework for assessing health indices, *J Chron Dis* 38(1):27–36, 1985.
61. Tang K, Beaton DE, Lacaille D, et al.: Sensibility of five at-work productivity measures was endorsed by patients with osteoarthritis or rheumatoid arthritis, *J Clin Epidemiol* 66(5):546–556, 2013.
62. Auger C, Demers L, Swaine B: Making sense of pragmatic criteria for the selection of geriatric rehabilitation measurement tools, *Arch Gerontol Geriatr* 43(1):65–83, 2006.
63. McDowell I, Jenkinson C: Development standards for health measures, *J Health Serv Res Policy* 1(4):238–246, 1996.
64. Hawkins M, Elsworth GR, Osborne RH: Application of validity theory and methodology to patient-reported outcome measures (PROMs): building an argument for validity, *Qual Life Res* 27(7):1695–1710, 2018.
65. Edwards MC, Slagle A, Rubright JD: Fit for purpose and modern validity theory in clinical outcomes assessment, *Qual Life Res* 27:1711–1720, 2018.
66. Tennant A, Conaghan PG: The Rasch measurement model in rheumatology: what is it and why use it? When should it be applied, and what should one look for in a Rasch paper? *Arthritis Rheum* 57(8):1358–1362, 2007.
67. Edelen MO, Reeve BB: Applying item response theory (IRT) modelling to questionnaire development, evaluation and refinement, *Qual Life Res* 16:5–18, 2007.
68. Sawatzky R, Chan EKH, Zumbo BD, et al.: Montreal Accord on patient reported outcomes (PORs) use series—Paper 7: modern perspectives on measurement validation emphasize justification of internces based on patient–reported outcome scores, *J Clin Epidemiol* 89:154–159, 2017.
69. Hays RD, Revicki D: Reliability and validity (including responsiveness). In Fayers P, Hays R, editors: *Assessing quality of life in clinical trials: methods and practice*, ed 2, New York, 2005, Oxford University Press, pp 25–39.
70. Stratford PW, Binkley JM: Applying the results of self-report measures to individual patients: an example using the Roland-Morris Questionnaire, *J Orthop Sports Phys Ther* 29(4):232–239, 1999.
71. Beaton DE, Bombardier C, Katz JN, et al.: A taxonomy for responsiveness, *J Clin Epidemiol* 54(12):1204–1217, 2001.
72. Deyo RA, Centor RM: Assessing the responsiveness of functional scales to clinical change: an analogy to diagnostic test performance, *J Chronic Dis* 39(11):897–906, 1986.
73. Buchbinder R, Bombardier C, Yeung M, et al.: Which outcome measures should be used in rheumatoid arthritis clinical trials? *Arthritis Rheum* 38(11):1568–1580, 1995.
74. Verhoeven A, Boers M, van der Linden S: Responsiveness of the core set, response criteria, and utilities in early rheumatoid arthritis, *Ann Rheum Dis* 59:966–974, 2000.
75. Tubach F, Wells GA, Ravaud P, et al.: Minimal clinically important difference, low disease activity state and patient acceptable symptom state: methodological issues, *J Rheumatol* 32(10):2025–2029, 2005.
76. Tubach F, Ravaud P, Baron G, et al.: Evaluation of clinically relevant states in patient reported outcomes in knee and hip osteoarthrits: the patient acceptable symptom state, *Ann Rheum Dis* 64:34–37, 2005.
77. Wells GA, Boers M, Shea B, et al.: Minimal disease activity for rheumatoid arthritis: a preliminary definition, *J Rheumatol* 32(10):2016–2024, 2005.
78. Boers M, Anderson JJ, Felson D: Deriving an operational definition of low disease activity state in rheumatoid arthritis, *J Rheumatol* 30(5):1112–1114, 2003.
79. Tubach F, Dougados M, Falissard B, et al.: Feeling good rather than feeling better matters more to patients, *Arthritis Rheum* 55(4):526–530, 2006.
80. Beaton DE, Boers M, Wells GA: Many faces of the minimal clinically important difference (MCID): a literature review and directions for future research, *Curr Opin Rheumatol* 14:109–114, 2002.
81. Tubach F, Ravaud P, Baron G, et al.: Evaluation of clinically relevant changes in patient reported outcomes in knee and hip osteoarthritis: the minimal clinically important improvement, *Ann Rheum Dis* 64:29–33, 2005.
82. Salaffi F, Stancati A, Silvestri CA, et al.: Minimal clinically important changes in chronic musculoskeletal pain intensity measures on a numerical rating scale, *Eur J Pain* 8:283–291, 2004.
83. Angst F, Aeschlimann A, Stucki G: Smallest detectable and minimal clinically important differences of rehabilitation intervention with their implications for required sample sizes using WOMAC and SF-36 quality of life measurement instruments in patients with osteoarthritis of the lower extremities, *Arthritis Care Res* 45:384–391, 2001.
84. Wyrwich KW, Norquist JM, Lenderking WR, et al.: Methods for interpreting change over time in patient-reported outcome measures, *Qual Life Res* 22:475–483, 2013.
85. Copay AG, Eyberg B, Chung AS, et al.: Minimum clinically important difference: current trends in the orthopaedic literature part ii: lower extremity, *J Bone Joint Surg Rev* 6(9):e1, 2018.
86. Farrar JT, Dworkin RH, Max MB: Use of the cumulative proportion of responders analysis graph to present pain data over a range of cut-off points: making clinical trial data more understandable, *J Pain Symp Management* 31(4):369–377, 2006.
87. Van Gestel AM, Prevoo MLL, Van't Hof MA, et al.: Development and validation of the European League Against Rheumatism response criteria for rheumatoid arthritis, *Arthritis Rheum* 39:34–40, 1996.
88. Jacobson NS, Roberts LJ, Berns SB, et al.: Methods for defining and determining the clinical significance of treatment effects: description, application, alternatives, *J Consult Clin Psychol* 67(3):300–307, 1999.
89. Oude Voshaar MAH, Das Gupta Z, Bijlmsa JWJ, et al.: The International Consortium for Health Outcome Measurement (ICHOM) Set of outcomes for people living with inflammatory arthritis: consensus from an international working group, *Arthritis Care Res*, 2018; electronic publication ahead of print.
90. Prevoo MLL, Van't Hof MA, Kuper HH, et al.: Modified disease activity scores that include twenty-eight-joint counts. Development and validation in a prospective longitudinal study of patients with rheumatoid arthritis, *Arthritis Rheum* 38(1):44–48, 1995.
91. Felson DT, Smolen J, Wells G: American College of Rheumatology/European League against Rheumatism preliminary definition of remission in rheumatoid arthritis for clinical trials, *Ann Rheum Dis In press*, 2010.
92. Garrett S, Jenkinson T, Kennedy LG, et al.: A new approach to defining disease status in ankylosing spondylitis: the BATH ankylosing spondylitis disease activity index, *J Rheumatol* 21(12):2286–2291, 1994.
93. Bingham CO, Pohl C, Woodworth TG, et al.: Developing a standardized definition for disease "flare" in rheumatoid arthritis (OMERACT 9 Special Interest Group), *J Rheumatol* 36(10):2335–2341, 2009.

94. Farrar JT, Portenoy RK, Berlin JA, et al.: Defining the clinically important difference in pain outcome measures, *Pain* 88(3):287–294, 2000.
95. Hawker GA, Mian S, Kendzerska T, et al.: Measures of adult pain: visual analog scale for pain (VAS Pain), numeric rating scale for pain (NRS Pain), McGill pain questionnaire (MPQ), Short-Form McGill Pain Questionnaire (SF-MPQ), chronic pain grade scale (CPGS), Short Form-36 Bodily Pain Scale (SF-36 BPS), and Measure of Intermittent and Constant Osteoarthritis Pain (ICOAP), *Arthritis Care Res (Hoboken)* 63(Suppl 11):S240–S252, 2011.
96. Kirwan JR, Newman S, Tugwell PS, et al.: Progress on incorporating the patient perspective in outcome assessment in rheumatology and the emergence of life impact measures at OMERACT 9, *J Rheumatol* 36(9):2071–2076, 2009.
97. Gossec L, Dougados M, Rincheval N, et al.: Elaboration of the preliminary Rheumatoid arthritis impact of disease (RAID) score: a EULAR initiative, *Ann Rheum Dis* 68(11):1680–1685, 2009.
98. Kirwan JR, Newman S, Tugwell PS, et al.: Patient perspective on outcomes in rheumatology—a position paper for OMERACT 9, *J Rheumatol* 36(9):2067–2070, 2009.
99. Wells GA, Li T, Kirwan JR, et al.: Assessing quality of sleep in patients with rheumatoid arthritis, *J Rheumatol* 36(9):2077–2086, 2009.
100. Linde L, Sorensen J, Osterfaard M, et al.: Health related quality of life: validity, reliability and responsiveness of the SF-36, 15D, EQ-5D, RAQoL, and HAQ in patients with rheumatoid arthritis, *J Rheumatol* 35(8):1528–1537, 2008.
101. Beaton DE, Bombardier C, Hogg-Johnson SA: Measuring health in injured workers: a cross-sectional comparison of five generic health status instruments in workers with musculoskeletal injuries, *Am J Ind Med* 29(6):618–631, 1996.
102. Beaton DE, Hogg-Johnson S, Bombardier C: Evaluating changes in health status: reliability and responsiveness of five generic health status measures in workers with musculoskeletal disorders, *J Clin Epidemiol* 50(1):79–93, 1997.
103. Feeny D: Preference-based measures: utility and quality-adjusted life years. In Fayers P, Hays R, editors: *Assessing quality of life in clinical trials: methods and practice*, ed 2, New York, 2005, Oxford University Press, pp 405–429.
104. Brazier J, Roberts J, Deverill M: The estimation of a preference-based measure of health from the SF-36, *J Health Econ* 21(2):271–292, 2002.
105. Trenaman L, Boonen A, Guillemin F, et al.: OMERACT quality-adjusted life years (QALY) working group: Do current QALY measures capture what matters to patients? *J Rheumatol* 44(12):1899–1903, 2017.
106. White DK, Wilson JC, Keysor JJ: Measures of adult general functional status: SF-36 physical functioning subscale (PF-10), health assessment questionnaire (HAQ), modified health assessment questionnaire (MHAQ), Katz index of independence in activities of daily living, functional independence measure (FIM), and osteoarthritis-function-computer adaptive test (OA-Function-CAT), *Arth Care and Res* 63(S11):S308–S324, 2011.
107. Lorig KR, Holman HR: Self-management education: history, definitions, outcomes, and mechanisms, *Ann Behav Med* 26(1):1–7, 2003.
108. Lorig K, Chastain RL, Ung E, et al.: Development and evaluation of a scale to measure perceived self-efficacy in people with arthritis, *Arthritis Rheum* 32(1):37–44, 1989.
109. Kristjansson E, Tugwell PS, Wilson AJ, et al.: Development of the effective musculoskeletal consumer scale, *J Rheumatol* 34:1392–1400, 2007.
110. Santesso N, Rader T, Wells GA, et al.: Responsiveness of the Effective Consumer Scale (EC-17), *J Rheumatol* 36(9):2087–2091, 2009.
111. Beaton D, Bombardier C, Escorpizo R, et al.: Measuring worker productivity: frameworks and measures, *J Rheumatol* 36(9):2100–2109, 2009.
112. Jolles BM, Buchbinder R, Beaton DE: A study compared nine patient-specific indices for musculoskeletal disorders, *J Clin Epidemiol* 58(8):791–801, 2005.
113. Lassere M, Johnson K, Van Santen S, et al.: Generic patient self-report and investigator report instruments of therapeutic safety and tolerability, *J Rheumatol* 32:2033–2036, 2005.
114. Mokkink LB, deVet HCW, Prinsen CAC, et al.: COSMIN risk of bias checklist for systematic reviews of patient-reported outcome measures, *Qual Life Res* 27(5):1171–1179, 2018.
115. Sajobi TT, Brahmbatt R, Lix LM, et al.: Scoping review of response shift methods: current reporting practices and recommendations, *Qual Life Res* 27(5):1133–1146, 2018.
116. Schwartz C, Sprangers M, Fayers P: Response shift: you know it's there but how do you capture it? Challenges for the next phase of research. In Fayers P, Hays R, editors: *Assessing quality of life in clinical trials: methods and practice*, ed 2, New York, 2005, Oxford University Press, pp 275–290.
117. Kirkham JJ, Clarke M, Williamson PR: A methodological approach for assessing the uptake of core outcome sets using ClinicalTrials.gov: findings from a review of randomized controlled trials of rheumatoid arthritis, *BMJ* 357:j2262, 2017.

37 Biomarkers in Rheumatology

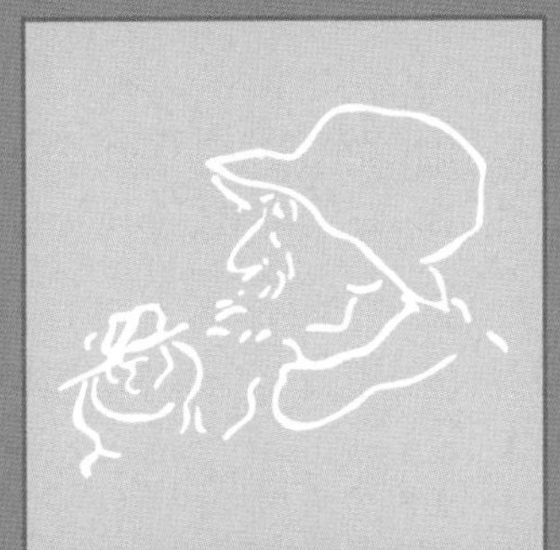

MICHAEL J. TOWNSEND, SALOUMEH K. FISCHER, AND ANDREW C. CHAN

KEY POINTS

Biomarkers are objective measurements that can assist in the diagnosis (e.g., anti-citrullinated protein antibodies in rheumatoid arthritis [RA]), prognosis (e.g., copy number of human leukocyte antigen [HLA]-DR subregion shared epitope in RA), and monitoring activity of diseases (e.g., complement or double-strand DNA autoantibodies in systemic lupus erythematosus [SLE]).

Biomarkers are often used to aid development of therapeutics to assess effects on target pathway modulation, as surrogate endpoints for clinical efficacy, or as predictors of adverse events.

Discovery and development of biomarkers for clinical utility is a complex and challenging process requiring considerations of many factors that affect their reliability and reproducibility.

Co-development of companion diagnostics with therapeutics requires a high degree of coordination so that qualified and validated assays are in place in time for each phase of therapeutic development.

In osteoarthritis (OA), biomarkers to identify patients at high-risk for cartilage loss as well as for predicting future cartilage loss will greatly aid development of disease-modifying OA drugs.

In RA, biomarkers to identify pre-RA patients with high risk to develop clinical RA, to identify patient subsets that have greater clinical benefit with targeted therapeutics, and to predict patients with greater bone and cartilage loss would advance disease understanding and development of therapeutics.

In SLE, biomarkers that predict disease activity and end-organ involvement will greatly aid patient care.

Biomarker Definitions and Applications

Biomarkers or biologic markers represent objective measurements of a patient at a given time. They are widely used in medicine for the diagnosis, prognosis, and monitoring disease activity. In drug discovery and development, they are often used to predict the degree of pharmacologic activity by a therapeutic candidate and as surrogate endpoints for potential toxicities and clinical efficacy. Use of surrogate biomarkers to establish therapeutic efficacy in registrational trials is also an accepted route for accelerated regulatory approval for therapeutics.[1]

The definition of biomarkers has evolved over the past decades. In 1993, the International Programme on Chemical Safety defined biomarker to include "any measurement reflecting an interaction between a biological system and a potential chemical, physical or biological hazards (including) functional and physiological, biochemical at the cellular level, or a molecular interaction."[2] In 2001, a Biomarkers Definitions Working Group commissioned by the National Institutes of Health (NIH) broadened its definition as "a characteristic that is objectively measured and evaluated as an indicator of normal biological processes, pathogenic processes, or pharmacologic responses to a therapeutic intervention."[3] Biomarkers have evolved to be important tools that have significant potential to guide both clinical management and development of therapeutics. In 2016, the Food and Drug Administration (FDA)-NIH collaboratively published The **B**iomarkers, **E**ndpoint**S**, and other **T**ools (BEST) Resource glossary to promote the consistent use of biomarker terms and concepts.[4] BEST defines a biomarker as "a defined characteristic that is measured as an indicator of normal biological processes, pathogenic processes, or responses to an exposure or intervention, including therapeutic interventions." They can aid in the diagnosis of disease (diagnostic), determine the potential for developing the disease (susceptibility/risk), assess the status of disease (monitoring), predict the future course of disease (prognostic), evaluate target engagement in response to a therapeutic (pharmacodynamic response), identify responders and nonresponders (predictive and complementary), and safety. Definitions of each biomarker category are listed in Table 37.1 and schematized in Fig. 37.1.

Defining Patient Heterogeneity

A major challenge in biomarker discovery and translation into clinical practice is disease heterogeneity. Most rheumatic diseases, historically considered monotypic, actually are comprised of multiple molecularly driven pathogenic pathways, though they share a common clinical presentation. In contrast, inherited monogenic diseases, such as hemophilia A, have a common pathogenic cause due to factor VIII (fVIII) deficiency and can be uniformly diagnosed by measuring fVIII levels and treated with fVIII replacement. In addition, the concept that one biomarker can be predictive in defining a patient population in heterogeneous clinical syndromes may need to be replaced by an integrative approach that includes multiple biomarkers, possibly involving more than one technology platform. For example, rheumatoid arthritis (RA) is a common rheumatic disease. That only approximately one-third of patients achieve improvement of their ACR50 scores with targeted therapies underscores the complex and multiple pathogenic

TABLE 37.1 BEST Definition of Biomarkers[4]

Categories of Biomarkers	Definition
Diagnostic	Detect or confirm presence of a disease or condition
Susceptibility/risk	Predicts potential for developing a disease or medical condition in a patient who is currently asymptomatic
Monitoring	Serially assesses disease status or exposure to a medical product or an environmental agent
Prognostic	Identifies likelihood of a clinical event, disease recurrence, or disease progression
Pharmacodynamic response	Demonstrates a biologic or biochemical response has occurred in an individual who has been exposed to a medical product or an environmental agent
Predictive	Identification of individuals who are more likely than similar individuals without the biomarker to experience an effect from exposure to a medical product or an environmental agent
Safety	Predicts likelihood, presence, or extent of an adverse effect

causes of this disease.[5] Accordingly, considerable research has focused on understanding patient disease heterogeneity, identification of markers associated with patient subsets that may reflect their underlying disease pathogenesis, and biomarkers that predict therapeutic responses. The ability to match therapy and patient, coined *personalized* or *precision medicine,* can have profound benefits for patients to provide them with the most effective therapy and avoid potential toxicities associated with ineffective therapies, as well as for the economics of health care. However, the discovery of such biomarkers and their transfer to clinical practice remains a significant challenge.

Pitfalls in Translation From Biomarker Discovery to Clinical Utility

Challenges With Biomarker Discovery and Qualification

Discovery and implementation of biomarkers in clinical practice require both analytical method validation and clinical qualification. Analytical method validation is the process of assessing the assay, its performance characteristics, and the optimal conditions that will ensure assay reproducibility and accuracy. Clinical qualification is the process of linking a biomarker with biologic processes and clinical endpoints.[6] Progress in the introduction of new biomarkers into clinical practice has been slow and underscores the multiple challenges of discovery, analytical validation, and clinical qualification of biomarkers.

While there has been a myriad of proposed biomarkers, only a few useful biomarkers have been successfully validated for routine clinical practice.[7] Contributing to the high failure rate is the poor clinical characteristics and qualification of the biomarkers of interest. A qualified biomarker must have adequate sensitivity (be able to correctly identify a high proportion of true positive rate) and specificity (be able to correctly identify a high proportion of true negative rate). Qualification not only requires appropriate bioanalytical methods, but also sufficient sample size; statistical analysis; availability of appropriately age-, sex-, and ethnicity-matched samples; information on sample collection, processing, and storage; and detailed knowledge of disease duration, severity, and medications associated with each sample. Each of these parameters will be discussed later.

Biomarker Assay Qualification and Validation

A critical component of biomarker development is the availability of reliable biomarker assays. Biomarker development often fails early in discovery not because of the underlying science, but due to poor assay choice and inappropriate assay validation.[7] Assay qualification/validation is complex and depends on the context of use (COU) of the biomarker and requires a fit-for-purpose strategy. In addition, the level of biomarker assay validation/qualification can differ between predictive biomarkers intended for clinical decision making and those intended for investigative work to support drug development. While both qualification and validation of analytical methods are designed to prove that the method is suitable for its intended purpose, they differ in terms of the depth and robustness of the evaluation. Qualifications are often sufficient for methods used for investigative evaluations. However, if the biomarker is used for clinical decision making or as a diagnostic associated with a therapeutic (e.g., dosing decisions, safety evaluations, and/or patient selection as with diagnostic markers), the method also needs to be validated.

A number of factors can impact the quality of bioanalytical assays that contribute to the challenges of biomarker discovery and translation to the clinic. It is therefore essential that the assay qualification used includes assessment of the following parameters: (1) precision-closeness in data from replicate determinations of the same sample under normal assay conditions; (2) analytical measurement range, which is the concentrations of analyte or assay values between the low and high limits of quantitation for which there is suitable level of precision, accuracy, and linearity; (3) sensitivity, which is the smallest concentration of analyte that can be measured accurately and precisely; (4) parallelism, which is assessment of the effects of dilution on quantitation of endogenous analyte(s) and confirmation of similar performance of calibrators and endogenous analyte in the assay; (5) selectivity/specificity, which is the ability to assess the target analyte in matrices (e.g., serum, plasma, synovial fluid, or urine) without interference from matrix components. A method that is selective for an analyte or group of analytes is said to be specific, (6) accuracy, which is the degree of closeness of the determined value to the nominal or known true value, and (7) stability of analytes and assay components to ensure short- and long-term reproducibility.

Biomarker qualification includes establishing that the analytical performance characteristics of a biomarker are acceptable for the proposed COU. This includes pre-analytical considerations including sample type, sample collection times, sample stability, study design, and biologic variability of the biomarker in the populations of interest. Research grade assays with well-characterized reagents are typically used in the biomarker discovery phase, but often are expensive, time consuming, and typically not automated to enable application in the clinical commercial setting. Commercial kits are an attractive option, but there are no currently harmonized qualification criteria for kit manufacturers.

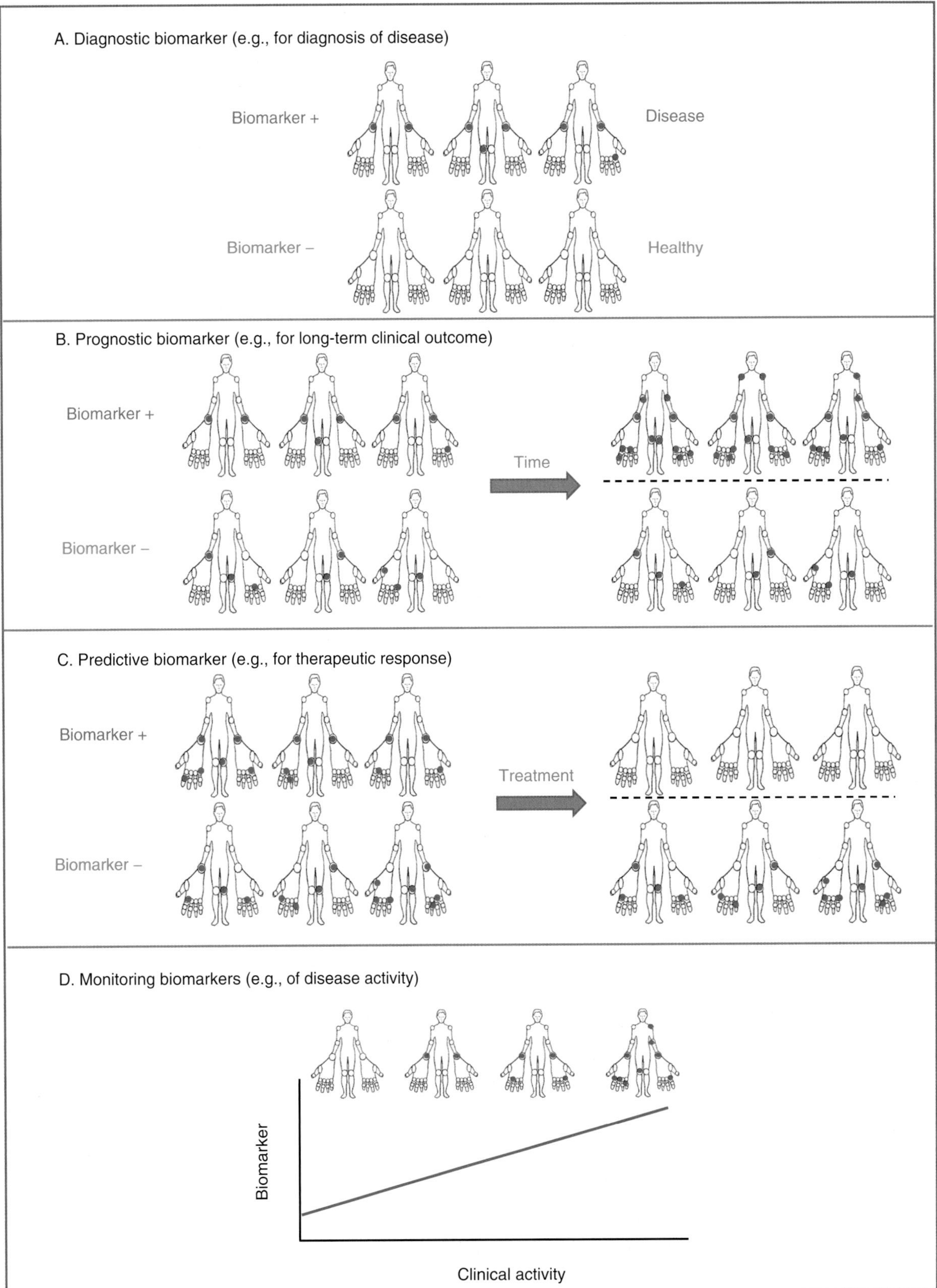

• **Fig. 37.1** Schematic representation of various types of biomarkers. *Red* denotes active joint inflammation in joint count activity diagrams. (A) Diagnostic biomarkers are utilized to aid diagnosis of a disease by distinguishing between biomarker-positive patients and biomarker-negative healthy individuals (or patients with a different disease). (B) Prognostic biomarkers identify patients at baseline that in time will develop a more severe disease. (C) Predictive biomarkers identify patients prior to treatment that will have greater benefit with a specific treatment. (D) Monitoring biomarkers correlate with disease activity.

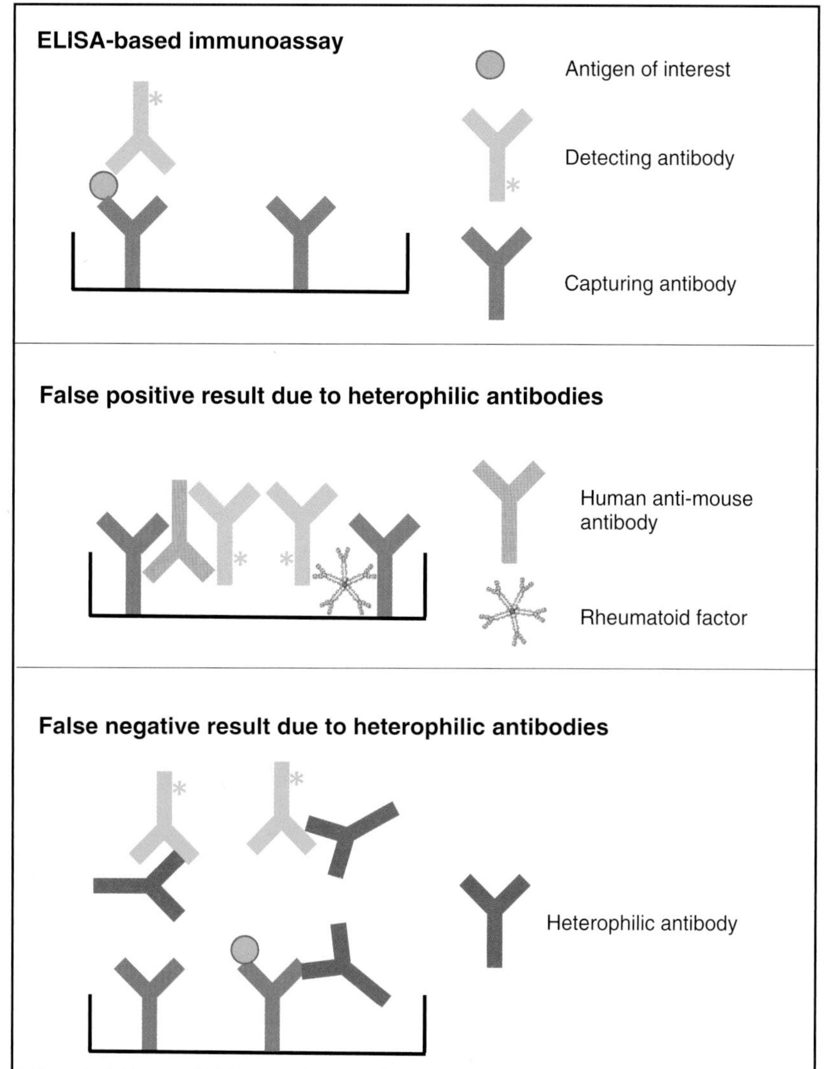

• **Fig. 37.2** Assay interference by heterophilic antibodies. *Top panel*: Standard schema for Enzyme-Linked ImmunoSorbent Assays (ELISA). *Middle panel*: Heterophilic antibodies (e.g., human anti-mouse antibodies or rheumatoid factor) can bind to Fc domains of the ELISA, capturing and detecting antibodies to result in a false-positive assay reading. *Bottom panel*: Heterophilic antibodies can bind Fab domains of ELISA, capturing or detecting antibodies to interfere with binding of antigen or detecting antibody to result in a false-negative assay reading.

Sample Matrices and Assay Interference

Biomarkers are often measured in readily available matrix such as serum, plasma, and synovial fluid, and hence have to be qualified for the disease-specific matrix, rather than buffer or samples from healthy volunteers. Matrix interference is defined as "the effect of a substance present in the sample that alters the correct value of the result."[8] These interferences are due to interactions between constituents in the sample with one or more reagent components and can be analyte-dependent (caused by matrix components) or analyte-independent (caused by assay components).

Analyte-dependent interference is often caused by endogenous substances including natural, polyreactive antibodies, autoantibodies (heterophiles) such as rheumatoid factor (RF), or human anti-animal antibodies (e.g., human anti-mouse antibodies [HAMA]). These interferences can alter the measurable concentration of the analyte or alter antibody binding causing erroneous results.[9–11] Using sera containing high titers of Fc-reactive heterophilic antibodies (HA), 21 of 170 immunoassay kits tested, including commercially available clinical assays covering 19 analytes, were susceptible to interference from heterophilic antibodies.[9] Presence of RF or HA can augment (positive interference) or inhibit (negative interference) antigen detection by binding the capturing or detecting antibody (Fig. 37.2). RF interference has been reported in a multitude of immunoassay measurements, including tacrolimus, cytokines (IL1β, IL4, IL6, and IL8), thyroid stimulating hormone, free thyroxine, mast cell tryptase, prostate specific antigen, and CA 19-9.[11–14] HA interference can be reduced or eliminated through the use of HA inhibitors such as HeteroBlock, an immunoglobulin-inhibiting reagent to quench HA activity,[12] or elimination of the Fc domain of capture or detection antibodies through use of $F(ab')_2$ fragments[15] or single-chain fragments (scFv).

Analyte-independent interference can also compromise biomarker assay integrity. As one recent example, biotin or vitamin B7 is a common dietary supplement that can exceed the daily recommended dose (30 μg) by more than 300-fold and is also given at a daily dose of 300 mg in clinical trials of the progressive form of multiple sclerosis. Presence of biotin can interfere with biotin-streptavidin based diagnostic immunoassays.[16] Biotin interference can result in either falsely high or falsely low results and has been reported to confound measurements of thyroid function tests (fT3, fT4, and TSH), estradiol, progesterone, NB-terminal pro-hormone of brain natriuretic peptide, digoxin, and troponin.[17] The FDA recently released an FDA Safety Communication[18] to raise awareness of this underrecognized analyte-independent interference complicating immunoassay performance.

Impact of Patient Selection on Validation of Biomarkers

Following biomarker discovery, rigor in biomarker validation in a well-designed independent validation patient data set is requisite for success in the clinical setting. Factors to consider in choosing the validation patient population include ensuring a diverse population that reflects the intended use of the biomarker; a balanced population in regards to age, sex, and ethnicity; as well as consideration of variables including alcohol consumption, tobacco use, body mass index, physical activity, and use of medications. The impact of age and sex on erythrocyte sedimentation rate (ESR) and C-reactive protein (CRP) levels is well recognized in rheumatology.[19–21] These factors can have profound impact on the qualification and interpretation of the biomarker or when setting limits for diagnosis.

Pre-analytical Variables

Pre-analytical variables also need to be carefully controlled especially in early phases of biomarker development. These include specimen collection, processing, storage, shipment, and handling, which can introduce inconsistency into assay results, either systematically or randomly, compromising reproducibility. A classic example involves the importance of temperature in sample handling, processing, and storage of blood samples when assessing complement function and levels.[22] All of these parameters must be established, remain consistent during all phases of biomarker development, and be amenable to real-world practice.

Surrogate Biomarkers

Primary endpoints are typically utilized to establish clinical effectiveness of investigational therapies. In RA, primary efficacy endpoints in clinical response and physical function can be assessed by American College of Rheumatology (ACR) response criteria or Disease Activity Score 28 (DAS28) and Health Assessment-Disability Index (HAQ-DI), respectively. Additional endpoints include prevention of structural damage progression supported by radiographic evidence and clinical remission based on durability of the remission response.[23] In systemic lupus erythematosus (SLE), primary efficacy endpoints in clinical response to support development of therapeutics include reduction in disease activity using a disease activity index, complete clinical response/remission, reduction in flare or increase in time to flare, reduction in concomitant steroid use, and treatment of acute clinical manifestations.[24] Many of these endpoints require prolonged clinical study. An alternative to these clinical endpoints is the use of "surrogate" endpoints. Surrogates are biomarkers that are an indirect measure, including physical signs of disease and laboratory measurements and radiographic tests that are expected to predict clinical benefit or harm. There are numerous advantages for use of surrogate biomarker endpoints, including smaller sized or shorter duration clinical studies resulting in cost- and time-savings, as well as the more quantitative nature of many surrogate biomarkers, as compared to clinical endpoints.

While surrogate biomarkers offer significant advantages, their ability to reliably predict clinical efficacy adds uncertainty in the regulatory process. Surrogate biomarkers that strongly correlate with clinical efficacy measures, but are not in the disease causal pathway, are fraught in their translation to clinical efficacy endpoints. Validating a surrogate endpoint requires providing evidence, often from randomized controlled clinical trials, that the surrogate endpoint reliably predicts a clinically meaningful endpoint.[25] Surrogate endpoints are an accepted route for regulatory approval by the FDA. As examples, forced expiratory volume in 1 second (FEV1) is an accepted surrogate for drug approval in asthma, chronic obstructive pulmonary disease, and cystic fibrosis. Among rheumatic disorders, serum uric acid is an accepted surrogate for uric acid lowering agents for patients with gout. Surrogate endpoints are most likely to translate and correlate with clinical endpoints when there is a comprehensive understanding of disease pathophysiology and clarity in the mechanism of action of the investigational therapy. However, even when the biomarker is within the pathophysiologic pathway of the disease, its use cannot anticipate off-target effects of the intervention. A classic example is the use of ventricular ectopic contractions as a surrogate for cardiovascular mortality of antiarrhythmic therapies. While encainide and flecainide were approved by the FDA based on their ability to reduce arrhythmias, the Cardiac Arrhythmia Suppression Trial subsequently demonstrated that more patients died in the treatment groups when compared to placebo.[26,27] Hence, regulatory approval using efficacy assessments based on surrogate endpoints is more susceptible to failure in translating into an acceptable therapeutic benefit-to-risk ratio.

Companion Diagnostics Versus CLIA Regulatory Routes

In vitro diagnostic products intended for clinical use are regulated by the Federal Food, Drug, and Cosmetic Act or the Clinical Laboratory Improvement Amendments (CLIA) of 1988. In both cases, the regulatory path is based on the diagnostic complexity and the level of control required to assure their safety and effectiveness. Categorization of complexity is based on operational knowledge, training and experience required, stability of diagnostic reagents and materials, complexity of operational steps, stability and availability of calibration materials, ease of troubleshooting and equipment maintenance, and degree of interpretation and judgment required.

An in vitro companion diagnostic (IVCDx) is a diagnostic test (e.g., biomarkers) predictive of treatment response and co-developed with a therapeutic product. The first IVCDx was the HercepTest™, measuring expression of human epidermal growth factor receptor 2 (HER-2) in breast cancer, that stratified patients more likely to have a therapeutic response to trastuzumab (Herceptin). To date, there are less than 50 FDA IVCDx tests approved with a companion therapeutic. Co-development of IVCDx and therapeutic requires early discovery of the diagnostic biomarker, clinical validation of the proposed biomarker in phase II studies, and subsequent confirmation of the biomarker in phase III or registrational trials (Fig. 37.3). In parallel, development of prototype tests, analytical validation, and clinical confirmation of the IVCDx test development is required. The importance of the coordinated development of therapeutic and companion diagnostics has been recognized by the FDA with its recent guidance on in vitro companion diagnostic devices.[28]

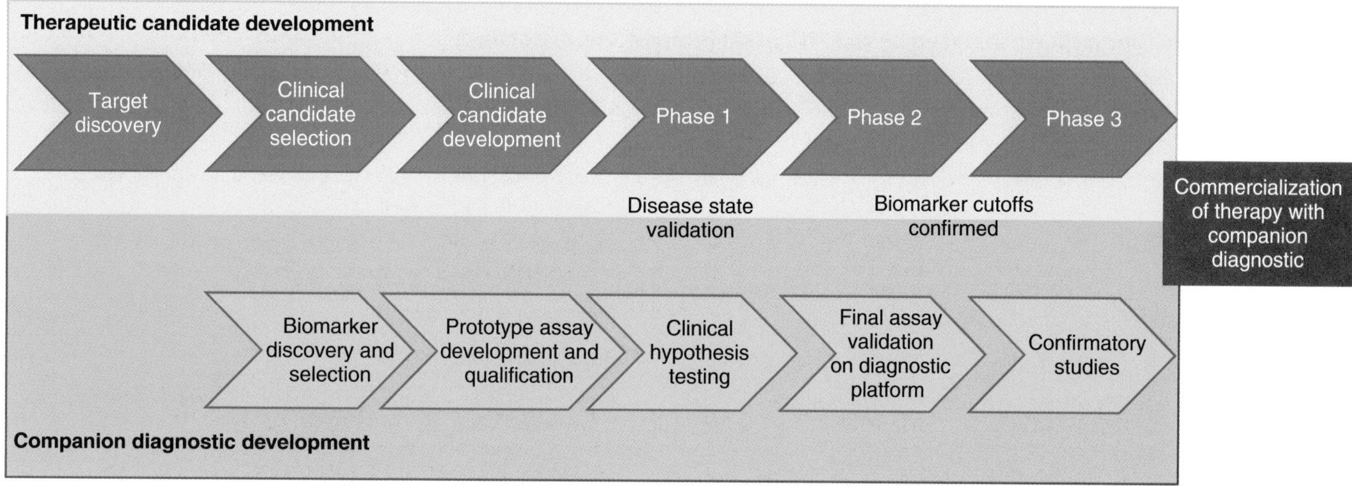

• **Fig. 37.3** Schematic for parallel development of therapeutic *(top)* and companion diagnostic *(bottom)*. During each phase of clinical development, the parallel activities for companion diagnostic development need to be timed appropriately so that assay development, qualification, and verification are ready for preclinical and clinical studies and regulatory filing. Misalignment of readiness and timing of this process will result in delays in either therapeutic or diagnostic development.

Safety Biomarkers

Adverse reactions (ADRs) occur with all drugs and are one of the leading causes of illness and death associated with prescription medications. ADRs are estimated to occur in a significant minority of all hospitalized patients, resulting in more than 2 million cases of ADRs annually, including approximately 100,000 incidences of death in the United States.[29] Although the factors that predispose individuals to develop ADRs remain largely unknown for most cases, it is believed that genetic predisposition can contribute. Significant efforts are being made to understand interindividual genetic differences with a goal to develop personalized, genetic-based strategies that will optimize and improve safety of therapeutics.[30] Examples include primaquine-induced hemolytic anemia, thioridazine-induced QT prolongation, voriconazole-induced hepatotoxicity, carbamazepine-induced skin injury, and statin-induced muscle toxicity.[31,32] In the case of statins, a small percentage of patients develop myopathy, myositis, and, rarely, rhabdomylolysis.[33] Statin dose, patient age, and concomitant medications, including HIV protease inhibitors, gemfibrozil, and amiodarone, are associated with increased risk. Pharmacogenetic studies have identified single-nucleotide polymorphisms (SNPs) in *SLCO1B1* that encode OATP1B1, a component of the solute carrier organic ion transporter system, which controls statin metabolism and increases the risk of myositis.[34] Odds ratio for myopathy is 4.5 (95% confidence interval [CI] 2.6 to 7.7) per copy of the C allele (prevalence 0.15) and 16.9 (95% CI, 4.7 to 61.1) in CC compared with TT homozygotes. These data have resulted in formal prescribing recommendations for simvastatin based on the myopathy risk categories defined by SLCO1B1 genotype.[35] Polymorphisms in additional genes, including *ABCB1, ABCG2, CYP3A4, HMGCR, CETP, GATM*, and *COQ2*, have also been identified and ongoing research may evolve multigene risk score modeling for statin-associated toxicities.[36,37]

Despite the long clinical experience with low-dose methotrexate in RA, ~4% of patients experience severe gastrointestinal and hepatobiliary toxicity.[38] As such, significant efforts have been expended on assessing biomarker predictors of methotrexate-associated toxicities.[39] Clinical and laboratory biomarkers, to date, have been poor predictors of methotrexate toxicity, although pre-existing conditions of obesity and organ system comorbidities contribute to toxicity risk. Extensive pharmacogenetic studies have been performed implicating variants in multiple genes involved in methotrexate transport and metabolism, but there has not been, to date, successful replication of these variants to support clinical adoption.[39]

Biomarkers in Rheumatic Diseases

In the remainder of this chapter, we highlight the application of biomarkers in three diseases: OA, RA, and SLE. In each disease, biomarkers can address a different need. In OA, the availability of prognostic biomarkers to identify patients at high-risk for cartilage loss and reliable surrogates for long-term cartilage loss will greatly aid development of disease-modifying OA drugs. In RA, prognostic biomarkers that identify presymptomatic patients, enable a better understanding of patient heterogeneity, or predict patients at greater risk for radiographic progression would greatly advance disease understanding and aid therapeutic development (Fig. 37.1B). Predictive biomarkers that predict greater therapeutic responses would improve patient outcomes (Fig. 37.1C). In SLE, biomarkers that predict disease activity and end-organ involvement would greatly aid clinical care (Fig. 37.1A and D).

Biomarkers in Osteoarthritis

OA is a heterogenous progressive inflammatory and degradative clinical syndrome affecting all components of the synovial joint, organ-cartilage, menisci, periarticular ligaments, synovium, and subchondral bone (see Chapters 104-106). Progressive disease results in synovial joint collapse, pain, and physical disability. Present day diagnosis remains, however, far from a cellular, molecular, or biochemical basis, but is based on radiographic evidence of disease and clinical symptoms. In addition, regulatory guidance for development of disease-modifying osteoarthritis drugs (DMOAD) remains focused on demonstration of benefit in slowing knee or hip joint space narrowing (JSN) using conventional radiography and improvement in pain and function.[40]

TABLE 37.2 **Selected Biomarkers Analyzed by the FNIH/OAI Biomarker Consortium**

Biomarker	Source	Biologic Process
Collagen Degradation		
Collagen I (CI), collagen 2 (2C), collagen IIC (2C)	Serum and urine	Neoepitope of Type I and II collagens created at their C-terminus following cleavage by collagenases
Collagen 2-1 NO2	Serum and urine	Oxidation related nitrated form of Type II alpha 1 collagen reflective of inflammation and collagen degradation
C-terminal telopeptide of Type I collagen (CTX-I)	Serum	Degradation of Type I collagen
N-terminal telopeptide of Type I collagen (NTX-1)	Serum and urine	Degradation of Type I collagen
Type IIA collagen propeptide (PIIANP)	Serum	N-propeptide of Type IIA collagen found in cartilage and vitreous humor of the eye
C-terminal cross-linked telopeptide of Type II collagen (CTX-II)	Urine	Degradation of Type II collagen, a major constituent of cartilage
Nonisomerized C-terminal telopeptide of Type I collagen (α CTX-1)	Urine	Degradation of nonisomerized newly formed bone collagen
β-isomerized fragment of Type I collagen (CTX-1β)	Urine	Degradation of Type I collagen
Synthetic Pathways		
Procollagen II C-propeptide (CPII)	Serum	Synthesis of Type II collagen
Chondroitin sulfate 846 (CS846)	Serum	Synthesis of aggregan
Extra-cellular Matrix		
Cartilage oligomeric matrix protein (COMP)	Serum	Extra-cellular matrix protein found in cartilage, synovium, and tendon
Hyaluronic acid	Serum	Glycosaminoglycan found in connective tissue
Matrix metalloproteinase 3 (MMP3)	Serum	Zinc-dependent MMP involved in degradation of ECM proteins

Development and validation of biomarkers in the diagnosis, prognosis, and treatment of OA are critically important. Because OA is a slow "degenerative" process, and development of DMOADs is likely to be more effective during the early phases of disease prior to significant synovial joint organ damage, prognostic biomarkers that identify patients at high risk for disease progression and joint damage would be a significant advance (see Fig. 37.1B). Quantitation of biomarkers of synovial inflammation, cartilage metabolism, and subchondral and bone marrow health that correlate longitudinally with disease progression (see Fig. 37.1D) would enable development of surrogates for clinical progression to monitor patient's progress and response to therapeutic intervention. The high prevalence of OA provides a large population of patients to facilitate biomarker discovery, but is counterbalanced by the challenges of the gradual nature of disease progression and patient heterogeneity.

To facilitate and accelerate this undertaking, the Foundation of the National Institutes of Health/Osteoarthritis Initiative (FNIH/OAI) consortium created in 2002 the Consortium OA Biomarkers Project to identify prognostic markers to measure early structural and symptomatic changes in knee OA (KOA) and to predict treatment responses. The OAI was a 4-year longitudinal observational study of KOA with annual measurements of clinical status, knee imaging, and collection of biochemical biomarkers. It enrolled ~4800 participants aged 45 to 79 years with follow-up data for up to 8 years.[41] Twelve discovery biomarkers, which were subsequently increased to 18, were chosen to assess bone and cartilage synthesis and degradation (Table 37.2).[42,43]

To further facilitate the utilization of biomarkers, the NIH/NIAMS-funded OA Biomarkers Network proposed the BIPED biomarker classification. This classification refers to different categories of biomarkers to assess **B**urden of disease (severity or extent of disease), **I**nvestigative (markers for which there are insufficient data to permit inclusion into one of the other categories), **P**rognostic (ability to predict future OA in healthy individuals or progression of OA with established diagnosis), **E**fficacy of intervention (markers associated with clinical or radiographic OA outcome) and **D**iagnostic (markers that classify individuals with OA). **S**afety was added later to give rise to the BIPEDS classification to include biomarkers for toxicities.[44,45]

Biochemical Biomarkers

Significant efforts have been made in discovery of biochemical biomarkers to assess burden of disease, prognosis, and diagnosis of disease progression. Markers of bone turnover (serum total osteocalcin, urine CTX-I, and serum CTX-I), cartilage turnover (serum PIIANP, uCTX-II, and serum cartilage oligomeric matrix protein [COMP]), and synovial components (U-Glc-Gal-PYD derived and serum hyaluronic acid) are associated with knee and hip OA. In addition, changes in these biomarkers are also associated with radiographic KOA/HOA progression.[46–53] In a nested case-control study of 194 case knees with clinically relevant OA progression (assessed by both pain and JSN) and 406 comparator nonprogressors (lacking pain and JSN in case or contralateral knees), baseline uCTXII and uCTXIα were both associated with case status over the 48 month study period.[43] Moreover, time-integrated concentrations (TIC) over a 24 month period of eight biomarkers (sCTXI, sHA, sNTXI, uC2C-HUSA, uCTXII, uNTXI, uCTXIα, and uCTXIβ) were associated with case status, but the combination of TIC over a 24 month period of uCTX-II, sHA, and sNTX-1 proved to be the most predictive.[43]

Complementing the discovery of biochemical biomarkers, imaging has been an intense area of investigation as a diagnostic platform for OA (see Chapter 61). While the present FDA-approved endpoint is JSN as assessed by conventional radiography, this approach is limited by its slow, minimal, and variable decrements in population studies as well as insensitivity to detect small changes in cartilage. In earlier disease, however, baseline JSN and osteophytes assessed by conventional radiography do not independently predict cartilage volume loss over a 10 year period when adjusted for MRI-assessed co-pathologies.[54] Further refinements, such as the femorotibial angle adjusted for mechanical alignment, have demonstrated promise in predicting cartilage loss over 1 or 2 years and may improve the use of conventional radiography as a predictive diagnostic.[55]

Imaging

The ability of MRI to assess total joint morphology including quantitation of cartilage morphometry (i.e., surface area and thickness), subchondral bone marrow lesions (BMLs) indicative of high bone turnover, osteophytes that may be hidden at the intracondylar femoral notch in KOA and not detected by conventional radiography, meniscal morphology, and synovitis affords greater sensitivity in detecting the earliest changes of OA when compared to standard radiographs. In the Framingham Osteoarthritis observational study of 710 participants with "normal" weight bearing posteroanterior knee radiographs, in which 29% of participants reported knee pain within the month prior to enrollment, 89% of knees had at least one MRI abnormality, with osteophytes, cartilage damage, and BMLs being the three most common findings.[56] The greater sensitivity and quantitative capabilities of MRI to assess multiple joint processes have prompted its inclusion in the FNIH OA Biomarker Consortium.[57,58] The contributions of each structural component as assessed by MRI are an area of intense investigation, with the goal of identifying early predictors of radiographic OA and disease progression. In KOA, presence of synovitis, effusions, meniscal lesions and extrusions, BMLs, or cartilage volume/thickness have been reported to be associated with cartilage volume loss and development of incident radiographic OA over time.[54,59–64] Moreover, total lesion load has been demonstrated to be more predictive than any specific structural feature in radiographic OA development.[65]

Correlations between biochemical markers and MRI changes have been an area of intense investigation as they may provide important insights into the underlying pathogenic cellular processes that drive OA. In a study of 600 OAI participants, all six biochemical markers (sCTX-I, sNTX-I, uNTX-I, uCTX-II, uCTX1α, and uCTX1β) measured were associated with the presence of BMLs. However, none were predictive of changes in BMLs or osteophytes over a 24 month period.[66] In addition, in the Rotterdam cohort, sCOMP (serum cartilage oligomeric protein), CRP, and uCTXII, as well as new novel biomarkers, sC1M (connective tissue type I collagen turnover) and sCRPM (matrix metalloproteinase-dependent degradation of C-reactive protein), were associated with incidence and progression of radiographic OA over a 5 year period.[67]

Finally, the application of biochemical and imaging biomarkers to drug development has been limited, in part, due to the paucity of potent and effective DMOADs. Ongoing and additional investigation to define and validate biochemical and imaging markers to predict disease progression will be vital for successful drug development in OA.

Biomarkers in Rheumatoid Arthritis

As RA is a progressive and disease that causes joint damage, a significant effort has been made to identify patients at risk of developing clinical disease as well as defining clinical features and biomarkers of patients who have the greatest risk of bone erosion and cartilage damage.[68] Several such biomarkers are well supported from a multitude of clinical studies, have well-validated assays available, and so are widely used in clinical practice. Early identification of disease and initiation of treatment are associated with diminished structural damage and a higher likelihood of achieving clinical remission.[69] Therefore, much effort is also being focused on determining the pre-clinical state of disease, sometimes termed pre-RA, where disease processes are already active even though the patient has yet to fulfill formal RA clinical diagnostic criteria. Parallel efforts have been expended on monitoring disease activity using biomarkers in the context of drug treatment and to understand disease heterogeneity by identifying biomarkers that predict responses to targeted therapies in patient subsets.

Autoantibodies in Rheumatoid Arthritis

Autoantibodies have long been appreciated as a dominant diagnostic feature of RA. We refer readers to Chapter 59 for detailed descriptions of RF, anti-citrullinated protein antibody (ACPA), anti-carbamylated (CarP), and antimutated citrullinated vimentin (anti-MCV) autoantibodies as diagnostic and prognostic biomarkers for RA and pre-RA. In addition to their associations with disease risk, diagnosis, and prognosis, autoantibodies have been assessed for their relationship with treatment outcome. Clinical response to methotrexate was observed to be higher in ACPA-positive versus ACPA-negative undifferentiated RA patients.[69] Mixed results have been observed when assessing the ability of autoantibodies to predict responses to biologic agents. RF positivity is associated with better clinical outcomes to rituximab (anti-CD20 antibody) and tocilizumab (anti-IL-6R antibody), but not with agents blocking TNF or abatacept (CTLA4-Fc, co-stimulation blocking antibody).[70,71] Similarly, ACPA status as a predictor of TNF blockade response has been examined in multiple studies, but no consistent effect has been identified.

More instructive results have come from studies of rituximab and abatacept. Systematic analyses and meta-analyses of the pivotal trials of rituximab indicated more robust clinical responses in patients who were seropositive for RF and/or ACPA antibodies, although this effect was greatest in patients who were also refractory to anti-TNF therapies.[72–74] Consistent findings have also been made in studies utilizing registries, where the presence of autoantibodies was associated with greater clinical responses to rituximab.[75] Clinical response to abatacept has also been reported to be greater in patients who are ACPA-positive.[76] The AMPLE (Abatacept Versus Adalimumab Comparison in Biologic-Naive RA Subjects with Background Methotrexate) study demonstrated that the greatest decrease in DAS28-CRP scores after treatment with abatacept, but not adalimumab, was observed in patients with the highest ACPA titers.[77] Several studies of abatacept-treated patients have also suggested a relationship between post-treatment reduction of ACPAs and clinical response.[72] In contrast, while rituximab decreases RF and ACPA titers as well as synovial plasma cells,[78] reduction in RF/APCA was not correlated with clinical outcome.[72]

Prognostic and Diagnostic Biomarkers of Structural Damage in Rheumatoid Arthritis

A major consequence of the inflammatory reaction in RA is erosion of bone and destruction of cartilage. The long-term goal for RA treatment is preservation of joint integrity and function. The current gold standard methodology used to measure bone and cartilage damage is conventional radiography allowing binary assessment of the presence of erosive disease; radiologist-based quantitative assessment of bone erosions; and JSN using validated and health authority-accepted Sharp Score or its modifications, van der Heijde Sharp score (vdH-S), or Genant-Sharp score (G-S).[79] However, the rate of structural damage progression varies widely between patients so identifying patients with rapid progressive joint disease is critical both for clinical practice and for design of clinical studies of therapies assessing joint health. As less than 50% of patients have worsening Sharp score over the course of 1 year,[80] assessing the effect of therapies on radiographic progression has typically required large clinical trials over multiple years. Efforts have therefore been made to identify biomarkers, including genetic markers, proteins in blood or urine, or MRI imaging that reflect turnover of bone and cartilage. Rigorous criteria for such structural damage biomarkers have been proposed by an OMERACT (Outcome Measures in Rheumatology) task force, including evidence that the biomarker reflects tissue remodeling derived from pre-clinical models, production of the biomarker in joint tissue, and correlation of biomarkers with other surrogates of bone and cartilage damage.[81]

Genetics

Because risk of structural damage progression is partially (~50%) genetically heritable,[82,83] the identified genetic variants have only a few reproducible effects on structural progression risk. HLA-DRB "shared epitope" (SE) is associated with RA risk, disease severity, erosive disease, and presence of ACPA. In contrast, analysis of ACPA-negative patients did not identify variants in HLA as being risk factors[84] and raises the possibility that the relationship observed for SE alleles and radiographic risk may be indirect and partly driven by their association with ACPA status. Many other genetic variants have been studied either as part of genome-wide association studies or by a candidate gene approach, but further studies have not replicated them and/or have a small effect on joint damage risk. Results from several meta-analyses have identified statistically significant and replicable associations with radiographic progression in several genes associated with inflammation and autoimmunity as well as bone and cartilage turnover (Table 37.3).[83]

Of note, a genetic interaction was observed between *DKK1* and *SOST* (sclerostin, a negative regulator of the Wnt pathway) where individuals carrying variants in both genes had more severe radiographic progression. In addition, the *DKK1* variants were also associated with protein quantitative trait loci (pQTL), as they affected the blood levels of the corresponding protein.[85] However, at present, the small effect sizes of these variants on progression risk likely precludes them being clinically useful decision-making tools.

TABLE 37.3 List of Genetic Variants Associated With Radiographic Progression in Rheumatoid Arthritis

	Gene	Variants	Effect of Minor Allele(s) on Joint Radiographic Severity
Immune genes	*HLA-DRB1*[86–88]	SE alleles	Destruction
	CD40[89]	rs4810485	Destruction
	IL2RA[90]	rs2104286	Protection
	IL4R[91,92]	rs1119132 rs1805011	Destruction
	IL10[83,93,94]	rs1800896	Protection
	IL15[95]	rs7667746 rs7665842 rs4371699	Destruction
Bone and cartilage turnover	*OPG*[96]	rs1485305	Destruction
	DKK1[85]	rs1896368 rs1896367 rs1528873	Destruction Protection Destruction
	GRZB[97]	rs8192916	Destruction
	MMP3[98,99]	5A/6A	Destruction
	MMP9[100]	rs11908352	Destruction

Protein Biomarkers

Additional efforts have gone into assessing protein biomarkers of radiographic progression risk. These include indicators of inflammation and bone/cartilage turnover. As discussed previously, autoantibodies (in particular, ACPA) have consistent associations with risk of progression. General inflammatory biomarkers such as the acute phase reactants CRP and ESR are associated with a small (~20%) progression risk.[101] A wide variety of other immune and inflammatory proteins have also been noted to be elevated in disease and correlated with disease activity metrics,[102] but their clinical utility for assessing disease activity and treatment outcome is not clear. For example, baseline serum TNF, IL-6, or IL-1 levels receiving therapies targeted against those respective cytokines have not been predictive of clinical response.[103] A more systemic approach has been taken to define a composite biomarker score of 12 serum proteins that correlates with components of the DAS28 score, an imaging-based assessment of joint inflammation and predictive for radiographic progression.[104] However, recent assessment of these biomarkers in the AMPLE trial has shown poor correlation of these biomarkers with clinical disease activity as assessed by the Clinical Disease Activity Index (CDAI), Simplified Disease Activity Index (SDAI), and DAS28-CRP.[105] Demonstration of robust clinical utility for measuring blood inflammatory proteins beyond acute phase reactants thus remains elusive at present.

A substantial effort has also been focused on biomarkers of bone and cartilage turnover, though none have emerged with sufficient sensitivity, specificity, and dynamic range for clinical decision making. Elevation of serum MMP3, implicated in destruction of cartilage and bone, is associated with joint damage progression, and further increase with course of disease.[83,106] uCTX-II has been associated with prediction of joint damage in the context of MMP3,[107] while serum COMP, a chondrocyte marker, is elevated in patients with severe erosive disease.[108] The PYD collagen marker is elevated in both joints and serum of RA patients, and is predictive of joint destruction in both early and established RA.[109] The ratio of RANKL (a pro-osteoclast cytokine) to OPG (a decoy receptor for RANKL) may provide an indicator of osteoblast and osteoclast balance and has been demonstrated to be predictive of greater joint destruction.[110,111] uCTX-I, a marker of collagen turnover, is associated with the degree of bone damage across multiple studies, and importantly, this marker predicts severity independently of other known factors such as autoantibodies and acute phase reactants.[112,113] Serum CTX-I is also superior to COMP, RANKL/OPG ratio, and other cartilage biomarkers as associating with 10 year changes in radiographic scores.[114] Many additional biomarkers including proteolytic products have been described but their clinical utility requires additional investigation.[115]

Imaging

As in OA, imaging technologies beyond conventional radiography, such as MRI and Power Doppler Ultrasound, are being widely implemented in clinical practice and therapeutic agent trials.[83] Bone marrow edema assessed by MRI consistently predicts radiographic progression out to several years.[83] Significant efforts are being expended to standardize a validated MRI scoring system for use in clinical studies (OMERACT Rheumatoid Arthritis Magnetic Resonance Imaging scoring system [RAMRIS]),[116] and use of this technology may influence the design of future RA clinical trials for new therapeutic agents. As in OA, a more sensitive short-term method that can predict long-term radiographic progression would shorten the duration of clinical studies and minimize time of placebo exposure for patients in clinical trials.

Emerging Rheumatoid Arthritis Biomarkers

Biomarkers in Synovial Biopsies

Beyond serum biomarkers, efforts are being expended in assessing additional measures of disease activity and treatment response using new technologies focused on the synovial end-organ.[117] Synovial biopsy is a recent addition to the technology armamentarium for RA biomarker discovery with the potential to aid disease diagnosis, determine prognosis, and obtain an early read on therapeutic treatment benefit. Biopsies, often guided by ultrasound imaging, coupled with histologic, cellular, immunohistochemical, and transcriptomic analysis have provided significant pathophysiologic insights into RA. We direct the reader to Chapter 56 for a more detailed technologic discussion on synovial biopsies.

Assessment of synovial tissues of autoantibody-positive pre-clinical RA patients has suggested that an increase in CD3$^+$ T cell infiltration in knee synovium may be predictive of development of clinical symptoms.[118] Examination of synovium from early-RA patients has provided evidence for oligoclonal T cell expansion, presence of epigenetic changes in fibroblast-like synoviocytes (FLS), and elevation of macrophage-associated chemokines indicative of evolving inflammation in the synovial tissue.[119,120] Correspondingly, peripheral blood naïve T cells share hypermethylation sites in their genomic DNA with those found in FLS, which could enable development of peripheral blood epigenetic biomarkers that reflect synovial pathology.[121] Elevation of synovial B cell and macrophage markers as well as increased Jun-N-terminal kinase (JNK) pathway activity are useful for distinguishing RA from non-RA or undifferentiated arthritis patients.[119] Elevation in synovial proangiogenic factors and their receptors has also been demonstrated to distinguish patients with erosive versus nonerosive RA.[119] Histologic features of the synovium such as presence of lymphocyte aggregates or elevated T cell infiltrates do not by themselves clearly delineate a clinical subset of RA, but are associated with elevated disease activity such as DAS28 score, presence of autoantibodies, and elevation of cytokine expression.[122] While baseline synovial lymphoid aggregates are associated with longer duration of disease and less clinical improvement with therapy, a reduction in synovial lymphoid aggregates following anti-TNF therapy was associated with a better clinical response.[123]

Studies have also linked cellular and molecular synovial heterogeneity with responses to therapeutics.[124] Patients with B and T lymphocyte synovial infiltration, accompanied by presence of synovial lymphoid aggregates (termed *lymphoid phenotype*), have greater clinical responses to rituximab. Conversely, patients with significant myeloid cell infiltration (termed *myeloid phenotype*) have greater clinical improvement with anti-TNF therapies.[125] In contrast, patients who have low levels of inflammatory (lymphocytic or myeloid) infiltrates in their synovial tissue (termed *fibroid phenotype*) have poor response to B cell-targeted therapy and are characterized by lower levels of acute phase reactants.[126] Multiple studies have also underscored the importance of synovial macrophages as biomarkers of disease activity and treatment response. Presence of synovial CD68$^+$ sublining macrophages is correlated with disease activity, and their diminishment is strongly linked to clinical improvement for multiple therapies.[127] These findings, coupled with robustness of this tissue biomarker across multiple study centers, have led to the suggestion that CD68 expression in synovial tissue may serve as a surrogate biomarker for therapeutic efficacy of novel anti-rheumatic agents in RA patients.[128]

Analyses of synovial tissue have also been utilized in evaluating pharmacodynamic responses to experimental therapies. Treatment with the Janus Kinase inhibitor tofacitinib decreases synovial tissue levels of the phosphorylated forms of STAT1 and STAT3 (substrates of JAKs), and these decreases correlate with clinical improvement.[129] Recent and future advances in technologies including single cell isolation, transcriptomics, and proteomics will continue to advance our ability to obtain additional insights into patient disease pathogenesis and heterogeneity.[130] With increased access and potential adaptation of synovial biopsies into clinical practice, biopsies may evolve to serve as a rich source of biomarkers in clinical practice.[117]

Blood Transcriptomic Biomarkers

Efforts have also been expended in assessing the transcriptome in whole blood from RA patients. These analyses are challenging, as the synovial end-organ pathophysiology is diluted in the blood resulting in weaker signals. However, some examples of blood transcriptional biomarkers impact clinical outcome in a consistent manner across multiple studies. A biomarker signature comprised of genes induced by type I interferons (IFNs) termed *interferon gene signature* (IGS) (further described later in the SLE biomarkers section) can be detected in pre-clinical RA and is elevated in 20% to 65% of established RA patients,[131,132] although variation in IGS depending on disease stage, course, and co-medications complicates interpretation of IGS in RA.[133] In established RA, an elevated IGS has been reported to be associated with a poorer clinical response to initial therapy in treatment-naïve patients, good clinical response to anti-TNF or tocilizumab therapy, and, conversely, a poorer clinical response to rituximab.[134–138] A transcriptional biomarker surrogate for plasmablast numbers, IgJ, also defined a 25% subgroup of RA patients with decreased clinical responses to rituximab across multiple studies.[139] Transcriptional profiles may be of utility for monitoring responses to drug treatment. Gene modules, reflecting immune system lineages and profiles, reproducibly decrease in response to anti-TNF therapy and correlate with clinical outcome.[140] However, these modules have not, to date, predicted therapeutic outcome, and in general whole blood transcriptional biomarkers have not offered sufficient robustness and reproducibility to be useful for clinical decision making.

Biomarkers in Systemic Lupus Erythematosus

SLE is a complex and heterogeneous disease affecting multiple organ systems, with varied and irregular progression and episodic disease flares. Much attention has been paid to defining biomarkers that are diagnostic of disease subphenotypes, monitor disease activity, predict flare, and assess treatment response. We refer readers to Chapters 58, 84, and 85 for detailed descriptions. While the presence of a multitude of autoantibodies has long been recognized as a hallmark of the disease, no single autoantibody has emerged to be absolutely predictive of disease activity or therapeutic response. Of note, in two phase 3 trials of belimumab (a therapeutic antibody against BAFF, a B-cell survival factor), high titers of anti-dsDNA antibodies were associated with SLE flare within 1 year in the placebo arm.[141] Clinical response to belimumab was greatest in patients with positive anti-dsDNA status and belimumab treatment reduced anti-dsDNA titers.[142] Corticosteroids also reduce anti-dsDNA titers and decrease flare incidence.[143] In contrast, while rituximab also decreased anti-dsDNA autoantibodies, decreased anti-cardiolipin antibodies, and normalized serum complement levels in lupus nephritis patients, these improvements were not associated with clinical improvement.[144]

Type 1 Interferon Pathway Biomarkers in Systemic Lupus Erythematosus

Another hallmark of SLE is elevated systemic activity of the type 1 interferon (IFN) pathway. Type 1 IFNs comprise a family of related cytokines (12 IFNα subtypes, IFNβ, IFNε, IFNκ, and IFNω) that act through the IFNα receptor (IFNAR) complex and primarily amplify immune responses important for antipathogen immunity. Two key cell types that produce large quantities of type 1 IFN, particularly IFNα and IFNβ, are plasmacytoid dendritic cells and monocytes. In SLE, ongoing production of type 1 IFNs is driven by activation of intra-cellular nucleic acid sensors such as Toll-like receptors (TLRs) and other pattern-recognition receptors that are normally utilized for microbial infection, but in SLE are likely triggered by immune complexes containing self-nucleic acids.[145] Additionally, genetic loci linked to the IFN pathway, *IRF5, TYK2, STAT4,* and *TLR7*, are associated with SLE risk.[146] Elevated expression of IGS is observed in ~50% to 75% of adult SLE patients and in ~90% of pediatric SLE patients, as well as in RA (as described earlier), Sjögren's syndrome, systemic sclerosis (SSc), and early arthritis.[147–149] The IGS is diminished after therapeutic treatment of type 1 IFN-targeting agents, and in the case of anifrolumab (anti-IFNαR1), the highest clinical benefit was seen in IGS-high SLE patients.[150,151] The IGS was initially reported to be associated with disease severity and particularly with CNS and renal manifestations.[152] However, later reports did not find a strong relationship of IGS to clinical activity measures such as SELENA-SLEDAI or BILAG, but instead associated it with anti-dsDNA, hypocomplementemia, and elevation of BAFF levels.[153] Longitudinal assessments of IGS have shown that the biomarker is fairly stable over time but has not demonstrated strong clinical utility in predicting disease flare or reflecting acute changes in disease activity.[154,155] Beyond the IGS, type 1 IFN-regulated serum chemokines, CXCL10, CCL2, and CCL19, have also been reported to have stronger relationships with disease activity and flare, albeit with variable concordance across patients, raising the possibility that biomarkers of downstream IFN activation may have clinical utility in monitoring SLE patients.[156]

Emerging Biomarkers in Systemic Lupus Erythematosus

In addition to the IGS, transcriptomic signatures derived from peripheral blood of 158 pediatric SLE patients defined specific immune lineage gene modules that tracked with disease activity.[157] A plasmablast gene signature, reflecting elevations of this immune lineage in the blood of patients, correlated best with overall disease activity defined using SLEDAI, while a neutrophil gene signature specifically correlated with nephritis clinical manifestations. Hence, assessment of a "molecular fingerprint" in SLE patients could define disease state and associated end-organ involvement that may be helpful in monitoring and treating SLE patients.

An emerging paradigm for pathophysiology that drives disease pathophysiology in lupus are neutrophil extra-cellular traps (NETs), which are structures produced by neutrophils undergoing a special form of cell death in response to inflammation. NETs play a key role in pathogen defense, but have also been implicated in multiple autoimmune diseases including SLE, where they are produced by the low-density granulocytes (LDGs) that are elevated in SLE.[158] These NETs contain high levels of autoantigens and immune-stimulatory molecules that can trigger elevated autoimmune inflammation in organs where NETs are deposited, including skin and kidney. NET or LDG components could potentially serve as biomarkers reflective of pathogenic neutrophil activity in SLE patients, especially given the link described above between neutrophil signatures and renal disease.

Urinary biomarkers, in addition to standard clinical assessments such as glomerular filtration rate and histologic assessment of renal biopsies, have been an area of intense investigation. Urinary MCP1 and TWEAK levels, biomarkers reflective of inflammation, both correlate with disease activity and subsequent renal flare. Markers of renal epithelial activation and damage such as neutrophil gelatinase-associated lipocalin and vascular cell adhesion molecule 1 (VCAM1) are also elevated in lupus nephritis and correlate with disease activity. Urinary levels of post-translationally modified proteins, shed podocytes, and microRNAs are also currently being investigated.[159–161] However, these markers have not yet been implemented into standard clinical practice and will require further validation studies with standardized assays.

Next Horizons for Biomarkers

Biomarkers, as reviewed in this chapter, will increasingly influence diagnosis, prognosis, therapeutic response, and understanding disease pathogenesis of rheumatic disorders.

Reclassifying Disease

Biomarkers that reflect underlying disease pathophysiology may alter our definition of rheumatic diseases from a constellation of clinical symptoms and diagnostic biomarkers to a molecular reclassification of diseases. As an example, while the IGS, as described earlier, is elevated in a subset of SLE and RA patients, the IGS is also elevated in patients with noncutaneous SSc, a subset of patients with early SSc, limited cutaneous SSc, and diffuse cutaneous SSc.[148] In SSc, the IGS is also elevated in patients without clinical fibrosis and is associated with elevated BAFF levels and collagen type III synthesis.[148] Rare monogenic disorders termed *Type I interferonopathies* with constitutive activation of the Type I IFN axis can present with a diverse multitude of systemic auto-inflammatory and autoimmune manifestations.[162] The presence of an elevated IGS may signify a common pathophysiologic pathway across a multitude of different clinical rheumatic disorders with different, but overlapping, clinical features. In turn, elevated IGS may permit reclassification of clinical diseases (e.g., IGS-high RA, SLE, and SSc patients) into a spectrum of molecular disorders that underscore dysregulation of type I interferons and go beyond Type I interferonopathies to not only provide a molecular definition of IFN-driven disorders, but also to identify patients that may be potential responders to IFN-targeted therapies.

Enabling Personalized Health Care

Advances in methodologies to increase assay sensitivity combined with new technologic platforms and -omics have and will continue to increase our abilities to determine protein, metabolites, genetic, epigenetic, transcriptomic, and biome-based biomarkers from blood, stool, tissue, or other end-organ fluids. Advances and standardization of imaging modalities and emerging mobile health sensors will further enhance our diagnostic capabilities. The regulatory landscape to facilitate biomarker-based therapeutics will likely also evolve with these technologic advances. Complementing these technologic advances is the widespread adoption of electronic medical records (EMRs), which affords an opportunity to collect and analyze clinical phenotypic, epidemiologic, biomarker data, medications, and outcomes on a longitudinal basis on large patient populations. In addition, there are various efforts in data-sharing projects and collaborations that can answer many questions that would otherwise be difficult to resolve using the data sets of each individual company/lab alone. Usefulness of this abundance of data requires our ability to generate, annotate, and standardize high quality data as well as appropriate analytical software and end-user browser capabilities to enable clinicians and scientists to answer clinical and scientific questions. Machine-assisted learning will undoubtedly also play an important role in discovery and clinical care management. As one recent example, models generated through machine learning of retinal photographs can predict sex and age with extremely high accuracy, and smoking status, systolic blood pressure, and major adverse cardiac events with somewhat lesser accuracy.[163] These emerging capabilities from disparate fields will enable physicians and scientists to query medical conditions and manage patients with tools unimagined.

Full references for this chapter can be found on ExpertConsult.com.

Selected References

1. *The Food and Drug Modernization Act of 1997*, Title 21 Code of Federal Regulations, 1997.
2. WHO: WHO International Programme on Chemical Safety Biomarkers and risk assessment: concepts and principles, http://www.inchem.org/documents/ehc/ehc/ehc155.htm. 1993.
3. Group BDW: Biomarkers and surrogate endpoints: preferred definitions and conceptual framework, *Clin Pharmacol Ther* 69(3):89–95, 2001.
4. FDA-NIH Biomarker Working Group. BEST (Biomarkers, EndpointS, and other Tools) Resource. Silver Spring (MD); 2016.
5. Bluett J, Barton A: Precision medicine in rheumatoid arthritis, *Rheum Dis Clin North Am* 43(3):377–387, 2017.
6. Wagner JA: Overview of biomarkers and surrogate endpoints in drug development, *Dis Markers* 18(2):41–46, 2002.
7. Drucker E, Krapfenbauer K: Pitfalls and limitations in translation from biomarker discovery to clinical utility in predictive and personalised medicine, *EPMA J* 4(1):7, 2013.
8. Kroll MH, Elin RJ: Interference with clinical laboratory analyses, *Clin Chem* 40(11 Pt 1):1996–2005, 1994.
9. Bolstad N, Warren DJ, Bjerner J, et al.: Heterophilic antibody interference in commercial immunoassays; a screening study using paired native and pre-blocked sera, *Clin Chem Lab Med* 49(12):2001–2006, 2011.
10. Mongolu S, Armston AE, Mozley E, et al.: Heterophilic antibody interference affecting multiple hormone assays: Is it due to rheumatoid factor? *Scand J Clin Lab Invest* 76(3):240–242, 2016.
11. Bartels EM, Falbe Watjen I, Littrup Andersen E, et al.: Rheumatoid factor and its interference with cytokine measurements: problems and solutions, *Arthritis* 2011:741071, 2011.
12. Todd DJ, Knowlton N, Amato M, et al.: Erroneous augmentation of multiplex assay measurements in patients with rheumatoid arthritis due to heterophilic binding by serum rheumatoid factor, *Arthritis Rheum* 63(4):894–903, 2011.
13. Emerson JF, Lai KKY: Endogenous antibody interferences in immunoassays, *Lab Med* 44(1):69–73, 2013.
14. Barcelo Martin B, Marquet P, Ferrer JM, et al.: Rheumatoid factor interference in a tacrolimus immunoassay, *Ther Drug Monit* 31(6):743–745, 2009.
15. Bjerner J, Nustad K, Norum LF, et al.: Immunometric assay interference: incidence and prevention, *Clin Chem* 48(4):613–621, 2002.
16. Li D, Radulescu A, Shrestha RT, et al.: Association of biotin ingestion with performance of hormone and nonhormone assays in healthy adults, *JAMA* 318(12):1150–1160, 2017.
17. Willeman T, Casez O, Faure P, et al.: Evaluation of biotin interference on immunoassays: new data for troponin I, digoxin, NT-Pro-BNP, and progesterone, *Clin Chem Lab Med* 55(10):e226–e229, 2017.
18. Communication FS. The FDA Warns that Biotin May Interfere with Lab Tests: FDA Safety Communication. 2017. https://www.fda.gov/MedicalDevices/Safety/AlertsandNotices/ucm586505.htm (accessed November 28 2017).
19. Siemons L, Ten Klooster PM, Vonkeman HE, et al.: How age and sex affect the erythrocyte sedimentation rate and C-reactive protein in early rheumatoid arthritis, *BMC Musculoskelet Disord* 15:368, 2014.
20. Bennett MR, Ma Q, Ying J, et al.: Effects of age and gender on reference levels of biomarkers comprising the pediatric Renal Activity Index for Lupus Nephritis (p-RAIL), *Pediatr Rheumatol Online J* 15(1):74, 2017.
21. Majka DS, Deane KD, Parrish LA, et al.: Duration of preclinical rheumatoid arthritis-related autoantibody positivity increases in subjects with older age at time of disease diagnosis, *Ann Rheum Dis* 67(6):801–807, 2008.
22. Yang S, McGookey M, Wang Y, et al.: Effect of blood sampling, processing, and storage on the measurement of complement activation biomarkers, *Am J Clin Pathol* 143(4):558–565, 2015.

23. Guidance for Industry. Rheumatoid Arthritis: Developing Drug Products for Treatment. 2013. Docket Number FDA-2013-D-0571.
24. Guidance for Industry. Systemic Lupus Erythematosus—Developing Medical Products for Treatment. 2010. https://www.fda.gov/downloads/Drugs/GuidanceComplianceRegulatoryInformation/Guidances/ucm072063.pdf (accessed November 20th 2018).
25. Fleming TR, Powers JH: Biomarkers and surrogate endpoints in clinical trials, *Stat Med* 31(25):2973–2984, 2012.
26. Cardiac Arrhythmia Suppression Trial I: Preliminary report: effect of encainide and flecainide on mortality in a randomized trial of arrhythmia suppression after myocardial infarction, *N Engl J Med* 321(6):406–412, 1989.
27. Echt DS, Liebson PR, Mitchell LB, et al.: Mortality and morbidity in patients receiving encainide, flecainide, or placebo. The Cardiac Arrhythmia Suppression Trial, *N Engl J Med* 324(12):781–788, 1991.
28. In vitro companion diagnostic devices. Guidance for industry and food and drug administration staff. 2014.
29. Lazarou J, Pomeranz BH, Corey PN: Incidence of adverse drug reactions in hospitalized patients: a meta-analysis of prospective studies, *JAMA* 279(15):1200–1205, 1998.
30. Crews KR, Hicks JK, Pui CH, et al.: Pharmacogenomics and individualized medicine: translating science into practice, *Clin Pharmacol Ther* 92(4):467–475, 2012.
31. Wilke RA, Lin DW, Roden DM, et al.: Identifying genetic risk factors for serious adverse drug reactions: current progress and challenges, *Nat Rev Drug Dis* 6(11):904–916, 2007.
32. Becquemont L: Pharmacogenomics of adverse drug reactions: practical applications and perspectives, *Pharmacogenomics* 10(6):961–969, 2009.
33. Pasternak RC, Smith Jr SC, Bairey-Merz CN, et al.: ACC/AHA/NHLBI Clinical Advisory on the Use and Safety of Statins, *Circulation* 106(8):1024–1028, 2002.
34. Group SC, Link E, Parish S, et al.: SLCO1B1 variants and statin-induced myopathy—a genomewide study, *N Engl J Med* 359(8):789–799, 2008.
35. Wilke RA, Ramsey LB, Johnson SG, et al.: The clinical pharmacogenomics implementation consortium: CPIC guideline for SLCO1B1 and simvastatin-induced myopathy, *Clin Pharmacol Ther* 92(1):112–117, 2012.
36. Canestaro WJ, Austin MA, Thummel KE: Genetic factors affecting statin concentrations and subsequent myopathy: a HuGENet systematic review, *Genet Med* 16(11):810–819, 2014.
37. Kitzmiller JP, Mikulik EB, Dauki AM, et al.: Pharmacogenomics of statins: understanding susceptibility to adverse effects, *Pharmgenomics Pers Med* 9:97–106, 2016.
38. Salliot C, van der Heijde D: Long-term safety of methotrexate monotherapy in patients with rheumatoid arthritis: a systematic literature research, *Ann Rheum Dis* 68(7):1100–1104, 2009.
39. Romao VC, Lima A, Bernardes M, et al.: Three decades of low-dose methotrexate in rheumatoid arthritis: can we predict toxicity? *Immunol Res* 60(2-3):289–310, 2014.
40. Guidance for Industry. Clinical development programs for drugs, devices, and biological products intended for the treatment of osteoarthritis (OA). Guidance for Industry Clinical development programs for drugs, devices, and biological products intended for the treatment of osteoarthritis (OA). Rockville, MD; 1999.
41. Lester G: Clinical research in OA—the NIH Osteoarthritis Initiative, *J Musculoskelet Neuronal Interact* 8(4):313–314, 2008.
42. Hunter DJ, Nevitt M, Losina E, et al.: Biomarkers for osteoarthritis: current position and steps towards further validation, *Best Pract Res Clin Rheumatol* 28(1):61–71, 2014.
43. Kraus VB, Collins JE, Hargrove D, et al.: Predictive validity of biochemical biomarkers in knee osteoarthritis: data from the FNIH OA Biomarkers Consortium, *Ann Rheum Dis* 76(1):186–195, 2017.
44. Bauer DC, Hunter DJ, Abramson SB, et al.: Classification of osteoarthritis biomarkers: a proposed approach, *Osteoarthritis Cartilage* 14(8):723–727, 2006.
45. Kraus VB, Burnett B, Coindreau J, et al.: Application of biomarkers in the development of drugs intended for the treatment of osteoarthritis, *Osteoarthritis Cartilage* 19(5):515–542, 2011.
46. Garnero P, Piperno M, Gineyts E, et al.: Cross sectional evaluation of biochemical markers of bone, cartilage, and synovial tissue metabolism in patients with knee osteoarthritis: relations with disease activity and joint damage, *Ann Rheum Dis* 60(6):619–626, 2001.
47. Sharif M, George E, Shepstone L, et al.: Serum hyaluronic acid level as a predictor of disease progression in osteoarthritis of the knee, *Arthritis Rheum* 38(6):760–767, 1995.
48. Kluzek S, Bay-Jensen AC, Judge A, et al.: Serum cartilage oligomeric matrix protein and development of radiographic and painful knee osteoarthritis. A community-based cohort of middle-aged women, *Biomarkers* 20(8):557–564, 2015.
49. Sasaki E, Tsuda E, Yamamoto Y, et al.: Serum hyaluronic acid concentration predicts the progression of joint space narrowing in normal knees and established knee osteoarthritis—a five-year prospective cohort study, *Arthritis Res Ther* 17:283, 2015.
50. Garnero P, Conrozier T, Christgau S, et al.: Urinary type II collagen C-telopeptide levels are increased in patients with rapidly destructive hip osteoarthritis, *Ann Rheum Dis* 62(10):939–943, 2003.
51. Van Spil WE, Welsing PM, Bierma-Zeinstra SM, et al.: The ability of systemic biochemical markers to reflect presence, incidence, and progression of early-stage radiographic knee and hip osteoarthritis: data from CHECK, *Osteoarthritis Cartilage* 23(8):1388–1397, 2015.
52. Sharif M, Kirwan J, Charni N, et al.: A 5-yr longitudinal study of type IIA collagen synthesis and total type II collagen degradation in patients with knee osteoarthritis—association with disease progression, *Rheumatology (Oxford)* 46(6):938–943, 2007.
53. Reijman M, Hazes JM, Bierma-Zeinstra SM, et al.: A new marker for osteoarthritis: cross-sectional and longitudinal approach, *Arthritis Rheum* 50(8):2471–2478, 2004.
54. McBride A, Khan HI, Aitken D, et al.: Does cartilage volume measurement or radiographic osteoarthritis at baseline independently predict ten-year cartilage volume loss? *BMC Musculoskelet Disord* 17:54, 2016.
55. Moyer R, Wirth W, Duryea J, et al.: Anatomical alignment, but not goniometry, predicts femorotibial cartilage loss as well as mechanical alignment: data from the Osteoarthritis Initiative, *Osteoarthritis Cartilage* 24(2):254–261, 2016.
56. Guermazi A, Niu J, Hayashi D, et al.: Prevalence of abnormalities in knees detected by MRI in adults without knee osteoarthritis: population based observational study (Framingham Osteoarthritis Study), *BMJ* 345:e5339, 2012.
57. Peterfy CG, Schneider E, Nevitt M: The osteoarthritis initiative: report on the design rationale for the magnetic resonance imaging protocol for the knee, *Osteoarthritis Cartilage* 16(12):1433–1441, 2008.
58. Conaghan PG, Hunter DJ, Maillefert JF, et al.: Summary and recommendations of the OARSI FDA osteoarthritis Assessment of Structural Change Working Group, *Osteoarthritis Cartilage* 19(5):606–610, 2011.
59. Felson DT, Niu J, Neogi T, et al.: Synovitis and the risk of knee osteoarthritis: the MOST Study, *Osteoarthritis Cartilage* 24(3):458–464, 2016.
60. Niu J, Felson DT, Neogi T, et al.: Patterns of Coexisting Lesions Detected on Magnetic Resonance Imaging and Relationship to Incident Knee Osteoarthritis: The Multicenter Osteoarthritis Study, *Arthritis Rheumatol* 67(12):3158–3165, 2015.
61. Roubille C, Raynauld JP, Abram F, et al.: The presence of meniscal lesions is a strong predictor of neuropathic pain in symptomatic knee osteoarthritis: a cross-sectional pilot study, *Arthritis Res Ther* 16(6):507, 2014.

62. Garnero P, Peterfy C, Zaim S, et al.: Bone marrow abnormalities on magnetic resonance imaging are associated with type II collagen degradation in knee osteoarthritis: a three-month longitudinal study, *Arthritis Rheum* 52(9):2822–2829, 2005.
63. Stefanik JJ, Gross KD, Guermazi A, et al.: The relation of MRI-detected structural damage in the medial and lateral patellofemoral joint to knee pain: the Multicenter and Framingham Osteoarthritis Studies, *Osteoarthritis Cartilage* 23(4):565–570, 2015.
64. Eckstein F, Collins JE, Nevitt MC, et al.: Brief report: cartilage thickness change as an imaging biomarker of knee osteoarthritis progression: data from the foundation for the national institutes of health osteoarthritis biomarkers consortium, *Arthritis Rheumatol* 67(12):3184–3189, 2015.
65. Roemer FW, Kwoh CK, Hannon MJ, et al.: What comes first? Multitissue involvement leading to radiographic osteoarthritis: magnetic resonance imaging-based trajectory analysis over four years in the osteoarthritis initiative, *Arthritis Rheumatol* 67(8):2085–2096, 2015.
66. Deveza LA, Kraus VB, Collins JE, et al.: Association between biochemical markers of bone turnover and bone changes on imaging: data from the osteoarthritis initiative, *Arthritis Care Res (Hoboken)* 69(8):1179–1191, 2017.
67. Hosnijeh FS, Siebuhr AS, Uitterlinden AG, et al.: Association between biomarkers of tissue inflammation and progression of osteoarthritis: evidence from the Rotterdam study cohort, *Arthritis Research & Therapy* 18:81–90, 2016.
68. Mankia K, Emery P: Preclinical rheumatoid arthritis: progress toward prevention, *Arthritis Rheumatol* 68(4):779–788, 2016.
69. van Dongen H, van Aken J, Lard LR, et al.: Efficacy of methotrexate treatment in patients with probable rheumatoid arthritis: a double-blind, randomized, placebo-controlled trial, *Arthritis Rheum* 56(5):1424–1432, 2007.
70. Maneiro RJ, Salgado E, Carmona L, et al.: Rheumatoid factor as predictor of response to abatacept, rituximab and tocilizumab in rheumatoid arthritis: systematic review and meta-analysis, *Semin Arthritis Rheum* 43(1):9–17, 2013.
71. Salgado E, Maneiro JR, Carmona L, et al.: Rheumatoid factor and response to TNF antagonists in rheumatoid arthritis: systematic review and meta-analysis of observational studies, *Joint Bone Spine* 81(1):41–50, 2014.
72. Martin-Mola E, Balsa A, Garcia-Vicuna R, et al.: Anti-citrullinated peptide antibodies and their value for predicting responses to biologic agents: a review, *Rheumatol Int* 36(8):1043–1063, 2016.
73. Lal P, Su Z, Holweg CT, et al.: Inflammation and autoantibody markers identify rheumatoid arthritis patients with enhanced clinical benefit following rituximab treatment, *Arthritis Rheum* 63(12):3681–3691, 2011.
74. Isaacs JD, Cohen SB, Emery P, et al.: Effect of baseline rheumatoid factor and anticitrullinated peptide antibody serotype on rituximab clinical response: a meta-analysis, *Ann Rheum Dis* 72(3):329–336, 2013.
75. Chatzidionysiou K, Lie E, Nasonov E, et al.: Highest clinical effectiveness of rituximab in autoantibody-positive patients with rheumatoid arthritis and in those for whom no more than one previous TNF antagonist has failed: pooled data from 10 European registries, *Ann Rheum Dis* 70(9):1575–1580, 2011.
76. Gottenberg JE, Ravaud P, Cantagrel A, et al.: Positivity for anti-cyclic citrullinated peptide is associated with a better response to abatacept: data from the 'Orencia and Rheumatoid Arthritis' registry, *Ann Rheum Dis* 71(11):1815–1819, 2012.
77. Sokolove J, Schiff M, Fleischmann R, et al.: Impact of baseline anti-cyclic citrullinated peptide-2 antibody concentration on efficacy outcomes following treatment with subcutaneous abatacept or adalimumab: 2-year results from the AMPLE trial, *Ann Rheum Dis* 75(4):709–714, 2016.
78. Thurlings RM, Vos K, Wijbrandts CA, et al.: Synovial tissue response to rituximab: mechanism of action and identification of biomarkers of response, *Ann Rheum Dis* 67(7):917–925, 2008.
79. Strand V, Kingsbury SR, Woodworth T, et al.: OMERACT 10 Sharp Symposium: important findings in examination of imaging methods for measurement of joint damage in rheumatoid arthritis, *J Rheumatol* 38(9):2009–2013, 2011.
80. van der Heijde D: Impact of imaging in established rheumatoid arthritis, *Best Pract Res Clin Rheumatol* 17(5):783–790, 2003.
81. Syversen SW, Landewe R, van der Heijde D, et al.: Testing of the OMERACT 8 draft validation criteria for a soluble biomarker reflecting structural damage in rheumatoid arthritis: a systematic literature search on 5 candidate biomarkers, *J Rheumatol* 36(8):1769–1784, 2009.
82. Knevel R, Grondal G, Huizinga TW, et al.: Genetic predisposition of the severity of joint destruction in rheumatoid arthritis: a population-based study, *Ann Rheum Dis* 71(5):707–709, 2012.
83. Krabben A, Huizinga TW, Mil AH: Biomarkers for radiographic progression in rheumatoid arthritis, *Curr Pharm Des* 21(2):147–169, 2015.
84. de Rooy DP, Tsonaka R, Andersson ML, et al.: Genetic factors for the severity of ACPA-negative rheumatoid arthritis in 2 cohorts of early disease: a genome-wide study, *J Rheumatol* 42(8):1383–1391, 2015.
85. de Rooy DP, Yeremenko NG, Wilson AG, et al.: Genetic studies on components of the Wnt signalling pathway and the severity of joint destruction in rheumatoid arthritis, *Ann Rheum Dis* 72(5):769–775, 2013.
86. Goronzy JJ, Matteson EL, Fulbright JW, et al.: Prognostic markers of radiographic progression in early rheumatoid arthritis, *Arthritis Rheum* 50(1):43–54, 2004.
87. Kaltenhauser S, Wagner U, Schuster E, et al.: Immunogenetic markers and seropositivity predict radiological progression in early rheumatoid arthritis independent of disease activity, *J Rheumatol* 28(4):735–744, 2001.
88. van der Helm-van Mil AH, Huizinga TW, Schreuder GM, et al.: An independent role of protective HLA class II alleles in rheumatoid arthritis severity and susceptibility, *Arthritis Rheum* 52(9):2637–2644, 2005.
89. van der Linden MP, Feitsma AL, le Cessie S, et al.: Association of a single-nucleotide polymorphism in CD40 with the rate of joint destruction in rheumatoid arthritis, *Arthritis Rheum* 60(8):2242–2247, 2009.
90. Knevel R, de Rooy DP, Zhernakova A, et al.: Association of variants in IL2RA with progression of joint destruction in rheumatoid arthritis, *Arthritis Rheum* 65(7):1684–1693, 2013.
91. Krabben A, Wilson AG, de Rooy DP, et al.: Association of genetic variants in the IL4 and IL4R genes with the severity of joint damage in rheumatoid arthritis: a study in seven cohorts, *Arthritis Rheum* 65(12):3051–3057, 2013.
92. Marinou I, Till SH, Moore DJ, et al.: Lack of association or interactions between the IL-4, IL-4Ralpha and IL-13 genes, and rheumatoid arthritis, *Arthritis Res Ther* 10(4):R80, 2008.
93. Huizinga TW, Keijsers V, Yanni G, et al.: Are differences in interleukin 10 production associated with joint damage? *Rheumatology (Oxford)* 39(11):1180–1188, 2000.
94. Marinou I, Healy J, Mewar D, et al.: Association of interleukin-6 and interleukin-10 genotypes with radiographic damage in rheumatoid arthritis is dependent on autoantibody status, *Arthritis Rheum* 56(8):2549–2556, 2007.
95. Knevel R, Krabben A, Brouwer E, et al.: Genetic variants in IL15 associate with progression of joint destruction in rheumatoid arthritis: a multicohort study, *Ann Rheum Dis* 71(10):1651–1657, 2012.
96. Knevel R, de Rooy DP, Saxne T, et al.: A genetic variant in osteoprotegerin is associated with progression of joint destruction in rheumatoid arthritis, *Arthritis Res Ther* 16(3):R108, 2014.
97. Knevel R, Krabben A, Wilson AG, et al.: A genetic variant in granzyme B is associated with progression of joint destruction in rheumatoid arthritis, *Arthritis Rheum* 65(3):582–589, 2013.

98. Dorr S, Lechtenbohmer N, Rau R, et al.: Association of a specific haplotype across the genes MMP1 and MMP3 with radiographic joint destruction in rheumatoid arthritis, *Arthritis Res Ther* 6(3):R199–207, 2004.
99. Mattey DL, Nixon NB, Dawes PT, et al.: Association of matrix metalloproteinase 3 promoter genotype with disease outcome in rheumatoid arthritis, *Genes Immun* 5(2):147–149, 2004.
100. de Rooy DP, Zhernakova A, Tsonaka R, et al.: A genetic variant in the region of MMP-9 is associated with serum levels and progression of joint damage in rheumatoid arthritis, *Ann Rheum Dis* 73(6):1163–1169, 2014.
101. Knevel R, van Nies JA, le Cessie S, et al.: Evaluation of the contribution of cumulative levels of inflammation to the variance in joint destruction in rheumatoid arthritis, *Ann Rheum Dis* 72(2):307–308, 2013.
102. Altobelli E, Angeletti PM, Piccolo D, et al.: Synovial fluid and serum concentrations of inflammatory markers in rheumatoid arthritis, psoriatic arthritis and osteoarthitis: a systematic review, *Curr Rheumatol Rev* 13(3):170–179, 2017.
103. Cuppen BV, Welsing PM, Sprengers JJ, et al.: Personalized biological treatment for rheumatoid arthritis: a systematic review with a focus on clinical applicability, *Rheumatology (Oxford)* 55(5):826–839, 2016.
104. Segurado OG, Sasso EH: Vectra DA for the objective measurement of disease activity in patients with rheumatoid arthritis, *Clin Exp Rheumatol* 32(5 Suppl 85):S-29-34, 2014.
105. Fleischmann R, Connolly SE, Maldonado MA, et al.: Brief report: estimating disease activity using multi-biomarker disease activity scores in rheumatoid arthritis patients treated with abatacept or adalimumab, *Arthritis Rheumatol* 68(9):2083–2089, 2016.
106. Tchetverikov I, Lard LR, DeGroot J, et al.: Matrix metalloproteinases-3, -8, -9 as markers of disease activity and joint damage progression in early rheumatoid arthritis, *Ann Rheum Dis* 62(11):1094–1099, 2003.
107. Young-Min S, Cawston T, Marshall N, et al.: Biomarkers predict radiographic progression in early rheumatoid arthritis and perform well compared with traditional markers, *Arthritis Rheum* 56(10):3236–3247, 2007.
108. Lindqvist E, Eberhardt K, Bendtzen K, et al.: Prognostic laboratory markers of joint damage in rheumatoid arthritis, *Ann Rheum Dis* 64(2):196–201, 2005.
109. Krabben A, Knevel R, Huizinga TW, et al.: Serum pyridinoline levels and prediction of severity of joint destruction in rheumatoid arthritis, *J Rheumatol* 40(8):1303–1306, 2013.
110. Geusens PP, Landewe RB, Garnero P, et al.: The ratio of circulating osteoprotegerin to RANKL in early rheumatoid arthritis predicts later joint destruction, *Arthritis Rheum* 54(6):1772–1777, 2006.
111. van Tuyl LH, Voskuyl AE, Boers M, et al.: Baseline RANKL:OPG ratio and markers of bone and cartilage degradation predict annual radiological progression over 11 years in rheumatoid arthritis, *Ann Rheum Dis* 69(9):1623–1628, 2010.
112. Garnero P, Gineyts E, Christgau S, et al.: Association of baseline levels of urinary glucosyl-galactosyl-pyridinoline and type II collagen C-telopeptide with progression of joint destruction in patients with early rheumatoid arthritis, *Arthritis Rheum* 46(1):21–30, 2002.
113. Jansen LM, van der Horst-Bruinsma I, Lems WF, et al.: Serological bone markers and joint damage in early polyarthritis, *J Rheumatol* 31(8):1491–1496, 2004.
114. Syversen SW, Goll GL, van der Heijde D, et al.: Cartilage and bone biomarkers in rheumatoid arthritis: prediction of 10-year radiographic progression, *J Rheumatol* 36(2):266–272, 2009.
115. Karsdal MA, Woodworth T, Henriksen K, et al.: Biochemical markers of ongoing joint damage in rheumatoid arthritis—current and future applications, limitations and opportunities, *Arthritis Res Ther* 13(2):215, 2011.
116. Ostergaard M, Peterfy CG, Bird P, et al.: The OMERACT Rheumatoid Arthritis Magnetic Resonance Imaging (MRI) scoring system: updated recommendations by the OMERACT MRI in Arthritis Working Group, *J Rheumatol* 44(11):1706–1712, 2017.
117. Humby F, Romao VC, Manzo A, et al.: A multicenter retrospective analysis evaluating performance of synovial biopsy techniques in patients with inflammatory arthritis: arthroscopic versus ultrasound-guided versus blind needle biopsy, *Arthritis Rheumatol* 70(5):702–710, 2018.
118. de Hair MJ, van de Sande MG, Ramwadhdoebe TH, et al.: Features of the synovium of individuals at risk of developing rheumatoid arthritis: implications for understanding preclinical rheumatoid arthritis, *Arthritis Rheumatol* 66(3):513–522, 2014.
119. Orr C, Vieira-Sousa E, Boyle DL, et al.: Synovial tissue research: a state-of-the-art review, *Nat Rev Rheumatol* 13(10):630, 2017.
120. Whitaker JW, Shoemaker R, Boyle DL, et al.: An imprinted rheumatoid arthritis methylome signature reflects pathogenic phenotype, *Genome Med* 5(4):40, 2013.

38 Occupational and Recreational Musculoskeletal Disorders

RICHARD S. PANUSH

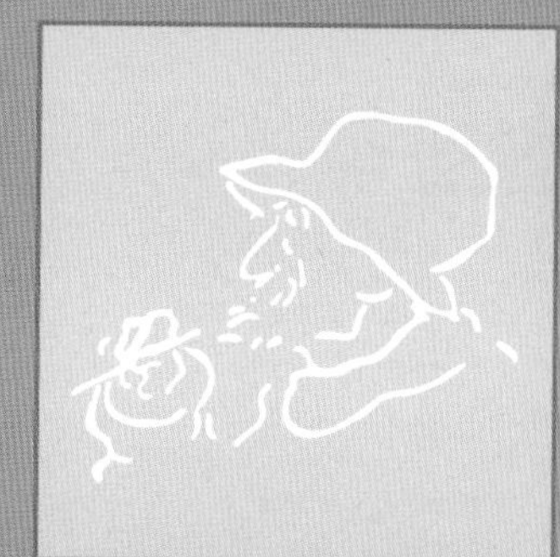

KEY POINTS

- Some occupational and recreational activities are linked with musculoskeletal syndromes or disorders that cause neck pain; shoulder, elbow, hand, or wrist pain or tendinitis; carpal tunnel syndrome; and hand-arm vibration syndrome.
- The intuitive concepts of so-called *cumulative trauma disorders* and *repetitive strain disorders* have poor support in the literature. Causal relationships between most occupations or activities and these "syndromes" have not been well established.
- Some activities and mechanical stresses have been associated with osteoarthritis at certain sites. For example, the hips of farmers, the knees of workers whose jobs involve frequent bending of the knees, and the hands of workers who perform repetitive tasks with their hands.
- Certain rheumatic disorders have been related to environmental or occupational risks.
- Putting a normal joint through its physiologic range of motion is not necessarily harmful for an otherwise healthy individual. However, if the joint, motion, stress, or biomechanics are not normal, there may be a risk of harm to the joint.
- Most healthy people comfortably engaging in reasonable recreational activities can do so without evidence of lasting soft tissue or articular damage. Runners, who have been best studied, exemplify this principle. Conversely, people who exercise with pain, effusions, underlying joint pathology, or abnormal or unusual biomechanics, or as professional or elite athletes may be at increased risk of joint injury.
- Performing artists, vocalists, dancers, and musicians have a risk of soft tissue and joint injury analogous to that of athletes.

"The diseases of persons incident to this craft arise from three causes: first constant sitting, second the perpetual motion of the hand in the same manner, and thirdly the attention and application of the mind. … Constant writing also considerably fatigues the hand and whole arm…."

RAMAZZINI, 1713[1]

"When job demands … repeatedly exceed the biomechanical capacity of the worker, the activities become trauma-inducing. Hence, traumatogens are workplace sources of biomechanical strain that contribute to the onset of injuries affecting the musculoskeletal system."

NATIONAL INSTITUTE FOR OCCUPATIONAL SAFETY AND HEALTH, 1986[2]

Introduction

The possible associations of certain occupational and recreational activities with musculoskeletal disorders are not as clear as had once been thought. Conventional wisdom was that "wear and tear" from at least some activities led to reversible or irreversible damage to the musculoskeletal system.[2–5] Despite the intuition that work or recreational activities might cause rheumatic and musculoskeletal syndromes, this putative relationship is controversial and likely seriously flawed. Many of the available data have confounding aspects, as will be discussed in this chapter.

Occupation-Related Musculoskeletal Disorders

Many presumptive work-related musculoskeletal disorders have been described, some of which are presented in Table 38.1.[1–8] Although the appealing and suggestive names invite conclusions of causal association, these have not been demonstrated.[1–8] Work-related musculoskeletal injuries comprise at least 50% of nonfatal injury cases resulting in days away from work.[9] The cost of work-related disability from musculoskeletal disorders has been equivalent to approximately 1% of the United States' gross national product, making these entities of considerable societal interest.[10] Worldwide ergonomic (occupational) disability from low back pain in 2010 was estimated to affect as much as 26% of the population.[11] Industries with the highest rates of musculoskeletal disorders were meatpacking, knit-underwear manufacturing, motor vehicle manufacturing, poultry processing, mail and message distribution, health assessment and treatment, construction, butchery, food processing, machine operation, dental hygiene and dentistry, data entry, hand grinding and polishing, carpentry, industrial truck and tractor operation, nursing assistance, housecleaning, and, worldwide, agriculture. Associations between work-related musculoskeletal syndromes and age, sex, fitness, and weight have been imprecise.[6–8,11]

TABLE 38.1 Reported Occupation-Related Musculoskeletal Syndromes

Cherry pitter's thumb	Gamekeeper's thumb
Staple gun carpal tunnel syndrome	Espresso maker's wrist
Bricklayer's shoulder	Espresso elbow
Carpenter's elbow	Pizza maker's palsy
Janitor's elbow	Poster presenter's thumb
Stitcher's wrist	Rope maker's claw hand
Cotton twister's hand	Telegraphist's cramp
Writer's cramp	Waiter's shoulder
Bowler's thumb	Ladder shins
Jeweler's thumb	Tobacco primer's wrist Carpet layer's knee

From Mani L, Gerr F: Work-related upper extremity musculoskeletal disorders. *Primary Care* 27:845–864, 2000; and Colombini D, Occhipinti E, Delleman N, et al: Exposure assessment of upper limb repetitive movements: a consensus document developed by the Technical Committee on Musculoskeletal Disorders of International Ergonomics Association endorsed by International Commission on Occupation Health. *G Ital Med Lav Ergon* 23:129–142, 2000.

TABLE 38.2 Selected Literature Describing Regional Occupation-Related Musculoskeletal Syndromes

Syndrome	No. of Epidemiologic Studies	Odds Ratio/ Relative Risk
Neck pain	26	0.7-6.9
Shoulder tendinitis	22	0.9-13
Elbow tendinitis	14	0.7-5.5
Hand-wrist tendinitis	16	0.6-31.7
Carpal tunnel syndrome	22	1-34
Hand-arm vibration syndrome	8	0.5-41

A number of work-related regional musculoskeletal syndromes have been described. These syndromes include disorders of the neck, shoulder, elbow, hand and wrist, lower back, and lower extremities[7] (Table 38.2); some of these syndromes are discussed in greater detail in other chapters. Neck musculoskeletal disorders are associated with repetition, forceful exertion, and constrained or static postures.[12] Shoulder musculoskeletal disorders occur with work at or above shoulder height, lifting of heavy loads, static postures, hand-arm vibration, and repetitive motion. For elbow epicondylitis, risk factors are overexertion of finger and wrist extensors with the elbow in extension, as well as posture. Hand-wrist tendinitis and work-related carpal tunnel syndrome were noted with repetitive work, forceful activities, flexed wrists, and duration of continual effort.[1,7] Hand-arm vibration syndrome (Raynaud-like phenomenon)[13] has been linked to the intensity and duration of exposure to vibration. Work-related lower back disorders are associated with repetition, the weight of objects lifted, twisting, poor biomechanics of lifting, and particularly agriculture.[11,14] Other risk factors for work-related musculoskeletal disorders involving the back include awkward posture, high static muscle load, high-force exertion at the hands and wrists, sudden applications of force, work with short cycle times, little task variety, frequent tight deadlines, inadequate rest or recovery periods, high cognitive demands, little control over work, a cold work environment, localized mechanical stresses to tissues, and poor spinal support.[1]

Rehabilitation for these so-called occupational musculoskeletal disorders requires collaboration by workers, employers, insurers, and health professionals. The process has been divided into phases of protection from and resolution of symptoms, restoration of strength and dynamic stability, and return to work.

Not long ago, the prevailing view was that many musculoskeletal disorders were consistently and predictably work related. That understanding has been questioned and is now perceived more critically.[2,15–21] Much published information (see Table 38.2) about occupational musculoskeletal disorders is now considered flawed. The quality of this information was uneven and perhaps poor in some instances. Definitions of musculoskeletal disorders were imprecise. Diagnoses, by rheumatologic standards, were infrequent. Studies were usually not prospective, and selection and recall biases were present. Inferential observations were made, and investigators had difficulty quantifying activities and defining health effects. Outcome measures varied. The quality of reported observations was uneven. Psychological influences and secondary gain were often ignored. Claims, anecdotal, and survey data were often used without validation of subjective complaints. Quantification of putative causative factors was difficult. Indeed, a review of this literature concluded that none of the published studies satisfactorily established a causal relationship between work and distinct medical entities.[18] In fact, certain experiences argued powerfully against the notion of work-related musculoskeletal disorders. In Lithuania, for example, where insurance was limited and disability was not a societal expectation or entitlement, "whiplash" from auto accidents did not exist.[17] Similarly, when legislation for compensability was made more stringent in Australia, an epidemic of whiplash and repetitive-strain injuries abated.[19,20] In the United States as well, expressed symptoms correlated closely with the likelihood of obtaining compensation.[22] In other instances it was found that ergonomic interventions had no effect on alleged work-related symptoms, and close analysis of epidemics of work-related musculoskeletal disorders revealed serious inconsistencies.[15] A Japanese study found no relationship between physical activity and musculoskeletal pain.[23] Interestingly, another report described familial linkage to chronic musculoskeletal pain.[24] Thus the Industrial Injuries Committee of the American Society for Surgery of the Hand and the American Society for Surgery of the Hand, the Working Group of the British Orthopaedic Association, and the World Health Organization[2,15,18,19] have all stated that current data do not support a causal relationship between specific work activities and the development of well-recognized disease entities; in addition, they have noted that these had become socio-political problems and urged restraint in considering regulations regarding these so-called *entities.*[16] Hadler has written particularly forcefully that popular notions about work-related musculoskeletal disorders have been based on inadequate science.[2,15]

An appreciation of the importance of psychosocial factors influencing work disability has emerged. These factors include lack of job control, fear of layoff, monotony, job dissatisfaction, unsatisfactory performance appraisals, distress and unhappiness with co-workers or supervisors, repetitive tasks, duration of the work day, poor quality of sleep, perceptions of air quality and ergonomics, poor coping abilities, divorce, low income, less education, poor social support, presence of chronic disease, self-rated perception of poor air quality, and poor office ergonomics.[2,15–22,25,26] This situation is reminiscent of the story of silicone breast implants and their presumed association with rheumatic disease, where—as seems to be the case for work-related musculoskeletal disorders—there was a coalescence of naïvely simplistic assumptions, untested hypotheses, confusion between the repetition of hypotheses and their scientific validation, media exaggeration, and public advocacy intertwined with politics and governmental regulatory agencies, confounding compensatory rewards, litigation, and inadequate science. All these elements perverted the silicone breast implant story[27] and may have confused the interpretation of evidence-based work-related musculoskeletal disorders as well. More good quality, standardized investigation is necessary to learn about work-related musculoskeletal disorders and to clearly identify the circumstances in which they occur. Work-related musculoskeletal disorders exist, but they are less pervasive and less noxious than had been thought.

Occupation-Related Rheumatic Diseases

Associations between occupations and well-defined rheumatic disorders are clearer than those involving broader musculoskeletal disorders. This discussion recapitulates the simplistic perception that joints deteriorate with use. However, this notion is neither necessarily logical nor correct.

Osteoarthritis

Is osteoarthritis (OA) caused, at least in part, by mechanical stress? OA is presented in Chapters 104 to 106; however, brief consideration of the role of certain occupational and recreational activities is within the scope of this discussion. One analytic approach to determining a possible relationship between activity and joint disease is to consider the epidemiologic evidence that degenerative arthritis may follow repetitive trauma. Most investigations of the pathogenesis of OA include a role for "stress."[28–41] Several studies have suggested an increased prevalence of OA of the elbows, knees, and spine in miners[32–34]; of the knees in floor layers and in other occupations requiring kneeling; of the knees in shipyard workers and a variety of occupations involving knee bending; of the shoulders, elbows, wrists, and metacarpophalangeal joints in pneumatic drill operators[35]; of the intervertebral disks, distal interphalangeal joints, elbows, and knees in dockworkers[33]; of the hands in cotton workers,[36] diamond cutters,[32,37] seamstresses,[37] and textile workers[15,38]; of the knees and hips in farmers; and of the spine in foundry workers[40,41] (Table 38.3). Population studies have noted increased hip OA in farmers, firefighters, mill workers, dockworkers, female mail carriers, unskilled manual laborers, fishermen, and miners and have reported increased knee OA in farmers, firefighters, construction workers, house and hotel cleaners, craftspeople, laborers, and service workers.[40,41] Activities leading to an increased risk for premature OA involved power gripping, carrying, lifting, increased physical loading, increased static loading, kneeling, walking, squatting, and bending.[40,41] Recent studies and systematic reviews have confirmed that heavy lifting and crawling and sometimes climbing were associated with knee and hip OA; individual studies were variable, often small, and with interpretive limitations.[42] The effect of body mass index (BMI) in work-related OA appeared to predispose toward the development of knee OA, with primarily valgus malalignment.[43,44] Systematic review and meta-analysis concluded that data supported risk of OA from activities involving heavy or manual work (average relative risk [RR], 1.45; range, 1.20 to 1.76), elite sports (RR, 1.72; range, 1.35 to 2.20), kneeling (RR, 1.30; range, 1.03 to 1.63), squatting (RR, 1.40; range, 1.21 to 1.61), lifting/carrying (RR, 1.58; range, 1.28 to 1.94), climbing stairs (RR, 1.29; range, 1.08 to 1.55), standing work (RR, 1.11; range, 0.81 to 1.51), and knee bending/straining (RR, 1.60; range, 1.15 to 2.21).[45] A common

TABLE 38.3 Occupational Physical Activities and Possible Associations With Osteoarthritis

Occupation	Involved Joints	Risk of OA
Miner[33,34,40,41]	Elbow, hip, knee, spine	Increased
Pneumatic driller[35,47]	Shoulder, elbow, wrist, MCP joint	Increased/none
Dockworker[33,39–41]	Intervertebral disk, DIP joint, elbow, hip, knee	Increased
Cotton mill worker[36]	Hand	Increased
Diamond worker[32,37]	Hand	Increased
Shipyard laborer[40,41]	Knee	Increased
Foundry worker[40,41]	Lumbar spine	Increased
Seamstress[37]	Hand	Increased
Textile worker[38]	Hand	Increased
Manual laborer[39–41,45]	MCP joint, hip	Increased
Occupations requiring knee bending[39–41,45]	Knee	Increased
Farmer[39–41]	Hip, knee	Increased
Firefighter[39–41]	Hip, knee	Increased
Millworker[39–41]	Hip	Increased
Female mail carrier[39–41]	Hip	Increased
Fisherman[39–41]	Hip	Increased
Construction worker[39–41]	Knee	Increased
House and hotel cleaner[39–41]	Knee	Increased
Craftperson[39–41]	Knee	Increased
Service worker[39–41]	Knee	Increased
Heavy lifter[42]	Hip, knee	Increased
Crawling[42]	Hip, knee	Increased
Kneeling[45]	Knee	Increased
Squatting[45]	Knee	Increased
Lifting/carrying[45]	Knee	Increased
Climbing stairs[45]	Knee	Increased
Standing work[45]	Knee	Increased

DIP, Distal interphalangeal; *MCP*, metacarpophalangeal; *OA*, osteoarthritis.

theme for occupational activities leading to knee OA was cumulative joint loading.[46] Bending was associated with MRI abnormalities in cartilage of asymptomatic people,[47] as was physical activity, assessed by objective measures[48–50]; injuries accelerated progression of knee OA.[51]

Studies of skeletons of several populations have suggested that age at onset, frequency, and location of osteoarthritic changes were directly related to the nature and degree of physical activities.[52] However, not all these studies adhered to contemporary standards, nor have they been confirmed. One report, for example, failed to find an increased incidence of OA in pneumatic drill users and criticized inadequate sample sizes, lack of statistical analyses, and omission of appropriate control populations in previous reports.[34] The investigators further commented that earlier work was "frequently misinterpreted" and that their studies suggested that "impact, without injury or preceding abnormality of either joint contour or ligaments, is unlikely to produce osteoarthritis."[35]

Do epidemiologic studies of OA implicate physical or mechanical factors related to disease predisposition or development? The first national Health and Nutrition Examination Survey of 1971 to 1975 (HANES I) and the Framingham studies explored cross-sectional associations between radiographic OA of the knee and possible risk factors.[39–44,53] Strong associations were noted between knee OA and obesity and occupations involving the stress of knee bending, but not all habitual physical activities and leisure-time physical activities (e.g., running, walking, team sports, racquet sports, and others) were linked with knee OA[28–30,54–56]; indeed, certain activities and/or exercise regimens may be protective[57–59] (see Chapter 104 for a more detailed discussion of the pathogenesis of OA.)

Other Occupational Rheumatologic Disorders

Certain rheumatic diseases other than repetitive strain or cumulative trauma disorders have been associated with occupational risks. Reports have been made of reflex sympathetic dystrophy after trauma; Raynaud's phenomenon with vibration or exposure to chemicals (particularly polyvinyl chloride); autoimmune disease from teaching at a school, farming, occupations with exposure to animals and pesticides, mining, use of a textile machine, and decorating operations[41,60]; scleroderma from exposure to chemicals, silica, and solvents and with use of vibrating tools[61,62]; scleroderma-like syndromes from exposure to rapeseed oil and L-tryptophan[62,63]; systemic lupus erythematosus (SLE) from exposure to the sun, silica, mercury, pesticides, nail polish, paints, dye, canavanine, hydrazine, solvents,[64,65] trauma and post-traumatic stress disorder,[66] oral contraceptives, cigarette smoking,[67–69] and with shiftwork and patient contact[70]; lupus, scleroderma, and Paget's disease from exposure to pets[71]; granulomatous vasculitis from exposure to mercury, lead,[72] and inhaled antigens[73]; primary systemic vasculitis from farming, exposure to silica and solvents, and allergy[74]; anti-synthetase syndrome from exposure to dust, gas, and fumes[75]; arthritis in patients with psoriasis from infections requiring antibiotics and in people who have performed heavy lifting[76] and following trauma[77]; spondyloarthropathy from stressful events[78]; gout (saturnine) and hyperuricemia with lead intoxication[79]; juvenile idiopathic arthritis with cigarette smoke exposure during pregnancy[80]; juvenile dermatomyositis with tobacco and air pollution exposure during pregnancy[81]; and rheumatoid arthritis (Caplan's syndrome) with silica exposure, farming, mining, quarrying, electrical work, construction and engine operation, nursing, religious, juridical, and other social science–related work, smoking, traffic and pollution, insecticides, periodontal disease,[82–84] and potential noxious airborne agents[85] (Table 38.4).

TABLE 38.4 Other Reported Occupation-Related Rheumatic Diseases

Disease or Syndrome	Occupation or Risk Factor
Reflex sympathetic dystrophy	Trauma
Raynaud's phenomenon	Vibration Chemicals (polyvinyl chloride)
Autoimmune disease[41,60]	Teaching at a school
Scleroderma[61,62]	Chlorinated hydrocarbons Organic solvents Silica
Vasculitis[72–74]	Mercury, lead, silica, solvents, allergy, inhaled antigens
Scleroderma-like syndromes[62,63]	Rapeseed oil L-Tryptophan
Anti-synthetase syndrome[75]	Dust, gas, fume exposure
Systemic lupus erythematosus[65–71]	Canavanine, hydrazine, mercury, pesticides, solvents, shift work, patient contact, trauma, post-traumatic stress disorder, oral contraceptives, cigarette smoke
Lupus, scleroderma, and Paget's disease[71]	Pet ownership
Rheumatoid arthritis (Caplan's syndrome)[82,83,85]	Silica, insecticides, traffic, pollution, smoking, periodontal disease, potential noxious airborne agents
Arthritis in people with psoriasis[76,77]	Heavy lifting, infection requiring antibiotic treatment, trauma
Spondyloarthritis[78]	Stressful events
Gout (saturnine)[79]	Lead
Juvenile idiopathic arthritis[80]	Cigarette smoke exposure during pregnancy
Juvenile dermatomyositis[81]	Tobacco and air pollution during pregnancy

Recreation- and Sports-Related Musculoskeletal Disorders

Do recreational or sports-related activities lead to musculoskeletal disorders?[86–111] Some suggest that the risk of joint degeneration is increased by participation in sports that have high impact levels with torsional loading. The presence of prior joint injury, surgery, arthritis, joint instability and/or malalignment, neuromuscular disturbances, and muscle weakness also predispose to higher risks of joint damage during sports participation.[84] People with sports injuries to the anterior cruciate and medial collateral ligaments (such as from downhill skiing and football) frequently experienced the chondromalacia patellae and radiographic abnormalities of OA (20% to 52%).[28–30] Retrospective studies found that OA was associated with varus deformity, previous meniscectomy, and relative body weight.[86,87,112] Both partial and total meniscectomies have been linked with degenerative changes. Early joint stabilization and direct meniscus repair surgery may decrease the incidence of premature OA. Observations like these support the concept that abnormal biomechanical forces, either congenital or secondary to joint injury, are important factors in the development of exercise-related OA.[28–30] Other observations include certain physical characteristics of the participant, biomechanical and biochemical factors, age, sex, hormonal influences, nutrition, characteristics of the playing surface (when applicable), unique features of particular sports, and duration and intensity of exercise participation, as has been reviewed extensively elsewhere.[28–30] It is increasingly recognized that biomechanical factors have an important role in the pathogenesis of OA, as has been presented.

Is regular participation in physical activity associated with degenerative arthritis? Several animal studies (of tentative scientific relevance, but of interest) have suggested a possible relationship between exercise and OA. For example, some state that the husky breed of dog has increased hip and shoulder arthritis associated with pulling sleds, that tigers and lions develop foreleg OA related to sprinting and running, and that racehorses and workhorses develop OA in the forelegs and hind legs, respectively, consistent with their physical stress patterns.[28,30] In rabbits with experimentally induced arthritis in one hind limb, progressive OA did not develop when they exercised on treadmills, but OA did develop in sheep with normal health who walked on concrete. Other studies found that OA did not develop in dogs (beagles) who ran 4 to 20 km a day,[28–30] that lifelong physical activity (running) protected mice from OA,[113] that running 30 km in 3 weeks or 55 km in 6 weeks induced OA in rats,[114] that running exacerbated induced OA in other rats,[115] and that running was salutary for rats with collagen-induced arthritis.[116] Although these observations were not entirely consistent, they suggested that physical activities in some circumstances might predispose to degenerative joint disease.

Human studies have provided pertinent observations[28–30] (Table 38.5). Wrestlers were reported to have an increased incidence of OA of the lumbar spine, cervical spine, and knees; boxers, of the carpometacarpal joints; parachutists, of knees, ankles, and spine, which was not confirmed; cyclists, of the patella; cricketers, of the fingers; and basketball and volleyball players, of the knees.[28–30,43] In addition, athletes involved in sports requiring repetitive overhead throwing such as baseball, tennis, volleyball, and swimming were reported to have an increased incidence of early glenohumeral arthritis[90]; people with meniscal and anterior cruciate ligament injuries incurred in youth-related sports were reported to have an increased incidence of knee OA[91]; soccer players were reported to have an increased incidence of OA of the talar joint, ankle, cervical spine, knee, and hip[28–30,92–95,112]; and OA of the hips and knees of elite athletes from impact sports.[96] Studies of American football players have suggested that they are susceptible to OA of the knees, particularly those who sustained knee injuries while playing football.[31] Among football players (average age, 23 years) competing for a place on a professional team, 90% had radiographic abnormalities of the foot or ankle, compared with 4% of an age-matched control population; linemen had more changes than did ball carriers or linebackers, who in turn had more changes than did flankers or defensive backs. All athletes who had played football for 9 years or longer had abnormal radiographic findings.[28–31,91] Most of these studies were deficient in several respects: criteria for OA (or "osteoarthrosis," "degenerative joint disease," or "abnormality") were not always clear, specified, or consistent; duration of follow-up was often not indicated or was inadequate to determine the risk of musculoskeletal problems at a later age; intensity and duration of physical activity were variable and difficult to quantify;

TABLE 38.5 Sports Participation and Alleged Associations With Osteoarthritis

Sport	Site (Joint)	Risk
Ballet[28–30]	Talus Ankle Cervical spine Hip Knee Metatarsophalangeal joint	Possibly to probably increased depending on type, intensity, and duration of participation
Baseball[28–30]	Elbow Shoulder	
Boxing[28–30]	Hand (carpometacarpal joints)	
Cricket[28–30]	Finger	
Cycling[28–30]	Finger	
American football[28–30,112]	Ankle Foot Knee Spine	
Gymnastics[28–30,112]	Elbow Shoulder Wrist Hip Knee	
Lacrosse[28–30]	Ankle Knee	
Martial arts[28–30]	Spine	
Parachuting[28–30]	Ankle Knee Spine	
Rugby[28–30]	Knee	
Running (see Table 38.6)[28–30,96,98,104,105,110–112,118,119]	Knee Hip Ankle	Small
Soccer[28–30,95,96,110,112]	Ankle-foot Hip Knee Talus Talofibular	
Weightlifting[28–30]	Spine	
Wrestling[28–30]	Cervical spine Elbow Knee	

selection bias toward people exercising or participating versus those not exercising or participating was not weighted; other possible risk factors and predispositions to musculoskeletal disorders were rarely considered; studies were not always properly controlled, and examinations were not always "blind"; little information regarding nonprofessional, recreational athletes was available; and little clinical information about functional status was provided.[28–30,88,89,112]

A number of studies have examined a possible relationship between running and OA. Uncontrolled observations generally suggested that runners without underlying biomechanical problems of the lower extremity joints did not develop arthritis at a different rate from a normal population of nonrunners. However, people who had underlying articular biomechanical abnormalities from a previously injured joint (and perhaps elite athletes, particularly women) appeared to be at greater risk for the subsequent development of OA. Early studies showed that groups of long-duration, high-mileage runners and nonrunning control subjects had a comparable (and low) prevalence of OA and suggested that recreational running need not inevitably lead to OA.[117] These observations have generally now been confirmed by the original authors in long-term follow-up studies[98] and by other investigators[28–30,88,89,92,97–99,104,111,117] and in comprehensive reviews[101,112,118] (Table 38.6). Eight- and 9-year follow-up observations were supportive; most of the original runners were still running, with a prevalence of OA that was comparable with that of the control subjects.[89] Perhaps even more significant was the growing evidence that running and other aerobic exercise protected against the development of disability and early mortality.[97] In another study,[98] former college varsity long-distance runners were compared with former college swimmers; no association was found between moderate levels of running or number of years running and the development of symptomatic OA. Other authors have concluded that running in and of itself does not cause OA; rather, prior injuries and anatomic variances were directly responsible for some of the changes.[28–30,117] Prospective studies have found that runners were not at risk for the development of premature OA of the knees.[98–103] Runners had hip replacements less frequently than did other people (perhaps related to lower BMIs).[104] However, another recent study found that running 20 miles per week was associated with 2.4 hazard ratio for OA for men younger than 50 years.[105] The most recent reports confirmed no increased risk of symptomatic knee OA in self-selected runners, as compared with nonrunners.[119–121]

Studies examining hip OA in former athletes[106–110] noted that former champion distance runners had no more clinical or radiographic evidence of OA than did nonrunners.[106] However, another study found more radiographic changes due to degenerative hip disease in former national team long-distance runners than in bobsled competitors and control subjects.[122] In all the subjects studied, age and mileage run in 1973 were strong predictors of radiographic evidence of hip OA; for runners, running pace in 1973 was the strongest predictor of subsequent radiographic evidence of hip OA in 1988. These authors concluded that high-intensity, high-mileage running should not be dismissed as a risk factor for premature OA of the hip. Other reports found that former top-level soccer players and weightlifters, but not runners, were at risk for the development of knee OA,[92,109] but it was suggested elsewhere that former athletes seemed to be disproportionately represented in hospital admissions for OA of hip, knee, or ankle.[109] A questionnaire of former elite and track-and-field athletes noted they had increased hip OA.[108] Similarly, radiographic OA of the hip and knee was reported in women who were formerly runners and tennis players.[109] Other investigators reported no correlation between OA and running but rather with other sports, particularly soccer and tennis (where knee injuries were prevalent).[110] It was speculated that peak load per unit distance (stride and short duration of ground contact) may explain the fewer injuries and reduced prevalence of OA in running compared with certain other sports.[111]

It is of interest that physical activity is now recommended as a valuable therapeutic modality for certain people with rheumatic diseases.[123,124] It may be pertinent to note the confounding effect of obesity on the expression of rheumatic disorders like rheumatoid arthritis and SLE (see Chapter 39).[125,126]

Cross-sectional studies on the effect of weight-bearing exercise on the development of OA of the hip, knee, or ankle and foot must be interpreted with caution. The radiographic scoring methods used by each group of investigators differ, and their reliability has not been adequately tested. This information is important when the major end points in the studies are radiographic features of OA.

Performing Arts–Related Musculoskeletal Disorders

Musculoskeletal problems are common among performing artists. Performing artists—particularly musicians and dancers—have unique medical and musculoskeletal problems that merit special consideration. Injuries that might be trivial to others may be catastrophic to such artists. These injuries are usually associated with overuse—the consequences of tissues stressed beyond anatomic or normal physical limits. Understanding the technical requirements and biomechanics required in the performance of a craft (art), as well as the lifestyle required to pursue a successful career in these fields, should help physicians appreciate causative factors that lead to these injuries.

The following principles are important in treating such patients:

- Musculoskeletal problems constitute the bulk of health issues for these people.
- Performing artists are usually wary of consulting with physicians and skeptical of their expertise.
- An appropriate evaluation should be carried out by someone knowledgeable about the technical and biomechanical requirements of the patient's craft(s)/art(s). The evaluation should consider instrument(s), instrument usage, travel with instruments, shoes, performance surface and setting, practice and performance routines, repertoire, coaches and training/trainers, and lifestyle and psychological factors, as appropriate.
- Evaluation should include attention to joint laxity and other physical features of the artist, as well as to their relationship to performance, considering the entities encountered as listed in Table 38.7.[122,127–130] The evaluation should assess muscle tension and fatigue. Patients should demonstrate how they use an instrument while both the actively moving body parts and the relatively immobilized parts are examined.[122,131,132]
- Inquiry should be made about all prescription and nonprescription therapies, nutritional and exercise practices, and non-mainstream (so-called *complementary* and/or *alternative*) treatments.

TABLE 38.6 Studies of Running and Risk of Developing Osteoarthritis

No. of Runners	Mean Age (yr)	Mean No. of Years Running	Miles/Wk	Comments
319	NA	NA	NA	OA noted more frequently in former runners (with underlying anatomic "tilt" abnormality—epiphysiolysis) than in nonathletes[27–29]
74	56	21	NA	Champion distance runners had no more hip OA than did nonrunners in their sixth decade[27–29]
32	NA	NA	NA	Radiographic findings of runners' hips and knees were similar to those of control subjects[27–29]
20	35	13	48	OA occurred in runners with underlying anatomic (biomechanical) abnormality[107]
504	57	9-15	18-19	No association between moderate long-distance running and future development of OA (of hip and knees)[101]
17	53	12	28	Comparable low prevalence of lower extremity OA in runners and nonrunners[97]
41	58	9	5 h/wk	No differences between runners and control subjects in cartilage loss, crepitus, joint stability, or symptoms[88]
498	59	12	27	No differences between groups in conditions thought to predispose to OA and musculoskeletal disability[27–29]
27	42	NA	61	More radiographic changes of hip OA in former Swiss national team long-distance runners than in bobsledders and control subjects; few runners had clinical symptoms of OA; no difference in ankle joints[106,107]
30	58	40	12-24	No clinical or radiographic differences in hips, knees, and ankles between runners and nonrunners[102]
114	50-80	NA	NA	Unvalidated questionnaire reported threefold increase of hip arthrosis in former athletes[108]
342	NA	NA	NA	More former athletes hospitalized with hip OA than expected[103]
28	60	32	NA	Women soccer players and weightlifters, nonrunners were at risk of premature OA[92]
16	63	22	22	8-yr follow-up of original observations made in 1986 still found no differences between runners and nonrunners[117]
35	60	10-13	23-28	Running did not appear to influence the development of radiographic OA (with possible exception of spur formation in women)[89]
16,691 subjects	40% > 50	Variable		>20 miles/wk was associated (2000) with 2.4 hazard ratio for OA in men[105]
1/45	58	18	183.5 h/wk	No increased OA in runners[98]
NA	NA	NA	NA	Comprehensive literature review of in vitro, animal, and human studies; "Low-and moderate-volume runners appear to have no more risk of developing OA than nonrunners. The existing literature is inconclusive (for)... high-volume running..."[118]
74,752	46	13	<1.8 – >5.4 METhr/d	Fewer hip and knee replacements in runners[104]
778	62	NA	NA	No increase in symptomatic knee OA in runners compared with nonrunners[119]

METhr/d, Metabolic equivalent hours per day; *NA,* not available; *OA,* osteoarthritis.

- Clinicians must have an understanding of and sympathy for the unique expectations of these performers and expertise in assessing their medical problems and developing treatment plans.
- Prevention should be emphasized—ensuring performance ability, promoting endurance and conditioning, facilitating good posture, protecting joints, maintaining proper ergonomics, and establishing appropriate exercise regimens.[131,132]
- Therapeutic interventions will usually be conservative.

Instrumentalists

The frequency of musculoskeletal problems in musicians rivals the frequency of disability in athletes. Up to 82% of orchestral musicians have experienced medical problems (mainly musculoskeletal) related to their occupation. Up to 76% of musicians have reported

TABLE 38.7 **Musculoskeletal and Rheumatic Disorders Associated With Overuse in Performing Artists**

Instrument	Affliction (Common Name)
Piano, keyboard[135]	Myalgias Tendinitis Synovitis Contractures Nerve entrapment Median nerve (carpal tunnel–pronator syndrome) Ulnar nerve Brachial plexus Posterior interosseous branch of radial nerve Thoracic outlet syndrome Motor palsies Osteoarthritis
Strings	
Violin, viola[135]	Myalgias Tendinitis Epicondylitis Cervical spondylosis Rotator cuff tears Thoracic outlet syndrome Temporomandibular joint syndrome Motor palsies Garrod's pads Nerve entrapment Ulnar Interosseous
Cello[135]	Myalgias Tendinitis Epicondylitis Low back pain Nerve entrapment Motor palsies Thoracic outlet syndrome
Bass[135]	Low back pain Myalgias Tendinitis Motor palsies
Viola de gamba[135]	Saphenous nerve compression (gamba leg)
Harp[135]	Tendinitis Nerve entrapment
Woodwinds	
Clarinet and oboe[135]	First web space muscle strain Tendinitis Motor palsies
Flute[135]	Myalgias Spine pain Temporomandibular joint syndrome Tendinitis Nerve entrapment Digital Posterior interosseous Thoracic outlet syndrome
Brass	
Trumpet, cornet[135]	Motor palsies Orbicularis oris rupture (Satchmo's syndrome)
English horn[135]	de Quervain's tenosynovitis
French horn[135]	Motor palsies
Saxophone[135]	Thoracic outlet syndrome
Percussion	Osteoarthritis
Drums[135]	Tendinitis Myalgias Nerve entrapment
Cymbals[135]	Bicipital tenosynovitis (cymbal player's shoulder)
Miscellaneous	
Guitar, strings[135]	Tendinitis Synovitis Motor palsies
Congas[135]	Pigmenturia
Spoons[135]	Tibial stress fracture (spoon player's tibia)

a musculoskeletal issue that is grave enough to influence their ability to perform.[122,133] Woodwind players and female instrumentalists seem to be affected more often compared with other types of other instrumentalists and male artists, respectively. Muscle-tendon overuse or repetitive stress injuries, nerve entrapment problems, and focal dystonias are most common (see Table 38.7).[122,127]

The causes of, mechanisms of, and therapies for these musculoskeletal problems are unclear. Overuse, tendinitis, cumulative trauma disorder, repetitive motion disorder, occupational cervicobrachial disorder, and regional pain syndrome have been considered critical risk factors in the development of joint laxity in musicians.[133] Joint laxity declined with age and was associated with sex, starting earlier in men but persisting in women through their mid-40s. The presence or absence of hypermobility at certain sites was associated with musicians' reports of associated symptoms. Hypermobility in musicians might produce advantages or disadvantages, depending on the site of the laxity and the instrument played.[134] Paganini, with his long fingers and reported hyperextensibility, had a wider finger reach on the violin than his contemporaries, but he may have had a predisposition to OA because of this. Of interest and seemingly unexplained was the high frequency of symptoms among women (68% to 84%); perhaps this finding is related to their higher incidence of hypermobility.[133] Stress also likely contributes to motor function problems such as occupational cramps; dealing with this issue often requires the best efforts of a team of physicians and therapists.[133–136]

Vocal Artists

Musculoskeletal problems among singers have not been addressed extensively. The frequency of musculoskeletal problems was the same in both instrumentalists and opera singers. However, singers had more hip, knee, and foot joint complaints, perhaps reflecting the effects of prolonged standing.[135]

Dancers

Dance has been viewed as a demanding art form. Classical ballet ranked first in activities generating physical and mental stress, followed by professional football and professional hockey. The dancer and athlete have much in common, but important differences in training and performance technique influence the nature of their injuries. Other important sociocultural differences affect their care. Professional dancers (as well as musicians and vocalists) traditionally have not been convinced that most physicians know how to effectively approach the unique issues of dance and music. Injured dancers seeking care have often been told that the treatment is to stop dancing. Others, seeking assistance with weight control, have been told to gain weight. Dancers frequently underreport their injuries and seek care from nonmedical therapists.

The incidence of reported dance-related injuries ranged from 17% to 95%.[137] The majority of injuries involved the foot, ankle, and knee. It is difficult to generalize about dance injuries because "dance" and its training, performance, and settings are so variable. Most injuries are from overuse and are rarely catastrophic, regardless of the style or setting.[133] The distribution of injuries is strongly influenced by the type and style of dance and the age and sex of the population.[134,138] A better understanding of the technical and aesthetic requirements of a dance, as well as the biomechanics involved to perform these requirements, is necessary to appreciate the type of injuries that can be sustained by dancers. For example, ballet dancers in companies whose choreography emphasizes bravura technique with big jumps and balances are more likely to experience Achilles tendinitis than are those in companies that do not have this emphasis. Men are more likely to have back injuries because of the requisite jumping and lifting, whereas women who dance *en pointe* are more prone to toe, foot, and ankle problems. Also in ballet, the most important physical feature is proper turnout of the hip, which requires maximal external rotation of the lower extremity that can result in hyperlordosis of the lumbar spine, valgus heel with forefoot pronation, and external rotation of the knee.[137,139]

Tendinitis of the flexor hallucis longus tendon, commonly known as dancer's tendinitis, may be confused with posterior tibial tendinitis because of the location of pain at the posteromedial ankle. Other dancer- and environment-related factors that increase the risk of dance-related injuries include nutritional status, improper support from footwear and floors, and their rehearsal and performance schedules.[137,139] Most dance shoes do not have a shock-absorbing sole, and some dances may be performed barefoot.[139] Traditionally constructed with paper, glue, and satin or canvas or leather, ballet pointe shoes tend to soften once broken in, thus contributing to ankle injury. Intensive rehearsals before and during the opening months of a performance season and pressures to return to work quickly after an injury must also be considered in the care of dancers.[133,139] Touring companies may encounter nonflexible surfaces, including concrete, predisposing to shin splints and stress fractures. Stress fractures may be associated with the pressure to maintain a certain weight, resulting in amenorrhea, disordered eating, and low bone density. Physicians caring for dancers, particularly ballet dancers at any level, must be aware of the aesthetic pressures for extreme leanness and the potential health consequences. Unfortunately, the dance world is not lacking in other serious medical problems including mental illness, drug abuse, and HIV infection.[133]

Full references for this chapter can be found on ExpertConsult.com.

Selected References

1. Buckle PW: Work factors and upper limb disorders, *BMJ* 315:1360, 1997.
2. Hadler NM: Repetitive upper-extremity motions in the workplace are not hazardous, *J Hand Surg [Am]* 22(19), 1997.
3. Yassi A: Work-related musculoskeletal disorders, *Curr Opin Rheumatol* 12:124–130, 2000.
4. Schouten SAG, de Bie RA, Swaen G: An update on the relationship between occupational factors and osteoarthritis of the hip and knee, *Curr Opin Rheumatol* 14:89–92, 2002.
5. Mani L, Gerr F: Work-related upper extremity musculoskeletal disorders, *Prim Care* 27:845–864, 2000.
6. Colombini D, Occhipinti E, Delleman N, et al.: Exposure assessment of upper limb repetitive movements: a consensus document developed by the technical committee on musculoskeletal disorders of International Ergonomics Association endorsed by International Commission on Occupation Health, *G Ital Med Lav Ergon* 23:129–142, 2000.
7. Hales TR, Bernard BP: Epidemiology of work-related musculoskeletal disorders, *Orthop Clin North Am* 27:679, 1996.
8. Malchaire N, Cook N, Vergracht S: Review of the factors associated with musculoskeletal problems in epidemiologic studies, *Arch Occup Environ Health* 74:79–90, 2001.
9. American Academy of Orthopedic Surgeons: *The burden of musculoskeletal diseases in the United States: prevalence, societal and economic cost,* Rosemont, Ill, 2008, American Academy of Orthopedic Surgeons, pp 130–137.
10. Harrington JM: Occupational medicine and rheumatic diseases, *Br J Rheumatol* 36:153, 1997.
11. Driscoll T, Jacklyn G, Orchard J, et al.: The global burden of occupationally related low back pain: estimates from the global Burden of Disease 2010 study, *Ann Rheum Dis* 73:975–981, 2013.
12. Descatha A, Albo F, Leclerc A, et al.: Lateral epicondylitis and physical exposure at work? A review of prospective studies and meta-analysis, *Arthritis Care Res* 68:1681–1687, 2016.
13. Hadler NM: Vibration white finger revisited, *J Occup Environ Med* 41:772, 1998.
14. Viikari-Juntura ERA: The scientific basis for making guidelines and standards to prevent work-related musculoskeletal disorders, *Ergonomics* 40(1097), 1997.
15. Hadler NM: *Occupational musculosketal disorders*, ed 3, Philadelphia, 2004, Lippincott Williams & Wilkins.
16. Lister GD: Ergonomic disorders [editorial], *J Hand Surg [Am]* 353(20), 1995.
17. Schrader H, Obelieniene D, Bovim G, et al.: Natural evolution of late whiplash syndrome outside the medicolegal context, *Lancet* 347:1207, 1996.
18. Vender MI, Kasdan ML, Truppa KL: Upper extremity disorders: a literature review to determine work-relatedness, *J Hand Surg [Am]* 20:534, 1995.
19. Reilly PA, Travers R, Littlejohn GO: Epidemiology of soft tissue rheumatism: the influence of the law [editorial], *J Rheumatol* 18:1448, 1991.
20. Bell DS: "Repetition strain injury": an iatrogenic epidemic of simulated injury, *Med J Aust* 151:280, 1989.
21. Davis TR: Do repetitive tasks give rise to musculoskeletal disorders? *Occup Med* 49:257–258, 1999.
22. Higgs PE, Edwards D, Martin DS, et al.: Carpal tunnel surgery outcomes in workers: effect of workers' compensation status, *J Hand Surg [Am]* 20:354, 1995.

23. Kamada M, Kitayuguchi J, Lee IM, et al.: Relationship between physical activity and chronic musculoskeletal pain among community-dwelling Japanese adults, *J Epidemiol* 24:474–483, 2014.
24. Lier R, Nilsen TIL, Mork PJ: Parental chronic pain in relation to chronic pain in their adult offspring: family-linkage within the HUNT study, Norway, *BMC Public Health* 14:797, 2014.
25. Macfarlane GJ, Pallewatte N, Paudyal P, et al.: Evaluation of work-related psychosocial factors and regional musculoskeletal pain: results from a EULAR task force, *Ann Rheum Dis* 68:885–891, 2009.
26. Harkness EF, Macfarlane GJ, Nahit E, et al.: Mechanical injury and psychosocial factors in the work place predict the onset of widespread body pain: a two-year prospective study among cohorts of newly employed workers, *Arthritis Rheum* 50:1655–1664, 2004.
27. Angell M: *Science on trial: the clash of medical evidence and the law in the breast implant case*, New York, 1997, Norton.
28. Panush RS, Lane NE: Exercise and the musculoskeletal system, *Baillieres Clin Rheumatol* 8:79, 1994.
29. Panush RS: Physical activity, fitness, and osteoarthritis. In Bouchard C, Shephard RJ, Stephens T, editors: *Physical activity, fitness, and health: international proceedings and consensus statement*, Champaign, Ill, 1994, Human Kinetics, pp 712–723.
30. Panush RS: Does exercise cause arthritis? Long-term consequences of exercise on the musculoskeletal system, *Rheum Dis Clin North Am* 16:827, 1990.
31. Golightly YM, Marshall SW, Callahan LF, et al.: Early-onset arthritis in retired National Football League players, *J Phys Act Health* 6:638, 2009.
32. Kellgren JH, Lawrence JS: Radiological assessment of osteoarthrosis, *Ann Rheum Dis* 16:494, 1957.
33. Lawrence JS: Rheumatism in coal miners. III. Occupational factors, *Br J Ind Med* 12:249, 1955.
34. Kellgren JH, Lawrence JS: Osteoarthritis and disc degeneration in an urban population, *Ann Rheum Dis* 12(5), 1958.
35. Burke MJ, Fear EC, Wright V: Bone and joint changes in pneumatic drillers, *Ann Rheum Dis* 36:276, 1977.
36. Lawrence JS: Rheumatism in cotton operatives, *Br J Ind Med* 18:270, 1961.
37. Tempelaar HHG, Van Breeman J: Rheumatism and occupation, *Acta Rheumatol* 4:36, 1932.
38. Hadler NM, Gillings DB, Imbus HR: Hand structure and function in an industrial setting: the influence of the three patterns of stereotyped, repetitive usage, *Arthritis Rheum* 21:210, 1978.
39. Anderson J, Felson DR: Factors associated with knee osteoarthritis (OA) in the HANES I survey: evidence for an association with overweight, race and physical demands of work, *Am J Epidemiol* 128:179, 1988.
40. Felson DT, Zhang Y, Hannan MT, et al.: Risk factors for incident radiographic knee osteoarthritis in the elderly: the Framingham Study, *Arthritis Rheum* 40:728, 1997.
41. Felson DT, Zhang Y: An update on the epidemiology of knee and hip osteoarthritis with a view to prevention, *Arthritis Rheum* 41:1343, 1998.
42. Allen KD, Chen JC, Callahan LF, et al.: Associations of occupational tasks with knee and hip osteoarthritis: the Johnston county osteoarthritis project, *J Rheumatol* 37:842–850, 2010.
43. Vrezas I, Elsner G, Bolm-Audorff U, et al.: Case-control study of knee osteoarthritis and lifestyle factors considering their interaction with physical workload, *Int Arch Occup Environ Health* 83:291–300, 2010.
44. Niu J, Zhang YQ, Torner J, et al.: Is obesity a risk factor for progressive radiographic knee osteoarthritis? *Arthritis Rheum* 61:329–335, 2009.
45. McWilliams DF, Leeb SG, Doherty M, et al.: Occupational risk factors for osteoarthritis of the knee: a meta-analysis, *Osteoarthritis Cartilage* 19:829–839, 2011.
46. Exxat AM, Cibere J, Koehoorn M, et al.: Association between cumulative joint loading from occupational activities and knee osteoarthritis, *Arthritis Care Res* 65:1634–1642, 2013.
47. Virayavanich W, Alizai H, Baum T, et al.: Association of frequent knee bending activity with focal knee lesions detected with 3T magnetic resonance imaging: data from the Osteoarthritis Initiative, *Arthritis Care Res* 65:1441–1448, 2013.
48. Dore DA, Winzenberg TM, Ding C, et al.: The association between objectively measured physical activity and knee structural change using MRI, *Ann Rheum Dis* 72:1170–1175, 2013.
49. Lin W, Alizai H, Joseph GB, et al.: Physical activity in relation to knee cartilage T2 progression measured with 3 T MRI over a period of 4 years: data from the Osteoarthritis Initiative, *Osteoarthritis Cartilage* 21:1558–1566, 2013.
50. Mosher TJ, Liu Y, Torok CM, et al.: Functional cartilage MRI T2 mapping: evaluating the effect of age and training on knee cartilage response to running, *Osteoarthritis Cartilage* 18:358–364, 2009.
51. Driban JB, Eaton CB, Lo GH, et al.: Knee injuries are associated with accelerated knee osteoarthritis progression: data from the Osteoarthritis Initiative, *Arthritis Care Res* 66:1673–1679, 2014.
52. Molleson T: The eloquent bones of Abu Hureyra, *Sci Am* 271:70–75, 1994.
53. Felson DT: Developments in the clinical understanding of osteoarthritis, *Arthritis Res Ther* 11:203, 2009.
54. Wang Y, Simpson JA, Wluka AE, et al.: Is physical activity a risk factor for primary knee or hip replacement due to osteoarthritis? A prospective cohort study, *J Rheumatol* 38:350–357, 2011.
55. Lohmander LS, Gerhardsson de Verdier M, Rollof J, et al.: Incidence of severe knee and hip osteoarthritis in relation to different measures of body mass: a population-based prospective cohort study, *Ann Rheum Dis* 68:490–496, 2009.
56. Felson DT, Niu J, Clancy M, et al.: Effect of recreational physical activities on the development of knee osteoarthritis in older adults of different weights: the Framingham Study, *Arthritis Rheum* 57(6–12), 2007.
57. Abbasi J: Can exercise prevent knee osteoarthritis, *JAMA* 318(22):2169–2171, 2017.
58. Wallace IJ, Worthington S, Felson DT, et al.: Knee osteoarthritis has doubled in prevalence since the mid-20th century, *Proc Natl Acad Sci U S A* 114(35):9332–9336, 2017.
59. Qin J, Barbour KE, Nevitt MC, et al.: Objectively measured physical activity and risk of knee osteoarthritis, *Med Sci Sports Exerc* 50, 2018. 377-283.
60. Gold LS, Ward MH, Dosemeci M, et al.: Systemic autoimmune disease mortality and occupational exposures, *Arthritis Rheum* 56:3189–3201, 2007.
61. Mora GF: Systemic sclerosis: environmental factors, *J Rheumatol* 36:2383–2396, 2009.
62. Nietert PJ, Silver RM: Systemic sclerosis: environmental and occupational risk factors, *Curr Opin Rheumatol* 12:520–526, 2000.
63. Dospinescu P, Jones GT, Basu N: Environmental risk factors in systemic sclerosis, *Curr Opin Rheumatol* 25:179–183, 2013.
64. Parks CG, Cooper GS, Nylander-French LA, et al.: Occupational exposure to crystalline silica and risk of systemic lupus erythematosus: a population-based, case-control study in the southeastern United States, *Arthritis Rheum* 46:1840–1850, 2002.
65. Cooper GS, Wither J, Bernatsky S, et al.: Occupational and environmental exposures and risk of systemic lupus erythematosus: silica, sunlight, solvents, *Rheumatology (Oxford)* 49:2172–2180, 2010.
66. Roberts AL, Malspeis S, Bubzansky LD, et al.: Association of trauma and posttraumatic stress disorder with incident systemic lupus erythematosus in a longitudinal cohort of women, *Arthritis Rheum* 69(11):2162–2169, 2017.
67. Barbhaiya M, Tedeschi SK, Lu B, et al.: Cigarette smoking and the risk of systemic lupus eryuthematosus, overall and by anti-double stranded DNA antibody subtype, in the Nurses' Health Study cohorts, *Ann Rheum Dis* 77:196–202, 2018.

68. Orione MAM, Silva CA, Sallum AME, et al.: Risk factors for juvenile dermatomyositis: exposure to tobacco and air pollutants during pregnancy, *Arthritis Care Res* 66:1571–1575, 2014.
69. Gulati G, Brunner HI: Environmental triggers in systemic lupus erythematosus, *Seminars Arthritis Rheum* 47:710–717, 2018.
70. Cooper GS, Parks CG, Treadwell EL, et al.: Occupational risk factors for the development of systemic lupus erythematosus, *J Rheumatol* 31:1928–1933, 2004.
71. Panush RS, Levine ML, Reichlin M: Do I need an ANA? Some thoughts about man's best friend and the transmissibility of lupus, *J Rheumatol* 27:287–291, 2000.
72. Albert D, Clarkin C, Komoroski J, et al.: Wegener's granulomatosis: possible role of environmental agents in its pathogenesis, *Arthritis Rheum* 51:656–664, 2004.
73. Stamp L, Chapman PT, Francis J, et al.: Association between environmental exposures and granulomatosis with polyangiitis in Canterbury, New Zealand, *Arthritis Res Ther* 17:333–340, 2015.
74. Lane SE, Watts RA, Bentham G, et al.: Are environmental factors important in primary systemic vasculitis? A case control study, *Arthritis Rheum* 48:814–823, 2003.
75. Labirua-Iturburu A, Selva-O'Callaghan A, Zock JP, et al.: Occupational exposure in patients with the antisynthetase syndrome, *Clin Rheumatol* 33:221–225, 2014.
76. Eder L, Law T, Chandran V, et al.: Association between environmental factors and onset of psoriatic arthritis in patients with psoriasis, *Arthritis Care Res* 63:1091–1097, 2011.
77. Thorarensen SM, Lu N, Agdie A, et al.: Physical trauma recorded in primary care is associated with the onset of psoriatic arthritis among patients with psoriasis, *Ann Rheum Dis* 76(3):521–525, 2016.
78. Zeboulon-Ktorza N, Boelle PY, Nahal RS, et al.: Influence of environmental factors on disease activity in spondyloarthritis: a prospective cohort study, *J Rheumatol* 40:469–475, 2013.
79. Shadick NA, Kim R, Weiss S, et al.: Effect of low level lead exposure on hyperuicemia and gout among middle-aged and elderly men, *J Rheumatol* 27:1708–1712, 2000.
80. Franca CMP, Sallum AME, Braga ALF, et al.: Risk factors associated with juvenile idiopathic arthritis: exposure to cigarette smoke and air pollution from pregnancy to disease diagnosis, *J Rheumatol* 45(2):248–256, 2018.
81. Orione MAM, Silva CA, Sallum AME, et al.: Risk factors for juvenile dermatomyositis: exposure to tobacco and air pollutants during pregnancy, *Arthritis Care Res* 66:1571–1575, 2014.
82. Sverdrup B, Kallberg H, Bengtsson C, et al.: Association between occupational exposure to mineral oil and rheumatoid arthritis: results from the Swedish EIRA case-control study, *Arthritis Res Ther* 7:R1296–R1303, 2005.
83. Li X, Sundquist J, Sundquist K: Socioeconomic and occupational risk factors for rheumatoid arthritis: a nationwide study based on hospitalizations in Sweden, *J Rheumatol* 35:986–991, 2008.
84. Karlson EW, Deane K: Environmental and gene-environment interactions and risk of rheumatoid arthritis, *Rheum Dis Clin N Am* 38:405–426, 2012.
85. Ilar A, Alfredsson L, Wieberyt P, et al.: Occupation and risk of developing rheumatoid arthritis: results from a population-based case-control study, *Arthritis Care Res* 70:499–509, 2018.
86. Buckwalter JA, Martin JA: Sports and osteoarthritis, *Curr Opin Rheumatol* 16:634–639, 2004.
87. Videman T: The effect of running on the osteoarthritic joint: an experimental matched-pair study with rabbits, *Rheumatol Rehabil* 21(1):1–8, 1982.
88. Lane NE, Bloch DA, Jones HH, et al.: Long-distance running, bone density and osteoarthritis, *JAMA* 255:1147–1151, 1986.
89. Lane NE, Oehlert JW, Bloch DA, et al.: The relationship of running to osteoarthritis of the knee and hip and bone mineral density of the spine: 9 year longitudinal study, *J Rheumatol* 25:334–341, 1998.
90. Reineck JR, Krishnan SG, Burkhead WZ: Early glenohumeral arthritis in the competing athlete, *Clin Sports Med* 27:803–819, 2008.
91. Maffulli N, Longo UG, Gougoulias N, et al.: Long-term health outcomes of youth sports injuries, *Br J Sports Med* 44:21–25, 2010.
92. Kujala UM, Kettunen J, Paananen H, et al.: Knee osteoarthritis in former runners, soccer players, weight lifters, and shooters, *Arthritis Rheum* 38:539–546, 1995.
93. Lohmander LS, Ostenberg A, Englund M, et al.: High prevalence of knee osteoarthritis, pain, and functional limitations in female soccer players twelve years after anterior cruciate ligament injury, *Arthritis Rheum* 50:3145–3152, 2004.
94. Elleuch MH, Guermazi M, Mezghanni M, et al.: Knee osteoarthritis in 50 former top-level soccer players: a comparative study, *Ann Readapt Med Phys* 51:174–178, 2008.
95. Kuijt MT, Inklaar H, Gouttebarge V, et al.: Knee and ankle osteoarthritis in former elite soccer players: a systematic review of the recent literature, *J Sci Med Sport* 15:480–487, 2012.
96. Tveit M, Rosengren BE, Nilsson JA, et al.: Former male elite athletes have a higher prevalence of osteoarthritis and arthoplasty in the hip and knee than expected, *Am J Sports Med* 40:527–533, 2012.
97. Panush RS, Schmidt C, Caldwell J, et al.: Is running associated with degenerative joint disease? *JAMA* 255:1152–1154, 1986.
98. Chakravarty F, Hubert HB, Lingala V, et al.: Long distance running and knee osteoarthritis. A prospective study, *Am J Prev Med* 35:133–138, 2008.
99. Wang WE, Ramey DR, Schettler JD, et al.: Postponed development of disability in elderly runners: a 13-year longitudinal study, *Arch Intern Med* 162:2285–2294, 2002.
100. Fries JF, Singh G, Morfeld D, et al.: Running and the development of disability with age, *Ann Intern Med* 121:502–509, 1994.
101. Sohn RS, Micheli LJ: The effect of running on the pathogenesis of osteoarthritis of the hips and knees, *Clin Orthop Relat Res* 198:106–109, 1985.
102. Konradsen L, Hansen EM, Søndergaard L: Long distance running and osteoarthrosis, *Am J Sports Med* 18:379–381, 1990.
103. Kujala UM, Kapriio J, Samo S: Osteoarthritis of weight-bearing joints in former elite male athletes, *BMJ* 308:231–234, 1994.
104. Williams PT: Effects of running and walking on osteoarthritis and hip replacement risk, *Med Sci Sports Exerc* 45:1292–1297, 2013.
105. Cheng Y, Macera CA, Davis DR, et al.: Physical activity and self-reported, physician-diagnosed osteoarthritis: is physical activity a risk factor? *J Clin Epidemiol* 53:315–322, 2000.
106. Marti B, Knobloch M, Tschopp A, et al.: Is excessive running predictive of degenerative hip disease? Controlled study of former elite athletes, *BMJ* 299:91–93, 1989.
107. Marti B, Biedert R, Howald H: Risk of arthrosis of the upper ankle joint in long distance runners: controlled follow-up of former elite athletes, *Sportverletz Sportschaden* 4:175–179, 1990.
108. Vingard E, Sandmark H, Alfredsson L: Musculoskeletal disorders in former athletes. A cohort study in 114 track and field champions, *Acta Orthop Scand* 66:289–291, 1995.
109. Specter TD, Harris PA, Hart DJ, et al.: Risk of osteoarthritis associated with long-term weight-bearing sports, *Arthritis Rheum* 39:988–995, 1996.
110. Thelin N, Holmberg S, Thelin A: Knee injuries account for the sports-related increased risk of knee osteoarthritis, *Scand J Med Sci Sports* 16:329–333, 2006.
111. Miller RJ, Edwards WB, Brandon SCE, et al.: Why don't most runners get knee osteoarthritis. A case for per-unit-distance loads, *Med Sci Sports Exerc* 46:572–579, 2014.
112. Richmond SA, Fukuchi RK, Ezzat A, et al.: Are joint injury, sport activity, physical activity, obesity, or occupational activities predictors for osteoarthritis. A systematic review, *J Orthop Sports Phys Ther* 43:515–533, 2013.
113. Hubbard-Turner T, Guderian S, Turner MJ: Lifelong physical activity and knee osteoarthritis development in mice, *Int J Rheum Dis* 18:33–39, 2015.

114. Beckett J, Schultz M, Tolbert D, et al.: Excessive running induces cartilage degeneration in knee joints and alters gait of rats, *J Orthop Res* 30:1604–1610, 2012.
115. Siebelt M, Groen HC, Koelwijn SJ, et al.: Increased physical activity severely induces osteoarthritic changes in knee joints with papain induced sulfate-glycosaminoglycan depleted cartilage, *Arthritis Res Ther* 16:R32, 2014.
116. Shimonumura S, Inoue H, Nakagawa S, et al.: Treadmill running ameliorates destruction of articular cartilage and subchondral bone, not only synovitis, in a rheumatoid arthritis rat model, *Int J Mol Sci* 19(6), 2018. pii: E1653.
117. Panush RS, Hanson CS, Caldwell JR, et al.: Is running associated with osteoarthritis? An eight-year follow-up study, *J Clin Rheum* 1(35), 1995.
118. Hansen P, English M, Willick SE: Does running cause osteoarthritis in the hip or knee? *PM&R* 4:S117–S121, 2012.
119. Lo GH, Dribabn JB, Kriska AM, et al.: Is there an association between a history of running and symptomatic knee osteoarthritis? A cross-sectional study from the Osteoarthritis Initiative, *Arthritis Care Res* 69:183–191, 2017.
120. Roberts WO: Running causes knee osteoarthritis: myth or misunderstanding, *Br J Sports Med* 52:900142, 2018.

39

Cardiovascular Risk in Inflammatory Rheumatic Disease

CYNTHIA S. CROWSON, SHERINE E. GABRIEL, AND ANNE GRETE SEMB

KEY POINTS

Excess rates of cardiovascular disease (CVD) have been reported among patients with a variety of inflammatory rheumatic diseases.

CVD mortality and morbidity—in particular, ischemic heart disease and heart failure—are significantly higher among people with rheumatoid arthritis (RA) and/or systemic lupus erythematosus (SLE), and other autoimmune disorders, when compared with people in the general population of the same age who do not have these diseases.

Although the prevalence of some traditional CVD risk factors is elevated in people with inflammatory rheumatic diseases, these elevations alone do not adequately explain the excess CVD risk.

The systemic inflammation and immune dysfunction that characterize rheumatic diseases appear to be a major driver of the increased CVD risk in these patients.

The relationship between rheumatic drugs and CVD risk is difficult to disentangle because of confounding by indication/contraindication.

Introduction

For nearly half a century, excess rates of cardiovascular (CV) disease (CVD) have been reported among people with inflammatory rheumatic diseases.[1–3] More recently, the discovery of the inflammatory and immune mechanisms underlying atherosclerosis has spurred renewed interest in the association between CVD risk and the rheumatic diseases. In this chapter, we review biologic mechanisms underlying CVD comorbidity in the rheumatic diseases and discuss the risks of these diseases, especially in rheumatoid arthritis (RA) and systemic lupus erythematosus (SLE). We also discuss the contribution of traditional and nontraditional CVD risk factors (CVDRFs) to the observed excess CVD risk.

Biologic Mechanisms: Relationship Between Inflammation and Cardiovascular Disease

Over the past two decades there has been mounting evidence in support of the inflammatory hypothesis of atherothrombosis. Many cytokines have been implicated, such as IL-1, IL-6, and TNF. For example, the pro-inflammatory cytokine, IL-1β, plays multiple roles in the development of atherosclerotic plaques, such as the induction of pro-coagulant activity, the promotion of monocyte and leukocyte adhesion to vascular endothelial cells, and the growth of vascular smooth muscle cells.[4–6] Activation of IL-1β stimulates the downstream IL-6 receptor signaling pathway, which has also been implicated as a potential causal pathway for atherothrombosis (Fig. 39.1).[7,8] The Canakinumab Anti-Inflammatory Thrombosis Outcomes Study (CANTOS) recently provided clinical evidence for a role for inflammation in atherthrombosis.[9] In CANTOS, 10,061 patients with a previous myocardial infarction (MI) and a high-sensitivity C-reactive protein (CRP) (hsCRP) level of 2 mg/L or more were randomly assigned to one of three doses of Canakinumab (an IL-1 inhibitor) or to placebo. Results, after median follow-up of 3.7 years, showed that anti-inflammatory therapy that targeted IL-1β with Canakinumab significantly reduced hsCRP, and the 150 mg dose resulted in a significantly lower incidence of recurrent CV events when compared to placebo. Thus, despite an inconsistent dose response, CANTOS favors a causative role for inflammation in atherothrombosis.

Rheumatologic diseases have long been viewed as a "natural experiment" in the interplay between chronic inflammation and CVD. Thus, the study of CVD in rheumatology may elucidate the fundamental mechanisms by which inflammation accelerates the development of atherosclerosis and heart disease. RA is the most common and best studied of the autoimmune rheumatic diseases. The immune underpinnings of CVD and of RA share many similarities. Circulating acute-phase reactants, such as CRP, are elevated in people with RA and are risk markers for heart disease in the general population. Emerging evidence suggests that T lymphocytes play a crucial pathogenic role in both RA and CVD.[10,11] The major risk gene for RA, *HLA-DRB1*, predisposes the patient to disease by promoting the selection and survival of autoreactive $CD4^+$ T cells. *HLA-DRB1* alleles are also associated with increased risk of MI and various forms of non–RA-associated heart disease. T cells isolated from the joints of patients with RA have enhanced production of interferon (IFN)-γ and IL-17, which presumably mediate chronic inflammation.[12,13] The proven efficacy of antagonizing T cell co-stimulation is perhaps the most compelling evidence that T cells are pathogenic in RA.[14] Similarly, percutaneous

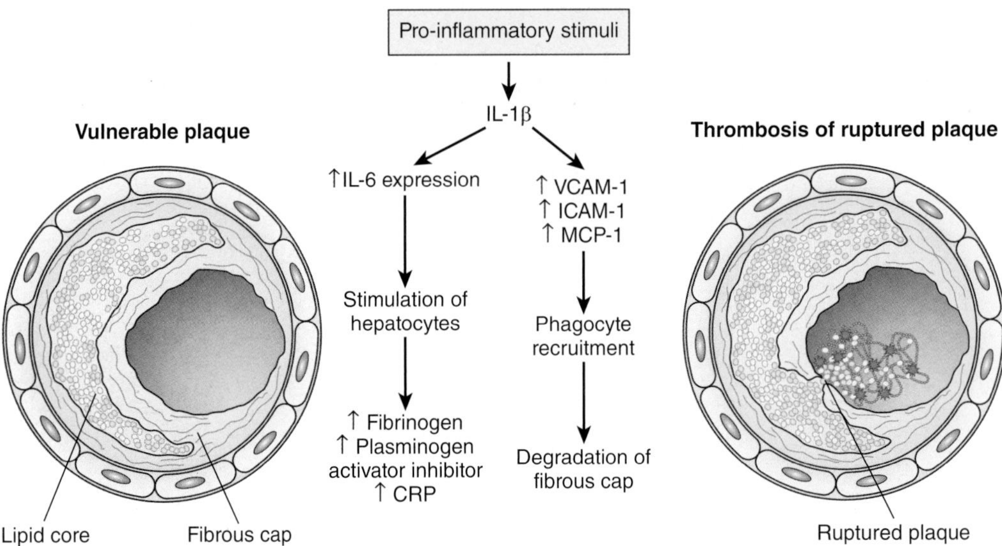

• **Fig. 39.1** Role of inflammation in plaque rupture: in atherosclerosis, inflammatory cells and accumulation of lipids can lead to the formation of lipid-rich core within the intima of arteries. As the lipid core expands, the intima thins, creating a vulnerable fibrous cap between the lipid core and lumen of the artery. Pro-inflammatory stimuli initiate a cascade of events, which activate IL-Iβ. IL-Iβ stimulates adhesion molecules, including intercellular adhesion molecule (ICAM)-1 and vascular cell adhesion molecule (VCAM)-1, and chemokines, such as monocyte chemoattractant protein (MCP)-1, which are involved in inflammatory cardiovascular disease (CVD). IL-Iβ also induces expression of IL-6, which stimulates hepatocytes to synthesize prothrombotic acute phase reactants, including fibrinogen, plasminogen activator inhibitor, and CRP. Phagocytes recruited by MCP-1 disrupt the atherosclerotic plaque by producing proteolytic enzymes, which degrade the collagen that support the plaque's protective fibrous cap, leaving it prone to rupture. When the plaque ruptures, blood comes in contact with prothrombotic factors and coagulates. Activation of the coagulation cascade, through contact with the intimal space, prompts thrombus formation. If the vessel is sufficiently and persistently occluded by the thrombus, vascular events, such as a myocardial infarction (MI) can result. (From Martinez BK, White CM. The Emerging Role of Inflammation in Cardiovascular Disease. *Annals Pharmacotherapy* 52(8):801-809, 2018.)

stents that elute T cell inhibiting drugs (e.g., sirolimus) prevent in-stent re-stenosis and repeat re-vascularization in people with coronary artery disease (CAD).[15]

In people with either RA or CVD, CD4+ T cells characteristically lose expression of the co-stimulatory molecule, CD28, which ordinarily provides the "second signal" required for T cell activation. So-called *CD28^null^* T cells are believed to have undergone reprogramming, leading to premature senescence.[16,17] Expansion of these senescent T cells among people with RA is associated with extra-articular inflammatory manifestations, including vasculitis, lung disease, as well as CAD.[16,17] In the setting of heart disease, $CD28^{null}$ T cells are identified in atherosclerotic plaque, where they are believed to contribute to the inflammatory process by producing cytokines and by killing vascular smooth muscle cells.[18] Interestingly, *HLA-DRB1*, the aforementioned RA-risk gene, also predisposes to expansion of $CD28^{null}$ T cells in RA and in CAD.[19]

Premature senescence of T cells in RA appears to be caused by fundamental defects in the hematopoietic system. $CD34^+$ hematopoietic progenitor cells have accelerated telomere erosion, a sign of senescence.[20] Naïve T cells in people with RA also are prematurely aged, with increased fragility and damage of their DNA because of insufficient activity of basic DNA repair enzymes.[21] Similarly, telomere shortening in hematopoietic progenitor cells correlates with myocardial dysfunction in people with CAD.[22] The onset of both RA and CVD coincides with the loss of thymic emigration of naïve T cells in the fifth decade, which suggests T cell senescence may contribute to the pathogenesis of both of these age-associated conditions. In the foreseeable future, rejuvenation of senescent T cells with use of new drugs, which restore genomic repair and integrity, has the potential to be an effective strategy for the prevention and treatment of CVD.[23]

Cardiovascular Morbidity and Mortality in Rheumatoid Arthritis and Systemic Lupus Erythematosus

Rheumatoid Arthritis

Ischemic Heart Disease in Rheumatoid Arthritis

Patients with RA are at increased risk of ischemic heart disease (IHD).[3,24–26] Data from the Rochester Epidemiology Project have shown that, in the 2-year period immediately preceding the fulfillment of the American College of Rheumatology (ACR) 1987 criteria, people with RA were more likely to experience hospitalization for MI (odds ratio [OR], 3.17; 95% confidence interval [CI], 1.16 to 8.68) and unrecognized ("silent") MI (OR, 5.86; 95% CI, 1.29 to 26.64) than age- and sex-matched control subjects. The increased risk of unrecognized MI persisted after the diagnosis of RA (hazard ratio [HR], 2.13; 95% CI, 1.13 to 4.03). One group[27] failed to demonstrate a statistically significant elevated increase in MI, angina, or heart failure (HF) prior to the onset of symptoms in two large Swedish cohorts, although trends toward such elevation were reported. As in studies of mortality, these results suggest that accelerated atherosclerosis begins at the onset of RA symptoms, or even earlier, and not at the time of diagnosis or later in the disease course. In a recent study of 11,782

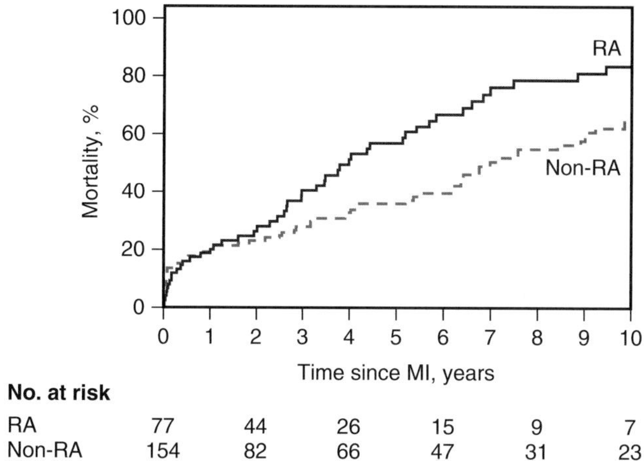

• **Fig. 39.2** Cumulative incidence of mortality after myocardial infarction (MI) among 77 patients with rheumatoid arthritis (RA) and 154 patients without RA (55 deaths in patients with RA; 85 deaths in patients without RA; log-rank *P* = 0.036). (From McCoy SS, Crowson CS, Maradit-Kremers H, et al: Longterm outcomes and treatment after myocardial infarction in patients with rheumatoid arthritis. *J Rheumatology* 40:605–610, 2013.)

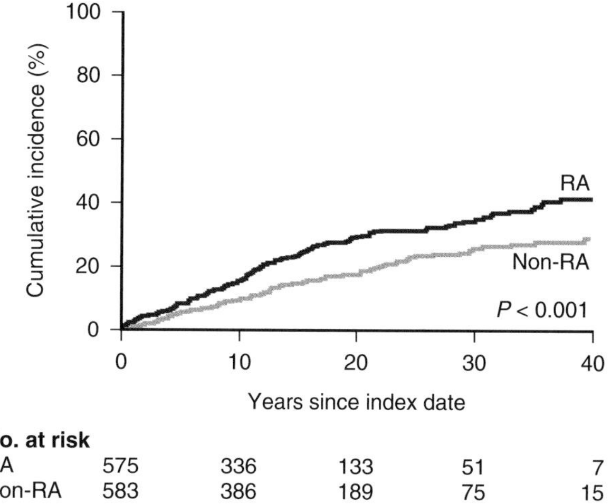

• **Fig. 39.3** Comparison of the cumulative incidence of congestive heart failure in the rheumatoid arthritis (RA) cohort and the non-RA cohort according to the number of years after the index date and adjusting for the competing risk of death. (From Nicola PJ, Maradit-Kremers H, Roger VL, et al: The risk of congestive heart failure in rheumatoid arthritis: a population-based study over 46 years. *Arthritis Rheum* 52:412–420, 2005. Permission to reprint from John Wiley & Sons.)

patients with RA and 57,973 age- and sex-matched general population controls, the risk for IHD was significantly higher among RA patients in comparison to controls, independent of traditional CV risk factors.[28]

Patterns of clinical care and outcome after MI may vary in people with RA when compared with the general population. Some evidence suggests that, although patients with RA receive MI care similar to care received by patients without RA, they experience higher rates of HF and death after sustaining an MI (Fig. 39.2).[26,29,30] However, other investigators have reported that patients with RA who experience acute MI receive acute reperfusion and secondary prevention medications (e.g., β-blockers and lipid-lowering agents) less frequently than do control subjects.[31] Among patients with MI, those with RA were more likely to undergo thrombolysis and percutaneous coronary intervention (PCI) but were less likely to receive medical therapy and/or coronary artery bypass grafting.[32] Patients with RA may have an in-hospital survival advantage, particularly those undergoing medical therapy and PCI, although potential confounding could not be ruled out.

Heart Failure in Rheumatoid Arthritis

People with RA are at increased risk of developing HF compared with the general population.[33,34] In the Rochester RA cohort, the cumulative incidence of HF (defined according to the Framingham criteria) at 30-year follow-up was 34%, compared with 25% in the non-RA cohort (Fig. 39.3).[34] Even after adjustment for demographics, CV risk factors, and IHD, patients with RA had almost twice the risk of developing HF as subjects without RA (HR, 1.87; 95% CI, 1.47 to 2.39). This increased risk of HF appeared to be predominant in the subgroup of patients with rheumatoid factor (RF) who were RF^+; the HR in RF^+ patients was 2.59 with a 95% CI of 1.95 to 3.43, whereas the HR in RF^- patients was 1.28 with a 95% CI of 0.93 to 1.78. These findings were confirmed in a recent large analysis of two contemporary cohorts of Swedish RA subjects that included 45,982 patients with established RA and 12,943 patients with new onset RA matched 1:10 to general population comparator subjects.[35] Patients with RA are at an increased risk for HF that cannot be explained by

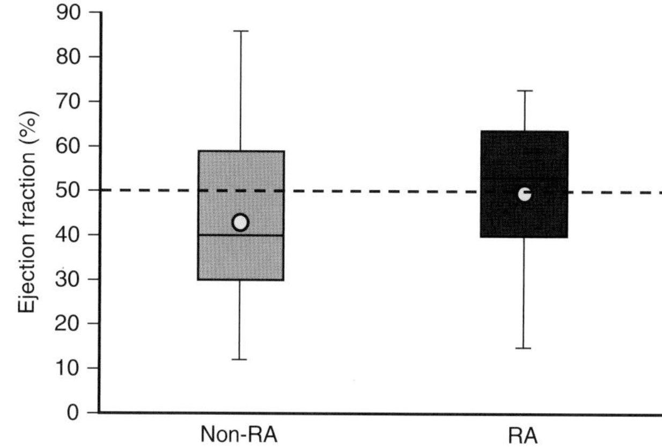

• **Fig. 39.4** Distribution of ejection fraction (EF) between patients with and without rheumatoid arthritis (RA) at the onset of heart failure. Data are presented as box plots, with the *boxes* representing the 25th to 75th percentiles, the *vertical lines* representing the 10th and 90th percentiles, the *circles* representing the means, the *lines within the boxes* representing the medians, and the *broken line* representing the 50% EF reference. (From Davis JM, Roger VL, Crowson CS, et al: The presentation and outcome of heart failure in patients with rheumatoid arthritis differs from that in general population. *Arthritis Rheum* 58:2603–2611, 2008. Permission to reprint from John Wiley & Sons.)

their increased risk of IHD; this increased risk occurred early and was associated with RA severity. Disease activity and health assessment have been associated with reduced left ventricular systolic myocardial function in RA patients.[36]

The clinical presentation of HF in patients with RA differs from that of HF in patients without RA.[37] Patients with RA who have HF are less likely to be obese or hypertensive or have clinical IHD. Moreover, patients with RA who have HF are less likely to have typical signs and symptoms. Importantly, the proportion of patients with HF who have preserved ejection fraction (HFpEF) (EF >50%) is significantly higher among patients who have RA compared with patients who do not have RA (Fig. 39.4).[37]

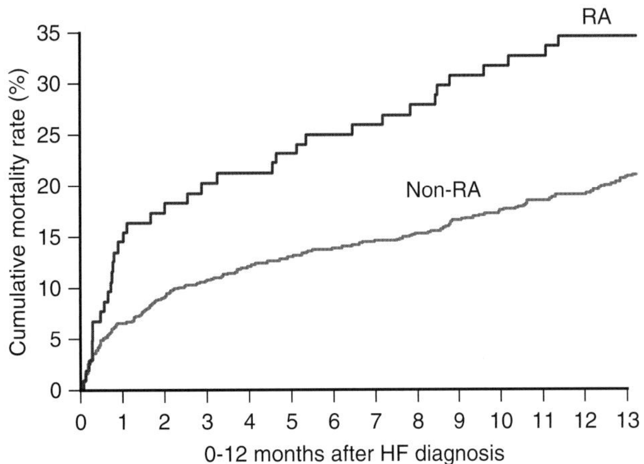

• **Fig. 39.5** Mortality through 1 year after the onset of heart failure (HF) in the rheumatoid arthritis (RA) and non-RA cohorts. (From Davis JM, Roger VL, Crowson CS, et al: The presentation and outcome of heart failure in patients with rheumatoid arthritis differs from that in general population. *Arthritis Rheum* 58:2603–2611, 2008. Permission to reprint from John Wiley & Sons.)

Patients with RA who have HF tend to undergo less aggressive investigation and be managed less aggressively than patients without RA.[37] Finally, patients with RA who have HF also appeared to have poorer outcomes (Fig. 39.5), experiencing approximately twice the risk for death in the period immediately after HF identification compared with patients who do not have RA.[38]

Cardiovascular Mortality in Rheumatoid Arthritis

Mortality of patients with established RA is higher than that of the general population. A meta-analysis of 24 mortality studies in people with RA, which were published between 1970 and 2005, reported a weighted combined all-cause standardized mortality ratio (met-SMR) of 1.50 (95% CI, 1.39 to 1.61) with similar increases for IHD (met-SMR, 1.59; 95% CI, 1.46 to 1.73) and stroke (met-SMR, 1.52; 95% CI, 1.40 to 1.67) and for men (met-SMR, 1.45) and women (met-SMR, 1.58).[39–41] Approximately 50% of all deaths in subjects with RA are attributable to CV causes, including IHD and stroke,[42] and CVD appears to occur earlier in people with RA. A large community-based prospective cohort study that used UK Biobank data confirmed higher rates of CVD-related mortality in multiple inflammatory conditions, including RA, which reported, once again, that these events can occur early in the disease course.[43] The latter observation is consistent with the recent hypothesis of accelerated aging in people with RA.[44] Moreover, people with RA frequently experience "silent" IHD and/or silent MI—that is, showing no symptoms at all before a sudden cardiac death. Sudden cardiac deaths are almost twice as common in patients with RA as in the general population (HR, 1.99; 95% CI, 1.06 to 3.55).[24]

The excess CVD mortality related to RA may be confined to, or at least be substantially higher in, subjects who are RF+.[45–47] The link may be even stronger with anti-citrullinated protein antibody (ACPA) positivity.[48] As might be expected, the relative risk (RR) of CVD mortality is highest in younger age groups (i.e., people younger than 55 years of age) and in women, whereas the attributable risk is highest in the oldest age groups and in men.[25,46,49]

Controversy persists regarding how soon after symptom onset the excess CVD mortality risk becomes apparent and/or whether there is a secular trend toward improving CVD mortality in people with RA (as is seen in the general population). This controversy may, in part, be explained by differences in the period of follow-up—that is, follow-up starting from the time of symptom onset, from a physician's diagnosis of RA, or from the date of fulfillment of ACR criteria or other diagnostic criteria. The latter may not occur until some years after the first symptoms appear. In the Norfolk Arthritis Register (NOAR), the excess CVD mortality is detectable beginning around 7 years after symptom onset.[45] In a Dutch inception cohort of 1049 patients with RA recruited between 1985 and 2007, excess mortality became apparent at around 10 years after diagnosis (with all subjects having <1 year symptom duration).[50] Emerging evidence indicates that mortality may be improving among people with RA, but CV mortality has also improved in the general population; thus, the relative increase in CV mortality has not changed over time.[51] A meta-analysis that included 17 studies (91,916 patients) also showed no trend toward improving CVD mortality with time.[52]

Systemic Lupus Erythematosus

Ischemic Heart Disease in Systemic Lupus Erythematosus

Accelerated atherosclerosis and an increased risk of CAD are well established in SLE.[53–58] The prevalence of atherosclerotic vascular events varies from 1.8% early in the course of the disease to more than 27% later in the course of SLE.[57] The majority of studies reported increased risk of MI ranging from twofold to greater than 10-fold in various SLE patient groups compared with the general population.[56,57,59] This increased RR of MI is particularly apparent in younger patients with SLE. The most striking example comes from the University of Pittsburgh lupus cohort, in which women with SLE aged 35 to 44 years were more than 50 times more likely to have an MI when compared with women without SLE in the Framingham Offspring study (RR, 52.43; 95% CI, 21.6 to 98.5).[57] Furthermore, the majority (67%) of women with SLE were younger than 55 years of age at the time of their first cardiac event. In addition, a more than twofold increased risk of hospitalizations for MI have been reported in young women with SLE between the ages of 18 and 44 years compared with people without SLE (OR, 2.27; 95% CI, 1.08 to 3.46).[60,61] As in RA, it appears that the increased risk of CVD among people with SLE may begin before the diagnosis of SLE (OR, 3.7; 95% CI, 1.8 to 7.9); a recent report in a population-based study of 70 patients who had SLE compared with 2565 patients who did not have SLE supported similar findings.[62] A recent study showed promising results for CV magnetic resonance (CMR) as a tool to detect subclinical cardiac involvement in SLE.[63] The risk of CVD and mortality also increased 10-fold among women with SLE who had successful deliveries, despite the rarity of CVD among women of reproductive age.[64]

In a recent study of patients undergoing coronary revascularization procedures, no significant differences were found in the mean percentage of coronary stenosis and total occlusion in subjects with and without SLE.[65] Except for the increased likelihood of lesions confined to the left anterior descending artery in subjects with SLE versus subjects without SLE (42% versus 19%; $P = 0.003$), the pattern of coronary involvement, including artery dominance and prevalence of multivessel disease, appeared similar in subjects with SLE versus subjects without SLE. However, the study reported significantly worse CV outcomes at 1 year after PCI in subjects with SLE versus subjects without SLE, including higher risk of MI (16% versus 5%; $P = 0.01$)

and repeat PCI (31% versus 12%; $P = 0.009$) in people with SLE, even after adjustment for important covariates.[60,65] Given the increased vulnerability of atherosclerotic plaque in people with SLE, which is associated with the risk of occlusive events irrespective of the size of the plaque, these findings suggest an increased risk of unfavorable CV events in people who had SLE compared with people who did not have SLE with a seemingly similar pattern of coronary involvement.[66]

A large population-based study from 1996 to 2000 of patients hospitalized in California with acute MI showed that in-hospital mortality and length of stay were essentially similar in patients who had SLE compared with patients who did not have SLE; the study adjusted for age, race, ethnicity, type of medical insurance, and Charlson Index.[61] In contrast, data from the 1993-2002 U.S. Nationwide Inpatient Sample showed significantly increased rates of in-hospital mortality (RR, 1.46; 95% CI, 1.31 to 1.61) and prolonged hospitalization (RR, 1.68; 95% CI, 1.43 to 2.04) for acute MI in people who had SLE compared with control subjects; this study adjusted for age, sex, race/ethnicity, income, and HF.[60] Differences in methodology (e.g., a smaller sample size, older age of patients and controls in the earlier study, potential ascertainment bias, and a shorter observation period in the later study) may partially explain these contrasting results.[67] Considering the presence of myocardial involvement, chronic systemic inflammation, vasculitis, and hyperviscosity syndrome in SLE, worse outcomes after acute coronary events and associated interventions can reasonably be expected.[67] Further study is required.

Heart Failure in Systemic Lupus Erythematosus

The risk of HF and related hospitalization in people with SLE appears to be substantially increased.[60,61] In particular, young women with SLE between the ages of 18 and 44 years have more than a 2.5-fold increased risk of hospitalization for HF compared with people who do not have SLE, even after adjustment for age, race, insurance status, hospital characteristics, and the presence of hypertension (HT), diabetes mellitus (DM), and chronic renal failure.[69] The nature of HF in SLE is likely multifactorial and only partly attributable to atherosclerosis.[70,71] The presentation of HF in people with SLE may vary from severe overt HF to insidious myocardial involvement.[70–74] Finally, mortality in patients with SLE who have HF is significantly higher than in patients without HF (18% versus 6%, $P < 0.001$) and approximates 3.5-fold compared with patients who have HF in the general population.[60,70]

Cardiovascular Mortality in Systemic Lupus Erythematosus

Mortality in SLE appears to follow a bimodal pattern, with an early peak in mortality (within 1 year of diagnosis) and a later peak occurring more than 5 years after diagnosis. Reported survival in the first 5 years of SLE has improved considerably from about 50% in the 1950s to greater than 90% in the 1990s.[75] However, this improvement may be due, at least in part, to earlier diagnosis and improved ascertainment of mild cases. In the Toronto lupus cohort of 1241 patients recruited between 1970 and 2005, the SMR improved from 13.84 (95% CI, 9.78 to 19.76) during 1970-1978 for those who entered the cohort in that decade to 3.81 (95% CI, 1.98 to 7.32) during 1997-2005 in people who entered the cohort in that period.[76] The SMR during 1997-2005 was very similar for patients regardless of their disease duration; it ranged from 3.23 for those who had entered the cohort in 1970-1978 to 3.93 for those who had entered the cohort in 1988-1996. Similarly, evidence from Olmsted County showed an SMR of 2.70 with significant improvement in survival in recent decades.[77] In a study of 434 female patients with SLE from Seoul, Korea, who were followed up from 1992 to 2002, the SMR was 3.02 (95% CI, 1.45 to 5.55).[78] A recent population-based cohort study of 70 patients with incident SLE in 1991-2008 reported nearly twofold increased mortality and increased CVD rates. In addition, increased mortality and CVD event rates were found perioperatively in women with SLE who were undergoing surgical procedures, even for low-risk procedures (OR, 1.54; 95% CI, 1.00 to 2.37).[79] A community-based prospective cohort study from UK showed increased CV-related mortality in SLE and emphasized the public health value of early screening and effective preventive strategies.[43]

Risk Factors for Cardiovascular Disease

Evidence for the pivotal role of inflammation in driving increased CVD risk in people with RA is compelling. Yet, despite improved control of inflammation, CVD risk among people with RA remains elevated. Moreover, the identification of clinically valuable biomarkers of CVD risk in people with RA remains elusive.[80] In the next sections, we highlight recent evidence and discussions regarding the relative contribution of traditional and nontraditional risk factors (e.g., markers of inflammation and RA features) toward the excess CVD risk in people with RA and suggest directions for future research.[81]

Traditional Cardiovascular Risk Factors in Rheumatoid Arthritis: Occurrence and Impact

In the general population, five major CVDRFs (i.e., HT, elevated total cholesterol (TC) levels, smoking, obesity, and DM) account for 80% of the risk for MI[82] and half of the CV mortality.[83] Moreover, a recent meta-analysis found that these five major CVDRFs also increased the risk of CVD in patients with RA.[84] One possible explanation for the increase in CVD in people with RA could be that the traditional CVDRFs are more common in people with RA or that they are as common but more deleterious. The five CVDRFs (i.e., HT, elevated TC, smoking, obesity, and DM) were comparable across patients with RA, ankylosing spondylitis (AS), and psoriatic arthritis (PsA), except for more HT and obesity in the older age categories.[85] In addition, the excess CVD risk may also be explained by the adverse impact of the inflammatory and immune changes of RA on the vessel wall. It is most likely, however, that traditional risk factors and inflammation are intimately interconnected and perhaps act synergistically (Fig. 39.6).[86] Indeed, one study showed that progression of a new CVD event in subjects with early RA may be predicted by traditional CVDRFs but precipitated by high disease activity.[87]

Smoking in People With Rheumatoid Arthritis

The link between tobacco smoking and CVD events is well known and is identified both in the general population as well as in patients with RA.[84,88] Smoking is a known risk factor for the development of RA, in particular RF^+ and $ACPA^+$ RA.[89] In a meta-analysis of four case-control studies of traditional CVDRFs in RA that included 1415 patients with RA, the prevalence of smoking was found to be significantly higher than in control subjects (OR, 1.56; 95% CI, 1.35 to 1.80).[90] A known interaction

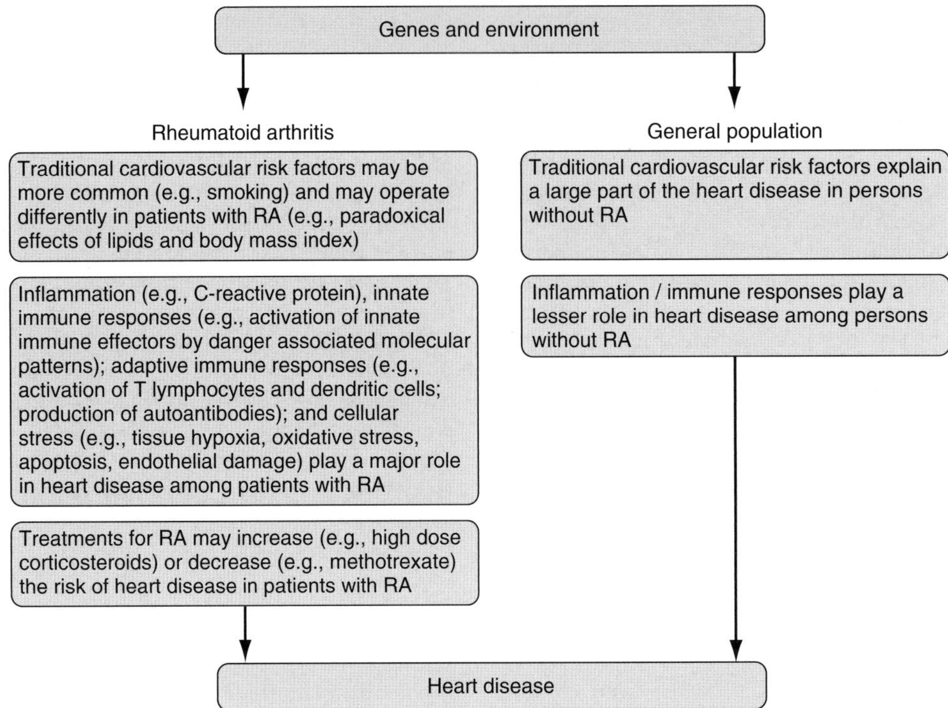

• **Fig. 39.6** Why do patients with rheumatoid arthritis (RA) develop heart disease? Determinants of heart disease in patients with RA differ from the general population. (From Crowson CS, Liao KP, Davis JM, et al: Rheumatoid arthritis and cardiovascular disease. *Am Heart J* 166:622–628, 2013. Permission to reprint from Elsevier.)

exists between smoking, *HLA-DR1* shared epitope (SE) alleles, and the production of ACPA[91] and between smoking, ACPA, and the SE in premature CVD mortality in RA.[92]

Hypertension in Rheumatoid Arthritis

HT is common in people with RA, but it remains unclear whether it is more common than in the general population. Whereas some studies have found HT to be an important risk factor for CVD in people with RA,[93] a recent meta-analysis of seven case-control studies (1053 patients with RA) found the prevalence of HT to be the same in people with RA as in control subjects (OR, 1.09; 95% CI, 0.91 to 1.31).[90] However, evidence exists for underdiagnosis and undertreatment of HT in people with RA.[94] Multiple other factors may influence blood pressure control in people with RA, including physical inactivity, obesity, specific genetic polymorphisms, smoking, and some anti-rheumatic medications, including nonsteroidal anti-inflammatory drugs (NSAIDs), corticosteroids, leflunomide, and cyclosporine.

Lipids in People With Rheumatoid Arthritis

There is a complex relationship between low-density lipoprotein cholesterol (LDL-C), high-density lipoprotein cholesterol (HDL-C), and risk of CVD, and this is nonlinear in RA-patients and not different from non-RA people[95] (Fig. 39.7A). RA patients have lower lipid levels related to disease activity/inflammation (Fig. 39.7B).[96] Effective treatment has an "adverse" effect on lipids manifest as level increases[97] (Fig. 39.7C). Knowing that high cholesterol level is a major risk factor for future CVD and has a high weight in CVD risk calculators, this may make it difficult to predict the risk for future CVD in RA patients.[98] Serum levels of TC and LDL-C decline during the 3- to 5-year period prior to RA incidence,[99] and lower total and LDL-C levels are associated with higher CVD risk.[98] Suppression of total and LDL-C levels during acute or chronic high-grade inflammation is well described, as is a proportionately greater suppression of HDL-C, which resulted in a disadvantageous TC: HDL-C ratio.[100] This phenomenon may explain why hyperlipidemia (i.e., high TC or LDL-C) appears to be less common in people who have RA compared with subjects who do not.[96,101,102] Indeed, even among patients who sustained a previous MI, those with RA had significantly lower levels of total and LDL-C than did those without.[103] Dyslipidemia (i.e., alterations of individual lipid components and their ratios as defined by specific criteria) may affect up to half of all people with RA.[104] A recent meta-analysis showed that RA is associated with an abnormal lipid pattern, principally low levels of HDL-C.[105] *In vitro*, animal model and *in vivo* human studies clearly demonstrate that the interplay between inflammation and lipid components is far more complex than simple alterations of their serum levels (Fig. 39.8).[106]

Inflammation-induced alterations of the structure and function of lipid molecules require further study, specifically in people with RA and in the context of disease control through nonbiologic and biologic disease-modifying anti-rheumatic drugs (DMARDs).[107] Several studies suggest anti-rheumatic therapy effects on lipid levels, including glucocorticoids, hydroxychloroquine, gold, and cyclosporine, as well as the biologics, which include TNF inhibitors, rituximab, and tocilizumab.[108] However, these studies are of short duration, and more research is needed. Multiple other factors are involved in lipid regulation and function, including physical activity, adiposity, diet, alcohol intake, and smoking. However, their effects have not been assessed in sufficient detail in people with RA. Similarly, the importance of genetic regulation of lipid metabolism, particularly in the context of gene-environment interactions, has not been addressed in the RA population. This factor may be particularly important because lipid alterations appear to pre-date the diagnosis of RA.[109] Although the relationships between lipids and CVD in RA are complex, the value of primary lipid screening in people with RA is undisputed. Unfortunately, evidence suggests an unacceptable low rate of primary lipid screening and of statin use in people with RA.[104,110–112]

Diabetes Mellitus and Metabolic Syndrome in Rheumatoid Arthritis

The prevalence of DM has increased in patients with RA in comparison with control subjects.[90] Likewise, patients with RA were significantly more likely to have metabolic syndrome than were subjects who did not have RA.[113,114] Abdominal obesity, antihypertensive medication, disease activity, and use of corticosteroids all affect glucose metabolism in RA.[115] On the other hand, use of hydroxychloroquine reduces the risk of developing DM in people with RA by approximately 77%.[116] Epidemiologic studies on RA and non-RA subjects indicate that RA patients and diabetics have twice the risk of CVD compared to non-diabetic, non-RA individuals, and that DM accounts for 3% to 10% of CVD events.[117–119]

Body Composition/Obesity in Rheumatoid Arthritis

High body mass index (BMI) signifies excess weight and is a surrogate marker for elevated adipose tissue. BMI ≥25 kg/m^2 and ≥30 kg/m^2 is the standard definition for overweight and obesity, respectively. Globally, the World Health Organization (WHO) estimates that 650 million of the adult populations in 2016 were obese (13% of the worldwide population).[120] Interestingly, there are profound differences across regions, as prevalence of obesity varies from 5% in South East Asian populations to 29% in USA.[121] Inflammatory joint disease patients may be at increased risk of unwanted weight gain due to physical inactivity and prolonged used of corticosteroids.[122]

One study[123] reported a "paradoxical effect of BMI on survival in people with RA," demonstrating that as BMI declined, so did survival probability among study subjects with RA. Among people without RA, low BMI is not associated with increased risk of CV death. However, among patients with RA, low BMI,

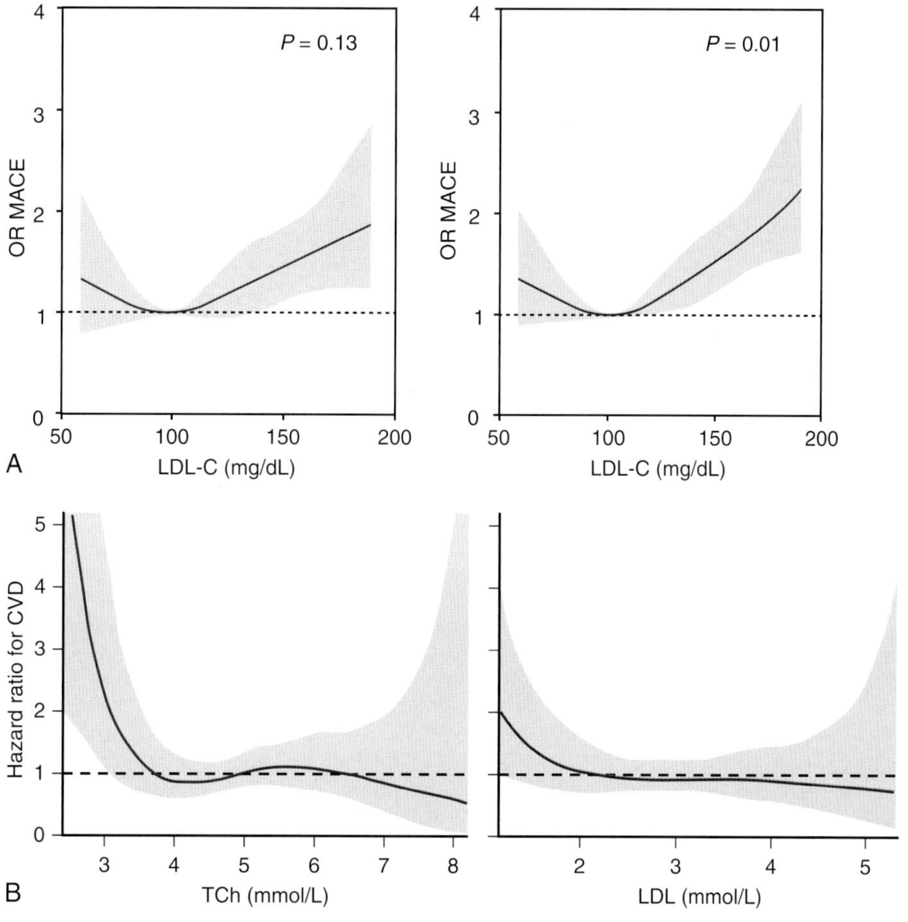

• **Fig. 39.7** (A) The complex relationship between LDL-C, HDL-C, and risk of CVD was non-linear in RA patients and not different from non-RA subjects. P-values indicate the significance of association in tests for linearity in the RA and no-RA cohorts. (From Liao K, et al. Association Between Lipid Levels and Major Adverse Cardiovascular Events in Rheumatoid Arthritis Compared to Non–Rheumatoid Arthritis Patients. *Arthritis Rheumatol* 2015;67:2004-10.) (B) Hazard ratios for cardiovascular disease (CVD) in rheumatoid arthritis (RA; *solid lines*) according to total cholesterol (TCh; *left panel*) and low density lipoprotein cholesterol (LDL-C) *(right panel)*. Shaded areas represent 95% confidence intervals. (From Myasoedova E, Crowson CS, Maradit-Kremers H, et al: Lipid paradox in rheumatoid arthritis: the impact of serum lipid measures and systemic inflammation on the risk of cardiovascular disease. *Ann Rheumatic Dis* 70:482–487, 2011. Permission to reprint from BMJ Publishing Group LTD.)

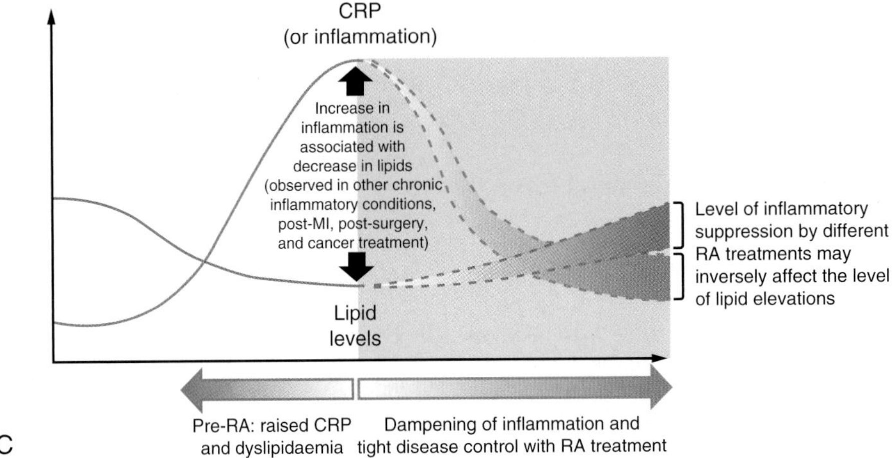

• **Fig. 39.7 cont'd** (C) Representation of the inverse relationship between changes in inflammatory and lipid parameters The paradigm by which an increase in the inflammatory burden in RA is associated with the lowering of lipid levels has also been noted in other chronic inflammatory conditions, after MI, after surgery, and in cancer treatment. In RA, a reduction of inflammation through treatment with traditional and/or biologic DMARDs is reflected in elevations in lipid levels. Data, although limited, suggest the extent to which lipid levels change may be different between RA therapies; however, further studies are required to fully ascertain the relationship between suppression of inflammation, lipid elevations, and future cardiovascular (CV) risk. *CRP,* C-reactive protein; *MI,* myocardial infarction. (From Choy E, Ganeshalingam K, Semb AG, et al: Cardiovascular risk in rheumatoid arthritis: recent advances in the understanding of the pivotal role of inflammation, risk predictors and the impact of treatment. *Rheumatology (Oxford)* Dec;53(12):2143-54, 2014.)

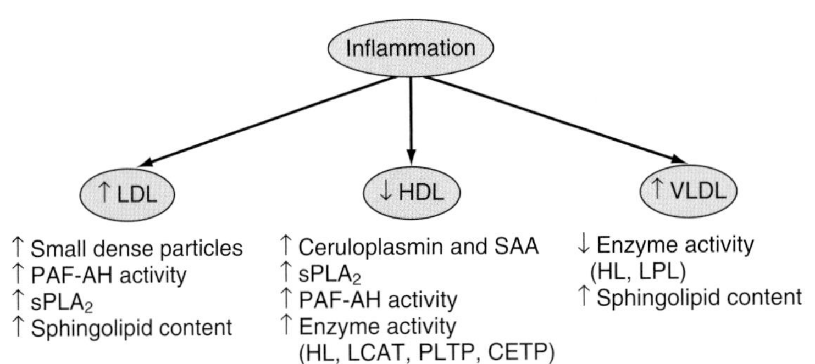

• **Fig. 39.8** The effects of inflammation on lipid and function. *CETP,* Cholesterol ester transfer protein; *HDL,* high-density lipoprotein; *HL,* hepatic lipase; *LCAT,* lecithin cholesterol acyltransferase; *LDL,* low-density lipoprotein; *LPL,* lipoprotein lipase; *PAF-AH,* platelet-activating factor acetylhydrolase; *PLTP,* phospholipid transfer protein; *SAA,* serum amyloid A; *$sPLA_2$,* secretory phospholipase A; *VLDL,* very low density lipoprotein. (From Toms TE, Symmons DP, Kitas GD: Dyslipidaemia in rheumatoid arthritis: the role of inflammation, drugs lifestyle and genetic factors. *Curr Vasc Pharmacol* 8:301–326, 2010. Reproduced with permission of BENTHAM SCIENCE PUBLISHERS LTD. in the format Book via Copyright Clearance Center.)

which may indicate uncontrolled active systemic inflammation, is associated with a threefold increased risk of CV death[124] even after adjustment for cardiac history, smoking, DM, HT, and malignancy.

Obesity is associated with the development of RA.[125,126] Obesity is also associated with an increased frequency of traditional CV risk factors in patients with RA.[127] In particular, abdominal fat is associated with insulin resistance and inflammatory load in patients with RA, and new evidence indicates that in such patients, abdominal fat is distributed differently between the visceral and subcutaneous compartments, with visceral fat more strongly associated with cardiometabolic risk.[128,129] Adipose tissue is metabolically active and, through a network of adipocytokines, regulates not only energy intake and expenditure but also inflammation.

Regardless, attentive management of obesity in inflammatory rheumatic diseases is warranted because obesity increases the risk of developing other CVDRFs (e.g., HT, DM, and hypercholesterolemia)[130–132] and because it induces a pro-inflammatory state characterized by impaired anti-inflammatory treatment response.[133,134] Interventions to reverse cachexia and to control obesity in people with RA have been inadequately studied.

Nontraditional Cardiovascular Risk Factors in Rheumatoid Arthritis: Occurrence and Impact

Rheological characteristics, such as whole blood viscosity, plasma viscosity, erythrocyte deformability, aggregation, and erythrocyte nitric oxide (NO) production, have been increasingly linked to CVD risk in the general population[135–137]; one study reports similar

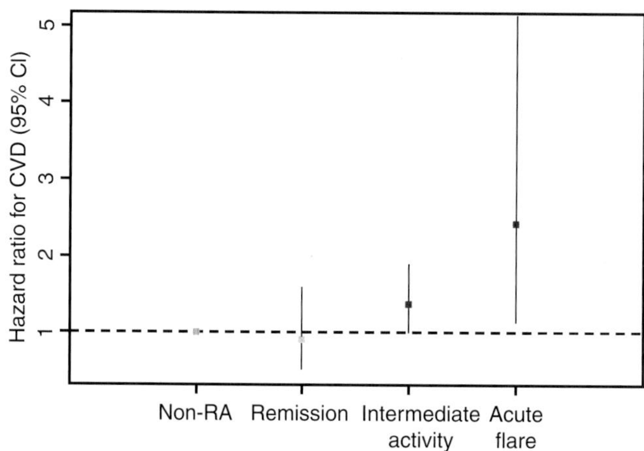

• **Fig. 39.9** Cardiovascular disease (CVD) risk depending on the level of rheumatoid arthritis (RA) disease activity in patients with RA as compared with the non-RA subjects adjusted for age, sex, calendar year, and cardiovascular (CV) risk factors. (From Myasoedova E, Chandran A, Ilhan B, et al: The role of rheumatoid arthritis [RA] flare and cumulative burden of RA severity in the risk of cardiovascular disease. *Ann Rheum Dis* 75:560-565, 2016.)

findings in patients with RA.[138] Likewise, cytokines, such as IL-17, IL-6, and TNF,[139,140] as well as wider cytokine/chemokine profiles, may play a role.[141] Hyperuricemia and vitamin D deficiency may also be independent risk factors for CVD in patients with RA, but it is unclear whether uric acid lowering therapies or vitamin D supplementation reduce the CVD risk.[142,143] Hyperhomocysteinemia is twice as common in patients with RA as in the general population and can increase CVD risk in RA.[144] Folic acid supplementation prevents increases in homocysteine levels, but it has not prevented CVD in the general population or in patients with RA.[145] Chronic kidney disease and osteoporotic fractures were also associated with increased CVD risk among patients with RA.[146,147]

The Impact of Rheumatoid Arthritis Disease Activity and Severity on Cardiovascular Co-morbidity

A number of studies have linked CVD risk with markers of RA disease activity, such as CRP and erythrocyte sedimentation rate (ESR).[24,148] In a study of 231 male veterans with RA, a baseline disease activity score (DAS28) greater than or equal to 5.1 predicted CV events (HR, 1.3; 95% CI, 1.1 to 1.6).[149] Markers of disease severity, such as RF, ACPA, physical disability, destructive changes on joint radiographs, rheumatoid nodules, vasculitis, and rheumatoid lung disease, are statistically significant and associated with increased risk of CV events and/or death even after adjustment for traditional CV risk factors.[48,150–154] RA flares have been associated with an increased risk of CVD, whereas patients in remission were found to have CVD risks similar to subjects without RA (Fig. 39.9).[150] A large international cohort of patients with RA demonstrated that 30% of CVD events were attributable to RA characteristics.[151] Thus, RA characteristics should play an important role in efforts to reduce CVD risk in RA.

Medications and Cardiovascular Risk

Medications used for the treatment of rheumatic diseases may also affect CVD risk. Because of the common use of NSAIDs, and concerns surrounding CVD risk with their use, this subject has been extensively studied. Although some evidence indicates that NSAID use is not associated with increased CVD risk in people with RA,[155] a meta-analysis of 31 trials in 116,429 patients concluded that there was little evidence to suggest that any of the investigated drugs (i.e., naproxen, ibuprofen, diclofenac, celecoxib, etoricoxib, rofecoxib, or lumiracoxib) were not safe in relation to CVD.[156] In contrast, use of DMARDs (methotrexate and hydroxychloroquine in particular) and/or biologic agents may decrease CVD risk[157–162] This outcome likely reflects effective long-term control of systemic inflammation. Although these findings are intriguing, they cannot be considered definitive evidence that these agents reduce CVD risk because of confounding by indication and/or contra-indication. Reports of the effect of corticosteroids on CVD risk are conflicting, but low doses (<7.5 mg/day) may be beneficial and high doses may be detrimental.[163–165] Statins have established effectiveness in the primary prevention of CV events in the general population and at-risk subpopulations (e.g., patients with DM). These agents have both lipid modifying and anti-inflammatory effects.[166] The Justification for the Use of Statins in Primary Prevention: an Intervention Trial Evaluating Rosuvastatin (JUPITER) demonstrated improved CVD outcomes in patients with elevated CRP and normal lipids.[167]

Traditional and Nontraditional Cardiovascular Risk Factors in Systemic Lupus Erythematosus

Patients with SLE have an increased prevalence of several traditional CVDRFs, including sedentary lifestyle, elevated very LDL-C and triglycerides, smoking, premature menopause, chronic renal impairment, HT, hyper-homocystinemia, metabolic syndrome, and insulin resistance.[168–173] Nonetheless, traditional CV risk factors cannot alone explain the observed excess risk of premature and accelerated CVD in patients with SLE. Nontraditional risk factors are also major contributors to this excess risk. The most reproducible, nontraditional CVDRFs in patients with SLE include disease activity, disease duration, and corticosteroid use. The genetics of CVD in patients with SLE have not been clearly elucidated, but predictor single nucleotide polymorphisms that also confer risk of thrombosis in the general population may play a role.[174] Several biomarkers have been associated with CVD risk in SLE, including antiphospholipid (aPL) antibodies, autoantibodies directed against apolipoprotein A, HDL-C, heat shock protein,[175–178] as well as pro-inflammatory HDL-C and high-sensitivity CRP. IFNs have received attention as mediators of disease pathogenesis and even as treatment targets in SLE. It is now increasingly recognized that by promoting endothelial injury and failed repair during SLE disease flares, IFNs may also have a profound impact on CVD risk.[179,180] SLE therapeutics likely have mixed effects on CVD risk. Although it is well known that long-term corticosteroid use increases CVD risk in patients with SLE, it is also clear that aggressive immunosuppressive and anti-inflammatory therapy correlates with reduced CVD burden.[58] Among all SLE therapeutics, the strongest evidence for a vasculo-protective effect exists with antimalarial agents.[181] These agents are associated with reduced vascular stiffness, decreased carotid plaque, and lower cholesterol levels. They also have a protective effect on thrombovascular events.[182,183] Although some evidence suggests that mycophenolate mofetil may also protect against CVD in patients with SLE, these findings are less consistent than those reported with antimalarial drugs.[184] Despite this large and growing body of evidence regarding risk factors for CVD in patients with SLE, no randomized controlled trials (RCTs) have been performed to test preventive CVD strategies in this patient population. Thus, management of risk factors must be individualized for each patient who has SLE, with prompt treatment of modifiable traditional risk factors (including use of statins, where indicated), careful monitoring of SLE therapeutics, and aggressive treatment of the underlying disease process.

Cardiovascular Mortality, Morbidity, and Risk Factors in Other Rheumatic Diseases

Ankylosing Spondylitis

Although the risk of CVD in people with AS has not been as well defined as in people with RA, mortality was increased for male and female patients with AS, and predictors of death within the AS cohort included socioeconomic status, general comorbidities, and hip replacement surgery.[185–187] Moreover, patients with AS are at a 30% to 50% increased risk of incident CV events. When compared to patients with RA, this level of increase was similar for stroke, but only half as high for acute coronary syndromes (ACS) and thrombotic events.[188] Both recording of CVDRFs and CVD prevention is low in patients with AS.[189]

Psoriasis and Psoriatic Arthritis

Both psoriasis and PsA are associated with an increased risk of CVD relative to the general population. The prevalence of traditional CV risk factors has been demonstrated to be higher among patients with psoriasis, but even after adjusting for these variables, the risk of IHD remains high (OR, 1.78; 95% CI, 1.51 to 2.11); recent studies suggest that psoriasis may be an independent risk factor for MI.[190–192] People with PsA are more likely to have evidence of pre-clinical atherosclerosis and are at increased risk of CVD relative to the general population.[193–196] Among 648 patients with PsA enrolled in the University of Toronto database, the risk of MI (standardized prevalence ratio 2.57; 95% CI, 1.73 to 3.80) and angina (standardized prevalence ratio 1.97; 95% CI, 1.24 to 3.12) was significantly higher than that of the general population, with increased risk seen in patients with more severe psoriasis.[197]

Patients with AS, PsA, and spondyloarthropathy (SpA) are at increased risk for acute coronary syndrome and stroke events, which emphasizes the importance of identification of and intervention against CV risk factors in SpA patients.[198] Increased awareness for cardiac arrhythmia is warranted in patients with SpA.

Giant Cell Arteritis, Takayasu's Arteritis and Polymyalgia Rheumatica

Whether the risk of CVD is increased among patients with giant cell arteritis is less clear. Two population-based studies reported twofold to threefold increased risk, and two other population-based studies reported no increased risk.[199–202] The risk of CVD among patients with Takayasu's arteritis has not been well studied. CV risk factors are more common, and CV event rates appear to be elevated in patients with Takayasu's arteritis.[203] A few studies have reported increased risks for CVD in patients with polymyalgia rheumatica, which are similar to the risk levels reported in other inflammatory diseases.[204,205] However, two recent systematic reviews found high heterogeneity between studies, suggesting that more research is needed to definitively determine whether the risk of CVD is increased among patients with polymyalgia rheumatica.[206,207]

Antineutrophil Cytoplasmic Antibodies (ANCA)-Associated Vasculitis

ANCA-associated vasculitis is a heterogenous group of diseases including granulomatosis with polyangiitis (GPA, formerly Wegener's granulomatosis), microscopic polyangiitis (MPA), and eosinophilic granulomatosis with polyangiitis (EGPA, formerly Churg-Strauss syndrome). A population-based study demonstrated a threefold increased risk of CVD and an eightfold increased risk of cerebrovascular events in patients with ANCA-associated vasculitis without increased prevalence of CV risk factors compared to the general population.[208] Other studies have also reported increased risks for CVD in patients with ANCA-associated vasculitis.[209–211]

Dermatomyositis and Polymyositis

Because large epidemiologic studies of CVD risk in patients with myositis are lacking, the frequency of CVD in patients with myositis is not clear, but cardiac involvement is well recognized as a clinically important manifestation of myositis.[212] A recent report that utilized the Nationwide Inpatient Sample found that one-fifth of dermatomyositis hospitalizations in the United States were associated with an atherosclerotic CV diagnosis or procedure; the report also found that patients with dermatomyositis and CVD have twice the risk of in-hospital death compared with control subjects and patients who have dermatomyositis without CVD.[213] Two Canadian studies found increased rates of MI among patients with dermatomyositis and polymyositis compared with the general population of Canada.[214,215]

Osteoarthritis

Although osteoarthritis is the most common rheumatic disease, very little is known about the link between osteoarthritis and CVD. Osteoarthritis may be associated with an increased risk of CVD because of its associated synovial inflammation and muscle weakness or because it leads to less physical activity and to NSAID use, which are all associated with increased risk of CVD.[216] Although one study[216] found modestly increased risks of IHD (RR, 1.30; 95% CI, 1.19 to 1.42) and HF (RR, 1.15; 95% CI, 1.04 to 1.28) in patients with osteoarthritis, another study found no evidence of increased risks for CVD and reported that disability rather than osteoarthritis was responsible for increased CVD risk in patients with osteoarthritis.[217] One group[218] found that patients with more severe osteoarthritis were at higher risk for CV events than those with milder disease.

Pediatric-Onset Rheumatologic Diseases

CVD has been difficult to study in patients with pediatric-onset rheumatologic disease, such as juvenile idiopathic arthritis, pediatric-onset SLE, and juvenile dermatomyositis, this is because CV events are rare at young ages.[219] Surrogate measures of CVD, such as flow-mediated dilatation, carotid intima media thickness, and pulse wave velocity, have recently been used to explore CVD in children with pediatric-onset rheumatologic diseases. Studies of these measures of subclinical CVD and of lipids have shown increased levels among children with juvenile idiopathic arthritis, pediatric-onset SLE, and juvenile dermatomyositis.[220–224] It is likely that these patients will experience significant CVD morbidity and mortality in adulthood, despite the fact that one study of juvenile idiopathic arthritis, which had an average of 29 years of follow-up, did not demonstrate a significantly increased risk for CV events.[225] More studies are needed to better define the increased risk of CVD among patients with pediatric-onset rheumatologic diseases, to design and test preventive strategies to circumvent this eventuality, and to improve the long-term outcomes of these patients. Although data on the increased risk of CVD among patients with less widely studied inflammatory rheumatic diseases are still emerging, CVD has been recognized as an important contribution to increased mortality and morbidity in this patient population and represents an area of ongoing research.[226]

Managing Cardiovascular Risk in Rheumatic Disease

Coordinating Care: Cardiology and Rheumatology

Despite the large and growing body of knowledge showing increased risk of CVD in people with RA and other rheumatic diseases, even when controlling for traditional CV risk factors,[56,227] little translation into clinical care has occurred. Inflammation and immune mechanisms underlie the atherosclerotic process.[228] Because traditional risk factors alone do not explain the elevated CVD risk in patients with rheumatic diseases, addressing control of inflammation is essential to decrease the CVD risk.[97]

Thus, close collaboration between the rheumatologist and the cardiologist is vital.[229–231] Not only does the rheumatologic condition need to be treated aggressively to decrease the inflammatory burden but the traditional CV risk factors must also be identified and appropriately treated. Specialized CV clinics that specifically address the needs of rheumatologic patients allow these patients to be followed up in a more rigorous fashion, with more uniform evaluation and longitudinal follow-up. Examples of such clinics include the Preventive Cardio-Rheuma clinic at the Department of Rheumatology at Diakonhjemmet Hospital in Norway and the Cardio-Rheum clinic at the Division of Cardiovascular Diseases at Mayo Clinic in Rochester, Minnesota. Both models represent deep and ongoing collaborations between the clinical disciplines of rheumatology and preventive cardiology. Integral to both models are (1), extensive patient and provider education regarding CVD risk in the unique setting of autoimmune diseases, such as RA; (2), comprehensive CVD risk assessment including history, physical examination, and use of relevant risk assessment scores, as well as noninvasive and (when indicated) invasive measurement techniques; and (3), development and monitoring of an aggressive plan for CVD risk reduction, considering not only traditional CVD risks but also tight control of systemic inflammation and RA disease management. Each program also includes a clinical research component aimed at continually evaluating and improving the preventive care paradigms.

Cardiovascular Disease Risk Assessment

Risk Calculators

As previously noted, both traditional and nontraditional risk factors affect the development of CVD in people with RA and SLE. Traditional CV risk factors alone cannot account for the increased risk of CVD in these patients.[56,232] This information, together with the findings that traditional CV risk factors behave differently in patients with inflammatory rheumatic diseases compared with the general population, suggests that risk scores based on traditional CV risk factors alone are unlikely to accurately estimate CVD risk in these patients. Indeed, risk calculators (e.g., Framingham) have underestimated CVD risk twofold in patients with RA.[227] The Systematic COronary Risk Evaluation (SCORE), QRISK II, and Reynolds CVD risk calculators also underestimate future CV events in patients with RA, except for those in the highest risk classes.[226,227,233] In the latest European Society of Cardiology guidelines for CVD prevention,[234] immunologic diseases, such as RA, were, for the first time, mentioned and categorized as a CV risk factor and have similarly been included in the latest version of the United Kingdom CV risk calculator, the QRISK II.[235] The European League Against Rheumatism (EULAR) recognizes that patients with inflammatory joint diseases have increased risk for CVD and make recommendations for management of CV risk factors, which they base largely on expert consensus.[226] The EULAR task force recommended a multiplication factor of 1.5 to the calculated CVD risk by SCORE for all patients with RA. This multiplier and the other RA-specific risk calculators have not demonstrated improved prediction accuracy compared to risk calculators used in the general population.[236,237] Further development of accurate CVD risk assessment tools for RA and SLE are needed to allow incorporation of inflammatory and disease-related factors that may help predict CVD in these patients.

Risk Scores and Risk Markers: Biomarkers and Tests for Subclinical Disease

One reason for underestimation of CVD risk in people with RA may be the high frequency of asymptomatic atherosclerosis,[238–241] which is easily visualized upon ultrasound of the carotid arteries. In addition, carotid artery plaques in patients with RA are predictors of a future acute coronary syndrome.[242] RA-specific factors, such as disease duration and disease activity, have been associated with plaque size and vulnerability in patients with RA. Moreover, in the recent European guidelines on CVD prevention,[234] the presence of carotid artery plaques is considered a CVD equivalent, which suggests that including ultrasound of carotid arteries in the CVD risk evaluation (class: IIa, level of evidence: B, GRADE: strong) would increase the proportion of correct risk stratification.[240,243] Due to the high pre-test probability for detection of carotid artery plaques by use of ultrasound in patients with RA, and the clinical consequence of indication for statin treatment if a carotid plaque is present, this procedure could be of additional value for CVD risk evaluation. Ultrasound of the carotid arteries to identify atherosclerosis has reclassified a considerable proportion of patients with RA into a more appropriate CVD risk group in accordance with current guidelines.[244]

Other tests for subclinical disease that might be useful for assessing CVD risk in patients with RA include aortic pulse wave velocity and lipoprotein(a).[245] Soluble biomarkers are also appealing because they are typically less costly and have more widespread availability.[80] However, they also may be more difficult to interpret in patients with rheumatic disease because of their dual association with CVD and rheumatic disease (Fig. 39.10).[80]

In conclusion, available CVD risk calculators developed for the general population inaccurately estimate CVD risk in patients with RA but currently represent the best utility for CVD risk evaluation in these patients.

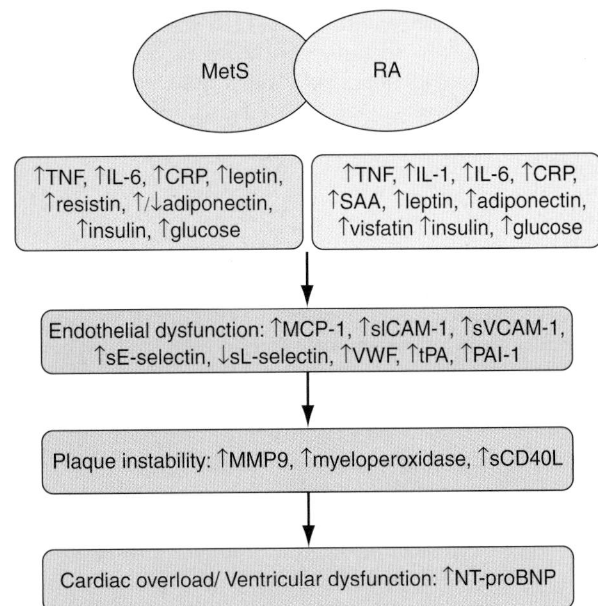

• **Fig. 39.10** Key soluble biomarkers that are associated with different stages of the atherosclerotic pathway in the metabolic syndrome and rheumatoid arthritis (RA). *CRP,* C-reactive protein; *MCP,* monocyte chemotactic protein; *MetS,* metabolic syndrome; *MMP,* matrix metalloproteinase; *NT-proBNP,* N-terminal pro–brain natriuretic peptide; *PAI-1,* plasminogen activator inhibitor-1; *SAA,* serum amyloid A; *sICAM,* soluble intercellular adhesion molecule; *sVCAM,* soluble vascular cell adhesion molecule; *TNF,* tumor necrosis factor; *tPA,* tissue plasminogen activator; *VWF,* von Willebrand factor. (From Kozera L, Andrews J, Morgan AW: Cardiovascular risk and rheumatoid arthritis-the next step: differentiating true soluble biomarkers of cardiovascular risk from surrogate measures of inflammation. *Rheumatology* 50:1944–1954, 2011. Permission to reprint from Oxford University Press.)

Managing CVD Risk in Patients With Rheumatic Disease

Both in Europe and in the United States, patients with RA are significantly less likely to receive CVD preventive measures compared with the general population.[246] A study showed that despite receiving similar treatment, patients with RA who had an MI experienced worse long-term outcomes than did patients with an MI who did not have RA.[30] This deficiency in CVD risk management is amply confirmed in an investigation of CV risk factor control in 836 patients with RA by one study.[247] Among the most striking observations is that in the 644 patients without established CVD or DM, inadequate blood pressure and lipid control was documented in 36% and 55% of the participants, respectively. Findings from a preventive cardio-rheuma clinic revealed that 63% of the patients referred were in need of CVD preventive medical intervention.[241]

Compounding the uncertainties surrounding management of CVD risk, no evidence is available regarding CVD preventive treatment effects in patients with RA. To date, there is a lack of published prospective RCTs in RA, which compare either different primary prevention strategies (e.g., lipid-lowering or anti-hypertensive medications) or the effects of the different anti-rheumatic drugs using CVD outcomes as the primary endpoint. Such trials require a high number of patients to be monitored for lengthy periods; these studies have high costs. Promising results from a post hoc analysis of two large statin trials with CVD endpoints showed that effects on lipid reduction and CVD events by statins were comparable in patients with and without inflammatory joint diseases, including RA.[248] A large RCT regarding statin versus placebo (Trial of Atorvastatin for the Primary Prevention of CVD Events in patients with RA [TRACE RA], including >3000 patients with RA) was recently prematurely terminated because of a low incidence of the primary CVD endpoint and because power was inadequate to be able to reach a clear conclusion.

An important CV risk factor in the general population is lipid levels, although lipid levels appear to be less important for patients with inflammatory rheumatic diseases.[98] However, meta-analyses of RCTs have shown that patients in the general population benefit from lipid-lowering treatment regardless of baseline lipid levels.[249] Clinical experience regarding use of CVD preventive medications in inflammatory joint diseases is scarce. Experience from a preventive cardio-rheumatology clinic for patients with inflammatory joint diseases revealed that lipid targets were attained using fewer than three consultations in 90% of the patients without serious adverse events.[241] These results indicate that treating patients who have RA with statins and achieving recommended lipid goals is safe. Prospective, longitudinal data are needed to demonstrate whether patients with RA need to achieve the same low lipid targets as people without RA, or if a relatively smaller or larger reduction in lipids will result in the same CVD protection as in people without RA.

Modern RA therapy and the multiple comorbidities lead to polypharmacy, thus increasing the possibility of drug to drug interactions with CVD preventive medications, such as statins. Interaction between anti-rheumatic treatments, such as NSAIDs and synthetic or biologic DMARDs, with CVD preventive medications is also an area of uncertainty. Although neither inflammation (by CRP or ESR levels) nor anti-rheumatic medications, such as NSAIDS, prednisolone, or synthetic- or biologic-DMARDs, influenced the dose of statin needed to obtain lipid recommended targets.[250] The influence of statins on clinical response and B cell depletion after rituximab treatment in people with RA is inconclusive.[251,252] An increased CVD risk associated with NSAID use is recognized in the general population,[156,253] but in a recent Danish nationwide study, the CVD risk associated with use of NSAIDs in people with RA was modest and significantly lower than in people without RA.[254] Furthermore, NSAIDs interfere with the thrombocyte inhibitory effect of aspirin, which complicates secondary CVD prevention.[255] Observational studies have provided indications that use of synthetic and biologic DMARDs is associated with reduced CVD risk in people with RA.[158,160] However, it is unknown whether this effect is related to the reduction in inflammation opposing the increased levels of atherogenic lipids that occur with biologic DMARDs and improvement of HDL function.[256] Studies to clarify these issues are needed.

CVD prevention in patients with RA is fraught with concerns of drug- and disease-related complexities. Therapies of rheumatic conditions have evolved enormously in the past two decades, as have CVD prevention strategies. The available literature suggests substantial underuse of CVD preventive pharmacotherapy in the general population.[257,258] More than half of all patients did not reach their LDL treatment goals in general practice. These findings are also supported by the Eurospire IV report, which indicates that clinical implementation of secondary prevention treatments remains suboptimal.[259] Similar undertreatment and failure to obtain recommended lipid and blood pressure targets have been shown in patients with RA.[260] Efforts to address the high CVD risk in patients with rheumatic disease should be a focus in the cardiology community and among rheumatologists. It is hoped that such a focus will result in more patients with RA being evaluated for CVD risk and the institution of preventive measures when necessary.

There are several new medications for CVD prevention; the most promising are alirocumab/evolocumab (proprotein convertase subtilisin/kexin type 9 [PCSK9] inhibitors), which are recommended for patients with primary hypercholesterolemia who do not achieve lipid goals with statins.[261] An interesting clinical indication is statin intolerance, but until now, alirocumab was only tested in addition to statin medication.

Patient Awareness of Cardiovascular Disease Risk

Communicating future risk and the need for preventive treatment is one of the most challenging aspects of the patient/health professional interaction. Awareness of patients about their CVD risk is important for successful implementation of preventive strategies related to lifestyle modifiable CV risk factors.[262] Although such programs for assessing CVD risk in people with RA have been developed, it will take a great effort to fully disseminate them. These strategies include education of health care professionals, written material, and online and group education of patients and their families. Even starting with simple information and brochures as a precursor to implementing a full education program is a step forward. It is of the utmost importance for patients with rheumatic diseases to understand that effective CVD risk management comprises not only adequate treatment of conventional CV risk factors but also tight control of the rheumatic disease activity.

Conclusion

CVD remains a major problem for people with systemic inflammatory diseases. Systemic inflammation and its interplay with traditional and nontraditional CV risk factors appear to have a major role. Future work should focus on further delineating the underlying biologic mechanisms involved, developing and evaluating risk assessment tools and biomarkers, and developing prevention and treatment strategies specific to rheumatic disease populations. Optimal control of traditional risk factors is imperative but insufficient to reduce CVD risk for people with rheumatic diseases. Tight control of systemic inflammation will be required for optimal results.

Full references for this chapter can be found on ExpertConsult.com.

Selected References

1. Cobb S, Anderson F, Bauer W: Length of life and cause of death in rheumatoid arthritis, *N Engl J Med* 249:553–556, 1953.
2. Urowitz MB, Bookman AA, Koehler BE, et al.: The bimodal mortality pattern of systemic lupus erythematosus, *Am J Med* 60:221–225, 1976.
9. Ridker PM, Everett BM, Thuren T, et al.: for the CANTOS group: Antiinflammatory therapy with canakinumab for atherscle-rotic disease, *N Engl J Med* 377:1119–1131, 2017.
11. McInnes IB, Schett G: The pathogenesis of rheumatoid arthritis, *N Engl J Med* 365:2205–2219, 2011.
12. Eid RE, Rao DA, Zhou J, et al.: Interleukin-17 and interferon-gamma are produced concomitantly by human coronary artery-infiltrating T cells and act synergistically on vascular smooth muscle cells, *Circulation* 119:1424–1432, 2009.
14. Kremer JM, Genant HK, Moreland LW, et al.: Effects of abatacept in patients with methotrexate-resistant active rheumatoid arthritis: a randomized trial, *Ann Intern Med* 144:865–876, 2006.
15. Schomig A, Dibra A, Windecker S, et al.: A meta-analysis of 16 randomized trials of sirolimus-eluting stents versus paclitaxel-eluting stents in patients with coronary artery disease, *J Am Coll Cardiol* 50:1373–1380, 2007.
16. Gerli R, Schillaci G, Giordano A, et al.: CD4+CD28- T lymphocytes contribute to early atherosclerotic damage in rheumatoid arthritis patients, *Circulation* 109:2744–2748, 2004.
18. Nakajima T, Schulte S, Warrington KJ, et al.: T-cell-mediated lysis of endothelial cells in acute coronary syndromes, *Circulation* 105:570–575, 2002.
19. Sun W, Cui Y, Zhen L, et al.: Association between HLA-DRB1, HLA-DRQB1 alleles, and CD4(+)CD28(null) T cells in a Chinese population with coronary heart disease, *Mol Biol Rep* 38:1675–1679, 2011.
20. Colmegna I, Diaz-Borjon A, Fujii H, et al.: Defective proliferative capacity and accelerated telomeric loss of hematopoietic progenitor cells in rheumatoid arthritis, *Arthritis Rheum* 58:990–1000, 2008.
21. Shao L, Fujii H, Colmegna I, et al.: Deficiency of the DNA repair enzyme ATM in rheumatoid arthritis, *J Exp Med* 206:1435–1449, 2009.
22. Spyridopoulos I, Hoffmann J, Aicher A, et al.: Accelerated telomere shortening in leukocyte subpopulations of patients with coronary heart disease: role of cytomegalovirus seropositivity, *Circulation* 120:1364–1372, 2009.
23. Weyand CM, Fujii H, Shao L, et al.: Rejuvenating the immune system in rheumatoid arthritis, *Nat Rev Rheumatol* 5:583–588, 2009.
24. Maradit-Kremers H, Crowson CS, Nicola PJ, et al.: Increased unrecognized coronary heart disease and sudden deaths in rheumatoid arthritis: a population-based cohort study, *Arthritis Rheum* 52:402–411, 2005.
27. Holmqvist ME, Wedren S, Jacobsson LT, et al.: No increased occurrence of ischemic heart disease prior to the onset of rheumatoid arthritis: results from two Swedish population-based rheumatoid arthritis cohorts, *Arthritis Rheum* 60:2861–2869, 2009.
30. McCoy SS, Crowson CS, Maradit-Kremers H, et al.: Longterm outcomes and treatment after myocardial infarction in patients with rheumatoid arthritis, *J Rheumatol* 40:605–610, 2013.
31. Van Doornum S, Brand C, Sundararajan V, et al.: Rheumatoid arthritis patients receive less frequent acute reperfusion and secondary prevention therapy after myocardial infarction compared with the general population, *Arthritis Res Ther* 12:R183, 2010.
32. Francis ML, Varghese JJ, Mathew JM, et al.: Outcomes in patients with rheumatoid arthritis and myocardial infarction, *Am J Med* 123:922–928, 2010.
34. Nicola PJ, Maradit-Kremers H, Roger VL, et al.: The risk of congestive heart failure in rheumatoid arthritis: a population-based study over 46 years, *Arthritis Rheum* 52:412–420, 2005.
37. Davis 3rd JM, Roger VL, Crowson CS, et al.: The presentation and outcome of heart failure in patients with rheumatoid arthritis differs from that in the general population, *Arthritis Rheum* 58:2603–2611, 2008.
38. Davis JM, Crowson CS, Maradit Kremers H, et al.: Mortality following heart failure is higher among rheumatoid arthritis subjects compared to non-RA subjects, *Arthritis Rheum* 54:S387, 2006.
39. Avina-Zubieta JA, Choi HK, Sadatsafavi M, et al.: Risk of cardiovascular mortality in patients with rheumatoid arthritis: a meta-analysis of observational studies, *Arthritis Rheum* 59:1690–1697, 2008.
42. Maradit-Kremers H, Nicola PJ, Crowson CS, et al.: Cardiovascular death in rheumatoid arthritis: a population-based study, *Arthritis Rheum* 52:722–732, 2005.
44. Crowson CS, Liang KP, Therneau TM, et al.: Could accelerated aging explain the excess mortality in patients with seropositive rheumatoid arthritis? *Arthritis Rheum* 62:378–382, 2010.

45. Goodson NJ, Wiles NJ, Lunt M, et al.: Mortality in early inflammatory polyarthritis: cardiovascular mortality is increased in seropositive patients, *Arthritis Rheum* 46:2010–2019, 2002.
46. Naz SM, Farragher TM, Bunn DK, et al.: The influence of age at symptom onset and length of followup on mortality in patients with recent-onset inflammatory polyarthritis, *Arthritis Rheum* 58:985–989, 2008.
47. Gonzalez A, Icen M, Kremers HM, et al.: Mortality trends in rheumatoid arthritis: the role of rheumatoid factor, *J Rheumatol* 35:1009–1014, 2008.
48. Farragher TM, Goodson NJ, Naseem H, et al.: Association of the HLA-DRB1 gene with premature death, particularly from cardiovascular disease, in patients with rheumatoid arthritis and inflammatory polyarthritis, *Arthritis Rheum* 58:359–369, 2008.
50. Radovits BJ, Fransen J, Al Shamma S, et al.: Excess mortality emerges after 10 years in an inception cohort of early rheumatoid arthritis, *Arthritis Care Res (Hoboken)* 62:362–370, 2010.
51. Dadoun S, Zeboulon-Ktorza N, Combescure C, et al.: Mortality in rheumatoid arthritis over the last fifty years: systematic review and meta-analysis, *Joint Bone Spine* 80:29–33, 2013.
52. Meune C, Touze E, Trinquart L, et al.: Trends in cardiovascular mortality in patients with rheumatoid arthritis over 50 years: a systematic review and meta-analysis of cohort studies, *Rheumatology (Oxford)* 48:1309–1313, 2009.
56. Esdaile JM, Abrahamowicz M, Grodzicky T, et al.: Traditional Framingham risk factors fail to fully account for accelerated atherosclerosis in systemic lupus erythematosus, *Arthritis Rheum* 44:2331–2337, 2001.
57. Manzi S, Meilahn EN, Rairie JE, et al.: Age-specific incidence rates of myocardial infarction and angina in women with systemic lupus erythematosus: comparison with the Framingham Study, *Am J Epidemiol* 145:408–415, 1997.
60. Shah MA, Shah AM, Krishnan E: Poor outcomes after acute myocardial infarction in systemic lupus erythematosus, *J Rheumatol* 36:570–575, 2009.
61. Ward MM: Outcomes of hospitalizations for myocardial infarctions and cerebrovascular accidents in patients with systemic lupus erythematosus, *Arthritis Rheum* 50:3170–3176, 2004.
62. Bartels CM, Buhr KA, Goldberg JW, et al.: Mortality and cardiovascular burden of systemic lupus erythematosus in a US population-based cohort, *J Rheumatol* 41:680–687, 2014.
64. Wu LS, Tang CH, Lin YS, et al.: Major adverse cardiovascular events and mortality in systemic lupus erythematosus patients after successful delivery: a population-based study, *Am J Med Sci* 347:42–49, 2014.
65. Maksimowicz-McKinnon K, Selzer F, Manzi S, et al.: Poor 1-year outcomes after percutaneous coronary interventions in systemic lupus erythematosus: report from the National Heart, Lung, and Blood Institute Dynamic Registry, *Circ Cardiovasc Interv* 1:201–208, 2008.
66. Von Feldt J: Premature atherosclerotic cardiovascular disease and systemic lupus erythematosus from bedside to bench, *Bull NYU Hosp Jt Dis* 66:184–187, 2008.
68. Nikpour M, Urowitz MB, Gladman DD: Epidemiology of atherosclerosis in systemic lupus erythematosus, *Curr Rheumatol Rep* 11:248–254, 2009.
69. Ward MM: Premature morbidity from cardiovascular and cerebrovascular diseases in women with systemic lupus erythematosus, *Arthritis Rheum* 42:338–346, 1999.
75. Haque S, Bruce IN: Cardiovascular outcomes in systemic lupus erythematosus: big studies for big questions, *J Rheumatol* 36:467–469, 2009.
76. Urowitz MB, Gladman DD, Tom BD, et al.: Changing patterns in mortality and disease outcomes for patients with systemic lupus erythematosus, *J Rheumatol* 35:2152–2158, 2008.
77. Uramoto KM, Michet CJ, Thumboo J, et al.: Trends in the incidence and mortality of systemic lupus erythematosus (SLE)—1950–1992, *Arthritis Rheum* 42:46–50, 1999.
78. Chun BC, Bae SC: Mortality and cancer incidence in Korean patients with systemic lupus erythematosus: results from the Hanyang lupus cohort in Seoul, Korea, *Lupus* 14:635–638, 2005.
79. Yazdanyar A, Wasko MC, Scalzi LV, et al.: Short-term perioperative all-cause mortality and cardiovascular events in women with systemic lupus erythematosus, *Arthritis Care Res* 65:986–991, 2013.
80. Kozera L, Andrews J, Morgan AW: Cardiovascular risk and rheumatoid arthritis—the next step: differentiating true soluble biomarkers of cardiovascular risk from surrogate measures of inflammation, *Rheumatology (Oxford)* 50:1944–1954, 2011.
82. Yusuf S, Hawken S, Ounpuu S, et al.: Effect of potentially modifiable risk factors associated with myocardial infarction in 52 countries (the INTERHEART study): case-control study, *Lancet* 364(9438):937–952, 2004.
86. Crowson CS, Liao KP, Davis 3rd JM, et al.: Rheumatoid arthritis and cardiovascular disease, *Am Heart J* 166:622–628, 2013.
90. Boyer JF, Gourraud PA, Cantagrel A, et al.: Traditional risk factors in rheumatoid arthritis: a meta-analysis, *Joint Bone Spine* 78:179–183, 2011.
91. Klareskog L, Catrina AI, Paget S: Rheumatoid arthritis, *Lancet* 373:659–672, 2009.
94. Panoulas VF, Douglas KM, Milionis HJ, et al.: Prevalence and associations of hypertension and its control in patients with rheumatoid arthritis, *Rheumatology (Oxford)* 46:1477–1482, 2007.
98. Myasoedova E, Crowson CS, Kremers HM, et al.: Lipid paradox in rheumatoid arthritis: the impact of serum lipid measures and systemic inflammation on the risk of cardiovascular disease, *Ann Rheum Dis* 70:482–487, 2011.
99. Myasoedova E, Maradit Kremers H, Fitz-Gibbon P, et al.: Lipid profile improves with the onset of rheumatoid arthritis, *Ann Rheum Dis* 68(Suppl 3):78, 2009.
100. Hahn BH, Grossman J, Chen W, et al.: The pathogenesis of atherosclerosis in autoimmune rheumatic diseases: roles of inflammation and dyslipidemia, *J Autoimmun* 28:69–75, 2007.
103. Semb AG, Holme I, Kvien TK, et al.: Intensive lipid lowering in patients with rheumatoid arthritis and previous myocardial infarction: an explorative analysis from the incremental decrease in endpoints through aggressive lipid lowering (IDEAL) trial, *Rheumatology (Oxford)* 50:324–329, 2011.
104. Toms TE, Panoulas VF, Douglas KM, et al.: Statin use in rheumatoid arthritis in relation to actual cardiovascular risk: evidence for substantial undertreatment of lipid-associated cardiovascular risk? *Ann Rheum Dis* 69:683–688, 2010.
105. Steiner G, Urowitz MB: Lipid profiles in patients with rheumatoid arthritis: mechanisms and the impact of treatment, *Semin Arthritis Rheum* 38:372–381, 2009.
106. Toms TE, Symmons DP, Kitas GD: Dyslipidaemia in rheumatoid arthritis: the role of inflammation, drugs, lifestyle and genetic factors, *Curr Vasc Pharmacol* 8:301–326, 2010.
107. Kitas GD, Gabriel SE: Cardiovascular disease in rheumatoid arthritis: state of the art and future perspectives, *Ann Rheum Dis* 70:8–14, 2011.
108. van Sijl AM, Peters MJ, Knol DL, et al.: The effect of TNF-alpha blocking therapy on lipid levels in rheumatoid arthritis: a meta-analysis, *Semin Arthritis Rheum* 41:393–400, 2011.
111. Bartels CM, Kind AJ, Everett C, et al.: Low frequency of primary lipid screening among Medicare patients with rheumatoid arthritis, *Arthritis Rheum* 63:1221–1230, 2011.
113. Crowson CS, Myasoedova E, Davis 3rd JM, et al.: Increased prevalence of metabolic syndrome associated with rheumatoid arthritis in patients without clinical cardiovascular disease, *J Rheumatol* 38:29–35, 2011.
115. Dessein PH, Joffe BI: Insulin resistance and impaired beta cell function in rheumatoid arthritis, *Arthritis Rheum* 54:2765–2775, 2006.
116. Wasko MC, Hubert HB, Lingala VB, et al.: Hydroxychloroquine and risk of diabetes in patients with rheumatoid arthritis, *JAMA* 298:187–193, 2007.

123. Escalante A, Haas RW, del Rincon I: Paradoxical effect of body mass index on survival in rheumatoid arthritis: role of comorbidity and systemic inflammation, *Arch Intern Med* 165:1624–1629, 2005.
124. Maradit Kremers HM, Nicola PJ, Crowson CS, et al.: Prognostic importance of low body mass index in relation to cardiovascular mortality in rheumatoid arthritis, *Arthritis Rheum* 50:3450–3457, 2004.
125. Symmons DP, Bankhead CR, Harrison BJ, et al.: Blood transfusion, smoking, and obesity as risk factors for the development of rheumatoid arthritis: results from a primary care-based incident case-control study in Norfolk, England, *Arthritis Rheum* 40:1955–1961, 1997.
127. Stavropoulos-Kalinoglou A, Metsios GS, Panoulas VF, et al.: Associations of obesity with modifiable risk factors for the development of cardiovascular disease in patients with rheumatoid arthritis, *Ann Rheum Dis* 68:242–245, 2009.
129. Giles JT, Allison M, Blumenthal RS, et al.: Abdominal adiposity in rheumatoid arthritis: association with cardiometabolic risk factors and disease characteristics, *Arthritis Rheum* 62:3173–3182, 2010.
135. Koenig W, Sund M, Filipiak B, et al.: Plasma viscosity and the risk of coronary heart disease: results from the MONICA-Augsburg Cohort Study, 1984 to 1992, *Arterioscler Thromb Vasc Biol* 18:768–772, 1998.
138. Santos MJ, Pedro LM, Canhao H, et al.: Hemorheological parameters are related to subclinical atherosclerosis in systemic lupus erythematosus and rheumatoid arthritis patients, *Atherosclerosis* 219:821–826, 2011.
139. Marder W, Khalatbari S, Myles JD, et al.: Interleukin 17 as a novel predictor of vascular function in rheumatoid arthritis, *Ann Rheum Dis* 70:1550–1555, 2011.
149. Banerjee S, Compton AP, Hooker RS, et al.: Cardiovascular outcomes in male veterans with rheumatoid arthritis, *Am J Cardiol* 101:1201–1205, 2008.
155. Goodson NJ, Brookhart AM, Symmons DP, et al.: Non-steroidal anti-inflammatory drug use does not appear to be associated with increased cardiovascular mortality in patients with inflammatory polyarthritis: results from a primary care based inception cohort of patients, *Ann Rheum Dis* 68:367–372, 2009.
156. Trelle S, Reichenbach S, Wandael S, et al.: Cardiovascular safety of non-steroidal anti-inflammatory drugs: network meta-analysis, *Br Med J* 342:c7086, 2011.
173. Gustafsson JT, Simard JF, Gunnarsson I, et al.: Risk factors for cardiovascular mortality in patients with systemic lupus erythematosus, a prospective cohort study, *Arthritis Res Ther* 14:R46, 2012.
174. Kaiser R, Li Y, Chang M, et al.: Genetic risk factors for thrombosis in systemic lupus erythematosus, *J Rheumatol* 39:1603–1610, 2012.
175. Ames PR, Margarita A, Alves JD: Antiphospholipid antibodies and atherosclerosis: insights from systemic lupus erythematosus and primary antiphospholipid syndrome, *Clin Rev Allergy Immunol* 37:29–35, 2009.
178. Thacker SG, Zhao W, Smith CK, et al.: Type I interferons modulate vascular function, repair, thrombosis, and plaque progression in murine models of lupus and atherosclerosis, *Arthritis Rheum* 64:2975–2985, 2012.
181. Selzer F, Sutton-Tyrrell K, Fitzgerald S, et al.: Vascular stiffness in women with systemic lupus erythematosus, *Hypertension* 37:1075–1082, 2001.
183. Jung H, Bobba R, Su J, et al.: The protective effect of antimalarial drugs on thrombovascular events in systemic lupus erythematosus, *Arthritis Rheum* 62:863–868, 2010.
184. van Leuven SI, van Wijk DF, Volger OL, et al.: Mycophenolate mofetil attenuates plaque inflammation in patients with symptomatic carotid artery stenosis, *Atherosclerosis* 211:231–236, 2010.
192. Gelfand JM, Neimann AL, Shin DB, et al.: Risk of myocardial infarction in patients with psoriasis, *JAMA* 296:1735–1741, 2006.
196. Jamnitski A, Symmons D, Peters MJ, et al.: Cardiovascular comorbidities in patients with psoriatic arthritis: a systematic review, *Ann Rheum Dis* 72:211–216, 2013.
197. Gladman DD, Ang M, Su L, et al.: Cardiovascular morbidity in psoriatic arthritis, *Ann Rheum Dis* 68:1131–1135, 2009.
199. Tomasson G, Peloquin C, Mohammad A, et al.: Risk for cardiovascular disease early and late after a diagnosis of giant-cell arteritis: a cohort study, *Ann Intern Med* 160:73–80, 2014.
200. Uddhammar A, Eriksson AL, Nystrom L, et al.: Increased mortality due to cardiovascular disease in patients with giant cell arteritis in northern Sweden, *J Rheumatol* 29:737–742, 2002.
201. Udayakumar PD, Chandran AK, Crowson CS, et al.: Cardiovascular risk and acute coronary syndrome in giant cell arteritis: a population based retrospective cohort study, *Arthritis Care Res (Hoboken)* 67:396–402, 2015.
204. Hancock AT, Mallen CD, Muller S, et al.: Risk of vascular events in patients with polymyalgia rheumatica, *CMAJ* 186:495–501, 2014.
206. Hancock AT, Mallen CD, Belcher J, et al.: Association between polymyalgia rheumatica and vascular disease: a systematic review, *Arthritis Care Res* 64:1301–1305, 2012.
213. Linos E, Fiorentino D, Lingala B, et al.: Atherosclerotic cardiovascular disease and dermatomyositis: an analysis of the Nationwide Inpatient Sample survey, *Arthritis Res Ther* 15:R7, 2013.
214. Tisseverasinghe A, Bernatsky S, Pineau CA: Arterial events in persons with dermatomyositis and polymyositis, *J Rheumatol* 36:1943–1946, 2009.
216. Rahman MM, Kopec JA, Anis AH, et al.: Risk of cardiovascular disease in patients with osteoarthritis: a prospective longitudinal study, *Arthritis Care Res* 65:1951–1958, 2013.
218. Hawker GA, Croxford R, Bierman AS, et al.: All-cause mortality and serious cardiovascular events in people with hip and knee osteoarthritis: a population based cohort study, *PLoS One* 9:e91286, 2014.
219. Barsalou J, Bradley TJ, Silverman ED: Cardiovascular risk in pediatric-onset rheumatological diseases, *Arthritis Res Ther* 15:212, 2013.
221. Schanberg LE, Sandborg C, Barnhart HX, et al.: Premature atherosclerosis in pediatric systemic lupus erythematosus: risk factors for increased carotid intima-media thickness in the atherosclerosis prevention in pediatric lupus erythematosus cohort, *Arthritis Rheum* 60:1496–1507, 2009.
226. Agca R, Heslinga SC, Rollefstad S, et al.: EULAR recommendations for cardiovascular disease risk management in patients with rheumatoid arthritis and other forms of inflammatory joint disorders: 2015/2016 update, *Ann Rheum Dis* 76:17–28, 2017.
227. Crowson CS, Matteson EL, Roger VL, et al.: Usefulness of risk scores to estimate the risk of cardiovascular disease in patients with rheumatoid arthritis, *Am J Cardiol* 110:420–424, 2012.
228. Hansson GK: Inflammation, atherosclerosis, and coronary artery disease, *N Engl J Med* 352:1685–1695, 2005.
230. Tyrrell PN, Beyene J, Feldman BM, et al.: Rheumatic disease and carotid intima-media thickness: a systematic review and meta-analysis, *Arterioscler Thromb Vasc Biol* 30:1014–1026, 2010.
231. Friedewald VE, Ganz P, Kremer JM, et al.: AJC editor's consensus: rheumatoid arthritis and atherosclerotic cardiovascular disease, *Am J Cardiol* 106:442–447, 2010.
234. Perk J, De Backer G, Gohlke H, et al.: European Guidelines on cardiovascular disease prevention in clinical practice (version 2012): The Fifth Joint Task Force of the European Society of Cardiology and Other Societies on Cardiovascular Disease Prevention in Clinical Practice (constituted by representatives of nine societies and by invited experts), *Atherosclerosis* 223:1–68, 2012.
235. Hippisley-Cox J, Coupland C, Vinogradova Y, et al.: Predicting cardiovascular risk in England and Wales: prospective derivation and validation of QRISK2, *BMJ* 336:1475–1482, 2008.
241. Rollefstad S, Kvien TK, Holme I, et al.: Treatment to lipid targets in patients with inflammatory joint diseases in a preventive cardio-rheuma clinic, *Ann Rheum Dis* 72:1968–1974, 2013.
246. Lindhardsen J, Ahlehoff O, Gislason GH, et al.: Initiation and adherence to secondary prevention pharmacotherapy after myocardial infarction in patients with rheumatoid arthritis: a nationwide cohort study, *Ann Rheum Dis* 71:1496–1501, 2012.
247. Primdahl J, Clausen J, Horslev-Petersen K: Results from systematic screening for cardiovascular risk in outpatients with rheumatoid arthritis in accordance with the EULAR recommendations, *Ann Rheum Dis* 72:1771–1776, 2013.

248. Semb AG, Kvien TK, DeMicco DA, et al.: Effect of intensive lipid-lowering therapy on cardiovascular outcome in patients with and those without inflammatory joint disease, *Arthritis Rheum* 64:2836–2846, 2012.
249. Mihaylova B, Emberson J, Blackwell L, et al.: The effects of lowering LDL cholesterol with statin therapy in people at low risk of vascular disease: meta-analysis of individual data from 27 randomised trials, *Lancet* 380:581–590, 2012.
251. Arts EE, Jansen TL, Den Broeder A, et al.: Statins inhibit the antirheumatic effects of rituximab in rheumatoid arthritis: results from the Dutch Rheumatoid Arthritis Monitoring (DREAM) registry, *Ann Rheum Dis* 70:877–878, 2011.
252. Das S, Fernandez Matilla M, Dass S, et al.: Statins do not influence clinical response and B cell depletion after rituximab treatment in rheumatoid arthritis, *Ann Rheum Dis* 72:463–464, 2013.
254. Lindhardsen J, Gislason GH, Jacobsen S, et al.: Non-steroidal anti-inflammatory drugs and risk of cardiovascular disease in patients with rheumatoid arthritis: a nationwide cohort study, *Ann Rheum Dis* 73:1515–1521, 2014.
255. Meek IL, Vonkeman HE, Kasemier J, et al.: Interference of NSAIDs with the thrombocyte inhibitory effect of aspirin: a placebo-controlled, ex vivo, serial placebo-controlled serial crossover study, *Eur J Clin Pharmacol* 69:365–371, 2013.
258. Reiner Z, De Bacquer D, Kotseva K, et al.: Treatment potential for dyslipidaemia management in patients with coronary heart disease across Europe: findings from the EUROASPIRE III survey, *Atherosclerosis* 231:300–307, 2013.

40

Cancer Risk in Rheumatic Diseases

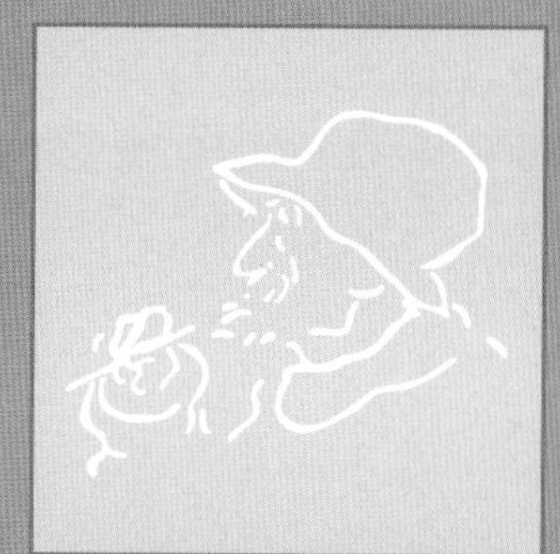

ERIC L. MATTESON

KEY POINTS

Risk of malignancy, especially lymphoproliferative malignancy, is increased in autoimmune rheumatic diseases.

The occurrence of cancer in patients with rheumatic diseases adversely affects quality of life and life expectancy compared with the general population.

This risk is related to the pathobiology of the underlying rheumatic disease, including the inflammatory burden, immunologic defects such as overexpression of *Bcl-2* oncogenes, traditional risk factors such as smoking, and, in some cases, associated viral infection.

Several of the immunomodulatory treatments used in the management of autoimmune disease, especially chemotherapeutic agents, are associated with an increased risk of cancer.

The decision to use immunomodulating therapies in patients with rheumatic disease must take into account host and environmental risk factors for cancer. Effective screening and monitoring strategies can markedly reduce the risk of cancer in these patients.

Introduction

Systemic rheumatic diseases have been associated with an increased risk of development of malignancy. This increased risk is the result of fundamental underlying immunologic effects of autoimmunity on cancer risk and on the risk of cancers associated with drug treatments for rheumatic diseases.

Accelerated growth of cancer cells in immunodeficient mice and increased risk of cancer in heavily immunosuppressed transplant patients have shaped the perception of the immune system as a potent barrier against neoplasms.[1,2] It might be expected that immunosuppressive treatment would inevitably result in effects favoring malignant cell growth. However, emerging evidence supports the seemingly paradoxical notion, perhaps formulated first by Rudolph Virchow in 1863, that inflammation is a critical component of cancer initiation and progression, and that reduction of systemic inflammation may reduce cancer risk in these conditions.[3]

Assessment of cancer risk in rheumatic diseases must be weighed against the lifetime risk of developing cancer, which is approximately 20% in Western Europe and North America, with 5% of the general population having current cancer or a history of cancer.[4] Approximately 1 in 10 women will develop breast cancer, and as many as one in eight men will develop prostate cancer, 1 in 25 colorectal cancer, 1 in 40 lung cancer, and approximately 1 in 100 lymphoma or other lymphoproliferative malignancy.[4]

The combination of increased risk for some and decreased risk for other types of cancers in different rheumatic diseases may result in a neutral effect for malignancies in general, emphasizing why, from a clinical standpoint, it is important to identify risks pertaining to specific cancers, which may be uncommon. The statistical approach for capturing differences in sparse event data, particularly when malignancy is not a prespecified study outcome, and assumptions of proportional hazards models and stable frequencies of events over time for a nonlinear risk such as cancer can lead to major errors in interpretation.

Malignancy in Autoimmune Rheumatic Diseases

Several of the rheumatic diseases appear to be associated with increased risk of malignancy, particularly lymphoproliferative disorders. A list of rheumatic diseases that have been associated with malignancy is provided in Table 40.1. A global assessment of susceptibility to Hodgkin's lymphoma using population-based linked registry data from Sweden and Denmark identified significantly increased risks of Hodgkin's lymphoma associated with a personal history of autoimmune disorders, including rheumatoid arthritis (odds ratio [OR], 2.7; 95% confidence interval [CI], 1.9 to 4.0), systemic lupus erythematosus (SLE) (OR, 5.8; 95% CI, 2.2 to 15.1), sarcoidosis (OR, 14.1; 95% CI, 5.4 to 36.8), and immune thrombocytopenic purpura (OR, ∞; $P = .022$).[5] A statistically significant increase in the risk of Hodgkin's lymphoma was associated with family histories of sarcoidosis (OR, 1.8; 95% CI, 1.01 to 3.1) and ulcerative colitis (OR, 1.6; 95% CI, 1.02 to 2.6).[5]

The occurrence of cancer has a profound effect on the already compromised quality of life of patients with rheumatic diseases and may affect survivorship and influence treatment decisions. A population-based study of cancer survival in patients with inflammatory arthritis from Great Britain suggests decreased survival compared with the general population.[6] Survivorship related to the occurrence of cancer in this population was unrelated to disease-modifying anti-rheumatic drug (DMARD) exposure.[6]

TABLE 40.1 **Rheumatic Diseases Associated With Malignancy**

Connective Tissue Disease	Malignancy	Associated Factors	Clinical Alert
Dermatomyositis	Lymphoproliferative disorders; ovarian, lung, and gastric cancers in Western populations; nasopharyngeal carcinoma in Asian populations	Older age, normal creatinine kinase levels, presence of cutaneous vasculitis; antibody specificities to transcription intermediary factor 1γ and nuclear matrix protein-2	Malignancy evaluation needs to be tailored to individual patient's age, symptoms, and signs
Rheumatoid arthritis	Lymphoproliferative disorders, lung cancer	Presence of paraproteinemia, greater disease severity, longer disease duration, immunosuppression, Felty's syndrome	Rapidly progressive; refractory flare in long-standing rheumatoid disease may suggest an underlying malignancy
Seronegative spondyloarthritis	Most studies show no increased risk. Lymphoproliferative disorder risk higher in Taiwan	Risk highest in first 3 years of disease (Taiwan)	
Systemic lupus erythematosus (SLE)	Lymphoproliferative disorders, solid malignancy including thyroid and renal cancer; skin		Non-Hodgkin's lymphoma should be considered in SLE patients who develop adenopathy or masses; lymphoma of the spleen is another cause of splenic enlargement in SLE
Systemic sclerosis (scleroderma)	Alveolar cell carcinoma Nonmelanoma skin cancer Adenocarcinoma of the esophagus	Pulmonary fibrosis, interstitial lung disease Areas of scleroderma and fibrosis in the skin Barrett's metaplasia Presence of anti-RNA polymerase III	Annual chest radiograph after fibrosis is detected Change in skin features or poorly healing lesions should be evaluated If indicated, esophagoscopy and biopsy of distal esophageal constricting lesions
ANCA-associated vasculitis	Lymphoproliferative disorders, bladder, liver, lung		Hematuria or hemoptysis may be due to active disease or cancer, associated especially with cyclophosphamide treatment

Rheumatoid Arthritis

KEY POINTS

Rheumatoid arthritis is associated with a greater than twofold increased risk of lymphoma. This risk is higher in patients with high disease activity and with more severe disease, including extra-articular involvement.

The risk of solid malignancies is variable, with an increased risk of lung cancer and likely melanoma, with decreased risks of colorectal cancer and cancers of the urogenital tract in men and women.

A considerable body of evidence supports rheumatoid arthritis as a pathogenic factor in the development of lymphoma. A standardized incidence ratio (SIR) of 2.4 for lymphoma was described in a population of more than 20,000 Danish patients, as was an increased risk of twofold increased risk in U.S. patients.[7–9]

In many studies, the risk of cancer is particularly increased early in the disease course, and cancer risk appears to be greater in patients who have persistently high disease activity, high cumulative disease activity, and more severe disease, and in those who have positive rheumatoid factor (SIR, 3.6; 95% CI, 1.3 to 7.8).[10,11] The unadjusted OR for average disease activity comparing highest versus lowest quartile was 71.3 (95% CI, 24.1 to 211.4), and the OR for cumulative disease activity of the 10th decile versus the first decile was 61.6 (95% CI, 21.0 to 181.0) in a case-control registry study from Sweden.[11]

Extra-articular disease of rheumatoid arthritis, particularly Felty's syndrome and Sjögren's syndrome, confers a further increased risk of non-Hodgkin's lymphoma; one study of 906 men with rheumatoid arthritis revealed a twofold increase in total cancer incidence among patients with rheumatoid arthritis who have Felty's syndrome.[12] Large granular T cell leukemia (T-LGL) may rarely occur in association with rheumatoid arthritis.[13] T-LGL in rheumatoid arthritis usually is chronic and rarely becomes aggressive.

Contemporary studies continue to show that patients with rheumatoid arthritis are at higher risk for some cancers. A meta-analysis of 21 publications from 1990 to 2007 combined with an updated analysis of nine studies from 2008 through 2014 summarized the risk of malignancy in patients with rheumatoid arthritis.[9] The risk of lymphoma was increased and is reported to be from almost a doubling (SIR 1.7) to 12-fold increase, with greater risks of Hodgkin's and non-Hodgkin's lymphoma. The total pooled SIR (95% CI) for all studies for this period was 2.08 (1.80 to 2.39) for malignant lymphoma, 3.29 (2.56 to 4.22) for Hodgkin's disease, and 1.95 (1.70 to 2.24) for non-Hodgkin's lymphoma.[9] The risk of lung cancer was increased with an SIR of 1.64 (95% CI, 1.51 to 1.79), as was the risk of melanoma (SIR 1.23; 95% CI, 1.01 to 1.49).[14] The risk of colorectal cancer was decreased (SIR, 0.78; 95% CI, 0.71 to 0.86), as was the risk of breast cancer (SIR, 0.86;

95% CI, 0.73 to 1.01). The overall risk for malignancy is about 10% higher than the general population, SIR 1.09 (95% CI, 1.06 to 1.13). The lower risk of colorectal cancer may be attributable to the use of long-term nonsteroidal anti-inflammatory agents in patients with rheumatoid arthritis.[14] The overall increased risk of cancer in patients with rheumatoid arthritis was largely driven by increased risks of lymphoproliferative cancers.

In summary, cancer is frequent in the general population and is at least as common among patients with rheumatoid arthritis. Following a diagnosis of rheumatoid arthritis at the typical age of 55 years, one in five patients will be diagnosed with cancer; however, in the great majority of patients, the cancer cannot be linked to rheumatoid arthritis or to its treatment but rather reflects the background cancer risk.

Systemic Lupus Erythematosus

KEY POINTS

The risk of lymphoma is at least twofold increased in systemic lupus erythematosus (SLE).

Risks of solid malignancy, including lung, thyroid, and kidney cancers, and of skin cancer are increased overall in SLE, although rates of cervix and prostate cancers appear to be somewhat lower. Breast cancer risk has been reported to be increased in some studies and decreased in others.

The risk of at least certain malignancies appears to be increased in patients with SLE. A large multinational study across 30 centers including 16,409 patients observed for 121,283 (average 7.4) person-years reported 644 cancers.[15] Overall, a small increased risk was estimated across all cancers (SIR, 1.14; 95% CI, 1.05, 1.23).The risk of hematologic malignancies was increased (SIR, 3.02; 95% CI, 2.48, 3.63), particularly non-Hodgkin's lymphoma (SIR, 4.39; 95% CI, 3.46, 5.49) and leukemia. The risk is especially high for diffuse large B cell lymphoma, often of aggressive subtypes.[16] In addition, increased risks of cancer of the vulva (SIR, 3.78; 95% CI 1.52, 7.78), lung (SIR, 1.30; 95% CI, 1.04, 1.60), thyroid (SIR, 1.76; 95% CI, 1.13, 2.61), and possibly liver (SIR, 1.87; 95% CI, 0.97, 3.27) were suggested. Cancer risk was lower for breast (SIR, 0.73; 95% CI, 0.61–0.88), endometrial (SIR, 0.44; 95% CI, 0.23–0.77), and possibly ovarian cancers (SIR, 0.64; 95% CI, 0.34–1.10).[17]

Patients with SLE in a California statewide patient hospital discharge database from 1991 to 2001 were followed using Cancer Registry data to compare observed versus expected numbers of cancers based on age, sex, and specific incidence rates in the California population.[18] A total of 30,478 SLE patients were observed for 157,969 person-years. There were a total of 1273 cancers for an overall significantly increased cancer risk (SIR, 1.14; 95% CI, 1.07 to 1.20). Patients with SLE had higher risks of vagina/vulva (SIR, 3.27; 95% CI, 2.41 to 4.31) and liver cancers (SIR, 2.70; 95% CI, 1.54 to 4.24). Also, elevated risks of lung, kidney, and thyroid cancers and hematopoietic malignancies were observed with lower rates of screenable cancers, including breast cancer, cervix cancer, and prostate cancer. Drug effects were not assessed.[18]

The origin of any risk of the development of malignant disorders in SLE remains unclear, although it does not appear to be related to the use of immunosuppressive or cytotoxic agents; most cohorts are too small to allow detection of a statistically meaningful risk increase in rare events over short periods of observation. Race and ethnicity have not been identified as major factors in cancer risk in SLE.[19] Anti-malarial drug use does not appear to affect the relative risk of malignancy, as was postulated in early studies.[17]

Risk factors for the development of hematologic malignancies may relate to inflammatory burden and disease activity, immunologic defects and overexpression of *Bcl-2* oncogenes, and viruses, especially Epstein-Barr virus (EBV).[20] A nested case-control study that included 6438 patients with SLE linked to the national cancer registry in Sweden found that leukopenia, independent of immunosuppressive treatment, was a risk factor for developing these leukemias. Bone marrow investigation was suggested for SLE patients with long-standing leukopenia and anemia.[21] Disease characteristics predisposing to non-Hodgkin's lymphoma include longer disease duration and increased disease activity with moderately severe end-organ damage.[22]

Women with SLE, likely out of concern for treatment side effects and effects of pregnancy on disease control, are less often exposed to oral contraceptives and are more likely to be nulliparous, which may affect their malignancy risk. On the other hand, the possibly increased breast cancer risk suggests that other, poorly understood factors may increase this risk in women with SLE, whereas at least one study suggested that patients with SLE are less likely than healthy women to undergo breast cancer screening.[23] Patients with SLE also appear to be less likely to undergo routine Pap testing. Increased prevalence of human papillomavirus infection and immunosuppression have been implicated in the apparently increased prevalence of abnormal Pap smears and cervical dysplasia in patients with SLE.[24]

Women with SLE may be at higher risk of lung cancer, for which smoking is a predictor.[20] Similar to rheumatoid arthritis, smoking is a risk factor for developing both SLE and lung cancer, reflecting a complex interplay of disease susceptibility factors.

Systemic Sclerosis (Scleroderma)

KEY POINTS

Risks of lymphoma, skin cancer, and lung cancer are markedly increased in scleroderma.

Scleroderma-related risk factors for malignancy include esophageal disease related to Barrett's esophagus and lung cancer related to pulmonary fibrosis.

The risk of malignancy in patients with scleroderma appears to be increased in most reviews and reports, although at least one population-based study failed to detect increased risk.[25,26] A meta-analysis of six population-based cohort studies reported a standardized incidence ratio of 1.41 (95% CI, 1.18, 1.68) for cancer overall, with no difference between limited and diffuse cutaneous scleroderma.[27] The highest SIRs for individual cancers are those for lung cancer, with an incidence ratio of up to 7.8, and non-Hodgkin's lymphoma, with an incidence rate ratio (IRR) of 9.6.

A population-based disease registry and cancer registry retrospective cohort linkage study from Sweden following patients from 1965 to 1983 revealed an SIR of 1.5 for overall cancer, with highest rates for lung cancer (SIR, 4.9), skin cancer (SIR, 4.2), hepatoma (SIR, 3.3), and hematopoietic malignancies (SIR, 2.3).[28] A cohort study of patients followed from 1987 to 2002 revealed a similar magnitude of increased overall risk of malignancy (SIR, 1.55) with the observation of markedly increased risks of oropharyngeal cancer (SIR, 9.63; 95% CI, 2.97 to 16.3) and esophageal cancer (SIR, 15.9; 95% CI, 4.2 to 27.6).[28] Esophageal disease related to systemic sclerosis is the likely reason for the increased incidence of Barrett's esophagus, which has been reported to be present in 12.7% of patients with scleroderma.[29]

A high rate of abnormal Pap tests in women with onset of scleroderma before the age of 50 has been reported, with a lifetime prevalence by self-report of 25.4% (95% CI, 20.9 to 30.4) compared with a self-reported prevalence of abnormal Pap tests in the general Canadian population of 13.8% (95% CI, 11.6 to 16.4). A significant relationship was found between self-reported abnormal Pap tests and diffuse disease and younger age at disease onset.[30]

Lung cancer has been reported to account for up to 30% of all cancers in patients with scleroderma; it is thought to be related to fibrosis. The relationship to smoking is uncertain and studies are contradictory, with some reporting a link and others failing to find a link to smoking.[26,28,31]

The mechanisms of malignancy in scleroderma are largely unexplored. Risk factors for development of malignancy in patients with scleroderma may be related to inflammation and fibrosis of affected organs. The link to smoking is controversial.[27,31] As in some other autoimmune rheumatic diseases, the risk appears higher early in the disease, and patients who are older at the time of diagnosis may be at higher risk as well.[28,32] Presence of anti-RNA polymerase III is associated with a twofold increased risk of cancer at scleroderma onset compared to anti-centromere antibodies. Some patients with scleroderma harbor autoantibodies to RPC1, an RNA polymerase subunit encoded by the *POLR3A* gene that may drive both cancer and the disease.[33] In contrast to systemic sclerosis, localized scleroderma, including morphea and linear scleroderma, has not been associated with increased risk of cancer.[34]

Idiopathic Inflammatory Myopathy

KEY POINTS

The risk of cancer in patients with idiopathic inflammatory myopathies is about five to seven times higher than in the general population.

Malignancy is strongly associated with dermatomyositis and, if present, is often detectable at disease outset. Antibody specificities to TIF1γ and NXP-2 antibodies are strongly associated with cancer risk.

The most common malignancies in inflammatory myositis are adenocarcinomas.

Suspicion for cancer should be high, especially in patients with active muscle and skin inflammation but normal creatine kinase levels, age over 50 years, and periungual erythema.

Both dermatomyositis and polymyositis occurring in adults have been associated with malignancies. The link to malignancy in newly diagnosed patients with dermatomyositis is strongest, although in neither condition is the origin of the association well understood. The association between malignancy and polymyositis and inclusion body myositis is less strong.

The incidence of cancer occurring in patients with inflammatory myositis is approximately two to five times higher than in the general population.[35] A meta-analysis of 20 publications reported a pooled relative risk of malignancy for patients with polymyositis of 1.62 (95% CI, 1.19, 2.04); for dermatomyositis 5.50 (4.31, 6.70), and dermatomyositis/polymyositis (3.02, 5.12).[36] The prevalence of malignancy is about 25%; cancers are reported more frequently in dermatomyositis, occurring in 6% to 60% of patients, and in 0 to 28% of patients with polymyositis. In dermatomyositis, over 80% of patients with malignancy have autoantibodies specific for nuclear matrix protein 2 (NXP-2) or transcription intermediary factor 1γ (TIF 1γ), which confers a 27-fold increased risk for cancer; however, a sizable proportion do not manifest cancer.[37]

In most studies, cancers manifest within 2 years before or after the initial diagnosis of inflammatory myopathy.[38,39] Inflammatory myopathies may initially manifest with the recurrence of a previously diagnosed cancer. A previously diagnosed but inactive inflammatory myopathy may become reactivated with occurrence of a cancer, supporting the hypothesis of autoantigens as drivers of the inflammatory disease.

The strength of the association between malignancy and inflammatory myositis varies. An older study done at the Mayo Clinic failed to reveal an increased risk of malignancy in patients with inflammatory myopathy, and a more recent registry study from Sweden of 788 patients diagnosed with dermatomyositis or polymyositis between 1963 and 1987 revealed that 15% of 392 patients with dermatomyositis had cancer diagnosed concurrently with or after the diagnosis of dermatomyositis, with a relative risk of cancer of 2.4 (95% CI, 1.6 to 3.6) for males and 3.4 (95% CI, 2.4 to 4.7) for females.[38,40] Of 396 patients with polymyositis, 9% had cancer at or after the time of diagnosis of polymyositis, with the relative risk of 1.8 for development of cancer (95% CI, 1.1 to 2.7) in males and 1.7 (95% CI, 1.0 to 2.5) in females.

A population-based retrospective cohort study from Victoria, Australia, of 537 patients with biopsy-proven dermatomyositis and polymyositis reported a relative risk for malignancy in dermatomyositis compared with polymyositis of 2.4 (95% CI, 1.3 to 4.2) with a higher SIR for dermatomyositis than polymyositis (6.2 vs. 2.0).[39] Finally, ORs for association of cancer with dermatomyositis from a large meta-analysis were reported to be 4.4, and for polymyositis, 2.1.[41]

A wide range of malignancies is associated with dermatomyositis and polymyositis. The most common malignancies in populations of Northern European descent are adenocarcinomas of the cervix, lungs, ovaries, pancreas, bladder, and stomach, which account for more than two-thirds of these cancers.[36,40,41] In patients from Southeast Asia, a higher proportion of nasopharyngeal cancers are found, followed by lung cancer.[42]

The association of cancer is less well understood for more unusual forms of inflammatory myopathies. Amyopathic dermatomyositis, a rare form of dermatomyositis with typical cutaneous but no muscle involvement, can be associated with the development of cancer, but the frequency of this condition is low, so that no stable estimates of cancer risk are available.[43] Inclusion body myositis has not been well studied for the same reasons, although the overall risk of cancer of 2.4 suggests a possible link.[39]

It is likely that relevant antigens are expressed in the underlying tumor and affected muscle. Myositis-specific antigens develop during the process of regeneration in patients who have myositis; these are the same antigens expressed in some cancers known to be associated with the development of inflammatory myopathies.[44] This relationship is supported by the finding that antibodies to NXP-2 or TIF 1γ are present in most (83%) patients with cancer-associated dermatomyositis.[35] A link between malignancy and inflammatory myositis is further supported by observations that in many cases, myositis improves after removal of the malignancy.[45]

Clinical disease characteristics that may portend higher malignancy risk include active inflammatory disease with normal serum levels of creatine kinase, distal extremity weakness, pharyngeal and diaphragmatic involvement, and leukocytoclastic vasculitis.[46,47] Other independent risk factors for the development of cancer in patients who have dermatomyositis in one study of 92 patients included age at diagnosis greater than 52 years (hazard ratio [HR], 7.24; 95% CI, 2.35 to 22.41), rapid onset of skin and/or muscle symptoms (HR, 3.11; 95% CI, 1.07 to 9.02), periungual erythema (HR, 3.93; 95% CI, 1.16 to 13.24), low baseline level of complement factor C4 (HR, 2.74; 95% CI, 1.11 to 6.75), and possibly topoisomerase I.[48,49] A low baseline lymphocyte count was a protective factor for malignancy (HR, 0.33; 95% CI, 0.14 to 0.80), although the number of assessable patients was small.[48]

Sjögren Syndrome

KEY POINTS

The risk of lymphoproliferative cancers, especially various types of lymphoma, is at least sixfold increased in patients with primary Sjögren's syndrome.

Immunologic perturbations, including *p35* mutations and B cell activation, as well as *Helicobacter pylori*, are likely predisposing risk factors.

Patients with primary Sjögren's syndrome are at increased risk of lymphoproliferative diseases. A systematic review of 14 studies involving more than 14,523 patients with pSS reported significantly increased risks of overall cancer (pooled RR, 1.53; 95% CI, 1.17 to 1.88), non-Hodgkin's lymphoma (pooled RR, 13.76; 95% CI, 8.53 to 18.99), and thyroid cancer (pooled RR, 2.58; 95% CI, 1.14, 4.03).[50] Individual studies report that the relative risk for the development of lymphoproliferative disorders in these patients ranges from 6 to 44 in individual studies, and a meta-analysis of cohort studies reported a pooled SIR of 18.8.[51] Lymphoproliferative disorders eventually occur in between 4% and 10% of patients with primary Sjögren syndrome, with a lifetime risk of non-Hodgkin's lymphoma of about 5%.[8,51–54]

In addition to non-Hodgkin's lymphoma, forms of lymphoproliferative disease seen in patients with Sjögren's syndrome include low-grade B cell lymphoma and diffuse large B cell lymphoma, including follicular center lymphoma. Less commonly seen lymphoproliferative diseases include lymphocytic leukemia, Waldenström's macroglobulinemia, and multiple myeloma.[53] The risk of other cancers does not appear to be particularly high in patients with Sjögren's syndrome.[53,54] The development of lymphoma and malignancy in patients with Sjögren's syndrome does not appear to affect or cause mortality.[8,54]

The pathoetiology of lymphoproliferative diseases occurring in patients with Sjögren's syndrome is unclear. It is likely that the B cell activation characteristic of Sjögren's syndrome is a predisposing risk factor. Most lymphomas in Sjögren's syndrome appear to arise from lymphoepithelial sialadenitis or benign lymphoepithelial lesions, perhaps associated with *p35* mutations.[55] Infectious agents such as hepatitis C and Epstein-Barr virus have been implicated, although the nature of this relationship remains speculative. *Helicobacter pylori* is associated with MALT (mucosa-associated lymphoid tissue) lymphoma in Sjögren's syndrome.[56]

Appropriate evaluation in symptomatic patients should include diagnostic testing for *H. pylori* in this setting.[57] The link of cancer in Sjögren's syndrome to the proto-oncogene *Bcl-2* translocation is, as yet, not clearly defined but may be helpful for early detection of malignancy.[58]

Vasculitis

KEY POINT

It is unclear whether the risk of cancer development is increased in vasculitis independent of drug treatment effects.

Vasculitis as a paraneoplastic syndrome may be present in about 8% of patients with malignancy.[59] Not as well studied is the risk of primary malignancy in patients with vasculitis. Most cases appear to be related to treatment, although one study using the Danish Cancer Registry suggested an increased risk of nonmelanoma within 2 years of the vasculitis diagnosis in anti-neutrophil cytoplasmic antibody (ANCA)-associated vasculitis (AAV) (granulomatosis with polyangiitis [GPA]) (OR, 4.0; 95% CI, 1.4 to 12).[60]

Current data do not support a link between AAV (GPA) and malignancy as a trigger for vasculitis, or the vasculitis itself as a trigger for malignancy, independent of treatment effects. However, data from several studies suggest a standardized incidence ratio of cancer in AAV of 1.6 to 2.0 compared to the general population and a possibly higher risk in GPA than in microscopic polyangiitis (MPA).[61]

The risk of malignancy among patients with giant cell arteritis was not increased in a population-based study of 204 patients with giant cell arteritis and 407 age- and sex-matched controls.[62]

Seronegative Spondyloarthritis

KEY POINT

The overall risk of cancer does not appear to be increased in the seronegative spondyloarthropathies.

The risk of cancer among patients with spondyloarthropathies is not as well studied as that of patients with rheumatoid arthritis and other connective tissue diseases. A cohort study of 665 patients from Canada with psoriatic arthritis revealed an SIR for all cancers of 0.98 (95% CI, 0.77 to 1.24) without evidence of increase in cancer type–specific SIR for hematologic, lung, or breast cancer.[63]

Most studies of patients with ankylosing spondylitis report no increased risk of cancer. These include a Swedish national cohort and population-based cohort study of patients with ankylosing spondylitis from Australia.[64,65] In contrast, an increased rate of cancer in Asians with ankylosing spondylitis was reported using national health insurance system data in Taiwan. Matching each of 5452 patients with four comparators, the SIR for all cancers was 1.15 (95% CI, 1.03 to 1.27).[66]

SIR was highest for hematologic malignancy 2.10 (1.32, 3.19). The cancer risk was reported to be higher in the first 3 years following diagnosis of ankylosing spondylitis.[66]

Cancer Risks Associated With Anti-rheumatic Drug Therapies

KEY POINTS

The effect on cancer risk of therapies used in the treatment of autoimmune rheumatic diseases can be difficult to separate from the underlying risk intrinsic to the diseases themselves.

Nonsteroidal anti-inflammatory drugs and glucocorticosteroids have not been associated with increased risk of cancer.

The risk of cancer with chemotherapeutic drugs is greatest in patients who have had the highest cumulative exposure to these agents.

Chronic active inflammation is related to increased risk of lymphoma in RA. Effective management of the underlying disease may reduce this risk.

Assessment of risk associated with both nonbiologic and biologic DMARDs is challenging because of the overall generally high burden of cancer in the population, the variable rheumatic disease–related cancer risk, and the potential risk of cancer associated with agents used to treat them. Disease severity may be a risk factor for developing cancer, introducing confounding or channeling bias if patients with severe disease are treated more intensively with immunomodulatory agents. The sequential and combined use of immunomodulatory agents further complicate the assessment of risk related to individual agents. A further concern, as with all immunosuppressive drugs, is the oncogenic potential of immunosuppressive therapies in patients who have a preexistent or concurrent cancer, and whether such patients should be treated with DMARDs, and if so, which DMARDs should be given. Major guidelines for management of rheumatic diseases lack recommendations for DMARD use in patients with preexisting malignancies[67,68]

Nonsteroidal anti-inflammatory agents and glucocorticosteroids do not appear to be associated with increased risk of malignancy in patients with rheumatoid arthritis or other rheumatic diseases.[69] In a large population-based cohort study from Sweden, a total duration of oral corticosteroid treatment of less than 2 years was not associated with lymphoma risk (OR, 0.87; 95% CI, 0.51 to 1.5), whereas treatment lasting longer than 2 years was associated with a lower lymphoma risk (OR, 0.43; 95% CI, 0.26 to 0.72).[70] The duration of rheumatoid arthritis at initiation of oral corticosteroids did not affect lymphoma risk. Whether this observed reduced lymphoma risk may be due to decreased disease activity, is a generic effect of corticosteroids, or is specific to rheumatoid arthritis is uncertain.[70]

Nonbiologic DMARD Therapy

KEY POINTS

The nonbiologic disease-modifying anti-rheumatic drugs gold, hydroxychloroquine, penicillamine, and sulfasalazine are not associated with increased risk of cancer.

The risk of lymphoma, especially B cell lymphoma, may be increased with methotrexate. Some patients may experience regression with discontinuation of methotrexate.

Use of azathioprine is associated with increased risk of lymphoma, and alkylating agents are particularly associated with increased risk of several types of malignancies, including bladder and lung cancer and leukemia in patients treated with cyclophosphamide.

The nonbiologic (nb-)DMARDs sulfasalazine and hydroxychloroquine and gold and penicillamine do not appear to be associated with increased risk of cancer. Radiation is no longer used for the treatment of rheumatic diseases and will not be further addressed. Although no increase in cancer occurrence has been reported, a paucity of data is available regarding the long-term risks of malignancies occurring with leflunomide.[71]

All of the anti-metabolites used in prevention of transplant rejection and treatment of cancer have tumorigenic potential and, in general, may, or do, confer an increased risk of malignancy. The risk of cancer is increased with chemotherapeutic nb-DMARDs, particularly cyclophosphamide, and the risk of certain cancers, particularly lymphoproliferative disorders, may be increased with the use of other nb-DMARDs, such as azathioprine, methotrexate, and cyclosporine, although data are relatively sparse. Data regarding cancer risk in rheumatic diseases in patients treated with mycophenolate mofetil are few, although cancers clearly do occur in patients treated with this drug.[72]

Overall risk for cancer in patients with rheumatoid arthritis treated with nb-DMARDs was found to be 28% higher compared to the general population in a review of 3771 patients from the British Society for Rheumatology Biologics Register.[73] The cancer risk appears to be greatest in patients who have had highest cumulative exposure to DMARDs, compared with patients with less than 1 year of exposure (SIR, 4.82).[74] Exposure to azathioprine, cyclosporine, or cyclophosphamide increased the relative risk for cancer 65% in the British study, although only 367 patients had taken one of these drugs.[73]

Methotrexate

The overall malignancy risk attributable to methotrexate treatment in patients with rheumatic diseases does not appear to be increased, although numerous studies suggest that the risk of lymphoproliferative disease may be increased.

Most cases of methotrexate-associated lymphomas reported in the literature are B cell lymphomas, often with extranodal involvement.[75] Assays for EBV in one study revealed that 7 of 17 patients (41%) were positive.[75] Further evidence supporting a link between methotrexate use and the development of lymphoma comes from observations of spontaneous remission of B cell lymphoma in 8 of 50 cases, including four that were positive for EBV.[75] This suggests that methotrexate may potentiate persistent immunologic stimulation, clonal selection, and malignant transformation of B cells by direct oncogenic action, decreased apoptosis of infected B cells, and decreased natural killer cell activity.[75]

Azathioprine

The use of azathioprine may be associated with increased risk of lymphoproliferative disorders. Studies from a Canadian azathioprine registry revealed increased rates of lymphoproliferative disorders in patients with rheumatoid arthritis compared with the general population (SIR, 8.05).[76] A study from Britain also revealed a markedly increased risk of development of lymphoma in rheumatoid arthritis patients treated with azathioprine, with an estimated one case of lymphoma per 1000 patient-years of azathioprine treatment.[77] Risk was highest in patients on higher daily doses of azathioprine of up to 300 mg per day.

The risk of leukemia in patients with SLE treated with azathioprine has been generally reported as not increased, although one study reported an increase in risk.[78] In up to 24 years of longitudinal follow-up, 5.4% of patients treated with azathioprine developed malignancies, none of which were lymphomas, compared with 6.7% of patients who had never received azathioprine, three of whom developed lymphoma.[78]

Cyclosporine

Relatively few patients with rheumatic diseases treated with cyclosporine have been followed for protracted periods, making assessment of malignancy risk in these patients difficult. Similar to methotrexate, cyclosporine has been associated with the development of EBV-associated lymphomas in a few patients with rheumatoid arthritis.[79] A retrospective study aggregating experience from clinical trials of more than 1000 patients with rheumatoid arthritis treated with cyclosporine failed to demonstrate an increased risk of malignancy, at least beyond that seen with other DMARDs.[80]

Alkylating Agents

The use of alkylating agents in patients with rheumatoid arthritis, SLE, and vasculitis has been associated with an increase in non-Hodgkin's lymphoma, leukemia, skin cancer, bladder cancer, and solid malignancies.[81,82] Considerably more experience with cyclophosphamide than chlorambucil has been documented in these diseases.

Cyclophosphamide use in rheumatic diseases is associated with an overall increased risk of developing malignancy of between 1.5 and 4.1, compared with controls. This risk is best studied in AAV (especially necrotizing GPA), in which risk is highest for bladder cancers (SIR, 4.8), leukemia (SIR, 5.7), and lymphoma (SIR, 4.2). Bladder cancer is a particular concern, and patients who have been treated with higher doses over longer periods and those who smoke appear to be at especially high risk.[82] Bladder cancer related to cyclophosphamide use may occur within 1 year of initiation of therapy and up to 15 years or longer after discontinuation of cyclophosphamide treatment.[82]

Increased risk of hemorrhagic cystitis of the urinary bladder or development of bladder cancer is due to cyclophosphamide metabolites, especially acrolein. For this reason, current recommendations are to attempt to restrict the use of cyclophosphamide to 6 months or less, and to use it only in life-threatening or organ-threatening disease. The risk of bladder cancer, although probably not the overall malignancy risk, may be less with the use of pulse intravenous cyclophosphamide than with daily oral administration. Some authors advocate concurrent administration of mesna, which inactivates acrolein in the urine. Mesna may be administered intravenously at the time of pulse cyclophosphamide dosing, or by mouth daily, although this is rarely done because of its disagreeable taste.

Biologic Response Modifiers

KEY POINTS

The overall risk of a first, or second cancer associated with biologics used in the treatment of rheumatoid arthritis does not appear to be markedly increased from baseline cancer risk in these patients.

The risk of skin cancer, especially nonmelanoma skin cancer, does appear to be somewhat increased by about 1.5-fold in patients treated with anti–tumor necrosis factor therapy.

Biologic response modifiers target specific pathways involved in the pathogenesis of some rheumatic diseases such as rheumatoid arthritis and spondyloarthritis. The term *targeted* should not imply absolute selectivity between physiologic and pathologic processes with these drugs. It is speculative that the risk of malignancy with use of biologics therapy may be related to the specific biologic mechanisms of the drug. However, a review of 63 randomized clinical trials with 29,423 patients on abatacept, adalimumab, anakinra, certolizumab, etanercept, golimumab, infliximab, rituximab, and tocilizumab for at least 6 months' duration did not find a significantly increased risk of malignancy.[83] An important aspect of all randomized clinical trials of biologics is the exclusion of patients with a history of cancer, sometimes excepting nonmelanoma skin cancer (NMSC).

Anti–tumor Necrosis Factor Agents

Since their introduction, anti-TNF agents have been studied over a wide range of indications. The concern regarding cancer arises from animal models of TNF action, in vitro studies, and studies in humans suggesting that TNF is important in cancer initiation and promotion; indeed, anti-TNF agents may even be beneficial for patients with cancers, although clinical evidence of such a benefit is lacking.[84] An interesting observation of regression of non–small cell lung cancer in a patient receiving anti-TNF therapy has been reported, which adds to the biologic plausibility of a connection between anti-TNF therapies and malignancy in individual patients who may have particular susceptibility.[85]

Cancer does not occur more frequently in patients on anti-TNF agents compared with patients on nb-DMARDs.[86–90] Lymphoma also does not occur more frequently.[87–91] Nonmelanoma skin cancer (NMSC) does not occur more frequently,[88,90,92,93] while melanoma may occur more frequently.[9,94] Table 40.2 contains a list of meta-analyses and cohort studies undertaken to explore anti-TNF treatment and solid cancers, lymphoma NMSC, and melanoma in rheumatoid arthritis.

The possibly increased risk of cancer early after the start of anti-TNF therapy may be a factor in meta-analyses of randomized clinical trials, which have suggested a possibly increased risk of cancer in patients with rheumatoid arthritis treated with these agents. One meta-analysis of nine randomized clinical trials including infliximab and adalimumab found an OR of 2.4 for developing any malignancy for patients receiving infliximab or adalimumab compared with patients receiving placebo.[95] A meta-analysis of randomized controlled trials (RCTs) including 15,418 patients on anti-TNF agents and 7486 randomized to comparators could not refute or verify that individual anti-TNF therapies affect the short-term clinical emergence of cancer.[96]

A pooled analysis of RCT using etanercept, infliximab, or adalimumab attempted to distinguish between the effects of recommended versus higher doses of anti-TNF on the development of malignancy, excluding nonmelanoma skin cancers. Exposure-adjusted analysis revealed ORs of 1.21 (95% CI, 0.79 to 4.28) and 3.04 (95% CI, 0.05 to 9.68) in patients treated with recommended and high doses of anti-TNF agents, respectively.[97]

Results of larger observational studies have not replicated the increased risk of malignancy observed with meta-analytical approaches. In the Swedish Biologics Registry, overall cancer risk was similar in anti-TNF–treated patients with rheumatoid arthritis compared with three different control cohorts.[86] In this database, no trend toward increased cancer incidence was noted with longer duration of TNF exposures. Studies from other databases including the German and British Biologic Registries and North American cohort and administrative databases have detected no significant safety signals with respect to overall cancer risk.[88,89,98,99]

TABLE 40.2 Summary of Observational Studies of Malignancies Occurring in Patients With Rheumatoid Arthritis Treated With Antinecrosis Factor Agents

Study, Reference Number	Registry	Intervention	Control nb-DMARDs	Control/ General Population	Adjusted Hazards Ratio (Intervention vs. Comparator/ Control)	Adjusted Hazards Ratio (Intervention vs. General Population)	Risk of Bias
All Types of Cancer							
Askling, 2009[91]	ARTIS	3 TNFi	nb-DMARDs	General population	TNFi vs. pts starting MTX: 1.0 (0.8, 1.2): TNFi vs./nb-DMARDs combination therapy to 1.0 (0.7, 1.4)	1.1 (1.0, 1.3)	Low
Strangfeld, 2010[89]	RABBIT	3 TNFi + anakinra	nb-DMARDs	General population	TNFi vs. nb-DMARDs 0.7 (0.4, 1.1); ANA vs. nb-DMARDs 1.4 (0.6, 3.5)	0.8 (0.5, 1.0)	Low
Carmona, 2011[87]	BIOBADASER	3 TNFi	nb-DMARDs	General population	0.5 (0.1, 2.5)	0.7 (0.5, 0.9)	Low
Haynes 2013[88]	Claim database	3 TNFi	nb-DMARDs	N/A	0.8 (0.6, 1.1); ever-analysis 0.9 (0.8, 1.1)	N/A	Moderate
Patients With History of Cancer							
Dixon, 2010[99]	BSRBR	3 TNFi	nb-DMARDs	N/A	0.5 (0.1, 2.2); censoring after first cancer 0.5 (0.1, 2.2)	N/A	Low
Dreyer, 2018[101]	DANBIO	5 TNFi + rituximab, abatacept, OR tocilizumab	Nb-DMARDs	Danish Cancer Registry	1.11 (0.74, 1.67) ever; 1.13 (0.71, 1.80) after first cancer	N/A	Low
Lymphoma							
Askling, 2009[64]	ARTIS	3 TNFi	nb-DMARDs	General population	1.4 (0.8, 2.1)	2.7 (1.8, 4.1)	Low
Carmona, 2011[87]	BIOBADASER	3 TNFi	nb-DMARDs	General population	N/A	Hodgkin's, 5.3 (0.1, 29.5); non-Hodgkin's, 1.5 (0.31, 4.4)	Low
Haynes, 2013[88]	Claim database	3 TNFi	nb-DMARDs	N/A	0.8 (0.3, 2.1), ever-analysis 1.3 (0.7, 2.2); any lymphoma or leukemia: 0.7 (0.3, 1.5); ever-analysis 1.0 (0.6, 1.6)	N/A	Moderate
Nonmelanoma Skin Cancer							
Amari, 2011[92]	Claim database	3 TNFi	nb-DMARDs	N/A	1.4 (1.2, 1.6); TNFi vs. MTX 1.4 (1.2, 1.7)	N/A	Moderate
Mercer, 2012[73]	BSRBR	3 TNFi	nb-DMARDs	General population	BCC 1.0 (0.5, 1.7), SCC 1.2 (0.4, 3.8); 1st cancer per subject BCC 0.8 (0.5, 1.5)	1.7 (1.4, 2.0)	Low
Haynes, 2013[88]	Claim database	3 TNFi	nb-DMARDs	N/A	0.8 (0.5, 1.4); ever-analysis 1.1 (0.8, 1.5)	N/A	Moderate

TABLE 40.2 Summary of Observational Studies of Malignancies Occurring in Patients With Rheumatoid Arthritis Treated With Antinecrosis Factor Agents—cont'd

Study, Reference Number	Registry	Intervention	Control nb-DMARDs	Control/ General Population	Adjusted Hazards Ratio (Intervention vs. Comparator/ Control)	Adjusted Hazards Ratio (Intervention vs. General Population)	Risk of Bias
Solomon 2014[112]	CORONA	3 TNFi rituximab abatacept	MTZ	N/A	0.4 (0.1, 1.2) 0.7 (0.0, 13.6) 15.3 (2.1, 114)[a]	N/A	Low
Melanoma							
Raaschou, 2013[94]	ARTIS	5 TNFi	nb-DMARDs	N/A	1.5 (1.0, 2.2)	N/A	Low

[a]Based on two cases.*ANA,* Anakinra; *ARTIS,* Swedish Biologics Register; *BCC,* basal cell carcinoma; *BIOBADASER,* Spanish Biologics Register; *BSRBR,* British Society of Rheumatology Biologics Register; *CORRONA,* Consortium of Rheumatology Researchers of North America; *DANBIO,* Danish Biologics Registry; *MTX,* methotrexate; *nb-DMARDs,* conventional synthetic nonbiologic disease-modifying antirheumatic drugs; *N/A,* not available; *pts.,* patients; *RABBIT,* German Biologics Register; *SCC,* squamous cell carcinoma; *TNFi,* tumor necrosis factor inhibitor.

Modified from Ramiro S, Sepriano A, Chatzidionysiou K, et al: Safety of synthetic and biological DMARDs: a systematic literature review informing the 2016 update of the EULAR recommendations for management of rheumatoid arthritis. *Ann Rheum Dis* 76:1093, 2017.

Use of anti-TNF agents may be associated with increased risk of nonmelanoma skin cancer. An OR for nonmelanoma skin cancer of 1.5 (95% CI, 1.2 to 1.8) was reported from the U.S. National Databank of Rheumatic Diseases.[98] A cohort study from this population suggested that the combination of anti-TNF plus methotrexate versus control was associated with a higher risk of nonmelanoma skin cancer (HR, 1.97; 95% CI, 1.51 to 2.58) compared with an HR of 1.24 (95% CI, 0.97 to 1.58) in patients receiving anti-TNF monotherapy versus controls, while a study using a large clinical database found no difference in risk of nonmelanoma skin cancer in patients on anti-TNF compared to those on methotrexate.[98,100] The possible potentiating effects of combination therapies for the development of cancers is perhaps underlined by observations from a randomized clinical trial of 180 patients with ANCA-associated GPA vasculitis. The occurrence of solid and skin malignancies in the group assigned to etanercept was increased above that expected from treatment with cyclophosphamide alone.[100]

Discordant results regarding cancer risk are likely explained by different patient populations and differing drug exposures. Meta-analyses of clinical trials generally reflect relatively short-term effects but offer the advantage of randomization, which should largely neutralize the variability introduced by individual comorbidities and previous drug exposures; long-term observational studies place more emphasis on mid- and long-term results. In either case, if cancer events occur in a nonlinear fashion with early dropout of individuals at risk for cancer, a conclusive analysis, even after several years of follow-up, may be unable to capture such a signal.

A crucial clinical question is whether patients with pre-existent cancers should be exposed to anti-TNF or other immunomodulatory therapies. Patients with pre-existent malignancies are generally excluded from clinical trials, and in clinical practice, clinicians may be reluctant to treat such patients with anti-TNF therapy, resulting in channeling of treatment with these agents toward low-risk cohorts. Thus far, two registry and two population-based studies have failed to detect an increased risk of recurrent or second cancer in patients treated with anti-TNF agents.[86,99,101,102] However, relatively few events were included in these analyses, so definite conclusions about overall or cancer-specific risks in individual patients cannot be drawn, although the most recent population-based study from Sweden reported not only no increase in overall cancer risk, but also no difference in mortality between patients with previous cancer who had been exposed to anti-TNF compared to non-anti–TNF exposed patients.[102]

Rituximab

B cells appear to be involved in generation of antitumor responses and are important in maintaining inflammatory states, which promote carcinogenesis and tumor growth. The absence of B cells, for example, in hypogammaglobulinemia, has not been associated with increased susceptibility to cancers, and B cell depletion with rituximab slows the growth of solid nonhematopoietic murine tumors.[103]

Pooled analysis of safety data from patients with rheumatoid arthritis treated with rituximab in RCT with more than 5000 patient-years of exposure revealed an incidence of malignancy excluding nonmelanoma skin cancer of 0.84 per 1000 patient-years (SIR, 1.05; 95% CI, 0.76 to 1.42).[104] The incidence appeared to be stable over multiple courses of rituximab, and no unusual pattern of malignancy type was observed.

Abatacept

Abatacept is a fusion protein consisting of the extra-cellular domain of human cytotoxic T lymphocyte–associated antigen-4 (CTLA-4) linked to the Fc portion of human immunoglobulin. CTLA-4–mediated T cell suppression has been suggested to be important in the pathogenesis of several types of malignancies, especially malignant melanoma.[105] Because abatacept blocks the same signal that new anticancer treatments based on this interaction are intended to enhance, theoretically a potentially increased risk of malignancies may be seen with the use of this biologic. So far, however, no signal for increased malignancy risk including lung cancers has been noted in patients treated with this agent.[83,106]

Tocilizumab

Tocilizumab is a humanized monoclonal antibody to the IL-6 receptor. IL-6 has an important role in inflammation and in the promotion of various types of malignancies, including suppression of apoptosis, promotion of angiogenesis, and induction of genes that mediate cell proliferation.[107]

Data from studies of rheumatoid arthritis, the disease in which experience with this agent is most extensive, so far have not revealed any signals of an increased incidence of cancer.[83] Labeling information for tocilizumab contains a general statement that "treatment with immunosuppressants may result in an increased risk of cancer," but no specific warnings are included.

Anakinra

The IL-1 receptor antagonist, anakinra, has been best studied in rheumatoid arthritis. As is the case for most studies of biologic response modifiers, methotrexate usually has been administered concomitantly. The case rate for the development of malignant lymphoma with anakinra is 0.12 cases per 100 patient-years, with eight cases of lymphoma observed among 5300 patients with rheumatoid arthritis treated with this drug in clinical trials for a mean of 15 months.[108] This represents a 3.6-fold higher than expected rate of lymphoma compared with the general population. The SIR for lymphoma in this study (3.71; 95% CI, 0.77 to 11.0) is consistent with ORs from other studies of patients with rheumatoid arthritis. A number of solid tumors have also been reported with this agent.[83]

Tofacitinib

Like most other disease-modifying anti-rheumatic drugs, the janus kinase 3-inhibitor tofacitinib carries an FDA black box warning regarding the potential risk for malignancy. To date, no signals of increased malignancy risk have emerged from 19 trials including 6194 patients.[109,110]

Cancer Screening in Patients With Rheumatic Disease

Evidence of cancer risk in patients with rheumatic diseases forms the basis for clinically useful recommendations regarding cancer screening. First, with respect to management of the inflammatory disease, it is imperative to achieve optimal disease control and the lowest level of clinical disease activity possible using the least intensive treatment regimen available. Second, patients for whom immunomodulatory therapy, including nb-DMARDs and biologic DMARDs, is being contemplated should undergo routine cancer screening that is appropriate to their age, sex, familial cancer burden, and risk factors such as smoking. Third, because cancers may develop at an accelerated rate in the first few months to the first year or so of treatment, patients should be seen at frequent intervals and closely questioned and examined for signs and symptoms of malignancy, especially during this initial treatment period, and throughout the course of their disease.

Routine blood counts and differential blood cell counts should be performed at the initiation of treatment and as appropriate for the specific drug therapy used. Age- and sex-appropriate cancer screening for colorectal cancer, prostate cancer, breast cancer, and cervical cancer is advisable. In patients with particularly high cancer risk, such as dermatomyositis, assessment for tumor markers such as CA-125 and radiographic imaging of chest, abdomen, and pelvis may be appropriate yearly in the first year or two of the disease, and then as otherwise clinically indicated.[111]

Patients taking alkylating agents such as cyclophosphamide may be at particularly high risk of cancer. These patients certainly should undergo routine cancer screening Pap smears and urinalyses for at least 15 years from cyclophosphamide therapy. With these considerations, the morbidity and mortality experienced by patients with rheumatic disease can be favorably managed.

Conclusion

Assessment of risk for malignancy in patients with rheumatic diseases is complex. Some rheumatic diseases such as dermatomyositis and Sjögren's syndrome appear to confer a particularly high risk of cancers, particularly lymphoproliferative disorders. Many of these diseases are relatively rare, so that large patient cohorts required for more precise assessment of risk are not available or must be studied over long periods of time to develop stable risk estimates.

Malignancy and perineoplastic syndrome should be considered when patients present with musculoskeletal symptoms caused by an underlying malignancy, or noted as symptoms and signs associated with the presence of an underlying malignancy in a patient with a preexistent autoimmune disease.

Most of the agents used in the treatment of these diseases are purposefully employed to modulate the immune response, and some, including the alkylating agents, are known carcinogens. Others may modulate immune response to decrease tumor surveillance. Further complicating the assessment are the individual susceptibility host factors, including the presence of oncogenic genes such as *Blc*-2, and family history and environmental factors such as viruses, which may enhance the carcinogenic potential of the treatments.

Recommendations for treatment must include a general understanding of the disease and treatment-related malignancy and individualized discussion with the patient regarding risks and benefits of treatment as they relate to disease activity and severity and, most importantly, patient preference.

The references for this chapter can also be found on ExpertConsult.com.

References

1. Shankaran V, Ikeda H, Bruce AT, et al.: IFN gamma and lymphocytes prevent primary tumour development and shape tumour immunogenicity, *Nature* 410:1107, 2001.
2. Vajdic CM, McDonald SP, McCredie MR, et al.: Cancer incidence before and after kidney transplantation, *JAMA* 296:2823, 2006.
3. Balkwill F, Mantovani A: Inflammation and cancer: back to Virchow? *Lancet* 357:539, 2001.
4. Ljung R, Talbäck M, Haglund B, et al.: *Cancer incidence in Sweden 2005*, Stockholm, 2007, National Board of Health and Welfare.
5. Landgren O, Engels EA, Pfeiffer RM, et al.: Autoimmunity and susceptibility to Hodgkin lymphoma: a population-based case-control study in Scandinavia, *J Natl Cancer Inst* 98:1321, 2006.
6. Franklin J, Lunt M, Bunn D, et al.: Influence of inflammatory polyarthritis on cancer incidence and survival: results from a community-based prospective study, *Arthritis Rheum* 56:790, 2007.
7. Mellemkjaer L, Linet MS, Gridley G, et al.: Rheumatoid arthritis and cancer risk, *Eur J Cancer* 32:1753, 1996.
8. Wolfe F, Michaud K: Lymphoma in rheumatoid arthritis: the effect of methotrexate and anti-tumor necrosis factor therapy in 18,572 patients, *Arthritis Rheum* 50:1740, 2004.
9. Simon TA, Thompson A, Gandhi KK, et al.: Incidence of malignancy in adult patients with rheumatoid arthritis: a meta-analysis, *Arthritis Res Ther* 17:212, 2015.

10. Franklin J, Lunt M, Bunn D, et al.: Incidence of lymphoma in a large primary care derived cohort of cases of inflammatory polyarthritis, *Ann Rheum Dis* 65:617, 2006.
11. Baecklung E, Iliadou A, Askling J, et al.: Association of chronic inflammation, not its treatment, with increased lymphoma risk in rheumatoid arthritis, *Arthritis Rheum* 54:692, 2006.
12. Gridley G, Klippel JH, Hoover RN, et al.: Incidence of cancer among men with Felty syndrome, *Ann Intern Med* 120:35, 1994.
13. Lamy T, Loughran Jr TP: Current concepts: large granular lymphocyte leukemia, *Blood Rev* 13:230, 1999.
14. Berkel H, Holcombe RF, Middlebrooks M, et al.: Nonsteroidal anti-inflammatory drugs and colorectal cancer, *Epidemiol Rev* 18:205, 1996.
15. Bernatsky S, Ramsey-Goldman R, Labrecque J, et al.: Cancer risk in systemic lupus: an updated international multi-centre cohort study, *J Autoimmun* 42:130, 2013.
16. Lofstrom B, Backlin C, Sundstrom C, et al.: A closer look at non-Hodgkin's lymphoma cases in a national Swedish systemic lupus erythematosus cohort: a nested case-control study, *Ann Rheum Dis* 66:1627, 2007.
17. Xu Y, Wiernik PH: Systemic lupus erythematosus and B-cell hematologic neoplasm, *Lupus* 10:841, 2001.
18. Parikh-Patel AR, White H, Allen M, et al.: Cancer risk in a cohort of patients with systemic lupus erythematosus (SLE) in California, *Cancer Causes Control* 19:887, 2008.
19. Bernatsky S, Boivin JF, Joseph L, et al.: Race/ethnicity and cancer occurrence in systemic lupus erythematosus, *Arthritis Rheum* 53:781, 2005.
20. Gayed M, Bernatsky S, Ramsey-Goldman R, et al.: Lupus and cancer, *Lupus* 18:479, 2009.
21. Lofstrom B, Backlin C, Sundstrom C, et al.: Myeloid leukemia in systemic lupus erythematosus: a nested case-control study based on Swedish registers, *Rheumatology* 48:1222, 2009.
22. King JK, Costenbader KH: Characteristics of patients with systemic lupus erythematosus (SLE) and non-Hodgkin's lymphoma (NHL), *Clin Rheumatol* 26:1491, 2007.
23. Bernatsky SR, Cooper GS, Mill C, et al.: Cancer screening in patients with systemic lupus erythematosus, *J Rheumatol* 33:45, 2006.
24. Dhar JP, Kmak D, Bhan R, et al.: Abnormal cervicovaginal cytology in women with lupus: a retrospective cohort study, *Gynecol Oncol* 82(4), 2001.
25. Rosenthal AK, McLaughlin JK, Linet MS, et al.: Scleroderma and malignancy: an epidemiological study, *Ann Rheum Dis* 52:531, 1993.
26. Chatterjee S, Dombi GW, Severson RK, et al.: Risk of malignancy in scleroderma: a population-based cohort study, *Arthritis Rheum* 52:2415, 2005.
27. Onishi A, Sugiyama D, Kumagai S, et al.: Cancer incidence in systemic sclerosis: meta-analysis of population-based cohort studies, *Arthritis Rheum* 65:1913, 2013.
28. Derk CT, Rasheed M, Artlett CM, et al.: A cohort study of cancer incidence in systemic sclerosis, *J Rheumatol* 33:1113, 2006.
29. Wipff J, Allanore Y, Soussi F, et al.: Prevalence of Barrett's esophagus in systemic sclerosis, *Arthritis Rheum* 52:2882, 2005.
30. Bernatsky S, Hudson M, Pope J, et al.: Reports of abnormal cervical cancer screening tests in systemic sclerosis, *Rheumatology* 48:149, 2009.
31. Pontifex EK, Hill CL, Roberts-Thomson P: Risk factors for lung cancer in patients with scleroderma: a nested case-control study, *Ann Rheum Dis* 66:551, 2007.
32. Moinzadeh P, Fonseca C, Hellmich M, et al.: Association of anti-RNA polymerase III autoantibodies and cancer in scleroderma, *Arthritis Res Ther* 16:R53, 2014.
33. Joseph CG, Farah E, Shah AA: Association of the autoimmune disease scleroderma with an immunologic response to cancer, *Science* 343:152, 2014.
34. Rosenthal AK, McLaughlin JK, Gridley G, et al.: Incidence of cancer among patients with systemic sclerosis, *Cancer* 76:910, 1995.
35. Fiorentino DF, Chung LS, Christopher-Stine L, et al.: Most patients with cancer-associated dermatomyositis have antibodies to nuclear matrix protein NXP-2 or transcription intermediary factor 1γ, *Arthritis Rheum* 65:2954, 2013.
36. Yang Z, Lin F, Qin B, et al.: Polymyositis/dermatomyositis and malignancy risk: a metaanalysis study, *J Rheumatol* 42:282, 2015.
37. Shah AA, Casciola-Rosen L, Rosen A: Cancer-induced autoimmunity in the rheumatic diseases, *Arthritis Rheumatol* 67:317, 2015.
38. Sigurgeirsson B, Lindelof B, Edhag O, et al.: Risk of cancer in patients with dermatomyositis or polymyositis, *N Engl J Med* 326:363, 1992.
39. Buchbinder F, Forbes A, Hall S, et al.: Incidence of malignant disease in biopsy-proven inflammatory myopathy, *Ann Intern Med* 134:1087, 2001.
40. Lakhanpal S, Bunch TW, Ilstrup DM, et al.: Polymyositis-dermatomyositis and malignant lesions: does an association exist? *Mayo Clin Proc* 61:645, 1986.
41. Zantos D, Zhang Y, Felson D, et al.: The overall and temporal association of cancer with polymyositis and dermatomyositis, *J Rheumatol* 21:1855, 1994.
42. Huang YL, Chen YJ, Lin MW, et al.: Malignancies associated with dermatomyositis and polymyositis in Taiwan: a nationwide population-based study, *Br J Dermatol* 161:854, 2009.
43. Bendewald MJ, Wetter DA, Li X, et al.: Incidence of dermatomyositis and clinically amyopathic dermatomyositis: a population-based study in Olmsted County, *Arch Dermatol* 146:26, 2010.
44. Casciola-Rosen L, Nagaraju K, Plotz P, et al.: Enhanced autoantigen expression in regenerating muscle cells in idiopathic inflammatory myopathy, *J Exp Med* 201:591, 2005.
45. Hidano A, Kaneko K, Arai Y, et al.: Survey of the prognosis for dermatomyositis with special reference to its association with malignancy and pulmonary fibrosis, *J Dermatol* 13:233, 1986.
46. Fudman EJ, Schnitzer TJ: Dermatomyositis without creatine kinase elevation: a poor prognostic sign, *Am J Med* 80:329, 1986.
47. Hunger RE, Durr C, Brand CU: Cutaneous leukocytoclastic vasculitis in dermatomyositis suggests malignancy, *Dermatology* 202:123, 2001.
48. Fardet L, Dupuy A, Gain M, et al.: Factors associated with underlying malignancy in a retrospective cohort of 121 patients with dermatomyositis, *Medicine* 88:91, 2009.
49. Rothfield N, Kurtzman S, Vazquez-Abad D, et al.: Association of anti-topoisomerase I with cancer, *Arthritis Rheum* 35:724, 1992.
50. Liang Y, Yang Z, Qin B, et al.: Primary Sjögren's syndrome and malignancy risk: a systematic review and meta-analysis, *Ann Rheum Dis* 73:1151, 2014.
51. Smedby KE, Hjalgrim H, Askling J, et al.: Autoimmune and chronic inflammatory disorders and risk of non-Hodgkin's lymphoma by subtype, *J Natl Cancer Inst* 98:51, 2006.
52. Nocture G, Mariette X: Sjögren syndrome-associated lymphomas: an update on pathogenesis and management, *Br J Haematol* 168:317, 2015.
53. Pertovaara M, Pukkala E, Laippala P, et al.: A longitudinal cohort study of Finnish patients with primary Sjögren's syndrome: clinical, immunological, and epidemiological aspects, *Ann Rheum Dis* 60:467, 2001.
54. Theander E, Henriksson G, Ljungbery O, et al.: Lymphoma and other malignancies in primary Sjögren's syndrome, *Ann Rheum Dis* 65:796, 2006.
55. Tapinos NI, Polihronis M, Moutsopoulos HM, et al.: Lymphoma development in Sjögren's syndrome: novel p53 mutations, *Arthritis Rheum* 42:1466, 1999.
56. Voulgarelis M, Moutsopoulos HM: Mucosa-associated lymphoid tissue lymphoma in Sjögren's syndrome: risks, management, and prognosis, *Rheum Dis Clin N Am* 34:921, 2008.

57. Raderer M, Osterreicher C, Machold K, et al.: Impaired response of gastric MALT-lymphoma to Helicobacter pylori eradication in patients with autoimmune disease, *Ann Oncol* 12:937, 2001.
58. Takacs I, Zeher M, Urban L, et al.: Frequency and evaluation of (14;18) translocations in Sjögren's syndrome, *Ann Hematol* 79:444, 2000.
59. Gonzalez-Gay MA, Garcia-Porrua C, Salvarani C, et al.: Cutaneous vasculitis and cancer: a clinical approach, *Clin Exp Rheumatol* 18:305, 2000.
60. Faurschou M, Mellemkjaer L, Sorensen IJ, et al.: Cancer preceding Wegener's granulomatosis: a case-control study, *Rheumatology* 48:421, 2009.
61. Shang W, Ning Y, Xu X, et al.: Incidence of cancer in ANCA-associated vasculitis: a meta-analysis of observational studies, *PLoS One* 10:e0126016, 2015.
62. Kermani TA, Schäfer VS, Crowson CS, et al.: Malignancy risk in patients with giant cell arteritis: a population-based cohort study, *Arthritis Care Res* 62:149, 2010.
63. Rohekar S, Tom B, Hassa A, et al.: Prevalence of malignancy in psoriatic arthritis, *Arthritis Rheum* 58:82, 2007.
64. Askling J, Klareskog L, Blomqvist P, et al.: Risk for malignant lymphoma in ankylosing spondylitis: a nationwide Swedish case-control study, *Ann Rheum Dis* 65:1184, 2006.
65. Oldroyd J, Schachna L, Buchbinder R, et al.: Ankylosing spondylitis patients commencing biologic therapy have high baseline levels of comorbidity: a report from the Australian Rheumatology Association database, *Int J Rheumatol* 10:1155, 2009.
66. Chang C-C, Chang C-W, Nguyen P-AA, et al.: Anklyosing spondylitis and the risk of cancer, *Oncology Let* 14:1315, 2017.
67. Singh JA, Saag KG, Bridges Jr SL, et al.: American College of Rheumatology guideline for the treatment of rheumatoid arthritis, *Arthritis Rheumatol* 68(1):2016, 2015.
68. Smolen JS, Landewé R, Bijlsma J, et al.: EULAR recommendations for the management of rheumatoid arthritis with synthetic and biological disease-modifying antirheumatic drugs: 2016 update, *Ann Rheum Dis* 76(9), 2017.
69. Bernatsky S, Lee JL, Rahme E, et al.: Non-Hodgkin's lymphoma-meta-analyses of the effects of corticosteroids and non-steroidal anti-inflammatories, *Rheumatology (Oxford)* 46:690, 2007.
70. Hellgren K, Iliadou A, Rosenquist R, et al.: Rheumatoid arthritis, treatment with corticosteroids and risk of malignant lymphomas: results from a case-control study, *Ann Rheum Dis* 69:654, 2010.
71. Initial scientific discussion for the approval of Arava (PDF file). www.ema.europa.eu/docs/en_GB/document_library/EPAR_Scientific_Discussion/human/000235/WC500026286.pdf.
72. Dasgupta N, Gelber AC, Racke F, et al.: Central nervous system lymphoma associated with mycophenolate mofetil in lupus nephritis, *Lupus* 14:910, 2005.
73. Mercer LK, Davies R, Galloway JB, et al.: Risk of cancer in patients receiving non-biologic disease-modifying therapy for rheumatoid arthritis compared with the UK general population, *Rheumatology* 52:91, 2013.
74. Asten P, Barrett J, Symmons D, et al.: Risk of developing certain malignancies is related to duration of immunosuppressive drug exposure in patients with rheumatic diseases, *J Rheumatol* 26:1705, 1999.
75. Georgescu L, Quinn GC, Schwartzman S, et al.: Lymphoma in patients with rheumatoid arthritis: association with the disease state or methotrexate treatment, *Semin Arthritis Rheum* 26:794, 1997.
76. Matteson EL, Hickey AR, Maguire L, et al.: Occurrence of neoplasia in patients with rheumatoid arthritis enrolled in a DMARD registry: rheumatoid arthritis azathioprine registry Steering Committee, *J Rheumatol* 18:809, 1991.
77. Silman AJ, Petrie J, Hazleman B, et al.: Lymphoproliferative cancer and other malignancy in patients with rheumatoid arthritis treated with azathioprine: a 20-year follow-up study, *Ann Rheum Dis* 47:988, 1988.
78. Nero P, Rahman A, Isenberg DA, et al.: Does long-term treatment with azathioprine predispose to malignancy and death in patients with systemic lupus erythematosus? *Ann Rheum Dis* 63:325, 2004.
79. Zijlmans JM, van Rijthoven AW, Kluin PM, et al.: Epstein-Barr virus-associated lymphoma in a patient with rheumatoid arthritis treated with cyclosporine, *N Engl J Med* 326:1363, 1992.
80. Arellano F, Krupp P: Malignancies in rheumatoid arthritis patients treated with cyclosporin A, *Br J Rheumatol* 32(Suppl 1):72, 1993.
81. Vasquez S, Kavanaugh AF, Schneider NR, et al.: Acute non-lymphocytic leukemia after treatment of systemic lupus erythematosus with immunosuppressive agents, *J Rheumatol* 19:1625, 1992.
82. Radis CD, Kahl LE, Baker GL, et al.: Effects of cyclophosphamide on the development of malignancy and on long-term survival in patients with rheumatoid arthritis: a 20-year follow-up study, *Arthritis Rheum* 38:1120, 1995.
83. Lopez-Olivo MA, Tayar JH, Martinez-Lopez, et al.: Risk of malignancies in patients with rheumatoid arthritis treated with biologic therapy: a meta-analysis, *JAMA* 308:898, 2012.
84. Madhusudan S, Muthuramalingam SR, Braybrooke JP, et al.: Study of etanercept, a tumor necrosis factor-alpha inhibitor, in recurrent ovarian cancer, *J Clin Oncol* 23:5950, 2005.
85. Lees CW, Ironside J, Wallace WA, et al.: Resolution of non-small-cell lung cancer after withdrawal of anti-TNF therapy, *N Engl J Med* 359:320, 2008.
86. Askling J, van Vollenhoven RF, Granath F, et al.: Cancer risk in patients with rheumatoid arthritis treated with anti-tumor necrosis factor alpha therapies: does the risk change with the time since start of treatment? *Arthritis Rheum* 60(3180):87, 2009.
87. Carmona L, Abasolo L, Descalzo MA, et al.: Cancer in patients with rheumatic diseases exposed to TNF antagonists, *Semin Arthritis Rheum* 41:71, 2011.
88. Haynes K, Beukelman T, Curtis JR, et al.: Tumor necrosis factor alpha inhibitor therapy and cancer risk in chronic immune-mediated diseases, *Arthritis Rheum* 65:48, 2013.
89. Strangfeld A, Hierse F, Rau R, et al.: Risk of incident or recurrent malignancies among patients with rheumatoid arthritis exposed to biologic therapy in the German Biologics register RABBIT, *Arthritis Res Ther* 12:R5, 2010.
90. Ramiro S, Sepriano A, Chatzidionysiou K, et al.: Safety of synthetic and biological DMARDs: a systematic literature review informing the 2016 update of the EULAR recommendations for management of rheumatoid arthritis, *Ann Rheum Dis* 76:1093, 2017.
91. Askling J, Baecklund E, Granath F, et al.: Anti-tumour necrosis factor therapy in rheumatoid arthritis and risk of malignant lymphomas: relative risks and time trends in the Swedish Biologics Register, *Ann Rheum Dis* 68:648, 2009.
92. Amari W, Zeringue AL, McDonald JR, et al.: Risk of non-melanoma skin cancer in a national cohort of veterans with rheumatoid arthritis, *Rheumatology* 50:1431, 2011.
93. Mercer LK, Green AC, Galloway JB, et al.: The influence of anti-TNF therapy upon incidence of keratinocyte skin cancer in patients with rheumatoid arthritis: longitudinal results from the British Society for Rheumatology Biologics Register, *Ann Rheum Dis* 71:869, 2012.
94. Raaschou P, Simaard JF, Holmqvist M, et al.: Rheumatoid arthritis, anti-tumour necrosis factor therapy, and risk of malignant melanoma: nationwide population based prospective cohort study from Sweden, *BMJ* 346:f1939, 2013.
95. Bongartz T, Sutton AJ, Sweeting MJ, et al.: Anti-TNF antibody therapy in rheumatoid arthritis and the risk of serious infections and malignancies: systematic review and meta-analysis of rare harmful effects in randomized controlled trials, *JAMA* 295:2275, 2006.
96. Askling J, Fahrbach K, Nordstrom B, et al.: Cancer risk with numor necrosis factor alpha (TNF) inhibitors: meta-analysis of randomized controlled trials of adalimumab, etanercept, and infliximab using patient level data, *Pharmacoepi Drug Safety* 20:119, 2011.

97. Leombruno JP, Einarson TR, Keystone EC, et al.: The safety of anti-tumor necrosis factor treatments in rheumatoid arthritis: meta and exposure adjusted pooled analysis of serious adverse events, *Ann Rheum Dis* 68:1136, 2009.
98. Wolfe F, Michaud K: Biologic treatment of rheumatoid arthritis and the risk of malignancy: analyses from a large US observational study, *Arthritis Rheum* 56:2886, 2007.
99. Dixon WG, Watson KD, Lunt M, et al.: The influence of anti-tumor necrosis factor therapy on cancer incidence in patients with rheumatoid arthritis who have had a prior malignancy: results from the British Society for Rheumatology Biologics Register, *Arthritis Rheum* 62:775, 2010.
100. Stone JH, Holbrook JT, Marriott MA, et al.: Solid malignancies among patients in the Wegener's granulomatosis etanercept trial, *Arthritis Rheum* 54:1608, 2006.
101. Dreyer L, Cordtz RL, Hansen IMJ, et al.: Risk of second malignant neoplasm and mortality in patients with rheumatoid arthritis treated with biological DMARDs: a Danish population-based cohort study, *Ann Rheum Dis* 77:510, 2018.
102. Raashow P, Söderling J, Turesson C, et al.: Tumor necrosis factor inhibitors and cancer recurrence in Swedish patients with rheumatoid arthritis: a nationwide population-based cohort study, *Ann Intern Med* 169:291, 2018.
103. Kim S, Fridlender ZG, Dunn R, et al.: B-cell depletion using an anti-CD20 antibody augments anti-tumor immune responses and immunotherapy in non-hematopoietic murine tumor models, *J Immunother* 31:446, 2008.
104. Van Vollenhoven RF, Emery P, Bingham 3rd CO, et al.: Long term safety of patients receiving rituximab in rheumatoid arthritis clinical trials, *J Rheumatol* 37:558, 2010.
105. O'Day SJ, Hamid O, Urba WJ, et al.: Targeting cytotoxic T-lymphocyte antigen-4 (CTLA-4): a novel strategy for the treatment of melanoma and other malignancies, *Cancer* 110:2614, 2007.
106. Simon TA, Smitten AL, Franklin J, et al.: Malignancies in the rheumatoid arthritis abatacept clinical development programme: an epidemiological assessment, *Ann Rheum Dis* 68:1819, 2009.
107. Becker C, Fantini MC, Schramm C, et al.: TGF-beta suppresses tumor progression in colon cancer by inhibition of IL-6 trans-signaling, *Immunity* 21:491, 2004.
108. Fleischmann RM, Tesser J, Schiff MH, et al.: Safety of extended treatment with anakinra in patients with rheumatoid arthritis, *Ann Rheum Dis* 65:1006, 2006.
109. Cohen SB, TanakaY Mariette X: Long-term safety of tofacitinib for the treatment of rheumatoid arthritis up to 8.5 years: integrated analysis of data from the global clinical trials, *Ann Rheum Dis* 76:1253, 2017.
110. Mariette X, Chen C, Biswas P, et al.: Lymphoma in the tofacitinib rheumatoid arthritis clinical development program, *Arthritis Care Res* 70:685, 2018.
111. Chow WH, Gridley G, Mellemkjaer L, et al.: Cancer risk following polymyositis and dermatomyositis: a nationwide cohort study in Denmark, *Cancer Causes Control* 6(9), 1995.
112. Solomon DH, Kremer JM, Fisher m, et al.: Comparative cancer risk associated with methotrexate, other non-biologic and biologic disease-modifying anti-rheumatic drugs, *Semin Arthritis Rheum* 43:489, 2014.

41 Introduction to Physical Medicine and Rehabilitation

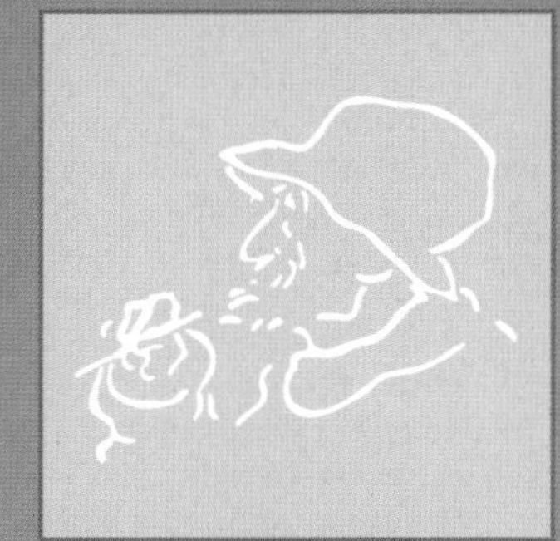

SARA J. CUCCURULLO, JACLYN JOKI, AND OFURE LUKE

KEY POINTS

- Physical medicine and rehabilitation (PM&R) uses a multidisciplinary approach to maximize quality of life and improve function.
- Coordinated care of the rheumatologic patient should co-exist between the medical and rehabilitation teams.
- The goals of rehabilitation are to alleviate pain, prevent joint deformity, conserve energy, and restore and/or maintain function.
- Rest, exercise, physical modalities, and orthoses are treatment options to reduce pain and improve function.
- Assistive and adaptive devices, as well as home and environmental modifications, can improve activities of daily living and facilitate integration within the community.
- Patient-centered comprehensive care, including education, is essential to help patients achieve their individual goals.

Introduction

Physical medicine and rehabilitation (PM&R), also known as *physiatry*, is an American Board of Medical Specialties specialty focused on enhancing and restoring functional ability and quality of life. PM&R physicians treat people with physical impairments or disabilities that affect the neurologic, musculoskeletal, and cardiopulmonary systems. The goals of PM&R are to maximize independence with activities of daily living (ADLs) and mobility, optimize quality of life, minimize dysfunction, and prevent further functional decline.

Physiatrists, alongside an extensive rehabilitation team, can offer comprehensive, patient-centered care focused on prevention and early recognition and treatment of impairments. Rheumatologic conditions frequently impair musculoskeletal function. Early in many rheumatologic disease processes, inflammation and pain can lead to limited joint mobility. As time passes, joint instability, weakness, and deformity increase the degree of disability, impacting functional mobility, self-care, and vocational and recreational activities. Care is goal-oriented and individualized and uses a multidisciplinary team that includes but is not limited to physical, occupational, and speech therapists; social workers; and psychologists. Education of both the patient and their caregivers is essential.

Rehabilitation Interventions

Goals of rehabilitation interventions include pain management, joint preservation, and maintenance of function and mobility. Pain control can be achieved though interventions that reduce inflammation and stabilize joints. Individualized exercise programs can maintain and restore strength and range of motion (ROM). Joint protection measures can help to minimize inflammation and allow for participation in daily activities. The rehabilitation team can assist with adapting to functional impairments and integrating within the community. Physical therapists assist by providing functional restoration using ROM, strengthening, and endurance exercises, as well as balance, transfer, and ambulation training. Occupational therapists can provide additional services for self-care activities, home management skills and modifications, vocational training, and education for energy conservation.

Rest

Generally, three forms of rest have been used by individuals with arthritic conditions. Depending on the acuity and severity of inflammation or injury, complete (systemic) bed rest, local joint rest, or short rest periods throughout the day may be utilized. Complete bed rest for several days to weeks in combination with analgesic medications was a widely accepted treatment regimen for rheumatoid arthritis (RA) from the 1950s through the mid 1980s.[1,2] However, the approach to management has evolved to include the early initiation of disease modifying anti-rheumatic drugs (DMARDs) and appropriate exercise and mobilization to prevent the adverse effects of prolonged bed rest. Local rest for inflamed joints with the use of nighttime splints and immobilizers can help to reduce inflammation and pain.[3] Short rest periods throughout the day ranging from 20 to 30 minutes at a time may be used to manage joint inflammation and generalized fatigue in patients with inflammatory arthritis.[4]

Exercise

Immobilization secondary to arthritis can lead to declines in muscle strength by as much as 40% after one week.[5] Exercise programs are prescribed for patients with arthritis and inflammatory conditions in order to build muscle strength and endurance, improve aerobic capacity, increase and maintain ROM, increase bone density, and improve overall function and well-being.

Exercise for the acutely inflamed joint can be achieved with twice daily passive ROM within the tolerable range to prevent joint contracture. More active regimens include isometric, isotonic, and isokinetic exercises. During isometric exercise, muscle force is generated with no visible joint movement (i.e., plank hold). Isometric exercises cause the least amount of intra-articular inflammation, bone destruction, and pressure.[6] For this reason, isometric strengthening is preferred in an acute flare. During isotonic exercise, muscle force is generated with visual joint movement, variable speed, and constant weight through ROM (i.e., lifting free weights). Isotonic contraction can be incorporated for patients without acute inflammation because they are able to tolerate changes in muscle length and joint position with a fixed load. During isokinetic exercise, muscle force is generated with visible joint movement, constant speed, and variable external resistance (i.e., Nautilus, Cybex machine). Isokinetic contraction is not recommended for patients with arthritis unless there is excellent joint preservation, as it usually requires maximal force of contraction.

Patients with RA may suffer muscle loss and a reduced endurance of up to 50%.[7] Recent literature has shown that a combined strength and endurance training program can result in significant improvements in cardiorespiratory endurance and muscle strength in patients with RA.[8] Enhanced physical fitness as a result of these programs also leads to improved functional ability and positive changes in body composition.

Stretching is utilized to maintain and/or increase ROM and prevent contractures. Passive stretching is recommended for patients severely weakened by active disease. Active assistive stretching in which the patient initiates muscle contraction and receives assistance from a therapist or assistive device can be used once pain and inflammation have decreased. Active stretching is done in the absence of pain.

The benefits of aquatic therapy for this patient population are numerous. They include increased joint and muscle support due to the buoyancy of water, increased resistance to movement secondary to the viscosity of water, and sensory input from water temperature and pressure, which may decrease pain.[9]

Physical Modalities

Therapeutic heat can be applied through various devices and techniques for pain relief. It is generally used for subacute and chronic processes. Superficial heating modalities include hot packs, paraffin baths (Fig. 41.1), heating pads, hydrotherapy, fluidotherapy, and radiant heat. Deep heating modalities include ultrasound, short wave diathermy, and microwave diathermy. Heating increases extensibility of collagen tissue at higher temperatures and can improve joint mobility.[10] Contraindications to heat therapy include ischemia (arterial insufficiency), bleeding disorders (hemophilia) or hemorrhage, impaired sensation, inability to communicate or respond to pain, malignancy, acute trauma or inflammation, scar tissue formation, edema, atrophic skin, and poor thermal regulation.

Therapeutic cold is the preferred modality in the acutely inflamed joint. Benefits include decreases in the inflammatory response, spasticity,[11] pain, and muscle spasms. This is accomplished through modalities such as cold packs, ice massage, and cold baths. Precautions and contraindications for cold therapy include cold intolerance or hypersensitivity to cold (Raynaud's phenomenon), arterial insufficiency, impaired sensation, and cognitive and communication deficits.

Clinical uses for electrotherapy include pain management and muscle stimulation. Transcutaneous nerve stimulation (TENS) uses a pocket-sized programmable device to apply an electrical signal through lead wires and electrodes attached to the patient's skin at the site of pain. It provides symptomatic pain relief by stimulating nerve fibers. Neuromuscular electrical stimulation (NMES) involves applying electrical stimulation above the motor threshold to induce a muscle contraction. NMES strengthens muscles and maintains muscle mass after immobilization.[4]

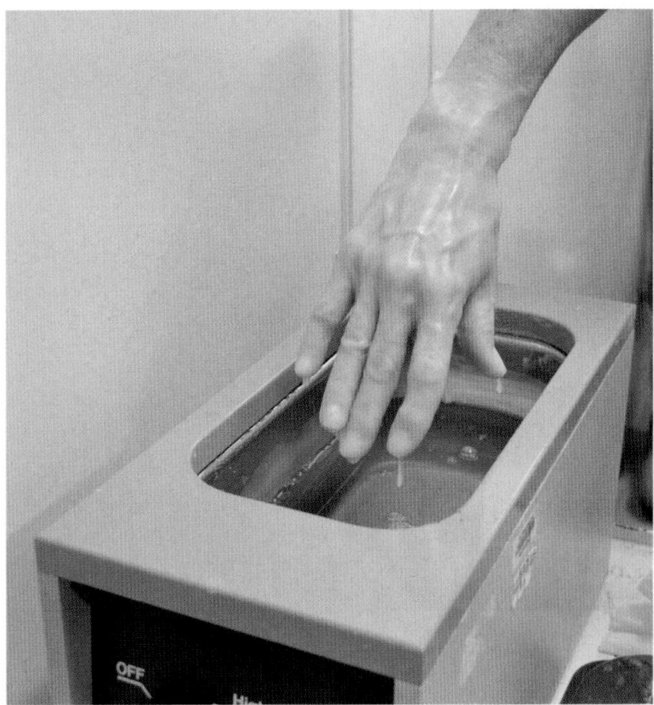

• **Fig. 41.1** Paraffin wax bath.

Orthoses

An orthosis or brace is an external device applied to body parts to provide benefits including but not limited to reduction in pain, prevention or correction of a deformity, support/stability, and improvement of function.

Upper extremity orthoses are used in the hand and wrist to immobilize painful joints in early RA, carpal tunnel syndrome, first carpometacarpal (CMC) osteoarthritis, and de Quervain's extensor tenosynovitis.[4] These orthoses are designed to provide pain relief and reduce inflammation[12] of affected joints while allowing for mobility of unaffected surrounding joints (Figs. 41.2 and 41.3).

Lower extremity orthoses are used to control abnormalities of the knee, foot, and ankle, including knee instability, quadriceps weakness, ligamentous laxity, excess pronation at the subtalar joint, and plantar fasciitis. Shoe modifications can be made to accommodate joint deformities of the toes such as hallux valgus.

Spinal orthoses are used to provide support and limit motion, thus decreasing pain. These orthoses are available in varying degrees of motion restriction depending on the level of spinal instability.

Assistive Devices and Home/Environmental Modifications

Many patients with rheumatologic diseases develop some level of disability. The use of assistive devices for ambulation (canes and walkers), safe transfers, and activities of daily living (built up

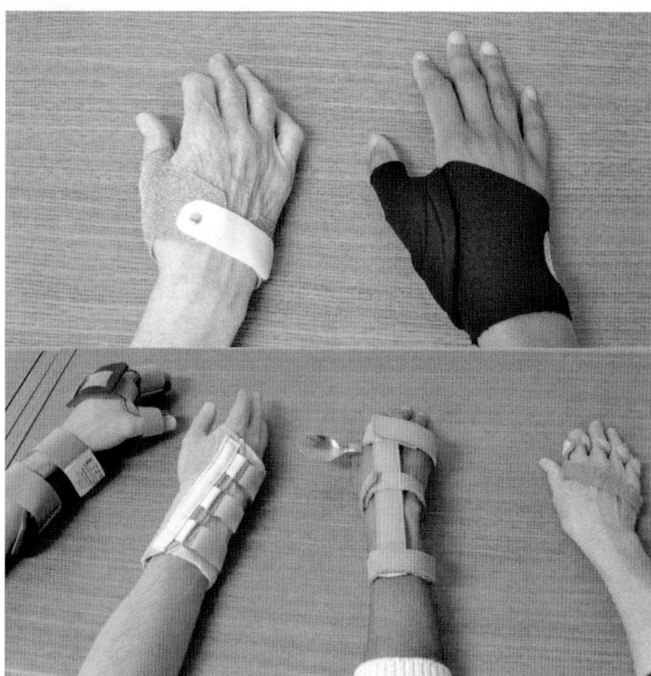

• **Fig. 41.2** Wrist and hand orthoses. *Top from left to right,* Custom-molded short opponens orthosis, prefabricated soft neoprene hand orthosis. *Bottom from left to right,* Resting wrist and hand orthosis, functional wrist splint, ADL splint with utensil holder/universal cuff, ulnar deviation correction splint.

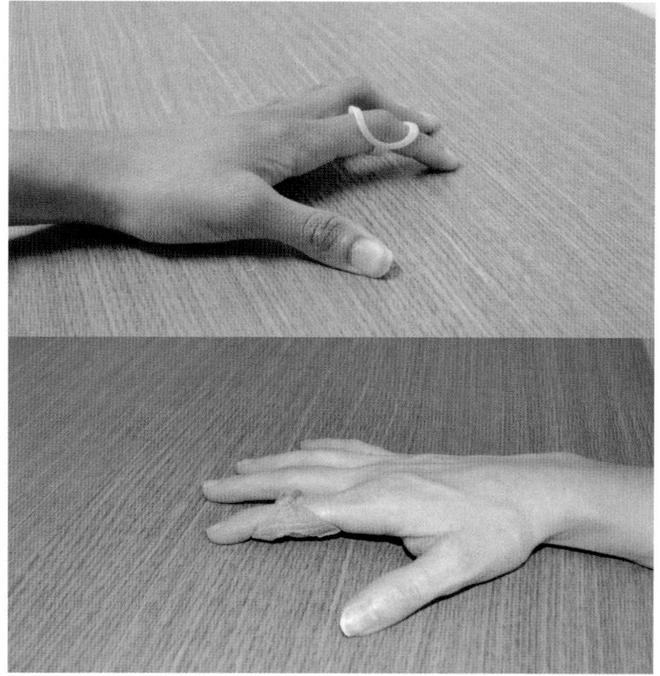

• **Fig. 41.3** Finger orthoses. *Top,* Swan neck splint. *Bottom,* Boutonnière splint.

handles for feeding, button hooks, hook and loop fastening shoes) compensate for limited ROM and pain while promoting independence for patients with arthritis. Home modifications, including the installation of grab bars in the bathroom, chair lifts, and ramps may be necessary to ensure safety (Figs. 41.4, 41.5, 41.6 and 41.7).

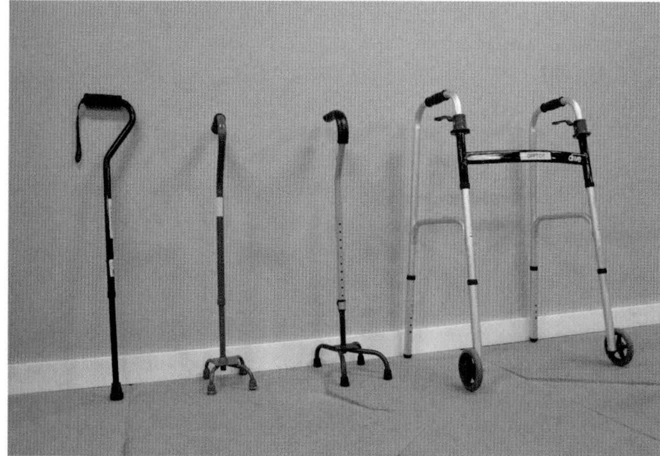

• **Fig. 41.4** Gait aids. *From left to right,* Straight cane, narrow base quad cane, wide base quad cane, rolling walker.

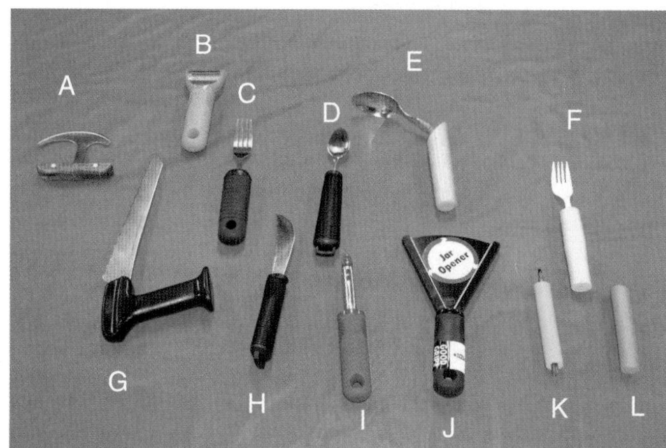

• **Fig. 41.5** Utensils with adaptive or built up handles to facilitate ADLs. (A) Rocker knife. (B) Peeler with built up handle. (C) Fork with built up handle. (D) Spoon with built up handle. (E) Adjustable angle spoon. (F) Fork with built up foam handle. (G) Right angle knife. (H) Rocker knife with built up handle. (I) Peeler with built up handle. (J) Jar opener. (K) Pen with built up foam handle. (L) Foam tubing to use with existing utensils (different sizes available).

Procedural Interventions

Patients with pain due to joint diseases may benefit from minimally invasive procedures such as intra-articular corticosteroid and/or anesthetic injections.[13] Additionally, therapeutic drainage of effusions may provide short-term relief. Surgical intervention, such as total joint replacements, synovectomies, and joint arthrodesis, may be indicated after failing less invasive and conservative measures.

Patient Education

Clear and consistent communication between physicians, patients, and their family members is key for optimal care. Patients should be educated on proper physical activity, methods to protect their joints from further damage, and techniques to conserve energy to maximize function and minimize fatigue. It is important to address psychosocial sequelae of the disease process including anxiety, depression, negative self-image, and sexual adjustment.

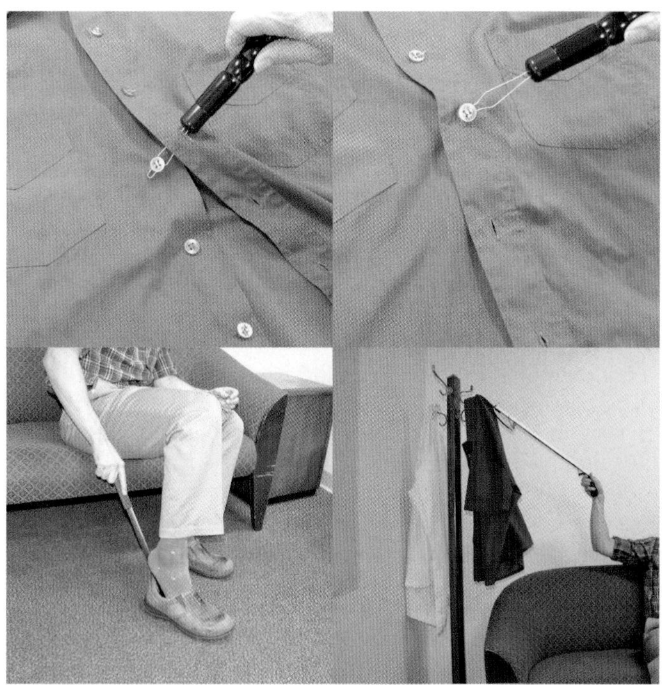

• **Fig. 41.6** *Top,* A button hook device can assist with independent buttoning of clothing if dexterity is impaired. *Bottom left,* Long-handled shoe horn. *Bottom right,* Long-handled reacher.

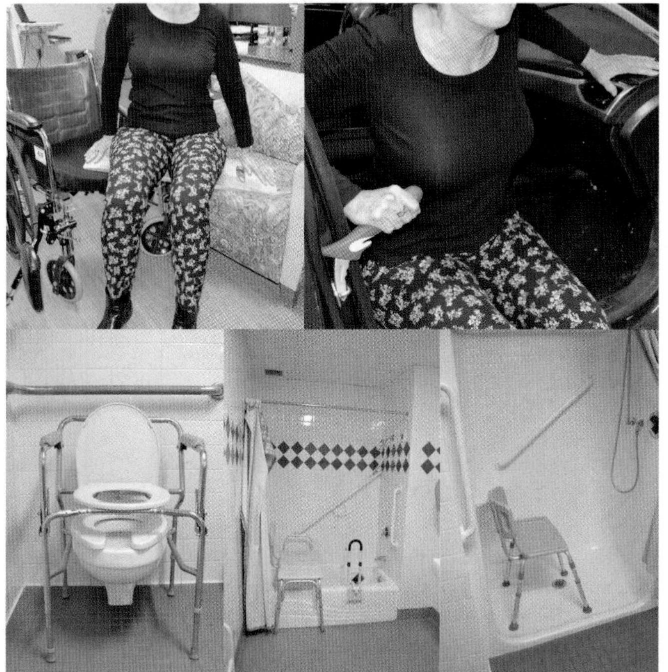

• **Fig. 41.7** Assistive and adaptive equipment, home modifications. *Top left,* Transfer board. *Top right,* Adaptive device used to assist with transfers in and out of a vehicle. *Bottom left,* A three-in-one commode, which can be used as a bedside commode, a raised toilet seat, or a shower chair. *Bottom middle,* Shower bench and removable/adjustable bathtub handrail. *Bottom right,* Walk-in shower with shower chair. Note the additional grab bars and removable hand-held shower heads present in the bathrooms.

Vocational Aspects

Patients wishing to resume working or begin the search for employment may benefit from workplace evaluations to ensure maximum efficiency. A vocational rehabilitation assessment will take into account level of education, physical function, work history, and social and psychological status, which can facilitate successful reintegration into the workplace environment.

Specific Disorders

Rheumatoid Arthritis

Rheumatoid arthritis (RA) is a chronic and systemic inflammatory disease that affects the joints and their surrounding structures. It may additionally present with extra-articular manifestations. Depending on the severity of progression, the disease process can result in varying degrees of functional decline, disability, and psychological impairment. Early aggressive pharmacologic management, along with an early functional assessment and multidisciplinary rehabilitation team approach, improves clinical outcomes.[14]

Prior to initiating a treatment regimen, it is important to be aware of comorbid conditions that may dictate the type, frequency, and intensity of activity. Such entities include but are not limited to atlantoaxial subluxation, joint sepsis, cardiopulmonary complications, diffuse vasculitis, Felty's syndrome, and neuropathy. Once these comorbid conditions are evaluated and adequately addressed, a comprehensive rehabilitation program can be safely prescribed, including rest, exercise, modalities, orthoses, adaptive and assistive devices, procedural interventions, and education.

Shoulder Rheumatoid Arthritis

RA of the shoulder damages the glenohumeral joint and surrounding tendons, bursae, ligaments, and capsule. Glenohumeral arthritis leading to limited internal rotation is an early finding in RA, while proximal subluxation of the humeral head is a later finding.[15] Rotator cuff injuries, including superior subluxation, tears, and fragmentation of the tendons, occur as a result of erosion of the greater tuberosity. Adhesive capsulitis, or shortening and fibrosis of the glenohumeral joint capsule, can result from shoulder pain, inflammation, and limited joint movement. Subacromial and subdeltoid bursitis, as well as bicipital tendonitis, are also seen in shoulder RA.

Localized rest can be used for the acutely inflamed joint through immobilization and with twice-daily full and slow passive range of motion (PROM) to prevent joint contracture and loss of mobility. Once pain and inflammation are controlled, Codman/pendulum and wall walking exercises can assist with shoulder flexion and internal and external rotation. Isometric strengthening, focused on the deltoid, biceps, and triceps, can be added to the regimen. The use of TENS significantly increases ROM more than heat combined with exercise and manipulation.[16] For pain control, intra-articular corticosteroid joint injections are a consideration. The combination of steroid injection with a therapy program appears more effective than therapy or injections alone in the recovery of ROM.[17] Finally, arthroplasty may be an option prior to the occurrence of end-stage joint erosion and soft-tissue contraction.

Elbow Rheumatoid Arthritis

Studies have shown that 51% to 61% of individuals with RA have elbow involvement with destruction and erosions occurring at the humeroulnar and humeroradial joints.[18] This greatly affects function and activities of daily living, as elbow flexion, extension, and lateral stability may be compromised. Lateral and medial epicondylitis are commonly diagnosed among this patient population.[4] Patients may experience severe cubitus valgus deformity, leading to ulnar neuropathy, and in rare cases, attrition rupture of the ulnar nerve.[19] Subcutaneous nodules and olecranon bursitis are associated conditions.

Although relative rest is required for the acutely inflamed joint, a physical therapy exercise regimen consisting of eccentric strengthening may decrease pain in patients suffering from lateral epicondylitis. The literature shows that deep heating through ultrasonography provides modest pain reduction over the course of 1 to 3 months.[20] The use of iontophoresis in conjunction with topical nonsteroidal anti-inflammatory drugs (NSAIDs) with 10 to 20 treatments over the course of 2 to 4 weeks has also conferred some benefit in subjective function and pain reduction.[21] The use of an inelastic, nonarticular, proximal forearm strap (tennis elbow orthosis) may decrease pain. For patients suffering from olecranon bursitis, the use of a cushioned pad that conforms to the elbow contours may relieve pressure. Prior to attempting corticosteroid injection for olecranon bursitis, it is important to obtain a culture to rule out infection.[4] Local corticosteroid injection for lateral epicondylitis has demonstrated benefits in pain reduction and grip strength for up to 2 to 6 weeks.[20] Open or arthroscopic synovectomy may be required for severe elbow involvement if medical and conservative management fails. Total elbow replacement is an effective procedure for end-stage disease,[22] and anterior transposition of the ulnar nerve with or without total elbow arthroplasty is a consideration for those with ulnar neuropathy.[19]

Wrist Rheumatoid Arthritis

Synovial proliferation at the wrist leads to increased pressure and damage to the surrounding ligaments, tendons, and cartilage. Weakness of the extensor carpi ulnaris, ulnar, and radial collateral ligaments causes the wrist to deviate radially. The increased torque of the stronger ulnar finger flexors leads to ulnar deviation of the fingers at the metacarpophalangeal (MCP) joints.[15] Synovial inflammation at the ulnar styloid can lead to destruction of the ulnar collateral ligament, which causes the ulnar head to spring up dorsally and "float."[4] Flexor tenosynovitis in early RA can cause significant hand pain and weakness and may be confused with de Quervain's disease. Median nerve compression may lead to bilateral carpal tunnel syndrome.

The wrist may be immobilized acutely with a resting wrist splint. Gentle stretching and ROM prevent contracture while adequate strengthening of the musculature surrounding the joint promote optimal joint stability.[23] Local cryotherapy causes a temporary decrease in intra-articular joint temperature, lasting up to 3 hours and offering pain relief in patients with active disease.[24] Although there is insufficient evidence demonstrating the effectiveness of wrist orthoses in pain reduction or increased grip strength in RA, many patients prefer wearing them as an external stabilizer.[25] An ulnar deviation correction splint may be used to limit ulnar deviation at the MCP while still allowing for MCP flexion and extension (see Fig. 41.2). Corticosteroid injections to the wrist joint may provide temporary pain relief. *Arthrodesis*, or surgical immobilization of a joint through fusion of adjacent bone structures, is a last resort after failure of conservative management.

Hand Rheumatoid Arthritis

Several hand deformities may occur as a result of RA. A boutonnière deformity is initially caused by proximal interphalangeal (PIP) joint synovitis and results when there is weakness or rupture of the terminal portion of the extensor hood, which holds the lateral bands in place, at the PIP joint. The lateral bands then sublux downward from above the axis of the PIP joint to below the axis, and they become flexors at the PIP joint. The PIP joint protrudes through the split tendon and the distal phalanx hyperextends. The end result is MCP hyperextension, PIP flexion, and distal interphalangeal (DIP) hyperextension. Treatment includes the use of a boutonnière ring splint, which immobilizes the PIP in extension and prevents flexion through a three-point pressure system (see Fig. 41.3).

A swan neck deformity commonly occurs secondary to synovitis at the MCP, PIP, or DIP (rare) joints. Flexor tenosynovitis leads to MCP flexion contracture, and contracture of the lumbricals and interossei of the hand cause PIP hyperextension. Contracture of the deep finger flexor muscles and tendons causes DIP flexion. This results in MCP flexion contracture, PIP hyperextension, and DIP flexion. Treatment includes a swan neck ring splint, which prevents PIP joint hyperextension through a three-point pressure system, while allowing for full PIP and DIP flexion (see Fig. 41.3).

Other complications of hand RA include intrinsic hand muscle weakness, which leads to decreased grip strength and resorptive arthropathy, where digits are shortened and phalanges appear retracted with skin folds.

Rehabilitation efforts are focused on a ROM program to stretch affected intrinsic hand muscles and an exercise regimen to increase grip strength, including mobility exercises and strengthening exercises against resistance provided by therapeutic putty, bands, or balls.[26] Cold therapy applied through a cold pack, ice, or cryotherapy is preferred in active joint inflammation. Superficial moist heat should be avoided in acutely inflamed joints, as it increases collagenase enzyme activity, which leads to increased joint destruction. Thermotherapy can be applied as a hot pack, paraffin wax (see Fig. 41.1), fluidotherapy, or hydrotherapy. Evidence suggests that there may be some benefit, including pain reduction from the application of paraffin wax nonacutely prior to engaging in exercise in patients with hand RA.[27] The use of a nighttime hand positioning splint can both reduce pain and improve pinch and grip strength in patients with RA.[3] While there is no evidence that splinting will stop hand deformities, stabilization of the MCP combined with an exercise program may help prevent or slow the progression.[15] Patients with severe hand involvement may require the use of a built-up handle to increase dexterity and reduce effort (see Fig. 41.5). Universal cuffs can also be used for assistance with ADLs (see Fig. 41.2).

Hip Rheumatoid Arthritis

There is hip involvement in about 50% of patients with RA.[28] While synovitis of the hip can cause pain radiating to the groin, trochanteric bursitis can present with pain over the lateral thigh with radiation to the buttock, anterior thigh, knee, or low back. *Protrusio acetabuli*, or collapse of the femoral head and inward bulging of the acetabulum into the pelvic cavity, can be seen in 5% of patients with RA.[4] Hip effusions, synovial cysts, and joint damage all contribute to reduction of internal rotation, which is an early finding.

During acute inflammation, the hip joint should be rested in a functional position of at least 45 degrees of abduction without any flexion.[29] ROM and stretching can address tight internal and external rotators, extensors, abductors, and the tensor fascia lata. Isometric strengthening exercises of the hip abductors and extensors can be added to the regimen. The use of deep heating ultrasound should be avoided in acute disease, as it can increase joint temperature and aggravate the existing inflammatory process. Assistive devices are used to maintain independence and self-efficiency. The proper use of a cane on the contralateral side can provide a 50% reduction in loading over the hip joint.[29] Corticosteroid injections may provide relief for trochanteric bursitis. Synovectomy may be helpful if the disease is limited to the synovium. Patients that have failed conservative management may be considered for total hip arthroplasty to relieve pain and restore joint ROM.

Knee Rheumatoid Arthritis

Symmetric involvement at the knees is common and can result in quadriceps atrophy, which causes increased force through the patella. The increase in force leads to increased intra-articular pressure, which pushes synovial fluid into the popliteal space, causing popliteal or Baker's cyst formation. Loss of full knee extension with subsequent knee flexion contracture may occur. Involvement of the surrounding ligaments and tendons can lead to joint instability and varus and valgus deformity.

Knee joint rest should take place in a functional position with the knees fully extended to avoid flexion contracture with at least once-daily gentle ROM.[29] It is important to stretch the hamstring muscles regularly. Quadriceps strengthening can be accomplished through isometric exercises in acutely inflamed joints and isotonic exercises with light weights if disease activity is low. There is some evidence to suggest that hydrotherapy or aquatic therapy can help to reduce pain and improve overall health in patients with RA, compared to no intervention.[30] The benefits of aquatic therapy include improvements in function and muscle strength using the buoyancy and resistance of water. Cold modalities can be applied acutely, and heat is reserved for subacute and chronic management. Knee orthoses or braces can be used to help control edema, ligamentous instability, significant quadriceps weakness, or recurvatum. Intra-articular corticosteroid injection of the knee to address pain is a common procedure. Synovectomy may be attempted if conservative measures are ineffective. Although total knee arthroplasty has proven to be the most successful intervention to reduce knee pain and improve physical function, complications following the procedure may occur secondary to poor healing tendencies of the soft tissues and severe pre-operative joint deformity.[31]

Foot and Ankle Rheumatoid Arthritis

RA of the foot and ankle can lead to painful and disabling joint deformities, antalgic gait patterns, and difficulty performing ADLs. Patients with RA can acquire a planovalgus foot deformity, which can cause increased tibial nerve traction or entrapment and subsequent tarsal tunnel syndrome. Painful hallux valgus deformities can occur along with metatarsal head subluxation and hammer-toe abnormalities. Patients may suffer from heel pain secondary to heel spurs, retrocalcaneal bursitis, and/or superficial calcaneal bursitis. Rheumatoid nodules overlying a bony protuberance or the Achilles tendon can rub against footwear and cause friction and skin irritation. Plantar fasciitis and tenosynovitis are other associated conditions.

Joint rest during acute inflammation should be done with the feet in a neutral position. ROM and stretching with either passive or active movement of the ankle joint is appropriate for contracted Achilles tendons and metatarsal phalangeal (MTP) and interphalangeal (IP) joints. There is evidence that hydrotherapy decreases pain and improves function and health-related quality of life.[32] Thermotherapy modalities, including contrast and paraffin wax baths, can be applied locally or through whole-body submersion in conjunction with other therapies. For painful metatarsal head subluxation, hallux valgus deformity, and hammer-toe abnormalities, adequate footwear is essential and includes shoes with an extra-depth toe box and a firm heel counter, lace-up style upper, and custom-molded inserts. Plantar fasciitis can be treated with night splints and corticosteroid injections. Risks associated with corticosteroid injections include tendon rupture, fat pad necrosis, and osteonecrosis. Debridement of hyperkeratotic tissue or hard callus overlying hammer toes, rheumatoid nodules, and subluxed metatarsal heads may be necessary. For advanced disease, ankle arthrodesis and total ankle replacement are two surgical options. Hindfoot fusions limit lateral motions of the foot, which makes it difficult to ambulate on uneven surfaces. Patients with forefoot deformities may opt for surgical management of hallux valgus or hammer toe deformities.

Cervical Spine Rheumatoid Arthritis

The most common abnormality of the spine in RA is ventral atlantoaxial (AA) subluxation, which is considered present if the atlantodental interval (ADI), or the horizontal distance between the anterior arch of the atlas and the dens of the axis, exceeds 3 mm in adults or 4 mm in children.[33] It occurs secondary to inflammatory pannus formation, ligamentous destruction, and bone softening. Patients may present with difficulty raising the head to the neutral position after looking downward. Atlantoaxial instability may cause pain and progressive neurologic injury secondary to myelopathy. Surgical reduction and fixation of the atlantoaxial joint is indicated in these patients.

RA patients, including those with no evidence of cervical spine involvement, should obtain pre-operative cervical spine flexion-extension radiographs to ensure that there is no cervical instability prior to receiving general anesthesia.[15] Signs of spinal cord injury, such as pain, paresthesias, and neurologic symptoms should be closely monitored in RA patients with AA subluxation and intervened on early by obtaining neurosurgical consultation to prevent more devastating neurologic compromise.

Osteoarthritis

Osteoarthritis (OA) is the most common form of arthritis. OA can occur in any joint but is most common in the knee, hip, hand, foot, and spine.[34] OA is often associated with pain symptoms, muscle weakness, loss of joint range of motion, and impaired functional mobility and ADLs. Symptoms can limit ability to perform daily activities, such as stair climbing, walking, and doing household chores.[35] In elderly people, OA is the most common cause of disability.[36]

Altered or abnormal joint biomechanics increase joint vulnerability and OA. Biomechanical changes may result from articular surface abnormalities, joint dysplasia, joint instability or malalignment, disturbances of joint innervation (proprioception), ligament and muscle issues, and muscle strength and endurance limitations.[37] A comprehensive rehabilitation program for patients with OA should include interventions to reduce joint pain, maintain and improve joint mobility, reduce physical disability and improve quality of life, limit the progression of joint damage, and educate patients about the nature of the disorder and its management.[38]

Hip and Knee Osteoarthritis

OA involvement of the large weight bearing joints of the lower extremities can cause significant pain, limited mobility, and impaired function. Pain and muscle weakness may cause gait abnormalities. An antalgic gait (limp) is an abnormal gait pattern in which stance time on a painful limb is decreased, stride length for the contralateral limb is shortened, and double-limb support time is increased. Depression and anxiety may impact an individual's pain experience and ability to cope with the pain, weakness, and impaired physical function.[37] Additionally individuals may attempt to avoid movement and activity for fear it will cause pain, which can result in adverse outcomes, including reduced muscle mass, increased pain and inactivity, generalized deconditioning, functional decline, and poor general health.

Optimal management of hip and knee OA requires an initial assessment, individualized treatment, and comprehensive care.[36] Relative rest with the reduction of adverse mechanical factors, as well as avoiding excess joint loading and painful motions, may be helpful initially, but complete rest and joint immobilization are not recommended for OA. Therapeutic exercise including physical therapy is one of the most effective interventions for OA. Barriers in regards to willingness or ability to participate should be investigated to improve compliance and optimize response to treatment.

Regular exercise should be encouraged, including regular low impact aerobic cardiovascular exercise, muscle strengthening, and ROM or flexibility exercises.[38,39] Exercise can be used to prevent the occurrence of OA or to treat OA in those with an established diagnosis. Joint ROM deficits are commonly seen in OA. In the hip, loss of internal rotation is the earliest sign, followed by restricted abduction and flexion. In the knee, there is usually loss of terminal knee extension, but flexion may also be limited. It is important to assess and treat joints above, below, and contralateral to the involved joint for any ROM deficits as well. A flexibility program often starts with gentle movement of joints through the currently available ROM to prevent loss. Stretching is initiated to increase ROM. Patients should be taught a proper stretching program (slow, gentle, and sustained stretching), while avoiding sudden, jerky, or ballistic stretching.[37]

The quadriceps muscles are important in OA. Quadriceps weakness is a predictor of lower limb functional limitations and disability.[40] Quadriceps weakness is associated with an increased risk of worsening knee pain and knee joint space narrowing in women.[41,42] Quadriceps strengthening is a therapy goal and can be done using isometric or isotonic exercises. Isotonic and closed chain exercises can allow for greater resistance and strengthening; however, exercises should be done within a pain-free range. It may be necessary to start with isometric exercises initially with a goal to progress to isotonic and functional exercises.[37]

Aerobic cardiovascular exercise with minimal impact including walking, cycling, or aquatic therapy is recommended for patients with OA. This activity may be started initially as part of a formal physical therapy program, but the goal is for it to be continued as part of a long-term home exercise program, achieving at least 30 minutes of moderate activity on most days. If land-based exercises cannot be tolerated due to symptoms, consider aquatic therapy. Water reduces the joint loading forces and the mechanical burden on the hip and knee joints, improving exercise tolerance and participation with benefits including management of metabolic syndrome, improvement of muscle function, and improvement of osteoarthritis index.[43] Patient preference should be taken into consideration when developing an exercise program to facilitate compliance. Exercise should be started at a level within the individual's capabilities and built up as tolerated. When initiating an exercise program, initial instruction is required; 12 or more supervised sessions were more effective than fewer sessions.[36] Research regarding the effects of exercise for individuals with OA of the hip and knee showed improvements in pain and physical function. For OA of the knee, improved quality of life was also demonstrated with exercise.[44,45] High impact aerobic conditioning exercises, including running and jogging on dry land, are not recommended in patients with lower extremity arthritis as they involve repetitive joint motion and loading with limited benefits in regards to improving strength and function with daily activities.[4]

Heat and cryotherapy are used widely in the management of patients with OA and are frequently recommended in existing guidelines; however, there is limited supporting evidence for their efficacy.[38] Therapeutic heat can be applied using hydrotherapy, hydrocollator packs, or paraffin. Heat can improve muscle and tendon flexibility, enhance stretching, promote relaxation, and provide pain relief.[37] Ice massage and cold packs improve ROM, function, and knee strength and decrease swelling, but did not significantly reduce pain.[46] TENS provides short-term efficacy of 2 to 4 weeks in providing clinically significant pain relief in patients with knee OA.[38] Medical literature shows little or no support for the use of electrical stimulation, iontophoresis, or therapeutic ultrasound in OA patients.

Orthotic options for knee OA include valgus unloading braces and lateral wedged insoles for symptomatic medial compartment knee OA, which is the most common site of involvement. Lower limb OA orthoses provide joint support and stability while attempting to relieve pain and prevent further joint injury. A knee brace for medial compartment OA is a three-point system with a valgus force applied that unloads the medial compartment.[37] Lateral wedge insoles in the treatment of medial knee OA was associated with reduced NSAID usage and improved treatment compliance compared to the control group.[47] There is limited evidence that braces and lateral wedges may provide benefit in knee OA.[48]

Assistive devices, including canes and walkers, are used to offload involved lower extremity joints. Canes should be used in the contralateral hand and walkers are often preferable for those with bilateral disease (see Fig. 41.4). Assessment and instruction on the use of walking aids by physical or occupational therapists is important to ensure that the patient is utilizing the most appropriate device, has the device adjusted to the proper height, and is using the device in a manner that avoids excessive loading of upper extremities. Knee and hip OA patients may additionally benefit from occupational therapy if lower extremity dressing, bathing, or home safety is impacted by limited lower limb ROM. Occupational therapy can help maximize independence and function for dressing by instructing the proper use of assistive devices including long-handled reachers, sock donners, long-handled shoe horns, and elastic shoe laces (see Fig. 41.6). Occupational therapists can recommend home modifications and durable medical equipment that may provide benefit and increase safety, including raised toilet seats, handrails for bathrooms and stairs, and tub benches or walk-in showers and shower chairs (see Fig. 41.7).

If noninvasive approaches and medications are not adequately controlling symptoms, minimally invasive procedures such as drainage of effusion, steroid and lidocaine injections, or viscosupplementation injections can be considered. Surgical treatments, including replacement arthroplasties and joint fusions, can be considered in patients that have failed more conservative treatment options.

Education is essential in the management of hip and knee OA. Obesity is associated with OA, and weight reduction can help prevent the onset of OA and alleviate symptoms. Effective weight loss interventions typically include dietary modifications, exercise programs, behavioral reinforcements, weight maintenance programs, physician support, and weight loss support groups.[37] Physical disability can be significantly improved in overweight patients with knee OA with weight loss >5% achieved within a 20-week period (>0.25% reduction per week).[49] Physical and occupational therapists can provide further education, including activity modification and joint protection strategies. The Arthritis Foundation is a not-for-profit organization and can be a great educational resource for the public, patients, and their caregivers. This group helps individuals improve quality of life and provides support through its educational and community-based programs.

Shoulder Osteoarthritis

Shoulder OA is often associated with shoulder pain, restricted ROM, and muscle weakness. There is typically loss of external rotation and abduction. Pain is usually worse at ROM extremes. Joint restrictions are seen with both active and passive ROM. Acromioclavicular (AC) joint OA may also be present. Degenerative changes of the shoulder, suboptimal biomechanics, and repetitive overhead activities can be associated with additional shoulder pathology, including subacromial impingement syndrome and chronic partial and full thickness rotator cuff tears. OA of the shoulder and other degenerative shoulder pathology cause impairments in upper extremity strength, endurance, and flexibility. Limitations in the ability to reach overhead and internally or externally rotate can negatively impact daily activities, including hair and/or teeth brushing, upper body dressing, and reaching for items overhead.[50]

Rehabilitation programs are designed to improve pain while maintaining and restoring function. Treatment should be implemented early in the course of disease to avoid significant loss of ROM and the muscle atrophy that can develop due to pain inhibition and disuse. In the acute phase, relative rest is utilized and activities that aggravate the symptoms should be avoided. The goal is to reduce pain and inflammation. Modalities, including therapeutic ultrasound and iontophoresis, can be utilized to assist with pain control. Rehabilitation programs should be designed to stabilize and strengthen the shoulder musculature to reestablish nonpainful scapulohumeral ROM and retard muscle atrophy of the entire upper extremity. Supervised physical or occupational therapy focus on improving upper extremity ROM and proprioception, strengthening of the rotator cuff and scapular stabilizers, and addressing the entire upper extremity kinetic chain.[51]

For patients who continue to have significant symptoms despite noninvasive treatment, injection options may provide benefit. Improved pain control and subsequent increased function may be achieved with use of periarticular injections for subacromial bursitis and rotator cuff tendinopathy and intra-articular injections for glenohumeral and AC joint arthritis. If conservative treatment options fail to adequately improve pain, surgical options, including joint debridement or shoulder arthroplasty, may be indicated.[50]

Hand Osteoarthritis

OA of the hands can involve the PIP, DIP, and CMC joints. Bouchard's nodes can be seen at the PIP joints and Heberden's nodes at the DIP joints. The first CMC joint is the primary joint for symptomatic OA of the thumb, as this articulation is the primary site of mobility of the thumb. Rest with immobilization of this joint can improve pain symptoms and allow for continued functional use. Orthotic treatment of the thumb can be used to stabilize the base of the first metacarpal and inhibit CMC joint motion during grip and pinching activities. Orthotic treatments for this condition include custom-made long opponens wrist hand orthoses (WHO), WHOs with thumb spica, custom-molded thermoplastic short opponens hand orthoses, and prefabricated soft neoprene hand orthoses with CMC motion resist (see Fig. 41.2). These splints all stabilize the CMC joint in abduction while allowing IP motion of the thumb. Orthotic treatment can be an effective option for decreasing pain with functional use.[52] The short opponens hand orthosis, which allows wrist and MCP motion, is reported as more effective in providing pain relief than the more traditional long opponens WHO, which stabilizes and prevents wrist and MCP joint motion. In a study comparing custom-made thermoplastic short opponens splints versus prefabricated neoprene short opponens splints, both showed to be effective treatment techniques for relieving pain, controlling subluxation forces, and improving ADLs. Patients, however, preferred the soft neoprene splint over the hard custom-made splint, perceiving that it provided greater support and pain relief while allowing more motion, given the softer and less restrictive material.[53]

Rehabilitation for hand OA typically involves utilization of occupational therapy to assist with pain, disability, and weakness associated with hand OA. Therapists can make recommendations and train patients on the use of adaptive and assistive equipment. These devices can improve independence with activities that require grip strength or dexterity, including jar opening, buttoning, and holding utensils (see Fig. 41.5 and Fig. 41.6). Ergonomic modifications may be helpful in work and home environments to minimize upper extremity overuse injuries.[37] Home modifications such as changing doorknobs to levers may also be recommended. Therapeutic modalities such as paraffin baths, contrast baths, and ice massages are modalities that may provide some benefit with symptom relief. Joint injections may help reduce inflammation and improve pain in acutely inflamed joints, and surgical interventions for joint immobilization may be indicated for patients who have failed conservative treatment options.[54]

Foot Osteoarthritis

Patients with OA often have foot problems, which commonly include first MTP joint involvement with hallux valgus, hallux rigidus, and metatarsal head calluses.[4] Education, including proper fitting shoes, may help prevent secondary complications such as pain, skin breakdown and wounds from deformities, poor fitting footwear, and sensory and healing impairment from comorbid medical conditions such as peripheral vascular disease or diabetes. Shoe modifications may include a high toe box for hammer toes, a wide toe box for bunion/hallux valgus, or a soft toe box to adjust for deformities.[55]

Footwear interventions are associated with improvements in foot pain and function in individuals with first MTP joint OA. A rocker-sole shoe allows for smoother progression of the center of gravity over the stance foot, reduction of forefoot joint loading, and a decrease in the amount of first MTP dorsiflexion required. Improvement in patient reported outcomes has been shown with the use of rocker-sole shoes.[56] Injection and surgical options may be considered if there is continued difficulty despite more conservative interventions.

Spondyloarthropathies

The spondyloarthritides consist of a group of disorders, including ankylosing spondylitis (AS), reactive arthritis, psoriatic

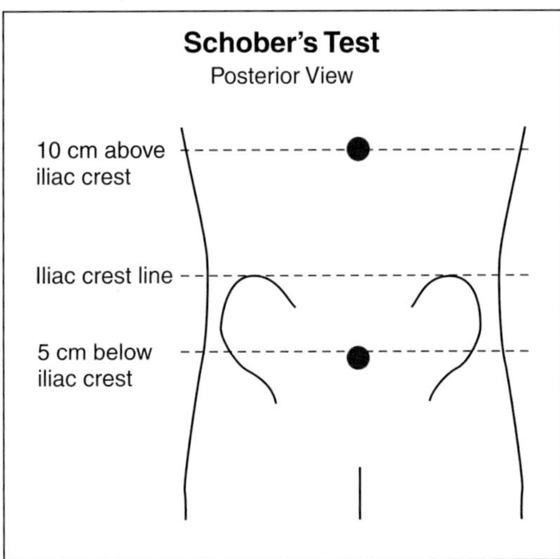

• **Fig. 41.8** Schober's test. (From Cuccurullo, S. J. [Ed.]: [2019]. *Physical Medicine and Rehabilitation Board Review*, Fourth Edition. New York, NY: Demos Medical Publishing, an imprint of Springer Publishing Company.)

arthritis, inflammatory bowel disease-related arthritis, and undifferentiated spondyloarthritis. Involvement of the axial skeleton, enthesopathy, and extra-articular manifestations are common in these disorders. Many result in disability from the loss of spinal mobility and decreased pulmonary function. Although available management includes NSAIDs, DMARDs, and drugs that inhibit TNF, several rehabilitation interventions have been used to reduce pain, encourage functional independence, and preserve joint alignment and posture.[4]

AS is the most common of the seronegative spondyloarthritides. Sacroiliitis is the hallmark of the disease, and it is also associated with decreased lumbar lordosis, increased thoracic kyphosis, and cervical ankylosis. Schober's test is used to detect the limitation of forward flexion and hyperextension of the lumbar spine. While standing erect, place a landmark midline at a point 5 cm below the iliac crest line and 10 cm above the iliac crest midline at the spinous process. On forward flexion the line should increase by greater than 5 cm to a total of 20 cm or more (from 15 cm). Any increase less than 5 cm is considered a restriction (Fig. 41.8). Respiratory restriction with limited chest expansion secondary to ankylosis of costochondral joints also occurs once there is thoracic spine involvement, which includes the costovertebral, costosternal, manubriosternal, and sternoclavicular joints, leading to restrictive lung disease. Normal chest expansion after maximal inhalation is 7 to 8 cm as measured at the nipple line.[15] In patients with AS, if the chest expansion is less than 7 to 8 cm, there is a risk of developing restrictive lung disease. Once this lung pattern ensues, chest expansion decreases and patients are at risk for developing diaphragmatic breathing.

Patients are encouraged to maintain adequate posture, sleep in the prone position, and use a firm mattress to prevent spine flexion contractures.[15] A 2008 Cochrane review and subsequent 2012 update on the effects of physical therapy interventions on pain, stiffness, spinal mobility, and physical function concluded that an individual home-based or supervised exercise program is better than no intervention at all and supervised group physical therapy is better than home exercise.[57,58] Other therapy interventions are aimed at increasing spine mobility through the use of extension-based exercises and swimming for overall aerobic conditioning. A 2009 randomized controlled study demonstrated that swimming and walking increased functional capacity and had beneficial effects on the quality of life and pulmonary functions of patients with AS.[59] Patients are also encouraged to practice deep breathing exercises to maintain chest expansion and to take appropriate measures for smoking cessation. Assistive devices such as long-handled reachers and shoe-horns may be useful in performing ADLs for patients with limited neck and spine movement (see Fig. 41.6).

Fluoroscopy-guided intra-articular corticosteroid injections for sacroiliitis are regarded as safe, rapid, and effective.[60] For patients with advanced disease, surgical procedures such as total hip replacement or hip resurfacing have shown significant pain relief and good restoration of function and mobility.[57] Spinal vertebral osteotomy to resolve kyphotic deformity can give superb functional results by restoring balance and horizontal vision, although it is accompanied by severe risks.[57]

Patients must be educated about the risk of cervical spine fracture and subsequent spinal cord injury (SCI), as the likelihood of SCI is 11.4 times higher in those with AS than those without it.[4] Counseling on fall prevention, avoidance of contact sports, and appropriate home modifications is emphasized to minimize risks.

Systemic Lupus Erythematous

Systemic lupus erythematous (SLE) is an autoimmune chronic inflammatory disease. In SLE, joint pain and arthritis usually involve smaller peripheral joints (fingers, wrist, elbows, toes, ankles, knees) in association with more generalized systemic symptoms, including fatigue, depression, and decreased endurance.

Deformities of the hand are secondary to ligamentous laxity with ulnar subluxation of MCP joints and hyperextension of the thumb at the IP joints (Jaccoud's arthritis). Synovitis may contribute to joint pain and swelling. There can also be osteonecrosis, which can occur at the MCP heads or other joints, including the shoulder, hip, and knee. There may be muscle involvement with myositis or myopathy with inhibition of proximal muscle contraction and movement, weakness, and painful or easily fatigable muscles. SLE is associated with premature atherosclerosis, hypercoagulable states, vasculitis, and secondary complications from the disease, including vision loss, interstitial lung disease, myocardial infarction, renal failure, and strokes.[61] Extra-articular manifestations should be taken into consideration when initiating a comprehensive rehabilitation program.

For severe new-onset SLE or severe systemic acute flares, several days of bed rest may be indicated. In general, however, local rest of acutely or subacutely inflamed joints with splinting can help reduce pain and minimize generalized deconditioning and muscle mass loss associated with complete bed rest. Patients with SLE may experience fatigue, muscle weakness, disruption of sleep-wake cycle, cognitive difficulty, psychomotor slowing, and depression with significant functional impairment and disability.[62,63] Fatigue, deconditioning, and disability can improve with rehabilitation interventions. Exercise can be an important part of rehabilitation management of SLE patients with fatigue. Supervised graded cardiovascular exercise is particularly important with recommendations including biking, walking, interval training, and aerobic exercise. Benefits include improvements in endurance, aerobic capacity, fatigue, physical function, quality of life, and depression.[64]

If edema is present, management of edema with compression pumps and garments may be used. Modalities for pain control may include heat, cold, TENS, and acupuncture or acupressure. Referral to an occupational therapist or hand therapist can be helpful for SLE patients with impaired hand function that interferes with ADLs. Intrinsic muscle stretching exercises can help prevent deformities. Orthoses can be used to reduce joint subluxations, stabilize joints, and prevent the development of contractures. Assistive devices such as a cane can be used on the contralateral side to offload hip and knee joints with avascular necrosis. In SLE, articular surfaces are typically preserved, and management targets soft tissues and may include steroid injections. A surgical option of joint replacement can be indicated if conservative treatment is unsuccessful for osteonecrosis.

Fatigue is common and education, including energy conservation training and efforts to improve sleep-wake cycles, can be useful for fatigue management. Functional positioning is important to minimize contractures. Speech therapy can be utilized to provide education on strategies to enhance memory. Family education and support group utilization can improve compliance with treatment programs.[4]

Juvenile Idiopathic Arthritis

Children and adolescents can have arthritic conditions, which can have a significant impact on their day-to-day activities. Juvenile idiopathic arthritis (JIA) is arthritis of unknown etiology and includes a collection of heterogeneous diseases. These conditions can cause osteopenia/osteoporosis, joint-space narrowing, loss of cartilage, bony erosions, intra-articular bony ankyloses, growth disturbances, joint subluxation, soft tissue swelling, synovial thickening, and effusion. Extra-articular manifestations include rash, pericardial effusion, decreased aerobic capacity, iritis, and blindness.

Children are at risk to develop cervical spine stiffness, spinal flexion contracture, fusion, and loss of extension.[65] Restricted shoulder mobility, flexion contractures at the elbows and wrists, and involvement of the small joints of the hand can occur.[66] Patients may experience acute lower extremity muscle spasms, rapid formation of hip flexion contracture, valgus knee deformity, and leg length discrepancy resulting in a pelvic tilt and scoliosis as an adult.[67] In the mouth and jaw, there may be involvement of the mandibular head and temporomandibular joint (TMJ) with limitation of mouth opening and micrognathia.[68] Pre-operative evaluation of the TMJ and cervical spine is needed to assess for limited ROM with dynamic radiographs.

Rest is not specifically recommended, and encouragement should be provided for continued activities with the exception of contact sports during active flares. Patients and their families should be educated regarding proper positioning at night with the use of a single thin pillow to prevent neck flexion contractures and periods of prone lying to maintain hip extension.[4] Exercise, including physical and occupational therapy, is aimed at pain management and optimization of musculoskeletal function to maintain and improve flexibility, balance, strength, and quality of life.[69] ROM exercises and stretching should be used to prevent joint contractures. Patients with JIA have been found to have a lower cardiopulmonary exercise capacity compared to their healthy peers, and evidence suggests that the combination of ROM exercises and regular aerobic exercise may offer improvements in cardiopulmonary capacity.[70]

Orthoses can be used to prevent contracture and improve ROM. For wrist flexion contractures, cock-up resting splints at night or serial casting can be utilized. A resting splint that includes the hand and wrist can be used if there is PIP involvement; however, this type of splint is passive and is not designed for use with functional activities[4] (see Fig. 41.2). If IP joint contractures are present, a dynamic outrigger splint can be used during the day. An adjustable hinge splint may be used for the acutely inflamed elbow joint. For an acutely inflamed knee joint, a posterior resting splint at night can help prevent contracture. Leg length discrepancies should be addressed and corrected with a shoe insert or a built-up shoe if the correction required is greater than ⅜ inch.[4] A desk with a tilt top may be beneficial to maintain ideal spine posture and reduce neck pain.

Intra-articular corticosteroid injections are most commonly used in oligoarticular JIA; however, they may be used in other subtypes of JIA during active disease.[71] Surgical management of disease that is not responsive to conservative therapies includes joint resurfacing, joint arthroplasty for severe deformities, synovectomy, correction of uveitis, limb length discrepancy surgery, and limb and mandibular osteotomy.

Alternative, Innovative, and Emerging Therapeutic Approaches

The joint pain, stiffness, muscle aches, weakness, fatigue, and depression that can be associated with various rheumatologic diseases often lead to a reduction in activity level and exercise participation as well as gait and balance problems. Early disease diagnosis, management, and treatment may help reduce the debilitating nature of many rheumatologic diseases. It is important to help facilitate and maintain regular physical activity if possible.

In addition to traditional rehabilitation management, alternative exercise modalities may be of benefit. For example, tai chi uses slow and controlled body movements that involve components of posture and strength to achieve a state of balance.[72] Several studies have demonstrated the beneficial effects of tai chi, including improved balance and dynamic stability, increased strength, improved ability to perform ADLs, and overall improvements in psychological well-being.[73] Yoga focuses on the use of breathing, body poses, and meditation to improve balance and strength, and it may be beneficial to decrease pain as well. In particular, studies have shown that patients with OA experienced a reduction in knee pain after participating in yoga.[73]

The use of various forms of technology can allow for improvements in gait and balance to prevent secondary complications such as injury and falls. There is a growing body of work focusing on the use of wearable and ambient sensors in the early detection of functional impairments and disability in older adults and individuals with chronic conditions.[74] These wearable sensors may be in the form of wristbands and shoe insoles that provide vibratory feedback for awareness of positioning, gait and balance improvement, and fall prevention.[75,76]

Exercise using computer and gaming technology can offer cost-effective, home-based interventions to address balance, motor skills, and physical fitness in older adults.[72] Virtual reality and robotic devices create simulated environments that provide users with visual and tactile feedback and strategies to improve movement. Further advancements in technology may provide future therapeutic options.

Another emerging therapeutic approach in the management of OA involves using modified footwear to improve function in patients with knee pain secondary to OA. An ongoing clinical trial is investigating specialized footwear that promotes exercise and improves abnormal biomechanics to reduce osteoarthritic knee pain. This home-based program will be evaluated as a conservative option that may supplement and/or replace traditional treatment modalities for painful knee OA. Continuation of this clinical trial will determine the effectiveness of this therapeutic approach.[77]

Further advancements in medicine and technology will hopefully continue to minimize the disability caused by rheumatologic disease. The goal is to allow people to remain active and functional in an effort to prevent muscular atrophy, deconditioning, and other complications of immobility.

Conclusion

Patients with rheumatologic diseases can benefit from a multidisciplinary approach to treatment, including input and coordinated care from both the medical and rehabilitation teams. Successful rehabilitation plans are individualized and require clinical assessments of both medical and functional status. The goal of rehabilitation is to improve quality of life through pain alleviation, prevention of joint deformity, and maximization of function. In conjunction with pharmacotherapy, recommended rehabilitation interventions include rest, exercise, physical modalities, orthoses, assistive and adaptive equipment, and joint injections. It is essential to educate patients and provide ongoing support during the course of their treatment for optimal outcomes.

The references for this chapter can also be found on ExpertConsult.com.

References

1. Upchurch K, Kay J: Evolution of treatment for rheumatoid arthritis, *Rheumatology* 51(6):vi28–vi36, 2012.
2. Sokka T, Envalds M, Pincus T, et al.: Treatment of rheumatoid arthritis: a global perspective on the use of antirheumatic drugs, *Mod Rheumatol* 18(3):228–239, 2008.
3. Silva AC, Jones A, Silva PG, et al.: Effectiveness of a night-time hand positioning splint in rheumatoid arthritis: a randomized controlled trial, *J Rehabil Med* 40(9):749–754, 2008.
4. Joe GO, Hicks JE, Gerber LH, et al.: Rehabilitation of the patient with rheumatic diseases. In Frontera WR, DeLisa JA, Gans BM, et al.: *Physical medicine and rehabilitation: principles and practice*, ed 5, vol. I. Philadelphia, 2010, Lippincott Williams & Wilkins Health, pp 1034–1065.
5. Topp R, Ditmyer M, King K, et al.: The effect of bed rest and potential of prehabilitation on patients in the intensive care unit, *AACN Clinical Issues* 13(2):263–276, 2002.
6. Anwer S, Alghadir A: Effect of isometric quadriceps exercise on muscle strength, pain, and function in patients with knee osteoarthritis: a randomized controlled study, *J Phys Ther Sci* 26(5):745–748, 2014.
7. Ekdahl C, Broman G: Muscle strength, endurance, and aerobic capacity in rheumatoid arthritis: a comparative study with healthy subjects, *Ann Rheum Dis* 51(1):35–40, 1992.
8. Strasser B, Leeb G, Strehblow C, et al.: The effects of strength and endurance training in patients with rheumatoid arthritis, *Clin Rheumatol* 30(5):623–632, 2011.
9. Wang T, Belza B, Thompson E, et al.: Effects of aquatic exercise on flexibility, strength and aerobic fitness in adults with osteoarthritis of the hip or knee, *J Adv Nurs* 57(2):141–152, 2007.
10. Oosterveld F, Rasker J: Treating arthritis with locally applied heat or cold, *Semin Arthritis Rheum* 24(2):82–90, 1994.
11. Price R, Lehmann J, Boswell-Bessette S, et al.: Influence of cryotherapy on spasticity at the human ankle, *Arch Phys Med Rehabil* 74(3):300–304, 1993.
12. Stenger AA, vanLeeuwen MA, Houtman PM, et al.: Early effective suppression of inflammation in rheumatoid arthritis reduces radiologic progression, *Br J Radiol* 37:1157–1163, 1998.
13. Maarse W, Watts A, Bain G, et al.: Medium-term outcome following intra-articular corticosteroid injection in first cmc joint arthritis using fluoroscopy, *Hand Surg* 14(2n03):99–104, 2009.
14. Scholten C, Brodowicz T, Graninger W, et al.: Persistent functional and social benefit 5 years after a multidisciplinary arthritis training program, *Arch Phys Med Rehabil* 80(10):1282–1287, 1999.
15. Nucatola TR, Freeman ED, Brown DP, et al.: Rheumatology. In Cuccurullo SJ, editor: *Physical medicine and rehabilitation board review*, ed 3, New York, 2015, Demos Medical, pp 101–147.
16. Page P, Labbe A: Adhesive capsulitis: use the evidence to integrate your interventions, *N Am J Sports Phys Ther* 5(4):266–273, 2010.
17. D'Orsi GM, Via AG, Frizziero A, et al.: Treatment of adhesive capsulitis: a review, *Muscles Ligaments Tendons J* 2(2):70–78, 2012.
18. Lehtinen JT, Kaarela K, Ikavalko M, et al.: Incidence of elbow involvement in rheumatoid arthritis. A 15 year endpoint study, *J Rheumatol* 28(1):70–74, 2001.
19. Ochi K, Ikari K, Momohara S, et al.: Attrition rupture of ulnar nerve in an elbow of a patient with rheumatoid arthritis, *J Rheumatol* 41(10):2085, 2014.
20. Johnson GW, Cadwaller K, Scheffel SB, et al.: Treatment of lateral epicondylitis, *Am Fam Physician* 76:843–853, 2007.
21. Bisset L, Paungmali A, Vicenzino B, et al.: A systematic review and meta-analysis of clinical trials on physical interventions for lateral epicondylalgia, *Br J Sports Med* 39:411–422, 2005.
22. Dyer G, Blazar PE: Rheumatoid elbow, *Hand Clin* 27(1):43–48, 2011.
23. Cooney JK, Law R, Matschke V, et al.: Benefits of exercise in rheumatoid arthritis, *J Aging Res*14, 2011. Article ID: 681640.
24. Hirvonen HE, Mikkelsson MK, Kautiainen H, et al.: Effectiveness of different cryotherapies on pain and disease activity in active rheumatoid arthritis. A randomized single blinded controlled trial, *Clin Exp Rheumatol* 24:295–301, 2006.
25. Egan M, Brosseau L, Farmer M, et al.: Splints and orthosis for treating rheumatoid arthritis, *Cochrane Database Syst Rev* 4:2001.
26. Lamb SE, Williamson EM, Heine PJ, et al.: Exercises to improve function of the rheumatoid hand (sarah): a randomised controlled trial, 385(9966):421–429, 2014.
27. Ayling J, Marks R: Efficacy of paraffin wax baths for rheumatoid arthritic hands, *Physiotherapy J* 86(4):190–201, 2000.
28. Duthie RB, Harris CM: A radiographic and clinical survey of the hip joint in sero-positive arthritis, *Acta Orthop Scand* 40:346–364, 1969.
29. Kavuncu V, Evcik D: Physiotherapy in rheumatoid arthritis, *MedGenMed* 6(2):3, 2004.
30. Al-Qubaeissy KY, Fatoye FA, Goowin PC, et al.: The effectiveness of hydrotherapy in the management of rheumatoid arthritis: as systematic review, *Musculoskeletal Care* 11(1):3–18, 2012.
31. Lee JK, Choi CH: Total knee arthroplasty in rheumatoid arthritis, *Knee Surg Relat Res* 24(1):1–6, 2012.
32. Anain JM, Bojrab AR, Rhinehart FC, et al.: Conservative treatments for rheumatoid arthritis in the foot and ankle, *Clin Podiatr Med Surg* 27:193–207, 2010.
33. Heary RF, Yanni DS, Halim AY, et al.: Rheumatoid arthritis. In Benzel EC, Steinmetz MP, editors: *Benzel's spine surgery: techniques, complication avoidance, and management*, ed 4, Philadelphia, 2017, Elsevier, pp 843–859.
34. Woolf AD, Pfleger B: Burden of major musculoskeletal conditions, *Bull World Health Organ* 81:646–656, 2003.
35. Bijlsma JW, Berenbaum F, Lafeber FP, et al.: Osteoarthritis: an update with relevance for clinical practice, *Lancet* 377:2115–2126, 2011.
36. Fernandes L, Hagen KB, Bijlsma JWJ, et al.: EULAR recommendations for the non-pharmacological core management of hip and knee osteoarthritis, *Ann Rheum Dis* 72:1125–1135, 2013.
37. Stitik TP, Kim JH, Stiskal D, et al.: Osteoarthritis. In ed 5, Frontera WR, DeLisa JA, Gans BM, et al.: *Physical medicine and rehabilitation: principles and practice*, vol. I. Philadelphia, 2010, Lippincott Williams & Wilkins Health, pp 782–809.
38. Zhang W, Moskowitz RW, Nuki G, et al.: OARSI recommendations for the management of hip and knee osteoarthritis, Part II:

OARSI evidence-based, expert consensus guidelines, *Osteoarthritis Cartilage* 16:137–162, 2008.
39. Zhang W, Nuki G, Moskowitz RW, et al.: OARSI recommendations for the management of hip and knee osteoarthritis Part III: changes in evidence following systematic cumulative update of research published through January 2009, *Osteoarthritis Cartilage* 18:476–499, 2010.
40. McAlindon TE, Cooper C, Kirwan JR, et al.: Determinants of disability in osteoarthritis of the knee, *Ann Rheum Dis* 52(4):258–262, 1993.
41. Segal NA, Glass NA, Torner J, et al.: Quadriceps weakness predicts risk for knee joint space narrowing in women in the MOST cohortOsteoarthritis and Cartilage, 18(6):769–775, 2010.
42. Glass NA, Torner JC, Frey Law LA, et al.: The relationship between quadriceps muscle weakness and worsening of knee pain in the MOST cohort: a 5-year longitudinal study, *Osteoarthritis Cartilage* 21(9):1154–1159, 2013.
43. Ha GC, Yoon JR, Yoo CG, et al.: Effects of 12-week aquatic exercise on cardiorespiratory fitness, knee isokinetic function, and Western Ontario and McMaster University osteoarthritis index in patients with knee osteoarthritis women, *J Exerc Rehabil* 14(5):870–876, 2018.
44. FransenM, McConnell S, Harmer AR, et al.: Exercise for osteoarthritis of the knee, *Cochrane Database Syst Rev* 1:CD004376, 2015.
45. Fransen M, McConnell S, Hernandez-Molina G, et al.: Exercise for osteoarthritis of the hip, *Cochrane Database Syst Rev* (4), 2014. Art. No.: CD007912.
46. Brosseau L, Yonge KA, Robinson V, et al.: Thermotherapy for treatment of osteoarthritis, *Cochrane Database Syst Rev* 4:CD004522, 2003.
47. Pham T, Maillefert JF, Hudry C, et al.: Laterally elevated wedged insoles in the treatment of medial knee osteoarthritis. A two-year prospective randomized controlled study, *Osteoarthritis Cartilage* 12:46–55, 2004.
48. Brouwer RW, Jakma TS, Verhagen AP, et al.: Braces and orthoses for treating osteoarthritis of the knee, *Cochrane Database Syst Rev* (1)CD004020, 2005.
49. Christensen R, Bartels EM, Astrup A, et al.: Effect of weight reduction in obese patients diagnosed with knee osteoarthritis: a systematic review and meta-analysis, *Ann Rheum Dis* 66:433–439, 2007.
50. Stretanski MF: Shoulder arthritis. In Frontera WR, Silver JK, Rizzo TD, editors: *Essentials of physical medicine and rehabilitation: musculoskeletal disorders, pain, and rehabilitation*, ed 3, Philadelphia, PA, 2015, Elsevier Saunders, pp 97–102.
51. Brown DP, Freeman ED, Cuccurullo SJ, et al.: Musculoskeletal medicine. In Cuccurullo SJ, editor: *Physical medicine and rehabilitation board review*, ed 3, New York, 2015, Demos Medical, pp 149–340.
52. Hovorka C, Acker D: Orthotic treatment considerations for arthritis and overuse syndromes in the upper Limb. In Webster JB, Murphy DP, editors: *Atlas of orthoses and assistive devices*, ed 5, Philadelphia, 2019, Elsevier, pp 176–197.
53. Weiss S, Lastayo P, Mills A, et al.: Splinting the degenerative basal joint: custom-made or prefabricated neoprene? *J Hand Ther* 17(4):401–406, 2004.
54. Ring D: Hand osteoarthritis. In Frontera WR, Silver JK, Rizzo TD, editors: *Essentials of physical medicine and rehabilitation: musculoskeletal disorders, pain, and rehabilitation*, ed 4, Philadelphia, PA, 2015, Elsevier Saunders, pp 160–164.
55. Uustal H, Baerga E, Joki J, et al.: Prosthetics and Orthotics. In Cuccurullo SJ, editor: *Physical medicine and rehabilitation board review*, ed 3, New York, 2015, Demos Medical, pp 471–549.
56. Frecklington M, Dalbeth N, McNair P, et al.: Footwear interventions for foot pain, function, impairment and disability for people with foot and ankle arthritis: a literature review, *Semin Arthritis Rheum* 47(6):814–824, 2018.
57. Dagfinrud H, Kvien TK, Hagen KB, et al.: Physiotherapy interventions for ankylosing spondylitis, *Cochrane Database Syst Rev* CD002822, 2008.
58. Van den Berg Rosaline, Xenofon Baraliakos, Braun Jürgen, et al.: First update of the current evidence for the management of ankylosing spondylitis with non-pharmacological treatment and nonbiologic drugs: a systematic literature review for the ASAS/EULAR management recommendations in ankylosing spondylitis, *Rheumatology* 51(8):1388–1396, 2012.
59. Karapolat H, Eyigor S, Zoghi M, et al.: Are swimming or aerobic exercise better than conventional exercise in ankylosing spondylitis patients? A randomized controlled study, *Eur J Phys Rehabil Med* 45(4):449–457, 2009.
60. Karabacakoglu A, Karaköse S, Ozerbil OM, et al.: Fluoroscopy-guided intraarticular corticosteroid injection into the sacroiliac joints in patients with ankylosing spondylitis, *Acta Radiol* 43(4):425–427, 2002.
61. Chinratanalab S, Sergent J: Systemic lupus erythematosus. In Frontera WR, Silver JK, Rizzo TD, editors: *Essentials of physical medicine and rehabilitation: musculoskeletal disorders, pain, and rehabilitation*, ed 3, Philadelphia, PA, 2015, Elsevier Saunders, pp 878–884.
62. Tayer WG, Nicassio PM, Weisman MH, et al.: Disease status predicts fatigue in systemic lupus erythematosus, *J Rheumatol* 28(9):1999–2007, 2001.
63. Tench C, Bentley D, Vleck V, et al.: Aerobic fitness, fatigue, and physical disability in systemic lupus erythematosus, *J Rheumatol* 29(3):474–481, 2002.
64. Carvalho MR, Sato EI, Tebexreni AS, et al.: Effects of supervised cardiovascular training program on exercise tolerance, aerobic capacity, and quality of life in patients with systemic lupus erythematosus, *Arthritis Rheum* 53(6):838–844, 2005.
65. Hospach T, Maier J, Peter Muller-Abt, et al.: Cervical spine involvement in patients with juvenile idiopathic arthritis-mri follow-up study, *Pediatric Rheumatol* 12(9), 2014.
66. Al-Matar MJ, Petty RE, Tucker LB, et al.: The early pattern of joint involvement predicts disease progression in children with oligoarticular (pauciarticular) juvenile rheumatoid arthritis, *Arthrit Rheumatol* 46(10):2708–2715, 2002.
67. Davidson J, Cleary AG, Bruce C, et al.: Disorders of bones, joints and connective tissues. In McIntosh N, Helms PJ, Smyth RL, et al.: *Forfar & Arneil's textbook of pediatrics*, ed 7, Edinburgh, 2008, Churchill Livingstone Elsevier, pp 1385–1415.
68. Ringold S, Cron RQ: The temporomandibular joint in juvenile idiopathic arthritis: frequently used and frequently arthritic, *Pediatric Rheumatol* 7(11), 2009.
69. Kuntze G, Nesbitt C, Whittaker J, et al.: Exercise therapy in juvenile idiopathic arthritis: a systematic review and meta-analysis, *Arch Phys Med Rehabil* 99(1):178–193, 2016.
70. Apti MD, Kasapçopur Ö, Mengi M, et al.: Regular aerobic training combined with range of motion exercises in juvenile idiopathic arthritis, *BioMed Res Int* 2014: 2014. Article ID 748972, 6 pages.
71. Ruth NM, Passo MH: Juvenile idiopathic arthritis: management and therapeutic options, *Ther Adv Musculoskelet Dis* 4(2):99–110, 2012.
72. Khanuja K, Joki J, Bachman G, et al.: Gait and balance in the aging population: fall prevention using innovation and technology, *Maturitas* 110:51–56, 2018.
73. Field T: Knee osteoarthritis pain in the elderly can be reduced by massage therapy, yoga and tai chi: a review, *Complement Ther Clin Pract* 22:87–92, 2016.
74. Patel S, Hyung P, Paolo B, et al.: A review of wearable sensors and systems with application in rehabilitation, *J Neuroeng. Rehabil.* 9:21, 2012.
75. Danielsen A, Olofsen H, Bremdal BA, et al.: Increasing fall risk awareness using wearables: a fall risk awareness protocol, *J Biomed Inf* 63:184–194, 2016.
76. Lipsitz L, Lough M, Niemi J, et al.: A shoe insole delivering subsensory vibratory noise improves balance and gait in healthy elderly people, *Arch Phys Med Rehabil* 96:432–439, 2015.
77. The Effect of AposTherapy on Knee Pin (AposKnee). (2017). Retrieved from https://clinicaltrials.gov/ct2 (Identification No. NCT03171168).

42 Pregnancy and Rheumatic Diseases

LISA R. SAMMARITANO AND BONNIE L. BERMAS

KEY POINTS

With careful planning and a team approach, most women with rheumatic diseases can have successful pregnancies.

For best maternal and fetal outcome, patients with rheumatic diseases should conceive in periods of low disease activity and while on medications considered compatible with pregnancy.

Rheumatology patients should undergo pre-pregnancy assessment to assess disease severity and activity, medication safety, and relevant autoantibodies.

Not all anti-rheumatic medications can be used during pregnancy or breastfeeding, but recent data provide guidance for many commonly used medications.

Use of effective and safe contraception is critical for rheumatic disease patients, especially those taking teratogenic medications or with severe or active disease.

Introduction

The predominance of many rheumatic diseases in women during their reproductive years makes management of pregnancy an important component of the comprehensive care of these patients. Advancements in disease therapies and identification of risk factors for poor pregnancy outcome allow many more patients to safely pursue pregnancy. In order to best counsel and manage pregnant patients with rheumatic diseases, rheumatologists should be familiar with basic pregnancy-related changes and their interplay with disease manifestations and be knowledgeable about use of medications compatible with pregnancy and breastfeeding.

Interplay of Rheumatic Disease and Pregnancy Physiology

KEY POINTS

Normal pregnancy induces multiple physiologic changes that often impact manifestations of rheumatic diseases.

Hypertensive diseases of pregnancy may complicate pre-existing rheumatic disease and be difficult to differentiate from active rheumatic disease.

Understanding potential interactions between pregnancy and rheumatic disease requires a basic knowledge of pregnancy physiology. Pregnancy affects the maternal immune system in multiple ways to ensure fetal survival. In brief, cell-mediated immunity decreases, immunoglobulin secretion increases, and pregnancy-specific proteins suppress lymphocyte function. The dominant T helper 2 cell cytokine profile may have varying implications for different autoimmune diseases.[1]

During normal pregnancy, a majority of the organ systems experience some degree of change. Intravascular volume increases by 30% to 50% and may be poorly tolerated by patients with significant renal or cardiac compromise. The glomerular filtration rate (GFR) increases by 50%; as a result, patients with pre-existing proteinuria experience increased urinary protein excretion. Pregnancy induces a prothrombotic state, and the combination of estrogen-induced hypercoagulability, venous stasis, and compression by the gravid uterus elevates the risk of venous thromboembolism by a factor of five. Red blood cell mass increases to a lesser extent than plasma volume, resulting in anemia that is secondary to hemodilution. Elevated progesterone levels decrease gastrointestinal motility and sphincter tone: in conjunction with uterine compression, these changes result in gastric reflux in 80% of pregnant women. Slowed intestinal transit time contributes to an exacerbation of constipation in illnesses such as systemic sclerosis. Pregnancy-related rashes may occasionally be confused with autoimmune disease skin manifestations. A more common problem is facial and palmar erythema caused by pregnancy-induced vasodilatation mimicking inflammatory rash. Chloasma gravidarum, an estrogen-induced facial hyperpigmentation, may similarly suggest a malar rash. Hormone-induced ligamentous laxity often causes arthralgias. Finally, reversible bone loss occurs with both pregnancy and lactation; this is especially worrisome for patients with pre-existing osteopenia or osteoporosis[2] (Table 42.1).

Hypertensive disorders complicate as many as 10% of pregnancies in the general obstetric population and are more common in patients with rheumatic disorders. They are a major cause of maternal, fetal, and neonatal complications. Gestational hypertension and pre-eclampsia are both more common among women with systemic lupus erythematosus (SLE) and among women with renal disease of any etiology. The hypertension, proteinuria, renal insufficiency, and edema associated with pre-eclampsia can mimic a flare of rheumatic disease. Eclampsia, which includes seizures and rarely stroke, may be confused with central nervous system inflammation or ischemia. HELLP (hemolysis, elevated liver enzymes, low platelets) syndrome, a variant of severe pre-eclampsia, may similarly suggest active inflammatory disease.

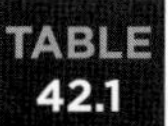

TABLE 42.1 Pregnancy Symptoms and Complications That Can Mimic or Exacerbate Rheumatic Disease

Pregnancy Manifestations	SLE	APS	Inflammatory Arthritis	Systemic Sclerosis	Vasculitis
Normal Pregnancy					
Skin					
Hypervascularity (malar or palmar erythema)	Malar flush, cutaneous vasculitis			Telangiectasias	Cutaneous vasculitis
Chloasma gravidarum	Malar rash				
Edema	Nephrotic syndrome	DVT	Periarticular inflammation	Early disease edema	Nephritis/renal vasculitis
Renal					
Proteinuria, lower GFR	Nephritis	APS Nephropathy		Renal crisis	Nephritis/Renal vasculitis
Heme					
Elevated WBC	Infection (especially if immunosuppressive therapy)				Active vasculitis
Anemia	Active disease				
Elevated ESR	Active disease				
Hypercoagulability	Increases already present risk, especially for APS				
GI					
Delayed motility				Worsening GI symptoms	
Musculoskeletal					
Arthralgia from ligamentous laxity	Arthralgia from active disease		Arthralgia from active disease		
SI joint/low back pain			Mimic/worsen axial arthritis pain		
Lowered bone density	Exacerbates low bone density associated with disease or therapy				
Abnormal Pregnancy					
Transient osteoporosis of hip	Avascular necrosis or hip arthritis				
Rash	Active disease				Active disease
HTN	Active disease			Active disease	
Pre-eclampsia	Nephritis	Nephropathy CAPS		Renal crisis	Nephritis/vasculitis
HELLP	Flare	CAPS		Renal crisis	Flare
Eclampsia	CNS Lupus	CNS thrombosis CAPS			CNS vasculitis

APS, Antiphospholipid syndrome; *CAPS*, catastrophic antiphospholipid syndrome; *CNS*, central nervous system; *DVT*, deep vein thrombosis; *ESR*, erythrocyte sedimentation rate; *GFR*, glomerular filtration rate; *GI*, gastrointestinal; *HELLP*, hemolysis, elevated liver enzymes, low platelet count; *HTN*, hypertension; *SLE*, systemic lupus erythematosus; *WBC*, white blood cell count.

General Principles of Pregnancy and Rheumatic Disease: Pre-pregnancy Assessment

KEY POINTS

Women with rheumatic diseases should aim to conceive during a period of inactive disease when possible for optimal pregnancy outcome.

Preconception evaluation should include assessment for disease damage, current disease activity, safety of medications for pregnancy, and aPL, anti-Ro/SS-A, and anti-La/SS-B antibodies.

General principles of pregnancy management for rheumatic disease patients include a structured pre-pregnancy assessment for risk for maternal and obstetric complications, communication of risk and prognosis through counseling, and coordinated rheumatology and obstetric care. Assessment of rheumatic disease patients considering pregnancy should follow the same protocol regardless of the specific diagnosis (Table 42.2). Determination of risk should include the identification of serious disease-related organ damage that might affect the patient's ability to safely carry a pregnancy, an evaluation of current and recent disease activity, a review of medication safety, and a serologic evaluation for autoantibodies associated with adverse maternal, fetal, or neonatal outcome.

TABLE 42.2 Checklist for Pre-pregnancy Assessment

No severe disease related damage (e.g., renal, cardiac, vascular)
Quiescent disease activity
Stable for 6 months on pregnancy-compatible medications
APL screening
Anti-SSA/Ro, SSB/La screening
Counseling regarding risks of disease, autoantibodies, medications and potential long-term risks

APL, Antiphospholipid antibody.

Severe Disease Damage

Severe manifestations of disease damage may preclude pregnancy. These include severe cardiomyopathy, cardiac valve disease, pulmonary arterial hypertension (PAH), neurologic manifestations, and renal insufficiency. The most important predictors of permanent renal disease in pregnant women with chronic kidney disease (CKD) are GFR <40 mL/min/1.73 m^2 and proteinuria greater than 1 g/24 hours.[3] The potential complications associated with severe chronic disease manifestations make pregnancy extremely high risk for these patients. If such patients are intent on having a biologic child, it may be appropriate to consider the safety of in vitro fertilization (IVF) with a surrogate.

Disease Activity

Active disease increases the risk of adverse pregnancy outcomes in almost every immune-mediated rheumatic disease. Active patients should defer pregnancy if possible, use suitable contraception, and be treated aggressively: when disease has been inactive for approximately 6 months, they should be reassessed.[4] Even in RA, disease activity during pregnancy is associated with a small increase in the risk of lower birth weight and pre-term delivery.[5]

Medication Review

If disease is inactive and there is no indication of severe damage, it is appropriate to assess the patient's present medical regimen. When current medications are contraindicated for use in pregnancy, one option is to taper and discontinue the current medications, allowing an appropriate period of time for high-risk medications to leave the system and for disease to demonstrate stability. The other option is to change to medications compatible with pregnancy and observe for stability on the new regimen.

Assessment of Autoantibodies

Assessment of relevant autoantibodies helps determine the type and frequency of pregnancy monitoring and the need for potential additional therapy; it also helps inform both physician and patient regarding risk. All patients with SLE, and any rheumatic disease patient with an adverse obstetric history or history of thrombosis, should be evaluated for the presence of antiphospholipid antibodies (aPL). Patients with SLE, RA, undifferentiated connective tissue disease (UCTD), and Sjögren's syndrome should be evaluated for the presence of anti-Ro/SS-A and La/SS-B antibodies.

Counseling

The full reproductive spectrum from fertility through lactation should be reviewed during the preconception visit. Education should include the risks of pregnancy for the individual patient given her particular clinical profile and underlying diagnosis and is based on damage, disease activity, renal function, aPL, anti-Ro/SS-A and La/SS-B, and medications. Each patient and her partner need to understand the risk to her health, the anticipated pregnancy outcome, and the potential risk to offspring (most commonly pre-term birth or small size for dates, which may have long-term health implications). The necessary follow-up and monitoring during pregnancy should be considered, as well as assurance of neonatal supportive care if complications develop. Long-term outcomes of children born to mothers with rheumatic disease have received recent attention. Children of both SLE and antiphospholipid syndrome (APS) patients are thought to have a slightly increased risk for developmental disability; thus these children should be monitored accordingly.[6]

Systemic Lupus Erythematosus

KEY POINTS

There is a higher risk of pre-eclampsia, pre-term delivery, fetal loss, and low birth weight infants in SLE patients.

SLE can flare up during pregnancy, especially in patients with pre-existing renal disease and highly active disease at the time of conception.

Anti-malarial medications should be continued during SLE pregnancy; prednisone and prednisolone may be used when necessary, as may azathioprine, cyclosporine, and tacrolimus.

SLE has its peak incidence in women in their reproductive years; thus co-existing pregnancy in this patient population is a frequent occurrence. Fertility is generally unimpaired in SLE patients in the absence of severe disease activity or history of cyclophosphamide administration.

Maternal Outcomes

For many years it was thought that patients with SLE would worsen during pregnancy, and most patients were counseled against becoming pregnant. Recent advances in management and a better understanding of pregnancy risk assessment have dramatically changed the recommendations and outlook for patients with SLE. At present, the majority of women with SLE can anticipate successful pregnancies resulting in a healthy baby. Nonetheless, patients can have flares during pregnancy and do experience a higher incidence of pregnancy-related complications. The data on whether SLE significantly worsens during pregnancy or remains stable are variable,[7,8] likely reflecting a lack of uniformity in the definition of disease flare, differing patient populations, lack of control groups, and varied medication use. Most agree that patients with active disease in the 6 months before conception are at greatest risk for flare during pregnancy, and flares during pregnancy are likely to mirror disease manifestations present prior to conception.[9] The overall flare rate in patients with active disease in the preconception period is estimated at 60%, whereas pregnancy flare rates may be as low as 10% in those with quiescent disease.[10]

TABLE 42.3 Differentiating Systemic Lupus Erythematosus Flare During Pregnancy From Pre-eclampsia

Systemic Lupus Erythematosus Flare	Pre-eclampsia or HELLP
Low white blood cell count	Normal to high white blood cell count
Occasional thrombocytopenia	Possible thrombocytopenia
Normal liver function tests	Elevated liver function tests
Elevated blood pressure	Elevated blood pressure
Proteinuria	Proteinuria
Cellular urine with red blood cells and casts	Acellular urine
Normal uric acid	Elevated uric acid
Low complement levels	Normal to elevated complement levels
Increased anti-dsDNA levels	No change in dsDNA levels
Other clinical signs of disease activity (rash, arthritis, etc.)	No additional signs of disease activity

dsDNA, Double-stranded DNA; *HELLP,* hemolysis, elevated liver enzymes, low platelet count.

In the PROMISSE (Predictors of Pregnancy Outcome: Biomarkers in Antiphospholipid Antibody Syndrome and Systemic Lupus Erythematosus) study, a multicenter prospective observational study of pregnant patients with stable SLE at conception, the rate of mild to moderate lupus flare was 15% and the risk of severe flare was 5%.[11]

Women with SLE have a two to fourfold increase in the rate of pregnancy complications. Pre-eclampsia will develop up to 25% of women with SLE,[12] and early onset pre-eclampsia (≤34 weeks gestation) is almost eight times more common in women with SLE than in the general population.[13] Distinguishing a lupus flare from pre-eclampsia is challenging. In general, one expects laboratory and clinical evidence suggesting active disease in a lupus flare, whereas pre-eclampsia is more likely associated with stable disease parameters and an acellular urine despite presence of proteinuria (Table 42.3). Differentiation is important because pre-eclampsia is managed with expectant delivery, whereas lupus flares are managed with medication. In reality, management often includes treatment for both because differentiation may be impossible and disease flare and pre-eclampsia may co-exist. In addition to the higher rate of pre-eclampsia, one-third of pregnancies in SLE patients are complicated by pre-term birth and one-third are delivered by Cesarean section.[12]

Fetal and Neonatal Outcomes

Fetal loss rate in SLE pregnancies, as manifested by combined miscarriage and still-birth rates, approaches 20%.[14] Risk factors for adverse pregnancy outcomes (APO), including fetal loss, intrauterine growth restriction (IUGR), and pre-term delivery, are varied but numerous studies suggest they fall into one of several categories: presence of active SLE, presence of renal disease, and presence of aPL (Table 42.4).[11,12,15] In addition, non-Caucasian patients have a higher risk of APO.[11] Patients with anti-Ro/SS-A and anti-La/SS-B antibodies are at risk for giving birth to children with neonatal lupus and congenital complete heart block.[16]

TABLE 42.4 Risk Factors for Adverse Pregnancy Outcomes in Systemic Lupus Erythematosus Patients

Active SLE	
High lupus disease activity (PGA)	Prednisone use
High DNA/low complements	Thrombocytopenia
Renal Disease	
Prior or active nephritis	Proteinuria > 1 gm
Hypertension	
Antiphospholipid Antibody (LAC)	

LAC, Lupus anticoagulant; *PGA,* patient global assessment; *SLE,* systemic lupus erythematosus.

TABLE 42.5 Pre-pregnancy Laboratory Work-up for Systemic Lupus Erythematosus

Complete blood count with differential and platelets
Complete metabolic panel
Urinalysis including microscopic analysis
Spot protein/creatinine urine ratio or 24-hour urine collection for protein[a]
Complement levels (C3, C4)
Anti-dsDNA level
Anti-Ro/SS-A and Anti-La/SS-B antibodies
Antiphospholipid antibodies: Anti-cardiolipin antibodies, anti-beta-2 glycoprotein I antibodies, and lupus anticoagulant
Uric acid

[a]As appropriate.

Management

Patients with SLE should be co-managed by a rheumatologist and a maternal-fetal medicine physician. Before pregnancy, patients should have a baseline evaluation including history, physical examination, and laboratory testing as summarized in Table 42.5. Laboratory testing should be repeated at least once per trimester with the exception of aPL and anti-Ro/SSA and anti-La/SSB antibodies. SLE patients should be maintained on anti-malarial medication throughout pregnancy because studies suggest benefits for both mother and neonate.[17] Patients with active disease or severe disease-related damage should be counseled against pregnancy. Low-dose aspirin is recommended for all SLE patients as pre-eclampsia prophylaxis because SLE is considered a significant risk factor for pre-eclampsia.[18] Those with co-existing APS are managed as outlined below. Ideally, patients should have well-controlled disease on low-risk medications for 6 months prior to attempting conception. Disease flares are managed with non-fluorinated glucocorticoids and, if necessary, the introduction of immunosuppressive agents compatible with pregnancy.

Overlap Syndromes and Undifferentiated Connective Tissue Disease

KEY POINTS

Patients with overlap syndromes or undifferentiated connective tissue disease are likely to have uncomplicated pregnancies unless accompanied by pulmonary hypertension or progression to more well-defined systemic rheumatic disease.

Overlap syndromes, sometimes referred to as *mixed connective tissue disease* (MCTD), has many clinical features in common with SLE. *Undifferentiated connective tissue disease* (UCTD) is the terminology applied to patients who have autoantibodies and clinical findings suggestive of rheumatologic disease but who cannot be classified with a specific disorder. Fertility is not reduced in women with overlap syndromes or UCTD.

Maternal Outcomes

Limited data are available on pregnancy outcomes in women with these disorders. In a series of ten patients with overlap syndromes, three had flares during pregnancy.[19] Flares included proteinuria, myositis, synovitis, and serositis. Pulmonary arterial hypertension (PAH) may develop in pregnant overlap syndrome patients; thus pre-pregnancy echocardiogram screening for PAH should be considered. In 25 reported UCTD pregnancies, six patients had flares, and symptoms meeting criteria for a new SLE diagnosis developed in one patient.[20]

Fetal and Neonatal Outcomes

There is no reported increase in fetal loss in women with overlap syndromes.[21] In general, patients with MCTD and UCTD have good pregnancy outcomes, although they should be monitored for disease flares and progression to other systemic rheumatic diseases.

Sjögren's Syndrome

KEY POINTS

Mothers who are anti-Ro/SS-A and anti-La/SS-B antibody-positive are recommended to have serial fetal echocardiograms to assess for development of congenital heart block; hydroxychloroquine may have a protective effect.

Although there are no reports of diminished fertility in patients with Sjögren's syndrome, some women experience dyspareunia because of vaginal dryness related to exocrine dysfunction.

Maternal Outcomes

Although case reports describe new onset renal disease and pericarditis in women with Sjögren's syndrome during pregnancy,[22] no large-scale studies document a pregnancy-associated increase in disease activity.

Fetal and Neonatal Outcomes

Case-control studies have suggested an increased risk of adverse pregnancy outcomes, including fetal loss, in women with Sjögren's syndrome, but not all studies confirm this.[23,24] Sixty percent of patients with Sjögren's syndrome have anti-Ro/SS-A and anti-La/SS-B antibodies. These antibodies confer risk for the development of congenital complete heart block (CHB) (2%) and neonatal lupus manifestations, including reversible thrombocytopenia or leukopenia, transaminitis, and photosensitive rash in their offspring (7% to 16%).[25]

Management

Antibody-positive women should undergo screening fetal echocardiograms between 16 and 26 weeks of pregnancy to monitor for the development of CHB. No data support a specific frequency of monitoring, but weekly monitoring has been suggested for women at highest risk, such as those with a history of a prior affected child, as their risk for complete heart block in a subsequent pregnancy is 18%.[25] Fluorinated glucocorticoids and intravenous immunoglobulin (IVIG) have been used in an effort to prevent development of CHB when first or second degree heart block is detected, but controlled studies have failed to demonstrate efficacy. Preliminary data suggest that hydroxychloroquine (HCQ) may reduce CHB risk[26] and delay or reduce risk of cutaneous manifestations.[27] A prospective study is in progress.

Antiphospholipid Antibody

KEY POINTS

Presence of lupus anticoagulant is the most important risk factor for adverse pregnancy outcome in aPL-positive women.

Standard prophylactic therapy for obstetric antiphospholipid syndrome is a combination of low-dose aspirin and low-dose heparin (low-molecular-weight heparin or unfractionated heparin).

The presence of antiphospholipid antibody (aPL) is a risk factor for pregnancy loss and other adverse pregnancy outcomes, especially when present in association with SLE. Clinical criteria for obstetric antiphospholipid syndrome (OB-APS) include pregnancy loss (three or more consecutive losses at less than 10 weeks of gestation or one or more losses on or after 10 weeks of gestation) or delivery at less than 34 weeks of gestation because of pre-eclampsia, IUGR, or fetal distress. Laboratory criteria include persistent lupus anticoagulant (LAC) or persistent moderate to high titer IgG or IgM isotypes of anti-cardiolipin (aCL) or anti–beta-2-glycoprotein I (aβ2GPI) antibodies.[28] Importantly, other causes of pregnancy loss must be ruled out with appropriate evaluation. When considering a diagnosis of OB-APS, all three criteria aPL (LAC, aCL, and aβ2GPI) should be tested. The usefulness of alternative (noncriteria) aPL testing is uncertain.

The potential effect of aPL on fertility has been controversial, with the concern that aPL may interfere with implantation, particularly after IVF. Nevertheless, the Practice Committee of the American Society for Reproductive Medicine has released guidelines based on extensive literature review, which state that there is no indication to check aPL as part of a fertility work-up or to treat aPL-positive women for the purpose of improving IVF cycle outcome.[29]

Maternal Outcomes

Maternal complications associated with OB-APS include pregnancy loss, pre-eclampsia, eclampsia, and HELLP syndrome. Antiphospholipid antibody associated with HELLP syndrome generally occurs early (at 28 to 36 weeks), with hepatic infarction in one-third of cases and frequent progression to other thrombotic complications.[30] Other maternal complications include thrombosis (including catastrophic APS) and severe third-trimester thrombocytopenia.

Fetal and Neonatal Outcomes

The most frequent neonatal complications are premature birth and IUGR. Premature births are more common in patients who have both APS and SLE. In primary APS pregnancies, risk factors for poor neonatal outcome are similar to predictors for adverse pregnancy outcomes overall and include LAC, triple antibody positivity (defined as presence of LAC, aCL, and aβ2GPI), and history of vascular thrombosis. Patients with previous pregnancy morbidity alone without history of thrombotic manifestations may have a more favorable neonatal outcome.[31] Transplacental passage of anti-cardiolipin antibody has been documented, but thrombosis in the fetus or neonate is rare. Neonatal APS has been reported in less than 20 infants, and many infants had additional thrombotic risk factors, such as indwelling catheters.[32]

Management

Effective management of the aPL-positive patient during pregnancy requires assessment of risk for adverse pregnancy outcome and appropriate fetal monitoring in the third trimester. In the prospective multicenter PROMISSE study, LAC was identified as the most important risk factor for adverse pregnancy outcome in 144 aPL-positive women. Multivariate analysis showed the relative risk for adverse pregnancy outcome with presence of LAC to be 12.15 (95% CI 2.92 to 50.54, $P = 0.0006$).[33] Other independent risk factors included younger age, history of thrombosis, and SLE. Importantly, aCL and aβ2GPI status were not independently associated with adverse pregnancy outcome in this study. Triple aPL positivity has been suggested as an important risk factor in other cohorts, however,[31] and presence of low complement levels may also be associated with increased risk.[34]

A 1992 prospective study by one group first showed that low-dose heparin plus low-dose aspirin is equal in efficacy to prior therapy with corticosteroids plus low-dose aspirin, with fewer side effects.[35] This combination remains the standard of care, alongside either low-molecular-weight heparin (LMWH) or unfractionated heparin (UF). Meta-analyses of treatment trials confirm the benefit of combination therapy; however, controversy continues regarding the details of the efficacy of this therapy. One analysis of five studies with 334 primary APS patients suggested success rates of 75% for combination therapy versus 56% for low-dose aspirin alone[36]; another meta-analysis found combination therapy to be effective for early, but not late, losses and found UF, but not LMWH, to improve outcomes.[37] Second-line therapy for treatment failure is usually the addition of IVIG based on case reports, although randomized treatment trials do not support benefit.[38] Preliminary data suggest a possible benefit of adding HCQ to standard therapy for primary APS patients.[39] Future therapies based on murine models may include complement[40] or TNF inhibitors.[41] No strong data currently exist to support aspirin plus heparin treatment of obstetric patients with asymptomatic aPL antibodies, but low-dose aspirin therapy is generally recommended for all patients with positive aPL as pre-eclampsia prophylaxis.[18] Patients with previous thrombosis require therapeutic dosing of heparin throughout pregnancy, with a change from warfarin either preconception or before 6 weeks of gestation, to avoid warfarin embryopathy. Heparin dosing usually requires adjustment later in pregnancy because of increased clearance, and LMWH is frequently changed to UF near term because of its shorter half-life. Fetal monitoring with nonstress tests, Doppler studies, or serial ultrasound is routine in the third trimester. Postpartum anticoagulation should be continued for 6 to 12 weeks for patients with OB-APS. Recommendations for long-term thrombosis prophylaxis in patients with OB-APS without a history of thrombosis are lacking, although one large observational cohort study reported an increased risk for subsequent deep vein thrombosis and stroke in these women.[42]

Inflammatory Arthritis

KEY POINTS

- RA tends to improve during pregnancy.
- Active RA during pregnancy can result in lower birth weight infants.
- Preconception planning for inflammatory arthritis patients may require medication adjustments; anti-malarials and sulfasalazine can potentially be continued, methotrexate and leflunomide must be discontinued, and recent data suggest TNF inhibitors may be continued if necessary.

Rheumatoid Arthritis

Rheumatologists are frequently required to manage RA during pregnancy and, less commonly, to manage pregnancy in women with psoriatic arthritis (PsA) and the spondyloarthropathies (SpA). Smaller family size has been reported in women with RA diagnosed before childbearing.[43] Decreased family size is likely multifactorial and may include delays in conception because of disease activity or medication adjustment. Reduced fertility does not seem to be related to ovarian function because anti-Müllerian hormone levels (a marker of ovarian reserve) are normal.[44] Prolonged time-to-pregnancy in RA may relate to patients being older or nulliparous, having higher disease activity, using nonsteroidal anti-inflammatory drugs (NSAIDs), or using prednisone >7.5 mg daily.[45]

Maternal Outcomes

Clinically meaningful remission in RA during pregnancy may be difficult to define, in part because inflammatory markers, including erythrocyte sedimentation rate (ESR) and C-reactive protein (CRP), are elevated in healthy pregnancies and do not provide a good reflection of disease activity. Although early reports suggested approximately 70% of RA patients entered remission during pregnancy,[46] a 2008 study that used the Disease Activity Scale (DAS) 28 found that only 48% of RA patients improved.[47] Patients who are negative for anti-citrullinated protein antibodies (ACPAs) and rheumatoid factor (RF) are more likely to remit.[48]

Fetal and Neonatal Outcomes

RA does not appear to increase the rate of fetal loss during pregnancy.[49] Nevertheless, even after controlling for medication use, women with active RA during pregnancy are at increased risk for giving birth to small for gestational age infants and for pre-term delivery.[5,50]

Minimizing disease activity during pregnancy appears to be important for optimal fetal outcome.

Psoriatic Arthritis and Ankylosing Spondylitis

Some, but not all, case series suggest pregnancy-associated remission rates for PsA are similar to those for RA.[51] Results are more disparate for pregnancy in spondyloarthropathies. One survey of 649 women with ankylosing spondylitis (AS) found that roughly one-third of patients worsened, one-third stayed the same, and one-third improved during pregnancy.[52] Cesarean section rates may be as high as 58% in the spondyloarthropathies, with a reported miscarriage rate of 15% and a slightly increased rate of pre-term delivery.[53,54]

Management

Teratogenic medications such as methotrexate and leflunomide must be discontinued before pregnancy; current evidence suggests that other medications such as anti-malarials and sulfasalazine may be continued. Recent evidence suggests that TNF inhibitors may be continued during pregnancy through the second trimester in women with active disease. NSAIDs and glucocorticoids may be used sparingly during pregnancy, but NSAIDs must be stopped during the third trimester due to concern for premature closure of the ductus arteriosis. Evaluation of cervical spine stability and hip range of motion is suggested before delivery.

Inflammatory Myositis

KEY POINTS

Quiescent disease at conception is associated with better pregnancy outcomes for idiopathic inflammatory myopathy patients.

Corticosteroids, intravenous immunoglobulin, and azathioprine are useful for idiopathic inflammatory myopathy flares during pregnancy.

Idiopathic inflammatory myopathies (IIM) include polymyositis (PM), dermatomyositis (DM), juvenile myositis (JM), and inclusion body myositis (IBM). Because the age of onset is bimodal, either in childhood or older adulthood, it is uncommon for patients to have pregnancies after the diagnosis of adult-onset myositis, and data are limited. One series found myositis developed in only 14% of patients before or during the childbearing years[55]; another recent series reported 8 in 51 patients with pregnancies following diagnosis.[56] There are no data on fertility in patients with IIM.

Maternal Outcomes

Pregnancies have been reported during both quiescent and active periods of disease, and a number of reports have described new onset disease during or immediately after pregnancy.[55,57] New disease onset during pregnancy is often acute and severe, and rhabdomyolysis and myoglobinuria have been reported.[57] Risk of flare during pregnancy for patients in remission before conception is low.[56] Although disease with onset during pregnancy has a more severe course, maternal outcome is good overall for patients with IIM, and maternal mortality is rare.

Fetal and Neonatal Outcomes

Neonatal outcomes are best for patients with pre-existing disease who are in remission at the time of conception, with no increased risk for fetal loss. Active disease early in the pregnancy has an adverse effect on fetal and neonatal outcomes, whereas a flare later in pregnancy generally does not. Neonatal outcomes are worst for patients with new onset disease during pregnancy, with only a 38% survival rate. In addition to fetal loss, prematurity, and IUGR, other uncommon fetal outcomes have been reported. Two infants with elevated creatinine kinase (CK) levels at birth were born to mothers with IIM.[58]

Management

Patients with IIM are most likely to have successful pregnancies if disease is quiescent before conception.[59] No evidence supports prophylactic corticosteroid treatment, but careful follow-up with prompt treatment of even mild disease flares may improve pregnancy outcome. IVIG has been used successfully with disease onset in the first trimester.[60] Azathioprine may be considered, either alone or in combination with IVIG.

Systemic Sclerosis

KEY POINTS

Systemic sclerosis patients with active renal disease, PAH, or significant cardiac compromise should avoid pregnancy because of high risk for poor maternal outcome.

Systemic sclerosis patients with early diffuse disease should generally defer pregnancy due to a higher risk of scleroderma renal crisis.

Systemic sclerosis (SSc) is an uncommon disease with a predilection for women during the fifth to sixth decade of life; as a result, there is limited information on this disorder during pregnancy. Nevertheless, as more women extend childbearing into their forties, pregnancy issues in SSc become more relevant. Data on whether SSc impacts fertility are conflicting. One retrospective study reports a greater than twofold incidence of infertility before diagnosis,[61] but another study did not find decreased fertility.[62]

Maternal Outcomes

Raynaud's phenomenon generally improves in SSc pregnancy because of increased blood flow to the periphery, whereas gastroesophageal reflux often worsens because of diaphragmatic relaxation. Skin disease does not progress.[63] Patients with early diffuse SSc and active skin thickening may have a higher risk of scleroderma renal crisis during pregnancy.[64] Management of renal crisis during pregnancy is challenging because angiotensin-converting enzyme (ACE)-inhibitors and angiotensin receptor blockers (ARBs) are contraindicated; however, when life-threatening disease occurs, these medications should be used. Scleroderma renal crisis may be difficult to differentiate from pre-eclampsia. Patients with pre-existing PAH are at very high risk for serious pregnancy complications: fluid shifts during pregnancy and especially during delivery may lead to right heart failure and, in some instances, death. In general, these patients should be counseled to avoid pregnancy.

Fetal Outcomes

Retrospective studies reveal a twofold increase in spontaneous abortion rate in women who are subsequently diagnosed with SSc,[65] and women with SSc have higher rates of pre-term delivery. Other reported complications include IUGR and low birth weight infants.[63]

Management

Given the potential for renal crisis, SSc patients should be followed by a rheumatologist and a maternal-fetal medicine specialist. Patients with PAH should be counseled about the high risk of maternal morbidity and mortality. Those with pre-existing renal disease should have their disease well-controlled on medications compatible with pregnancy.

Vasculitis

KEY POINTS

Pregnancy outcome in Takayasu's arteritis patients is largely determined by the presence of hypertension and pre-existing vascular damage. Aortic valve disease and the presence of aortic or renal aneurism are contraindications to becoming pregnant.

Patients with medium and small vessel vasculitides are likely to have safe and successful pregnancies if conception is during a period of disease remission.

Pregnancy in Behçet's disease has a variable effect on disease activity, but overall, fetal/neonatal outcomes are good.

Medical management for patients with vasculitis during pregnancy may involve corticosteroids, azathioprine, IVIG, and rarely, cyclophosphamide in the second or third trimester for life-threatening disease. Rituximab may also be considered for severe disease flares.

There are a limited number of reported cases of pregnancy in systemic vasculitis, in part due to both the older age of onset and male predominance. The available literature suggests active disease at the time of conception or new disease onset during pregnancy carries the most serious prognosis for maternal health and pregnancy outcome. Presence of vasculitis activity and end-organ damage may both affect pregnancy outcome. There are no data on fertility in these patients. In general, women who conceive after the diagnosis of any vasculitis report higher rates of pregnancy loss and pre-term delivery.[66] Flares of vasculitis activity during pregnancy vary from 18% to 50%.[66,67] A prospective series reported rates of miscarriage to be 20%; premature rupture of the membranes (PROM), 33%; and pre-term delivery, 50%.[67]

Large Vessel Vasculitis: Takayasu's Arteritis

Takayasu's arteritis is unique among the vasculitides in that it most commonly affects young women. Pregnancy complications are more commonly the result of vascular damage rather than disease activity, and pregnancy and maternal outcomes are optimized in patients with fewer damaged vessels. Risk of hypertension, pre-eclampsia, and IUGR is high, but likelihood of relapse of active vasculitis is low. In a large systematic review of 214 pregnancies in Takayasu's patients, pre-eclampsia occurred in 45% and pre-term delivery occurred in 16% of pregnancies. Although pregnancy did not affect disease activity, pre-existing aortic valve disease or aortic or renal artery aneurysm conferred high risk for maternal mortality.[68] Another case series reported serious maternal complications of congestive heart failure, renal insufficiency, and cerebral hemorrhage. Smoking and disease activity were significantly associated with increased risk of obstetric and maternal complications.[69] In one study, patients with renal artery involvement had a lower likelihood of adverse pregnancy outcomes if intervention (angioplasty or bypass graft) was performed prior to pregnancy.[70] Neonatal effects include low birth weight, premature delivery, and IUGR in as many as 40% of newborns, but favorable outcome overall is seen in 85%.[71]

Risk of complications such as cerebral hemorrhage or infarction in patients with Takayasu's arteritis is greatest at delivery because of fluctuations in regional blood flow. Monitoring of central aortic blood pressure is recommended for patients with severe vascular disease, with cautious use of epidural anesthesia to circumvent blood pressure vacillations.

Medium Vessel Vasculitis: Polyarteritis Nodosa

The earliest reports of polyarteritis nodosa (PAN) in pregnancy suggested high rates of maternal mortality. New onset disease during pregnancy mimicked pre-eclampsia, and diagnosis was delayed in most cases.[72] Recent reports of pregnancies in established disease suggest better outcomes during periods of remission.[73] Fetal outcome overall is good. Because new onset disease is most often in the third trimester or postpartum period, the risk to the pregnancy is primarily that of prematurity and low birth weight rather than fetal loss. Infants with transient cutaneous vasculitis have been reported.[74] Management includes use of corticosteroid and immunosuppressive medications.

Anti-neutrophil Cytoplasmic Antibody–Associated Vasculitis

In granulomatosis with polyangiitis (GPA), there is a 25% relapse rate during pregnancy, but a high rate of successful pregnancy outcome. As with PAN, adverse outcome is more likely in those with active or new manifestation of disease during pregnancy. Because most cases of new diagnoses have been in the third trimester, most of these pregnancies result in live-born births but pre-term deliveries. Quiescent disease at conception yields better outcomes.[75–77] Successful case reports describe the use of IVIG, azathioprine, and plasma exchange. Rarely, critically ill patients have been treated with cyclophosphamide in the second or third trimester with good neonatal outcome.[75] Severe subglottic stenosis may complicate delivery and require temporary tracheotomy to protect the airway.

Eosinophilic granulomatosis with polyangiitis (EGPA) case reports suggest maternal morbidity to be lower than in PAN.[78] Microscopic polyangiitis in pregnancy has rarely been reported, including a neonate with (transplacental) myeloperoxidase (MPO) antibodies, pulmonary hemorrhage, and renal disease.[79]

Behçet's Disease

There are contradictory reports of pregnancy effects on disease activity in patients with Behçet's disease. A literature review including 220 pregnancies found improved disease activity in 63% of cases and relapse in 28% of cases.[80] Necrotizing neutrophilic vasculitis in two placentas has been described.[81] Pregnancy outcome overall is good, with a miscarriage rate of 20%. Infants with pustulonecrotic skin lesions have been described[82] and there is a potential increased risk of thrombosis.[83]

Medications During Pregnancy and Breastfeeding

KEY POINTS

NSAID use should be minimized during early pregnancy and should be discontinued after 30 weeks of gestation because of the risk of premature closure of the ductus arteriosus.

The nonfluorinated glucocorticoids prednisone and prednisolone are the preferred corticosteroids for use during pregnancy because of their low placental transfer. The lowest dose possible should be used to control disease activity.

Hydroxychloroquine, sulfasalazine, azathioprine, 6-mercaptopurine, cyclosporine, tacrolimus, and IVIG are compatible with pregnancy.

TNF inhibitors can be used when needed to control active inflammatory arthritis. They should be discontinued after the second trimester if possible to minimize immunosuppression in the newborn. Avoid live vaccines for 6 months in infants exposed to biologics during pregnancy.

Other biologics such as abatacept, tocilizumab, belimumab, and rituximab can be used up until conception.

Methotrexate, leflunomide, thalidomide, mycophenolate mofetil, and cyclophosphamide should be avoided during pregnancy and lactation.

For other small molecules such as kinase inhibitors, limited data exist regarding their safety during pregnancy and lactation. These agents should be avoided until safety data are available.

Medication management during the preconception period for men and women and for women during pregnancy and lactation is challenging as not all medications can be safely used. In women with rheumatic diseases who desire pregnancy and require medication treatment, the potential risks of medication to the developing fetus and newborn must be weighed against the benefits of disease control. When assessing any medication, risk must be measured against the reported background congenital anomaly rate of approximately 3%. Limited information exists regarding drug safety in pregnancy. In an attempt to address this issue, the Food and Drug Administration (FDA) recently changed their labeling system. The former system utilized a graded system of A, B, C, D, and X, which incorrectly implied an increased risk with ascending letter grade rather than what it truly was: a reflection of the type (animal or human) and quality of data. The new labeling format is more clearly reflective of existing data and includes information for females and males of reproductive potential during the preconception period, pregnancy, and lactation.[84] Ideally, medications should be adjusted in women before conception, but inadvertent exposure to teratogenic medications does occur. If this happens, the patient should be referred to maternal-fetal medicine or genetics specialists for counseling and should be encouraged to enroll in appropriate registries such as the Organization of Teratology Information Specialists, or OTIS (http://www.mothertobaby.org/). If available, high-resolution fetal ultrasound should be performed to assess for detectable anomaly.

Although the benefits of breastfeeding extend to both the mother and the infant, drugs are transferred to breast milk by diffusion: nonprotein bound, low-molecular-weight, nonionized, and lipid-soluble medications are most likely to enter breast milk.[85] Limited data are available on the safety of paternal exposure to medication, but most medications are compatible with male exposure in the preconception period. There are no data to suggest that paternal use of medication postconception portends any risks to the developing fetus.[86] A summary of potential drug use in men and women who want to conceive and in women during pregnancy and lactation is shown in Table 42.6.

Aspirin, Nonsteroidal Anti-inflammatory Medications, and Cyclooxygenase-2 Inhibitors

High-dose aspirin and NSAIDs are teratogenic in animals, but congenital anomalies have not been reported in humans.[87] NSAIDs can cause premature closure of the ductus arteriosus in the third trimester and should be discontinued by 30 weeks of gestation. Both NSAIDs and cyclooxygenase (COX)-2 inhibitors can potentially interfere with implantation and ovulation and should be avoided during a conception cycle.[88] Some data suggest that NSAIDs and COX-2 inhibitors increase risk of spontaneous abortion during the first trimester.[89] Although findings are inconclusive, it seems reasonable to minimize the use of these medications during pregnancy. NSAIDs cross into breast milk at a very low concentration; thus these medications are thought to be compatible with nursing. Mothers of jaundiced infants should avoid those medications metabolized by the liver, and all NSAIDs should be avoided in lactating mothers whose infants have thrombocytopenia.

Glucocorticoids

The nonfluorinated glucocorticoids prednisone and prednisolone, which are typically used in the management of rheumatologic diseases, cross the placenta in low concentrations. In contrast, fluorinated glucocorticoids such as betamethasone readily cross the placenta to reach the developing fetus.[90] Recent evidence suggests that there is no increased rate of congenital anomalies after in utero glucocorticoid exposure.[91] Glucocorticoid use throughout pregnancy increases risk of pre-term delivery, small-for-gestational age infants, maternal hypertension, and gestational diabetes. Prednisone and prednisolone cross into breast milk in very low concentrations[92] and can be used in lactating women. When the dose is greater than 20 mg per day, avoiding breastfeeding within 4 hours of drug administration is recommended.

Anti-malarial Agents

Studies have not demonstrated an increased risk of teratogenicity in human pregnancy.[93] Importantly, no ocular toxicity was found on examination of 588 neonates exposed to these medications in utero.[94] Anti-malarials cross into breast milk at a low concentration, but exposed neonates showed no ocular toxicity.[95] Thus these medications are considered to be compatible with nursing.

Sulfasalazine

Although sulfasalazine and its metabolites do cross the placenta, large case series have not shown evidence for teratogenicity.[96] Sulfasalazine interferes with folic acid absorption, and thus pregnant women on this medication should take additional folic acid. Sulfasalazine appears in breast milk in significant concentrations. A single case of bloody diarrhea in a breastfed infant has been reported,[97] but this medication is considered compatible with

TABLE 42.6 Risks of Rheumatic Disease Medications During Pregnancy and Lactation

Drug	Maternal	Fetal	Lactation
Minimal Risk			
Hydroxychloroquine	None	None	Compatible
Sulfasalazine	Additional folic acid required as absorption is decreased	None	Compatible-one case of bloody diarrhea reported in neonate
IVIG	Risk of hepatitis C	Risk of hepatitis C	Compatible
Unfractionated heparin	Bleeding	None	Compatible
LMW heparin	Bleeding	None	Compatible
Aspirin (low-dose)	Bleeding	None	Compatible
Low to Moderate Risk			
NSAIDs	Interferes with ovulation and implantation, possible increase in first trimester pregnancy losses	Safe; discontinue after 30 weeks of gestation because of increased risk of premature closure of the ductus arteriosus	Compatible but avoid NSAIDs with long half-life and enterohepatic circulation
Prednisone and Prednisolone	PROM, gestational diabetes, hypertension	Possible No increase in congenital anomalies	Compatible but at dosing greater than 20 mg a day, discard breast milk for 4 hours after dose
Azathioprine 6-Mercaptopurine Cyclosporine A Tacrolimus	None None Renal Insufficiency None	Transplant and IBD literature endorse the safety of these immunosuppressives during pregnancy. All increase the risk of PROM, SGA, IUGR	Low risk Low risk Low risk Low risk
Etanercept Adalimumab Infliximab Golimumab Certolizumab	None None None None None		TNF inhibitors: Low concentration in breast milk—low risk
Colchicine	None	Limited studies in FMF suggest that this medication can be used during pregnancy	
High Risk			
Methotrexate		Embryotoxic and Teratogenic	Avoid
Leflunomide		Congenital anomalies reported	Avoid
Cyclophosphamide	Maternal infection	Teratogenic	Avoid
Mycophenolate Mofetil		Congenital anomalies reported	Avoid
Warfarin	Bleeding	Teratogenic	Avoid
Unknown Risk			
Rituximab			Avoid
Abatacept			Avoid
Tocilizumab			Avoid
Anakinra			Avoid
Belimumab			Avoid
Tofacitinib			Avoid

FMF, Familial Mediterranean fever; *IBD,* inflammatory bowel disease; *IUGR,* intrauterine growth retardation; *IVIG,* intravenous immunoglobulin; *LMW,* low-molecular-weight; *NSAIDS,* nonsteroidal anti-inflammatory drugs; *PROM,* premature rupture of the membranes; *SGA,* small for gestational age newborns; *TNF,* tumor necrosis factor.

Modified from Bermas BL: The medical management of the rheumatology patient during pregnancy. In *Contraception and Pregnancy in Patients with Rheumatic Disease.* New York, Springer, 2014, p. 275.

nursing. Because the active metabolite of sulfasalazine can displace bilirubin, women nursing premature infants or infants with hyperbilirubinemia should avoid this medication.

Immune Modulating Therapies

Methotrexate is both teratogenic and abortogenic and is contraindicated during pregnancy. In humans, methotrexate exposure during pregnancy, particularly between 6 and 8 weeks of gestation, can lead to craniofacial and limb malformations as well as significant developmental delays.[98] In women, methotrexate should be discontinued 1 to 3 months prior to conception. Limited data suggest that methotrexate is poorly transmitted into breast milk; however, current recommendations are to avoid use in lactating women.

Cyclophosphamide is extremely teratogenic and is contraindicated during pregnancy, although there are rare successful case reports of use during the third trimester for the management of vasculitis.[99] It is contraindicated in nursing women.

Although leflunomide is considered a potent teratogen in rodents, recent studies suggest early exposure results in few anomalies in humans.[100] Current recommendations are to either stop this medication 2 years before conception or to treat the patient with a cholestyramine washout to remove active metabolites in anticipation of pregnancy. No data exist as to whether leflunomide crosses into breast milk in significant concentrations. Nevertheless, given its long half-life, leflunomide should be avoided in lactating women.

Large transplant registries have followed thousands of pregnancies in which the mother is taking azathioprine and 6-mercapto purine and there is not an increased rate of congenital anomalies in exposed infants.[101] Minimal levels of these drugs are found in breast milk[102]; thus use of these medications in nursing mothers of full-term infants is low risk, although testing for thiopurine *S*-methyltransferase (TPMT) levels in the newborn may be considered. Cyclosporine does not carry an increased risk of congenital anomalies. Although only low levels of this medication have been found in breast milk, a single breastfed infant was found to have a therapeutic level after nursing.[103] Tacrolimus has been used in the management of lupus nephritis, and this medication is considered compatible with pregnancy.[104] Little tacrolimus is transferred into breast milk and thus breastfeeding may be low risk for the neonate.[105] Mycophenolate mofetil, although a cornerstone of lupus nephritis management, has been associated with patterns of congenital anomalies and is contraindicated during pregnancy and breastfeeding.[106]

Intravenous Immunoglobulin

Limited information exists on the safety of IVIG during pregnancy, but no cases of congenital anomalies have been reported; it is considered compatible with pregnancy and lactation.

Tumor Necrosis Factor Inhibitors

Most TNF inhibitors are not actively transported through the placenta until 15 weeks of gestation, when elevated levels in cord blood can be found. While there were early reports of a potential pattern of congenital anomalies in women exposed to TNF inhibitors during pregnancy, subsequent data did not substantiate these findings. Significant data support the use of these medications through the first two trimesters of pregnancy.[91] PEGylated forms (those linked to a polyethylene glycol, or PEG, chain) cross the placenta in very limited amounts and may be used throughout pregnancy.[107] A 3-month-old infant of a mother treated with infliximab throughout pregnancy died of disseminated infection after Bacille-Calmette-Guérin (BCG) immunization;[108] thus current suggestions aim to discontinue the IgG1-construct TNF inhibitors by the third trimester of pregnancy and to avoid immunizations with live vaccines for 6 months in exposed infants. Transfer of TNF inhibitors into breast milk is minimal. These agents are considered compatible with breastfeeding.[109]

Other Biologic Agents

Limited information exists on the safety of other biologic medications during pregnancy. One large series of 153 pregnancies in rituximab-exposed fetuses demonstrated that the congenital malformation rate was similar to the background rate.[110] There are varied recommendations by manufacturers as to when these medications should be discontinued prior to pregnancy, with ranges from a few months (belimumab, abatacept, tocilizumab) to a year (rituximab); however, given that little IgG crosses the placenta before 12 weeks of gestation, it seems unlikely that significant amounts of biologic agents would reach the developing fetus if medication were discontinued at the time of conception.

Other Medications

Anticoagulation is the mainstay of therapy for the management of APS during pregnancy. Although warfarin is contraindicated during pregnancy because of its teratogenicity, heparin and LMWH are considered compatible with pregnancy and lactation. Too little information exists on the newer anticoagulants to assess their safety during pregnancy and lactation. Colchicine is rarely used during pregnancy; however, available data suggest that use during pregnancy does not cause congenital anomalies.[111] ACE inhibition and ARBs are contraindicated during pregnancy and lactation because of the risk of oligohydramnios and renal failure in the newborn; transition to another anti-hypertensive in advance of conception is recommended.

Paternal Medication Use

KEY POINTS

Cyclophosphamide and thalidomide should be avoided in men planning for pregnancy.

Sulfasalazine may affect spermatogenesis, and semen analysis should be considered if there is a delay in conception.

There are two main issues regarding paternal exposure to medications. The first is use of medication in men planning to conceive, and the second is medication use after conception has occurred. The latter concern is generally thought to be hypothetical and not a significant risk; the dose of medication transferred to the mother via semen and available for placenta transfer is negligible.[86] There are two medications that are contraindicated in men planning to conceive: thalidomide and cyclophosphamide. Detectable levels of thalidomide have been measured in semen and so paternal use should be avoided given its strong potential as a human teratogen. Cyclophosphamide induces germ cell damage in animals, so it is recommended to discontinue this medication in men planning to conceive.[112] Sulfasalazine may cause abnormalities in sperm count and function, and semen analysis should be considered if there is a delay in conception; however, it has not been associated with teratogenicity.[91] Other medications including NSAIDs, anti-malarials, TNF inhibitors, the immunosuppressive agents azathioprine and 6-mercaptopurine, cyclosporine, mycophenolate mofetil, and tacrolimus are all considered compatible with paternal use.[91] Reassuringly, recent data suggest that paternal exposure to methotrexate does not cause teratogenicity; therefore this medication does not need to be discontinued in men wanting to conceive.[113,114] There are no data on the safety of abatacept, belimumab, tocilizumab, ustekinumab, secukinumab, or the small molecules such as tofacitinib, baracitinib, and apremilast for men wanting to conceive.

Pregnancy-Related Issues for Rheumatic Disease Patients

Contraception

KEY POINTS

Contraceptive options should be discussed with all female patients of reproductive age, with recommendations tailored to the individual patient's medical and social situation.

Combined hormonal contraceptives may be used in stable SLE patients but are contraindicated in patients with positive aPL. Levonorgestrel IUDs or progesterone subdermal implants are good alternatives for most aPL-positive patients.

Rheumatic disease patients are strongly advised to use contraception to avoid pregnancy if they have severe disease-related damage, active disease, or are taking teratogenic medications. In practice, however, rheumatic disease patients underutilize effective contraception. In a series of 97 SLE patients at risk for pregnancy, 23% had unprotected sex "most of the time."[115] In another series, 55% of those who used contraceptives were using less effective barrier methods, even those on teratogenic medications.[116] Efforts at formalizing patient education to improve physician and patient awareness of effective contraception include educational materials, the use of institutional quality indicators, and adherence to FDA recommendations.

Contraceptive Methods

Currently available contraceptives include barrier methods, hormonal contraceptives, intrauterine devices (IUDs), and subdermal implants. In general, long-acting reversible contraceptives such as IUDs or subdermal implants have the greatest efficacy, followed by other hormonal contraceptives; barrier or natural methods of contraception are least effective, although barrier methods may reduce the risk of sexually transmitted diseases.

IUDs generally contain either progesterone (levonorgestrel) or copper. They have a low risk of infection for most patients; however, patients treated with immunosuppressive medications have not been specifically studied. Reassuringly, studies show no increased infection risk in women infected with HIV.[117]

Hormonal contraceptives may be combined estrogen-progesterone or progesterone-only. Combined hormonal contraceptives include the pill, transdermal patch, and vaginal ring. Serious side effects include a three to five times increase in the risk of venous thromboembolism and two times increase in stroke risk. Common medications, including warfarin and mycophenolate, may interact with these agents. In the past, concern about estrogen-induced flares has limited use of combined oral contraceptives in patients with SLE; however, prospective controlled studies in women with mild or stable disease activity showed no increased risk of flares with combined oral contraceptive (COC) use.[118,119] Oral contraceptives containing the progestin drospirenone may increase potassium levels and should be used with caution in patients with nephritis or on ACE-inhibitors. While the vaginal ring provides equal or lower estrogen levels than the pill, the patch provides 60% greater estrogen levels, raising concern for increased thrombosis risk. Estrogen-containing contraceptives are not advised for use in aPL-positive patients.

Progesterone-only contraceptives include oral and intramuscular preparations, IUDs, and the subdermal etonogestrel implant. Prolonged depot medroxyprogesterone acetate (DMPA) may decrease bone density due to inhibition of ovulation: it is best avoided in corticosteroid-treated patients or patients with low bone density. Progesterone-only contraceptives represent a good option for aPL-positive patients: the risk for thromboembolism is low and they generally decrease menstrual bleeding, a potential benefit for patients on anti-coagulation. Emergency contraception is an option for all rheumatic disease patients and includes the copper IUD, prescription progesterone-receptor modulators, and over-the-counter levonorgestrel. Levonorgestrel is effective, convenient, and not contraindicated in patients with thrombophilia or cardiovascular disease.

Contraceptive choice in patients with rheumatic disease is challenging but important. The progesterone IUD or subdermal implant is preferable for most patients. Ultimately, decisions regarding contraceptive method in patients must take into account not only the risk of the method but also the risk of unplanned pregnancy, the ease of use, the efficacy of each method, and the patient's values and preferences (Table 42.7).

Fertility and Assisted Reproductive Techniques

KEY POINTS

Measures to preserve fertility in rheumatology patients include use of leuprolide during treatment with cyclophosphamide and embryo or oocyte cryopreservation.

Risk of lupus flare and thrombosis are concerns for SLE and aPL/APS patients undergoing ovarian induction/in vitro fertilization; careful management generally results in successful outcomes.

Fertility is generally unimpaired by rheumatic diseases, with important exceptions. Patients treated with cyclophosphamide (CYC) are at risk for gonadal failure, especially with older age and greater cumulative dose.[120] Active disease, high-dose corticosteroid, and chronic renal failure may adversely affect the hypothalamic-pituitary-ovarian axis. Tests of ovarian reserve include follicle-stimulating hormone (FSH), antral follicle count, and anti-Müllerian hormone level.

Prevention of medication-induced infertility is important. Concurrent treatment with a long-acting GnRH analogue (e.g., leuprolide) may decrease risk of premature ovarian failure in

TABLE 42.7 **Benefits and Risks of Contraceptive Methods for Rheumatic Disease Patients**

	Copper IUD	LNG IUD	Progestin Pill	DMPA	Progestin Implant	Comb OC	Vaginal Ring	Patch
Frequency	10 years; Insertion by MD	3-5 years; Insertion by MD	Daily oral; Take same time each day	Every 3 months; Injection by MD	3 years; Insertion by MD	Daily; oral	Monthly	Weekly
Relevant Side Effects	Increased cramps/ bleeding	Little to no systemic progestin effects Decreased cramps, bleeding	Break-through bleeding	Delayed return to fertility Decreased bone density	Rapid return to fertility No effect on bone density	Prothrombotic effect Frequent medication interactions May increase bone density		
Rheumatic Disease-Related Concerns	Uncertain, but unlikely increased infection risk in immunosuppressed patients[a] LNG IUD decreases menstrual bleeding in anticoagulated patients No significant thrombosis or lupus flare risk		Decreased menstrual bleeding No significant thrombosis or lupus flare risk	Decreased menstrual bleeding No sig lupus flare risk Sig risk of osteoporosis; avoid in RA or steroid-treated patients; possible thrombosis risk	Decreased menstrual bleeding No significant thrombosis or lupus flare risk	No increased risk of flare in stable SLE Increased risk thrombosis: Avoid with (+) aPL	Similar estrogen levels to OC Increased risk thrombosis: Avoid with (+) aPL	Higher estrogen levels than OC Increased risk thrombosis: Avoid with (+) aPL

[a]Avoid if patient has multiple sexual partners.

aPL, Antiphospholipid antibody; *DMPA*, depot medroxyprogesterone acetate; *IUD*, intrauterine device; *LNG IUD*, levonorgestrel intrauterine device; *OC*, oral contraceptive; *RA*, rheumatoid arthritis.

CYC-treated patients, although long-term data are limited.[121] Embryo and oocyte cryopreservation are good options for preserving fertility in patients who are stable enough to undergo ovarian hyperstimulation but are not able or ready to pursue pregnancy. For male patients, sperm cryopreservation prior to CYC therapy is encouraged.

Common assisted reproduction techniques include ovarian induction (OI), with or without IVF, and embryo transfer. IVF cycles require more aggressive hyperstimulation with surgical extraction of oocytes, fertilization, and reimplantation. Although rare, ovarian hyperstimulation syndrome (OHSS) is an important complication that results in capillary leak with pleural effusion and ascites; severe OHSS increases risk for thrombosis and renal compromise, particular issues of concern for rheumatic disease patients. Important risks relate to the elevated estrogen levels and include lupus flare and thrombosis.[122–124] SLE patients with OI/IVF–induced flare generally have good outcomes.

Thrombosis in aPL-positive or APS patients undergoing OI/IVF appears to be rare, although most reported patients have been treated empirically with aspirin or LMWH. Data do not support aPL as a cause of failed IVF or infertility, and so anticoagulation is not indicated to improve IVF cycle outcome but should be considered as thromboprophylaxis.[29] Pre-IVF assessment should mimic the pre-pregnancy evaluation for rheumatic disease patients. OI/IVF should be planned for patients with stable inactive disease on medications compatible with pregnancy. Prophylactic anticoagulation with heparin or LMWH is mandatory for confirmed APS patients, and reproductive medicine specialists may choose to modify the hormonal protocol to limit peak estrogen levels.

Conclusion

Caring for women with rheumatic disease throughout their reproductive lifespans is both challenging and rewarding. The American College of Rheumatology has released a comprehensive guideline for the management of reproductive health in rheumatic and musculoskeletal disease patients; detailed recommendations based on GRADE methodology provide guidance for decisions regarding contraception, assisted reproductive technology, fertility preservation with use of cyclophosphamide, use of hormone replacement therapy, and management and medication use in pregnancy and breastfeeding.[125] In summary, all reproductive-aged rheumatic disease patients on potentially teratogenic medications need to be counseled about effective contraceptive methods. In patients who are treated with cyclophosphamide, it is important to discuss fertility-sparing approaches before the initiation of therapy. Common principles of reproductive care for rheumatic disease patients considering pregnancy, regardless of specific diagnosis, include identifying the limited number of patients with severe disease-related damage who should avoid pregnancy, counseling patients to conceive when disease has been stable and inactive on medications considered low risk for pregnancy, and assessing particular risk factors for outcome, such as antiphospholipid and anti-Ro/SS-A and anti-La/SS-B antibodies. Finally, a plan for medication use in the case of disease flare during or after pregnancy should be agreed upon by the patient and treating clinician at the onset of pregnancy. With careful planning, most women with rheumatic disorders can anticipate a successful pregnancy with a good outcome.

The references for this chapter can also be found on ExpertConsult.com.

References

1. Betz AG: Immunology: tolerating pregnancy, *Nature* 490(7418): 47–48, 2012.
2. Branch DW, Wong LF: Normal pregnancy, pregnancy complications, and obstetric management. In Sammaritano LR, Bermas BL, editors: *Contraception and pregnancy in patients with rheumatic disease*, New York, 2014, Springer, pp 31–62.
3. Imbasciati E, Gregorini G, Cabiddu G, et al.: Pregnancy in CKD stages 3 to 5: fetal and maternal outcomes, *Am J Kidney Dis* 49(6):753–762, 2007.
4. Chakravarty EF, Colón I, Langen ES, et al.: Factors that predict prematurity and preeclampsia in pregnancies that are complicated by systemic lupus erythematosus, *Am J Obstet Gynecol* 192(6):1897–1904, 2005.
5. Wallenius M, Skomsvoll JF, Irgens LM, et al.: Pregnancy and delivery in women with chronic inflammatory arthritides with a specific focus on first birth, *Arthritis Rheum* 63(6):1534–1542, 2011.
6. Nalli C, Iodice A, Reggia R, et al.: Long-term outcome of children of rheumatic disease patients. In Sammaritano LR, Bermas BL, editors: *Contraception and pregnancy in patients with rheumatic disease*, New York, 2014, Springer, pp 289–303.
7. Lockshin MD: Pregnancy does not cause systemic lupus erythematosus to worsen, *Arthritis Rheum* 32(6):665–670, 1989.
8. Petri M, Howard D, Repke J: Frequency of lupus flare in pregnancy. The Hopkins lupus pregnancy center experience, *Arthritis Rheum* 34(12):1538–1545, 1991.
9. Tedeschi SK, Guan H, Fine A, et al.: Organ-specific systemic lupus erythematosus activity during pregnancy is associated with adverse pregnancy outcomes, *Clin Rheumatol* 35(7):1725–1732, 2016.
10. Ruiz-Irastorza G, Lima F, Alves J, et al.: Increased rate of lupus flare during pregnancy and the puerperium: a prospective study of 78 pregnancies, *Br J Rheumatol* 35(2):133–138, 1996..
11. Buyon JP, Kim MY, Guerra MM, et al.: Predictors of pregnancy outcomes in patients with lupus: a cohort study, *Ann Intern Med* 163(3):153–163, 2015.
12. Clowse MEB, Jamison M, Myers E, et al.: A national study of the complications of lupus in pregnancy, *Am J Obstet Gynecol* 199(2):127.e1–127.e6, 2008.
13. Simard JF, Arkema EV, Nguyen C, et al.: Early-onset preeclampsia in lupus pregnancy, *Paediatr Perinat Epidemiol* 31(1):29–36, 2017.
14. Yasmeen S, Wilkins EE, Field NT, et al.: Pregnancy outcomes in women with systemic lupus erythematosus, *J Matern Fetal Med* 10(2):91–96, 2001.
15. Kim MY, Guerra MM, Kaplowitz E, et al.: Complement activation predicts adverse pregnancy outcome in patients with systemic lupus erythematosus and/or antiphospholipid antibodies, *Ann Rheum Dis* 77(4):549–555, 2018.
16. Mendez B, Saxena A, Buyon JP: Neonatal lupus. In Sammaritano LR, Bermas BL, editors: *Contraception and pregnancy in patients with rheumatic disease*, New York, 2014, Springer, pp 251–272.
17. Clowse MEB, Magder L, Witter F, et al.: Hydroxychloroquine in lupus pregnancy, *Arthritis Rheum* 54(11):3640–3647, 2006.
18. ACOG Committee Opinion No. 743, *Obstet Gynecol* 132(1):e44–e52, 2018.
19. Kitridou RC: Pregnancy in mixed connective tissue disease, *Rheum Dis Clin North Am* 31(3):497–508, 2005. vii.
20. Mosca M, Neri R, Strigini F, et al.: Pregnancy outcome in patients with undifferentiated connective tissue disease: a preliminary study on 25 pregnancies, *Lupus* 11(5):304–307, 2002.
21. Lundberg I, Hedfors E: Pregnancy outcome in patients with high titer anti-RNP antibodies. A retrospective study of 40 pregnancies, *J Rheumatol* 18(3):359–362, 1991.
22. Mutsukura K, Nakamura H, Iwanaga N, et al.: Successful treatment of a patient with primary Sjögren's syndrome complicated with pericarditis during pregnancy, *Intern Med* 46(14):1143–1147, 2007.
23. De Carolis S, Salvi S, Botta A, et al.: The impact of primary Sjogren's syndrome on pregnancy outcome: our series and review of the literature, *Autoimmun Rev* 13(2):103–107, 2014.
24. Ballester C, Grobost V, Roblot P, et al.: Pregnancy and primary Sjögren's syndrome: management and outcomes in a multicentre retrospective study of 54 pregnancies, *Scand J Rheumatol* 46(1):56–63, 2017.
25. Izmirly PM, Rivera TL, Buyon JP: Neonatal lupus syndromes, *Rheum Dis Clin North Am* 33(2):267–285, 2007.
26. Izmirly PM, Kim MY, Llanos C, et al.: Evaluation of the risk of anti-SSA/Ro-SSB/La antibody-associated cardiac manifestations of neonatal lupus in fetuses of mothers with systemic lupus erythematosus exposed to hydroxychloroquine, *Ann Rheum Dis* 69(10):1827–1830, 2010.
27. Barsalou J, Costedoat-Chalumeau N, Berhanu A, et al.: Effect of in utero hydroxychloroquine exposure on the development of cutaneous neonatal lupus erythematosus, *Ann Rheum Dis* 77(12):1742–1749, 2018.
28. Miyakis S, Lockshin MD, Atsumi T, et al.: International consensus statement on an update of the classification criteria for definite antiphospholipid syndrome (APS), *J Thromb Haemost* 4(2):295–306, 2006.
29. Practice committee of the American Society for Reproductive Medicine: Anti-phospholipid antibodies do not affect IVF success, *Fertil Steril* 90:S172–S173, 2008.
30. Appenzeller S, Souza FHC, Wagner Silva de Souza A, et al.: HELLP syndrome and its relationship with antiphospholipid syndrome and antiphospholipid antibodies, *Semin Arthritis Rheum* 41(3):517–523, 2011.
31. Ruffatti A, Tonello M, Visentin MS, et al.: Risk factors for pregnancy failure in patients with anti-phospholipid syndrome treated with conventional therapies: a multicentre, case-control study, *Rheumatology (Oxford)* 50(9):1684–1689, 2011.
32. Boffa M-C, Lachassinne E: Infant perinatal thrombosis and antiphospholipid antibodies: a review, *Lupus* 16(8):634–641, 2007.
33. Lockshin MD, Kim M, Laskin CA, et al.: Prediction of adverse pregnancy outcome by the presence of lupus anticoagulant, but not anticardiolipin antibody, in patients with antiphospholipid antibodies, *Arthritis Rheum* 64(7):2311–2318, 2012.
34. De Carolis S, Botta A, Santucci S, et al.: Complementemia and obstetric outcome in pregnancy with antiphospholipid syndrome, *Lupus* 21(7):776–778, 2012.
35. Cowchock FS, Reece EA, Balaban D, et al.: Repeated fetal losses associated with antiphospholipid antibodies: a collaborative randomized trial comparing prednisone with low-dose heparin treatment, *Am J Obstet Gynecol* 166(5):1318–1323, 1992.
36. Mak A, Cheung MWL, Cheak AAC, et al.: Combination of heparin and aspirin is superior to aspirin alone in enhancing live births in patients with recurrent pregnancy loss and positive anti-phospholipi dantibodies: a meta-analysis of randomized controlled trials and meta-regression, *Rheuatology* 49(2):281–288, 2010.
37. Ziakas PD, Pavlou M, Voulgarelis M: Heparin treatment in antiphospholipid syndrome with recurrent pregnancy loss: a systematic review and meta-analysis, *Obstet Gynecol* 115(6):1256–1262, 2010.
38. Branch DW, Peaceman AM, Druzin M, et al.: A multicenter, placebo-controlled pilot study of intravenous immune globulin treatment of antiphospholipid syndrome during pregnancy.

The Pregnancy Loss Study Group, *Am J Obstet Gynecol* 182(1 Pt 1):122–127, 2000.
39. Ruffatti A, Tonello M, Hoxha A, et al.: Effect of additional treatments combined with conventional therapies in pregnant patients with high-risk antiphospholipid syndrome: a multicentre study, *Thromb Haemost* 118(4):639–646, 2018.
40. Salmon JE, Girardi G, Holers VM: Activation of complement mediates antiphospholipid antibody-induced pregnancy loss, *Lupus* 12(7):535–538, 2003.
41. Berman J, Girardi G, Salmon JE: TNF-alpha is a critical effector and a target for therapy in antiphospholipid antibody-induced pregnancy loss, *J Immunol* 174(1):485–490, 2005.
42. Gris JC, Bouvier S, Molinari N, et al.: Comparative incidence of a first thrombotic event in purely obstetric antiphospholipid syndrome with pregnancy loss: the NOH-APS observational study, *Blood* 119(11):2624–2632, 2012.
43. Clowse MEB, Chakravarty E, Costenbader KH, et al.: Effects of infertility, pregnancy loss, and patient concerns on family size of women with rheumatoid arthritis and systemic lupus erythematosus, *Arthritis Care Res (Hoboken).* 64(5):668–674, 2012.
44. Brouwer J, Laven JSE, Hazes JMW, et al.: Levels of serum anti-Müllerian hormone, a marker for ovarian reserve, in women with rheumatoid arthritis, *Arthritis Care Res (Hoboken).* 65(9):1534–1538, 2013.
45. Brouwer J, Hazes JMW, Laven JSE, et al.: Fertility in women with rheumatoid arthritis: influence of disease activity and medication, *Ann Rheum Dis* 74(10):1836–1841, 2015.
46. Persellin RH. The effect of pregnancy on rheumatoid arthritis. *Bull Rheum Dis* 27(9):922-927..
47. de Man YA, Dolhain RJEM, van de Geijn FE, et al.: Disease activity of rheumatoid arthritis during pregnancy: results from a nationwide prospective study, *Arthritis Rheum* 59(9):1241–1248, 2008.
48. de Man YA, Bakker-Jonges LE, Gorberth CM, et al.: Women with rheumatoid arthritis negative for anti-cyclic citrullinated peptide and rheumatoid factor are more likely to improve during pregnancy, whereas in autoantibody-positive women autoantibody levels are not influenced by pregnancy, *Ann Rheum Dis* 69(2):420–423, 2010.
49. Ostensen MHG: A prospective clinical study of the effect of pregnancy on rheumatoid arthritis and ankylosing spondylitis, *Arthritis Rheum* 26(9):1155–1159, 1983.
50. Bharti B, Lee SJ, Lindsay SP, et al.: Disease severity and pregnancy outcomes in women with rheumatoid arthritis: results from the organization of teratology information specialists autoimmune diseases in pregnancy project, *J Rheumatol* 42(8):1376–1382, 2015.
51. Mouyis MA, Thornton CC, Williams D, et al.: Pregnancy outcomes in patients with psoriatic arthritis, *J Rheumatol* 44(1):128–129, 2017.
52. Ostensen M, Ostensen H: Ankylosing spondylitis—the female aspect, *J Rheumatol* 25(1):120–124, 1998.
53. Jakobsson GL, Stephansson O, Askling J, et al.: Pregnancy outcomes in patients with ankylosing spondylitis: a nationwide register study, *Ann Rheum Dis* 75(10):1838–1842, 2016.
54. Zbinden A, van den Brandt S, Østensen M, et al.: Risk for adverse pregnancy outcome in axial spondyloarthritis and rheumatoid arthritis: disease activity matters, *Rheumatology (Oxford)* 57(7):1235–1242, 2018.
55. Silva CA, Sultan SM, Isenberg DA: Pregnancy outcome in adult-onset idiopathic inflammatory myopathy, *Rheumatology (Oxford)* 42(10):1168–1172, 2003.
56. Iago PF, Albert SOC, Andreu FC, et al.: Pregnancy in adult-onset idiopathic inflammatory myopathy. Report from a cohort of myositis patietns from a single center, *Semin Arthritis Rheum* 44(2):234–240, 2014.
57. Kofteridis DP, Malliotakis PI, Sotsiou F, et al.: Acute onset of dermatomyositis presenting in pregnancy with rhabdomyolysis and fetal loss, *Scand J Rheumatol* 28(3):192–194, 1999.
58. Messina S, Fagiolari G, Lamperti C, et al.: Women with pregnancy-related polymyositis and high serum CK levels in the newborn, *Neurology* 58(3):482–484, 2002.
59. Zhong Z, Lin F, Yang J, et al.: Pregnancy in polymyositis or dermatomyositis: retrospective results from a tertiary centre in China, *Rheumatology (Oxford)* 56(8):1272–1275, 2017.
60. Williams L, Chang PY, Park E, et al.: Successful treatment of dermatomyositis during pregnancy with intravenous immunoglobulin monotherapy, *Obstet Gynecol* 109(2 Pt2):561–563, 2007.
61. Englert H, Brennan P, McNeil D, et al.: Reproductive function prior to disease onset in women with scleroderma, *J Rheumatol* 19(10):1575–1579, 1992.
62. Steen VD, Medsger TA: Fertility and pregnancy outcome in women with systemic sclerosis, *Arthritis Rheum* 42(4):763–768, 1999.
63. Taraborelli M, Ramoni V, Brucato A, et al.: Brief report: successful pregnancies but a higher risk of preterm births in patients with systemic sclerosis: an Italian multicenter study, *Arthritis Rheum* 64(6):1970–1977, 2012.
64. Steen VD, Conte C, Day N, et al.: Pregnancy in women with systemic sclerosis, *Arthritis Rheum* 32(2):151–157, 1989.
65. Silman AJ, Black C: Increased incidence of spontaneous abortion and infertility in women with scleroderma before disease onset: a controlled study, *Ann Rheum Dis* 47(6):441–444, 1988.
66. Clowse MEB, Richeson RL, Pieper C, Vasculitis Clinical Research Consortium, et al.: Pregnancy outcomes among patients with vasculitis, *Arthritis Care Res (Hoboken)* 65(8):1370–1374, 2013.
67. Pagnoux C, Le Guern V, Goffinet F, et al.: Pregnancies in systemic necrotizing vasculitides: report on 12 women and their 20 pregnancies, *Rheumatology (Oxford)* 50(5):953–961, 2011.
68. Gatto M, Iaccarino L, Canova M, et al.: Pregnancy and vasculitis: a systematic review of the literature, *Autoimmun Rev* 11(6–7):A447–A459, 2012.
69. Comarmond C, Mirault T, Biard L, et al.: Takayasu arteritis and pregnancy, *Arthritis Rheumatol (Hoboken, NJ)* 67(12):3262–3269, 2015.
70. Singh N, Tyagi S, Tripathi R, et al.: Maternal and fetal outcomes in pregnant women with Takayasu aortoarteritis: does optimally timed intervention in women with renal artery involvement improve pregnancy outcome? *Taiwan, J Obstet Gynecol* 54(5):597–602, 2015.
71. Khandelwal M, Lal N, Fischer RL, et al.: Takayasu arteritis and pregnancy, *Obstet Gynecol Surv* 64(4):258–272, 2009.
72. Burkett G, Richard R: Polyarteritis nodosa and pregnancy, *Obs Gynecol* 59(2):252–254, 1982.
73. Owen J, Hauth JC: Polyarteritis nodosa in pregnancy: a case report and brief literature review, *Am J Obstet Gynecol* 160(3):606–607, 1989.
74. Stone MS, Olson RR, Weismann DN, et al.: Cutaneous vasculitis in the newborn of a mother with cutaneous polyarteritis nodosa, *J Am Acad Dermatol* 28(1):101–105, 1993.
75. Auzary C, Huong DT, Wechsler B, et al.: Pregnancy in patients with Wegener's granulomatosis: report of five cases in three women, *Ann Rheum Dis* 59(10):800–804, 2000.
76. Tuin J, Sanders JSF, de Joode AAE, et al.: Pregnancy in women diagnosed with antineutrophil cytoplasmic antibody-associated vasculitis: outcome for the mother and the child, *Arthritis Care Res (Hoboken)* 64(4):539–545, 2012.
77. Croft AP, Smith SW, Carr S, et al.: Successful outcome of pregnancy in patients with anti-neutrophil cytoplasm antibody-associated small vessel vasculitis, *Kidney Int* 87(4):807–811, 2015.
78. Priori R, Tomassini M, Magrini L, et al.: Churg-Strauss syndrome during pregnancy after steroid withdrawal, *Lancet (London, England)* 352(9140):1599–1600, 1998.

79. Schlieben DJ, Korbet SM, Kimura RE, et al.: Pulmonary-renal syndrome in a newborn with placental transmission of ANCAs, *Am J Kidney Dis* 45(4):758–761, 2005.
80. Doria A, Bajocchi G, Tonon M, et al.: Pre-pregnancy counselling of patients with vasculitis, *Rheumatology (Oxford)* 47(Suppl 3):iii13–5, 2008.
81. Hwang I, Lee CK, Yoo B, et al.: Necrotizing villitis and decidual vasculitis in the placentas of mothers with Behçet disease, *Hum Pathol* 40(1):135–138, 2009.
82. Fam AG, Siminovitch KA, Carette S, et al.: Neonatal Behçet's syndrome in an infant of a mother with the disease, *Ann Rheum Dis* 40(5):509–512, 1981.
83. Iskender C, Yasar O, Kaymak O, et al.: Behçet's disease and pregnancy: a retrospective analysis of course of disease and pregnancy outcome, *J Obstet Gynaecol Res* 40(6):1598–1602, 2014.
84. Bermas BL, Tassinari M, Clowse M, et al.: The new FDA labeling rule: impact on prescribing rheumatological medications during pregnancy, *Rheumatology (Oxford)* 57(Suppl 5):v2–v8, 2018.
85. Neville MC: Anatomy and physiology of lactation, *Pediatr Clin North Am* 48(1):13–34, 2001.
86. Colie CF: Male mediated teratogenesis, *Reprod Toxicol* 7(1):3–9, 1993.
87. van Gelder MMHJ, Roeleveld N, Nordeng H: Exposure to non-steroidal anti-inflammatory drugs during pregnancy and the risk of selected birth defects: a prospective cohort study, *PLoS One* 6(7):e22174, 2011.
88. Pall M, Fridén BE, Brännström M: Induction of delayed follicular rupture in the human by the selective COX-2 inhibitor rofecoxib: a randomized double-blind study, *Hum Reprod* 16(7):1323–1328, 2001.
89. Nakhai-Pour HR, Broy P, Sheehy O, et al.: Use of nonaspirin non-steroidal anti-inflammatory drugs during pregnancy and the risk of spontaneous abortion, *CMAJ* 183(15):1713–1720, 2011.
90. Blanford AT, Murphy BE: In vitro metabolism of prednisolone, dexamethasone, betamethasone, and cortisol by the human placenta, *Am J Obstet Gynecol* 127(3):264–267, 1977.
91. Flint J, Panchal S, Hurrell A, et al.: BSR and BHPR guideline on prescribing drugs in pregnancy and breastfeeding-part I: standard and biologic disease modifying anti-rheumatic drugs and corticosteroids, *Rheumatology (Oxford)* 55(9):1693–1697, 2016.
92. Ost L, Wettrell G, Björkhem I, et al.: Prednisolone excretion in human milk, *J Pediatr* 106(6):1008–1011, 1985.
93. Costedoat-Chalumeau N, Amoura Z, Huong DLT, et al.: Safety of hydroxychloroquine in pregnant patients with connective tissue diseases. Review of the literature, *Autoimmun Rev* 4(2):111–115, 2005.
94. Osadchy A, Ratnapalan T, Koren G: Ocular toxicity in children exposed in utero to antimalarial drugs: review of the literature, *J Rheumatol* 38(12):2504–2508, 2011.
95. Motta M, Tincani A, Faden D, et al.: Follow-up of infants exposed to hydroxychloroquine given to mothers during pregnancy and lactation, *J Perinatol* 25(2):86–89, 2005.
96. Mogadam M, Dobbins WO, Korelitz BI, et al.: Pregnancy in inflammatory bowel disease: effect of sulfasalazine and corticosteroids on fetal outcome, *Gastroenterology* 80(1):72–76, 1981.
97. Branski D, Kerem E, Gross-Kieselstein E, et al. Bloody diarrhea-a possible complication of sulfasalazine transferred through human breast milk. *J Pediatr Gastroenterol Nutr* 5(2):316–317.
98. Feldkamp M, Carey JC: Clinical teratology counseling and consultation case report: low dose methotrexate exposure in the early weeks of pregnancy, *Teratology* 47(6):533–539, 1993..
99. Fields CL, Ossorio MA, Roy TM, et al.: Wegener's granulomatosis complicated by pregnancy. A case report, *J Reprod Med* 36(6):463–466, 1991.
100. Cassina M, Johnson DL, Robinson LK, et al.: Pregnancy outcome in women exposed to leflunomide before or during pregnancy, *Arthritis Rheum* 64(7):2085–2094, 2012.
101. Radomski JS, Ahlswede BA, Jarrell BE, et al.: Outcomes of 500 pregnancies in 335 female kidney, liver, and heart transplant recipients, *Transplant Proc* 27(1):1089–1090, 1995.
102. Gardiner SJ, Gearry RB, Roberts RL, et al.: Exposure to thiopurine drugs through breast milk is low based on metabolite concentrations in mother-infant pairs, *Br J Clin Pharmacol* 62(4):453–456, 2006.
103. Moretti ME, Sgro M, Johnson DW, et al.: Cyclosporine excretion into breast milk, *Transplantation* 75(12):2144–2146, 2003.
104. Kainz A, Harabacz I, Cowlrick IS, et al.: Analysis of 100 pregnancy outcomes in women treated systemically with tacrolimus, *Transpl Int* 13(Suppl 1):S299–300, 2000.
105. Bramham K, Chusney G, Lee J, et al.: Breastfeeding and tacrolimus: serial monitoring in breast-fed and bottle-fed infants, *Clin J Am Soc Nephrol* 8(4):563–567, 2013.
106. Perez-Aytes A, Ledo A, Boso V, et al.: In Utero exposure to mycophenolate mofetil: a characteristic phenotype? *Am J Med Genet A* 146A(1):1–7, 2008.
107. Mahadevan U, Wolf DC, Dubinsky M, et al.: Placental transfer of anti-tumor necrosis factor agents in pregnant patients with inflammatory bowel disease, *Clin Gastroenterol Hepatol* 11(3):286–292, 2013; quiz e24.
108. Cheent K, Nolan J, Shariq S, et al.: Case report: fatal case of disseminated BCG infection in an infant born to a mother taking infliximab for Crohn's disease, *J Crohns Colitis* 4(5):603–605, 2010.
109. Raja H, Matteson EL, Michet CJ, et al.: Safety of tumor necrosis factor inhibitors during pregnancy and breastfeeding, *Transl Vis Sci Technol* 1(2):6, 2012.
110. Chakravarty EF, Murray ER, Kelman A, et al.: Pregnancy outcomes after maternal exposure to rituximab, *Blood* 117(5):1499–1506, 2011.
111. Diav-Citrin O, Shechtman S, Schwartz V, et al.: Pregnancy outcome after in utero exposure to colchicine, *Am J Obstet Gynecol* 203(2):144.e1–144.e6, 2010.
112. Anderson D, Bishop JB, Garner RC, et al.: Cyclophosphamide: review of its mutagenicity for an assessment of potential germ cell risks, *Mutat Res* 330(1–2):115–181, 1995.
113. Weber-Schoendorfer C, Hoeltzenbein M, Wacker E, et al.: No evidence for an increased risk of adverse pregnancy outcome after paternal low-dose methotrexate: an observational cohort study, *Rheumatology (Oxford)* 53(4):757–763, 2014.
114. Eck LK, Jensen TB, Mastrogiannis D, et al.: Risk of adverse pregnancy outcome after paternal exposure to methotrexate within 90 days before pregnancy, *Obstet Gynecol* 129(4):707–714, 2017.
115. Schwarz EB, Manzi S: Risk of unintended pregnancy among women with systemic lupus erythematosus, *Arthritis Rheum* 59(6):863–866, 2008.
116. Yazdany J, Trupin L, Kaiser R, et al.: Contraceptive counseling and use among women with systemic lupus erythematosus: a gap in health care quality? *Arthritis Care Res (Hoboken)* 63(3):358–365, 2011.
117. Stringer EM, Kaseba C, Levy J, et al.: A randomized trial of the intrauterine contraceptive device vs hormonal contraception in women who are infected with the human immunodeficiency virus, *Am J Obstet Gynecol* 197(2), 2007. 144.e1-8.
118. Petri M, Kim MY, Kalunian KC, et al.: Combined oral contraceptives in women with systemic lupus erythematosus, *N Engl J Med* 353(24):2550–2558, 2005.
119. Sánchez-Guerrero J, Uribe AG, Jiménez-Santana L, et al.: A trial of contraceptive methods in women with systemic lupus erythematosus, *N Engl J Med* 353(24):2539–2549, 2005.
120. Boumpas DT, Austin HA, Vaughan EM, et al.: Risk for sustained amenorrhea in patients with systemic lupus erythematosus receiving intermittent pulse cyclophosphamide therapy, *Ann Intern Med* 119(5):366–369, 1993.

121. Dooley MA, Nair R: Therapy insight: preserving fertility in cyclophosphamide-treated patients with rheumatic disease, *Nat Clin Pract Rheumatol* 4(5):250–257, 2008.
122. Guballa N, Sammaritano L, Schwartzman S, et al.: Ovulation induction and in vitro fertilization in systemic lupus erythematosus and antiphospholipid syndrome, *Arthritis Rheum* 43(3):550–556, 2000.
123. Bellver J, Pellicer A: Ovarian stimulation for ovulation induction and in vitro fertilization in patients with systemic lupus erythematosus and antiphospholipid syndrome, *Fertil Steril* 92(6):1803–1810, 2009.
124. Orquevaux P, Masseau A, Le Guern V, et al.: In vitro fertilization in 37 women with systemic lupus erythematosus or antiphospholipid syndrome: a series of 97 procedures, *J Rheumatol* 44(5):613–618, 2017.
125. Sammaritano LR, Bermas BL, Chakravarty EE, et al.: 2020 American College of Rheumatology Guideline for the Management of Reproductive Health in Rheumatic and Musculoskeletal Diseases. *Arthritis Rheumatol* 2020.

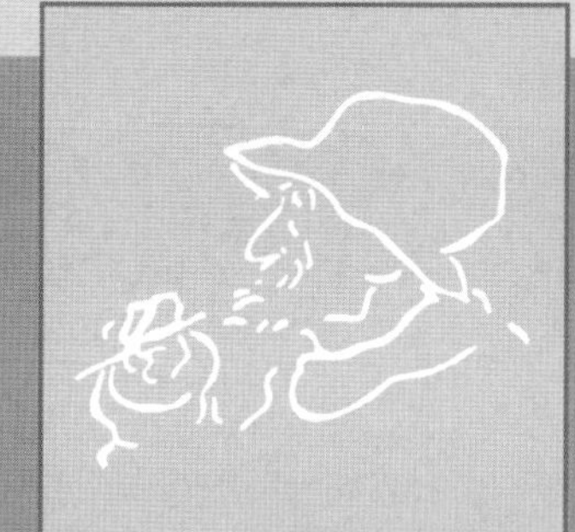

43 History and Physical Examination of the Musculoskeletal System

JOHN M. DAVIS III, KEVIN G. MODER, AND GENE G. HUNDER

KEY POINTS

A detailed and accurate history is crucial to make the correct diagnosis in patients with musculoskeletal diseases.

The primary symptoms of musculoskeletal disease are pain, joint stiffness, swelling, limitation of motion, weakness, fatigue, and loss of function.

An understanding of the anatomy, the planes of motion, and, particularly, the configuration of the synovial lining is imperative for proper physical diagnosis of musculoskeletal diseases.

It is important to record qualitative and quantitative aspects of the joint examination to monitor disease activity in patients with inflammatory arthropathies.

Early recognition of how patients' psychosocial factors affect their musculoskeletal symptoms and musculoskeletal examination enhances clinical assessment.

History in a Patient With Musculoskeletal Disease

An accurate and comprehensive history of a patient's musculoskeletal symptoms is crucial to make a correct diagnosis. This history must include a precise understanding of what the patient means by his or her description of symptoms. The physician must obtain a detailed account of symptom onset, location, patterns of progression, and severity, as well as exacerbating and alleviating factors and associated symptoms. The relationship of the symptoms to psychosocial stressors is important and should be determined. The impact of the symptoms on all aspects of the patient's functioning must be assessed to guide therapy.

The effects of current or previous therapy on the course of the illness are helpful in efforts to understand current symptoms. Response to anti-inflammatory or glucocorticoid medications may suggest an inflammatory origin. Such responses are not specific to inflammatory rheumatic diseases, however, and must be considered in light of the entire history and physical examination. The physician must assess compliance with therapies for musculoskeletal diseases. Noncompliance with the recommended treatment must be differentiated from treatment failure as the explanation for the patient's lack of improvement.

While the physician is taking the patient's history, the patient provides verbal and nonverbal clues to the nature of the illness and how the patient has responded to it. Patients with early rheumatoid arthritis (RA) may hold their hands in a flexed posture to minimize intra-articular pressure and pain. Some patients may be overly concerned, whereas others may seem inappropriately indifferent to their symptoms. The physician must appreciate the patient's understanding of the illness and attitudes toward it to begin effective treatment.

Pain

Pain is the most common symptom that brings a patient with musculoskeletal diseases to the physician. Pain is a subjective hurting sensation or experience that is described in various terms, often of actual or perceived physical damage. Pain is a complex sensation that is difficult to define, qualify, and measure. The patient's pain may be modified by emotional factors and previous experiences.

The character of the pain usually is best defined early in the interview because this can be helpful in categorizing the patient's complaints. Aching in a joint area suggests an arthritic disorder, whereas burning or numbness in an extremity may indicate a neuropathy. Descriptions of pain as "excruciating" or "intolerable" when the patient is otherwise able to function provide a clue that emotional or psychosocial factors are contributing to or amplifying the symptoms.

The physician must elicit the distribution of the patient's pain and determine whether this fits with anatomic structures. Patients describe their pain location in terms of body part names, but frequently the terms are used in a nonanatomic manner. Patients frequently complain of "hip" pain when they are actually referring to pain in the low back, buttock, or thigh. The interviewer must attempt to clarify this complaint by asking the patient to point to the area of pain with one finger. Pain localized in the distribution of a joint or joints likely reflects an articular disorder. Pain may localize to bursae, tendons, ligaments, or nerves, implying disorders of these structures. In contrast to superficial structures, deep structures often give rise to poorly localizing pain. Similarly, pain arising from small, peripheral joints is often more focal than pain arising from proximal, large joints, such as the shoulders and hips. Pain that is widespread, is vaguely described, and does not respect anatomic distributions generally suggests a chronic pain syndrome, such as fibromyalgia or psychiatric disease.

The severity of the pain should be assessed. A common approach is to ask the patient to describe the level of pain on a numeric scale of intensity from 0 (no pain) to 10 (very severe pain). To monitor disease activity of inflammatory arthritis, measuring pain on a visual analogue scale by having the patient mark the severity of pain during the past week on a 100-mm line can be helpful. Similar scales are used in validated instruments, such as the McGill Pain Questionnaire.

The physician must determine what exacerbates and alleviates the pain. Joint pain present at rest but worse with movement suggests an inflammatory process, whereas pain that occurs primarily with activity and is relieved by rest usually indicates a mechanical disorder such as degenerative arthritis. Timing of pain symptoms during the day and night also provides important information, as discussed in the next section.

Stiffness

Stiffness is a common complaint among patients with arthritis. What is meant by stiffness varies from patient to patient, however. Some patients may use the term *stiffness* to refer to pain, soreness, weakness, fatigue, or limitation of motion.[1] Rheumatologists generally use the term *stiffness* to describe discomfort and limitation when the patient attempts to move the joints after a period of inactivity. This "gel" phenomenon occurs usually after an hour or more of inactivity. The duration of stiffness related to inactivity varies, with mild stiffness lasting minutes and severe stiffness lasting hours.

Morning stiffness is an early feature of inflammatory arthropathies and is particularly noted in RA and polymyalgia rheumatica, in which morning stiffness may last for several hours. The absence of morning stiffness does not exclude inflammatory arthritis, but its absence is uncommon. A useful question to assess morning stiffness is this: "In the morning, how long does it take for your joints to limber up to as good as they are going to get for the day?" Morning stiffness associated with non-inflammatory joint diseases, such as degenerative arthritis, generally is of short duration (usually <30 minutes) and is less severe than stiffness of inflammatory joint disease. Additionally, the degree of stiffness in non-inflammatory joint diseases is related to the extent of use of the damaged joint: stiffness is worse after excessive use, generally improving within several days to the baseline level. Morning stiffness is not specific for inflammatory arthropathies and may be described by patients with fibromyalgia or chronic idiopathic pain syndromes, neurologic disorders such as Parkinson's disease (although generally without limbering up), and sleep-related breathing disorders.

Limitation of Motion

Limitation of motion is a common complaint among patients with articular disorders. This complaint must be differentiated from stiffness, which usually is transient and variable, whereas limitation of motion secondary to joint disease is generally fixed and varies less with time. The interviewer should determine the extent of disability resulting from the restriction in joint motion. The duration of the restriction in joint motion frequently predicts the likelihood of improvement with interventions such as oral and intra-articular glucocorticoids or physical therapy. Determining the rapidity of onset of the limitation of motion may be helpful in the differential diagnosis; abrupt onset of the limitation of motion suggests a structural derangement such as a tendon rupture or torn knee cartilage, whereas insidious onset of restricted joint motion is more common with inflammatory joint disease.

Swelling

Joint swelling is an important symptom in patients with rheumatic diseases. The presence of true joint swelling narrows the differential diagnosis in a patient with arthralgia. To determine whether the swelling is related to joint synovitis as opposed to soft tissue conditions, clarifying the anatomic location and distribution of the swelling is key. Diffuse soft tissue swelling can occur because of venous or lymphatic obstruction, soft tissue injury, or obesity. The description of swelling in patients with such conditions usually is ill defined or is not in a distribution of particular joints, bursae, or tendons. Obese patients may interpret normal adipose tissue over the medial aspect of the elbow, the knee, or the lateral aspect of the ankle as joint swelling. In contrast, patients with inflammatory arthritis may describe swelling of joints in a distribution typical of a specific disease—symmetric swelling of the metacarpophalangeal joints and wrists in RA, or swelling of several toes and a knee in psoriatic arthritis.

It is useful to delineate the onset and progression of swelling and the factors that influence it. Swelling of a joint resulting from synovitis or bursitis frequently is associated with discomfort with motion because of tension on the inflamed tissues. If swollen tissues are periarticular, however, no discomfort may be present with joint motion because the inflamed tissues are not stressed. Swelling of a confined structure, such as a synovial cavity or bursa, is most painful when it has developed acutely, whereas a similar degree of swelling that has developed slowly often is much more tolerable.

Weakness

Weakness is another common complaint that can be associated with myriad different subjective meanings. True weakness is the loss of muscle power. When present, it is demonstrable on physical examination.

The temporal course of weakness is important to the differential diagnosis. Weakness of sudden onset without trauma often indicates a neurologic disorder, such as an acute cerebrovascular event, which generally results in a fixed, nonprogressive deficit. Weakness of insidious onset more often suggests a muscle disease, such as an inflammatory myopathy (e.g., polymyositis). The latter tends to be ongoing and progressive. Weakness that is intermittent suggests a disorder of the neuromuscular junction, such as myasthenia gravis. Patients with this disease may describe muscle fatigue with activity as opposed to true weakness.

The physician should determine the distribution of the patient's weakness. Proximal weakness that is bilateral and symmetric suggests an inflammatory myopathy. In contrast, inclusion body myositis causes an asymmetric and more distal weakness. The presence of a unilateral or isolated deficit generally indicates a neurogenic origin. Distal weakness, in the absence of joint findings, generally indicates a neurologic disorder such as peripheral neuropathy. Patients with peripheral neuropathies also complain of pain and sensory symptoms, such as paresthesias. In contrast, patients with inflammatory myopathy often present with painless weakness.

Inquiring about the patient's family history may provide valuable information. A history of other family members with similar symptoms may increase the likelihood that the patient has a hereditary disorder, such as muscular dystrophy or familial neuropathy.

It also is important to review medication taken recently or currently. Many medications, including corticosteroids and lipid-lowering agents, can cause muscle injury. Less commonly, environmental exposure can lead to symptoms of weakness. Heavy metal poisoning causes a peripheral neuropathy. Dietary exposure also should be investigated, such as eating undercooked pork as a source of trichinosis. Excessive alcohol intake has been associated with neuropathy and myopathy.

Taking a complete review of systems is helpful in evaluating a patient with weakness. Constitutional symptoms, such as weight loss and night sweats, may indicate the presence of a malignancy as the cause of generalized weakness. Rash, arthralgia, or Raynaud's phenomenon may prompt further testing for a connective tissue disease.

Fatigue

Patients with musculoskeletal disorders frequently complain of fatigue. Fatigue can be defined as an inclination to rest even though pain and weakness are not limiting factors. Fatigue after varying degrees of activity that is relieved by rest is normal. Patients with rheumatic diseases experience fatigue even without activity. Fatigue generally improves as the systemic rheumatic disease improves. Malaise frequently occurs with, but is not synonymous with, fatigue. Malaise indicates the lack of well-being that often occurs at the onset of an illness. Fatigue and malaise may occur in the absence of identifiable disease, and psychosocial factors, anxiety, or depression may account for the symptoms.

Loss of Function

The comprehensive history should include an assessment of the patient's ability to perform activities of daily living, as loss of function is a common manifestation of musculoskeletal disease with serious impact on health and quality of life. The extent of disability may vary from loss of the ability to use one finger joint because of arthritis to complete physical incapacitation resulting from severe inflammatory polyarthritis. Irrespective of the cause, loss of physical function often has a profound impact on patient social activities, exercise routine, work capacity, and even basic self-care. Assessing for the presence and degree of functional disability is important to evaluate the severity of illness and in making treatment recommendations, particularly in RA, in which disability is among the strongest predictors of long-term outcomes and mortality.[2–4]

Functional capacity is assessed first by asking general questions about the patient's ability to perform daily activities, including grooming, dressing, bathing, eating, walking, climbing stairs, opening doors, carrying objects, and so forth. A report of a specific loss of function, such as difficulty opening a milk carton, should be investigated further to clarify why the task is difficult, which will inform the differential diagnosis and guide clinical examination. This information will also yield important information for management, such as opportunities for physical and occupational therapy, use of splints/braces, and so forth. Overall functional capacity may be evaluated with the use of an instrument such as the Health Assessment Questionnaire (see Chapter 36), which is widely used in research and in the clinic to monitor changes in physical function in response to therapy among patients with RA and other rheumatic diseases.

Systematic Method of Examination

The musculoskeletal examination should be a systematic, thorough assessment of the status of the joints, periarticular soft tissues, tendons, ligaments, bursae, and muscles. Rheumatologists commonly begin by examining the upper extremities followed by the trunk and lower extremities, but many routines may be effective provided that a systematic, consistent approach is used. Gentle handling of tender and painful joints enhances cooperation by the patient and allows an accurate evaluation of the joints.

The general aim of the examination of the joints is to detect abnormalities in structure and function. Key signs of articular disease include swelling, tenderness, limitation of motion, crepitus, deformity, and instability.

General Observation

A general examination of the patient should be performed to look for any signs of systemic illness. This should include an examination of the skin, noting signs of pallor (which may suggest anemia), nodules (which may suggest RA or gout), or rashes (which may suggest lupus, vasculitis, or dermatomyositis). The patient should be appropriately undressed for examination. The physician should assess gait by asking the patient to walk in the examining room or down the hallway, because an antalgic gait may be seen in various musculoskeletal disorders of the spine or lower extremities, and various gait disorders may occur in neuromuscular diseases. The ability of the patient to arise and transfer to the examining table should also be evaluated, as this will provide information on pain, proximal muscle strength, and overall physical function. The patient should be assessed for appearance of the muscles, including bulk, tone, and tenderness. Muscle bulk should be compared on one side of the body with the other to look for any asymmetry, hypertrophy, or atrophy. The patient's manner and body language may provide information on his or her mood and anxiety level, which merits consideration in evaluating pain and tenderness.

Swelling

Swelling around a joint may be caused by intra-articular effusion, synovial proliferation, periarticular subcutaneous tissue inflammation, bursitis, tendinitis, bony enlargement, or extra-articular fat pads. A keen understanding of the anatomic configuration of each joint's synovial membrane is crucial in differentiating soft tissue swelling secondary to a joint effusion from swelling of periarticular tissues. First, the examiner should inspect the joints for visible evidence of swelling, such as loss of normal landmarks or contours. It is frequently helpful to visually compare the same joints on both sides of the body to detect subtle evidence of swelling and to appreciate symmetry.

Second, the examiner should palpate each joint. The normal synovial membrane is too thin to palpate, whereas the thickened synovial membrane in many chronic inflammatory arthritides, such as RA, may have a "doughy" or "boggy" consistency. In some joints, such as the knee, the extent of the synovial cavity can be delineated on physical examination by compressing the fluid into one of the extreme synovial recesses. The edge of the resulting bulge may be palpated more easily. If this palpable edge is within the anatomic confines of the synovial membrane and disappears on release of compression, the distention usually represents synovial effusion; if it persists, it is an indication of a thickened synovial membrane. Reliable differentiation between synovial membrane thickening and effusion is not always possible by physical examination, however. Ultrasonography is used increasingly as an extension of the physical examination, allowing the examiner to differentiate between synovial proliferation and effusion.

Tenderness

In the musculoskeletal examination, tenderness is unusual discomfort when the physician palpates and puts pressure on articular and periarticular tissues. Localizing the tenderness to palpation may assist the examiner in determining whether the pathology is intra-articular or periarticular in location, such as a fat pad, tendon attachment, ligament, bursa, muscle, or skin. It can be useful to palpate structures that are not involved to assess the importance of tenderness. Finding tender joints in a patient who also has numerous other myofascial tender points is less of a concern for arthritis than finding tender joints in a patient with no extra-articular tenderness.

Limitation of Motion

Limitation of motion is a common manifestation of articular disease; the examiner must know the normal type and range of motion for each joint. Comparison of the affected joint with an unaffected joint of the opposite extremity is useful to evaluate individual variation. Restricted joint motion may be caused by changes in the joint itself or in periarticular structures. To distinguish these possibilities, it is crucial to compare the passive with the active range of motion. If the passive range of motion is greater than the active range of motion, the restriction may be the result of pain, weakness, or the state of articular or periarticular structures. It also is important to distinguish muscle tension from a true limitation of joint motion, emphasizing the importance of ensuring relaxation of the patient. Pain that occurs with attempts to move a joint passively to the limit of range of motion in one plane is referred to as *stress pain*. Pain in the joint with attempted active or passive range of motion usually indicates an abnormality in the joint.

Crepitus

Crepitus is a palpable or audible grating or crunching sensation produced by motion. This sensation may or may not be accompanied by discomfort. Crepitus occurs when roughened articular or extra-articular surfaces are rubbed together by active motion or by manual compression. Fine crepitus often is palpable over joints involved by chronic inflammatory arthritis and usually indicates roughening of the opposing cartilage surfaces as a result of erosion or the presence of granulation tissue. Coarse crepitus may be caused by inflammatory or non-inflammatory arthritis. Bone-on-bone crepitus produces a higher-frequency, palpable, audible squeak. Crepitus from within a joint should be differentiated from cracking or popping sounds caused by the slipping of ligaments or tendons over bony surfaces during motion. The latter phenomena are usually less contributory to the diagnosis of joint disease and may be heard over normal joints. In scleroderma, a distinct, coarse, creaking, leathery crepitus may be palpable or audible over tendon sheaths.

Deformity

Deformity of the joints may manifest as a bony enlargement, articular subluxation, contracture, or ankylosis in nonanatomic positions. Deformed joints usually do not function normally, frequently restrict activities, and may be associated with pain, especially with overuse. Occasionally, a deformed joint may function well but is a cosmetic concern. Joint deformities may be reversible or irreversible. Multiple swan neck deformities of the fingers that can be corrected with manipulation may indicate Jaccoud's arthropathy of lupus. In contrast, hand deformities in RA generally are not correctable.

Instability

Joint instability is present when the joint has greater than normal movement in any plane. *Subluxation* refers to a joint in which there is partial displacement of the articular surfaces but still some joint surface-to-surface contact. A dislocated joint has lost all cartilage surface-to-surface contact. Instability is best determined by supporting the joint between the examiner's hands and stressing the adjacent bones in directions in which the normal joint does not move. The patient must be relaxed during the examination because muscle tension may stabilize an otherwise unstable joint. A knee with a deficient ligament might appear stable if the patient contracts the quadriceps muscles during evaluation.

Other Aspects of the Examination

Examinations of the cervical spine and low back are discussed in Chapters 48 and 50.

Recording the Joint Examination

Documentation of the joint examination is important for making decisions about therapy, monitoring the activity of arthritis, and determining the efficacy of interventions. Many different recording methods have been described. Abbreviations for each joint can be used, such as *PIP* for the proximal interphalangeal joints. The S-T-L system has been used historically to record the degree of swelling (S), tenderness (T), and limitation of motion (L) of each joint on the basis of a quantitative estimate of gradation.[5] This method remains useful but is used less commonly today because of increasing reliance on electronic medical records. It is easier to describe joint findings in narrative form, for example, "there is 2+ swelling of the second and third metacarpophalangeal (MCP) joints," where grade 0 indicates no swelling, grade 1 indicates palpable synovial thickening, grade 2 indicates loss of normal joint contours, and grade 3 indicates frank cystic swelling of the MCP joint. An alternative method is to record joint examination findings by using a schematic skeleton or homunculus.

Joint counts are standard assessments to monitor the activity of inflammatory arthritides in practice and in clinical trials.[6] For monitoring disease activity of RA, a 28-joint count for tenderness and swelling has been recommended. To assess the tender joint count, the examiner documents which joints the patient indicates are painful on palpation with enough pressure to blanch the nail bed of the examiner's thumb and index fingers. To assess the swollen joint count, the examiner documents which joints have palpable soft tissue swelling or fluctuance, excluding joints affected only by deformity or bony hypertrophy. The 28-joint count[7] includes the shoulders, elbows, wrists, first to fifth MCP joints, first to fifth proximal interphalangeal joints, and knees on both sides of the body. Compared with more extensive joint counts, the 28-joint count has the advantage of being quick and easy to perform; however, it is limited by the fact that the ankles and metatarsophalangeal joints are not included, so active disease in the feet may be underestimated. The 28-joint count is used to calculate the Disease Activity Score 28 (DAS28),[8] which is a validated instrument used to monitor disease activity.

The function of the joints in normal use is not captured by assessments of tenderness, swelling, or range of motion, so other examination techniques are necessary. Other tests are available that attempt to measure joint function by assessing the patient's ability to perform a coordinated task (e.g., shoulder arc of motion, measuring the 50-foot walk time). The results of such functional tests may vary, however. Biologic factors, such as circadian changes in joint size and grip strength among rheumatoid patients observed during a 24-hour interval, contribute to variability.

Interpreting the Joint Examination

The physician must understand the significance of specific joint findings, both their presence and absence, to make appropriate treatment decisions. As with any diagnostic assessment, the accuracy and reliability of the joint examination are important considerations. With regard to accuracy in detecting physical signs of inflammatory synovitis, numerous studies have shown that joint examination is far less sensitive in detecting synovitis or effusions than high-resolution ultrasonography or MRI.[9–11] Although it is true that swollen joints are more specific for active synovitis, recent clinical studies have suggested that joint tenderness has similar value compared with swelling in predicting the progression of radiographic joint damage.[12] Demonstrable physical signs of arthritis may be particularly subtle for patients with early disease.[13] Considering that MRI bone marrow edema is a predictor of radiographic damage, it is notable that one study reported that 35% to 57% of joints with bone marrow edema were negative for physical signs of synovitis.[14] In contrast, among patients with obesity, the finding of a clinically swollen joint is less likely to reflect true synovitis compared to imaging as the gold standard, which could lead to overestimation of disease activity among obese patients.[15] Thus the examiner must consider the physical findings in view of the complete history of joint symptoms to make an accurate diagnosis, assess prognosis, and prescribe management. Ultrasound examination can also be useful in clarifying the interpretation of joint pathology and enhancing confidence in clinical decisions about therapies (see Chapter 44).[16]

The joint examination is also affected by variability. For observations such as joint tenderness or grip strength, interobserver variability usually is greater than intraobserver variability. Considerable intraobserver variability may be noted in observations of the same patient, even during a short interval. Interobserver reliability, in general, is higher for joint-line tenderness than for swelling and is specifically related to the underlying disease, such as higher reliability of the examination for joint swelling in RA than in psoriatic arthritis.[11]

Examination of Specific Joints

Temporomandibular Joint

The temporomandibular joint is formed by the condyle of the mandible and the fossa of the temporal bone just anterior to the external auditory canal. It is difficult to visualize swelling of this joint. The examiner may palpate the joint by placing a finger just anterior to the external auditory canal and asking the patient to open and close the mouth and to move the mandible from side to side.[17] The presence of synovial thickness or swelling of minimal or moderate degree can be detected most easily if the synovitis is unilateral or asymmetric compared with the other side. To assess vertical movement of the temporomandibular joint, the examiner should ask the patient to open the mouth maximally and then measure the distance between the upper and lower incisor teeth, normally 3 to 6 cm. Lateral movement can be determined by using incisor teeth as landmarks. Audible or palpable crepitus or clicking may be present in patients with and without evidence of severe arthritis.

Many arthritides can affect the temporomandibular joints, including juvenile and adult RA. Micrognathia may develop in children in whom these joints are affected, as a result of arrested bone growth of the mandible. Arthralgias of the temporomandibular joint may develop in patients without inflammatory arthritis, consistent with temporomandibular joint syndrome (see Chapter 54). This syndrome is thought by some investigators to result from bruxism and is likely to be a form of myofascial pain, similar to fibromyalgia.

Cricoarytenoid Joints

The paired cricoarytenoid joints are formed by the articulation of the base of the small pyramidal arytenoid cartilage and the upper posterolateral border of the cricoid cartilage. The vocal ligaments (true vocal cords) are attached to the arytenoid cartilages. The cricoarytenoid joints are diarthrodial joints that normally move medially and laterally and rotate during opening and closing of the vocal cords. Examination of these joints is performed by direct or indirect laryngoscopy. Erythema, swelling, and lack of mobility during phonation may result from inflammation of the joints. The cricoarytenoid joints may be involved in RA, trauma, and infection. Involvement in RA is more common than is clinically apparent. Symptoms may include hoarseness or a sense of fullness or discomfort in the throat, which is worse on speaking or swallowing. Severe airway obstruction may occur in rare cases.

Sternoclavicular, Manubriosternal, and Sternocostal Joints

The medial ends of the clavicles articulate on each side of the sternum at its upper end to form the sternoclavicular joints. The articulations of the first ribs and the sternum (sternocostal joints) are immediately caudal. The articulation of the manubrium and the body of the sternum is at the level of attachment of the second costal cartilage to the sternum. The third through seventh sternocostal joints articulate distally along the lateral borders of the sternum. The sternoclavicular joints are the only articulations in this group that are always diarthrodial; the others are amphiarthroses or synchondroses. The sternoclavicular joints are the only true points of articulation of the shoulder girdle with the trunk. These joints are just beneath the skin; synovitis usually is visible and palpable. These joints have only slight movement, which cannot be accurately measured.

The sternoclavicular joints are commonly involved by ankylosing spondylitis, RA, and degenerative arthritis, although this involvement is often subclinical. The sternoclavicular joint may be the site of septic arthritis, especially in injection drug users. These joints should be examined for tenderness, swelling, and bony abnormalities. Tenderness of the manubriosternal or sternocostal joints is much more frequent than actual swelling. Tenderness of these joints without actual swelling has been termed *costochondritis;* if actual swelling is present, *Tietze's syndrome* may be the term used.

Acromioclavicular Joint

The acromioclavicular joint is formed by the lateral end of the clavicle and the medial margin of the acromion process of the scapula. Arthritis of the acromioclavicular joint is most commonly attributable to trauma leading to degenerative arthritis. Bony enlargement of this joint is typically observed, but soft tissue swelling is not usually visible or palpable. Tenderness or pain with adduction of the arm across the chest indicates pathology of the acromioclavicular joint. Movement of this joint occurs with shoulder motion but is difficult to measure accurately. The acromioclavicular joint may be involved by RA or spondyloarthropathies, although these often are not severe enough to come to clinical attention.

Shoulder

See Chapter 49 for a detailed description

Elbow

The elbow joint is composed of three bony articulations (Fig. 43.1). The principal articulation is the humeroulnar joint, which is a hinge joint. The radiohumeral and proximal radioulnar articulations allow rotation of the forearm.

To examine the elbow joint, the examiner places his or her thumb between the patient's lateral epicondyle and the olecranon process in the lateral para olecranon groove and places one or two fingers in the corresponding groove medial to the olecranon. The examiner relaxes and passively moves the elbow through flexion, extension, and rotation. The examiner should examine the skin around the elbow joint carefully, noting abnormalities such as psoriatic plaques, rheumatoid nodules, or tophi. It is useful to palpate the olecranon bursa carefully to exclude the presence of small nodules or tophi. Limitation of motion and crepitus should be noted. Synovial swelling is most easily palpated because it bulges under the examiner's thumb when the elbow is passively extended. The synovial membrane sometimes can be palpated over the posterior aspect of the joint between the olecranon process and the distal humerus. Synovitis or effusion generally results in limitation of elbow extension.

The olecranon bursa overlies the olecranon process of the ulna. Olecranon bursitis is common after chronic local trauma and in rheumatic diseases, including RA and gout. A septic olecranon bursitis may occur. A patient who has olecranon bursitis usually presents with a swelling over the olecranon process, which is often tender and may be erythematous. Sometimes a large collection of fluid over the area is palpable as a cystic mass, often requiring aspiration and drainage. There is generally no pain with elbow movement.

The medial and lateral epicondyles of the humerus are the sites of attachment of the common flexor and extensor tendons,

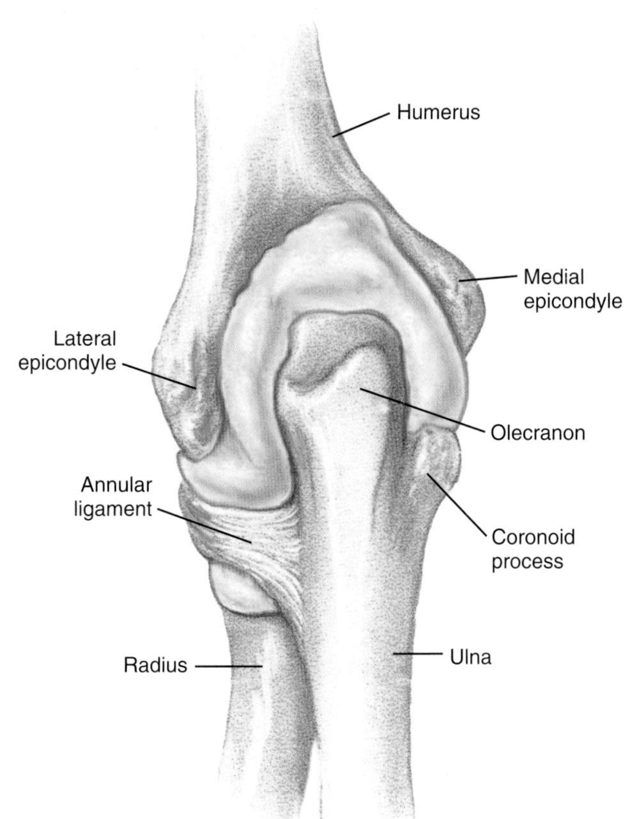

• **Fig. 43.1** Diagram of the elbow. Posterior aspect of the elbow joint shows radius and ulna in extension and the distribution of the synovial membrane in distention. (From Polley HF, Hunder GG: *Rheumatologic interviewing and physical examination of the joints*, ed 2, Philadelphia, 1978, WB Saunders. With permission from the Mayo Foundation for Medical Education and Research.)

controlling hand and wrist motion. Tenderness at the epicondyles without swelling or other signs of inflammation may indicate overuse tendinopathy, termed *lateral epicondylitis* (tennis elbow) and *medial epicondylitis* (golfer's elbow). In lateral epicondylitis, discomfort can be elicited by resisted supination of the forearm or resisted extension of the pronated wrist.[18] In medial epicondylitis, discomfort can be elicited by resisted flexion of the supinated wrist.

To assess motor function of the elbow, flexion and extension can be assessed. The principal flexors of the elbow are the biceps brachii (nerve roots C5 and C6), brachialis (C5 and C6), and brachioradialis (C5 and C6) muscles. The principal extensor of the elbow is the triceps brachii muscle (C7 and C8). Occasionally, a patient may rupture the attachment site of one of the heads of the biceps, resulting in visible and palpable muscle swelling on the anterior upper arm.

Wrist and Carpal Joints

The wrist is a complex joint formed by many articulations between the radius, the ulna, and the carpal bones. The true wrist or radiocarpal articulation is a biaxial ellipsoid joint formed proximally by the distal end of the radius and the triangular fibrocartilage and distally by a row of three carpal bones: scaphoid (navicular), lunate, and triquetrum (triangular). The distal radioulnar joint is a uniaxial pivot joint. The midcarpal joints are formed by the

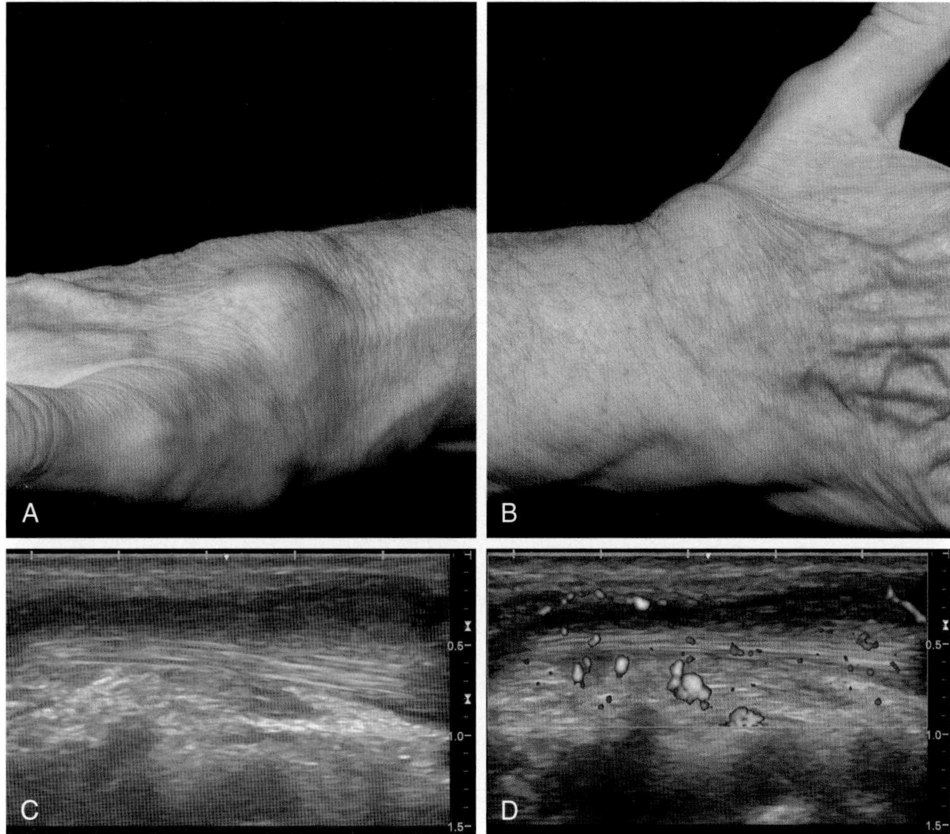

• **Fig. 43.2** Tenosynovitis of the wrist. (A) Radial and (B) dorsal views of the wrist in a patient with rheumatoid arthritis. Note the localized swelling at the dorsoradial aspect of the wrist. Sonographic evaluation of this patient revealed evidence of (C) hypoechoic thickening of the third dorsal extensor compartment with (D) hyperemia as detected by power Doppler signal, consistent with active inflammatory tenosynovitis.

junction of the proximal and distal rows of the carpal bones. The midcarpal and carpometacarpal articular cavities often communicate. The intercarpal joints refer to the articulations between individual carpal bones.

Movements of the wrist include flexion (palmar flexion), extension (dorsiflexion), radial deviation, ulnar deviation, and circumduction. Pronation and supination of the hand and forearm occur primarily at the proximal and distal radioulnar joints. The only carpometacarpal joint that moves to a notable degree is the carpometacarpal joint of the thumb. This joint is saddle-shaped and moves in three planes. Crepitus at this joint is common because it is frequently involved in degenerative arthritis.

The wrist normally can be extended to 70 to 80 degrees and flexed to 80 to 90 degrees. Ulnar and radial deviation should allow 50 degrees (ulnar) and 20 to 30 degrees (radial) of movement. Loss of extension is the most incapacitating functional impairment of wrist motion.

The long flexor tendons of the forearm musculature cross the volar aspect of the wrist and are enclosed in the flexor tendon sheath under the flexor retinaculum (transverse carpal ligament). The flexor retinaculum and the underlying carpal bones form the carpal tunnel. The median nerve passes through the carpal tunnel superficial to the flexor tendons. The extensor tendons of the forearm musculature are enclosed by six synovial lined compartments.

The palmar aponeurosis (fascia) spreads out into the palm from the flexor retinaculum. Dupuytren's contracture, a fibrosing condition, affects the palmar aponeurosis, which becomes thickened and contracted and may draw one or more fingers into flexion at the MCP joint. The fourth finger is frequently affected first.

Swelling of the wrist may be caused by effusion, synovial proliferation, or both, of the tendon sheaths (tenosynovitis), the wrist joint, or a combination thereof. When swelling is attributable to tenosynovitis, swelling is localized to the distribution of a particular tendon sheath or compartment (i.e., ulnar swelling attributable to tenosynovitis of the flexor carpi ulnaris tendon), tends to be more localized, and moves with flexion and extension of the fingers (Fig. 43.2). Articular swelling tends to be more diffuse and protrudes anteriorly and posteriorly from under the tendons (Fig. 43.3).

Synovitis of the wrist is best detected by palpation of the dorsal aspect of the joint. Accurate localization of the synovial margins is difficult because of structures overlying the volar and dorsal aspects of the wrist. To examine the wrist, the examiner should palpate the joint gently between the thumbs dorsally and the fingers on the volar aspect. Thickening or frank synovial proliferation of the synovium should be noted. When this thickening or proliferation is severe, the range of motion of the wrist joint frequently is limited and associated with stress pain.

A ganglion is a cystic enlargement arising from a joint capsule. Ganglions characteristically occur at the volar or dorsal aspect of the wrist between the tendons.

Subluxation of the ulna may develop as a result of severe chronic inflammatory arthritis. The subluxated ulna appears as a prominence on the dorsomedial wrist. Chronic irritation of the extensor tendons, primarily the fourth and fifth finger extensor tendons, may cause these tendons to rupture.

"Trigger fingers" secondary to stenosing tenosynovitis can be detected by palpating crepitus or nodules along the tendons in the palm while the patient slowly flexes and extends the fingers.[19] The patient usually gives a history of the affected finger catching or locking with movement.

Tenosynovitis of the first extensor compartment, which encloses the abductor pollicis longus and extensor pollicis brevis muscles of the thumb, is known as de Quervain's tenosynovitis. Patients complain of pain at the radial aspect of the wrist. Tenderness may be elicited by palpating near the radial styloid process. The examiner performs the Finkelstein test for de Quervain's tenosynovitis by asking the patient to make a fist with the thumb enclosed in the palm of the hand, then to move the wrist into ulnar deviation. Severe pain over the radial styloid is a positive finding, often indicating stretching of the thumb tendons in a stenosed tendon sheath.

Carpal tunnel syndrome results from pressure on the median nerve in the carpal tunnel. Carpal tunnel syndrome is discussed in detail in Chapter 53.

Muscle function of the wrist may be measured by testing flexion and extension and supination and pronation of the forearm. The principal flexors of the wrist are the flexor carpi radialis (nerve roots C6 and C7) and flexor carpi ulnaris (C8 and T1) muscles. Each of these muscles can be tested separately. This testing can be accomplished if the examiner provides resistance to flexion at the base of the second metacarpal bone in the direction of extension and ulnar deviation in the case of the flexor carpi radialis muscle and resistance at the base of the fifth metacarpal in the direction of extension and radial deviation in the case of the flexor carpi ulnaris muscle. The principal extensors of the wrist are the extensor carpi radialis longus (C6 and C7), extensor carpi radialis brevis (C6 and C7), and extensor carpi ulnaris (C7 and C8) muscles. The radial and ulnar extensor muscles can be tested separately. The principal supinators of the forearm are the biceps brachii (C5 and C6) and supinator (C6) muscles. The principal pronators of the forearm are the pronator teres (C6 and C7) and pronator quadratus (C8 and T1) muscles.

Metacarpophalangeal and Proximal and Distal Interphalangeal Joints

The MCP joints are hinge joints. Lateral collateral ligaments that are loose in extension tighten in flexion, preventing lateral movement of the digits. The extensor tendons that cross the dorsum of each joint strengthen the articular capsule. When the extensor tendon of the digit reaches the distal end of the metacarpal head, it is joined by fibers of the interossei and lumbricales muscles and expands over the entire dorsum of the MCP joint and onto the dorsum of the adjacent phalanx. This expansion of the extensor mechanism is known as the *extensor hood.*

The proximal and distal interphalangeal joints also are hinge joints. The ligaments of the interphalangeal joints resemble those of the MCP joints. When the fingers are flexed, the bases of the

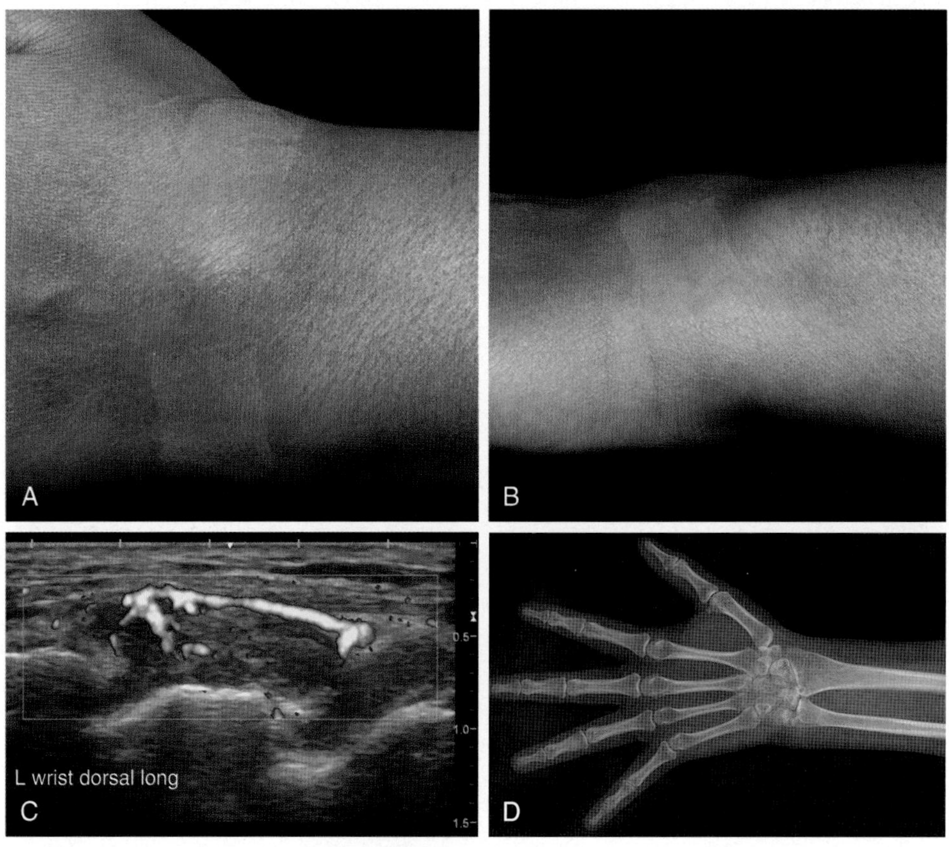

• **Fig. 43.3** Synovitis of the wrist. (A) Dorsal and (B) radial views of the wrist in another patient with rheumatoid arthritis. Note diffuse swelling through the dorsal recess of the wrist. (C) Sonographic evaluation reveals hypoechoic thickening and power Doppler hyperemia. (D) Corresponding plain radiograph of the wrist demonstrates carpal erosions and joint space narrowing.

proximal phalanges slide toward the palmar side of the heads of the metacarpal bones. The metacarpal heads form the rounded prominences of the knuckles, with the metacarpal joint spaces situated about 1 cm distal to the apex of the prominences.

To examine the MCP joints, the examiner may use either a two- or four-finger technique. In the two-finger technique, the examiner uses both thumbs to palpate the medial and lateral aspects of the dorsal joint line and recesses of each joint in 30 to 45 degrees of flexion (Fig. 43.4).[20] The skin on the palmar surface of the hand is thick and covers a fat pad between it and the MCP joint. This makes palpation of the palmar surface of the joint difficult, but some examiners also palpate the volar aspects of the joint using one or two other fingers of either hand. In the dorsal four-finger technique, the examiner supports one finger at a time using her or his third through fifth fingers of the dominant hand (Fig. 43.5).[20] Then, the examiner uses the thumb and index fingers of both hands to palpate the dorsal recesses of the MCP joint and assess for bogginess or ballottement of the soft tissues. The dorsal four-finger technique may have greater sensitivity and negative predictive value for clinical synovitis as compared to the historical two-finger technique and correlates better to ultrasonographic findings.[20] It is especially helpful in examining the small joints to compare one with another to detect subtle synovitis. Gentle lateral compression with force applied at the base of the second and fifth metacarpophalangeal joints (the squeeze test) often elicits pain if synovitis is present.

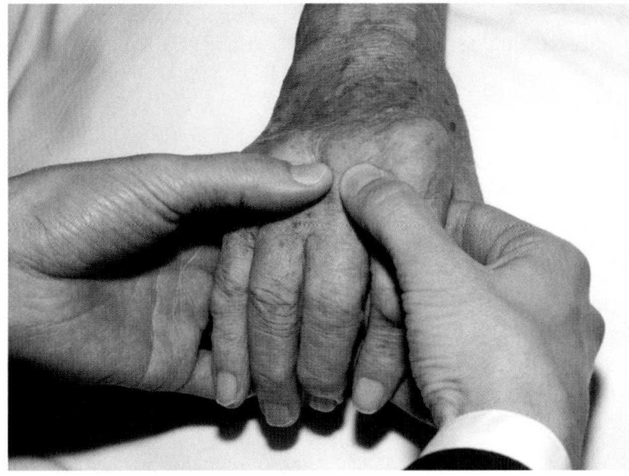

• **Fig. 43.4** The two-finger technique is the conventional technique for palpation of metacarpophalangeal joints for synovitis. The technique is performed with the metacarpophalangeal joint in 30 to 45 degrees of flexion. The examiner's thumbs palpate the medial and lateral aspects of the dorsal joint line while the forefingers palpate the volar aspects of the joint.

The proximal and distal interphalangeal joints are best examined by palpating gently over the lateral and medial aspects of the joint, where the flexor and extensor tendons do not interfere with assessment of the synovial membrane. Alternatively, the joint can be compressed anteroposteriorly by the thumb and index finger of one of the examiner's hands, while the other thumb and index finger palpate for synovial distention medially and laterally. The Bunnell test is useful in differentiating synovitis of the proximal interphalangeal joints from tightening of the intrinsic muscles (see Chapter 53).

Swelling of the fingers may result from articular or periarticular causes. Synovial swelling usually produces symmetric enlargement of the joint itself, whereas extra-articular swelling may be diffuse and may extend beyond the joint space. Asymmetric enlargement, involving only one side of the digit or joint, is less common and usually indicates an extra-articular process. Diffuse swelling of an entire digit, known by the terms *dactylitis* and *sausage digit,* may result from tenosynovitis and is seen most commonly in the spondyloarthropathies, such as reactive arthritis or psoriatic arthritis. Rheumatoid nodules are firm periarticular swellings that frequently overlie the joints or bony prominences in patients with chronic rheumatoid disease. Chronic swelling with distention of the metacarpophalangeal joints tends to produce stretching and laxity of the articular capsule and ligaments. This laxity, combined with muscle imbalance and other forces, eventually results in the

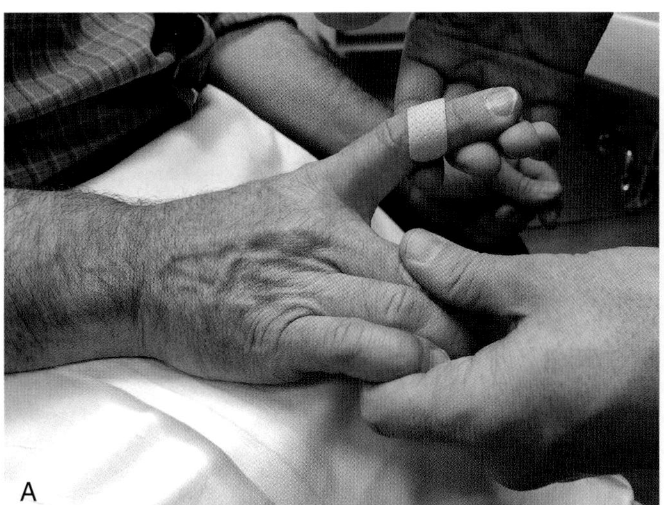

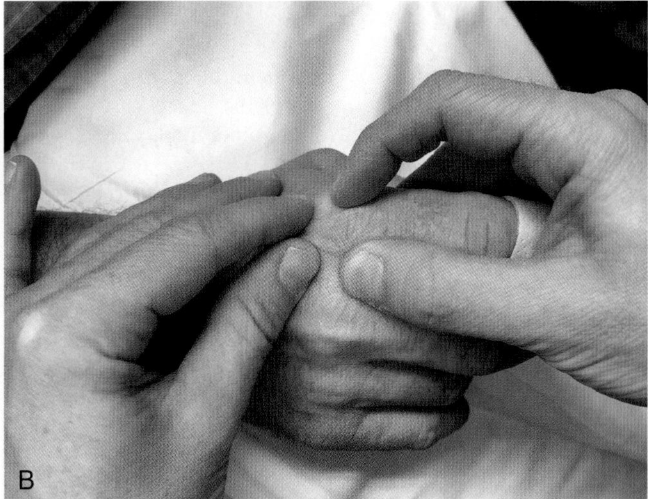

• **Fig. 43.5** The dorsal four-finger technique is an alternative technique for palpation of metacarpophalangeal joints for synovitis. (A) The finger is supported using the third to fifth fingers of the examiner's dominant hand in approximately 45 degrees of extension. (B) The thumb and index fingers of both hands palpate the dorsal surfaces of the metacarpophalangeal joint both at the distal joint line and proximal synovial recess, forming a "diamond" shape. The examiner notes synovial thickening and effusion by ballottement.

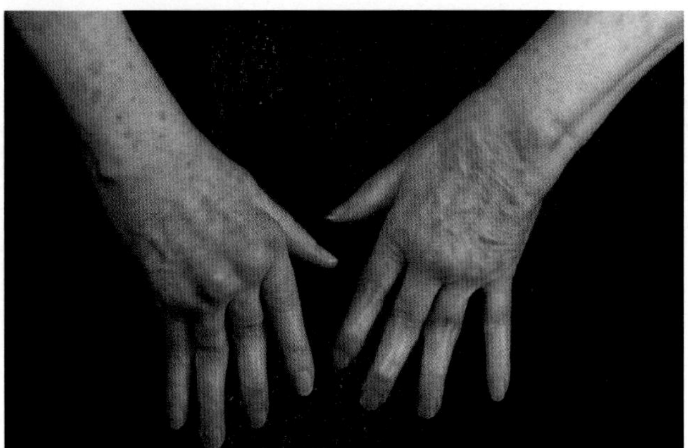

• **Fig. 43.6** Destructive rheumatoid arthritis. Chronic synovial pannus formation involves the metacarpophalangeal joints of both hands and both wrist joints. Subluxation and ulnar deviation are present in the right hand metacarpophalangeal joints. Swan neck deformities are present in the right third through fifth and left second through fourth digits.

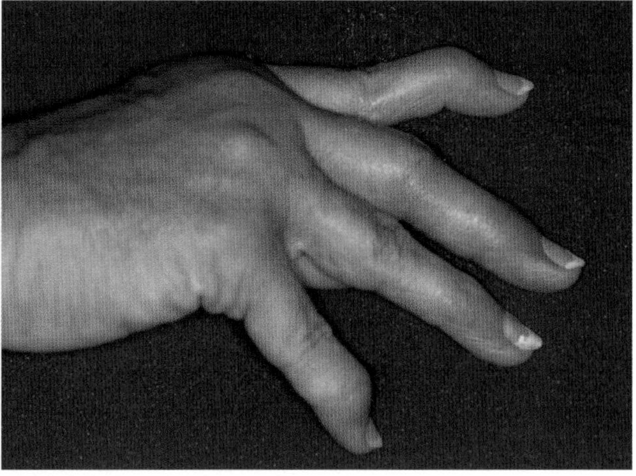

• **Fig. 43.7** Swan neck deformity in a patient with psoriatic arthritis. Note hyperextension of the proximal interphalangeal joint and hyperflexion of the distal interphalangeal joint of the second digit. Also note the psoriatic changes of the third and fourth fingernails.

extensor tendons of the digits slipping off the metacarpal heads to the ulnar sides of the joints. The abnormal pull of the displaced tendons is one of the factors that cause ulnar deviation of the fingers in chronic inflammatory arthritis (Fig.43.6).

Swan neck deformity describes a finger with a flexion contracture of the MCP joint, hyperextension of the proximal interphalangeal joint, and flexion of the distal interphalangeal joint. These changes are produced by contraction of the interossei and other muscles that flex the MCP joints and extend the proximal interphalangeal joints. This deformity is characteristic of RA but may be seen in other chronic arthritides (Fig. 43.7).

Boutonnière deformity describes a finger with a flexion contracture of the proximal interphalangeal joint associated with hyperextension of the distal interphalangeal joint. The deformity is common in RA and occurs when the central slip of the extensor tendon of the proximal interphalangeal joint becomes detached from the base of the middle phalanx, allowing palmar dislocation of the lateral bands. The dislocated bands cross the fulcrum of the joint and act as flexors instead of extensors of the joint.

Another abnormality is telescoping or shortening of the digits produced by resorption of the ends of the phalanges secondary to destructive arthropathy. This may be seen in the arthritis mutilans form of psoriatic arthritis. Shortening of the fingers is associated with wrinkling of the skin over involved joints and is called *opera-glass hand* or *la main en lorgnette.*

A mallet finger results from avulsion or rupture of the extensor tendon at the level of the distal interphalangeal joint. With this deformity, the patient is unable to extend the distal phalanx, which remains in a flexed position. This deformity frequently results from traumatic injuries.

The Murphy sign is a test for lunate dislocation. The patient is asked to make a fist. The third metacarpal head usually is more prominent than the second and fourth. If the third metacarpal is level with the second and fourth, the finding is positive for lunate dislocation.

Involvement of the distal interphalangeal joints in RA is uncommon. Bony hypertrophy and osteophyte formation are commonly seen, however, at the distal and proximal interphalangeal joints in patients with osteoarthritis. Enlarged, bony, hypertrophic distal interphalangeal joints are called *Heberden nodes,* whereas similar changes at the proximal interphalangeal joints are called *Bouchard nodes.* These usually are easily differentiated from the synovitis of inflammatory arthritis because, on palpation, the enlargement is hard or bony. In addition, signs of inflammation are minimal. Heberden and Bouchard nodes should be easily distinguished from rheumatoid nodules, but patients occasionally confuse these when describing swellings over joints. The examiner should be aware of other causes of joint enlargement or nodules on the hands, including tophaceous gout (Fig. 43.8) and, rarely, multicentric reticulohistiocytosis. The first carpometacarpal joint also is often affected in osteoarthritis (Fig. 43.9).

The patient's fingernails should be inspected for evidence of clubbing or other abnormalities. Often in patients with psoriatic arthritis, ridging, onycholysis, or nail pitting is present. Occasionally, patients with osteoarthritis develop a groove deformity of the nail on a digit with a Heberden node. (This nail deformity has been called a *Heberden node nail.*) The abnormality is believed to occur secondary to synovial cyst encroachment on the nail bed by the evolving osteoarthritis process. With time, the nail may return to normal.

A crude but sometimes useful assessment of hand function can be made by asking the patient to make a fist. An estimate of the patient's ability to form a full fist can be recorded as a percentage fist, with 100% a complete fist. A fist of 75% indicates that the patient can touch the palm with the fingertips. The ability to oppose fingers, especially the thumb, is crucial to hand function because of the necessity to grasp or at least pinch for objects. If the patient is unable to form a full fist, the ability or inability to pinch or oppose fingers can be demonstrated by asking the patient to pick up a small object.

Strength of the hands can be assessed crudely by asking the patient to grip firmly two or more of the examiner's fingers. More accurate measures of grip strength can be made by using a dynamometer or by having the patient squeeze a partially inflated sphygmomanometer (at 20 mm Hg). It sometimes is useful to test the strength of the fingers separately. The prime movers of flexion of the second through fifth MCP joints are the dorsal and palmar interossei muscles (nerve roots C8 and T1). The lumbricales muscles (C6, C7, and C8) flex the MCP joints when the proximal phalangeal joints are extended. The flexors of the proximal interphalangeal joints are the flexor digitorum

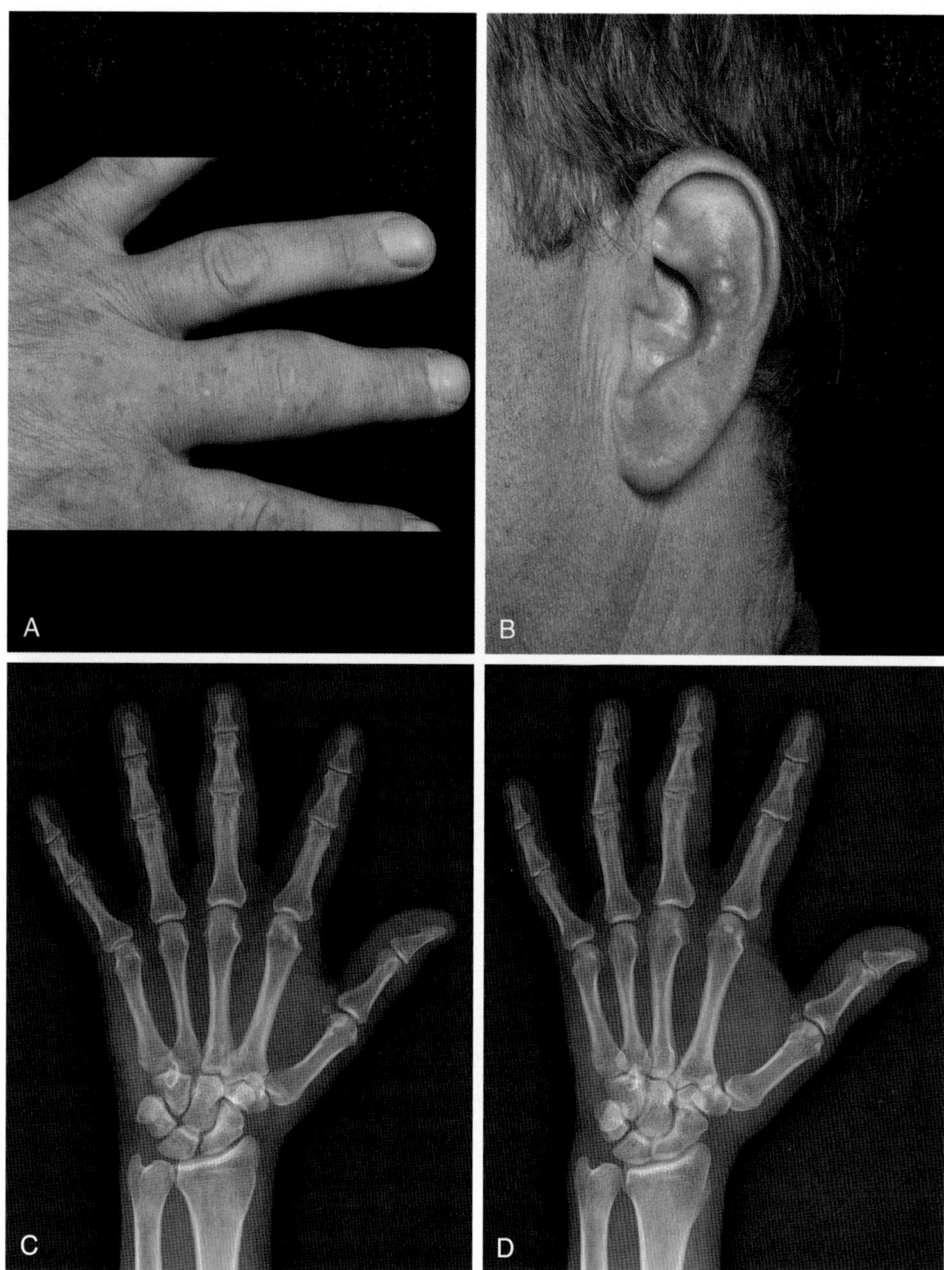

• **Fig. 43.8** Gout. (A) Note the swelling and enlargement of the left third proximal interphalangeal joint in a patient with crystal-proven gout. (B) The same patient was found to have a tophus in the left ear. (C) and (D) The corresponding posteroanterior and oblique radiographs of the hands demonstrate soft tissue swelling and increased density about the left third proximal interphalangeal joint likely due to tophaceous deposits.

superficialis muscles (C7, C8, and T1), and the flexor of the distal interphalangeal joints is the flexor digitorum profundus muscle (C7, C8, and T1).

The prime extensors of the MCP and interphalangeal joints of the second through fifth fingers are the extensor digitorum communis (nerve roots C6, C7, and C8), extensor indicis proprius (C6, C7, and C8), and extensor digiti minimi (C7) muscles. The interossei and lumbricales muscles simultaneously flex the MCP joints and extend the interphalangeal joints. The dorsal interossei (C8 and T1) and abductor digiti minimi (C8) muscles abduct the fingers, whereas the palmar interosseous muscles adduct the fingers.

The thumb is moved by several muscles. The prime flexor of the first MCP joint is the flexor pollicis brevis muscle (nerve roots C6, C7, C8, and T1). The prime flexor of the interphalangeal joint is the flexor pollicis longus muscle (C8 and T1). The MCP joint of the thumb is extended by the extensor pollicis brevis muscle, and the prime extensor of the interphalangeal joint is the extensor pollicis longus muscle (C6, C7, C8, and C9).

The principal abductors of the thumb are the abductor pollicis longus (nerve roots C6 and C7) and the abductor pollicis brevis (C6 and C7) muscles. Motion occurs primarily at the carpometacarpal joint. The principal adductor of the thumb is the adductor pollicis muscle (C8 and T1). Motion occurs primarily at the carpometacarpal joint. The principal movers in opposition of the thumb and fifth fingers are the opponens pollicis (C6 and C7) and opponens digiti minimi (C8 and T1) muscles.

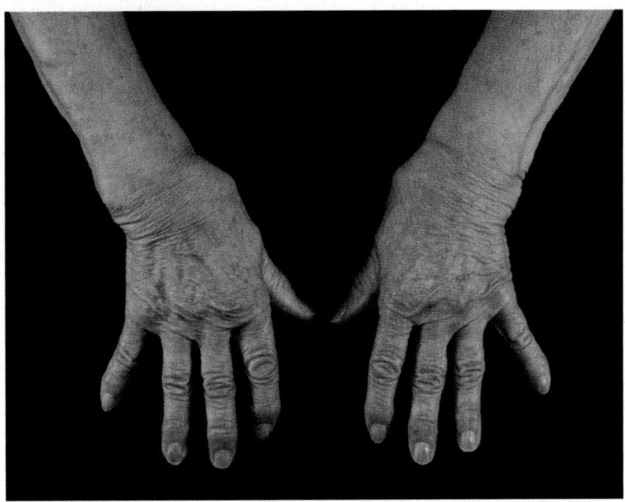

• **Fig. 43.9** Osteoarthritis of the hands. Note the advanced hypertrophic enlargement at the base of both thumbs. Both second distal interphalangeal joints are notable for advanced bony enlargement, and more moderate changes are seen in the other interphalangeal joints.

Hip

The hip is a spheroidal or ball-and-socket joint formed by the rounded head of the femur and the cup-shaped acetabulum (see Chapter 51). Stability of the joint is ensured by the fibrocartilaginous rim of the glenoid labrum and the dense articular capsule and surrounding ligaments, including the iliofemoral, pubofemoral, and ischiocapsular ligaments that reinforce the capsule. Support also is provided by the powerful muscle groups that surround the hip. The principal hip flexor is the iliopsoas muscle assisted by the sartorius and rectus femoris muscles. Hip adduction is accomplished by the three adductors (longus, brevis, and magnus) plus the gracilis and pectineus muscles. The gluteus medius is the major hip abductor, whereas the gluteus maximus and hamstrings extend the hip. Several clinically important bursae are found around the hip joint. Anteriorly, the iliopsoas bursa lies between the psoas muscle and the joint surface. The trochanteric bursa lies between the gluteus maximus muscle and the posterolateral greater trochanter, and the ischiogluteal bursa overlies the ischial tuberosity.

Examination of the hip should begin by observation of the patient's stance and gait. The patient should stand in front of the examiner so that the anterior iliac spines are visible. Pelvic tilt or obliquity may be present and related to structural scoliosis, anatomic leg-length discrepancy, or hip disease.

Hip contractures may result in abduction or adduction deformities. To compensate for an adduction contracture, the pelvis is tilted upward on the side of the contracture. This allows the legs to be parallel during walking and weight bearing. With a fixed abduction deformity, the pelvis becomes elevated on the normal side during standing or walking. This elevation causes an apparent shortening of the normal leg and forces the patient to stand or walk on the toes of the normal side or to flex the knee on the abnormal leg. Viewed from behind with the legs parallel, the patient with hip disease and an adducted hip contracture may have asymmetric gluteal folds secondary to pelvic tilt, with the diseased side elevated. In this situation, the patient is unable to stand with the foot of the involved leg flat on the floor. In abduction contracture, the findings are reversed; with both legs extended and parallel, the uninvolved side is elevated.

A hip flexion deformity commonly occurs in diseases of the hip. Unilateral flexion of the hip in the standing position reduces weight bearing on the involved side and relaxes the joint capsule, causing less pain. This posture is best noted by observing the patient from the side. A hyperlordosis curve of the lumbar spine compensates for lack of full hip extension.

Gait should be assessed in the patient with possible hip joint disease. With a normal gait, the abductors of the weight-bearing leg contract to hold the pelvis level or to elevate the non–weight-bearing side slightly. Two abnormalities of gait may be commonly observed in patients with hip disease. The most common abnormality seen with a painful hip is the antalgic (limping) gait. With this gait, the individual leans over the diseased hip during the phase of weight bearing on that hip, placing the body weight directly over the joint to avoid painful contraction of the hip abductors. With a Trendelenburg gait, with weight bearing on the affected side, the pelvis drops and the trunk shifts to the normal side. Although the antalgic gait is frequently seen with painful hips, and the Trendelenburg gait is seen in patients with weak hip abductors, these gaits are not specific, and either may occur as a result of hip pain from one of several causes. A mild Trendelenburg gait is seen often in healthy individuals.

The Trendelenburg test assesses the stability of the hip, together with the ability of the hip abductor muscle to stabilize the pelvis on the femur.[21] It is a measure of the gluteus medius hip abductor strength. The patient is asked to stand while bearing weight on only one leg. Normally, the abductors hold the pelvis level or the nonsupported side slightly elevated. If the non–weight-bearing side drops, the test is positive for weakness of the weight-bearing side hip abductors, especially the gluteus medius muscle. This test is nonspecific and may be used in primary neurologic or muscle disorders and in hip diseases that lead to weakness of the hip abductors.

The motion of the hip should be assessed with the patient in the supine position. Range of motion of the hip includes flexion, extension, abduction, adduction, internal and external rotation, and circumduction. The degree of flexion permitted varies with the manner with which it is assessed. When the knee is held flexed at 90 degrees, the hip normally flexes to an angle of 120 degrees between the thigh and the long axis of the body. If the knee is held in extension, the hamstrings limit hip flexion to approximately 90 degrees. The presence of a hip flexion contracture is suggested by the persistence of lumbar lordosis and pelvic tilt, which masks the contracture by allowing the involved leg to remain in contact with the examination table. The Thomas test shows the flexion contracture. With this test, the opposite hip is fully flexed to flatten the lumbar lordosis and fix the pelvis. The patient's involved leg should be extended toward the examination table as far as possible. Flexion contracture of the diseased hip becomes more obvious and can be estimated in degrees from full extension. Measurement for leg-length discrepancy is performed with the patient in a supine position and the legs fully extended. Each leg is measured from the anterior superior iliac spine to the medial malleolus. A difference of 1 cm or less is unlikely to cause any abnormality of gait and may be considered normal. In addition to true leg-length asymmetries, apparent leg-length discrepancies may result from pelvic tilt or abduction or adduction contractures of the hip.

Abduction is measured with the patient in a supine position and the leg in an extended position, perpendicular to the pelvis. Pelvic stabilization is achieved by the examiner placing an arm across the pelvis with the hand on the opposite anterior iliac spine. With the other hand, the examiner grasps the patient's ankle and abducts the leg until the pelvis begins to move. Abduction to approximately 45 degrees is normal. It is helpful to compare one side with the other because the normal range of motion may vary. Alternatively, the examiner could stand at the foot of the table, grasp both of the patient's ankles, and simultaneously abduct both legs. Abduction is commonly limited in hip joint disease. The examiner assesses adduction by grasping the patient's ankle and raising the leg off the examination table by flexing the hip enough to allow the tested leg to cross over the opposite leg. Normal adduction is approximately 2 to 30 degrees. Hip rotation may be tested with the hip and knee flexed to 90 degrees or with the leg extended. Normal hip external rotation and internal rotation are observed to 45 and 40 degrees, respectively. The difference in rotation between the flexed and extended hip is attributable to increased stabilization of the joint by surrounding ligaments in the extended position. Rotation decreases with extension. To test hip rotation, the examiner grasps the extended leg above the ankle and rotates it externally and internally from the neutral position. Limitation of internal rotation of the hip is a sensitive indicator of hip joint disease.

Extension is tested with the patient in the prone position. Estimating hip extension can be difficult because some of the apparent motion arises from hyperextension of the lumbar spine, pelvis rotation, motion of the buttock soft tissue, and flexion of the opposite hip. The pelvis and the lumbar spine can be partially immobilized by the examiner placing an arm across the posterior iliac crest and the lower lumbar spine. The examiner places the other hand under the thigh with the knee flexed and hyperextends the thigh. Normal extension ranges from 10 to 20 degrees. Limitation of extension often occurs secondary to a hip flexion contracture.

Swelling around the hip only rarely can be discerned on examination. The flexion abduction external rotation (FABER) test, also known as the *Patrick* test, is a commonly used screening test for intra-articular hip pathology.[22] To perform this test, the examiner has the patient lie in a supine position with the foot ipsilateral to the test hip, resting on the contralateral knee. The examiner then slowly lowers the patient's test leg toward the examining table, applying gentle pressure to the knee of the test hip and the contralateral anterior superior iliac spine. Normally, the test leg will fall at least parallel to the opposite leg. The FABER test is considered positive when the maneuver reproduces the patient's pain. Although very sensitive for hip joint disease, this test is not specific because a positive test may indicate iliopsoas tightness or sacroiliac joint disease.

The iliotibial band is a part of the fascia lata that extends from the iliac crest, sacrum, and ischium over the greater trochanter to the lateral femoral condyle, tibial condyle, and fibular head, and along the lateral intermuscular system, separating the hamstrings from the vastus lateralis muscle. The tensor fasciae latae muscle may produce an audible snap while it slips over the greater trochanter if the weight-bearing leg moves from hip flexion and adduction to a neutral position, as when climbing stairs. Most commonly observed in young women, the snapping hip usually does not cause severe pain. The Ober test evaluates the iliotibial band for contracture. The patient lies on the side, with the lower leg flexed at the hip and knee. The examiner abducts and extends the upper leg with the knee flexed at 90 degrees. The hips should be slightly extended to allow the iliotibial band to pass over the greater trochanter. The examiner slowly lowers the patient's limb with the muscles relaxed. A positive test result indicative of an iliotibial band contracture occurs if the leg does not fall back to the level of the tabletop.

A common cause of lateral hip pain is trochanteric bursitis. Patients with this condition often complain of pain and tenderness when they attempt to lie on the affected side or climb stairs. The greater trochanter should be palpated for tenderness and compared with the opposite side. In trochanteric bursitis, this area is usually exquisitely tender. The pain of trochanteric bursitis is aggravated by actively resisted abduction of the hip. Aching and tenderness over the buttock area may be secondary to an ischial bursitis. Other causes of lateral and posterior hip (buttock) discomfort include pain at muscle and tendon insertion sites.

Anterior hip and groin pain may be secondary to hip abnormality, most commonly degenerative arthritis. The examiner should take note of decreased range of motion in these patients. Other causes include iliopsoas bursitis, in which swelling and tenderness may be noted in the middle third of the inguinal ligament lateral to the femoral pulse. This pain is aggravated by hip extension and is reduced by flexion. The bursitis may be a localized problem or may represent extension of hip synovitis. It usually is impossible to distinguish between a localized bursitis and an extension of hip synovitis on the basis of the physical examination. If the patient has tenderness in the region of the iliopsoas bursa, but no swelling is palpable, the examiner should consider tendinitis of the iliopsoas muscle. The inguinal region should be palpated for other abnormalities, such as hernias, femoral aneurysms, adenopathy, tumor, and psoas abscess or masses.

Muscle strength testing should include the hip flexors, extensors, abductors, and adductors. The primary hip flexor is the iliopsoas muscle (nerve roots L2 and L3). Flexion may be tested with the patient sitting at the edge of a table. The examiner exerts downward pressure against the thigh proximal to the knee while the patient attempts to flex the hip. The pelvis may be stabilized by the examiner's other hand placed on the ipsilateral iliac crest. Alternatively, with the patient supine and holding the leg in 90 degrees of flexion at the hip, the examiner may attempt to straighten the hip.

Hip extension is tested with the patient lying prone. The primary hip extensor is the gluteus maximus muscle (L5 and S1). With the patient's knee flexed to remove hamstring action, the patient is instructed to extend the hip and thigh off the surface of the table while the examiner places a forearm across the posterior iliac crest to stabilize the pelvis and applies downward pressure to prevent the lateral trunk muscles from elevating the pelvis and leg off the table.

Abduction may be tested with the patient prone or supine. The patient should abduct the thigh and leg against resistance from the examiner applied at the midthigh level.

The primary adductor is the adductor longus muscle (nerve roots L3 and L4). The examiner holds the upper leg proximal to the knee in slight abduction, while the patient resists and attempts to adduct the leg. Testing for abduction and adduction also may be done in the two legs simultaneously. The patient lies supine with the legs fully extended and the hips moderately abducted. To test abduction, the patient actively pushes out against the examiner's resistance against the lateral malleoli. Adduction is tested by movement against resistance at the medial malleoli.

Knee

The knee is a compound condylar joint with three articulations: the patellofemoral and the lateral and medial tibiofemoral condyles with their fibrocartilaginous menisci. The knee is stabilized by its articular capsule, the patellar ligament, medial and lateral collateral ligaments, and anterior and posterior cruciate ligaments. The collateral ligaments provide medial and lateral stability, whereas the cruciatus provide anteroposterior and rotatory stability. Normal knee motion is a combination of flexion or extension and rotation. With flexion, the tibia internally rotates, and with extension, it externally rotates on the femur. The surrounding synovial membrane is the largest of the body's joints; it extends 6 cm proximal to the joint as the suprapatellar pouch beneath the quadriceps femoris muscle. Several important bursae are found around the knee, including the superficial prepatellar bursa, the superficial and deep infrapatellar bursae, the pes anserine bursa distal to the medial tibial plateau, and the posterior medial semimembranosus and posterolateral gastrocnemius bursae. Knee extension is primarily mediated by the quadriceps femoris muscle; knee flexion is mediated by the hamstrings. The biceps femoris muscle externally rotates the lower leg on the femur, whereas the popliteus and semitendinosus muscles mediate internal rotation.

In taking the history of a patient with knee complaints, the examiner should ask the patient about symptoms of knee locking, catching, or giving way. *Locking* is the sudden loss of ability to extend the knee; it usually is painful and may be associated with an audible noise, such as a click or pop. It often implies extensive intra-articular abnormality, including loose bodies or cartilaginous tears. *Catching* refers to a subjective sensation of the patient that the knee might lock; the patient may experience a momentary interruption in the smooth range of motion of the joint but is able to continue with normal motion after this brief hesitation. Catching usually implies less abnormality than true locking and may occur in various pathologic conditions. True give-way indicates that the knee actually buckles and gives out in certain positions or with certain activities. It is important to elicit details of the patient history to verify this common subjective complaint. Patients often experience a sensation that the knee will give out when it actually does not. Other patients say their knees are "giving out" to describe severe pain that necessitates stopping an activity. True give-way implies severe intra-articular abnormality, such as an unstable joint from ligamentous injury or incompetence.

Examination of the knees should always include observation of the patient while standing and walking (see Chapter 51). Deviation of the knees, including genu varum (lateral deviation of the knee joint with medial deviation of the lower leg), genu valgum (medial deviation of the knee with lateral deviation of the lower leg), and genu recurvatum (hyperextension deformity of the knee), is most easily evaluated with the patient standing. The patient also should be observed ambulating for evidence of gait abnormalities.

Inspection should be done with the patient standing and supine. It is essential to compare side to side, noting any asymmetry that may be caused by swelling or muscle atrophy. Suprapatellar swelling with fullness of the distal anterior thigh that obliterates the normal depressed contours along the sides of the patella usually indicates knee joint effusion or synovitis. Localized swelling over the surface of the patella is generally secondary to prepatellar bursitis. Patellar alignment should be noted, including high-riding or laterally displaced patellae. The examiner also should inspect the knee from behind to identify popliteal swelling caused by a popliteal or Baker cyst, most commonly caused by medial semimembranosus bursal swelling. If the calves appear asymmetric, calf circumference should be measured and compared bilaterally. Popliteal cysts may rupture and dissect down into the calf muscles, resulting in enlargement and palpable fullness. Edema may be present if the cyst causes secondary venous or lymphatic obstruction. Acute rupture and dissection of a popliteal cyst can mimic thrombophlebitis, with local pain, heat, redness, and swelling. This is probably a more common cause of unilateral calf swelling in patients with RA than is deep venous thrombosis. The two conditions may be difficult to distinguish on physical examination alone.

Quadriceps femoris muscle atrophy usually develops in chronic arthritis of the knee. Atrophy of the vastus medialis muscle is the earliest change and may be appreciated by comparing the two thighs for medial asymmetry and circumference. Measurement of the thigh circumference should be performed at 15 cm above the knee to avoid spurious results due to suprapatellar effusions.

Palpation of the knee should be performed with the joint relaxed. This usually is best accomplished with the patient supine and the knees fully extended and not touching. Palpation should begin over the anterior thigh approximately 10 cm above the patella. To identify the superior margin of the suprapatellar pouch, which is an extension of the knee joint cavity, the examiner should palpate the anterior thigh, moving distally toward the knee. Swelling, thickening, nodules, loose bodies, tenderness, and warmth should be noted. A thickened synovial membrane has a boggy, doughy consistency, which differs from the surrounding soft tissue and muscle. It usually is palpated earlier over the medial aspect of the suprapatellar pouch and the medial tibiofemoral joint. To enhance detection of knee fluid, any fluid in the suprapatellar pouch is compressed with the palm of the hand placed just proximal to the patella. The synovial fluid forced into the inferior distal articular cavity is palpated with the opposite thumb and index finger laterally and medially to the patella. If the examiner alternates compression and release of the suprapatellar pouch, the synovial thickening can be differentiated from a synovial effusion. An effusion intermittently distends the joint capsule under the thumb and index finger of the opposite hand, whereas synovial thickening does not.

The examiner should not compress the suprapatellar pouch too firmly or push the tissues distally because the patella or normal soft tissue, including the fat pads, fills the palpated space and could be misinterpreted as synovitis or joint swelling. With a large effusion, the patella can be balloted by pushing it posteriorly against the femur with the right forefinger, while maintaining suprapatellar compression with the left hand.

At the other extreme, effusions of 4 to 8 mL can be detected by eliciting the bulge sign. This test is performed with the patient's knee extended and relaxed. The examiner strokes or compresses the medial aspect of the knee proximally and laterally with the palm of a hand to move fluid from the area. The lateral aspect of the knee is tapped or stroked, and a fluid wave or bulge appears medially (Fig. 43.10). A so-called *spontaneous bulge sign* occurs if, on compression along the medial side of the joint space, fluid reaccumulates with no pressure or compression along the lateral side of the joint.

The medial and lateral tibiofemoral joint margins are palpated for tenderness and bony lipping or exostosis, as can be seen in degenerative joint disease. Joint margins can be palpated easily with the hip flexed to 45 degrees, the knee flexed to 90 degrees, and the foot resting on the examining table. Tenderness localized over the medial or lateral joint margins may represent articular

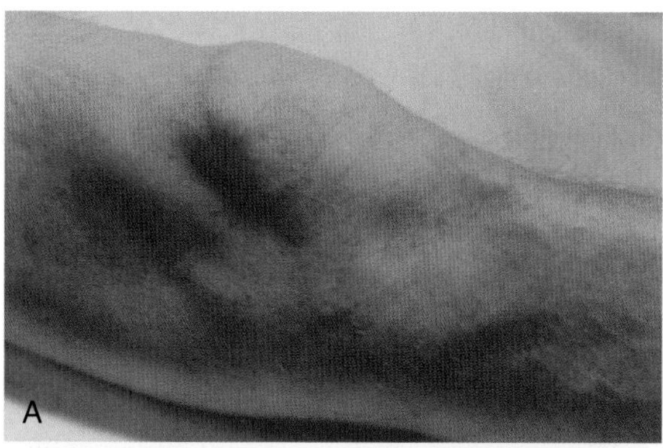

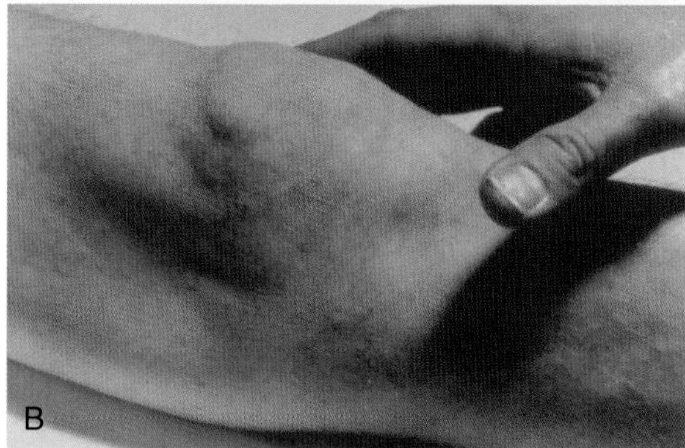

• **Fig. 43.10** Demonstration of the bulge sign for a small synovial knee effusion. The medial aspect of the knee has been stroked to move the synovial fluid from this area *(shaded depressed area in A)*. (B) Shows a bulge in the previously depressed area after the lateral aspect of the knee has been tapped.

cartilage disease, medial or lateral meniscal abnormality, or medial or lateral collateral ligament injury. Other causes of tenderness include pathologic conditions in the underlying bony structures.

Bursitis is another cause of localized tenderness around the knee; the two most common sites are the pes anserine and the prepatellar bursae. Exquisite local tenderness usually can be elicited if bursitis is present. Mild swelling also may be appreciated. Occasionally, the prepatellar bursa can become quite swollen. It is important not to interpret this swelling mistakenly as knee joint synovitis. The two can be differentiated because the bursal margins can be outlined by palpation; other features of true joint effusion, such as the bulge sign, are absent.

Patellofemoral malalignment is another common cause of knee pain. It is more common in female patients because of the wider Q angle caused by the broader female pelvis. The Q angle is the angle formed between the quadriceps and the patellar tendon. Patients with patellofemoral disease may complain of stiffness in the knee after a period of flexion (the moviegoer sign) or may have particular difficulty with stair climbing. Some patients may experience a sensation of catching as the patella moves over the distal femur. Patellar palpation is best performed with the knee extended and relaxed. The patella is compressed and moved so that its entire articular surface comes into contact with the underlying femur. Slight crepitation may be observed in many normally functioning knees. Pain with crepitation may suggest patellofemoral degenerative arthritis or chondromalacia patellae.

Retropatellar pain occurring with active knee flexion and extension and secondary to patellofemoral disease may be differentiated from tibiofemoral articular pain. To test this, the examiner should attempt to lift the patella away from the knee, while passively moving the knee through the range of motion. Painless motion during this maneuver indicates that the patellofemoral joint is the likely source of the pain. In addition, the "patellar grind" test is useful in patients with extensive patellofemoral abnormality. In this test, the examiner compresses the patella distally away from the femoral condyles, while instructing the patient to contract the quadriceps isometrically. Sudden patellar pain and quadriceps relaxation indicate a positive test result. This test has frequent false-positive results, however.

Patellar stability should be assessed. The Fairbanks apprehension test is done with the patient supine, the quadriceps relaxed, and the knee in 30 degrees of flexion. The examiner slowly pushes the patella laterally. A sudden contraction of the quadriceps and a distressed reaction from the patient constitute a positive apprehension test result. A patient who has had previous patellar dislocations usually has a positive apprehension test result. The patella also can be examined for subluxation while the knee is moved through a range of motion from full flexion to extension.

The normal knee range of motion should be from full extension (0 degrees) to full flexion of 120 to 150 degrees. Some normal individuals may be able to hyperextend to 15 degrees. Loss of full extension that is generally reversible and pain with extension or when straightening the knee frequently occurs with a knee joint effusion, synovitis, or both.[23] However, permanent loss of extension caused by flexion contracture is a common finding that accompanies chronic arthritis of the knee. In advanced arthritis, such as in some cases of RA, posterior subluxation of the tibia on the femur may be observed.

Testing for ligamentous and meniscal derangements is covered in Chapter 51.

Muscle strength testing includes testing flexion supplied by the hamstrings (i.e., the biceps femoris, semitendinosus, and semimembranosus) (nerve roots L5 to S3) and extension supplied by the quadriceps femoris (L2, L3, and L4). The hamstrings are best tested with the patient prone and attempting to move the knee from 90 degrees to maximal flexion. The ankle should be kept in a neutral position or dorsiflexed to remove gastrocnemius action. With the leg externally rotated, the biceps femoris, which inserts on the fibula and lateral tibia, is primarily tested, whereas flexion with internal rotation tests the semitendinosus and semimembranosus muscles, which insert on the medial side of the tibia. Extension is tested with the patient sitting upright with the knee fully extended. The examiner stabilizes the thigh with downward pressure just proximal to the knee and places downward pressure at the ankle to test the knee extensors.

Ankle

The true ankle is a hinged joint, and movement is limited to plantar flexion and dorsiflexion. It is formed by the distal ends of the tibia and fibula and the proximal aspect of the body of the talus. Inversion and eversion occur at the subtalar joint (see Chapter 52). The tibia forms the weight-bearing portion of the ankle joint, whereas the fibula articulates on the side of the tibia. The malleoli of the tibia and fibula extend downward beyond the weight-bearing part of the joint and articulate with the sides of the talus. The malleoli provide medial and lateral stability by enveloping the talus in a mortise-like fashion. The articular capsule of the ankle is lax on the anterior and posterior aspects of the joint, allowing extension and flexion, but it is tightly bound bilaterally by ligaments. The synovial membrane of the ankle on the inside of the capsule usually does not communicate with any other joints, bursae, or tendon sheaths.

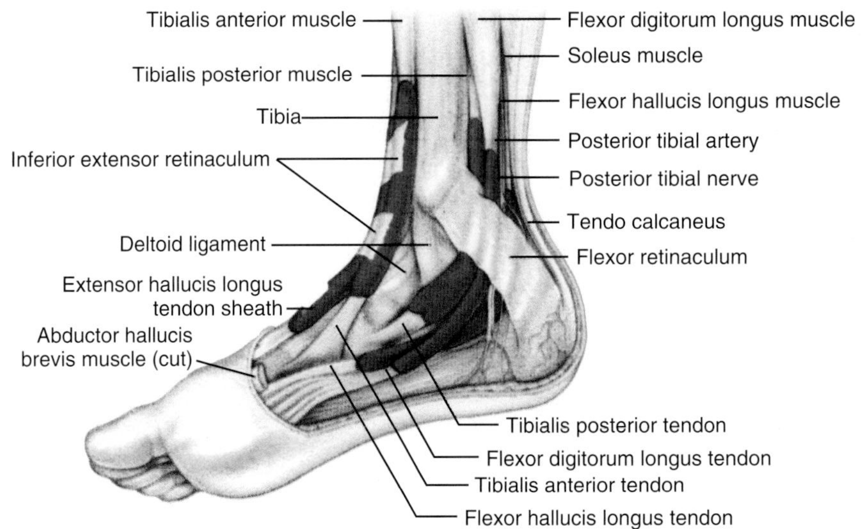

• **Fig. 43.11** Diagram of the ankle. Medial aspect of the ankle shows the relationship among tendons, ligaments, artery, and nerve. (From Polley HF, Hunder GG: *Rheumatologic interviewing and physical examination of the joints*, ed 2. Philadelphia, 1978, WB Saunders. With permission from the Mayo Foundation for Medical Education and Research.)

The medial and lateral ligaments surrounding the ankle contribute to medial and lateral stability of the joint. The deltoid ligament, the only ligament on the medial side of the ankle, is a triangle-shaped fibrous band that resists eversion of the foot. It may be torn in eversion sprains of the ankle. The lateral ligaments of the foot consist of three distinct bands forming the posterior talofibular, the calcaneofibular, and the anterior talofibular ligaments. These ligaments may be injured in inversion sprains of the ankle.

All tendons crossing the ankle joint lie superficial to the articular capsule and are enclosed in synovial sheaths for part of their course across the ankle. On the anterior aspect of the ankle, the tendons and the synovial tendon sheaths of the tibialis anterior, extensor digitorum longus, peroneus tertius, and extensor hallucis longus muscles overlie the articular capsule and synovial membrane. On the medial side of the ankle, posterior and inferior to the medial malleolus, lie the flexor tendons and tendon sheaths of the tibialis posterior, flexor digitorum longus, and flexor hallucis longus muscles (Fig. 43.11). All three of these muscles plantar flex and supinate the foot. The tendon of the flexor hallucis longus is located more posteriorly than the other flexor tendons and lies beneath the Achilles tendon for part of its course. The calcaneus tendon (Achilles tendon), the common tendon of the gastrocnemius and soleus muscles, inserts into the posterior surface of the calcaneus, where it is subject to external trauma, various inflammatory reactions, and irritations from bone spurs beneath it. On the lateral aspect of the ankle, posterior and inferior to the lateral malleolus, a synovial sheath encloses the tendons of the peroneus longus and peroneus brevis. These muscles extend the ankle (plantar flex) and evert (pronate) the foot. Each of the tendons adjacent to the ankle may be involved separately in traumatic or disease processes.

Synovial swelling of the ankle joint is most likely to cause fullness over the anterior or anterolateral aspect of the joint because the capsule is more lax in this area. Mild swelling of the joint may not be apparent on inspection because of the many structures crossing the joint superficially. Efforts should be made to differentiate superficial linear swelling localized to the distribution of the tendon sheaths from more diffuse fullness and swelling attributable to involvement of the ankle joint. Swelling of the heels may be observed from behind the standing patient and may be caused by enthesitis of the Achilles tendon insertion, which can occur in spondyloarthropathies (Fig. 43.12).

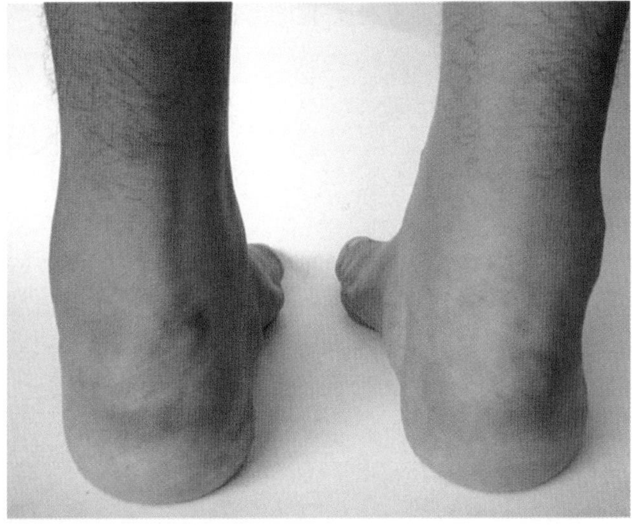

• **Fig. 43.12** Diffuse swelling of the posterior aspect of the feet, including the ankles and the Achilles, peroneal, and tibial posterior tendons, in a 12-year-old-boy with undifferentiated SpA. (From Burgos-Vargas R. The juvenile-onset spondyloarthritides. In: Weisman MH, van der Heijde D, Reveille JD, editors. Ankylosing spondylitis and the spondyloarthropathies. St. Louis: Mosby; 2006.)

It is difficult to observe synovitis of the intertarsal joints. Intertarsal joint synovitis may produce an erythematous puffiness or fullness over the dorsum of the foot.

From the normal position of rest in which there is a right angle between the leg and the foot, labeled 0 degrees, the ankle normally allows approximately 20 degrees of dorsiflexion and approximately 45 degrees of plantar flexion. Inversion and eversion of the foot occur mainly at the subtalar and other intertarsal joints. From the normal position of the foot, the subtalar joint normally permits approximately 20 degrees of eversion and 30 degrees of inversion. To test the subtalar joint, the examiner grasps the calcaneus with a hand and attempts to invert and evert it, holding the ankle motionless.

A general assessment of muscular strength of the ankle can be obtained by asking the patient to walk on toes and on heels. If the patient can walk satisfactorily on the toes and on the heels, the muscle strength of the flexors and extensors of the ankle can be considered normal. If this cannot be accomplished, it is desirable to test the muscles individually.

The principal flexors of the ankle are the gastrocnemius (nerve roots S1 and S2) and the soleus (S1 and S2) muscles. The principal extensor (dorsiflexors) of the ankle is the tibialis anterior muscle (L4, L5, and S1). The tibialis posterior muscle (L5 and S1) is the principal inverter. To test the tibialis posterior muscle, the foot should be in plantar flexion. The examiner applies graded resistance on the medial border of the forefoot while the patient attempts to invert the foot. The principal everters of the foot are the peroneus longus (L4, L5, and S1) and peroneus brevis (L4, L5, and S1) muscles.

Foot

See Chapter 52 for a detailed description

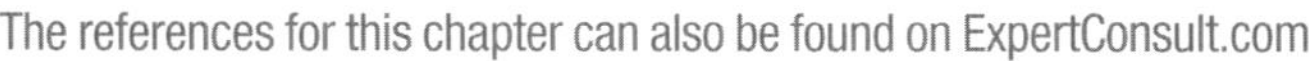
The references for this chapter can also be found on ExpertConsult.com

References

1. Woolf AD: How to assess musculoskeletal conditions: history and physical examination, *Best Pract Res Clin Rheumatol* 17:381–402, 2003.
2. Leigh JP, Fries JF: Mortality predictors among 263 patients with rheumatoid arthritis, *J Rheumatol* 18:1307–1312, 1991.
3. Wolfe F, Michaud K, Gefeller O, et al.: Predicting mortality in patients with rheumatoid arthritis, *Arthritis Rheum* 48:1530–1542, 2003.
4. Farragher TM, Lunt M, Bunn DK, et al.: Early functional disability predicts both all-cause and cardiovascular mortality in people with inflammatory polyarthritis: results from the Norfolk Arthritis Register, *Ann Rheum Dis* 66:486–492, 2007.
5. Polley HF, Hunder GG: *Rheumatologic interviewing and physical examination of the joints*, ed 2, Philadelphia, 1978, WB Saunders.
6. Sokka T, Pincus T: Quantitative joint assessment in rheumatoid arthritis, *Clin Exp Rheumatol* 23:S58–S62, 2005.
7. Fuchs HA, Brooks RH, Callahan LF, et al.: A simplified twenty-eight-joint quantitative articular index in rheumatoid arthritis, *Arthritis Rheum* 32:531–537, 1989.
8. Prevoo ML, van't Hof MA, Kuper HH, et al.: Modified disease activity scores that include twenty-eight-joint counts: development and validation in a prospective longitudinal study of patients with rheumatoid arthritis, *Arthritis Rheum* 38(44–48), 1995.
9. Brown AK, Quinn MA, Karim Z, et al.: Presence of significant synovitis in rheumatoid arthritis patients with disease-modifying antirheumatic drug-induced clinical remission: evidence from an imaging study may explain structural progression, *Arthritis Rheum* 54:3761–3773, 2006.
10. Szkudlarek M, Klarlund M, Narvestad E, et al.: Ultrasonography of the metacarpophalangeal and proximal interphalangeal joints in rheumatoid arthritis: a comparison with magnetic resonance imaging, conventional radiography and clinical examination, *Arthritis Res Ther* 8:R52, 2006.
11. Stone MA, White LM, Gladman DD, et al.: Significance of clinical evaluation of the metacarpophalangeal joint in relation to synovial/bone pathology in rheumatoid and psoriatic arthritis detected by magnetic resonance imaging, *J Rheumatol* 36:2751–2757, 2009.
12. Klarenbeek NB, Guler-Yuksel M, van der Heijde DM, et al.: Clinical synovitis in a particular joint is associated with progression of erosions and joint space narrowing in that same joint, but not in patients initially treated with infliximab, *Ann Rheum Dis* 69:2107–2113, 2010.
13. Wakefield RJ, Green MJ, Marzo-Ortega H, et al.: Should oligoarthritis be reclassified? Ultrasound reveals a high prevalence of subclinical disease, *Ann Rheum Dis* 63:382–385, 2004.
14. Krabben A, Stomp W, Huizinga TW, et al.: Concordance between inflammation at physical examination and on MRI in patients with early arthritis, *Ann Rheum Dis* 74:506–512, 2015.
15. Bauer EM, Ben-Artzi A, Duffy EL, et al.: Joint-specific assessment of swelling and power Doppler in obese rheumatoid arthritis patients, *BMC Musculoskeletal Disorders* 18(1):99, 2017.
16. Ceponis A, Onishi M, Bluestein HG, et al.: Utility of the ultrasound examination of the hand and wrist joints in the management of established rheumatoid arthritis, *Arthritis Care Res* 66:236–244, 2014.
17. Doherty M, Hazleman BL, Hutton CW, et al.: *Rheumatology examination and injection techniques*, ed 2, London, 1999, WB Saunders.
18. Malanga GA, Nadler SF: *Musculoskeletal physical examination: an evidence-based approach*, Philadelphia, 2006, Mosby.
19. Moore G: *Atlas of the musculoskeletal examination*, Philadelphia, 2003, American College of Physicians.
20. Omair MA, Akhavan P, Naraghi A, et al.: The dorsal 4-finger technique: a novel method to examine metacarpophalangeal joints in patients with rheumatoid arthritis, *The Journal of Rheumatology* 45(3):329–334, 2018.
21. Waldman SD: *Physical diagnosis of pain: an atlas of signs and symptoms*, Philadelphia, 2006, Saunders.
22. Maslowski E, Sullivan W, Forster Harwood J, et al.: The diagnostic validity of hip provocation maneuvers to detect intra-articular hip pathology, *PM R* 2:174–181, 2010.
23. Berlinberg A, Ashbeck EL, Roemer FW, et al.: Diagnostic performance of knee physical exam and participant-reported symptoms for MRI-detected effusion-synovitis among participants with early or late stage knee osteoarthritis: data from the Osteoarthritis Initiative. *Osteoarthritis Cartilage* 27:80–89, 2019.

44

Ultrasound in Rheumatology

EUGENE Y. KISSIN, PAUL J. DEMARCO, AND AMY C. CANNELLA

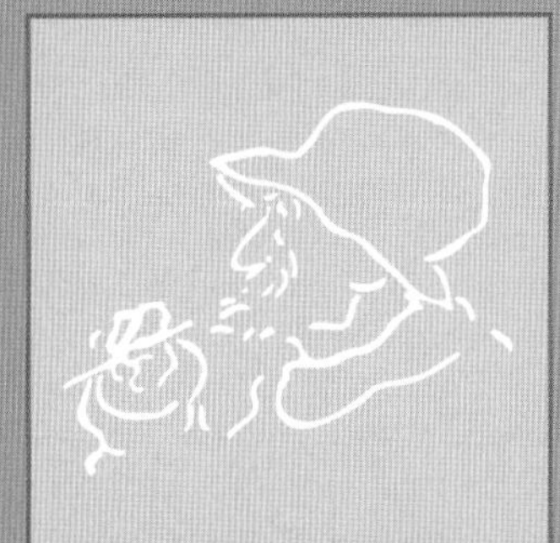

KEY POINTS

- Ultrasound in Rheumatology (RhUS) is utilized by rheumatologists both diagnostically and therapeutically.
- RhUS can assess inflammatory and non-inflammatory conditions of the joints and peri-articular structures.
- Power and color power Doppler (PD/CPD) allows for detection of inflammatory changes that are not apparent on physical examination and can guide management decisions.
- RhUS is evolving to include other organ systems involved in rheumatic diseases, such as salivary glands and blood vessels.
- Utilizing RhUS for invasive procedures, such as aspiration and injection of joints, bursa, and tendon sheaths, allows improved precision and increases patient satisfaction.
- RhUS is a safe, reliable, and inexpensive alternative to other imaging modalities.

Introduction

Ultrasonography (US) uses nonionizing sound waves to produce two- or three-dimensional (2D or 3D) grayscale images. The first US descriptions of normal and abnormal musculoskeletal tissues were published in 1958 and 1972, respectively.[1,2] The use of color power Doppler for synovitis was first described in 1994.[3] Annual publications on musculoskeletal ultrasound (MSUS) have increased exponentially in the past 3 decades.[4]

As with other specialties, such as Orthopedics, PM&R, Radiology, and Podiatry, the use of US has gained increasing acceptance in the field of rheumatology.[5,6] US in Rheumatology or Rheumatologic Ultrasound (RhUS) has several distinct advantages over other imaging modalities. Properly employed, RhUS is fast, safe (no ionizing radiation or contrast), noninvasive, and relatively inexpensive. Multiple regions and tissue types can be imaged statically or dynamically, with immediate comparison to the contralateral side. US machine technology and image quality have improved rapidly, allowing for improved visualization of structures and detection of Doppler signal. Utilization of RhUS has good acceptability and high satisfaction scores for both patients and referring providers.[7]

RhUS has evolved beyond the musculoskeletal system to include additional organ systems involved in rheumatic disease, including the lungs, blood vessels, skin, and salivary glands. Point-of-care (POC) bedside RhUS allows the rheumatology provider to combine a deep understanding of the pathobiology of rheumatic diseases with real-time dynamic imaging, allowing for immediate diagnostic confirmation, intervention, or follow-up of therapy.[8] RhUS has become a powerful addition to the diagnostic and therapeutic skills of the rheumatology provider. Applications of RhUS include the diagnosis of inflammatory and non-inflammatory rheumatic disease, the assessment of an individual's response to treatment, and guidance for procedures.[9–11]

Despite the known benefits of RhUS, the results are operator dependent, with relatively high upfront costs for equipment and training. Although competency in RhUS is not currently a requirement for rheumatology training in the United States or most European countries,[12,13] there has been a marked increase in educational opportunities with incorporation of RhUS into training programs and clinical practice.[14–19]

Technical Aspects

US is an operator-dependent modality. Picture quality and image interpretation depend significantly on the grade of the equipment, the technical conditions of the examination, and the skills and experience of the sonographer. Three- and four-dimensional (4D) US, elastosonography, and fusion imaging hold promise for further improvement in utility.[20] 3D-US has the potential to improve standardization and reduce the duration of the examination. Longitudinal, transverse, and coronal planes, with 3D reconstruction of the target area, can be acquired in a few seconds.[21] Elastosonography evaluates tissue elasticity, with potential applications in assessment of skin (systemic sclerosis), tendon integrity and stiffness, soft tissue infiltration (salivary glands), and subcutaneous nodules. Fusion imaging simultaneously compares and maps an US image onto other preacquired modalities, such as CT or MRI.

Physics

Sound moves best through solids and liquids, and less effectively through gas (air). Appropriate conduction of sound relies on a continuous liquid medium (gel) from the transducer surface to the skin surface. A sound wave will travel to a point where it encounters an object and is absorbed or reflected away from or back to the source, depending on the depth and tissue type. The US transducer initiates an image by sending a "pulse" of sound, dependent on the chosen frequency. The further the sound wave travels, the less energy it sustains over the distance. This phenomenon is known as the attenuation of sound. Different tissue types have varying abilities to absorb, scatter, and reflect sound. Furthermore, particular tissue structures will create distinct echo signals, or echotextures.[22] The US frequencies used for medical imaging will be completely reflected by bone or other calcium-laden structures, such that no anatomy can be discerned deep to such structures with a resulting artifact.

In reality, an US transducer spends more time "listening" for returning sound echoes than generating the initial sound pulse. The variance in returning echoes differentiates between tissue type, and the software component of the machine "un-codes" this information to generate a 2D or 3D image on the screen. The composite event of sound generation, sound reflection, and detection of returning sound waves allows for the construction of images, mapping to anatomic and histologic changes in the tissue region of interest.[23]

Skin and soft tissues are the standard for echogenicity and are seen as medium gray and described as "isoechoic." An object that strongly reflects a sound wave, such as bone, is referred to as "hyperechoic," and seen in grayscale as bright images that are brighter than soft tissue. Conversely, an object that does not reflect sound at all, or rather allows sound to pass through it essentially without reflection, is referred to as "anechoic" on grayscale, and these images are dark. Fluid-filled structures, such as simple joint effusions, blood vessels, and ganglion cysts do not reflect sound and are seen as anechoic structures. Objects that have a lower capacity to reflect sound, such as fat, are referred to as "hypoechoic" and seen as a darker gray.

Knobology

Understanding the basic setting options on the standard US machine is critical to generate quality diagnostic images. The following summaries are provided as an overview of terms.[24]

Frequency refers to the sound wave cycles per second, or Hertz. The frequency of the transducer can be adjusted and is chosen because of the thickness and location of the tissue of interest, including the needed sound wave depth of penetration. A higher frequency will travel a shorter distance, require less energy, and provide superior resolution. A lower frequency can be used to penetrate further into a structure but sacrifices resolution. Therefore, imaging the superficial structures of the skin is best performed in the higher frequency range (14 to 25 MHz). Low-frequency transducers (2 to 5 MHz) are used to explore deep targets (e.g., the hip and sacroiliac joints), while medium-frequency transducers (6 to 13 MHz) are the best choice to explore large joints (the shoulder, knee, and elbow).

Gain, in grayscale, refers to the brightness or darkness of the image on the computer screen and is only an enhancement of the already acquired image. Gain can also be applied to the use of color or power Doppler to regulate the scope and breadth of tissue movement. Gain is akin to the volume switch on an amplifier. For example, when the gain is increased, it can create sound (and image) distortion, but when the gain is decreased, it can fail to project sound (or create an image) and lose detail. In US, gain is usually best set in a mid-range, around 50%, for optimum image generation.

Time gain compensation is a variant of the gain control and adjusts the brightness at a specific region of the image, while compensating for the attenuation effect in tissue as the sound moves through tissue and returns to the US transducer.

Depth control predicts the distance viewed. Sound may continue to a depth beyond the scope of the chosen field of view. Depth should always be adjusted to locate the deepest hyperechoic structure. In RhUS, the sonographer is usually looking to orient the image by locating the bone. The depth control will create a "shallow" or "deep" field, and display the visualized level on the US screen. Some machines will adjust the frequency based on the chosen depth, while other machines will "detect" sound to the chosen depth.

Focus is the region of maximized resolution to distinguish two objects at the level or region of interest. Each level of interest is commonly referred to as a "focal point." Some US machines allow for the placement of multiple focal points on the same image. Designation of multiple focal points will sacrifice frame rate and can result in lower temporal resolution and thus should be limited to one or two.

Color Doppler and ***power Doppler*** US explore blood perfusion, and may play a key role in the monitoring of inflammatory disease activity and the assessment of response to therapy.[25] Power Doppler (PD) has greater sensitivity than color Doppler to detect blood flow, but only the latter provides information on flow direction and velocity. US contrast agents can enhance the detection of tissue vascularity with Doppler US and may improve detection of subclinical synovitis.[26]

Doppler performance depends on the machine's adjustable pulse repetition frequency (PRF) setting. A medium to high PRF range is typically chosen for standard imaging of vasculature. However, in RhUS, a lower PRF, between 400 and 1000 Hz or 0.4 and 1.0 kHz, is used to detect low blood flow states seen in the microvasculature of inflamed synovium. An individual machine's PD imaging requires standardization of signal and control, which can be accomplished by adjusting the settings to demonstrate digital (finger) pulp blood flow.

Artifacts

US interpretation requires the sonographer to comprehend the physics of sound, recognize patient anatomy, and interpret a screen image based upon the acquisition process. ***Artifact*** refers to nonanatomic variances in the screen image, resulting from the process of image generation. The ability to avoid or utilize artifacts is critical to proper image generation and interpretation. The following terms describe common sonographic artifacts.[27]

Anisotropy (Fig. 44.1) results from the redirection of sound waves that travel to a structure but do not directly reflect back to the transducer, suggesting there is no structure in the region of interest. Tendon imaging is classically affected by this artifact, as the highly ordered structure of the tendon will reflect sound waves back to the transducer only when the sound waves are perpendicular. Tendon orientation at an angle to the transducer surface will direct sound away from the tendon and not back to the "listening" transducer, resulting in an anechoic appearing area where the tendon should be. The tendon will reappear after repositioning the transducer parallel to the tendon, resulting in a perpendicular sound wave.

Shadowing (Fig. 44.2) is a phenomenon where an US wave cannot penetrate through an object, with complete reflection back to the probe. The area deep or posterior to an impenetrable object

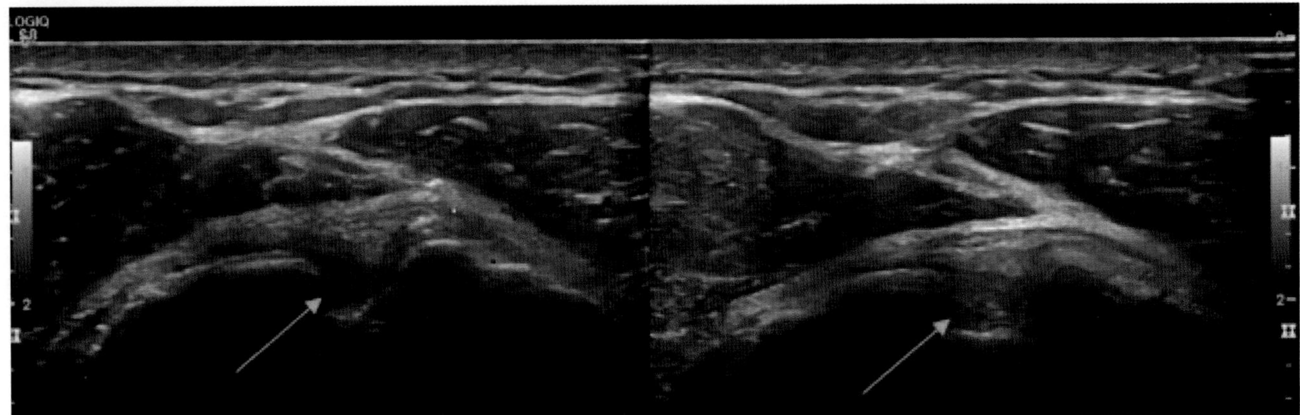

• **Fig. 44.1** Anisotropy of the biceps tendon in the transverse view. These images are taken in the same footprint. The tendon on the left demonstrates anisotropy, appearing anechoic *(arrow)* and can be interpreted incorrectly as absent; the tendon on the right is normal *(arrow)*.

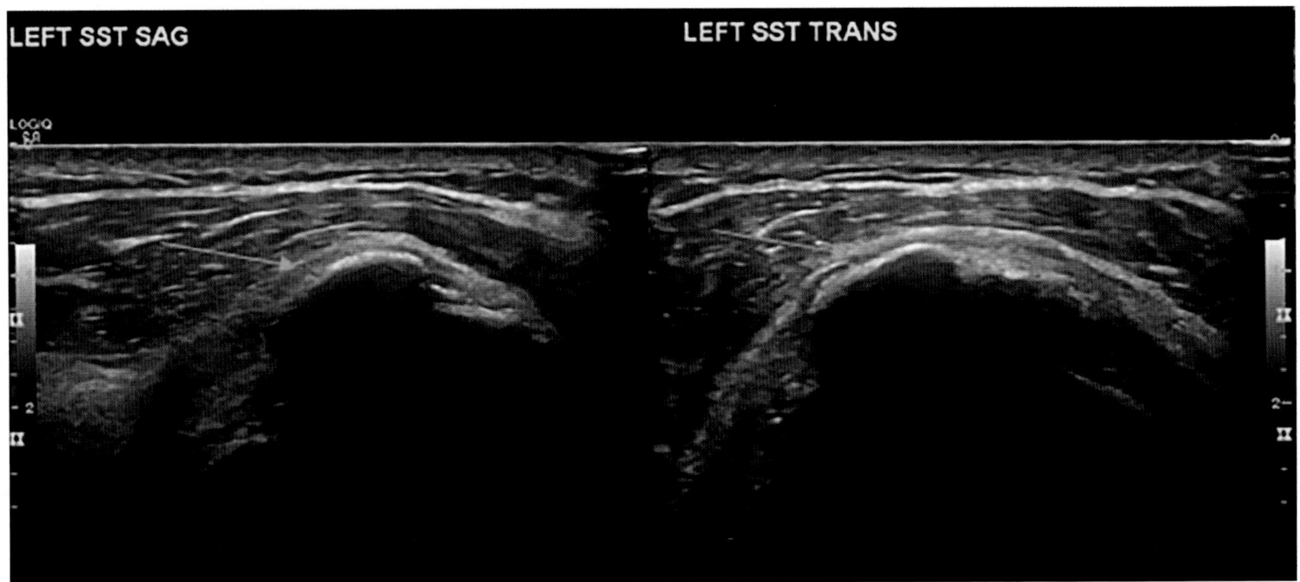

• **Fig. 44.2** Shadowing by a calcium deposit in the supraspinatus tendon *(arrows)*. The tendon is seen on the sides of the calcium deposit. The region posterior or deep to the tendon is anechoic from shadowing. The bone borders on the lower portion of the screen define the humeral head.

is shadowed, appearing anechoic and obscured from view. Bone or calcific tendon deposits classically demonstrate shadowing.

This ***posterior acoustic shadowing*** is also referred to as ***attenuation artifact***. A variation of this effect occurs when imaging a rounded structure, such as a tendon. The edges of the tendon can appear anechoic when followed deep into the area of imaging, which is called ***lateral edge shadowing***.

Increased through-transmission is the opposite of shadowing. This phenomenon occurs when a fluid-filled structure allows an increased transmission of sound and results in the structures deep to the region appearing more intense, hyperechoic, or brighter than the adjacent tissue at the same depth. It is also referred to as ***posterior acoustic enhancement***.

Reverberation artifact (Fig. 44.3) occurs when an object reflects sound so strongly that the sound wave bounces between

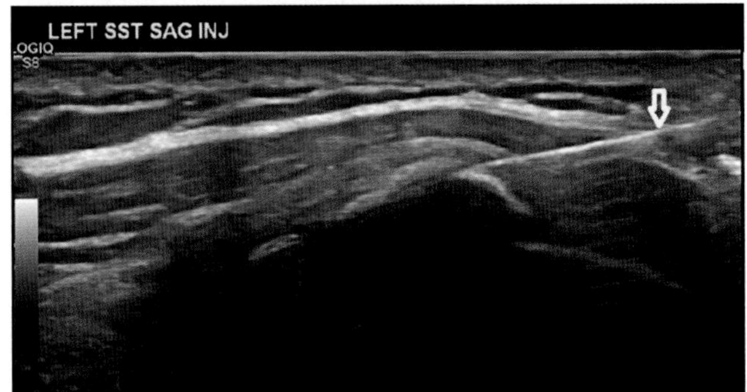

• **Fig. 44.3** This image shows needle *(arrow)* barbatage of a calcium deposit in the supraspinatus tendon. Note the serial linear images appearing below the needle as a manifestation of reverberation artifact.

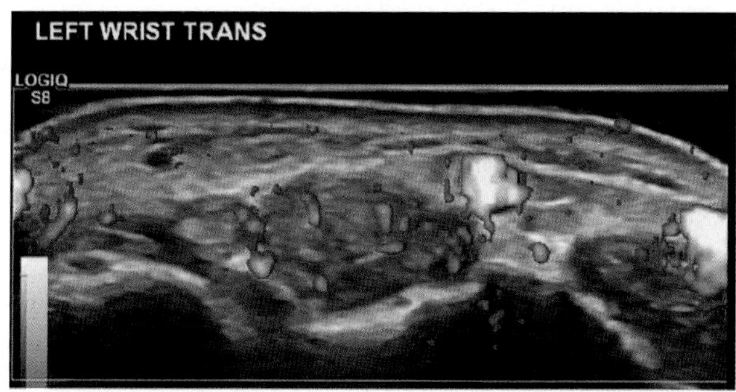

• **Fig. 44.4** In this transverse view of the wrist, there is compartment IV tenosynovitis, and adjacent blood vessels on the radial side of the image show color signal outside of the blood vessels. The vessel furthest to the right shows color flow in the extensor carpi radialis brevis (ECRB) tendon, which is only present due to blooming artifact.

the probe and the object repeatedly. The time differential required for this event results in the US creating an image of the same structure at increasing depths, in parallel to the initial structure. An injection needle, metal joint replacement, or joint hardware can create reverberation artifacts.

Reverberation artifact is similar to a ***mirror image***. The mirror image effect is noted when Doppler reflects sound strongly enough to allow repeated echoes back and forth between the transducer and the object, and the time delay allows the computer to generate the same Doppler image near or below the object. This may be seen when a Doppler image appears below bone.

An ***interface sign*** is a bright slender region at the site where tissue planes with differing impedance meet, such as soft tissue or fluid with cartilage. The resulting normal bright region is referred to as the ***cartilage interface sign***, which is often confused with the "double contour sign" of gout.

The ***blooming artifact*** (Fig. 44.4) results when the gain on a Doppler image is increased to the point that the color or power flow appears outside the region of motion, and makes the area of interest, such as a blood vessel, appear larger. Blooming results when the computer places a color signal directly below (or above) a vessel, obscuring the vessel walls and borders. Blooming artifact is minimized by reducing the Doppler gain, resulting in Doppler interpretation of motion only inside the structure of interest.

Examination Technique

US examination technique relies on proper positioning of the patient, the examiner, and the US transducer. Without attention to all three factors, the resulting images may not optimally demonstrate the tissues being studied.

Transducer Positioning

The transducer should be held at the base, the part of the transducer that touches the patient's skin, in order to keep the sonographer's hand in contact with the patient. Anchoring the scanning hand to the patient allows stabilization and the use of proprioception to minimize unintended movements of the transducer while the examiner is looking at the machine monitor. By simultaneously touching the transducer and the patient's skin, the sonographer can control the amount of applied pressure and avoid accidental compression of structures, such as superficial tendon sheaths and bursa. Sonopalpation, varying transducer pressure over a structure, can allow most fluid collections to be distinguished from surrounding hypoechoic tissue.

Certain US probe manipulations such as "fish-tailing," "rocking," and "heel-toeing" help overcome imaging difficulties. "Fish-tailing" keeps one edge of the transducer fixed in place, while sweeping the other edge from side to side to align the transducer with a structure. "Rocking" tilts the transducer along its short axis, while "heel-toeing" tilts the transducer along its long axis. Both maneuvers are used to direct the US waves at 90 degrees relative to smooth surfaces such as bone and tendons to maximize sound reflection back to the transducer, thereby avoiding anisotropic artifact.

Conventions for Imaging Orientation

Conventions exist for image orientation that can vary by specialty. Most rheumatology sonographers position the transducer so that the left side of the image corresponds to either the proximal or the medial portion of the body in anatomic position. For example, the ulna is medial and the radius is lateral. Conventions for scanning orientation reduce the time required for image labeling, confusion in image review, and image interpretation at a later time. If scanning conventions are not utilized, the image orientation should be labeled.

Examiner Positioning

Subtle transducer movements can lead to significant changes in the image. The sonographer should position the structure to be scanned between themselves and the US monitor, in order to reduce any head or body motion required to look from the patient to the monitor. This position also leads to sound ergonomic positioning for the sonographer, reducing neck, arm, and back discomfort. In order to reduce transducer cord pull, it can be wrapped around the scanning hand, while keeping the other hand free for equipment or patient manipulation. Alternatively, the transducer cord can be hung around the examiner's neck, but this practice is considered less hygienic. The scanning hand should be properly supported by a solid surface at the wrist and elbow whenever possible to minimize unintended fine motions, thus reducing Doppler artifact and allowing for more sensitive Doppler settings.

Patient Positioning

Patient positioning depends on the goal of the scan. For example, a tendon should be scanned at maximal length to identify a tear but should be relaxed to detect hyperemia through Doppler.

There are specific positioning techniques for each body region and target structure. For example, dynamic imaging, with flexion and extension, can localize flexor tendon sheath abnormalities and pulley constriction in the hands. External rotation of the shoulder can help visualize both glenohumeral joint effusions and subluxation of the biceps tendon.

There are also some specialized positions for US scanning to improve the acoustic window onto a structure of interest. For example, the "Crass" position (arm internally rotated with the patient's hand against the lower back) allows imaging of the longest region of the supraspinatus tendon in longitudinal view but can be uncomfortable and might hide the most medial fibers of the tendon from view. The "modified Crass" position (arm adducted and shoulder flexed with the elbow straight back) is usually better tolerated, and allows visualization of the rotator cuff interval and medial fibers of the supraspinatus tendon in transverse view.

Limited Versus Comprehensive Studies

Performance of the US examination can be subdivided into limited and comprehensive exams. Limited scans are performed to identify abnormalities of a single structure, such as nerve compression or a tendon tear. Comprehensive scans attempt to answer questions about a region, such as identification of the cause of wrist pain. A comprehensive study may include assessment of multiple tissues types, including synovium, tendon, bone, ligament, muscle, nerve, and blood vessels, with multiple views in orthogonal planes. A limited study may only assess one tissue type and contain fewer views. Pathology should always be shown in orthogonal views.

Ultrasound in Rheumatology Definitions

In 2005, the Outcome Measures in Rheumatology (OMERACT) ultrasound (US) working group (WG) set forth six provisional definitions for US lesions considered to represent a core set of pathophysiologic manifestations of rheumatic disease.[28] These definitions have become fundamental to OMERACT methodology for developing and validating US as a disease outcome measurement instrument across the domains of inflammatory and structural damage. US has become increasingly utilized in many rheumatic disease states, and in 2019 the OMERACT US WG sought to refine the original US definitions and scoring systems for synovitis, enthesitis, tenosynovitis, and tendon damage[29] (Table 44.1).

The 2005 definition of synovitis included both synovial effusion and synovial hypertrophy, and presence of either one or both could indicate synovitis.[28] The revised definition of US-detected synovitis delineates synovial hypertrophy in a semiquantitative graded B-mode feature and a graded Doppler mode feature. Hypoechoic synovial hypertrophy must be present for defining US-detected synovitis and grading Doppler activity. The new definition eliminates synovial effusion, as it was not reliable and frequently detected in healthy subjects. However, the definition of synovitis in children includes hypoechoic synovial hypertrophy or the presence of synovial effusion.

The term enthesopathy was utilized in the 2005 definitions, but is now exclusively reserved for mechanically related tendinopathy. The current definition of enthesitis is a hypoechoic and/or thickened insertion of the tendon close to the bone that exhibits Doppler signal if active and that may show erosions, enthesophytes, and calcifications as a sign of structural damage.

Tenosynovitis is defined as abnormal anechoic or hypoechoic (relative to tendon fibers) tendon sheath widening, which can be related to abnormal tenosynovial fluid and/or hypertrophy. If sheath widening is seen on B-mode imaging, Doppler should be employed and, when present, visible in two perpendicular planes within the peri-tendinous synovial sheaths and exclude normal feeding vessels. Tendon damage is a structural lesion of tendon morphology and only defined in B-mode.

There was not an update to the original definition of a bone erosion, which remains an intra- and/or extra-articular discontinuity of the bone surface and must be seen in perpendicular planes. Further work will focus on refinement of the etiology of the lesion.

As part of this work, scoring systems were also developed for synovitis, enthesitis, tenosynovitis, and tendon damage. In addition to validation of the original US-detected pathology definitions, the 2019 OMERACT update defined the most common inflammatory and structural elementary lesions, and they are summarized in Table 44.1.

Rheumatoid Arthritis

Rheumatoid arthritis (RA) can result in synovial and tenosynovial inflammation, as well as damage to bone and tendons. As most of the pathology lies in peripheral joints and structures, US is particularly well suited to help with the diagnosis and evaluation of this condition. The submillimeter tissue resolution that can be obtained with US imaging in the superficial joints of the hands and feet allow the sonographer to identify synovial cavity abnormalities and distinguish synovial hypertrophy from effusion. US imaging is more sensitive and specific for synovial abnormalities than clinical examination and can, via Doppler, detect subclinical hyperemia, a marker for disease activity. This increased sensitivity can lead to an earlier diagnosis of RA.[30] Furthermore, sonography can identify signs of bone and tissue damage from the inflammatory process earlier than can be appreciated on plain film radiographs.[31,32] However, the high sensitivity should be treated with consideration to avoid over-attribution of nutrient vessels as bone erosions.[33] In addition, US evaluation has been employed to evaluate RA disease activity, especially when there is a discrepancy between patient-reported symptoms and physical exam findings. Finally, US may help establish disease remission, or lack thereof, in patients who are clinically quiescent.

Diagnosis

US identification of subclinical synovial or tenosynovial hypertrophy and hyperemia in an asymptomatic seropositive patient predicts the development of clinical synovitis within the next 2 years (odds ratio of 13) (Fig. 44.5).[34] In seronegative patients, hand and wrist US Doppler signal increases the chances of a clinical diagnosis of RA within a year. Baseline US Doppler assessment of wrist synovitis is a better predictor for RA than the 2010 American College of Rheumatology/European League Against Rheumatism (ACR/EULAR) criteria[35] and can increase the accuracy of these criteria compared to clinical joint exam.[36] Alternatively, one-third of patients with a clinical diagnosis of inflammatory arthritis are not found to have sonographic evidence for synovitis.[37]

US can detect tenosynovitis in RA. Extensor carpi ulnaris grayscale and Doppler abnormality by US are found in over 50% of early RA patients prior to diagnosis, compared with less than 20% in those who had an alternate diagnosis or whose arthritis resolved.[38] However, Doppler signal in the tendon sheaths or joints of the fingers predicts development of RA less strongly than anti-citrullinated peptide antibody (ACPA) positivity.

The size and location of erosions can help in the diagnosis of RA. Erosions of >2.5 mm are 68% specific for RA in comparison with PsA, gout, osteoarthritis (OA), and healthy controls. If the erosions occur in the ulnar styloid, second metacarpophalangeal (MCP), or fifth metatarsal phalangeal (MTP) joint, the specificity increases to 87%.[39] Erosions lose specificity when the size is ≤2 mm.[40]

US can aid in the diagnosis of subcutaneous nodules. By US, finger tendon nodules have been found to occur in as many as 16% of patients with RA.[41] RA nodules tend to be homogeneous,

TABLE 44.1 2019 OMERACT Definitions of US-Detected Pathologies with Inflammatory and Structural Elementary Lesions (IEL and SEL)

Pathology	Definition
Synovitis	Definition: Presence of a hypoechoic synovial hypertrophy regardless of the presence of effusion or any grade of Doppler signal **IEL:** SH is presence of abnormal hypoechoic synovial tissue within the capsule that is not displaceable and poorly compressible and may exhibit Doppler signal
Enthesitis	Definition: Hypoechoic and/or thickened insertion of the tendon close to the bone which exhibits Doppler signal if active and that may show erosions, enthesophytes/calcifications as sign of structural damage **IEL:** Increased thickness of tendon at enthesis; hypoechoic tendon at enthesis; Doppler signal <2 mm from bony surface **SEL:** Calcifications/enthesophytes at enthesis; erosions at enthesis
Tenosynovitis	Definition: Abnormal anechoic and/or hypoechoic (relative to tendon fibers) tendon sheath widening which can be related to abnormal tenosynovial fluid and/or hypertrophy; Doppler signal can be considered if seen in two perpendicular planes, within the peri-tendinous synovial sheath, excluding normal feeding vessels; Doppler mode should be used only if the tendon shows peritendinous synovial sheath widening on B-mode **IEL:** Tenosynovial hypertrophy is the presence of abnormal hypoechoic (relative to tendon fibers) tissue within the synovial sheath that is not displaceable and poorly compressible, and seen in two perpendicular planes; it may exhibit Doppler
Tendon damage	Definition: Internal and/or peripheral focal tendon defect (i.e., absence of fibers) in the region enclosed by tendon sheath, seen in two perpendicular planes; the grade of tendon damage should be assessed in both planes
Erosion	Definition: Intra- and/or extra-articular discontinuity of bone surface (visible in two perpendicular planes)
Pediatric synovitis	Definition: Presence of hypoechoic synovial hypertrophy or the presence of synovial effusions
Osteoarthritis osteophytes	**SEL:** Step-up bony prominence at the bony margin that is visible in two perpendicular planes
Osteoarthritis hyaline cartilage damage	**SEL:** Loss of anechoic structure and/or thinning of cartilage layer, and irregularities and/or sharpness of at least one cartilage margin
Gout double contour sign	**SEL:** Abnormal hyperechoic band over the superficial margin of the articular hyaline cartilage, independent of the angle of insonation; may be either irregular or regular, continuous or intermittent, and can be distinguished from the cartilage interface sign
Gout tophus	**SEL:** Circumscribed, inhomogeneous, hyperechoic and/or hypoechoic aggregation (with or without posterior acoustic shadow), which may be surrounded by a small anechoic rim
Gout aggregates	**SEL:** Heterogenous hyperechoic foci that maintain their high degree of reflectivity with minimization of gain or change of insonation angle; occasionally may generate posterior acoustic shadow
CPPD fibrocartilage	**SEL:** Hyperechoic deposits of variable shape, localized within fibrocartilage, that remain fixed or move with fibrocartilage during dynamic assessment
CPPD hyaline cartilage	**SEL:** Hyperechoic deposits of variable size and shape, without posterior shadowing, located within hyaline cartilage, that remain fixed and move with the hyaline cartilage during dynamic assessment
CPPD tendon	**SEL:** Hyperechoic linear structure(s) generally without posterior shadow, localized within the tendon and remain fixed and move with the tendon during dynamic assessment
CPPD synovial fluid	**SEL:** Hyperechoic deposits of variable size, localized within the synovial fluid, without posterior shadowing, and mobile along with joint movement and probe pressure
Halo sign	**IEL:** Homogeneous, hypoechoic wall thickening, well delineated towards the luminal side, visible in two perpendicular planes, most commonly concentric in transverse scan
Compression sign	**IEL:** Thickened arterial wall remains visible under compression, i.e., the echogenicity contrasts hypoechogenic due to vasculitic vessel wall thickening in comparison to mid/hyperechoic surrounding tissue

CPPD, Calcium pyrophosphate deposit; *IEL,* inflammatory elementary lesion; *SEL,* structural elementary lesion; *SH,* synovial hypertrophy.
Adapted from OMERACT definitions for ultrasonographic pathology and elementary lesions of rheumatic diseases.[29]

with a central well-defined hypoechoic area representing necrosis. This is in contrast to tophi, which can be multilobular with a heterogenous echotexture and a hypoechoic or anechoic rim. Tophi may also have adjacent bone erosions.[42]

US assists in the diagnosis of shoulder pain. In contrast to degenerative shoulder conditions, PD signal is frequently detected inside the biceps tendon sheath in patients with RA.[43] Bilateral synovial, tenosynovial, or bursal effusions occur in 76% of patients with polymyalgia rheumatic (PMR) in comparison to 12% of patients with RA, while effusion in one shoulder and at least one hip occurs in 48% of patients with PMR but only 4% of patients with RA.[44]

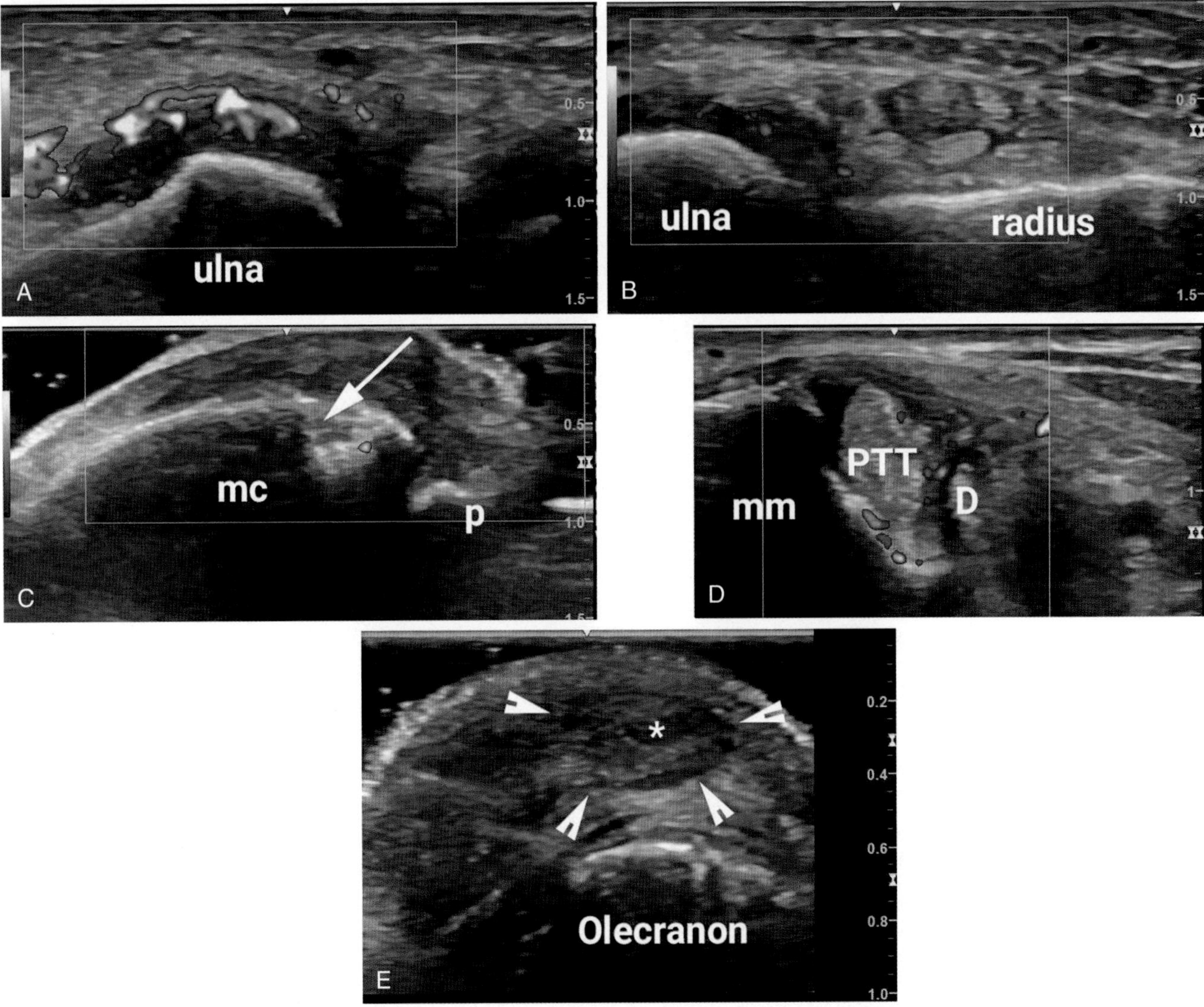

• **Fig. 44.5** Ultrasound findings in rheumatoid arthritis (RA). (A) Dorsal longitudinal and transverse (B) view of a distal ulna with hypoechoic synovial tissue and prominent Doppler signal indicating severe hyperemia. (C) Longitudinal view of the MCP joint demonstrates an erosion *(arrow)* of the dorsal aspect of the distal metacarpal (mc), just proximal to the phalanx (p), positive Doppler signal suggests that the erosive process remains active. (D) Transverse view of the posterior tibial tendon (PTT), and flexor digitorum (D) over the medial malleolus (mm) of the tibia shows hyperemia of inflamed tissue. (E) Rheumatoid nodule *(arrowheads)* over the olecranon with hypoechoic, necrotic center (*), a distinguishing feature of a rheumatoid nodule on US.

Monitoring

US has been validated as a measure of RA disease activity.[45] A 12-joint assessment for effusion, synovitis, and PD signal is the smallest number of joints, which will maximize correlation with clinical measures of disease activity.[46]

However, a seven-joint US assessment can reliably reflect a therapeutic effect of disease-modifying anti-rheumatic drug (DMARD) or biologic therapy for RA.[47] The 22-joint, 12-joint, and 7-joint US assessments all have similar sensitivity to change.[48] US shows reduction in RA pannus in response to treatment.[49] Finally, US can detect continued disease activity as measured by increased Doppler signal within synovium in patients in clinical remission.[50] Thus the more sensitive simplified disease activity index (SDAI) definition of remission correlates better with a lack of Doppler signal by US than the less sensitive disease activity index 28 (DAS-28).[50]

US may assist in monitoring RA disease activity when standard measures are less useful. For example, IL-6 inhibition therapy reduces C-reactive protein (CRP) and can artificially lower DAS-28 CRP. PD US can measure the changes in joint inflammation after treatment of both IL-6 and TNF inhibition, allowing valid comparison between agents.[51]

In patients treated with anti-IL-6 combination therapy, persistent power Doppler signal is associated with the development of erosions, even if clinical features of synovitis as measured by DAS-28 improve.[52,53]

Concomitant fibromyalgia (FMS) can skew measures of RA disease activity, but a seven-joint Doppler US assessment correlates with clinical disease activity scores in patients with RA, but not in patients with both RA and FMS.[54,55] In patients with similar objective evidence of RA activity, DAS-28, SDAI, and Crohn's Disease Activity Index were all higher in the RA plus FMS group, but the two groups had no significant differences in either gray-scale US7 or power Doppler US7 scores.

Using US assessment of RA activity to help determine escalation of therapy doubled the percentage of patients receiving either combination DMARD therapy or treatment with a TNF inhibitor.[56] Similarly, more patients randomized to US-driven tight disease control strategies received biologic therapy compared with placebo (29% vs. 17%), but disease activity, remission, and erosion outcomes were similar in the two groups.[57] Therefore, the routine use of US assessment to inform treatment decisions in RA has not been established.

Predicting Outcome

US findings in the synovium may help predict future disease activity and resulting tissue damage. In symptomatic patients with RA on methotrexate, both synovial hypertrophy and Doppler signal in the synovium predicts progression in total sharp scores.[58] Correlation between joint Doppler score and DAS at 1 year is greater than erythrocyte sedimentation rate, CRP, or tender or swollen joint counts. PD signal also predicts radiographic progression[59] and may be superior to MRI bone marrow edema.[60] However, in patients on treatment with anti-TNF inhibitors, baseline Doppler activity does not predict future erosion.[59]

In patients in clinical remission, persistent Doppler signal has been found to be associated with continued structural deterioration.[61] In fact, US Doppler is a better predictor of radiographic progression than low-field MRI. However, the degree of structural progression in patients in clinical remission, but with persistent Doppler signal, is mild, and less than 2% of joints in patients in clinical remission developed erosions overall.[62]

US of patients in clinical remission may also help predict the loss of disease control. A number of studies have shown that Doppler signal in RA remission indicates more than a two-fold increased risk of loss of disease control compared to patients who do not have Doppler signal.[63,64] A meta-analysis of five studies using positive Doppler signal to predict an RA flare found an OR of 3.2.[65] Others have found that while US can help predict flare of disease at a group level, it did little to help predict flare at an individual level. US did not increase the clinician's ability to predict which individual would flare after stopping a TNF inhibitor.[66]

Osteoarthritis

OA has multiple definitions based on site of involvement and etiology of the damage. Based on clinical and conventional radiographic findings, the ACR classification criteria for OA of the knee and hip have not been revised since 1986 and 1991, respectively.[67,68] In a 2008 review of 25 different classification criteria studies for knee OA, it was found that most utilize clinical signs and symptoms with laboratory and conventional radiographs (CR), while no studies use MRI or US.[69] US abnormalities that can be observed in OA include cartilage changes, osteophytes, synovial effusion, and synovial proliferation.[70] The ability of US to identify characteristic joint abnormalities in OA that cannot be seen by CR makes it particularly suited for use in the diagnosis of pain and mechanical symptoms in multiple joint regions.[10]

Diagnosis

US can provide reliable information about structural changes of the articular cartilage.[70] Normal hyaline cartilage is a homogeneous hypo- to anechoic layer delineated by two thin, sharp, and hyperechoic margins, and are similar across anatomic sites. Cartilage thickness, which can be reproducibly measured by US, is variable depending on the joint region. The earliest US features of OA include loss of the thin and sharp contour of the outer border of the cartilage and increased cartilage echogenicity with patchy or diffuse loss of clarity.[71] Variable changes in cartilage thickness are detectable in patients at different stages of disease, and quantification of cartilage thickness may have diagnostic and prognostic value.

Joint effusions are commonly found in patients with OA, and can easily be detected as an anechoic fluid collection. Non-homogeneous echogenicity of the fluid may give clues to the duration and etiology. For example, echoic spots with or without acoustic shadowing may suggest proteinaceous material, cartilage fragments, aggregates of crystals, or calcified loose bodies. Fine particulate debris can be seen after long-standing or repeated joint effusions or after intra-articular corticosteroid injections.[70] Popliteal cysts can be seen in knee OA, and US provides structural details about the content of the cyst, its communication with the joint space, its architecture, and the possible compression of adjacent vascular structures.[70] US is particularly useful in aspiration of the cyst to assure distance from the popliteal artery and navigation through possible multiloculated anatomy.

Alteration of the subchondral bone, ranging from a tiny irregularity of the bone profile to multiple erosions, can be detected in areas that appear normal on CR in both erosive and nonerosive OA. Osteophytes are the most frequent and characteristic abnormalities of the bone profile in patients with OA, and are easily detected as irregularities of the bone contour with posterior acoustic shadow.[70]

In 2018, EULAR published recommendations for the use of imaging in the clinical management of peripheral joint OA.[74] They recommended that imaging, including US, is not required to make a diagnosis in patients with a typical clinical presentation of OA. In an atypical presentation, imaging is recommended to confirm the diagnosis of OA and/or to make an alternative or additional diagnosis. US may play a significant role in this latter recommendation, as it can delineate inflammatory from non-inflammatory conditions.

Monitoring

It is widely accepted that US can demonstrate changes in synovial thickness, effusion size, and popliteal cyst size.[75] However, reproducibility data are scarce and no consensus on scoring systems exist. Quantitative assessment of cartilage is restricted to thickness, as total volumes cannot be measured. More work is required to develop standardized definitions of pathology and to demonstrate the validity of US in OA.[76]

EULAR recommends that routine imaging for follow-up of OA is not warranted unless there is rapid progression of symptoms or a change in clinical characteristics to denote an additional diagnosis.[74] Very few studies including US have examined the correlation between the change in imaging features with symptoms or relevant clinical or therapeutic outcomes. EULAR further recommended that if imaging is needed, CR should be used before other modalities. US can be used if additional soft tissue imaging is required.

Predicting Outcome

The role of US in the prediction of the natural history of OA progression and treatment response to therapy, excluding intra-articular injection, is unknown. In patients with OA of the hand, the presence of inflammatory features such as power Doppler signal, synovial thickening, and effusions are strongly associated with radiologic progression in the subsequent 2 years.[73] However, due to insufficient and inconsistent data across multiple trials, EULAR recommends against using imaging features to predict noninterventional treatment response.[74]

In OA, US-guided procedures improve injection accuracy when compared with blind procedures but do not improve outcomes. Therefore, EULAR recommends image guidance, particularly US, to improve accuracy of intra-articular therapies in joints that are difficult to assess due to location, degree of deformity, or obesity.[74] Although US can be an effective tool in the diagnosis of OA when other diagnostic possibilities exist, its added value for the monitoring and prognosis of OA is yet to be defined.

Crystalline Arthropathy

US is increasingly used to identify disorders associated with crystalline deposition affecting cartilage, synovium, and tendons. Due to its high resolution and sonic reflectivity, even small deposits of monosodium urate (MSU) and calcium pyrophosphate (CPPD) crystals can be detected by US, with an otherwise normal CR.[77,78] The potential of US in crystalline arthropathy is related to operator experience and quality of the equipment, and proper machine settings are critical.[79]

Gout

Diagnosis

The US appearance of urate crystal aggregates can vary from homogeneously punctate to sharply defined hyperechoic densities of variable size, eventually appearing as dense tophaceous material with posterior acoustic shadows.[77,80] MSU crystals deposit on the surface of articular cartilage and result in hyperechoic enhancement of the superficial margin. This homogeneous thickening or areas of focal deposition is referred to as the double contour sign.[77] Differing from the normal cartilage interface, the echogenicity of MSU crystal layering is not dependent on the angle of insonation, and the full chondrosynovial interface can be seen. When MSU aggregates occur, sonopalpation can cause them to move and give rise to a "snowstorm" appearance.[77] Bone erosions are common in gout and differ from RA by their location, shape (oval), well-defined borders, and adjacent tophaceous materials.[81]

When tophi are present they can be soft or hard based on sonopalpation. Soft tophi vary in echogenicity, while hard tophi generate a hyperechoic band and acoustic shadow. MSU may also deposit in tendons as micro-deposits, which are ovoid-shaped hyperechoic densities, or tophus, which are hypoechoic aggregates with occasional hyperechoic spots and can evolve to hyperechoic bands with acoustic shadowing[77] (Fig. 44.6).

Despite general consensus regarding definitions of gout lesions, MSU deposition has a predilection for certain tissue types and structures. The assessment of the radiocarpal joint, patellar and triceps tendons for hyperechoic aggregates, and the first metatarsal, talar, second metacarpal, and femoral cartilage for a double contour sign yields a sensitivity of 84.6% and a specificity of 83.3% for the diagnosis of gout.[82] However, a universally adopted standardized scanning technique for a core set of joints is still needed.[83]

Because MSU aggregates are radiolucent, US is superior to detecting MSU compared with CR. Dual energy CT (DECT) has comparable sensitivity for the detection of gouty arthritis.[84] In 2015, the ACR/EULAR Gout Classification Criteria were published.[85] Imaging features of this criteria included urate deposition identified by US as a double contour sign or by DECT or by CR identified erosions. All were given an equal weight of 4, with a total score of ≥8 to needed classify an individual as having gout.

Although US is a valuable tool in the diagnosis of gout, questions remain regarding validation of US as an OMERACT outcome measure.[83] In 2016, a systematic literature search was performed to define imaging modalities as potential OMERACT outcome measures in gout based on the detection of three domains: urate deposition, joint damage, and inflammation. Seventy-eight articles were identified that included CR, US, conventional CT, DECT, and MRI.[86] Twenty-nine articles assessed US for urate deposition (double contour sign and tophus), damage (erosion), and inflammation (synovial hypertrophy and Doppler signal). US was the only imaging modality to clearly and reliably identify the double contour sign, and was comparable to DECT and MRI for the identification of tophus. US identified more erosions than CR, but MRI identified more erosions than US when CR was normal. No data were found to assess inflammation and Doppler signal in gout; however, MRI did identify more synovial pannus compared to US. The authors concluded that no single imaging modality was superior to fulfill all aspects of the OMERACT filter for any domain; however, US was found to be very promising for the detection of urate deposition and joint damage.

Monitoring

Tophus size can be reported by longest diameter and total volume, and US measurement is comparable to MRI.[80] Unlike physical measurement techniques, US can assess subcutaneous and intra-articular tophi.[80,87] Tophi measurement by US is sensitive to change, with reduction in tophi size seen in patients who normalize serum urate levels.[80] Disappearance of the double contour sign has also been described with normalization of serum urate levels.[88,89]

Predicting Outcome

The prognostic value of US findings in gout is not known.

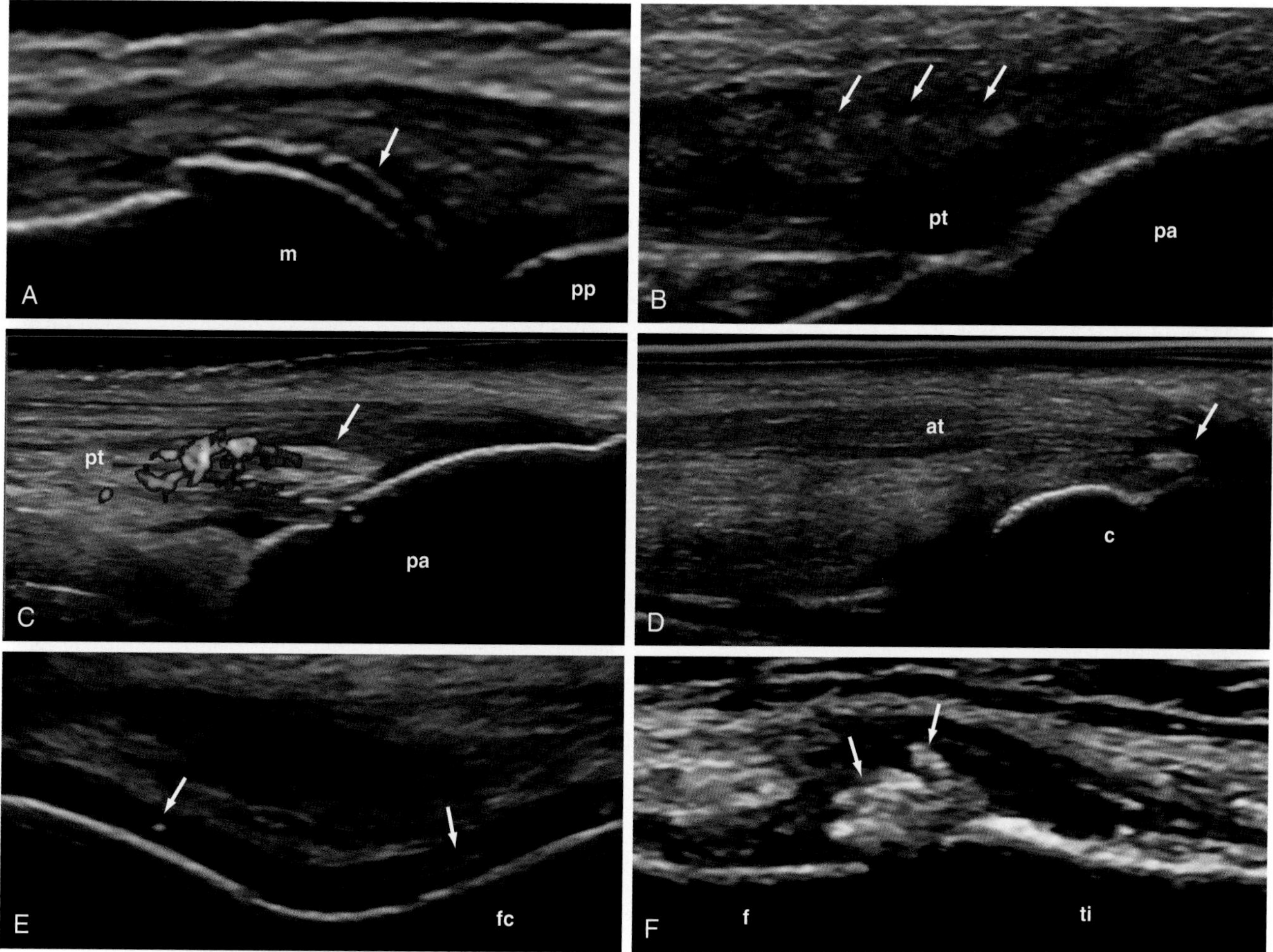

• **Fig. 44.6** Gout and calcium pyrophosphate dihydrate (CPPD) crystal deposition disease (ultrasonography). (A-C) Gout. (A) Chronic gout. Metacarpophalangeal joint (longitudinal scan with fingers in full flexion): hyperechoic enhancement of the chondrosynovial interface *(arrow)* caused by monosodium urate crystal deposition. (B) Distal patellar enthesis (longitudinal anterior scan): intratendinous monosodium urate deposits *(arrows).* (C) Distal patellar enthesis (longitudinal anterior scan): tophaceous deposits *(arrow)* surrounded by power Doppler signal. (D-F) CPPD crystal deposition disease. (D) Achilles tendon *(at)* (longitudinal scan): intratendinous linear hyperechoic deposits without acoustic shadow *(arrow).* (E) Femoral hyaline cartilage (transverse scan): calcium pyrophosphate deposits within the hyaline cartilage *(arrows).* (F) Knee (longitudinal lateral scan): diffuse meniscal calcification *(arrows). c,* Calcaneus; *f,* femur; *fc,* femoral condyle; *m,* metacarpal head; *pa,* patella; *pp,* proximal phalanx; *pt,* patellar tendon; *ti,* tibia. (From Østergaard M, et al. Imaging in rheumatic diseases. In Firestein GF, et al. (eds): *Kelley & Firestein's Textbook of Rheumatology, Tenth Edition*. Elsevier, Philadelphia, 2017.)

Calcium Pyrophosphate Dihydrate Crystal Deposition

Diagnosis

The US appearance of Calcium Pyrophosphate Dihydrate Crystal Deposition (CPPD) crystal aggregates range from tiny circumscribed hyperechoic spots to extended deposits with or without acoustic shadow.[77,78,90] CPPD aggregates differ from MSU as they lie primarily within the geometric middle of the hyaline cartilage and can reach large dimensions. They are described by sparkling reflectivity, allowing visualization of even minimal aggregates within cartilage. Within fibrocartilage, they appear as hyperechoic rounded or amorphous-shaped aggregates that correlate with their radiographic appearance. Hyperechoic aggregates can also be seen in synovial fluid that are typically rounded in shape with a sharply defined border (see Fig. 44.6). CPPD deposits linearly within the fibrillary echotexture of tendons, but can be punctate and can give rise to posterior acoustic shadowing.

In 2011, EULAR appointed a task force to produce evidence-based recommendations for the terminology and diagnosis of CPPD.[91] One of the final 11 recommendations was that US can demonstrate CPPD in peripheral joints with excellent sensitivity and specificity, possibly better than those of CR. US of the knee had a sensitivity and specificity of 87% and 96%, respectively, for CPPD crystals in the synovial fluid.[92] Though no standardized systematic assessment for CPPD exists, some authors advocate including the knee as it has the highest probability to be positive for CPPD aggregates.[79] Using synovial fluid crystal identification as a gold standard, US has a sensitivity of 100% compared with 82% with CR.[78] US was not found to be as useful for imaging CPPD in deep structures, such as the spine.

More recently, a meta-analysis reviewed published studies seeking to validate US definitions of elementary findings and evaluate US diagnostic accuracy in CPPD.[90] Thirty-one articles were chosen to define elementary lesions and the definitions are included in the previous paragraphs. Thirteen studies were chosen for diagnostic accuracy. For studies looking at the entire patient, US had a pooled sensitivity of 89% (95% CI 72% to 97%) and pooled specificity of 94% (95% CI 87% to 98%). These values changed when looking at individual joints, tissue types, and reference standards.

The reliability of OMERACT US definitions for CPPD has also been evaluated.[93] Using a web-based exercise grading static images yielded high kappa values for intra- and interobserver values for all sites examined. However, with a patient-based exercise, inter-reader agreement was only acceptable for the acromioclavicular joint and triangular fibrocartilage. These results suggest the US definitions are reliable, but the scanning method must be further refined.

Monitoring

Data are not available to assess the role of US in monitoring CPPD arthropathy.

Predicting Outcome

The prognostic value of US findings is not known.

Spondyloarthropathy

US evaluation may be even more helpful in patients with seronegative spondyloarthropathies (SpA) than in patients with RA, as the technique offers additional objective evidence of disease where serologic confirmation is lacking.[94] While the role of US in assessment of axial disease is minimal, other features, such as peripheral enthesitis, extensor tendon inflammation, and distal interphalangeal (DIP) abnormalities can be reliably detected (Fig. 44.7). Enthesitis is seen as hypoechoic and/or thickened tendon at its insertion on bone that exhibits Doppler signal if active, and which may show erosions and enthesophytes/calcifications as signs of structural damage.[95] Tendon thickness, hyperemia, bursitis, erosion, and enthesophytes are determinants of most enthesitis scoring systems, with assessments done at the quadriceps tendon, inferior pole of patella, tibial tuberosity, superior (Achilles) calcaneus, and plantar aponeurosis. Some include the lateral and medial epicondyles and triceps insertion.[96]

Doppler signal at the enthesis can be graded on a semiquantitative scale, and numerous Doppler grading scales exist.[97,98]

Diagnosis

Among patients with ankylosing spondylitis (AS), almost all (97%) will have at least one entheseal abnormality by US, compared with 64% by clinical exam.[99] Erosions are seen in 10% of entheseal sites in patients with AS. Importantly, enthesitis is not specific for SpA, also seen in degenerative/metabolic causes,[100] but it can be diagnostically helpful if seen in a young patient with back pain.

Isolated enthesitis and extensor hand tendon MCP paratenon Doppler signal may help distinguish patients with psoriatic arthritis (PsA) from those with RA.[101–103] Central slip enthesitis, soft tissue edema around the flexor tendon, and paratenon hyperemia are four times more common in PsA patients compared to RA. Conversely, erosions of the MCP or PIP joints are three times more common in early seropositive RA than in early PsA.[103]

While both PsA and RA affect synovial and tenosynovial structures in the digits, PsA is more likely to affect the extrasynovial structures such as the extensor tendon, capsule, and periosteum.[104] The Belgrade Ultrasound Enthesis Score (BUSES), a cumulative score of enthesis thickness, fibrillar echogenicity and pattern, enthesophytes, Doppler, and erosion at six sites, was able to differentiate enthesitis from SpA versus RA and/or mechanical disease.[105]

While US evaluation may help differentiate PsA from RA, it has not been found to distinguish DIP changes of PsA from nodal OA.[106]

Monitoring

There is a lack of consensus on which composite score is most useful for assessing PsA, but the PsASon22 has been found to be sensitive to change over time.[107] US enthesitis as measured by the Madrid Sonography Index (MASEI) correlates with both peripheral and axial CR damage, and can help differentiate PsA from healthy controls.[108] TNF inhibition reduces both grayscale and Doppler semiquantitative synovitis scores.[109] More research is needed before standardized, reliable, and responsive US outcome measures in PsA are available.

Predicting Outcome

In comparison to healthy controls, a subclinical enthesitis composite score is greater in patients with psoriasis, but this has not been found to predict the development of PsA over 3.5 years.[110] However, US may be useful in predicting maintenance of disease remission in patients with PsA. Flare within 6 months occurred in almost a quarter of PsA patients in clinical remission but with subclinical Doppler signal in at least one joint, compared with less than 10% of patients without subclinical Doppler.[111] Although US does not reliably predict the development of PsA in patients with psoriasis, it may have a role in prediction of flare for those whose PsA is in remission.

Polymyalgia Rheumatica

Polymyalgia rheumatica (PMR) is characterized by pain and morning stiffness of the shoulder and hip girdles, representing bursitis and synovitis. PMR is associated with giant-cell arteritis (GCA), with 40% to 60% of GCA patients having PMR and 16% to 21% of PMR patients having GCA.[112] Therefore, a comprehensive assessment of inflammatory status in PMR patients is crucial.[113] US evaluation in PMR should include the shoulder and hip regions. The shoulder structures that should be examined include the glenohumeral (GH) joint, subacromial/subdeltoid (SAD) bursa, and long head of the biceps tendon (LBT). Evaluation of the hip should include the hip joint and peri-articular bursal structures.

Diagnosis

Multiple inflammatory findings around the shoulder and hip girdle have been reported in PMR.[114] A recent review of 12 published studies identified GH synovitis, SAD bursitis, LBT tenosynovitis, hip synovitis, and trochanteric bursitis as the main

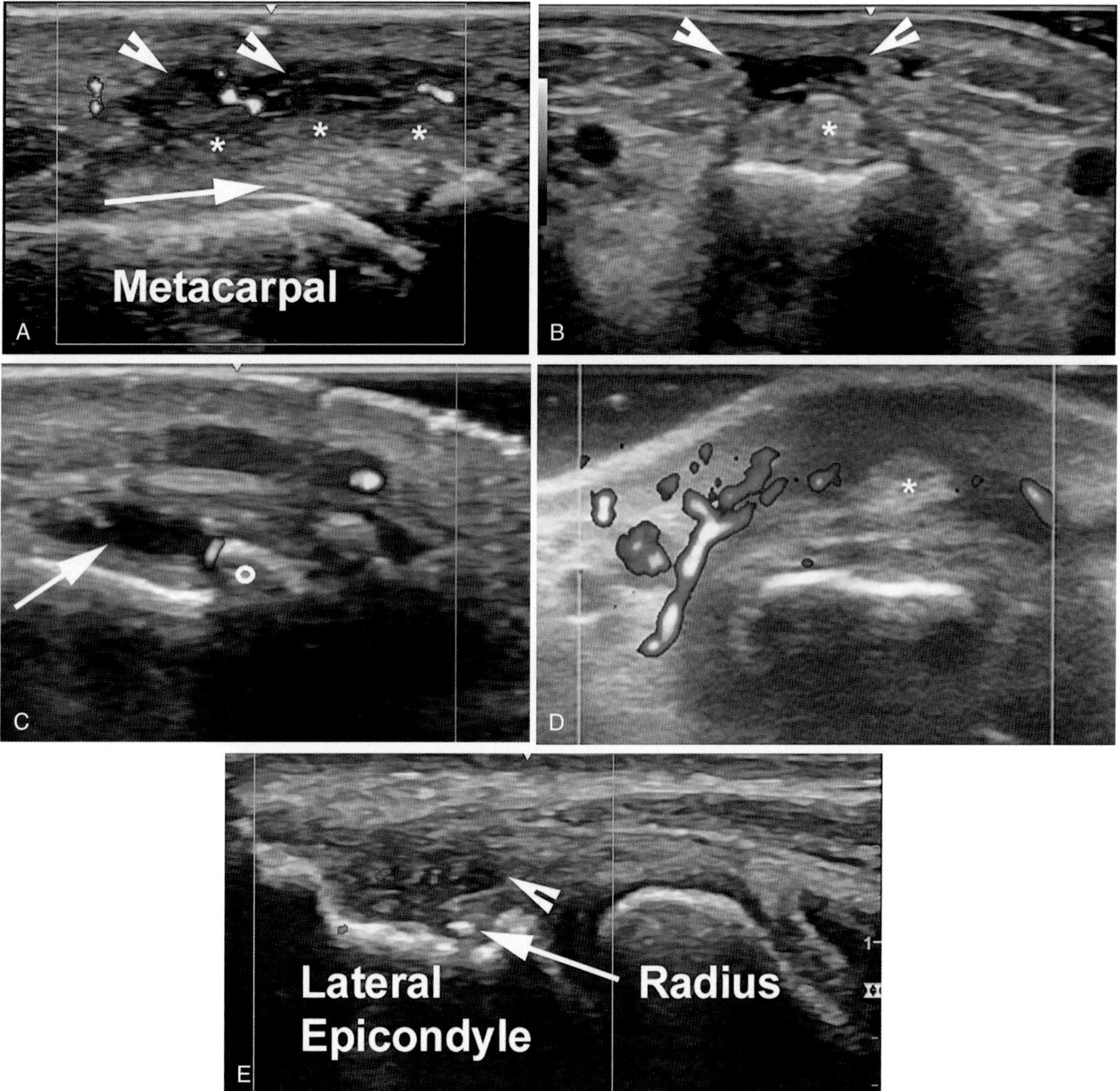

• **Fig. 44.7** US findings in SpA. (A) Dorsal longitudinal view of MCP shows hypoechoic swelling of the paratenon *(arrowheads)* dorsal to the extensor tendon (*) with grade 1 Doppler signal and non-distended synovial reflection *(arrow)* of the MCP joint. (B) Dorsal transverse view of MCP in (A) with paratenon swelling and effusion *(arrowhead)* dorsal to the tendon (*). (C) Longitudinal view of DIP joint shows Doppler signal at the proximal osteophyte (o) as well as a small joint effusion *(arrow),* which could be seen in either psoriatic arthritis or erosive osteoarthritis. (D) Transverse view of MCP shows more extensive Doppler signal in the soft tissues and paratenon over and to the sides of an extensor tendon (*). (E) Lateral longitudinal view of the elbow shows lateral epicondylitis in a patient with SpA with transition from normal to hypoechoic enthesis fibers *(arrowhead),* mild Doppler signal in the enthesis and at the bone surface, and a calcification casting a shadow on the epicondyle *(arrow);* the surface of the epicondyle is irregular but without definitive erosion.

inflammatory findings.[113] SAD bursitis is noted to be the inflammatory hallmark. When compared with MRI as a gold standard for SAD and trochanteric bursitis, US had a sensitivity of 96% and 100%, respectively.[115,116]

In 2012, a provisional classification criterion for PMR was developed by a collaborative initiative between EULAR and the ACR.[117] This group developed a classification criteria scoring algorithm with and without US. When US is available and included, a diagnosis is made with a total of ≥5 out of 8 possible points. Two points are denoted for US findings as follows: one point is given for unilateral shoulder findings and at least one hip finding, and one point is given for bilateral shoulder findings.

Monitoring

US has shown a decrease in SAD bursa involvement with the initiation of glucocorticoid (GC) therapy.[114,118] Although a parallel decrease is seen in clinical, laboratory, and US parameters, US inflammatory findings have similar or better sensitivity to change than clinical or laboratory parameters. US may be a valuable additional tool to assess response to therapy.

Predicting Outcome

US with power Doppler can identify patients who will have relapsing disease.[118] Patients with a positive baseline PD signal have higher acute phase reactants and frequency of relapse compared with those without PD signal. This effect is greater with bilaterally positive PD signal and is independent of other clinical demographic and laboratory parameters. Over half of patients deemed in clinical remission may have persistent inflammation by US criteria, primarily in the extra-articular synovial structures of the shoulders. This finding predicts disease relapse similar to a positive PD signal at baseline.

Giant Cell Arteritis

Giant cell arteritis (GCA) causes inflammation of the medium to large arteries.[119] The diagnosis has been traditionally established by clinical and laboratory findings and supported with a temporal artery (TA) biopsy. TA biopsy is dependent on the length of the segment sampled, the timing of the biopsy to the initiation of treatment, and unilateral versus bilateral sampling. The "gold standard" for diagnosis is biopsy, which can have false negative results due to skip lesions and be associated with significant morbidity.[120]

The first report of US imaging of the temporal arteries as a surrogate for temporal artery biopsy was in 1997.[121] Current EULAR recommendations emphasize early imaging in a setting of high clinical suspicion to replace biopsy, and for TA US to be the first imaging modality.[122] When properly employed, vascular US can rival the diagnostic utility of temporal artery biopsy.[123]

Vascular US relies on specific settings to optimize the image collection, including grayscale (frequency, focus, depth, B-mode gain, line density, frame rate, etc.) and color Doppler (frequency, PRF, wall filter, color box, color flow gain, flow direction).[124] A standard linear probe with a grayscale frequency of 15 MHz or greater and a color Doppler frequency with a vascular preset is a minimum requirement. TA branches are best imaged with a higher frequency (≥15 MHz), and a compact linear or "hockey stick" probe is recommended.

Diagnosis

There are four cardinal US features of vascular change in patients with giant cell arteritis, including (1) wall thickening, or the halo sign, (2) noncompressibility, (3) stenosis, and (4) occlusion.[125] The wall thickening (halo sign) appears as a hypoechoic rim and is felt to represent cellular infiltrates and edema in the vascular media, intima, and adventitia (Figs. 44.8 through 44.10), noted both on biopsy and on correlating positron emission tomography (PET)-CT imaging. This inflammatory response results in vessel wall stiffness, resisting collapse during direct sonopalpation, and noncompressibility of the artery segment.

Multiple studies have confirmed the utility of US for the diagnosis of GCA with a sensitivity of 68% to 87% and specificity of 82% to 96%. Specificity approaches 100% in the presence of bilateral halo signs.[126–128] A positive compression sign has excellent inter-observer agreement and has a sensitivity of 75% to 79% and a specificity of 100% for the diagnosis of GCA.[129] Vessel stenosis and occlusion can also be seen by US but do not add to the diagnostic sensitivity and specificity of the halo sign coupled with the noncompressibility of the interrogated artery.[124]

US for GCA relies on imaging vessels other than the TAs. A typical bilateral evaluation includes the temporal, with the frontal and parietal branches, the carotid, and the axillary arteries. Imaging should include orthogonal planes, and the compression maneuver is typically performed in the transverse view[130] (Fig. 44.11). Imaging multiple bilateral vessels leads to marked improvements in both sensitivity and specificity, when compared with clinical or pathologic diagnosis.[123,131]

The concept of a fast-track outpatient clinic for the early identification of GCA through the use of US has been piloted at some centers and has been effective in earlier diagnosis with less permanent vision loss.[132]

Monitoring

The role of US in detecting disease remission and flare has yet to be defined. The duration of US findings after corticosteroid therapy initiation has been assessed and is variable.[133] Given the differences in the vascular sites assessed, US evidence of vessel inflammation with a graded loss of the halo response can be seen for up to 16 to 56 days after steroid exposure, with the average duration of approximately 21 days.[124,134]

The data underscore the exciting potential for US evaluation in the early diagnosis of GCA but, as a relatively new modality, it is underutilized.[124]

Predicting Outcome

The role of US in predicting outcome in GCA has yet to be defined.

Sjögren's Syndrome

US has been recognized as a useful modality for evaluating soft tissues of the head and neck, including the salivary glands.[135–137] US of the salivary glands for the diagnosis of Sjögren's syndrome (SS) has an evidence level of grade B.[10] It compares favorably with scintigraphy, MRI, and CT imaging, yet the role of salivary gland US in clinical practice as well as in clinical research continues to evolve.[138]

The general approach to imaging salivary glands (Figs. 44.12 and 44.13) focuses on a bilateral assessment of the parotid and submandibular glands.[137] The parotid gland lies anterior to the external ear and the sternocleidomastoid but extends along the mandible into the retromandibular fossa. The submandibular gland is rostral to the retromandibular fossa as well as the angle of the mandible, and lies more caudally, further into the soft tissues of the neck.

Salivary glands without pathology have a homogeneous echostructure with a parenchymal echogenicity similar to the thyroid gland. Pathologic findings in a salivary gland include spherical infiltrates and tubular dilatations, and orthogonal views should be obtained to characterize the geometric nature of visualized abnormalities. Conventional US machine presets for imaging thyroid tissue provide maximal image quality, and most authors suggest a 5 to 12 MHz linear transducer for image production.[135–137] Salivary gland imaging assesses parenchymal homogeneity and the presence or absence of increased blood flow. The salivary glands

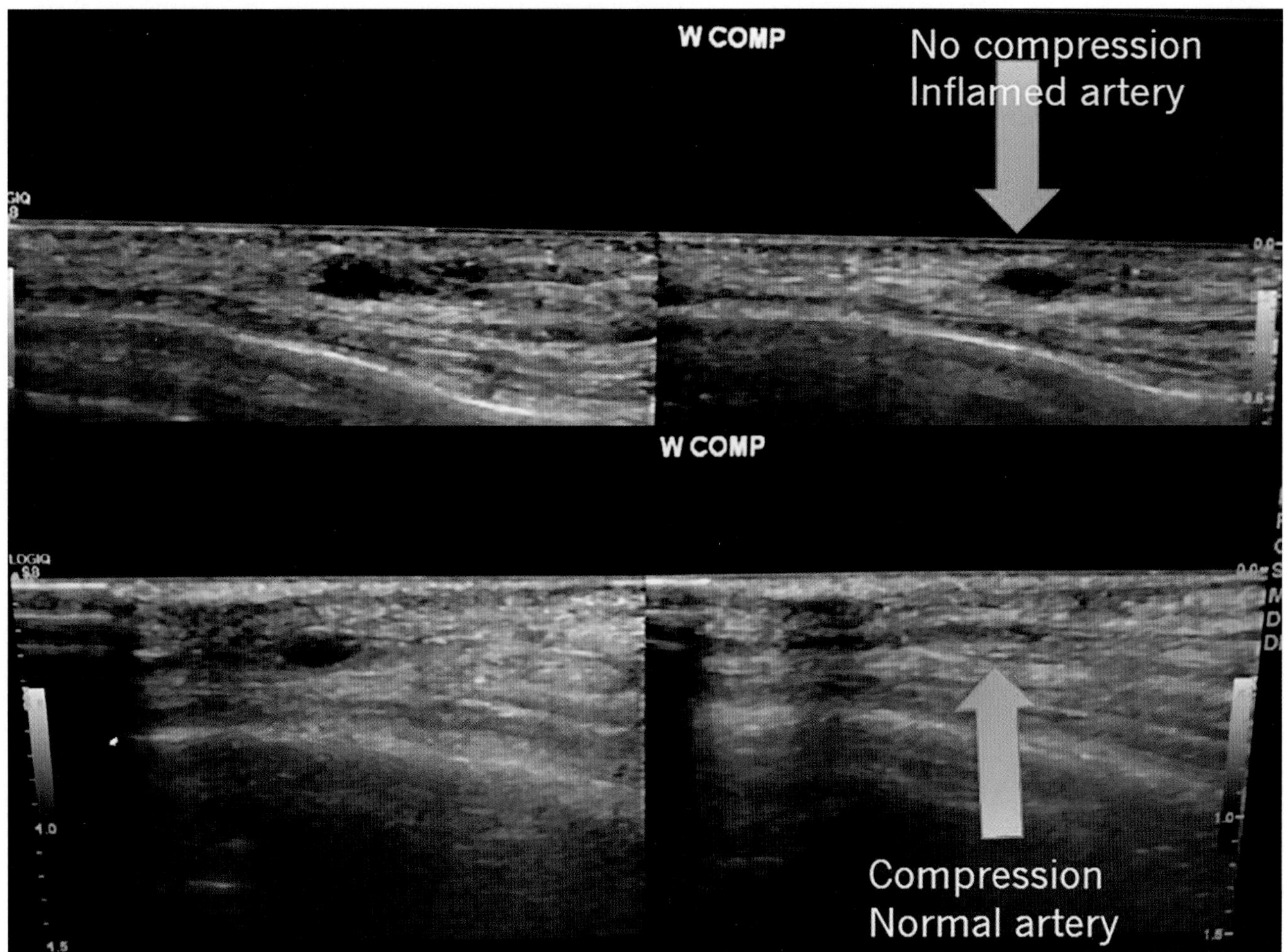

• **Fig. 44.8** Compression of temporal artery. The upper images demonstrate the compression of the temporal artery before and after sonopalpation, where the artery sustains its lumen; it represents an inflamed artery (in this case, confirmed by biopsy). The lower images demonstrate the opposite effect, where the artery demonstrates compression with sonopalpation; it represents an uninvolved artery (in this case, also confirmed by biopsy).

are usually associated with lymph nodes, and these should also be assessed during the examination.

Measuring the speed of sound conduction through tissue, elastography provides a qualitative visual or quantitative measurement of tissue compliance, compressibility, or "elasticity" and may provide new insights into salivary gland function.[139,140] The elastic properties of a tissue can be assessed by direct compression of tissue, strain, or shear wave elastography. The latter has been postulated to be of use to evaluate infiltrative disorders, such as the glandular infiltration seen in SS[141] (Fig. 44.14).

Diagnosis

On B-mode imaging, heterogenous glandular parenchyma with scattered multiple small oval, hypoechoic, or anechoic regions are the typical findings noted in SS (Fig. 44.15).[135] Echogenic bands were found in one study to distinguish primary from secondary SS.[142] The visualized hypoechoic or anechoic areas may represent lymphocytic infiltrates, dilated ducts, or vasculature, suggesting a role for Doppler during routine assessment.[135] Acutely symptomatic or inflamed salivary glands in SS can show an increased vascular pattern (see Fig. 44.15).

Glandular changes of inhomogeneity, hypoechoic, and anechoic regions can be seen in a variety of pathologic states beyond SS.[135] SS patients can develop salivary gland infections and sialoliths, which may be seen during routine US assessment.

When compared with controls, US has diagnostic sensitivity and specificity of 88.8% and 84.6%, respectively, for primary SS and 53.8% and 92.2%, respectively, for secondary SS, with moderate inter-rater reliability.[143,144]

A review of 31 studies on behalf of the US-pSS Study Group concluded that US has proven its usefulness in detecting typical structural abnormalities in SS and may become a first-line imaging tool.[145] No uniform definitions of US pathology and consensus-based scoring systems have been adopted, though many have been published and compare favorably with current diagnostic criteria.[142,143,146,147]

The acute inflammation of SS can increase salivary gland vascularity and result in positive Doppler signal.[148] Higher elastography scores correlate better with gland dysfunction than B-mode US in subjects with SS compared with asymptomatic subjects.[141] Higher strain wave patterns in parotid glands have also been reported in SS subjects over controls.[149–151] Elastography and B-mode scores correlate with duration of illness.[152] Combining B-mode and

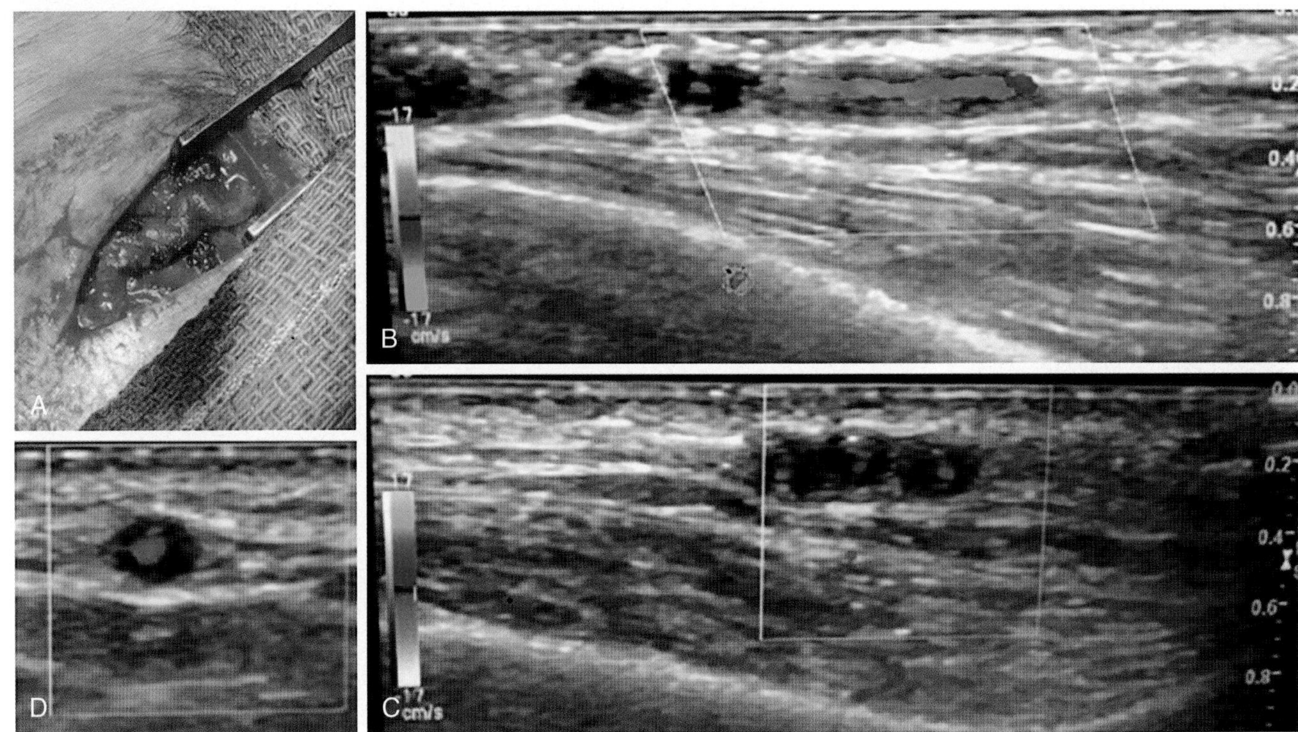

• **Fig. 44.9** Study of tortuous temporal artery. (A) View of temporal artery during surgical excision for biopsy. (B) Both long and transverse view, resulting from interrogation at the base of the artery with halo sign. (C) Series of 3 halo signs resulting from interrogation of the middle region of the tortuous artery. (D) Halo sign, isolated region of the artery.

shear wave readings for diagnostic purposes provides improved ability to discern SS from sicca alone.[153]

Monitoring

Monitoring of therapeutic interventions may be possible with US, which identifies improvement in glandular echotexture and Doppler resistive indices in patients treated with rituximab compared with placebo.[154–156]

Predicting Outcome

Salivary gland scores have been associated with systemic disease including skin vasculitis, higher disease activity, CD4 lymphopenia, and may be a marker for lymphoma development in patients with primary SS.[157] In RA, salivary gland US changes correlated with sicca symptoms, more active measures of RA disease activity, and poorer oral health.[158]

Sclerosing Diseases

Over the past few decades US imaging has been investigated in the evaluation of fibrosing diseases, including scleroderma, eosinophilic fasciitis, and complications of diabetes mellitus, as this technology allows visualization of the extra-cellular matrix accumulation typical of these conditions.

Use in Diagnosis, Monitoring, and Predicting Outcome

Diabetic complications of carpal tunnel syndrome (CTS), stenosing tenosynovitis, Dupuytren's contracture, and cheiroarthropathy can all be evaluated with US. In CTS, the median nerve is typically swollen proximal to the point of impingement by and flattening deep to the flexor retinaculum, with bowing of the retinaculum itself.[159] In stenosing tenosynovitis, US findings include nodular thickening of the A1 pulley, disorganization of the flexor tendon fibers, thickening of the tendon distal to the pulley, and loss of normal tendon sliding with finger flexion on dynamic imaging.[160,161] In patients with diabetic hand syndrome (cheiroarthropathy), flexor tendon sheaths in the hands are also an average of three times thicker than age-matched healthy controls,[162] while the skin in the arms is 50% thicker than in controls.[163]

US measured skin is also thickened in scleroderma, and this thickness correlates with clinical skin scores.[164–166] With increased disease duration, skin thickness and dermal echogenicity increase.[165] Scleroderma produces a characteristic sclerotic tenosynovitis, with a characteristic hyperechoic tenosynovium. Unlike RA patients, it is characterized by an alternating hypo- and hyperechoic pattern.[167,168] Unlike other inflammatory forms of arthritis, extensor tendons (78%) are more commonly affected than flexor tendons (22%).[168] While synovitis and calcinosis are common, joint erosions have been reported in only 2% to 11% of patients with systemic sclerosis.[169] Thus, in comparison to RA, scleroderma is more likely to cause extensor tendon sclerosing tenosynovitis, and less likely to cause synovitis, especially with high Doppler signal and associated erosion (Fig. 44.16). US can also be employed to detect ulnar artery occlusion, a risk factor for the development of digital ulceration in scleroderma.[170]

US can be used for evaluation of scleroderma lung disease. In comparison to high resolution CT and CR, US has a sensitivity of 92% and 48% and specificity of 71% and 91%, respectively, for the detection of interstitial lung disease.[171] Many other studies report similar results, but there have not been studies

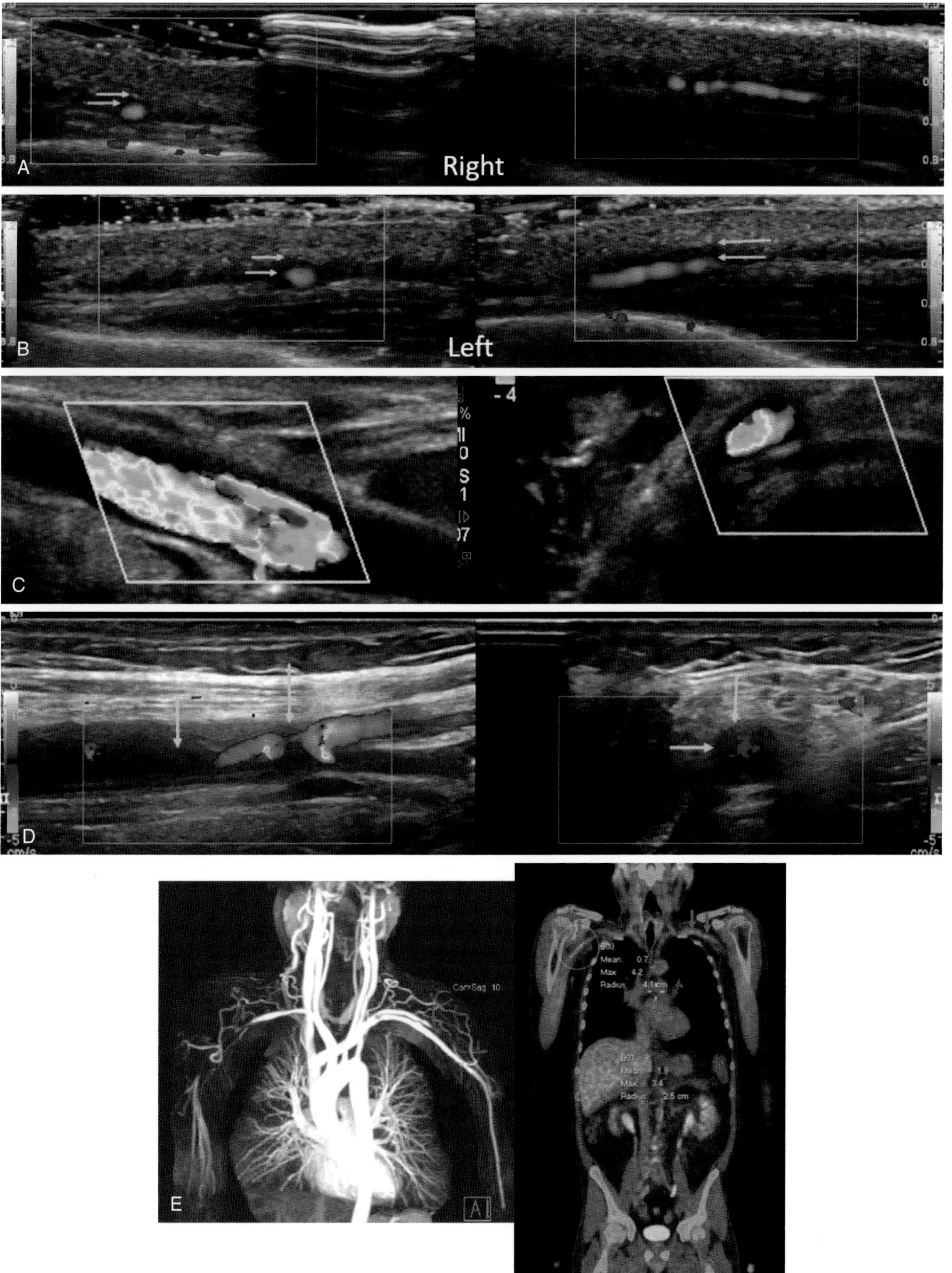

• **Fig. 44.10** Study of diffuse vascular involvement in giant cell arteritis. (A and B) Normal right temporal artery, two views (A), and left temporal artery, two views, both showing positive halo sign, confirmed as vasculitis on biopsy (B). (C and D) A normal right axillary artery, two views (C) and right axillary artery, two views, showing stenoses and halo sign (D). (E) Positron emission tomography (PET)-CT imaging from patient in B and D with FDG uptake (inflammation) at the axillary artery region identified by ultrasound *(red arrows)*.

demonstrating that US can be used to evaluate response to treatment or distinguish ground glass opacities (inflammatory) from "honey combing" (fibrotic) changes as seen on CT scan.[172]

Eosinophilic fasciitis (EF) can also be evaluated with US and is characterized by loss of compressibility of the hypodermal fat layer.[173] Numerous case reports describe thickening of the subdermal fascia fibers, hyperechogenicity of the deep dermal tissue, and hypoechoic rims about the affected tendons.[174]

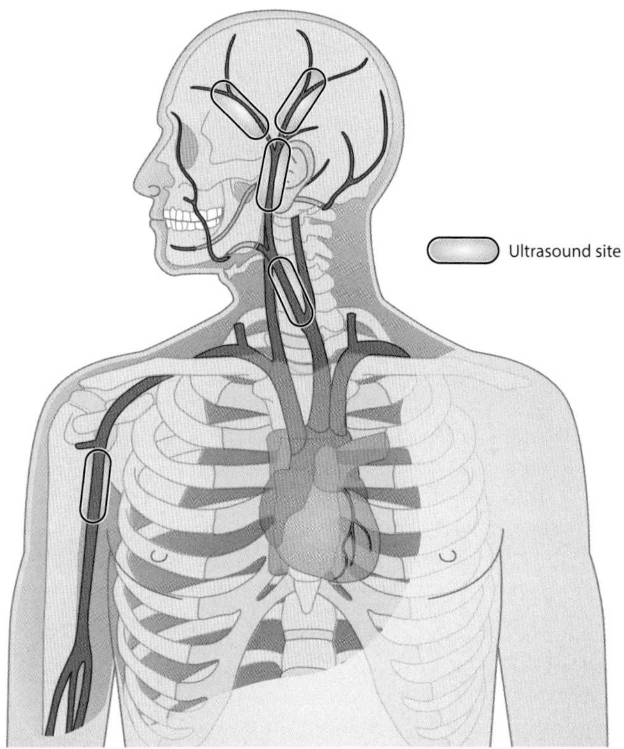

• **Fig. 44.11** Illustration of ultrasound sites for the evaluation of vasculitis. Probe position is demonstrated only in the long plane, but orthogonal planes are recommended to demonstrate all normal and abnormal findings. Three branches of the temporal artery (main, frontal, parietal branches), carotid artery, and axillary views are shown. Unilateral imaging is shown, but bilateral views are recommended.

Non-inflammatory Conditions

US has shown great promise in the diagnosis of multiple localized inflammatory and non-inflammatory musculoskeletal conditions, such as entrapment neuropathies, tendon and ligament disease, bursitis, plantar fasciitis, and nodules.

Nerves

The nerves most commonly evaluated by US include the median, ulnar, suprascapular, and peroneal nerves, though US evaluation is not limited to these four nerves. CTS is caused by compression of the

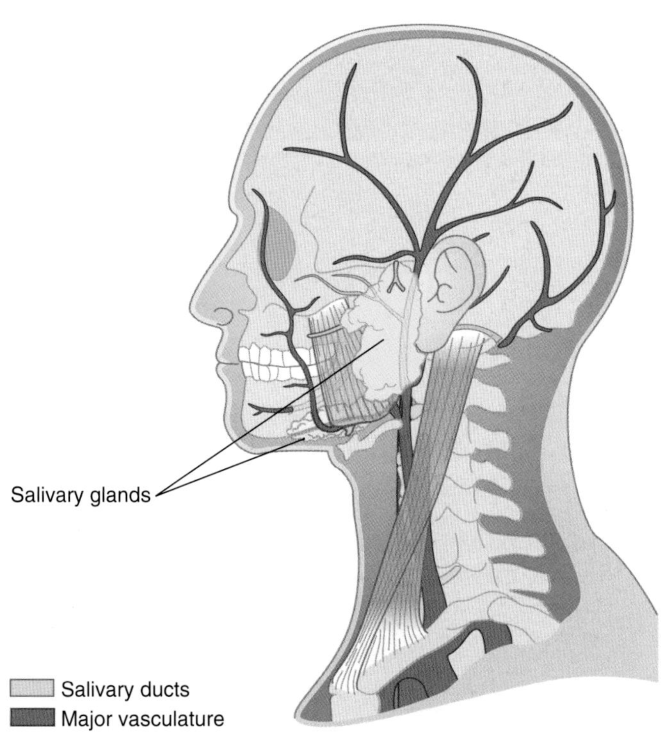

• **Fig. 44.12** Anatomy of the salivary gland. Yellow represents major salivary glands and green represents ducts leading away from glands. Red is the pathway of major vasculature.

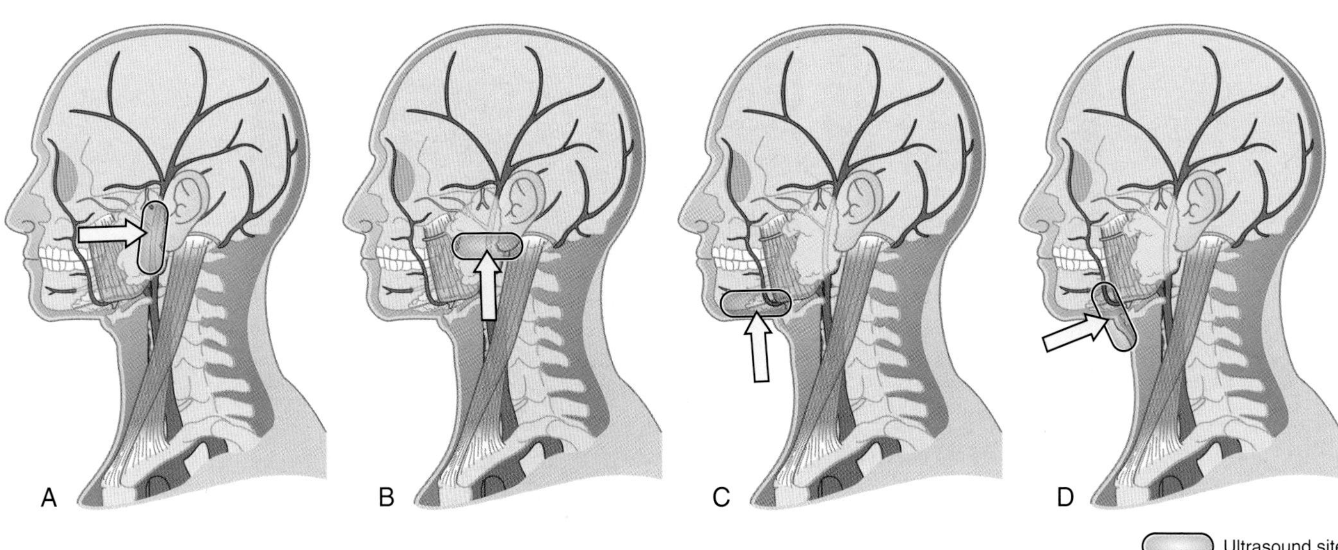

• **Fig. 44.13** Probe position during salivary gland imaging. (A) Parotid gland, long view. (B) Parotid gland, transverse view. (C) Submandibular gland, long view. (D) Submandibular gland, transverse view.

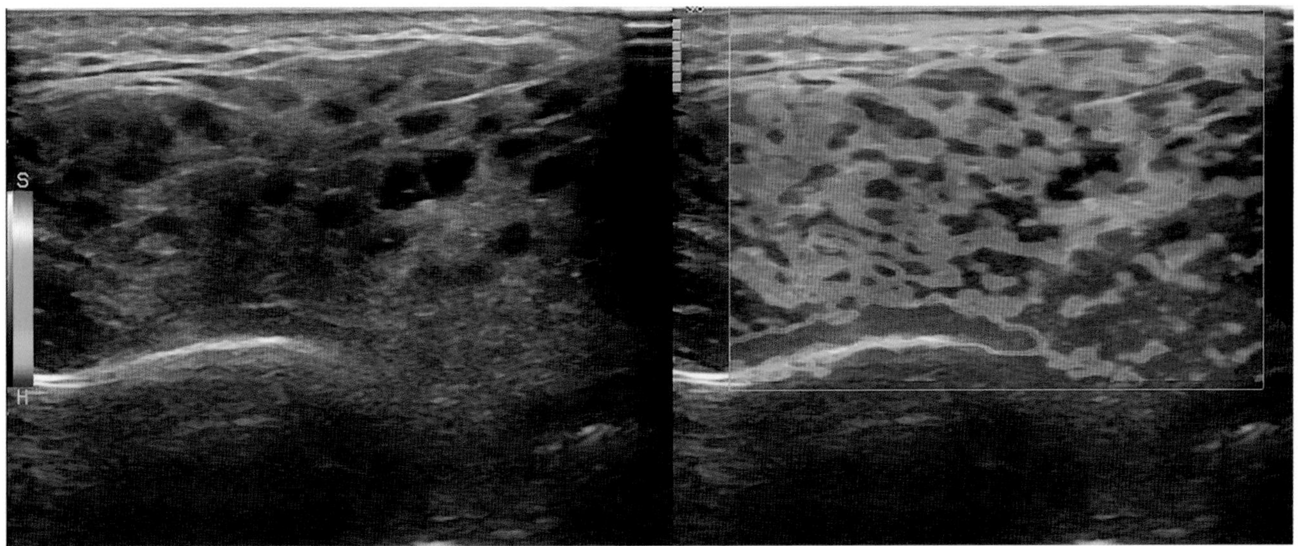

• **Fig. 44.14** Left parotid gland in transverse view with strain elastography. *Left* image is grayscale image and right image is same site with elastography. *Blue* represents areas of least compressibility ("hard" or "H" on the accompanying scale) and *red* represents areas of greatest compressibility ("soft" or "S" on the accompanying scale). Note that *blue areas* correspond with anechoic areas in this figure but also in areas outside of the salivary gland, near the bone; this underscores the importance of a grayscale image for immediate comparison to the strain elastograph.

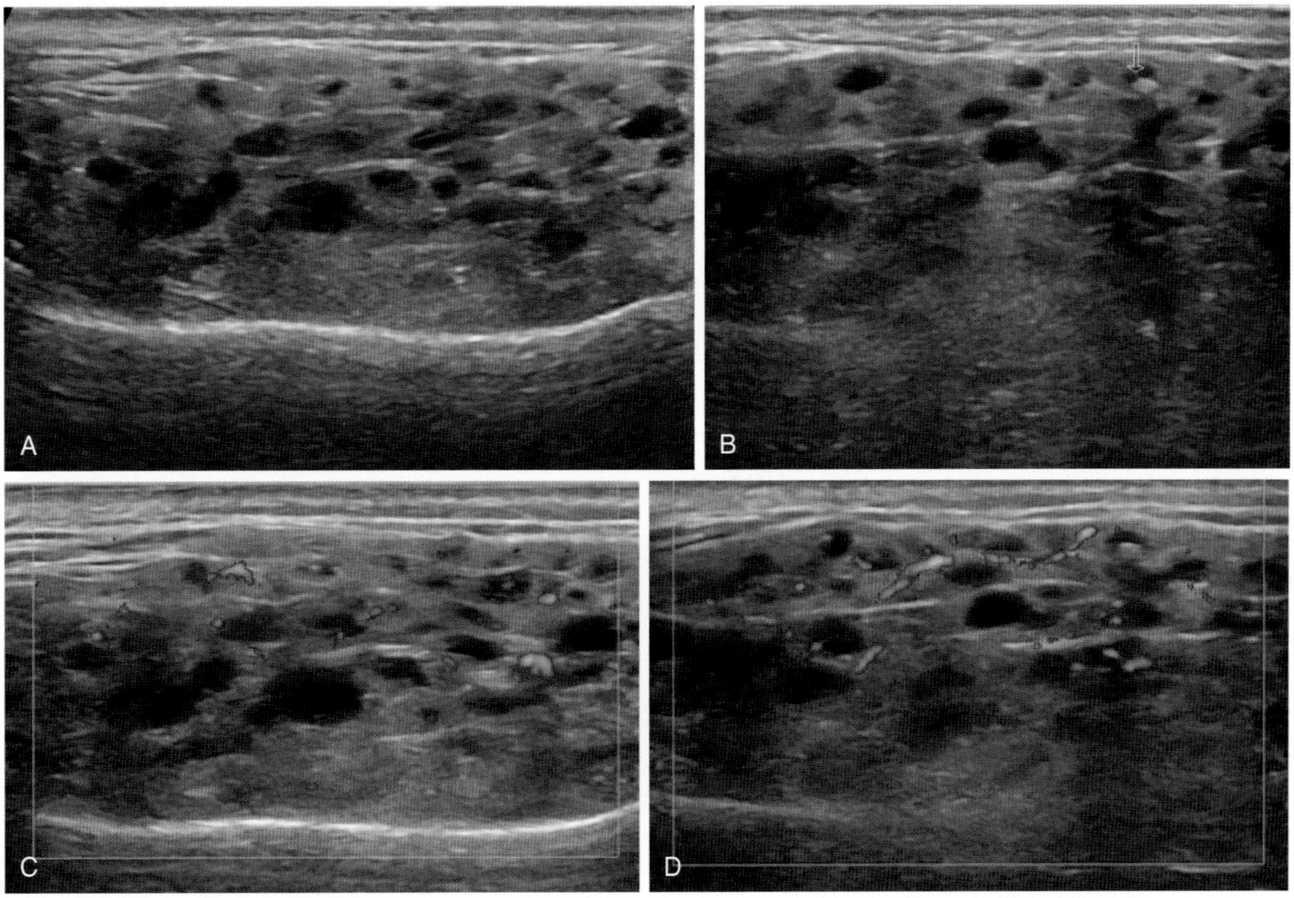

• **Fig. 44.15** The parotid gland demonstrates characteristic anechoic oval changes that are a combination of dilated ducts and immune infiltrates in a patient fulfilling ACR criteria for Sjögren's syndrome. (A) Left parotid longitudinal view. (B) Right parotid gland longitudinal view with evidence of a sialolith *(arrow)* within a dilated salivary gland duct with characteristic shadow artifact. (C) Left parotid longitudinal view with power Doppler showing scattered activity, suggestive of parenchymal inflammation. (D) Right parotid gland longitudinal view with power Doppler showing diffuse signal more characteristic of inflammation due to sialolith in contrast to C.

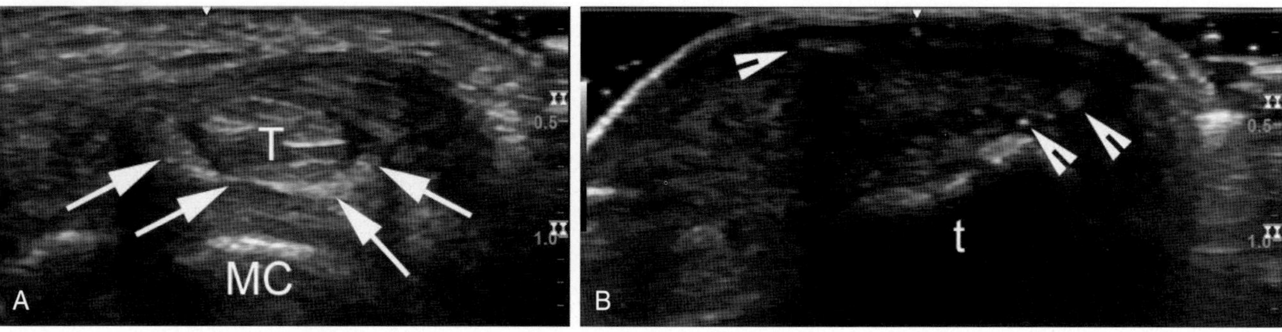

• **Fig. 44.16** Ultrasound changes characteristic of scleroderma. (A) Volar transverse view of MCP (MC) where the flexor tendon (T) is surrounded by a thick hyperechoic tenosynovium *(arrows);* (B) volar transverse view of digital tuft (t) shows hyperechoic deposits of varying size *(arrowheads)* due to calcifications, the largest of which cause soft tissue shadowing deep to the lesion.

median nerve by the flexor retinaculum of the wrist and can be seen with inflammatory and mechanical conditions. Classically diagnosed via electrodiagnostic (EDX) studies, US has emerged as a potential diagnostic tool, allowing visualization of the swollen nerve just proximal to the mechanical compression. Multiple studies have been published showing US sensitivity of up to 94% and specificity of up to 98% for the diagnosis of CTS when measuring median nerve cross-sectional area at the level of the carpal tunnel inlet.[175] However, the wide variation of sensitivity and specificity reported in the literature has prevented meaningful analysis of US as a screening or confirmatory tool in the diagnosis of CTS when compared to EDX studies. Both US and EDX are highly operator dependent and, although EDX is considered the gold standard, it is normal in 16% to 34% of patients with clinically defined disease and has a sensitivity and specificity of 69% and 97%, respectively.[176,177]

In 2011 and 2012, meta-analyses were done to look at the diagnostic accuracy of US versus EDX testing.[175,178] The 2011 meta-analysis studies included varied on reference group (clinical versus EDX testing), US derived median nerve cross-sectional area (CSA), and measurement location. Although US performed well, with composite sensitivity and specificity of 77.6% and 86.8%, it was not superior to EDX or clinical examination. Thus, US may not completely replace EDX but may be considered an alternative as a first-line confirmatory test.

The 2012 meta-analysis looked at median nerve CSA compared with EDX.[178] For a CSA of 9.5 to 10.5 mm^2, the pooled sensitivity and specificity were found to be 84% and 78%, respectively. For a CSA of 7.0 to 8.5 mm^2, the pooled sensitivity was 94%, and for a CSA of 11.5 to 13.0 mm^2, the pooled specificity was 97%. The authors concluded that US could not replace EDX, but rather was complementary.

No consensus method exists for a reference standard for US diagnosis of CTS, and studies have examined US diagnosis based on median nerve inlet and outlet measurements.[179] The outlet level measurement was defined as the location at the level of the hook of the hamate, and the inlet level was defined as the location at the pisiform or the proximal margin of the flexor retinaculum. US measurement of the CSA of the median nerve at the inlet level was found to be a useful strategy for diagnosis of CTS and had better accuracy than outlet-level measurements. The pooled sensitivity and specificity of the inlet measurement was 81% and 84%, respectively. The authors were not able to identify an optimal cutoff threshold for the CSA but presented a 95% CI of 9.0 to 12.6 mm^2 for inlet level diagnosis. US is a reasonable first-line test in patients with clinical symptoms of CTS and can aid in diagnosis of median nerve compression, diagnosis of potential etiologies for CTS (wrist synovitis, etc), and guide therapeutic intervention (injection), all in one setting (Fig. 44.17).

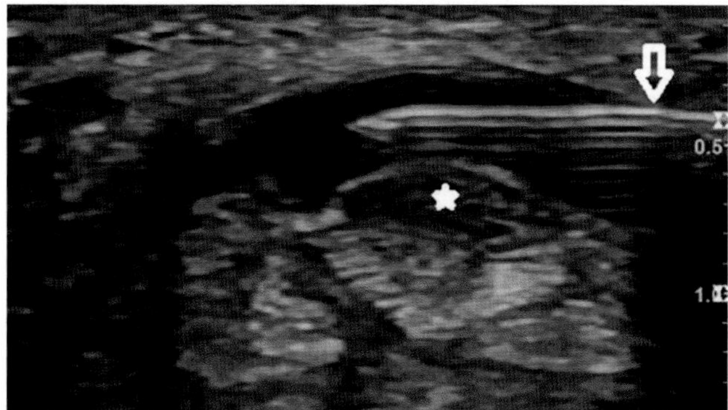

• **Fig. 44.17** This transverse view of the volar wrist shows a carpal tunnel injection with the needle *(arrow)* just above the median nerve *(star)* and deep to the flexor retinaculum. The needle displays posterior reverberation artifact.

US has been utilized to look at ulnar nerve entrapment. Cubital tunnel syndrome refers to compression of the ulnar nerve at the elbow level. Sites of compression include the cubital tunnel inlet, the medial epicondyle, and cubital tunnel outlet. US findings of ulnar neuropathy at the elbow include changes in echotexture, diameter CSA, and swelling ratio.[180] Subluxation of the ulnar nerve can also occur at the area and is seen in dynamic scanning in up to 23% of healthy controls.[181]

It is unclear where the CSA of the ulnar nerve in the elbow should be measured, and there is no consensus on the diagnostic CSA. A recent meta-analysis showed that the ulnar nerve CSA rarely exceeded 10 mm^2 in healthy controls.[182] The between-group differences in the CSA in patients with cubital tunnel syndrome is most significant at the medial epicondyle, just before the cubital tunnel outlet. Overall, US was found to have a pooled sensitivity and specificity of 85% and 91%, respectively, when using an ulnar nerve CSA of ≥10 mm^2.

US can also be used for diagnosis of less common nerve entrapments. Tibial nerve entrapment can occur at the posteromedial tarsal tunnel, a fibrous and osseous tunnel situated posteriorly and inferiorly to the medial malleolus with a proximal and distal floor. US reliably identifies pathology of the tarsal tunnel, including nerve compression from various etiologies.[183]

The suprascapular nerve arises from the C5 and C6 roots and travels deep to the trapezius toward the posterior shoulder along the border of the scapula. It is visible on US as it traverses through the suprascapular notch, deep to the superior transverse scapular ligament, and travels with the artery and vein. It provides motor innervation to the supra- and infraspinatus muscles and sensory innervation to the acromioclavicular and glenohumeral (GH) joints. US guided injection in this area can be used to treat intractable shoulder pain, or the nerve can become compressed by a labral cyst, which requires aspiration.[184]

Tendon

Inflammatory and non-inflammatory tendon pathology can be reliably identified on both B-mode and power Doppler US and includes tendinopathy, full or partial tears, and tenosynovitis. Disorders of the rotator cuff (RC) are common and associated with substantial disability. Certain RC diagnoses require surgical intervention, while others are treated conservatively. US provides the potential for immediate bedside evaluation that is significantly more cost effective than MRI. US performs as well as MRI and MRI arthrogram (MRA) in the diagnosis of full thickness tears of the RC, with a sensitivity of 90% to 91% and specificity of 86% to 90%.[185] For partial thickness RC tear, US and MRI were similar, with sensitivity of 67% to 68%, but MRA had a sensitivity of 83%. There was no difference seen in specificity between the three modalities at 93% to 94%. RC tendinopathy by US had an overall sensitivity of 79% and specificity of 94%.

Calcific tendonitis of the shoulder is a painful disorder characterized by deposits of calcium hydroxyapatite or carbonate apatite crystals in the RC tendons or SAD bursa. The disease may subside spontaneously with conservative treatment or be prolonged and require intervention, including surgery, US-guided barbatage/needling (UGN), or extracorporeal shock wave therapy (ESWT).[186] US has a dual role in the diagnosis and treatment of calcific tendonitis of the shoulder. Most commonly located in the supraspinatus tendon, calcium deposits in the resting phase appear as hyperechoic and arc shaped with posterior acoustic shadowing, and in the resolving phase as fragmented/punctate, cystic, and nodular with increased Doppler signal.[187]

UGN involves the use of local anesthesia and subsequent repeated needling of the calcific deposit with simultaneous lavage and removal of calcium. UGN can lead to disappearance of the calcium and significant pain relief, with few reported side effects.[188]

Bursa

A bursa is an extra-articular sac that exists in areas of high friction to promote tissue movement and can be classified into native and non-native types.[189] Native bursa have a synovial membrane, and the non-native or adventitial bursa occur secondary to friction and do not have a synovial lining but can develop inflammation from increased vascular permeability. Bursal distention may be caused by simple fluid, appearing anechoic on US, or complex fluid, appearing heterogenous with variable echogenicity. Bursa may also be distended by synovitis, which lacks compressibility in comparison to fluid. Similar to joint effusions and synovitis, US imaging of the bursa does not have distinct features, and clinical and laboratory findings should be used in combination with imaging to guide the diagnosis.[189]

Superficial bursa and joint recesses are most amenable to US evaluation, including the knee joint's supra-patellar and gastrocnemio-semimembranosus recesses. When distended, the latter bursa is referred to as a Baker cyst. When evaluating bursa for pathology, it is essential to understand the anatomy and scan any associated joint for primary pathology. For example, SAD bursa effusion may be seen as a result of GH pathology and a complete tear of the rotator cuff.

Fascia

Plantar fasciitis is a common cause of heel pain and results from micro-trauma due to repetitive overload of the plantar connective tissue, which over time leads to an inflammatory response, pain, and discomfort.[190] US findings include plantar fascia thickening, with any thickness >4.0 mm considered abnormal. Additional findings include abnormal echogenicity and vascularity, bony spurs, perifascial fluid, and bioconvexity of the fascia at the origin compared with the middle and distal third. US has a high level of agreement with MRI and elastography in the diagnosis of plantar fasciitis.[190]

Nodules

Nodules are described under RA diagnosis.

Pediatric Rheumatology

Because US can visualize soft tissues without radiation, it is an ideal modality to assist in the evaluation of the pediatric patient. The changing anatomic and physiologic milestones of musculoskeletal development mandate a comprehensive understanding of normal US anatomy appearance by age group prior to the diagnosis of pathology in the pediatric population.[191]

The unique US appearance of the articular cartilage, epiphysis, metaphysis, growth plates, and joint space have to be considered by age group.[192] Pivotal work in this field has been done by OMERACT members to yield definitions of sonographic findings in healthy children.[192] The epiphyseal ossification center appears as a hyperechoic structure that may have a smooth or irregular surface, within a cartilage system. The joint capsule appears as a hyperechoic structure that can (but does not have to) appear over bone, cartilage, and other intra-articular tissues of the joint. The synovial membrane in a healthy child is not visualized using conventional US. The ossified portion of articular bone is detected as a hyperechoic linear region that may have interruptions at the growth plates and at ossification center junctions. Hyaline cartilage presents as well-defined, noncompressible anechoic structure that may contain bright echoes or dots, which are vascular channels in developing cartilage.[193] Standardized views have been established for the knee, ankle, wrist, and second metacarpophalangeal joints.[194]

In the pediatric population, the fat pad is an intra-articular structure with a heterogenous echotexture and potential normal vascularity.[193] Intra-articular blood flow has also been established in younger children, particularly in the epiphyseal cartilage, as well as around the healthy joint.[194] Patterns vary by site, as well as by view. In the knee region, for example, this vasculature could be seen parallel to the periosteum, within the femoral physis, as well as surrounding the parapatellar recess. The initial OMERACT definitions were revised to recognize the physiologic vascularity that can be detected at any age during growth and development and distinguish the normal vascular pattern from the pathologic vascular flow that can be seen in an adult patient.[193] Vascular patterns and joint ossification have also been validated for intrareader reliability.[195]

Synovitis has been established to include both synovial fluid and hypertrophy, with Doppler signals required to be localized only in the region of synovial hypertrophy.[196] Feeding vessels may have enhanced presence during joint hyperemia, but this observation requires further study to be incorporated in routine assessment. Joint effusion demonstrates compressibility. In juvenile idiopathic arthritis (JIA), clinically inactive joints have been shown by US to have synovitis but did not predict flare.[197]

Entheseal disease is characteristic of some forms of JIA.[198] Normal entheseal thickness is symmetric and correlates more with weight than age. Asymmetric findings can be helpful in unilateral symptoms. Elastography may prove beneficial in the evaluation of entheseal disease, but requires further study.[199]

Ultrasound in Rheumatology Intervention

US use for guidance of needle placement was first reported in 1981 for aspiration of a septic shoulder and is one of the most obvious advantages of RhUS.[200] US guided needle placement results in superior injection accuracy, efficacy, and humanity. The latter refers to the immediate visualization of a target with accurate needle placement to reduce patient discomfort.

Traditionally, most joint and soft tissue injections are guided by landmark palpation. Notable exceptions include the hip joint and a popliteal cyst. Using US guidance, these procedures can now be done by the clinician at the bedside, without radiation exposure. The decision to use US guidance as opposed to palpation guidance for other sites can be determined by the likelihood for success based on patient factors, the added efficacy for an accurate injection of medication, and the likelihood of causing less pain.

Preparation for an US guided procedure requires proper positioning of the patient, equipment, and provider to minimize the effort required for the procedure and maximize comfort for both the patient and the provider.

There are several approaches for US guided procedures.

For direct in-plane guidance, the sonographer finds the target, stabilizes the transducer, and inserts the needle in the same direction and deep to the long axis of the transducer. The entire length of the needle is seen as it traverses the tissues and until the needle tip enters the target (Fig. 44.18). For direct out-of-plane guidance, the sonographer finds the target, stabilizes the probe, and inserts the needle perpendicular to the direction of the transducer. The core of the needle appears as a bright dot in the tissue when it crosses the plane of the transducer (see Fig. 44.18). For indirect guidance, the sonographer finds the target and marks its location on the overlying skin, while noting the depth of the target. The transducer is removed, and the needle is inserted to the marked depth.

The direct in-plane technique may be preferable, as it allows for needle visualization throughout the entire path from the subcutaneous to the target tissue. The needle trajectory can be adjusted as the needle is advanced to help ensure accurate placement with one pass through the tissues. The direct out-of-plane technique can confirm accurate needle placement but cannot ensure that other sensitive tissues are not injured by the needle prior to reaching the target and does not allow for real time trajectory adjustment. The indirect technique can help target the tissue of interest but does not help steer the needle around sensitive tissues or confirm that the needle is being placed accurately. The indirect and direct out-of-plane approaches require less training and skill than the direct in-plane technique.

Pitfalls

Inexperienced sonographers inaccurately and preferentially focus attention on the US screen, and thus do not ascertain correct needle-transducer alignment (see Fig. 44.18). The needle and transducer should be aligned in two directions, including a "bird's eye view" and "shot gun view" before looking at the screen and advancing the needle. Subtle unintended motion of the transducer can result in loss of visualization of the needle and/or the target. It is critical that the transducer hand be anchored on the patient while viewing the intended target for the benefit of sonographer proprioception and to tether the transducer to the skin, avoiding unwanted motion and site contamination.

In the early stages of using US guidance, thinking in 3D space while looking at a 2D screen may be a challenge, resulting in inaccurate needle adjustments. This problem can be overcome by practicing needle manipulation under US guidance in model systems, such as firm tofu, gelatin cups, chicken, or other meat.

Needle visualization difficulties can stem from faulty beam angles. If a needle is lined up exactly with the transducer but the transducer is angled ("rocking") a few degrees off to one side, the needle will not be seen. It is best to point the transducer straight in/down (perpendicular to the skin) to avoid this potential problem.

If the needle angle into the tissues is greater than 45 degrees, sound beams may be reflected away from the transducer and reduce needle visualization (see Fig. 44.18). Several mechanisms exist to facilitate needle visualization for steep trajectory injections. Tissue motion can be used as a surrogate for the needle. Doppler can identify needle motion during advancement, regardless of the trajectory, and can accentuate medication flowing out of the needle tip (see Fig. 44.18). Special "echogenic" needles exist but are relatively expensive. An equally echogenic thicker gauge needle may be easier to align than a thinner needle. Finally, beam steering settings exist on many US machines that direct the sound waves toward the needle with the resulting echoes more likely to bounce back to the transducer.

Tissue invagination may occur when the needle contacts the synovial or tenosynovial lining surrounding an effusion and give a false appearance of needle penetration. A test injection with lidocaine will help verify accurate needle placement.

Minimizing the depth setting in some machines reduces the field of view at the edges, and can lead to difficulty finding the needle tip. The equipment should be tested to determine the depth setting at which the most lateral transducer edge is still visualized.

Accuracy

US guided knee injections are more accurate than those by palpation guidance (96% vs. 80%, respectively).[201] US guided acromioclavicular and GH joint injections are also superior to palpation guided.[202–204] For ankle injections, accuracy ranged from 58% to 100% for landmark guided, compared with 100% for US guided.[205]

Efficacy

There is good evidence that US guided injections are more efficacious than landmark guided injections.[206] A meta-analysis on randomized knee injection studies showed decreased pain scores (by 16%) 2 weeks after injection for the US versus landmark guided injections.[201] Comparing three studies of injection efficacy for pain after SAD bursa injections, the standard mean difference was 1.47 in favor of the US group.[202] Similarly, in a meta-analysis of four studies comparing the efficacy of corticosteroid injections for wrist joints, the mean visual analogue scale (VAS) pain reduction was 1.0 additional point for US compared with landmark guided injections.[207] In summary, US guided joint injections do seem to improve efficacy as well as accuracy, with the improvement in efficacy ranging around 20%.

Procedural Pain

Performance of US guided injections, especially those with the direct in-plane approach, can reduce procedural pain in a number of ways. First, the needle can be directed away from sensitive structures, like minor nerves and vessels that lie between the skin and the target structure. Second, the clinician injects local anesthetic before sensitive synovial membrane punctures. Third,

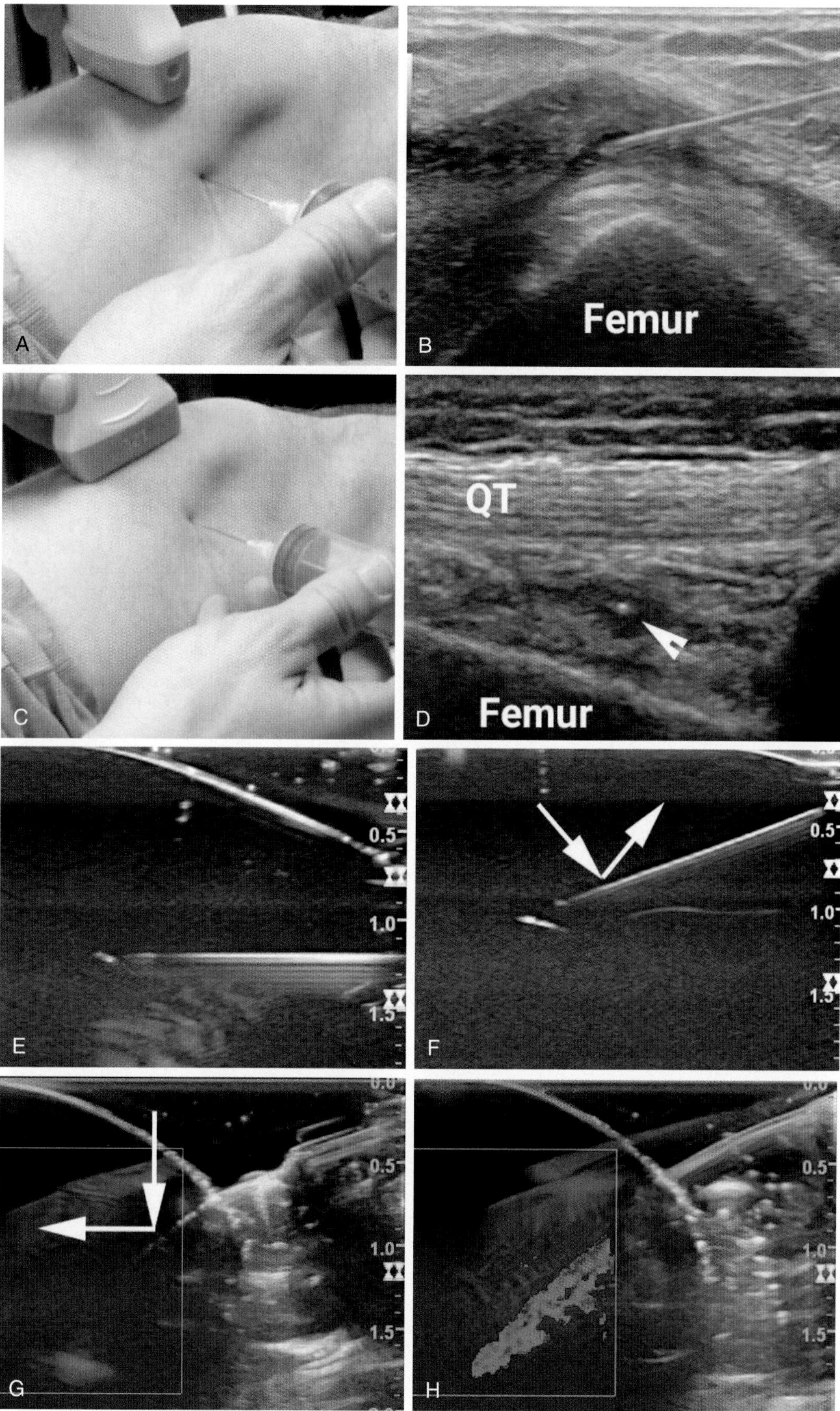

• **Fig. 44.18** Common injection techniques. The relationship between the needle and the transducer during direct in-plane needle guidance (A) and indirect out-of-plane needle guidance (C) with the resulting image of the long axis of a needle (B) and short axis of the needle *(arrowhead)* (D) entering the synovial cavity of the knee above the femur within the synovial cavity deep to the quadriceps tendon (QT) and superficial to the femur. (E-F) The needle parallel to the transducer is easily seen (E), while increasing needle angle of tissue penetration creates difficulties in visualizing the needle as the sound beams are reflected by the needle away from the transducer (G) (*arrows* represent sound direction), and employing beam steering (F) helps to fix this problem. (H) Doppler imaging can help visualize a needle that is inserted too steeply to be easily seen otherwise.

the needle can be passed through the synovial lining quickly and without "overshooting" into the back layer of synovium or into nearby bone. US guided procedural pain scores among three studies investigating this issue were 2.24 points lower than landmark guided procedures on a 10-point scale.[201]

The available literature regarding US guidance of needle placement for joint and soft tissue procedures has been evaluated by a number of societies. The American Medical Society for Sports Medicine issued a position statement stating that "ultrasound guided injections into inflamed or painful joints are more accurate, less painful, more efficacious, and less expensive than landmark guided injections."[206] Similarly, the ACR report on reasonable use of US stated that, "It is reasonable to use MSUS to guide articular and periarticular aspiration or injection at sites that include the synovial, tenosynovial, bursal, peritendinous, and perientheseal areas," with a grade A level of evidence.[10]

Conclusion

Imaging in rheumatic disease has undergone significant change in the past 2 decades. CR, once the cornerstone of diagnostic imaging, has been enhanced and in certain cases replaced by newer imaging modalities. A recent review of imaging in rheumatic disease summarized current literature for three common disease states.[208] In RA, both US and MRI are more sensitive than clinical examination to identify minimal synovitis, can predict progression to clinical RA in ACPA-positive patients, and can detect subclinical synovitis to predict flare. Both modalities may be used to predict treatment response and disease activity. In PsA, US can visualize the peripheral joints and entheses better than clinical examination, can show subclinical enthesitis and synovitis in patients with psoriasis but without arthritis, and can predict structural damage based on changes in synovitis or enthesitis after treatment. For OA, US does show characteristic changes but adds little at this time to the current clinical practice unless there is an atypical presentation or the diagnosis is in question.

Novel US applications are appearing frequently, and its use has expanded beyond the musculoskeletal system. US criteria inclusion into diagnostic and classification criteria is on the rise, and a critical mass of rheumatologists is being trained to utilize and harness the potential of this rapid, safe, inexpensive, and powerful imaging modality.

Full references for this chapter can be found on ExpertConsult.com.

Selected References

4. Thiele R: Ultrasonography applications in diagnosis and management of early rheumatoid arthritis, *Rheum Dis Clin N Am* 38:259–275, 2012.
8. Cannella A, Kissen E, Torralba K, et al.: Evolution of musculoskeletal ultrasound in the United States: implementation and practice in rheumatology, *Arthritis Care Res* 66:7–13, 2014.
9. Klauser A, Tagliafico A, Allen G, et al.: Clinical indications for musculoskeletal ultrasound: a Delphi-based consensus paper of the European Society of Musculoskeletal Radiology, *Eur Radiol* 22:1140–1148, 2012.
10. McAlindon T, Kissin E, Nazarian L, et al.: American College of Rheumatology report on reasonable use of musculoskeletal ultrasonography in rheumatology clinical practice, *Arthritis Care Res* 64:1625–1640, 2012.
11. Naredo E, Bijlsma J: Becoming a musculoskeletal ultrasonographer, *Best Prac Res Clin Rheum* 23:257–267, 2009.
22. Smith J, Finnoff JT: Diagnostic and interventional musculoskeletal ultrasound: part 2. Clinical applications. *PM R* 1:162–177, 2009.
23. Smith J, Finnoff JT: Diagnostic and interventional musculoskeletal ultrasound: part 1. Fundamentals. *PM R* 1:64–75, 2009.
24. Brull R, Macfarlane AJ, Tse CC: Practical knobology for ultrasound-guided regional anesthesia, *Reg Anesth Pain Med* 35:S68–S73, 2010.
27. Taljanovic MS, Melville DM, Scalcione LR, et al.: Artifacts in musculoskeletal ultrasonography, *Semin Musculoskelet Radiol* 18:3–11, 2014.
28. Wakefield R, Balint P, Szkudlarek M, et al.: Musculoskeletal ultrasound including definitions for ultrasonographic pathology, *J Rheumatol* 32:2485–2487, 2005.
29. Bruyn GA, Iagnocco A, Naredo E, et al.: OMERACT definitions for ultrasonographic pathology and elementary lesions of rheumatic disorders fifteen years on, *J Rheumatol* 46:1388–1393, 2019.
35. Ji L, Deng X, Geng Y, et al.: The additional benefit of ultrasonography to 2010 ACR/EULAR classification criteria when diagnosing rheumatoid arthritis in the absence of anti-cyclic citrullinated peptide antibodies, *Clini Rheumatol* 36:261–267, 2017.
44. Macchioni P, Boiardi L, Catanoso M, et al.: Performance of the new 202 EULAR/ACR classification criteria for polymyalgia rheumatica: comparison with the previous criteria in a single-centre study, *Ann Rheum Dis* 73:1190–1193, 2014.
48. Iagnocco A, Naredo E, Wakefield R, et al.: Responsiveness in rheumatoid arthritis. A report from the OMERACT 11 ultrasound workshop, *J Rheumatol* 41:379–382, 2014.
60. Brown AK, Conaghan PG, Karim Z, et al.: An explanation for the apparent dissociation between clinical remission and continued structural deterioration in rheumatoid arthritis, *Arthritis Rheum* 58:2958–2967, 2008.
62. Kawashiri SY, Suzuki T, Nakashima Y, et al.: Ultrasonographic examination of rheumatoid arthritis patients who are free of physical synovitis: power Doppler subclinical synovitis is associated with bone erosion, *Rheumatology (Oxford)* 53:562–569, 2014.
65. Nguyen H, Ruyssen-Witrand A, Gandjbakhch F, et al.: Prevalence of ultrasound-detected residual synovitis and risk of relapse and structural progression in rheumatoid arthritis patients in clinical remission: a systematic review and meta-analysis, *Rheumatology (Oxford)* 53:2110–2118, 2014.
74. Sakellariou G, Conaghan PG, Zhang W, et al.: EULAR recommendations for the use of imaging in the clinical management of peripheral joint osteoarthritis, *Ann Rheum Dis* 76:1484–1494, 2017.
77. Grassi W, Meenagh G, Pascual E, et al.: "Crystal clear"-sonographic assessment of gout and calcium pyrophosphate deposition disease, *Semin Arthritis Rheum* 36:197–202, 2006.
79. Grassi W, Okano T, Filippucci E: Use of ultrasound for diagnosis and monitoring of outcomes in crystal arthropathies, *Curr Opin Rheumatol* 27:147–155, 2015.
82. Naredo E, Uson J, Jimenez-Palop M, et al.: Ultrasound-detected musculoskeletal urate crystal deposition: which joints and what findings should be assessed for diagnosing gout? *Ann Rheum Dis* 73:1522–1528, 2014.
83. Terslev L, Gutierrez M, Schmidt WA, et al.: Ultrasound as an outcome measure in gout. A validation process by the OMERACT Ultrasound Working Group, *J Rheumatol* 42:2177–2181, 2015.
85. Neogi T, Jansen TL, Dalbeth N, et al.: 2015 gout classification criteria: an American College of Rheumatology/European League Against Rheumatism collaborative initiative, *Ann Rheum Dis* 74:1789–1798, 2015.
86. Durcan L, Grainger R, Keen HI, et al.: Imaging as a potential outcome measure in gout studies: a systematic literature review, *Semin Arthritis Rheum* 45:570–579, 2016.
90. Filippou G, Adinolfi A, Iagnocco A, et al.: Ultrasound in the diagnosis of calcium pyrophosphate dihydrate deposition disease. A systematic literature review and a meta-analysis, *Osteoarthritis Cartilage* 24:973–981, 2016.

91. Zhang W, Doherty M, Bardin T, et al.: European League against Rheumatism recommendations for calcium pyrophosphate deposition. Part I: terminology and diagnosis, *Ann Rheum Dis* 70:563–570, 2011.
93. Filippou G, Scire CA, Adinolfi A, et al.: Identification of calcium pyrophosphate deposition disease (CPPD) by ultrasound: reliability of the OMERACT definitions in an extended set of joints-an international multiobserver study by the OMERACT Calcium Pyrophosphate Deposition Disease Ultrasound Subtask Force, *Ann Rheum Dis* 77:1194–1199, 2018.
97. Balint PV, Terslev L, Aegerter P, et al.: Reliability of a consensus-based ultrasound definition and scoring for enthesitis in spondyloarthritis and psoriatic arthritis: an OMERACT US initiative, *Ann Rheum Dis* 77:1730–1735, 2018.
102. Gutierrez M, Filippucci E, Salaffi F, et al.: Differential diagnosis between rheumatoid arthritis and psoriatic arthritis: the value of ultrasound findings at metacarpophalangeal joints level, *Ann Rheum Dis* 70:1111–1114, 2011.
106. Yumusakhuylu Y, Kasapoglu-Gunal E, Murat S, et al.: A preliminary study showing that ultrasonography cannot differentiate between psoriatic arthritis and nodal osteoarthritis based on enthesopathy scores, *Rheumatology (Oxford)* 55:1703–1704, 2016.
110. Tinazzi I, McGonagle D, Biasi D, et al.: Preliminary evidence that subclinical enthesopathy may predict psoriatic arthritis in patients with psoriasis, *J Rheumatol* 38:2691–2692, 2011.
113. Iagnocco A, Finucci A, Ceccarelli F, et al.: Musculoskeletal ultrasound in the evaluation of polymyalgia rheumatica, *Med Ultrason* 17:361–366, 2015.
117. Dasgupta B, Cimmino MA, Kremers HM, et al.: 2012 Provisional classification criteria for polymyalgia rheumatica: a European League Against Rheumatism/American College of Rheumatology collaborative initiative, *Arthritis Rheum* 64:943–954, 2012.
121. Schmidt WA, Kraft HE, Vorpahl K, et al.: Color duplex ultrasonography in the diagnosis of temporal arteritis, *N Engl J Med* 337:1336–1342, 1997.
122. Dejaco C, Ramiro S, Duftner C, et al.: EULAR recommendations for the use of imaging in large vessel vasculitis in clinical practice, *Ann Rheum Dis* 77:636–643, 2018.
124. Monti S, Floris A, Ponte C, et al.: The use of ultrasound to assess giant cell arteritis: review of the current evidence and practical guide for the rheumatologist, *Rheumatology (Oxford)* 57:227–235, 2018.
125. Schmidt WA: Ultrasound in the diagnosis and management of giant cell arteritis, *Rheumatology (Oxford)* 57:ii22–ii31, 2018.
129. Aschwanden M, Imfeld S, Staub D, et al.: The ultrasound compression sign to diagnose temporal giant cell arteritis shows an excellent interobserver agreement, *Clin Exp Rheumatol* 33:S-113–S-115, 2015.
131. Diamantopoulos AP, Haugeberg G, Hetland H, et al.: Diagnostic value of color Doppler ultrasonography of temporal arteries and large vessels in giant cell arteritis: a consecutive case series, *Arthritis Care Res* 66:113–119, 2014.
132. Diamantopoulos AP, Haugeberg G, Lindland A, et al.: The fast-track ultrasound clinic for early diagnosis of giant cell arteritis significantly reduces permanent visual impairment: towards a more effective strategy to improve clinical outcome in giant cell arteritis? *Rheumatology (Oxford)* 55:66–70, 2016.
138. Luciano N, Ferro F, Bombardieri S, et al.: Advances in salivary gland ultrasonography in primary Sjogren's syndrome, *Clin Exp Rheumatol* 36(Suppl 114):159–164, 2018.
140. Martire MV, Santiago ML, Cazenave T, et al.: Latest advances in ultrasound assessment of salivary glands in Sjogren syndrome, *J Clin Rheumatol* 24:218–223, 2018.
141. Dejaco C, De Zordo T, Heber D, et al.: Real-time sonoelastography of salivary glands for diagnosis and functional assessment of primary Sjogren's syndrome, *Ultrasound Med Biol* 40:2759–2767, 2014.
142. Cornec D, Jousse-Joulin S, Pers JO, et al.: Contribution of salivary gland ultrasonography to the diagnosis of Sjogren's syndrome: toward new diagnostic criteria? *Arthritis Rheum* 65:216–225, 2013.
144. Damjanov N, Milic V, Nieto-Gonzalez JC, et al.: Multiobserver reliability of ultrasound assessment of salivary glands in patients with established primary Sjogren syndrome, *J Rheumatol* 43:1858–1863, 2016.
145. Jousse-Joulin S, Milic V, Jonsson MV, et al.: Is salivary gland ultrasonography a useful tool in Sjogren's syndrome? A systematic review, *Rheumatology (Oxford)* 55:789–800, 2016.
155. Fisher BA, Everett CC, Rout J, et al.: Effect of rituximab on a salivary gland ultrasound score in primary Sjogren's syndrome: results of the TRACTISS randomised double-blind multicentre substudy, *Ann Rheum Dis* 77:412–416, 2018.
164. Kissin EY, Schiller AM, Gelbard RB, et al.: Durometry for the assessment of skin disease in systemic sclerosis, *Arthritis Rheum* 55:603–609, 2006.
167. Elhai M, Guerini H, Bazeli R, et al.: Ultrasonographic hand features in systemic sclerosis and correlates with clinical, biologic, and radiographic findings, *Arthritis Care Res* 64:1244–1249, 2012.
169. Cuomo G, Zappia M, Abignano G, et al.: Ultrasonographic features of the hand and wrist in systemic sclerosis, *Rheumatology (Oxford)* 48:1414–1417, 2009.
171. Vizioli L, Ciccarese F, Forti P, et al.: Integrated use of lung ultrasound and chest x-ray in the detection of interstitial lung disease, *Respiration* 93:15–22, 2017.
173. Kissin EY, Garg A, Grayson PC, et al.: Ultrasound assessment of subcutaneous compressibility: a potential adjunctive diagnostic tool in eosinophilic fasciitis, *J Clin Rheumatol* 19:382–385, 2013.
175. Fowler JR, Gaughan JP, Ilyas AM: The sensitivity and specificity of ultrasound for the diagnosis of carpal tunnel syndrome: a meta-analysis, *Clin Orthop Relat Res* 469:1089–1094, 2011.
178. Descatha A, Huard L, Aubert F, et al.: Meta-analysis on the performance of sonography for the diagnosis of carpal tunnel syndrome, *Semin Arthritis Rheum* 41:914–922, 2012.
179. Torres-Costoso A, Martinez-Vizcaino V, Alvarez-Bueno C, et al.: Accuracy of ultrasonography for the diagnosis of carpal tunnel syndrome: a systematic review and meta-analysis, *Arch Phys Med Rehabil* 99:758–765.e10, 2018.
182. Chang KV, Wu WT, Han DS, et al.: Ulnar nerve cross-sectional area for the diagnosis of cubital tunnel syndrome: a meta-analysis of ultrasonographic measurements, *Arch Phys Med Rehabil* 99:743–757, 2018.
184. Strakowski JA: Ultrasound-guided peripheral nerve procedures, *Phys Med Rehabil Clin N Am* 27:687–715, 2016.
185. Roy JS, Braen C, Leblond J, et al.: Diagnostic accuracy of ultrasonography, MRI and MR arthrography in the characterisation of rotator cuff disorders: a systematic review and meta-analysis, *Br J Sports Med* 49:1316–1328, 2015.
186. Merolla G, Singh S, Paladini P, et al.: Calcific tendinitis of the rotator cuff: state of the art in diagnosis and treatment, *J Orthop Traumatolo* 17:7–14, 2016.
190. Radwan A, Wyland M, Applequist L, et al.: Ultrasonography, an effective tool in diagnosing plantar fasciitis: a systematic review of diagnostic trials, *Int J Sports Phys Ther* 11:663–671, 2016.
191. Bruyn GA, Naredo E, Iagnocco A, et al.: The OMERACT ultrasound Working Group 10 years on: update at OMERACT 12, *J Rheumatol* 42:2172–2176, 2015.
192. Roth J, Jousse-Joulin S, Magni-Manzoni S, et al.: Definitions for the sonographic features of joints in healthy children, *Arthritis Care Res* 67:136–142, 2015.
193. Collado P, Windschall D, Vojinovic J, et al.: Amendment of the OMERACT ultrasound definitions of joints' features in healthy children when using the Doppler technique, *Pediatr Rheumatol Online J* 16:23, 2018.
194. Collado P, Vojinovic J, Nieto JC, et al.: Toward standardized musculoskeletal ultrasound in pediatric rheumatology: normal age-related ultrasound findings, *Arthritis Care Res* 68:348–356, 2016.

196. Roth J, Ravagnani V, Backhaus M, et al.: Preliminary definitions for the sonographic features of synovitis in children, *Arthritis Care Res* 69:1217–1223, 2017.
201. Wu T, Dong Y, Song H, et al.: Ultrasound-guided versus landmark in knee arthrocentesis: a systematic review, *Semin Arthritis Rheum* 45:627–632, 2016.
206. Finnoff JT, Hall MM, Adams E, et al. American Medical Society for Sports Medicine (AMSSM) position statement: interventional musculoskeletal ultrasound in sports medicine. *PM R* 7:151–168.e2, 2015.
207. Dubreuil M, Greger S, LaValley M, et al.: Improvement in wrist pain with ultrasound-guided glucocorticoid injections: a meta-analysis of individual patient data, *Semin Arthritis Rheum* 42:492–497, 2013.

45

Evaluation of Monoarticular and Polyarticular Arthritis

RONALD F. VAN VOLLENHOVEN

KEY POINTS

The differential diagnosis of arthritis is extensive.

Diagnosing arthritis depends on an accurate medical history, a thorough physical examination, and appropriately chosen laboratory and imaging investigations.

The cause of arthritis may be revealed by associated symptoms and signs in other organ systems.

In acute monoarthritis, synovial fluid analysis is the most valuable laboratory test.

Laboratory testing and imaging, when used correctly, can lead to rapid diagnostic certainty in many cases.

An early (presumptive) diagnosis and appropriate management will contribute to better outcomes.

"For the physician, it is essential to recognize what diseases are and whence they come; which are long and which are short; which are in the process of changing into others; which are major and which are minor."

HIPPOCRATES

Introduction

Diagnosing patients with musculoskeletal symptoms remains one of the rheumatologist's core responsibilities. Although in the general field of medicine significant advances have been made by using sophisticated laboratory analyses and imaging modalities, in rheumatology making correct diagnoses remains as much an art as a science, today as in the days of Hippocrates. In case of a monoarticular presentation with a serious consideration of infectious (septic) arthritis, evaluation is urgent to prevent permanent joint damage. But even for patients with polyarthritis, a purposeful and expeditious diagnostic workup has gained in importance as the benefits of early intervention have been identified for some specific diagnoses, most notably rheumatoid arthritis (RA).

This chapter will review the current state of the art of diagnosing mono- and polyarthritis in adults (the evaluation of children with joint symptoms is discussed in Chapter 113), with special reference to the proper use of laboratory testing and imaging but without detracting from the central role of a detailed history and a thorough physical examination.

Approach to the Patient With Arthritis

Monoarthritis Versus Oligo- and Polyarthritis

In practice, the approach to the patient presenting with signs of inflammation in a single joint, monoarthritis, is often quite different from the approach taken when several joints are inflamed simultaneously (oligo- or polyarthritis). This is particularly true in the acute care setting where the consideration of infectious (septic) arthritis is paramount: a delay in diagnosis and treatment can lead to severe consequences for the patient: a prolonged disease course, irreversible damage to the joint, other morbidities, and even mortality. Thus, the sudden onset of monoarthritis in a synovial joint is a significant clinical event, and each case of monoarthritis requires immediate investigation and treatment to limit pain and prevent joint destruction. For this reason, and because the initial differentiation between inflammation versus injury may at times be unclear, the care responsibility for patients with monoarthritis may be organized differently from the care for those with multiple inflamed joints. For example, the former patients may be triaged primarily to orthopedic urgent care and the latter to medical urgent care. Nonetheless, the distinctions are not absolute. An acute monoarthritis can be the first manifestation of a systemic rheumatologic disease, while an oligo- or polyarthritis may on rare occasions be septic. In the following, the differential diagnosis will therefore be discussed simultaneously for mono-, oligo-, and polyarthritis, pointing out how the likelihood of each possible diagnosis is influenced by the presentation.

History

Obtaining a thorough history remains a *sine qua non* for diagnosis, even in the age of high-tech investigations. The "seven dimensions" of the history of present illness as encountered in documentation guidelines—location, quality, quantity, duration, context, modifying factors, and associations—all provide clues to the diagnosis. The location of the symptoms makes it clear whether we are dealing with a monoarticular, oligoarticular, or polyarticular disease, but patients may sometimes focus on just one particularly bothersome joint even though additional joints are inflamed.

The quality of the symptoms may provide some information; for example, pain associated with persistent morning stiffness is a notable feature of inflammation, whereas the gel phenomenon—a more short-lived stiffness when first starting to move—is typical of osteoarthritis (OA). Obviously, it is important to ascertain the severity of the symptoms. Asking the patient about the duration of symptoms, how they first started, how they fluctuate during the day, and what (s)he has done to find relief will come quite naturally. It may be less intuitive, but at least as important, to ask specifically about other symptoms, including fever and weight loss, gastrointestinal symptoms, skin rashes and mucosal lesions, ophthalmologic issues, and urogenital symptoms. The probable cause of the arthritis frequently becomes obvious after associated features that the patient often does not believe are important have been elicited by the clinician. Likewise, one must investigate risk factors for infectious causes of arthritis, such as possible exposures to pathogenic organisms, risk of sexually acquired infections, and recent travel to tropical countries or to areas where Lyme disease is endemic. Routinely inquiring about these types of exposures minimizes the risk of missing an important clue. Many clinicians now use a standardized form to collect this information in advance of the patient encounter.

Physical Examination

Rheumatologists take pride in their ability to detect inflammation by simple clinical means, but they must hone this skill continuously. An inflamed joint is typically swollen, and upon palpation the swelling is soft rather than hard. Synovial swelling may be quite obvious in some cases but is harder to establish in others. Even experienced joint assessors will not always agree where to draw the line between swollen and not swollen. In one study, six rheumatologists achieved complete agreement in only about 70% of cases,[1] and other studies have also highlighted the lack of complete agreement between experienced specialists. Fortunately, one such study also showed that specific training improves consistency.[2] Because it may not be in the patient's interest to define joints as swollen in borderline cases, I generally teach my fellows to be restrained in assessing joint swelling. One study suggested that the "squeeze test"—that is, pain on lateral compression of the metacarpophalangeal (MCP) or metatarsophalangeal joints—was more specific than other tests for arthritis, but a recent study found a low sensitivity for this test.[3,4]

In addition to swelling ("tumor") and tenderness ("dolor"), inflamed joints may exhibit other classic signs of inflammation. Redness ("rubor") is frequently seen over joints that are affected by highly acute inflammation, such as septic arthritis or gout, but is seen only rarely in RA and other autoimmune inflammations. Warmth ("calor") is more confidently assessed in larger than in smaller joints but may be a useful clue, especially in the knees, where the normal temperature gradient—with the knee being slightly cooler than the proximal musculature—may be reversed. Finally, impaired function is an almost universal finding in inflamed joints, and here it is important to distinguish between true limitations in range of motion (contractures) and limitations solely caused by pain.

The proper technique for examining joint swelling has been a matter of some discussion. The European League Against Rheumatism (EULAR) has published a set of recommendations for examining the joints, along with instructional images; its handbook may serve as a good starting point for learning joint examination or for achieving standardization across different sites. Inflamed large joints often have palpable effusions, and in the knee the signs of "fluid wave" and "ballottement" can be elicited in the case of moderate or large effusions. In the initial workup of the patient with polyarthritis, a detailed examination and documentation of the individual inflamed joints, including those in the feet, will be necessary to document the range of movement (predictably decreased in the inflamed joint) or early anatomic changes. Moreover, when first evaluating a patient, a full joint examination must be performed, whereas for follow-up purposes a more limited but standardized joint examination is recommended. For patients with polyarthritis it may be practical to use the standardized 28-joint count, where the MCP and proximal interphalangeal (PIP) joints of both hands, the wrist, elbows, shoulders, and knees are examined.[5] It is good practice to document such a standardized joint examination in the medical record for most visits. The more extensive 44-joint count and the even more comprehensive systematic joint count based on 68 joints are rarely used in practice for long-term follow-up of patients with arthritis.

Perhaps the two most useful pieces of information gained from the physical examination of the affected joints are the nature of the swelling (assuming swelling is present) and the pattern of joint involvement. Synovial inflammation is palpated as a soft, doughy swelling around the joint line, obstructing the possibility of feeling the two apposed bony edges. In contrast, hypertrophy emanating from these bony edges, such as occurs in OA, is palpated as a hard structure. Patterns of joint involvement that are easily recognized and usually point at the correct diagnosis are the symmetric involvement of wrists, MCP and PIP joints of the hands, and the corresponding joints in the feet, suggesting RA; the asymmetric involvement of predominantly the lower extremity larger joints in reactive arthritis and spondyloarthritis (SpA); and involvement of multiple distal interphalangeal (DIP) joints in OA but also in some patients with psoriatic arthritis (PsA), who may also have prominent nail changes. The typical pattern of joint involvement in various conditions is summarized in Table 45.1. The important distinction between RA and OA is further illustrated in Fig. 45.1.

The spine must be examined, even if no symptoms are reported, in order to detect early signs of axial involvement in SpA. Deep palpation of the large muscle groups around the shoulders and hips sometimes reveals exquisite tenderness, which, together with the patient's age of 50 years or older and a high erythrocyte sedimentation rate (ESR), might suggest a diagnosis of polymyalgia rheumatica (PMR), in which case some peripheral joint arthritis also may be present.

Furthermore, a general examination should be performed with special attention to the skin and integuments (psoriasis and nail pitting in PsA), mucous membranes (ulcers in reactive arthritis, Behçet's disease, or systemic lupus erythematosus [SLE]), lymph glands, salivary glands, thyroid, heart, lungs, eyes, and other organs based on specific suspicion.

Laboratory Investigation

After a comprehensive history and physical examination, a laboratory workup will most likely be needed. Although some tests can be ordered "routinely," clearly many tests should be ordered on the basis of the possible differential diagnosis at this stage, at which time most often the possibilities already have been narrowed down considerably.

Inflammation can be reflected by several routine measures, including leukocytosis and neutrophilia, normocytic anemia ("of chronic disease"), and thrombocytosis. The latter in particular may be a strong indicator of systemic inflammation of significant duration and severity. Systemic disease involvement is assessed by renal, liver, muscle, or bone biochemical screening and protein electrophoresis. Raised uric acid levels suggest a diagnosis of gout. In acute hemarthrosis, a platelet count, international normalized ratio (INR), and clotting studies are warranted. The ESR is typically elevated in patients with inflammation, although it lacks specificity or sensitivity for any single diagnosis, and the same applies to the C-reactive protein (CRP). A normal ESR or CRP argues against infectious causes but does not preclude a rheumatologic diagnosis, whereas extremely high ESR or CRP values should trigger suspicion of a more serious disease underlying the arthritis.

Blood cultures are mandatory in patients with suspected septic arthritis and should precede antibiotic prescription. Testing for

TABLE 45.1 Typical Distribution of Joint Involvement in Common Forms of Polyarthritis

	Rheumatoid Arthritis	Osteoarthritis	Psoriatic Arthritis	Gout/Pseudogout
Large weight-bearing joints	Knees and ankles, usually symmetric; hips rarely	Hips, knees, ankles	Knees and ankles, usually asymmetric	Knees and ankles; wrists in pseudogout
Small joints	MCP and PIP joints in the hands; MTP joints in the feet	DIP, PIP, and first CMC joints in the hands; first MTP joint in the feet	Frequently DIP joints along with nail involvement; other small joints	Small joints of the feet; MCP joints in pseudogout
Spine	Cervical spine	Cervical spine and LS spine	LS spine and SI joints	No

CMC, Carpometacarpal; *DIP*, distal interphalangeal; *LS*, lumbo-sacral; *MCP*, metacarpophalangeal; *MTP*, metatarsophalangeal; *PIP*, proximal interphalangeal; *SI*, sacroiliac.

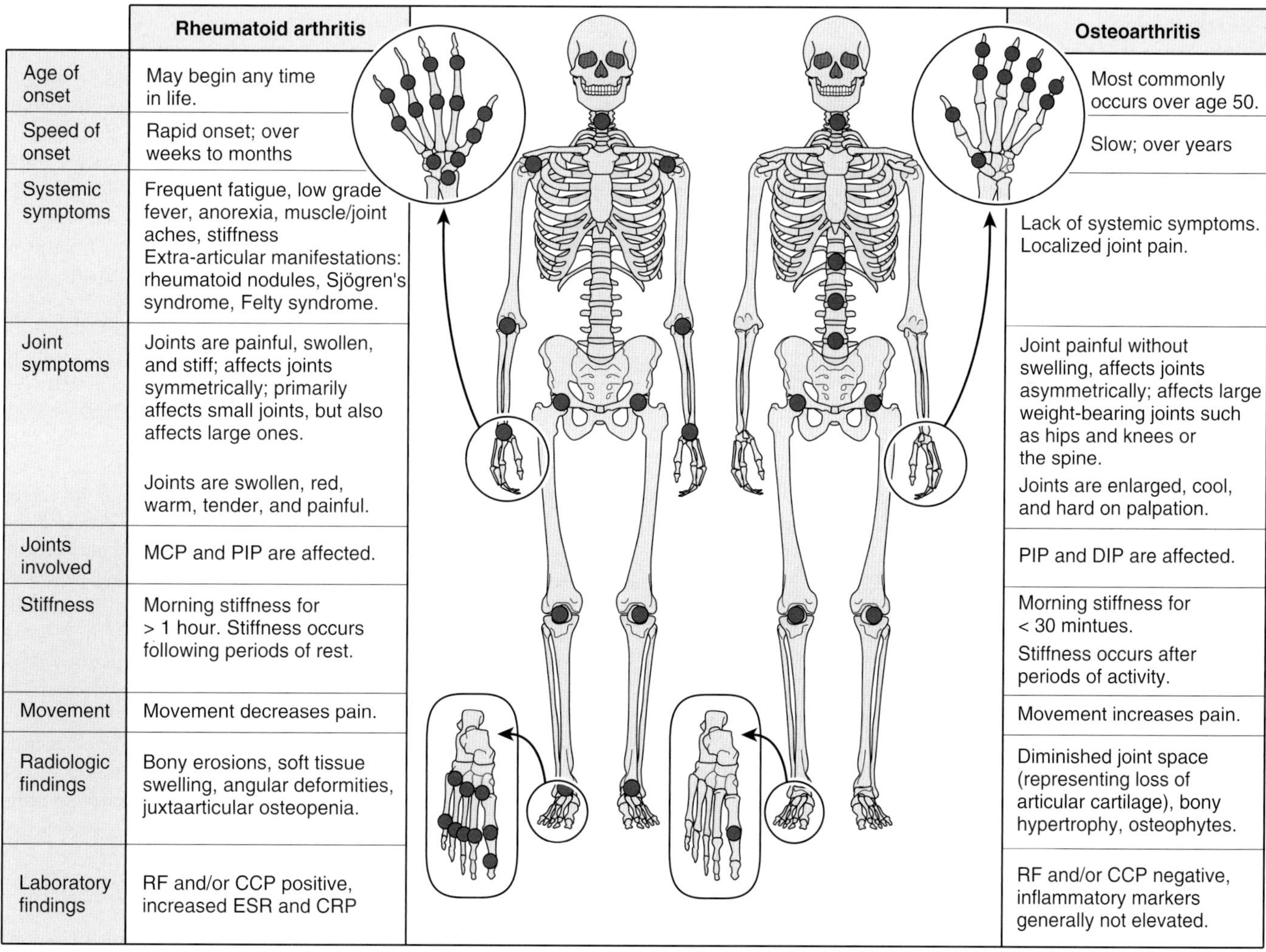

• **Fig. 45.1** The typical distribution of joint involvement in rheumatoid arthritis and osteoarthritis. Hips can be involved in late rheumatoid arthritis as well. *CCP*, Cyclic citrullinated peptide; *CRP*, C-reactive protein; *DIP*, distal interphalangeal; *ESR*, erythrocyte sedimentation rate; *MCP*, metacarpophalangeal; *PIP*, proximal interphalangeal; *RF*, rheumatoid factor. (From O'Dell JR. Rheumatoid arthritis: the clinical picture. In: Koopman WJ, ed. Arthritis and Allied Conditions: A Textbook of Rheumatology, 14th ed. Philadelphia: Lippincott Williams & Wilkins, 2001 p. 1154.)

specific infectious causes of polyarthritis can and should also be performed on the basis of clinical suspicion and only in relevant situations. This could in appropriate situations include testing for hepatitis virus, HIV, and various other viruses (IgG and IgM antibodies) the antistreptolysin-O test (ASOT), and serologic testing for Lyme disease or for enteric and urogenital pathogens.

Serologic autoantibody testing is one of the rheumatologist's most treasured domains. The demonstration of rheumatoid factors (IgM antibodies binding to IgG; RF) in the 1940s was one of the first indications that RA was an autoimmune disease,[6,7] a concept considered inadmissible for many decades. RFs are indeed commonly seen in RA but are not more than 60% to 70% sensitive, and in the setting of an undiagnosed polyarthritis, the test must be interpreted with caution because several viral and bacterial infections can cause polyarthritis with a positive RF, including parvovirus and hepatitis B and C. Moreover, RF can be positive in a wide range of rheumatologic diseases—not only RA but also Sjögren's syndrome, scleroderma, SLE, and vasculitis, for example. Nonetheless, in an early undifferentiated arthritis clinic, the presence of RF conferred a considerably increased risk of the development of persistent disease and radiologic damage.[8–12] In other words, although RF is useful in the diagnostic process, it must not be relied upon blindly; and once the diagnosis of RA is established, the presence of RF suggests a worse prognosis.

More recently, it has become standard to test for antibodies against citrullinated proteins using an assay based on cyclic citrullinated peptides (CCPs). The test is therefore often called the anti-CCP test, but the antibodies that are detected are more properly called anti-citrullinated protein antibodies (ACPA) because the CCP is a laboratory construct that does not exist in nature. Regardless, anti-CCP or ACPA are about equally sensitive for RA as RF but are much more specific.[11,13] Combined testing for RF and ACPA is the current standard for evaluating a patient with polyarthritis when RA is a possible diagnosis, and the specificity of the combined positivity was indeed 100% in one study, although of course the sensitivity was reduced.[13]

Other serologic tests can be useful in the evaluation of the patient with polyarthritis but must be interpreted with even greater caution. Anti-nuclear antibodies (ANAs) are positive in many autoimmune diseases, as well as in various infections, malignancies, drug-induced conditions, and so on. When ANAs are tested by immunofluorescence on human cell lines, they can be helpful in that a negative test provides a strong argument against a diagnosis of SLE, whereas a positive test will allow further testing for more specific autoantibodies (but does not prove that the patient has any particular disease). ANA by enzyme-linked immunosorbent assay (ELISA) methods may have more false-negative results. Antibodies against extractable nuclear antigens (ENAs) can point in the direction of various systemic inflammatory diseases, whereas anti-Ro/La (SS-A/SS-B) will point to Sjögren's syndrome, and anti-neutrophil cytoplasmic antibodies (ANCA) will point to systemic vasculitis. Other relevant blood tests may include thyroid function tests, ferritin, angiotensin-converting enzyme, and vitamin D levels.

Urine

The urinary tract can be a source of Gram-negative bacteria in septic arthritis in the elderly. Significant proteinuria and/or hematuria and red cell casts indicate renal damage in SLE, vasculitis, or subacute bacterial endocarditis.

Genetic Testing

The HLA-B27 gene marker is found in approximately 3% to 8% of the population, but it is found in more than 90% of patients with ankylosing spondylitis and in 50% to 80% of patients with other SpAs. Some say that the HLA-B27 test is not useful because of the prevalence of this gene marker in healthy people, but this argument does not do justice to the subtle "probabilistic" process of diagnosis; in the right clinical setting, a positive HLA-B27 test can raise the diagnostic likelihood from modest to high. Moreover, the HLA-B27 test only needs to be performed once over the lifetime of the patient, making it a rather cost-effective way to obtain an additional diagnostic clue.

Few other genetic tests have become useful in rheumatology practice. Determining whether the patient has the "shared epitope" (a constellation of HLA-DR genes that confer an elevated risk for RA) is not yet part of standard care. The *HFE* gene is linked to hereditary hemochromatosis and can be performed in the right clinical setting. Rare genetic disorders are associated with fever syndromes or vasculitis-mimickers where arthritis is part of the clinical picture. Without a doubt the list of such diseases will increase in the future.

Synovial Fluid Analysis

If at all possible, synovial fluid should be obtained and analyzed in the initial workup of arthritis, and even more so in acute presentations and/or in monoarthritis. The fluid should be analyzed for color and cloudiness (Table 45.2). Microscopy should be used to characterize the predominant cells. Crystal arthritis can be definitively diagnosed by using polarized light analysis to demonstrate intra-cellular crystals of uric acid or calcium pyrophosphate dihydrate (CPPD), although the latter can be difficult to detect. Identification of bacteria following synovial fluid culture can provide results even when a Gram stain is negative. *Neisseria* organisms are fastidious with low yields from culture, but PCR can detect *Neisseria*-specific DNA.

Most rheumatologists measure synovial fluid white cell counts, which may help differentiate inflammatory from non-inflammatory presentations but does not reliably differentiate between inflammation and infection. Thus, the fluid from an inflamed but aseptic joint typically is yellow and turbid and contains 5000 to 50,000 white cells/mm^3, mostly neutrophils. Higher leukocyte counts suggest bacterial infection but may also occur in crystal diseases, whereas lower counts would be expected in degenerative diseases. Low synovial fluid glucose and high lactate and procalcitonin are found in septic arthritis, but evidence that these can distinguish infectious from inflammatory arthritis in a clinically meaningful way is limited. Bacterial identification in synovial fluid from patients with septic arthritis can be inhibited by prior antibiotic use, and hence a careful medication history should be elicited.

The presence of large amounts of blood in the synovial fluid (hemarthrosis) suggests trauma or, more rarely, inherited/acquired clotting abnormalities, intra-articular hemangiomas, or pigmented villonodular synovitis (PVNS).

Imaging and Additional Diagnostic Procedures

Although conventional radiography is not often the key to making a diagnosis in the patient with arthritis, ordering radiographs of affected joints may nonetheless be useful. Plain radiographs identify soft tissue swelling, calcium in periarticular tissues, fractures, local bone disease, and loose bodies, as well as destructive changes

TABLE 45.2 Synovial Fluid Characteristics in Clinical Situations, With Imaging and Investigation Techniques to Identify the Cause

Diagnosis	Cells	Microorganisms	Appearance	Imaging Modality	Comments
Bacterial arthritis	Neutrophils, 10,000->100,000	Gram stain usually positive	Turbid/pus	May need ultrasound to aspirate dryness	Systemic symptoms, Gram stain, blood and synovial fluid culture
Gonococcal arthritis	Neutrophils, 10,000-100,000	Gram stain usually positive	Turbid/pus	May need ultrasound to aspirate dryness	Systemic symptoms, Gram stain, blood and synovial fluid culture
Crystal arthritis	Neutrophils, 10,000->100,000	—	Turbid/pus	Radiographs, CPPD	Presence of appropriate crystals Acute serum urate unreliable
Tuberculous arthritis	Mononuclear 5000-50,000	Acid-fast stain often negative, may need to culture synovial tissue	Turbid/pus		At-risk population; Ziehl-Neelsen stain biopsy may be necessary
Inflammatory monoarthropathies	Neutrophils 5000-50,000	—	Slightly turbid	Ultrasound/MRI for early synovitis and erosions	Serum autoantibodies such as RF, ACPA, ANA
Osteoarthritis	Mononuclear 0-2000	—	Clear	Radiographic changes	Usually non-inflammatory CPPD may be present
Internal derangement	Red blood cells	—	Clear/turbid	MRI	Arthroscopy may be necessary
Trauma	Red blood cells	—	Clear/turbid	Radiographs	Tc bone scan may aid diagnosis if radiograph normal
Ischemic necrosis		—		MRI in early disease	XR abnormal only in advanced cases
Uncommon Causes					
Sarcoidosis	Mononuclear, 5000-20,000	—		CXR	
PVNS	Red blood cells	—	Turbid	Ultrasound and MRI	Synovial biopsy essential
Charcot's	Mononuclear, 0-2000	—		Radiographs	CPPD may be present
Lyme disease	Neutrophils, 0-5000	—	Clear/turbid		SF eosinophilia may be found Serology for *Borrelia*
Amyloid	Mononuclear, 2000-10,000	—	Turbid		Synovial biopsy for Congo red stain

ACPA, Anti-citrullinated protein antibody; *ANA*, anti-nuclear antibody; *CPPD*, calcium pyrophosphate dehydrate deposition; *CXR*, chest radiograph; *PVNS*, pigmented villonodular synovitis; *RF*, rheumatoid factor; *SF*, synovial fluid; *Tc*, technetium; *XR*, radiograph.

in long-standing arthritides. Such findings provide diagnostic clues and, in addition, radiographs may provide an indication of the severity of inflammation (juxta-articular osteopenia) and form a baseline for future evaluation. In some cases they may establish the diagnosis, such as when typical erosions are found and the diagnosis of RA can be made. Typical "clues" on plain radiographs are summarized in Table 45.3.

CT scanning better identifies fractures, bone diseases, and intra-abdominal and chest pathology. It is useful when MRI is contraindicated. In acute arthritis, CT scanning can show osteomyelitis in addition to acute inflammation.

MRI has become an important diagnostic modality in musculoskeletal diseases and has largely replaced CT, conventional tomography, and scintigraphy in this setting. MRI combines several favorable attributes: It is noninvasive and carries minimal risk; it offers unparalleled structural detail in soft tissues; and it can be adapted to demonstrate inflammation, such as by T2 weighting, fluid-attenuated inversion recovery (FLAIR) sequencing, and the use of contrast media. The disadvantages of MRI are that it is quite time consuming for the patient and may be associated with physical and psychological discomfort (e.g., lying still in an uncomfortable position and claustrophobia); the images it provides are not as good for bone as for other tissues; only a relatively limited region can be imaged at one time; and both acquisition and pass-through costs are very high. Some of these disadvantages are lessened for low-magnetic-strength "office" MRI.[14] With use of a device that can be operated easily in a general practice setting, images of reasonable quality can be obtained and at a lower cost. However, the region that can be imaged is small, and image acquisition time is significantly longer. Based on all these considerations, when initially evaluating a patient with polyarthritis, the use of MRI will only rarely be indicated.

Use of musculoskeletal ultrasound examination (MSUS) has been increasing rapidly in the past several years. MSUS combines several attractive features: It is easily accommodated in the practice setting and even adds to the patient-physician interaction, images of good quality can be obtained and evaluated in real time based on the clinical situation, inflammation is readily detected with use of Doppler technology, and the costs are surmountable. Inflammation is easily identified using MSUS, as demonstrated in Fig. 45.2. Distinct disadvantages of MSUS are that it requires an experienced physician or physician assistant to perform the procedure, it remains rather more subjective compared with MRI, and soft tissue structures can be "hidden" from view by overlying bone. Nonetheless, MSUS has increasingly become a valuable tool in rheumatology practice. Sensitivity and specificity are similar to MRI.[15–17] Moreover, when assessing patients with polyarthritis, MSUS has proven useful to increase the diagnostic certainty on the part of the rheumatologist, both in terms of establishing that polyarthritis is truly present[18] in cases where there may be doubt, and in establishing a more definitive diagnosis.[19]

Arthrography (i.e., imaging the internal joint structure after injection of a radiopaque solution) is rarely used today, but when MRI is not possible it can be useful for demonstrating damaged structures of the larger joints.

Bone scanning with technetium-labeled methylene diphosphonate identifies osteoid osteomas, bone sarcomas, bony metastases, osteomyelitis, and stress fractures not seen on plain radiographs. Bone scintigraphy is helpful when excluding bone and joint disorders in patients with chronic pain syndromes. Although not specific in acute arthritis, bone scans show differences in the pattern of joint involvement between inflammatory conditions and OA. Labeled white cell scans can identify areas of infection, especially when the source of infection is uncertain in patients with septic arthritis.

Optical imaging, using light in or near the visible wave-length range, has been developed as a diagnostic tool for evaluating the hands. Fluorescence optical imaging ("Rheumascan") is based on the intravenous injection of a fluorochrome that emits ultraviolet light, after which false-color images of the hands are produced indicating areas of increased perfusion. It has been used at some European centers, and several studies have demonstrated that it has similar sensitivity and specificity to MSUS.[20–22] However, its use is limited to the hands, and the injection can in rare instances cause allergic reactions. Optical spectral transmission ("Hand-Scan") uses visible light, the scatter of which is analyzed to measure increased perfusion (i.e., inflammation) of the small joints. Analysis of the PIP joints with this device correlated well with clinical assessment,[23] and it performed similarly to ultrasound in assessing the PIP and metacarpophalangeal joints of the fingers.[24] It was also used to guide treatment in a tight-control study.[25] This procedure is easy for the patient and very safe. Neither of these two devices is yet available in the United States.

TABLE 45.3 Clues to Diagnosis on Plain Film Radiographs

Finding	Disease Suggested
Juxta-articular osteopenia	Early RA
Joint-space narrowing	RA, PsA, or OA
Subchondral sclerosis	OA
Eburnation	OA
Entheseal calcifications	PsA, SpA
Bony erosions	RA, gout
Osteophytes	OA
Chondrocalcinosis	Pseudogout

OA, Osteoarthritis; *PsA*, psoriatic arthritis; *RA*, rheumatoid arthritis; *SpA*, spondyloarthropathy.

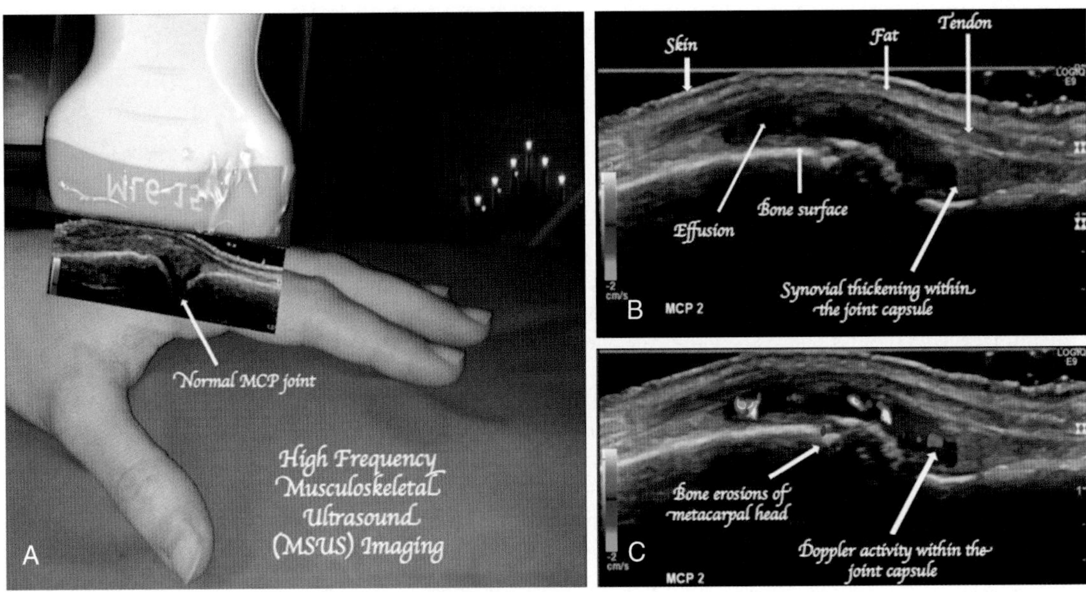

• **Fig. 45.2** Musculoskeletal ultrasound examination can complement the clinical examination (see Chapter 44). (A) The normal metacarpophalangeal (MCP) joint. (B) Synovial thickening in "grayscale" mode and an effusion. (C) A distinct Doppler signal in the synovium, indicating inflammation. (Original photographs courtesy Mr. Yogan Kisten, the Karolinska Institute.)

Synovial or Bone Biopsy

Arthroscopic synovial biopsy is rarely necessary, but in tuberculosis, sarcoidosis, amyloid, pigmented villonodular synovitis, lipoma arborescens, and foreign body synovitis it is required for diagnosis. Proteomic and genomic assays have begun to show between-patient differences in the synovium from chronic arthritides, raising hopes that synovial biopsy may be used to support more personalized treatment in the future. Bone biopsy may be needed to identify tumors and may demonstrate underlying abnormalities in nonresolving osteomyelitis.

Differential Diagnosis

The differential diagnosis of arthritis is large; however, information that is readily available at the initial presentation will in many cases narrow the diagnosis to a limited number of possibilities. Thus, when in early spring polyarthritis of recent onset is seen in a young woman and is associated with febrile symptoms and a maculopapular rash, a viral diagnosis is likely, and parvovirus B19 infection is a good guess. In contrast, if a middle-aged man being treated with hemodialysis wakes up one night with a single hot, red, and swollen joint at the base of the big toe, it does not take an expert diagnostician to suspect gout. Nonetheless, surprises do occur, and it remains important to consider the entire spectrum of possible diagnoses when first evaluating the patient. Table 45.4 lists a comprehensive differential diagnosis of arthritis. The most important disease categories to be considered are outlined in the following sections.

Bacterial Infections

Bacterial joint infection (i.e., septic arthritis) is one of the prime considerations in a sudden-onset strongly inflammatory presentation in a single joint. It is a medical emergency because the mortality rate is between 7% and 15%.[26,27] Large limb joints are most frequently involved, usually associated with underlying OA or inflammatory arthropathies, especially RA.[28] Patients are particularly at risk after joint surgery, including arthroplasty and intra-articular injection, as are patients with distant infections.[29] Patients with underlying disease affecting the immune response or those taking drugs that impair immune function are also at risk,[30] as are the elderly and those living in deprived socioeconomic circumstances.

Most patients experience an acute, painful, swollen monoarthritis, but up to 10% of patients with septic arthritis may present with polyarticular infection. An identifiable distant site of infection may be found at presentation, fever occurs in more than 50% of cases, and sweats/rigors in approximately 30%.[26] When patients are first seen, ESR and CRP are almost invariably raised, but approximately 35% of all septic arthritis patients do not have a raised blood white cell count. When infection is in the context of underlying RA, this figure rises to 50%. Impaired renal and liver function when the patient is first examined predicts a poorer outcome. Plain radiographs can show soft tissue swelling but are usually normal at first examination. Ultrasound can localize synovitis and fluid collection to target aspiration, while MRI may be required to demonstrate osteomyelitis.

Synovial fluid is usually cloudy or even purulent. High levels of synovial leukocytes are seen but fail to differentiate between septic arthritis and inflammatory arthritis of other causes. Studies assessing the use of other serum and synovial fluid markers, such as procalcitonin, IL-6, and TNF have been performed with varying success.[31] Synovial fluid Gram stain should be done immediately and the fluid sent for culture.[32] However, this detects the organism in only approximately 50% of cases. Because blood cultures may identify bacteria in patients in whom synovial fluid culture is negative, these should always be done in parallel, and if clinical suspicion for infection is high, antibiotics should be initiated before culture results are available. Organisms detected most commonly include staphylococci (*Staphylococcus aureus*, with an increasing prevalence of methicillin-resistant strains,[33] and *Staphylococcus species*), streptococci, and Gram-negative bacteria. Prompt intervention can reduce mortality[34]; the joint must be aspirated daily to dryness, which may require orthopedic intervention.

Importantly, no difference in outcome is seen for patients with culture-proven septic arthritis compared with patients in whom a clinical diagnosis of septic arthritis is made but in whom bacteria cannot be isolated.[33] Hence normal investigations at first examination should not delay treatment in the presence of a strong clinical suspicion.

Some bacterial joint infections behave atypically, including those with *Neisseria gonorrhoeae* and Lyme arthritis. These infections may cause small-joint polyarthritis in a relatively early phase, which is believed to be a result of the dissemination of immune complexes into the joints rather than to direct infection.[35]

Neisseria infection should be suspected in sexually active patients who are seen with migratory small joint arthritis or arthralgias, tenosynovitis, skin rashes, and vesicles. Untreated Neisseria infection can also lead to destructive arthritis. Most patients are febrile with a raised acute phase response and blood leukocytosis, but, as with other bacterial causes of septic arthritis, these may be normal at presentation.[36] Investigations should include swabs from the urethra, cervix, pharynx, and rectum, inoculated immediately on Thayer-Martin medium. In contrast with other bacterial infections, polymerase chain reaction (PCR) has been used on synovial fluid to improve diagnostic results.[37]

Lyme Disease

Patients with Lyme disease typically live in, or travel through, at-risk geographic areas and may present with expanding erythematous rashes (typically erythema migrans) after a tick bite resulting from *Borrelia* infection, usually *Borrelia burgdorferi*. The rash can be absent in as many as 30% of patients.[38] The infection may cause polyarthritis in an early phase of the infection; as with Neisseria, both direct infection of the joints by *Borrelia burgdorferi* and an autoimmune reaction triggered by that organism may play a role. Large joint monoarthritis develops a few weeks after initial infection,[39] associated with a high ESR and CRP.

Specific IgG antibodies, detected 4 weeks after infection, are diagnostic. Low levels of rheumatoid factor and ANAs can be detected. Synovial fluid contains polymorphs, and *Borrelia* organisms may be cultured, but PCR of synovial fluid for *Borrelia* DNA represents a superior test.[40]

Plant Thorn Synovitis

Foreign bodies, including plant thorns, can cause inflammation in intra-articular and tendon synovial tissue in hands or feet. Sometimes the antecedent history of penetrating injury is absent. Ultrasound, CT, and MRI are helpful in localizing foreign bodies, and synovial biopsy can make the diagnosis.[41] Synovial fluid can be

TABLE 45.4 The Differential Diagnosis of Polyarthritis

Disease Category	Specific Disease	Mono-, Oligo-, or Polyarthritis (Most Common Presentation)
Infections		
Viral	Parvovirus B19	Poly
	Rubella virus	Poly
	Hepatitis A, B, C	Poly
	HIV	Oligo, poly
	Alphaviruses, including Chikungunya infection	Poly
Bacterial	Gram-positive and gram-negative infections	Mono, occasionally oligo/poly
	Initial phase of gonorrhea	Poly
	Later phase of gonorrhea	Mono
	Early phase of Lyme arthritis	Poly
	Later phase of Lyme arthritis	Oligo, mono
Diseases Triggered by Infection but Presumed to Be Autoimmune		
Reactive arthritis	After urogenital infections (*Chlamydia* and *Ureaplasma*); after gastrointestinal infections (*Yersinia*, *Shigella*, *Campylobacter*, and *Salmonella*)	Mono, oligo, poly
Acute rheumatic fever	After infection with group A streptococcus	Oligo
Autoimmune Diseases		
Primary arthritides	Rheumatoid arthritis	Poly
	Psoriatic arthritis	Oligo, poly
	Spondyloarthropathies	Oligo, poly
	Juvenile inflammatory arthritis	Mono, oligo, poly
Transient and recurring polyarthritides	Palindromic rheumatism	Poly
	Recurrent symmetric seronegative synovitis with pitting edema (RS3PE syndrome)	Poly
Systemic autoimmune disease	Systemic lupus erythematosus	Poly
	Mixed connective tissue disease	Poly
	Primary Sjögren's syndrome	Poly
	Progressive systemic sclerosis and limited scleroderma	Poly
	Behçet's disease	Oligo, poly
	Sarcoidosis	Oligo, poly
	Vasculitis	Poly
Autoinflammatory diseases	Adult-onset Still's disease	Oligo, poly
	Familial Mediterranean fever and other cryopyrin-associated fever syndromes	Poly
	Various genetic autoinflammatory conditions usually manifested first in childhood	Poly
Degenerative diseases	Includes erosive inflammatory osteoarthritis	Poly
Osteoarthritis		
Hypertrophic osteoarthropathy		Poly
Osteonecrosis		Mono, oligo

TABLE 45.4 The Differential Diagnosis of Polyarthritis—cont'd

Disease Category	Specific Disease	Mono-, Oligo-, or Polyarthritis (Most Common Presentation)
Metabolic Diseases		
Thyroid diseases	Hypothyroidism	Mono, oligo
Hemochromatosis	Hyperthyroidism (Grave's disease; early phase of Hashimoto's disease)	Oligo, poly
Hemoglobinopathies	Sickle cell anemia	Oligo, poly
Hemochromatosis	Thalassemia	Oligo, poly
Crystal diseases	Gout	Mono (initial), oligo, poly (late stage)
	Pseudogout	Mono, oligo, poly
Deposition diseases	Glycogen storage diseases; amyloid deposition in primary amyloidosis; mucopolysaccharidoses; light- and heavy-chain deposition diseases; others	Oligo, poly
Drug-Induced Diseases		
Vasculitic drug reactions, serum sickness		Poly

sparse and, although usually sterile, may be infected with *Enterobacter agglomerans*, a Gram-negative bacillus commonly found in soil.[42]

Mycobacteria

Monoarthritis resulting from tuberculosis, frequently including atypical forms,[43] should be considered in at-risk populations and people with a relevant social history. Synovial fluid contains mononuclear cells, but synovial biopsy and culture may be required to identify organisms. The same holds true for joint infection with atypical mycobacteria, seen mostly in immunocompromised individuals. A reactive arthritis (Poncet's disease) can occur after tuberculosis infection elsewhere and may also follow viral and fungal infections.

Whipple's Disease

Up to 60% of patients with Whipple's disease experience migratory large joint monoarthritis or oligoarthritis.[44] Blood tests show a high acute phase response with leukopenia, whereas synovial fluid usually shows a high leukocyte count. The diagnosis is based on histologic analysis of jejunal or synovial biopsy and molecular biologic tests for *Tropheryma whippelii*.[44]

Several other bacterial infections may also lead to rheumatic syndromes through mechanisms other than direct infection of the joints. A classic finding in rheumatic fever after infection with group A streptococcus is a migratory aseptic arthritis of the large joints (discussed further in Chapter 122), and various gram-negative infections of the gastrointestinal system (e.g., *Shigella* and *Campylobacter*) and genitourinary tract (e.g., *Chlamydia* and *Ureaplasma*) may trigger reactive arthritis (see Chapter 81).

Viral Infections

Many different viral infections can cause transient and self-limiting polyarthritis. One may suspect that the relatively common occurrence of transient polyarthritis without further explanation usually represents viral infection, even if it is not so diagnosed. Viral arthritis is usually a symmetric polyarthritis of the small joints in the hands and feet and may therefore trigger a workup for early RA. As indicated previously, viral and some bacterial infections may cause a false-positive RF, adding to the diagnostic challenge; the fact that the anti-CCP test is more specific for RA may help in these instances.

The following viral infections are important to consider in the evaluation of polyarthritis:

- Parvovirus B19, which occurs seasonally and often appears in teenagers or young adults, is sometimes severe enough to trigger suspicions of RA. The discovery that this infection can be associated with transient positivity for RF led to speculation that parvovirus might be the cause of RA.[45] Later studies clearly ruled out that possibility.[46,47] The course of parvovirus arthritis is self-limiting, but treatment may be needed for several days or weeks.[48]
- Although rubella virus infection has become uncommon as a result of vaccination, it may nonetheless be encountered from time to time in young adults. Rubella virus infection is self-limiting and usually mild, but the diagnosis is important when pregnancy is an issue.[49]
- Hepatitis virus infection: Each of the hepatitis viruses can cause polyarthritis as the first and sometimes only clinical manifestation.[50–52] The fact that RF can be positive in individuals with viral hepatitis may lead even experienced clinicians astray.[53]
- HIV infection may cause polyarthritis, which may be the first manifestation of HIV.[54] Because early diagnosis and treatment is very important, this disease must always be considered. In contrast to most types of viral arthritis, HIV-related polyarthritis can be severe.[55]
- Alphavirus infections, including Chikungunya arthritis: In tropical countries, several alphaviruses (i.e., viruses belonging to the family of togaviruses and the class of arboviruses that are transmitted by mosquitoes) are not uncommonly encountered. These infections with fanciful names such as Chikungunya[56] ("bending up" in the Akonde language), Sindbis,[57]

and O'nyong-nyong[58] (meaning "severe joint pain" in the East African Acholi language) are not always self-limiting and may sometimes be destructive. Ross River virus arthritis in Australia is also caused by an alphavirus.[59] Until recently these types of viral arthritis were rarely encountered in practice outside tropical regions, but a remarkable change in the epidemiology of Chikungunya virus arthritis is taking place. As recently as 2013, this virus gained a foothold in the Caribbean region, where more than a million people are since estimated to have been infected.[60] Frequent travel between that region and North America is now making Chikungunya infection in general, and Chikungunya arthritis more specifically, a diagnosis to be reckoned with in daily practice in the United States and Canada. Moreover, evidence indicates that the virus is adapting to mosquito strains that are ubiquitous in the United States, so the infection may become endemic in the United States as well. Chikungunya infection almost invariably causes moderate or severe myalgias and arthralgias that frequently persist weeks or months after other signs of the acute infection have subsided.[61–63] Frank arthritis may also be seen, usually in a small joint pattern that is difficult to differentiate from seronegative RA.[64] Recent studies have highlighted the frequent development of long-lasting symptoms in these patients.[65]

Malignancy-Associated Polyarthritis

Although direct invasion of the joint by tumor cells or metastases is very rare, polyarthritis can be a paraneoplastic phenomenon.[66] Relatively little is known about the epidemiology or pathophysiology of this entity. Diagnostic clues may be the rapid onset of a fulminant polyarthritis and associated symptoms such as weight loss and diffuse pain; in the absence of an obvious clue, these cases can be diagnostically very challenging.[67]

Crystal-Associated Polyarthritis

Gout

Podagra is the classic monoarthritis of the first metatarsophalangeal joint. Patients tend to be obese males, aged 45 to 60 years with hypertension, and consumers of excess alcohol.[68] However, post-menopausal females with low estrogen and who take loop diuretics for hypertension are also predisposed to gout. Usually gout progresses from recurrent monoarticular episodes to oligoarticular (2 to 3 joints) and then polyarticular phases, especially when left untreated. The initial locations of the gout attack are usually the feet, ankles, and knees, but the later polyarticular manifestations may also involve the upper extremities. Thus, gout in the polyarticular phase can sometimes mimic RA, and this may be particularly important to consider if patients are partially treated with nonsteroidal anti-inflammatory drugs (NSAIDs).

Fever is present in 34% of patients, especially in polyarticular presentations.[69] In acute settings, blood leukocytes, ESR, and CRP are raised, and to this extent gout mimics septic arthritis. Serum uric acid may be raised, but levels are normal in 33% of patients during acute attacks.[70] Renal and liver function should be assessed. Negatively birefringent needle-shaped uric acid crystals located intra-cellularly in synovial fluid leukocytes (or tophi aspirates) confirm the diagnosis.[71] Synovial fluid should be examined for bacteria to exclude concomitant septic arthritis.

Routine radiographs frequently show no bony abnormalities but may identify erosions after repeated or prolonged attacks. Ultrasound and dual-energy CT (DECT) are superior imaging techniques compared with conventional radiographs.[72] A double-contour sign overlying cartilage is suggestive of gout on ultrasound. Cortical erosions, however, may be more clearly identified on MRI.[73]

Pseudogout, more properly called acute calcium pyrophosphate (CPP) crystal arthritis, occurs mostly in elderly people and affects the knees and ankles but also the joints of the toes, and even the joints of the wrists and hands; thus it can mimic many other diseases. It is rare in patients younger than 50 years, and the initial symptom is usually monarticular inflammation, most common at the knees and wrists, often with concomitant OA. Acute attacks often occur following a trigger such as infection, trauma, or surgery.[74] It can also occur in relation to specific metabolic diseases, such as hemochromatosis and primary hyperparathyroidism. Calcinosis of cartilage and periarticular tissues can be seen on radiographs and ultrasound, with ultrasound the more sensitive modality. Synovial fluid microscopy demonstrates rhomboid-shaped crystals at ×400 magnification, and this remains the diagnostic gold standard.[75] Culture should be undertaken to exclude co-existent septic arthritis. Repeat imaging (e.g., using MRI) may be necessary to formally exclude bone injury if clinical suspicion exists.

Calcium Phosphate Crystal Arthritis

Intra-articular deposits of basic calcium phosphate crystals, most importantly calcium hydroxyapatite, may cause an acute on chronic inflammatory arthritis in older female patients with OA, with severe destruction usually on the dominant side (Milwaukee shoulder).[76] The effusion is not inflammatory, but synovial fluid can be viscous and blood stained and may contain calcium aggregates and cartilage fragments. Plain radiographs show upward shoulder dislocation. CT is superior to a radiograph in identifying calcification.

Calcium hydroxyapatite deposition in periarticular tissues may also cause acute calcific periarthritis or tendonitis, rare clinical manifestations including peripheral nerve and spinal cord compression, and pseudotumoral deposition.[77]

Cholesterol Crystal Arthritis

Cholesterol crystals have been reported in synovial fluid, albeit rarely, and often in association with inflammatory arthropathies. Whether these large rhomboid-shaped crystals are truly a separate cause of synovial inflammation remains a subject for speculation.

Degenerative Arthritis

Although OA is considered a degenerative disease, some inflammation is often detected in the affected joint. Less commonly, overt clinical inflammation is present, and the moniker "erosive-inflammatory OA," although not very well defined, is used.[78,79] The presentation in this case may be a true polyarthritis, although the experienced clinician will have little difficulty recognizing this entity, based on the distribution (predominantly the distal and proximal interphalangeal joints and frequently the first carpometacarpal joint) and typical bony hypertrophy around the affected joints.

A history of intra-articular fracture or recurrent occupational-related injury (e.g., carpet fitter's knee) can lead to a more localized OA. In younger patients with hip OA, slipped epiphysis, congenital dislocation, or avascular necrosis may antedate disease. Blood investigations will usually be normal, and provided there are no additional pathologies, synovial fluid shows a non-inflammatory leukocyte level. Plain radiographs usually confirm the diagnosis in established disease, but ultrasound and MRI can clarify the extent of inflammation. In the presence of inflammatory symptoms, it is important to exclude crystal deposition and/or infection.

Neuropathic arthropathy (Charcot's joint) should be suspected in patients in whom there is a monoarthritis in the distal lower limb with severe OA on plain radiograph in association with demonstrable peripheral neuropathy. The reduced incidence of syphilis means that diabetes mellitus is the most common cause of peripheral neuropathy in the Western world.[80]

Benign Tumors Causing Arthritis

Patients with primary or secondary tumors in periarticular tissues present with monoarthritis and are usually diagnosed by routine radiographs and/or MRI. Lipoma arborescens is a benign tumor, often presenting with knee swelling, in which synovium is replaced by mature fat cells. This tumor is more widely recognized with the increased use of MRI, which shows villous proliferation and characteristic features similar to subcutaneous fat.[81]

Patients with synovial osteochondromatosis often present with symptoms of pain and locking in the large joints, predominantly hips and knees. Synovial fluid is pale in color with few cells. Plain radiographs show calcification in synovial tissues, and synovial histology after biopsy shows the formation of osteocartilaginous bodies in the synovial membrane.[82]

Pigmented villonodular synovitis (PVNS) is a benign tumor of the synovium that may cause arthritis. If clinical suspicion is aroused by recurrent blood-stained effusions that are resistant to local interventions such as glucocorticoid injection, further investigation by MRI may be done, but synovial biopsy is essential for pathologic confirmation.[83]

Trauma and Internal Derangement

Trauma, either acute or after repeated injury, is the most common cause of acute monoarticular pain, especially in the knee and the ankle. In the knee, torn menisci or loose bodies in the synovial fluid may wedge between articulating surfaces and lead to sudden and painful locking and weakness when walking, which the patient describes as "giving way." Examination for other ligament damage is important, with use of tests for cruciate or collateral knee ligament stability. Careful attention to inversion and eversion stability of the ankle is also essential for evaluating monoarticular pain in that area. Plain radiographs may demonstrate abnormal architecture, dislocation, or loose bodies, but MRI is diagnostically superior and will usually establish the cause of a trauma-related diagnosis. If MRI is impossible, arthrography may be required to assess the hip for damage, particularly to establish tears in the acetabular labrum.

Stress fractures can cause monoarticular or periarticular pain on weight bearing and occur after repeated minor trauma (e.g., march fracture of the metatarsal) or may occur secondary to underlying local or systemic bone disease, particularly in sedentary individuals and those on prolonged bisphosphonate therapy.[84] These fractures can be missed on standard radiographs; thus CT, MRI, or bone scintigraphy are helpful in the context of persistent localizing regional articular pain.

Osteonecrosis can occur in patients with connective tissues diseases, particularly when receiving high-dose glucocorticoids. Other causes of osteonecrosis include decompression sickness, hemoglobinopathies, and patients with hyperlipidemia, hyperuricemia, or high alcohol consumption. History is of monoarticular pain, and examination can be normal, but early MRI is diagnostic while plain radiographs are often unremarkable.

Metabolic Diseases

Metabolic diseases such as hemochromatosis may cause progressive degenerative and inflammatory changes in multiple joints.[85] Abnormal liver function and iron saturation tests are found in association with sequence variations in the *HFE* gene, which regulates iron transport, and in more chronic cases osteophytes occur in the MCPs of the second and third fingers. The arthropathy associated with alkaptonuria affects the spine and large joints with degenerative arthritis on radiographs. Discoloration of ear cartilage and sclera is diagnostic. A polyarticular presentation may on occasion be encountered in primary amyloidosis[86] and in other deposition diseases as well.[87–89] Both hypothyroidism and hyperthyroidism may be associated with a range of musculoskeletal symptoms,[90,91] mono- or oligoarticular arthritis of the large joints with large effusions being most typical of hypothyroidism[92] and muscular symptoms of hyperthyroidism[93]; however, frank polyarthritis occasionally may be seen in both conditions. A seronegative erosive arthritis with inflammatory synovial fluid and lymphocytic infiltrate on biopsy may occur after jejunoileal surgery for obesity,[94] but to date arthropathies are not a significant problem after less invasive gastric banding surgery.[95]

Diabetic Cheiroarthropathy

Diabetes mellitus is associated with a painful syndrome of the hands, characterized by thickened connective tissues and restricted range of motion rather than true arthritis. Fibrosis resulting from microvascular disease is the most likely underlying pathology. If similar symptoms occur in the shoulder, it is also named the diabetic hand-shoulder syndrome.

Autoimmune Diseases

Autoimmune inflammation of the joints is the most important concern for the rheumatologist when evaluating a patient with new-onset polyarthritis. In addition to diseases in which arthritis is the dominant manifestation, such as RA, PsA, and peripheral SpA, consideration must be given to the systemic inflammatory diseases for which arthritis may be the first presenting manifestation, including SLE, systemic vasculitis, Sjögren's syndrome, progressive systemic sclerosis, Behçet's disease, sarcoidosis, and others. In these diseases there usually is an oligo- or polyarthritis with moderate inflammatory signs primarily in the small joints, and with pain that may be more pronounced than the physical findings would suggest. Deformities are rarely seen in SLE (Jaccoud's arthropathy). Some patients with celiac disease may present with short-lived peripheral joint oligoarthritis.[96]

Transient syndromes in which prominent polyarthritis is self-limiting but recurrent include palindromic rheumatism[97] and the syndrome of recurrent symmetric seronegative synovitis with peripheral edema (RS3PE syndrome).[98]

Autoinflammatory diseases with high fever, skin rashes, lymphadenopathy, and polyarthritis are more commonly diagnosed in the pediatric population but can on occasion become manifest first in adults. Important considerations in the patient with polyarthritis and fever are adult-onset Still's disease and cryopyrin-associated periodic syndromes, including familial Mediterranean fever.

Drug-Induced Arthritis and Serum Sickness

Classic descriptions of drug-induced vasculitis or "serum sickness" include polyarthritis, which may variably be inflammatory and oligoarticular or polyarticular.[99] The clinical setting is usually sufficient to make the diagnosis, and the course is self-limiting. Check-point inhibitors, which in recent years have emerged as highly effective medications in some types of cancer, are associated with a plethora of autoimmune manifestations, including polyarthritis in a pattern similar to RA.[100,101]

Formal Criteria and Their Role in Clinical Diagnosis

"Classification criteria" have been developed for many rheumatologic diseases, perhaps most notably for RA. These criteria were developed originally to achieve uniformity between clinicians in different health care settings, regions, or countries, and primarily so for epidemiologic or other research purposes. They were explicitly not developed as diagnostic criteria. Nonetheless, the very existence of these criteria has led to changes in the way RA and other rheumatologic diseases are perceived, and many clinicians do, in fact, rely on the classification criteria for making clinical diagnoses. The most recent classification criteria for RA, which were developed internationally under the auspices of the American College of Rheumatology (ACR) and the EULAR, were quite significantly different from previous versions[102] (Table 45.5). First, it was recognized that if a radiograph showed incontrovertible evidence for RA, then the diagnosis could be made and no other evidence was needed. Unfortunately, the criteria did not make it entirely clear exactly how certain the radiographic evidence would have to be, and most radiologists agree that there can be considerable variations in the interpretations of radiographic findings.

When radiographic evidence is lacking, the classification of RA is based on a system of points, where the number and nature of the inflamed joints, combined with several other characteristics, determines whether the patient "has" or "does not have" RA. It remains critically important to emphasize that these criteria were benchmarked on the opinions of expert clinicians and had sensitivity and specificity in the 90% range, indicating that in 1 in 10 patients, an experienced clinician will disagree with the criteria. This is not to belittle the importance of these criteria but to underscore that their use should not replace the clinical judgment of a competent specialist.

Similar considerations apply to other rheumatologic diagnoses, with the added caveat that classification criteria for diseases such as PsA,[103] ankylosing spondylitis,[104] and gout[105] usually achieve sensitivity and specificity lower than that for RA.

TABLE 45.5 The 2010 American College of Rheumatology/European League Against Rheumatism Classification Criteria for Rheumatoid Arthritis[a]

Criteria	Score
Joint involvement	
2-10 large joints	1
1-3 small joints (with or without involvement of large joints)	2
4-10 small joints (with or without involvement of large joints)	3
>10 joints (with at least 1 small joint)	5
Serology (at least 1 test result is needed for classification)	
Negative RF and negative ACPA	0
Low-positive RF or low-positive ACPA	2
High-positive RF or high-positive ACPA	3
Acute-phase reactants	
Normal CRP and normal ESR	0
Abnormal CRP or abnormal ESR	1
Duration of symptoms	
<6 wk	0
≥6 wk	1

A score of 6 or greater is needed for classification of a patient as having definite rheumatoid arthritis.

[a]Target population (patients who can be evaluated using these criteria): those who have *at least one joint with definite clinical synovitis* (swelling), with the synovitis not better explained by another disease.

If incontrovertible radiographic evidence of rheumatoid arthritis exists, the diagnosis can be made even if the criteria provided are not fulfilled.

If a patient has previously fulfilled the criteria for rheumatoid arthritis, the diagnosis is maintained even if the criteria are not fulfilled on current re-examination.

ACPA, Anti-citrullinated protein antibodies; *CRP*, C-reactive protein; *ESR*, erythrocyte sedimentation rate; *RF*, rheumatoid factor.

Preliminary Diagnoses, Working Diagnoses, Presumptive Treatments, Reassessments, and Future Perspectives

Even after applying all possible diagnostic acumen and each and every available test, the diagnosis may not be entirely clear. All clinicians are familiar with the fact that medical diagnostics remains, to some extent, a probabilistic venture. Nonetheless, there comes a point where a preliminary diagnosis must be made, the patient must be informed, and a course of treatment must be chosen. This situation poses some challenges in terms of patient-physician communication. Understandably, clinicians may not want to appear uncertain when speaking with their patients, but nonetheless, it may be better to be frank and say something to the effect that, "I think it is likely that you have X, but we cannot be certain. There are no further tests right now to be done, and I propose that we start treatment with Y. We will reassess in a few weeks' or months' time."

Most important, a time point for reassessment must be chosen. This point could be a few weeks or several months into the future, depending on the situation, but by explicitly marking this point, the patient will have greater acceptance if a preliminary diagnosis must be revised.

Modern rheumatologic diagnostics, applied in the setting of a clinic with experienced specialists, will achieve a final diagnosis in 60% to 90% of patients presenting with new-onset polyarthritis.[106,107] It does seem likely that further advances can be made in diagnosing specific rheumatologic disorders earlier, especially RA; the interest in this possibility is based not only on the desire to achieve an expeditious diagnosis but also on the potential for very early intervention, taking advantage of a presumed "window of opportunity" and thereby achieving better long-term results for the patient.[108] However, if this earlier diagnosis is to be achieved, it may well have to done in the pre-clinical phase, before the patient actually has clinically detectable arthritis.

The references for this chapter can also be found on ExpertConsult.com.

References

1. Gormley G, Steele K, Gilliland D, et al.: Can rheumatologists agree on a diagnosis of inflammatory arthritis in an early synovitis clinic? *Ann Rheum Dis* 60:638–639, 2001.
2. Grunke M, Antoni CE, Kavanaugh A, et al.: Standardization of joint examination technique leads to a significant decrease in variability among different examiners, *J Rheumatol* 37:860–864, 2010.
3. Quinn MA, Green MJ, Conaghan P, et al.: How do you diagnose rheumatoid arthritis early? *Best Pract Res Clin Rheumatol* 15:49–66, 2001.
4. van den Bosch WB, Mangnus L, Reijnierse M, et al.: The diagnostic accuracy of the squeeze test to identify arthritis: a cross-sectional cohort study, *Ann Rheum Dis* 74:1886–1889, 2015.
5. Smolen JS, Breedveld FC, Eberl G, et al.: Validity and reliability of the twenty-eight-joint count for the assessment of rheumatoid arthritis activity, *Arthritis Rheum* 38:38–43, 1995.
6. Rose HM, Ragan C, et al.: Differential agglutination of normal and sensitized sheep erythrocytes by sera of patients with rheumatoid arthritis, *Proc Soc Exp Biol Med* 68:1–6, 1948.
7. Pike RM, Sulkin SE, Coggeshall HC: Concerning the nature of the factor in rheumatoid-arthritis serum responsible for increased agglutination of sensitized sheep erythrocytes, *J Immunol* 63:447–463, 1949.
8. Visser H, le Cessie S, Vos K, et al.: How to diagnose rheumatoid arthritis early: a prediction model for persistent (erosive) arthritis, *Arthritis Rheum* 46:357–365, 2002.
9. Jansen LM, van der Horst-Bruinsma IE, van Schaardenburg D, et al.: Predictors of radiographic joint damage in patients with early rheumatoid arthritis, *Ann Rheum Dis* 60:924–927, 2001.
10. Hulsemann JL, Zeidler H: Undifferentiated arthritis in an early synovitis out-patient clinic, *Clin Exp Rheumatol* 13:37–43, 1995.
11. Rantapaa-Dahlqvist S, de Jong BA, Berglin E, et al.: Antibodies against cyclic citrullinated peptide and IgA rheumatoid factor predict the development of rheumatoid arthritis, *Arthritis Rheum* 48:2741–2749, 2003.
12. Tunn EJ, Bacon PA: Differentiating persistent from self-limiting symmetrical synovitis in an early arthritis clinic, *Br J Rheumatol* 32:97–103, 1993.
13. Raza K, Breese M, Nightingale P, et al.: Predictive value of antibodies to cyclic citrullinated peptide in patients with very early inflammatory arthritis, *J Rheumatol* 32:231–238, 2005.
14. Schiff MH, Hobbs KF, Gensler T, et al.: A retrospective analysis of low-field strength magnetic resonance imaging and the management of patients with rheumatoid arthritis, *Curr Med Res Opin* 23:961–968, 2007.
15. Szkudlarek M, Narvestad E, Klarlund M, et al.: Ultrasonography of the metatarsophalangeal joints in rheumatoid arthritis: comparison with magnetic resonance imaging, conventional radiography, and clinical examination, *Arthritis Rheum* 50:2103–2112, 2004.
16. Szkudlarek M, Klarlund M, Narvestad E, et al.: Ultrasonography of the metacarpophalangeal and proximal interphalangeal joints in rheumatoid arthritis: a comparison with magnetic resonance imaging, conventional radiography and clinical examination, *Arthritis Res Ther* 8:R52, 2006.
17. Hoving JL, Buchbinder R, Hall S, et al.: A comparison of magnetic resonance imaging, sonography, and radiography of the hand in patients with early rheumatoid arthritis, *J Rheumatol* 31:663–675, 2004.
18. Matsos M, Harish S, Zia P, et al.: Ultrasound of the hands and feet for rheumatological disorders: influence on clinical diagnostic confidence and patient management, *Skeletal Radiol* 38:1049–1054, 2009.
19. Rezaei H, Torp-Pedersen S, Af Klint E, et al.: Diagnostic utility of musculoskeletal ultrasound in patients with suspected arthritis—a probabilistic approach, *Arthritis Res Ther* 16:448, 2014.
20. Werner SG, Langer HE, Ohrndorf S, et al.: Inflammation assessment in patients with arthritis using a novel in vivo fluorescence optical imaging technology, *Ann Rheum Dis* 71:504–510, 2012.
21. Werner SG, Langer HE, Schott P, et al.: Indocyanine green-enhanced fluorescence optical imaging in patients with early and very early arthritis: a comparative study with magnetic resonance imaging, *Arthritis Rheum* 65:3036–3044, 2013.
22. Kisten Y, Gyori N, Af Klint E, et al.: Detection of clinically manifest and silent synovitis in the hands and wrists by fluorescence optical imaging, *RMD Open* 1:e000106, 2015.
23. Meier AJ, Rensen WH, de Bokx PK, et al.: Potential of optical spectral transmission measurements for joint inflammation measurements in rheumatoid arthritis patients, *J Biomed Opt* 17:081420, 2012.
24. van Onna M, Ten Cate DF, Tsoi KL, et al.: Assessment of disease activity in patients with rheumatoid arthritis using optical spectral transmission measurements, a non-invasive imaging technique, *Ann Rheum Dis* 75:511–518, 2016.
25. Nair SC, Welsing PM, Jacobs JW, et al.: Economic evaluation of a tight-control treatment strategy using an imaging device (handscan) for monitoring joint inflammation in early rheumatoid arthritis, *Clin Exp Rheumatol* 33:831–838, 2015.
26. Margaretten ME, Kohlwes J, Moore D, et al.: Does this adult patient have septic arthritis? *JAMA* 297:1478–1488, 2007.
27. Gupta MN, Sturrock RD, Field M: A prospective 2-year study of 75 patients with adult-onset septic arthritis, *Rheumatology (Oxford)* 40:24–30, 2001.
28. Goldenberg DL: Septic arthritis, *Lancet* 351:197–202, 1998.
29. Weston VC, Jones AC, Bradbury N, et al.: Clinical features and outcome of septic arthritis in a single UK Health District 1982-1991, *Ann Rheum Dis* 58:214–219, 1999.
30. Edwards CJ, Cooper C, Fisher D, et al.: The importance of the disease process and disease-modifying antirheumatic drug treatment in the development of septic arthritis in patients with rheumatoid arthritis, *Arthritis Rheum* 57:1151–1157, 2007.
31. Talebi-Taher M, Shirani F, Nikanjam N, et al.: Septic versus inflammatory arthritis: discriminating the ability of serum inflammatory markers, *Rheumatol Int* 33:319–324, 2013.
32. Coakley G, Mathews C, Field M, et al.: BSR & BHPR, BOA, RCGP and BSAC guidelines for management of the hot swollen joint in adults, *Rheumatology (Oxford)* 45:1039–1041, 2006.
33. Gupta MN, Sturrock RD, Field M: Prospective comparative study of patients with culture proven and high suspicion of adult onset septic arthritis, *Ann Rheum Dis* 62:327–331, 2003.
34. Mathews CJ, Weston VC, Jones A, et al.: Bacterial septic arthritis in adults, *Lancet* 375:846–855, 2010.
35. Lightfoot Jr RW, Gotschlich EC: Gonococcal disease, *Am J Med* 56:327–356, 1974.
36. Wise CM, Morris CR, Wasilauskas BL, et al.: Gonococcal arthritis in an era of increasing penicillin resistance. Presentations and outcomes in 41 recent cases (1985-1991), *Arch Intern Med* 154:2690–2695, 1994.
37. Liebling MR, Arkfeld DG, Michelini GA, et al.: Identification of Neisseria gonorrhoeae in synovial fluid using the polymerase chain reaction, *Arthritis Rheum* 37:702–709, 1994.

38. Schutzer SE, Berger BW, Krueger JG, et al.: Atypical erythema migrans in patients with PCR-positive Lyme disease, *Emerg Infect Dis* 19:815–817, 2013.
39. Steere AC: Lyme disease, *N Engl J Med* 345:115–125, 2001.
40. Nocton JJ, Dressler F, Rutledge BJ, et al.: Detection of Borrelia burgdorferi DNA by polymerase chain reaction in synovial fluid from patients with Lyme arthritis, *N Engl J Med* 330:229–234, 1994.
41. Tung CH, Chen YH, Lan HH, et al.: Diagnosis of plant-thorn synovitis by high-resolution ultrasonography: a case report and literature review, *Clin Rheumatol* 26:849–851, 2007.
42. Baskar S, Mann JS, Thomas AP, et al.: Plant thorn tenosynovitis, *J Clin Rheumatol* 12:137–138, 2006.
43. Hsiao CH, Cheng A, Huang YT, et al.: Clinical and pathological characteristics of mycobacterial tenosynovitis and arthritis, *Infection* 41:457–464, 2013.
44. Schneider T, Moos V, Loddenkemper C, et al.: Whipple's disease: new aspects of pathogenesis and treatment, *Lancet Infect Dis* 8:179–190, 2008.
45. Luzzi GA, Kurtz JB, Chapel H: Human parvovirus arthropathy and rheumatoid factor, *Lancet* 1:1218, 1985.
46. Hajeer AH, MacGregor AJ, Rigby AS, et al.: Influence of previous exposure to human parvovirus B19 infection in explaining susceptibility to rheumatoid arthritis: an analysis of disease discordant twin pairs, *Ann Rheum Dis* 53:137–139, 1994.
47. Harrison B, Silman A, Barrett E, et al.: Low frequency of recent parvovirus infection in a population-based cohort of patients with early inflammatory polyarthritis, *Ann Rheum Dis* 57:375–377, 1998.
48. Gran JT, Johnsen V, Myklebust G, et al.: The variable clinical picture of arthritis induced by human parvovirus B19. Report of seven adult cases and review of the literature, *Scand J Rheumatol* 24:174–179, 1995.
49. Smith CA, Petty RE, Tingle AJ: Rubella virus and arthritis, *Rheum Dis Clin North Am* 13:265–274, 1987.
50. Inman RD: Rheumatic manifestations of hepatitis B virus infection, *Semin Arthritis Rheum* 11:406–420, 1982.
51. Ramos-Casals M, Font J: Extrahepatic manifestations in patients with chronic hepatitis C virus infection, *Curr Opin Rheumatol* 17:447–455, 2005.
52. Schiff ER: Atypical clinical manifestations of hepatitis A, *Vaccine* 10(Suppl 1):S18–S20, 1992.
53. Holborow EJ, Asherson GL, Johnson GD, et al.: Antinuclear factor and other antibodies in blood and liver diseases, *Br Med J* 1:656–658, 1963.
54. Brancato L, Itescu S, Skovron ML, et al.: Aspects of the spectrum, prevalence and disease susceptibility determinants of Reiter's syndrome and related disorders associated with HIV infection, *Rheumatol Int* 9:137–141, 1989.
55. Calabrese LH: The rheumatic manifestations of infection with the human immunodeficiency virus, *Semin Arthritis Rheum* 18:225–239, 1989.
56. Ali Ou Alla S, Combe B: Arthritis after infection with Chikungunya virus, *Best Pract Res Clin Rheumatol* 25:337–346, 2011.
57. Laine M, Luukkainen R, Toivanen A: Sindbis viruses and other alphaviruses as cause of human arthritic disease, *J Intern Med* 256:457–471, 2004.
58. Rwaguma EB, Lutwama JJ, Sempala SD, et al.: Emergence of epidemic O'nyong-nyong fever in southwestern Uganda, after an absence of 35 years, *Emerg Infect Dis* 3:77, 1997.
59. Fraser JR: Epidemic polyarthritis and Ross River virus disease, *Clin Rheum Dis* 12:369–388, 1986.
60. Weaver SC, Lecuit M: Chikungunya virus and the global spread of a mosquito-borne disease, *N Engl J Med* 372:1231–1239, 2015.
61. Burt FJ, Rolph MS, Rulli NE, et al.: Chikungunya: a re-emerging virus, *Lancet* 379:662–671, 2012.
62. Burt F, Chen W, Mahalingam S: Chikungunya virus and arthritic disease, *Lancet Infect Dis* 14:789–790, 2014.
63. Javelle E, Ribera A, Degasne I, et al.: Specific management of post-chikungunya rheumatic disorders: a retrospective study of 159 cases in Reunion Island from 2006-2012, *PLoS Negl Trop Dis* 9:e0003603, 2015.
64. Miner JJ, Aw Yeang HX, Fox JM, et al.: Brief report: chikungunya viral arthritis in the United States: a mimic of seronegative rheumatoid arthritis, *Arthritis Rheumatol* 67:1214–1220, 2015.
65. Chang AY, Encinales L, Porras A, et al.: Frequency of chronic joint pain following chikungunya virus infection: a Colombian cohort study, *Arthritis Rheumatol* 70:578–584, 2018.
66. Libera I, Gburek Z, Klus D: [Pseudorheumatoid paraneoplastic syndrome], *Reumatologia* 19:305–309, 1981.
67. Meyer B, Goldsmith E, Mustapha M: An internist's dilemma: differentiating paraneoplastic from primary rheumatologic disease, *Minn Med* 97:47, 2014.
68. Zhang W, Doherty M, Pascual E, et al.: EULAR evidence based recommendations for gout. Part I: diagnosis. Report of a task force of the Standing Committee for International Clinical Studies Including Therapeutics (ESCISIT), *Ann Rheum Dis* 65:1301–1311, 2006.
69. Ho Jr G, DeNuccio M: Gout and pseudogout in hospitalized patients, *Arch Intern Med* 153:2787–2790, 1993.
70. Urano W, Yamanaka H, Tsutani H, et al.: The inflammatory process in the mechanism of decreased serum uric acid concentrations during acute gouty arthritis, *J Rheumatol* 29:1950–1953, 2002.
71. Jordan KM, Cameron JS, Snaith M, et al.: British Society for Rheumatology and British Health Professionals in Rheumatology guideline for the management of gout, *Rheumatology (Oxford)* 46:1372–1374, 2007.
72. Sivera F, Andres M, Carmona L, et al.: Multinational evidence-based recommendations for the diagnosis and management of gout: integrating systematic literature review and expert opinion of a broad panel of rheumatologists in the 3e initiative, *Ann Rheum Dis* 73:328–335, 2014.
73. Ogdie A, Taylor WJ, Weatherall M, et al.: Imaging modalities for the classification of gout: systematic literature review and meta-analysis, *Ann Rheum Dis* 74:1868–1874, 2015.
74. Richette P, Bardin T, Doherty M: An update on the epidemiology of calcium pyrophosphate dihydrate crystal deposition disease, *Rheumatology (Oxford)* 48:711–715, 2009.
75. Ivorra J, Rosas J, Pascual E: Most calcium pyrophosphate crystals appear as non-birefringent, *Ann Rheum Dis* 58:582–584, 1999.
76. Dieppe PA, Doherty M, Macfarlane DG, et al.: Apatite associated destructive arthritis, *Br J Rheumatol* 23:84–91, 1984.
77. Ea HK, Liote F: Diagnosis and clinical manifestations of calcium pyrophosphate and basic calcium phosphate crystal deposition diseases, *Rheum Dis Clin North Am* 40:207–229, 2014.
78. Utsinger PD, Resnick D, Shapiro RF, et al.: Roentgenologic, immunologic, and therapeutic study of erosive (inflammatory) osteoarthritis, *Arch Intern Med* 138:693–697, 1978.
79. Punzi L, Frigato M, Frallonardo P, et al.: Inflammatory osteoarthritis of the hand, *Best Pract Res Clin Rheumatol* 24:301–312, 2010.
80. Armstrong DG, Todd WF, Lavery LA, et al.: The natural history of acute Charcot's arthropathy in a diabetic foot specialty clinic, *Diabet Med* 14:357–363, 1997.
81. Vilanova JC, Barcelo J, Villalon M, et al.: MR imaging of lipoma arborescens and the associated lesions, *Skeletal Radiol* 32:504–509, 2003.
82. Davis RI, Hamilton A, Biggart JD: Primary synovial chondromatosis: a clinicopathologic review and assessment of malignant potential, *Hum Pathol* 29:683–688, 1998.
83. Sharma H, Rana B, Mahendra A, et al.: Outcome of 17 pigmented villonodular synovitis (PVNS) of the knee at 6 years mean follow-up, *Knee* 14:390–394, 2007.
84. Rizzoli R, Akesson K, Bouxsein M, et al.: Subtrochanteric fractures after long-term treatment with bisphosphonates: a European Society on Clinical and Economic Aspects of Osteoporosis and Osteoarthritis, and International Osteoporosis Foundation Working Group Report, *Osteoporos Int* 22:373–390, 2011.

85. de Seze S, Solnica J, Mitrovic D, et al.: Joint and bone disorders and hypoparathyroidism in hemochromatosis, *Semin Arthritis Rheum* 2:71–94, 1972.
86. Katoh N, Tazawa K, Ishii W, et al.: Systemic AL amyloidosis mimicking rheumatoid arthritis, *Intern Med* 47:1133–1138, 2008.
87. McAdam LP, Pearson CM, Pitts WH, et al.: Papular mucinosis with myopathy, arthritis, and eosinophilia. A histopathologic study, *Arthritis Rheum* 20:989–996, 1977.
88. Rivest C, Turgeon PP, Senecal JL: Lambda light chain deposition disease presenting as an amyloid-like arthropathy, *J Rheumatol* 20:880–884, 1993.
89. Husby G, Blichfeldt P, Brinch L, et al.: Chronic arthritis and gamma heavy chain disease: coincidence or pathogenic link? *Scand J Rheumatol* 27:257–264, 1998.
90. Dux S, Pitlik S, Rosenfeld JB: Pseudogouty arthritis in hypothyroidism, *Arthritis Rheum* 22:1416–1417, 1979.
91. Vague J, Codaccioni JL: [Rheumatic manifestations developing in association with hyperthyroidism; 5 case reports on scapulohumeral periarthritis], *Ann Endocrinol (Paris)* 18:737–744, 1957.
92. Dorwart BB, Schumacher HR: Joint effusions, chondrocalcinosis and other rheumatic manifestations in hypothyroidism. A clinicopathologic study, *Am J Med* 59:780–790, 1975.
93. Segal AM, Sheeler LR, Wilke WS: Myalgia as the primary manifestation of spontaneously resolving hyperthyroidism, *J Rheumatol* 9:459–461, 1982.
94. Delamere JP, Baddeley RM, Walton KW: Jejuno-ileal bypass arthropathy: its clinical features and associations, *Ann Rheum Dis* 42:553–557, 1983.
95. Brancatisano A, Wahlroos S, Brancatisano R: Improvement in comorbid illness after placement of the Swedish Adjustable Gastric Band, *Surg Obes Relat Dis* 4:S39–46, 2008.
96. Lubrano E, Ciacci C, Ames PR, et al.: The arthritis of coeliac disease: prevalence and pattern in 200 adult patients, *Br J Rheumatol* 35:1314–1318, 1996.
97. Wingfield A: Palindromic rheumatism, *Br Med J* 2:157, 1945.
98. McCarty DJ, O'Duffy JD, Pearson L, et al.: Remitting seronegative symmetrical synovitis with pitting edema. RS3PE syndrome, *JAMA* 254:2763–2767, 1985.
99. Keith JR: The treatment of serum sickness occurring in diphtheria, *Br Med J* 2:105, 1911.
100. Smith MH, Bass AR: Arthritis after cancer immunotherapy: symptom duration and treatment response, *Arthritis Care Res (Hoboken)* 71:362–366, 2019.
101. Tocut M, Brenner R, Zandman-Goddard G: Autoimmune phenomena and disease in cancer patients treated with immune checkpoint inhibitors, *Autoimmun Rev* 17:610–616, 2018.
102. Aletaha D, Neogi T, Silman AJ, et al.: Rheumatoid arthritis classification criteria: an American College of Rheumatology/European League Against Rheumatism collaborative initiative, *Ann Rheum Dis* 69(2010):1580–1588, 2010.
103. Tillett W, Costa L, Jadon D, et al.: The ClASsification for Psoriatic ARthritis (CASPAR) criteria—a retrospective feasibility, sensitivity, and specificity study, *J Rheumatol* 39:154–156, 2012.
104. Rudwaleit M, Khan MA, Sieper J: The challenge of diagnosis and classification in early ankylosing spondylitis: do we need new criteria? *Arthritis Rheum* 52:1000–1008, 2005.
105. Taylor WJ, Fransen J, Dalbeth N, et al.: Performance of classification criteria for gout in early and established disease, *Ann Rheum Dis*, 2014.
106. van der Horst-Bruinsma IE, Speyer I, Visser H, et al.: Diagnosis and course of early-onset arthritis: results of a special early arthritis clinic compared to routine patient care, *Br J Rheumatol* 37:1084–1088, 1998.
107. Wolfe F, Ross K, Hawley DJ, et al.: The prognosis of rheumatoid arthritis and undifferentiated polyarthritis syndrome in the clinic: a study of 1141 patients, *J Rheumatol* 20:2005–2009, 1993.
108. Mottonen TT, Hannonen PJ, Boers M: Combination DMARD therapy including corticosteroids in early rheumatoid arthritis, *Clin Exp Rheumatol* 17:S59–S65, 1999.

46 Skin and Rheumatic Diseases

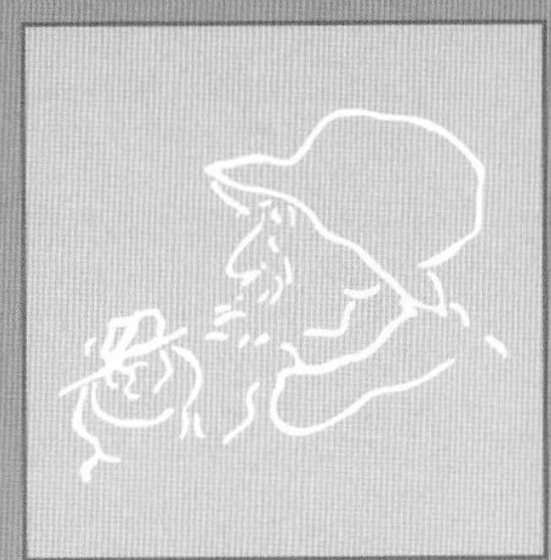

DAVID F. FIORENTINO AND VICTORIA P. WERTH

KEY POINTS

The skin is often affected in rheumatic diseases, and many patients present with skin findings.

Accurate diagnosis of cutaneous lesions requires knowledge of the differential diagnosis, understanding of when and when not to obtain additional studies (e.g., biopsy), and the ability to interpret the results in the context of the clinical presentation.

Skin biopsy findings of inflammatory conditions are often not definitively diagnostic.

Diagnosis of Skin Lesions Associated With Rheumatic Diseases

The skin is a highly visible organ that is frequently affected in rheumatic diseases, and the presence of skin lesions may be helpful diagnostically. Certain caveats are worth noting before discussing the specifics. First, a major pitfall for the nondermatologist in evaluating skin lesions is incomplete knowledge of the entities in the differential diagnosis. For example, malar erythema occurs frequently in patients with systemic lupus erythematosus (SLE), but the differential diagnosis for malar erythema is rather extensive and includes conditions that are much more prevalent than lupus (e.g., rosacea), as well as conditions that are far less prevalent (e.g., Rothmund-Thomson syndrome). Patients frequently have more than one skin condition, which often makes diagnosis more challenging.

Another caveat for the nondermatologist concerns skin biopsy. The ability to determine when a skin biopsy might be diagnostically useful in many cases requires a great deal of specialized knowledge, as does the interpretation of pathology reports. It is often the case with inflammatory skin conditions that the microscopic findings are actually less diagnostically specific than the clinical examination. Unfortunately, it is common for a pathology report to list a diagnosis with no context to help the clinician understand how definitive the findings were. For example, a skin biopsy report may list psoriasis as the final diagnosis, but, depending on the specific case, the unstated additional possibilities may include nummular dermatitis, atopic dermatitis, seborrheic dermatitis, lichen simplex chronicus, dermatophytosis, or drug eruption. Particularly with regard to inflammatory skin conditions, a working knowledge of both dermatopathology and dermatology and placement of the histologic findings in the context of the clinical presentation may be necessary for the clinician to arrive at the correct diagnosis.

The above considerations notwithstanding, it is useful for the physician caring for patients with rheumatic diseases to be well versed in their cutaneous manifestations. In this chapter, we provide an overview of these manifestations, as well as a perspective on diagnosis and differential diagnosis. Therapy is discussed briefly in conditions in which treatment may be specifically directed toward the skin lesions. Etiology and pathogenesis of these diseases are covered elsewhere in this text.

Psoriasis

KEY POINTS

Psoriasis is associated with multiple comorbidities beyond the skin and joints, including atherosclerosis.

The major phenotypes of psoriasis are chronic plaque, guttate, localized pustular, generalized pustular, and erythroderma. Chronic plaque and guttate are the most common phenotypes.

Pustular psoriasis, unstable/advancing psoriasis, and plaque psoriasis likely all have different pathogenic pathways and might respond differently to targeted therapies.

Guttate psoriasis may occur a few weeks after a streptococcal infection.

Nail changes are common but are not specific for psoriasis.

Systemic corticosteroids should be avoided in psoriasis, if possible, because severe flaring may occur upon tapering.

Skin findings of reactive arthritis include circinate balanitis, keratoderma blenorrhagica, oral mucosal erosions, and psoriasiform plaques.

Skin biopsy cannot distinguish between psoriasis and reactive arthritis.

Psoriasis is one of the most common inflammatory skin diseases, affecting approximately 2% of the general population.[1] Women and men are affected equally. Psoriasis can manifest at any age, but onset usually occurs between 18 and 39 years of age or between 50 and 69 years of age. Psoriasis is less common in children than in adults, and onset in childhood portends more severe disease. There is a wide range of severity of skin lesions, from a few relatively asymptomatic plaques to extensive, disabling disease. The onset may be at any time during life. Once present, it may exhibit exacerbations and remissions, but it does not tend to resolve permanently.

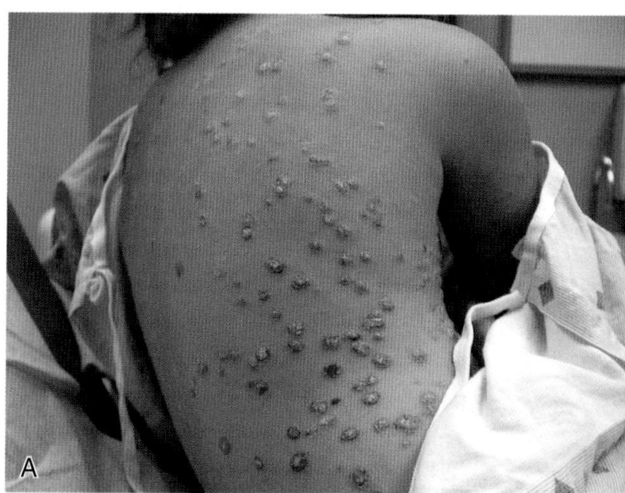

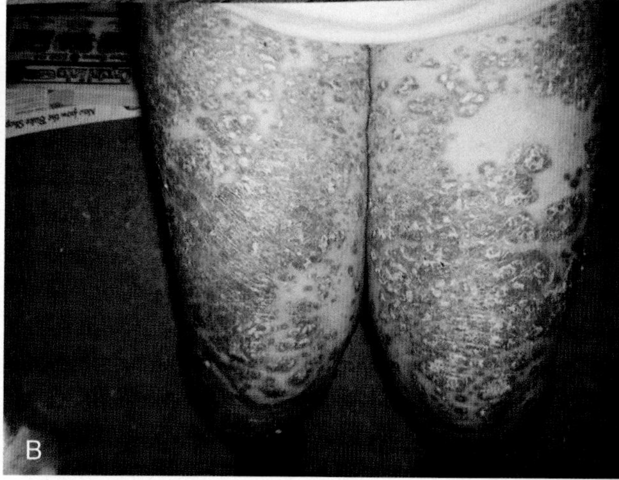

• **Fig. 46.1** (A) Guttate psoriasis resembles "drops" of discrete scaly papules with erythema, often on the trunk. (B) Plaque psoriasis with thick micaceous scale on the thighs. (A, Courtesy Dr. Nicole Rogers, Tulane University School of Medicine, New Orleans; B, courtesy Dr. Abby Van Voorhees, University of Pennsylvania.)

Psoriasis is clearly more than a skin disease, and has been associated with an increased prevalence of atherosclerosis and systemic and vascular inflammation with cardiovascular disease being the leading cause of death.[2] Other comorbidities include psoriatic arthritis, associated autoimmune diseases, hypertension, diabetes, dyslipidemia, obesity, metabolic syndrome, depression, addictive habits like smoking and alcohol use, and non-alcoholic steatohepatitis.

There are three distinct inflammatory pathways that drive different clinical expressions of psoriasis: the IL-17/23 axis, most important in plaque psoriasis; the interferon (IFN) pathway, which is active in early/acute and unstable psoriasis; and the IL-36/IL-1 pathway, important in pustular psoriasis.[3] For example, mutations in the IL-36 receptor antagonist (IL-36RN) gene are associated with pustular psoriasis, but not typical plaque-type psoriasis.[4]

Skin lesions of psoriasis characteristically are sharply demarcated plaques with silvery scale and underlying erythema, although there may be a paucity of scale if the lesions have been partially treated or if they occur in intertriginous areas. When the scale is removed, pinpoint bleeding may be observed (Auspitz sign). Lesions may occur in areas of trauma (Koebner phenomenon) such as in surgical scars. In some cases lesions contain small pustules.

General phenotypes of psoriasis are chronic plaque, guttate, localized pustular, generalized pustular, and erythrodermic.[1] Chronic plaque and guttate psoriasis are the most common, and generalized pustular psoriasis and erythroderma are typically the most disabling and even life threatening. Chronic plaque psoriasis lesions are often relatively large in diameter and occur preferentially on elbows, knees, scalp, genitalia, lower back, and the gluteal cleft, although they may occur in many other locations. It is quite common for only one area of skin, such as the scalp, to be affected. Guttate lesions are relatively small in diameter and are usually quite numerous, distributed preferentially on the trunk and proximal extremities (Fig. 46.1). Guttate psoriasis occurs relatively commonly in children and young adults, often manifesting a few weeks after a streptococcal infection.

Nail changes are common, occurring in approximately half of patients, and are often mistaken for fungal infection. Findings include pitting, onycholysis ("oil spots"), dystrophy of nails, and loss of the nail plate. These changes are not specific for psoriasis. Notably, pitting may occur as a result of trauma. Nail changes are more frequent in patients with arthritis of the distal interphalangeal joints.[5]

Arthritis occurs more often in patients with severe cutaneous disease, but cutaneous disease need not be present at all. Remissions and exacerbations of arthritis do not correlate well with remissions and exacerbations of skin disease. The presence of psoriatic skin lesions may be helpful in supporting a diagnosis of psoriatic arthritis, although many patients with psoriasis have joint disease unrelated to psoriasis.

The physician usually makes the diagnosis of psoriatic skin disease on clinical grounds alone, largely on the basis of the morphology and distribution of lesions. The differential diagnosis may be extensive and includes in selected cases nummular eczema, seborrheic dermatitis, candidiasis (in intertriginous areas), pityriasis rubra pilaris, Bowen's disease or Paget's disease (for isolated plaques), drug eruption, pityriasis rosea, pityriasis lichenoides, dermatophytosis, lichen planus, secondary syphilis, parapsoriasis, cutaneous lupus (especially subacute cutaneous lupus erythematosus [SCLE]), and dermatomyositis. In cases in which the diagnosis is not clear cut, biopsy may be helpful. The histologic findings may range from virtually diagnostic for psoriasis to merely consistent with but not diagnostic. Histologically, psoriasis cannot generally be distinguished from the skin lesions seen in reactive arthritis.

Common topical therapies include corticosteroids, vitamin D analogues, salicylic acid, calcineurin inhibitors, and, less commonly, tar, anthralin, and retinoids.[1] Phototherapy with sunlight, narrow-band ultraviolet B (UVB), 308-nm excimer laser, or, less commonly, psoralen ultraviolet A (PUVA)-range is still an effective therapy for many patients. Common traditional systemic therapies include methotrexate, acitretin, and fumarates (in Europe), while cyclosporine is less commonly used and only to gain rapid control of disease.[6] Apremilast is a phosphodiesterase-4 inhibitor that is used for both skin and joint disease. The biologic therapies have emerged as the most effective therapies for skin and joint disease, and include TNF inhibitors, IL-12/23 dual inhibitors, IL-17 antagonists, and IL-23 inhibitors.[6] Although topical corticosteroids are an acceptable treatment for many patients, systemic

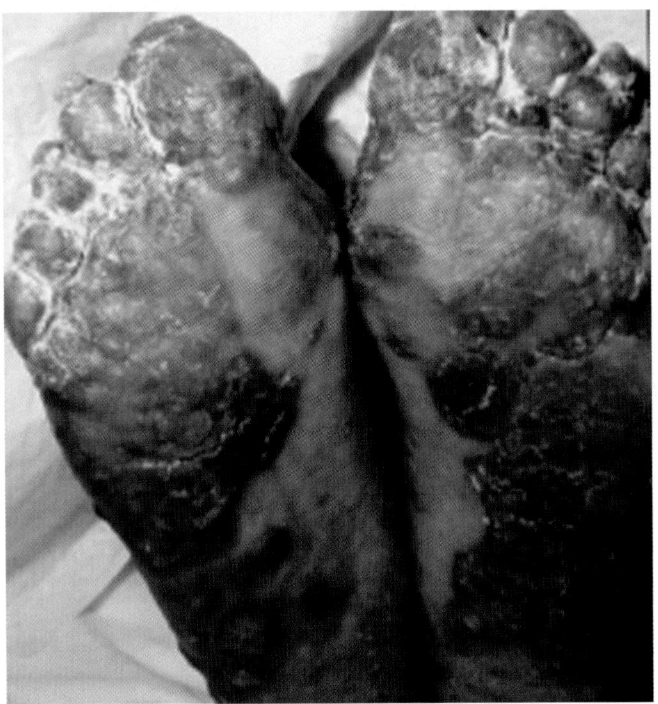

• **Fig. 46.2** Reactive arthritis with keratoderma blennorrhagica of the feet.

corticosteroids are avoided for the treatment of cutaneous disease, in particular because of the observation of severe flaring of psoriasis following withdrawal of systemic corticosteroids.

Reactive Arthritis

Circinate balanitis is the most common of the characteristic mucocutaneous lesions of reactive arthritis, occurring in 50% of men.[7] Small, painless, erythematous papules and pustules coalesce to form well-demarcated, serpiginous erosive or crusted plaques on the glans penis and around the urethral meatus. In uncircumcised men, the appearance is more often that of erosion rather than crust because the moisture and trauma minimize the formation of crust. In circumcised men, crusting may be more obvious than erosion. Women develop similar lesions of ulcerative vulvitis, with well-demarcated, erythematous plaques.

Lesions that are initially similar to the small erythematous papules, vesicles, and pustules of the genital region may develop on the palms and, particularly, the soles in approximately 10% of patients 1 to 2 months after development of reactive arthritis.[7] With time, these lesions, termed *keratoderma blennorrhagica,* tend to become markedly hyperkeratotic (Fig. 46.2). They may coalesce into large plaques or generalized hyperkeratosis involving the entire plantar surface, or they may remain discrete, erythematous, hyperkeratotic papules a few millimeters in diameter.

Erythematous, scaly plaques indistinguishable from psoriasis, may appear elsewhere on the skin, including the scrotum, scalp, elbows, and knees. When lesions occur around the nails, it is common for there to be hyperkeratosis underneath the nails. Pitting is not typical of reactive arthritis, but thickening, ridging, or shedding of the nail plate may occur. Painless erosions, macules, and papules of the oral mucosa are relatively common on the tongue, buccal mucosa, and palate, with circinate lesions having the appearance of geographic tongue. Erythema nodosum is an uncommon manifestation, occurring more commonly in women and especially linked to *Yersinia* infections.

The diagnosis of the cutaneous lesions is usually made on a clinical basis. Skin biopsy may be helpful in excluding many entities in the differential diagnosis, but in general, it cannot exclude psoriasis. Unfortunately, the major condition in the differential diagnosis of the skin lesions is usually psoriasis. One somewhat distinguishing histologic feature is that the older lesions of keratoderma blennorrhagica may have a considerably thickened stratum corneum, corresponding to the markedly hyperkeratotic papules seen grossly.

For the genital lesions, conditions to consider in the differential diagnosis may include candidiasis, psoriasis, dermatitis, Bowen's disease, Paget's disease, squamous cell carcinoma, Zoon's balanitis, erosive lichen planus, lichen sclerosus (balanitis xerotica obliterans), aphthosis, fixed drug eruption, and certain infectious diseases. The differential diagnosis for lesions on the soles and palms may include psoriasis, hereditary or acquired hyperkeratosis of the palms and soles, pustular eruption of the palms and soles, pompholyx, scabies, and dermatophytosis. The differential diagnosis for oral lesions may include geographic tongue, lichen planus, candidiasis, aphthae, and autoimmune bullous diseases.

The approach to treatment of skin lesions is similar to that for psoriasis, particularly in cases in which the lesions are persistent. Choice of topical therapies may be somewhat limited because of the sites involved. The oral mucosa is a difficult site to deliver medication topically, and the genital area may develop irritant reactions to certain topical medications. Often, topical corticosteroids are preferred for both areas because of low potential for irritation and the availability of topical preparations designed for these sites, but topical calcineurin inhibitors can also be tried. In the genital area, superinfection with *Candida* may occur, and concurrent therapy with a topical or systemic anticandidal medication may be necessary on occasion.

Rheumatoid Arthritis

KEY POINTS

Skin findings associated with RA are characteristically granulomatous or neutrophilic.

The major granulomatous cutaneous finding is the rheumatoid nodule. The major neutrophilic conditions are vasculitis, Sweet's syndrome, and pyoderma gangrenosum.

Sweet's syndrome and pyoderma gangrenosum are part of a group of noninfectious inflammatory conditions called ***neutrophilic dermatoses.*** These conditions may be associated with internal diseases, including rheumatic diseases.

Interstitial granulomatous dermatitis (IGD) and palisaded neutrophilic and granulomatous dermatitis (PNGD) are rare conditions that may be associated with RA or other rheumatic diseases. It is not clear whether IGD and PNGD are distinct entities or variants of the same condition.

The cutaneous eruptions of juvenile idiopathic arthritis and adult-onset Still's may be similar to viral exanthems or drug eruptions, but they are distinctive in that they clear completely between episodes.

The major skin manifestations associated with rheumatoid arthritis (RA) generally fall under granulomatous lesions, exemplified by the rheumatoid nodule, and neutrophilic lesions, exemplified by vasculitis and pyoderma gangrenosum.

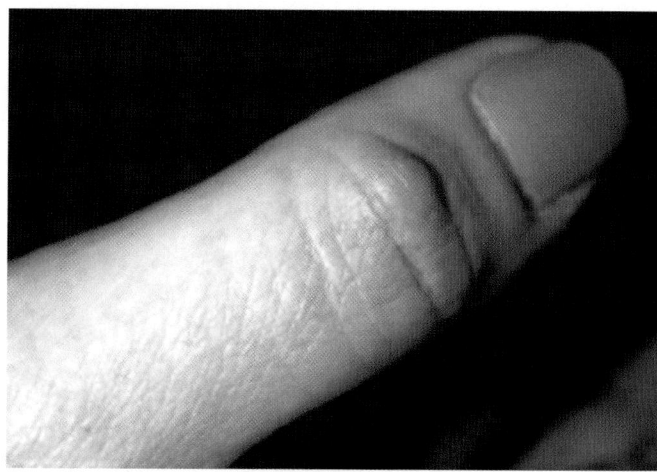

• **Fig. 46.3** Rheumatoid nodule over the extensor tendon of the distal interphalangeal joint.

Rheumatoid nodules are the most common cutaneous manifestations of RA.[8] They occur more often in seropositive patients and correlate somewhat with higher rheumatoid factor titers, more severe arthritis, and increased risk for vasculitis. Nodules are usually relatively deep, firm, and painless and tend to develop over areas of pressure and trauma, such as the extensor forearms, fingers, olecranon processes, ischial tuberosities, sacrum, knees, heels, and posterior scalp (Fig. 46.3). In patients who wear glasses, nodules may develop under the bridge or nosepieces. In most cases, rheumatoid nodules are in the subcutaneous tissue and/or deep dermis, but occasionally they may occur more deeply or more superficially.

Clinically, depending on the presentation, numerous entities may be in the differential diagnosis, including infections, inflammatory disorders, and benign tumors. If needed, biopsy of a nodule may be quite helpful in establishing the diagnosis. Rheumatoid nodules exhibit a distinctive histologic finding called necrobiosis, a fibrinoid degeneration of the connective tissue, surrounded by palisaded histiocytes. Rheumatoid nodules and synovia contain significant amounts of citrullinating peptidyl arginine deiminases 2, 3, and 4 and homocitrullination-facilitating neutrophil myeloperoxidase enzymes. This could explain the levels of citrulline and homocitrulline in seropositive RA rheumatoid nodule necrotic tissue.[9] Necrobiosis is also a characteristic feature of granuloma annulare and necrobiosis lipoidica diabeticorum. Although necrobiosis lipoidica diabeticorum is easily distinguished from rheumatoid nodule clinically, the subcutaneous variant of granuloma annulare may be difficult to distinguish, both clinically and histologically.

The term *rheumatoid nodulosis* has been used to describe an entity characterized by subcutaneous rheumatoid nodules, cystic bone lesions, rheumatoid factor positivity, and arthralgias in patients with little or no evidence of systemic manifestations of RA or erosive joint disease.[10] Older males are preferentially affected.

The development of nodules in RA patients undergoing treatment with methotrexate has been noted by several observers and termed *accelerated rheumatoid nodulosis*.[11] The nodules are newly appearing and occur preferentially on the hands. There are also case reports of the phenomenon in RA patients treated with etanercept and tocilizumab.[12]

The other major type of cutaneous lesion associated with RA is neutrophil predominant. Rheumatoid vasculitis occurs more frequently in patients who are seropositive and have rheumatoid nodules, and it often occurs relatively late in the course of the disease.[13] Vessels of any size may be affected. In the skin, vasculitis may appear as purpuric papules and macules, nodules, ulcerations, or infarcts. Bywaters lesions are periungual or digital pulp purpuric papules that represent a small vessel vasculitis but are not necessarily associated with vasculitic lesions elsewhere. The incidence of rheumatoid vasculitis is decreasing with earlier treatment and more effective therapies for RA, but the mortality rate is still high.[14]

The differential diagnosis of purpuric or petechial lesions may include stasis dermatitis, Schamberg's purpura, platelet dysfunction, petechial drug eruptions, viral exanthems, emboli, thromboses, and sludging. Of these, Schamberg's purpura, a relatively common condition unassociated with systemic disease, is probably the most frequently confused with small vessel vasculitis. Skin biopsy may be helpful in establishing the diagnosis of vasculitis, particularly if an early lesion is sampled, although rheumatoid vasculitis cannot be distinguished histologically from many other causes of small vessel vasculitis. Immunofluorescent examination of an early lesion may be helpful in ruling out immunoglobulin (Ig)A-predominant vasculitis. The differential diagnosis of ulcers and infarcts is extensive. Biopsy is often unrewarding because nonspecific changes present in established lesions may make interpretation difficult, but on occasion biopsy of ulcers or infarcts may result in a definitive diagnosis of vasculitis.

The neutrophilic dermatoses are a group of diseases inflammatory rather than infectious in origin, typified by pyoderma gangrenosum and Sweet's syndrome. These conditions have been associated with a variety of extracutaneous diseases, including RA. The classic pyoderma gangrenosum lesion is a rapidly appearing, large, destructive ulcer in which the border is undermined. The classic lesion of Sweet's syndrome is an erythematous, edematous plaque with a surface often described as mammillated, pseudovesicular, or microvesicular. Clinical appearances intermediate between these two have been described. For pyoderma gangrenosum, the differential diagnosis is usually that of conditions causing leg ulcer, and the diagnosis is mainly clinical, with biopsy primarily serving to exclude some of the other entities under consideration. For Sweet's syndrome, the differential diagnosis may include infections, halogenoderma, and other neutrophilic dermatoses. Biopsy often provides helpful supporting evidence. The mainstay of therapy for acute lesions of both conditions is systemic corticosteroids. For more persistent lesions, a variety of options may be considered, cyclosporine and infliximab being two of the more common. Colchicine, dapsone, or potassium iodide may be first-line therapies in patients with infections or contraindications to corticosteroids.[15]

The term *rheumatoid neutrophilic dermatitis* has been given to describe chronic, erythematous, urticarial-like plaques that occur primarily on the distal arms.[16] Clinically and histologically, rheumatoid neutrophilic dermatitis is similar to Sweet's syndrome and may be a variant of it.

Palisaded neutrophilic and granulomatous dermatitis (PNGD) of connective tissue disease is an unusual condition or set of conditions for which consistent terminology is still evolving. As the name implies, the major bases for diagnosis of this entity are the histologic appearance and the occurrence in a patient with connective tissue disease, often RA.[17] The clinical appearance ranges from erythematous or flesh-colored papules that appear primarily on fingers and elbows to erythematous or flesh-colored linear cords on the trunk. Some authors classify the latter as interstitial granulomatous dermatitis with cutaneous cords or interstitial granulomatous dermatitis with arthritis (IGDA). Treatment of PNGD and IGDA can be challenging. PNGD may respond to dapsone or sulfapyridine. IGDA can be treated with anti-malarials or immunosuppressives, but evidence is based on case reports and small case series. Patients can progress to a severe deforming arthritis. In some cases, granuloma annulare and rheumatoid nodule may be in the differential diagnosis.

Juvenile Rheumatoid Arthritis/Still's Disease

The majority of patients with classic Still's disease manifest an exanthematous eruption coincident with daily fever spikes.[18] The lesions are evanescent, usually nonpruritic, erythematous macules occurring over the trunk, extremities, and face. The differential diagnosis includes viral exanthem, drug eruption, familial periodic fever syndromes, and rheumatic fever. It is not unusual for exanthems of any type to be more prominent during fevers, but it is not expected that viral exanthems and drug eruptions will clear completely between fever spikes. However, it should be noted that the eruption of erythema infectiosum (fifth disease) due to parvovirus B19 may resolve completely but reappear when the skin temperature rises, as with warm baths or exercise. Adult-onset Still's disease is also typified by an evanescent erythematous, sometimes salmon-colored, eruption over the trunk and extremities, associated with high fever. Skin biopsy may be nonspecific. Some patients with adult-onset Still's disease have more persistent, pruritic lesions. The chronic lesions have been described as hyperpigmented plaques with a linear and rippled morphology. These lesions may exhibit a distinctive histology consisting of dyskeratotic keratinocytes in the upper epidermis, along with increased dermal mucin.[19] Subcutaneous nodules may develop in both juvenile-onset and adult-onset Still's disease. The lesions tend to occur at the same sites of the body as do rheumatoid nodules in RA, but histologically they appear similar to nodules of rheumatic fever. Nonsteroidal anti-inflammatory drugs (NSAIDs) and glucocorticoids are first-line treatment, especially for musculoskeletal manifestations and fever. Methotrexate, azathioprine, and leflunomide are often used as steroid-sparing agents. Intravenous immunoglobulin, anti-TNF, and anti-IL-6 agents control the disease in nonresponders to conventional therapy. Treatment with IL-1 inhibitors has been successful.[20]

Lupus Erythematosus

KEY POINTS

- Patients with lupus erythematosus can have a wide variety of lupus-specific and lupus-nonspecific skin lesions.
- Nonspecific skin lesions are more frequently seen in patients who have systemic lupus erythematosus or overlap syndromes.
- Acute cutaneous lupus erythematosus is associated with a high risk for significant systemic disease.
- Patients who present with other lupus-specific skin lesions have a low risk for moderate or severe systemic disease.
- Subacute cutaneous lupus erythematosus is associated with antibodies to Ro/SSA and is frequently drug induced. They can have a +SSA/SSB autoantibody independent of having Sjögren's syndrome.
- Neonatal lupus is associated with maternal IgG autoantibodies to Ro/SSA. Clinical findings may include cutaneous lesions, cardiac disease (usually complete heart block), hepatobiliary disease, or hematologic cytopenias.
- The major skin findings in patients with Sjögren's syndrome consist of dryness and sequelae of dryness of the skin and mucous membranes. Vasculitis is also a relatively common finding.
- Some patients with Sjögren's syndrome have subacute cutaneous lupus lesions or an annular erythematous eruption.

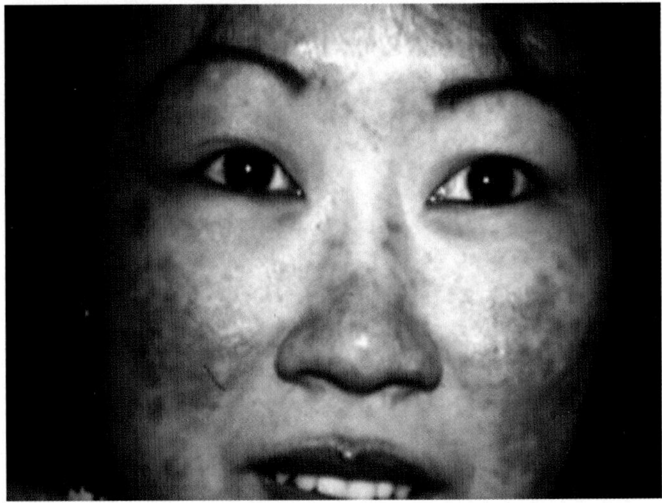

• **Fig. 46.4** Acute malar rash in a butterfly distribution in systemic lupus erythematosus.

The skin is involved at some time in the course of disease in the majority of patients with lupus erythematosus (LE), and skin lesions may be important in establishing the diagnosis. Some skin lesions are highly likely to be associated with "systemic" (i.e., extracutaneous) disease, whereas others may or may not be associated with extracutaneous disease. The phenomenon of lupus skin lesions occurring in the absence of systemic disease has previously been termed *discoid lupus* by some. However, dermatologists use this term to denote a specific type of skin lesion, regardless of presence or absence of systemic disease. It is the latter meaning of discoid lupus to which we refer in this chapter.

Lupus-Specific Skin Lesions

James Gilliam classified cutaneous lesions as specific or nonspecific for lupus, with discoid lupus lesions an example of the former and palpable purpura an example of the latter.[21] Although this division of lesions is useful, sometimes a lupus-specific lesion occurs in a patient who has a primary autoimmune disease other than LE. For example, SCLE lesions may occur in patients whose primary condition is Sjögren's syndrome, and discoid lesions may be seen in a variety of conditions, such as mixed connective tissue disease. Many of the lupus-specific skin lesions can occur in patients who have no evidence of extracutaneous disease.

The characteristic morphologies of the various lupus-specific skin lesions are largely a function of the depth and intensity of the inflammatory infiltrate, presence or absence of epidermal basal cell damage, involvement of hair follicles, abundance of dermal mucin, and tendency to scar. In practice, there may be some overlap of these features, and there may be more than one type of lesion present in a given patient, which makes classification difficult. Also the exact subtype may not be clear early on in the disease. Because therapy for most of the lupus-specific lesions is similar, it is not always important to distinguish among the various types of lesions. However, it can be useful to identify conditions that are more likely to scar, to target more aggressive therapy, and to identify conditions that are highly likely or highly unlikely to be associated with systemic disease.

Acute cutaneous lupus (ACLE) lesions are typified by malar erythema, the classic butterfly rash (Fig. 46.4). The inflammation tends to be superficial, with little propensity to scar. Precipitation

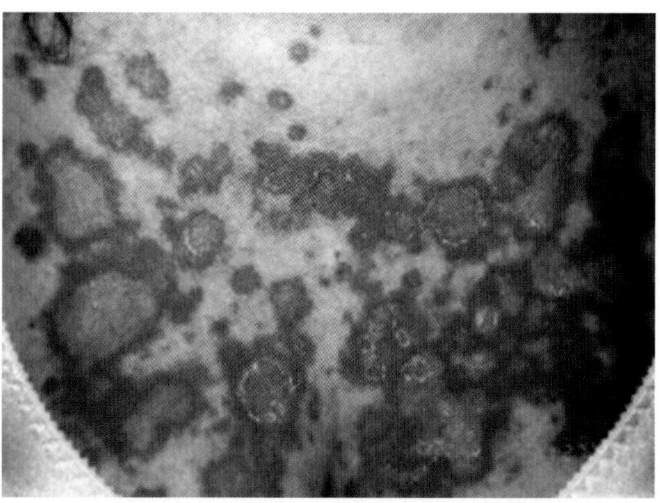

• **Fig. 46.5** Subacute cutaneous lupus erythematosus: annular-polycyclic type.

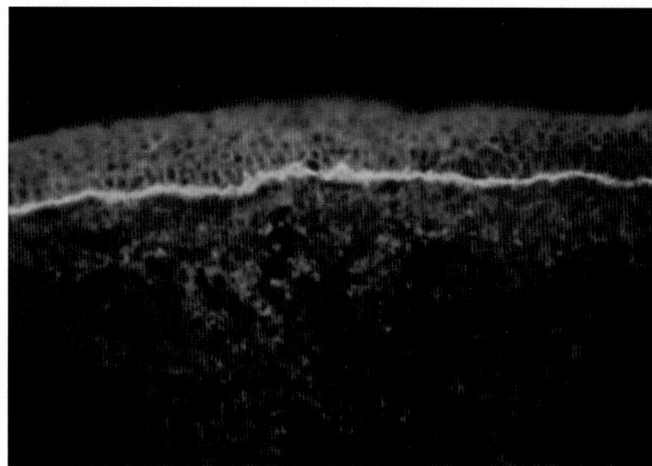

• **Fig. 46.6** Direct immunofluorescence (lupus band test) demonstrating IgG deposits at the dermal-epidermal junction.

or exacerbation of lesions by sun exposure is common, and lesions tend to be distributed on the sun-exposed face, neck, extensor arms, and dorsal hands, where the skin over the knuckles is relatively spared. Often the lesions are quite transient, but they may be persistent. When the face is severely affected, facial edema may be prominent. Oral lesions are often present concurrently. Acute eruptions with considerable focal basal cell damage can result in erythematous papules with dusky centers that clinically mimic erythema multiforme. The major importance of recognition of ACLE is its strong association with systemic disease. The differential diagnosis of malar rash may include several conditions. In some cases, the facial rash of ACLE may be difficult to distinguish from rosacea. Seborrheic dermatitis, atopic dermatitis, and photosensitive eruptions, such as polymorphous light eruption and drug-induced photosensitivity, may also be considered. Dermatomyositis (DM) may cause a photosensitive facial erythema with edema similar to ACLE, although the erythema tends to be more violaceous. Persistent lesions on the neck and arms may be indistinguishable from SCLE. Discoid lupus lesions occasionally appear in a butterfly distribution, where they can result in disfiguring scarring. Skin biopsy is usually not performed on malar erythema because of its transient character, the scar resulting from biopsy, and the availability of other means of establishing the diagnosis of SLE. If a biopsy is done, it should be noted that DM and SCLE cannot be distinguished from ACLE by histology, and, also, that skin biopsy findings are sometimes nonspecific.

SCLE is a photosensitive eruption usually associated with anti-Ro/SSA autoantibodies.[22] Lesional morphology is of two main types: annular erythematous plaques and scaly erythematous psoriatic plaques. Lesions are distributed over sun-exposed skin of the arms, upper trunk, neck, and sides of the face (Fig. 46.5). Inexplicably, the midfacial area is usually uninvolved. Fair-skinned individuals are preferentially affected. Lesions may resolve with hypopigmentation or even depigmentation, but they rarely scar. Several drugs, particularly hydrochlorothiazide, proton pump inhibitors, and terbinafine, have been reported to induce SCLE.[23,24] The risk for systemic disease is not fully known, but perhaps 15% of patients with SCLE have or will develop significant systemic disease, often SLE, Sjögren's syndrome, or an overlap of the two disorders. Depending on the morphology of the lesions and the clinical presentation, the differential diagnosis may include psoriasis, tinea, polymorphous light eruption, reactive erythema, and erythema multiforme. Skin biopsy for routine histology is often helpful in establishing the diagnosis. The characteristic finding of skin biopsy for immunofluorescence is a particulate deposition of IgG in the epidermis (Fig. 46.6), both in lesions and uninvolved skin.[25] This pattern can be reproduced in animal models by infusing anti-Ro, and thus immunofluorescence results provide information that duplicates serologic testing for anti-Ro.[26] The particulate epidermal pattern seen in normal skin does not indicate an increased risk for SLE. However, increased risk is indicated by the finding of granular deposits of IgG at the dermal-epidermal junction of normal skin (the nonlesional lupus band test). It should be noted that many immunofluorescence laboratories do not routinely report particulate epidermal staining.

Discoid lupus erythematosus (DLE) lesions are the most common of the persistent lupus-specific skin lesions. Population-based studies indicate that cutaneous lupus, to include DLE and SCLE, has an incidence similar to that of SLE.[27,28] Active DLE lesions are erythematous papules and plaques that, when palpated, may feel indurated because of the substantial numbers of inflammatory cells that infiltrate the dermis. Involvement of hair follicles may be grossly evident as follicular plugs and scarring alopecia. Dyspigmentation is common, often with hypopigmentation or even depigmentation in the center and hyperpigmentation at the periphery (Fig. 46.7). Visible scale is common, and occasionally the epidermis is thickened in a clinical variant called *hypertrophic DLE.* In established lesions, scarring may be disfiguring. Lesions tend to occur on the scalp, ears, and face but may be widespread and occasionally involve mucosal surfaces. It is unusual to have lesions below the neck in the absence of lesions above the neck. Sun exposure may exacerbate DLE in some cases, but the presence of lesions in sun-protected areas of the scalp and ears and the frequent absence of a history of photosensitivity indicates that sun exposure is probably not a trigger in every instance. There are case reports of squamous cell carcinoma developing in patients with established DLE lesions. In a patient who presents with DLE lesions only, the risk for development of moderate to severe systemic symptoms is probably approximately 5% to 10%, although mild systemic symptoms such as arthralgias are relatively common. As many as 15% to 20% may meet the criteria for SLE, but many do so solely on the basis of mucocutaneous findings.[29] The differential diagnosis of DLE lesions is often that of conditions that exhibit intense lymphocytic or granulomatous infiltrates such as

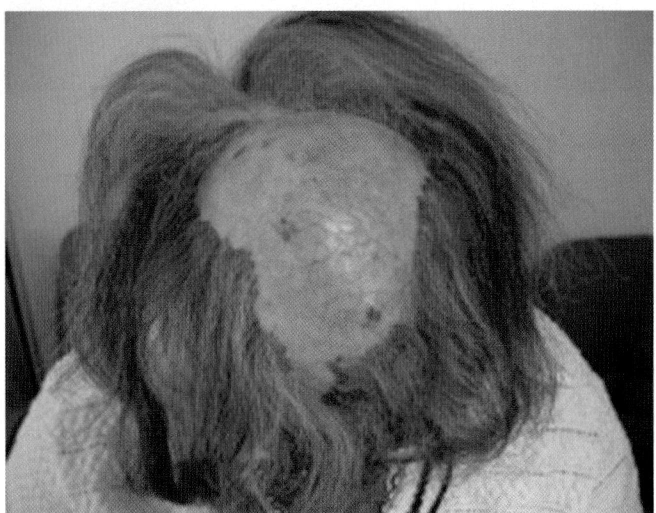

• **Fig. 46.7** Discoid lupus erythematosus of the scalp, with scarring alopecia and central hypopigmentation. (Courtesy Dr. Nicole Rogers, Tulane University School of Medicine, New Orleans.)

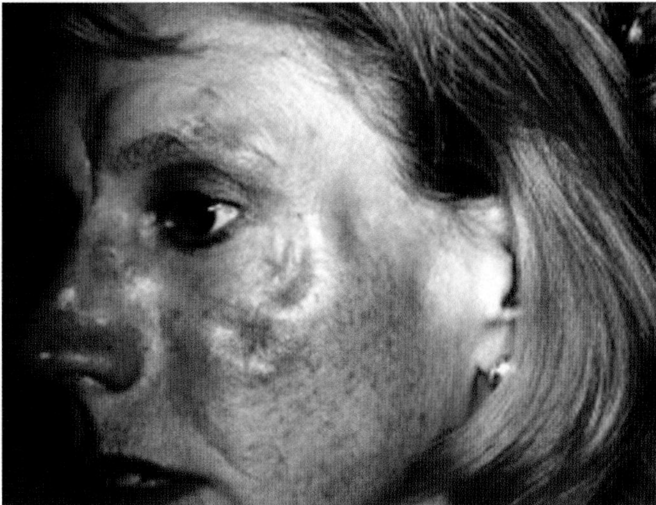

• **Fig. 46.8** Lupus profundus (panniculitis) with extensive atrophy.

sarcoid, Jessner's lymphocytic infiltrate, granuloma faciale, polymorphous light eruption, lymphocytoma cutis, and lymphoma cutis. In the scalp, lichen planopilaris and other scarring alopecias may be considered. Skin biopsy for routine histology often establishes the diagnosis definitively. In more difficult cases, biopsy for immunofluorescence may provide additional supporting diagnostic information. Lesions are expected to have granular deposits of immunoglobulins (Ig) at the dermal-epidermal junction. Unless there is concomitant systemic disease, normal skin is expected not to have Ig deposits.

Tumid lupus (TLE) skin lesions are similar to DLE lesions in that they are erythematous indurated papules and plaques with a substantial lymphocytic infiltrate. Unlike DLE, though, the lesions do not exhibit epidermal abnormalities, follicular involvement, or scarring. Considerable mucin is present in the dermis, which gives the lesions a somewhat boggy look and feel. In some reports, lesions are most common on the face and may be reproduced by phototesting.[30] The risk for SLE appears to be low, and Ig deposits are not generally present in skin biopsies. Jessner's lymphocytic infiltrate and other lymphocytic and granulomatous infiltrative conditions (see earlier) are in the differential diagnosis. Skin biopsy for routine histology is valuable in establishing the diagnosis, with the exception of reliably distinguishing TLE from Jessner's lymphocytic infiltrate. Some have argued that Jessner's lymphocytic infiltrate and TLE are one and the same, and it might reasonably be argued that what is called TLE is not appropriately classified as a form of chronic cutaneous LE but rather as an independent entity. However, the presence of TLE lesions in some patients with lupus is evidence to the contrary.

Lupus panniculitis (LEP) lesions have inflammation in the subcutaneous tissue, resulting in deep indurated plaques that become disfiguring, depressed areas (Fig. 46.8). Usual sites of involvement are the face, scalp, upper trunk, breasts, upper arms, buttocks, and thighs. The risk for SLE is not known precisely, but clearly some patients with LEP have or will develop SLE. The differential diagnosis is that of the panniculitides, but the distribution exhibited in LEP is unusual for most other conditions that cause panniculitis. The correlation of clinical with histologic findings usually establishes the diagnosis. Lupus panniculitis needs to be differentiated from panniculitic lymphoma, which can be a mimicker.[31]

Some unusual variants of cutaneous lupus are chilblain lupus (red or dusky plaques on colder areas of skin, such as fingers, toes, nose, elbows, knees, and lower legs), cutaneous lupus/lichen planus overlap, and a bullous eruption associated with autoantibodies to type VII collagen or other basement membrane zone proteins. Not all bullae related to lupus are due to autoantibodies to basement membrane proteins, however. It is not unusual for bullae to develop in the patient simply from intensive destruction of the basal cell layer in ACLE, SCLE, or, rarely, DLE.

Treatment of the lupus-specific lesions is relatively similar for most of the subtypes, with some exceptions and modifications.[32] Sun protection is critical for lesions that are initiated or exacerbated by sun exposure. Many or most patients underestimate the amount of sunscreen they need to apply, the potential damage of the seemingly minimal exposure one has in the course of day-to-day activities, and the value of protective clothing. Tobacco use appears to be an exacerbating factor and can prevent response to therapy.[33] Topical therapy is often used to avoid side effects of systemic medications or to provide adjunctive therapy, although topical agents are unlikely to be beneficial if the disease process is deep, as in panniculitis. Topical or intralesional corticosteroids are the most often used local therapy, but there are some reports of benefit from topical calcineurin inhibitors and topical retinoids. The first-line systemic medication for cutaneous lupus is anti-malarial therapy, most often hydroxychloroquine. For skin disease not responsive to hydroxychloroquine, changing to chloroquine or adding quinacrine has been helpful in some patients.[34] For anti-malarial-resistant skin disease, a wide variety of medications have been used, but there is no clear second choice when patients have not responded to anti-malarials. When evaluating response to therapy, it is important for the clinician to distinguish active disease, as manifested by erythema or development of new lesions, from "damage," as exemplified by scarring or dyspigmentation. Although dapsone is arguably not helpful in most types of cutaneous lupus, it may be helpful in neutrophil-predominant bullous eruptions.[35] Measures to keep the skin warm may be useful for chilblains lupus.

Nonspecific Cutaneous Lesions

A wide variety of lupus nonspecific skin lesions has been reported. Many of these, such as vasculitic lesions, are cutaneous clues to the possibility of extracutaneous disease. Livedo reticularis is noteworthy in this regard. The net-like erythema of livedo reticularis is a vascular phenomenon caused by lowered oxygenation at the periphery of the area supplied by a particular vessel. This can simply be due to vasoconstriction, such as occurs in a cold environment, and thus can be a benign finding. If livedo is more prominent than usual, not corrected by warming, and persistent, it can indicate lowered flow caused by pathology such as vasculitis, atherosclerotic disease, or sludging. In lupus, livedo reticularis may be a sign of the presence of antiphospholipid antibodies.[36]

Other lupus nonspecific skin lesions include Raynaud's phenomenon, palmar erythema, periungual telangiectasia, alopecia, erythromelalgia, papulonodular mucinosis, and anetoderma. Sclerodactyly, calcinosis, and rheumatoid nodules have been reported but may be more likely in overlap syndromes than in SLE.

Neonatal Lupus Syndrome

Neonatal lupus erythematosus (NLE) is associated with maternal IgG autoantibodies to Ro/SSA, La/SSB, and rarely U1RNP.[37,37a] Affected children may have cutaneous lesions, cardiac disease (notably complete heart block and/or cardiomyopathy), hepatobiliary disease, or hematologic cytopenias. Most children have only one or two features of the disease. Similar to the anti-Ro/SSA–associated SCLE of adults, the skin lesions are often photosensitive, have relatively superficial inflammatory infiltrates, and do not tend to scar. The lesions usually appear in infants at a few weeks of age but have been noted at birth in several cases. The natural history of the skin disease is that the lesions last for weeks or months and resolve spontaneously, usually leaving no residuum. In a few cases, persistent telangiectasias have been noted. Individual lesions appear as erythematous annular papules or plaques. Lesions are usually more numerous and more intensely inflamed on the face and scalp, but may additionally occur on the patient's trunk and extremities. Confluent periorbital erythema, which gives the appearance of an erythematous mask, is common and diagnostically helpful. Even though the skin disease resolves and most children without extracutaneous involvement remain otherwise healthy, there is a possibility that children who have had NLE are at increased risk for autoimmune disease later in childhood.[38]

Differential diagnosis of the skin lesions may include reactive erythema, drug eruption, erythema multiforme, and urticaria. Annular NLE lesions usually have little or no scale, unlike the annular lesions of tinea. In areas where there is intense destruction of the basal cell layer, lesions may be crusted and look similar to bullous impetigo. Treatment of skin lesions consists largely of sun protection and mild topical steroids.

The pathogenesis of lupus is covered elsewhere, but it is noteworthy that SCLE-like, anti-Ro/SSA–associated skin lesions may occur in neonates, but other lupus-specific skin lesions do not appear to be maternally transmissible.

Sjögren's Syndrome

The most common mucocutaneous findings of Sjögren's syndrome are related to glandular dysfunction.[39] Lacrimal gland dysfunction causes dryness and irritation of the eyes and can lead to keratitis and corneal ulceration. Salivary gland dysfunction causes dry mouth and may result in angular cheilitis and numerous dental caries. Vaginal xerosis may cause burning and dyspareunia. The skin may be dry, cracked, and pruritic. Mildly dry mucous membranes and even severely dry skin may be present in a substantial percentage of healthy individuals who live in dry climates, thus the findings should be interpreted in the context of the setting. In Japanese patients with Sjögren's syndrome, an annular erythema has been described that is somewhat reminiscent of annular SCLE or annular lesions of NLE, although more indurated.[40]

Vasculitis is a relatively common finding. In one series of 558 patients with primary Sjögren's syndrome, 52 had vasculitis, typically involving the small vessels. In most cases, lesions were purpuric, but in some, urticarial vasculitis was the clinical presentation. Patients with cutaneous evidence of vasculitis generally had more severe systemic disease.[41]

Dermatomyositis

KEY POINTS

- Patients with DM may present with only skin or skin and lung involvement in the absence of muscle disease.
- Skin biopsies are important to rule out other diseases that can mimic DM, such as psoriasis, eczema, acne rosacea, or other photosensitive disorders including polymorphous light eruption. Clinical-pathologic correlation is critical because skin biopsies of cutaneous lupus and DM can be identical.
- DM-associated antibodies can be helpful in making a diagnosis of DM, stratifying risk for internal malignancy and interstitial lung disease, and counseling patients regarding disease course.
- Patients with mechanic's hands are more likely to have interstitial lung disease. All patients with DM should have screening pulmonary function tests.
- Patients with anti-MDA5 antibodies have a characteristic cutaneous phenotype of palmar papules (inverse Gottron papules), skin ulcers, and alopecia and need to be recognized as they are at high risk of interstitial lung disease.
- All patients with a recent diagnosis of DM should be screened for internal malignancy, and patients with cutaneous necrosis, anti-TIF1-γ, or anti-NXP2 antibodies are at higher risk for malignancy.

Skin findings in DM are important in diagnosis, subclassifying patients, and assessing systemic risk. The most recently published classification criteria for myositis recognize the importance of skin disease in diagnosing DM and also include clinically amyopathic (CADM) patients.[42] CADM refers to the group of patients with biopsy-proven cutaneous findings of DM that never manifest clinical weakness or elevated muscle enzymes, but may have subclinical muscle abnormalities on electromyogram, MRI, or muscle biopsy studies.[43] It is estimated that CADM patients comprise 20% of the total DM population.

Cutaneous Manifestations of Dermatomyositis

DM skin inflammation encompasses a wide variety of manifestations, many of which are often misdiagnosed or overlooked.[44] The major finding is that of macular and/or papular violaceous erythema, which often occurs in stereotypical sites, many of which are photodistributed. The most common of these include Gottron's papules (Fig. 46.9), which are papules and/or plaques over the interphalangeal and/or metacarpophalangeal joints. Gottron's sign refers to similar lesions, often macular, over bony extensor surfaces (e.g., elbows, knees, malleoli). Other characteristic areas for violaceous erythema of DM include heliotrope rash (Fig. 46.10), V-neck, and shawl sign, representing macular erythema involving periorbital region, chest, and upper back, respectively. Additional common areas for erythema include the lateral upper arm, lower lateral back (often reticulated), medial

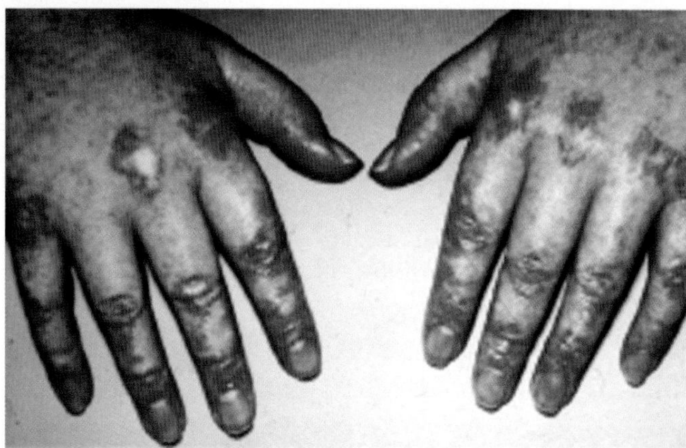

• **Fig. 46.9** Gottron's papules over the interphalangeal joints in dermatomyositis.

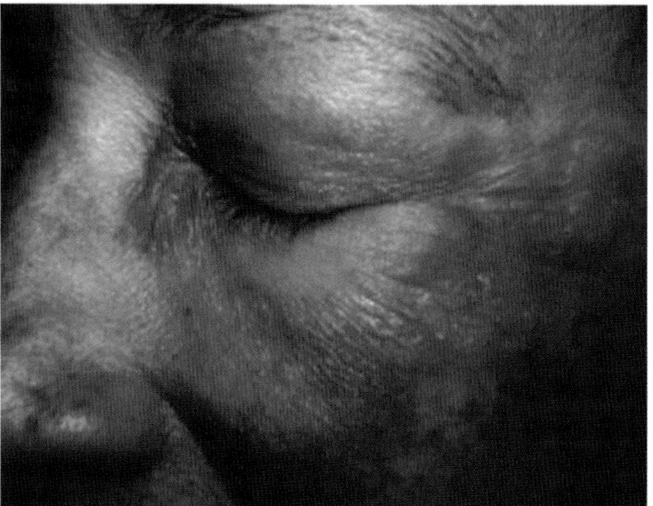

• **Fig. 46.10** Heliotrope eruption of dermatomyositis with characteristic edema.

wrist, and lateral thighs (the so-called *holster sign*). Some patients can present with a diffuse photodistributed erythema and even erythroderma.

Other cutaneous findings in DM include alopecia, which is more commonly diffuse and nonscarring but can also be focal. Cuticular overgrowth and/or hemorrhages and periungual edema and/or telangiectasias are often commonly seen, and patients often complain of periungual tenderness. Hyperkeratosis of the palmar and lateral surfaces of the fingers, called *mechanic's hands,* can be seen and is associated with anti-synthetase autoantibodies and interstitial lung disease.[45] Rarely, patients can have a panniculitis, presenting as subcutaneous plaques and nodules that often calcify. Vasculopathy, with livedo reticularis, ulceration, or painful palmar papules, can occur. Itching can result in excoriations and lichenification and is particularly seen on the scalp. Other morphologic findings include red-on-white, representing erythematous, telangiectatic macules (often follicular) on a background of ivory white skin.[46] Oral lesions are commonly seen, including the ovoid palatal patch, which is a semicircular erythematous patch on either side of the midline of the posterior palate, characteristically admixed with white macular discoloration.[47] Other oral mucosal findings include gingival telangiectasias (noted above) as well as more classic lichen planus-like lesions around the gingiva and/or buccal mucosa.

Several cutaneous findings represent long-term damage. These lesions include post-inflammatory hyperpigmentation, poikiloderma, calcinosis, lipoatrophy, and depressed scars.[44] Calcinosis is most frequent on the extremities in DM, in contrast to systemic sclerosis in which digital calcinosis is most frequent.[48] *Poikiloderma* is a descriptive term for a pattern of finely mottled white areas and brown pigmentation, telangiectasia, and atrophy.

Skin biopsy from a patient with cutaneous DM can be identical to that seen with cutaneous lupus erythematosus, although classically lesions tend to have less inflammation and increased vascular damage and dilation.[49] Immunofluorescence studies may be useful in distinguishing from cutaneous lupus—in DM, C5b-9 complement components (forming the membrane attack complex) are deposited in and around the dermal vessels, and a strong lupus band (strong, linear IgG, IgM, and complement deposition along the basement membrane) is not seen.[50]

Autoantibodies in Dermatomyositis

In recent years, the targets for several circulating autoantibodies have been characterized in DM patients (Table 46.1).[51] These antibodies tend to be mutually exclusive, are present in at least 80% of DM patients, are generally not found in other rheumatic disorders or healthy controls, and are associated with distinct clinical and laboratory features. Anti-synthetase antibodies (e.g., anti-Jo1 and others) are associated with interstitial lung disease (ILD), Raynaud's, and arthritis, and the rash tends to be mild in these patients, with predominantly mild facial, neck, and hand involvement. Anti-Mi2 antibodies are associated with muscle disease, high creatine kinase (CK) values, absence of ILD, and UV exposure.[51] The rash tends to be severe with "classic" photodistributed features, also including cuticular hemorrhage, and it is responsive to therapy but tends to relapse when treatment is withdrawn.

Anti-TIF-1γ antibodies comprise the most common serologic subgroup in the United States and are associated with increased risk of internal malignancy. These patients can be clinically amyopathic but even with severe muscle involvement tend to have relatively modest CK values. The rash is typically severe and chronic, often photodistributed, and can involve all of the classic skin sites—the ovoid palatal patch and red-on-white discoloration are commonly seen in this subgroup. Anti-NXP2 antibodies are also variably associated with cancer, as well as a distinctive myalgia, dysphagia (which is often severe), peripheral edema, distal weakness, and calcinosis. Finally, anti-MDA5 antibodies are associated with increased risk of ILD (which can be rapidly progressive and fatal, occurring more commonly in Asians), as well as arthritis, which is often severe and chronic. These patients have a distinctive mucocutaneous phenotype that includes tender palmar papules (also called inverse Gottron's papules), cutaneous ulceration, severe alopecia, and oral sensitivity and ulcers.

Diagnosis and Management

A diagnosis of DM is made by clinical-pathologic correlation and does not need to include muscle disease. In terms of the skin findings, the differential diagnosis includes lupus erythematosus, psoriasis, mixed connective tissue disease, seborrheic dermatitis, acne rosacea, phototoxic/photoallergic drug eruption, and polymorphous light eruption. There are currently no validated cutaneous criteria for diagnosing DM, and the presence of one of the DM-associated autoantibodies can be useful in making the diagnosis. Patients with DM frequently experience a delay in obtaining a diagnosis, and the presence of photosensitivity, malar rash, oral

TABLE 46.1 Dermatomyositis (DM)-Associated Autoantibodies[51]

AUTOANTIGEN			AUTOANTIBODY	
Symbol	**Name**	**Cellular Location**	**Prevalence**	**Associated Clinical Features**
Mi-2	Nucleosome-remodeling deacetylase complex	Nuclear	2%-38% (Adult DM) 4%-10% (JDM)	Classic photodistributed rash
MDA-5 CADM-140 IFIH1	Melanoma differentiation-associated gene 5	Cytoplasmic	0%-13% (Caucasian) 11%-57% (Asian) 7%-12% (JDM)	Interstitial lung disease Alopecia Arthritis Clinically amyopathic Cutaneous ulcers Mechanic's hands Painful palmar papules
NXP-2 MJ MORC3	Nuclear matrix protein	Nuclear	14%-25% (Caucasian) 2%-5% (Asian) 20%-25% (JDM)	Malignancy Peripheral edema Dysphagia/myalgia/distal weakness Calcinosis
Tlf-1γ 155/140 TRIM33	Transcription intermediary factor 1γ	Nuclear	38%-41% (Caucasian) 7%-14% (Asian) 20%-32% (JDM)	Malignancy Classic photodistributed rash Ovoid palatal patch Red-on-white
SAE1/2	Small ubiquitin-like modifier 1 activating enzyme	Nuclear	5%-10% (Caucasian) 1%-3% (Asian) <1% (JDM)	Dysphagia Classic photodistributed rash Cutaneous ulcers Dark red/violaceous rash
ASAs	Aminoacyl tRNA synthetases	Cytoplasmic		Interstitial lung disease
Jo-1	Histidyl-tRNA synthetase		5%-20%	Arthritis
PL-12	Alanyl-tRNA synthetase		~3%	Mechanic's hands
PL-7	Threonyl-tRNA synthetase		~2%	
EJ	Glycyl-tRNA synthetase		~1%	
OJ	Isoleucyl-tRNA synthetase		~1%	
KS	Asparaginyl-tRNA synthetase		<1%	
Zo	Phenylalanyl-tRNA synthetase		<1%	
Ha/YRS	Tyrosyl-tRNA synthetase		<1%	

JDM, Juvenile dermatomyositis.

ulcers, and a positive anti-nuclear antibody (ANA) test results in a frequent misdiagnosis of SLE.[43] Once a diagnosis is made, the clinician should screen for ILD and internal malignancy. ILD is present in 15% to 50% of patients, can be mild, chronic, or rapidly progressive, and typically presents in the first 1 to 2 years following symptom DM onset.[52] Patients should be screened for ILD with pulmonary function testing followed by high resolution chest CT evaluation for any patient with a forced vital capacity or diffusion capacity less than 70% to 80% of that predicted. The risk of internal malignancy is elevated in DM, with most of the risk surrounding the first 1 to 3 years surrounding DM onset.[53] There are currently no official guidelines for how to screen DM patients for malignancy, though studies suggest that age-appropriate screening, while appropriate, is probably not sensitive enough; CT scans or alternatively PET-CT scans could be considered, at least once in a patient with a diagnosis of DM in the past 1 to 3 years.[54] Of note, patients with ADM appear to have similar incidence of pulmonary involvement and internal malignancy as those with classic DM.

Certain skin findings can indicate systemic risk in DM. Mechanic's hands (mentioned above) are associated with ILD, especially when the hand involvement is diffuse and comprises overt scaling of the palms and digits.[55] Cutaneous ulcers can be associated with interstitial lung disease, mostly due to their association with anti-MDA5 antibodies. However, this finding is not specific, although the presence of ulcers within the anti-MDA5 group increases the risk for ILD.[56] Palmar papules (inverse Gottron's papules), especially those that are tender and/or ulcerate, have a strong association with anti-MDA5 antibodies and therefore ILD. Patients with these findings, with or without concomitant severe arthritis and alopecia, should also be suspected of having increased risk of anti-MDA5 antibodies and ILD. Cutaneous necrosis has been commonly associated with internal malignancy, as has rapid onset or fulminant skin disease, in addition to the traditional risk factors of increased age, male sex, and severe dysphagia.[57] Interestingly, mechanic's hands (along with Jo1 antibodies, Raynaud's, arthritis, and ILD) are protective for malignancy.[57]

The patients with both skin and muscle disease frequently experience resolution of their muscle disease after aggressive treatment with glucocorticoids, with or without immunosuppressives.[58] Immunosuppressives such as methotrexate, azathioprine, or mycophenolate mofetil can be of additive benefit for patients with resistant skin disease. Intravenous immunoglobulin (IVIG) is an effective therapy for skin and muscle disease. Calcineurin inhibitors, such as cyclosporine or tacrolimus, are often used, especially in patients with ILD.[59] Rituximab can be used to manage refractory muscle disease and is currently being studied for ILD. Recent reports suggest that janus kinase (JAK) inhibition may be a useful treatment for skin, muscle, and/or joint disease.[60] Patients with CADM or residual skin disease after treatment often benefit from hydroxychloroquine, although it should be noted that an increased risk of cutaneous hypersensitivity to hydroxychloroquine has been reported in the DM population.[61] Patients who do not improve with a single anti-malarial can benefit from the addition of quinacrine or a switch from hydroxychloroquine to chloroquine.[62]

Morphea, Systemic Sclerosis, and Other Sclerosing Conditions

KEY POINTS

- Morphea occurs as circumscribed, generalized, linear, or mixed forms.
- Linear forms of the disease occur more often in children, and on the head can present as hemifacial atrophy or en coup de sabre.
- In morphea it is important to distinguish activity (erythema, expansion of growth, pruritus) from damage (sclerosis, hyperpigmentation, atrophy).
- The cutaneous induration with systemic sclerosis, especially limited cutaneous systemic sclerosis (lcSSc), can be very subtle, and other cutaneous features (nailfold capillary changes, digital pitted scars, matted telangiectasias) as well as other clinical and laboratory features may be required for diagnosis.
- Eosinophilic fasciitis involves the fascia below the fat and can be associated with eosinophils in the tissue and is more responsive to glucocorticoids than other sclerosing disorders of the skin.
- Some fibrosing conditions, including scleromyxedema and scleredema, are associated with monoclonal gammopathies.
- Nephrogenic systemic fibrosis is related to gadolinium exposure in patients with decreased renal function. The histology is indistinguishable from scleromyxedema.

TABLE 46.2 Sclerosing Disorders of the Skin[63]

Immune-mediated/inflammatory	Eosinophilic fasciitis Graft vs. host disease
Sclerodermiform mucinoses	Scleromyxedema Scleredema adultorum Buschke Nephrogenic systemic fibrosis (or nephrogenic fibrosing dermopathy)
Genetic	Progeroid disorders (progeria, acrogeria, Werner's syndrome) Scleroatrophic Huriez syndrome (OMIM 181600) Stiff skin syndrome (or congenital facial dystrophy) (OMIM 184900) Winchester syndrome (OMIM 277950) GEMSS syndrome (OMIM 137765) Pachydermoperiostosis (OMIM 167100)
Drug-induced and toxic	Bleomycin Pentazocine Eosinophilia-myalgia syndrome (L-tryptophan) Toxic-oil syndrome (aniline-denaturated rapeseed oil) Post-radiation fibrosis Docetaxel (taxotere) Melphalan Uracyl-tegafur Local injection of vitamin K, corticosteroids, vitamin B_{12} Intramuscular injection of pentazocin Amines: bromocriptine, appetite suppressants; carbidopa; epoxy resin: bis (4-amino-3-methylcyclohexyl); methane Solvents Silica Vinyl chloride disease
Metabolic	Porphyria cutanea tarda Diabetic stiff-hand syndrome (diabetic cheiroarthropathy)
Panniculitis (panniculitides)/vascular	Lipodermatosclerosis
Paraneoplastic disorders	POEMS syndrome Lung cancer, carcinoid, plasma cell dyscrasia, cancer of the ovary, cervix, breast, esophagus, stomach, nasopharynx, melanoma, and sarcoma

GEMSS, Glaucoma, ectopia, microspherophakia, stiff joints, short stature; *OMIM,* Online Mendelian Inheritance in Man; *POEMS,* Polyneuropathy, organomegaly, endocrinopathy, monoclonal gammopathy, and skin changes.

There are multiple scenarios in which patients can present with sclerosing plaques of the skin (Table 46.2).[63] A careful medical history will usually help with diagnosis, including infection, environmental exposures (radiation, medication, or other toxins), and cancer. The most common entities are discussed below.

Morphea

Morphea, also called localized scleroderma, is classified into linear, generalized, plaque (circumscribed), and mixed forms. Linear type is the most common form in children and is typically chronic,

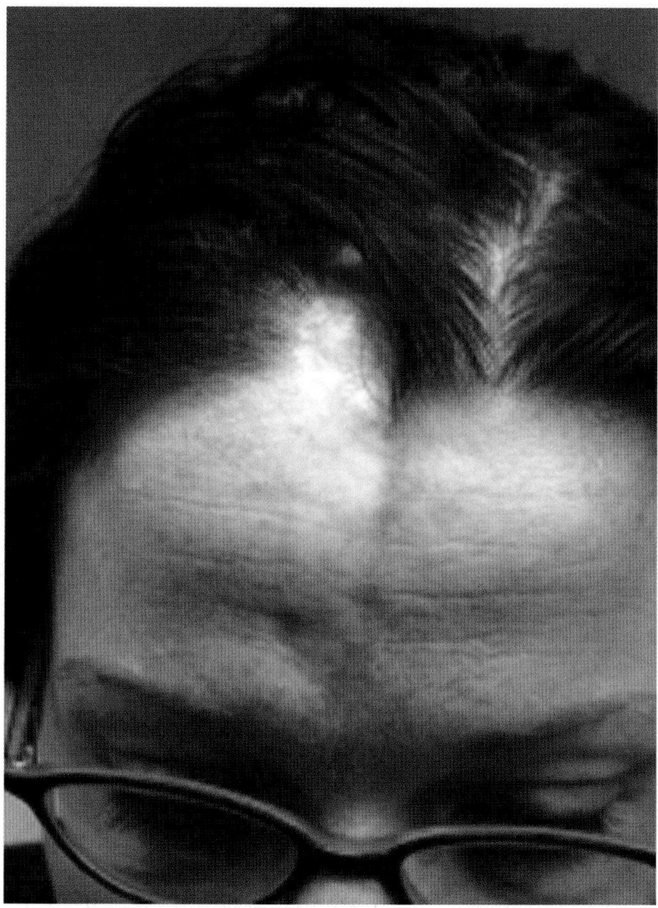

• **Fig. 46.11** Linear scleroderma of the forehead. (Courtesy Dr. Victoria Werth, University of Pennsylvania Department of Dermatology and Philadelphia Veterans Administration Medical Center, Philadelphia.)

while plaque and generalized forms occur commonly in adults and can often have remissions in 3 to 5 years.[64] Two disorders that are often considered as variants of linear scleroderma (and more common in children) include facial hemiatrophy, otherwise known as *Parry-Romberg syndrome*, and *en coup de sabre* (Fig. 46.11). Both PRS and ECDS can be accompanied by neurologic, ocular, and dental abnormalities. Eosinophilic fasciitis (EF) is considered by some a deeper form of morphea, which typically involves acute onset (often following exercise) of deep, symmetric induration of the fascia involving the limbs and less commonly the neck and trunk but sparing the hands and feet.[65] If not accompanied by more superficial dermal involvement, the overlying skin itself is typically soft with underlying firmness at the level of the muscle and fascia.

Active morphea lesions present with inflammation in the form of erythema and induration, often accompanied by pain and pruritus.[66] Inactive lesions reveal sclerosis, hyperpigmentation, and/or atrophy that can involve the epidermis, dermis, and subcutaneous tissue. Damage from unchecked activity in morphea can cause cosmetic sequelae such as hair loss and subcutaneous atrophy, as well as functional impairment, including joint contracture. Morphea can involve the dermis ("superficial morphea") or deeper structures of the subcutis and even fascia and muscle (morphea profunda). Deep inflammatory lesions are poorly circumscribed erythematous plaques with variable amounts of edema and induration. Morphea can have different presentations, including an overlap with lichen sclerosus et atrophicus, in which there can be "cigarette paper" atrophy, follicular plugging, and/or flat-topped papules that coalesce to form a white plaque, sometimes combined with a deeper morphea lesion. Morphea often appears following trauma to the skin—triggers include radiation, surgery, insect bites, or injections.

Linear scleroderma is frequently located on the lower limbs, upper limbs, frontal head area, and anterior trunk. It is frequently unilateral and can result in joint deformity, joint contractures, and limb atrophy. Some cases are associated with seizures or other focal neurologic symptoms. Parry-Romberg syndrome can occur in the first or second decade of life and leads to unilateral facial atrophy in 95% of people, and can involve deeper subcutaneous muscle and bony structures—the overlying skin is mobile. The *en coup de sabre* variant occurs as a linear indurated plaque along the paramedian forehead and/or scalp. Patients can have seizures, headaches, visual changes, trigeminal neuralgia, atrophy of the salivary glands, and hemiatrophy of the tongue on the same side as the facial atrophy. Any reparative surgical treatment should be timed to occur no sooner than 1 year after cessation of the ongoing atrophic process.

Morphea must be differentiated from systemic sclerosis (SSc), which is usually not a problem in the majority of cases. Morphea patients will not have sclerodactyly, digital ulcers and/or pitted scars, calcinosis, periungual telangiectasias, salt and pepper pigmentary changes, Raynaud's, or SSc-specific autoantibodies that are all typically seen in SSc. They also typically lack the internal involvement of SSc, although some patients experience arthralgia/arthritis, including a "dry" (non-inflammatory) synovitis that can lead to fibrosis of the joint capsule, fascia, and tendon. Many other mimics of morphea exist.[66] At the early inflammatory stages these include lichen sclerosus, mycosis fungoides, stasis dermatitis, and lipodermatosclerosis, while later sclerotic disease can mimic radiation-induced morphea, injection-induced morphea-like lesions, morphea-like Lyme disease (seen in Europe), eosinophilia-myalgia syndrome, toxic oil syndrome, scleredema, scleromyxedema, and nephrogenic systemic fibrosis (NSF). Late stage, atrophic disease, as well as PRS can be confused with traumatic fat atrophy, lipodystrophy, and even late, atrophic forms of panniculitis (e.g., lupus panniculitis).

ANAs are positive 18% to 68% of the time in morphea but are of unclear clinical value.[66] A peripheral eosinophilia and hypergammaglobulinemia can be seen, especially in those with concomitant eosinophilic fasciitis.[65] Rheumatoid factor can be positive and is associated with increased risk of arthritis. A skin biopsy is not universally required to make the diagnosis in typical cases, but will show a superficial and deep perivascular infiltrate composed of lymphocytes and plasma cells, and also typically thickened and homogenized collagen bundles at the papillary and reticular dermis. The role of MRI is increasingly being evaluated to assess extent of disease (and looking for underlying myositis) as well as looking for CNS involvement in linear forms involving the head and neck.[66]

Treatment of morphea can include topical corticosteroids and/or calcineurin inhibitors, or calcipotriene for localized disease that is limited to the dermis. More widespread dermal disease will require other modalities, including phototherapy (UVA1 preferred over UVB), and, for deeper and/or linear lesions, methotrexate with or without systemic corticosteroids, or mycophenolate mofetil.[66]

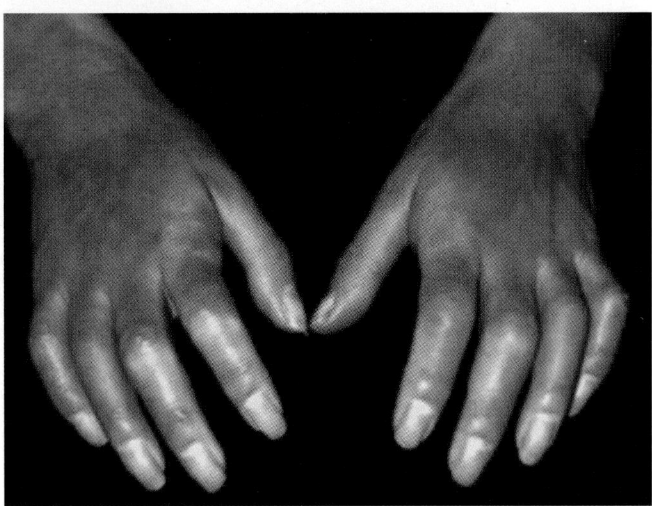

• **Fig. 46.12** Sclerodactyly with flexion contractures.

Systemic Sclerosis

With the realization that degree of cutaneous fibrosis in SSc can often be very subtle, new classification criteria were published in 2013 that included the three cardinal aspects of disease (vasculopathy, fibrosis, and autoantibodies) and were designed to classify patients with lcSSc that would not have otherwise been recognized.[67] Patients with lcSSc have cutaneous sclerosis that is limited to the limbs, distal to the elbows and knees, and face.[68] The skin involvement can range from severe sclerodactyly (Fig. 46.12) and skin sclerosis to very subtle disease consisting only of puffy fingers or even near clinical absence of induration. These patients often have anti-centromere autoantibodies, but can also have anti-Scl70 as well as nucleolar antibodies (Th/To, PM-Scl). Patients with diffuse cutaneous systemic sclerosis (dcSSc) have induration of the skin that extends proximal to the elbows and knees, also typically on the trunk as well, as well as facial involvement.[68] Patients with early dcSSc frequently have recent onset of Raynaud's, acute onset, tendon friction rubs, and severe pruritus, and often have anti–Scl-70, anti–RNA polymerase III, or anti-fibrillarin (U3RNP) antibodies.[68] Digital ulcers are seen in 32% to 58% of patients (more commonly in those with early or diffuse disease), either on the digital pulp (often presenting as a hyperkeratotic, wart-like, painful lesion that resolves with a pitted scar) or over the interphalangeal or metacarpophalangeal joints.[68] Digital ulcers can also present as hyperkeratotic lesions beneath the distal nailplate that often resolve with a scar (so-called *inverse pterygium*). Digital ischemia can also be subtle, manifesting only as distal pulp tenderness with subtle hyperkeratosis ("hardening") of the skin. Matted (square) telangiectasias can often be seen on the palms, chest, face, lips, and tongue, and high numbers can indicate increased risk for pulmonary arterial hypertension. Dyspigmentation is commonly seen, and can range from a diffuse or photo-accentuated hyperpigmentation, to vitiligo-like areas with follicular hyperpigmentation ("salt and pepper"), to streaky or reticulate hyperpigmentation. Calcinosis occurs in 10% to 25% of patients, commonly on the hands and elbows but can be more generalized, and may be seen in areas of trauma (thumb > 5th digit) and is associated with digital ischemia, calcinosis, and osteoporosis.[68]

Therapies used for cutaneous sclerosis in SSc include methotrexate and mycophenolate mofetil, while cyclophosphamide is typically reserved for those with severe lung disease. There are mixed data regarding the success of rituximab and IVIG for skin sclerosis. Recently, immunoablation with autologous stem cell rescue has demonstrated beneficial effects on sclerosis and mortality.[69] Trials are evaluating the role of abatacept, tocilizumab, and lenabasum (cannabinoid agonist). Treatment of Raynaud's phenomenon is covered elsewhere. For digital ulcers, patients can benefit from phosphodiesterase-5 inhibitors such as sildenafil, endothelin receptor antagonists (e.g., bosentan or ambrisentan), as well as IV iloprost or other prostacyclins for severe cases.[68] Use of digital sympathectomy can be very helpful for digital ulcers in the hands of an experienced hand surgeon.[70] In addition, botulinum toxin has been successfully used for Raynaud's and digital ulcerations.[71] Calcinosis remains a difficult condition to treat, and successful outcomes with warfarin, calcium channel blockers, minocycline, bisphosphonates, IVIG, colchicine, and sodium thiosulfate have been reported.

Eosinophilic Fasciitis

EF involves inflammation of the fascia overlying muscle and results in abrupt onset of edema and deep induration of the extremities.[65] It typically is symmetric and involves all four extremities but rarely the trunk. In the edematous phase the skin may have a *peau d'orange* appearance, and a "groove sign" can be seen with arm elevation, marking collapse of superficial veins. The dermis and subcutaneous fat can also be involved. In contrast to SSc, the digits are typically spared, there is no Raynaud's or nailfold capillary changes, and the ANA is usually negative. There is often a rapid onset of disease activity, particularly following physical exertion. A contaminant of L-tryptophan was associated with an EF-like disease in the early 1990s. Approximately 30% to 40% of EF patients have concurrent plaque morphea.

Diagnosis is normally based on a deep, usually excisional biopsy of the skin that includes fascia. There are inflammatory cells among collagen bundles, thickening of collagen, sclerosis of the dermis and fat/fascia, and absent sweat glands and hair. MRI of active EF demonstrates thickening of the fascia overlying the muscle, hyperintense signal within the fascia on fluid-sensitive sequences, and fascial enhancement after IV contrast. Evidence supports early treatment to prevent fibrosis and contractures.[65] Systemic corticosteroids are the first line therapy, with at least 3 to 6 months of moderate-to-high dose therapy. Agents such as methotrexate and mycophenolate mofetil are effective steroid sparing agents with long-term therapy.

Scleromyxedema

Scleromyxedema is a rare disorder of middle age that is a primary cutaneous mucinosis.[63] It has gradual onset and consists of diffuse 2 to 3 mm flesh-colored papules that can coalesce. It almost always involves the hands and face, especially the glabella and ears, giving rise to "leonine facies," which eventually generalizes. It is associated with systemic issues, including dysphagia and esophageal dysmotility, arthralgia in 25%, myopathy in 10% to 50%, and Raynaud's in 10% of patients. Peripheral nervous system involvement can cause carpal tunnel or a peripheral sensorimotor neuropathy, while CNS involvement manifests as seizures, memory loss, unsteady gait, or strokes. A dermato-neuro syndrome can be seen in patients with frank encephaolopathy. Ninety percent of patients have a monoclonal gammopathy, most frequently IgGλ, but occasionally IgGκ.[63]

Skin biopsy shows mucin deposition and a proliferation of fibroblasts in the upper dermis. Treatment now includes IVIG as first-line therapy, with thalidomide or lenalidomide and prednisone as common alternatives. Historically the disease has been also treated with PUVA, systemic retinoids, plasmapheresis, photopheresis, low-dose melphalan, and high-dose dexamethasone. Successful therapy with bortezomib and autologous stem cell transplantation has been reported.[63]

Scleredema

Scleredema is another primary disorder of mucin deposition in the dermis.[72] It usually starts as asymptomatic, nonpitting woody induration of the posterior neck, which then spreads to the upper back and shoulders, but can extend down to involve much of the trunk, upper arms, and neck. It rarely involves the face and spares the hands and feet. This condition can be one of the most restrictive of the sclerosing disorders, with patients complaining of movement restriction, even including the muscles of mastication. The disease classically is divided into three types: the first is the most common, occurring in 25% to 50% of cases, and occurring in the setting of diabetes (usually poorly controlled and more commonly in men); the second follows an acute onset, and is associated with upper respiratory tract infections (often streptococcal) and typically resolves over time; the third is associated with blood dyscrasias (usually a paraproteinemia) that follows a chronic, progressive course.[72] Skin biopsy shows increased dermal mucin deposition but also abnormally swollen collagen bundles that can also involve the subcutis—there is no proliferation of fibroblasts or inflammatory cells. Patients rarely experience systemic symptoms, most commonly esophageal (dysphagia) and cardiac. Treatment is notoriously unsuccessful, with spotty reports of success using phototherapy (UVA or UVA), electron beam therapy, extracorporeal photopheresis, traditional DMARDs, tamoxifen, colchicine, or IVIG.

Nephrogenic Systemic Fibrosis

NSF is a relatively recently described illness that occurs in patients with renal disease; most of the patients have undergone dialysis for renal failure.[73] NSF presents as either a morphea-like disease or a more diffuse acral sclerosis. Morphea-like presentations include ill-defined indurated plaques, with islands of sparing and finger-like projections that involve lower more than upper extremities. More diffuse confluent acral sclerosis, sometimes with truncal involvement, can occur. There are often yellow plaques on the conjunctiva. Patients can experience pain, severe itching, joint contractures, fibrosis and calcification of the skin, subcutaneous tissue, fascia, muscle, myocardium, lungs, renal tubules, and testes. Patients typically do not have Raynaud's syndrome. Skin biopsy is identical to that seen with scleromyxedema, with stellate fibroblasts, glycosaminoglycans, and thickening of collagen.[73,74] There is no proven effective therapy, and prognosis depends on the extent, rapidity of skin involvement, and severity of the systemic disease. Treatments that have been reported to potentially help include plasmapheresis, IVIG, immunosuppressives, glucocorticoids, IFN-α, thalidomide, PUVA, UVA1, photopheresis, and imatinib mesylate.[73] Exposure to unstable gadolinium-based contrast agents (GBCA) is now clearly associated with NSF.[75] Newer professional and regulatory guidelines have been established that all include screening for renal insufficiency in all patients for whom gadolinium-based contrast agents are contemplated, and it is recommended that high-risk patients avoid certain agents that are unstable. Data support that combined use of screening and avoidance of unstable types of GBCA has reduced the incidence of NSF.[76]

Primary Vasculitis Involving the Skin

KEY POINTS

In cutaneous diseases, the term ***vasculitis*** is typically reserved for lesions that histologically show damage to vessel walls and a neutrophilic infiltrate.

Cutaneous vasculitis can be a skin manifestation of predominantly systemic disease, a skin-limited form of a disease that is typically systemic, or one of a number of unique disorders only described in skin that have no systemic counterpart.

The major determinant of the clinical appearance of vasculitis on the skin is the size of the vessel affected.

A characteristic lesion of cutaneous small vessel vasculitis is palpable purpura in dependent areas of the body. It is common for the majority of lesions to be nonpalpable.

Medium-sized vasculitis can present with livedo reticularis, retiform purpura, subcutaneous nodules, ulcers, or cutaneous necrosis/gangrene.

Small vessel vasculitis includes both ANCA-associated vasculitis (AAV) as well as immune complex vasculitis that can be systemic or skin-predominant.

AAV, cryoglobulinemic vasculitis, although classified as small vessel vasculitis, can commonly involve medium-sized vessels as well.

Systemic corticosteroids are not routinely indicated for skin-limited disease.

Primary vasculitis of the skin, or cutaneous vasculitis, takes three forms: (1) the skin manifestations of a systemic vasculitis; (2) a skin-limited or skin-predominant form of a recognized systemic vasculitis; (3) a single organ vasculitis (SOV) that represents a disease with essentially no known systemic counterpart in terms of clinical and/or laboratory manifestations.

Nomenclature and Classification for Cutaneous Vasculitis

The Chapel Hill Consensus Conference (CHCC) of 2012 is the most widely adopted classification system for vasculitis and is discussed elsewhere in this text. Because this system did not deal with special forms of cutaneous vasculitis or forms of skin-predominant and skin-limited versions of the systemic forms, an international consensus group mostly of dermatologists proposed an addendum to the CHCC system that provides a framework for subclassification and nomenclature of vasculitis that is expressed in the skin (Table 46.3).[77]

Cutaneous Vasculitis Involving Predominantly Small-Sized Vessels

Vasculitis that affects small vessels (arterioles, postcapillary venules, and/or capillaries) typically presents with purpura (sometimes palpable) and/or petechiae, although urticaria and/or vesicles can also be seen. Although involving predominantly small vessels, some forms can more rarely involve the small arteries and even rarely medium-sized arteries of the deep dermis/subcutis. It has the

TABLE 46.3 **Classification of Cutaneous Vasculitis**[77]

	SKIN INVOLVEMENT STATUS	
CHCC 2012 Vasculitis Category, Name	**Cutaneous Component of Systemic Vasculitis**	**Skin-Limited or Skin-Dominant Variant**
Large vessel vasculitis		
Takayasu's arteritis	No	No
Giant cell arteritis	Rare	No
Medium vessel vasculitis		
Polyarteritis nodosa	Yes	Yes
Kawasaki's disease	No	No
Small vessel vasculitis		
Microscopic polyangiitis	Yes	Yes
Granulomatosis with polyangiitis	Yes	Yes
Eosinophilic granulomatosis with polyangiitis	Yes	Yes
Anti–glomerular basement membrane disease	No	No
Cryoglobulinemic vasculitis	Yes	Yes
IgA vasculitis (Henoch-Schönlein)	Yes	Yes
Hypocomplementemic urticarial vasculitis (anti-C1q vasculitis)	Yes	Yes
Variable vessel vasculitis		
Behçet's disease	Yes	Yes
Cogan's syndrome	Rare	No
Vasculitis associated with systemic disease		
SLE, rheumatoid arthritis, sarcoidosis, etc	Yes	Yes
Vasculitis associated with probable etiology		
Drugs, infections, sepsis, autoimmune diseases, etc.	Yes	Yes
Cutaneous SOV (not included in CHCC 2012)		
IgM/IgG vasculitis	No (not observed yet)	Yes (as SOV)
Nodular vasculitis (erythema induratum of Bazin)	No	Yes (as SOV)
Erythema elevatum et diutinum	No	Yes (as SOV)
Hypergammaglobulinemic macular vasculitis	No	Yes (as SOV)
Normocomplementemic urticarial vasculitis	No	Yes (as SOV)

CHCC, Chapel Hill Consensus Conference; *SOV*, single organ vasculitis.

characteristic histologic findings of fibrinoid necrosis of vessel walls, a neutrophil-predominant infiltrate, and leukocytoclasis (i.e., fragmented nuclei resulting from degeneration of neutrophils).[78] The lesions are typically described as palpable, but in practice the majority of the lesions are nonpalpable.[79] The usual diameter of the purpuric papules is approximately 0.3 to 0.6 cm, although smaller and larger lesions may be observed (Fig. 46.13). Discrete lesions have a round shape, and the center may look dusky, pustular, or ulcerated, or it may appear as a hemorrhagic vesicle. Larger ulcerations may occur when lesions coalesce. Particularly in larger lesions, the devitalized tissue may be a focus for secondary bacterial infection.

The differential diagnosis of purpuric or petechial lesions may include stasis dermatitis, pigmented purpuric dermatosis, platelet dysfunction or deficiency, petechial drug eruptions, viral exanthems, emboli (cholesterol, septic), thromboses, and sludging.[79] Skin biopsy is often helpful in establishing the diagnosis of small vessel vasculitis, especially if an early lesion is sampled. Immunofluorescence of an early lesion may establish whether the vasculitis is IgA-predominant.

Leg elevation, compression stockings, and reduction of activity may be helpful in management of all types of small-vessel vasculitis. NSAIDs or antihistamines are sometimes used. Systemic corticosteroids are not routinely indicated for skin-limited disease. For patients with persistent disease confined to the skin, colchicine and dapsone have each been used with some success.[79]

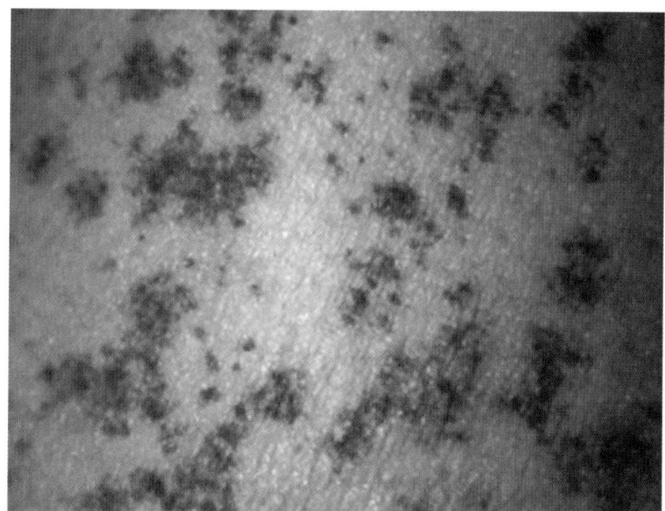

• **Fig. 46.13** Leukocytoclastic vasculitis demonstrating nonblanching, purpuric macules.

In terms of classification of small vessel vasculitis, these include two main groups: ANCA-associated vasculitis (AAV) and immune complex vasculitis (SVV) (see Table 46.3).[77]

ANCA-Associated Vasculitis

AAVs were discussed earlier in the text, and all can be associated with cutaneous findings, most commonly palpable purpura, but small- or medium-sized involvement can be seen.[80] GPA can involve the oral mucosa and cause "strawberry gingivitis," and nasal involvement can cause saddle nose deformity. Histology of all AAV skin lesions can show small- or medium-sized vessel disease, as well as extravascular, nonvasculitic granulomatous inflammation (for GPA and EGPA). Extravascular granulomatous inflammation may be more likely to occur in nonpurpuric papules or nodules than in palpable purpura. Patients with eosinophilic granulomatosis with polyangiitis characteristically present with respiratory symptoms, but skin lesions are common during the vasculitic phase of the disease.[80] Hemorrhagic lesions range from petechiae to palpable purpura to ecchymosis, cutaneous nodules with or without ulceration, subcutaneous nodules, and nonspecific erythematous eruptions are most common.

Hypereosinophilic syndrome may share clinical and laboratory features with eosinophilic granulomatosis with polyangiitis, but vasculitis is not characteristic. Also, many AAVs with skin-limited involvement involve drug-induced cases—common causes being propylthiouracil, minocycline, hydralazine, or levamisole-adulterated cocaine.

Immune Complex Vasculitis

Immune complex vasculitis includes cryoglobulinemic vasculitis (CV), IgA vasculitis (Henoch-Schönlein), and hypocomplementemic urticarial vasculitis (HUV). These lesions tend to occur in dependent areas (e.g., lower legs), with the exception of HUV. Koebnerization, the appearance of lesions along lines of trauma, such as scratches, is sometimes observed. Extensive involvement of vessels beyond small vessels (e.g., postcapillary venules) is not seen in the immune complex cutaneous vasculitidies except for CV.[77]

IgA vasculitis (HSP) is the most common form of vasculitis in children, but can be seen in adults. It typically presents with round, purpuric papules, but it can also be associated with retiform purpura.[81] In the latter case of retiform purpura, other forms of vasculitis or occlusive vasculopathy should be considered in the differential diagnosis. Skin biopsies show IgA1 deposition in the vessels, and the presence of eosinophils is associated with decreased risk of renal disease.[82] Urticarial vasculitis with normal complement levels (NUV) is now considered a skin-limited SOV.[77] Patients present with urticarial papules and plaques, typically on the trunk and extremities. These often can be contrasted with classic urticaria because they are present longer than 24 hours, leave behind pigmentation and/or faint purpuric erythema, and can burn instead of itch. This condition is often associated with SLE or Sjögren's disease, as well as hepatitis C, monoclonal gammopathy, or other lymphoid malignancy. HUV has the same skin findings but is associated with an increased risk of systemic symptoms. At the severe end of this spectrum is HUV syndrome (HUVS), in which patients have many features of SLE, but also angioedema, obstructive pulmonary disease, and anti-C1q antibodies. The entity that is now called *IgM/IgG immune complex vasculitis* represents small vessel disease that rarely, if ever, is associated with systemic disease.[77] This disease has previously been termed *hypersensitivity vasculitis* or *idiopathic cutaneous leukocytoclastic vasculitis*.

CV can be systemic or skin-limited and is often associated with hepatitis C infection. It is most often seen in type II (less often type III) mixed cryoglobulinemia, while patients with type I monoclonal cryoglobulinemia may more often have purpura caused by occlusive vasculopathy rather than a true vasculitis. CV typically presents with palpable purpura with a predilection for the lower extremities, but less commonly can also involve medium-sized vessels resulting in livedo reticularis, acrocyanosis, leg ulcers, and digital ulceration or gangrene. Raynaud's is present in 20% to 50% of cases, and arthralgia and weakness are commonly also seen.

Erythema elevatum diutinum is an unusual form of small vessel vasculitis (now considered a single organ vasculitis by CHCC) that is characterized by erythematous or violaceous papules, plaques, and nodules over the dorsal hands, ears, knees, heels, and buttocks.[83] In the clinical differential diagnosis are Sweet's syndrome, multicentric reticulohistiocytosis, sarcoidosis, and lymphoma, among others. With time, fibrosis often occurs. Established lesions may be disfiguring and may have an appearance somewhat reminiscent of keloids. Although significant extracutaneous involvement is not expected and many patients are otherwise well, erythema elevatum diutinum has been reported in association with various autoimmune, infectious, and hematologic conditions, including streptococcal infection, paraproteinemia, inflammatory bowel disease, RA, SLE, and HIV. For active skin lesions, dapsone is the usual treatment.[83] Intralesional corticosteroids are sometimes used for fibrotic lesions.

Nodular vasculitis (erythema induratum of Bazin), another SOV of the skin, is a lobular panniculitis with vasculitis in the subcutaneous fat. It is associated with tuberculosis in many cases, and it involves both small- and medium-sized vessels. Hypergammaglobulinemic purpura of Waldenstrom is also an SOV characterized by relapsing episodic crops of purpura of the lower extremities. It is associated with hypergammaglobulinemia (usually polyclonal) as well as other autoimmune diseases, especially Sjögren's syndrome.

Acute hemorrhagic edema of childhood is an uncommon but generally benign and self-limited form of vasculitis usually occurring in children younger than 2 years, commonly preceded by an upper respiratory infection or medication.[84] The clinical appearance may be dramatic, with large purpuric plaques on the face, ears, and extremities. On the basis of the appearance of the skin lesions, meningococcemia is sometimes suspected, but the child with acute hemorrhagic edema appears relatively healthy. Generally there is no extracutaneous involvement. Treatment is symptomatic.

Cutaneous Vasculitis Involving Predominantly Medium-Sized Vessels: Polyarteritis Nodosa

This group of diseases is characterized by involvement of predominantly medium-sized arteries, although small and large arteries are more rarely affected. Clinical manifestations of medium-sized vessel involvement include livedo reticularis, retiform purpura, dermal nodules, ulcers, and cutaneous necrosis/digital infarction. It includes both cutaneous manifestations of classic polyarteritis nodosa (PAN) as well as cutaneous PAN. Cutaneous PAN (also called *cutaneous arteritis*) is a chronic, relapsing vasculitis that typically involves the extremities—most commonly the legs, ankles, and feet.[85] It typically presents with subtle dermal nodules, more rarely ulcerations, often on a background of localized livedo reticularis centered about the anterior leg or ankles. Although associated with Crohn's disease, streptococcal infections (especially in children), and hepatitis B and C, most commonly it is idiopathic.[85] Perhaps 80% of patients have circulating IgM antiphosphatidylserine-prothrombin complex antibodies.[86] Cutaneous PAN can involve peripheral nerves adjacent to the skin lesions (unlike in classic PAN in which nervous system involvement is diffuse), although it is unclear if this is due to direct vasculitic involvement. A macular form has been recently described (macular lymphocytic arteritis), although it is controversial if this represents a separate entity or is a reparative form of cutaneous PAN.[87] Cutaneous PAN differs from the cutaneous manifestations of classic PAN in that it is more chronic and the skin manifestations more stereotypical.[77] Reports of cutaneous PAN developing into classic PAN are extraordinarily rare. Recently, patients with loss-of-function mutations in the gene adenosine deaminase 2 (ADA2) present with skin manifestations similar to those of cutaneous PAN, with patients having both skin-limited as well as systemic vasculitis as well as features of immunodeficiency and hematologic abnormalities.[88] It is unclear what percentage of patients with cutaneous PAN harbor ADA2 mutations, but it is reasonable to consider screening patients with cutaneous PAN (especially those with recurrent infections or cytopenias) for this abnormality.

The main differential diagnosis for medium-sized vasculitis of the skin depends on the clinical manifestations. With the more typical presentation of livedo and nodules or ulcerations, the most important diagnostic entity to rule out would be an occlusive vasculopathy. This group of disorders is large, and includes livedoid vasculopathy, genetic thrombotic diseases (such as protein C/S deficiency), calciphylaxis, Burger's disease, type I cryoglobulinemia, antiphospholipid antibodies, arteriosclerosis, and venous disease. Predominant ulceration without livedo should also prompt consideration of atypical or fungal infection, venous or arterial disease, and pyoderma gangrenosum. Clinically, panniculitides such as erythema nodosum and erythema induratum may be considered in cases limited to nodules without livedo.

Therapy is typically conservative and may consist of intralesional corticosteroids, NSAIDs, low-dose methotrexate, dapsone, or, occasionally, systemic corticosteroids.

Large Vessel Vasculitis

Skin findings of temporal arteritis (giant cell arteritis) consist mainly of palpable temporal arteries, skin tenderness in the area, and scalp nodules or ulcerations. Skin lesions in patients with Takayasu's arteritis may include Raynaud's phenomenon, livedo reticularis, ulcerated nodules, subcutaneous nodules, and pyoderma gangrenosum-like ulcers. Skin biopsy is generally not performed in these conditions.

Infections

KEY POINTS

- Infections frequently occur on the skin and can mimic autoimmune skin diseases.
- Skin biopsies can help confirm some types of skin infections, and some require a skin biopsy for culture to determine the organism and drug sensitivity.

Patients with many infectious diseases present with both skin and rheumatologic findings.[89] This section will highlight a few examples.

Lyme Borreliosis

Borrelia burgdorferi, the causative agent of Lyme disease in North America, is associated with erythema migrans (EM). In Europe the related genospecies *Borrelia afzelii* is associated with both EM and acrodermatitis chronica atrophicans (ACA), and several European studies have found compelling evidence for *B. afzelii* infection in patients with morphea.[90] There has been rare or no similar association of *Borrelia* with morphea in the United States and other countries.[91] Hematogenous dissemination from the initial skin site is believed to cause secondary skin lesions and extracutaneous manifestations, and only certain subtypes of *B. burgdorferi* are associated with dissemination.

EM is the first manifestation of Lyme disease in 60% to 80% of people and occurs at the site of the tick bite.[92] At the time of the skin lesion, which occurs within a few days to a month after the bite, the spirochetes enter the circulation and disseminate. The skin findings may be associated with fever, chills, fatigue, headache, neck stiffness, myalgias, arthralgias, conjunctivitis, erythematous throat, and regional or generalized lymphadenopathy. The lesions of EM begin as red macules that become papular and then expand into an erythematous, annular plaque (Fig. 46.14). Two forms of EM exist. In one, there is an expanding red plaque with varying intensities of redness within the plaque. In the second, there is a target, with a central red plaque surrounded by normal-appearing skin, which in turn is surrounded by another band of erythema. They can enlarge rapidly, and multiple lesions resulting from hematogenous spread are seen 17% of the time. While the lesion enlarges, the central erythema can fade. The central portion of the lesion may be edematous, vesicular, urticarial, or crusted. Triangular and elongated oval lesions have been described, but circular lesions are most frequent. The most common locations are the inguina, axillae, abdomen, and behind the knees. EM lesions are usually asymptomatic but can be pruritic or painful. Untreated EM lesions resolve in a median of 28 days, with a range from 1 day

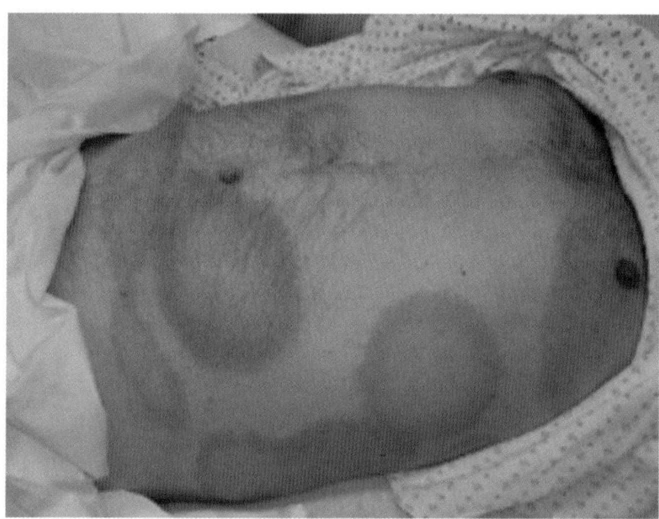

• **Fig. 46.14** Lyme disease with characteristic erythematous, annular plaques. (Courtesy Dr. Joshua Levin, University of Pennsylvania Department of Dermatology, Philadelphia.)

to 14 months. Resolution is within a few days after treatment with antibiotics such as doxycycline or penicillin.

ACA is associated with late-stage Lyme disease. It occurs mainly in women between the ages of 40 and 70 years. The lesions begin on an extremity, usually the lower leg or foot as a bluish-red edematous plaque. Fibrous bands may develop, especially on the ulnar and tibial regions, and fibrous nodules may form near joints. Regional lymphadenopathy is often present. Over many years, the skin becomes atrophic.[93] *B. burgdorferi* has been isolated from the skin of patients with ACA.[94]

Parvovirus

The skin findings of patients seen with parvovirus B19 include an erythematous "slapped cheeks" appearance; a lacy, reticulated proximal extremity rash; a febrile petechial eruption; and papular-purpuric gloves and socks syndrome (PPGSS). The infection is self-limited and generally resolves spontaneously within 1 to 2 weeks. Laboratory findings may include mild or severe leukopenia, transient neutropenia or relative neutrophilia, eosinophilia, and mild thrombocytopenia. Adults who are infected often contract the virus from infected children and commonly present with systemic disease, including arthropathy and a flu-like illness, and with additional skin lesions of periflexural pattern and purpura.[95]

Atypical Infections: *Mycobacterium marinum*

Many types of mycobacteria, atypical mycobacteria, and deep fungal infections can affect skin and joints. *Mycobacterium marinum* is an example and can be acquired through exposure to fresh water, salt water, fish tanks, swimming pools, fish or aquatic exposures, timber cuts, or splinters. The incubation period is usually about 3 weeks, although much longer periods are possible. The disease often occurs after inoculation into abrasions or after penetrating injuries to the fingers and hands. This is an indolent disease, with nodules or ulcerated plaques, occasionally with extension to deep tissue. Common areas of involvement are the fingers, dorsum of the hands, and knees. The lesions can be localized or sporotrichoid (25%), with dissemination 2% of the time.

Panniculitis

KEY POINTS

There are many causes and types of panniculitis. Some are associated with systemic conditions and require a careful history and physical examination, along with a skin biopsy, to determine the cause.

Diseases such as amyloidosis and sarcoidosis can involve the skin and can be diagnosed with the help of a skin biopsy. A diagnosis of these diseases in the skin should prompt a search for systemic involvement. Treatment is determined by the cause of the disease and the organs involved.

Panniculitis refers to a group of diseases that manifest as inflammation or alterations in the subcutaneous fat. The complexity of etiologies for even one form of panniculitis, such as erythema nodosum, the relative rarity of most forms of panniculitis, and the number of different panniculitides has slowed progress in elucidating pathogenesis. The etiologies for many panniculitides are still poorly understood.

Panniculitis may be primary without an identifiable cause, or secondary. Common secondary causes of panniculitis include infection, trauma, pancreatic disease, immunodeficiency states, malignancies, and connective tissue disease. Erythema nodosum remains the most common form of panniculitis, and although there is a long list of diseases and medications with which it is associated, it is frequently not associated with an identifiable underlying condition. Some underlying conditions associated with erythema nodosum include inflammatory bowel disease; sarcoidosis; malignancies such as leukemia and lymphoma; infections (bacteria, *Yersinia, Rickettsiae*, chlamydial, spirochetal, and protozoal disease); pregnancy; drugs (sulfonamides and contraceptives); and autoimmune diseases such as Behçet's disease (BD), Sjögren's syndrome, reactive arthritis, and SLE.[96]

Although the understanding of lobular panniculitis has expanded, cases that were lumped into the wastebasket diagnosis of "Weber-Christian" disease are now recognized to be clearly definable and separate entities, such as lupus panniculitis, cytophagic histiocytic panniculitis, subcutaneous panniculitis-like T cell lymphoma, α_1-anti-trypsin deficiency, factitial panniculitis, traumatic panniculitis, calciphylaxis, and drug-induced.[97,98] Infections are recognized as a trigger of panniculitis, as exemplified by erythema nodosum caused by streptococcal infection; hepatitis B or C associated with polyarteritis nodosa; infectious panniculitides, often in immunocompromised hosts; and most recently, some cases of erythema induratum/nodular vasculitis associated with *Mycobacterium tuberculosis*.[99] In addition, atypical infections can themselves cause lesions that resemble panniculitis.

An understanding of the heterogeneity of lymphomas that involve the fat is still evolving, but advances in differentiating various histologic and clinical outcomes are occurring.[100] Some patients thought to have lupus panniculitis on the basis of cytopenias and laboratory tests are actually diagnosed with subcutaneous lymphoma after careful review of their pathology.[100,101]

Patients with panniculitis frequently have erythematous tender nodules, and the clinical presentation frequently is not specific enough to allow for determination of the exact subtype of

TABLE 46.4 Classification of Panniculitis

I. Without prominent vasculitis
   A. Septal inflammation
      1. Lymphocytic and mixed: erythema nodosum and variants
      2. Granulomatous: palisaded granulomatous diseases, sarcoidosis, subcutaneous infection: tuberculosis, syphilis
      3. Sclerotic: scleroderma, eosinophilic fasciitis, lipodermatosclerosis, toxins
   B. Lobular inflammation
      1. Neutrophilic: infection, ruptured folliculitis and cysts, pancreatic fat necrosis
      2. Lymphocytic: lupus panniculitis, poststeroid panniculitis, lymphoma/leukemia
      3. Macrophagic: histiocytic cytophagic panniculitis
      4. Granulomatous: erythema induratum/nodular vasculitis, palisaded granulomatous diseases, sarcoidosis, Crohn's disease
      5. Mixed inflammation with many foam cells: α_1-anti-trypsin deficiency, Weber-Christian disease, traumatic fat necrosis
      6. Eosinophilic: eosinophilic panniculitis, arthropod bites, parasites
      7. Enzymatic fat necrosis: pancreatic enzyme panniculitis
      8. Crystal deposits: sclerema neonatorum, subcutaneous fat necrosis of the newborn, gout, oxalosis
      9. Embryonic fat pattern: lipoatrophy, lipodystrophy

II. With prominent vasculitis (septal or lobular)
   A. Neutrophilic: leukocytoclastic vasculitis, subcutaneous polyarteritis nodosa, thrombophlebitis, ENL
   B. Lymphocytic: nodular vasculitis, perniosis, angiocentric lymphomas
   C. Granulomatous: nodular vasculitis/erythema induratum, ENL, granulomatosis with polyangiitis, Churg-Strauss allergic granulomatosis

III. Mixed patterns

ENL, Erythema nodosum leprosum.

panniculitis without a biopsy. Patients with panniculitis can have associated symptoms such as low-grade fevers, fatigue, arthralgias, and myalgias.

An adequate skin biopsy, often involving an elliptical excision, is essential to properly diagnose the various entities that fall into the category of panniculitis (Table 46.4). Panniculitis is typically classified into four main subgroups: septal, lobular, mixed panniculitis, and panniculitis with vasculitis, and the exact nature of the cellular infiltrate also contributes to a proper diagnosis. There is no question that these overall categorizations help to narrow the differential in any given case, but at times there are overlapping features or reaction patterns that do not allow for a specific diagnosis. Clinical-pathologic correlation is important, as emphasized by a published review that has an expanded and useful classification of panniculitis.[102]

Anecdotes exist about the efficacy of combination antimalarials, such as hydroxychloroquine and quinacrine, in treating subcutaneous sarcoid, but no studies exist that support definitive recommendations. Reports on the use of newer therapies, such as mycophenolate mofetil and thalidomide, to treat inflammatory causes of panniculitis, such as nodular panniculitis and erythema nodosum, are already in the literature, and indicate that these drugs will likely evolve to be useful for these conditions.[103,104] The effectiveness of these and more established drugs, such as NSAIDs, anti-malarials, and methotrexate, need to be studied, and outcomes will hopefully be more systematically evaluated.

Relapsing Polychondritis

The diagnosis of relapsing polychondritis (RP) is based on the typical clinical manifestations, with auricular findings seen in 90% of patients. Nasal and respiratory tract chondritis can occur, along with nonerosive inflammatory arthritis, cardiac valvular insufficiency, vasculitis, and eye and audiovestibular involvement. The estimated prevalence of 3.5 per million makes controlled trials nearly impossible. The etiology is unknown, but the pathogenesis appears to be mediated by an immune reaction to type II collagen. Clinical skin manifestations include inflammation of the ear, with sparing of the earlobe. Diagnosis includes the presence of a positive serum antibody test to type II collagen and a wedge biopsy that shows cartilage necrosis and perichondral inflammation with lymphocytes and histiocytes. Involvement of other cartilage areas, including the upper airway, should be assessed. Glucocorticoids are the therapeutic choice for reducing the inflammatory process in patients with RP. For patients with sustained disease, many immunosuppressive drugs have been used as steroid-sparing agents. There have been reports of response to TNF inhibitors, rituximab, tocilizumab, and abatacept in patients otherwise refractory to therapy.[105]

Infiltrative Diseases

Amyloid

Type AL amyloidosis (primary amyloidosis) is rare, with an incidence of less than one per 100,000 individuals. Skin lesions may occur in as many as 40% of these patients. Skin lesions can be an early sign of the disease and may include purpura, petechiae, and ecchymosis caused by infiltration of blood vessels by amyloid. Other skin findings include alopecia, plaques, and nodules, often found on flexor surfaces, the face, or the buccal mucosa. Bullae and nail dystrophy are occasionally seen. Diagnosis is confirmed by biopsy of lesional or nonlesional skin, along with urine and serum for immunoelectrophoresis to confirm the presence of a circulating monoclonal protein. Skin biopsy shows Congo-red positive, homogeneous, hyaline, fibrillary deposits. Treatment includes autologous stem cell transplantation, with approximately 50% of patients achieving prolonged remission with such therapy. Other effective therapies include the combination of melphalan with high-dose dexamethasone, thalidomide, proteasome inhibitors, and stem cell transplant in conjunction with melphalan.[106,107] The prognosis depends on the stage at the time of diagnosis, which emphasizes the importance of recognizing the disease.

Sarcoidosis

Cutaneous involvement occurs in 20% to 25% of sarcoidosis cases and is most likely to be seen early in the disease. Cutaneous lesions can be classified as nonspecific, typically erythema nodosum, and as specific or granulomatous. Erythema nodosum occurs frequently as part of Löfgren's syndrome, with bilateral hilar lymphadenopathy and acute iridocyclitis. This variant has a good prognosis and resolves in 80% of patients within 2 years. The skin lesions of sarcoidosis generally have no prognostic significance or correlation with disease activity. Skin involvement has no effect on the course of the disease, and the number of skin lesions does not correlate with systemic disease. Skin plaques tend to be more persistent and are commonly associated with chronic forms of the disease. Lupus pernio (Fig. 46.15), with violaceous

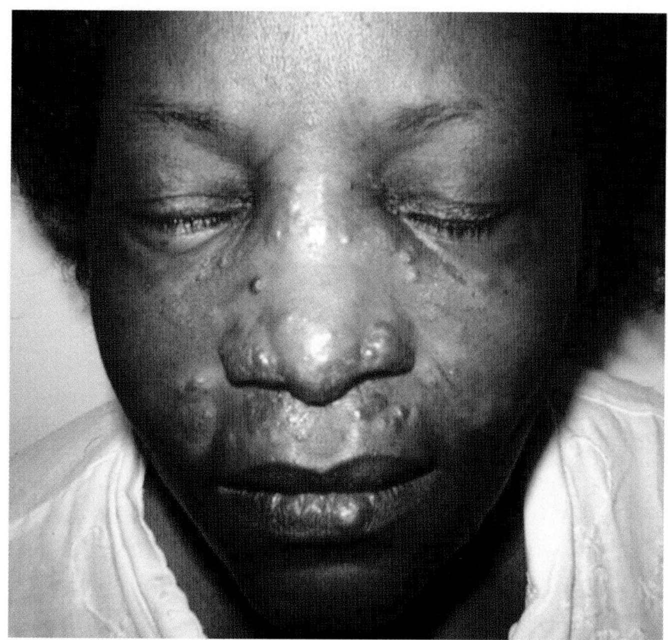

• **Fig. 46.15** Sarcoidosis with "apple-jelly" plaques on the face and lupus pernio, or nasal rim lesions.

plaques on the nose, ears, cheeks, lips, and fingers, is often seen in long-standing sarcoidosis and is associated with upper airway involvement and pulmonary fibrosis.[108] Other forms of cutaneous sarcoidosis include papules, follicular papules, subcutaneous nodules, ulcerative lesions, alopecia, and ichthyosis. Cutaneous sarcoid can arise in scars. Because of the many types of presentation, diagnosis can be challenging, and a skin biopsy is necessary to confirm the clinical suspicion. Mimickers of papules include xanthelasma, rosacea, trichoepithelioma, syphilis, LE, and granuloma annulare. Plaques can resemble lupus vulgaris, necrobiosis lipoidica, morphea, leprosy, *Leishmania,* or lupus erythematosus. Nodules can resemble lymphoma or other types of panniculitis. Treatment of cutaneous sarcoidosis depends on the degree of systemic involvement. Clearly, patients who need prednisone for systemic disease often experience improvement of their cutaneous sarcoid. Patients with isolated skin disease or systemic disease that does not require aggressive therapy can benefit from topical or intralesional corticosteroids, topical tacrolimus, minocycline, hydroxychloroquine, combination anti-malarials with hydroxychloroquine and quinacrine, or chloroquine. If anti-malarials are not adequate, then methotrexate or oral retinoids may be used. There have been case reports and small case series of successful therapy with thalidomide and TNF inhibitors, as well as laser remodeling of lupus pernio. There is some concern that TNF inhibitors and IFN-α therapy may induce sarcoidosis.

Miscellaneous Skin Diseases and Arthritis

KEY POINTS

There are a number of autoinflammatory diseases, including Behçet's disease, familial Mediterranean fever, and cryopyrin-associated periodic syndromes, that involve mutations of the inflammasome and can be treated with cytokine inhibitors.

Behçet's Disease

BD is most prevalent in the Middle East and the Far East. Human leukocyte antigen (HLA)-B5 and HLA-B51 genes are important in the pathogenesis of the disease. The criteria for BD include recurrent oral and genital ulcers, eye lesions (uveitis or retinal vasculitis), characteristic skin lesions, and a positive pathergy test.[109] The pathergy test involves use of a sterile needle to prick the forearm. The results are positive when the puncture causes an aseptic erythematous nodule or pustule that is more than 2 mm in diameter at 24 to 48 hours. A diagnosis is made if patients have recurrent oral ulceration plus at least two of the other findings without other clinical explanations. Skin lesions include erythema nodosum, pseudofolliculitis, or papulopustular lesions or acneiform nodules in postadolescents. Oral ulcers are painful and occur on the gingiva, tongue, and buccal and labial mucosa. Genital ulcers, usually larger and deeper than oral ulcers, are typically on the scrotum and penis in men and the vulva in women. Venous involvement, including superficial thrombophlebitis and deep venous thrombosis, can occur. On skin biopsy, small vessel vasculitis is common. Ulcer treatment includes topical corticosteroids, colchicine, thalidomide, interferon-α, TNF inhibitors or apremilast, and there are some reports of biologics, including inhibitors of IL-1, IL-12/23, being helpful.[110] Systemic corticosteroids are prescribed for unresponsive erythema nodosum.

Familial Mediterranean Fever

Familial Mediterranean fever (FMF) is an autosomal recessive disease that tends to affect certain ethnic groups, including Sephardic Jews, Arabs, Armenians, and Turks. There is a mutation on the short arm of chromosome 16, and the mutant protein pyrin likely plays an inhibitory role in the control of inflammation.[111,112] It is characterized by recurrent, self-limited attacks of peritonitis, pleuritis, and synovitis. Erysipelas-like erythema (ELE) is the pathognomonic skin manifestation. This is characterized by tender erythematous and well-demarcated plaques, usually located on the lower legs.[113] They may be triggered by physical effort and subside spontaneously within 48 to 72 hours of bed rest. Fever and leukocytosis may accompany this condition. Other associated skin findings include Henoch-Schönlein purpura; nonspecific purpura; erythema of the face, trunk, or palm; angioneurotic edema; Raynaud's phenomenon; pyoderma; and subcutaneous nodules. Secondary generalized amyloidosis may lead to chronic renal failure and death if not recognized. Skin biopsy shows edema of the superficial dermis and sparse perivascular infiltrate composed of a few lymphocytes, neutrophils, and nuclear dust, without vasculitis. Direct immunofluorescence shows deposits of C3 in the wall of small superficial vessels. Early treatment with colchicine, which prevents or diminishes the frequency and severity of the inflammatory episodes, can be beneficial. Refractory patients may benefit from IL-1 blockade.[114]

Multicentric Reticulohistiocytosis

Multicentric reticulohistiocytosis (MRH) is a rare condition of unknown etiology that most frequently occurs in Caucasian women in their fifth and sixth decades. There is destructive symmetric arthritis, with arthritis mutilans developing in approximately 45% of cases, associated with cutaneous papulonodular lesions. Skin findings include cutaneous red-to-brown papules or nodules, typically on the face, dorsum of the fingers, and over the proximal and distal interphalangeal joints, but they can be in a more generalized distribution. A rarer presentation includes photodistributed erythema, often with targeting over joints, which masquerades as DM.[115] Diagnosis is made by skin biopsy, which shows infiltration of histiocytes and multinucleated giant cells. These changes can be seen in a variety of tissues, including the heart, lungs, skeletal muscle, and gastrointestinal tract. The differential diagnosis of skin disease includes other infiltrative processes, such as sarcoidosis and even leprosy. Treatment recommendations, based on mostly small case reports, include glucocorticoids and methotrexate, cyclophosphamide, and finally chlorambucil if the condition is unresponsive.[116] Cyclosporine, TNF inhibitors, and bisphosphonates have also been used with reported benefit.[117] In approximately one-third of patients, MRH may precede or follow an underlying malignancy. Reported associated malignancies include breast, cervix, colon, stomach, lung, larynx, ovary, lymphoma, leukemia, sarcoma, melanoma, mesothelioma, and metastatic cancer of unknown primary.

Cryopyrin-Associated Periodic Syndromes

Cryopyrin-associated periodic syndromes (CAPS) are inherited autoinflammatory conditions characterized by recurrent bouts of systemic inflammation related to inappropriate activation of the innate immune system. The syndrome encompasses a continuum of three diseases. The mildest is familial cold autoinflammatory syndrome (FCAS). Patients with FCAS present with recurrent, cold-induced episodes of fever, urticaria-like rash, arthralgia, and conjunctivitis. Patients with Muckle–Wells syndrome (MWS) have an intermediate phenotype. In MWS, the disease tends to be chronic, with fever, rash, and arthritis or arthralgia; sensorineural hearing loss; and AA amyloidosis in adulthood. The most severe is neonatal-onset multisystem inflammatory disease (NOMID), also referred to as *chronic infantile neurologic cutaneous articular* (CINCA) syndrome. In CINCA/NOMID, fever is rare. Patients present with an early onset, intermittent, urticaria-like rash, and neurosensory involvement. Hypertrophic arthropathy with contractures and bone deformity can occur in severely affected patients with CINCA/NOMID. CAPS are caused by dominantly inherited or de novo gain-of-function mutations within the *NLRP3* gene. Somatic mutations have been recently described in CINCA/NOMID germline-mutation–negative patients. *NLRP3* encodes cryopyrin, a cytosolic protein complex that controls activation of caspase-1, which then activates IL-1β. Mutations in *NLRP3* are associated with overactivation of the inflammasome and thus overexpression of IL-1β. Inhibition of IL-1β can dramatically improve all the clinical manifestations related to this type of inflammation.[118] Isolated reports also suggest that TNF inhibitors and thalidomide can be beneficial therapeutically in these patients.

Interferon-Associated Genetic Syndromes

Interferons modulate innate (autoinflammatory) effects. Patients with these syndromes have monogenic defects leading to increased type I interferons and share clinical, histologic, and functional features. The syndromes include the proteasome defect–associated autoinflammatory disease CANDLE, Aicardi–Goutières syndrome, *TREX1*-mediated familial chilblain lupus, and stimulators of interferon genes (STING)–associated vasculopathy of infancy. Patients with these conditions have a vasculopathy early in life, granulocyte precursors in the skin, and a prominent interferon-response-gene signature in the peripheral blood and with variable B-cell activation.[119]

Full references for this chapter can be found on ExpertConsult.com.

Selected References

1. Greb JE, Goldminz AM, Elder JT, et al.: Psoriasis, *Nat Rev Dis Primers.* 2:16082, 2016.
2. Takeshita J, Grewal S, Langan SM, et al.: Psoriasis and comorbid diseases: epidemiology, *J Am Acad Dermatol* 76(3):377–390, 2017.
3. Conrad C, Gilliet M: Psoriasis: from pathogenesis to targeted therapies, *Clin Rev Allergy Immunol* 54(1):102–113, 2018.
4. Marrakchi S, Guigue P, Renshaw BR, et al.: Interleukin-36-receptor antagonist deficiency and generalized pustular psoriasis, *N Engl J Med* 365(7):620–628, 2011.
5. Tan AL, Benjamin M, Toumi H, et al.: The relationship between the extensor tendon enthesis and the nail in distal interphalangeal joint disease in psoriatic arthritis—a high-resolution MRI and histological study, *Rheumatology (Oxford)* 46(2):253–256, 2007.
6. Kaushik SB, Lebwohl MG: Review of safety and efficacy of approved systemic psoriasis therapies, *Int J Dermatol* 58(6):649–658, 2019.
7. Chua-Aguilera CJ, Moller B, Yawalkar N: Skin manifestations of rheumatoid arthritis, juvenile idiopathic arthritis, and spondyloarthritides, *Clin Rev Allergy Immunol* 53(3):371–393, 2017.
8. Sayah A, English 3rd JC: Rheumatoid arthritis: a review of the cutaneous manifestations, *J Am Acad Dermatol* 53(2):191–209, 2005. .
9. Turunen S, Huhtakangas J, Nousiainen T, et al.: Rheumatoid arthritis antigens homocitrulline and citrulline are generated by local myeloperoxidase and peptidyl arginine deiminases 2, 3 and 4 in rheumatoid nodule and synovial tissue, *Arthritis Res Ther* 18(1):239, 2016.
10. Maldonado I, Eid H, Rodriguez GR, et al.: Rheumatoid nodulosis: is it a different subset of rheumatoid arthritis? *J Clin Rheumatol* 9(5):296–305, 2003.
11. Ahmed SS, Arnett FC, Smith CA, et al.: The HLA-DRB1*0401 allele and the development of methotrexate-induced accelerated rheumatoid nodulosis: a follow-up study of 79 Caucasian patients with rheumatoid arthritis, *Medicine (Baltimore)* 80(4):271–278, 2001.
12. Talotta R, Atzeni F, Batticciotto A, et al.: Accelerated subcutaneous nodulosis in patients with rheumatoid arthritis treated with tocilizumab: a case series, *J Med Case Rep* 12(1):154, 2018.
13. Vollertsen RS, Conn DL, Ballard DJ, et al.: Rheumatoid vasculitis: survival and associated risk factors, *Medicine (Baltimore)* 65(6):365–375, 1986.
14. Watts RA, Scott DG: Vasculitis and inflammatory arthritis, *Best Pract Res Clin Rheumatol* 30(5):916–931, 2016.
15. Schadt CR, Callen JP: Management of neutrophilic dermatoses, *Dermatol Ther* 25(2):158–172, 2012.
16. Brown TS, Fearneyhough PK, Burruss JB, et al.: Rheumatoid neutrophilic dermatitis in a woman with seronegative rheumatoid arthritis, *J Am Acad Dermatol* 45(4):596–600, 2001.
17. Sangueza OP, Caudell MD, Mengesha YM, et al.: Palisaded neutrophilic granulomatous dermatitis in rheumatoid arthritis, *J Am Acad Dermatol* 47(2):251–257, 2002.
18. Schneider R, Passo MH: Juvenile rheumatoid arthritis, *Rheum Dis Clin North Am* 28(3):503–530, 2002.
19. Woods MT, Gavino AC, Burford HN, et al.: The evolution of histopathologic findings in adult Still disease, *Am J Dermatopathol* 33(7):736–739, 2011.
20. Colafrancesco S, Priori R, Valesini G, et al.: Response to interleukin-1 inhibitors in 140 Italian patients with adult-onset Still's disease: a multicentre retrospective observational study, *Front Pharmacol* 8:369, 2017.
21. Gilliam JN, Sontheimer RD: Distinctive cutaneous subsets in the spectrum of lupus erythematosus, *J Am Acad Dermatol* 4(4):471–475, 1981.

22. Sontheimer RD, Maddison PJ, Reichlin M, et al.: Serologic and HLA associations in subacute cutaneous lupus erythematosus, a clinical subset of lupus erythematosus, *Ann Intern Med* 97(5):664–671, 1982.
23. Gronhagen CM, Fored CM, Linder M, et al.: Subacute cutaneous lupus erythematosus and its association with drugs: a population-based matched case-control study of 234 patients in Sweden, *Br J Dermatol* 167(2):296–305, 2012.
24. Sandholdt LH, Laurinaviciene R, Bygum A: Proton pump inhibitor-induced subacute cutaneous lupus erythematosus, *Br J Dermatol* 170(2):342–351, 2014.
25. David-Bajar KM, Bennion SD, DeSpain JD, et al.: Clinical, histologic, and immunofluorescent distinctions between subacute cutaneous lupus erythematosus and discoid lupus erythematosus, *JInvestDermatol* 99:251, 1992.
26. Lee LA, Gaither KK, Coulter SN, et al.: Pattern of cutaneous immunoglobulin G deposition in subacute cutaneous lupus erythematosus is reproduced by infusing purified anti-Ro (SSA) autoantibodies into human skin-grafted mice, *J Clin Invest* 83(5):1556–1562, 1989.
27. Durosaro O, Davis MD, Reed KB, et al.: Incidence of cutaneous lupus erythematosus, 1965-2005: a population-based study, *Arch Dermatol* 145(3):249–253, 2009.
28. Gronhagen CM, Fored CM, Granath F, et al.: Cutaneous lupus erythematosus and the association with systemic lupus erythematosus: a population-based cohort of 1088 patients in Sweden, *Br J Dermatol* 164(6):1335–1341, 2011.
29. Wieczorek IT, Propert KJ, Okawa J, et al.: Systemic symptoms in the progression of cutaneous to systemic lupus erythematosus, *JAMA Dermatol* 150(3):291–296, 2014.
30. Kuhn A, Richter-Hintz D, Oslislo C, et al.: Lupus erythematosus tumidus—a neglected subset of cutaneous Lupus erythematosus: report of 40 cases.[see comment], *ArchDermatol* 136:1033, 2005.
31. Bosisio F, Boi S, Caputo V, et al.: Lobular panniculitic infiltrates with overlapping histopathologic features of lupus panniculitis (lupus profundus) and subcutaneous T-cell lymphoma: a conceptual and practical dilemma, *Am J Surg Pathol* 39(2):206–211, 2015.
32. Chang J, Werth VP: Therapeutic options for cutaneous lupus erythematosus: recent advances and future prospects, *Expert Rev Clin Immunol* 12(10):1109–1121, 2016.
33. Piette EW, Foering KP, Chang AY, et al.: Impact of smoking in cutaneous lupus erythematosus, *Arch Dermatol* 148(3):317–322, 2012.
34. Chang AY, Piette EW, Foering KP, et al.: Response to antimalarial agents in cutaneous lupus erythematosus: a prospective analysis, *Arch Dermatol* 147(11):1261–1267, 2011, .
35. Hall RP, Lawley TJ, Smith HR, et al.: Bullous eruption of systemic lupus erythematosus. Dramatic response to dapsone therapy, *Ann Intern Med* 97(2):165–170, 1982.
36. Frances C, Piette JC: The mystery of Sneddon syndrome: relationship with antiphospholipid syndrome and systemic lupus erythematosus, *J Autoimmun* 15(2):139–143, 2000.
37. Lee LA: Transient autoimmunity related to maternal autoantibodies: neonatal lupus, *Autoimmun Rev* 4(4):207–213, 2005.
38. Martin V, Lee LA, Askanase AD, et al.: Long-term followup of children with neonatal lupus and their unaffected siblings, *Arthritis Rheum* 46(9):2377–2383, 2002.
39. Jhorar P, Torre K, Lu J: Cutaneous features and diagnosis of primary Sjogren syndrome: an update and review, *J Am Acad Dermatol* 79(4):736–745, 2018.
40. Nishikawa T, Provost TT: Differences in clinical, serologic, and immunogenetic features of white versus Oriental anti-SS-A/Ro-positive patients, *J Am Acad Dermatol* 25(3):563–564, 1991. PubMed PMID: 1918496.
41. Ramos-Casals M, Anaya JM, Garcia-Carrasco M, et al.: Cutaneous vasculitis in primary Sjogren syndrome: classification and clinical significance of 52 patients, *Medicine (Baltimore)* 83(2):96–106, 2004.
42. Lundberg IE, Tjarnlund A, Bottai M, et al.: International Myositis Classification Criteria Project Consortium, The Euromyositis Register, and The Juvenile Dermatomyositis Cohort Biomarker Study and Repository: 2017 European League against rheumatism/American College of Rheumatology classification criteria for adult and juvenile idiopathic inflammatory myopathies and their major subgroups, *Ann Rheum Dis* 76(12):1955–1964, 2017.
43. Concha JSS, Tarazi M, Kushner CJ, et al.: The diagnosis and classification of amyopathic dermatomyositis: a historical review and assessment of existing criteria, *Br J Dermatol* 180(5):1001–1008, 2019.
44. Sontheimer RD: Cutaneous features of classic dermatomyositis and amyopathic dermatomyositis, *CurrOpinion Rheumatol* 11:475, 1999. PubMed PMID: 2659.
45. Zhang L, Wu G, Gao D, et al.: Factors associated with interstitial lung disease in patients with polymyositis and dermatomyositis: a systematic review and meta-analysis, *PLoS One* 11:e0155381, 2016.
46. Fiorentino DF, Kuo K, Chung L, et al.: Distinctive cutaneous and systemic features associated with antitranscriptional intermediary factor-1gamma antibodies in adults with dermatomyositis, *J Am Acad Dermatol* 72(3):449–455, 2015.
47. Bernet LL, Lewis MA, Rieger KE, et al.: Ovoid palatal patch in dermatomyositis: a novel finding associated with anti-TIF1gamma (p155) antibodies, *JAMA Dermatol* 152(9):1049–1051, 2016.
48. Balin SJ, Wetter DA, Andersen LK, et al.: Calcinosis cutis occurring in association with autoimmune connective tissue disease: the Mayo Clinic experience with 78 patients, 1996-2009, *Arch Dermatol* 148(4):455–462, 2012.
49. Crowson AN, Magro CM: The role of microvascular injury in the pathogenesis of cutaneous lesions of dermatomyositis, *Hum Pathol* 27(1):15–19, 1996.
50. Magro CM, Crowson AN: The immunofluorescent profile of dermatomyositis: a comparative study with lupus erythematosus, *J Cutan Pathol* 24(9):543–552, 1997.
51. Wolstencroft PW, Fiorentino DF: Dermatomyositis clinical and pathological phenotypes associated with myositis-specific autoantibodies, *Curr Rheumatol Rep* 20(5):28, 2018.
52. Connors GR, Christopher-Stine L, Oddis CV, et al.: Interstitial lung disease associated with the idiopathic inflammatory myopathies: what progress has been made in the past 35 years? *Chest* 138(6):1464–1474, 2010.
53. Olazagasti JM, Baez PJ, Wetter DA, et al.: Cancer risk in dermatomyositis: a meta-analysis of cohort studies, *Am J Clin Dermatol* 16(2):89–98, 2015.
54. Leatham H, Schadt C, Chisolm S, et al.: Evidence supports blind screening for internal malignancy in dermatomyositis: data from 2 large US dermatology cohorts, *Medicine (Baltimore)* 97(2):e9639, 2018.
55. Sato Y, Teraki Y, Izaki S, et al.: Clinical characterization of dermatomyositis associated with mechanic's hands, *J Dermatol* 39(12):1093–1095, 2012.
56. Narang NS, Casciola-Rosen L, Li S, et al.: Cutaneous ulceration in dermatomyositis: association with anti-melanoma differentiation-associated gene 5 antibodies and interstitial lung disease, *Arthritis Care Res (Hoboken)* 67(5):667–672, 2015.
57. Lu X, Yang H, Shu X, et al.: Factors predicting malignancy in patients with polymyositis and dermatomyostis: a systematic review and meta-analysis, *PLoS One* 9(4):e94128, 2014.
58. Femia AN, Vleugels RA, Callen JP: Cutaneous dermatomyositis: an updated review of treatment options and internal associations, *Am J Clin Dermatol* 14(4):291–313, 2013.
59. Kurita T, Yasuda S, Amengual O, et al.: The efficacy of calcineurin inhibitors for the treatment of interstitial lung disease associated with polymyositis/dermatomyositis, *Lupus* 24(1):3–9, 2015.
60. Kahn JS, Deverapalli SC, Rosmarin DM: JAK-STAT signaling pathway inhibition: a role for treatment of discoid lupus erythematosus and dermatomyositis, *Int J Dermatol* 57(8):1007–1014, 2018.

61. Pelle MT, Callen JP: Adverse cutaneous reactions to hydroxychloroquine are more common in patients with dermatomyositis than in patients with cutaneous lupus erythematosus, *Arch Dermatol* 138(9):1231–1233, 2002.
62. Ang GC, Werth VP: Combination antimalarials in the treatment of cutaneous dermatomyositis: a retrospective study, *Arch Dermatol* 141(7):855–859, 2005.
63. Ferreli C, Gasparini G, Parodi A, et al.: Cutaneous manifestations of scleroderma and scleroderma-like disorders: a comprehensive review, *Clin Rev Allergy Immunol* 53(3):306–336, 2017.
64. Fett N, Werth VP: Update on morphea: part I. Epidemiology, clinical presentation, and pathogenesis, *J Am Acad Dermatol* 64(2):217–228, 2011.
65. Mazori DR, Femia AN, Vleugels RA: Eosinophilic fasciitis: an updated review on diagnosis and treatment, *Curr Rheumatol Rep* 19(12):74, 2017.
66. Florez-Pollack S, Kunzler E, Jacobe HT, et al.: Current concepts, *Clin Dermatol* 36(4):475–486, 2018.
67. van den Hoogen F, Khanna D, Fransen J, et al.: 2013 classification criteria for systemic sclerosis: an American College of Rheumatology/European League against Rheumatism collaborative initiative, *Arthritis Rheum* 65(11):2737–2747, 2013.
68. Pearson DR, Werth VP, Pappas-Taffer L: Systemic sclerosis: Current concepts of skin and systemic manifestations, *Clin Dermatol* 36(4):459–474, 2018.
69. Spierings J, van Rhijn-Brouwer FCC, van Laar JM: Hematopoietic stem-cell transplantation in systemic sclerosis: an update, *Curr Opin Rheumatol* 30(6):541–547, 2018.
70. Momeni A, Sorice SC, Valenzuela A, et al.: Surgical treatment of systemic sclerosis—is it justified to offer peripheral sympathectomy earlier in the disease process? *Microsurgery* 35(6):441–446, 2015.
71. Motegi SI, Uehara A, Yamada K, et al.: Efficacy of botulinum toxin B injection for Raynaud's phenomenon and digital ulcers in patients with systemic sclerosis, *Acta Derm Venereol* 97(7):843–850, 2017.
72. Yaqub A, Chung L, Rieger KE, et al.: Localized cutaneous fibrosing disorders, *Rheum Dis Clin North Am* 39(2):347–364, 2013.
73. Bernstein EJ, Schmidt-Lauber C, Kay J: Nephrogenic systemic fibrosis: a systemic fibrosing disease resulting from gadolinium exposure, *Best Pract Res Clin Rheumatol* 26(4):489–503, 2012.
74. Kucher C, Xu X, Pasha T, et al.: Histopathologic comparison of nephrogenic fibrosing dermopathy and scleromyxedema, *J Cutan Pathol* 32(7):484–490, 2005.
75. Daftari Besheli L, Aran S, Shaqdan K, et al.: Current status of nephrogenic systemic fibrosis, *Clinical Radiology* 69:661–668, 2014.
76. Bruce R, Wentland AL, Haemel AK, et al.: Incidence of nephrogenic systemic fibrosis using Gadobenate Dimeglumine in 1423 patients with renal insufficiency compared with Gadodiamide, *Invest Radiol* 51(11):701–705, 2016.
77. Sunderkotter CH, Zelger B, Chen KR, et al.: Nomenclature of cutaneous vasculitis: Dermatologic addendum to the 2012 revised international Chapel Hill consensus conference nomenclature of Vasculitides, *Arthritis Rheumatol* 70(2):171–184, 2018.
78. Carlson JA: The histological assessment of cutaneous vasculitis, *Histopathology* 56(1):3–23, 2010.
79. Fiorentino DF: Cutaneous vasculitis, *J Am Acad Dermatol* 48(3):311–340, 2003.
80. Marzano AV, Raimondo MG, Berti E, et al.: Cutaneous manifestations of ANCA-associated small vessels vasculitis, *Clin Rev Allergy Immunol* 53(3):428–438, 2017.
81. Piette WW, Stone MS: A cutaneous sign of IgA-associated small dermal vessel leukocytoclastic vasculitis in adults (Henoch-Schonlein purpura), *Arch Dermatol* 125(1):53–56, 1989. PubMed PMID: 2642681.
82. Poterucha TJ, Wetter DA, Gibson LE, et al.: Histopathology and correlates of systemic disease in adult Henoch-Schonlein purpura: a retrospective study of microscopic and clinical findings in 68 patients at Mayo Clinic, *J Am Acad Dermatol* 68(3):420–424 e3, 2013.
83. Momen SE, Jorizzo J, Al-Niaimi F: Erythema elevatum diutinum: a review of presentation and treatment, *J Eur Acad Dermatol Venereol* 28(12):1594–1602, 2014.
84. Fiore E, Rizzi M, Simonetti GD, et al.: Acute hemorrhagic edema of young children: a concise narrative review, *Eur J Pediatr* 170(12):1507–1511, 2011.
85. Morgan AJ, Schwartz RA: Cutaneous polyarteritis nodosa: a comprehensive review, *Int J Dermatol* 49(7):750–756, 2010.
86. Kawakami T, Yamazaki M, Mizoguchi M, et al.: High titer of anti-phosphatidylserine-prothrombin complex antibodies in patients with cutaneous polyarteritis nodosa, *Arthritis Rheum* 57(8):1507–1513, 2007.
87. Buffiere-Morgado A, Battistella M, Vignon-Pennamen MD, et al.: Relationship between cutaneous polyarteritis nodosa (cPAN) and macular lymphocytic arteritis (MLA): Blinded histologic assessment of 35 cPAN cases, *J Am Acad Dermatol* 73(6):1013–1020, 2015.
88. Meyts I, Aksentijevich I: Deficiency of adenosine deaminase 2 (DADA2): Updates on the phenotype, genetics, pathogenesis, and treatment, *J Clin Immunol* 38(5):569–578, 2018.
89. Khan-Sabir SM, Werth VP: Infectious diseases that affect the skin and joint. In Sontheimer RD, Provost TT, editors: *Cutaneous manifestations of rheumatic diseases*, Philadelphia, 2004, Lippincott Williams & Wilkins, p 242.
90. Fujiwara H, Fujiwara K, Hashimoto K, et al.: Detection of Borrelia burgdorferi DNA (B garinii or B afzelii) in morphea and lichen sclerosus et atrophicus tissues of German and Japanese but not of US patients, *Arch Dermatol* 133(1):41–44, 1997. PubMed PMID: 9006371.
91. Tolkki L, Hokynar K, Meri S, et al.: Granuloma annulare and morphea: correlation with Borrelia burgdorferi infections and Chlamydia-related bacteria, *Acta Derm Venereol* 98(3):355–360, 2018.
92. Steere AC: Diagnosis and treatment of Lyme arthritis, *Med Clin North Am* 81(1):179–194, 1997. PubMed PMID: 9012760.
93. Aberer E, Breier F, Stanek G, et al.: Success and failure in the treatment of acrodermatitis chronica atrophicans, *Infection* 24(1):85–87, 1996.
94. Asbrink E, Hovmark A: Successful cultivation of spirochetes from skin lesions of patients with erythema chronicum migrans Afzelius and acrodermatitis chronica atrophicans, *Acta Pathol Microbiol Immunol Scand B* 93(2):161–163, 1985.
95. Mage V, Lipsker D, Barbarot S, et al.: Different patterns of skin manifestations associated with parvovirus B19 primary infection in adults, *J Am Acad Dermatol* 71(1):62–69, 2014.
96. Psychos DN, Voulgari PV, Skopouli FN, et al.: Erythema nodosum: the underlying conditions, *Clin Rheumatol* 19(3):212–216, 2000.
97. White Jr JW, Winkelmann RK: Weber-Christian panniculitis: a review of 30 cases with this diagnosis, *J Am Acad Dermatol* 39(1):56–62, 1998.
98. Borroni G, Torti S, D'Ospina RM, et al.: Drug-induced panniculitides, *G Ital Dermatol Venereol* 149(2):263–270, 2014.
99. Magalhaes TS, Dammert VG, Samorano LP, et al.: Erythema induratum of Bazin: Epidemiological, clinical and laboratorial profile of 54 patients, *J Dermatol* 45(5):628–629, 2018.
100. LeBlanc RE, Tavallaee M, Kim YH, et al.: Useful parameters for distinguishing subcutaneous panniculitis-like T-cell lymphoma from lupus erythematosus panniculitis, *Am J Surg Pathol* 40(6):745–754, 2016.
101. Arps DP, Patel RM: Lupus profundus (panniculitis): a potential mimic of subcutaneous panniculitis-like T-cell lymphoma, *Arch Pathol Lab Med* 137(9):1211–1215, 2013.
102. Peters MS, Su WP: Panniculitis. *Dermatol Clin.* 10(1):37–57, 1992.
103. Enk AH, Knop J: Treatment of relapsing idiopathic nodular panniculitis (Pfeifer-Weber-Christian disease) with mycophenolate mofetil, *J Am Acad Dermatol* 39(3):508–509, 1998.

104. Calderon P, Anzilotti M, Phelps R: Thalidomide in dermatology. New indications for an old drug, *Int J Dermatol* 36(12):881–887, 1997. PubMed PMID: 9466191.
105. Rednic S, Damian L, Talarico R, et al.: Relapsing polychondritis: state of the art on clinical practice guidelines, *RMD Open* 4(Suppl 1):e000788, 2018.
106. Vaxman I, Gertz M: Recent advances in the diagnosis, risk stratification, and management of systemic light-chain amyloidosis, *Acta Haematol* 141(2):93–106, 2019.
107. Merlini G, Dispenzieri A, Sanchorawala V, et al.: Systemic immunoglobulin light chain amyloidosis, *Nat Rev Dis Primers* 4(1):38, 2018.
108. Wanat KA, Rosenbach M: Cutaneous sarcoidosis, *Clin Chest Med* 36(4):685–702, 2015.
109. Criteria for diagnosis of Behcet's disease. International study group for Behcet's disease, *Lancet* 335(8697):1078–1080, 1990.
110. Leccese P, Ozguler Y, Christensen R, et al.: Management of skin, mucosa and joint involvement of Behcet's syndrome: a systematic review for update of the EULAR recommendations for the management of Behcet's syndrome, *Semin Arthritis Rheum* 48(4):752–762, 2019.
111. Ancient missense mutations in a new member of the RoRet gene family are likely to cause familial Mediterranean fever. The International FMF Consortium, *Cell* 90(4):797–807, 1997.
112. Pras E, Aksentijevich I, Gruberg L, et al.: Mapping of a gene causing familial Mediterranean fever to the short arm of chromosome 16, *N Engl J Med* 326(23):1509–1513, 1992.
113. Azizi E, Fisher BK: Cutaneous manifestations of familial Mediterranean fever, *Arch Dermatol* 112(3):364–366, 1976.
114. Ozen S, Bilginer Y: A clinical guide to autoinflammatory diseases: familial Mediterranean fever and next-of-kin, *Nat Rev Rheumatol* 10(3):135–147, 2014.
115. Hsiung SH, Chan EF, Elenitsas R, et al.: Multicentric reticulohistiocytosis presenting with clinical features of dermatomyositis, *J Am Acad Dermatol* 48(Suppl 2):S11–S14, 2003.
116. Liang GC, Granston AS: Complete remission of multicentric reticulohistiocytosis with combination therapy of steroid, cyclophosphamide, and low-dose pulse methotrexate. Case report, review of the literature, and proposal for treatment, *Arthritis Rheum* 39(1):171–174, 1996.
117. Selmi C, Greenspan A, Huntley A, et al.: Multicentric reticulohistiocytosis: a critical review, *Curr Rheumatol Rep* 17(6):511, 2015.
118. Levy R, Gerard L, Kuemmerle-Deschner J, et al.: Phenotypic and genotypic characteristics of cryopyrin-associated periodic syndrome: a series of 136 patients from the Eurofever Registry, *Ann Rheum Dis* 74(11):2043–2049, 2015.
119. Liu Y, Jesus AA, Marrero B, et al.: Activated STING in a vascular and pulmonary syndrome, *N Engl J Med* 371(6):507–518, 2014.

47 The Eye and Rheumatic Diseases

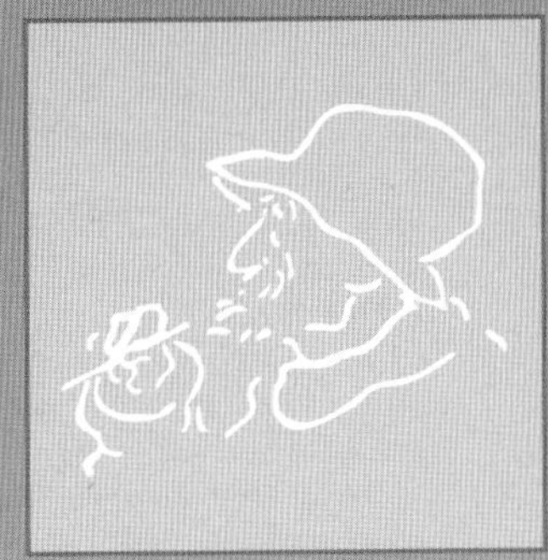

JAMES T. ROSENBAUM

KEY POINTS

- Symptoms of uveitis vary widely based on the location of the inflammation within the eye and the suddenness of onset.
- Ankylosing spondylitis is the systemic rheumatic disease most often associated with uveitis in North America and Europe.
- During a lifetime, acute anterior uveitis develops in about 40% of patients with ankylosing spondylitis.
- The uveitis associated with human leukocyte antigen (HLA)-B27 tends to be unilateral, recurrent, and sudden in onset. Recurrences sometimes affect the opposite eye.
- Sarcoidosis frequently manifests as uveitis.
- Most patients with retinal vasculitis do not have systemic vasculitis.
- Many patients with scleritis have a systemic disease, such as rheumatoid arthritis.
- Anti-neutrophilic cytoplasmic antibody testing helps identify a subset of patients with severe scleritis.
- Granulomatosis with polyangiitis is the rheumatic disease that most frequently involves the orbit.
- Anterior ischemic optic neuropathy is the most common ocular manifestation of giant cell arteritis.
- Most patients with visual loss resulting from optic nerve ischemia do not have arteritis.

Introduction

Virtually all of the systemic inflammatory diseases that require rheumatologic care affect the eye or its surrounding structures. Table 47.1 presents the prototypic ocular manifestations of rheumatoid arthritis, systemic lupus erythematosus, Sjögren's syndrome, spondyloarthropathies, vasculitides including granulomatosis with polyangiitis and giant cell arteritis (also known as *temporal arteritis*), scleroderma, Behçet's disease, relapsing polychondritis, and dermatomyositis. Each of these diseases is addressed elsewhere in this text. This chapter focuses on specific ocular structures—the uvea, cornea, orbit, and optic nerve—and illustrates how inflammation of each might relate to an autoimmune or inflammatory process.

Ocular Anatomy and Physiology

A diagram of the eye is shown in Fig. 47.1. The eye is a tiny but elegantly complex structure. The anterior segment of the eye includes the cornea, which is avascular and transparent when healthy. The lens also is an avascular structure. The anterior chamber is filled with aqueous humor, which has homology to cerebrospinal fluid. When the blood-aqueous barrier is intact, the aqueous humor contains no leukocytes and very little protein. The blood-aqueous barrier, which resembles the blood-synovial barrier, is disrupted in anterior uveitis. In this case, a routine, noninvasive biomicroscopic or slit lamp examination would reveal leukocytes and increased protein in the anterior chamber. An ophthalmologist has the opportunity to observe two universal hallmarks of inflammation noninvasively.

The term *uvea* derives from the Latin word for "grape." The anterior uvea includes the iris and the ciliary body. The aqueous humor is synthesized by the ciliary body. The posterior portion of the uvea is the choroid, which is a highly vascular tissue just posterior to the retina. Any portion of the uveal tract can become inflamed, and adjacent tissue also is frequently inflamed. Anatomic subsets of uveitis include anterior uveitis, which consists of iritis or iridocyclitis (ciliary body inflammation); intermediate uveitis, in which leukocytes are present within the vitreous humor; and posterior uveitis, in which the choroid and the retina are inflamed. Panuveitis occurs when all portions of the uveal tract are inflamed. An attempt has been made to standardize the nomenclature used to describe uveitis by the Standardization of Uveitis Nomenclature Working Group[1]; however, ambiguities persist because, at present, not all ophthalmologists follow these definitions.

Signs and symptoms of uveitis depend on the portion of the uveal tract that is affected. An anterior uveitis, especially if it begins suddenly, is associated with redness, pain, and photophobia. Visual loss varies and often is due to macular edema, if present (Figs. 47.2 and 47.3). An intermediate uveitis usually causes floaters as a result of leukocytes that enter the visual axis, although most floaters are due to aging or other changes within the vitreous humor. Posterior uveitis by itself does not usually produce pain or redness. Visual loss depends on the location and extent of the inflammatory process.

The outer tunic of the eye is known as the *sclera*. At the front of the eye, the sclera meets the cornea at a tissue known as the *limbus*. The most interior layer of the eye is an extension of the brain that responds to visual signals; this is called the *retina*. The eye shares some common features with joints, including the presence of hyaluronic acid, which occurs primarily in the vitreous humor and in the presence of type II collagen; however, ocular inflammation is not a reported accompaniment of collagen-induced arthritis. Aggrecan is a proteoglycan present both in the eye and in joints. An autoimmune response to aggrecan in BALB/c mice can produce both arthritis and uveitis.[2]

TABLE 47.1 Most Characteristic Ocular Findings of Selected Rheumatic Diseases

Disease	Most Characteristic Ocular Findings
Rheumatoid arthritis	Sicca Scleritis
Systemic lupus erythematosus	Sicca Cotton-wool spots
Sjögren's syndrome	Sicca
Spondyloarthritis	Acute anterior uveitis
Granulomatosis with polyangiitis	Scleritis Orbital inflammation
Giant cell arteritis	Anterior ischemic optic neuropathy
Scleroderma	Sicca
Behçet's disease	Uveitis, retinal arteritis
Relapsing polychondritis	Scleritis, episcleritis, uveitis
Dermatomyositis	Heliotrope eyelids

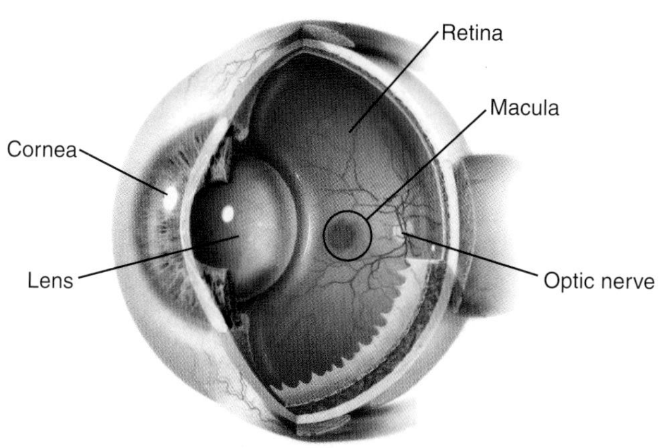

• **Fig. 47.1** Diagram of the eye.

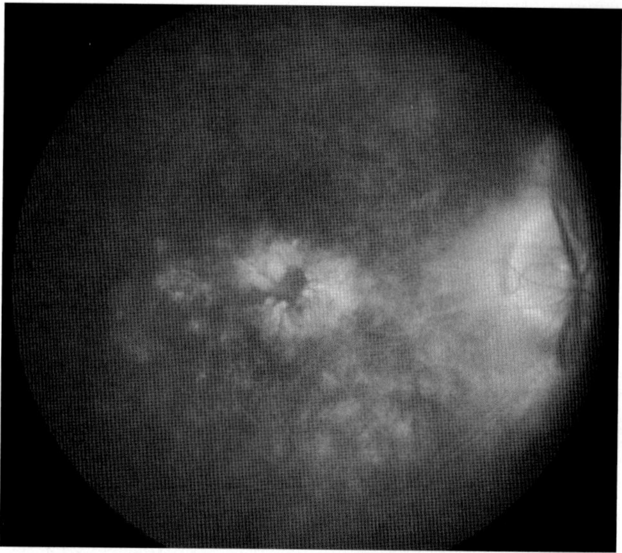

• **Fig. 47.2** A fluorescein angiogram. The normal macula is avascular and does not stain with fluorescein dye. This patient has macular edema, as indicated by the donut-shaped pattern of dye in the *center of the photo*. The optic nerve is at the *3-o'clock position* in the photo. Macular edema can complicate uveitis, even anterior uveitis.

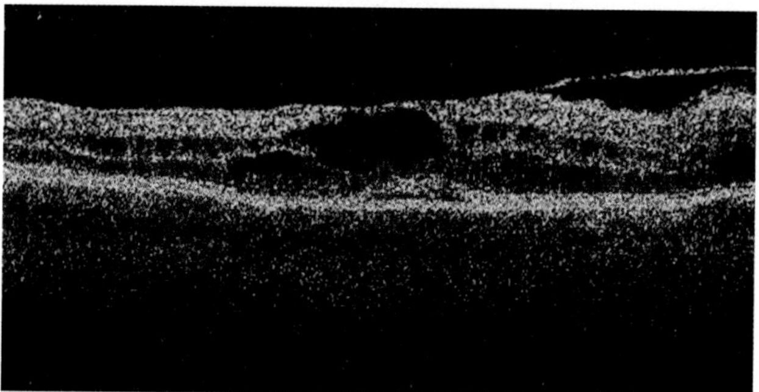

• **Fig. 47.3** Optical coherence tomography produces precise imaging of the retinal structure. The ovoid black hole in the *center of the image* is due to macular edema, a major cause of visual loss in patients with uveitis.

Because uveitis and arthritis co-exist in multiple diseases, it is logical to seek the mechanism for this co-existence. It is likely that the mechanism for one disease, such as ankylosing spondylitis, might differ from the mechanism that explains the co-existence of eye and joint disease in Blau syndrome or in juvenile idiopathic arthritis (JIA). In a disease such as reactive arthritis, bacterial products might be trapped in synovium, where they become the target of an immune response. A similar pathogenesis in the iris is difficult to prove because of a relative inability to obtain a biopsy specimen of uveal tissue while it is inflamed; however, many microbial products are inflammatory within the eye.[3] Because the eye and joints share specific antigens such as aggrecan, an autoimmune response could also account for the simultaneous inflammation of uvea and joints.

Ocular Immune Response

The eye generally is regarded as an immune privileged site.[4] From a teleologic perspective, many scientists believe that the eye has developed mechanisms to avoid becoming inflamed because of the consequences that inflammation has for visual acuity. Similar to the brain, the internal portion of the eye has no lymphatics, although the conjunctiva on the ocular surface has lymphatic drainage. Portions of the eye—the cornea and the lens—are avascular. The aqueous humor contains several factors that are known to be immunosuppressive, including transforming growth factor-β and α-melanocyte-stimulating hormone. Several tissues within the eye express ligands that promote apoptosis, including TNF-related apoptosis-inducing ligand (TRAIL) and Fas ligand. If a soluble antigen is injected into the anterior chamber, a cellular immune response is suppressed. This phenomenon is known as *anterior chamber–associated immune deviation* (ACAID). These factors are important to consider in the effort to understand why the eye sometimes is targeted as part of an immune or inflammatory disease.

In several mouse models,[5,6] the microbiome is a major factor that contributes to uveitis. Scientists suspect that the microbiome contributes to the development of noninfectious causes of uveitis in humans as well.[3]

TABLE 47.2 Differential Diagnosis of Uveitis

Differential Diagnosis of Uveitis
Infections—toxoplasmosis, syphilis, herpes simplex, herpes zoster, and cytomegalovirus
Systemic, immune-mediated diseases
Masquerade syndromes, such as lymphoma
Syndromes confined to the eye, such as pars planitis, birdshot chorioretinopathy, and serpiginous choroiditis

TABLE 47.3 Immune-Mediated Diseases Most Often Associated With Uveitis

Immune-Mediated Diseases Most Often Associated With Uveitis
Ankylosing spondylitis
Behçet's disease
Drug/hypersensitivity reactions
Familial granulomatous synovitis
Inflammatory bowel disease
Interstitial nephritis
Juvenile idiopathic arthritis
Multiple sclerosis
Neonatal-onset multisystem inflammatory disease
Psoriatic arthritis
Reactive arthritis
Sarcoidosis
Sweet's syndrome
Systemic lupus erythematosus
Vasculitis, especially Cogan's syndrome and Kawasaki's disease
Vogt-Koyanagi-Harada syndrome

Uveitis

Rheumatologists may be consulted to identify a systemic disease in a patient with uveitis, and a rheumatologist often is asked to assist in the management of immunosuppression in select patients with uveitis. In some referral practices for patients with uveitis, 40% of patients might have an associated systemic illness. Table 47.2 lists the differential diagnoses of uveitis. The immunologic diseases most likely to be associated with uveitis are listed in Table 47.3.

The most common systemic illness associated with uveitis in most North American practices is ankylosing spondylitis. From an epidemiologic perspective, anterior uveitis is more common than posterior or intermediate uveitis.[7]

About 50% of people with acute anterior uveitis are positive for human leukocyte antigen (HLA)-B27.[8] The uveitis associated with HLA-B27 is almost always unilateral, recurrent, of relatively short duration (<3 months per attack), resolves completely between attacks, and is associated with reduced intraocular pressure (in contrast to herpes simplex, which can cause recurrent anterior uveitis associated with increased intraocular pressure).[9] Hypopyon or pus in the anterior chamber sometimes is present in patients with HLA-B27–associated uveitis (Fig. 47.4). Recurrent episodes can affect the contralateral eye, but simultaneous bilateral involvement is rare. Many studies have tried to address the question of how frequently a patient with HLA-B27–associated anterior uveitis has an associated spondyloarthropathy. A wide range of answers has been suggested, and the percentage depends on the definition of spondyloarthropathy; however, one reasonable estimate is that 80% of HLA-B27^{+} patients with acute anterior, unilateral uveitis have associated spondyloarthropathy.[10] A study from the emergency department in Dublin, Ireland[11] and a collaboration between rheumatologists and ophthalmologists in Spain[12] showed convincingly that the spondyloarthropathy associated with acute anterior uveitis is frequently not diagnosed.

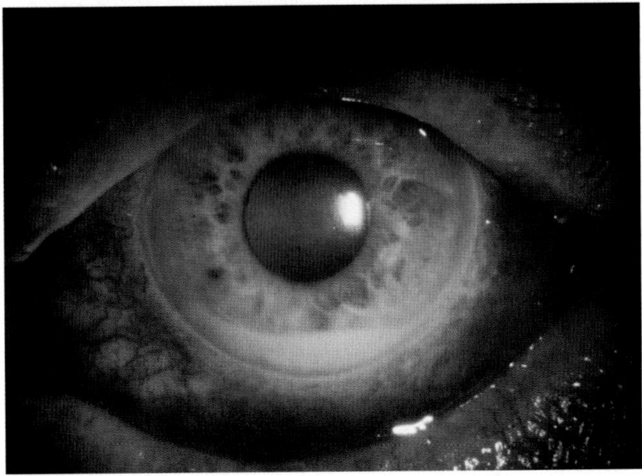

• **Fig. 47.4** The creamy material at the bottom of the pupil is an accumulation of leukocytes, which is also known as a *hypopyon*.

The uveitis associated with reactive arthritis is indistinguishable from the uveitis associated with ankylosing spondylitis. In either of these entities, acute anterior uveitis develops in about 40% of patients during a lifetime. Although conjunctivitis is part of the classic triad of reactive arthritis (in association with arthritis and nongonococcal urethritis), conjunctivitis is uncommon in ankylosing spondylitis. A genome-wide screen for susceptibility genes for acute anterior uveitis identified loci that predispose patients to ankylosing spondylitis; the screens also identified loci that seem to be unassociated with susceptibility to ankylosing spondylitis.[13]

Uveitis develops in approximately 5% of people with inflammatory bowel disease and in 7% of people with psoriatic arthritis. Although some of these people have disease that is unilateral, anterior, and recurrent, many have disease that is bilateral, chronic in duration, and posterior to the lens.[14,15] About half of all patients with Crohn's disease or psoriatic arthritis and uveitis are positive for HLA-B27.

Sarcoidosis is the second most common systemic disease associated with uveitis, at least in North America; in some geographic areas, it might be more common than spondyloarthritis. Sarcoidosis is promiscuous within the eye, meaning that it can affect a wide range of structures, including the orbit, lacrimal gland, anterior uvea, vitreous humor, choroid, retina, or optic nerve. Ocular inflammation with sarcoidosis frequently is termed *granulomatous* because large collections of cells deposit on the back of the cornea (Fig. 47.5). A retinal vasculitis can be a prominent feature of sarcoidosis, even though systemic vasculitis is not a typical feature of the disease; this phenomenon results in part from the manner in which vasculitis is diagnosed in the retina.

Histologic evidence of vessel wall destruction is rarely obtained because of the morbidity associated with a retinal biopsy. Instead, retinal vasculitis is diagnosed on the basis of perivascular sheathing

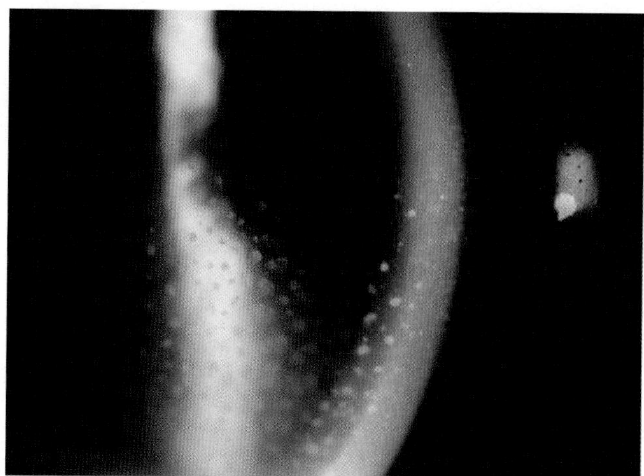

• **Fig. 47.5** Keratic precipitates. The white dots result from concretions of cells depositing against the corneal endothelium. These keratic precipitates are large and usually are described as granulomatous even though a granuloma is not present histologically.

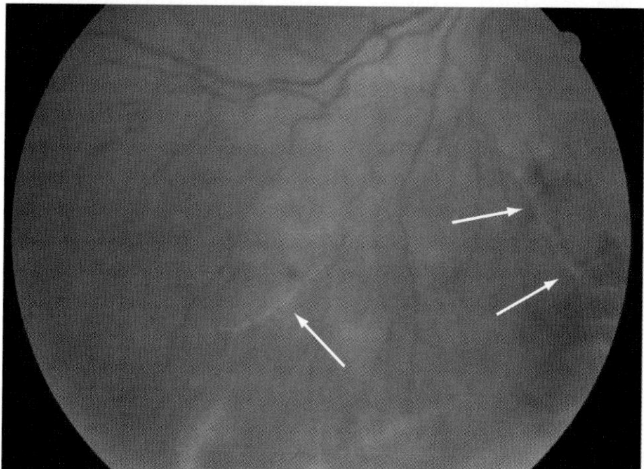

• **Fig. 47.6** Retinal vasculitis. *Arrows* indicate areas of vascular sheathing or occlusion.

along a vessel, as seen on funduscopic examination (Fig. 47.6), intraretinal hemorrhages that must be secondary to vascular injury, and fluorescein angiography indicating increased vascular permeability.[16] Most rheumatologists find the term *retinal vasculitis* misleading since it does indicate vessel wall disruption. In addition, the classic systemic vasculitides, such as polyarteritis nodosa and granulomatosis with polyangiitis, are rarely associated with retinal vasculitis.[17]

Initially, sarcoidosis frequently manifests as an ocular problem.[18] An ocular symptom is the initial manifestation almost as frequently as a pulmonary symptom. Sarcoidosis frequently involves the conjunctiva, which is an accessible tissue for biopsy confirmation of the diagnosis. In most series of patients with uveitis, about 30% of patients have uveitis that defies placement within a diagnostic category.[19] Many of these patients may have sarcoidosis that is difficult to find outside the eye. The sensitivity and specificity of studies (e.g., a serum angiotensin-converting enzyme level or gallium scan for sarcoid that is primarily ocular) are unknown. I consider obtaining a chest CT scan to look for symmetric hilar adenopathy in any patient who has uveitis of unknown origin.[20] The therapeutic implications of the result of the scan must be balanced against the cost and potential harm from radiation exposure. Several studies evaluated cardiac rhythm after establishing a diagnosis of ocular

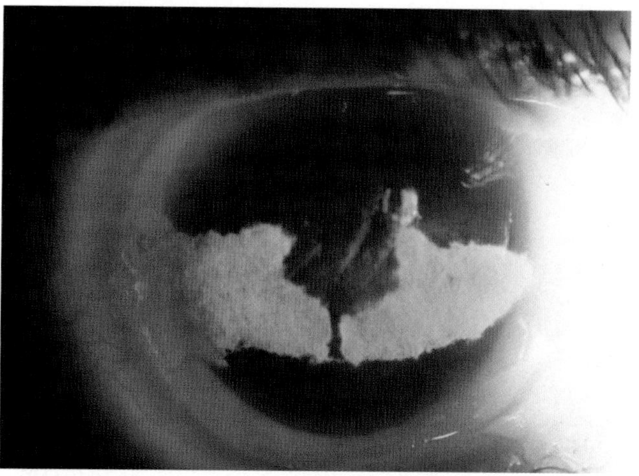

• **Fig. 47.7** Band keratopathy is illustrated by calcific patches stretching across the cornea.

sarcoid.[20a] These studies concluded that the identification of ocular sarcoid occasionally led to potentially life-saving intervention to prevent arrhythmia secondary to cardiac sarcoidosis.[4]

JIA comprises several different diseases. Patients with juvenile ankylosing spondylitis resemble their adult counterparts in that a sudden-onset, unilateral anterior uveitis can develop. The subset of JIA that is most classically associated with uveitis tends to be female, with onset of arthritis between the ages of 2 years and 8 years.[22] The joint disease is pauciarticular, and most patients test positive for anti-nuclear antibodies. The uveitis tends to have an insidious onset, such that pain and redness are almost always absent. Joint disease can be minimal as well, and some patients are not diagnosed until a visual screening examination is performed when starting school. The eye disease usually is bilateral and very persistent, although remissions have been well described. Band keratopathy, which is the deposition of calcium superficially in the cornea, is a well-known and frequent complication of this form of uveitis (Fig. 47.7). Patients may also experience glaucoma and posterior *synechiae,* a term that describes adhesions of the iris to the lens.

Other forms of uveitis associated with joint disease include Behçet's disease, relapsing polychondritis, and vasculitis (e.g., Cogan's syndrome and Kawasaki's disease). In Behçet's disease, the symptom of uveitis often "drives" the therapy; it is often the manifestation that most often requires systemic immunotherapy.[23] Eye inflammation usually is bilateral and recurrent. In contrast to the recurrences typical of ankylosing spondylitis, recurrences of uveitis with Behçet's disease usually do not have complete resolution between attacks. A hallmark of Behçet's disease–associated uveitis is a retinal vasculitis. Retinal arteries are especially prone to be affected. The visual prognosis with Behçet's disease can be grim, and blindness is a frequent concomitant of untreated ocular disease.

Relapsing polychondritis can impact almost any portion of the eye, including the episclera, sclera, and uveal tract.[24] Ocular inflammation is common.

Cogan's syndrome is classically defined as sensorineural hearing loss with corneal disease, especially interstitial keratitis. This definition usually is broadened to include any ocular inflammatory process, such as uveitis or scleritis. Although uveitis can occur with polyarteritis or with granulomatosis with polyangiitis, scleral disease is typical. In contrast, anterior uveitis in association with conjunctivitis is present in most patients with Kawasaki's disease.

Uveitis and arthritis occasionally can result from an infection such as Whipple's disease or Lyme disease. Uveal involvement with Lyme disease has been described but is extremely rare.

TABLE 47.4 **Some Causes of Red Eyes: A Comparison**

	Conjunctivitis	Episcleritis	Scleritis
Discomfort	Scratchy	Scratchy	Pain
Redness	Diffuse, includes palpebral conjunctivae of lids	Diffuse or a sector, spares palpebral conjunctivae	Diffuse or a sector, spares palpebral conjunctivae
Causes	Allergy, viral, chemical irritant	Usually idiopathic but presumed immune response	Usually idiopathic but presumed immune response; can be an infection
Relation to systemic disease	Rare	Rare	Common (approximately 40%)

Some autoinflammatory diseases are associated with uveitis. Autoinflammatory diseases are characterized by widespread inflammation in the absence of detectable autoantibodies. Many autoinflammatory syndromes respond dramatically to inhibition of IL-1. Blau syndrome, which also is known as *familial granulomatous synovitis,* results from a single base change in the nucleotide-binding domain of the *NOD2* gene, which used to be known as *CARD15* or *NLRC2*.[25] Polymorphisms elsewhere in this same gene predispose patients to Crohn's disease. Blau syndrome is characterized by childhood onset of uveitis, arthritis, and dermatitis. Inflammation in additional organ systems also has been described. The disease is autosomal dominant. The histopathology of affected skin or joint can present with noncaseating granuloma, as in sarcoidosis. Lung involvement has not been described in Blau syndrome, however. Gene sequencing has shown that many patients thought to have so-called early-onset sarcoidosis actually have new mutations in the *NOD2* gene.[26]

Neonatal-onset multisystem inflammatory disease (NOMID), which also is known as *chronic infantile neurologic cutaneous articular syndrome* (CINCA), is an autosomal dominant autoinflammatory syndrome. Ocular involvement in NOMID is more variable than in Blau syndrome. Characteristic findings include papilledema and uveitis.[21]

Treatment of uveitis depends on multiple factors, such as severity, location within the eye, patient preference, and the specific diagnosis (e.g., Behçet's disease might be especially responsive to infliximab[27] or interferon alpha[27]). For noninfectious causes of uveitis that involve the anterior portion of the eye, treatment usually begins with topical corticosteroids and, often, dilating drops to prevent posterior synechiae and to relieve spasm of the ciliary muscle. Periocular or intraocular corticosteroid injections, usually with triamcinolone, are given for inflammation posterior to the lens that is not responding to topical medication. Local corticosteroids can increase intraocular pressure, induce cataracts, interfere with the response to infection, and delay wound healing. A long-lasting corticosteroid surgical implant containing fluocinolone has been approved by the U.S. Food and Drug Administration.[28] A cataract develops in all patients who elect to receive this type of therapy if the lens has not already been surgically removed, and glaucoma develops in most patients, with many people requiring surgery to control the intraocular pressure. Intravitreal corticosteroid therapy can also be given in the form of dexamethasone or fluocinolone in a slow-release formulation, or triamcinolone can be injected intravitreally.

Systemic immunosuppressive therapy generally is reserved for patients with active, noninfectious causes of inflammation. For systemic immunosuppression to be indicated, the inflammation usually is bilateral and severe enough to interfere with activities of daily living. A variety of immunomodulatory medications have been tried to treat intraocular inflammation,[29] including azathioprine, chlorambucil, cyclophosphamide, cyclosporine, daclizumab, infliximab, methotrexate, mycophenolate mofetil, and tacrolimus. In 2017, adalimumab became the first noncorticosteroid medication approved by the Food and Drug Administration for the treatment of uveitis. The approval is for noninfectious intermediate, posterior, or panuveitis on the basis of two well-designed clinical trials called Visual I and Visual II.[30,31] Infliximab is especially useful in the treatment of Behçet's disease and approved for this indication in Japan.[27] A third study with adalimumab established its efficacy in the treatment of the chronic anterior uveitis that can accompany JIA.[32] In most instances, clinicians treat uveitis with an indicated biologic only if other therapies, such as local corticosteroids, oral corticosteroids, and/or an anti-metabolite have been tried and have failed.[33] The optimal choice of therapy depends on many factors, not the least of which is the empiric result of any therapeutic approach. Maintaining a treatment for uveitis usually requires some efficacy in association with good tolerability. In this regard, at least one study found methotrexate to be superior to other anti-metabolites.[34] Because of the range of diseases being treated and the range of clinical response, room for many options exists in the therapeutic armamentarium of a uveitis clinic.

The optimal therapy for uveitis presumably depends on the underlying cause of the uveitis. The approach to uveitis in association with JIA should differ from the approach to uveitis resulting from Vogt-Koyanagi-Harada syndrome. However, the relative rarity of uveitis is such that few studies have been performed on specific forms. For JIA-associated uveitis, many clinicians follow the algorithm of using topical therapy with prednisolone acetate initially and adding methotrexate if the inflammation is not controlled by drops used up to three times per day. If methotrexate does not help gain control of the inflammation, a monoclonal antibody to TNF is generally added to the regimen, as noted earlier.

Scleritis and Corneal Melt

Many diseases cause a red eye, including conjunctivitis, keratitis, iritis, acute closed-angle glaucoma, episcleritis, and scleritis. Conjunctivitis is compared with episcleritis and scleritis in Table 47.4. A rheumatologist should refer patients with red eyes to an ophthalmologist if the problem is associated with pain, photophobia, or a change in visual acuity. Patients with persistent redness should also be referred.

Scleritis often is divided into five categories: diffuse anterior, nodular, necrotizing, scleromalacia perforans, and posterior (Fig. 47.8). Each of the first three categories results in a red, painful eye. Pain is more variable in scleromalacia perforans, in which a nodule pathologically similar to a rheumatoid nodule forms in the

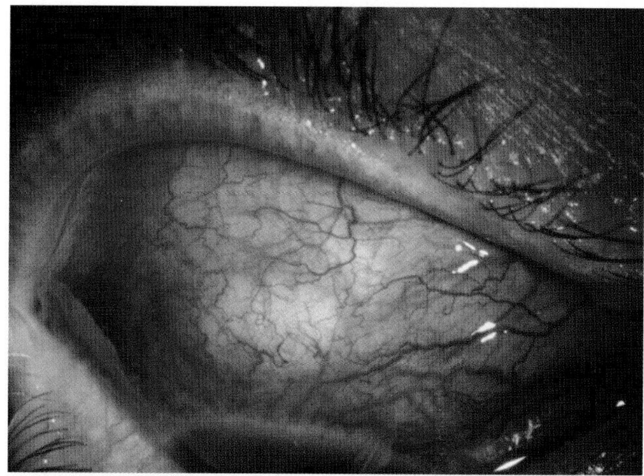

• **Fig. 47.8** A scleral nodule. Active scleritis is present superior to the limbus. In this patient, scleritis has taken on a nodular configuration.

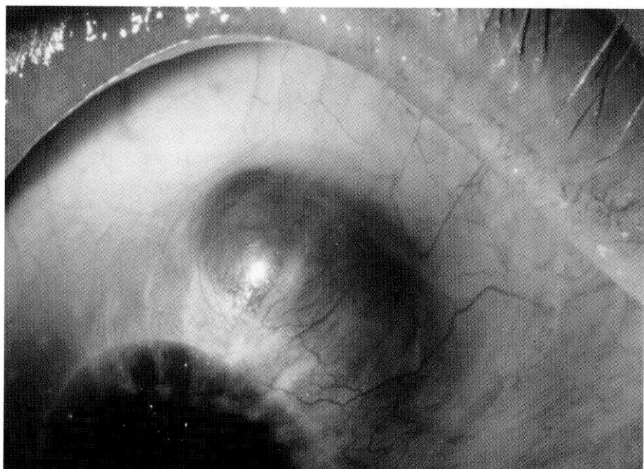

• **Fig. 47.9** Scleromalacia has resulted in ulceration of the sclera and a bluish appearance.

sclera (Fig. 47.9). Pain also varies with posterior scleritis; because the sclera extends back to the optic nerve, posterior scleritis can occur in a localized fashion that does not lead to a red eye. Because of the risk of perforation, the sclera is not normally biopsied, but biopsy studies have indicated that scleritis is often a vasculitis of scleral tissue.[35]

Patients with scleritis can experience complications within the eye, including uveitis, glaucoma, optic nerve edema, and retinal or choroidal distortion. A corneal melt or peripheral thinning of the cornea sometimes develops in people with severe scleritis and represents a potentially blinding complication of the disease (Fig. 47.10).

About 40% of patients with scleritis have an associated systemic illness.[35,36] The most common of such illnesses are limited granulomatosis with polyangiitis and rheumatoid arthritis. Generally, the associated rheumatoid arthritis is long standing and seropositive. Patients may have associated nodules, vasculitis, or pleuropericarditis. They have a shortened life expectancy compared with other patients with rheumatoid arthritis.[37] It is unusual for scleritis to be an initial manifestation of rheumatoid arthritis.

Granulomatosis with polyangiitis is commonly associated with scleritis. In contrast to rheumatoid arthritis, scleritis can be the initial manifestation of granulomatosis with polyangiitis. Obtaining

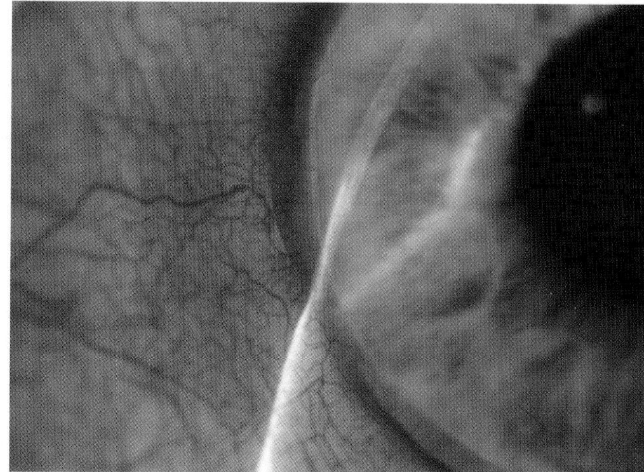

• **Fig. 47.10** Corneal melt. The white light of the slit lamp beam narrows over the peripheral cornea, where the tissue is thin.

anti-neutrophilic cytoplasmic antibody serology for any patient who presents with scleritis without an obvious systemic disease association is appropriate. Other systemic associations with scleritis include inflammatory bowel disease, relapsing polychondritis, other vasculitides such as giant cell arteritis, and ankylosing spondylitis. Infections are a rare but possible cause of scleritis. Tophaceous gout also has been reported as an unusual cause of scleritis.

Scleritis tends to be a painful and persistent disease that often lasts for years. In contrast, episcleritis involves more superficial tissue and is usually transient. Episcleritis may be a feature of rheumatoid arthritis, although many patients with episcleritis may not have any associated systemic illness. Complications within the eye, such as glaucoma or uveitis, are absent. Mild discomfort, rather than frank pain, is the usual presenting symptom. In contrast to scleritis, patients with episcleritis have vessels that constrict completely after 2.5% phenylephrine is placed on the surface of the eye.[37a]

Some patients with scleritis, especially those who do not have an associated systemic illness, are treated adequately with an oral nonsteroidal anti-inflammatory drug. Some experts treat scleritis with locally injected corticosteroids, but this approach should be avoided if the sclera is thin (a sign of necrotizing disease). In addition, corticosteroids have the theoretical risk of promoting thinning. The usual option for patients who do not respond to nonsteroidal anti-inflammatory drugs is oral prednisone. Some patients can be effectively treated with low doses of prednisone, but many patients require the addition of an anti-metabolite as a steroid-sparing drug. Scleritis usually responds to treatment of the underlying disease if an associated disease is present. Thus, control of rheumatoid arthritis or inflammatory bowel disease usually results in control of associated scleritis. Rituximab is reportedly effective for the majority of patients with scleritis who fail to respond to anti-metabolite therapy.[38]

Orbital Disease

Graves' disease, the most common orbital inflammatory disease, generally results in an orbital myositis that can be identified on imaging, such as CT, ultrasound, or MRI. From a rheumatologic perspective, granulomatosis with polyangiitis is the disease that most commonly affects the orbit. The inflammation can be extremely painful and may result in blindness. Orbital inflammation sometimes is more recalcitrant to therapy than other aspects of granulomatosis with polyangiitis. A small series suggested that rituximab may be efficacious in patients with granulomatosis with polyangiitis, including those with orbital involvement.[39]

Orbital pseudotumor, or nonspecific orbital inflammatory disease, is a diagnosis of exclusion. It is made on the basis of objective orbital swelling as documented by imaging and a biopsy that shows an inflammatory process that cannot be ascribed to another process, such as Graves' disease. A biopsy specimen of the orbit is not always obtained, but it can be useful in ruling out lymphoma or a metastatic malignancy as the cause of the proptosis. Methotrexate is a therapeutic option to treat nonspecific orbital inflammation.[40] Another systemic disease that commonly affects the orbit is sarcoidosis. Rituximab has been used successfully to treat orbital inflammation that is refractory to anti-metabolite therapy.[36]

Optic Neuritis

Optic nerve disease can result from many insults, including toxins (some of which are medications), vascular insufficiency (such as the insufficiency that occurs as a result of atherosclerotic disease or giant cell arteritis), and immunologic attack. The immune-mediated disease that most commonly affects the optic nerve is multiple sclerosis. This demyelinating condition generally starts suddenly in one eye with pain, an afferent pupillary defect, loss of color vision, and visual field loss typical of optic nerve disease. Initially, the optic nerve may show papilledema, or it may appear normal if the inflammation is retrobulbar. Over several weeks, the affected nerve usually becomes pale.

Demyelinating disease affecting the optic nerve generally is not treated by a rheumatologist. On rare occasions, however, patients with optic nerve disease have inflammation that might require long-term immunosuppression. These patients carry a diagnosis labeled variously as *autoimmune optic neuropathy* or, sometimes, *steroid-sensitive optic neuropathy*. This diagnosis is clinically distinct from optic neuritis associated with multiple sclerosis because MRIs of the head do not indicate a demyelinating process; the disease is often bilateral, the kinetics of the inflammation are different from that of multiple sclerosis, and the disease usually responds to oral corticosteroids. In most centers, a neuro-ophthalmologist would be involved in establishing this diagnosis.[40a] Systemic lupus erythematosus and sarcoidosis may affect the optic nerve in this way, but many patients with the diagnosis of steroid-sensitive optic neuropathy do not have an associated systemic illness. Therapy with an alkylating agent or an anti-metabolite can be beneficial for many patients with this entity.[41,42]

Rheumatologists should also be familiar with the syndrome of neuromyelitis optica (NMO). This condition usually associates with detectable antibodies to aquaporin 4.[43] The classic syndrome manifests as optic neuropathy in association with transverse myelitis.[44] The spinal cord involvement should span the length of 3 or more vertebral bodies.

Sudden blindness is arguably the most feared consequence of giant cell arteritis. This disease is characterized by granulomatous inflammation of multiple vessels above the waist. These vessels frequently include the temporal artery and the posterior ciliary arteries. Inflammation in these latter vessels leads to anterior ischemic optic neuropathy (AION), which is ischemia of the optic nerve that manifests as sudden visual loss (Fig. 47.11). Giant cell arteritis also can affect the central retinal artery, which may result in blindness. In this condition, the funduscopic appearance of the eye presents with a markedly reduced arteriolar flow and a cherry-red spot in the macula. Giant cell arteritis can cause diplopia by affecting circulation to extraocular muscles.

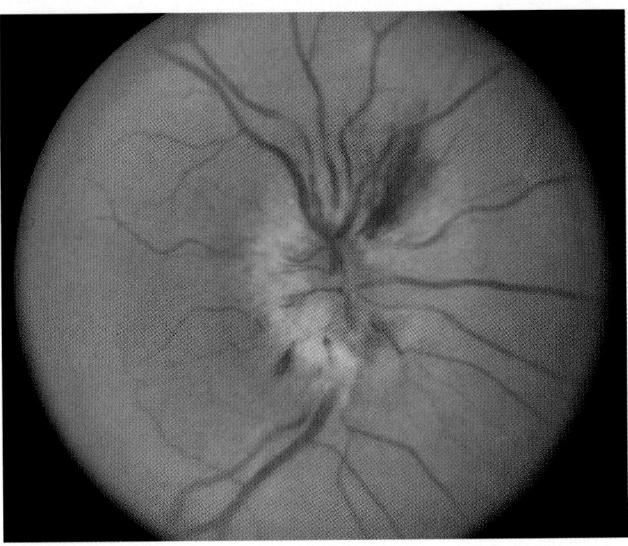

• **Fig. 47.11** Anterior ischemic optic neuropathy resulting from giant cell arteritis. The optic nerve is swollen, and surrounding hemorrhages are evident.

The visual loss associated with giant cell arteritis is frequently labeled *arteritic AION* to distinguish it from the more common nonarteritic AION, which usually is attributable to small vessel atherosclerosis.[44a] Patients with arteritic AION typically are older than 50 years and have an erythrocyte sedimentation rate greater than 50 mm/hr. Many patients with arteritic AION have associated symptoms of polymyalgia rheumatica, jaw claudication, scalp tenderness, or temporal artery tenderness. The biopsy specimen of the temporal artery presents with vasculitis in about 80% of patients with giant cell arteritis if an adequate length of vessel is sampled. Approximately 15% of patients with giant cell arteritis might have a negative biopsy specimen of the artery because the disease either spared this vessel or has a sufficiently patchy distribution so the biopsy specimen did not reveal it.[40a] Patients with nonarteritic AION tend to have small optic nerve cups.[44a,44b]

Medication-Related Ocular Toxicity

A variety of medications have the potential to cause uveitis. These medications include rifabutin,[45] intravenously administered bisphosphonates,[46] moxifloxacin,[47] TNF inhibitors,[48] and ipilumumab.[49]

Rheumatologists need to be especially aware of the potential for anti-malarial agents to cause retinal toxicity. The widespread use of optical coherence tomography (OCT) has resulted in the ability to image retinal layers accurately, quickly, and noninvasively. Although hydroxychloroquine was once considered to be a rare cause of retinal toxicity, OCT studies now report that retinal toxicity is roughly 7.5% among people who take hydroxychloroquine (Fig. 47.12).[43] The American Academy of Ophthalmology revised its recommendations to monitor for anti-malarial toxicity.[50] The likelihood of toxicity relates to both dosage and duration of therapy.[51] The dosage should be reduced in the setting of concomitant tamoxifen therapy or if renal disease is present.[50] The dosage should not exceed 5 mg/kg/day of actual body weight.[52] After an initial examination, routine examinations can be deferred until usage reaches 5 years. A dilated examination, a visual field test, and an OCT are often the modalities used to monitor for toxicity.[52]

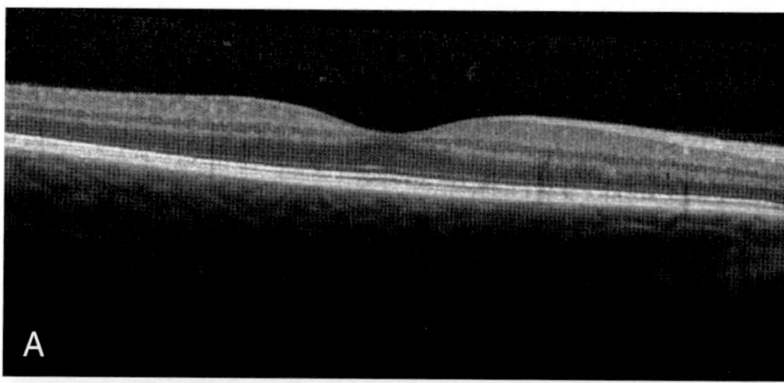

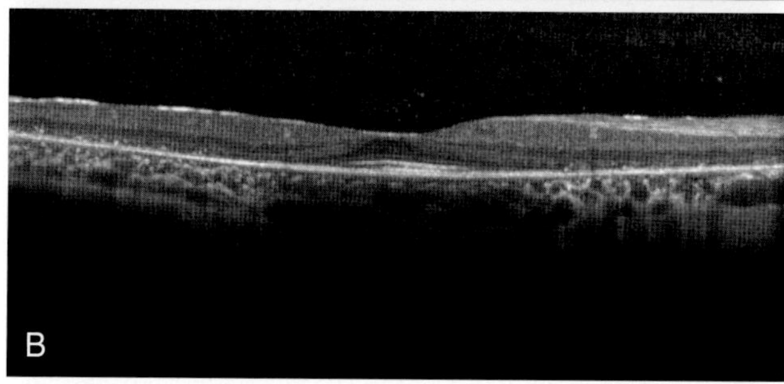

• **Fig. 47.12** Optical coherence tomography (OCT) demonstrating characteristic changes from anti-malarial toxicity. (A) An OCT of a normal retina. The "valley" at the *center* of the image is the macula. (B) Characteristic changes from hydroxychloroquine toxicity. The thinning of the outer nuclear layer in the fovea results in a configuration sometimes called the "flying saucer sign." (Photograph courtesy Mark Pennesi.)

Conclusion

In some ways, from a rheumatologist's perspective, the eye is a microcosm of the body. Its complex structures frequently reflect inflammation elsewhere. Treatment of many forms of ocular inflammation requires collaboration between a rheumatologist and an ophthalmologist.

The references for this chapter can also be found on ExpertConsult.com.

References

1. Jabs DA, Nussenblatt RB, Rosenbaum JT: Standardization of Uveitis Nomenclature Working Group. Standardization of uveitis nomenclature for reporting clinical data. Results of the first international workshop, *Am J Ophthalmol* 140(3):509–516, 2005. PMID: 16196117.
2. Rosenzweig HL, Martin TM, Planck SR, et al.: Anterior uveitis accompanies joint disease in a murine model resembling ankylosing spondylitis, *Ophthalmic Res* 40(3-4):189–192, 2008. PMID: 18421237.
3. Allensworth JJ, Planck SR, Rosenbaum JT, et al.: Investigation of the differential potentials of TLR agonists to elicit uveitis in mice, *J Leukoc Biol* 90(6):1159–1166, 2011. Epub 2011/09/22. PMID: 21934069; PMC3236551.
4. Niederkorn JY: See no evil, hear no evil, do no evil: the lessons of immune privilege, *Nat Immunol* 7(4):353–359, 2006.
5. Horai R, Zarate-Blades CR, Dillenburg-Pilla P, et al.: Microbiota-dependent activation of an autoreactive T cell receptor provokes autoimmunity in an immunologically privileged site, *Immunity* 43(2):343–353, 2015. PMID: 26287682; 4544742.
6. Nakamura YK, Metea C, Karstens L, et al.: Gut microbial alterations associated with protection from autoimmune uveitis, *Invest Ophthalmol Vis Sci* 57(8):3747–3758, 2016. PMID: 27415793; PMC4960998.
7. Gritz DC, Wong IG: Incidence and prevalence of uveitis in Northern California; the Northern California Epidemiology of Uveitis Study, *Ophthalmology* 111(3):491–500, 2004.
8. Brewerton DA, Webley M, Ward AM: Acute anterior uveitis and the fourteenth chromosome, *Advances Inflam Res* 9:225–229, 1985.
9. Rosenbaum JT: Characterization of uveitis associated with spondyloarthritis, *J Rheumatol* 16(6):792–796, 1989. Epub 1989/06/01. PMID: 2778762.
10. Brewerton DA, Caffrey M, Nicholls A, et al.: Acute anterior uveitis and HL-A 27, *Lancet* 302(7836):994–996, 1973. Epub 1973/11/03. PMID: 4127279.
11. Haroon M, O'Rourke M, Ramasamy P, et al.: A novel evidence-based detection of undiagnosed spondyloarthritis in patients presenting with acute anterior uveitis: the DUET (Dublin Uveitis Evaluation Tool), *Ann Rheum Dis* 74(11):1990–1995, 2015. PMID: 24928841.
12. Juanola X, Loza Santamaria E, Cordero-Coma M, et al.: Description and prevalence of spondyloarthritis in patients with anterior uveitis: The SENTINEL interdisciplinary collaborative project, *Ophthalmology* 123(8):1632–1636, 2016. PMID: 27084561.
13. Martin TM, Zhang G, Luo J, et al.: A locus on chromosome 9p predisposes to a specific disease manifestation, acute anterior uveitis, in ankylosing spondylitis, a genetically complex, multisystem, inflammatory disease, *Arthritis Rheum* 52(1):269–274, 2005. PMID: 15641041.
14. Paiva ES, Macaluso DC, Edwards A, et al.: Characterisation of uveitis in patients with psoriatic arthritis, *Ann Rheum Dis* 59(1):67–70, 2000. Epub 2000/01/11. PMID: 10627431; PMC1752985.
15. Lyons JL, Rosenbaum JT: Uveitis associated with inflammatory bowel disease compared with uveitis associated with spondyloarthropathy, *Arch Ophthalmol* 115(1):61–64, 1997. PMID: 9006426.
16. Rosenbaum JT, Robertson JE, Watzke RC: Retinal vasculitis: a primer, *West J Med* 154:182–185, 1991.
17. Rosenbaum JT, Ku J, Ali A, et al.: Patients with retinal vasculitis rarely suffer from systemic vasculitis, *Semin Arthritis Rheum* 41(6):859–865, 2012. Epub 2011/12/20. PMID: 22177107.
18. Obenauf CD, Shaw HE, Sydnor CF, et al.: Sarcoidosis and its ophthalmic manifestations, *Am J Ophthalmol* 86(5):648–655, 1978. PMID: 568886.
19. Rosenbaum JT: Uveitis. An internist's view, *Arch Intern Med* 149(5):1173–1176, 1989. Epub 1989/05/01. PMID: 2719509.
20. Kaiser PK, Lowder CY, Sullivan P, et al.: Chest computerized tomography in the evaluation of uveitis in elderly women, *Am J Ophthalmol* 133(4):499–505, 2002.

20a. Han YS, Rivera-Grana E, Salek S, et al.: Distinguishing uveitis secondary to sarcoidosis from idiopathic disease: cardiac implications, *JAMA Ophthalmol* 136(2):109–115, 2018.

21. Dollfus H, Hafner R, Hofmann HM, et al.: Chronic infantile neurological cutaneous and articular/neonatal onset multisystem inflammatory disease syndrome: ocular manifestations in a recently recognized chronic inflammatory disease of childhood, *Arch Ophthalmol* 118(10):1386–1392, 2000. PMID: 11030821.
22. Petty RE, Smith JR, Rosenbaum JT: Arthritis and uveitis in children. A pediatric rheumatology perspective, *Am J Ophthalmol* 135(6):879–884, 2003.
23. Yazici H, Pazarli H, Barnes CG, et al.: A controlled trial of azathioprine in Behcet's syndrome, *N Engl J Med* 322(5):281–285, 1990. PMID: 2404204.
24. Isaak BL, Liesegang TJ, Michet Jr CJ: Ocular and systemic findings in relapsing polychondritis, *Ophthalmology* 93(5):681–689, 1986. PMID: 3523358.
25. Miceli-Richard C, Lesage S, Rybojad M, et al.: CARD15 mutations in Blau syndrome, *Nat Genet* 29(1):19–20, 2001. PMID: 11528384.
26. Rose CD, Doyle TM, McIlvain-Simpson G, et al.: Blau syndrome mutation of CARD15/NOD2 in sporadic early onset granulomatous arthritis, *J Rheumatol* 32(2):373–375, 2005. PMID: 15693102.
27. Sfikakis PP, Theodossiadis PG, Katsiari CG, et al.: Effect of infliximab on sight-threatening panuveitis in Behcet's disease, *Lancet* 358(9278):295–296, 2001.

28. Lim LL, Smith JR, Rosenbaum JT: Retisert (Bausch & Lomb/Control Delivery Systems), *Curr Opin Investig Drugs* 6(11):1159–1167, 2005. Epub 2005/11/30. PMID: 16312138.
29. Jabs DA, Rosenbaum JT, Foster CS, et al.: Guidelines for the use of immunosuppressive drugs in patients with ocular inflammatory disorders: recommendations of an expert panel, *Am J Ophthalmol* 130:492–513, 2000.
30. Jaffe GJ, Dick AD, Brezin AP, et al.: Adalimumab in patients with active noninfectious uveitis, *N Engl J Med* 375(10):932–943, 2016. PMID: 27602665.
31. Nguyen QD, Merrill PT, Jaffe GJ, et al.: Adalimumab for prevention of uveitic flare in patients with inactive non-infectious uveitis controlled by corticosteroids (VISUAL II): a multicentre, double-masked, randomised, placebo-controlled phase 3 trial, *Lancet* 388(10050):1183–1192, 2016. PMID: 27542302.
32. Ramanan AV, Dick AD, Jones AP, et al.: Adalimumab plus methotrexate for uveitis in juvenile idiopathic arthritis, *N Engl J Med* 376(17):1637–1646, 2017. PMID: 28445659.
33. Dick AD, Rosenbaum JT, Al-Dhibi HA, et al.: Fundamentals of care for uveitis international consensus G. Guidance on noncorticosteroid systemic immunomodulatory therapy in noninfectious uveitis: Fundamentals Of Care for UveitiS (FOCUS) Initiative, *Ophthalmology* 125(5):757–773, 2018. Epub 2018/01/10. PMID: 29310963.
34. Baker KB, Spurrier NJ, Watkins AS, et al.: Retention time for corticosteroid-sparing systemic immunosuppressive agents in patients with inflammatory eye disease, *Br J Ophthalmol* 90(12):1481–1485, 2006. PMID: 16914474; 1857545.
35. Riono WP, Hidayat AA, Rao NA: Scleritis: a clinicopathologic study of 55 cases, *Ophthalmology* 106(7):1328–1333, 1999.
36. Akpek EK, Thorne JE, Qazi FA, et al.: Evaluation of patients with scleritis for systemic disease, *Ophthalmology* 111(3):501–506, 2004. PMID: 15019326.
37. Foster CS, Forstot SL, Wilson LA: Mortality rate in rheumatoid arthritis patients developing necrotizing scleritis or peripheral ulcerative keratitis, *Ophthalmology* 91:1253–1263, 1984.
37a. Smith JR, Mackensen F, Rosenbaum JT: Therapy insight: scleritis and its relationship to systemic autoimmune disease, *Nat Clin Pract Rheumatol* 3(4):219–226, 2007.
38. Suhler EB, Lim LL, Beardsley RM, et al.: Rituximab therapy for refractory scleritis: results of a phase I/II dose-ranging, randomized, clinical trial, *Ophthalmology*, 2014. PMID: 24953794.
39. Keogh KA, Wylam ME, Stone JM, et al.: Induction of remission by B lymphocyte depletion in eleven patients with refractory antineutrophil cytoplasmic antibody-associated vasculitis, *Arthritis Rheum* 52(1):262–268, 2005.
40. Smith JR, Rosenbaum JT: A role for methotrexate in the management of non-infectious orbital inflammatory disease, *Br J Ophthalmol* 85(10):1220–1224, 2001.
40a. Petzold A, Plant GT. Chronic relapsing inflammatory optic neuropathy: a systematic review of 122 cases reported, *J Neurol* 261(1):17–26, 2014.
41. Maust HA, Foroozan R, Sergott RC, et al.: Use of methotrexate in sarcoid-associated optic neuropathy, *Ophthalmology* 110(3):559–563, 2003. Epub 2003/03/08. PMID: 12623821.
42. Rosenbaum JT, Simpson J, Neuwelt EM: Successful treatment of optic neuritis in association with systemic lupus erythematosus using intravenous cyclophosphamide, *Br J Ophthalmol* 81:130–132, 1997.
43. Hamid SHM, Whittam D, Mutch K, et al.: What proportion of AQP4-IgG-negative NMO spectrum disorder patients are MOG-IgG positive? A cross sectional study of 132 patients, *J Neurol* 264(10):2088–2094, 2017. Epub 2017/08/26. PMID: 28840314; PMC5617862.
44. Bruscolini A, Sacchetti M, La Cava M, et al.: Diagnosis and management of neuromyelitis optica spectrum disorders—An update, *Autoimmun Rev* 17(3):195–200, 2018. Epub 2018/01/18. PMID: 29339316.
44a. Hayreh SS: Ischemic optic neuropathy, *Prog Retin Eye Res* 28(1):34–62, 2009.
44b. Gonzalez-Gay MA, Garcia-Porrua C, Llorca J, et al.: Biopsy-negative giant cell arteritis: clinical spectrum and predictive factors for positive temporal artery biopsy, *Semin Arthritis Rheum* 30(4):249–256, 2001.
45. Havlir D, Torriani F, Dube M: Uveitis associated with rifabutin prophylaxis, *AnncInt Med* 121:510–512, 1994.
46. Macarol V, Fraunfelder FT: Pamidronate disodium and possible ocular adverse drug reactions, *Am J Ophthalmol* 118:220–224, 1994.
47. Eadie B, Etminan M, Mikelberg FS: Risk for uveitis with oral moxifloxacin: a comparative safety study, *JAMA Ophthalmol*, 2014. PMID: 25275293.
48. Taban M, Dupps WJ, Mandell B, et al.: Etanercept (Enbrel)-associated inflammatory eye disease: case report and review of the literature, *Ocul Immunol Inflamm* 14(3):145–150, 2006. Epub 2006/06/13. PMID: 16766397.
49. Della Vittoria Scarpati G, Fusciello C, Perri F, et al.: Ipilimumab in the treatment of metastatic melanoma: management of adverse events, *OncoTargets and Therapy* 7:203–209, 2014. PMID: 24570590; 3933725.
50. Marmor MF, Kellner U, Lai TY, et al.: Recommendations on screening for chloroquine and hydroxychloroquine retinopathy (2016 revision), *Ophthalmology* 123(6):1386–1394, 2016. PMID: 26992838.
51. Melles RB, Marmor MF: The risk of toxic retinopathy in patients on long-term hydroxychloroquine therapy, *JAMA Ophthalmol* 132(12):1453–1460, 2014. PMID: 25275721.
52. Marmor MF, Kellner U, Lai TY, et al.: Revised recommendations on screening for chloroquine and hydroxychloroquine retinopathy. *Ophthalmol* 118(2):415–422. PMID: 21292109.

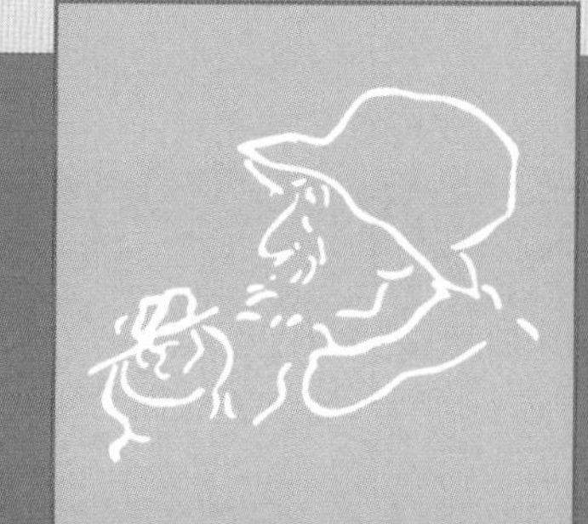

48 Neck Pain

JENNIFER KOSTY, RANI NASSER, RAUL A. VASQUEZ, CYRUS C. WONG, AND JOSEPH S. CHENG

KEY POINTS

- Neck pain is a ubiquitous condition associated with enormous medical and legal costs.
- Physicians need to differentiate causes of neck pain that can be managed conservatively from causes that require more aggressive treatments.
- Knowledge of the anatomy helps with the diagnosis and the differentiation of symptoms from a musculoskeletal, neurogenic, or vascular cause.
- The history and clinical examination help focus the differential diagnosis and identify the origin of the neck pain based on the anatomy and physiology.
- Indicated imaging studies, neurophysiologic procedures, and laboratory studies aid in diagnosis and in determining a treatment plan for the patient's symptoms.
- In the absence of spinal instability, neurologic deficit, infectious process, or neoplastic process, the patient may benefit from conservative treatment with recovery expected in time.

Epidemiology

Pain is an evolutionary protective mechanism to prevent further tissue damage. Neck pain is a ubiquitous condition with a lifetime prevalence of 67% to 71%.[1] The annual total cost for neck and low back pain corresponds to 1% of the gross national product in Sweden, with direct health-service costs representing only a small fraction of this percentage.[2–4] The medical and legal expenses associated with neck pain can be enormous, such as in whiplash injuries, which can result in $29 billion in costs annually in the United States alone.[5]

Neck pain may originate from various anatomic structures, including paraspinal soft tissues, the intervertebral joints and disk, compression of the spinal cord or nerve roots, and referred visceral pain. The cause of neck pain has a wide differential diagnosis, which can include trauma, degenerative changes, infection, autoimmune disorders, and lifestyle modifiable factors like smoking.[6–11]

The perception and resultant reporting of this pain varies significantly based on cultural and social circumstance. Honeyman and Jacobs[12] noted that Australian Aborigines significantly underreport pain and are rarely disabled by pain. Social circumstances also play an important role in an individual's ability to cope with and overcome neck pain. Studies have demonstrated worse outcomes after diskectomy for patients with a workers' compensation claim or litigation surrounding their condition.[13] These studies indicate nonorganic contributions to neck pain for secondary gain. Fortunately, most episodes of acute neck pain resolve with the "tincture of time" and patient education.

Physicians need to be able to differentiate causes of neck pain that can be managed with a conservative approach from those that require more aggressive treatments. An understanding of the anatomy and physiology and their association with the pathogenesis of neck pain provides the basis for obtaining a thorough history, physical examination, and ancillary data with the ultimate goal of effective treatment.

Anatomy

The cervical spine consists of seven vertebrae (C1 through C7) (Fig. 48.1). The bony anatomy of the atlas (C1) and axis (C2) are unique, whereas C3 to C7 demonstrate fairly consistent anatomy.[1] The atlas has no vertebral body; its lateral masses articulate with the skull's occipital condyles, forming the atlanto-occipital joints, which are supported by the anterior and posterior occipital membranes.[14] The atlanto-occipital joint is responsible for approximately 50% of the total flexion and extension in the neck and 50% of the rotatory motion. The axis (C2) has the *dens*, an odontoid peg that projects upward and anterior to articulate with the posterior aspect of the anterior arch of the atlas. The principal stabilizer of the odontoid to the anterior arch of the atlas is the transverse ligament, with the alar and apical ligaments acting as secondary stabilizers. C2 is a true synovial joint and thus is susceptible to inflammatory processes such as RA. Both the atlanto-occipital joint and the atlanto-axial joint lack an intervertebral disc, making them exceptionally prone to instability from destructive inflammatory arthritides.[15]

The subaxial cervical spine consists of the C3 through C7 vertebrae, which all demonstrate fairly similar anatomy. Each vertebra consists of a body, two interconnecting pedicles, two lateral masses, two transverse processes, two lamina, and spinous processes. The transverse and spinous processes project outward, providing attachment for ligaments and muscles and creating a moment arm to facilitate motion. The spinous processes of C3 through C6 are bifid, whereas the C7 spinous process usually is not bifid. The C7 spinous process is large and is the most prominent and easily palpable spinous process below C2.

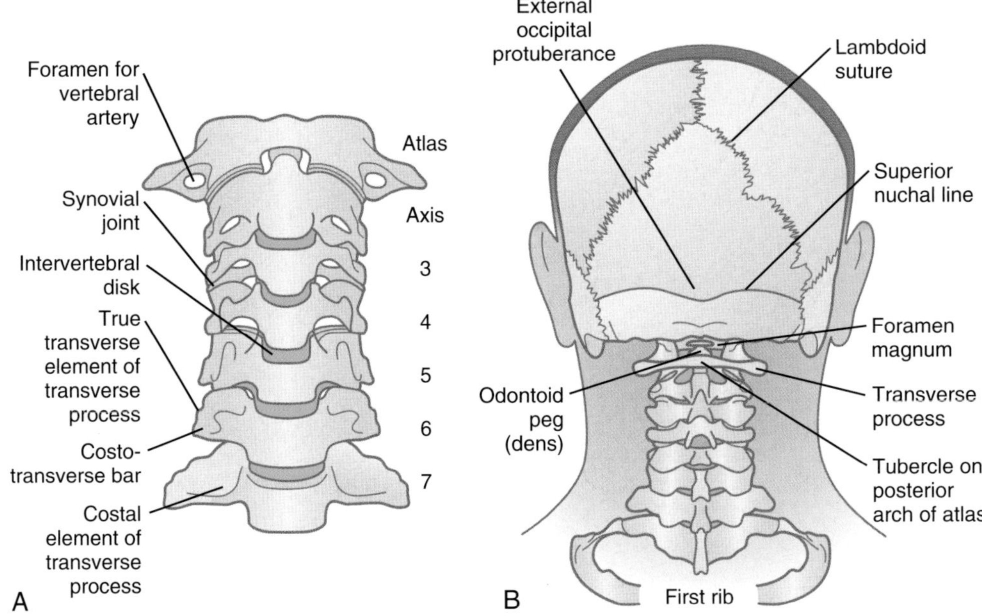

• **Fig. 48.1** Cervical spine anatomy. (A) Anterior view. (B) Posterior view.

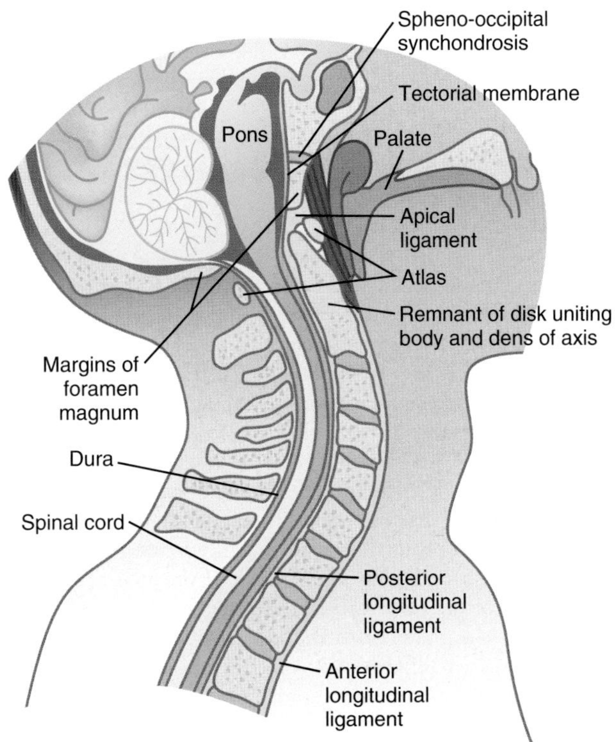

• **Fig. 48.2** Cervical spine anatomy: sagittal view.

Five articulations are found between each vertebra from C2 through C7, including the intervertebral disk, two uncovertebral joints, and two facet (zygoapophyseal) joints. The facet joints are true apophyseal joints with hyaline cartilage articulations, intervening menisci, synovial lining, and a joint capsule. This composition makes them susceptible to degenerative changes and systemic arthritides. The cartilage and synovial lining are aneural, whereas the joint capsule is highly innervated by the dorsal primary ramus. The facet joints are angled approximately 45 degrees from the transverse plane, articulating in concert with the uncovertebral joints and ligaments.

The intervertebral disks increase in size from C2 downward, giving the cervical spine its characteristic lordotic shape. Each disk consists of an outer annulus fibrosus and an inner nucleus pulposus, as well as a cephalad and caudal end plate. The annulus fibrosus consists of type I collagen, which gives form to the disk and provides tensile strength. It is innervated by the sinuvertebral nerve, formed by branches of the ventral nerve root and the sympathetic plexus.[16] The nucleus pulposus consists of type II collagen and proteoglycans, which interact with water to resist compressive stress. The pressure within the disk is highest with flexion, which may explain why individuals with a disk herniation find this position most uncomfortable.[17] Disk degeneration with aging includes loss of water content with resultant loss of height, annular tears, and myxomatous changes, increasing the risk of disk herniation. This process typically occurs in the posterolateral aspect of the disk, medial to the uncovertebral joints, where the posterior longitudinal ligament is not present and the annulus fibrosus is at its weakest.

The spinal column is supported by an interplay of ligaments and muscles (Fig. 48.2). The anterior longitudinal ligament and posterior longitudinal ligament course along the anterior and posterior aspect of the vertebral bodies, with the anterior longitudinal ligament resisting hyperextension and the posterior longitudinal ligament resisting hyperflexion. The ligamentum flavum joins the laminae of adjacent vertebra and with degeneration may buckle and thicken, resulting in spinal canal stenosis and the potential for cord impingement. In a similar manner, the interspinous ligament joins the spinous process of adjacent vertebrae. The supraspinous ligament originates as the nuchal ligament at the occiput and extends caudally as an aponeurosis until it attaches to the tip of the spinous processes of C7 and then continues to the lumbar region. Fourteen paired anterior, lateral, and posterior muscles help orchestrate the complex movements of the neck.

A brief review of the spinal cord and nerve roots is beneficial and assists in performing a thorough evaluation. In general, the

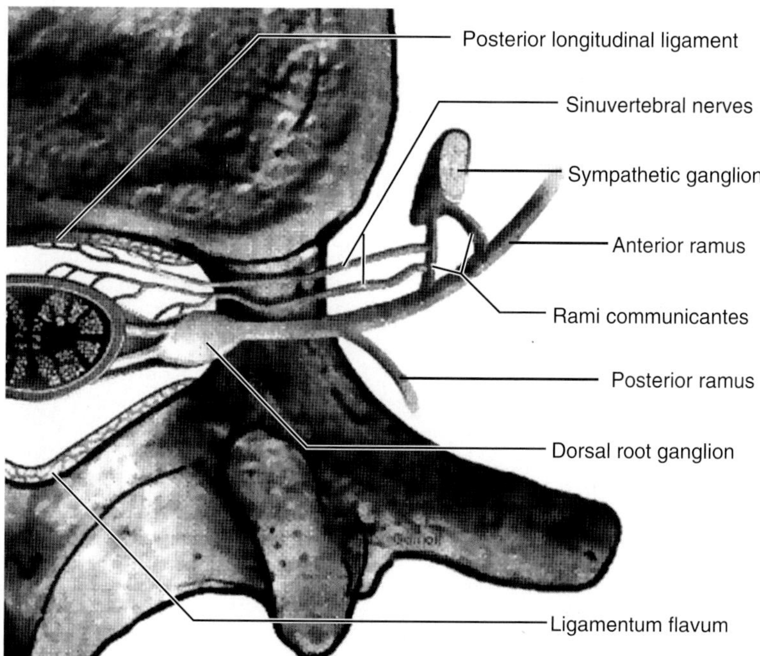

• **Fig. 48.3** Cervical spine anatomy. (From Levin KH, editor: *Neck and back pain: continuum 7 [No. 1].* Philadelphia, 2002, Lippincott Williams & Wilkins, p 9.)

spinal cord is divided into the posterior column, the lateral column, and the anterior column. The posterior column mediates proprioceptive, vibratory, and tactile sensation; the lateral column is a conduit for motor fibers, along with pain and temperature sensation from the contralateral side of the body; and the anterior column conveys crude touch sensation. Humans have a total of eight cervical nerve roots as the dorsal and ventral roots converge to form the spinal nerve within the vertebral foramen. Cervical nerve roots enter the intervertebral foramina by passing over the top of the corresponding pedicle, except the C8 cervical nerve, which lies between C7 and T1. Therefore a C5-C6 posterolateral disk herniation will affect the C6 nerve root. The nerve root occupies approximately one-third of the foramen (Fig. 48.3). The space available for the nerve root is decreased with neck extension and degenerative changes and increased with neck flexion.

The anterior spinal artery arises from the vertebral arteries and supplies the majority of the spinal cord, excluding the posterior columns. The posterior columns receive their blood supply from the two posterior spinal arteries, which originate from either the inferior cerebellar artery or the vertebral arteries. The vertebral arteries arise from the subclavian arteries and course cephalad through the C6 transverse foramen, passing anterior to the emerging cervical nerve root at each level. They pass behind the lateral mass of C1 and enter the foramen magnum. Diseases such as arterial dissection can be associated with severe neck pain and impairment of blood flow through the vertebral artery and can result in posterior circulation signs that include nystagmus, vertigo, drop attacks, dysarthria, and visual impairment. These symptoms are often associated with head position, and if a critical reduction of blood flow occurs, it can result in a cerebellar infarction.

The cervical spine is the most mobile segment of the spine; it has approximately 90 degrees of motion in flexion and extension, with three-fourths of this mobility due to extension (Table 48.1). The maximal range of motion in the sagittal plane within the subaxial spine is at the C5-C6 level, making it a common site of disk degeneration. Rotation encompasses approximately 80 to 90 degrees of motion, with 50% of this motion occurring at the atlanto-axial joint. Much like extension, rotation also reduces the cross-sectional area of the spinal canal. The cervical spine demonstrates 30 degrees of lateral mobility in each direction, which typically occurs with some degree of rotation as a result of the orientation of the facet joints.

Axial Neck Pain

Axial neck pain may originate from any tissue that receives innervation, including the zygoapophyseal joints, cervical disks, vertebral periosteum, posterior neck muscles, cervical dura mater, occipito-atlanto-axial joints, and the vertebral artery. The cause of neck pain may include degenerative, traumatic, malignant, infectious, and systemic inflammatory processes, as well as smoking. The most direct supporting data available link zygoapophyseal joints and cervical disks to the origin of axial neck pain. Provocative injections into the facet joint in asymptomatic volunteers invoke a reproducible pattern of occipital or axial neck pain.[18] This pattern of pain can be accurately diagnosed and treated, for at least a short period, with anesthetic injections targeted at the joint capsule itself or by blocking its respective dorsal primary ramus.[19–21] Degenerative arthritis within the upper cervical spine can manifest as suboccipital headaches, termed *cervicogenic headaches*, which are thought to result from irritation of the greater occipital nerve. Typically arthritis within the atlanto-occipital joints is made worse with provocative neck flexion and extension, whereas atlanto-axial arthritis is made worse with rotation. This phenomenon is supported by a study that found that this pattern of pain was reproduced when asymptomatic volunteers underwent injections at the atlanto-occipital and atlanto-axial joints.[22] Relief of suboccipital pain can be obtained by fluoroscopically guided injection of corticosteroid into the diseased joint, or fusion of these joints in recalcitrant cases.

The cervical disk is a more controversial source of axial neck pain, with pain occurring as a result of insult of the highly innervated

TABLE 48.1 Age and Normal Cervical Movement

Age (yr)	Flexion-Extension (degrees)	Lateral Rotation (degrees)	Lateral Flexion (degrees)
<30	90	90	45
31–50	70	90	45
>50	60	90	30

annulus fibrosis. This idea is based on provocative diskography, whereby a diseased disk is fluoroscopically injected to a given pressure. A positive test occurs when there is reproduction of pain in reliable patterns. To be a true positive, also known as a *concordant study*, an adjacent normal disk should not produce pain when injected. Using this method, several studies have implicated cervical disks as a source of axial neck pain.[16,23,24] Even with use of careful technique, a false-positive finding can occur, and it is not unusual to have a nonconcordant study with multiple disks eliciting a pain response despite being normal.[16] Interventions directed at treating the disk for isolated axial neck pain have been found to be unpredictable, despite the fact that the cervical disk likely contributes to axial neck pain.

Myofascial pain due to irritation of the muscles in the neck region can contribute to axial neck pain. Patients with chronic myofascial pain have a lower level of high-energy phosphates in the involved muscle tissue.[25] Myofascial pain can be the original source of neck pain or, more commonly, a manifestation of postural adaptations, compensatory overuse of normal tissue that remains after the injured structure heals, and lifestyle habits like smoking. A more generalized form of myofascial pain is fibromyalgia, a widespread disorder defined by diffuse pain that affects all four quadrants of the body, with at least 11 of 18 pressure points being positive. Patients have associated symptoms of fatigue, cognitive difficulties, irritable bowel syndrome, and a nondermatomal pattern of dysesthesias, weakness, and parasthesias.[26]

Systemic inflammatory arthropathies causing neck pain typically demonstrate the classic pattern of morning stiffness, polyarticular involvement, rigidity, and associated cutaneous manifestations. Rheumatoid arthritis (RA) often involves the cervical spine, initially causing stiffness and later causing pain and potentially leading to instability. After the hands and feet, the cervical spine is the most common site of disease involvement in RA.[27] The upper cervical spine is most commonly involved (occiput to C2), followed by the subaxial cervical spine (C3 to C7). The likelihood of developing cervical spine disease can be predicted by the amount of rheumatoid changes seen in the hands and feet. Basilar invagination is one such manifestation, in which the C1 lateral masses erode, allowing the odontoid peg to settle into the foramen magnum and place pressure on the brain stem with the potential for instantaneous death. The atlanto-axial joint can also demonstrate instability with the potential for neurologic injury. Because of these potential catastrophic complications, dynamic radiographs of the cervical spine should be obtained prior to any procedure requiring intubation. The seronegative spondyloarthropathies that can manifest with neck pain include ankylosing spondylitis, psoriatic arthritis, and reactive arthritis. Psoriatic arthritis will manifest with skin lesions before the development of arthritis in 70% of patients, and reactive arthritis rarely involves the cervical spine.

Ankylosing spondylitis often affects the entire axial skeleton with limitation of lumbar motion and chest expansion and later involvement of the cervical spine. In progressive patterns the cervical spine will take on a kyphotic deformity, and as the spine fuses it biomechanically becomes similar to a long bone. As such, minor trauma with neck pain should be taken very seriously in these patients. Even in the face of negative plain radiographs, these patients should undergo an extensive workup with a CT scan, observe strict spine precautions with appropriate neutral alignment according to their baseline spinal curvature, and undergo frequent neurologic evaluations to assess for development of an epidural hematoma.

Infection and neoplasms can cause axial neck pain through bone destruction, with irritation of vertebral body periosteal nerves and altered biomechanics on the facet joints and cervical disks. The onus is on the clinician to identify these patients at the initial visit because a delay in diagnosis can have catastrophic consequences. Red flags for axial neck pain that require further workup at the initial presentation include elderly patients or patients with a history of malignancy, immunocompromised patients, fevers, chills, unexplained weight loss, fatigue, nighttime awakening, recent antecedent bacteremia, and severe nonmechanical neck pain.[26]

Patients who have undergone previous cervical spine surgery should be evaluated for the presence of a pseudoarthrosis or iatrogenic instability. A *pseudoarthrosis* is failure of an attempted arthrodesis or fracture to fully heal with bridging bone. These patients describe a "honeymoon" period in which they do well for 3 to 6 months after surgery but then experience worsening axial neck and interscapular pain with associated headaches. Pseudoarthrosis can be diagnosed on plain radiographs with evidence of hardware loosening or movement on dynamic images. A CT scan with coronal and sagittal reconstructions should be obtained to more definitively diagnose a pseudoarthrosis. Once a pseudoarthrosis has been diagnosed, a surgical consult should be obtained, a bone metabolic workup should be undertaken, and the patient should be counseled on smoking cessation, given the deleterious effect of nicotine and carbon monoxide on bone healing. An additional cause of neck pain after surgery is iatrogenic instability, whereby the surgery itself creates pathologic motion. This condition requires a surgical consultation to determine if stabilization is warranted.

Radiculopathy and Myelopathy

The clinician must determine if there is evidence of nerve root compression, termed *radiculopathy*, versus a spinal cord compression, termed *myelopathy*. Cervical spondylosis and changes within the disk may cause loss of height with posterior bulging of the disk into the spinal canal and foramen. As the disk collapses, the posterior soft tissue structures, including the ligamentum flavum and facet joint capsule, buckle inward, further compromising the spinal canal and neural foramen. Pressure that was once dispersed throughout the disk is then transferred to the facet joints and uncinate processes, resulting in the development of bone overgrowth or osteophytes, which place extrinsic pressure on the nerve root or spinal cord.

Radiculopathy is a problem with the peripheral nervous system that affects the exiting nerve root. With radiculopathy, mechanical distortion of the nerve occurs, leading to increased vascular permeability, resulting in chronic edema and eventually fibrosis. This condition leads to hypersensitivity of the nerve root with an inflammatory response mediated by chemicals released from the cell bodies of sensory neurons and the cervical disk.[28] Compression of the dorsal root ganglion is believed to be especially important in producing radicular pain.[29] Clinically, this compression presents with pain in a dermatomal distribution, which is easily identifiable for roots C5-T1. Dermatomes for the higher cervical nerve roots, including C3 and C4, are along the posterior scapula and should not be confused with isolated axial neck pain.[30] Minor symptoms that are tolerable may be treated with conservative care, but persistent compression on a nerve root can lead to sensory loss and weakness. Disabling deficits should be treated operatively given that prolonged nerve compression can result in irreversible changes. In patients without a neurologic deficit, it is reasonable to expect a good outcome with conservative care.[31]

Myelopathy is a problem with the CNS and is a clinical presentation of long tract signs from compression of the spinal cord. Factors that contribute to the development of myelopathy include a congenitally narrow spinal canal, dynamic cord compression, dynamic thickening of the spinal cord, and vascular changes. The anterior-posterior diameter in the subaxial spine for a normal adult measures 17 to 18 mm, with diameters of less than 13 mm considered congenitally stenotic. The cord measures 10 mm. The shape of the spinal cord deformity has a high association with development of myelopathy because patients with a banana-shaped cord on axial views had evidence of myelopathy 98% of the time.[32] Ono and associates[33] described a ratio whereby the anterior-posterior diameter of the spinal cord is divided by the transverse diameter of the cord. Patients with a ratio of less than 0.40 tended to have severe neurologic deficits.[33] Certain patients may have dynamic cord compression with signs and symptoms of myelopathy only during neck flexion and extension. The space available for the cord is decreased during neck extension because of infolding of the ligamentum flavum and overlapping of the lamina. Also during extension, the spinal cord shortens as the distance from the skull base to the cervical spine is lengthened, effectively increasing cord diameter and making it more prone to compression by the posterior structures. In flexion, the cord lengthens and drapes over anterior degenerated disks and osteophytes.[34]

Myelopathy can be exacerbated by altered biomechanics from degenerated segments. For example, when a given level stiffens, the level above can become hypermobile.[35] A certain subset of patients can experience myelopathy in the absence of mechanical compression, which has been attributed to ischemic insult.[36] Despite the prevalent theory of ischemia, the precise molecular mechanisms that contribute to the development of myelopathy are not completely known. Some studies have debated the role of ischemia, proposing a complex cascade of bimolecular events that leads to the disease.[37] Patients with mild cases of myelopathy that do not affect activities of daily living can be closely monitored.[38] Patients with more severe deficits or progressive deficits tend to deteriorate over time with conservative care, and it is recommended that these patients undergo surgery to decompress the spinal cord.[39]

Infection and Neoplasm

Outside the degenerative cascade, infection and neoplasm can be the source of axial neck pain or neurologic deficit. In terms of infection, several entities are often seen: diskitis, osteomyelitis, and epidural abscess. Risk factors for infections of the spine include immunosuppression, intravenous drug use, and alcohol abuse, among others. Infection can also spread after lumbar puncture or epidural anesthesia.

The most common symptoms of spinal infection include excruciating pain and tenderness, accompanied by constitutional symptoms such as fever, night sweats, and lethargy. Disease progression may eventually lead to neurologic deficits such as motor deficits, sensory loss, and bowel/bladder dysfunction. Neurologic deficits are more common with epidural abscesses and are less commonly seen with osteomyelitis and diskitis. Whether CT or MRI scans are performed, contrast is needed in the setting of infection. MRI best evaluates epidural abscesses, but if no deficit is seen, CT may help with evaluating the bony destruction and mechanical instability.

The most common organisms seen in spinal infections include *Staphylococcus aureus,* streptococcus, *Escherichia coli, Pseudomonas aeruginosa* (especially in intravenous drug abusers), and *Haemophilus influenza* (pediatric diskitis). In 29% to 50% of the cases an organism is not identified, especially when antibiotics have been started.[40]

Diskitis and osteomyelitis often can be treated nonsurgically. Long-term treatment with antibiotics in combination with bracing can treat the underlying infection and avoid progressive deformity.[40] The antibiotics used most often include vancomycin, rifampin, and a third-generation cephalosporin for 4 to 6 weeks with or without an oral agent. These patients are watched closely for progression of disease—that is, worsening pain or neurologic deficit—and also are monitored with serial inflammatory markers, such as erythrocyte sedimentation rate (ESR) and C-reactive protein (CRP). Because of the nature of the antibiotics and the prolonged treatment time, kidney function must be monitored as well. Refractory infections and/or suspected instability cases should be referred for a surgical consultation.

Because of their proximity to the spinal cord and high chance for rapid neurologic deterioration, epidural abscesses have a lower threshold for surgical treatment, and a surgical consultation should always be considered.[40–43] Nonsurgical management is indicated in the neurologically intact patient with a small abscess or in patients too unstable for surgery.[40] In the setting of a progressive deficit or large abscess, the main goals of surgery are to decompress the neural elements and disrupt the abscess capsule, which helps with antibiotic penetration and infection control.

Neoplasms represent another source of neck pain. Similar to infection, neoplastic processes cause axial neck pain through bone destruction and irritation of periosteal nerves and altered biomechanics of facet joints and the anterior column, leading to progressive cervical kyphosis. The spine is the most frequent site of bone metastases, and spinal metastases will develop in 5% to 10% of patients with cancer.[44–47] Common tumors that metastasize to the spine are lung, breast, and prostate. Multiple myeloma may also involve the spine. A smaller percentage of cervical spine tumors are primary spine tumors. Spine tumors are often classified based on location: extradural, intradural-extramedullary, or intramedullary. Extradural tumors include schwannomas and neurofibromas; intradural-extramedullary tumors include myxopapillary ependymomas, meningiomas, and schwannomas; and intramedullary tumors include astrocytomas, gangliogliomas, and ependymomas. Tumors can also arise from vertebrae and include plasmacytoma, giant cell tumors, osteochondroma, osteoid osteoma, osteoblastoma, hemangioma, aneurysmal bone cyst, chondrosarcoma, osteosarcoma, and Ewing sarcoma. MRI with contrast is the imaging modality of choice to visualize the tumor. Consultation with a spine surgeon should be requested in all neoplasm cases.

Treatment of spinal tumors is based on tumor disease, neural compression, and the presence of instability. The main driver of treatment in terms of tumor biology is its radiosensitivity. Radiosensitive tumors can be emergently treated with radiation even in the setting of compression of neural elements. The most common radiosensitive tumors include lymphoma and multiple myeloma. Stereotactic radiation is becoming increasingly popular as a method of maximizing radiation to the surrounding tumor without damaging the sensitive spinal elements.[48–51] For metastatic spinal tumors causing spinal cord compression, the standard of treatment is surgical decompression followed by radiation.[52]

Clinical Features

In terms of functional anatomic pathways, neck pain is mediated via somatic or autonomic pathways.[53] Somatic pain, the most common, is perceived in dermatomes, myotomes, or sclerotomes. Pain originating in the autonomic pathway, or sympathetic nervous system, may fall into somatic segmental distributions, vascular supply distributions, peripheral nerve distributions, or nonconforming patterns. Because pain mediation pathways may have significant overlap, additional clinical information regarding characteristics of the neck pain along with diagnostic studies will complement the determination of the pain origin.

Patient History

Neck pain is the most common symptom of cervical spine disease, and correctly characterizing it helps to identify conditions requiring immediate treatment. Important characteristics to note include onset, distribution, frequency, duration, quality, aggravating factors, and the presence of neurologic symptoms. In general, pain that is present only intermittently may be indicative of instability or motion, whereas constant and increasing pain is a source of concern for a mass effect. The new onset of generalized neck pain that is of relatively short duration is likely related to benign disease, including muscle strain, whereas a longer duration of symptoms indicates significant or progressive disease. A well-localized quality of pain indicates specific nerve root irritation, whereas poorly defined pain may derive from irritation of deep connective tissue structures such as muscle, joint, bone, or disk. Aggravating and relieving factors may help elucidate biomechanical changes in the cervical spine that are contributing to the symptomatology.

Localized axial neck pain is commonly reported as originating posteriorly with extension into the shoulder or occiput. Localized pain of myofascial origin may worsen with neck flexion, whereas diskogenic neck pain will worsen with neck extension or rotation. Referred pain to the occiput usually indicates pathologic changes in the upper cervical spine and may radiate down the neck and to the ear. Shoulder girdle pain develops as a result of postural adaptations from initial neck pain symptoms. It is not uncommon for pain to be referred from the shoulder, heart, lungs, viscera, or temporomandibular joint to the neck region because of overlapping nerve distribution. Symptoms may arise as a result of irritation or activation of receptors directly, as with articular pain, pseudoarticular pain, vascular pain, cervicogenic headaches, pseudoangina pectoris, eye and ear symptoms, and throat symptoms.

Articular symptoms arise from innervation to the facet and uncovertebral joints, causing local pain and stiffness. Patients often state that their symptoms are made worse with inactivity and describe feelings of clicking, grating, or "sand" in the neck. Pseudoarticular pain may be felt in the shoulder and elbow, with the true disease originating from the neck. Vascular symptoms result from compression of the vertebral artery by osteophytes or a protruding disk. Symptoms may intensify with neck movement or certain postures. Tenosynovitis and tendonitis may involve the rotator cuff and tendons about the elbow, wrist, or hand. Stenosis or fibrosis of tendon sheaths or palmar fascia may be present, along with trigger points over the affected joints, giving a false impression of local disease.[54]

Localization of Pain Generators

Pain may be somatic or autonomic and is not always felt in precise anatomic zones. Overlapping sensory supplies may be present, as well as radiation in spinal segments by recruitment within the spinal column, causing difficulty in localization. Somatic pain is caused by cervical nerve root irritation. It is the most common type of pain, and diabetics are more susceptible to this nerve root irritation. Neurologic deficits correspond with the offending disk level in 80% of patients.[55]

Neuralgic and myalgic pain describes symptoms resulting from compression of different areas of the nerve root. Neuralgic pain originates from irritation of the dorsal sensory root and has a "lightning" or "electric" sensation that tends to be dermatomal and associated with numbness and paresthesias. The pain tends to present more proximally, with paresthesias more distally. Myalgic pain occurs with irritation of the ventral motor root. This pain is described as a deep, boring, and unpleasant sensation that tends to be poorly localized because of its referral to sclerotomal areas. These sensations conform to the areas of muscles that are innervated by the compressed nerve root. Autonomic-mediated symptoms result in dizziness, blurring of vision, tinnitus, retroocular facial pain, and jaw pain.

It is important to determine if the axial neck pain is isolated or if there is associated radiating pain, weakness, changes in sensation, or alterations in proprioception. The compression of a nerve root often can be localized by identifying the distribution of pain, paresthesia, or weakness as it follows segmental distribution of that respective nerve root (Table 48.2). Sensory loss may be described by the patient in precise terms with a description of numbness. Alternatively the patient may have vague symptoms of swelling or bogginess to the skin. If the face, head, or tongue is involved, the upper three nerve roots of the cervical plexus may be affected. Numbness of the neck, shoulder, arm, forearm, or fingers indicates involvement of C5-T1. Weakness, as with sensory changes, occurs in a graded fashion depending on the amount of compression on the nerve root. This weakness presents clinically with an obvious functional deficit or more subtle findings, made obvious only after repetitive testing. The clinician must be attuned to these subtle complaints of weakness, which may be described by the patient as a feeling of heaviness of the limbs, early fatigue, or insufficient power in the grip. If obvious atrophy is present in a muscle, then more than one nerve root is affected because of the evolutionary benefit of multiple levels of innervation for a given muscle. Alterations in proprioception are due to compression of the dorsal column of the spinal cord and will be described by the patient as symptoms of clumsiness, with reports of tripping or dropping objects. This presentation raises concern for the more ominous condition of myelopathy, which is secondary to spinal cord compression.

Cervical spinal disease classically causes isolated axial neck pain or a radicular pain that radiates to the shoulder or down the upper extremity (Table 48.3). Less commonly it can be the cause of headache, pseudoangina pectoris, and otolaryngologic sensations. Cervicogenic occipital headaches can be compounded by adaptive

TABLE 48.2 **Cervical Nerve Root Segments and Corresponding Clinical Signs**

Nerve Root	Symptom	Correlate
C3	Suboccipital pain with extension to the back of the ear	If C3, C4, and C5 are all involved, paradoxical breathing might occur
C4	Pain from the caudal aspect of the neck to the superior aspect of shoulder	
C5	Numbness over the shoulder and down the lateral aspect of the arm to the mid portion; the deltoid muscle may be weak, and the biceps reflex may be affected	
C6	Radiating pain and numbness down the lateral aspect of the arm and forearm to the thumb and index finger ("six shooter"); weakness in wrist extension, elbow flexion, and supination; diminished brachioradialis and biceps reflex	Sensory component can mimic carpal tunnel syndrome
C7	Numbness and pain down the posterior aspect of the arm and forearm to the long finger; weakness in the triceps, wrist flexion, and finger extensors	Most frequent; posterior interosseous nerve entrapment can mimic motor component, but no sensory deficits are present
C8	Pain and numbness down the medial aspect of the arm and forearm into the 4th and 5th digits; weakness in the flexor digitorum profundus to IF and LF and FPL	AIN entrapment can mimic motor component of C8 or T1; however, sensory changes and involvement of thenar muscles will not be present; ulnar nerve entrapment will spare short thenar muscles with the exception of ADP; does not involve FPL or FDP to IF and LF
T1		

ADP, Adductor pollicis; *AIN*, anterior interosseous nerve; *FDP*, flexor digitorum profundus; *FPL*, flexor pollicis longus; *IF*, index finger; *LF*, long finger.

TABLE 48.3 **Cervical Nerve Root Pain Referral Pathways**

Location of Pain	Source
Upper posterolateral cervical region	C0-C1, C1-C2, C2-C3
Occipital region	C2-C3, C3
Upper posterior cervical region	C2-C3, C3-C4, C3
Middle posterior cervical region	C3-C4, C4-C5, C4
Lower posterior cervical region	C4-C5, C5-C6, C4, C5
Suprascapular region	C4-C5, C5-C6, C4
Superior angle of scapula	C6-C7, C6, C7
Midscapular region	C7-T1, C7

changes in the posterior occipital muscles and often spread to the eye region, manifesting as a dull rather than a pulsating pain. These headaches are unique in that they are aggravated by neck movements. They typically have migraine-like symptoms, including phonophobia or photophobia.

Pseudoangina pectoris has been reported as a result of cervical spinal disease and can be confused with angina pectoris or breast pain in women (Fig. 48.4). In the presence of a C6-C7 lesion, neuralgic or myalgic pain may be present along with tenderness in the precordium or scapular region. Differentiation of heart disease from symptoms associated with C6-C7 dysfunction is made on the basis of muscle weakness, fasciculations, sensory changes, or reflex changes. Differentiation of these two diseases may be difficult when true angina and pseudoangina co-exist in the same patient.[56]

Cervical spinal disease may manifest in the form of eye, ear, and throat symptoms (see Fig. 48.3). Eye and ear symptoms may arise from irritation of the plexuses surrounding the vertebral and internal carotid arteries. Eye symptoms can present with blurring of vision relieved by changing neck position, increased tearing, orbital and retro-orbital pain, and descriptions of eyes being "pulled backward" or "pushed forward." Altered equilibrium with associated gait disturbances may result from irritation of surrounding sympathetic plexus or vertebral insufficiency. Hearing can be affected with tinnitus and altered auditory acuity. Throat symptoms, including dysphagia, may be related to anterior vertebral osteophytes that cause direct compression, as well as cranial nerve and sympathetic nerve communications.

Symptoms of dyspnea and cardiac arrhythmia and drop attacks may have a cervical spinal origin. Dyspnea can be related to a deficit in C3-C5 innervation of the diaphragm. Cardiac palpitations and tachycardia resulting from cervical spine disease can be differentiated from other causes by the fact that these symptoms are associated with unusual positions or hyperextension of the neck. This presentation is caused by irritation of C4 innervation of the diaphragm and pericardium or irritation of the cardiac sympathetic nerve supply. Drop attacks suggest posterior circulation insufficiency, resulting in an abrupt loss of proprioception without the loss of consciousness.

Myelopathy, or spinal cord compression, initially presents with subtle complaints of hand clumsiness or difficulty with balance. Patients report worsening handwriting in the past few months or difficulty buttoning shirts. Patients also may have nausea and emesis caused by equilibrium dysfunction. Paresthesias and dysesthesias may be present, often involving bilateral upper extremities and not following a dermatomal distribution. This presentation is often mistaken for peripheral neuropathy or carpal tunnel syndrome but should be considered when bilateral extremity symptoms are present. As the disease progresses over time, more advanced manifestations occur, including most commonly weakness in the triceps, hand intrinsic, and hip flexors. Late manifestations include spasticity, as well as bowel and bladder dysfunction.

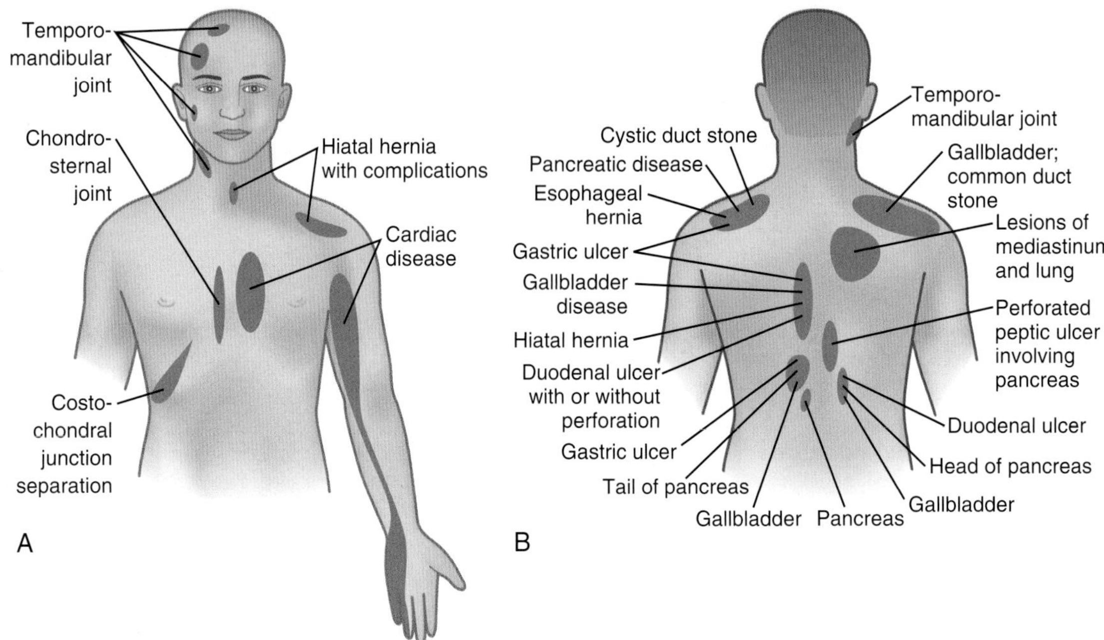

• **Fig. 48.4** Patterns of referred pain. (A) Anterior distribution. (B) Posterior distribution.

Finally, neck pain may present concomitant with systemic disease with varied symptoms that require further investigation. Examples include inflammatory arthritides, infection or tumor, multiple sclerosis, subacute combined degeneration, or syrinx. Inflammatory arthritides often present with morning stiffness, polyarticular involvement, or cutaneous manifestations. Fever, weight loss, or night pain points to an infectious or neoplastic cause. A Pancoast's tumor is a neoplastic process of the apical portion of the lung that can cause a mass effect on the caudal cervical nerve roots. This tumor should always be considered in a person with radicular symptoms and a history of smoking, with workup including a chest radiograph. Idiopathic brachial plexus neuritis, formerly known as *Parsonage-Turner syndrome*, is caused by viral infection of the brachial plexus that presents with severe arm pain involving multiple nerve roots. The classic presentation is weakness and variable deficits after the acute phase of severe pain resolves. Subacute combined degeneration from B_{12} deficiency is a consideration when greater sensory deficit is present in the lower extremities.

Clinical Examination

A careful clinical examination provides additional focus to the differential diagnosis. The clinical examination begins by broadly observing the patient's gait, as well as his or her head and neck posture. Results of further palpation, range of motion testing, and a neurologic examination for motor signs, reflexes, sensory signs, autonomic signs, and articular signs are assessed (Table 48.4).

Careful palpation with knowledge of key anatomic bony and soft tissue landmarks in the cervical spine may localize pain to a particular cervical level and location. Anteriorly or anterolaterally, the transverse process of C1 is palpated between the angle of the jaw and the styloid process. C3 is identified by palpation of the hyoid bone. C4-C5 is at the level of the thyroid cartilage, and C6 is at the level of the cricoid ring and the carotid tubercle. In the process of examining the neck, the sagittal balance with retention or loss of normal cervical lordosis also should be noted. Posteriorly and posterolaterally, the occiput, inion, superior nuchal line, mastoid processes, and spinous processes of C2 and C7-T1 are palpable.

Soft tissues about the anterior and posterior triangles of the neck, occipital region, and posterior paraspinal muscles are examined. The sternocleidomastoid muscle is involved with whiplash injuries, whereby abrupt hyperextension of the neck occurs. The muscle may be tender to palpation, or the patient may be splinting the neck with the head turned away from the injured muscle. This posturing of the neck is termed *torticollis,* and the clinician should remember that the head is turned away from the side of the involved sternocleidomastoid. Flexion injuries may traumatize the trapezius muscle. Midline cervical tenderness is more of a concern for ligament injury, whereas paraspinal muscle tenderness is typically a more benign process.[57] The greater occipital nerves are located lateral to the inion and may be involved in traumatic inflammation associated with flexion or extension injuries resulting in suboccipital headaches. Skin markings or visible trauma should be noted at this time.

Range of motion examination may reveal pain or limitations in flexion-extension, lateral bending, and rotation. Flexion limitation may be assessed by placing fingers between the patient's chin and sternum at maximum flexion, with 50% the motion occurring at the occiput-C1 joint and the remaining 50% distributed over C2-C7. If the patient is unable to place the chin on the chest, the interval should be measured. One finger width shows a limitation of 10 degrees, whereas three fingers' width indicates a 30-degree limitation in flexion. Upon extension the distance between the base of the occiput and the spinous process of T1 should be measured. Lateral flexion should allow the ear to touch the shoulder, with motion being shared across all cervical vertebrae. Upon rotation, the chin should touch the shoulder, with 50% of rotation occurring at C1-C2 and the remaining 50% distributed in the subaxial spine between C3-C7. A natural decrease in range of motion occurs with age, even in healthy individuals.[58]

Range of motion tests the ligaments, capsules, and fascia; it is reduced in the presence of cervical spinal muscular spasm or pain. Patients with degenerative changes of the cervical spine have back pain with decreased range of motion of the cervical spine without resistance. The most common findings due to changes in the

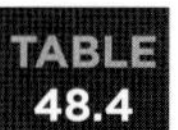

Nerves and Tests of Principal Muscles

Nerve	Nerve Roots	Muscle	Test
Accessory	Spinal	Trapezius	Elevation of shoulders
			Abduction of the scapula
	Spinal	Sternocleidomastoid	Tilting of the head to the same side with rotation to the opposite side
Brachial plexus		Pectoralis major	
	C5, C6	Clavicular part	Adduction of the arm
	C7, C8, T1	Sternocostal part	Adduction, forward depression of the arm
	C5, C6, C7	Serratus anterior	Fixation of the scapula during forward thrusting of the arm
	C4, C5	Rhomboid	Elevation and fixation of the scapula
	C4, C5, C6	Supraspinatus	Abduction of arm initiated
	(C4), C5, C6	Infraspinatus	External rotation of the arm
	C6, C7, C8	Latissimus dorsi	Adduction of horizontal, externally rotated arm, coughing
Axillary	C5, C6	Deltoid	Lateral and forward elevation of the arm to the horizontal position
Musculocutaneous	C5, C6	Biceps	Flexion of the supinated forearm
		Brachialis	
Radial	C6, C7, C8	Triceps	Extension of the forearm
	C5, C6	Brachioradialis	Flexion of the semiprone forearm
	C6, C7	Extensor carpi radialis longus	Extension of the wrist to the radial side
Posterior interosseous	C5, C6	Supinator	Supination of the extended forearm
	C7, C8	Extensor digitorum	Extension of the proximal phalanges
	C7, C8	Extensor carpi ulnaris	Extension of the wrist to the ulnar side
	C7, C8	Extensor indicis	Extension of the proximal phalanx of the index finger
	C7, C8	Abductor pollicis longus	Abduction of the first metacarpal in plane at a right angle to the palm
	C7, C8	Extensor pollicis longus	Extension of the first interphalangeal joint
	C7, C8	Extensor pollicis brevis	Extension of the first metacarpophalangeal joint
Median	C6, C7	Pronator teres	Pronation of the extended forearm
	C6, C7	Flexor carpi radialis	Flexion of the wrist to the radial side
	C7, C8, T1	Flexor digitorum superficialis	Flexion of the middle phalanges
	C8, T1	Flexor digitorum profundus (lateral part)	Flexion of the terminal phalanges, index, and middle fingers
	C8, T1	Flexor pollicis longus (anterior interosseous nerve)	Flexion of the distal phalanx, thumb
	C8, T1	Abductor pollicis brevis	Abduction of the first metacarpal in plane at right angle to the palm
	C8, T1	Flexor pollicis brevis	Flexion of the proximal phalanx, thumb
	C8, T1	Opponens pollicis	Opposition of the thumb against the fifth finger
	C8, T1	First and second lumbricals	Extension of the middle phalanges while the proximal phalanges are fixed in extension
Ulnar	C7, C8	Flexor carpi ulnaris	Observation of tendons during testing of abductor digiti minimi
	C8, T1	Flexor digitorum profundus (medial part)	Flexion of distal phalanges of the ring and little fingers
	C8, T1	Hypothenar muscles	Abduction and opposition of the little finger
	C8, T1	Third and fourth lumbricals	Extension of the middle phalanges while the proximal phalanges are fixed in extension
	C8, T1	Adductor pollicis	Adduction of the thumb against the palmar surface of the index finger
	C8, T1	Flexor pollicis brevis	Flexion of the proximal phalanx, thumb
	C8, T1	Interossei	Abduction and adduction of the fingers

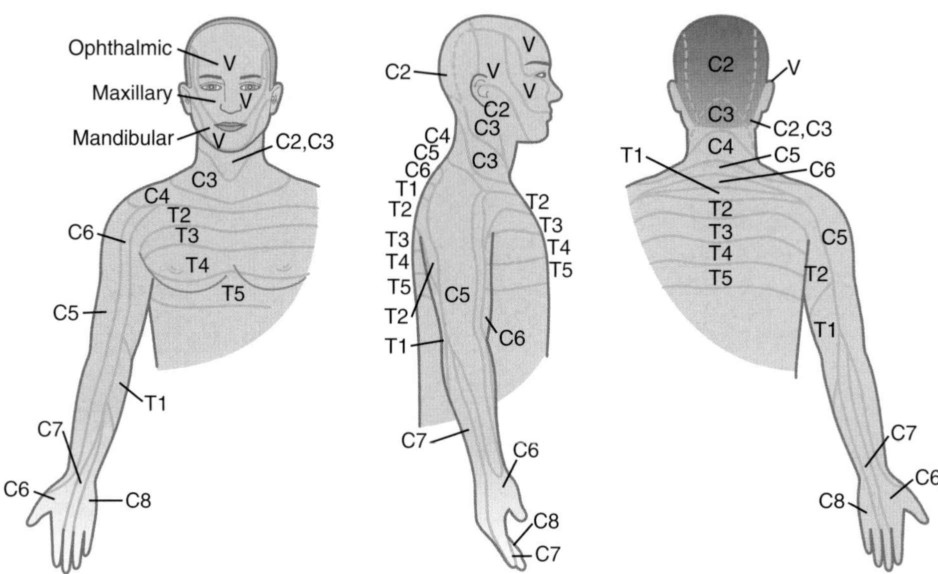

• **Fig. 48.5** Dermatome distributions. Dermatome distribution of nerve fibers from C1 through T5, carrying senses of pain, heat, cold, vibration, and touch to the head, neck, arm, hand, and thoracic area. The sclerotomes and myotomes are similar but show some overlap. Pain arising from structures deep to the deep fascia (myotome and sclerotome) does not precisely follow the dermatome distribution.

cervical spine articulations are (in order): restriction of movement with or without pain, pain upon movement, and local tenderness. Lateral flexion is the earliest and most impaired movement in degenerative diseases, with rotation first impaired in RA because of involvement of the odontoid peg. A uniformly stiff neck may be caused by diffuse idiopathic skeletal hyperostosis, which is present in a quarter of elderly patients but also may be due to ankylosing spondylosis or recent trauma to the neck.[59] If articular signs are found, the examiner must evaluate the entire vertebral column and peripheral joints for evidence of further arthritis and search for extra-articular manifestations.

Motion against resistance testing is performed after active and passive range of motion is established. Muscle groups tested include the flexors and extensors of the neck. In testing flexor muscles, a hand is placed between the forehead and chest. The primary flexor is the sternocleidomastoid muscle, with secondary flexors being the three scalene muscles and small pre-vertebral muscles. Extensor muscles are tested by placing a hand on the shoulder and head for resistance. Primary extensors include the paravertebral extensor mass, splenius, semispinalis capitis, and trapezius. Secondary flexors include the small intrinsic muscles of the neck. Rotators are examined by placing a hand on the shoulder and chin for resistance. The sternocleidomastoid muscle and the intrinsic muscles of the neck provide rotational force. Motion against resistance testing should include an active maximum effort strength testing to the extremes of flexion, extension, and rotation to assess muscle strength. Causes of decreased range of motion of the cervical spine include joint locking and bony ankylosis from degenerative changes or arthritides, fibrous contractures, muscle spasm, and splinting over painful joints, as well as nerve root or spinal cord compression or irritation. Decreased range of motion in the presence of pain or weakness warrants further investigation.

Sensation for light touch, pinprick, temperature, and proprioception should be performed. These tests are admittedly subjective, and therefore both extremities should be compared to assess differences in sensation. Comparing an unaffected area such as the face to the area of decreased sensation can also be helpful. Pinprick can be performed using a sterile needle and temperature using an alcohol pad; these methods assess the functioning of the spinothalamic tract that traverses the anterolateral aspect of the spinal cord. Light touch and proprioception assess functioning of the posterior spinal column.

Dermatomes are anatomically distributed, as noted in Fig. 48.5. The lower extremities demonstrate a unique dermatomal map that correlates with embryologic development, in which the limb starts in a supinated position and with longitudinal growth pronates. Perineal sensation and rectal tone are important to examine because an abnormality may indicate compression of the spinal cord or cauda equina, requiring immediate surgical intervention. Isolating the level of disease can be challenging at times. Nerve roots with proximal compression are more susceptible to distal compression. When the nerve is compressed both proximally and distally, it is called a *double crush phenomenon*. The cervical spine should always be considered as the potential etiology in patients who present with symptoms of carpal or cubital tunnel syndrome and peripheral neuropathy. Ancillary imaging and nerve conduction studies can help elucidate the cause.

After palpation, range of motion testing, and assessment of sensation, muscle strength testing is continued for localization of any positive findings. Lower motor neuron disease is indicated by weakness, hypotonia, and fasciculations. Upper motor neuron disease is indicated by spasticity. Motor function should be graded using the standard 0-5 nomenclature: grade 0, no function; 1, a trace of function; 2, full range of joint motion with gravity eliminated; 3, antigravity function; 4, function against slight resistance; and 5, normal strength against resistance (Table 48.5). If weakness is present, a more focused examination should be performed to look at other muscles innervated by that same nerve root.

Deep tendon stretch reflexes should be performed and graded from 0 to 3, as follows: 0, no response; 1, hyporeflexive; 2, normal; and 3, hyper-reflexive. C5 is tested by striking the biceps tendon; C6, the brachioradialis; C7, the triceps; L4, the patellar tendon; and S1, the Achilles tendon. To facilitate reflex testing, it may be helpful to use muscle loading or Jendrassik's maneuver (performed by having the patient flex both sets of fingers into a hook-like form, interlock the hands, and then pull apart). This technique

TABLE 48.5 Strength Grading in Motor Examination

0	No function with total paralysis
1	Trace movement with palpable or visible contraction
2	Full range of joint motion with gravity eliminated
3	Active movement against gravity
4	Active movement against slight resistance
5	Normal strength

creates a diversion to help relax the patient and better assess lower extremity reflexes. If difficulty with reflex testing persists, one must ensure that no peripheral neuropathy is present. In addition to deep tendon reflex testing, the abdominal reflex, Babinski test, and bulbocavernosus test should also be assessed.

Provocative tests that can be helpful in confirming compressive extradural monoradiculopathy include Spurling's test, the arm abduction test, and the axial compression and traction test. All of these tests are meant to change the diameter of the neural foramen, thus increasing or decreasing the symptoms, respectively. Spurling's test is performed by having the patient extend his or her neck and rotate toward the side of pain. The test is positive if the radicular pain is made worse in this position and indicates foraminal stenosis with potential compression of a nerve root. The arm abduction sign is positive if the patient's pain is relieved by placing the hand on the affected side, on top of the head.[60] The axial compression test is performed by pressing on top of the patient's head with the neck in the neutral position, with a positive result if the radicular symptoms are exacerbated by this maneuver and relieved by placing traction on the head and opening up the foramina.

Provocative tests that are helpful in diagnosing myelopathy include the presence of Hoffmann's sign, the finger escape sign, the abnormal grip-release test, and Lhermitte's sign. A positive (pathologic) Hoffmann's sign is performed by holding the middle finger extended and suddenly extending the distal interphalangeal joint, resulting in flexion of the index finger and thumb. A positive finger escape sign occurs when a person cannot hold all of the fingers in an adducted and extended position without the ulnar two digits falling into flexion and abduction over time. The grip-release test reveals an inability to rapidly open and close a fist because of weakness and spasticity of the hand. Lhermitte's sign evaluates changes in the spinal cord itself and occurs when the patient's neck is forcefully flexed, resulting in electric-like shocks that travel down the arms and legs. This reaction indicates changes in the white matter of the spinal cord and may be a result of cervical myelopathy or multiple sclerosis.

Diagnostic Evaluation

After completing the history and clinical examination, performing indicated imaging studies, neurophysiologic procedures, and laboratory studies may aid in completing the differential diagnosis and treatment plan for the patient's neck pain. Cervical radiographs often show degenerative changes in asymptomatic people in their sixties.[61] In the absence of trauma, constitutional symptoms, or worsening neurologic deficit, 4 to 6 weeks of conservative care for neck pain is indicated prior to obtaining radiographs.[62] Dynamic radiographs should also be used for screening patients with RA prior to endotracheal intubation, given the risk of cervical instability. One study demonstrated that 61% of patients with RA had evidence of instability defined by at least 3 mm of atlanto-axial subluxation on pre-operative screening radiographs.[63]

In the presence of significant degenerative changes and end plate osteophytes, CT myelography can be helpful in further characterizing the bony involvement. CT myelography should be thought of as a complimentary test to MRI.[64] It should only be used as the primary test to evaluate neural involvement when MRI is contraindicated because MRI is superior for evaluating spinal cord changes such as syringomyelia, myelomalacia, or neoplasm.[65] MRI scanning is indicated for progressive neurologic deficit, disabling weakness, or long tract signs and is recommended for patients with persistent cervical radiculopathy after 6 weeks of conservative care.[62] The addition of gadolinium contrast enhancement is helpful in evaluating infection and neoplasm and differentiating scarring from recurrent disk herniation in patients who have undergone previous spinal surgery. MRI results must be correlated with physical examination findings, given that asymptomatic volunteers have been found to have abnormal cervical spine MRI findings.[53] Increased signal on the T2 sequence can be representative of a spectrum of disease from edema to myelomalacia and syrinx formation. Therefore the presence of increased signal within the spinal cord warrants a surgical consultation and operative intervention if the examination and history correlate, or close follow-up at a minimum. If the MRI findings do not correlate with the history and physical examination findings, further studies may be required, such as CT myelography. CT myelography is superior at detecting bony foraminal stenosis. Nuclear bone scanning techniques, including the single photon emission computerized tomography scans, have been used to identify and characterize acuity in occult fractures, periosteal injury, and post-traumatic osteoarthritis in the absence of positive radiograph findings.[66]

Neurophysiologic procedures are indicated when the clinical examination and imaging studies fail to correlate or when there is conflicting information. Electromyography (EMG), nerve conduction studies, and somatosensory evoked responses help differentiate cervical spine disorders from peripheral nerve entrapment syndromes and help in differentiating intrinsic joint disease from a radiculopathy. These tests are complementary to plain radiographs and an MRI scan or CT myelogram.

Neck pain is typically a result of mechanical causes, and laboratory studies generally are not helpful in its diagnosis. Nevertheless, laboratory studies can be critical in ruling out infection, neoplasm, and systemic arthritides. ESR indirectly measures the acute-phase response with a high sensitivity but low specificity. Patients younger than 50 years should have an ESR less than 20 mm/hour, with the accepted normal range increasing as the patient ages. Values greater than 100 are seen with infection and neoplasm, whereas less dramatic elevations are seen with RA and after surgery.[67] CRP is an acute-phase reactant synthesized by the liver, with elevations peaking by day 2 of the inciting event and returning to normal within 3 to 7 days of removing the insult.[68] The complete blood cell count with differential and a spinal tap can also be helpful if meningitis is a concern.

Differential Diagnosis and Treatment

Using the combination of history, physical examination, and diagnostic studies is detrimental to establish the differential diagnosis of benign axial neck pain, radiculopathy, myelopathy, infection, neoplasm, systemic arthritides, and referred pain (Table 48.6). Most axial neck pain is self-limiting and will resolve with appropriate conservative care.[69] Axial neck pain with associated

TABLE 48.6 Differential Diagnosis of Common Causes of Axial Neck Pain

Etiology	Cause	Characteristics	Physical Exam	Treatment
Trauma	Irritation of muscles, facets, intervertebral discs, and ligaments (i.e., "whiplash") Bony fractures	History of trauma Neck stiffness Pain worsens with movement May have accompanying neurologic deficits	Guarding of the neck muscles leading to reduced ROM Severe midline tenderness with fractures Moderate tenderness with whiplash type injuries Neurologic deficit	Physical therapy and anti-inflammatories may be beneficial in the case of whiplash Bracing may be necessary for minor fractures Surgical intervention may be necessary for instability or neurologic compression
Degenerative changes (non-neuropathic)	Irritation of zygoapophyseal (facet) joints Irritation of cervical discs	Often chronic in nature Pain radiates to shoulders Suboccipital headaches Facet pain improves with injections targeting the joint capsule or block of dorsal primary ramus	Limited neck range of motion Facet pain worsened by palpation of paraspinal region Discogenic pain worsened by midline palpation Discogenic pain worsened with neck extension and rotation	Physical therapy, anti-inflammatories Medial branch blocks or radiofrequency ablation for facet pain Surgical intervention may be considered if instability or deformity is present
Cervical radiculopathy	Herniated cervical disc Spondylosis Noncompressive pathologies (diabetes, herpes zoster, etc.)	Sharp, shooting pain Radiation into the associated dermatome	Positive Spurling's sign Numbness, tingling, and/or pain in associated dermatomes Weakness in associated myotomes	Physical therapy, anti-inflammatories, oral steroids, and epidural steroid injections Surgery for failure of conservative therapy or if weakness is present
Cervical stenosis	Spondylosis Congenitally narrow canal Postsurgical Traumatic Rheumatologic	Often accompanied by myelopathy (deterioration in fine motor skills, gait and balance disturbances, incontinence, etc.)	Broad-based, spastic gait Hyperreflexia Weakness Positive Hoffman's sign	Symptomatic treatment may be beneficial in the absence of a neurologic deficit Surgical intervention warranted in the presence of neurologic deficits or hyperreflexia
Myofascial pain	Chronic irritation of neck muscles May be due to postural or biomechanical imbalance, trauma, emotional stress, and endocrine or hormone abnormalities	Dull and persistent pain without clear exacerbating or alleviating factors Sometimes worsened with neck flexion May be associated with fibromyalgia	Patient may have trigger points, or palpable muscle bands that refer pain when pressure is applied	Physical therapy and anti-inflammatories Psychotherapy Trigger point injections
Rheumatologic disease Rheumatoid arthritis (RA) Ankylosing spondylitis (AS) Others	Joint inflammation Cervical stenosis Musculoskeletal strain from cervicothoracic kyphotic deformity in AS	Morning stiffness and rigidity RA may lead to atlanto-axial instability AS may lead to cervicothoracic kyphosis	Additional symptoms related to systemic disorder	Physical therapy and anti-inflammatories may be considered to alleviate symptoms Surgery may be necessary to address instability or deformity
Infection Osteomyelitis Diskitis Epidural abscess	Bone destruction Irritation of periosteal nerves Instability Altered biomechanics	Severe neck pain that is present at rest and worsened with movement Signs/symptoms of infection Pts with history of IVDU or immunocompromise	Severe pain that is worsened with movement Neurologic deficits may be due to epidural abscess Stigmata of bacteremia	IV antibiotics Surgery may be necessary in the presence of an epidural abscess Bracing may offer symptomatic relief

TABLE 48.6 Differential Diagnosis of Common Causes of Axial Neck Pain—cont'd

Etiology	Cause	Characteristics	Physical Exam	Treatment
Neoplasm Metastatic tumors Multiple myeloma/ plasmacytoma Primary bone tumors	Bone destruction Irritation of periosteal nerves Mechanical instability	Neck pain worsens with movement Pain awakens patient from sleep Systemic symptoms such as unexplained weight loss, anorexia, malaise, etc.	Severe neck tenderness Neck pain worsens with movement Neurologic deficits present from epidural tumor	Symptomatic treatment with anti-inflammatories and pain medications Radiation Surgical intervention may be warranted for decompression and/or stabilization
Vascular Cervical carotid dissection	Traumatic or spontaneous tear in the tunica intima Blood enters the space between the inner and outer wall	Sudden onset Tearing sensation Headache Facial or eye pain Pulsatile tinnitus Ischemic events	Horner's syndrome Carotid bruit Expanding hematoma Neurologic deficit	Anti-platelet agents, anti-coagulants, stenting
Postsurgical Pseudoarthrosis (failed fusion) Postsurgical iatrogenic instability	Hardware loosening Instability due to disruption of disc and joints	Improvement in neck pain after surgery ("honeymoon period") with worsening neck and interscapular pain	Painful range of motion in the neck History of cervical surgery	Revision surgical procedure

radiculopathy also has a fairly benign course, with 75% of patients having only one recurrence or mild symptoms at 19-year follow-up with conservative treatment.[70] Patients with isolated neck pain and a negative radiographic and laboratory workup are best treated with a multimodal approach. During the acute phase, patients can be treated with a soft collar to reduce inflammation, but the collar should not be worn for more than 2 weeks to avoid deconditioning. Multimodal treatments have been found to be the most effective at treating axial neck pain, including proprioceptive training, exercises with resisted strengthening, muscle relaxants, and NSAIDs.[71–76] Evidence is inconclusive as to the effectiveness of radiofrequency denervation of facet joints, acupuncture, transcutaneous electrical nerve stimulation unit, iontophoresis, EMG biofeedback, or local injections for treatment of axial neck pain.[77–80]

Cervical traction may be prescribed, with a typical regimen of 3.5 to 4.5 kg for 15- to 20-minute sessions with the device at 20 to 25 degrees of flexion. This treatment, however, has only shown short-term relief of radicular symptoms.[81] Fluoroscopically guided interlaminar and transforaminal epidural steroids are effective at treating lumbar radiculopathy, but not in the cervical spine.[82] Cervical injections carry a higher risk, with complications in up to 16% of patients, including neurologic deficits.[83,84] Given these increased risks with epidural steroid injections in the cervical spine, a more conservative approach should be taken in prescribing this treatment modality. Atlanto-axial facet joint osteoarthritis may be treated successfully with a facet block and NSAIDs. If conservative therapy with NSAIDs fails, a fusion may be indicated.

In addition to degenerative changes to the cervical spine, trauma, and acute disk herniation, more insidious causes of neck pain exist, such as schwannomas, Pancoast's tumor, brachial plexus neuritis, and complex regional pain syndrome. Schwannomas, if intradural, may involve a sensory nerve root, causing dermatomal pain along with a myelopathy or radiculopathy from compression. Pancoast's tumor involving the lung apex may cause caudal cervical nerve root and sympathetic changes in addition to nerve root or brachial plexus compression. Brachial plexus neuritis (Parsonage-Turner syndrome), which is of viral origin, causes severe arm pain followed by weakness and then pain resolution followed by a return of arm strength. This condition may progress to complex regional pain syndrome in a small number of cases associated with diffuse burning pain along with autonomic changes, including discoloration of the skin.

Follow-up and vigilance are in order because a progressive neurologic deficit, segmental instability, or persistent radicular symptoms for at least 6 weeks may be indications for surgical intervention. In a prospective randomized study comparing surgery, physical therapy, and cervical collar use for long-standing cervical radiculopathy, no difference between the three groups was found at 12 months.[85] Cervical myelopathy with very mild deficits can be followed closely; however, the natural course of the illness is long periods of stability with episodes of deterioration. Definitive indications for surgery include the presence of myelopathy for 6 months or longer, progression of signs or symptoms, difficulty walking, or change in bowel or bladder function. Surgery is directed at decompressing the spinal cord and preventing further deterioration rather than improving neurologic deficits.

Systemic arthritides, infection, and tumors can affect the cervical spine with variable neurologic and constitutional symptoms. RA typically causes atlanto-axial subluxation, atlanto-axial impaction, and subaxial subluxation (Table 48.7) Surgical stabilization is indicated with progressive neurologic deficit, persistent axial neck pain with radiographic evidence of instability, canal diameter of less than or equal to 14 mm (posterior atlanto-dens interval), and odontoid migration of greater than or equal to 5 mm above McGregor's line. In the setting of atlanto-axial subluxation or subaxial subluxation, the involved levels are fused posteriorly and atlanto-axial impaction should be treated with occipitocervical fusion.[15] Patients with rheumatoid disease who have evidence

TABLE 48.7 Rheumatologic Disorders Causing Neck Pain

Rheumatoid arthritis
• Without disease of the C1-C2 joint
• With structural cervical abnormalities
  • C1-C2 subluxation
  • C1-C2 facet involvement

Spondyloarthropathies • Ankylosing spondylitis • Reactive arthritis • Psoriatic arthritis • Enteropathic arthritis
Polymyalgia rheumatica
Osteoarthritis
Fibromyalgia
Nonspecific musculoskeletal pain
Miscellaneous spondyloarthropathies • Whipple's disease • Behçet's disease • Paget's disease • Acromegaly • Ossification of the posterior longitudinal ligament • Diffuse idiopathic skeletal hyperostosis

of instability demonstrate radiographic progression over time, but this progression correlates poorly with neurologic outcome.[86] Regardless, these patients require close follow-up given that once myelopathy develops, most patients die within 1 year.[87]

Ankylosing spondylitis commonly affects the cervical spine, resulting in a kyphotic deformity over time with altered biomechanics, which has implications in the setting of trauma. The kyphotic deformity can have significant functional implications as the person's gaze moves toward the floor, making interaction with the surrounding world difficult. Corrective osteotomies are available but carry the risk of neurologic deficit and intra-operative bleeding. Nevertheless, earlier diagnosis and treatment with tumor necrosis factor blocking agents may reduce the instance of cervical deformity in this disease.[88]

Infection and neoplastic processes both can cause destruction with mechanical or nonmechanical neck pain, constitutional symptoms, and variable neurologic deficit. The goal is similar with eradication of the infection or tumor, decompression if a neurologic deficit exists, and stabilization of the spinal column.

In summary, a careful history, physical examination, and ancillary studies can help one arrive at a fairly narrow differential diagnosis. In the absence of spinal instability, neurologic deficit, or an infectious or neoplastic process, the patient may benefit from conservative treatment with expectant recovery using "tincture of time."

 The references for this chapter can also be found on ExpertConsult.com.

References

1. Nachemson AL, Jonsson E, editors: *Neck and back pain: the scientific evidence of causes, diagnosis, and treatment*, Philadelphia, 2000, Lippincott Williams & Wilkins.
2. Andersson HI, Ejlertsson G, Leden I, et al.: Chronic pain in a geographically defined general population: studies of differences in age, gender, social class, and pain localization, *Clin J Pain* 9:174–182, 1993.
3. Hansson EK, Hansson TH: The costs for persons sick-listed more than one month because of low back or neck problems. A two-year prospective study of Swedish patients, *Eur Spine J* 14:337–345, 2005.
4. Mäkelä M, Heliövaara M, Sievers K, et al.: Prevalence, determinants, and consequences of chronic neck pain in Finland, *Am J Epidemiol* 134:1356–1367, 1991.
5. Freeman MD, Croft AC, Rossignol AM, et al.: A review and methodologic critique of the literature refuting whiplash syndrome, *Spine* 24:86–96, 1999.
6. Boshuizen HC, Verbeek JH, Broersen JP, et al.: Do smokers get more back pain? *Spine* 18:35–40, 1993.
7. Andersson H, Ejlertsson G, Leden I: Widespread musculoskeletal chronic pain associated with smoking. An epidemiological study in a general rural population, *Scand J Rehabil Med* 30:185–191, 1998.
8. Zvolensky MJ, McMillan K, Gonzalez A, et al.: Chronic pain and cigarette smoking and nicotine dependence among a representative sample of adults, *Nicotine Tob Res* 11:1407–1414, 2009.
9. McLean SM, May S, Klaber-Moffett J, et al.: Risk factors for the onset of non-specific neck pain: a systematic review, *J Epidemiol Community Health* 64:565–572, 2010.
10. Mitchell MD, Mannino DM, Steinke DT, et al.: Association of smoking and chronic pain syndromes in Kentucky women, *J Pain* 12:892–899, 2011.
11. Gill DK, Davis MC, Smith AJ, et al.: Bidirectional relationships between cigarette use and spinal pain in adolescents accounting for psychosocial functioning, *Br J Health Psychol* 19:113–131, 2014.
12. Honeyman PT, Jacobs EA: Effects of culture on back pain in Australian Aboriginals, *Spine* 21:841–843, 1996.
13. Klekamp J, McCarty E, Spengler DM: Results of elective lumbar discectomy for patients involved in the workers' compensation system, *J Spinal Disord* 11:277–282, 1998.
14. Daniels DL, Williams AL, Haughton VM: Computed tomography of the articulations and ligaments at the occipito-atlantoaxial region, *Radiology* 146:709–716, 1983.
15. Kim DH, Hilibrand AS: Rheumatoid arthritis in the cervical spine, *J Am Acad Orthop Surg* 13:463–474, 2005.
16. Bogduk N, Aprill C: On the nature of neck pain, discography and cervical zygapophysial joint pain, *Pain* 54:213–217, 1993.
17. Nachemson AL: Disc pressure measurements, *Spine* 6:93–97, 1981.
18. Dwyer A, Aprill C, Bogduk N: Cervical zygapophyseal joint pain patterns: I. A study in normal volunteers, *Spine* 15:453–457, 1990.
19. Aprill C, Dwyer A, Bogduk N: Cervical zygapophyseal joint pain patterns: II. A clinical evaluation, *Spine* 15:458–461, 1990.
20. Bogduk N, Marsland A: The cervical zygapophyseal joints as a source of neck pain, *Spine* 13:610–617, 1988.
21. Cavanaugh JM, Lu Y, Chen C, et al.: Pain generation in lumbar and cervical facet joints, *J Bone Joint Surg Am* 88(Suppl 2):63–67, 2006.
22. Dreyfuss P, Michaelsen M, Fletcher D: Atlantooccipital and lateral atlanto-axial joint pain patterns, *Spine* 19:1125–1131, 1994.
23. Grubb SA, Kelly CK: Cervical discography: clinical implications from 12 years of experience, *Spine* 25:1382–1389, 2000.
24. Schellhas KP, Smith MD, Gundry CR, et al.: Cervical discogenic pain: prospective correlation of magnetic resonance imaging and discography in asymptomatic subjects and pain sufferers, *Spine* 21:300–311, 1996, discussion 311–312.
25. Bengtsson A, Henriksson KG, Larsson J: Reduced high-energy phosphate levels in the painful muscles of patients with primary fibromyalgia, *Arthritis Rheum* 29:817–821, 1986.
26. Dreyer SJ, Boden SD: Laboratory evaluation in neck pain, *Phys Med Rehabil Clin N Am* 14:589–604, 2003.
27. Crockard HA: Surgical management of cervical rheumatoid problems, *Spine* 20:2584–2590, 1995.
28. Cooper RG, Freemont AJ, Hoyland JA, et al.: Herniated intervertebral disc-associated periradicular fibrosis and vascular abnormalities occur without inflammatory cell infiltration, *Spine* 20:591–598, 1995.
29. Chabot MC: The pathophysiology of axial and radicular neck pain, *Semin Spine Surg* 7:2–8, 1995.

30. An HS, Riley III LH, editors: *An atlas of surgery of the spine*, London, 1998, Martin Dunitz Ltd.
31. Truumees E: Cervical spondylotic myelopathy and radiculopathy, *Instr Course Lect* 29:339–360, 2000.
32. Houser OW, Onofrio BM, Miller GM, et al.: Cervical spondylotic stenosis and myelopathy: evaluation with computed tomographic myelography, *Mayo Clin Proc* 69:557–563, 1994.
33. Ono K, Tada K, Yamamoto T: Cervical myelopathy secondary to multiple spondylotic protrusions: a clinicopathologic study, *Spine* 2:109–125, 1977.
34. Breig A, Turnbull I, Hassler O: Effects of mechanical stresses on the spinal cord in cervical spondylosis, *J Neurosurg* 25:45–56, 1966.
35. Mihara H, Ohnari K, Hachiya M, et al.: Cervical myelopathy caused by C3-C4 spondylosis in elderly patients: a radiographic analysis of pathogenesis, *Spine* 25:796–800, 2000.
36. Ferguson RJ, Caplan LR: Cervical spondylotic myelopathy, *Neurol Clin* 3:373–382, 1985.
37. Karadimas SK, Gatzounis G, Fehlings MG: Pathobiology of cervical spondylotic myelopathy, *Eur Spine J* 24(Suppl 2):132–138, 2015.
38. Nurick S: The pathogenesis of the spinal cord disorder associated with cervical spondylosis, *Brain* 95:87–100, 1972.
39. Sampath P, Bendebba M, Davis JD, et al.: Outcome of patients treated for cervical myelopathy: a prospective, multicenter study with independent clinical review, *Spine* 25:670–676, 2000.
40. Vaccaro AR, Anderson D: *Decision making in spinal care*, New York, 2007, Thieme.
41. Byrne TN, Waxman SG, Benzel EC: *Diseases of the spine and spinal cord*, Oxford, 2000, Oxford UP.
42. Darouiche RO: Spinal epidural abscess, *N Engl J Med* 355:2012–2020, 2006.
43. Shah NH, Roos KL: Spinal epidural abscess and paralytic mechanisms, *Curr Opin Neurol* 26:314–317, 2013.
44. Aebi M: Spinal metastasis in the elderly, *Eur Spine J* 12(Suppl 2):S202–S213, 2003.
45. Parkin DM, Pisani P, Ferlay J: Global cancer statistics, *CA Cancer J Clin* 49:33–64, 1999.
46. Patil CG, Lad SP, Santarelli J, et al.: National inpatient complications and outcomes after surgery for spinal metastasis from 1993-2002, *Cancer* 110:625–630, 2007.
47. Yoshihara H, Yoneoka D: Trends in the surgical treatment for spinal metastasis and the in-hospital patient outcomes in the United States from 2000 to 2009, *Spine* 14:1844–1849, 2014.
48. Gerszten PC, Mendel E, Yamada Y: Radiotherapy and radiosurgery for metastatic spine disease: what are the options, indications, and outcomes? *Spine* 34:S78–S92, 2009.
49. Harel R, Angelov L: Spine metastases: current treatments and future directions, *Eur J Cancer* 46:2696–2707, 2010.
50. Laufer I, Iorgulescu JB, Chapman T, et al.: Local disease control for spinal metastases following "separation surgery" and adjuvant hypofractionated or high-dose single-fraction stereotactic radiosurgery: outcome analysis in 186 patients, *J Neurosurg Spine* 18:207–214, 2013.
51. Sahgal A, Bilsky M, Chang EL, et al.: Stereotactic body radiotherapy for spinal metastases: current status, with a focus on its application in the postoperative patient, *J Neurosurg Spine* 14:151–166, 2011.
52. Patchell RA, Tibbs PA, Regine WF, et al.: Direct decompressive surgical resection in the treatment of spinal cord compression caused by metastatic cancer: a randomised trial, *Lancet* 366:643–648, 2005.
53. Romanelli P, Esposito V: The functional anatomy of neuropathic pain, *Neurosurg Clin N Am* 15:257–268, 2004.
54. Mackley RJ: Role of trigger points in the management of head, neck, and face pain, *Funct Orthod* 7:4–14, 1990.
55. Henderson CM, Hennessy RG, Shuey Jr HM, et al.: Posterior-lateral foraminotomy as an exclusive operative technique for cervical radiculopathy: a review of 846 consecutively operated cases, *Neurosurgery* 13:504–512, 1983.
56. Frøbert O, Fossgreen J, Søndergaard-Petersen J, et al.: Musculo-skeletal pathology in patients with angina pectoris and normal coronary angiograms, *J Intern Med* 245:237–246, 1999.
57. Hoffman JR, Mower WR, Wolfson AB, et al.: National Emergency X-Radiography Utilization Study Group validity of a set of clinical criteria to rule out injury to the cervical spine in patients with blunt trauma, *N Engl J Med* 343:94–99, 2000.
58. Sforza C, Grassi G, Fragnito N, et al.: Three-dimensional analysis of active head and cervical spine range of motion: effect of age in healthy male subjects, *Clin Biomech* 17:611–614, 2002.
59. Weinfeld RM, Olson PN, Maki DD, et al.: The prevalence of diffuse idiopathic skeletal hyperostosis (DISH) in two large American Midwest metropolitan hospital populations, *Skeletal Radiol* 26:222–225, 1997.
60. Davidson RI, Dunn EJ, Metzmaker JN: The shoulder abduction test in the diagnosis of radicular pain in cervical extradural compressive monoradiculopathies, *Spine* 6:441–446, 1981.
61. Gore DR, Sepic SB, Gardner GM: Roentgenographic findings of the cervical spine in asymptomatic people, *Spine* 11:521–524, 1986.
62. Levine MJ, Albert TJ, Smith MD: Cervical radiculopathy: diagnosis and nonoperative management, *J Am Acad Orthop Surg* 4:305–316, 1996.
63. Collins DN, Barnes CL, FitzRandolph RL: Cervical spine instability in rheumatoid patients having total hip or knee arthroplasty, *Clin Orthop Relat Res* 272:127–135, 1991.
64. Modic MT, Masaryk TJ, Mulopulos GP, et al.: Cervical radiculopathy: prospective evaluation with surface coil MR imaging, CT with metrizamide, and metrizamide myelography, *Radiology* 161:753–759, 1986.
65. Modic MT, Ross JS, Masaryk TJ: Imaging of degenerative disease of the cervical spine, *Clin Orthop Relat Res* 239:109–120, 1989.
66. Seitz JP, Unguez CE, Corbus HF, et al.: SPECT of the cervical spine in the evaluation of neck pain after trauma, *Clin Nucl Med* 20:667–673, 1995.
67. Waddell G: An approach to backache, *Br J Hosp Med* 28:187–190, 1982.
68. Kushner HL: Acute phase response, *Clin Aspects Autoimmunity* 3:20–30, 1989.
69. Gore DR, Sepic SB, Gardner GM, et al.: Neck pain: a long-term follow-up of 205 patients, *Spine* 12:1–5, 1987.
70. Saal JS, Saal JA, Yurth EF: Nonoperative management of herniated cervical intervertebral disc with radiculopathy, *Spine* 21:1877–1883, 1996.
71. Beebe FA, Barkin RL, Barkin S: A clinical and pharmacologic review of skeletal muscle relaxants for musculoskeletal conditions, *Am J Ther* 12:151–171, 2005.
72. Bronfort G, Evans R, Nelson B, et al: A randomized clinical trial of exercise and spinal manipulation for patients with chronic neck pain. *Spine* 26:788–797, discussion 798–799, 2001.
73. Gross AR, Kay T, Hondras M, et al.: Manual therapy for mechanical neck disorders: a systematic review, *Man Ther* 7:131–149, 2002.
74. Kay TM, Gross A, Goldsmith C, et al.: Exercises for mechanical neck disorders, *Cochrane Database Syst Rev* 3:CD004250, 2005.
75. Taimela S, Takala EP, Asklof T, et al.: Active treatment of chronic neck pain, *Spine* 25:1021–1027, 2000.
76. Waling K, Sundelin G, Ahlgren C, et al.: Perceived pain before and after three exercise programs: a controlled clinical trial of women with work-related trapezius myalgia, *Pain* 85:201–207, 2000.
77. Dagenais S, Haldeman S, Wooley JR: Intraligamentous injection of sclerosing solutions (prolotherapy) for spinal pain: a critical review of the literature, *Spine J* 5:310–328, 2005.
78. Irnich D, Behrens N, Molzen H, et al.: Randomised trial of acupuncture compared with conventional massage and "sham" laser acupuncture for treatment of chronic neck pain, *BMJ* 322:1574–1578, 2001.
79. Kroeling PL, Gross AR, Goldsmith CH, et al.: A Cochrane review of electrotherapy for mechanical neck disorders, *Spine* 30:E641–E648, 2005.
80. Niemisto L, Kalso E, Malmivaara A, et al.: Radiofrequency denervation for neck and back pain. A systematic review of randomized controlled trials, *Cochrane Database Syst Rev* 1:CD004058, 2003.

81. Carette S, Fehlings MG: Clinical practice. Cervical radiculopathy, *N Engl J Med* 353:392–399, 2005.
82. Riew KD, Yin Y, Gilula L, et al.: The effect of nerve-root injections on the need for operative treatment of lumbar radicular pain: a prospective, randomized, controlled, double-blind study, *J Bone Joint Surg Am* 82-A:1589–1593, 2000.
83. Abbasi AL, Malhotra G, Malanga G, et al.: Complications of interlaminar cervical epidural steroid injections: a review of the literature, *Spine* 32:2144–2151, 2007.
84. Malhotra GL, Abbasi A, Rhee M: Complications of transforaminal cervical epidural steroid injections, *Spine* 34:731–739, 2009.
85. Truumees E: Cervical spondylotic myelopathy and radiculopathy, *Instr Course Lect* 29:339–360, 2000.
86. Pellicci PM, Ranawat CS, Tsairis P, et al.: A prospective study of the progression of rheumatoid arthritis of the cervical spine, *J Bone Joint Surg Am* 63:342–350, 1981.
87. Marks JS, Sharp J: Rheumatoid cervical myelopathy, *Q J Med* 50:301–319, 1989.
88. Mansour M, Cheema GS, Naguwa SM, et al.: Ankylosing spondylitis: a contemporary perspective on diagnosis and treatment, *Semin Arthritis Rheum* 36:210–223, 2007.

49 Shoulder Pain

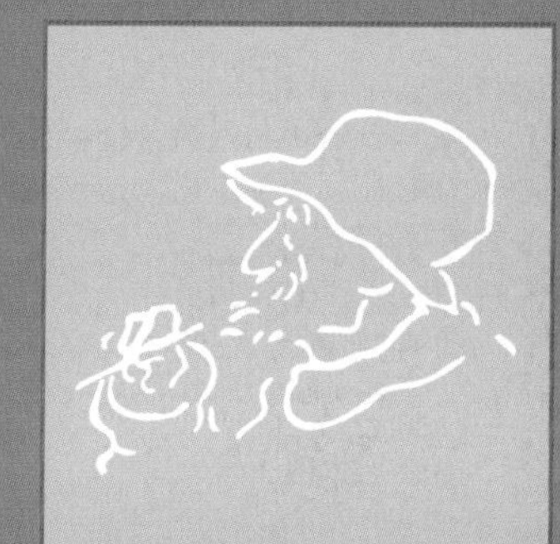

SCOTT DAVID MARTIN AND THOMAS S. THORNHILL

KEY POINTS

Comprehension of functional anatomy allows diagnosis of most causes of shoulder pain upon clinical examination.

History and clinical examination aided by ancillary tests will usually guide application of the most appropriate treatment for shoulder pain.

The differential diagnosis of shoulder pain includes common local disorders (e.g., of tendons and adjacent structures) and consideration of causes arising from distant anatomic sites via referred pain-mediated pathways.

A variety of specific diagnostic tests can greatly aid in the diagnosis of shoulder pain.

Most causes of shoulder pain can be treated with a structured physical therapy program. Successful treatment programs can benefit potential surgical candidates, including those who fail to respond to conservative treatment.

Systemic arthropathies occasionally present with shoulder disease and often involve the shoulder over time. Early assessment in such patients is essential.

Introduction

Shoulder pain, which is one of the most common musculoskeletal maladies, may arise from diverse causes. Accurate diagnosis of shoulder pain is made difficult by the unique anatomy and position of the shoulder, which serves as a link between the upper extremity and the thorax. One of the most complex and mobile joints of the body, the shoulder is traversed by muscle, tendon, and bone and is surrounded by major neurovascular structures, all of which may serve as potential sources of local and referred pain.

Determining the source of shoulder pain is essential in order to recommend the proper method of treatment. The examining physician must be able to differentiate the occurrence of shoulder pain caused by intrinsic or local factors, extrinsic or remote factors, or a combination of the two. Intrinsic factors originate from the shoulder girdle and include glenohumeral and periarticular disorders, whereas extrinsic factors occur outside of the shoulder girdle with secondary referral of pain to the shoulder (Table 49.1). An example of an extrinsic factor is left shoulder pain as the initial presentation of coronary artery disease. Hepatic, gallbladder, and splenic disease also may manifest initially as shoulder pain.

Accurate evaluation, diagnosis, and treatment require a thorough understanding of shoulder anatomy, including pain referral patterns. A complete and systematic physical examination is crucial for an accurate diagnosis. During the initial evaluation, care must be taken to discern all possible causes of shoulder pain. The final diagnosis may require repeated office examinations and correlation of diagnostic tests with symptoms, along with response to selective injections. Improvements in diagnostic tests, such as MRI, CT-arthrography, ultrasonography, and electromyography (EMG), have facilitated early diagnosis of shoulder pain and have provided a better understanding of shoulder disease. This chapter provides practical guidelines for the diagnosis and treatment of painful shoulder disorders that may be encountered in a rheumatology or general practice. A detailed analysis of shoulder problems and information on the treatment of major trauma are beyond the scope of this chapter and have been addressed by other authors.

Anatomy and Function

Because of the shoulder's complexity, clinicians treating shoulder pain must have an understanding of the structural and functional anatomy of this joint. The shoulder is the most mobile joint of the body, although this mobility is gained at the sacrifice of stability. Only 25% of the humeral head surface has contact with the glenoid at any time. The labrum increases the contact area of the articular surface and confers stability to the joint.[1] Lesions of the labrum may result from instability, and the type of lesion may indicate the type of instability. Labral tears also may be a source of pain from internal derangement of the shoulder.[2] Joint stability is provided by a thin capsule and by the glenohumeral ligaments, which are thickenings of the capsule anteriorly, posteriorly, and inferiorly.[1] Anterior stability is predominantly conferred by the anterior band of the inferior glenohumeral ligament.

The rotator cuff, which provides dynamic stability of the joint, is composed of four musculotendinous units: the supraspinatus, infraspinatus, and teres minor posteriorly, and the subscapularis anteriorly. The shoulder consists of three joints: the acromioclavicular (AC), sternoclavicular, and glenohumeral joints, and two gliding planes—the scapulothoracic and subacromial surfaces.

Fig. 49.1 shows the musculoskeletal and topographic localization of pain associated with common shoulder disorders. Fig. 49.2 shows the relationship of the three posterior rotator cuff muscles coursing anteriorly underneath the acromion to insert on the greater tuberosity. The subscapularis, the only anterior rotator cuff muscle, inserts on the lesser tuberosity. By understanding the relationship between the rotator cuff and the subacromial region, bounded inferiorly by the humeral head and superiorly by the undersurface of the acromion, the clinician can visualize the problems of impingement syndrome and administer an injection into this space with accuracy. Knowledge of the route of the tendon of the long head of the biceps through the bicipital groove and onto the superior aspect of the glenoid helps in understanding

TABLE 49.1 Common Causes of Shoulder Pain

Common Causes of Shoulder Pain
Intrinsic Causes
Periarticular Disorders
Rotator cuff tendinitis or impingement syndrome
Calcific tendinitis
Rotator cuff tear
Bicipital tendinitis
Acromioclavicular arthritis
Glenohumeral Disorders
Inflammatory arthritis
Osteoarthritis
Osteonecrosis
Cuff arthropathy
Septic arthritis
Glenoid labral tears
Adhesive capsulitis
Glenohumeral instability
Extrinsic Causes
Regional Disorders
Cervical radiculopathy
Brachial neuritis
Nerve entrapment syndromes
Sternoclavicular arthritis
Reflex sympathetic dystrophy
Fibrositis
Neoplasms
Renal osteodystrophy
Miscellaneous
• Gallbladder disease
• Splenic trauma
• Subphrenic abscess
• Myocardial infarction
• Thyroid disease
• Diabetes mellitus

bicipital tendinitis. Before attempting to diagnose and treat shoulder pain, the clinician should review in detail one of the many sources describing the structural and functional relationships of the shoulder girdle.[3,4]

Diagnosis

Clinical Evaluation of the Shoulder

Accurate diagnosis and successful treatment of a shoulder disorder begin with a thorough history and physical examination. Most of the information needed to make a correct diagnosis can be elicited with basic clinical skills, rather than by relying on expensive and highly technologic investigative aids when it will not affect the treatment plan.[5] Diagnostic tests should be used only to confirm an established diagnosis or to assist in cases with a challenging presentation.

History

When establishing a diagnosis, it is important to consider the patient's age and chief reason for presenting. The differential diagnosis of shoulder pain in a 70-year-old sedentary person is entirely different from that in a 20-year-old athlete. Did the pain occur slowly over time, or suddenly after a particular event? Gradual onset of pain over the anterolateral or deltoid region that is increased with forward elevation of the shoulder, along with nocturnal pain, suggests impingement with rotator cuff tendinopathy. The presence of significant weakness with pain upon engaging in overhead actions suggests impingement with a rotator cuff tear. Pain and weakness also may be noted upon reaching behind the back with the shoulder in extension and external rotation, as when reaching into the back seat of a car. Initiating factors relative to the onset of symptoms should be elicited, and any history of shoulder pain or trauma should be carefully documented.

Pain intensity, character, location, and periodicity and aggravating or alleviating factors should be assessed. Pain should be graded on a visual analog scale of 0 to 10, with 0 indicating no pain and 10 indicating the worst pain the patient has ever experienced. Another indication of the severity of pain is disruption of sleep; the patient should be asked if the pain prevents sleep or awakens the patient and if he or she can lie on the affected shoulder. The patient also should be asked if the pain is sharp or dull. Sharp, burning pain over the top of the shoulder indicates a neurogenic origin, whereas a dull, aching pain over the lateral deltoid suggests rotator cuff disease with impingement. The location or distribution of the pain should be identified: Is it local around the shoulder girdle, or does the pain radiate down the arm? Is concomitant sensory loss or weakness present? Periodicity of the pain as constant or intermittent should be determined, along with factors that aggravate or alleviate the pain. Pain caused by rotator cuff tendinopathy usually is exacerbated by repetitive activities that involve the elbow away from the side of the body.

Any history of neck pain should be considered, along with a history of radicular pain. Radicular-type pain frequently extends below the elbow and is associated with sensory loss and weakness. Pain located in the paracervical region may indicate a cervical origin, or it can be localized to the trapezius. Trapezial pain often is associated with shoulder pain and results from the patient trying to favor the shoulder. Assuming a military brace position may produce fatigue, spasm, and trigger points of the trapezius and levator scapulae muscle.

Any pertinent medical history, such as a history of malignancy, should be considered. Neurologic, visceral, and vascular disease can produce referred pain to the shoulder and should always be considered, especially in a patient with painless range of motion.

Physical Examination

Proper physical examination of the shoulder includes close inspection of the shoulder girdle from the front and back. The evaluation is started by standing behind the patient, who has both shoulders exposed. The normal shoulder is always inspected and compared with the injured shoulder. Examination can be performed with the patient in the sitting or standing position. Contour and symmetry are observed and compared between shoulders, and any atrophy or asymmetry in shoulder position or level is assessed. Spinatus muscle atrophy may result from disuse, chronic cuff tear, or suprascapular or brachial neuropathy.[6] If scapular winging is evident, the patient should be asked to perform a wall push-up, which accentuates winging.

Range of motion should be carefully recorded, along with notation of any absence of rhythmic shoulder motion or excessive scapulothoracic motion that may compensate for the lack of glenohumeral motion. Internal rotation of the shoulder is checked by having the patient reach behind his or her back with the thumb while the examiner notices the vertebral level. Loss of internal rotation is seen early with shoulder pain and usually indicates some tightness of the posterior shoulder capsule, also called

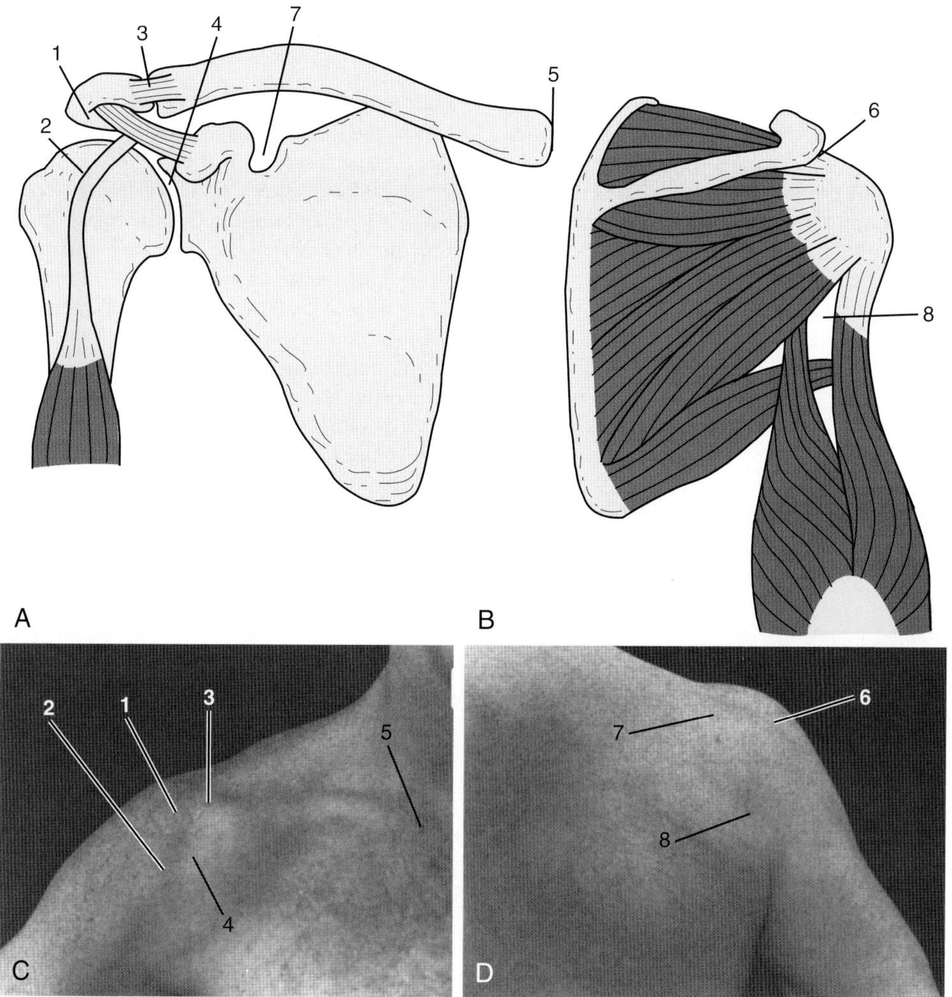

• **Fig. 49.1** Musculoskeletal (A and B) and topographic (C and D) areas localizing pain and tenderness associated with specific shoulder problems. *1,* Subacromial space (rotator cuff tendinitis/impingement syndrome, calcific tendinitis, and rotator cuff tear). *2,* Bicipital groove (bicipital tendinitis, biceps tendon subluxation, and tear). *3,* Acromioclavicular joint. *4,* Anterior glenohumeral joint (glenohumeral arthritis, osteonecrosis, glenoid labrum tears, and adhesive capsulitis). *5,* Sternoclavicular joint. *6,* Posterior edge of acromion (rotator cuff tendinitis, calcific tendinitis, and rotator cuff tear). *7,* Suprascapular notch (suprascapular nerve entrapment). *8,* Quadrilateral space (axillary nerve entrapment). These areas of pain and tenderness frequently overlap.

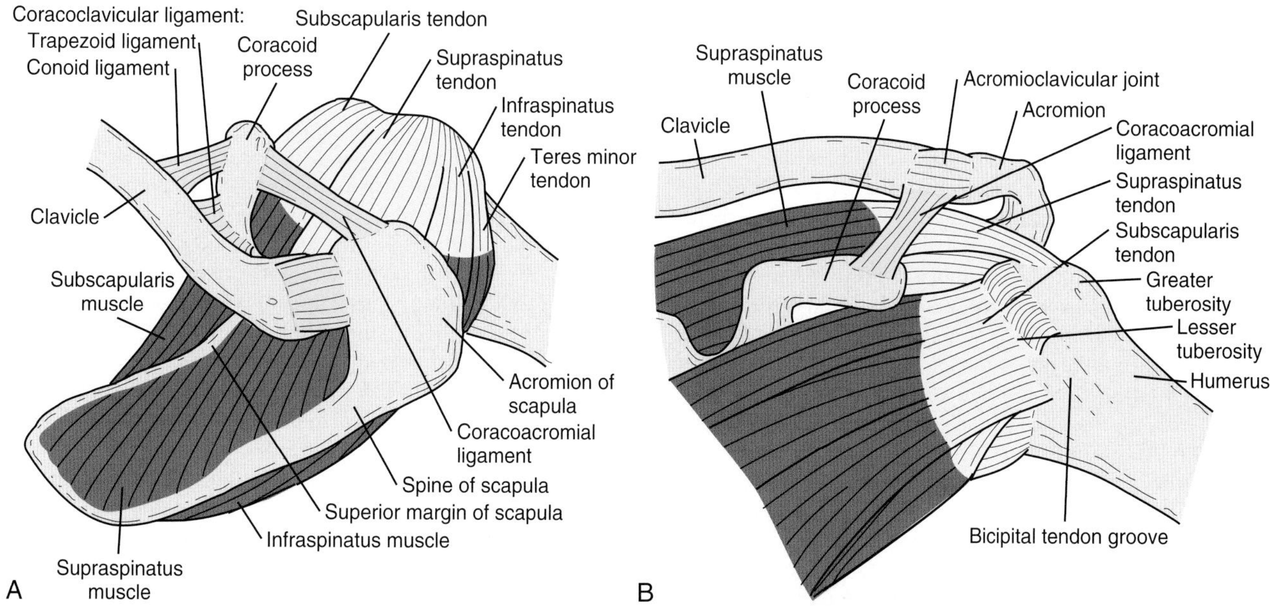

• **Fig. 49.2** (A) Superior view of the rotator cuff musculature as it courses anteriorly underneath the coracoacromial arch to insert on the greater tuberosity. (B) Anterior view of the shoulder reveals the subscapularis, which is the only anterior rotator cuff muscle inserting on the lesser tuberosity. It internally rotates the humerus and provides dynamic anterior stability to the shoulder. (From *The Ciba collection of medical illustrations,* Volume 8, Part I. Netter Illustration from www.netterimages.com. Copyright Elsevier Inc. All rights reserved.)

GIRD (glenohumeral internal rotation deficit). The biceps tendon is palpated, along with the coracoid, lesser and greater tuberosities, and the posterior cuff, and any tenderness is gauged (Fig. 49.3A). Tenderness upon palpation of the long head of the biceps is frequently associated with rotator cuff tendinopathy and tenderness of the greater tuberosity. Any spasm or tenderness of the trapezius or levator scapulae may be associated with rotator cuff or cervical spine disease. Cervical range of motion is evaluated, and the paracervical muscles are palpated. Paracervical tenderness and limited range of motion of the neck may indicate cervical spondylosis or neurogenic disease. A Spurling test is performed by flexing the neck laterally while applying axial compression to the skull. Pain that radiates to the ipsilateral shoulder is considered a positive test result and indicates radiculopathy.

To elicit the impingement sign, the shoulder is elevated passively in forward flexion while the scapula is depressed with the opposite hand, forcing the greater tuberosity against the anterior acromion and producing pain in cases of impingement (see Fig. 49.3B).[7] This maneuver also may be painful in the presence of conditions such as adhesive capsulitis, glenohumeral and AC arthritis, glenohumeral instability, and calcific tendinitis. A dynamic impingement test, known as the circumduction-adduction shoulder maneuver (also called the Clancy test), is 95% sensitive and 95% specific for diagnosing rotator cuff tendinopathy, including partial tears.[8] The test is performed with the patient in the standing position, with the head turned to the contralateral shoulder. The affected shoulder is circumducted and adducted across the body to shoulder level while the elbow is kept in extension, the shoulder is in internal rotation, and the thumb is pointing toward the floor (see Fig. 49.3C). In this position, the patient is instructed to resist maximally as a uniform downward force is applied to the extended arm by the examiner. The test result is considered positive if pain or weakness is elicited during the maneuver, with pain localized to the anterolateral aspect of the shoulder. A strong positive correlation of pain and weakness is noted with a complete cuff tear.[8]

The sternoclavicular and AC joints should be observed for prominences and palpated for stability and tenderness. Many patients with impingement have tenderness upon direct downward palpation of the AC joint as a result of impingement on the cuff from undersurface osteophytes of the distal clavicle.[3,6]

AC joint tenderness also may result from primary AC joint arthrosis and should be differentiated by physical examination, including the cross-chest adduction test and O'Brien's test.[9] Radiographic evidence of AC joint arthrosis is common in patients older than 40 years, but this condition usually is not painful.[10]

The cross-chest adduction test or the horizontal adduction test is performed by forward flexing the shoulder 90 degrees with subsequent cross-chest adduction of the arm (see Fig. 49.3D). Pain localized to the AC joint is considered a positive test result. If pain occurs posteriorly over the shoulder, a tight posterior capsule with impingement is suspected. O'Brien's test is performed by forward flexing the arm 90 degrees and adducting the arm 10 degrees out of the sagittal plane of the body. The first part of the test is performed with the hand maximally pronated with the thumb pointed down. In this position, the patient is asked to resist as the examiner applies a downward force on the arm. If the test elicits pain, the patient is asked if the pain is on top of the shoulder or deep inside. Pain localized to the top of the shoulder indicates AC joint pain, and pain deep inside the shoulder indicates a superior labrum anterior posterior (SLAP) lesion. In the second part of the test, the patient is asked to supinate the hand maximally, while the examiner applies a downward force to the arm. If the patient notices significantly less pain, the test result is positive for a SLAP lesion. If the pain is unchanged and is located on top of the shoulder, the test result is positive for AC joint disease.[9]

If the cause of AC joint tenderness is still in question, a lidocaine injection should be administered. The clinician should carefully avoid injecting the lidocaine into the subacromial space by advancing the needle too far inferiorly through the AC joint, which can lead to a false interpretation. Painful degenerative changes of the AC joint may exist concomitantly with subacromial impingement and should be evaluated thoroughly when surgical treatment (i.e., distal clavicle excision) is being considered.[11]

In patients with pain out of proportion to objective findings, other causes of shoulder pain should be sought, including calcific tendinitis, infection, reflex sympathetic dystrophy, and fracture. Patients with significant wasting of the supraspinatus and infraspinatus muscles and posterior shoulder pain, especially younger patients, may have suprascapular neuropathy or brachial neuropathy (Parsonage-Turner syndrome).[6,12]

Patients with chronic cuff disease frequently have variable disuse atrophy of the supraspinatus and infraspinatus fossae. In cases of chronic massive cuff tears, atrophy and weakness can be severe. Strength testing of external rotation should be performed with the elbow at the side and supported by the examiner; the patient is asked to attempt external rotation of the shoulder from a neutral position (0 degrees of adduction) while the examiner applies resistance (see Fig. 49.3E).[13] Weakness in this position may suggest a tear of the infraspinatus tendon. Abduction strength testing against resistance is performed with the shoulder in 30 degrees of forward flexion and 90 degrees of abduction and with the thumb pointed toward the floor (see Fig. 49.3F).[14,15] Weakness in this position may suggest a tear of the supraspinatus tendon. A lift-off test should be performed with the shoulder in internal rotation; the patient is asked to try to hold his or her hand away from the back. Inability to do so indicates a subscapularis tear.

If impingement is suspected after a thorough physical examination, an impingement test should be performed with injection of 5 mL of a local anesthetic into the subacromial space.[16,17] Before the test is performed, the patient is asked to grade the pain during the impingement signs on a visual analog scale of 0 to 10, with 0 equal to no pain and 10 equal to the most severe pain the patient has ever experienced. The injection may be performed anteriorly, laterally, or posteriorly, depending on the physician's preference. Ten minutes after injection of a local anesthetic into the subacromial space, the patient should be re-examined and asked to grade the pain again on the same visual analog scale. A 50% or greater reduction in pain is thought to be a positive test result for impingement; otherwise, an alternative cause of shoulder pain should be sought, or inadequate placement of the anesthetic should be suspected. If the AC joint is thought to be contributing to the shoulder pain, 1 to 2 mL of a local anesthetic should be injected into the joint, and the shoulder should be re-examined. When subacromial impingement and the AC joint are thought to be contributing to shoulder pain, serial injections during separate office visits may be required to evaluate the shoulder while minimizing discomfort to the patient.[10]

In cases of suspected bicipital tendinitis, Speed's test is performed by having the patient flex the shoulder and extend the elbow while a downward force is applied to the arm. The production of pain over the long head of the biceps is a positive test result and suggests bicipital tendinitis.

Upper extremity strength testing should be performed and compared with the contralateral side so that any atrophy is

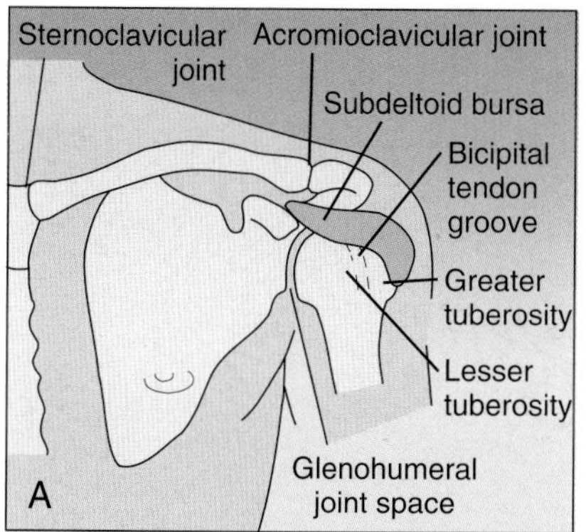

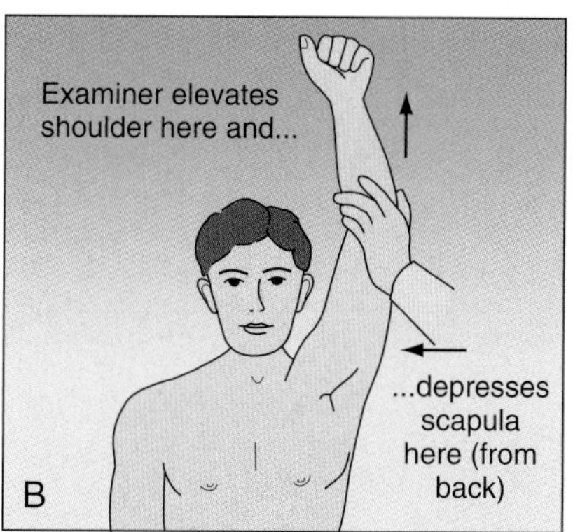

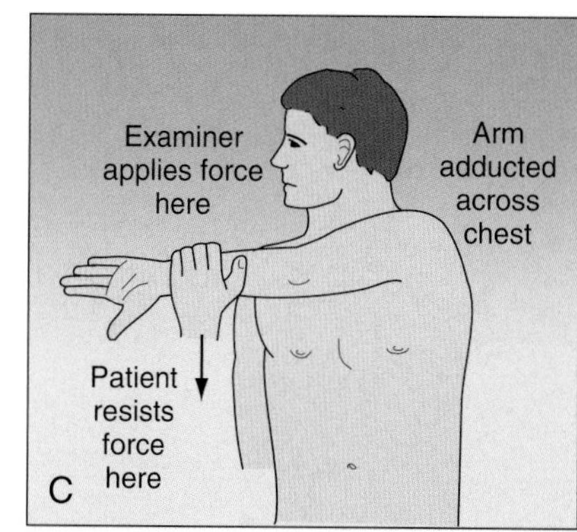

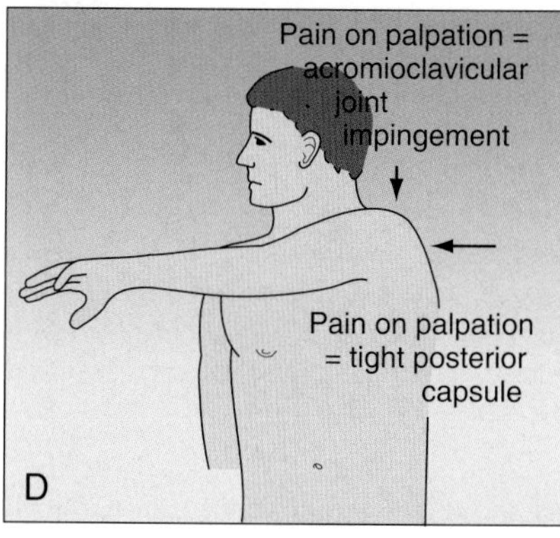

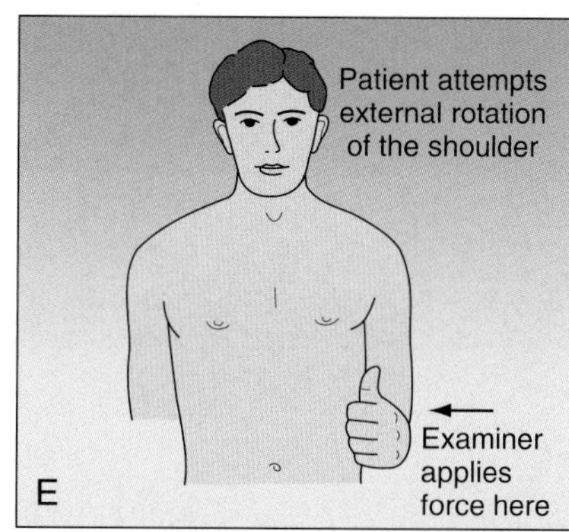

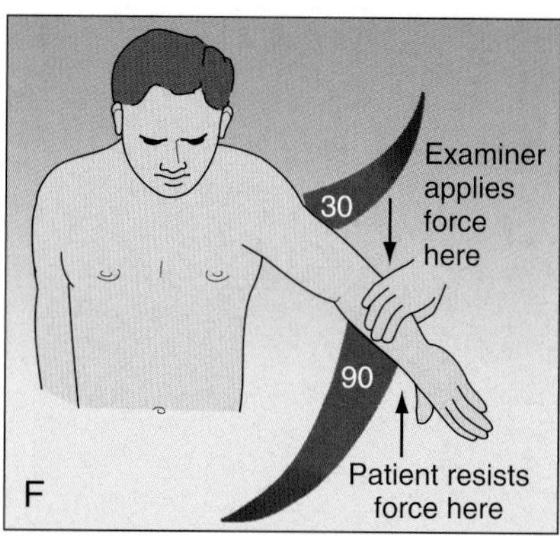

• **Fig. 49.3** (A) Tenderness upon palpation of trigger points may help localize the site of disease. Tenderness upon palpation of the long head of the biceps and greater tuberosity suggests impingement with possible cuff tendinopathy. (B) To elicit the impingement sign, the shoulder is elevated in forward flexion while the scapula is depressed with the opposite hand, forcing the greater tuberosity and the rotator cuff against the anterior acromion and producing pain when impingement exists. Relief of pain after injection of local anesthetics (i.e., the impingement test) provides additional evidence of subacromial disease. (C) The Clancy test is performed with the patient standing and with the head turned toward the contralateral shoulder. The affected shoulder is circumducted and adducted across the body to shoulder level, keeping the elbow in extension with the arm internally rotated with the thumb pointed toward the floor. In this position, the patient is asked to resist maximally as a uniform downward force is applied to the extended arm by the examiner. Production of pain or weakness localized to the anterior lateral portion of the shoulder is considered a positive test result. (D) The test is performed by forward flexion of the arm at 90 degrees and subsequent cross-chest adduction of the arm. Pain localized to the acromioclavicular joint is considered a positive test result. (E) The test is performed with the patient's elbow flexed at 90 degrees and held at the patient's side by the examiner. The patient is asked to attempt external rotation of the shoulder from a neutral position (0 degrees of adduction) as the examiner applies resistance to the forearm. Strength is compared with that of the contralateral arm. (F) Abduction strength testing is performed with the patient's shoulder in 30 degrees of forward flexion and 90 degrees of abduction and with the thumb pointed toward the floor. The patient is asked to resist as the examiner exerts a downward force on the abducted arm. Strength is compared with the contralateral shoulder. (From Martin TL, Martin SD: Rotator cuff tendinopathy. *Hosp Med* 12:23–31, 1998.)

detected. Grip strength is checked, and the hands are examined carefully for evidence of intrinsic atrophy. The biceps (C5), triceps (C7), and brachioradialis (C6) reflexes are checked for symmetry and briskness.

Light touch sensory testing should be conducted, and the dermatomal distribution of any deficits that may suggest that cervical radiculopathy should be identified. The cervical, supraclavicular, axillary, and epitrochlear regions should be palpated for enlarged lymph nodes, which may suggest malignancy.

Imaging

Radiographic Assessment

For nontraumatic painful shoulder evaluation, standard radiographic profiles are used. An impingement series should be obtained that includes anteroposterior views with a 30-degree caudal tilt (Rockwood view), an outlet view (scapular Y with a 10- to 15-degree caudal tilt), and an axillary view. Internal and external rotational views may be obtained if calcific tendinitis or instability is suspected. The Rockwood view can reveal any osteophytes off the anterior acromion and AC joint.[18] In cases of traumatic injury, a trauma series is obtained that includes a true anteroposterior view, a scapular Y view, and an axillary view. The axillary view is useful in assessing posterior or anterior subluxation of the humeral head and assessment of joint space narrowing. Additional views, such as the West Point view, which evaluates the glenoid for evidence of a bony Bankart lesion, or the Styker notch view, which assesses the humeral head for a Hill-Sachs lesion, may be obtained to assist in the evaluation if the diagnosis of instability is in doubt. Secondary impingement-type rotator cuff tendinitis

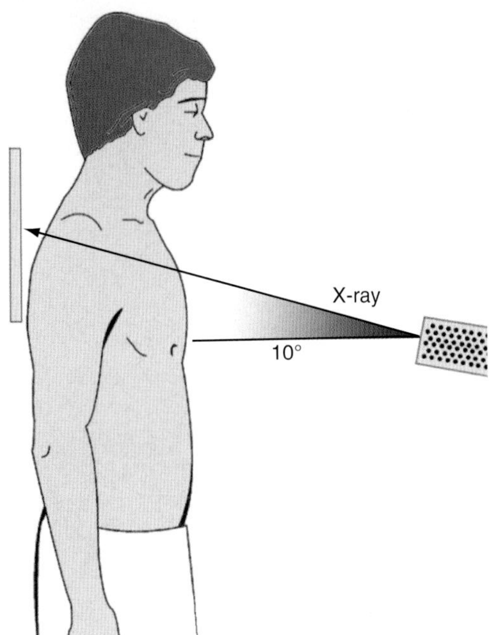

• **Fig. 49.4** The Zanca view of the acromioclavicular joint is obtained with a 10-degree cephalic tilt and 50% penetrance. (From Rockwood CA Jr, Young DC: Disorders of the acromioclavicular joint. In Rockwood CA Jr, Matsen TA III, editors: *The shoulder*. Philadelphia, 1985, WB Saunders, pp 413–476.)

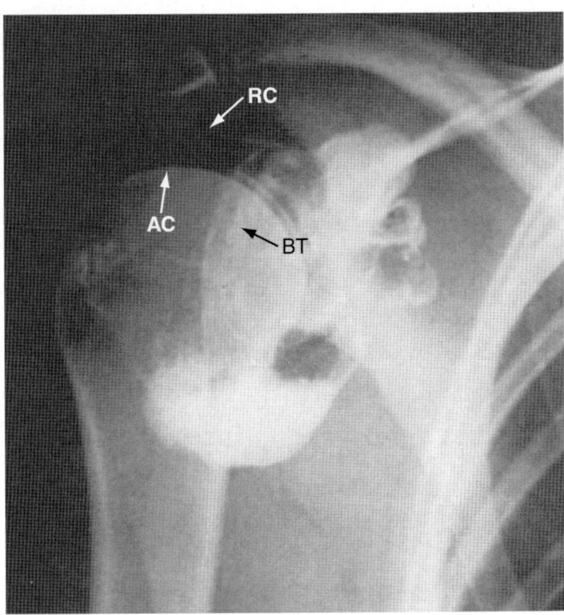

• **Fig. 49.5** Normal double-contrast arthrography shows the inferior edge of the rotator cuff (RC) as it courses through the subacromial space to the greater tuberosity, the tendon of the long head of the biceps (BT), and the articular cartilage of the humeral head (AC).

may be caused by increased anterior translation with subluxation of the humeral head. In such cases, an axillary view or fluoroscopy can help show the subluxation.[19,20]

When AC joint disease is suspected, a 10-degree, cephalic tilt view of the AC joint at 50% penetrance, as described by Zanca,[21] should be obtained (Fig. 49.4). Stress views of the AC joint may be obtained by strapping 5- to 10-lb weights to the patient's forearms and determining AC separation. Comparing the coracoclavicular distance of both shoulders may be helpful. When clinically indicated, cervical spine radiographs should be obtained to exclude cervical spondylosis as a cause of shoulder pain, especially when radicular symptoms of numbness or tingling are present.

Scintigraphy

Technetium 99m (Tc 99m) methyl diphosphonate (MDP) or gallium may be of diagnostic help in evaluating skeletal lesions in the area of the shoulder joint. Bone scans generally are not helpful in the diagnosis of non-neoplastic or noninfectious shoulder disease.

Scintigraphy may have a role in identifying patients with complete rotator cuff tears that evolved to cuff-tear arthropathy. This distinction is important because patients with complete rotator cuff tears may do well, whereas patients who experience progressive changes of cuff-tear arthropathy have progressive arthritis, pain, and significant functional impairment. Synovitis or calcium pyrophosphate deposition disease may be an important factor in the pathogenesis of cuff-tear arthropathy. In such cases, scintigraphy may show the increased blood flow and blood pooling associated with chronic synovitis.

Arthrography

Double-contrast arthrotomography (DCAT) can be used to evaluate problems of the rotator cuff, glenoid labrum, biceps tendon, and shoulder capsule.[22–25] Fig. 49.5 shows normal DCAT of the shoulder. Rotator cuff tears can be shown by single-contrast or double-contrast studies. Proponents of double-contrast arthrography believe that the extent of the tear, the preferred surgical approach, and the quality of the rotator cuff tissue are best determined by double-contrast studies.[22–27] Arthrography without MRI or CT can be misleading and may result in underestimation of the extent of a rotator cuff tear. Multidetector CT can enhance the accuracy of diagnosing labral and rotator cuff tears, especially in patients for whom MRI is not possible (Fig. 49.6).

Tears of the glenoid labrum without shoulder dislocation are sources of anterior shoulder pain in athletes.[2] Glenoid labrum tears (Fig. 49.7), with or without associated glenohumeral subluxation, frequently can be identified by DCAT.[25,26] One study[28] described 55 patients who underwent DCAT followed by diagnostic shoulder arthroscopy. DCAT predicted the arthroscopic findings in 76% of anterior labrum studies and 96% of posterior labrum studies. This test was 100% sensitive and 94% specific in diagnosing complete rotator cuff tears. Partial rotator cuff tears identified at arthroscopy were missed in 83% of patients who underwent DCAT. Investigators believed that DCAT was more effective in diagnosing intra-articular and cuff disease in cases of instability than when pain alone was the presenting diagnosis.[28]

Shoulder arthrography can confirm a diagnosis of adhesive capsulitis by showing a contracted capsule with an obliterated axillary recess (Fig. 49.8). The use of subacromial bursography has been beneficial in visualizing the outer surface of the rotator cuff and the subacromial space in cases of impingement.[29,30] Fukuda and associates[31] reported a small series of younger patients (average age, 41.8 years) who underwent subacromial bursography after a negative glenohumeral arthrographic result. These patients showed pooling of contrast medium on the bursal side of a tear, which was confirmed at the time of surgery. Subacromial bursography is not routinely used diagnostically and, in our opinion, it is of little value in planning surgical procedures.

Computed Tomography

CT is helpful in evaluating the musculoskeletal system, and CT combined with contrast arthrography (CT-arthrography) has

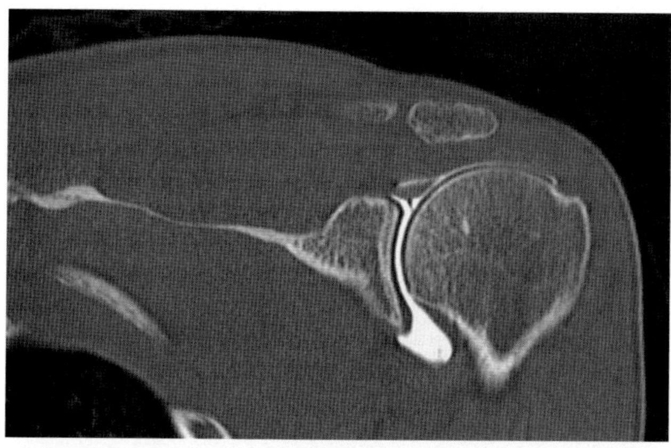

• **Fig. 49.6** Multidetector CT reveals a superior labral tear of the shoulder.

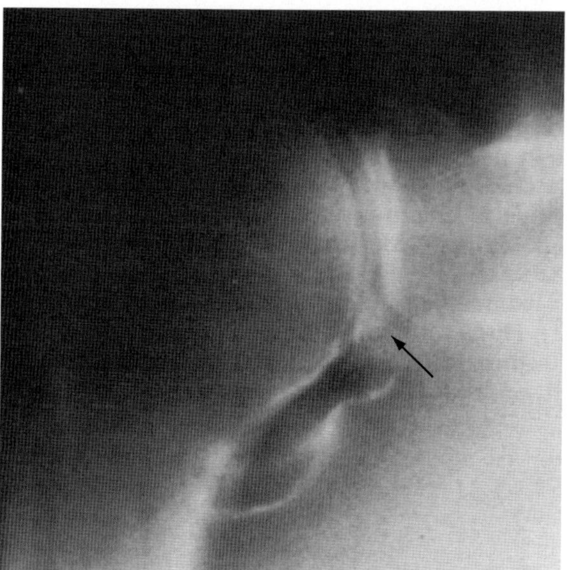

• **Fig. 49.7** Double-contrast arthrotomography shows a tear of the anterior-inferior portion of the glenoid labrum *(arrow)*.

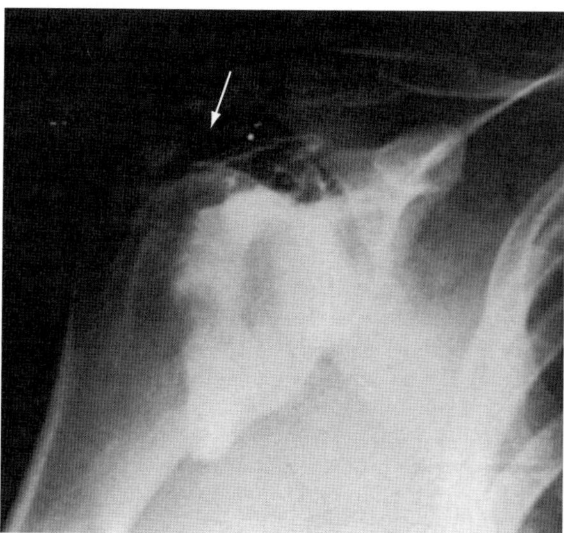

• **Fig. 49.8** Double-contrast arthrography of a patient with calcific tendinitis *(arrow)* and adhesive capsulitis. Notice the contracted capsule with diminution of the synovial space and obliteration of the axillary recess.

become a major diagnostic tool for the evaluation of glenoid labrum tears, loose bodies, and chondral lesions (Fig. 49.9). One study[32] reported using CT-arthrography in an evaluation of shoulder derangement and found 95% accuracy of CT-arthrography for investigating lesions of the labrum and articular surface.[33] More recently, multidetector CT-arthrography scans have been used to evaluate partial cuff tears (Fig. 49.10A), cystic lesions (see Fig. 49.10B), and calcific tendinopathy (see Fig. 49.10C).

Ultrasonography

Technologic improvements in ultrasound equipment have led to improved ultrasound study of the rotor cuff. The technique is noninvasive and rapid and involves no radiation exposure.[28–30,34] The cuff is examined in the horizontal and transverse planes with the arm in different positions to allow visualization of various areas of the cuff. These techniques generally provide visualization of the distal cuff, where most rotator cuff tears are located. Fig. 49.11 shows normal and abnormal ultrasound images of the rotator cuff in longitudinal and transverse planes.

Several studies report high sensitivity and specificity for the diagnosis of a rotator cuff tear by ultrasound.[30–32,34] The specificity and sensitivity of the procedure are reported to be greater than 90% as determined by arthrographic and surgical correlations.[32,34] This technique has also been used for the post-operative evaluation of a rotator cuff repair and for evaluation of abnormalities of the biceps tendon.[33,35–38]

Gardelin and Perin[39] reported ultrasound to be 96% sensitive in determining rotator cuff and biceps tendon disease. Mack and associates[35] found ultrasound to be valuable in evaluating post-operative patients with recurrent shoulder symptoms. One prospective study[37] compared ultrasound with MRI and arthrography in evaluating rotator cuff lesions in 24 shoulders. Ultrasound identified 14 of 15 torn cuffs, MRI identified 10 of 15, and arthrography identified 15 of 15.[37] Ultrasound identified 7 of 9 intact rotator cuffs, whereas MRI was accurate in 8 of 9 intact cuffs.[37] Another study[40] found ultrasound to be as accurate as MRI in the diagnosis of humeral head defects and joint effusions but inferior to MRI in the diagnosis of labrum lesions, rotator cuff lesions, subacromial spurs, and synovial inflammatory disease. In the hands of an experienced sonographer, ultrasound may be the most cost-effective test for the initial evaluation of a rotator cuff injury, but most surgeons require CT-arthrography or MRI confirmation before beginning surgical exploration.[35,37,39–41]

Magnetic Resonance Imaging

MRI has been used to diagnose partial-thickness and full-thickness rotator cuff tears (Fig. 49.12), biceps tendon tears, impingement of the rotator cuff, synovitis, articular cartilage damage, and labral disease associated with glenohumeral instability.[42–44] In rheumatoid arthritis (RA), MRI is reported to be more sensitive than plain radiographs in determining soft tissue abnormalities and osseous abnormalities of the glenoid and humeral head.[45]

One of the most valuable diagnostic uses of MRI is in rotator cuff disease. Morrison and Offstein[46] studied 100 patients with chronic subacromial impingement syndrome using arthrography and MRI. MRI was 100% sensitive but only 88% specific in confirming arthrography-proven rotator cuff tears. Nelson and associates[47] studied 21 patients with shoulder pain and found MRI to be more accurate than CT-arthrography or ultrasound in identifying partial-thickness cuff tears. These investigators also reported

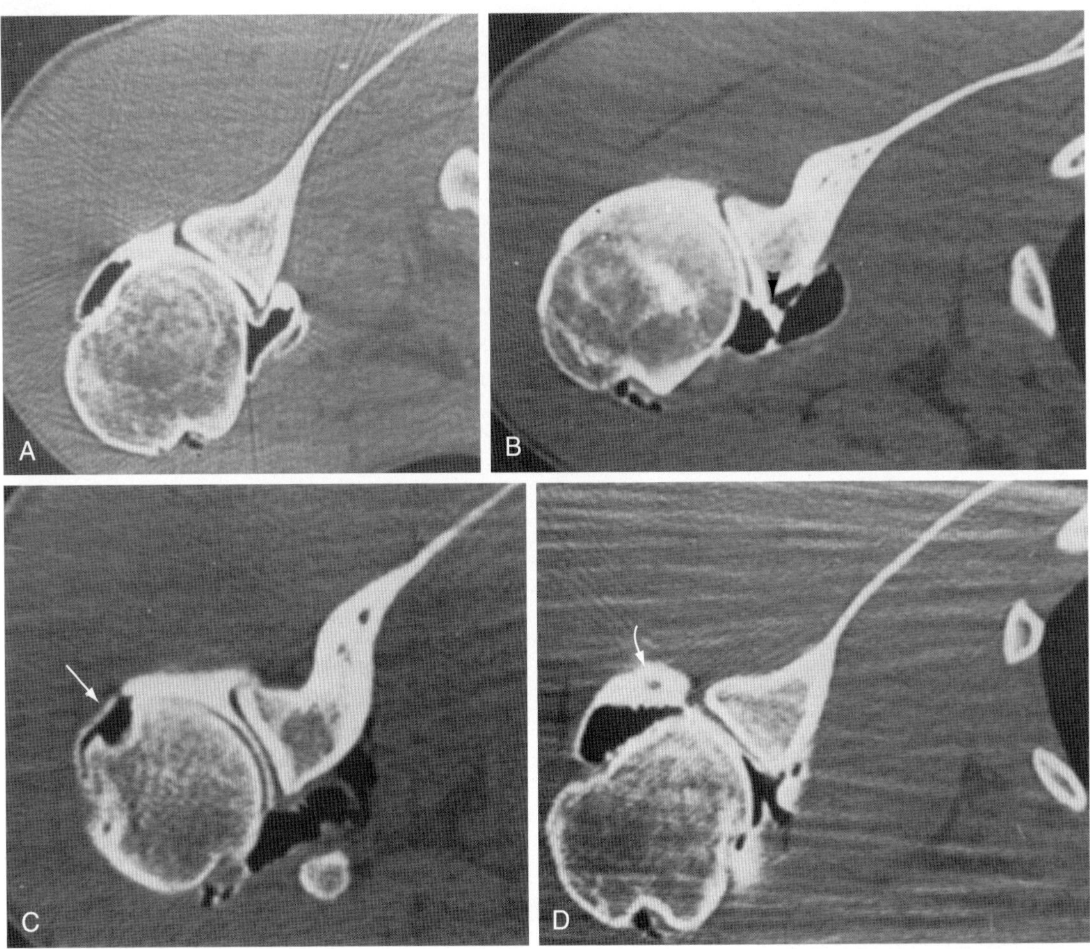

• **Fig. 49.9** CT–arthrography of the shoulder. (A) Normal findings. (B) A tear of the anterior glenoid labrum. (C) A large defect of the articular surface of the posterior portion of the humeral head (Hill-Sachs lesion) *(arrow).* (D) A loose body in the posterior recess *(arrow).*

MRI to be as accurate as CT-arthrography in the diagnosis of abnormalities of the glenoid labrum.[47]

Characteristic MRI findings in people with rotator cuff tears include a hypointense gap within the supraspinatus muscle tendon complex on T1-weighted films, absence of a demonstrable supraspinatus tendon with narrowing of the subacromial space, and an increased signal within the supraspinatus tendon on T2-weighted images.[48] A report[49] of 170 MRI studies found that T1-weighted images were highly sensitive for identifying abnormalities within the supraspinatus tendon but that T2-weighted images were required to differentiate tendinitis from a small supraspinatus tendon tear. However, large full-thickness tears could be identified on T1- and T2-weighted images. Fig. 49.13 depicts common shoulder disease as seen by MRI. Compared with scintigraphy, MRI is almost as sensitive and more specific in the diagnosis of osteonecrosis and neoplastic lesions in the shoulder area.

Arthroscopy

The use of arthroscopy for the diagnosis of shoulder disease increased in the 1980s, in part because of its accuracy, which was far greater than that of clinical examination and better than the accuracy of other diagnostic modalities of the time. With technologic advances in fiberoptics, video output, and arthroscopic instrumentation, the use of arthroscopy to diagnose and treat shoulder problems exponentially increased to include procedures previously used only for open techniques.[50]

Compared with DCAT, arthroscopy is more accurate in the diagnosis of intra-articular lesions associated with a painful shoulder.[28] An additional benefit is that arthroscopy can be used to diagnose and treat shoulder problems of the glenohumeral joint and the subacromial region. With increased accuracy of MRI-arthrography in detecting partial cuff tears and labral lesions, diagnostic shoulder arthroscopy has become less common in the absence of clear indications and specific treatment plans. In combination with a detailed history and physical examination, and along with examination under the effects of anesthesia, shoulder arthroscopy has been helpful in the diagnosis of chronic instability patterns of the glenohumeral joint.[50–53]

The indications and usefulness of shoulder arthroscopy in the treatment of common pathologic conditions have continued to increase as the technology improves and as understanding of the pathophysiology of shoulder problems grows. Shoulder arthroscopy has been used routinely to confirm and treat SLAP lesions, labral tears, partial cuff tears, refractory adhesive capsulitis, partial biceps tendon tears, and multidirectional instability. Other conditions that are routinely treated arthroscopically include rotator cuff tears, glenohumeral instability, AC joint disease, loose bodies, sepsis, osteochondritis dissecans, synovitis, chondral lesions, subacromial impingement, and calcific tendinitis.[2,11,50,53]

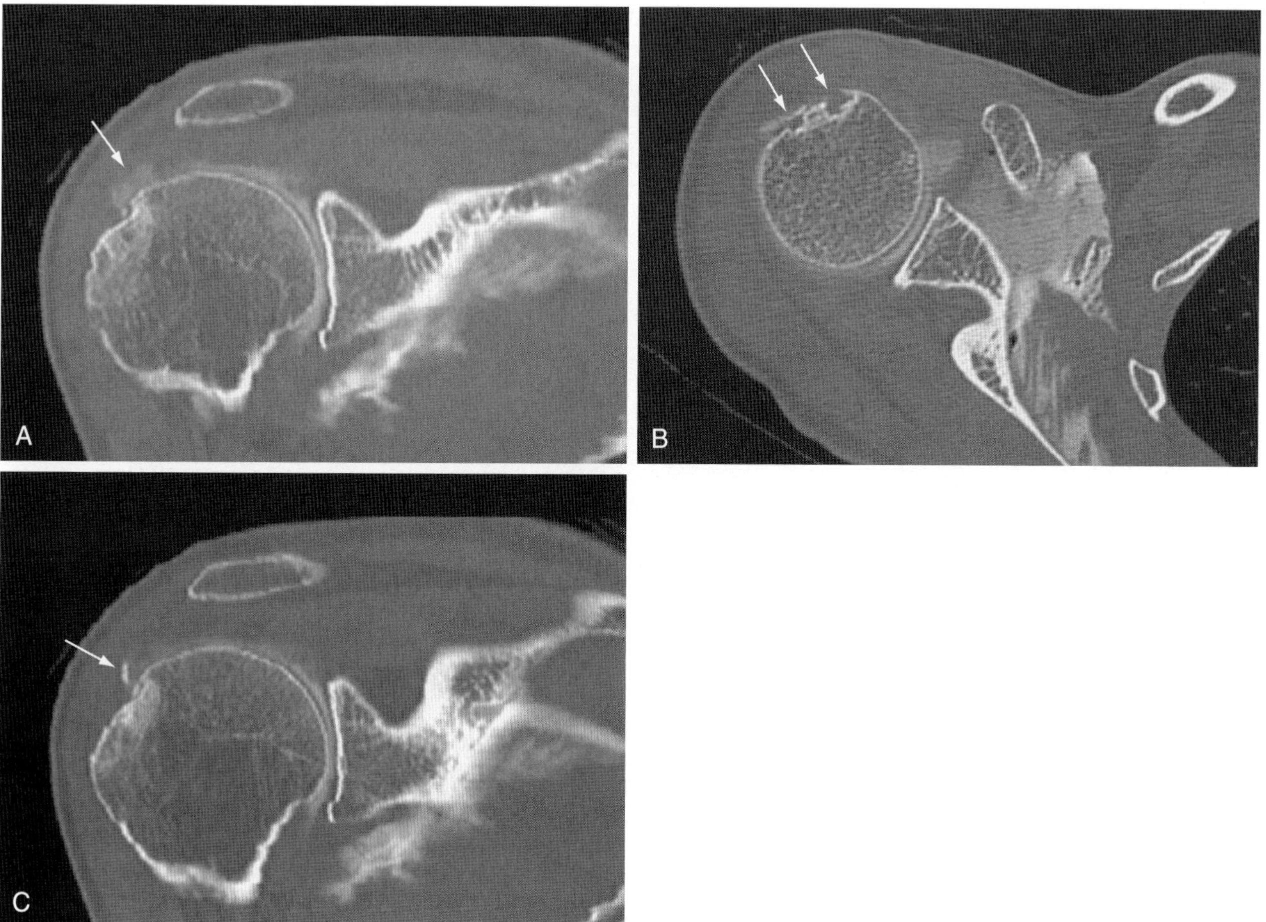

• **Fig. 49.10** Multidetector CT–arthrography. (A) A partial rotator cuff tear (coronal view) *(arrow)*. (B) Cystic humeral head erosions with calcification (axial view) *(arrows)*. (C) Calcification within rotator cuff tendon (coronal view) *(arrow)*.

Electromyography and Nerve Conduction Velocity Studies

EMG and nerve conduction velocity studies can help differentiate shoulder pain from pain of neurogenic origin. They also may be beneficial in determining the localization of neurogenic pain to a particular cervical root, the brachial plexus, or a peripheral nerve.[54,55]

Injection

Injection of local anesthetics and glucocorticoids is a useful technique for the diagnosis and treatment of shoulder pain.[56] The physician must have a thorough understanding of the anatomy of the shoulder girdle and a presumptive diagnosis to direct the injection properly. Injection of referred pain areas may be misleading. In a patient with lateral arm pain resulting from deltoid bursal involvement from calcific tendinitis of the supraspinatus tendon, the injection should be directed to the subacromial space, rather than the area of referred pain in the deltoid muscle. It is often better to use a posterior or lateral subacromial approach when performing an injection for rotator cuff tendinitis in a patient with anterior impingement symptoms because it is easier to enter the subacromial region posteriorly or laterally, and this approach is less traumatic for contracted anterior structures.

The instillation of rapidly acting local anesthetics can be beneficial in determining the source of shoulder pain. Obliteration of pain by injection of a local anesthetic along the bicipital groove can confirm a diagnosis of bicipital tendinitis. The use of local anesthetics is less helpful when the subacromial space is injected because of its extensive communication with the remainder of the shoulder girdle, but relief of symptoms after such an injection can exclude pain from conditions such as cervical radiculopathy or entrapment neuropathy.

Diagnostic Tests

Table 49.2 lists reimbursement and charges for various shoulder diagnostic tests based on 2014 Medicare fee schedules and 2014 charges at a single institution. The choice of a specific test depends on its sensitivity, specificity, and cost-benefit analysis. History and physical examination are the most important factors in establishing diagnosis of the painful shoulder. Plain radiographs (three views) should be the first radiographic tests performed. Although they are not as sensitive as the more sophisticated tests, plain radiographs can identify arthritic change, calcific tendinitis, established osteonecrosis, and most neoplasms.

If intra-articular disease (e.g., a labrum tear, capsular tear, loose body, or chondral defect) is suspected, MRI-arthrography is preferable to CT-arthrography. In diagnosing acute rotator cuff tears in a younger patient, ultrasound is the most cost-effective test to confirm a clinical suspicion. In cases of impingement syndrome, MRI is sensitive, but it is difficult to differentiate tendinitis,

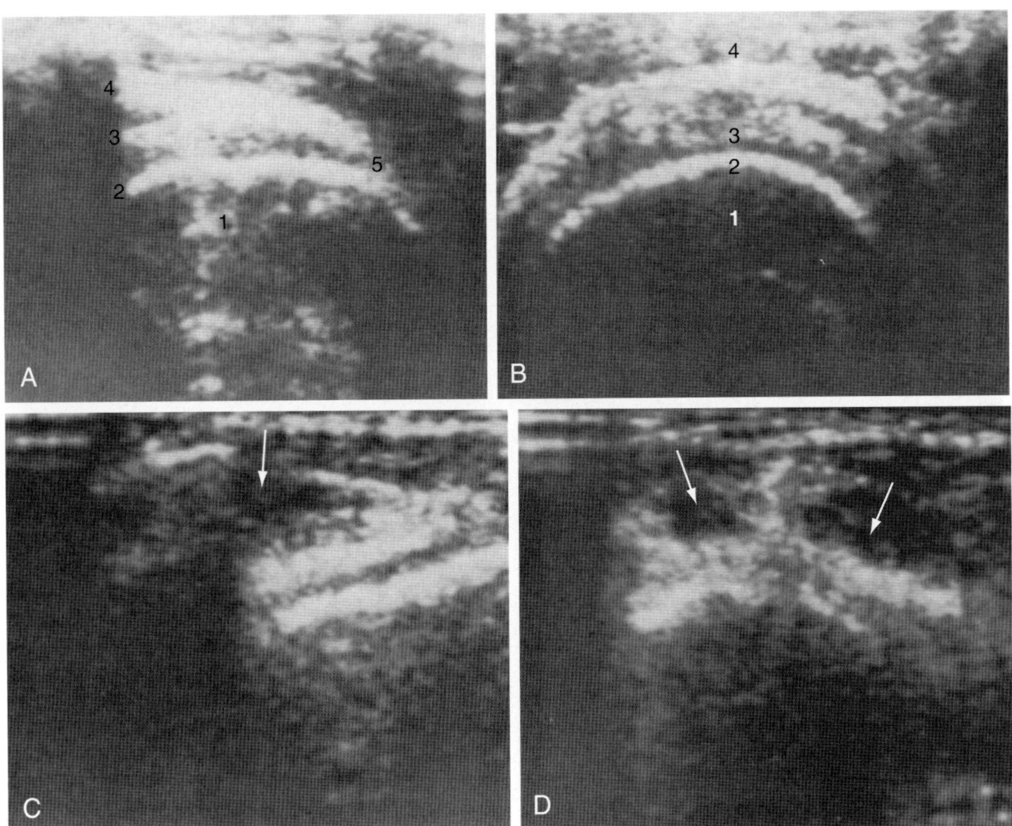

• **Fig. 49.11** (A) A normal longitudinal view of the rotator cuff by ultrasound shows the humeral head *(1),* the superior articular surface *(2),* the rotator cuff *(3),* the deltoid tendon *(4),* and tapering of the cuff to its insertion on the greater tuberosity *(5).* (B) A transverse view of a normal intact rotator cuff covering the humeral head. (C) A rotator cuff tear showing a hypoechoic area *(arrow)* on a longitudinal view. (D) A rotator cuff tear showing a hypoechoic area *(arrows)* on a transverse view.

partial tears, and small complete tears without MRI-arthrography. Orthopedic surgeons prefer use of MRI-arthrography for verification of labral tears or partial rotator cuff tears. In the case of a suspected full-thickness rotator cuff tear, MRI is preferred to determine the size of the tear, the amount of muscle atrophy and tendon retraction, and the quality of remaining tissue for repair.

Intrinsic Factors Causing Shoulder Pain

Periarticular Disorders

Shoulder Impingement and Rotator Cuff Tendinopathy

One of the most common nontraumatic causes of shoulder pain is impingement with rotator cuff tendinopathy. In 1972 Neer[7] described his results of 100 anatomic shoulder dissections and coined the term *impingement syndrome.* Impingement may be defined as the encroachment of the acromion, coracoacromial ligament, coracoid process, or AC joint on the rotator cuff as it passes beneath them during glenohumeral motion. The function of the posterior rotator cuff is to abduct and externally rotate the humerus. The cuff with the biceps tendon serves as a humeral head depressor to maintain the head centered within the glenoid fossa as the cuff and to use the deltoid to elevate the arm.[57–59]

Controversy continues, however, as to the exact cause of impingement—that is, whether it is a primary, intrinsic, degenerative event within the tendon with superior migration of the head on arm elevation and secondary impingement on the acromion, or purely mechanical attrition of the tendon with primary impingement against the acromion. The mechanical impingement of the rotator cuff may be influenced by variations in the shape and slope of the acromion.[60,61] The supraspinatus outlet may become narrowed from proliferative spur formation of the acromion or degenerative changes in the AC joint. These changes, along with intrinsic degenerative changes of the rotator cuff, may lead to a rotator cuff tear, but the exact pathogenesis remains controversial. Many studies have found a strong correlation between degenerative hypertrophic spur formation, with its resulting narrowing of the supraspinatus outlet, and the presence of full-thickness cuff tears,[7,17,62–69] but clinical studies have failed to confirm whether hypertrophic changes in the coracoacromial arch are caused by the cuff lesions or whether these changes themselves cause the lesions.

Neer[7] developed a staging system for the description of impingement lesions of the shoulder. A stage I lesion involves edema and hemorrhage of the rotator cuff and typically is found in people younger than 25 years who are active in athletics that involve repetitious overhead activities. The condition usually responds to conservative treatment that includes rest, anti-inflammatory medication, and physical therapy. Stage II lesions usually occur in people in their 30s or 40s and represent the biologic response of fibrosis and thickening of the tendon after repeated episodes of mechanical impingement over time. Lesions are treated conservatively, as in stage I, but attacks may recur. If symptoms persist despite adequate conservative management for longer than 6 to 12 months, surgical intervention is warranted. Stage III

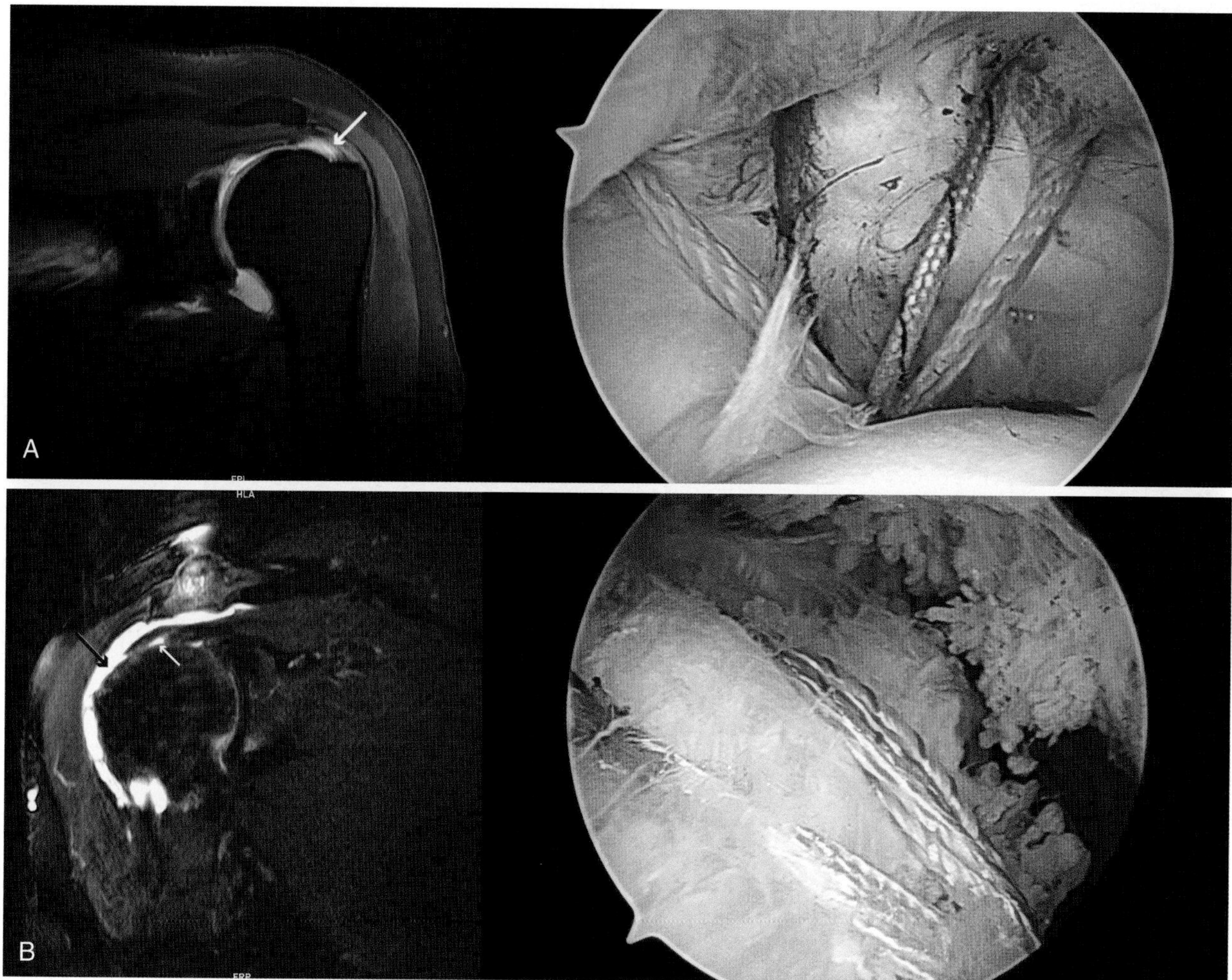

• **Fig. 46.12** (A, *left*) MRI–arthrogram coronal view of a partial-thickness rotator cuff tear *(white arrow)*. (A, *right*) Transtendinous repair of partial-thickness rotator cuff tear as viewed from the articular side. (B, *left*) MRI–arthrogram coronal view of a full-thickness rotator cuff tear *(black arrow)*. Part of the tendon is seen still attached to the anterior tendon footprint *(white arrow)*. (B, *right*) Repair of full-thickness rotator cuff tear as viewed from the bursal side.

lesions involve rotator cuff tears, biceps tendon rupture, and bone changes, and they rarely occur before age 40 years. Patients may present with pain, weakness, or supraspinatus atrophy, depending on the chronicity of the tear. Surgical treatment depends on the patient's age, loss of function, weakness, and pain.

Patients usually present to the clinician with a report of pain that has failed to resolve after a variable period. Pain can be sudden and incapacitating in cases of traumatic cuff tears, or more commonly it may manifest as a dull ache in cases of chronic impingement. Pain usually is located over the anterior and lateral aspects of the shoulder and may radiate into the lateral deltoid. It may worsen after sleeping on the affected extremity and is exacerbated by overhead activity. Tenderness on palpation may be elicited over the greater tuberosity and the long head of the biceps within the bicipital groove, indicating an associated biceps tendinitis. In cases with concomitant degenerative changes in the AC joint, tenderness may be noted on palpation over the AC joint, as an offending osteophyte impinges on the rotator cuff beneath.

The impingement sign as described by Neer[7] (Fig. 49.14) is useful in the diagnosis of rotator cuff tendinopathy. The patient often describes a catch as the arm is brought into the overhead position. The patient may be observed to raise the arm by abduction and external rotation to clear the greater tuberosity of the acromion, bypassing the painful area. A typical painful arc usually occurs between 70 and 110 degrees of abduction. Neer[7] also described an impingement test that involves injection of lidocaine into the subacromial bursa. Relief of pain is a positive impingement test result and usually indicates rotator cuff origin of the shoulder pain.

Radiographs in the early stages of cuff tendinopathy may be normal or may reveal a hooked acromion. As the disease progresses, sclerosis, cyst formation, and sclerosis of the anterior third of the acromion and the greater tuberosity may be observed. An anterior acromial traction spur may appear on the undersurface of the acromion lateral to the AC joint and represents contracture of the coracoacromial ligament. Late radiographic findings include narrowing of the acromiohumeral gap, superior subluxation of the humeral head in relation to the glenoid, and erosive changes in the anterior acromion.[70] Arthrography, MRI, and ultrasound may be helpful in diagnosing a full-thickness tear of the rotator cuff in association with stage III disease. In some cases of chronic large rotator cuff tears, proximal migration of the humeral head leads to a pattern of degenerative arthritis termed *cuff-tear arthropathy*.

The choice of treatment and, frequently, its result are functions of the stage of the impingement and the response to pain. In stage

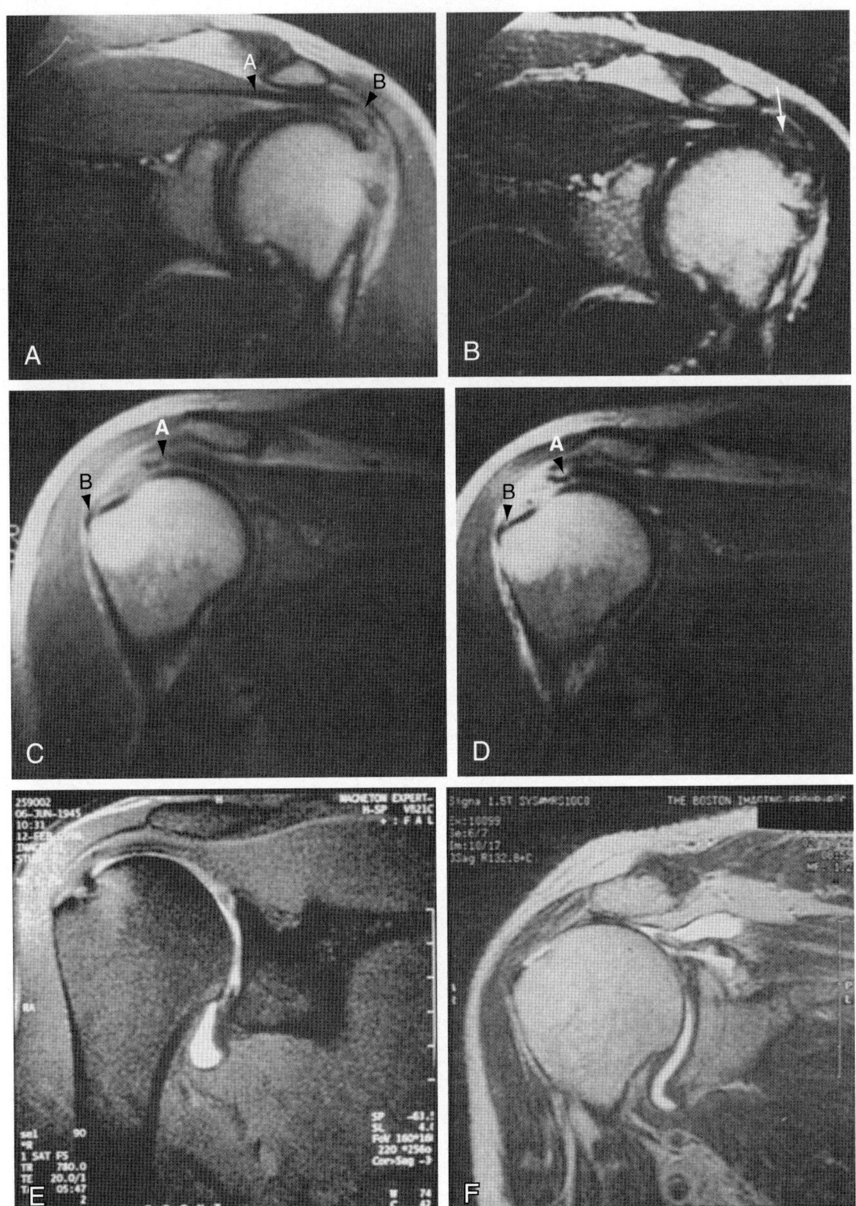

• **Fig. 49.13** (A) An MRI proton density–weighted coronal view shows the supraspinatus tendon as a black band *(A)* that has an increased signal as it nears insertion on the greater tuberosity *(B)*. (B) A similar view with a T2-weighted image shows increased signal as gray *(arrow)*, indicating a partial-thickness tear or tendinitis. (C) MRI proton density–weighted coronal view shows abrupt end of supraspinatus tendon as it courses right to left *(A)*. From A to B is an area of increased signal followed by a short portion of tendon *(B)* inserting at the greater tuberosity. (D) A similar view on a T2-weighted image shows increased signal as white (fluid density), indicating fluid in the gap of a complete rotator cuff tear. (E) MR arthrography shows a normal rotator cuff. (F) MR arthrography shows a chronic cuff tear with retraction.

I disease, in which little mechanical impingement occurs, most patients respond to rest. It is important to avoid immobilizing the shoulder for any period because contraction of the shoulder capsule and periarticular structures can produce an adhesive capsulitis. After a period of rest, a progressive program of stretching and strengthening exercises generally restores the shoulder to normal function. Use of aspirin and other nonsteroidal anti-inflammatory drugs (NSAIDs) may shorten the symptomatic period. Modalities such as ultrasound, neuroprobe, and transcutaneous electrical nerve stimulation generally are not helpful. Patients with stage I or II disease may have a dramatic response to local injection of glucocorticosteroids and local anesthetic agents. For stage II disease in which fibrosis and thickening occur anteriorly, it is frequently better to perform the injection with a posterior approach. We prefer a combination of 3 mL of 1% lidocaine, 3 mL of 0.5% bupivacaine, and 20 mg of triamcinolone. This injection combines a short-acting anesthetic to help confirm the diagnosis, a longer-acting anesthetic for analgesic purposes, and a steroid preparation in a depot form.

An integrated program of occupational and physical therapy often precludes the need for surgery in patients with stage II disease. Job modification for people with impingement syndrome

TABLE 49.2 Relative Costs of Shoulder Diagnostic Procedures in 2014 in the United States

Procedure	Initial Fee (USD)	Technical Fee (USD)	Interpretation Fee (USD)
Medicare B Fee Schedule			
Initial office visit (30 min)	108.18		
Plain radiography (3 views)		91.36	29.36
Arthrography		340.49	72.78
MRI		492.63	86.33
CT		287.65	61.79
Institutional Charges			
Initial office visit (30 min)	394.00		
Plain radiography (3 views)		436.00	35.00
Arthrography		625.00	302.00
MRI		4785.00	350.00
CT		2184.00	181.00

USD, U.S. dollars.

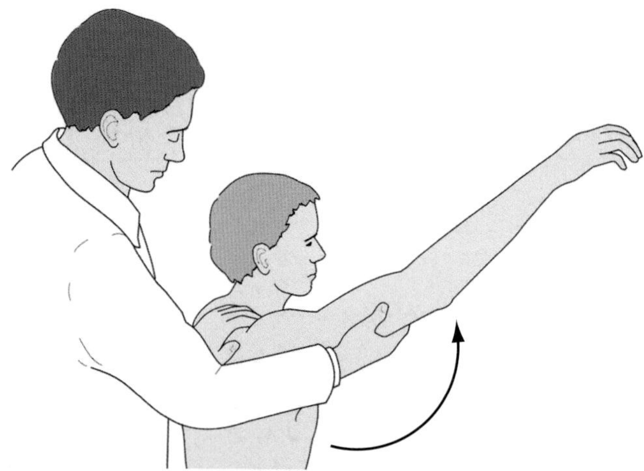

• **Fig. 49.14** The impingement sign is elicited by forced forward elevation of the arm. Pain results as the greater tuberosity impinges on the acromion. The examiner's hand prevents scapular rotation. This maneuver may be positive in other periarticular disorders. (From Neer CS II: Impingement lesions. *Clin Orthop Relat Res* 173:70, 1983.)

caused by overuse may alleviate symptoms. Businesses are becoming increasingly aware of the cost savings associated with proper job ergonomics.[71,72]

The initial rehabilitation in stage II impingement consists of cessation of repetitive overhead activity. Use of ice, NSAIDs, and local injections also may be beneficial. Initial physical therapy includes passive, active-assisted, and active range of motion combined with stretching and mobilization exercises to prevent contracture. As pain and inflammation subside, isometric or isotonic exercises are used to strengthen the rotator cuff musculature. Isokinetic training at variable speeds and in variable positions is instituted before the patient is allowed to return to full activity. For patients with a job-related injury, it is crucial to review and modify job mechanics to prevent recurrent episodes that can cause further disability and may precipitate the need for surgery.[71]

Neer[17] suggested that a patient with refractory stage II disease may respond to division of the coracoacromial ligament and bursectomy of the subacromial bursa. Open anterior acromioplasty as described by Neer has become accepted as the procedure of choice for stage II and III impingement lesions, with many investigators reporting high success rates in treating impingement syndrome and rotator cuff tears.[70,73–75] Reported results show good and excellent relief of symptoms in 71% to 87% of patients treated with the open surgical procedure.[76–79]

In 1985 Ellman[51] described the technique of arthroscopic subacromial decompression. His initial results[52] and the results of others are comparable with those of open surgical techniques.[53,80] Arthroscopic subacromial decompression has become a widely accepted treatment for refractory stage II and III impingement lesions. The procedure can be performed as outpatient surgery, and because no deltoid is detached, as with the open technique, the procedure facilitates rehabilitation and increases overall recovery rates. A recent Cochrane review did not support performance of subacromial decompression in the treatment of impingment.[81]

Calcific Tendinitis

Calcific tendinitis is a painful condition around the rotator cuff that is associated with deposition of calcium salts, primarily hydroxyapatite.[82–84] The cause of calcific tendinitis is unknown. The commonly accepted cause is degeneration of the tendon, which leads to calcification through a dystrophic process.[84] A common clinicopathologic correlation is seen in three distinct phases of the disease process: the precalcific or formative phase, which can be relatively painless; the calcific phase, which tends to be quiescent and may last months to years; and the resorptive or postcalcific phase, which tends to be painful, as calcium crystals are resorbed.[82] Although calcific tendinitis is more common in the right shoulder, at least a 6% incidence of bilaterality has been reported. Patients with bilateral shoulder involvement often have the syndrome of calcific periarthritis, in which calcium hydroxyapatite crystals are found at multiple sites.[85] Patients usually present with impingement-type pain in the affected shoulder during overhead activity. The pain may seem to be out of proportion to any objective physical findings. The patient may describe difficulty sleeping on the shoulder and trouble falling asleep. Symptoms may last a few weeks or a few months.

The incidence of calcific tendinitis among asymptomatic people varies from 2.7% to 20% in the literature. Most calcification occurs in the supraspinatus tendon, and 57% to 76.7% of patients are women. The average age of patients is 40 to 50 years.[82,86]

Codman[87] pointed out the localization of calcification within the tendon of the supraspinatus. He provided a detailed description of the symptoms and the natural history of this condition. In describing the phases of pain, spasm, limitation of motion, and atrophy, he noted the lack of correlation between symptoms and the size of the calcific deposit. According to Codman,[87] the natural history includes degeneration of the supraspinatus tendon, calcification, and eventual rupture into the subacromial bursa. During the latter phase, pain and decreased motion can lead to adhesive capsulitis (see Fig. 49.8).

Several factors may affect localization of calcium within the supraspinatus. Many patients have an early stage of impingement that compresses the supraspinatus tendon on the anterior portion of the acromion.[7,17] This long-standing impingement may lead to local degeneration of tendon fibers. In patients without impingement, localization of calcium within the supraspinatus may be related to the blood supply of the rotator cuff, which normally is derived from an anastomotic network of vessels from the greater tuberosity or from the bellies of the short rotator muscles.[83] The watershed of these sources is just medial to the tendinous attachment of the supraspinatus.[88] Rathburn and Macnab[89] referred to this watershed as the critical zone and pointed out that during abduction this area was rendered ischemic.

Treatment of calcific tendinitis depends on the clinical presentation and the presence of associated impingement. Patients can have an acute inflammatory reaction that may resemble gout. The acute inflammation can be treated with a local glucocorticoid injection, NSAIDs, or both. Ultrasound may be beneficial. If impingement is associated, treatment depends on the stage at presentation. The radiographic appearance of the calcification can direct and perhaps predict the response to therapy. In the resorptive state, deposits appear floccular, suggesting that the process is in the phase of repair and that a conservative program is indicated.

Patients with discrete calcification and perhaps associated adhesive capsulitis (see Fig. 49.8) may be at a stable phase, in which calcium produces a mechanical block and is unlikely to be resorbed. For these patients, mechanical removal of calcific deposits and correction of associated pathologic lesions may be necessary.[90–92] Percutaneous disruption of calcified areas may be performed using a needle directed by fluoroscopy. This technique allows lavage and injection, but it does not treat associated impingement. Subacromial arthroscopy allows mechanical débridement of calcific deposits under direct visualization. This technique can be combined with arthroscopic removal of the inflamed bursa and decompression of associated impingement. Improved results have been noted with complete removal of calcific deposits.[93] In many cases of refractory calcific tendinitis associated with impingement, open or arthroscopic acromioplasty, subacromial bursectomy, and decompression are indicated.

Rotator Cuff Tear

Pathophysiology. Spontaneous tear of the rotator cuff in an otherwise healthy person is rare.[17] It can occur in patients with RA or systemic lupus erythematosus as part of the pathologic process with invasion from underlying pannus. Metabolic conditions such as renal osteodystrophy and agents such as glucocorticoids occasionally are associated with cuff tears. Most patients report a traumatic episode, such as falling on an outstretched arm or lifting a heavy object. The usual presenting symptoms are pain and weakness of abduction and external rotation. Crepitus and even a palpable defect may be associated with the tear. Long-standing tears generally are associated with atrophy of the supraspinatus and infraspinatus muscles. It may be difficult to differentiate painful tendinitis from a partial-thickness or a small full-thickness cuff tear.

The exact cause of cuff tendinopathy continues to be controversial.[88,92,94,95] Most likely, the pathophysiology involves a combination of factors, including decreased vascularity and cellularity of the tendon, along with changes in the collagen fibers of the tendon that occur with aging.

Loss of motion with subsequent capsular tightness, particularly in the posterior capsule, may lead to cephalad migration of the humeral head, with subsequent impingement of the cuff under the coracoacromial arch.[96] Rehabilitation exercises focus on regaining a normal range of motion. To achieve full, painless motion, the normal relationship of glenohumeral to scapulothoracic motion must be achieved.[14,15,97]

Diagnosis—History. Patients with nontraumatic tears of the rotator cuff report symptoms of chronic impingement. Loss of motion and a feeling of stiffness are often noted with extremes of motion, along with difficulty during activities of daily living, such as combing one's hair, hooking a bra strap, putting on a shirt or coat, and reaching into the back pocket. In chronic cases of cuff tendinopathy, loss of motion usually occurs. Limitation of internal rotation caused by posterior capsular contracture occurs initially and is often associated with posterior shoulder pain with adduction of the ipsilateral shoulder. Further shoulder impingement occurs with forward flexion because of superior migration of the humeral head against the anterior inferior acromion. This upward translation is analogous to the action of a yo-yo climbing on a string.[96,98] Over time, loss of forward flexion, abduction, and external rotation occurs with passive and active motion of the shoulder.

Diagnosis—Imaging. In acute cases, a history of trauma, such as a fall onto the affected shoulder, may be reported. In cases involving an anterior shoulder dislocation with subsequent profound weakness of the rotator cuff, a large cuff tear or a greater tuberosity avulsion should be suspected, in addition to axillary nerve palsy. In younger patients, traumatic failure of the cuff under tensile overload may result in cuff failure caused by forced adduction of the affected shoulder or active abduction against resistance, and this outcome may occur with traumatic dislocation. Repetitive tensile overload also can result in partial rotator cuff tears in an athlete whose sport entails repetitive overhead actions.

Plain radiographs are used in the initial evaluation of impingement-type shoulder pain with cuff tendinopathy. An impingement series should be ordered, including an anteroposterior radiograph with a 30-degree cephalic tilt (the Rockwood view), which can reveal osteophytes of the anterior os acromion and AC joint; a scapular Y view with a 10-degree cephalic tilt (the supraspinatus outlet view), which can evaluate the type of acromion and reveal anterior and AC osteophytes; and an axillary view, which can evaluate the acromion for possible os acromiale. Calcific deposits within the rotator cuff tendon can be viewed best with rotational anteroposterior radiographs. Cuff arthropathy should be suspected if the acromial-humeral distance is less than 7 mm, or with the presence of cyst formation within the greater tuberosity, humeral head osteopenia, sclerosis around the greater tuberosity, or humeral head collapse. In advanced stages of cuff arthropathy, complete loss of glenohumeral joint space may be seen with superior migration and abutment of the humeral head against the undersurface of the acromion.[57]

In the past, shoulder arthrography was considered the "gold standard" for diagnosing full-thickness and partial-thickness rotator cuff tears, with greater than 90% sensitivity and specificity.[31,99] Currently, arthrography with CT or MRI is routinely used to diagnose rotator cuff disease, including full-thickness and partial-thickness tears.

Ultrasonography has been accurate in the diagnosis of full-thickness rotator cuff tears.[37,100–103] Ultrasonography offers the advantages of being inexpensive and noninvasive, but disadvantages include unproven effectiveness in determining subacromial impingement, capsular and labral abnormalities, and partial cuff tears. The procedure and its results are technician dependent.

Ultrasonography may have a useful role in determining the postoperative integrity of the cuff repair or following progression of a cuff tear over time.[36]

MRI has been invaluable in evaluating rotator cuff tears. The sensitivity and specificity of MRI for diagnosing full-thickness cuff tears are 100% and 95%.[104] With the use of gadolinium or saline solution, partial tears that are otherwise difficult to detect with conventional imaging can be detected.

Diagnosing cuff tears with MRI usually is based on discontinuity of the tendon on T1-weighted images and consistency with fluid signal on T2-weighted images. Ancillary findings include fluid in the subacromial space on T2-weighted images, loss of the subacromial fat plane on T1-weighted images, and proliferative spur formation of the acromion or AC joint. Large, chronic cuff tears also may be associated with cephalad migration of the humeral head and fatty atrophy of the supraspinatus muscle. Periarticular soft tissues, including the capsulolabral complex and the biceps tendon, as well as the rotator cuff, can be thoroughly examined. The degree of tear and tendon retraction and evidence of muscle atrophy can be evaluated, all of which are crucial in preoperative planning for possible cuff repair.

Treatment—Nonsurgical. Codman and Akerson[62] recommended early operative repair for acute full-thickness rotator cuff tears and reported the first documented repair in 1911. McLaughlin[64] recommended early repair in cases of grossly displaced tuberosity fractures or massive tears. Several other clinical studies have supported the concept that a full-thickness tear does not preclude good shoulder function. DePalma[105] reported that 90% of patients with rotator cuff tears responded to conservative measures, such as rest, analgesics, anti-inflammatory agents, and physiotherapy.

The reported percentage of patients responding to nonsurgical treatment in the literature varies from 33% to 90%.[4,16,106] Conservative treatment includes pain control with NSAIDs, ultrasound, application of heat before shoulder stretching and exercise, and application of ice after overhead activity. Deep massage therapy is used to reduce trigger point tenderness within the trapezius, levator scapulae, and periscapular muscles. Patients taking anti-inflammatory medications on a long-term basis are monitored periodically for evidence of gastrointestinal bleeding and for hepatic or renal toxicity. Opiate-based drugs are used only in the acute setting, such as after a fall, or in the perioperative period.

Steroid and local anesthetic injections are used when the patient has significant pain that prohibits rehabilitation. Injections may be repeated once every 3 months if needed; injection into the cuff tendon is to be avoided. If the patient fails to improve after 3 months of conservative treatment or does not continue to improve after three sequential injections, surgical options should be discussed.

The mainstay of conservative therapy is exercise. Rehabilitation stresses pain relief with exercises aimed at restoring shoulder motion and strengthening remaining cuff muscles, deltoid muscles, and scapular stabilizers. Therapy can be divided into three phases. The goals of the initial phase of therapy are to relieve pain and restore shoulder motion. Motion therapy includes pendulum exercises, passive motion with use of a wand with assistance of the uninvolved shoulder, an overhead pulley system, and posterior capsular stretching. The arc of motion is gradually increased and is guided by the patient's discomfort to avoid painful impingement arcs.

The second phase of therapy is entered after the patient has return of motion and little discomfort with overhead activity. Emphasis is placed on strengthening the remaining rotator cuff musculature and deltoid and periscapular muscles. Strengthening with elastic surgical tubing provides variable degrees of resistance, depending on the size of the tubing. Initial strengthening is performed out of the impingement arc (with 70 to 120 degrees of shoulder flexion). The goal of this phase is to strengthen the shoulder to prevent dynamic proximal humeral migration with impingement during active shoulder elevation.[57,60] Normal shoulder kinematics rely on combined and synchronous glenohumeral flexion and scapular rotation.[58,92] In addition to strengthening the cuff and deltoid, the scapular rotators, including the trapezius and the serratus anterior muscles, are emphasized.[107]

After the patient has successfully completed phase two of the rehabilitation program with minimal symptoms and good shoulder function, the final phase is entered. Phase three is characterized by a gradual return to normal overhead activities, including work and sporting activities. This part of the rehabilitation program should be tailored to the individual patient's needs and the demands placed on the shoulder.

Treatment—Surgical. A Cochrane review of the effectiveness of surgery for rotator cuff disease failed to reach any firm conclusions about the effectiveness or safety of rotator cuff surgery.[108]

Severity and duration of pain are the primary indications for surgical intervention in a rotator cuff tear. Other factors important in surgical decision making include shoulder dominance, activity level, physiologic age, acuteness of the tear, degree of the tear, loss of function, the amount of tendon retraction, and fatty atrophy of the remaining cuff musculature.

A systematic review of indications for rotator cuff surgery found that earlier surgical intervention may be needed for patients with cuff tears who have weakness and significant functional disability. In addition, older chronologic age did not portend a worse outcome; however, pending workman's compensation claims negatively affected treatment results.[109]

Acute Tears. Acute tears of the rotator cuff can be treated with conservative measures of periscapular and cuff strengthening along with capsular stretching to restore motion. Early surgical intervention should be considered in a young patient, especially an athlete whose sport entails repetitive overhead actions. Conservative shoulder rehabilitation should be maintained for 3 to 6 months before a decision is made regarding surgery for an older sedentary patient, in whom functional results without surgery may be acceptable. Many older patients may function well with chronic cuff tears, but they may become debilitated if an acute tear is superimposed on chronic changes. Surgical intervention may be required in these cases to return the patient to baseline function by repairing the acute tear and attempting to repair the chronic tear if possible.

Chronic Tears. For elderly patients whose pain and weakness do not create a functional problem, a conservative program is preferable for chronic tears. Pain that is unresponsive to conservative management is the main indication for surgery in an older patient with a chronic rotator cuff tear. In these cases, surgery should be considered on an individual basis after at least 3 months of conservative treatment, including subacromial steroid injection. In a recent systematic review, favorable improvement was noted in clinical outcome scores and patient satisfaction for rotator cuff repair in patients over 65 years.[110]

If the cuff tear is massive and irreparable, débridement and subacromial decompression may provide good pain relief without extensive surgery and prolonged immobilization.[52,80,111–115] In a younger patient with a chronic tear and weakness, surgery to repair

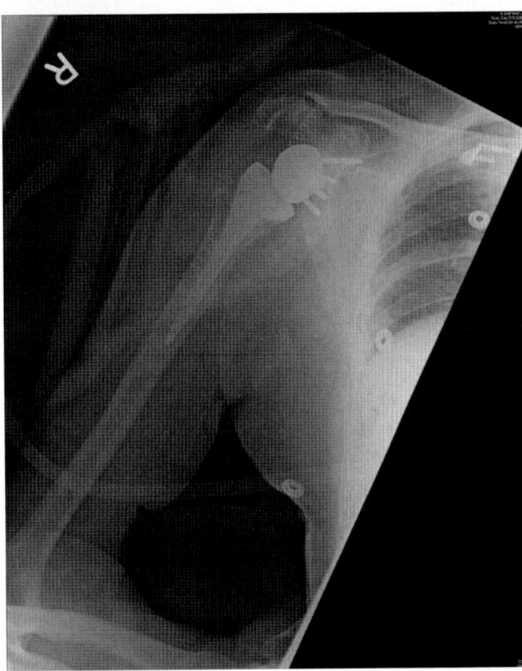

• **Fig. 49.15** Reverse total shoulder replacement in a 72-year-old man who had severe cuff arthropathy.

the cuff may be indicated to improve strength and prevent further extension of the tear.[113] In cases of rotator cuff arthropathy with glenohumeral joint degeneration, a reverse total shoulder replacement may be indicated. This type of total shoulder replacement reverses the normal relationship between scapular and humeral components, moving the center of rotation medially and distally to increase the lever arm length of the deltoid muscle. The deltoid compensates for the deficient rotator cuff, allowing as near-normal function as possible (Fig. 49.15). Reverse total shoulder arthroplasty may be considered for the treatment of irreparable rotator cuff tear with disability and no glenohumeral arthritis.[116]

Economic Aspect of Rotator Cuff Repair. With the recent shift of health care management toward reducing costs and efficient treatment, rotator cuff repairs have become an area of consideration. Evaluation fees, including visit and imaging fees, have gradually increased in recent years, generating a larger burden on both the health care system and the economy at large. A common aspect of health care costs that is not taken into consideration is the opportunity cost faced by patients when they choose to seek and follow medical advice. To fully understand the scope of the financial impact of rotator cuff repair, indirect costs such as travel costs to and from medical facilities, missed wages, decrease in labor and productivity, and disability support must be added into the equation. Indirect costs, combined with the increased costs reflected in Table 49.2, can show the real fiscal significance.

In subsequent debates it has been argued whether operative treatment is superior to nonoperative treatment, with both sides utilizing hidden costs as the deciding factor. One group[117] published a study showcasing this exact quandary of operative versus nonoperative treatment in cost reduction and societal benefit. The investigators utilized a decision-based, semirandom optimization framework, the Markov decision process, in comparing the repair of full-thickness tears to nonoperative management after an assumed failure of a course of nonoperative therapy. Patients in the model were reimbursed by the standards of average Medicare payouts at the time and several indirect costs, such as those previously mentioned, were used as measuring points. The results showed a significant cost efficacy at any age with repair, with a substantial impact on patients younger than 40 years because of their increased earning potential and financial activity.[117] Although the savings margin was increased for all ages, it was much more reduced in people older than 70 years. The total savings calculated was approximately $3.44 billion, and the authors commented that although surgery is not indicated for all cases, it assisted with the global costs of rotator cuff tear management.

A more recent level I study conducted in Norway included 103 patients randomized into nonoperative or operative management for both full- and partial-thickness tears not exceeding 3 cm.[118] Although this study did not focus on the economic aspect of care, the results favored operative management and by doing so indicated certain financial benefits. The two major areas in which operative treatment excelled and had a meaningful influence were in quality of life as measured by several outcome measures and rate of retearing and persistent tears during a 5-year period. The assumption can be made that with increased quality of life and decreased symptomatic retearing, patients most likely stayed on disability for shorter periods and fewer resources were allocated to symptom assessment and treatment.

Although these studies highlight certain aspects of the economics of rotator cuff repair, several limitations must be considered, such as sample size, assumptions made to develop the logic model, and financial motivation. At present there is still a dearth of analysis with regard to the fiscal environment surrounding health care costs for people undergoing management of symptomatic rotator cuff tears.

Bicipital Tendonitis and Rupture

The long head of the biceps passes through the bicipital groove, crosses over the humeral head, and inserts on the superior rim of the glenoid (see Fig. 49.1A).[119] The biceps tendon aids in flexion of the forearm, supination of the pronated forearm if the elbow is flexed, and forward elevation of the shoulder.[4] Bicipital tendinitis, subluxation or dislocation of the biceps tendon within the bicipital groove, and rupture of the long head of the biceps generally are associated with anterior shoulder pain.

Bicipital tendinitis is sometimes an associated feature of a rotator cuff tear. The rotator cuff tear compromises centering of the humeral head on the glenoid. This compromise results in increased mechanical loading of the long head of the biceps, which initiates a hypertrophic tendonitis.[120]

Dislocation of the long head of the biceps usually is combined with a lesion of the subscapularis tendon.[10] Isolated rupture of the long head of the biceps tendon is rare when the rotator cuff is intact. Rupture of the long head of the biceps is common, however, when a co-existing rotator cuff tear is present.[121] The effects of rotator cuff tear and concomitant biceps tendon rupture on strength can be substantial.[10]

Early phases of bicipital tendinitis are associated with hypervascularity, edema of the tendon, and tenosynovitis.[122] Persistence of this process leads to adhesions between the tendon and its sheath, along with impairment of the normal gliding mechanism in the groove. Stretching of the adhesions may be associated with chronic bicipital tendonitis.[123] The diagnosis of bicipital tendonitis is based on localization of tenderness. It is often confused with impingement symptoms and is frequently seen with an impingement syndrome.[22] Isolated bicipital tendinitis can be differentiated by the fact that the tender area migrates with the bicipital groove as the arm is abducted and externally rotated.

Many eponyms are associated with tests to identify bicipital tendinitis.[4] Yergason's supination sign refers to pain in the bicipital groove when the examiner resists supination of the pronated forearm with the elbow at 90 degrees. Ludington's sign refers to pain in the bicipital groove when the patient interlocks the fingers on top of the head and actively abducts the arms.

Biceps tendon rupture can occur in some patients who report no history of shoulder pain. Patients often report an acute onset of pain and ecchymosis around the anterior shoulder and sagging of the biceps muscle belly. In these cases, a concomitant rotator cuff injury should be excluded by clinical examination. More often, the biceps tendon rupture is preceded by painful shoulder symptoms that often improve or disappear after the rupture.[123]

Treatment generally is conservative and consists of rest, analgesics, NSAIDs, and local injection of glucocorticoids. The use of ultrasound and a neuroprobe is more beneficial in this condition than in isolated rotator cuff tendinitis. Patients with refractory bicipital tendonitis and recurrent symptoms of subluxation are treated by arthroscopic biceps tenodesis or open tenodesis—that is, opening the bicipital groove and resecting the proximal portion of the tendon with tenodesis of the distal portion into the groove or beneath the pectoralis tendon.

Acromioclavicular Disorders

The AC joint is a common source of shoulder pain. Acute causes of AC joint pain are often related to direct trauma of the affected shoulder that may result in a distal clavicle injury with an intra-articular chondral fracture, or in AC joint instability from ligamentous disruption.

Post-traumatic distal clavicle osteolysis, with resorption of the distal clavicle, may ensue 4 weeks after a shoulder injury, leading to AC joint pain.[124] Osteolysis may be caused by microfracture of the subchondral bone and subsequent attempts at repair.[125] Other authors believe the cause to be an autonomic nerve dysfunction affecting the blood supply to the clavicle. The increased blood supply leads to resorption of bone from the distal clavicle.[126] More commonly, chronic osteolysis results from repetitive microtrauma to the AC joint from activities such as weight lifting, gymnastics, and swimming.[125,127,128]

The underlying pathophysiology is believed to be an inflammatory process caused by stress fracture of the subchondral bone with hyperemic resorption of the distal clavicle.[125,129] Other causes of osteolysis include rheumatoid arthrosis, hyperparathyroidism, and sarcoidosis, which should be considered in the differential diagnosis, especially in bilateral cases.[124] Patients with atraumatic osteolysis of the distal clavicle should be forewarned that bilateral involvement may occur; an incidence of 70% was reported for one study with long-term follow-up.[130] Other chronic causes of AC pain include idiopathic, intra-articular disk disease, post-traumatic degenerative arthrosis from joint incongruity, primary degenerative arthrosis, and RA.

Evaluation should always include a detailed history, physical examination, and radiographic evaluation. A history of trauma to the AC joint from a direct fall or blow to the ipsilateral shoulder may be reported. Less commonly, the AC joint may have been injured indirectly, as during a fall on the outstretched arm with forces transmitted through the arm to the AC joint.[131] Patients with osteolysis of the distal clavicle sometimes report a history of acute trauma, although the more common cause is repetitive microtrauma to the AC joint caused by activities such as weight lifting or gymnastics.[124,127,128]

Patients frequently report having pain over the AC joint when adducting the ipsilateral shoulder, such as during a golf swing or when buckling a seat belt. Often, pain occurs when the patient sleeps on the affected shoulder. Athletes may experience AC joint pain when bench pressing and when performing push-ups and dips.[130,132,133] Pain and weakness of the affected shoulder also may be experienced with forward flexion and adduction of the arm.

On physical examination, a visible step-off may be observed between the medial acromion and the distal clavicle, indicating a probable AC separation. Pain usually can be elicited on direct palpation of the AC joint and is made worse by a cross-arm adduction maneuver. This test is performed by internally rotating the arm, which is maximally adducted across the chest, and is considered positive if pain is produced in the AC joint (see Fig. 49.3D). Pain also may be elicited by moving the arm from a horizontally abducted position to the extended position and upon maximal internal rotation of the shoulder.[132,134] These tests cause rotation and compression of the AC joint and are sensitive but less specific. They also may be positive with other disorders of the shoulder, such as posterior capsular stiffness.[135]

Frequently, AC joint pain co-exists with subacromial impingement and rotator cuff disease. In these cases, impingement signs are positive, and rotator cuff weakness may be present. Otherwise, no muscle weakness should be detectable on manual resistance testing, and no evidence of muscle atrophy should be found.[130,135,136] The AC joint and the subacromial space may require injection on separate occasions to determine the true source of the symptoms. Some physicians have noticed an association of AC joint symptoms with shoulder instability.[130] Glenohumeral motion can vary, depending on chronicity and isolation of the problem to the AC joint. In isolated cases, some loss of internal rotation of the affected shoulder may be caused by pain.

Radiographs should include anteroposterior views of the shoulder in the scapular plane in neutral, internal, and external rotation; a transcapular Y view; an axillary view; and a 15-degree cephalic tilt view of the AC joint at 50% penetrance, as described by Zanca (see Fig. 49.4).[21] Stress views may be obtained by strapping 5- to 10-lb weights to the forearms and determining AC separation. Comparing the coracoclavicular distance of both shoulders also may be helpful. When clinically indicated, cervical spine radiographs should be obtained to exclude cervical spondylosis.

Radiographic evaluation may reveal AC joint arthrosis with microcystic changes in the subchondral bone, sclerosis, osteophytic lipping, and joint space narrowing.[137] In cases of osteolysis, radiographs may reveal loss of subchondral bone detail with microcystic appearances in the subchondral region of the distal clavicle and osteopenia of the lateral one-third of the clavicle.[124,125,127,128] In late stages of osteolysis, resorption of the distal end of the clavicle results in marked widening of the AC joint and sometimes complete resorption of the distal clavicle. AC separation may be evident with widening of the coracoclavicular distance and post-traumatic ossification of the coracoclavicular ligaments.

AC symptoms do not always correlate with the radiographic appearance of the joint. DePalma[138] found AC joint degeneration to be an age-related process, with symptoms not always correlating with radiographic findings of AC joint arthrosis.[21] AC joint pain may occur despite normal findings of radiographs.[139]

A Tc 99m phosphate bone scan may assist in the diagnosis, revealing increased uptake in the distal clavicle and the medial acromion.[125] In cases of atraumatic osteolysis of the distal clavicle, increased uptake may be isolated to the distal clavicle, but in approximately 50% of cases, scintigraphic activity of the adjacent medial acromion is increased.[130] The bone scan may reveal pathologic changes in the AC joint when plain radiographs appear normal.

In selected cases, MRI can be valuable in determining a diagnosis and evaluating the glenohumeral and subacromial regions for co-existing disease (Fig. 49.16). AC joint involvement may reveal increased fluid with synovitis, soft tissue enlargement, and periarticular ossifications with encroachment on underlying bursal and cuff tissue.

Patients with AC joint pain usually respond well to nonoperative treatment; however, complete relief of symptoms may require an extended period. Conservative therapy includes application of heat, use of NSAIDs, steroid injections, shoulder rehabilitation, and avoidance of painful positions and activities. Steroid injections are repeated at 3-month intervals if painful conditions persist.

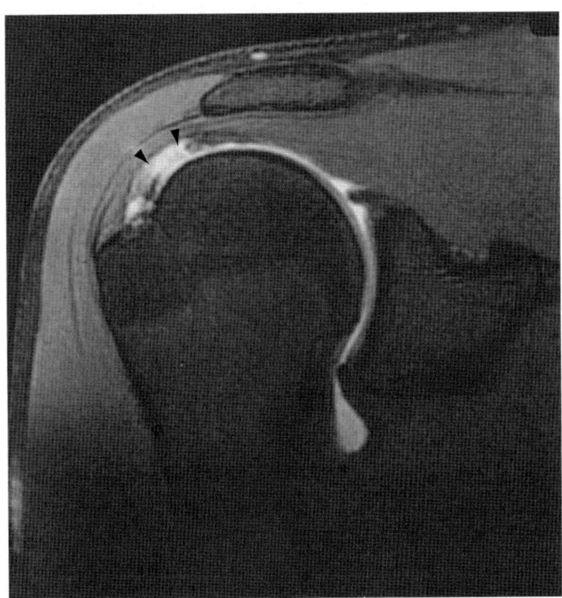

• **Fig. 49.16** Sagittal section MRI of the shoulder in a 32-year-old weight lifter with shoulder pain. A fat-suppressed proton density fast spin-echo image shows a bursal-side high-grade partial cuff tear *(arrowheads)*.

Open resection of the distal clavicle for chronic AC joint pain was initially reported by Gurd[140] and by Mumford,[141] both with good results. Since that time, other surgeons have reported similar good results with open resection; however, significant morbidity, such as disruption of the deltotrapezial fascia and anterior deltoid rupture, can occur.[124,137,139,142] Arthroscopic resection of the distal clavicle has been described with results similar to those of open resection with lower complication rates.[11,129,134,136,143–146]

Glenohumeral Disorders

The various arthritides that affect the shoulder joint are discussed in detail in other chapters. They are presented here to address aspects that are unique to the glenohumeral joint. The usual presentation of intra-articular disorders consists of pain with motion and symptoms of internal derangement, such as locking and clicking. Pain is generalized throughout the shoulder girdle and sometimes is referred to the neck, back, and upper arm. The usual response to pain includes decreased glenohumeral motion and substitution with increased scapulothoracic mobility. Patients with adequate elbow and scapulothoracic motion require little glenohumeral motion for activities of daily living, and patients with glenohumeral arthrodesis can achieve adequate function.[147,148] The response to pain consists of diminution of motion and secondary soft tissue contractures with muscle atrophy. With increasing weakness and involvement of adjacent joints, pain, limitation of motion, and weakness can cause a substantial functional deficit.

Inflammatory Arthritis

Although the most common inflammatory arthritis involving the shoulder joint is RA, other systemic disorders such as systemic lupus erythematosus, psoriatic arthritis, ankylosing spondylitis, reactive arthritis, and scleroderma may cause glenohumeral degeneration. Motion is limited by splinting of the joint with secondary soft tissue contractures or by primary soft tissue involvement with scarring or rupture. Plain radiographs confirm glenohumeral involvement (Fig. 49.17A). Narrowing of the glenohumeral joint space may occur, with erosion and cyst formation and without significant sclerosis or osteophytes. As the disease progresses, superior and posterior erosion of the glenoid with proximal subluxation of

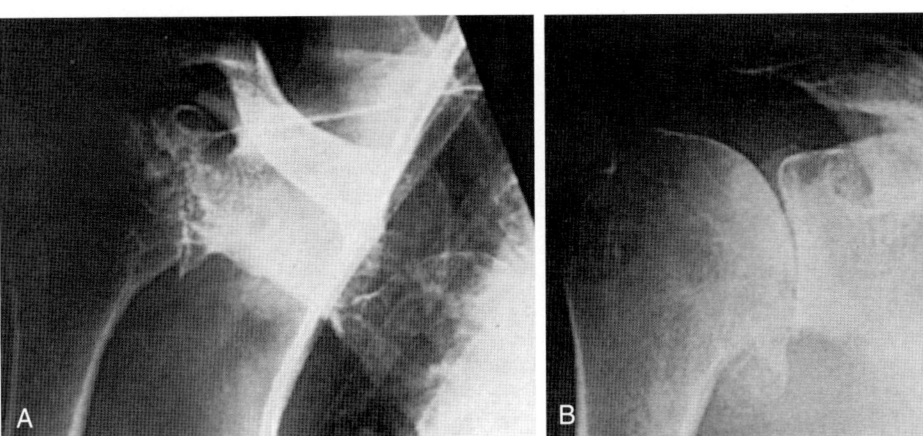

• **Fig. 49.17** Plain radiographs. (A) Rheumatoid arthritis with loss of joint space, cyst formation, glenohumeral erosion, and early proximal subluxation of the humerus, indicating a rotator cuff tear. (B) Osteoarthritis with narrowing of the glenohumeral joint space, sclerosis, and osteophyte formation. Notice the preservation of the subacromial space, suggesting an intact rotator cuff.

the humeral head may occur. Eventually, secondary degenerative changes and even osteonecrosis of the humeral head may occur.

Treatment is initially conservative and is directed toward controlling pain, inducing a systemic remission, and maintaining joint motion through physical therapy. The use of intra-articular glucocorticoids may be beneficial in controlling local synovitis. In RA, the involvement of periarticular structures with subacromial bursitis and rupture of the rotator cuff magnifies the functional deficit. When synovial cartilage interactions produce significant symptoms and radiographic changes that cannot be controlled by conventional therapy, glenohumeral replacement should be considered.

When following up on a patient with RA who has shoulder involvement, the rheumatologist should assess range of motion carefully and obtain radiographs periodically. Patients with progressive loss of motion or radiographic destruction should be referred for evaluation for possible surgical treatment. The treatment of choice is an unconstrained total shoulder arthroplasty.[149,150] Total shoulder arthroplasty is best performed in patients with RA before end-stage bony erosion and soft tissue contractions have occurred.[151,152] Acute inflammatory arthritis of the glenohumeral joint may be associated with gout, pseudogout, hydroxyapatite deposition of renal osteodystrophy, and recurrent hemophilic hemarthrosis.

Osteoarthritis

Osteoarthritis of the glenohumeral joint is less common than that in the hip, its counterpart in the lower extremity; this condition is caused by non–weight-bearing characteristics of the shoulder joint and the distribution of forces throughout the shoulder girdle. Osteoarthritis is divided into conditions associated with high unit loading of articular cartilage and conditions in which an intrinsic abnormality within the cartilage causes abnormal wear at normal loads. Because the shoulder is normally a non–weight-bearing joint and is not usually susceptible to repeated high loading, the presence of osteoarthritis of the glenohumeral joint should alert the physician to consider other factors. Has the patient engaged in unusual activities, such as boxing, heavy weight lifting, construction, or long-term use of a pneumatic hammer? Has some disorder, such as epiphyseal dysplasia, created joint incongruity with high unit loading of the articular cartilage? Is this a neuropathic process caused by diabetes, syringomyelia, or leprosy? Have associated hemochromatosis, hemophilia, or gout altered the ability of articular cartilage to withstand normal loading? Is unrecognized chronic dislocation responsible?

Pain is the usual presentation, but generally it is not as acute or it may be associated with the spasm seen in inflammatory conditions. Plain radiographs show narrowing of the glenohumeral joint, osteophyte formation, sclerosis, and some cyst formation (see Fig. 49.17B). Because the rotator cuff usually is intact, less bone erosion of the glenoid and proximal subluxation of the humerus is noted. Patients with osteoarthritis of the glenohumeral joint frequently do well with functional adjustments and conservative therapy. Analgesics and NSAIDs may provide symptomatic relief. The use of glucocorticoid injections is less beneficial, unless evidence of synovitis is observed. Patients with severe involvement who fail to respond to conservative therapy are best treated with shoulder arthroplasty.

Osteonecrosis

Osteonecrosis of the shoulder refers to necrosis of the humeral head seen in association with a variety of conditions. Symptoms are due to synovitis and joint incongruity resulting from resorption, repair, and remodeling.

The most common cause of osteonecrosis of the shoulder is avascularity resulting from a fracture through the anatomic neck of the humerus.[153] Fracture through this area disrupts intramedullary and capsular blood supplies to the humeral head.[154] Another common cause of osteonecrosis of the shoulder is oral steroid therapy provided in conjunction with organ transplantation, systemic lupus erythematosus, or asthma. Other conditions associated with osteonecrosis of the humeral head include hemoglobinopathies, pancreatitis, and hyperbarism.

Early diagnosis is difficult because the presence of symptoms is often delayed. Bone scans may be helpful in early cases, before radiographic changes are evident. MRI is highly sensitive and is more specific than scintigraphy. Plain radiographs show progressive phases of necrosis and repair. In early stages, the films may be normal or may show osteopenia or bone sclerosis. A crescent sign representing subchondral fracture or demarcation of the necrotic segment appears during the reparative process. Patients who fail to undergo remodeling show collapse of the humeral head with secondary degenerative changes. A considerable discrepancy is often noted between symptoms and radiographic involvement. Patients with extensive bone changes may be asymptomatic. Treatment should be directed by the patient's symptoms rather than by the radiographs and is similar to that provided for osteoarthritis. Arthroscopy occasionally is helpful by removing loose chondral fragments and débriding chondral incongruities.[155] Patients with severe symptoms that cannot be controlled by conservative means are best treated with unconstrained shoulder arthroplasty, hemiarthroplasty, or resurfacing arthroplasty.[149]

Cuff-Tear Arthropathy

In 1873 Adams described the pathologic changes that characterize RA of the shoulder and a condition that since that time has been referred to as "Milwaukee shoulder" or cuff-tear arthropathy.[156] McCarty called the condition Milwaukee shoulder and reported that factors predisposing to this syndrome included deposition of calcium pyrophosphate dihydrate crystals, direct trauma, chronic joint overuse, chronic renal failure, and denervation.[157,158] Patients with Milwaukee shoulder have elevated levels of synovial fluid 5-nucleotidase activity and elevated levels of synovial fluid inorganic pyrophosphate and nucleotide pyrophosphohydrolase activity.[159]

One study[158] reported a similar condition in which untreated massive tears of the rotator cuff with proximal migration of the humeral head are associated with erosion of the humeral head. Erosion of the humeral head differs from that seen in other arthritides and is presumed to be caused by a combination of mechanical and nutritional factors acting on the superior glenohumeral cartilage.

Patients with cuff-tear arthropathy present a difficult therapeutic problem because bone erosion and disruption of the cuff jeopardize the functional result from an unconstrained prosthesis.[151] Hemiarthroplasty or a reverse total shoulder arthroplasty may be indicated.[160,161] The major challenge in treating cuff-tear arthropathy is to determine which patients with massive rotator cuff tears will proceed to the syndrome of cuff-tear arthropathy. Patients with massive rotator cuff tears in whom localized calcium pyrophosphate disease develops may be predisposed to further proximal migration and further joint destruction. This situation poses a dilemma for the treating physician. Many patients with massive rotator cuff tears remain stable and require little or no treatment. Occasionally, symptomatic patients can be treated by arthroscopic débridement of the cuff tear. In a recent study, patients who had massive rotator cuff tears without arthritis did well when treated with reverse total shoulder arthroplasty.[116] It is crucial to define the patient who will proceed to the syndrome of cuff-tear arthropathy. If crystal deposition disease predisposes patients to proximal migration and joint destruction, joint aspiration with crystal analysis and scintigraphy to determine synovial reaction may be helpful diagnostic tools.

One study[162] followed up 22 patients with massive rotator cuff tears who were treated conservatively. Radiographic findings included narrowing of the acromiohumeral interval and degenerative changes in the humeral head, tuberosities, acromion, AC joint, and glenohumeral joint. Five of seven patients followed up for longer than 8 years progressed to cuff-tear arthropathy. Investigators concluded that progressive radiographic changes were associated with repetitive use of the arm in elevation, rupture of the long head of the biceps, impingement of the humeral head against the acromion, and weakness of external rotation.[162]

Septic Arthritis

Septic arthritis can masquerade as any of the conditions classified as periarticular or glenohumeral disorders. Sepsis must be included in any differential diagnosis of shoulder pain because early recognition and prompt treatment are necessary to achieve a good functional result. The diagnosis is confirmed by joint aspiration with synovial fluid analysis and culture. Cultures should include aerobic, anaerobic, mycobacterial, and fungal studies.

Labral Tears

The glenoid labrum increases the depth of the glenoid and serves as an anchor for the attachment of the glenohumeral ligaments. Historically, labral tears have been difficult to diagnose. Findings on physical examination can be confused with impingement and rotator cuff tendinopathy and bicipital tendinitis. Diagnosis can be confirmed with MRI-arthrography, CT-arthrography, and DCAT.[25] Arthroscopy has greatly increased our knowledge of the glenoid labrum in normal and pathologic situations and has aided clinicians in the diagnosis and treatment of labral lesions.

Labral tears can be divided into tears associated with symptoms of internal derangement and tears associated with anterior or posterior instability. A soft tissue Bankart lesion is associated with a tear of the anterior band of the inferior glenohumeral ligament and with anterior instability. Isolated labral tears that do not involve detachment of the ligaments can cause internal derangement and may have an arthroscopic appearance similar to that of a meniscal tear of the knee.

Andrews and associates[2] first described lesions of the anterior superior labrum in athletes whose sport entails throwing; these lesions were often associated with biceps tendon tears (10%), which may result from traction of the biceps tendon. Another study[163] introduced the term *SLAP lesion* in 1990 to describe an injury involving the long head of the biceps tendon and the superior portion of the glenoid labrum.

The long head of the biceps tendon originates at the supraglenoid tubercle and the glenoid labrum in the superior-most portion of the glenoid. The major portion of the tendon blends with the posterior superior aspect of the labrum. The most common mechanism of a SLAP injury is a fall onto an outstretched arm with the shoulder in abduction and slight forward flexion.[163] The lesion also can result from acute traction on the arm and from an abduction and external rotation mechanism.[164,165]

Patients usually report pain with overhead activities and a frequent catching or popping sensation in the shoulder. The most reliable diagnostic test is O'Brien's test. The test is performed against resistance with the arm in forward flexion and with the elbow extended and the forearm pronated. In the second part of the test, the arm is supinated. Less pain during the latter part of the test suggests a SLAP lesion.[163] The most accurate diagnostic test is MRI-arthrography with gadolinium.[166] Treatment for symptomatic SLAP lesions is surgical in symptomatic young athletes and conservative in non-athletes.

Adhesive Capsulitis

Adhesive capsulitis, or frozen shoulder syndrome (FSS), is a condition characterized by limited motion of the shoulder joint with pain at the extremes of motion. It was first described by Putman[167] in 1882 and later by Codman.[87] The initial presentation is pain that is generalized and is referred to the upper arm, back, and neck. As pain increases, loss of joint motion ensues. The process generally is self-limiting and in most cases resolves spontaneously within 10 months, unless an underlying problem is present.

The exact cause of FSS is unknown.[92,168] It is frequently associated with conditions such as diabetes mellitus, parkinsonism, thyroid disorders, and cardiovascular disease. When one of these conditions exists, a history of some mild trauma that initiated the frozen shoulder is often reported. Major skeletal trauma and soft tissue injury may co-exist with FSS. It also may be seen with a variety of other conditions, including apical lung tumor, pulmonary tuberculosis, and cervical radiculopathy, as well as after myocardial infarction.[169–171] In one review of FSS, three of 140 patients with this syndrome had local primary invasive neoplasms.[172] Another study described three patients with adhesive capsulitis who subsequently were found to have a neoplastic lesion of the midshaft of the humerus.[173] In a high-risk patient with an underlying disorder, even minor surgery or trauma in a remote location, such as the hand, can precipitate FSS.

The pathophysiology involves a diffuse inflammatory synovitis with subsequent adherence of the capsule and loss of the normal axillary pouch and joint volume, which leads to significant loss of motion. Capsular contracture is thought to result from adhesion of the capsular surfaces or fibroblastic proliferation in response to cytokine production.[168,174,175] The condition is common in women in their 40s and 50s. Typically, the patient relays a history of diffuse, dull aching around the shoulder, with weakness and loss of motion occurring over a few months.

Usually, three distinct clinical stages of the syndrome can be identified. Stage one is the painful inflammatory or freezing phase. During this stage, pain is severe, is exacerbated by any attempts at movement, and usually lasts a few weeks or months. The patient usually feels most comfortable with the arm at the side in an adducted and internally rotated position. Phase two, the adhesive or stiffening phase, generally lasts 4 to 12 months. Pain is usually minimal during this phase, although periscapular symptoms may develop from compensatory motion to achieve elevation of the arm. The third phase of the syndrome is the resolution or thawing phase, which may last 5 to 26 months. During this time, pain eases and motion slowly improves, although some patients may improve dramatically over a short period.[176]

In the early stages, any attempts at motion may produce severe pain and associated weakness. The syndrome usually is associated with a prolonged period of immobilization.[177] Pain at night is common, along with an inability to sleep on the associated shoulder; these findings are similar to those of impingement syndrome.

In patients with a history of minimal or no trauma and FSS, a metabolic cause should be excluded. A complete blood cell count, erythrocyte sedimentation rate, serum chemistry, and thyroid function tests are performed as a screening panel. Further testing is performed if results suggest that the patient may have a systemic illness. Plain radiographs should include true anteroposterior, axillary, and scapular Y views of the shoulder. In patients with no underlying detectable illness and a negative workup, a Tc 99m pertechnetate scan may show increased uptake in FSS but, more important, it is used to exclude occult lesions or metastasis.[178]

A literature review reveals a multitude of treatment options, along with significant deficits on accurate reporting of disease staging with response to treatment.[179]

Treatment of FSS is mainly conservative and consists of intra-articular injections, application of heat, gentle stretching, NSAIDs, and modalities such as transcutaneous electrical nerve stimulation. The disease usually is self-limited, and after the painful phase it is not severely disabling. Communication between the physician and the patient, together with a thorough explanation of the condition, is essential, because resolution of the syndrome occurs slowly. Closed manipulation and surgery (open and arthroscopic) are reserved for patients whose condition is recalcitrant to conservative measures or for whom the diagnosis is in question. Paramount in the prevention of FSS is avoiding overimmobilization with a minor shoulder injury, in addition to careful identification of patients at risk for FSS.

Fareed and Gallivan[180] reported good results with hydraulic distention of the glenohumeral joint using local anesthetic agents. Rizk and associates[181] conducted a prospective, randomized study to assess the effects of steroid or local anesthetic injection in 48 patients with FSS. No significant difference in outcome was noted between people who received intrabursal or intra-articular injection. Steroid with lidocaine offered no advantage compared with lidocaine alone in restoring shoulder motion. However, transient pain relief occurred in two-thirds of patients treated with steroids.[181]

General anesthesia occasionally is indicated for closed manipulation. Hill and Bogumill[182] reported the results of manipulation of 17 frozen shoulders in 15 patients who did not respond to physical therapy. On average, 78% of people who were working before their shoulder problems returned to work 2.6 months after manipulation. Investigators concluded that manipulation allowed patients to return to a normal lifestyle and to work sooner than the reported natural history of the condition.[182] Surgical intervention for adhesive capsulitis should be limited to treatment of an underlying problem, such as calcific tendinitis or an impingement syndrome and failure to respond to a prolonged period of conservative treatment.

Glenohumeral Instability

Glenohumeral instability is a pathologic condition that manifests as pain associated with excessive translation of the humeral head on the glenoid during shoulder motion. Instability can range from excessive laxity with episodes of subluxation to frank dislocation of the joint. Traumatic dislocation of the glenohumeral joint reveals characteristic clinical and radiographic findings that are beyond the scope of this chapter and have been reviewed in detail elsewhere.[183] The most common type of instability is anterior, although posterior and multidirectional laxity of the shoulder is increasingly recognized as a cause of shoulder pain. Anterior dislocation usually occurs with the arm in an abducted and externally rotated position, and the diagnosis is usually obvious. Posterior dislocation is frequently associated with convulsive disorders or unusual trauma with the arm in a forward flexed and internally rotated position. The diagnosis is often missed and should always be suspected in the patient who is unable to rotate the arm externally after trauma.

Recurrent subluxation without dislocation may be difficult to diagnose and may mistakenly be identified as impingement with chronic cuff tendinitis. An athlete whose sport entails overhead actions may experience repetitive stresses to the shoulder, causing microtrauma to the static stabilizers. One study[19] described a syndrome of shoulder pain in athletes who engage in overhead activities or throwing that manifests as impingement but is caused by anterior subluxation of the joint, with the humeral head impinging on the anterior aspect of the coracoacromial arch. Another study[184] underscored this distinction by dividing the causes of rotator cuff tendinitis into primary impingement of the tendon on the coracoacromial arch and anterior subluxation with secondary impingement in young athletes performing overhead movements. Another study[185] described intra-articular impingement between the undersurface of the rotator cuff (supraspinatus and infraspinatus) and the posterior superior glenoid rim and labrum. This "internal impingement" usually is observed in athletes who engage in overhead activities and have subtle anterior glenohumeral instability, and it results in tendonitis or partial tears of the rotator cuff (see Fig. 49.17).

The diagnosis of glenohumeral instability with subluxation in one or multiple directions is made with the combination of a detailed history and physical examination and the use of adjuncts, such as arthrography, CT, MRI, and arthroscopy with examination under the effects of anesthesia. The syndrome of multidirectional instability has been recognized in patients with symptomatic inferior instability, in addition to anterior or posterior instability. Approximately 50% of affected patients have evidence of generalized laxity. Frequently, the syndrome occurs in young athletic patients who are loose jointed, oftentimes affecting the dominant arm of pitchers, racket sports players, and swimmers. In these types of athletes, repetitive microtrauma may cause stretching of the shoulder, resulting in a large capsular pouch without labral detachment. A traumatic event may damage the shoulder, resulting in the syndrome of multidirectional instability and a Bankart lesion.[186]

The most common manifestation in these patients is pain, which often is mistakenly considered to be rotator cuff tendonitis. The patient may relate a history of minor trauma causing acute pain and a "dead arm" syndrome lasting minutes or hours. Other associated symptoms include a sense of instability, weakness, and radicular symptoms suggestive of neuropathy. Few or no positive physical findings may be associated with chronic subluxation or multidirectional instability. The patient may have signs of generalized ligamentous laxity, and pain may be reproduced by subluxating the glenohumeral joint in multiple directions. One particularly helpful sign of inferior laxity is the sulcus sign, which refers to the subacromial indentation that occurs when longitudinal traction is applied to the humerus with the arm at the side. This sign occurs with inferior translation of the humeral head. Because this syndrome frequently occurs in athletes with highly developed musculature around the shoulder girdle, physical findings of subluxation may be difficult to reproduce in the office setting.

Plain radiographs are generally normal, although some inferior subluxation may be shown on stress radiographs obtained with the use of weights. Special radiographs, as discussed previously, may show a Bankart lesion (i.e., avulsion of the anterior inferior glenoid rim) or a Hill-Sachs lesion (i.e., osteochondral defect of the posterior humeral head) with subluxation of the humeral head in front of the anterior glenoid rim. CT-arthrography or MRI-arthrography may show increased capsular volume, a labral detachment, or a Hill-Sachs lesion (see Fig. 49.9). When surgery is indicated, examination under the effects of anesthesia and shoulder arthroscopy may assist in diagnosing the primary direction of instability in the syndrome of multidirectional instability. In selected patients with traumatic anterior dislocation who have no history of multidirectional instability, arthroscopic stabilization may be performed with stabilization of the capsulolabral complex.

Treatment of patients with chronic subluxation or the syndrome of multidirectional instability is first directed toward prolonged rehabilitation. Activities that stress the shoulder and produce symptoms are avoided. Strengthening exercises of the shoulder girdle may control symptoms, dynamically stabilizing the glenohumeral joint, and may obviate the need for surgical intervention. If a conservative treatment program fails, surgery is performed on the side associated with the greatest clinical instability. Stabilization is directed toward tightening of the capsular structures to stabilize the glenohumeral joint.[186,187]

Extrinsic or Regional Factors Causing Shoulder Pain

Because the shoulder girdle connects the thorax with the upper extremity, and because major neurovascular structures pass in proximity to the joint, shoulder pain can be a hallmark of many nonarticular conditions.

Cervical Radiculopathy

Cervical disease may manifest with associated shoulder pain. The area of referred pain has a dermatomal pattern, consistent with the distribution of dermatomal nerve roots. Isolation of the pain usually defines the exact location of associated cervical disease. Pain can be differentiated from shoulder pain on the basis of history, physical examination, EMG, cervical radiographs, and myelography or MRI when indicated. Because conditions causing cervical neck pain and conditions causing shoulder pain, such as calcific tendinitis and cervical radiculopathy, may co-exist, it often is difficult to distinguish which lesion is responsible for the symptoms. These conditions often can be differentiated by injection of local anesthetics to block certain components of the pain.

The thoracic outlet is an interval created by the anterior and middle scalene muscles and the first rib through which the brachial plexus and vessels pass to the arm. In thoracic outlet syndrome, compression of these nerves and vessels often manifests as vague shoulder pain with numbness of the ipsilateral fourth and fifth digits. Cervical rib or hypertrophy of the scalene muscles can be related to the onset of pain.[188–190] The occurrence of pain also has been related to scapular ptosis, poor posture, and clavicular fracture with malunion or copious formation of callus.

Brachial Neuritis

In the 1940s Spillane[191] and Parsonage and Turner[192,193] described a painful condition of the shoulder associated with limitation of motion. As pain subsided and motion improved, muscle weakness and atrophy became apparent. The deltoid, supraspinatus, infraspinatus, biceps, and triceps are the most frequently involved muscles,[194] although diaphragmatic paralysis also has been reported.[193,195] The cause is unclear, but the clustering of cases suggests a viral or postviral syndrome.[192,193] Occasionally, an associated influenza-like syndrome or previous vaccination has been reported.[194]

One study[196] described acute brachial neuropathy in athletes. Findings that suggest an acute brachial neuropathy include acute onset of pain without trauma; persistent, severe pain that continues despite rest; and patchy neurologic signs. The diagnosis is confirmed by EMG and nerve conduction studies.[196] The prognosis for recovery is excellent, although full recovery may take 2 to 3 years. Tsairis and associates[197] reported 80% recovery within 2 years and more than 90% recovery by the end of 3 years.

Nerve Entrapment Syndromes

Peripheral compression neuropathies of the upper extremities may produce referral pain to the shoulder. Distant compression neuropathies, such as carpal tunnel (median nerve) and cubital tunnel (ulnar nerve) syndromes, may manifest with concomitant and separate shoulder impingement with rotator cuff disease. Associated numbness and paresthesias with mapping of the dermatomal distribution and with peripheral neuropathy often direct the examiner to the appropriate diagnosis. Patients often give a history of dropping objects and a feeling of clumsiness with the affected hand. A Tinel's sign may be elicited over the region of entrapment at the elbow or wrist. Provocative maneuvers such as Phalen's test may be positive and usually indicate median nerve compression at the wrist. Diminished vibratory sensation is an early finding in the disease and is easily reproducible,[198,199] whereas decreased two-point discrimination and intrinsic atrophy are late findings of peripheral compression neuropathy.[198]

The diagnosis usually can be made by clinical examination with exclusion of other possible causes. EMG and nerve conduction velocity tests may reveal slowed conduction and latency at appropriate compression points to aid in diagnosis. Spinal accessory nerve injury with subsequent denervation of the trapezius may cause weakness and pain in the shoulder consistent with impingement. The injury can occur from traction injury to the neck or a direct blow or pressure to the base of the neck. Iatrogenic nerve injury may result from surgical procedures on the neck such as lymph node biopsy.[200] The injury produces weakness in shoulder abduction with associated pain that radiates from the neck into the trapezius and shoulder. Subsequent atrophy of the trapezius may lead to dissymmetry and ptosis of the involved shoulder, with narrowing of the supraspinatus outlet and secondary impingement with shoulder pain. Definitive diagnosis can be made by EMG examination.

Early treatment is conservative. If return of function is not evident at 6 months, surgical exploration of the nerve with possible tendon transfers may be indicated.[201]

Injury to the long thoracic nerve (cervical fifth, sixth, and seventh roots) can lead to scapular winging. The resultant scapular dysrhythmia and weakness can lead to a painful shoulder that may mimic rotator cuff disease.[200] Patients also report pain and discomfort with active forward flexion of the shoulder. Patients who remain symptomatic after conservative treatment may require surgery for scapulothoracic fusion or tendon transfer with use of the pectoralis major or minor to stabilize the scapula.[202,203]

In quadrilateral space syndrome, the axillary nerve is compressed by fibrous bands in the quadrilateral space.[200,204,205] This syndrome typically occurs when the arm is held in abduction and external rotation, with subsequent tightening of fibrous bands across the nerve.[206] It is most commonly seen in the dominant shoulder of young athletic individuals such as pitchers, tennis players, and swimmers who function with an excessive amount of overhead activity. Pain may occur throughout the shoulder girdle and may radiate down the arm in a nondermatomal pattern. Findings of neurologic and EMG testing may be normal. Diagnosis often is made by an arteriogram of the subclavian artery. A positive arteriogram reveals compression of the posterior humeral circumflex artery as it traverses the quadrangular space when the arm is in the abducted and externally rotated position. Surgical intervention may be required to release the fibrotic bands or the tendon of the teres minor if the patient does not respond to conservative treatment.[200,207]

Suprascapular nerve entrapment syndrome can be caused by a traction lesion resulting from repetitive overhead activities, a compression lesion, or both, involving the nerve; it is caused by tethering of the nerve at the suprascapular notch by the suprascapular ligament or at the spinoglenoid notch by the transverse ligament. Suprascapular nerve entrapment syndrome also can result from direct compression of a space-occupying lesion, such as a ganglion or a lipoma. One study[208] described variations in size and shape of the suprascapular notch that may predispose the nerve to entrapment. Several authors have noted an association of suprascapular neuropathy with massive rotator cuff tears, presumably resulting from a traction injury to the nerve.[209,210]

The resulting suprascapular neuropathy produces pain in the posterolateral aspect of the shoulder that may radiate into the ipsilateral extremity, shoulder, or side of the neck. Although this condition is uncommon, it can have a prolonged and disabling course when it is not diagnosed. Because the suprascapular nerve has no cutaneous innervation, no numbness, tingling, or paresthesias are associated with this condition. Weakness is usually noted in abduction and external rotation, and significant atrophy is often observed at diagnosis. The pain frequently is described as a deep burning or aching that can be well localized and often can be elicited by palpation over the region of the suprascapular notch. Any activity that brings the scapula forward, such as reaching across the chest, may aggravate the pain.[211] The location of pain and other symptoms can mimic more common entities, such as impingement, rotator cuff disease, cervical disk disease, brachial neuropathy, biceps tendinitis, thoracic outlet syndrome, AC disease, and instability of the shoulder.[212]

One study[213] reported the efficacy of MRI in the diagnosis of suprascapular nerve entrapment as a result of space-occupying lesions. Definitive diagnosis is made with EMG and nerve conduction studies. EMG changes usually reveal spontaneous activity in the muscle at rest and fibrillations indicating motor atrophy and denervation. Nerve conduction studies may reveal slowing across the site of entrapment. As with axillary nerve entrapment, the syndrome is often associated with young, athletic people who engage in excessive overhead activity.[214] It also has been associated with trauma.[212,215,216]

Lack of consensus continues regarding the optimal treatment of suprascapular neuropathy.[1,212,214,217–219] Post and Grinblat[217] reported good to excellent results with surgical treatment in 25 of 26 cases. No difference in residual atrophy and in strength deficits has been shown, however, for operative and nonoperative treatments. Another study[214] evaluated 96 top-level volleyball players from the 1985 European Championships and found that 12 had isolated suprascapular neuropathy with atrophy of the infraspinatus of the dominant shoulder. All players were unaware of any impairment, however, and played without limitations. After a space-occupying lesion has been excluded, a 6-month trial of conservative treatment may be indicated for some people. If the entrapment does not improve or if symptoms worsen with conservative treatment, surgical decompression for pain relief is warranted; however, resolution of atrophy and strength gains can vary.[212]

Sternoclavicular Arthritis

Occasionally, traumatic, nontraumatic, or infectious conditions can cause pain in the area of the sternoclavicular joint (see Fig. 49.1). The most common problem involves ligamentous injury and painful subluxation or dislocation, which can be diagnosed by palpable instability and crepitus over the sternoclavicular joint. Radiographic sternoclavicular views may show dislocation.[220]

Inflammatory arthritis of the sternoclavicular joint has been associated with RA, psoriatic arthritis, ankylosing spondylitis, and septic arthritis. The association of palmoplantar pustulosis with sternoclavicular arthritis has been reported.[221] Seven of 15 patients who underwent biopsy for this condition had cultures positive for *Propionibacterium acnes*, suggesting an infectious origin of the condition.[221]

Two other conditions involving the sternoclavicular joint are Tietze's syndrome, a painful, nonsuppurative swelling of the joint and adjacent sternochondral junctions, and Friedrich's syndrome, a painful osteonecrosis of the sternal end of the clavicle.[4] Condensing osteitis of the clavicle is a rare benign idiopathic lesion of the medial one-third of the clavicle. This condition, which is better described as aseptic enlarging osteosclerosis of the clavicle, is most commonly seen in middle-aged women and manifests as a tender swelling over the medial one-third of the clavicle.[222]

Reflex Sympathetic Dystrophy

Since its original description by Mitchell[223] in 1864, reflex sympathetic dystrophy (RSD) has remained a poorly understood and frequently overlooked condition. Its cause is unknown but may be related to sympathetic overflow or short-circuiting of impulses through the sympathetic system. Any clinician who deals with painful disorders must be familiar with the diagnosis and treatment of this condition. Bonica's[224] excellent review covers the clinical presentation, various stages of the disease, and the importance of early intervention to ensure a successful outcome.

RSD has been called causalgia, shoulder-hand syndrome, and Sudeck's atrophy, which has caused some confusion. It is generally associated with minor trauma and is to be differentiated from causalgia, which involves trauma to major nerve roots.[223] RSD is divided into three phases, which are important in determining appropriate treatment.[224] Phase one is characterized by sympathetic overflow with diffuse swelling, pain, increased vascularity, and radiographic evidence of demineralization. If left untreated for 3 to 6 months, the condition may progress to phase two, which is characterized by atrophy. The extremity may now be cold and shiny, with atrophy of the skin and muscles. Phase three refers to progression of trophic changes, with irreversible flexion contracture and a pale, cold, painful extremity. It has been speculated that phase one is related to peripheral short-circuiting of nerve impulses, phase two represents short-circuiting through the internuncial pool in the spinal cord, and phase three is controlled by higher thalamic centers.[224,225]

Steinbrocker[226] reported that recovery is possible as long as vasomotor activity with swelling and hyperemia is evident. After the trophic phase two or three is established, the prognosis for recovery is poor. Prompt recognition of the syndrome is important because early intervention to control pain is mandatory. Careful supervision and reassurance are crucial because many of these patients are emotionally labile as a result of the pain or an underlying problem. The syndrome may be reversed to a remarkable degree by a sympathetic block. Patients who receive transient relief from sympathetic blockade may be helped by surgical sympathectomy.

Neoplasms

Primary and metastatic neoplasms may cause shoulder pain by direct invasion of the musculoskeletal system or by compression with referred pain.[2,227] Primary tumors are more likely to occur in younger individuals. More common lesions have a typical distribution, such as the predilection of a chondroblastoma for the proximal humeral epiphysis or an osteogenic sarcoma for the metaphysis.[228] The differential diagnosis of spontaneous onset of shoulder pain in older individuals should include metastatic lesions and myeloma. Neoplasms are best identified by plain radiographs, MRI, Tc 99m MDP scintigraphy, and CT.

Neoplasms also may involve the shoulder region through metastases to the region. An associated history of carcinomas should alert the examiner to the possibility of a bone tumor, especially in patients who have had malignancies with a predilection for metastasis to bone (e.g., thyroid, renal, lung, prostate, and breast malignancies). Pain often is present at rest and is exacerbated at night. Atypical pain distribution that is not relieved by injection without specific dermatomal distribution should alert the examiner to other underlying possibilities. Plain radiographs should be evaluated thoroughly for any cortical destruction and for lytic lesions.

Pancoast syndrome or apical lung tumor may manifest as shoulder pain or cervical radiculitis caused by invasion of the brachial plexus or invasion of C8 or T1 roots.[229–231] With invasion of the cervical sympathetic chain, the patient also may experience Homer's syndrome.

Miscellaneous Conditions

With increasing numbers of patients undergoing long-term maintenance hemodialysis, a shoulder pain syndrome known as dialysis shoulder arthropathy has been described. This syndrome consists of shoulder pain, weakness, loss of motion, and functional limitation. The cause and pathogenesis of this syndrome are unclear, although rotator cuff disease, pathologic fracture, bursitis, and local amyloid deposition have been implicated as causative factors.[232] Surgical or necropsy data are insufficient to confirm a specific diagnosis. Patients generally respond poorly to local measures of injection, application of heat, and NSAIDs, but their condition may improve with correction of underlying metabolic disorders, such as osteomalacia and secondary hyperparathyroidism.

In patients older than 50 years who have bilateral shoulder pain and stiffness, polymyalgia rheumatica should be considered as a diagnosis. This condition is twice as common among females and is almost exclusively found in white people.[233] Most patients have sedimentation rates greater than 40 mm/hr and respond to low doses of corticosteroids.[234]

Full references for this chapter can be found on ExpertConsult.com.

Selected References

1. O'Brien SJ, Arnoczky SP, Warren RF: Developmental anatomy of the shoulder and anatomy of the glenohumeral joint. In Rockwood CA, Matsen III FA, editors: *The shoulder*, Philadelphia, 1990, WB Saunders.
2. Andrews JR, Carson W, McLeod W: Glenoid labrum tears related to the long head of the biceps, *Am J Sports Med* 13:337, 1985.
3. Bateman E: *The shoulder and neck*, ed 2, Philadelphia, 1978, WB Saunders.
4. Post M: *The shoulder: surgical and non-surgical management*, Philadelphia, 1988, Lea & Febiger.
5. Cortes A, Quinlan NJ, Nazal MR, et al.: A value-based care analysis of magnetic resonance imaging in patients with suspected partial rotator cuff tears and the implicated role of conservative management, *J Shoulder and Elbow Surg* 28(11):2153–2160, 2019.
6. Martin SD, Warren RF, Martin TL, et al.: The non-operative management of suprascapular neuropathy, *J Bone Joint Surg Am* 79:1159, 1997.
7. Neer II CS: Anterior acromioplasty for the chronic impingement syndrome in the shoulder: a preliminary report, *J Bone Joint Surg Am* 54:41, 1972.
8. Martin SD, Al-Zahrani SM, Andrews JR, et al.: *The circumduction adduction shoulder test*, Atlanta, February 22, 1996, Presented at Sixty-Third Annual Meeting of the American Academy of Orthopedic Surgeons.
9. O'Brien SJ, Pagnani MJ, McGlynn SR, et al.: *A new and effective test for diagnosing labral tears and AC joint pathology*, Atlanta, February 22, 1996, Presented at Sixty-Third Annual Meeting of the American Academy of Orthopedic Surgeons.
10. DePalma AF: Surgical anatomy of the acromioclavicular and sternoclavicular joints, *Surg Clin North Am* 43:1540, 1963.
11. Martin SD, Baumgarten T, Andrews JR: Arthroscopic subacromial decompression with concomitant distal clavicle resection, *J Bone Joint Surg Am* 85:328, 2001.
12. Dillin L, Hoaglund FT, Scheck M: Brachial neuritis, *J Bone Joint Surg Am* 67:878, 1985.
13. Kelly BT, Kadrmas WR, Speer KP: The manual muscle examination for rotator cuff strength, *Am J Sports Med* 24:581, 1996.
14. Saha AK: *Theory of shoulder mechanism*, Springfield, IL, 1961, Charles C Thomas.
15. Saha AK: Mechanics of elevation of glenohumeral joint: its application in rehabilitation of flail shoulder in upper brachial plexus injuries and poliomyelitis and in replacement of the upper humerus by prosthesis, *Acta Orthop Scand* 44:668, 1973.
16. Brown JT: Early assessment of supraspinatus tears: procaine infiltration as a guide to treatment, *J Bone Joint Surg Br* 31:423, 1949.
17. Neer CS: Impingement lesions, *Clin Orthop Relat Res* 173:70, 1983.
18. Rockwood CA: The role of anterior impingement in lesions of the rotator cuff, *J Bone Joint Surg Am* 62:274, 1980.
19. Jobe FW, Kvitne RS, Giangarra CE: Shoulder pain in the overhead or throwing athlete: the relationship of anterior instability and rotator cuff impingement, *Orthop Rev* 18:963, 1989.
20. Dalton SE, Snyder SJ: Glenohumeral instability, *Baillieres Clin Rheumatol* 3:511, 1989.
21. Zanca P: Shoulder pain: involvement of the acromioclavicular joint (analysis of 1000 cases), *AJR Am J Roentgenol* 112:493, 1971.
22. Goldman AB: *Shoulder arthrography*, Boston, 1982, Little, Brown.
23. Goldman AB, Ghelman B: The double contrast shoulder arthrogram: a review of 158 studies, *Radiology* 127:655, 1978.
24. Mink J, Harris E: Double contrast shoulder arthrography: its use in evaluation of rotator cuff tears, *Orthop Trans* 7:71, 1983.
25. Braunstein EM, O'Connor G: Double-contrast arthrotomography of the shoulder, *J Bone Joint Surg Am* 64:192, 1982.
26. Ghelman B, Goldman AB: The double contrast shoulder arthrogram: evaluation of rotator cuff tears, *Radiology* 124:251, 1977.

27. Goldman AB, Ghelman B: The double contrast shoulder arthrogram, *Cardiology* 127:665, 1978.
28. Kneisl JS, Sweeney HJ, Paige ML: Correlation of pathology observed in double contrast arthrotomography, *Arthroscopy* 4:21, 1988.
29. Strizak AM, Danzig L, Jackson DW, et al.: Subacromial bursography, *J Bone Joint Surg Am* 64:196, 1982.
30. Lie S: Subacromial bursography, *Radiology* 144:626, 1982.
31. Fukuda H, Mikasa M, Yamanaka K: Incomplete thickness rotator cuff tears diagnosed by subacromial bursography, *Clin Orthop Relat Res* 223:51, 1987.
32. Rafii M, Minkoff J, Bonana J, et al.: Computed tomography (CT) arthrography of shoulder instabilities in athletes, *Am J Sports Med* 16:352, 1988.
33. Crass JR, Craig EV, Bretzke C, et al.: Ultrasonography of the rotator cuff, *Radiographics* 5:941, 1985.
34. el Khoury GY, Kathol MH, Chandler JB, et al.: Shoulder instability: impact of glenohumeral arthrotomography on treatment, *Radiology* 160:669, 1986.
35. Mack LA, Matsen FA, Kilcoyne RF, et al.: US evaluation of the rotator cuff, *Radiology* 157:206, 1985.
36. Harryman DT, Mack LA, Wang KA, et al.: *Integrity of the postoperative cuff: ultrasonography and function*, New Orleans, February 9, 1990, Presented at Fifty-Seventh Annual Meeting of the American Academy of Orthopedic Surgeons.
37. Hodler J, Fretz CJ, Terrier F, et al.: Rotator cuff tears: correlation of sonic and surgical findings, *Radiology* 169:791, 1988.
38. Middleton WD, Edelstein G, Reinus WR, et al.: Ultrasonography of the rotator cuff: technique and normal anatomy, *J Ultrasound Med* 3:549, 1984.
39. Gardelin G, Perin B: Ultrasonics of the shoulder: diagnostic possibilities in lesions of the rotator cuff, *Radiol Med (Torino)* 74:404, 1987.
40. Vestring T, Bongartz G, Konermann W, et al.: The place of magnetic resonance tomography in the diagnosis of diseases of the shoulder joint, *Fortschr Geb Rontgenstr Neuen Bildgeb Verfahr* 154:143, 1991.
41. Ahovuo J, Paavolainen P, Slatis P: Diagnostic value of sonography in lesions of the biceps tendon. *Clin Orthop Relat Res* 202:184, 1986.
42. Zlatkin MB, Reicher MA, Kellerhouse LE, et al.: The painful shoulder: MRI imaging of the glenohumeral joint, *J Comput Assist Tomogr* 12:995, 1988.
43. Meyer SJ, Dalinka MK: Magnetic resonance imaging of the shoulder, *Orthop Clin North Am* 21:497, 1990.
44. Seeger LL, Gold RH, Bassett LW: Shoulder instability: evaluation with MR imaging, *Radiology* 168:696, 1988.
45. Kieft GJ, Dijkmans BA, Bioem JL, et al.: Magnetic resonance imaging of the shoulder in patients with rheumatoid arthritis, *Ann Rheum Dis* 49(7), 1990.
46. Morrison DS, Offstein R: The use of magnetic resonance imaging in the diagnosis of rotator cuff tears, *Orthopedics* 13(633), 1990.
47. Nelson MC, Leather GP, Nirschl RP, et al.: Evaluation of the painful shoulder: a prospective comparison of magnetic resonance imaging, computerized tomographic arthrography, *J Bone Joint Surg Am* 73:707, 1991.
48. Reeder JD, Andelman S: The rotator cuff tear: MR evaluation, *Magn Reson Imaging* 5:331, 1987.
49. Seeger LL, Gold RH, Bassett LW, et al.: Shoulder impingement syndrome: MR findings in 53 shoulders, *AJR Am J Roentgenol* 150:343, 1988.
50. Ogilvie-Harris DJ, D'Angelo G: Arthroscopic surgery of the shoulder, *Sports Med* 9:120, 1990.
51. Ellman H: Arthroscopic subacromial decompression, *Orthop Trans* 9(49), 1985.
52. Ellman H: Arthroscopic subacromial decompression: analysis of one- to three-year results, *Arthroscopy* 3(173), 1987.
53. Paulos LE, Franklin JL: Arthroscopic shoulder decompression development and application: a five year experience, *Am J Sports Med* 17:235, 1990.
54. Nakano KK: *Neurology of musculoskeletal and rheumatic disorders*, Boston, 1979, Houghton Mifflin.
55. Leffert RD: Brachial plexus injuries, *N Engl J Med* 291:1059, 1974.
56. Buchbinder R, Gren S, Youd J: Corticosteroid injections for shoulder pain, *Cochrane Database Syst Rev* 1:CD004016, 2003.
57. Altchek DW, Schwartz E, Warren RF, et al.: *Radiologic measurement of superior migration of the humeral head in impingement syndrome*, New Orleans, February 11, 1990, Presented at the Sixth Open Meeting of the American Shoulder and Elbow Surgeons.
58. Inman VT, Saunders JB, Abbott LC: Observations on the functions of the shoulder joint, *J Bone Joint Surg Am* 26(1), 1944.
59. Poppen NK, Walker PS: Normal and abnormal motion of the shoulder, *J Bone Joint Surg Am* 58:195, 1976.
60. LU Bigliani, Morrison D, April EW: The morphology of the acromion and its relationship to rotator cuff tears, *Orthop Trans* 10(228), 1986.
61. Morrison DS, LU Bigliani: The clinical significance of variations in acromial morphology, *Orthop Trans* 11:234, 1987.
62. Codman E, Akerson TB: The pathology associated with rupture of the supraspinatus tendon, *Ann Surg* 93:354, 1911.
63. Fukuda H, Hamada K, Yamanaka K: Pathology and pathogenesis of bursal side rotator cuff tears: views from enbloc histological sections, *Clin Orthop Relat Res* 254:75, 1990.
64. McLaughlin HL: Lesions of the musculotendinous cuff of the shoulder. I. The exposure and treatment of tears with retraction, *J Bone Joint Surg Am* 26:31, 1944.
65. Neer II CS, Flatow EL, Lech O: *Tears of the rotator cuff: long term results of anterior acromioplasty and repair*, Atlanta, February 1988, Presented at Fourth Open Meeting of the American Shoulder and Elbow Surgeons.
66. Ogata S, Uhthoff HK: Acromial enthesopathy and rotator cuff tears: a radiographic and histologic postmortem investigation of the coracoacromial arch, *Clin Orthop Relat Res* 254:39, 1990.
67. Olsson O: Degenerative changes in the shoulder joint and their connection with shoulder pain: a morphological and clinical investigation with special attention to the cuff and biceps tendon, *Acta Chir Scand* 181(Suppl):1, 1953.
68. Ozaki J, Fujimoto S, Nakagawa Y, et al.: Tears of the rotator cuff of the shoulder associated with pathologic changes of the acromion: a study in cadavers, *J Bone Joint Surg Am* 70:1224, 1988.
69. Skinner HA: Anatomical consideration relative to ruptures of the supraspinatus tendon, *J Bone Joint Surg Br* 19(137), 1937.
70. Jackson DW: Chronic rotator cuff impingement in the throwing athlete, *Am J Sports Med* 4:231, 1976.
71. Ellman H: Occupational supraspinatus tendinitis: the rotator cuff syndrome, *Ugeskr Laeger* 151:2355, 1989.
72. Scheib JS: Diagnosis and rehabilitation of the shoulder impingement syndrome in the overhand and throwing athlete, *Rheum Dis Clin North Am* 16:971, 1990.
73. Hawkins RJ, Kennedy JC: Impingement syndrome in athletes, *Am J Sports Med* 8:151, 1980.
74. McShane RB, Leinberry CF, Fenlin JM: Conservative open anterior acromioplasty, *Clin Orthop Relat Res* 223:137, 1987.
75. Rockwood CA, Lyons FA: Shoulder impingement syndrome: diagnosis, radiographic evaluation, and treatment with a modified Neer acromioplasty, *J Bone Joint Surg Am* 75:1593, 1993.
76. Hawkins RJ, Brock RM, Abrams JS, et al.: Acromioplasty for impingement with an intact rotator cuff, *J Bone Joint Surg Br* 70:797, 1988.
77. Stuart MJ, Azevedo AJ, Cofield RH: Anterior acromioplasty for treatment of the shoulder impingement syndrome, *Clin Orthop Relat Res* 260(195), 1990.
78. LU Bigliani, D'Alesandro DF, Duralde XA, et al.: Anterior acromioplasty for subacromial impingement in patients younger than 40 years of age, *Clin Orthop Relat Res* 246:111, 1988.
79. Bjorkheim JM, Paavolainen P, Ahovuo J, et al.: Surgical repair of the rotator cuff and the surrounding tissues: factors influencing the results, *Clin Orthop Relat Res* 236:148, 1988.

80. Levy HJ, Gardner RD, Lemak LJ: Arthroscopic subacromial decompression in the treatment of full-thickness rotator cuff tears, *Arthroscopy* 7(8), 1991.
81. Karjalainen TV, et al.: *Chochrane database of systematic reviews*, 2019.
82. McKendry RJR, Uhthoff HK, Sarkar K, et al.: Calcifying tendinitis of the shoulder: prognostic value of clinical, histologic, and radiographic features in 57 surgically treated cases, *J Rheumatol* 9:75, 1982.
83. Uhthoff HK, Sarkar K, Maynard JA: Calcifying tendinitis, a new concept of its pathogenesis, *Clin Orthop Relat Res* 118:164, 1976.
84. Sarkar K, Uhthoff HK: Ultrastructure localization of calcium in calcifying tendinitis, *Arch Pathol Lab Med* 102:266, 1978.
85. Hayes CW, Conway WF: Calcium hydroxyapatite deposition disease, *Radiographics* 10(1031), 1990.
86. Vebostad A: Calcific tendinitis in the shoulder region: a review of 43 operated shoulders, *Acta Orthop Scand* 46:205, 1975.
87. Codman EA: *The shoulder: rupture of the supraspinatus tendon and other lesions in or about the subacromial bursa*, Boston, 1934, Thomas Todd.
88. Moseley HF, Goldie I: The arterial pattern of the rotator cuff of the shoulder, *J Bone Joint Surg Br* 45:780, 1963.
89. Rathburn JB, Macnab I: The microvascular pattern of the rotator cuff, *J Bone Joint Surg Br* 52:540, 1970.
90. Bosworth BM: Calcium deposits in the shoulder and subacromial bursitis: a survey of 12,122 shoulders, *JAMA* 116:2477, 1941.
91. Bosworth BM: Examination of the shoulder for calcium deposits, *J Bone Joint Surg Am* 23:567, 1941.
92. DePalma AF, Kruper JS: Long term study of shoulder joints afflicted with and treated for calcified tendonitis, *Clin Orthop Relat Res* 20:61, 1961.
93. Rizzello G, Franceschi F, Ruzzini L, et al.: Arthroscopic management of calcific tendinopathy of the shoulder, *Bull NYU Hosp Jt Dis* 67:330, 2009.
94. Linblom K: Arthrography and roentgenography in ruptures of the tendon of the shoulder joint, *Acta Radiol* 20:548, 1939.
95. Swiontkowski M, Iannotti JP, Herrmann HJ, et al.: Intraoperative assessment of rotator cuff vascularity using laser Doppler flowmetry. In Post M, Morrey BE, Hawkins RJ, editors: *Surgery of the shoulder*, St Louis, 1990, Mosby, pp 208–212.
96. Matsen III FA, Arntz CT: Subacromial impingement. In Rockwood Jr CA, Matsen III FA, editors: *The shoulder*, Philadelphia, 1990, WB Saunders, pp 623–646.
97. Neer II CS, Poppen NK: Supraspinatus outlet, *Orthop Trans* 11:234, 1987.
98. Clark J, Sidles JA, Matsen FA: The relationship of the glenohumeral joint capsule to the rotator cuff, *Clin Orthop Relat Res* 254:29, 1990.
99. Samilson RL, Raphael RL, Post L, et al.: Arthrography of the shoulder, *Clin Orthop Relat Res* 20:21, 1961.
100. Collins RA, Gristina AG, Carter RE, et al.: Ultrasonography of the shoulder, *Orthop Clin North Am* 18:351, 1987.
101. Crass JR, Craig EV, Feinberg SB: Ultrasonography of rotator cuff tears: a review of 500 diagnostic studies, *J Clin Ultrasound* 16:313, 1988.
102. Crass JR, Craig EV, Feinberg SB: The hyperextended internal rotation view in rotator cuff ultrasonography, *J Clin Ultrasound* 15:415, 1987.
103. Mack LA, Gannon MK, Kilcoyne RF, et al.: Sonographic evaluation of the rotator cuff: accuracy in patients without prior surgery, *Clin Orthop Relat Res* 234:21, 1988.
104. Iannotti JP, Zlatkin MB, Esterhai JL, et al.: Magnetic resonance imaging of the shoulder: sensitivity, specificity, and predictive value, *J Bone Joint Surg Am* 73(17), 1991.
105. DePalma AF: *Surgery of the shoulder*, ed 2, Philadelphia, 1973, JB Lippincott.
106. Wolfgang GL: Surgical repair of tears of the rotator cuff of the shoulder: factors influencing the result, *J Bone Joint Surg Am* 56(14), 1974.
107. Jobe FW, Moynes DR: Delineation of diagnostic criteria and a rehabilitation program for rotator cuff injuries, *Am J Sports Med* 10:336, 1982.
108. Coghlan JA, Buchbinder R, Green S, et al.: Surgery for rotator cuff disease, *Cochrane Database Syst Rev* 1:CD005619, 2009.
109. Oh L, Wolf B, Hall M, et al.: Indications for rotator cuff repair, *Clin Orthop Relat Res* 455:52, 2007.
110. Silva BM, Cartucho A, Sarmento M, et al.: Surgical treatment of rotator cuff tears after 65 years of age: a systematic review, *Acta Med. Port* 30(4), 2017.
111. Earnshaw P, Desjardins D, Sakar K, et al.: Rotator cuff tears: the role of surgery, *Can J Surg* 25:60, 1982.
112. Rockwood CA, Williams GR, Burkhead WZ: *Debridement of massive, degenerative lesions of the rotator cuff*, Anaheim, CA, March 10, 1991, Presented at Seventh Open Meeting of the American Shoulder and Elbow Society Surgeons.
113. Martin SD, Andrews JR: *The rotator cuff: open and miniopen repairs*, Palm Desert, CA, June 26, 1994, Presented at American Orthopaedic Society for Sports Medicine 20th Annual Meeting.
114. Rockwood Jr CA: The shoulder: facts, confusion and myths, *Int Orthop* 15:401, 1991.
115. Steffens K, Konermann H: Rupture of the rotator cuff in the elderly, *Z Gerontol* 20:95, 1987.
116. Mulieri P, Dunning P, Klein S, et al.: Reverse shoulder arthroplasty for the treatment of irreparable rotator cuff tear without glenohumeral arthritis, *J Bone Joint Surg Am* 92:2544, 2010.
117. Mather RC, Koenig L, Acevedo D, et al.: The societal and economic value of rotator cuff repair, *J Bone Joint Surg Am* 95:1993–2000, 2013.
118. Moosmayer S, Lund G, Seljom US, et al.: Tendon repair compared with physiotherapy in the treatment of rotator cuff tears: a randomized controlled study in 103 cases with a five-year follow-up, *J Bone Joint Surg* 96:1504–1514, 2014.
119. Goss CM: *Gray's anatomy of the human body*, ed 28, Philadelphia, 1966, Lea & Febiger.
120. Neer CS, Craig EV, Fukuda H: Cuff tear arthropathy, *J Bone Joint Surg Am* 65:1232, 1983.
121. Neer II CS, LU Bigliani, Hawkins RJ: Rupture of the long head of the biceps related to subacromial impingement, *Orthop Trans* 1:111, 1977.
122. Crenshaw AH, Kilgore WE: Surgical treatment of bicipital tendonitis, *J Bone Joint Surg Am* 48:1496, 1966.
123. Hitchcock HH, Bechtol CO: Painful shoulder: observations on the role of the tendon of the long head of the biceps brachii in its causation, *J Bone Joint Surg Am* 30:263, 1948.

50 Low Back Pain

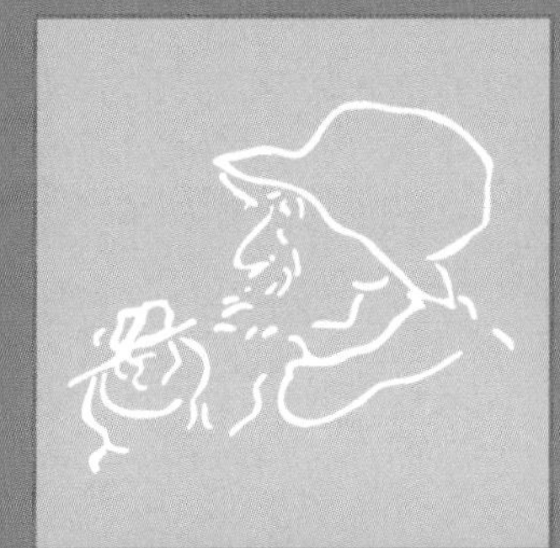

RAJIV DIXIT

KEY POINTS

- Low back pain (LBP) affects as many as 80% of individuals, and degenerative changes of the lumbar spine is the most common cause.
- More than 90% of these patients are mostly pain free within 8 weeks, although recurrences are common.
- The initial evaluation should focus on identification of the few patients with neurologic involvement, fracture, or possible systemic disease (infection, malignancy, or spondyloarthritis) because they may need urgent or specific intervention.
- Psychosocial and other factors that predict risk of chronic disabling LBP should be assessed.
- Early imaging is rarely indicated in the absence of significant neurologic involvement, trauma, or suspicion of systemic disease.
- Imaging abnormalities, often the result of age-related degenerative changes, should be carefully interpreted because they are frequently present in asymptomatic individuals.
- A precise pathoanatomic diagnosis with identification of the pain generator cannot be made in up to 85% of patients.
- Persistent LBP should be treated with an individually tailored program that includes analgesia, core strengthening, stretching, aerobic conditioning, loss of excess weight, and patient education.
- Intensive multidisciplinary rehabilitation with an emphasis on cognitive-behavioral therapy should be strongly considered if conservative measures fail.
- There is no evidence for the effectiveness of epidural corticosteroid injections in patients without radiculopathy secondary to disk herniation.
- A large number of injection techniques, physical therapy modalities, and nonsurgical interventional therapies lack evidence of efficacy.
- The major indication for back surgery is presence of a serious or progressive neurologic deficit.
- In the absence of neurologic deficits, back surgery, especially spinal fusion for degenerative changes, is not more effective than conservative care.

Epidemiology

Low back pain (LBP) is one of the most common conditions encountered in clinical medicine. It affects the area between the lower rib cage and gluteal folds.

LBP is uncommon in the first decade of life, but prevalence increases steeply during the teenage years. Around 40% of 9 to 18 year olds report having LBP.[1] The prevalence increases with age until between 60 and 69 years, then gradually declines.[1,2] LBP is more common in women.

An estimated 65% to 80% of the population will experience LBP during their lifetime. In 2015 the global point prevalence of activity limiting LBP was 7.3%, implying that 540 million people were affected at any one time. LBP is now the number one cause of disability globally, the most prevalent chronic pain syndrome, and the leading cause of limitation of activity in patients younger than 45 years. In the United States LBP accounts for more lost work days than any other occupational condition.[1]

The natural history of LBP, especially the duration and chronicity, is somewhat controversial. Back pain is increasingly understood as a long-lasting condition with a variable course rather than episodes of unrelated occurrences. Acute LBP improves substantially in most patients within 4 weeks, and more than 90% are better at 8 weeks.[3,4] However, two-thirds of the patients still report low grade discomfort at 3 and 12 months.[1] Recurrences of acute LBP are common and also tend to be brief. It is estimated that about a third of people will have a recurrence within a year of recovering from a previous episode.[5] Chronic persistent, and at times disabling, LBP (affected by a range of biophysical, psychological, and social factors) develops in the remaining 7% to 10%. These individuals with chronic pain are largely responsible for the high costs associated with LBP.

Expenditures on spinal conditions in the United States have significantly increased in recent years, despite little change in the health status among people who experience these conditions.[6] The general consensus is that approximately $90 billion is spent on the diagnosis and management of LBP, and an additional $10 to $20 billion is attributed to economic losses in productivity each year.[6–8]

A number of risk factors have been associated with LBP, including heredity (with recent identification of genetic variants associated with chronic LBP[9]), psychosocial factors, heavy lifting, obesity, pregnancy, weaker trunk strength, cigarette smoking, and low income and educational status.[10] Persistence of disabling LBP has been associated with the presence of maladaptive pain coping behavior, nonorganic signs, functional impairment, poor general health status, and psychiatric comorbidities.[11]

Anatomy

The lumbar spine is composed of five vertebrae. Each vertebra consists of a body anteriorly and a neural arch that encloses the spinal canal posteriorly (Fig. 50.1). Their cartilaginous end plates cover the superior and inferior surfaces of the vertebral body.

Adjacent vertebrae are united by an intervertebral disk. The outer circumference of the disk is made up of concentric layers of dense, tough fibrous tissue, the annulus fibrosus. The annulus encloses a shock-absorbing gelatinous nucleus pulposus. In addition to the anteriorly placed diskovertebral joint (formed by the

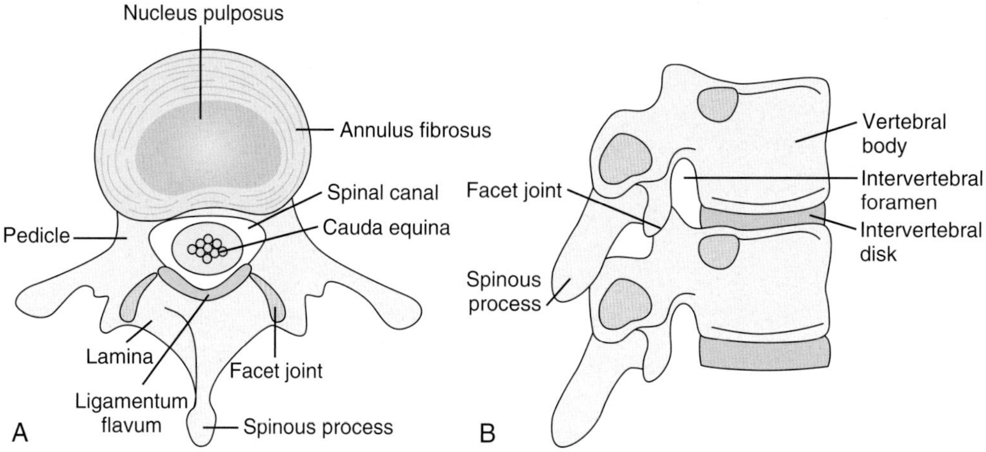

• **Fig. 50.1** Anatomy of the lumbar spine. (A) Cross-sectional view through a lumbar vertebra. (B) Lateral view of the lumbar spine.

intervertebral disk and adjacent vertebrae), at each level of the lumbar spine, there are two posterolaterally placed synovial facet (apophyseal) joints. These are formed by articulation of the superior and inferior articular processes of adjacent vertebrae.

The vertebral column is further stabilized by ligaments and paraspinal muscles (erector spinae, trunk, and abdominal muscles). The anterior and posterior longitudinal ligaments run the length of the spinal column. They anchor the anterior and posterior vertebral body surfaces and intervertebral disks. The ligamentum flavum interconnects the laminae, whereas the interspinous and supraspinous ligaments interconnect the spinous processes. The intertransverse ligaments interconnect the transverse processes.

The sacroiliac joints join the spinal column to the pelvis. The anterior and inferior part of the joint is lined with synovium, whereas the posterior and superior part is fibrous. There is little or no movement at the sacroiliac joint.

The spinal canal in the lumbar region contains the cauda equina (the bundle of lumbar and sacral nerve roots that occupy the vertebral canal below the cord), blood vessels, and fat. Because the spinal cord ends at the L1 level, cord compression is generally not a feature of lumbar pathology. At each level a pair of nerve roots leaves the spinal canal and exits through the intervertebral foramina.

TABLE 50.1 Red Flags for Potentially Serious Underlying Causes of Low Back Pain

Spinal Fracture
Significant trauma
Prolonged glucocorticoid use
Age >50 yr
Infection or Cancer
History of cancer
Unexplained weight loss
Immunosuppression
Injection drug use
Nocturnal pain
Age >50 yr
Cauda Equina Syndrome
Urinary retention
Overflow incontinence
Fecal incontinence
Bilateral or progressive motor deficit
Saddle anesthesia
Spondyloarthritis
Severe morning stiffness
Pain improves with exercise, not rest
Pain during second half of night
Alternating buttock pain
Age <40 yr

Clinical Evaluation

LBP is a symptom, not a disease, and can result from several different known or unknown abnormalities or diseases. The spectrum of clinical presentation is broad. Many individuals will have self-limited episodes of acute LBP that resolve without specific treatment, whereas others may be seen with chronic LBP with periods of acute exacerbation. A thorough history is the most important part of the clinical evaluation of these patients. Imaging is often unnecessary.

History

The major focus in the initial evaluation of a patient with LBP is to identify the small fraction[12] (<5%) of patients who may have neural compression, fracture, or underlying systemic disease (infection, malignancy, or spondyloarthritis) as the cause of back pain. These patients require early diagnostic testing (mostly imaging) and may require specific treatment (e.g., antibiotics for vertebral osteomyelitis) or urgent treatment (e.g., surgical decompression in a patient with major or progressive neural compression). As such, clues to the presence of the previously mentioned conditions[13–15] (Table 50.1), often referred to as "red flags," should be carefully sought. The prevalence of serious spine disorders is low, and the sensitivity and specificity of individual red flags to detect these is also low. As a result, recent studies have highlighted the limited predictive value of individual red flags, and suggested that performing imaging with the presence of any one red flag would result in unnecessarily high rates of imaging. It has therefore been suggested that use of imaging should be guided by the full clinical picture and observations over time, rather than by the uncritical use of individual red flags. The presence of multiple red flags generates higher predictive values.[16] It is also important to look for any social or psychological distress, such as job dissatisfaction, pursuit of disability compensation, and depression, that may amplify or prolong the pain.[15]

Mechanical LBP is due to an anatomic or functional abnormality in the spine that is not associated with inflammatory, infectious, or neoplastic disease. It typically increases with physical activity and upright posture and tends to be relieved by rest and recumbency. More than 95% of LBP is mechanical,[12] and degenerative change in the lumbar spine is the most common cause of mechanical LBP.[13] Severe and acute mechanical LBP in a post-menopausal woman would suggest a vertebral compression fracture secondary to osteoporosis. Nocturnal pain suggests the possibility of underlying infection or neoplasm as the cause of LBP.

Inflammatory LBP, as seen in the spondyloarthritides, usually has an insidious onset and is more common in patients younger than 40 years.[17] It is associated with marked morning stiffness that usually lasts for more than 30 minutes. The pain frequently improves with exercise but not with rest. Pain is often worse during the second half of the night, and some patients complain of alternating buttock pain. It should, however, be noted that new-onset inflammatory back pain progresses to spondyloarthritis only in a minority of patients. The fact that inflammatory back pain often resolves may explain the difference between the prevalence of inflammatory back pain (3% to 6%) and the prevalence of spondyloarthritis (0.4% to 1.3%).[18] Recent data also suggest that the association between a history of inflammatory back pain and the finding of axial inflammation on MRI is weak. This, to some degree, compromises the use of a history of inflammatory back pain as a marker of axial inflammation.[19]

It is important to ask the patient if the back pain radiates into the lower extremities, suggesting neurogenic claudication (pseudoclaudication) secondary to spinal stenosis or sciatica (usually secondary to a herniated disk or spinal stenosis). Young adults are more likely to be seen with the clinical syndrome of disk herniation, and elderly patients are more likely to be seen with the clinical features of spinal stenosis. Sciatica results from nerve root compression and causes radicular pain. There is often no specific precipitating event. It has been proposed that because the term sciatica has been used inconsistently for different types of leg and back pain it should be replaced by the term radicular pain. Radicular pain has a dermatomal distribution with leg pain generally worse than back pain. The pain (often accompanied by paresthesias) usually radiates to a level below the knee and often to the foot or ankle. The pain may be lancinating, shooting, and sharp in quality and frequently worsens during coughing, sneezing, Valsalva maneuver, and almost always with the straight leg raise test. Radicular pain may be accompanied by radiculopathy characterized by a variable combination of findings that include the presence of weakness, loss of sensation, or loss of reflexes associated with a particular nerve root. Radicular pain should be differentiated from non-neurogenic sclerotomal pain. This pain can arise from pathology within the disk, facet joint, or lumbar paraspinal muscles and ligaments. Similar to radicular pain, sclerotomal pain is often referred into the lower extremities, but unlike radicular pain, sclerotomal pain is nondermatomal in distribution, is usually dull in quality, and the pain usually does not radiate below the knee or have associated paresthesias. Most radiant pain is sclerotomal.[13] Bowel or bladder dysfunction should suggest the possibility of the cauda equina syndrome.

Physical Examination

A physical examination usually does not lead to a specific diagnosis. Nevertheless, a general physical examination including a careful neurologic examination may help identify those few but critically important cases of LBP that are secondary to a systemic disease or have clinically significant neurologic involvement (see Table 50.1).

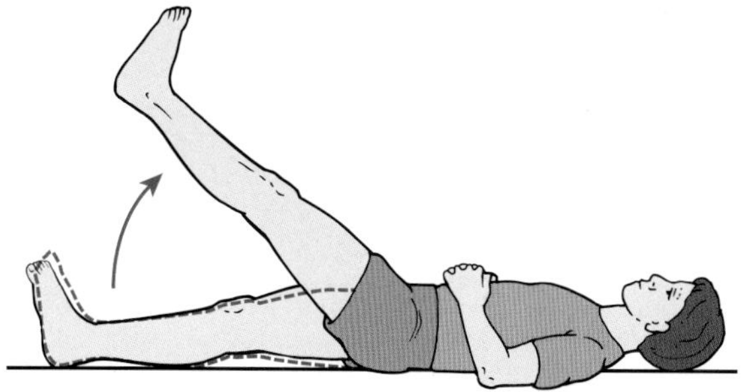

• **Fig. 50.2** Straight leg–raising test. A very sensitive test for nerve root impingement at the L4-5 or L5-S1 level.

Inspection may reveal the presence of scoliosis. This can be either structural or functional. A structural scoliosis is associated with structural changes of the vertebral column and sometimes the rib cage as well. In adults structural scoliosis is usually secondary to degenerative changes, although some adults may have a history of adolescent idiopathic scoliosis. With forward flexion, structural scoliosis persists. In contrast, functional scoliosis, which usually results from paravertebral muscle spasm or leg length discrepancy, usually disappears. A tuft of hair in the lumbar spine region may indicate a congenital structural abnormality such as spina bifida occulta.

Palpation can detect paravertebral muscle spasm. This often leads to loss of the normal lumbar lordosis. Point tenderness on percussion over the spine has sensitivity but not specificity for vertebral osteomyelitis. A palpable step-off between adjacent spinous processes suggests spondylolisthesis.

Limited spinal motion (flexion, extension, lateral bending, and rotation) is not associated with any specific diagnosis because LBP from any cause may limit motion. Range-of-motion measurements, however, can help in monitoring treatment.[10] Chest expansion of less than 2.5 cm has specificity but not sensitivity for ankylosing spondylitis.[17]

The hip joints should be examined for any decrease in range of motion because hip arthritis, which normally causes groin pain, may occasionally refer pain to the back. Trochanteric bursitis with tenderness over the greater trochanter of the femur can be confused with LBP. The presence of more widespread tender points, especially in a female patient, suggests the possibility that LBP may be secondary to fibromyalgia.

A complete neurologic examination should be performed because neurologic abnormalities in the upper extremities, such as hyper-reflexia, may indicate a more proximal etiology of a patient's lower extremity complaints. In patients with a history of LBP that radiates into the lower extremities (radicular pain, pseudoclaudication, or referred sclerotomal pain), a straight leg–raising test (Fig. 50.2) should be performed. With the patient lying on his or her back, the examiner places the heel in the palm of his or her hand and progressively raises the patient's leg with the knee fully extended. This movement places tension on the sciatic nerve (that originates from L4, L5, S1, S2, and S3) and thereby stretches the nerve roots (especially L5, S1, and S2). If any of these nerve roots is already irritated, such as by impingement from a herniated disk, further tension on the nerve root by straight leg raising will result in radicular pain that extends below the knee. The test is positive if

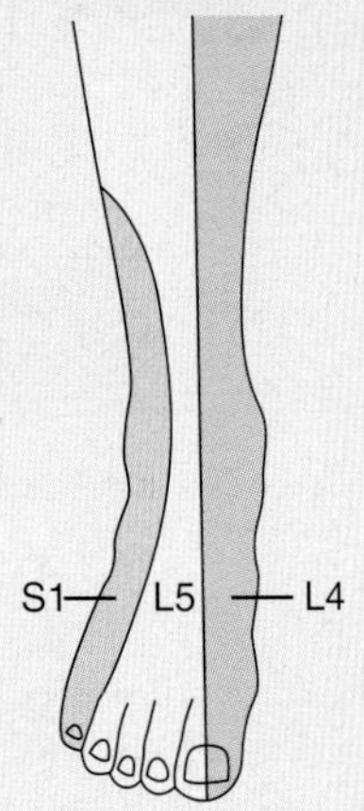

Lower extremity dermatome	Disk	Nerve root	Motor loss	Sensory loss	Reflex loss
S1, L5, L4	L3-4	L4	Dorsiflexion of foot	Medial foot	Knee
	L4-5	L5	Dorsiflexion of great toe	Dorsal foot	None
	L5-S1	S1	Plantarflexion of foot	Lateral foot	Ankle

• **Fig. 50.3** Neurologic features of lumbosacral radiculopathy.

radicular pain is produced when the leg is raised between 30 and 70 degrees. Dorsiflexion of the ankle further stretches the sciatic nerve and increases the sensitivity of the test. Pain experienced in the posterior thigh or knee during straight leg raising is generally from hamstring tightness and does not represent a positive test. The straight leg–raising test is sensitive (91%) but not specific (26%) for clinically significant disk herniation at the L4-5 or L5-S1 level (the sites of 95% of clinically meaningful disk herniations). False-negative tests are more frequently seen with herniation above the L4-5 level. The straight leg–raising test is usually negative in patients with spinal stenosis. The crossed straight leg–raising test (with radicular pain reproduced when the opposite leg is raised) is highly specific but insensitive for a clinically significant disk herniation.[10,15,20,21]

The neurologic evaluation (Fig. 50.3) of the lower extremities in a patient with radicular pain can often identify the specific nerve root involved. As a general rule of thumb, if a disc herniation results in nerve root compression the more caudal nerve root is usually impinged. Therefore, for example, L4-5 disk herniation will likely result in L5 nerve root impingement rather than L4 nerve root impingement. The evaluation should include motor testing with focus on dorsiflexion of the foot (L4), great toe dorsiflexion (L5), and foot plantar flexion (S1); determination of knee (L4) and ankle (S1) deep tendon reflexes; and tests for dermatomal sensory loss. The inability to toe walk (mostly S1) and heel walk (mostly L5) indicates muscle weakness. Muscle atrophy can be detected by circumferential measurements of the calf and thigh at the same level bilaterally.[10]

Clinically significant disk herniation at the L1-2, L2-3, or L3-4 levels is seen infrequently. It may be detected by the femoral nerve stretch test. With the patient lying prone, the knee is passively flexed to its maximum and then the hip is passively extended. The test is positive if the patient experiences anterior thigh pain. Because a tight rectus femoris can also produce anterior thigh pain with this maneuver, it is important to perform the test on both sides and compare the symptoms.

Patients involved with litigation or with psychological distress occasionally exaggerate their symptoms. They may display nonorganic signs where the objective findings do not match the subjective complaints, such as with nonanatomic motor or sensory loss. A number of tests to detect this have been described by one study.[22] The most reproducible tests are the presence of superficial tenderness, over-reaction during the examination, and observation of a discrepancy in the straight leg–raising test done in the seated and supine positions.

Diagnostic Tests

Imaging

There is concern about overuse of lumbar spine imaging, especially in the United States where imaging capacity is high. Indiscriminate spine imaging leads to a low yield of clinically useful findings, a high yield of misleading findings, radiation exposure, and costs.[16] The major function of diagnostic testing, especially imaging, is the early identification of pathology in those few patients who have evidence of a major or progressive neurologic deficit, and those in whom an underlying systemic disease or vertebral fracture is suspected (see Table 50.1). Otherwise, imaging is not required unless significant symptoms persist beyond 6 to 8 weeks. This approach avoids unnecessary early testing because more than 90% of the patients will have largely recovered by 8 weeks.[10,12] Furthermore, neither MRI nor plain radiographs obtained early in the course of LBP evaluation improves clinical outcome, predicts recovery course, or reduces the overall cost of care.[2,23]

A significant problem with all imaging studies is that many of the anatomic abnormalities identified in patients with LBP are also commonly present in asymptomatic individuals and are frequently unrelated to the back pain.[13] Often these abnormalities result from age-related degenerative changes, which begin to appear even in early adulthood and are among the earliest degenerative changes in the body.[24] Although clinically challenging and sometimes impossible, one should refrain from making causal inferences based solely on imaging abnormalities in the absence of corresponding clinical findings because this may lead to unnecessary, invasive, and costly interventions.[25,26]

Given the weak association between imaging abnormalities and symptoms, it is not surprising that in as many as 85% of patients a precise pathoanatomic diagnosis with identification of the pain generator cannot be made.[15] Patients should understand that the reason for imaging is to rule out serious conditions and that common degenerative findings are expected. Ill-considered attempts to make a diagnosis on the basis of imaging studies may falsely reinforce the suspicion of serious disease (leading to "fear avoidance" behavior), magnify the importance of nonspecific findings, and label patients with spurious diagnoses.

Plain radiographs and MRI are the major modalities used in the evaluation of patients with LBP. In patients with persistent LBP of greater than 6 to 8 weeks' duration despite standard therapies, radiography may be a reasonable first option if there are no symptoms suggesting radiculopathy or spinal stenosis.[27] Standing anteroposterior and lateral views are usually adequate. Oblique views substantially increase radiation exposure and add little new diagnostic information. Gonadal radiation in a woman from a two-view radiograph of the lumbar spine is equivalent to radiation exposure from a chest radiograph taken daily for more than 1 year.[27]

Abnormalities on radiography, such as single-disk degeneration, facet joint degeneration, Schmorl's nodes (protrusion of the nucleus pulposus into the spongiosa of a vertebra), spondylolysis, mild spondylolisthesis, transitional vertebrae (the "lumbarization" of S1 or "sacralization" of L5), spina bifida occulta, and mild scoliosis, are equally prevalent in individuals with and without LBP.[12,13,28]

MRI without contrast is generally the best initial test for patients with LBP who require advanced imaging. It is the preferred modality for the detection of spinal infection and cancers, herniated disks, and spinal stenosis.[12] MRI testing for LBP should largely be limited to patients in whom there is a suspicion of systemic disease (such as infection or malignancy), for the pre-operative evaluation of patients who are surgical candidates on clinical grounds[15,27] (e.g., the presence of a significant or progressive neurologic deficit), or for those patients with radiculopathy who are candidates for epidural corticosteroids.[27] Disk abnormalities are commonly noted on MRI studies but often have little or no relationship with the patient's symptoms. A disk bulge is a symmetric, circumferential extension of disk material beyond the interspace. A disk herniation is a focal or asymmetric extension. Herniations are subdivided into protrusions and extrusions. Protrusions are broad-based, whereas extrusions have a "neck" so that the base is narrower than the extruded material. Bulges (52%) and protrusions (27%) are common in asymptomatic adults, but extrusions are rare.[12] MRI with the intravenous contrast agent gadolinium may be useful for the evaluation of patients with prior back surgery (with no hardware present) to help in the differentiation of scar tissue from recurrent disk herniation.

The presence of bone marrow edema on MRI of the sacroiliac joints is often considered a hallmark of axial spondyloarthritis. However, low-grade bone marrow edema (that fulfills the existing definitions of sacroiliitis) may be seen in healthy individuals (25.5%), patients with chronic mechanical LBP (10.6%), long distance runners (16.7%), and women with postpartum back pain (57.1%). The presence of deep bone marrow edema and joint erosions are, however, significantly more specific for axial spondyloarthritis.[29,30]

MRI is generally preferred versus CT scanning in the evaluation of patients with LBP. However, when bone anatomy is critical, CT is superior. This is particularly true when spondylolysis is suspected as this may not be well seen with MRI. Unlike MRI, CT can safely be done in patients with a ferromagnetic implant such as a cardiac pacemaker. In patients with metal hardware (anterior or posterior spinal fusion) CT (or CT myelography) is usually superior to MRI to assess hardware position or fractures close to the hardware.

Nuclear medicine bone scanning with technetium-99m is used primarily to detect infection, bony metastases, or occult fractures. Bone scans have limited specificity due to poor spatial resolution, and thus abnormal findings often require further confirmatory imaging such as MRI.

Electrodiagnostic Studies

Electrodiagnostic studies can be helpful in the evaluation of some patients with lumbosacral radiculopathy. The main procedures are electromyography and nerve conduction studies. When used in combination they provide information regarding the integrity of spinal nerve roots and their connection with the muscles they innervate. These studies can confirm nerve root compression and define the distribution and severity of involvement. Whereas studies such as MRI can only provide anatomic information, electrodiagnostic studies provide physiologic information that may support or refute the findings on imaging. Electrodiagnostic testing is therefore mostly considered in patients with persistent disabling symptoms of radiculopathy in which there is discordance between the clinical presentation and findings on imaging. Electromyography and nerve conduction studies can also be helpful in differentiating the limb pain of peroneal nerve palsy or lumbosacral plexopathy from that of L5 radiculopathy. These studies are also useful to evaluate possible factitious weakness. Electrodiagnosis is unnecessary in a patient with an obvious radiculopathy. It should be noted that electromyographic changes depend on the development of muscle denervation following nerve injury and may not be detected for 2 to 3 weeks after the injury. In contrast, nerve conduction tests become abnormal immediately after nerve damage. Another limitation is that electromyographic abnormalities may persist for more than a year following decompressive surgery.[31]

Laboratory Studies

Laboratory studies are used mostly in identifying patients with systemic causes of LBP. A patient with normal blood cell counts, erythrocyte sedimentation rate, and radiographs of the lumbar spine is unlikely to have underlying infection or malignancy as the cause of LBP.[32]

Differential Diagnosis

LBP usually originates from pathology within the lumbar spine or associated muscles and ligaments (Table 50.2). Rarely, pain is referred to the back from visceral disease. In the vast majority of patients with LBP, the pain is mechanical.[15] Degenerative change in the lumbar spine is the largest contributor to the mechanical causes of LBP[12] (see Table 50.2) and indeed the most commonly identified cause of back pain.

Lumbar Spondylosis

The current common usage of the term *lumbar spondylosis* incorporates degenerative changes in both the anteriorly placed disk-overtebral joints and the posterolaterally placed facet joints.[10] These degenerative or osteoarthritic changes are seen radiographically as disk or joint-space narrowing, subchondral sclerosis, and osteophytosis (Fig. 50.4).

Imaging evidence of lumbar spondylosis is common in the general population, increases with age, and may be unrelated to back symptoms. Radiographic abnormalities such as single-disk degeneration, facet joint degeneration, Schmorl's nodes, mild spondylolisthesis, and mild scoliosis are equally prevalent in people with and without back pain.[33] The situation is further complicated by the observation that patients with severe mechanical LBP may have minimal radiographic changes, and conversely patients with advanced changes may be asymptomatic.

The clinical spectrum of mechanical LBP is wide. Patients may present with acute LBP (with recurrent attacks in some),

TABLE 50.2 Causes of Low Back Pain

Mechanical
Lumbar spondylosis[a]
Disk herniation[a]
Spondylolisthesis[a]
Spinal stenosis[a]
Fractures (mostly osteoporotic)
Nonspecific (idiopathic)
Neoplastic
Primary
Metastatic
Inflammatory
Spondyloarthritis
Infectious
Vertebral osteomyelitis
Epidural abscess
Septic diskitis
Herpes zoster
Metabolic
Osteoporotic compression fractures
Paget's disease
Referred Pain to Spine
From major viscera, retroperitoneal structures, urogenital system, aorta, or hip

[a]Related to degenerative changes.

whereas chronic LBP (often with periods of acute exacerbation) may develop in others. Somatic referral may lead to sclerotomal pain that radiates into the buttocks and lower extremities. Lumbar spondylosis predisposes patients to intervertebral disk herniation, spondylolisthesis, and spinal stenosis. Overall, degenerative changes of the lumbar spine are the most common cause of back pathology and pain.

In some patients with facet joint osteoarthritis the pain may radiate into the buttock and posterior thigh, be alleviated with forward flexion, and be exacerbated by bending ipsilateral to the involved joint or by lumbar hyperextension (facet syndrome). The facet joints are innervated by the medial branches of the dorsal rami. The prevalence of facet syndrome in patients with LBP using local anesthetic nerve blockade (medial branch block), and using pain relief as a criterion standard, is 25% to 40%.[34] However, in clinical practice it is difficult to isolate symptoms specifically to facet joint osteoarthritis, and its true prevalence as a pain generator remains controversial.

The terms internal disk disruption and diskogenic LBP are used interchangeably and remain controversial diagnoses[20] when diagnosed by provocative diskography. Following contrast injection into several disks in sequence, the radiographic appearance and induced pain at each level are assessed. If injection into a disk reproduces a patient's usual LBP, the test is considered positive. Advocates of this technique interpret a positive diskogram as defining the particular disk as the primary pain generator, and spinal fusion or disk arthroplasty is frequently recommended.[2] However, injection into a disk can simulate the quality and location of pain known not to originate from that disk.[35] Furthermore, diskographic abnormalities and induced pain are frequently seen in asymptomatic people and, more importantly, the diskogenic

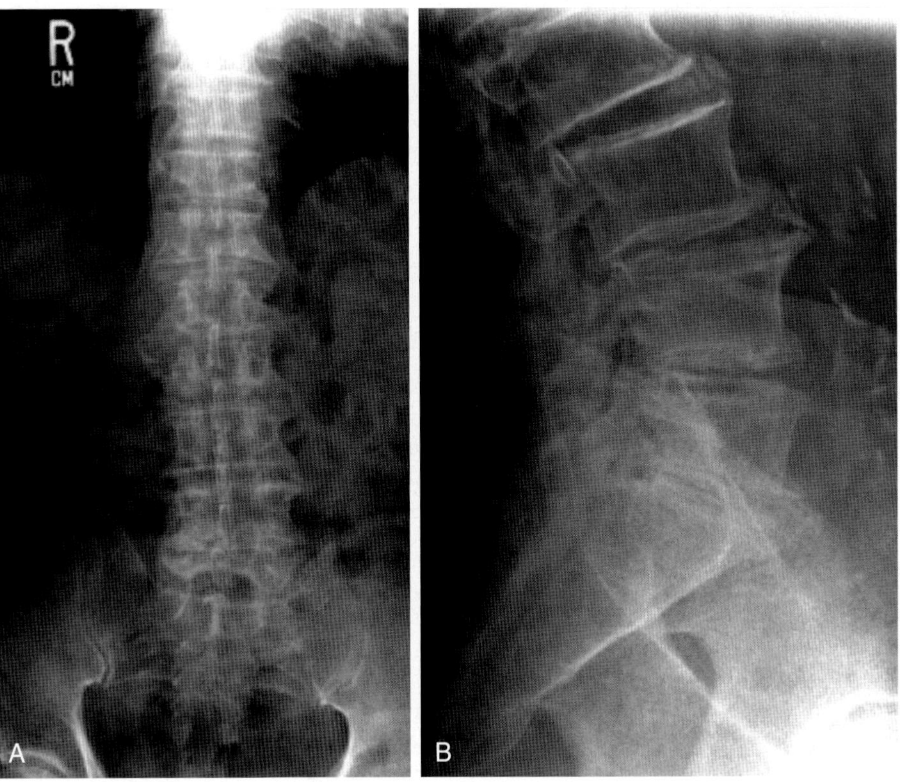

• **Fig. 50.4** Lumbar spondylosis. Anteroposterior (A) and lateral (B) radiographs of the lumbar spine show the cardinal features of disk-space narrowing, marginal osteophytes, and end-plate sclerosis. (Courtesy Dr. John Crues, University of California, San Diego.)

pain attributed to disk disruption frequently improves spontaneously.[12,15] Finally, long-term follow-up of patients who have undergone diskography has led to a concern that the procedure itself may lead to accelerated disk degeneration and disk herniation.[36] Therefore the clinical importance and appropriate management of this condition when diagnosed by diskography remains unclear.

Modic changes are signal changes related to spinal degeneration in the vertebral endplate and adjacent bone marrow that are commonly reported following lumbar MRI. Modic type I changes are secondary to marrow edema and inflammation, Modic type II changes represent fatty replacement of marrow, and Modic type III changes reflect subchondral bone sclerosis.[37,38] The prevalence of these changes, which may progress or regress over time, increases with age and appears to be associated with degenerative disk changes.[39] Modic changes are present in 20% to 40% of LBP patients but may be seen in as many as 10% of asymptomatic adults.[37,38] The clinical usefulness with regard to selecting treatment options of these signal changes is unclear.[40]

Focal high signal in the posterior annulus fibrosus as seen on T2-weighted MRI images, sometimes referred to as a *high-intensity zone,* is believed to represent tears in the annulus fibrosus and to correlate with positive findings on provocative diskography.[12] The high prevalence of high-intensity zones in asymptomatic individuals limits its clinical value.[41]

Spinal instability is seen in some patients with lumbar spondylosis. It is identified by demonstrating abnormal vertebral motion (anteroposterior displacement or excessive angular change of adjacent vertebrae) on lateral radiographs in flexion and extension. However, such spinal motion may be seen in asymptomatic people and its natural history and relationship to the causation of LBP is unclear. Thus the diagnosis of spinal instability (in the absence of fractures, infection, neoplastic disease, or spondylolisthesis) as a cause of LBP and its treatment by spinal fusion remains controversial.

Disk Herniation

Intervertebral disk herniation occurs when the nucleus pulposus in a degenerated disk prolapses and pushes out the weakened annulus, usually posterolaterally where the annulus fibrosus is thinner. Imaging evidence of disk abnormalities has a high prevalence in the general population, and disk bulges and herniations are common in asymptomatic adults.[42] Occasionally, however, the herniated disk can cause nerve root impingement that leads to lumbosacral radiculopathy (Figs. 50.5 and 50.6). A herniated intervertebral disk is the most common cause of radicular pain in young adults.[12]

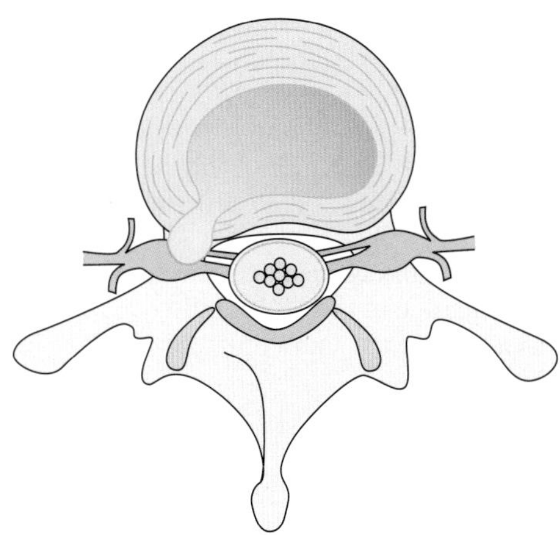

• **Fig. 50.5** Schematic drawing showing posterolateral disk herniation resulting in nerve root impingement.

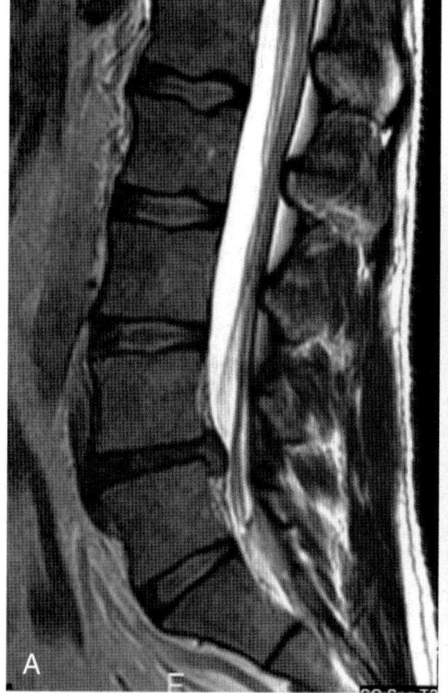

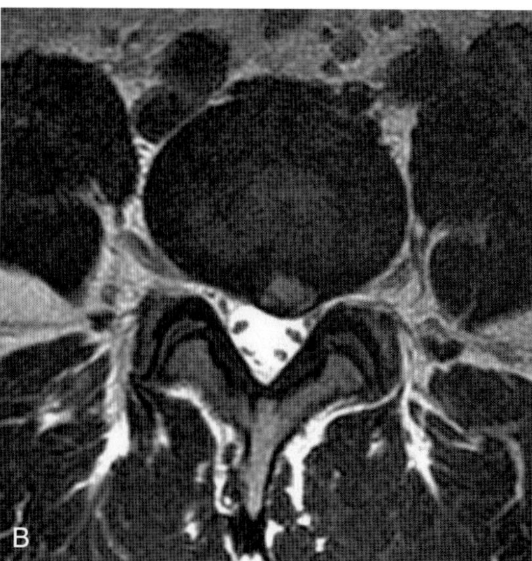

• **Fig. 50.6** Lumbar disk extrusion. (A) The sagittal T2-weighted MRI shows an extruded disk at the L4-5 level. (B) The axial image through the L4-5 level shows disk extrusion to the left side of the neural canal and compressing the traversing L5 nerve root in the left lateral recess. (Courtesy Dr. John Crues, University of California, San Diego.)

TABLE 50.3 Spectrum of Signs and Symptoms of Cauda Equina Syndrome

Altered/reduced urinary sensation
Loss of desire to void or poor stream
Sexual dysfunction
Saddle area anesthesia
Bilateral (or unilateral) sciatica
Motor weakness of lower extremities
Urinary and/or fecal incontinence
Loss of rectal tone
Absent voluntary anal contraction

Neuroradiologic studies affirm that 85% of cases of radicular pain are associated with a herniated intervertebral disk.[43]

The lumbosacral spine is susceptible to disk herniation because of its mobility. Seventy-five percent of flexion and extension occurs at the lumbosacral joint (L5-S1), and 20% occurs at L4-5[44] (with more torsion at the L4-5 level). Probably related to this, 90% to 95% of clinically significant compressive radiculopathies occur at these two levels.[15]

The frequency of disk herniation increases with age. The peak frequency of herniation at the L5-S1 and L4-L5 levels is between the ages of 44 and 50 years, with a progressive decline in frequency thereafter.[45]

The genesis of sciatica is felt to have both a mechanical (disk material impinging on a nerve root) and biologic component. Inflammation, vascular invasion, immune responses, and an array of cytokines have been implicated.

The clinical features of disk herniation resulting in lumbosacral radiculopathy have already been discussed (see history, physical examination, and Fig. 50.3). It should be noted that immediate imaging is unnecessary in patients without a clinically significant neurologic deficit and no red flags to suggest an underlying systemic pathology (see Table 50.1). L1 radiculopathy is rare, and patients are seen with symptoms of pain, paresthesias, and sensory loss in the inguinal region.[46] L2, L3, and L4 radiculopathies are uncommon and more likely to be seen in older patients with lumbar spinal stenosis.

The natural history of disk herniation is favorable, with progressive improvement expected in most patients. Sequential MRI studies reveal that the herniated portion of the disk regresses with time, and there is partial or complete resolution in a majority of cases after 6 to 12 months.[15,47,48] The condition of patients who have motor deficits secondary to herniated disks also improve over time. In one study 81% of patients with initial paresis had recovered without surgery after 1 year.[49] Even a sequestered fragment (piece of herniated material that breaks off and is free in the epidural space) tends to be reabsorbed with time.[50] Only approximately 10% of patients have sufficient pain after 6 weeks of conservative care, and for this group, decompressive surgery is considered.[15]

Rarely, a large midline disk herniation, usually L4-5,[13] compresses the cauda equina, resulting in cauda equina syndrome. Patients usually are seen with LBP, bilateral radicular pain, and bilateral motor deficits with leg weakness. Physical examination findings are often asymmetric. Sensory loss in the perineum (saddle anesthesia) is common.[15] The cardinal clinical feature is urinary retention with overflow incontinence (sensitivity 90%, specificity 95%).[51] Fecal incontinence may also occur. The spectrum of signs and symptoms are presented in Table 50.3. Other causes of cauda equina syndrome include neoplasia, epidural abscess, hematoma, and rarely lumbar spinal stenosis. Cauda equina syndrome is a surgical emergency because neurologic results are affected by the time to decompression.[10] Whenever possible, the cauda equina syndrome should be recognized before established incontinence because, once urinary retention has occurred, the prognosis is worse.[52]

Spondylolisthesis

Spondylolisthesis is the anterior displacement of a vertebra on the one beneath it. There are two major types: isthmic and degenerative. Traumatic spondylolisthesis (following high impact trauma) and pathologic spondylolisthesis (such as secondary to a lytic tumor) occur infrequently.

Isthmic spondylolisthesis (Fig. 50.7), most commonly seen at the L5-S1 level, is caused by bilateral spondylolysis. Spondylolysis is a unilateral or bilateral defect in the pars interarticularis that is most commonly seen at L5. It is typically a fatigue fracture acquired early in life that is more commonly seen in boys. It is usually an overuse injury although it may present following an acute overload. It occurs most frequently in athletes whose sport involves repetitive spinal loads. Based on CT imaging the prevalence of spondylolysis in adults is 11.5%, nearly twice the prevalence of plain radiograph–based studies.[53] Spondylolysis progresses to spondylolisthesis in approximately 15% of patients.[54]

Degenerative spondylolisthesis (Fig. 50.8) develops in some patients with severe degenerative changes with subluxation at the facet joints allowing anterior or posterior movement of one vertebra over another. It is usually seen in an older age group (typically older than 60 years), is more common in women, most frequently involves the L4-5 level, and rarely exceeds 30% of vertebral width.[13]

Most patients, especially those with a minor degree of spondylolisthesis, are asymptomatic. Some may complain of an aching mechanical LBP. Neurologic complications may occur in some with greater degrees of spondylolisthesis. Nerve root impingement is more likely to be seen in patients with isthmic spondylolisthesis (especially L5 nerve root), whereas in degenerative spondylolisthesis the more likely clinical presentation is of spinal stenosis. Rarely, extreme slippage results in cauda equina syndrome. In view of its potential dynamic nature, spondylolisthesis may be missed if standing radiographs are not obtained.

Spinal Stenosis

The diagnosis of the clinical syndrome of lumbar spinal stenosis requires both the presence of characteristic symptoms and signs as well as imaging confirmation of narrowing of the lumbar spinal canal or foramina.[55] Radiographic lumbar spinal stenosis is defined as a narrowing of the central spinal canal, its lateral recesses, and neural foramina that diminishes space available for neural and vascular elements. It may result in a compression of lumbosacral nerve roots. Spinal stenosis can occur at one or multiple levels, and the narrowing may be asymmetric. It is important to recognize that 20% to 30% of asymptomatic adults older than 60 years have imaging evidence of spinal stenosis.[56] The prevalence of symptomatic lumbar spinal stenosis is not established. A Japanese study of subjects with a mean age of 66 reported the prevalence of symptomatic spinal stenosis to be 9.3%.[57] Lumbar spinal stenosis is the most frequent indication for spinal surgery in patients older than 65 years.

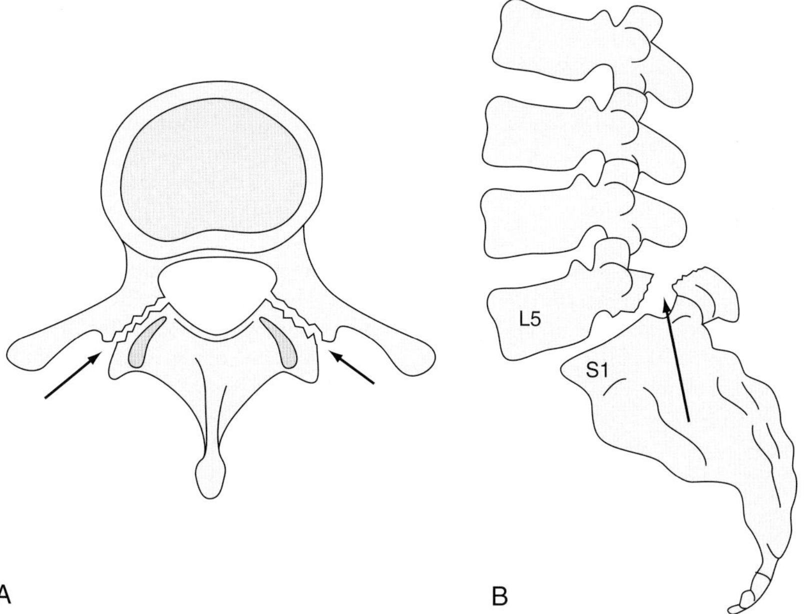

• **Fig. 50.7** (A) Spondylolysis with bilateral defects in the pars interarticularis *(arrows).* (B) Spondylolysis of the L5 vertebra *(arrow)* resulting in isthmic spondylolisthesis at L5-S1.

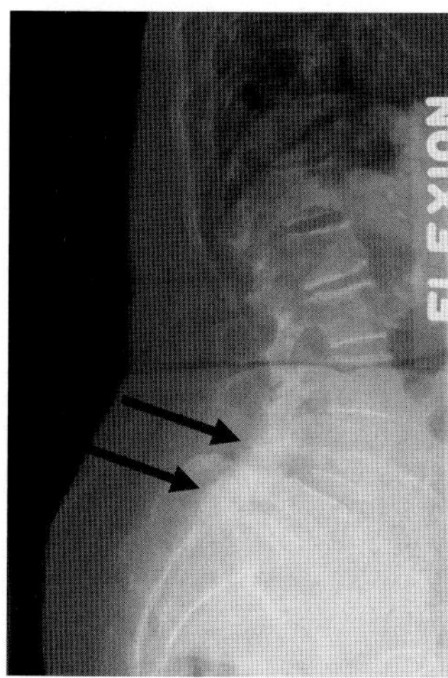

• **Fig. 50.8** Lumbar spondylolisthesis. Lateral radiograph of the lumbar spine showing grade 1 anterolisthesis at the levels of L4-5 and L5-S1 *(arrows)* related to severe degenerative changes of the facet joints. (Courtesy Thomas Link, MD, University of California, San Francisco.)

TABLE 50.4 Causes of Lumbar Spinal Stenosis

Congenital
Idiopathic
Achondroplastic
Acquired
Degenerative
Hypertrophy of facet joints
Hypertrophy of ligamentum flavum
Disk herniation
Spondylolisthesis
Scoliosis
Iatrogenic
Postlaminectomy
Postsurgical fusion
Miscellaneous
Paget's disease
Fluorosis
Diffuse idiopathic skeletal hyperostosis
Ankylosing spondylitis

Congenital idiopathic spinal stenosis (Table 50.4) is not uncommon and results from congenitally short pedicles. These patients tend to become symptomatic early (in the third to fifth decade of life) when superimposed mild degenerative changes that would normally be tolerated result in sufficient further narrowing of the spinal canal to cause symptoms.[56]

Degenerative changes are the cause of spinal stenosis in the vast majority of cases. The intervertebral disk loses height while it degenerates. This results in a bulging or buckling of the now redundant and often hypertrophied ligamentum flavum into the posterior part of the canal. Any herniation of the degenerated disk narrows the anterior part of the canal, whereas hypertrophied facets and osteophytes may compress nerve roots in the lateral recess or intervertebral foramen (Figs. 50.9 and 50.10). Any degree of spondylolisthesis will further exacerbate spinal canal narrowing. There is evidence that genetic factors influence disk degeneration and spinal canal dimensions and thereby contribute to the development of lumbar spinal stenosis.[58]

The hallmark of spinal stenosis is neurogenic claudication (pseudoclaudication). The symptoms of neurogenic claudication are usually bilateral but often asymmetric. The patient's primary complaint is of pain in the buttocks, thighs, and legs. The buttock pain is sometimes described as a burning sensation. The pain may be accompanied by paresthesias. Neurogenic claudication is induced by standing erect or walking and relieved by sitting or flexing forward. This forward flexion increases the spinal canal dimensions, and may lead to the patient adopting a simian stance.

It is therefore not surprising that these patients often feel relief by stooping forward while holding onto a shopping cart (the "shopping cart sign"), and may exhibit surprising endurance while pedaling a stationary bicycle. Symptoms of neurogenic claudication probably represent intermittent mechanical and ischemic disruption of lumbosacral nerve root function.[59] The patients also often have a sense of weakness in the lower extremities. Unsteadiness of gait, related to compression of proprioceptive fibers, is a frequent complaint. The finding of a wide-based gait in a patient with LBP has more than 90% specificity for lumbar spinal stenosis.[60] Intermittent priapism with walking has been described.[61] Factors that favor a diagnosis of neurogenic claudication versus vascular claudication include preservation of pedal pulses, provocation of symptoms by standing erect just as readily as by walking, relief of symptoms with flexion of the spine, and location of maximal discomfort in the thighs rather than the calves. Whereas central canal stenosis predominantly results in neurogenic claudication, lateral canal stenosis may result in a radiculopathy.

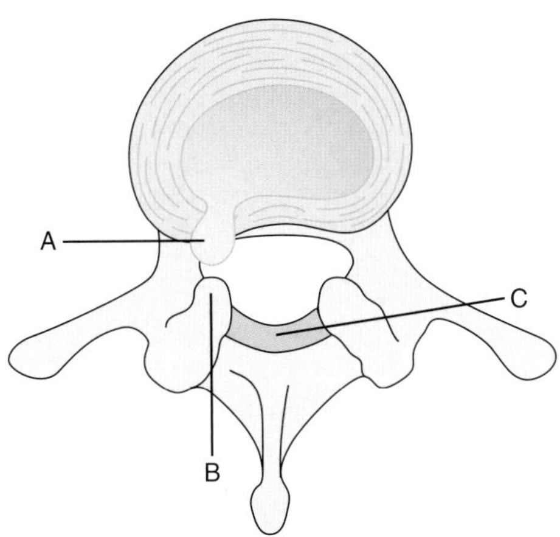

• **Fig. 50.9** Spinal stenosis secondary to a combination of disk herniation *(A)*, facet joint hypertrophy *(B)*, and hypertrophy of the ligamentum flavum *(C)*.

The physical examination of a patient with lumbar spinal stenosis is often unimpressive.[10] Severe neurologic deficits are uncommon. Lumbar range of motion may be normal or reduced, and the result of straight leg raising is usually negative. An abnormal Romberg test is seen in some patients. Deep tendon reflexes and vibration sense may be reduced. Mild diffuse weakness in the lower extremities may be present in others. The significance of these findings is often difficult to determine in elderly patients. However, in a few patients with spinal stenosis, a fixed nerve root injury may occur, resulting in a lumbosacral radiculopathy or, rarely, a cauda equina syndrome.

An uncommon presentation, resulting from spinal stenosis between T12 and L2, is of the conus medullaris syndrome. This produces a mixed picture of a myelopathy and nerve root compression from a combination of upper and lower motor neuron involvement (unlike the cauda equina syndrome, which results from lower motor neuron deficits). Bowel and bladder dysfunction is commonly present in both the cauda equina and conus medullaris syndromes. Both require urgent surgical consultation.

The diagnosis of lumbar spinal stenosis is most often suspected when a history of neurogenic claudication is elicited. The diagnosis is best confirmed by MRI.

Spinal stenosis is generally an indolent condition in which the symptoms evolve gradually and the natural history is benign. In a study of patients with lumbar spinal stenosis followed up for 49 months without surgical intervention, symptoms remained unchanged in 70%, improved in 15%, and worsened in 15%.[62] As such, prophylactic surgical intervention is not warranted.[56]

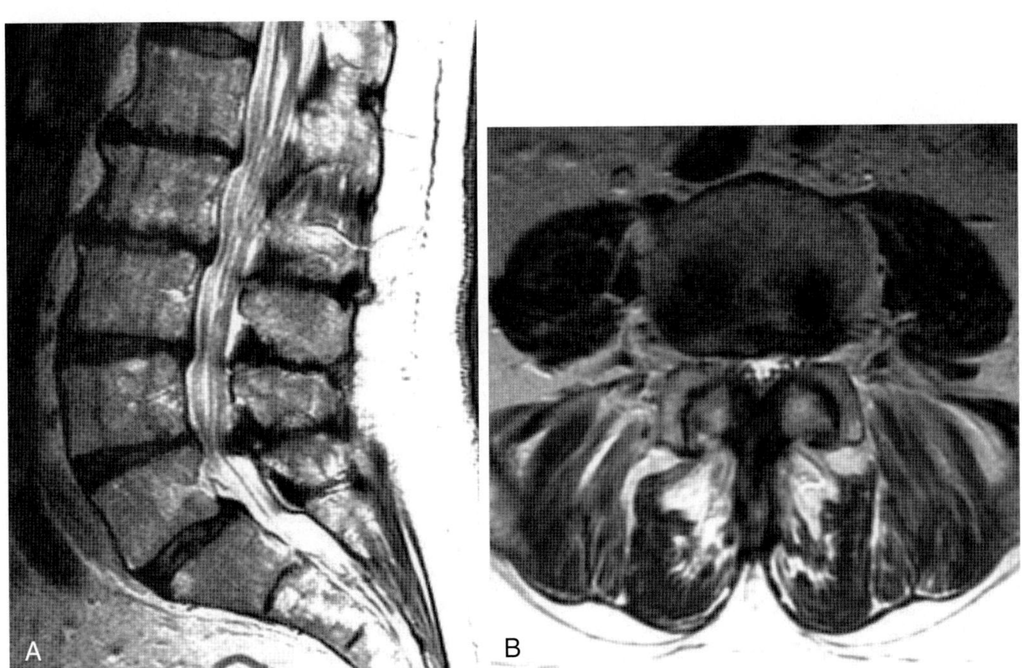

• **Fig. 50.10** Degenerative spinal stenosis. (A) The sagittal T2-weighted MRI shows decreased anteroposterior diameter of the neural canal at the L4-5 level due to redundancy of the ligamentum flavum. (B) The axial image through the L4-5 disk shows decreased cross-sectional area of the thecal sac from hypertrophic changes of the facet joints posterolateral to the thecal sac. (Courtesy Dr. John Crues, University of California, San Diego.)

Diffuse Idiopathic Skeletal Hyperostosis

Diffuse idiopathic skeletal hyperostosis (DISH) is characterized by calcification and ossification of paraspinous ligaments and the entheses.[63] It is a non-inflammatory condition of unknown etiology that is not associated with human leukocyte antigen (HLA)-B27 positivity.

DISH has been associated with obesity, diabetes mellitus, and acromegaly.[64] It is rarely diagnosed before 30 years, is more commonly seen in men, and the prevalence rises with age.[65]

The thoracic spine is most commonly involved, although the cervical and lumbar regions may also be affected. Ossification of the anterior longitudinal ligament is best seen on a lateral radiograph of the thoracic spine. The ossification, together with bridging enthesophytes in the spine, give the appearance of flowing wax (Fig. 50.11) on the anterior and right lateral aspects of the spine. Involvement of the left lateral aspect in patients with situs inversus has led to speculation that the descending aorta plays a role in the location of the calcification. Intervertebral disk spaces and facet joints are preserved (unless there is co-existing lumbar spondylosis), and the sacroiliac joints appear normal. This helps to differentiate DISH from spondylosis and the spondyloarthritides. Skeletal hyperostosis resembling DISH has been described in patients with long-term exposure to retinoids (retinoid hyperostosis) such as with isotretinoin therapy for acne.[66] Almost any extraspinal osseous or articular site may be affected.[67] Irregular new bone formation ("whiskering") is often best seen at the iliac crests, ischial tuberosities, and femoral trochanters. Ossification of tendons and ligaments at sites of attachment (such as the patella, olecranon process, and calcaneus) and periarticular osteophytes (such as the lateral acetabulum and inferior portion of the sacroiliac joint on pelvic radiographs) may also be seen. Severe ligamentous calcification may be seen in the sacrotuberous and iliolumbar ligaments, and heterotopic bone formation following hip replacement in patients with DISH has been described.[68]

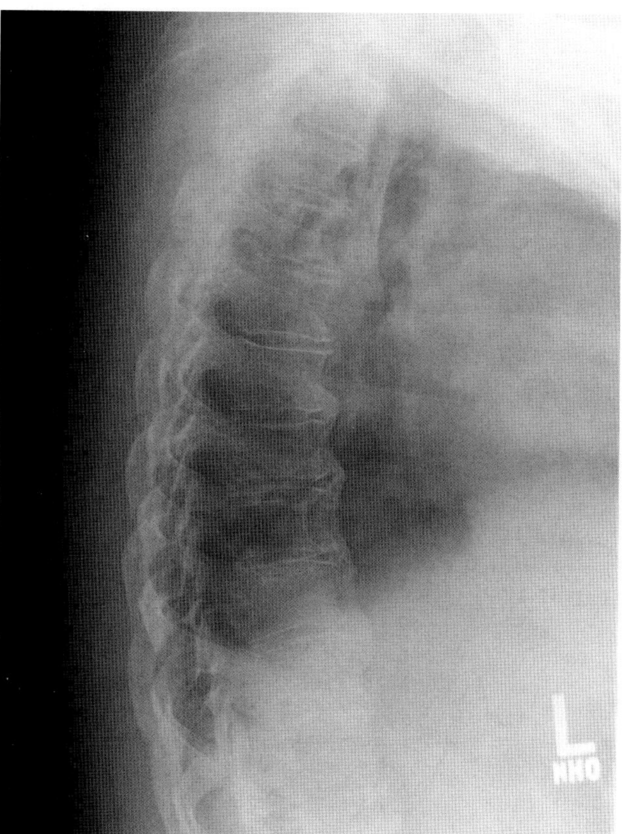

• **Fig. 50.11** Diffuse idiopathic skeletal hyperostosis. Lateral radiograph of the thoracic spine demonstrating bridging syndesmophytes, maintained disk spaces, and no fusion of the facet joints. (Courtesy Thomas Link, MD, University of California, San Francisco.)

DISH may be entirely asymptomatic. The most common complaint encountered is of pain and stiffness involving the spine, often the thoracic region. Usually there is only a moderate limitation of spinal motion. The loss of lateral spinal flexion is particularly notable in some patients. Extensive ossification of the anterior longitudinal ligament, together with large anterior enthesophytes, may occasionally compress the esophagus and cause dysphagia.[63] Ossification of the posterior longitudinal ligament is predominantly seen in the cervical spine and may occur either as a discrete disorder or as part of DISH. This can rarely lead to cervical myelopathy. Pain and tenderness may be present at the entheses, and these patients may have findings of lateral or medial humeral epicondylitis, Achilles tendinitis, or plantar fasciitis.

If treatment of DISH is necessary at all, it is symptomatic. Most patients respond to acetaminophen, nonsteroidal anti-inflammatory drugs (NSAIDs), and judicious use of glucocorticoid injections for painful enthesopathy.

Nonspecific Low Back Pain

This is defined as pain in the low back that has no identifiable cause (identification of the pain generator) and no clear association with a specific, serious underlying anatomic impairment or disease process.[69]

This condition is also referred to as *idiopathic LBP*. As mentioned earlier, a precise pathoanatomic diagnosis, with identification of the pain generator, cannot be made in as many as 85% of the patients. This is largely because of the nonspecific nature of the symptoms in patients with LBP, and the weak association of these symptoms with findings on imaging. Thus terms such as lumbago, strain, and sprain have come into use. Strain and sprain have never been histologically characterized. Therefore nonspecific LBP is a more accurate label for these patients who have a mostly self-limited syndrome of acute mechanical LBP. The severity of pain can vary from mild to severe, and whereas sometimes the back pain develops immediately after a traumatic event such as lifting a heavy object or a twisting injury, other patients may simply wake up with LBP. Most patients are better within 1 to 4 weeks[4] but remain susceptible to similar future episodes. Chronic nonspecific LBP develops in less than 10% of patients. These individuals are however largely responsible for the high cost associated with LBP.

Patients with nonspecific LBP are managed conservatively with a goal to relieve pain and restore function.

Neoplasm

Neoplasms are an uncommon, but nevertheless important, cause of LBP. In a primary care setting, neoplasia accounts for less than 1% of cases of LBP.[15]

In a large prospective study of patients in a walk-in clinic, a history of cancer, unexplained weight loss, failure to improve after 1 month of conservative therapy, and age older than 50 years were each associated with a higher likelihood for cancer.[70] By far the most important predictor for the likelihood of underlying cancer as the cause of LBP was a prior history of cancer.

The typical patient with LBP secondary to spinal malignancy presents with a persistent and progressive pain that is not alleviated by rest and is often worse at night. In some patients a spinal mass can result in a lumbosacral radiculopathy or cauda equina syndrome. Acute LBP may be the presentation in a patient with a pathologic compression fracture. Rarely, leptomeningeal carcinomatosis (in patients with breast cancer, lung cancer, lymphoma, or leukemia) may present with a lumbosacral polyradiculopathy.[71]

Most cases result from involvement of the spine by metastatic carcinoma (especially prostate, lung, breast, thyroid, gastrointestinal, or kidney) or multiple myeloma. Vertebral metastases occur in 3% to 5% of people with cancer, and 97% of spinal tumors are metastatic disease. Metastatic vertebral lesions, more commonly seen in the thoracic spine, account for 39% of bony metastases in patients with primary neoplasms.[72] Spinal cord tumors, primary vertebral tumors, and retroperitoneal tumors may in rare cases be the cause of LBP.[15]

Osteoid osteoma, a benign tumor of bone, typically presents with LBP in the second or third decade of life. The pain is often accompanied by a functional scoliosis secondary to paravertebral spasm. Patients may be seen with pain even before the osteoid osteoma is visible radiographically. Osteoid osteomas predominantly involve the posterior elements of the spine, usually the neural arch. A sclerotic lesion measuring less than 1.5 cm with a lucent nidus is pathognomonic.[73] A bone scan, CT scan, or MRI should be ordered if an osteoid osteoma is suspected but not detected on radiography. Symptoms can often be controlled by NSAIDs, presumably because the nidus produces high levels of prostaglandins. Surgical resection is an option for intolerable pain. Osteoid osteomas spontaneously resolve during the course of several years.[74]

Plain radiographs are less sensitive than other imaging tests in detecting neoplastic lesions because approximately 50% of trabecular bone must be lost before a lytic lesion is visible.[12] Metastatic lesions may be lytic (radiolucent), blastic (radiodense), or mixed. The majority of metastases are osteolytic. Vertebral bodies are primarily involved (Fig. 50.12) because of their rich blood supply associated with red marrow, and unlike infections, the disk space is usually spared. It should be noted that a purely lytic lesion such as multiple myeloma will not be detected by a bone scan. MRI offers the greatest sensitivity and specificity in the evaluation of spinal tumors and is generally the modality of choice.

Radiation therapy is usually helpful in controlling the pain related to skeletal metastases. Decompressive surgery is often required if the spinal mass results in a nerve root compression syndrome.

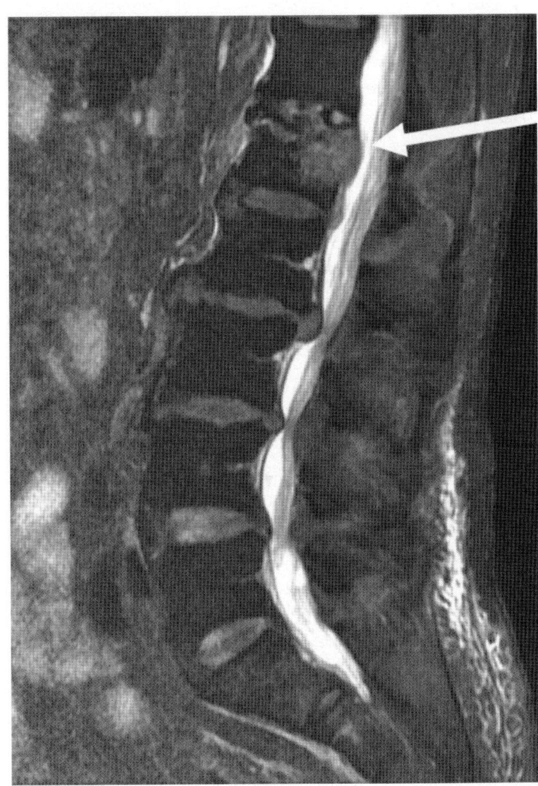

• **Fig. 50.12** Vertebral metastasis. Sagittal T2-weighted fat saturated fast spin echo sequence image of the lumbar spine demonstrating a L1 vertebral bone metastasis *(arrow)* typically located in the posterior aspect of the vertebral body with a convex posterior border. (Courtesy Thomas Link, MD, University of California, San Francisco.)

Infection

Vertebral osteomyelitis (spinal osteomyelitis, spondylodiskitis) may be acute (usually pyogenic) or chronic (pyogenic, fungal, or granulomatous). Acute vertebral osteomyelitis evolves during a period of a few days or weeks and is the major focus of this discussion.

Vertebral osteomyelitis usually results from hematogenous seeding, direct inoculation at the time of spinal surgery, or contiguous spread from an infection in the adjacent soft tissue. The lumbar spine is the most common site of vertebral osteomyelitis, followed by the thoracic and cervical spine.[75] *Staphylococcus aureus* is the most common microorganism (accounting for more than 50% of cases), followed by *Escherichia coli.* Coagulase-negative staphylococci and *Propionibacterium acnes* are almost always the cause of exogenous osteomyelitis after spinal surgery, particularly if internal fixation devices are used.[75]

A source of infection is detected in approximately half the cases, with endocarditis diagnosed in as many as a third of cases of vertebral osteomyelitis.[75] Other common sites for the primary focus of infection are the urinary tract, skin, soft tissue, a site of vascular access, bursitis, or septic arthritis.[76] Most patients with hematogenous pyogenic vertebral osteomyelitis have underlying medical disorders, such as diabetes, coronary artery disease, immunosuppressive disorders, malignancy, and renal failure.[75,76] Intravenous drug abuse is also a risk factor for vertebral osteomyelitis.

Vertebral osteomyelitis may be complicated by an epidural or paravertebral abscess. This may result in neurologic complications. Back pain is the initial symptom in most patients.

The back pain usually starts insidiously and progressively worsens over several weeks. The pain tends to be persistent, present at rest, exacerbated by activity, and at times well localized. Point tenderness on percussion over the spine has sensitivity but not specificity for vertebral osteomyelitis. Fever is present in only approximately half of the patients,[75] in part because most patients are using analgesic medications. Because most cases of vertebral osteomyelitis result from hematogenous seeding, the dominant manifestations initially may be of the primary infection. An epidural abscess may result in a radiculopathy or cauda equina syndrome.

Leukocytosis is seen in only approximately two-thirds of the patients. However, almost all the patients have increases in the erythrocyte sedimentation rate and C-reactive protein, with the latter best correlating with clinical response to therapy.[76] Blood

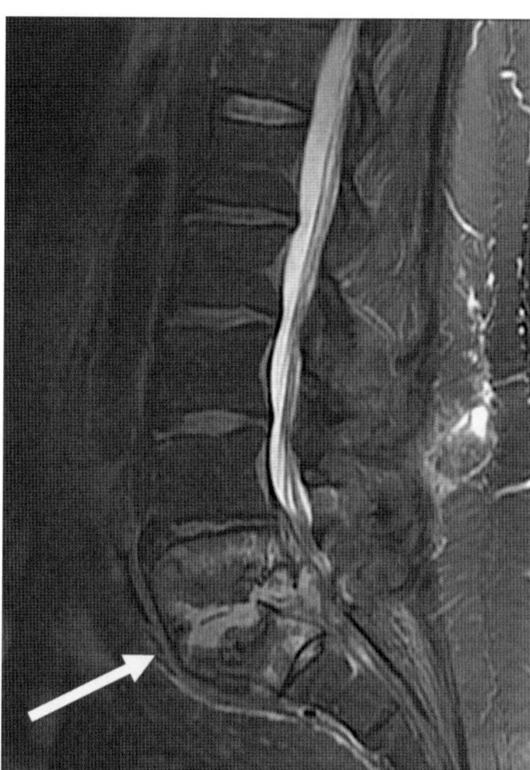

• **Fig. 50.13** Lumbar vertebral osteomyelitis. Sagittal T2-weighted fat saturated fast spin echo sequence image demonstrating severe L5-S1 osteomyelitis with diskitis *(arrow)* with destruction of the endplates, fluid in the disk space and epidural extension of the infection. Also note bone marrow edema pattern in the entire L5 and S1 vertebral bodies. (Courtesy Thomas Link, MD, University of California, San Francisco.)

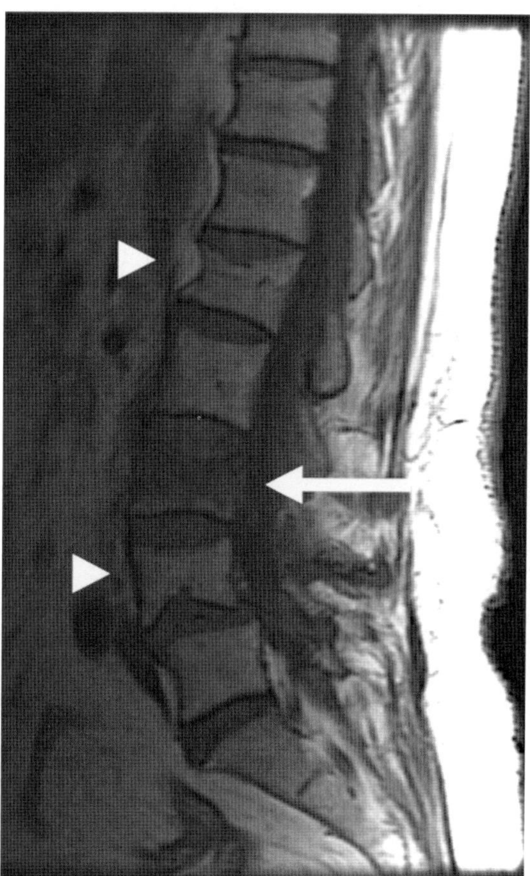

• **Fig. 50.14** Osteoporotic fractures. Sagittal T1-weighted fast spin echo image demonstrating chronic fractures at L1 and L4 *(arrowheads)* and more acute fracture at L3 *(arrow)* with bone marrow edema pattern. (Courtesy Thomas Link, MD, University of California, San Francisco.)

cultures are positive in up to 50% to 70% of patients. If blood cultures are negative in a patient suspected of having vertebral osteomyelitis, a bone biopsy (CT-guided or open) with appropriate culture studies and histopathologic analysis is indicated.

Plain radiography is usually the initial imaging study. Radiographic changes, however, occur relatively late and are nonspecific. Typically there is loss of disk height and loss of cortical definition followed by bony lysis of adjacent vertebral bodies. MRI is the most sensitive and specific imaging technique to detect spinal infections. The classic finding of pyogenic osteomyelitis is involvement of two vertebral bodies with their intervening disk (Fig. 50.13).[12] In a patient with neurologic impairment, MRI should be done early to rule out an epidural abscess. Whenever possible, anti-microbial therapy should be directed against an identified susceptible pathogen. Empiric anti-microbial therapy, pending culture results, is warranted in cases of neurologic compromise and sepsis. Empiric treatment, based on the most likely organism to cause infection, is also warranted when cultures are negative but there is a high index of suspicion. There are no data from randomized, controlled trials to guide decisions about specific anti-microbial regimens or the duration of therapy.[76] Intravenous therapy of at least 4 to 6 weeks, and possibly additional oral antibiotic therapy, is usually recommended. Surgery may be necessary to drain an abscess, although CT-guided catheter drainage may be sufficient in some cases. Surgical débridement is always required when infection is associated with a spinal implant with removal of the implant whenever possible.[76]

Tuberculosis and nontubercular granulomatous infections (blastomycosis, cryptococcosis, actinomycosis, coccidioidomycosis, and brucellosis) of the spine should be considered in the appropriate clinical and geographic setting.

Lumbar nerve roots are commonly involved in patients with herpes zoster. In most cases a single unilateral dermatome is involved. Pain is often severe and may precede the appearance of a maculopapular rash that evolves into vesicles and pustules.

Pyogenic sacroiliitis is rare. Patients, often children or young adults, present with back pain that may radiate into the buttock or posterior thighs. The sacroiliac joints are usually tender to palpation. MRI is the most sensitive imaging modality. Immediate CT-guided needle biopsy and culture, followed by appropriate antibiotic therapy, will usually produce an excellent outcome.[77]

Inflammation

The spondyloarthritides cause inflammatory LBP (see Table 50.1) and are discussed in detail elsewhere (see Chapters 79 to 83).

Metabolic Disease

The major consideration in this category is the occurrence of acute mechanical LBP secondary to a vertebral compression fracture (Fig. 50.14) in a patient with osteoporosis (see Chapter 107). Most patients are post-menopausal women.

Paget's disease of bone (see Chapter 107) is most often detected in an asymptomatic patient by the incidental finding of either an elevated alkaline phosphatase or characteristic radiographic abnormality. The spine is the second most commonly affected site after the pelvis. Within the spine, the L4 and L5 vertebrae are most commonly involved.[78] Paget's disease of the spine may involve single or multiple levels. The vertebral body is almost always involved together with a variable portion of the neural arch. Radiographically, Paget's disease is seen as areas of enlargement of the bone with thickened, coarsened trabeculae. Usually a mixed picture of sclerotic and lytic Paget's disease is encountered. The vertebrae may enlarge, weaken, and fracture. LBP may occur because of the pagetic process itself (with periosteal stretching and vascular engorgement), microfractures, overt fractures, secondary osteoarthritis of the facet joints, spondylolysis with or without spondylolisthesis, or sarcomatous transformation (rare).[78] Neurologic complications secondary to Paget's disease of the lumbar spine include sciatica secondary to nerve root impingement, spinal stenosis, and, rarely, cauda equina syndrome.

Visceral Pathology

Disease in organs that share segmental innervation with the spine can cause pain to be referred to the spine. In general, pelvic diseases refer pain to the sacral area, lower abdominal diseases to the lumbar area, and upper abdominal diseases to the lower thoracic spine area. Local signs of disease, such as tenderness to palpation, paravertebral muscle spasm, and increased pain on spinal motion, are absent.

Vascular, gastrointestinal, urogenital, or retroperitoneal pathology may on occasion cause LBP. A partial list of causes includes an expanding aortic aneurysm, pyelonephritis, ureteral obstruction due to renal stones, chronic prostatitis, endometriosis, ovarian cysts, inflammatory bowel disorders, colonic neoplasms, and retroperitoneal hemorrhage (usually in a patient taking anti-coagulants).

Most abdominal aortic aneurysms are asymptomatic but may become painful as they expand. Aneurysmal pain is usually a harbinger of rupture. Rarely, the aneurysm may develop leakage. This produces severe pain with abdominal tenderness. Most patients with aortic dissection present with a sudden onset of severe "tearing" pain in the chest or upper back. Pain originating from a hollow viscus such as the ureter or colon is often colicky.

Miscellaneous

LBP may be part of the clinical spectrum in innumerable conditions. It would not be practical or useful to discuss all of these entities here. Considered next are some of the more important or controversial causes of LBP.

The piriformis syndrome is thought to be an entrapment neuropathy of the sciatic nerve related to anatomic variations in the muscle-nerve relationship or to overuse. The piriformis is a narrow muscle that originates from the anterior part of the sacrum and inserts into the greater trochanter. It is an external rotator of the hip. The sciatic nerve underlies the piriformis muscle. There is, however, debate about the existence of the piriformis syndrome as a discrete entity because of the lack of objective, validated, and standardized tests. The diagnosis is clinical. Patients complain of pain and paresthesias in the gluteal region that may radiate down the leg to the foot. Some patients describe aggravation of pain after sitting. Unlike sciatica from lumbosacral nerve root compression, the pain is not restricted to a specific dermatome. The straight leg–raising test is usually negative. There may be tenderness over the sciatic notch. Physical examination maneuvers for the diagnosis of piriformis syndrome are based on the notion that stretching the irritated piriformis muscle may provoke sciatic nerve compression. This can be done by internally rotating the hip (Freiburg's sign) or by flexion, adduction, and internal rotation (FAIR maneuver) of the hip. Physical therapy that focuses on stretching the piriformis muscle and NSAIDs are generally the treatments offered. In refractory patients injections into the muscle under fluoroscopic or ultrasonographic guidance are sometimes used. Local anesthetic, corticosteroid, and botulinum toxin injections have been used. Support for any of these treatments is weak.[43]

The diagnosis of sacroiliac joints as the source of LBP, in patients without spondyloarthritis, remains controversial. Sacroiliac joint dysfunction is a term used to describe pain in the sacroiliac region related to abnormal sacroiliac joint movement or alignment. However, tests of pelvic symmetry or sacroiliac joint movement have low intertester reliability, and fluoroscopically guided sacroiliac joint injections have been unreliable in diagnosis and treatment.[43,79] Radiographic degenerative changes of the sacroiliac joint are often noted in the evaluation of patients with LBP. Whether these changes are the primary cause of the back pain remains unresolved.[80]

Lumbosacral transitional vertebrae include sacralization of the lowest lumbar vertebral body (assimilation of L5 to the sacrum resulting in four lumbar vertebrae and an enlarged sacral segment) and lumbarization of the uppermost sacral segment (assimilation of S1 to lumbar spine resulting in six lumbar vertebrae and a shortened sacral segment). These common variants can be seen in 15% to 35% of the general population.[81] The association of these variants with LBP remains controversial.

A "back mouse" is a mobile subcutaneous fibro-fatty nodule in the lumbosacral area. The nodule may be tender. Although there are case reports of patients with LBP and "back mice,"[82] the association with LBP remains unproven.

Epidural lipomatosis may be seen in obese patients, but it is more commonly seen as a rare side effect of long-term use of corticosteroids. There is an increase in epidural adipose tissue that causes a narrowing of the spinal canal. This is usually an incidental finding, although it may lead to compression of neural structures.

LBP during pregnancy is common. The pain usually starts between the fifth and seventh months of pregnancy.[83] The etiology of LBP in pregnancy is unclear. Biomechanical, hormonal, and vascular factors have been implicated. Most women have resolution of their pain postpartum.

Fibromyalgia (see Chapter 55) and polymyalgia rheumatica (see Chapter 93) are two frequently encountered rheumatologic conditions in which LBP may be a prominent part of the clinical syndrome.

Treatment

Specific treatment is available only for the small fraction of patients with LBP who have either evidence of clinically significant neural compression or an underlying systemic disease (cancer, infection, visceral disease, and spondyloarthritis). In the vast majority of patients with LBP, either the precise pathoanatomic cause (i.e., the pain generator) cannot be determined or, when the cause is determined, no specific treatment is available. These patients are managed with a conservative program centered on analgesia, education, and physical therapy. Currently a greater emphasis is placed on education, self-management, physical and psychological therapies, and less emphasis on pharmacologic, invasive interventional, and surgical procedures. The goal of treatment is relief of pain and restoration of function. Surgery is rarely necessary (Fig. 50.15).

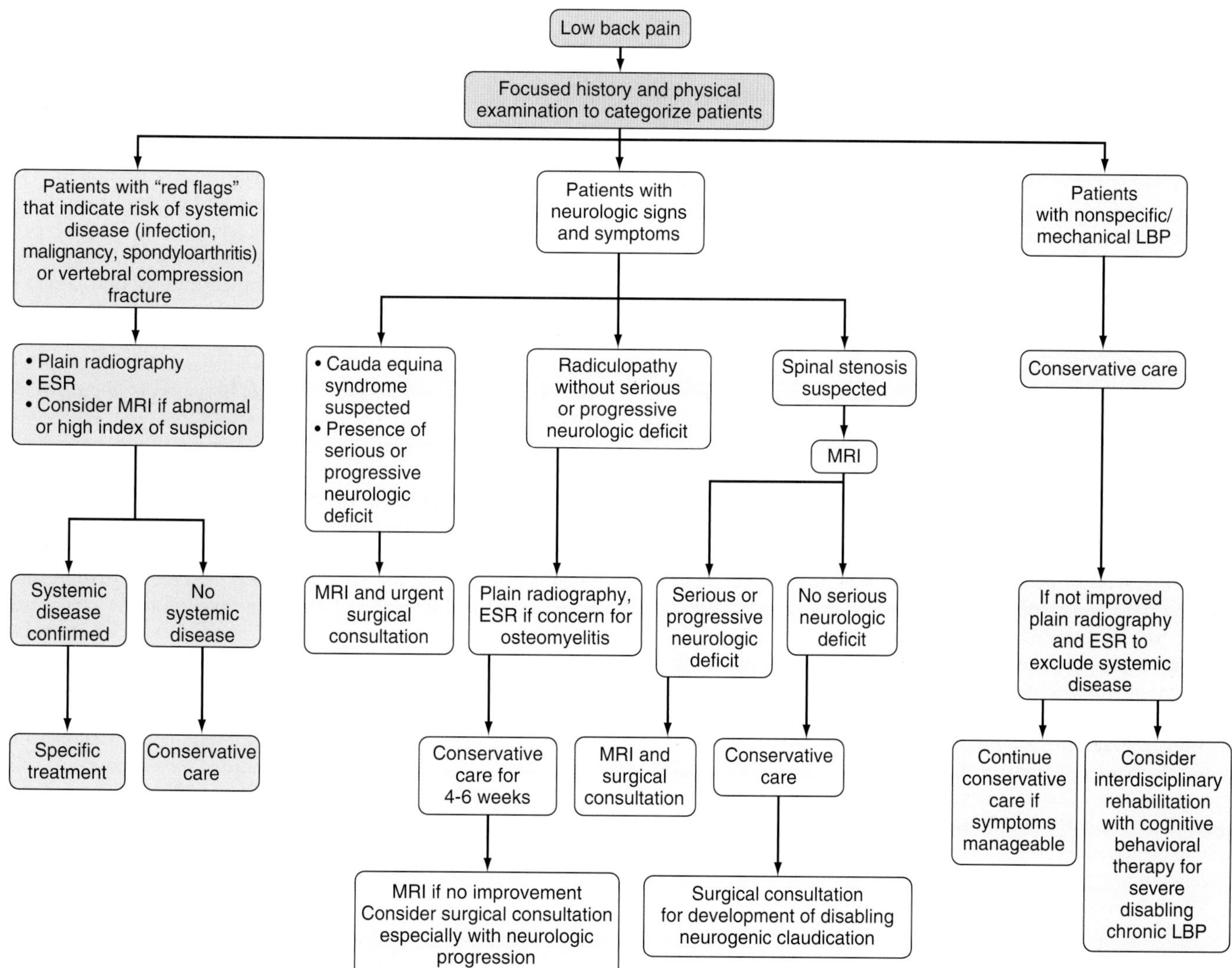

• **Fig. 50.15** Algorithm for the differential diagnosis and treatment of low back pain. *ESR,* Erythrocyte sedimentation rate; *LBP,* low back pain.

One should be wary of the proliferation of unproven medical, surgical, and alternative therapies. Most have not been rigorously tested in well-designed randomized controlled trials. Uncontrolled studies can produce a misleading impression of efficacy because of fluctuating symptoms and the largely favorable natural history of LBP in most patients.

For management purposes, patients with LBP are considered to have either acute LBP (duration <3 months), chronic LBP (duration >3 months), or a nerve root compression syndrome.

Acute Low Back Pain

The typical patient seeks medical attention for sudden onset of severe mechanical LBP. Examination usually reveals paravertebral muscle spasm, which often results in loss of the normally present lumbar lordosis and a severe decrease in range of motion secondary to pain. The prognosis for acute LBP is excellent. Indeed, only approximately a third of these patients seek medical care, and more than 90% recover substantially or completely within 8 weeks or less.[84]

Patients with acute LBP are advised to stay active and continue ordinary daily activities within the limits permitted by pain. This leads to more rapid recovery than bed rest.[85] Bed rest of more than 1 or 2 days is discouraged.

Pharmacologic therapy is used for symptomatic relief and does not affect recovery time. Unfortunately, no medication consistently results in large average benefits on pain, and evidence of beneficial effects on function is even more limited.[8] In spite of limited efficacy it is reasonable to use NSAIDS as first line analgesics, taking into account the patient's age and risk for gastrointestinal, liver, and cardio-renal toxicity. Acetaminophen is an ineffective analgesic in patients with LBP.[86–88] Short-term use of short-acting opioids is reasonable in patients with severe disabling LBP or in those at high risk of complications because of NSAIDs. Muscle relaxants such as cyclobenzaprine and tizanidine may be tried as second line pharmacologic therapy for short-term symptomatic relief but have a high prevalence of adverse effects, including drowsiness and dizziness.[8] It is unclear whether these medications truly relax muscles or if their effects are related to sedation or other nonspecific effects. Benzodiazepines have similar efficacy to muscle relaxants for short-term pain relief but are associated with risks for abuse, addiction, and tolerance.[27] There is no convincing evidence for the efficacy of systemic corticosteroids in patients with acute LBP with or without radicular symptoms.[89]

Back exercises are not helpful in the acute phase, and a physical therapy referral is usually unnecessary in the first month. Later, an individually tailored program that focuses on core strengthening, stretching exercises, aerobic conditioning, functional restoration, loss of excess weight, and education is recommended to prevent recurrences.[10,15,86] The purpose of back exercises is to stabilize the spine by strengthening trunk muscles. Flexion exercises strengthen the abdominal muscles, and extension exercises strengthen the paraspinal muscles. Numerous exercise programs have been developed and appear to be equally effective.

Patient education, including the use of education booklets, is recommended by most guidelines.[27] However, in a recent randomized clinical trial in adults with acute LBP, adding intensive patient education (an effective approach in patients with chronic LBP) to first-line care of patients was no better at improving pain outcomes than a placebo intervention (that nevertheless included brief advice and education).[89] The information provided should include causes of LBP, basic anatomy, favorable natural history, minimal value of diagnostic testing, importance of remaining active, effective self-care options, and coping techniques.

Spinal manipulation is provided mainly by chiropractors and osteopaths. It may involve low-velocity mobilization or manipulation with a high-velocity thrust that stretches spinal structures beyond the normal range and is frequently accompanied by a cracking or popping sound. For acute LBP, current evidence suggests that manipulative therapy is no more effective than conventional medical therapy.[27] There is no evidence that ongoing manipulation reduces the risk of recurrence of LBP.[90]

Given that most patients with acute LBP improve over time regardless of treatment, it is reasonable to select nonpharmacologic treatment with superficial heat (moderate-quality evidence), massage, acupuncture, or spinal manipulation (low-quality evidence).[87]

There is insufficient evidence to recommend the use of corsets and braces.[27] Traction provides no significant benefit for LBP patients with or without sciatica.[91]

Epidural corticosteroid injections have gained remarkable, but unjustified, popularity. The rationale for their use is that the genesis of radicular pain, when a herniated disk impinges on a nerve root, is at least partly related to locally induced inflammation. There is evidence of a small treatment benefit compared with placebo injection for short-term relief of leg pain in patients with radiculopathy resulting from a herniated nucleus pulposus.[92,93] However, epidural corticosteroid injections offer no significant functional benefit, nor do they reduce the need for surgery. It is important to note that there is no convincing evidence for the effectiveness of epidural corticosteroid injections in LBP patients without radiculopathy, in patients with spinal stenosis and neurogenic claudication,[94,95] or for failed back surgery syndrome. Nonetheless, most of the use of epidural steroid injections occurs in these situations of questionable benefit.[96] The U.S. Food and Drug Administration (FDA) has not approved the use of epidural corticosteroid injections. In April 2014 the FDA issued a drug safety communication requiring label changes to warn of rare but serious neurologic problems (including loss of vision, stroke, and death) after epidural corticosteroid injections. This safety issue is unrelated to the contamination of compounded corticosteroid injections products used for epidural injections that was reported in 2012.

A variety of other injection therapies with glucocorticoids or anesthetic agents, often in combination, are used in individuals with LBP with or without radicular pain and other symptoms in the leg. These include injection of trigger points, ligaments, sacroiliac joints, facet joints, and intradiskal steroid injections. There is no convincing evidence of the efficacy of these interventions.[97,98] Medial branch block for presumed facet joint pain and nerve root blocks for therapeutic or diagnostic purposes are also not recommended.[98] Unfortunately, these invasive and expensive procedures are commonly used in interventional pain clinics.

A number of physical therapy modalities are currently used in the treatment of patients with subacute and chronic LBP. These include transcutaneous electrical nerve stimulation (TENS), percutaneous electrical nerve stimulation, interferential therapy, low-level laser therapy, shortwave diathermy, and ultrasound. There is insufficient evidence of efficacy to recommend their use.

Vertebral compression fractures secondary to osteoporosis are common. There is resolution of pain with fracture healing within a few weeks in most patients. Vertebroplasty and balloon kyphoplasty are invasive and expensive procedures that are used to treat persistent pain associated with these fractures. Both procedures involve the percutaneous placement of needles into the vertebral body through or lateral to the pedicles, as well as the injection of bone cement to stabilize the fracture. Kyphoplasty differs from vertebroplasty in that the cement is injected into a void in the vertebral body created by inflation of a balloon. Several early studies had suggested a positive treatment effect for vertebroplasty.[99] However, two blinded, randomized, placebo-controlled trials of vertebroplasty for painful osteoporotic spinal fractures found no beneficial effect of vertebroplasty compared with a sham procedure.[100,101] A subset analysis of data from these trials, and results from another randomized and sham controlled clinical trial, confirmed that the lack of benefit from vertebroplasty extended to patients with pain of recent onset (0 to 9 weeks) and to those with severe pain.[102,103] Therefore, on the basis of current evidence, the routine use of vertebroplasty or indeed kyphoplasty for relief of pain from osteoporotic compression fractures cannot be justified.[104]

Chronic Low Back Pain

The clinical spectrum in patients with chronic LBP is wide. Some complain of severe, unrelenting pain, but most have a nagging mechanical LBP that may radiate into the buttocks and upper thighs. Patients with chronic LBP may experience periods of acute exacerbation. These exacerbations are managed according to the principles discussed earlier. A significant number of patients with chronic LBP remain functional and continue working, but overall, the results of treatment are unsatisfactory, and complete relief of pain is unrealistic for most. There is evidence that in a subset of patients with chronic LBP a pattern of augmented CNS pain processing (similar to fibromyalgia) is present, suggesting a component of "centralized pain."[105] A systematic review identified moderate evidence that patients with chronic LBP show structural brain differences in specific cortical and subcortical areas and altered functional connectivity in pain related areas following painful stimulation.[106] These patients are more likely to have poor treatment outcomes. Patients with chronic LBP are largely responsible for the high costs associated with LBP. It is therefore incumbent on physicians who treat these patients to judiciously use proven therapies.

For patients with chronic LBP clinicians should initially select nonpharmacologic treatment including education, exercise (with a focus on core strengthening and flexibility), aerobic conditioning, and loss of excess weight. Multidisciplinary rehabilitation including cognitive-behavioral therapy should be considered if the more conservative measures mentioned fail.

For most patients the initiation of pharmacologic therapy is with NSAIDs. They may provide some degree of analgesia, but the evidence for their long-term efficacy is not compelling. Acetaminophen is ineffective. Randomized clinical trial results do not support initiation of opioid therapy for moderate to severe chronic LBP. Treatment with opioids is not superior to treatment with nonopioid medications (mostly NSAIDs) for improving pain related function over 12 months.[107] Opioid analgesics are an option when used judiciously in a minority of patients with severe disabling pain. Because of substantial risks, including aberrant drug-related behaviors with long-term use in patients vulnerable to abuse or addiction, potential benefits and harms of opioid analgesics should be carefully weighed before starting therapy.[27,108] The co-prescribing of opioids and benzodiazepines should be avoided. There is no evidence that long-acting, around-the-clock dosing is more effective than short-acting or as-needed dosing, and continuous exposure to opioids could induce tolerance and lead to dose escalations.[8] Tramadol (a weak opioid) and duloxetine (a serotonin-norepinephrine reuptake inhibitor) may be considered for second line therapy. There is moderate-quality evidence that these agents achieved small to moderate improvement in pain intensity and function compared with placebo.[89,109,110] Muscle relaxants are not recommended for long-term use in patients with chronic stable LBP. Low-dose tricyclic anti-depressants have inconsistent benefits in patients with chronic LBP, and adverse side effects are common.[8] There is no evidence of efficacy of selective serotonin reuptake inhibitors for LBP. Depression is, however, common in patients with chronic LBP and should be treated appropriately. There is insufficient evidence to recommend antiepileptic medications, such as gabapentinoids (gabapentin and pregabalin) and topiramate, for pain relief in patients with LBP with or without radiculopathy.[8,111,112]

An individually tailored physical therapy program and patient education, as discussed in the earlier section on the treatment of acute LBP, are particularly important aspects in the management of a patient with chronic LBP. The use of physical therapy modalities (as discussed earlier) is also not recommended for patients with chronic LBP. Lumbar supports and traction are ineffective. For most patients with LBP a medium-firm mattress or a back-conforming mattress (waterbed or foam) may be superior to a firm mattress.[113,114]

A large number of other nonpharmacologic treatments have been evaluated for chronic LBP. The studies reveal that for acupuncture and mindfulness-based stress reduction (moderate-quality evidence), tai chi, yoga, motor control exercise, progressive relaxation, electromyography biofeedback, low-level laser therapy, operant therapy, and spinal manipulation (low-quality evidence) there is a small to moderate effect on pain and function.[88,115–119]

There has been a proliferation of nonsurgical interventional therapies for back pain. Various injection therapies (such as injections of trigger points, facet joints, and nerve root blocks) as discussed under the treatment of acute LBP, lack convincing evidence of efficacy and as such are also not recommended in the treatment of patients with chronic LBP.

Radiofrequency denervation aims to prevent the conduction of nociceptive impulses through the use of an electric current that damages the pain-conducting nerve. It has been used most frequently for treatment of presumed facet joint pain after a positive response to a diagnostic medial branch block. In the United States facet joint interventions in Medicare recipients increased from approximately 425,000 interventions in 2000 to 2.2 million interventions in 2013.[120] There is a lack of convincing evidence about the long-term effectiveness of this invasive procedure.[98] A recent randomized clinical trial concluded that radiofrequency denervation combined with a standardized exercise program resulted in no clinically important improvement in chronic LBP compared with a standardized exercise program alone.[120] Intradiskal electrothermal therapy (IDET) and percutaneous intradiskal radiofrequency thermocoagulation (PIRFT) involve placement of an electrode into the intervertebral disk of patients with presumed diskogenic pain and using electric or radiofrequency current to provide heat to thermocoagulate and shrink intradiskal tissue and destroy nerves. Current evidence does not support the use of IDET or PIRFT.[98,121] Prolotherapy (also referred to as *sclerotherapy*) involves repeated injections of an irritant sclerosing agent into ligaments and tendinous attachments. It is based on the hypothesis that back pain in some patients stems from weakened ligaments, and repeated injections of a sclerosing agent will strengthen the ligaments and reduce pain. On the basis of trial data, a guideline from the American Pain Society recommends against prolotherapy for chronic LBP.[98]

Spinal cord stimulation is a procedure involving the placement of electrodes, percutaneously or by laminotomy, in the epidural space adjacent to the area of the spine presumed to be the source of pain and applying an electric current in order to achieve neuromodulatory effects.[98] Power for the spinal cord stimulator is supplied by an implanted battery or transcutaneously through an external radiofrequency transmitter. Spinal cord stimulation is associated with a greater likelihood for pain relief compared with reoperation or conventional medical management in patients with failed back surgery syndrome with persistent radiculopathy.[98] At present there is no good evidence for the use of spinal cord stimulation for chronic LBP not related to the failed back surgery syndrome with radiculopathy. Approximately a third of the patients involved in studies have experienced a complication following spinal cord stimulation implantation, including electrode migration, infection, wound breakdown, and lead- and generator pocket–related complications.[98]

Intraspinal drug infusion systems, with use of a subcutaneously implanted pump with attached catheter, have been used in some patients with chronic intractable LBP for the intrathecal delivery of analgesics, usually morphine. Adequate evidence to support this intervention is not available.

Chronic LBP is a complex condition that involves biologic, psychological, and environmental factors. For patients with persistent and disabling nonradicular LBP despite recommended non-multidisciplinary therapies, the clinician should strongly consider intensive multidisciplinary rehabilitation with an emphasis on cognitive-behavioral therapy.[99] Multidisciplinary rehabilitation (also called *interdisciplinary therapy*) is an intervention that combines and coordinates physical, vocational, and behavioral components and is provided by multiple health professionals with different clinical backgrounds. Cognitive-behavioral therapy is a psychotherapeutic intervention that involves working with cognitions to change emotions, thoughts, and behaviors. There is strong evidence of improved function and moderate evidence of pain improvement with intensive multidisciplinary rehabilitation programs.[35,87] The problem lies in the limited availability and affordability of multidisciplinary rehabilitation programs. Functional restoration (also called *work hardening*) is an intervention that involves simulated or actual work in a supervised environment to enhance job performance skills and improve strength, endurance, flexibility, and cardiovascular fitness in injured workers. When combined with a cognitive-behavioral component, functional restoration is more effective than standard care alone to reduce time lost from work.[116]

As previously discussed, the precise identification of the pain generator in an LBP patient with degenerative changes involving the lumbar spine and no radicular pain is usually not possible in contradistinction to the patient with radicular symptoms. It is therefore not surprising that, as a general rule, the results of back surgery are disappointing when the goal is relief of back pain rather than relief of radicular symptoms resulting from neurologic compression. As such, the role of surgical treatment for chronic disabling LBP without neurologic involvement in patients with degenerative disease remains controversial. The most common surgery performed is spinal fusion. In spite of the unclear efficacy, rates of spinal fusion surgery for this indication are rapidly increasing. Interbody fusion is achieved from either a posterior or an anterior approach or both combined for a circumferential fusion. All fusion techniques involve placement of a bone graft between the vertebrae. Instrumentation refers to the use of hardware, such as screws, plates, or cages, that serve as an internal splint while the bone graft heals. Bone morphogenetic proteins are sometimes used to speed fusion. The rationale for fusion is based on its successful use at painful peripheral joints.

The current evidence is that for nonradicular back pain with degenerative changes, fusion is no more effective than intensive interdisciplinary rehabilitation but is associated with small to moderate benefits compared with standard nonsurgical care.[122] Furthermore, the majority of patients who undergo surgery do not experience an optimal outcome defined as no pain, discontinuation or occasional pain medication use, and return of high-level function.[99]

Lumbar disk replacement with a prosthetic disk is a newer alternative to fusion. Disk replacement is approved in the United States for patients with disease limited to one disk between L3-S1 and no spondylolisthesis or neurologic deficit. Approval was based on data showing efficacy equal to that of spinal fusion. This may be faint praise, given the controversy regarding the efficacy of spinal fusion for lumbar disk disease. No data support the hypothetical advantage that, unlike spinal fusion, prosthetic disks will protect adjacent levels from further degeneration by preserving motion. At present there is insufficient evidence regarding the long-term benefits and risk of disk replacement to support its recommendation.

Most patients with LBP, including those with neurogenic signs and symptoms, do not require surgical treatment.

Spine Patient Outcomes Research Trial

The precise role of surgery in the care of patients with LBP and neurogenic signs and symptoms is often unclear and controversial. This prompted the National Institute of Arthritis and Musculoskeletal and Skin Diseases (NIAMS) to fund three large parallel randomized[123–126] Spine Patient Outcomes Research Trial (SPORT) studies in an effort to assess the role of surgery in patients with lumbar disk herniation, lumbar degenerative spondylolisthesis with spinal stenosis, or lumbar spinal stenosis. Of note, in each of these milestone studies, all the patients had radicular leg pain with associated neurologic signs or neurogenic claudication. Patients with serious or progressive neurologic deficits require urgent surgical decompression and, as such, were excluded from all the SPORT studies. Each study included a randomly assigned cohort and an observational cohort. Patients in the observational cohort declined to be randomly assigned in favor of designating their own treatment, but agreed to undergo follow-up according to the same protocol. The primary study outcomes were measures of pain, physical function, and disability during a 2-year period. All three studies were compromised by high rates of crossover (as much as 50%) between the assigned treatment, surgical or nonsurgical, in both cohorts. This has caused concern over the validity of the conclusions.

The first study[123,124] in patients with lumbar disk herniation looked at surgical (diskectomy) versus nonoperative treatment (physical therapy, education, NSAIDs if tolerated) in patients with persistent radicular symptoms despite nonoperative treatment for at least 6 weeks. Both treatment groups improved substantially; the intent-to-treat analysis showed no significant difference in the randomly assigned cohort.[123] Greater improvement with surgery was reported in the observational cohort.[124] However, nonrandomly assigned comparisons of self-reported outcomes are subject to potential confounding and must be interpreted cautiously.

In the second study, in patients with lumbar degenerative spondylolisthesis and spinal stenosis, with persistent neurologic symptoms for at least 12 weeks, the intent-to-treat analyses for the randomly assigned cohort showed no significant differences between the surgical (decompressive laminectomy with or without fusion) and usual nonsurgical treatment. The nonrandomly assigned "as treated" comparison that combined both cohorts showed greater improvement in the surgical group. "As treated" analyses are significantly confounded and should be interpreted with caution.[127]

In the final study[126] for patients with lumbar spinal stenosis without spondylolisthesis, with persistent neurologic symptoms for at least 12 weeks, both the intent-to-treat and "as treated" analyses showed a significant advantage favoring surgery (posterior decompressive laminectomy).

SPORT data also revealed that, in general, spinal surgery improves leg pain more than LBP, and benefits of surgery diminish with time.[128–130]

Disk Herniation

Patients with a herniated disk with radicular pain secondary to nerve root compression should be treated nonsurgically, as described in the section on acute LBP, unless they have a serious or progressive neurologic deficit. Only approximately 10% of patients have sufficient pain after 6 weeks of conservative care that surgery is considered.[15] A decision to continue with nonsurgical therapy beyond 6 weeks in these patients does not increase the risk for paralysis or cauda equina syndrome.[99] Surgery in these patients is associated with moderate short-term (through 6 to 12 weeks) benefits compared with nonsurgical therapy, although differences in outcome diminish with time and are generally no longer present after 1 to 2 years.[92,99]

Open diskectomy or microdiskectomy (currently the standard surgical procedure) is the usual surgery performed on patients with serious or progressive neurologic deficit or electively on patients with persistent disabling pain secondary to radiculopathy (Table 50.5). Open diskectomy generally involves a laminectomy, whereas microdiskectomy, by using a smaller incision and an operating microscope, involves a unilateral hemilaminotomy to remove the disk fragment compressing the nerve root. There are no clear differences in the outcome between open diskectomy and microdiskectomy. Newer minimally invasive approaches show a trend towards earlier and better pain relief but require longer operating times and are associated with a higher rate of rerupture of the disk.[78,122,131]

TABLE 50.5 Indications for Surgical Referral

Disk Herniation
Cauda equina syndrome (emergency)
Serious neurologic deficit
Progressive neurologic deficit
Longer than 6 weeks of disabling radiculopathy (elective)
Spinal Stenosis
Serious neurologic deficit
Progressive neurologic deficit
Persistent and disabling pseudoclaudication (elective)
Spondylolisthesis
Serious or progressive neurologic deficit

Epidural corticosteroid injections may offer a small treatment benefit for short-term relief of radicular pain but do not offer significant functional benefit and do not reduce the need for surgery.[93]

There is no convincing evidence of efficacy for the uses of systemic corticosteroids or gabapentinoids (gabapentin and pregabalin) in patients with radiculopathy.

Anti-TNF therapy has been investigated in patients with lumbar radiculopathy.

There is biologic plausibility for its potential efficacy in sciatica because TNF is an important mediator of nerve root inflammation, central sensitization, and neuropathic pain.[132] However, there have been conflicting results in small randomized control trials looking at patients with radiculopathy. The addition of a short course of subcutaneous adalimumab to the treatment regimen of patients with acute sciatica resulted in a small decrease in leg pain and fewer surgical procedures.[133] However, another trial found no difference between intravenous infliximab and a saline infusion.[134] In a three-group trial, leg pain appeared to be reduced more with epidural steroids than with epidural etanercept or saline.[135] The results of the etanercept group were no better than the saline group. Yet a trial that used the transforaminal approach to deliver epidural etanercept concluded that etanercept reduced both leg and back pain compared with placebo.[132]

Spinal Stenosis

It is critical to understand the natural history of degenerative lumbar spinal stenosis before making treatment decisions. The symptoms of spinal stenosis remain stable for years in most patients and may improve in some. Dramatic improvement is uncommon. Even when symptoms progress, there is little likelihood of rapid deterioration of neurologic function. Therefore conservative nonoperative treatment is a rational choice for most patients.

There is a paucity of good data to guide the conservative management of lumbar spinal stenosis. Physical therapy is the mainstay of management, but evidence for the efficacy of specific standardized regimens is not available. Most regimens include core strengthening, stretching, aerobic conditioning, loss of excess weight, and patient education. Exercises that involve lumbar flexion, such as bicycling, are better tolerated. Strengthening of abdominal muscles may be helpful by promoting lumbar flexion and reducing lumbar lordosis. Lumbar corsets that maintain slight flexion may provide symptomatic relief. They should only be used for a limited number of hours a day to avoid atrophy of paraspinal muscles.

NSAIDs and tramadol are often used for symptomatic relief of pain.

Lumbar epidural corticosteroid injections are used on the assumption that symptoms may result from inflammation at the interface between the nerve root and compressing tissues.[56] To assess this potential for efficacy, a double-blind placebo controlled, randomized trial[95] was carried out in patients with lumbar spinal stenosis and associated moderate to severe leg pain. There was no significant difference between patients assigned to epidural injections of glucocorticoids plus lidocaine and those assigned to lidocaine alone with regards to the co-primary outcomes of functional disability or pain intensity. Based on this well-designed study, the routine use of epidural corticosteroids in patients with lumbar spinal stenosis cannot be recommended.

Surgery is indicated for the few patients with lumbar spinal stenosis who have a serious or progressive neurologic deficit. However, most surgery for lumbar spinal stenosis is elective. The indication for elective surgery is to relieve persistent and disabling symptoms of neurogenic claudication that have not responded to conservative care. In patients without fixed neurologic deficits, delayed surgery produces similar benefits to surgery selected as the initial treatment.[56,136] The surgical goal is to decompress the central spinal canal and the neural foramina to eliminate pressure on the nerve roots. This is accomplished by laminectomy, partial facetectomy of hypertrophied facet joints, and excision of the hypertrophied ligamentum flavum and any protruding disk material. Two recent randomized controlled trials clearly show that for most patients with lumbar spinal stenosis, with or without degenerative spondylolisthesis, surgery should be limited to decompression.[137,138] The addition of instrumented fusion for the treatment of spinal stenosis is no longer the best practice. Its use should be restricted to patients who have proven spinal instability as confirmed on flexion-extension radiographs.[139] Unfortunately, there is an alarming increase in spinal fusion surgery with routine use of complex fusion techniques in the absence of evidence of greater efficacy. The techniques include instrumentation, bone graft augmentation with bone cement and human bone morphogenetic proteins, and combined anterior and posterior fusion (often at multiple levels). These techniques are associated with increased perioperative mortality, major complications, re-hospitalization, and cost in the absence of evidence of greater efficacy.[140–142]

Overall, for patients with spinal stenosis, with or without spondylolisthesis, who have disabling symptoms of neurogenic claudication despite conservative care, there is some evidence to support the effectiveness of decompressive laminectomy in reducing pain and improving function through 1 to 2 years.[56,99,122,126] Beyond this time frame, the benefits appear to diminish and reoperations are frequently necessary. Given all this, patient preferences should weigh heavily in the decision of whether to have surgery for lumbar spinal stenosis.[143]

A less invasive alternative to decompressive laminectomy is the implantation of a titanium interspinous spacer at one or two vertebral levels. This spacer distracts adjacent spinous processes and thereby imposes lumbar flexion, which in turn potentially increases the spinal canal dimensions. There is preliminary evidence of efficacy in patients with one- or two-level spinal stenosis, without spondylolisthesis, and with a history of relief of neurogenic claudication with flexion.[122] It is at present unclear how this newer procedure compares with the standard surgical approach.

Spondylolisthesis

The vast majority of patients with spondylolisthesis and chronic LBP are treated conservatively. Rarely, a patient may need decompression surgery if a serious or progressive neurologic deficit develops from nerve root impingement or disabling pseudoclaudication secondary to spinal stenosis develops in the patient. A randomized trial involving patients with isthmic spondylolisthesis and disabling isolated LBP or sciatica for at least a year suggested fusion surgery produced better results than nonsurgical care,[144] although the differences in outcome narrowed during a 5-year follow-up period.[145] As discussed earlier, in most patients with degenerative lumbar spondylolisthesis and spinal stenosis decompressive surgery alone without instrumented fusion is the recommended surgical treatment.

Outcome

The natural history of most patients with acute LBP is favorable. There is substantial improvement in pain and function within a month in the majority of patients, although two-thirds of the patients still report low grade discomfort at 3 and 12 months,[4] and more than 90% are better at 8 weeks.[5] Only approximately a third of patients with acute LBP seek medical care. Presumably, the rest improve on their own. Relapses, which also tend to be brief, are common and may affect as many as 40% of patients within 6 months.

Improvement is also the norm for patients with sciatica secondary to a herniated disk.[146] A third of these patients are significantly better in 2 weeks, and 75% improve after 3 months.[12] Only approximately 10% of these patients ultimately undergo surgery.

The symptoms of spinal stenosis tend to remain stable in 70% of patients, improve in 15%, and worsen in 15%.[62] Disabling symptoms of neurogenic claudication secondary to spinal stenosis can be relieved by decompressive surgery, but the benefits of surgery often diminish with time.

The 7% to 10% of patients in whom chronic pain develops are largely responsible for the high costs associated with LBP and remain a major challenge. Factors that predict persistence of chronic disabling LBP include maladaptive pain coping behaviors, presence of nonorganic signs, functional impairment, poor general health status, psychiatric comorbidities, job dissatisfaction, disputed compensation claims, and a high level of "fear avoidance" (an exaggerated fear of pain leading to avoidance of beneficial activities).[35,147]

Conclusion

Of the general population, 80% will experience LBP. Of these patients, 90% will be largely pain free within 8 weeks. Degenerative change in the lumbar spine is the most commonly identified cause of LBP. The initial evaluation of LBP should focus on identifying the few patients with significant neurologic involvement, fracture, or systemic disease (infection, malignancy, or spondyloarthritis) because they may need urgent or specific intervention. Early imaging is rarely indicated in the absence of trauma, significant neurologic involvement, or suspicion of systemic disease. Imaging abnormalities, often the result of age-related degenerative changes, should be carefully interpreted because they are frequently present in asymptomatic individuals. A precise pathoanatomic diagnosis with identification of the pain generator cannot be made in 85% of patients. Regardless, most patients with the largely self-limited syndrome of acute LBP will only require reassurance, education, and simple analgesics. The management of patients with chronic LBP remains a challenge and complete relief of pain is an unrealistic goal for most. Patients with chronic LBP benefit from an initial program of core strengthening, stretching, aerobic conditioning, loss of excess weight, and education. Long-term opioid therapy is strongly discouraged. Intensive interdisciplinary rehabilitation with an emphasis on cognitive-behavioral therapy should be strongly considered if conservative measures fail. Epidural corticosteroids have a small treatment benefit, and their use should be restricted to patients with radiculopathy resulting from disk herniation. A large number of injection techniques, physical therapy modalities, and nonsurgical interventional therapies lack evidence of efficacy. Decompressive surgery is indicated for serious or progressive neurologic deficit and is rarely needed.

Rates of back surgery (including spinal fusion) in the United States are the highest in the world and continue to rise rapidly.[122] This increase continues in spite of the fact that the role of surgery in the management of patients without serious or progressive neurologic deficit remains controversial. Randomized trials incorporating a sham operation may be the only way to resolve the controversy. Such trials may be justifiable because genuine clinical equipoise exists among clinicians about the merits of the intervention, the surgery is often not performed for a life-threatening condition, the primary outcomes are subjective, and the rate of complications is high.[127,142]

There continues to be a proliferation and increasing utilization of expensive but unproven interventional and alternative therapies. Whenever possible, these need to be subjected to randomized, placebo-controlled trials. This is the only truly valid means to assess the efficacy of interventions for subjective outcomes such as pain. Once the efficacy has been established, these treatments should be further subjected to "comparative effectiveness research" to determine how these effective interventions compare with each other.[148]

Protection of the public from unproven or harmful approaches to managing LBP requires that governments and health care leaders tackle entrenched and counterproductive reimbursement strategies, vested interests, and financial and professional incentives that maintain the status quo.[149] A major barrier to changing clinical pathways relates to current models of health care reimbursements, which reward volume rather than quality, perversely providing remuneration not for how effectively patients are treated, but for how much they are treated.[150]

A promising new approach for the management of LBP in primary care involves stratified care according to the estimated risk of poor prognosis by using a validated and simple screening method that involves the use of a short self-completed questionnaire. Patients are allocated into three different risk-defined groups (low, medium, and high) and treated according to three treatment pathways matched to the risk groups. This resulted in better clinical and economic outcomes than did nonstratified conventional care.[151] This strategy should be further explored and confirmed in different settings.

Evidence-based clinical practice guidelines regarding indications for tests or treatment at specific steps in the care of patients with LBP exist in many countries. They are intended to provide a cost-effective road map for rational and efficient care. The implementation of these guidelines, however, remains a challenge. Avenues that will facilitate this implementation should be explored.

Full references for this chapter can be found on ExpertConsult.com.

Selected References

1. Hartvigsen J, Hancock MJ, Kongsted A, et al.: What low back pain is and why we need to pay attention, *The Lancet* 391:2356–2367, 2018.
2. Hoy D, Brooks P, Blyth F, et al.: The epidemiology of low back pain, *Best Pract Res Clin Rheumatol* 24:769–781, 2010.
4. Dunn KM, Hestback L, Cassidy JD: Low back pain across the life course, *Best Pract Res Clin Rheum* 27:591–600, 2013.
5. daSilva T, Mills K, Brown BT, et al.: Risk of recurrence of low back pain: a systematic review, *J Orthop Sports Phys Ther* 47:305–313, 2017.
6. Martin B, Deyo R, Mirza S, et al.: Expenditures and health status among adults with back and neck problems, *JAMA* 299:656–664, 2008.
7. Davis M, Onega T, Weeks W, et al.: Where the United States spends its spine dollars, *Spine* 37:1693–1701, 2012.
8. Chou R: Pharmacological management of low back pain, *Drugs* 70(4):384–402, 2010.
9. Suri P, Palmer MR, Tsepilov YA, et al.: Genome-wide meta-analysis of 158,000 individuals of European ancestry indentifies three loci associated with chronic back pain, *PLoS Genet* 14(9):e1007601, 2018.
10. Dixit RK: Approach to the patient with low back pain. In Imboden J, Hellmann D, Stone J, editors: *Current diagnosis and treatment in rheumatology*, ed 2, New York, 2007, McGraw-Hill, pp 100–110.
11. Chou R, Shekelle P: Will this patient develop persistent disabling low back pain? *JAMA* 303(13):1295–1302, 2010.
12. Jarvik JG, Deyo RA: Diagnostic evaluation of low back pain with emphasis on imaging, *Ann Intern Med* 137:586–597, 2002.
13. Dixit RK, Schwab JH: Low back and neck pain. In Stone JH, editor: *A clinician's pearls and myths in rheumatology*, New York, 2009, Springer.
14. Dixit RK, Dickson DJ: Low back pain. In Adebajo A, editor: *ABC of rheumatology*, ed 4, Hoboken, NJ, 2010, Wiley-Blackwell.
16. Deyo R, Jarvik J, Chou R: Low back pain in primary care, *BMJ* 349:4266–4271, 2014.
17. Gran JT: An epidemiological survey of the signs and symptoms of ankylosing spondylitis, *Clin Rheumatol* 4:161–169, 1985.
18. Wang R, Crowson CS, Wright K, et al.: Clinical evolution in patients with new onset inflammatory back pain: a population-based cohort study, *Arthritis Rheumatol* 70(7):1049–1055, 2018.
19. Arnbak B, Jurik AG, Jensen TS, et al.: Association between inflammatory back pain characteristics and magnetic resonance imaging findings in the spine and sacroiliac joints, *Arthritis Care Res* 70(2):244–251, 2018.
23. Chou R, Fu R, Carrino JA, et al.: Imaging strategies for low back pain: systematic review and meta-analysis, *Lancet* 373:463–472, 2009.
25. Chou R, Qaseem A, Owens D, et al.: Diagnostic imaging for low back pain: advice for high-value health care from the American College of Physicians, *Ann Intern Med* 154:181–189, 2011.
26. Webster B, Choi Y, Bauer A, et al.: The cascade of medical services and associated longitudinal costs due of nonadherent magnetic resonance imaging for low back pain, *Spine* 39:1433–1440, 2014.
27. Chou R, Qaseem A, Snow V, et al.: Diagnosis and treatment of low back pain: a joint clinical practice guideline from the American College of Physicians and the American Pain Society, *Ann Intern Med* 147(7):478–491, 2007.
29. Winter J, Hooge M, Sande M, et al.: Magnetic resonance imaging of the sacroiliac jonts indicating sacroiliitis according to the assessment of spondyloarthritis international society definition in healthy individuals, runners, and women with postpartum back pain, *Arthritis Rheumatol* 70(7):1042–1048, 2018.
30. Weber U, Jurik AG, Zejden A, et al.: Frequency and anatomic distribution of magnetic resonance imaging features in the sacroiliac joints of young athletes. Exploring 'background noise' toward a data driven definition of sacroiliitis in early spondyloarthritis, *Arthritis Rheumatol* 70(5):736–745, 2018.
34. Manchikanti L, Pampati V, Fellows B, et al.: The diagnostic validity and therapeutic value of lumbar facet joint nerve blocks with or without adjuvant agents, *Current Review of Pain* 4(5):337–344, 2000.
35. Carragee EJ: Persistent low back pain, *N Engl J Med* 352(18):1891–1898, 2005.
36. Carragee E, Don A, Hurwitz E, et al.: 2009 ISSLS Prize Winner: does discography cause accelerated progression of degeneration changes in the lumbar disc. A ten-year matched cohort study, *Spine* 34:2338–2345, 2009.
37. Zhang Y, Zhao C, Jiang L, et al.: Modic changes: a systematic review of the literature, *Eur Spine J* 17:1289, 2008.
38. Jensen T, Karppineu J, Sorensen J, et al.: Vertebral end plate signal changes (Modic change): a systematic literature review of prevalence and association with non-specific low back pain, *Eur Spine J* 17:1407, 2008.
39. Hulton M, Bayer G, Powell J: Modic vertebral body changes: the natural history as assessed by consecutive magnetic resonance imaging, *Spine* 36:2304, 2011.
40. Jensen R, Leboeuf-Yde C: Is the presence of modic changes associated with the outcomes of different treatments? A systematic critical review, *BMC Musculoskelet Disord* 12:183–191, 2011.
43. Ropper AH, Zafonte RD: Sciatica. *N Engl J Med* 372:1240–1248, 2015.
46. Tarulli AW, Raynor EM: Lumbosacral radiculopathy, *Neurol Clin* 25:387, 2007.
48. Panagopoulos J, Hush J, Steffens D, et al.: Do MRI findings change over a period of up to 1 year in patients with low back pain? *Spine* 42(7):504–512, 2017.
49. Deyo RA, Mirza SK: Herniated lumbar intervertebral disk, *N Engl J Med* 374:1763–1772, 2016.
50. Oegema TR: Intervertebral disc herniation: does the new player up the ante? *Arthritis Rheum* 62:1840–1842, 2010.
51. Abraham JL: Assessment and treatment of patients with malignant spinal cord compression, *J Support Oncol* 2:88–91, 2004.
52. Lavy C, James A, Wilson-MacDonald J, et al.: Cauda equine syndrome, *BMJ* 338:b936, 2009.
53. Kalichman L, Kim D, Guermazi A, et al.: Spondylolysis and spondylolisthesis: prevalence and association with low back pain in the adult community-based population, *Spine* 34(2):199–205, 2009.
55. Tomkins-Lane C, Melloh M, Lurie J, et al.: Consensus on the clinical diagnosis of lumbar spinal stenosis: results of an international Delphi study, *Spine* 41:1239–1246, 2016.
56. Katz JN, Harris MB: Lumbar spinal stenosis, *N Engl J Med* 358(8):818–825, 2008.
57. Ishimoto Y, Yoshimura N, Muraki S, et al.: Prevalence of symptomatic lumbar spinal stenosis and its association with physical performance in a population-based cohort in Japan: the Wakayama Spine Study, *Osteoarthritis Cartilage* 20(10):1103–1108, 2012.
58. Battie MC, Ortega-Alonso A, Niemelainen R, et al.: Lumbar spinal stenosis is a highly genetic condition partly mediated by disc degeneration, *Arthritis Rheumatol* 66(12):3505–3510, 2014.
61. Suri P, Rainville J, Kalichman L, et al.: Does this older adult with lower extremity pain have the clinical syndrome of lumbar spinal stenosis? *JAMA* 304:2628–2636, 2010.
65. Kiss C, O'Neill TW, Mituszova M, et al.: The prevelance of diffuse idiopathic skeletal hyperostosis in a population-based study in Hungary, *Scand J Rheumatol* 31:226, 2002.
69. O'Connell NE, Cook CE, Wand BM, et al.: Clinical guidelines for low back pain: a critical review of concensus and inconsistencies across three major guidelines, *Best Pract Res Clin Rheumatol* 30:968–980, 2016.
75. Mylona E, Samarkos M, Kakalou E, et al.: Pyogenic vertebral osteomyelitis: a systemic review of clinical characteristics, *Semin Arthritis Rheum* 39:10–17, 2009.
76. Zimmerli W: Vertebral osteomyelitis, *N Engl J Med* 362(11):1022–1029, 2010.

77. Attarian D: Septic sacroiliitis: the overlooked diagnosis, *J South Orthop Assoc* 10(1):57–60, 2001.
78. Dell'Atti C, Cassar-Pullicino VN, Lalam RK, et al.: The spine in Paget's disease, *Skeletal Radiol* 36:609–626, 2007.
80. Riddle DL, Freburger JK: Evaluation of the presence of sacroiliac joint region dysfunction using a combination of tests: a multicenter intertester reliability study, *Phys Ther* 82:772, 2002.
81. O'Shea FD, Boyle E, Salonen DC, et al.: Inflammatory and degenerative sacroiliac joint disease in a primary back pain cohort, *Arthritis Care Res* 62:447–454, 2010.
82. Konin G, Walz D: Lumbosacral transitional vertebrae: classification, imaging findings, and clinical relevance, *Am J Neuroradiol* 31(10):1778–1786, 2010.
83. Curtis P, Gibbons G, Price F: Fibro-fatty nodules and low back pain. The back mouse masquerade, *J Fam Pract* 49:345, 2000.
85. Coste J, Delecoeuillerie G, Cohen deLara A, et al.: Clinical course and prognostic factors in acute low back pain: an inception cohort study in primary care practice, *BMJ* 308:577, 1994.
86. Malmivaara A, Hakkinen U, Aro T, et al.: The treatment of acute low back pain—bed rest, exercises, or ordinary activity? *N Engl J Med* 332(6):351–355, 1995.
87. Williams C, Maher C, Latimer J, et al.: Efficacy of paracetamol for acute low back pain: a double blind, randomized controlled trial, *Lancet* 384:1586–1596, 2014.
88. Qaseem A, Wilt TJ, McLean RM, et al.: Noninvasive treatments for acute, subacute, and chronic low back pain: a clinical practice guideline from the American College of Physicians, *Ann Intern Med* 166(7):514–530, 2017.
89. Chou R, Deyo R, Friedly J, et al.: Systemic pharmacologic therapies for low back pain: a systematic review for an American College of Physicians Clinical Practice Guideline, *Ann Intern Med* 166(7):480–492, 2017.
90. Traeger AC, Lee H, Hubscher M, et al.: Effect of intensive patient education versus placebo patient education on outcomes in patients with acute low back pain, *JAMA Neurol.* Published Online November 5, 2018.
91. Cherkin DC, Deyo RA, Battie M, et al.: A comparison of physical therapy, chiropractic manipulation, and provision of an educational booklet for the treatment of patients with low back pain, *N Engl J Med* 339:1021–1029, 1998.
92. Clarke JA, van Tulder MW, Blomberg SE, et al.: Traction for low back pain with or without sciatica, *Cochrane Database Syst Rev* 23:CD003010, 2007.
93. Carette S, Leclaire R, Marcouxs S, et al.: Epidural corticosteroid injections for sciatica due to herniated nucleus pulposus, *N Engl J Med* 336(23):1634–1640, 1997.
94. Pinto R, Maher C, Ferreira M, et al.: Epidural corticosteroid injections in the management of sciatica. A systematic review and meta-analysis, *Ann Intern Med* 157:865–877, 2012.
95. Friedly J, Comstock B, Turner J, et al.: A randomized trial of epidural glucocorticoid injections for spinal stenosis, *N Engl J Med* 371:11–21, 2014.
96. Chou R, Hashimoto R, Friedly F, et al.: Epidural corticosteroid injections for radiculopathy and spinal stenosis: a systematic review and meta-analysis, *Ann Intern Med* 163(5):373–381, 2015.
97. Friedly J, Deyo R: Imaging and uncertainty in the use of lumbar epidural steroid injections, *Arch Intern Med* 172(2):142–143, 2012.
98. Chou R, Atlas SJ, Stanos SP, et al.: Nonsurgical interventional therapies for low back pain. A review of the evidence for an American Pain Society Clinical Practice Guideline, *Spine* 34(10):1078–1093, 2009.
99. Chou R, Loeser JD, Owens DK, et al.: Interventional therapies, surgery, and interdisciplinary rehabilitation for low back pain. An evidence based clinical practice guideline from the American Pain Society, *Spine* 34(10):1066–1077, 2009.
100. Weinstein JN: Balancing science and informed choice in decisions about vertebroplasty, *N Engl J Med* 361(6):619–621, 2009.
101. Kallmes DF, Comstock BA, Heagerty PJ, et al.: A randomized trial of vertebroplasty for osteoporotic spinal fractures, *N Engl J Med* 361(6):569–579, 2009.
102. Buchbinder R, Osborne RH, Ebeling PR, et al.: A randomized trial of vertebroplasty for painful osteoporotic vertebral fractures, *N Engl J Med* 361(6):557–568, 2009.
103. Staples M, Kallmes D, Comstock B, et al.: Effectiveness of vertebroplasty using individual patient data from two randomized placebo controlled trials: meta-analysis, *BMJ* 343:d3952, 2011.
104. Firanescu CE, deVries J, Lodder P, et al.: Vertebroplasty versus sham procedure for painful acute osteoporotic vertebral compression fractures (VERTOS IV) randomized sham controlled clinical trial, *BMJ* 361:k1551, 2018.
105. McCullough B, Comstock B, Deyo R, et al.: Major medical outcomes with spinal augmentation vs conservative therapy, *JAMA Intern Med* 173(16):1514–1521, 2013.
106. Brummett C, Goesling J, Tsodikov A, et al.: Prevalence of the fibromyalgia phenotype in patients with spine pain presenting to a tertiary care pain clinic and the potential treatment implications, *Arthritis Rheum* 65(12):3285–3292, 2013.
107. Kregel J, Meeus M, Malfliet A, et al.: Structural and functional brain abnormalities in chronic low back pain: a systematic review, *Semin Arthritis Rheum* 45:229–237, 2015.
108. Krebs EE, Gravely A, Nugent S, et al.: Effect of opioid vs non-opioid medications on pain-related function in patients with chronic back pain or hip pain or knee osteoarthritis pain. The SPACE randomized clinical trial, *JAMA* 319(9):872–882, 2018.
109. Martell BA, O'Connor PG, Kerns RD, et al.: Systematic review: opioid treatment for chronic back pain: prevalence, efficacy, and association with addiction, *Ann Intern Med* 146:116–127, 2007.
110. Skljarevski V, Desaiah D, Liu-Seifert H, et al.: Efficacy and safety of duloxetine in chronic low back pain, *Spine* 35(13):E578–E585, 2010.
111. Skljarevski V, Ossanna M, Liu-Seifert H, et al.: A double-blind, randomized trial of duloxetine versus placebo in the management of chronic low back pain, *Eur J Neurol* 16(9):1041–1048, 2009.
112. Mathieson S, Chiro M, Maher CG, et al.: Trial of pregabalin for acute and chronic sciatica, *N Engl J Med* 376(12):1111–1120, 2017.
113. Attal N, Barrot M: Is pregabalin ineffective in acute or chronic sciatica? *N Engl J Med* 376(12):1169–1170, 2017.
114. Kovacs FM, Abraira V, Pena A, et al.: Effect of firmness of mattress on chronic non-specific low back pain: randomized, double-blind, controlled, multicentre trial, *Lancet* 362:1599, 2003.
115. Bergholdt K, Fabricius RN, Bendix T: Better backs by better beds? *Spine* 33:703, 2008.
116. Chou R, Huffman LH: Nonpharmacologic therapies for acute and chronic low back pain: a review of the evidence for an American Pain Society/American College of Physicians Clinical Practice Guideline, *Ann Intern Med* 147(7):492–514, 2007.
117. Franke H, Franke J, Fryer G: Osteopathic manipulative treatment for nonspecific low back pain: a systematic review and meta-analysis, *BMC Musculoskelet Disord* 15:286, 2014.
118. Tilbrook H, Cox H, Hewitt C, et al.: Yoga for chronic low back pain. A randomized trial, *Ann Intern Med* 155:569–578, 2011.
119. Sherman K, Cherkin D, Wellman R, et al.: A randomized trial comparing yoga, stretching, and a self-care book for chronic low back pain, *Arch Intern Med* 171(22):2019–2026, 2011.
120. Juch JNS, Maas ET, Ostelo RWJG, et al.: Effect of radiofrequency denervation on pain intensity among patients with chronic low back pain: the mint randomized clinical trials, *JAMA* 318(1):68–81, 2017.
121. Urrutia G, Kovacs F, Nishishinya MD, et al.: Percutaneous thermocoagulation intradiscal techniques for discogenic low back pain, *Spine* 32:1146, 2007.
122. Chou R, Baisden J, Carragee EJ, et al.: Surgery for low back pain. A review of the evidence for an American pain society clinical practice guideline, *Spine* 34(10):1094–1109, 2009.

123. Weinstein J, Tosteson T, Lurie J, et al.: Surgical vs nonoperative treatment for lumbar disk herniation. The Spine Patient Outcomes Research Trial (SPORT): a randomized trial, *JAMA* 296:2441–2450, 2006.
124. Weinstein J, Lurie J, Tosteson T, et al.: Surgical vs nonoperative treatment for lumbar disk herniation. The Spine Patient Outcomes Research Trial (SPORT): observational cohort, *JAMA* 296:2451–2459, 2006.
125. Weinstein J, Lurie J, Tosteson T, et al.: Surgical versus nonsurgical treatment for lumbar degenerative spondylolisthesis, *N Engl J Med* 356(22):2257–2270, 2007.
126. Weinstein J, Tosteson T, Lurie J, et al.: Surgical versus nonsurgical treatment for lumbar spinal stenosis, *N Engl J Med* 358(8):794–810, 2008.
127. Flum D: Interpreting surgical trials with subjective outcomes, *JAMA* 296(20):2483–2485, 2006.
128. Freedman MK, Hilibrand AS, Blood EA, et al.: The impact of diabetes on the outcome of surgical and nonsurgical treatment of patients in the spine patients outcome research trial, *Spine* 36(4):290–307, 2011.
129. Pearson A, Blood E, Lurie J, et al.: Predominant leg pain is associated with better surgical outcomes in degenerative spondylolisthesis and spinal stenosis: results from the Spine Patient Outcomes Research Trial (SPORT), *Spine* 36(3):219–229, 2011.
130. Lurie JD, Toste4son TD, Abdu WA, et al.: Long-term outcomes of lumbar spinal stenosis: eight-year results of the spine patient outcome research trial (SPORT), *Spine* 40(2):63–76, 2015.
131. Peul WC, van Houwelingen HC, van den Hout WB, et al.: Surgery versus prolonged conservative treatment for sciatica, *N Engl J Med* 356:2245–2256, 2007.
132. Freeman B, Ludbrook G, Hall S, et al.: Randomized, double-blind, placebo-controlled, trial of transforaminal epidural etanercept for the treatment of symptomatic lumbar disc herniation, *Spine* 38(23):1986–1994, 2013.
133. Genevay S, Viatte S, Finckh A, et al.: Adalimumab in severe and acute sciatica, *Arthritis Rheum* 62:2339–2346, 2010.
134. Korhonen T, Karppinen J, Paimela L, et al.: The treatment of disc-herniation-induced sciatica with infliximab: one-year follow-up results of FIRST II, a randomized controlled trial, *Spine* 31(24):2759–2766, 2006.
135. Cohen S, White R, Kurihara C, et al.: Epidural steroids, etanercept, or saline subacute sciatica, *Ann Intern Med* 156:551–559, 2012.
136. Amundsen T, Weber H, Nordal JH, et al.: Lumbar spinal stenosis: conservative or surgical management? A prospective 10 year study, *Spine* 25:1424, 2000.
137. Forsth P, Olafsson G, Carlsson T, et al.: A randomized, controlled trial of fusion surgery for lumbar spinal stenosis, *N Engl J Med* 374(15):1413–1423, 2016.
138. Ghogawala Z, Dziura J, Butler WE, et al.: Laminectomy plus fusion versus laminectomy alone for lumbar spondylolisthesis, *N Engl J Med* 374(15):1424–1434, 2016.
139. Peul WC, Moojen WA: Fusion for lumbar spinal stenosis—safeguard or superfluous surgical implant? *N Engl J Med* 374(15):1478–1479, 2016.
140. Carragee EJ: The increasing morbidity of elective spinal stenosis surgery. Is it necessary? *JAMA* 303(13):1309–1310, 2010.
141. Deyo RA, Mirza SK, Martin BI, et al.: Trends, major medical complications, and charges associated with surgery for lumbar spinal stenosis in older adults, *JAMA* 303(13):1259–1265, 2010.
142. Deyo RA, Nachemson A, Mirza S: Spinal fusion surgery—the case for restraint, *N Engl J Med* 350(7):722–726, 2004.
143. Katz JN: Surgery for lumbar spinal stenosis: informed patient preferences should weigh heavily, *Ann Intern Med* 162:518–519, 2015.
144. Moller H, Hedlund R: Surgery versus conservative management in adult isthmic spondylolisthesis—a prospective randomized study: part 1, *Spine* 25:1711–1715, 2000.
145. Ekman P, Moller H, Hedlund R: The long-term effect of posterolateral fusion in adult isthmic spondylolisthesis: a randomized controlled study, *Spine J* 5(1):36–44, 2005.
146. Vroomen P, deKrom M, Knottnerus JA: Predicting the outcome of sciatica at short-term follow-up, *Br J Gen Pract* 52:119, 2002.
147. Chou R, Shekelle P: Will this patient develop persistent disabling low back pain? *JAMA* 303(13):1295–1302, 2010.
148. Carey T: Comparative effectiveness studies in chronic low back pain, *Arch Intern Med* 171(22):2026–2027, 2011.
149. Buchbinder R, Van Tulder Mauritis, Oberg B, et al.: Low back pain: a call for action, *The Lancet* 391:2384–2389, 2018.
150. Foster NE, Anema JR, Cherkin D, et al.: Prevention and treatment of low back pain: evidence challenges, and promising directions, *Lancet* 391:2368–2383, 2018.
151. Hill J, Whitehurst D, Lewis M, et al.: Comparison of stratified primary care management for low back pain with current best practice (Star T back): a randomized controlled trial, *Lancet* 378:1560–1571, 2013.

51 Hip and Knee Pain

JAMES I. HUDDLESTON, III, AND STUART GOODMAN

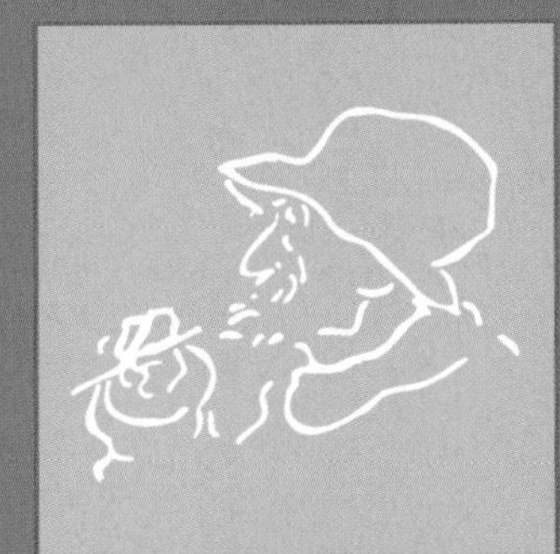

KEY POINTS

- The clinician should be able to narrow the differential diagnosis of hip or knee pain down to two to three diagnoses after the history and physical examination. Imaging studies should be used to confirm the diagnosis.
- The initial imaging study ordered should be conventional radiographs.
- Many of the vital structures in the knee can be palpated easily or examined with provocative tests.
- A knee effusion is often associated with internal derangement.
- The clinician should suspect a torn meniscus if a patient has an effusion, joint line tenderness, and pain with hyperextension and hyperflexion.
- Patients with osteoarthritis often report stiffness and pain with activity.
- Inflammatory arthritis should be considered when a patient continues to experience pain despite resting the joint.
- Groin pain with internal rotation of the hip is considered to be due to hip disease until proven otherwise.
- Concurrent hip and lumbosacral disease is common.

Introduction

Musculoskeletal pain affects one-third to one-half of the general population.[1,2] A substantial increase in the burden of musculoskeletal disease is expected in the next decade as the "Baby Boomers" reach middle age and beyond. This increased burden is exemplified by the increasing prevalence of hip and knee replacement operations. By 2020 there will be over 500,000 primary total hip replacements and 1,300,000 primary total knee replacements performed in the United States annually.[3] The prevalence of revision total knee and total hip arthroplasty procedures is rising as well.[4] The hip and knee joints are two of the most commonly affected sites of musculoskeletal pain, with the prevalence of hip pain ranging from 8% to 30% in people 60 years and older[5,6] and the prevalence of knee pain ranging from 20% to 52% in individuals 55 years and older. In general, women experience more musculoskeletal pain than men do.[7] Geographic and ethnic variations in the rates of both hip and knee pain also exist. For example, there tends to be significantly less hip and knee pain with decreasing latitude, as well as significantly less hip pain and osteoarthritis, in China than in the United States.[8–15]

When evaluating reports of knee or hip pain, knowledge of the anatomy of these joints is necessary to formulate a differential diagnosis. Given the thin soft tissue envelope around the knee and the fact that knee pain is rarely referred, the pain generators around the knee often can be elucidated with a complete history and thorough physical examination. Diagnosis of hip pain may be more challenging because the joint is deeper and the region is not infrequently the site of referred pain from the spine. An understanding of the basic biomechanics of these joints is also important in formulating a differential diagnosis because certain activities are likely to cause specific injuries.

Knee Pain

History

A detailed history is perhaps the most important step in accurately diagnosing the cause of knee pain. Knee complaints generally fall into two broad categories: pain or instability. Pain may arise from injury to the articular surfaces (e.g., osteoarthritis, inflammatory arthritis, osteochondral defects, and osteochondritis desiccans), torn menisci, quadriceps and patella tendon tears, bursitis, nerve damage, fractures, neoplasia, or infection. Referred pain from the hip or spine is less common. Instability is usually episodic and stems from injuries to the quadriceps-patellar extensor mechanism, collateral ligaments, or cruciate ligaments. It is important to distinguish true instability from the common complaint of "giving way" because the latter is usually due to a robust pain response rather than specific structural disease.

People in certain age groups tend to experience similar injuries. Ligament injuries, acute meniscus tears, and patellofemoral problems are frequently encountered in patients younger than 40 years. In contrast, degenerative conditions such as osteoarthritis and degenerative meniscal lesions tend to occur more frequently in older people.

The location and character of the pain are particularly important when evaluating knee pain because many of the structures vital to proper knee function are subcutaneous and can be palpated easily. The knee can be conceptualized as three separate compartments—medial, lateral, and patellofemoral. Each compartment should be examined separately. The patient should be able to point to the exact area where the pain is most severe. The time of onset of the pain should be determined. Osteoarthritis and inflammatory arthritis tend to have an insidious onset, whereas injuries to menisci and ligaments are usually associated with a traumatic event. Knowing the details of a traumatic event will be helpful. For example, a twisting injury, especially one sustained with a flexed knee, suggests a meniscus tear, whereas a noncontact knee injury associated with change of direction is more likely to produce a tear of the anterior cruciate ligament (ACL). Pain from degenerative arthritis tends to be associated with stiffness, is generally worse with ongoing activity during the day, and is exacerbated by activities such as exercise, stair climbing, getting up from a chair, and getting in and out of a car.

The presence or absence of knee swelling is an important part of the history because knee effusions (i.e., fluid in the knee joint) usually accompany internal derangement. An effusion also may be present with synovitis, osteoarthritis, inflammatory arthritis, fractures, infection, and neoplasms. Distinguishing between soft tissue swelling around the knee, synovial thickening, and a true knee effusion is critical and is described in the following text. The timing or onset of the swelling is also important for determining the diagnosis. An acute cruciate or collateral ligament injury or osteochondral fracture usually presents with an acute hemarthrosis (occurring within an hour), whereas an effusion associated with arthritis tends to be more insidious in nature.

One common symptom is *locking*. In a younger patient, locking may be due to a displaced meniscal tear. In older patients who have degenerative arthritis, locking is often due to loose bodies. It is important to distinguish between true locking and diminished range of motion due to pain (so-called *pseudolocking*) because this distinction will determine which imaging studies are most appropriate.

Timing of the pain with activity is also important for making the correct diagnosis. Meniscus tears and ligament injuries leading to instability will be particularly troublesome with activities such as walking on uneven surfaces and stairs, movements requiring knee flexion, and pivoting. Osteoarthritis tends to be exacerbated by all load-bearing activities and relieved by rest.

The clinician also should explore the patient's exercise tolerance and ability to perform activities of daily living. These details may give insight into the severity of the injury and also will guide treatment. Important details include the use of ambulatory assist devices (e.g., a cane, crutches, walker, brace, or wheelchair), walking tolerance, and capability for other exercises (e.g., physical therapy).

A history of any previous treatments rendered also should be recorded. A patient's response to physical therapy, analgesics, nonsteroidal anti-inflammatory drugs, nutritional supplements (such as glucosamine and chondroitin), intra-articular injections of corticosteroids or hyaluronic acid derivatives, and any operative treatments will lend further insight into the accurate diagnosis and have implications for treatment once the diagnosis has been confirmed.

After obtaining a detailed history, the clinician should be able to formulate a differential diagnosis with a short list of potential conditions. This information should then allow the physician to concentrate on specific aspects of a focused physical examination that will lead to confirmation of the diagnosis.

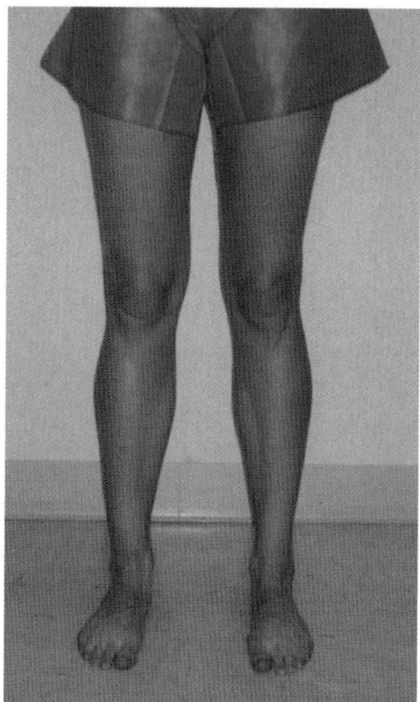

• **Fig. 51.1** Assessment of coronal alignment.

Physical Examination

General

After a brief overall assessment of the patient, the physical examination should begin with observation of the patient's lower extremity coronal alignment and leg lengths. Patients should stand with their legs slightly apart while they face the examiner (Fig. 51.1). A goniometer is then used to measure the varus/valgus alignment of the knees. Evaluation of leg lengths should be performed with step blocks of known sizes. The total height of the blocks needed to make the iliac crests level with the floor is equivalent to the leg length discrepancy (Fig. 51.2).

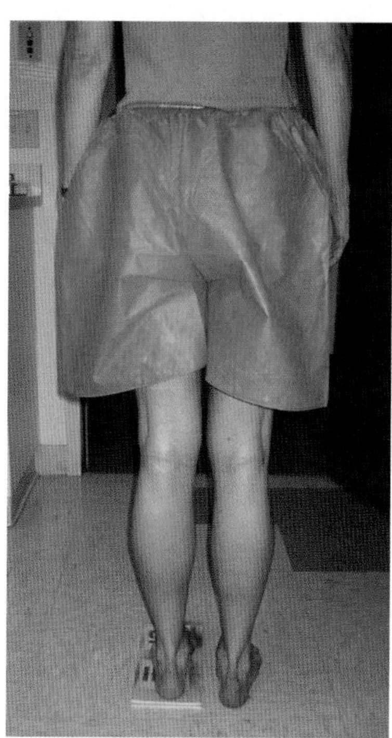

• **Fig. 51.2** The total height of the blocks needed to make the iliac crests level is equal to the length discrepancy.

Gait is examined next. Although a comprehensive discussion of gait analysis is beyond the scope of this chapter, all clinicians should routinely make a few basics observations when evaluating patients with a knee problem. *Antalgic gaits* (i.e., a shortened stance phase) and thrusts are commonly seen. Any disorder that causes lower extremity pain may cause an antalgic gait. Seen in the stance phase of gait, thrusts may be due to a progressive angular deformity as a result of degenerative changes or chronic ligamentous instability. Medial thrusts result from medial collateral ligament and/or posteromedial capsular laxity. Lateral thrusts arise from lateral collateral ligament or posterolateral corner laxity (Fig. 51.3). Patients also may thrust into recurvatum (the so-called *back-knee deformity*) as a result of posterior capsular laxity or quadriceps weakness.

The patient should then transfer to the examination table for evaluation in a comfortable supine position. The examination should proceed with inspection and palpation prior to performing any provocative maneuvers. A pillow should be placed under the knee if full extension is not possible because of pain (e.g., as a result of fractures, displaced meniscus tears, or a large effusion). If the patient has no known pre-existing disease, the contralateral knee can serve as an adequate control. The lower extremity should be

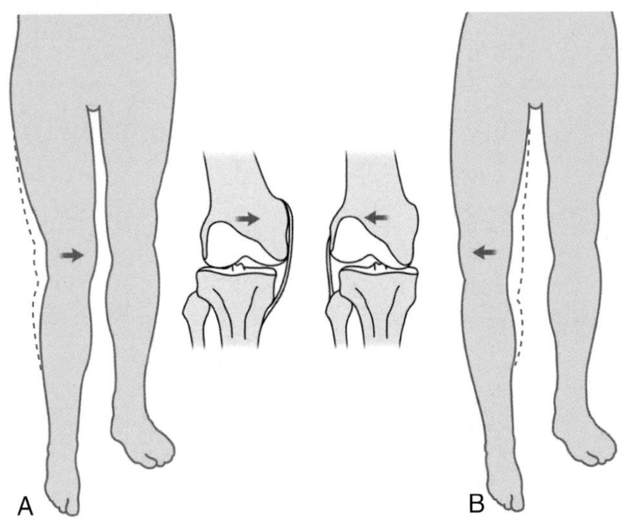

• **Fig. 51.3** The femur shifts medially during a medial thrust (A) and laterally during a lateral thrust (B).

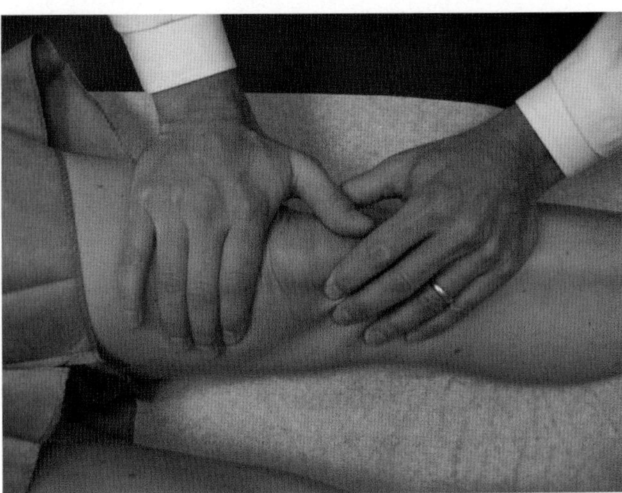

• **Fig. 51.5** Small effusions can be appreciated by the "milking" of fluid into the suprapatellar pouch.

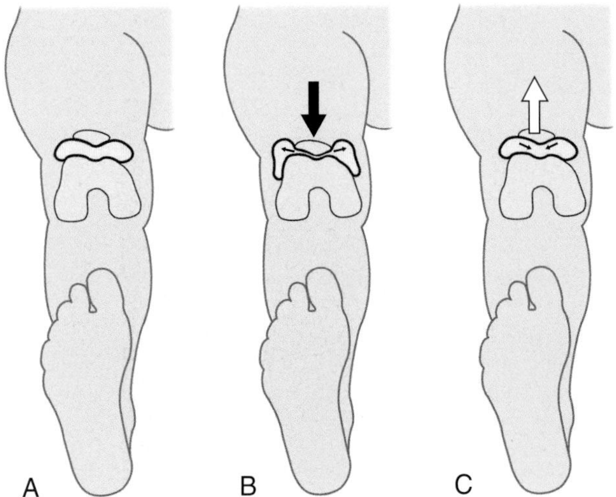

• **Fig. 51.4** Large effusions can be detected by "balloting" the patella with the knee in extension.

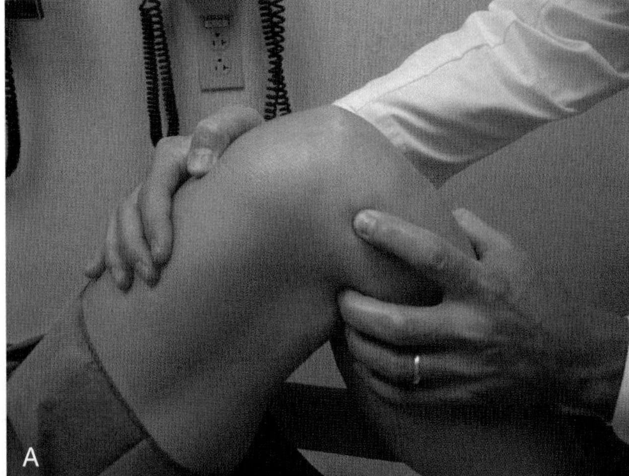

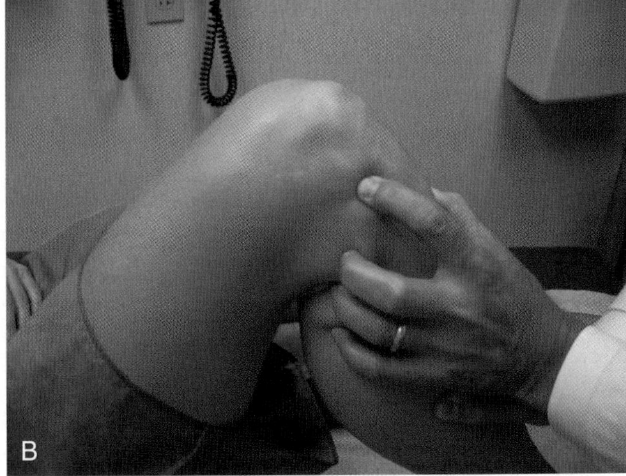

• **Fig. 51.6** Palpation of the medial (A) and lateral (B) joint lines.

inspected for any skin lesions, areas of ecchymosis, or surgical scars. Quadriceps atrophy should be noted, and a tape measure should be used to record thigh circumference. It is good practice to measure the thigh circumference at the same distance from the patella or joint line in each knee. The presence of an effusion, which will be seen as fullness or swelling in the suprapatellar pouch, should be noted. The effusion should be confirmed by ballottement of the patella (Fig. 51.4). Small effusions will require "milking" of the fluid upward into the suprapatellar pouch, which will allow for quantification of the amount of fluid (Fig. 51.5). The active and passive range of motion of both knees should be recorded with a goniometer.

The examiner should then proceed with palpation of all structures of the knee. It is important to perform this palpation in a systematic manner to ensure completeness. Palpation should be gentle but firm enough to detect subtle disease. Structures to be palpated include the quadriceps tendon, the patella (superior and inferior poles), the pes anserinus bursa, the medial (Fig. 51.6A) and lateral (Fig. 51.6B) joint lines, the origins and insertions of the collateral ligaments, the tibial tubercle, and the popliteal fossa. Fullness in the posterior knee may be indicative of a Baker's cyst.

Ligaments

Injuries to the collateral or cruciate ligaments may lead to knee instability. It is important to mention that for each translational and rotational motion of the knee, both primary and secondary restraints exist. When a primary restraint is disrupted, motion will

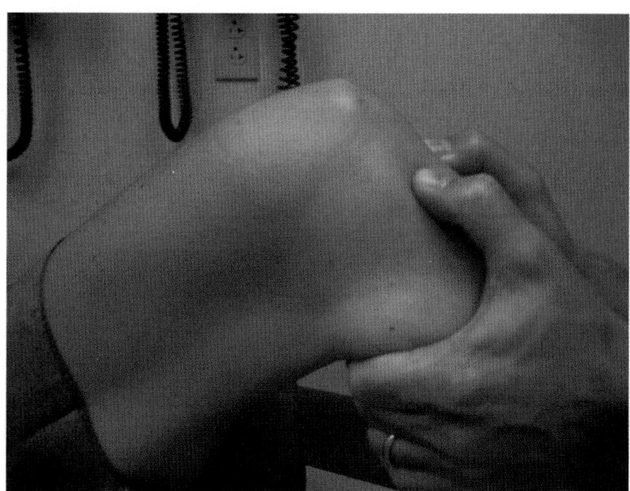

• **Fig. 51.7** The anterior drawer test is performed by subluxating the tibia anteriorly with the knee in 90 degrees of flexion. The amount of anterior translation (mm) is noted. The endpoint is characterized as "soft" or "hard."

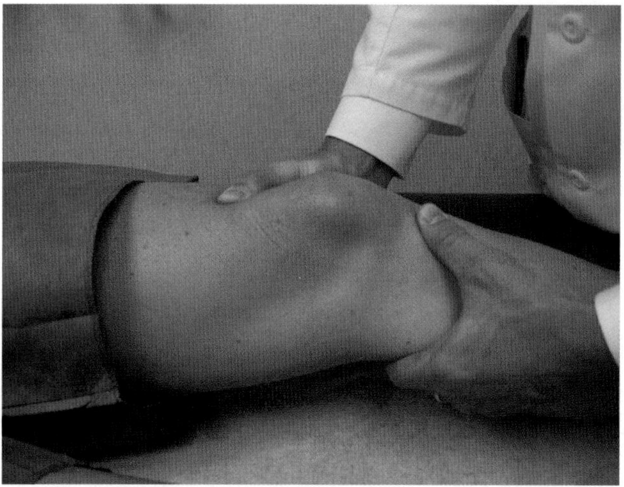

• **Fig. 51.8** The Lachman test is performed by applying an anterior force on the tibia while stabilizing the femur with the knee in 30 degrees of flexion.

be limited by the secondary restraint. If a secondary restraint is injured and the primary restraint remains intact, then motion will not be abnormal. For example, the ACL is the primary restraint to anterior translation of the tibia, and the medial meniscus is the secondary restraint. ACL disruption will lead to a significant increase in anterior tibial translation. This translation will be increased if the patient has undergone a prior medial menisectomy.[16]

The collateral ligaments can be examined with stress applied in the coronal plane. They should be examined both in full extension and in 30 degrees of flexion to remove the influence of the cruciate ligaments and the capsular restraints. With the patient in a supine position, a varus force is applied across the knee to test the lateral collateral ligament and a valgus force is applied across the knee to evaluate the medial collateral ligament.

The ACL is one of the most frequently injured structures in the knee. ACL insufficiency is also common in patients with advanced osteoarthritis. Common mechanisms of injury include a direct blow to the lateral side of the knee (the "clipping" injury in football causing the triad of medial collateral ligament, ACL, and medial meniscus injuries[17]), as well as noncontact injuries that occur during cutting, pivoting, and jumping.[18] Patients often report an audible "pop" accompanied by the acute onset of knee swelling. Multiple tests have been described to evaluate the ACL. The most sensitive tests for diagnosis of an ACL injury include the anterior drawer, Lachman,[19] and pivot-shift tests.[20,21] All three tests are performed with the patient in the supine position. The anterior drawer test is performed with the knee flexed to 90 degrees. The examiner places his or her hands on the posterior surface of the proximal tibia and subluxates the tibia anteriorly (Fig. 51.7). Any gross movement of the tibia that is different from the contralateral side is considered abnormal. The Lachman test is performed with the knee in 30 degrees of flexion (to remove the contribution of secondary restraints). The examiner applies an anterior force on the tibia while stabilizing the femur with his or her contralateral hand. Any increase in anterior tibial translation relative to the contralateral side is considered abnormal (Fig. 51.8). The pivot-shift test is performed with the knee in extension. The examiner holds the tibia in slight internal rotation and applies a valgus stress while the knee is slowly flexed. This combination of forces should cause the tibia to subluxate anteriorly if the ACL is injured. The test is positive if the tibia reduces with a "clunk" or a "glide" at 20 to 40 degrees of flexion (Fig. 51.9).

The posterior cruciate ligament (PCL) is the strongest ligament in the knee,[22,23] and thus injuries to the PCL are usually a result of significant knee trauma. The "dashboard" injury is a common mechanism for PCL injury and occurs during a motor vehicle accident when the flexed knee strikes the dashboard (Fig. 51.10). The PCL can be evaluated with the posterior drawer, posterior sag, and quadriceps active tests. All tests are performed with the patient in the supine position. The posterior drawer test is performed with the knee in 90 degrees of flexion. The examiner applies a posteriorly directed force to the tibia. Placement of one's thumb tips at the anterior joint line permits quantification of any abnormal translation (Fig. 51.11). The posterior sag test is positive when the tibia subluxates posteriorly with the knee at 90 degrees of flexion. Loss of the medial tibial step-off at the joint line should alert the examiner to a PCL injury (Fig. 51.12).[22] This test is usually positive in the chronic setting or after inducement of anesthesia in the acute setting. The quadriceps active test is performed with the knee in 60 degrees of flexion. The patient is asked to extend the knee while keeping his or her foot on the examination table. Reduction of the tibia will be seen in a positive test.[24]

Injuries to the PCL are often accompanied by injuries to the posterolateral corner, a complex structure that functions as both a static and a dynamic stabilizer of the knee.[23] It is composed of the lateral collateral ligament, the popliteofibular ligament, the popliteomeniscal attachment, the arcuate ligament, and the popliteus tendon and muscle.[25] Injuries to the posterolateral corner and/or the PCL can be examined with the dial test (Fig. 51.13). The posterolateral corner structures restrain external rotation at 30 degrees of flexion, whereas the PCL restrains external rotation at 90 degrees of flexion. An increase of external rotation at 90 degrees of flexion without an increase in external rotation at 30 degrees of flexion suggests an isolated PCL injury. An increase of external rotation at 30 degrees of flexion without an increase at 90 degrees of flexion suggests an isolated injury to the posterolateral corner. Increased external rotation at both 30 and 90 degrees of flexion suggests combined PCL and posterolateral corner injuries.

Menisci

Traumatic and degenerative meniscal injuries are among the most common knee injuries. The menisci are considered the shock-absorbing cartilages of the knee and also provide rotational and translational restraint. The medial meniscus tends to be more

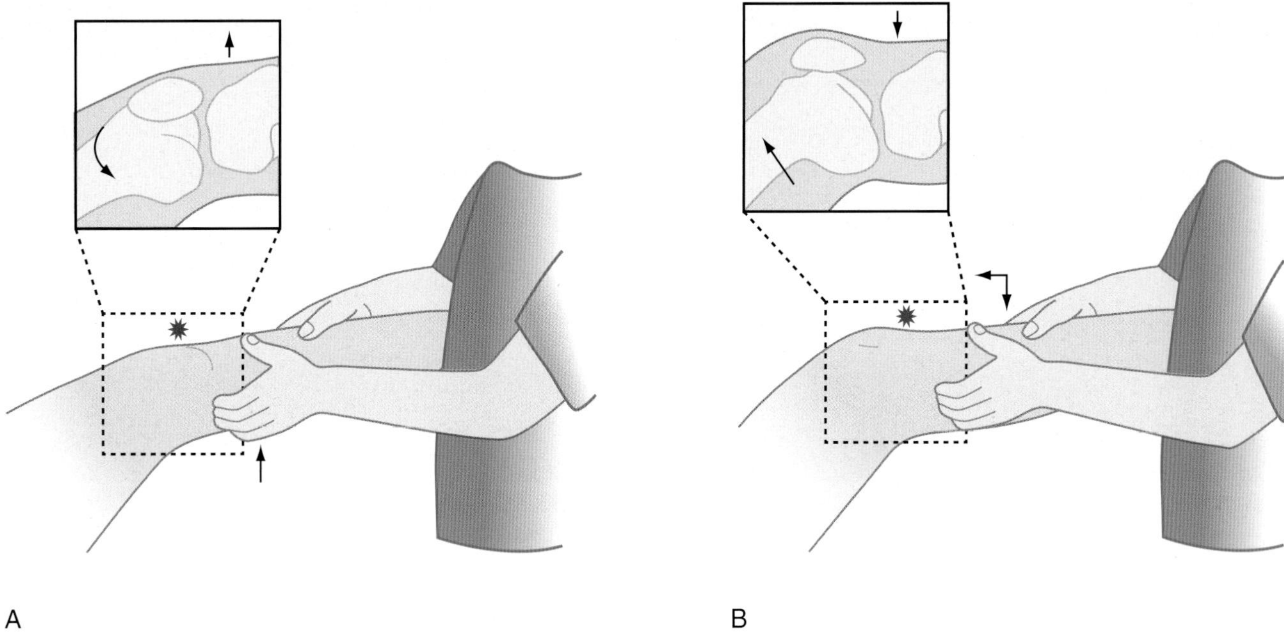

• **Fig. 51.9** The pivot shift test is positive if the tibia reduces with a "clunk" or a "glide" at 20 to 40 degrees of flexion.

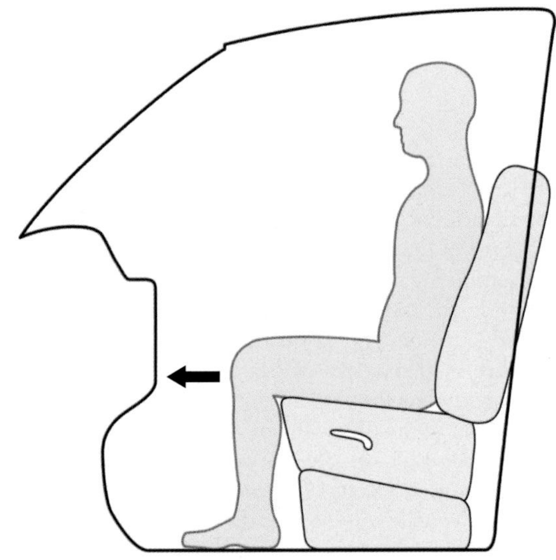

• **Fig. 51.10** An injury to the posterior cruciate ligament can occur when the tibia strikes the dashboard, causing the tibia to subluxate posteriorly on the femur.

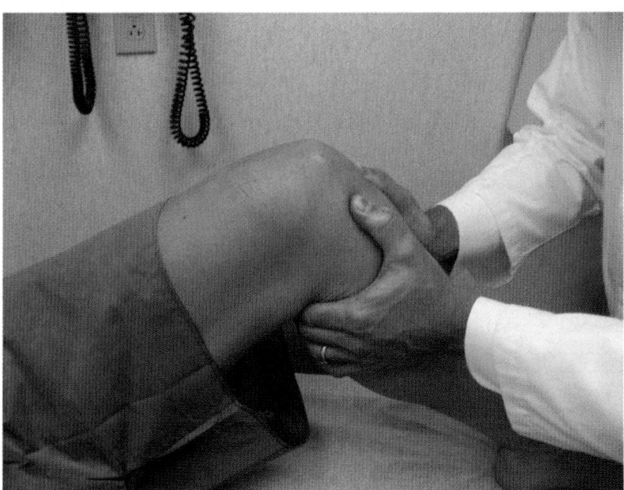

• **Fig. 51.11** The posterior drawer test is performed by subluxating the tibia posteriorly with the knee in 90 degrees of flexion. The amount of posterior translation (mm) is noted. The endpoint is characterized as "soft" or "hard."

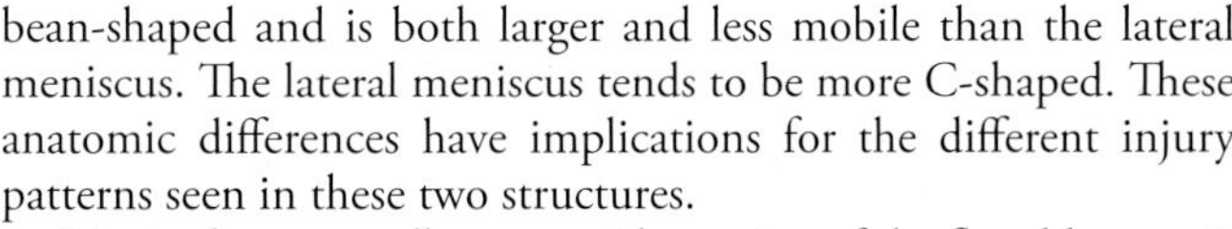

bean-shaped and is both larger and less mobile than the lateral meniscus. The lateral meniscus tends to be more C-shaped. These anatomic differences have implications for the different injury patterns seen in these two structures.

Meniscal tears usually occur with rotation of the flexed knee as it moves into extension. Tears of the medial meniscus are more common than tears of the lateral meniscus, likely because of the relative lack of mobility of the medial meniscus.[26] Patients frequently report "locking" and "clicking" or a sense of something not being right with the knee, which usually results from displacement of the torn meniscus during motion. Common physical findings include pain with hyperflexion and with hyperextension, joint line tenderness, and an effusion. Many provocative tests have been described to diagnose meniscal tears. The McMurray[27] and Apley compression[28] tests are frequently performed, although they lack sensitivity and specificity. The flexion McMurray test is performed with the patient supine and the hip and knee flexed to 90 degrees. A compressive and rotational force is applied to the knee as it is moved from a flexed to an extended position. The test is positive if the patient reports pain (Fig. 51.14). The Apley compression test is performed with the patient prone and the knee flexed to 90 degrees. When the test is positive, the patient will report pain with rotation of the tibia. An arthroscopic photograph in Fig. 51.15 shows a tear in the posterior horn of the medial meniscus.

Quadriceps Tendon

Injuries to the quadriceps tendon are most common in the sixth and seventh decades of life. Patients with systemic lupus erythematosus, renal failure, endocrinopathies, diabetes, and various other systemic inflammatory and metabolic diseases tend to be at a higher risk for these injuries. The occurrence of quadriceps tendon rupture after total knee arthroplasty is a rare complication (with an incidence of 0.1%), but when it occurs it is devastating.[29] Patients usually present with intense anterior knee pain after experiencing an eccentric quadriceps contraction during a fall or twisting injury. Physical examination reveals a palpable defect in the tendon, an effusion resulting from hemarthrosis, and hypermobility of the patella. Patients usually will not be able to fully extend their knee (Fig. 51.16).

Patella Tendon

Problems with the infrapatellar tendon include tendonitis and rupture. Tendonitis is usually an overuse injury and is often associated with jumping, changes in activity level, and eccentric contractions during falls. Patients exhibit tenderness at their tibial tubercle or at the inferior pole of their patella. Rupture of the patella tendon usually occurs in patients younger than 40 years and is associated with chronic patella tendonitis. Patients usually present with anterior knee pain and the inability to extend their knee.

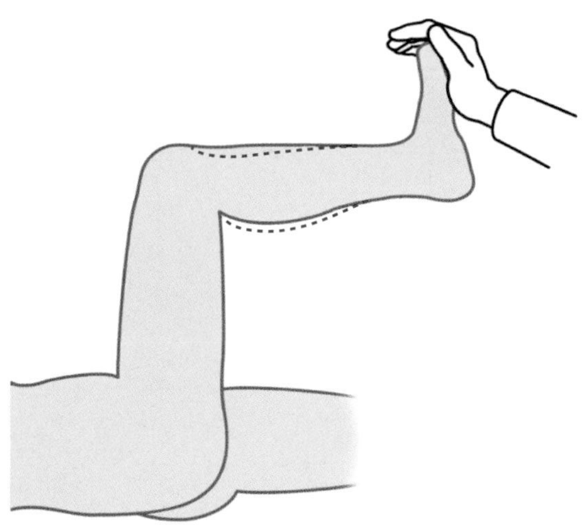

• **Fig. 51.12** The posterior sag test is positive when the tibia subluxates posteriorly with the knee at 90 degrees of flexion.

Patellofemoral Pain

People who report having anterior knee pain are commonly seen by orthopedic surgeons. Anterior knee pain is more common in women and accounts for up to 25% of all sports-related knee injuries.[30] A variety of factors contribute to the biomechanics of the patellofemoral joint, including overuse, the depth of the trochlea, the shape of the patella, quadriceps strength, the line of pull of the quadriceps relative to the patella tendon (the Q angle), the length of the patella tendon, the shape of the femoral condyles, and the articular cartilage. Abnormalities of any of these factors may contribute to this pain syndrome, and successful treatment is possible only with correct identification of any contributing factors.

Physical examination of the patellofemoral joint begins with an analysis of coronal alignment of the knee because any valgus deformity may contribute to lateral subluxation. The height of the patella relative to the tibial tubercle should be noted (patella alta or baja). The J sign is present when the patella slides laterally at terminal extension, indicating excessive pull of the vastus lateralis. The vastus medialis obliquus is the primary stabilizer against lateral pull by the vastus lateralis. With the knee extended and the quadriceps relaxed, the examiner should make note of any patellar tilt. Any crepitus, either audible or palpable, should be noted as well. Crepitus is common in patients with osteoarthritis. A Q angle greater than 15 degrees in women and greater than 8 to 10 degrees in men is considered abnormal.[30] Patellar mobility should be assessed using a quadrant system for passive mediolateral displacement of the patella relative to the trochlear groove. The normal patella should not be displaced medially or laterally beyond the second quadrant. Any abnormality in mobility may stem from changes in the tightness of the retinaculum. The apprehension test is performed by attempting to subluxate the patella with the knee in extension. The test is positive when it elicits pain and an unwillingness to allow the examiner to move the patella laterally (Fig. 51.17).

At the conclusion of the history and physical examination, the astute clinician should have formulated a short list of possible

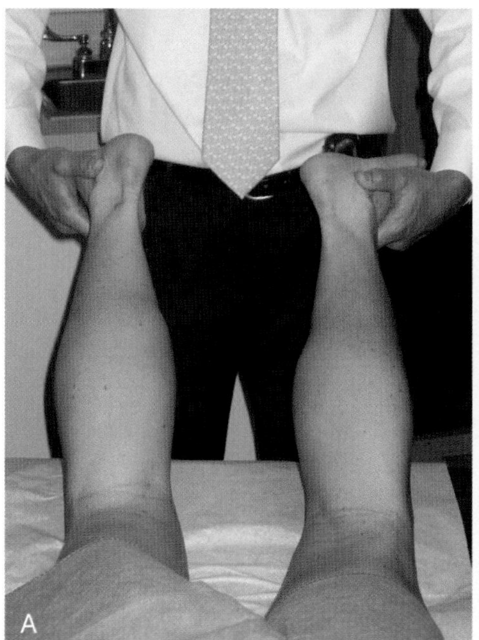

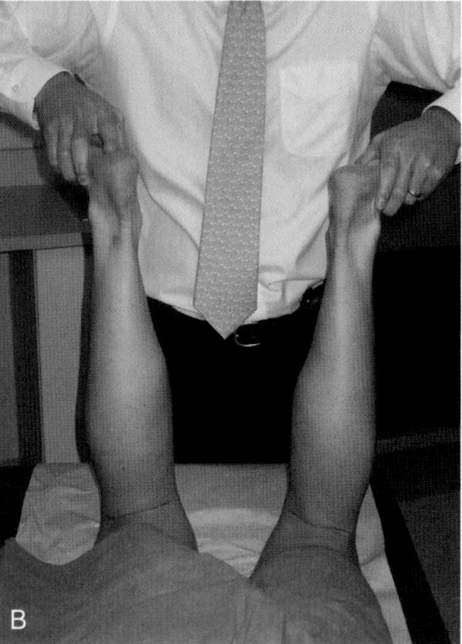

• **Fig. 51.13** The degree of tibial external rotation is measured in the dial test.

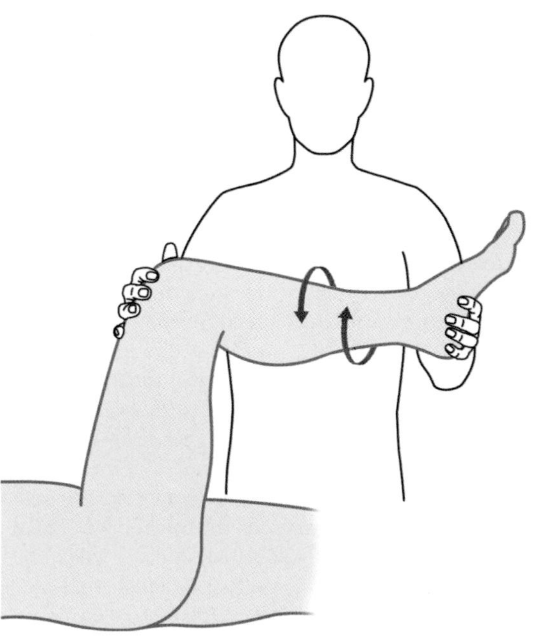

• **Fig. 51.14** A positive flexion McMurray test may indicate a torn meniscus.

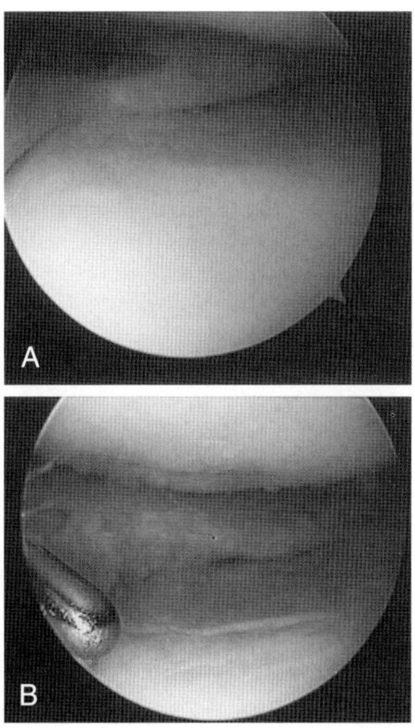

• **Fig. 51.15** An arthroscopic photograph of a tear in the posterior horn of the medial meniscus before (A) and after (B) debridement.

diagnoses. With this list in mind, the appropriate imaging studies can now be obtained. The goal of the initial imaging studies should be to confirm the diagnosis with the most appropriate and least-expensive study. Advanced imaging studies should not replace a thorough history and physical examination.

Imaging

Conventional Radiographs

Conventional radiographs are usually the first study obtained after knee injury and should be read in a systematic fashion. Soft tissues should be evaluated before examining the bony structures.

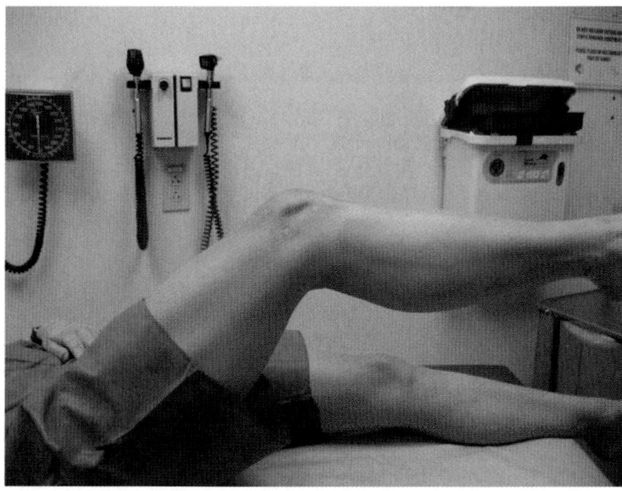

• **Fig. 51.16** An extensor lag due to a complete tear in the quadriceps tendon.

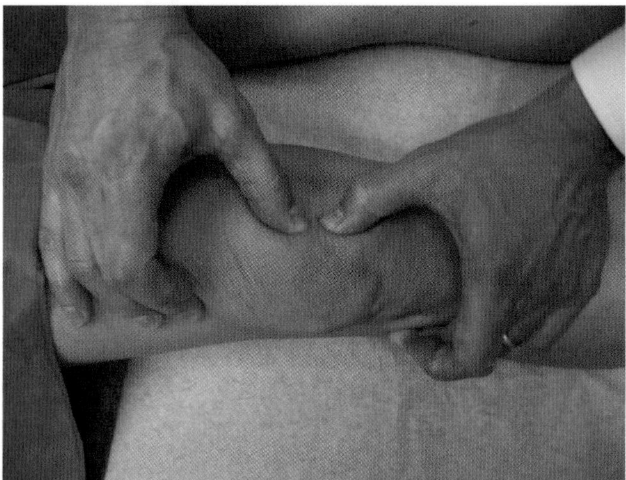

• **Fig. 51.17** The apprehension test is positive when subluxation of the patella causes pain.

Findings should be described in terms of radiolucent and radiopaque lines. Only after the findings have been described should the interpretation phase begin. Bypassing the description and proceeding directly to interpretation is a natural tendency, but if this tendency is followed, it is likely that certain findings will be missed or dismissed prematurely.

The basic radiographic evaluation of the knee consists of standing anteroposterior (AP) weight-bearing, lateral, and Merchant's views. The AP view permits evaluation of coronal alignment and the height of the tibiofemoral joint spaces. The normal coronal alignment of the knee should be 5 to 7 degrees of anatomic (tibiofemoral) valgus. The lateral tibiofemoral joint space should be wider than the medial tibiofemoral joint space in a normal knee. The presence of marginal osteophytes, joint space narrowing, subchondral sclerosis, and cystic change can be seen in the presence of osteoarthritis (Fig. 51.18). Periarticular osteopenia, concentric joint space narrowing, and a paucity of osteophytes are commonly seen in people with inflammatory arthritis (Fig. 51.19). The lateral radiograph allows for evaluation of an effusion, patella tendon length, and the quadriceps tendon. The Merchant's view, which is taken tangential to the patellofemoral joint,[31] permits detection of patellofemoral arthritis and malalignment.

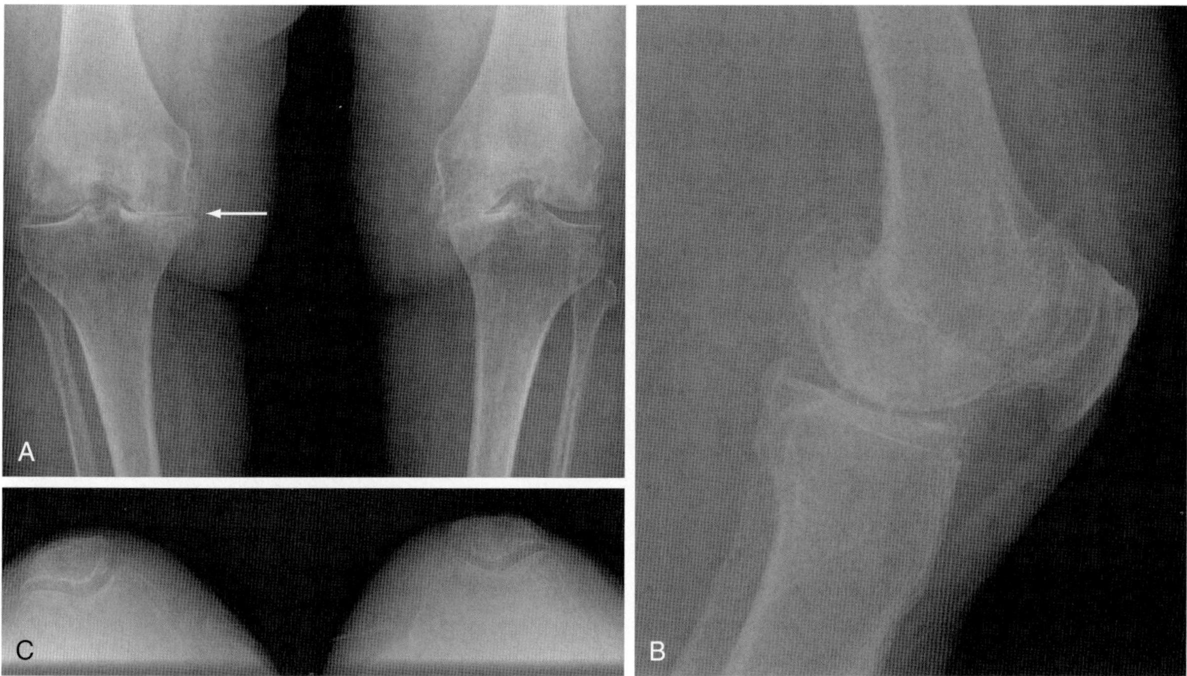

• **Fig. 51.18** Standing anteroposterior (A), lateral (B), and Merchant's (C) views of an osteoarthritic knee.

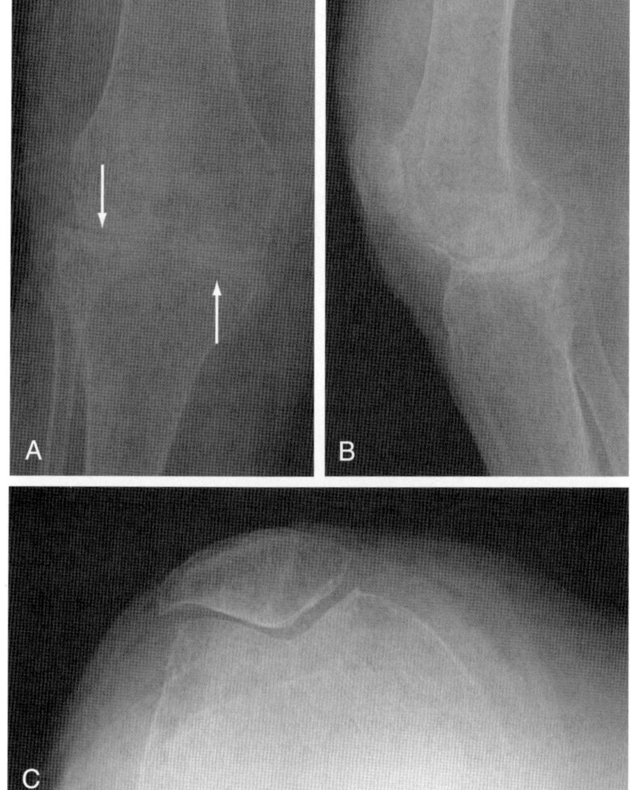

• **Fig. 51.19** Standing anteroposterior (A), lateral (B), and Merchant's (C) views of the knee in a patient with rheumatoid arthritis.

Additional views include a posteroanterior (PA) standing view with the knees flexed approximately 45 degrees, the tunnel or intercondylar notch view, and the 36-inch AP standing view of bilateral lower extremities. The flexed PA standing view is taken with the radiographic beam directed 10 degrees caudad from anterior to posterior, which permits evaluation of the posterior femoral condyles for joint space narrowing.[32] The tunnel view is obtained with the knee flexed and the radiographic beam directed inferiorly at an angle perpendicular to the tibial plateau. It is useful in detecting posterior tibiofemoral joint space narrowing, tibial spine fractures, loose bodies, and osteochondral lesions on the medial aspect of the femoral condyles. The 36-inch standing view is used for determining the mechanical axis of the lower extremity, as well as for evaluating any deformity that may be present. The normal mechanical axis is a straight line joining the center of the hip, knee, and ankle joints. Surgeons use it for pre-operative planning and post-operative evaluation in total knee arthroplasty, as well as for the planning of distal femoral and proximal tibia osteotomies in arthritis surgery.

Computed Tomography

CT has largely been replaced by MRI in evaluation of routine knee problems. CT is now used primarily for detection of bony tumors and in the trauma setting for detection of subtle fractures that are not easily visualized with conventional radiographs, as well as for a more thorough evaluation of intra-articular fractures. In cases of distal femoral or proximal tibia fractures, CT is used to help the surgeon plan operative treatment. CT is also used to assess axial alignment of the femoral and tibial components in cases of painful total knee arthroplasty.[33,34]

Ultrasound

The use of ultrasound has become more common in the diagnosis and treatment of knee disorders. Some clinicians use ultrasound routinely in both hospital and office settings to assist in arthrocentesis of the knee. Ultrasound is an attractive imaging modality because of its low cost, real-time capabilities and portability. The ability to perform provocative maneuvers during sonography is particularly appealing. Ultrasound can easily and reliably detect joint effusions and popliteal cysts (Fig. 51.20), as well as quadriceps and patella tendon disruptions. Ultrasound reportedly can detect a 1 mm increase in joint fluid.[35]

Nuclear Scintigraphy

Nuclear scintigraphy is very sensitive but not specific and is used to detect areas of increased osseous remodeling. It requires clinical correlation and should be used in conjunction with other imaging modalities. Technetium phosphate compounds are injected intravenously. Approximately 50% of the tracer is excreted by the kidneys, and the remainder is taken up in areas of increased osseous turnover. Imaging of the skeleton is typically performed 2 to 3 hours after injection because this delay allows for maximum contrast between the soft tissues and the skeletal structures while still providing for an adequate photon count.[36]

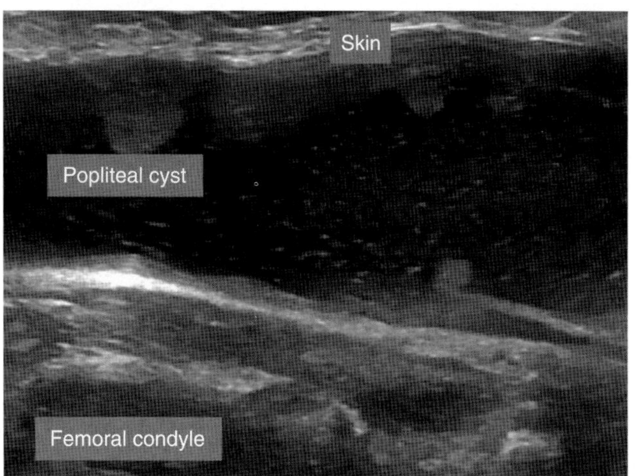

• **Fig. 51.20** This ultrasound image shows a large popliteal cyst in a patient with symptomatic knee osteoarthritis that was treated with aspiration and injection of corticosteroid.

Three-phase bone scanning can yield additional information. The three phases include an angiographic pool, followed by a blood pool and bone imaging. The angiographic phases allow for the detection of regional hyperemia. This technique has been reported to have greater specificity and can be used in cases of suspected osteomyelitis, osteonecrosis, stress fracture, and implant loosening.[36] Increased radionuclide uptake can be seen for up to 12 to 18 months after total knee arthroplasty. Asymmetric uptake in one area around the prosthesis should raise the question of loosening or periprosthetic fracture (Fig. 51.21).[37,38] The addition of labeled leukocytes to the technetium-99m sulfur colloid yields an 80% sensitivity and 100% specificity for diagnosing infection.[39]

Magnetic Resonance Imaging

MRI has supplanted many imaging modalities because of its direct multiplanar capabilities and superior soft tissue contrast. Nevertheless, MRI should not be the initial imaging modality for evaluation of hip and knee pain, as it is costly and often unnecessary. Although conventional radiographs remain the gold standard for defining osseous structures, MRI provides excellent visualization of articular cartilage, the cruciate ligaments, the collateral ligaments, the patella tendon, the quadriceps tendon, and the menisci (Fig. 51.22). It is also highly sensitive for detecting bone marrow edema (contusion), stress fractures, and mass lesions. Use of the "two-slice touch" rule has improved the sensitivity and specificity of MRI in accurately diagnosing meniscal tears. This rule classifies a meniscus as torn if two or more MR images show abnormal findings and as possibly torn if only one MR image shows an abnormal finding. Using fast spin-echo imaging, the sensitivity and specificity for diagnosing medial and lateral meniscal tears was 95% and 85%, and 77% and 89%, respectively, translating to a positive predictive value of 91% to 94% for medial meniscus tears and 83% to 96% for lateral meniscus tears.[40]

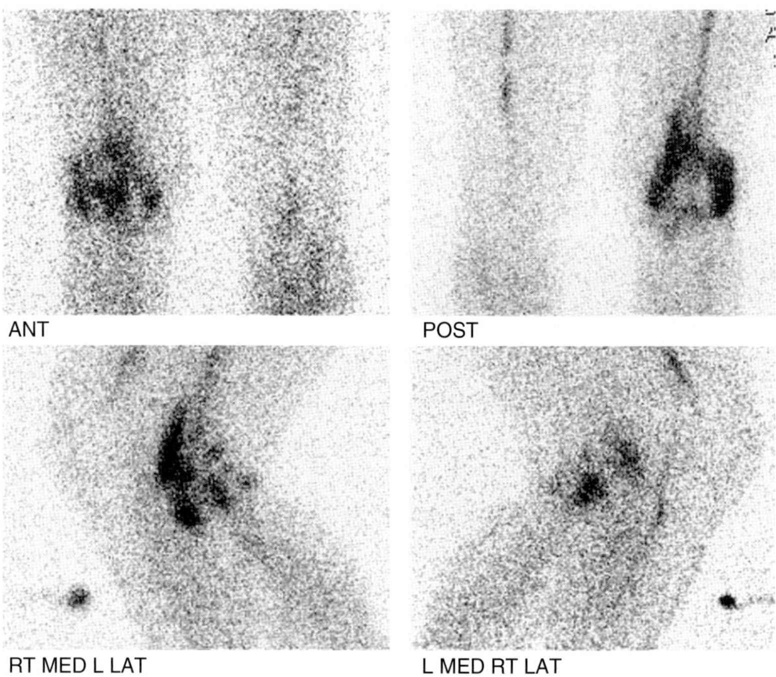

• **Fig. 51.21** A bone scan reveals an increased uptake of radiotracer around the distal femur in this patient with an infected total knee arthroplasty and septic loosening of his femoral component. *ANT,* Anterior; *L MED RT LAT,* left medial right lateral; *POST,* posterior; *RT MED L LAT,* right medial left lateral.

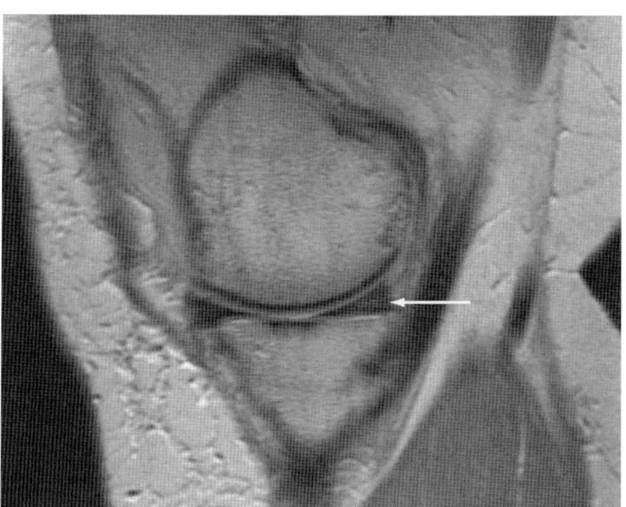

• **Fig. 51.22** This sagittal MRI shows linear signal change extending to the meniscal surface consistent with a tear *(arrow)* in the posterior horn of the medial meniscus.

Common Disorders in the Differential Diagnosis of Knee Pain

General

Although many diseases exist that may involve the knee, a limited number of them are encountered frequently. In evaluating knee pain, the clinician should be familiar with osteoarthritis; rheumatoid arthritis; inflammatory arthritis associated with the seronegative spondyloarthropathies; tears of the menisci, ligaments, and tendons; osteochondritis desiccans; osteochondral fractures; fractures; referred pain from the hip (such as with slipped capital femoral epiphysis in adolescents); vascular claudication; neurogenic claudication; complex regional pain syndrome; sarcoma; metastases; and infection. While infection is not a common source of native hip or knee pain, its prevalence as a cause of pain around hip and knee replacements is increasing.[41]

Bursitis

The prepatellar bursa lies between the retinaculum and the subcutaneous fat and runs from the patella to the tibial tubercle. The bursa may become inflamed and fill with fluid when exposed to a direct blow or repetitive microtrauma (e.g., kneeling). Patients with prepatellar bursitis present with anterior knee pain upon flexion and a fluctuant mass over the anterior knee. If the area becomes warm, tender to palpation, and erythematous, septic bursitis should be ruled out with aspiration. The pes anserinus bursa, located over the insertions of the sartorius, gracilis, and semitendinosus muscles on the proximal medial tibia, can also be a source of knee pain if it is inflamed.

Neoplasia

Tumors in the area of the knee are often diagnosed after trauma prompts medical evaluation. Pain at night, pain at rest, and constitutional symptoms should alert the clinician to consider the appropriate workup. Some of the benign tumors seen in the area of the knee include enchondroma, pigmented villonodular synovitis, osteochondromatosis, and giant cell tumor. Malignant tumors seen in the area of the knee include but are not limited to metastases, osteosarcoma, Ewing's sarcoma, chondrosarcoma, and malignant fibrous histiocytoma.

Popliteal Cysts

A popliteal cyst, originally called a Baker's cyst, is a synovial fluid-filled mass located in the popliteal fossa. The most common synovial popliteal cyst is considered to be a distension of the bursa located beneath the medial head of the gastrocnemius muscle. Usually, in an adult patient, an underlying intra-articular disorder (osteoarthritis) is present. In children, the cyst can be isolated and the knee joint can be normal. Patients usually present with episodic posterior knee pain.[42] The diagnosis is made by ultrasonography or MRI. Treatment options include benign neglect, aspiration, surgical excision, or removal of the underlying disease process (arthritis) with knee arthroplasty.

Hip Pain

History

Obtaining an accurate history is an important initial step in formulating a differential diagnosis for patients who present with hip pain. In general, more conditions should be considered in the differential diagnosis for hip pain than for knee pain, because the hip is a common site for referred pain from lumbosacral and intrapelvic disease. A detailed, comprehensive history will direct the clinician to a focused physical examination.

Most patients who present with hip disease report having pain. It is important to define the exact location of the pain because "hip" pain may refer to discomfort in the groin, lateral thigh, or buttock. Pain in the groin or medial thigh region is usually due to hip disease and is believed to arise from irritation of the capsule and/or synovial lining.[43] Pain generated in the lumbosacral spine may be referred to the buttocks and/or lateral thigh.[44] Lateral thigh pain may stem from so-called *trochanteric bursitis* (usually abductor tendonitis) as well. Activities or positions that aggravate and relieve the pain should be explored. The severity, frequency, and patterns of radiation of the pain also should be evaluated. It is not uncommon for knee pain to be generated from the hip joint. Metastatic and primary tumors that occur in the pelvic and proximal thigh regions should always be included in the differential diagnosis. Intrapelvic disease from the prostate, seminal vesicles, hernias, ovaries, gastrointestinal system, and vasculature should also be considered.[45,46]

Knowledge of the patient's general level of functioning is important, because this information will lend insight into the severity of the disease and may influence treatment. Patients with hip disease may have difficulty trimming their toenails, donning shoes and socks, and using stairs. Walking tolerance and use of assist devices also should be recorded. The Harris Hip Score and the Western Ontario and McMaster Universities (WOMAC) Osteoarthritis Index are two rating scales that are widely used to assess function in this patient population.[47,48]

The patient should be asked about any hip problems that he or she encountered in childhood. Diseases such as developmental dysplasia, slipped capital femoral epiphysis, Legg-Calvé-Perthes disease, polio, and trauma may lead to osteoarthrosis later in life.[49–51] The patient should be asked about any treatment rendered for these diseases as well.

Osteoarthritis and inflammatory arthritis are two common causes of hip pain. In general, pain from osteoarthritis is exacerbated by activity and relieved by rest. Mild arthritis of the hip may not become symptomatic until a certain activity level is reached. Stiffness (usually from synovitis) is also commonly reported with both degenerative and inflammatory arthritis. When the hip pain

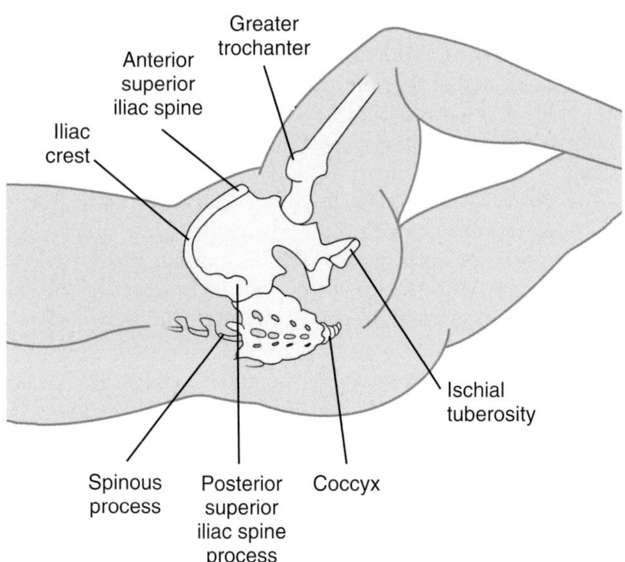

• **Fig. 51.23** The bony landmarks on the pelvis that can be palpated during physical examination.

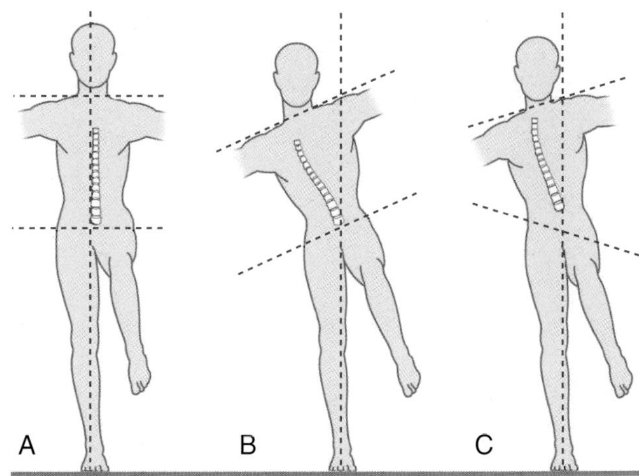

• **Fig. 51.24** Physical examination of abductor function: (A) Normal single-legged stance. (B) Positive Trendelenburg lurch and negative Trendelenburg's sign. (C) Positive Trendelenburg lurch with pelvic obliquity and leaning over the involved hip to shift the body's center of gravity.

continues despite a trial of rest, an underlying inflammatory or infectious process should be considered.

Any previous treatments for hip pain should be discussed. The patient's response to nonsteroidal anti-inflammatory medications, nutritional supplements (such as chondroitin and glucosamine), physical therapy, corticosteroid injections, local anesthetic injections, hyaluronic acid injections, ultrasound, and operative interventions should be recorded. Lastly, a more general medical history should be explored. The physician should be aware of alcoholism, neuromuscular disorders, smoking history, and general support systems.

Physical Examination

The physical examination of the patient with hip pain begins as the clinician observes the patient for the first time. Ease of rising from a chair, postures, and walking speed all provide insight into the extent of a patient's disability. A general evaluation of the patient's spine, lower extremity alignment, and leg lengths is performed next. With the examiner behind the patient, the spine is examined for coronal and sagittal balance. The patient is asked to touch his or her toes. A rib hump indicates the presence of scoliosis. Any gross deformity of the spine will alert the examiner to the potential of a pelvic obliquity and resultant leg length discrepancy.

The overall coronal alignment of the lower extremities is evaluated next. If a leg length discrepancy is detected, blocks can be used, as discussed previously, to determine the amount of apparent inequality. If the leg length discrepancy is due to a fixed pelvic obliquity from lumbosacral disease, blocks may not be able to level the pelvis. Previous surgical scars in the area of the hip should be noted. Palpation of the bony landmarks (iliac crest, anterior superior iliac spine, posterior superior iliac spine, ischial tuberosity, coccyx, spinous processes, and greater trochanter) should be performed (Fig. 51.23). The femoral neck is located approximately three fingerbreadths below the anterior superior iliac spine.

A basic evaluation of gait should be performed. Although gait analysis is a complex science, all clinicians should feel comfortable evaluating patients for common abnormalities. The patient with hip pain may present with an antalgic gait. The severity of the limp should be classified as mild, moderate, or severe. Mild limps can only be detected by trained observers. Moderate limps will be noticed by the patient. A severe limp will be readily apparent and have a significant impact on the speed of ambulation. Common causes of a limp include pain and abductor (gluteus medius and gluteus minimus) weakness; differentiating between these two causes of limp is an important part of the physical examination.

The patient with abductor dysfunction will likely have an abductor or Trendelenburg lurch.[52] With a Trendelenburg lurch, the patient compensates for abductor dysfunction by leaning over the involved hip to shift the body's center of gravity in that direction (Fig. 51.24). If a patient has a Trendelenburg lurch, the clinician should proceed to evaluate for Trendelenburg's sign. A positive Trendelenburg's sign occurs when the pelvis tilts toward the unsupported side during a one-legged stance. This test is best performed with the examiner behind the patient. Causes of abductor weakness are numerous and may include a contracted or shortened gluteus medius, coxa vara, fracture, dysplasia, neurologic conditions (e.g., superior gluteal nerve injury, radiculopathy, poliomyelitis, myelomeningocele, and spinal cord lesions), and slipped capital femoral epiphysis.

The patient is then asked to lay supine on the examination table. The range of motion of both hips should be evaluated by recording flexion, extension, adduction, abduction, internal rotation in extension, and external rotation in extension. Hip extension is best evaluated with the patient in the prone position. Normal range of motion values include 100 to 135 degrees for flexion (the knee should be flexed to relax the hamstrings), 15 to 30 degrees for extension, 0 to 30 degrees for adduction, 0 to 40 degrees for abduction, 0 to 40 degrees for internal rotation, and 0 to 60 degrees for external rotation. Motion is often limited in cases of deformity (such as limited internal rotation in slipped capital femoral epiphysis) and advanced osteoarthritis. Internal rotation and abduction are usually the first motions to be limited in osteoarthritis. Motion will be painful in patients with synovitis as well. Areas that are painful should be palpated.

A series of special tests can be performed to evaluate for subtle muscle contractures and limitation of motion. The presence of a hip flexion contracture is common in patients with moderate to severe hip disease and can be quantified with the Thomas test (Fig. 51.25).[53] This test is performed by having the patient bring his or her thighs to the chest while in the supine position. This maneuver allows for flattening of the spine, and the hip to be evaluated is allowed to extend to neutral. If the patient is unable to reach neutral, the amount of flexion contracture is recorded. The Ober test measures tightness of the iliotibial band. The patient lies on the unaffected side and the examiner helps the patient abduct the hip with the hip extended and the knee flexed to 90 degrees. The leg is slowly released from abduction to neutral, and the hip will remain abducted if contracture of the iliotibial band occurs. Ely's test can detect a tight rectus femoris. The knee is passively flexed with the patient in the prone position. If the rectus femoris is tight, the ipsilateral hip will spontaneously flex. If the rectus femoris is normal, the hip will remain flush with the examination table.

Patients occasionally report a "snapping" sensation in their hip. Although it may be difficult for the clinician to reproduce the snapping, patients may be able to demonstrate it by flexing and internally rotating their hip. Extra-articular causes of hip snapping include a thickened iliotibial band snapping over the greater trochanter, the iliopsoas tendon gliding over the iliopectineal eminence, the long head of the biceps tendon rubbing on the ischial tuberosity, and the iliofemoral ligament rubbing on the femoral head. Intra-articular causes of snapping hip syndrome include loose bodies and large labral tears.

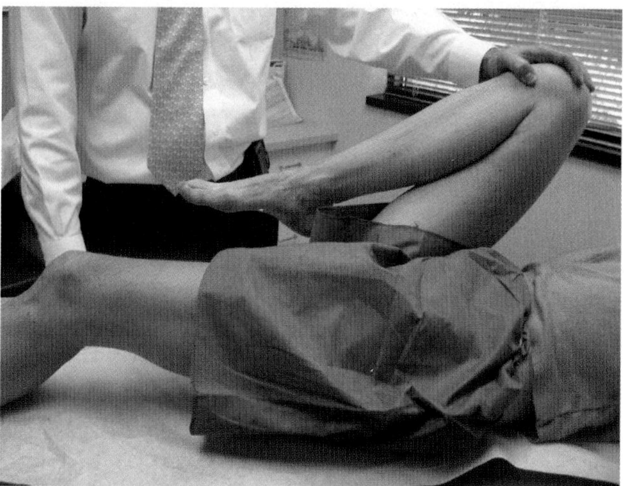

• **Fig. 51.25** In the Thomas test, a hip flexion contracture is measured by flexing the contralateral hip to eliminate compensatory lumbar lordosis. The ipsilateral hip is then allowed to extend with gravity. The angle between the examination table and the thigh is the degree of flexion contracture.

In addition to using blocks with the patient standing, leg lengths can be measured while the patient is in the supine position (Fig. 51.26). The *apparent* leg length is the distance from the umbilicus to the medial malleolus. The *true* leg length is measured from the anterior superior iliac spine to the medial malleolus. Pelvic obliquity and abduction/adduction of the hip will create an apparent leg-length discrepancy.

Sacroiliac disease should be included in the differential diagnosis of hip pain. Although multiple provocative tests have been described to elicit sacroiliac disease, the FABER (flexion, abduction, and external rotation) test (also known as Patrick's test) can help distinguish between hip and sacroiliac joint disease. With the patient supine, the clinician has the patient place his/her hip in the FABER position. The clinician then presses the flexed knee and the contralateral anterior superior iliac spine toward the floor. Pain in the buttocks suggests sacroiliac joint disease, whereas pain in the groin points to hip disease. If the sacroiliac joint is implicated, it is recommended that multiple other provocative tests be performed. Sacroiliac joint disease is the likely pain generator when three or more of the following tests are positive: the distraction, thigh thrust, compression, sacral thrust, Gaenslen's, and FABER tests.[54,55]

The acetabular labrum is drawing attention as a previously underappreciated cause of hip pain. Clinical presentation of a labral tear of the acetabulum may be variable, and the diagnosis is often delayed. Patients usually see multiple providers before the diagnosis is confirmed. In a series of 66 patients with arthroscopically confirmed tears of the acetabular labrum, 92% reported groin pain, 91% had activity-related pain, 71% reported pain at night, 86% described the pain as moderate to severe, and 95% had a positive impingement sign. The authors recommended that

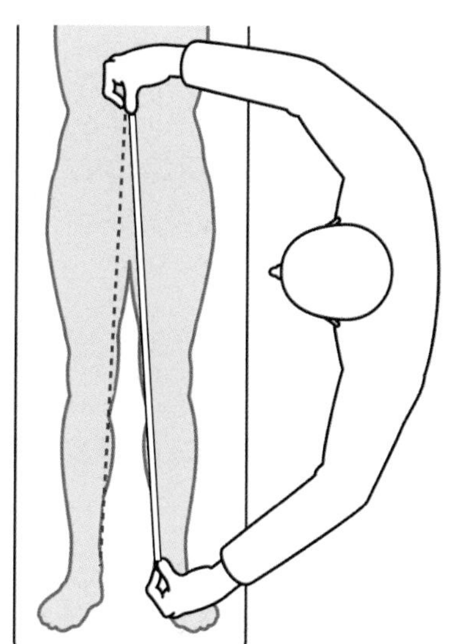

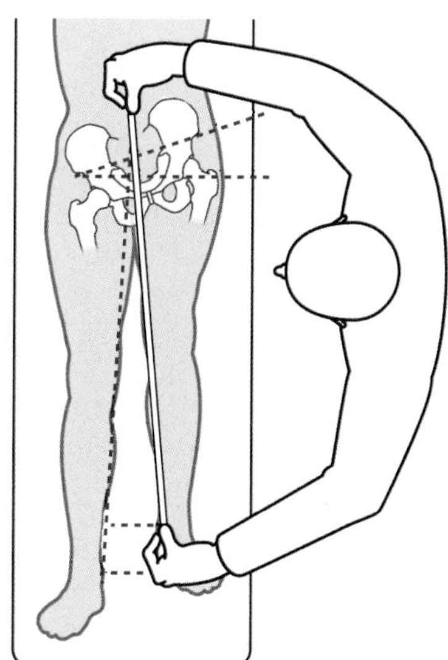

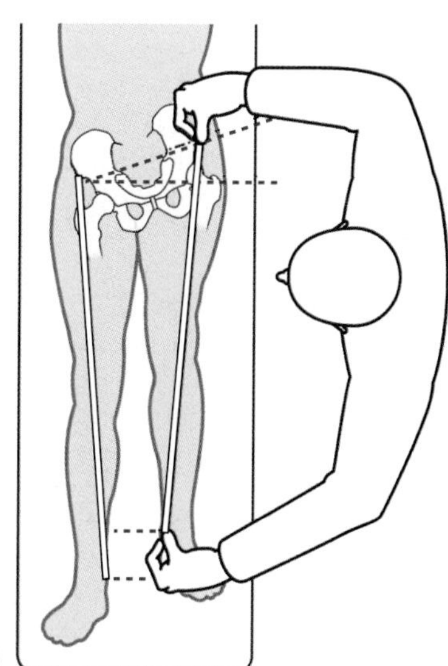

• **Fig. 51.26** Measurement of leg lengths. (A) The apparent leg length is the distance from the umbilicus to the medial malleolus. (B) Pelvic obliquity causing an apparent leg-length discrepancy. (C) The true leg length is the distance from the anterior superior iliac spine to the medial malleolus.

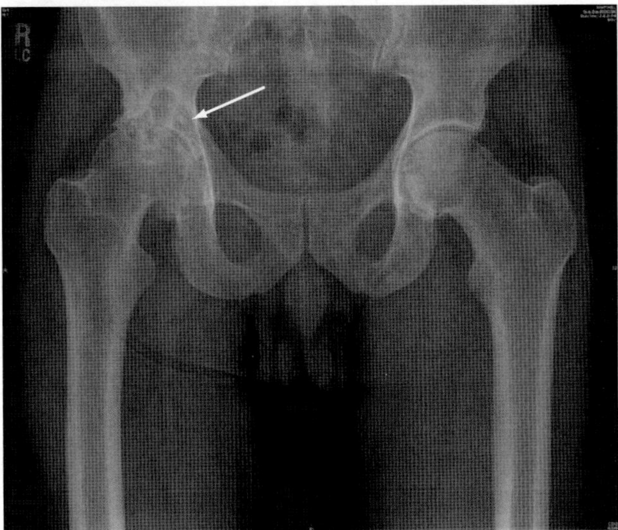

• **Fig. 51.27** An anteroposterior pelvis demonstrates the characteristic joint space narrowing, cystic changes, and osteophytes seen in osteoarthritis.

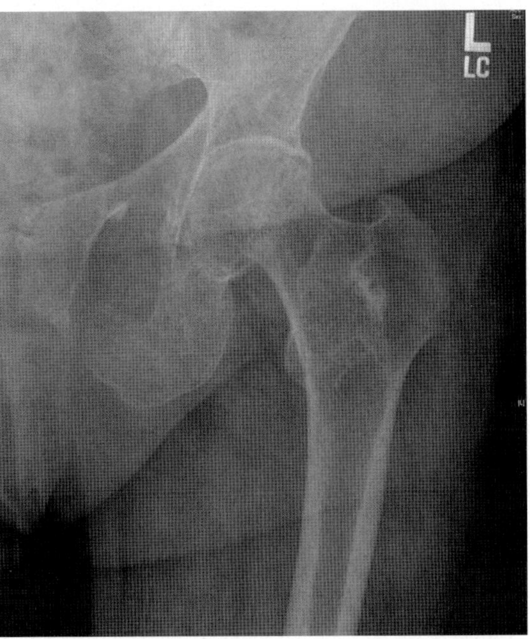

• **Fig. 51.28** An anteroposterior hip demonstrating the characteristic concentric joint space narrowing, paucity of osteophytes, and periarticular osteopenia seen in rheumatoid arthritis.

a diagnosis of acetabular labral tear be suspected in young, active patients reporting groin pain with or without trauma.[56] The positive impingement test helps confirm the diagnosis of a labral tear. The test is positive if the patient experiences groin pain with the hip flexed, adducted, and internally rotated. The positive predictive value of this test ranges from 0.91 to 1.00 in six different studies.[57–62]

A thorough evaluation of the neurovascular system should be completed after the musculoskeletal portion of the physical examination for the hip or knee is completed. This evaluation should include palpation or Doppler evaluation of the femoral, popliteal, dorsalis pedis, and posterior tibial arteries, as indicated. Strength testing with resisted isometric movements for each muscle in the lower extremity should also be performed, with 5 being normal strength, 4 being full motion against gravity and against some resistance, 3 being fair motion against gravity, 2 being movement only with gravity eliminated, 1 being evidence of muscle contraction but no joint motion, and 0 being no evidence of contractility. Sensation in the lower extremity should be evaluated by assessing for light touch and/or appreciation of pinprick in a dermatomal distribution. Patellar and ankle reflexes should be tested. Lastly, the examiner should test for any abnormal clonus and Babinski reflexes as indicated.

Imaging

Conventional Radiographs

Plain radiographs remain the primary diagnostic imaging tool for the evaluation of hip disease. All other imaging modalities should be viewed as complementary to conventional radiographs. A standard screening series includes a low AP pelvis (Fig. 51.27), an AP hip (Fig. 51.28), a frog-lateral view, and a cross-table lateral view. The frog-lateral view provides a lateral of the proximal femur and is useful for detecting femoral head collapse (as seen in osteonecrosis; Fig. 51.29). Numerous other special radiographs of the hip may be obtained, some of which include Judet 45-degree oblique views and the false profile view. Judet views allow for easier visualization of the anterior (obturator oblique) and posterior (iliac oblique) columns. The false profile view allows for evaluation of the anterior bony coverage of the femoral head in cases of acetabular dysplasia. Developmental dysplasia of the hip is common, and special views are generally not routinely recommended prior to referral to an orthopedic surgeon (Fig. 51.30).

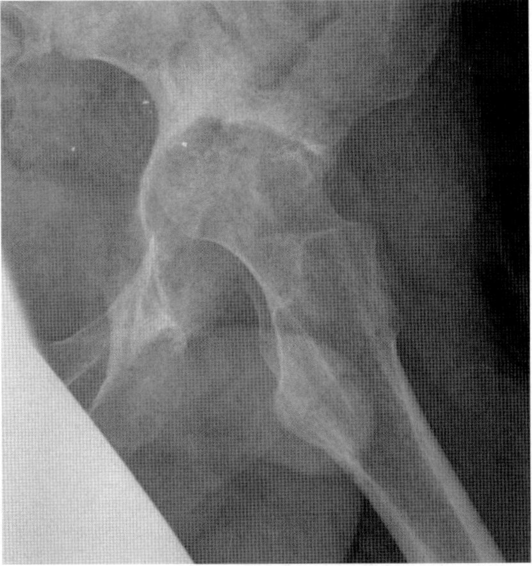

• **Fig. 51.29** A frog-lateral radiograph demonstrating femoral head collapse from osteonecrosis.

Computed Tomography

CT is used for assessment of acetabular fractures, acetabular nonunion, femoral head fractures, subtle femoral neck fractures, neoplasia, and bone stock in the revision total hip arthroplasty setting. Because of its limited soft-tissue contrast, CT has largely been replaced by MRI for detailed evaluation of the soft tissues around the hip.

Nuclear Scintigraphy

The role of bone scanning in the evaluation of hip disease is similar to its role in the assessment of knee pain. It should always be used in conjunction with other imaging modalities because of its limited specificity (Fig. 51.31).

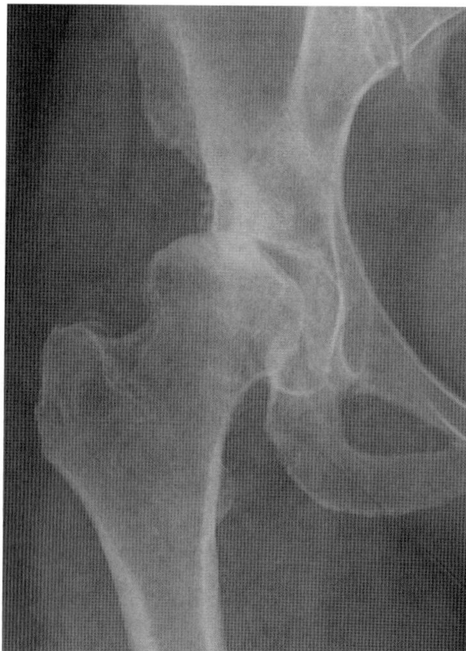

• **Fig. 51.30** An anteroposterior hip radiograph demonstrates osteoarthrosis from developmental dysplasia. The up-sloping lateral edge of the acetabulum is characteristic for developmental dysplasia of the hip.

Magnetic Resonance Imaging

MRI provides unprecedented detail of the soft tissues around the hip joint. MRI is now commonly used for diagnosis of osteonecrosis, labral disease, neoplasia, effusion, synovitis, loose bodies, tendonitis, transient osteoporosis of the hip, occult femoral neck fractures, bone edema, gluteus medius tendon avulsions, and nerve injury. MR arthrography of the hip joint is useful for identifying gluteus medius tendon avulsion after total hip arthroplasty (Fig. 51.32) and for detecting labral tears. One study showed a 92% sensitivity for the detection of labral tears using MR arthrography.[63] Delayed gadolinium-enhanced MRI of cartilage, a technique designed to measure early arthritis in the hip joint, is now being used clinically in the management of hip dysplasia.[64] Despite the tremendous diagnostic capabilities of MRI, its ability to detect bony disease is limited. As such, conventional radiographs remain the imaging modality of choice for the screening of hip disease.

Ultrasound

The use of ultrasound for the diagnosis and treatment of hip disorders is common. Some clinicians use ultrasound routinely in the office setting. Common hip conditions that are often managed with ultrasound-guided injections and/or aspirations include osteoarthritis, septic arthritis (Fig. 51.33), iliopsoas tendonitis, adverse local tissue reaction associated with metal-on-metal articulating total hip arthroplasties, and trochanteric bursitis.

Hip Arthrography

Hip arthrography is useful for detecting avulsions of the gluteus medius tendon from the greater trochanter and for differentiating intra-articular hip disease from lumbosacral disease. In one study, intra-articular anesthetic injection was 90% accurate in predicting intra-articular disease as confirmed by hip arthroscopy.[65] Anesthetic arthrogram of the hip has shown a 95% positive predictive value and a 67% negative predictive value for pain relief after total hip arthroplasty in patients with concurrent hip and lumbar osteoarthritis.[66]

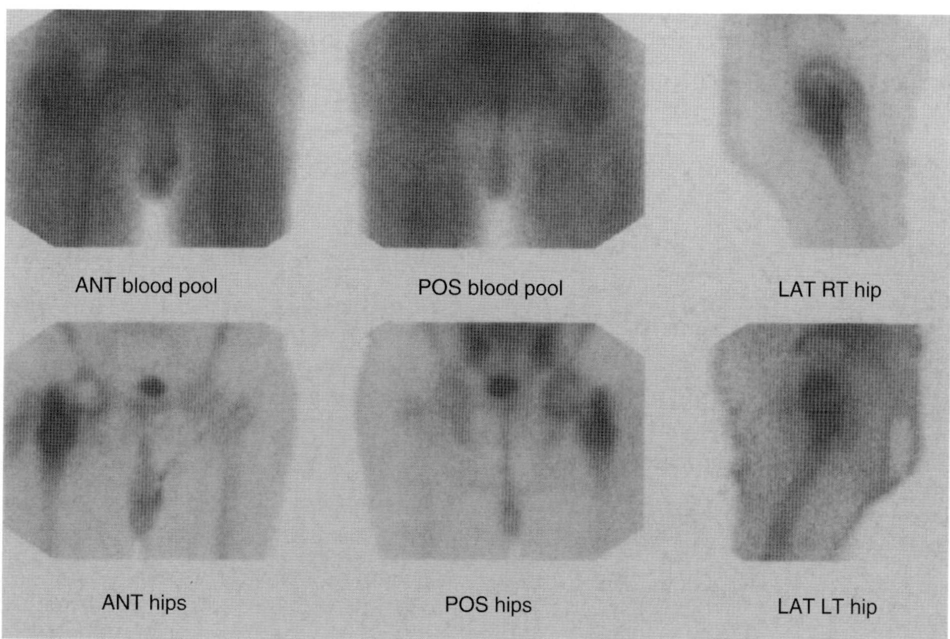

• **Fig. 51.31** This bone scan shows an increased radiotracer uptake at the proximal femur. The patient presented with activity-related thigh pain 1 year after undergoing primary cementless total hip arthroplasty. History, physical examination, and conventional radiographs suggested failure of osseointegration. At the time of surgery, the femoral component was found to be grossly loose. *ANT,* Anterior; *LAT,* lateral; *LT,* left; *POS,* posterior; *RT,* right.

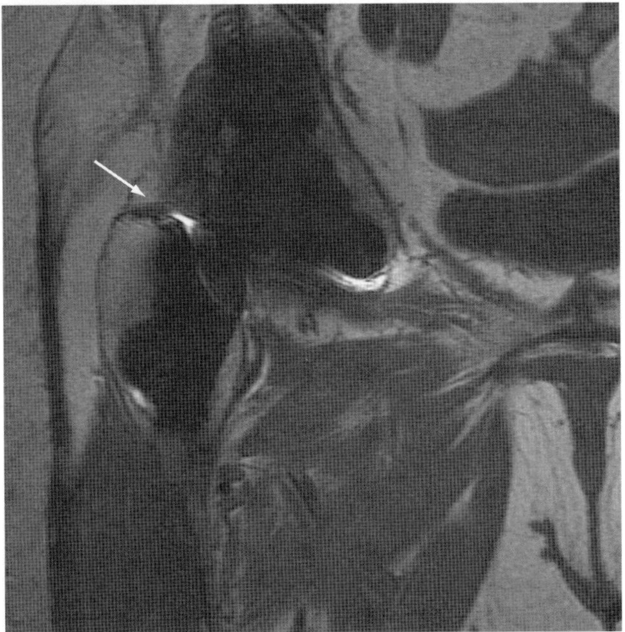

• **Fig. 51.32** This short tau inversion recovery coronal MRI shows a complete avulsion of the gluteus medius tendon from its insertion on the greater trochanter. Note the signal change along the lateral aspect of the greater trochanter, consistent with accumulation of intra-articular gadolinium at the site where the gluteus medius tendon should be.

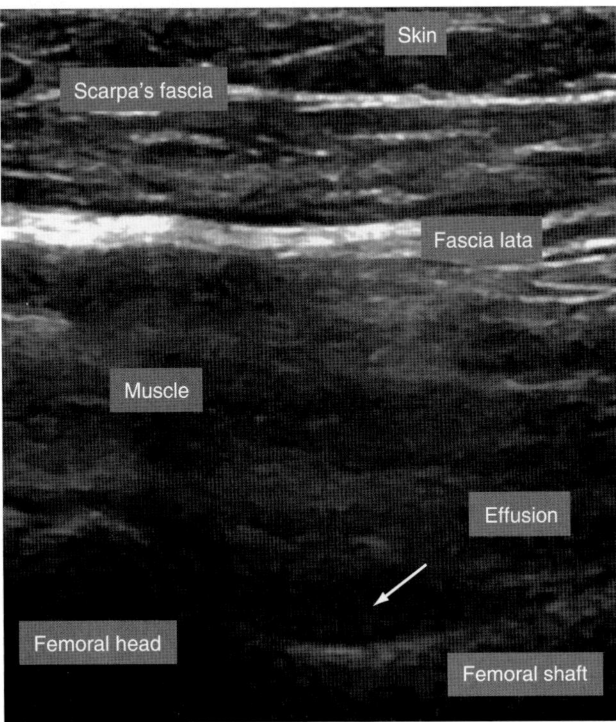

• **Fig. 51.33** This ultrasound image depicts a small hip effusion in a 9-year-old girl who was evaluated for toxic synovitis versus septic arthritis. Ultrasound images from the asymptomatic, contralateral hip showed comparable amounts of fluid, arguing against septic arthritis.

Common Disorders in the Differential Diagnosis of Hip Pain

Common causes of hip pain are numerous, and a detailed discussion of these causes is beyond the scope of this chapter. The differential diagnosis of hip pain should include osteoarthrosis (most frequently from developmental dysplasia, Legg-Calvé-Perthes disease, or slipped capital femoral epiphysis), inflammatory arthritis, osteonecrosis, fractures (acetabulum, femoral head, femoral neck, intertrochanteric, or subtrochanteric), trochanteric bursitis, femoroacetabular impingement, tears of the acetabular labrum, transient osteoporosis of the proximal femur, infection, snapping hip syndrome, osteitis pubis, neoplasia (osteosarcoma, chondrosarcoma, pigmented villonodular synovitis, osteochondromatosis, malignant fibrous histiocytoma, or metastases), inguinal hernia, or referred pain (lumbosacral spine, sacroiliac joint, prostate, seminal vesicles, uterus, ovaries, and lower gastrointestinal tract). This list can be efficiently narrowed down by taking a detailed history, performing a comprehensive examination of the musculoskeletal and neurovascular systems, and obtaining the appropriate imaging studies.

The references for this chapter can also be found on ExpertConsult.com.

References

1. Mallen CD, Peat G, Thomas E, et al.: Is chronic musculoskeletal pain in adulthood related to factors at birth? A population-based case-control study of young adults, *Eur J Epidemiol* 21:237–243, 2006.
2. Peat G, McCarney R, Croft P: Knee pain and osteoarthritis in older adults: a review of community burden and current use of primary health care, *Ann Rheum Dis* 60:91–97, 2001.
3. Kurtz SM, Ong KL, Lau E, et al.: Impact of the economic downturn on total joint replacement demand in the United States: updated projections to 2021, *J Bone Joint Surg* 96(8):624–630, 2014.
4. Ong KL, Mowat FS, Chan N, et al.: Economic burden of revision hip and knee arthroplasty in Medicare enrollees, *Clin Orthop Relat Res* 446:22–28, 2006.
5. Aoyagi K, Ross PD, Huang C, et al.: Prevalence of joint pain is higher among women in rural Japan than urban Japanese-American women in Hawaii, *Ann Rheum Dis* 58:315–319, 1999.
6. Jacobsen S, Sonne-Holm S, Soballe K, et al.: Radiographic case definitions and prevalence of osteoarthrosis of the hip: a survey of 4,151 subjects in the Osteoarthritis Substudy of the Copenhagen City Heart Study, *Acta Orthop Scand* 75:713–720, 2004.
7. Helme RD, Gibson SJ: The epidemiology of pain in elderly people, *Clin Geriatr Med* 17:417–431, 2001.
8. Chen J, Devine A, Dick IM, et al.: Prevalence of lower extremity pain and its association with functionality and quality of life in elderly women in Australia, *J Rheumatol* 30:2689–2693, 2003.
9. Felson DT: Epidemiology of hip and knee osteoarthritis, *Epidemiol Rev* 10:1–28, 1988.
10. Felson DT: An update on the pathogenesis and epidemiology of osteoarthritis, *Radiol Clin North Am* 42:1–9, 2004. v.
11. Felson DT, Nevitt MC: Epidemiologic studies for osteoarthritis: new versus conventional study design approaches, *Rheum Dis Clin North Am* 30:783–797, 2004. vii.
12. Gelber AC, Hochberg MC, Mead LA, et al.: Joint injury in young adults and risk for subsequent knee and hip osteoarthritis, *Ann Intern Med* 133:321–328, 2000.
13. Horvath G, Than P, Bellyei A, et al.: Prevalence of musculoskeletal symptoms in adulthood and adolescence (survey conducted in the Southern Transdanubian region in a representative sample of 10.000 people), *Orv Hetil* 147:351–356, 2006.

14. Leveille SG, Zhang Y, McMullen W, et al.: Sex differences in musculoskeletal pain in older adults, *Pain* 116:332–338, 2005.
15. Zeng QY, et al.: Low prevalence of knee and back pain in southeast China; the Shantou COPCORD study, *J Rheumatol* 31:2439–2443, 2004.
16. Butler DL, Noyes FR, Grood ES: Ligamentous restraints to anterior-posterior drawer in the human knee. A biomechanical study, *J Bone Joint Surg Am* 62:259–270, 1980.
17. O'Donoghue DH: Surgical treatment of fresh injuries to the major ligaments of the knee, *J Bone Joint Surg Am* 32A:721–738, 1950.
18. Griffin LY, et al.: Noncontact anterior cruciate ligament injuries: risk factors and prevention strategies, *J Am Acad Orthop Surg* 8:141–150, 2000.
19. Torg JS, Conrad W, Kalen V: Clinical diagnosis of anterior cruciate ligament instability in the athlete, *Am J Sports Med* 4:84–93, 1976.
20. Bach Jr BR, Warren RF, Wickiewicz TL: The pivot shift phenomenon: results and description of a modified clinical test for anterior cruciate ligament insufficiency, *Am J Sports Med* 16:571–576, 1988.
21. Noyes FR, Grood ES, Cummings JF, et al.: An analysis of the pivot shift phenomenon. The knee motions and subluxations induced by different examiners, *Am J Sports Med* 19:148–155, 1991.
22. Harner CD, Hoher J: Evaluation and treatment of posterior cruciate ligament injuries, *Am J Sports Med* 26:471–482, 1998.
23. Harner CD, Xerogeanes JW, Livesay GA, et al.: The human posterior cruciate ligament complex: an interdisciplinary study. Ligament morphology and biomechanical evaluation, *Am J Sports Med* 23:736–745, 1995.
24. Fanelli GC: Posterior cruciate ligament injuries in trauma patients, *Arthroscopy* 9:291–294, 1993.
25. Watanabe Y, Moriya H, Takahashi K, et al.: Functional anatomy of the posterolateral structures of the knee, *Arthroscopy* 9:57–62, 1993.
26. Andrews JR, Norwood Jr LA, Cross MJ: The double bucket handle tear of the medial meniscus, *J Sports Med* 3:232–237, 1975.
27. McMurray T: The semilunar cartilages, *Br J Surg* 29:407, 1941.
28. Apley A: The diagnosis of meniscus injuries: some new clinical methods, *J Bone Joint Surg Br* 29:78, 1929.
29. Dobbs RE, Hanssen AD, Lewallen DG, et al.: Quadriceps tendon rupture after total knee arthroplasty. Prevalence, complications, and outcomes, *J Bone Joint Surg Am* 87:37–45, 2005.
30. Fredericson M, Yoon K: Physical examination and patellofemoral pain syndrome, *Am J Phys Med Rehabil* 85:234–243, 2006.
31. Merchant AC: Classification of patellofemoral disorders, *Arthroscopy* 4:235–240, 1988.
32. Messieh SS, Fowler PJ, Munro T: Anteroposterior radiographs of the osteoarthritic knee, *J Bone Joint Surg Br* 72:639–640, 1990.
33. Barrack RL, Schrader T, Bertot AJ, et al.: Component rotation and anterior knee pain after total knee arthroplasty, *Clin Orthop Relat Res* 392:46–55, 2001.
34. Berger RA, Rubash HE: Rotational instability and malrotation after total knee arthroplasty, *Orthop Clin North Am* 32:639–647, 2001.
35. van Holsbeeck M, Introcaso JH: Musculoskeletal ultrasonography, *Radiol Clin North Am* 30:907–925, 1992.
36. Palmer EL, Scott SA, Strauss HW: Bone imaging. In Palmer EL, Scott JA, Strauss HW, editors: *Practical nuclear medicine*, Philadelphia, 1992, WB Saunders, pp 121–183.
37. Duus BR, Boeckstyns M, Kjaer L, et al.: Radionuclide scanning after total knee replacement: correlation with pain and radiolucent lines. A prospective study, *Invest Radiol* 22:891–894, 1987.
38. Kantor SG, Schneider R, Insall JN, et al.: Radionuclide imaging of asymptomatic versus symptomatic total knee arthroplasties, *Clin Orthop Relat Res* 260:118–123, 1990.
39. Palestro CJ, Swyer AJ, Kim CK, et al.: Infected knee prosthesis: diagnosis with In-111 leukocyte, Tc-99m sulfur colloid, and Tc-99m MDP imaging, *Radiology* 179:645–648, 1991.
40. De Smet AA, Tuite MJ: Use of the "two-slice-touch" rule for the MRI diagnosis of meniscal tears, *AJR Am J Roentgenol* 187:911–914, 2006.
41. Parvizi J, Gerhke T, et al.: International consensus meeting on musculoskeletal infection, *J Orthop Res* 37(5):2019, 2018.
42. Fritschy D, Fasel J, Imbert JC, et al.: The popliteal cyst, *Knee Surg Sports Traumatol Arthrosc* 14:623–628, 2006.
43. Kellgren JH, Samuel EP: The sensitivity and innervation of the articular capsule, *J Bone Joint Surg Br* 32:84, 1950.
44. Offierski CM, MacNab I: Hip-spine syndrome, *Spine* 8:316–321, 1983.
45. Dewolfe VG, Lefevre FA, Humphries AW, et al.: Intermittent claudication of the hip and the syndrome of chronic aorto-iliac thrombosis, *Circulation* 9:1–16, 1954.
46. Leriche R, Morel A: The syndrome of thrombotic obliteration of the aortic bifurcation, *Am Surg* 127:193, 1948.
47. Bellamy N, Buchanan WW, Goldsmith CH, et al.: Validation study of WOMAC: a health status instrument for measuring clinically important patient relevant outcomes to antirheumatic drug therapy in patients with osteoarthritis of the hip or knee, *J Rheumatol* 15:1833–1840, 1988.
48. Harris WH: Traumatic arthritis of the hip after dislocation and acetabular fractures: treatment by mold arthroplasty. An end-result study using a new method of result evaluation, *J Bone Joint Surg Am* 51:737–755, 1969.
49. Harris WH: Etiology of osteoarthritis of the hip, *Clin Orthop Relat Res* 213:20–33, 1986.
50. Millis MB, Murphy SB, Poss R: Osteotomies about the hip for the prevention and treatment of osteoarthrosis, *Instr Course Lect* 45:209–226, 1996.
51. Millis MB, Poss R, Murphy SB: Osteotomies of the hip in the prevention and treatment of osteoarthritis, *Instr Course Lect* 41:145–154, 1992.
52. Trendelenburg F: Trendelenburg's Test: 1895, *Dtsch Med Wschr (RSM translation)* 21:21–24, 1895.
53. Thomas H: *Hip, knee and ankle*, Dobbs, 1976, Liverpool.
54. Laslett M: Pain provocation tests for diagnosis of sacroiliac joint pain, *Aust J Physiother* 52:229, 2006.
55. Laslett M, Aprill CN, McDonald B: Provocation sacroiliac joint tests have validity in the diagnosis of sacroiliac joint pain. *Arch Phys Med Rehabil* 87:874, author reply 874–875, 2006.
56. Burnett RS, Della Rocca GJ, Prather H, et al.: Clinical presentation of patients with tears of the acetabular labrum, *J Bone Joint Surg Am* 88:1448–1457, 2006.
57. Beaule P, Zaragoza E, Motamedi K, et al.: Three-dimensional computed tomography of the hip in the assessment of femoracetabular impingement, *J Orthop Res* 23:1286–1292, 2005.
58. Beck M, Leunig M, Parvizi J, et al.: Anterior femoroacetabular impingement. Part II. Midterm results of surgical treatment, *Clin Orthop* 418:67–73, 2004.
59. Burnett RSJ, Della Rocca GJ, Prather H, et al.: Clinical presentation of patients with tears of the acetabular labrum, *J Bone Joint Surg* 88A:1448–1457, 2006.
60. Ito K, Leunig M, Ganz R: Histopathologic features of the acetabular labrum in femoroacetabular impingement, *Clin Orthop* 429:262–271, 2004.
61. Kassarjian A, Yoon LS, Belzile E, et al.: Triad of MR arthrographic findings in patients with cam-type femoroacetabular impingement, *Radiology* 236:588–592, 2005.
62. Keeney JA, Peelle MW, Jackson J, et al.: Magnetic resonance arthrography versus arthroscopy in the evaluation of articular hip pathology, *Clin Orthop* 429:163–169, 2004.
63. Toomayan GA, Holman WR, Major NM, et al.: Sensitivity of MR arthrography in the evaluation of acetabular labral tears, *AJR Am J Roentgenol* 186:449–453, 2006.
64. Cunningham T, Jessel R, Zurakowski D, et al.: Delayed gadolinium-enhanced magnetic resonance imaging of cartilage to predict early failure of Bernese periacetabular osteotomy for hip dysplasia, *J Bone Joint Surg Am* 88:1540–1548, 2006.
65. Byrd JW, Jones KS: Diagnostic accuracy of clinical assessment, magnetic resonance imaging, magnetic resonance arthrography, and intra-articular injection in hip arthroscopy patients, *Am J Sports Med* 32:1668–1674, 2004.
66. Illgen 2nd RL, Honkamp NJ, Weisman MH, et al.: The diagnostic and predictive value of hip anesthetic arthrograms in selected patients before total hip arthroplasty, *J Arthroplasty* 21:724–730, 2006.

52

Foot and Ankle Pain

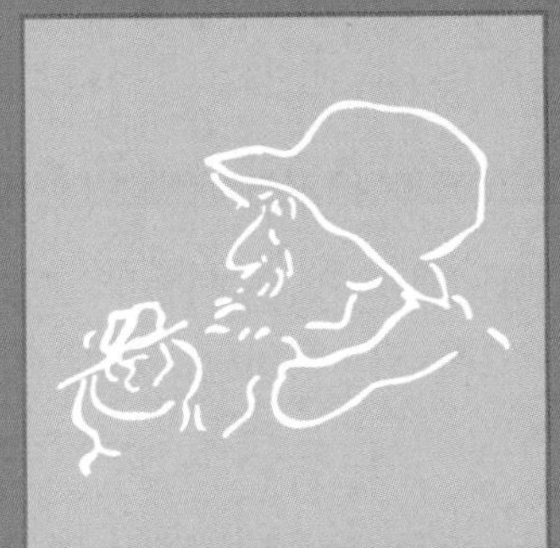

CHRISTOPHER P. CHIODO, MARK D. PRICE, AND ADAM P. SANGEORZAN

KEY POINTS

The differential diagnosis for foot and ankle pain is vast. Localizing symptoms by anatomic region helps narrow this differential.

On physical examination, most structures in the foot and ankle are immediately subcutaneous and readily palpable.

Beyond medications, useful nonoperative treatments include bracing, shoe wear modification, orthoses, and physical therapy.

Most surgical procedures in foot and ankle surgery fall into one of the following categories: arthrodesis, arthroplasty, corrective osteotomy, ostectomy, tendon débridement and transfer, and synovectomy. Patient compliance and soft tissue integrity are important factors when considering surgery.

Advances in medical management now make joint-sparing procedures possible in many patients with inflammatory arthritis who previously would have required arthrodesis.

Introduction

Foot and ankle pain are independent risk factors for locomotor instability, impaired balance, and increased risk for falling, as well as compromised functional activities of daily living.[1–5] Foot and ankle pain affect approximately one in five middle-aged to older individuals. Interference with daily activities occurs in one-half to one-third of affected individuals but is rarely disabling outside the context of rheumatoid arthritis. Foot and ankle pain are significantly more common in women, a finding that has been attributed to gender-specific footwear. The differential diagnosis of foot and ankle pain is vast and includes disorders of tendons, ligaments, muscle, bone, joints, periarticular structures, nerves, and vessels, as well as referred pain (Table 52.1). One of the most common causes of pain of the foot and ankle is osteoarthritis (OA). Although OA is the most prevalent joint disease, its pathophysiology remains poorly understood. Ankle and foot OA results from damage and loss of the articular cartilage, which can cause inflammation, stiffness, pain, swelling, deformity, and limitation of function, such as walking or standing. Osteophyte formation can also lead to mechanical impingement. In the foot, OA most commonly occurs in the big toe (hallux), the midfoot, and ankle. In the early stages, pain may occur only at the beginning and at the end of an activity, but as the condition progresses it can become constant and occur even while the individual is at rest.

The ankle is a complex joint that is subject to enormous force during daily activities and in sports, especially running. It is also the joint most commonly injured in the human body and is subject to sprains, fractures, and chondral injuries. This combination of factors predisposes the ankle joint to degenerative changes, although the risk is lower than in other weight-bearing joints such as the hip and knee. The ankle also rarely develops arthritic changes without an identifiable cause. The most common cause of ankle OA is trauma, including both fracture and ligamentous injury with subsequent chronic instability. Other causes of OA are abnormal mechanics (flat feet and high-arched feet) and, less commonly, systemic diseases such as hemochromatosis.

Foot and ankle pain is the presenting complaint in approximately 15% to 20% of newly diagnosed rheumatoid arthritis (RA) patients.[6] Further, of those patients already diagnosed with RA, the prevalence of foot and ankle involvement is greater than 90%.[7]

The clinician should begin the evaluation of the rheumatoid foot and ankle with a thorough history and physical examination. The location, timing, and duration of symptoms can help to establish a specific diagnosis and guide the subsequent course of treatment. Radiographs and advanced imaging modalities provide useful adjuncts to the evaluation of specific foot and ankle pathologies.

The treatment of the rheumatoid foot and ankle is aimed at both alleviating pain and preserving function (i.e., maintaining the ambulatory status of the patient). Initial nonoperative treatment includes medical management, physical therapy, shoe wear modification, orthotics, and bracing. These measures provide substantial relief for many patients. For recalcitrant symptoms, surgical intervention may be necessary. Most surgical procedures fall into one of the following general categories: arthrodesis (joint fusion), arthroplasty (joint replacement), corrective osteotomy, ostectomy, and synovectomy (joint or tendon).

Functional Anatomy and Biomechanics

The ankle, or tibiotalar joint, is composed of the articulation between the foot (talus) and the lower leg (distal tibia and fibula). Its primary motion is plantarflexion and dorsiflexion in the sagittal plane. In addition, the articulation between the distal tibia and fibula allows a lesser amount of internal and external rotation to occur in the axial, or transverse, plane.

The foot may be loosely divided into three anatomic regions: forefoot, midfoot, and hindfoot. The forefoot consists of the toes and metatarsal bones, along with the metatarsophalangeal (MTP) and interphalangeal (IP) joints. The tarsometatarsal

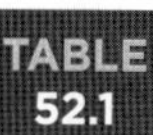

Differential Diagnosis of Foot and Ankle Pain

Tendon, Ligament, and Muscle
Ankle or foot ligament tear or attenuation
Chronic joint instability secondary to ligament compromise
Joint impingement caused by ligamentous tear and/or hypertrophy
Sinus tarsi pathology
Achilles tendon pathology
Achilles tendon rupture
Plantar fasciitis
Posterior tibial tendon dysfunction (usually with adult acquired flatfoot)
Flexor hallucis longus tenosynovitis and stenosis
Tibialis anterior tendon tear
Peroneus tendon pathology
Bone
Acute fractures of the ankle or foot
Stress fractures
Freiberg's infraction (osteonecrosis of the second metatarsal head)
Osteonecrosis of talus and navicular
Sesamoid bone pathology
Metatarsal overload (metatarsalgia)
Joint
Osteoarthritis
Gout
Rheumatoid arthritis
Other inflammatory arthritides
Charcot neuroarthropathy
Osteochondral lesion of the talus
Joint impingement (bone, synovitis, or ligamentous hypertrophy)
Hammer toe, claw toe, and mallet toe deformities
Hallux rigidus
Nerve Compression
Tarsal tunnel syndrome
Anterior tarsal tunnel syndrome (involvement of deep peroneal nerve under the superficial fascia of the ankle)
Morton's neuroma
Vessels
Vasculitis
Atherosclerosis
Compartment syndrome
Neuropathic and referred pain
Neuropathy
Spinal pathology
Complex regional pain syndrome

Courtesy of Dr. George Raj, No Surgical Spine and Joint Clinic, PS, Bellingham, Wash.

(TMT) joints connect the forefoot to the midfoot, which comprises the three cuneiform bones, the navicular, and the cuboid. Finally, the hindfoot, located below the ankle, consists of the talus and calcaneus. The joints of the hindfoot include the talocalcaneal (subtalar), talonavicular, and calcaneocuboid articulations.

Forefoot and midfoot motion is primarily plantarflexion and dorsiflexion in the sagittal plane, with some secondary pronation and supination in the coronal plane and abduction/adduction in the axial plane. Motion in the hindfoot is primarily composed of inversion/eversion in the coronal plane, with secondary internal/external rotation in the axial plane and plantarflexion/dorsiflexion in the sagittal plane.

Knowledge of these anatomic divisions is important because radiographs often demonstrate polyarticular disease in patients with RA. An intimate understanding of the local anatomy is an essential resource for the physician to establish an accurate diagnosis and formulate an appropriate treatment plan.

Diagnostic Evaluation

Physical Examination

The physician should begin a thorough physical examination of the foot and ankle with gait analysis, even if by simply observing the patient enter the examination room. Normal human gait is divided into two phases. The stance phase is the weight-bearing portion of the gait cycle and comprises roughly 60% of normal walking. This phase begins with heel-strike and then extends through foot-flat to toe-off motion. Meanwhile, the swing phase of gait extends from toe-off to heel-strike and comprises the remaining 40% of the gait cycle.

Patients with an "antalgic" gait pattern will have a shortened stance phase on the side of the affected limb while they attempt to more quickly transfer their weight to the nonpainful limb. In addition to an antalgic gait, foot and ankle pain often results in the avoidance of ground contact with the painful part of the foot. A further problem noted in stance phase is dynamic collapse of the medial longitudinal arch, most apparent at foot-flat and toe-off.

During the swing phase of gait, a "steppage" gait may be noted. This type of gait is characterized by excessive hip and knee flexion, to allow the foot to clear the ground in the setting of a footdrop. In patients with RA, it may be caused by attritional rupture of the anterior tibialis tendon, which is the main dorsiflexor of the ankle.

After gait analysis, the physician inspects the foot and ankle, both with the patient in the sitting and standing position. The location of swelling is usually well correlated with the joint(s) involved (e.g., the ankle vs. the talocalcaneal joint). Deformity should also be noted. Commonly seen deformities in patients with RA include hallux valgus, or bunion (Fig. 52.1); hammertoes; and flatfoot deformity (characterized by hindfoot valgus/forefoot abduction). Callosities develop over regions of increased pressure and are associated with deformity and fat pad atrophy. Rheumatoid nodules can appear anywhere on the foot but are often found in areas of repetitive trauma (i.e., at the site of irritation from a tight shoe counter). Similarly, ulcerations may appear in areas of increased pressure or repeated injury. Finally, wear patterns on shoes should also be noted. As Hoppenfeld observed[8]: "A deformed foot can deform any good shoe; in fact, in many cases the shoe is a literal showcase for certain disorders."

After inspection of the foot and ankle, the physician performs range-of-motion analysis. Passive range of motion of the ankle is normally between 10 and 20 degrees of dorsiflexion and 40 and 50 degrees of plantarflexion. Normal hindfoot inversion and eversion are approximately 20 and 10 degrees, respectively. The first MTP joint should have approximately 45 degrees of "plantarflexion" (flexion) and 70 to 90 degrees of "dorsiflexion" (extension). Deviations from these norms should be noted as part of the standard workup.

Next, the physician thoroughly palpates the foot and ankle. The dorsum of the foot and ankle has little overlying musculature. As such, many of the bones and tendons are immediately subcutaneous and a great deal of information can be gained from palpating these structures. It is helpful to palpate the foot and ankle by anatomic location (i.e., forefoot, midfoot, hindfoot, and anterior and posterior ankle).

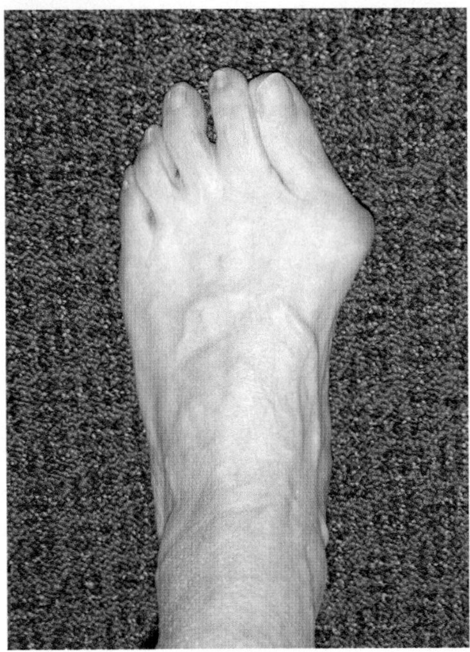

• **Fig. 52.1** Clinical photograph of hallux valgus deformity.

TABLE 52.2 Anatomic Basis of Common Causes of Foot and Ankle Pain

Location	Pathology/Dysfunction
Forefoot	Arthritis/synovitis Hallux valgus Hammertoes, claw toes, and mallet toes Morton's neuroma Metatarsophalangeal arthritis/synovitis/instability Osteonecrosis of the second metatarsal head (Freiberg's)
Midfoot	Arthritis/synovitis, stress fracture, osteonecrosis (navicular)
Hindfoot	Arthritis/synovitis Hindfoot valgus deformity Stress fracture Plantar fasciitis
Anterior ankle	Arthritis, synovitis, impingement, osteochondral defect
Central ankle	Osteochondral lesion Stress fracture
Posterior ankle	Achilles tendinitis/tendinosis Retrocalcaneal bursitis Achilles rupture Stress fracture
Posterolateral ankle	Peroneal tendinitis, tear, instability
Posteromedial ankle	Posterior tibial tendinitis/dysfunction Flexor hallucis longus/flexor digitorum longus tendinitis Tarsal tunnel syndrome

In the forefoot, the first metatarsal head and MTP joint can be palpated at the base of the hallux, at the medial aspect of the "ball" of the foot. Proceeding laterally, the physician can then sequentially palpate the lesser metatarsal heads and MTP joints. In patients with RA, such palpation often reveals tenderness, synovitis, and bursal swelling. In the second and third MTP joints, sagittal plane instability often results from attenuation of the plantar joint capsule. This condition can be appreciated by gently translating the second and third toes dorsally.

In the hindfoot, the calcaneus is readily palpable, and its various parts can be palpated individually. A stress fracture should always be considered in patients with RA. Further, tenderness over the posterior aspect of the bone may indicate Achilles tendon pathology, while pain over the medial tubercle (palpable on the medial plantar surface) may indicate plantar fasciitis. Tenderness over the "sinus tarsi" of the hindfoot (located laterally, just anterior and distal to the tip of the fibula) usually indicates talocalcaneal joint pathology. Posterolateral tenderness most often indicates peroneal tendon pathology. Finally, posteromedial tenderness may be secondary to tenosynovitis, posterior tibial tendinosis, and tarsal tunnel syndrome (usually secondary to adjacent tenosynovitis).

In the ankle joint proper, tenderness over the anterior joint line usually correlates with ankle joint pathology including arthritis, synovitis, impingement, and osteochondral defect (OCD). In contrast, deep posterior pain may or may not correlate with tenderness and may indicate a posterior OCD or posterior impingement, such as from an os trigonum.

A more detailed description of these conditions and their correlation with anatomic location is provided later in the chapter and in Table 52.2.

Imaging

Despite the abundant availability of advanced imaging modalities such as MRI and CT, radiographs remain the imaging mainstay in the evaluation of foot and ankle pain. Weight-bearing images should be obtained whenever possible because joint space narrowing and deformity may not be apparent in non–weight-bearing images. Standard images consist of weight-bearing anteroposterior, lateral, and oblique views of the foot and anteroposterior, mortise, and lateral views of the ankle. Further radiographic findings of RA include periarticular erosions and osteopenia.

MRI provides reliable imaging of soft tissue structures and can be a useful tool in the evaluation of the rheumatoid foot and ankle. Early in the course of RA, MRI allows one to look for signs of the disease such as synovitis, tenosynovitis, periarticular edema, and bursitis.[9] Later, MRI is useful in assessing disease progression and extent of joint involvement, as well as in distinguishing between tendon rupture and tendinitis/tendinopathy (Fig. 52.2).

CT scan[10] and nuclear scintigraphy[11] are also used in the evaluation of foot and ankle pain. For example, either method can be quite helpful in post-operative evaluation in fusion surgery. Ultrasound is gaining utility as a method to evaluate joint inflammation as well as tendon integrity. There is no radiation involved, and the procedure is now frequently performed in the office setting. However, the results are sometimes operator- and technique-dependent with minimization of artifacts being of utmost concern. In addition, ultrasound may be difficult to use in pre-operative planning because important landmarks are often not included, and overall alignment of the foot and ankle cannot be appreciated.[12]

Anesthetic arthrograms are an extremely useful adjunct in diagnosing foot and ankle pain in patients with RA. Given the

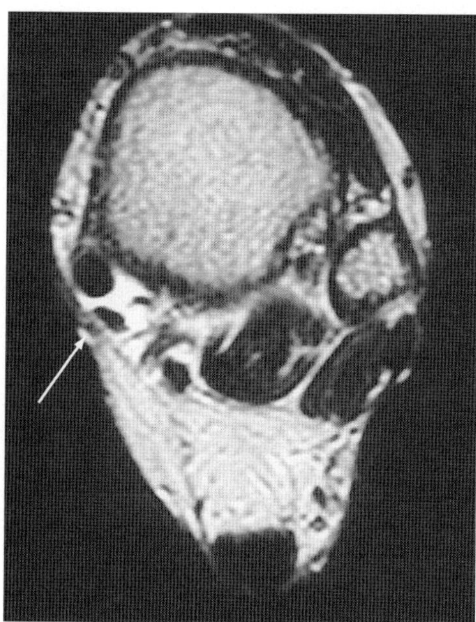

• **Fig. 52.2** Axial MRI of ankle demonstrating posterior tibial tendon degeneration and synovitis *(arrow)*.

complex and crowded geometry of the foot and the propensity of RA to affect multiple joints and tendons, it is often difficult to determine whether the pain is articular and, if so, which joint is symptomatic. With an anesthetic arthrogram, a mixture of steroid, anesthetic, and contrast material is injected under fluoroscopic guidance into a suspect joint. This allows the clinician to more precisely determine whether or not the injected joint is a significant pain generator. Again, this is especially helpful in the foot and ankle, where multiple joints are in close proximity and may be simultaneously diseased.[13]

Differential Diagnosis of Ankle Pain

From a diagnostic standpoint, it is useful for the clinician to conceptualize ankle pain on the basis of anatomic location. This approach applies to patients with virtually any form of ankle or foot pain. RA will be used to illustrate how to formulate a differential diagnosis and treatment plan while taking into account how advances in medical management temper disease and "allow" patients to develop other, non-inflammatory disorders.

Anterior Ankle Pain

Anterior ankle pain, in patients both with and without RA, is most often the result of intra-articular pathology. Anteriorly, the ankle joint is not shielded by the malleoli and is immediately subcutaneous. Further, the anterior extensor tendons are typically not prone to the development of tendinitis and tendinosis.

In early RA, synovitis can cause anterior joint line pain, swelling, and tenderness. Clinically, this results in symptoms of "impingement." Specifically, patients will note pain with ankle dorsiflexion, such as when they walk up stairs or an incline. On physical examination, there may be anterior tenderness and/or pain with terminal passive dorsiflexion. Anterior osteophyte formation may produce even more pronounced impingement symptoms, although such osteophytes are more commonly seen with OA and longstanding ankle instability.

Central Joint Pain

Two other causes of central ankle pain, stress fracture and OCD, should be considered. Stress fractures are commonly seen in patients with periarticular and generalized osteopenia. An OCD is a focal defect in the articular cartilage and subchondral bone. These lesions are encountered more commonly in patients without inflammatory arthritis. In the setting of RA, their presence may represent an early manifestation of RA or a separate pathologic process.

Posterior Ankle and Hindfoot Pain

Posterior ankle and hindfoot pain usually originates from the Achilles tendon, its insertion onto the calcaneal tuberosity, and two associated bursae in this region. The Achilles tendon is the largest tendon in the body but lacks a true synovial lining. As such, isolated Achilles tendinitis is uncommon. In most instances, Achilles pain results from degenerative tendinosis, with or without an overlying tendinitis. Although associated spur formation is common, it is important to remember that Achilles spurs are a manifestation of a disease process. As such, surgeries directed at spur excision also frequently entail tendon débridement and reconstruction, as well as tendon transfer.

The Achilles tendon is associated with two bursae. The retrocalcaneal bursa is a larger structure that lies deep in the Achilles. Inflammation of this structure often accompanies Achilles tendinitis/tendinosis. It may also be irritated by an enlarged posterior superior calcaneal tuberosity, sometimes referred to as *Haglund's deformity*. Less commonly, a more superficial, immediately subcutaneous bursa can develop with irritation from ill-fitting shoes with a tight counter ("pump bump").

Posterior ankle pain may also be attributed to posterior joint pathology such as an OCD of the talus. If symptoms are worsened with plantarflexion of the ankle, posterior impingement from synovitis or os trigonum syndrome should be considered.

Medial and Lateral Ankle Pain

As with anterior, central, and posterior ankle pain, the origin of medial or lateral ankle pain is also anatomically based.

On the medial side, pain directly over the medial malleolus should alert the clinician to the possibility of a stress fracture. Pain anterior to the medial malleolus is usually articular in nature. Pain posterior to the medial malleolus is often caused by inflammation and/or degeneration of the posteromedial flexor tendons. These include the posterior tibial tendon and the flexor hallucis longus and flexor digitorum longus tendons. The posterior tibial tendon is the largest and strongest of the posteromedial flexor tendons. Its primary function is to invert the hindfoot and thus support the medial longitudinal arch of the foot. Long-standing synovitis and dysfunction of this tendon may ultimately lead to collapse of the arch and the development of an acquired flatfoot deformity.

On the lateral side of the ankle, pain directly over the lateral malleolus may be caused by a stress fracture. This is especially relevant in the setting of hindfoot valgus and a flatfoot, which will increase fibular loading. Similar to the medial side, pain anterior to the lateral malleolus is usually articular in nature. Finally, pain posterior to this lateral malleolus is usually indicative of peroneal tendon pathology. In patients with RA, the peroneal tendons may be affected by tenosynovitis, longitudinal "split" tears, and chronic tendon instability. With the latter, the tendons sublux over the posterolateral edge of the fibula, causing pain as well as attritional tearing. These patients will often describe "popping" of the tendons out of place, and can sometimes demonstrate tendon dislocation with resisted eversion of the foot.

Differential Diagnosis of Foot Pain

Typically, the forefoot is the most common site of involvement early in the course of diseases such as RA, but can also occur in patients with gout and OA.[14] The pathogenesis of forefoot pain and deformity in the rheumatoid forefoot is inflammation and progressive synovitis that eventually leads to a capsular distention at the MTP joints and attenuation of the plantar plates.[15] Eventually it progresses to loss of collateral ligament stability and, finally, destruction of the articular cartilage and bone (Fig. 52.3A and B). Clinically, this typically manifests as hallux valgus and dorsal subluxation or dislocation of the lesser toe MTP joints with a hallux valgus deformity, and presents in the patient as metatarsalgia.

In the lesser MTP joints, such loss of stability leads to progressive deformity secondary to ligamentous attenuation combined with the standard forces on the forefoot. Muscle imbalance and dorsiflexion forces during the toe-off phase of gait cause progressive subluxation and even dorsal dislocation of the MTP joints. With these changes, the metatarsal head is prone to forming keratotic skin lesions that can ultimately ulcerate. Muscle imbalance can also lead to the development of painful hammertoe and claw toe deformities that can exert a plantar-directed force that further exacerbates symptomatic metatarsalgia. Lesser MTP joint subluxation occurs in up to 70% of cases, with a concomitant incidence of pressure sores in approximately 30% of those patients.

In the hallux, RA can cause both articular erosions and loss of capsular integrity that often results in the development of a hallux valgus deformity or bunion (see Fig. 52.1). The progression of this deformity may be further accelerated by loss of support from the adjacent lesser MTP joints. The incidence of hallux valgus deformity in patients with RA is up to 70%.

The midfoot is a less common site of involvement in the rheumatoid foot. Radiographically there can be erosions; however, the prevalence of symptoms is often quite low. The most frequent site of involvement is the first TMT joint. The symptoms seen here, though, may not be from rheumatoid synovitis per se, as seen in the forefoot. Rather, pain may also be due to hindfoot and hallux valgus deformities that lead to increased stresses across the TMT joint. Eventually this increased stress can lead to dorsiflexion of the first TMT joint and resultant lesser toe TMT joint abduction and dorsiflexion, thereby leading to pain in the dorsomedial midfoot. In addition, progressive biomechanical changes can lead to OA of the midfoot TMT joints, causing discomfort and pain with weight bearing.

The three joints of the hindfoot (talonavicular, talocalcaneal, and calcaneocuboid) are commonly affected by RA. Although these joints are affected at different rates, the overall prevalence of hindfoot involvement in patients with RA is between 21% and 29%. The talonavicular joint is most often affected, followed by the talocalcaneal and then calcaneocuboid joints. Further, the hindfoot becomes more symptomatic and involved the longer the duration of RA. The incidence of hindfoot deformity in patients diagnosed with RA for less than 5 years is 8% and increases to 25% in patients with RA for longer than 5 years.[16] Clinically, patients with talocalcaneal or calcaneocuboid involvement will complain of lateral hindfoot pain. Meanwhile, arthritis and synovitis of the talonavicular joint are manifested by dorsal or medial pain.

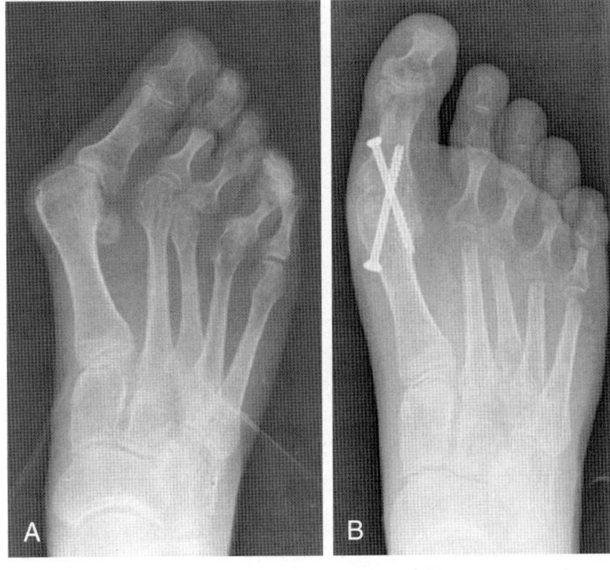

• **Fig. 52.3** Pre-operative (A) and post-operative (B) anteroposterior radiographs of hallux valgus deformity with lesser metatarsophalangeal joint erosions treated by fusion and lesser metatarsal head resections.

The deformity most often seen in patients with hindfoot RA is an acquired flatfoot deformity, characterized by heel valgus and forefoot abduction. This usually results from articular deformity and instability, but may also be caused by tenosynovitis and tendinosis of the posterior tibial tendon, the main dynamic supporter of the longitudinal arch of the foot. Typically, symptoms start with posteromedial ankle pain and swelling along the course of the posterior tibial tendon with lateral pain only developing with progressive deformity and bony impingement.

Nonoperative Treatment

Medical management remains the cornerstone of treatment for many forms of foot and ankle arthritis. In fact, many of the current recommendations for operative treatment may soon be modified given the alteration of disease progression with current medical regimens for RA.[17] The most common medical management still consists of nonsteroidal anti-inflammatory drugs (NSAIDs), steroids, and disease-modifying anti-rheumatic drugs (DMARDs) and, more recently, biologic therapies. Although each of these drug classes has done much to alleviate patient suffering, they are not without impact on the surgical management of rheumatic disease. There is concern about lower fusion rates in the setting of NSAIDs and increased infection rates in the setting of steroids or DMARDs.[18,19] Moreover, patients who have been on chronic steroids are at risk for post-operative adrenal insufficiency and may require perioperative corticosteroids.[20] Close communication and collaboration between the rheumatologist and surgeon are essential to good outcomes.

Footwear modification can often have profound benefits for patients. Shoes should be examined in the clinic to be sure that they can accommodate a patient's deformity. Patients often feel best in shoes with a deep, wide toe-box, a firm heel counter, and soft heel. Well-constructed walking or jogging shoes usually provide sufficient room for mild to moderate deformities. It is helpful to provide patients with a list of suitable manufacturers when making such recommendations.

Often it is necessary to prescribe a custom orthotic insert for those with more moderate deformities. Typically the insole of the shoe must be removed to make room for the orthotic. Again, most walking or jogging shoes will suffice. In general, custom orthotics can be divided into rigid, semirigid, and softer accommodative devices. Rigid and semirigid orthotics are usually used to correct supple deformities and should be used with caution in patients with RA.[21] More commonly, patients benefit from accommodative orthotics (i.e., orthotics made of softer material that can be molded to "accommodate" a deformity).[22] These can then be further modified by incorporating a "relief" under a deformity, thereby further unloading it. When referring patients to a specialist for orthotics, it is best to provide the orthotist with a prescription that includes the patient's precise diagnosis (e.g., RA or OA with metatarsalgia), as well as the type of orthotic and any modifications desired (e.g., a "custom accommodative orthotic with a relief under the lesser metatarsal heads").[23]

Finally, injections of a mixture of anesthetic and corticosteroid to areas of inflammation or bursitis are useful to treat both inflammatory and non-inflammatory conditions affecting the foot and ankle. In the foot and ankle, however, such injections must be judiciously used. Most important, injections into and around tendons should be avoided. Because of the forces associated with weight bearing and ambulation, these tendons are under substantial load. The injection of a corticosteroid directly into or even near a tendon can adversely affect the biomechanical properties of the tendon and can ultimately lead to rupture.[24] In fact, steroid injection into the plantar fascia is the primary risk factor for chronic plantar fascia rupture.[25] A further precaution is to avoid corticosteroid injections into the lesser MTP when there is evidence of joint instability (manifested by valgus or varus deviation on radiographs or sagittal plane instability on physical examination). Such injections can lead to further attenuation of the joint capsule and can result in frank joint dislocation.

Operative Treatment

If symptoms persist despite nonoperative management, surgical intervention should be considered. Two important factors must be taken into account when deciding whether or not to proceed with surgery. First, the soft tissues and vascular status must be carefully assessed. Both may be compromised and could negatively affect outcome. Second, the ability of patients to comply with the postoperative regimen (e.g., the ability to use crutches and not bear weight if necessary) must be considered. Even limited noncompliance can lead to a poor outcome, especially in fusion surgery.

As noted earlier, most surgical procedures fall into one of the following categories: arthrodesis (joint fusion), arthroplasty (joint replacement), corrective osteotomy, ostectomy, and synovectomy (joint or tendon).

Arthrodesis

Arthrodesis remains a surgical cornerstone for the rheumatoid foot and ankle. With an arthrodesis procedure, the two sides of the joint are roughened with a burr or small chisel. Next, the two bones to be fused are compressed and fixed together, usually with one or more screws (see Fig. 52.3B). In the weeks and months after surgery, the body is "tricked" into thinking that there is a fracture present at the fusion site and heals this with bone. As such, the two bones become one and are considered fused. Fusion surgery offers reliable pain relief in the majority of patients. One obvious concern with fusion surgery is the loss of motion. For the patient, however, this usually results in only mild functional compromise. Further, to the untrained eye, the patient has a remarkably minor change in gait.

Commonly performed fusions in patients with RA include ankle arthrodesis, isolated hindfoot fusions, triple arthrodesis, midfoot arthrodesis, and arthrodesis of the first MTP joint. A triple arthrodesis involves fusion of the talocalcaneal, talonavicular, and calcaneocuboid joints. Together, these joints allow coronal plane motion and thereby are most important when an individual is walking on uneven ground.

Arthrodesis is still commonly performed in patients with RA of the ankle. If there is minimal deformity and no loss of bone stock, ankle fusion surgery may be performed arthroscopically or through a "mini open" approach. These techniques involve less soft tissue dissection and stripping, thereby minimizing loss of bony perfusion. Nevertheless, the time period for which the patient must avoid bearing weight (from 6 to 12 weeks) remains the same. The success rate of ankle fusion surgery in patients with RA is generally 85% or greater. Although the osteopenia associated with the disease can compromise fixation, it can also theoretically enhance fusion because less sclerotic subchondral bone is present.

In the hindfoot, fusion surgery may be performed on one or more of the three joints of this part of the foot (i.e., the talocalcaneal, talonavicular, and calcaneocuboid joints). If only one of these joints is diseased, an isolated fusion of this joint is acceptable.[26] This reduces surgical morbidity and the extent of the procedure. Nevertheless, with fusion of just one of the joints of the hindfoot, motion in the other joints is reduced.[27] If more than one joint is diseased, a "double" or "triple" arthrodesis is necessary.

In the midfoot, fusion surgery results in negligible loss of motion because the joints of the midfoot normally have less than 10 degrees of motion. In a patient with both OA and inflammatory arthritis, symptomatology is most often limited to the medial (first through third) TMT joints. The lateral (fourth and fifth) TMT joints are infrequently symptomatic, even in the setting of advanced radiographic changes.

Finally, in the forefoot, fusion surgery is indicated only for the first MTP joint. This procedure is used for both arthrosis and advanced hallux valgus (bunion) deformities. When the first MTP joint is fused, it is positioned in a slightly dorsiflexed position to assist ambulation. With MTP fusion in 47 patient feet, Coughlin[28] reported 96% good to excellent results and 100% fusion at an average 6.2-year follow-up.

In summary, fusion surgery generally provides reliable pain relief and a stable, plantigrade foot. Nevertheless, the loss of motion of the fused joint can lead to increased motion and altered biomechanics at adjacent joints. This result ultimately may lead to arthritic changes in these joints.[29] Further, fusion surgery may lead to subtle, albeit real, changes in gait.[30] Finally, the minimal ramifications of fusing just one joint may become much greater in the setting of a subsequent fusion in either the ipsilateral or contralateral limb. However, patients with bilateral ankle or combined ankle and hindfoot fusions have been found to have mostly satisfactory outcomes in short and midterm follow up (1 to 4 years) with minimal need for further joint fusions.[31,32]

Arthroplasty

Concerns regarding fusion have driven many to work toward improving joint replacement surgery (arthroplasty) in the foot and ankle. Most notably, total ankle replacement surgery has evolved and is now a viable alternative to arthrodesis. Nevertheless, although there are many orthopedic surgeons who perform ankle replacement surgery, there are still some who do not or who do so on a limited basis. The U.S. Food and Drug Administration currently approves seven ankle prostheses for implantation. Robust long-term survival data as published for hip and knee arthroplasty are not yet available.

The main advantage of ankle arthroplasty is preservation of motion. Its main two disadvantages are technical complexity and the difficulty with subsequent fusion if the procedure fails. In general, ankle replacement surgery is indicated for middle-aged and elderly individuals with low functional demands and minimal deformity. Two other indications especially pertinent in patients with ankle arthritis include (1) bilateral disease and (2) concomitant ipsilateral hindfoot disease or pre-existing arthrodesis. The paradox of ankle replacement surgery is that ankle replacement is contraindicated in young patients, for whom preservation of motion is most important. On the other hand, arthroplasty is more commonly performed in older patients, for whom preservation of motion is less important and who might do fine with a fusion. Nevertheless, total ankle replacement surgery continues to evolve, and reported success rates with modern designs continue to improve[33,34] (Fig. 52.4). In one large study, arthroplasty has superior functional outcome score improvements as compared to arthrodesis, particularly when newer generation implants were used.[35]

In the foot, arthroplasty is performed by some surgeons for the first MTP joint. Results from the relevant literature are still somewhat conflicted, however. Earlier silicone-based implants for first MTP arthroplasty have unacceptably high rates of implant failure and loosening secondary to synovitis from polymeric silicone (Silastic) particle wear.[36–38] Direct comparison of metal articulated arthroplasty to fusion favors fusion.[39] Further, advanced deformity, often present in patients with RA, is considered a relative contraindication to first MTP joint arthroplasty.

Nevertheless, new implant designs may hold increased promise. A recent randomized controlled trial comparing a polyvinyl alcohol hydrogel implant to first MTP fusion showed equivalent pain and functional outcomes at 2 years.[40] A subsequent study showed 96% implant survival at 5 years, suggesting that the new implant may be a reasonable alternative in patients who desire to preserve motion.[41]

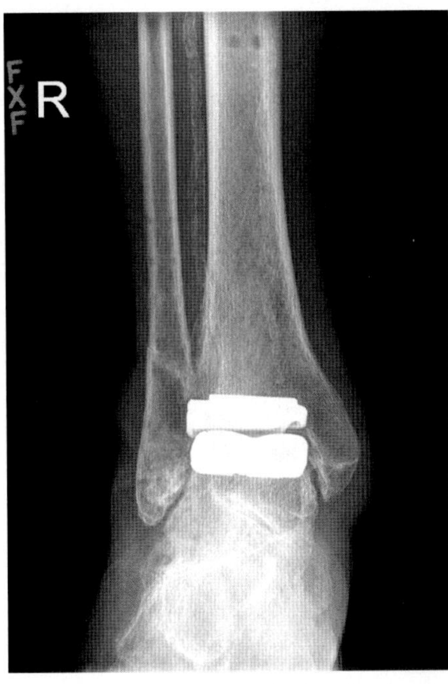

• **Fig. 52.4** Anteroposterior radiograph of total ankle arthroplasty.

Osteotomy

Corrective osteotomies are used for two primary reasons in the treatment of RA: to correct deformity, to redistribute forces on a joint or the terminal aspect of a bone, or both.

Examples of osteotomies to correct deformity include calcaneal osteotomies for pes planovalgus and metatarsal osteotomies for hallux valgus. Previously, patients with RA and concomitant pes planovalgus or hallux valgus underwent fusion surgery. However, with advances in medical management of the disease, it is not unreasonable to attempt joint preservation surgery in patients who have mild to moderate disease, healthy soft tissues, and flexible deformities.

Examples of osteotomies to redistribute forces include tibial osteotomies in the setting of eccentric ankle arthritis and metatarsal osteotomies in the setting of metatarsal overload and metatarsalgia. Patients requiring surgery for ankle RA previously underwent fusion surgery only, while patients requiring surgery for metatarsalgia underwent metatarsal head resection. Again, however, advances in medical management of the disease allow joint preservation osteotomies to be considered. This is especially the case for metatarsalgia, which is common in patients with RA, yet increasingly does not entail frank dislocation or articular erosion.

Ostectomy

Although more commonly seen in patients with OA, some patients with RA may present with symptoms of mechanical ankle impingement arising from anterior bone spurs. In cases without global joint destruction, surgical resection of the spurs, or cheilectomy, is a reasonable treatment. Although no studies have examined cheilectomy in RA specifically, patients with less severe erosive changes tend to be more satisfied with the results of cheilectomy.[42]

Synovectomy

For those patients with inflammatory arthritis resistant to medical management and nonoperative treatment, synovectomy can provide a period of pain relief for many patients.[43,44] It is thought that early synovectomy of either the affected joint or tendon may help halt the progress of joint destruction. Joint synovectomy is indicated in those who have failed medical management yet still have a relatively preserved articular surface. This may be performed arthroscopically or open through a traditional arthrotomy. Otherwise, synovectomy of the affected tendons allows some preservation of function.

Conclusion

Foot and ankle pain is a prevalent and potentially debilitating problem. Unfortunately, many forms of arthritis, including RA, establish a vicious cycle of foot and ankle pain and altered biomechanics. Synovitis and articular erosions lead to both pain and deformity. A proper history and physical examination are essential for establishing an anatomic diagnosis. Although advanced imaging modalities such as MRI and CT can be useful as adjuncts, radiography remains the gold standard. Nonoperative modalities such as medications, bracing, physical therapy, orthotics, and footwear modification are able to relieve pain and maintain function for many. For recalcitrant symptoms, substantial relief may be afforded by surgical intervention in the form of arthrodesis, arthroplasty, osteotomy, ostectomy, or synovectomy.

The references for this chapter can also be found on ExpertConsult.com.

References

1. Bowling A, Grundy E: Activities of daily living: changes in functional ability in three samples of elderly and very elderly people, *Age Ageing* 26(2):107–114, 1997.
2. Keysor JJ, Dunn JE, Link CL, et al.: Are foot disorders associated with functional limitation and disability among community-dwelling older adults? *J Aging Health* 17(6):734–752, 2005.
3. Menz HB, Morris ME, Lord SR: Foot and ankle characteristics associated with impaired balance and functional ability in older people, *J Gerontol A Biol Sci Med Sci* 60(12):1546–1552, 2005.
4. Menz HB, Morris ME, Lord SR: Foot and ankle risk factors for falls in older people: a prospective study, *J Gerontol A Biol Sci Med Sci* 61(8):866–870, 2006.
5. Peat G, Thomas E, Wilkie R, et al.: Multiple joint pain and lower extremity disability in middle and old age, *Disabil Rehabil* 28(24):1543–1549, 2006.
6. Vanio E: Rheumatoid foot. Clinical study with pathological and roentgenological comments, *Ann Chir Gynaecol Fenniae* 45(S): 1–107, 1956.
7. Flemming A, Crown JM, Corbett M: Early rheumatoid disease. I. Onset, *Ann Rheum Dis* 35:357–360, 1976.
8. Hoppenfeld S: *Physical examination of the spine and extremities*, Norwalk, Conn, 1976, Appleton and Lange.
9. Boutry N, Flipo RM, Cotton A: MR imaging appearance of rheumatoid arthritis in the foot, *Semin Musculoskelet Radiol* 9:199–209, 2005.
10. Seltzer SE, Weismann BN, Braunstein EM, et al.: Computed tomography of the hindfoot with rheumatoid arthritis, *Arthritis Rheum* 28:1234–1242, 1985.
11. Groshar D, Gorenberg M, Ben-Haim S, et al.: Lower extremity scintigraphy: the foot and ankle, *Semin Nucl Med* 28:62–77, 1998.
12. Riente L, Delle Sedie A, Iagnocco A, et al.: Ultrasound imaging for the rheumatologist. V. Ultrasonography of the ankle and foot, *Clin Exp Rheumatol* 24:493–498, 2006.
13. Khoury NK, el Khoury GY, Saltzman CL, et al.: Intrarticular foot and ankle injections to identify source of pain before arthrodesis, *AJR Am J Roentgenol* 167:669–673, 1996.
14. Vidigal E, Jacoby RK, Dixon AS, et al.: The foot in chronic rheumatoid arthritis, *Ann Rheum Dis* 34:292–297, 1975.
15. Jaakkola JI, Mann RA: A review of rheumatoid arthritis affecting the foot and ankle, *Foot Ankle Int* 25:866–874, 2004.
16. Spiegel TM, Spiegel JS: Rheumatoid arthritis in the foot and ankle—diagnosis, pathology and treatment, *Foot Ankle* 2:318–324, 1982.
17. Matteson EL: Current treatment strategies for rheumatoid arthritis, *Mayo Clin Proc* 75:69–74, 2000.
18. Conn DL, Lim SS: New role for an old friend: prednisone is a disease-modifying agent in early rheumatoid arthritis, *Curr Opin Rheumatol* 15:192–196, 2003.
19. Mohan AK, Cote TR, Siegel JN, et al.: Infectious complications of biologic treatment of rheumatoid arthritis, *Curr Opin Rheumatol* 15:179–184, 2003.
20. Coursin DB, Wood KE: Corticosteroid supplementation for adrenal insufficiency, *JAMA* 287:236–240, 2002.
21. Clark H, Rome K, Plant M, et al.: A critical review of foot orthoses in the rheumatoid arthritic foot, *Rheumatology* 45:139–145, 2006.
22. Woodburn J, Barker S, Helliwell PS: A randomised controlled trial of foot orthoses in rheumatoid arthritis, *J Rheumatol* 29:1377–1383, 2002.
23. Magalhaes E, Davitt M, Filho DJ, et al.: The effect of foot orthoses in rheumatoid arthritis, *Rheumatology* 45:449–453, 2006.
24. Hugate R, Pennypacker J, Saunders M, et al.: The effects of intratendinous and retrocalcaneal intrabursal injections of corticosteroid on the biomechanical properties of rabbit Achilles tendons, *J Bone Joint Surg Am* 86:794–801, 2004.
25. Lee HS, Jeong JJ, et al.: Risk factors affecting chronic rupture of the plantar fascia, *Foot Ankle Int* 35:258–263, 2014.
26. Chiodo CP, Martin T, Wilson MG: A technique for isolated arthrodesis for inflammatory arthritis of the talonavicular joint, *Foot Ankle Int* 21:307–310, 2000.
27. Astion DJ, Deland JT, Otis JC, et al.: Motion of the hindfoot after simulated arthrodesis, *J Bone Joint Surg Am* 79:241–246, 1997.
28. Coughlin M: Rheumatoid forefoot reconstruction. A long term follow-up study, *J Bone Joint Surg Am* 82:322–341, 2000.
29. Coester LM, Saltzman CL, Leupold J, et al.: Long-term results following ankle arthrodesis for post-traumatic arthritis, *J Bone Joint Surg Am* 83:219–228, 2001.
30. Thomas R, Daniels TR, Parker K: Gait analysis and functional outcomes following ankle arthrodesis for isolated ankle arthritis, *J Bone Joint Surg Am* 88:526–535, 2006.
31. Henricson A, Carlsson A, et al.: Bilateral arthrodesis of the ankle joint: Self-reported outcomes in 35 patients from the Swedish Ankle Registry, *J Foot Ankle Surg* 55:1195–1198, 2016.
32. Houdek M, Turner N, et al.: Radiographic and functional outcomes following bilateral ankle fusions, *Foot Ank Int* 35(12):1250–1254, 2014.
33. Daniels TR, Mayich DJ, Penner MJ: Intermediate to long-term outcomes of total ankle replacement with the Scandinavian Total Ankle Replacement (STAR), *J Bone Joint Surg Am* 97(11):895–903, 2015.
34. Saltzman CL, Mann RA, Ahrens JE, et al.: Prospective controlled trial of STAR total ankle replacement versus ankle fusion: initial results, *Foot Ankle Int* 30:579–596, 2009.
35. Benich MR, Sangeorzan BJ: Comparison of treatment outcomes of arthrodesis and two generations of ankle replacement implants, *J Bone Joint Surg Am 1* 99(21):1792–1800, 2017.
36. Deheer PA: The case against first metatarsal phalangeal joint implant arthroplasty, *Clin Podiatr Med Surg* 23:709–723, 2006.
37. Bommireddy R, Singh SK, Sharma P, et al.: Long term followup of Silastic joint replacement of the first metatarsophalangeal joint, *Foot* 12:151–155, 2003.
38. Shankar NS: Silastic single-stem implants in the treatment of hallux rigidus, *Foot Ankle Int* 16:487–491, 1995.
39. Gibson JN, Thomson C: Arthrodesis or total replacement arthroplasty for hallux rigidus: a randomized controlled trial, *Foot Ank Int* 26(9):680–690, 2005.
40. Baumhauer JF, Daniels T: Prospective, randomized, multi-centered clinical trial assessing safety and efficacy of a synthetic cartilage implant versus first metatarsophalangeal arthrodesis in advance hallux rigidus, *Foot Ank Int* 37(5):457–469, 2016.
41. Daniels T, Glazebrook M: Midterm outcomes of polyvinyl alcohol hydrogel hemiarthroplasty of the first metatarsophalangeal joint in advanced hallux rigidus, *Foot Ankle Int* 38(3):243–247, 2017.
42. Hattrup SJ, Johnson KA: Subjective results of hallux rigidus treatment with cheilectomy, *Clin Orthop Relat Res* 226:182–191, 1988.
43. Aho H, Halonen P: Synovectomy of the MTP joints in rheumatoid arthritis, *Acta Orthop Scand Suppl* 243(1), 1991.
44. Tokunaga D, Hojo T, Takatori R, et al.: Posterior tibial tendon tenosynovectomy for rheumatoid arthritis: a report of three cases, *Foot Ankle Int* 27:465–468, 2006.

53 Hand and Wrist Pain

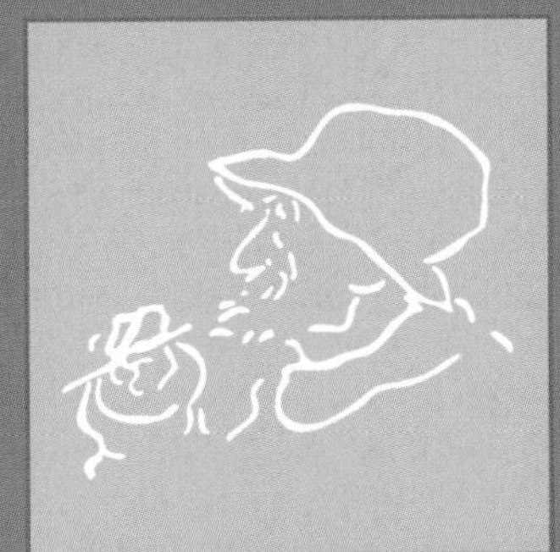

KENNETH W. DONOHUE, FELICITY G. FISHMAN, AND CARRIE R. SWIGART

KEY POINTS

- Patients with carpal tunnel syndrome typically present with nocturnal paresthesia and may have intermittent pain or paresthesia during the day.
- Ganglia are mucin-filled cysts arising from joint capsules or tendon sheaths. If they are painful, treatment with corticosteroid injections may be attempted. Recurrence is common and surgical excision may be necessary.
- De Quervain's disease, which is inflammation of the first dorsal compartment tendons (extensor pollicis brevis and abductor pollicis longus), is common in women and is associated with repetitive lifting activities, such as caring for an infant.
- Painful osteoarthritis involving the carpometacarpal joint of the thumb can often be treated successfully with splinting and nonsteroidal anti-inflammatory medication.
- Trigger fingers, caused by thickening of the A1 retinacular pulley in the palm, can usually be treated with corticosteroid injections.

Introduction

The multiple functions that the hand performs in daily life are usually taken for granted until the hand becomes affected by disease or injury. Depending on the nature of the disorder, patients have different adaptive capacities. Patients presenting with pain and dysfunction of the hand, wrist, or both represent a wide spectrum, diverse in age, occupations, and avocations. These patients have a broad range of medical conditions that may or may not be related to their current problem. Each patient has a different story to tell about his or her hand and wrist and why he or she is seeking treatment. It is the clinician's role to sort out these various factors, some of which may seem confounding, and determine the most appropriate diagnosis and treatment strategy.

This chapter presents guidelines that are useful in the evaluation of patients presenting with hand and wrist pain. Discussion of all of the various conditions that can affect the hand and wrist is beyond the scope of this chapter. Instead, this chapter highlights the most common disorders seen by general clinicians and hand surgeons. The conditions are grouped by their anatomic area to include pain localized to the volar, dorsal, radial, or ulnar wrist; the base of the thumb; and the palm and digits.

Patient Evaluation

Anatomy

The complex anatomy of the hand and wrist involves many structures that interact in close proximity to one another. Several different disorders can manifest with similar symptom patterns despite varying diagnoses. Precise knowledge of the anatomy of the hand and wrist helps to focus the diagnosis as a nerve, tendon, ligament, bone, or joint problem. The history of the illness, examination, and appropriate diagnostic tests help confirm the diagnosis. Several common sites of pain in the hand and wrist and their corresponding diagnoses are illustrated in Fig. 53.1. Pain in one location can have multiple causes depending on the patient profile and the history of the problem. A thorough review of the pertinent regional anatomy is important to help differentiate the many possible causes of hand and wrist pain.

History

Important patient factors include age, sex, hand dominance, occupation, hobbies, and sports. It is important to ask about recent trauma or activities that may have instigated the patient's symptoms. Next, questions about the duration, frequency, intensity, and quality of pain should be addressed. The pain of degenerative arthritis is often described as a localized, aching pain that is always present. In contrast, tendinitis is often associated with sharp, diffuse pain, which is only present with activity. Rheumatoid arthritis (RA) manifests initially with hand and wrist involvement in 25% of patients and is characterized by bilateral hand and wrist involvement with joint effusion and morning stiffness. Peripheral nerve entrapment, such as carpal tunnel syndrome, is associated with nighttime paresthesia that the patient may describe as feeling like "pins and needles." Trigger finger involves painful locking of the digits that is usually worse in the morning and improves throughout the day. Activities that provoke pain should also be noted. Arthritis at the base of the thumb is often aggravated by opening jars, turning doorknobs, and doing needlework or other hobbies.

Physical Examination

A thorough examination of the involved extremity and comparison with the uninvolved extremity are essential. Attention should be directed to abnormalities of the more proximal joints of the elbow and shoulder and the cervical spine. As the differential diagnosis narrows, the examination should be tailored to include or eliminate any possible systemic causes. As with other musculoskeletal examinations, the range of motion of the involved joints should be observed and compared with the opposite side. Any difference between active and passive motion should be noted. Careful palpation for the site of maximal tenderness is important

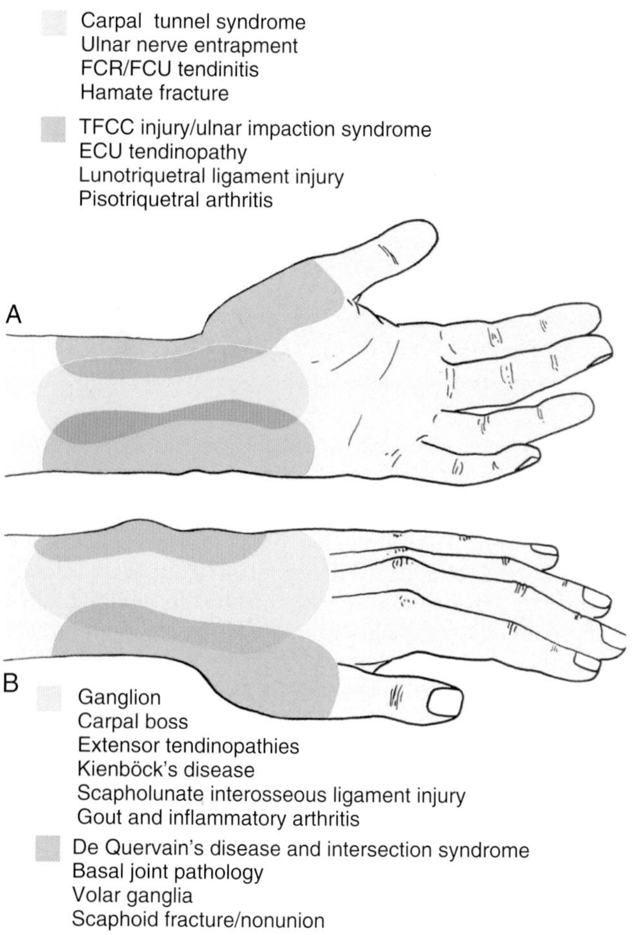

A

Carpal tunnel syndrome
Ulnar nerve entrapment
FCR/FCU tendinitis
Hamate fracture

TFCC injury/ulnar impaction syndrome
ECU tendinopathy
Lunotriquetral ligament injury
Pisotriquetral arthritis

B

Ganglion
Carpal boss
Extensor tendinopathies
Kienböck's disease
Scapholunate interosseous ligament injury
Gout and inflammatory arthritis

De Quervain's disease and intersection syndrome
Basal joint pathology
Volar ganglia
Scaphoid fracture/nonunion

• **Fig. 53.1** (A) Palmar and ulnar view of the hand and wrist with areas of pain and tenderness marked with their corresponding leading differential diagnoses. (B) Dorsal and radial view of the hand and wrist with areas of pain and tenderness marked with their corresponding leading differential diagnoses. *ECU,* Extensor carpi ulnaris; *FCR,* flexor carpi radialis; *FCU,* flexor carpi ulnaris; *TFCC,* triangular fibrocartilage complex.

in differentiating the source of the pain. Measurements of grip and pinch strength are also helpful in many situations as a diagnostic aid and a baseline measurement to follow for improvement. Many provocative maneuvers are useful in differentiating causes of pain; these maneuvers are discussed later in the chapter.

Imaging Studies

Technologic advances have increased the availability of imaging studies for the hand and wrist. Improvements in MRI resolution using small joint coils allow for more precise imaging of small structures in the hand and wrist. Ultrasound allows for dynamic assessment of tendon and nerve issues. With the multitude of ancillary studies available, it is important to be selective in using these tools. With cost containment in mind, imaging studies should be used most often to confirm a diagnosis rather than to find one. An understanding of the advantages and limitations of each tool is necessary to enable them to be used appropriately.

Among the available tools, plain radiographs are the easiest to perform and most readily available. A routine hand or wrist series, including anteroposterior, lateral, and oblique views, is a useful screening tool but often lacks the required specificity. Depending on the suspected diagnosis, many special views are available. These views are discussed later in this chapter with the specific diagnoses to which they pertain.

When further detail of the bony anatomy is required, CT is currently the best available tool. The most common uses for CT in the hand and wrist include evaluation of intra-articular fractures of the distal radius and metacarpals, scaphoid fractures and non-unions, and intraosseous cysts or tumors.[1,2]

Advances in ultrasound and MRI technology have enhanced our ability to evaluate the soft tissue structures of the hand and wrist. Smaller ultrasound probes with higher resolution have made it possible to visualize and differentiate structures such as flexor tendons, ganglion cysts, and ligaments. MRI technology is constantly improving, providing new uses in the hand and wrist. By altering the parameters of this test, information about anatomy and physiology can be obtained.[3] Specific uses of these tests and others, such as arthrography, ultrasound, and bone scans, are addressed with the diagnoses for which they are most useful.

Additional Diagnostic Tests

Neurodiagnostic Tests

Neurodiagnostic tests, including nerve conduction studies and electromyography, are useful in the diagnosis of suspected neurologic disorders of the upper extremity. Specifying the type and nature of the examination required enhances the information gained by these studies. If a nerve compression syndrome such as carpal or cubital tunnel syndrome is suspected, nerve conduction studies may be sufficient without the added cost and patient discomfort of formal electromyographic testing. Nerve conduction studies evaluate the speed of conduction of motor and sensory nerves across a set distance at a specific location and compare this speed with established normal values. A decrease in the speed of nerve conduction, as evidenced by an increase in the latency, is seen with localized nerve compression and is shown in several different nerves concomitantly in demyelinating diseases such as multiple sclerosis. When more severe nerve injuries are suspected or if there is clinical evidence of muscle weakness or atrophy, an electromyogram can be useful to evaluate the extent of the process or rule out a myopathic process.[4]

Injections and Aspirations

The use of injections and aspirations can be therapeutic and diagnostic. Corticosteroids can be administered selectively in conjunction with a local anesthetic for more lasting relief and in some cases can be curative.[5–11] Some of the most common sites for injection are the A1 pulley region of the finger for trigger finger, the carpal canal for carpal tunnel syndrome, and the first dorsal compartment of the wrist for de Quervain's disease.

Aspiration of joints or other fluid collections, such as ganglia, can yield vital diagnostic information and be therapeutic. If infection is suspected, aspiration should be used to obtain a sample of joint fluid for gram stain, cell count, and culture. Diagnoses such as gout and pseudogout can be confirmed by crystal analysis under polarized light. Many ganglia and retinacular cysts can be treated temporarily or permanently with simple aspiration.[12,13]

The accuracy of injections and aspirations can be increased with the use of ultrasound. This modality can aid in the injection of symptomatic trigger fingers, de Quervain's tenosynovitis, and carpal tunnel syndrome. Ultrasound-guided injections were found to be in the tendon sheath 70% of the time versus 15% of the time when ultrasound was not used.[14,15] Joint injections or aspirations, as well as aspiration of ganglia, can also be greatly aided by ultrasound guidance.[16]

Arthroscopy

Direct visualization of a joint via arthroscopy can be an invaluable diagnostic tool. Despite the increasing sensitivity of imaging techniques such as MRI, arthroscopy provides a dynamic evaluation that static imaging cannot provide.[17] Since the first published report of a series of cases by investigators in 1988,[18] it has become the "gold standard" for evaluation of chronic wrist pain.[19–21] With new surgical techniques being developed, surgeons often can proceed directly to the definitive treatment using arthroscopy entirely or in part.[22–27]

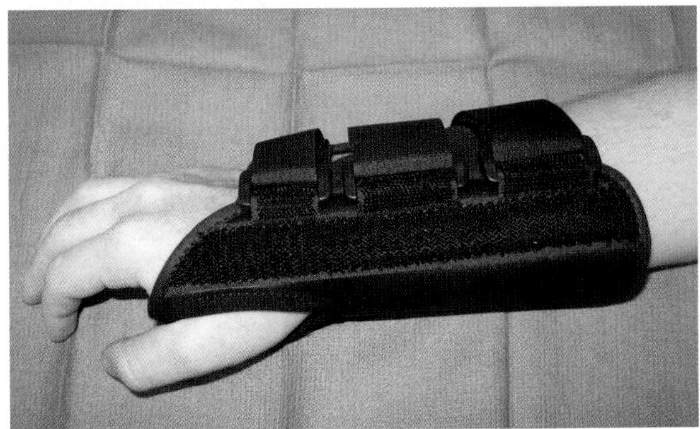

• **Fig. 53.2** Typical night splint used to treat carpal tunnel syndrome.

Common Causes of Hand and Wrist Pain

Wrist Pain: Palmar

Carpal Tunnel Syndrome

Carpal tunnel syndrome (CTS) is the most commonly diagnosed compression neuropathy in the upper extremity. It usually occurs as an isolated phenomenon, but symptoms of CTS can accompany many systemic diseases, such as congestive heart failure, multiple myeloma, and tuberculosis.[28–31] More commonly, CTS is associated with conditions such as pregnancy, diabetes, obesity, RA, and gout.[32–42]

The classic constellation of symptoms consists of nocturnal paresthesia in the affected digits; paresthesia or hypoesthesia in the thumb, index, and long fingers; and weakness or clumsiness of the hand. Patients often report forearm and elbow pain that is aggravated by activities but is poorly localized and aching in nature. Occasionally, more proximal symptoms such as shoulder pain are the main presenting complaint.[43] Past reports have indicated a 3 : 1 prevalence of CTS in women. Approximately half of patients are aged 40 to 60 years, although occasionally CTS has been diagnosed in children.[44,45]

The diagnosis of CTS is usually clinical. Tinel's sign, shown by radiating paresthesia in the median nerve distribution with gentle percussion over the volar wrist, indicates nerve irritation. Reproduction of symptoms with wrist flexion, as described by Phalen,[46] and with the carpal compression test, as described by Durkan,[47] is more specific.[48] Decreased sensibility and thenar atrophy are late signs seen in people with advanced median nerve entrapment. Bilateral electrodiagnostic tests, specifically nerve conduction velocity testing, should be used to confirm the diagnosis, particularly in patients claiming a compensable injury or in patients with atypical signs or symptoms. Prolonged motor and sensory latencies across the carpal canal confirm pathologic compression of the median nerve.[49–51] In patients with classic clinical findings, a study found that CTS could be diagnosed with a high degree of accuracy on clinical grounds alone and that the addition of electrodiagnostic tests did not increase the accuracy.[52] When attempting to differentiate CTS from more proximal nerve entrapments such as cervical root compression or thoracic outlet syndrome, the addition of electromyography of the cervical paraspinal muscles and proximal conduction tests (H reflex, f waves) can be useful.[53]

Conservative treatment for CTS consists of splinting the wrist in a neutral position and considering oral nonsteroidal anti-inflammatory drugs (NSAIDs) for pain control. Splinting should be used sparingly during the workday to prevent secondary muscle weakness and fatigue and is best prescribed to prevent provocative wrist positioning at night. The splint should not hold the wrist in extension beyond 10 degrees (Fig. 53.2). "Off the shelf" splints often need to be manipulated to neutral or 10 degrees of extension before being provided to the patient. Although splinting may be beneficial for relief of symptoms in cases of mild compression, its long-term effectiveness is limited.[54] The use of vitamin B_6 (100 to 200 mg/day) has been helpful in some cases, but its efficacy has not been confirmed in a randomized trial. The popularity of corticosteroid injections in the treatment of CTS has waxed and waned during the past half century. Although it is quite effective in the short term, the long-term efficacy is mixed.[55–57] In addition, injections have been associated with exacerbation of the condition and permanent median nerve injury if performed incorrectly.[58,59] For these reasons, injections are most often indicated in cases when the condition is thought to be temporary, such as with pregnancy, or if surgery must be deferred because of a medical condition or major life event.

Surgical release is indicated for patients with confirmed CTS who have not responded to a course of conservative treatment. In patients who exhibit late findings of objective sensory loss or thenar atrophy, early surgery should be recommended. The incision for a modern carpal tunnel release is not more than 3 cm long and parallels the skin creases of the palm (Fig. 53.3).

Ulnar Nerve Entrapment: Cubital Tunnel Syndrome

Entrapment of the ulnar nerve as it passes through the cubital tunnel just posterior to the medial epicondyle of the elbow can manifest with symptoms localized to the ulnar border of the hand. Medial forearm pain and irritability of the ulnar nerve at the elbow may be present as well. Presenting symptoms usually consist of paresthesia, numbness, or both in the small and ring fingers. Percussion of the nerve in the cubital tunnel elicits Tinel's sign. Prolonged elbow flexion reproduces the symptoms. In contrast to CTS, it is not unusual for patients to present with early atrophy of the intrinsics, which is most easily appreciated in the first dorsal interosseous muscle.

Electrodiagnostic studies can help confirm the diagnosis and differentiate cubital tunnel syndrome from more distal compression of the ulnar nerve in Guyon's canal (discussed in a later section). If malalignment of the elbow is present or the patient relates a history of childhood trauma, radiographs should be obtained to rule out a supracondylar or epicondylar malunion. So-called tardy ulnar nerve palsy can develop years after a supracondylar fracture of the elbow.[60]

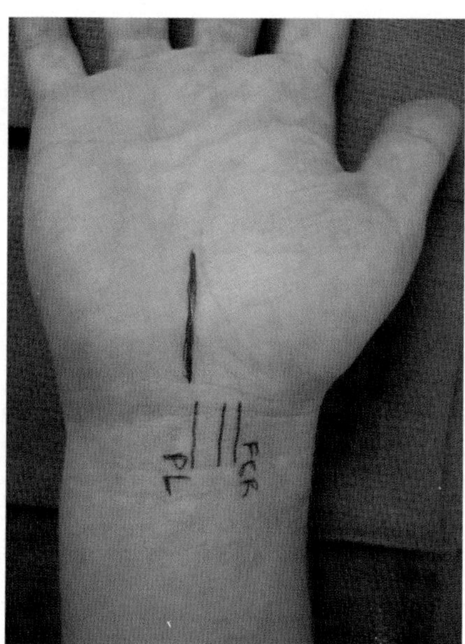

• **Fig. 53.3** Usual incision used for release of the carpal tunnel. Note its position just ulnar to the course of the palmaris longus tendon (PL) and the relative position of the flexor carpi radialis tendon (FCR).

Conservative treatment includes strategies to help the patient avoid having the elbow flexed for prolonged periods, particularly at night. Soft or semirigid elbow splints prevent elbow flexion beyond 50 to 70 degrees. NSAIDs can be beneficial in acute or traumatic cases. Surgical decompression of the nerve is indicated when a person does not obtain relief from splinting and activity modification or when clinical or electrodiagnostic evidence of muscle denervation is present.

Ulnar Nerve Entrapment: Guyon's Canal

In 1861 Guyon[61] published a description of the contents of an anatomic canal at the wrist. The distal branches of the ulnar nerve and the ulnar artery pass through this space. As it exits the canal, the ulnar nerve divides into its sensory and motor branches. Compression of the nerve within or proximal to the canal usually manifests with a combination of sensory and motor symptoms in the ulnar nerve distribution. Patients report numbness and paresthesia of the palmar aspect of the ring and small fingers. Motor symptoms are usually described as a cramping weakness with grasping and pinching. As with median neuropathy, atrophy of the intrinsics and objective sensory loss are late findings.

In contrast to carpal tunnel syndrome, in which patients usually have an ill-defined onset of symptoms, ulnar nerve compression in the canal of Guyon is often of more acute onset. It can be associated with repeated blunt trauma,[62–64] a fracture of the hamate or the metacarpal bases, or occasionally a fracture of the distal radius.[65,66] Space-occupying lesions such as a ganglion, lipoma, or anomalous muscle can also cause compression.[67–71] Because of the difference in etiology, this nerve entrapment syndrome often is not amenable to conservative treatment. If an anatomic lesion such as a fracture or a mass is present, it must be addressed. If repetitive blunt trauma is the cause, without associated fracture or arterial thrombosis, splinting and activity modification can alleviate the symptoms.

Flexor Carpi Radialis and Flexor Carpi Ulnaris Tendinitis

Similar to other tendinopathies around the wrist, irritation of the wrist flexors occurs with stress of the wrist in a particular position. Activities that require forced wrist flexion for prolonged periods or with repetition put patients at risk for inflammation around the flexor carpi radialis tendon,[72] the flexor carpi ulnaris tendon, or both. The condition manifests with tenderness along the course of the tendon, especially near its insertion. Wrist flexion against resistance with radial or ulnar deviation reproduces the symptoms. Treatment consists of splinting and rest, elimination of activities that cause pain, and use of oral NSAIDs. Injection of a corticosteroid into the flexor carpi radialis or flexor carpi ulnaris sheath may be curative. Sharp pain that is associated with an intense inflammatory localized reaction is suggestive of calcific tendinitis and is most commonly seen around the flexor carpi ulnaris tendon.[73,74] If calcific tendinitis is suspected, a plain radiograph can be useful in confirming the diagnosis, but the calcification may not become apparent until 7 to 10 days after the onset of symptoms.

Hamate Fracture

An uncommon and underdiagnosed cause of palmar pain in young, active people is a fracture of the hook of the hamate. These fractures can occur from a fall on an extended wrist, from a "dubbed" golf shot, or from forcefully striking a ball with a club or bat. Plain radiographs of the wrist are usually read as normal. Pain in the base of the palm overlying the hamate is the most common presenting symptom. Often the pain is present only with the activity that caused the fracture. Because of the proximity of the ulnar nerve, patients can also have sensory and motor symptoms of distal ulnar neuropathy. Occasionally, in the acute setting, vascular complaints such as cold intolerance or frank ischemia from ulnar artery thrombosis can be the presenting condition. Fracture of the hamate hook has also been reported to cause rupture of flexor tendons if left untreated.[75]

A carpal tunnel radiographic view, obtained with the wrist in a hyperextended position, may show the fracture (Fig. 53.4A). Alternatively, a selective CT scan through the hamate is a more accurate way to confirm the diagnosis (Fig. 53.4B).[76] If diagnosed within 2 to 3 weeks of injury, casting should be attempted to allow the fracture to heal.[77] If casting fails to achieve healing or if the fracture is diagnosed late, surgical treatment is indicated; most authors favor excision of the hook, followed by a gradual return to activities.[78–81]

Wrist Pain: Dorsal

Ganglion

Ganglia account for 50% to 70% of all soft tissue tumors of the hand and wrist. Of these, 60% to 70% occur around the dorsal wrist. These mucin-filled cysts usually arise from an adjacent joint capsule or tendon sheath. The most common site of origin in the wrist is the scapholunate ligament. Although most ganglia occur as a well-circumscribed and obvious soft mass, some are evident only with the wrist in marked volar flexion. As a result of their characteristic appearance, ganglia usually are not misdiagnosed but should be differentiated from the less well-demarcated swelling of extensor tenosynovitis, lipomas, and other hand tumors. Plain radiographs are typically normal but occasionally show an intraosseous cyst or an osteoarthritic joint. Some ganglia may not be clinically apparent and are known as *occult ganglia*. Ultrasound and MRI are useful in the diagnosis of these ganglia.[82,83]

Not all ganglia are painful. Patients may present with reports of wrist weakness or simply because of the cosmetic appearance of the cyst. In approximately 10% of cases, evidence of associated trauma to the wrist is seen. The ganglia may appear suddenly or develop over many months. Intermittent complete resorption followed by reappearance months or years later is common.

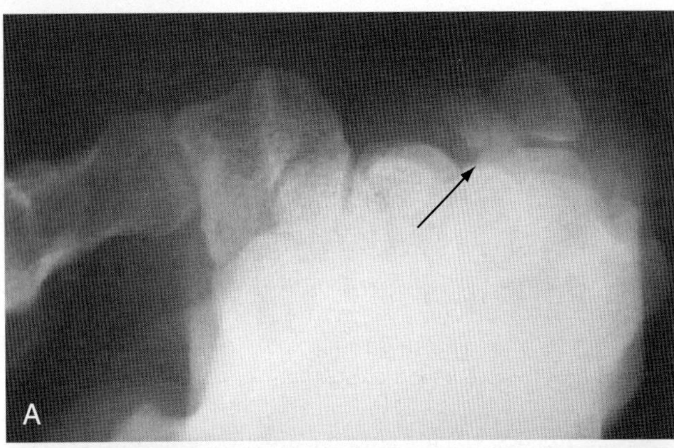

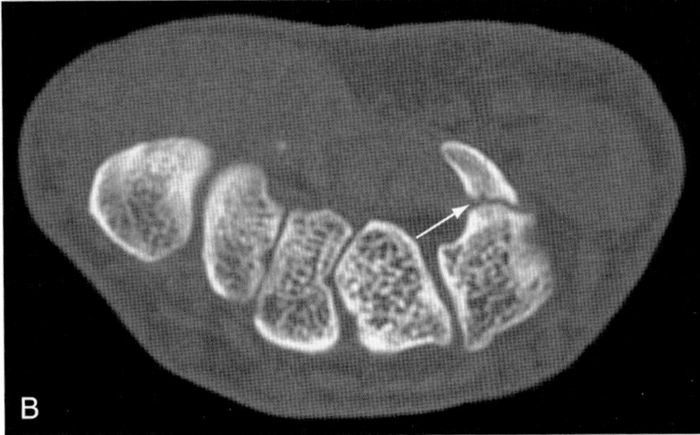

• **Fig. 53.4** (A) Carpal tunnel view radiograph showing a hamate hook fracture *(arrow)*. (B) Coronal CT scan showing the same hamate hook fracture *(arrow)*.

Most conservative measures such as splinting and rest have only a temporary effect on ganglia. They tend to diminish in size with rest and enlarge with increased activity. Spontaneous rupture is common, and, at one time, attempting to rupture the cyst with a heavy object, such as a large book, was recommended as treatment. Aspiration can be performed but has mixed results because of the thick gelatinous nature of the fluid within the cyst. Even if adequate decompression of the cyst can be achieved, reaccumulation of the fluid usually occurs. Aspiration in conjunction with irrigation or injection of corticosteroids can be effective in alleviating the symptoms for varying periods.[12,13,84]

Occasionally a ganglion can interfere with the function of the wrist by limiting motion, especially in extension. Pressure of the mass on the terminal branches of the posterior interosseous nerve may be painful. Excision is generally curative but may result in short-term stiffness and some loss of terminal flexion as a result of surgical scarring. Occasionally a patient desires excision of the cyst for cosmetic reasons. With proper excision, recurrence is less than 10%,[85–87] but when the dissection is incomplete and fails to identify the origin of the cyst, recurrence rates can reach 50%. Arthroscopic resection is a safe and effective method of treating dorsal wrist ganglia.[26,27]

Carpal Boss

Often confused with a dorsal ganglion, the carpal boss is a bony, nonmobile prominence on the dorsum of the wrist. It is an osteoarthritic spur that forms at the second or third carpometacarpal joints.[88] The boss is most evident with the wrist in volar flexion. The vast majority are asymptomatic, but some people may present with pain and localized tenderness over the prominence. The condition is twice as common in women as in men, and most patients are in their 20s to 30s. Radiographs are best taken with the hand and wrist in 30 to 40 degrees of supination and 20 to 30 degrees of ulnar deviation to put the bony prominence on profile (the *carpal boss view*).[89] Conservative treatment consists of rest, immobilization, NSAIDs, and occasionally injection with corticosteroids. If persistently painful despite these measures, surgical excision of the boss may be necessary but is associated with a prolonged recovery and continued symptoms in a high percentage of patients.

Extensor Tendinopathies

The extensor pollicis longus (EPL) tendon can be irritated as it passes around Lister's tubercle. In contrast to other tendinopathies around the wrist, this condition carries a significant risk of tendon rupture. Early diagnosis and sometimes urgent operative treatment are necessary to prevent this complication. Localized pain, swelling, and tenderness are the hallmarks of this condition, and, similar to other tendinopathies, initial treatment consists of decreased activity and splinting. A short course of oral anti-inflammatory medication can be useful in decreasing symptoms. Diagnostic injections with lidocaine can help differentiate the condition from other causes of wrist pain, but corticosteroid injections are not routinely used in this condition because of a propensity for the EPL to rupture in chronic cases.

Patients may present with a rupture of the EPL without antecedent pain or swelling. It is well-known that EPL rupture is associated with fractures of the distal radius that likely occur as a result of a relative "watershed zone" of vascular supply within its tight retinacular sheath as it passes around Lister's tubercle of the distal radius. Tendon rupture most often occurs with minimally displaced or nondisplaced fractures and can occur several weeks or months after the original injury.[90–93] People with RA and systemic lupus erythematosus are especially prone to rupture of the EPL and other tendons.

Kienböck's Disease

Kienböck's disease is named for Dr. Robert Kienböck,[94] who in 1910 first described what he postulated were avascular changes in the lunate. Nearly a century later, the cause of this disease remains unclear; it is likely multifactorial. Kienböck's disease should be suspected when a young adult presents with pain and stiffness of the wrist and swelling and tenderness around the region of the dorsal lunate. An increased propensity of the disease occurs among patients with an ulna that is anatomically shorter than the radius (so-called ulnar negative variance). Radiographs are needed to confirm and stage the process. Kienböck's disease is staged by the degree of fragmentation and collapse of the lunate, associated osteoarthritis, and carpal collapse in a system originally proposed by Stahl.[95] In this system, the earliest sign of the disease is a linear or compression fracture in the lunate. Later stages show sclerosis of the lunate, followed by lunate collapse and a loss of carpal height. In the final stage, the carpus shows signs of diffuse osteoarthritis with complete collapse and fragmentation of the lunate (Fig. 53.5). With the increased sensitivity of MRI, it is possible to identify avascular changes within the lunate before they become evident on plain radiographs. These avascular changes are referred to as "stage zero" Kienböck's disease.

The treatment for Kienböck's disease is largely surgical. Based on the stage of the disease and the postulated cause, several surgical procedures have been described. In early stages of the disease, when lunate collapse is minimal and no osteoarthritis is present,

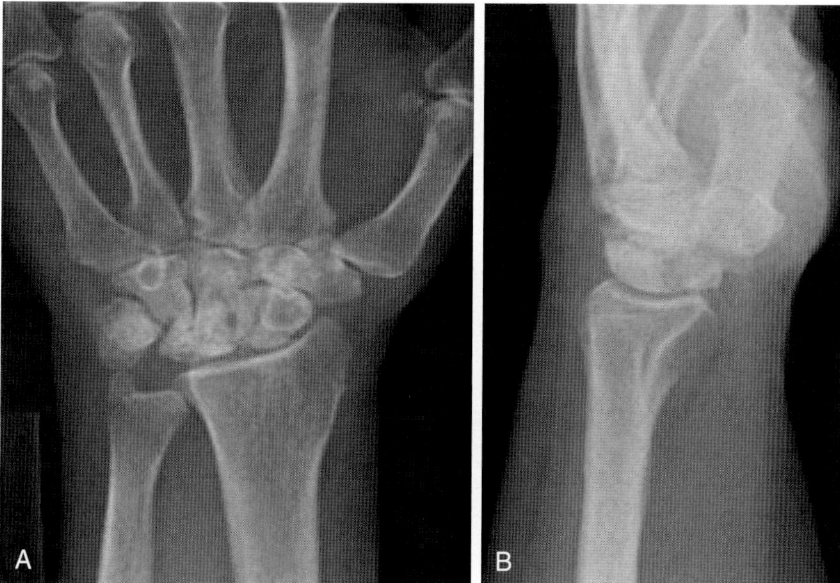

• **Fig. 53.5** Advanced Kienböck's disease, showing carpal collapse, intercarpal and radiocarpal arthrosis, and fragmentation of the lunate. (A) Posteroanterior view. (B) Lateral view.

the goal of surgery is to "unload" the lunate by redistributing articular contact forces and allowing it to revascularize.[96–99] The most common procedure is a radial shortening osteotomy that is performed to neutralize the ulnar variance. In later stages, various intercarpal arthrodeses have been used to readjust and maintain carpal height and alignment.[100–102] More recently, microsurgical techniques have been used to revascularize the lunate with promising early results.[103]

Scapholunate Interosseous Ligament Injury

The interosseous ligament between the scaphoid and the lunate is a stout structure, especially dorsally, and usually requires a significant force to cause disruption. The typical mechanism of injury is a fall onto the outstretched hand with the wrist extended. Early diagnosis is essential to prevent the late sequelae of carpal collapse. The key radiographic features of scapholunate dissociation (scapholunate interval widening) are shown in Fig. 53.6. The anteroposterior view shows the scapholunate interval better than the posteroanterior view.[104] Early surgical intervention is recommended with the goals of maintaining carpal alignment and preventing an otherwise inevitable progression to carpal collapse and degenerative arthritis.

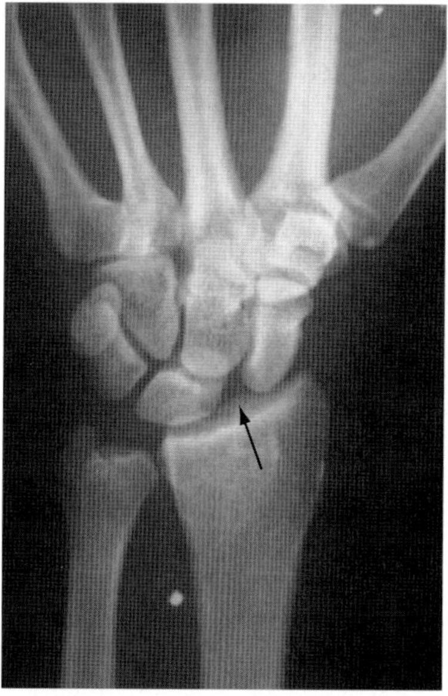

• **Fig. 53.6** Anteroposterior radiograph of the wrist showing scapholunate interosseous space widening *(arrow)* and scaphoid foreshortening associated with scapholunate interosseous ligament disruption.

Gout and Inflammatory Arthritis

All of the inflammatory arthritides, including the crystal arthropathies, can manifest as dorsal wrist pain. Approximately 25% of patients with a diagnosis of RA present initially with hand and wrist symptoms. The reader is referred to Chapters 94 to 96 for further details.

Wrist Pain: Ulnar

Triangular Fibrocartilage Complex Injury and Ulnocarpal Impaction Syndrome

One of the most complex and confusing areas of the wrist from a diagnostic standpoint is the articulation of the ulna with the carpus. The triangular fibrocartilage complex (TFCC), so named by Palmer and Werner,[105] comprises the articular disk itself and the immediately surrounding ulnocarpal ligaments. It can be injured by a variety of acute and chronic mechanisms. Hyperpronation and hypersupination of the carpus during forceful activities are the usual causes of acute injuries, whereas repetitive pronation and supination more often cause attritional changes in the TFCC.

The radius and ulna must remain congruent through a 190-degree arc.[106] Limitation of motion and pain with pronation and supination are consistent with a tear of the supporting ligaments and resultant distal radioulnar joint (DRUJ) instability. If a sufficient portion of the stability has been lost, the ulna appears clinically dislocated or subluxated, and forearm rotation is severely limited. Lateral radiographs of the wrist in neutral and full pronation and supination generally are not specific enough to confirm ulnar subluxation. To evaluate better the congruency of the DRUJ

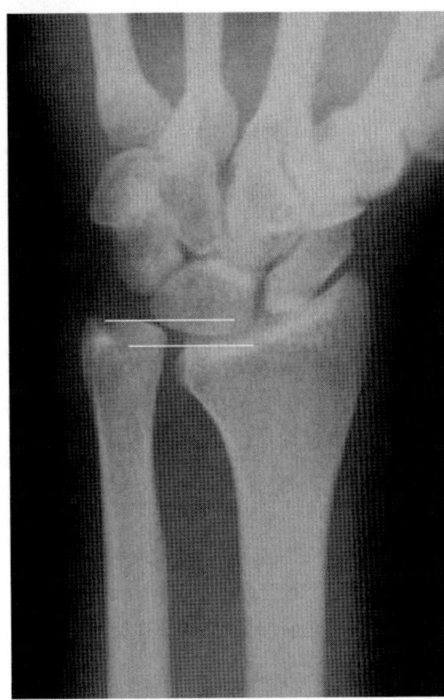

• **Fig. 53.7** Posteroanterior radiograph of the wrist in neutral forearm rotation showing the method of measuring ulnar variance by drawing tangential lines to the distal ulna and distal radius. The space between these lines in millimeters is the ulnar variance. A positive value indicates that the ulnar length is greater than the radial length.

through its range of motion and to assess for subtle subluxations, CT can be performed on both wrists simultaneously in positions of neutral, full pronation, and full supination.[107–110]

Tears of the TFCC may manifest with painful clicking during wrist rotation. Patients generally have localized tenderness on the midaxial border of the wrist and directly beneath the extensor carpi ulnaris tendon. If forced ulnar deviation of the wrist or gripping reproduces the patient's symptoms, a degenerative tear of the central portion of the TFCC is more likely. The degenerative tear is frequently a component of the ulnocarpal impaction syndrome, a condition associated with higher than normal loads on the ulnar carpus secondary to a congenitally positive ulnar variance.

Plain radiographs are most useful in determining ulnar variance and for ruling out fractures or arthritis as a cause of ulnar wrist pain. Because of the variable relationship of the radius and ulna depending on forearm rotation, it is important to take standardized films when measuring ulnar variance.[111,112] A posteroanterior view of the wrist with the shoulder abducted to 90 degrees and the elbow flexed to 90 degrees shows the DRUJ in neutral forearm rotation and is easily reproducible (Fig. 53.7). Because the ulna lengthens relative to the radius during power grip, a radiograph in the same position during maximal grip best shows impaction of the ulna on the carpus.

Ancillary studies for TFCC tears include three-compartmental arthrography and MRI. In arthrography, sequential injections of radiopaque dye are performed into the carpal joint, midcarpal joint, and DRUJ. The test is considered positive when the dye is seen leaking from one compartment to another. The site of the leak determines the location of the torn structure.[113] Several studies, however, have shown that age-related attritional tears occur in the TFCC and other ligamentous structures of the wrist.[114–116] Technologic advancements in MRI have improved the ability to visualize and diagnose abnormalities in the TFCC. MRI can be combined with arthrography to better visualize the TFCC and the intrinsic wrist ligaments. Peripheral detachments and central degenerative tears of the TFCC can be visualized. MRI remains highly operator dependent and technique dependent, and the studies should be interpreted in the context of the findings on physical examination.[117]

Patients presenting with pain localized to the ulnar side of the wrist often respond to simple splinting and rest. This conservative treatment and NSAIDs can be used effectively while a workup is in progress. A course of rest and splinting, followed by a gradual return to activities, may completely alleviate ulnar-sided symptoms.

Despite the advancements in imaging techniques, there is often no substitute for direct visualization of the ulnocarpal joint, DRUJ, or both. Arthroscopy has become an invaluable diagnostic and surgical tool. Tears of the TFCC can be visualized and their clinical significance better determined. Arthroscopy, performed in conjunction with fluoroscopy, can assess for instability of the DRUJ, intercarpal joints, or both. Several surgical procedures can now be performed entirely or in part through the arthroscope.[118,119]

Extensor Carpi Ulnaris Tendinitis and Subluxation

The extensor carpi ulnaris tendon can become irritated with forced pronation/supination activities, such as putting topspin on a tennis ball. In severe cases the tendon can become unstable around the ulnar head as its restraining dorsal retinaculum becomes increasingly lax. Patients report pain with forceful rotation of the forearm, and sometimes an associated snapping of the extensor carpi ulnaris (ECU) tendon is present. Early treatment consists of immobilization of the wrist and forearm to prevent rotation. Anti-inflammatory oral medication or a cortisone injection can help decrease the inflammation more quickly. After an adequate period of rest, if the acute inflammation resolves but the ECU tendon continues to be unstable, surgery may be indicated to reconstruct or release the sheath at the wrist.

Pisotriquetral Arthritis

Degenerative changes in the pisotriquetral articulation are usually post-traumatic in nature. Patients may recall a fall onto the extended wrist with direct trauma to the ulnar side of the palm. Affected individuals present with pain during passive wrist hyperextension and exacerbation with flexion against resistance. Tenderness and often crepitus occurs with palpation of the pisotriquetral joint. As with many joints, splinting, NSAIDs, and occasionally injection with corticosteroid and lidocaine are the mainstays of conservative treatment. If this approach is inadequate to control the symptoms, surgical resection of the pisiform is indicated.

Wrist Pain: Radial and Thumb

De Quervain's Disease and Intersection Syndrome

One of the most common sites of tendon irritation around the wrist is in the first dorsal extensor compartment, a phenomenon known as de Quervain's disease. The tendons involved are the extensor pollicis brevis (EPB) and the abductor pollicis longus (APL). At the level of the radial styloid, these two tendons pass through an osteoligamentous tunnel composed of a shallow groove in the radius and an overlying ligament. Anatomic studies have shown that a high percentage of patients have a divided first dorsal compartment, with separate compartments for the EPB and APL slips, and this feature can account for failure of conservative treatment and injections.[120–122]

People with de Quervain's disease are typically women in their 30s and 40s, although the condition can develop in men and women at any age. De Quervain's disease is the most common tendinopathy to develop in postpartum women because of the specific hand and wrist position requirements in the care of an infant. Any activity requiring repeated thumb abduction and extension in combination with wrist radial and ulnar deviation can aggravate this problem. Patients report pain along the course of these tendons with grasping activities. Clinically, tenderness is present along the affected compartment, and swelling may be present over the radial styloid. In severe cases, a creaking sound can be elicited with movement of the involved tendons. Finkelstein's test of forced ulnar deviation of the wrist with the thumb clasped in the fisted palm is pathognomonic of the condition.[123,124]

A less common condition that may occur in the same general location in the wrist is intersection syndrome. Although initially attributed to friction between the first and second dorsal compartment tendons, Grundberg and Reagan[125] subsequently showed that the condition represented a tendinopathy of the radial wrist extensors within the second dorsal compartment.

The primary treatment for de Quervain's disease and intersection syndrome is rest with splinting. For de Quervain's disease, the wrist should be held in slight extension and the thumb abducted in a thumb spica splint to the level of the interphalangeal joint. Immobilization of the wrist alone, in approximately 15 degrees of extension, is usually adequate for intersection syndrome. The addition of a 2- to 4-week course of anti-inflammatory medication can also be helpful. Phonophoresis with a cortisone cream and injection of the compartment with cortisone are second-line treatments if immobilization alone fails to provide adequate relief. Injection of corticosteroid into the affected first dorsal compartment is curative for de Quervain's disease in approximately 75% of patients.[126] Surgery may be indicated for patients who do not respond to a course of conservative treatment, including injection. For de Quervain's disease and intersection syndrome, surgery consists of releasing the stenotic retinacular sheath of the involved compartment.

Basal Joint Arthropathy

Inflammation and pain related to the carpometacarpal joint of the thumb are common and can occur at any age. In younger patients, instability secondary to ligamentous laxity is associated with joint subluxation and abnormal cartilage wear and may lead to pain with mechanical activities. In women older than 45 years, studies show that 25% have radiographic evidence of degeneration of the basal joint.[127,128] Patients generally present with pain at the base of the thumb, which is worsened by pinch activities. They often report difficulty with tasks such as opening jars and bottles or turning doorknobs and keys. The thumb carpometacarpal joint may be swollen and subluxed and is generally tender to palpation. The joint should be assessed for the presence of increased laxity by manual subluxation of the base of the metacarpal out of the trapezial "saddle" with radial and volar force. With advanced degenerative disease, crepitus is sometimes appreciated.

Radiographs should be obtained to determine the stage of the disease. The addition of a basal joint posteroanterior stress film, in which the patient presses the tips of the thumbs together firmly with the nail plates facing up, is helpful in assessing joint subluxation (Fig. 53.8). The most commonly used staging system, which was developed by Eaton and Glickel,[129] is based on the degree of involvement of the trapeziometacarpal joint and whether the scaphotrapezial joint is involved.[129] Advancing stages show increased subluxation of the basal joint with development of joint space narrowing, osteophytes, and subchondral cysts.

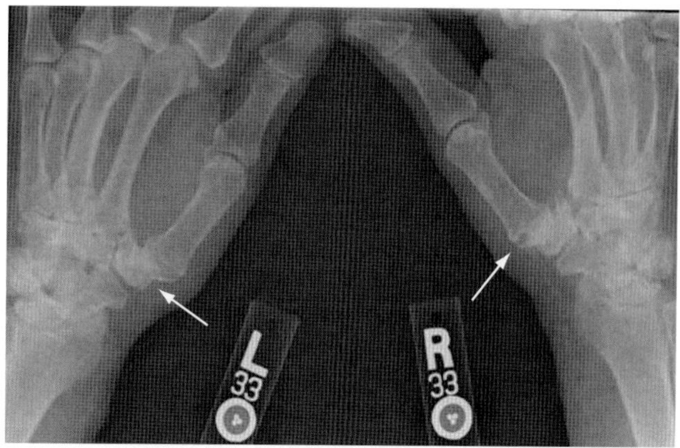

• **Fig. 53.8** Basal joint stress radiograph showing stage 3 degeneration of the left thumb and stage 4 degeneration of the right thumb.

Regardless of the stage of the disease, the first line of treatment is immobilization of the thumb carpometacarpal joint, leaving the interphalangeal joint free. Splinting alleviates the symptoms of carpometacarpal joint inflammation in more than 50% of patients.[130] NSAIDs can be a useful adjunct. Injections of a corticosteroid are effective, usually for just a limited time. Although therapy for thenar muscle strengthening has been advocated, especially in early stages, its benefits are minimal, and occasionally it can aggravate the problem.

Many people are able to manage their symptoms with a combination of splinting, medications, corticosteroid injections, and activity modification. The most effective splints are those that are custom made of a moldable plastic material. They may be hand based as shown in Fig. 53.9 or forearm based to immobilize the wrist as well. If these various nonoperative treatments are insufficient, surgery may be indicated. In people with advanced degenerative changes and those whose symptoms continue to interfere sufficiently with their daily activities, surgery to replace the joint with a prosthetic device or to excise the trapezium and reconstruct the soft tissue supports is indicated.

Thumb Metacarpophalangeal Joint Injuries and Instability

The metacarpophalangeal (MCP) joint of the thumb is primarily stabilized by the radial and ulnar collateral ligaments, which provide radioulnar and dorsal stability.[131,132] Ulnar collateral ligament (UCL) injuries result from a sharp radial deviation of the thumb MCP joint, whereas radial collateral ligament (RCL) injuries are generally the product of a sudden adduction of the MCP joint. A complete rupture of the UCL and retraction of the ligament proximal to the adductor aponeurosis is referred to as a *Stener lesion*. In this situation, the UCL cannot reapproximate to the anatomic origin of the ligament. Acute UCL injuries are often termed *skier's thumb*, whereas chronic attritional ruptures are described as *gamekeeper's thumb*. RCL injuries occur less commonly than UCL injuries and are estimated to comprise only 10% to 42% of collateral injuries to the thumb.[133]

Radiographic evaluation and physical examination remain the mainstays for diagnosis of an RCL or UCL injury. Stress views of the MCP joint can be performed and may demonstrate asymmetry of the joint space. Physical examination, including stress testing of the MCP joint, can determine a partial versus complete

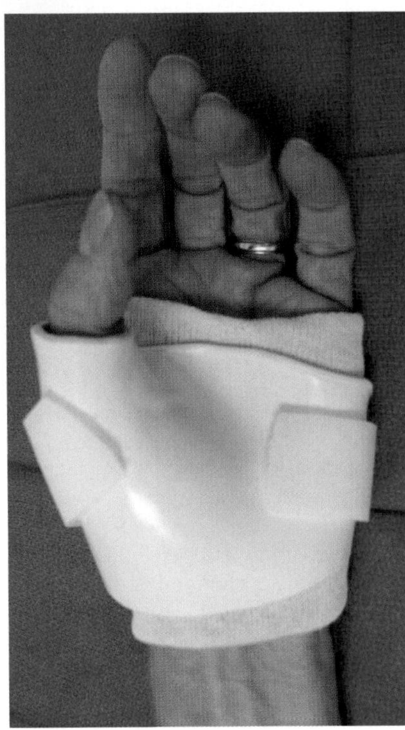

• **Fig. 53.9** Typical hand-based custom-molded splint used in the treatment of symptomatic basal joint arthritis. The thumb interphalangeal joint and wrist are left free to improve the patient's function while wearing the splint.

tear. Physical examination in the acute setting may be aided by administration of plain lidocaine into the MCP joint to help decrease patient discomfort and anxiety. A 30-degree overall laxity of the affected thumb MCP joint or a 15-degree difference from the contralateral thumb is considered predictive of disruption of the collateral ligament.[134,135]

Nonoperative treatment is successful for the majority of acute UCL and RCL tears. Partial tears of the UCL, with a firm endpoint detected on physical examination, can be immobilized for 2 to 6 weeks in a thumb-spica cast or thermoplastic splint, which can result in a stable, minimally symptomatic joint. Partial or complete tears of the RCL can be similarly treated with immobilization. If gross instability of the MCP joint is present on stress testing with no firm endpoint or if a Stener lesion is suspected, these injuries are best treated with surgical intervention.[132,135]

Volar Ganglion

Another common location for ganglia is the radial side of the volar wrist. Ganglia typically originate from the scaphotrapezial joint but become superficial and are clinically evident at or near the distal wrist crease over the flexor carpi radialis tendon. Volar ganglia can occur in close proximity to the radial artery and should be differentiated from a radial artery aneurysm. Aspiration, if attempted, should be performed carefully to avoid vascular injury, and surgery should be preceded by performance of an Allen test to document patent ulnar arterial flow. Volar ganglia are associated with a higher recurrence rate and a higher complication rate than their dorsal counterparts.[136]

Scaphoid Fracture With Nonunion

Occasionally a young or middle-aged patient presents with a nonunited scaphoid fracture with no recollection of a traumatic incident. When evaluating a relatively young patient with pain at the base of the thumb, wrist swelling in the region of the anatomic snuffbox, and a decreased range of motion of the wrist, plain radiographs and a specialized ulnar-deviation "navicular" radiograph should be obtained to rule out scaphoid disease. In patients in whom a scaphoid nonunion has been present for a significant period, secondary changes in carpal alignment and joint degeneration have usually occurred. Although treatment with splint or cast immobilization can be attempted, surgical repair of the scaphoid or another wrist salvage procedure is usually required.

Distal Radius Fractures

Distal radius fractures often occur as a result of a fall on an outstretched hand. Patients with a distal radius fracture generally present with a history of recent trauma with subsequent pain, swelling, ecchymosis, and often an obvious deformity of the affected wrist. The median nerve and carpal tunnel are in close anatomic proximity to the fracture site, and the patient may describe paresthesia in addition to pain. Radiographs of the wrist will demonstrate the degree of displacement and whether the fracture is extra-articular or intra-articular. Although many distal radius fractures can be treated successfully with closed reduction and immobilization (generally performed in the setting of the emergency department or urgent care facility), a fivefold increase in the operative treatment of distal radius fractures in elderly individuals from 1996 to 2005 has recently been reported.[137] The vast majority of distal radius fractures are still treated nonoperatively, but improvements in orthopedic implants have led to an increasing trend toward operative fixation of these injuries.

Palm

Trigger Finger

Painful clicking and locking of the digits in flexion is one of the most common causes of pain in the hand. This condition, caused by a thickening of the A1 retinacular pulley in the palm, is commonly known as *trigger finger*. The thumb is the most commonly affected digit, followed by the ring and long fingers.[138] Patients may present with isolated activity-related pain in the proximal interphalangeal joint without frank clicking or locking. Early clicking is felt as a snapping sensation during digital motion and is frequently worse upon awakening. As the condition progresses, the digital range of motion can be reduced and secondary proximal interphalangeal joint contractures develop. The final stage is a locked trigger finger that cannot be straightened actively.

Primary trigger finger is the most common type and is found most often in middle-aged individuals. Triggering of the thumb is four times more frequent in women than in men.[5] Secondary triggering is seen in association with such diseases as RA, diabetes, and gout. In this type, trigger fingers are often multiple and can co-exist with other stenosing tendinopathies, such as de Quervain's disease or CTS. Congenital or developmental triggering can be identified in children and is much less common. Similar to its presentation in adults, the thumb is most commonly affected, but in contrast to adults, triggering often presents with the interphalangeal joint locked in flexion.

Nonoperative treatment of this condition consists primarily of splinting and local steroid injections. Splinting is most effective at night to prevent the digit from locking. In adults, injection of steroid into the tendon sheath is quite effective (Fig. 53.10).[5,6,139] Injection is used infrequently in infants or children. When nonoperative treatments fail to give lasting relief, surgical treatment

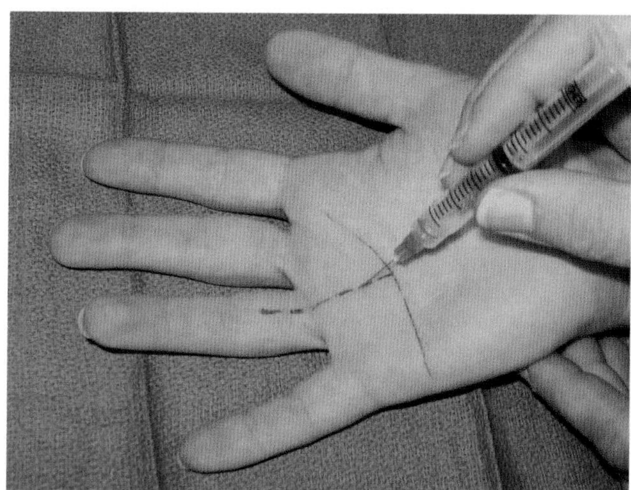

• **Fig. 53.10** Technique for injecting a trigger finger. The *solid line* denotes the distal palmar crease. The *dashed line* indicates the midline of the digit. The needle enters at an angle of between 45 and 60 degrees.

consists of longitudinal division of the A1 pulley at the level of the metacarpal head, which is a simple procedure that yields reliable results with few complications.

Retinacular Cysts

Retinacular ganglion cysts can occur in conjunction with a triggering digit or in isolation. These cysts are located at the base of the digit over the A1 pulley as a discrete, firm, pea-sized nodule. They originate from the flexor tendon sheath or annular pulleys and contain synovial fluid. Patients usually report pain when gripping objects or with direct pressure over the cyst. A retinacular cyst is most easily treated initially by needle decompression, with care taken to avoid injury to the sensory nerves that lie immediately adjacent to the flexor tendon and associated cyst. Approximately 50% recur after aspiration, and surgical resection may be required.

Digits

Mallet Finger

Mallet finger refers to a loss of terminal extension of the distal interphalangeal joint of the digit and can be classified as bony or soft tissue depending on where the disruption in the extensor mechanism occurred. Mallet fingers can occur with minimal trauma, such as tucking in bed sheets, and may not be recalled by the patient, which sometimes leads to a delay in diagnosis and treatment. When a person presents with a digit that droops at the distal interphalangeal joint and cannot be actively extended but has full passive motion, a radiograph should be obtained to determine if there is an associated fracture of the distal phalanx. An extension splint is the treatment of choice for bony and soft tissue mallet fingers. The distal interphalangeal (DIP) joint should be held in full extension, and care should be taken not to force the DIP joint into hyperextension to prevent dorsal skin ischemia and necrosis. Splinting is performed full time for 6 to 8 weeks. The patient should not remove the splint for showering or any other activity but may change the splint carefully for skin care, provided that the joint is maintained in extension. Proximal interphalangeal flexion exercises are initiated from the outset and are important to help reset the tension in the extensor mechanism. Gentle DIP flexion exercises are begun at 8 weeks, and splinting is decreased to nighttime between 8 and 10 weeks. Patients usually can expect

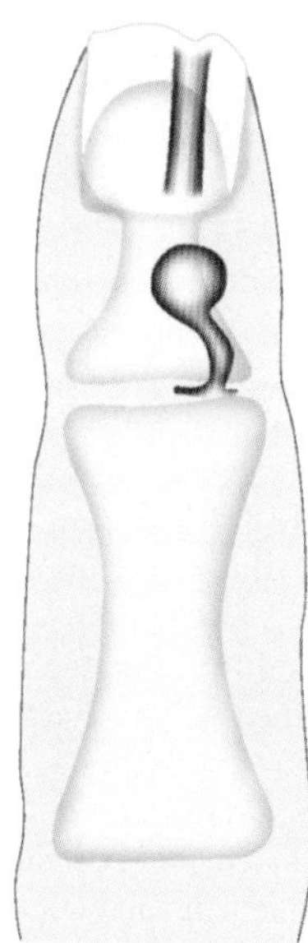

• **Fig. 53.11** Dorsal view of a digit with an as yet clinically unapparent mucous cyst and the corresponding groove deformity of the nail plate.

a small extension lag, on the order of 5 degrees, and a return of most of their flexion.

Osteoarthritis of the Digits

Osteoarthritis of the interphalangeal (IP) joints is extremely common in older people and is most often manifested as Heberden's nodes of the DIP joint. Despite gross deformities, pain and dysfunction may be minimal. A mucous cyst may appear in association with degenerative arthritis. Mucous cysts appear on the dorsum of the joint and can cause nail growth deformities as a result of pressure on the germinal matrix (Fig. 53.11). The changes in nail growth may precede clinical detection of the cyst. These cysts should not be aspirated with a needle because of the close proximity of the DIP joint and the risk of secondary joint infection. Treatment consists of DIP joint immobilization to control symptoms or surgical excision of the cyst and, in particular, the underlying osteophytic spurs.

Tumors

Benign bone tumors, such as simple bone cysts and enchondromas, are common in the phalanges. These tumors usually cause no symptoms and frequently are diagnosed as incidental findings on routine hand radiographs. Enchondromas are most commonly located in the metaphysis of the proximal phalanx and may lead to fracture with minimal trauma as a result of weakening of the bone structure. If a pathologic fracture occurs, nonoperative treatment is indicated until the fracture heals. The bone tumor subsequently can be addressed with curettage and bone grafting. Occasionally, because of malalignment, earlier surgical intervention becomes necessary.

Many soft tissue tumors can occur in the hand and digits. Some common benign tumors are giant cell tumors of the tendon sheath, lipomas, and glomus tumors. Lipomas and giant cell tumors of the tendon sheath manifest clinically as painless, slow-growing masses in the palm and digits. Surgical excision is necessary for diagnosis. Glomus tumors arise from the pericytes in the fingertip or subungual area and typically present with intermittent sharp pain in the fingertip. These vascular tumors become intensely symptomatic when the hand is exposed to cold temperatures because of abnormal arteriovenous shunting through the hypertrophic glomus system. Surgical excision is generally curative and should be preceded by MRI to rule out multifocal sites.

Infection

The most common infection in the hand is the paronychia. It involves the fold of tissue surrounding the fingernail. *Staphylococcus aureus* is the usual pathogen, introduced by a hangnail, a manicure instrument, or nail biting. Patients present with an exquisitely painful and erythematous swelling involving a part of the nail fold. Occasionally, the infection can progress to surround the nail in a horseshoe fashion and undermine the nail plate. If seen early, within the first 24 to 48 hours, oral antibiotics and local treatment of the finger with warm soaks can be effective. Superficial abscesses can be drained with a sharp blade through the thin skin without requiring local anesthesia. Larger or more chronic infections require surgical drainage.

An infection of the distal pulp of the fingertip, known as a *felon,* is a particular problem in diabetic patients. This infection differs from other subcutaneous infections because of the vertical fibrous septa that divide and stabilize the pulp of the fingertip. Often patients have had some recent penetrating injury in the area. Because of the tightly constrained area of the infection, patients present with an intensely painful fingertip. There may be an area of "pointing" over the abscess. Surgical drainage is required, followed by soaks and oral antibiotics, and intravenous antibiotics are generally recommended in diabetic patients.

Although similar in appearance to a paronychia, herpetic whitlow is caused by herpes simplex virus and must be differentiated from other fingertip infections because of a radically different treatment protocol.[140,141] Whitlow was common among dental hygienists before the widespread use of gloves for all health care workers. It is now most commonly seen in children. As with bacterial infections, the area becomes painful and erythematous; local tenderness is much less severe, however. Diagnosis is ascertained by clinical presentation and history. Vesicles that are seen early can be ruptured for fluid analysis and viral culture. Nonoperative treatment with oral anti-viral agents is recommended.

Other hand and digit infections, such as suppurative flexor tenosynovitis, deep space infections of the palm, pyogenic arthritis, infections from bite wounds, and osteomyelitis, should be evaluated initially with radiographs of the hand and appropriate blood work. If possible, antibiotics should be withheld until definitive cultures are obtained from the affected area. Antibiotics should be administered intravenously, and the hand and wrist should be immobilized. Most infections of this nature require surgical drainage for definitive treatment.

Full references for this chapter can be found on ExpertConsult.com.

Selected References

1. Metz VM, Gilula LA: Imaging techniques for distal radius fractures and related injuries, *Orthop Clin North Am* 24:217–228, 1993.
2. Larsen CF, Brondum V, Wienholtz G, et al.: An algorithm for acute wrist trauma: a systematic approach to diagnosis, *J Hand Surg Br* 18:207–212, 1993.
3. Schreibman KL, Freeland A, Gilula LA, et al.: Imaging of the hand and wrist, *Orthop Clin North Am* 28:537–582, 1997.
4. Kaufman MA: Differential diagnosis and pitfalls in electrodiagnostic studies and special tests for diagnosing compressive neuropathies, *Orthop Clin North Am* 27:245–252, 1996.
5. Marks MR, Gunther SF: Efficacy of cortisone injection in treatment of trigger fingers and thumbs, *J Hand Surg Am* 14:722–727, 1989.
6. Newport ML, Lane LB, Stuchin SA: Treatment of trigger finger by steroid injection, *J Hand Surg Am* 15:748–750, 1990.
7. Freiberg A, Mulholland RS, Levine R: Nonoperative treatment of trigger fingers and thumbs, *J Hand Surg Am* 14:553–558, 1989.
8. Gelberman RH, Aronson D, Weisman MH: Carpal tunnel syndrome: results of a prospective trial of steroid injection and splinting, *J Bone Joint Surg* 62:1181–1184, 1980.
9. Avci S, Yilmaz C, Sayli U: Comparison of nonsurgical treatment measures for de Quervain's disease of pregnancy and lactation, *J Hand Surg Am* 27:322–324, 2002.
10. Lane LB, Boretz RS, Stuchin SA: Treatment of de Quervain's disease: role of conservative management, *J Hand Surg Am* 26:258–260, 2001.
11. Taras JS, Raphael JS, Pan WT, et al.: Corticosteroid injections for trigger digits: is intrasheath injection necessary? *J Hand Surg Am* 23:717–722, 1998.
13. Richman JA, Gelberman RH, Engber WD, et al.: Ganglions of the wrist and digits: results of treatment by aspiration and cyst wall puncture, *J Hand Surg Am* 12:1041–1043, 1987.
14. Easterling KJ, Wolfe SW: Wrist arthroscopy: an overview, *Contemp Orthop* 24:21–30, 1992.
19. Adolfsson L: Arthroscopy for the diagnosis of post-traumatic wrist pain, *J Hand Surg Am* 17:46–50, 1992.
20. Koman LA, Poehling GG, Toby EB, et al.: Chronic wrist pain: indications for wrist arthroscopy, *Arthroscopy* 6:116–119, 1990.
22. DeSmet L, Dauwe D, Fortems Y, et al.: The value of wrist arthroscopy: an evaluation of 129 cases, *J Hand Surg Am* 21:210–212, 1996.
23. Kelly EP, Stanley JK: Arthroscopy of the wrist, *J Hand Surg* 15:236–242, 1990.
24. Poehling GP, Chabon SJ, Siegel DB: Diagnostic and operative arthroscopy. In Gelberman RH, editor: *The wrist: master techniques in orthopedic surgery*, New York, 1994, Raven Press, pp 21–45.
25. Bienz T, Raphael JS: Arthroscopic resection of the dorsal ganglia of the wrist, *Hand Clin* 15:429–434, 1999.
26. Luchetti R, Badia A, Alfarano M, et al.: Arthroscopic resection of dorsal wrist ganglia and treatment of recurrences, *J Hand Surg Br* 25:38–40, 2000.
27. Ho PC, Griffiths J, Lo WN, et al.: Current treatment of ganglion of the wrist, *Hand Surg* 6:49–58, 2001.
31. Mayers LB: Carpal tunnel syndrome secondary to tuberculosis, *Arch Neurol* 10:426, 1964.
32. Champion D: Gouty tenosynovitis and the carpal tunnel syndrome, *Med J Aust* 1:1030, 1969.
33. Gould JS, Wissinger HA: Carpal tunnel syndrome in pregnancy, *South Med J* 71:144–145, 1978.
34. Green EJ, Dilworth JH, Levitin PM: Tophacceous gout: an unusual cause of bilateral carpal tunnel syndrome, *JAMA* 237:2747–2748, 1977.
36. Massey EW: Carpal tunnel syndrome in pregnancy, *Obstet Gynecol Surg* 33:145, 1978.
37. Michaelis LS: Stenosis of carpal tunnel, compression of median nerve, and flexor tendon sheaths combines with rheumatoid arthritis elsewhere, *Proc R Soc Med* 43:414, 1950.
39. Phillips RS: Carpal tunnel syndrome as manifestation of systemic disease, *Ann Rheum Dis* 26(59), 1967.
40. Stallings SP, Kasdan ML, Soergel TM, et al.: A case-control study of obesity as a risk factor for carpal tunnel syndrome in a population of 600 patients presenting for independent medical examination, *J Hand Surg Am* 22:211–215, 1997.
41. Karpitskaya Y, Novak CB, Mackinnon SE: Prevalence of smoking, obesity, diabetes mellitus, and thyroid disease in patients with carpal tunnel syndrome, *Ann Plast Surg* 48:269–273, 2002.
42. Mondelli M, Giannini F, Giacchi M: Carpal tunnel syndrome incidence in a general population, *Neurology* 58:289–294, 2002.

45. al-Qattan MM, Thomson HG, Clarke HM: Carpal tunnel syndrome in children and adolescents with no history of trauma, *J Hand Surg Br* 21:108–111, 1996.
46. Phalen GS: Spontaneous compression of the median nerve at the wrist, *JAMA* 145:1128, 1951.
47. Durkan JA: A new diagnostic test for carpal tunnel syndrome, *J Bone Joint Surg* 73:535–538, 1991.
45. González del Pino J, Delgado-Martinez AD, González González I, et al.: Value of the carpal compression test in the diagnosis of carpal tunnel syndrome, *J Hand Surg Am* 22:38–41, 1997.
50. Ludin HP, Lütschg J, Valsangiacomo F: Comparison of orthodromic and antidromic sensory nerve conduction, 1: normals and patients with carpal tunnel syndrome, *EEG EMG* 8:173, 1977.
51. Richier HP, Thoden U: Early electroneurographic diagnosis of carpal tunnel syndrome, *EEG EMG* 8:187, 1977.
52. Szabo RM, Slater Jr RR, Farver TB, et al.: The value of diagnostic testing in carpal tunnel syndrome, *J Hand Surg Am* 24:704–714, 1999.
53. Melvin JL, Schuckmann JA, Lanese RR: Diagnostic specificity of motor and sensory nerve conduction variables in the carpal tunnel syndrome, *Arch Phys Med Rehabil* 54:69, 1973.
54. Gerritsen AAM, deVet HCW, Scholten RJPM, et al.: Splinting vs surgery in the treatment of carpal tunnel syndrome: a randomized controlled trial, *JAMA* 288:1245–1251, 2002.
55. Gonzalez MH, Bylak J: Steroid injection and splinting in the treatment of carpal tunnel syndrome, *Orthopedics* 24:479–481, 2001.
58. Linskey ME, Segal R: Median nerve injury from local steroid injection for carpal tunnel syndrome, *Neurosurgery* 26:512–515, 1990.
60. Ogino T, Minami A, Fukada K: Tardy ulnar nerve palsy caused by cubitus varus deformity, *J Hand Surg Am* 11:352–356, 1986.
62. Blunden R: Neuritis of deep branch of the ulnar nerve, *J Bone Joint Surg* 40:354, 1958.
64. Uriburu IJF, Morchio FJ, Marin JC: Compression syndrome of the deep branch of the ulnar nerve (piso-hamate hiatus syndrome), *J Bone Joint Surg* 58:145–147, 1976.
65. Poppi M, Padovani R, Martinelli P, et al.: Fractures of the distal radius with ulnar nerve palsy, *J Trauma* 18:278–279, 1978.
66. Vance RM, Gelberman RH: Acute ulnar neuropathy with fractures at the wrist, *J Bone Joint Surg* 60:962–965, 1978.
67. Jeffery AK: Compression of the deep palmar branch of the ulnar nerve by an anomalous muscle, *J Bone Joint Surg* 53:718–723, 1971.
68. Kalisman M, Laborde K, Wolff TW: Ulnar nerve compression secondary to ulnar artery false aneurysm at the Guyon's canal, *J Hand Surg Am* 7:137–139, 1982.
70. Richmond DA: Carpal ganglion with ulnar nerve compression, *J Bone Joint Surg* 45:513–515, 1963.
71. Toshima Y, Kimata Y: A case of ganglion causing paralysis of intrinsic muscles innervated by the ulnar nerve, *J Bone Joint Surg* 43:153, 1961.
72. Bishop AT, Gabel G, Carmichael SW: Flexor carpi radialis tendonitis, part I: operative anatomy, *J Bone Joint Surg* 76:1009–1014, 1994.
73. Carroll RE, Sinton W, Garcia A: Acute calcium deposits in the hand, *JAMA* 157:422–426, 1955.
74. Moyer RA, Bush DC, Harrington TM: Acute calcific tendonitis of the hand and wrist: a report of 12 cases and a review of the literature, *J Rheumatol* 16:198–202, 1989.
75. Yang SS, Kalainov DM, Weiland AJ: Fracture of the hook of hamate with rupture of the flexor tendons of the small finger in a rheumatoid patient: a case report, *J Hand Surg Am* 21:916–917, 1996.
76. Kato H, Nakamura R, Horii E, et al.: Diagnostic imaging for fracture of the hook of the hamate, *Hand Surg* 5:19–24, 2000.
77. Whalen JL, Bishop AT, Linscheid RL: Nonoperative treatment of acute hamate hook fractures, *J Hand Surg Am* 17:507–511, 1992.
78. Bishop AT, Bechenbaugh RD: Fracture of the hamate hook, *J Hand Surg Am* 13:863–868, 1988.
79. Carter PR, Eaton RG, Littler JW: Ununited fracture of the hook of the hamate, *J Bone Joint Surg Am* 59:583–588, 1977.
80. Stark HH, Chao EK, Zemel NP, et al.: Fracture of the hook of the hamate, *J Bone Joint Surg* 71:1202–1207, 1989.
82. Cardinal E, Buckwalter KA, Braunstein EM, et al.: Occult dorsal carpal ganglion: comparison of US and MR imaging, *Radiology* 193:259–262, 1994.
83. Vo P, Wright T, Hayden F, et al.: Evaluating dorsal wrist pain: MRI diagnosis of occult dorsal wrist ganglion, *J Hand Surg Am* 20:667–670, 1995.
84. Zubowicz VN, Ishii CH: Management of ganglion cysts of the hand by simple aspiration, *J Hand Surg Am* 12:618–620, 1987.
85. Angelides AC, Wallace PF: The dorsal ganglion of the wrist: its pathogenesis, gross and microscopic anatomy, and surgical treatment, *J Hand Surg Am* 1:228–235, 1976.
86. Clay NR, Clement DA: The treatment of dorsal wrist ganglia by radical excision, *J Hand Surg Am* 13:187–191, 1988.
87. Janzon L, Niechajev IA: Wrist ganglia: incidence and recurrence rate after operation, *Scand J Plast Reconstr Surg* 15:53–56, 1981.
88. Angelides AC: Ganglions of the hand and wrist. In Green DP, editor: *Operative hand surgery*, New York, 1993, Churchill Livingstone.
89. Cuono CB, Watson HK: The carpal boss: surgical treatment and etiological considerations, *Plast Reconstr Surg* 63:88–93, 1979.
90. Bonatz E, Dramer TD, Masear VR: Rupture of the extensor pollicis longus tendon, *Am J Orthop* 25:118–122, 1996.
91. Stahl S, Wolff TW: Delayed rupture of the extensor pollicis longus tendon after nonunion of a fracture of the dorsal radial tubercle, *J Hand Surg Am* 13:338–341, 1988.
92. Hove LM: Delayed rupture of the thumb extensor tendon: a 5-year study of 18 consecutive cases, *Acta Orthop Scand* 65:199–203, 1994.
93. Dawson WJ: Sports-induced spontaneous rupture of the extensor pollicis longus tendon, *J Hand Surg Am* 17:457–458, 1992.
95. Stahl F: On lunatomalacia (Keinböck's disease): clinical and roentgenological study, especially on its pathogenesis and late results of immobilization treatment, *Acta Chir Scand* 126(Suppl):1–133, 1947.
96. Wada A, Miura H, Kubota H, et al.: Radial closing wedge osteotomy for Kienböck's disease: an over 10 year clinical and radiographic follow-up, *J Hand Surg Br* 27:175–179, 2002.
97. Wintman BI, Imbriglia JE, Buterbaugh GA, et al.: Operative treatment with radial shortening in Kienböck's disease, *Orthopedics* 24:365–371, 2001.
98. Quenzer DE, Dobyns JH, Linscheid RL, et al.: Radial recession osteotomy for Kienböck's disease, *J Hand Surg Am* 22:386–395, 1997.
99. Nakamura R, Imaeda T, Miura T: Radial shortening for Kienböck's disease: factors affecting the operative result, *J Hand Surg Am* 15:40–45, 1990.
100. Oishi SN, Muzaffar AR, Carter PR: Treatment of Kienböck's disease with capitohamate arthrodesis: pain relief with minimal morbidity, *Plast Reconstr Surg* 109:1293–1300, 2002.
101. Watson HK, Monacelli DM, Milford RS, et al.: Treatment of Kienböck's disease with scaphotrapezio-trapezoid arthrodesis, *J Hand Surg Am* 21:9–15, 1996.
102. Chuinard RG, Zeman SC: Kienböck's disease: an analysis and rationale for treatment by capitate-hamate fusion, *Orthop Trans* 4(18), 1980.
104. Thompson TC, Campbell Jr RD, Arnold WD: Primary and secondary dislocation of the scaphoid bone, *J Bone Joint Surg* 46:73–82, 1964.
106. King GJ, McMurtry RY, Rubenstein JD, et al.: Kinematics of the distal radioulnar joint, *J Hand Surg Am* 11:798–804, 1986.
107. Burk Jr DL, Karasick D, Wechsler RJ: Imaging of the distal radioulnar joint, *Hand Clin* 7:263–275, 1991.
109. Mino DE, Palmer AK, Levinsohn EM: The role of radiography and computerized tomography in the diagnosis of subluxation and dislocation of the distal radioulnar joint, *J Hand Surg Am* 8:23–31, 1983.

110. Mino DE, Palmer AK, Levinsohn EM: Radiography and computerized tomography in the diagnosis of incongruity of the distal radioulnar joint: a prospective study, *J Bone Joint Surg* 67:247–252, 1985.
111. Steyers CM, Blair WF: Measuring ulnar variance: a comparison of techniques, *J Hand Surg Am* 14:607–612, 1989.
114. Mikic ZD: Age changes in the triangular fibrocartilage of the wrist joint, *J Anat* 126:367–384, 1978.
116. Palmer AK, Levinsohn EM, Kuzma GR: Arthrography of the wrist, *J Hand Surg Am* 8:18–23, 1983.
117. Potter HG, Asnis-Ernberg L, Weiland AJ, et al.: The utility of high-resolution magnetic resonance imaging in the evaluation of the triangular fibrocartilage complex of the wrist, *J Bone Joint Surg* 79:1675–1684, 1997.
118. Feldon P, Terronon AL, Belsky MR: The wafer procedure: partial distal ulnar resection, *Clin Orthop* 275:124–129, 1992.
119. de Araujo W, Poehling GG, Kuzma GR: New Tuohy needle technique for triangular fibrocartilage complex repair: preliminary studies, *Arthroscopy* 12:699–703, 1996.
120. Lacey 2nd T, Goldstein LA, Tobin CE: Anatomical and clinical study of the variations in the insertions of the abductor pollicis longus tendon, associated with stenosing tendovaginitis, *J Bone Joint Surg Am* 33:347–350, 1951.
121. Leao L: De Quervain's disease: a clinical and anatomical study, *J Bone Joint Surg* 40:1063–1070, 1958.
122. Strandell G: Variations of the anatomy in stenosing tenosynovitis at the radial styloid process, *Acta Chir Scand* 113:234–240, 1957.
123. Finkelstein H: Stenosing tendovaginitis at the radial styloid process, *J Bone Joint Surg* 12:509–540, 1930.
124. Pick RY, De Quervain's disease: a clinical triad, *Clin Orthop* 143:165–166, 1979.
125. Grundberg AB, Reagan DS: Pathologic anatomy of the forearm: intersection syndrome, *J Hand Surg Am* 10:299–302, 1985.
126. Weiss AP, Akelman E, Tabatabai M: Treatment of de Quervain's disease, *J Hand Surg Am* 19:595–598, 1994.
127. Kelsey JL, Pastides H, Kreiger N, et al.: *Arthritic disorders, upper extremity disorders: a survey of their frequency and cost in the United States*, St. Louis, 1980, CV Mosby.
128. Armstrong AL, Hunter JB, Davis TRC: The prevalence of degenerative arthritis of the base of the thumb in post-menopausal women, *J Hand Surg Am* 19:340–341, 1994.
129. Eaton RG, Glickel SZ: Trapeziometacarpal osteoarthritis: staging as a rationale for treatment, *Hand Clin* 3:455–469, 1987.

54 Temporomandibular Joint Pain

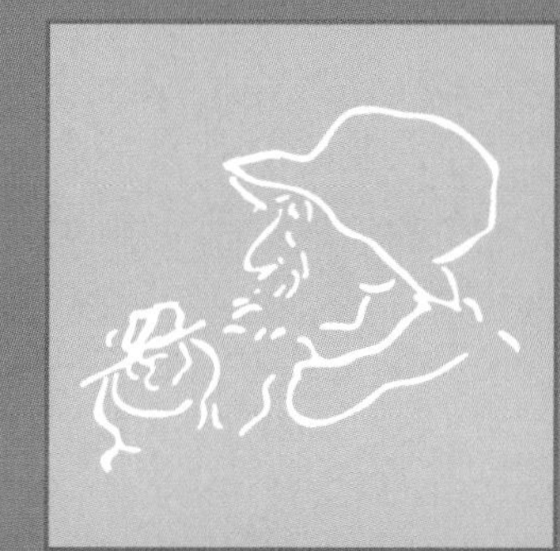

DANIEL M. LASKIN

KEY POINTS

- Temporomandibular joint (TMJ) pain must be distinguished from pain that more commonly arises from the muscles of mastication (myofascial pain), which can produce similar signs and symptoms.
- TMJ pain also must be distinguished from pain that originates in the ear or parotid gland.
- TMJ pain and masticatory muscle pain usually are accompanied by limitation of mouth opening, but pain arising from the ear or parotid gland is not.
- Most major systemic arthropathies can also involve the TMJ and thereby give rise to pain and limited jaw movement.
- Displacement of the intra-articular disk in the TMJ produces pain that is accompanied by a clicking or popping sound or the sudden onset of jaw locking.

Introduction

Pain in the temporomandibular joint (TMJ) region is a commonly encountered symptom that affects more than 10 million people in North America, and is universally recognized across populations worldwide as a significant health care burden. Because of its diverse causes, however, proper diagnosis and treatment may be difficult to achieve. Because of the proximity of the ear and parotid gland and the similar nature of pain arising from these areas, pathologic conditions involving these structures are often confused with conditions arising in the TMJ. Pain that occurs in the adjacent muscles of mastication, also a frequently encountered situation, not only is similar to TMJ pain in character and location but also is associated with jaw dysfunction, a common finding with painful conditions directly involving the TMJ. For these reasons, knowledge of the various painful conditions occurring in the TMJ region is essential to establishing a correct diagnosis.

Because patients with primary TMJ disease often have secondary myofascial pain in the muscles of mastication, and because secondary TMJ disease can develop in patients with primary myofascial pain, the generally accepted term used to describe this overlapping group of conditions is *temporomandibular disorders*. These conditions are subdivided for the purposes of diagnosis and treatment into conditions that primarily involve the TMJ (TMJ problems) and conditions that primarily involve the muscles of mastication (myofascial pain and dysfunction [MPD], masticatory myalgia). From a diagnostic standpoint, it is important to consider the numerous conditions that mimic the temporomandibular disorders or MPD by producing similar signs and symptoms (Tables 54.1 and 54.2).

Table 54.3 lists the various pathologic entities that commonly involve the TMJ. Although a variety of conditions are known, only three types are considered to generally produce pain: the various arthritides, derangements of the intra-articular disk, and certain neoplasms.

Arthritis of the Temporomandibular Joint

Arthritis is the most common painful condition affecting the TMJ. Although osteoarthritis and rheumatoid arthritis are encountered most frequently, cases of infectious arthritis, metabolic arthritis, and TMJ involvement as part of the spondyloarthropathies are also seen in practice. Traumatic arthritis is another relatively common occurrence.

Osteoarthritis

Osteoarthritis is the most common type of arthritis involving the TMJ and the most frequent cause of pain in that region. Clinical symptoms of the disease have been reported in 16% of the general population,[1] but radiographic features have been found in 44% of asymptomatic individuals.[2] Although the TMJ is not a weight-bearing joint in the same sense as the joints of the long bones, the stresses associated with such parafunctional habits as clenching and grinding of the teeth are sufficient to contribute to similar degenerative changes in some patients.[3] Acute and chronic trauma and derangements of the intra-articular disk also are common causes of secondary degenerative arthritis.

Clinical Findings

Primary osteoarthritis, which is usually seen in older individuals, is insidious in its onset; it generally produces only mild discomfort, and individuals rarely complain about the condition. Secondary osteoarthritis usually occurs in younger patients (20 to 40 years old) and tends to be painful. In contrast to primary degenerative joint disease and rheumatoid arthritis, it often is limited to only one TMJ, although it may become bilateral in the late stages, and involvement of other joints is uncommon. The condition is characterized by TMJ pain that is increased by function, joint tenderness, limitation of mouth opening, and occasional clicking and popping sounds. In the late stages, crepitation may be noted in the joint.

TABLE 54.1 Differential Diagnosis of Nonarticular Conditions Mimicking Temporomandibular Joint Pain or Myofascial Pain in the Masticatory Muscles

Disorder	Jaw Limitation	Muscle Tenderness	Diagnostic Features
Pulpitis	No	No	Mild to severe ache or throbbing; intermittent or constant; aggravated by thermal change; pain eliminated by dental anesthesia; positive radiographic findings (dental caries)
Pericoronitis	Yes	Possible	Persistent mild to severe ache; difficulty swallowing; possible fever; local inflammation; pain relieved with dental anesthesia
Otitis media	No	No	Moderate to severe earache; constant pain; fever; usually history of upper respiratory infection; no temporomandibular joint tenderness
Parotitis	No	No	Constant aching pain, worse when eating; feeling of pressure in ears; absent salivary flow; ear lobe elevated; suppuration from duct
Sinusitis	No	No	Constant aching or throbbing; worse with change of head position; nasal discharge; often maxillary molar pain not relieved by dental anesthesia
Trigeminal neuralgia	No	No	Sharp stabbing pain of short duration; trigger zone; pain follows nerve pathway; older patient age group; pain often relieved by dental anesthesia
Atypical (vascular) neuralgia	No	No	Diffuse throbbing or burning pain of long duration; often associated autonomic symptoms; no pain relief with dental anesthesia
Temporal arteritis	No	No	Constant throbbing preauricular pain; artery prominent and tender; low-grade fever; may have visual problems; elevated erythrocyte sedimentation rate
Trotter's syndrome	Yes	No	Aching pain in ear, side of face, and lower jaw; deafness; nasal obstruction; cervical lymphadenopathy
Eagle's syndrome	No	No	Mild to sharp stabbing pain in ear, throat, and retromandible; provoked by swallowing, turning head, carotid compression; usually post tonsillectomy; styloid process >2.5 cm

Modified from Laskin DM, Block S: Diagnosis and treatment of myofascial pain dysfunction (MPD) syndrome. *J Prosthet Dent* 56:75–84, 1986.

TABLE 54.2 Differential Diagnosis of Nonarticular Conditions Producing Limitation of Mandibular Movement

Disorder	Jaw Limitation	Muscle Tenderness	Diagnostic Features
Odontogenic infection	Yes	Yes	Fever; swelling; positive dental radiographic findings; tooth tender to percussion; pain relieved and movement improved with dental anesthesia
Nonodontogenic infection	Yes	Yes	Fever; swelling; negative dental findings on radiograph; dental anesthesia may not relieve pain or improve jaw movement
Myositis	Yes	Yes	Sudden onset; jaw movement associated with pain; areas of muscle tenderness; usually no fever
Myositis ossificans	No	No	Palpable nodules seen as radiopaque areas on radiograph; involvement of nonmasticatory muscles
Neoplasia	Possible	Possible	Palpable mass; regional nodes may be enlarged; may have paresthesia; radiograph may show bone involvement
Scleroderma	No	No	Skin hard and atrophic; mask-like facies; paresthesia; arthritic joint pain; widening of periodontal ligament
Hysteria	No	No	Sudden onset after psychological trauma; no physical findings; jaw opens easily under general anesthesia
Tetanus	Yes	No	Recent wound; stiffness of neck; difficulty swallowing; spasm of facial muscles; headache
Extrapyramidal reaction	No	No	Patient on antipsychotic drug or phenothiazine tranquilizer; hypertonic movement; lip smacking; spontaneous chewing motions
Depressed zygomatic arch	Possible	No	History of trauma; facial depression; positive radiographic findings
Osteochondroma of coronoid process	No	No	Gradual limitation of mouth opening; jaw may deviate to unaffected side; possible clicking sound on jaw movement; positive radiograph findings

Modified from Laskin DM, Block S: Diagnosis and treatment of myofascial pain dysfunction (MPD) syndrome. *J Prosthet Dent* 56:75–84, 1986.

TABLE 54.3 Differential Diagnosis of Temporomandibular Joint (TMJ) Diseases

Disorder	Jaw Limitation	Muscle Tenderness	Diagnostic Features
Agenesis	No	Yes	Congenital; usually unilateral; mandible deviates to affected side; unaffected side of face long and flat; severe malocclusion; often ear abnormalities; radiograph shows condylar deficiency
Condylar hypoplasia	No	No	Congenital or acquired; affected side has short mandibular body and ramus, fullness of face, deviation of chin; body of mandible elongated and face flat on unaffected side; malocclusion; radiograph shows condylar deformity, antegonial notch
Condylar hyperplasia	No	No	Facial asymmetry with deviation of chin to unaffected side; cross-bite malocclusion; prognathic appearance; lower border of mandible often convex on affected side; radiograph shows symmetric enlargement of condyle
Neoplasia	Possible	Yes	Mandible may deviate to affected side; radiographs show enlarged, irregularly shaped condyle or bone destruction, depending on type of tumor; unilateral condition
Infectious arthritis	Yes	No	Signs of infection; may be part of systemic disease; radiograph may be normal early, later can show bone destruction; fluctuance may be present; pus may be obtained on aspiration; usually unilateral
Rheumatoid arthritis	Yes	Yes	Signs of inflammation; findings in other joints (hands, wrists, feet, elbows, ankles); positive laboratory test results; retarded mandibular growth in children; anterior open bite; radiograph shows bone destruction; usually bilateral
Spondyloarthropathies			
Psoriatic arthritis	Yes	Yes	Presence of cutaneous psoriasis; nail dystrophy; involvement of distal interphalangeal joints; radiograph shows condylar erosion; negative for rheumatoid factor
Ankylosing spondylitis	Yes	Yes	Frequent involvement of the spine and sacroiliac joint; extra-articular manifestations of spondylitis include iritis, anterior uveitis, aortic insufficiency, and conduction defects; erosive condylar changes; TMJ ankylosis may occur
Metabolic arthritis			
Gout	Yes	Yes	Usually sudden onset; often monoarticular; commonly involves great toe, ankle, and wrist; joint swollen, red, and tender; increased serum uric acid; late radiographic changes
Pseudogout	Yes	Yes	Generally unilateral; TMJ may be only joint involved; joint frequently swollen; presence of intra-articular calcification; may be a history of trauma
Traumatic arthritis	Yes	Yes	History of trauma; radiograph normal except for possible widening of joint space; local tenderness; usually unilateral
Degenerative arthritis	Yes	Yes	Unilateral joint tenderness; often crepitus; TMJ may be only joint involved; radiograph may be normal or show condylar flattening, lipping, spurring, or erosion
Ankylosis	Yes	Yes	Usually unilateral, but can be bilateral; may be history of trauma; young patient may show retarded mandibular growth; radiographs show loss of normal joint architecture
Internal disk derangement	Yes	Yes	Pain exacerbated by function; clicking on opening or opening limited to <25 mm with no click; positive MRI findings; may be history of trauma; usually unilateral

Modified from Laskin DM, Block S: Diagnosis and treatment of myofascial pain dysfunction (MPD) syndrome. *J Prosthet Dent* 56:75–84, 1986.

Imaging Findings

The earliest radiologic feature of osteoarthritis of the TMJ, whether primary or secondary, is subchondral sclerosis in the mandibular condyle. If the condition progresses, condylar flattening and marginal lipping may be noted. In the later stages, erosion of the cortical plate, osteophyte formation, or both may occur. Breakdown of the subcortical bone occasionally may result in the formation of so-called *bone cysts*. Although changes in the articular fossa generally are not as severe as changes in the condyle, cortical erosion can sometimes be seen. Narrowing of the joint space also occurs in the late stages; this is indicative of concomitant degenerative changes and thinning of the intra-articular disk. Although changes in the TMJ usually can be seen on plain radiographs, sagittal and coronal CT scans are the preferred modality to image the bony structures.

Diagnosis

The diagnosis of osteoarthritis is made on the basis of the patient's history and the clinical and radiographic findings. The patient often reports a history of trauma or parafunctional oral habits. Involvement is generally unilateral, and no significant changes are observed in any of the other joints. The pain tends to be well localized, and the TMJ is often tender to palpation.

Treatment

Treatment of degenerative arthritis of the TMJ is usually medical, as in other joints of the body. Treatments involve patient use of nonsteroidal anti-inflammatory drugs, application of heat, the eating of a soft diet, limitation of jaw function, and use of a bite appliance to control parafunction if the patient has a chronic habit of clenching or grinding the teeth. Arthrocentesis is helpful.[4,5] Physical therapy with thermal agents, ultrasound, and iontophoresis can also be beneficial, and isotonic and isometric exercises are used to improve joint stability after the acute symptoms have subsided. The use of intra-articular steroid injections is controversial; they should be used only in patients with acute symptoms that do not respond to other forms of medical management. Because of the potentially damaging effects of multiple steroid injections,[4,6] they should be limited to no more than three or four single injections given at 3-month intervals. Intra-articular injection of high-molecular-weight sodium hyaluronate given twice, 2 weeks apart, has essentially the same therapeutic effect as a steroid injection, without the potential adverse effects.[5,7]

When the acute symptoms have been controlled, therapy is directed toward control of factors that might contribute to the degenerative process. Unfavorable loading of the joint is eliminated by replacement of missing teeth to establish a good, functional occlusion; correction of any severe dental malrelations through orthodontics or orthognathic surgery; and continued use of a bite appliance at night to control teeth-clenching or teeth-grinding habits.[6,8]

For patients in whom medical management for 3 to 6 months fails to relieve the symptoms, surgical management may be indicated. Surgery involves removal of the minimal amount of bone necessary to produce a smooth articular surface. Unnecessary removal of the entire cortical plate, as occurs with the so-called *condylar shave* procedure or high condylotomy, can lead to continuation of the resorptive process in some instances, and should be avoided if possible.

Rheumatoid Arthritis

More than 50% of patients with rheumatoid arthritis have involvement of the TMJ.[9] Although the TMJ may be affected early in the course of the disease, other joints in the body usually are involved first. The approximate female-to-male ratio is 3 : 1. TMJ involvement may also characterize juvenile inflammatory arthritis. In children, destruction of the mandibular condyle by the disease process results in growth retardation and facial deformity characterized by a severely retruded chin. Fibrous or bony ankylosis is a possible sequel at all ages.

Clinical Findings

Patients with rheumatoid arthritis of the TMJ have bilateral pain, tenderness, swelling in the preauricular region, and limitation of mandibular movement. These symptoms are characterized by periods of exacerbation and remission. Joint stiffness and pain are usually worse in the morning and decrease during the day. The limitation in mandibular movement worsens as the disease progresses; an anterior open bite may also develop in the patient.

Imaging Findings

Although radiographic changes may not be noted in the early stages of the disease, approximately 50% to 80% of patients show bilateral evidence of demineralization, condylar flattening, and bone erosion while the disease progresses, so the articular surface appears irregular and ragged. Erosion of the glenoid fossa also may be seen. Narrowing of the joint space is caused by destruction of the intra-articular disk. With continued destruction of the condyle, loss of ramus height can lead to contact of only the posterior teeth and an anterior open bite. Increasingly, MRI is used as an additional modality for the detection of articular damage, synovitis, or both, or of involvement of adnexal structures.

Diagnosis

Rheumatoid arthritis is diagnosed on the basis of the patient's history, clinical and radiographic findings, and confirmatory laboratory tests. Distinguishing features for rheumatoid arthritis and degenerative arthritis of the TMJ are shown in Table 54.3.

Treatment

Treatment of rheumatoid arthritis of the TMJ is similar to that provided for other joints.[7,10] Anti-inflammatory drugs are used during the acute phases, and mild jaw exercises are used to prevent excessive loss of motion when acute symptoms subside. In severe cases, disease-modifying drugs, such as methotrexate, and biologic agents, including TNF inhibitors, abatacept, tocilizumab, and etanercept may be used pending systemic presentation. Orthognathic surgery may be necessary in patients with an anterior open bite after the disease goes into remission, or in patients in whom ankylosis develops after that condition is corrected.

Spondyloarthropathies

In addition to the adult and juvenile forms of rheumatoid arthritis, psoriatic arthritis, ankylosing spondylitis, and reactive arthritis can also involve the TMJ.[8–13]

Psoriatic Arthritis

Psoriatic arthritis occurs in approximately one-third of patients who have cutaneous psoriasis (see Chapter 77). This disorder has a sudden onset, can be episodic in nature, and may show spontaneous remission.[9,12] Often only one TMJ is involved. Symptoms include TMJ pain and tenderness, restricted jaw movement, and crepitation, mimicking the symptoms of rheumatoid arthritis.[9,12] Radiographic changes are nonspecific and cannot be distinguished easily from those of other types of arthritis, particularly rheumatoid arthritis and ankylosing spondylitis.[13,14] They usually involve erosive changes in the condyle and glenoid fossa associated with extreme narrowing of the joint space.[11,15,16] In severe cases, ankylosis may develop, reflected occasionally in new bone formation at earlier stages.[12,17]

The physician usually diagnoses psoriatic arthritis on the basis of the triad of psoriasis, radiographic evidence of erosive arthritis, and a negative serologic test for rheumatoid factor. Even in the presence of a rash, however, the diagnosis cannot be absolutely confirmed. The differential diagnosis always should include rheumatoid arthritis, reactive arthritis, ankylosing spondylitis, and gout.

Treatment of psoriatic arthritis of the TMJ is as described in Chapter 77 and is driven essentially by the imperative to treat the systemic inflammatory disease process.[13,18–21] In particular, given the recent advances in this field, especially with the advent of IL-17 and IL-23 targeting agents, it will be important to establish that local benefits in the TMJ accrue with the commencement of these agents. Surgery is necessary if ankylosis occurs.

Ankylosing Spondylitis

TMJ involvement develops in approximately one-third of patients with ankylosing spondylitis several years after onset of the disease. Pain and limitation of jaw movement are the most common symptoms, and ankylosis can develop in advanced cases.[8,11,14,22] On radiographic examination, approximately 30% of patients show erosive changes in the condyle and fossa and narrowing of the joint space.[15,23] In long-standing cases, a more florid osteophytic response is sometimes seen during quiescent periods. The severity of the changes seems to be related to the severity of the disease. Treatment of ankylosing spondylitis of the TMJ is generally medical and is part of the total management of the patient; as with psoriatic arthritis it will be important to establish that TMJ involvement is amenable to such systemic medical therapy. This should be especially borne in mind when considering the range of joint assessments currently performed to monitor therapy, which often do not include the TMJ region. Moreover, some of the newer agents being introduced seem to have regional variation in their depth of response. For example, IL-23 inhibitors are effective in peripheral synovitis and enthesitis but appear not to be effective in axial disease. Physical therapy is used to improve jaw mobility, and a bite appliance is used, when indicated, to reduce parafunctional stress on the joint. If ankylosis develops, surgery is the treatment of choice.[24]

Reactive Arthritis

Reactive arthritis of the temporomandibular joint is more common in males than in females. It is characterized by recurrent pain, swelling, and limitation of mouth opening.[25] Radiographically, condylar erosion may be evident.[26] Treatment is similar to that of the other seronegative spondyloarthropathies, consisting of nonsteroidal anti-inflammatory drugs, intra-articular steroids, and disease-modifying drugs. If a specific triggering bacterial infection can be identified, an appropriate antibiotic should be prescribed.

Traumatic Arthritis

Acute trauma to the mandible that does not result in a fracture can still produce injury to the TMJ. When this occurs in a child, it is essential to warn the parents about the possibility of future retardation of mandibular growth and associated facial deformity resulting from damage to the articular cartilage, which is an important growth site.[16,27]

Traumatic arthritis is characterized by TMJ pain and tenderness and limitation of jaw movement. The resultant inflammation and occasional hemarthrosis can lead to loss of tooth contact on the affected side. Frequently, bruises or lacerations are apparent at the site of the initial injury. No radiographic changes may be seen, or widening of the joint space may be produced by intra-articular edema or hemorrhage. In some instances, radiographs may show an intracapsular fracture that was not recognized on clinical examination.

Treatment of traumatic arthritis consists of the use of nonsteroidal anti-inflammatory drugs, application of heat, a soft diet, and initial restriction of jaw movement. When acute symptoms subside, range-of-motion exercises should be used to avoid fibrous ankylosis.

Infectious Arthritis

Infectious arthritis rarely involves the TMJ. Although it can affect the joint as part of such systemic diseases as gonorrhea, syphilis, tuberculosis, and Lyme disease,[17,18,28,29] the most common way is by direct extension of an adjacent infection of dental, parotid gland, or otic origin.[19,30] Occasionally, it also may occur from localization of blood-borne organisms in the joint after a traumatic injury or by direct involvement through a penetrating wound.[20,30] The most common pathogens are *Staphylococcus aureus, Haemophilus influenzae,* and *Streptococcus* species.[31]

Clinical Findings

Infectious arthritis generally results in unilateral pain, tenderness, swelling, and redness in the region of the TMJ. Chills, fever, sweating, and systemic findings characteristic of the specific type of infection are also present. Often the patient's teeth cannot be occluded because of swelling within the joint. In pyogenic forms of infectious arthritis, fluctuation may be noted in the joint region. Patients with Lyme disease show characteristic skin lesions and, often, positive serology.[18,29]

Imaging Findings

Radiographic findings are usually normal in early stages of the disease because of lack of bony involvement, but the intra-articular accumulation of pus or inflammatory exudate may cause separation of articulating surfaces, which can be detected on MRI. Later, depending on the severity and chronicity of the infection, varying degrees of bony destruction, ranging from damage to the articular surface of the mandibular condyle to extensive osteomyelitis, may be seen. In the late stages, fibrous or bony ankylosis may occur. In children, infectious arthritis can affect growth of the condyle, resulting in facial asymmetry.

Treatment

Treatment of infectious arthritis includes the use of appropriate antibiotics, proper hydration, control of pain, and limitation of jaw movement. Arthrocentesis with Ringer's solution one to three times weekly until acute symptoms subside has also been recommended.[32] Suppurative infections may require aspiration, incision and drainage, or sequestrectomy. When bone loss is extensive, reconstructive procedures may be necessary. In children in whom mandibular growth has been affected, a costochondral graft can be used to correct facial asymmetry and re-establish growth of the mandible.

Metabolic Arthritis

Metabolic arthritis, which can accompany gout or pseudogout (calcium pyrophosphate dehydrate arthropathy) (see Chapters 101, 102), is rare in the TMJ.[21,33]

Gout

Gouty arthritis of the TMJ occurs most frequently in men older than 40 years and is usually preceded by involvement of one or more joints of the feet or hands. The attack usually occurs suddenly, and the joint becomes swollen, painful, red, and tender. Recovery may occur in a few days, and remission can last for months to years.

When attacks are infrequent, radiographic changes may not be noted for a long time. Because so few cases have been reported, the precise radiographic changes that occur have not been well documented. Calcified areas in the disk, destruction of the hard tissues of the joint, condylar exostoses and spurring, and the presence of tophi have been described.[21,33–35] The initial approach to treatment of gout involving the TMJ is medical. If symptoms are not controlled, however, surgical débridement of the joint and arthroplasty may be indicated.

Pseudogout

Calcium pyrophosphate dihydrate arthropathy (pseudogout) in the TMJ clinically mimics gout, and the mandibular condyle may show degenerative and erosive changes radiographically. In the primary form, which is usually seen in older patients, intra-articular calcification is noted (chondrocalcinosis), and diffuse calcification occurs in the intra-articular disk.[21–25,36–39] Similar changes are seen in the secondary form, but it occurs in younger patients and frequently is preceded by a history of trauma. Fine-needle aspiration can help distinguish pseudogout from gout. In gout, under polarizing microscopy, the crystals are needle shaped and there is negative birefringence; in pseudogout, the crystals are rhomboid/rod shaped and weakly birefringent.

Just as in gout of the TMJ, the initial treatment of pseudogout is medical, and surgery is reserved for patients in whom such treatment is ineffective.

Internal Derangements

Internal derangements are a common cause of pain in the TMJ. They represent a disturbance in the normal anatomic relationship between the intra-articular disk and the condyle, resulting in interference with the smooth movement of the joint.

Clinical Findings

Three stages of internal derangement have been identified: (1) a painless incoordination phase, in which a momentary catching sensation is felt during mouth opening; (2) anterior disk displacement with reduction into the normal position during mouth opening, which is characterized by a clicking or popping sound (Fig. 54.1); and (3) anterior disk displacement without reduction on attempted mouth opening, which is characterized by restriction of jaw movement, or locking (Fig. 54.2). Joint pain in patients with anterior disk displacement, with or without reduction, is caused by condylar compression of the highly innervated retrodiskal tissue that occupies the glenoid fossa when the intra-articular disk assumes a more forward position, and by the accompanying inflammation.

Etiology

The three main causes of internal derangement of the intra-articular disk are trauma, abnormal functional loading of the joint, and degenerative joint disease.[26,40] Although some clinicians believe that occlusal factors also play a role in causing internal derangements, no conclusive studies have shown such a relationship.

Acute macrotrauma is probably the most common cause of internal derangement. Among the events thought to cause macrotrauma are a blow to the jaw, endotracheal intubation, cervical traction, and iatrogenic stretching of the joint during dental

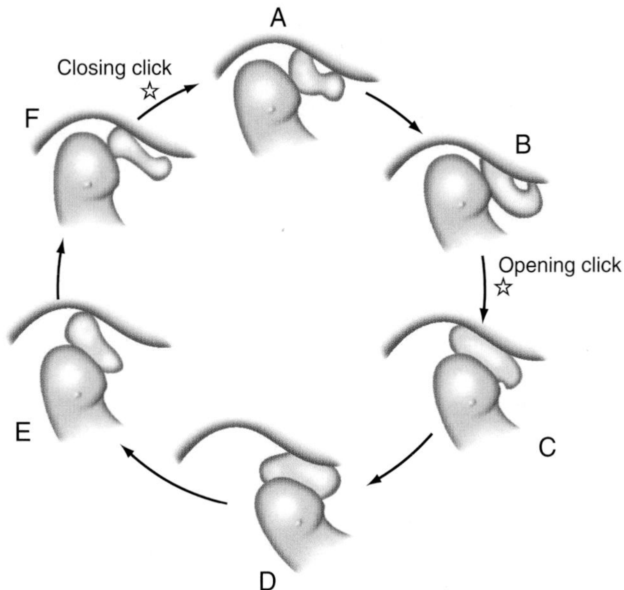

• **Fig. 54.1** (A-F) Anterior displacement of the intra-articular disk with reduction on opening of the mouth. A clicking or popping sound occurs as the disk returns to its normal position in relation to the condyle. During closure, the disk again becomes anteriorly displaced, sometimes accompanied by a second sound (reciprocal click). (Modified from McCarty W: Diagnosis and treatment of internal derangements of the articular disc and mandibular condyle. In Solberg WK, Clark GT, editors: *Temporomandibular joint problems: biologic diagnosis and treatment*, Chicago, 1980, Quintessence, p 155.)

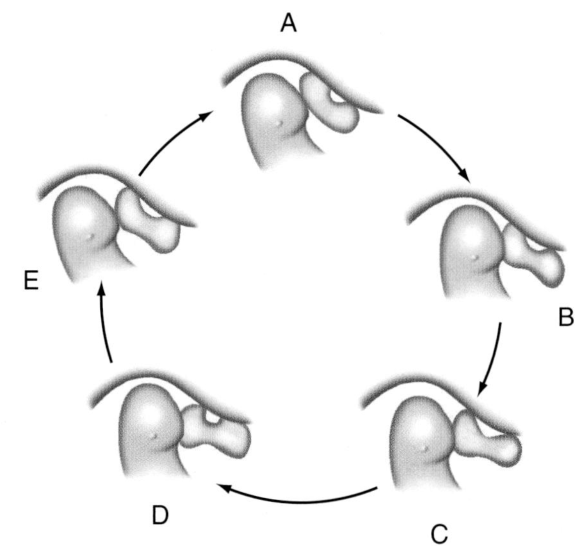

• **Fig. 54.2** (A-E) Anterior displacement of the intra-articular disk without reduction on attempted mouth opening. The displaced disk acts as a barrier and prevents full translation of the condyle. (Modified from McCarty W: Diagnosis and treatment of internal derangements of the articular disc and mandibular condyle. In Solberg WK, Clark GT, editors: *Temporomandibular joint problems: biologic diagnosis and treatment*. Chicago, 1980, Quintessence, p 151.)

or oral surgical procedures. Although whiplash injuries have frequently been implicated in the development of internal derangement, a study of 155 patients with this type of injury showed that clicking in the TMJ immediately after the automobile accident developed in only one patient.[27,41] At 1 month of follow-up, two additional patients of the 129 contacted experienced clicking, but at 1 year, no additional patients of the 104 contacted had developed clicking. Although internal derangements of the TMJ can be caused by a whiplash injury, the incidence seems to be low.

Whether a patient manifests alterations in the articular surface leading to a catching or binding sensation, anterior disk displacement with reduction on mouth opening (clicking or popping), or anterior disk displacement without reduction during mouth opening (locking) after trauma to the TMJ depends on the severity of the injury. Although associated traumatic arthritis causes pain during function in each of these instances, the pain is more severe in the last two conditions because of compression of retrodiskal tissue, which is now located in the articular zone.

Functional overloading of the TMJ, associated with the habit of chronic teeth clenching, is another frequent cause of internal derangements. Although the TMJ is constructed for eccentric movements, it is not constructed for the constant isometric loading and unloading that occurs during this activity. Such parafunction affects the lubrication of the joint and alters the articular surfaces, introducing friction between the disk and the condyle that leads to degenerative changes in the articular surfaces and results in gradual anterior displacement of the disk.[26,28,40,42]

Degenerative joint disease may precede the development of an internal derangement, or it may occur after the development of an internal derangement. In the first instance, changes in the character of the articulating surfaces result in an inability of the parts to glide smoothly over each other, gradually leading to forward displacement of the disk, which normally rotates posteriorly during mouth opening. In the second instance, the displaced disk results in an altered relationship between articulating components of the joint, which leads to degenerative changes in these structures. In patients in whom the condition causing the degenerative joint disease is still active, whether primarily or secondarily, both the causative condition and the disk derangement must be treated for the problem to be resolved completely.

Imaging Findings

Depending on the cause of the internal derangement and its duration, radiographs may or may not show any evidence of degenerative joint disease. MRI shows anterior disk displacement in the closed mouth position, as well as a return to a normal disk relationship during mouth opening, in patients with clicking and popping. In patients with locking, however, the disk remains in the anterior position on attempted mouth opening, and movement of the condyle is limited. In a small group of patients with locking, MRI showed the intra-articular disk in normal position when the teeth were in occlusion, rather than in anterior displacement, and no change in disk position occurred when the patient attempted to open the mouth.[29,43] In such cases, adhesion of the disk to the articular eminence prevents translation of the condyle. These patients differ from those with anteriorly displaced, nonreducing disks in that they do not have a history of TMJ clicking that precedes the sudden onset of locking.

Treatment

Initial treatment of patients with painful clicking or popping in the TMJ consists of a nonsteroidal anti-inflammatory drug; a soft, nonchewy diet; and use of a bite-opening appliance to reduce compression of retrodiskal tissue (Fig. 54.3). A muscle relaxant drug can be added to the regimen if the patient has associated

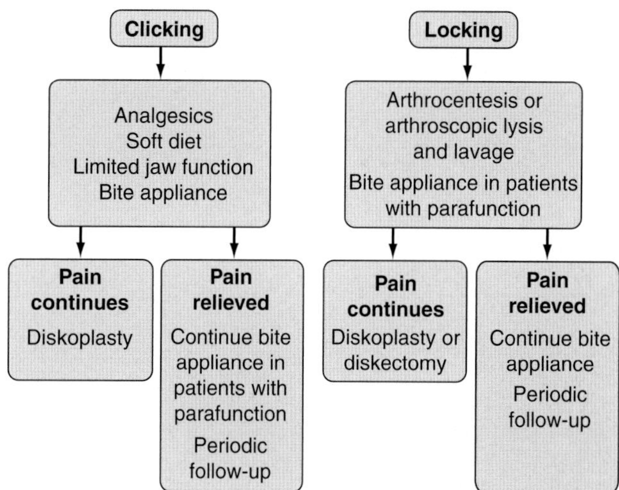

• **Fig. 54.3** Management of internal derangements of the temporomandibular joint. Patients with painful clicking or locking are treated medically initially, whereas patients with locking require surgical intervention.

myofascial pain. When the pain has stopped, no further treatment is generally necessary, although joint noise may still be present. In patients who have teeth-clenching and -grinding habits, however, use of a bite appliance is indicated at night to control these habits and prevent recurrence of the pain.

A long-term follow-up study (1 to 15 years) of 190 patients with a history of clicking treated by such conservative nonsurgical modalities, which are not directed specifically to the problems of joint noise or disk displacement, showed that the condition worsened in only 1% of patients, indicating that it is permissible to observe individuals with painless clicking as long as they remain otherwise asymptomatic.[30,44]

In patients with pain and clicking in the TMJ that is unresponsive to nonsurgical management, the disk should be repositioned arthroscopically or by open surgery (diskoplasty). Patients with parafunctional habits should continue the use of a bite appliance when sleeping. In patients with locking (anterior disk displacement without reduction), whether painful or not, treatment is urgent because if the condition is left untreated for a long time, subsequent management can be complicated by further degenerative changes in the disk and condyle that make disk salvage (diskoplasty) impossible. Initial treatment involves joint lavage and lysis of adhesions by arthrocentesis or arthroscopically. The former involves the establishment of inlet and outlet portals in the upper joint space with hypodermic needles, irrigation with lactated Ringer's solution to remove inflammatory tissue breakdown products and cytokines, and lysis of adhesions by hydraulic distention and manual manipulation of the joint (Fig. 54.4).[31,45]

The results of arthrocentesis parallel those achieved with arthroscopic lysis and lavage, and the procedure is less invasive. Although neither of these procedures restores the disk to its normal position, they do restore disk and joint mobility, and they reduce pain and improve function in most patients.[32,33,46,47] In these patients, the retrodiskal tissue within the joint undergoes fibrosis and acts as a pseudodisk. It is important that patients who have teeth-grinding or -clenching habits are prescribed a bite appliance post-operatively to wear while sleeping.

In patients who do not respond favorably to arthrocentesis or arthroscopy, the displaced disk should be repositioned by an open operation. If the disk is extremely deformed and cannot be repositioned, or if a large, nonrepairable perforation in the disk or a tear

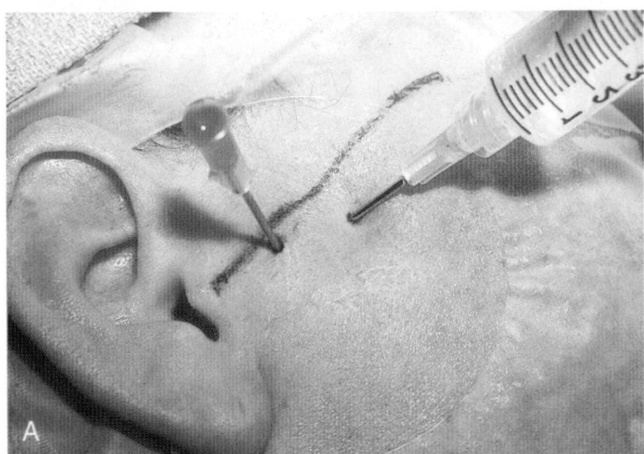

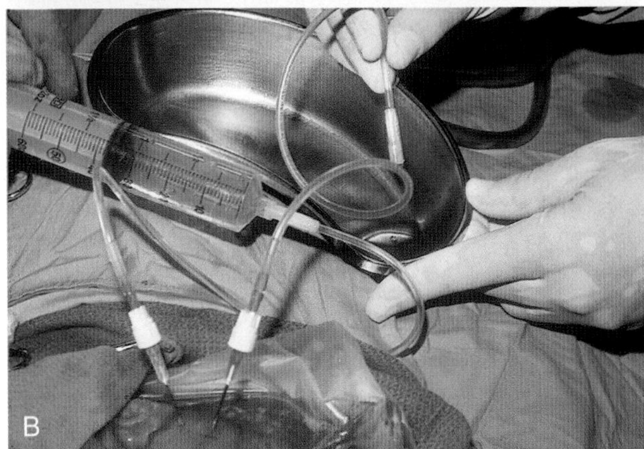

• **Fig. 54.4** Temporomandibular joint arthrocentesis. (A) Hypodermic needles inserted into the upper joint space to allow lavage of the joint. (B) Joint is being irrigated with lactated Ringer's solution.

in the retrodiskal tissue is present, the disk should be removed. Although autogenous auricular cartilage or dermal grafts, or temporalis muscle flaps, have been used as disk replacements, results have been unpredictable.[31,45,48] More recent long-term studies have shown that most patients can tolerate a diskless joint.[34,49] Currently, no acceptable alloplastic substitutes for the disk are available.

Neoplasms

Although primary neoplasms involving the TMJ are uncommon, they must be considered in the differential diagnosis of painful conditions affecting this region.[35,36,50,51] Chondroma, osteochondroma, and osteoma are the most frequently encountered benign tumors, but isolated cases of fibro-osteoma, myxoma, fibrous dysplasia, giant cell reparative granuloma, aneurysmal bone cyst, synovioma, synovial chondromatosis, chondroblastoma, osteoblastoma, glomus tumor, and synovial hemangioma have been reported. Malignant tumors of the TMJ are even rarer, with infrequent reports of fibrosarcoma, chondrosarcoma, synovial fibrosarcoma, osteosarcoma, malignant fibrous histiocytoma, malignant schwannoma, leiomyosarcoma, and multiple myeloma. The TMJ can also be invaded by neoplasms from the cheek, the parotid gland, the external auditory canal, and the adjacent ramus of the mandible. Metastasis to the condyle from distant neoplasms in the breast, lung, prostate, colon, thyroid gland, liver, stomach, and kidney has been described.

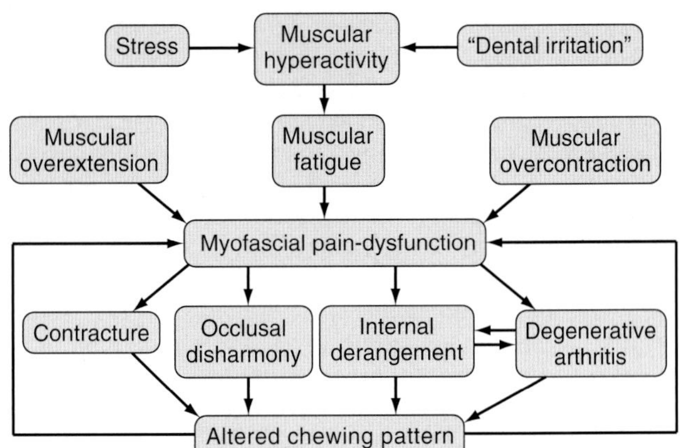

• **Fig. 54.5** Causes of myofascial pain and dysfunction. Although the diagram shows three pathways, the one involving psychological stress is most common. The mechanism by which stress leads to myofascial pain and dysfunction is termed the *psychophysiologic theory.* (Modified from Laskin DM: Etiology of the pain-dysfunction syndrome. *J Am Dent Assoc* 79:147–153, 1969. Copyright 1969, American Dental Association. Reprinted by permission of ADA Publishing Co.)

Tumors of the TMJ can cause pain, limitation of jaw movement, deviation of the mandible to the affected side on attempted mouth opening, and difficulty in occluding the teeth. Depending on the nature of the condition, radiographs may show bony deformation, apposition, or resorption. A biopsy is necessary to establish a definitive diagnosis.

Myofascial Pain and Dysfunction

Mastictory muscle myofascial pain and dysfunction (MPD) is considered a psychophysiologic disease that primarily involves the muscles of mastication, not the TMJ. Women are affected more frequently than men; the ratio in various reports ranges from 3:1 to 5:1. Although the condition can occur in children, the incidence seems to be greatest in adults 20 to 40 years old. MPD is frequently confused with painful conditions that affect the TMJ, such as degenerative arthritis or internal derangements; patients with primary MPD can develop these diseases secondarily, and patients with primary joint disease can develop secondary MPD. Enhanced understanding of the causes and pathogenesis of this condition makes its diagnosis easier and its treatment more effective.[37,38,52,53]

Etiology

Psychological stress has been suggested as an important contributing factor in the development of MPD (psychophysiologic theory).[39,54,55] It is hypothesized that in most patients, stress-related, centrally induced increases in muscle activity, frequently combined with the presence of parafunctional habits such as clenching or grinding of the teeth, may result in associated muscle fatigue, pain, and limited mouth opening.[40,54] Nevertheless, similar symptoms have occasionally been seen to result from muscle overextension, muscle overcontraction, or trauma (Fig. 54.5). A counter-theory (the pain adaptation theory of Lund)[56] has been proposed to suggest that pain in the masticatory muscles leads to a reduction rather than an increase in muscle activity as a protective mechanism, and this reduction causes the limitation in mouth opening; however, this theory does not explain the origin of the pain. Despite extensive research, the cause of myofascial pain and dysfunction remains unknown.

Clinical Findings

Pain of unilateral origin is the most common symptom of MPD. In contrast to the pain associated with joint disease, which is well localized, the pain of muscle origin is more diffuse. The patient generally is unable to identify accurately the specific site involved; this can serve as an important diagnostic criterion in distinguishing between muscle and joint disorders.

Depending on the muscle involved, the pain associated with MPD may be described by the patient in various ways. The masseter is the muscle most frequently involved, and the patient usually refers to the pain as a *jaw ache*. The temporalis is the next most commonly involved muscle; it produces pain on the side of the head, which is interpreted by the patient as a headache. Involvement of the lateral pterygoid muscle produces earache or a deep pain behind the eye, whereas medial pterygoid involvement causes discomfort on swallowing and the feeling of a painful, swollen gland beneath the angle of the mandible. Medial pterygoid involvement can cause stuffiness or a full feeling in the ear.

The pain associated with MPD is usually constant, but it is often more severe on arising in the morning or may worsen gradually as the day progresses. Pain generally is exacerbated by jaw function, especially during such activities as eating and excessive talking. Myofascial pain tends to be regional rather than local, and patients with a long-standing problem may complain that pain in the facial region has spread to the cervical area and later to the shoulders and back.

Tenderness in the muscles of mastication, another common finding, can be used to confirm the source of the pain in muscles that are accessible to palpation (masseter, temporalis, and medial pterygoid). Although muscle tenderness usually is not reported by the patient, this symptom can be elicited easily by the examiner. The most frequent sites of tenderness are near the angle of the mandible, in the belly and the posterosuperior aspect of the masseter, in the anterior temporal region, and over the temporal crest on the anterior aspect of the coronoid process. The location of some of the tender areas suggests that tendons may also be a source of pain and tenderness.

Limitation of mandibular movement is the third cardinal symptom of MPD. It manifests as an inability to open the mouth as wide as usual and as a deviation of the mandible to the affected side when mouth opening is attempted. Lateral excursion to the unaffected side is also reduced. The limitation of mandibular movement usually is correlated with the amount of pain present.

A clicking or popping sound in the TMJ is another finding in some patients with MPD. This is not a cardinal sign, however, because it occurs only in patients with a chronic teeth-clenching habit, which gradually produces frictional changes in the joint and subsequent disk displacement.[26,40] The presence of joint sounds alone is insufficient to allow a diagnosis of MPD. Joint sounds must be accompanied by myofascial pain and tenderness in the masticatory muscles that began before the onset of the joint noise. Such patients must be distinguished from patients with a primary internal derangement, in whom muscle splinting produces myofascial pain and tenderness after the onset of the joint noise. The history and differences in physical findings are helpful in making this distinction.

In addition to the three cardinal symptoms of pain, muscle tenderness, and limitation of mouth opening, patients with MPD usually have no clinical or radiographic evidence of pathologic changes in the TMJ. These negative characteristics are important for the physician in establishing the diagnosis because they confirm that the primary site of the problem is not the articular structures.

Diagnosis

Because the cardinal signs and symptoms of MPD are similar to those produced by such organic problems involving the TMJ as degenerative joint disease and internal disk derangement and by a variety of nonarticular conditions (see Tables 54.1 and 54.2), diagnosis of this condition can be difficult. To make a diagnosis, the physician needs a careful patient history and a thorough clinical evaluation. Periapical radiographs of the teeth and a screening radiograph (panoramic) of the TMJs can be helpful to eliminate dental problems or gross joint disease. If screening views of the TMJs show some abnormality, CT scans are usually advisable for confirmation. MRI also can be useful in determining the position of the disk when an internal derangement of the TMJ is being considered. Depending on the suspected condition, other radiographic views of the head and neck and scintigraphy may be needed to establish a final diagnosis.

Certain laboratory tests may be helpful in some instances. These include a complete blood cell count if an infection is suspected; serum calcium, phosphorus, and alkaline phosphatase measurements for possible bone disease; serum uric acid determination for gout; serum creatinine and creatine kinase levels to detect muscle disease; and erythrocyte sedimentation rate, rheumatoid factor, latex fixation, and anti-nuclear antibody tests for suspected rheumatoid arthritis. Electromyography can be used to evaluate muscle function. Psychological evaluation and psychometric testing are good research tools, but they have little diagnostic value other than to identify the presence of associated abnormal behavioral characteristics.

Fibromyalgia is a condition that sometimes is confused with myofascial pain, particularly when MPD involves several regions in addition to the face. Although fibromyalgia may eventually develop in a small subset of patients with MPD, these are probably distinct conditions.[41,57] Table 54.4 lists the distinguishing characteristics of myofascial pain versus fibromyalgia.

TABLE 54.4 Distinguishing Features of Myofascial Pain and Fibromyalgia

	Myofascial Pain	Fibromyalgia
Patient age distribution	20-40 years	20-50 years
Sex distribution	Mainly women	Mainly women
Distribution of pain	Localized; usually unilateral	Generalized; bilaterally symmetric
Tender points	Few	Multiple
Trigger points	Uncommon	Common
Fatigue	Localized muscle fatigue	Generalized fatigue
Sleep disturbance	Common	Common

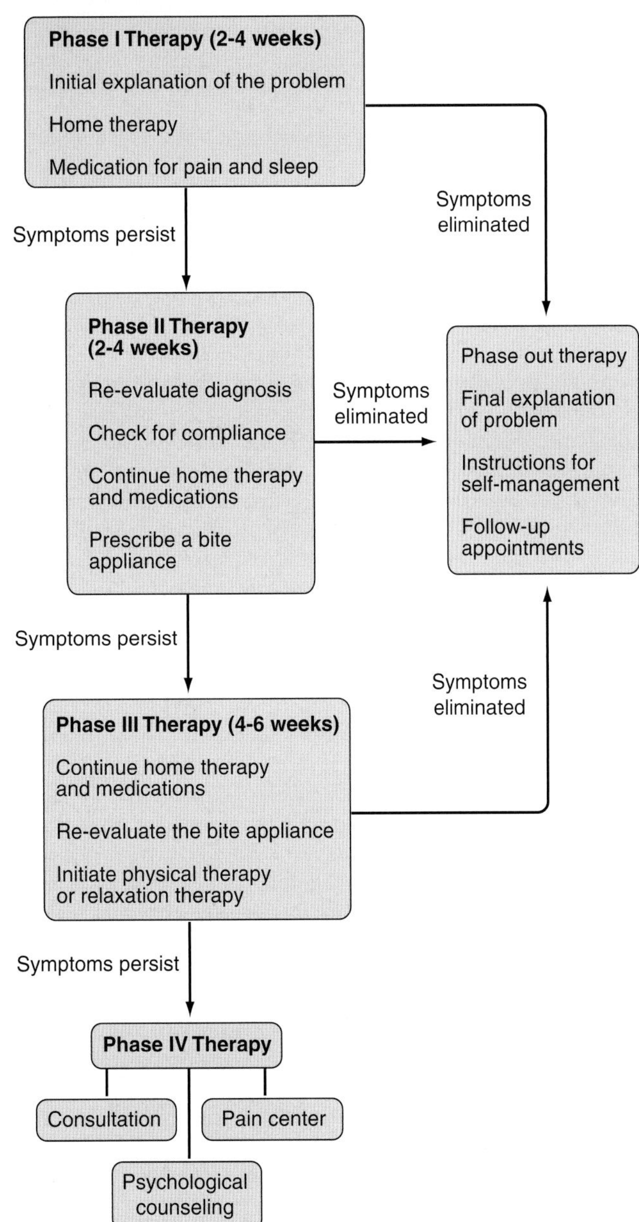

• **Fig. 54.6** Management of myofascial pain and dysfunction. The treatments are divided into four phases. If the symptoms are eliminated in any of the first three phases, the ongoing therapy is gradually phased out, and the patient is instructed in continued self-management of the condition. (Modified from Laskin DM, Block S: Diagnosis and treatment of myofascial pain dysfunction [MPD] syndrome. *J Prosthet Dent* 56:75–84, 1986.)

Treatment

Treatment of MPD is divided into four phases.[42,58] When a definitive diagnosis is made, phase I therapy should be started (Fig. 54.6). Phase I therapy initially involves providing the patient with some understanding of the problem. Because patients often have difficulty accepting a psychophysiologic explanation for their condition, the physician's discussion with the patient should deal first with the issue of muscle fatigue as the cause of the pain and dysfunction, and delay consideration of the role of stress and psychological factors until the symptoms have improved and the patient's confidence has been gained. Associating the symptoms to the specific masticatory muscles from which they arise helps the patient understand the reason for the type and location of the pain—headache from the temporalis muscle, jaw ache from the masseter muscle, discomfort on swallowing and stuffiness in the ear from the medial pterygoid muscle, and earache and pain behind the eye from the lateral pterygoid muscle.

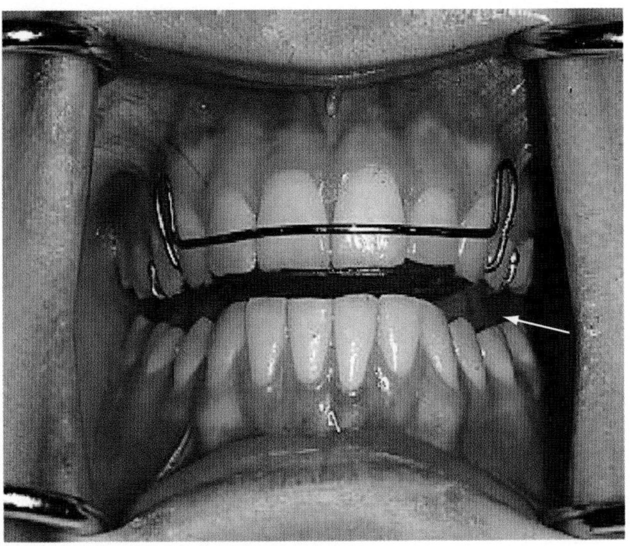

• **Fig. 54.7** Hawley-type maxillary bite appliance. Only the anterior teeth contact the appliance, and space between the posterior teeth is evident *(arrow).*

In addition to the initial explanation, the patient should be counseled regarding home therapy. This counseling includes recommendations to avoid clenching and grinding of the teeth, to eat a soft diet, to use moist heat and massage on the masticatory muscles, and to limit jaw movement. A nonsteroidal anti-inflammatory drug should be prescribed for the pain. In patients who have problems sleeping, a small dose of amitriptyline at bedtime is helpful to improve sleep and reduce parafunction.

Approximately 50% of these patients experience resolution of their symptoms within 2 to 4 weeks with phase I therapy. For patients whose symptoms persist, phase II therapy is initiated. Home therapy and medications are continued, and a bite appliance is made for the patient. Although numerous types have been used, the Hawley-type maxillary appliance is probably the most effective because it prevents contact of the posterior teeth and thus prevents most forms of parafunctional activity (Fig. 54.7).[43,59] The appliance generally is worn at night, but it can be worn for 5 to 6 hours during the day, if necessary. The appliance should not be worn continuously, however, because the posterior teeth may supraerupt in some patients.

With phase II therapy, another 20% to 25% of patients become symptom free in 2 to 4 weeks. When the patient becomes symptom free, the medications are stopped first, and use of the bite appliance is discontinued next. If the patient has a return of symptoms, and the appliance is worn only at night, its use can be continued indefinitely.

Patients who do not respond to the use of a bite appliance are entered into phase III treatment for 4 to 6 weeks. In this phase, physical therapy (heat, massage, ultrasound, and electrogalvanic stimulation)[60] or relaxation therapy (electromyographic biofeedback and conditioned relaxation)[61] is added to the regimen. No evidence shows that one form of treatment is better than the other, and either can be used first. If one is unsuccessful, the other can be tried. Phase III therapy usually helps another 10% to 15% of patients.

If all of these approaches fail, and no question arises about the correctness of the diagnosis, psychological counseling is recommended. This counseling involves helping patients to identify possible stresses in their lives and learn to cope with such situations. If the diagnosis is in doubt, the patient should be referred first for appropriate dental and neurologic consultation and re-evaluation. Another alternative is to refer patients with recalcitrant MPD to a TMJ center or pain clinic because such patients generally require a multidisciplinary approach for successful treatment.

Conclusion

Successful management of patients with temporomandibular disorders depends on an accurate diagnosis of the disorder and use of the proper therapy based on the physician's understanding of the cause of the patient's condition. Of particular importance is distinguishing patients with MPD, who constitute the majority of patients encountered and who are not surgical candidates, from patients with TMJ disease, who frequently require surgical treatment. Even in the latter group, many commonly encountered conditions, such as arthritis and internal disk derangements, often respond to nonsurgical therapy, and this type of treatment should be given a fair trial before more aggressive management is considered.

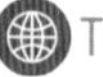 The references for this chapter can also be found on ExpertConsult.com.

References

1. Merjersjo C: Therapeutic and prognostic considerations in TMJ osteoarthrosis: a literature review and a long-term study in 11 subjects, *J Craniomandib Pract* 5:70, 1987.
2. Madsen B: Normal variations in anatomy, condylar movements and arthrosis frequency of the TMJs, *Acta Radiol* 4:273, 1966.
3. Milam SB, Zardeneta G, Schmitz JP: Oxidative stress and degenerative temporomandibular joint disease, *J Oral Maxillofac Surg* 56:214, 1998.
4. Manfredini D, Bonnini S, Arboretti R, et al.: Temporomandibular joint osteoarthritis: an open label trial of 76 patients treated with arthrocentesis and hyaluronic acid injections, *Int J Oral Maxillofac Surg* 38:827, 2009.
5. Onder ME, Tuz HH, Kocyigit D, et al.: Long-term results of arthrocentesis in degenerative temporomandibular disorders, *Oral Surg Oral Med Oral Pathol Radiol Endod* 107(1), 2008.
6. Haddad IK: Temporomandibular joint osteoarthritis: histopathological study of the effects of intra-articular injection of triamcinolone acetonide, *Saudi Med J* 21:675, 2000.
7. Bjornland T, Gjaerum AA, Moystad A: Osteoarthritis of the temporomandibular joint: an evaluation of the effects and complications of corticosteroid injection compared with injection with sodium hyaluronate, *J Oral Rehabil* 34:583, 2007.
8. Abubaker AO, Laskin DM: Nonsurgical management of arthritis of the temporomandibular joint, *Oral Maxillofac Surg Clin N Am* 7(1), 1995.
9. Bessa-Nogueira RV, Vasconcelos BC, Duarte AP, et al.: Targeted assessment of the temporomandibular joint in patients with rheumatoid arthritis, *J Oral Maxillofac Surg* 66:1804, 2008.
10. Zide MF, Carlton D, Kent JH: Rheumatoid arthritis and related arthropathies: systemic findings, medical therapy, and peripheral joint surgery, *Oral Surg Oral Med Oral Pathol* 61:119, 1986.
11. Davidson C, Wojtulewsky JA, Bacon PA, et al.: Temporomandibular joint disease in ankylosing spondylitis, *Ann Rheum Dis* 34:87, 1975.
12. Wilson A, Braunwald E, Issilbacker KJ: Psoriatic arthropathy of the temporomandibular joint, *Oral Surg Oral Med Oral Pathol* 70:555, 1990.
13. Kononen M: Radiographic changes in the condyle of the temporomandibular joint in psoriatic arthritis, *Acta Radiol* 28:185, 1987.
14. Wenneburg B, Kononen M, Kallenberg A: Radiographic changes in the temporomandibular joint of patients with rheumatoid arthritis, psoriatic arthritis, ankylosing spondylitis, *J Craniomandib Disord* 4(35), 1990.
15. Miles DA, Kaugers GA: Psoriatic involvement of the temporomandibular joint: literature review and report of two cases, *Oral Surg Oral Med Oral Pathol* 71:770, 1991.
16. Lundberg M, Ericsson S: Changes in the temporomandibular joint in psoriasis arthropathica, *Acta Derm Venereol* 47:354, 1967.
17. Koorbusch GF, Zeitler DL, Fotos PG, et al.: Psoriatic arthritis of the temporomandibular joint with ankylosis, *Oral Surg Oral Med Oral Pathol* 71:267, 1991.
18. de Viam K, Laries RJ: Update in treatment options for psoriatic arthritis, *Expert Rev Clin Immunol* 5:779, 2009.
19. Alstergren P, Larsson PT, Kopp S: Successful treatment with multiple intra-articular injections of infliximab in a patient with psoriatic arthritis, *Scand J Rheumatol* 37:155, 2008.
20. Lamazza L, Guerra F, Messina AM, et al.: The use of etanercept as a non-surgical treatment for temporomandibular joint psoriatic arthritis: a case report, *Aust Dent J* 54:161, 2009.
21. Salvarini C, Cantini F, Olivieri I: Disease-modifying antirheumatic drug therapy for psoriatic arthritis, *Clin Exp Rheumatol* 20(Suppl 28):S71, 2002.
22. Wenneberg B: Inflammatory involvement of the temporomandibular joint: diagnostic and therapeutic aspects and a study of individuals with ankylosing spondylitis, *Swed Dent J Suppl* 20(1), 1983.
23. Wenneberg B, Hollender L, Kopp S: Radiographic changes in the temporomandibular joint in ankylosing spondylitis, *Dentomaxillofac Radiol* 12:25, 1983.
24. Manemi RV, Fasanmade A, Revington PJ: Bilateral ankylosis of the jaw treated with total alloplastic replacement using the TMJ concepts system in a patient with ankylosing spondylitis, *Br J Oral Maxillofac Surg* 47:159, 2009.
25. Kononen M: Signs and symptoms of craniomandibular disorders in men with Reiter's disease, *J Craniomandib Disord* 6:247, 1992.
26. Kononen M, Kovero O, Wenneberg B, et al.: Radiographic signs in the temporomandibular joint in Reiter's disease, *J Orofac Pain* 16:143, 2002.
27. Harris S, Rood JP, Testa HJ: Post-traumatic changes of the temporomandibular joint by bone scintigraphy, *Int J Oral Maxillofac Surg* 17:173, 1988.
28. Hanson TL: Pathological aspects of arthritides and derangements. In Sarnat BG, Laskin DM, editors: *The temporomandibular joint: a biological basis for clinical practice*, ed 4, Philadelphia, 1992, Saunders, pp 165–182.
29. Lesnicar DG, Zerdoner D: Temporomandibular joint involvement caused by *Borrelia burgdorferi*, *J Craniomaxillofac Surg* 35:397, 2007.
30. Leighly SM, Spach DH, Myall RW, et al.: Septic arthritis of the temporomandibular joint: review of the literature and report of two cases in children, *Int J Oral Maxillofac Surg* 22:292, 1993.
31. Cai XY, Yang C, Zhang ZY, et al.: Septic arthritis of the temporomandibular joint: a retrospective review of 40 cases, *J Oral Maxillofac Surg* 68:731, 2010.
32. Cai XY, Yang C, Chen MJ, et al.: Arthroscopic management of septic arthritis of the temporomandibular joint, *Oral Surg Oral Med Oral Pathol Oral Radiol Endod* 109(24), 2010.
33. Gross BD, Williams RB, DiCosimo CT, et al.: Gout and pseudogout of the temporomandibular joint, *Oral Surg Oral Med Oral Pathol* 63:551, 1987.
34. Barthelemy I, Karanas Y, Sannajust JP, et al.: Gout of the temporomandibular joint: pitfalls in diagnosis, *J Craniomaxillofac Surg* 29:307, 2001.

35. Suba Z, Takacs D, Gyulai-Gaal S, et al.: Tophaceous gout of the temporomandibular joint: a report of 2 cases, *J Oral Maxillofac Surg* 67:1526, 2009.
36. Nakagawa Y, Ishibashi K, Kobayoshi K, et al.: Calcium phosphate deposition disease in the temporomandibular joint: report of two cases, *J Oral Maxillofac Surg* 57:1357, 1999.
37. Chuong R, Piper MA: Bilateral pseudogout of the temporomandibular joint: report of a case and review of the literature, *J Oral Maxillofac Surg* 53:691, 1995.
38. Aoyama S, Kino K, Amagosa T, et al.: Differential diagnosis of calcium pyrophosphate dihydrate deposition of the temporomandibular joint, *Br J Oral Maxillofac Surg* 38:550, 2000.
39. Ascani G, Pieramici MD, Fiosa A, et al.: Pseudogout of the temporomandibular joint: a case report, *J Oral Maxillofac Surg* 66:386, 2008.
40. Laskin DM: Etiology and pathogenesis of internal derangements of the temporomandibular joint, *Oral Maxillofac Surg Clin N Am* 6:217, 1994.
41. Heise AP, Laskin DM, Gervin AS: Incidence of temporomandibular joint symptoms following whiplash injury, *J Oral Maxillofac Surg* 50:825, 1992.
42. Nitzan DW: The process of lubrication impairment and its involvement in temporomandibular disk displacement: a theoretical concept, *J Oral Maxillofac Surg* 59:36, 2001.
43. Nitzan DW, Samson B, Better H: Long-term outcome of arthrocentesis for sudden-onset persistent, severe closed lock of the temporomandibular joint, *J Oral Maxillofac Surg* 55:151, 1997.
44. Greene CS, Laskin DM: Long-term status of TMJ clicking in patients with myofascial pain and dysfunction, *J Am Dent Assoc* 117:461, 1988.
45. Laskin DM: Surgical management of internal derangements. In Laskin DM, Greene CS, Hylander WL, editors: *Temporomandibular disorders: an evidence-based approach to diagnosis and treatment*, Chicago, 2006, Quintessence, pp 469–481.
46. Dimitroulis G: A review of 55 cases of chronic closed lock treated with temporomandibular joint arthroscopy, *J Oral Maxillofac Surg* 60:519, 2002.
47. Carvajal W, Laskin DM: Long-term evaluation of arthrocentesis for treatment of internal derangement of the temporomandibular joint, *J Oral Maxillofac Surg* 58:852, 2000.
48. Kramer A, Lee JJ, Bierne OR: Meta-analysis of TMJ discectomy with and without autogenous/alloplastic interpositional materials: comparison analysis of functional outcomes, *J Oral Maxillofac Surg* 62(Suppl 1):49, 2004.
49. Eriksson L, Westesson PL: Discectomy as an effective treatment for painful temporomandibular joint internal derangement: a 5 year clinical and radiographic follow-up, *J Oral Maxillofac Surg* 59:750, 2001.
50. Stern D: Benign and malignant tumors. In Laskin DM, Greene CS, Hylander WL, editors: *Temporomandibular disorders: an evidence-based approach to diagnosis and treatment*, Chicago, 2006, Quintessence, pp 319–333.
51. Clayman L: Surgical management of benign and malignant neoplasms. In Laskin DM, Greene CS, Hylander WL, editors: *Temporomandibular disorders: an evidence-based approach to diagnosis and treatment*, Chicago, 2006, Quintessence, pp 509–532.
52. Laskin DM: Diagnosis and etiology of myofascial pain and dysfunction, *Oral Maxillofac Surg Clin N Am* 7:73, 1995.
53. Clark GT: Treatment of myogenous pain and dysfunction. In Laskin DM, Greene CS, Hylander WL, editors: *Temporomandibular disorders: an evidence-based approach to diagnosis and treatment*, Chicago, 2006, Quintessence, pp 483–500.
54. Laskin DM: Etiology of the pain-dysfunction syndrome, *J Am Dent Assoc* 59:147, 1969.
55. Dworkin SF: Psychological and psychosocial assessment. In Laskin DM, Greene CS, Hylander WL, editors: *Temporomandibular disorders: an evidence-based approach to diagnosis and treatment*, Chicago, 2006, Quintessence, pp 203–217.
56. Lund JP, Donga R, Widmer CG, et al.: The pain-adaptation model: a discussion of the relationship between chronic musculoskeletal pain and motor activity, *Can J Physiol Pharmacol* 69:683, 1991.
57. Cimino R, Michelotti A, Stradi R, et al.: Comparison of the clinical and psychologic features of fibromyalgia and masticatory myofascial pain, *J Orofac Pain* 12(35), 1998.
58. Laskin DM, Block S: Diagnosis and treatment of myofascial pain-dysfunction (MPD) syndrome, *J Prosthet Dent* 56:75, 1986.
59. Clark GT, Minakuchi H: Oral appliances. In Laskin DM, Greene CS, Hylander WL, editors: *Temporomandibular disorders: an evidence-based approach to diagnosis and treatment*, Chicago, 2006, Quintessence, pp 377–390.
60. Feine JS, Thomason M: Physical medicine. In Laskin DM, Greene CS, Hylander WL, editors: *Temporomandibular disorders: an evidence-based approach to diagnosis and treatment*, Chicago, 2006, Quintessence, pp 359–379.
61. Ohrbach R: Biobehavioral therapy. In Laskin DM, Greene CS, Hylander WL, editors: *Temporomandibular disorders: an evidence-based approach to diagnosis and treatment*, Chicago, 2006, Quintessence, pp 391–402.

Websites

www.nicdr.nih.gov—General information, clinical trials, and sponsored research in TMJ and related areas.
www.aaoms.org—General information about TMJ surgery.
www.tmj.org—Advocate group that provides general information for patients.

55 Fibromyalgia

LESLIE J. CROFFORD

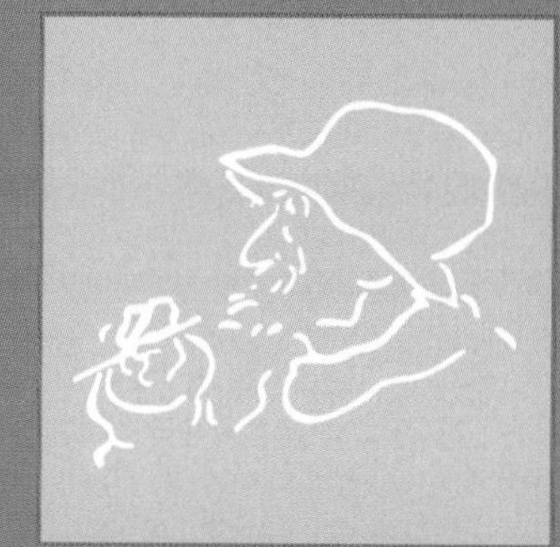

KEY POINTS

Fibromyalgia (FM) is a disorder of centrally amplified and maintained musculoskeletal pain with objective evidence of altered pain processing in the spinal cord and brain.

Although pain is the defining symptom of FM, fatigue, unrefreshing sleep, cognitive complaints, depression, and anxiety also have a significant impact on health-related quality of life.

The diagnosis of FM relies on patient report using one of several valid criteria sets.

Patients with other rheumatic diseases have a higher prevalence of FM than the general population, and the presence of comorbid FM affects assessment of disease activity.

It is important to identify FM to develop an overall treatment plan that addresses the mechanisms responsible for musculoskeletal pain in each patient.

Introduction

Fibromyalgia (FM) is a disorder characterized by chronic widespread musculoskeletal pain often associated with debilitating fatigue, unrefreshing sleep, cognitive complaints, depression, and anxiety.[1] Patients with FM have evidence of disordered sensory processing as manifested by widespread allodynia (i.e., pain elicited by an innocuous stimulus that is not usually painful) and hyperalgesia (i.e., exaggerated pain elicited by a noxious stimulus). Patients often have a personal and family history of regional or visceral pain, such as migraine or tension headaches, temporomandibular disorder, irritable bowel syndrome, interstitial cystitis, pelvic pain syndromes, and depression or anxiety.[1,2] A careful history typically reveals a pain-prone phenotype with musculoskeletal pain as only one of the affected body regions.[1] Genetic vulnerability to FM and other disorders characterized by amplified pain is associated with polymorphisms in genes involving pain transmission, neurotransmitter, and stress-response pathways.[3,4] It is thought that in vulnerable people, triggering events involving activation of sensory nociceptors lead to long-term changes in pain transmission and descending inhibitory pathways.[3] This concept of centrally maintained or amplified pain as the central physiologic alteration in FM has led to treatment strategies that differ from traditional anti-inflammatory or analgesic approaches to musculoskeletal pain.[1] Cognitive and emotional factors also play a significant role in the impact of FM on health, requiring the clinician to address the patient's beliefs and behaviors that augment pain symptoms. In some patients, a multidisciplinary approach to treatment will provide significant benefits.[5]

Because the diagnosis of FM relies solely on patient report, and all of the symptoms of FM exist in a continuum in healthy people, significant controversy has existed regarding the legitimacy of FM as a medical illness.[6] What is clear is that pain reports of people with FM are associated with activation of areas in the brain associated with pain transmission, which advanced neuroimaging studies determine.[7] Thus, objective evidence of the subjective report of pain exists. From a practical perspective, the treating clinician should be able to identify the symptoms of FM, sort through the differential diagnosis, understand its relationship to comorbid rheumatic diseases, assist the patient in distinguishing central pain from mechanical or inflammatory pain, and provide management approaches that address the patient's symptoms.

Historical Perspective

Descriptions of patients with symptoms of FM in the medical literature go back centuries. In early descriptions, the condition was often called *muscular rheumatism,* which distinguished it from *articular rheumatism*.[8] In 1815, Dr. William Balfour, a surgeon from Edinburgh, described nodules and suggested that inflammation in muscle connective tissue was the cause for nodules and pain. He also first reported focal tenderness, referred to as *tender points*, in 1824. Sir William Gowers coined the term *fibrositis* in 1904, sharing in the belief that patients experienced inflammation of fibrous connective tissue that led to tender points in patients with muscular rheumatism.[9]

An interesting historical treatise by Dr. Philip Hench and Edward Boland published in 1946 described the management of rheumatic diseases in U.S. Army soldiers and provides insights that remain relevant in more modern times.[10] They reported that muscular rheumatism occurred in 13% of soldiers from the First World War (April 1, 1917 to December 31, 1919). Specialized rheumatism centers were established in the 1940s for soldiers of the Second World War. Hench and Boland published the incidence of rheumatic diseases in the first 1000 cases and differentiated *psychogenic rheumatism* (which occurred in 20% of cases) from *fibrositis*, which included regional syndromes, such as bursitis and tendonitis, in 13.4% of cases. Hench and Boland noted that most of the patients sent to these specialized centers with muscular rheumatism did not have myositis or fibrositis; instead, the patients had psychogenic rheumatism, which the researchers considered a psychoneurosis manifested by musculoskeletal complaints. They went on to state that primary fibrositis "puts its victims at the mercy of changes in external environment: thus weather, heat, cold, humidity, rest, exercise, etc. characteristically influences most of them for better or for worse."[10] On the other hand, they stated that psychogenic rheumatism "puts its victims at the mercy of changes in the internal environment: thus, their symptoms may vary with mood or psyche, pleasure, excitement, mental distraction, worry, or fatigue."[10]

The description of psychogenic rheumatism included an attitude that was tense, anxious, defensive, and antagonistic. The chief symptoms were described as burning, tightness, weakness, numbness, tingling, or tired sensations that were often continuous day and night. They also describe severe fatigue causing disability, worsening of symptoms during and after exercise, and a "touch me not" reaction to examination. Psychotherapy was the preferred treatment approach for these patients. Patients with fibrositis, on the other hand, were treated with physical rehabilitation. In evaluating outcome, 82% of patients with primary fibrositis returned to duty, compared with only 64% of patients with psychogenic rheumatism.[10] In our current understanding, FM likely represents a combination of primary fibrositis and psychogenic rheumatism, with both conditions having a component of central pain amplification but diverging in the psychological and behavioral responses to pain.

Dr. Hugh Smythe provided the first modern description of widespread pain and tender points in the 1970s.[11] The term *fibromyalgia* was adopted soon thereafter because pathologic studies consistently fail to find evidence of inflammation in tender areas, calling into question the underlying hypothesis of the fibrositis construct. In 1981, Dr. Muhammad Yunus published a more comprehensive description of the symptoms and signs of FM,[12] which was recognized as a diagnosis by the American Medical Association in 1987. Yunus made the relevant comment that many patients with fibrositis syndrome, fibromyositis, FM, myofibrositis, interstitial myofibrositis, myofascial pain syndrome, myofascitis, muscular rheumatism, nonarticular rheumatism, and tension rheumatism were also diagnosed with the separate entity of psychogenic rheumatism.

Research intended to ascribe an etiology to FM began when Dr. Harvey Moldofsky reported abnormalities in polysomnographic studies of people with FM in 1975, reporting intrusion of alpha or waking frequency waves in regions of delta or slow wave sleep now known to be nonspecific.[13] The American College of Rheumatology (ACR) published classification criteria for FM in 1990 relying on the presence of widespread pain and the presence of a specific number of tender points. The availability of these criteria had the effect of allowing researchers from around the world to identify a more homogenous group of patients for research. Since their publication, investigators have identified a number of other potential mechanisms associated with FM, which may be responsible for symptoms.[14] In 2007, the U.S. Food and Drug Administration (FDA) approved pregabalin, an agent also approved for neuropathic pain, for treatment of FM. This step was followed by approval of the dual norepinephrine-serotonin reuptake inhibitors duloxetine and milnacipran for treatment of FM.[15]

Throughout the history of FM, controversy has existed regarding the veracity of patients' complaints and their reported impact on function.[6] The controversy has become somewhat contentious in the era of disability and the increased cost of FDA-approved medications. However, identifying FM and understanding the recent advances in mechanisms associated with development of central pain amplification has significant benefits that allow clinicians to educate patients about their symptoms and utilize tested therapies. With respect to the presence of psychogenic rheumatism in these patients, the most current approach to patients with FM who have excessive thoughts, feelings, and behaviors that are distressing and disruptive to daily life would be to consider an additional diagnosis of somatic symptom disorder, the new terminology in the *Diagnostic and Statistical Manual of Mental Disorders* (DSM-5) that replaces somatization disorder, hypochondriasis, pain disorder, and undifferentiated somatoform disorder. This way of approaching patients separates the neurobiologic changes resulting in widespread pain amplification from the emotional and behavioral response to these symptoms. Considering both these aspects of FM, which occur in differing proportions in individual patients, may assist the clinician in developing a treatment plan.

Diagnostic Criteria

All of the validated criteria sets for FM include a requirement for chronic musculoskeletal pain. The ACR 1990 criteria focus on the widespread nature of the musculoskeletal pain, requiring that pain be present on both sides of the body, above and below the waist, and including the neck, back, or chest. A demonstration of the presence of widespread allodynia also was required, which was accomplished by a physical examination of 18 defined areas that should be painful with mechanical pressure, at a minimum of 11 sites (Table 55.1).[14] The tender point examination has been controversial for several reasons, including differences in the ability to detect tenderness in men compared with women when using this examination. Another criticism of the ACR 1990 criteria is the absence of other important symptoms, such as fatigue and unrefreshing sleep.

In 2010, a new preliminary criteria set was published that eliminates the requirement for a physical examination. It relies on the patient's report of the number of painful areas to define a widespread pain index (WPI), and incorporates a symptom severity score (SSS) in recognition of the other symptoms of FM.[16] The criticism of the 2010 criteria, as well as a modification published in 2011 intended for use in epidemiologic studies,[17] is the loss of the requirement that the pain be widespread (as defined in the 1990 criteria) and the potential expansion of the prevalence of FM by including people with a lower level of pain symptoms, with a possible bias toward people with somatic symptom disorder. Thus, a further revision of classification criteria published in 2016 again requires pain to be dispersed in different regions much as the 1990 criteria (Table 55.2).[18]

Other criteria sets have been published that include other configurations of symptoms and signs, but the basic clinical manifestations remain unchanged.[19,20] There have been efforts to define criteria more useful in clinical practice using a diagnostic system that would be clinically useful and consistent across chronic pain disorders.[21] The FM criteria developed for this initiative endorse pain as the defining characteristic, and in studies using large population-based datasets with more than 25,000 subjects, the authors determined that multisite pain in 6 or more out of 9 possible sites (see Fig. 55.2) plus moderate to severe sleep problems or fatigue for at least 3 months, would identify people with FM.[22,23] Features not included in the core criteria but supportive of the diagnosis included the following: tenderness, cognitive complaints, musculoskeletal stiffness, and environmental sensitivity or hypervigilance.[22] The implications of the changing definitions of criteria include differences in the prevalence, potential differences in heterogeneity of research populations, and impact on the population studied in clinical trials.

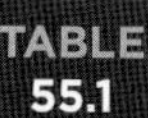

TABLE 55.1 American College of Rheumatology 1990 Criteria for the Classification of Fibromyalgia[a]

1. History of Widespread Pain

Definition: Pain is considered widespread when all of the following are present: pain in the left side of the body, pain in the right side of the body, pain above the waist, and pain below the waist. In addition, axial skeletal pain (cervical spine or anterior chest or thoracic spine or low back) must be present. In this definition, shoulder and buttock pain is considered as pain for each involved side. "Low back" pain is considered lower segment pain.

2. Pain in 11 of 18 Tender Point Sites Upon Digital Palpation

Definition: Pain, upon digital palpation, must be present in at least 11 of the following 18 sites:

- Occiput: bilateral, at the suboccipital muscle insertions
- Low cervical: bilateral, at the anterior aspects of the intertransverse spaces at C5-C7
- Trapezius: bilateral, at the midpoint of the upper border
- Supraspinatus: bilateral, at origins, above the scapula spine near the medial border
- Second rib: bilateral, at the second costochondral junctions, just lateral to the junctions on upper surfaces
- Lateral epicondyle: bilateral, 2 cm distal to the epicondyles
- Gluteal: bilateral, in upper outer quadrants of buttocks in anterior fold of muscle
- Greater trochanter: bilateral, posterior to the trochanteric prominence
- Knee: bilateral, at the medial fat pad proximal to the joint line

Digital palpation should be performed with an approximate force of 4 kg.

For a tender point to be considered "positive," the subject must state that the palpation was painful. "Tender" is not to be considered "painful."

[a]For classification purposes, patients will be said to have fibromyalgia (FM) if both criteria are satisfied. Widespread pain must have been present for at least 3 months. The presence of a second clinical disorder does not exclude the diagnosis of FM.

From Wolfe F, Smythe HA, Yunus MB, et al: The American College of Rheumatology 1990 Criteria for the Classification of Fibromyalgia. Report of the Multicenter Criteria Committee. *Arthritis Rheum* 33:160-172, 1990.

Epidemiology

A number of epidemiologic studies have been performed using different ways to identify patients with FM. The first major study was conducted in Wichita, Kansas, using a population-based mail screening followed by physician assessment using ACR 1990 criteria.[24] In that study, the overall prevalence was 2%, with 3.4% of women and 0.5% of men diagnosed with FM. A recent meta-analysis that included 65 studies and more than 3 million people reported FM prevalence as 2.64% (95% confidence interval [CI] 2.10 to 3.18) in the EURO region, 2.41% (95% CI 1.69 to 3.23) in the AMRO region, and 1.78% (95% CI 1.65 to 2.91) total. The estimated total prevalence in women is 3.98% (95% CI 2.80 to 5.20) and 0.01% (95% CI –0.04 to 0.06) in men. Publications date, diagnostic method, and World Health Organization (WHO) region did not influence the heterogeneity of the results.[25] The prevalence of FM appears to increase with age to about 70 years of age, after which it decreases slightly.[24,26] FM can be diagnosed in children—usually in adolescents, and most commonly in girls.[27] The prevalence of FM in children is approximately 1.5% across studies.[27] The prevalence of FM is generally greater in clinical settings than in epidemiologic studies. A meta-analysis estimated the total prevalence of FM in internal medicine and rheumatology practices at 15.20% (95% CI 13.60 to 16.90).[25]

The incidence of FM is not easily determined; however, one study, which used an *International Classification of Diseases, Ninth Revision* (ICD-9) coding insurance claims database (containing 62,000 nationwide enrollees per year between 1997 and 2002), found an age-adjusted incidence of 11.28 per 1000 person-years

TABLE 55.2 2016 Revisions to the 2010/2011 Diagnostic Criteria for Fibromyalgia

Criteria

A patient satisfies diagnostic criteria for fibromyalgia (FM) if the following three conditions are met:

1. WPI ≥7 and SSS ≥5 OR WPI of 4-6 and SSS ≥9
2. Generalized pain, defined as pain in at least 4 of 5 regions, must be present. Jaw, chest, and abdominal pain are not included in generalized pain definition.
3. Symptoms have been generally present for at least 3 months.A diagnosis of FM is valid irrespective of other diagnoses. A diagnosis of FM does not exclude the presence of other clinically important illnesses.

Ascertainment

1. **Widespread pain index (WPI):** note the number areas in which the patient has had pain during the past week. In how many areas has the patient had pain? Score will be between 0 and 19.

Left upper region (Region 1)	Right upper region (Region 2)	Axial region (Region 5)
Jaw, left[a]	Jaw, right[a]	Neck
Shoulder girdle, left	Shoulder girdle, right	Upper back
Upper arm, left	Upper arm, right	Lower back
Lower arm, left	Lower arm, right	Chest[a]
		Abdomen[a]
Left lower region (Region 3)	**Right lower region (Region 4)**	
Hip (buttock, trochanter), left	Hip (buttock, trochanter), right	
Upper leg, left	Upper leg, right	
Lower leg, left	Lower leg, right	

2. Symptom severity scale (SSS) score:
   - Fatigue
   - Waking unrefreshed
   - Cognitive symptoms

For each of the 3 previously mentioned symptoms:

- 0 = No problem
- 1 = Slight or mild problems; generally mild or intermittent
- 2 = Moderate; considerable problems; often present and/or at a moderate level
- 3 = Severe: pervasive, continuous, life-disturbing problems

The SSS score is the sum of the severity of the three symptoms (fatigue, waking unrefreshed, and cognitive symptoms) (0-9) plus sum (0-3) of the number of the following symptoms the patient has been bothered by that occurred during the previous 6 months:
(1) Headaches (0-1)
(2) Pain or cramps in lower abdomen (0-1)
(3) Depression (0-1)
The final score is between 0 and 12.

The fibromyalgia severity (FS) scale[b] is the sum of the WPI and SSS

[a]Not included in generalized pain definition.

[b]The FS scale is also known as the polysymptomatic distress (PSD) scale.

Adapted from Wolfe F, Clauw DJ, Fitzcharles MA, et al: 2016 revisions to the 2010/2011 fibromyalgia diagnostic criteria. *Semin Arthritis Rheum* 46:319-329, 2016.

for females and 6.88 cases per 1000 person-years in males.[28] In the UK, a study conducted in primary care practices reported an annual incidence of 35 cases per 100,000 people between 1990 and 2001.[29] A more recent update found an annual incidence of 33.3 cases (95% CI 32.8 to 33.8) per 100,000 between 2001 to 2013. The incidence of FM increased with age until 59 years of age, and then it fell. The incidence was approximately sixfold higher in females as compared with males. They also reported a 40% increase in incidence among those in the most deprived segment of the population compared with the least deprived.[30] In a cohort of approximately 1000 patients in the early stage of arthritis who were followed up by rheumatologists, the incidence of FM was 6.77 per 100 person-years in the first year after the diagnosis. The incidence declined to 3.58 per 100 person-years in the second year.[31]

Clinical Features

In clinical settings, patients often report that they have pain "all over their body." They often have difficulty precisely localizing the pain and may describe it as moving from place to place. Patients often describe the pain as "deep," originating in muscles or bones. Patients may use many different pain descriptors, including "throbbing," "stabbing," and "burning." Pain is typically present on most days almost all day, although the intensity may wax and wane. Patients often describe tenderness to light touch or pressure. Pain is typically exacerbated by physical activity, and some patients report that it is worsened with changes in the weather. In addition to pain, patients report muscular stiffness, tightness, and weakness.[32]

The main purpose of the physical examination is to evaluate the patient for other conditions that cause musculoskeletal pain. Patients with FM exhibit tenderness that can be identified by tender point examination. Tender point sites represent specific areas of muscle, tendon, and fat pads that are more tender to palpation than surrounding sites. Sites selected as part of the ACR 1990 criteria represent tender point sites that best discriminate between patients with and without FM. To test for pain with digital palpation, the ACR 1990 criteria indicate that the examiner should press with an approximate force of 4 kg.[14] The patient should report pain in response to this level of pressure, which, in practice, is approximately the force it takes for the thumbnail to blanche.

In addition to the usual musculoskeletal and connective tissue examination, it is useful to evaluate patients, particularly young patients, for joint hypermobility.[33,34] There are indications that FM may be more common among patients with these findings, and physical measures may be quite useful in management of patients with these associations. If regional pain disorders, such as bursitis, tendonitis, or arthritis, can be identified during the physical examination, treatment of these potentially exacerbating pain generators may help with the more widespread pain. Certainly, any mechanical or inflammatory conditions with the potential to cause musculoskeletal pain should be identified and treated.

The pain of FM is often accompanied by other pain amplification syndromes (Table 55.3). These syndromes often have been present for many years and, as with FM, they may wax and wane over time. It may be important for the patient to understand the genetic and physiologic relationships between these diagnoses. In addition, it is clinically important to determine which symptoms have the greatest impact on the patient. Symptom domains have been evaluated by patient and physician Delphi exercises and were generally concordant (Table 55.4).[32] Assessing these clinical concerns may help the clinician prioritize management strategies. For

TABLE 55.3 Fibromyalgia-Associated Pain Amplification Syndromes

Temporomandibular disorder
Tension and migraine headaches
Irritable bowel syndrome and other functional gastrointestinal disorders
Interstitial cystitis/irritable bladder
Dysmenorrhea and other pelvic pain syndromes
Vulvodynia

TABLE 55.4 Patient-Reported Outcomes (PROs) in Fibromyalgia

PRO Concept	Patient Domains[a]	Clinician Domains and Measures[b]
Pain	Pain or physical discomfort Joints aching or pain Stiffness Feeling tender where touched	Pain Patient global status Clinician global status Tender point intensity
Treatment side effects	Problems with medication (e.g., medication adverse effects or reliance on medications)[c]	Adverse effects
Mobility	Difficulty moving, walking, or exercising	Physical function HRQOL
Cognition	Problems with attention or concentration Disorganized thinking Memory problems	Dyscognition HRQOL
Energy	Lack of energy or fatigue Having to push yourself to do things	Fatigue HRQOL
Impact on daily living	Limited in doing normal daily life and household activities Ability to make plans, accomplish goals, or complete tasks Being sensitive to outside factors Unpredictability of symptoms	HRQOL
Emotional well-being	Depression Having to push yourself to do things Frustration[c] Irritability[c]	Depression Anxiety HRQOL
Sleep	Impact on sleep (e.g., difficulty falling asleep, saying asleep, or getting up in the morning)	Sleep quality HRQOL

[a]Most important fibromyalgia (FM) symptoms based on a Delphi exercise involving 100 patients with FM and conducted at four different sites in the United States. The original 104 items were extracted from patient focus groups and then consolidated and reduced according to pretest rankings before being tested by Delphi.

[b]Clinician Delphi exercise involving 23 clinicians and outcome filtered through Outcome Measures in Rheumatology Clinical Trials VII (OMERACT VII) FM workshop attendees.

[c]Included based on pretest priority rankings.

HRQOL, Health-related quality of life; *PRO*, patient-reported outcomes.

From Mease PJ, Arnold LM, Crofford LJ, et al: Identifying the clinical domains of fibromyalgia: contributions from clinician and patient Delphi exercises. *Arthritis Rheum* 59:952-960, 2008.

example, if sleep is a major contributor to symptoms, the patient may be counseled on sleep hygiene or, if appropriate, screened for restless leg syndrome or sleep apnea and then referred for evaluation and management of sleep disorder.[35] Similarly, if depression or anxiety is a major contributor to the overall symptom complex, then attention should be given to management of these concerns.[36] Cognitive impairment may be of major importance to patients, particularly in the workplace.[37,38] These complaints have validity when studied carefully, with abnormalities in executive function and divided attention identified in FM patients. Fatigue may be the most difficult symptom to evaluate and treat because it may be due to deconditioning, depression, disrupted sleep, medication adverse effects, or comorbid conditions.

Differential Diagnosis and Comorbidities

A strategy for diagnosing FM is in Fig. 55.1.[39] Common conditions that should be considered in the differential diagnosis are in Table 55.5. Most of these conditions should be identified by careful history and physical examination with selected laboratory tests. Medications that may be associated with FM mimics, such as statins, should be noted. Physical findings that should prompt additional testing include prominent focal abnormalities on neurologic examination, such as weakness, numbness, joint inflammation, fever, rash, skin ulcers, or alopecia.[22,39] Hypothyroidism can be excluded using laboratory tests. Seronegative spondyloarthropathies may have elevated inflammatory markers and abnormal results of imaging studies. Patients with seronegative spondyloarthropathies also typically report that their pain lessens with exercise. In older patients, polymyalgia rheumatic should be excluded using laboratory testing. Screening questions for major depressive disorder should be undertaken. If the history and physical examination suggest inflammatory arthritis or a systemic autoimmune disease, appropriate laboratory and serologic testing should be undertaken. It is not useful to perform repeat diagnostic testing, particularly if symptoms have been

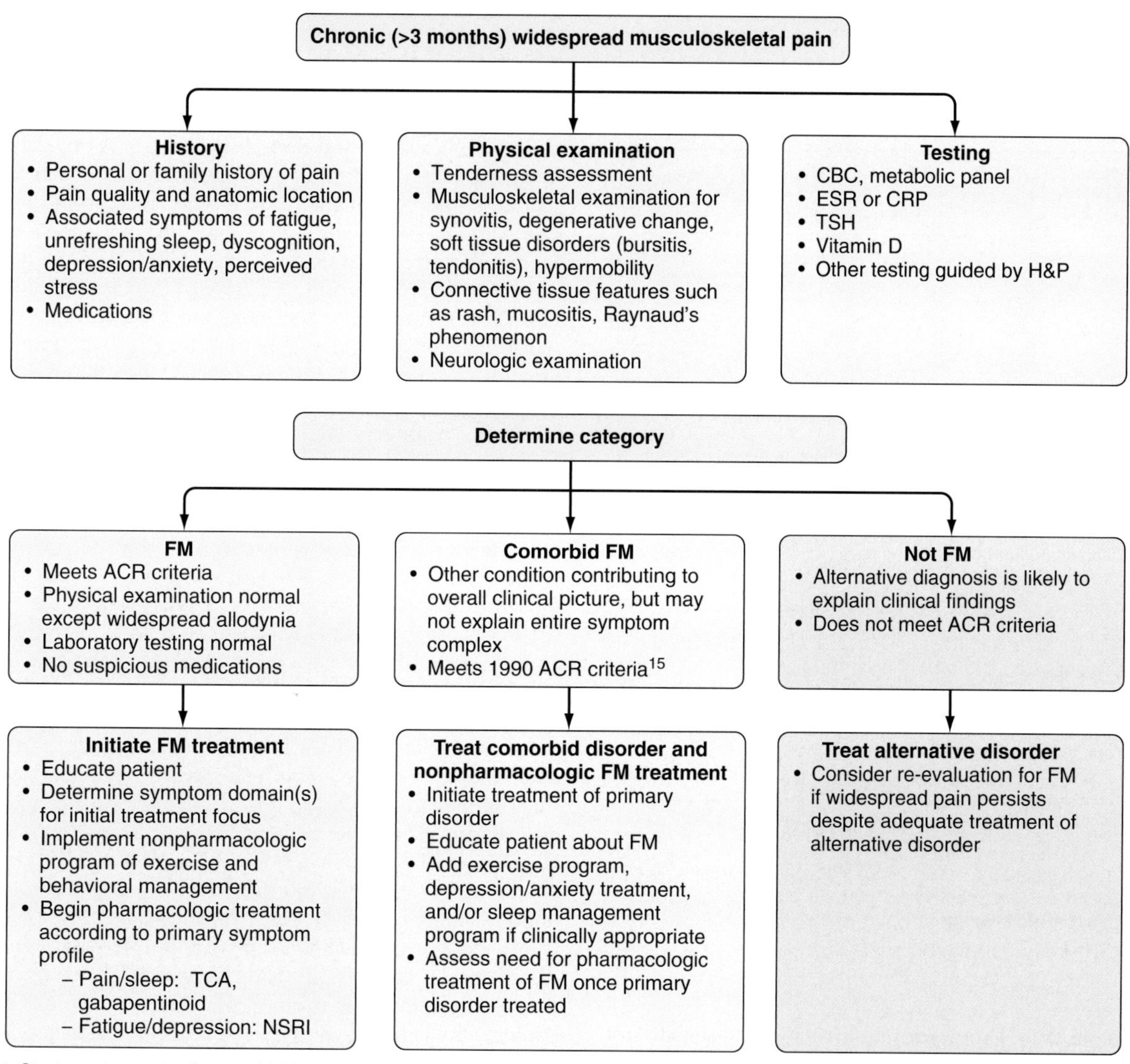

• **Fig. 55.1** Strategy for evaluation and initial management of patients with chronic widespread musculoskeletal pain. After initial evaluation, patients may be diagnosed with fibromyalgia (FM), FM comorbid with another diagnosis, or not FM. The figure presents strategies for initial management of each category. *ACR*, American College of Rheumatology; *CBC*, complete blood cell count; *CRP*, C-reactive protein; *ESR*, erythrocyte sedimentation rate; *H&P*, history and physical examination; *NSRI*, norepinephrine serotonin reuptake inhibitor; *TCA*, tricyclic anti-depressants; *TSH*, thyroid-stimulating hormone.

TABLE 55.5 **Differential Diagnosis of Diffuse Myalgias**

Diagnosis	Findings[a]
Inflammatory	
Polymyalgia rheumatica	Elevated ESR and/or CRP
Seronegative spondyloarthropathies	Abnormal imaging
Connective tissue diseases	Positive serologies
Systemic vasculitis	Systemic inflammation, end-organ damage
Infectious	
Hepatitis C	Positive antibodies
HIV	Positive antibodies
Lyme disease	Positive antibodies
Parvovirus B19	Positive antibodies
Epstein-Barr virus	Positive antibodies
Non-inflammatory	
Degenerative joint/spine disease	Abnormal imaging
Fibromyalgia	Widespread allodynia/hyperalgesia
Myofascial pain	Localized allodynia/hyperalgesia
Joint hypermobility	Joint hypermobility
Metabolic myopathies	Abnormal muscle biopsy
Endocrine	
Hypo- or hyperthyroidism	Abnormal thyroid function tests
Hyperparathyroidism	Elevated serum calcium
Addison's disease	Abnormal serum cortisol
Vitamin D deficiency	Low serum vitamin D
Neurologic Diseases	
Multiple sclerosis	Abnormal neurologic examination and imaging
Neuropathic pain	Reasonable cause or abnormal imaging
Psychiatric Diseases	
Major depressive disorder	Positive depression screening
Drugs	
Statins	History of exposure
Aromatase inhibitors	History of exposure

[a]Recommended routine testing includes ESR or CRP and thyroid-stimulating hormone. Other diagnostic testing should be guided by risk profile and history and physical examination. Repeated diagnostic testing is discouraged.

CRP, C-reactive protein; *ESR,* erythrocyte sedimentation rate.

present for more than 1 to 2 years and if the symptoms do not change.

FM is frequently comorbid with other rheumatologic diseases and identifying central pain amplification has important implications for evaluation and treatment of comorbid conditions. In a recent study of 835 patients, the prevalence of FM was 13.4% in 67 patients with systemic lupus erythematosus, 12.6% in 119 patients with ankylosing spondylitis, 12% in 25 patients with Sjögren's syndrome, 10.1% in 238 patients with osteoarthritis, 6.9% in 29 patients with polymyalgia rheumatica, and 6.6% in 197 patients with rheumatoid arthritis. Significant correlations were found between disease activity indexes and FM Impact Questionnaire (FIQ) scores for most rheumatologic patients.[40] A systematic review and meta-analysis found the pooled prevalence of FM is 21% in RA, 13% in ankylosing spondylitis, and 18% in psoriatic arthritis. In all cases, concomitant FM related to a higher disease activity score of odds ratio (OR) 1.24 for disease activity score 28 (DAS28) and OR of 2.22 for Bath Ankylosing Spondylitis Disease Activity Index (BASDAI).[41] Using more objective criteria for synovitis, such as ultrasound, in these patients may be required to determine if treatment of rheumatoid arthritis should be accelerated.

Other comorbidities are frequent in patients with FM. Patients with FM have a significantly higher prevalence of visceral pain syndromes, regional pain syndromes, and mood disorders. In one study using an ICD-9 coding insurance claims database containing 62,000 nationwide enrollees, patients with FM were between two and seven times more likely to have comorbid depression, anxiety, headache, irritable bowel syndrome, chronic fatigue syndrome, systemic lupus erythematosus, and rheumatoid arthritis.[28] In a study from the United Kingdom primary care dataset of people eventually diagnosed with FM, visit rates were highest for depression, fatigue, chest pain, headache, and sleep disturbance.[42] A population-based study from the Swedish Twin Registry, which evaluated 44,897 people, found substantial co-occurrence for chronic widespread pain with chronic fatigue (OR, 23.53; 95% CI, 19.67 to 18.16), depressive symptoms (OR, 5.26; 95% CI, 4.75 to 5.82), and irritable bowel syndrome (OR, 5.17; 95% CI, 4.55 to 5.88).[43] Using a co-twin analysis, the associations remained for chronic fatigue and irritable bowel syndrome but not for depressive symptoms. In a rheumatology practice, patients with FM were found to have high lifetime rates of migraine, irritable bowel syndrome, chronic fatigue syndrome, major depression, and panic disorder.[44]

FM is frequently identified in patients seen primarily for interstitial cystitis, irritable bowel syndrome, migraine and other forms of headache, temporomandibular disorder, multiple chemical sensitivities, and chronic fatigue syndrome. In a systematic review from 2001 of the aforementioned conditions, it was noted that there were many similarities in case definition and symptoms and that the proportion of patients with an unexplained clinical condition meeting criteria for a second unexplained condition was striking.[45] Psychiatric conditions associated with FM include major depressive disorder, bipolar disorder, anxiety disorders, including panic disorder, post-traumatic stress disorder, social phobia, and obsessive compulsive disorder, and substance abuse disorder.[46] Evidence from a prospective population-based cohort study of more than 500,000 people conducted in southern Sweden over 10 years showed that the incidence rate ratio of developing mental illness after FM was 4.05 (95% CI 3.58 to 4.59) and FM after mental illness was 5.54 (95% CI 4.99 to 6.16). These data confirm a bidirectional relationship between pain and mental illness.[47]

Should a patient with FM have multiple pain amplification disorders or a comorbidity, the clinician will need to determine if he or she should be treated as having one disorder of central etiology or whether there is a clinical reason for diagnosis of multiple different disorders. Many of the medications and nonpharmacologic treatments for these conditions overlap. To avoid use of multiple medications, if a single agent can be used—for example, an agent with anti-depressant activity—it may be possible to treat comorbidities and FM.

The revised Fibromyalgia Impact Questionnaire

Domain 1 directions: For each of the following nine questions, check the one box that best indicates how much your fibromyalgia made it difficult to do each of the following activities over the past 7 days:

Brush or comb your hair	No difficulty	□ □ □ □ □ □ □ □ □ □ □	Very difficult
Walk continuously for 20 minutes	No difficulty	□ □ □ □ □ □ □ □ □ □ □	Very difficult
Prepare a homemade meal	No difficulty	□ □ □ □ □ □ □ □ □ □ □	Very difficult
Vacuum, scrub, or sweep floors	No difficulty	□ □ □ □ □ □ □ □ □ □ □	Very difficult
Lift and carry a bag full of groceries	No difficulty	□ □ □ □ □ □ □ □ □ □ □	Very difficult
Climb one flight of stairs	No difficulty	□ □ □ □ □ □ □ □ □ □ □	Very difficult
Change bed sheets	No difficulty	□ □ □ □ □ □ □ □ □ □ □	Very difficult
Sit in a chair for 45 minutes	No difficulty	□ □ □ □ □ □ □ □ □ □ □	Very difficult
Go shopping for groceries	No difficulty	□ □ □ □ □ □ □ □ □ □ □	Very difficult

Domain 2 directions: For each of the following two questions, check the one box that best describes the overall impact of your fibromyalgia over the past 7 days:

Fibromyalgia prevented me from accomplishing goals for the week	Never	□ □ □ □ □ □ □ □ □ □ □	Always
I was completely overwhelmed by my fibromyalgia symptoms	Never	□ □ □ □ □ □ □ □ □ □ □	Always

Domain 3 directions: For each of the following 10 questions, check the one box that best indicates the intensity of your fibromyalgia symptoms over the past 7 days:

Please rate your level of pain	No pain	□ □ □ □ □ □ □ □ □ □ □	Unbearable pain
Please rate your level of energy	Lots of energy	□ □ □ □ □ □ □ □ □ □ □	No energy
Please rate your level of stiffness	No stiffness	□ □ □ □ □ □ □ □ □ □ □	Severe stiffness
Please rate the quality of your sleep	Awoke rested	□ □ □ □ □ □ □ □ □ □ □	Awoke very tired
Please rate your level of depression	No depression	□ □ □ □ □ □ □ □ □ □ □	Very depressed
Please rate your level of memory problems	Good memory	□ □ □ □ □ □ □ □ □ □ □	Very poor memory
Please rate your level of anxiety	Not anxious	□ □ □ □ □ □ □ □ □ □ □	Very anxious
Please rate your level of tenderness to touch	No tenderness	□ □ □ □ □ □ □ □ □ □ □	Very tender
Please rate your level of balance problems	No imbalance	□ □ □ □ □ □ □ □ □ □ □	Severe imbalance
Please rate your level of sensitivity to loud noises, bright lights, odors, and cold	No sensitivity	□ □ □ □ □ □ □ □ □ □ □	Extreme sensitivity

Scoring: Step 1. Sum the scores for each of the three domains (function, overall, and symptoms).
Step 2. Divide domain 1 score by three, divide domain 2 score by one (that is, it is unchanged), and divide domain score 3 by two.
Step 3. Add the three resulting domain scores to obtain the total revised Fibromyalgia Impact Questionnaire score.

• **Fig. 55.2** The revised Fibromyalgia Impact Questionnaire (FIQR) assesses functional status as well as the overall impact and fibromyalgia (FM) symptoms.[50] The FIQR total score can be used as an outcome measure in clinical studies. The FIQR function score and the symptom scores can be used individually to determine severity. Paper and online versions perform similarly, and the FIQR performs similarly to its original version.

Assessment of Severity

Symptom severity, physical function, and disability are key status and outcome variables in people with FM. In the clinic, numeric ratings for pain and fatigue along with a measure of functional status, including those routinely used for rheumatic diseases, such as one of the Health Assessment Questionnaires (HAQs) instruments, work very well in patients with FM.[48,49] The revised FIQ (FIQR) addresses all of these core domains, as well as FM impact and several other symptoms (see Fig. 55.2).[50] The ACR 2010 criteria modified for epidemiologic studies provide another measure of FM severity; it is called the FM Symptom Scale or Polysymptomatic Distress Scale, and it combines the WPI and the modified SSS into a continuous score.[16,17]

For research purposes, the Outcome Measures in Rheumatoid Arthritis Clinical Trials (OMERACT) FM working group has recommended that the domains of pain, fatigue, sleep, depression, physical function, quality of life, multidimensional function, patient's global impression of change, tenderness, cognitive complaints, anxiety, and stiffness be assessed.[51]

Mechanisms of Disease

The two intrinsic mechanisms associated with the risk of developing chronic painful musculoskeletal disorders, including FM, are pain amplification and psychological distress.[52] Pain amplification may be related to sensitization of afferent pathways in the peripheral or CNS that process coded pain information or impairment in the inhibitory systems of the CNS.[7] Psychological factors include enhanced somatic awareness or the perception and interpretation of sensory information, anxiety, depression, perceived stress, and catastrophizing.[53] It is likely that genetic vulnerability coupled with environmental triggers are required to produce the clinical phenotype. The specific environmental triggers may include nonspecific behavioral factors, such as smoking and obesity, stress exposures, and nociceptive musculoskeletal pain. The combination of risk factors is likely to vary among people who meet the definition of FM.

Genetic Risk

A number of studies have demonstrated the importance of genetics in the susceptibility of FM and other syndromes that are often comorbid with FM.[2,4,54] A study of familial aggregation reported that first-degree relatives of FM probands are far more likely to have FM (OR, 8.5; 95% CI, 2.8 to 26; $P < 0.001$).[2] Twin studies have estimated that the contribution of genetic factors to chronic widespread musculoskeletal pain load on two latent traits are best explained by both affective and sensory components.[55] These twin studies suggest a modest genetic influence with concordance for chronic widespread pain, with concordance for monozygotic female twins of 30%, and for dizygotic female twins of 16%.[56]

It is unlikely that a specific gene or set of genes is associated with FM. Rather, similar to autoimmune diseases, there are more general vulnerability genes that interact with environmental exposures to lead to clinical expression of pain conditions. Thus, most of the genes associated with FM have also been reported in association with other clinically defined pain syndromes. For example, two major neurotransmitter pathways have been repeatedly associated with musculoskeletal pain.[52] The first is the adrenergic pathway, in which *COMT*, the gene encoding the enzyme catechol-*O*-methyltransferase that is responsible for the catabolism of catechol neurotransmitters, such as epinephrine, norepinephrine, and dopamine, is most frequently associated with chronic musculoskeletal pain conditions.[3,52] Additional genetic variation in the β2-adrenergic receptor gene has been associated with an increased risk of FM and chronic widespread pain.[57] The second pathway associated with chronic pain syndromes is the serotonin pathway. Specific genes include the 5-hydroxytryptamin receptor 2A *(HTR2A)* and 5HT transporter *(SLC6A4)*.[58–60] A 44–base pair insertion/deletion polymorphism in the promoter region of *SLC6A4* is most frequently associated with risk of chronic pain conditions, including FM.[3] Both of these genetic pathways are also associated with several *endophenotypes* or intermediate measurable phenotypes that are present in patients with FM. These endophenotypes include autonomic dysregulation, altered pain processing and modulation, sleep dysfunction, and anxiety, in the case of the adrenergic pathway.[3] Personality and affective traits, such as somatic awareness, depression, and anxiety, have also been associated with genetic variation in the serotonin pathway.[3]

Candidate gene analysis of patients, who carried the diagnosis of FM, identified pathways also including genes within the biogenic amine and adrenergic pathways, as well as a cannabinoid receptor.[4] A genome-wide linkage scan study of families with FM identified chromosome 17p11.2-q11.2, a region that contains the serotonin transporter gene *(SLC6A4)* and the transient receptor potential vanilloid channel 2 gene *(TRPV2)*.[54] At this time, there are no validated genetic variants specific to FM.

Central Pain Amplification and Peripheral Pain Generators

Several lines of evidence support the concept of central pain amplification (also called central sensitization), which is generally interpreted as a change in the relationship between stimulus intensity and the perception of the stimulus as noxious or painful.[61] In patients with FM, stimuli usually perceived as innocuous are perceived as painful (allodynia), and painful stimuli are given a higher pain rating (hyperalgesia).[62,63] During central sensitization, second-order and higher-order neurons exhibit transcriptional and translational events that lead to heightened sensitivity.

Most of the data supporting central sensitization are generated through psychophysical testing using different types of stimuli, such as pressure or heat. The investigator may use either a subjective report of pain or an objective measure, such as brain imaging. One experimental paradigm called *wind-up* or *temporal summation of pain* measures the change in pain intensity after repeated applications of a sensory stimulus.[64] Healthy people will experience an increase in pain in response to identical stimulus intensity if the stimulus is presented with a short interstimulus interval. Patients with FM report the same wind-up phenomenon with longer interstimulus intervals, which is interpreted to mean that patients with FM have presensitized pain transmission neurons.[65,66] Patients with FM also have a delayed recovery to baseline, termed *aftersensations*, which correlates with clinical pain intensity.[66] A newer dynamic psychophysical approach using slow repeated evoked stimuli where a train of low intensity stimuli of five-second duration with a thirty-second interstimulus interval was evaluated in FM and compared with healthy controls and patients with RA.[67,68] This method exhibits excellent overall diagnostic accuracy, sensitivity, and specificity for FM, thus it is suggested to be a potential measure of central sensitization.

Studies have also implicated a deficiency in descending inhibitory control of noxious stimulation in people with FM. Normally, endogenous inhibitory mechanisms are activated in response to nociceptive stimuli and involve serotonergic, noradrenergic, and opioidergic inhibitory pathways. People with FM exhibit reduction in the activity of these pathways.[69] Positron emission tomographic (PET) scanning has demonstrated alterations in mu-opioid receptor availability and increased dopamine activity in people with FM, both of which could indicate alteration of normal pain inhibitory pathways.[70,71] It is difficult to know whether activation of afferent pain pathways, deficiency of descending pathways, or both explain enhanced pain perception in a given person.

Disagreement exists regarding the role of peripheral nociceptive input in the cause and maintenance of FM, although the increased prevalence of FM in people with other rheumatic diseases provides an argument that persistent peripheral pain generators may be an important risk factor contributing to the phenotypic changes in pain transmission neurons.[72] Other triggering events, such as certain types of infections, trauma, or psychological stress, have been proposed.[73,74] Pain is localized to muscle tissues in virtually all people with FM. Abnormalities in muscle tissues have been reported, including altered metabolisms by phosphorus-31 magnetic resonance spectroscopy (MRS).[75] Some data implicate muscle microcirculation and muscle mitochondria in FM.[63,76,77] Reports have been made of small fiber neuropathies in people with FM, which are thought potentially to be a source of persistent nociceptive input.[78–80] However, it may be that this is a nonspecific finding that has been reported in different pain and nonpain conditions.[81]

Functional neuroimaging has contributed much to the understanding of FM and, because the outcome is objective, it has clearly confirmed the validity of patient reports. One of the first studies to address this issue demonstrated that greater regional cerebral blood flow receiving pain pathway input was related to the patient's report of pain rather than to the stimulus intensity.[82] Other neuroimaging techniques have emerged and have provided information in FM and other chronic pain states.[83] Using proton MRS (^{1}H-MRS), people with FM were found to have low levels of *N*-acetyl-aspartate, a metabolite believed to be a marker of neuronal density and viability, which perhaps indicated loss of neural function and activity in the hippocampus.[83] Also using ^{1}H-MRS, it was found that the main excitatory neurotransmitter, glutamate/glutamine, was elevated in the posterior insular cortex, and a decrease in the signal correlated with improvements in pain.[84,85]

Other brain regions of people with FM, including the amygdala, posterior cingulate, and ventral lateral prefrontal cortex, had elevated levels of glutamate/glutamine, which suggested a possible role for this neurotransmitter in pain and perhaps other symptoms of FM.[83] Additional neuroimaging techniques, which included resting state functional connectivity, have also found abnormalities in patients with FM. These techniques explore connectivity to the brain network maintaining ongoing resting brain activity, which is known as the *default mode network*. Patients with FM demonstrate alterations to functional connectivity with regions important for pain and cognitive and emotional processing.[86–89] Recent imaging techniques have allowed evaluation of glial activation using a PET probe that binds to a protein upregulated in activated glia with suggestions of widespread activation of microglia in FM.[90]

Altered peripheral and cerebrospinal fluid levels of neurotrophins, chemokines, and cytokines have also been reported in people with FM.[63] Mechanisms for the effects of these substances in explaining the pathophysiology of FM remain undetermined. However, the concept that activation of glial cells by cytokines and chemokines may accompany activation of pain transmission neurons can be demonstrated in animal models.[91]

Stress Response Systems

A number of studies suggest abnormalities of stress-response systems—the hypothalamic-pituitary-adrenal (HPA) axis and autonomic nervous system—in people with FM. It is unclear whether these abnormalities are a cause or a consequence of FM. Genetic studies implicating genes in these pathways suggest that lack of resiliency in these pathways may provide a measure of vulnerability, but other studies implicate exposure to acute or chronic stress as a triggering mechanism. One study of patients, without chronic widespread pain but who were at risk based on high rates of psychological distress and somatization, provided evidence that HPA axis dysfunction may precede the development of chronic pain[92] and that HPA axis dysfunction associated with the subsequent development of chronic widespread pain.[93] There is a striking lack of consistency in the specific HPA axis measures associated with FM.

Many studies, however, consistently demonstrate alterations of measures of autonomic function, especially heart rate variability. According to evidence, these alterations demonstrate predominance of the sympathetic nervous system, a characteristic shared by other pain amplification syndromes.[94] Other studies are interpreted as demonstrating stronger parasympathetic decline, which is a finding associated with the tendency to exhibit defensive behaviors.[95] Many of the changes to autocrine function are shared among disorders with centrally maintained pain.

Social and Psychological Factors

Life Stress and Socioeconomic Factors

In many longitudinal epidemiologic studies, chronic pain and other somatic symptoms can be predicted by childhood abuse and traumas, low educational attainment, social isolation, depression, and anxiety.[96] In a population-based study to determine psychosocial factors that predicted new-onset chronic widespread pain, investigators identified a random sample of subjects from sociodemographically disparate backgrounds; they then identified more than 3000 patients who did not have pain at baseline and more than 300 patients who had new widespread musculoskeletal pain at follow-up.[97] The strongest predictors were premorbid somatic symptoms, illness behaviors, and sleep problems. In another community-based study, perceived physical and emotional trauma as precipitating factors for FM were associated with health care seeking rather than pain severity.[98]

Lower socioeconomic status predicts greater symptom severity and functional impairment in people with FM, even controlling for levels of pain, depression, and anxiety.[99] The biopsychosocial model of pain posits that pain experience and its impact on the individual is a function of interacting combinations of nociceptive input; psychological processes, including beliefs; coping repertoire and mood; and environmental contingencies that would include family, community, and cultural rules or expectations.[100] All of these factors are likely to play a key role in the clinical expression and health impact of FM.

Personality, Cognitive, and Psychological Factors

People with FM may have a specific personality profile characterized, for example, by high levels of neuroticism. Several studies have been conducted using a standard five-factor personality scale (extraversion vs. introversion, agreeableness vs. antagonism, conscientiousness/control vs. impulsivity, neuroticism vs. emotional stability, and openness to new experience/intellect vs. closed-mindedness). One study showed that patients with FM were not different from patients with other rheumatic pain conditions or other chronic illnesses.[101] Furthermore, the scores fell within the normal range for the general population. However, a cluster of patients with FM was identified with a personality profile (high neuroticism and lower extraversion) that reflects a proneness to experience emotional distress, a difficulty for positive emotion, and a tendency to ineffective use of emotional regulation processes rather exhibiting rumination and maladaptive behaviors. The patients in this cluster also exhibited more psychosocial problems.[101] Another study showed FM patients had higher scores on agreeableness, neuroticism, and openness than the scores with other rheumatic disease taken as a whole. Their scores were not different from those of patients with RA. High neuroticism and low conscientiousness were associated with a high level of chronic pain across rheumatic diseases.[102] It is suggested that the association between high neuroticism and worse health outcomes in FM is mediated through depression and anxiety, which suggests that personality may modulate coping with stress.[103] A recent meta-analysis that focused on personality across pain states found that in studies using Cloninger's Temperament and Character Inventory, higher harm avoidance and lower self-directedness may be the most distinguishing personality feature of chronic pain sufferers.[104] High harm avoidance refers to a tendency to be fearful, pessimistic, sensitive to criticism, and requiring high levels of reassurance. This personality is also seen in those patients with anxiety and depression. Low self-directedness often manifests as difficulty with defining and setting meaningful goals, low motivation, and problems with adaptive coping.

Another way of stratifying patients is the psychological and behavioral response to chronic pain. People with FM have been characterized and divided into groups that predict outcome based on psychological characteristics.[105] People classified as *dysfunctional* exhibit the highest pain intensity, interference, and distress and the lowest control and activity levels. The *adaptive coper* groups report the lowest levels of pain and interference as well as the highest activity levels. The *interpersonally distressed* patients report high levels of affective distress and more negative spousal responses to pain.

It is likely that important relationships exist between psychological and physiologic pathways in people with FM. This likelihood is certainly not surprising because regulation of domains characterized as psychological and physiologic use common mediators. For example, in a recent study of people with FM, investigators performed a cluster analysis based on pain characteristics and cognitive, affective, and behavioral responses to pain and stress.[106] The study demonstrated that psychophysiologic responses of blood pressure, heart rate, and skin conductance were associated with specific types of psychological coping and psychiatric diagnoses.

Treatment Approaches

The most recent guidelines for FM treatment are from the European League Against Rheumatism (EULAR) and include pharmacologic and nonpharmacologic approaches.[107] Unanimous expert opinion recommends prompt diagnosis and providing the patient with information. Management should be aimed at improving health-related quality of life and should focus first on nonpharmacologic modalities.[107]

Education and Self-Management

Treatment guidelines for people with FM emphasize the need to incorporate principles of self-management.[19,107,108] Making the diagnosis of FM provides an intellectual framework for educating patients about their symptoms and engaging them as an active participant in the treatment plan (Fig. 55.3).[19] Providing the diagnosis can provide relief from health-related anxiety, and no studies have suggested that labeling with FM is harmful for health or health care expenditures.[109,110] Educating patients regarding the physiology of chronic pain in FM, as well as the importance of nonpharmacologic therapies for its management, is likely to be beneficial. One key goal is to assist the patient in differentiating peripheral pain generators from the centrally maintained diffuse pain. In addition, educating patients about which treatment is intended to target which pain symptom may help with adherence and satisfaction with treatment. For example, nonsteroidal anti-inflammatory drugs (NSAIDs) or disease-modifying agents may be intended for peripheral mechanical or inflammatory pain but would not be expected to effectively treat FM pain.[108]

A comparison of network meta-analyses of different treatment strategies found that multicomponent therapies incorporating pharmacologic therapies with aerobic exercise and cognitive behavioral therapy (CBT) seem most promising.[111] Many of the nonpharmacologic strategies useful for FM may not be available locally but lend themselves to internet-based programs or written materials.[19] The provider and patient should collaborate to prioritize individual treatment goals and develop a plan to achieve those goals. Focusing on longer term goals, although acknowledging that FM symptoms tend to wax and wane in response to both external and internal environmental stressors, is advised.

Exercise and Body-Based Therapies

A number of systematic reviews have been conducted to assess the benefits of exercise for people with FM.[112–114] Reviews of trials with almost 2500 participants conclude that aerobic exercise

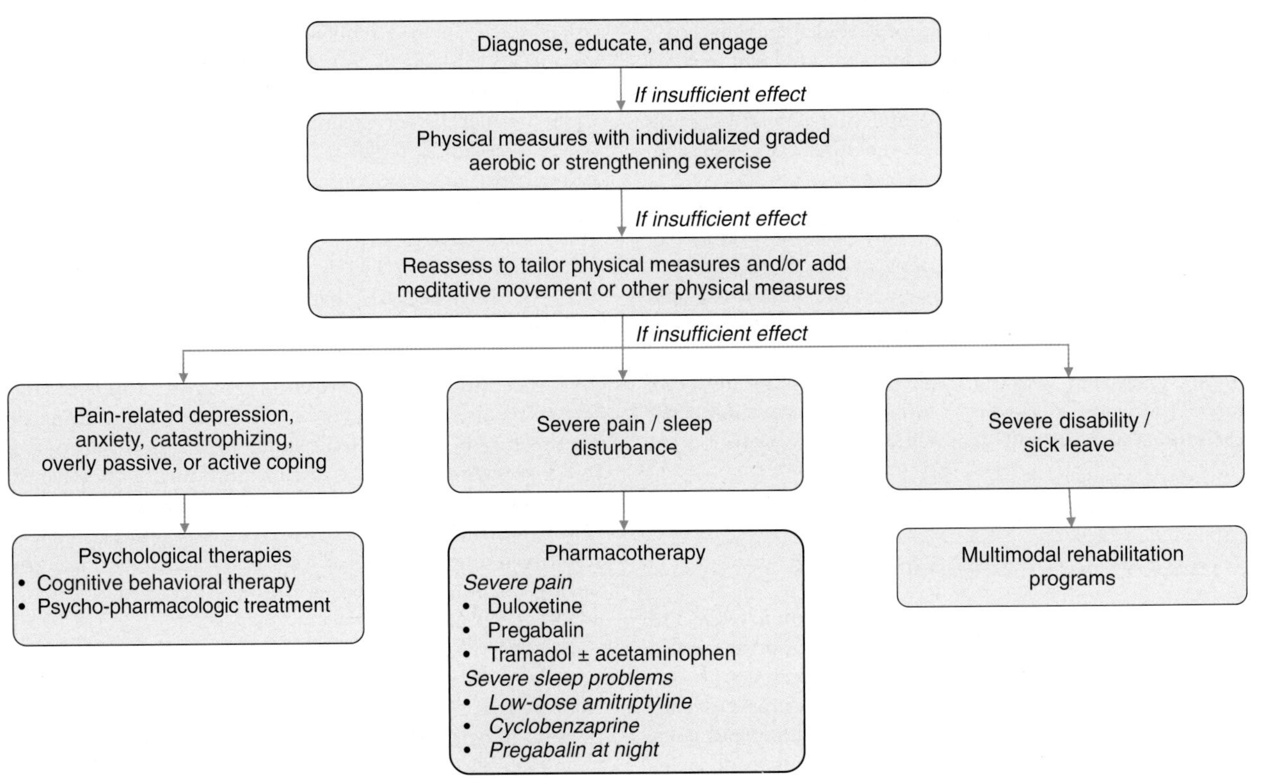

• **Fig. 55.3** Approach to fibromyalgia (FM) management. (Modified from Macfarlane GJ, Kronisch C, Dean LE et al: EULAR revised recommendations for the management of fibromyalgia. *Ann Rheum Dis* 76:318-328, 2017.)

is associated with improvements in pain reduction and physical function. Resistance training also resulted in pain reduction. Insufficient evidence exists to prefer one modality over another.[107] In evaluating exercise interventions, a recent umbrella systematic review synthesized physical activity interventions for adults with FM and focused on four outcomes: pain, multidimensional function, physical function, and adverse effects.[115] The researchers found positive results of diverse exercise interventions for all outcomes and no adverse effects. The variability of the interventions did not allow for recommendations regarding the mode of exercise or the frequency, intensity, and duration of treatments. It is not possible to rigorously determine whether land- or water-based exercise is superior. All major outcomes, including function, pain, stiffness, muscle strength, and fitness, improved after aquatic exercise training compared with control subjects; however, the quality of the evidence was rated as low to moderate; however, land-based training was superior to aquatic training for improving muscle strength.

Meditative movements, including tai chi, yoga, qigong, and a variety of other movement therapies, have also been reported to be safe and effective for overall symptoms and physical functioning in people with FM.[116] A comparative effectiveness study compared supervised aerobic exercise to one of four classic Yang style supervised tai chi interventions and found that tai chi treatment, administered with the same intensity and duration (24 weeks twice weekly), had greater benefit. Longer duration of tai chi demonstrated greater improvement.[117] In general, active physical exercise strategies of any type will be helpful. Finding the exercise to which the patient is most likely to adhere will be the most important factor.

More passive strategies may be useful as an adjunct but should not replace active physical exercise. A meta-analysis of balneotherapy and hydrotherapy reported evidence for a small reduction in pain and a small improvement in health related to quality of life, although the investigators recommend that high-quality studies with larger sample sizes be performed.[118] Acupuncture has been compared with sham acupuncture, and a meta-analysis including nine trials concluded that there was not enough evidence to prove the efficacy of acupuncture therapy compared with sham acupuncture.[119] The most recent treatment guidelines concluded there was little understanding of the active component of acupuncture and provided a weak recommendation for use.[107] Transcutaneous electric nerve stimulation (TENS) was studied as an adjunct treatment for pain and fatigue in women with FM in a large randomized, placebo-controlled trial, which demonstrated reduction in exercise-induced pain and other FM symptoms as well as a marked improvement in global disease symptoms.[120] Nonpharmacologic therapies have been tested and found to have insufficient evidence to recommend their use for FM including biofeedback, hypnotherapy, and massage. Chiropractic and homeopathy received a rating of "strong against" in EULAR guidelines.[107]

Cognitive Behavioral Therapy

CBT includes interventions that are based on the basic premise that chronic pain is maintained by cognitive and behavioral factors and that psychological treatment leads to changes in these factors through training in specific techniques.[121] These interventions would include cognitive restructuring and behavioral training, such as relaxation and social skills training. An updated systematic review and meta-analysis demonstrated the CBTs were superior to controls of all types in pain relief of 50% or greater, improvement in health-related quality of life of 20% of greater, and in reducing negative mood, disability, and fatigue.[122] Mindfulness-based stress reduction is a cognitive therapy that helps people self-manage and reframe worrisome and intrusive thoughts through mindfulness meditation. This technique reduced perceived stress, sleep disturbance, and symptom severity, although there was no improvement in pain or physical functioning in a randomized, controlled clinical trial.[123] Operant behavioral treatment focuses on the modification of pain behavior by increasing activity levels, reducing health care-seeking behavior, and reducing pain-reinforcing behaviors in significant relationships.[122] Overall, CBT is recommended for treatment of FM, although the quality of individual trials is low. However, the benefits were sustained long-term.[107]

Pharmacologic Approaches

The major classes of drugs useful for patients with FM are anti-depressants, particularly those with mixed reuptake inhibition of serotonin and norepinephrine, such as duloxetine, milnacipran, and other agents useful for neuropathic pain, such as gabapentin and pregabalin (Table 55.6).[107] Evidence-based guidelines have been formulated by the American Pain Society (2004),[124] EULAR (2007, 2017),[107,125] the Association of the Scientific Medical Societies in Germany (2008),[126] and the Canadian National Fibromyalgia Guideline Advisory Panel (2012),[108] among others. These guidelines emphasize the need for selecting a treatment approach based on predominant symptoms and initiating treatment in low doses with slow dose escalation.

Drugs with anti-depressant activity have been a mainstay for FM treatment. Comparisons of older and newer agents have not found large differences in treatment effects, although adverse effect profiles differ.[127] Older agents, such as amitriptyline and cyclobenzaprine, may improve a wide range of symptoms, although adverse effects, such as dry mouth, weight gain, constipation, and sedation may limit their tolerability.[127] Selective serotonin reuptake inhibitors typically have not been as useful as mixed reuptake inhibitors with respect to analgesic activity, although they are helpful for symptoms of depression and anxiety.[1] Older agents, such as fluoxetine, paroxetine, sertraline, and venlafaxine, which are not as serotonin selective, are favored over newer, more serotonin-specific agents, such as citalopram and escitalopram. These drugs are associated with nausea, sexual dysfunction, weight gain, and sleep disturbance. The norepinephrine serotonin reuptake inhibitors duloxetine and milnacipran are approved by the FDA for treatment of FM. The addition of norepinephrine reuptake inhibition is important for achieving analgesic efficacy.[128] Two systematic reviews of the heterocyclic anti-depressant mirtazapine differed in their conclusions of the utility of this agent in FM. One review cited potential harms, and the other review emphasized cost-effectiveness.[129,130] Time to effect for anti-depressants is generally 2 to 4 weeks; thus, dose adjustment and assessment of efficacy after institution of treatment should be performed within several months. Providers are cautioned to ensure that high doses or combinations of anti-depressants and concomitant medications or supplements do not result in the serotonin syndrome, which can cause agitation, tachycardia, hypertension, sweating/shivering, diarrhea, muscle rigidity, fever, seizures, and even death.

In general, agents tested and used for neuropathic pain have been more useful in FM than agents targeting peripheral mechanical and inflammatory sources of pain. Gabapentin and pregabalin are both approved by the FDA for use in postherpetic neuralgia and painful diabetic neuropathy. Although only pregabalin has

TABLE 55.6 **EULAR REVISED (2016) Recommendations for the Management of Fibromyalgia**

Recommendation	Level of Evidence	Grade	Strength of Recommendation	Agreement (%)
Overarching Principles				
Optimal management requires prompt diagnosis and assessment of pain, function, and psychosocial context Recognition as a complex and heterogeneous condition Gradual approach	IV	D		100
Management should aim at improving HRQL balancing benefit and risk of treatment Initial management should focus on nonpharmacologic treatment	IV	D		100
Specific Recommendations				
Nonpharmacologic management				
Aerobic and strengthening exercise	Ia	A	Strong for	100
Cognitive behavioral therapies	Ia	A	Weak for	100
Multicomponent therapies	Ia	A	Weak for	93
Defined physical therapies: acupuncture or hydrotherapy	Ia	A	Weak for	93
Meditative movement therapies (qigong, yoga, tai chi) and mindfulness-based stress reduction	Ia	A	Weak for	71-73
Pharmacologic management				
Amitriptyline (at low dose)	Ia	A	Weak for	100
Duloxetine or milnacipran	Ia	A	Weak for	100
Tramadol	Ib	A	Weak for	100
Pregabalin	Ia	A	Weak for	94
Cyclobenzaprine	Ia	A	Weak for	75

HRQOL, Health-related quality of life.
Modified from Macfarlane GJ, Kronisch C, Dean LE, et al: EULAR revised recommendations for the management of fibromyalgia. *Ann Rheum Dis* 76:318-328, 2017.

been approved by the FDA for use in FM, a study of gabapentin found that it also was effective.[131–133] Both gabapentin and pregabalin bind to a receptor subunit, the α2δ subunit of a calcium channel on the cell surface of neurons, to inhibit excitatory neurotransmitters.[128] There are pharmacokinetic and pharmacodynamic advantages for pregabalin, which may make dosing somewhat simpler than for gabapentin; however, the mechanism of actions for these drugs is the same. Both drugs may reduce pain, improve sleep, and improve health-related quality of life; however, they have substantial adverse effects, including dizziness, grogginess, weight gain, and edema of the extremities.[134] Other anticonvulsant agents have less evidence to support their use in people with FM.

Three agents are approved by the FDA for FM. With regard to efficacy and harms, indirect comparisons demonstrate that pregabalin, duloxetine, and milnacipran are superior to placebo for all outcomes of interest (pain, fatigue, sleep disturbance, depressed mood, and reduced health-related quality of life) except pregabalin for depressed mood, duloxetine for fatigue, and milnacipran for sleep disturbance. Adjusted indirect comparisons indicated no significant differences between these drugs for achieving 30% pain relief or for dropout rates due to adverse events.[134]

Cannabinoids are used by people with many forms of chronic pain. A systematic review of smoked cannabis, cannabis extracts, nabilone, and dronabinol suggests modest efficacy in people with FM and other chronic pain conditions.[135] NSAIDs are not effective treatments for central pain, although they may be helpful in treating inflammatory or mechanical peripheral pain generators, which contribute to the overall burden of pain. Tramadol, with or without acetaminophen, has been studied in people with FM, although there is increasing concern that opioids are less effective than previously thought, and their risk-benefit profile is worse than that of other classes of analgesics.[1] A Cochrane review found no evidence to support the use of oxycodone for treatment of FM.[136] Treatment recommendations from professional societies uniformly advise against the use of strong opioids in people with FM.[107] This recommendation is based, at least in part, on mechanistic studies demonstrating elevated cerebrospinal fluid enkephalins and evidence that mu-opioid receptors are either occupied or downregulated in the brains of people with FM.[83] Low-dose naltrexone has been evaluated in very small trials and is thought to, perhaps, act on glial cells rather than on neurons.[137,138] A single systematic review of five studies investigating the narcolepsy drug sodium oxybate in FM reported small effect sizes on pain, sleep, and fatigue[139]; however, safety concerns led to refusal to approve this agent by the European Medicines Agency and the FDA. EULAR guidelines have given a strong recommendation against use of this drug in FM.[107]

Practical Advice

Developing a set of key talking points for FM patients may be helpful to providers. For example, it is often helpful to educate patients about the waxing and waning nature of FM and ask that they make note of their personal triggers so that they better understand the linkage between environment, behaviors, and FM symptoms. Reassuring patients that the pain they are experiencing is due to altered neurophysiology of pain processing rather than tissue destruction may relieve anxiety. Making the point that research has discovered the close links between pain pathways and other cognitive or emotional pathways in the brain may help the patient understand these relationships in their own experience of FM.

It is essential to engage the patient in setting their individual treatment plan and expectations. Developing a set of personalized functional goals may assist providers and patients to assess progress. People with FM are likely to benefit from multimodal treatment that includes nonpharmacologic treatment, especially if one component includes exercise or meditative movement. Patients should be involved in choosing nonpharmacologic strategies that will be most accepted and that are practical to employ. In addition to general nonpharmacologic approaches, it may be useful to target specific symptoms, such as sleep, with efforts to improve sleep hygiene and regulation of circadian rhythms.[19]

In practice, it is crucial that patients be informed that there is no pharmacologic treatment that can alleviate the symptoms of FM. A general rule is that effective medications only improve pain by 30% to 50% in only 30% to 50% of patients, which includes the placebo response rate. Little information is available about combinations of approved medications, although patients with FM often use multiple medications.[140] In general, efforts should be made to consolidate treatments and use the fewest number of medications possible.

Many drugs and alternative therapies are used by people who have FM and other forms of chronic musculoskeletal pain. Widespread use of nonapproved treatments reflects the generally poor effectiveness and tolerability of currently available drugs. For any treatment of FM, there is also likely to be a significant placebo effect in addition to the specific efficacy of a therapeutic agent. It is certainly reasonable to work with patients on individual "n-of-1" trials, although it is important to assess both efficacy and harm and to discontinue use of ineffective medications or treatments with adverse effects.

Outcome

The outcome of FM can be studied in terms of the change in the level of symptoms, use of services, and work disability. In a 2006 study intended to assess utilization of health services, 2260 patients, who were seen in a primary care setting and newly diagnosed with FM, were studied from 10 years before until 4 years after FM diagnosis.[42] Patients with FM had considerably higher rates of visits, prescriptions, and testing from at least 10 years prior to diagnosis compared with control subjects, and these rates accelerated to twice the numbers of visits and prescriptions at the time of diagnosis. Visit rates were highest for depression, fatigue, chest pain, headache, and sleep disturbance. After diagnosis, visits for most symptoms and health care use markers declined, but within 2 to 3 years, most visits rose to levels at or higher than those at diagnosis. The authors concluded that being diagnosed with FM may help patients cope with some symptoms, but the diagnoses had a limited impact on health care resource use in the longer term. In another longitudinal study, of 1555 patients with FM observed semiannually for up to 11 years; there was minimal improvement in symptoms overall. These data suggested that the course of FM was one of continuous, high levels of self-reported symptoms and distress.[141] Taken as a whole, although some patients improve, data tend to suggest minimal improvement in most cases despite treatment.

A study of patients with juvenile FM (JFM) was recently reported. In this study, patients with JFM and healthy control subjects were assessed approximately 6 years after diagnosis and with an average age of 21 years. Patients with JFM had more pain, poorer physical function, and greater anxiety and depression than did healthy control subjects. More than 80% of patients with JFM continued to experience symptoms into adulthood, and more than half met the criteria for FM at follow-up. Those who met adult FM criteria exhibited the highest levels of physical and emotional impairment.[27]

Overall, patients with FM typically have a lifelong problem with chronic pain. Assisting patients in the self-management of their symptoms, reducing health care–seeking behaviors, and improving healthy behaviors are important goals of treatment. Perhaps the most important function of the rheumatologist is to confirm the diagnosis and determine if the patient has a comorbid rheumatic condition that should be treated. If FM is complicating another rheumatic condition, specific management of FM may improve overall health outcomes.

Full references for this chapter can be found on ExpertConsult.com.

Selected References

1. Clauw DJ: Fibromyalgia: a clinical review, *JAMA* 311(15):1547–1555, 2014.
2. Arnold LM, Hudson JI, Hess EV, et al.: Family study of fibromyalgia, *Arthritis Rheum* 50:944–952, 2004.
3. Diatchenko L, Fillingim RB, Smith SB, et al.: The phenotypic and genetic signatures of common musculoskeletal pain conditions, *Nature Rev Rheum* 9(6):340–350, 2013.
4. Smith SB, Maixner DW, Fillingim RB, et al.: Large candidate gene association study reveals genetic risk factors and therapeutic targets for fibromyalgia, *Arthritis Rheum* 64(2):584–593, 2012.
5. Arnold LM, Bradley LA, Clauw DJ, et al.: Multidisciplinary care and stepwise treatment for fibromyalgia, *J Clin Psych* 69(12):e35, 2008.
6. Wolfe F, Walitt B: Culture, science and the changing nature of fibromyalgia, *Nature Rev Rheumatol* 9(12):751–755, 2013.
7. Clauw DJ, Arnold LM, McCarberg BH: The science of fibromyalgia, *Mayo Clinic Proc* 86(9):907–911, 2011.
8. Inanici F, Yunus MB: History of fibromyalgia: past to present, *Curr Pain Headache Rep* 8:369–378, 2004.
14. Wolfe F, Smythe HA, Yunus MB, et al.: The American College of Rheumatology 1990 criteria for the classification of fibromyalgia, *Arthritis Rheum* 33:160–172, 1990.
15. Clauw DJ: Pain management: fibromyalgia drugs are 'as good as it gets' in chronic pain, *Nature Rev Rheumatol* 6(8):439–440, 2010.
16. Wolfe F, Clauw DJ, Fitzcharles MA, et al.: The American College of Rheumatology preliminary diagnostic criteria for fibromyalgia and measurement of symptom severity, *Arthritis Care Res* 62(5):600–610, 2010.
17. Wolfe F, Clauw DJ, Fitzcharles MA, et al.: Fibromyalgia criteria and severity scales for clinical and epidemiological studies: a modification of the ACR Preliminary Diagnostic Criteria for Fibromyalgia, *J Rheumatol* 38(6):1113–1122, 2011.

18. Wolfe F, Clauw DJ, Fitzcharles MD, et al.: Revisions to the 2010/2011 fibromyalgia diagnostic criteria, *Semin Arthritis Rheum* 46(2016):319–329, 2016.
19. Arnold LM, Clauw DJ, Dunegan LJ, et al.: A framework for fibromyalgia management for primary care providers, *Mayo Clinic Proc* 87(5):488–496, 2012.
20. Bennett RM, Friend R, Marcus D, et al.: Criteria for the diagnosis of fibromyalgia: validation of the modified 2010 preliminary American College of Rheumatology criteria and the development of alternative criteria, *Arthritis Care Res* 66:1364–1373, 2014.
22. Arnold LM, Bennett RM, Crofford LJ, et al.: AAPT diagnostic criteria for fibromyalgia, *J Pain* 2018.
23. Dean LE, Arnold LM, Crofford L, et al.: Impact of moving from a widespread to multisite pain definition on other fibromyalgia symptoms, *Arthritis Care Res* 69:1878–1886, 2018.
24. Wolfe F, Ross K, Anderson J, et al.: The prevalence and characteristics of fibromyalgia in the general population, *Arthritis Rheum* 38:19–28, 1995.
25. Heidari F, Afshari M, Moosazadeh M: Prevalence of fibromyalgia in general population and patients, a systematic review and meta-analysis, *Rheumatol Int* 37:1527–1539, 2017.
26. White KP, Speechley M, Harth M, et al.: The London Fibromyalgia Epidemiology Study: the prevalence of fibromyalgia syndrome in London, Ontario, *J Rheumatol* 26(7):1570–1576, 1999.
27. Kashikar-Zuck S, Cunningham N, Sil S, et al.: Long-term outcomes of adolescents with juvenile-onset fibromyalgia in early adulthood, *Pediatrics* 133(3):e592–600, 2014.
28. Weir PT, Harlan GA, Nkoy FL, et al.: The incidence of fibromyalgia and its associated comorbidities: a population-based retrospective cohort study based on International Classification of Diseases, 9th Revision codes, *J Clin Rheumatol* 12(3):124–128, 2006.
29. Gallagher AA, Thomas JM, Hamilton WT, et al.: Incidence of fatigue symptoms and diagnoses presenting in UK primary care from 1990 to 2001, *J R Soc Med* 97:571–575, 2004.
30. Collin SM, Bakken IJ, Nazareth I, et al.: Trends in the incidence of chronic fatigue syndrome and fibromyalgia in the UK, 2001-2013: a Clinical Practice Research Datalink study, *J R Soc Med* 110:231–244, 2017.
31. Lee YC, Lu G, Boire G, et al.: Incidence and predictors of secondary fibromyalgia in an early arthritis cohort, *Ann Rheum Dis* 72:949–954, 2013.
32. Mease PJ, Arnold LM, Crofford LJ, et al.: Identifying the clinical domains of fibromyalgia: contributions from clinician and patient Delphi exercises, *Arthritis Rheum* 59:952–960, 2008.
33. Gedalia A, Press J, Klein M, et al.: Joint hypermobility and fibromyalgia in schoolchildren, *Ann Rheum Dis* 52:494–496, 1993.
34. Di Stefano G, Celletti C, Baron R, et al.: Central sensitization as the mechanism underlying pain in joint hypermobility syndrome/Ehlers-Danlos syndrome, hypermobility type, *Eur J Pain* 20:1319–1325, 2016.
35. Civelek GM, Ciftkaya PO, Karatas M: Evaluation of restless legs syndrome in fibromyalgia syndrome: an analysis of quality of sleep and life, *J Back Musculoskelet Rehabil* 27:537–544, 2014.
36. Arnold LM, Bradley LA, Clauw DJ, et al.: Evaluating and diagnosing fibromyalgia and comorbid psychiatric disorders, *J Clin Psych* 69(10):e28, 2008.
37. Kravitz HM, Katz RS: Fibrofog and fibromyalgia: a narrative review and implications for clinical practice, *Rheumatology Int* 35:1115–1125, 2015.
38. Glass JM: Cognitive dysfunction in fibromyalgia and chronic fatigue syndrome: new trends and future directions, *Curr Rheumatol Rep* 8:425–429, 2006.
39. Arnold LM, Clauw DJ, McCarberg BH: Improving the recognition and diagnosis of fibromyalgia, *Mayo Clinic Proc* 86(5):457–464, 2011.
40. Haliloglu S, Carlioglu A, Akdeniz D, et al.: Fibromyalgia in patients with other rheumatic diseases: prevalence and relationship with disease activity, *Rheumatology Int* 34(9):1275–1280, 2014.
41. Duffield SJ, Miller N, Zhao S, et al.: Concomitant fibromyalgia complicating chronic inflammatory arthritis: a systematic review and meta-analysis, *Rheumatology (Oxford)* 57:1453–1460, 2018.
42. Hughes G, Martinez C, Myon E, et al.: The impact of a diagnosis of fibromyalgia on health care resource use by primary care patients in the UK: an observational study based on clinical practice, *Arthritis Rheum* 54:177–183, 2006.
43. Kato K, Sullivan PF, Evengard B, et al.: Chronic widespread pain and its comorbidities: a population-based study, *Arch Intern Med* 166:1649–1654, 2006.
47. Bondesson D, Larrosa Pardo F, Stigmar K, et al.: Comorbidity between pain and mental illness—Evidence of a bidirectional relationship, *Eur J Pain* 22:1304–1311, 2018.
48. Wolfe F, Michaud K, Pincus T: Development and validation of the health assessment questionnaire II: a revised version of the health assessment questionnaire, *Arthritis Rheum* 50:3296–3305, 2004.
50. Bennett RM, Friend R, Jones KD, et al.: The revised Fibromyalgia Impact Questionnaire (FIQR): validation and psychometric properties, *Arthritis Res Ther* 11:R120, 2009.
51. Choy EH, Arnold LM, Clauw DJ, et al.: Content and criterion validity of the preliminary core dataset for clinical trials in fibromyalgia syndrome, *J Rheumatol* 36(10):2330–2334, 2009.
52. Diatchenko L, Slade GD, Nackley AG, et al.: Genetic basis for individual variations in pain perception and the development of a chronic pain condition, *Hum Mol Genet* 14:135–143, 2005.
54. Arnold LM, Fan J, Russell IJ, et al.: The fibromyalgia family study: a genome-wide linkage scan study, *Arthritis Rheum* 50:944–952, 2013.
55. Kato K, Sullivan PF, Evengard B, et al.: A population-based twin study of functional somatic syndromes, *Psychol Med* 39:497–505, 2009.
61. Geisser ME, Casey KL, Brucksch CB, et al.: Perception of noxious and innocuous heat stimulation among healthy women and women with fibromyalgia: association with mood, somatic focus, and catastrophizing, *Pain* 102:243–250, 2003.
62. Staud R, Rodriguez ME: Mechanisms of disease: pain in fibromyalgia syndrome, *Nat Clin Pract Rheumatol* 2:90–98, 2006.
63. Staud R: Peripheral pain mechanisms in chronic widespread pain, *Best Practice Res Clin Rheumatol* 25:155–164, 2011.
67. de la Coba R, Bruehl S, Moreno-Padilla M, et al.: Responses to slowly repeated evoked pain stimuli in fibromyalgia patients: Evidence of enhanced pain sensitization, *Pain Med* 18:1778–1786, 2017.
68. de la Coba R, Bruehl S, Galvez-Sanchez CM, et al.: Slowly repeated evoked pain as a marker of central sensitization in fibromyalgia: Diagnostic accuracy and reliability in comparison with temporal summation of pain, *Psychosom Med* 80:573–580, 2018.
69. Julien N, Goffaux P, Arsenault P, et al.: Widespread pain in fibromyalgia is related to a deficit of endogenous pain inhibition, *Pain* 114:295–302, 2005.
70. Harris RE, Clauw DJ, Scott DJ, et al.: Decreased central mu-opioid receptor availability in fibromyalgia, *J Neurosci* 27:10000–10006, 2007.
72. Phillips K, Clauw DJ: Central pain mechanisms in chronic pain states—maybe it is all in their head, *Best Practice Res Clin Rheumatol* 25(2):141–154, 2011.
73. Buskila D, Atzeni F, Sarzi-Puttini P: Etiology of fibromyalgia: the possible role of infection and vaccination, *Autoimmun Rev* 8:41–43, 2008.
74. Buskila D, Neumann L, Vaisberg G, et al.: Increased rates of fibromyalgia following cervical spine injury, *Arthritis Rheum* 40:446–452, 1997.
75. Park JH, Phothimat P, Oates CT, et al.: Use of P-31 magnetic resonance spectroscopy to detect metabolic abnormalities in muscles of patients with fibromyalgia, *Arthritis Rheum* 41:406–413, 1998.

76. Shang Y, Gurley K, Symons B, et al.: Noninvasive optical characterization of muscle blood flow, oxygenation, and metabolism in women with fibromyalgia, *Arthritis Res Ther* 14:F236, 2012.
77. Srikuea R, Symons B, Long DE, et al.: Association of fibromyalgia with altered skeletal muscle characteristics which may contribute to postexertional fatigue in postmenopausal women, *Arthritis Rheum* 65:519–528, 2013.
78. Caro XJ, Winter EF: Evidence of abnormal epidermal nerve fiber density in fibromyalgia: clinical and immunologic implications, *Arthritis Rheum* 66:1945–1954, 2014.
79. Doppler K, Rittner HL, Deckart M, et al.: Reduced dermal nerve fiber diameter in skin biopsies of patients with fibromyalgia, *Pain* 156:2319–2325, 2015.
80. Oaklander AL, Herzog ZD, Downs HM, et al.: Objective evidence that small-fiber polyneuropathy underlies some illnesses currently labeled as fibromyalgia, *Pain* 154:2310–2316, 2013.
82. Gracely RH, Petzke F, Wolf JM, et al.: Functional magnetic resonance imaging evidence of augmented pain processing in fibromyalgia, *Arthritis Rheum* 46:1333–1343, 2002.
83. Napadow V, Harris RE: What has functional connectivity and chemical neuroimaging in fibromyalgia taught us about the mechanisms and management of "centralized" pain? *Arthritis Res Ther* 16:425, 2014.
84. Harris RE, Sundgren PC, Craig AD, et al.: Elevated insular glutamate in fibromyalgia is associated with experimental pain, *Arthritis Rheum* 60:3146–3152, 2009.
85. Harte SE, Clauw DJ, Napadow V, et al.: Pressure Pain Sensitivity and Insular Combined Glutamate and Glutamine (Glx) Are Associated with Subsequent Clinical Response to Sham But Not Traditional Acupuncture in Patients Who Have Chronic Pain, *Medical Acupuncture* 25(2):154–160, 2013.
86. Napadow V, Kim J, Clauw DJ, et al.: Decreased intrinsic brain connectivity is associated with reduced clinical pain in fibromyalgia, *Arthritis Rheum* 64(7):2398–2403, 2012.
87. Ichesco E, Schmidt-Wilcke T, Bhavsar R, et al.: Altered resting state connectivity of the insular cortex in individuals with fibromyalgia, *J Pain* 15(8):815–826 e1, 2014.
88. Lazaridou A, Kim JC, M C, Loggia ML, et al.: Effects of cognitive-behavioral therapy (CBT) on brain connectivity supporting catastrophizing in fibromyalgia, *Clin J Pain* 33:215–221, 2017.
89. Fallon N, Chiu Y, Nurmikko T, et al.: Functional connectivity with the default mode network is altered in fibromyalgia patients, *PLoS One* 11:e159198, 2016.
90. Albrecht DS, Forsberg A, Sandstrom A, et al.: Brain glial activation in fibromyalgia—A multi-site positron emission tomography investigation, *Brain Behav Immun* 75:72–83, 2019.
93. McBeth J, Silman AJ, Gupta A, et al.: Moderation of psychosocial risk factors through dysfunction of the hypothalamic-pituitary-adrenal stress axis in the onset of chronic widespread musculskeletal pain: findings of a population-based prospective cohort study, *Arthritis Rheum* 56:360–371, 2007.
94. Martinez-Martinez LA, Mora T, Vargas A, et al.: Sympathetic nervous system dysfunction in fibromyalgia, chronic fatigue syndrome, irritable bowel syndrome, and interstitial cystitis: a review of case-control studies, *J Clin Rheumatol* 20:146–150, 2014.
95. Eisenlohr-Moul TA, Crofford LJ, Howard TW, et al.: Parasympathetic reactivity in fibromyalgia and temporomandibular disorder: associations with sleep problems, symptoms severity, and functional impairment, *J Pain* 16:247–257, 2015.
96. Nicholl BI, Macfarlane GJ, Davies KA, et al.: Premorbid psychosocial factors are associated with poor health-related quality of life in subjects with new onset of chronic widespread pain—results from the EPIFUND study, *Pain* 141:119–126, 2009.
97. Gupta A, Silman AJ, Ray D, et al.: The role of psychosocial factors in predicting the onset of chronic widespread pain: results from a prospective population-based study, *Rheumatol (Oxford)* 46:666–671, 2007.
99. Fitzcharles MA, Rampakakis E, Ste-Marie PA, et al.: The association of socioeconomic status and symptom severity in persons with fibromyalgia, *J Rheumatol* 41(7):1398–1404, 2014.
100. Turk DC, Adams LM: Using a biopsychosocial perspective in the treatment of fibromyalgia patients, *Pain Manag* 6:357–369, 2016.
101. Torres X, Bailles E, Valdes M, et al.: Personality does not distinguish people with fibromyalgia but identified subgroups of patients, *Gen Hosp Psych* 35:640–648, 2013.
102. Bucourt E, Martaille V, Mulleman D, et al.: Comparison of the Big Five personality traits in fibromyalgia and other rheumatic diseases, *Joint Bone Spine* 84:203–207, 2017.
103. Seto A, Han X, Price LL, et al.: The role of personality in patient with fibromyalgia, *Clin Rheumatol* 38:149–157, 2019.
104. Naylor A, Boag S, Gustin SM: New evidence for a pain personality? A critical review of the last 120 years of pain and personality, *Scand J Pain* 17:58–67, 2017.
105. Thieme K, Turk DC, Flor H: Responder criteria for operant and cognitive-behavioral treatment of fibromyalgia syndrome, *Arthritis Rheum* 57:830–836, 2007.
106. Thieme K, Turk DC, Gracely RH, et al.: The relationship among psychological and psychophysiological characteristics of fibromyalgia patients, *J Pain* 16:186–196, 2015.
107. Macfarlane GJ, Kronisch C, Dean LE, et al.: EULAR revised recommendations for the management of fibromyalgia, *Ann Rheum Dis* 76:318–328, 2017.
108. Fitzcharles MA, Ste-Marie PA, Goldenberg DL, et al.: 2012 Canadian Guidelines for the diagnosis and management of fibromyalgia syndrome: executive summary, *Pain Res Management* 18(3):119–126, 2013.
109. Annemans L, Wessely S, Spaepen E, et al.: Health economic consequences related to the diagnosis of fibromyalgia syndrome, *Arthritis Rheum* 58:895–902, 2008.
110. White KP, Nielson WR, Harth M, et al.: Does the label "fibromyalgia" alter health status, function, and health service ulitlization? A prospective, within-group comparison in a community cohort of adults with chronic widespread pain, *Arthritis Rheum* 47:260–265, 2002.
111. Nuesch E, Hauser W, Bernardy K, et al.: Comparative efficacy of pharmacological and non-pharmacological interventions in fibromyalgia syndrome: network meta-analysis, *Ann Rheum Dis* 72:955–962, 2013.
113. Busch AJ, Schachter CL, Overend TJ, et al.: Exercise for fibromyalgia: a systematic review, *J Rheumatol* 35:1130–1144, 2008.
115. Bidonde J, Busch AJ, Bath B, et al.: Exercise for adults with fibromyalgia: an umbrella systematic review with synthesis of best evidence, *Curr Rheumatol Rev* 10:45–79, 2014.
116. Mist SD, Firestone KA, Jones KD: Complementary and alternative exercise for fibromyalgia: a meta-analysis, *J Pain Res* 6:247–260, 2013.
117. Wang C, Schmid CH, Fielding RA, et al.: Effect of tai chi versus aerobic exercise for fibromyalgia: comparative effectiveness randomized controlled trial, *BMJ Open* 360:k851, 2018.
118. Naumann J, Sadaghiani C: Therapeutic benefit of balneotherapy and hydrotherapy in the management of fibromyalgia syndrome: a qualitative systematic review and meta-analysis of randomized controlled trials, *Arthritis Res Ther* 16:R141, 2014.
119. Yang B, Yi G, Hong W, et al.: Efficacy of acupuncture on fibromyalgia syndrome: a meta-analysis, *J Tradit Chin Med* 34:381–391, 2014.
120. Noehren B, Dailey DL, Rakel BA, et al.: Effect of transcuteneous electrical nerve stimulation on pain, function, and quality of life in fibromyalgia: a double-blind randomized clinical trial, *Phys Ther* 95:129–140, 2015.
122. Bernardy K, Klose P, Welsch P, et al.: Efficacy, acceptability and safety of cognitive behavioral therapies in fibromyalgia syndrome—A systematic review and meta-analysis of randomized controlled trials, *Eur J Pain* 22:242–260, 2018.

123. Cash E, Salmon P, Weissbecker I, et al.: Mindfulness meditation alleviates fibromyalgia symptoms in women: results of a randomized clinical trial, *Ann Behav Med* 49:310–330, 2015.
124. Goldenberg DL, Burckhardt C, Crofford L: Management of fibromyalgia syndrome, *JAMA* 292(19):2388–2395, 2004.
125. Carville SF, Arendt-Nielsen S, Bliddal H, et al.: EULAR evidence-based recommendations for the management of fibromyalgia syndrome, *Ann Rheum Dis* 67:537–541, 2008.
126. Hauser W, Arnold B, Eich W, et al.: Management of fibromyalgia syndrome—an interdisciplinary evidence-based guideline, *Ger Med Sci* 6:Doc14, 2008.
127. Hauser W, Petzke F, Uceyler N, et al.: Comparative efficacy and acceptability of amitriptyline, duloxetine and milnacipran in fibromyalgia syndrome: a systematic review with meta-analysis, *Rheumatology (Oxford)* 50:532–543, 2011.
128. Schmidt-Wilcke T, Clauw DJ: Fibromyalgia: from pathophysiology to therapy, *Nature Rev Rheumatol* 7(9):518–527, 2011.
129. Ottman AA, Warner CB, Brown JN. The role of mirtazapine in patients with fibromyalgia: a systematic review, *Rheumatol Int* 18;38:2217–2224.
131. Crofford LJ, Rowbotham MD, Mease PJ, et al.: Pregabalin for the treatment of fibromylagia syndrome: results of a randomized, double-blind, placebo-controlled trial, *Arthritis Rheum* 52:1264–1273, 2005.
132. Arnold LM, Goldenberg DL, Stanford SB, et al.: Gabapentin in the treatment of fibromyalgia: a randomized, double-blind, placebo-controlled, multicenter trial, *Arthritis Rheum* 56:1336–1344, 2007.
133. Hauser W, Bernardy K, Uceyler N, et al.: Treatment of fibromyalgia syndrome with gabapentin and pregabalin—a meta-analysis of randomized controlled trials, *Pain* 145:69–81, 2009.
134. Hauser W, Petzke F, Sommer C: Comparative efficacy and harms of duloxetine, milnacipran, and pregabalin in fibromyalgia syndrome, *J Pain* 11:505–521, 2010.
135. Hauser W, Petzke F, Fitzcharles MA: Efficacy, tolerability and safety of cannabis-based medicines for chronic pain management—An overview of systematic reviews, *Eur J Pain* 22:455–470, 2018.
136. Gaskell H, Moore RA, Derry S, et al.: Oxycodone for pain in fibromyalgia in adults, *Cochrane Database Syst Rev* 9:CDO12329, 2016.
137. Metyas S, Chen CL, Yeter K, et al.: Low dose naltrexone in the treatment of fibromyalgia, *Curr Rheumatol Rev* 14:177–180, 2018.
138. Younger J, Noor N, McCue R, et al.: Low-dose naltrexone for the treatment of fibromyalgia: findings of a small, randomized, double-blind, placebo-controlled, counterbalanced, crossover trial assessing daily pain levels, *Arthritis Rheum* 65:529–538, 2013.
139. Russell IJ, Holman AJ, Swick TJ, et al.: Sodium oxybate reduces pain, fatigue, and sleep disturbance and improves functionality in fibromyalgia: results from a 14-week, randomized, double-blind, placebo-controlled study, *Pain* 152:1007–1017, 2011.
140. Vincent A, Whipple MO, McAllister SJ, et al.: A cross-sectional assessment of the prevalence of multiple chronic conditions and medication use in a sample of community-dwelling adults with fibromyalgia in Olmsted County, Minnesota, *BMJ Open* 5:e006681, 2015.
141. Walitt B, Fitzcharles MA, Hassett AL, et al.: The longitudinal outcome of fibromyalgia: a study of 1555 patients, *J Rheumatol* 38(10):2238–2246, 2011.

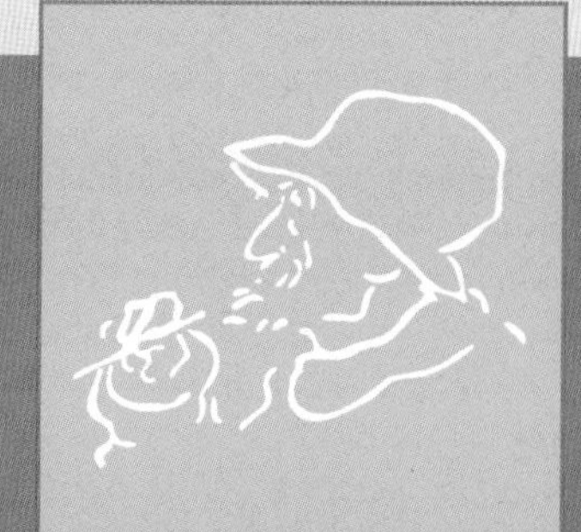

56 Synovial Fluid Analyses, Synovial Biopsy, and Synovial Pathology

HANI S. EL-GABALAWY AND STACY TANNER

KEY POINTS

Analysis of synovial fluid samples by leukocyte count, cytology, polarized microscopy, Gram stain, and culture provides key diagnostic information, particularly in acute monoarthritis.

Synovial biopsy performed by using closed needle techniques or arthroscopy may provide valuable diagnostic information, particularly in persistent monoarthritis.

Although the histopathologic features of synovitis are generally nonspecific, some synovial diseases can be diagnosed with small synovial tissue biopsies.

Analysis of synovial tissue using immunohistology and other molecular techniques has increased understanding of the mechanisms of synovitis.

Sequential analysis of synovial tissue samples in the context of therapeutic trials provides unique information regarding the effects of treatment on the target organ.

Introduction

Analysis of synovial fluid and synovial tissue obtained from diseased joints provides important diagnostic information in specific clinical settings and is valuable in addressing a spectrum of research questions about the pathogenesis and mechanisms of rheumatic diseases. Many peripheral joints are readily accessible to sampling of both synovial fluid effusions and synovial tissue, although the knee is the most frequently sampled joint. The techniques used to obtain and analyze synovial fluid and tissue samples are discussed in this chapter.

Synovial Fluid Analysis

Synovial Fluid in Health

Under normal conditions, a small volume of synovial fluid is present in each joint, forming a thin interface between the surfaces of the articular cartilage and providing for friction-free movement of these surfaces. In a large joint such as the knee, the volume of synovial fluid is estimated to be less than 5 mL. Moreover, intra-articular pressure is typically subatmospheric. Compositionally, normal synovial fluid is an ultrafiltrate of plasma to which proteins and proteoglycans are added by fibroblast-like synoviocytes in the lining layer. Most of the small-molecular-weight solutes such as O_2, CO_2, lactate, urea, creatinine, and glucose diffuse freely through the fenestrated endothelium of the synovium and are normally present at levels comparable with plasma levels. Evidence for active transport of glucose has been found. The total protein concentration of normal synovial fluid is 1.3 g/dL. The concentration of individual plasma proteins is inversely proportional to the molecular size, with small proteins such as albumin present at approximately 50% of plasma levels, and large proteins such as fibrinogen, macroglobulins, and immunoglobulins present at low levels. In contrast to this selective entry on the basis of size, clearance of synovial fluid proteins through the synovial lymphatics is unrestricted by size. Hyaluronan is the major proteoglycan synthesized by synovial cells and secreted into synovial fluid. Hyaluronan is highly polymerized and reaches molecular weights exceeding one million Daltons, which gives this fluid its characteristic viscosity. The hyaluronan also acts to retain small molecules in the synovial fluid. The lubricating capacity of the synovial fluid is attributed to a glycoprotein called *lubricin.*[1] This molecule has been fully characterized on the basis of the study of individuals with mutations of the *PRG4* gene, which encodes for its production.[2] These mutations result in an autosomal recessive loss-of-function disorder called the *camptodactyly–arthropathy–coxa vara–pericarditis syndrome,* which features a progressive, non-inflammatory arthropathy characterized by severe cartilage destruction associated with proliferation of synovial lining cells. The role of lubricin in maintaining the health of the cartilage has been further demonstrated in a murine knockout model.[3]

Accumulation of Synovial Effusions

Synovial fluid and its contents are cleared through the synovial lymphatics by a process that is aided by joint motion. Excess fluid can accumulate in any diarthrodial joint as a result of many processes, including non-inflammatory, inflammatory, and septic disorders. In addition, overt hemarthroses can result from both traumatic and nontraumatic disorders. The most important mechanism contributing to the accumulation of joint effusions is an increase in synovial microvascular permeability. This permeability allows for an increase in the efflux of plasma proteins, particularly larger proteins, which in turn increases osmotic pressure and contributes to the effusion. Leukocytes accumulate in the fluid after transmigration through the endothelium, stimulated by chemokines produced in the synovium. The capacity of synovial lymphatics to clear proteins, cells, and debris is rapidly exceeded, which in turn contributes to their accumulation in the synovial compartment.

Arthrocentesis

Most peripheral joints are readily accessible for diagnostic arthrocentesis, and the procedure can be performed in almost any ambulatory care setting equipped for sterile procedures. Joints that are less accessible because of their deeper location, such as the hip, may require an imaging technique that uses fluoroscopy or ultrasound to guide the needle and ensure accurate placement. Details of techniques used for arthrocentesis are described in Chapter 57. Because the ease with which joint fluid is aspirated depends on the gauge of the needle that is used, physicians should attempt arthrocentesis with a needle of adequate gauge, particularly in the larger joints. Moreover, high-suction gradients created by large syringes should be avoided, because they may actually reduce a physician's ability to successfully aspirate synovial fluid. Difficulty in aspiration of synovial fluid may stem from a number of intra-articular factors, including viscosity, the presence of debris such as rice bodies, and loculation of fluid into inaccessible areas. Instillation of a small amount of sterile saline may help to obtain enough fluid for culture in situations in which infection is highly suspected, yet direct aspiration is difficult.

Once obtained, it is important to analyze aspirated synovial fluid samples as quickly as possible to avoid spurious results. Ideally, leukocyte count and differential should be performed on fresh specimens. If the specimen cannot be analyzed quickly and short-term storage is needed, the specimen should be kept at 4° C. An aliquot preferably should be placed in ethylenediaminetetraacetic acid (EDTA) or heparin to prevent clotting. Delays in analysis longer than 48 hours should be avoided. A simplified algorithm for analyzing synovial fluid samples is shown in Fig. 56.1.

Gross Examination

The physician can get a first impression of the nature of the synovial fluid when fluid enters the syringe during the arthrocentesis procedure itself. For example, the viscosity of the fluid is apparent during this step. As has been mentioned, normal synovial fluid is highly viscous because of its hyaluronan content and forms a long string when a drop is expressed from the end of the needle. With increasing levels of inflammation associated with recruitment and activation of leukocytes in the synovial cavity, the hyaluronan is digested, resulting in loss of viscosity that is appreciated as a reduction in the "stringiness" of the fluid. Large pieces of debris such as rice bodies, thought to arise from detached ischemic synovial villi, may be visible while they are aspirated. These can cause sudden arrests in the flow of fluid into the syringe, requiring manipulation and redirection of needle placement.

Inspection of the aspirated synovial fluid can yield other important diagnostic information. For example, floridly purulent fluid will be completely opaque because of the very high number of leukocytes present, but synovial fluid that is transparent to the point at which printed text can be read through it is seen in non-inflammatory settings. Inflammatory synovial fluid of the type that would be aspirated from an individual with active rheumatoid arthritis (RA) appears cloudy and translucent. The degree of translucency depends on the intensity of the inflammatory response and the concentration of leukocytes in the sample. Synovial fluid from patients with ochronosis may have a speckled appearance, and particulate debris from joint prostheses may be visible on gross inspection.

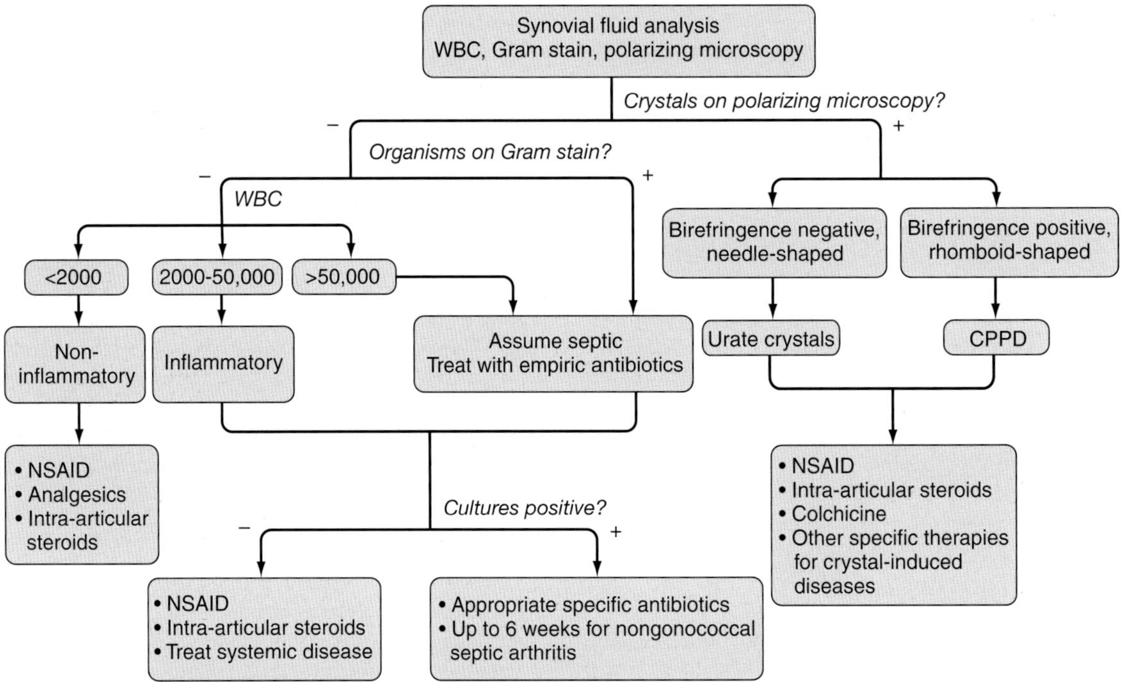

• **Fig. 56.1** A simplified algorithm for analyzing synovial fluid samples and initiating a plan of management. *CPPD*, Calcium pyrophosphate dihydrate; *NSAID*, nonsteroidal anti-inflammatory drug; *WBC*, white blood cell; –, negative test; +, positive test.

During the arthrocentesis procedure, the physician may have an important challenge in determining whether the presence of blood in the aspirated synovial fluid indicates a hemarthrosis or, alternatively, is a result of trauma from the procedure itself. In the latter case, the blood may remain unmixed with the synovial fluid and appear as red streaks in an otherwise yellow fluid. In the case of hemarthroses, the synovial fluid is generally homogeneously bloody and does not form a clot. The causes of frank hemarthrosis are varied and include trauma, pigmented villonodular synovitis, tumors, hemophilia, and other bleeding disorders or anticoagulant therapy, Charcot joint, and, occasionally, intense inflammation from a chronic arthropathy such as RA or psoriatic arthritis.

Leukocyte Count

Analysis of leukocyte counts and cytology provide important diagnostic information regarding the cause of a synovial effusion (Table 56.1). A fresh specimen should be placed in a heparinized tube for rapid analysis and, if the fluid is particularly viscous, it may need to be diluted in normal saline before counting. Normal synovial fluid contains fewer than 180 nucleated cells/mm^3, most of which originate as desquamated synovial lining cells. The leukocyte count broadly classifies synovial fluids as non-inflammatory (<2000 cells/mm^3), inflammatory (2000 to 50,000 cells/mm^3), and septic (>50,000 cells/mm^3). During a traumatic tap where circulating leukocytes may be introduced into the specimen along with large numbers of red blood cells, corrective calculations can be employed to account for these leukocytes.[4] These definitions provide broad guidelines to help narrow the differential diagnosis rather than representing inherent biologic properties of the fluid.

The most common causes of non-inflammatory synovial fluids are mechanical derangements of the joint and osteoarthritis. Other causes include endocrinopathies such as acromegaly and hyperparathyroidism; inherited disorders such as ochronosis, hemophilia (which can also present with hemarthrosis), Ehlers-Danlos syndrome, Wilson's disease, and Gaucher's disease; acquired disorders such as Paget's disease, avascular necrosis, and osteochondritis dissecans; and an uncommon condition called *intermittent hydrarthrosis,* in which joints become effused in a cyclic manner. At the other extreme, leukocyte counts of 50,000 to 300,000 cells/mm^3 are most commonly associated with septic arthritis and should prompt the clinician to empirically treat the individual as such until this diagnosis is excluded with a high degree of certainty, which typically requires definitive culture results and, possibly, repeat aspiration. Leukocyte counts exceeding 50,000 cells/mm^3 are often seen in acute crystal-induced arthritis, particularly gout. Inflammatory cell counts between 3000 and 50,000 cells/mm^3 are seen in a wide spectrum of articular disorders, including many cases of septic arthritis. Thus, most patients with acute attacks of gout and pseudogout, active RA, reactive arthritis, and psoriatic arthritis, as well as patients with gonococcal arthritis and other nonpyogenic forms of septic arthritis, will typically present with synovial fluid cell counts in this range (see Table 56.1).

Synovial Fluid Cytology

Characterization of the cells present in synovial fluid is an important diagnostic step that the examiner can achieve initially by performing cytology on a wet mount of the synovial fluid. To perform the wet mount analysis, the examiner places a drop of synovial fluid on a clean glass slide, which then is covered by a coverslip and examined under low- and high-power light microscopy. In addition to leukocytes, and in the case of traumatic taps or hemarthroses, or large numbers of erythrocytes, wet mount may reveal the presence of clumps of fibrin and crystals, cartilage and synovium fragments, and lipid droplets. These can all appear as amorphous material, and care should be taken to avoid assuming their composition without further characterization.

TABLE 56.1 Characteristics of Synovial Fluid

	Appearance	Viscosity	Cells per mm^3	% PMNs	Crystals	Culture
Normal	Transparent	High	<200	<10%	Negative	Negative
Osteoarthritis	Transparent	High	200-2000	<10%	Occasional calcium pyrophosphate and hydroxyapatite crystals	Negative
Rheumatoid arthritis	Translucent	Low	2000-50,000	Variable	Negative	Negative
Psoriatic arthritis	Translucent	Low	2000-50,000	Variable	Negative	Negative
Reactive arthritis	Translucent	Low	2000-50,000	Variable	Negative	Negative
Gout	Translucent to cloudy	Low	200->50,000	>90%	Needle-shaped, negatively birefringent monosodium urate monohydrate crystals	Negative
Pseudogout	Translucent to cloudy	Low	200-50,000	>90%	Rhomboid, positively birefringent calcium pyrophosphate crystals	Negative
Bacterial arthritis	Cloudy	Variable	2000->50,000	>90%	Negative	Positive
PVNS	Hemorrhagic or brown	Low	—	—	Negative	Negative
Hemarthrosis	Hemorrhagic	Low	—	—	Negative	Negative

PMNs, Polymorphonuclear neutrophils; *PVNS,* pigmented villonodular synovitis.

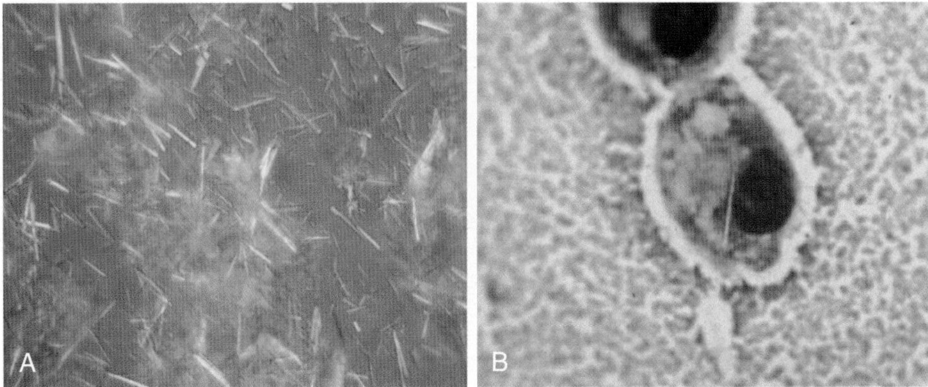

• **Fig. 56.2** (A) Urate crystals in the tophus from a patient with gouty arthritis. Crystals are negatively birefringent and needle shaped. (B) Intra-cellular urate crystal as seen on Wright stain. (Courtesy H. Ralph Schumacher, Jr.)

Characterization of synovial fluid leukocytes is best achieved by staining a dried smear of the fluid. Wright stain is most commonly used for this purpose. The phenotype and morphology of the leukocytes can then be assessed under high power by using oil immersion. Septic-range synovial fluid containing more than 50,000 cells/mm^3 is almost always associated with a high preponderance of polymorphonuclear leukocytes, often greater than 90%. Monocytes and lymphocytes predominate in the synovial fluid of patients with viral arthritis, lupus, and other connective tissue diseases. Synovial fluid samples from patients with active RA, reactive arthritis, psoriatic arthritis, and acute attacks of crystal-induced arthritis typically demonstrate a preponderance of polymorphonuclear leukocytes, although fluids from patients with early-stage RA may have a low leukocyte count with primarily mononuclear cells. The presence of large numbers of "ragocytes," which are granulocytes that have engulfed immune complexes, is associated with active RA, and their presence may indicate an unfavorable prognosis in this disease.[5] Reiter's cells represent cytophagocytic mononuclear cells that have phagocytized apoptotic polymorphonuclear leukocytes. This may represent a pathway by which autolysis and release of damaging mediators from the latter cells are avoided.[6] The presence of Reiter's cells is not specific for reactive arthritis, nor indeed for spondyloarthropathies in general. Occasionally, eosinophils will predominate in the synovial fluid, which may be associated with parasitic infection, urticaria, or hypereosinophilic syndrome. It has been suggested that cytocentrifugation of synovial fluid is the optimum method for performing cytopathology, although the cost-effectiveness of this technique is questionable in most clinical settings.

Wet Smear Analysis by Polarized Microscopy

A search for crystals by using polarized microscopy is particularly valuable in the diagnosis of acute monoarthritis or oligoarthritis, in which gout and pseudogout are often on the differential diagnosis. In such a clinical situation, if indeed the absence of pathogenic crystals in synovial fluid can be established, the likelihood of septic arthritis increases, prompting the initiation of intravenous antibiotics and potentially necessitating a hospital admission. Thus the rapid and accurate diagnosis of a crystal-induced process can prevent a costly and unnecessary sequence of events. It is helpful if the individual or the team that performs the arthrocentesis can also rapidly examine the specimen by polarized microscopy. For this procedure, the examiner requires a functional polarizing microscope, as well as adequate experience in the identification of crystals using this technique. This is particularly important in the case of calcium pyrophosphate crystals, which are notoriously difficult to detect.

The examiner should take care that the slide and the coverslip are free of dust, talc, and other particulate matter. Crystals present in the specimen rotate the light in such a way that they appear as bright objects in an otherwise dark field. Birefringent debris frequently are scattered throughout the slide and should not be mistaken for crystals.

The first-order red compensator is usually inserted immediately below the upper filter and serves to block out green light. Birefringent material in the specimen appears as a bright yellow or blue color in the red field generated by the first-order compensator. While birefringent crystals are rotated relative to the axis of the first-order compensator, the color changes from yellow to blue, or vice versa. Crystals that are yellow when oriented parallel to the axis of the compensator are negatively birefringent, and those that are blue are positively birefringent.

Identification of crystals in synovial fluid is greatly facilitated by a detailed examination of the specimen, under both low and high power, using the approach previously described. A combination of morphology and birefringence serves to identify the crystals. Monosodium urate (MSU) crystals, as shown in Fig. 56.2, are the easiest to identify because the crystal load is typically high during an acute attack of gout. A good degree of concordance between laboratories in the identification of MSU crystals has been shown.[7–9] These crystals appear as strongly negatively birefringent needle-shaped objects, many of which are intra-cellular, having been phagocytized by synovial fluid leukocytes. In contrast, the calcium pyrophosphate dihydrate (CPPD) crystals seen during attacks of pseudogout tend to be smaller, rhomboid-shaped objects that are weakly positively birefringent, as shown in Fig. 56.3. Because the CPPD crystal load during an attack of pseudogout tends to be relatively low, and because CPPD crystals are only weakly birefringent, it is important to examine all areas of the specimen on the microscope slide, and possibly to prepare a second wet mount to exclude or confirm this diagnosis. Concordance between laboratories in the recognition of CPPD is substantially lower than in the case of MSU crystals.[7–9] A particularly challenging situation arises when intra-cellular crystals cannot be identified, yet birefringent extra-cellular objects resembling crystals are seen scattered throughout the slide. This may be caused by powder from gloves or dirt on the slides.

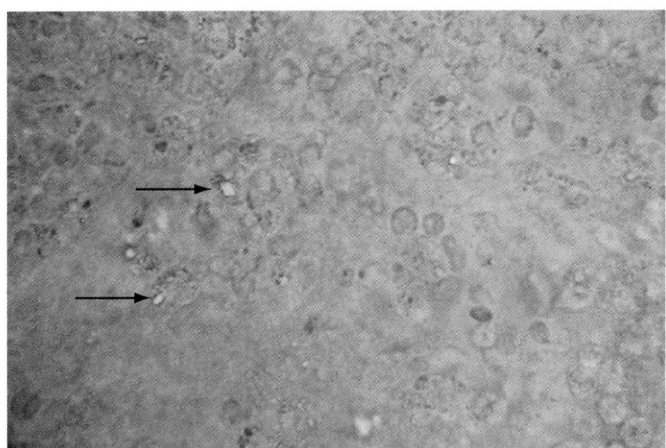

• **Fig. 56.3** Calcium pyrophosphate crystals in the synovial fluid from a patient with pseudogout. Crystals are positively birefringent and rhomboid shaped *(arrows).* (Courtesy H. Ralph Schumacher, Jr.)

As with other analyses on the synovial fluid, the examiner should perform wet mount preparation and analysis as quickly as possible, although identification of crystals can still be successful after prolonged storage of specimens. The crystal load decreases substantially as the acute inflammatory attack subsides, thus making a specific diagnosis more difficult when the attack begins to subside. Urate crystals have been detected in synovial fluid between attacks of gout.

Deposits of hydroxyapatite or basic calcium phosphate are present within the joint and in periarticular locations such as around the shoulder area and are associated with osteoarthritis. These crystals have been implicated in a particularly destructive syndrome that has been named *Milwaukee shoulder.*[10] Hydroxyapatite can be detected in synovial fluid, but because these crystals are generally nonbirefringent, it is not possible to detect them by polarized microscopy. A useful and rapid method with which to detect hydroxyapatite and other calcium-containing crystals such as octacalcium and tricalcium phosphate is to stain the fluid with alizarin red S stain and look for clumps of crystals under routine light microscopy (Fig. 56.4). These crystals have also been identified using electron microscopy, although this method is rarely available to the practicing clinician.

Synovial cholesterol crystals appear as flat, plate-like structures with notched corners (Fig. 56.5), and lipid crystals have the appearance of Maltese crosses. Both can be strongly birefringent, both negatively and positively. Corticosteroid crystals can be highly birefringent and mimic urate or CPPD crystals. Large amounts of lipid in the synovial fluid can be visible on gross examination. The significance of these crystals in synovial fluid is unclear, but it is unlikely that they are pathogenic in most cases.

Detection of Microorganisms by Gram Stain, Culture, and Polymerase Chain Reaction Analysis of Synovial Fluid

A wide spectrum of organisms can cause septic arthritis, but the most common pathogens are Gram-positive bacteria such as staphylococci and streptococci. Because septic arthritis causes rapid destruction of the joint, and because it can spread hematogenously to other areas and is associated with significant mortality, it is imperative that a specific diagnosis be made as quickly as possible, and that empiric therapy with broad-spectrum antibiotics be started until this diagnosis can be confirmed or excluded.

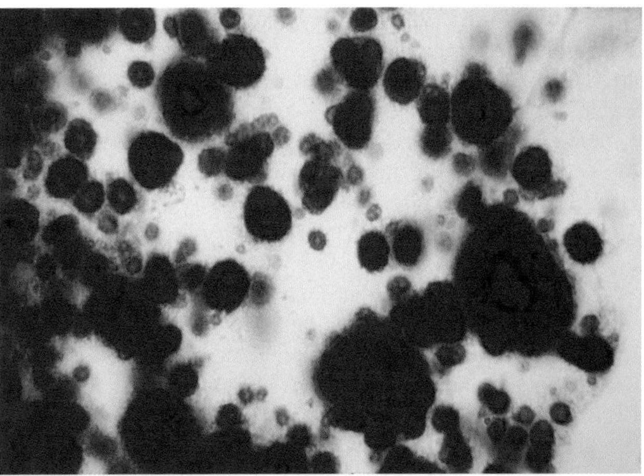

• **Fig. 56.4** Clumps of calcium hydroxyapatite crystals demonstrated by using alizarin red staining. Crystals are nonbirefringent. (Courtesy H. Ralph Schumacher, Jr.)

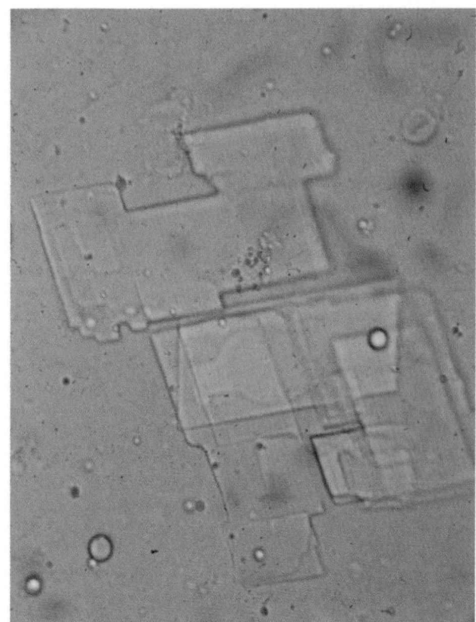

• **Fig. 56.5** Cholesterol crystals in a synovial fluid sample. (Courtesy H. Ralph Schumacher, Jr.)

A Gram stain performed on fresh synovial fluid will identify an organism in an estimated 50% of cases of septic arthritis,[11] with the highest sensitivity for Gram-positive organisms. Moreover, the specificity of a positive Gram stain approaches 100%. Clearly, this indicates that the positive predictive value for the Gram stain is very high, and that the negative predictive value is substantially lower. The gold standard for diagnosing septic arthritis is still bacteriologic culture, which has a sensitivity of 75% to 95% and a specificity of 90% in cases of nongonococcal septic arthritis.[12,13] The use of blood culture bottles further increases the yield of positive synovial cultures.[14] Bacteriologic cultures are the only studies that provide a guide for specific anti-microbial therapy. Because the sensitivity of bacteriologic cultures declines dramatically after antibiotic therapy is instituted, it is important that the clinician perform arthrocentesis before any antibiotics are administered. Cultures should be performed even when uric acid or other crystals are demonstrated in the synovial fluid because gout and septic arthritis can co-exist.[15] In the case of gonococcal arthritis, the sensitivity of bacteriologic culture, even if performed on a sample collected by using appropriate media, is low, with an estimate of less than 10%.

Polymerase chain reaction (PCR) carries a high degree of sensitivity and specificity for the detection of microorganisms in synovial fluid and tissue, even in individuals who are culture negative.[16] Most bacteria can be detected on the basis of amplifying specific sequences in their ribosomal RNA (16S rRNA). PCR is now the procedure of choice for diagnosing gonococcal arthritis[17,18] and is a highly sensitive and specific method of detecting tuberculous arthritis, although, as discussed later, analysis of synovial tissue is better than analysis of synovial fluid for making this diagnosis.[19,20] PCR is also a method of verifying the successful elimination of the offending organism in cases of septic arthritis.[21,22]

The sensitivity and specificity of PCR in detecting synovial microorganisms should be balanced against the biologic significance of a positive test. Contaminants are easily detected by using this method, and highly stringent conditions for sample collection are required to prevent false-positive tests. Moreover, PCR studies of synovial fluid and tissue from a spectrum of chronic forms of arthritis, including RA, osteoarthritis, reactive arthritis, and undifferentiated arthritis, have indicated the presence of microorganisms in a significant number of specimens.[23,24] The biologic significance of these findings and the potential role of bacterial DNA or cell wall fragments in the pathogenesis of these arthropathies remain unclear.

Biochemical Analysis of Synovial Fluid

A number of widely available biochemical tests may add to the diagnostic impression of aspirated synovial fluid samples, although lack of specificity of these biochemical analyses tends to limit their value.[13,25] Testing for synovial fluid glucose, protein, and lactate dehydrogenase (LDH) has long been included in routine practice, and values obtained should be compared with serum values. Samples from septic arthritis typically exhibit very low glucose, low pH, and high lactate levels; these levels are indicative of a switch to anaerobic metabolism. Highly inflammatory synovial fluids from RA exhibit a similar profile, along with high protein and LDH levels. Levels of pressure of oxygen (pO_2) in the blood are often in the hypoxic range in RA synovial fluids and are correlated with increased lactate and levels of pressure of carbon dioxide (pCO_2) in the blood.[26,27] A prospective study conducted to evaluate these tests in a spectrum of inflammatory and non-inflammatory disorders demonstrated considerable variability in each diagnostic category, which limits their clinical utility.[25]

Serologic testing of synovial fluid to detect rheumatoid factor, anti-nuclear antibodies, and complement levels has been suggested as a method that can be used to confirm a diagnosis of RA or other connective tissue diseases. In particular, RA synovial fluids may be positive for rheumatoid factor even when serum is not,[28] and complement levels are typically low as a result of consumption by immune complexes. These findings are not sufficiently sensitive or specific to be of value on a routine clinical basis.

Synovial Fluid Analysis in Arthritis Research

The ease with which synovial fluid is aspirated from many inflamed joints has allowed a wide spectrum of research studies to be conducted on this biologic material. In research settings, cells in synovial fluid samples are typically separated by centrifugation, and cellular and noncellular components of the fluid are analyzed separately. Detailed analysis of the phenotype and functional properties of synovial fluid leukocytes has been particularly informative in RA and reactive arthritis research, in which immunophenotyping of lymphocyte subpopulations has provided important clues to the pathogenesis of these diseases. In the case of reactive arthritis, in which triggering organisms are often identified, the proliferative and cytokine responses of synovial fluid lymphocytes to antigens derived from *Chlamydia, Yersinia,* and other pathogens have been elucidated.[29,30] Synovial fluid T cells from reactive arthritis patients are biased toward production of T helper (Th)2 cytokines such as IL-10 and IL-4, whereas synovial fluid T cells from patients with RA are Th1 biased and exhibit defects in Th2 differentiation.[31–33]

Analysis of the noncellular portion of synovial fluid has provided important information regarding a spectrum of soluble molecules, including cytokines and growth factors,[34] extra-cellular matrix proteins, autoantibodies, and therapeutic drug levels. Moreover, broad-based proteomic studies of synovial fluid with the use of fractionation techniques and mass spectrometry are beginning to provide novel approaches to understanding pathogenesis and prognosis in arthropathies such as RA.[35]

Synovial Biopsy

Sampling of synovial tissue is a direct approach to defining the pathologic processes that cause swollen, painful joints. In clinical settings, it can be particularly valuable in evaluating an undiagnosed persistent monoarthritis when other investigations, including synovial fluid analysis, have failed to provide a specific diagnosis. In research settings, analysis of synovial tissue samples has dramatically improved our understanding of the pathogenetic mechanisms underlying RA, spondyloarthropathies, and other chronic articular disorders. More recently, synovial biopsy has been explored as a method for defining the target tissue response to therapeutic agents, particularly targeted biologic therapies.

Blind Percutaneous Synovial Biopsy

Percutaneous needle biopsy is most commonly performed according to the method originally described by Parker and Pearson,[36,37] utilizing a biopsy needle that now carries their name. Percutaneous synovial biopsy is most often performed on the knee joint, although the technique can readily be adapted for use in other joints such as the wrist, elbow, ankle, or shoulder. A modification of the original Parker-Pearson needle has facilitated synovial biopsy of small hand joints such as metacarpophalangeal and proximal interphalangeal joints.[38] The technique for Parker-Pearson synovial biopsy uses a 14 gauge needle with a lateral aperture just proximal to the inserted end of the needle. This lateral opening features a sharp cutting edge for severing trapped synovial tissue that is captured by applying suction with a 3 to 5 mL syringe. With this approach, multiple 1 to 3 mm samples are obtained by angling the trocar in several directions. This also serves to minimize the sampling error involved. Synovial samples are typically pink and are easily removed with a slight twisting motion. Because of the blind nature of the procedure, samples of fat, muscle, or fibrous tissue may be obtained and need to be separated from true synovial samples.

Percutaneous synovial biopsy is easily performed in most ambulatory care settings with the use of relatively inexpensive equipment, and recently ultrasound guidance has improved the yield. The overall morbidity of the procedure is low and is comparable with that of arthrocentesis, with perhaps a slightly higher rate of hemarthrosis. The risk of hemarthrosis can be minimized if the patient does not bear weight for a few hours after the procedure. The main disadvantage of the procedure is its blind nature. In comparison with visually guided arthroscopy, samples derived from the interface between synovium and adjacent cartilage are underrepresented when the blind procedure is used.[39,40] As discussed later, this drawback is particularly relevant to a number of research questions.

Arthroscopically Guided Synovial Biopsy

Arthroscopy is widely used by orthopedic specialists for the diagnosis and treatment of a variety of articular disorders, particularly mechanical derangements of intra-articular structures such as cruciate ligaments and menisci. During the past two decades, the arthroscopic procedure has been adapted for diagnostic synovial biopsies in settings that do not require a fully equipped operating theater and general anesthetic. In most cases, intra-articular local anesthesia suffices for the procedure, although conscious sedation may be required in some individuals. The procedure is well tolerated and is associated with low morbidity, although the risks to the patient of hemarthrosis and infection after the procedure are slightly higher than that of percutaneous needle biopsy. The patient should be instructed to minimize weight bearing for 24 to 48 hours after the procedure.

The primary advantage of arthroscopy is its ability to visually guide the biopsy procedure. This permits macroscopic evaluation of the synovium and sampling of areas that appear to be severely affected by the pathologic process, and it allows for sampling of the interface between inflamed synovium and adjacent cartilage. This interface is an area of particular interest for understanding the pathogenesis of destructive arthropathies such as RA.[39] As with samples obtained by percutaneous synovial biopsy, individual samples are allocated for specific laboratory studies depending on the clinical or research question under investigation.

Ultrasound Guided Synovial Biopsy

Advances in ultrasound imaging and widespread use of ultrasound in rheumatology has facilitated the adoption of ultrasound guided synovial biopsies. In a typical procedure, local anesthesia is administered to soft tissues and the joint space; afterwards, a core needle biopsy, typically 14 to 18 gauge, under transverse ultrasound guidance is used to retrieve multiple samples of synovium (Fig. 56.6). In larger joints such as the knee, a coaxial needle may be used for repeated entries via a single skin incision. Similar to the Parker-Pearson method, this allows for sampling of small, medium, or large joints in an outpatient setting with the advantage of direct visualization of the synovium being targeted for biopsy.

Ultrasound guided biopsy is successful in retrieving tissue amenable for histopathologic characterization and RNA extraction. The thickness of the synovium on gray-scale ultrasound is the most important independent predictor of synovial tissue quantity and quality as compared with power Doppler signal and size of the biopsied joint.[41] When compared with other techniques such as blind needle biopsy and arthroscopic synovial biopsy, ultrasound guided biopsy is more effective than blind needle biopsy in attaining synovial tissue in small joints.[42]

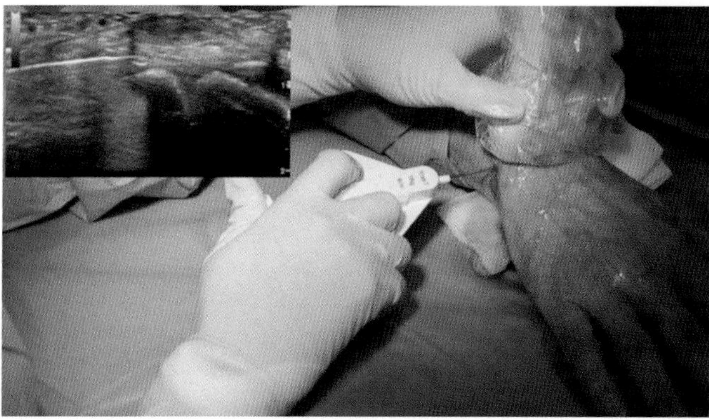

• **Fig. 56.6** Ultrasound guided synovial biopsy. Insert shows the needle traversing the scapholunate joint and entering synovial tissue. (From Kelly S, Humby F, Filer A, et al.: Ultrasound-guided synovial biopsy: a safe, well-tolerated and reliable technique for obtaining high-quality synovial tissue from both large and small joints in early arthritis patients. *Ann Rheum Dis* 2015;74[3]:611-7.)

Processing Synovial Tissue Samples

An adequate number of individual synovial specimens must be allocated for routine light microscopy with the use of formalin fixation and paraffin embedding. This provides the highest-quality sections for hematoxylin and eosin (H&E) histologic analysis, and it allows the most accurate delineation of pathologic processes within tissue. Although formalin-fixed sections can be used in some cases for immunohistology, formalin fixation alters the conformation of many protein antigens, making them inaccessible for specific identification by immunohistology. Many of the molecular markers used to analyze diseased synovium, including cell surface markers, cytokines, adhesion molecules, and proteases, require that tissue samples be snap frozen in a suitable mounting medium, such as optimal cutting temperature compound, and then sectioned with the use of a cryostat. The sections can be processed by using antigen-specific monoclonal or polyclonal antibodies and color development achieved by one of several immunofluorescence or immunoperoxidase methods. Typically, a nuclear counterstain is also used to assist in orientation of the tissue—hematoxylin in the case of immunoperoxidase studies. If only formalin-fixed, paraffin-embedded tissue is available, an alternative method for detecting antigens that are sensitive to formalin fixation is antigen retrieval.

Several antigen retrieval methods are available, including enzymatic and thermal methods,[43] which have been used to successfully retrieve a spectrum of antigens from archival synovial tissue samples for immunohistologic studies, although the quality of the tissue sections often deteriorates after antigen retrieval. A number of double-staining immunohistology techniques have been developed for simultaneous evaluation of the expression of two markers in the same tissue section, although these techniques are labor intensive and often require considerable experimentation to generate good stains.[44] Formalin fixation dissolves crystals, and if this is a diagnostic consideration, the specimen should be fixed in ethanol.

The sensitivity and specificity of molecular DNA and RNA techniques provide unprecedented opportunities to explore the pathogenesis of synovial disorders. Although these studies can be carried out on very small quantities of tissue, examiners need to take great care in handling and processing tissue samples to prevent degradation of the nucleic acids, particularly with RNA when

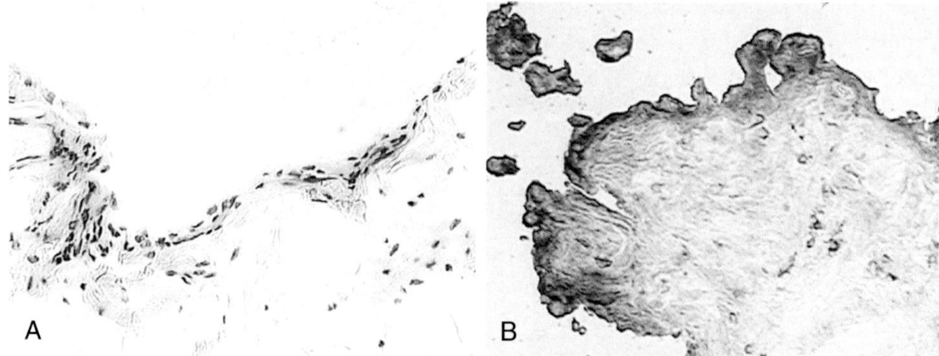

• **Fig. 56.7** Normal synovium. (A) A lining layer one to two cells deep that is composed of macrophage-like synoviocytes (type A) and fibroblast-like synoviocytes (type B). (B) Normal synovium stained for the enzyme uridine diphosphoglucose dehydrogenase, an indicator of hyaluronan synthesis by fibroblast-like synoviocytes.

RNase enzymes are ubiquitous and can rapidly degrade the small quantity of RNA present in a tissue sample. As discussed later, the search for microbial DNA and RNA has been of particular interest in attempts to understand the cause and pathogenesis of reactive arthritis, RA, and other forms of chronic synovitis of unknown cause. Techniques used to analyze human gene expression in small tissue samples have rapidly progressed. This has enabled the detection and quantitation of multiple mRNA transcripts in very small quantities of biopsy material, in many cases without the need for amplification.[45,46]

Synovial Pathology

Synovial Membrane in Healthy Individuals

A detailed description of the composition of normal synovium is provided in Chapter 2. Histologically, the normal synovial lining layer is one to three cells thick and is composed of closely associated macrophage-like (type A) and fibroblast-like synoviocytes (type B) that are not separated from the underlying stroma by a basement membrane, as is the case with a true epithelium. In many areas, visible gaps in this lining layer allow small molecules to easily diffuse through the extra-cellular matrix into the synovial fluid. The two types of lining layer synoviocytes are distinct and can be differentiated on the basis of ultrastructural and immunohistologic features. Macrophage-like synoviocytes are myeloid in origin, as they exhibit the morphologic characteristics of phagocytic cells and express macrophage markers such as CD68, CD14, and FcγRIIIa. Fibroblast-like synoviocytes are synthetic cells of mesenchymal origin that are the primary source of hyaluronan and other proteoglycans found in normal synovial fluid. They express CD55 (decay-accelerating factor [DAF]), high levels of vascular cell adhesion molecule (VCAM)-1, and the enzyme uridine diphosphoglucose dehydrogenase (UDPGD), which is involved in the synthesis of hyaluronan and has been detected by cytochemical methods (Fig. 56.7). Fibroblast-like synoviocytes also uniquely express cadherin-11, a specialized adhesion molecule that is involved in homotypic aggregation of these cells and that contributes to maintaining the integrity of the synovial lining layer.[47] Quantitatively, most of the cells in the normal synovial lining layer are type B cells. The underlying stroma features a rich network of capillaries with fenestrated endothelium in the immediate sublining area that serve to maintain the health and viability of adjacent cartilage. Larger arterioles and venules can be found deeper in the synovial stoma. The synovial microvasculature is surrounded by loose connective tissue, which also incorporates the synovial lymphatics that serve to drain this tissue. The synovium of completely asymptomatic individuals commonly exhibits a modest infiltrate of T lymphocytes that are occasionally organized in perivascular aggregates, although B cells are not seen.[48]

Synovial Histopathology in the Evaluation of Monoarthritis

Pathologic analysis of synovial tissue samples can be of considerable value in certain clinical settings. Nevertheless, the histopathologic interpretation of synovial biopsy specimens is often nondiagnostic and lacks specificity.[49] Pathologic analysis of synovial samples from patients with undiagnosed monoarthritis may be of particular value. The presence of large numbers of neutrophils in the synovial tissue stroma is highly suggestive of septic arthritis, and in such cases Gram stain may reveal bacteria in the tissue. Because septic arthritis is usually acute in onset, synovial biopsy is rarely required, and the diagnosis can be made by analyzing synovial fluid as described previously. Gonococcal arthritis may require synovial biopsy for diagnosis (Fig. 56.8). A mononuclear cell infiltrate, on the other hand, is more consistent with a chronic inflammatory process and has a wide differential diagnosis, as described previously. The presence of granulomas supports a diagnosis of tuberculous arthritis or sarcoidosis, both of which cause chronic monoarthritis. The synovial granulomas of tuberculosis (TB) may be caseating or noncaseating, and staining of the tissue for acid-fast bacilli, culture, and molecular probing can yield a definitive diagnosis in an estimated 50% of cases. Similarly, a spectrum of fungal infections can be diagnosed by using similar approaches, but special stains such as a Gomori stain may be required. The diagnosis of sarcoid arthropathy is suspected in synovial specimens with noncaseating granulomas in cases where mycobacterial or fungal infection has been excluded.

Pigmented villonodular synovitis (Video 56.1) is an important consideration in individuals with chronic monoarthritis of a large joint such as the knee or hip. This disorder has a characteristic MRI appearance caused by hemosiderin deposits in the synovium and large cystic lesions in adjacent bone. Histopathologic analysis of the synovium can confirm this diagnosis and demonstrates a diffusely hypervascular proliferative lesion with mononuclear cells

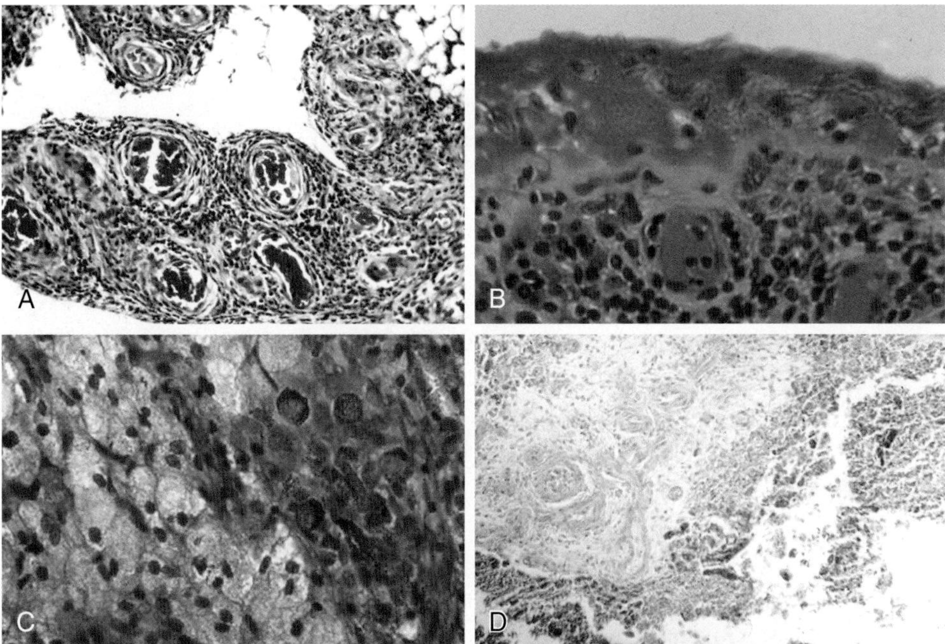

• **Fig. 56.8** (A) Synovial pathology of gonococcal arthritis. A marked infiltrate with polymorphonuclear leukocytes and vascular congestion is present. (B) Synovial pathology of scleroderma shows loss of the lining layer with surface fibrin deposition and mononuclear inflammation in sublining areas. (C) Pigmented nodular synovitis with hemosiderin deposits and foamy cells. (D) Amyloidosis with deposits on the synovial surface, Congo red stain. (A-D, Courtesy H. Ralph Schumacher, Jr.)

of the monocyte/macrophage lineage, foamy multinucleated cells resembling osteoclasts, and hemosiderin deposits[50] (see Fig. 56.8). Synovial sarcomas are rare tumors that must be diagnosed on the basis of synovial pathology.

Synovial Histopathology in the Evaluation of Polyarthritis

In current clinical practice, the availability of well-validated diagnostic criteria and specific serologic tests, combined with a relative lack of specificity in synovial histopathologic features, limits the clinical utility of synovial pathology in the differential diagnosis of oligoarthritis and polyarthritis. On the other hand, analysis of synovial tissue samples obtained in the context of research studies from patients with RA and various spondyloarthropathies has dramatically enhanced our understanding of the cellular and molecular mechanisms of these disorders. This is reflected in a large body of literature published during the past three decades.[39,51]

RA synovium has been the most extensively studied histopathologically, and a detailed discussion of RA synovitis can be found in Chapters 76 and 77. The two characteristic features seen in RA synovitis are hyperplasia of the lining layer and infiltration of the sublining stroma with mononuclear cells (Fig. 56.9). The surface of the lining layer is often covered with fibrin deposits generated from activation of the fibrinolytic system in inflammatory synovial fluid. Occasionally, the synovial lining layer is completely denuded and is replaced by a dense fibrin cap. In highly inflamed tissues, fibrin deposits extend deeply into the sublining stroma, which may be edematous because of the marked increase in vascular permeability. The earliest synovial changes in RA appear to feature microvascular abnormalities,[52] and mononuclear cell infiltrates have been detected in asymptomatic joints of patients with RA.[53,54] These features are nonspecific and are seen in the synovium of acutely inflamed joints from a spectrum of disorders, including reactive arthritis and psoriatic arthritis.

In RA, the mononuclear cell infiltrate in the sublining stroma can be diffuse but more commonly is arranged in perivascular aggregates that resemble lymphoid follicles (see Fig. 56.9). Although the presence of lymphoid aggregates in the synovial membrane is typical of RA, this histopathologic feature is by no means unique to RA synovitis.[55–58] Lymphoid follicles are typically located near vessels with tall endothelium, which are termed *high endothelial venules;* these vessels specialize in the recruitment of lymphocytes (Fig. 56.10). Multinucleated giant cells are occasionally seen in RA synovium (Fig. 56.11), and some tissues demonstrate granuloma formation. Finally, synovial tissue obtained at the time of joint arthroplasty often exhibits extensive fibrosis and may be indistinguishable from arthroplasty samples obtained from patients with osteoarthritis.

The synovial histopathology of psoriatic arthritis, ankylosing spondylitis, and reactive arthritis has been compared with that of RA.[59,60] In all cases, a similar spectrum of inflammatory cell populations has been identified, but several subtle and potentially important differences have been observed. Overall, synovial histologic and immunohistologic features of psoriatic arthritis, both oligo- and polyarticular, resemble those of other spondyloarthropathies to a greater extent than RA (see Synovial Immunohistology section below).[60] Comparative studies have suggested that synovial lesions in psoriatic arthritis are more vascular than those of RA, with more tortuosity of the synovial microvasculature.[61,62] This is evident both macroscopically and microscopically. Moreover, lymphoid aggregates of various sizes were identified in 25 of 27 synovial tissue samples from patients with psoriatic arthritis, and 13 of 27 had large organized aggregates with all of the features of ectopic lymphoid neogenesis that have been associated with RA synovitis.[55] Studies of synovium from the peripheral joints of

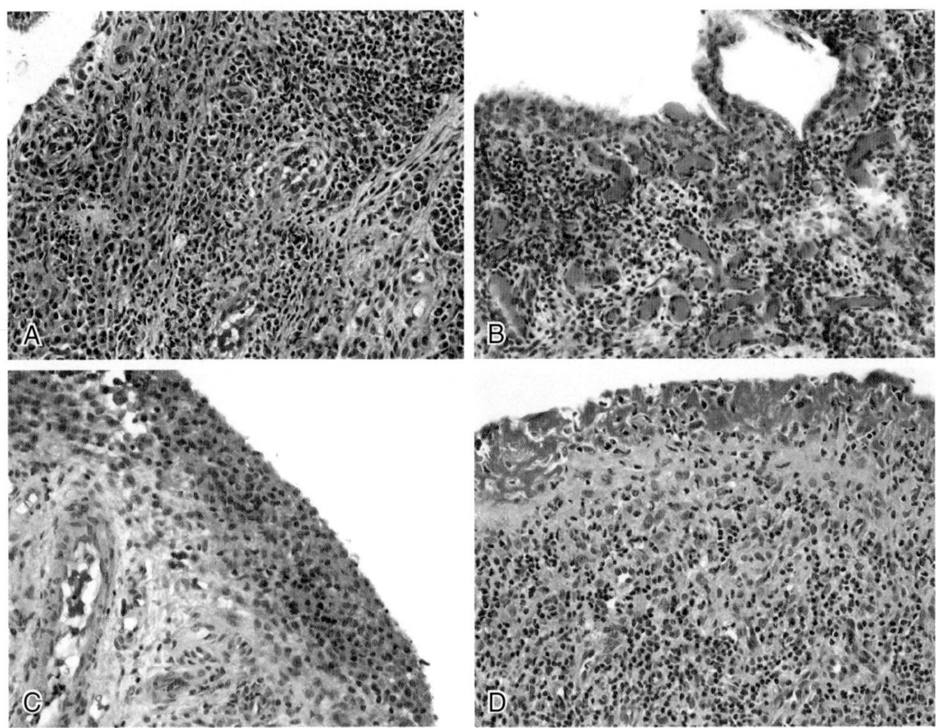

• **Fig. 56.9** Histopathology of rheumatoid arthritis synovitis. (A) Lymphoid aggregate. (B) Diffuse lymphocytic infiltrate. (C) Hyperplasia of the lining layer. (D) Fibrin cap replacing a denuded lining layer.

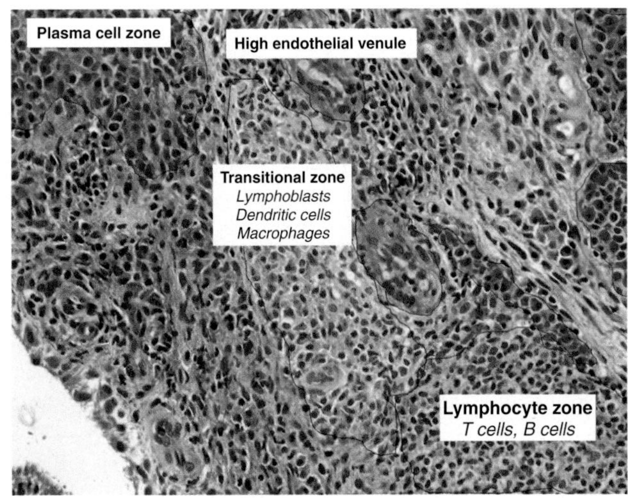

• **Fig. 56.10** Microarchitecture of rheumatoid arthritis synovial lymphoid aggregates.

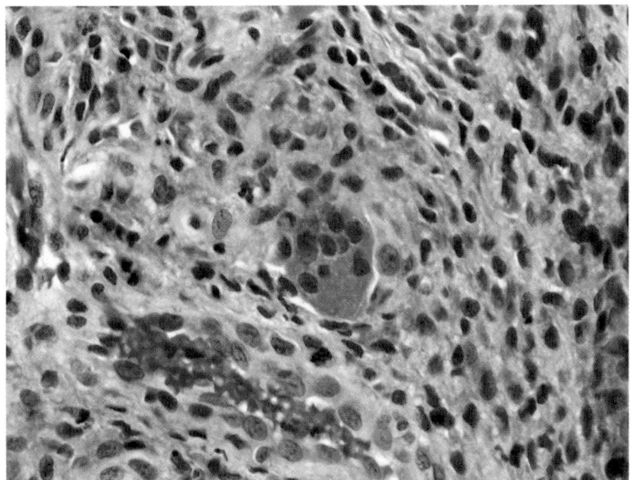

• **Fig. 56.11** Multinucleated giant cell in a patient with rheumatoid arthritis.

ankylosing spondylitis patients have revealed intense infiltrates of lymphocytes, plasma cells, and lymphocytic aggregates.[63,64] Comparisons made between the synovial lesions seen in patients with reactive arthritis and those seen in patients with early-stage RA of similar disease duration suggest that reactive arthritis synovia are less infiltrated with B lymphocytes, plasma cells, and macrophages.[65,66] Synovium from patients with osteoarthritis often features the presence of lymphocyte aggregates, although these tend to be small and less well developed than those seen in RA.[57]

The synovium of lupus patients showed synovial hyperplasia, inflammatory infiltrates, vascular proliferation, edema and congestion, fibrinoid necrosis and intimal fibrous hyperplasia of blood vessels, and superficial fibrin deposits, although these changes were quantitatively modest compared with those of RA.[67] In early scleroderma, the lining layer was seen to be thin with deposits of fibrin and stromal lymphocytes and plasma cells,[68] and similar changes were seen in patients with dermatomyositis and polymyositis[69] (see Fig. 56.8). A recent study comparing the immunopathologic features of early untreated Behçet's disease with those of psoriatic arthritis noted that although a similar degree of inflammation was seen in the two disorders, synovitis in Behçet's disease demonstrated higher numbers of neutrophils and T cells than were seen in psoriatic synovitis.[70]

In patients with chronic crystal arthropathies, large deposits of birefringent material can be detected in the synovium.[71] Amyloid arthropathy can be diagnosed by demonstrating amyloid deposits in the synovium with Congo red staining (see Fig. 56.8). The

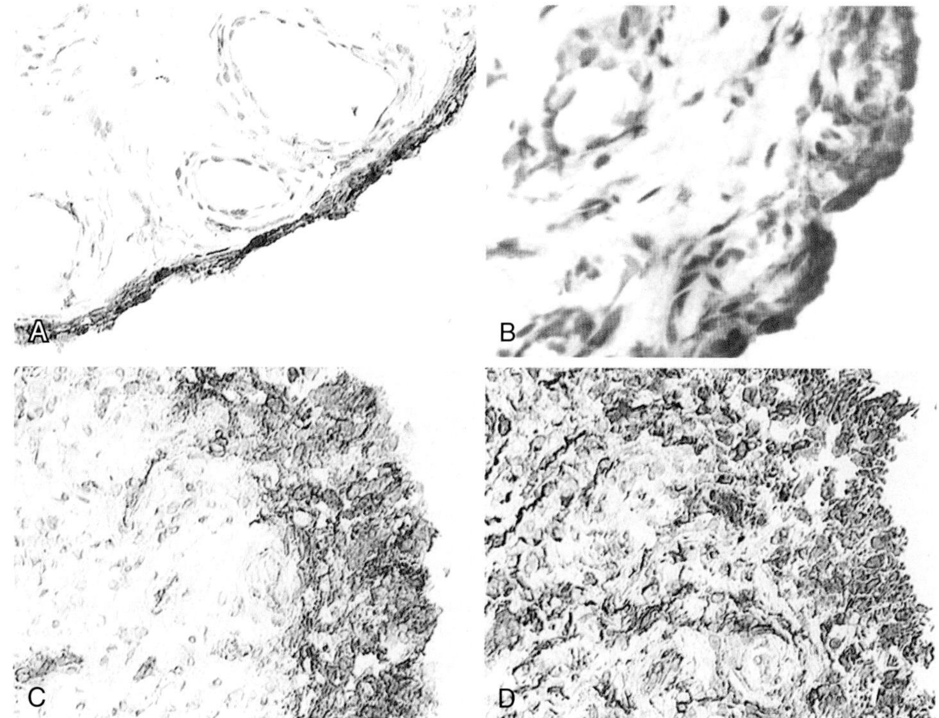

• **Fig. 56.12** (A-D) Immunoperoxidase staining *(brown color)* of normal synovium and rheumatoid arthritis (RA) synovium for CD55 (fibroblast-like synoviocytes) and CD68 (macrophage-like synoviocytes). Both subsets of lining cells are increased in the hyperplastic lining layer of RA synovium.

synovium in ochronosis contains brownish shards of cartilage.[72] Multicentric reticulohistiocytosis can be diagnosed pathologically by the presence of large foamy cells and multinucleated cells in the synovium. In arthritis of hemochromatosis, the synovium exhibits brown hemosiderin deposits in the lining cells, and CPPD crystals can also be observed.[73]

Synovial Immunohistology

Sampling Error and Quantitative Analysis

Immunohistology utilizes specific monoclonal or polyclonal antibodies with well-defined molecular targets and is an effective tool for analyzing the cellular and molecular features of the synovium. As the field has progressed during the past two decades, it has become clear that algorithms for generating reproducible quantitative data from immunohistologically stained sections are required. Moreover, approaches are needed for minimizing the sampling bias that is inherent in biopsy-based studies.[74] Studies have suggested that if six or more individual specimens from different parts of the joint are examined, variance is reduced to less than 10% for T cell and activation markers.[75] Furthermore, synovial inflammatory features are similar in areas adjacent to and distant from the pannus cartilage junction, with the possible exception of macrophage numbers, which tend to be higher in adjacent areas.[76,77]

Various methods have been proposed by which quantitative data for immunohistologically stained synovial tissue sections can be generated.[78,79] The easiest and least costly method is to generate semiquantitative scores of staining intensity (e.g., on a 0 to 3 scale) from multiple areas of the tissue, and on the basis of these to obtain an average score for the entire tissue. The reliability and reproducibility of this method are increased if two observers score the tissue sections independently and a final average of the scores is generated. Computer-assisted image analysis involves capturing images from multiple areas of the tissue samples to which color-specific quantitative software algorithms are then applied. This method generates the greatest quantity of reproducible data but requires expensive equipment and certain levels of operator skill. Furthermore, differences in the background staining intensity of individual sections can make this type of analysis technically difficult.

Synovial Lining Cell Layer

Compared with normal synovium, the lining layer in RA and other forms of chronic inflammatory arthritis is often hyperplastic, resulting from an increase in both type A and type B cells, as indicated by an increase in CD68 and CD55 staining, respectively (Fig. 56.12). Macrophage-like synoviocytes are likely recruited from the blood and then migrate through the synovial stroma and ultimately are retained in the lining layer in close association with fibroblast-like synoviocytes. The increase in fibroblast-like synoviocytes might be related more to defects in apoptosis than to recruitment or local proliferation. Expression of several families of adhesion molecules by both types of lining cells results in their close association and modulates their activation status. These include β1 and β2 integrins and their respective immunoglobulin supergene family ligands, particularly intercellular adhesion molecule (ICAM)-1 and VCAM-1.[80–82] Cadherin-11 expressed by fibroblast-like cells likely plays a key role in the adhesive interactions that sustain the lining layer hyperplasia.[47] This adhesion molecule is widely expressed in the lining layer of normal cells, as is shown in Fig. 56.13. The relationship between fibroblast-like synoviocytes in the lining layer and other populations of mesenchymal cells in the sublining stroma remains uncertain. Immunohistology indicates that expression of CD55, VCAM-1, and

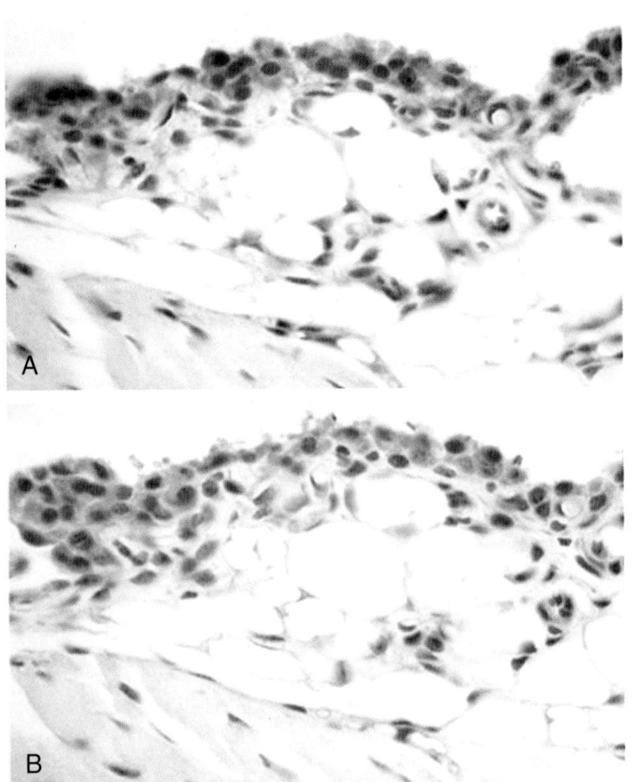

• **Fig. 56.13** Immunohistochemical staining for cadherin-11 in the normal synovial lining layer *(brown color)* (A). Control staining is shown in (B). (From Lee DM, Kiener HP, Agarwal SK, et al.: Cadherin-11 in synovial lining formation and pathology in arthritis. *Science* 315:1006–1010, 2007.)

cadherin-11 is primarily seen in the lining cell layer with minimal evidence of expression in sublining fibroblast populations. Similarly, our understanding of the relationship between lining layer macrophage-like cells and sublining macrophages is incomplete, and both express widely used macrophage markers such as CD68 and CD14. Macrophage-like lining cells preferentially express FcγRIIIa receptors, which may serve to localize immune complexes to the synovium.[83]

Functionally, the lining cell layer in chronic inflammatory arthropathies such as RA and psoriatic arthritis typically has the appearance of being activated. Human leukocyte antigen (HLA)-DR is highly expressed, particularly by macrophage-like cells, which may suggest a role for these cells in antigen presentation.[84] Several studies have indicated that cells in the lining layer are the principal source of cartilage-degrading proteases, particularly matrix metalloproteinase (MMP)-1 and MMP-3[85,86] (Fig. 56.14). The lining layer is generally less hyperplastic in spondyloarthropathies such as psoriatic arthritis and reactive arthritis compared with RA.[60,64,87] Less is known about the functional state of the lining cells in these disorders, although it is likely that differences compared with RA are quantitative rather than qualitative.

Synovial Lymphocytes and Plasma Cells

A predominance of CD3⁺ T cells is found in the synovial tissues of patients with RA and spondyloarthropathies, and the CD4/CD8 ratio is 4 : 1 or greater in the lymphocytic aggregates but is lower in more diffuse infiltrates. Moreover, the CD4 cells in the aggregates also express CD27,[88] which facilitates B cell help. Considerable attention has been paid to whether the infiltrating T cells in RA and other arthropathies are primarily Th1 (interferon [IFN]-γ producing) or Th2 (IL-4 producing) biased, but

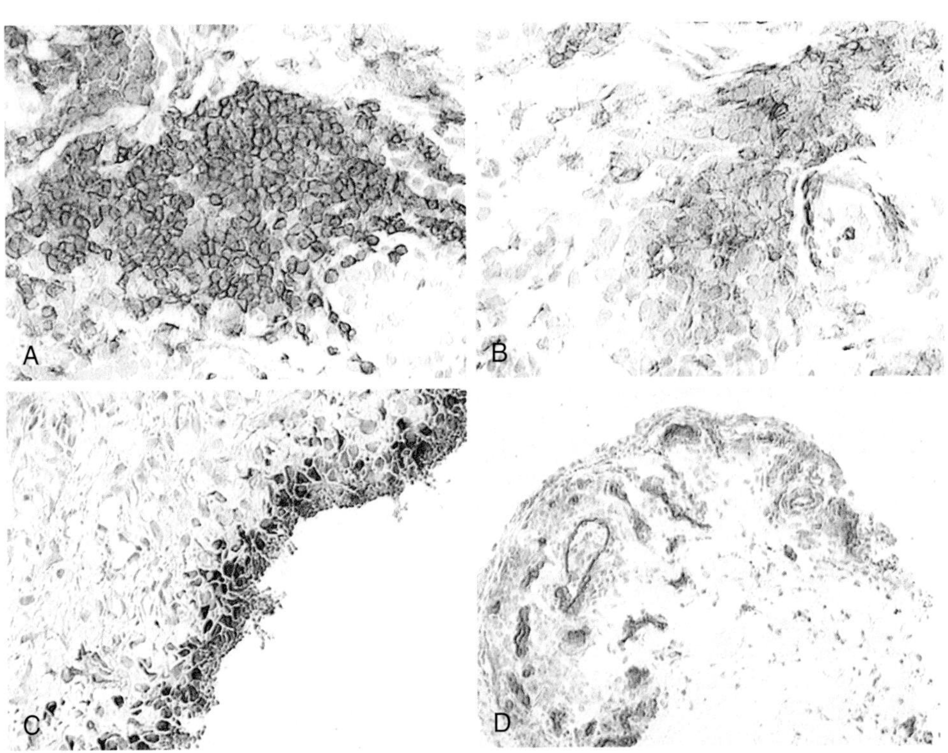

• **Fig. 56.14** Immunoperoxidase staining *(brown color)* of rheumatoid arthritis synovium. (A) T lymphocytes. (B) B lymphocytes. (C) Matrix metalloproteinase-1. (D) $\alpha_v\beta_3$ integrin (angiogenic vessels).

the data in this area have been inconsistent. Until recently, it was suggested that T cells in synovium from patients with RA are more Th1 biased compared with those in synovium from patients with spondyloarthropathies, with a higher Th1/Th2 cytokine ratio.[89] Identification of a third subset of Th cells that express IL-17 and play a central role in chronic inflammatory disorders has necessitated a revision in the role that T cells play in synovitis.[90,91] The presence of IL-17, IL-1β, and TNF in RA synovium was found to be predictive of progressive damage.[92] Furthermore, a subset of CD4 T cells expressing CD25 and the gene *FoxP3,* so-called *regulatory T cells* (Tregs), are now known to play a regulatory role in antigen-specific T cell expansion. Although Tregs are readily detected in the joints of patients with RA and other inflammatory arthropathies, their suppressor function appears to be defective in this microenvironment.[93–96] It has been suggested that CD8 T cells are needed to maintain the structure of ectopic lymphoid-like structures in RA synovium, even though the numbers of these T cells typically are substantially lower than the numbers of CD4$^+$ cells.[97]

B cells are identified by expression of CD19 and CD20 and are particularly abundant in tissues that exhibit large lymphoid aggregates with germinal centers. B cells typically are found in close association with CD4$^+$ T cells in these aggregates (see Fig. 56.10). Experiments in severe combined immunodeficiency (SCID) mice suggest that B cells may be critical for maintaining the microarchitecture of synovial lymphoid follicles and for T cell activation.[98] Memory B cells are efficient antigen-presenting cells, and rheumatoid factor–producing B cells are well suited for capturing a wide spectrum of antigens in immune complexes.

The areas surrounding the lymphoid aggregates are often densely infiltrated with sheets of CD38$^+$ plasma cells. Analysis of V gene variants and rearrangements in B cells and plasma cells in both RA and reactive arthritis synovium indicates that plasma cells from a particular aggregate are clonally related, suggesting that their terminal differentiation occurred in the synovial microenvironment.[99] Synovial plasma cells actively synthesize immunoglobulin, some of which result in the production of autoantibodies such as anticitrulline antibodies, which recognize local citrullinated antigens.[100–102] As stated previously, plasma cell infiltrates are also seen in psoriatic arthritis, ankylosing spondylitis, and reactive arthritis synovium, although a systematic analysis of synovial samples from patients with early arthritis has suggested that their presence is most suggestive of RA.[65] One study found that intra-cellular citrullinated proteins were detected in RA but not in spondylarthropathy synovium.[60] In contrast, another study found that the presence of citrullinated proteins was not specific for RA synovitis.[103]

The areas immediately adjacent to the dense lymphoid aggregates, which comprise primarily CD4$^+$ T cells and B cells, have been called *transitional zones*[104,105] (see Fig. 56.10). These areas feature a lower CD4/CD8 ratio and appear to be particularly active immunologically. Transitional areas are rich in macrophages and interdigitating dendritic cells, both of which are highly efficient antigen-presenting cells. Lymphoblasts, in particular CD8$^+$ T cells, are seen to be present in close proximity to antigen-presenting cells.

Natural killer cells can be identified by cell surface markers, expression of granzymes, and functional assays. Several studies have suggested an expansion of subsets of natural killer cells in RA synovial tissue and synovial fluids.[106–108] Mast cells are abundant in RA synovium and co-localize with inflammatory mediators and proteases in the synovial microenvironment.[109,110]

Synovial Sublining Macrophages and Dendritic Cells

Macrophages are present in the sublining areas of healthy and chronically inflamed synovium and are particularly abundant in the sublining stroma of RA synovium. Indeed, when markers such as CD68 and CD14 are used to study highly inflamed tissues, no clear distinction can be made between the sublining macrophage population and the macrophage-like synoviocytes present in the hyperplastic lining layer, although expression of complement receptor for C3b and iC3b was unique for lining macrophages.[111] Studies that used various macrophage markers suggest that recently migrated macrophages in perivascular areas express CD163 brightly, in addition to expressing CD68 and CD14, whereas macrophages in large lymphocytic aggregates and in the lining layer are less likely to express CD163. CD163$^+$ macrophages, which have recently been called M2 macrophages, were found to be more abundant in spondylarthropathy than in RA synovium.[60] The functional correlates of these phenotypic differences remain unclear.[112–114] M1 macrophages, which produce TNF and IL-1β, are more abundant in RA and are under-represented in psoriatic arthritis and other spondyloarthropathies in which M2 macrophages are more abundant.[114] Furthermore, the number of macrophages in RA synovium, primarily of the M1 subset, correlates well with the destructive potential of the synovitis, as evidenced by erosive radiographic damage.[115–117] This may reflect the highly activated status of these cells, which serve as the principal source of synovial TNF and IL-1β. A body of evidence has suggested that populations of synovial macrophages serve as osteoclast precursors that mature in the synovial microenvironment and then directly mediate erosive damage to adjacent bone.[118,119]

Mature dendritic cells are the most efficient and potent of the antigen-presenting cells, and are found abundantly in inflamed synovium in close contact with T lymphocytes.[120,121] Two major subsets of dendritic cells have been described: myeloid dendritic cells (mDCs) and plasmacytoid dendritic cells (pDCs). They can be identified by immunohistology as stellate cells with dendrites that express high levels of HLA-DR and co-stimulatory molecules such as CD80, CD83, and CD86. mDCs express CD11c and CD1c, and pDCs express CD304.[122] One study suggested that, compared with psoriatic synovitis, RA synovium is particularly enriched in pDCs.[122] Detailed studies that have examined the expression of chemokines involved in dendritic cell migration and recruitment suggest that a substantial proportion of dendritic cells in the synovium arrive in an immature state and subsequently undergo maturation within the synovial microenvironment in a T cell–rich area.[120,121] Follicular dendritic cells in the germinal centers of large lymphocytic aggregates express the markers CD16, FDC, and VCAM-1.

Synovial Microvasculature, Endothelium, and Stromal Mesenchymal Cells

The stromal elements in RA are often expanded in parallel with the inflammatory cell infiltration. The microvasculature appears to be markedly increased, particularly in the deep sublining areas, and this expansion is presumed to relate to local stimulation of angiogenesis (see Fig. 56.14). Morphometric studies have suggested that the number of vessels immediately adjacent to the lining layer is actually reduced compared with normal tissue.[123] This situation, combined with the metabolic demands of this tissue, may actually produce a relatively ischemic and hypoxic

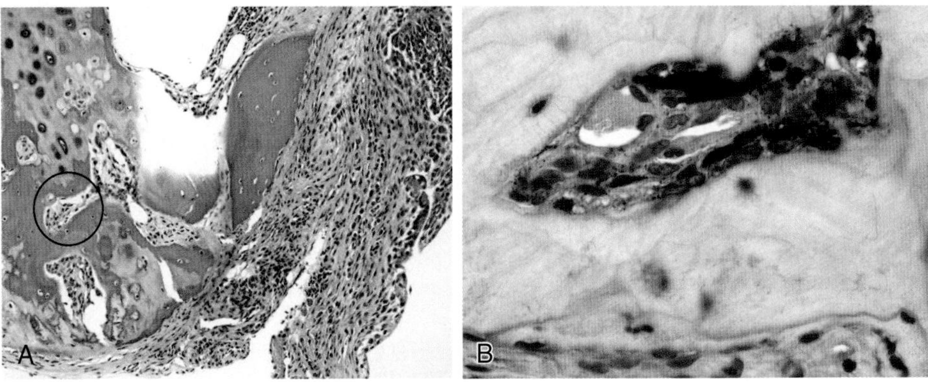

• **Fig. 56.15** Interface between pannus tissue and bone in a patient with rheumatoid arthritis. (A) The synovial lesion is invading adjacent bone (see *circle*). (B) Staining for tartrate-resistant acid phosphatase in the circled area demonstrates the presence of osteoclasts.

environment, which is reflected in the biochemical properties of RA synovial fluid.[124] Immunohistologic studies have indicated that the molecular consequences of hypoxia, particularly expression of hypoxia-inducible factor-1α (HIF-1α), a key regulator of the cellular hypoxic response, are increased in RA synovitis.[125,126] Investigators that have directly measured synovial tissue pO_2 by using arthroscopic probes have confirmed the hypoxic nature of RA synovitis.[127–129] The synovial endothelium in RA and other inflammatory arthropathies is activated by pro-inflammatory mediators in the microenvironment to express adhesion molecules such as E-selectin, ICAM-1, and VCAM-1, which are involved in the recruitment of inflammatory cells.[130]

Synovium-Cartilage-Bone Interface

The interface between inflamed synovium and adjacent cartilage and bone in RA and other chronic arthropathies is a site of particular interest because much of the articular damage occurs in these areas. In RA, this destructive synovial tissue is called *pannus,* which may spread to cover most of the surface of the cartilage and invade the bone in bare areas at the joint margin (Fig. 56.15). Pannus has been pathologically characterized primarily from samples obtained at the time of joint arthroplasty, although arthroscopic studies at earlier stages of disease have attempted to characterize synovial samples adjacent to this area. Immunohistology suggests that synovial macrophages and fibroblasts are abundant at the pannus-cartilage interface, and that high levels of proteases are expressed by these cells. At the interface between pannus and bone, substantial numbers of multinucleated osteoclasts can be identified morphologically and by specific markers such as calcitonin receptors, cathepsin K, and staining for tartrate-resistant acid phosphatase[131] (see Fig. 56.15). Moreover, expression of receptor activator of nuclear factor-κB (NF-κB) ligand (RANKL), a key cytokine in osteoclastogenesis, was prominent in these areas.[132]

Synovial Biopsy and Pathology as Research Tools for Clinical Biomarker Development

Multiple academic rheumatology centers have used arthroscopic or needle synovial biopsy and quantitative immunohistology as research tools with which to develop a better understanding of disease pathogenesis. In recent years, there has been a focus on the early clinical and pre-clinical stages of RA and other forms of chronic inflammatory arthritis, in the hope of devising interventions that could achieve long-term remissions and even disease prevention. In the case of RA, it is now well established that circulating autoantibodies such as RF and anti-CCP precede clinical disease onset, often by several years.[133] What is less clear is the stage where the synovium becomes engaged in the immune-inflammatory process. To address this question, synovial biopsy studies were undertaken in autoantibody-positive individuals at high risk for RA, but without clinical evidence of synovitis.[134,135] These studies failed to demonstrate significant inflammatory changes in the pre-clinical synovial samples, although there were subtle T cell infiltrates in the synovium of individuals who subsequently developed RA. These findings suggest that it is unlikely that a prolonged sub-clinical synovitis stage precedes clinical detectable joint inflammation in RA.

In individuals with established inflammatory arthritis, analysis of the synovial lesions could provide informative biomarkers for predicting the impact of therapeutic interventions in RA and other forms of inflammatory arthritis. Such studies may be particularly valuable in predicting the effects of the expanding arsenal of targeted biologic therapies, in which the molecular target and the biologic basis of the mechanism of action are well defined.[136–149] To test this hypothesis, a recent study developed a classification paradigm for RA synovial phenotypes based on gene expression profiling and immunohistology, and found that these synovial phenotypes could be used as a source of biomarkers that correlated with response to biologic therapeutics.[145] Using a statistical classification algorithm derived from the synovial gene expression profile and concordant immunohistologic pattern of synovitis, the study identified four distinct phenotypes: lymphoid, myeloid, low inflammatory, and fibroid. These phenotypes, in particular the lymphoid versus myeloid patterns, had a modest correlation with response to infliximab treatment in a post-hoc analysis of a synovial biopsy-based clinical trial, with good responders significantly more likely to express the myeloid, M1 macrophage-dominated phenotype.[140,141]

Representative soluble biomarkers were identified from the gene sets expressed by the myeloid versus lymphoid phenotype (the latter dominated by T and B lymphocyte-associated genes). These biomarkers were sICAM-1 for the myeloid phenotype and CXCL13 for the lymphoid phenotype. The serum levels of these biomarkers were found to be correlated with the clinical response to either adalimumab, a TNF inhibitor, or tocilizumab, an IL-6 receptor inhibitor, in a randomized clinical trial.[146] These results, derived from group level analyses, are encouraging, but it is too early to know how effective this approach will be in predicting response to therapeutic strategies on an individual level. They do demonstrate that synovial tissue analysis is a potentially important source of clinically relevant biomarkers.

This appealing proposition is currently hindered by several important considerations. First, the arthroscopic equipment, expertise, and infrastructure needed to undertake these studies remain limited to a small number of centers. Second, considerable concern has arisen regarding the issue of sampling bias in these studies, particularly because serial biopsies are compared in the same individual. As has been discussed, various approaches are used to minimize this bias, including systematic sampling of the same areas of the joint, computerized image analysis of multiple representative tissue samples, quantification of an adequate number of microscopic fields, and utilization of quantitative PCR and proteomic techniques to assess overall levels of specific molecules.

Conclusion

Analysis of synovial fluid and tissue samples provides valuable diagnostic information in specific clinical settings. In cases in which septic or crystal-induced arthritis is suspected, as in acute monoarthritis, synovial fluid analysis is critical for the diagnosis. In cases of undiagnosed chronic monoarthritis, synovial biopsy may provide definitive evidence of conditions such as TB, sarcoidosis, and pigmented villonodular synovitis.

Systematic analysis of synovial tissue in RA and other forms of inflammatory arthritis, particularly with the use of immunohistology, has provided a wealth of information concerning the cellular and molecular mechanisms that sustain synovial lesions. Research protocols are currently exploring the utility of synovial biopsy in predicting response to anti-rheumatic therapies.

Full references for this chapter can be found on ExpertConsult.com.

Selected References

1. Swann DA, Slayter HS, Silver FH: The molecular structure of lubricating glycoprotein-I, the boundary lubricant for articular cartilage, *J Biol Chem* 256:5921–5925, 1981.
2. Marcelino J, Carpten JD, Suwairi WM, et al.: CACP, encoding a secreted proteoglycan, is mutated in camptodactyly-arthropathy-coxa vara-pericarditis syndrome, *Nat Genet* 23:319–322, 1999.
3. Rhee DK, Marcelino J, Baker M, et al.: The secreted glycoprotein lubricin protects cartilage surfaces and inhibits synovial cell overgrowth, *J Clin Invest* 115:622–631, 2005.
4. Ghanem E, Houssock C, Pulido L, et al.: Determining "true" leukocytosis in bloody joint aspiration, *J Arthroplasty* 23(2):182–187, 2008.
5. Davis MJ, Denton J, Freemont AJ, et al.: Comparison of serial synovial fluid cytology in rheumatoid arthritis: delineation of subgroups with prognostic implications, *Ann Rheum Dis* 47:559–562, 1988.
6. Jones ST, Denton J, Holt PJ, et al.: Possible clearance of effete polymorphonuclear leucocytes from synovial fluid by cytophagocytic mononuclear cells: implications for pathogenesis and chronicity in inflammatory arthritis, *Ann Rheum Dis* 52:121–126, 1993.
7. von Essen R, Hölttä AM: Quality control of the laboratory diagnosis of gout by synovial fluid microscopy, *Scand J Rheumatol* 19:232–234, 1990.
8. Schumacher Jr HR, Sieck MS, Rothfuss S, et al.: Reproducibility of synovial fluid analyses: a study among four laboratories, *Arthritis Rheum* 29:770–774, 1986.
9. Hasselbacher P: Variation in synovial fluid analysis by hospital laboratories, *Arthritis Rheum* 30:637–642, 1987.
10. Garancis JC, Cheung HS, Halverson PB, et al.: "Milwaukee shoulder"—association of microspheroids containing hydroxyapatite crystals, active collagenase, and neutral protease with rotator cuff defects. III. Morphologic and biochemical studies of an excised synovium showing chondromatosis, *Arthritis Rheum* 24:484–491, 1981.
11. Faraj AA, Omonbude OD, Godwin P: Gram staining in the diagnosis of acute septic arthritis, *Acta Orthop Belg* 68:388–391, 2002.
12. Shmerling RH: Synovial fluid analysis: a critical reappraisal, *Rheum Dis Clin North Am* 20:503–512, 1994.
14. von Essen R, Holtta A: Improved method of isolating bacteria from joint fluids by the use of blood culture bottles, *Ann Rheum Dis* 45:454–457, 1986.
15. Yu KH, Luo SF, Liou LB, et al.: Concomitant septic and gouty arthritis—an analysis of 30 cases, *Rheumatology (Oxford)* 42:1062–1066, 2003.
16. Jalava J, Skurnik M, Toivanen A, et al.: Bacterial PCR in the diagnosis of joint infection, *Ann Rheum Dis* 60:287–289, 2001.
17. Muralidhar B, Rumore PM, Steinman CR: Use of the polymerase chain reaction to study arthritis due to *Neisseria gonorrhoeae*, *Arthritis Rheum* 37:710–717, 1994.
18. Liebling MR, Arkfeld DG, Michelini GA, et al.: Identification of *Neisseria gonorrhoeae* in synovial fluid using the polymerase chain reaction, *Arthritis Rheum* 37:702–709, 1994.
19. van der Heijden IM, Wilbrink B, Schouls LM, et al.: Detection of mycobacteria in joint samples from patients with arthritis using a genus-specific polymerase chain reaction and sequence analysis, *Rheumatology (Oxford)* 38:547–553, 1999.
20. Titov AG, Vyshnevskaya EB, Mazurenko SI, et al.: Use of polymerase chain reaction to diagnose tuberculous arthritis from joint tissues and synovial fluid, *Arch Pathol Lab Med* 128:205–209, 2004.
21. Canvin JM, Goutcher SC, Hagig M, et al.: Persistence of *Staphylococcus aureus* as detected by polymerase chain reaction in the synovial fluid of a patient with septic arthritis, *Br J Rheumatol* 36:203–206, 1997.
22. van der Heijden IM, Wilbrink B, Vije AE, et al.: Detection of bacterial DNA in serial synovial samples obtained during antibiotic treatment from patients with septic arthritis, *Arthritis Rheum* 42:2198–2203, 1999.
23. Wilkinson NZ, Kingsley GH, Jones HW, et al.: The detection of DNA from a range of bacterial species in the joints of patients with a variety of arthritides using a nested, broad-range polymerase chain reaction, *Rheumatology (Oxford)* 38:260–266, 1999.
24. van der Heijden IM, Wilbrink B, Tchetverikov I, et al.: Presence of bacterial DNA and bacterial peptidoglycans in joints of patients with rheumatoid arthritis and other arthritides, *Arthritis Rheum* 43:593–598, 2000.
25. Shmerling RH, Delbanco TL, Tosteson AN, et al.: Synovial fluid tests: what should be ordered? *JAMA* 264:1009–1014, 1990.
26. Treuhaft PS, McCarty DJ: Synovial fluid pH, lactate, oxygen and carbon dioxide partial pressure in various joint diseases, *Arthritis Rheum* 14:475–484, 1971.
27. Lund-Olesen K: Oxygen tension in synovial fluids, *Arthritis Rheum* 13:769–776, 1970.
28. Lettesjo H, Nordstrom E, Strom H, et al.: Autoantibody patterns in synovial fluids from patients with rheumatoid arthritis or other arthritic lesions, *Scand J Immunol* 48:293–299, 1998.
29. Thiel A, Wu P, Lauster R, et al.: Analysis of the antigen-specific T cell response in reactive arthritis by flow cytometry, *Arthritis Rheum* 43:2834–2842, 2000.
30. Mertz AK, Ugrinovic S, Lauster R, et al.: Characterization of the synovial T cell response to various recombinant *Yersinia* antigens in *Yersinia enterocolitica*-triggered reactive arthritis: heat-shock protein 60 drives a major immune response, *Arthritis Rheum* 41:315–326, 1998.
31. Davis LS, Cush JJ, Schulze-Koops H, et al.: Rheumatoid synovial CD4+ T cells exhibit a reduced capacity to differentiate into IL-4-producing T-helper-2 effector cells, *Arthritis Res* 3:54–64, 2001.

32. Yin Z, Braun J, Neure L, et al.: Crucial role of interleukin-10/interleukin-12 balance in the regulation of the type 2 T helper cytokine response in reactive arthritis, *Arthritis Rheum* 40:1788–1797, 1997.
33. Dolhain RJ, van der Heiden AN, ter Haar NT, et al.: Shift toward T lymphocytes with a T helper 1 cytokine-secretion profile in the joints of patients with rheumatoid arthritis, *Arthritis Rheum* 39:1961–1969, 1996.
34. Raza K, Falciani F, Curnow SJ, et al.: Early rheumatoid arthritis is characterized by a distinct and transient synovial fluid cytokine profile of T cell and stromal cell origin, *Arthritis Res Ther* 7:R784–R795, 2005.
35. Liao H, Wu J, Kuhn E, et al.: Use of mass spectrometry to identify protein biomarkers of disease severity in the synovial fluid and serum of patients with rheumatoid arthritis, *Arthritis Rheum* 50:3792–3803, 2004.
37. Schumacher Jr HR, Kulka JP: Needle biopsy of the synovial membrane—experience with the Parker-Pearson technic, *N Engl J Med* 286:416–419, 1972.
39. Tak PP, Bresnihan B: The pathogenesis and prevention of joint damage in rheumatoid arthritis: advances from synovial biopsy and tissue analysis, *Arthritis Rheum* 43:2619–2633, 2000.
40. Youssef PP, Kraan M, Breedveld F, et al.: Quantitative microscopic analysis of inflammation in rheumatoid arthritis synovial membrane samples selected at arthroscopy compared with samples obtained blindly by needle biopsy, *Arthritis Rheum* 41:663–669, 1998.
41. Kelly S, Humby F, Filer A, et al.: Ultrasound-guided synovial biopsy: a safe, well-tolerated and reliable technique for obtaining high-quality synovial tissue from both large and small joints in early arthritis patients, *Ann Rheum Dis* 74(3):611–617, 2015.
42. Humby F, Romao VC, Manzo A, et al.: A multicenter retrospective analysis evaluating performance of synovial biopsy techniques in patients with inflammatory arthritis: arthroscopic versus ultrasound-guided versus blind needle biopsy, *Arthritis Rheumatol* 70(5):702–710, 2018.
43. Shi SR, Cote RJ, Taylor CR: Antigen retrieval techniques: current perspectives, *J Histochem Cytochem* 49:931–937, 2001.
46. van der Pouw Kraan TC, van Gaalen FA, Kasperkovitz PV, et al.: Rheumatoid arthritis is a heterogeneous disease: evidence for differences in the activation of the STAT-1 pathway between rheumatoid tissues, *Arthritis Rheum* 48:2132–2145, 2003.
47. Lee DM, Kiener HP, Agarwal SK, et al.: Cadherin-11 in synovial lining formation and pathology in arthritis, *Science* 315:1006–1010, 2007.
48. Singh JA, Arayssi T, Duray P, et al.: Immunohistochemistry of normal human knee synovium: a quantitative study, *Ann Rheum Dis* 63:785–790, 2004.
50. Darling JM, Goldring SR, Harada Y, et al.: Multinucleated cells in pigmented villonodular synovitis and giant cell tumor of tendon sheath express features of osteoclasts, *Am J Pathol* 150:1383–1393, 1997.
52. Schumacher HR, Kitridou RC: Synovitis of recent onset: a clinicopathologic study during the first month of disease, *Arthritis Rheum* 15:465–485, 1972.
53. Kraan MC, Versendaal H, Jonker M, et al.: Asymptomatic synovitis precedes clinically manifest arthritis, *Arthritis Rheum* 41:1481–1488, 1998.
54. Soden M, Rooney M, Cullen A, et al.: Immunohistological features in the synovium obtained from clinically uninvolved knee joints of patients with rheumatoid arthritis, *Br J Rheumatol* 28:287–292, 1989.
55. Canete JD, Santiago B, Cantaert T, et al.: Ectopic lymphoid neogenesis in psoriatic arthritis, *Ann Rheum Dis* 66:720–726, 2007.
56. van de Sande MG, Thurlings RM, Boumans MJ, et al.: Presence of lymphocyte aggregates in the synovium of patients with early arthritis in relationship to diagnosis and outcome: is it a constant feature over time? *Ann Rheum Dis* 70:700–703, 2011.
57. Haywood L, McWilliams DF, Pearson CI, et al.: Inflammation and angiogenesis in osteoarthritis, *Arthritis Rheum* 48:2173–2177, 2003.
58. Thurlings RM, Wijbrandts CA, Mebius RE, et al.: Synovial lymphoid neogenesis does not define a specific clinical rheumatoid arthritis phenotype, *Arthritis Rheum* 58:1582–1589, 2008.
59. Baeten D, Kruithof E, De Rycke L, et al.: Diagnostic classification of spondylarthropathy and rheumatoid arthritis by synovial histopathology: a prospective study in 154 consecutive patients, *Arthritis Rheum* 50:2931–2941, 2004.
60. Kruithof E, Baeten D, De Rycke L, et al.: Synovial histopathology of psoriatic arthritis, both oligo- and polyarticular, resembles spondyloarthropathy more than it does rheumatoid arthritis, *Arthritis Res Ther* 7:R569–R580, 2005.
61. Reece RJ, Canete JD, Parsons WJ, et al.: Distinct vascular patterns of early synovitis in psoriatic, reactive, and rheumatoid arthritis, *Arthritis Rheum* 42:1481–1484, 1999.
64. Cunnane G, Bresnihan B, FitzGerald O: Immunohistologic analysis of peripheral joint disease in ankylosing spondylitis, *Arthritis Rheum* 41:180–182, 1998.
65. Kraan MC, Haringman JJ, Post WJ, et al.: Immunohistological analysis of synovial tissue for differential diagnosis in early arthritis, *Rheumatology (Oxford)* 38:1074–1080, 1999.
66. Smeets TJ, Dolhain RJ, Breedveld FC, et al.: Analysis of the cellular infiltrates and expression of cytokines in synovial tissue from patients with rheumatoid arthritis and reactive arthritis, *J Pathol* 186:75–81, 1998.
67. Natour J, Montezzo LC, Moura LA, et al.: A study of synovial membrane of patients with systemic lupus erythematosus (SLE), *Clin Exp Rheumatol* 9:221–225, 1991.
68. Schumacher Jr HR: Joint involvement in progressive systemic sclerosis (scleroderma): a light and electron microscopic study of synovial membrane and fluid, *Am J Clin Pathol* 60:593–600, 1973.
69. Schumacher HR, Schimmer B, Gordon GV, et al.: Articular manifestations of polymyositis and dermatomyositis, *Am J Med* 67:287–292, 1979.
70. Canete JD, Celis R, Noordenbos T, et al.: Distinct synovial immunopathology in Behçet disease and psoriatic arthritis, *Arthritis Res Ther* 11:R17, 2009.
71. Beutler A, Rothfuss S, Clayburne G, et al.: Calcium pyrophosphate dihydrate crystal deposition in synovium: relationship to collagen fibers and chondrometaplasia, *Arthritis Rheum* 36:704–715, 1993.
72. Schumacher HR, Holdsworth DE: Ochronotic arthropathy. I. Clinicopathologic studies, *Semin Arthritis Rheum* 6:207–246, 1977.
73. Schumacher Jr HR: Ultrastructural characteristics of the synovial membrane in idiopathic haemochromatosis, *Ann Rheum Dis* 31:465–473, 1972.
76. Smeets TJ, Kraan MC, Galjaard S, et al.: Analysis of the cell infiltrate and expression of matrix metalloproteinases and granzyme B in paired synovial biopsy specimens from the cartilage-pannus junction in patients with RA, *Ann Rheum Dis* 60:561–565, 2001.
77. Kirkham B, Portek I, Lee CS, et al.: Intraarticular variability of synovial membrane histology, immunohistology, and cytokine mRNA expression in patients with rheumatoid arthritis, *J Rheumatol* 26:777–784, 1999.
78. Cunnane G, Bjork L, Ulfgren AK, et al.: Quantitative analysis of synovial membrane inflammation: a comparison between automated and conventional microscopic measurements, *Ann Rheum Dis* 58:493–499, 1999.
80. El-Gabalawy H, Canvin J, Ma GM, et al.: Synovial distribution of alpha d/CD18, a novel leukointegrin: comparison with other integrins and their ligands, *Arthritis Rheum* 39:1913–1921, 1996.
81. El-Gabalawy H, Gallatin M, Vazeux R, et al.: Expression of ICAM-R (ICAM-3), a novel counter-receptor for LFA-1, in rheumatoid and nonrheumatoid synovium: comparison with other adhesion molecules, *Arthritis Rheum* 37:846–854, 1994.

82. El-Gabalawy H, Wilkins J: Beta 1 (CD29) integrin expression in rheumatoid synovial membranes: an immunohistologic study of distribution patterns, *J Rheumatol* 20:231–237, 1993.
83. Edwards JC, Blades S, Cambridge G: Restricted expression of Fc gammaRIII (CD16) in synovium and dermis: implications for tissue targeting in rheumatoid arthritis (RA), *Clin Exp Immunol* 108:401–406, 1997.
85. Firestein GS, Paine MM, Littman BH: Gene expression (collagenase, tissue inhibitor of metalloproteinases, complement, and HLA-DR) in rheumatoid arthritis and osteoarthritis synovium: quantitative analysis and effect of intraarticular corticosteroids, *Arthritis Rheum* 34:1094–1105, 1991.
86. Cunnane G, FitzGerald O, Hummel KM, et al.: Collagenase, cathepsin B and cathepsin L gene expression in the synovial membrane of patients with early inflammatory arthritis, *Rheumatology (Oxford)* 38:34–42, 1999.
89. Canete JD, Martinez SE, Farres J, et al.: Differential Th1/Th2 cytokine patterns in chronic arthritis: interferon gamma is highly expressed in synovium of rheumatoid arthritis compared with seronegative spondyloarthropathies, *Ann Rheum Dis* 59:263–268, 2000.
91. Chabaud M, Durand JM, Buchs N, et al.: Human interleukin-17: a T cell-derived proinflammatory cytokine produced by the rheumatoid synovium, *Arthritis Rheum* 42:963–970, 1999.
92. Kirkham BW, Lassere MN, Edmonds JP, et al.: Synovial membrane cytokine expression is predictive of joint damage progression in rheumatoid arthritis: a two-year prospective study (the DAMAGE study cohort), *Arthritis Rheum* 54:1122–1131, 2006.
93. Ruprecht CR, Gattorno M, Ferlito F, et al.: Coexpression of CD25 and CD27 identifies FoxP3+ regulatory T cells in inflamed synovia, *J Exp Med* 201:1793–1803, 2005.
94. van Amelsfort JM, Jacobs KM, Bijlsma JW, et al.: CD4(+)CD25(+) regulatory T cells in rheumatoid arthritis: differences in the presence, phenotype, and function between peripheral blood and synovial fluid, *Arthritis Rheum* 50:2775–2785, 2004.
95. de Kleer IM, Wedderburn LR, Taams LS, et al.: CD4+CD25bright regulatory T cells actively regulate inflammation in the joints of patients with the remitting form of juvenile idiopathic arthritis, *J Immunol* 172:6435–6443, 2004.
96. Cao D, Malmstrom V, Baecher-Allan C, et al.: Isolation and functional characterization of regulatory CD25brightCD4+ T cells from the target organ of patients with rheumatoid arthritis, *Eur J Immunol* 33:215–223, 2003.
97. Kang YM, Zhang X, Wagner UG, et al.: CD8 T cells are required for the formation of ectopic germinal centers in rheumatoid synovitis, *J Exp Med* 195:1325–1336, 2002.
98. Takemura S, Klimiuk PA, Braun A, et al.: T cell activation in rheumatoid synovium is B cell dependent, *J Immunol* 167:4710–4718, 2001.
99. Kim HJ, Krenn V, Steinhauser G, et al.: Plasma cell development in synovial germinal centers in patients with rheumatoid and reactive arthritis, *J Immunol* 162:3053–3062, 1999.
100. Masson-Bessiere C, Sebbag M, Girbal-Neuhauser E, et al.: The major synovial targets of the rheumatoid arthritis-specific antifilaggrin autoantibodies are deiminated forms of the alpha- and beta-chains of fibrin, *J Immunol* 166:4177–4184, 2001.
101. Masson-Bessiere C, Sebbag M, Durieux JJ, et al.: In the rheumatoid pannus, anti-filaggrin autoantibodies are produced by local plasma cells and constitute a higher proportion of IgG than in synovial fluid and serum, *Clin Exp Immunol* 119:544–552, 2000.
103. Vossenaar ER, Smeets TJ, Kraan MC, et al.: The presence of citrullinated proteins is not specific for rheumatoid synovial tissue, *Arthritis Rheum* 50:3485–3494, 2004.
106. Dalbeth N, Callan MF: A subset of natural killer cells is greatly expanded within inflamed joints, *Arthritis Rheum* 46:1763–1772, 2002.
107. Tak PP, Kummer JA, Hack CE, et al.: Granzyme-positive cytotoxic cells are specifically increased in early rheumatoid synovial tissue, *Arthritis Rheum* 37:1735–1743, 1994.
108. Goto M, Zvaifler NJ: Characterization of the natural killer-like lymphocytes in rheumatoid synovial fluid, *J Immunol* 134:1483–1486, 1985.
109. Woolley DE, Tetlow LC: Mast cell activation and its relation to proinflammatory cytokine production in the rheumatoid lesion, *Arthritis Res* 2:65–74, 2000.
110. Tetlow LC, Woolley DE: Mast cells, cytokines, and metalloproteinases at the rheumatoid lesion: dual immunolocalisation studies, *Ann Rheum Dis* 54:896–903, 1995.
111. Tanaka M, Nagai T, Tsuneyoshi Y, et al.: Expansion of a unique macrophage subset in rheumatoid arthritis synovial lining layer, *Clin Exp Immunol* 154:38–47, 2008.
113. Fonseca JE, Edwards JC, Blades S, et al.: Macrophage subpopulations in rheumatoid synovium: reduced CD163 expression in CD4+ T lymphocyte-rich microenvironments, *Arthritis Rheum* 46:1210–1216, 2002.
114. Vandooren B, Noordenbos T, Ambarus C, et al.: Absence of a classically activated macrophage cytokine signature in peripheral spondylarthritis, including psoriatic arthritis, *Arthritis Rheum* 60:966–975, 2009.
115. Cunnane G, FitzGerald O, Hummel KM, et al.: Synovial tissue protease gene expression and joint erosions in early rheumatoid arthritis, *Arthritis Rheum* 44:1744–1753, 2001.
116. Mulherin D, FitzGerald O, Bresnihan B: Synovial tissue macrophage populations and articular damage in rheumatoid arthritis, *Arthritis Rheum* 39:115–124, 1996.
117. Yanni G, Whelan A, Feighery C, et al.: Synovial tissue macrophages and joint erosion in rheumatoid arthritis, *Ann Rheum Dis* 53:39–44, 1994.
119. Gravallese EM, Manning C, Tsay A, et al.: Synovial tissue in rheumatoid arthritis is a source of osteoclast differentiation factor, *Arthritis Rheum* 43:250–258, 2000.
120. Page G, Miossec P: Paired synovium and lymph nodes from rheumatoid arthritis patients differ in dendritic cell and chemokine expression, *J Pathol* 204:28–38, 2004.
121. Page G, Lebecque S, Miossec P: Anatomic localization of immature and mature dendritic cells in an ectopic lymphoid organ: correlation with selective chemokine expression in rheumatoid synovium, *J Immunol* 168:5333–5341, 2002.
122. Lebre MC, Jongbloed SL, Tas SW, et al.: Rheumatoid arthritis synovium contains two subsets of CD83-DC-LAMP-dendritic cells with distinct cytokine profiles, *Am J Pathol* 172:940–950, 2008.
123. Stevens CR, Blake DR, Merry P, et al.: A comparative study by morphometry of the microvasculature in normal and rheumatoid synovium, *Arthritis Rheum* 34:1508–1513, 1991.
125. Hitchon C, Wong K, Ma G, et al.: Hypoxia-induced production of stromal cell-derived factor 1 (CXCL12) and vascular endothelial growth factor by synovial fibroblasts, *Arthritis Rheum* 46:2587–2597, 2002.
126. Hollander AP, Corke KP, Freemont AJ, et al.: Expression of hypoxia-inducible factor 1alpha by macrophages in the rheumatoid synovium: implications for targeting of therapeutic genes to the inflamed joint, *Arthritis Rheum* 44:1540–1544, 2001.
127. Ng CT, Biniecka M, Kennedy A, et al.: Synovial tissue hypoxia and inflammation in vivo, *Ann Rheum Dis* 69:1389–1395, 2010.
128. Kennedy A, Ng CT, Biniecka M, et al.: Angiogenesis and blood vessel stability in inflammatory arthritis, *Arthritis Rheum* 62:711–721, 2010.
129. Biniecka M, Kennedy A, Fearon U, et al.: Oxidative damage in synovial tissue is associated with in vivo hypoxic status in the arthritic joint, *Ann Rheum Dis* 69:1172–1178, 2010.
131. Gravallese EM, Harada Y, Wang JT, et al.: Identification of cell types responsible for bone resorption in rheumatoid arthritis and juvenile rheumatoid arthritis, *Am J Pathol* 152:943–951, 1998.
132. Pettit AR, Walsh NC, Manning C, et al.: RANKL protein is expressed at the pannus-bone interface at sites of articular bone erosion in rheumatoid arthritis, *Rheumatology (Oxford)* 45:1068–1076, 2006.

136. Vos K, Thurlings RM, Wijbrandts CA, et al.: Early effects of rituximab on the synovial cell infiltrate in patients with rheumatoid arthritis, *Arthritis Rheum* 56:772–778, 2007.
139. Pontifex EK, Gerlag DM, Gogarty M, et al.: Change in CD3 positive T-cell expression in psoriatic arthritis synovium correlates with change in DAS28 and magnetic resonance imaging synovitis scores following initiation of biologic therapy—a single centre, open-label study, *Arthritis Res Ther* 13:R7, 2011.
140. Lindberg J, Wijbrandts CA, van Baarsen LG, et al.: The gene expression profile in the synovium as a predictor of the clinical response to infliximab treatment in rheumatoid arthritis, *PLoS ONE* 5:e11310, 2010.
141. Klaasen R, Thurlings RM, Wijbrandts CA, et al.: The relationship between synovial lymphocyte aggregates and the clinical response to infliximab in rheumatoid arthritis: a prospective study, *Arthritis Rheum* 60:3217–3224, 2009.
143. Wijbrandts CA, Remans PH, Klarenbeek PL, et al.: Analysis of apoptosis in peripheral blood and synovial tissue very early after initiation of infliximab treatment in rheumatoid arthritis patients, *Arthritis Rheum* 58:3330–3339, 2008.
144. van Kuijk AW, Gerlag DM, Vos K, et al.: A prospective, randomised, placebo-controlled study to identify biomarkers associated with active treatment in psoriatic arthritis: effects of adalimumab treatment on synovial tissue, *Ann Rheum Dis* 68:1303–1309, 2009.
145. Vergunst CE, Gerlag DM, Dinant H, et al.: Blocking the receptor for C5a in patients with rheumatoid arthritis does not reduce synovial inflammation, *Rheumatology (Oxford)* 46:1773–1778, 2007.
148. Thurlings RM, Vos K, Wijbrandts CA, et al.: Synovial tissue response to rituximab: mechanism of action and identification of biomarkers of response, *Ann Rheum Dis* 67:917–925, 2008.
149. Kavanaugh A, Rosengren S, Lee SJ, et al.: Assessment of rituximab's immunomodulatory synovial effects (ARISE trial). 1. Clinical and synovial biomarker results, *Ann Rheum Dis* 67:402–408, 2008.

57 Arthrocentesis and Injection of Joints and Soft Tissues

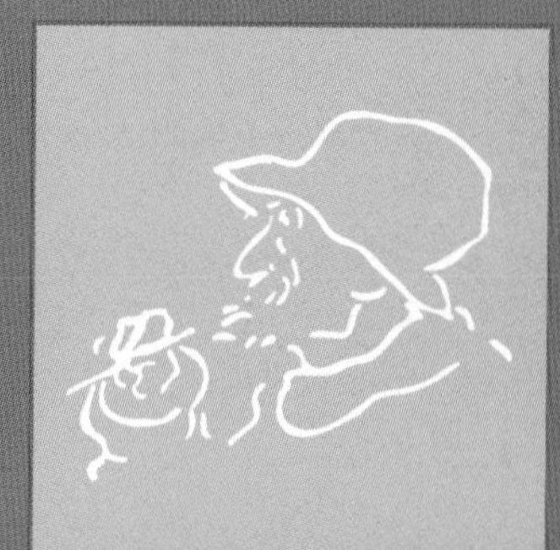

AHMED S. ZAYAT, ANDREA DI MATTEO, AND RICHARD J. WAKEFIELD

KEY POINTS

- Arthrocentesis (i.e., joint aspiration) is a key diagnostic procedure in rheumatology, especially for an acutely hot and swollen joint.
- Injection of joints and soft tissues can be an effective primary or adjuvant therapeutic approach for some rheumatic and musculoskeletal disorders.
- Knowledge of joint anatomy and supervised training are essential for safe practice.
- The right indication, proper technique, and good postinjection care improve procedure outcome.
- Procedure techniques vary between clinicians. However, certain anatomic facts and best practice techniques should always be considered.
- Ultrasound guidance can be used if available and if a blinded procedure has been deemed to be unsuccessful or is considered overly challenging at outset.
- For some anatomic sites, however, an ultrasound-guided procedure may be the preferred first-line approach.

Introduction

Arthrocentesis and injection of joints and soft tissues are the most common interventional procedures performed by rheumatologists and other health care clinicians who treat musculoskeletal disorders. When performing these procedures, there is an implicit assumption that the operator is adequately trained, the procedure is being done for the right reasons, the needle is delivered to the intended site, the correct therapy is given, and most importantly, patient safety is maintained during and after the procedure.

The placement of a needle into musculoskeletal tissue is usually done for three reasons: (1) to allow the withdrawal of fluid for diagnostic and therapeutic reasons, (2) to allow the accurate placement of local therapies, and (3) to perform a biopsy. The last reason will not be discussed in this chapter. Corticosteroids and local anesthetics remain the most common agents administered into joints and soft tissues.

To perform any interventional procedures, a good knowledge of relevant anatomy is important, as is the training of the operator. Accurate and efficient placement of a needle improves patient satisfaction, minimizes patient pain and other potential complications, and maximizes the potential outcome. Although needle interventions are traditionally done in a blinded manner (with the exception of some fluoroscopic-guided procedures), ultrasound-guided procedures are increasingly used by rheumatologists. Ultrasound has the advantage of validating the need for the procedure (by providing evidence of the presence of inflammation) especially when physical examination findings are uncertain. It also provides real-time visualization of the needle tip, which allows more accurate placement and avoidance of important neurovascular structures. However, this technique requires an additional skillset and more time than a blinded procedure. It may, therefore, be reasonable to restrict the use of ultrasound for joints that have not responded to a previous blinded injection and for those that are conventionally difficult to inject using a blinded approach (e.g., the hip joint). Recommendations for the steroid preparation and doses are provided. However, there are regional and national differences in the type of steroid and doses. Clinicians should refer to local guidelines for additional information.

Indications, Contraindications, and Potential Complications of Arthrocentesis and Soft Tissue Injections

A wide range of indications exist for arthrocentesis and injections of joints and soft tissues. The most common indication for arthrocentesis is diagnostic joint fluid aspiration. This is a crucial procedure to rule out septic arthritis and is usually in the context of a hot, swollen joint. Joint aspiration provides fluid for both macroscopic inspection (e.g., pus or hemarthrosis) and laboratory analysis (Table 57.1), the latter may identify crystals (usually urate or calcium pyrophosphate) and/or infection. Joint aspiration and drainage also may provide symptomatic relief by reducing pain from joint capsule distension. Joint injections are usually reserved for a single or few joints, although they may be used for a polyarthritis when systemic treatment fails or is not indicated. They may also be indicated in osteoarthritis (OA), which presents most commonly in the knee, first carpometacarpal (CMC) joint, proximal interphalangeal (PIP) joint, ankle, and midfoot. In inflammatory conditions, steroid joint injections tend to be more efficacious and longer lasting than in

TABLE 57.1 **Macroscopic and Microscopic Appearances of Synovial Fluid in Different Conditions**

Diagnosis	Appearance	Viscosity	Special Findings	Cellularity
Normal	Clear-yellow	High		Few cells & little debris
Inflammatory arthritis	Cloudy	Low		>90% polymorphs
Osteoarthritis	Clear-yellow	Very high to low (if inflammatory)		<50% polymorphs
Gout	Cloudy	Mild low	Monosodium urate crystals (needle-like)	>90% polymorphs
Pseudogout	Cloudy	Mild low	Calcium pyrophosphate crystals (rhomboid)	>90% polymorphs
Septic arthritis	Turbid or purulent	Low	Culture positive	>90% polymorphs
Hemoarthrosis	Red	High	Blood	Blood

OA, where the effects may be short lived or nonexistent.[1] Steroids aim to help reduce pain and swelling and improve range of movement. In addition to joints, they are also indicated for a range of soft tissue conditions with a presumed inflammatory component, such as tenosynovitis, trigger finger, enthesopathy, bursitis, adhesive capsulitis, and entrapment neuritis (e.g., carpal tunnel syndrome).

When performing such procedures, it is essential to check for contraindications and to warn the patient about potential complications (Table 57.2). The clinician will need to weigh the benefit of the procedure against any risks, such as infection and bleeding. Introducing infection into a joint should be of concern especially if the patient is immunocompromised, has a septicemia, or has evidence of a local infection around the area. A needle should never be inserted into or around a prosthetic joint unless it is done in a meticulously clean environment. It is our practice to refer to the orthopedic surgeons in these cases. Similarly, injecting near to previous surgical metal work may also impose a risk and should be discussed with colleagues before proceeding. The risk of bleeding from the procedure is also an important consideration. This is dependent on the site being injected and the use of any anticoagulant. Most MSK injections are considered low risk as they are generally superficial and can be compressed if needed. An exception would be the hip, for which we would advocate an image guided injection.

The use of anticoagulants, such as warfarin are a concern; however, the risk of bleeding is low as long as the internalized normalized ratio (INR) remains in the therapeutic range.[2] In the UK, there is a widely held belief that an INR of 2.5 represents a safe upper limit, but a higher INR (e.g., up to 3.5) is probably also safe. The direct oral anticoagulants (DOACs) also appear to be safe for joint injections, and a recent study recommended that there is no need to stop them.[3] Patients that have existing bleeding disorders, such as hemophilia or von Willebrand's disease, should receive appropriate factor replacement therapy before the injection. With respect to steroid injections, risks include leakage of steroid into the dermis and subcutaneous tissues, which may result in fat atrophy and depigmentation. This can be unsightly and is more likely to occur with stronger and longer lasting steroid preparations (e.g., triamcinolone hexacetonide), and when clinicians administer soft tissue injections (e.g., for de Quervain's tenosynovitis), in which case a shorter acting steroid is preferred. Care with steroids should also be taken when patients are taking HIV protease inhibitor drugs. Both drugs compete with the CYP34A pathway; consequently, steroid is competitively inhibited such that it is not metabolized, and Cushing's syndrome may result.

Drugs and Preparations Used for Injection

Over the years, different preparations have been investigated for potential intra-articular use, which range from the very early trials of ethiodized oil injection (poppy seed oil) and jodipin (product of sesame oil),[4,4a] to biologic therapies, and the recent intra-articular injections of cultured stem cells.[5] However, crystalline corticosteroid preparations continue to have the best evidence in reducing joint inflammation and reducing pain.[6] Local anesthetics are often used in conjunction with corticosteroids to provide immediate relief of symptoms and to help identify the site of the symptoms by observing whether the area, to which the anesthetic is applied, shows immediate relief of symptoms. Methylprednisolone acetate and triamcinolone acetonide are the most commonly used crystalline corticosteroids for treating joints; each treatment provided similar outcomes in some studies.[7] In contrast, triamcinolone hexacetonide has a slightly higher side effect profile but is more effective for some joints and in juvenile idiopathic arthritis (JIA).

Hydrocortisone is a weaker preparation of corticosteroid that is most often used for soft tissue or small joint injections. Hydrocortisone is soluble, therefore it is removed from the tissue quickly and has a reduced risk of skin depigmentation or fat atrophy. However, it tends to be less effective, and the effects are shorter lived than with methylprednisolone and triamcinolone. In this chapter, some suggestions for the type of preparation and the dose are provided. This preparation is used less often and longer lasting corticosteroids are more prevalent. However, the specific clinical circumstances, relative risks, and relative benefits of long-acting and short-acting agents should be considered for each patient.

Some clinicians prefer not to mix corticosteroid with local anesthetics because this may lead to precipitation of the corticosteroid or have a putative chondrotoxic effect *in vitro*.[8,9] However, anecdotal evidence suggests that mixing lidocaine with crystalline corticosteroid is a common practice with no increased procedure risk. Premixed preparations are currently available from manufacturers. Lidocaine hydrochloride (1% and 2%) and bupivacaine HCl (0.25% and 5%) are the most commonly used local anesthetics. Lidocaine starts acting within 30 seconds, and the effect lasts up to 1 hour. It is useful for painful procedures and for testing for accurate placement of the injection. However, if a longer local anesthetic effect is required (e.g., for a suprascapular nerve block), bupivacaine starts to act after 30 minutes, and the effect can last as long as 8 hours. This longer effect can also be useful if the patient has previously reported a postinjection pain flare up. Worldwide,

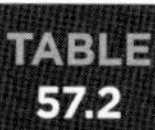

TABLE 57.2 Important Considerations for Joint Injections

Considerations Pre-joint Injection

Avoid performing joint injections in the following situations (if you have any clinical suspicion, do not inject with corticosteroid; discuss procedure with colleagues when necessary):

- Prosthetic joint (needs to be done by orthopedic surgeon in a sterile environment)
- Cellulitis or leg ulcers on same limb, psoriasis, or eczema at injection site
- Systemic infection
- Raised internalized normalized ratio (INR) outside normal therapeutic range; joint aspiration and injections appear to be safe in patients receiving direct oral anticoagulant therapy[10]
- Bleeding disorders (including low platelets)
- Drug allergy to any drug being injected
  Some orthopedic specialists do not want patients to have joint injections for at least 3 months before joint replacement

Always consider and explain potential complications before the procedure:

- Postinjection flare (uncommon and can occur after a few hours, or as long as 24 to 48 hours after injection)
- Septic arthritis (rare, incidence increases in the elderly or immunocompromised)
- Bleeding (avoid deep joints and use of large-gauge needles if patient is on warfarin)
- Tendon rupture (do not inject against resistance, do not inject Achilles tendon)
- Fat and skin atrophy and depigmentation of the skin around the injection site (avoid injecting superficial structures with potent corticosteroids preparations)
- Misplaced intravascular injection (always aspirate before injecting)
- Neurovascular damage (always know the anatomic landmarks of these structures before injecting)
- Cartilage damage (may occur with multiple, frequent injections)
- Allergic reaction to local anesthesia (check allergy history)
- Flushing and/or palpitations (within 24 hours of injection from systematic absorption of steroid)
- Possible transient increase in blood glucose level if patient has diabetes mellitus

Postinjection Care Advice

- Use a dressing to cover the wound postinjection. Advise to keep area clean.
- Rest (minimal duties) for at least 24 hours after procedure.
- Provide advice: area may flare for 48 hours postinjection, although this is uncommon; tell patient to report to doctor immediately if patient feels unwell or is concerned, but advise patient that symptoms are likely to settle within 24 to 48 hours.

many rheumatologists use hyaluronic acid derivatives to treat OA affected joints. These are believed to act by replacing the synovial fluid in the joint and to function as a lubricant, shock absorber, and anti-inflammatory agent. They have been reported to be useful for relatively longer-lasting pain relief in OA.[10]

Procedures Description

Clinicians need to perform joint aspiration and injections using considered and specific approaches for good localization of the needle and reduced risk of complications (Table 57.3). Clinicians often use varied approaches and different preparations. These descriptions, therefore, reflect the authors' own practices, but the general principles we

TABLE 57.3 Elements Required for Successful Injection

Choose a quiet and uninterrupted environment.
Always use aseptic technique. Mark before cleaning. Once the injection area is cleaned, do not touch it unless complete asterile conditions apply.
Always aspirate before injecting to avoid intravascular placement of a large volume of lidocaine or crystalline steroid.
Never force an injection against resistance to avoid risk of tendon/ligament rupture.
If difficulty is encountered or there is resistance to injection, withdraw slightly and change the needle direction.
Always document procedure in patient notes. Documentation should include confirmation of verbal/written consent, patient understanding of potential complications, confirmation of aseptic approach, and drug used.

describe in the text should still apply for the procedure to be safe and effective. Ultrasound-guided procedures are not always performed according to the anatomic landmarks used by the blind method, but the principles remain the same. The techniques described will be divided into procedures for intra-articular and for soft tissue injections. The technique for each procedure will be described for both upper and lower limbs, beginning with the distal and moving to the proximal joints. When ultrasound is the preferred technique, this approach will be described accordingly. The images in this chapter only show the hand that is used to hold the needle. In practice, the other hand is used to hold the position of the joint steady.

Upper Limb Injections

Proximal Interphalangeal Joint

This joint is easier to inject if it is clinically swollen. The aim of an intra-articular injection is to place the needle tip somewhere within the joint cavity enclosed by the capsule but not specifically within the joint space (i.e., directly between the bones). This is the same principle for the distal interphalangeal (DIP) joint and all the injections described in the chapter.

Materials needed for the procedure are a 25-gauge needle, a 2 mL syringe (an insulin syringe can be used as well), and a preparation of a longer-acting corticosteroid, such as triamcinolone acetonide, triamcinolone hexacetonide, or methylprednisolone, 5 to 10 mg (±0.2 mL 2% lidocaine).

The procedure is as follows:

1. Palpate and mark the PIP joint space medial or lateral to the extensor tendon on the dorsal aspect of the finger. Flexing and extending the joint may facilitate the identification of the joint line.
2. Insert the needle obliquely to the skin from the dorsolateral or mediolateral position with the tip of the needle passing under the extensor tendon (Fig. 57.1). The choice of needle approach may depend on the handedness of the operator or the physical characteristics of the joint. Aim to have the needle tip stop just proximal to the joint line. Aspirate and then slowly inject the syringe contents. The capsule of the joint should be felt to slowly distend with the opposite hand. If the joint has significant bony swelling, which clinicians may encounter in cases of osteophytosis, then an ultrasound-guided injection may be the better first line approach. Follow the general postinjection care steps.

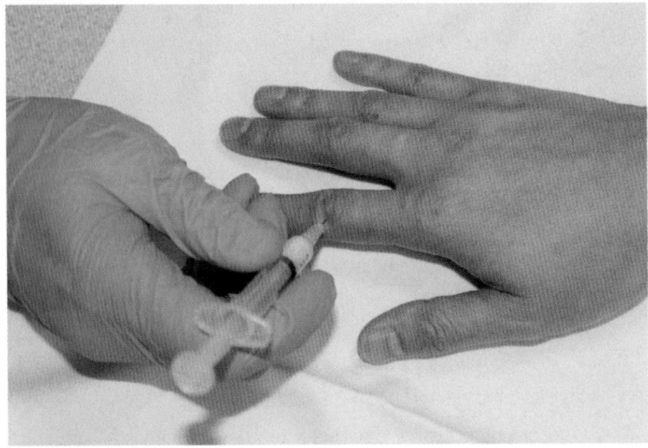

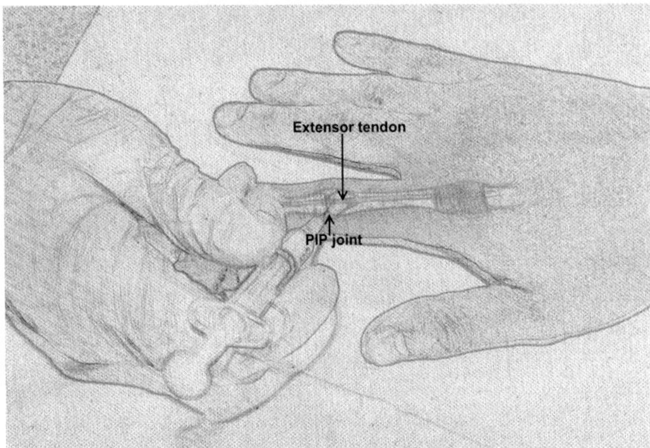

• **Fig. 57.1** Proximal interphalangeal (PIP) joint injection.

Metacarpophalangeal (MCP) Joint

Materials needed for the procedure are a 25-gauge needle, a 2 mL syringe (an insulin syringe can be used as well), and a preparation of methylprednisolone, 5 to 10 mg (±0.2 mL 2% lidocaine).

The procedure is as follows:

1. Palpate and mark the MCP joint space dorsomedial or dorsolateral to the extensor tendon from the dorsal side. A dorsoradial approach is preferred for the second MCP joint.
2. With the joint slightly flexed, the needle is inserted below the extensor tendon inside the joint capsule, as with the PIP joint (Fig. 57.2). Aspirate, and then slowly inject the syringe contents. Follow the general postinjection care steps.

Wrist Joint

Aspiration of the wrist may be undertaken to exclude a septic or crystal arthritis (Table 57.4). It is often more successful than aspirations of the PIP joint or the MCP joint because of the potentially larger quantity of fluid. However, clinical examination does not easily differentiate synovial hypertrophy from effusion; sometimes, an ultrasound can be useful to confirm the presence and location of fluid especially when the analysis of fluid is critical for management. The wrist is a common joint to be injected in inflammatory arthritis but is less common in OA. The best entry for needle placement is the gap between the third (extensor pollicis longus) and fourth extensor tendon (extensor digitorum communis and extensor indicis proprius) compartments (Figs. 57.3 and 57.4A).

Materials needed for the procedure are a 25-gauge needle, a 2 mL syringe (an insulin syringe can be used as well), and a preparation of a longer-acting corticosteroid, such as triamcinolone acetonide, triamcinolone hexacetonide, or methylprednisolone, 10 mg (±0.2 mL 2% lidocaine).

The procedure is as follows:

1. Palpate the joint line by flexing and extending the wrist. A gap can be identified between the second and third extensor tendon compartments, just ulnar and slightly distal to Lister's tubercle (dorsal prominence of the distal radius).
2. Insert the needle perpendicular to skin at the joint line. Aspirate and then slowly inject the syringe volume. Follow the general postinjection care steps.

For ultrasound-guided injection, the gap between the fourth and fifth extensor tendon compartments can also be used (see Fig. 57.4).

Elbow Joint Injection

When you perform the procedure, you should be aware of the ulnar nerve, which lies medially (on the ulnar side) and passes through the ulnar groove between the medial epicondyle and olecranon process. Thus, a radial approach is highly recommended.

Materials needed for the procedure are a 23-gauge needle, a 5 mL syringe, and a preparation of a longer-acting corticosteroid, such as triamcinolone acetonide, triamcinolone hexacetonide, or methylprednisolone, 10 to 40 mg (±2 mL 1% lidocaine).

The procedure is as follows:

1. Place the patient in supine position with the elbow flexed at 90 degrees over the chest.
2. Palpate and mark the cleft between the lateral epicondyle and olecranon process. Insert the needle perpendicular to the skin, radial to the triceps tendon, and aim distally (Fig. 57.5). Aspirate and then slowly inject the syringe. Follow the general postinjection care steps.
3. Injection medial to the olecranon process should be avoided (caution: ulnar nerve).

Shoulder Joint (Glenohumeral) Injection

Shoulder OA, rheumatoid arthritis (RA) (or other inflammatory arthritis), and frozen shoulder are the main indications for glenohumeral injections. We prefer injecting from the posterior aspect because there is less risk of damaging neurovascular structures compared to the anterior aspect. (Fig. 57.6).

Materials needed for the procedure are a 21-gauge needle, a 5 mL syringe, and a preparation of a longer-acting corticosteroid, such as triamcinolone acetonide, triamcinolone hexacetonide, or methylprednisolone, 20 to 60 mg (±1 mL 1% lidocaine).

The procedure is as follows:

1. Place the patient in a sitting position with his/her back to you.
2. Palpate the joint space 2 to 3 cm inferior and medial to the acromial tip. Internally and externally rotating the shoulder may help confirm the joint line. Advance the needle in an anterior direction. Ensure the plunger has very little or no resistance when injecting. Try to aspirate before slowly injecting the syringe. Follow the general postinjection care steps.

Acromioclavicular Joint

The acromioclavicular joint (ACJ) is synovial-lined and has a very small joint space. We recommend taking a few moments to locate

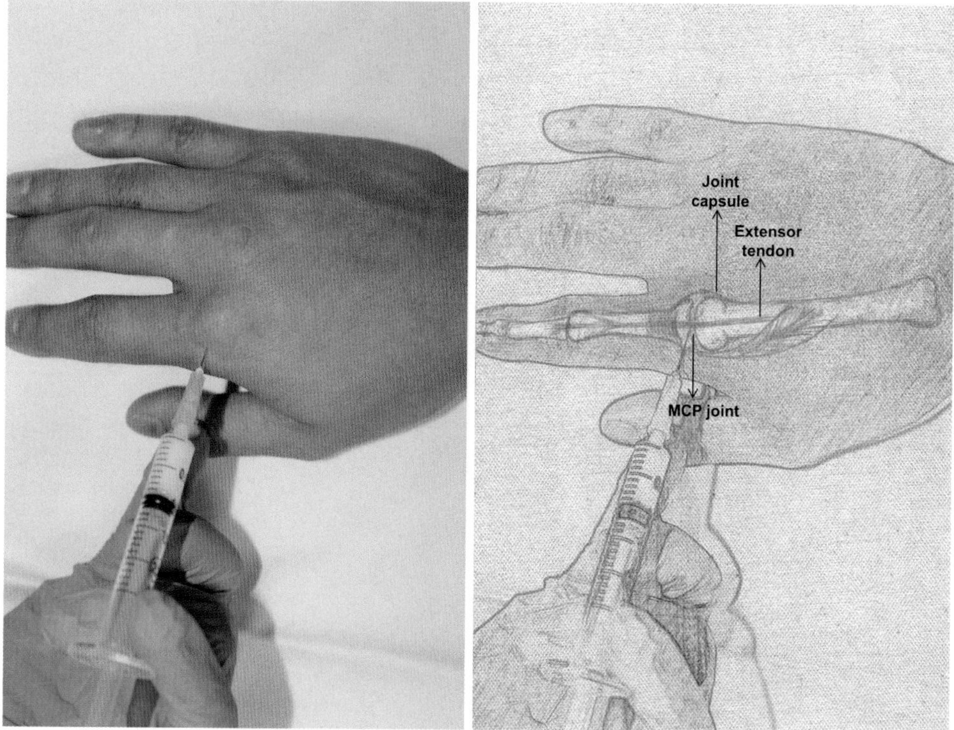

• **Fig. 57.2** Metacarpophalangeal (MCP) joint injection.

TABLE 57.4 Considerations for Possible Crystal Arthropathies

If infection is considered, send fluid to laboratory in a plain universal container—mark as *urgent*, contact laboratory asking for urgent microscopy/culture; subsequently, positively seek result.
Negative result for crystals from laboratory does not rule out crystal disease. Fluid should be analyzed within 3-4 hours due to degradation of crystals.
Clinicians should check for crystals if possible. Monosodium urate crystals are needle-shaped and negatively birefringent; however, calcium pyrophosphate crystals are short, thick, and negatively birefringent.

the joint line before injecting. Direct or indirect ultrasound guidance can help ensure the correct placement of the injection, especially if there is suspected osteophytosis or loss of joint space, or if the patient's body habitus means that the joint line is difficult to locate.

Materials needed for the procedure are a 25-gauge needle, a 2 mL syringe (an insulin syringe can be used as well), and a preparation of a longer-acting corticosteroid, such as triamcinolone acetonide, triamcinolone hexacetonide, or methylprednisolone, 10 mg (±0.2 mL 2% lidocaine).

The procedure is as follows:

1. Palpate and mark the ACJ.
2. Insert the needle directing inferiorly (from above) and slightly posteriorly, aiming towards the center of the joint space (Fig. 57.7). The joint is surrounded by tough ligaments and capsule that may produce some initial resistance to the needle. Aspirate and then slowly inject the syringe. Follow the general postinjection care steps.

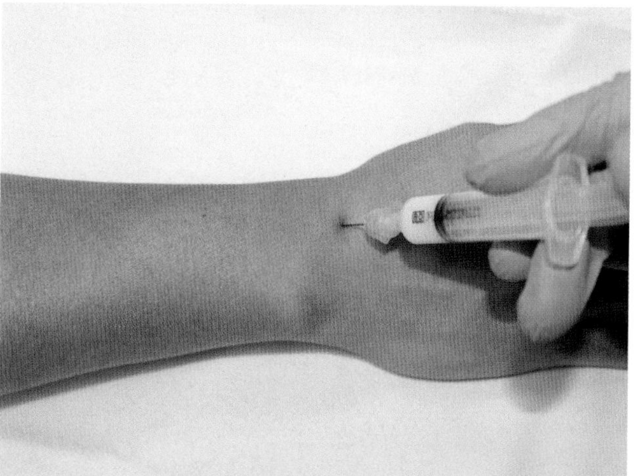

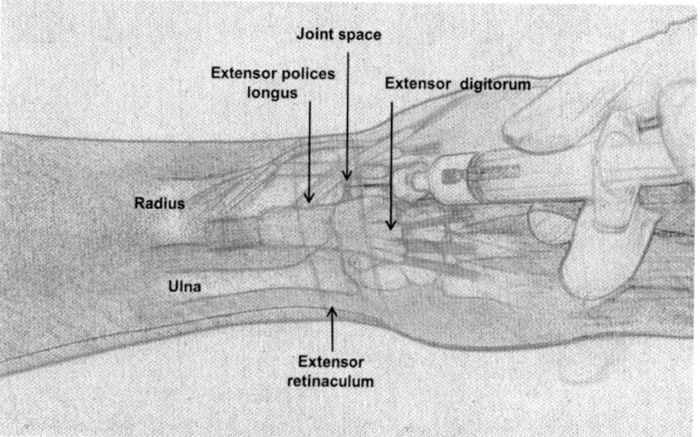

• **Fig. 57.3** Wrist joint injection.

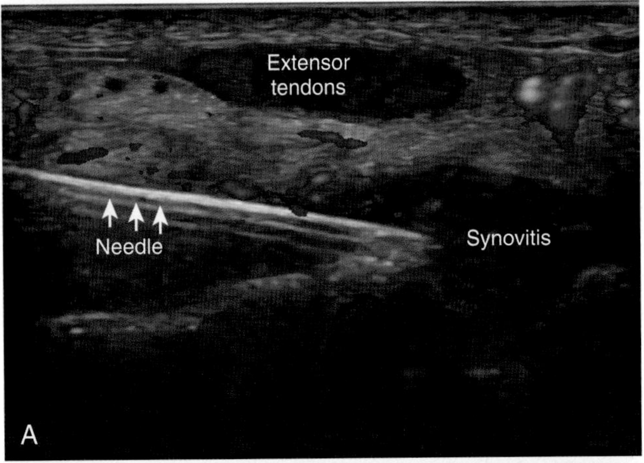

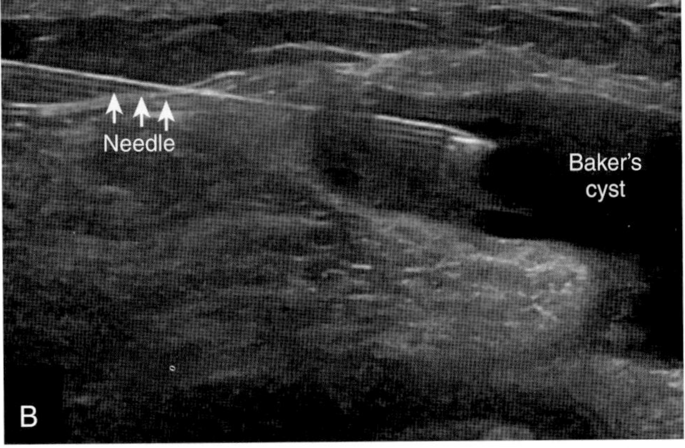

• **Fig. 57.4** Ultrasound image. (A) Wrist joint. (B) Baker's cyst injection.

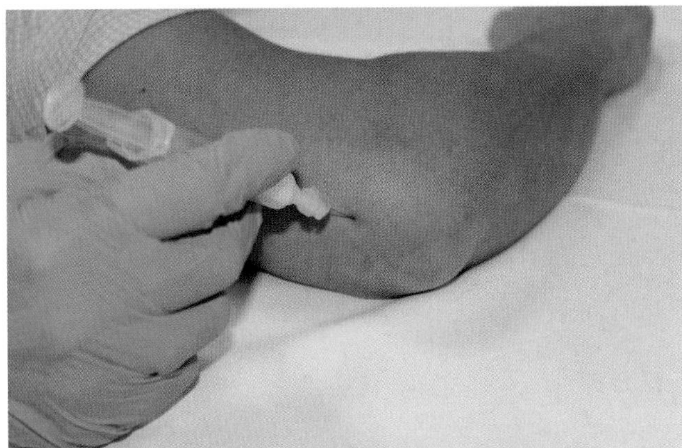

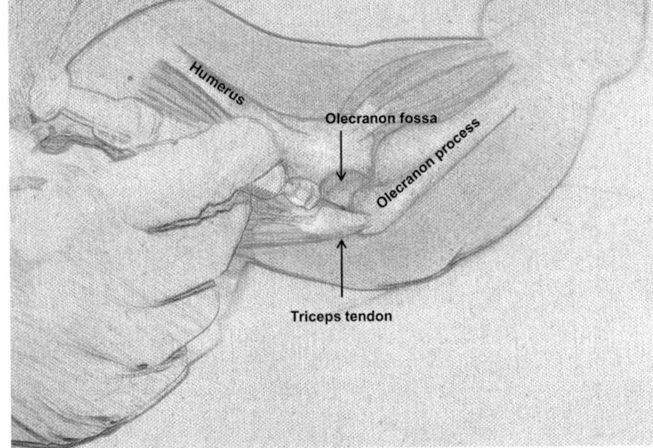

• **Fig. 57.5** Elbow joint injection.

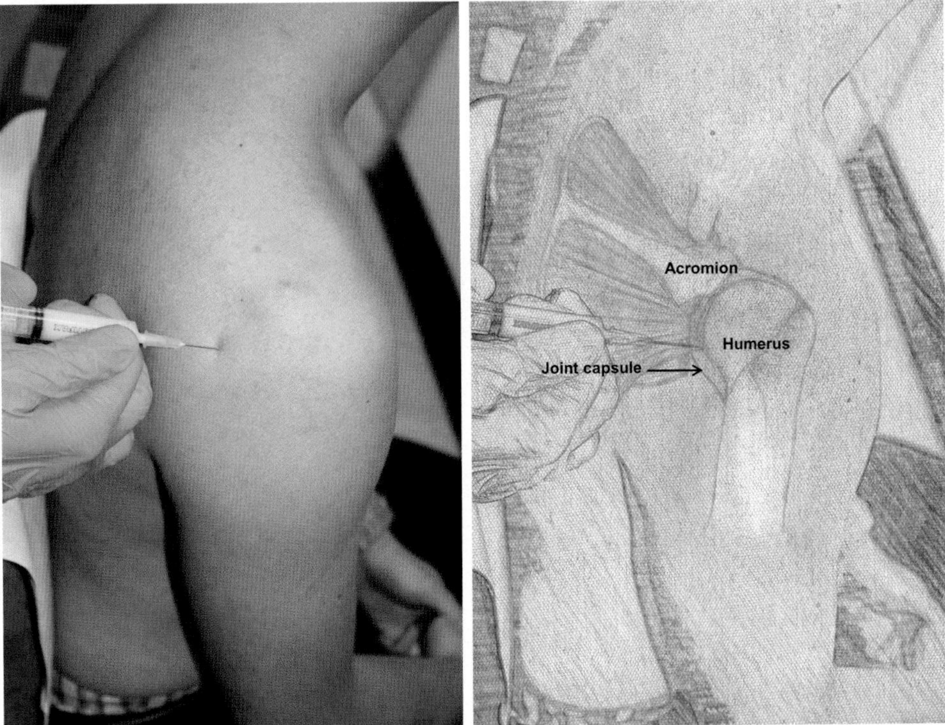

• **Fig. 57.6** Shoulder joint (glenohumeral) injection.

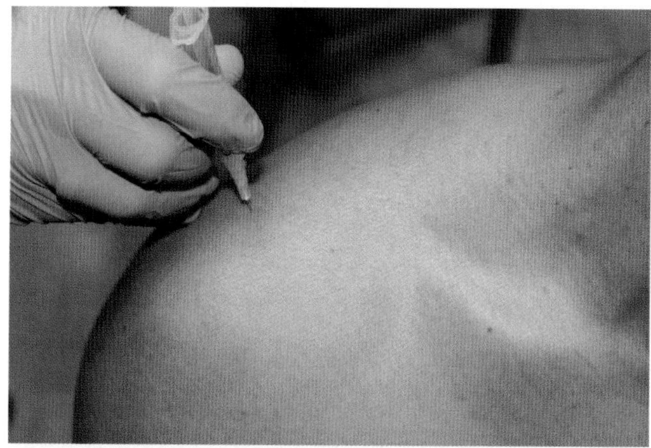

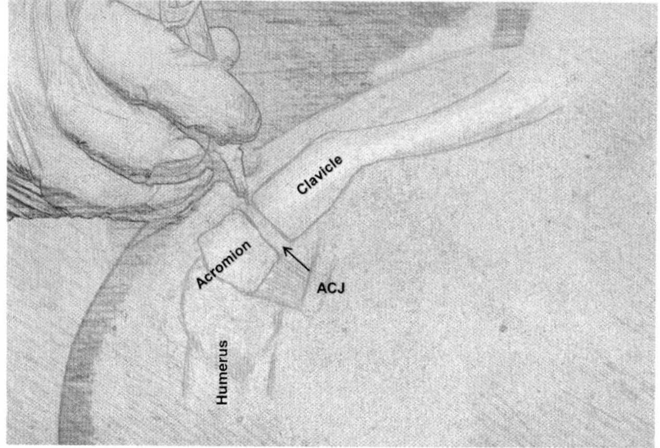

• **Fig. 57.7** Acromioclavicular joint injection.

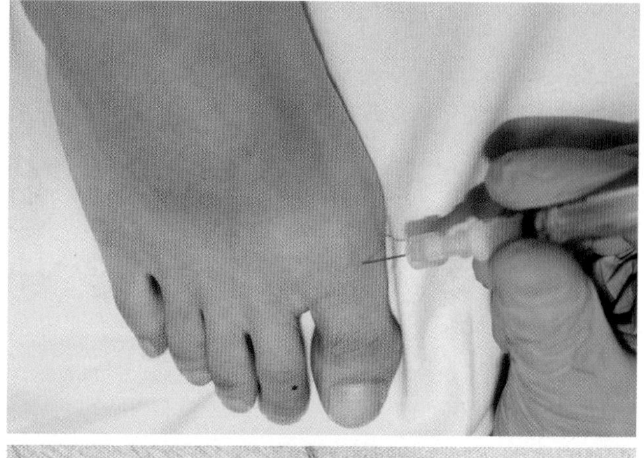

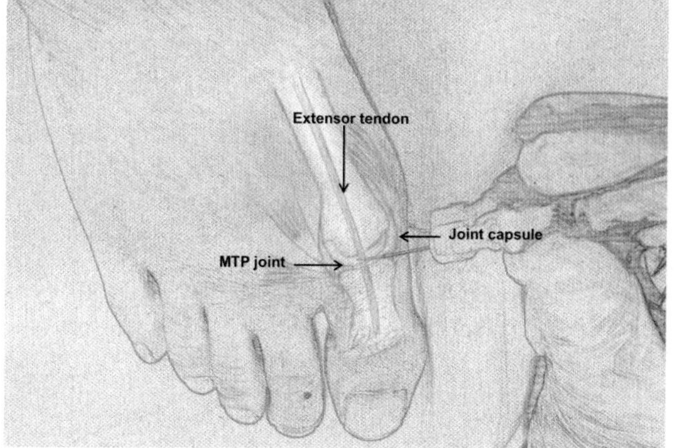

• **Fig. 57.8** Metatarsophalangeal (MTP) joint injection.

Lower Limbs Injections

Metatarsophalangeal Joint

Injection and aspiration of metatarsophalangeal (MTP) joints is often used for gout diagnosis (joint fluid analysis) and treatment and reduction of OA-related symptoms. The first MTP joint is the most commonly affected in gout.

Materials needed for the procedure are a 25-gauge needle, a 2 mL syringe (an insulin syringe can be used as well), and a preparation of a longer-acting corticosteroid, such as triamcinolone acetonide, triamcinolone hexacetonide, or methylprednisolone, 5 to 10 mg (±0.2 mL 2% lidocaine).

The procedure is as follows:

1. Palpate and mark the MTP joint space medial or lateral to the extensor tendon from the dorsal side. A dorsomedial approach is preferred for the first MTP procedure.
2. Insert the needle perpendicular to the skin with the MTP joints slightly in plantar flexion. Aim to place the needle under the extensor tendon (Fig. 57.8). Aspirate and then slowly inject the syringe. Follow the postinjection care steps.

Midfoot Joints (Talonavicular and Navicular Cuneiform)

Direct or indirect ultrasound guidance is preferred for these joints because they are narrow and difficult to locate by palpation, especially if co-existent OA is present. In indirect placement, the place of entry can be identified and marked by using a surgical marker in both longitudinal and transverse ultrasound view. A cross-mark can be made where the two lines meet. After the probe is removed, the needle can be inserted into the center of the cross-mark.

Ankle (Tibiotalar) Joint

Both anterior and posterior approaches for a blind ankle joint injection can be used. However, the anterior approach, is easier and less painful and will be described in this chapter. The clinician performing the ankle injection needs to be aware of specific anatomic structures to help identify the correct location, reduce the risk of complications, and improve the outcome of the procedure. One important structure is the dorsalis pedis artery that lies just lateral to the extensor hallucis tendon (EHL) at the ankle level. The EHL can be identified when the big toe is extended. The clinician is advised to palpate the artery to avoid injecting it. The deep peroneal nerve, which innervates the leg muscles that raise the feet and toes during walking, runs medial to the EHL, crosses behind the tendon 1 to 1.5 cm proximal to the ankle, and is located lateral to the EHL tendon at ankle joint space level. Because of these anatomic structures, we recommend making the injection medial to the EHL (between the tibialis anterior tendon).

Materials needed for the procedure are a 23-gauge needle, a 5 mL syringe, and a preparation of a longer-acting corticosteroid, such as triamcinolone acetonide, triamcinolone hexacetonide, or methylprednisolone, 10 to 40 mg (±2 mL 1% lidocaine).

The procedure is as follows:

1. Place the patient in the supine position with ankle in dorsal extension.

2. Identify the joint line by asking the patient to flex and extend the joint. The joint can be more proximal than expected by just looking at the surface anatomy, thus palpation is strongly recommended.
3. Insert the needle between the tibialis anterior tendon (the tendon just medial to the EHL). Direct the needle posterior-laterally tangent to the curve of the talus (Fig. 57.9). Aspirate and then slowly inject the syringe. Follow the general postinjection care steps.

Subtalar Joint

The subtalar joint is the articulation between the talus and calcaneus (calcaneal bone). This injection can be difficult if done blind because the joint is very narrow and covered with a thick capsule. Thus, ultrasound guidance is generally recommended. However, if ultrasound is not available, and the operator is less experienced, the anterior lateral approach into the sinus tarsi is often used because it is easy to identify, and there is a reduced risk of damaging neurovascular structures. Although not strictly part of the articulation of the subtalar joint, the sinus tarsi offers a route of communication into the joint. The talocalcaneal ligament is inside the joint, which can produce resistance to the needle during the procedure. The procedure, which we will define shortly, is the more conventional approach.

Materials needed for the procedure are a 23-gauge needle, a 5 mL syringe, and a preparation of a longer-acting corticosteroid, such as triamcinolone acetonide or triamcinolone hexacetonide or methylprednisolone, 10 to 40 mg (±2 mL 1% lidocaine).

The procedure is as follows:

1. Place the patient in supine position and the ankle in the inversion position.
2. Identify the joint line by eversion and inversion of the joint. The joint line is found anterior and inferior to lateral malleoli.
3. Insert the needle perpendicular to the skin in the direction of the medial malleolus for approximately 1 inch (Fig. 57.10). Insert the needle through the resistance of the talocalcaneal ligament until you feel the tissue give; this indicates that you are in the joint space. Aspirate and then slowly inject the syringe. If you feel high resistance to the plunger, it means you are still in the ligament. Push the needle further until you can easily inject the plunger. Follow the postinjection care steps.

Knee Joint

This is one of the most commonly performed procedures. It is usually indicated for aspirations of joint fluid for diagnostic purposes or as treatment for knee synovitis associated with inflammatory arthritis, such as crystal arthropathy, or secondary to OA. When performing a knee injection, the clinician should aim to inject the distal suprapatellar pouch (SPP) rather than the tibiofemoral joint per se. The SPP is a large, bursa-like structure that extends out from the knee joint from under the upper half of the patella. It then passes proximally under the quadriceps tendon and quadriceps muscle.

Materials needed for the procedure are a 21-gauge needle, 5 mL syringe (a long needle is needed in cases of obesity), and a preparation of a longer-acting corticosteroid, such as triamcinolone acetonide, triamcinolone hexacetonide, or methylprednisolone, 20 to 80 mg (±3 mL 1% lidocaine).

The procedure is as follows:

1. Place patient in supine position with the knee in a relaxed and slightly flexed position (the knee can be supported with a rolled towel or pillow to help with relaxing).

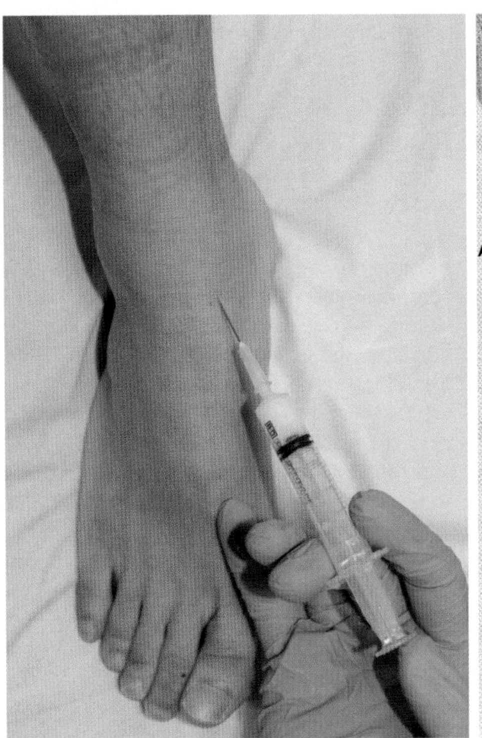

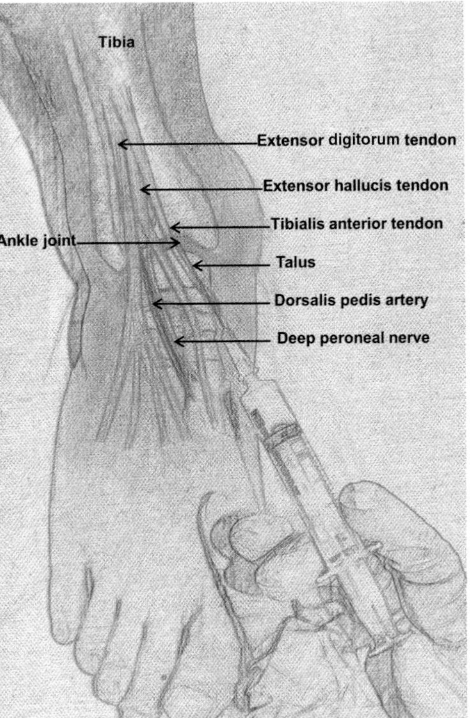

• **Fig. 57.9** Ankle (tibiotalar) joint injection.

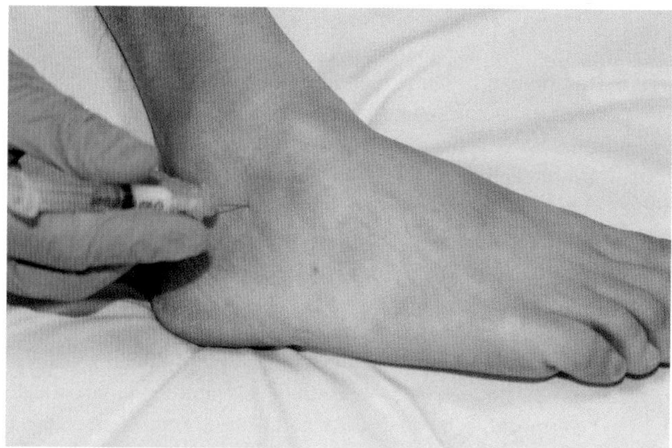

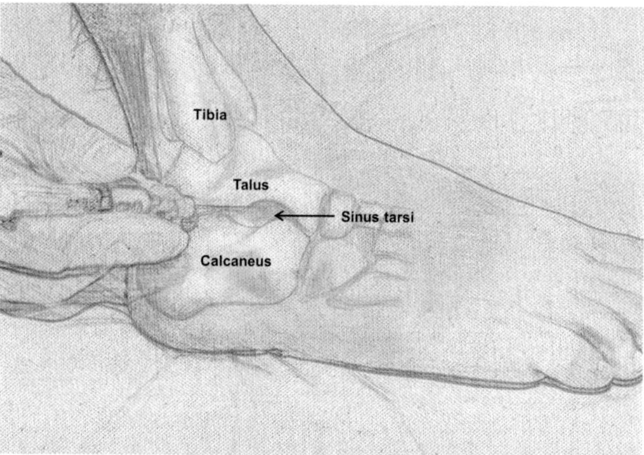

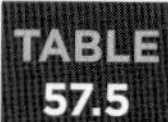

• **Fig. 57.10** Subtalar joint injection.

2. Palpate either the lateral or medial border of the patella. Identify the point at which the proximal one-third meets the distal two-thirds. Insert the needle under the patella in a slightly cranial position toward the SPP, just proximal to the upper pole of the patella (Fig. 57.11). Aspirate and then slowly inject the syringe contents. Follow the general postinjection care steps.

For Baker's cysts, an injection can be delivered either into the knee joint (as written above) or directly into the cyst using ultrasound guidance. In this way, the popliteal artery can be avoided (see Fig. 57.4B; Table 57.5).

Soft Tissue Injections: Upper Limbs

Tendon Sheath and Trigger Finger

Digital flexor tenosynovitis is a common condition associated with inflammatory arthropathies. Triggering may present with flexor tenosynovitis or, more commonly, as a result of thickened finger pulleys, which present at the A1 level in particular.

TABLE 57.5 Considerations for Suspected Septic Arthritis

Sometimes in septic arthritis, gout, or hemoarthrosis, the pus or synovial fluid can be very thick and, therefore, difficult to aspirate; in this case, use larger-bore needles and/or ultrasound guidance to allow the withdrawal of the knee content.
If no fluid is obtained and an infected joint is strongly suspected, consider injecting the joint with saline (lavage) and re-aspirating.

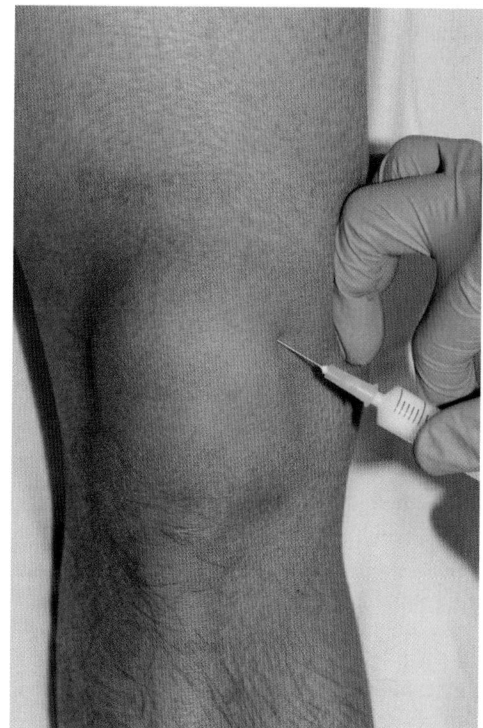

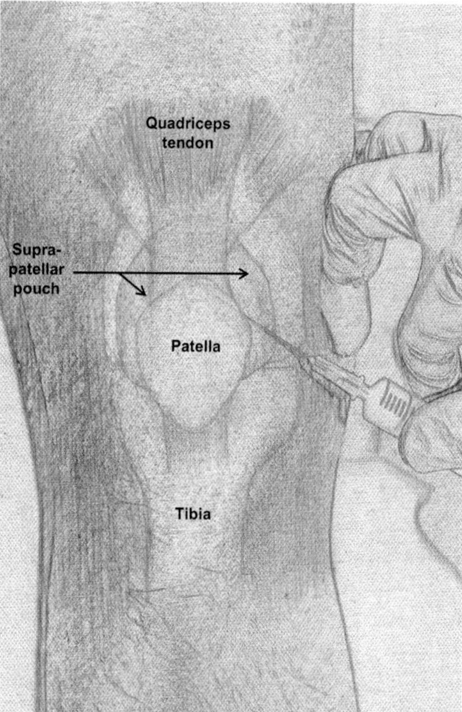

• **Fig. 57.11** Knee joint injection.

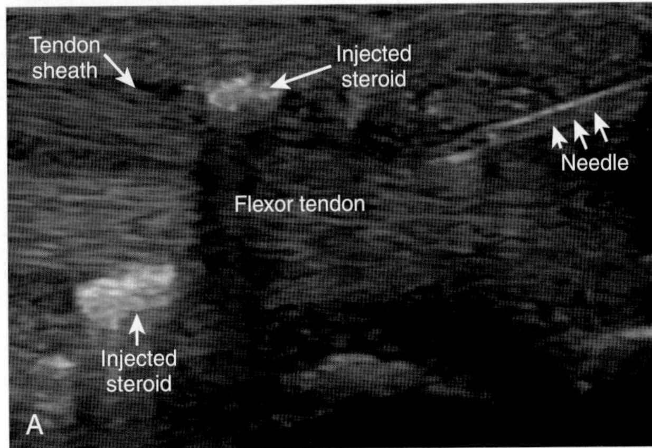

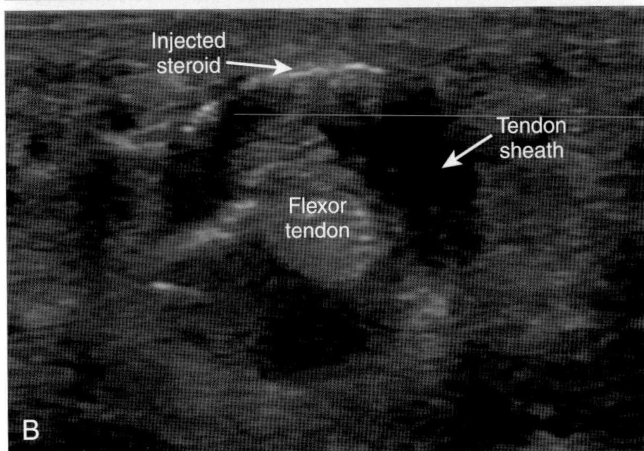

• **Fig. 57.12** Ultrasound-guided tendon sheath injection. (A) Longitudinal view. (B) Transverse view.

Conventionally, tenosynovitis and trigger finger are treated by a flexor tendon sheath injection; although, for the latter, targeted injections around the A1 pulley under ultrasound guidance may be the preferred method. Use of ultrasound also has the added advantage of confirming the correct diagnosis before injection.

Materials needed are a 25-gauge needle, a 2 mL syringe, and a preparation of a longer-acting corticosteroid, such as triamcinolone acetonide, triamcinolone hexacetonide (5 mg). We recommend methylprednisone over triamcinolone because this is potentially less harmful for tendons.

The procedure is as follows:

1. Position the patient's palm facing upward with the fingers extended.
2. Insert the needle with a 30 degree inclination distal to the crease over the MCP joint, and advance it proximally; aim toward the tendon and reduce the angle between the needle and the skin to as close to a parallel position as possible without touching skin.
3. Try to inject while advancing. Once the needle is inside the tendon sheath, the resistance to the plunger will disappear.

For an ultrasound-guided procedure, visualize the tendon on longitudinal view (Fig. 57.12). Insert the needle from a proximal (or distal) position to the probe, directing it to the region of interest where the whole length of needle can be visualized, and the location of injection can be allocated in real time. Proceed as we described previously.

Carpal Tunnel

This procedure can be beneficial in cases of mild to moderate sensory carpal tunnel syndrome that do not respond to conservative therapies, such as splints. It can also be indicated when surgical release cannot be done because of long wait times or patient preference. The median nerve lies below the palmaris longus tendon, which can be used as a landmark for this procedure. The clinician can visualize the palmaris longus tendon by asking the patient to oppose the thumb and little finger. It is anatomically absent in 14% of the population.[11]

Materials needed for the procedure are a 25-gauge needle, a 2 mL syringe, and a preparation of a longer-acting corticosteroid, such as triamcinolone acetonide, triamcinolone hexacetonide, methylprednisone (5 to 10 mg).

The procedure is as follows:

1. Place the patient's palm facing upward.
2. Insert the needle at an angle of approximately 45 degrees at the distal palmar crease toward the index finger and below the palmaris longus tendon (from the ulnar side) (Fig. 57.13). If the patient feels any paresthesia, withdraw the needle slightly and reposition it because this can be an indication of penetration of the median nerve.

For ultrasound-guided procedures, a transverse view of the median nerve should be obtained. Insert the needle from the ulnar side toward the median nerve. The clinician should be able to visualize the whole length of needle in real time. Be careful not to penetrate the nerve. Inject the corticosteroid close to the median nerve under the flexor retinaculum.

De Quervain's Tendonitis

This procedure is indicated for treatment of inflammation of the abductor pollicis longus and the extensor pollicis brevis common sheath. This procedure is best performed under direct ultrasound guidance. We do not recommend triamcinolone due to its greater risk of skin side effects.

Materials needed for the procedure are a 25-gauge needle, a 2 mL syringe, and a preparation of a longer-acting corticosteroid such methylprednisone (5 to 10 mg).

The procedure is as follows:

1. Locate and mark the tendons by asking the patient to extend and abduct the thumb. The tendon sheath can be swollen, which helps direct the position of the needle.
2. Insert the needle just distal to radial styloid near the base of thumb and advance it proximally along the line of the tendon sheath, directing it toward the radial styloid.

For ultrasound guidance, the approach is similar to the tendon sheath injection, which we described previously.

Tennis Elbow Injection

This injection can be indicated for lateral epicondylitis (tendinopathy of the forearm of common extensor tendon origin) in combination with or after failure of conservative management treatment, such as physiotherapy.

Materials needed are a 23-gauge needle, a 5 mL syringe, and a preparation of a longer-acting corticosteroid, such as triamcinolone acetonide, triamcinolone hexacetonide, or methylprednisone, 10 to 40 mg (±1 mL 1% lidocaine).

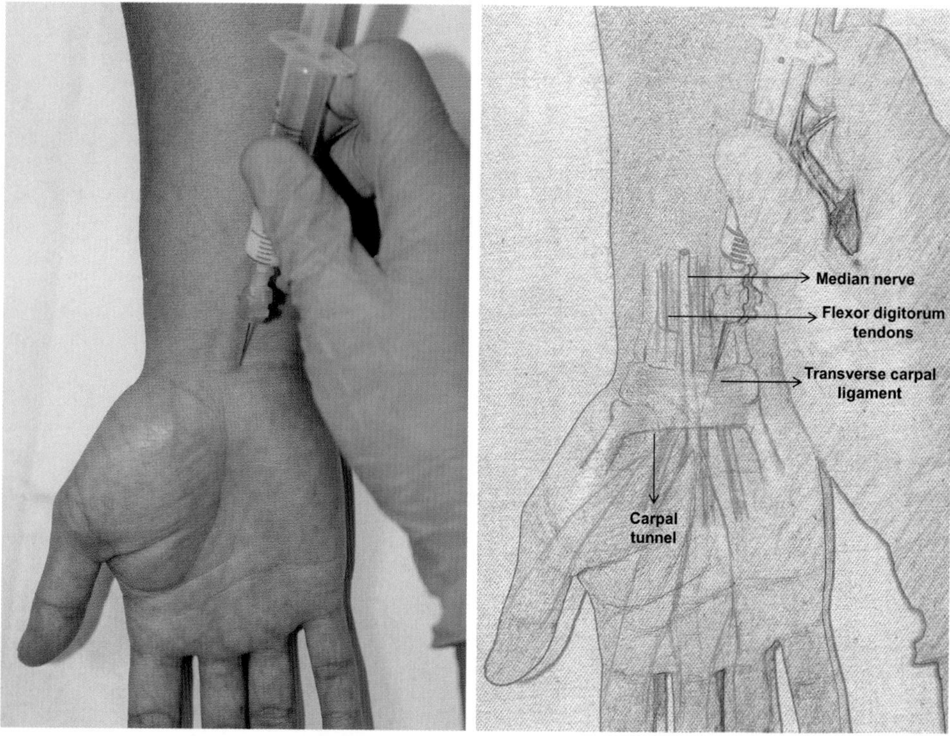

• **Fig. 57.13** Carpal tunnel injection.

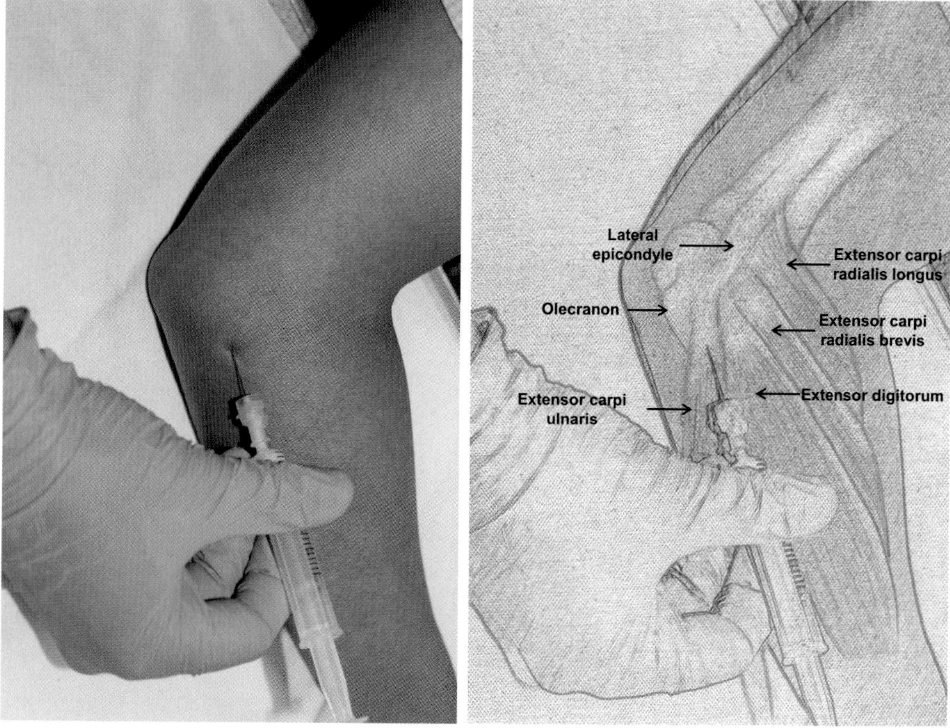

• **Fig. 57.14** Tennis elbow injection.

The procedure is as follows:

1. Place the patient in a supine position, with the elbow flexed to 90 degrees and placed over the chest.
2. Locate the most tender point at the level of the insertion of the common extensor tendons on the lateral epicondyle. (Fig. 57.14). Insert the needle until the bone surface is reached, withdraw slightly, and then inject.

Subacromial Bursa

This injection can be indicated for treatment of subacromial bursitis, impingement syndrome, rotator cuff tendinopathy, adhesive capsulitis, and calcific tendonitis. Both the anti-inflammatory effects of steroid and the hydrodistension of the capsule and bursa may have roles in relief of symptoms.

Materials needed for the procedure are a 21-gauge needle, a 5 mL syringe, and a preparation of a longer-acting corticosteroid, such as triamcinolone acetonide, triamcinolone hexacetonide, or methylprednisone, 20 to 40 mg (±3 mL 1% lidocaine).

The procedure is as follows:

1. While the patient's arm is in internal rotation, feel the depression below the acromial process posterior-laterally with your thumb.
2. Insert the needle, aiming to position it slightly anterior and inferior to the acromial process, directing it toward the coracoid process (Fig. 57.15). Little or no resistance should be encountered while injecting the plunger because the subacromial bursa has a potentially large space.

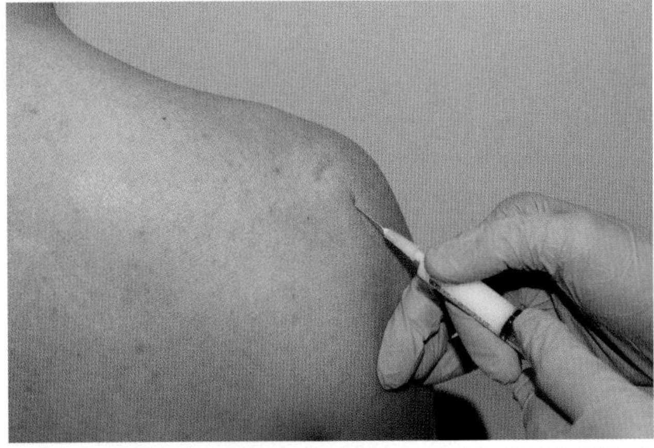

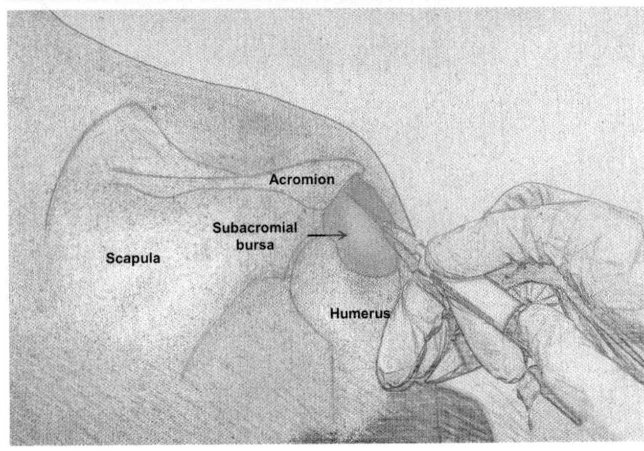

• **Fig. 57.15** Subacromial bursa injection.

Soft Tissue Injections: Lower Limbs

Morton's Neuroma Injection

Morton's neuroma is a benign neuroma of an intermetatarsal plantar nerve. Patients are seen with a pain between the third and fourth toes (the most commonly affected area) and/or with a feeling similar to a pebble in the shoe. Morton's neuroma can be confirmed with a click sound on MTP squeeze (Mulder's sign) or by ultrasound examination.

Materials needed for the procedure are a 25-gauge needle, a 2 mL syringe, and a preparation of a longer-acting corticosteroid, such as methylprednisone, 10 to 20 mg (±5 mL, 2% lidocaine).

The procedure is as follows:

1. Palpate and mark the place of entry, which should be halfway between the MTP heads and one-half inch proximal from the web space from the dorsal side (Fig. 57.16).
2. Insert the needle perpendicular to the skin and advance it through the resistance of the transverse tarsal ligament. A give sensation is felt when the needle passes through the ligament.

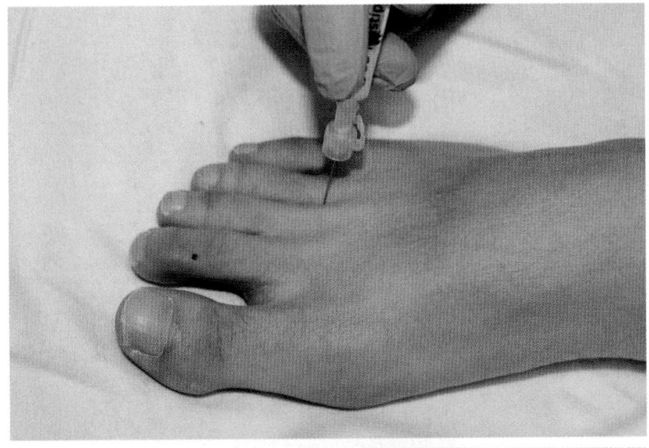

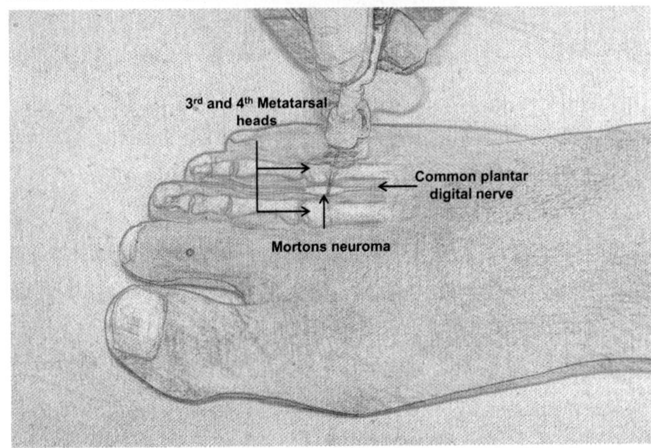

• **Fig. 57.16** Morton's neuroma injection.

Plantar Fascia Injection

Plantar fasciitis injections are indicated if conservative (physical) interventions fail (e.g., stretching exercises and insoles). The injection is usually very painful and may lead to fat pad atrophy, which reduces shock absorption. Rupture of plantar fascia is also a reported complication. For these reasons, we do not recommend frequent injections or injection of the fat pad directly at the foot base.

Materials needed for the procedure are a 23-gauge needle, a 5 mL syringe, and a preparation of a longer-acting corticosteroid, such as methylprednisone, 20 to 40 mg (±2 mL, 1% lidocaine).

The procedure is as follows:

1. Place the patient in lateral decubitus position on the affected side, with the lower leg extended and the upper leg flexed at the hip and knee.
2. Palpate the medial calcaneal tuberosity and mark the maximum tender point. Insert the needle medially perpendicular to the skin and slightly distal to the medial calcaneal tuberosity (Fig. 57.17). Advance the needle until it touches the bony surface.
3. Aspirate and then slowly inject the syringe. Follow the postinjection care steps.

For an ultrasound-guided procedure, a transverse view of the plantar fascia at the area just distal to the calcaneal tuberosity should be obtained. Insert the needle from the medial aspect, where its whole length and the location of the injection can be visualized in real time. Proceed as described in the preceding text.

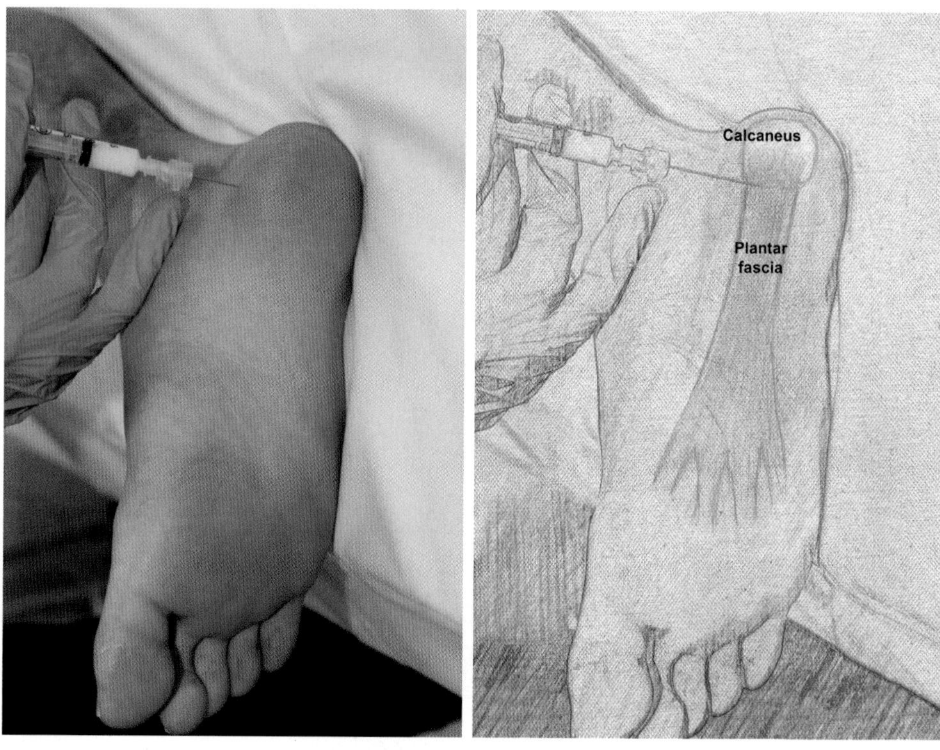

• **Fig. 57.17** Plantar fascia injection.

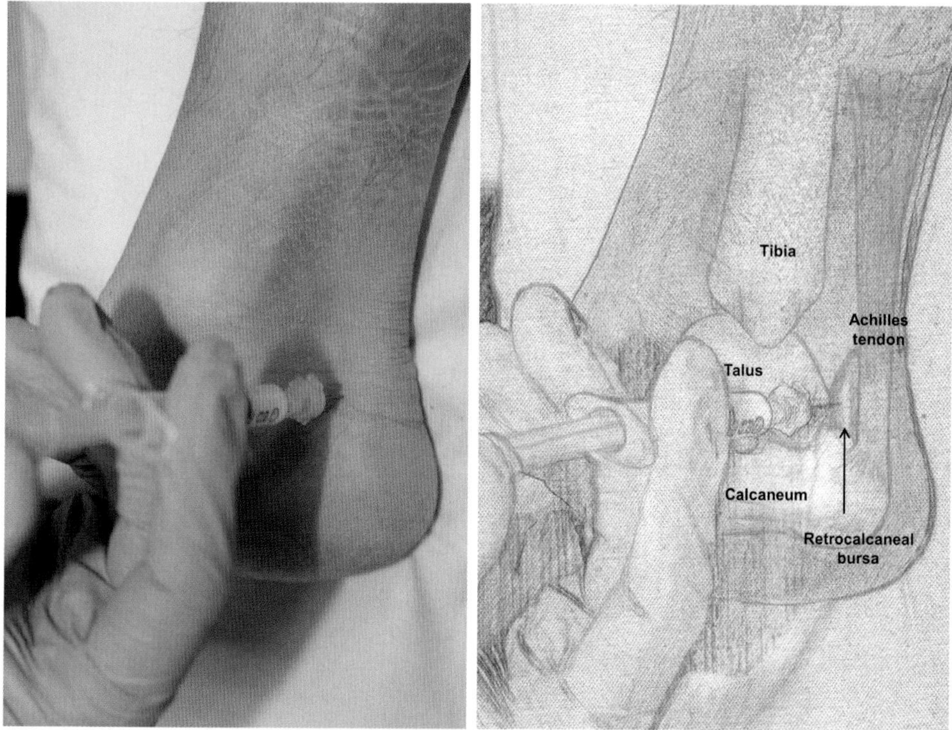

• **Fig. 57.18** Retrocalcaneal bursa injection.

Retrocalcaneal Bursa

This procedure is best performed under ultrasound guidance; however, it still can be done without imaging assistance if ultrasound is not available.

Materials needed for the procedure are a 23-gauge needle, a 5 mL syringe, and a preparation of methylprednisone, 20 mg (±1 mL, 1% lidocaine).

The procedure is as follows:

1. Mark the spot in front on the skin overlying the Achilles tendon just proximal to the calcaneus.
2. Insert the needle from the medial or lateral side, perpendicular to the skin at the marked spot for approximately 1.5 cm (Fig. 57.18). Never inject against resistance.

For ultrasound-guided procedures, place the Achilles tendon in a transverse view at the area where the retrocalcaneal bursa can

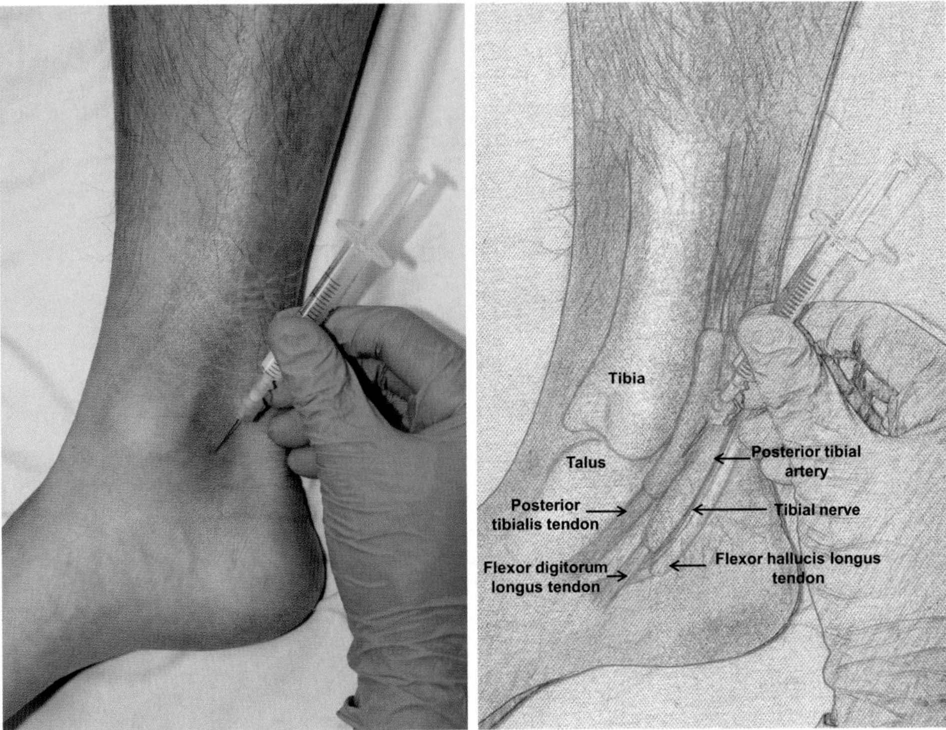

• **Fig. 57.19** Tibialis posterior and peroneal tendon-sheaths injection.

be visualized. Insert the needle from the medial or lateral aspects where the whole length of needle can be visualized, and the location of injection can be seen in real time. Proceed as described in the preceding text.

Tibialis Posterior and Peroneal Tendon-Sheaths

This procedure is best done under ultrasound guidance. However, a blinded procedure can be performed if swelling of the tendon sheaths is very visible, can be identified, and can be injected.

Materials needed for the procedure are a 25-gauge needle, a 2 mL syringe (an insulin syringe can be used as well), and a preparation of hydrocortisone, 25 mg/mL or methylprednisolone (10 to 20 mg).

The procedure is as follows:

Posterior tibialis tendon sheath

1. Palpate the medial malleolus and identify the pulsation of the posterior tibial artery. Mark the line of the posterior tibial artery to avoid it.
2. Insert the needle just posterior to the level of the distal end of the medial malleolus (Fig. 57.19). The tibialis posterior tendon is the first structure posterior to the medial malleolus (lateral malleoli for the peroneal tendon sheath injection). The needle needs to be directed proximally in a 45 degree angle on an artificial line, which extends from the big toe to the heel and follows the path of the tendon. Aspirate and then slowly withdraw the syringe. The tendon sheath may form a sausage-like swelling depending on the injection volume. Follow the postinjection care steps.

Peroneal tendons

1. Palpate the lateral malleolus. The peroneal tendon sheaths lie behind it and lie adjacent to each other. Do not inject the tendon sheath unless the sheath is clearly swollen. Otherwise, you should request an ultrasound examination.
2. Insert the needle just posterior to the level of the distal end of the lateral malleolus using a similar technique to that of the medial ankle tendons. Aspirate and then slowly withdraw the syringe. The tendon sheath may form a sausage-like swelling depending on the injection volume. Follow the postinjection care steps.

Tarsal Tunnel Syndrome Injection

This injection is indicated for tarsal tunnel syndrome, which is an entrapment of the posterior tibial nerve in the tarsal tunnel. Patients with tarsal tunnel syndrome can be seen with numbness and tingling in the medial third of the plantar area. Posterior tibial nerve pathology can be confirmed with nerve conduction studies. In our practice, it is a relatively rare injection. An ultrasound-guided injection would help reduce the risk of damaging the neurovascular bundle.

Materials needed for the procedure are a 25-gauge needle, a 2 mL syringe (an insulin syringe can be used as well), and a preparation of hydrocortisone, 25 mg/mL, or methylprednisolone (10 to 20 mg).

The procedure is as follows:

1. Palpate the medial malleoli and identify the pulsation of the posterior tibial artery. Mark the line of the posterior tibial artery to avoid it.
2. Insert the needle posterior to the medial malleoli and anterior to posterior tibial artery (Fig. 57.20). The needle should be inserted parallel to the skin, directed distally in a 45 degree angle on an artificial line extending from the big toe to the heel. Aspirate and then slowly inject the syringe. Follow the general postinjection care steps.

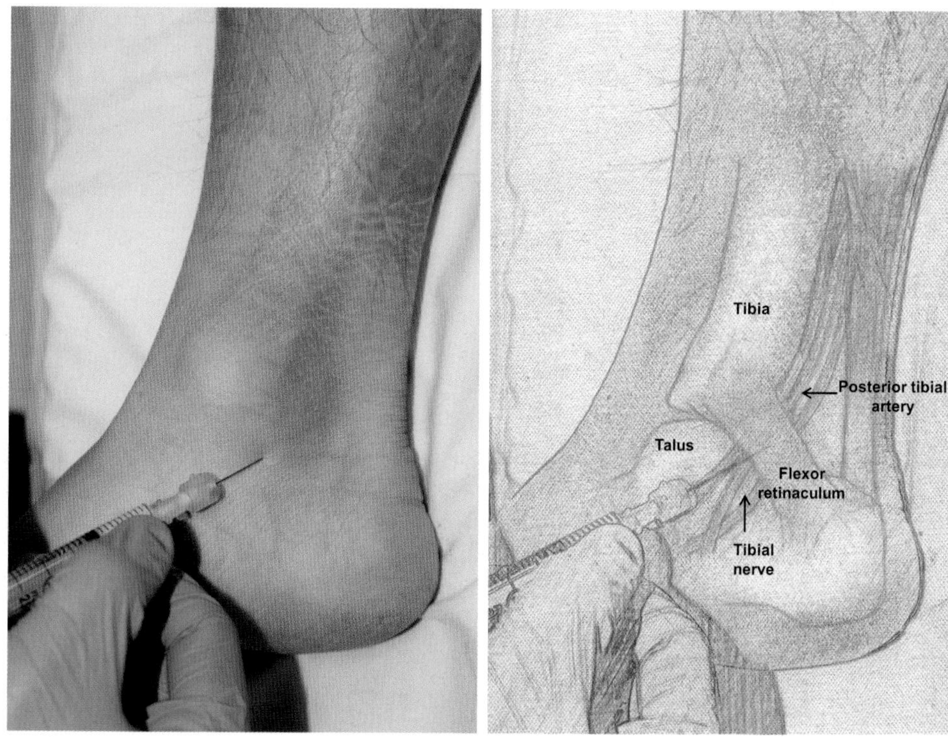

• **Fig. 57.20** Tarsal tunnel injection.

Trochanteric Bursa

"Trochanteric bursitis," now often referred to as greater trochanteric pain syndrome, is a common condition. Patients often describe hip pain over the greater trochanter area, which associates with severe tenderness when they lie (e.g., at night) on the affected side. It may be associated with tightness of the iliotibial band. Recent imaging evidence suggests the pain in this condition is multifactorial with tendinopathy of the gluteal tendons more common than bursitis. The greater trochanter can be identified as a bony prominence on palpation of the lateral aspect of the femur.

Materials needed for the procedure are a 23-gauge (long 2-inch) needle, a 5 mL syringe, and a preparation of a longer-acting corticosteroid like triamcinolone acetonide, triamcinolone hexacetonide, or methylprednisone, 40 mg (±2 mL, 1% lidocaine).

The procedure is as follows:

1. Ask the patient to lie on his/her side, with the affected side facing upward.
2. Palpate and mark the most tender point over the greater trochanter area.
3. Insert the needle perpendicular to the skin until it reaches the hard bony surface of the greater trochanter, withdraw the needle slightly, aspirate, and then inject. Follow the general postinjection care steps.

Conclusion

Arthrocentesis and joint and soft tissue injections are a key part of rheumatology management with respect to diagnosis and treatment. These procedures can be safe and effective as long as certain key points are considered. The correct indication, knowledge of anatomy, right technique, and use of correct medications can all impact the outcome of the procedure. Appropriate documentation, patient education about potential complications, and postinjection care all help improve patient satisfaction and minimize complaints. In general, injections work better for conditions of an inflammatory cause, whereas in OA, the benefits are for 6 to 12 weeks if they work. For soft tissue problems, the role of injections is less proven and place the patient at a higher risk of local complications. We, therefore, recommend an exploration of conservative approaches first unless the patient requires a prompter resolution of symptoms; steroids may resolve symptoms quicker and in the short term, whereas physical therapies may be more helpful longer term.

As long as the technique that is used is safe and the operator is suitably trained, there is no one way to best perform an injection. In our practice, ultrasound is increasingly used to guide procedures especially in joints that may be difficult to aspirate or inject using a conventional blinded technique.

The references for this chapter can also be found on ExpertConsult.com.

References

1. Ahmed I, Gertner E: Safety of arthrocentesis and joint injection in patients receiving anticoagulation at therapeutic levels, *Am J Med* 125(3):265–269, 2012.
2. Yui JC, Preskill C, Greenlund LS: Arthrocentesis and joint injection in patients receiving direct oral anticoagulants, *Mayo Clin Proc* 92(8):1223–1226, 2017.
3. Stefanich RJ: Intraarticular corticosteroids in treatment of osteoarthritis, *Orthop Rev* 15(2):65–71, 1986.
4. Fletcher E: The treatment of osteoarthritis by intra-articular injection of lipiodol and gomenol, *Postgrad Med J* 19(213):193–197, 1943.

4a. Bokarewa M, Tarkowski A: Local infusion of infliximab for the treatment of acute joint inflammation, *Ann Rheum Dis* 62:783–784, 2003.

5. Peeters CM, Leijs MJ, Reijman M, et al.: Safety of intra-articular cell-therapy with culture-expanded stem cells in humans: a systematic literature review, *Osteoarthr Cartil* 21(10):1465–1473, 2013.
6. Gray RG, Gottlieb NL: Intra-articular corticosteroids. An updated assessment, *Clin Orthop Relat Res* (177):235–263, 1983.
7. Pyne D, Ioannou Y, Mootoo R, et al.: Intra-articular steroids in knee osteoarthritis: a comparative study of triamcinolone hexacetonide and methylprednisolone acetate, *Clin Rheumatol* 23(2):116–120, 2004.
8. Braun HJ, Wilcox-Fogel N, Kim HJ, et al.: The effect of local anesthetic and corticosteroid combinations on chondrocyte viability, *Knee Surg Sports Traumatol Arthrosc* 20(9):1689–1695, 2012.
9. Seshadri V, Coyle CH, Chu CR: Lidocaine potentiates the chondrotoxicity of methylprednisolone, *Arthroscopy* 25(4):337–347, 2009.
10. Bellamy N, Campbell J, Robinson V, et al.: Viscosupplementation for the treatment of osteoarthritis of the knee, *Cochrane Database Syst Rev* (2):CD005321, 2006.
11. Sebastin SJ, Puhaindran ME, Lim AY, et al.: The prevalence of absence of the palmaris longus—a study in a Chinese population and a review of the literature, *J Hand Surg Br* 30(5):525–527, 2005.

58 Anti-nuclear Antibodies

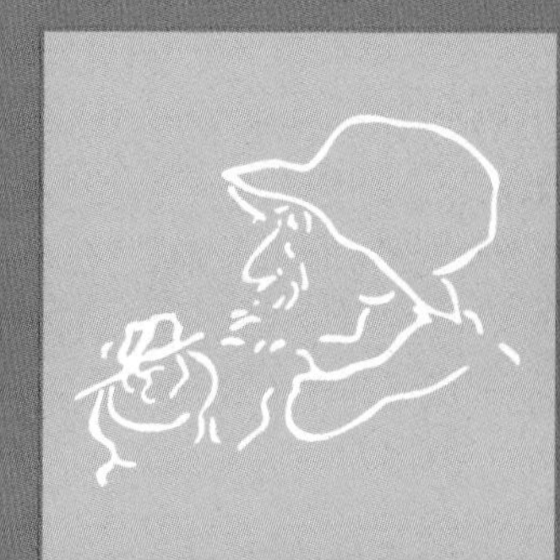

STANFORD L. PENG AND JOSEPH E. CRAFT

KEY POINTS

Among the rheumatic diseases, anti-nuclear antibodies (ANAs) are characteristic of systemic lupus erythematosus (SLE), systemic sclerosis, inflammatory myositis, and primary Sjögren's syndrome. Their presence is required for the diagnosis of some syndromes, such as drug-induced lupus. Fluorescent ANA testing is appropriate as a screening test when such diseases are suspected.

Key ANA specificities in SLE include anti–double-stranded DNA, which corresponds to renal disease and overall disease activity; antiribosomal P, which corresponds to neuropsychiatric manifestations and renal disease; anti-Ro/SS-A and anti-La/SS-B, which associate with cutaneous and neonatal lupus; and anti-Sm, which is considered SLE-specific without clear clinical disease manifestation correlates.

Key ANA specificities in systemic sclerosis include anti-kinetochore (anti-centromere), which corresponds to CREST (calcinosis, Raynaud's phenomenon, esophageal dysmotility, sclerodactyly, and telangiectasias) manifestations; anti–Scl-70 (topoisomerase I) and anti–RNA polymerase III, which are associated with diffuse cutaneous disease and pulmonary fibrosis and accelerated risk of cancer-associated systemic sclerosis; and anti–polymyositis (PM)-Scl (exosome), which is found in myositis–systemic sclerosis overlap.

Key ANA specificities in inflammatory myositis include anti-synthetase, such as antihistidyl transfer RNA synthetase (e.g., Jo-1), which is associated with the poor-prognosis anti-synthetase syndrome, and anti–Mi-2 (nucleosome remodeling-deacetylase complex), which is associated with dermatologic manifestations.

Key ANA specificities in primary Sjögren's syndrome (pSS) include anti-Ro/SS-A and anti-La/SS-B, also found in mothers of children with neonatal lupus, and in asymptomatic mothers of children with neonatal lupus.

Although many ANA specificities are generally considered disease or manifestation specific, exceptions are notoriously common, confounded by the observation that many autoantibodies are present at low frequencies in healthy people and/or exacerbated by other inflammatory conditions.

Ideally, testing of individual ANA specificities should be performed only in the context of clinical signs that correlate with antibody-disease associations (e.g., anti-DNA for lupus nephritis), but the growing availability and implementation of ANA panels in many clinical laboratories often result in the availability of specific ANA tests in settings of uncertain clinical significance. As a result, ANA and ANA specificity testing is insufficient to establish or refute diagnoses.

Introduction

Anti-nuclear antibodies (ANAs) include a wide diversity of autoantibodies directed against multiple intra-cellular antigens, classically consisting of nuclear specificities such as DNA or small nuclear ribonucleoproteins (snRNPs), but later expanding to include various other cell components including the mitotic spindle apparatus, cytosol, cytoplasmic organelles, and cell membranes.[1] The ANA diseases (Table 58.1) include syndromes characterized by an unusually high prevalence of ANAs, often screened for by the fluorescent ANA (FANA) test: systemic lupus erythematosus (SLE), systemic sclerosis (SSc), and mixed connective tissue disease (MCTD). The prevalence of ANAs in polymyositis (PM), dermatomyositis (DM), and primary Sjögren's syndrome (pSS) is somewhat lower than in the other ANA diseases, but these conditions are often grouped together because they share several target antigens and therefore presumably also share similar fundamental etiologies. For decades, ANA testing has been an important diagnostic and prognostic tool for these connective tissue diseases (CTDs), and it has become a routine assay in the evaluation of patients with suspected autoimmune disease by both specialists and primary care providers. However, ANAs also arise in a variety of infectious, inflammatory, and neoplastic diseases, as well as in healthy people, and thus some knowledge regarding their intricacies and the limitations of the assays is required for appropriate clinical utilization.

History

KEY POINT

ANAs are most well known as diagnostic aids for rheumatic and sometimes other autoimmune diseases; however, their importance extends to their targets, which often play critical roles in cellular homeostasis.

The first formal report of an ANA-related phenomenon is attributed to the 1948 description of lupus erythematosus (LE) cells in SLE bone marrow. These cells were soon discovered to be polymorphonuclear leukocytes that had engulfed the denatured nucleus of a cell injured by anti-DNA autoantibodies, and were often sought in the diagnosis of SLE and drug-induced lupus, as well as pSS and rheumatoid arthritis (RA).[2] Assessment of LE cells was a cumbersome technique, though, and in 1957,

TABLE 58.1 Diseases and Related Conditions Associated With Anti-nuclear Antibodies

Condition	Patients With ANAs (%)
Diseases for Which ANA Testing Is Helpful for Diagnosis	
Systemic lupus erythematosus	99-100
Systemic sclerosis	97
Polymyositis/dermatomyositis	40-80
Primary Sjögren's syndrome	48-96
Diseases in Which ANA Is Required for the Diagnosis	
Drug-induced lupus	100
Mixed connective tissue disease	100
Autoimmune hepatitis	100
Diseases in Which ANA May Be Useful for Prognosis	
Juvenile idiopathic arthritis	20-50
Antiphospholipid antibody syndrome	40-50
Raynaud's phenomenon	20-60
Some Diseases for Which ANA Is Typically Not Useful	
Discoid lupus erythematosus	5-25
Fibromyalgia	15-25
Rheumatoid arthritis	30-50
Relatives of patients with autoimmune diseases	5-25
Multiple sclerosis	25
Idiopathic thrombocytopenic purpura	10-30
Thyroid disease	30-50
Patients with silicone breast implants	15-25
Infectious diseases	Varies widely
Malignancies	Varies widely
Healthy ("Normal") Individuals	
≥1:40	20-30
≥1:80	10-12
≥1:160	5
≥1:320	3

ANA, Anti-nuclear antibody.

Modified from Kavanaugh A, Tomar R, Reveille J, et al.: Guidelines for clinical use of the antinuclear antibody test and tests for specific autoantibodies to nuclear antigens, American College of Pathologists. *Arch Pathol Lab Med* 124:71-81, 2000.

FANA testing was introduced as a more sensitive assay for SLE and related diseases.[3] Finer distinction of autoantibody reactivities detected by FANA testing led to the description of multiple specificities that continue to be well known today, such as Smith (Sm) antigen, nuclear ribonucleoprotein (nRNP), and Ro/Sjögren's syndrome (SS-A) and La/SS-B specificities, which gained further biologic prominence with the demonstration that their autoantigens play prominent roles in cellular homeostasis (Table 58.2). Many biochemical and cell biology studies have consequently been aided by ANAs as research reagents, and subsequent investigations continue to identify many additional ANA autoantigens.

Relevance of Anti-nuclear Antibodies to Disease Pathogenesis

KEY POINT

ANAs may contribute to disease pathogenesis by producing directly toxic or other pro-inflammatory effects upon binding to their autoantigens.

Several ANAs have long been suspected to play a role in the pathogenesis of disease. Anti-DNA antibodies, for instance, are thought to promote inflammation in SLE nephritis via immune complex deposition, direct binding to cross-reactive glomerular antigens, and/or intra-cellular penetration and induction of cellular toxicity.[4] Similarly, ribonucleoprotein antibodies such as anti-Ro/SS-A, anti-La/SS-B, and anti-Sm have been implicated in the pathogenesis of cutaneous or cardiac manifestations by penetrating live cells and/or binding to exposed antigens in the skin and/or heart.[5] Sera containing anti–Scl-70 (topoisomerase I) activity can induce high levels of interferon (IFN)-α, correlating with diffuse cutaneous scleroderma and lung fibrosis,[6] and anti-Jo-1- or anti-Ro/SSA-positive sera from myositis patients have been demonstrated to induce type I IFN and/or ICAM-1 on endothelial cells.[7,8]

However, autoantibodies alone fail to account for disease pathogenesis. Induction of type I IFN activity by anti-Ro/SS-A–containing sera, for instance, appears restricted to patients with SLE or pSS, not those who are asymptomatic.[9] This phenomenon, interestingly, may reflect additional biologic issues among or effects of the autoantigens themselves, such as novel conformations or epitopes: for example, a proteolytically sensitive conformation of histidyl-transfer RNA (tRNA) synthetase, the target of pulmonary fibrosis–related Jo-1–specific antibodies, has been described in the lung,[10] and an apoptope (i.e., an epitope expressed on apoptotic cells) of Ro/SS-A may be specific to SLE, suggesting a unique role of apoptosis in disease pathogenesis.[11] The autoantigens themselves may have unique biologic functions: 60 kDa Ro/SS-A, for instance, may serve as a receptor for the antiphospholipid-related β2-glycoprotein I, and this dynamic may account for differences in Ro antibody pathogenicity.[12] In addition, many autoantigens likely have intrinsic pro-inflammatory properties, such as the stimulation of innate inflammation by DNA and RNA via Toll-like receptors (TLRs) 3, 7, and 9 or other intra-cellular nucleic-acid binding receptors,[13] or the induction of smooth muscle responses by the centromere protein CENP-B via CCR3.[14] Interestingly, apparent remission of SLE in a patient has been correlated with loss of TLR responsiveness, antibody deficiency, and disappearance of anti-DNA, supporting such concepts.[15] Thus the pathogenesis of the connective tissue diseases appears to reflect a complex interplay between direct inflammatory or other biologic effects of the autoantigens, as well as the consequences of the autoantibody responses.

TABLE 58.2 Diagnostic Characteristics of the Anti-nuclear Antibodies

Specificity	Target Autoantigen(s) (Function)	ANA Pattern(s)	Other Tests	Disease Associations
Nuclear				
Chromatin-associated antigens				
DNA				
	ds-DNA	Rim, homogeneous	RIA, ELISA, CIF, Farr	SLE
	ss-, ds-DNA	Rim, homogeneous	RIA, ELISA, CIF	SLE
	ss-DNA	Undetectable	ELISA	SLE, DIL, RA
Histone	H1, H2A/B, H3, H4	Homogeneous, rim	IB, RIA, ELISA	SLE, DIL, RA, PBC, SSc
	H3 (nucleosome structure)	Large speckles		SLE, UCTD
Kinetochore (centromere)	CENP-A, -B, -C, and/or -D (mitotic spindle apparatus)	Speckles[a]	IF, ELISA	SSc, SLE, pSS
Ku	Regulatory subunit (Ku70/80) of DNA-dependent protein kinase (DNA break repair)	Diffuse-speckled nuclear or nucleolar[a]	ID, IPP, IB	SLE, PM/SSc overlap
PCNA/Ga/LE-4	PCNA (DNA scaffold)	Nuclear/nucleolar speckles[a]	ELISA, ID, IB, IPP	SLE
DEK	DEK autoantigen			SLE, JIA, SSc (transcriptional regulation)
Dense fine speckle 70 (DFS70)	Lens epithelium derived growth factor (LEDGF) and/or DNA binding transcription coactivator p75	Dense fine speckle	IF, IB	(absence of systemic auto-immune disease)
Spliceosome components		Speckled	ID, ELISA, IB, IPP	
Sm	Sm core B'/B, D, E, F, and G			SLE
RNP, nRNP	U1 snRNP 70K, A, and C			SLE, MCTD
	U2 snRNP			SLE, MCTD, overlap
	U4/U6 snRNP			pSS, SSc
	U5 snRNP			SLE, MCTD
	U7 snRNP			SLE
	U11 snRNP			SSc
	SR (splicing of pre-mRNA)		ELISA, IB, IPP	SLE
Other Ribonucleoproteins				
Ro/SS-A	Ro (ribosomal RNA processing)	Speckled or negative	ID, ELISA, IB, IPP	pSS, SCLE, NLE, SLE, PBC, SSc
La/SS-B/Ha	La (ribosomal RNA processing)	Speckled	ID, ELISA, IB, IPP	pSS, SCLE, NLE, SLE
RNA helicase A	RNA helicase A	?	IP	SLE
TIA-1, TIAR	TIA-1, TIAR	?	IB, IPP	SLE, SSc
Mi-2	NuRD complex (transcription regulation)	Homogeneous	ID, IPP	DM
p80-coilin	Coiled bodies	Speckled		pSS
MA-I	Mitotic apparatus	Speckled[a]		pSS, SSc
Nucleolar				
RNA polymerases (RNAP)		Punctate	IPP, IB	
	RNAP I	Nucleolar		SSc
	RNAP II	Nuclear/nucleolar[b]		SSc, SLE, overlap
	RNAP III (RNA transcription)	Nuclear/nucleolar[b]		SSc

Continued

TABLE 58.2 **Diagnostic Characteristics of the Anti-nuclear Antibodies—cont'd**

Specificity	Target Autoantigen(s) (Function)	ANA Pattern(s)	Other Tests	Disease Associations
Ribosomal RNP	Ribosomal RNPs (protein translation)	Nucleolar, cytoplasmic	ID, IB, IPP, ELISA	SLE
Topoisomerase I (Scl-70)	Topoisomerase I (DNA gyrase)	Diffuse, grainy nuclear or nucleolar	ID, IB, ELISA	SSc
Topoisomerase II	Topoisomerase II (DNA gyrase)	?	ELISA	SSc
U3 snoRNP (fibrillarin)	U3 snoRNP (ribosomal RNA processing)	Clumpy	IB, IPP	SSc
Th snoRNP (RNase MRP)	RNase MRP (mitochondrial RNA processing)	Diffuse with sparse nuclear	IPP	SSc
NOR 90 (hUBF)	hUBF (ribosomal RNA transcription)	10-20 discrete spots or nuclear[a]	IB, IPP	SSc
PM-Scl (PM-1)	Exosome (RNA processing/degradation)	Homogeneous nuclear or nucleolar	ID, IPP, IB	PM, DM, SSc, overlap
Nucleobindin-2 (Wa)	Nucleobindin-2	?	ELISA	SSc, SLE, PM/DM
Cytoplasmic				
tRNA Synthetases				
Jo-1	$tRNA^{His}$	Diffuse	ID, IPP, IB, ELISA, AAI	PM, DM
PL-7	$tRNA^{Thr}$	Diffuse	ID, IPP, IB, ELISA, AAI	PM, DM
PL-12	$tRNA^{Ala}$	Diffuse	ID, IPP, IB, ELISA, AAI	PM, DM
EJ	$tRNA^{Gly}$	Diffuse	ID, IPP, IB, ELISA, AAI	PM, DM
OJ	$tRNA^{Ile}$	Diffuse	ID, IPP, IB, ELISA, AAI	PM, DM
KS	$tRNA^{Asn}$	Diffuse	ID, IPP, IB, ELISA, AAI	UCTD, ?
Mas	$tRNA^{[Ser]Sec}$ (protein translational machinery)	?	IPP	myositis
Fodrin	α- and/or β-Fodrin (cytoskeletal component)	Diffuse subplasmalemmal	ELISA	pSS
Signal recognition particle	Signal recognition particle (transmembrane protein handling)	?	IPP, IB	PM
Eukaryotic initiation factor 2B (eIF2B)	Eukaryotic initiation factor 2B (eIF2B) (protein translation)	?	IB, IPP	SSc
KJ	Translational apparatus	?	ID, IB	Myositis
Calponin-3	Calponin-3 pSS, SLE, IIM (cytoskeletal)	?	IB, ELISA	
Elongation factor 1α (Fer)	Elongation factor 1α (protein translation)	?	IPP	Myositis

[a]Cell cycle–dependent.

[b]May also stain nucleoli because of an association with antibodies to RNA polymerase I.

AAI, Aminoacylation inhibition; *ANA,* anti-nuclear antibody; *CENP,* centromere protein; *CIF,* Crithidia luciliae immunofluorescence; *DIL,* drug-induced lupus erythematosus; *DM,* dermatomyositis; *ds,* double stranded; *ELISA,* enzyme-linked immunosorbent assay; *Farr,* Farr radioimmunoassay; *hUBF,* human upstream binding factor; *IB,* immunoblot; *ID,* immunodiffusion; *IF,* immunofluorescence; *IPP,* immunoprecipitation; *MCTD,* mixed connective tissue disease; *mRNA,* messenger RNA; *NLE,* neonatal lupus erythematosus; *NOR,* nuclear organizer region; *nRNP,* nuclear ribonucleoprotein; *NuRD,* nucleosome remodeling-deacetylase; *overlap,* overlap syndromes; *PBC,* primary biliary cirrhosis; *PCNA,* proliferating cell nuclear antigen; *PM,* polymyositis; *PM-Scl,* polymyositis scleroderma; *pSS,* primary Sjögren's syndrome; *RA,* rheumatoid arthritis; *RIA,* radioimmunoassay; *RNAP,* RNA polymerase; *RNase,* ribonuclease; *RNP,* ribonucleoprotein; *SCLE,* subacute cutaneous lupus erythematosus; *SLE,* systemic lupus erythematosus; *Sm,* Smith; *SnRNP,* small nuclear ribonucleoprotein; *SR,* serine/arginine splicing factors; *ss,* single stranded; *SSc,* systemic sclerosis; *TIA-1,* T cell intracytoplasmic antigen 1; *TIAR,* TIA-1–related protein; *tRNA,* transfer RNA; *UCTD,* undifferentiated connective tissue disease.

Modified from Fritzler MJ: Immunofluorescent antinuclear antibody test. In Rose NR, De Macario EC, Fahey JL, et al., editors: *Manual of clinical laboratory immunology,* Washington, DC, 1992, American Society for Microbiology. p 724.

Methods of Detection

KEY POINTS

The gold standard screening test for ANAs is the fluorescent ANA (FANA) test.

Many antibody tests, including ANA screening in some laboratories, are performed via enzyme-linked immunosorbent or other solid-phase assay affording high throughput; however, such techniques may result in lower accuracy.

Optimal clinical interpretation of ANA tests requires knowledge of the technique(s) used in each specific case.

Immunofluorescence

The FANA provides a rapid yet highly sensitive screening method for ANA detection and remains the gold standard for initial clinical testing.[1] Here, test sera at varying dilutions (typically serially increasing by twofold) are incubated with substrate cells, and bound antibodies are detected by fluorescein-conjugated anti-human IgG, followed by visualization via a fluorescence microscope. Results typically are reported by two parameters: pattern and titer, with any pattern of reactivity at a titer of 1:40 or greater generally considered positive. The former parameter includes one or more morphologic descriptors that typically reflect the localization of the respective autoantigen(s) (see Table 58.2; Figs. 58.1 and 58.2). Titer is generally reported as the last dilution at which an ANA pattern is detectable, but such an assessment has been considered somewhat imprecise and subjective, and interlaboratory standardization has not been widely instituted. Attempts to standardize the protocol have included computer-based fluorescent image quantification, subjective optical scales, and the use of standardized sera to define international units (IU/mL), which can vary by laboratory.

As such, FANA results must always be interpreted in light of the techniques used by the individual laboratory. Cultured cell lines such as HEp-2 cells have remained a gold standard substrate because of their higher concentration of nuclear and cytoplasmic antigens and standardization of use, but some laboratories continue to use heterogeneous substrates, such as rodent liver or kidney tissues, which possess the advantage of eliminating interference from blood-group antibodies, heterophile antibodies, or passenger viruses but may exhibit lower sensitivity of some cell cycle–dependent antigens such as Ro/SS-A. Additional issues that may contribute to variability in FANA results include differences in reagents and instruments, such as the quality of the fluorescein-conjugated anti-human IgG, specific reference sera, and the microscope used.[16]

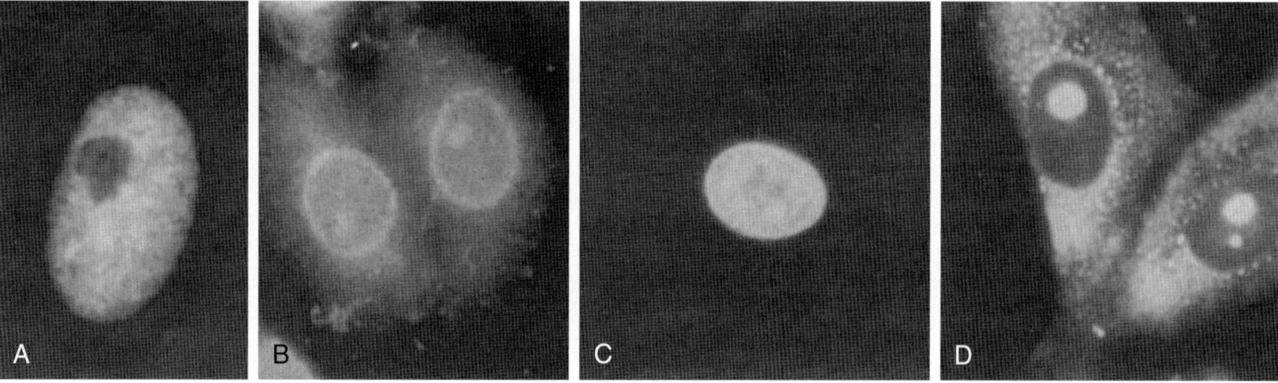

• **Fig. 58.1** The fluorescent anti-nuclear antibody test: specificities of systemic lupus erythematosus. (A) Speckled nuclear pattern of anti-Sm antibodies. (B) Nuclear rim pattern of anti–DNA antibodies. (C) Homogeneous nuclear pattern of anti-DNA antibodies. (D) Discrete cytoplasmic and nucleolar pattern of antiribosome antibodies. (A, From the Clinical Slide Collection on the Rheumatic Diseases, copyright 1991; used by permission of the American College of Rheumatology.)

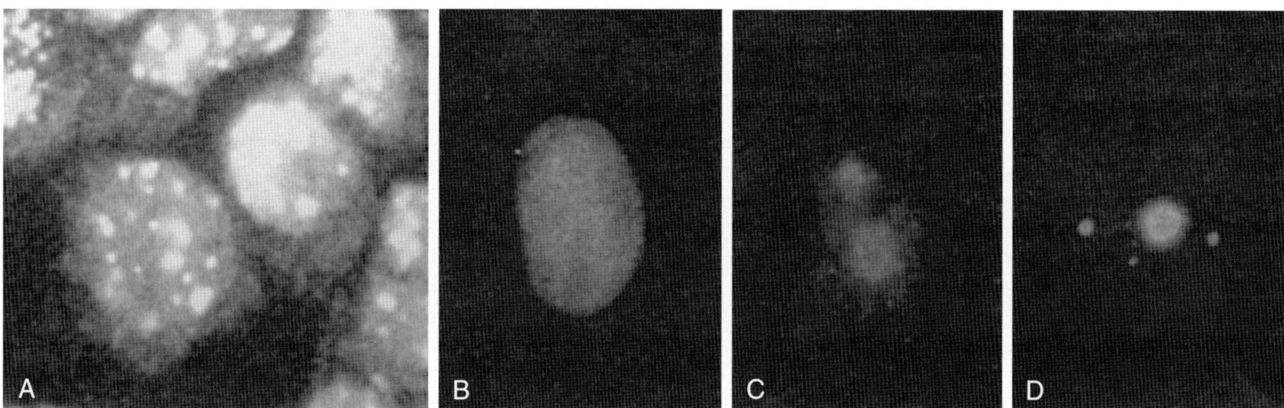

• **Fig. 58.2** The fluorescent anti-nuclear antibody test: specificities of systemic sclerosis. (A) Discrete speckled nuclear pattern of anti-kinetochore (centromere) antibodies. (B) Grainy nuclear and nucleolar pattern of anti-topoisomerase I (Scl-70) antibodies. (C) Diffuse nucleolar and sparse nucleoplasm pattern of anti-Th (ribonuclease mitochondrial RNA processing complex, 7-2) antibodies. (D) Punctate nucleolar staining of anti–RNA polymerase antibodies. (A, From the Clinical Slide Collection on the Rheumatic Diseases, copyright 1991; used by permission of the American College of Rheumatology.)

Enzyme-Linked Immunosorbent Assay

Enzyme-linked immunosorbent assays (ELISAs) provide highly sensitive and rapid techniques for the detection of autoantibodies. They are commonly used for the detection of specific ANAs, such as anti-DNA and extractable nuclear antigen (ENA) autoantibodies (anti-Sm, anti-Ro/SS-A, anti-La/SS-B, and anti-RNP), often in a "reflex" manner upon detection of a positive screening FANA test. With this technique, test sera are incubated in wells precoated with purified target antigen, and bound antibodies are detected via an enzyme-conjugated anti-human immunoglobulin antibody, followed by color visualization with the appropriate enzyme substrate. The popularity of this technique has further resulted from the commercial availability of ELISA kits and the ability to perform these assays on a multiplex platform, enabling large numbers of clinical specimens to be processed quickly at reasonably low cost. As a result, many laboratories also use such solid-phase immunoassays instead of FANA for the screening ANA test; however, this practice is limited by the number of displayed autoantigens (typically 8 to 10), resulting in reduced sensitivity compared with FANA.[17] Conversely, because the ELISA technique can denature autoantigens, ELISAs may produce false-positive results, and confirmation may warrant further testing, which is not always clinically available. Recognition of the local technique used for the detection of ANAs is therefore often important for their optimal clinical application in diagnosis and/or prognosis.

Anti-DNA Antibody Tests

Anti-DNA antibodies warrant special consideration because of their wide range of autoantigenic epitopes and their assay difficulties.[4] Antibodies that recognize denatured single-stranded (ss) DNA, which are less specific for rheumatic disease, bind the free purine and pyrimidine base sequences; SLE-specific antibodies that recognize native, double-stranded (ds)DNA bind the deoxyribose phosphate backbone or the rarer, conformation-dependent left-handed helical Z-form. Two methods to ensure the use of native dsDNA in anti-DNA tests include digestion with S1 nuclease, which removes overhanging ssDNA ends, and chromatography on a hydroxyapatite column, which separates ss segments from dsDNA. Unfortunately, despite such efforts, native DNA may spontaneously denature, especially when bound to plastic ELISA plates; this effect may account for some reports of a relative lack of specificity of anti-dsDNA antibodies for SLE.

The Farr radioimmunoassay, which remains the gold standard for DNA antibody testing, involves the binding of autoantibodies to radiolabeled dsDNA in solution. Precipitation of the antibody-DNA complexes by ammonium sulfate allows a quantification of the percentage of incorporated (antibody-bound) radioactive dsDNA. Normal sera typically bind a small fraction of added DNA (usually less than 20%), whereas SLE sera often bind nearly 100% of added DNA. However, the specificity of this assay still depends on the quality of dsDNA and the removal of contaminating ssDNA. Also, because of the involvement of radioactivity, the Farr assay is not routinely used in clinical laboratories.

The *Crithidia* test provides an inherently reliable dsDNA substrate that is more often clinically available. Here, the hemoflagellate *C. luciliae* serves as a substrate for indirect immunofluorescence. Its kinetoplast, a modified giant mitochondrion, contains a concentrated focus of stable, circularized dsDNA, without contaminating RNA or nuclear proteins, providing a sensitive and specific immunofluorescence substrate by which to establish anti-dsDNA activity. Thus, together, ELISAs, *C. luciliae* immunofluorescence, and possibly Farr radioimmunoassay tests provide effective, complementary mechanisms to distinguish anti-ssDNA and anti-dsDNA.

Other Assays

Several additional assays for the determination of ANA specificity include the immunodiffusion and counterimmunoelectrophoresis techniques, two relatively insensitive assays used in many historical clinical studies associating ANA specificities (especially ENAs) with disease manifestations and outcome; immunoprecipitation and immunoblot, two sensitive and specific assays predominantly confined to research settings; and enzyme inhibition assays (e.g., inhibition of topoisomerase I by anti–Scl-70 and inhibition of RNA splicing by anti-snRNP), which include highly specialized techniques to characterize ANA functionally. Such assays have not achieved widespread use in clinical diagnostic laboratories because of their cumbersome and/or highly specialized natures, but are worth recognizing for their common research applications.

Interpretation of the FANA

KEY POINT

Although the FANA pattern and titer may provide some insight into the specific autoantigen(s) targeted, as well as the potential likelihood of connective tissue disease, in a given patient such correlations should only guide, not absolutely determine, clinical decisions.

Pattern

Patterns of staining by FANA are often reported as homogeneous, speckled, or rim/peripheral when nuclear staining is present but may also be reported as cytoplasmic, centromere, or nucleolar, reflecting the intra-cellular localization of the target antigen(s) (see Table 58.2; see Figs. 58.1 and 58.2). The presence of unusual patterns may be particularly helpful in appropriate clinical settings, such as the presence of a centromere pattern in a patient with features of SSc, suggesting anti-kinetochore antibodies, or a cytoplasmic pattern in a patient with features of myositis, suggesting anti-tRNA synthetase antibodies.[18] Conversely, the dense fine speckle (DFS70) pattern, associated with reactivity to lens epithelium derived growth factor (LEDGF) and/or DNA binding transcription coactivator p75, has been recognized to associate with the lack of systemic autoimmune rheumatic disease, but unfortunately the pattern can often be confused with the more well-known speckled pattern, and specific testing for this autoantigen(s) is not widely available.[19] Indeed, consensus remains lacking regarding whether or not to report unusual patterns as ANA positive or negative.[20] As a result, the presence or absence of patterns is not always highly accurate in predicting specificity, and non-nuclear patterns may not be reported at all by some laboratories, including rare patterns such as nuclear dot, Golgi, or antimitochondrial antibodies.[21] Furthermore, the role of the FANA pattern in predicting target autoantigen specificities has been largely supplanted in some clinical laboratories by widely available autoantigen-specific ELISAs. As a result, the presence of any such pattern is evidence in an appropriate clinical setting of non–organ-specific autoimmunity, which may warrant further evaluation; however, a specific pattern may be available and useful in certain cases.

Titer

Although the widely accepted cutoff for FANA positivity has remained 1:40, greater clinical significance has generally been thought to correlate with higher titers,[16] and in fact a minimum titer of 1:80 has been proposed for the inclusion of lupus patients in clinical trials.[22] Healthy people, usually older and female people, or relatives of people with connective-tissue diseases may produce positive FANAs at a frequency sometimes exceeding 30% (see Table 58.1).[23,24] Although these people often possess titers of less than 1:320 with homogeneous and/or dense fine speckled staining patterns, many subjects possess higher titers yet remain clinically asymptomatic for years, and occasional patients with SLE may demonstrate negative FANAs, which perhaps is a more frequent observation if they possess isolated anti-Ro/SS-A or anti-ssDNA antibodies and/or if the laboratory uses rat or mouse tissues.[25] As a result, the presence of high- versus low-titer FANA results may not be of sufficient clinical significance to warrant subsequent evaluation. Rather, a positive screening FANA of any titer requires clinical correlation.

Diseases Associated With Anti-nuclear Antibodies

KEY POINTS

- Key ANA specificities in SLE include anti-dsDNA, which corresponds to renal disease and overall disease activity; antiribosomal P, which corresponds to neuropsychiatric manifestations and renal disease; anti-Ro/SS-A and anti-La/SS-B, which are associated with cutaneous and neonatal lupus; and anti-Sm, which is considered SLE specific without clear clinical disease manifestation correlation.
- Key ANA specificities in systemic sclerosis include anti-kinetochore (anti-centromere), which corresponds to CREST (calcinosis, Raynaud's phenomenon, esophageal dysmotility, sclerodactyly, and telangiectasias) manifestations; anti–Scl-70 (topoisomerase I) and anti-RNA polymerase III, which are associated with diffuse cutaneous disease and pulmonary fibrosis; and anti–PM-Scl (exosome), which is found in myositis–systemic sclerosis overlap.
- Key ANA specificities in inflammatory myositis include anti-histidyl-tRNA synthetase (e.g., Jo-1), which is associated with the poor prognosis anti-amino acyl tRNA synthetase syndrome, and anti–Mi-2 (nucleosome remodeling-deacetylase complex), which is associated with dermatologic manifestations.
- Key ANA specificities in primary Sjögren's syndrome include anti-Ro/SS-A and anti-La/SS-B, found also in mothers of children with neonatal lupus, and in asymptomatic mothers of children with neonatal lupus.

Systemic Lupus Erythematosus

ANAs remain a hallmark of SLE. Some past studies have reported FANA frequencies as low as 90%, but the test is positive in more than 99% of patients with the use of current methods.[26] SLE often evokes autoantibodies against a wide range of antigens in many cellular locations, but the majority of SLE autoantigens reside in the nucleus and may be broadly categorized into chromatin-associated versus ribonucleoprotein antigens (Tables 58.2 and 58.3).[27]

Chromatin-Associated Antigens

Anti-DNA. Although antibodies against DNA remain one of the most widely recognized specificities in SLE, antibodies against its more physiologic forms—such as nucleosomes or chromatin—are more prevalent and probably relevant to pathogenesis.[28,29] Nonetheless, most clinical literature remains linked to classic anti-dsDNA antibodies (see anti-DNA antibody tests discussed earlier); many diseases exhibit anti-ssDNA activity, but only SLE sera characteristically possess high-titer anti-dsDNA and/or anti–Z-DNA activity, as characterized by positive Farr or Crithidia assays seen in approximately 73% of patients, in contrast to low titers seen often in pSS, RA, other disorders, and healthy people.[30] In SLE, anti-DNA antibodies strongly correlate with nephritis and disease activity, in contrast to other ANA specificities.[4,31] In some settings, drug-induced anti-DNA antibodies are observed, such as during therapy with some TNF inhibitors, although they do not necessarily correlate with clinical manifestations of CTD or response to TNF inhibitor therapy.[32]

Some anti-DNA antibodies may cross-react with other autoantigens, explaining correlation with other end-organ manifestations, such as the neuronal *N*-methyl-D-aspartate (NMDA) receptor or ribosomal P antigens for CNS disease.[33,34] Such findings suggest that the immunologically relevant antigen for anti-DNA antibodies may not in fact be DNA. As a result, the presence of anti-DNA activity should always prompt consideration of renal disease, but the presence of anti-DNA activities does not always indicate lupus nephritis, and vice versa. Indeed, in inconsistent clinical settings, anti-dsDNA antibodies have low prognostic value.[35]

Anti-histone (Nucleosome). Anti-histone antibodies target the protein components of nucleosomes, the DNA-protein complexes that form the substructure of transcriptionally inactive chromatin. They are common in SLE, associate with anti-dsDNA, and are particularly characteristic of and sensitive for drug-induced lupus, where they associate with anti-ssDNA.[29] However, they are commonly seen in other rheumatic diseases, including myositis and SSc, as well as chronic infections, such as Epstein-Barr virus, and as a result clinical correlations for anti-histone antibodies have not been consistent.

Other Chromatin-Associated Autoantigens. Other chromatin-associated autoantigens in SLE include several specificities also observed in other rheumatic and nonrheumatic diseases with still somewhat undefined clinical significance. For instance, autoantibodies against Ku, the catalytic subunit of the DNA-dependent protein kinase implicated in DNA repair and V(D)J recombination, have been associated with a number of clinical manifestations, but only inconsistently.[36] Other chromatin-associated autoantigens include proliferating cell nuclear antigen (PCNA), which participates in a scaffold to facilitate DNA replication, recombination, and repair; DEK, a nuclear phosphoprotein involved in transcriptional regulation, modulation of chromatin architecture, DNA replication, and messenger RNA processing; and RNA polymerase II, which transcribes some snRNA genes, as well as all protein-encoding genes, both of which remain of uncertain clinical correlation.

Ribonucleoproteins

Anti-small Nuclear Ribonucleoproteins. In SLE, the most well-described snRNP autoantibodies include the Sm and U1 snRNP (RNP) specificities, which target the RNAs or proteins of the spliceosome, a complex of RNP particles involved in the pre-messenger (m)RNA splicing.[37] These particles include the U1, U2, U4/U6, U5, U7, U11, and U12 snRNPs, each of which consists of its respective uridine-rich ("U") snRNA and a set of polypeptides, including a common core of "Sm" polypeptides (B/B', D1, D2, D3, E, F, and G), as well as particle-specific

TABLE 58.3 **Anti-nuclear Antibodies in Systemic Lupus Erythematosus[a]**

Antibody Specificity	Prevalence (%)	SLE-Specific?	Major Disease Associations
Chromatin-Associated Antigens			
Chromatin	**80-90**	In high titer	
dsDNA	**70-80**	In high titer	**Renal LE, overall disease activity**
Histone	**50-70**	No	**Drug-induced lupus, anti-DNA**
	H1, H2B > H2A > H3 > H4		
Ku	**20-40**	No	Overlap
RNA polymerase II	9-14	Relatively (SLE and overlap)	
Kinetochore	6	No	
PCNA	3-6	No	
Ribonucleoprotein Components			
snRNPs			
Sm core	**20-30**	Yes	
U1 snRNP	**30-40**	No	
U2 snRNP	15		
U5 snRNP	?		
U7 snRNP	?		
Ro/SS-A	**40**	No	**Cutaneous LE** **Neonatal LE and CHB**
La/SS-B	**10-15**	No	**Neonatal LE**
Ribosomes			
P0, P1, P2 protein	**10-20**	Yes	**Neuropsychiatric LE**
28S rRNA	?		
S10 protein	?		
L5 protein	?		
L12 protein	?		
SR proteins	50-52		
Proteasome	58		
TNF TRs	61		Nephritis
RNA helicase A	6		
RNA	?		
Ki-67	?		

[a]Shown are the major anti-nuclear antibody specificities described in systemic lupus erythematosus, along with estimated prevalence and disease associations (*bold* indicates data supported by multiple studies). See text for details.

CHB, Congenital heart block; *dsDNA,* double-stranded DNA; *LE,* lupus erythematosus; *PCNA,* proliferating cell nuclear antigen; *pSS,* primary Sjögren's syndrome; *rRNA,* ribosomal RNA; *SLE,* systemic lupus erythematosus; *Sm,* Smith; *snRNP,* small nuclear ribonucleoprotein; *SR,* serine/arginine splicing factors; *TNF TRs,* tumor necrosis factor translational regulators, including T cell intracytoplasmic antigen-1 and TIA-1–related protein.

polypeptides.[38] Anti-Sm antibodies, which target proteins of the Sm core, the B/B', and one of the D polypeptides, as well as the Sm-like LSm4, appear in only 20% to 30% of patients with SLE but are considered specific for the diagnosis[39]; however, their presence has only inconsistently been associated with specific disease activity and/or prognosis. In contrast, anti–U1 snRNP (nuclear RNP or U1 RNP) autoantibodies, which target the 70K, A, or C polypeptides specific to the U1 snRNP, occur in 30% to 40% of patients with SLE but are not specific for SLE and likewise have been only variably associated with several disease manifestations.[40] Several other snRNP antibodies have been described in SLE, often in overlap syndromes—for example, U2, U5, or U7 snRNP–specific—although their clinical correlations also remain inconsistent.[38]

TABLE 58.4 **Anti-nuclear Antibodies in Systemic Sclerosis**[a]

Antibody Specificity	Prevalence (%)	SSc-Specific?	Mutually Exclusive?	Major Disease Associations
Kinetochore (centromere)	**22-36**	Relatively	Yes	**CREST**
Topoisomerase I	**22-40**	Relatively	Yes	**Diffuse cutaneous disease Pulmonary fibrosis**
Topoisomerase II	22			
RNA polymerases	**4-23**			
RNA polymerases I		Relatively	Yes	Renal crisis
RNA polymerase II		No		Overlap
RNA polymerases III		Relatively	Yes	Renal crisis, diffuse disease
B23 nuclear phospho-protein	11			
U3 snoRNP (fibrillarin)	6-8			
Th snoRNP (RNase MRP, 7-2 RNA)	**4-16**			Limited cutaneous disease
U11/U12 RNP	3			Pulmonary fibrosis
PM-Scl	**2-5**	No		**Myositis-SSc overlap**
Sp1	?	No		
NOR 90 (hUBF)	?	No		

[a]Shown are the major anti-nuclear antibody specificities described in systemic sclerosis, along with estimated prevalence and disease associations (*bold* indicates data supported by multiple studies). Anti-nuclear antibody specificities whose incidences are thought to be "mutually exclusive" of each other in systemic sclerosis are indicated. See text for details.

CREST, Calcinosis, Raynaud's phenomenon, esophageal dysmotility, sclerodactyly, and telangiectasias; *hUBF,* human upstream binding factor; *MRP,* mitochondrial RNA processing complex; *NOR,* nucleolar organizer region; *PM-Scl,* polymyositis scleroderma; *RNase,* ribonuclease; *snoRNP,* small nucleolar ribonucleoprotein; *SSc,* systemic sclerosis.

Anti-Ro/SS-A and La/SS-B. The RNP particles anti-Ro/SS-A and La/SS-B, which are part of a macromolecular complex that predominantly processes RNA polymerase III transcripts, often have been associated with pSS and the neonatal lupus syndrome, as well as ANA-negative SLE (especially anti-Ro/SS-A: see the previous discussion of FANA). Some, but not all, studies have indicated that anti-Ro may segregate among rheumatic diseases based on subunit specificities; for example, Ro52 without Ro60 specificities correlates with pSS, whereas Ro60, perhaps specifically a Ro60 apoptope, with or without Ro52 specificities, correlates with other CTDs, including SLE.[41] In SLE, anti-Ro associates with several manifestations, especially skin disease (cutaneous lupus, chilblains, and photosensitivity) and sicca symptoms, but also the neonatal lupus syndrome, including congenital heart block, anti-La, rheumatoid factor, pulmonary disease, complement (especially C4) deficiencies, thrombocytopenia, lymphopenia, and cardiac fibroelastosis. In comparison, anti-La correlates with late-onset SLE, secondary SS, the neonatal lupus syndrome, and protection from anti-Ro–associated nephritis.[42]

Antiribosome. The most well-studied antiribosome antibodies in SLE, antiribosomal P protein (anti-P), target the P0, P1, and P2 proteins of the large 60S ribosome subunit. Although they occur in only a minority of patients, they are considered highly specific for SLE and are particularly specific for neuropsychiatric lupus, classically psychosis,[43] perhaps in relationship to cross-reactivity to neuronal antigens like neuronal surface P antigen.[44] Correlations with active disease, renal disease, liver and hematologic disease, alopecia, anti-Sm, anti-DNA, and anticardiolipin antibodies have also been reported.[45] Other less prevalent antiribosomal antibodies target ribosomal (r)RNA, such as the 28S rRNA, or other ribosomal proteins, such as the S10, L5, and L12 subunit proteins, although their clinical significance remains unclear.[46]

Other ANAs in SLE. Many other SLE ANA specificities have been described, some of which apparently are quite prevalent, such as the SR splicing factors, proteasome, and TNF translational regulator or RNA helicase A specificities. Many such specificities continue to lack clear clinical context, although preliminary analyses indicate some correlation, such as Ki-67 with sicca or RNA with overlap syndromes. Others remain of interest because of their connection with other diseases, such as perinuclear anti-neutrophil cytoplasmic antigens, topoisomerase I, or kinetochore specificities.

Systemic Sclerosis (Scleroderma)

ANAs against certain chromatin and nucleolar antigens characterize the autoantibody response in SSc. Positive FANAs, sometimes speckled in appearance, appear in up to 97% of sera, although percentages vary depending on the substrate used for detection. Unlike SLE sera, however, SSc sera typically, but not always, contain monospecific autoantibody specificities, targeting such structures as the kinetochore, topoisomerase I, or RNA polymerases, and/or typically fall into autoantibody clusters that may have distinct clinical and serologic associations (Tables 58.2 and 58.4).[47–49]

Anti-kinetochore (Centromere) and Anti-topoisomerase I

Anti-kinetochore (centromere) and anti-topoisomerase I specificities constitute major diagnostic tools in the subclassification of SSc. Originally named *anti-centromere,* anti-kinetochore targets at least four centromere (kinetochore) antigens (CENPs) of the mitotic spindle apparatus that promote chromosome separation during mitosis: CENP-B (the predominant kinetochore autoantigen), CENP-A, CENP-C, and CENP-D. As such, these specificities require mitotically active cells for robust detection, accounting for some ANA-negative SSc findings. Their clinical significance has been extensively studied and is heavily associated with Raynaud's phenomenon (RP) and CREST (calcinosis, RP, esophageal dysmotility, sclerodactyly, and telangiectasias), in which up to 98% of patients have anti-kinetochore antibodies. In contrast, anti-topoisomerase I (Scl-70) autoantibodies, which predominantly target the catalytic region of DNA helicase topoisomerase I, generally predict diffuse cutaneous disease with proximal skin involvement and pulmonary fibrosis.[50] However, approximately 40% of all patients with SSc lack either antibody,[51] and a minority (<1%) possess both antibodies,[48] such that, although clinically useful for disease classification and prognosis, they may not be used for definitive diagnoses.

Anti-RNA Polymerases

Anti–RNA polymerase (RNAP) antibodies, which target the eukaryotic RNA polymerases (see the section on SLE: Anti–RNAP), are associated with diffuse cutaneous involvement. Although anti–RNAP II antibodies appear in other diseases, such as SLE or overlap syndrome, and may be associated with other autoantibody specificities against Ku or RNPs, anti–RNAP I and III antibodies appear to be specific for SSc, and they may be useful for the prediction of renal crisis. RNAP III antibodies in particular may predict diffuse cutaneous SSc, including higher skin score, tendon friction rubs, and renal crisis, and are associated with an increased risk of cancer, particularly of the lung.[52,53]

Anti–polymyositis Scleroderma

Anti–polymyositis scleroderma (anti–PM-Scl) antibodies target the PM-Scl-75 and PM-Scl-100 components of the exosome, an exoribonuclease complex that regulates rRNA.[54] Responses against PM-Scl-75 alone appear more common among patients with diffuse SSc, whereas overlap syndromes are typically associated with responses against both components.[55] Its presence associates with myositis-SSc overlap without SLE features: 50% of anti–PM-Scl antibody–positive patients have the overlap, whereas 25% of the patients with the overlap have the antibody.[56,57]

Other SSc-Related ANAs

Several other specificities have been described in SSc, with possible prognostic implications, including (1) anti-fibrillarin, which targets a component of the U3 small nucleolar (sno) RNP and may associate with diffuse disease, including internal organ or skeletal muscle involvement or pulmonary hypertension; (2) anti-topoisomerase II, which appears to associate with pulmonary hypertension, as well as localized scleroderma; (3) anti-Th (Th snoRNP, mitochondrial RNA processing ribonuclease [RNase]), which may predict pulmonary hypertension, limited cutaneous disease, puffy fingers, small-bowel involvement, hypothyroidism, and reduced arthritis or arthralgias; (4) antibodies against the nuclear phosphoprotein B23, which appear to associate with pulmonary hypertension and anti-fibrillarin antibodies; (5) antibodies against the RNAP II transcription activator Sp1, which seem to correlate with RP and other signs of undifferentiated CTDs; (6) TNF translational regulator specificities, which may associate with lung involvement; (7) anti-U11/U12 RNP antibodies, which appear to correlate with pulmonary fibrosis; and (8) anti–nucleolar organizer region (NOR) 90 (human upstream binding factor). Other ANAs described in SSc include several specificities characteristically observed in other CTDs, such as histone, Ku, Ro, tRNA, snRNP, and anti-neutrophil cytoplasmic antibody (ANCA), although their clinical relevance in SSc remains unclear.

Inflammatory Muscle Diseases

Inflammatory muscle diseases comprise a diverse group of illnesses often characterized by autoantibody responses against cytoplasmic antigens. Although between 40% and 80% of patients with polymyositis/dermatomyositis (PM/DM) have positive ANA, as many as 90% of patients with all types of inflammatory muscle diseases have autoantibodies to cellular antigens.[58] Myositis autoantibodies are generally categorized into myositis-specific autoantibodies (MSAs), which are considered exclusive to inflammatory myositis, and those associated with overlap syndromes that include myositis (Tables 58.2 and 58.5).

Myositis-Specific Autoantibodies

The most well-characterized MSAs include the anti-amino acyl tRNA synthetases, which target different aminoacyl-tRNA synthetases.[59] Some of these antibodies target the tRNA anticodon loop, enabling them to inhibit enzymatic activity. The individual prevalence of these antibodies varies, but their clinical associations remain similar: Although PM appears more commonly with anti–Jo-1, and DM is more common with the other synthetases, these specificities together correlate with the "anti-synthetase syndrome," which includes interstitial lung disease, arthritis, RP, "mechanic's hands," hyperkeratotic lines, sclerodactyly, facial telangiectasia, calcinosis, and sicca, generally with a relatively poor prognosis.[60] Recent studies have suggested that anti–Jo-1 antibody levels may correlate with disease activity, as well as the IFN-γ–inducible chemokines CXCL9 and CXCL10.[61] Nonetheless, other disease associations have been reported that are distinct from the anti-synthetase syndrome; for example, one study has associated anti–threonyl-tRNA synthetase antibodies with fetal loss and severe relapsing myositis.[62] A relatively rare activity, anti-KS, has been described against the asparaginyl-tRNA synthetase in a few patients with interstitial lung disease and inflammatory arthritis or undifferentiated CTD,[63] and PL-7 antibodies may correlate with milder muscle disease.[64]

Other MSAs include specificities against Mi-2, a component of the nucleosome remodeling–deacetylase (NuRD) complex involved in chromatin remodeling and transcription regulation, which associates with DM and dermatologic manifestations such as the "shawl" and "V" signs and ultraviolet light exposure,[65] and Mas, a UGA suppressor serine tRNA that carries selenocysteine (tRNA$^{[Ser]Sec}$). Antibodies against the signal recognition particle, the cytoplasmic RNP that translocates nascent proteins across the endoplasmic reticulum, have been reported to be MSAs that associate with acute, severe, treatment-resistant disease; however, findings of recent studies are conflicting.[66] Other specificities, like anti-p155 (transcriptional intermediary factor [TIF1]-γ), anti-p140 (MJ, nuclear matrix protein NXP-2), and anti–CADM-140, represent novel MSAs useful in the distinction of cancer-associated myositis.

TABLE 58.5 Anti-nuclear Antibodies in Inflammatory Muscle Diseases

Antibody Specificity	Prevalence (%)	Disease Specificity	Major Disease Associations
Anti-amino acyl tRNA synthetases			**Anti-amino acyl synthetase syndrome**
Histidyl (Jo-1)	**20-30**	Myositis	
Threonyl (PL-7)	1-5	Myositis	
Alanyl (PL-12)	1-5	Myositis	
Glycyl (EJ)	1-5	Myositis	
Isoleucyl (OJ)	1-5	Myositis	
Asparaginyl (KS)	?	Overlap	
Selenocysteine (Mas)	1-2	Myositis	?
Mi-2	**8 (15-20% of DM)**	Myositis[a]	**Dermatologic involvement**
Signal recognition particle	4	No	
KJ	<1	Myositis[a]	
Proteasome	62	No	
Histone	17	No	
RNPs		No	
U1 snRNP	12		MCTD features
U2 snRNP	3		
Ro	10		
La	?		
PM-Scl	8	Overlap	Overlap
Elongation factor 1α (Fer)	1	No	
Histone	?	No	
Ku	?	Overlap	
U3 snoRNP	?	Overlap	

Shown are the major anti-nuclear antibody specificities described in inflammatory myositis, along with estimated prevalence and disease associations (*bold* indicates data supported by multiple studies). See text for details.

[a]Often referred to as myositis-specific autoantibodies (MSAs).

DM, Dermatomyositis; *MCTD,* mixed connective tissue disease; *RNP,* ribonucleoprotein; *snRNP,* small nuclear ribonucleoprotein; *snoRNP,* small nucleolar ribonucleoprotein; *tRNA,* transfer RNA.

Myositis Overlap Autoantibodies

The most well-described myositis overlap–associated ANAs include snRNP and PM-Scl specificities. In myositis, anti-snRNP antibodies typically target U1 snRNP, although a few anti-Sm and anti–U2 snRNP specificities have been described (see SLE: Anti-snRNP). The former tend to associate with features of MCTD, including SLE-myositis overlap, myositis-SSc overlap, and undifferentiated features (RP, puffy fingers, and arthritis) later progressing to myositis, possibly responding to corticosteroids,[67] whereas anti–U2 snRNP associates with myositis and sclerodactyly, sometimes with SLE, and usually without interstitial lung disease.[38] Anti–PM-Scl antibodies associate with myositis-SSc overlap without SLE features (50% of anti–PM-Scl antibody–positive patients have overlap, whereas 25% of patients with overlap have the antibody), and they also associate with arthritis, DM skin lesions, calcinosis, mechanic's hands, and eczema.[56] Other antibodies associated with myositis in overlap syndromes include several specificities found in other diseases, such as Ku, found more commonly in SLE and SSc, and U3 snoRNP (fibrillarin), which is associated with myositis in SSc, especially of the diffuse type. Several other specificities have also been described in inflammatory myositis, although their clinical significance remains largely undefined (see Table 58.5).

Primary Sjögren's Syndrome

In individuals with pSS, reported incidences of positive FANAs range widely, reflecting differences in study populations and disease criteria, and they depend heavily on the inclusion or exclusion of secondary, CTD-related disease, which increases the likelihood and amplitude of positive tests.[68] Thus, although ANA positivity as low as 40% has been reported, many studies report frequencies of 90% to 96%,[69] with a diverse range of autoantibodies, including both ubiquitous (Tables 58.2 and 58.6) and tissue-specific reactivities, such as anti-thyroid, gastric parietal cell, and muscarinic receptor. Such issues hinder interpretation of disease associations and disease specificities of ANAs in pSS.

Of the pSS ANA specificities, the most well-characterized remain Ro (SS-A) and La (SS-B), two nuclear RNPs involved in RNA metabolism (see SLE: anti-Ro/SS-A and anti-La/SS-B),[70] as well as fodrin (nonerythroid spectrin), a cytoskeletal heterodimer composed of α and β subunits that are structurally and functionally similar to erythroid spectrin. Anti-Ro antibodies appear in approximately 40% to 95% of patients with pSS, are associated with a number of extraglandular manifestations, including serologic association with anti-La and rheumatoid factor, and, interestingly, may result from genetically linked alternative mRNA processing of Ro.[71] Similarly, anti-La antibodies appear in as many as 87% of patients with pSS and are also associated with extraglandular manifestations and serologic association with anti-Ro and rheumatoid factor.[21] Antibodies against α-fodrin have been detected in 64% to 67% of patients,[72] but they are relatively uncommon in other CTDs such as SLE. Preliminary analyses suggest some extraglandular and serologic associations. In contrast, antibodies against β-fodrin have been described in as many as 70% of patients, but clinical associations have not been reported.[73] Several other specificities have been reported in pSS in a significant proportion (>3%) of patients, including antibodies against MA-I, a 200 kDa protein localized to the mitotic apparatus in dividing cells (which may be identical to NuMA); p80-Coilin, an 80 kDa protein associated with nuclear coiled bodies (although this antibody might not be CTD specific); as well as specificities characteristically found in other rheumatic diseases, such as kinetochore and perinuclear ANCAs, although their clinical importance remains uncertain (see Table 58.6).

Overlap Syndromes

Overlap syndromes of CTD remain matters of nosological debate, but virtually all investigators concur that ANAs are universal in these

TABLE 58.6 **Anti-nuclear Antibodies in Primary Sjögren's Syndrome**[a]

Antibody Specificity	Prevalence (%)	SS-Specific?	Major Disease Associations
Ro/SS-A	**40-95**	No	**Neonatal LE and CHB**
La/SS-B	**80-90**	No	**Neonatal LE**
Fodrin	**64-100**	Possibly	
α-fodrin	64-67 (100 in pediatric?)		
β-fodrin	70		
Proteasome	39	No	
Pyruvate dehydrogenase	27	No	
p-ANCA	11-40	No	
Calponin-3	11	No	
MA-I	8	Possibly	
Mitochondrial	6.6	No	
pp75 (Ro-associated protein)	6	No	
Kinetochore	4	No	
p80-coilin	4	Possibly	

[a]Shown are the major anti-nuclear antibody specificities described in primary Sjögren's syndrome, along with estimated prevalence and disease associations (*bold* indicates data supported by multiple studies). See text for details.

CHB, Congenital heart block; *LE*, lupus erythematosus; *p-ANCA*, peripheral anti-neutrophil cytoplasmic antibody; *pSS*, primary Sjögren's syndrome.

conditions.[74] Indeed, since the initial formal description of MCTD in 1972, the presence of anti–U1 snRNP antibodies has been consistently required for classification and/or diagnosis, with associated ANA titers typically exceeding 1:1000 and often 1:10,000.[75] However, several investigations have noted that many such patients experience manifestations, both clinical and serologic, that allow the diagnosis of a defined CTD, such as SLE, RA, SSc, or PM/DM,[76] and therefore the accuracy of specific clinical associations of specific ANAs in "overlap" settings is hindered by issues of disease classification. Therefore, in such instances, it seems most reasonable to base the importance of individual autoantibody specificities upon their primary disease association, despite the lack of definitive, well-codified evidence (e.g., anti-topoisomerase I as predictive of eventual diffuse SSc-like skin disease or pulmonary fibrosis, or anti-dsDNA for lupus-like glomerulonephritis).

Other Conditions

In contrast to the traditional ANA diseases, the presence of a positive ANA in other diseases remains largely unhelpful for diagnosis, although in RP, juvenile idiopathic arthritis (JIA), and antiphospholipid antibody syndrome (APS), it can aid prognosis (see Table 58.1). In RP, a positive result increases the likelihood, from 19% to 30%, of the development of a systemic rheumatic disease, including SLE, RA, and SSc, whereas a negative result decreases the likelihood to approximately 7%, which is often helpful for patient reassurance.[77] In JIA, ANA positivity may predict the development of uveitis,[78] and in APS, it may predict the development or presence of underlying SLE.[79] Other conditions in which ANAs have been found include other rheumatic diseases such as the vasculitides or sarcoidosis; autoimmune diseases such as multiple sclerosis or inflammatory illnesses such as inflammatory bowel disease; and an ever-growing list of additional conditions, including dermatologic, infectious, psychiatric, neurologic, and cardiovascular diseases.

Clinical Utility of Anti-nuclear Antibody Testing

The ANAs encompass a wide range of nuclear, nucleolar, and cytoplasmic autoantigen specificities. Within the ANA diseases, including SLE, SSc, PM/DM, pSS, and MCTD, many autoantibodies possess unique rheumatologic associations, but the specificity of these associations has diminished over recent years as assay sensitivity has increased, resulting in the detection of these specificities in rheumatic and nonrheumatic diseases. Consequently, tests for ANAs have only an adjunct role in the diagnosis of rheumatic disease, but still may aid the clinical evaluation of patients in the context of their particular disease.

Fig. 58.3 describes an algorithm for the rheumatologic evaluation of a patient for ANAs. In most clinical laboratories, the FANA serves as a screening test, with a positive result often prompting "cascade" testing by the laboratory and/or ordering physician for specific autoantibody specificities, such as anti-dsDNA, anti-Ro/SS-A, anti-La/SS-B, anti-RNP, and anti-Sm.[1] A negative or low-titer FANA in the setting of a low clinical suspicion of rheumatic disease usually indicates the absence of significant ANAs and argues against the diagnosis of one of the ANA diseases (see Table 58.1)[80]; however, if the clinical picture strongly suggests CTD, further investigation may involve specific assays for antigens that are often FANA negative, such as Ro/SS-A, Jo-1, or phospholipids. On the other hand, because some specific ANAs possess diagnostic significance, positive FANA results usually warrant follow-up with specialized assays,

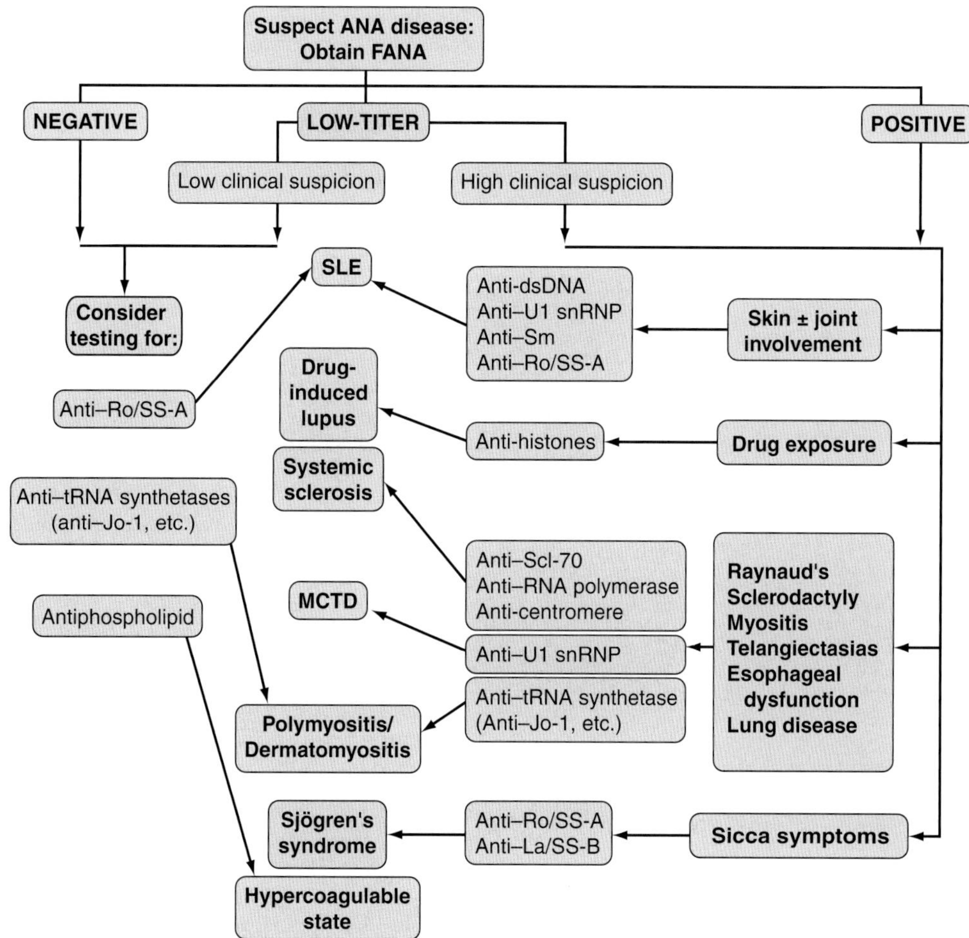

• **Fig. 58.3** Algorithm for the use of anti-nuclear antibodies (ANAs) in the diagnosis of connective tissue disorders. See text for details. *anti-tRNA,* Anti–amino acyl transfer RNA; *dsDNA,* double-stranded DNA; *FANA,* fluorescent anti-nuclear antibody; *MCTD,* mixed connective tissue disease; *SLE,* systemic lupus erythematosus; *snRNP,* small nuclear ribonucleoprotein; *SS,* Sjögren's syndrome.

but only in the setting of strong clinical suspicion, because the positive predictive value of an ANA in the absence of other clinical signs of CTD is low, in part because ANAs may precede clinical disease by many years,[81,82] and in part because of the relatively high incidence of ANA in healthy people.[23] Thus, if SLE features are present, further work may focus on anti-DNA, anti-Sm, anti–RNP/U1 snRNP, and anti-Ro antibodies. Similarly, if MCTD, pSS, SSc, or polymyositis are suspected, the serum may be tested, respectively, for anti–U1 snRNP; anti-Ro or anti-La; anti-topoisomerase I, anti-centromere, or anti-nucleoli; or anti–amino acyl tRNA synthetases. If these tests are negative in the setting of high clinical suspicion, repeat testing at a later date may be warranted because titers of such autoantibodies can fluctuate over time, irrespective of disease course.[83] Positive results in these more specialized assays do not alone signify specific diseases, but rather add weight to diagnoses that should throughout the evaluation rely heavily on other clinical information. Indeed, many clinical and research studies upon which autoantibody-disease associations have been developed often utilized highly refined detection methods, such as immunoprecipitation or immunoblot, which are generally unavailable in routine clinical laboratory testing. Thus the relevance of many antibody-test results in specific clinical settings continues to require careful, individualized interpretation by the referring physician.[84]

The references for this chapter can also be found on ExpertConsult.com.

References

1. Agmon-Levin N, Damoiseaux J, Kallenberg C, et al.: International recommendations for the assessment of autoantibodies to cellular antigens referred to as anti-nuclear antibodies, *Ann Rheum Dis* 73:17–23, 2014.
2. Tan EM: The L.E. cell and its legacy. 1948, *Clin Exp Rheumatol* 16:652–658, 1998.
3. Friou GJ: Clinical application of lupus serum nucleoprotein reaction using fluorescent antibody technique, *J Clin Invest* 36:890, 1957.
4. Hahn BH: Antibodies to DNA, *N Engl J Med* 338:1359–1368, 1998.
5. Deng SX, Hanson E, Sanz I: In vivo cell penetration and intracellular transport of anti-Sm and anti-La autoantibodies, *Int Immunol* 12:415–423, 2000.
6. Kim D, Peck A, Santer D, et al.: Induction of interferon-α by scleroderma sera containing autoantibodies to topoisomerase I: association of higher interferon-alpha activity with lung fibrosis, *Arthritis Rheum* 58:2163–2173, 2008.
7. Barbasso Helmers S, Englund P, Engström M, et al.: Sera from anti-Jo-1-positive patients with polymyositis and interstitial lung disease induce expression of intercellular adhesion molecule 1 in human lung endothelial cells, *Arthritis Rheum* 60:2524–2530, 2009.

8. Eloranta ML, Barbasso Helmers S, Ulfgren AK, et al.: A possible mechanism for endogenous activation of the type I interferon system in myositis patients with anti-Jo-1 or anti-Ro 52/anti-Ro 60 autoantibodies, *Arthritis Rheum* 56:3112–3124, 2007.
9. Niewold TB, Rivera TL, Buyon JP, et al.: Serum type I interferon activity is dependent on maternal diagnosis in anti-SSA/Ro-positive mothers of children with neonatal lupus, *Arthritis Rheum* 58:541–546, 2008.
10. Levine SM, Raben N, Xie D, et al.: Novel conformation of histidyl-transfer RNA synthetase in the lung: the target tissue in Jo-1 autoantibody-associated myositis, *Arthritis Rheum* 56:2729–2739, 2007.
11. Reed JH, Jackson MW, Gordon TP: A B cell apotope of Ro 60 in systemic lupus erythematosus, *Arthritis Rheum* 58:1125–1129, 2008.
12. Reed JH, Giannakopoulos B, Jackson MW, et al.: Ro 60 functions as a receptor for β(2)-glycoprotein I on apoptotic cells, *Arthritis Rheum* 60:860–869, 2009.
13. McCormack WJ, Parker AE, O'Neill LA: Toll-like receptors and NOD-like receptors in rheumatic diseases, *Arthritis Res Ther* 11:243, 2009.
14. Robitaille G, Christin MS, Clement I, et al.: Nuclear autoantigen CENP-B transactivation of the epidermal growth factor receptor via chemokine receptor 3 in vascular smooth muscle cells, *Arthritis Rheum* 60:2805–2816, 2009.
15. Visentini M, Conti V, Cagliuso M, et al.: Regression of systemic lupus erythematosus after development of an acquired toll-like receptor signaling defect and antibody deficiency, *Arthritis Rheum* 60:2767–2771, 2009.
16. Kavanaugh A, Tomar R, Reveille J, et al.: Guidelines for clinical use of the antinuclear antibody test and tests for specific autoantibodies to nuclear antigens. American College of Pathologists, *Arch Pathol Lab Med* 124:71–81, 2000.
17. American College of Rheumatology: Position statement. Methodology of testing for antinuclear antibodies. Available at http://www.rheumatology.org/Portals/0/Files/Methodology%20of%20Testing%20Antinuclear%20Antibodies%20Position%20Statement.pdf, 2009.
18. Mariz HA, Sato EI, Barbosa SH, et al.: Pattern on the antinuclear antibody-HEp-2 test is a critical parameter for discriminating antinuclear antibody-positive healthy individuals and patients with autoimmune rheumatic diseases, *Arthritis Rheum* 63:191–200, 2011.
19. Mahler M, Fritzler MJ: The clinical significance of the dense fine speckled immunofluorescence pattern on HEp-2 cells for the diagnosis of systemic autoimmune diseases, *Clin Dev Immunol* 2012:494356, 2012.
20. Damoiseaux J, von Mühlen CA, Garcia-De La Torre I, et al.: International consensus on ANA patterns (ICAP): the bumpy road towards a consensus on reporting ANA results, *Auto Immun Highlights* 7:1, 2016.
21. Vermeersch P, Bossuyt X: Prevalence and clinical significance of rare antinuclear antibody patterns, *Autoimmun Rev* 12:998–1003, 2013.
22. Willems P, De Langhe E, Westhovens R, et al.: Antinuclear antibody as entry criterion for classification of systemic lupus erythematosus: pitfalls and opportunities, *Ann Rheum Dis* 78:e76, 2019.
23. Tan EM, Feltkamp TE, Smolen JS, et al.: Range of antinuclear antibodies in "healthy" individuals, *Arthritis Rheum* 40:1601–1611, 1997.
24. Satoh M, Chan EK, Ho LA, et al.: Prevalence and sociodemographic correlates of antinuclear antibodies in the United States, *Arthritis Rheum* 64:2319–2327, 2012.
25. Abeles AM, Abeles M: The clinical utility of a positive antinuclear antibody test result, *Am J Med* 126:342–348, 2013.
26. Cross LS, Aslam A, Misbah SA: Antinuclear antibody-negative lupus as a distinct diagnostic entity—does it no longer exist? *QJM* 97:303–308, 2004.
27. To CH, Petri M: Is antibody clustering predictive of clinical subsets and damage in systemic lupus erythematosus? *Arthritis Rheum* 52:4003–4010, 2005.
28. Bizzaro N, Villalta D, Giavarina D, et al.: Are anti-nucleosome antibodies a better diagnostic marker than anti-dsDNA antibodies for systemic lupus erythematosus? a systematic review and a study of metanalysis, *Autoimmun Rev* 12:97–106, 2012.
29. Rekvig OP, van der Vlag J, Seredkina N: Review: antinucleosome antibodies: a critical reflection on their specificities and diagnostic impact, *Arthritis Rheumatol* 66:1061–1069, 2014.
30. Kavanaugh AF, Solomon DH: American College of Rheumatology ad hoc committee on immunologic testing guidelines: guidelines for immunologic laboratory testing in the rheumatic diseases: anti-DNA antibody tests, *Arthritis Rheum* 47:546–555, 2002.
31. Yung S, Chan TM: Mechanisms of kidney injury in lupus nephritis—the role of anti dsDNA antibodies, *Front Immunol* 6:475, 2015.
32. Williams EL, Gadola S, Edwards CJ: Anti-TNF-induced lupus, *Rheumatology* 48:716–720, 2009.
33. Lapteva L, Nowak M, Yarboro CH, et al.: Anti-*N*-methyl-D-aspartate receptor antibodies, cognitive dysfunction, and depression in systemic lupus erythematosus, *Arthritis Rheum* 54:2505–2514, 2006.
34. Harrison MJ, Ravdin LD, Lockshin MD: Relationship between serum NR2a antibodies and cognitive dysfunction in systemic lupus erythematosus, *Arthritis Rheum* 54:2515–2522, 2006.
35. Compagno M, Jacobsen S, Rekvig OP, et al.: Low diagnostic and predictive value of anti-dsDNA antibodies in unselected patients with recent onset of rheumatic symptoms: results from a long-term follow-up Scandinavian multicentre study, *Scand J Rheumatol* 42:311–316, 2013.
36. Belizna C, Henrion D, Beucher A, et al.: Anti-Ku antibodies: clinical, genetic and diagnostic insights, *Autoimmun Rev* 9:691–694, 2010.
37. Migliorini P, Baldini C, Rocchi V, et al.: Anti-Sm and anti-RNP antibodies, *Autoimmunity* 38:47–54, 2005.
38. Peng SL, Craft J: Spliceosomal snRNPs autoantibodies. In Peter JB, Shoenfeld Y, editors: *Autoantibodies*, Amsterdam, 1996, Elsevier, p 774.
39. Benito-Garcia E, Schur PH, Lahita R, et al.: Guidelines for immunologic laboratory testing in the rheumatic diseases: anti-Sm and anti-RNP antibody tests, *Arthritis Rheum* 51:1030–1044, 2004.
40. Sato T, Fujii T, Yokoyama T, et al.: Anti-U1 RNP antibodies in cerebrospinal fluid are associated with central neuropsychiatric manifestations in systemic lupus erythematosus and mixed connective tissue disease, *Arthritis Rheum* 62:3730–3740, 2010.
41. Schulte-Pelkum J, Fritzler M, Mahler M: Latest update on the Ro/SS-A autoantibody system, *Autoimmunity Rev* 8:632–637, 2009.
42. St Clair EW: Anti-La antibodies, *Rheum Dis Clin North Am* 18:359–376, 1992.
43. Hanly JG, Urowitz MB, Siannis F, et al.: Autoantibodies and neuropsychiatric events at the time of systemic lupus erythematosus diagnosis: results from an international inception cohort study, *Arthritis Rheum* 58:843–853, 2008.
44. Segovia-Miranda F, Serrano F, Dyrda A, et al.: Pathogenicity of lupus anti-ribosomal P antibodies: role of cross-reacting neuronal surface P antigen in glutamatergic transmission and plasticity in a mouse model, *Arthritis Rheumatol* 67:1598–1610, 2015.
45. do Nascimento AP, Viana Vdos S, Testagrossa Lde A, et al.: Antibodies to ribosomal P proteins: a potential serologic marker for lupus membranous glomerulonephritis, *Arthritis Rheum* 54:1568–1572, 2006.
46. Elkon KB, Bonfa E, Brot N: Antiribosomal antibodies in systemic lupus erythematosus, *Rheum Dis Clin North Am* 18:377–390, 1992.
47. Nihtyanova SI, Denton CP: Autoantibodies as predictive tools in systemic sclerosis, *Nat Rev Immunol* 6:112–116, 2010.
48. Heijnen IA, Foocharoen C, Bannert B, et al.: Clinical significance of coexisting antitopoisomerase I and anticentromere antibodies in patients with systemic sclerosis: a EUSTAR group-based study, *Clin Exp Rheumatol* 31:96–102, 2013.
49. Patterson KA, Roberts-Thomson PJ, Lester S, et al.: Interpretation of an extended autoantibody profile in a well-characterized australian systemic sclerosis (scleroderma) cohort using principal components analysis, *Arthritis Rheumatol* 67:3234–3244, 2015.
50. Reveille JD, Solomon DH: American College of Rheumatology ad hoc committee of immunologic testing guidelines: evidence-based

guidelines for the use of immunologic tests: anticentromere, Scl-70, and nucleolar antibodies, *Arthritis Rheum* 49:399–412, 2003.
51. Spencer-Green G, Alter D, Welch HG: Test performance in systemic sclerosis: anti-centromere and anti-Scl-70 antibodies, *Am J Med* 103:242–248, 1997.
52. Meyer O, De Chaisemartin L, Nicaise-Roland P, et al.: Anti-RNA polymerase III antibody prevalence and associated clinical manifestations in a large series of French patients with systemic sclerosis: a cross-sectional study, *J Rheumatol* 37:125–130, 2010.
53. Sobanski V, Dauchet L, Lefevre G, et al.: Prevalence of anti-RNA polymerase III antibodies in systemic sclerosis: new data from a French cohort and a systematic review and meta-analysis, *Arthritis Rheumatol* 66:407–417, 2014.
54. Raijmakers R, Renz M, Wiemann C, et al.: PM-Scl-75 is the main autoantigen in patients with the polymyositis/scleroderma overlap syndrome, *Arthritis Rheum* 50:565–569, 2004.
55. Hanke K, Bruckner CS, Dahnrich C, et al.: Antibodies against PM/Scl-75 and PM/Scl-100 are independent markers for different subsets of systemic sclerosis patients, *Arthritis Res Ther* 11:R22, 2009.
56. Oddis CV, Okano Y, Rudert WA, et al.: Serum autoantibody to the nucleolar antigen PM-Scl. clinical and immunogenetic associations, *Arthritis Rheum* 35:1211–1217, 1992.
57. D'Aoust J, Hudson M, Tatibouet S, et al.: Clinical and serologic correlates of anti-PM/Scl antibodies in systemic sclerosis: a multicenter study of 763 patients, *Arthritis Rheumatol* 66:1608–1615, 2014.
58. Love LA, Leff RL, Fraser DD, et al.: A new approach to the classification of idiopathic inflammatory myopathy: myositis-specific autoantibodies define useful homogeneous patient groups, *Medicine* 70:360–374, 1991.
59. Mahler M, Miller FW, Fritzler MJ: Idiopathic inflammatory myopathies and the anti-synthetase syndrome: a comprehensive review, *Autoimmun Rev* 13:367–371, 2014.
60. Imbert-Masseau A, Hamidou M, Agard C, et al.: Antisynthetase syndrome, *Joint Bone Spine* 70:161–168, 2003.
61. Richards TJ, Eggebeen A, Gibson K, et al.: Characterization and peripheral blood biomarker assessment of anti-Jo-1 antibody-positive interstitial lung disease, *Arthritis Rheum* 60:2183–2192, 2009.
62. Satoh M, Ajmani AK, Hirakata M, et al.: Onset of polymyositis with autoantibodies to threonyl-tRNA synthetase during pregnancy, *J Rheumatol* 21:1564–1566, 1994.
63. Hirakata M, Suwa A, Nagai S, et al.: Anti-KS: identification of autoantibodies to asparaginyl-transfer RNA synthetase associated with interstitial lung disease, *J Immunol* 162:2315–2320, 1999.
64. Yamasaki Y, Yamada H, Nozaki T, et al.: Unusually high frequency of autoantibodies to PL-7 associated with milder muscle disease in Japanese patients with polymyositis/dermatomyositis, *Arthritis Rheum* 54:2004–2009, 2006.
65. Love LA, Weinberg CR, McConnaughey DR, et al.: Ultraviolet radiation intensity predicts the relative distribution of dermatomyositis and anti-Mi-2 autoantibodies in women, *Arthritis Rheum* 60:2499–2504, 2009.
66. Kao AH, Lacomis D, Lucas M, et al.: Anti-signal recognition particle autoantibody in patients with and patients without idiopathic inflammatory myopathy, *Arthritis Rheum* 50:209–215, 2004.
67. Lundberg I, Nennesmo I, Hedfors E: A clinical, serological, and histopathological study of myositis patients with and without anti-RNP antibodies, *Sem Arthritis Rheum* 22:127–138, 1992.
68. Solomon DH, Kavanaugh AJ, Schur PH, et al.: Evidence-based guidelines for the use of immunologic tests: antinuclear antibody testing, *Arthritis Rheum* 47:434–444, 2002.
69. Harley JB, Alexander EL, Bias WB, et al.: Anti-Ro (SS-A) and anti-La (SS-B) in patients with Sjögren's syndrome, *Arthritis Rheum* 29:196–206, 1986.
70. Hernandez-Molina G, Leal-Alegre G, Michel-Peregrina M: The meaning of anti-Ro and anti-La antibodies in primary Sjögren's syndrome, *Autoimmun Rev* 10:123–125, 2011.
71. Nakken B, Jonsson R, Bolstad AI: Polymorphisms of the Ro52 gene associated with anti-Ro 52-kd autoantibodies in patients with primary Sjögren's syndrome, *Arthritis Rheum* 44:638–646, 2001.
72. Haneji N, Nakamura T, Takio K, et al.: Identification of α-fodrin as a candidate autoantigen in primary Sjögren's syndrome, *Science* 276:604–607, 1997.
73. Kuwana M, Okano T, Ogawa Y, et al.: Autoantibodies to the amino-terminal fragment of β-fodrin expressed in glandular epithelial cells in patients with Sjögren's syndrome, *J Immunol* 167:5449–5456, 2001.
74. Smolen JS, Steiner G: Mixed connective tissue disease: to be or not to be? *Arthritis Rheum* 41:768–777, 1998.
75. Greidinger EL, Hoffman RW: Autoantibodies in the pathogenesis of mixed connective tissue disease, *Rheum Dis Clin North Am* 31:437–450, 2005.
76. van den Hoogen FH, Spronk PE, Boerbooms AM, et al.: Long-term follow-up of 46 patients with anti-(U1)snRNP antibodies, *Br J Rheumatol* 33:1117–1120, 1994.
77. Koenig M, Joyal F, Fritzler MJ, et al.: Autoantibodies and microvascular damage are independent predictive factors for the progression of Raynaud's phenomenon to systemic sclerosis: a twenty-year prospective study of 586 patients, with validation of proposed criteria for early systemic sclerosis, *Arthritis Rheum* 58:3902–3912, 2008.
78. Nordal EB, Songstad NT, Berntson L, et al.: Biomarkers of chronic uveitis in juvenile idiopathic arthritis: predictive value of antihistone antibodies and antinuclear antibodies, *J Rheumatol* 36:1737–1743, 2009.
79. Petri M: Diagnosis of antiphospholipid antibodies, *Rheum Dis Clin North Am* 20:443–469, 1994.
80. Thomson KF, Murphy A, Goodfield MJ, et al.: Is it useful to test for antibodies to extractable nuclear antigens in the presence of a negative antinuclear antibody on Hep-2 cells? *J Clin Pathol* 54:413, 2001.
81. Arbuckle MR, McClain MT, Rubertone MV, et al.: Development of autoantibodies before the clinical onset of systemic lupus erythematosus, *N Engl J Med* 349:1526–1533, 2003.
82. Theander E, Jonsson R, Sjöström B, et al.: Prediction of Sjögren's syndrome years before diagnosis and identification of patients with early onset and severe disease course by autoantibody profiling, *Arthritis Rheumatol* 67:2427–2436, 2015.
83. Faria AC, Barcellos KS, Andrade LE: Longitudinal fluctuation of antibodies to extractable nuclear antigens in systemic lupus erythematosus, *J Rheumatol* 32:1267–1272, 2005.
84. Illei GG, Klippel JH: Why is the ANA result positive? *Bull Rheum Dis* 48:1–4, 1999.

59

Autoantibodies in Rheumatoid Arthritis

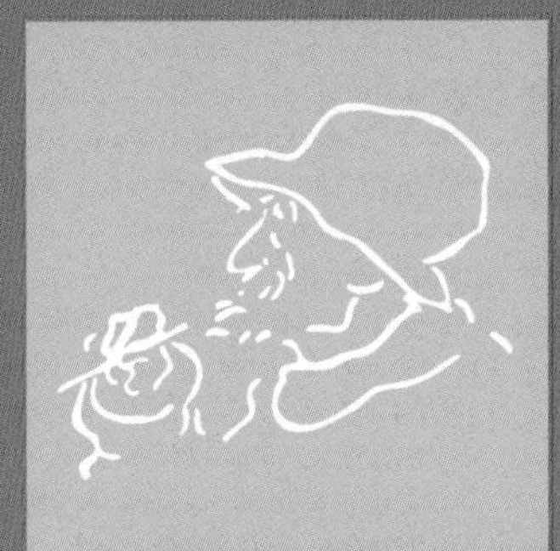

ERIKA DARRAH, ANTONY ROSEN, AND FELIPE ANDRADE

KEY POINTS

- Autoantibodies in rheumatoid arthritis (RA) have diagnostic and prognostic value.
- Autoantibodies precede the onset of clinical RA, which supports their potential role in disease pathogenesis and as important tools for defining pathogenic pathways in this disease.
- An increasing number of autoantibody specificities have been defined in RA, which include components involved in the process of citrullination (both enzymes and substrates), chemically modified autoantigens (carbamylated and malondialdehyde-acetaldehyde [MAA] adducts), and unmodified (native) proteins.
- Anti-citrullinated protein antibodies (ACPAs) are hallmarks of the immune response in RA.
- ACPAs identify an autoimmune process in RA that is linked to genetic factors, such as *HLA-DRβ1* alleles (collectively referred to as *shared epitope alleles*) and polymorphisms in the *PTPN22* gene, as well as environmental factors, such as smoking and infection.
- Autoantibodies targeting citrullinating enzymes (i.e., peptidylarginine deiminases [PADs]) are also found in patients with RA.
- Anti-PAD4 antibodies are associated with more severe disease, making them useful as possible diagnostic and prognostic tools.
- Anti-PAD2 and anti-RA33 (heterogeneous nuclear ribonucleoprotein A2/B1) antibodies are associated with milder forms of RA.
- Rheumatoid factors (RFs) are autoantibodies that recognize the Fc portion of immunoglobulin G molecules and were the first autoantibodies described in RA.
- Although RFs have limited specificity for RA, they are useful markers of more severe disease.

Introduction

Autoantibodies have proven to be very useful tools for diagnosis and prediction in autoimmune rheumatic diseases. Emerging data from several autoimmune diseases have demonstrated that the clinical evolution of disease from the pre-clinical phase to overt clinical disease is marked by a change in the specificity of the immune response with autoantibodies directed against distinct antigenic targets at different disease phases. Whereas numerous autoimmune rheumatic diseases traditionally have been marked by highly phenotype-specific autoantibody responses (e.g., anti–double-stranded DNA antibodies in systemic lupus erythematosus [SLE] and high-titer anti-topoisomerase-1 antibodies in diffuse scleroderma), the discovery of highly specific autoantibody markers of rheumatoid arthritis (RA) lagged significantly behind these other diseases. During the past two decades, enormous progress has occurred in this area, largely fueled by the discovery that citrullinated proteins are specific targets of autoantibodies in RA. This finding has highlighted post-translational modifications (PTMs) as critical antigenic determinants targeted by autoantibodies in RA, which has led to the identification of novel autoantibody systems and pathogenic mechanisms in this disease.

It is now recognized that autoantibodies in RA target a large and diverse group of proteins (Table 59.1), which appear to reflect distinct pathogenic mechanisms and contribute to the marked clinical heterogeneity among patients with RA. In this chapter, we will review the known autoantibodies in RA with emphasis on discrete subgroups of autoantibodies that have distinct value for diagnosis, prognosis, and identifying pathogenic pathways. These subsets include citrullination-associated autoantibodies, antibodies to chemically modified proteins, and autoantibodies that are shared with other autoimmune and inflammatory diseases. The implications of these specificities for diagnosis and prediction of disease outcome, as well as for understanding pathogenic events in RA, will be highlighted.

Citrullination-Associated Autoantibodies

Citrulline residues in proteins are generated post-translationally through the deimination of arginine residues. This process, known as *citrullination*, is mediated by peptidylarginine deiminase (PAD) enzymes (Fig. 59.1A). Patients with RA can develop antibodies to the products of citrullination (i.e., citrullinated proteins) as well as the PAD enzymes themselves (i.e., PAD2 and PAD4). Among autoantibodies found in RA patients, citrullination-associated antibodies have the highest specificity for RA, making them unique clinical tools for disease diagnosis. These antibodies also provide clues into disease mechanisms, which suggests that understanding the process of citrullination and factors that lead to the reversal of immunologic tolerance to these proteins may provide a foundation for understanding the etiology of RA.

Antibodies to Citrullinated Proteins

Discovery of Autoantibodies to Citrullinated Antigens

The discovery of a novel type of autoantibody, by Nienhuis and Mandema in 1964, revolutionized the study of autoantibodies in RA (Fig. 59.2).[1] These investigators identified autoantibodies that

TABLE 59.1 **Autoantibodies in Rheumatoid Arthritis (RA)**

Subgroup	Antibody Type	Type of PTM	Antigen Generation	Antigen(s)	Prevalence of Autoantibodies
Citrullination-associated antibodies	ACPA[a]	Citrullination	Enzymatic • Conversion of arginine residues to citrulline by PAD enzymes	Vimentin, fibronectin, actin, HSP90, histones, α-enolase, eEF1a, CAP-1, CapZalpha-1, asporin, cathepsin D, histamine receptor, PDI, ER60 precursor, ALDH2, collagen type-I and II, eIF4GI, aldolase, PGK1, calreticulin, HSP60, FUSE-BP1 and 2, ApoE, MNDA, hnRNP-A2/B1 (RA33)[39–55]	Up to 80%[31,59,60]
	Anti-PAD2	None	Unknown	PAD2	18.5%[145]
	Anti-PAD4	None	Unknown	PAD4	23%-45%[147,148]
	Anti-PAD3/PAD4	None	Unknown	PAD4 (cross-reacts with PAD3)	10%-12%[151–154]
Antibodies to chemically modified antigens	Anti-CarP	Carbamylation	Nonenzymatic • Reaction of cyanate with lysine residues resulting in homocitrulline	Alpha-1-anti-trypsin Others unknown	45%[223]
	Anti-MAA	MAA adducts	Nonenzymatic • Peroxidation of membrane lipids generate reactive aldehydes that modify lysine residues generating MAA adducts	Unknown	~70% IgA[229] ~90% IgG ~40% IgM
Nonspecific RA antibodies	RF	None	Unknown	IgG (Fc)	50%-90%[59]
	Anti-RA33	None	Unknown	hnRNP-A2/B1	15%-35%[44,165,267]
	Anti-G6PI	None	Unknown	G6PI	12%-29%[276,277,279]

ACPA, Anti-citrullinated protein antibody; *ALDH2,* mitochondrial aldehyde dehydrogenase; *ApoE,* apolipoprotein E; *CAP1,* adenylyl cyclase-associated protein 1; *CapZalpha-1,* F-actin capping protein alpha-1 subunit; *CarP,* carbamylated protein; *eEF1a,* elongation factor 1-alpha; *eIF4GI,* eukaryotic translation initiation factor-4G1; *ER60,* endoplasmic reticulum resident protein 60 precursor; *FUSE-BP,* far upstream element binding protein; *G6PI,* glucose-6-phosphate isomerase; *hnRNP,* heterogeneous nuclear ribonucleoprotein; *HSP,* heat shock protein; *Ig,* immunoglobulin; *MAA,* malondialdehyde-acetaldehyde; *MNDA,* myeloid nuclear differentiation antigen; *PAD,* peptidylarginine deiminase; *PDI,* protein disulfide-isomerase; *PGK1,* phosphoglycerate kinase-1; *PTM,* post-translational modification.

[a]Detected by the anti-CCP assay

stained keratohyalin granules surrounding the nucleus in cells of human buccal mucosa, which they called *antiperinuclear factor* (APF). APF antibodies were found in 49% to 91% of patients with RA,[1–5] and had a reported disease specificity of 73% to 99%.[1,4–7] The assay was difficult to standardize because of variability in the staining of buccal mucosal cells from different donors,[8–11] and the assay did not find its way into routine clinical practice. However, the striking specificity of APF antibodies for RA suggested that the assay might be reporting on RA-specific pathogenic pathways. Later, it was found that RA sera recognized antigens in the stratified squamous layer of esophageal epithelium—a staining pattern they termed *antikeratin antibodies* (AKAs) (see Fig. 59.2).[12] Subsequent iterations of this assay utilized other forms of stratified squamous epithelium, including human skin.[13] Although the AKA assay also had very good specificity for RA, it was of limited sensitivity[14–17] and not particularly convenient or easy to standardize. Thus, neither assay was broadly used in the clinical diagnostic arena. Nonetheless, these assays provided a framework for antigen discovery that would later lead to highly specific and convenient tools for RA diagnosis and classification.

These advances came from studies which demonstrated that a neutral/acidic isoform of filaggrin (filament-aggregating protein) was the target of AKAs in human epidermis,[18] and that APF and AKAs were the same autoantibody (see Fig. 59.2).[19] Filaggrin is produced during the late stages of terminal differentiation of epithelial cells. It is synthesized as a heavily phosphorylated precursor protein called profilaggrin.[20] Profilaggrin is deposited in granules, and filaggrin is released by proteolytic cleavage during differentiation of the cells. Coincident with cleavage, the protein is dephosphorylated, and a significant proportion (~20%) of the arginine residues are deiminated (i.e., converted to citrulline)[21,22] in a reaction mediated by the PAD enzymes (see the section "Citrullinated Autoantigen Generation in Rheumatoid Arthritis").[23] Because RA sera appeared to specifically target the neutral isoform of filaggrin

A. Citrullination

PAD + Ca^{2+}

H_2N NH NH_2 Protein H_2O NH_3 O NH NH_2 Protein

Peptidyl-arginine Peptidyl-citrulline

B. Carbamylation

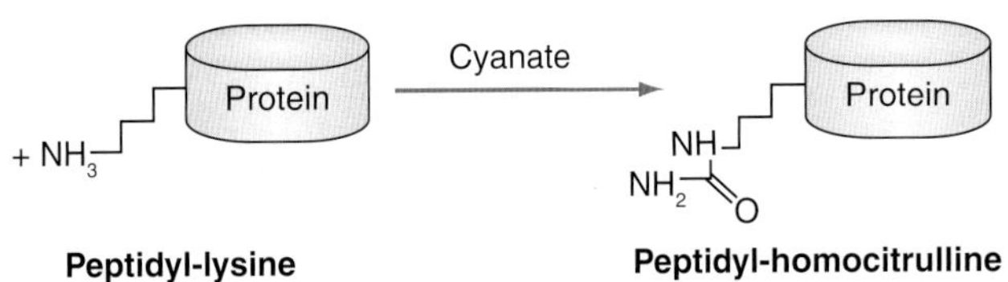

Peptidyl-lysine Peptidyl-homocitrulline

C. MAA adducts

AA + MDA FAAB MDHDC

+ NH_3 Protein Protein CH_3 Protein

Primary amine Malondialdehyde acetaldehyde adducts (MAA)

• **Fig. 59.1** Post-translational modifications targeted by autoantibodies in RA. (A) During citrullination, the calcium-dependent peptidylarginine deiminase (PAD) enzymes deiminate arginine residues in proteins, which results in the generation of citrulline residues and ammonia. (B) Carbamylation results from the reaction of cyanate with the primary amine group of peptidyl-lysine that converts to peptidyl-homocitrulline. (C) MAA adducts (FAAB, 2-formyl-3-[alkylamino] butanal and MDHDC [4-methyl-1,4-dihydropyridine-3,5-dicarbaldehyde]) generate from the reaction of malondialdehyde–acetaldehyde (MDA) and acetaldehyde (AA) with primary amine groups of amino acid residues, preferentially peptidyl-lysine.

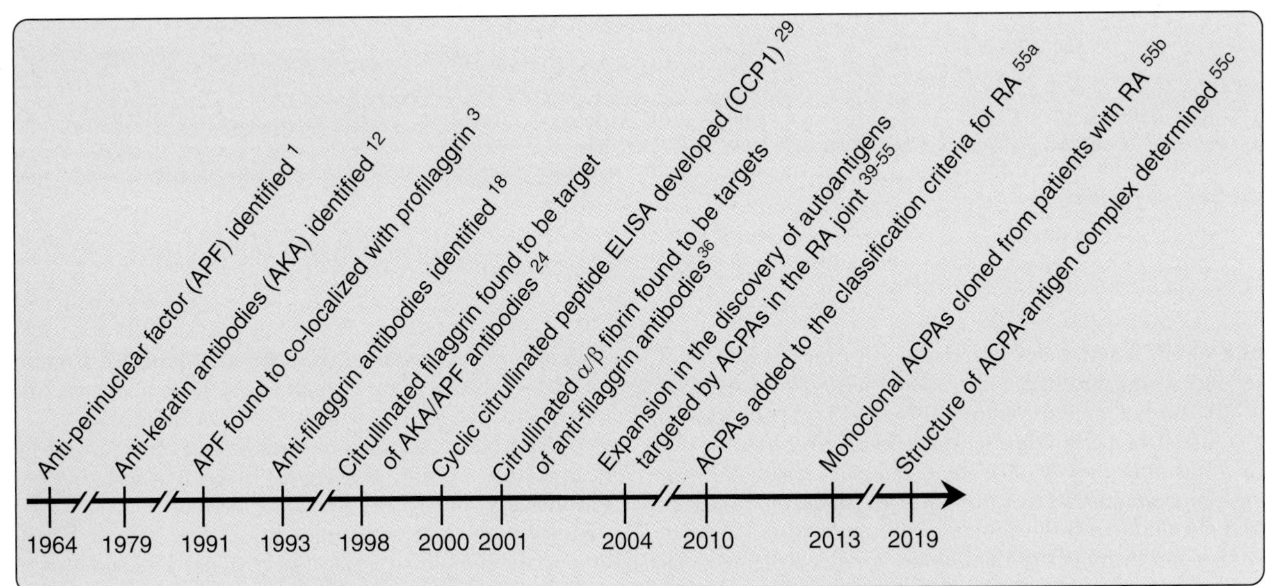

• **Fig. 59.2** A timeline of the discovery of anti-citrullinated protein antibodies in RA. *CCP1,* Cyclic citrullinated peptide; *ELISA,* enzyme-linked immunosorbent assay.

(which is present and citrullinated in fully differentiated squamous epithelia), studies were done to address whether RA sera, which were positive in the AKA/APF assays, specifically recognized citrullinated peptides.[24] Thus, regions within the deduced amino acid sequence of human profilaggrin, which had a high antigenicity index and the largest number of arginine residues, were selected to generate synthetic peptides where arginine residues were substituted with citrulline. Using these citrullinated peptides, investigators demonstrated that AKA/APF antibodies are directed against citrullinated filaggrin (see Fig. 59.2). It is important to highlight that antibodies against citrullinated proteins in RA do not recognize free citrulline but only peptidyl-citrullines within the context of peptides or protein sequences.

These initial studies became the basis for the major discovery that protein sequences containing citrulline residues are some of the most prominent targets for autoantibodies in RA. However, because the epidermis is not a target of rheumatoid inflammation, and there is no evidence that profilaggrin is expressed in articular tissues, this molecule was unlikely to be the driver of the autoantibody response in the RA joint. This, together with the observations that antibodies reactive to citrullinated filaggrin were enriched in synovial tissue compared with the serum or synovial fluid[25] and that these antibodies were synthesized locally by plasmacytes within the rheumatoid pannus,[26] suggested that the primary antigen(s) recognized by these antibodies were enriched in the RA synovium. The relevance of filaggrin in RA is, therefore, largely historic and unlikely to be of pathogenic relevance. Instead, its conformation and high content of citrulline residues made it an excellent surrogate with which to detect antibodies against citrullinated molecules. Many other citrullinated autoantigens found in the rheumatoid joint, which are currently being characterized, are much more likely to be of pathogenic relevance (see "Anti-Citrullinated Protein Autoantibodies [ACPA]").

The Anti–cyclic Citrullinated Peptide (Anti-CCP) Antibody Assay

In the initial characterization of AKA/APF antibodies, a single C-terminal peptide derived from filaggrin (amino acids 306 to 324) was used to generate nine variants in which five arginine residues were changed to citrullines, either individually or in pairs, and immunoreactivity to these peptides was assayed by enzyme-linked immunosorbent assay (ELISA).[24] Interestingly, although the peptides were almost identical (the only difference being that the citrulline residues had different positions within the peptide), remarkable differences were found in the serum reactivity toward each peptide (from 20% to 48% positivity), which suggested that, although citrullination played a critical role in antigen recognition by AKA/APF antibodies, the modification was not the only determinant that influenced antibody binding. The data rather suggested that AKA/APF represented a pool of antibodies with slightly different specificities, which recognized citrulline residues within the larger context of their surrounding amino acids. Indeed, when data from all peptides were pooled, assay sensitivity increased to 76%.[24]

Because peptides often adopt a β-turn conformation within the antibody–peptide complex,[27] cysteine-bridged cyclic peptides have been shown to mimic the β-turn structure of the original antigenic determinant and bind with enhanced affinity to antibodies.[28] Therefore, a cyclic citrullinated peptide of filaggrin was generated by substituting the terminal serine residues with cysteines and cyclizing the peptide through the formation of a disulfide bond. When they compared this cyclic citrullinated peptide (later named *CCP1*) to its linear counterpart, it was demonstrated that the cyclic structure increased the sensitivity of the assay (68% vs. 49%, without affecting specificity).[24,29] In 2000, CCP1 became the antigen for the first generation of ELISAs designed to detect antibodies against citrullinated autoantigens in the research setting (see Fig. 59.2), which led to the term *anti–cyclic citrullinated peptide (anti-CCP) antibodies*.[29]

As a single antigen, CCP1 was specific for RA but was less sensitive than assays that used a combination of linear peptides (i.e., 76% vs. 68%).[24] This prompted the development of libraries of CCPs that were used to construct the second-generation anti-CCP assay (CCP2), which was introduced for aiding in the diagnosis of RA in 2003[30] and broadly adopted for clinical use.[31,32] Later, a third generation assay (CCP3) was made available for the laboratory diagnosis of RA. CCP3 reportedly recognizes additional citrullinated epitopes not identifiable with CCP2. Studies directly comparing second- and third-generation assays found them to perform very similarly,[33,34] with a slightly increased sensitivity of CCP3 in one study (e.g., sensitivities of 82.9% vs. 78.6% for CCP2, with specificities in the 93% to 94% range) (see Table 59.1).[34]

Anti-citrullinated Protein Autoantibodies (ACPA)

The finding that autoantibodies in RA recognize peptide sequences containing citrulline residues and that filaggrin was unlikely to be the physiologic target of these antibodies prompted the search for the primary protein targets of the antibodies detected by the anti-CCP assay. It was proposed that the identification of antibodies to specific citrullinated antigens might aid patient subtyping (compared with the general anti-CCP assay), as well as provide novel insights into disease etiology and pathogenesis. With the initial discovery of antibodies to specific citrullinated protein antigens, the term *anti-citrullinated protein autoantibodies (ACPAs)*[35] was introduced to refer to RA autoantibodies detected using citrullinated proteins/peptides from putative RA-associated autoantigens, instead of filaggrin-derived or commercial CCPs. This is also the term now used to describe antibodies to citrullinated antigens that arise in patients with RA because anti-CCP antibodies are only those detected by the CCP assay.

Using protein extracts from rheumatoid synovial membranes and affinity purified anti-citrullinated filaggrin antibodies, it was shown that RA synovial tissue contains several citrullinated proteins, including the α and β chains of fibrin (ogen), which were identified as the first local targets for ACPAs in RA synovial tissue (see Fig. 59.2).[36] Because circulating fibrinogen is not citrullinated, the presence of citrullinated fibrin in the rheumatoid synovium strongly suggested that citrullination occurs *in situ* after fibrin deposition through the activity of locally expressed PAD enzymes. This proposal (i.e., that the joint is a site at which autoantigen citrullination occurs in RA) has been further supported and extended to many other citrullinated RA autoantigens.[37]

Using proteomic approaches and the analysis of antigens from different sources (e.g., RA pannus and synovial fluid), several additional citrullinated autoantigen candidates have also been identified. These include the following: vimentin,[38,39] fibronectin,[40] actin,[41] heat shock protein (HSP)90,[42] histones,[43] heterogeneous nuclear ribonucleoprotein (hnRNP)-A2/B1 (i.e., RA33),[44] α-enolase, elongation factor-1α, adenylyl cyclase–associated protein-1,[45] F-actin capping protein α-1 subunit, asporin, cathepsin D, histamine receptor, protein disulfide-isomerase, endoplasmic reticulum resident protein 60 (ER60) precursor, mitochondrial aldehyde dehydrogenase,[46] collagen type I[47] and II,[48] eukaryotic translation initiation factor 4G1,[49] aldolase, phosphoglycerate kinase-1 (PGK1), calreticulin, HSP60, the far upstream element binding proteins (FUSE-BP) 1 and 2,[50] apolipoprotein E, and myeloid nuclear differentiation antigen (see Table 59.1).[51]

Although this group of citrullinated antigens represents proteins that are recognized by RA antibodies, the number of citrullinated proteins found in the rheumatoid joint is more extensive and includes more than 100 molecules that have not yet been characterized.[51–55] Together, this set of proteins is referred to as the *RA citrullinome*. Whether unique ACPAs exist for each one of these molecules or whether only a few citrullinated autoantigens within the RA citrullinome are responsible for driving the complete ACPA response in RA is still unknown.

Among ACPAs, the best clinically and pathogenically characterized are antibodies to fibrinogen, vimentin, collagen type II, and α-enolase. ELISA-based assays have been developed using citrullinated proteins (e.g., fibrinogen) or citrullinated peptides (e.g., vimentin, collagen type II, and α-enolase) derived from these putative RA autoantigens to detect ACPAs. In the case of vimentin, the citrullinated sequence from a mutated isoform isolated from RA synovial fluid (named mutated citrullinated vimentin [MCV]) has been more commonly used in place of the native sequence.[56] Although it was proposed that the detection of ACPAs targeting single antigens might provide additional diagnostic or prognostic information compared to the anti-CCP ELISA, studies addressing this question remain inconclusive. The anti-CCP assay, therefore, remains the preferred test to identify the presence of antibodies against citrullinated proteins in the clinical setting.

Because individual ACPAs appear to have limited clinical utility in RA, a multiplex assay was created to detect multiple ACPAs simultaneously (e.g., custom Bio-Plex bead-based autoantibody assays in which antigens are conjugated to spectrally distinct beads).[57] This assay is slightly more sensitive than the anti-CCP ELISA, detecting ACPAs in approximately 10% of patients negative for anti-CCPs (representing 3.7% of the total patient cohort),[58] a difference that might be explained by the array of peptides used in the assay. In addition, the bead-based multiplex assay has been useful to define the epitope spreading of ACPAs in pre-clinical RA (see "Pre-Clinical Detection of Antibodies to Citrullinated Proteins").[57] Although the multiplex assay provides additional information with regard to unique ACPA specificities, it is unclear whether this information offers any significant advantage over the anti-CCP assay for RA diagnosis or prognosis.

Clinical Relevance of Antibodies to Citrullinated Proteins

The clinical importance of autoantibodies against citrullinated antigens in RA stems from the following favorable features:

- *ACPAs have high sensitivity and specificity for the diagnosis of RA.* In systematic reviews and meta-analyses, ACPA positivity is as sensitive as, but more specific than, rheumatoid factor (RF) in distinguishing RA from other forms of inflammatory arthritis (see "Rheumatoid Factor").[31,59,60]
- *The presence of ACPAs is an important predictor of RA development.* RA developed within 3 years in more than 90% of patients with undifferentiated arthritis who tested positive for ACPA, in contrast to only 25% of the patients who tested negative for ACPA.[61]
- *ACPA positivity is associated with a more severe and destructive disease course.* Some investigators have shown that both RF and ACPAs are independent predictors of severity, whereas others have shown that ACPAs rather than RF are the better predictor of radiographic progression,[62–69] particularly in patients who were seronegative for RF.[69]
- *ACPAs are associated with RA-related interstitial lung disease (ILD) and cardiovascular disease (CVD).*[70–76] ILD and CVD are extra-articular manifestations with high mortality in people with RA. Although the mechanistic significance of these associations is still unclear, one possibility is that these antibodies are markers of systemic inflammation, which plays a role in mediating lung and cardiovascular damage. Alternatively, the observation that citrullination occurs in lung, myocardium, and atherosclerotic plaque[77–80] has suggested that these antibodies may be directly pathogenic, targeting extra-articular tissues, which contain citrullinated antigens. The presence of ACPAs in patients who have ILD but do not have RA is intriguing and has focused attention on the lung as a possible extra-articular site where RA may be initiated (see "Environmental Factors Linked to the Development of Citrullination-Associated Autoantibodies").[81,82]

The early and accurate diagnosis of RA, together with effective treatment with disease-modifying anti-rheumatic drugs (DMARDs), decreases accrual of joint damage in RA. Because ACPAs are markers of disease severity and are detectable early in the disease course, they are powerful tools to classify patients with early stage inflammatory arthritis who will benefit from treatment.[83–85]

Pre-clinical Detection of Antibodies to Citrullinated Proteins

Recent studies have demonstrated that autoantibodies may precede the onset of clinical disease in both tissue-specific and systemic autoimmune diseases, including RA.[86–93] Although defining events prior to clinical onset is challenging, two major study designs have been used to examine the relationship between the appearance of autoantibodies and disease development. These include: (1) retrospective analysis of autoantibodies in stored blood samples collected prior to disease onset (e.g., blood banks or military cohorts) and (2) prospective studies examining emergence of autoantibodies and disease in high-risk people (often first-degree relatives of affected individuals).[94,95]

Analysis of stored pre-clinical blood samples has established that autoantibodies precede RA diagnosis in many people who subsequently develop RA, often by 2 to 6 years.[92,93,96,97] In several studies, 20% to 60% of patients with RA were RF-positive prior to diagnosis, and 30% to 60% of patients were positive for ACPAs.[92,93,96,97] In one study, pre-clinical ACPA positivity was strongly associated with the presence of radiographic erosions at or after RA diagnosis, whereas RF was not.[97] The evolution of autoantibody epitope spreading in pre-clinical RA has been addressed using a multiplex assay to detect ACPAs to multiple protein antigens.[57] This study confirmed that ACPA positivity predicts progression to RA in asymptomatic people and showed that the number of ACPA specificities accumulate over time during the pre-clinical phase of the disease.[57] Moreover, the expansion of the ACPA response precedes the elevation of many inflammatory cytokines, including TNF, IL-6, IL-12p70, and interferon (IFN)-γ, which suggests that ACPAs may be a driving force of the inflammatory process in RA.[57]

Analyses of unaffected first-degree relatives of patients with RA have also shown an increased prevalence of positivity for ACPAs in this group compared to healthy controls.[98–100] Moreover, reactivity to multiple ACPAs, and the presence of an increasing number of ACPAs in this group at risk for RA, is more likely associated with signs of joint inflammation and progression to RA.[98–100]

Together, these data highlight that the development of autoimmunity against citrullinated antigens is often asymptomatic and generally precedes the onset of clinical disease. This pre-clinical phase is potentially of great importance; it may identify people who have important precursor conditions for the subsequent development of RA.[100a] The pre-clinical phase could represent a unique therapeutic opportunity. The subsequent events that convert this RA precursor into a chronic, self-sustaining process are not yet known, but defining them is of great importance.

Citrullinated Autoantigen Generation in Rheumatoid Arthritis

Peptidylarginine Deiminase Enzymes

Citrulline is not part of the natural pool of amino acids used during translation of RNA to protein; therefore, citrulline residues need to be generated post-translationally once the protein has been synthesized. This process, termed *deimination* or *citrullination*, is mediated by the calcium-dependent PAD enzymes. PADs target arginine residues in proteins and mediate hydrolysis of the arginine guanidinium side chain, which results in the generation of citrulline residues and ammonia (see Fig. 59.1A). The PADs belong to a larger group of guanidino-modifying enzymes called the *amidinotransferase* (AT) *superfamily*.[101,102] This superfamily of enzymes is expressed both in prokaryotes and eukaryotes and includes the arginine deiminases, the dimethylarginine dimethylaminohydrolases, and the dihydrolases.[102] Importantly, unlike arginine deiminases and the bacterial PAD from *Porphyromonas gingivalis (P. gingivalis)*[103] that can catalyze free L-arginine, mammalian PADs can only catalyze arginine residues in the context of peptides or proteins.

Five PAD enzymes have been identified in mammals, and the *PADI* genes are located in a single cluster on chromosome 1p36.1.[23,104] For historical reasons, these isozymes have been designated PAD1 to PAD4 and PAD6. Human PAD4 was initially named *PAD5*[105] but was later renamed *PAD4* to reflect the fact that it is a true ortholog of mouse PAD4. PAD1-3 are classically viewed as cytosolic enzymes, while PAD4 is primarily expressed in the nucleus. However, recent evidence suggests a more complex picture, with surface expression of PAD4[106] and nuclear or secreted PAD2 reported in certain cell types.[106,107] The PADs are highly conserved and share 50% to 55% sequence identity,[108] but they exhibit distinct substrate preferences and tissue expression.[23,109] PAD1 is primarily expressed in uterus and skin. PAD2 is more widely expressed in muscle, skin, brain, spleen, secretory glands, monocytes, and neutrophils. PAD3 is largely expressed in skin. PAD4 is expressed in hematopoietic cells (e.g., neutrophils and monocytes), and PAD6 is broadly expressed in germ cells, peripheral blood leukocytes, the lungs, the small intestine, the liver, the spleen, and in skeletal muscle.[23,109,110] PAD2 and PAD4 have gained prominence as potential candidates that drive citrullination of self-antigens in RA due to their prominent expression in rheumatoid synovial tissue and fluid.[37,111,112]

Peptidylarginine Deiminase Structure, Activity, and Regulation

The three-dimensional structure of PAD4[108,113] and PAD2[114] has been solved and is likely representative of the broader family. PAD2 and PAD4 are homodimers formed by head-to-tail contact between the N-terminal domain of one molecule and the C-terminal domain of the second. Five and six Ca^{2+}-binding sites were identified in the structure of PAD4 and PAD2, respectively, with Ca^{2+} binding inducing conformational changes required to generate the active site cleft. In both enzymes, two calcium-binding sites in the C-terminal domain are required for catalysis, and the other sites appear to regulate protein interactions and enzyme activity. Interestingly, the calcium binding residues are highly conserved among PADs, except for PAD6,[108] which lacks some of these sites; the catalytic cysteine is also different in PAD6. Consistent with these observations, PAD6 is the only PAD member with no demonstrable citrullination activity.[115]

Unlike many other PTMs, citrullination appears to be an irreversible process, and enzymes that convert citrullinated proteins back to their native peptidylarginine containing forms have not been discovered.[116] The mechanisms involved in the clearance or turn-over of citrullinated proteins in cells also remain unknown. Because citrullination reduces the net charge of proteins by neutralizing one positive charge per arginine residue modified, it can increase protein hydrophobicity, lead to protein unfolding, and alter intra- and inter-molecular interactions.[117] These structural changes can lead to alterations in protein activity, most commonly a loss of function.[117–122] Given that citrullinated proteins are prominent targets of autoantibodies in RA, the mechanisms that control excessive citrullination of physiologic targets or citrullination of nonphysiologic substrates are important to define.

The activity of the PAD enzymes and generation of citrullinated proteins can be regulated at multiple levels. One regulatory component is calcium.[123,124] The binding of calcium ions to PAD4 induces a conformational change that generates the active form of the enzymes.[108] Although this requires millimolar amounts of calcium in vitro,[124,125] PAD activation in cells is observed under physiologic nanomolar calcium concentrations.[107,121,126–128] This suggests that physiologic calcium conditions are suboptimal but may select for high efficiency substrates and limit aberrant citrullination events. Another important regulatory component of PAD activity is the oxidative environment.[123,124] Reducing conditions, like those present in the cytoplasm, are necessary to maintain PAD activity due to the presence of free thiol cysteine in the active site required for catalysis.[129] Since the extra-cellular environment is oxidizing,[130] this may protect against aberrant extracellular citrullination by inactivating PADs that leak from activated or dying cells. Similarly, the importance of reactive oxygen species (ROS) in controlling PAD activity has been recently underscored by the finding that ROS generated by nicotinamide adenine dinucleotide phosphate (NADPH) oxidase inhibits the catalytic activity of PAD2 and PAD4.[131] The activity of the PADs may also be negatively regulated through autocitrullination because the enzymes can citrullinate themselves as well as substrates. This has been described for PADs 1, 2, 3, and 4.[132,133] In the case of PAD4, direct citrullination of arginines surrounding the active site appears to have a major impact on activity and substrate binding. This principle is similar to other enzymes, where automodification (e.g., autophosphorylation) alters enzymatic function. Although there are multiple natural mechanisms that inhibit PAD activity, the accumulation of citrullinated proteins in the RA joint demonstrates that these regulatory mechanisms are incompletely effective in patients with RA (see "Mechanisms for Citrullination-Associated Autoantigen Production in the Rheumatoid Joint").

Peptidylarginine Deiminases in Rheumatoid Arthritis

Evidence suggests that PAD2 and PAD4 are the predominant PAD enzymes responsible for the generation of citrullinated autoantigens in RA.[37,111,112] These PAD isoforms are found in the tissue and fluid of inflamed RA joints, and both enzymes citrullinate proteins that are targeted by ACPAs.[41,134,135] In addition, polymorphisms in the genes encoding PAD2 and PAD4 (*PADI2* and *PADI4*, respectively) are independently associated with RA development, particularly in Asian populations.[136–139] Two common haplotypes of the *PADI4* gene were initially identified[136] and designated *susceptible* or *nonsusceptible* based on their relative frequencies in patients with RA versus control subjects. Although the susceptible haplotype generates a PAD4 molecule containing three amino acid substitutions in the N-terminal region (i.e., Gly55-Ser, Val82-Ala, and Gly112-Ala), current evidence suggests that these changes have no effect on the function of the protein.[132,140] Changes in messenger RNA stability of the susceptible *PADI4* have been reported but they are not associated with changes in enzyme level. Furthermore, the polymorphisms appear to affect conformation only within the N-terminal domain but not the active site located in the C-terminal domain.[140] As such, the PAD4 genotype may exert its effects on RA disease susceptibility as a consequence of its immunogenicity rather than its enzyme activity.[132] Consistent with this hypothesis is the observation that, in addition to its ability to citrullinate RA autoantigens, PAD4 itself is an RA autoantigen (see "Antibodies to Peptidylarginine Deiminase Enzymes").[141,142] Moreover, it is noteworthy that the *PADI4* susceptible gene appears to contribute to the development and progression of RA regardless of ACPA status,[143,144] which supports the notion that the susceptible variant may drive RA susceptibility through other mechanisms besides the production of citrullinated autoantigens.

Antibodies to Peptidylarginine Deiminase Enzymes

In addition to their prominent enzymatic role in the generation of citrullinated autoantigens, PAD2 and PAD4 are targeted by autoantibodies in unique subsets of patients with RA.[141,142,145] Although PADs can citrullinate themselves,[132,133] antibodies to the PADs are distinct from ACPAs in that antibody recognition is independent of citrullination status.[146] As has been observed for ACPAs, anti-PAD4 antibodies are present in a subset of individuals pre-clinically, prior to the onset of any disease symptoms.[90] Interestingly, in a cohort of Caucasian patients with RA who had established disease, the susceptible PAD4 haplotype was strikingly associated with PAD4 autoantibodies, even though the association of the susceptible haplotype with RA development has not been observed in Caucasian populations.[141] The sensitivity of PAD4 antibodies for RA ranges between 23% and 45%, with a specificity of greater than 95% (see Table 59.1).[147,148] Importantly, PAD4 autoantibodies are strongly associated with ACPAs, and are independently associated with the presence of radiographic joint damage in multiple studies. Anti-PAD4 antibodies are also associated with the progression of erosive disease that persists despite treatment with TNF inhibitors.[149,150] However, a recent study has shown that these antibodies predict a more favorable response to treatment escalation in patients who failed first-line DMARD therapy.[151]

A subset of anti-PAD4 antibodies that cross-react with the PAD3 isoenzyme has been identified in 10% to 12% of patients with RA (see Table 59.1).[151–154] Anti-PAD3/PAD4 cross-reactive antibodies were most strongly associated with severe progressive joint damage and the highest risk of RA-associated ILD.[152,155] The risk for ILD was significantly augmented in patients who were past or present cigarette smokers,[154] yet a history of cigarette smoking was not associated with the development of anti-PAD4 or anti-PAD3/4 antibodies.[154] This suggests a two-hit model of lung damage in which anti-PAD3/PAD4 antibodies may synergize with smoking to induce more severe lung disease (see "Environmental Factors Linked to Citrullination-Associated Autoantibodies"). These antibodies also have the unique ability to enhance PAD4 enzyme activity upon binding, which may play a novel role in the pathogenesis of RA (see "The Origin and Pathogenesis of Citrullination-Associated Antibodies").

PAD2 has recently been identified as a target of autoantibodies in 18.5% of RA patients from a single cohort (see Table 59.1).[145] In contrast to anti-PAD4 or anti-PAD3/PAD4 antibodies, anti-PAD2 antibodies were found in patients with milder disease, including fewer swollen joints over time, less risk of RA-associated ILD, and a lower likelihood of progressive radiographic joint damage. These antibodies were not associated with other RA serologies, such as ACPA, RF, or anti-PAD3/PAD4 antibodies. Although antibodies to the PAD enzymes are not yet used in the clinical setting, this study suggested that when used together, anti-PAD2 and anti-PAD3/4 antibodies may provide prognostic value in predicting patients who will progress in their erosive joint disease over time.[145]

The Etiology and Pathogenesis of Citrullination-Associated Autoantibodies

Although the etiology of RA remains to be defined, the presence of citrullination-associated autoantibodies in the pre-clinical phase of the disease suggests that dysregp-ulated citrullination is an important event during disease initiation.[100a] This notion has sparked the idea that environmental factors that dysregulate citrullination may promote the breech of tolerance to citrullination-associated antigens and promote the development of autoantibodies in genetically susceptible hosts (Fig. 59.3).[100a] There is evidence that this leads to the establishment of feed-forward loops of disease propagation in the joint, in which ongoing immune responses drive the continued generation and release of PAD enzymes and citrullinated autoantigens (Fig. 59.4).[155a]

Genetic Factors Linked to the Development of Citrullination-Associated Autoantibodies

Although the association of specific human leukocyte antigen–DR *(HLA-DR)* alleles (which encode for HLA class II antigen-presenting molecules) and RA has been known for decades,[156] the relationship between genetics and the development of RA autoantibodies is just beginning to be elucidated. A subset of *HLA-DRB1* alleles termed the *shared epitope (SE) alleles* includes *HLA-DRB1*0101, *0102, *0401, *0404, *0405, *0408, *0410, *1001,* and **1402.* SE alleles are named due to the presence of a similar amino acid sequence (QRRAA, QKRAA, or RRRAA) at position 70–74 of the β-chain in the peptide-binding groove.[157] Although early studies identified SE alleles as inherited risk factors for RA development, the discovery of ACPAs revealed that SE was most strongly associated with ACPA-positive RA (see Fig. 59.3).[158] This is supported mechanistically by structural studies, which have shown that SE-containing HLA molecules

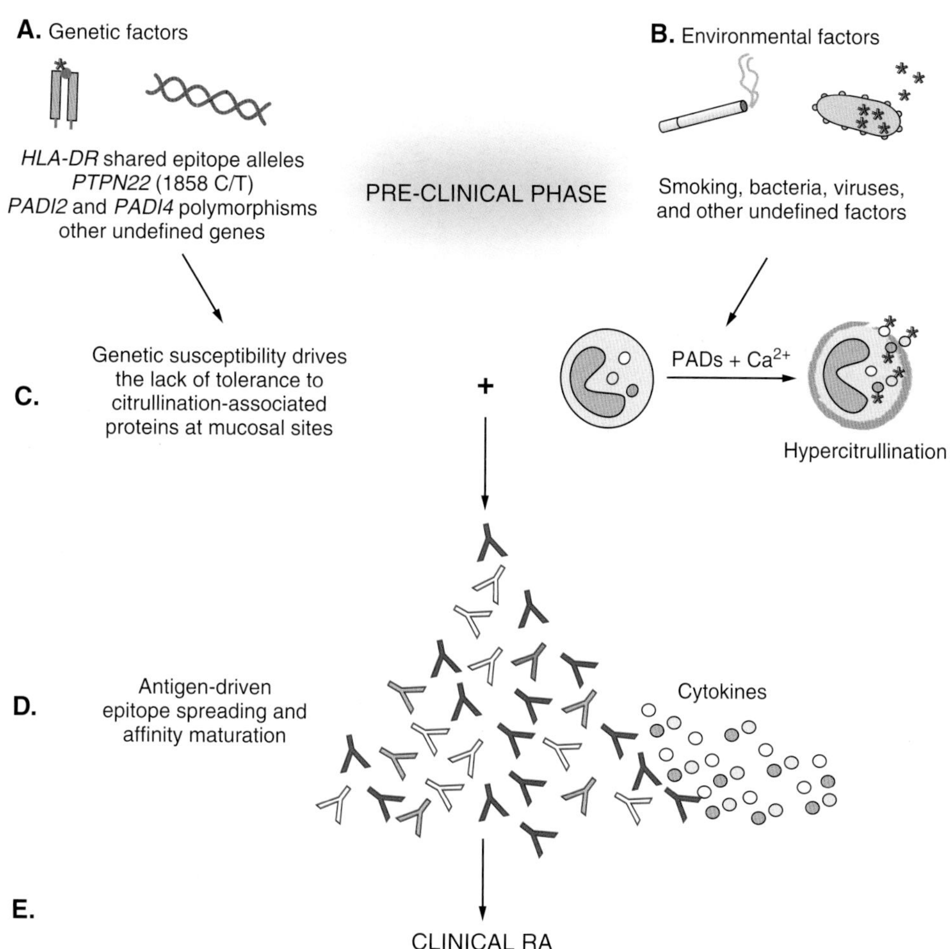

• **Fig. 59.3** Genetic and environmental factors initiate the development of citrullination-associated autoantibodies in pre-clinical RA. (A) Genetic factors have been identified that predispose an individual to the development of RA, including *HLA-DRB1*-shared epitope alleles and single-nucleotide polymorphisms in *PTPN22*, *PADI2*, and *PADI4*. (B) Environmental factors, such as smoking and infection, can induce the enhanced production of citrullination-associated autoantigens at mucosal sites (e.g., oral mucosa, lung, and gastrointestinal tract) by inducing recruitment, death, or activation of peptidylarginine deiminase (PAD)-expressing cells.[116] Membranolytic pathways induced by bacterial or host pore-forming proteins, uniquely, induce neutrophil hypercitrullination, which generates a pattern of citrullinated antigens similar to those found in the RA joint.[52,191] (C) Although this process is likely normal and self-limited in the majority of the cases, some genetically susceptible individuals may have the risk of developing autoantibodies against components involved in the process of citrullination (e.g., PAD4 and citrullinated proteins). This phase is likely asymptomatic because the autoantibodies are low-titer, may not be pathogenic, and likely target a limited number of citrullinated antigens.[57,208] (D) The presence of autoantibodies may persist for several months to decades, during which a transition phase may occur. This phase is characterized by the development of affinity-matured autoantibodies and an accumulation of multiple anti-citrullinated protein antibody (ACPA) specificities, which reflect the process of antigen-driven epitope spreading.[57] The expansion of the autoantibody response closely correlates with the appearance of pre-clinical inflammation that includes the elevation of inflammatory cytokines, such as tumor necrosis factor (TNF), IL-6, IL-12p70, and interferon (IFN)-γ.[57] Moreover, ACPAs acquire a pro-inflammatory Fc glycosylation phenotype prior to the onset of RA.[208] Together, the changes in the autoantibody response and the elevation in cytokines predict the imminent onset of clinical RA.[57,208] (E) When autoantibodies and cytokines overcome counter-regulatory mechanisms, the clinical phase is likely initiated.

preferentially bind citrullinated peptides over their arginine-containing counterparts.[159,160] Furthermore, there appears to be a gene dosage effect on the relative risk of ACPA development with an odds ratio of 3.3 to 4.7 for patients with one SE allele and an odds ratio of 11.8 to 13.3 for patients with two SE alleles.[61,158,161] Together, the combination of ACPAs and SE carriage is strongly associated with future onset of RA.[162] Interestingly, smoking modulates the genetic association of SE alleles with ACPA development (see "Environmental Factors Linked to the Development of Citrullination-Associated Autoantibodies" section).[163] Beyond the SE model, recent genome-wide association studies have suggested that unique polymorphisms that encode key amino acids in the peptide binding grooves of HLA-DRβ1 (at positions 11, 71, and 74), HLA-B (at position 9) and HLA-DPβ1 (at position 9) may explain most of the association between the HLA locus and ACPA–positive RA.[164]

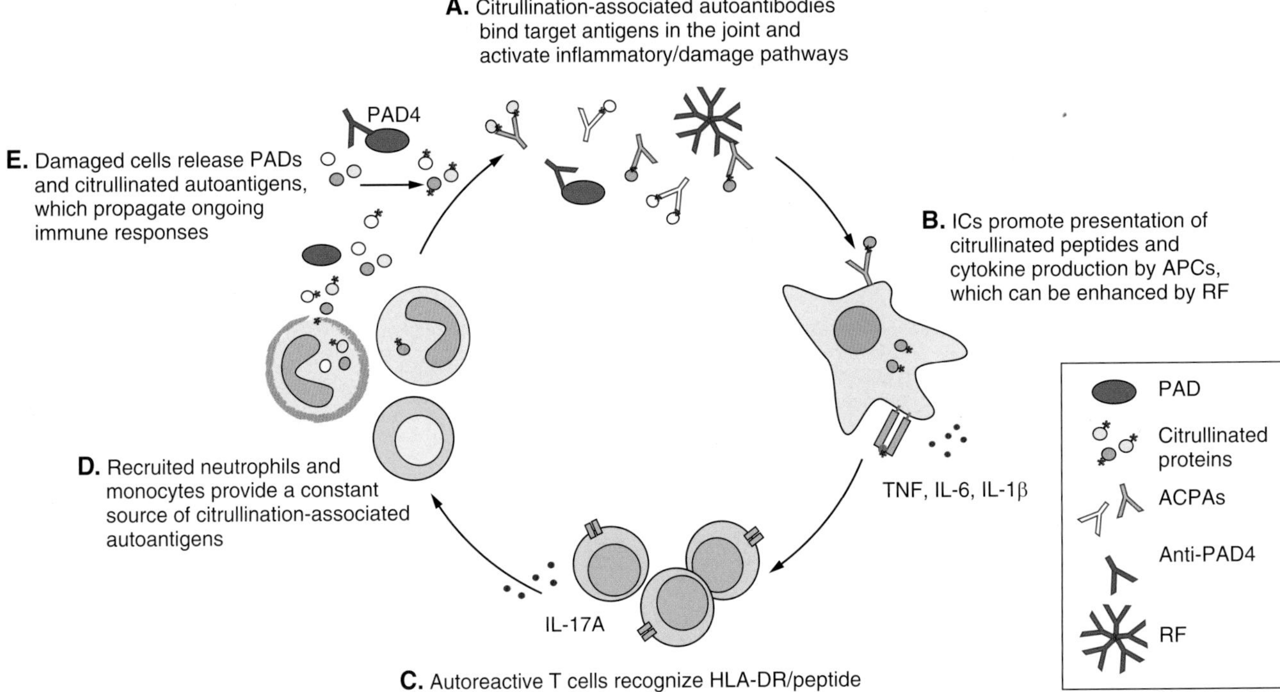

• **Fig. 59.4** A feed-forward model of RA pathogenesis: A pivotal role for citrullination-associated antibodies. Once initiated, the immune response drives a feed-forward loop of target tissue destruction and disease propagation resulting in the development of clinically apparent RA. (A) Citrullination-associated autoantibodies bind to citrullinated proteins and peptidylarginine deiminase (PAD) enzymes in the joint and activate inflammatory pathways or induce damage. This is mediated by the formation of immune complexes (ICs), which can fix complement or induce damage to antigen-expressing cells via cellular and humoral immunity.[203,280] (B) ICs are recognized by antigen-presenting cells (APCs), including dendritic cells and macrophages, and drive presentation of citrullinated peptides and production of pro-inflammatory cytokines (e.g. tumor necrosis factor (TNF), interleukin (IL)-6, and IL-1β).[202,204–206] Rheumatoid factor (RF) can bind ICs and further amplify these immune responses.[262–264] (C) Autoreactive T cells mediate tissue destruction via the cytotoxic-granule pathway, by secreting cytokines, and by recruiting/activating inflammatory cells.[281] (D) Neutrophils and monocytes, which are enriched in PAD enzymes,[38,41] are recruited to the joint. PAD activity and generation of citrullinated proteins is induced by immune effector pathways, which drive activation and death of PAD-expressing cells.[38,52,217] (E) Damaged cells release PADs and citrullinated proteins into the RA joint, which provides a continued source of citrullination-associated autoantigens to propagate the immune response.[116] Anti-PAD4 antibodies may further amplify this process by stabilizing and activating extra-cellular PAD4.[152]

In addition to HLA alleles, a single-nucleotide polymorphism in the *PTPN22* gene *(1858C/T)* is also associated with ACPAs with an odds ratio of 3.80 (see Fig. 59.3).[165] *PTPN22* encodes for protein tyrosine phosphatase non-receptor type 22 and is associated with several autoimmune disorders, including RA.[166] The combination of *PTPN22 1858C/T* genotype and ACPAs is 100% specific for RA and confers a relative risk of 130.03. The 1858C/T polymorphism is not associated with RF isotypes and appears to act independently of SE alleles.[165] Genetic factors, such as the SE and *PTPN22,* may, therefore, play a role in the pre-clinical phase of RA, which predisposes individuals to the generation of ACPAs and susceptibility to the overt disease phenotype.

Environmental Factors Linked to the Development of Citrullination-Associated Autoantibodies

Although abundant citrullination is found in RA synovial tissue, once disease is established, it is unknown whether abnormal synovial citrullination precedes the onset of clinical RA, which is a requisite to explain the presence of ACPAs long before the onset of clinical disease. Although such evidence will be very challenging to obtain, data suggest that the joint is not the only possible site of abnormal citrullination that might initiate the RA-specific immune responses to citrullination-associated autoantigens. There is growing support for the hypothesis that aberrant protein citrullination and breach of immunologic tolerance to citrullinated antigens initially occurs at mucosal sites, such as the oral mucosa, the lungs, and the gastrointestinal tract.[167–169] In support of this hypothesis, ACPAs of the immunoglobulin (Ig)A class (an isotype associated with mucosal immunity) are found in about one-third of patients with recent-onset RA[170]; and ACPAs can be detected in the sputum of individuals at risk of developing RA (e.g., RA-free first-degree relatives).[171] If the lung is an initial site of ACPA production, it is postulated that joints only become targeted secondarily after the immune response is initiated as a consequence of an inflammatory event triggered by a common environmental exposure, such as infection, inflammation, or smoking (see Fig. 59.3).[167–169]

Smoking is the most widely studied environmental factor linked to RA and ACPA development. A history of smoking in patients with SE alleles (see "Genetic Factors Linked to the

Development of Citrullination-Associated Autoantibodies") has been linked to the development of ACPA-positive RA in some populations,[163,172–174] but there is growing appreciation that this relationship is nuanced. Whereas *HLA-DRB1*04* alleles have been primarily associated with ACPA production,[175–177] in smokers, *HLA-DRB1*0101*, **0102*, and **1001* alleles demonstrate the strongest association with ACPAs.[163] In addition, certain ACPA fine specificities and specific ACPA isotypes may be responsible for driving this association.[178,179] Study of smokers without RA has shown that cigarette smoking increased expression of PAD2 with a modest increase in protein citrullination in the lungs.[77] ACPAs can also be found in patients with ILD who do not have RA,[81,82] which further suggests smoking may play a role in generating or sustaining autoantibodies to citrullinated proteins. Interestingly, despite the strong relationship between ACPAs and anti-PAD4 antibodies, the development of anti-PAD4 antibodies is independent of smoking history,[154] which suggests a role for other environmental factors in the development of these antibodies.

Infection, particularly at mucosal sites, may represent another factor associated with autoantibody development in RA. Tantalizing similarities and epidemiologic associations exist between periodontitis and RA, including the presence of bone erosions, association with similar SE alleles and smoking, and enrichment of severe periodontal disease in patients with RA.[168,180–183] These connections have focused attention on the study of oral pathogens as potential triggers of autoimmunity in RA.[190a] The identification of a bacterial PAD from *P. gingivalis* (termed PPAD) led to the initial hypothesis that infection with this periodontal pathogen may be etiologically linked to RA.[103,184] Although some studies supported the idea that PPAD can citrullinate autoantigens targeted by ACPAs,[185] the pattern of citrullination induced by this enzyme (i.e., C-terminal citrulline residues) is not characteristic in proteins recognized by ACPAs, which target citrulline residues within protein sequences (i.e., endocitrullination).[24] An alternative mechanism, which has been proposed for the involvement of PPAD in RA pathogenesis, is citrullinating its own bacterial products, which may act as the inciting citrullinated antigens. Although initial studies suggested that autocitrullination of PPAD may be relevant in this regard,[186] further studies by mass spectrometry and crystal structure analysis of PPAD isolated from *P. gingivalis* have not supported this hypothesis.[187–189] Nevertheless, it is possible that other bacterial or host proteins citrullinated by PPAD in *P. gingivalis* may be relevant as initiating antigens.[190,190a]

The periodontal microenvironment in patients with periodontitis is highly enriched in citrullinated proteins, mimicking patterns of endocitrullination generated by PADs in the RA joint.[191] This has suggested that the citrullinome in periodontitis is generated by the abnormal activation of host (rather than bacterial) PAD enzymes. Among different microbial species associated with severe periodontitis, *Aggregatibacter actinomycetemcomitans (Aa)* was identified as the only pathogen that could reproduce the citrullinome found in periodontitis and RA.[191] However, in contrast to *P. gingivalis,* in which citrullination is attributed to its own PAD, *Aa* does not encode a PAD enzyme. Instead, the bacterium secretes a pore-forming toxin (leukotoxin A) that targets neutrophils, inducing prominent calcium influx, osmotic lysis, and hyperactivation of PAD enzymes.[191] This dysregulated PAD activation was shown to induce global citrullination of a wide range of proteins in the neutrophil, a process termed *cellular hypercitrullination*.[52,191] Mechanistically, this process is similar to host immune-effector pathways in the RA joint (see "Mechanisms for Citrullination-Associated Autoantigen Production in the Rheumatoid Joint").[52,192] If tolerance is broken to the citrullinated products of *Aa*-induced hypercitrullination, this process may initiate the subsequent production of ACPAs.[116,191,193] Importantly, as other bacterial species also produce pore-forming toxins,[194] it is possible that a similar mechanism may also be relevant to other pathogens at various mucosal sites, including the lung and gut.[116,192]

Although no evidence exists that viral proteins are citrullinated in vivo, a subset of ACPA-positive RA sera has been demonstrated to cross-react with synthetic citrullinated peptides from Epstein-Barr virus EBNA-1 and human papilloma virus (HPV)-47 $E2_{345-362}$ proteins.[195,196] Defining the kinetics of appearance of these antibodies during disease development, and demonstrating directly that these modified proteins are generated during natural infection, will be important to determine if this cross-reactivity is relevant to RA pathogenesis.

These gene-environment interactions, playing out in microenvironments outside the joint, add important dimensions to the framework within which RA pathogenesis must be investigated and understood. Although it is possible that none of the mechanisms currently defined represent a unifying mechanism of RA pathogenesis, the broader view of potential immunizing environments and the search for a frequent worldwide environmental exposure are of great importance.

Origin and Pathogenesis of Citrullination-Associated Antibodies

Despite the recognized importance of citrullination-associated antibodies in RA, the molecular features and direct pathogenic consequences of such antibodies are only beginning to be defined. Important insights into their development and inflammatory effects have been gained through the study of single antibody-expressing cells from patients with RA. Although initial studies suggested that ~25% of synovial IgG-expressing B cells are specific to citrullinated antigens in ACPA-positive RA,[197] further studies have shown that this number was overestimated and may actually be ~4%.[198–201] Overall, the study of monoclonal ACPAs derived from single cells isolated from patients with RA has revealed that these antibodies are enriched in somatic mutations.[55b,201,202] Structural analysis of monoclonal ACPAs has confirmed that citrulline is the major determinant of antibody binding to citrullinated peptides.[55c] Together, this supports the notion that ACPAs are produced by constant exposure to abnormally citrullinated autoantigens.

Mechanistically, in vitro evidence suggests that ACPAs can activate both the classic and alternative pathways of complement,[203] and that ACPA immune complexes drive macrophages to produce TNF via engagement of Fcγ receptors and Toll-like receptor 4 (see Fig. 59.4).[202,204–206] Moreover, recent evidence also indicates that distinct glycosylation patterns in ACPAs may influence pathogenicity of these antibodies.[207,208] Monoclonal antibodies to citrullinated collagen type II generated by immunization in mice can cause arthritis by cross-reactivity to joint cartilage.[209] However, these findings have not been reproduced using ACPAs derived from patients with RA. Although some studies have suggested that RA-derived monoclonal ACPAs can induce pain in mice and osteoclast activation in vitro,[210,211] these findings have been questioned because later studies showed that monoclonals used in these experiments appear to have no specificity for citrullinated residues.[198,199] Therefore, whether ACPAs may be pathogenic in vivo still remains an open question.

Anti-PAD4 monoclonal autoantibodies have been derived from PAD4-specific memory B cells isolated from patients with RA. Analysis of these antibodies has suggested that they arise from PAD4-reactive precursors, implying that defective checkpoints in B cell tolerance are likely involved in the initial production of these antibodies.[212] Nevertheless, autoantibodies to PAD4 have evidence of somatic hypermutation, which suggests that in patients with RA, these antibodies have undergone antigen-driven affinity maturation. Although ACPAs and anti-PAD4 autoantibodies appear to originate by different mechanisms,[155a] the chronic exposure to immunogenic self-antigens appears to be a common driver.

Functional analysis of RA-derived monoclonal anti-PAD4 autoantibodies showed that, like polyclonal IgG from RA patients with anti-PAD3/PAD4 antibodies (see "Anti–Peptidylarginine Deiminase Antibodies"),[152,212] they were able to increase PAD4-citrullination activity at low-calcium concentrations. Biochemical studies have revealed that this enhancement is mediated by an interaction with structural epitopes at calcium-binding sites at the interface between the N- and C-terminal domains. This suggests that anti-PAD4 antibodies could possess the unique ability to propagate the generation of citrullinated proteins in the RA joint (see Fig. 59.4) (see "Mechanisms for Citrullination-Associated Autoantigen Production in the Rheumatoid Joint"), but further in vitro and in vivo characterization is needed to determine the full pathogenic potential of anti-PAD4 antibodies in patients with RA.

Mechanisms for Citrullination-Associated Autoantigen Production in the Rheumatoid Joint

Once citrullinated-associated autoantibody responses are formed, the propagation of inflammation in the RA joint requires the continued generation of citrullinated antigens and presence of active PAD enzymes (see Fig. 59.4). Analysis of synovial fluid and cells suggests that dysregulated PAD activation with ongoing protein citrullination occurs both intra- and extra-cellularly in the RA joint.[51–55,116] Several PAD-expressing cells (e.g., immune cells and synoviocytes) and distinct mechanisms of cell death (including autophagy, neutrophil extra-cellular traps [NETs], necrosis, and cytolysis induced by pore-forming proteins) have been implicated in the production of citrullinated autoantigens in RA by inducing intra-cellular PAD activation and the release of PADs into the extra-cellular environment.[116] In this regard, recent studies have implicated neutrophils as a major source of intra-cellular citrullination and soluble PADs for extra-cellular citrullination.[41,52,116,213] These cells represent one of the most abundant cell types in RA synovial fluid and constitutively express several PADs.[214]

Two mechanisms have been proposed to drive the cellular generation of RA autoantigens in neutrophils: (1) formation of NETs,[213] an anti-microbial form of cell death, in which granule proteins and chromatin are extruded from the cell and form extra-cellular fibers that bind pathogens[215]; and (2) membranolytic damage mediated by pore-forming proteins.[52,191] NET formation is increased in the joints of patients with RA and may be a relevant source of inflammatory signals through the extra-cellular redistribution of intra-cellular antigens.[213] Although these may include citrullinated autoantigens, a growing body of data has demonstrated that the formation of NETs is a complex process, which results from the activation of different pathways that can be triggered by a broad range of stimuli, only some of which are associated with citrullination of a limited number of substrates (mainly histones).[52,192,216] Hence, even though NETs in RA may be associated with PAD4 activation, the contribution of this process to generating the RA citrullinome is unclear.[155a,192] Thus, although citrullination and the formation of NETs may be increased in the RA joint, and NETs may contribute to RA pathogenesis,[213] these processes may not necessarily be directly associated.[155a]

As described (see "Environmental Factors Linked to the Development of Citrullination-Associated Autoantibodies"), bacterial toxins have the capacity to activate PADs and induce hypercitrullination, which could initiate the production of ACPAs at extra-articular sites. Host pore-forming proteins, such as perforin and the membrane attack complex (MAC) of complement, may be responsible for sustaining the production of citrullinated autoantigens in the joints of patients with RA.[52] These host effector pathways are active in the RA joint, and have been demonstrated to be potent activators of PADs and efficient inducers of the neutrophil hypercitrullination that mirrors the RA joint citrullinome.[52,191]

In addition to neutrophils, monocytes and fibroblast-like synoviocytes (FLS) can also generate citrullinated autoantigens as result of autophagy.[217] However, this process does not lead to hypercitrullination, but rather to the citrullination of α-enolase and vimentin. Interestingly, increased expression of autophagy markers correlates with ACPA titers, which suggests that autophagy may contribute to generation of these citrullinated antigens in patients with RA.[217]

The discovery that fibrinogen is heavily citrullinated in the RA joint provided initial evidence that citrullination can also occur extra-cellularly.[36] Soluble PAD2 and PAD4 have been detected in the synovial fluid from patients with RA,[37,125] which suggests that these enzymes are released from activated or dying cells, most likely neutrophils.[218] In this regard, a recent report showed that neutrophils constitutively secrete PAD2 and express a fraction of PAD4 on their cell surfaces, which can be upregulated after cell activation.[106] Although regulatory mechanisms exist to limit aberrant PAD activity (see "Peptidylarginine Deiminase Structure, Activity, and Regulation"), accumulation of PAD enzymes in the inflamed RA joint could overcome these inhibitory factors. For example, although the oxidizing extra-cellular environment is inhospitable to PAD activity, a continued supply of active PADs release from neutrophils infiltrating the inflamed RA joint could fuel the generation of citrullinated proteins. Autoantibodies to the PAD enzymes themselves may also support extra-cellular PAD activity by stabilizing the active conformation of PAD4. Human anti-PAD4 monoclonal and anti-PAD3/PAD4 cross-reactive autoantibodies also enhanced PAD4 enzymatic activity by lowering the amount of calcium needed for catalysis into the physiologic range.[152,212] Thus, PAD4 released during neutrophil activation or death may encounter anti-PAD4 antibodies in the synovial fluid with the capacity to sustain enzymatic activity, which may contribute to extra-cellular citrullinated autoantigen generation in RA. Together, the presence of effector pathways that drive hypercitrullination and the extra-cellular release of citrullinated antigens and PADs likely create a feed-forward loop, which keeps a constant production of autoantigens for B cell stimulation, autoantibody production, immune complex formation, and tissue damage (see Fig 59.4).

Antibodies to Chemically Modified Antigens

Antibodies to Carbamylated Proteins (Anti-CarP)

Carbamylation or homocitrullination is a nonenzymatic post-translational process in which lysine residues are converted to homocitrulline. This process results from the reaction of cyanate or carbamyl phosphate with the primary amine of lysine residues (see Fig. 59.1B).[219,220] Cyanate is present in the body in equilibrium with urea; therefore, carbamylation accumulates in conditions that enhance cyanate levels, such as uremia, inflammation, and cigarette smoking.[221] Carbamyl phosphate is generated from ammonia and bicarbonate by the catalytic activity of carbamoyl phosphate synthases.[219] Although homocitrulline is one methylene group longer than citrulline, these amino acids are similar in structure (see Fig. 59.1B). Because of this structural similarity, it was hypothesized that carbamylated proteins may be relevant to the lack of tolerance to citrullinated antigens in RA.[222] In support of this hypothesis, initial studies demonstrated that mice immunized with carbamylated peptides developed erosive arthritis.[222] Moreover, these mice became susceptible to a more aggressive form of erosive arthritis after a subsequent intra-articular injection of citrullinated peptides. Although the significance of these interesting findings were not pursued experimentally, they sparked interest in defining whether patients with RA have antibodies to carbamylated proteins.[223] Using carbamylated–fetal calf serum and carbamylated-fibrinogen as surrogate antigens in ELISA assays, IgG and IgA antibodies recognizing homocitrulline-containing proteins (thereafter *anti-carbamylated protein [anti-CarP]* antibodies), were identified in more than 40% of patients with RA (see Table 59.1).[223] Although homocitrulline structurally resembles citrulline, the finding that anti-CarP IgG and IgA antibodies are present in approximately 35% of ACPA-negative patients, and that these antibodies are predictive of a more severe disease course independent of ACPA status, has suggested that these antibodies are not merely cross-reactive between the two PTMs.[223] Moreover, anti-CarP antibodies appear many years before the diagnosis of RA and predict the development of RA independent of ACPAs in patients with arthralgia.[224–226] Although the mechanism by which carbamylated antigens are generated in RA is still unknown, it is possible that inflammation may be the trigger of enhanced carbamylation in this disease. Here, myeloperoxidase (MPO) released from neutrophils in the RA joint may promote the conversion of thiocyanate to cyanate, further enhancing carbamylation.[221,227] Nevertheless, despite the growing interest in anti-CarP antibodies, a major caveat is that their primary protein targets in RA are still unknown. Recently, alpha-1-anti-trypsin was found to be carbamylated in synovial fluid from an RA patient and recognized more strongly by RA patient sera compared to control sera.[228] Additional studies are needed to define the specific set of carbamylated autoantigens targeted in RA and their presence in RA target tissue in order to better understand the clinical significance and pathogenic role of anti-CarP antibodies in RA.

Antibodies to Malondialdehyde-Acetaldehyde Adducts (Anti-MAA)

Malondialdehyde-acetaldehyde (MAA) adducts are the most recently described target of anti-PTM antibodies in RA.[229] Similar to carbamylation, the generation of MAA is nonenzymatic and involves the preferential modification of the primary amine of lysine residues. During oxidative stress caused by a variety of stimuli, including inflammation and exposure to alcohol, ROS triggers peroxidation of membrane lipids, resulting in the formation of malondialdehyde (MDA) and acetaldehyde (AA),[230–233] which react with proteins and further result in the formation of stable MDA-AA protein adducts, referred to as *MAA* (see Fig. 59.1C).[234,235] These adducts have been implicated in contributing to inflammation and cellular injury associated with cardiovascular and alcoholic liver disease.[230–232] Interestingly, RA synovial tissue, but not tissue from patients with osteoarthritis, is enriched in MAA-modified proteins. Anti-MAA antibodies are currently detected using MAA-modified albumin as a surrogate antigen,[229] and the specific proteins containing MAA-modifications, which are targeted in patients with RA, are unknown.

Although anti-MAA antibodies are strongly associated with ACPA and RF, it is interesting that anti-MAA antibodies of the IgG isotype are found in 88% of patients who are negative for ACPAs,[229] which suggests that these may be useful biomarkers, particularly in people with ACPA$^-$ RA (see Table 59.1). However, whether this antibody system is clinically relevant in RA remains to be defined. In this regard, it is important to highlight that anti-MAA antibodies are not specific for RA but have also been found in patients with osteoarthritis, SLE, alcohol-induced liver disease, diabetes, and CVD.[236–239] Therefore, these antibodies may not exclusively be markers of joint damage but may be generated as a result of comorbidities associated with RA. Future studies defining the targets of anti-MAA antibodies in patients with RA are warranted to understand the role of this antibody system in RA.

Mechanistic Implications of Antibodies to Post-translationally Modified Proteins

The finding that people with RA have antibodies targeting different PTMs is intriguing and unlikely to be accidental. Because neutrophils produce all components (i.e., PADs, MPO, and ROS) required to generate the current set of modified autoantigens targeted by autoantibodies in RA (i.e., ACPAs, anti-CarP, and anti-MAA, respectively), these distinct antibody systems may indeed represent markers of a common pathogenic event driven by neutrophils. This would potentially place these cells at the center of autoantigen production in RA pathogenesis[240]; confirmation of this hypothesis would have important implications for future anti-neutrophil therapies in this disease.

Nonspecific Rheumatoid Arthritis Autoantibodies

Rheumatoid Factor

RFs are autoantibodies that target the Fc region of IgG. Besides their potential relevance to autoimmune disease pathogenesis, RFs hold a special place in rheumatology because they were the first autoantibodies discovered in the autoimmune rheumatic diseases. In 1940, Erik Waaler found that sera from patients with RA inhibited the hemolysis of antibody-sensitized sheep erythrocytes, and instead, caused marked agglutination of these cells.[241] He also noted that this effect was thermostable and associated with the globulin fraction of the serum, which demonstrated that it was not dependent on complement activation. It was suggested that this process resulted from the existence of a factor (called *the agglutination activating factor* but later called *rheumatoid factor*), which was increased in patients with RA.[241] Nevertheless, despite the high prevalence of a positive agglutination reaction in sera from patients with RA (35% positive), Waaler did not consider it of diagnostic value for RA because some patients with other diseases (e.g., cancer and infections) were also positive (~5%).[241] Later, this phenomenon was rediscovered in 1948 by Rose and colleagues while performing complement fixation tests for rickettsialpox, and they suggested the potential of this test in the diagnosis of RA.[242] These assays were later shown to detect IgM antibodies recognizing the Fc portion of IgG.[243–246] Numerous modifications of the agglutination assay have evolved (called the *Waaler-Rose agglutination test*), which lead to the use of IgG-coated latex beads instead of sheep erythrocytes.[247,248] Subsequent developments established RF assays in radioimmunoassay, ELISA, and nephelometry formats, with increased convenience but similar performance in terms of sensitivity and specificity.

RFs are positive in ~70% of RA patients but have lower specificity for RA compared to ACPAs (85% vs. 95%, respectively) (see Table 59.1).[59] RFs may be positive in healthy control subjects (1% in younger people and up to 5% in people older than 70 years of age) and in patients with numerous other non-RA diseases (including other rheumatic diseases, such as Sjögren's syndrome and cryoglobulinemia), as well as chronic infections.[249–251] The pretest probability of diagnosing RA, therefore, greatly influences the performance of the RF test; the sensitivities and specificities are both in the 50% to 90% range, but this depends on the patient groups studied.[252,253] The existence of IgG and IgA RFs and evidence of somatic hypermutation have suggested that some RFs in RA are T cell-dependent.[254,255] Although some studies have suggested that IgG and IgA RFs increase the specificity of RFs for RA,[256] a recent meta-analysis showed that assays of the different RF isotypes performed very similarly in terms of sensitivity and specificity to standard RF assays.[59]

Importantly, patients with RA also vary in terms of timing of the appearance of RF. RF precedes symptomatic disease in a significant subpopulation[86,257–259] and follows disease onset with variable kinetics in other patients. Indeed, earlier onset of RF in patients with RA has been associated with more severe disease, which highlights a possible contribution of these antibodies to disease amplification.[260] The observation that RF only appears after disease onset in some patients suggests that it may mark distinct, sequential events in pathogenesis, which are very close together in the subgroup in whom RF occurs early, or that are separated in time in patients in whom RF follows symptoms. The mechanisms that drive the production of RF in people with RA are not fully understood. The presence of somatic hypermutation in RFs and the evidence that these antibodies are produced by plasma cells in the rheumatoid synovium have suggested that the RF response is driven locally by antigen.[254,255] However, it is still unclear how IgG becomes a target of the autoimmune response in the rheumatoid joint. In contrast to other autoantigens in RA, there is no evidence that the IgG targeted by RFs requires modification (e.g., PTM) for antibody recognition. Nevertheless, it is still possible that the initial events that break tolerance to IgG may be initiated through an abnormally modified molecule, which also occurs for other autoantigens in RA. The possible mechanisms whereby RF may play an amplifying role in RA are numerous; they include formation of immune complexes, amplification of cellular antigen capture, signaling, effector functions, and others (see Fig. 59.4).[261] More recently, in vitro studies have suggested that RFs increase the capacity of ACPA immune complexes to activate complement and stimulate pro-inflammatory cytokine production by macrophages.[262–264] Thus, although RF may not be specific for RA, these autoantibodies may enhance the pathogenicity of RA-specific autoantibodies, such as ACPAs.

Anti-RA33 Autoantibodies

Anti-RA33 antibodies were discovered in 1989 as a novel autoantibody specificity, which recognized a nuclear protein with an apparent molecular mass of 33 kDa.[265] These autoantibodies were detected in 35% of patients with RA but were also detected in a small number of patients who had other autoimmune or degenerative rheumatic disorders (see Table 59.1). In later studies, the RA33 antigen was identified as the A2/B1 protein of the heterogeneous nuclear ribonucleoprotein complex (hnRNP-A2/B1).[266] Further characterization of this antibody showed that it was not specific to RA but was also found in approximately 20% of patients with SLE and in 40% to 60% of patients with mixed connective tissue disease (MCTD).[267,268] However, in SLE and MCTD, anti-RA33 usually occurred together with antibodies to U1–small nuclear ribonucleoproteins (snRNPs) or Smith (Sm) antigen. Therefore, anti-RA33 without concomitant anti–U1 snRNP autoantibodies were found to have specificity of 96% for RA.[267] Additionally, anti-RA33 antibodies in RA, SLE, and MCTD are distinguished by their recognition of different conformation-dependent epitopes in hnRNP-A2/B1.[269] Moreover, in the absence of RF and ACPAs, anti-RA33 antibodies in patients with very early arthritis (<3 months' duration) are associated with a relatively mild, nonerosive disease course; this may potentially help identify patients with a good prognosis who will respond well to treatment with DMARDs.[270] In addition, stimulation assays using hnRNP-A2 protein induced T cell proliferation in almost 60% of patients with RA but only 20% of the control subjects, with substantially stronger responses in patients with RA.[271] Interestingly, immunohistochemical analyses have revealed pronounced overexpression of hnRNP-A2 in synovial tissue of patients with RA, which places the antigen at sites of disease in RA.

An intriguing feature of RA33 is that this antigen is also citrullinated in the RA joint and is a target of ACPAs in RA.[44] Thus, patients with RA can have antibodies to both the native and citrullinated forms of RA33. Moreover, four transcript variants encoded by the same gene have been identified in cells from RA synovial fluid (designated *hnRNP-A2, B1, A2b, and B1b*), with *hnRNP-B1b* being most strongly recognized.[44] In a single cohort, antibodies against citrullinated *hnRNP-B1b* were identified in 44% of patients with RA, whereas antibodies against the native protein were detected in 10.7% of patients. Only 6% of patients with RA had both antibody specificities.[44] The presence of autoantibodies against the same antigen in two different forms (i.e., native and citrullinated) may reflect an evolving immune response to structural immunogenic changes in autoantigens that occur during the development of the disease.

Anti-glucose-6-Phosphate Isomerase Antibodies

Glucose-6-phosphate isomerase (G6PI) is another autoantigen of potential interest in RA, and is a glycolytic enzyme residing in the cytoplasm of all cells. Anti-G6PI antibodies were first discovered in the K/BxN mouse model of arthritis, in which pathogenic Igs that recognize G6PI are formed.[272–274] These antibodies are directly pathogenic in mice because passive transfer of anti-G6PI antibodies alone can induce arthritis to healthy recipients.[275] The pathogenic potential of this antibody prompted its study in human RA. However, although initial studies reported a high frequency of such antibodies in sera of patients with RA,[276] these results have been the subject of debate.[277–279] Overall, anti-G6PI antibodies are found in 12% to 29% of patients with RA in different cohorts and are more prevalent in patients with active disease (see Table 59.1). Patients with psoriatic arthritis, undifferentiated arthritis, and spondylarthropathy also develop anti-G6PI antibodies at similar frequencies (12% to 25%), and similar titers are detected in a proportion (5% to 10%) of control subjects or patients with Crohn's disease or sarcoidosis.[279] The potential relevance of these antibodies in RA is still uncertain.

Conclusion

The autoantibody repertoire in patients with RA is diverse, and new antigen specificities continue to be discovered. Autoantibodies in RA are important tools for disease diagnosis and for identifying clinically informative patient subgroups. They are also serologic clues for understanding disease pathogenesis. Autoantibodies identified to date, fall into three major categories: citrullination-associated autoantibodies, antibodies to chemically modified proteins, and those that recognize largely native proteins that are shared with other diseases. Although antigens targeted by these autoantibody families are not specific to the RA joint, understanding the generation of these antigens and defining the genetic and environmental factors linked to autoantibody development offers valuable insight into disease mechanism. To date, citrullination-associated antibodies are the most specific for the diagnosis of RA, and specific genetic and environmental factors associated with their development have been defined. The discovery of these antibodies has identified dysregulated protein citrullination as a key pathogenic mechanism and potential therapeutic target in this disease. Similar studies of other RA autoantibodies and their target antigens at sites of disease initiation and propagation may enable the development of additional novel strategies for the treatment and prevention of RA.

Full references for this chapter can be found on ExpertConsult.com.

Selected References

1. Nienhuis RL, Mandema E: A new serum factor in patients with rheumatoid arthritis; the antiperinuclear factor, *Ann Rheum Dis* 23:302–305, 1964.
2. Sondag-Tschroots IR, Aaij C, Smit JW, et al.: The antiperinuclear factor. 1. The diagnostic significance of the antiperinuclear factor for rheumatoid arthritis, *Ann Rheum Dis* 38:248–251, 1979.
3. Hoet RM, Boerbooms AM, Arends M, et al.: Antiperinuclear factor, a marker autoantibody for rheumatoid arthritis: colocalisation of the perinuclear factor and profilaggrin, *Ann Rheum Dis* 50:611–618, 1991.
4. Janssens X, Veys EM, Verbruggen G, et al.: The diagnostic significance of the antiperinuclear factor for rheumatoid arthritis, *J Rheumatol* 15:1346–1350, 1988.
5. Cassani F, Ferri S, Bianchi FB, et al.: Antiperinuclear factor in an Italian series of patients with rheumatoid arthritis, *Ric Clin Lab* 13:347–352, 1983.
6. Berthelot JM, Maugars Y, Audrain M, et al.: Specificity of antiperinuclear factor for rheumatoid arthritis in rheumatoid factor-positive sera, *Br J Rheumatol* 34:716–720, 1995.
7. Manera C, Franceschini F, Cretti L, et al.: Clinical heterogeneity of rheumatoid arthritis and the antiperinuclear factor, *J Rheumatol* 21:2021–2025, 1994.
8. Youinou P, Le GP, Dumay A, et al.: The antiperinuclear factor. I. Clinical and serologic associations, *Clin Exp Rheumatol* 8:259–264, 1990.
9. Youinou P, Seigneurin JM, Le GP, et al.: The antiperinuclear factor. II. Variability of the perinuclear antigen, *Clin Exp Rheumatol* 8:265–269, 1990.
10. Youinou P, Le GP: The reliability of the antiperinuclear factor test despite the inconstancy of the targeted antigens, *J Rheumatol* 21:1990–1991, 1994.
11. Aggarwal R, Liao K, Nair R, et al.: Anti-citrullinated peptide antibody assays and their role in the diagnosis of rheumatoid arthritis, *Arthritis Rheum* 61:1472–1483, 2009.
12. Young BJ, Mallya RK, Leslie RD, et al.: Anti-keratin antibodies in rheumatoid arthritis, *Br Med J* 2:97–99, 1979.
13. Scott DL, Delamere JP, Jones LJ, et al.: Significance of laminar antikeratin antibodies to rat oesophagus in rheumatoid arthritis, *Ann Rheum Dis* 40:267–271, 1981.
14. Miossec P, Youinou P, Le GP, et al.: Clinical relevance of antikeratin antibodies in rheumatoid arthritis, *Clin Rheumatol* 1:185–189, 1982.
15. Ordeig J, Guardia J: Diagnostic value of antikeratin antibodies in rheumatoid arthritis, *J Rheumatol* 11:602–604, 1984.
16. Vincent C, Serre G, Lapeyre F, et al.: High diagnostic value in rheumatoid arthritis of antibodies to the stratum corneum of rat oesophagus epithelium, so-called 'antikeratin antibodies', *Ann Rheum Dis* 48:712–722, 1989.
17. Paimela L, Gripenberg M, Kurki P, et al.: Antikeratin antibodies: diagnostic and prognostic markers for early rheumatoid arthritis, *Ann Rheum Dis* 51:743–746, 1992.
18. Simon M, Girbal E, Sebbag M, et al.: The cytokeratin filament-aggregating protein fillagrin is the target of the co-called "antikeratin antibodies," autoantibodies specific for rheumatoid arthritis, *J Clin Invest* 92:1387–1393, 1993.
19. Sebbag M, Simon M, Vincent C, et al.: The antiperinuclear factor and the so-called antikeratin antibodies are the same rheumatoid arthritis-specific autoantibodies, *J Clin Invest* 95:2672–2679, 1995.
20. Markova NG, Marekov LN, Chipev CC, et al.: Profilaggrin is a major epidermal calcium-binding protein, *Mol Cell Biol* 13:613–625, 1993.
21. Senshu T, Akiyama K, Kan S, et al.: Detection of deiminated proteins in rat skin: probing with a monospecific antibody after modification of citrulline residues, *J Invest Dermatol* 105:163–169, 1995.
22. Senshu T, Kan S, Ogawa H, et al.: Preferential deimination of keratin K1 and filaggrin during the terminal differentiation of human epidermis, *Biochem Biophys Res Commun* 225:712–719, 1996.
23. Vossenaar ER, Zendman AJ, van Venrooij WJ, et al.: PAD, a growing family of citrullinating enzymes: genes, features and involvement in disease, *BioEssays* 25:1106–1118, 2003.
24. Schellekens GA, de Jong BA, van den Hoogen FH, et al.: Citrulline is an essential constituent of antigenic determinants recognized by rheumatoid arthritis-specific autoantibodies, *J Clin Invest* 101:273–281, 1998.
25. Baeten D, Peene I, Union A, et al.: Specific presence of intracellular citrullinated proteins in rheumatoid arthritis synovium: relevance to antifilaggrin autoantibodies, *Arthritis Rheum* 44:2255–2262, 2001.
26. Masson-Bessiere C, Sebbag M, Durieux JJ, et al.: In the rheumatoid pannus, anti-filaggrin autoantibodies are produced by local plasma cells and constitute a higher proportion of IgG than in synovial fluid and serum, *Clin Exp Immunol* 119:544–552, 2000.
27. Dyson HJ, Wright PE: Antigenic peptides, *FASEB J* 9:37–42, 1995.
28. Dorow DS, Shi PT, Carbone FR, et al.: Two large immunogenic and antigenic myoglobin peptides and the effects of cyclisation, *Mol Immunol* 22:1255–1264, 1985.

29. Schellekens GA, Visser H, de Jong BA, et al.: The diagnostic properties of rheumatoid arthritis antibodies recognizing a cyclic citrullinated peptide, *Arthritis Rheum* 43:155–163, 2000.
30. Lee DM, Schur PH: Clinical utility of the anti-CCP assay in patients with rheumatic diseases, *Ann Rheum Dis* 62:870–874, 2003.
31. van Venrooij WJ, Zendman AJ: Anti-CCP2 antibodies: an overview and perspective of the diagnostic abilities of this serological marker for early rheumatoid arthritis, *Clin Rev Allergy Immunol* 34:36–39, 2008.
32. van Gaalen FA, Visser H, Huizinga TW: A comparison of the diagnostic accuracy and prognostic value of the first and second anti-cyclic citrullinated peptides (CCP1 and CCP2) autoantibody tests for rheumatoid arthritis, *Ann Rheum Dis* 64:1510–1512, 2005.
33. Lutteri L, Malaise M, Chapelle JP: Comparison of second- and third-generation anti-cyclic citrullinated peptide antibodies assays for detecting rheumatoid arthritis, *Clin Chim Acta* 386:76–81, 2007.
34. dos Anjos LM, Pereira IA, d'Orsi E, et al.: A comparative study of IgG second- and third-generation anti-cyclic citrullinated peptide (CCP) elisas and their combination with IgA third-generation CCP elisa for the diagnosis of rheumatoid arthritis, *Clin Rheumatol* 28:153–158, 2009.
35. Vincent C, Nogueira L, Clavel C, et al.: Autoantibodies to citrullinated proteins: ACPA, *Autoimmunity* 38:17–24, 2005.
36. Masson-Bessiere C, Sebbag M, Girbal-Neuhauser E, et al.: The major synovial targets of the rheumatoid arthritis-specific antifilaggrin autoantibodies are deiminated forms of the alpha- and beta-chains of fibrin, *J Immunol* 166:4177–4184, 2001.
37. Kinloch A, Lundberg K, Wait R, et al.: Synovial fluid is a site of citrullination of autoantigens in inflammatory arthritis, *Arthritis Rheum* 58:2287–2295, 2008.
38. Vossenaar ER, Radstake TR, van der HA, et al.: Expression and activity of citrullinating peptidylarginine deiminase enzymes in monocytes and macrophages, *Ann Rheum Dis* 63:373–381, 2004.
39. Vossenaar ER, Despres N, Lapointe E, et al.: Rheumatoid arthritis specific anti-Sa antibodies target citrullinated vimentin, *Arthritis Res Ther* 6:R142–R150, 2004.
40. van Beers JJ, Willemze A, Stammen-Vogelzangs J, et al.: Anti-citrullinated fibronectin antibodies in rheumatoid arthritis are associated with human leukocyte antigen-DRB1 shared epitope alleles, *Arthritis Res Ther* 14:R35, 2012.
41. Darrah E, Rosen A, Giles JT, et al.: Peptidylarginine deiminase 2, 3 and 4 have distinct specificities against cellular substrates: novel insights into autoantigen selection in rheumatoid arthritis, *Ann Rheum Dis* 71:92–98, 2012.
42. Harlow L, Rosas IO, Gochuico BR, et al.: Identification of citrullinated hsp90 isoforms as novel autoantigens in rheumatoid arthritis-associated interstitial lung disease, *Arthritis Rheum* 65:869–879, 2013.
43. Dwivedi N, Upadhyay J, Neeli I, et al.: Felty's syndrome autoantibodies bind to deiminated histones and neutrophil extracellular chromatin traps, *Arthritis Rheum* 64:982–992, 2012.
44. Konig MF, Giles JT, Nigrovic PA, et al.: Antibodies to native and citrullinated RA33 (hnRNP A2/B1) challenge citrullination as the inciting principle underlying loss of tolerance in rheumatoid arthritis, *Ann Rheum Dis* 75:2022–2028, 2016.
45. Kinloch A, Tatzer V, Wait R, et al.: Identification of citrullinated alpha-enolase as a candidate autoantigen in rheumatoid arthritis, *Arthritis Res Ther* 7:R1421–R1429, 2005.
46. Matsuo K, Xiang Y, Nakamura H, et al.: Identification of novel citrullinated autoantigens of synovium in rheumatoid arthritis using a proteomic approach, *Arthritis Res Ther* 8:R175, 2006.
47. Suzuki A, Yamada R, Ohtake-Yamanaka M, et al.: Anti-citrullinated collagen type I antibody is a target of autoimmunity in rheumatoid arthritis, *Biochem Biophys Res Commun* 333:418–426, 2005.
48. Burkhardt H, Sehnert B, Bockermann R, et al.: Humoral immune response to citrullinated collagen type II determinants in early rheumatoid arthritis, *Eur J Immunol* 35:1643–1652, 2005.
49. Okazaki Y, Suzuki A, Sawada T, et al.: Identification of citrullinated eukaryotic translation initiation factor 4G1 as novel autoantigen in rheumatoid arthritis, *Biochem Biophys Res Commun* 341:94–100, 2006.
50. Goeb V, Thomas-L'Otellier M, Daveau R, et al.: Candidate autoantigens identified by mass spectrometry in early rheumatoid arthritis are chaperones and citrullinated glycolytic enzymes, *Arthritis Res Ther* 11:R38, 2009.
51. van Beers JJ, Schwarte CM, Stammen-Vogelzangs J, et al.: The rheumatoid arthritis synovial fluid citrullinome reveals novel citrullinated epitopes in apolipoprotein E, myeloid nuclear differentiation antigen, and beta-actin, *Arthritis Rheum* 65:69–80, 2013.
52. Romero V, Fert-Bober J, Nigrovic PA, et al.: Immune-mediated pore-forming pathways induce cellular hypercitrullination and generate citrullinated autoantigens in rheumatoid arthritis, *Sci Transl Med* 5, 2013. 209ra150.
53. Tutturen AE, Fleckenstein B, de Souza GA: Assessing the citrullinome in rheumatoid arthritis synovial fluid with and without enrichment of citrullinated peptides, *J Proteome Res* 13:2867–2873, 2014.
54. Wang F, Chen FF, Gao WB, et al.: Identification of citrullinated peptides in the synovial fluid of patients with rheumatoid arthritis using LC-MALDI-TOF/TOF, *Clin Rheumatol* 35:2185–2194, 2016.
55. Tilvawala R, Nguyen SH, Maurais AJ, et al.: The rheumatoid arthritis-associated citrullinome, *Cell Chem Biol*, 2018.
56. Bang H, Egerer K, Gauliard A, et al.: Mutation and citrullination modifies vimentin to a novel autoantigen for rheumatoid arthritis, *Arthritis Rheum* 56:2503–2511, 2007.
57. Sokolove J, Bromberg R, Deane KD, et al.: Autoantibody epitope spreading in the pre-clinical phase predicts progression to rheumatoid arthritis, *PLoS One* 7:e35296, 2012.
58. Wagner CA, Sokolove J, Lahey LJ, et al.: Identification of anti-citrullinated protein antibody reactivities in a subset of anti-CCP-negative rheumatoid arthritis: association with cigarette smoking and HLA-DRB1 'shared epitope' alleles, *Ann Rheum Dis* 74:579–586, 2015.
59. Nishimura K, Sugiyama D, Kogata Y, et al.: Meta-analysis: diagnostic accuracy of anti-cyclic citrullinated peptide antibody and rheumatoid factor for rheumatoid arthritis, *Ann Intern Med* 146:797–808, 2007.
60. Sun J, Zhang Y, Liu L, et al.: Diagnostic accuracy of combined tests of anti cyclic citrullinated peptide antibody and rheumatoid factor for rheumatoid arthritis: a meta-analysis, *Clin Exp Rheumatol* 32:11–21, 2014.
61. van Gaalen FA, Linn-Rasker SP, van Venrooij WJ, et al.: Autoantibodies to cyclic citrullinated peptides predict progression to rheumatoid arthritis in patients with undifferentiated arthritis: a prospective cohort study, *Arthritis Rheum* 50:709–715, 2004.
62. Jansen LM, van Schaardenburg D, van der Horst-Bruinsma I, et al.: The predictive value of anti-cyclic citrullinated peptide antibodies in early arthritis, *J Rheumatol* 30:1691–1695, 2003.
63. Nell VP, Machold KP, Stamm TA, et al.: Autoantibody profiling as early diagnostic and prognostic tool for rheumatoid arthritis, *Ann Rheum Dis* 64:1731–1736, 2005.
64. Vencovsky J, Machacek S, Sedova L, et al.: Autoantibodies can be prognostic markers of an erosive disease in early rheumatoid arthritis, *Ann Rheum Dis* 62:427–430, 2003.
65. Mewar D, Coote A, Moore DJ, et al.: Independent associations of anti-cyclic citrullinated peptide antibodies and rheumatoid factor with radiographic severity of rheumatoid arthritis, *Arthritis Res Ther* 8:R128, 2006.
66. Syversen SW, Gaarder PI, Goll GL, et al.: High anti-cyclic citrullinated peptide levels and an algorithm of four variables predict radiographic progression in patients with rheumatoid arthritis: results from a 10-year longitudinal study, *Ann Rheum Dis* 67:212–217, 2008.
67. De RL, Peene I, Hoffman IE, et al.: Rheumatoid factor and anti-citrullinated protein antibodies in rheumatoid arthritis: diagnostic value, associations with radiological progression rate, and extra-articular manifestations, *Ann Rheum Dis* 63:1587–1593, 2004.

68. Turesson C, Jacobsson LT, Sturfelt G, et al.: Rheumatoid factor and antibodies to cyclic citrullinated peptides are associated with severe extra-articular manifestations in rheumatoid arthritis, *Ann Rheum Dis* 66:59–64, 2007.
69. Quinn MA, Gough AK, Green MJ, et al.: Anti-CCP antibodies measured at disease onset help identify seronegative rheumatoid arthritis and predict radiological and functional outcome, *Rheumatology (Oxford)* 45:478–480, 2006.
70. Kelly CA, Saravanan V, Nisar M, et al.: Rheumatoid arthritis-related interstitial lung disease: associations, prognostic factors and physiological and radiological characteristics—a large multicentre UK study, *Rheumatology (Oxford)* 53:1676–1682, 2014.
71. Giles JT, Danoff SK, Sokolove J, et al.: Association of fine specificity and repertoire expansion of anticitrullinated peptide antibodies with rheumatoid arthritis associated interstitial lung disease, *Ann Rheum Dis* 73:1487–1494, 2014.
72. Aubart F, Crestani B, Nicaise-Roland P, et al.: High levels of anti-cyclic citrullinated peptide autoantibodies are associated with co-occurrence of pulmonary diseases with rheumatoid arthritis, *J Rheumatol* 38:979–982, 2011.
73. Zhu J, Zhou Y, Chen X, et al.: A metaanalysis of the increased risk of rheumatoid arthritis-related pulmonary disease as a result of serum anticitrullinated protein antibody positivity, *J Rheumatol* 41:1282–1289, 2014.
74. Giles JT, Malayeri AA, Fernandes V, et al.: Left ventricular structure and function in patients with rheumatoid arthritis, as assessed by cardiac magnetic resonance imaging, *Arthritis Rheum* 62:940–951, 2010.
75. Marasovic-Krstulovic D, Martinovic-Kaliterna D, Fabijanic D, et al.: Are the anti-cyclic citrullinated peptide antibodies independent predictors of myocardial involvement in patients with active rheumatoid arthritis? *Rheumatology (Oxford)* 50:1505–1512, 2011.
76. Lopez-Longo FJ, Oliver-Minarro D, De lT I, et al.: Association between anti-cyclic citrullinated peptide antibodies and ischemic heart disease in patients with rheumatoid arthritis, *Arthritis Rheum* 61:419–424, 2009.
77. Makrygiannakis D, Hermansson M, Ulfgren AK, et al.: Smoking increases peptidylarginine deiminase 2 enzyme expression in human lungs and increases citrullination in BAL cells, *Ann Rheum Dis* 67:1488–1492, 2008.
78. Giles JT, Fert-Bober J, Park JK, et al.: Myocardial citrullination in rheumatoid arthritis: a correlative histopathologic study, *Arthritis Res Ther* 14:R39, 2012.
79. Bongartz T, Cantaert T, Atkins SR, et al.: Citrullination in extra-articular manifestations of rheumatoid arthritis, *Rheumatology (Oxford)* 46:70–75, 2007.
80. Sokolove J, Brennan MJ, Sharpe O, et al.: Brief report: citrullination within the atherosclerotic plaque: a potential target for the anti-citrullinated protein antibody response in rheumatoid arthritis, *Arthritis Rheum* 65:1719–1724, 2013.
81. Gizinski AM, Mascolo M, Loucks JL, et al.: Rheumatoid arthritis (RA)-specific autoantibodies in patients with interstitial lung disease and absence of clinically apparent articular RA, *Clin Rheumatol* 28:611–613, 2009.
82. Fischer A, Solomon JJ, Du Bois RM, et al.: Lung disease with anti-CCP antibodies but not rheumatoid arthritis or connective tissue disease, *Respir Med* 106:1040–1047, 2012.
83. Visser K, Verpoort KN, van DH, et al.: Pretreatment serum levels of anti-cyclic citrullinated peptide antibodies are associated with the response to methotrexate in recent-onset arthritis, *Ann Rheum Dis* 67:1194–1195, 2008.
84. Farragher TM, Lunt M, Plant D, et al.: Benefit of early treatment in inflammatory polyarthritis patients with anti-cyclic citrullinated peptide antibodies versus those without antibodies, *Arthritis Care Res (Hoboken)* 62:664–675, 2010.
85. Braun-Moscovici Y, Markovits D, Zinder O, et al.: Anti-cyclic citrullinated protein antibodies as a predictor of response to anti-tumor necrosis factor-alpha therapy in patients with rheumatoid arthritis, *J Rheumatol* 33:497–500, 2006.
86. Nielen MM, van SD, Reesink HW, et al.: Specific autoantibodies precede the symptoms of rheumatoid arthritis: a study of serial measurements in blood donors, *Arthritis Rheum* 50:380–386, 2004.
87. Kurki P, Aho K, Palosuo T, et al.: Immunopathology of rheumatoid arthritis. Antikeratin antibodies precede the clinical disease, *Arthritis Rheum* 35:914–917, 1992.
88. Arbuckle MR, James JA, Kohlhase KF, et al.: Development of anti-dsDNA autoantibodies prior to clinical diagnosis of systemic lupus erythematosus, *Scand J Immunol* 54:211–219, 2001.
89. Arbuckle MR, McClain MT, Rubertone MV, et al.: Development of autoantibodies before the clinical onset of systemic lupus erythematosus, *N Engl J Med* 349:1526–1533, 2003.
90. Kolfenbach JR, Deane KD, Derber LA, et al.: Autoimmunity to peptidyl arginine deiminase type 4 precedes clinical onset of rheumatoid arthritis, *Arthritis Rheum* 62:2633–2639, 2010.
91. Eriksson C, Kokkonen H, Johansson M, et al.: Autoantibodies predate the onset of systemic lupus erythematosus in northern Sweden, *Arthritis Res Ther* 13:R30, 2011.
92. Kokkonen H, Mullazehi M, Berglin E, et al.: Antibodies of IgG, IgA and IgM isotypes against cyclic citrullinated peptide precede the development of rheumatoid arthritis, *Arthritis Res Ther* 13:R13, 2011.
93. Rantapaa-Dahlqvist S, de Jong BA, Berglin E, et al.: Antibodies against cyclic citrullinated peptide and IgA rheumatoid factor predict the development of rheumatoid arthritis, *Arthritis Rheum* 48:2741–2749, 2003.
94. Deighton CM, Walker DJ, Griffiths ID, et al.: The contribution of hla to rheumatoid arthritis, *Clin Genet* 36:178–182, 1989.
95. McDonagh JE, Walker DJ: Incidence of rheumatoid arthritis in a 10-year follow-up study of extended pedigree multicase families, *Br J Rheumatol* 33:826–831, 1994.
96. Berglin E, Johansson T, Sundin U, et al.: Radiological outcome in rheumatoid arthritis is predicted by presence of antibodies against cyclic citrullinated peptide before and at disease onset, and by IgA-RF at disease onset, *Ann Rheum Dis* 65:453–458, 2006.
97. Majka DS, Deane KD, Parrish LA, et al.: Duration of preclinical rheumatoid arthritis-related autoantibody positivity increases in subjects with older age at time of disease diagnosis, *Ann Rheum Dis* 67:801–807, 2008.
98. Arlestig L, Mullazehi M, Kokkonen H, et al.: Antibodies against cyclic citrullinated peptides of IgG, IgA and IgM isotype and rheumatoid factor of IgM and IgA isotype are increased in unaffected members of multicase rheumatoid arthritis families from northern Sweden, *Ann Rheum Dis* 71:825–829, 2012.
99. Ioan-Facsinay A, Willemze A, Robinson DB, et al.: Marked differences in fine specificity and isotype usage of the anti-citrullinated protein antibody in health and disease, *Arthritis Rheum* 58:3000–3008, 2008.
100. Young KA, Deane KD, Derber LA, et al.: Relatives without rheumatoid arthritis show reactivity to anti-citrullinated protein/peptide antibodies that are associated with arthritis-related traits: studies of the etiology of rheumatoid arthritis, *Arthritis Rheum* 65:1995–2004, 2013.
101. Shirai H, Blundell TL, Mizuguchi K: A novel superfamily of enzymes that catalyze the modification of guanidino groups, *Trends Biochem Sci* 26:465–468, 2001.
102. Thompson PR, Fast W: Histone citrullination by protein arginine deiminase: is arginine methylation a green light or a roadblock? *ACS Chem Biol* 1:433–441, 2006.
103. McGraw WT, Potempa J, Farley D, et al.: Purification, characterization, and sequence analysis of a potential virulence factor from Porphyromonas gingivalis, peptidylarginine deiminase, *Infect Immun* 67:3248–3256, 1999.
104. Chavanas S, Mechin MC, Takahara H, et al.: Comparative analysis of the mouse and human peptidylarginine deiminase gene clusters reveals highly conserved non-coding segments and a new human gene, *PADI6 Gene* 330:19–27, 2004.

105. Nakashima K, Hagiwara T, Yamada M: Nuclear localization of peptidylarginine deiminase V and histone deimination in granulocytes, *J Biol Chem* 277:49562–49568, 2002.
106. Zhou Y, Chen B, Mittereder N, et al.: Spontaneous secretion of the citrullination enzyme PAD2 and cell surface exposure of PAD4 by neutrophils, *Front Immunol* 8:1200, 2017.
107. Cherrington BD, Morency E, Struble AM, et al.: Potential role for peptidylarginine deiminase 2 (PAD2) in citrullination of canine mammary epithelial cell histones, *PLoS One* 5:e11768, 2010.
108. Arita K, Hashimoto H, Shimizu T, et al.: Structural basis for Ca(2+)-induced activation of human PAD4, *Nat Struct Mol Biol* 11:777–783, 2004.
109. Witalison EE, Thompson PR, Hofseth LJ: Protein arginine deiminases and associated citrullination: physiological functions and diseases associated with dysregulation, *Curr Drug Targets* 16:700–710, 2015.
110. Esposito G, Vitale AM, Leijten FP, et al.: Peptidylarginine deiminase (PAD) 6 is essential for oocyte cytoskeletal sheet formation and female fertility, *Mol Cell Endocrinol* 273:25–31, 2007.
111. Foulquier C, Sebbag M, Clavel C, et al.: Peptidyl arginine deiminase type 2 (PAD-2) and PAD-4 but not PAD-1, PAD-3, and PAD-6 are expressed in rheumatoid arthritis synovium in close association with tissue inflammation, *Arthritis Rheum* 56:3541–3553, 2007.
112. Chang X, Yamada R, Suzuki A, et al.: Localization of peptidylarginine deiminase 4 (PADI4) and citrullinated protein in synovial tissue of rheumatoid arthritis, *Rheumatology (Oxford)* 44:40–50, 2005.
113. Arita K, Shimizu T, Hashimoto H, et al.: Structural basis for histone N-terminal recognition by human peptidylarginine deiminase 4, *Proc Natl Acad Sci U S A* 103:5291–5296, 2006.
114. Slade DJ, Fang P, Dreyton CJ, et al.: Protein arginine deiminase 2 binds calcium in an ordered fashion: implications for inhibitor design, *ACS Chem Biol* 10:1043–1053, 2015.
115. Raijmakers R, Zendman AJ, Egberts WV, et al.: Methylation of arginine residues interferes with citrullination by peptidylarginine deiminases in vitro, *J Mol Biol* 367:1118–1129, 2007.
116. Darrah E, Andrade F: Rheumatoid arthritis and citrullination, *Curr Opin Rheumatol* 30:72–78, 2018.
117. Tarcsa E, Marekov LN, Mei G, et al.: Protein unfolding by peptidylarginine deiminase. substrate specificity and structural relationships of the natural substrates trichohyalin and filaggrin, *J Biol Chem* 271:30709–30716, 1996.
118. Inagaki M, Takahara H, Nishi Y, et al.: Ca2+-dependent deimination-induced disassembly of intermediate filaments involves specific modification of the amino-terminal head domain, *J Biol Chem* 264:18119–18127, 1989.
119. Wang Y, Wysocka J, Sayegh J, et al.: Human PAD4 regulates histone arginine methylation levels via demethylimination, *Science* 306:279–283, 2004.
120. Proost P, Loos T, Mortier A, et al.: Citrullination of CXCL8 by peptidylarginine deiminase alters receptor usage, prevents proteolysis, and dampens tissue inflammation, *J Exp Med* 205:2085–2097, 2008.

60 Acute Phase Reactants

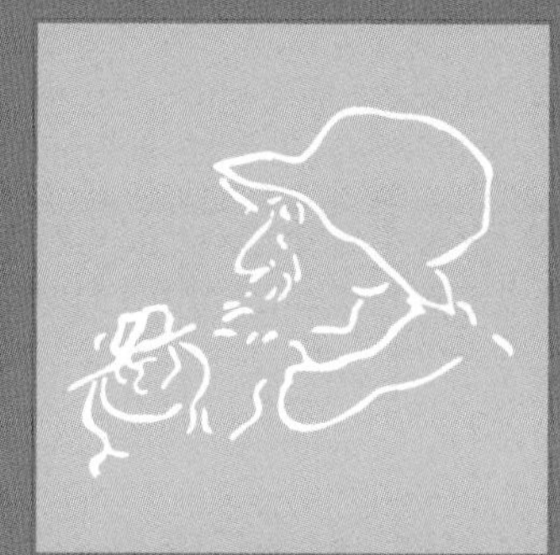

REBECCA HABERMAN, CESAR E. FORS NIEVES, BRUCE N. CRONSTEIN, AND AMIT SAXENA

KEY POINTS

Inflammation comprises a complex and highly variable set of processes that represent a response to tissue damage from infection or injury.

The acute phase response, a major accompaniment of inflammation, is induced by inflammation-associated cytokines and includes a reorchestration of acute phase protein synthesis by the liver.

The erythrocyte sedimentation rate (ESR), the most commonly used clinical measure of inflammation, depends on numerous physical and chemical characteristics of blood, many of which are not related to inflammation.

The quintessential acute phase protein, C-reactive protein (CRP), not only offers biomarker utility in the clinic, but it also plays a role in host defense by recognition of biologic substrates, activation of the complement pathway, and by binding to leukocytes.

Cytokines, chemokines, adhesion molecules, and other products of activated inflammatory cells are secreted during inflammation and play roles in the inflammatory response, but several problems limit the clinical usefulness of their quantitation for routine clinical purposes.

CRP and ESR may reflect disease activity and correlate with disease prognosis in rheumatoid arthritis but generally are not helpful for differential diagnosis.

Although CRP and ESR correlate with clinical activity in many inflammatory rheumatic diseases, the absent or modest CRP response seen in some patients with active systemic lupus erythematosus remains unexplained.

Minor elevations of CRP, within the normal population reference range, are associated with increased risk of myocardial infarction but are nonspecific (especially in patients with rheumatic disease). Minor CRP elevation is associated with well-recognized risk factors for cardiovascular disease, which may explain its predictive value.

Introduction

The inflammatory response is the body's natural defense against unchecked tissue damage from infection or injury. It occurs during the acute phase of an inciting event and, if the stimulus is not eliminated, in a chronic, putatively healing stage. When excessive or uncontrollfed, these responses have the potential to cause significant harm to the host through processes such as autoimmune diseases, allergic reactions, and septic shock.

The concept of inflammation itself has evolved over thousands of years. Celsus first described the cardinal signs of redness, swelling, heat, and pain in the first century AD. The fifth sign, loss of function, is often attributed to Galen's work in the second century.[1] Since that time, countless advances have been made in the understanding of inflammation, from histologic findings of inflammatory cells within tissues, to the discovery of hematologic and soluble mediators such as cytokines and complement. Also, the molecular signaling pathways that drive both its protective effects and the inappropriate injurious responses have been elucidated (see Chapters 20, 27, 28).

With increasing insight into mechanisms of the inflammatory response has come an appreciation of its significant complexity. Molecular and microscopic processes are different during acute and chronic stages, and diverse responses are induced by various types of exogenous and endogenous stimuli (e.g., bacteria, viruses, parasites, crystals, allergens, and ischemia). More recently, the role of the milieu of the inflammatory response, especially at the level of the vascular endothelium, has taken on considerable importance.[2] Furthermore, inherent redundancies of functions have been noted, as have interactions between the mediators of inflammation that allow for a broad, effective response, but these redundancies make it difficult to understand the pathways of inflammation in a linear fashion. These intricacies have resulted in a vague definition and on continued reliance on the final downstream macroscopic cardinal signs to tie together all of the ongoing processes. It is these same intricacies that have made evaluation of inflammation through laboratory tests imprecise.

Basic hematologic abnormalities may give clues to the presence of inflammation, but different patterns are often associated with underlying causes and are not universally found. Leukocytosis can be seen in infections, acute crystal diseases, and some autoimmune disorders such as adult Still's disease. Anemia is often associated with certain diseases that cause chronic inflammation, such as rheumatoid arthritis (RA). Reactive thrombocytosis occurs secondary to the release of cytokines after an inciting infectious or inflammatory event, and the role of platelets and platelet-derived mediators in stimulating inflammation has been described at the molecular level.[3]

Laboratory tests most commonly used by physicians to obtain information about the extent of inflammation are those that measure the acute phase reaction. In response to injury, local inflammatory cells secrete cytokines that influence the liver to increase or decrease production of various proteins. The erythrocyte sedimentation rate (ESR) has been the classic marker of inflammation, with serum C-reactive protein (CRP) taking on an increasingly prominent role. Other novel inflammatory markers such as procalcitonin have been recognized, but their clinical utility has yet to be fully determined.

CRP elevations, especially minor ones, have been noted in numerous conditions that traditionally have not been considered inflammatory, most significantly involving the cardiovascular system. This has shed light on subclinical inflammation as a possible factor in the pathogenesis of a number of nonrheumatologic diseases.

Acute Phase Response

Within minutes of tissue injury, activation of the innate immune system induces cytokine production that results in a multisystem acute phase response involving the liver, vascular system, bone marrow, and CNS.[4,5] Many elements of the reaction can be regarded as part of the innate response and are defensive or adaptive in nature.[6] Murine studies suggest that as much as 7% of the regulatory gene pool undergoes significant changes in expression during inflammation, and that induction of liver acute phase genes is mediated by the transcription factor signal transducer and activator of transcription 3 (STAT3).[7–9]

Although the acute phase response can trigger numerous neuroendocrine, hematopoietic, and metabolic effects, the changes in plasma proteins synthesized by hepatocytes are monitored as signs of underlying inflammation (Tables 60.1 and 60.2). An acute phase protein is one in which the plasma concentration changes from baseline by at least 25% during inflammation; responses vary in terms of concentration and kinetics (Fig. 60.1).[10] CRP and serum amyloid A (SAA) levels increase more than 1000-fold during acute infection and peak at 2 to 3 days. Concentrations of other proteins peak at longer periods and can range from a 50% increase in complement and ceruloplasmin, to a several-fold amplification in haptoglobin, fibrinogen, α1-proteinase inhibitor, and α1-acid glycoprotein. Other proteins are negative acute phase proteins, the concentrations of which fall during the inflammatory response. These include anti-thrombin III, protein S, prealbumin, albumin, transferrin, and apolipoprotein A-I.[4,5]

Hepatic stimulation of acute phase proteins is induced by cytokines released by activated monocytes, macrophages, neutrophils, natural killer (NK) cells, and endothelial cells acting at the front lines of the inflammatory response. The main cytokine influencing the liver is IL-6, once called the *hepatocyte-stimulating factor.* It likely mediates protein expression via the Janus kinase (JAK) and STAT3 pathways, as well as C/EBP family members and Rel proteins (nuclear factor-κB [NF-κB]).[9,11] During initial stages, IL-1 and TNF synergize with IL-6 and trigger further IL-6 production, but their roles are limited.[12] The soluble IL-6 receptor amplifies IL-6 effects both locally and systemically. IL-6 also performs a protective role during disease, inducing the expression of an IL-1 receptor antagonist.[13]

Acute phase protein levels are not uniform in their expression; this is likely related to the underlying pathophysiologic state and is regulated by different combinations and interactions of cytokines.[4] The roles of the acute phase proteins themselves will be discussed throughout the chapter but have been found to include direct involvement in host defense by activation of the complement, proteinase inhibition, and antioxidant activity.[14] However, some of the described in vitro effects of proteins may not be relevant in vivo.

Erythrocyte Sedimentation Rate

Although ESR is an indirect screen for elevated concentrations of acute phase proteins, it has been the most widely used marker of inflammation for almost a century. Measurement of ESR is performed when blood is placed in a vertical tube and the rate of fall of erythrocytes is measured. The ancient Greeks recognized increased red blood cell (RBC) sedimentation as a way to detect "bad bodily humors," but our modern understanding and use of RBC sedimentation as a test date back to the German scholar Fahraeus in 1918.[15] He determined that certain plasma proteins, especially fibrinogen, are able to lower the electrostatic charge on RBC surfaces so they can aggregate, form rouleaux, and fall faster.

Several factors are involved in acceleration of ESR. Asymmetric plasma proteins, such as fibrinogen and, to a lesser extent, alpha$_2$, beta, and gamma globulins decrease the negative charge of erythrocytes (zeta potential) that prevents rouleaux formation. Red cell factors themselves play a role as changes in plasma ratios in anemic states also favor rouleaux. However, microcytosis, polycythemia, and abnormally shaped RBCs (e.g., sickle cells and spherocytes) hinder aggregation and lower the ESR.[16] Conditions that elevate fibrinogen, even if they are not necessarily considered inflammatory, can raise ESR. These include pregnancy, diabetes, end-stage renal disease, and heart disease. Major increases in the concentration of a single molecular species, such as a monoclonal immunoglobulin in multiple myeloma, also cause increased sedimentation.[17] The ESR is elevated in obesity, as is CRP, presumably as a result of IL-6 secretion by adipocytes.[18] Factors such as glucocorticoids, cryoglobulinemia, hypofibrinogenemia, and hyperviscosity lower the value.[5] The physiochemical dynamics that allow for sedimentation have been a continued source of debate, with disparate models presented to explain how proteins on cell surfaces interact to cause RBC aggregation.[19]

Although novel and rapid tests for ESR have proven promising, the International Committee for Standardization in Hematology continues to recommend the Westergren technique of testing anti-coagulated blood.[20–23] Reference ranges are established locally, but the usual accepted upper limits of normal are 15 mm/hr for males and 20 mm/hr for females; however, the ESR increases with age and varies by race, which calls the reliability of the test into question.[24] A simple formula for calculating the upper limit of normal ESR at any age has been used regularly: in men, age in years divided by two; in women, 10 plus age in years divided by two. Despite the ability to control for age, other limitations of the test have been noted and are listed in Table 60.3. The relative virtues of CRP determination have diminished some of the importance of ESR, but it remains an easy, inexpensive test with a wealth of background literature. Therefore the ESR continues to play a prominent role in clinical practice.

C-Reactive Protein

CRP is an acute phase protein, the serum concentration of which reflects ongoing inflammation better than other tests in most, but not all, diseases.[25] CRP was identified in 1930, when sera

TABLE 60.1 Human Acute Phase Proteins

Plasma Proteins That Increase in Inflammation	
Complement System	
	C3
	C4
	C9
	Factor B
	C1 inhibitor
	C4b-binding protein
	Mannose-binding lectin
Coagulation and fibrinolytic system	
	Fibrinogen
	Plasminogen
	Tissue plasminogen activator
	Urokinase
	Protein S
	Vitronectin
	Plasminogen-activator inhibitor 1
Anti-proteases	
	α-Protease inhibitor
	α-Anti-chymotrypsin
	Pancreatic secretory trypsin inhibitor
	Inter-α-trypsin inhibitors
Transport proteins	
	Ceruloplasmin
	Haptoglobin
	Hemopexin
Participants in inflammatory responses	
	Secreted phospholipase A2
	Lipopolysaccharide-binding protein
	Interleukin-1–receptor antagonist
	Granulocyte colony-stimulating factor
Others	
	C-reactive protein
	Serum amyloid A
	α-Acid glycoprotein
	Fibronectin
	Ferritin
	Angiotensinogen
Plasma Proteins That Decrease in Inflammation	
	Albumin
	Transferrin
	Transthyretin
	α-HS glycoprotein
	Alpha-fetoprotein
	Thyroxine-binding globulin
	Insulin-like growth factor I
	Factor XII

HS, Heremans-Schmid.

From Gabay C, Kushner I: Acute-phase proteins and other systemic responses to inflammation. *N Engl J Med* 340:448–454, 1999.

obtained from patients with *Streptococcus* pneumonia infection were found to contain a protein that could bind to the "C" polysaccharide of the bacterial cell wall. This protein circulates as a 115 kDa pentamer of noncovalently linked 23 kDa subunits, which has been highly conserved during hundreds of millions of years of evolution. In contrast to immunoglobulins and complement components, CRP deficiency in humans has not been described. Genome-wide associated studies performed recently have shown that at least seven distinct loci are involved in the basal expression of CRP,[26–28] which is upregulated upon stimulation by the transcription factors C/EBP and Rel.[29] It is present in trace concentrations in the plasma of all humans (roughly 1 mg/L, with higher concentrations in women and the elderly). Plasma CRP is synthesized by hepatocytes, although other sites of local production and possibly minimal secretion have been suggested.

The precise function of CRP is unknown and may be varied, but it exhibits important recognition and activation capabilities, and it binds to numerous ligands.[30] CRP recognizes phosphocholine, phospholipids, fibronectin, chromatin, and histones, all of which are exposed at sites of tissue damage and by apoptotic cells; CRP may target them for clearance.[31] CRP bridges the gap between innate and adaptive immunity by activating the classic complement pathway and interacting with cells of the immune system through binding of Fcγ receptors.[32,33] CRP induces inflammatory cytokines, tissue factors, and shedding of the IL-6 receptor, all of which result in a complement-dependent increase in tissue damage.[31] Other CRP functions are anti-inflammatory, including promotion of the non-inflammatory clearance of apoptotic cells and prevention of neutrophil adhesion to the endothelium.[33,34] Thus CRP may play many pathophysiologic roles during the course of the inflammatory process.[14,35]

After an acute inflammatory stimulus, CRP concentration increases rapidly and peaks at 2 to 3 days at levels that reflect the extent of tissue injury. If the stimulus has been removed, serum CRP levels drop rapidly, with a half-life of roughly 19 hours.[36] Persistent elevations in CRP are seen in chronic inflammatory or infectious states such as active RA or pulmonary tuberculosis, and may be observed also in extensive malignant disease.

Immunoassays and laser nephelometry are used at modest cost to quantify serum CRP levels. Most healthy adults have levels less than 0.3 mg/dL. The significance of minor elevations in CRP is a subject of debate and will be discussed subsequently. However, usual methods of CRP determination are less precise at concentrations in the range of 0.3 to 1 mg/dL, so high-sensitivity (hs) CRP methods are used to accurately measure these levels. Generally, concentrations greater than 1 mg/dL reflect clinically

TABLE 60.2 Additional Acute Phase Phenomena

Neuroendocrine Changes
Fever, somnolence, and anorexia
Increased secretion of corticotropin-releasing hormone, corticotropin, and cortisol
Increased secretion of arginine vasopressin
Decreased production of insulin-like growth factor I
Increased adrenal secretion of catecholamines
Hematopoietic Changes
Anemia of chronic disease
Leukocytosis
Thrombocytosis
Metabolic Changes
Loss of muscle and negative nitrogen balance
Decreased gluconeogenesis
Osteoporosis
Increased hepatic lipogenesis
Increased lipolysis in adipose tissue
Decreased lipoprotein lipase activity in muscle and adipose tissue
Cachexia
Hepatic Changes
Increased metallothionein, inducible nitric oxide synthase, heme oxygenase, manganese superoxide dismutase, and tissue inhibitor of metalloproteinase-1
Decreased phosphoenolpyruvate carboxykinase activity
Changes in Nonprotein Plasma Constituents
Hypozincemia, hypoferremia, and hypercupremia
Increased plasma retinol and glutathione concentrations

From Gabay C, Kushner I: Acute-phase proteins and other systemic responses to inflammation. *N Engl J Med* 340:448–454, 1999.

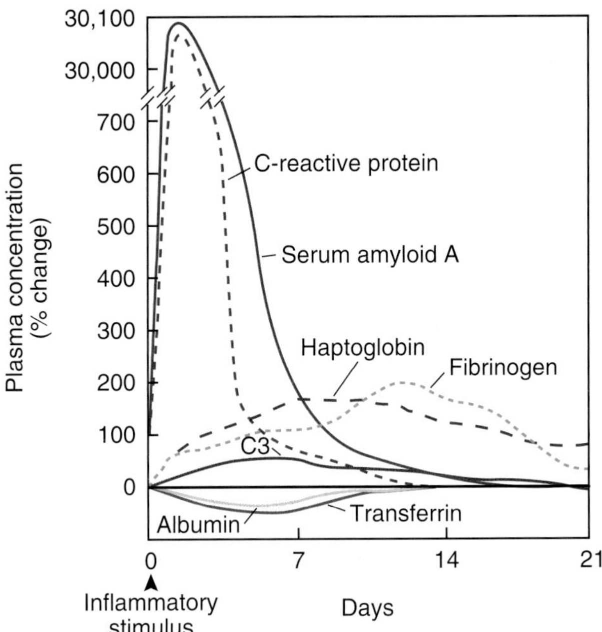

• **Fig. 60.1** Typical plasma acute phase protein changes after a moderate inflammatory stimulus. Several patterns of response are seen: major acute phase protein, increase 100-fold (e.g., C-reactive protein, serum amyloid A); moderate acute phase protein, increase twofold to fourfold (e.g., fibrinogen and haptoglobin); minor acute phase protein, increase 50% to 100% (e.g., complement C3); and negative acute phase protein, decrease (e.g., albumin, transferrin). (Modified from Gitlin JD, Colten HR: Molecular biology of the acute-phase plasma proteins. In Pick E, Landy M, editors: *Lymphokines*, vol 14, San Diego, 1987, Academic Press, pp 123–153.)

significant inflammatory disease.[10,37] Concentrations of 1 to 10 mg/dL can be considered to represent moderate increases, and concentrations greater than 10 mg/dL show marked increases. Most patients with extremely high levels (e.g., >15 mg/dL) have bacterial infection. One study found that in patients with CRP concentrations greater than 50 mg/dL, infection was present in 88% of participants.[38] Clinical conditions associated with varying degrees of elevation of CRP are listed in Table 60.4, and the range of CRP concentrations in many rheumatologic diseases is shown in Fig. 60.2.

Several limitations associated with the use of C-reactive protein measurement must be acknowledged. No uniformity in reporting concentrations has been noted between laboratories, and values can be conveyed in mg/L, µg/mL, or mg/dL. Similar to ESR, population studies show a skewed, rather than gaussian, distribution, which renders parametric statistical tests inappropriate for interpretation of CRP data. Population differences in CRP levels in the United States have been reported between sexes and among racial groups. This is presumably also prevalent as an issue in practice in other populations globally. Elevation of CRP in the elderly may represent age-related disorders, the pathogenesis of which may involve low-grade inflammation, which complicates the issue of what levels are considered normal.[39]

Procalcitonin

Procalcitonin (PCT), a propeptide of calcitonin, has recently received increased attention as a useful measure to differentiate between acute bacterial infection and other inflammatory and febrile syndromes. Normally produced in the C-cells of the thyroid gland, PCT is usually cleaved into calcitonin, katacalcin, and an N-terminal residue. Under normal circumstances, PCT is not released into the bloodstream; however, during severe infection, plasma levels can increase dramatically.[40,41] Interestingly, this does not lead to an increase in plasma calcitonin levels or activity. At this time, the exact site of PCT production, as well as its pathophysiologic role during infection and sepsis, remains uncertain.[42]

In healthy humans, PCT levels are undetectable or are very low (<0.1 ng/mL). During systemic bacterial infection, PCT levels can increase to higher than 100 ng/mL. Currently available diagnostic tests measure the calcitonin/N-ProCT part of the protein and therefore only a fragment of the 114 to 116 amino acid chain of the prohormone. A useful reference range to exclude sepsis and systemic inflammation is less than or equal to 0.2 ng/mL. Plasma levels of greater than or equal to 0.5 ng/mL should be interpreted as abnormal and suggest sepsis. After reaching peak levels, circulating PCT has a half-life of approximately 22 to 35 hours in serum, and its concentration declines with a 50% plasma-disappearance rate of roughly 1 to 1½ days. It is worth noting that in patients with severe renal dysfunction these rates may be prolonged, but accumulation does not occur.[43]

TABLE 60.3 Comparison of Erythrocyte Sedimentation Rate and C-Reactive Protein

	Erythrocyte Sedimentation Rate	C-Reactive Protein
Advantages	Much clinical information in the literature Might reflect overall health status	Rapid response to inflammatory stimuli Wide range of clinically relevant values are detectable Unaffected by age and sex Reflects value of a single acute phase protein Can be measured on stored sera Measurement is precise and reproducible
Disadvantages	Affected by red blood cell morphology Affected by anemia and polycythemia Reflects levels of many plasma proteins, not all of which are acute phase proteins Responds slowly to inflammatory stimuli Requires fresh sample May be affected by drugs	Not sensitive to changes in SLE disease activity

TABLE 60.4 Conditions Associated With Elevated C-Reactive Protein Levels

Normal or Minor Elevation (<1 mg/dL)
Vigorous exercise
Common cold
Pregnancy
Gingivitis
Seizures
Depression
Insulin resistance and diabetes
Several genetic polymorphisms
Obesity
Moderate Elevation (1 to 10 mg/dL)
Myocardial infarction
Malignancies
Pancreatitis
Mucosal infection (bronchitis, cystitis)
Most systemic autoimmune diseases
Rheumatoid arthritis
Marked Elevation (>10 mg/dL)
Acute bacterial infection (80% to 85%)
Major trauma
Systemic vasculitis

In differentiating between infection and other sources of inflammation, studies have shown that elevated serum levels of PCT have a significantly higher specificity for infection than ESR and CRP.[44–48] PCT has been studied extensively as a clinical tool to facilitate the decision as to when to start and stop anti-bacterial agents in patients with pneumonia,[49,50] and it has also shown promise in differentiating between infectious and noninfectious causes of fever after orthopedic surgery, in which ESR and CRP levels can be difficult to interpret.[51–53] For all of these reasons, it remains an intriguing clinical tool for use in patients with fevers in the setting of autoimmune disease who are commonly on immunosuppressive medications and at higher risk of infection.

As a biomarker for infection in autoimmune diseases, the role of PCT has not yet been fully established. In contrast to CRP, PCT levels are not elevated in the majority of cases of noninfectious inflammation or nonbacterial infection. High PCT levels in patients with autoimmune disorder are more likely to denote a concomitant bacterial or fungal infection than inflammation from the autoimmune disease itself.[44,48,54] However, exceptions to this rule include some vasculitis syndromes such as Kawasaki's disease, Goodpasture's syndrome, adult-onset Still's disease,[55,56] and granulomatosis with polyangiitis,[57] for which observational studies have demonstrated elevated levels of PCT in patients without evidence of bacterial infection. For the differentiation between infection and systemic lupus erythematosus flare[58–62] as well as for the differentiation between infection and an acute gout flare,[63,64] data are mixed, and no definitive statement regarding the usefulness of PCT can be made at this time.

Calprotectin

Fecal calprotectin is increasingly used in the diagnosis of inflammatory bowel disease (IBD). Calprotectin is a calcium and zinc binding protein (heterodimer of S100A8/S100A9) found mainly in neutrophils, accounting for up to 60% of cytosolic proteins.[65] It is located in a lesser extent in monocytes and macrophages.[66] With the recruitment of leukocytes at the gut mucosa with inflammation, calprotectin is released into the epithelial space. The calprotectin level correlates with granulocyte migration through the gut wall as evidenced by the excretion of indium-111-labeled neutrophilic granulocytes.[67] The exact role of calprotectin is unknown, but it may possess bactericidal and fungicidal properties. It can also act as an endogenous ligand of Toll-like receptor 4, leading to pro-inflammatory effects such as the upregulation of IL-6.[68–72]

Calprotectin is found in blood, saliva, urine, synovial fluid, and stool. It is most commonly found in the feces where concentrations are generally higher than in other bodily fluids and the protein can stay stable at room temperature for up to 7 days.[68,73] While the normal range for fecal calprotectin is usually reported at 10 to 50 to 60 µg/mg, the exact range is assay dependent. The normal range also varies with age; those at the extremes of life, particularly children younger than 5 years old, have higher levels that are considered normal.[74,75] In

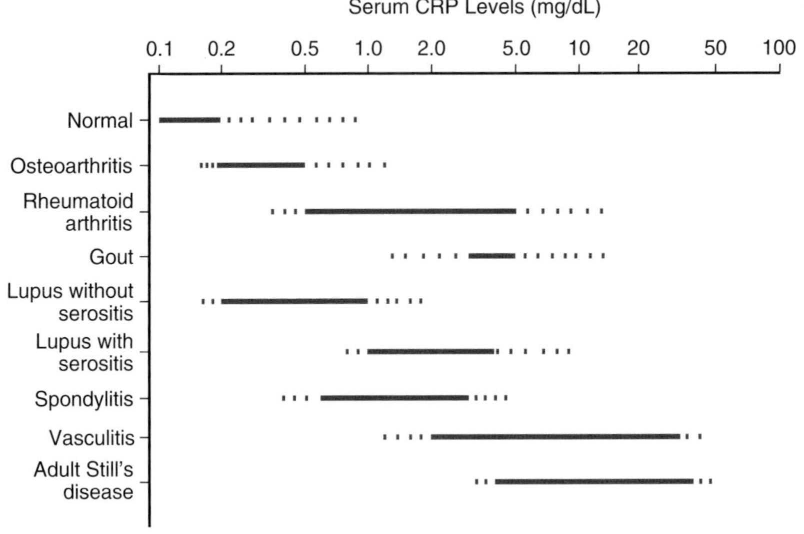

• **Fig. 60.2** Range of C-reactive protein (CRP) levels in rheumatic disease. Authors' estimates of expected levels of CRP (mg/dL) in certain rheumatic diseases.

young children, this difference is thought to be secondary to increased permeability of the intestinal mucosa and differences in the gut flora.

Calprotectin is now well established in distinguishing between IBD and nonorganic disease (such as irritable bowel syndrome) with recent meta-analyses showing a sensitivity of 72% to 95% and a specificity of 74% to 96%.[76–78] Calprotectin can also be used to monitor disease activity in IBD. Fecal calprotectin levels correlate with clinical and endoscopic disease activity[79–81] and are useful in predicting relapse in patients with known disease.[82] However, calprotectin is not specific to IBD. Increased calprotectin levels are seen in other causes of gut inflammation such as with the use of nonsteroidal anti-inflammatory drugs (NSAIDs) or aspirin,[83,84] colorectal cancer,[85] gastrointestinal infections,[86,87] and diverticulitis.[88,89] Furthermore, dietary fiber intake and physical activity may also affect measured levels of calprotectin.[75]

Calprotectin elevations are also seen in other autoimmune disorders. In RA, high calprotectin levels are found both in synovial fluid, likely produced by the pannus, and in the serum as compared with patients with osteoarthritis.[90,91] Furthermore, serum and synovial fluid calprotectin levels are higher in rheumatoid factor (RF) and anti-cycle citrullinated peptide (anti-CCP) positive patients,[31] correlate with disease activity scores such as the DAS28,[91,92] and are independent predictors of erosive progression and therapeutic response.[93] Calprotectin levels are also elevated in the serum and synovial fluid of patients with axial spondyloarthritis and correlate with effective therapy.[94] Patients with psoriasis alone produce elevated levels of calprotectin from keratinocytes, but have lower levels than comparable patients with psoriatic arthritis, underlying the importance of the synovium in calprotectin production.[95] Spondyloarthritis has also been associated with increased fecal calprotectin,[96] however this is likely reflective of the subclinical gut inflammation rather than the joint inflammation itself.[97,98]

Systemic lupus erythematosus (SLE) has also been associated with higher levels of calprotectin and with disease activity and flares.[99,100] Additionally, adult-onset Still's disease,[101] gout,[102] Sjögren's syndrome,[103] scleroderma,[103] Behçet's disease,[104] and ANCA-associated vasculitis[105,106] have all been associated with higher levels of calprotectin.

Other Acute Phase Proteins

Measurement of other acute phase proteins has been of limited value clinically because their responses to tissue injury are often slower, and the magnitude of concentration change is smaller than with CRP. SAA, a circulating family of proteins produced by hepatocytes, adipocytes, macrophages, and fibroblast-like synoviocytes, has been correlated with disease activity in a number of inflammatory disorders.[107] However, reliable testing for acute phase SAA is not widely available, and data about levels expected in disease are limited. Serum ferritin is moderately increased, triggered by cytokines such as IL-1, IL-6, IL-18, and TNF. Levels are frequently high in adult-onset Still's disease and SLE, and they correlate with disease activity.[108,109] Hepcidin, a liver-derived anti-microbial peptide and regulator of iron homeostasis, is induced by inflammation, and by IL-6 in particular.[110] Its levels rise in parallel with ferritin, and it is important in the development of anemia of chronic disease, acting as a negative regulator of iron absorption and macrophage iron release teleologically, to deprive microbes of iron.[111] Transferrin, which binds and transports iron, is a negative acute phase protein.

Apolipoprotein A-I, the principal protein constituent of high-density lipoprotein (HDL), is another negative acute phase protein. In chronic inflammatory diseases such as RA and SLE, decreased levels may contribute to increased risk of thrombotic events.[112,113] Serum albumin and prealbumin (transthyretin) are also negative acute phase proteins, although their measurement is not more helpful in diagnosis or prognosis than standard tests.[114] Serum complement fractions become depressed when the system is activated in certain autoimmune disorders but otherwise rise during the acute phase response.

Cytokines

Although not acute phase proteins in the classic sense, cytokines display the most striking acute phase behavior of any circulating proteins. IL-6 responds dramatically to tissue injury, with concentration changes that are faster and greater than those of CRP or SAA. Acute inflammation and chronic inflammation have been associated with increases in IL-6, and serum levels of this cytokine have been correlated with the severity and course of disease in RA, juvenile arthritis, ankylosing spondylitis, and polymyalgia

TABLE 60.5 Products of Inflammatory, Endothelial, and Resident Target Tissue Cells/Matrix

Cytokines and Related Molecules
Cytokines
IL-1
IL-6
IL-12
IFN-α
TNF
Granulocyte-macrophage colony-stimulating factor
IL-1 receptor antagonist
Products of Inflammatory and Endothelial Cells
Calprotectin von Willebrand factor
Soluble adhesion molecules (e.g., sVCAM and sE-selectin)
Hyaluronic acid
Collagen and aggrecan degradation products
Osteocalcin

sVCAM, Soluble vascular cell adhesion molecule.

rheumatica (PMR).[115,116] It is also more sensitive than ESR for detecting disease activity in giant cell arteritis (GCA).[117] IL-6 levels may be useful in monitoring inflammation if hepatocytes are damaged to the point that they are not able to synthesize acute phase proteins.[4] Knowledge of soluble IL-6 receptor levels may also be helpful in this regard. The importance of cytokines such as TNF, IL-1, and IL-6 has been inferred by the successful reduction of inflammation by their therapeutic inhibitors. Certain diseases, such as the TNF receptor–associated periodic syndrome (TRAPS) and the autoinflammatory syndromes that involve mutations of the inflammasome controlling IL-1, point to the importance of these cytokines (see Chapter 31).

Increased levels of several other cytokines and circulating cytokine receptors have been associated with inflammation or disease activity as well (Table 60.5).[117,118] Different patterns of cytokine responses have been reported in different diseases, suggesting that cytokine determinations are potentially useful clinically.[119,120] However, their quantitation presents several problems related to their short plasma half-lives, the presence of blocking factors and natural inhibitors, and other technical considerations.[121] At present, high costs, limited availability, and the absence of standardization discourage the measurement of plasma cytokines and their receptors in clinical practice.

Acute Phase Reactants in the Management of Rheumatic Diseases

Measurement of ESR and CRP has no role in the diagnosis of any particular disease, including RA, osteoarthritis, SLE, PMR, GCA, or other inflammatory arthropathies. However, these measurements can be clinically helpful in three ways: (1) in evaluating the extent or severity of inflammation, (2) in monitoring changes in disease activity over time, (3) and in assessing prognosis.

Rheumatoid Arthritis

ESR and CRP cannot be used definitively in the diagnosis of RA, because 45% of patients may have normal serum levels at presentation,[122] and these parameters represent part of the diagnostic syndrome or classification criteria sets. These tests are more appropriately applied in RA for monitoring disease activity and evaluating response to therapy in the context of other clinical modalities. Although ESR traditionally has been more widely used for these purposes, many studies have suggested that CRP levels correlate better with disease activity.[123] Some recent reports state that CRP levels may overestimate disease response compared with ESR; others claim that differences between the two are minimal.[123–125] The existence of patients with depressed CRP concentrations caused by carrying low-CRP–associated genetic variants must be taken into account when this test is used universally.[126] Matrix metalloproteinase (MMP)-3, pro-MMP-3, and soluble E-selectin have also been proposed as markers for RA disease activity. Their measurements correlate with CRP levels but do not provide more information than is provided by standard tests.[127–129]

CRP levels average 2 to 3 mg/dL in adult patients with RA who have moderate disease activity.[130] However, variation is considerable. At least 5% to 10% of patients have values in the normal range, whereas a few patients with severe disease activity have levels greater than 10 mg/dL. ESR values have been found to remain stable over the years.[131] ESR and CRP have long been used to follow the response to therapy; in general, effective disease-modifying anti-rheumatic drug therapy decreases CRP levels by approximately 40%. Inhibition of joint damage by these agents usually is accompanied by marked improvement in acute phase reactants. Progression of joint damage can occur while the patient is on therapy, however, despite decreases in ESR and CRP.[132] Even more striking improvement has been seen with biologic agents introduced since the 1990s, providing objective laboratory support for the encouraging clinical responses observed. In early reports of anti-TNF therapy, CRP and SAA levels declined by 75% and 85%, respectively, in approximately 1 week.[133] Treatment with abatacept, the T cell CD80/CD86:CD28 co-stimulation modulator, resulted in significant decreases in CRP at both 90 and 360 days of therapy.[134] Tofacitinib, a JAK inhibitor, also appeared to effectively decrease DAS28-ESR scores in RA patients in clinical trials; therefore it may be a useful tool to monitor disease activity.[135] In one study, failure to suppress CRP levels 2 weeks after initiation of infliximab therapy identified most patients who would prove to be clinical nonresponders after 12 weeks.[136] In contrast to traditional disease-modifying anti-rheumatic drugs, TNF inhibitors have been found to inhibit joint damage even while clinical activity, reflected by CRP levels, remains high.[137] Tocilizumab, a human IL-6 receptor antibody, improves RA by inhibiting effects of the cytokine. However, because of its mechanism of action, inflammatory markers such as ESR and CRP drop to negative values, so that tracking them may not reflect the actual effect of the drug but rather its pharmacodynamic effects on IL-6 mediated hepatocyte activation; care must be taken, therefore, when monitoring disease activity during tocilizumab therapy.[138,139]

ESR and CRP also have value as prognostic indicators in RA. Elevated acute phase reactant levels are associated with early synovitis and erosions as detected by MRI, with inflammatory cellular infiltrates in synovium, and with osteoclastic activation and reduced bone mineral density.[140–142] CRP predicts radiographic progression, as do ESR and the matrix metalloproteinases MMP-3 and MMP-1.[127,128,143–145] Finally, and perhaps most important, acute phase reactants correlate with work disability on long-term follow-up and predict progression to major joint replacement.[146,147] As in the normal population, CRP levels are associated with death from cardiovascular disease.[148] In patients with RA in whom heart failure developed, ESR was higher during the 6-month period immediately preceding the onset of heart failure than earlier in its course.[149]

Serum or synovial fluid levels of many other tissue products (see Table 60.5) have been correlated with clinical measures of disease activity, severity, and radiographic damage.

Newer quantitative and objective assays that incorporate some of the measures previously mentioned as well as other novel ones have recently come into the market to aid in the management and earlier diagnosis of patients with RA. The multibiomarker disease activity (MBDA) test is comprised of 12 different serum markers. It is increasingly popular and has correlated with DAS28 scores,[150] predicts radiologic joint damage,[151] and improves prediction of relapse.[102] It has recently been adjusted for body mass index (BMI). It could play a significant role in the future management and study of RA; however, more studies are required to determine their clinical usefulness across different mechanistic interventions.

Systemic Lupus Erythematosus

Although serum levels of CRP often parallel disease activity in autoimmune disorders, it has been recognized that SLE is an exception.[152] Although marked CRP responses are seen in subsets of patients, such as those with serositis or chronic synovitis, many (e.g., patients with nephritis) show mild or no elevation during periods of activity.[153–155] Serum levels of SAA are also relatively low in comparison with those of patients with RA, which may explain why rates of secondary amyloidosis are decreased in these patients.[156] In contrast, ESR correlates with disease activity and accrued tissue damage in SLE.[157] Fibrinogen levels increased over time in patients, regardless of disease activity.[158] Data are insufficient to evaluate the potential use of some of the other newer markers described previously, including PCT, but many SLE patients with normal CRP levels show elevated IL-6 concentrations.[159] Therefore a deficiency in IL-6 does not explain the muted CRP response in SLE.

Although the concomitant decrease in SAA may point against it, several investigations have raised the possibility that low CRP levels may be related to the pathogenesis of SLE: (1) an association has been noted between SLE and a genetic polymorphism associated with low CRP levels; (2) it has been observed that low CRP levels may contribute to defective clearance of autoantigens during apoptosis; (3) and the therapeutic efficacy of CRP has been reported in mouse models of SLE.[153,160–163] Recent studies have also raised the possibility that type I interferon (IFN), which is expressed significantly in SLE, may inhibit CRP expression.[164,165]

Substantial CRP elevation in SLE patients is more likely to result from superimposed infection than from activation of lupus. CRP levels greater than 6 mg/dL in these patients should serve as an impetus to exclude the possibility of infection, just as they should in other diseases.[10] Such levels should not be regarded as proof of infection, however; as indicated earlier, marked CRP elevation related to active SLE can be seen in the absence of infection.

Carotid plaque and intima-media wall thickness, correlates of atherosclerotic vascular disease, have been found in association with minor CRP elevation in women with SLE, as they have in patients with RA.[166,167] (see Chapter 39 for detailed discussion)

Polymyalgia Rheumatica and Giant Cell Arteritis

The diagnosis of PMR or GCA is supported by an elevated ESR, often greater than 100 mm/hr. However, such elevation is no longer regarded as a sine qua non of these disorders; continuing reports suggest that 10% to 20% of patients with PMR can have a "normal" ESR, depending on which value is taken as the limit of normal. Such patients tend to have fewer systemic symptoms and less severe, less frequent anemia.[168] They have the same frequency of positive temporal artery biopsy results, however, as patients with elevated ESR.[169,170]

Only approximately 5% of patients with GCA had ESR values less than 40 mm/hr; these patients had fewer visual and systemic symptoms than patients with high ESR values.[171] In contrast to these findings, ESR and CRP were found to be significantly lower in patients with ocular involvement, most commonly in the range of 70 mm/hr to 100 mm/hr. Patients with ESR greater than 100 mm/hr had decreased incidence of visual ischemic events.[172–174]

In PMR and GCA, CRP and ESR have been regarded in the past as equally valuable in assessing disease activity. However, recent reports suggest that CRP is more sensitive for both conditions and should be included routinely in the diagnostic workup.[170,175,176] The report that IL-6 is more sensitive than ESR for indicating disease activity in GCA is of particular interest.[177] Subsets of patients with PMR who have persistently elevated levels of CRP and IL-6 despite corticosteroid treatment have a higher risk of relapse.[172] A polymorphism at the IL-6 gene promoter has characterized these PMR patients with persistently elevated levels of the cytokine.[178] This connection is underlined by the effectiveness of tocilizumab, an IL-6 receptor inhibitor, in the treatment of GCA.[179]

Clinical manifestations of disease, even in the presence of a normal ESR or CRP level, should not be ignored. Furthermore, extreme elevation of the ESR in the absence of symptoms of PMR or GCA should raise suspicion of other disorders, such as infection, malignancy, or renal disease. PCT levels in patients with PMR or GCA are usually normal according to a French prospective study. Elevated PCT levels in these patients with a normal temporal artery biopsy would be suggestive of an alternate diagnosis.[180]

Numerous markers of endothelial perturbation, although not acute phase reactants in the strict sense, are elevated in plasma in various inflammatory disorders of vessels, particularly PMR, GCA, and other vasculitides.[181] These molecules include von Willebrand factor, thrombomodulin, some vasoactive prostanoids, and a variety of adhesion molecules, such as vascular cell adhesion molecule-1.

Adult-Onset Still's Disease

Markedly elevated concentrations of ferritin, disproportionately high compared with those of other acute phase reactants, have long been noted in adult-onset Still's disease but are not specific.[182] Only a small percentage, commonly less than 20%, of ferritin is glycosylated in adult-onset Still's disease, a criterion included in proposed classification criteria for this condition.[183,184] Concentrations of serum IL-18 were extremely elevated in patients with active adult-onset Still's disease compared with those of patients with other connective tissue diseases or of healthy individuals and were correlated with serum ferritin values and disease severity.[185] The cytokine profile in the sera of patients suggests a type 1 T helper (Th) cell response, with significantly higher levels of TNF, IL-6, and IL-8, in addition to IL-18.[55] The role of IL-1 has been inferred from significant improvement in disease activity by the IL-1 receptor antagonist, anakinra.[186,187] It has been suggested that IFN-α may be responsible for the hyperferritinemia of adult-onset Still's disease.[182] CRP levels are usually markedly elevated in this disease, and PCT levels have also been found to be disproportionately elevated without evidence of acute bacterial infection in these patients.[55,56]

Extremely elevated ferritin levels have been found in macrophage activation syndrome (MAS), and 40% of individuals with this condition meet the criteria for adult-onset Still's disease, suggesting to some that the two disorders are not distinct entities, but rather exist on a spectrum.[188–190] Recently, the measurement of IL-2 soluble receptors, heterotrimeric transmembrane proteins upregulated on activated T cells, have been used to aid in the diagnosis of MAS and may have better diagnostic value than ferritin.[191] Further investigation into normal ranges and diagnostic utility are still needed.

Axial Spondyloarthritis

Axial spondyloarthritis, mostly studied as ankylosing spondylitis, ordinarily does not lead to a substantial increase in ESR or CRP. Median ESR and CRP levels are 13 mm/hr and 1.6 mg/dL, respectively, in patients with only spinal involvement, and 21 mm/hr and 2.5 mg/dL in patients with peripheral involvement or associated IBD.[192] Treatment with infliximab led to an average decrease of 75% in CRP concentration after 12 weeks. Patients with lower CRP levels showed little improvement, however, raising the possibility that patients with higher CRP values show better responses to anti-TNF treatment than patients with lower CRP levels.[193–195] High-sensitivity CRP may better correlate with clinical disease activity compared with standard CRP testing.[196] It has been reported that levels of IL-8, IL-17, and IL-23 are elevated in the serum of patients with active ankylosing spondylitis, and polymorphisms in the IL-23 receptor gene are associated with the disease.[197–199]

Osteoarthritis

Minor CRP elevations of 0.3 to 1.0 mg/dL have been reported in patients with osteoarthritis, particularly those with progressive joint damage.[200] However, no evidence supports this association independent of BMI, because obesity is a common accompaniment of osteoarthritis.[201] Although local inflammation likely plays a role in the pathogenesis of osteoarthritis, systemic inflammation likely does not. However, CRP levels are higher in patients with erosive osteoarthritis of the hand than in those with nonerosive osteoarthritis.[202]

Other Rheumatic Diseases

Acute phase markers are elevated in numerous rheumatic diseases while the inflammatory cascade commences. Elevated ESR and CRP can be found in systemic vasculitides, crystal arthropathies, psoriatic and reactive arthritides, and infectious joint diseases.[203–206] Monitoring for elevated SAA levels has been proposed as a tool for diagnosis and medication adjustment in familial Mediterranean fever,[207] although this test is not widely available, limiting its utility. CRP is often normal in patients with primary Sjögren's syndrome, and those with elevated responses do not differ clinically from patients with normal levels.[208] Oligoarticular-onset juvenile idiopathic arthritis is classically considered as not associated with elevated inflammatory markers, although they are present in patients most at risk for systemic disease.[209]

Practical Use of Acute Phase Reactants

In the past, rheumatologists were found to use the ESR more than twice as frequently as they did CRP levels,[210] although ESR reflects many complex, poorly understood changes in the physical and chemical characteristics of blood not associated with inflammation. As indicated earlier, the reference normal values for ESR are unclear. It is well established that mean ESR values increase substantially with age and differ between men and women. Difficulties associated with interpretation of the ESR and an increasingly positive clinical experience with CRP suggest that rheumatologists may benefit from relying more on CRP than ESR testing.[211] No single ideal test can be used to evaluate the acute phase response, however.

Discrepancies between ESR and CRP may result from effects of blood constituents that are not related to inflammation, but that can influence the ESR. In fact, up to 12% of hospitalized patients have a discordant ESR and CRP.[212] In addition, patterns of acute phase protein changes differ in different conditions.[4] ESR may be markedly elevated in many patients with active SLE, whereas the CRP is normal. Undoubtedly, numerous other clinical situations exist in which similar discrepancies occur. Renal insufficiency and transient ischemic attacks, for example, may be more associated with high ESR and low CRP levels, while myocardial infarctions are more associated with high CRP and low ESR.[212,213]

Although a falsely high ESR has many non-inflammatory physicochemical causes (some known and many unknown), CRP values greater than 1 mg/dL almost invariably reflect a clinically significant inflammatory process. In light of these considerations, many authors believe that several tests, rather than a single test, should be performed and interpreted in their clinical context. It has been suggested that ESR, which is associated with anemia and immunoglobulin levels, may reflect general severity in RA, whereas CRP is a better test of active inflammation per se.[214]

C-Reactive Protein and Health: Associations With Nonrheumatologic Conditions

Although most ostensibly healthy individuals have CRP concentrations of 0.3 mg/dL or less, some have concentrations greater than 1 mg/dL. Such minor CRP elevation has long been attributed to trivial tissue injury or to minimal inflammatory processes, such as gingivitis. However, recent data indicate that CRP concentrations between 0.3 and 1 mg/dL have clinical relevance. This finding has led to an explosion of published literature measuring CRP levels in cardiac, neurologic, neoplastic, pulmonary, and even psychiatric disease.[215–219] The foundation of these investigations is the well-established notion that when a high-sensitivity CRP assay is used, serum CRP levels greater than 0.3 mg/dL indicate increased relative risk of atherogenesis and future myocardial infarction.[220] The statistical strength of this is as robust as, but not more robust than, established risk factors such as hypertension, diabetes, and hypercholesterolemia.[221–223] The primary unanswered questions remain: Why does CRP predict myocardial infarction? Is it a pathogenic mediator itself?

The observation that CRP is associated with many non-inflammatory conditions (e.g., low levels of physical activity, low intake of fruits and vegetables, a variety of other "unhealthy" diets, smoking, hypertension, obesity, sleep deprivation, and low alcohol intake) indicates that classic inflammation does not invariably underlie a CRP response.[224] Many of these CRP-associated conditions are known to be risk factors for cardiovascular disease, confounding the situation and suggesting that CRP predicts myocardial infarction because of its association with these risk factors. In addition, elevated CRP may not reflect inflammation, but rather a response to the presence of distressed, metabolically disturbed cells.[224] This reverse causation offers a potential explanation of the laboratory result, because atherosclerosis might trigger an elevation in CRP.

Nevertheless, CRP has been known for many years to bind to low-density lipoprotein (LDL) and to activate complement—a potentially pro-inflammatory response; it has also been detected in atherosclerotic plaques.[163,225–227] These observations have raised the possibility that CRP may play a direct causal role in coronary heart disease. Proatherogenic effects secondary to CRP injections given to mice, however, may have been caused by contaminants in commercial CRP preparations, not by CRP itself.[228] Because statin drugs lower CRP and LDL, some consider their effects to provide indirect evidence of a causal role of CRP. In the justification for the use of statins in prevention, in an intervention trial evaluating rosuvastatin (JUPITER), patients with normal LDL and elevated CRP were prescribed rosuvastatin, 20 mg daily, or placebo, and were followed prospectively. Those in the treatment arm had significant reductions in major cardiovascular events.[229] However, whether the effects of the study can be solely dependent on CRP reduction remains unclear; alternative explanations have been suggested, including the question of the importance of lowering LDL even among patients with healthy levels.[230] Whether to target CRP levels or use them as a screening tool in cardiovascular disease is an ongoing topic of intense debate.

Because no CRP inhibitor drugs are available to directly measure the effect of lowering the protein, recent studies have centered on observing patients with genetic variations that result in different baseline levels of CRP. To date, results have been conflicting with regard to the role of genetically determined CRP levels in coronary heart disease.[231–235]

Epidemiologic studies that describe an association of CRP levels with morbidity and mortality in many chronic diseases, and even in normal aging, have become a cottage industry. It is important to remember that these are observational population studies. Although such associations may have broad and intriguing implications, particularly at a societal level, they reflect probabilities. This limits their clinical value when they are applied to individual patients.

Full references for this chapter can be found on ExpertConsult.com.

Selected References

1. van den Tweel JG, Taylor CR: A brief history of pathology: preface to a forthcoming series that highlights milestones in the evolution of pathology as a discipline, *Virchows Arch* 457(1):3–10, 2010.
2. Biedermann BC: Vascular endothelium: checkpoint for inflammation and immunity, *News Physiol Sci* 16:84–88, 2001.
3. Gawaz M, Langer H, May AE: Platelets in inflammation and atherogenesis, *J Clin Invest* 115(12):3378–3384, 2005.
4. Gabay C, Kushner I: Acute-phase proteins and other systemic responses to inflammation, *N Engl J Med* 340(6):448–454, 1999.
5. Dayer E, Dayer JM, Roux-Lombard P: Primer: the practical use of biological markers of rheumatic and systemic inflammatory diseases, *Nat Clin Pract Rheumatol* 3(9):512–520, 2007.
6. Yoo JY, Desiderio S: Innate and acquired immunity intersect in a global view of the acute-phase response, *Proc Natl Acad Sci U S A* 100(3):1157–1162, 2003.
7. Desiderio S, Yoo JY: A genome-wide analysis of the acute-phase response and its regulation by Stat3beta, *Ann N Y Acad Sci* 987:280–284, 2003.
8. Alonzi T, Maritano D, Gorgoni B, et al.: Essential role of STAT3 in the control of the acute-phase response as revealed by inducible gene inactivation [correction of activation] in the liver, *Mol Cell Biol* 21(5):1621–1632, 2001.
9. Quinton LJ, Jones MR, Robson BE, et al.: Mechanisms of the hepatic acute-phase response during bacterial pneumonia, *Infect Immun* 77(6):2417–2426, 2009.
10. Morley JJ, Kushner I: Serum C-reactive protein levels in disease, *Ann N Y Acad Sci* 389:406–418, 1982.
11. Heinrich PC, Castell JV, Andus T: Interleukin-6 and the acute phase response, *Biochem J* 265(3):621–636, 1990.
12. Xing Z, Gauldie J, Cox G, et al.: IL-6 is an antiinflammatory cytokine required for controlling local or systemic acute inflammatory responses, *J Clin Invest* 101(2):311–320, 1998.
13. Jones SA, Horiuchi S, Topley N, et al.: The soluble interleukin 6 receptor: mechanisms of production and implications in disease, *FASEB J* 15(1):43–58, 2001.
14. Volanakis JE: Human C-reactive protein: expression, structure, and function, *Mol Immunol* 38(2-3):189–197, 2001.
15. Bedell SE, Bush BT: Erythrocyte sedimentation rate. From folklore to facts, *Am J Med* 78(6 Pt 1):1001–1009, 1985.
16. Vajpayee N, Gragam SS, Bem S: Basic examination of blood and bone marrow. In McPherson RA, Pincus MR, editors: *Henry's clinical diagnosis and management by labratory methods*, ed 21, Philidelphia, 2007, Saunders Elsevier, pp 465–466.
17. Sox Jr HC, Liang MH: The erythrocyte sedimentation rate. Guidelines for rational use, *Ann Intern Med* 104(4):515–523, 1986.
18. Bastard JP, Maachi M, Van Nhieu JT, et al.: Adipose tissue IL-6 content correlates with resistance to insulin activation of glucose uptake both in vivo and in vitro, *J Clin Endocrinol Metab* 87(5):2084–2089, 2002.
19. Neu B, Meiselman HJ: Red blood cell aggregration. In Baskurt OK, Meiselman HJ, editors: *Handbook of hemorheology and hemodynamics*, ed 1, Amsterdam, 2007, IOS Press, pp 114–115.
20. Cha CH, Park CJ, Cha YJ, et al.: Erythrocyte sedimentation rate measurements by TEST 1 better reflect inflammation than do those by the Westergren method in patients with malignancy, autoimmune disease, or infection, *Am J Clin Pathol* 131(2):189–194, 2009.
21. ICSH recommendations for measurement of erythrocyte sedimentation rate: International Council for Standardization in Haematology (Expert Panel on Blood Rheology), *J Clin Pathol* 46(3):198–203, 1993.
22. Jou JM, Lewis SM, Briggs C, et al.: ICSH review of the measurement of the erythocyte sedimentation rate, *Int J Lab Hematol* 33(2):125–132, 2011.
23. Kratz A, Plebani M, Peng M, et al.: ICSH recommendations for modified and alternate methods measuring the erythrocyte sedimentation rate, *Int J Lab Hematol* 39(5):448–457, 2017.
24. Osei-Bimpong A, Meek JH, Lewis SM: ESR or CRP? A comparison of their clinical utility, *Hematology* 12(4):353–357, 2007.
25. Pepys MB, Hirschfield GM: C-reactive protein: a critical update, *J Clin Invest* 111(12):1805–1812, 2003.
26. Ridker PM, Pare G, Parker A, et al.: Loci related to metabolic-syndrome pathways including LEPR, HNF1A, IL6R, and GCKR associate with plasma C-reactive protein: the Women's Genome Health Study, *Am J Hum Genet* 82(5):1185–1192, 2008.
27. Reiner AP, Barber MJ, Guan Y, et al.: Polymorphisms of the HNF1A gene encoding hepatocyte nuclear factor-1 alpha are associated with C-reactive protein, *Am J Hum Genet* 82(5):1193–1201, 2008.
28. Kathiresan S, Larson MG, Vasan RS, et al.: Contribution of clinical correlates and 13 C-reactive protein gene polymorphisms to interindividual variability in serum C-reactive protein level, *Circulation* 113(11):1415–1423, 2006.
29. Cha-Molstad H, Young DP, Kushner I, et al.: The interaction of C-Rel with C/EBPbeta enhances C/EBPbeta binding to the C-reactive protein gene promoter, *Mol Immunol* 44(11):2933–2942, 2007.
30. Black S, Kushner I, Samols D: C-reactive protein, *J Biol Chem* 279(47):48487–48490, 2004.

31. Griselli M, Herbert J, Hutchinson WL, et al.: C-reactive protein and complement are important mediators of tissue damage in acute myocardial infarction, *J Exp Med* 190(12):1733–1740, 1999.
32. Du Clos TW, Mold C: C-reactive protein: an activator of innate immunity and a modulator of adaptive immunity, *Immunol Res* 30(3):261–277, 2004.
33. Gershov D, Kim S, Brot N, et al.: C-reactive protein binds to apoptotic cells, protects the cells from assembly of the terminal complement components, and sustains an antiinflammatory innate immune response: implications for systemic autoimmunity, *J Exp Med* 192(9):1353–1364, 2000.
34. Zouki C, Beauchamp M, Baron C, et al.: Prevention of in vitro neutrophil adhesion to endothelial cells through shedding of L-selectin by C-reactive protein and peptides derived from C-reactive protein, *J Clin Invest* 100(3):522–529, 1997.
35. Mortensen RF: C-reactive protein, inflammation, and innate immunity, *Immunol Res* 24(2):163–176, 2001.
36. Vigushin DM, Pepys MB, Hawkins PN: Metabolic and scintigraphic studies of radioiodinated human C-reactive protein in health and disease, *J Clin Invest* 91(4):1351–1357, 1993.
37. Macy EM, Hayes TE, Tracy RP: Variability in the measurement of C-reactive protein in healthy subjects: implications for reference intervals and epidemiological applications, *Clin Chem* 43(1):52–58, 1997.
38. Vanderschueren S, Deeren D, Knockaert DC, et al.: Extremely elevated C-reactive protein, *Eur J Intern Med* 17(6):430–433, 2006.
39. Woloshin S, Schwartz LM: Distribution of C-reactive protein values in the United States, *N Engl J Med* 352(15):1611–1613, 2005.
40. Jacobs JW, Lund PK, Potts Jr JT, et al.: Procalcitonin is a glycoprotein, *J Biol Chem* 256(6):2803–2807, 1981.
41. Snider Jr RH, Nylen ES, Becker KL: Procalcitonin and its component peptides in systemic inflammation: immunochemical characterization, *J Investig Med* 45(9):552–560, 1997.
42. Assicot M, Gendrel D, Carsin H, et al.: High serum procalcitonin concentrations in patients with sepsis and infection, *Lancet* 341(8844):515–518, 1993.
43. Meisner M: Update on procalcitonin measurements, *Ann Lab Med* 34(4):263–273, 2014.
44. Wu JY, Lee SH, Shen CJ, et al.: Use of serum procalcitonin to detect bacterial infection in patients with autoimmune diseases: a systematic review and meta-analysis, *Arthritis Rheum* 64(9):3034–3042, 2012.
45. Wacker C, Prkno A, Brunkhorst FM, et al.: Procalcitonin as a diagnostic marker for sepsis: a systematic review and meta-analysis, *Lancet Infect Dis* 13(5):426–435, 2013.
46. Schuetz P, Albrich W, Mueller B: Procalcitonin for diagnosis of infection and guide to antibiotic decisions: past, present and future, *BMC Med* 9:107, 2011.
47. Riedel S: Procalcitonin and the role of biomarkers in the diagnosis and management of sepsis, *Diagn Microbiol Infect Dis* 73(3):221–227, 2012.
48. Shi Y, Peng JM, Hu XY, et al.: The utility of initial procalcitonin and procalcitonin clearance for prediction of bacterial infection and outcome in critically ill patients with autoimmune diseases: a prospective observational study, *BMC Anesthesiol* 15:137, 2015.
49. Christ-Crain M, Jaccard-Stolz D, Bingisser R, et al.: Effect of procalcitonin-guided treatment on antibiotic use and outcome in lower respiratory tract infections: cluster-randomised, single-blinded intervention trial, *Lancet* 363(9409):600–607, 2004.
50. Christ-Crain M, Stolz D, Bingisser R, et al.: Procalcitonin guidance of antibiotic therapy in community-acquired pneumonia: a randomized trial, *Am J Respir Crit Care Med* 174(1):84–93, 2006.
51. Hunziker S, Hugle T, Schuchardt K, et al.: The value of serum procalcitonin level for differentiation of infectious from noninfectious causes of fever after orthopaedic surgery, *J Bone Joint Surg Am* 92(1):138–148, 2010.
52. Glehr M, Friesenbichler J, Hofmann G, et al.: Novel biomarkers to detect infection in revision hip and knee arthroplasties, *Clin Orthop Relat Res* 471(8):2621–2628, 2013.
53. Ingber RB, Alhammoud A, Murray DP, et al.: A systematic review and meta-analysis of procalcitonin as a marker of postoperative orthopedic infections, *Orthopedics* 41(3):e303–e309, 2018.
54. Buhaescu I, Yood RA, Izzedine H: Serum procalcitonin in systemic autoimmune diseases—where are we now? *Semin Arthritis Rheum* 40(2):176–183, 2010.
55. Chen DY, Chen YM, Ho WL, et al.: Diagnostic value of procalcitonin for differentiation between bacterial infection and non-infectious inflammation in febrile patients with active adult-onset Still's disease, *Ann Rheum Dis* 68(6):1074–1075, 2009.
56. Scire CA, Cavagna L, Perotti C, et al.: Diagnostic value of procalcitonin measurement in febrile patients with systemic autoimmune diseases, *Clin Exp Rheumatol* 24(2):123–128, 2006.
57. Moosig F, Csernok E, Reinhold-Keller E, et al.: Elevated procalcitonin levels in active Wegener's granulomatosis, *J Rheumatol* 25(8):1531–1533, 1998.
58. Lanoix JP, Bourgeois AM, Schmidt J, et al.: Serum procalcitonin does not differentiate between infection and disease flare in patients with systemic lupus erythematosus, *Lupus* 20(2):125–130, 2011.
59. Kim HA, Jeon JY, An JM, et al.: C-reactive protein is a more sensitive and specific marker for diagnosing bacterial infections in systemic lupus erythematosus compared to S100A8/A9 and procalcitonin, *J Rheumatol* 39(4):728–734, 2012.
60. Bador KM, Intan S, Hussin S, et al.: Serum procalcitonin has negative predictive value for bacterial infection in active systemic lupus erythematosus, *Lupus* 21(11):1172–1177, 2012.
61. Liu LN, Wang P, Guan SY, et al.: Comparison of plasma/serum levels of procalcitonin between infection and febrile disease flare in patients with systemic lupus erythematosus: a meta-analysis, *Rheumatol Int* 37(12):1991–1998, 2017.
62. Serio I, Arnaud L, Mathian A, et al.: Can procalcitonin be used to distinguish between disease flare and infection in patients with systemic lupus erythematosus: a systematic literature review, *Clin Rheumatol* 33(9):1209–1215, 2014.
63. Choi ST, Song JS: Serum procalcitonin as a useful serologic marker for differential diagnosis between acute gouty attack and bacterial infection, *Yonsei Med J* 57(5):1139–1144, 2016.
64. Zhang J, Liu J, Long L, et al.: [Value of procalcitonin measurement in the diagnosis of bacterial infections in patients with fever and flare of chronic gouty arthritis], *Zhonghua Yi Xue Za Zhi* 95(31):2556–2559, 2015.
65. Hsu K, Champaiboon C, Guenther BD, et al.: Anti-infective protective properties of S100 calgranulins, *Antiinflamm Antiallergy Agents Med Chem* 8(4):290–305, 2009.
66. Dale I, Brandtzaeg P, Fagerhol MK, et al.: Distribution of a new myelomonocytic antigen (L1) in human peripheral blood leukocytes. Immunofluorescence and immunoperoxidase staining features in comparison with lysozyme and lactoferrin, *Am J Clin Pathol* 84(1):24–34, 1985.
67. Roseth AG, Schmidt PN, Fagerhol MK: Correlation between faecal excretion of indium-111-labelled granulocytes and calprotectin, a granulocyte marker protein, in patients with inflammatory bowel disease, *Scand J Gastroenterol* 34(1):50–54, 1999.
68. Acevedo D, Salvador MP, Girbes J, et al.: Fecal calprotectin: a comparison of two commercial enzymoimmunoassays and study of fecal extract stability at room temperature, *J Clin Med Res* 10(5):396–404, 2018.
69. Vogl T, Tenbrock K, Ludwig S, et al.: Mrp8 and Mrp14 are endogenous activators of Toll-like receptor 4, promoting lethal, endotoxin-induced shock, *Nat Med* 13(9):1042–1049, 2007.
70. Nishikawa Y, Kajiura Y, Lew JH, et al.: Calprotectin induces IL-6 and MCP-1 production via toll-like receptor 4 signaling in human gingival fibroblasts, *J Cell Physiol* 232(7):1862–1871, 2017.

71. Ehrchen JM, Sunderkotter C, Foell D, et al.: The endogenous Toll-like receptor 4 agonist S100A8/S100A9 (calprotectin) as innate amplifier of infection, autoimmunity, and cancer, *J Leukoc Biol* 86(3):557–566, 2009.
72. Ma L, Sun P, Zhang JC, et al.: Proinflammatory effects of S100A8/A9 via TLR4 and RAGE signaling pathways in BV-2 microglial cells, *Int J Mol Med* 40(1):31–38, 2017.
73. Naess-Andresen CF, Egelandsdal B, Fagerhol MK: Calcium binding and concomitant changes in the structure and heat stability of calprotectin (L1 protein), *Clin Mol Pathol* 48(5):M278–M284, 1995.
74. D'Angelo F, Felley C, Frossard JL: Calprotectin in daily practice: where do we stand in 2017? *Digestion* 95(4):293–301, 2017.
75. Poullis A, Foster R, Shetty A, et al.: Bowel inflammation as measured by fecal calprotectin: a link between lifestyle factors and colorectal cancer risk, *Cancer Epidemiol Biomarkers Prev* 13(2):279–284, 2004.
76. Gisbert JP, McNicholl AG: Questions and answers on the role of faecal calprotectin as a biological marker in inflammatory bowel disease, *Dig Liver Dis* 41(1):56–66, 2009.
77. van Rheenen PF, Van de Vijver E, Fidler V: Faecal calprotectin for screening of patients with suspected inflammatory bowel disease: diagnostic meta-analysis, *BMJ* 341:c3369, 2010.
78. von Roon AC, Karamountzos L, Purkayastha S, et al.: Diagnostic precision of fecal calprotectin for inflammatory bowel disease and colorectal malignancy, *Am J Gastroenterol* 102(4):803–813, 2007.
79. Sipponen T, Karkkainen P, Savilahti E, et al.: Correlation of faecal calprotectin and lactoferrin with an endoscopic score for Crohn's disease and histological findings, *Aliment Pharmacol Ther* 28(10):1221–1229, 2008.
80. Sipponen T, Savilahti E, Kolho KL, et al.: Crohn's disease activity assessed by fecal calprotectin and lactoferrin: correlation with Crohn's disease activity index and endoscopic findings, *Inflamm Bowel Dis* 14(1):40–46, 2008.
81. D'Haens G, Ferrante M, Vermeire S, et al.: Fecal calprotectin is a surrogate marker for endoscopic lesions in inflammatory bowel disease, *Inflamm Bowel Dis* 18(12):2218–2224, 2012.
82. Tibble JA, Sigthorsson G, Bridger S, et al.: Surrogate markers of intestinal inflammation are predictive of relapse in patients with inflammatory bowel disease, *Gastroenterology* 119(1):15–22, 2000.
83. Meling TR, Aabakken L, Roseth A, et al.: Faecal calprotectin shedding after short-term treatment with non-steroidal anti-inflammatory drugs, *Scand J Gastroenterol* 31(4):339–344, 1996.
84. Tibble JA, Sigthorsson G, Foster R, et al.: High prevalence of NSAID enteropathy as shown by a simple faecal test, *Gut* 45(3):362–366, 1999.
85. Moris D, Spartalis E, Angelou A, et al.: The value of calprotectin S100A8/A9 complex as a biomarker in colorectal cancer: a systematic review, *J BUON* 21(4):859–866, 2016.
86. Chen CC, Huang JL, Chang CJ, et al.: Fecal calprotectin as a correlative marker in clinical severity of infectious diarrhea and usefulness in evaluating bacterial or viral pathogens in children, *J Pediatr Gastroenterol Nutr* 55(5):541–547, 2012.
87. Shastri YM, Bergis D, Povse N, et al.: Prospective multicenter study evaluating fecal calprotectin in adult acute bacterial diarrhea, *Am J Med* 121(12):1099–1106, 2008.
88. Tursi A: Biomarkers in diverticular diseases of the colon, *Dig Dis* 30(1):12–18, 2012.
89. Tursi A, Brandimarte G, Elisei W, et al.: Faecal calprotectin in colonic diverticular disease: a case-control study, *Int J Colorectal Dis* 24(1):49–55, 2009.
90. Berntzen HB, Olmez U, Fagerhol MK, et al.: The leukocyte protein L1 in plasma and synovial fluid from patients with rheumatoid arthritis and osteoarthritis, *Scand J Rheumatol* 20(2):74–82, 1991.
91. Drynda S, Ringel B, Kekow M, et al.: Proteome analysis reveals disease-associated marker proteins to differentiate RA patients from other inflammatory joint diseases with the potential to monitor anti-TNFalpha therapy, *Pathol Res Pract* 200(2):165–171, 2004.
92. Hammer HB, Odegard S, Fagerhol MK, et al.: Calprotectin (a major leucocyte protein) is strongly and independently correlated with joint inflammation and damage in rheumatoid arthritis, *Ann Rheum Dis* 66(8):1093–1097, 2007.
93. Abildtrup M, Kingsley GH, Scott DL: Calprotectin as a biomarker for rheumatoid arthritis: a systematic review, *J Rheumatol* 42(5):760–770, 2015.
94. Kane D, Roth J, Frosch M, et al.: Increased perivascular synovial membrane expression of myeloid-related proteins in psoriatic arthritis, *Arthritis Rheum* 48(6):1676–1685, 2003.
95. Aochi S, Tsuji K, Sakaguchi M, et al.: Markedly elevated serum levels of calcium-binding S100A8/A9 proteins in psoriatic arthritis are due to activated monocytes/macrophages, *J Am Acad Dermatol* 64(5):879–887, 2011.
96. Duran A, Kobak S, Sen N, et al.: Fecal calprotectin is associated with disease activity in patients with ankylosing spondylitis, *Bosn J Basic Med Sci* 16(1):71–74, 2016.
97. Cypers H, Varkas G, Beeckman S, et al.: Elevated calprotectin levels reveal bowel inflammation in spondyloarthritis, *Ann Rheum Dis* 75(7):1357–1362, 2016.
98. Klingberg E, Strid H, Stahl A, et al.: A longitudinal study of fecal calprotectin and the development of inflammatory bowel disease in ankylosing spondylitis, *Arthritis Res Ther* 19(1):21, 2017.
99. Haga HJ, Brun JG, Berntzen HB, et al.: Calprotectin in patients with systemic lupus erythematosus: relation to clinical and laboratory parameters of disease activity, *Lupus* 2(1):47–50, 1993.
100. Soyfoo MS, Roth J, Vogl T, et al.: Phagocyte-specific S100A8/A9 protein levels during disease exacerbations and infections in systemic lupus erythematosus, *J Rheumatol* 36(10):2190–2194, 2009.
101. Guo Q, Zha X, Li C, et al.: Serum calprotectin—a promising diagnostic marker for adult-onset Still's disease, *Clin Rheumatol* 35(1):73–79, 2016.
102. Kienhorst LB, van Lochem E, Kievit W, et al.: Gout is a chronic inflammatory disease in which high levels of interleukin-8 (CXCL8), myeloid-related protein 8/myeloid-related protein 14 complex, and an altered proteome are associated with diabetes mellitus and cardiovascular disease, *Arthritis Rheumatol* 67(12):3303–3313, 2015.
103. Kuruto R, Nozawa R, Takeishi K, et al.: Myeloid calcium binding proteins: expression in the differentiated HL-60 cells and detection in sera of patients with connective tissue diseases, *J Biochem* 108(4):650–653, 1990.
104. Oktayoglu P, Mete N, Caglayan M, et al.: Elevated serum levels of calprotectin (MRP8/MRP14) in patients with Behcet's disease and its association with disease activity and quality of life, *Scand J Clin Lab Invest* 75(2):106–112, 2015.
105. Pepper RJ, Hamour S, Chavele KM, et al.: Leukocyte and serum S100A8/S100A9 expression reflects disease activity in ANCA-associated vasculitis and glomerulonephritis, *Kidney Int* 83(6):1150–1158, 2013.
106. Pepper RJ, Draibe JB, Caplin B, et al.: Association of serum calprotectin (S100A8/A9) level with disease relapse in proteinase 3-anti-neutrophil cytoplasmic antibody-associated vasculitis, *Arthritis Rheumatol* 69(1):185–193, 2017.
107. Cunnane G, Grehan S, Geoghegan S, et al.: Serum amyloid A in the assessment of early inflammatory arthritis, *J Rheumatol* 27(1):58–63, 2000.
108. Efthimiou P, Paik PK, Bielory L: Diagnosis and management of adult onset Still's disease, *Ann Rheum Dis* 65(5):564–572, 2006.
109. Nishiya K, Hashimoto K: Elevation of serum ferritin levels as a marker for active systemic lupus erythematosus, *Clin Exp Rheumatol* 15(1):39–44, 1997.
110. Nemeth E, Valore EV, Territo M, et al.: Hepcidin, a putative mediator of anemia of inflammation, is a type II acute-phase protein, *Blood* 101(7):2461–2463, 2003.
111. Andrews NC: Anemia of inflammation: the cytokine-hepcidin link, *J Clin Invest* 113(9):1251–1253, 2004.

112. Lahita RG, Rivkin E, Cavanagh I, et al.: Low levels of total cholesterol, high-density lipoprotein, and apolipoprotein A1 in association with anticardiolipin antibodies in patients with systemic lupus erythematosus, *Arthritis Rheum* 36(11):1566–1574, 1993.
113. Park YB, Lee SK, Lee WK, et al.: Lipid profiles in untreated patients with rheumatoid arthritis, *J Rheumatol* 26(8):1701–1704, 1999.
114. Myron Johnson A, Merlini G, Sheldon J, et al.: Scientific division committee on plasma proteins IFoCC, laboratory M. Clinical indications for plasma protein assays: transthyretin (prealbumin) in inflammation and malnutrition, *Clin Chem Lab Med* 45(3):419–426, 2007.
115. Tutuncu ZN, Bilgie A, Kennedy LG, et al.: Interleukin-6, acute phase reactants and clinical status in ankylosing spondylitis, *Ann Rheum Dis* 53(6):425–426, 1994.
116. Uddhammar A, Sundqvist KG, Ellis B, et al.: Cytokines and adhesion molecules in patients with polymyalgia rheumatica, *Br J Rheumatol* 37(7):766–769, 1998.
117. Luqmani R, Sheeran T, Robinson M, et al.: Systemic cytokine measurements: their role in monitoring the response to therapy in patients with rheumatoid arthritis, *Clin Exp Rheumatol* 12(5):503–508, 1994.
118. Pountain G, Hazleman B, Cawston TE: Circulating levels of IL-1beta, IL-6 and soluble IL-2 receptor in polymyalgia rheumatica and giant cell arteritis and rheumatoid arthritis, *Br J Rheumatol* 37(7):797–798, 1998.
119. Gabay C, Cakir N, Moral F, et al.: Circulating levels of tumor necrosis factor soluble receptors in systemic lupus erythematosus are significantly higher than in other rheumatic diseases and correlate with disease activity, *J Rheumatol* 24(2):303–308, 1997.
120. Gabay C, Gay-Croisier F, Roux-Lombard P, et al.: Elevated serum levels of interleukin-1 receptor antagonist in polymyositis/dermatomyositis. A biologic marker of disease activity with a possible role in the lack of acute-phase protein response, *Arthritis Rheum* 37(12):1744–1751, 1994.

61 Imaging in Rheumatic Diseases

MIKKEL ØSTERGAARD, HO JEN, JACOB L. JAREMKO, AND ROBERT G.W. LAMBERT

KEY POINTS

Practical use of imaging in inflammatory joint diseases

A. Peripheral joints

Use in clinical practice:

- To establish a diagnosis of RA, PsA, or JIA: radiography, MRI, ultrasonography
- To assist with the diagnostic workup in suspected, but not definite, inflammatory joint disease and early, unclassified adult or pediatric inflammatory joint disease (by detection of presence/absence of synovitis, enthesitis, bone erosion, etc.): radiography, MRI, ultrasonography
- To monitor disease activity: MRI, ultrasonography
- To monitor structural joint damage: radiography, MRI
- To assist with the prognostic stratification of patients with early RA: radiography, MRI, ultrasonography[a], DXR[a]
- To help define the presence or absence of true remission: MRI, ultrasonography
- To guide aspirations and injections in joints, bursae, and tendon sheaths: ultrasonography

Use in clinical research:

- To assess structural joint damage in RA trials: radiography, MRI
- To assess the anti-inflammatory effectiveness of a new compound: MRI, ultrasonography
- For pretrial selection of the patients most likely to progress ("enrichment"): radiography, MRI

B. Axial joints

Use in clinical practice:

- To establish a diagnosis of AS/SpA/axial involvement of JIA: radiography and MRI
- To monitor disease activity: MRI
- To monitor structural joint damage: radiography, MRI, CT[b]

Use in clinical research:

- To assess structural progression in AS/SpA/JIA trials: radiography, MRI
- To assess the anti-inflammatory effectiveness of a new compound: MRI
- For pretrial selection of the patients most likely to progress: radiography, MRI

[a]*Promising, but more data needed*

[b]*CT allows this but cannot be used due to radiation exposure*

Introduction

For decades, imaging in rheumatology was synonymous with conventional radiography (radiography, X-ray). However, new imaging modalities including MRI and ultrasonography and new nuclear medicine techniques have dramatically increased the amount and scope of information obtainable by imaging. In rheumatology, imaging may be used for multiple reasons that include establishing or confirming the diagnosis, determining extent of disease, monitoring change in disease (e.g., activity and structural damage), selecting patients for specific therapies (e.g., surgery or injections), identifying complications of disease or treatment, and assessing therapeutic efficacy in trials. These entirely different contexts may favor different imaging approaches.

The present chapter focuses on the inflammatory joint diseases, such as rheumatoid arthritis (RA), psoriatic arthritis (PsA), ankylosing spondylitis (AS), other types of axial spondyloarthritis (SpA), gout, juvenile idiopathic arthritis (JIA), and osteoarthritis (OA). The reader is kindly referred to the chapters on the individual diseases for imaging aspects of other rheumatologic diseases, and to textbooks of musculoskeletal radiology[1] for a more detailed description of the different imaging modalities, including the technical aspects. This chapter outlines the virtues of radiographs and describes their current major importance in diagnosis and follow-up of rheumatologic diseases, but also, by putting emphasis on newer imaging modalities, particularly MRI and ultrasonography, stresses that rheumatology has entered a time of exciting and expanding therapeutic as well as imaging possibilities.

Radiography

KEY POINTS

Relatively inexpensive, easily available and reliable.

Provides information on bone damage and indirectly, through joint space narrowing, on cartilage damage, but is neither sensitive nor specific for soft-tissue change.

Findings are important parts of the classification criteria for many rheumatic diseases, including RA, AS, SpA, PsA, and OA.

Should most often be the first imaging investigation in arthritis, as significance of positive and negative findings is well known.

Can be used to follow structural damage progression in inflammatory and degenerative joint diseases, but less sensitive to change than MRI.

Main disadvantage is low sensitivity, particularly for soft tissue changes.

Particularly insensitive for early arthritis in children due to incomplete ossification.

The first roentgen ray image was an "x-ray" of the hand. Since then, imaging of musculoskeletal structures has always been an important role of conventional radiography (x-rays).[1] The simple radiography is relatively cheap, available worldwide, and produces an image that is almost identical regardless of technical parameters or whether the image is analogue or digital. The reliability of the image means that, despite the limitations of radiography, advances in clinical practice can rely on the "good old x-ray" knowing that it is largely independent of technologic advance. For many years to come, radiographs will appear much the same.

Technical Aspects

The conventional radiography is a two-dimensional summation image that is dependent on variable absorption of x-rays by different tissues for its inherent contrast. It has a very high spatial resolution that is rarely surpassed by other modalities, but radiography only offers high contrast between a limited number of structures—bone (calcium), soft tissue, and air. Fat is visible as a separate density, but the distinction between soft tissue and fat is often subtle and radiography cannot distinguish between the other soft tissues because cartilage, muscle, tendon, ligament, synovium, and fluid all appear to be the same density. These characteristics give the radiography its inherent advantages and disadvantages.[1,2]

In its favor, the radiography shows skeletal structure very well, and because it is a summation image, it allows excellent overall assessment of skeletal trauma and alignment. The limited number of images produced facilitates rapid review and the high bone-soft tissue contrast often produces radiographic manifestations of disease in specific patterns that make the test particularly useful in daily clinical practice. The biggest disadvantage of radiography is its inherent lack of soft tissue contrast, making it insensitive for the detection of soft tissue abnormalities. The first radiographic sign of inflammatory arthritis may be permanent structural damage (bony erosion), and in degenerating joints, cartilage damage is not usually visualized until sufficient overall cartilage loss allows approximation of the bone ends, resulting in "joint space narrowing."

Most imaging records are now digitally archived, and this has promoted the widespread adoption of digital radiography. Two beneficial effects of using digital image acquisition are the development of tomosynthesis and radiogrammetry (see later). The planar images created by tomosynthesis resemble conventional tomography. However, whereas conventional tomography required multiple exposures and high radiation dose, a stack of thin slice digital tomographic images can be reconstructed from a single tomosynthesis exposure with only slight increase in radiation dose compared to a digital radiography. Tomosynthetic thin image-slices allow detection of more subtle radiographic abnormalities that may otherwise be obscured by the complex anatomy of overlying structures. Tomosynthesis is more accurate for detecting bone erosion than radiography and has similar sensitivity to CT and MRI for detection of erosion in the hands and feet of patients with RA.[3–5]

Although radiographs use ionizing radiation, they should be regarded as relatively safe, especially in older patients. An exception may be spine radiography where doses are higher in order to penetrate the trunk and, in a younger population, MRI offers a safer and more informative alternative. In most examinations, two or more projections are required to adequately visualize the joint in question, and radiographic quality is improved by strict adherence to standard imaging protocols.

Rheumatoid Arthritis

RA is the archetypal inflammatory joint disease and primarily targets synovium and peripheral joints. It is a systemic inflammatory disorder in which the typical clinical manifestations are usually symmetrical and so the radiographic signs usually follow this pattern. As in all of radiology, the observed distribution of disease is often characteristic of the underlying cause, and in RA, the metacarpophalangeal (MCP) and proximal interphalangeal (PIP) joints of the hands and the wrists and the metatarsophalangeal (MTP) joints of the feet are most often involved.[1,2]

Juxta-articular osteoporosis is a characteristic feature of RA best seen in early disease in small peripheral joints. Later, generalized osteoporosis is usually present and is exacerbated by disuse. Erosion of bone (Fig. 61.1) is a characteristic feature of RA and usually appears first at the margins of the joint where the proliferating synovium lies directly on the surface of the bone between the edge of the cartilage-covered articular surface and the capsular attachment—the "bare areas." These marginal erosions may be subtle and first appear as disruption of the thin white cortical line, especially at the radial aspect of the metacarpal heads where they may be best seen on dedicated radiographic projections such as the ball-catcher's view of the hands. These erosive changes are a good indication of the aggressiveness of the arthritis. In large joints, synovial proliferation may be very severe before bony erosion is detectable on radiography. This is especially notable in the knee where pain and swelling due to arthritis and bursitis occur long before erosion. In addition to bare-area erosions, two other types of erosions have been described in RA. Compressive erosion refers to remodeling of inflamed and osteoporotic bone with gradual invagination of one bone into another typified by protrusio acetabuli of the hip (Fig. 61.1E). Surface erosion of bone may also be seen usually resulting from inflammation of an adjacent tendon sheath, and a typical location for this is at the outer margin of the ulnar styloid process secondary to extensor carpi ulnaris tenosynovitis.

Joint space involvement is characteristic in RA.[1,2] In many cases, the inflammatory processes result in progressive destruction of articular cartilage, which in turn causes the radiographic finding of concentric joint space narrowing. This is usually diffuse in RA as all the cartilage is involved at the same time, and this feature may allow differentiation from the focal or asymmetric type of joint space loss that occurs with degenerative disorders. Occasionally cartilage destruction precedes synovial erosion of bone. Continued cartilage damage may result in partial or complete fibrous ankylosis but progression to bony ankylosis is uncommon although it may occur in end-stage disease in the wrist or midfoot. Subchondral radiolucent areas are common in RA and are often referred to as cysts, geodes, or pseudocysts. They may develop as a result of intraosseous extension of pannus, injury to the bone of any kind, or true intraosseous rheumatoid nodules. Mechanical factors accentuate their development, and very large cystic lesions may be seen in the elbow, femoral neck, or knee and occasionally precipitate pathologic fractures.

Symmetric soft tissue swelling around the small joints of the hands or feet is often the first clinical and radiographic sign of RA. The soft tissue swelling is caused by joint effusion, synovial proliferation, and periarticular inflammation, but the radiographic

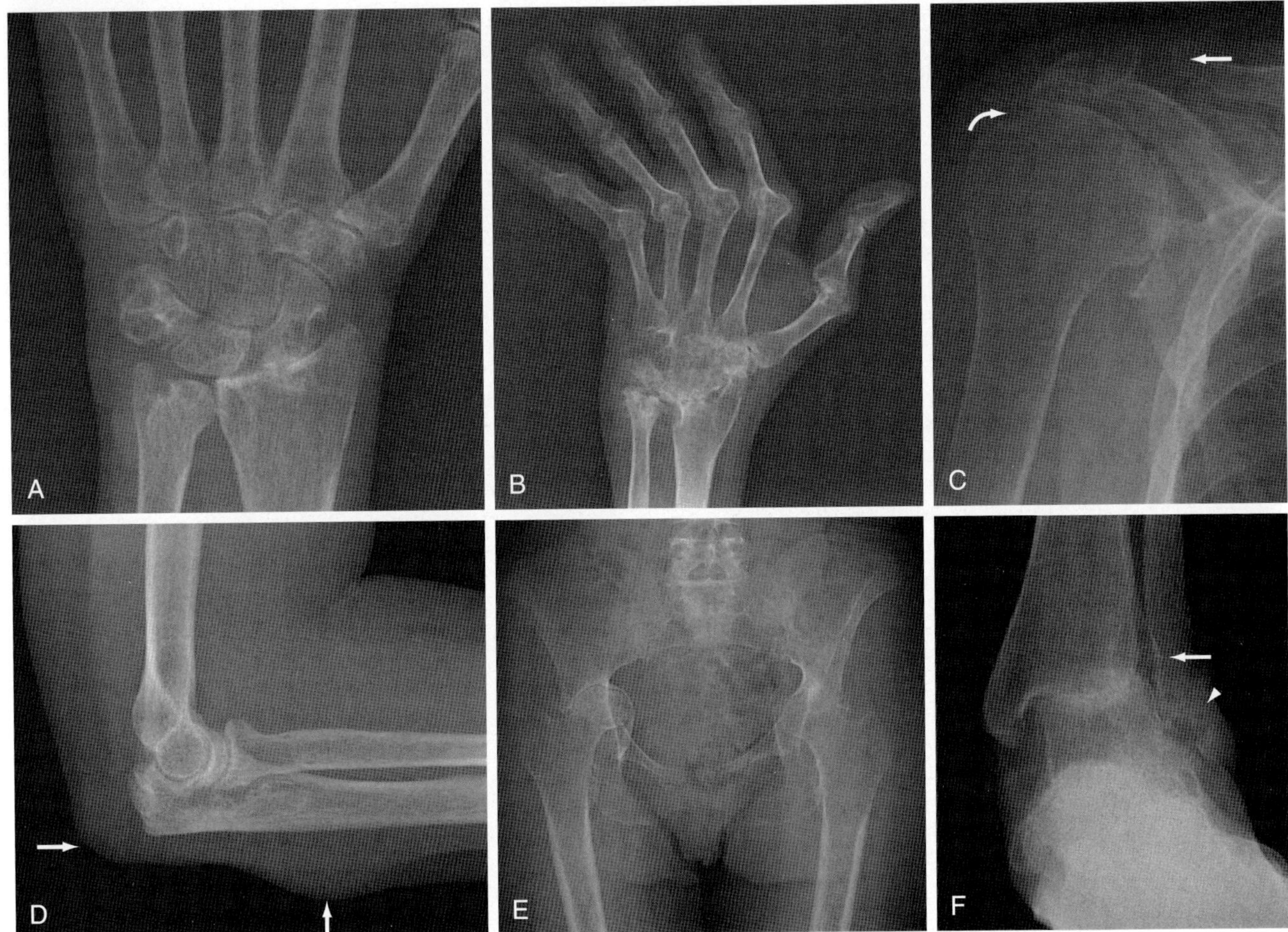

• **Fig. 61.1** Rheumatoid arthritis (radiography). (A) Multiple typical bone erosions are seen (e.g., in triquetrum, pisiform, scaphoid, radius, and ulnar styloid process). Diffuse cartilage loss also is evident in the radiocarpal compartment. (B) Severe ulnar deviation is present at the metacarpophalangeal joints with extensive erosions. Severe erosion and bony ankylosis are seen in the wrist. (C) Posterior oblique view of a shoulder shows severe glenohumeral joint space narrowing with marginal erosion and cystic change of the humeral head adjacent to the greater tuberosity *(curved arrow)*. Elevation of the humeral head with respect to the glenoid indicates chronic rotator cuff tear. Tapering of the distal end of the clavicle and widening of the acromioclavicular joint *(straight arrow)* are also evident. (D) Rheumatoid nodules appearing as lobulated subcutaneous soft tissue swellings *(arrows)* at the extensor surface of the elbow and forearm. (E) Bilateral protrusio acetabuli. The medial acetabular margins protrude into the pelvis. Severe accompanying cartilage loss has occurred. (F) Ankle with diffuse loss of cartilage space with erosions of the fibula *(arrow and arrowhead)*. The hindfoot is in valgus alignment.

findings are nonspecific, and radiographs are much less sensitive for such changes than MRI and ultrasonography. Eccentric soft tissue swelling may be due to adjacent bursitis, tenosynovitis, or rheumatoid nodules. Involvement of tendons and tendon sheaths is common; however, the soft-tissue changes are usually poorly visualized and so are of lesser diagnostic importance.

Joint malalignment and deformity (Fig. 61.1) are very common in RA and occur due to laxity and disruption of capsule, ligaments, and tendons. The deformities are most characteristic in the hand, wrist, foot, and neck. Note that these malalignments may be transient and can reduce when positioning for the radiographs. Late disease is associated with severe deformity as seen in arthritis mutilans.[1,2]

Spine

Cervical spine involvement is common in RA and merits specific attention. It occurs mainly after several years of disease in rheumatoid–factor-positive patients with severe peripheral RA, and may cause severe pain, instability, and, ultimately, spinal cord compression.[6] Prevalences of radiologic cervical involvement up to 70% have been reported, but are much lower in recent studies in accordance with the fact that intensive disease-modifying anti-rheumatic drug (DMARD) therapy has reduced cervical radiologic progression.[7]

The upper cervical region is most affected although abnormalities throughout the cervical spine are frequent (Fig. 61.2). Upper cervical changes include odontoid process (dens) erosion and atlantoaxial subluxations. Anterior subluxation of the atlas is most common and is caused by laxity or rupture of the transverse ligament. Vertical subluxation (known as cranial settling) is now seldom seen, but the dens may protrude through the foramen magnum causing compression of neurologic structures.[1] Subaxial manifestations include abnormalities of apophyseal and discovertebral joints, with varying degrees of bone erosion, joint space narrowing, and subluxation/dislocation of facet joints, as well as disc space narrowing and spinous process erosion. Subaxial subluxations may also lead to neurologic deficits.[1]

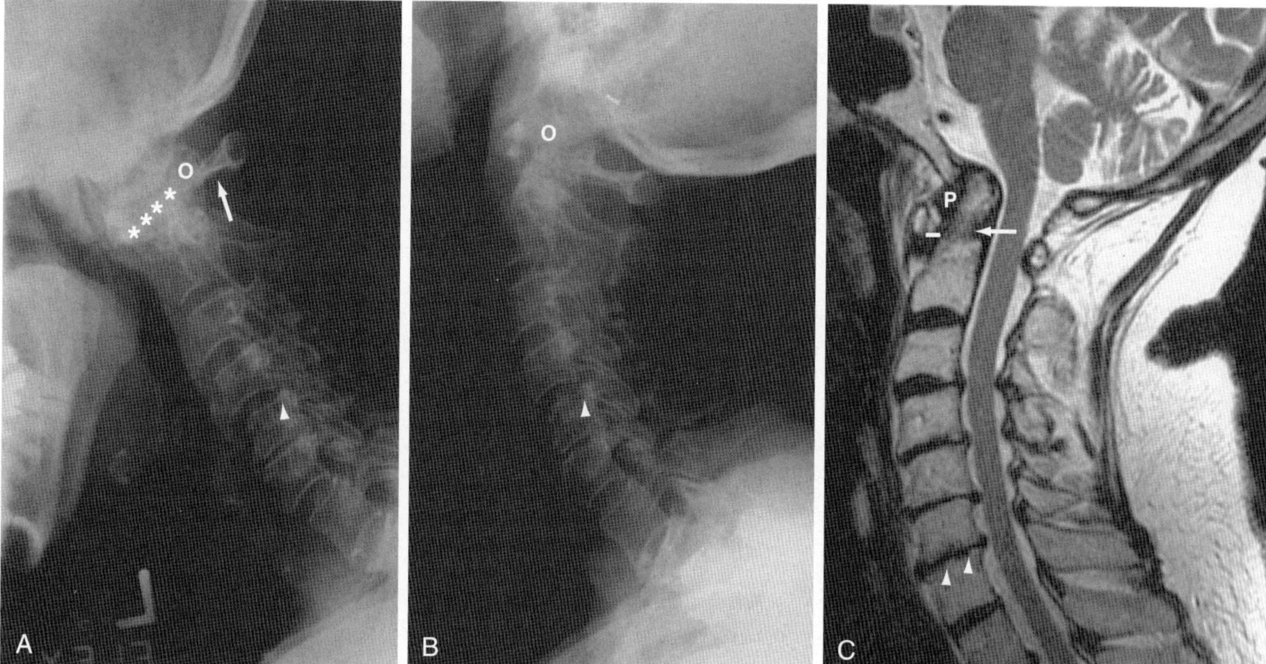

• **Fig. 61.2** Cervical spine in rheumatoid arthritis (RA) (radiography). (A and B) Anterior atlantoaxial subluxation in RA. (A) Lateral radiography in flexion shows severe anterior atlantoaxial subluxation with a wide anterior atlantodental interval *(asterisks)* and a decreased posterior atlantodental interval *(arrow)*. (B) Almost complete reduction of subluxation is noted on the lateral view in extension. There also is subaxial subluxation at the level of C4-C5 *(arrowhead)* with erosive changes in various facet joints. *O*, Odontoid. (C) T2-weighted sagittal magnetic resonance (MR) image in RA shows low signal periodontoid pannus (P). The odontoid process appears irregular secondary to erosions *(arrow)*. The atlantodental distance shows mild widening *(solid line)*. There also is vertical subluxation without signs of cord compression. The anterior subarachnoid space is compromised by disk protrusions at multiple levels. Small erosions *(arrowheads)* are seen at the vertebral end plates at the C6-C7 level.

Adequate radiographic evaluation of the cervical spine requires lateral views in flexion and extension and should be performed in all RA patients with neck pain. The flexion-extension views are especially important for demonstration of the degree of atlantoaxial instability. MRI is useful for supplementary information on cervical spine involvement (Fig. 61.2C), including spinal cord compression (see MRI section).

Use in Diagnosis, Monitoring, and Prognosis

Diagnosis. Characteristic radiographic findings are part of the American College of Rheumatology (ACR) 1987 classification criteria for RA.[8] Radiography also has a role in the recent ACR/European League Against Rheumatism (EULAR) 2010 classification criteria, as patients who display bone erosions typical for RA plus at least one clinically swollen joint fulfill the criteria and are classified as RA.[9,10] Radiographs can be helpful in the differentiation from other joint conditions including OA, psoriatic arthritis, and neoplasm.[2] EULAR recommendations for the use of imaging, including radiographs, in the clinical management of RA have recently been published (Table 61.1)[11]

Monitoring. In routine clinical management and in clinical trials of RA, radiographic evaluation focuses on joint space narrowing and bone erosions in hands, wrists, and forefeet as measures of structural joint damage.[12–14] Validated scoring methods of radiolographic damage (the Larsen method and the Sharp method and their modifications) are available and extensively used in clinical trials.[13–15] The van der Heijde and Genant modifications of the Sharp score are generally considered the methods most sensitive to change, but are also the most time consuming.[16] For clinical practice, the less time-consuming simple erosion narrowing score (SENS), based on counting joints with bone erosion and joints with joint space narrowing, is available,[17,18] but is seldom used.

Prognosis. Early bone erosion correlates with poor long-term radiographic and functional outcome,[19] and early progression in radiographic erosion is related to future impairment in physical function.[20] In early undifferentiated arthritis, the presence of radiographic erosion increases the risk of developing persistent arthritis.[21] However, radiographic erosions are only present in a minority of patients with early RA, with reported prevalences of 8% to 40% at 6 months,[22–26] and the absence of erosion in early disease is not necessarily associated with good outcomes, so, at this stage, radiography is not effective for identifying future "nonprogressors," that is, patients who will not show increasing structural joint damage.[27]

Ankylosing Spondylitis

AS is the archetypal inflammatory joint disease that primarily targets fibrocartilage and the axial skeleton. Cartilaginous joints and sites of enthesis (tendon and ligament insertion) are involved early, and the characteristic involvement of the axial skeletal includes a predilection for the sacroiliac joints and all the articulations and entheses of the spine.

Sacroiliac Joints

Erosion and ankylosis of the sacroiliac joints are the hallmarks of spondyloarthritis.[1,28] Sacroiliitis is usually the first manifestation and is characteristically bilateral and symmetrical in AS.[29,30] Early radiographic findings predominate on the iliac side of the cartilage compartment with erosion of subchondral bone causing

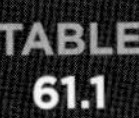

TABLE 61.1 **EULAR Recommendations for the Use of Imaging in the Clinical Management of Rheumatoid Arthritis[a]**

EULAR Recommendations for the Use of Imaging in the Clinical Management of Rheumatoid Arthritis[a]
When there is diagnostic doubt, conventional radiography, ultrasonography, or MRI can be used to improve the certainty of a diagnosis of RA in addition to clinical criteria alone.[b]
The presence of inflammation seen with ultrasonography or MRI can be used to predict the progression to clinical RA from undifferentiated inflammatory arthritis.
Ultrasonography and MRI are superior to clinical examination in the detection of joint inflammation; these techniques should be considered for more accurate assessment of inflammation. Conventional radiography of the hands and feet should be used as the initial imaging technique to detect damage. However, ultrasonography and/or MRI should be considered if conventional radiographs do not show damage and may be used to detect damage at an earlier time point (especially in early-stage RA).
MRI bone edema is a strong independent predictor of subsequent radiographic progression in early RA, and should be considered as a prognostic indicator. Joint inflammation (synovitis) detected by MRI or ultrasonography as well as joint damage detected by conventional radiographs, MRI, or ultrasonography can also be considered for the prediction of further joint damage.
Inflammation seen on imaging may be more predictive of a therapeutic response than clinical features of disease activity; imaging may be used to predict response to treatment.
Given the superior detection of inflammation by MRI and ultrasonography versus clinical examination, they may be useful in monitoring disease activity.
The periodic evaluation of joint damage, usually by radiographs of the hands and feet, should be considered. MRI (and possibly ultrasonography) is more responsive to change in joint damage and can be used to monitor disease progression.
Monitoring of functional instability of the cervical spine by lateral radiography obtained in flexion and neutral positions should be performed in patients with clinical suspicion of cervical involvement. When radiography is positive or specific neurologic symptoms and signs are present, MRI should be performed.
MRI and ultrasonography can detect inflammation that predicts subsequent joint damage, even when clinical remission is present and can be used to assess persistent inflammation.

[a]Recommendations are based on data from imaging studies that have mainly focused on the hands (particularly wrists, metacarpophalangeal, and proximal interphalangeal joints). There are few data with specific guidance on which joints to image.[8]

[b]In patients with at least one joint with definite clinical synovitis, which is not better explained by another disease.

EULAR, European League Against Rheumatism; *RA,* rheumatoid arthritis.

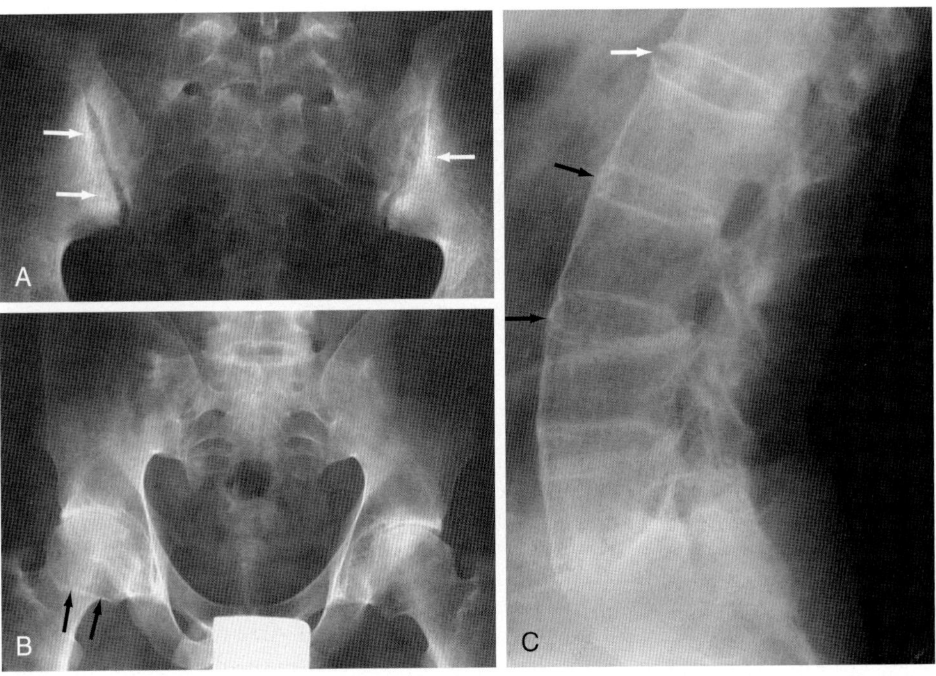

• **Fig. 61.3** Ankylosing spondylitis (radiography). (A) Sclerosis *(arrows)* is seen along the iliac sides of the sacroiliac joints along with loss of portions of the iliac subchondral bone indicating erosion. (B) Bilateral hip joint space narrowing is present. A ring of osteophytes is noted at the synovial insertion *(arrows)* on each femoral head. The sacroiliac joints are fused (ankylosis). (C) Syndesmophytes *(black and white arrows),* some of which extend from the edge of one vertebral body to the next (bridging syndesmophytes, ankylosis; *black arrows*), are seen in this lateral view of the spine.

loss of definition of the articular surfaces usually accompanied by variable degrees of adjacent osteoporosis and surrounding reactive sclerosis. Bone erosion may result in the radiographic observation of focal joint space widening (Fig. 61.3A) and, as the disease progresses, definition of the joint is completely lost with radiographic superimposition of erosion, sclerosis, and new bone formation, which fills in the erosions and the original cartilaginous "joint space." The joint may disappear completely in late disease

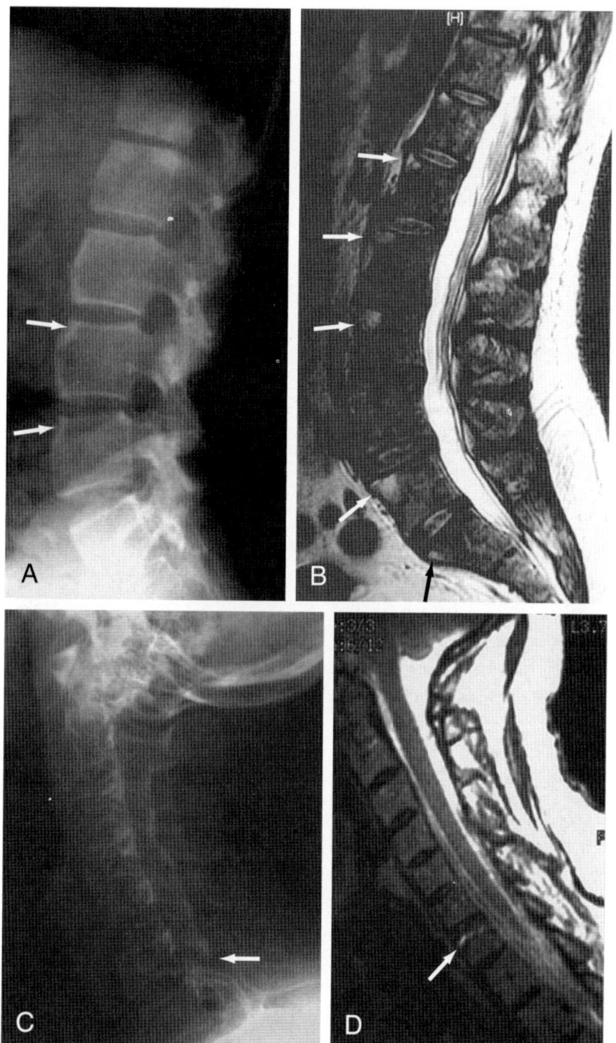

• **Fig. 61.4** Ankylosing spondylitis (radiography and MRI). (A) Lateral radiography of the spine shows marked erosion at the vertebral margins has produced straight or slightly convex anterior vertebral surfaces ("squaring"). New bone formation has resulted in "shiny corners" *(arrows)*. The facet joints are fused. (B) Sagittal fast spin echo T2-weighted MR image in another patient shows bone marrow edema at the anterosuperior corners of the vertebral bodies *(arrows)*, corresponding to early osteitis. (C and D) Fracture in ankylosing spondylitis. (C) Radiography shows disruption of the previously fused C6-C7 facet joints *(arrow)* and slight anterior subluxation. (D) Sagittal T2-weighted MR image confirms a high signal fracture line *(arrow)* through the superior aspect of C7.

with ankylosis and remodeling of the bone (Fig. 61.3B). The ligamentous compartment of the sacroiliac joint is frequently affected by bony erosion and entheseal proliferation although these may be hard to see radiographically.[29,30]

Spine

Traditional descriptions of the initial sites of spinal involvement are enormously influenced by the inability of radiography to adequately visualize many parts of the spine. Radiographic reports indicate that the lumbosacral and thoracolumbar junctions are first affected, whereas the MRI literature clearly indicates a predilection for early involvement of the mid-thoracic spine, an area that is extremely difficult to evaluate radiographically. The cervical spine is rarely affected first, but this can occur occasionally in women, and spinal disease rarely occurs in the absence of significant sacroiliac joint involvement.

The early radiographic manifestations of AS in the spine are most often due to enthesitis at the corners of the discovertebral joints.[29] Focal sclerosis (a "shiny corner") and erosion (a "Romanus lesion") develop at the attachment of the annulus fibrosis to the anterior corner of the vertebral endplate and are characteristic features of early AS (Fig. 61.4A).[31] The anterior borders of vertebrae may appear straight or "squared" due to periosteal proliferation of new bone filling in the normal concavity or erosion at the anterosuperior and anteroinferior vertebral margins. This observation is much easier to make in the lumbar spine where normal vertebrae are always concave anteriorly in comparison to the thoracic and cervical spine, where the normal contour is much more variable and may be square or occasionally convex.

The hallmark of spinal disease in AS is the development of characteristic bony spurs, syndesmophytes (Fig. 61.3C). These start as thin, vertically oriented projections of bone that develop due to ossification within the outer fibers of the annulus fibrosus of the intervertebral disc. Syndesmophytes are radiographically visible on the anterior and lateral aspects of the spine starting from the corner of the vertebra. Progressive growth will bridge the intervertebral disk causing ankylosis, and extensive syndesmophyte formation produces a smooth, undulating spinal contour, known as the *bamboo spine.* The syndesmophytes that characterize AS must be differentiated from other spinal and paraspinal bone formations. Degenerative bony spurring in spondylosis deformans arises several millimeters from the discovertebral junction, is typically triangular in shape, and has a horizontally oriented segment of variable length at the point of origin. In diffuse idiopathic skeletal hyperostosis (DISH), bone formation in the anterior longitudinal ligament results in a flowing pattern of ossification that is usually thick and the sacroiliac joints are not involved.

Erosion of the vertebral endplate is common in later stages of AS and may be focal or diffuse. It is also seen when pseudoarthrosis develops following a fracture in a previously ankylosed spine. Changes in the apophyseal joints are common and start with ill-defined erosion and sclerosis but may be hard to see. Capsular ossification or intra-articular bony ankylosis frequently occurs in late disease (Fig. 61.4). The ankylosed spine is very susceptible to fractures (Fig. 61.4C and D), which should always be suspected in case of unexplained pain exacerbations. Enthesitis at the interspinous and supraspinous ligamentous attachments is very common, with bone formation causing whiskering and interspinous ankylosis.

Use in Diagnosis, Monitoring, and Prognosis

While the modified New York Criteria are actually classification criteria, these criteria are the most commonly used criteria for the diagnosis of AS and are based on clinical features and radiographic sacroiliitis.[28] According to these criteria AS may be diagnosed if, in addition to one clinical criterion, grade 2 sacroiliitis (minimal sacroiliitis: loss of definition of the joint margins, minimal sclerosis, joint space narrowing, and erosions) or higher occurs bilaterally, grade 3 (moderate sacroiliitis: definite sclerosis on both sides of the joint, erosions, and loss of joint space), or grade 4 (complete bony ankylosis) occurs unilaterally.[28] Due to the requirement for these radiographic structural changes, the duration of disease before diagnosis has been a median of 7 to 10 years.[32] The definitions of radiographic changes according to the New York Criteria are included in the Assessment of Spondyloarthritis International Society (ASAS) classification criteria for axial spondyloarthritis,[33] the European Spondyloarthritis Study Group (ESSG) criteria for spondyloarthritis,[34] and in the modified New York Criteria.[28] EULAR recommendations for the use of imaging, including radiography, in the diagnosis and clinical management of SpA have recently become available (Table 61.2).[35]

Radiography of the spine is not included in the classification criteria but may be useful to follow structural disease progression in patients with spinal involvement. The bone changes seen in patients with axial SpA develop slowly and are often not present in patients with early disease, and generally only minor changes can be observed in the first several years. Different scoring methods, all based on assessment of lateral views, have been developed to quantify changes in the spine of patients with AS: the Stoke AS Spine Score (SASSS), Bath AS Radiology Index (BASRI), and the modified Stoke AS Spine Score (mSASSS). A comparative study of the three methods concluded that all measures were reliable but mSASSS was more sensitive to change.[36] These spine scores are primarily used in clinical research.

Psoriatic Arthritis

The presentation of PsA is quite variable but often distinctive. Peripheral joint involvement is common and up to half of patients with PsA have evidence of joint damage on radiographs within 2 years of presentation.[37] The hand and wrist are most often involved and are affected in up to three-quarters of PsA patients, but the pattern of joint involvement varies from patient to patient and also over time in individual patients. Radiographic appearances are usually asymmetrical and may have a ray distribution with the affected joints involving a single digit, including the distal interphalangeal (DIP) joints (Fig. 61.5), which are seldom involved in RA. Clinically this manifests as dactylitis and is a common early presentation of PsA. Osteoporosis is frequently absent, with the propensity for bone proliferation a distinguishing feature of PsA. This may be in the form of periostitis of the shafts of the phalanges, which is sometimes the first radiographic manifestation, or irregular bony spurring at joints or entheses. Fluffy new bone formation adjacent to marginal joint erosions may result in a particularly characteristic "whiskering" appearance. Severe marginal erosion of the heads of metacarpals or phalanges may produce the appearance of a whittled pencil and if combined with deep central erosion of phalangeal bases this is referred to as the *pencil-in-cup* appearance. Ankylosis of joints occurs frequently in advanced disease. Large joints are less often affected when the findings are usually similar to those of RA. Spinal involvement is frequent in PsA. It may be seen in early disease and sacroiliitis may be demonstrable in up to 75% of the patients.[38] The changes may be extensive and are more likely to be asymmetrical than in AS.

Use in Diagnosis, Monitoring, and Prognosis

While RA is characterized by mainly osteo-destructive lesions, in PsA there are both osteo-destructive and osteo-proliferative manifestations, which may even co-exist not only in the same patient, but also in the same joint.[39] In particular the osteo-proliferative lesions on radiography are characteristic, and are included in the new classification criteria (CASPAR) for PsA.[40] The presence of juxta-articular new bone formation appearing as ill-defined ossification near joint margins (but excluding osteophytes) on radiographs of the hand or foot is one of five criteria.[40]

Structural joint damage on conventional radiography is an important outcome measure in PsA. Different radiographic scoring methods of peripheral joints have been developed, for example, the Sharp-van der Heijde modified scoring method for PsA, which is a detailed scoring system for evaluating erosions and joint space narrowing, while osteolysis and pencil-in-cup phenomena are assessed separately.[16] Scoring systems are primarily used in clinical trials. No specific scoring systems for spine and sacroiliac joints in PsA exist, but axial involvement in PsA can be monitored as in AS (as discussed previously).

Gout

A variety of microcrystals can deposit in and around the joints and induce an inflammatory response. In this chapter, the characteristics of gout, that is, arthritis related to monosodium urate deposition, and of calcium pyrophosphate dihydrate (CPPD) crystal deposition disease will be presented, whereas the reader is referred to chapters on the individual diseases for description of the remaining

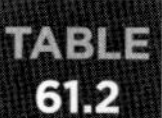

TABLE 61.2 EULAR Recommendations for the Use of Imaging in the Diagnosis and Management of Spondylarthritis in Clinical Practice

Axial SpA: Diagnosis

A. In general, conventional radiography of the sacroiliac joints is recommended as the first imaging method to diagnose sacroiliitis as part of axial SpA. In certain cases, such as young patients and those with short symptom duration, MRI of the sacroiliac joints is an alternative first imaging method.
B. If the diagnosis of axial SpA cannot be established based on clinical features and conventional radiography, and axial SpA is still suspected, MRI of the sacroiliac joints is recommended. On MRI, both active inflammatory lesions (primarily bone marrow edema) and structural lesions (such as bone erosion, new bone formation, sclerosis, and fat infiltration) should be considered. MRI of the spine is not generally recommended to diagnose axial SpA.
C. Imaging modalities other than conventional radiography and MRI are generally not recommended in the diagnosis of axial SpA.[a]

Peripheral SpA: Diagnosis

When peripheral SpA is suspected, ultrasonography or MRI may be used to detect peripheral enthesitis, which may support the diagnosis of SpA. Furthermore, ultrasonography or MRI might be used to detect peripheral arthritis, tenosynovitis, and bursitis.

Axial SpA: Monitoring Activity

MRI of the sacroiliac joints and/or the spine may be used to assess and monitor disease activity in axial SpA, providing additional information on top of clinical and biochemical assessments. The decision on when to repeat MRI depends on the clinical circumstances. In general, STIR sequences are sufficient to detect inflammation and the use of contrast medium is not needed.

Axial SpA: Monitoring Structural Changes

Conventional radiography of the sacroiliac joints and/or spine may be used for long-term monitoring of structural damage, particularly new bone formation, in axial SpA. If performed, it should not be repeated more frequently than every second year. MRI may provide additional information.

Peripheral SpA: Monitoring Activity

Ultrasonography and MRI may be used to monitor disease activity (particularly synovitis and enthesitis) in peripheral SpA, providing additional information on top of clinical and biochemical assessments. The decision on when to repeat ultrasonography/MRI depends on the clinical circumstances. Ultrasonography with high-frequency color or power Doppler is sufficient to detect inflammation, and the use of ultrasonography contrast medium is not needed.

Peripheral SpA: Monitoring Structural Changes

In peripheral SpA, if the clinical scenario requires monitoring of structural damage, then conventional radiography is recommended. MRI and/or ultrasonography might provide additional information.

Axial SpA: Predicting Outcome/Severity

In patients with AS (not nr-axSpA), initial conventional radiography of the lumbar and cervical spine are recommended to detect syndesmophytes, which predict development of new syndesmophytes. MRI (vertebral corner inflammatory or fatty lesions) may also be used to predict development of new radiographic syndesmophytes.

Axial SpA: Predicting Treatment Effect

Extensive MRI inflammatory activity (bone marrow edema), particularly in the spine in AS patients, might be used as a predictor of good clinical response to anti-TNF treatment in axial SpA. Thus, MRI might aid in the decision of whether to initiate anti-TNF therapy, in addition to clinical examination and CRP.

Spinal Fracture

When spinal fracture in axial SpA is suspected, conventional radiography is the recommended initial imaging method. If conventional radiography is negative, CT should be performed. MRI is an additional imaging method to CT, which can also provide information on soft tissue lesions.

Osteoporosis

In axial SpA patients without syndesmophytes in the lumbar spine on conventional radiography, osteoporosis should be assessed by hip DXA and AP-spine DXA. In patients with syndesmophytes in the lumbar spine on conventional radiography, osteoporosis should be assessed by hip DXA, supplemented by either spine DXA in lateral projection or possibly QCT of the spine.

AP-spine, Anterior-posterior spine; *AS,* ankylosing spondylitis; *CRP,* C-reactive protein; *DXA,* dual-energy x-ray absorptiometry; *EULAR,* European League Against Rheumatism; *nr-axSpA,* nonradiographic axial spondyloarthritis; *SIJ,* sacroiliac joints; *SOR,* strength of recommendation; *SpA,* spondyloarthritis; *STIR,* short tau inversion recovery; *TNF,* tumor necrosis factor.

[a]CT may provide additional information on structural damage if conventional radiography is negative and MRI cannot be performed. Scintigraphy and ultrasonography are not recommended for diagnosis of sacroiliitis as part of axial SpA.

From Mandl P, Navarro-Compan V, Terslev L, et al.: EULAR recommendations for the use of imaging in the diagnosis and management of spondyloarthritis in clinical practice. *Ann Rheum Dis* 74:1327–1339, 2015.

conditions, such as calcium hydroxyapatite crystal deposition disease, hemochromatosis, ochronosis, and Wilson's disease.

Radiography is not helpful in the diagnosis in acute gouty arthritis as the findings are limited to the soft tissues and are nonspecific. Chronic tophaceous gout is an asymmetrical arthritis that frequently affects the feet, hands, wrists, elbows, and knees. The most common site of involvement is the first MTP joint (Fig. 61.6). The radiologic changes in long-standing gout are related to tophi and their effect on soft tissue and bone.[41]

Tophi appear as eccentric, nodular soft tissue masses around the joints with an amorphous increased density or patchy calcification.[41] Intraosseous tophi cause well-marginated subchondral cystic lucencies or intraosseous calcifications. Erosion of the adjacent bone is common at either the periosteal or endosteal surface. The erosions may be intra-articular,

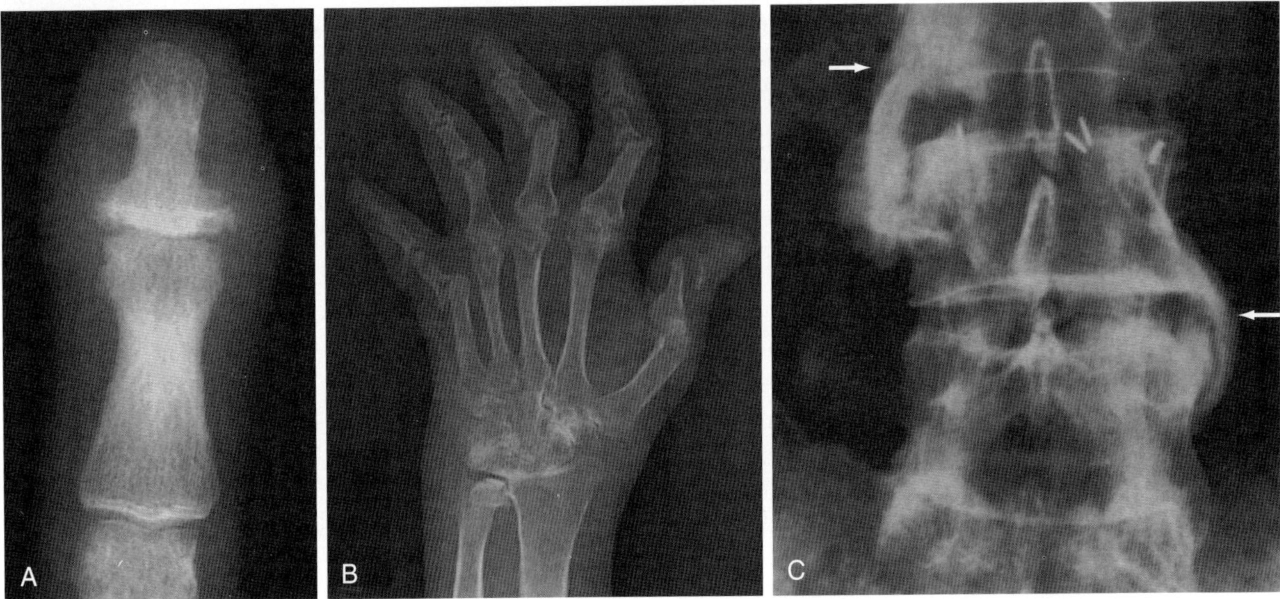

• **Fig. 61.5** Psoriatic arthritis (radiography). (A) Distal interphalangeal joint with classic radiographic findings, including soft tissue swelling, bone erosions with accompanying bone proliferation, and lack of osteoporosis. (B) Arthritis mutilans resulting from psoriatic arthritis with destructive changes and joint deformity of the hand and pancompartmental ankylosis of the wrist. (C) Psoriatic spondylitis. Thick asymmetric paravertebral ossifications *(arrows)*, which are characteristic of psoriatic spondylitis and reactive arthritis. (From Resnick D, Niwayama G: *Diagnosis of Bone and Joint Disorders.* Philadelphia, 1988, WB Saunders.)

para-articular, or remote from the joint and are typically well defined with smooth sclerotic borders. An overhanging margin of bone at the edge of the erosion is a characteristic feature of gout. The joint space and bone density are usually preserved until late in the disease. Bursal inflammation commonly produces soft tissue swelling around the olecranon and in a prepatellar location.

Use in Diagnosis, Monitoring, and Prognosis

The 1977 Criteria for the Classification of Acute Arthritis of Primary Gout[42] include the conventional radiographic features of asymmetric swelling and subcortical cysts without erosion. However, conventional radiographic features of acute gout have low clinical utility due to lack of sensitivity and specificity. In the chronic phase the characteristic pattern with asymmetrical, erosive polyarticular disease and tophi appearing as nodular soft tissue masses with amorphous increased density or patchy calcification may be diagnostically useful.

A specific gout radiographic scoring method has been developed and validated and may improve sensitivity to change in longitudinal studies.[43] However, radiography is not a sensitive method for monitoring gout manifestations compared to ultrasonography and MRI, because inflammatory changes and tophi volumes cannot be assessed.[44]

Calcium Pyrophosphate Dihydrate Crystal Deposition Disease

The term *CPPD crystal deposition disease* refers to a variety of clinical situations including asymptomatic crystal deposition, pseudogout, pyrophosphate arthropathy, and other, less frequent presentations, such as pseudo-RA. *Chondrocalcinosis* is a general term that refers to calcification of hyaline or fibrocartilage regardless of its etiology (Fig. 61.7).

The acute attack of pseudogout is often a monoarthropathy, and typical radiographic findings of soft tissue swelling and joint effusion are nonspecific mimicking gout and infection. Often chondrocalcinosis is not radiographically visible. The radiographic changes in more chronic pyrophosphate arthropathy are very similar to OA, with joint space narrowing, sclerosis, and subchondral cysts, with or without intra-articular or periarticular calcinosis.[45]

The patellofemoral joint and, in contrast to OA, radiocarpal and the second to third MCP joints, are typical sites of involvement in pyrophosphate arthropathy. The distribution is usually bilateral and may be symmetrical, whereas OA is uncommon in MCP joints, and when they are affected by OA the distribution is rarely symmetrical and often unilateral. In addition to the usual target sites, arthritic changes may be observed in non–weight-bearing joints and the sacroiliac joints.[46]

Pyrophosphate arthropathy may be associated with extensive and rapid subchondral bone collapse and fragmentation with intra-articular loose bodies, resembling neuropathic osteoarthropathy (pseudo-Charcot). Tumorous CPPD crystal deposits that resemble gouty tophi are observed occasionally, most frequently in digits, and are referred to as tophaceous pseudogout.[47]

Septic Arthritis

Septic arthritis is usually monoarticular and typically associated with rapid onset of symptoms, systemic illness, obvious local clinical signs, and laboratory evidence of acute inflammation. The earliest clinical sign is symmetrical soft tissue swelling around a joint due to soft tissue edema, hypertrophied synovium, and joint effusion. However, this may be hard to discern on radiography, and periarticular osteopenia may be the first radiographic feature. Initial widening of the joint space may be seen such as in septic arthritis of the pediatric hip. Marginal erosions develop

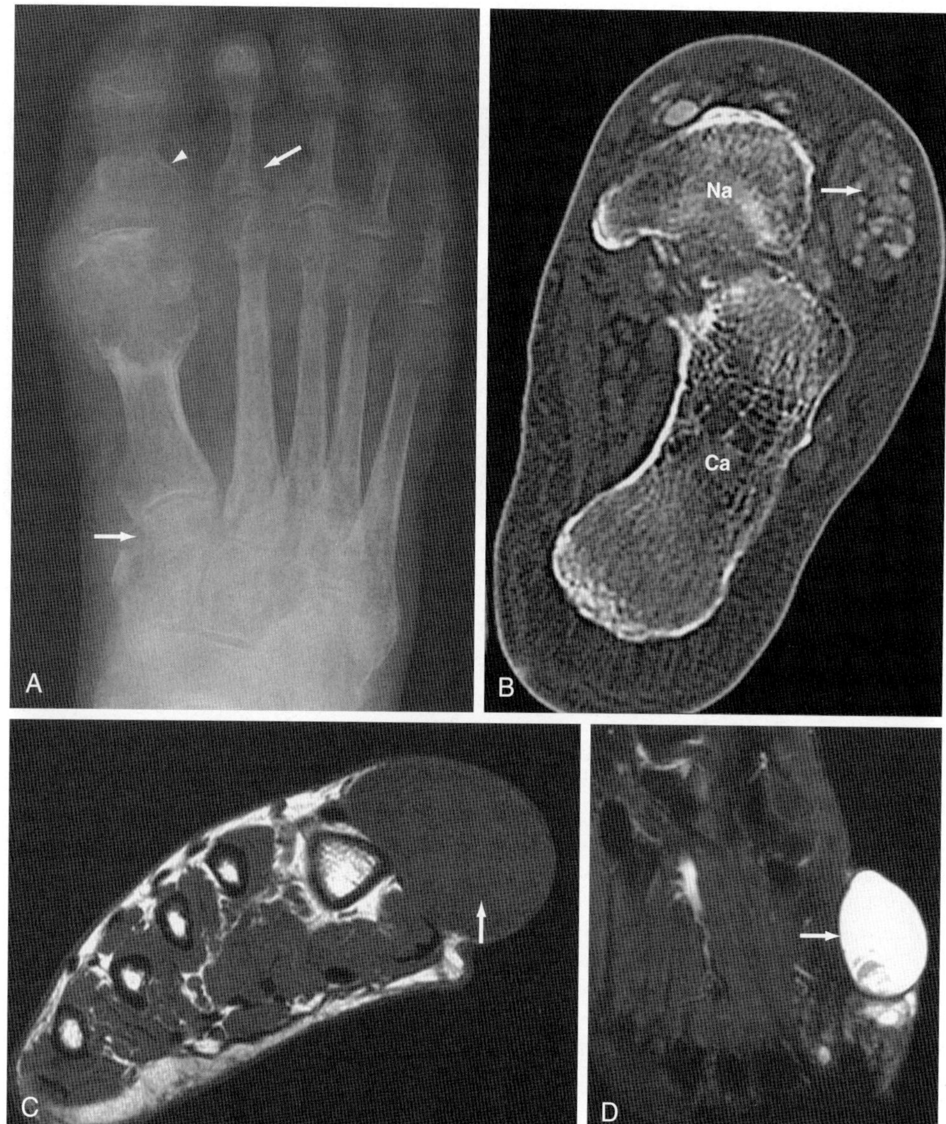

• **Fig. 61.6** Tophaceous gout (radiography, CT, and MRI). (A) Radiography of forefoot in tophaceous gout. Extensive bone destruction is seen at the first metatarsophalangeal (MTP) joint with overhanging edges *(arrowhead)* and soft tissue swelling. Smaller erosions are present involving the first tarsometatarsal and second MTP joints *(arrows)*. (B) CT scan shows hyperdense tophus around the extensor digitorum muscle *(arrow)*, with smaller deposits around the other extensor tendons. Axial precontrast (C) and coronal short tau inversion recovery (D) MR images show a large tophus *(arrow)* medial to the first metatarsal bone. *Ca,* Calcaneus; *Na,* navicular. (C and D, Courtesy Professor Fiona McQueen, Auckland, New Zealand.)

quickly and have a very similar appearance to other forms of erosive inflammatory arthritis. As the infection progresses, hyaline cartilage and the subchondral cortex are rapidly destroyed with progressive narrowing of the joint space (Fig. 61.8). In late stages, ankylosis of the joint may be seen. Adjacent osteomyelitis occurs with increasing frequency as the infection becomes chronic. With granulomatous infections, the characteristic triad (Phemister's triad) of radiographic findings are marked osteoporosis, marginal erosions, and absent or mild joint space narrowing. Periostitis and bone production are less common.

Use in Diagnosis, Monitoring, and Prognosis

Radiography should be routinely performed but is insensitive for diagnosis. When there is clinical suspicion of septic arthritis, joint aspiration should be performed without delay.

The utility of radiography is limited in septic arthritis with immediate joint aspiration (directly or by image guided techniques) required for early diagnosis and more advanced imaging techniques required for assessment of associated osteomyelitis or other complications.[48] However, radiography should still be routinely performed as it may assist in interpretation of other studies and still offers a satisfactory overall assessment of bone morphology and background disease.

Osteoarthritis

OA primarily targets hyaline cartilage, and its distribution is profoundly influenced by mechanical factors. OA is typically asymmetrical in distribution both within and between joints. The most characteristic sites of OA include the hips, knees (Fig. 61.9), proximal and distal

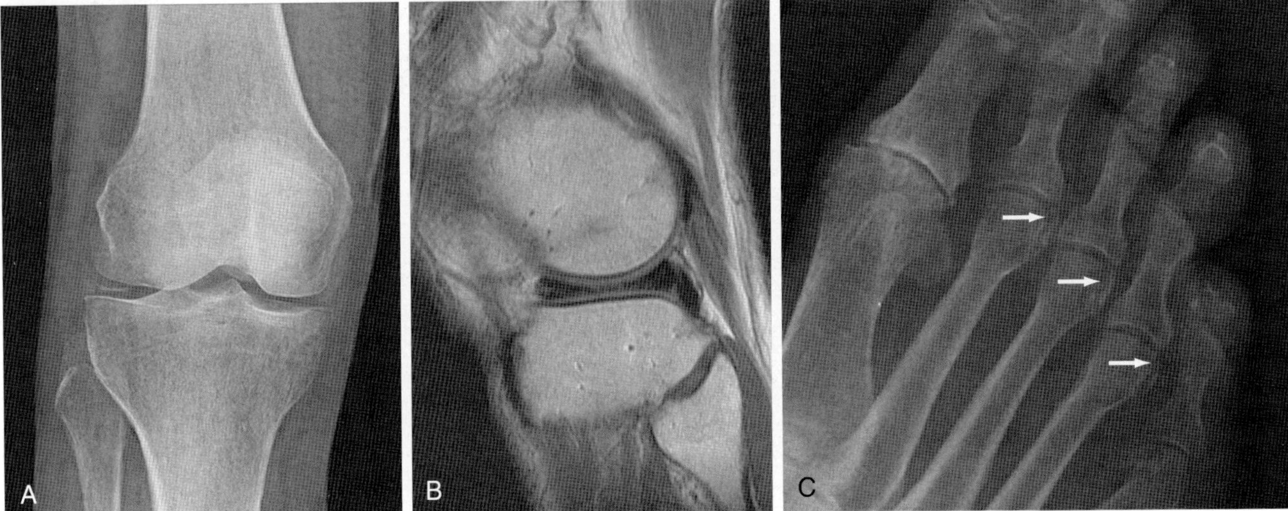

• **Fig. 61.7** Calcium pyrophosphate dihydrate crystal deposition disease (radiography and MRI). Radiography of the knee (A) shows linear calcification within the lateral meniscus, whereas sagittal proton density MRI (B) of the same patient shows increased signal within the lateral meniscus, corresponding to chondrocalcinosis. (C) Radiography of forefoot shows cartilaginous and capsular calcifications *(arrows)* within second through fourth metatarsophalangeal joints. A nondisplaced fracture of the fourth metatarsal neck is noted.

interphalangeal joints of the hand, first carpometacarpal and trapezioscaphoid joints of the wrist (Fig. 61.10), and first metatarsophalangeal joints.[1]

Joint space narrowing due to thinning of hyaline cartilage is a key feature of OA. Unlike the inflammatory arthropathies, the resultant narrowing of the radiographic joint space is asymmetrical with cartilage thinning more pronounced in areas subject to greater mechanical stress such as in one compartment of the knee. Accurate assessment of cartilage loss is hugely influenced by radiographic projection, particularly in the lower limbs. Sensitive detection of cartilage thinning requires apposition of the most affected surfaces, which requires the joint to be optimally positioned with sufficient mechanical stress to bring the surfaces into contact. In the knee for example, angular deformity tends to reduce on supine radiography and severe cartilage loss, may not be detected at all (see Fig. 61.9). Bilateral weight bearing projections are more consistent for the detection and measurement of cartilage loss, and the erect extended anterior-posterior (AP) view has been established as the preferred projection for diagnostic utility. However, no view is completely reliable until there is global loss of cartilage in late disease. Weight bearing in flexion is the most sensitive projection for cartilage thinning in the knee and the most reliable for detection of change, although the ideal degree of flexion for a specific individual varies depending on the distribution of cartilage loss (see Fig. 61.9).[49,50]

Osteophytes are the most characteristic abnormality of OA, being more specific than joint space narrowing, and are often the first radiographic sign of the disease. They start as osseous metaplasia of the hyaline cartilage best seen at the articular margins but also occur centrally on the articular surface. They can become large and often dominate the radiographic appearance. Thus, osteophytes are the key criterion to define presence of OA.[51]

Bone density is usually normal or sclerotic. Bone erosion does not occur except at the articular surface in late disease or occasionally earlier in the IP joints in inflammatory OA. The radiographic appearance of periarticular soft tissues is relatively normal in OA. Synovitis and effusion do occur but only rarely dominate the radiographic presentation. Some deformity is common but tends to occur in particular joints such as the thumb and knee. The deformity is primarily due to the asymmetric loss of cartilage and bone resulting in malalignment or subluxation.

Use in Diagnosis, Monitoring, and Prognosis

Conventional radiography is the standard method for diagnosis and follow-up of OA. Radiographic changes are key in the ACR criteria for classification of OA. A patient with radiographic osteophytes, knee pain, and either age older than 50 years, stiffness less than 30 minutes, or crepitus should be classified as OA.[51] However, newer imaging modalities, in particular MRI, are providing additional information that is used in clinical trials and for understanding the disease.

Various scoring systems have been developed to grade the severity of OA. Among the most well known is the Kellgren and Lawrence five point scale, which has been widely used in OA research studies.[52] Further atlas-based scoring systems have been developed that provide more accurate discrimination between individual radiographic features of OA.[52,53] Whichever system is used, the reliability is variable. In addition, quantitative measurement of joint space width as a surrogate for cartilage thickness has been employed in research studies, particularly in cases of knee OA but also in the hip and hand, and is subject to the limitations as discussed above.

Juvenile Idiopathic Arthritis (JIA)

JIA is the most common rheumatic disease of childhood,[54] with seven subtypes defined by the International League of Associations for Rheumatology (ILAR)[55] representing a heterogeneous set of chronic arthropathies with overlapping genetic predispositions.[56] JIA was previously misleadingly known as juvenile rheumatoid arthritis (JRA). The pattern of involvement of the polyarticular rheumatoid-factor-positive subtype does bear some resemblance to RA, but other subtypes

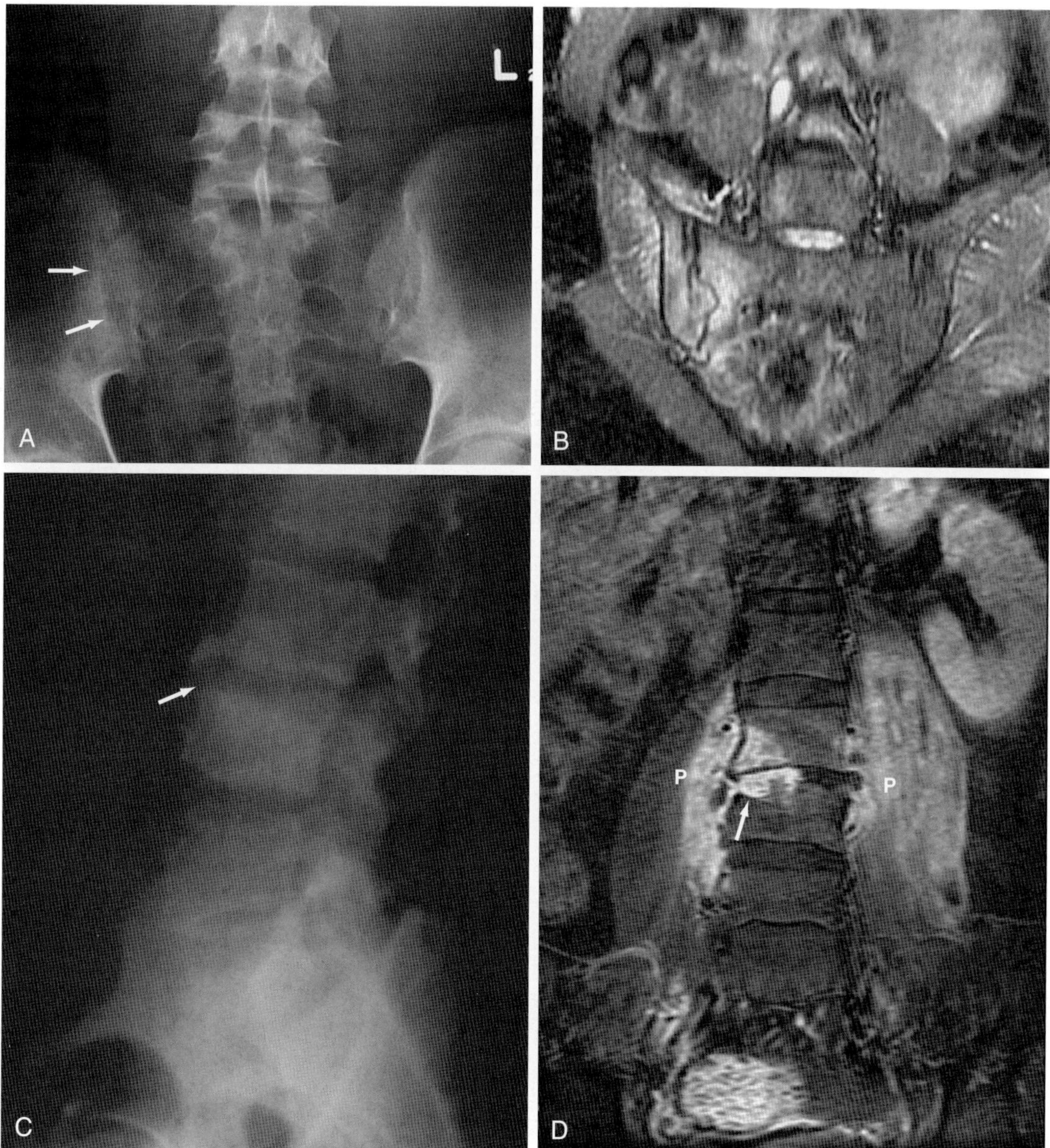

• **Fig. 61.8** Septic arthritis (radiography and MRI). (A) Radiography in anteroposterior view of sacroiliac joints shows destruction of the right sacroiliac joint as part of septic arthritis *(arrows).* (B) In another patient, short tau inversion recovery (STIR) coronal MRI through sacroiliac joints shows erosive changes in the right sacroiliac joint with extensive bone marrow edema. (C and D) Tuberculous spondylitis. (C) Radiography of the lumbar spine in lateral view shows disk space narrowing at the L3-L4 level with destructive changes involving the superior end plate of the L4 vertebral body *(arrow).* (D) Coronal STIR MRI of the lumbar spine of the same patient confirms focal destruction of the L4 vertebral body *(arrow)*. Enlargement of both psoas muscles (P) with increased signal is noted, owing to paraspinal extension of the infection.

do not. JIA can involve just one joint (oligoarticular), multiple joints (polyarticular), primarily the axial skeleton such as spine and sacroiliac joints (enthesitis-related or undifferentiated subtype), and other organs including the skin (psoriatic arthritis), serosa, spleen, and lymphatic tissue (systemic subtype).[54] The exact imaging features of arthropathy seen at a particular joint in JIA are less important than a broader overview of the distribution of joint involvement in the body over time, and patterns of extra-articular involvement. Particularly because many articular structures are not yet ossified in children, radiographs may appear normal until late in the disease course.[57] Rather than the erosions seen in adults, in children many radiographic changes relate to chronic hyperemia from articular inflammation, such as periarticular bony overgrowth seen as widening or squaring of structures such as tibial spines or carpal bones (Fig. 61.11).

Use in Diagnosis, Monitoring, and Prognosis

Radiographic abnormalities indicate that structural damage has occurred in JIA and are insensitive for early disease.[57] An unexplained effusion, features of overgrowth (bony deformity, joint space loss), and/or erosions in one or more joints suggest the possibility of JIA. The Sharp/van der Heijde scoring system, which quantifies radiographic wrist involvement by characterizing joint space narrowing

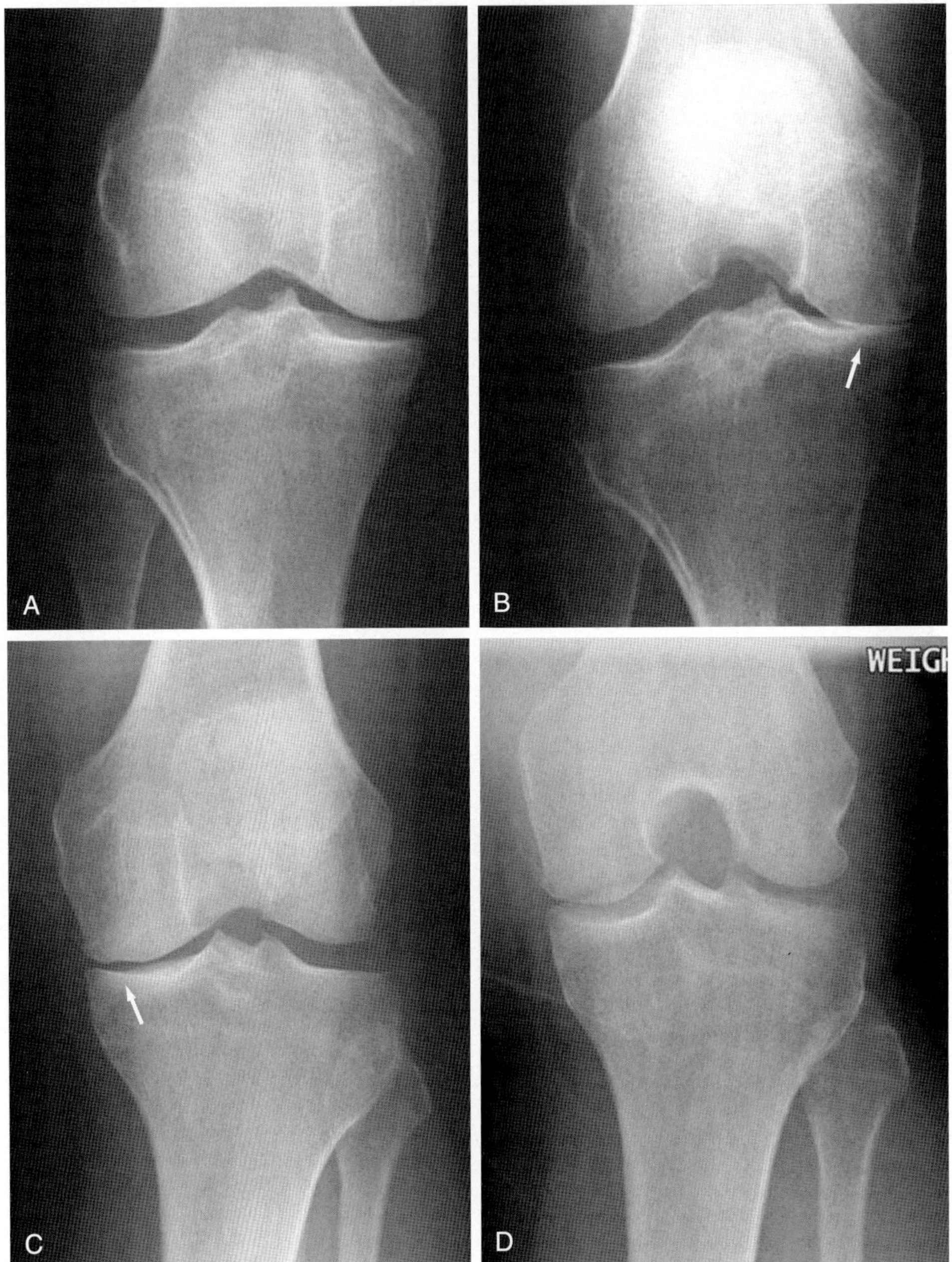

• **Fig. 61.9** Osteoarthritis of the knee (radiographs). Nonweight-bearing radiographs of the knee frequently underestimate the severity of cartilage loss. A 59-year-old man with pain and suspected osteoarthritis had supine anteroposterior (AP) (A) and erect weight-bearing AP (B) radiographs of the knee. The supine view demonstrates mild osteophytosis and possible subtle joint space narrowing in the medial compartment, whereas on the weight-bearing view, severe medial joint space narrowing is present, indicating severe cartilage damage *(arrow)*. Usually the weight-bearing semi-flexed view is most sensitive to joint space narrowing (cartilage loss) but this is unpredictable. In a 53-year-old man, the erect AP view (C) shows more severe joint space narrowing *(arrow)* than is seen on the weight-bearing semi-flexed view (D).

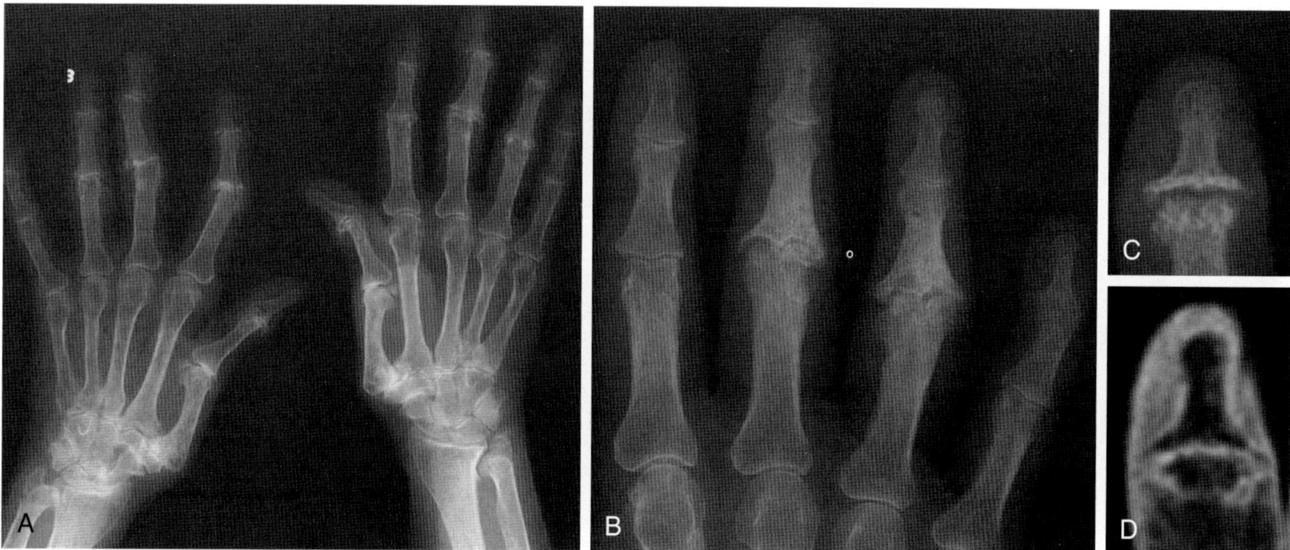

• **Fig. 61.10** Osteoarthritis of the hand (radiography and MRI). (A) Radiography shows asymmetric cartilage space narrowing at the proximal and distal interphalangeal joints, the first carpometacarpal joints, and the scaphoid-trapezium-trapezoid articulations. Subluxation at the first carpometacarpal joint and secondary hyperextension at the metacarpophalangeal joints are characteristic deformities of osteoarthritis. (B) "Gull wing" deformities in erosive osteoarthritis. Cartilage loss and bone remodeling at the third and fourth proximal interphalangeal joints produce a gull wing appearance. Radiography (C) and coronal MRI (D) of the distal interphalangeal joint show osteophyte and central erosions/collapse of the bone plate, representing severe osteoarthritis. (C and D Courtesy Dr. Ida Haugen, Oslo, Norway.)

and erosion or deformity at multiple sites for a maximum score of 330, has been used to assess progression of JIA at the wrists.[58]

Computed Tomography

KEY POINTS

Tomographic radiographic imaging technique that visualizes calcified tissue with high resolution, and a standard reference for detecting bone destructions.

Mainly useful for detection of bone abnormalities in the axial skeleton, i.e., erosions, sclerosis, new bone formation, and fractures.

More sensitive for these purposes than X-ray and in most occasions MRI.

The role in the axial skeleton is limited by a relative high amount of ionizing radiation.

Rarely used in clinical practice unless X-ray is unclear and MRI is unavailable.

The main disadvantages are the low sensitivity for soft tissue changes and the high exposure to ionizing radiation.

CT has been available for 40 years, and each decade has brought further development in computing and engineering that has resulted in remarkable changes in the technology. Although still limited in soft-tissue contrast, CT offers fast and reliable acquisition, high resolution, and multiplanar capabilities that have enhanced its use in recent years. The modern CT scanner is a remarkable tool that will likely have an increasingly important role in arthritis imaging in the future.

Technical Aspects

CT image acquisition is no longer restricted to the axial plane of imaging, and its multiplanar capability is so versatile that many CT scans of the body are now interpreted primarily from thin slice coronal or sagittal reconstructions in the same way as MRI. Unlike MRI, there are no absolute contraindications to CT and scans are so fast that patient motion is rarely a problem and patient tolerance is excellent. Spatial resolution is high, usually higher than MRI, and contrast resolution between soft tissue and bone is unsurpassed by any other modality. However, despite these advantages, the application of CT in arthritis imaging still has flaws that prevent its universal application. Firstly, CT is constrained in the same way as radiography by its limited soft-tissue contrast capability. Secondly, ionizing radiation is used with increasing dose proportional to size of body part and requirements for spatial detail. While this is not a problem with the more distal extremities as the exposure doses are smaller and the tissue more radio resistant, it remains an issue for spine, hip, and shoulder CT. Consequently, in most routine clinical situations, radiography provides sufficient information of a similar nature to CT for clinical decision making and radiography is cheaper than CT and readily available; ultrasonography is a better and cheaper way to visualize and quantify superficial soft-tissue pathology; and MRI offers superior soft-tissue contrast and bone marrow imaging. However, the technology continues to evolve and low-dose CT (LDCT) is becoming more common with iterative reconstruction techniques that reduce the radiation exposure by about 80%.[59] Exposure dose from LDCT of the sacroiliac joints is similar to radiography and should probably replace radiography as a first line test in many cases.[60]

LDCT can quantify bone formation in the spine, which is undetectable with radiography,[61] and cone-beam CT is a new technology that can detect bone erosion in extremities at extremely low dose.[62]

Dual energy CT (DECT) allows the separation of calcium-containing bone from the soft-tissue components, thereby allowing detection of soft-tissue changes that were previously invisible

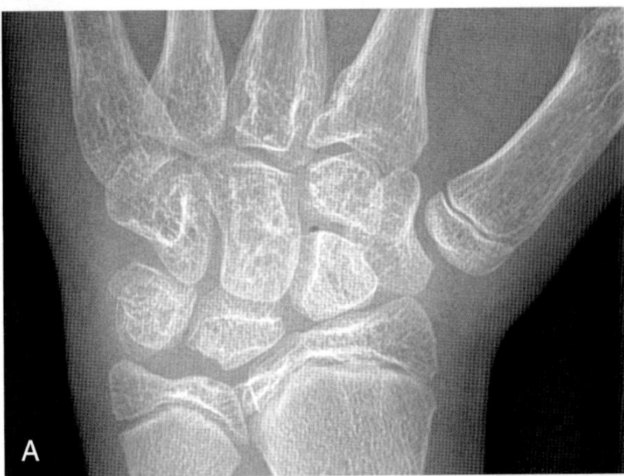

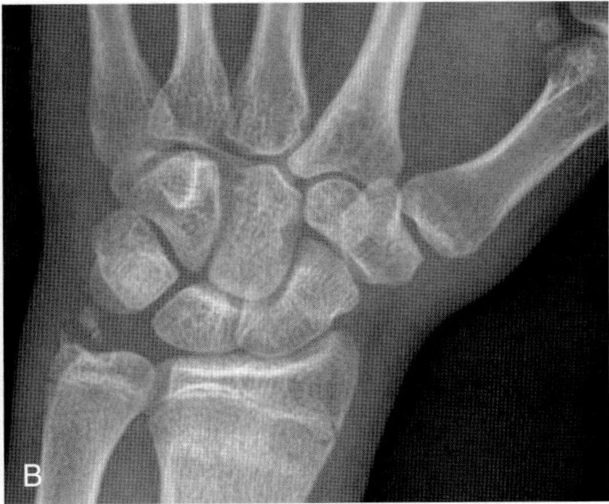

• **Fig. 61.11** Radiography in patients with juvenile idiopathic arthritis (JIA). Left wrist radiographs in (A) 14-year-old girl with long-standing JIA, (B) 15-year-old girl with an ulnar styloid fracture and no known arthropathy, for comparison. In (A), note the contour deformities of carpal bones, particularly the lunate and scaphoid, relative widening/expansion of distal radial and ulnar articular surfaces, ulnar subluxation of the carpus so that much of the lunate overlies the ulna, and heterogeneous bone density. There are no erosions or carpal fusion; the findings are likely mainly due to overgrowth from chronic hyperemia.

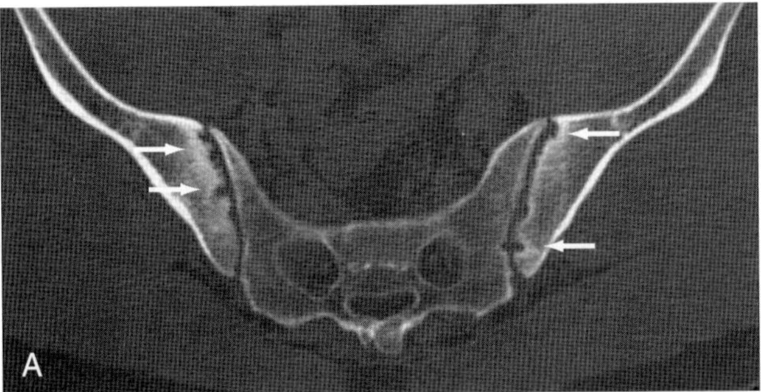

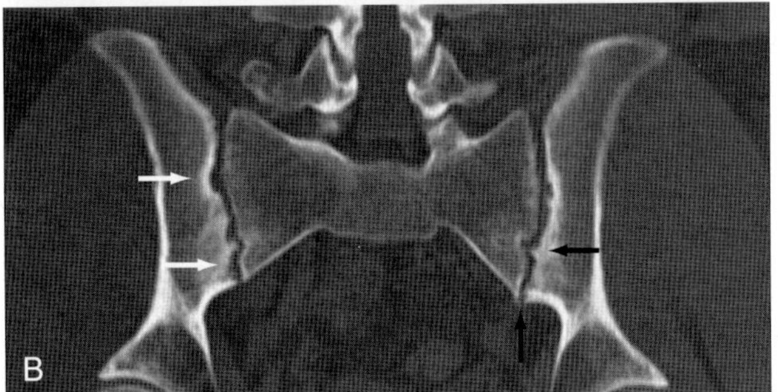

• **Fig. 61.12** Bone erosion in sacroiliac joints in spondyloarthritis (CT). Coronal (A) and axial (B) CT images of the sacroiliac joints in a patient with spondyloarthritis. Bone erosions *(white arrows)* and mild sclerosis and new bone formation *(black arrows)* are seen.

with CT. For example, it has recently been reported that DECT can detect bone marrow edema (BME) with good reliability.[63,64]

DECT can also be used for analysis of composition of some specific tissues, most particularly urate crystals, which can be detected in bone and soft tissues (see later).

Rheumatoid Arthritis

The exquisite inherent contrast between bone and soft tissue that is afforded by CT makes it a gold standard reference for the detection of bone erosion, and as such CT is ideally suited to the investigation of erosion in inflammatory arthritides. Modern CT with isotropic voxel acquisition and three-dimensional visualization allows accurate detection and quantification of bone erosion with good intraobserver agreement, whereas radiography is limited by its two-dimensional projection and superimposition of structures. However, CT is very limited in ability to visualize soft-tissue changes, and even with contrast enhancement and complex subtraction techniques CT is still inferior to MRI and ultrasonography for assessment of synovial changes such as thickening and hyperemia. Furthermore, detection of erosion on CT and MRI shows very good agreement, although CT is slightly more sensitive.[65,66]

Use in Diagnosis, Monitoring, and Prognosis

CT is not currently used in routine clinical practice for the diagnosis of RA. However, it could be potentially useful for diagnosis as CT appears to be the most sensitive technique for detection of erosion,[65,66] and CT of the feet is very simple with very low radiation dose. CT is used for problem solving in specific cases, such as examination of the cervical spine if MRI is unavailable or contraindicated.

The use of CT for longitudinal assessment of damage progression has potential merit.[66,67] A problem with CT in comparison to MRI or ultrasonography is its inability to demonstrate improvement in soft-tissue pathology. No CT data are available for prognosis in RA. The current use of CT in RA is very limited, but it has detected erosion reliably,[68] scoring systems are in development,[69] and CT can detect and quantify repair of erosion.[70]

Ankylosing Spondylitis/Axial Spondyloarthritis

CT allows visualization of the same pathologic processes as conventional radiography—erosion, osteoporosis/sclerosis, and new bone formation/ankylosis—with the added benefit of multiplanar imaging free from superimposition of overlying structures (Fig. 61.12).

In AS, the pathologic processes start in bone marrow and at sites of enthesis. However, CT has poor ability to detect soft-tissue change and is usually normal until structural damage is present. CT can detect osteoporosis or osteosclerosis quite well, but these changes are very nonspecific. The primary value of CT in AS is its ability to detect and clearly define erosion of bone at any joint or enthesis. New bone formation is also well visualized in the form of syndesmophytes, ligamentous ossification, and periarticular and intra-articular ankylosis, but the use for CT in this regard is limited. CT can show these findings equally well in the axial and peripheral skeleton but is used primarily in areas where radiographic visualization or interpretation is problematic.

Use in Diagnosis, Monitoring, and Prognosis

Diagnosis. The diagnosis of AS is primarily based on the radiographic observation of bilateral moderate or unilateral severe sacroiliitis. When good quality radiographs of the sacroiliac joints are normal or radiographic changes meet diagnostic criteria, there is no role for CT. Early detection of AS is better done by MRI. However, CT of the sacroiliac joints is much easier to interpret than radiography, which is notoriously subject to poor observer reliability. When the radiographic findings are unclear, CT will usually resolve this uncertainty. Because CT shows bone erosion in exquisite detail, CT may also have a role to play in the further investigation of MRI equivocal findings. It should be noted that classification criteria for AS depend on radiographic findings and more recently MRI but not CT specifically. In the spine, CT is useful in the diagnosis of complications of late disease such as spondylodiscitis or spinal fracture when patients may be unable to tolerate MRI due to pain or spinal deformity.

Monitoring Disease Activity and Damage. CT has no role in monitoring disease activity or damage at this time because although DECT can show BME, it is not yet widely available and has relatively high radiation dose. Studies have shown that quantitative measurement of syndesmophyte formation in the spine is reliable and significantly more sensitive to change than assessment by radiography,[71] and this has been reproduced at lower radiation exposure levels.[61] Consequently, LDCT could have an important future in the monitoring of structural damage progression in the spine.

Prognosis. The prognostic value of CT findings of sacroiliitis requires further investigation.

Psoriatic Arthritis

CT is rarely used for the investigation of PsA, and very little data are published on this topic. It has been confirmed that, in comparison to radiography, CT is much more sensitive for the detection of small foci of erosion or proliferation of the small bones of the hand.[72,73] CT was highly reliable for the detection of erosion but less so for proliferation, and neither radiography nor CT detected significant change in the bone findings in this short trial. In the peripheral skeleton, it would be expected that the application of CT for PsA would be similar to RA, and in the axial skeleton, use of CT would be similar to AS. In both cases, use of CT is limited by inability to directly visualize inflammation in soft tissue, and although it has superior ability versus radiography to detect bone erosion and proliferation, in most circumstances the extra radiation dose is not warranted.

Use in Diagnosis, Monitoring, and Prognosis

CT visualizes bone erosion and bone proliferation but no systematic studies of specific diagnostic utility or prognostic value have been performed. Because of radiation concerns, CT is not used for disease monitoring in PsA.

Gout

CT allows clear visualization of bone erosion, and recent developments in technology offer exciting prospects for crystal imaging. Acute and chronic tophaceous gout is associated with deposition of urate crystals in soft tissues and the development of tophi. Chronic tophi are often partially calcified and all CT scanners are sensitive for the deposition of calcium in soft tissues (see Fig. 61.6). The condition frequently involves intraosseous deposition of crystals and this is much better visualized on CT than radiography.[74] CT shows soft-tissue swelling due to tophi quite well, and as anatomical bone detail is very good on CT, erosions are clearly delineated. DECT is a new technologic development whereby images can be reconstructed based on a two-material decomposition algorithm that can separate calcium from monosodium urate (Fig. 61.13).[75] DECT has been used to show that monosodium urate (MSU) crystals are frequently present in joints affected by radiographic damage in gout, which supports the concept that MSU crystals interact with articular tissues contributing to the development of structural joint damage.[76]

Use in Diagnosis, Monitoring, and Prognosis

CT visualizes bone erosions and tophi, but few systematic studies of specific diagnostic utility have been performed. Until recently, CT had no role in the diagnosis of acute gout, prior to the development of bone erosions or tophi, as it does not provide imaging of synovitis, tenosynovitis, or osteitis. However, CT scanning with DECT is a recent technical development that can accurately detect the presence of monosodium urate with about 90% sensitivity and 80% specificity and with excellent reader reliability.[77,78] The sensitivity is less in subjects with acute gout, but DECT is quite specific in this group, whereas specificity drops when concomitant OA is present. The greatest diagnostic utility of DECT would appear to be in acute gout in small joints where the differential diagnosis is septic arthritis and joint fluid is unobtainable or fluid microscopy fails to demonstrate monosodium urate crystals. DECT was initially limited to CT scanners that had dual-source technology; however, software has been developed that now permits DECT on single source scanners with good reliability,[79] and DECT is likely to become widely available in the near future.

CT, including DECT, is reliable for monitoring tophus size.[44,80] A bone erosion scoring method has recently been developed.[81] These methods may be useful in trials.

Calcium Pyrophosphate Dihydrate Crystal Deposition Disease

CT is not used in the management of uncomplicated peripheral CPPD, although calcifications can be visualized. CPPD can involve the cervical spine and cause neck pain. In such patients, CT may visualize CPPD deposition at the craniovertebral junction, often in the transverse ligament of atlas (crowned dens syndrome).[82,83] Calcific deposits may also be found in other peri-odontoid structures and the ligamenta flava in some patients, as may osseous abnormalities of the odontoid process, such as subchondral cysts or erosions. CT may also be used for verifying the presence of calcifications at other rare locations, for example, the temporomandibular joints.[84] In peripheral joints, CT can accurately depict the distribution of CPPD crystals and has confirmed that, in fact, soft-tissue deposition outside cartilaginous structures is common, especially so in ligaments and joint capsule.[85]

Septic Arthritis

CT is rarely used for the investigation of septic arthritis. Acute septic arthritis of large joints is a surgical emergency, and while

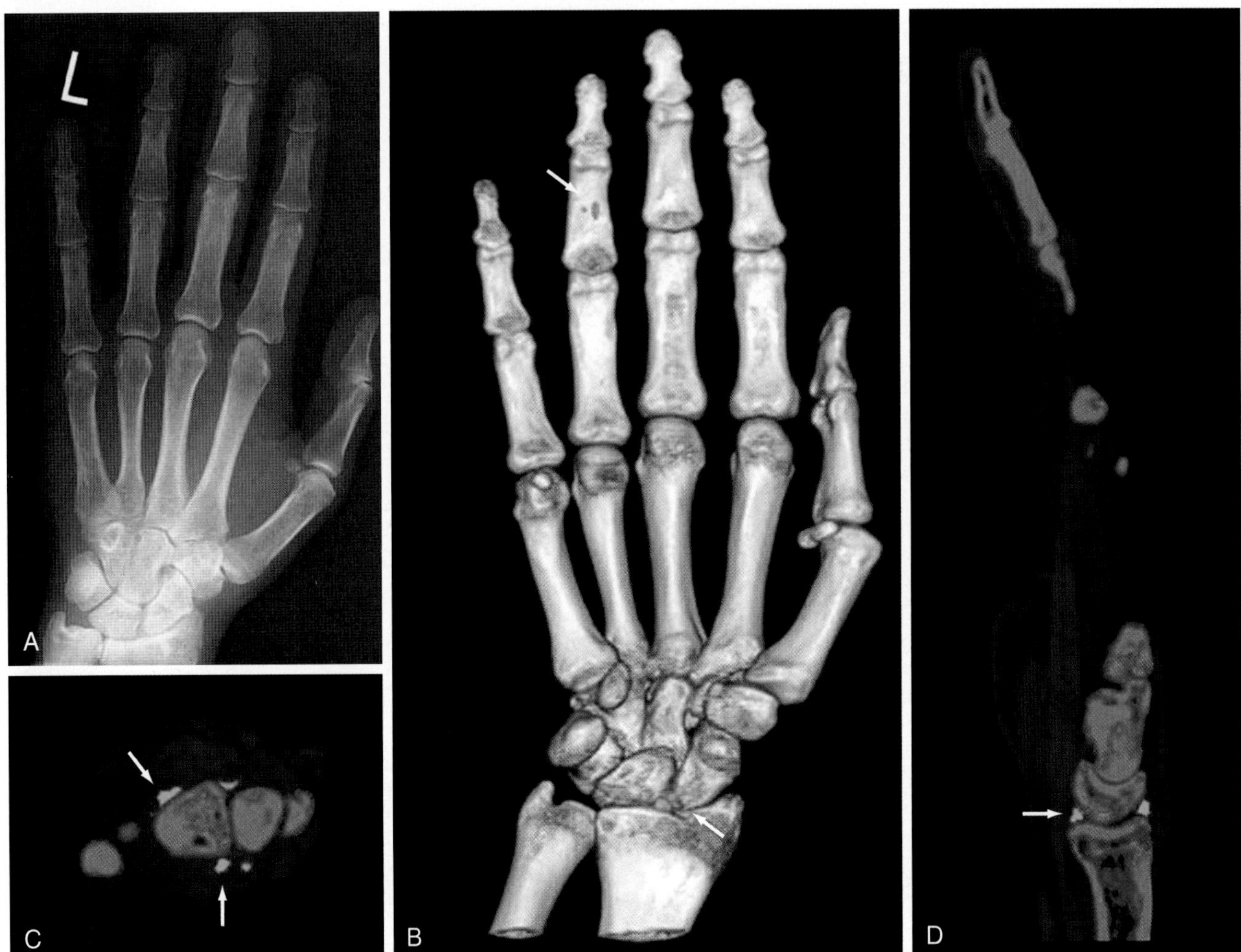

• **Fig. 61.13** Gout (radiography and dual-energy CT scan). Radiography (A) and dual-energy CT scans (B-D) of left hand and wrist of a 39-year-old male patient with recent-onset bilateral pain in hands and wrists. Radiography (A) and laboratory investigations were all normal. Dual-energy CT was performed and confirmed the presence of sodium urate crystals in the left wrist and one finger. Left wrist aspirate was attempted but was unsuccessful. The patient responded well to treatment for gout. Imaging findings: After processing of CT data with an algorithm specific for detection of urate crystals (Siemens, Erlangen), the urate crystals are displayed green *(arrows)* on three-dimensional anterior (B), two-dimensional transverse (C), and two-dimensional sagittal (D) reconstructions.

radiography, fluoroscopy, and ultrasonography may be useful for either diagnosis or image-guided aspiration, there is no use for CT in the peripheral skeleton. In chronic septic arthritis and infectious discitis, CT may be used to investigate complications, particularly osteomyelitis. However, MRI or a variety of scintigraphic studies are generally preferred.[48] In complex cases where MRI scanning is problematic, contrast-enhanced CT can be very useful to detect abscess formation in deep soft-tissues that are not easily assessed by ultrasonography, and CT guidance may be preferred for spine biopsy.

Osteoarthritis

Even though CT can detect bone changes more accurately than radiography, such as osteophytes,[86] overall it offers little additional diagnostic utility in peripheral joints. It generally has poor soft-tissue contrast capability, hyaline cartilage cannot be directly visualized, and spatial resolution of bone detail is inferior to radiography. It may be used in specific problem-solving situations where anatomy is complex and/or poorly visualized on radiography, such as in the lumbar spine facet joints, but this is not usually the case in the peripheral joints. CT is occasionally used to assess extent of disease, such as in the orthopedic assessment of large joints where detailed evaluation of bone morphology may be required preoperatively. CT scanning with intra-articular contrast material (CT arthrography) may be the single most accurate modality for detecting cartilage thinning, fissuring, flaps, or volume[87] (Fig. 61.14), and loose intra-articular bodies. This requires both a minimally invasive procedure and radiation exposure and is not widely used. Experimentally, CT arthrography can detect changes related to alteration of the glycosaminoglycan (GAG) content of hyaline cartilage[88] and it correlates well with gadolinium-enhanced MRI estimates of cartilage damage, but neither modality correlates with arthroscopic findings in early disease.[89] CT arthrography may be used as a problem-solving tool in patients who are not able to undergo MRI.

Use in Diagnosis, Monitoring, and Prognosis

CT is not currently used in routine clinical practice for the diagnosis of OA, it has no role for monitoring disease as it cannot

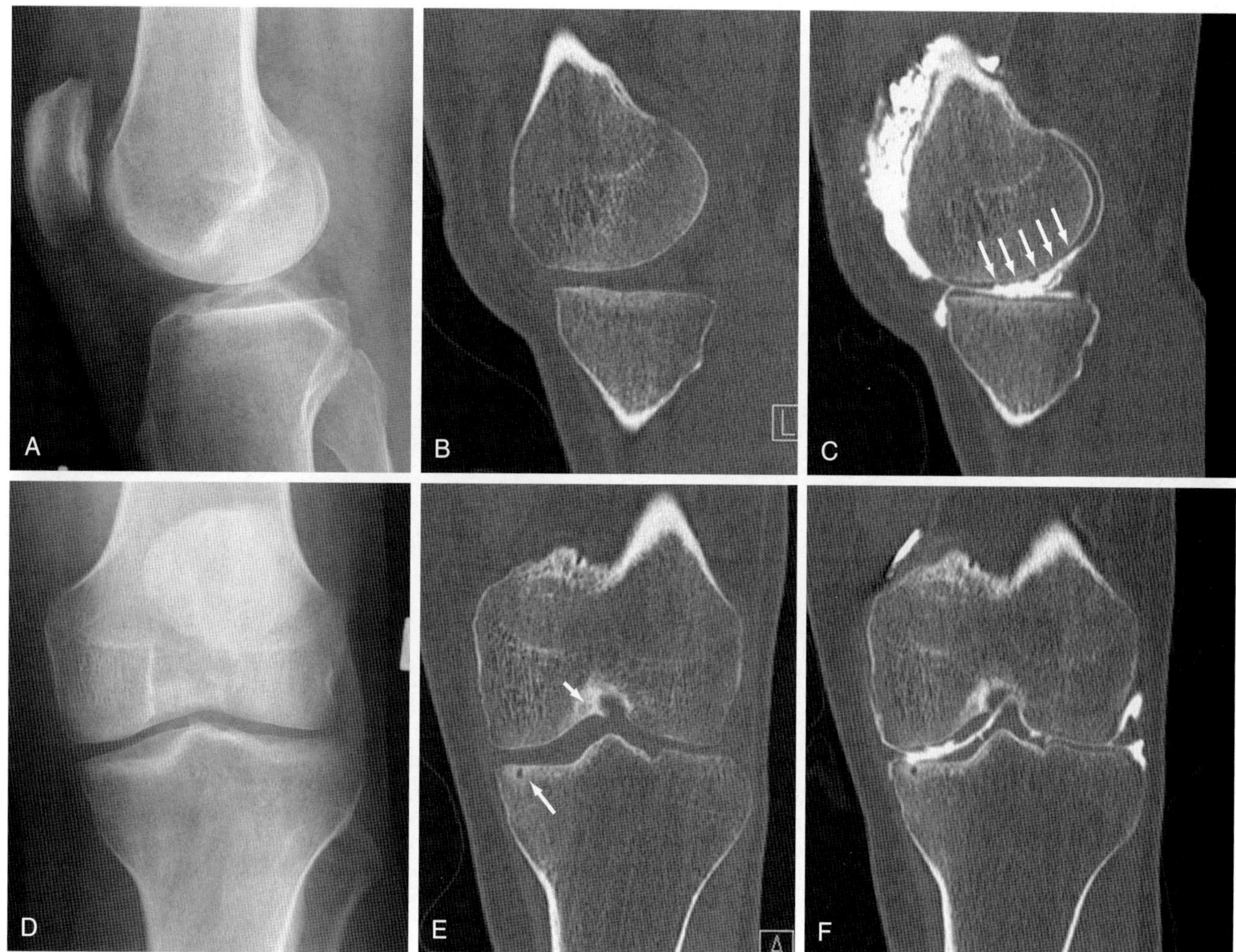

• **Fig. 61.14** Radiography, CT, and CT arthrogram of the knee in a 46-year-old male patient with unexplained pain and locking. Initial radiographs (A and D) appear near normal with preserved joint space, a tiny osteophyte arising from the medial tibial spine, and no other definite abnormality. CT scan with sagittal (B) and coronal (E) reconstructions confirms the presence of osteophytosis *(short arrow)* and a small subchondral cyst *(long arrow)* but shows no definite chondral changes. CT arthrogram with sagittal reconstruction (C) demonstrates several focal hyaline cartilage thinning *(arrows)* and a meniscal tear. On the coronal reconstruction (F), the tibial subchondral cyst is associated with complete loss of overlying hyaline cartilage.

quantify change in the target tissue (cartilage) without an invasive procedure, and there are no published data on the independent prognostic use of CT, as good quality radiography usually provides the same or more information.

Juvenile Idiopathic Arthritis

Because CT involves a relatively high ionizing radiation dose and cannot effectively evaluate cartilage, it has little role in JIA, except in surgical planning for complex structural deformities induced by chronic JIA.

Magnetic Resonance Imaging

KEY POINTS

Allows sensitive visualization and assessment of peripheral inflammatory and destructive joint and soft tissue involvement in a variety of degenerative and inflammatory rheumatic diseases.

By far the best available method for detecting and monitoring inflammation in the spine and sacroiliac joints in AS and other spondyloarthritides including JIA.

Allows monitoring of inflammatory soft-tissue changes (e.g., synovitis, tenosynovitis, and enthesitis) during treatment of adult and pediatric patients with peripheral inflammatory joint diseases.

Can contribute to earlier diagnosis of RA, SpA and JIA, through detection of early inflammatory changes.

Bone edema is uniquely visualized and provides prognostic information in RA, SpA, OA, undifferentiated inflammatory arthritis, and possibly other rheumatic arthritides such as JIA.

Main disadvantages are costs, lack of availability, and the potential need for sedation in young children

MRI provides multiplanar tomographical imaging with unprecedented soft tissue contrast, without the use of ionizing radiation, and allows assessment of all the structures involved in musculoskeletal diseases. MRI is more sensitive than clinical examination and radiography for detection of inflammation and damage in inflammatory and degenerative rheumatologic disorders in adults and children.

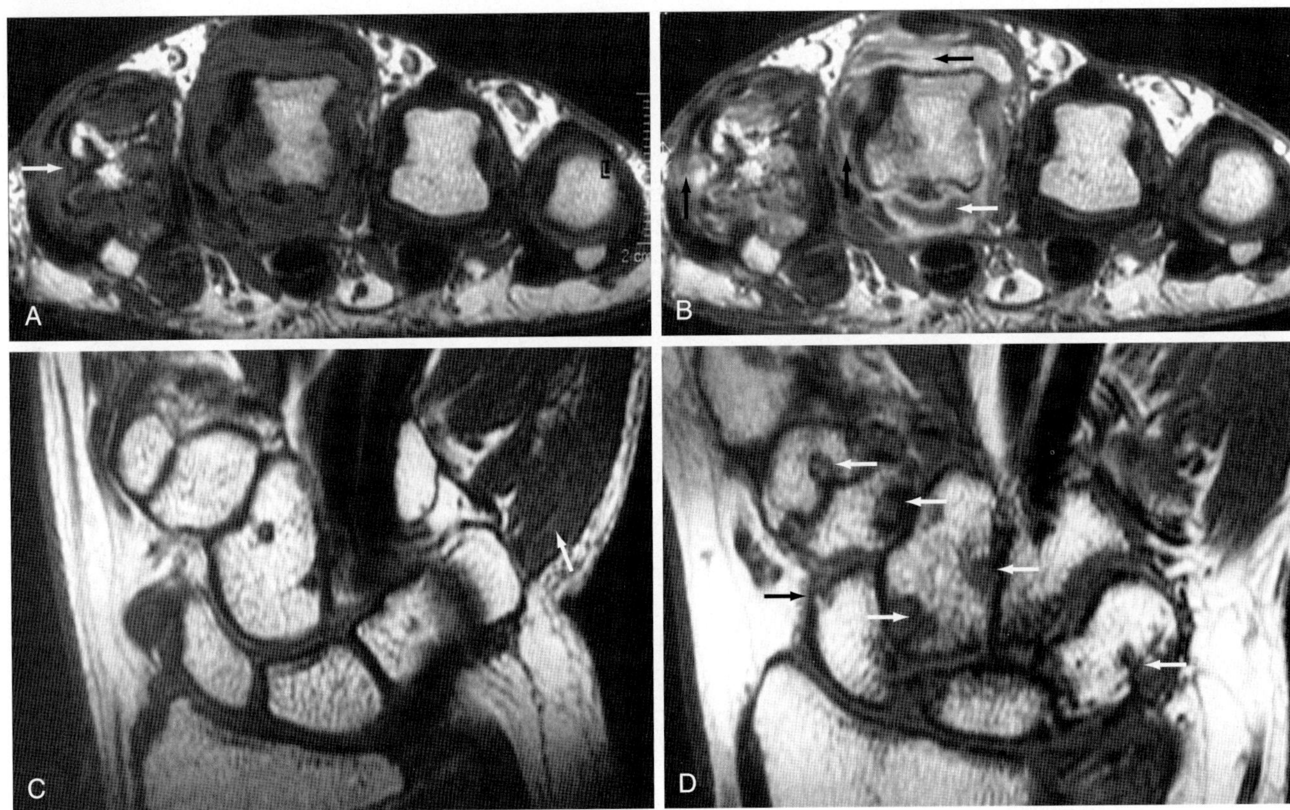

• **Fig. 61.15** Rheumatoid arthritis (MRI). Axial T1-weighted precontrast (A) and postcontrast (B) MRI of the second (left) through fifth (right) fingers at the level of the metacarpophalangeal joints in a patient with rheumatoid arthritis (RA). Synovitis (*black arrows* in B), joint effusion (*white arrow* in B), and severe bone erosion (*arrow* in A) are seen. Coronal T1-weighted precontrast MRI of the wrist (C) in another RA patient shows no bone erosions. Similar images 1 year later (D) show severe erosive progression (bone erosions marked by *arrows*).

Disadvantages of MRI include higher costs and lower availability than radiography, longer examination times, and, except when using the novel whole-body MRI technique, restriction to a limited anatomical area per session. It should be remembered, however, that costs of MRI are only a small fraction of the cost of biologic treatment or of the indirect costs of sick leaves and early retirements.

Preceded by a section on key technical aspects, the characteristics of MRI with respect to diagnosis, monitoring and prognosis, and clinical utility in RA, SpA, PsA, gout, OA, and JIA will be described in the following section.

Technical Aspects

T1-weighted (T1w) imaging sequences are favored by offering relatively short imaging times and good anatomical detail. Furthermore, after intravenous contrast (paramagnetic gadolinium compounds; Gd) injection these sequences visualize tissues with high perfusion and permeability, including the inflamed synovium. Fat and Gd-enhanced tissues have a high signal intensity on T1w images (Fig. 61.15). T2-weighted (T2w) images depict both fat and fluid/edematous tissues with a high signal intensity. These are used together with T1w images in degenerative spine disease. In inflammatory conditions T2w images with fat saturation (FS) (Fig. 61.16) are particularly useful, because the signal from fat is suppressed in such sequences, allowing detection of edematous tissue/fluid located in areas with fatty tissue, for example, bone marrow edema. FS requires a homogenous field and a high magnetic field strength, not available on low field (<1.0T) MRI units.

The STIR (short tau inversion recovery) technique, another fat-suppressed sequence based on relaxation time differences, can be acquired on low-field MRI and can provide information on bone marrow edema,[90] although with less detail.

Whereas MRI examination of axial joints requires whole-body MRI units, MRI of the peripheral joints can be performed with whole-body MRI units or dedicated extremity MRI units (E-MRI). E-MRI increases the potential for widespread rheumatologic use, through markedly lower costs, more comfortable patient positioning, and elimination of claustrophobia.

Some E-MRI units may provide information on synovitis and bone destructions not markedly inferior to what is obtained by standard sequences on high-field units,[90,91] but the performance of different machines varies, and for some units smaller field of view, longer imaging times, and lack of certain imaging techniques (particularly FS at low field) should be considered.[92]

The majority of MRI studies of the sacroiliac joint have used only one imaging plane (semi-coronal, i.e., parallel with the axis of the sacral bone). A supplementary T1w FS sequence may improve the evaluation of erosions,[93] and sequences designed for cartilage evaluation, for example, three-dimensional gradient echo sequences, may also be added.[94] To be maximally sensitive for changes in the ligamentous portion of the sacroiliac joints, imaging in the semi-axial plane is required.[93] This may therefore be recommended when MRI is used for diagnostic purposes, while it is probably not essential when used as an outcome measure in trials. While MRI on some indications (e.g., suspected disc herniation) should include axial images, MRI of the spine in SpA generally only involves sagittal images, but these

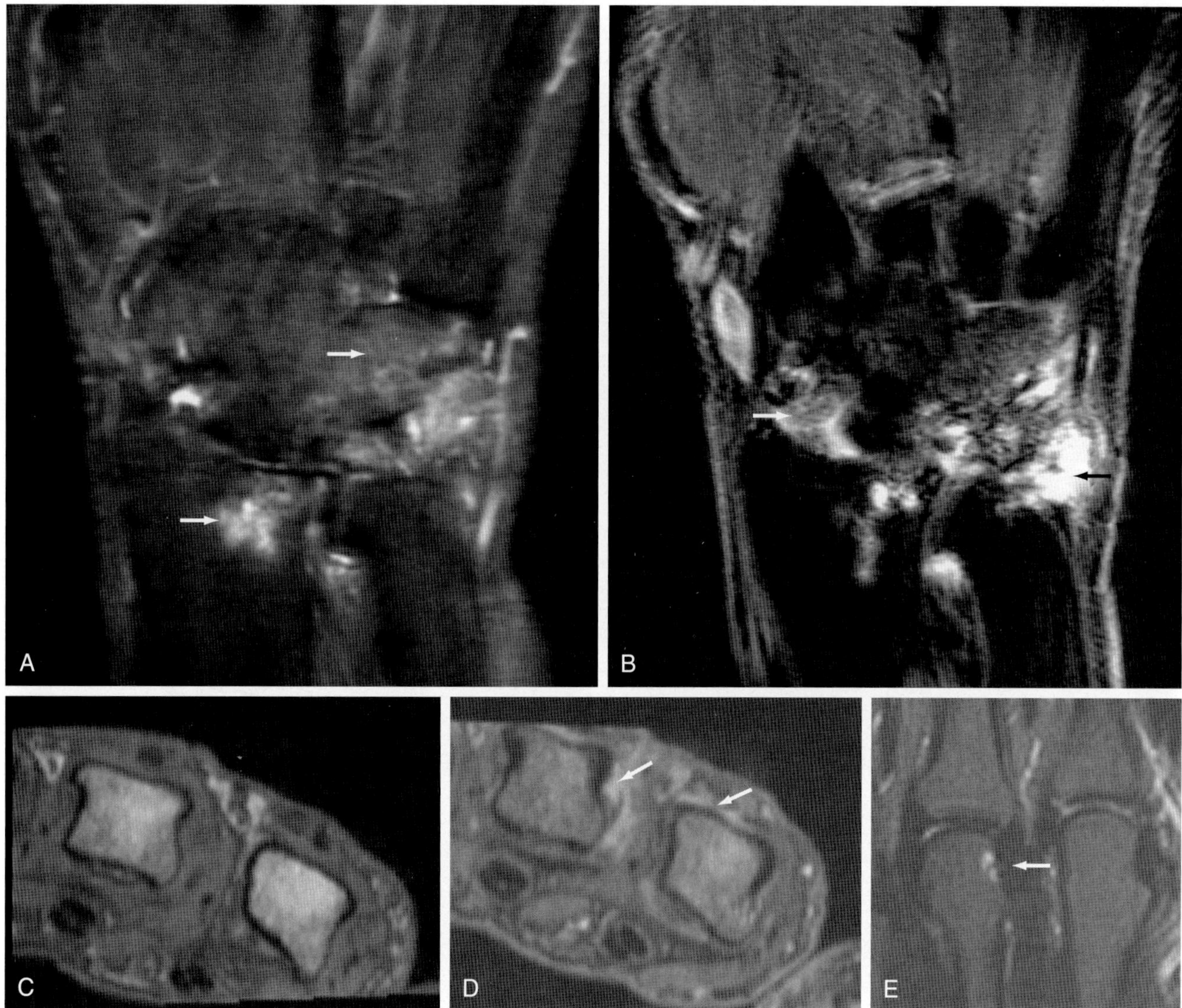

• **Fig. 61.16** Rheumatoid arthritis (RA) in clinical remission (MRI) and undifferentiated arthritis (MRI). (A and B) RA patient in clinical remission. Despite clinical remission, coronal short tau inversion recovery (STIR) (A) and postcontrast T1-weighted fat-suppressed (B) MRI show marked bone marrow edema (osteitis, *arrows* in A) and synovitis (*arrows* in B). (C-E) Patient with undifferentiated arthritis. Axial T1-weighted precontrast (C) and postcontrast (D) T1-weighted MRI views show synovitis in second and third metacarpophalangeal joints *(arrows)*, whereas the STIR sequence (E) shows bone edema *(arrow)*. Radiography was normal. One year later the patient had developed RA, according to the American College of Rheumatology 1987 criteria. (Courtesy Dr. Anne Duer-Jensen, Glostrup, Denmark.)

should extend sufficiently lateral to include the frequently involved facet, costo-vertebral, and costo-transversal joints.[95] Bone marrow abnormalities in both sacroiliac joints and spine are detected almost equally well with the STIR and contrast-enhanced T1w FS sequences in patients with SpA, so contrast injection is generally not needed for assessment of the axial skeleton.[96,97] However, contrast injection increases the sensitivity for synovitis in peripheral joints.[98] For evaluation of structural (sometimes referred to as chronic) changes such as bone erosion, new bone formation, and fat infiltrations, T1-weighted images are mandatory. A supplementary T1w FS sequence may improve the evaluation of erosions.[93] In peripheral as axial joints, specific sequences designed for cartilage optimal evaluation can be applied, for example, three-dimensional gradient echo sequences.[94]

New MRI techniques are being developed all the time, and a variety of sequences is now available for the detection of increased water content in bone marrow such as occurs with inflammation—so called *bone marrow edema* (BME)—including T2 with water excitation (WE), hybrid sequences, and chemical shift–based fat-water separation with the Dixon technique.[99] Each sequence has advantages, and disadvantages, and at this time it would appear that none of them consistently alters the diagnostic properties of MRI for the detection of BME. Most centers continue to use the more traditional T2FS or STIR sequences because almost all MRI scanners can perform these two sequences, they are generally reliable and fairly consistent across different manufacturers and magnetic field strengths.

The potential for molecular imaging with MRI is an exhilarating prospect for arthritis research and the future of clinical practice. Numerous techniques are being developed for evaluation of the chemical and biophysical structure of musculoskeletal tissues and particularly articular cartilage. Many publications now attest to the capabilities of T2 or T2* relaxation time mapping,[100,101] delayed Gadolinium Enhanced MRI of cartilage (dGEMRIC),[102,103]

T1ρ imaging (T1rho–T1 properties in the rotating frame of reference),[104,105] glycosaminoglycan chemical exchange saturation transfer (gagCEST),[106,107] diffusion tensor imaging (DTI),[108,109] and sodium MRI.[110,111] All of these MRI developments are highly technical, require dedicated software and/or hardware, and are challenging to perform consistently. Several have been proposed for use in clinical practice but none of them have established unequivocal utility beyond a standard set of high quality sequences.

Of these new developments, DTI may have the most promise (Fig. 61.17). DTI signal is dependent on water movement with one signal component dependent on the speed of water movement independent of direction—apparent diffusion coefficient

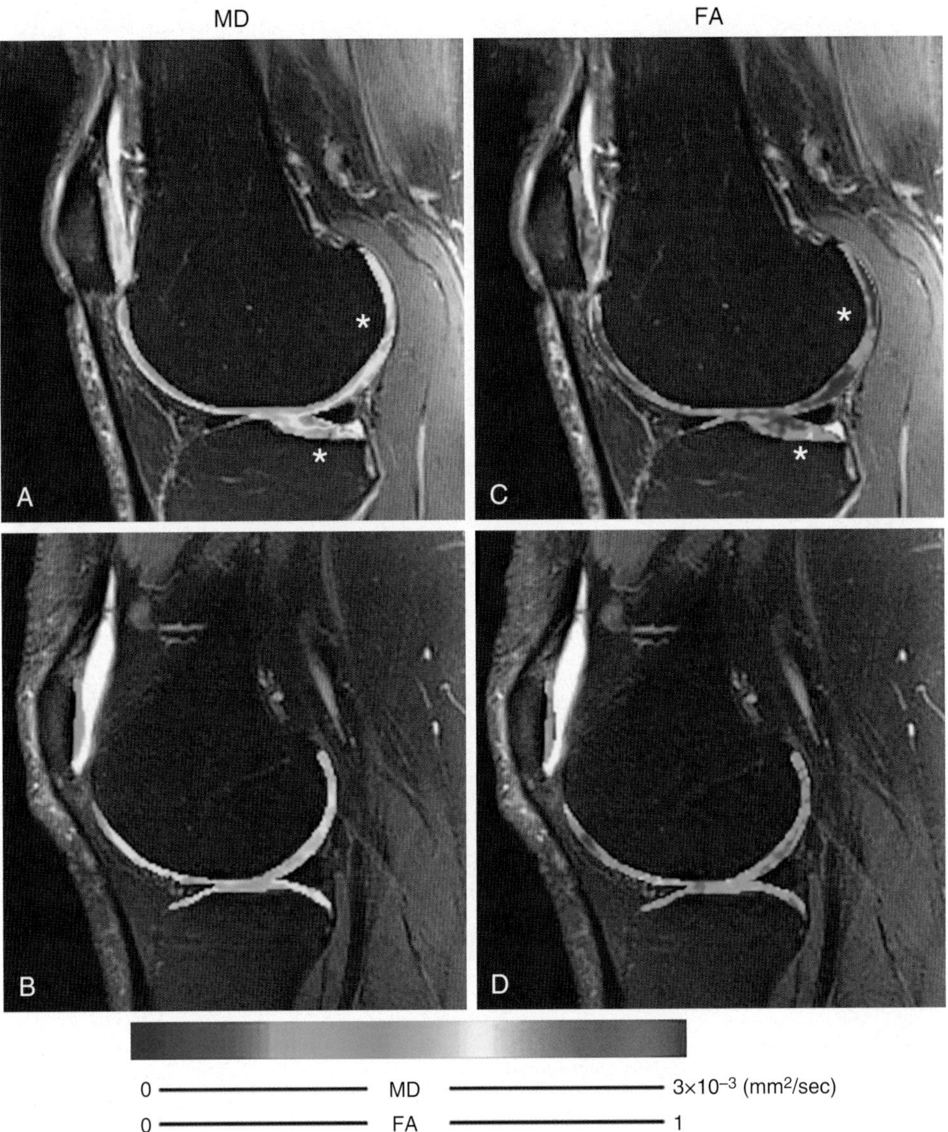

• **Fig. 61.17** Diffusion tensor imaging of hyaline cartilage. Sagittal MRI of the knee performed at 3 Tesla using a RAISED sequence (radial spin echo diffusion tensor imaging). Diffusion tensor imaging (DTI) is an MRI technique that displays intensity of signal, often using color scales, to represent specific properties of water within a tissue. It has two primary components that relate to water movement at the microscopic level. Mean diffusivity (MD) (A and C) is the mean of the apparent diffusion coefficients (ADC) and is representative of the degree (speed) of water movement (brighter = faster). Anisotropy is the property of being directionally dependent, and fractional anisotropy (FA) (B and D) records the degree to which the direction of water movement in a tissue is constrained by the microscopic architecture of the tissue (brighter = more directionally dependent and less random). Subject 1 (A and B) is a patient with Kellgren Lawrence grade 2 osteoarthritis (OA). Some of the water in the hyaline cartilage (adjacent to asterisks) is less tightly bound and so the MD of the cartilage appears more in the red end of the scale in comparison to subject B who is a healthy volunteer. Damage to the cartilage in early OA results in proteoglycan loss and the water in the cartilage is less tightly bound and so it can move faster. The structure of the collagen network may also be damaged in early OA and the FA map in subject 1 shows that some of the cartilage has less FA and appears as a darker blue (adjacent to *asterisks*) compared to the healthy volunteer (subject 2) (C and D). As the highly organized collagen network starts to break down, the motion of the water becomes more random and less directionally dependent. Using these measurements, DTI has the unique capacity to separately detect damage in hyaline cartilage to both collagen and proteoglycan. (Courtesy Dr. José Raya, New York, New York.)

(ADC)—creating an ADC map; and a second signal component dependent on the direction of water movement independent of speed—fractional anisotropy (FA)—creating an FA map. In cartilage the ADC is affected mostly by glycosaminoglycan concentration and distribution, whereas the FA is heavily dependent on the orientation and degree of organization of the collagen fibers. Consequently, DTI would seem to be capable of supplying all, or most, of the information available from all the other technologies combined.

Whole-body MRI is another technique in rapid development. It allows imaging of the entire body in one examination, and has been introduced as a potential method for simultaneous assessment of peripheral and axial joints and entheses in both RA (Fig. 61.18) and SpA/PsA (Fig. 61.19).[112,113] The method still

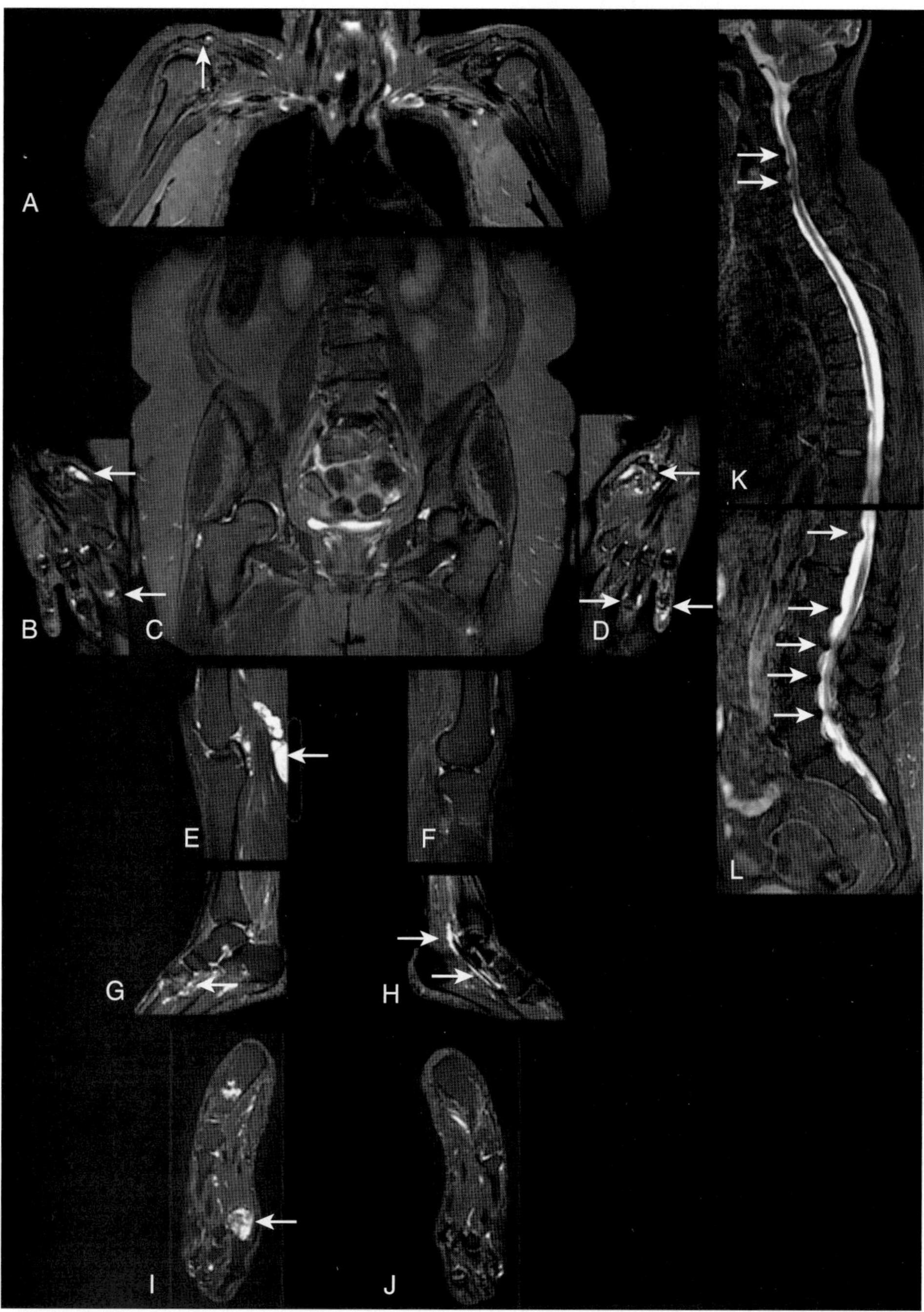

• **Fig. 61.18** Whole-body MRI (WBMRI) of patient with rheumatoid arthritis (RA) and osteoarthritis and degenerative disc disease. Short tau inversion recovery (STIR) MRI of the shoulder girdle (A), the right hand (B), the hips (C), the left hand (D), the right (E) and left (F) knee, the right (G) and left (H) ankle and midfoot, the right (I) and left (J) foot, and the upper (K) and lower (L) spine. MR images show mild inflammation of the right acromioclavicular joint (arrow in A), inflammation of the wrist, first carpometacarpal joints, several metacarpophalangeal and interphalangeal joints (*arrows* in B and D), a Baker's cyst in the right knee (*arrow* in E), inflammation in the right medial tarsometatarsal joint (*arrow* in G), tenosynovitis of the left flexor hallucis longus tendon (*arrows* in H), inflammation in the right first metatarsophalangeal joint (*arrow* in I), and several disc protrusions (*arrows* in K and L), but no spinal inflammation. The images were obtained in less than 45 minutes on a 3 Tesla MRI unit.

needs improved image quality and more validation, and it is not yet ready for routine clinical use in most centers. However, the method seems extremely promising, not the least in PsA, due to the diverse manifestations of the disease.[113–115]

MRI is very safe. It involves no ionizing radiation and thereby no associated increased risk of malignancies. Adverse reactions to gadolinium-based contrast agents (GBCAs) are infrequent. The frequency of adverse reactions requiring treatment is less than 1/1000. Postcontrast acute kidney insufficiency (previously called *contrast induced nephropathy*) is almost non-existent when approved doses are used. In 2006 it became clear that that there is a link between exposure to some less stable GBCA and the development of nephrogenic systemic fibrosis (NSF) in patients with reduced renal function or on dialysis.[116,117] NSF is a rare fibrosing condition that causes thickening and hardening of the skin and sometimes involves organs such as liver, lungs, and heart.[118,119] Since 2009 only two cases have been published, and NSF may be eliminated by the later-mentioned minimal use of the less stable GBCAs.[120]

Small amounts of gadolinium is deposited in bone, liver, and to a lesser extent, brain.[121] The clinical consequences of the deposition, if any, are still unknown. Gadolinium has also been demonstrated in small amounts in water (lakes, drinking water, waste water).[122]

In 2017, the European Medicines Agency (EMA) suspended the use of the linear (less stable) GBCA with the exceptions of gadobenate deglumine and gadoxetate disodium for liver imaging (there are no macrocyclic agents for liver imaging) and gadopentetae dimeglumine for arthrography (a very small amount of the

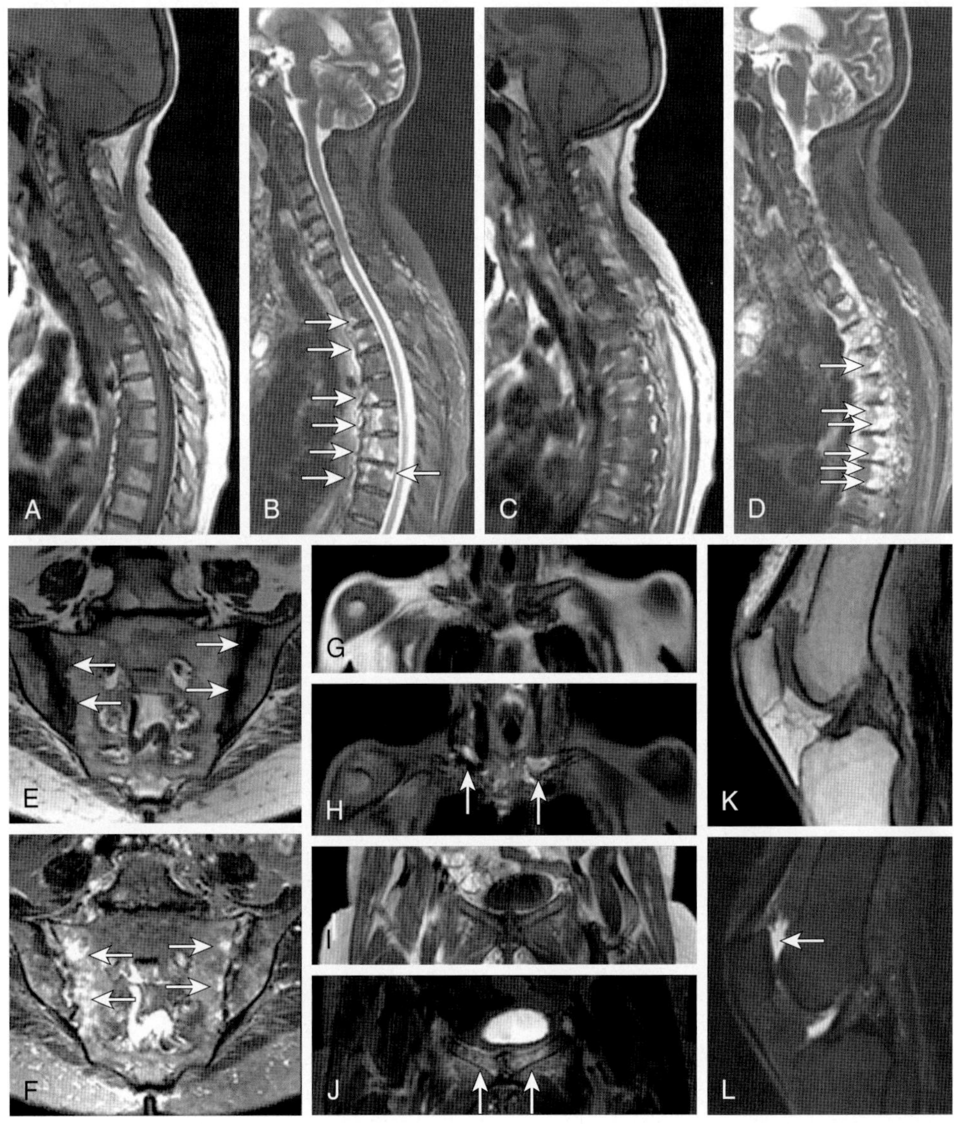

• **Fig. 61.19** Whole-body MRI (WBMRI) of patient with spondyloarthritis (SpA). T1-weighted (A, C, and every 2nd image thereafter) and short tau inversion recovery (STIR) (B, D, and every 2nd image thereafter) at before (A-L) and 4 months after (M-X) initiation of anti-tumor necrosis factor alpha (anti-TNF) therapy. Before anti-TNF initiation, MR images of the central (A and B) and lateral (C and D) cervical and thoracic spine show anterior corner inflammatory lesions (*arrows* in B) and inflammation in the pedicles and costovertebral joints (*arrows* in D). MRI of the sacroiliac joints (E and F), shoulder girdle (G and H), anterior pelvic girdle (I and J), and right knee (K and L) shows severe sacroiliac bone erosion (*arrows* in E), active sacroiliitis (*arrows* in F), sternoclavicular joint inflammation (*arrows* in H), inflammation of the pubic symphysis (*arrows* in J), and mild knee joint effusion/synovitis (*arrow* in L).

Continued

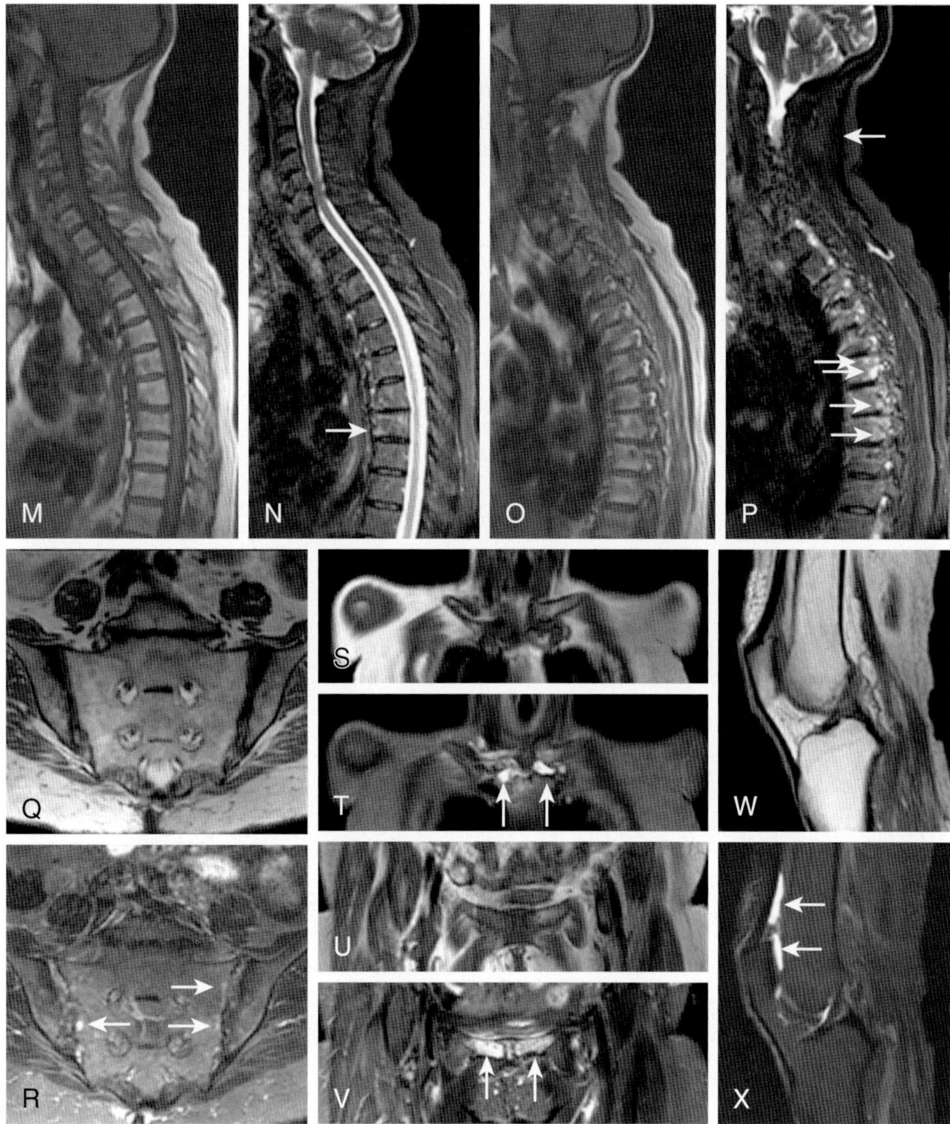

• **Fig. 61.19, cont'd** After 4 months of anti-TNF therapy, the corresponding images show almost no inflammatory activity in the spine (almost absent corner inflammatory lesions in N; less but still present costo-vertebral inflammation in P) and the sacroiliac joint (only minimal bone marrow edema in R). The inflammation in the sternoclavicular joints (*arrows* in T) and pubic symphysis (*arrows* in V) is by and large unchanged, and the amount of knee joint effusion/synovitis is somewhat increased (*arrows* in X). The images were obtained in less than 45 minutes on a 3 Tesla MRI unit.

contrast agent). EMA did not change the approved indications for the low-risk macrocyclic agents.

The European Society of Urogenital Radiology (ESUR) guidelines recommend that one never denies any patient a well-indicated enhanced MRI (ESUR, 2017 3201/id). Furthermore, one should use the lowest diagnostic dose of the generally approved macrocyclic GBCA, for example, gadoterate meglumine, gadoteridol, or gadobutrol (ESUR, 2017 3201/id). The pharmacokinetics and diagnostic performance of these agents are similar to those contraindicated. Therefore, it seems logical to use the low risk agents in every patient independent of renal function.

Rheumatoid Arthritis

The majority of MRI studies in RA have investigated knee, wrist, and finger joints. While the knee is an excellent model for methodological studies, the clinical value of MRI is mainly dependent on its power to evaluate wrists, hands, and feet, which is also the primary focus of this section. Reports on other peripheral joints are fewer and not essentially different. Definitions of key pathologies in RA and PsA are provided in Table 61.3.

MRI allows assessment of all the structures involved in RA, that is, synovial membrane, intra- and extra-articular fluid collections, cartilage, bone, ligaments, tendons, and tendon sheaths (see Fig. 61.15). MRI, histopathologic, and mini-arthroscopical signs of synovial inflammation are closely correlated.[124,125] MRI BME (see Fig. 61.15) represents inflammatory infiltrates in the bone marrow, that is, osteitis, as demonstrated by comparison with histologic samples obtained at surgery in RA patients.[126,127] Whereas erosions reflect bone damage that has already occurred, BME appears to represent the link between joint inflammation and bone destruction. A high level of agreement for detection of bone erosions in RA wrists and MCP joints (concordance at 77% to 90% of sites) between

TABLE 61.3 **MRI Definitions of Inflammatory and Structural Lesions in Rheumatoid Arthritis, Psoriatic Arthritis, and Axial Spondyloarthritis**

A. Peripheral Joints in Rheumatoid Arthritis (RA) and Psoriatic Arthritis (PsA)[c]

Inflammatory Lesions

Synovitis: An area in the synovial compartment that shows increased postgadolinium (postgadolinium [Gd]) enhancement[a] of a thickness greater than the width of the normal synovium.

[a]*Enhancement (signal intensity increase) is judged by comparison between T1-weighted (T1w) images obtained before and after intravenous (IV) Gd contrast.*

Tenosynovitis: Signal characteristics consistent with increased water content[a] or abnormal post-Gd enhancement[b] adjacent to a tendon, in an area with a tendon sheath.

[a]*High signal intensity on T2-weighted (T2w) fat-saturated (FS) and short tau inversion recovery (STIR) images, and low signal intensity on T1w images.*

[b]*Enhancement is judged by comparison between T1w images obtained before and after IV Gd contrast.*

Periarticular inflammation: Signal characteristics consistent with increased water content[a] or abnormal post-Gd enhancement[b] at extra-articular sites, including the periosteum ("periostitis") and the entheses ("enthesitis"), but not the tendon sheaths.[c]

[a]*High signal intensity on T2w FS and STIR images.*

[b]*Enhancement is judged by comparison between T1w images, obtained before and after IV Gd-contrast.*

[c]*Defined as tenosynovitis.*

Bone marrow edema: A lesion[a] within trabecular bone, with signal characteristics consistent with increased water content[b] and often with ill-defined margins.

[a]*May occur alone or surrounding an erosion or other bone abnormalities.*

[b]*High signal intensity on T2w FS and STIR images, and low signal intensity on T1w images.*

Structural Lesions

Bone erosion: A sharply marginated bone lesion, with typical signal characteristics,[a] which is visible in two planes with a cortical break seen in at least one plane.[b]

[a]*On T1w images: loss of normal low signal intensity of cortical bone and loss of normal high signal intensity of marrow fat.*

[b]*This appearance is nonspecific for focal bone loss. Other lesions such as bone cysts may mimic erosions.*

Joint space narrowing: Reduced joint space width compared with normal, as assessed in a slice perpendicular to the joint surface.

Bone proliferation: Abnormal bone formation in the periarticular region, such as at the entheses (enthesophytes) and across the joint (ankylosis).

B. Axial Disease: Ankylosing Spondylitis and Other Spondyloarthritides[d]

Inflammatory Lesions

Bone marrow edema: Increase in bone marrow signal[a] on STIR images.

Structural Lesions

Bone erosion: Full-thickness loss of dark appearance of the cortical bone and change in normal bright appearance of adjacent bone marrow on T1-weighted images.[b]

Fat infiltration: Focal increased signal in bone marrow on T1-weighted images.[b]

Bone spur: Bright signal on T1w images extending from the vertebral endplate towards the adjacent vertebra (spine).

Ankylosis: Bright signal on T1-weighted images extending across the sacroiliac joints or extending from one vertebra being continuous with the adjacent vertebra (spine).

[a]*Reference point for bone marrow signal on STIR images: Sacroiliac joints: the center of the sacrum at the same craniocaudal level; spine: the center of the vertebra, if normal. If not normal, the signal in the center of the closest available normal vertebra.*

[b]*Reference point for bone marrow signal on T1-weighted images: Sacral bone: the center of the sacrum at the same craniocaudal level; Iliac bone: normal iliac marrow at the same craniocaudal level; spine: the center of the vertebra, if normal. If not normal, the signal in the center of the closest available normal vertebra.*

[c]OMERACT (Outcome Measures in Rheumatology) MRI in inflammatory arthritis task force recommendations for MRI definitions of important pathologies in rheumatoid arthritis and peripheral psoriatic arthritis.[123,172]

[d]Canada-Denmark MRI Working Group and MORPHO group recommendations for MRI definitions of important pathologies in spine and sacroiliac joints in axial spondyloarthritis.[148,149,151]

MRI and CT, the gold standard reference for detection of bony destruction, documents that MRI erosions represent true bone damage.[65,128] MRI-assessed hand inflammation is documented to influence the function of the hand, and is independently associated with patient-reported overall physical impairment of the patient (the Health Assessment Questionnaire [HAQ]), global assessment of disease activity, and pain in early RA.[129–131]

In the cervical spine, the primary imaging modality is conventional radiography, but MRI can provide detailed information on bone and soft tissue abnormalities, which can be a valuable supplement to radiographic evaluation[132–138] (see Fig. 61.2C). MRI is able to directly visualize the pannus tissue, for example, around the odontoid process. Cord compression on MRI seems a better predictor for deterioration than initial clinical and plain radiographic features, supporting that MRI as the imaging method of choice for evaluation of spinal cord affection in RA.[139]

Use in Diagnosis, Monitoring, and Prognosis

Diagnosis. Two large follow-up studies of undifferentiated arthritis have documented an independent predictive value of MRI in the diagnosis of RA.[140,141] Presence of bone edema (see Fig. 61.16) had a positive predictive value of 86.1% for subsequent development of RA,[140] and a prediction model, including clinical hand arthritis, morning stiffness, positive RF, and MRI bone edema score in MTP and wrist joints correctly identified the development of RA or non-RA in 82% of patients.[141]

In the ACR/EULAR 2010 criteria for RA,[9] classification as definite RA is based on presence of definite clinical synovitis (swelling at clinical examination) in 1 or more joint, absence of an alternative diagnosis that better explains the synovitis, and achievement of a total score of 6 or more (of a possible 10) from the individual scores in four domains. In the joint involvement domain, which can provide up to five points of the six needed for an RA diagnosis, MRI and ultrasonographic synovitis count. In other words, MRI and ultrasonography can be used to determine the joint involvement.[9,142,143]

Monitoring Disease Activity and Structural Damage. Monitoring joint inflammation and destruction requires methods that are reproducible and sensitive to change. MRI allows quantitative (volume or, for synovitis, early contrast enhancement after intravenous contrast injection) as well as less detailed (qualitative: presence/absence; semiquantitative: scoring) evaluation of synovitis, bone edema, and bone erosions. In observational and randomized clinical trials, semiquantitative scoring by the OMERACT (Outcome Measures in Rheumatology) RA MRI scoring system (RAMRIS) has been the most frequently used system. It involves semiquantitative assessment of synovitis, bone erosions, and bone edema in RA hands and wrists, based on consensus MRI definitions of important joint pathologies and a "core set" of basic MRI sequences.[144]

The OMERACT erosion scores are closely correlated with erosion volumes estimated by MRI and CT. Good intra- and inter-reader reliability and a high sensitivity to change have been reported, demonstrating that the OMERACT RAMRIS system, after proper training and calibration of readers, is suitable for monitoring joint inflammation and destruction in RA.[145] A EULAR-OMERACT RA MRI reference image atlas has been developed, providing an easy-to-use tool for standardized RAMRIS scoring of MR images for RA activity and damage by comparison with standard reference images.[146] An MRI joint space narrowing scoring system to be used to assess cartilage damage as an adjunct to the RAMRIS system has subsequently been developed and validated.[147–149]

MRI allows more sensitive monitoring of inflammation[150] and bone erosion (see Fig. 61.15)[151–153] than clinical and radiographic assessments. A large study of 318 methotrexate-naïve patients demonstrated that inhibition of erosive progression by biologic therapy compared to placebo can be demonstrated by MRI using half the patients and half the follow-up time as by radiography,[153] and several randomized controlled trials have documented the superior ability of MRI to discriminate the ability of different therapies to inhibit progressive structural bone and cartilage damage.[154–157]

Prognosis. Several studies have demonstrated a predictive value of MRI pathology in wrist and/or MCP joints to radiographic progression. In particular, bone marrow edema (see Fig. 61.15) is now established as a strong independent predictor of subsequent radiographic progression in early RA.[158,159] Regression analyses in 3-year and 5-year follow-up in the two respective cohorts have documented that MRI-bone edema is a strong predictor of long-term radiographic progression.[160–162] Clinical trial data have confirmed this predictive value, and that early treatment-induced changes in BME and synovitis also predict the rate of future radiographic progression.[163] Small studies have indicated a relationship of baseline MRI findings with long-term functional disability[164] and tendon rupture at 6 years.[165]

Another issue of high clinical importance is whether MRI is useful in patients in clinical remission (see Fig. 61.16) to predict the disease course. MRI and ultrasonography synovitis are found frequently in patients in clinical remission,[166,167] and several studies have reported that baseline MRI and ultrasonography inflammation are significantly related to subsequent progressive structural damage.[168–170] In a recent study of routine care RA patients in sustained remission, successful tapering of biologic DMARD was independently predicted by 1 or less previous bDMARD, male sex, low baseline MRI combined inflammation score (synovitis, tenosynovitis, and BME), and/or combined damage score (erosion and joint space narrowing).[171]

Ankylosing Spondylitis/Axial Spondyloarthritis

MRI allows direct visualization of the abnormalities in peripheral and axial joints and entheses that occur in AS, PsA, and other forms of SpA. AS, which is thought to be the most common and most typical form of SpA, is dominated by axial disease manifestations in the spine and sacroiliac joints. In accordance with this, this section will mainly focus on the axial manifestations, while the PsA section later will deal with peripheral manifestations.

MRI is, through its ability to detect inflammatory changes in bone and soft tissues, the most sensitive imaging modality for recognizing early spine and sacroiliac joint changes in AS.[31,35,172] MRI findings indicating active disease in the sacroiliac joints (sacroiliitis) include juxta-articular BME and enhancement of the bone marrow and the joint space after intravenous contrast agent administration, while visible chronic changes include bone erosions, sclerosis, periarticular fatty tissue accumulation, bone spurs, and ankylosis (Fig. 61.20). Typical lesions of the spine, which indicate active disease, are spondylitis, spondylodiscitis (Fig. 61.21), and arthritis of the facet, costo-vertebral, and costo-transverse joints (Fig. 61.22).[31,172,173] Chronic changes, such as bone erosions, focal fat infiltration, bone spurs, and/or ankylosis (see Fig. 61.22)[174] frequently occur. Enthesitis is also common and may affect the interspinal and supraspinal ligaments and the inter-osseous ligaments in the retro-articular space of the sacroiliac joints. Some patients also have disease manifestations in peripheral joints and entheses, and these can be visualized by MRI.[31,172] Definitions of key pathologies in SpA are provided in Table 61.3. Table 61.2 lists the EULAR recommendations for use of imaging in the diagnosis and management of SpA.[35]

Use in Diagnosis, Monitoring, and Prognosis

Diagnosis. The introduction of MRI has resulted in a major improvement in the evaluation and management of patients with SpA. Diagnosis was previously dependent on presence of bilateral

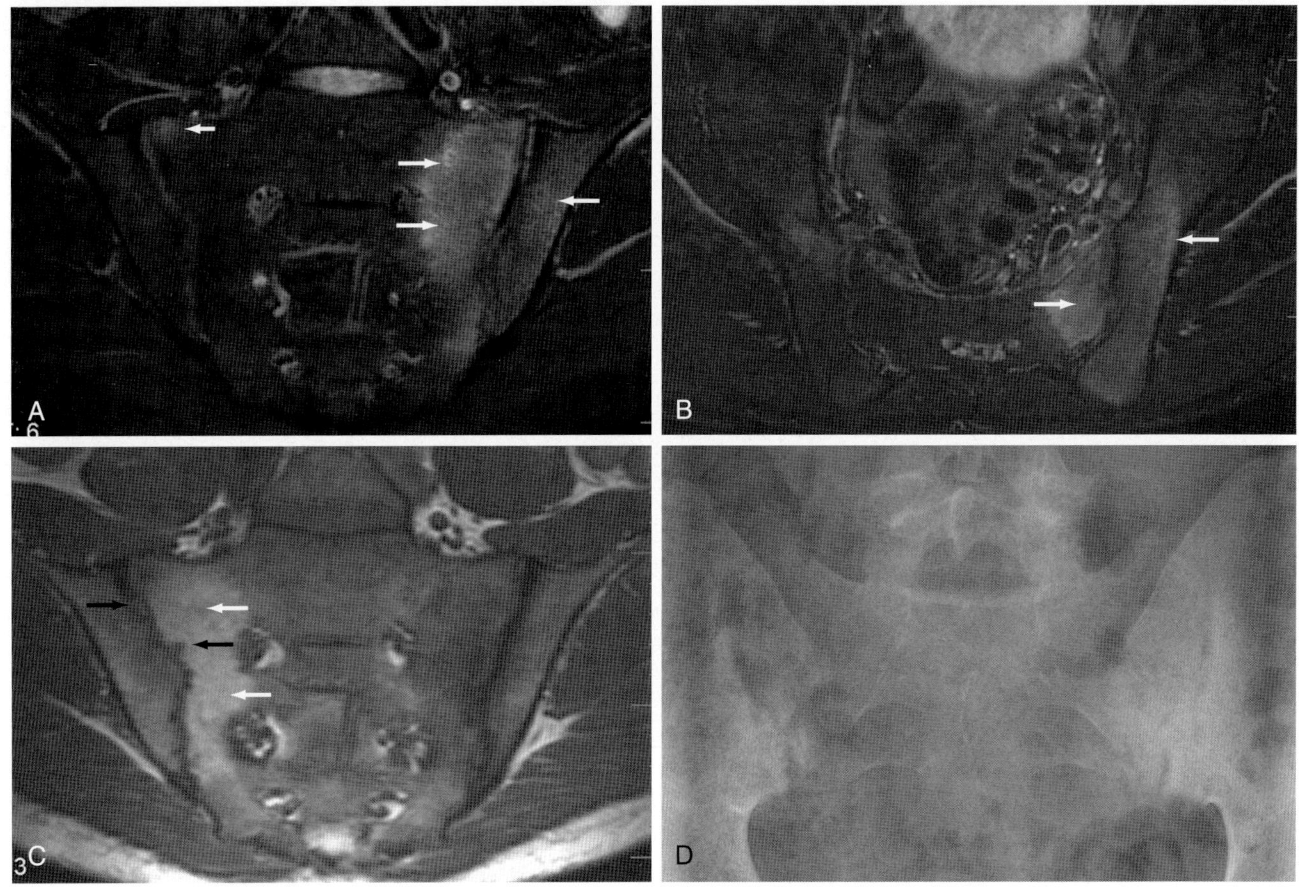

• **Fig. 61.20** Sacroiliitis in spondyloarthritis (MRI and radiography). MRI (A-C) and radiography (D) of the sacroiliac joints of a 26-year-old male with inflammatory back pain for 4 years. Semi-coronal (A) and semi-axial (B) short tau inversion recovery images show massive iliac and sacral bone edema around the left sacroiliac joint (i.e., demonstrate severe active sacroiliitis) (long arrows in A and B). Inflammation (sacroiliitis) is also present in the right sacroiliac joint (*short arrow* in A). T1-weighted semi-coronal image shows fat infiltration (*white arrows* in C) and bone erosion (*black arrows* in C). Anteroposterior radiography (D) shows bilateral mild sclerosis on the iliac side, and bilaterally the articular surface is less well defined than normal, consistent with erosion. However, this feature is exaggerated by overlying bowel gas. (Courtesy Dr. Susanne Juhl Pedersen, Glostrup, Denmark.)

moderate or unilateral severe radiographic sacroiliitis, as part of the modified New York criteria for AS.[28] This frequently delayed the diagnosis by 7 to 10 years.[32] Now, through the recent ASAS (ASsessment of SpondyloArthitis) classification criteria for axial SpA, MRI forms an integral part, as patients with active sacroiliitis on MRI (Fig. 61.23) plus one clinical feature (e.g., psoriasis, enthesitis, or uveitis; see ref. 33 for complete list), should be classified as axial SpA.[33] A consensus-based definition of the requirements to constitute active sacroiliitis, that is, fulfill the MRI criterion of the ASAS criteria ("a positive MRI") has been defined, and it is required that sacroiliac BME should be "highly suggestive of axSpA," and that BME should be present in 2 or more sites and/or in 2 or more consecutive slices.[175] Subsequent data have demonstrated that incorporating structural damage lesions (erosions) into the criteria would improve the diagnostic utility of MRI.[176–179] In contrast, sacroiliac joint fat lesions and/or spine lesions have not been documented to improve the diagnostic utility of MRI.[180,181] Recently an update from the ASAS MRI working group emphasized that subtle BME changes should not be over-interpreted, that determining their importance should never be made in isolation of the clinical context, and that presence or absence of structural changes, particularly erosions, should be taken into account in the case of subtle BME.[182] In accordance with this, recent data have found that BME that resemble milder degrees of inflammatory sacroiliitis can be observed in athletes and postpartum women.[183,184]

MRI and radiography of the sacroiliac joints were recently compared with CT as gold standard reference of structural changes in axial SpA patients. The sensitivity and specificity for structural changes were 0.85 and 0.92 for MRI while only 0.48 and 0.88 for radiography, documenting that even for structural changes MRI is superior to radiography.[185]

Monitoring Disease Activity and Damage. MRI can provide objective evidence of currently active inflammation in patients with SpA (see Fig. 61.21).[31,172] Until the introduction of MRI, disease activity assessment was restricted to patient-reported outcomes, such as the Bath Ankylosing Spondylitis disease activity index (BASDAI) and functional index (BASFI), because disease activity could not be assessed in a sensitive manner by biochemical (mainly C-reactive protein [CRP]) or physical evaluation.

Several systems for assessment of disease activity in the sacroiliac joints and in the spine have been proposed (see ref. 186 for details). Reproducible and responsive methods are available.[187] The sensitivity to change and discriminatory ability of the three

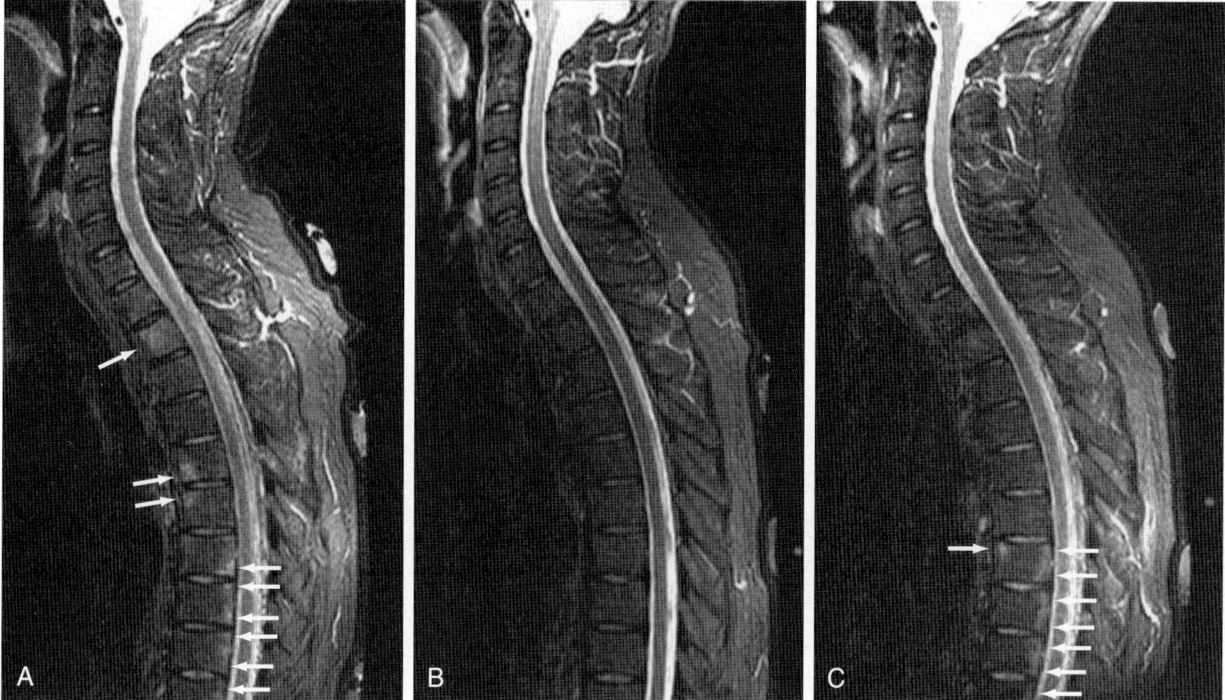

• **Fig. 61.21** Spine inflammation in ankylosing spondylitis (MRI). A 43-year-old man with HLA-B27 positive ankylosing spondylitis with deteriorating symptoms, including inflammatory back pain, had an MRI scan before starting biologic therapy. Baseline sagittal short tau inversion recovery (STIR) MRI (A) shows diffuse increased signal (edema) in the T2 vertebral body and multiple foci of corner inflammation anteriorly at T5 and 6, and posteriorly at T7, T8, T9, and T10 *(arrows)*. Other images confirmed extensive active inflammation in the spine. The patient responded very well, and after 6 months of therapy, a repeat STIR MRI (B) showed complete resolution of bone marrow inflammation. Subsequently, the patient experienced recurrence of symptoms, and a third MRI (C) was performed (2 months after anti-TNF-therapy was stopped). This MRI shows no edema at T5-T6, a conspicuous new lesion anteriorly at T7, and recurrent inflammation posteriorly in the lower thoracic spine *(arrows)*.

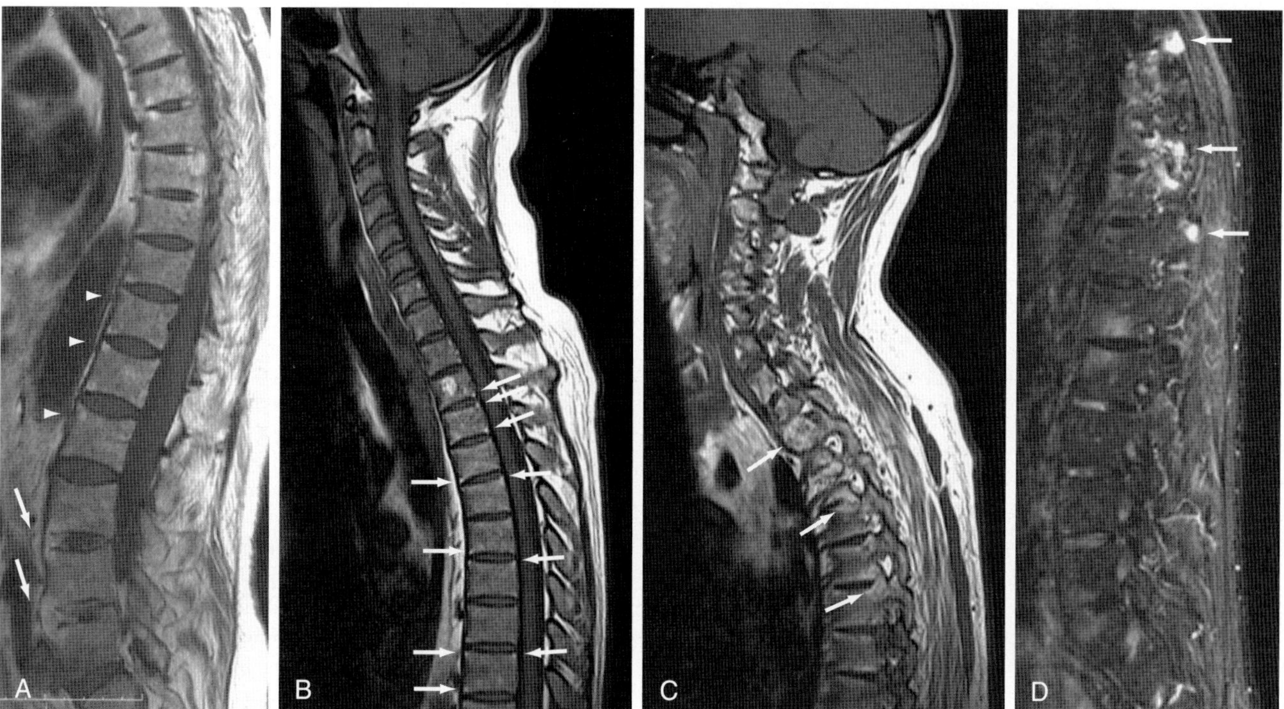

• **Fig. 61.22** The spine in ankylosing spondylitis (MRI). (A-C) T1-weighted sagittal MRI of three different patients with AS shows different structural lesions. (A) Fat infiltration *(arrowheads)* in the bone marrow of several lumbar vertebral corners and anterior fusion *(arrows)* at L3-L4 and L4-L5. (B) Fatty infiltration *(arrows)* in the bone marrow of multiple vertebral corners in the cervical spine, indicative of the diagnosis of spondyloarthritis. (C) Extensive increased marrow fat signal *(arrows)* crossing the costo-vertebral joints (thoracic ankylosis) is seen, as are changes in several facet joints and other posterior elements. (D) Sagittal short tau inversion recovery MRI shows intense inflammation in the bone marrow of the transverse processes and facet joints of the lower thoracic spine *(arrows)*, as well as less intense inflammation in several discovertebral joints.

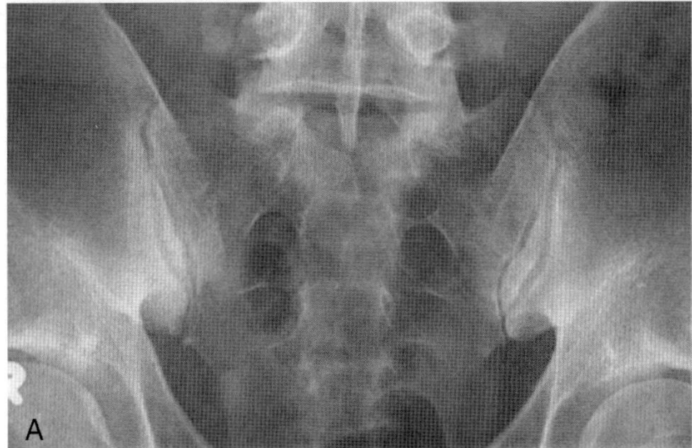

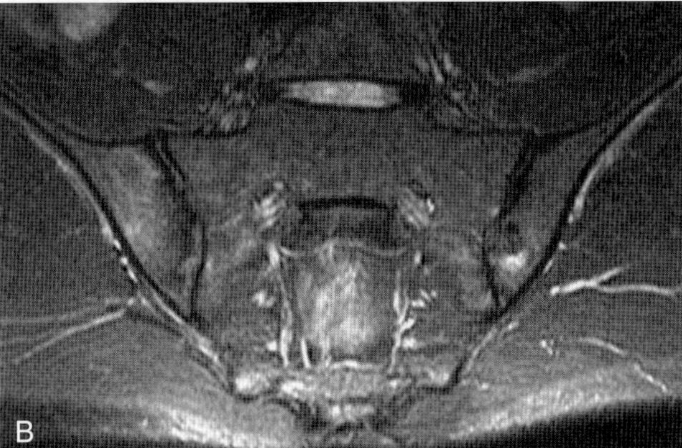

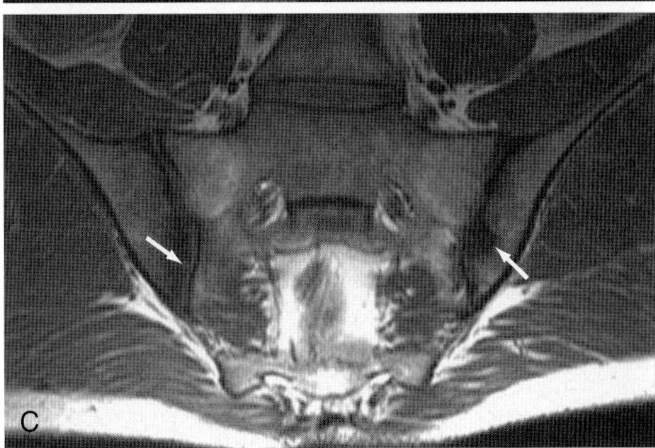

• **Fig. 61.23** Inflammatory back pain (radiography and MRI). A 31-year-old man with inflammatory back pain. (A) Radiography of the sacroiliac joints demonstrates only very subtle findings with possible sclerosis on the iliac side of the right sacroiliac joint and subtle spur formation at the inferior margin. (B and C) MRI at the same time shows obvious findings of spondyloarthritis with mild bilateral iliac inflammation on short tau inversion recovery (B) and multiple findings on T1-weighted images (C), including sclerosis most prominent on the right side and subchondral erosion *(arrows)*, which are very small on the right side and obvious on the left side.

most used spine scoring systems (the Ankylosing Spondylitis spine MRI-activity [ASspiMRI-a] score, the Berlin modification of the ASspiMRI-a score, and the Spondyloarthritis Research Consortium of Canada [SPARCC] scoring system)[188–190] have been demonstrated in clinical trials, and they have been tested against each other by the ASAS/OMERACT MRI in AS group.[187] All methods were feasible, reliable, sensitive to change, and discriminative. The SPARCC method had the highest sensitivity to change, as judged by Guyatt's effect size, and the highest reliability as judged by the inter-reader intra-class correlation coefficient (ICC).[187] Separate MRI assessment of different inflammatory and structural findings at distinct anatomical locations in each discovertebral allows studying the temporal and spatial course of the disease development,[173,174] and also separate analyses of various scores of articular, entheseal, and discovertebral components of the disease. This approach, the Canada-Denmark assessment system, may become increasingly important as drugs with different modes of action, and thereby potentially different effect on different aspects of the disease, are becoming available.[191,192] However, MRI for assessment of structural changes[174,188,193] is much less established than for assessment of inflammatory changes. Further validation of the methods for damage assessment is needed to clarify their clinical value.

Prognosis. Three spine studies have documented an association between the presence of BME at the anterior corners of the vertebrae on MRI and subsequent development of syndesmophytes on radiography after 2 years of follow-up. Presence as opposed to absence of MRI anterior corner inflammation provides relative risks of three to five for a new anterior radiographic syndesmophyte at that level.[194–196] The association was even more pronounced in those vertebral corners in which the inflammation had resolved following institution of anti-TNF therapy, possibly explained by TNF in an active inflammatory lesion restricting new bone formation, whereas reduction of TNF by applying a TNF-inhibitor allows tissue repair to manifest as new bone formation.[195,196] Fat infiltration in the vertebral corners seems to be a key intermediary in the process, as its development is linked to resolution of previous inflammation and to future development of syndesmophytes.[197,198]

One study suggests that in early inflammatory back pain, severe sacroiliac MRI BME together with HLA-B27 positivity is a strong predictor of future AS, whereas mild or no sacroiliitis, irrespective of HLA-B27 status, was a predictor of not developing AS.[199] Data on the value of MRI for predicting therapeutic response in SpA are very limited. A high spine MRI inflammation score and short disease duration are statistically significant predictors of clinical response (BASDAI improvement >50%) to anti-TNF therapy.[200,201] Further and larger studies are needed to clarify the role of MRI in the prediction of disease course and therapeutic response in clinical practice.

Psoriatic Arthritis

The clinical appearance of PsA is very diverse, involving the spine, sacroiliac joints, peripheral joints, and/or entheses, and accordingly MRI findings vary. PsA shares clinical manifestations with RA and SpA, and this also applies to its MRI features.[202] Peripheral PsA synovitis and erosions do not have disease-specific MRI features, and MRI bone edema can involve any bone. A general agreement on which joints to image to assess PsA activity and damage is not established, and possibly needs to be individualized, based on the disease pattern. Peripheral enthesitis is common in PsA and can be visualized and assessed by MRI.[203] Whole-body MRI, allowing imaging of both peripheral and axial joints and entheses of the entire body in one examination, may be a future solution to this, but still requires more validation.[113–115,204]

MRI can visualize both peripheral and axial musculoskeletal anatomy and PsA disease manifestations. Findings include synovitis, tenosynovitis, periarticular inflammation, enthesitis, bone edema, bone erosion, and bone proliferation (Fig. 61.24).[205–208] As in other types of SpA, enthesitis, dactylitis, and spondylitis can

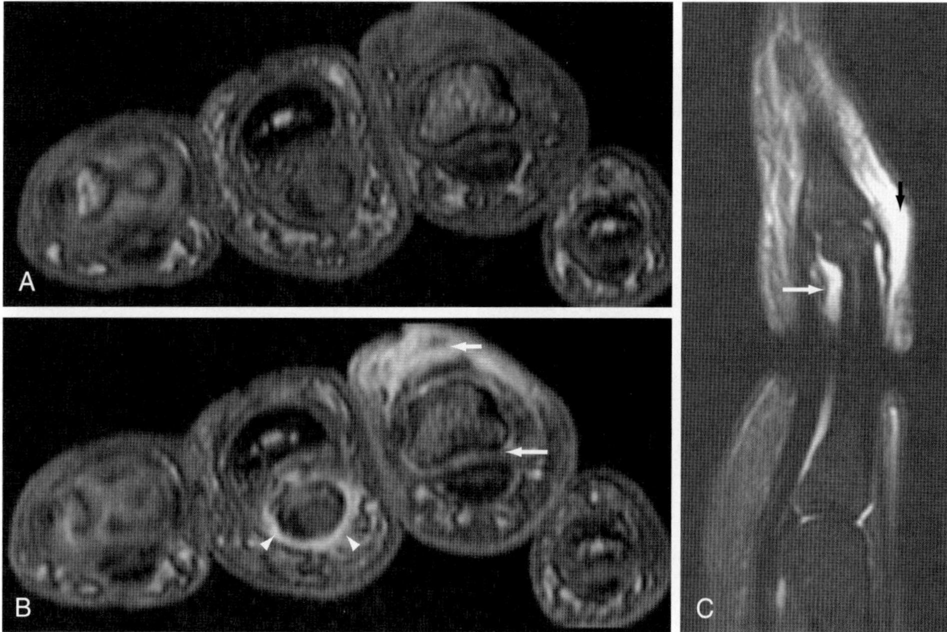

• **Fig. 61.24** Psoriatic arthritis (MRI). Axial T1-weighted precontrast (A) and postcontrast (B) MRI of the second (left) through fifth (right) fingers at the level of the fourth proximal interphalangeal joint and sagittal short tau inversion recovery MRI (C) of the fourth finger show mild synovitis (*long arrows* in B and C) and considerable periarticular inflammation (*short arrows* in B and C) around the fourth distal interphalangeal joint and tenosynovitis (*arrowheads* in B). (Courtesy Rene Poggenborg, Glostrup, Denmark.)

be seen. Dactylitis has shown on MRI to be a result of tenosynovitis with effusion, sometimes associated with diffuse soft tissue edema and/or synovitis in nearby finger or toe joints (Fig. 61.25).[209,210] There are few MRI studies in axial PsA, but findings are similar to AS findings, although more frequently asymmetric.[184,191,211–213]

The entheses have attracted attention as a possible primary location of disease.[214] Nail disease is common in PsA, and DIP joint inflammation on MRI has been described to extend to the nail bed.[215]

PsA can be clinically silent. In patients with psoriasis without arthritic signs or symptoms, pathologic findings on MRI (including periarticular edema, tendon sheath effusion, intra-articular effusion, synovial pannus, bone erosion, bone cysts, subchondral changes, and joint subluxation) have been reported in more than 2/3 (68% to 92%) versus none to 1/12 or less of healthy controls.[216–218] The clinical importance of these findings is not yet clarified.

Use in Diagnosis, Monitoring, and Prognosis

Diagnosis. As described previously, MRI can detect the different pathologies involved in PsA, and some MRI findings can be used to assist in differential diagnosis. BME in PsA is often close to entheses, in contrast to synovial attachments in RA and primarily subchondral areas in OA.[207] PsA is characterized by more prevalent diaphyseal bone marrow and/or enthesitis, soft-tissue inflammation, extracapsular inflammation, and involvement of primarily flexor tendons, in contrast to extensor tendons in RA.[219] Erosions in PsA often are located close to the collateral ligaments, while in OA they are mostly found centrally.[220] A comparative study found erosions to be more frequent in RA, and periostitis more frequent in PsA.[221] Studies on psoriasis patients who do not have clinical arthritis have indicated subclinical inflammation on MRI in both joints and entheses.[216,222] One of these studies found that patients with subclinical inflammation on MRI, in conjunction with arthralgia, had a high (55%) risk for later development of PsA, whereas patients without these had a low risk (15%).[222] Further studies to clarify the diagnostic role of MRI are needed.

Monitoring. Data on monitoring activity and damage are limited. Most studies only report qualitative MRI assessments of the different pathologies of PsA.[202] Quantitative assessment of contrast enhancement has been reported,[223,224] but is insufficiently validated for clinical use. Scoring systems of inflammation and damage have been developed,[205,225,226] with the OMERACT Psoriatic Arthritis Magnetic Resonance Image Scoring System (PsAMRIS) being the best validated, and with a documented good intra- and inter-reader reliability and, for inflammatory parameters (synovitis, tenosynovitis, periarticular inflammation), sensitivity to change.[205,227,228] Furthermore, enthesitis can be visualized, and preliminary validation of an assessment system has recently been done.[203,229] Whole-body MRI may in the future be the method of choice for monitoring peripheral and axial inflammation of joints and entheses.[115,230–232] The EULAR recommendations for the use of imaging in the diagnosis and management of SpA in clinical practice[35] support the use of MRI and/or ultrasonography for monitoring both disease activity and structural changes in peripheral SpA, as they may add additional information to clinical and biochemical examinations and radiography, respectively. There is, however, no evidence for or consensus on if and how often examinations should be repeated in routine clinical practice.[35]

Prognosis. BME on MRI has been found to be related to subsequent development of later erosions detected by CT,[73] but further longitudinal studies of the prognostic value of MRI findings in PsA are needed.

Gout

MRI can directly visualize the inflammatory (synovitis, tenosynovitis, bone edema, and soft tissue inflammation) and destructive (bone erosion) aspects of gout arthropathy.[44,233–235]

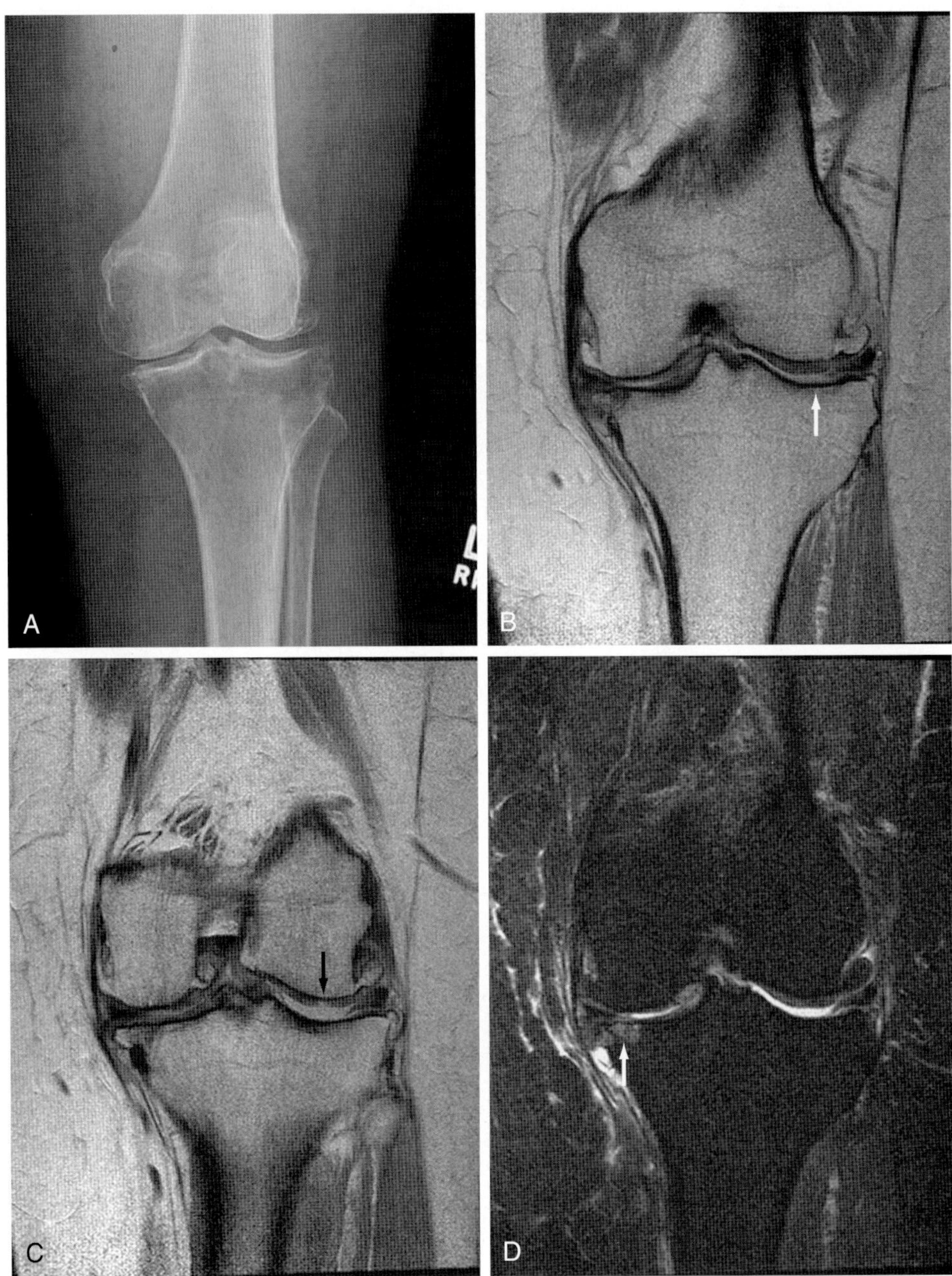

• **Fig. 61.25** Osteoarthritis of the knee (radiography and MRI). (A) Anteroposterior radiographic view of the left knee shows large osteophyte of the medial and lateral tibiofemoral joint and mild medial joint space narrowing. (B and C) Coronal proton density-weighted MRI confirms the presence of large osteophytes in the tibiofemoral joint, shows diffuse cartilage loss of the medial tibia and femur, and discloses a denuded bone with complete loss of cartilage in the lateral tibial plateau (*arrow* in B). A small focal cartilage defect of the lateral femoral condyle (*arrow* in C) is also evident. Both lateral and medial menisci are partially macerated, and a subluxation of the medial meniscus is seen, along with severe cartilage loss on the medial and lateral tibial plateau and the medial femoral condyle. (D) Coronal T2-weighted fat-suppressed MRI shows medial tibial plateau subchondral bone marrow edema (*arrow* in D). (Courtesy Professor Ali Guermazi, Boston, Mass.)

MRI can also visualize tophi and provide information on the inflammatory nature of these lesions, which cannot be appreciated from radiography or CT. On MRI, tophi typically exhibit low signal on T1w images, with varying postcontrast enhancement, and medium-high signal on T2w images, indicating the presence of cellular tissue surrounding or infiltrating the crystalline mass (see Fig. 61.6).[233,235] Calcification within the tophus can lead to regions of low signal on T2w images. Tophi are not always clinically detectable if the location is deep to the skin surface.

Use in Diagnosis, Monitoring, and Prognosis

Little evidence exists for the validity of MRI for diagnosing gout.[236] It is unclear at present how MRI performs compared to ultrasonography and other imaging modalities in the diagnosis of gout. In addition to the currently uncertain diagnostic accuracy of MRI, and the diagnostic accuracy of MRI-documented synovitis, bone erosion, and/or tophi against the gout classification, criteria have not yet been determined. Feasibility factors may limit the use of MRI as a diagnostic tool, particularly the prolonged scanning time and the cost. MRI is not included in the 2015 Gout classification criteria.[237] However, MRI can detect tophi, and the presence of these strongly suggests a diagnosis of gout, but joint aspirate confirmation of monosodium urate crystals is required as the differential diagnosis includes infection or other space-occupying lesions.

Monitoring gout by MRI could include assessment of joint inflammation, erosion progression, and extent/size of tophi (see Fig. 61.6). Tophus volume assessment by MRI has been reported to have a good intra- and inter-reader reproducibility and may be useful for this purpose in trials.[238] In contrast to RA, AS, and PsA, no MRI scoring system for overall assessment of gouty arthritis has yet been developed. The RA MRI scoring (RAMRIS) system was developed to monitor RA patients, but has been used to quantify bone erosions in gout, with good cross-sectional intra- and inter-reader agreement,[239] but no longitudinal data exist.[236]

The Gout MRI Cartilage Score (GOMRICS) has been developed to quantify cartilage damage in advanced gout. The GOMRICS was highly correlated with the Sharp van der Heijde total score (r = 0.80) and joint space narrowing score (r = 0.71), with moderate-good inter-reader reliability.[240] No longitudinal studies monitoring cartilage damage have been reported.[236]

Calcium Pyrophosphate Dihydrate Crystal Deposition Disease

MRI detects calcification of hyaline cartilage as an area of low signal intensity, especially on gradient echo images; meniscal chondrocalcinosis exhibits increased signal on T1-weighted and proton density images and may simulate meniscal degeneration or tear (see Fig. 61.7).[241] As in other diseases MRI is a sensitive method for subchondral cysts and inflammatory changes such as synovitis and effusion.

Septic Arthritis

The MRI appearance of septic arthritis is nonspecific, and similar findings can be observed in other inflammatory arthritides. Thus, in case of clinical suspicion of septic arthritis, a joint aspiration must be performed without delay to avoid irreversible articular damage. Characteristic findings are synovitis, joint effusion, and soft-tissue edema (see Fig. 61.8) followed by bone erosion and cartilage destruction. MRI may be helpful in diagnosing complications of septic arthritis, such as abscesses and osteomyelitis. It should be remembered that most of the individual findings on MRI are not specific and BME alone does not necessarily denote osteomyelitis.[242] Contrast enhanced MRI is particularly useful to identify abscess/necrosis in either soft tissue or bone that may confirm the diagnosis and/or requirement for surgical debridement. Investigation of the painful diabetic foot is a specific clinical presentation for which MRI may now be routinely performed to help distinguish between infection and trauma and to identify nonviable tissues, although scintigraphic studies also play an important role in these complex patients.[48]

Osteoarthritis

Based on the tomographic nature and ability to visualize cartilage, bone, and various soft tissues, MRI is well suited for assessment of inflammatory changes, structural and compositional changes in the cartilage, and other structural lesions in OA. The majority of studies have been undertaken in knee joints (see Fig. 61.25),[243] or more recently hip joints,[244,245] and also in small joints in the hand (see Fig. 61.10) in generalized OA.

MRI allows direct assessment of the thickness, surface contour, and internal architecture of articular cartilage in OA[246–248] (see Fig. 61.25), making staging and monitoring of OA development possible. Osteophytes at the joint margins or beneath the articular cartilage may be seen. Subchondral changes include bone edema, sclerosis, and bone cysts. MRI "bone marrow lesions" (sometimes referred to as *bone edema lesions*), which are areas with inhomogeneous, intermediate-low signal on T1w and high signal on water sensitive techniques (STIR/T2FS) (Fig. 61.26), have, by comparison with histologic samples obtained by surgery in advanced OA, shown trabecular microfracture and bone marrow fibrosis and/or necrosis, but limited interstitial edema.[249–252] Synovitis is seen frequently by MRI in OA, albeit to a lesser degree than in RA.[253] Synovitis scores obtained by contrast-enhanced MRI have demonstrated a good correlation with arthroscopic and microscopic synovitis scores.[254]

Use in Diagnosis, Monitoring, and Prognosis of Osteoarthritis

Diagnosis. The classification criteria for OA is based on clinical and conventional radiographic findings.[51] However, the use of MRI in the diagnosis of OA offers the advantage of sensitively depicting all the involved pathologic changes.

Monitoring. Various quantitative and semiquantitative techniques have been used to measure structural abnormalities and change on MRI in OA.[246] Quantitative measurements apply computer-aided image processing to quantitate various aspects, for example, volumes of cartilage, bone, bone marrow lesions, menisci, or synovium. These have been reported to have excellent reproducibility.[255] Measures of cartilage composition are also available, for example, quantification of glycosaminoglycan content.[247,248] Semiquantitative methods have been used to provide semiquantitative "multiple feature" ("whole-organ") assessments in the knee, based on conventional MRI acquisitions.[243,256–259] These measures have high reliability and better sensitivity to change than radiographic methods.[255] Other scoring systems focused on bone marrow lesion and effusion/synovitis as markers of active disease are being evaluated at the hip and knee.[244] A system for systematic assessment of hand OA has also been developed and validated.[260]

Prognosis. In a systematic literature review,[261] quantitative cartilage volume change and presence of cartilage defects or bone marrow lesions (bone edema) in three of three studies were significantly related to subsequent total knee replacement, that is, a predictive value was demonstrated.[262–264]

Furthermore, enlargements in bone marrow lesions have been demonstrated to be related to increased pain (and improvements in bone marrow lesions to decreased pain) in follow-up studies.[265,266] In contrast, inconsistent and generally weak relations between cartilage loss and symptom change, and a weak relation between change in synovitis and change in pain have been reported. Finally, the presence of meniscal damage, cartilage defects, and/or BMLs predicts subsequent MRI progression[261] or even progression to arthroplasty.[267]

Juvenile Idiopathic Arthritis

MRI is increasingly used to evaluate involvement of joints that are difficult to examine clinically or by ultrasonography in JIA, including sacroiliac joints,[268] hips[269] (Fig. 61.27), and TMJ.[270] MRI findings of inflammatory changes include BME, joint effusion, synovitis, and capsulitis, while findings of structural damage include deformity, erosions, periarticular fatty infiltration, cartilage loss, and fusion/ankylosis[268,271,272] (Fig. 61.28). Challenges in pediatric MRI in JIA include the need for anesthesia in younger children, volume averaging and image resolution in small joints, normal variants such as rim-like increased periarticular T2 signal at growing physes that

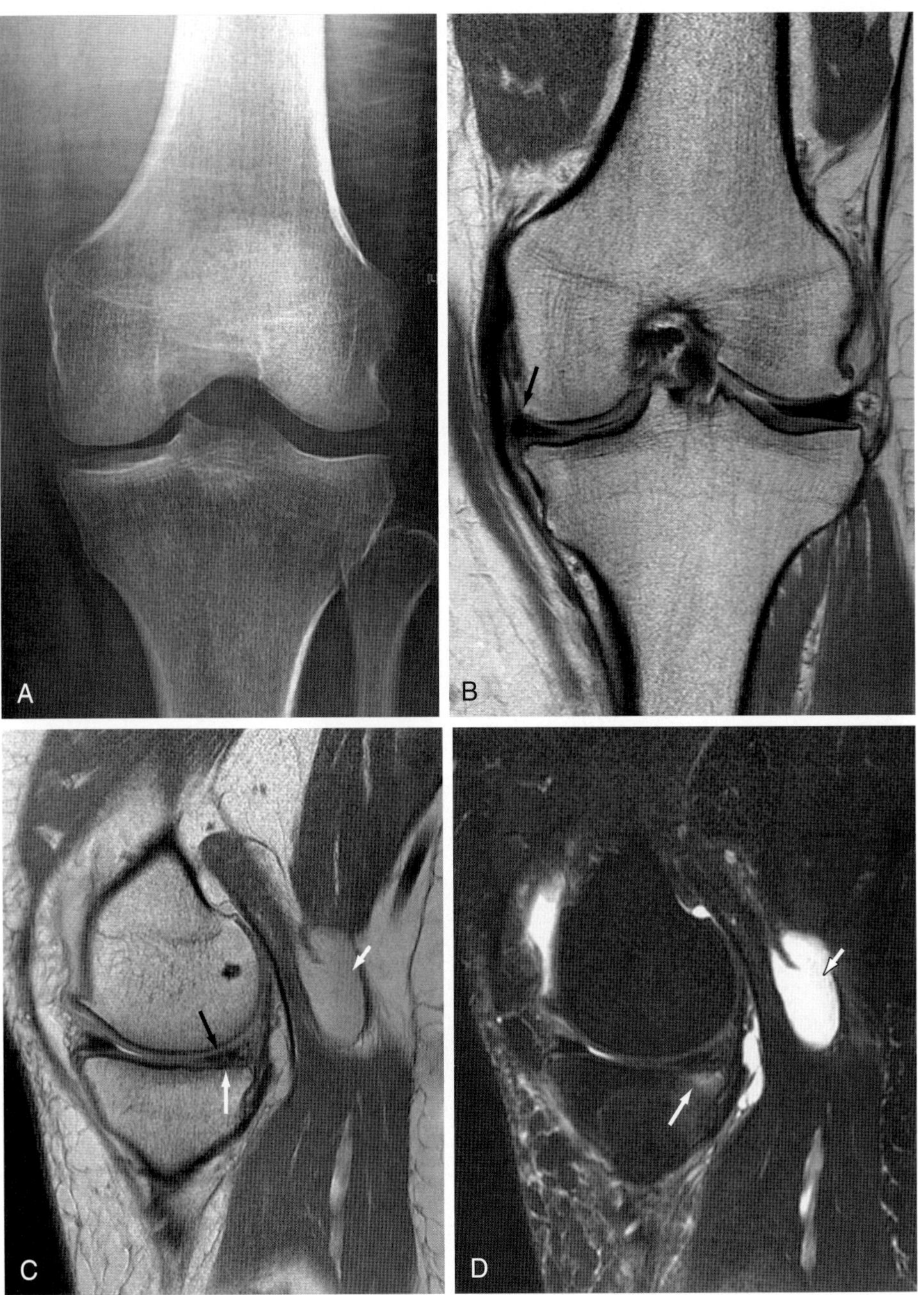

• **Fig. 61.26** Early osteoarthritis (OA) of the knee (radiography and MRI). Radiography (A) and MRI (B-D) of the knee with early OA. (A) Anteroposterior radiographic view shows an almost normal knee. The only possible abnormality is a tiny osteophyte at the medial tibial plateau. (B) Coronal proton density-weighted MRI shows a minimal medial meniscus subluxation *(arrow)*. (C) Sagittal proton density-weighted MRI shows partial maceration of the posterior horn of the medial meniscus *(black arrow)*, thinning of the cartilage at the posterior medial tibial plateau *(long white arrow)*, and a moderate sized Baker's cyst *(short white arrow)*. (D) Sagittal fat-suppressed T2-weighted MRI confirms the Baker's cyst *(short arrow)* and also shows subchondral bone marrow edema *(long arrow)* subjacent to the loss of cartilage at the posterior subregion of the medial tibial plateau. (Courtesy Professor Ali Guermazi, Boston, Mass.)

can mimic BME, and a lack of controlled studies of the diagnostic and prognostic significance of MRI features of JIA.

Use in Diagnosis, Monitoring, and Prognosis

As with adult spondyloarthropathy, sacroiliitis as a feature of axial JIA is increasingly evaluated by MRI. The MRI features with highest diagnostic utility for sacroiliitis are erosions and expert radiologist global impression,[268] or synovial enhancement if gadolinium is given.[271] MRI is much more reliable for diagnosis of sacroiliitis than radiography.[268,273] Attempts to apply and modify adult diagnostic criteria for sacroiliitis to pediatric MRI are currently being vigorously pursued.[274] Semiquantitative scoring systems are also in development for TMJ[272] and other joints such as the knee,[275] wrists, and whole-body MRI. Several of these scoring systems are currently undergoing reliability testing, and in the near future are likely to be available as a set of objective, reliable imaging biomarkers for evaluation of natural history and response to therapy in JIA. MRI findings may eventually form part of the diagnostic criteria for some aspects or subtypes of JIA.

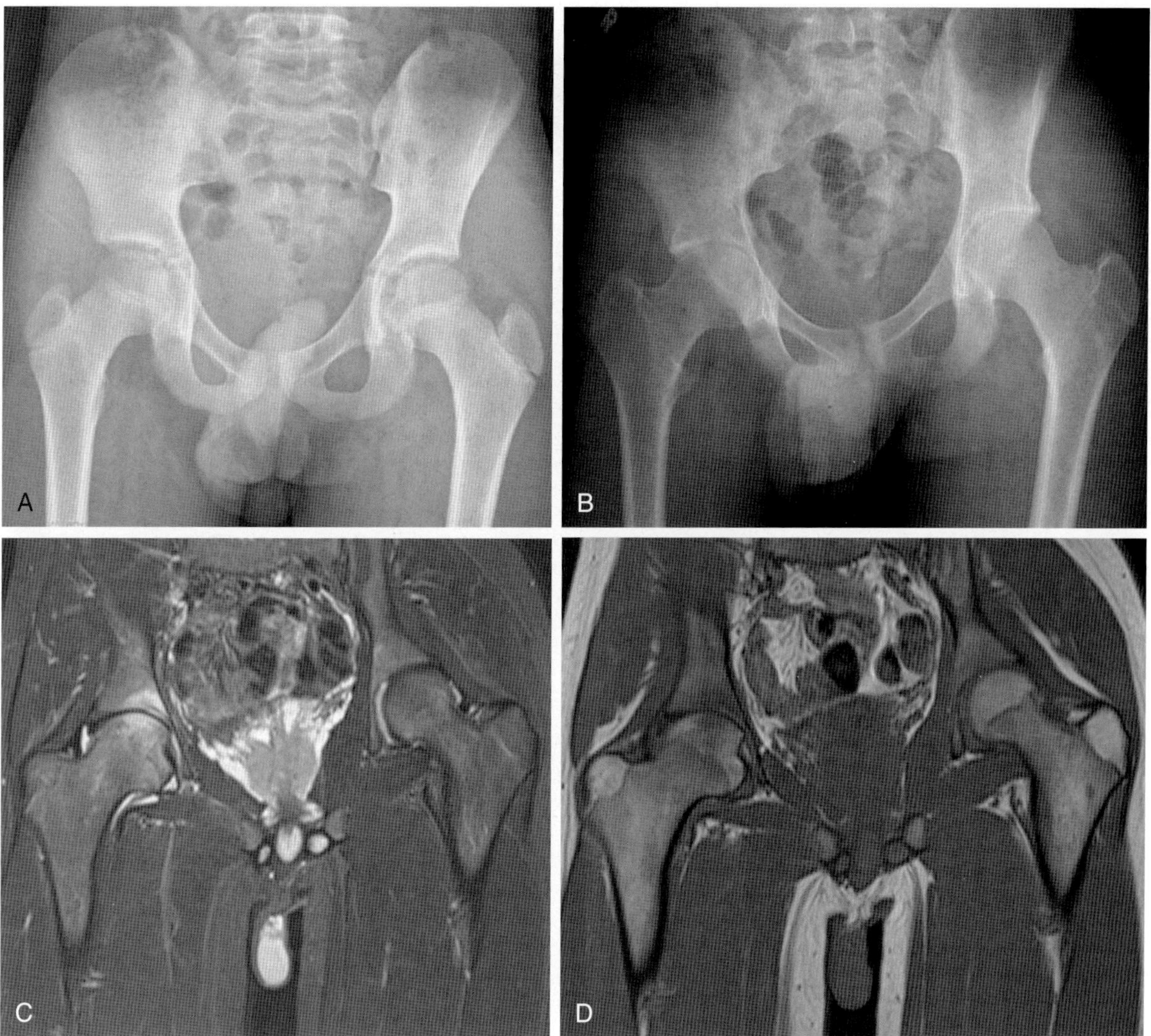

• **Fig. 61.27** Radiography and MRI of the hip in a child with juvenile idiopathic arthritis (JIA). Hip imaging in a teenaged boy whose family refused treatment for his polyarticular JIA for 8 years. (A) Frontal hip radiography at age 11 showing preserved joint spaces. (B) Frontal hip radiography at age 15, showing marked nearly symmetrical axial hip joint space loss, with coxa profunda developing on the right and periarticular osteopenia. (C) Coronal short tau inversion recovery and (D) coronal T1-weighted MRI at age 15, showing prominent marrow edema and a small effusion at the right hip with full thickness cartilage loss, as well as linear subchondral low signal on T1-weighted sequence concerning for a subchondral fracture. With modern biologic therapy, development of severe structural damage like this is becoming less common.

Other Imaging Modalities

Digital X-Ray Radiogrammetry (DXR)

KEY POINTS

Automated radiogrammetry from conventional hand X-rays provides an approximated bone mineral density (BMD).

Bone loss as measured by DXR-BMD may be useful for monitoring and predicting bone damage in RA.

Three types of bone loss are early features of rheumatoid arthritis: focal articular bone erosion, periarticular osteopenia, and systemic osteoporosis. Periarticular bone loss is frequently the earliest radiographic feature of RA, is associated with disease activity, and is known to precede bone erosions.[276] Radiographic osteopenia is, however, only detected if there is bone loss greater than 30%.[277]

Digital x-ray radiogrammetry (DXR) is a fully automated technique for performing radiogrammetry from standard hand radiographs to bridge the gap between radiogrammetry and bone densitometry. The DXR technology is based on a combined computerized radiogrammetric and textural analysis of the narrowest parts of the second, third, and fourth metacarpal bones. Based on cortical thickness (cm), porosity index, and an assumption of a constant bone density and elliptical bone, DXR calculates an approximated bone mineral density (BMD; g/cm^2).[278] Short-term precision of DXR-BMD (coefficient of variation [CV]) and long-term precision have been reported

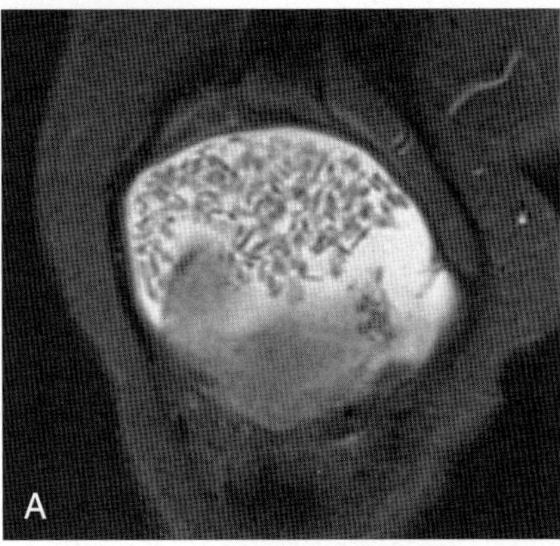
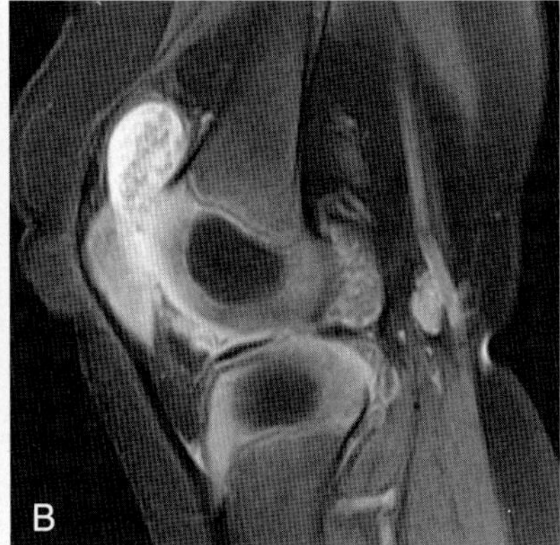
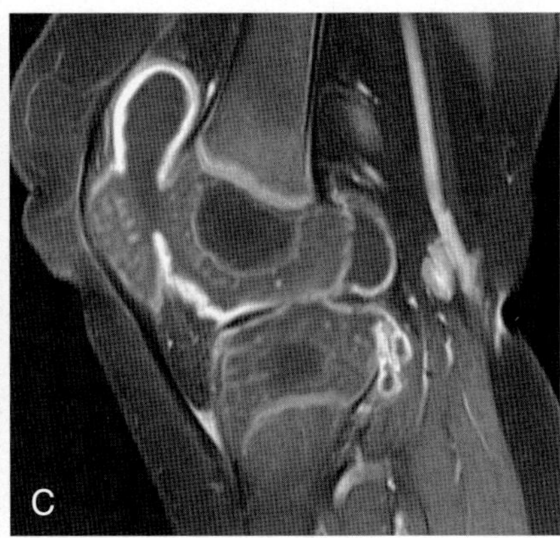

• **Fig. 61.28** MRI of the knee in a child with juvenile idiopathic arthritis (JIA). MRI of the right knee in an 18-month-old child with knee swelling and clinical risk factors for juvenile idiopathic arthritis (JIA). (A) Coronal STIR and (B) sagittal proton density-weighted fat saturated MR images through the knee show florid synovial thickening with innumerable rice bodies in a large effusion, but no bone marrow edema or periarticular edema. (C) Postgadolinium sagittal T1-weighted fat saturated image demonstrates thickened, avidly enhancing knee synovium and no abnormal bony enhancement. This pattern of florid synovitis with little involvement of bone or periarticular soft tissues is typical for JIA at peripheral joints. The case also highlights that JIA can occur in even very young children.

as 0.28% and 0.25%, respectively and the reproducibility as 0.05% to 0.27%.[279,280]

DXR is highly correlated with periarticular BMD measurements, and can therefore reflect periarticular bone loss even though it measures mid-shaft cortical bone.[281] DXR-BMD shows greater loss in RA patients with high levels of inflammation, positive rheumatoid factor, or positive anti-CCP. Further, measurements of DXR-BMD changes are significantly associated with progression of structural damage in early RA subjects.[282] Losses seen over 1 year with DXR-BMD are predictive of subsequent erosive development.[279] However, so far only changes in DXR-BMD are of predictive value, limiting its clinical applicability. DXR-BMD changes are also responsive to treatment interventions. During disease modifying treatment, DXR-BMD losses are less severe in patients responding to treatment than in those who do not.[279,281,282] This suggests that DXR-BMD may become a useful outcome measure and predictor of joint damage in RA clinical trials. However, its clinical usefulness and applicability have yet to be established.

Nuclear Medicine

KEY POINTS

- Provides not only morphologic but also physiologic information regarding the metabolic state of tissues.
- Nuclear medicine techniques can be fused with other imaging modalities (e.g., SPECT/CT) providing combined functional and anatomic information.
- PET can be useful for diagnosis and management of vasculitides, fever of unknown origin, and malignancies.
- Other imaging modalities are generally better suited than nuclear medicine for investigating inflammatory and degenerative rheumatic diseases in clinical practice.

Bone Scintigraphy (Planar)

Bone scintigraphy imaging can be planar (i.e., whole body and spot views) or tomographic (SPECT or SPECT/CT). This is analogous to the relationship between planar radiography (conventional radiographs) and CT.

As with all other modalities in diagnostic nuclear medicine, bone scintigraphy uses a physiologic approach to imaging bone or joint pathology. An organic analogue of phosphate (methylene diphosphonate [MDP] or hydroxymethylene diphosphonate [HDP]) is tagged with a standard radionuclide (99mTc). The combined tracer, 99mTc-MDP or 99mTc-HDP, is then administered intravenously. This organic phosphate analogue is distributed with a whole-body distribution proportional to regional perfusion. It is adsorbed onto the surface of osteoid, at the sites of active mineralization (calcium phosphate formation). At various times after tracer administration, nuclear medicine gamma cameras detect photons emitted by the decaying radionuclide, to form diagnostic images. The nature of the information depends on the time of image acquisition. In the first few minutes after administration, the images demonstrate arterial blood flow and relative blood pool distribution. By 3 hours, images reflect true tracer incorporation into osteoid. Tracer that is not incorporated into bone is eliminated by renal excretion. Residual free tracer within plasma and extra-cellular space account for blood pool and soft tissue activity. At 24 hours, clearance of physiologic tracer distribution in normal bone and soft tissue *amplifies* tracer retention in *pathologic* bone. Radionuclide decay of 99mTc (6 hour half-life) precludes any further imaging beyond 24 hours.

Because the delayed bone images (3 to 24 hours) provide an indirect measure of osteoblastic activity, bone scintigraphy is effectively an imaging map of bone metabolism.[283,284] Bone scintigraphy allows an opportunity to detect a pathologic condition that is associated with abnormal bone metabolism, particularly where there is *increased* osteoblastic activity. In theory, most bone and joint pathologies are associated with some degree of abnormal osteoblastic activity, even those that are primarily destructive or lytic. Sensitivity is limited by the volume of pathologic tissue, the relative intensity of the bone reaction, and physical constraints of photon detection. These parameters limit the spatial resolution.

Traditionally, bone scintigraphy has been used to diagnose and characterize a variety of bone and joint pathologies (traumatic, inflammatory, neoplastic, metabolic) (Fig. 61.29), particularly in the setting of negative plain radiographs. It has relatively high sensitivity in this regard.[285] Although many traditional uses for bone scintigraphy have been supplanted by anatomic modalities with greater spatial resolution such as MRI and CT, scintigraphy is still the imaging modality of choice for certain specific

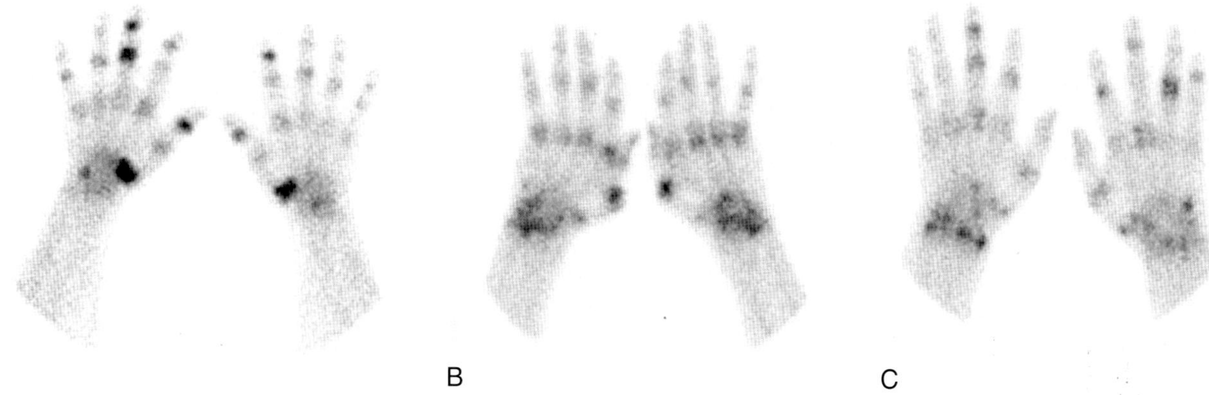

• **Fig. 61.29** Distributions of activity in osteoarthritis (OA), rheumatoid arthritis (RA), and psoriatic arthritis (PsA), on planar bone scintigraphy. (A) Primary OA. Severe activity is seen in the first carpometacarpal (CMC) joint bilaterally and in several proximal interphalangeal (PIP) and distal interphalangeal (DIP) joints. Mild/moderate activity is seen in the index DIP and thumb IP joints bilaterally. (B) RA. Symmetric activity is seen in the radiocarpal joints, and all MCP and PIP joints. (C) PsA. Bilateral asymmetric distribution is seen in the right radiocarpal and in bilateral PIP and DIP in different fingers. Note the ray distribution in the right third finger.

clinical problems (e.g., follow-up of osteoblastic bone metastases, diagnosis of shin splints, demonstration of reflex sympathetic dystrophy). Bone scintigraphy is complementary to anatomic modalities such as CT and MRI because it provides an alternate, functional view of bone pathology that may not be anatomically apparent.

Whole-body bone images are still an efficient means of observing systemic bone pathology such as widespread bony metastatic disease, metabolic bone disease, or bone marrow expansion. A traditional three-phase planar bone scan is similarly efficient at demonstrating *regional* pathology, such as type I chronic regional pain syndrome, with higher accuracy than MRI or plain radiography.[286]

From a rheumatology perspective, bone scintigraphy can demonstrate evidence of active arthritis (see Fig. 61.29).[287] The whole-body surveillance capability easily documents the specific distribution of an active systemic arthritis or other concurrent systemic pathology. This information can augment or complement a clinical rheumatologic impression. In the presence of anatomically established arthropathy, bone scintigraphy can distinguish a metabolically active from an inactive joint.[288] From an orthopedic standpoint, bone scintigraphy has the ability to demonstrate bone stress reactions, periosteal reactions, or fractures. This is sometimes valuable for orthopedic surgical management.[289]

In the evaluation of arthritides, scintigraphy can be a useful adjunct to clinical assessment, but should not be used routinely. Bone scans are more sensitive than conventional radiographs for detecting active bone pathology, but MRI is usually more sensitive and specific than bone scintigraphy, with the added advantage of not using ionizing radiation.[290–292] However, bone scintigraphy can provide a useful complementary role to MRI and other modalities for several clinical situations.

In addition to the use of ionizing radiation, costs, and limited spatial resolution, traditional planar bone scans have limited anatomic resolution, depending on the body part. Because the location of active pathology is often as important as its presence, this limitation has often reduced the specificity and overall accuracy of traditional planar bone scans.

Single-Photon-Emission Computer Tomography (SPECT) and SPECT-CT

SPECT (single photon emission tomography) uses the principle of tomography to generate cross-section images from multiple planar images. Tomographic bone scintigraphy imaging provides improved sensitivity for the detection pathologies such as active facet arthritis or spondylolysis.[293] However, precise anatomic location of the active pathology seen on conventional SPECT images (i.e., without concurrent CT) can be very difficult. This reduces its specificity. For example, facet arthritis versus active spondylolysis or other pathology in the posterior elements of a vertebral segment may be difficult to distinguish on SPECT imaging alone.[293]

SPECT/CT is an example of modern "fusion imaging." Other examples include positron emission tomography (PET)/CT and PET/MRI (see later). SPECT/CT is the acquisition of a CT study concurrent with the acquisition of a nuclear medicine SPECT study, while the patient remains in the same body position. This is performed by a single machine: a SPECT/CT capable gamma camera. The high resolution, anatomically specific CT images are then fused with the functional images from SPECT. The combined, "fused" images provide far greater diagnostic accuracy than either alone. It is an effective marriage of tomographic imaging between functional (SPECT) and anatomic (CT) images.

SPECT/CT has, as PET/CT, revolutionized nuclear medicine imaging. The traditional weakness of nuclear medicine imaging, lack of anatomic resolution, has been largely corrected by its fusion with CT. In addition to identifying a functionally active abnormality, SPECT/CT now allows its precise anatomic localization to the extent allowed by modern CT. The effect of this anatomic precision is a dramatic increase in the anatomic and overall diagnostic specificity of bone scintigraphy (and all other nuclear medicine modalities) when augmented with SPECT/CT. This improved specificity has been demonstrated for multiple medical problems such as infection, trauma, and tumor imaging.[294,295]

Previously obscure bone reactions on planar imaging can now be localized with anatomic precision using SPECT/CT. As a result, several bone and joint pathologies that were

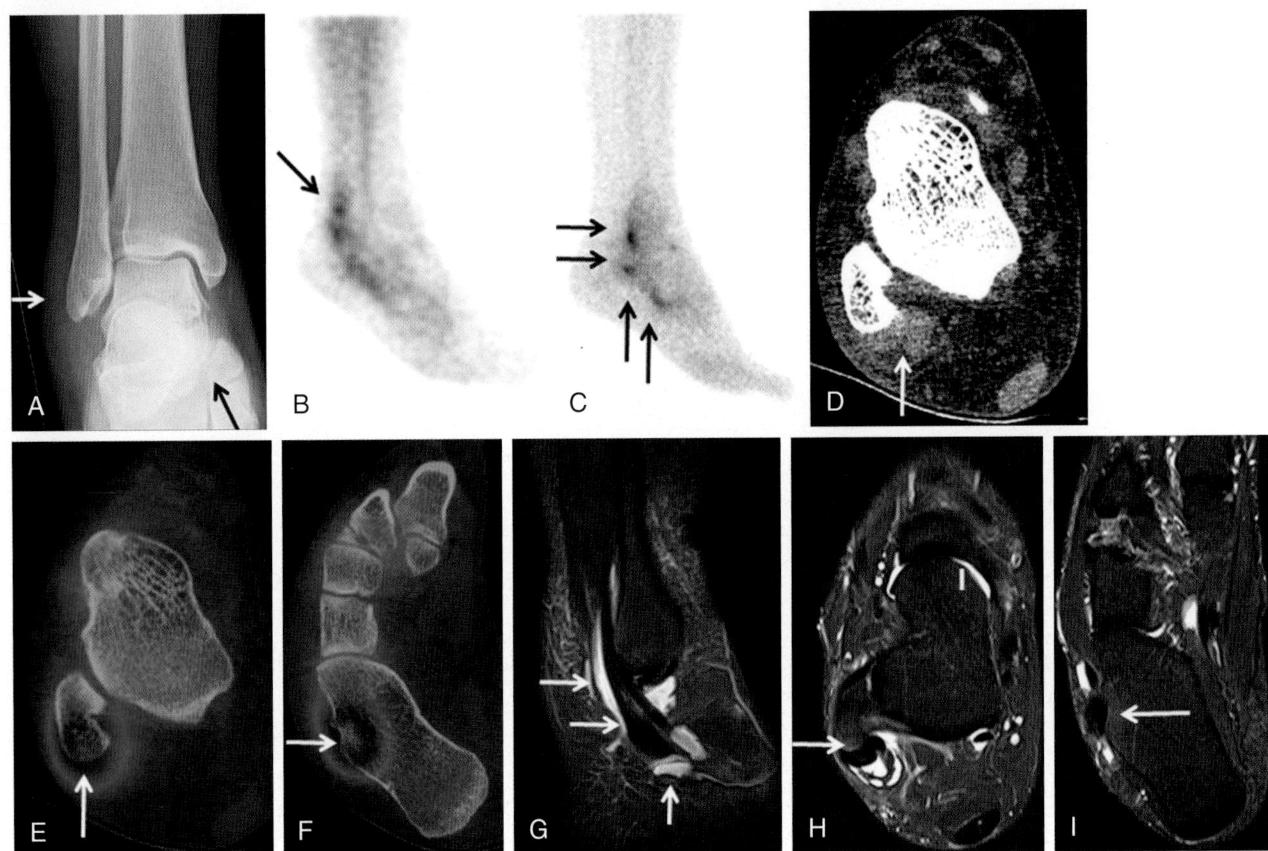

• **Fig. 61.30** Severe peroneus longus tendonopathy demonstrated on bone scan with single photon emission tomography/computed tomography (SPECT/CT). A 37-year-old female with atraumatic right lateral ankle pain and swelling. (A) Ankle radiography shows nonspecific swelling over lateral malleolus. Bone scan was performed to exclude stress fracture. (B) Blood pool image shows lateral hyperemia in a peculiar tubular distribution. (C) Delayed lateral planar bone image shows three distinct foci of bone reaction, which are anatomically localized by SPECT/CT. (D) The CT component of the SPECT/CT shows a swollen peroneal tendon complex. (E and F) The fused SPECT/CT images show bone reaction in the posterior surface of lateral malleolus (E), lateral surface of calcaneus posterior to peroneal tubercle (F), and inferior surface of cuboid (not included). All suggest severe peroneus longus tendonopathy. (G-I) Follow-up MRI of the ankle confirms severe peroneal tenosynovitis (G) with tendonosis and longitudinal split tear of the peroneus longus tendon. Reactive bone marrow edema is confirmed in the adjacent surfaces of lateral malleolus (H), lateral surface of calcaneus (I), and inferior surface of cuboid (not included).

not well seen on planar bone scintigraphy can now be diagnosed, for example, virtually all of the bony impingement syndromes.

There is an approximate congruence between BME seen on MRI and low-to-medium grade patches of bone reaction.[296,297] As a result, fused bone SPECT/CT images approach the diagnostic capabilities of MRI in certain situations. With SPECT/CT, certain soft tissue pathologies (severe tendonopathy [Fig. 61.30], subtle enthesitis, ligamentous injuries) which are not traditionally diagnosed with bone scintigraphy, can now be suggested by the combination of adjacent bone reaction on SPECT, and soft tissue findings on CT.

For assessment of arthropathy, SPECT/CT can occasionally diagnose a specific arthritis by the distribution of bone reaction and specific anatomic findings on CT, in both peripheral and axial joints (Figs. 61.31, 61.32, and 61.33). When SPECT/CT, as CT, is used in clinical practice, the radiation dose should be considered.

Augmented by SPECT/CT, contemporary bone scintigraphy will continue to play an important role in bone and joint imaging. This role could potentially grow, because its full diagnostic capability is not optimally used in clinical practice.

The current literature for bone scintigraphy with SPECT/CT imaging is still deficient. Multiple musculoskeletal pathologies now visible on bone SPECT/CT, which were previously visible only with conventional anatomic imaging (CT and MRI), have not yet been adequately documented in the nuclear medicine imaging literature. Multiple new signs and patterns of bone reaction, which can offer indirect diagnoses of soft tissue pathologies, have yet to be properly documented. Many of the current practicing interpreters of bone scintigraphy do not necessarily have the same degree of experience with diagnostic CT for musculoskeletal pathology, required to optimally extract the added information from SPECT/CT.

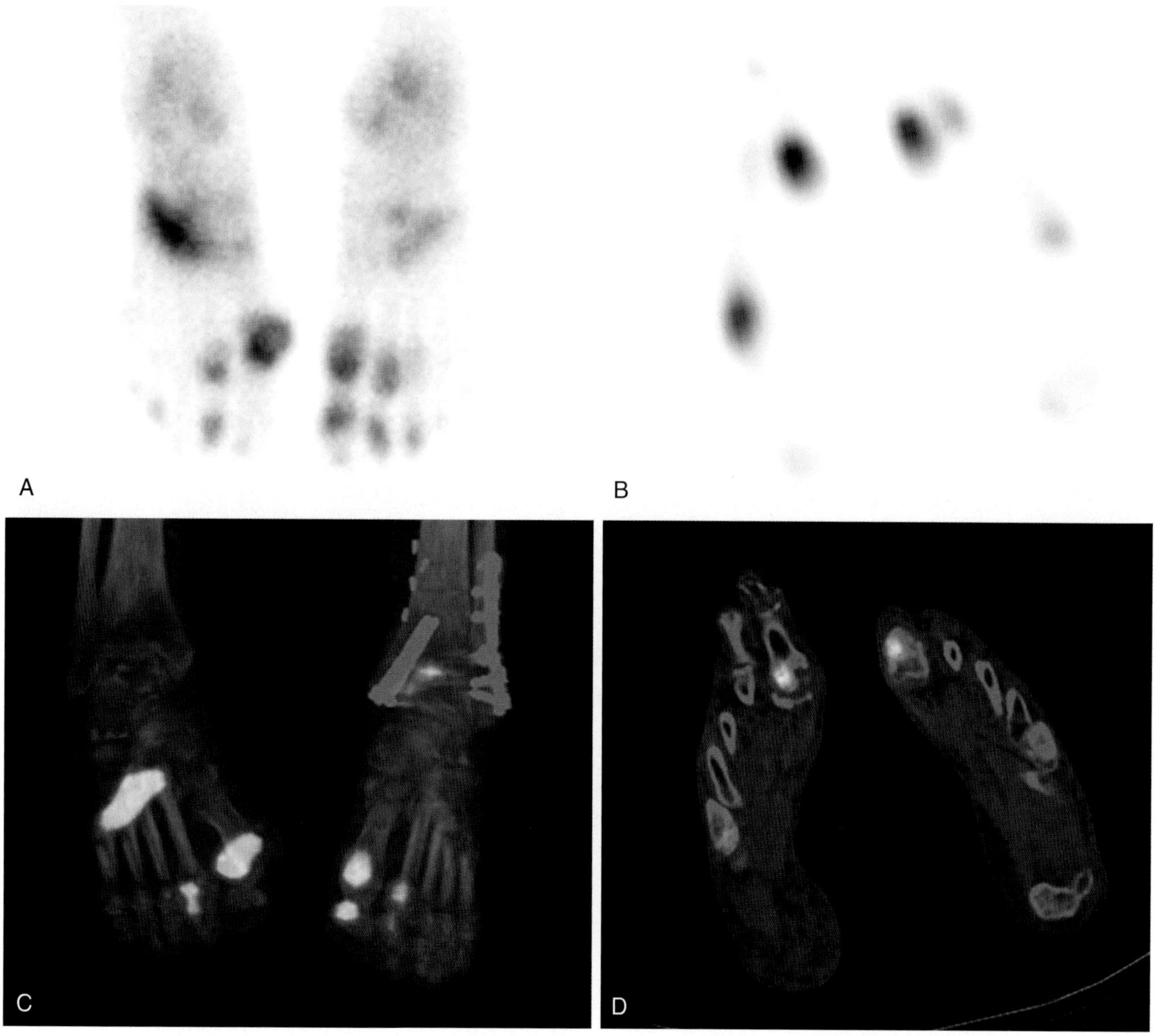

• **Fig. 61.31** Gout (single-photon emission computed tomography [SPECT]). A 72-year-old female patient with known gout and prior trauma was investigated for possible complications. Planar (A) and transverse SPECT (B) images show multifocal increased uptake. Three-dimensional fused SPECT-CT (C) and transverse two-dimensional SPECT-CT (D) images provide superior localization of scintigraphic activity corresponding to the joints most affected by gout.

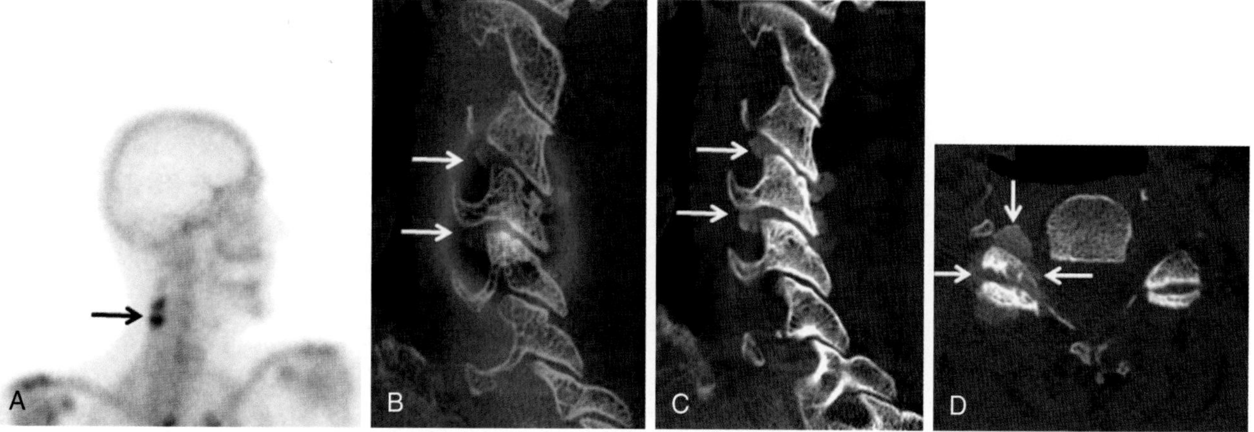

• **Fig. 61.32** Gout in cervical facet joint, visualized by single-photon emission computed tomography (SPECT). A 54-year-old male with unexplained neck pain and decreased range of motion. Bone scan with SPECT/CT was performed to confirm clinically suspected cervical facet arthrosis. (A) Planar spot image confirms active facet arthritis. SPECT/CT was performed for specific anatomic localization and potential steroid injection therapy. (B) The fused image from SPECT/CT localizes the arthritis to the right C3-4 and C4-5 facet joints. However, the high-resolution CT component of this scan (C and D) indicates that it is actually an erosive arthritis with bulky high volume intra-articular and periarticular calcific deposits. A history of gout was subsequently confirmed. (Courtesy Dr Ryan Hung, University of Alberta Hospitals, Edmonton, Canada.)

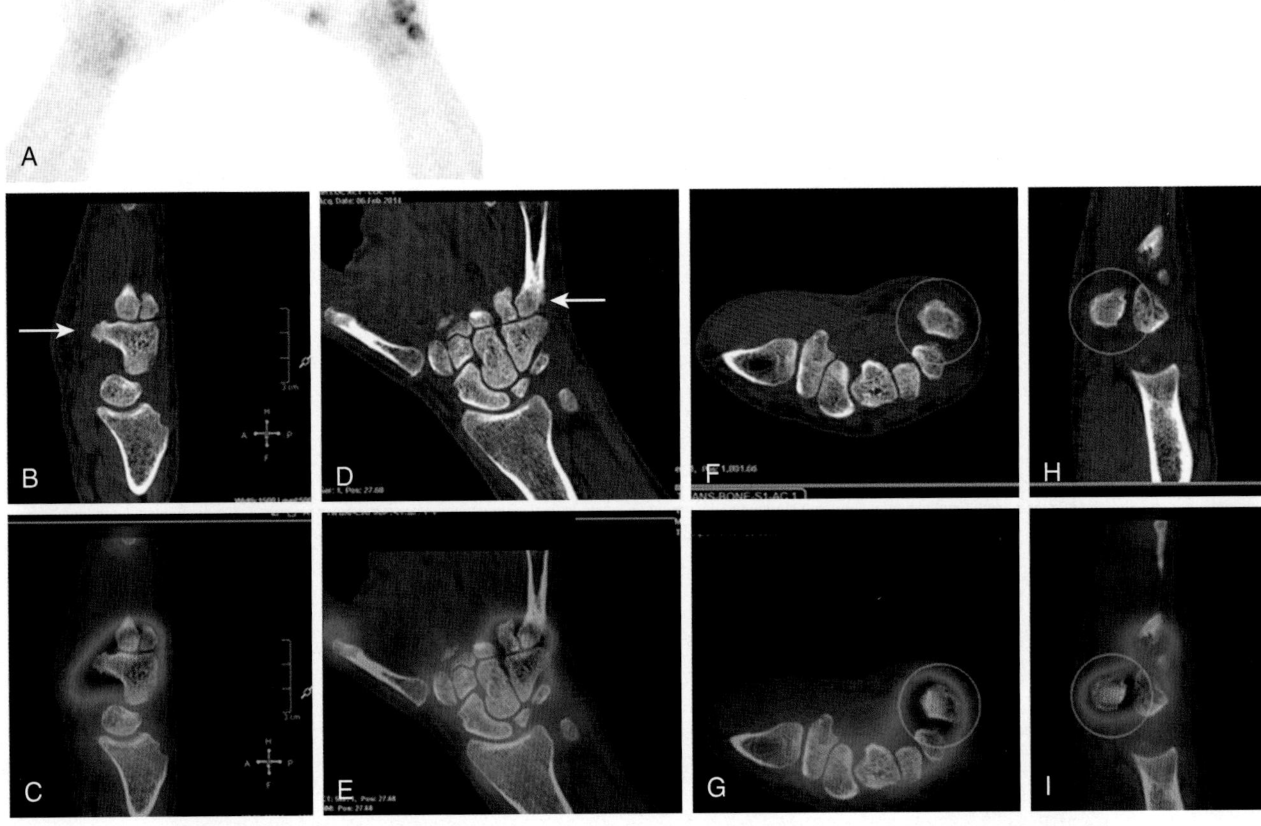

• **Fig. 61.33** Radiographically occult seronegative arthritis on single photon emission tomography/computed tomography (SPECT/CT). A 43-year-old man with pain in hands and feet for years, and normal radiographs. (A) Planar bone scintigraphy of the hands show a nonspecific pattern of bone reaction within the pisiform and several ulnar-sided carpal bones including the 4th and 5th carpometacarpal (CMC) joints. Planar bone scintigraphy images of the feet (not shown) suggested enthesopathy in the base of the left 5th metatarsal bone and synovitis in the right ankle. (B-I) SPECT/CT demonstrates active arthritis in the 4th and 5th CMC joints (C and E) and the pisiform (G and I), with glowing orange signal. Images B, D, F, and H are CT images in the sagittal (B and H), coronal (D), and axial (F) planes, and C, E, G, and I are the corresponding fused SPECT/CT images. Bone reactions on SPECT/CT include the hook of the hamate (*arrow* in B), the base of the 5th metacarpal (*arrow* in D), and the pisiform at the attachment of flexor carpi ulnaris tendon (*circle* in F), where the CT shows fine, fluffy, whisker-like enthesopathy. The distribution of findings on planar images and on SPECT/CT suggest the presence of a seronegative arthritis, which was subsequently serologically confirmed.

Because bone SPECT/CT imaging approaches the diagnostic capability of MRI for certain clinical situations, its clinical role is still evolving. For example, bone SPECT/CT imaging can be more useful in orthopedic management, where orthopedic surgeons are more comfortable using CT compared to MRI.[298]

Various tracers other than 99mTc-MDP are available for the purpose of detecting inflammatory pathologies. Options include ^{67}Ga citrate scan, ^{111}In white blood cell (WBC) scan, 99mTc WBC scan with or without concurrent bone imaging (Fig. 61.34), and 18F-fluorudeoxyglucose (FDG) PET.[285,299] These may assist with imaging workup of osteomyelitis or soft tissue infection.

Similar to planar bone scintigraphy, SPECT/CT technology can be used for each nuclear medicine tracer, providing the same degree of improved anatomic and diagnostic specificity.

The choice of imaging agent depends on the specific clinical scenario: native versus violated bone, axial versus peripheral skeleton, prosthetic infection, acute versus chronic infection, fever of unknown origin. A discussion of optimal inflammatory imaging for each clinical condition is beyond the scope of this discussion.

Positron Emission Tomography (PET)

Positron emission tomography (PET) is a functional imaging technique that enables metabolic mapping of tissues in vivo with positron-emitting radionuclides. 18F-Fluorudeoxyglucose (^{18}FDG) is the most commonly used radiopharmaceutical in PET because of its availability, favorable 110-minute half-life, and high uptake in most metabolically active tissues. When injected into the body, ^{18}FDG demonstrates sites of increased glucose metabolism,

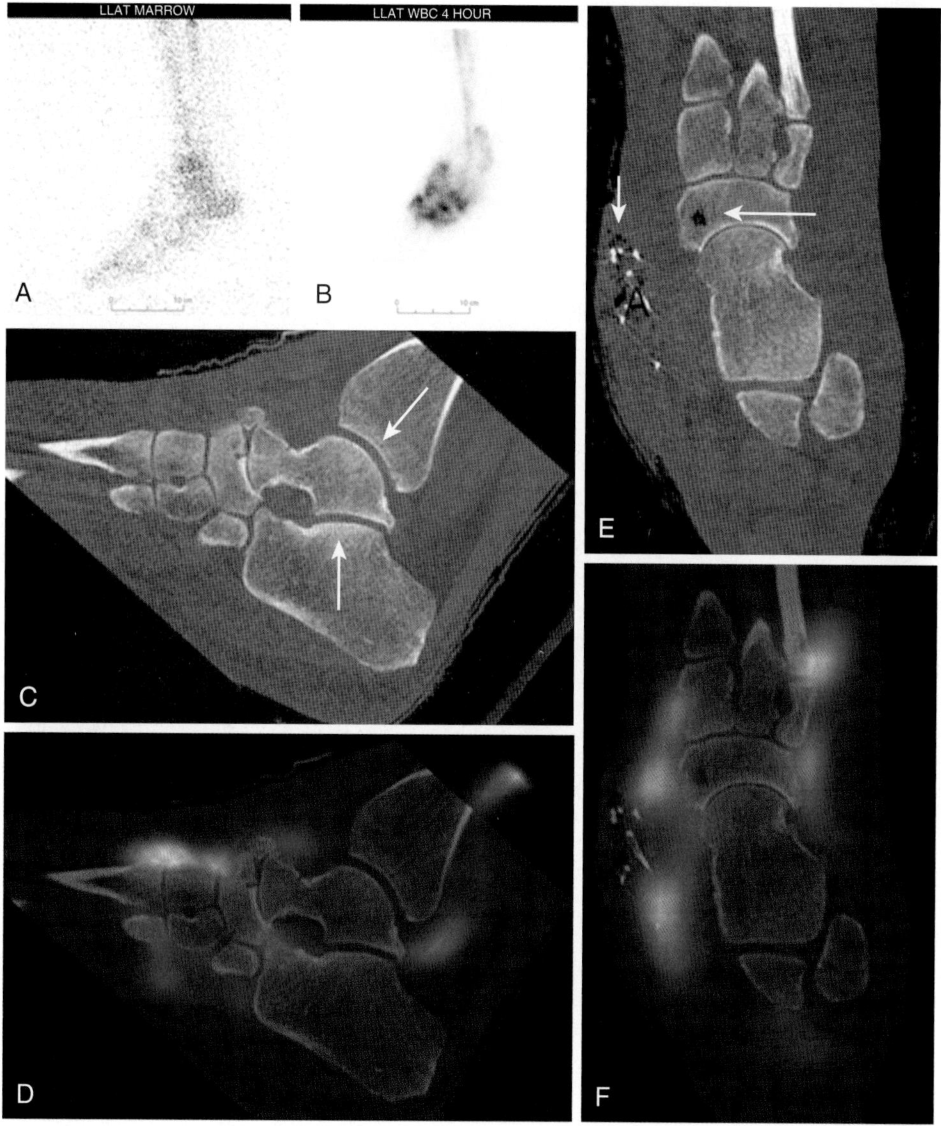

• **Fig. 61.34** Extensive septic arthritis of the midfoot demonstrated by planar white blood cell (WBC) bone scintigraphy and with single photon emission tomography/computed tomography (SPECT/CT). A 41-year-old male with soft tissue infection after minor surgery for removal of a small skin lesion in the dorsal/medial aspect of the midfoot. Extensive cellulitis was apparent clinically, along with a soft tissue abscess, which was surgically drained. Standard planar bone marrow image, using 99m Technetium-sulfur colloid tracer (A), and white blood cell (WBC) (B) image show intense, extensive WBC activity throughout the entire midfoot, with a bone and joint (rather than superficial soft tissue) distribution (B). This is grossly incongruous with the distribution of bone marrow (A), suggesting that the WBC distribution represents extensive septic arthritis. (C-F) Sagittal (C) and axial (E) CT and the corresponding SPECT/CT images (D and F), CT fused with WBC SPECT. SPECT/CT confirms deep midfoot infection, with septic arthritis and osteomyelitis. WBC activity (D and F) has an articular (faint), periarticular, and deep soft tissue distribution. The CT (E) shows medial soft tissue gas and speckled high density *(thick arrow)* in the site of surgical debridement. Intraosseous gas in the navicular (E, *long arrow*) demonstrates at least one site of contiguous osteomyelitis. WBC uptake is seen within most joints of the midfoot (D and F). Note the sparing of the ankle and posterior subtalar joints (C, *thin arrows*), because they do not anatomically communicate with the midfoot joints.

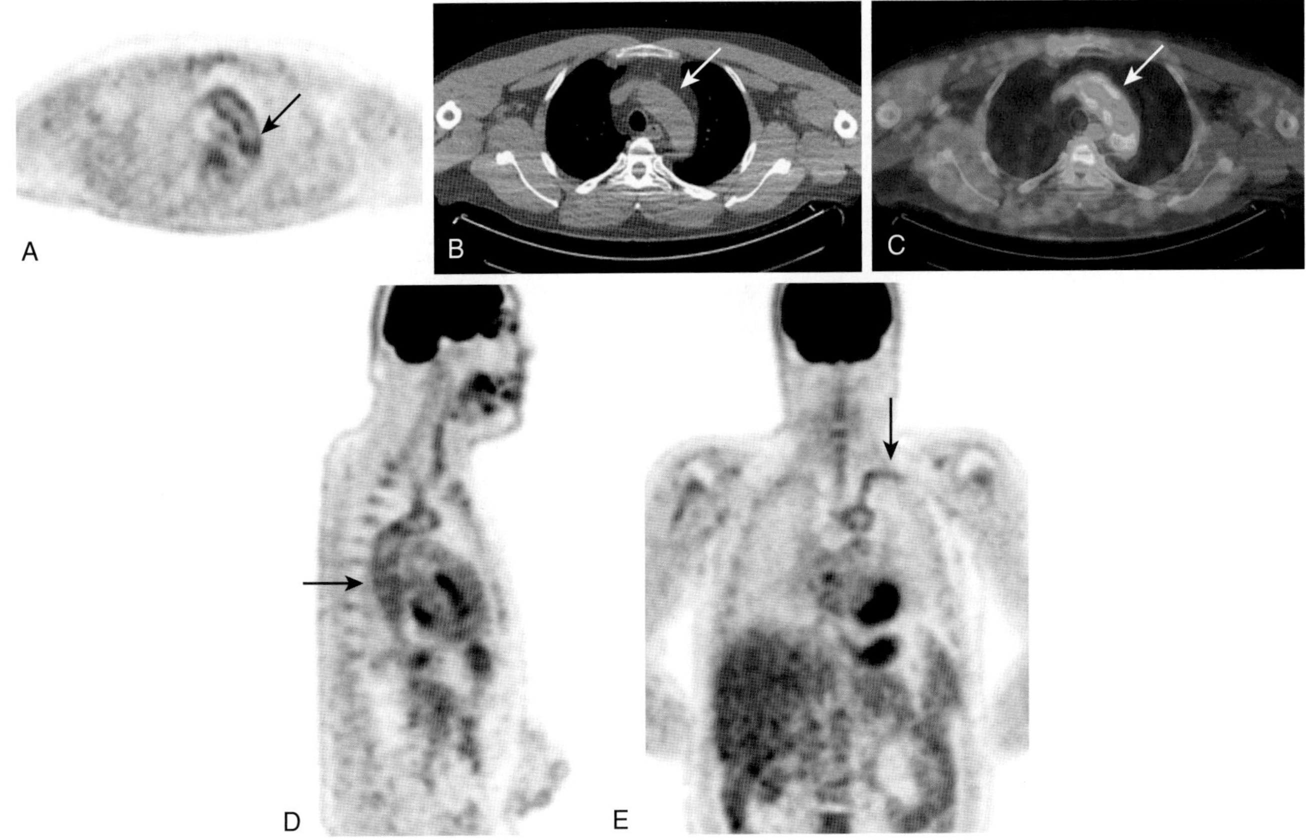

• **Fig. 61.35** Takayasu arteritis, visualized by positron emission tomography/computed tomography (PET/CT). A 46-year-old male with Takayasu arteritis receiving glucocorticoid therapy. An 18F-fluorudeoxyglucose (FDG) PET/CT scan was requested to document active vasculitis, because suboptimal therapy was suspected. (A-E) axial PET (A), CT (B), and PET/CT (C) and sagittal (D) and coronal (E) PET images. Moderately intense inflammation is present in the aortic arch (A-C) and descending aorta (D, *arrow*). Inflammation extends to the great vessels, including the left subclavian artery (E, *arrow*). These suggest persistent, active vasculitis.

thus identifying sites of metabolically active pathology in both bone and soft tissue. The metabolically active pathology can be malignant, inflammatory, or infectious. A PET scan is inherently tomographic and it has a slightly higher spatial resolution than a SPECT scan. A PET/CT scan acquires both a PET and CT scan concurrently on the same machine, allowing fusion of the two sets of images. Similar to SPECT/CT, the CT component of PET/CT provides a precise anatomic map, which is fused with the functional images of glucose metabolism provided by PET.

^{18}FDG PET/CT is most often used in oncology, where it has a well-established role for the diagnosis and clinical management of several malignancies. But ^{18}FDG PET/CT imaging is also useful for a variety of clinical problems in cardiology, neurology, and infectious diseases. For example, ^{18}FDG PET is now considered by many to be *the* diagnostic imaging test of choice for the assessment of fever of unknown origin.[300] ^{18}FDG PET has the highest overall sensitivity and specificity for the diagnosis of chronic osteomyelitis compared to bone scintigraphy, CT, and MRI.[301]

The uptake of ^{18}FDG, like many other nonspecific inflammatory tracers, can conveniently demonstrate the presence and distribution of systemic disease.[302] In rheumatology, ^{18}FDG-PET can be useful for the diagnosis and management of large vessel vasculitis, such as Takayasu's arteritis, and that associated with granulomatosis with polyangiitis (Wegener's), polyarteritis nodosa, giant cell arteritis, and polymyalgia rheumatic (Figs. 61.35 and 61.36).[299,303,304] ^{18}FDG uptake is strongly correlated with MRI synovitis in RA,[305] but the role, if any, in routine clinical management of inflammatory arthritides remains to be determined. Despite some overlap with findings of RA and vasculitis, ^{18}FDG PET/CT can diagnose polymyalgia rheumatica with variable sensitivity and reasonable specificity.[306,307]

^{18}F-flouride is a positron emitting bone tracer that can be used for PET/CT bone scintigraphy. This has superior skeletal kinetics and imaging characteristics compared to conventional ^{99m}Tc based bone scintigraphy.[308] It has better sensitivity, specificity, and accuracy in the evaluation of various benign and malignant bone diseases.[308,309] This is effectively a superior PET/CT version of a "bone scan." However, it is not yet in widespread clinical use and has not yet replaced the traditional, more widely accessible ^{99m}Tc-based bone scan. For some common clinical settings such as the detection of bone metastases in a low prevalence population, its technical superiority does not result in added clinical benefit.[310]

Conclusion

Imaging is an integral part of management of patients with rheumatic diseases. This chapter has outlined the status of imaging in rheumatic diseases, with a particular focus on inflammatory joint diseases. Please see the key point boxes for main messages.

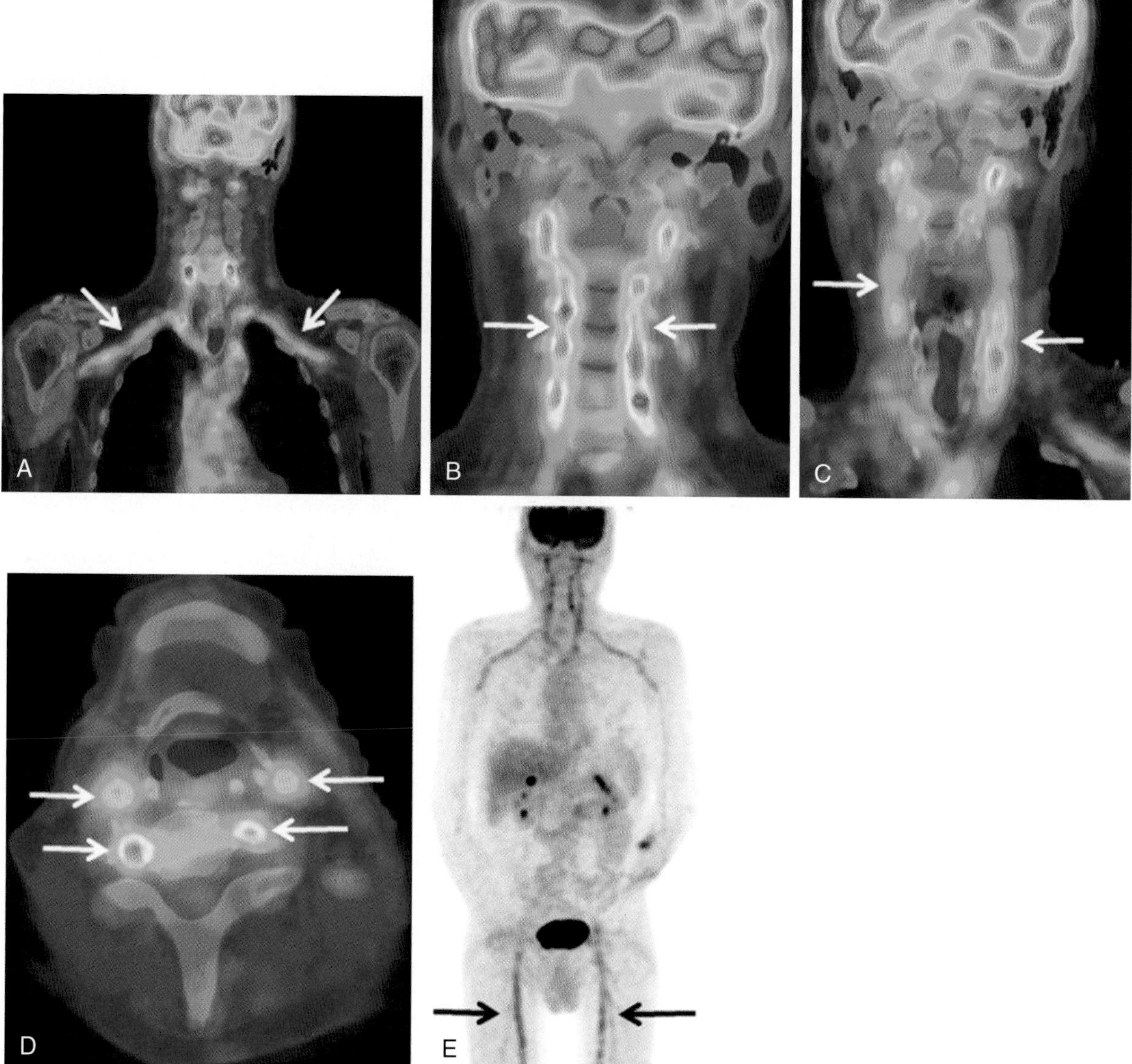

• **Fig. 61.36** Extensive severe large vessel vasculitis, visualized by positron emission tomography/computed tomography (PET/CT). A 67-year-old male, presenting with strokes. (A-C) Coronal fused images from an 18F-fluorudeoxyglucose (FDG) FDG PET/CT study shows intense hypermetabolism in bilateral subclavian (A), vertebral (B), and common carotid (C) arteries. (D) Axial fused images show bilateral carotid and vertebral artery disease. (E) Maximum intensity projection whole body image shows additional involvement of bilateral superficial femoral arteries, in addition to the upper body large vessels. (Courtesy of Dr Richard Coulden, University of Alberta Hospitals, Edmonton, Canada).

The chapter has explained the important role of conventional radiography, but also the exciting new opportunities to be gained with newer imaging techniques. The last decade has brought a vast amount of new knowledge that has dramatically changed the way we manage our patients with rheumatic diseases. It is exciting that with continued dedicated research and rapid technical development it is likely that even larger improvements may occur in the decade to come, for the benefit of our patients.

Full references for this chapter can be found on ExpertConsult.com.

Selected References

1. Resnick D: *Diagnosis of bone and joint disorders*, 4th ed., Philadelphia, 2002, WB Saunders.
2. Watt I: Basic differential diagnosis of arthritis, *Eur Radiol* 7:344–351, 1997.
3. Canella C, Philippe P, Pansini V, et al.: Use of tomosynthesis for erosion evaluation in rheumatoid arthritic hands and wrists, *Radiology* 258(1):199–205, 2011.
4. Aoki T, Fujii M, Yamashita Y, et al.: Tomosynthesis of the wrist and hand in patients with rheumatoid arthritis: comparison with radiography and MRI, *AJR Am J Roentgenol* 202(2):386–390, 2014.
5. Simoni P, Gerard L, Kaiser MJ, et al.: Use of tomosynthesis for detection of bone erosions of the foot in patients with established rheumatoid arthritis: comparison with radiography and CT, *AJR Am J Roentgenol* 205(2):364–370, 2015.
6. Halla JT, Hardin JG, Vitek J, et al.: Involvement of the cervical spine in rheumatoid arthritis, *Arthritis Rheum* 32(5):652–659, 1989.
7. Neva MH, Kauppi MJ, Kautiainen H, et al.: Combination drug therapy retards the development of rheumatoid atlantoaxial subluxations, *Arthritis Rheum* 43(11):2397–2401, 2000.

8. Arnett FC, Edworthy SM, Bloch DA, et al.: The American Rheumatism Association 1987 revised criteria for the classification of rheumatoid arthritis, *Arthritis Rheum* 31:315–324, 1988.
9. Aletaha D, Neogi T, Silman AJ, et al.: 2010 rheumatoid arthritis classification criteria: an American College of Rheumatology/European League Against Rheumatism collaborative initiative, *Ann Rheum Dis* 69(9):1580–1588, 2010.
10. van der Heijde D, van der Helm-van Mil AH, Aletaha D, et al.: EULAR definition of erosive disease in light of the 2010 ACR/EULAR rheumatoid arthritis classification criteria, *Ann Rheum Dis* 72(4):479–481, 2013.
11. Colebatch AN, Edwards CJ, Østergaard M, et al.: EULAR recommendations for the use of imaging of the joints in the clinical management of rheumatoid arthritis, *Ann Rheum Dis* 72(6):804–814, 2013.
12. American College of Rheumatology Subcommittee on Rheumatoid Arthritis Guidelines: Guidelines for the management of rheumatoid arthritis: 2002 Update, *Arthritis Rheum* 46(2):328–346, 2002.
13. Sharp JT, Young DY, Bluhm GB, et al.: How many joints in the hands and wrists should be included in a score of radiologic abnormalities used to assess rheumatoid arthritis? *Arthritis Rheum* 28:1326–1335, 1985.
14. Larsen A, Dale K, Eek M: Radiographic evaluation of rheumatoid arthritis and related conditions by standard reference films, *Acta Radiol Diagn* 18:481–491, 1977.
15. van der Heijde DMFM: Plain X-rays in rheumatoid arthritis: overview of scoring methods, their reliability and applicability, *Bailleres Clin Rheumatol* 10:435–453, 1996.
16. van der Heijde D: Quantification of radiological damage in inflammatory arthritis: rheumatoid arthritis, psoriatic arthritis and ankylosing spondylitis, *Best Pract Res Clin Rheumatol* 18(6):847–860, 2004.
17. van der Heijde D, Dankert T, Nieman F, et al.: Reliability and sensitivity to change of a simplification of the Sharp/van der Heijde radiological assessment in rheumatoid arthritis, *Rheumatology (Oxford)* 38(10):941–947, 1999.
18. Dias EM, Lukas C, Landewe R, et al.: Reliability and sensitivity to change of the Simple Erosion Narrowing Score compared with the Sharp-van der Heijde method for scoring radiographs in rheumatoid arthritis, *Ann Rheum Dis* 67(3):375–379, 2008.
19. Kaarela K: Prognostic factors and diagnostic criteria in early rheumatoid arthritis, *Scand J Rheumatol* 14(Suppl. 57):1–54, 1985.
20. Ødegård S, Landewe R, Van Der Heijde D, et al.: Association of early radiographic damage with impaired physical function in rheumatoid arthritis: a ten-year, longitudinal observational study in 238 patients, *Arthritis Rheum* 54(1):68–75, 2006.
21. Visser H, le Cessie S, Vos K, et al.: How to diagnose rheumatoid arthritis early: a prediction model for persistent (erosive) arthritis, *Arthritis Rheum* 46(2):357–365, 2002.
22. Nissilä M, Isomaki H, Kaarela K, et al.: Prognosis of inflammatory joint diseases. A three-year follow-up study, *Scand J Rheumatol* 12(1):33–38, 1983.
23. Möttönen TT: Prediction of erosiveness and rate of development of new erosions in early rheumatoid arthritis, *Ann Rheum Dis* 47(8):648–653, 1988.
24. van der Heijde DMFM, van Leeuwen MA, van Riel PLCM, et al.: Biannual radiographic assessments of hands and feet in a three-year prospective followup of patients with early rheumatoid arthritis, *Arthritis Rheum* 35:26–34, 1992.
25. McQueen FM, Stewart N, Crabbe J, et al.: Magnetic resonance imaging of the wrist in early rheumatoid arthritis reveals a high prevalence of erosion at four months after symptom onset, *Ann Rheum Dis* 57:350–356, 1998.
26. van der Heijde DMFM: Joint erosions and patients with early rheumatoid arthritis, *Br J Rheumatol* 34(suppl. 2):74–78, 1995.
27. Paulus HE, Oh M, Sharp JT, et al.: Correlation of single time-point damage scores with observed progression of radiographic damage during the first 6 years of rheumatoid arthritis, *J Rheumatol* 30(4):705–713, 2003.
28. van der Linden S, Valkenburg HA, Cats A: Evaluation of diagnostic criteria for ankylosing spondylitis. A proposal for modification of the New York criteria, *Arthritis Rheum* 27(4):361–368, 1984.
29. Berens DL: Roentgen features of ankylosing spondylitis, *Clin Orthop Relat Res* 74:20–33, 1971.
30. Resnick D, Niwayama G, Goergen TG: Comparison of radiographic abnormalities of the sacroiliac joint in degenerative disease and ankylosing spondylitis, *AJR Am J Roentgenol* 128(2):189–196, 1977.
31. Hermann KG, Althoff CE, Schneider U, et al.: Spinal changes in patients with spondyloarthritis: comparison of MR imaging and radiographic appearances, *Radiographics* 25(3):559–569, 2005.
32. Feldtkeller E, Khan MA, van der Heijde D, et al.: Age at disease onset and diagnosis delay in HLA-B27 negative vs. positive patients with ankylosing spondylitis, *Rheumatol Int* 23(2):61–66, 2003.
33. Rudwaleit M, van der Heijde D, Landewe R, et al.: The development of Assessment of SpondyloArthritis international Society classification criteria for axial spondyloarthritis (part II): validation and final selection, *Ann Rheum Dis* 68(6):777–783, 2009.
34. Dougados M, van der LS, Juhlin R, et al.: The European Spondylarthropathy Study Group preliminary criteria for the classification of spondylarthropathy, *Arthritis Rheum* 34(10):1218–1227, 1991.
35. Mandl P, Navarro-Compan V, Terslev L, et al.: EULAR recommendations for the use of imaging in the diagnosis and management of spondyloarthritis in clinical practice, *Ann Rheum Dis*, 2015 (Published online).
36. Wanders AJ, Landewe RB, Spoorenberg A, et al.: What is the most appropriate radiologic scoring method for ankylosing spondylitis? A comparison of the available methods based on the Outcome Measures in Rheumatology Clinical Trials filter, *Arthritis Rheum* 50(8):2622–2632, 2004.
37. Kane D, Stafford L, Bresnihan B, et al.: A prospective, clinical and radiological study of early psoriatic arthritis: an early synovitis clinic experience, *Rheumatology (Oxford)* 42(12):1460–1468, 2003.
38. Battistone MJ, Manaster BJ, Reda DJ, et al.: The prevalence of sacroilitis in psoriatic arthritis: new perspectives from a large, multicenter cohort. A Department of Veterans Affairs Cooperative Study, *Skeletal Radiol* 28(4):196–201, 1999.
39. van der Heijde D, Østergaard M: Assessment of disease activity and damage in inflammatory arthritis. In Bijlsma JWJ, editor: *The EULAR Compendium on Rheumatic Diseases*, London, United Lingdom, 2009, BMJ Publishing Group, pp 182–201.
40. Taylor W, Gladman D, Helliwell P, et al.: Classification criteria for psoriatic arthritis: development of new criteria from a large international study, *Arthritis Rheum* 54(8):2665–2673, 2006.
41. Cornelius R, Schneider HJ: Gouty arthritis in the adult, *Radiol Clin North Am* 26(6):1267–1276, 1988.
42. Wallace SL, Robinson H, Masi AT, et al.: Preliminary criteria for the classification of the acute arthritis of primary gout, *Arthritis Rheum* 20(3):895–900, 1977.
43. Dalbeth N, Clark B, McQueen F, et al.: Validation of a radiographic damage index in chronic gout, *Arthritis Rheum* 57(6):1067–1073, 2007.
44. Dalbeth N, McQueen FM: Use of imaging to evaluate gout and other crystal deposition disorders, *Curr Opin Rheumatol* 21(2):124–131, 2009.
45. Martel W, McCarter DK, Solsky MA, et al.: Further observations on the arthropathy of calcium pyrophosphate crystal deposition disease, *Radiology* 141(1):1–15, 1981.
46. Steinbach LS, Resnick D: Calcium pyrophosphate dihydrate crystal deposition disease revisited, *Radiology* 200(1):1–9, 1996.
47. Ishida T, Dorfman HD, Bullough PG: Tophaceous pseudogout (tumoral calcium pyrophosphate dihydrate crystal deposition disease), *Hum Pathol* 26(6):587–593, 1995.
48. Palestro CJ, Love C, Miller TT: Diagnostic imaging tests and microbial infections, *Cell Microbiol* 9(10):2323–2333, 2007.
49. Piperno M, Hellio Le Graverand MP, Conrozier T, et al.: Quantitative evaluation of joint space width in femorotibial osteoarthritis: comparison of three radiographic views, *Osteoarthritis Cartilage* 6(4):252–259, 1998.

50. Buckland-Wright JC, Macfarlane DG, Williams SA, et al.: Accuracy and precision of joint space width measurements in standard and macroradiographs of osteoarthritic knees, *Ann Rheum Dis* 54(11):872–880, 1995.
51. Altman R, Asch E, Bloch D, et al.: Development of criteria for the classification and reporting of osteoarthritis. Classification of osteoarthritis of the knee, *Arthritis Rheum* 8:1039–1049, 1986.
52. Kellgren JH, Lawrence JS: Radiological assessment of osteo-arthrosis, *Ann Rheum Dis* 16(4):494–502, 1957.
53. Scott Jr WW, Lethbridge-Cejku M, Reichle R, et al.: R eliability of grading scales for individual radiographic features of osteoarthritis of the knee. The Baltimore longitudinal study of aging atlas of knee osteoarthritis, *Invest Radiol* 28(6):497–501, 1993.
54. Gowdie PJ, Tse SM: Juvenile idiopathic arthritis, *Pediatr Clin North Am* 59(2):301–327, 2012.
55. Petty RE, Southwood TR, Manners P, et al.: International League of Associations for Rheumatology classification of juvenile idiopathic arthritis: second revision, Edmonton, 2001, *J Rheumatol* 31(2):390–392, 2004.
56. Cobb JE, Hinks A, Thomson W: The genetics of juvenile idiopathic arthritis: current understanding and future prospects, *Rheumatology (Oxford)* 53(4):592–599, 2014.
57. Damasio MB, de Horatio LT, Boavida P, et al.: Imaging in juvenile idiopathic arthritis (JIA): an update with particular emphasis on MRI, *Acta Radiol* 54(9):1015–1023, 2013.
58. Ravelli A, Ioseliani M, Norambuena X, et al.: Adapted versions of the Sharp/van der Heijde score are reliable and valid for assessment of radiographic progression in juvenile idiopathic arthritis, *Arthritis Rheum* 56(9):3087–3095, 2007.
59. Vardhanabhuti V, Riordan RD, Mitchell GR, et al.: Image comparative assessment using iterative reconstructions: clinical comparison of low-dose abdominal/pelvic computed tomography between adaptive statistical, model-based iterative reconstructions and traditional filtered back projection in 65 patients, *Invest Radiol* 49(4):209–216, 2014.
60. Chahal BS, Kwan ALC, Dhillon SS, et al.: Radiation exposure to the sacroiliac joint from low-dose CT compared with radiography, *AJR Am J Roentgenol* 211(5):1058–1062, 2018.
61. de Koning A, de Bruin F, van den Berg R, et al.: Low-dose CT detects more progression of bone formation in comparison to conventional radiography in patients with ankylosing spondylitis: results from the SIAS cohort, *Ann Rheum Dis* 77(2):293–299, 2018.
62. Aurell Y, Andersson M, Forslind K: Cone-beam computed tomography, a new low-dose three-dimensional imaging technique for assessment of bone erosions in rheumatoid arthritis: reliability assessment and comparison with conventional radiography—a BARFOT study, *Scand J Rheumatol* 47(3):173–164, 2019.
63. Jans L, De K I, Herregods N, et al.: Dual-energy CT: a new imaging modality for bone marrow oedema in rheumatoid arthritis, *Ann Rheum Dis* 77(6):958–960, 2018.
64. Wu H, Zhang G, Shi L, et al.: Axial spondyloarthritis: dual-energy virtual noncalcium CT in the detection of bone marrow edema in the sacroiliac joints, *Radiology* 290:157–164, 2019.
65. Døhn UM, Ejbjerg BJ, Court-Payen, et al.: Are bone erosions detected by magnetic resonance imaging and ultrasonography true erosions? A comparison with computed tomography in rheumatoid arthritis metacarpophalangeal joints, *Arthritis Res Ther* 8(4):R110, 2006.
66. Døhn UM, Ejbjerg B, Boonen A, et al.: No overall progression and occasional repair of erosions despite persistent inflammation in adalimumab-treated rheumatoid arthritis patients: results from a longitudinal comparative MRI, ultrasonography, CT and radiography study, *Ann Rheum Dis* 70(2):252–258, 2011.
67. Døhn UM, Boonen A, Hetland ML, et al.: Erosive progression is minimal, but erosion healing rare, in patients with rheumatoid arthritis treated with adalimumab. A 1 year investigator-initiated follow-up study using high-resolution computed tomography as the primary outcome measure, *Ann Rheum Dis* 68(10):1585–1590, 2009.
68. Barnabe C, Toepfer D, Marotte H, et al.: Definition for rheumatoid arthritis erosions imaged with high resolution peripheral quantitative computed tomography and interreader reliability for detection and measurement, *J Rheumatol* 43(10):1935–1940, 2016.
69. Scharmga A, Peters M, van den Bergh JP, et al.: Development of a scoring method to visually score cortical interruptions on high-resolution peripheral quantitative computed tomography in rheumatoid arthritis and healthy controls, *PLoS One* 13(7):e0200331, 2018.
70. Yue J, Griffith JF, Xiao F, et al.: Repair of bone erosion in rheumatoid arthritis by denosumab: a high-resolution peripheral quantitative computed tomography study, *Arthritis Care Res (Hoboken)* 69(8):1156–1163, 2017.
71. Tan S, Yao J, Flynn JA, et al.: Quantitative syndesmophyte measurement in ankylosing spondylitis using CT: longitudinal validity and sensitivity to change over 2 years, *Ann Rheum Dis* 74:437–443, 2015.
72. Poggenborg R, Bird P, Boonen A, et al.: Pattern of bone erosion and bone proliferation in psoriatic arthritis hands: a high-resolution computed tomography and radiography follow-up study during adalimumab therapy, *Scand J Rheumatol* 53:746–756, 2014.
73. Poggenborg RP, Wiell C, Boyesen P, et al.: No overall damage progression despite persistent inflammation in adalimumab-treated psoriatic arthritis patients: results from an investigator-initiated 48-week comparative magnetic resonance imaging, computed tomography and radiography trial, *Rheumatology (Oxford)* 53(4):746–756, 2014.
74. Gerster JC, Landry M, Dufresne L, et al.: Imaging of tophaceous gout: computed tomography provides specific images compared with magnetic resonance imaging and ultrasonography, *Ann Rheum Dis* 61(1):52–54, 2002.
75. Nicolaou S, Yong-Hing CJ, Galea-Soler S, et al.: Dual-energy CT as a potential new diagnostic tool in the management of gout in the acute setting, *AJR Am J Roentgenol* 194(4):1072–1078, 2010.
76. Dalbeth N, Aati O, Kalluru R, et al.: Relationship between structural joint damage and urate deposition in gout: a plain radiography and dual-energy CT study, *Ann Rheum Dis* 74:1030–1036, 2015.
77. Bongartz T, Glazebrook KN, Kavros SJ, et al.: Dual-energy CT for the diagnosis of gout: an accuracy and diagnostic yield study, *Ann Rheum Dis* 74:1072–1077, 2015.
78. Choi HK, Burns LC, Shojania K, et al.: Dual energy CT in gout: a prospective validation study, *Ann Rheum Dis* 71(9):1466–1471, 2012.
79. Kiefer T, Diekhoff T, Hermann S, et al.: Single source dual-energy computed tomography in the diagnosis of gout: Diagnostic reliability in comparison to digital radiography and conventional computed tomography of the feet, *Eur J Radiol* 85(10):1829–1834, 2016.
80. Dalbeth N, Clark B, Gregory K, et al.: Computed tomography measurement of tophus volume: comparison with physical measurement, *Arthritis Rheum* 57(3):461–465, 2007.
81. Dalbeth N, Doyle A, Boyer L, et al.: Development of a computed tomography method of scoring bone erosion in patients with gout: validation and clinical implications, *Rheumatology (Oxford)* 50(2):410–416, 2011.
82. Salaffi F, Carotti M, Guglielmi G, et al.: The crowned dens syndrome as a cause of neck pain: clinical and computed tomography study in patients with calcium pyrophosphate dihydrate deposition disease, *Clin Exp Rheumatol* 26(6):1040–1046, 2008.
83. Fenoy AJ, Menezes AH, Donovan KA, et al.: Calcium pyrophosphate dihydrate crystal deposition in the craniovertebral junction, *J Neurosurg Spine* 8(1):22–29, 2008.
84. Mikami T, Takeda Y, Ohira A, et al.: Tumoral calcium pyrophosphate dihydrate crystal deposition disease of the temporomandibular joint: identification on crystallography, *Pathol Int* 58(11):723–729, 2008.

85. Misra D, Guermazi A, Sieren JP, et al.: *CT imaging for evaluation of calcium crystal deposition in the knee: initial experience from the Multicenter Osteoarthritis (MOST) study*, Osteoarthritis Cartilage, 2014.
86. Chan WP, Lang P, Stevens MP, et al.: Osteoarthritis of the knee: comparison of radiography, CT, and MR imaging to assess extent and severity, *Am J Roentgenol* 157:799–806, 1991.
87. Vande Berg BC, Lecouvet FE, Poilvache P, et al.: Assessment of knee cartilage in cadavers with dual-detector spiral CT arthrography and MR imaging, *Radiology* 222(2):430–436, 2002.
88. Yoo HJ, Hong SH, Choi JY, et al.: Contrast-enhanced CT of articular cartilage: experimental study for quantification of glycosaminoglycan content in articular cartilage, *Radiology* 261(3):805–812, 2011.
89. Hirvasniemi J, Kulmala KA, Lammentausta E, et al.: In vivo comparison of delayed gadolinium-enhanced MRI of cartilage and delayed quantitative CT arthrography in imaging of articular cartilage, *Osteoarthritis Cartilage* 21(3):434–442, 2013.
90. Ejbjerg BJ, Narvestad E, Jacobsen S, et al.: Low cost, low field dedicated extremity MRI is highly specific and sensitive for synovitis and bone erosions in rheumatoid arthritis wrist and finger joints: comparison with conventional high field MRI and radiography, *Ann Rheum Dis* 64(9):1280–1287, 2005.
91. Taouli B, Zaim S, Peterfy CG, et al.: Rheumatoid arthritis of the hand and wrist: comparison of three imaging techniques, *AJR Am J Roentgenol* 182(4):937–943, 2004.
92. Duer-Jensen A, Ejbjerg B, Albrecht-Beste E, et al.: Does low-field dedicated extremity MRI (E-MRI) reliably detect bone erosions in rheumatoid arthritis? A comparison of two different E-MRI units and conventional radiography with high-resolution CT scanning, *Ann Rheum Dis* 68(8):1296–1302, 2009.
93. Madsen KB, Jurik AG: Magnetic resonance imaging grading system for active and chronic spondylarthritis changes in the sacroiliac joint, *Arthritis Care Res (Hoboken)* 62(1):11–18, 2010.
94. Puhakka KB, Melsen F, Jurik AG, et al.: MR imaging of the normal sacroiliac joint with correlation to histology, *Skeletal Radiol* 33(1):15–28, 2004.
95. Maksymowych WP, Crowther SM, Dhillon SS, et al.: Systematic assessment of inflammation by magnetic resonance imaging in the posterior elements of the spine in ankylosing spondylitis, *Arthritis Care Res (Hoboken)* 62(1):4–10, 2010.
96. Baraliakos X, Hermann KG, Landewe R, et al.: Assessment of acute spinal inflammation in patients with ankylosing spondylitis by magnetic resonance imaging: a comparison between contrast enhanced T1 and short tau inversion recovery (STIR) sequences, *Ann Rheum Dis* 64(8):1141–1144, 2005.
97. Madsen KB, Egund N, Jurik AG: Grading of inflammatory disease activity in the sacroiliac joints with magnetic resonance imaging: comparison between short-tau inversion recovery and gadolinium contrast-enhanced sequences, *J Rheumatol* 37(2):393–400, 2010.
98. Østergaard M, Conaghan PG, O'Connor P, et al.: Reducing invasiveness, duration, and cost of magnetic resonance imaging in rheumatoid arthritis by omitting intravenous contrast injection—Does it change the assessment of inflammatory and destructive joint changes by the OMERACT RAMRIS? *J Rheumatol* 36(8):1806–1810, 2009.
99. Del Grande F, Santini F, Herzka DA, et al.: Fat-suppression techniques for 3-T MR imaging of the musculoskeletal system, *Radiographics* 34(1):217–233, 2014.
100. Nieminen MT, Rieppo J, Toyras J, et al.: T2 relaxation reveals spatial collagen architecture in articular cartilage: a comparative quantitative MRI and polarized light microscopic study, *Magn Reson Med* 46(3):487–493, 2001.
101. Hesper T, Hosalkar HS, Bittersohl D, et al.: T2* mapping for articular cartilage assessment: principles, current applications, and future prospects, *Skeletal Radiol* 43(10):1429–1445, 2014.
102. Bashir A, Gray ML, Boutin RD, Burstein D: Glycosaminoglycan in articular cartilage: in vivo assessment with delayed Gd(DTPA)(2-)-enhanced MR imaging, *Radiology* 205(2):551–558, 1997.
103. Owman H, Ericsson YB, Englund M, et al.: Association between delayed gadolinium-enhanced MRI of cartilage (dGEMRIC) and joint space narrowing and osteophytes: a cohort study in patients with partial meniscectomy with 11 years of follow-up, *Osteoarthritis Cartilage* 22(10):1537–1541, 2014.
104. Duvvuri U, Charagundla SR, Kudchodkar SB, et al.: Human knee: in vivo T1(rho)-weighted MR imaging at 1.5 T—preliminary experience, *Radiology* 220(3):822–826, 2001.
105. Rautiainen J, Nissi MJ, Salo EN, et al.: Multiparametric MRI assessment of human articular cartilage degeneration: Correlation with quantitative histology and mechanical properties, *Magn Reson Med* 74:249–259, 2015.
106. Singh A, Haris M, Cai K, et al.: Chemical exchange saturation transfer magnetic resonance imaging of human knee cartilage at 3 T and 7 T, *Magn Reson Med* 68(2):588–594, 2012.
107. Rehnitz C, Kupfer J, Streich NA, et al.: Comparison of biochemical cartilage imaging techniques at 3 T MRI, *Osteoarthritis Cartilage* 22(10):1732–1742, 2014.
108. Raya JG, Dettmann E, Notohamiprodjo M, et al.: Feasibility of in vivo diffusion tensor imaging of articular cartilage with coverage of all cartilage regions, *Eur Radiol* 24(7):1700–1706, 2014.
109. Raya JG, Horng A, Dietrich O, et al.: Articular cartilage: in vivo diffusion-tensor imaging, *Radiology* 262(2):550–559, 2012.
110. Shapiro EM, Borthakur A, Gougoutas A, et al.: 23Na MRI accurately measures fixed charge density in articular cartilage, *Magn Reson Med* 47(2):284–291, 2002.
111. Feldman RE, Stobbe R, Watts A, et al.: Sodium imaging of the human knee using soft inversion recovery fluid attenuation, *J Magn Reson* 234:197–206, 2013.
112. Weckbach S: Whole-body MR imaging for patients with rheumatism, *Eur J Radiol* 70(3):431–441, 2009.
113. Weckbach S, Schewe S, Michaely HJ, et al.: Whole-body MR imaging in psoriatic arthritis: additional value for therapeutic decision making, *Eur J Radiol* 77(1):149–155, 2011.
114. Poggenborg RP, Pedersen SJ, Eshed I, et al.: Head-to-toe whole-body MRI in psoriatic arthritis, axial spondyloarthritis and healthy subjects: first steps towards global inflammation and damage scores of peripheral and axial joints, *Rheumatology (Oxford)* 54(6):1039–1049, 2015.
115. Poggenborg RP, Eshed I, Østergaard M, et al.: Enthesitis in patients with psoriatic arthritis, axial spondyloarthritis and healthy subjects assessed by 'head-to-toe' whole-body MRI and clinical examination, *Ann Rheum Dis* 74(5):823–829, 2015.
116. Grobner T: Gadolinium—a specific trigger for the development of nephrogenic fibrosing dermopathy and nephrogenic systemic fibrosis? *Nephrol Dial Transplant* 21(4):1104–1108, 2006.
117. Marckmann P, Skov L, Rossen K, et al.: Nephrogenic systemic fibrosis: suspected causative role of gadodiamide used for contrast-enhanced magnetic resonance imaging, *J Am Soc Nephrol* 17(9):2359–2362, 2006.
118. Thomsen HS, Reimer P: Intravascular contrast media for radiography, CT, MRI and ultrasound. In Adam A, Dixon AK, Gillard JH, Schafer-Prokop CM, editors: *Grainger & Allison's Diagnostic Radiology—a textbook of medical imaging*, Edinburgh, 2015, Churchill Livingstone Elsevier, pp 26–51.
119. Marckmann P, Skov L, Rossen K, et al.: Clinical manifestation of gadodiamide-related nephrogenic systemic fibrosis, *Clin Nephrol* 69(3):161–168, 2008.
120. Thomsen HS: NSF: still relevant, *J Magn Reson Imaging* 40(1):11–12, 2014.

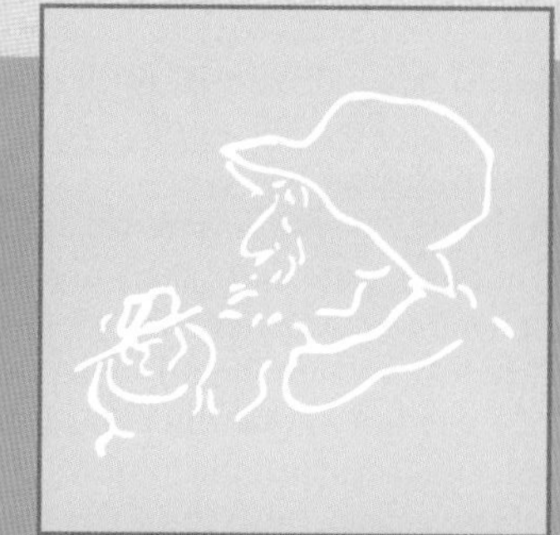

62 Therapeutic Targeting of Prostanoids

LESLIE J. CROFFORD

KEY POINTS

Nonsteroidal anti-inflammatory drugs (NSAIDs) are effective anti-inflammatory, antipyretic, and analgesic compounds.

There is little difference in the efficacy of the various NSAIDs, but the pharmacologic characteristics of individual drugs, including potency, half-life, and relative inhibition of cyclooxygenase (COX)-1 and COX-2, play important roles in toxicity.

Aspirin is an NSAID used in low doses to prevent cardiovascular disease. Taking aspirin and NSAIDs together is associated with increased toxicity in the gastrointestinal (GI) tract, and concomitant use of some NSAIDs with aspirin may be associated with aspirin resistance.

NSAIDs are associated with risk for GI ulceration and bleeding. Patient-specific risk factors for toxicity should be recognized so risk-reduction strategies can be implemented.

NSAIDs are associated with an elevated risk for cardiovascular disease. Clinicians should be aware of cardiovascular risk factors and either avoid prescribing NSAIDs or use intermittent dosing, low doses, or drugs with a short half-life.

Periodic assessment of blood pressure, hemoglobin, electrolytes, renal function, and liver function is advisable, particularly in elderly patients.

Introduction

The use of nonsteroidal anti-inflammatory drugs (NSAIDs) is ubiquitous in the practice of medicine because of their effectiveness as anti-inflammatory, analgesic, and antipyretic agents. NSAIDs differ widely in their chemical class but share the property of blocking production of prostaglandins (PGs). This effect is accomplished by inhibiting the activity of the enzyme PG G/H synthase (PGHS), also called *cyclooxygenase* (COX).

The clinical effects of NSAIDs are evaluated not only by their specific pharmacologic properties but also in terms of their effects on the different COX isoforms, COX-1 and COX-2. These isoforms serve different biologic functions in that COX-1 is expressed under basal conditions and is involved in the biosynthesis of PGs that serve homeostatic functions, whereas COX-2 expression is increased during inflammation and other pathologic situations. Inhibition of COX-2 by NSAIDs blocks PG production at sites of inflammation, whereas inhibition of COX-1 in certain other tissues, most importantly platelets and the gastroduodenal mucosa, can lead to common adverse effects of NSAIDs such as bleeding, bruising, and gastrointestinal (GI) ulceration.

In addition to their use in people with rheumatoid arthritis (RA) and osteoarthritis (OA), NSAIDs are widely used in the symptomatic management of acute and chronic pain associated with other rheumatic diseases. Aspirin, which has unique properties among NSAIDs, is used by millions of people for primary and secondary prevention of cardiovascular thrombosis. In light of the widespread use of these drugs for common diseases, which are likely to increase in prevalence with the aging of the population, it is critically important to appreciate the potential adverse events and drug interactions associated with NSAIDs.

This chapter analyzes aspirin and other NSAIDs on the basis of their chemical structure, pharmacologic properties, and relative inhibition of COX-1 and COX-2. Particular attention to potential adverse events of specific NSAIDs in individual patients will facilitate use of these drugs in the safest possible manner. Acetaminophen (known as *paracetamol* outside the United States), an antipyretic and analgesic drug without anti-inflammatory activity, inhibits COX enzymes via a different mechanism than NSAIDs and is also discussed.

History

Botanicals containing salicylates have been used since antiquity to treat pain, inflammation, and fever. About 3500 years ago, the Egyptian Ebers Papyrus recommended use of a decoction of dried myrtle leaves to be applied to the abdomen and back for relief of rheumatic pains. A thousand years later, Hippocrates recommended poplar tree juices for treatment of eye disease and willow bark to alleviate fever and the pain of childbirth. Throughout Roman times, the use of botanical treatments, including willow bark for pain and inflammation, was widespread. Plants containing salicylate were used medicinally in China and other parts of Asia. In addition, the curative effects of other botanicals were known to the indigenous populations of North America. Extracts of the autumn crocus plant containing colchicine were used for treatment of acute gout as early as the sixth century AD.[1]

The first modern description of the therapeutic application of plants containing salicylates was reported to the Royal Society of London by the Reverend Edward Stone, who provided an account of the successful use of dried willow bark for fever.[1] In this first "clinical trial," a pound of bark was dried, pulverized, and put into the tea, beer, or water of 50 people with fever. Stone found that one dram (1 dram = 1.8 g) cured their fever. In 1763, Stone wrote, "I have no other motives for publishing this valuable specific, than that it may have a fair and full trial in all its variety of circumstances and situations, and that the world may reap the benefits accruing from it."

In 1860 salicylic acid was chemically synthesized, which led to its widespread use as an external antiseptic, antipyretic, and analgesic.[1] The bitter taste of salicylic acid prompted the chemist Felix Hoffman to synthesize the more palatable acetylsalicylic acid (ASA). After a demonstration of its anti-inflammatory effects, Dr. Heinrich Dreser of Bayer introduced this compound into medicine in 1899 as aspirin, and it remains the most widely used drug in the world.[1] Salicylate was identified as the active ingredient of willow bark in 1929.

Phenylbutazone came into clinical practice in 1949 and was followed by indomethacin, fenamates, naproxen, and others. Despite the diversity of their chemical structures, these drugs shared therapeutic properties with aspirin. Furthermore, adverse events including gastric upset, GI ulceration and bleeding, hypertension, edema, and renal damage were shared by all these drugs. In 1971 it was discovered that these drugs all acted by inhibiting PG biosynthesis, thereby providing a unifying explanation of their therapeutic actions and a rationale for grouping them together as NSAIDs.[1]

COX was isolated in 1976 from the endoplasmic reticulum of PG-forming cells.[2,3] Several groups of investigators, however, speculated that there must be a second COX enzyme on the basis of observed biology. In 1990 investigators demonstrated that bacterial lipopolysaccharide (LPS) increased PG synthesis in human monocytes in vitro and in mouse peritoneal macrophages in vivo, but only the LPS-induced increase was inhibited by dexamethasone and required the de novo synthesis of "new" COX protein.[4] This observation was the foundation of the concept for "constitutive" and "inducible" forms of COX. Soon thereafter, a number of investigators working in different systems reported the discovery of an inducible second form of COX.[3] Investigators who proceeded to clone the gene and deduced its structure found that the gene product was homologous to COX but to no other known protein. The observation that glucocorticoids inhibited the expression of COX-2 after a pro-inflammatory stimulus represented a link between the anti-inflammatory actions of NSAIDs and corticosteroids.

Because of the prediction that inhibition of COX-2 would block PG biosynthesis participating in the inflammatory response but was not required for homeostasis, there was a tremendous effort to develop drugs that would selectively inhibit COX-2 without affecting COX-1 in the belief that these medications would provide clinical efficacy without adverse effects.[2,5] Identification of new drugs that differentially inhibited COX-2 over COX-1 was accomplished quickly as existing NSAIDs were tested on the two COX isoforms and crystal structures revealed differences in the protein structures on which new drug development could be based.[5,6]

One hundred years after aspirin was introduced and 10 years after the discovery of COX-2, the selective COX-2 inhibitors, celecoxib and rofecoxib, were developed. In clinical trials, the safety and efficacy profiles of these and related drugs showed promise, and the U.S. Food and Drug Administration (FDA) subsequently approved these COX-2–selective NSAIDs for treatment of arthritis and pain. After their introduction into clinical practice, however, it became clear that the most highly COX-2–selective NSAIDs, particularly rofecoxib, were more likely than traditional NSAIDs to be associated with adverse cardiovascular events.[7] This finding led to the voluntary withdrawal of rofecoxib and several other COX-2–selective NSAIDs from the market. Debate surrounding the relative risks of different NSAIDs to specific organ systems continues to the present day.

Mechanism of Action

Cyclooxygenase Inhibition

All of the NSAIDs are synthetic inhibitors of the COX active site, but subtle mechanistic differences in the manner in which individual NSAIDs interact and bind with the active site are responsible for some of the differences in their pharmacologic characteristics.[8] ASA is the only covalent, irreversible modifier of COX-1 and COX-2, whereas all of the other NSAIDs are competitive inhibitors, competing with arachidonic acid (AA) for binding in the active site. The competitive inhibitors are subdivided further on the basis of whether they bind to the COX active site in a time-dependent or time-independent manner.

Crystallographic studies have shown how ASA acetylates serine 530 of COX-1. Similar to other NSAIDs, ASA diffuses into the COX-1 active site at the mouth of the channel and travels to the constriction created by arginine 120, where it is in the best orientation to transacetylate serine 530, leading to the complete and irreversible inhibition of COX-1.[9] In COX-2, the channel of the active site is larger than COX-1, the orientation of ASA for serine 530 attack is not as good, and transacetylation efficiency for COX-2 is 10-fold to 100-fold less than for COX-1. ASA can also "trigger" COX-2 to alter its catalytic activity to produce 15 R-hydroxyeicosatetraenoic acid (HETE) and lipoxins from AA and to generate anti-inflammatory lipids from omega-3–polyunsaturated fatty acids (PUFA).[10]

The time it takes for an NSAID to inhibit the COX active site relative to how long it takes for it to leave the COX channel is a crucial factor in the inhibition of COX.[11] Drugs such as ibuprofen exhibit such rapid rates that they essentially inhibit COX instantly but can be removed from the COX active site just as quickly when drug levels decrease. Both COX monomers must be inhibited by ibuprofen to block catalytic activity.[12] Conversely, indomethacin and diclofenac are time-dependent allosteric inhibitors that require seconds to minutes to bind to the COX active site and need only block one of the COX monomers to completely inhibit catalytic activity.[12] These NSAIDs also need hours to exit the COX active site. Initially, most traditional time-dependent NSAIDs form a loose complex with the COX active site before a stronger interaction is established. This complex is limited by the time it takes the drug to become properly oriented within the COX channel at arginine 120, the constriction site in the COX channel. This orientation may involve a change in conformation to the "open state" to allow the drug to access the upper part of the COX catalytic site.

Drugs such as flurbiprofen and indomethacin form a salt bridge between the carboxylate moiety of the NSAID and the guanidinium moiety of arginine 120. Hydrophobic interactions between the aromatic rings and the hydrophobic amino acids in the channel aid binding. Such interactions at the constriction point of the channel completely block the entry of substrate to the active site.[13] Diclofenac interacts with serine 530, not arginine 120, but also blocks entry of substrate.[14]

COX-2 Selectivity

NSAIDs such as meloxicam, nimesulide, and etodolac show some selectivity for inhibiting COX-2 compared with COX-1. After the discovery of COX-2, efforts to further enhance COX-2 selectivity led to the development of celecoxib, rofecoxib, valdecoxib, etoricoxib, and lumiracoxib. The prototypical COX-2-selective NSAIDs, celecoxib and rofecoxib, are diaryl compounds

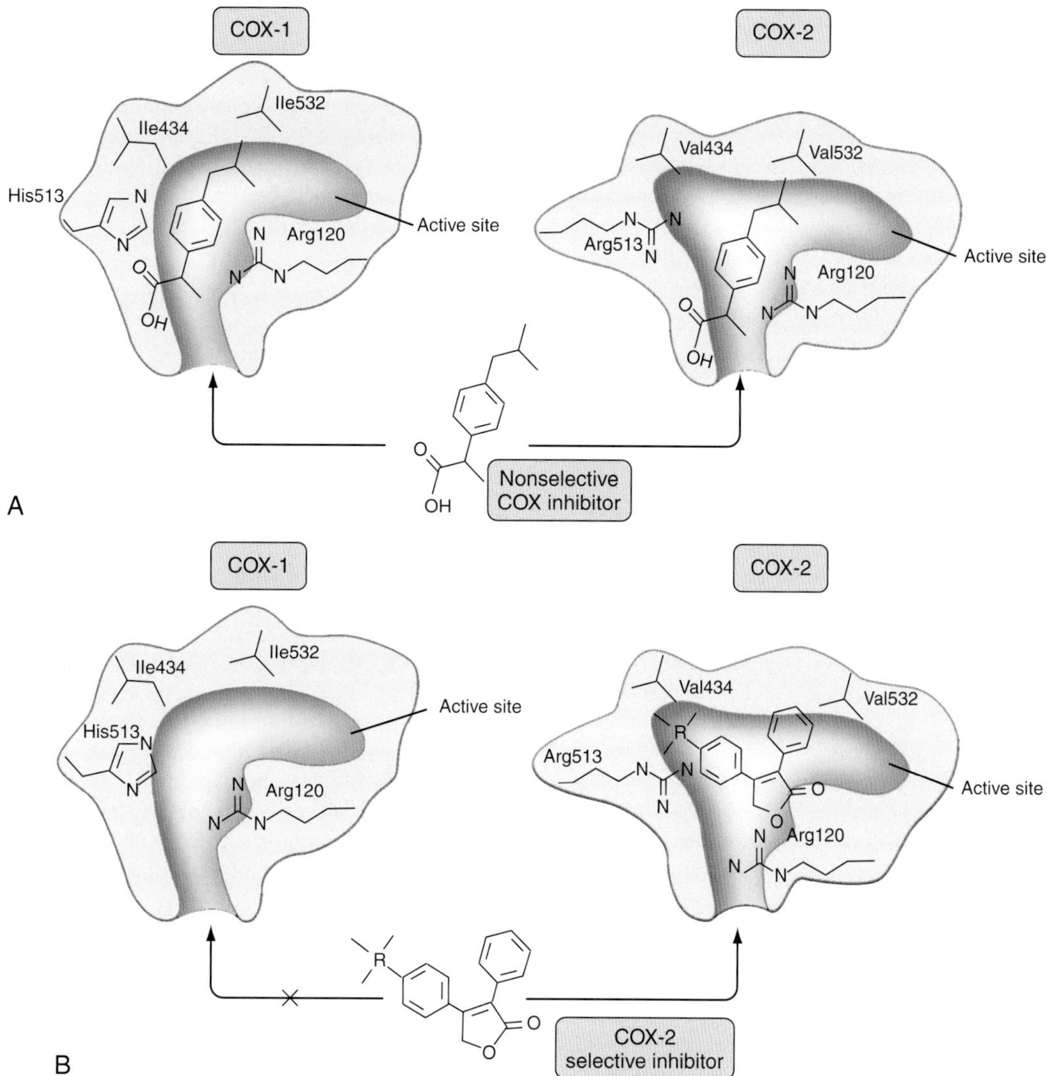

• **Fig. 62.1** Cyclooxygenase (COX)-1 and COX-2 substrate-binding channels. A schematic depiction of the structural differences between the substrate-binding channels of COX-1 and COX-2 that allowed the design of selective inhibitors. The amino acid residues, Val434, Arg513, and Val523, form a side pocket in COX-2 that is absent in COX-1. (A) Nonselective inhibitors have access to the binding channels of both isoforms. (B) The more voluminous residues in COX-1, Ile434, His513, and Ile532, obstruct access of the bulky side chains of the coxibs. (From Grosser T, Fries S, FitzGerald GA: Biological basis for the cardiovascular consequences of COX-2 inhibition: therapeutic challenges and opportunities. *J Clin Invest* 116:4–15, 2006.)

containing a sulfonamide (celecoxib) and methylsulfone (rofecoxib) rather than a carboxyl group. Both drugs are weak time-independent inhibitors of COX-1 but strong time-dependent inhibitors of COX-2 that require their entry into and stabilized binding in the catalytic pocket. Because these drugs lack a carboxyl group, arginine 120 is not involved, but multiple sites of hydrogen and hydrophobic binding stabilize drugs at the catalytic site. The sulfur-containing phenyl ring of COX-2–selective NSAIDs plays a pivotal role in binding stability by occupying the hydrophobic side pocket characteristic of the COX-2 catalytic site. If this side pocket is removed by mutagenesis, all isozyme selectivity is lost (Fig. 62.1).[6]

Most commonly, COX isozyme selectivity is defined by using the concentration of drug required to inhibit PG production by 50% (inhibitory concentration [IC]50). Ratios using values obtained for COX-1 IC50s compared with COX-2 IC50s can be calculated and used as a standard measure for comparing the degrees of selectivity of a particular NSAID for one or the other COX isoform.[15] PG assay systems can vary widely, however, making it difficult to directly compare results from studies using different assay systems. To circumvent such problems, most clinicians have accepted the use of the in vitro whole-blood assay to compare NSAID selectivities. In this system, COX-1 inhibition is assessed as a function of the reduction of thromboxane made by platelets after clot formation. Inhibition of COX-2 is based on the inhibition of prostaglandin E_2 (PGE_2) production in a heparinized blood sample after LPS stimulation. A COX-2–selective NSAID lacks inhibitory effect on platelet COX-1 at concentrations at or above those that maximally inhibit COX-2.[5,16]

Cyclooxygenase-Independent Mechanisms of Action

At high, nonphysiologic concentrations, some NSAIDs seem to elicit effects on cellular pathways in vitro that do not involve the inhibition of COX. Because of the high doses of drug required and the use of in vitro systems, the relevance of these effects to in vivo activity is uncertain. Some NSAIDs inhibit phosphodiesterases associated with the metabolism of cyclic adenosine monophosphate (cAMP), leading to increased intracellular cAMP levels and the subsequent general inhibition of peripheral blood lymphocyte responses to mitogen stimulation, monocyte and neutrophil migration, and neutrophil aggregation.[17] NSAIDs scavenge free radicals, inhibit superoxide production by polymorphonuclear neutrophils, reduce mononuclear cell phospholipase C activity, and inhibit inducible nitric oxide (NO) synthase activity. Sodium salicylate and ASA inhibit NF-κB activation, as do certain inactive enantiomers of flurbiprofen. Some reports indicate that other cell signaling molecules such as mitogen-activated protein kinases and the transcription factor activator protein (AP)-1 also may be modulated by NSAIDs. Some NSAIDs bind to and activate members of the peroxisome proliferator-activated receptor (PPAR) family and other intra-cellular receptors. PPAR activation is thought to mediate anti-inflammatory activities. Nonselective acidic NSAIDs, including salicylate, ibuprofen, and diclofenac, but not nonacidic drugs, activate adenosine monophosphate–activated protein kinase (AMPK).[18] Selective COX-2 inhibitors may have unique structural features that promote COX-independent activities such as cell-cycle regulation, apoptosis, and antiangiogenesis.[19]

Mechanism of Acetaminophen and Other Analgesic Antipyretic Drugs

Acetaminophen (paracetamol) and dipyrone relieve pain and fever, but they are not anti-inflammatory. The precise mechanisms by which these drugs elicit their effects remain unclear. In the 1970s it was proposed that acetaminophen worked by means of a "central" action by inhibiting COX activity primarily in the brain and not in peripheral tissues because they were not acidic and could cross the blood-brain barrier.[20] Acetaminophen does inhibit COX-1 and COX-2, but variably, in a manner dependent on cell and tissue type. Acetaminophen does not appear to inhibit by interacting with the COX active site; rather, it serves as a reducing co-substrate for the peroxidase site. The peroxide tone of cells and tissues in vivo may be responsible for inhibitor specificity, with platelets and activated macrophages being resistant to the action of acetaminophen and vascular endothelial cells being sensitive to its inhibitory effects on COX. Additionally the inhibitory potency of acetaminophen is determined by the concentration of the COX enzyme.[20] This phenomenon may be an additional factor for the lack of clinical anti-inflammatory effects, because inflammation is associated with a markedly increased expression of the COX-2 enzyme. With the discovery of a COX-1 splice variant and studies showing that it is both highly expressed in brain and more sensitive to inhibition by acetaminophen, some investigators proposed that the analgesic and antipyretic actions of acetaminophen could be explained by its ability to inhibit the COX-1 splice variants (called COX-3 by some investigators, despite the fact that this variant does not arise from a unique gene).[21] Nevertheless, more recent studies have rejected this mechanism as explanatory for the effects of acetaminophen.[20,22]

Salicylate has analgesic, antipyretic, and anti-inflammatory activity, but, similar to acetaminophen and in contrast to ASA, it is a poor COX inhibitor. Salicylate also inhibits COX activity if substrate levels are low, and it is also dependent on the oxidative state of the enzyme, suggesting that this drug may inhibit COX by redox-related mechanisms.[23]

Pharmacology and Dosing

Classification

NSAIDs are generally grouped according to their chemical structures, plasma half-life, and COX-1 versus COX-2 selectivity (Table 62.1 and Fig. 62.2). Table 62.1 presents a representative compilation of common NSAIDs, formulations, dosages, half-lives, and precautions. Structurally, most NSAIDs are organic acids with low pK values that lend themselves to their accumulation at sites of inflammation—areas that often exhibit lower pH values than do uninvolved sites. The persistence of NSAIDs in the synovial fluid is associated with a sustained therapeutic effect, despite relatively rapid clearance from the plasma, vascular wall, and kidneys.[24] Usually a direct relationship exists between low pK and a short half-life, but there are exceptions, such as nabumetone, which is nonacidic. Classifying NSAIDs on the basis of plasma half-life can be problematic for the treatment of joint inflammation, given the fact that these drugs tend to accumulate in synovial fluid, where the concentration of the drug may remain more stable than in the plasma. Short–half-life NSAIDs potentially could be given less frequently than indicated by their plasma half-life. NSAIDs exhibiting longer half-lives require more time to reach steady-state plasma levels. Drugs with a half-life greater than 12 hours can be given once or twice a day. Plasma levels increase for a few days to several weeks (depending on the specific half-life) but then tend to remain constant between doses. NSAIDs with longer half-lives also enable drug concentrations to equilibrate between the plasma and the synovial fluid, although total bound and unbound drug levels are usually lower in synovial fluid because less albumin is present in synovial fluid than in plasma. Nevertheless, NSAIDs with longer half-lives or extended-release formulation may be associated with an increased propensity to cause adverse effects.[25] COX-isozyme selectivity is likely to be a critically important factor in determining relative GI and cardiovascular risk, which also should be considered in addition to other pharmacologic properties for each NSAID.[15]

NSAID Metabolism

Almost all NSAIDs are more than 90% bound to plasma proteins. If total drug concentrations are increased beyond the point at which the binding sites on albumin are saturated, biologically active free drug concentrations increase disproportionately to the increasing total drug concentration. The clearance of NSAIDs is usually by hepatic metabolism, with production of inactive metabolites that are excreted in the bile and urine. Most NSAIDs are metabolized through the microsomal cytochrome P450-containing mixed-function oxidase system. NSAIDs are most often metabolized by CYP3A, CYP2C9, or both. Some NSAIDs, however, are metabolized by other cytosolic hepatic enzymes.

TABLE 62.1 Common Nonsteroidal Anti-inflammatory Drugs

Drug	Brand Names	Available Formulations (mg)	Maximal Daily Dose (mg)	Tmax (hr)	Half-life (hr)	Dose Adjustment or Special Precautions
Salicylic Acids						
Acetylsalicylic acid	Aspirin	Tablets: 81, 165, 325, 500, 650	3000	0.5	4-6	Decrease dose by 50% in patients with renal failure and hepatic insufficiency
		Children's: 81				
		Suppository: 120, 200, 300, 600				
Salsalate	Disalcid	Capsule: 500	3000	1.4	1	
	Amigesic	Tablet: 500, 750				
	Salflex					
Diflunisal	Dolobid	Tablets: 250, 500	1500	2-3	7-15	Decrease dose by 50% in patients with renal failure
Acetic Acids						
Diclofenac	Voltaren	Tablets: 25, 50, 75	225	1-2	2	Incidence of increased transaminase levels higher than with other NSAIDs
	Voltaren XR	Extended release: 100				
	Cataflam					
Diclofenac + misoprostol	Arthrotec	Tablets: 50 or 75 plus misoprostol 200 μg	200	1-2	2	Incidence of increased transaminase levels higher than with other NSAIDs
Indomethacin	Indocin	Caps: 25, 50	200	1-4	2-13	Approved for treatment of patent ductus arteriosus
	Indocin SR	Sustained release: 75				
		Oral suspension: 25 mg/5 mL				
		Suppositories: 50				
Sulindac	Clinoril	Tablets: 150, 200	400	2-4	16	Prodrug metabolized to active compound
						Decrease dose in patients with renal and liver disease and in elderly patients
Ketorolac	Toradol	IM/IV: 15 or 30 mg/mL	120 IV/IM	0.3-1	4-6	Decrease dose by 50% in patients with renal failure and in elderly patients
		Tablets: 10	40 mg PO			Do not use >5 days
Tolmetin	Tolectin	Tablets: 200, 600	1800	0.5-1	1-1.5	
		Caps: 400				
Etodolac	Lodine	Caps: 200, 300	1200	1-2	6-7	
	Lodine XL	Tablets: 400				
		Extended release: 400, 500, 600				
Propionic Acids						
Ibuprofen	Motrin	Tablets: 200 (OTC), 300, 400, 600, 800	3200	1-2	2	Avoid use in patients with severe hepatic disease
	Advil					
	Nuprin					
	Rufen					

Continued

TABLE 62.1 **Common Nonsteroidal Anti-Inflammatory Drugs—cont'd**

Drug	Brand Names	Available Formulations (mg)	Maximal Daily Dose (mg)	Tmax (hr)	Half-life (hr)	Dose Adjustment or Special Precautions
Naproxen	Naprosyn	Tablets: 125 (OTC), 250, 375, 500	1375	2-4	12-15	Decrease dose in patients with renal and liver disease and in elderly patients
	Aleve	Sustained release: 375, 500				
	Anaprox	Suspension: 125 mg/5 mL				
	EC-Naprosyn					
	Naprelan					
Fenoprofen	Nalfon	Caps: 200, 300, 600	3200	1-2	2-3	Idiosyncratic nephropathy more frequent than with other NSAIDs
Ketoprofen	Orudis	Tablets: 12.5 (OTC)	300	0.5-2	2-4	Decrease dose in patients with severe renal disease and hepatic disease and in elderly patients
	Oruvail	Caps: 25, 50, 75				
		Sustained release: 100, 150, 200				
Flurbiprofen	Ansaid	Tablets: 50, 100	300	1.5-2	3-4	
Oxaprozin	Daypro	Tablets: 600	1800 or 26 mg/kg/day	3-6	49-60	Decrease dose in patients with renal failure and patients who weigh <50 kg
Fenamic Acids						
Meclofenamate	Meclomen	Caps: 50, 100	400	0.5	2-3	
Oxicams						
Piroxicam	Feldene	Caps: 10, 20	20	2-5	3-86	Decrease dose in patients with hepatic disease and in elderly patients
Meloxicam	Mobic	Tab: 7.5, 15	15	5-6	20	
Nonacidic Compounds						
Nabumetone	Relafen	Tablets: 500, 750	2000	3-6	24	Food increases peak concentration
						Reduce dose in patients with renal disease
						Avoid in patients with severe liver disease
						Limit dose to 1 g/day in elderly patients
COX-2 Selective Inhibitors						
Celecoxib	Celebrex	Caps: 100, 200, 400	400 (800 mg in FAP)	3	11	Contraindicated in people with a sulfonamide allergy
Etoricoxib[a]	Arcoxia	Tablets: 60, 90, 120	120	1-1.5	22	Contraindicated in patients with severe renal or liver disease
						Caution in patients with mild to moderate disease

[a]Not approved by the U.S. Food and Drug Administration.

COX-2, Cyclooxygenase-2; *FAP*, familial adenomatous polyposis; *IM/IV*, intramuscular/intravenous; *OTC*, over the counter; *PO*, oral.

Salicylate Metabolism and Aspirin Resistance

Salicylates are acetylated (e.g., aspirin) or nonacetylated (e.g., sodium salicylate, choline salicylate, choline magnesium trisalicylate, and salicylsalicylic acid).[23] Although the nonacetylated salicylates are only weak inhibitors of COX in vitro, they are able to reduce inflammation in vivo. After oral administration, aspirin crosses the gastric or small bowel mucosa with a bioavailability of 40% to 50%.[26] There is substantial hydrolysis to salicylic acid by plasma and endothelial esterases before entering the systemic circulation. The plasma half-life is approximately 15 to 20 minutes across a range of doses. Approximately 50% of absorbed aspirin is conjugated

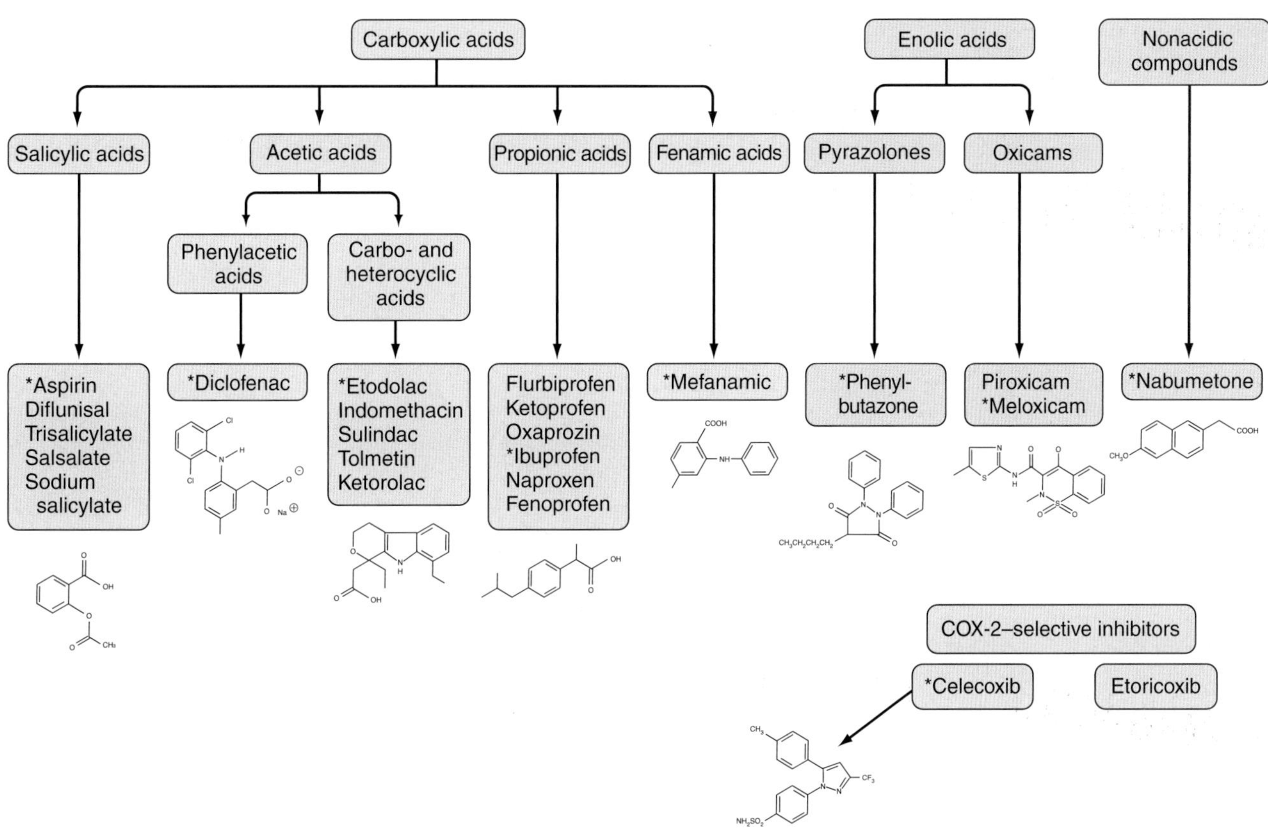

• **Fig. 62.2** Classification and representative structures of the traditional NSAIDs and cyclooxygenase-2 (COX-2)–selective NSAIDs. *Selected NSAID structure from each subclass.

during first-pass hepatic metabolism. Platelet COX-1 inhibition occurs primarily in the portal circulation. It is thought that more than 95% inhibition of COX-1-derived thromboxane A_2 (TXA_2) is necessary to inhibit platelet aggregation.

Differences in the formulation of salicylates affect the absorption properties but not bioavailability. Buffered aspirin tablets contain antacids that increase the pH of the microenvironment, whereas enteric coating slows absorption. The bioavailability of rectal aspirin suppositories increases with retention time. Salicylates primarily bind to albumin and rapidly diffuse into most body fluids. Salicylate is metabolized principally by the liver and excreted primarily by the kidney. In the kidney, salicylate and its metabolites are freely filtered by the glomerulus, then reabsorbed and secreted by the tubules. Salicylate serum levels usually do not correlate well with dosage, however, and small increases in dosage may result in disproportionate increases in serum levels. The drug clearance rate is a function of serum concentration. The primary factors regulating serum salicylate levels are urinary pH and metabolic enzyme activity.

The term *aspirin resistance* is broadly used to describe the failure of aspirin to prevent a thrombotic event, whether as a result of pharmacologic resistance to the anti-platelet effects of aspirin or the inability of aspirin to overcome thrombophilia in a given clinical setting.[27] A more precise definition centers on the biochemical determination using various ex vivo assays. The classification of aspirin resistance can be pharmacokinetic, where there is a failure of in vivo aspirin to inhibit aggregation and thromboxane formation that can be overcome by the addition of aspirin in vitro. This type of aspirin resistance may be overcome by increasing the dose. Pharmacodynamic resistance is a failure of both in vivo and in vitro aspirin to inhibit aggregation and thromboxane formation. Pseudoresistance is a failure of both in vivo and in vitro aspirin to inhibit aggregation, despite appropriate inhibition of thromboxane formation. Mechanisms for aspirin treatment resistance may include poor absorption due to drugs such as proton-pump inhibitors, esterase-mediated metabolism, NSAID interference with COX-1 binding or COX-1 polymorphisms, regeneration of platelet COX-1 or alternative sources of TXA_2, and TXA_2-independent platelet activation.[26]

Pharmacologic Variability

Different patients can respond to the same NSAID in a variety of ways, and the basis for this individual variability remains unclear. Several pharmacologic factors related to NSAIDs may influence this variability, such as dose response, plasma half-life, enantiomeric conversion, urinary excretion, and pharmacodynamic variation.[24] Other important drug factors include protein binding, the metabolic profile of the drug, and the percentage of the drug that is available as the active *(S)* enantiomer. Some NSAIDs exist as two enantiomers; these NSAIDs include the propionic acid derivatives ibuprofen, ketoprofen, and flurbiprofen, which exist as mixtures of inactive *(R)* and active *(S)* enantiomers. Naproxen is composed of the active *(S)* enantiomer. Conversion of the propionic acid NSAIDs from the inactive *(R)* enantiomer to the active *(S)* enantiomer occurs in vivo to various degrees, providing some basis for the variability in patient response. Genetic variability also exists in the cytochrome P450 metabolic enzymes, and consequently some people or ethnic groups metabolize drugs more slowly. For example, Asians frequently experience slow metabolism through the CYP2C9 pathway. A number of single-nucleotide polymorphisms in the genetic sequence of *CYP2C9* have been described, and the product of one of these altered genes, CYP2C9*2, is associated with reduced metabolism of celecoxib and an accompanying increase in plasma concentration of the drug.[24] Finally, the pharmacokinetics of some NSAIDs are affected by hepatic disease, renal disease, or old age.

Routes of Drug Delivery

NSAIDs are produced in a variety of dosage forms, including intravenous, slow-release, and sustained-release oral preparations; topical preparations in various forms, including gels and patches; and suppositories. Given the desire to reduce NSAID toxicity while preserving drug delivery to a specific site, efforts continue to alter drug formulation and delivery systems. Nanoparticles, liposomes, and microspheres are under investigation to allow dose reduction and specific targeting. Strategies for encapsulation must take into account selection of carrier type and encapsulation method, with most focused at the nanoscale (1 to 100 nm in at least one dimension).[28]

Topical NSAID formulations were developed to reduce systemic exposure while preserving efficacy. Diclofenac, for example, is available as a solution, gel, or patch. The systemic effects are directly proportional to the surface area, and this method of delivery results in a relatively stable systemic level of diclofenac compared with oral administration.[29]

Combination Drugs and Prodrugs

NSAIDs have also been combined with agents that have gastroprotective effects in the form of "polypills" that are currently available on the market. This strategy may increase compliance with effective protective agents, thereby reducing adverse effects in clinical practice. Combining diclofenac with the synthetic PGE_1 analogue misoprostol reduces the risk of NSAID-related peptic ulcerations and mucosal injury, but utility of the combination is often limited by misoprostol-induced cramping and diarrhea. In population-based studies, the combination pill was more effective than diclofenac and misoprostol co-prescription in preventing hospitalization for peptic ulcer disease or GI hemorrhage. The combination of enteric-coated naproxen and the proton pump inhibitor (PPI) esomeprazole, as well as combination ibuprofen with famotidine, into single pills has also been approved by the FDA.

Other strategies for improved safety have been tested, including NO- or H_2S-releasing NSAIDs, which are designed to release vasodilatory molecules that protect the gastrointestinal and/or cardiovascular systems from NSAID-related adverse effects. These compounds have not been approved by the FDA for treatment of arthritis. One agent, naproxcinod, was extensively studied in patients with OA, but failed to receive FDA approval for this indication as it failed to demonstrate noninferiority to naproxen.[30]

Therapeutic Effects

Anti-inflammatory Effects

NSAIDs are frequently used as first-line agents for the symptomatic relief of many different inflammatory conditions. In double-blind, randomized clinical trials of inflammatory arthritis, NSAIDs have been compared with placebo, aspirin, and each other. Clinical trials of NSAID efficacy in RA (and OA) usually employ a design whereby the current NSAID is discontinued and the patient must have an increase in symptoms or flare to enter the study. Although primary outcome measures have some variation, most include parameters that make up the American College of Rheumatology (ACR)20. Efficacy superior to that of placebo is easily demonstrated for NSAIDs within 1 to 2 weeks in patients with active RA who are not receiving corticosteroids or other anti-inflammatory medications.[31] Comparisons of adequate doses of traditional NSAIDs or COX-2–selective NSAIDs with one another almost always show comparable efficacy. Despite improvement in pain and stiffness with NSAIDs, these agents do not usually reduce acute phase reactants, nor do they modify radiographic progression. The anti-inflammatory effects of NSAIDs have also been demonstrated in rheumatic fever, juvenile RA, ankylosing spondylitis, gout, OA, and systemic lupus erythematosus (SLE). Although not as rigorously proven, their efficacy is also accepted in treatment of reactive arthritis, psoriatic arthritis, acute and chronic bursitis, and tendinitis.

Analgesic Effects

Virtually all NSAIDs relieve pain when used in doses substantially lower than those required to suppress inflammation. The analgesic action of NSAIDs is due to inhibition of PG production in peripheral tissues and in the CNS. In the periphery, PGs do not induce pain per se but rather sensitize peripheral nociceptors to the effects of mediators, such as bradykinin or histamine.[32] PGs released during inflammation or other trauma lower the activation threshold of tetrodotoxin-resistant sodium channels on sensory neurons. In the CNS, where NSAIDs and acetaminophen exert analgesic effects, PGs also play an important role in neuronal sensitization. COX-2 is constitutively expressed in the dorsal horn of the spinal cord, and its expression is increased during inflammation.[32] Centrally generated PGE_2 activates spinal neurons and also microglia that contribute to neuropathic pain.[33] Both COX-1 and COX-2 play a role in nociception as demonstrated by reductions in experimental pain in mice deficient in either COX-1 or COX-2.[34]

Antipyretic Effects

The NSAIDs and acetaminophen effectively suppress fever in humans and in animals included in experiments. Fever results from the production of PG, primarily PGE_2, from vascular endothelial cells via COX-2 and mPGES-1.[35] These PGs generate neuronal signals that activate the thermoregulatory center in the preoptic area of the anterior hypothalamus. PGE_2 synthesis is stimulated by endogenous (e.g., IL-1) or exogenous (e.g., LPS) pyrogens. Mice with a targeted deletion of either the COX-2 or mPGES-1 genes fail to develop fever in response to inflammatory stimuli.[36]

Little evidence suggests that any NSAID has superior efficacy as an antipyretic agent. In fever associated with viral illnesses, however, aspirin should be avoided because of the association with hepatocellular failure (Reye's syndrome).[37]

Disease and Symptom-Modifying Effects

There is little evidence that NSAIDs exert any disease-modifying effects in OA or RA, despite the effects of PG on multiple joint tissues and symptomatic improvement. A systematic review and meta-analysis of patients with knee osteoarthritis, which included 72 randomized controlled trials and more than 26,000 participants, concluded that NSAIDs demonstrate moderate, statistically significant effects on pain and function that peak at 2 weeks and begin to decline by 8 weeks. The magnitude of the effect on symptoms decreases over time, and GI adverse events are significantly increased as early as 4 weeks after initiation of treatment.[38] A recent review of NSAIDs in patients with OA concluded that there was no evidence of disease modification.[39] There is, however, some evidence that NSAIDs may reduce progression of spondyloarthritis.[40–42] A recent review examined the benefits and harms of NSAIDs in axial spondyloarthritis (axSpA), finding that high-quality evidence indicates that both traditional and COX-2 NSAIDs are efficacious for treating axSpA, and harms are not different from placebo in the short term. Furthermore, various NSAIDs are equally effective.[41] NSAIDs are recommended as first-line treatment for ankylosing spondylitis and nonradiographic axial spondyloarthritis.[43,44]

Other Therapeutic Effects

Anti-platelet Effects

Aspirin and traditional NSAIDs inhibit platelet COX-1 to variable degrees. Except for aspirin, inhibition of platelet aggregation is reversible and depends on the concentration of drug in the platelet. Aspirin acetylates platelet COX-1, which cannot be resynthesized. The antiaggregation effect of as little as 80 mg of aspirin can last for up to 4 to 6 days, until the bone marrow can synthesize new platelets.[45]

On the basis of accumulated data showing its benefits, the FDA has approved ASA for use in the secondary prevention of cardiovascular disease. Major trials have shown that meaningful decreases in nonfatal myocardial infarction (MI), nonfatal stroke, and death can be realized by daily administration of ASA of 75 to 325 mg. Major vascular events can be reduced by 10 to 20 events for every 1000 patients treated, at a cost of one to two major GI bleeds.[46]

In the Nurses Health Study of primary prevention of major vascular events, no reduction in rates of MI was observed with the use of ASA, 100 mg every other day, whereas rates of GI bleeding were increased. Stroke rates, however, were significantly reduced with use of this regimen.[47] Several additional large studies of primary prevention were published in 2018 that addressed the issue of primary prevention of cardiovascular events. A study of participants with a moderate to high risk of cardiovascular events was unable to find a significant reduction in incidence of first occurrence of confirmed myocardial infarction, stroke, cardiovascular death, unstable angina, or transient ischemic attack.[48] The study had lower than expected event rates, perhaps reflecting the modern approach to cardiovascular disease prevention. Another large study of participants with diabetes but no evident cardiovascular disease found a reduction of cardiovascular events over 7.4 years.[49] In patients older than 70, there was no benefit of aspirin for prevention of cardiovascular disease.[50] Nevertheless, a systematic review and meta-analysis that included more than 164,000 participants with more than a million participant-years of follow-up—and incorporated results of the recent studies—found a significant absolute risk reduction for composite cardiovascular outcomes of 38%.[51] All prevention studies demonstrate a significantly increased risk for gastrointestinal bleeding. Thus risk of both benefit and harms must be considered. The U.S. Preventive Services Task Force updated its recommendations for primary prevention of cardiovascular disease and colorectal cancer in 2016.[52] There was insufficient evidence to assess the balance of benefits and harms for individuals younger than 50 or older than 70 years of age, but they recommended initiating aspirin in adults aged 50 to 59 with a 10% or greater 10-year cardiovascular risk who are not at increased risk for bleeding, have a life expectancy of at least 10 years, and are willing to take low-dose aspirin daily for at least 10 years. Additionally, they stated that the decision to initiate low-dose aspirin in individuals aged 60 to 69 should be individualized according to whether there is a higher value on the potential benefits than the potential harms.

Cancer Chemoprevention

A large body of epidemiologic and animal studies provides evidence that a high-fat diet can be associated with a risk for cancer. AA, one of the major ingredients of animal fats, and the eicosanoids derived from AA are important contributors to the development of cancer.[53] Large-scale epidemiologic studies have long indicated that long-term NSAID use reduces the incidence of a variety of cancers, including colon, intestinal, gastric, breast, and bladder, by 40% to 50%.[53] Given the ability of NSAIDs to inhibit COX and PG production, the COX pathway immediately becomes implicated as playing an important role in the pathogenic process. It is well recognized that growth factors, tumor promoters, and oncogenes stimulate PG production via the induction of COX-2 and that human tumorigenic tissues exhibit increased COX activity compared with their normal, nontumorigenic counterparts. COX-2 is overexpressed in 80% of colorectal cancer tissues. Among the PGs, PGE_2 is most abundant in human neoplasms. The inducible mPGES-1 enzyme is highly expressed in tumors, and its absence suppresses intestinal tumorigenesis in animal models. Furthermore, the enzyme that metabolizes intra-cellular PGE_2, 15-hydroxyprostaglandin dehydrogenase, is ubiquitously lacking in tumors, and mice with a genetic deletion of this enzyme have accelerated tumorigenesis.[53] Many natural products, including resveratrol (red wine), catechins (green tea), and curcumin (saffron), also inhibit COX, which may be an important mechanism underlying their putative cancer-preventing effects.[54]

A retrospective cohort study shows that aspirin and traditional NSAIDs specifically reduce cancer risk in the subgroup of patients whose colon tumors express higher levels of COX-2.[55] In a meta-analysis of the effects of ASA (75 mg daily and upward without dose dependence) on cancer, allocation to receive aspirin reduced death due to cancer by more than 20%.[56] Upon analysis of individual patient data, a cancer death benefit was apparent only after 5 years of follow-up, and the benefit increased with scheduled duration of trial treatment. ASA effects appear to be greater on adenomatous cancer than on other cancer types. Other studies demonstrated a reduction in both the incidence of colorectal cancer and death from colorectal cancer, particularly for cancers of the proximal colon.[56] Long-term low-dose ASA use also appears to reduce the risk of prostate cancer.[57]

Clinical trials also demonstrated that traditional and COX-2–selective NSAIDs could cause regression of polyps in patients with familial adenomatous polyposis (FAP).[58] Celecoxib was subsequently approved by the FDA for reduction of polyps in patients with FAP. A prospective study of primary prevention for colorectal adenomas comparing eicosapentaenoic acid (EPA) with aspirin alone and in combination found that neither agent was associated with a reduction in the proportion of patients with at least one colorectal adenoma in individuals at high risk. There was, however, an effect on colorectal adenoma burden as measured by a reduction in the mean number of adenomas per participant.[59]

TABLE 62.2 Shared Toxicities of Nonsteroidal Anti-inflammatory Drugs

Organ System	Toxicity
Gastrointestinal	Dyspepsia Esophagitis Gastroduodenal ulcers Ulcer complications (bleeding, perforation, obstruction) Small bowel erosions and strictures Colitis
Renal	Sodium retention Weight gain and edema Hypertension Type IV renal tubular acidosis and hyperkalemia Acute renal failure Papillary necrosis Acute interstitial nephritis Accelerated chronic kidney disease
Cardiovascular	Heart failure Myocardial infarction Stroke Cardiovascular death
Hepatic	Elevated transaminases Reye's syndrome (aspirin only)
Asthma/allergic	Aspirin-exacerbated respiratory disease[a] (susceptible patients) Rash
Hematologic	Cytopenias
Neurologic	Dizziness, confusion, drowsiness Seizures Aseptic meningitis
Bone	Delayed healing

[a]Reduced risk in cyclooxygenase-2–selective NSAIDs.

Adverse Effects

NSAIDs share a common spectrum of clinical toxicities, although the frequency of particular adverse effects varies with the compound (Table 62.2). The hazard of individual NSAIDs is related to their pharmacologic characteristics, such as bioavailability and half-life, as well as their potency for inhibition of COX-1 and COX-2.[15,25,60]

Gastrointestinal Tract Effects

Gastrointestinal injury is by far the most common adverse event in individuals taking NSAIDs. NSAIDs cause GI injury through both topical and systemic effects. In addition to inhibiting COX-1 and COX-2, their physicochemical property of being lipid-soluble weak acids provides them with detergent action and interaction with phospholipids.[61] NSAIDs interact with the intestinal mucus layer and the cell surface phospholipid layer. Mucus acts as a lubricant between the surface epithelium and the luminal contents, restricting access of large hydrophilic molecules, digestive enzymes, and bacteria to the surface epithelium. Mucus also acts to buffer luminal acids in the stomach. The production and secretion of mucus is determined by interactions between luminal agents, such as acid, pepsin, and *Helicobacter pylori* in the stomach or bile and bacteria in the small bowel. Mucus also serves as a matrix for phospholipids that maintain GI integrity. Because NSAIDs decrease the hydrophobicity in GI mucosa, the protective functions of mucus are compromised.[61] NSAIDs also uncouple mitochondrial oxidative phosphorylation due to ion trapping, leading to reduction in ATP production and apoptosis of endothelial cells. COX-2-selective agents, such as celecoxib, do not uncouple oxidative phosphorylation.[61] In general, nonacidic NSAIDs such as nabumetone, etodolac, and celecoxib do not cause acute mucosal lesions. Esterification of acidic NSAIDs, as in the case of NO-NSAIDs, suppress mucosal injury.[62]

After a mucosal injury occurs, however, NSAIDs inhibit the early events necessary to repair superficial injury, as well as later events of cell proliferation and angiogenesis, leading to delayed ulcer healing through inhibition of COX-1 and COX-2.[63] The mechanism is likely related to reduced microvascular flow and mucus section and increased acid secretion.[61] Thus topical injury initiates the initial mucosal erosions by disrupting the gastric epithelial cell barrier, but PG depletion is essential for the development of clinically significant gastric and duodenal ulcers. The integrity of mucosal defense depends on generation of PGE_2 and PGI_2 from COX enzymes. COX-1 is abundantly expressed under basal conditions in gastric mucosa, whereas COX-2 is almost undetectable. Nevertheless, both COX-1 and COX-2 are rapidly upregulated after injury or when pre-existing ulcers are present,[64] which may explain the observation that concurrent *H. pylori* infection increases the risk of developing peptic ulcers and increases bleeding in people who use NSAIDs.[65]

It appears that concurrent COX-1 and COX-2 inhibition is associated with the highest propensity to develop gastric ulcers.[25] This clinical observation is consistent with animal studies whereby mice deficient for a single COX enzyme or treated with drugs that specifically inhibit either COX-1 or COX-2 do not develop ulceration. Severe gastric lesions are seen when both enzymes are simultaneously blocked. When the gastric mucosa is damaged, however, inhibition of either COX-1 or COX-2 is associated with the development of ulcers.[63] Traditional and COX-2–selective NSAIDs delay ulcer healing, with nonselective NSAIDs doing so to a greater degree.[66] It also should be noted that GI bleeding may be related to the combination of injury and inhibition of platelet aggregation, which is an additional factor in the propensity of aspirin and other nonselective NSAIDs to cause clinically apparent ulcers.[62,63] Risk factors for developing gastrointestinal toxicity are shown in Fig. 62.3.

Major Gastrointestinal Toxicity

Recent prospective trials have been conducted to determine the risk of clinically important GI toxicity, comparing celecoxib, a COX-2-selective NSAID, with traditional NSAIDs. A large (>8000 participants) prospective, randomized, open label, blinded endpoint study compared celecoxib with other NSAIDs for adjudicated upper and lower GI adverse events in OA patients.[67] Patients using aspirin were excluded and PPIs or H_2 blockers were used by discretion. Randomization was stratified by baseline *H. pylori* status, which was present in 33% of the participants. Clinically significant adverse outcomes were seen in 1.3% of patients randomized to celecoxib and 2.4% of patients randomized to other NSAIDs. These rates increased to 1.8% and 2.5% respectively, in *H. pylori*–positive patients. PPI or histamine-2 receptor antagonists (H2RA) were taken by approximately 22% of

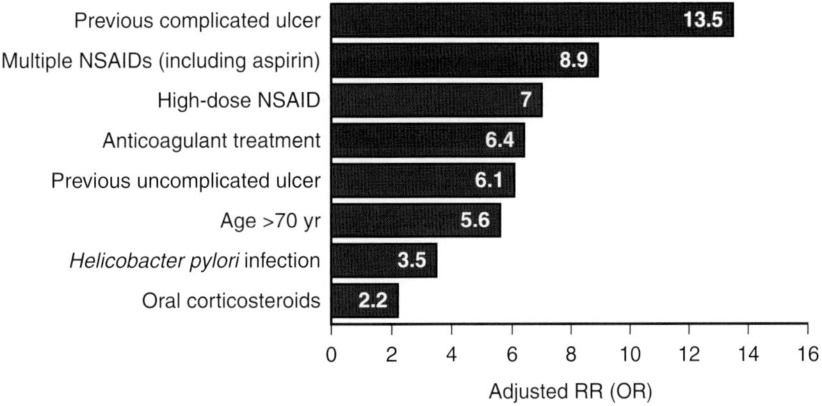

• **Fig. 62.3** Established risk factors for upper gastrointestinal bleeding associated with NSAID use. *OR,* Odds ratio; *RR,* relative risk. (Modified from Gutthann SP, García-Rodríguez LA, Raiford DS: Individual non-steroidal anti-inflammatory drugs and other risk factors for upper gastrointestinal bleeding and perforation. *Epidemiology* 8:18–24, 1997; Huang JQ, Sridhar S, Hunt RH: Role of Helicobacter pylori infection and non-steroidal anti-inflammatory drugs in peptic ulcer disease: a meta-analysis. *Lancet* 359:14–22, 2002; and Lanas A, García-Rodríguez LA, Arroyo MT, et al.: Risk of upper gastrointestinal ulcer bleeding associated with selective cyclooxygenase-2 inhibitors, traditional non-aspirin non-steroidal anti-inflammatory drugs, aspirin and combinations. *Gut* 55:1731–1738, 2006.)

participants in each group. The rates of clinically significant GI events and anemia were higher in the PPI groups, likely due to confounding by indication.

A very large (>20,000 participants), blinded, prospective safety study comparing celecoxib, naproxen, and ibuprofen, the Prospective Randomized Evaluation of Celecoxib Integrated Safety versus Ibuprofen or Naproxen (PRECISION) study, found hazard ratios of adjudicated clinically significant GI events in the intention-to-treat (ITT) population were not significantly different. Clinically important gastrointestinal events were defined as gastroduodenal hemorrhage; gastric outlet obstruction; perforation of the gastroduodenum, small bowel, or large bowel; or symptomatic gastric or duodenal ulcer. According to analysis of data while participants were on treatment or 30 days after, among the modified intention-to-treat (mITT) population, clinically significant events occurred in 0.34%, 0.73%, and 0.66% of those taking celecoxib, ibuprofen, and naproxen, respectively, with clinically significantly lower hazard ratios favoring celecoxib. In the PRECISION study, all participants were prescribed a PPI and the overall risk was low. The composite endpoint, which included clinically significant gastrointestinal events and iron deficiency anemia, demonstrated significantly fewer events in the celecoxib group in both the ITT and mITT analyses.[68–70]

In a very high-risk group of patients with endoscopy-documented upper gastrointestinal ulcers who were on NSAIDs and required aspirin for cardiovascular risk, a randomized double-blind trial demonstrated a cumulative incidence of recurrent bleeding over 18 months of 5.6% in patients randomized to celecoxib plus esomeprazole and 12.3% in patients randomized to naproxen plus esomeprazole. The crude hazard ratio was 0.44 (95% confidence interval [CI], 0.23 to 9.2). The adjudicated outcome was hematemesis or melena documented by the admitting physician, with ulcers or bleeding erosions confirmed by endoscopy or a decrease in hemoglobin of at least 2 g/cL in the presence of endoscopically proven ulcers or bleeding erosions. In this study, an additional 22 participants, 7 in each group, had lower gastrointestinal bleeding.[71]

Dyspepsia

Nonulcer dyspepsia is the most common adverse event (10% to 20%) associated with use of NSAIDs and may account for poor tolerability.[72] Dyspepsia is more often reported in younger than in older patients.[73] Although they are expected to reduce dyspepsia, COX-2–selective NSAIDs are also associated with a substantial level of adverse GI symptoms.[72] PPIs reduce dyspepsia in controlled trials.[66] Studies have shown that H2RAs are also effective for reducing dyspepsia.[74] Crucially from a clinical perspective, subjective symptoms of dyspepsia, fecal blood loss, and endoscopic findings correlate poorly. Furthermore, only a minority of patients with serious GI events report antecedent dyspepsia.[75]

Gastritis and Gastroduodenal Ulcer

Older studies, generally in individuals not using gastroprotective agents, demonstrated that up to 25% of long-term NSAID users will experience ulcer disease, and 2% to 4% of the ulcers will bleed or perforate. These GI events result in more than 100,000 hospital admissions annually in the United States and between 7000 and 10,000 deaths, especially in patients with the highest risk.[76] The risk for ulcer complications appears highest within the first 3 months of use but remains present with longer-term therapy. A meta-analysis of observational studies on NSAIDs and upper GI bleeding or perforation published between 2000 and 2008 demonstrated a relative risk of 4.50 (95% CI, 3.82 to 5.31) for traditional NSAIDs and 1.88 (95% CI, 0.96 to 3.71) for selective COX-2 inhibitors.[25] For traditional NSAIDs, low and medium doses were associated with a lower risk than were higher doses. Drugs with a long half-life or slow-release formulation were associated with higher risk, even accounting for dose.[25] Profound and coincident inhibition of both COX-1 and COX-2 using whole blood assay, as seen for ketorolac, piroxicam, naproxen, ketoprofen, and indomethacin, was associated with a relative risk of greater than 5 for GI bleeding and perforation.[25] The use of low-dose aspirin, even in the absence of other risk factors, increases risk for bleeding and death. Many patients taking low-dose aspirin may do so without the knowledge of their physician, and thus it is essential to query patients specifically on this point.

TABLE 62.3 Strategies for Gastrointestinal Risk Reduction[47]

Gastrointestinal Risk	Potential Strategies
Low risk	Intermittent NSAID use Low-dose NSAID
Moderate risk (1-2 risk factors) Age >65 yr High-dose NSAID Previous history of uncomplicated ulcer Concurrent use of aspirin, corticosteroids, or anti-coagulants	COX-2 selective NSAID Intermittent NSAID use NSAID + PPI NSAID + misoprostol NSAID + high-dose H2RA[a]
High risk >2 Risk factors History of previous complicated ulcer, especially recent	Alternative treatment COX-2–selective NSAID + PPI COX-2–selective NSAID + misoprostol
Helicobacter pylori positive	Consider eradication in moderate- to high-risk patients

[a]Less effective than PPI or misoprostol.

COX-2, Cyclooxygenase-2; *H2RA,* histamine-2 receptor antagonist; *NSAID,* nonsteroidal anti-inflammatory drug; *PPI,* proton pump inhibitor.

Patient-specific factors influence the overall risk for GI ulcers and ulcer complications (see Fig. 62.3).[76,77] A previous history of ulcer or ulcer complications is an important risk, especially if combined with other risks. Infection with *H. pylori* is likely to be associated with additive effect.[65] It remains unclear if eradication of *H. pylori* would be useful in the primary prevention of NSAID-induced ulcers, but it may be advantageous in patients requiring long-term use of NSAIDs.[76] Eradication alone is insufficient as a single strategy for secondary prevention of ulcer complications. This strategy appears to be most effective in reducing the bleeding risk of patients taking low-dose aspirin but is less useful than use of PPIs in patients taking NSAIDs.[76]

Table 62.3 provides recommendations for patients who need NSAIDs and have GI risks.[76] Misoprostol is effective in the reduction of gastroduodenal ulcers. Meta-analysis showed a reduction of 74% in gastric ulcers and 53% in duodenal ulcers when compared with placebo.[78] The effectiveness of misoprostol is comparable with the PPI lansoprazole.[79] Nevertheless, the high prevalence of abdominal cramping and diarrhea limit misoprostol use at full doses. For people who do not tolerate full doses (200 µg four times daily), lower doses of 400 to 600 µg/day may be useful and comparable with PPIs.

PPIs have been used extensively for prevention of NSAID-induced ulcers and are also used for ulcer healing. Their excellent tolerability and availability over the counter have led to their dominance as pharmacologic agents for preventing NSAID-induced gastroduodenal ulcers. Studies have shown a reduction in the endoscopic ulcer rate from 17% in patients taking traditional or COX-2–selective NSAIDs plus placebo to 5.2% and 4.6% in patients taking NSAIDs plus esomeprazole 20 mg or 40 mg, respectively.[80] As noted previously, a combination pill containing naproxen and esomeprazole has been approved for use. It may reduce noncompliance but will be associated with higher cost.

High-dose, twice-daily doses of H2RA reduce the risk of NSAID-induced endoscopic ulcers and are the least costly alternative. Nevertheless, these agents are inferior to PPIs and, as with PPIs, no randomized clinical outcome trials have been performed to evaluate the efficacy of H2RAs in long-term users of NSAIDs.[62]

Esophageal Injury

Aspirin and NSAIDs are associated with esophagitis as a result of mechanisms similar to those in the gastric mucosa.[81,82] Esophageal emptying may be slowed in elderly people, resulting in a prolonged exposure of the mucosa to the irritant action of aspirin and NSAIDs. Gastroesophageal reflux may be an aggravating factor and may lead to stricture formation. Bleeding also may complicate esophagitis. NSAIDs should be prescribed with caution in the presence of gastroesophageal reflux disease.

Small Bowel Injury

The availability of video capsule endoscopy (VCE) and balloon enteroscopy has advanced the ability to detect small intestinal lesions in patients taking NSAIDs. NSAIDs can cause a concentric "diaphragm-like" stricture in the small bowel, in addition to causing mucosal injury and bleeding. Two recent studies of patients taking NSAIDs for at least 3 months, using VCE, demonstrated a prevalence for small bowel injuries of 70% to 80%.[83] Furthermore, NSAID-induced small bowel injury is likely a common cause of obscure GI bleeding. NSAIDs that undergo enterohepatic circulation are likely to be associated with higher risk. Small bowel injury may be detected by anemia or symptoms of obstruction related to a stricture.[83] Strategies effective for gastroduodenal ulcers such as misoprostol or certain PPIs also may reduce the risk for small bowel mucosal injury. Strictures may require balloon endoscopy or surgical intervention.[83]

Colitis

NSAIDs cause erosions, ulcers, hemorrhage, perforations, strictures, and complications of diverticulosis in the large bowel.[84] NSAID-induced injury is more common in the right colon (80%) but can occur in the transverse and left colon. Suppositories containing NSAIDs can cause erosions, ulcers, and stenoses in the rectum. NSAID colonopathy is in the differential diagnosis of inflammatory bowel disease. Patients with NSAID-induced colonopathy are typically older, and the erosions are more likely to be transverse or circular.[85] There is also a concern that treatment with traditional and COX-2–selective NSAIDs may exacerbate inflammatory bowel disease.[86] NSAIDs are also implicated in the development of collagenous colitis.[87]

Renal Effects

PGs play a vital role in solute and renovascular homeostasis.[88] PGs are produced by both COX-1 and COX-2, generally in different locations within the kidney, and these PGs may play different physiologic roles in renal function.[89,90] COX-1 is highly expressed in the renal vasculature, glomerular mesangial cells, and collecting duct. COX-2 expression is restricted to the vasculature, cortical thick ascending limb (specifically in cells associated with the macula densa), and medullary interstitial cells. COX-2 expression in the macula densa increases in high-renin states (e.g., salt restriction, angiotensin-converting enzyme inhibition, and renovascular hypertension), and selective COX-2 inhibitors significantly decrease plasma renin levels and renal renin activity. COX-2 expression in the macula densa is reduced by angiotensin II and mineralocorticoids. Dehydration or hypertonicity appears to regulate COX-2 expression in the medullary interstitium. COX-2 is also necessary for normal renal development.

The PRECISION study demonstrated serious renal toxicity in 0.7%, 0.9%, and 1.1% of the celecoxib, naproxen, and ibuprofen groups respectively.[68]

Electrolyte Effects

PGs are known to regulate renal sodium resorption by their ability to inhibit active transport of sodium in both the thick ascending limb and the collecting duct and to increase renal water excretion by blunting the actions of vasopressin.[91] The cellular source of COX-2–derived prostanoids that promote natriuresis remains uncertain, but it is possible that they may in large part be derived from the medullary interstitial cells. Sodium retention has been reported in up to 25% of patients treated with NSAIDs and may be particularly apparent in patients who have an existing avidity for sodium, such as those with mild heart failure or liver disease.[91] Decreased sodium excretion in patients treated with NSAIDs can lead to weight gain and peripheral edema. This effect may be sufficiently important to cause clinically important exacerbations of congestive heart failure.

PGs stimulate renin release, which, in turn, increases secretion of aldosterone and, subsequently, potassium secretion by the distal nephron. For this reason, hyporeninemic hypoaldosteronism, which manifests as type IV renal tubular acidosis and hyperkalemia, may develop in patients treated with NSAIDs.[91] The degree of hyperkalemia is generally mild; however, patients with renal insufficiency or those who may otherwise be prone to hyperkalemia (e.g., patients with diabetes mellitus and those taking angiotensin-converting enzyme inhibitors or potassium-sparing diuretics) may be at greater risk.

Hypertension

NSAIDs may cause altered blood pressure, with average increases of mean arterial pressure of between 5 and 10 mm Hg. In addition, use of NSAIDs may increase the risk of initiating antihypertensive therapy in older patients, with the magnitude of increased risk being proportional to the NSAID dose.[92] Furthermore, in a large (n = 51,630) prospective cohort of women aged 44 to 69 years without hypertension in 1990, incident hypertension during the following 8 years was significantly more likely in frequent users of aspirin, acetaminophen, and NSAIDs.[93] NSAIDs can attenuate the effects of anti-hypertensive agents, including diuretics, angiotensin-converting enzyme inhibitors, and β-blockers, thus interfering with control of blood pressure.

Acute Renal Failure and Papillary Necrosis

Acute renal failure is an uncommon consequence of NSAID treatment. Acute renal failure occurs because of the vasoconstrictive effects of NSAIDs, and it is reversible. In most cases, renal failure occurs in patients who have a depleted actual or effective intravascular volume (e.g., congestive heart failure, cirrhosis, or renal insufficiency).[93] A marked reduction in medullary blood flow may result in papillary necrosis that may arise from apoptosis of medullary interstitial cells. Inhibition of COX-2 may be a predisposing factor.[90,94]

A recent systematic review and meta-analysis of studies evaluating NSAID risk of acute kidney injury in the general population estimated that the pooled odds ratio for current NSAID exposure is 1.73 (95% CI, 1.44 to 2.07) with a higher risk for older people. Eight of 10 studies showed a statistically significant association between NSAID exposure and acute kidney injury. In people with pre-existing chronic kidney disease, the pooled estimate odds ratio is 1.63 (95% CI, 1.22 to 2.19).[95]

Interstitial Nephritis

Another adverse renal effect resulting from NSAIDs involves an idiosyncratic reaction accompanied by massive proteinuria and acute interstitial nephritis. Hypersensitivity phenomena, such as fever, rash, and eosinophilia, may occur. This syndrome has been observed with most NSAIDs.

Chronic Kidney Disease

Use of analgesics, particularly acetaminophen and aspirin, has been associated with nephropathy that leads to chronic renal failure. In one large case-control study, the regular use of aspirin or acetaminophen was associated with a risk of chronic renal failure 2.5 times as high as that for nonuse, and the risk increased significantly with an increasing cumulative lifetime dose.[96] In subjects regularly using both acetaminophen and aspirin, the risk was also significantly increased compared with users of either agent alone. No association between the use of nonaspirin NSAIDs and chronic renal failure could be detected after adjusting for acetaminophen and aspirin use. Pre-existing renal or systemic disease was a necessary precursor to analgesic-associated renal failure, and people without pre-existing renal disease had only a small risk of end-stage renal disease.[96,97]

Cardiovascular Effects

The risk of adverse cardiovascular effects associated with NSAID use was not widely appreciated until COX-2–selective NSAIDs were introduced into clinical practice. Rofecoxib, a potent, highly specific COX-2 inhibitor with a long half-life, has a substantially increased risk of MI and stroke and was removed from the market because of this adverse effect.[7,60] The mechanisms for cardiovascular risks associated with all NSAIDs are likely related to an imbalance between complete inhibition of COX-1 and COX-2 across the dosing interval. The COX-1 isoform is responsible for the generation of platelet thromboxane A_2, which facilitates platelet aggregation and thrombus formation. To inhibit this activity, COX-1 must be inhibited by 95% or greater.[98] Anti-thrombotic PGI_2 synthesized by endothelial COX-2 is inhibited almost completely by both traditional and COX-2–selective NSAIDs. The relationship between excess cardiovascular risk for all NSAIDs, not only COX-2–selective NSAIDs, may be related to the degree of COX-2 inhibition absent complete inhibition of COX-1.[99] Investigators have shown that drugs that inhibit COX-2 less than 90% at therapeutic concentrations in the whole blood assay present a relative risk for MI of 1.18 (95% CI, 1.02 to 1.38), whereas drugs that inhibit COX-2 to a greater degree present a relative risk of 1.60 (95% CI, 1.41 to 1.81).[99]

Relative inhibition of the COX isoforms is not the only mechanism that contributes to cardiovascular hazard. Other actions of NSAIDs, including effects on blood pressure, endothelial function, and NO production, as well as other renal effects, may play a role in cardiovascular risks.[60,100,101] Multiple analyses have demonstrated that the risk for cardiovascular hazard is significantly higher in people with pre-existing coronary artery disease. Some NSAIDs, notably ibuprofen and naproxen, may interfere with the irreversible inhibition of platelet COX-1 by aspirin, thereby increasing the cardiovascular hazard in aspirin users.[99]

A number of large-scale randomized controlled trials comparing NSAIDs with placebo or with each other have been performed and analyzed to determine the risk of MI, stroke, cardiovascular death, death from any cause, and Anti-platelet Trialists' Collaboration (APTC) composite outcomes.[60] A large network meta-analysis of 31 trials with 116,429 patients and more than 115,000 patient-years of follow-up was reported. The authors concluded that there is little evidence that any NSAID is safe in cardiovascular terms, although naproxen is potentially the least harmful.[102] It appears from analyses of these aggregated clinical trials that all traditional and COX-2–selective NSAIDs except naproxen carry an excess risk of more than 30% compared with placebo.[60] Pairwise comparisons of the most commonly used traditional and COX-2–selective NSAIDs studied in clinical trials also suggest that naproxen may have lower cardiovascular risk.[60] Estimation of absolute risk was performed in another comprehensive meta-analysis of clinical trials.[103] Compared with placebo, allocation to a COX-2–selective NSAID (with celecoxib grouped together with rofecoxib and others) or diclofenac caused approximately three additional major vascular events per 1000 participants per year. One meta-analysis explored the effects of dose and dosing regimen in a pooled analysis of six randomized placebo-controlled trials of celecoxib.[104] Lower doses and once-daily regimens were associated with lower relative risks for the APTC outcomes. This finding confirms data from other studies that suggest that avoiding continuous interference with PG biosynthesis is associated with lower cardiovascular risk.[99]

Because clinical trials of NSAID efficacy have been underpowered to specifically address the relative cardiovascular risk of NSAIDs, investigators have turned to observational data sets. Using a large observational database with 8852 cases of nonfatal MI, a recent case-control study also identified a 35% increase in the risk of MI while using NSAIDs.[99] In a nationwide cohort of patients after MI, an increased risk of death or recurrent MI of approximately 50% for patients using NSAIDs was present at the beginning of treatment and persisted throughout the observation period.[105] The largest meta-analysis of observational studies available to date also clearly demonstrates that higher doses of NSAIDs, with the exception of naproxen, increased the risk of serious cardiovascular events.[106] The effect of dose and slow-release formulation demonstrated that risk was a direct consequence of prolonged drug exposure. It appears that the risk associated with these pharmacologic factors may be even more important than COX-2 specificity for most NSAIDs.[60,99]

More recently, large safety studies powered to determine if celecoxib was noninferior to naproxen and ibuprofen (PRECISION) or nonspecific NSAIDs, including ibuprofen, diclofenac, and "other" (the Standard Care Vs Celecoxib Outcome Trial [SCOT]) have been conducted.[68,107] PRECISION was conducted in patients at higher risk, and SCOT was conducted in patients free of pre-existing cardiovascular disease. For both studies, the APTC cardiovascular event rates were lower than predicted. In PRECISION, the APTC outcome occurred in 2.3%, 2.5%, and 2.7% in the celecoxib, naproxen, and ibuprofen ITT population, respectively, and 1.7%, 1.8%, and 1.9% in the mITT population. Noninferiority was demonstrated in both analyses for all treatment groups. The event rate for SCOT was 1.1% in both groups in the ITT and 0.95% and 0.86% in the celecoxib and nonspecific NSAID groups in the mITT. Noninferiority was also demonstrated in this trial. There have been concerns raised around both of these studies because the doses of the comparators were potentially not equipotent, with celecoxib used at the lower end of the dose range. Furthermore, there were substantial instances of participants in both studies discontinuing their assigned group.

A number of strategies have been suggested to mitigate cardiovascular risks associated with NSAID use (Table 62.4).[108] These recommendations take into account a patient's underlying risk, aspirin use, and the interaction between NSAIDs. In addition, the specific choice of NSAID should consider its pharmacologic properties.[60,99,109]

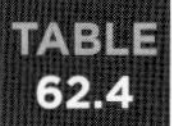

TABLE 62.4 Strategies for Reducing Cardiovascular Risk[a]

If using aspirin, take aspirin dose ≥2 hr before NSAID dose.[b]
Do not use NSAIDs within 3-6 mo of an acute cardiovascular event or procedure.
Carefully monitor and control blood pressure.
Use low-dose, short–half-life NSAIDs and avoid extended-release formulations.

[a]See refs 69, 100, and 108.

[b]Especially ibuprofen. Celecoxib does not appear to interfere with aspirin actions.

NSAID, Nonsteroidal anti-inflammatory drug.

Heart Failure

NSAIDs are associated with reduced sodium excretion, volume expansion, increased preload, and hypertension. As a result of these properties, patients with pre-existing heart failure are at risk of decompensation with a relative risk of 3.8 (95% CI, 1.1 to 12.7). After adjusting for age, sex, and concomitant medication, the relative risk was 9.9 (95% CI, 1.7 to 57.0).[110] Studies disagree as to whether NSAIDs are a risk for new episodes of heart failure, although elderly people may be at particular risk.[110,111] A recent study examining patients who survived first hospitalization for heart failure demonstrated increased risk of death with all NSAIDs at high doses and again demonstrated that lower doses reduced risk for all agents.[112]

Closure of the Ductus Arteriosus

The maintenance of an open ductus arteriosus and its closure during the postnatal period are regulated by PG. COX-1, COX-2, and EP_4-deficient mice die from neonatal circulatory failure because the ductus arteriosus remains open. It is inadvisable for pregnant women to take NSAIDs during the last trimester of pregnancy because of the risk of a persistently patent ductus arteriosus.

Hepatic Effects

Small elevations of one or more liver tests may occur in up to 15% of patients taking NSAIDs, and notable elevations of alanine aminotransferase or aspartate aminotransferase (approximately three or more times the upper limit of normal) have been reported in approximately 1% of patients in clinical trials of NSAIDs. Patients usually have no symptoms, and discontinuation or dose reduction generally results in normalization of the transaminase values, although rare, fatal outcomes have been reported with almost all NSAIDs. The NSAIDs that appear most likely to be associated with hepatic adverse events are diclofenac and sulindac.

In clinical trial reports to the FDA, 5.4% of patients with RA who were treated with aspirin experienced persistent elevations of results in more than one liver function test. In children with viral illnesses, hepatocellular failure and fatty degeneration (Reye's syndrome) are associated with aspirin ingestion.[37]

Asthma and Allergic Reactions

Asthma and Aspirin-Exacerbated Respiratory Disease

Up to 10% to 20% of the general asthmatic population, especially those with the triad of vasomotor rhinitis, nasal polyposis, and asthma, are hypersensitive to aspirin.[113] In these patients, ingestion of aspirin and nonspecific NSAIDs leads to severe exacerbations of asthma with naso-ocular reactions. These patients, who were formerly said to have aspirin-sensitive asthma, are now characterized as having aspirin-exacerbated respiratory disease (AERD) because they have chronic upper and lower respiratory mucosal inflammation, sinusitis, nasal polyposis, and asthma independent of their hypersensitivity reactions. The prevalence of AERD is reported in meta-analysis as 7.2% in the general asthmatic population, 14.9% among those with severe asthma, 9.7% of patients with nasal polyps, and 8.7% of patients with chronic sinusitis.[114] Production of protective PGs in the setting of AERD may be derived from COX-1, not COX-2. According to clinical trial evidence in patients with stable mild-to-moderate asthma with AERD, acute exposure to COX-2 inhibitors is safe, and selective NSAIDs exhibit a small risk. It is thought, therefore, that COX-2 inhibitors could be used in patients with AERD or in patients with general asthma unwilling to risk nonselective NSAID exposure,[115] but the fact that specific COX-2 inhibitors appear safe in people with AERD does not obviate the possibility that other hypersensitivity reactions may occur.

Allergic Reactions

A wide variety of cutaneous reactions have been associated with NSAIDs. Almost all of the NSAIDs have been associated with cutaneous vasculitis, erythema multiforme, Stevens-Johnson syndrome, or toxic epidermal necrolysis. NSAIDs are also associated with urticaria/angioedema and anaphylactoid or anaphylactic reactions. It should be especially noted that celecoxib and valdecoxib contain a sulfonamide group and should not be given to patients who report allergy to drugs containing sulfa.

Hematologic Effects

Aplastic anemia, agranulocytosis, and thrombocytopenia are rarely associated with NSAIDs, but they are prominent among the causes of deaths attributed to these drugs. Because of the risk of hematologic effects, phenylbutazone is no longer recommended for use in any condition in the United States and has been taken off the market.[116]

Central Nervous System Effects

Elderly patients may be particularly susceptible to developing cognitive dysfunction and other CNS effects, including headache, dizziness, depression, hallucination, and seizures, that are related to NSAIDs. Acute aseptic meningitis has been reported in patients with SLE or mixed connective tissue disease who were treated with ibuprofen, sulindac, tolmetin, or naproxen.

Effects on Bone

The complex effects of prostanoids on bone formation and remodeling have been appreciated for many years. It is now clear that COX-2 is required for many functions of both osteoblasts and osteoclasts.[117] COX-2 is rapidly inducible and highly expressed and regulated in osteoblasts. Parathyroid hormone (PTH) is a strong inducer of COX-2. The production of PG by osteoblasts is an important mechanism for the regulation of bone turnover.[117] The major effect of PGE_2 is considered to occur indirectly via upregulation of receptor activator of NF-κB ligand (RANKL) expression and by inhibition of osteoprotegerin (OPG) expression in osteoblastic cells, which facilitates osteoclastogenesis. Genetic deletion of *PTGS2* or COX-2–selective NSAIDs partially block the PTH- or 1,25-OH vitamin D–induced formation of osteoclasts in organ cultures. Recently a familial disorder, primary idiopathic hypertrophic osteoarthropathy, was found to be associated with a mutation in the enzyme 15-hydroxyprostaglandin dehydrogenase, the enzyme that inactivates PGE_2.[118] These patients have chronically elevated PGE_2 levels and digital clubbing with evidence of increased bone formation and resorption in the phalanges.

NSAIDs can inhibit experimental fracture healing and reduce formation of heterotopic bone in patients.[119] Given the effectiveness of NSAIDs as analgesics, it is important to understand the clinical concern regarding impaired fracture healing and NSAIDs. Surgeons often avoid NSAIDs because of their possible influence on bone healing. Nevertheless, there are few high-quality studies, and review articles come to conflicting conclusions regarding the safety of NSAIDs. Systematic reviews conclude that there is no strong evidence that NSAIDs used for pain after fracture osteosynthesis or spinal fusion surgery lead to an increased nonunion rate.[120]

The impact of NSAIDs on bone mineral density (BMD) also remains unclear.[119] In older men, daily use of COX-2–selective NSAIDs was associated with lower hip and spine BMD compared with nonusers, but in post-menopausal women not taking hormone replacement therapy, a higher BMD was found.[121] A study comparing the effects of different analgesics on bone mineral density did not show accelerated decline in new NSAID users.[122]

Effects on Ovarian and Uterine Function

PGs derived from COX-2 have been implicated as mediators in multiple stages of the female reproductive cycle. Induction of COX-2 immediately after the luteinizing hormone surge was the first observation involving the isoenzyme during a normal physiologic event. COX-2–derived PGs may signal the time of ovulation in mammals.[123,124] Studies using COX-2 null mice show reproductive failure at ovulation, fertilization, implantation, and decidualization.[125] COX-2–dependent prostanoid production probably leads to the generation of proteolytic enzymes that rupture the follicles. Continuous use of NSAIDs, especially potent selective COX-2 inhibitors, can induce luteinized unruptured follicle syndrome in women with inflammatory arthritis.[126] After fertilization, COX-2 also plays a role in embryo implantation in the myometrium.[125] PGs are important for inducing uterine contractions during labor. Murine studies have shown that the mechanism of uterine contraction involves fetal release of $PGF_{2\alpha}$, a compound that induces luteolysis. This pathway leads to reduced maternal progesterone levels, induction of oxytocin receptors in the myometrium, and parturition.

An analysis of time to pregnancy in women with RA showed that use of NSAIDS was associated with a longer time to pregnancy with a hazard ratio for occurrence of pregnancy of 0.66 (95% CI, 0.46 to 0.94).[127]

Salicylate Intoxication and Nonsteroidal Anti-inflammatory Drug Overdose

The new appearance of tachypnea, confusion, ataxia, oliguria, or a rising blood urea nitrogen/creatinine level in a patient, particularly an elderly patient, who takes aspirin or salicylates should suggest the possibility of salicylate intoxication.

In adults, metabolic acidosis is masked by hyperventilation because of the stimulation of respiratory centers, which is a direct effect of salicylates. Sudden increases in salicylate levels can occur even if there is no change in dose. This increase is particularly common in patients who experience acidosis from any cause, experience dehydration, or ingest other drugs that displace salicylate from protein-binding sites. Therapy consists of removing the residual drug from the GI tract, forced diuresis while maintaining the urinary pH in the alkaline range and with potassium replacement, or hemodialysis if diuresis is unsatisfactory. Vitamin K is recommended because large doses of salicylate may interfere with the synthesis of the vitamin K–dependent clotting factors.

Acute overdoses of NSAIDs are much less toxic than are overdoses of aspirin or salicylates. This subject has been most carefully evaluated for ibuprofen, prompted by its approval for over-the-counter sale to the general public. Symptoms with overdoses ranging up to 40 g include CNS depression, seizures, apnea, nystagmus, blurred vision, diplopia, headache, tinnitus, bradycardia, hypotension, abdominal pain, nausea, vomiting, hematuria, abnormal renal function, coma, and cardiac arrest. Treatment includes prompt evacuation of the stomach contents, observation, and administration of fluids.

Adverse Effects of Acetaminophen

Acetaminophen is used widely as the first-line treatment of pain, chiefly because it is viewed as effective and safer than NSAIDs. When used in doses of less than 2 g daily, there is little evidence of toxicity.[128] Acetaminophen-induced acute liver failure is a result of direct injury from the toxic metabolite, *N*-acetyl-*p*-benzoquinoneimine, a highly reactive electrophilic compound that depletes glutathione and subsequently accumulates in hepatocytes.[129] Acetaminophen is a highly predictable hepatotoxin with a threshold dose of 10 to 15 g in adults and 150 mg/kg in children (lower dosages have also been associated with hepatic injury). In the United States, acetaminophen overdoses are usually unintentional, with patients taking therapeutic doses of multiple acetaminophen-containing medications. Intentional self-poisoning with acetaminophen also remains an important problem. Acetaminophen is the most frequent cause of acute liver failure of any etiology in the United States and in most Western countries.[130] Treatment of acetaminophen overdose includes gastric lavage, activated charcoal, or induction of vomiting within the first 3 hours of injection. In addition, intensive support measures and early treatment with *N*-acetylcysteine, which replenishes glutathione, have reduced the mortality associated with acute acetaminophen toxicity. With high doses of acetaminophen, other toxicities may occur, including GI ulcers and bleeding.[131,132] Regular use of acetaminophen has also been associated with an increased risk for chronic renal failure.[96]

Effects of Concomitant Drugs, Diseases, and Aging

Because of the widespread use of prescription and nonprescription NSAIDs, ample opportunities exist for interaction with other drugs and for interactions with patient-specific factors.[133] Specific drug interactions are listed on the package inserts of individual agents.

Drug-Drug Interactions

Because most NSAIDs are extensively bound to plasma proteins, they may displace other drugs from binding sites or may themselves be displaced by other agents. Aspirin and other NSAIDs may increase the activity or toxicity of sulfonylurea, hypoglycemic agents, oral anti-coagulants, phenytoin, sulfonamides, and methotrexate by displacing these drugs from their protein-binding sites and increasing the free fraction of the drug in plasma.[133] NSAIDs may blunt the anti-hypertensive effects of β-blockers, angiotensin-converting enzyme inhibitors, and thiazides, leading to destabilization of blood pressure control.[134] An increased risk of GI toxicity is present when NSAIDs and selective serotonin reuptake inhibitors are taken concomitantly compared with taking either agent alone, and more than an additive risk occurs.[135]

Interactions between aspirin and NSAIDs, particularly ibuprofen, are related to blocking of the ability of aspirin to access the COX active site. This effect may be important when aspirin is used for the prevention of cardiovascular disease. It is prudent to recommend that aspirin be taken 2 hours before ingestion of ibuprofen.[108,136]

Drug-Disease Interactions

RA and other diseases (e.g., hepatic and renal disease) that decrease serum albumin concentrations are associated with increased concentrations of free NSAIDs. Hepatic and renal diseases also may impair drug metabolism or excretion and thereby increase the toxicity of a given dose of an NSAID to an individual patient. Renal insufficiency may be accompanied by accumulated endogenous organic acids that may displace NSAIDs from protein-binding sites.

Drug Reactions in Elderly People

Aging is accompanied by changes in physiology, resulting in altered pharmacokinetics and pharmacodynamics. Decreased drug clearance may be the consequence of reductions in hepatic mass, enzymatic activity, blood flow, renal plasma flow, glomerular filtration rate, and tubular function associated with aging. Elderly people are more likely to experience adverse GI and renal effects related to NSAIDs. The increased risk of cardiovascular disease in elderly patients raises concerns of accelerated MI or stroke. The use of aspirin for prevention of cardiovascular disease increases the toxicity of NSAIDs, and conversely the concomitant use of NSAIDs may increase aspirin resistance. Use of a PPI for gastroprotection may interfere with the efficacy of anti-platelet agents such as clopidogrel.[136] Elderly people have more illnesses than younger patients and therefore take more medications, increasing the possibility of drug-drug interactions. Older patients also may be more likely to self-medicate or make errors in drug dosing. For these reasons, frequent monitoring for compliance and toxicity should accompany the use of NSAIDs in this population.

Choosing Anti-inflammatory Analgesic Therapy

In choosing an NSAID for a particular patient, the clinician must consider efficacy, potential toxicity related to concomitant drugs and patient factors, and cost. Furthermore, patient preference for factors such as dosing regimen may be taken into account. In addition to choices from the perspective of the individual patient and physician, it may be important to take a broader view. Choice of anti-inflammatory analgesic therapy can also be considered from the perspective of health care institutions and payers. The symptoms and conditions for which NSAIDs are used are extraordinarily common. Consequently, the cost of NSAIDs as a proportion of total drug costs can be high when drugs are expensive. The increased cost of branded NSAIDs has an important pharmacoeconomic impact. On the other hand, adverse events can have important economic consequences, and improved safety may be cost-effective.

Choosing anti-inflammatory analgesic therapy has become increasingly complex with the increased understanding of associated toxicities. Prospectively considering the presence of GI and cardiovascular risk factors is essential when considering treatment options (Table 62.5). GI risks are well known, and strategies to prevent ulceration and bleeding are available. Many questions regarding the risk for cardiovascular events in patients using NSAIDs exist. In general, the data suggest that physicians should be cautious in using NSAIDs in patients with known cardiovascular disease. In patients with risks for NSAID toxicity, avoiding potent drugs with a long half-life or extended-release formulations is prudent. Intermittent dosing rather than continuous daily use reduces toxicity.

Absence of anti-inflammatory activity reduces the effectiveness of acetaminophen for diseases accompanied by a significant component of inflammation (e.g., RA and gout). However, acetaminophen is a safe and effective alternative for milder pain conditions, including OA. With respect to patient preference, a survey study demonstrated that only 14% of a large group of patients with rheumatic disease (n = 1799) who had RA, OA, or fibromyalgia preferred acetaminophen rather than NSAIDs, whereas 60% preferred NSAIDs.[137] In a head-to-head clinical trial of acetaminophen versus diclofenac plus misoprostol, patients in the diclofenac group had significantly greater improvement in pain scores. This finding was magnified in patients with more severe disease at baseline.[138]

Acetaminophen can be tried as the initial therapy in patients with mild to moderate pain for reasons of safety and cost. Nevertheless, a recent meta-analysis of the safety and efficacy of acetaminophen for spinal pain and OA found that this agent is ineffective in the treatment of low back pain and provides minimal short-term benefit for people with OA.[139] Furthermore, patients taking acetaminophen were nearly four times more likely to have abnormal results on liver function tests. If patients have moderate to severe symptoms or if evidence of inflammation is present, moving to treatment with NSAIDs may provide more rapid and effective relief.[140]

Conclusion

The strategy of blocking PG production by inhibiting the COX enzymes has provided relief from pain and inflammation for centuries. Given the proven importance of PG in this pathway and the advances in understanding the molecules involved, pharmacologic targeting of enzymes involved in biosynthesis, transport, or degradation may provide new therapeutic opportunities. Understanding and weighing the benefits and risks of each potential NSAID for each individual patient is essential to the appropriate use of these drugs.

Full references for this chapter can be found on ExpertConsult.com.

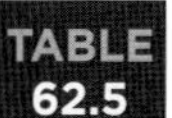

TABLE 62.5 Choosing Anti-inflammatory Analgesic Therapy

Risk Category	Treatment Recommendations
Low	
<65 yr No cardiovascular risk factors No requirement for high-dose or chronic therapy No concomitant aspirin, corticosteroids, or anti-coagulants	Traditional NSAID Shortest duration and lowest dose possible
Intermediate	
≥65 yr No history of previous complicated GI ulceration Low cardiovascular risk, may be using aspirin for primary prevention Requirement for chronic therapy and/or high-dose therapy	Traditional NSAID + PPI, misoprostol, or high-dose H2RA Once-daily celecoxib + PPI, misoprostol, or high-dose H2RA if taking aspirin If using aspirin, take a low dose (75-81 mg) If using aspirin, take a traditional NSAID ≥2 hr before aspirin dose
High	
Elderly, especially if frail or if hypertension, renal disease, or liver disease is present History of previous complicated ulcer or multiple GI risk factors History of cardiovascular disease and taking aspirin or another anti-platelet agent for secondary prevention History of heart failure	Use acetaminophen, <2 g/day Avoid chronic use of NSAIDs if at all possible: Use intermittent NSAID dosing Use low-dose, short–half-life NSAIDs Do not use an extended-release NSAID formulation If chronic NSAID use is required, consider: Once-daily celecoxib + PPI/misoprostol (GI > CV risk) Naproxen + PPI/misoprostol (CV > GI risk) Avoid use of a PPI if using an anti-platelet agent such as clopidogrel Monitor and treat blood pressure Monitor creatinine and electrolytes

CV, Cardiovascular; *GI,* gastrointestinal; *H2RA,* histamine-2-receptor antagonist; *NSAID,* non-steroidal anti-inflammatory drug; *PPI,* proton pump inhibitor.

Selected References

1. Vane JR, Botting RM: The history of anti-inflammatory drugs and their mechanism of action. In Bazan N, Botting J, Vane J, editors: *New targets in inflammation: inhibitors of COX-2 or adhesion molecules*, London, 1996, Kluwer Academic Publishers and William Harvey Press, pp 1–12.
2. Crofford LJ, Lipsky PE, Brooks P, et al.: Basic biology and clinical application of specific COX-2 inhibitors, *Arthritis Rheum* 43:4–13, 2000.
3. Simmons DL, Botting RM, Hla T: The biology of prostaglandin synthesis and inhibition, *Pharmacol Rev* 56:387–437, 2004.

4. Masferrer JL, Zweifel BS, Seibert K, et al.: Selective regulation of cellular cyclooxygenase by dexamethasone and endotoxin in mice, *J Clin Invest* 86:1375–1379, 1990.
5. FitzGerald GA, Patrono C: The coxibs, selective inhibitors of cyclooxygenase-2, *N Engl J Med* 345:433–442, 2001.
6. Kurumbail RA, Stevens AM, Gierse JK, et al.: Structural basis for selective inhibition of cyclooxygenase-2 by anti-inflammatory agents, *Nature* 384:644–648, 1996.
7. Juni P, Nartey L, Reichenbach S, et al.: Risk of cardiovascular events and rofecoxib: a cumulative metaanalysis, *Lancet* 364:2021–2029, 2004.
8. Llorens O, Perez JJ, Palomar A, et al.: Differential binding mode of diverse cyclooxygenase inhibitors, *J Mol Graph Model* 20:359–371, 2002.
9. Loll PJ, Picot D, Garavito RM: The structural basis of aspirin activity inferred from the crystal structure of inactivated prostaglandin H2 synthase, *Nat Struct Biol* 2:637–643, 1995.
10. Spite M, Serhan CN: Novel lipid mediators promote resolution of acute inflammation: impact of aspirin and statins, *Circ Res* 107:1170–1184, 2010.
11. Marnett LJ: Cyclooxygenase mechanisms, *Curr Opin Chem Biol* 4:545–552, 2000.
12. Sharma NP, Dong L, Yuan C, et al.: Asymmetric acetylation of the cyclooxygenase-2 homodimer by aspirin and its effects on the oxygenation of arachidonic, eicosapentaenoic, and docosahexaenoic acids, *Mol Pharmacol* 77:979–986, 2010.
13. Loll PJ, Picot D, Ekabo O, et al.: Synthesis and use of iodinated non-steroidal antiinflammatory drug analogs as cystallographic probes of the prostaglandin H2 synthase cyclooxygenase active site, *Biochemistry* 35:7330–7340, 1996.
14. Rowlinson SW, Keifer JR, Prusakiewicz JJ, et al.: A novel mechanism of cyclooxygenase-2 inhibition involving interactions with Ser-530 and Tyr-385, *J Biol Chem* 278:45763–45769, 2003.
15. Capone ML, Tacconelli S, Rodriguez LG, et al.: NSAIDs and cardiovascular disease: transducing human pharmacology results into clinical read-outs in the general population, *Pharmacol Rep* 62:530–535, 2010.
16. Capone ML, Tacconelli S, Di Francesco L, et al.: Pharmacodynamic of cyclooxygenase inhibitors in humans, *Prostaglandins Other Lipid Mediat* 82:85–94, 2007.
17. Tegeder I, Pfeilschifter J, Geisslinger G: Cyclooxygenase-independent actions of cyclooxygenase inhibitors, *FASEB J* 15:2057–2072, 2001.
18. King TS, Russe OQ, Moser CV, et al.: AMP-activated protein kinase is activated by non-steroidal anti-inflammatory drugs, *Eur J Pharmacol* 762:299–305, 2015.
19. Grosch S, Maier TJ, Schiffmann S, et al.: Cyclooxygenase-2 (COX-2)-independent anticarcinogenic effects of selective COX-2 inhibitors, *J Natl Cancer Inst* 98:736–741, 2006.
20. Aronoff DM, Oates JA, Boutaud O: New insights into the mechanism of action of acetaminophen: its clinical pharmacologic characteristics reflects its inhibition of the two prostaglandin H2 synthases, *Clin Pharmacol Ther* 79:9–19, 2006.
21. Chandrasekharan NV, Dai H, Roos KLT, et al.: COX-3, a cyclooxygenase-1 variant inhibited by acetaminophen and other analgesic/antipyretic drugs: cloning, structure, and expression, *Proc Natl Acad Sci U S A* 99:13926–13931, 2002.
22. Qin N, Zhang SP, Reitz TL, et al.: Cloning, expression, and functional characterization of human cyclooxygenase-1 splicing variants: evidence for intron 1 retention, *J Pharmacol Exp Ther* 315:1298–1305, 2005.
23. Aronoff DM, Boutaud O, Marnett LJ, et al.: Inhibition of prostaglandin H2 synthases by salicylate is dependent on the oxidative state of the enzymes, *Adv Exp Med Biol* 525:125–128, 2003.
24. Brune K, Patrignani P: New insights into the use of currently available non-steroidal anti-inflammatory drugs, *J Pain Res* 8:105–118, 2015.
25. Massó González EL, Patrignani P, Tacconelli S, et al.: Variability among nonsteroidal antiinflammatory drugs in risk of upper gastrointestinal bleeding, *Arthritis Rheum* 62:1592–1601, 2010.
26. Floyd CN, Ferro A: Mechanisms of aspirin resistance, *Pharmacol Ther* 141:69–78, 2014.
27. Airee A, Draper HM, Finks SW: Aspirin resistance: disparities and clinical implications, *Pharmacotherapy* 28:999–1018, 2008.
28. Badri W, Miladi K, Nazari QA, et al.: Encapsulation of NSAIDs for inflammation management: overview, progress, challenges and prospects, *Int J Pharmaceutics* 515:757–773, 2016.
29. Kienzler J-L, Gold M, Nollevaux F: Systemic bioavailability of topical diclofenac sodium gel 1% versus oral diclofenac sodium in healthy volunteers, *J Clin Pharmacol* 50:50–61, 2010.
30. Atkinson TJ, Fudin J, Jahn HL, et al.: What's new in NSAID pharmacotherapy: oral agents to injectables, *Pain Med* (Suppl 1):S11–17, 2013.
31. Hochberg MC: New directions in symptomatic therapy for patients with osteoarthritis and rheumatoid arthritis, *Semin Arthritis Rheum* 32:4–14, 2002.
32. Ito S, Okuda-Ashitaka E, Minami T: Central and peripheral roles of prostaglandins in pain and their interactions with novel neuropeptides nociceptin and nocistatin, *Neurosci Res* 41:299–332, 2001.
33. Kunori S, Matsumura S, Okuda-Ashtaka E, et al.: A novel role of prostaglandin E2 in neuropathic pain: blockade of microglial migration in the spinal cord, *Glia* 59:208–218, 2011.
34. Ballou LR, Botting RM, Goorha S, et al.: Nociception in cyclooxygenase isozyme-deficient mice, *Proc Natl Acad Sci U S A* 97:10272–10276, 2000.
35. Ek M, Engblom D, Saha S, et al.: Inflammatory response: pathway across the blood-brain barrier, *Nature* 410:430–431, 2001.
36. Engblom D, Saha S, Engström L, et al.: Microsomal prostaglandin E synthase-1 is the central switch during immune-induced pyresis, *Nat Neurosci* 6:1137–1138, 2003.
37. Belay ED, Bresee JS, Holman RC, et al.: Reye's syndrome in the United States from 1981 through 1997, *N Engl J Med* 340:1377–1382, 1999.
38. Osani MC, Vaysbrot EE, Ahou M, et al.: Duration of symptom relief and early trajectory of adverse events for oral NSAIDs in knee osteoarthritis: a systematic review and meta-analysis, *Arthritis Care Res* Mar 25, 2019. Epub ahead of print.
39. Nakata K, Hanai T, Take Y, et al.: Disease-modifying effects of COX-2 selective inhibitors and non-selective NSAIDs in osteoarthritis: a systematic review, *Osteoarthritis Cartilage* 26:1263–1273, 2018.
40. Wanders A, Heijde Dv, Landewe R, et al.: Nonsteroidal anti-inflammatory drugs reduce radiographic progression in patients with ankylosing spondylitis: a randomized clinical trial, *Arthritis Rheum* 52:1756–1765, 2005.
41. Kroon F, Landewe R, Dougados M, et al. Continuous NSAID use reverts the effects of inflammation on radiographic progression in patients with ankylosing spondylitis, *Ann Rheum Dis* 71: 1623–1629, 2012.
42. Sieper J, Listing J, Poddubnyy D, et al.: Effect of continuous versus on-demand treatment of ankylosing spondylitis with diclofenac over 2 years on radiographic progression of the spine: results from a randomized multicenter trial (ENRADAS), *Ann Rheum Dis* 75:1438–1443, 2016.
43. Braun J, van den Berg R, Baraliakos X, et al: 2010 update of the ASA/EULAR recommendations for the management of ankylosing spondylitis. *Ann Rheum Dis* 70:869-904, 2011.
44. Ward MM, Deodhar A, Akl EA, et al.: American College of Rheumatology/Spondylitis Association of America/Spondyloarthritis Research and Treatment Network 2015 recommendations for the treatment of ankylosing spondylitis and nonradiographic axial spondyloarthritis, *Arthritis Rheumatol* 68:282–298, 2016.

45. Patrono C: Aspirin as an antiplatelet drug, *N Engl J Med* 330:1287–1294, 1994.
46. US Preventative Health Task Force: Aspirin for the prevention of cardiovascular disease: U.S. Preventive Services Task Force recommendation statement, *Ann Intern Med* 150:1–37, 2009.
47. Ridker PM, Cook NR, Lee IM, et al.: A randomized trial of low-dose aspirin in the primary prevention of cardiovascular disease in women, *N Engl J Med* 354:1293–1304, 2005.
48. Gaziano JM, Brotons C, Coppolecchia R, et al.: Use of aspirin to reduce risk of initial vascular events in patients at moderate risk of cardiovascular disease (ARRIVE) a randomize, double-blind, placebo-controlled trial, *Lancet* 392:1036–1046, 2018.
49. ASCEND Study Collaborative Group, Bowman L, Mafham M, et al.: Effects of aspirin for primary prevention in persons with diabetes mellitus, *N Engl J Med* 379:1529–1539, 2018.
50. McNeil JJ, Wolfe R, Woods RL, et al.: Effect of aspirin on cardiovascular events and bleeding in the healthy elderly, *N Engl J Med* 379:1509–1518, 2018.
51. Zheng SL, Roddick AJ: Association of aspirin use for primary prevention with cardiovascular events and bleeding events. A systematic review and meta-analysis, *JAMA* 321(3):277–287, 2019.
52. Bibbins-Domingo K on behalf of the U.S. Preventive Services Task Force: Aspirin use for the primary prevention of cardiovascular disease and colorectal cancer: U.S. Preventive Services Task Force recommendation statement, *Ann Intern Med* 164:836–845, 2016.
53. Wang D, Dubois RN: Eicosanoids and cancer, *Nat Rev Cancer* 10:181–193, 2010.
54. Gupta SC, Kim JH, Prasad S, et al.: Regulation of survival, proliferation, invasion, angiogenesis, and metastases of tumor cells by modulation of inflammatory pathways by nutraceuticals, *Cancer Metastasis Rev* 29:405–434, 2010.
55. Chan AT, Ogino S, Fuchs CS: Aspirin and the risk of colorectal cancer in relation to the expression of COX-2, *N Engl J Med* 356:2131–2142, 2007.
56. Rothwell PM, Fowkes FG, Belkes JF, et al.: Effect of daily aspirin on long-term risk of death due to cancer: analysis of individual patient data from randomised trials, *Lancet* 377:31–41, 2010.
57. Salinas CA, Kwon EM, FitzGerald LM, et al.: Use of aspirin and other nonsteroidal antiinflammatory medications in relation to prostate cancer risk, *Am J Epidemiol* 172:578–590, 2010.
58. Phillips RK, Wallace MH, Lynch PM, et al.: A randomised, double blind, placebo controlled study of celecoxib, a selective cyclooxygenase 2 inhibitor, on duodenal polyposis in familial adenomatous polyposis, *Gut* 50:857–860, 2002.
59. Hull MA, Sprange K, Hepburn T, et al.: Eicosapentaenoic acid and aspirin, alone and in combination, for the prevention of colorectal adenomas (seafood Polyp Prevention trial): a multicenter, randomized, double-blind, placebo-controlled, 2 x 2 factorial trial, *Lancet* 392:2583–2594, 2018.
60. Trelle S, Reichenback S, Wandel S, et al.: Cardiovascular safety of non-steroidal anti-inflammatory drugs: network meta-analysis, *BMJ* 342:c7086, 2011.
61. Bjarnason I, Scarpignato C, Holmgren E, et al.: Mechanisms of damage to the gastrointestinal tract from nonsteroidal anti-inflammatory drugs, *Gastroenterology* 154:500–514, 2018.
62. Scarpignato C, Hunt RH: Nonsteroidal antiinflammatory drug-related injury to the gastrointestinal tract: clinical picture, pathogenesis, and prevention, *Gastroenterol Clin North Am* 39:433–464, 2010.
63. Musamba C, Pritchard DM, Pirmohamed M: Review article: cellular and molecular mechanisms of NSAID-induced peptic ulcers, *Aliment Pharmacol Ther* 30:517–531, 2009.
64. To KF, Chan FKL, Cheng AS, et al.: Up-regulation of cyclooxygenase-1 and -2 in human gastric ulcer, *Aliment Pharmacol Ther* 15:25–34, 2001.
65. Huang JX, Sridhar S, Hunt RH: Role of Helicobacter pylori infection and nonsteroidal anti-inflammatory drugs in peptic-ulcer disease: a meta-analysis, *Lancet* 359:14–22, 2002.
66. Dikman A, Sanyal S, Von Althann C, et al.: A randomized, controlled study of the effects of naproxen, aspirin, celecoxib or clopidogrel on gastroduodenal mucosal healing, *Aliment Pharmacol Ther* 29:781–791, 2009.
67. Cryer B, Li C, Simon LS, et al.: GI-REASONS: a novel 6-month, prospective, randomized, open-label, blinded endpoint (PROBE) trial, *Am J Gastroenterol* 108:392–400, 2013.
68. Nissen SE, Yeomans ND, Solomon DH, et al.: Cardiovascular safety of celecoxib, naproxen or ibuprofen for arthritis, *N Engl J Med* 375:2519–2529, 2016.
69. Yeomans ND, Graham DY, Husni ME, et al.: Randomised clinical trial: gastrointestinal events in arthritis patients treated with celecoxib, ibuprofen or naproxen in the PRECISION trial, *Aliment Pharmacol Ther* 47:1453–1463, 2018.
70. Solomon DH, Husni ME, Libby PA, et al.: The risk of major NSAID toxicity with celecoxib, ibuprofen, or naproxen: a secondary analysis of the PRECISION trial, *Am J Med* 130:1415–1422, 2017.
71. Chan FKL, Ching JYL, Tse YK, et al.: Gastrointestinal safety of celecoxib versus naproxen in patients with cardiothrombotic diseases and arthritis after upper gastrointestinal bleeding (CONCERN): an industry-independent, double-blind, double-dummy, randomized trial, *Lancet* 389:2375–2382, 2017.
72. Straus WL, Ofman JJ, MacLean C, et al.: Do NSAIDs cause dyspepsia? A meta-analysis evaluating alternative dyspepsia definitions, *Am J Gastroenterol* 97:1951–1958, 2002.
73. Hawkey CJ, Talley NJ, Scheiman JM, et al.: Maintenance treatment with esomeprazole following initial relief of non-steroidal anti-inflammatory drug-associated upper gastrointestinal symptoms: the NASA2 and SPACE2 studies, *Arthritis Res Ther* 7:R17, 2007.
74. Velduyzen van Zanten SJ, Chiba N, Armstrong D, et al.: A randomized trial comparing omeprazole, ranitidine, cisapride, or placebo in Helicobacter pylori negative, primary care patients with dyspepsia: the CADET-HN study, *Am J Gastroenterol* 100:1477–1488, 2005.
75. Singh G, Ramey DR, Morfeld D, et al.: Gastrointestinal tract complications of nonsteroidal anti-inflammatory drug treatment in rheumatoid arthritis: a prospective observational cohort study, *Arch Intern Med* 156:1530–1536, 1996.
76. Lanza PL, Chan FKL, Quigley EMM: Guidelines for prevention of NSAID-related ulcer complications, *Am J Gastroenterol* 104:728–738, 2009.
77. Lanas A: A review of the gastrointestinal safety data—a gastroenterologist's perspective, *Rheumatology (Oxford)* 49(Suppl 2):ii3–ii10, 2010.
78. Rostom A, Dube C, Wells G, et al.: Prevention of NSAID-induced gastroduodenal ulcers, *Cochrane Database Syst Rev* (4):CD002296, 2002.
79. Graham DY, Agrawal NM, Campbell DR, et al.: Ulcer prevention in long-term users of nonsteroidal anti-inflammatory drugs, *Arch Intern Med* 162:169–175, 2002.
80. Scheiman JM, Yeomans ND, Talley NJ, et al.: Prevention of ulcers by esomeprazole in at-risk patients using non-selective NSAIDs and COX-2 inhibitors, *Am J Gastroenterol* 101:701–710, 2006.
81. Lanas A: Nonsteroidal antiinflammatory drugs and cyclooxygenase inhibition in the gastrointestinal tract: a trip from peptic ulcer to colon cancer, *Am J Med Sci* 338:96–106, 2009.
82. Zografos GN, Geordiadou D, Thomas D, et al.: Drug-induced esophagitis, *Dis Esophagus* 22:633–637, 2009.
83. Higuchi K, Umegaki E, Watanabe T, et al.: Present status and strategy of NSAIDs-induced small bowel injury, *J Gastroenterol* 44:879–888, 2009.
84. Hawkey CJ: NSAIDs, coxibs, and the intestine, *J Cardiovasc Pharmacol* 47:S72–S75, 2006.
85. Stolte M, Hartmann FO: Misinterpretation of NSAID-induced colopathy as Crohn's disease, *Z Gastroenterol* 48:472–475, 2010.
86. Feagins LA, Cryer BL: Do non-steroidal anti-inflammatory drugs cause exacerbations of inflammatory bowel disease? *Dig Dis Sci* 55:226–232, 2010.

87. Milman M, Kraag G: NSAID-induced collagenous colitis, *J Rheumatol* 37:11, 2010.
88. Brater DC: Anti-inflammatory agents and renal function, *Semin Arthritis Rheum* 32:33–42, 2002.
89. FitzGerald GA: The choreography of cyclooxygenases in the kidney, *J Clin Invest* 110:33–34, 2002.
90. Harris RC, Breyer MD: Update on cyclooxygenase-2 inhibitors, *Clin J Am Soc Nephrol* 1:236–245, 2006.
91. Brater DC, Harris C, Redfern JS, et al.: Renal effects of COX-2 selective inhibitors, *Am J Nephrol* 21:1–15, 2001.
92. Gurwitz JH, Avorn J, Bonh RL, et al.: Initiation of antihypertensive treatment during nonsteroidal anti-inflammatory drug therapy, *JAMA* 272:781–786, 1994.
93. Dedier J, Stampfer MJ, Hankinson SE, et al.: Nonnarcotic analgesic use and the risk of hypertension in US women, *Hypertension* 40:604–608, 2002.
94. Akhund L, Quinet RJ, Ishaq S: Celecoxib-related renal papillary necrosis, *Arch Intern Med* 163:114–115, 2003.
95. Zhang X, Donnan PT, Bell S, et al.: Non-steroidal anti-inflammatory drug induced acute kidney injury in the community dwelling general population and people with chronic kidney disease: systematic review and meta-analysis, *BMC Nephrology* 18:256, 2017.
96. Fored CM, Ejerblad E, Lindblad P, et al.: Acetaminophen, aspirin, and chronic renal failure: a nationwide case-control study in Sweden, *N Engl J Med* 345:1801–1808, 2001.
97. Rexrode KM, Buring JE, Glynn RJ, et al.: Analgesic use and renal function in men, *JAMA* 286:315–321, 2001.
98. Reilly IA, FitzGerald GA: Inhibition of thromboxane formation in vivo and ex vivo: implications for therapy with platelet inhibitory drugs, *Blood* 69:180–186, 1987.
99. Garcia Rodriguez LA, Tacconelli S, Patrignani P: Role of dose potency in the prediction of risk of myocardial infarction associated with nonsteroidal anti-inflammatory drugs in the general populations, *J Am Coll Cardiol* 52:1628–1636, 2008.
100. FitzGerald GA: Coxibs and cardiovascular disease, *N Engl J Med* 351:1709–1711, 2004.
101. Harirforoosh S, Aghazadeh-Habashi A, Jamali F: Extent of renal effect of cyclo-oxygenase-2-selective inhibitors is pharmacokinetic dependent, *Clin Exp Pharmacol Physiol* 33:917–924, 2006.
102. Trelle S, Reichenbach S, Wandel S, et al.: Cardiovascular safety of non-steroidal anti-inflammatory drugs: network meta-analysis, *BMJ* 342:c7086, 2011.
103. Bhala N, Emberson J, Merhi A, et al.: Vascular and upper gastrointestinal effects of non-steroidal anti-inflammatory drugs: meta-analyses of individual participant data from randomised trials, *Lancet* 382:769–779, 2013.
104. Solomon SD, Wittes J, Finn PV, et al.: Cardiovascular risk of celecoxib in 6 randomized placebo-controlled trials: the cross trial safety analysis, *Circulation* 117:2104–2113, 2008.
105. Schjerning Olsen AM, Fosbol EL, Lindhardsen J, et al.: Duration of treatment with nonsteroidal anti-inflammatory drugs and impact on risk of death and recurrent myocardial infarction in patients with prior myocardial infarction: a nationwide cohort study, *Circulation* 123:2226–2235, 2011.
106. McGettigan P, Henry D: Cardiovascular risk with non-steroidal anti-inflammatory drugs: systematic review of population-based controlled observational studies, *PLoS Med* 8:e1001098, 2011.
107. MacDonald RM, Hawkey CJ, Ford I, et al.: Randomized trial of switching from prescribed non-selective non-steroidal anti-inflammatory drugs to prescribed celecoxib: the Standard care vs. Celecoxib Outcome Trial (SCOT), *Eur Heart J* 38:1843–1850, 2017.
108. Friedewald VE, Bennett JS, Christo JP, et al.: AJC Editor's consensus: selective and nonselective nonsteroidal anti-inflammatory drugs and cardiovascular risk, *Am J Cardiol* 106:873–884, 2010.
109. Grosser T, Ricciotti E, FitzGerald GA: The cardiovascular pharmacology of nonsteroidal anti-inflammatory drugs, *Trends Pharmacol Sci* 38:733–748, 2017.
110. Feenstra J, Heerdink ER, Grobbee DE, et al.: Association of nonsteroidal anti-inflammatory drugs with first occurrence of heart failure and with relapsing heart failure: the Rotterdam Study, *Arch Intern Med* 162:265–270, 2002.
111. Page J, Henry D: Consumption of NSAIDs and the development of congestive heart failure in elderly patients: an underrecognized public health problem, *Arch Intern Med* 160:777–784, 2000.
112. Gislason GH, Rasmussen JN, Abildstrom SZ, et al.: Increased mortality and cardiovascular morbidity associated with use of nonsteroidal anti-inflammatory drugs in chronic heart failure, *Arch Intern Med* 169:141–149, 2009.
113. White AA, Stevenson DD: Aspirin-exacerbated respiratory disease, *N Eng J Med* 379:1060–1070, 2018.
114. Rajan JP, Wineinger NE, Stevenson DD, et al.: Prevalence of aspirin-exacerbated respiratory disease among asthmatic patients: a meta-analysis of the literature, *J Allergy Clin Immunol* 135:676–681, 2015.
115. Morales DR, Lipworth JB, Guthrie B, et al.: Safety risks for patients with aspirin-exacerbated respiratory disease after acute exposure to selective nonsteroidal anti-inflammatory drugs and COX-2 inhibitors: meta-analysis of controlled clinical trials, *J Allergy Clin Immunol* 134:40–50, 2014.
116. Santana-Sahagun E, Weisman MH: Non-steroidal antiinflammatory drugs. In Harris ED, editor: *Kelley's textbook of rheumatology*, Philadelphia, 2000, Elsevier.
117. Blackwell KA, Raiz LG, Pilbeam CC: Prostaglandins in bone: bad cop, good cop? *Trends Endocrinol Metab* 21:294–301, 2010.
118. Uppal S, Diggle CP, Carr IM, et al.: Mutations in 15-hydroxyprostaglandin dehydrogenase cause primary hypertrophic osteoarthropathy, *Nat Genet* 40:789–793, 2008.
119. Einhorn TA: Do inhibitors of cyclooxygenase-2 impair bone healing? *J Bone Miner Res* 17:977–978, 2002.
123. Sirois J, Dore M: The late induction of prostaglandin G/H synthase in equine preovulatory follicles supports its role as a determinant of the ovulatory process, *Endocrinology* 138:4427–4434, 1997.

63 Glucocorticoid Therapy

MARLIES C. VAN DER GOES AND JOHANNES W.G. JACOBS

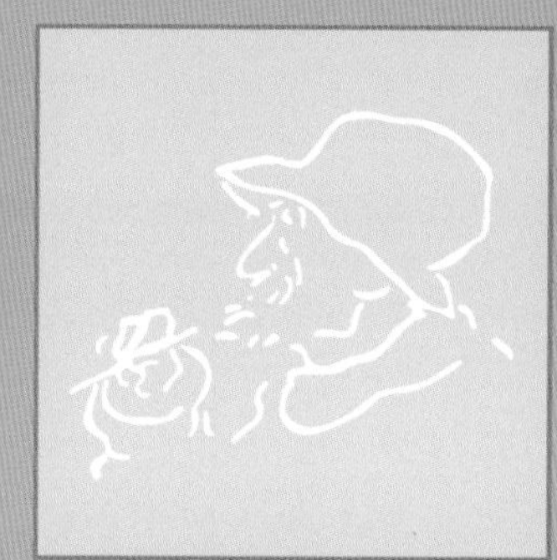

KEY POINTS

- The mode of action of glucocorticoids is based on interactions between the glucocorticoid receptor and genomic DNA and, in high dosages, might operate through nongenomic mechanisms.
- Glucocorticoids differ considerably in potency and biologic half-life.
- Cortisone and prednisone are biologically inactive and are converted in the liver into biologically active cortisol and prednisolone, respectively.
- Glucocorticoids continue to be the cornerstone of therapy of many rheumatic disorders. The risk of adverse effects of a glucocorticoid is dependent on the disease, comorbidities, dose, duration of therapy, and individual patient factors.
- Intralesional and intra-articular injections of a glucocorticoid can be very effective, and the risk of causing a local bacterial infection is very low.
- Low to moderate doses of prednisolone during pregnancy appear to be safe.
- New approaches are currently being investigated, such as selective glucocorticoid receptor agonists and liposomes containing glucocorticoids.

Introduction

Even though biologic drugs are increasingly being used, glucocorticoids are still anchor drugs in treatment strategies for patients with rheumatic disease. The first glucocorticoid to be isolated, in 1935, was the endogenous glucocorticoid hormone cortisone. It was synthesized in 1944 and subsequently became available for clinical use. In 1948 cortisone (at that time called *compound E*) was administered by the American physician Philip S. Hench to a 29-year-old woman with active rheumatoid arthritis (RA) of more than 4 years' duration. This nearly bedridden patient was able to walk after 3 days of treatment. Hench published this case of dramatic improvement in 1949[1] and, along with two colleagues, won the 1950 Nobel Prize in Physiology or Medicine. Later, chemical modification of endogenous steroids enabled production of synthetic glucocorticoids, some of which have proven to be effective anti-inflammatory and immunosuppressive substances with rapid effects.

When the wide array of potentially serious adverse effects became apparent in patients treated with supraphysiologic glucocorticoid dosages, enthusiasm for and use of glucocorticoids decreased. Nevertheless, they continue to be the cornerstone of therapy of many rheumatic disorders, including systemic lupus erythematosus (SLE), vasculitis, polymyalgia rheumatica, and myositis. In addition, the use of glucocorticoids in therapeutic strategies for patients with RA also has become generally accepted.[2] The estimated prevalence of the use of glucocorticoids in the general adult population in the United States for all medical indications is 1.2%; this percentage predominantly reflects chronic glucocorticoid use.[3]

Although knowledge about glucocorticoids has increased during the past several decades, much remains to be learned about the modes of actions of these drugs in rheumatic autoimmune disorders. It is hoped that the unraveling of these mechanisms may eventually lead to novel classes of therapy with fewer adverse effects, as well as to personalized medicine.[4]

Characteristics of Glucocorticoids

Structure

The precursor molecule of all steroid hormones is cholesterol, which is also a building block for vitamin D, cell membranes, and cell organelles (Fig. 63.1). Steroid hormones and cholesterol are characterized by a sterol skeleton consisting of three six-carbon hexane rings and one five-carbon pentane ring. The carbon atoms of this sterol nucleus are numbered in a specific sequence; the term *steroid* refers to this basic sterol nucleus (Fig. 63.2). No *qualitative* differences have been noted between the glucocorticoid effects of endogenous cortisol and exogenously applied synthetic glucocorticoids because these effects are, except for higher doses, predominantly genomic (i.e., mediated through the glucocorticoid receptor).[5] *Quantitative* differences, however, have been identified. The potency and other biologic characteristics of the glucocorticoids depend on structural differences in the steroid configuration. In the 1950s, when more potent synthetic steroid hormones were developed by chemical modification of endogenous steroids, research revealed numerous structural features essential for specific biologic activities. For instance, the 17-hydroxy, 21-carbon steroid configuration (see Fig. 63.2) is required for glucocorticoid activity through binding to the glucocorticoid receptor. The introduction of a double bond between the 1 and 2 positions of cortisol yields prednisolone, which has about four times more glucocorticoid activity than cortisol (Table 63.1). Addition of a six-methyl group to prednisolone yields methylprednisolone, which is about five times more potent than cortisol. All these glucocorticoids also have more or less a mineralocorticoid effect. The synthetic glucocorticoids triamcinolone and dexamethasone, meanwhile, have negligible mineralocorticoid activity.

Classification

Steroid hormones can be classified on the basis of their main function into sex hormones (male and female), mineralocorticoids,

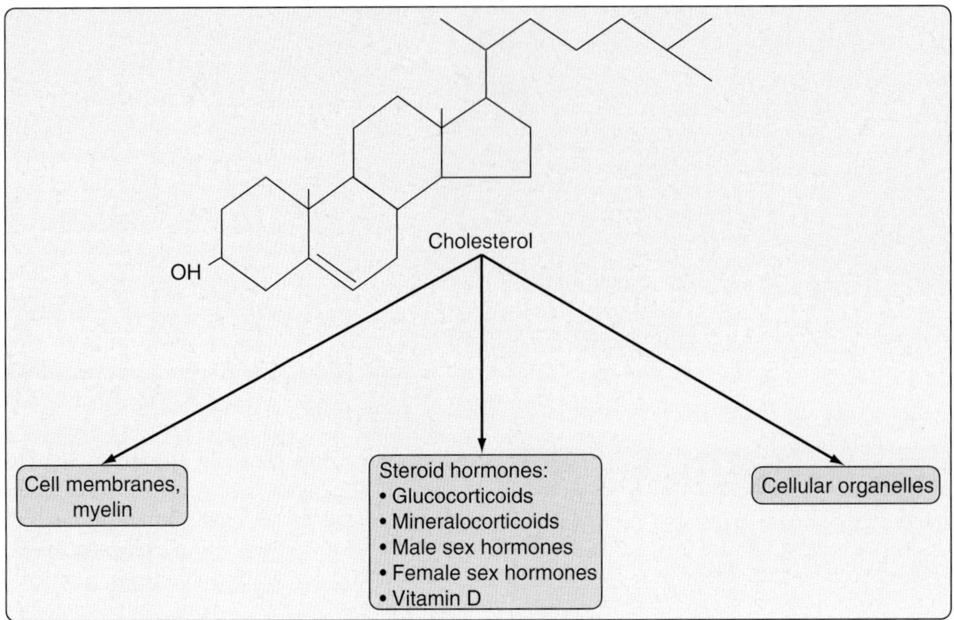

• **Fig. 63.1** Cholesterol as a building block for steroid hormones, vitamin D, cell membranes, and organelles.

and glucocorticoids (see Fig. 63.1). Sex hormones are synthesized mainly in the gonads but also in the adrenal cortex. Mineralocorticoids and glucocorticoids are synthesized only in the adrenal cortex; the terms *corticosteroid* and *corticoid* for these hormones refer to the adrenal cortex. Some glucocorticoids also have a mineralocorticoid effect and vice versa. The main endogenous mineralocorticoid is aldosterone, and the main endogenous glucocorticoid is cortisol (hydrocortisone). Although the classification of corticoids into mineralocorticoids and glucocorticoids is not absolute (see later), it is more precise to use the term *glucocorticoid* than the term *corticosteroid* when referring to one of the glucocorticoid compounds.[6]

Activation

Glucocorticoids with an 11-keto group, such as cortisone and prednisone, are prohormones that must be reduced in the liver to their 11-hydroxy configurations—cortisol and prednisolone, respectively—to become biologically active. For patients with severe liver disease, it is thus rational to prescribe prednisolone instead of prednisone. This formation of biologically active glucocorticoids from their inactive forms is promoted by the reductase action of the intra-cellular enzyme 11β-hydroxysteroid dehydrogenase (11β-HSD) type 1. The same enzyme can also promote the reverse reaction by dehydrogenation, leading to inactivation of active glucocorticoids. In contrast, 11β-HSD type 2 only has dehydrogenase activity, so it only catalyzes the conversion of active glucocorticoids to their inactive forms. In different tissues, local balance between the intra-cellular enzymes 11β-HSD type 1 and type 2 might modulate intra-cellular glucocorticoid concentrations and thus tissue sensitivity for glucocorticoids.[7] Synovial tissue metabolizes glucocorticoids via the two 11β-HSD enzymes, with the net effect being glucocorticoid activation. This endogenous glucocorticoid activation in the joint increases with joint inflammation and, vice versa, has an impact on local inflammation and on bone of the joint.[8]

Genomic and Nongenomic Modes of Action

Glucocorticoids at any therapeutically relevant dosage exhibit pharmacologic effects via classic genomic mechanisms. The lipophilic glucocorticoid passes across the cell membrane and attaches to the cytosolic glucocorticoid receptor. These glucocorticoid complexes then bind in the nucleus to glucocorticoid-responsive elements of genomic DNA or interact with nuclear transcription factors. This process takes time. When acting through genomic mechanisms, it takes at least 30 minutes before the clinical effects of a glucocorticoid begin to show.[9] Only when high doses are given, such as in pulse therapy, do nongenomic mechanisms also occur, by which glucocorticoids act within minutes. The response to high-dose pulse methylprednisolone therapy may be biphasic, consisting of an early, rapid, nongenomic effect and a more delayed and more sustained genomic effect.[10] Clinically, however, genomic and nongenomic effects cannot be separated.

Genomic Mechanisms

Most of the effects of glucocorticoids are exerted via genomic mechanisms by binding to the glucocorticoid receptor located in the cytoplasm of the target cells. Glucocorticoids are lipophilic and have a low molecular mass, and thus they can pass through the cell membrane easily. Next to the tissue-specific intra-cellular density of glucocorticoid receptors, the balance of intra-cellular 11β–HSDs (described earlier) probably determines the sensitivity of specific tissues for glucocorticoids.[7] Of the isoforms α and β of the glucocorticoid receptor, only the α isoform, commonly present in all target tissues, binds to glucocorticoids. This is a 94 kDa protein to which several heat shock proteins (chaperones) are bound. Binding of the glucocorticoid to this complex causes shedding of the chaperones. The resulting activated glucocorticoid receptor–glucocorticoid complex is rapidly translocated into the nucleus, where it binds as a dimer to specific consensus sites in the DNA (glucocorticoid-responsive elements) regulating (i.e., stimulating or suppressing) the transcription of a large variety of target

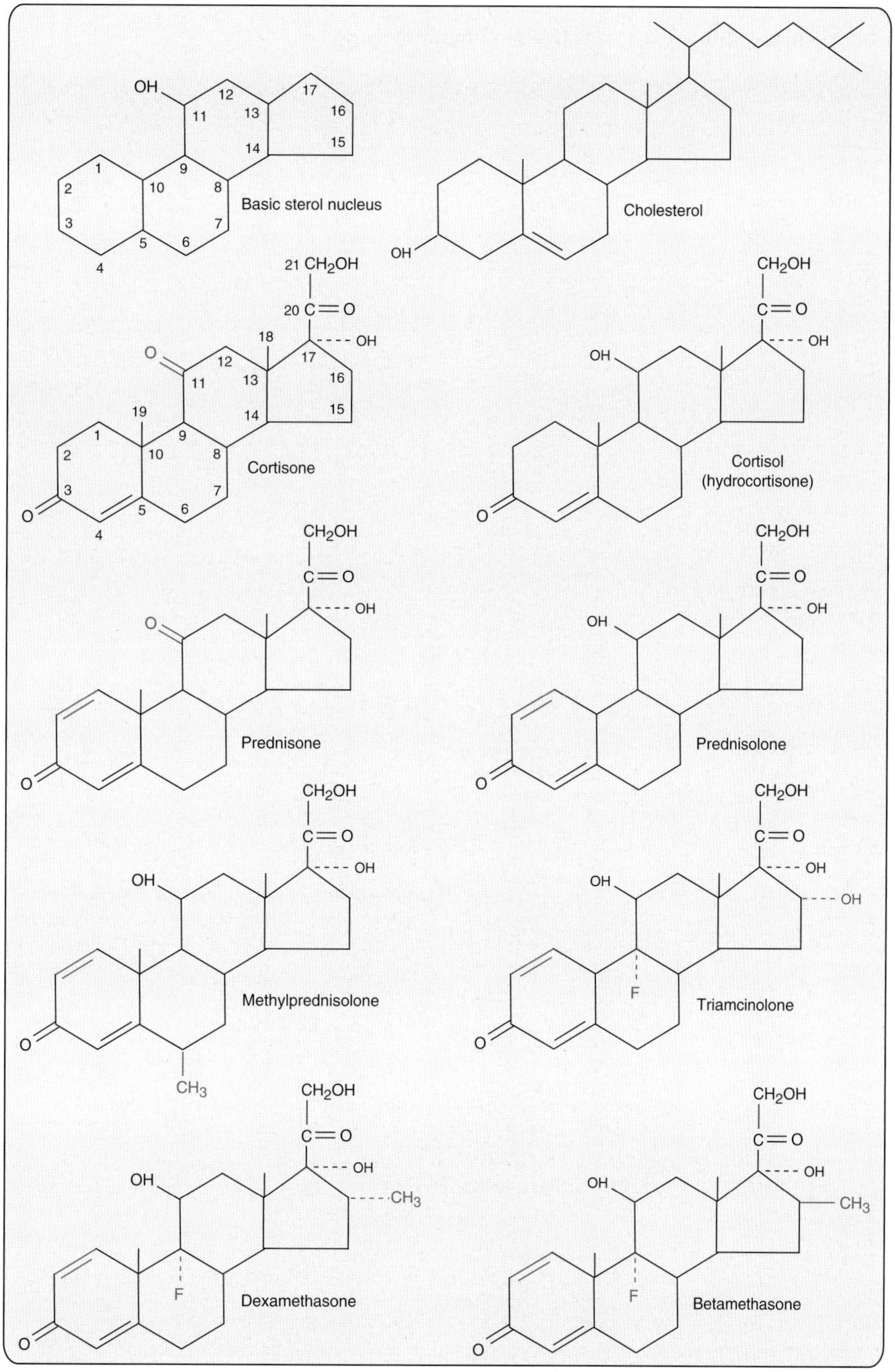

• **Fig. 63.2** Basic steroid configuration and structure of cholesterol and of natural and some synthetic glucocorticoids. Structural differences compared with cortisol, the endogenous active glucocorticoid, are shown in *red.*

genes. This process is termed *transactivation*. Activated glucocorticoid receptor–glucocorticoid complexes also, as monomers, interact with transcriptional factors (such as activator protein [AP]-1, interferon regulatory factor [IRF]-3, and nuclear factor-κB [NF-κB]), leading to inhibition of binding of these transcriptional factors to their consensus sites in the DNA.[11] This process, resulting in downregulation of predominantly pro-inflammatory protein synthesis, is called *transrepression* (Fig. 63.3).

The nature and availability of transcription factors may be pivotal in determining the differential sensitivity of different tissues to glucocorticoids because these factors play a crucial role in regulating the expression of a wide variety of pro-inflammatory

TABLE 63.1 **Pharmacodynamics of Glucocorticoids Used in Rheumatology**

	Equivalent Glucocorticoid Dose (mg)	Relative Glucocorticoid Activity	Relative Mineralocorticoid Activity[a]	Protein Binding	Half-Life in Plasma (hr)	Biologic Half-Life (hr)
Short-Acting						
Cortisone	25	0.8	0.8	–	0.5	8-12
Cortisol	20	1	1	++++	1.5-2	8-12
Intermediate-Acting						
Methylprednisolone	4	5	0.5	–	>3.5	18-36
Prednisolone	5	4	0.6	++	2.1-3.5	18-36
Prednisone	5	4	0.6	+++	3.4-3.8	18-36
Triamcinolone	4	5	0	++	2->5	18-36
Long-Acting						
Dexamethasone	0.75	20-30	0	++	3-4.5	36-54
Betamethasone	0.6	20-30	0	++	3-5	36-54

[a]Clinically; sodium and water retention, potassium depletion.

–, None; ++, high; +++, high to very high; ++++, very high.

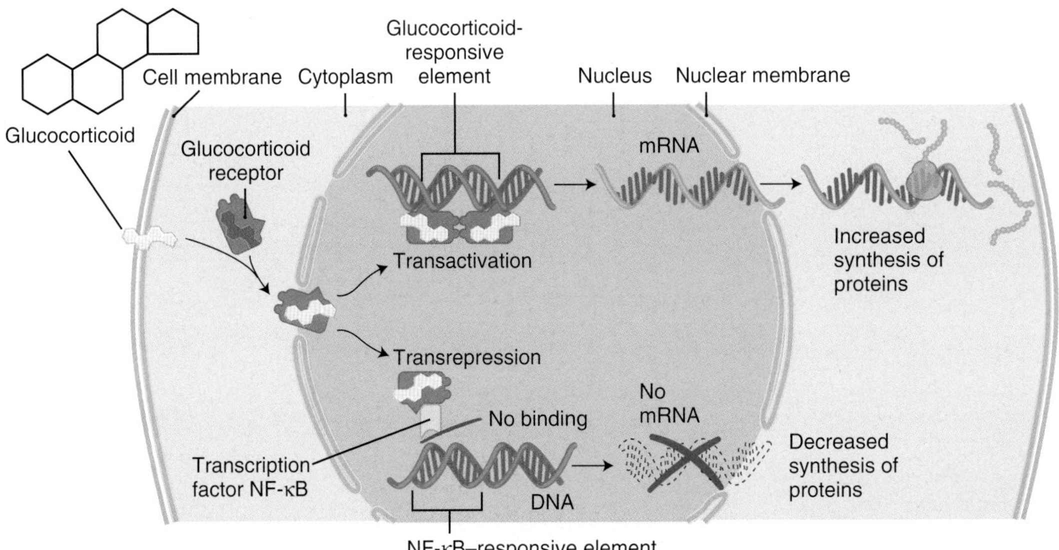

• **Fig. 63.3** Genomic action of glucocorticoids. Glucocorticoid binds to the glucocorticoid receptor (GCR) in the cytoplasm. This complex migrates into the nucleus. Activation of transcription (transactivation), by binding of GCR-glucocorticoid complex dimers to glucocorticoid-responsive elements of DNA, upregulates synthesis of regulatory proteins, thought to be responsible for metabolic effects and also some anti-inflammatory/immunosuppressive effects. Interaction of GCR-glucocorticoid complex monomers with pro-inflammatory transcription factors, such as activator protein-1, interferon regulatory factor-3, and nuclear factor-κB (NF-κB), leads to inhibition of binding of these transcriptional factors to their DNA consensus sites (for NF-κB: NF-κB–responsive elements). Thus the transcription of these pro-inflammatory transcription factors is repressed. This process is called "transrepression" and downregulates synthesis of predominantly inflammatory/immunosuppressive proteins. (Modified from Huisman AM, Jacobs JW, Buttgereit F, et al.: New developments in glucocorticoid therapy: selective glucocorticoid receptor agonists, nitrosteroids and liposomal glucocorticoids. *Ned Tijdschr Geneeskd* 150:476-480, 2006.)

genes induced by cytokines. The inhibited binding of transcriptional factors to DNA by glucocorticoids results in depressed expression of these genes and inhibition of their amplifying role in inflammation.

The hypothesis has been proposed that adverse effects of glucocorticoids may be based predominantly on transactivation, whereas the anti-inflammatory effects may be mostly due to transrepression. Better understanding of these molecular mechanisms could lead to the development of novel glucocorticoids, such as selective glucocorticoid receptor agonists, with a more favorable balance of transactivation and transrepression and, clinically, to a more favorable balance of metabolic and endocrine adverse effects and therapeutic effects.[11] However, although many immunosuppressive effects are based on transrepression, some effects are based on transactivation, such as glucocorticoid-induced gene transcription and protein synthesis of NF-κB inhibitor[12] and of lipocortin-1. Some immunosuppressive effects of glucocorticoids are not based on either transrepression or transactivation. Post-transcriptional mRNA destabilization resulting in decreased protein synthesis may also be an important anti-inflammatory mechanism of glucocorticoids. This mechanism has been proposed to mediate glucocorticoid-induced inhibition of the synthesis of IL-1, IL-6, granulocyte-macrophage colony-stimulating factor (GM-CSF), and inducible cyclooxygenase (COX)-2.[13] On the other hand, not all adverse effects are related to transactivation; increased risk of infection is associated with immunosuppression, primarily based on transrepression, which is also the mechanism of suppression of the hypothalamic-pituitary-adrenal (HPA) axis. Moreover, a study in a mouse strain with a deficiency to form dimer glucocorticoid receptor–glucocorticoid complexes, and thus with a transactivation deficiency, showed, along with a failure of glucocorticoids to exert a full anti-inflammatory response, classic adverse effects in these mice, such as osteoporosis.[14] These data challenge the concept of selective glucocorticoid receptor agonists[15]; furthermore, in an asthma trial, the effect of a selective glucocorticoid receptor agonist was disappointing.[16]

Nongenomic Mechanisms

Compared with genomic effects, nongenomic effects at high doses of glucocorticoids occur more rapidly—within minutes. One mechanism involves membrane-bound glucocorticoid receptors. Dexamethasone targets these receptors on T lymphocytes, which rapidly impairs T lymphocyte receptor signaling and immune response.[17] Nongenomic actions without involvement of glucocorticoid receptors occur via physicochemical interactions with biologic membranes, altering cell function. For instance, the resulting inhibition of calcium and sodium cycling across the plasma membrane of immune cells contributes to rapid immunosuppression and reduced inflammation.[5]

Glucocorticoid Effects on Hypothalamic-Pituitary-Adrenal Axis

Hypothalamic-Pituitary-Adrenal Axis and Inflammation

Pro-inflammatory cytokines (such as IL-1 and IL-6), eicosanoids (such as prostaglandin [PG]E_2), and endotoxins all activate corticotropin-releasing hormone (CRH) at the hypothalamic level and adrenocorticotropic hormone (ACTH) at the pituitary level. CRH also activates ACTH, and this activation stimulates the secretion of glucocorticoids by the adrenal glands, which is also stimulated by the inflammatory mediators previously mentioned (Fig. 63.4). In otherwise healthy people with severe infections or other major physical stress, cortisol production may increase to six times the normal amount.[18] In patients with chronic inflammatory diseases, such as active RA, this increase of cortisol driven by elevated cytokine levels might be inappropriately low,[19] meaning that cortisol levels, although normal or elevated in the absolute sense, are insufficient to control the inflammatory response. This is the concept of relative adrenal insufficiency.[19–22] Endogenous and exogenous glucocorticoids exert negative feedback control on the HPA axis *directly* by suppressing secretion of ACTH and CRH and also *indirectly* in inflammatory diseases by suppressing the release from inflammatory tissues of pro-inflammatory cytokines that stimulate secretion of ACTH and CRH (see Fig. 63.4). Sensitivity of the HPA axis for pro-inflammatory cytokines is probably decreased in people with RA.[23]

ACTH is secreted in brief, episodic bursts, resulting in relatively sharp increases in plasma concentrations of ACTH and cortisol, followed by slower declines in cortisol levels—the normal diurnal rhythm in cortisol secretion. Secretory ACTH episodic bursts increase in amplitude but not in frequency after 3 to 5 hours of sleep, reach a maximum in the hours before and the hour after awakening, decline throughout the morning, and are minimal in the evening. Cortisol levels are highest at about the time of awakening in the morning, are low in the late afternoon and evening, and reach their lowest level some hours after falling asleep (see Fig. 63.4). Glucocorticoids are not stored in the adrenal glands in great quantities; continuing synthesis and release are required to maintain basal secretion or to increase blood levels during stress. The total daily basal or physiologic secretion of cortisol in humans has been estimated to range from 5.7 to 10 $mg/m^2/day$.[24,25] Although during periods of physiologic stress the replacement dose should be higher (discussed later), this need would be covered in people with primary adrenal insufficiency by oral administration of 15 to 25 mg of cortisol,[24] equivalent to about 4 to 6 mg of prednisolone. This low daily cortisol production rate may explain the cushingoid symptoms and other adverse effects that are sometimes observed in patients with adrenal insufficiency who use glucocorticoids at doses previously regarded to be replacement doses (based on estimates of physiologic secretion of cortisol of 12 to 15 $mg/m^2/day$) but that are in fact supraphysiologic doses.

Tertiary Adrenal Insufficiency

Chronic suppression of the HPA axis by administration of exogenous glucocorticoids, as a result of negative feedback loops on CRH and ACTH (see Fig. 63.4), leads to failure of pituitary ACTH release and thus to partial functional adrenal atrophy with loss of cortisol secretory capability. Although this adrenal insufficiency is a result of the use of glucocorticoids (and thus is secondary to glucocorticoids) and although ACTH release is also directly inhibited by glucocorticoids, this adrenal insufficiency is often referred to as tertiary adrenal insufficiency, referring to the inhibition of CRH release.[26] The inner adrenal cortical zone (i.e., the fasciculate-reticularis zone) is the site of cortisol and adrenal androgen synthesis and is dependent on ACTH for structure and function. The outer cortical zone (glomerulosa zone) is involved in biosynthesis of mineralocorticoids (aldosterone) and is functionally independent of ACTH. It stays functionally intact. Patients

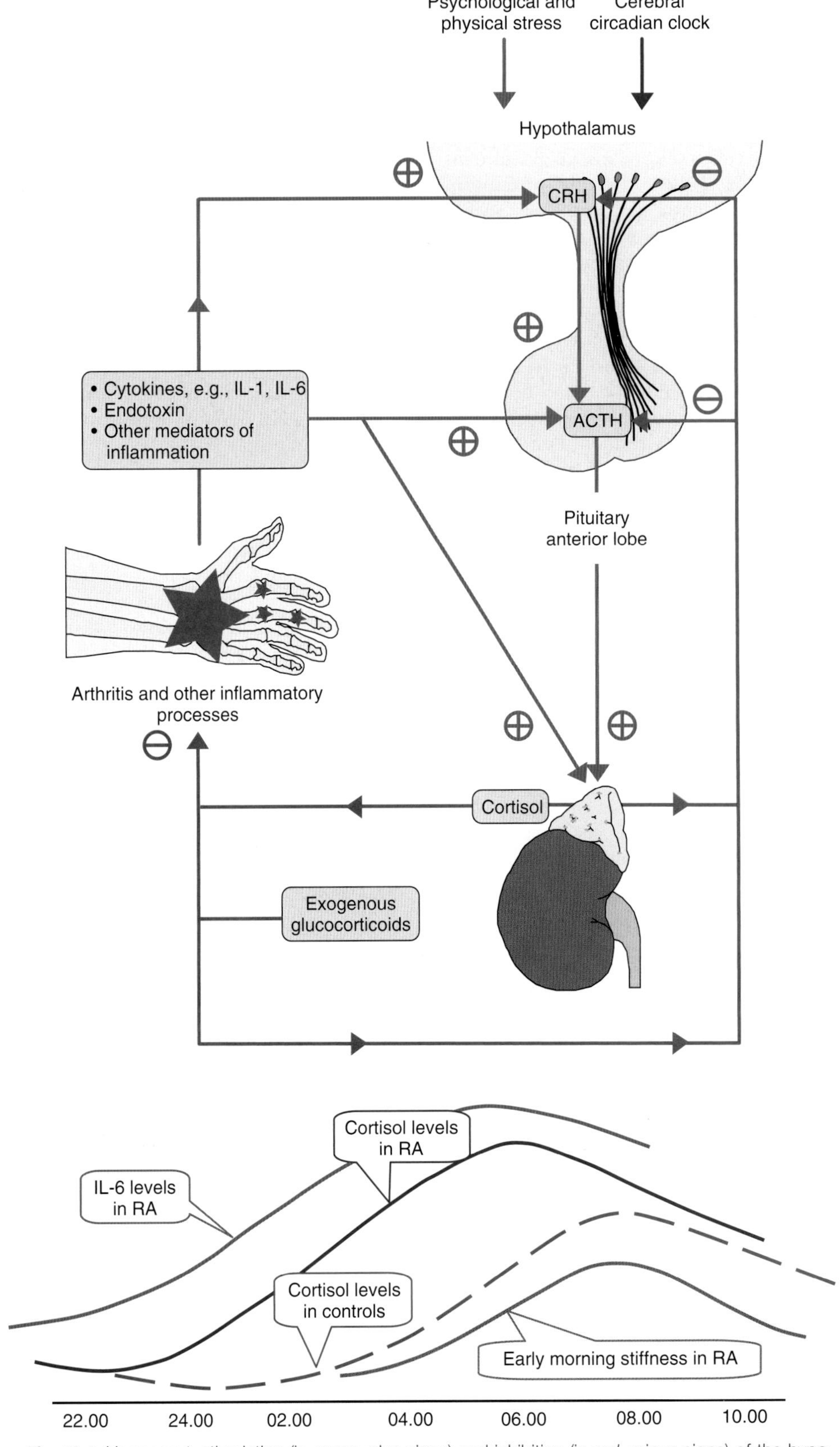

• **Fig. 63.4** *Upper part,* stimulation (in *green*, plus signs) and inhibition (in *red*, minus signs) of the hypothalamic-hypopituitary-adrenal axis. *Lower part,* hours on the x-axis; plasma cortisol levels in patients with rheumatoid arthritis (RA) show an earlier and higher circadian rise compared with that in healthy control subjects, possibly caused by the rise in the pro-inflammatory cytokine IL-6; this IL-6 rise is absent in healthy control subjects. IL-6 stimulates the hypothalamus and thus the release of cortisol, but probably also contributes to early morning stiffness and other inflammatory symptoms in (rheumatoid) arthritis. *ACTH,* Adrenocorticotropic hormone; *CRH,* corticotropin-releasing hormone.

experience a failure of pituitary CRH and ACTH release and adrenal responsiveness to ACTH. Serum cortisol, ACTH levels, and adrenal responsiveness to ACTH are low, but other pituitary axes function normally, in contrast to the situation in most primary pituitary disorders. Tertiary adrenal insufficiency generally has a less dramatic presentation than primary adrenal insufficiency because aldosterone levels, which are controlled predominantly by the renin-angiotensin system, are preserved; thus mineralocorticoid therapy is not necessary.

The duration of glucocorticoid therapy leading to suppression of the HPA axis depends on the dosage and the serum half-life of the glucocorticoid used, but it also varies among patients, probably because of individual differences in glucocorticoid sensitivity and rates of glucocorticoid metabolism. Reliable prediction of chronic suppression of the HPA axis and adrenal insufficiency on the patient level is not possible. This risk may be increased when glucocorticoids are used concomitantly with other steroid drugs, such as megestrol acetate and medroxyprogesterone, also inhibiting the HPA axis.[27]

The duration of the anti-inflammatory effect of one dose of a glucocorticoid approximates the duration of HPA suppression. After a single oral dose of 250 mg of hydrocortisone or cortisone, 50 mg of prednisone or prednisolone, or 40 mg of methylprednisolone, suppression for 1.25 to 1.5 days has been described. Duration of suppression after 40 mg of triamcinolone or 5 mg of dexamethasone was 2.25 and 2.75 days, respectively.[28] After intramuscular administration of a single dose of 40 to 80 mg of triamcinolone acetonide, the duration of HPA suppression is 2 to 4 weeks; after administration of 40 to 80 mg of methylprednisolone, suppression lasts 4 to 8 days.[28]

After 5 to 30 days of taking at least 25 mg of prednisolone or its equivalent daily, suppression of adrenal response (measured by a low-dose corticotropin test) was present in 34 of 75 patients studied (45%).[29] In these patients, a basal plasma cortisol concentration of less than 100 nmol/L was highly suggestive of adrenal suppression, whereas levels of basal cortisol greater than 220 nmol/L predicted a normal adrenal response in most, but not all, patients.

The risk of clinical (symptomatic) adrenal insufficiency is not negligible in patients on long-term low-dose or medium-dose therapy—for example, those who have had less than 10 mg of prednisolone or its equivalent per day in one dose in the morning. Investigators who performed a review of adrenal insufficiency stated that if the daily dose is 7.5 mg or more of prednisolone or its equivalent for at least 3 weeks, adrenal hypofunctioning should be anticipated, and acute cessation of glucocorticoid therapy in this situation could lead to problems.[18] In 21 patients with RA who were undergoing long-term glucocorticoid therapy (a mean daily dose of 6.7 mg prednisone equivalents), 52% had a normal (≥5 μg/dL) increase of serum cortisol after an intravenous 30-second bolus injection of 100 μg of human CRH, 33% had a subnormal response of cortisol, and 14% had no response at all.[30] Even patients who have received glucocorticoids for less than 3 weeks or have been treated with alternate-day prednisolone therapy do not have zero risk of suppression of the HPA axis, depending on the dose,[31,32] but the risk is low.

Thus adrenal suppression is difficult to predict, and it probably occurs frequently in daily practice.[33,34] It seems prudent to consider each patient who is undergoing chronic glucocorticoid therapy as being at risk for tertiary adrenal insufficiency. Nevertheless, after slow tapering, glucocorticoid therapy often can be stopped (if there is no indication for this therapy any longer); generally, adrenal function gradually recovers during the slow tapering period.

Glucocorticoid Effects on the Immune System

Glucocorticoids reduce activation, proliferation, differentiation, and survival of a variety of inflammatory cells, including macrophages and T lymphocytes, and promote apoptosis, especially in immature and activated T cells (Fig. 63.5). This activity is mediated mainly by changes in cytokine production and secretion. In contrast, B lymphocytes and neutrophils are less sensitive to glucocorticoids, and their survival may be increased by glucocorticoid treatment. The main effect of glucocorticoids on neutrophils seems to be inhibition of adhesion to endothelial cells. Glucocorticoids inhibit not only the expression of adhesion molecules but also the secretion of complement pathway proteins and prostaglandins. At supraphysiologic concentrations, glucocorticoids suppress fibroblast proliferation and IL-1 and TNF-induced metalloproteinase synthesis. By these effects, glucocorticoids may retard bone and cartilage destruction in inflamed joints of patients with early phase RA.[35,36]

Leukocytes and Fibroblasts

Administration of glucocorticoids leads to an increase in the total leukocyte count because of an increase of circulating neutrophil granulocytes in the blood, although the numbers of other leukocyte subsets in blood, such as eosinophil and basophil granulocytes, monocytes/macrophages (decreased myelopoiesis and bone marrow release), and T cells (redistribution effect), are decreased. Table 63.2 summarizes the effects of glucocorticoids on leukocyte subsets. The redistribution of lymphocytes, which is maximal 4 to 6 hours after administration of a single high dose of prednisone and returns to normal within 24 hours, has no clinical consequences. B cell function and immunoglobulin production are hardly affected. The effects of glucocorticoids on monocytes and macrophages, including decreased expression of class II major histocompatibility complex (MHC) molecules and Fc receptors, may increase susceptibility to infection, however.[37] Effects of glucocorticoids on fibroblasts include decreased proliferation and decreased production of fibronectin and prostaglandins.

Cytokines

The influence of glucocorticoids on cytokine production and action represents one of the major mechanisms of glucocorticoid action in chronic inflammatory diseases. Glucocorticoids exert potent inhibitory effects on the transcription and action of a large variety of cytokines. Most T helper (Th) type 1 pro-inflammatory cytokines are inhibited by glucocorticoids, including IL-1β, IL-2, IL-3, IL-6, TNF, and interferon-γ, along with IL-17 (associated with Th17 cells), and GM-CSF (see Fig. 63.5). In people with RA, these cytokines are considered to be responsible for synovitis, cartilage degradation, and bone erosion. Conversely, the production of Th2 cytokines, such as IL-4, IL-10, and IL-13, may be stimulated or not affected by glucocorticoids (see Fig. 63.5).[38] These cytokines have been related to the extra-articular features of erosive RA associated with B cell overactivity, such as immune complex formation and vasculitis. Activation of Th2 cells can suppress rheumatoid synovitis and joint destruction through release of the anti-inflammatory cytokines IL-4 and IL-10, which inhibit Th1 activity and downregulate monocyte and macrophage functions.[39]

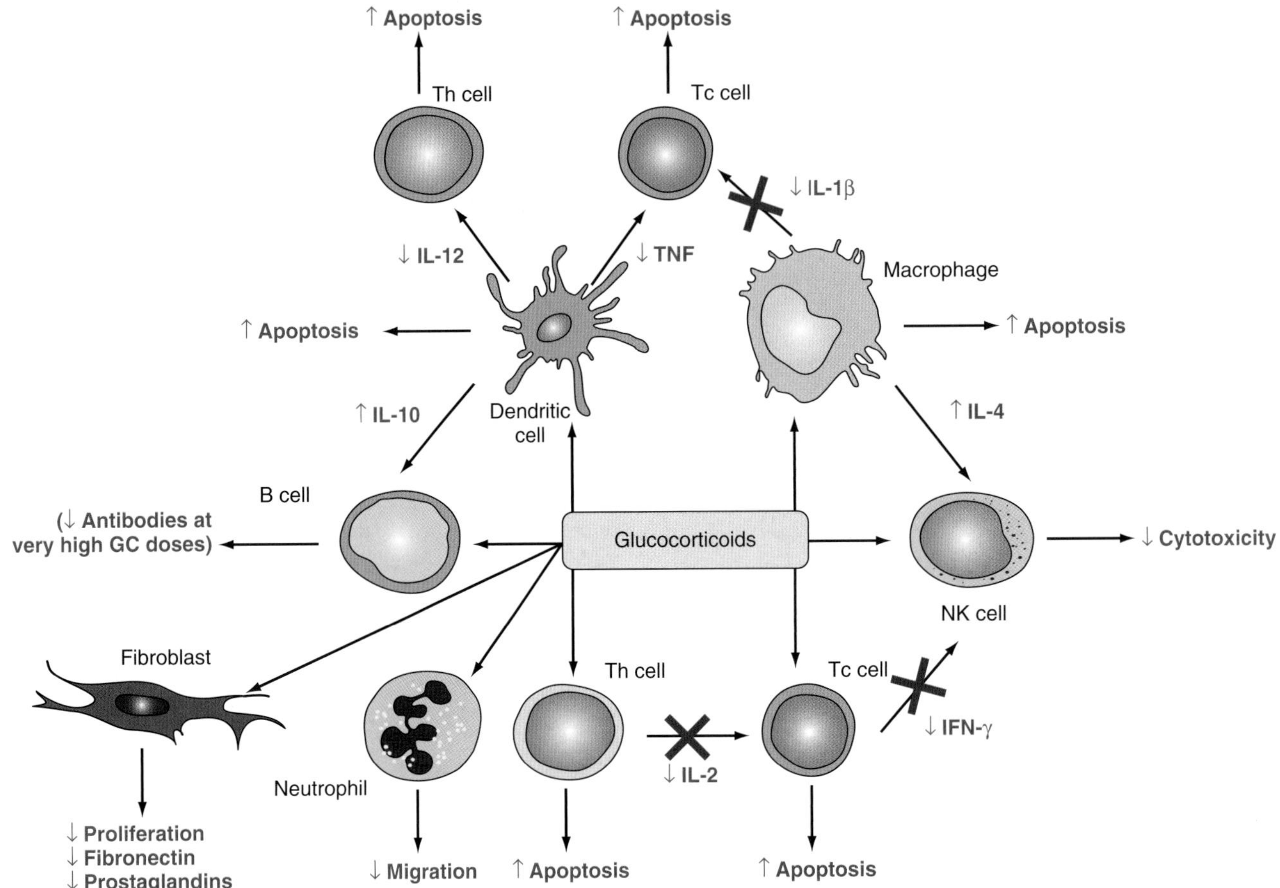

• **Fig. 63.5** Glucocorticoid (GC) effects (in *red*) on the interplay of inflammatory cells and cytokines. Glucocorticoids act on immune cells both directly and indirectly. The production of pro-inflammatory cytokines, such as IL-1β and tumor necrosis factor (TNF), is inhibited, and the production of anti-inflammatory cytokines, such as IL-10, by macrophages and dendritic cells is stimulated. Glucocorticoids promote apoptosis of macrophages, dendritic cells, and T cells. All these effects result in inhibition of immune responses. *IFN-γ,* Interferon-γ; *NK cell,* natural killer cell; *Tc,* cytotoxic T cell; *Th,* T helper cell. (Modified from Sternberg EM: Neural regulation of innate immunity: a coordinated nonspecific host response to pathogens. *Nat Rev Immunol* 6:318-328, 2006.)

TABLE 63.2 Anti-inflammatory Effects of Glucocorticoids on Immune Cells

Cell Type	Effects
Neutrophils	Increased in peripheral blood, decreased trafficking, relatively unaltered functioning
Macrophages and monocytes	Decreased in peripheral blood, decreased trafficking, decreased phagocytosis and bactericidal effects, inhibited antigen presentation, decreased cytokine and eicosanoid release
Lymphocytes	Decreased in peripheral blood, decreased trafficking, decreased cytokine production, decreased proliferation and impaired activation, little effect on immunoglobulin synthesis
Eosinophils	Decreased in peripheral blood, increased apoptosis
Basophils	Decreased in peripheral blood, decreased release of mediators of inflammation

Pro-inflammatory Enzymes

An important part of the inflammatory cascade is arachidonic acid metabolism, which leads to the production of prostaglandins and leukotrienes, most of which are strongly pro-inflammatory. Through the induction of lipocortin (an inhibitor of phospholipase A2), glucocorticoids reduce the formation of arachidonic acid metabolites. Glucocorticoids also inhibit the production of COX-2 and phospholipase A2 induced by cytokines in monocytes/macrophages, fibroblasts, and endothelial cells. In addition, glucocorticoids are potent inhibitors of the production of metalloproteinases in vitro and in vivo, especially collagenase and stromelysin, which are the main effectors of cartilage degradation induced by IL-1 and TNF.[40]

Adhesion Molecules and Permeability Factors

Pharmacologic doses of glucocorticoids markedly inhibit exudation of plasma and migration of leukocytes into inflammatory sites. Adhesion molecules play a central role in chronic inflammatory diseases by controlling the trafficking of inflammatory cells into sites of inflammation. Glucocorticoids reduce the expression of adhesion molecules through the inhibition of pro-inflammatory cytokines and by direct inhibitory effects on the expression of adhesion molecules, such as intercellular adhesion molecule (ICAM)-1 and E-selectin.[41] Chemotactic cytokines attracting immune cells to the inflammatory site, such as IL-8 and macrophage chemoattractant proteins, also are inhibited by glucocorticoids. Nitric oxide production in inflammatory sites is increased by pro-inflammatory cytokines, resulting in increased blood flow, exudation, and probably amplification of the inflammatory response. The inducible form of nitric oxide synthase by cytokines is potently inhibited by glucocorticoids.[42]

Pharmacology and Clinical Considerations

Pharmacokinetics

Apart from the steroid configuration, biologic characteristics of glucocorticoids also depend on whether they are in free form (as alcohol) or are chemically bound (as ester or salt). In their free form, glucocorticoids are virtually insoluble in water, so they can be used in tablets but not in parenteral preparations. For this reason, synthetic glucocorticoids are formulated as either organic esters or as salts. Esters, such as (di)acetate and (hex)acetonide, are lipid soluble but have limited water solubility and are suitable for oral use and intramuscular, intralesional, and intra-articular injection. Salts, such as sodium phosphate and sodium succinate, are generally more water soluble and thus are also suitable for intravenous use. Dexamethasone sodium phosphate can be used intravenously, whereas dexamethasone acetate cannot. When given intramuscularly, dexamethasone sodium phosphate is absorbed much faster from the injection site than dexamethasone acetate. If an immediate effect is required, dexamethasone sodium phosphate should be administered intravenously because it has a more rapid effect than the same preparation given intramuscularly. Intramuscular administration of dexamethasone acetate has the least rapid effect. For local use, less solubility means longer duration of the local effect, which generally is beneficial.

Water insolubility does not impair absorption from the digestive tract. Most orally administered glucocorticoids, whether in free form or as an ester or salt, are absorbed readily, probably within about 30 minutes. The bioavailability of prednisone and prednisolone is high. Commercially available oral and rectal prednisone and prednisolone preparations are considered approximately bioequivalent.

The affinity of the different glucocorticoids for various plasma proteins varies (see Table 63.1). Of cortisol in plasma, 90% to 95% is bound to plasma proteins, primarily transcortin (also called corticosteroid-binding globulin) and, to a lesser degree, albumin. Protein-bound cortisol is not biologically active, but the remaining 5% to 10% of free cortisol is biologically active. In contrast to methylprednisolone, dexamethasone, and triamcinolone, prednisolone has a high affinity for transcortin and competes with cortisol for this binding protein. Two-thirds of the other synthetic glucocorticoids with little or no affinity for transcortin are (weakly) bound to albumin, so about one-third circulates as free glucocorticoid.

Because only unbound glucocorticoids are pharmacologically active, patients with low levels of plasma proteins, such as albumin (e.g., because of liver diseases or chronic active inflammatory diseases), are more susceptible to effects and adverse effects of glucocorticoids. Dosage adjustment should be considered in these patients. In people with liver disease, an additional argument for dosage adjustment is reduced clearance of glucocorticoids (discussed later).

Glucocorticoids have biologic half-lives 2 to 36 times longer than their plasma half-lives (see Table 63.1). Because prednisolone has a plasma half-life of about 3 hours, it can be prescribed in a once-daily dose for most diseases. Maximal effects of glucocorticoids lag behind peak serum concentrations. Transcortin binds these compounds more strongly than does albumin. The plasma elimination of glucocorticoids predominantly bound to transcortin is in general slower than that of glucocorticoids predominantly bound to albumin or that of glucocorticoids that do not bind to plasma proteins. Transcortin binding is not a major determinant of biologic half-lives of glucocorticoids, but it is a major determinant of distribution to different compartments of the body and of binding to the cytosolic glucocorticoid receptor. Compared with cortisol, synthetic glucocorticoids have a lower affinity for transcortin but a higher affinity for the cytosolic glucocorticoid receptor. The affinity of prednisolone and triamcinolone for the glucocorticoid receptor is approximately two times higher, and for dexamethasone it is seven times higher. Before they have been chemically reduced, prednisone and cortisone have negligible glucocorticoid bioactivity because of their very low affinity for the glucocorticoid receptor.

Another important factor determining biologic half-lives of glucocorticoids is the rate of metabolism. Synthetic glucocorticoids are subject to the same reduction, oxidation, hydroxylation, and conjugation reactions as cortisol. Pharmacologically active glucocorticoids are metabolized primarily in the liver into inactive metabolites that are excreted by the kidneys; only small amounts of unmetabolized drug also are excreted in the urine. An inverse correlation has been found between prednisolone clearance and age, which means that a given dose may have a greater effect in older people.[43] Prednisolone clearance also is slower in African Americans compared with the clearance in Caucasians.[44] The serum half-life of prednisolone is 2.5 to 5 hours, but it is increased in patients with renal disease and liver cirrhosis and in elderly people. Prednisolone can be removed by hemodialysis, but, overall, the amount removed does not require dosage adjustment in patients undergoing hemodialysis. In patients with cirrhosis of the liver, the clearance of unbound steroid is about two-thirds of normal, a difference that should be taken into account with dosing.

Glucocorticoid Resistance

A small proportion of patients does not react favorably to glucocorticoids or even fails to respond to high doses. Furthermore, the susceptibility to adverse effects of glucocorticoids varies widely. Several different factors are involved in the variability of glucocorticoid sensitivity in patients with rheumatic diseases,[45–47] and an understanding of the mechanisms involved might eventually permit their modulation.

Hereditary glucocorticoid resistance (which is rare) and increased susceptibility to glucocorticoids have been related to specific polymorphisms of the glucocorticoid receptor gene. The glucocorticoid receptor exists as α and β isoforms, but only the α isoform binds glucocorticoids. The β isoform functions as an endogenous inhibitor of glucocorticoids and is expressed in several tissues. Glucocorticoid resistance has been associated with enhanced expression of this β receptor, but it is unlikely to be an important mechanism for glucocorticoid resistance because in most cells, apart from neutrophilic granulocytes, expression of the β receptor is much less than that of the α receptor.[45] The protein lipocortin-1 (or annexin-1) inhibits eicosanoid synthesis. Glucocorticoids are thought to stimulate lipocortin-1. In patients with RA, autoantibodies to lipocortin-1 have been described. The titers in these patients correlate with the levels of maintenance doses of glucocorticoids, suggesting that these antibodies may lead to glucocorticoid resistance.[48]

Glucocorticoids exert most of their immunosuppressive actions through inhibition of cytokine production; high concentrations of cytokines, especially IL-2, antagonize the suppressive effect of glucocorticoids in a dose-dependent manner.[49] The balance is usually in favor of glucocorticoids, but high local concentrations of cytokines may result in a localized glucocorticoid resistance that cannot be overridden by exogenous glucocorticoids. In addition, macrophage migration inhibitory factor may play a role in glucocorticoid resistance in RA. This pro-inflammatory cytokine is involved in TNF synthesis and T cell activation, suggesting a role in the pathogenesis of RA. Macrophage migration inhibitory factor is suppressed by higher concentrations of glucocorticoids, but it is induced by low concentrations, leading to stimulation of inflammation.[50] Other possible mechanisms of glucocorticoid resistance include activation of mitogen-activated protein kinase (MAPK) pathways by certain cytokines, excessive activation of transcription factor AP-1, reduced histone deacetylase-2 expression, and increased P-glycoprotein–mediated drug efflux.[45] Drugs also may play a role in glucocorticoid sensitivity and resistance (see next section, Drug Interactions).

Drug Interactions

Cytochrome P450 (CYP) is a family of isozymes responsible for the biotransformation of several drugs. Drug interactions can be based on induction or inhibition of these enzymes. Certain drugs (e.g., barbiturates, phenytoin, and rifampin), by inducing CYP isoenzymes (e.g., CYP3A4), increase the metabolism (breakdown) of synthetic and natural glucocorticoids, particularly by enhancing hepatic hydroxylase activity, thus reducing glucocorticoid concentrations (Fig. 63.6). Indeed, rifampin-induced nonresponsiveness to prednisone in inflammatory diseases has been described,[51,52] as has rifampin-induced adrenal crisis in patients receiving glucocorticoid replacement therapy.[53] Clinicians should consider increasing the dosage of glucocorticoids in patients who are concomitantly treated with these medications.

Conversely, concomitant use of glucocorticoids with inhibitors of the drug metabolizing CYP3A4 (e.g., ketoconazole, itraconazole, diltiazem, mibefradil, and grapefruit juice) decreases glucocorticoid clearance and leads to higher concentrations and prolonged biologic half-life of glucocorticoid drugs, thus increasing the risk of adverse effects.[27] On the other hand, antifungal therapies, especially ketoconazole, are known to interfere with endogenous glucocorticoid synthesis and therefore are also used, in doses of 400 to 1200 mg per day, to treat hypercortisolism.[27] Etomidate, a short-acting intravenous anesthetic agent used for the induction of general anesthesia and for sedation, can also lower cortisol levels, which could be clinically relevant in critically ill patients.[27] In general, however, even potent CYP3A4 inhibitors are probably not that important for prednisone and prednisolone metabolism; in addition, the effect of grapefruit juice intake is likely to be of limited clinical significance.[54]

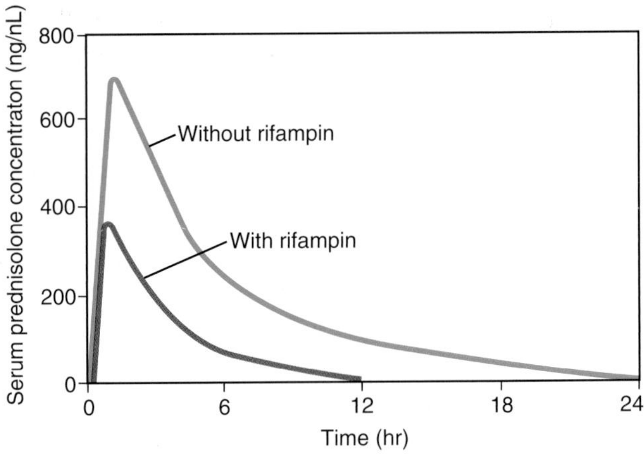

• **Fig. 63.6** Serum prednisolone concentration in time in one patient, after 0.9 mg/kg oral prednisone daily, in the presence and absence of therapy with rifampin. The *red* curve shows the concentration during a period of continuous administration of both prednisolone and rifampin. The *green* curve shows the concentration after a washout of rifampin of 4 weeks. Rifampin results in a reduced area under the curve, indicating reduced bioavailability of prednisolone during rifampin therapy.

Concomitant administration of prednisolone and cyclosporine may result in increased plasma concentrations of the former drug, whereas concomitant administration of methylprednisolone and cyclosporine may result in increased plasma concentrations of the latter drug. The mechanism involved is probably competitive inhibition of microsomal liver enzymes. Antibiotics such as erythromycin may increase plasma concentrations of glucocorticoids. Synthetic estrogens in oral contraceptives increase the level of transcortin and thus the total (sum of bound and unbound) glucocorticoid levels. Therefore, in women taking oral contraceptives, care is required in the interpretation of cortisol measurements, especially because adrenal insufficiency may be present even if total cortisol levels are within the normal range.[18] Next to glucocorticoids, other steroid drugs such as megestrol acetate and medroxyprogesterone inhibit the HPA axis[27]; this risk may be increased when used concomitantly with glucocorticoids. Sulphasalazine has been reported to increase the sensitivity of immune cells for glucocorticoids,[55] which might be beneficial. Mifepristone is an antiprogesterone drug and glucocorticoid receptor antagonist, and chlorpromazine inhibits glucocorticoid receptor–mediated gene transcription[56]; via these mechanisms, these drugs decrease the effect of glucocorticoids.

Glucocorticoid Therapy

Glucocorticoids are widely used in various dosages for several rheumatic diseases. Often it is unclear what is meant by semi-quantitative terms used for dosages, such as low or high. Based on pathophysiologic and pharmacokinetic data, standardization has been proposed to minimize problems in interpretation of these generally used terms (Table 63.3).[6]

Indications

For each disease, indications for glucocorticoid therapy are discussed in the specific chapters related to the disease. Glucocorticoids are anchor drugs of the therapeutic strategy in myositis, polymyalgia rheumatica, giant cell arteritis, and systemic vasculitis. In people with systemic sclerosis, glucocorticoids, especially in

TABLE 63.3 Classification of Glucocorticoid Dosages

Low dose	≤7.5 mg prednisone equivalents per day
Medium dose	>7.5 mg and ≤30 mg prednisone equivalents per day
High dose	>30 mg and ≤100 mg prednisone equivalents per day
Very high dose	>100 mg prednisone equivalents per day
Pulse therapy	≥250 mg prednisone equivalents per day for 1 day or a few days

high doses, are contraindicated because of the risk of scleroderma renal crisis, but they may be useful when myositis or interstitial lung disease complicates systemic sclerosis. For other diseases, glucocorticoids serve as adjunctive therapy or are not used at all. For instance, in people with RA, glucocorticoids are used almost exclusively as adjunctive therapy in combination with other disease-modifying anti-rheumatic drugs (DMARDs), described later. Although glucocorticoids are effective in reducing pain in inflammatory hand osteoarthritis (OA),[56a] they are not given to people with OA in daily practice, with the exception of an intra-articular injection if signs of synovitis of an osteoarthritic joint are present.[57] For generalized soft tissue disorders such as fibromyalgia, glucocorticoids are not indicated, and for localized soft tissue disorders, glucocorticoids should be used only for intralesional injection.[58]

Glucocorticoid Therapy in Rheumatoid Arthritis

Glucocorticoids are frequently prescribed for people with RA. Worldwide estimates of the percentages of patients with RA who are treated with glucocorticoids range from 15% to 90%.[59] The Consortium Of Rheumatology Researchers Of North America (CORRONA) registry, a U.S.-based longitudinal registry of patients with RA (n = 25,000) shows that about 30% of its RA patients uses a glucocorticoid.[1] In an older US study, 35.5% of 12,749 RA-patients were currently using glucocorticoids and the lifetime exposure was 65.5%.[2] Aims of this therapy are reduction of signs and symptoms and inhibition of the development of joint damage. A review of seven studies (including 253 patients) concluded that glucocorticoids, when administered for approximately 6 months, are effective for the treatment of RA.[60] After 6 months of therapy, the beneficial effects of glucocorticoids seem to diminish, but if this therapy is then tapered off and stopped, patients often—especially during the first months—experience aggravation of symptoms, which indicates that the glucocorticoid therapy was effective after all, and which partly can be ascribed to some grade of adrenal insufficiency by persistent suppression of the adrenal gland by the recent glucocorticoid therapy.

An inhibitory effect of glucocorticoids on progression of radiographic joint damage and functional deterioration has firmly been proven[3] in a randomized study with a tight control and treat-to-target design.[61] Nevertheless, it is still not known whether glucocorticoids can also inhibit progression of joint erosions and functional deterioration in established RA or for a treatment duration longer than 2 years. The joint-sparing effect of glucocorticoids probably is based on the inhibition of pro-inflammatory cytokines such as IL-1 and TNF,[62] which stimulate osteoblasts and T cells to produce the receptor activator of NF-κB (RANK) ligand. This ligand binds to RANK on osteoclast precursor cells and on mature osteoblasts, leading to activation of osteoclasts, which are responsible for bone resorption, periarticular osteopenia, and formation of bone erosions in RA. Furthermore, fibroblast proliferation and IL-1 and TNF-induced metalloproteinase synthesis are inhibited by glucocorticoids, retarding bone and cartilage destruction in inflamed joints of patients with early RA.[35,36,40]

Glucocorticoid Pulse Therapy

Glucocorticoid pulse therapy is used in rheumatology, especially for remission induction, treatment of flares of inflammatory rheumatic disorders and vasculitis, and severe complications of rheumatic diseases, such as visual loss in people with giant cell arteritis. Nevertheless, in 144 patients with biopsy-confirmed giant cell arteritis—91 with vision loss upon being seen initially and 53 without vision loss—no evidence was found that intravenous glucocorticoid pulse therapy (usually 150 mg dexamethasone sodium phosphate every 8 hours for 1 to 3 days) was more effective than high and very high doses of oral (80 to 120 mg) prednisone daily in preventing deterioration of vision.[63] In people with active RA, pulse therapy to induce remission is sometimes applied in the initiation phase of a (new) DMARD strategy to stabilize in the long term the remission induced by the pulse therapy. The beneficial effect of pulse therapy generally lasts about 6 weeks, with a large individual variation in the duration of the effect.[64] For this purpose, pulse therapy with schemes of 1000 mg of methylprednisolone per day intravenously for one or several days has been proven to be effective in many studies. Short-term effects of pulse therapy in patients with established, active RA at various dimensions of health status are very similar to long-term effects of effective conventional DMARD therapy, such as methotrexate, in patients with early phase RA.[65]

The risk of adverse effects of pulse therapy is not the same for all rheumatic disorders. Compared with patients with RA, patients with SLE more frequently experience osteonecrosis and psychosis as adverse effects of pulse therapy.[65] Osteonecrosis and psychosis also can be complications of SLE itself, however. Contraindications for pulse therapy are pregnancy and lactation, infections, current peptic ulcer disease, glaucoma, and insufficiently controlled hypertension and diabetes mellitus. In patients with well-controlled hypertension or diabetes mellitus or a family history of glaucoma, pulse therapy can be applied with checks of blood pressure, blood glucose levels, and eye pressure, respectively, before and during high-dose glucocorticoid therapy and pulse therapy.[66]

Glucocorticoid Tapering Regimens

Because of potential adverse effects, glucocorticoids usually are tapered off as soon as the disease being treated is under control. Tapering must be performed carefully to avoid recurrent activity of the disease and cortisol deficiency resulting from chronic HPA axis suppression. Gradual tapering permits recovery of the adrenal function. There is no best scheme for tapering glucocorticoids based on controlled, comparative studies. Tapering depends on the specific disease being treated; it also depends on the clinical response, current disease activity, and doses and duration of glucocorticoid therapy, which are all influenced by the individual patient's glucocorticoid sensitivity. Only generic guidelines can be offered. To taper the dose of prednisone, decrements of 5 to 10 mg every 1 to 2 weeks can be applied when the prednisone dose is

TABLE 63.4 Glucocorticoid Tapering Scheme to Provide to Patients[a]

	Monday	Tuesday	Wednesday	Thursday	Friday	Saturday	Sunday
Period 1	High	High	High	High	Low	High	High
Period 2	High	Low	High	High	High	Low	High
Period 3	High	Low	High	Low	High	Low	High
Period 4	Low	High	Low	High	Low	High	Low
Period 5	Low	High	Low	Low	Low	High	Low
Period 6	Low	Low	Low	High	Low	Low	Low
Period 7	Low	Low	Low	Low	Low	Low	Low
Duration of each period ____ week(s)[b]				Low = ____ mg/day[b] High = ____ mg/day[b]			

[a]At each consecutive period, which can last 1 week, 2 weeks, or more weeks, depending on clinical considerations, the number of days per period at which a low dose is taken increases by 1. After completion of period 7, the next step in tapering can be taken; the dose called "low" during the previous seven periods now is "high." In case of aggravation of symptoms, the patient should not diminish the dose and should contact the physician.

[b]To be filled out by the physician.

higher than 40 mg/day, followed by 5 mg decrements every 1 to 2 weeks at doses between 40 and 20 mg/day, and finally 1 to 2.5 mg/day decrements every 2 to 3 weeks at a prednisone dose of less than 20 mg/day. Another scheme is to taper 5 to 10 mg every 1 to 2 weeks down to 30 mg/day of prednisone, and when the dose is less than 20 mg/day, to taper 2.5 to 5 mg every 2 to 4 weeks down to 10 mg/day; thereafter, the dose may be tapered 1 mg each month or 2.5 mg (half a 5 mg tablet of prednisolone) each 7 weeks. For tapering steps over 7 weeks or a multiple number of 7 weeks, a printed schedule can be given to the patient, such as the one shown in Table 63.4, on which the doses and period of tapering should be filled out.

Stress Regimens and Perioperative Care

Patients taking low-dose glucocorticoid medication on a long-term basis have suppressed adrenal activity and should be advised to double their daily glucocorticoid dose, or increase the dose to 15 mg prednisolone or its equivalent, if they experience fever attributed to infection; they should also seek medical help. In the case of major surgery, given the unreliable prediction of adrenal suppression on the basis of the duration and dose of glucocorticoid therapy (see the section in this chapter on the effects of glucocorticoids on the HPA axis), many physicians recommend "stress doses" of glucocorticoids, also for patients with a low risk of adrenal suppression. The scheme of 100 mg of hydrocortisone administered intravenously just before the operation is performed, followed by an additional 100 mg every 6 hours for 3 days, is based on anecdotal information and is not always necessary.[67,68] A scheme with a lower dose, possibly reducing the risk of post-operative bacterial infectious complications, is to continuously infuse 100 mg of hydrocortisone intravenously the first day of surgery, followed by 25 to 50 mg of hydrocortisone every 8 hours for 2 or 3 days. Another option is to administer the usual dose of oral glucocorticoid orally or (the equivalent) parenterally on the day of surgery, followed by 25 to 50 mg of hydrocortisone every 8 hours for 2 or 3 days.

In cases of minor surgery, it is probably sufficient to double the oral dose or to increase the dose to 15 mg of prednisolone or its equivalent for 1 to 3 days. No comparative randomized studies on different perioperative glucocorticoid stress schemes have been published, however. Because aldosterone secretion is preserved in people with glucocorticoid-induced tertiary adrenal insufficiency, mineralocorticoid therapy is unnecessary, whereas it is necessary in people with primary adrenal insufficiency.

Pregnancy and Lactation

In pregnancy, two mechanisms protect the fetus from exogenous glucocorticoids. First, glucocorticoids bound to transport proteins cannot pass the placenta, in contrast to unbound glucocorticoids. Second, the enzyme 11β-HSD in the placenta, which catalyzes the conversion of active cortisol, corticosterone, and prednisolone into the inactive 11-dehydro-prohormones (cortisone, 11-dehydrocorticosterone, and prednisone), protects the fetus from glucocorticoids in the blood of the mother. The maternal-to-fetal prednisolone blood concentration ratio is about 10 : 1 as a result of these mechanisms. In contrast, dexamethasone has little or no affinity for transport proteins and is poorly metabolized by 11β-HSD in the placenta; the maternal-to-fetal dexamethasone blood concentration ratio is about 1 : 1.

If a pregnant woman must be treated with glucocorticoids, then prednisone, prednisolone, and methylprednisolone would be good choices; if the unborn child must be treated—for example, to treat congenital heart block associated with maternal Sjögren's syndrome—then fluorinated glucocorticoids, such as betamethasone or dexamethasone, would be indicated. The risk of adverse effects of antenatal exposure to glucocorticoids, such as reduced intrauterine growth and birth weight, neurocognitive adverse effects, and oral cleft, seems to be dependent on dose, duration of therapy, and stage of pregnancy. Several studies report conflicting results regarding the occurrence of these adverse effects,[69–71] but doses of glucocorticoid and indications for this therapy differ between studies. Furthermore, it is difficult to discriminate between negative effects and complications of the fetal condition treated and adverse effects of the glucocorticoid therapy. Avoidance of high doses (1 to 2 mg/kg prednisolone-equivalent) in the first trimester of pregnancy is advised,[72,73] whereas low to medium doses of prednisone seem to be safe.[73]

Early postnatal dexamethasone therapy for the prevention or treatment of chronic lung disease has had negative effects on neuromotor and cognitive function at school age.[74] Prednisolone and prednisone are excreted only in small quantities in breast milk.

Breastfeeding is generally considered safe for an infant whose mother is taking these drugs. The exposure of the infant seems further minimized if the infant is breastfed before the mother takes her daily dose, or if breastfeeding is avoided during the first 4 hours after the intake of prednisolone, because curves of milk and serum concentrations of prednisolone are similar in time.[73]

Intralesional and Intra-articular Glucocorticoid Injections

Injections with glucocorticoids are widely used for arthritis, tenosynovitis, bursitis, enthesitis, and compression neuropathies such as carpal tunnel syndrome.[58] Generally, the effect occurs within days; it can be long lasting, but if the underlying disease is active, the effect is of short duration. Administration of a local anesthetic concurrently with intra-articular or soft tissue injection of a glucocorticoid may provide immediate pain relief.

Soluble glucocorticoids (e.g., phosphate salts) have a more rapid onset of action and likely have less risk of subcutaneous tissue atrophy and depigmentation of the skin when given intralesionally. Insoluble glucocorticoids are longer acting and might decrease the soft tissue fibrous matrix to a greater extent than soluble glucocorticoids, so they should be used with caution in places with thin skin, especially in elderly patients and patients with peripheral vascular disease. Administration of insoluble glucocorticoids into deep sites is a safer approach. Short-acting soluble glucocorticoids can be mixed with long-acting insoluble glucocorticoids to combine rapid onset with long-acting effects.

The effect of an intra-articular glucocorticoid injection probably depends on several factors: the underlying disease (e.g., RA or OA), characteristics of the treated joint (e.g., size and weight bearing or non–weight bearing), the activity of arthritis, the volume of synovial fluid of the treated joint,[47] the application of arthrocentesis (synovial fluid aspiration) before injection, the choice and dose of the glucocorticoid preparation, the application of rest to the injected joint, and the injection technique. The effect of injections seems to be less favorable in OA compared with RA.[75] Arthrocentesis before injecting the glucocorticoid preparation reduces the risk for relapse of arthritis. Triamcinolone hexacetonide, which among the injectable glucocorticoids is the least soluble preparation, demonstrates the longest effect.

Theoretically, rest of the injected joint minimizes leakage of the injected glucocorticoid preparation to the systemic circulation (via the hyperemic, inflamed synovium by enhanced pressure in the joint during activity), minimizes the risk of cartilage damage, and optimizes the condition for repair of inflammatory tissue damage. Advice and procedures for the postinjection period in terms of activity vary from no restrictions to minimal activity of the injected joint for a couple of days to bed rest for 24 hours after injection of a knee joint or splinting of injected joints. Based on the literature, no definite evidence-based recommendation can be made, but it seems prudent to rest and not to overuse the injected joint for several days, even if pain is relieved.

It is recommended that intra-articular glucocorticoid injections be repeated no more than once every 3 weeks and be given no more frequently than three times a year in a weight-bearing joint (e.g., the knee) to minimize glucocorticoid-induced joint damage. This recommendation also seems sensible, but there is no definite clinical evidence to support it. As one would expect, accuracy of steroid placement influences the clinical outcome of glucocorticoid injections into the shoulder and probably into other joints as well.[76] This factor is important because it is estimated that a little more than half of shoulder injections are inaccurately placed.[76,77] The reported infection rate of joints after local injections with glucocorticoids is low, ranging from 1 case in 13,900 to 77,300 injections.[78,79] Introduction in the past of disposable needles and syringes has helped to reduce the risk of infection. In a 3-year prospective study in an urban area of 1 million people in the Netherlands, bacterial infections were detected in 214 joints (including 58 joints with a prosthesis or osteosynthetic material) of 186 patients; only 3 of these joint infections were attributed to an intra-articular injection.[80]

Other adverse effects of local glucocorticoid injections are systemic adverse effects of the glucocorticoid, such as disturbance of the menstrual pattern, hot flush–like symptoms the day of or the day after injection, and hyperglycemia in people with diabetes mellitus.[58] Local complications include subcutaneous fat tissue atrophy (especially after improper local injection), local depigmentation of the skin, tendon slip and rupture, and lesions to local nerves.[58]

Improving the Therapeutic Ratio of Glucocorticoids

Alternate-Day Regimens

For oral, long-term use of glucocorticoid therapy, alternate-day regimens have been devised in an attempt to alleviate adverse effects, such as HPA axis suppression. Alternate-day therapy consists of a single dose administered every other morning, which is usually equivalent to, or somewhat higher than, twice the usual or pre-established daily dose. The rationale for this regimen is that the body, including the HPA, exposed to exogenous glucocorticoid only on alternate days, may recover the other days. This rationale makes sense only for usage of a class and dosage of a glucocorticoid that suppresses the HPA axis activity for less than 36 hours after a single dose. Another prerequisite is that the patient should have a responsive HPA axis that has not been chronically suppressed by previous glucocorticoid regimens. The alternate-day schedule does not work in patients taking medium- or high-dose glucocorticoids on a long-term basis, which suppresses the HPA axis activity for longer than 36 hours.

Alternate-day therapy is unsuccessful in several inflammatory rheumatic diseases. Nowadays, alternate-day regimens are rarely used, except in patients with juvenile idiopathic arthritis, in whom alternate-day glucocorticoid usage results in less inhibition of body growth than is associated with daily usage.[81]

Glucocorticoid-Sparing Agents

For several inflammatory rheumatic diseases such as SLE, vasculitis, and myositis, early in the disease other immunosuppressive drugs such as hydroxychloroquine, methotrexate, and, for systemic vasculitis, cyclophosphamide often are added to therapy with glucocorticoids. For these indications, increasingly, biologic agents also are used.[82] Combination therapy is applied if it is known that the effect of the combination for the specific disease (e.g., systemic vasculitis) is better than that of glucocorticoids alone or if the disease (e.g., inflammatory myositis) seems resistant to the high initial doses of glucocorticoids.

If in a later stage of the disease immunosuppressive drugs are added to therapy with glucocorticoids to enable further reduction of the dose to decrease the risk of adverse effects, these immunosuppressive drugs are termed *glucocorticoid-sparing agents.* Azathioprine and methotrexate are often used for this purpose, although any drug that has an additive or synergistic effect in suppressing the disease activity, thus enabling reduction of the glucocorticoid dose, could be used as a glucocorticoid-sparing agent.

In people with polymyalgia rheumatica and giant cell arteritis, azathioprine, antimalarial agents, cyclosporine, dapsone, infliximab, adalimumab, leflunomide, and, most frequently, methotrexate have been tried as glucocorticoid-sparing agents; half of the six randomized trials on methotrexate support its use in this situation.[83–88] A meta-analysis showed a marginal benefit of methotrexate as a glucocorticoid-sparing agent in giant cell arteritis with respect to relapse (relative risk [RR] 0.85; 95% CI, 0.66 to 1.11) and no improved outcome associated with the use of other glucocorticoid-sparing agents.[89] In giant cell arteritis, the addition of tocilizumab (IL-6 receptor blockade) was superior to glucocorticoid monotherapy with regard to sustained glucocorticoid-free remission, and cumulative glucocorticoid exposure was significantly lower.[90] Because the effects of tocilizumab are more convincing than those of conventional glucocorticoid-sparing agents, the use of this biologic agent in giant cell arteritis is expected to be incorporated in updated treatment recommendations in the coming years, and the use of tocilizumab is expected to increase in clinical practice over the coming years. An important drawback is the suppression of laboratory inflammatory markers such as C-reactive protein by tocilizumab. This means that these markers are no longer a reliable indication of disease activity.

Modified-Release Prednisone

The inflammatory process and signs and symptoms of inflammatory rheumatic diseases generally have a diurnal rhythm. Early in the morning, patients experience the most extensive stiffness and other symptoms because of the circadian rhythm of cortisol (see Fig. 63.4). In patients with RA who have low or moderate disease activity, serum cortisol maximum and minimum levels shift to earlier times of the day and night, whereas in patients with RA who have high disease activity, the circadian rhythm is markedly reduced or even lost.

The timing of glucocorticoid administration may be important for efficacy and adverse effects. Older data in the literature on this topic were ambiguous.[91,92] More recently, a trial has been performed with a newly developed modified-release prednisone tablet that releases prednisone about 4 hours after ingestion.[93] When it was taken in the evening, thus synchronizing its prednisone release to circadian increases of pro-inflammatory cytokine concentrations, symptoms of RA early in the morning were lessened compared with the symptoms reported when the same dose of prednisone was taken via a normal tablet early in the morning. This 3-month double-blind trial included patients with RA who had a duration of morning stiffness of 45 minutes or longer, a pain score of 30 mm or more on a 100 mm visual analog scale, three or more painful joints, one or more swollen joints, an erythrocyte sedimentation rate (ESR) of 28 mm 1st hour or greater, or a C-reactive protein concentration 1.5 times or more the upper limit of normal, and who had been taking glucocorticoids at least 3 months, with a stable daily dose of 2 to 10 mg prednisolone-equivalent for at least 1 month. Patients were randomized in a double-dummy manner to continue their prednisone or to switch to modified-release prednisone. At the end of the trial, the difference in duration of morning stiffness was about 30 minutes in favor of the modified-release prednisone group. No differences were noted in the other clinical variables of disease activity between the two groups. The safety profile did not differ between treatments, and no statistical difference was found in HPA axis function.[30,94]

In an open-label observational study among 950 outpatients with RA who were being treated with glucocorticoids and were switching to modified-release prednisone, at assessment 4 months later, decreased disease activity was seen.[95] Longer-term benefits and risks of this preparation and application in other inflammatory rheumatic diseases have to be further investigated.[96]

Other Developments: Selective Glucocorticoid Receptor Agonists and Liposomes

Deflazacort,[97] an oxazoline derivative of prednisolone introduced in 1969, initially was thought to be as effective as prednisolone while inducing fewer adverse effects, but there is the issue of the real equivalence ratio compared with prednisolone,[98] and deflazacort has not represented a major breakthrough. Knowledge about the mechanisms of glucocorticoids (with the hypothesis that transrepression and transactivation lead, respectively, to predominantly beneficial effects and adverse effects; see earlier) led to the development of selective glucocorticoid receptor agonists.[99] Nevertheless, the underlying hypothesis was challenged,[15] and the effect of a selective glucocorticoid receptor agonist was disappointing.[16] A phase 2 study with fosdagrocorat demonstrated efficacy in RA with manageable adverse effects.[100] More studies are needed, especially on longer-term safety before such a drug will enter the market.

Glucocorticoid preparations releasing nitric oxide, the so-called *nitrosteroids*, could induce stronger anti-inflammatory effects because nitric oxide also has anti-inflammatory effects.[101] These drugs have yet to be tested in patients.

To overcome side effects and glucocorticoid resistance, new delivery vehicles have been developed, including PEGylated liposomes, polymeric micelles, polymer-drug conjugates, inorganic scaffolds, and hybrid nanoparticles.[102] Liposomes that contain glucocorticoids and are targeted to integrins that are expressed on endothelial cells at sites of inflammation have been studied; these liposomes deliver their glucocorticoids specifically at sites of inflammation.[103] Their selective biodistribution might allow for less frequent and lower dosing, which could result in an improved therapeutic ratio.[104] Clinical studies are needed to see if liposomal glucocorticoids will be effective in clinical rheumatologic practice.

In all, these new glucocorticoid developments, which seemed promising in the past, have not yet lived up to expectations or still must be tested in randomized clinical trials.

Another type of strategy to improve the clinical use of glucocorticoids has been the development of guidelines.[66,105,106]

Adverse Effects and Monitoring

A toxicity index score for DMARDs based on symptoms, laboratory abnormalities, and hospitalization data of 3000 patients with more than 7300 patient-years from the Arthritis, Rheumatism, and Aging Medical Information System (ARAMIS) database has been published.[107] Although this score has not been validated and is influenced by confounding-by-indication, it gives an impression of the relative toxicity of glucocorticoids. It is comparable with that of other immunosuppressive medications used in people with RA, such as methotrexate and azathioprine. A review also showed that the incidence, severity, and impact of adverse effects of low-dose glucocorticoid therapy in RA trials were modest and suggested that many of the well-known adverse effects of glucocorticoids probably are predominantly associated with high-dose treatment.[108]

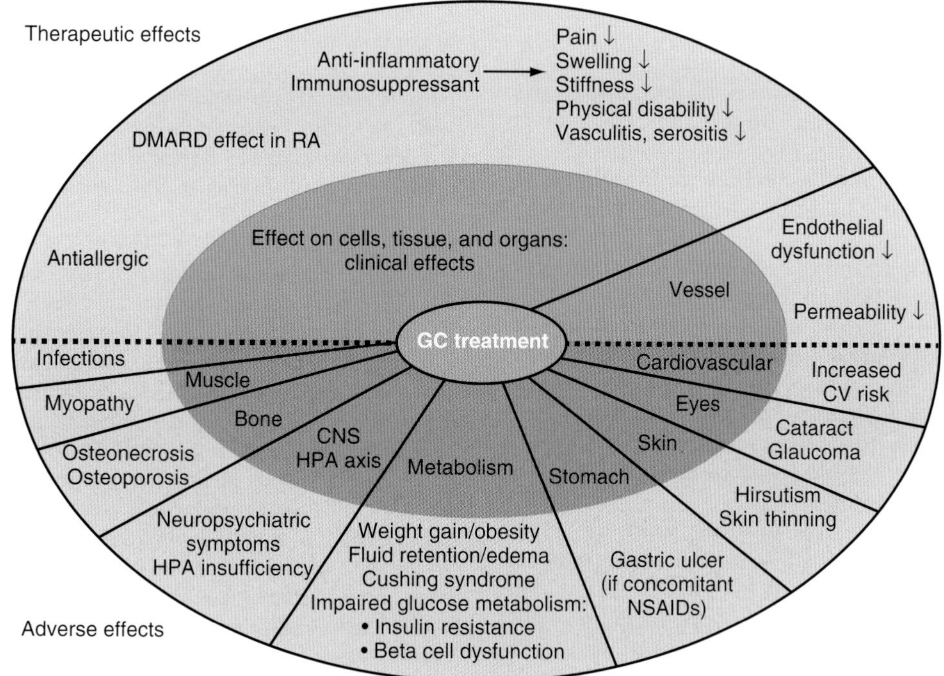

• **Fig. 63.7** The spectrum of effects of glucocorticoids (GCs) therapy. Beneficial effects are shown in the *green upper part* of the figure, and adverse effects in the *rose-colored lower part*. *CV,* Cardiovascular; *DMARD,* disease-modifying anti-rheumatic drug; *HPA,* hypothalamic-pituitary-adrenal; *NSAIDs,* nonsteroidal anti-inflammatory drugs; *RA,* rheumatoid arthritis. (Modified from Buttgereit F, Burmester GR, Lipworth BJ: Optimised glucocorticoids therapy: the sharpening of an old spear. *Lancet* 365:801-803, 2005.)

Because many questions remain to be answered, such as how the effect of glucocorticoids compares with that of high dosages of methotrexate or that of TNF inhibitors and for how long glucocorticoids should be prescribed and in what dosages, the final role of glucocorticoid therapy in RA has yet to be determined. Presently, guidelines on how to use (low-dose) glucocorticoids and how to monitor this therapy have been developed.[105,106]

Given the diversity of their mechanisms and sites of action, it is not surprising that glucocorticoids can cause a wide array of adverse effects (Figs. 63.7 and 63.8). Most of these adverse effects cannot be avoided, but the risk of most complications is dosage and time dependent, and minimizing the amount of glucocorticoids minimizes the risk of complications.[105] Dose-related patterns of adverse effects of glucocorticoids have been described.[109] Low-dose glucocorticoid therapy is safer than is commonly thought,[108] and medium- to long-term glucocorticoid therapy in people with RA is associated with limited toxicity compared with placebo,[110] but sensitivity for adverse effects varies among individuals. Clinical observations indicate some patients experience adverse effects after small doses of glucocorticoids, whereas other patients receive high doses without serious adverse effects. The apparent individual susceptibility to adverse effects does not seem to parallel the individual susceptibility to beneficial effects. Osteoporosis, diabetes, and cardiovascular diseases are ranked among the most worrisome adverse effects of glucocorticoids by both patients and rheumatologists.[111] The frequency and severity of glucocorticoid-related adverse effects, however, have seldom been studied systematically. A problem in interpreting results from nonrandomized studies examining glucocorticoid-related adverse effects is bias by indication. Patients with severe disease tend to receive glucocorticoids more frequently than do patients with less severe disease, and both the disease and the glucocorticoids can cause unfavorable signs and symptoms[112]; on the other hand, glucocorticoids decrease disease activity and thus influence the frequency and severity of disease-associated signs and symptoms (see Fig. 63.8). Longitudinal data analyses of patients using glucocorticoids at different dosages in time with repeated standardized assessments of disease activity and of other effects would be the best way to disentangle the intricate interaction between glucocorticoids, disease activity, disease-associated signs and symptoms, and glucocorticoid-induced adverse effects. In the coming years, more information on the benefits and risks of adding glucocorticoids to treatment strategies for RA in elderly patients is expected.[113,114]

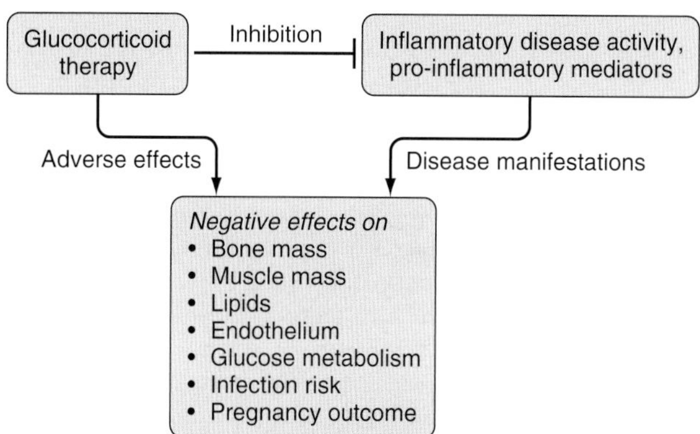

• **Fig. 63.8** Interplay of glucocorticoid therapy, the inflammatory disease, and negative effects, which can be adverse effects of glucocorticoids and negative effects of the disease itself. Inflammatory diseases have been proven to exert negative effects on bone mass, lipids, endothelium, glucose metabolism and insulin tolerance, infection risk, and pregnancy outcome. These negative effects also are attributed to (especially medium- and high-dose) glucocorticoids. Glucocorticoids suppress the inflammatory disease and thus also these negative disease-related effects.

Infections

All patients suffering from inflammatory rheumatic diseases are at increased risk for infections, and therefore influenza and 23-valent polysaccharide pneumococcal vaccination should be strongly considered.[115]

At high doses, glucocorticoids diminish neutrophil phagocytosis and bacterial killing in vitro, whereas in vivo, normal bactericidal and phagocytic activities are found. Monocytes are more susceptible; during treatment with medium to high doses of glucocorticoids, bactericidal and fungicidal activity in vivo and in vitro is reduced. These factors may influence the risk of infection. From epidemiologic studies, treatment with a daily dose of less than 10 mg of prednisolone or its equivalent seems to lead to no risk or only a slightly increased risk of infection, whereas if doses of 20 to 40 mg daily are used, an increased risk of infection is found (RR 1.3 to 3.6).[116] This risk increases with an increase of the dose and duration of treatment.[117]

In a meta-analysis of 71 trials involving more than 2000 patients with different diseases and who were taking different doses of glucocorticoids, an increased RR of infection of 2 was found. The risk varied according to the type of disease being treated. Five of these trials involved patients with rheumatic diseases and showed no increased risk (RR 1).[116] The same was found in a double-blind, placebo-controlled, 2-year trial in patients with early RA, in which the effect of 10 mg of prednisone daily was compared with that of placebo.[118] In a study, after adjustment for covariates, prednisone use increased the risk of hospitalization for pneumonia in a dose-dependent manner.[117] Another study applying a weighted cumulative-dose model found an elevated risk of serious infections among patients with RA aged 65 years or older, even with chronic low-dose glucocorticoid use; the risk increased with the dosage.[119] In a retrospective RA cohort of patients aged 66 years or older, a clear dose-dependent risk of infections was found, but bias could not be fully excluded, especially because surrogate markers for disease activity had been used as covariates in the analysis.[120] The study suggests, however, that seniors with RA in comparison with younger RA populations may have a higher infection risk related to glucocorticoid use.

Thus in patients treated with glucocorticoids, especially older patients and those who have comorbidities and are taking immunosuppressive co-medications, especially at high doses, clinicians should anticipate infections with usual and unusual organisms because glucocorticoids may blunt classic clinical features and thus delay diagnosis. For example, when applying a high dose of glucocorticoid treatment or when glucocorticoids are given to patients with lung disease, prophylactic treatment for *Pneumocystis jirovecii* should be considered because treatment with trimethoprim/sulfamethoxazole effectively decreases its incidence.[121]

Cardiovascular Adverse Effects

Mineralocorticoid Effects

Some glucocorticoids also have mineralocorticoid actions (see Table 63.1), including reduced excretion of sodium and chloride and increased excretion of potassium, calcium, and phosphate. This activity may lead to edema, weight gain, increased blood pressure, and cardiac problems. Heart failure can occur because of reduced excretion of sodium and chloride. Cardiac arrhythmia can be caused by increased excretion of potassium. Hypocalcemia can result in tetany and electrocardiographic changes. Glucocorticoids exhibit no direct effects on kidneys or on renal function.

Low doses of glucocorticoids are not a cause of hypertension, in contrast to higher doses.[122] No formal studies addressing the effects of glucocorticoids in previously hypertensive patients have been reported. Two randomized, controlled studies in patients with myocarditis and idiopathic cardiomyopathy showed no differences between placebo-treated or glucocorticoid-treated groups after 1 year or in survival at 2 and 4 years.[123,124]

Atherosclerosis and Dyslipidemia

Accelerated atherosclerosis and elevated cardiovascular risk have been reported in patients with inflammatory joint disorders.[125,126] The duration of the disease and the use of glucocorticoids are associated with increased cardiovascular mortality.[127] Glucocorticoids may enhance cardiovascular risk via their potentially deleterious effects on lipids,[128] glucose tolerance, insulin production and resistance, blood pressure, and obesity.[125]

These risk factors, however, do not seem to be adverse effects of low-dose glucocorticoids. Furthermore, atherosclerosis itself has been recognized as an inflammatory disease of arterial walls,[129] for which glucocorticoids may be beneficial.[130] Glucocorticoids have been found to inhibit macrophage accumulation in injured arterial walls in vitro, possibly resulting in attenuation of the local inflammatory response.[131] Low-dose glucocorticoids might also improve dyslipidemia associated with inflammatory disease.[125,132–134] Nevertheless, the effects on lipids and other cardiovascular risk factors of low-dose glucocorticoids in inflammatory diseases probably are different from those of medium and high doses of glucocorticoids[128] or of those of glucocorticoid therapy in people with non-inflammatory diseases. This variation, and the interplay of disease activity, glucocorticoids, and adverse effects (see Fig. 63.8), makes it difficult to judge the net adverse effects of glucocorticoids on cardiovascular risk and lipids.[135] The finding that a common haplotype of the glucocorticoid receptor gene is associated with heart failure and that this association is partly mediated by low-grade inflammation complicates this issue even more.[136]

In an RA cohort with prospective yearly data assessments, including 779 patients with a total of 7203 patient-years of observation, during which 237 patients died, Cox proportional hazards regression adjusted for potential confounders and for the propensity to receive glucocorticoids was used to assess the hazard ratio of glucocorticoid use for cardiovascular mortality.[137] Compared with no glucocorticoid use, daily doses up to 7 mg prednisolone equivalent were not associated with a statistically increased hazard rate; the hazard rate (95% CI) at 8 to 15 mg was 2.3 (1.4 to 3.8), and at 15 mg or more was 3.2 (1.1 to 9.0). Compared with no glucocorticoid use, cumulative doses up to 39 g were not associated with a statistically increased hazard rate; the hazard rate (95% CI) at 40 g or greater was 2.1 (1.3 to 3.3). Compared with no glucocorticoid use, cumulative doses per year up to 5.07 g were not associated with a statistically increased hazard rate; the hazard rate (95% CI) at 5.08 g or more per year was 2.4 (1.5 to 3.8).

Thus medium and high glucocorticoid doses and long duration of therapy, next to traditional cardiovascular risk factors, including comorbidities such as diabetes mellitus, duration and level of inflammatory disease activity, and co-therapies such as COX-2 selective NSAIDs, seem to be the most important cardiovascular risk factors.

Mortality

In a German biologics register, Cox regression was applied to investigate the impact of time-varying covariates (i.e., disease activity,

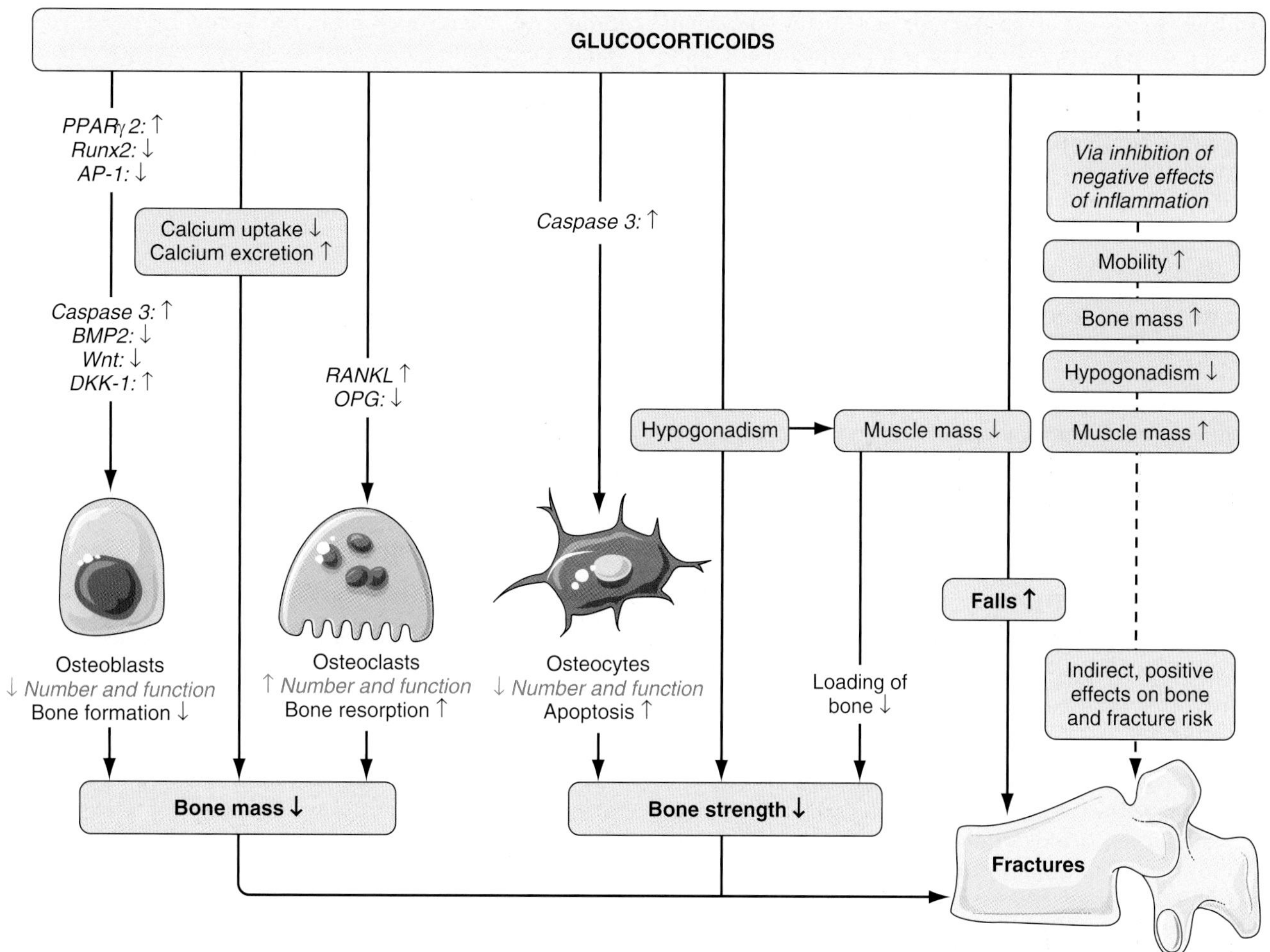

• **Fig. 63.9** Effects of glucocorticoids on fracture risk: negative effects as adverse effects of this medication and indirect positive effects as therapeutic effects, inhibiting the negative effects of the inflammatory disease.[140–143] *AP-1,* Activator protein-1 transcription factor complex, including Fos proteins; ↑ increase, stimulation, or upregulation; ↓ decrease, inhibition, or downregulation; *BMP2,* bone morphogenetic protein-2 of the group of BMPs that belong to the transforming growth factor-β superfamily, initiating bone formation; *Caspase 3,* a critical enzyme for apoptosis and cell survival; *DKK-1,* dickkopf-1, Wnt inhibitor; *OPG,* osteoprotegerin, the antiosteoclastic decoy receptor for RANKL; *PPARγ2,* nuclear receptor peroxisome proliferator-activated receptor-γ2 signaling; *RANKL,* ligand of receptor activator of nuclear factor-κB (RANK), differentiating and activating osteoclasts; *Runx2,* the Runx2 gene product, stimulating differentiation of mesenchymal cells into osteoblasts; *Wnt,* wingless type signaling pathway regulating bone homeostasis.

functional disability, treatment with glucocorticoids, and biologic or synthetic DMARDs) on mortality, after adjustment for age, sex, comorbid conditions, and smoking.[138] Disease activity was a clear risk factor for mortality because the risk increased with increasing disease activity. In addition, a dose-dependent risk was seen for glucocorticoid therapy with doses greater than 5 mg prednisone equivalents per day, with an adjusted hazard rate (95% CI) of 1.5 (1.1 to 2.0) for greater than 5 to 10 mg and of 2.0 (1.3 to 3.1) for greater than 10 to 15 mg. Although confounding cannot be fully excluded, similar results have been reported[139]; increased mortality seems to be primarily caused by infections and cardiovascular complications.

Skeletal Adverse Effects

Osteoporosis

Osteoporosis is a well-known adverse effect of glucocorticoids; however, the inflammatory disease for which glucocorticoids are given and, especially in inflammatory joint diseases, physical disability and reduced mobility as outcomes of the disease are also risk factors for osteoporosis. Thus glucocorticoids have, independent of the disease treated, negative effects on bone, but may as therapy for an inflammatory disease have positive effects on bone by suppressing the inflammatory disease and its negative consequences on bone (Fig. 63.9). For instance, suppressing proinflammatory cytokines such as IL-1 and TNF,[62] which stimulate osteoblasts and T cells to produce RANK-ligand, leading to activation of osteoclasts, indirectly has a positive effect on bone mass.

Whether a patient should be treated depends on fracture risk, effectiveness, safety, and the cost of the treatment. To estimate the risk of fractures for individual patients, several algorithms have been developed, such as the fracture risk in glucocorticoid-induced osteoporosis score (FIGS), which includes the glucocorticoid dosage taken, and fracture risk assessment (FRAX; https://www.shef.ac.uk/FRAX/),[144] for which adjustments also have been suggested for glucocorticoid dosages greater than 7.5 mg prednisone equivalents daily.[145]

To a large degree, osteoporosis can be prevented with calcium and vitamin D supplementation and a biphosphonate if indicated,[146] following national and international guidelines, which are periodically updated.[147,148] In specific circumstances, teriparatide and denosumab may be indicated.[147] Preventive and therapeutic management of glucocorticoid-induced osteoporosis is discussed in another chapter.

Osteonecrosis

High-dose glucocorticoids for longer periods are implicated as a cause for osteonecrosis, especially in young adults[149] and patients with SLE.[150] Vascular mechanisms seem to be involved. Ischemia may possibly be caused by microscopic fat emboli or impingement of the sinusoidal vascular bed by increased intraosseous pressure as a result of fat accumulation. An early symptom is diffuse pain, which becomes persistent and increases with activity. Most frequently, hip or knee joints are involved; ankle and shoulder joints are involved less frequently. For early assessment, MRI is the most sensitive investigation. Treatment in the early stage includes immobilization and decreased weight bearing. Surgical decompression, joint replacement, or both follow this treatment if needed. There are no preventive measures; awareness is the most important factor in early detection.

Myopathy

Weakness in proximal muscles, especially of the lower extremities, occurring within weeks to months after the onset of treatment with glucocorticoids or after an increase in the dosage may indicate steroid myopathy. It is often suspected but infrequently found; it occurs almost exclusively in patients treated with high dosages (>30 mg/day prednisolone or its equivalent). Diagnosis is clinical and can be confirmed by a muscle biopsy specimen that reveals atrophy of type II fibers and lack of inflammation; serum muscle enzymes are not elevated. Treatment is withdrawal of the glucocorticoid, if possible, and quite often a prompt decrease in symptoms occurs after withdrawal of the drug. A rare syndrome of rapid-onset, acute myopathy, occurring within days after the start of high-dose glucocorticoids or pulse therapy, has been described; muscle biopsy specimens show atrophy and necrosis of all muscle fibers.

Gastrointestinal Adverse Effects

Peptic Ulcer Disease

Data from the literature on upper gastrointestinal safety of oral glucocorticoids are inconclusive. The fact that glucocorticoids inhibit the production of COX-2 without hampering the production of COX-1 supports studies that found no increased risk. In other studies, a RR of serious upper gastrointestinal peptic complications of about 2 was found.[151,152] Combination with a nonselective NSAID or aspirin further elevates the RR of peptic ulcer disease and associated complications to about 4.[152,153] Thus, in the case of co-medication with an NSAID, one should consider co-treatment with a PPI or switch to a COX-1–sparing NSAID[108] if there is not a high risk of cardiovascular disease (clearly, an inflammatory disease is a moderate risk factor for cardiovascular disease in its own right[129]). In patients treated with glucocorticoids without concomitant use of NSAIDs, there is no indication for gastrointestinal protective agents unless other risk factors for peptic complications are present.

Other Gastrointestinal Adverse Effects

Although glucocorticoids usually are listed as one of the many potential causes of pancreatitis, evidence for such an association is weak and difficult to separate from the underlying disease, such as vasculitis or SLE.[154] The risk of asymptomatic and symptomatic colonization of the upper gastrointestinal tract with *Candida albicans* is increased in patients treated with glucocorticoids, especially when other risk factors are present, such as advanced age, diabetes mellitus, and concomitant use of other immunosuppressive agents. Glucocorticoids may mask symptoms and signs usually associated with the occurrence of intra-abdominal complications, such as perforation of the intestine and peritonitis, and can lead to a delay in diagnosis with, as a consequence, increased morbidity and mortality.

Ocular Adverse Effects

Cataract

Glucocorticoids especially tend to stimulate the formation of posterior subcapsular cataract,[155] but the risk of cortical cataract also seems to be increased, with an odds ratio (OR) of 2.6.[156] To some extent, the likelihood or severity of this adverse effect depends on the dose and duration of treatment. In patients treated with glucocorticoids on a long-term basis at a dosage of 15 mg or more of prednisone daily for 1 year, cataract is observed frequently; in patients receiving long-term therapy with less than 10 mg of prednisone daily, the percentage of cataract is less, but cataracts may develop at dosages of greater than 5 mg/day of prednisolone equivalent.[109] These cataracts are usually bilateral but progress slowly. They may cause glare disturbance but usually cause little visual impairment until the end stages.

Glaucoma

By increasing intraocular pressure, glucocorticoids may cause or aggravate glaucoma. Patients with a family history of open-angle glaucoma are probably prone to the development of this adverse effect, as are patients receiving high doses of glucocorticoids; checks of intraocular pressure are warranted. If ocular pressure is increased, patients need to be treated with medications that reduce this pressure, often for a prolonged period after stopping the glucocorticoid.[157] Topical application of a glucocorticoid in the eye has a more pronounced effect on intraocular pressure compared with systemic glucocorticoid therapy.[158]

Dermal Adverse Effects

Cushingoid habitus, easy bruising, skin atrophy, and impaired wound healing are skin-related adverse effects, which have been reported by RA patients while using glucocorticoids.[159] Physicians recognize ecchymoses and cushingoid habitus more often in these patients. Striae, acne, perioral dermatitis, hyperpigmentation, facial redness, mild hirsutism, and thinning of scalp hair are not correlated with glucocorticoid use in RA, but may be a problem if glucocorticoids are given in higher dosages or with longer duration.[109] Physicians often consider skin changes to be of minor clinical importance, but they may be disturbing to patients.[111] Many physicians can immediately recognize the skin of a patient who has been taking glucocorticoids on a long-term basis.

Endocrine Adverse Effects

Glucose Intolerance and Diabetes Mellitus

Glucocorticoids increase hepatic glucose production and induce insulin resistance by inhibiting insulin-stimulated glucose uptake and metabolism by peripheral tissues. Glucocorticoids probably also have a direct effect on the beta cells of the pancreas, resulting in enhanced insulin secretion during glucocorticoid therapy. It may take only a few weeks before glucocorticoid-induced hyperglycemia occurs in people taking low and medium glucocorticoid doses. In previously nondiabetic subjects, one case-controlled, population-based study suggested an OR of 1.8 for the need to initiate antihyperglycemic drugs during glucocorticoid therapy with doses of 10 mg or less of prednisolone or equivalent per day. This risk increased with higher daily doses of glucocorticoids. The OR was 3 for 10 to 20 mg, 5.8 for 20 to 30 mg, and 10.3 for 30 mg or more of prednisolone or its equivalent per day.[160]

It is likely that the risk is increased further in patients with other risk factors for diabetes mellitus, such as a family history of the disease, advanced age, obesity, and previous gestational diabetes. Postprandial hyperglycemia and only mildly elevated fasting glucose concentrations are characteristic of glucocorticoid-induced diabetes mellitus. Worsening of glycemic control in patients with established glucose intolerance or diabetes mellitus can be expected. Glucocorticoid-induced diabetes usually is reversible when the drug is discontinued, unless the patient had pre-existent clear glucose intolerance.

Increased Body Weight and Altered Fat Redistribution

Weight gain is an adverse effect of long-term glucocorticoid therapy that is of concern for patients and rheumatologists.[111,161] Weight gain is due to increased appetite and alterations in fat and glucose metabolism, resulting in an increase of total body and trunk fat. Nevertheless, weight gain associated with low-dose glucocorticoid therapy for inflammatory diseases seems minor[118,162] and might at least partly also be due to the effectiveness of treatment because active disease has been reported to induce weight loss, possibly as a result of cytokine effects and loss of appetite. In the Computer Assisted Management in Early Rheumatoid Arthritis (CAMERA)-II trial,[61] the extra weight gain in the prednisone strategy group seemed at least partly attributable to reduction of weight-loss–inducing disease activity, rather than being simply an adverse effect of prednisone.[49] Weight gain in patients with RA who are taking TNF inhibitor agents seems to be attributable to the same mechanism of efficient suppression of disease activity mechanisms.[163]

One of the most notable effects of long-term endogenous or exogenous glucocorticoid excess is the redistribution of body fat. A centripetal fat accumulation with thin extremities is a characteristic feature of patients exposed to long-term, high-dose glucocorticoids. Potential mechanisms include increased conversion of cortisone to cortisol in visceral adipocytes, hyperinsulinemia, and a change in expression and activity of adipocyte-derived hormones and cytokines, such as leptin and TNF.[164] Protein loss resulting in muscle atrophy also contributes to the change in body appearance.

Suppression of the Hypothalamic-Pituitary-Adrenal Axis

In the section on effects of glucocorticoids on the HPA axis, mechanisms of chronic suppression of the HPA axis by administration of exogenous glucocorticoids are described. In such a situation, acute discontinuation of glucocorticoid therapy may lead to acute adrenal insufficiency with possible circulatory collapse and death.[27,165] About 10 years after glucocorticoid therapy became available, the first well-documented case of adrenal insufficiency after withdrawal of exogenous glucocorticoid was reported.[166] Acute cessation of glucocorticoid therapy without tapering is indicated for corneal ulceration by herpes virus, which can lead rapidly to perforation of the cornea, and glucocorticoid-induced acute psychosis. In these patients, assessment of the adrenal responsiveness on a corticotropin test seems prudent. Not all patients with a blunted cortisol response have signs or symptoms of adrenal insufficiency, however.

Clinical signs and symptoms of chronic adrenal hypofunctioning are nonspecific and include fatigue and weakness, lethargy, orthostatic hypotension, nausea, loss of appetite, vomiting, diarrhea, arthralgia, and myalgia. These symptoms partially overlap glucocorticoid withdrawal symptoms and features of rheumatic diseases (e.g., polymyalgia rheumatica). When in doubt, measurements of serum cortisol levels and the corticotropin stimulation test are indicated. Because mineralocorticoid secretion remains intact via the renin-angiotensin-aldosterone axis, electrolyte disturbances such as hypokalemia are uncommon.

Adverse Behavioral Effects

Glucocorticoid treatment is associated with a variety of behavioral symptoms. Although most attention has been directed toward specific dramatic disturbances collectively described under the term *glucocorticoid psychosis,* less florid effects also occur that may cause distress to a patient and warrant medical attention.[111] Minor behavioral manifestations may also occur upon withdrawal of glucocorticoids.

Steroid Psychosis

Overt psychosis is rare and usually is associated with high-dose glucocorticoids or glucocorticoid pulse therapy, but psychosis may also be a complication of the disease itself, especially SLE. This situation makes it difficult to distinguish whether psychosis in an individual patient with SLE is a complication of the disease, the therapy, or both.

Isolated psychosis represents about 10% of glucocorticoid-related cases, but in most patients affective disorders are present as well. Around 40% of cases of glucocorticoid-induced psychosis manifests as depression, whereas mania, often dominated by irritability, is predominant in 30% of cases.[167] Psychotic symptoms usually start just after initiation of treatment (60% within the first 2 weeks and 90% within the first 6 weeks), and remission after drug dose reduction or withdrawal follows the same pattern. Although the data are largely anecdotal, people experiencing steroid psychosis frequently have had prior evidence of some dissociative symptoms. Occasionally, remission occurs without dose reduction.

Minor Mood Disturbances

Glucocorticoids have been associated with a wide variety of low-grade disturbances, such as depressed or elated mood (euphoria), insomnia, irritability, emotional instability, anxiety, memory failure, and other cognition impairments. Although the symptoms may not become severe enough for a specific diagnosis, they warrant attention—not only because they cause distress to the patient, but also because they may interfere with evaluation and treatment of the underlying disease. Most physicians recognize the occurrence of such symptoms in many patients treated with glucocorticoids; these symptoms may occur in varying degrees in up to 50% of treated patients within the first week. The exact incidence in patients with rheumatic disease who are exposed to the usual doses of glucocorticoids is unknown; most series dedicated to mood disturbances studied high doses.[168] It is important to inform patients about these minor mood disturbances before starting glucocorticoid therapy.[111]

Monitoring

Glucocorticoid-related adverse effects have seldom been studied systematically. The Glucocorticoid Toxicity index has been developed to assess the impact of glucocorticoid-associated morbidity and showed excellent reliability and validity.[169] Until new trials have been performed and toxicity is extensively studied and reported, recommendations based on the opinions of experts and patients are the best available. The conclusion for low-dose therapy is that, in daily practice, standard care monitoring for serious diseases warranting glucocorticoid therapy needs not be extended for patients undergoing low-dose glucocorticoid therapy, except for osteoporosis (for which national guidelines should be followed) and baseline assessments of fasting blood glucose and risk factors for glaucoma, next to a baseline check for ankle edema.[106] Of course, monitoring should be extended for medium and high dosages, to monitor not only for adverse effects of the glucocorticoid therapy but also for adverse effects of the concomitant medication and complications of the severe disease. For these glucocorticoid dosages, no monitoring guidelines yet exist, but there are recommendations on the management of medium- to high-dose glucocorticoid therapy in rheumatic diseases.[66] In these situations, next to good clinical practice, monitoring including, for instance, blood pressure measurements, checks of ocular pressure, and urine glucose seems to be particularly indicated. When performing clinical trials on glucocorticoids, it is advised that these drugs be monitored and reported in a more comprehensive manner and that more data on the spectrum, incidence, and severity of adverse events of glucocorticoids be sampled.[106] When applied prudently, glucocorticoids are still one of the most relevant therapeutic tools in clinical medicine of the 21st century.

Future Directions

Although biologic therapies are applied frequently in rheumatology, they have not replaced—and in the near future will not replace—glucocorticoids as anchor drugs in therapeutic strategies for autoimmune and inflammatory diseases and vasculitides. In contrast to their established use, there is a paucity of data on the spectrum, incidence, and severity of the adverse effects of glucocorticoids at different dosages and in different diseases, and collection of more data is needed.[106] Additional research into molecular mechanisms and genetic developments might in the future lead to new agents and personalized medicine,[4] but it appears that these developments still have a long way to go. With the exception of modified-release prednisone, new glucocorticoid developments that seemed promising in the past have not yet lived up to expectations or still need to be tested in randomized clinical trials.

Full references for this chapter can be found on ExpertConsult.com.

Selected References

1. Hench PS, Kendall EC, Slocumb CH, et al.: The effect of a hormone of the adrenal cortex (17-hydroxy-11-dehydrocorticosterone: compound E) and of pituitary adrenocorticotropic hormone on rheumatoid arthritis: preliminary report, *Proc Staff Meet Mayo Clin* 24:181–197, 1949.
2. Smolen JS, Landewe R, Breedveld FC, et al.: EULAR recommendations for the management of rheumatoid arthritis with synthetic and biological disease-modifying antirheumatic drugs, *Ann Rheum Dis* 69:964–975, 2010.
3. Overman RA, Yeh JY, Deal CL: Prevalence of oral glucocorticoid usage in the United States: a general population perspective, *Arthritis Care Res (Hoboken)* 65:294–298, 2013.
4. Burska AN, Roget K, Blits M, et al.: Gene expression analysis in RA: towards personalized medicine, *Pharmacogenomics J* 14:93–106, 2014.
5. Buttgereit F, Wehling M, Burmester GR: A new hypothesis of modular glucocorticoid actions: steroid treatment of rheumatic diseases revisited, *Arthritis Rheum* 41:761–767, 1998.
6. Buttgereit F, da Silva JA, Boers M, et al.: Standardised nomenclature for glucocorticoid dosages and glucocorticoid treatment regimens: current questions and tentative answers in rheumatology, *Ann Rheum Dis* 61:718–722, 2002.
7. Buttgereit F, Zhou H, Seibel MJ: Arthritis and endogenous glucocorticoids: the emerging role of the 11beta-HSD enzymes, *Ann Rheum Dis* 67:1201–1203, 2008.
8. Hardy R, Rabbitt EH, Filer A, et al.: Local and systemic glucocorticoid metabolism in inflammatory arthritis, *Ann Rheum Dis* 67:1204–1210, 2008.
9. Barnes PJ: Anti-inflammatory actions of glucocorticoids: molecular mechanisms, *Clin Sci (Lond)* 94:557–572, 1998.
10. Lipworth BJ: Therapeutic implications of non-genomic glucocorticoid activity, *Lancet* 356:87–89, 2000.
11. Rhen T, Cidlowski JA: Antiinflammatory action of glucocorticoids—new mechanisms for old drugs, *N Engl J Med* 353:1711–1723, 2005.
12. Almawi WY, Melemedjian OK: Negative regulation of nuclear factor-kappaB activation and function by glucocorticoids, *J Mol Endocrinol* 28:69–78, 2002.
13. Ristimaki A, Narko K, Hla T: Down-regulation of cytokine-induced cyclo-oxygenase-2 transcript isoforms by dexamethasone: evidence for post-transcriptional regulation, *Biochem J* 318(Pt 1):325–331, 1996.
14. Vandevyver S, Dejager L, Tuckermann J, et al.: New insights into the anti-inflammatory mechanisms of glucocorticoids: an emerging role for glucocorticoid-receptor-mediated transactivation, *Endocrinology* 154:993–1007, 2013.
15. Kleiman A, Tuckermann JP: Glucocorticoid receptor action in beneficial and side effects of steroid therapy: lessons from conditional knockout mice, *Mol Cell Endocrinol* 275:98–108, 2007.
16. Bareille P, Hardes K, Donald AC: Efficacy and safety of once-daily GW870086 a novel selective glucocorticoid in mild-moderate asthmatics: a randomised, two-way crossover, controlled clinical trial, *J Asthma* 50:1077–1082, 2013.
17. Harr MW, Rong Y, Bootman MD, et al.: Glucocorticoid-mediated inhibition of Lck modulates the pattern of T cell receptor-induced calcium signals by down-regulating inositol 1,4,5-trisphosphate receptors, *J Biol Chem* 284:31860–31871, 2009.
18. Cooper MS, Stewart PM: Corticosteroid insufficiency in acutely ill patients, *N Engl J Med* 348:727–734, 2003.
19. Neeck G: Fifty years of experience with cortisone therapy in the study and treatment of rheumatoid arthritis, *Ann N Y Acad Sci* 966:28–38, 2002.
20. Gudbjornsson B, Skogseid B, Oberg K, et al.: Intact adrenocorticotropic hormone secretion but impaired cortisol response in patients with active rheumatoid arthritis. Effect of glucocorticoids, *J Rheumatol* 23:596–602, 1996.

21. Chikanza IC, Petrou P, Kingsley G, et al.: Defective hypothalamic response to immune and inflammatory stimuli in patients with rheumatoid arthritis, *Arthritis Rheum* 35:1281–1288, 1992.
22. Radikova Z, Rovensky J, Vlcek M, et al.: Adrenocortical response to low-dose ACTH test in female patients with rheumatoid arthritis, *Ann N Y Acad Sci* 1148:562–566, 2008.
23. Bijlsma JW, Cutolo M, Masi AT, et al.: The neuroendocrine immune basis of rheumatic diseases, *Immunol Today* 20:298–301, 1999.
24. Arlt W: The approach to the adult with newly diagnosed adrenal insufficiency, *J Clin Endocrinol Metab* 94:1059–1067, 2009.
25. Debono M, Ross RJ, Newell-Price J: Inadequacies of glucocorticoid replacement and improvements by physiological circadian therapy, *Eur J Endocrinol* 160:719–729, 2009.
26. Charmandari E, Nicolaides NC, Chrousos GP: Adrenal insufficiency, *Lancet* 383:2152–2167, 2014.
27. Bornstein SR: Predisposing factors for adrenal insufficiency, *N Engl J Med* 360:2328–2339, 2009.
28. American Society of Health-System Pharmacists: *AHFS drug information*, Bethesda, MD, 2001, American Society of Health-System Pharmacists.
29. Henzen C, Suter A, Lerch E, et al.: Suppression and recovery of adrenal response after short-term, high-dose glucocorticoid treatment, *Lancet* 355:542–545, 2000.
30. Alten R, Doring G, Cutolo M, et al.: Hypothalamus-pituitary-adrenal axis function in patients with rheumatoid arthritis treated with nighttime-release prednisone, *J Rheumatol* 37:2025–2031, 2010.
31. Ackerman GL, Nolsn CM: Adrenocortical responsiveness after alternate-day corticosteroid therapy, *N Engl J Med* 278:405–409, 1968.
32. Schlaghecke R, Kornely E, Santen RT, et al.: The effect of long-term glucocorticoid therapy on pituitary-adrenal responses to exogenous corticotropin-releasing hormone, *N Engl J Med* 326:226–230, 1992.
33. Dinsen S, Baslund B, Klose M, et al.: Why glucocorticoid withdrawal may sometimes be as dangerous as the treatment itself, *Eur J Intern Med* 24:714–720, 2013.
35. Boumpas DT, Chrousos GP, Wilder RL, et al.: Glucocorticoid therapy for immune-mediated diseases: basic and clinical correlates, *Ann Intern Med* 119:1198–1208, 1993.
36. Kirwan JR, Bijlsma JW, Boers M, et al.: Effects of glucocorticoids on radiological progression in rheumatoid arthritis, *Cochrane Database Syst Rev* (1):CD006356, 2007.
37. Leonard JP, Silverstein RL: Corticosteroids and the haematopoietic system. In Lin AN, Paget SA, editors: *Principles of Corticosteroid Therapy*, New York, 2002, Arnold, pp 144–149.
38. Verhoef CM, van Roon JA, Vianen ME, et al.: The immune suppressive effect of dexamethasone in rheumatoid arthritis is accompanied by upregulation of interleukin 10 and by differential changes in interferon gamma and interleukin 4 production, *Ann Rheum Dis* 58:49–54, 1999.
39. Morand EF, Jefferiss CM, Dixey J, et al.: Impaired glucocorticoid induction of mononuclear leukocyte lipocortin-1 in rheumatoid arthritis, *Arthritis Rheum* 37:207–211, 1994.
40. DiBattista JA, Martel-Pelletier J, Wosu LO, et al.: Glucocorticoid receptor mediated inhibition of interleukin-1 stimulated neutral metalloprotease synthesis in normal human chondrocytes, *J Clin Endocrinol Metab* 72:316–326, 1991.
41. Cronstein BN, Kimmel SC, Levin RI, et al.: A mechanism for the antiinflammatory effects of corticosteroids: the glucocorticoid receptor regulates leukocyte adhesion to endothelial cells and expression of endothelial-leukocyte adhesion molecule 1 and intercellular adhesion molecule 991, *Proc Natl Acad Sci U S A* 89:9991–9995, 1992.
42. Di Rosa M, Radomski M, Carnuccio R, et al.: Glucocorticoids inhibit the induction of nitric oxide synthase in macrophages, *Biochem Biophys Res Commun* 172:1246–1252, 1990.
43. Tornatore KM, Logue G, Venuto RC, et al.: Pharmacokinetics of methylprednisolone in elderly and young healthy males, *J Am Geriatr Soc* 42:1118–1122, 1994.
44. Tornatore KM, Biocevich DM, Reed K, et al.: Methylprednisolone pharmacokinetics, cortisol response, and adverse effects in black and white renal transplant recipients, *Transplantation* 59:729–736, 1995.
45. Barnes PJ, Adcock IM: Glucocorticoid resistance in inflammatory diseases, *Lancet* 373:1905–1917, 2009.
46. Ramamoorthy S, Cidlowski JA: Exploring the molecular mechanisms of glucocorticoid receptor action from sensitivity to resistance, *Endocr Dev* 24:41–56, 2013.
47. Quax RA, Manenschijn L, Koper JW, et al.: Glucocorticoid sensitivity in health and disease, *Nat Rev Endocrinol* 9:670–686, 2013.
48. Podgorski MR, Goulding NJ, Hall ND, et al.: Autoantibodies to lipocortin-1 are associated with impaired glucocorticoid responsiveness in rheumatoid arthritis, *J Rheumatol* 19:1668–1671, 1992.
49. Jurgens MS, Jacobs JW, Geenen R, et al.: Increase of body mass index in a tight controlled methotrexate-based strategy with prednisone in early rheumatoid arthritis: side effect of the prednisone or better control of disease activity? *Arthritis Care Res (Hoboken)* 65:88–93, 2013.
50. van der Goes MC, Jacobs JW, Jurgens MS, et al.: Are changes in bone mineral density different between groups of early rheumatoid arthritis patients treated according to a tight control strategy with or without prednisone if osteoporosis prophylaxis is applied? *Osteoporos Int* 24:1429–1436, 2013.
51. Carrie F, Roblot P, Bouquet S, et al.: Rifampin-induced nonresponsiveness of giant cell arteritis to prednisone treatment, *Arch Intern Med* 154:1521–1524, 1994.
52. McAllister WA, Thompson PJ, Al Habet SM, et al.: Rifampicin reduces effectiveness and bioavailability of prednisolone, *Br Med J (Clin Res Ed)* 286:923–925, 1983.
53. Kyriazopoulou V, Parparousi O, Vagenakis AG: Rifampicin-induced adrenal crisis in addisonian patients receiving corticosteroid replacement therapy, *J Clin Endocrinol Metab* 59:1204–1206, 1984.
54. Varis T, Kivisto KT, Neuvonen PJ: Grapefruit juice can increase the plasma concentrations of oral methylprednisolone, *Eur J Clin Pharmacol* 56:489–493, 2000.
55. Oerlemans R, Vink J, Dijkmans BA, et al.: Sulfasalazine sensitises human monocytic/macrophage cells for glucocorticoids by upregulation of glucocorticoid receptor alpha and glucocorticoid induced apoptosis, *Ann Rheum Dis* 66:1289–1295, 2007.
56. Basta-Kaim A, Budziszewska B, Jaworska-Feil L, et al.: Chlorpromazine inhibits the glucocorticoid receptor-mediated gene transcription in a calcium-dependent manner, *Neuropharmacology* 43:1035–1043, 2002.
56a. Kroon FP, Kortekaas MC, Boonen A, et al.: Results of a 6-week treatment with 10 mg prednisolone in patients with hand osteoarthritis (HOPE): a double-blind, randomised, placebo-controlled trial, *Lancet* 2019.
57. Gaffney K, Ledingham J, Perry JD: Intra-articular triamcinolone hexacetonide in knee osteoarthritis: factors influencing the clinical response, *Ann Rheum Dis* 54:379–381, 1995.
58. Jacobs JW, Michels-van Amelsfort JM: How to perform local soft-tissue glucocorticoid injections? *Best Pract Res Clin Rheumatol* 27:171–194, 2013.
59. Sokka T, Toloza S, Cutolo M, et al.: Women, men, and rheumatoid arthritis: analyses of disease activity, disease characteristics, and treatments in the QUEST-RA study, *Arthritis Res Ther* 11:R7, 2009.
60. Criswell LA, Saag KG, Sems KM, et al.: Moderate-term, low-dose corticosteroids for rheumatoid arthritis, *Cochrane Database Syst Rev* 2:CD001158, 2000.
61. Bakker MF, Jacobs JW, Welsing PM, et al.: Low-dose prednisone inclusion in a methotrexate-based, tight control strategy for early rheumatoid arthritis: a randomized trial, *Ann Intern Med* 156:329–339, 2012.

62. Moreland LW, Curtis JR: Systemic nonarticular manifestations of rheumatoid arthritis: focus on inflammatory mechanisms, *Semin Arthritis Rheum* 39:132–143, 2009.
63. Hayreh SS, Zimmerman B: Visual deterioration in giant cell arteritis patients while on high doses of corticosteroid therapy, *Ophthalmology* 110:1204–1215, 2003.
64. Weusten BL, Jacobs JW, Bijlsma JW: Corticosteroid pulse therapy in active rheumatoid arthritis, *Semin Arthritis Rheum* 23:183–192, 1993.
65. Jacobs JW, Geenen R, Evers AW, et al.: Short term effects of corticosteroid pulse treatment on disease activity and the wellbeing of patients with active rheumatoid arthritis, *Ann Rheum Dis* 60:61–64, 2001.
66. Duru N, van der Goes MC, Jacobs JW, et al.: EULAR evidence-based and consensus-based recommendations on the management of medium to high-dose glucocorticoid therapy in rheumatic diseases, *Ann Rheum Dis* 72:1905–1913, 2013.
67. Salem M, Tainsh Jr RE, Bromberg J, et al.: Perioperative glucocorticoid coverage. A reassessment 42 years after emergence of a problem, *Ann Surg* 219:416–425, 1994.
68. Marik PE, Varon J: Requirement of perioperative stress doses of corticosteroids: a systematic review of the literature, *Arch Surg* 143:1222–1226, 2008.
69. Peltoniemi OM, Kari MA, Lano A, et al.: Two-year follow-up of a randomised trial with repeated antenatal betamethasone, *Arch Dis Child Fetal Neonatal Ed* 94:F402–F406, 2009.
70. Wapner RJ, Sorokin Y, Mele L, et al.: Long-term outcomes after repeat doses of antenatal corticosteroids, *N Engl J Med* 357:1190–1198, 2007.
71. Khalife N, Glover V, Taanila A, et al.: Prenatal glucocorticoid treatment and later mental health in children and adolescents, *PLoS One* 8:e81394, 2013.
72. Park-Wyllie L, Mazzotta P, Pastuszak A, et al.: Birth defects after maternal exposure to corticosteroids: prospective cohort study and meta-analysis of epidemiological studies, *Teratology* 62:385–392, 2000.
73. Temprano KK, Bandlamudi R, Moore TL: Antirheumatic drugs in pregnancy and lactation, *Semin Arthritis Rheum* 35:112–121, 2005.
74. Yeh TF, Lin YJ, Lin HC, et al.: Outcomes at school age after postnatal dexamethasone therapy for lung disease of prematurity, *N Engl J Med* 350:1304–1313, 2004.
75. Hepper CT, Halvorson JJ, Duncan ST, et al.: The efficacy and duration of intra-articular corticosteroid injection for knee osteoarthritis: a systematic review of level I studies, *J Am Acad Orthop Surg* 17:638–646, 2009.
76. Eustace JA, Brophy DP, Gibney RP, et al.: Comparison of the accuracy of steroid placement with clinical outcome in patients with shoulder symptoms, *Ann Rheum Dis* 56:59–63, 1997.
77. Jones A, Regan M, Ledingham J, et al.: Importance of placement of intra-articular steroid injections, *BMJ* 307:1329–1330, 1993.
78. Gray RG, Gottlieb NL: Intra-articular corticosteroids. An updated assessment, *Clin Orthop* 177:235–263, 1983.
79. Seror P, Pluvinage P, d'Andre FL, et al.: Frequency of sepsis after local corticosteroid injection (an inquiry on 1160000 injections in rheumatological private practice in France), *Rheumatology (Oxford)* 38:1272–1274, 1999.
80. Kaandorp CJ, Krijnen P, Moens HJ, et al.: The outcome of bacterial arthritis: a prospective community-based study, *Arthritis Rheum* 40:884–892, 1997.
81. Avioli LV: Glucocorticoid effects on statural growth, *Br J Rheumatol* 32(Suppl. 2):27–30, 1993.
82. Furst DE, Keystone EC, Fleischmann R, et al.: Updated consensus statement on biological agents for the treatment of rheumatic diseases, 992009, *Ann Rheum Dis* 69(Suppl. 1):i2–i29, 2010.
83. Ferraccioli G, Salaffi F, De Vita S, et al.: Methotrexate in polymyalgia rheumatica: preliminary results of an open, randomized study, *J Rheumatol* 23:624–628, 1996.
84. van der Veen MJ, Dinant HJ, Booma-Frankfort C, et al.: Can methotrexate be used as a steroid sparing agent in the treatment of polymyalgia rheumatica and giant cell arteritis? *Ann Rheum Dis* 55:218–223, 1996.
85. Jover JA, Hernandez-Garcia C, Morado IC, et al.: Combined treatment of giant-cell arteritis with methotrexate and prednisone. A randomized, double-blind, placebo-controlled trial, *Ann Intern Med* 134:106–114, 2001.
86. Spiera RF, Mitnick HJ, Kupersmith M, et al.: A prospective, double-blind, randomized, placebo controlled trial of methotrexate in the treatment of giant cell arteritis (GCA), *Clin Exp Rheumatol* 19:495–501, 2001.
87. Hoffman GS, Cid MC, Hellmann DB, et al.: A multicenter, randomized, double-blind, placebo-controlled trial of adjuvant methotrexate treatment for giant cell arteritis, *Arthritis Rheum* 46:1309–1318, 2002.
88. Caporali R, Cimmino MA, Ferraccioli G, et al.: Prednisone plus methotrexate for polymyalgia rheumatica: a randomized, double-blind, placebo-controlled trial, *Ann Intern Med* 141:493–500, 2004.
89. Yates M, Loke YK, Watts RA, et al.: Prednisolone combined with adjunctive immunosuppression is not superior to prednisolone alone in terms of efficacy and safety in giant cell arteritis: meta-analysis, *Clin Rheumatol* 33:227–236, 2014.
91. Arvidson NG, Gudbjornsson B, Larsson A, et al.: The timing of glucocorticoid administration in rheumatoid arthritis, *Ann Rheum Dis* 56:27–31, 1997.
92. Kowanko IC, Pownall R, Knapp MS, et al.: Time of day of prednisolone administration in rheumatoid arthritis, *Ann Rheum Dis* 41:447–452, 1982.
93. Derendorf H, Ruebsamen K, Clarke L, et al.: Pharmacokinetics of modified-release prednisone tablets in healthy subjects and patients with rheumatoid arthritis, *J Clin Pharmacol* 53:326–333, 2013.
94. Buttgereit F, Doering G, Schaeffler A, et al.: Efficacy of modified-release versus standard prednisone to reduce duration of morning stiffness of the joints in rheumatoid arthritis (CAPRA-1): a double-blind, randomised controlled trial, *Lancet* 371:205–214, 2008.
118. Van Everdingen AA, Jacobs JW, Siewertsz Van Reesema DR, et al.: Low-dose prednisone therapy for patients with early active rheumatoid arthritis: clinical efficacy, disease-modifying properties, and side effects: a randomized, double-blind, placebo-controlled clinical trial, *Ann Intern Med* 136:1–12, 2002.
162. Wassenberg S, Rau R, Steinfeld P, et al.: Very low-dose prednisolone in early rheumatoid arthritis retards radiographic progression over two years: a multicenter, double-blind, placebo-controlled trial, *Arthritis Rheum* 52:3371–3380, 2005.

64 Traditional DMARDs: Methotrexate, Leflunomide, Sulfasalazine, Hydroxychloroquine, and Combination Therapies

AMY C. CANNELLA AND JAMES R. O'DELL

KEY POINTS

Methotrexate is one of the most durable and frequently used disease-modifying anti-rheumatic drugs (DMARDs), for use as monotherapy or as the cornerstone of combination therapy for rheumatoid arthritis (RA).
Leflunomide, sulfasalazine, and hydroxychloroquine are effective therapies in RA and are commonly used in combination therapy.
Although the precise mechanisms of action of the traditional DMARDs are incompletely understood, most have both anti-inflammatory and immunomodulatory actions.
The choice of DMARD therapy should be tailored to the individual patient, with attention given to age, fertility plans, concomitant medications, and comorbidities.
Toxicity from DMARD therapy can cause significant morbidity and rarely mortality; thus appropriate dosing and monitoring for toxicity are essential.
Combination therapy in RA can be more effective than mono-DMARD therapy in groups of patients with early-stage and established RA.
The appropriate timing and combinations of DMARD therapy in individual patients are still not defined.

Methotrexate

KEY POINTS

An important mechanism of action for methotrexate (MTX) in addition to blocking dihydrofolate reductase is the increased release of adenosine, which is a potent inhibitor of inflammation.
MTX is polyglutamated in cells, and this is responsible for its long therapeutic effect.
The effects of MTX may be enhanced by splitting the dose (within a 12-hour window) when levels greater than 15 mg/week are used or by using a subcutaneous route of administration.
Combined use of folic acid with MTX abrogates some of the side effects of MTX without significantly decreasing its efficacy.
The dose of MTX must be adjusted for reduced renal function.
Although rare, MTX pneumonitis is a serious and potentially fatal complication of therapy.

Introduction

It would be difficult to overstate the importance of methotrexate (MTX) in contemporary management of rheumatic disease, particularly rheumatoid arthritis (RA). Because of its anti-proliferative effects, MTX was introduced in the 1950s to treat malignancy. The first reports of its use in rheumatic diseases were in the 1960s for psoriasis and RA.[1,2] With more experience in efficacy, dosing, and toxicity, MTX has become the disease-modifying anti-rheumatic drug (DMARD) of choice in the treatment of RA, and it is also used in many other rheumatic diseases.

Chemical Structure

MTX is a structural analogue of folic acid and has substitutions in the pteridine group and para-aminobenzoic acid structure (Fig. 64.1). The structure of folic acid (pteroylglutamic acid) consists of three elements: a multiring pteridine group linked to a para-aminobenzoic acid, which is connected to a terminal glutamic acid residue.

Actions of Methotrexate

Because MTX is a folate analogue, it enters cells via a reduced folate carrier (RFC). Leucovorin competes with MTX for uptake by using the same RFC; however, folic acid enters cells via another group of transmembrane receptors called *folate receptors* (FRs).[3] FRs may be upregulated in cells with increased metabolic activity, including synovial macrophages, and serve as a second conduit for MTX influx.[4,5] MTX efflux occurs via members of the adenosine triphosphate (ATP)-binding cassette (ABC) family of transporters, specifically ABCC1-4 and ABCG2.[6] Genetic polymorphisms may affect MTX transporter proteins (influx and efflux) and can result in a variable MTX response and toxicity profile.[6] Furthermore, multidrug-resistance proteins have been identified that transport MTX, folic acid, and leucovorin out of cells, leading to MTX resistance.[7]

Once inside the cell, naturally occurring folates as well as MTX undergo polyglutamation by the enzyme folyl-polyglutamyl synthetase (FPGS). Polyglutamation of MTX (MTX-PG) is essential to prevent efflux of MTX, which easily occurs in the monoglutaminated state. MTX-PG has several key inhibitory effects on intra-cellular enzymes, which result in its postulated anti-inflammatory and anti-proliferative (immunosuppressive) mechanisms: (1) inhibition of aminoimidazole carboxamide ribonucleotide (AICAR) transformylase (ATIC) results in increased intra-cellular and extra-cellular adenosine, (2) inhibition of thymidylate synthetase (TYMS) results in decreased pyrimidine synthesis, and (3) inhibition of dihydrofolate reductase (DHFR) results in inhibition of transmethylation reactions essential for cellular functioning (Fig. 64.2).

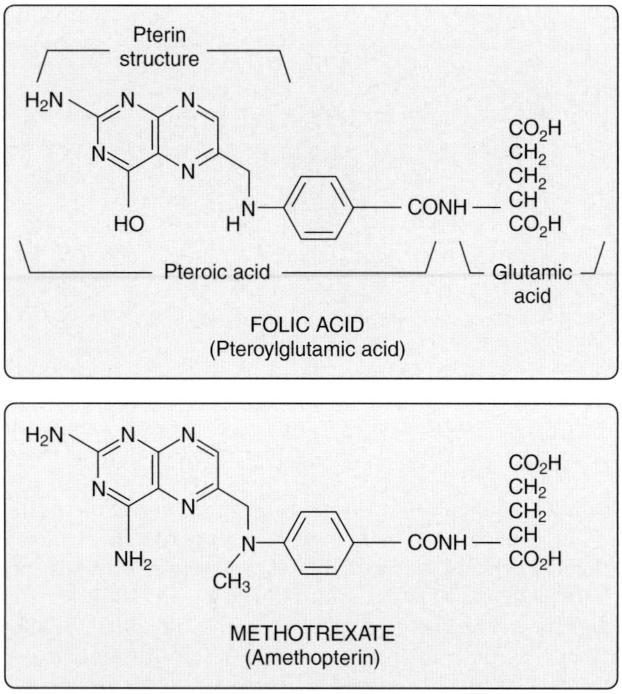

• **Fig. 64.1** Chemical structure of folic acid and methotrexate.

Inhibition of ATIC by MTX-PG leads to accumulation of AICAR and, ultimately, to increased levels of adenosine. Three possible mechanisms are postulated and likely work in combination: (1) AICAR inhibition of adenosine monophosphate (AMP) deaminase leads to excess production of adenosine from AMP, (2) AICAR inhibition of adenosine deaminase (ADA) leads to decreased breakdown of adenosine to inosine, and (3) AICAR stimulation of the ecto-5′-nucleotidase converts extra-cellular AMP to adenosine[8–10] (Fig. 64.3).

Adenosine, a purine nucleoside, has been termed a *retaliatory metabolite* because of its tissue protective functions after stressful injurious stimuli.[11] Adenosine, a potent inhibitor of inflammation,[11] induces vasodilation.[12,13] Adenosine's anti-inflammatory effects include regulation of endothelial cell inflammatory functions, including cell trafficking,[12,13] counter-regulation of neutrophils and dendritic cells,[11,14] and cytokine modulation of monocytes and macrophages.[11] Adenosine receptor ligation on monocytes and macrophages suppresses IL-12, a strong pro-inflammatory cytokine.[15] Adenosine also suppresses the pro-inflammatory mediators TNF, IL-6, IL-8, macrophage inflammatory protein (MIP)-1α, leukotriene (LT)B_4, and nitric oxide and enhances production of the anti-inflammatory mediators IL-10 and IL-1 receptor antagonist.[16–21] Furthermore, adenosine receptor–mediated processes result in inhibition of the synthesis of collagenase, including tissue inhibitors of metalloproteinases.[22] In sum, adenosine appears to promote a self-limiting, healthy immune response, hastening the transition from neutrophil-mediated

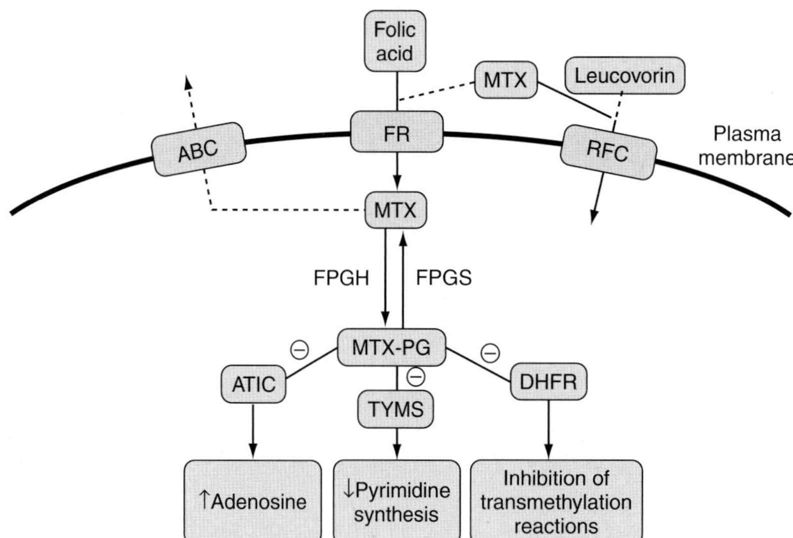

• **Fig. 64.2** Methotrexate (MTX) enters cells primarily via the reduced folate carrier (RFC) but can use the folate receptor (FR). Once inside the cell, it becomes polyglutamated and can interfere with several cellular enzymes, including 5-aminoimidazole-4-carboxamide ribonucleotide (AICAR) transformylase (ATIC), thymidylate synthetase (TYMS), and dihydrofolate reductase (DHFR). *ABC,* ATP-binding cassette; *FPGH,* folylpolyglutamate hydrolase; *FPGS,* folyl-polyglutamyl synthetase; *MTX-PG,* polyglutamation of MTX.

inflammation to a more efficient and highly specific dendritic cell–mediated response. Ultimately, adenosine leads to the resolution of inflammation by downregulation of macrophage activation and promotes a shift from a T helper (Th)1 cell to a Th2 cell response.[11]

Evidence that the anti-inflammatory effects of MTX are mediated through adenosine has accumulated in in vitro and in animal studies.[23] However, because of adenosine's short blood half-life of 2 seconds and MTX's long latent period for active metabolites that modulate adenosine, it has been difficult to demonstrate changes in blood adenosine levels directly related to MTX.[24] Recent evidence with use of forearm blood flow as a surrogate marker for adenosine release in patients with RA treated with MTX has shown that MTX inhibits deamination of adenosine and potentiates adenosine-induced vasodilation.[25] Demonstration of altered adenosine kinetics in patients treated with MTX coupled with adenosine's known anti-inflammatory effects lends further credence to the hypothesis that MTX increases extra-cellular adenosine, which likely mediates some of the anti-inflammatory effects of MTX.

In addition to vasodilation, adenosine's cardiovascular effects include negative inotropic and chronotropic cardiac effects, inhibition of vascular smooth muscle cell proliferation, presynaptic inhibition of sympathetic neurotransmitter release, and inhibition of thrombocyte aggregation.[26] Patients with RA have a higher incidence of cardiovascular disease than the general population.[27] MTX has been suggested to have a preferentially beneficial effect on cardiovascular mortality compared with other DMARDs in RA, and this effect likely occurs via adenosine modulation.[28]

The anti-inflammatory and anti-proliferative effects of MTX may be mediated through its inhibition of transmethylation reactions. Both MTX and MTX-PG inhibit DHFR, resulting in diminution of tetrahydrofolate (THF). THF acts as a proximal methyl donor for several reactions by donating the methyl group for the conversion of homocysteine to methionine. Methionine is then converted to S-adenosylmethionine (SAM), which acts as a methyl donor for the following: methylation of RNA, DNA, amino acids, proteins, and phospholipids, and synthesis of the polyamines spermidine and spermine. Upon demethylation of SAM to *S*-adenosylhomocysteine (SAH), SAH is converted to adenosine and homocysteine. Methylation products that are dependent upon SAM, and thus indirectly upon DHFR, to generate THF are required for cellular survival and function, although specific cellular dependence upon each varies[19] (see Fig. 64.3).

The role of polyamines deserves further discussion. Spermine and spermidine accumulate in urine,[29] in peripheral blood mononuclear cells,[30] and in synovial fluid and tissue[31] in patients with RA. Metabolism of polyamines by mononuclear cells gives rise to toxic agents, including ammonia and hydrogen peroxide, which may impair lymphocyte function.[32,33] Additionally, accumulation of polyamines in B cells is associated with enhanced production of rheumatoid factor (RF) in vitro, and incubation of these cells with MTX diminishes their ability to secrete both immunoglobulin and RF.[19] These effects are seen with high in vitro concentrations of MTX and may not translate into the in vivo therapeutic effects of MTX in RA.

In addition, MTX inhibits methylation of 2′-deoxyuridylate (dUMP) into 2′-deoxythymidylate (dTMP) by TYMS, resulting in a further mechanism for disruption of DNA synthesis and

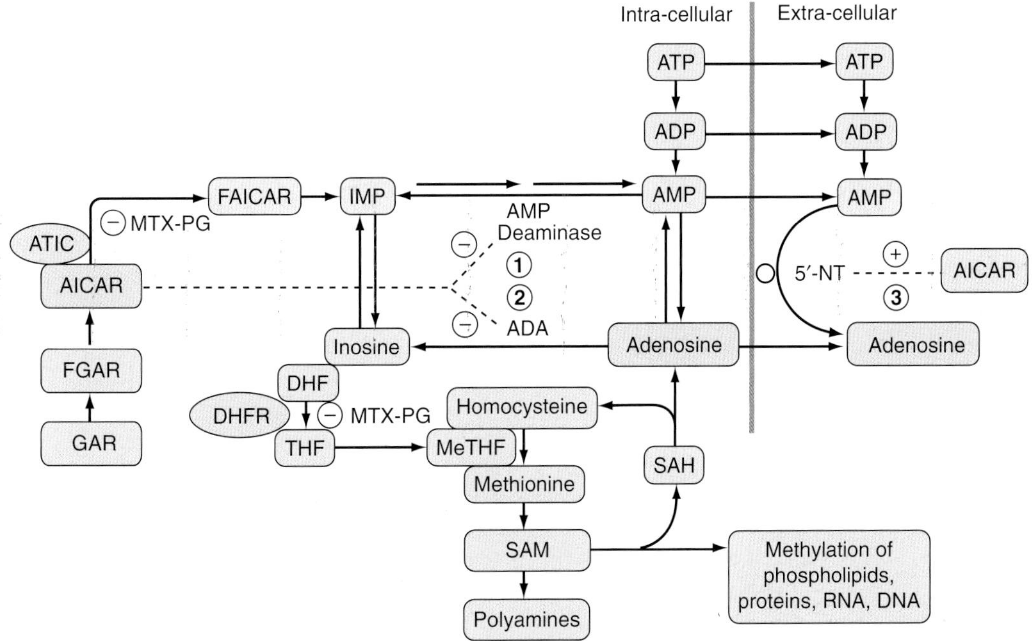

• **Fig. 64.3** Simplified schema of the effects of polyglutamation of methotrexate (MTX-PG) on intra-cellular and extra-cellular adenosine production and interference with intra-cellular transmethylation reactions. *Blue coloring* denotes important steps as discussed in the text. *ADA,* Adenosine deaminase; *ADP,* adenosine diphosphate; *AICAR,* 5-aminoimidazole-4-carboxamide ribonucleotide; *AMP,* adenosine monophosphate; *ATIC,* aminoimidazole carboxamide ribonucleotide transformylase; *ATP,* adenosine triphosphate; *DHF,* dihydrofolate; *DHFR,* dihydrofolate reductase; *FAICAR,* formyl-AICAR; *FGAR,* α-*N*-formylglycinamide ribonucleotide; *GAR,* β-glycinamide ribonucleotide; *IMP,* inosine monophosphate; *MeTHF,* methyltetrahydrofolic acid; *5′NT,* 5′-nucleotidase; *SAH,* S-adenosylhomocysteine; *SAM,* S-adenosylmethionine; *THF,* tetrahydrofolate.

proliferation of inflammatory cells. This effect has been shown in vitro in human peripheral blood mononuclear cells incubated with low concentrations of MTX.[34] Cell cycle disruption may lead to apoptosis of mononuclear cells via CD95 (APO-1/Fas) ligand-dependent[35] and ligand-independent mechanisms.[36]

Therefore, inhibition of transmethylation reactions may lead to MTX efficacy via anti-proliferative and anti-inflammatory mechanisms. Disruption of DNA, RNA, amino acid, and phospholipid synthesis results in its anti-proliferative effect, which may be mediated via cellular apoptosis. Decreased levels of polyamines may downregulate the production of toxic agents, as well as RF secretion, leading to its anti-inflammatory effect.

In theory, the anti-inflammatory and anti-proliferative properties of MTX already described should make it a potent inhibitor of the immune response that characterizes many rheumatic diseases. Indeed, MTX has become the cornerstone of therapy for RA and is efficacious in multiple other rheumatic diseases. Direct evidence for the immunomodulatory effects of MTX exists, whether studied in in vitro or in vivo systems.

Treatment with MTX modulates monocytic and lymphocytic cytokines and their inhibitors. MTX inhibits pro-inflammatory cytokine IL-1 secretion and induces the IL-1 receptor antagonist, effectively inhibiting cellular responses to IL-1.[37,38] Soluble TNF receptor (sTNFR p75) synthesis upregulation is also a result of MTX treatment from cultured monoblastic leukemia cells, which results in a diminished TNF inflammatory effect.[39] MTX also inhibits production and secretion of the pro-inflammatory cytokine, IL-6, by cultured human monocytes.[40,41] Reverse transcriptase polymerase chain reaction has been used to study the effects of MTX on gene expression for lymphocytic cytokines.[42,43] MTX increases anti-inflammatory Th2 cytokine (IL-4 and IL-10) gene expression and decreases pro-inflammatory Th1 cytokine (IL-2 and IFN-γ) gene expression in peripheral blood mononuclear cells (PBMCs) of patients with RA.[43]

Prostaglandins (PGs) and LTs are important mediators of joint destruction in RA. MTX modulates the inflammatory enzymes cyclooxygenase (COX) and lipoxygenase (LOX), and their products PG and LT. Thromboxane B_2 and prostaglandin E_2 activities were reduced in the whole blood of patients with RA treated with MTX when compared with healthy controls.[44] MTX also reduces LTB_4 synthesis by neutrophils, resulting in a decrease in total plasma LTB_4 levels in patients with RA treated weekly with MTX.[45] In addition to possible direct effects on COX and LOX, MTX exerts an inhibitory effect on neutrophil chemotaxis, which may result in a further reduction of these enzymes in sites of inflammation.[46]

Tissue destruction at sites of inflammation is thought to be related to increased synthesis and activity of proteolytic enzymes released by inflammatory cells, particularly in RA. MTX treatment reduces gene expression of collagenase, metalloproteinase-1, and stromelysin, and upregulates expression of tissue inhibitor of metalloproteinase (TIMP)-1.[47] MTX may exert direct effects on mRNA for certain enzymes, such as collagenase. MTX also likely exerts indirect effects on gene expression via upstream cytokine modulation (IL-1 and IL-6) in the case of matrix metalloproteinase (MMP)-1 and TIMP-1.[48]

Pharmacology

Absorption and Bioavailability

At low doses, MTX can be administered either orally or parenterally (subcutaneous [SQ] or intramuscular [IM]), and absorption is rapid, peaking at 1 to 2 or 0.1 to 1 hour, respectively. The absorption of low-dose oral MTX (<15 mg/week) can be variable, and once the oral dose exceeds 15 mg/week, absorption diminishes by as much as 30%.[49] Absorption is not reduced by concomitant food intake, except for milk, which may be inhibitory.[50] MTX absorption may be reduced in the setting of intestinal pathology, such as inflammatory bowel disease or malabsorptive conditions.

Orally administered MTX is absorbed via the gastrointestinal (GI) tract and passes through the liver via the portal vein; parenterally administered MTX passes through the liver via the hepatic artery. Systemic levels are higher for parentally administered MTX compared to orally administered MTX at equal dosing intervals. In addition, the bioavailability of single dose daily oral MTX plateaus at doses of 15 mg/week, whereas parenteral MTX has a linear increase in systemic levels with increasing dosages.[51] These higher systemic levels have not been associated with any increase in toxicity.[51,52] Although not prospectively studied in RA patients receiving long-term MTX treatment, the parenteral route should have diminished potential for hepatotoxicity. This effect has been seen in a retrospective study wherein more elevations in transaminases were noted when oral MTX was administered to the same individuals versus when given parenterally.[53] Equivalent MTX doses showed improved efficacy in RA clinical endpoints for parenteral versus orally administered MTX.[54]

Absorption of orally administered MTX plateaus above certain doses. Forty-one RA patients who received 10 mg/m^2 of oral MTX had a mean bioavailability of 70% with a range of 40% to 100%.[55] The mean absorption time was 1.2 hours. Four hours after MTX administration, synovial fluid concentrations equaled serum levels.[55] A recent study of high-dose oral MTX (median dose, 30 mg/week) has shown that mean bioavailability is improved by splitting the dose by 8 hours compared with one single dose (mean bioavailability of 0.9 and 0.76, respectively).[56] The pharmacokinetics of subcutaneous MTX are equivalent to those of IM MTX; maximum serum concentration is attained within 2 hours of injection by either route.[57] Also, the bioavailability is equivalent between tablets and orally administered parenteral solution.[58]

Distribution and Half-Life

MTX is 50% to 60% bound to plasma proteins and has a half-life of approximately 6 hours.[55] An increase in free MTX caused by displacement from albumin by more highly protein-bound drugs, such as aspirin, nonsteroidal anti-inflammatory drugs (NSAIDs), and sulfonamides can occur. This is generally of limited clinical significance with low MTX doses because the increase in free MTX is usually only modest.

MTX accumulates in third-space fluids, which can serve as a reservoir for redistribution into the circulation long after the last dose is administered.[59] Caution should be used when administering MTX to patients with pleural effusions or ascites. Furthermore, unexpectedly high levels of MTX have been seen in patients with bladder cancer who have undergone ileal conduit surgery because of enhanced intestinal absorption through the newly fashioned conduit.[60]

The biologically active form of MTX occurs after intra-cellular polyglutamation (MTX-PG). MTX undergoes up to five polyglutamations, and recent studies have looked at this aspect of MTX pharmacology. Once on a stable dose of MTX, the median time until 90% of the maximum steady-state concentration of MTX-PG was reached was found to be 27.5 weeks (range, 6.6 to 62.0 weeks).[61]

Elimination

Most MTX is excreted in the urine within the first 12 hours after administration, except for MTX-PG. MTX undergoes some hepatic metabolism by the enzyme aldehyde oxidase to the 7-hydroxymethotrexate metabolite; this metabolite has unknown significance in RA. MTX and metabolites are excreted by the kidney by glomerular filtration and proximal tubular secretion but also undergo distal tubular reabsorption. The estimated median half-life of elimination of MTX-PG is 3.1 weeks (range, 0.94 to 4.1 weeks), and MTX-PG is undetectable at 15 weeks.[61] MTX-PG_3 is the most common subtype seen (30% of total MTX-PG) and has a median half-life elimination of 4.1 weeks.

Indications

Rheumatoid Arthritis. The efficacy of MTX in RA has been clearly established. Four well-designed, blinded, placebo-controlled trials[62–65] published in 1984 and 1985 had a tremendous impact on the treatment of RA. These trials varied in design and duration: Two of these trials used oral MTX and two used IM MTX, two trials had a crossover and two were parallel, and the duration of treatment varied from 6 to 28 weeks. Although the design and duration of therapy in these trials varied, the conclusions did not, as all showed MTX to be superior to placebo in the short-term treatment of RA. A meta-analysis of these trials by one study[66] showed that MTX-treated patients had a 37% greater improvement in swollen joint and tender joint scores, a 39% greater improvement in joint pain, and a 46% greater improvement in morning stiffness. MTX was generally well tolerated in these trials; withdrawal rates ranged from 0% to 32% and were mostly related to minor toxicities (i.e., stomatitis and nausea). Taken together, the results of these trials firmly established MTX as an effective therapy for the treatment of RA.

Numerous trials have compared MTX with other DMARDs. A meta-analysis done by one study showed that MTX was superior to placebo, auranofin, and probably hydroxychloroquine (HCQ), and was comparable with penicillamine, sulfasalazine (SSZ), and IM gold.[67] No trial has ever suggested that any other synthetic DMARD is superior to MTX.

Accumulating evidence suggests that the short-term benefit of most DMARDs is not sustained, and few patients continue to take these drugs after 3 years.[68,69] MTX appears to have the best durability. Another study has shown that 60% of patients continued MTX at 5 years, compared with less than 25% for penicillamine, gold, HCQ, and azathioprine.[68] Of all the DMARDs, MTX appears to have the best efficacy-to-toxicity ratio.[67] However, despite all the favorable efficacy reports, MTX alone rarely induces remissions of RA, and it has become the cornerstone of combinations of DMARD therapies, as discussed later.[70,71]

Rheumatoid Arthritis–Related Conditions. MTX has been used successfully in treating Felty's syndrome[72] and the large granular lymphocyte syndrome when it is found in patients with RA.[73] Improvement in neutrophil count occurs within 4 to 8 weeks of MTX initiation in both cases. MTX has been used successfully in adult-onset Still's disease[74] and for the cutaneous vasculitis of RA.[75]

Juvenile Idiopathic Arthritis. MTX is efficacious in juvenile idiopathic arthritis. A definitive, randomized, placebo-controlled trial (RCT) demonstrated that MTX at a dose of 10.0 mg/m^2 was superior to 5.0 mg/m^2 or placebo.[76] Sixty-three percent of children receiving the higher dose (10.0 mg/m^2) of MTX improved, compared with 32% in the lower-dose group (5.0 mg/m^2) and 36% in the placebo group.

Psoriatic Arthritis (PsA). Numerous prospective and retrospective trials have showed a benefit for MTX in PsA.[77] The largest double-blind randomized trial compared weekly oral MTX with placebo and showed statistically significant results only for physician global assessment of arthritis activity and the amount of affected skin surface area; however, this study was small and may have been underpowered to detect differences in joint count, pain, and swelling.[78] Despite the paucity of randomized controlled trial data, MTX remains a commonly used systemic agent in the treatment of PsA.

Systemic Lupus Erythematosus (SLE). MTX is efficacious in controlling cutaneous and/or articular manifestations of SLE, particularly in disease resistant to anti-malarials or requiring high doses of systemic steroids.[79] Concomitant folic acid should be administered to abrogate the elevated levels of homocysteine that may be a side effect of MTX therapy and is considered a risk factor for cardiovascular disease in SLE. The role of MTX in treating more severe SLE involvement, including renal, hematologic, or CNS disease, has not yet been established.[80] Extreme caution should be used in patients with renal disease.

Vasculitis. MTX in conjunction with corticosteroids is efficacious in treating early and non–life-threatening granulomatosis with polyangiitis, including upper airway disease and mild renal disease.[81–84] In addition to induction of remission, MTX maintains remission in granulomatosis with polyangiitis, although physician vigilance for patient relapse is warranted.[85] Despite a lack of well-designed studies, MTX has been efficacious in corticosteroid-resistant Takayasu's arteritis[86] and in relapsing polychondritis.[87]

The use of MTX for polymyalgia rheumatica (PMR) and giant cell arteritis (GCA) has been controversial. Recently, RCTs of MTX in addition to corticosteroids in PMR and GCA have shown conflicting results.[88–91] Thus, the routine use of MTX in either PMR or GCA has not been adopted, but some advocate for its use in an effort to more rapidly taper corticosteroid use in patients with intolerable side effects.

Inflammatory Myopathies. A review of the published reports of MTX and the inflammatory myopathies polymyositis (PMS) and dermatomyositis (DMS) shows overall positive results.[92] However, despite the frequent use of MTX in the inflammatory myopathies, a recent Cochrane Database Review reveals a paucity of well-designed trials.[93]

Other Rheumatic Diseases. MTX has been used in systemic sclerosis. One RCT looking at MTX use in early systemic sclerosis[94] showed a trend in benefit for skin scores and pulmonary diffusion capacity and a significant benefit for physician global assessment; a second RCT in established systemic sclerosis[95] showed significant benefit for skin scores and total creatinine clearance. In addition, prospective trials have shown that MTX is efficacious in the treatment of corticosteroid-resistant multisystem sarcoidosis,[96,97] and a recent RCT showed that, if initiated early in sarcoidosis, MTX is an effective steroid-sparing agent.[98] MTX is also effective as primary treatment and as a corticosteroid-sparing agent in inflammatory ocular disease.[99,100] Finally, MTX in combination with corticosteroids is effective in the treatment of multicentric reticulohistiocytosis.[101]

Dose and Drug Administration

MTX is available as 2.5, 5, 7.5, 10, and 15 mg tablets, and as a solution of 25 mg/mL for SQ or IM injection. Recently, the U.S. Food and Drug Administration (FDA) has approved single- and multiple-use, prefilled auto-injection pens at various dosages.

In patients with normal renal function, the starting dose is usually 15 mg given as a single weekly dose, with a range of 5 to 25 mg weekly, and consideration should be given to initiation via the parenteral route for improved efficacy. More frequent administration is associated with a significantly increased risk of liver toxicity.[102] If the oral dose of MTX exceeds 15 mg, consideration should be given to splitting the dose, with each half given 6 to 12 hours apart, for improved absorption and bioavailability. The dosage of MTX can be escalated, usually every 4 to 8 weeks to 25 mg/week to achieve the desired clinical response. MTX may be administered orally via tablet or parenteral solution; the latter may be less costly. Because its oral bioavailability is variable and decreases at higher doses, parenteral MTX is generally recommended if patients have active disease despite oral doses at approximately 20 mg weekly. In fact, recent data have shown that parenteral MTX is clinically superior to orally administered MTX, and that this may be a preferred route of administration for initial therapy[103] or if oral MTX is not optimally effective.[54]

MTX is not directly toxic to the kidneys, but as the main mechanism of elimination is via the kidneys, it is contraindicated in patients with a GFR less than 30 mL/minute.[104] MTX may be used in patients with a GFR of 30 to 59 mL/minute, but it is prudent to initiate a lower dose and monitor carefully with subsequent dose escalations.

Because MTX works by interfering with folate-dependent pathways, a relative folate-deficient state can occur in individuals taking MTX. Concomitant administration of folic acid (1 to 3 mg/day) or folinic acid decreases the frequency of MTX side effects, including GI toxicity (nausea, vomiting, abdominal pain) and stomatitis. Supplementation of folic or folinic acid is protective against elevated transaminase concentrations, results in fewer toxicity-related withdrawals of MTX, and does not interfere with the efficacy of MTX.[105] Folic acid administration also decreases hyperhomocysteinemia in patients on MTX, and this may be important to help decrease the already high cardiovascular risk of patients with RA. There is insufficient evidence to suggest that one form of folate has clinical advantages versus the other, and because folic acid is widely available and less expensive, it has become the preferred agent for most.[105]

In the case of overdose leading to amino transferase elevations over three times the upper limits of normal and cytopenias, intravenous leucovorin should be given at a dose of 5 to 10 mg every 12 hours until the patient has recovered.

Measurement of MTX-PG levels is commercially available ($MTXGlu_n$). It would be valuable to have a marker to predict response and adverse events associated with MTX therapy, but mixed results have been obtained in the search for a trend in the dose-response relationship for $MTXGlu_n$ levels and RA disease activity. A recent study showed no relationship between $MTXGlu_n$ concentration and reduced disease activity in RA.[106] Furthermore, no relationship was identified between $MTXGlu_n$ levels and adverse events. Disease activity was influenced by red blood cell (RBC) folate level, and further study is warranted to determine whether this may serve as a marker for MTX efficacy.

Geriatric Patients

Patients older than 65 years represent a special subset of patients receiving pharmacotherapy. Pharmacokinetic profiles, including drug distribution, are changed in the elderly as the result of decreases in end-organ blood flow and lean body mass, decreased hepatic drug metabolism, and decreased renal drug excretion. Furthermore, these patients are more likely to have multiple comorbidities, polypharmacy, noncompliance, increased risk for dosage errors, and limited access to medication for financial reasons.[107]

In practice, recommended doses should be reduced when therapy is initiated and should be adjusted for renal function based on creatinine clearance (CrCl).[108] The serum creatinine may be a misleading measure of renal function in older patients because of an overall reduction in lean muscle mass. Dosing recommendations are as follows: initial doses should be approximately 5 to 7.5 mg/week and should not exceed 20 mg/wk. Dosage adjustments for CrCl are as follows: for a CrCl of 61 to 80 mL/min, reduce the dose by 25%; for a CrCl of 51 to 60 mL/min, reduce the dose by 30%; for a CrCl of 30 to 50 mL/min, reduce the dose by 50% to 80%; and for a CrCl less than 30 mL/min, avoid use[109] (Table 64.1).

Pediatric Patients

MTX is commonly used in the pediatric population (see Table 64.1). It can be given orally or SQ, with a starting dose of 0.3 to 1

TABLE 64.1 Special Considerations for DMARD Therapy

	Fertility	Pregnancy	Lactation	Elderly	Pediatrics
Methotrexate	W: no effect M: reversible sterility Stop 3 mo before conception	Contraindicated FDA category X; abortifacient; teratogenic	Contraindicated; present in breast milk	Lower initial dose (5-7.5 mg/wk); dose based on CrCl	Dosing based on weight
Leflunomide	No effect; test levels before conception; may require washout	Contraindicated FDA category X; embryolethal; teratogenic	Contraindicated; unknown concentrations in breast milk	No dosage adjustment required	Dosing based on weight
Sulfasalazine	W: no effect M: reversible sterility	Relatively safe; FDA category B, C	Relatively safe; present in breast milk	No dosage adjustment required	Dosing based on weight
Hydroxychloroquine	No effect	Relatively safe; FDA category C	Relatively safe; present in breast milk	No dosage adjustment required	Dosing based on weight

CrCl, Creatinine clearance; *FDA,* U.S. Food and Drug Administration; *M,* men; *W,* women.

mg/kg/dose once weekly. It is common to start at 0.3 mg/kg/dose and escalate to a dose of 25 mg/wk. It is suggested that at doses greater than 15 mg/week, parenteral application should be considered because of better bioavailability and tolerability. Guidelines for toxicity monitoring are similar to adult recommendations.

Toxicity

Despite initial concerns, when given once a week in doses used for rheumatic diseases and monitored correctly, MTX is very well tolerated. Some of the toxicities of MTX (e.g., stomatitis, nausea, and bone marrow depression) are dose dependent, appear to be related to folate deficiency, and respond to folate replacement. Other toxicities (e.g., pneumonitis) appear to be idiosyncratic or allergic and, in most cases, require discontinuation of MTX. Still other toxicities, such as liver fibrosis and cirrhosis, appear to be multifactorial and may depend on the presence of concomitant risk factors, total dose, and frequency of administration.

Gastrointestinal and Hepatic Side Effects

GI symptoms, including dyspepsia, nausea, and anorexia, are common, occurring in as many as 20% to 70% of patients within the first year of therapy.[110] These symptoms may be attenuated by adding folic acid or by changing to a parenteral dosing regimen.

The risk of significant liver toxicity appears to be low when MTX is given once weekly to patients who abstain from alcohol and are monitored carefully, and occurs in approximately one patient per 1000 after 5 years of use.[111] However, a review of a large North American database of patients with RA and PsA found that elevations in aspartate aminotransferase (AST)/alanine aminotransferase (ALT) greater than one time the upper limit of normal (ULN) occurred in 22% and 31% of patients taking MTX or MTX and leflunomide, respectively. Elevations greater than two times ULN occurred in 1% to 2% on monotherapy and in greater than 5% on combination therapy. Elevated liver function tests (LFTs) were more likely in patients with PsA.[112] Alcohol consumption, α_1–anti-trypsin deficiency, morbid obesity, diabetes, concomitant hepatotoxic drugs, and chronic hepatitis B or C have all been implicated as possible risk factors for MTX toxicity.[113]

Hematologic Side Effects

Bone marrow toxicity, in most cases, is dose dependent and responds to folic acid administration. Pancytopenia, leukopenia, anemia, and thrombocytopenia can occur, but are rare. Clinically significant pancytopenia may develop in as many as 1% to 2% of RA patients on MTX therapy.[114] Severe, life-threatening bone marrow toxicity can be treated with folinic acid (leucovorin) and, if necessary, granulocyte-stimulating factor (GSF). Because the elimination of MTX is dependent on the kidney, decreases in renal function may precipitate bone marrow toxicity in patients who have been previously stable. Additional risk factors include hypoalbuminemia, dosing errors, and concomitant use of probenecid or trimethoprim/sulfamethoxazole (TMP/SMX).

Pulmonary Side Effects

Five clinical pulmonary syndromes have been associated with MTX treatment: acute interstitial pneumonitis (hypersensitivity pneumonitis), interstitial fibrosis, noncardiogenic pulmonary edema (seen in high-dose treatment for malignancy with rare reports in RA), pleuritis and pleural effusions, and pulmonary nodules.[115] Time lapse from initiation of therapy to cumulative dose before the onset of pulmonary toxicity is extremely variable, at 1 to 480 weeks and 7.5 to 3600 mg of MTX, respectively.[115] MTX-induced pulmonary disease is rare and is difficult to quantify, but estimates suggest an incidence of 3.9 cases per 100 patient-years of MTX exposure and a prevalence of 2.1% to 5.5%.[116,117] A recent meta-analysis of MTX and lung disease in RA has shown a modest increased risk of all respiratory events (relative risk [RR], 1.10; 95% confidence interval [CI], 1.02 to 1.19) and respiratory infection (RR, 1.11; 95% CI, 1.02 to 1.21), but not an increased risk for death from lung disease (RR, 1.53; 95% CI, 0.46 to 5.01) or noninfectious respiratory events (RR, 1.02; 95% CI, 0.65 to 1.60) when compared with other DMARDs and biologic agents.[118]

Patients generally are seen with shortness of breath, tachypnea, dry cough, and fever. Chest radiographs most typically show a bilateral interstitial infiltrate (although this finding varies). Infectious causes, including opportunistic organisms, must always be ruled out. If routine evaluations for infection, including sputum studies, and for other medical conditions to explain the pulmonary symptoms are negative, bronchoscopy with bronchoalveolar lavage and transbronchial biopsy is recommended. If MTX pulmonary toxicity is suspected, MTX should be discontinued and supportive treatment initiated with the use of corticosteroids in more severe cases. Some patients with pulmonary toxicity have been successfully restarted on MTX,[119] but clinicians have reported mortality in up to 50% of re-treated patients.[59]

Factors that appear to predispose to MTX lung toxicity include age, blue collar occupation, smoking (in women), diabetes, pleuropulmonary rheumatoid disease, and skin rashes from MTX.[120]

Mucocutaneous Side Effects

The mucocutaneous toxicities of MTX, which have been reported to occur in up to one-third of patients, are dose dependent and respond to folate replacement. Patients generally report fairly minor oral ulcerations, but severe ulceration of the mouth, esophagus, bowel, and vagina can occur, especially at higher doses.

Malignancies

The induction of malignancies by MTX is a concern, and several studies have examined this question with conflicting conclusions. Recently, reports of lymphoma in MTX-treated patients with RA have appeared. Because the incidence of lymphoma is already increased in patients with RA,[121] these reports are difficult to interpret. The case for a causative role of MTX has been strengthened, however, because a number of these cases have been B cell lymphomas of the type commonly seen in association with immunosuppression (associated with Epstein-Barr virus) and that may regress after discontinuation of MTX.[122,123] Subsequently, lack of a causal relationship between MTX treatment and the development of lymphoma has been seen in two large series of RA patients—one prospective study[121] and one retrospective study.[124] The potential benefits of MTX for most RA patients thus far outweigh these statistically small risks.[125]

Miscellaneous

Methotrexate "Flu." Patients taking MTX may describe flu-like symptoms shortly after taking their weekly dose. Nausea, low-grade fevers, myalgias, and chills are the most common signs of the so-called MTX flu. These side effects usually respond to supplementation with folic acid, decreasing the dose, switching from oral to parenteral administration, or changing the time of the dose (so that the patient takes MTX right before going to bed).

Nodulosis. The development of, or increase in the number or size of, rheumatoid nodules has been reported to occur in patients with RA treated with MTX, with a prevalence of as much as 8%.[126] This may occur in rheumatoid factor–negative patients, and in those in whom the synovitis is under excellent control. The mechanism of this nodule formation has been suggested to be the result of an increase in adenosine, which appears to promote nodule formation.[127] Conversely, nodules have been reported to decrease during MTX therapy.

Vasculitis. Despite efficacy in the treatment of the cutaneous vasculitis associated with RA, leukocytoclastic vasculitis has also been attributed to MTX therapy.[128]

Fertility, Pregnancy, and Lactation

MTX does not seem to adversely affect female fertility but can cause reversible sterility in men.[129] Women and men should discontinue MTX for at least 3 months before attempting to conceive because of its large distribution and long half-life in the liver. Folic acid supplementation is essential before conception. MTX is included in the 1979 FDA Pregnancy Category Group of X and is contraindicated during pregnancy. The new FDA guidelines continue to recommend against the use of MTX in pregnancy. Women of childbearing age who are considered for MTX therapy should receive extensive counseling regarding teratogenic risk and should be placed and maintained on adequate contraception before therapy is begun. Toxicities include fetal abnormalities such as aminopterin syndrome (multiple craniofacial, limb, and CNS abnormalities)[130] and embryonic or fetal loss. MTX at high doses (1 mg/kg) is an effective abortifacient. MTX is also contraindicated during lactation because small amounts are excreted in breast milk and can accumulate in neonatal tissue (see Table 64.1).

Toxicity Monitoring

The American College of Rheumatology (ACR) has recently revised recommendations for the use of DMARDs, and these serve as an excellent resource.[104,131] Toxicities that require monitoring include myelosuppression, hepatotoxicity, and pulmonary toxicity. Baseline evaluation should include a complete blood count (CBC) with platelets, hepatitis B and C serology in high-risk patients, liver transaminases, and creatinine. Although these guidelines make no recommendations on the need for a baseline chest radiograph, this is a reasonable approach. Liver biopsies are not routinely recommended before MTX is initiated. The rare patients whom one wants to treat with MTX despite abnormalities in screening laboratory or other significant risk factors may require liver biopsy before MTX is initiated. In addition, biopsies are recommended only in those patients who continue to have enzyme abnormalities and for whom continuation of MTX therapy is contemplated.

Monitoring for toxicity should be done every 2 to 12 weeks and is based on the duration of therapy, with more frequent monitoring provided earlier in the course of treatment. Systems review and physical examination should include monitoring for symptoms or signs of myelosuppression (fever, infection, bruising, and bleeding), pulmonary toxicity (shortness of breath, cough, rales), GI intolerance (nausea, vomiting, diarrhea), and lymphadenopathy. Laboratory parameters that should be followed include a CBC with platelets, liver transaminases, and creatinine (Table 64.2).

TABLE 64.2 Safety Monitoring

	Baseline	Monitoring Interval <3 Months of Drug Therapy[a]	3-6 Months of Drug Therapy[a]	>6 Months of Drug Therapy[a]	Contraindications
MTX	CBC, LFT, Cr, HBV, HCV; vaccinate: influenza, *Pneumococcus,* HBV	Every 2-4 wk	Every 8-12 wk	Every 12 wk	Active infection, symptomatic pulmonary disease, WBC <3000/mm^3, Plt <50,000/mL^3, CrCl <30 mL/min, history of myelodysplasia or recent lymphoproliferative disorder, LFT >2 × ULN, acute or chronic HBV or HCV, pregnancy, lactation
Leflunomide	CBC, LFT, Cr, HBV, HCV; vaccinate: influenza, *Pneumococcus,* HBV	Every 2-4 wk	Every 8-12 wk	Every 12 wk	Active infection WBC <3000/mm^3, Plt <50,000/mL^3, history of myelodysplasia or recent lymphoproliferative disorder, LFT >2 × ULN, acute or chronic HBV or HCV, pregnancy, lactation
Sulfasalazine	CBC, LFT, Cr; vaccinate: influenza, *Pneumococcus*	Every 2-4 wk	Every 8-12 wk	Every 12 wk	Sulfa allergy, Plt <50,000/mL^3, LFT >2 × ULN, acute HBV/HCV, some classes of chronic HBV/HCV
Hydroxychloroquine	CBC, LFT, Cr; complete ophthalmologic examination within 1 year	None	None	None	History of vision changes attributed to 4-aminoquinolone derivatives, some classes of untreated HBV/HCV

[a]Monitoring at <3, 3-6, and >6 mo need only include CBC, LFT, and Cr.

CBC, Complete blood count; *Cr,* creatinine; *CrCl,* creatinine clearance; *HBV,* hepatitis B; *HCV,* hepatitis C; *LFT,* liver function test; *Plt,* platelets; *ULN,* upper limit of normal; *WBC,* white blood cell count.

From Saag K, Geng G, Patkar N: American College of Rheumatology 2008 recommendations for the use of nonbiologic and biologic disease-modifying anti-rheumatic drugs in rheumatoid arthritis. *Arthritis Rheum* 59:762–784, 2008.

It is important to consider vaccination status in any patient who is going to use MTX. RA patients have an increased incidence of death from pneumonia,[132] and MTX may reduce the immune response to pneumococcal antigen.[133] Thus any patient in whom MTX is going to be used should first receive the pneumococcal vaccination, with booster as appropriate. Vaccinations for hepatitis B virus for at-risk patients and yearly influenza vaccines are recommended as well. Caution should be exercised when administering live virus vaccinations to patients on MTX.

Drug Interactions and Contraindications

Drug Interactions

Drugs that are known hepatotoxins, such as SSZ, leflunomide, and azathioprine, may potentiate liver toxicity when used in combination. Organic acids, such as sulfonamides, salicylates, NSAIDs, penicillin G, piperacillin, and probenecid, competitively inhibit tubular secretion, and this delays MTX clearance.[134] MTX also undergoes distal tubular reabsorption, which may be enhanced by the addition of HCQ[135] and blocked by the addition of folic acid.[134] Drugs that affect renal function should be used with caution because of the renal clearance of MTX and, therefore, the increased risk of MTX toxicity that could occur because of decreased clearance.

Several of the aforementioned drugs deserve special mention. TMP-SMX at daily doses should be avoided or used with extreme caution because of possible hematologic toxicity with MTX. Mechanisms for this toxicity include an additive anti-folate effect from TMP, decreased MTX clearance because of inhibition of tubular secretion by SMX, and altered MTX plasma protein binding. NSAIDs are commonly used in patients with RA as adjunctive therapy. NSAIDs may increase MTX levels by displacing MTX from plasma proteins and limiting tubular secretion. Despite lack of a significant pharmacokinetic or clinical interaction between low-dose MTX and a variety of NSAIDs,[136] vigilance for MTX toxicity should increase whenever NSAID dosages are changed in patients on stable weekly doses of MTX. Low doses of aspirin used for cardiovascular prophylaxis are not likely to be of concern. Furthermore, probenecid should be avoided because it inhibits tubular secretion of MTX.

Contraindications

MTX should not be used in patients with severe renal, pulmonary, or hepatic impairment, pre-existing bone marrow suppression, alcoholic liver disease, or during pregnancy or breastfeeding. Ongoing or active infection is also a contraindication. In most cases, patients who desire to continue drinking alcohol should not be treated with MTX. Mild to moderate renal insufficiency is a relative contraindication, and use of MTX in these patients may require more vigilant toxicity monitoring (Table 64.3).

Leflunomide

KEY POINTS

- Leflunomide reversibly inhibits dihydroorotate dehydrogenase.
- Loading doses are not often used in clinical practice because of gastrointestinal toxicity.
- Because of enterohepatic recirculation, leflunomide has a very long half-life.
- Leflunomide is absolutely contraindicated in pregnancy, and levels must be checked with a washout protocol if needed before conception.
- Vigilance must be used for hepatotoxicity.

TABLE 64.3 Methotrexate, Leflunomide, Sulfasalazine, and Anti-malarials: Summary of Mechanism of Action, Efficacy, and Toxicity

	Proposed Mechanism of Action	Efficacy	Toxicity
Methotrexate	Inhibition of ATIC→↑ Adenosine Inhibition of TYMS→↓ Pyrimidine synthesis Inhibition of DHFR→↓ Transmethylation reactions	RA LGL/Felty's syndrome JIA PsA SLE Vasculitis	Nausea Hepatotoxicity Bone marrow suppression Pneumonitis MTXflu
Leflunomide	Inhibition of DHODH→↓ Pyrimidine synthesis Inhibition of tyrosine kinase→↓ Cell signal transduction	RA SLE PsA	Hepatotoxicity Diarrhea Weight loss
Sulfasalazine	Inhibition of arachidonic acid cascade Inhibition of ATIC→↑ Adenosine Multiple cellular effects Systemic effects via MALT	RA JIA Ankylosing spondylitis PsA Reactive arthritis	Nausea Headache Leukopenia Rash
Anti-malarials Hydroxychloroquine Chloroquine	↑ pH of subcellular vesicles→Interference with Ag processing and cell-mediated cytotoxicity Blocks TLR binding to nucleic acid to down regulate pro-inflammatory cytokine production	RA SLE Discoid lupus APS Sjögren's syndrome	Nausea Rash Neuromyopathy Retinopathy

Ag, Antigen; *APS,* antiphospholipid syndrome; *ATIC,* 5-aminoimidazole-4-carboxamide ribonucleotide (AICAR) transformylase; *DHFR,* dihydrofolate reductase; *DHODH,* dihydroorotate dehydrogenase; *JIA,* juvenile idiopathic arthritis; *LGL,* large granular lymphocyte; *MALT,* mucosa-associated lymphoid tissue; *MTX,* methotrexate; *PsA,* psoriatic arthritis; *RA,* rheumatoid arthritis; *SLE,* systemic lupus erythematosus; *TLR,* toll-like receptor; *TYMS,* thymidylate synthetase; ↑, increased; ↓, decreased; →, indicates the result.

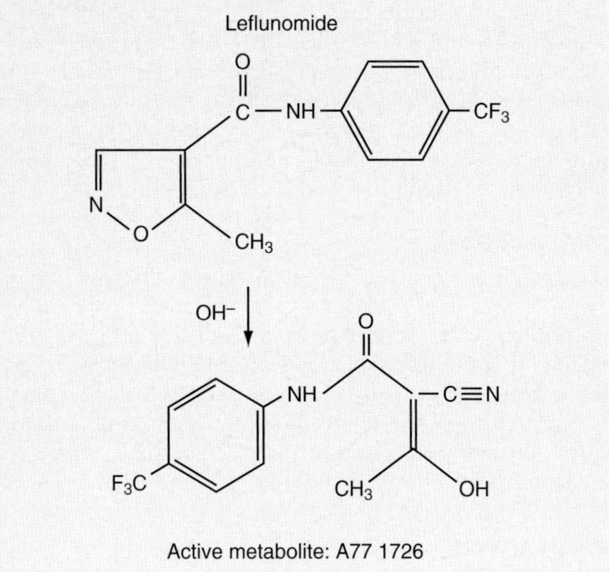

Leflunomide

OH⁻

Active metabolite: A77 1726

• **Fig. 64.4** Leflunomide is rapidly and completely metabolized to its active metabolite, A77 1726.

Leflunomide, an isoxazole derivative, is a synthetic DMARD approved for the treatment of RA. It emerged from a specific anti-inflammatory drug development program and has potent immunomodulatory effects.

Chemical Structure

Leflunomide is a low-molecular-weight isoxazole compound and is chemically unrelated to any previous immunosuppressant. Leflunomide is a prodrug and is rapidly and completely converted to its active metabolite, the malononitriloamide A77 1726. A77 1726 is also known as *teriflunomide* (Fig. 64.4).

Actions of Leflunomide

As with MTX, the precise mechanism of action responsible for the effects of leflunomide in rheumatic disease is not completely understood.[137] Leflunomide is immunomodulatory, with the net effect being a reduction in activated T lymphocytes. Its two in vitro mechanisms of action vary depending on concentration: (1) At the concentration of the active metabolite (A77 1726) achieved in patients, its major effect appears to be reversible inhibition of the enzyme dihydroorotate dehydrogenase (DHODH), which results in inhibition of pyrimidine synthesis; (2) at higher concentrations, A77 1726 also inhibits tyrosine kinases, interfering with cell signal transduction.[138]

Activation of T cells results in progression from the resting phase (G_0) to the G_1 phase, where ribonucleotides are synthesized, and then to the S phase, where cellular DNA is replicated in preparation for mitosis. T cell activation requires significant increases in de novo pyrimidine and purine biosynthesis. Sensors such as proto-oncogenes *(p53)* and checkpoints (cyclins C and D) in this pathway monitor the level of nucleotide pools and prevent damaged cells from replicating.[138]

Ribonucleotide uridine monophosphate (rUMP) is a precursor for the formation of pyrimidine nucleotides and thus is essential for both RNA and DNA synthesis. The steps in de novo rUMP synthesis are seen in Fig. 64.5. A critical step in this pathway is the generation of dihydroorotate in the cytoplasm with subsequent diffusion into the mitochondria, where the enzyme DHODH is located. DHODH converts dihydroorotate to orotate, and the latter diffuses back into the cytoplasm and is subsequently converted to rUMP and, ultimately, to RNA and DNA.

The first postulated mechanism of action of leflunomide consists of inhibition of DHODH by A77 1726, which lowers orotate levels and leads to a decrease in rUMP and subsequent nucleotide synthesis, resulting in T cell cycle arrest. This mechanism of action has been substantiated by experimental evidence. In vitro mitogen-stimulated activation of T cells is blocked by levels of A77 1726 that inhibit DHODH, and this inhibition can be reversed by the addition of uridine, suggesting that A77 1726 works by disruption of pyrimidine biosynthesis.[139,140] Further, the only enzyme inhibited by A77 1726 in this pathway, at concentration obtained in vivo, is DHODH.[141]

Evidence also exists to support that inhibition of DHODH produces an arrest of lymphocytes in the G_1 phase of the cell cycle.[142] If the level of ribonucleotides, including rUMP, falls below a critical point, cytoplasmic p53 activation occurs, and p53 will translocate to the nucleus and initiate cellular arrest by ultimately preventing transcription of cyclins D and E. In cultures of human T cells, A77 1726 depletes rUMP pools and results in an accumulation of nuclear p53 with resultant cell cycle arrest.[143] In comparison, treatment of cell lines lacking p53 with A77 1726 does not cause a G_1 phase arrest.[144]

Resting lymphocytes maintain ribonucleotide requirements largely through salvage pathways and are essentially unaffected by leflunomide.[145] Active, or autoimmune, lymphocytes rely on the de novo pathway and are affected by leflunomide. During the course of treatment with this slow-acting agent, autoimmune lymphocytes should be removed progressively.[138]

At higher concentrations, A77 1726 inhibits phosphorylation of tyrosine kinases that are critical for cell growth and differentiation of activated cells.[146,147] This inhibition has been proposed to partially or completely explain the anti-proliferative effects of leflunomide; however, it is unclear whether concentrations sufficient to achieve this effect are obtained in vivo.

Several other additional anti-inflammatory properties of leflunomide have been noted. Leflunomide has the ability to block the activation of nuclear factor-κB (NF-κB),[148] which regulates the expression of genes important in inflammatory processes, including those seen in inflammatory arthritis.[149] Ex vivo and in vitro studies in humans have shown that both leflunomide and MTX inhibit neutrophil chemotaxis, which may decrease the recruitment of inflammatory cells into the joints.[46] Leflunomide also decreases the ratio of MMP-1 to TIMP-1.[46] Finally, leflunomide alters the synthesis of cytokines by augmenting the immunosuppressive cytokine-transforming growth factor-β1 and suppressing the immunostimulatory cytokine IL-2.[150]

Pharmacology

Absorption and Bioavailability

The GI tract and the liver rapidly and completely convert ingested leflunomide into teriflunomide (A77 1726). Food does not interfere with absorption. Circulating teriflunomide is highly bound (>99%) to plasma proteins, predominantly albumin. Its plasma concentration is linearly correlated with a single oral dose over a range of 5 to 25 mg; steady state is reached in 7 weeks after daily dosing.[151]

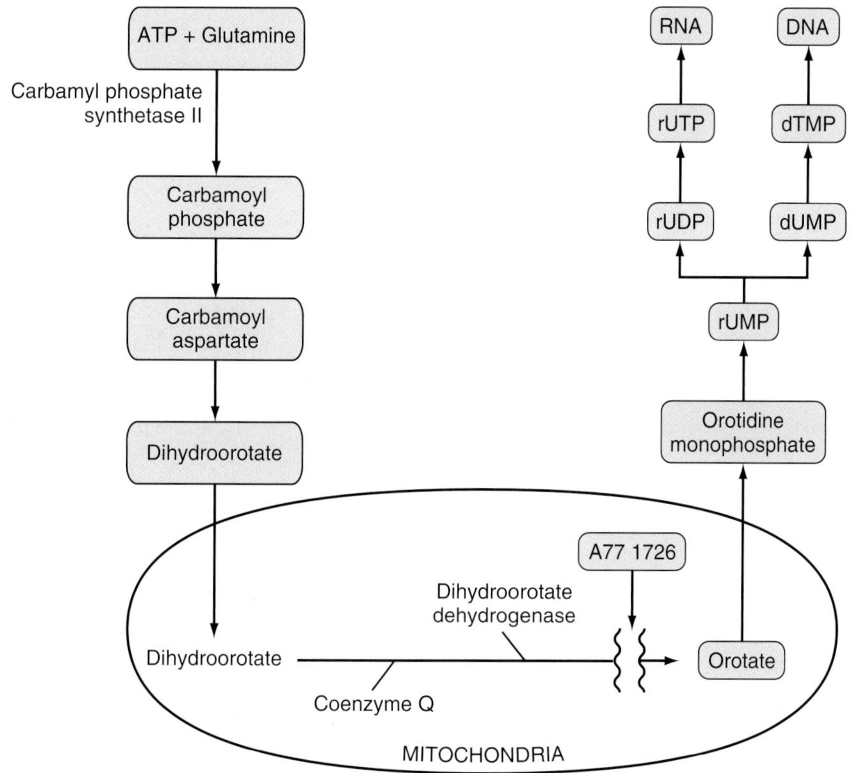

• **Fig. 64.5** The active metabolite of leflunomide, A77 1726, blocks the conversion of dihydroorotate to orotate within the mitochondria. *ATP,* Adenosine triphosphate; *dTMP,* 2-deoxythymidylate; *dUMP,* 2-deoxyuridylate; *rUDP,* ribonucleotide diphosphate; *rUMP,* ribonucleotide uridine monophosphate; *rUTP,* ribonucleotide triphosphate.

Distribution and Half-Life

Teriflunomide has a half-life of approximately 2 weeks (mean, 15.5 days),[151] with a low apparent volume of distribution. Although 90% of teriflunomide is excreted by 28 days, it undergoes extensive enterohepatic recirculation, and levels can be detectable for much longer periods.[151]

Elimination

In healthy individuals, the proportions excreted by the kidney and the gut are nearly equal. Because detectable teriflunomide may be present in the body months or years later, the ability to rapidly and effectively eliminate teriflunomide with cholestyramine is important. Oral administration of cholestyramine, 8 g three times daily for 11 days, can lower the apparent half-life of teriflunomide to 1 to 2 days.[152] Furthermore, activated charcoal, 50 g every 6 hours, can reduce plasma levels by 50% within 24 hours.[152]

Indications

Rheumatoid Arthritis. Leflunomide was first safe and effective in treating RA in a placebo-controlled, dose-ranging, 6-month trial.[151] Two pivotal trials, one in Europe and one in the United States, have compared leflunomide with SSZ and MTX. The European trial had three treatment arms: leflunomide (20 mg/day after a loading dose), SSZ (increased to 2 g/day), and placebo.[153] In this trial, both leflunomide and SSZ were superior to placebo in terms of swollen and tender joint counts, as well as physicians' and patients' overall assessments. It is important to note that both the leflunomide and SSZ groups reported significant effects on slowing of radiographic progression of disease compared with placebo. The U.S. trial compared patients treated with leflunomide (20 mg/day after a loading dose), MTX (7.5 to 15 mg/week), or placebo.[154] Again, both active drugs were found to be superior to placebo but not different from each other. Both leflunomide and MTX also slowed radiographic progression of disease compared with the placebo group. Another trial compared leflunomide (20 mg/day with loading) with MTX (10 to 15 mg/week) in a 1-year trial with a 1-year extension.[155] In this trial, MTX was statistically superior to leflunomide for the clinical outcomes measured, as well as the rate of radiographic progression after 2 years.

Other Rheumatic Diseases. Leflunomide has been reported to be effective in treating SLE. In a randomized, controlled trial, leflunomide was more effective than placebo in improving markers of lupus disease activity, and was safe and well tolerated.[156] A subsequent small, prospective, open-label trial of patients with lupus nephritis unresponsive to conventional therapy showed that leflunomide was efficacious and well tolerated.[157]

Leflunomide has been effective in treating PsA and psoriasis when compared with placebo.[158] In an open-label trial of AS, leflunomide was effective in treating peripheral arthritis, but axial symptoms did not improve.[159]

Both an open-label trial[160] and a randomized, controlled clinical trial[161] have shown the efficacy of leflunomide in maintaining remission in granulomatosis with polyangiitis after successful induction with cyclophosphamide. In the latter trial, leflunomide was superior to MTX in preventing relapse.

Leflunomide is also safe and effective in patients with juvenile idiopathic arthritis (JIA) who did not respond to or could not tolerate MTX.[162]

Dose and Drug Administration

Leflunomide is available in oral tablets at doses of 10, 20, and 100 mg. Oral leflunomide is rapidly metabolized to teriflunomide, which has a very long half-life; therefore, the standard recommendation had been to start therapy with a loading dose of 100 mg daily for 3 days, then switch to the standard maintenance dose of 20 mg daily. Despite this recommendation, many clinicians no longer prescribe a loading dose because it is believed to increase the drug's GI toxicity.[163] Also, it is common practice to decrease the dose to 10 mg daily if toxicity occurs, or if complete control of the disease can be maintained. Because of its long half-life, some clinicians give leflunomide less often (three to five times per week).

Geriatric Patients

No pharmacokinetic studies specific to geriatric patients have been done for leflunomide; hence dosing recommendations are the same as for the general population. No clinical experience in patients with renal insufficiency has been reported, so those patients should be monitored carefully (see Table 64.1).

Pediatric Patients

Although not approved in the United States to treat patients with JIA, leflunomide is used off-label for this condition at a dose of 10 to 20 mg/day. This dosing is often based on a patient's body weight. A recently published example of dosing by body weight is as follows: A patient weighing less than 20 kg receives 10 mg every other day, a patient weighing more than 20 kg but less than 40 kg receives 10 mg/day, and a patient weighing more than 40 kg receives 20 mg/day[164] (see Table 64.1).

Toxicity

For major controlled trials that have used leflunomide at a dose of 20 mg/day, the incidence of adverse events that resulted in trial withdrawal is shown in Table 64.4. Leflunomide-associated withdrawals (19%) were more frequent than those associated with MTX (14%) and placebo (8%), but were similar in frequency to those associated with SSZ (19%).

Gastrointestinal and Hepatic Side Effects

The most common side effect that limits the use of leflunomide is diarrhea, which responds to dose reduction and may be less common if the loading dose is not used. Abdominal pain, dyspepsia, and nausea from leflunomide appear to be slightly increased versus placebo rates.

Liver toxicity can occur in association with leflunomide administration. Data from a large U.S. cohort of RA and PsA patients show that elevations in ALT/AST levels greater than 1 × ULN occurred in 17% and elevations greater than 2 × ULN occurred in 1% to 2% of patients. Leflunomide given in combination with MTX resulted in ALT/AST elevations greater than 1 × ULN in 31% and greater than 2 × ULN in 5% of patients. Furthermore, this change in transaminases was more commonly seen in patients with PsA.[112] The European Agency for Evaluation of Medicinal Products (EMEA) reported 296 patients with hepatic abnormalities and 15 patients with liver failure and death while taking leflunomide.[165,166] The FDA reviewed adverse event reports between August 2002 and May 2009, and found 49 cases of severe liver injury, 14 of which resulted in death.[167] Most patients with hepatotoxicity have risk factors, including concomitant administration of another hepatotoxic agent or underlying liver disease.

TABLE 64.4 Leflunomide Trial Withdrawals for Adverse Events

	No. of Patients	Withdrawals
Leflunomide	816	154 (19%)
Methotrexate	680	94 (14%)
Sulfasalazine	133	25 (19%)
Placebo	210	16 (8%)

Cardiovascular Side Effects

Hypertension has consistently been reported to occur more frequently in leflunomide-treated compared with placebo-treated patients.[153,154] Additionally, elevation of cholesterol levels has been reported in association with leflunomide use.[168] Both of these effects should be monitored because of the excess cardiovascular mortality reported in patients with RA.

Miscellaneous

Dermatologic. Skin rashes have been reported, most commonly occurring between the second and fifth months of treatment and necessitating discontinuation of the drug. Severe skin reactions such as Stevens-Johnson syndrome or toxic epidermal necrolysis require leflunomide washout with cholestryramine.

An increased incidence of alopecia has been reported in clinical trials in association with leflunomide treatment.

Pulmonary. Recent reports have suggested that leflunomide can cause interstitial lung disease (ILD), usually within 3 months of starting therapy. Patients with pre-existing ILD are at highest risk for this potentially fatal complication.[169,170]

Hematologic. Rare cases of pancytopenia have been reported in post-marketing surveillance, primarily in patients with known risk factors for blood dyscrasias. An increased risk of lymphoproliferative disorders has not been associated with leflunomide.

Neurologic. CNS side effects such as dizziness, headaches, and parasthesias have been reported with leflunomide.[171] A sensory axonal neuropathy has also been seen with a reported prevalence of 1.4%.[171,172] In addition to discontinuation of leflunomide, cholestyramine washout may be useful.

Weight Loss. Significant weight loss has also been reported to occur in patients taking leflunomide.[173]

Fertility, Pregnancy, and Lactation

Although new data are emerging in humans that may show less fetal risk after exposure to leflunomide,[173a] it remains a 1979 FDA Pregnancy Category group X. Animal studies have demonstrated substantial teratogenic and embryolethal effects with small doses of leflunomide. Therefore, women of childbearing potential should be strongly counseled about this, and leflunomide should not be prescribed for women who are not practicing reliable birth control methods. A pregnancy test should be considered before therapy is initiated. Leflunomide excretion in milk is unknown; therefore, nursing mothers should not receive leflunomide.

It is critically important to note that teriflunomide, largely because of its enterohepatic recirculation, may remain in the body for years. Therefore, if a woman who has previously received leflunomide wishes to become pregnant, teriflunomide levels should be measured. Active elimination of leflunomide from the body should be considered for levels above 0.02 mg/L. This can be achieved by the oral administration of cholestyramine for 11 days (8 g, three times daily).[174] Before pregnancy is attempted, verification of levels below 0.02 mg/L should be confirmed on two separate occasions, at least 14 days apart, and the woman should then wait an additional three full menstrual cycles.[175] Patients may require more than one course of cholestyramine to achieve this level. Although no data exist, men wishing to father children should undergo the same washout procedure as women and should wait an additional 3 months after the second drug plasma level is verified to be below 0.02 mg/L (see Table 64.1). Studies are ongoing that are evaluating this risk. Due to the small number of subjects, caution is still advised.

Toxicity Monitoring

Similar to MTX, the ACR has published guidelines on the initiation and monitoring of leflunomide treatment.[104] Patients taking leflunomide should have a baseline CBC and liver enzyme monitoring, including AST, ALT, and albumin. Serum creatinine measurement is important because leflunomide is partially eliminated by the kidney. The frequency of monitoring depends on the duration of therapy (see Table 64.2). More frequent monitoring may be warranted if concomitant immunosuppressive agents, such as MTX, are given. If patients experience significant toxicity, a washout procedure is indicated to more rapidly eliminate the drug. Caution should be exercised when live virus vaccinations are administered to patients on leflunomide.

Drug Interactions and Contraindications

Drug Interactions

Cholestyramine interferes with enterohepatic recycling of leflunomide, resulting in lower serum concentrations. Concomitant use with hepatotoxic agents, including MTX, increases the risk of liver toxicity, and leflunomide must be used with caution and monitored judiciously. Rifampin may increase the serum concentration of teriflunomide. Leflunomide may potentiate warfarin therapy.

Contraindications

Leflunomide should not be used in patients with impaired liver function, severe renal impairment, bone marrow dysplasia, severe immunodeficiency, severe hypoproteinemia, or known hypersensitivity to the drug. The liver is involved in enterohepatic recirculation and biliary excretion; thus leflunomide use in liver disease is contraindicated. In renal insufficiency, the levels of circulating teriflunomide do not appear to be increased, but the component of free teriflunomide is increased and patients should be closely monitored. Leflunomide is contraindicated in the setting of serious infection and should be discontinued in patients with new or worsening pulmonary symptoms or rash. Leflunomide is absolutely contraindicated in pregnancy and breastfeeding (see Table 64.1).

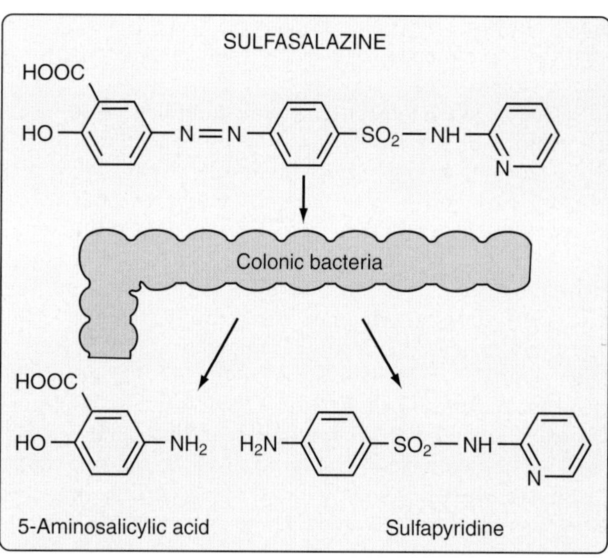

• **Fig. 64.6** Sulfasalazine and its major metabolites.

Sulfasalazine

KEY POINTS

Sulfasalazine (SSZ) has anti-microbial and anti-inflammatory properties, but the exact mechanism of action is unknown.

SSZ is commonly used as part of combination therapy for RA.

Gastrointestinal intolerance is a common side effect.

Although rare, surveillance for leukopenia is important early in the course of the treatment.

SSZ was the first agent to be synthesized specifically for rheumatoid arthritis in 1938, by Professor Nanna Svartz of Stockholm, in collaboration with the Swedish pharmaceutical company Pharmacia. The prevailing notion at that time was that RA was caused by infection, and SSZ was designed with both anti-inflammatory and anti-bacterial properties.

Chemical Structure

Salicylazosulfapyridine (SASP), now known as *sulfasalazine*, is a conjugate of the anti-inflammatory 5-aminosalicylic acid (5-ASA or *mesalamine*) and the anti-bacterial sulfapyridine joined by an azo bond (Fig. 64.6). The abbreviation *SASP* is still in use as an alternative to SSZ.

Actions of Sulfasalazine

Despite more than eight decades of use, the mechanism of action of SSZ in rheumatic disease still is not fully elucidated. When SSZ was designed, its anti-microbial properties were thought to be fundamentally important in the successful treatment of RA, which was postulated to be an enteropathic arthropathy. Through alteration of gut flora, SSZ may downregulate the immune response which leads to inflammatory arthritis. Although this hypothesis has never been disproved, this mechanism of action has fallen out of favor for several reasons. To date, no conclusive evidence has been found for an infectious cause of RA, other sulfonamides have failed to result in clinical improvement, and a relationship between gut flora and clinical response to SSZ is lacking.[176] Currently, SSZ is presumed to work via anti-inflammatory and immunomodulatory effects.

SSZ has been demonstrated in vitro to possess multiple anti-inflammatory properties. First, SSZ weakly inhibits the pro-inflammatory effects of the arachidonic acid cascade, with a slight inhibitory effect on prostaglandin E_2 synthetase activity,[177] as well as lipoxygenase products.[178] SSZ also downregulates neutrophil chemotaxis, migration, and proteolytic enzyme production and degranulation,[179,180] and inhibits neutrophil activation by decreasing the flux of second messengers involved in intra-cellular signal transduction.[181] Neutrophil migration to sites of inflammation can be downregulated by adenosine. SSZ inhibits folate-dependent enzymes, including ATIC and DHFR, resulting in increased adenosine release into the extra-cellular milieu.[182] One study[183] confirmed that SSZ, similar to MTX, modulates inflammation via increased adenosine release. This effect appears to be the result solely of SSZ because sulfapyridine and 5-ASA are inactive. SSZ is a more potent inhibitor of ATIC than MTX.

SSZ also possesses multiple immunomodulatory properties. In vitro, SSZ inhibits T cell proliferation, natural killer cell activity, and B cell activation, with resultant declines in immunoglobulin synthesis and RF production.[176] In all of these systems, sulfapyridine and 5-ASA are less active than SSZ. Cytokine profiles are also altered by SSZ, resulting in inhibition of the T cell cytokines IL-2[184] and IFN-γ,[185] and the monocyte/macrophage cytokines IL-1, TNF, and IL-6.[186,187] NF-κB is a key transcription factor that when active mediates the transcription of key cytokines, adhesion molecules, and chemokines essential to mounting an immune response. In vitro, SSZ, but not sulfapyridine or 5-ASA, inhibits NF-κB translocation to the nucleus.[188]

SSZ, more so than sulfapyridine, inhibits endothelial cell proliferation and angiogenesis, which likely contributes to the synovitis of RA.[189] The synovial fibroblast also plays a key role in the pathogenesis of RA, and SSZ inhibits fibroblast proliferation and metalloproteinase synthesis.[190] Finally, SSZ inhibits the formation of osteoclasts and may be anti-resorptive in RA.[191]

The active moiety of SSZ is controversial. The parent compound, SSZ, appears to have the most biologic activity when compared with sulfapyridine and 5-ASA. However, the SSZ levels needed in vitro to see the anti-inflammatory and immunomodulatory effects are far greater than those obtained in vivo. No demonstrable relationship has been shown between plasma SSZ, sulfapyridine, and 5-ASA levels that correlates with clinical efficacy, so serum levels may be irrelevant.[176] In an open, nonrandomized study comparing two groups of patients who received either sulfapyridine or 5-ASA in doses that would represent the molar equivalent of 2 g of SSZ, the group receiving sulfapyridine showed significant improvement in erythrocyte sedimentation rate (ESR) and in some clinical parameters, including grip strength and joint circumference.[192] Taken together, it would appear that both SSZ and sulfapyridine have a role in therapeutic efficacy for RA.

One potential site of action for SSZ that may explain its systemic action despite low serum levels is the mucosa-associated lymphoid tissue (MALT) in the small bowel.[176] In the gut lumen, the therapeutic concentration of SSZ is at least two times greater than in the serum, and drug concentration in the surrounding mucosal tissue is likely also high. The gut immune system is extensive, and active communication with the rest of the body occurs via migration and recirculation of activated lymphocytes.[176] Furthermore, a link between MALT and the joints has been suggested.[193] Evidence that some of the efficacy of SSZ may be mediated via MALT is described as follows. Treatment with SSZ decreases circulating immunoglobulin (Ig)A-producing cells and serum levels of IgA, correlating with disease improvement[194]; SSZ reduces gut mucosa lymphocytes in treated patients[195]; and SSZ modulates an immune response elicited by an oral antigen in mice and healthy volunteers.[196]

Pharmacology

Absorption and Bioavailability

Less than 30% of SSZ is absorbed by the small bowel; most undergoes enterohepatic circulation and is secreted unchanged in the bile, with a resulting bioavailability of 10%.[176] The steady-state serum concentration of SSZ is 5 μg/mL after an oral dose of 2 g/day. Most SSZ reaches the colon, where intestinal bacteria reduce the azo bond and release the two active components: sulfapyridine and 5-ASA.[197] Most of the sulfapyridine is absorbed from the colon (>90%) and appears in plasma 4 to 6 hours after an oral dose (steady-state serum concentration of 30 μg/mL after 2 g/day dose). Most of the 5-ASA (80% to 90%) remains in the bowel.[176] Sulfapyridine and SSZ are likely the active components in rheumatic disease, and 5-ASA is the active component in ulcerative colitis.[198]

The bioavailability of standard SSZ is similar to that of enteric-coated SSZ.[199] Administration of SSZ with food decreases the blood concentration of both SSZ and sulfapyridine.[200]

Distribution and Half-Life

Both SSZ and sulfapyridine are widely distributed in the body, with more than 99% and 50% to 70% plasma protein binding, respectively.[176,200] Serum and synovial concentrations are comparable.[201] The half-life of SSZ is 6 to 17 hours, with upper-range values characteristic of older patients, and the half-life of sulfapyridine is 8 to 21 hours, with upper-range values characteristic of slow acetylators.[202]

Elimination

Sulfapyridine is extensively metabolized in the liver by *N*-acetylation and ring hydroxylation with subsequent glucuronidations,[203] and because of genetic variations in acetylator phenotype, wide variability is seen among individuals.[202] Slow acetylators have a reduced clearance rate and higher serum sulfapyridine concentrations. Sulfapyridine is excreted in the urine, and 5-ASA is eliminated primarily in the feces. The small portion of 5-ASA that is absorbed is excreted in the urine as *N*-acetylmesalamine.[204]

Indications

Rheumatoid Arthritis. Multiple published trials since the early 1980s have shown significant benefit in both clinical and laboratory parameters for SSZ (2 to 3 g daily) versus placebo in the treatment of RA.[205] A meta-analysis of randomized controlled clinical trials of SSZ for the treatment of RA was published in 1999.[206] In this analysis, SSZ was compared with placebo and other single DMARD therapies, including HCQ, D-penicillamine (D-Pen), and gold sodium thiomalate or aurothioglucose. In trials of SSZ versus placebo, SSZ was superior to placebo in patient improvement in multiple clinical parameters. The withdrawal rate because of lack of efficacy was significantly greater in the placebo group than in the SSZ group; however, more patients in the SSZ group than in the placebo group withdrew because of adverse effects ($P < 0.0001$). No single DMARD emerged as clinically superior in this meta-analysis. Subsequent studies have demonstrated equivalent clinical efficacy with SSZ and MTX,[207,208] as well as with SSZ and leflunomide,[153] although a 2-year extension trial did show that beneficial effects are sustained to a greater extent with leflunomide than with SSZ.[209]

Spondyloarthropathies

Psoriatic Arthritis. A recently published systematic review of therapies for psoriatic arthritis looked at six randomized controlled trials comparing SSZ with placebo in PsA.[210] Results show that SSZ is efficacious in treating the peripheral arthritis of PsA, but does not appear to influence the axial manifestations.[211] Few data on the prevention of radiographic progression are available.

Ankylosing Spondylitis. A recent meta-analysis reviewed 11 trials that included 895 patients with AS treated with SSZ or placebo.[212] In all patients with AS, SSZ showed some benefit in reducing ESR and easing spinal stiffness. The authors concluded that SSZ may benefit patients at an early disease stage with a higher ESR and peripheral arthritis. This finding is in agreement with those of one group,[211] who found a significant benefit for SSZ in peripheral arthritis, but not in axial arthritis, in patients with AS.

Reactive Arthritis. Most cases of reactive arthritis (ReA) resolve spontaneously; others become chronic with peripheral or axial arthritis. In a randomized, controlled trial of 134 male veterans with ReA (predominantly peripheral arthritis) who were unresponsive to NSAIDs, SSZ was more effective than placebo.[213]

Inflammatory Bowel–Associated Arthritis. SSZ has been used effectively to treat ulcerative colitis and distal Crohn's disease. No randomized controlled trials have investigated SSZ in terms of peripheral or axial arthritis manifestations of these diseases, although SSZ is used in clinical practice for peripheral arthritis.

Juvenile Inflammatory Arthritis. SSZ is effective in polyarticular and pauciarticular JIA. A literature review in 2001[214] found reports of 550 patients with JIA (half with polyarticular and one-third with pauciarticular disease) treated with SSZ. Results showed at least some drug-associated benefit in all subtypes, with the best response noted in late-onset pauciarticular disease and the least benefit observed in systemic-onset disease. Toxicity and intolerance were similar to those noted with adult use of SSZ, except for a substantial incidence of serum sickness in patients with systemic-onset disease.

Dosing

SSZ is available in regular and enteric-coated tablets of 500 mg and in a suspension of 50 mg/mL. To minimize side effects, most clinicians will prescribe 500 mg daily and will escalate the dose by 500 mg/day every week to the standard dose of 1500 to 3000 mg, divided daily. Dose reduction may ameliorate side effects. Because SSZ can inhibit enzymes in the folate-dependent pathway, concomitant administration of folic acid may be beneficial.

Geriatric Patients

Dosing recommendations for SSZ in geriatric patients are the same as for the general adult population.[109] Studies of pharmacokinetics in the elderly have shown that although the elimination half-life is longer, it is primarily dependent on acetylator phenotype; however, the dose may be reduced for renal insufficiency[107] (see Table 64.1).

Pediatric Patients

In pediatric patients, SSZ is dosed initially at 10 to 12.5 mg/kg/day, with a weekly dose increase of 50 mg/kg/day in two divided doses, until a maintenance dose of 2 g/day is achieved. This can be increased to 3 g/day if no response is seen with lower doses (see Table 64.1).

Toxicity

In general, a majority of adverse effects from SSZ occur within the first several months of treatment and decrease with continued use.[215] The most common early adverse effects include GI effects, headache, dizziness, and rash. They tend to decrease with continued use.[200]

Gastrointestinal and Hepatic

Nausea and upper abdominal discomfort are the most common adverse effects with SSZ. Nausea frequently occurs with CNS effects, including dizziness and headache. In one large cohort of 1382 RA patients, GI/CNS effects were reported as transient in 8% of patients; SSZ was continued and in another 18% led to discontinuation of therapy.[216] Nausea is more common in patients who achieve higher sulfapyridine levels and in slow acetylators.[217] Diarrhea can occur, usually in the first several months. GI effects may be decreased by administration of enteric-coated preparations. Elevations in liver transaminases may occur and are usually transient. However, they may be accompanied by fever, rash, hepatomegaly, and, possibly, eosinophilia.[215]

Hematologic

Hematologic disturbances are rare, occurring in less than 3% of patients; they usually occur within the first 3 months.[200] The most common abnormalities include leukopenia, which usually reverses upon cessation of the drug, although some cases of fatal agranulocytosis have been reported, warranting continued surveillance.[218] Macrocytosis and hemolysis have been reported with SSZ; its use should be avoided in patients with glucose-6-phosphate dehydrogenase (G6PD) deficiency. Folic acid supplementation may be reasonable because of SSZ effects on folate metabolism. Thrombocytopenia is rare.

Dermatologic

Rashes occur in less than 5% of patients, usually in the first 3 months of therapy.[216] Rashes are usually maculopapular, pruritic, and generalized, although urticaria develops in some patients. Desensitization to SSZ has been reported.[219] Anecdotally, erythema multiforme, toxic epidermal necrolysis, and Stevens-Johnson syndrome have been rarely reported, but were not seen in the major clinical trials. Photosensitivity has also been reported. Patients in whom a rash develops while on SSZ should be cautioned to avoid other sulfonamide-containing agents, such as thiazide diuretics, celecoxib, and antibiotics.

Pulmonary

Pulmonary toxicity from SSZ is rare and manifests as reversible infiltrates with peripheral eosinophilia, cough, dyspnea, fever, and weight loss.[220] Pathology reveals an eosinophilic pneumonia with interstitial infiltrates with or without fibrosis. Most cases resolve with discontinuation of SSZ with or without corticosteroids.

Miscellaneous

Minor reactions, such as irritability, anxiety, headache, and difficulty sleeping, may occur.[215,216] Rare cases of drug-induced lupus,[221] hypogammaglobulinemia,[221] and aseptic meningitis have been reported.[222] Advise patients that they may experience orange discoloration of their urine, sweat, and tears.

Fertility, Pregnancy, and Lactation

No reports have described diminished fertility in women taking SSZ; however, men can have oligospermia, impaired sperm motility, and abnormal sperm morphology[223] that returns to normal 2 to 3 months after cessation of the drug. SSZ is considered 1979 FDA Category Group B, C for pregnancy. SSZ and sulfapyridine cross the placenta, and fetal concentrations are equivalent to maternal concentrations; however, SSZ does not seem to cause or increase fetal abnormalities or spontaneous abortions, and may be one of the DMARDs of first choice for treating rheumatic disease in women of childbearing age who are or wish to become pregnant.[129] Sulfapyridine is excreted into breast milk, and one report described a child in whom bloody diarrhea developed, which led the American Academy of Pediatrics to classify SSZ as a drug that must be given with caution to nursing women[129] (see Table 64.1).

Toxicity Monitoring

Most side effects from SSZ occur early in the course of treatment. The ACR guidelines recommend a baseline CBC with platelets, liver enzyme monitoring (including AST, ALT, and albumin), creatinine, and consideration for G6PD.[104] The frequency of monitoring depends on the duration of therapy (see Table 64.2). With the initiation of therapy, vigilance for leukopenia is warranted, for example, monitoring a CBC 1 week after each dose increase and frequent monitoring in the first 3 to 6 months of therapy. Vaccination with *Pneumococcus* should be given if appropriate at the initiation of therapy, and yearly influenza vaccination is recommended (see Table 64.2).

Drug Interactions and Contraindications

Drug Interactions

Few SSZ-drug interactions are known. SSZ may impair absorption of digoxin and decrease its bioavailability. Rarely, SSZ can increase the effects of oral hypoglycemics and the anti-coagulant effects of warfarin. Broad-spectrum antibiotics may alter gut flora and decrease the bioavailability of sulfapyridine and 5-ASA through reduced cleavage of the azo bond.

Contraindications

Patients with hypersensitivity to any component of SSZ, or with a sulfonamide or salicylate allergy, should not be prescribed SSZ. Caution should be used in patients with porphyria or GI or genitourinary obstruction. SSZ should not be used in thrombocytopenia, severe liver disease, and active viral hepatitis (see Table 64.2).

Anti-malarials

KEY POINTS

Hydroxychloroquine (HCQ) is a well-tolerated DMARD that is commonly used in systemic lupus erythematosus (SLE) and in combination therapy regimens for RA.

HCQ is more commonly used than chloroquine.

HCQ has a very long half-life, attributed to its affinity for melanin-containing cells in the skin.

Doses of HCQ should not exceed 5 mg/kg in chronic therapy to minimize the risk of retinal toxicity.

Although routine laboratory monitoring is not required, ophthalmologic screening is an essential component of toxicity monitoring.

Diabetic patients initiating HCQ should be instructed to follow blood sugars closely because of the hypoglycemic effects of the drug.

HCQ is considered safe in pregnancy; it is recommended that most pregnant patients with SLE remain on the drug to improve pregnancy outcomes.

The aminoquinolones, including quinine, were first derived from the bark of the Peruvian cinchona tree, and were originally used to treat malaria. Amelioration of rheumatic symptoms in World War II soldiers taking quinine and quinacrine sparked an interest in the possible effects of this class of drugs in the treatment of rheumatic disease. To reduce toxicity, the 4-aminoquinolines, chloroquine (CQ), and HCQ were developed. CQ and HCQ are the most common anti-malarials prescribed, although quinacrine is used occasionally.

Chemical Structure

HCQ and CQ are very similar in their chemical structure, differing only by the substitution of a hydroxyethyl group for an ethyl group on the tertiary amino nitrogen of the side chain of CQ. Quinacrine includes the CQ structure, although it is not a 4-aminoquinolone derivative (Fig. 64.7).

Actions of Hydroxychloroquine

Anti-malarial agents have both immunomodulatory and anti-inflammatory properties, although their precise mechanism of action in rheumatic disease is unknown. Because HCQ and CQ are weak bases, they can pass through cytoplasmic membranes into cytoplasmic vesicles and accumulate, thereby increasing the vesicle pH from approximately 4.0 to 6.0 and interfering with acid-dependent subcellular functions in what is referred to as *lysosomotropic activity.* This increased pH has several postulated immunoregulatory effects, including stabilization of lysosomal membranes, attenuation of antigen processing and presentation, and inhibition of cell-mediated cytotoxicity.[224,225] Macrophages and monocytes require precise pH concentrations for protein digestion and antigen processing, which is altered with an increased pH.[226] Furthermore, receptor assembly is disrupted, including the class II major histocompatibility complex (MHC) molecules, because a higher pH in the endoplasmic reticulum stabilizes the MHC protein with invariant chains and prevents their displacement by low-affinity autoantigens. This, combined with decreased membrane receptor recycling, leads to downregulation of antigen presentation.[224,226,227] Furthermore, anti-malarial treatment decreases circulating immune complexes.[228]

Anti-malarials also have inhibitory effects on macrophage production of pro-inflammatory cytokines, and one of the most important recent advances has been the identification of their antagonistic effect on the nucleic acid sensing Toll-like receptors (TLRs).[229] Endosomal TLRs are located within the cell and are germline coded during species evolution to recognize specific pathogenic molecular patterns. The nucleic acid sensing TLRs (TLR3, TLR7, TLR8, and TLR9) are located in the intra-cellular compartments to minimize

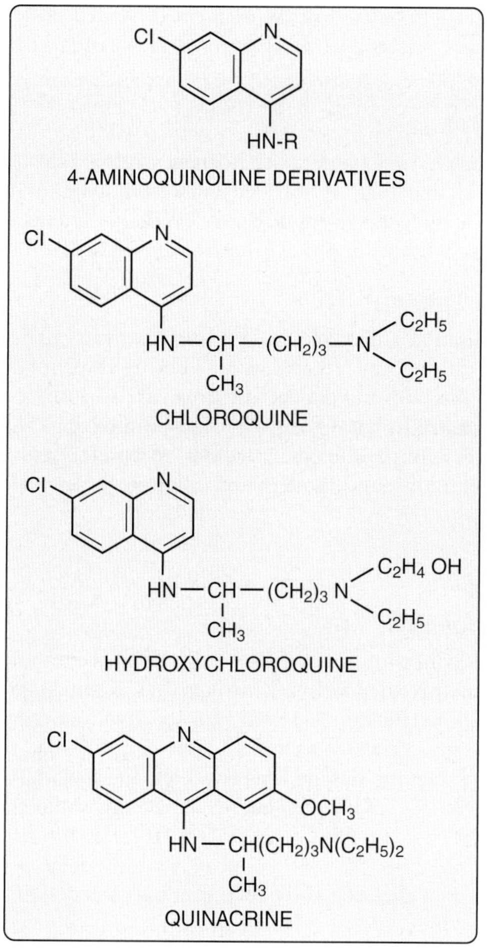

Cl N HN-R

4-AMINOQUINOLINE DERIVATIVES

Cl N HN—CH—$(CH_2)_3$—N C_2H_5 C_2H_5 CH_3

CHLOROQUINE

Cl N HN—CH—$(CH_2)_3$ N C_2H_4 OH C_2H_5 CH_3

HYDROXYCHLOROQUINE

Cl N OCH_3 HN—$CH(CH_2)_3N(C_2H_5)_2$ CH_3

QUINACRINE

• **Fig. 64.7** Chemical structures of anti-malarial drugs used to treat rheumatic disease and the basic structure of 4-aminoquinolones. *R* represents the side chain.

accidental exposure to self-nucleic acids. They should only be activated by the delivery of foreign nuclear material by the normal functioning immune system, leading to nuclear transcription of type 1 interferon and other pro-inflammatory cytokines.

Antibodies against nucleic acids is a hallmark of autoimmune conditions, suggesting ineffective clearance of nuclear debris from apoptotic cells. HCQ and CQ directly block TLR binding epitopes of nucleic acids, preventing the downstream pro-inflammatory cytokine production by macrophages to self-antigen. Masking nucleic acid binding to TLRs also downregulates IFNα production by plasmacytoid dendritic cells and mitigate the effects of neutrophils via extra-cellular traps (NETs).

In vitro evidence has shown that CQ inhibits IL-1 and IFN-γ production by monocytes and T cells in RA.[230] CQ also inhibits macrophage TNF mRNA transcription and endotoxin-induced secretion of TNF, IL-1, and IL-6.[231] Studies of HCQ have yielded conflicting results in terms of the ability to inhibit TNF, but HCQ blocks IL-1, IL-6, and IFN-γ production by monocytes.[232,233]

Apoptosis or cell death plays an important role in regulation of the immune system, and defects in apoptosis may allow for longevity and persistence of autoreactive lymphocyte clones and perpetuation of autoimmunity. Both CQ and HCQ upregulate apoptosis and may downregulate autoimmunity by elimination of autoreactive lymphocytes.[225] Furthermore, anti-malarials inhibit the proliferative response of human lymphocytes and natural killer cell activity.[234,235]

Anti-inflammatory properties of the anti-malarials include effects on the arachidonic acid cascade caused by downregulation of phospholipases A_2 and C, which contribute to the production of pro-inflammatory prostaglandins and lipid peroxidation.[236–238] Lipid peroxidation is thought to play a role in apoptosis, particularly in response to ultraviolet (UV)A and UVB irradiation.[239] Anti-malarial agents also have antioxidant properties and may protect against tissue damage from free radicals.[240]

Anti-malarials have several other beneficial effects relevant to rheumatic disease that warrant further discussion. First, they are photoprotective, and this is likely the result of locally induced anti-inflammatory effects.[225] Second, both HCQ and CQ inhibit platelet adhesion and aggregation, leading to an anti-thrombotic effect.[241,242] Third, HCQ and CQ favorably alter the lipid profile, with reductions in total cholesterol, triglycerides, very-low-density lipoproteins (VLDLs), and low-density lipoproteins (LDLs), particularly in patients on concomitant corticosteroid therapy.[225,243] Finally, HCQ and CQ have been reported to decrease plasma glucose levels through inhibition of insulin degradation in the Golgi apparatus.[225,244]

Pharmacology

Absorption and Bioavailability

HCQ and CQ are administered orally and are rapidly and completely absorbed, with the peak plasma concentration for both occurring within 8 hours.[245] Considerable variability in blood concentrations has been reported among patients treated with the same dose, but higher plasma levels do not correlate with a better therapeutic response.[225]

Distribution and Half-Life

Anti-malarials accrue in different concentrations in various tissue compartments. Relatively small concentrations, similar to those seen in the plasma, are contained in fat, bone, tendon, and brain. Increased concentrations are seen in the kidney, bone marrow, spleen, lungs, adrenal glands, and liver. The highest concentration occurs in melanin-containing cells, such as those in the skin and the retina.[246] In fact, the skin can serve as a long-term reservoir whereby the drug can exert its effect or toxicity even after it has been stopped.[225] The half-life of HCQ and CQ is 40 to 50 days, and plasma levels will increase gradually and equilibrate after 3 to 4 months.[247]

Elimination

Most of the absorbed drug is excreted in the urine unchanged, but some is metabolized to a desethyl derivative. The remainder is excreted in the feces.[248]

Indications

Rheumatoid Arthritis. The efficacy of anti-malarial agents in rheumatoid arthritis has been seen in their ability to control signs and symptoms of the disease[249–251]; however, they do not retard bone erosions.[252] In a meta-analysis of anti-malarials, HCQ was found to be less toxic but also less effective than CQ.[253] In comparison with other DMARDs, symptomatic efficacy is equal to or slightly less than that of other agents, and they have the slowest onset of action.[254] Anti-malarial agents are particularly suited for use in early, mild RA and in combination therapy.

Systemic Lupus Erythematosus. Although anti-malarials are not appropriate as monotherapy for severe manifestations of SLE, they are used frequently to control constitutional symptoms, arthritis, fever, fatigue, and rash. The most convincing data supporting the efficacy of anti-malarials in SLE come from studies in which the medication was discontinued in successfully treated patients. In one double-blind, placebo-controlled drug discontinuation study of 47 SLE patients in remission on HCQ, the risk of disease flare was increased by a factor of 2.5 in the placebo group.[255] Anti-malarials are particularly suited to treat SLE because of their photoprotective effects, and they are especially useful in dermatologic manifestations of SLE.

Discoid Lupus. Anti-malarials are effective in discoid lesions, with remission or major improvement reported in 60% to 90% of treated patients.[235] When HCQ or CQ treatment alone is unsuccessful, the addition of quinacrine may be helpful, but long-term use may be limited by the development of yellowish skin pigmentation.[256]

Antiphospholipid Antibody Syndrome. HCQ use is associated with a decreased incidence of thrombosis in patients with antiphospholipid (aPL) antibodies.[257] HCQ also diminishes thrombus size and time in mice injected with aPL antibodies, and reverses aPL antibody–mediated platelet activation.[258,259] Although clinical trials are needed to further establish efficacy, it is reasonable to consider the use of HCQ in patients with aPL antibody syndrome, especially if they are unable to tolerate high levels of anti-coagulation or if they develop thrombosis despite oral anti-coagulation.[260]

Sjögren's Syndrome. HCQ improved local eye and mouth symptoms, arthralgia, and myalgia in a prospective open-label study of patients with Sjögren's syndrome.[261] In addition to causing the immunomodulatory and anti-inflammatory effects discussed earlier, HCQ may inhibit glandular cholinesterase activity and enhance salivary gland secretion.[262]

Miscellaneous. Anti-malarials have been reported to be efficacious in small and uncontrolled trials for the treatment of palindromic rheumatism,[263] childhood SLE,[264] childhood dermatomyositis,[265] eosinophilic fasciitis,[266] and erosive osteoarthritis.[267] In a controlled trial of 17 patients, the arthritis of calcium pyrophosphate crystal deposition disease improved more in the HCQ than in the placebo group.[268]

Dosing

HCQ comes in 200-mg tablets, CQ is available in 250-mg and 500-mg tablets, and quinacrine is available from compounding pharmacies. To prevent ocular toxicity, dosing should be adjusted for weight. Previous dosing recommendations of 6.5 mg/kg of ideal body weight have been replaced by newer guidelines.[269,270,272] Current guidelines by The American Academy of Ophthalmology recommend a maximum daily dose for HCQ and CQ of ≤5.0 mg/kg and ≤2.3 mg/kg for real weight, respectively.[272] In practice, doses of HCQ rarely exceed 400 mg daily and doses of CQ rarely exceed 250 mg daily. HCQ and CQ are both cleared by the kidney and the liver. Diseases of either organ may lead to increased serum drug levels. To reduce the risk of retinal toxicity, dose adjustment is needed for a glomerular flow rate less than 60 mL/min (stage 3 or higher chronic kidney disease).[270]

Geriatric Patients

No specific pharmacokinetic studies have explored the use of anti-malarials in the elderly; thus dosing recommendations are the same as for the general population.[109] Elderly patients should be screened at baseline for pre-existing ocular disease (see Table 64.1).

Pediatric Patients

HCQ is used at a dose of 3 to 5 mg/kg/day, typically to a maximum of 400 mg/day. To achieve this dosing in younger children and using the 200-mg tablets, the drug can be dosed every other day. Alternatively, HCQ can be compounded in a 25 mg/mL suspension. Ophthalmologic screening recommendations are the same as for adults, and some rheumatologists prefer yearly screening (see Table 64.1).

Toxicity

Ophthalmologic

Early eye symptoms can include defects in accommodation or conversion or blurred vision, which resolves. Retinal toxicity is the most feared side effect. A recent retrospective case-control study found the prevalence of retinal toxicity to be 7.5% with the following risk factors: dosage level too high for weight (OR, 5.67; 95% CI, 4.14 to 7.7 for >5.0 mg/kg actual body weight); duration of use (OR, 3.22; 95% CI, 2.20 to 4.70 for >10 years); kidney disease (OR, 2.08; 95% CI, 1.44 to 3.01 for stage 3 or higher chronic kidney disease); and concurrent tamoxifen use (OR, 4.59; 95% CI, 2.05 to 10.27).[270] CQ has a higher risk of retinal toxicity than HCQ.[273] Within 10 years of use, the prevalence of retinal toxicity remained low (<2%) but rose to nearly 20% after 20 years of use.[270]

HCQ or CQ retinopathy is described as bilateral bull's eye maculopathy, with retinal pigment epithelial (RPE) cell depigmentation in the central macula and sparing of a small foveal island. Testing of the paracentral visual field can usually show toxicity before RPE changes are visible. When advanced, visual loss may be irreversible and may continue despite cessation of the drug because of its long half-life in the retina, so early detection is essential. CQ and HCQ can also cause corneal deposits, which can be associated with halos around lights and are benign and reversible.

Dermatologic

Rash is a common side effect leading to discontinuation of therapy. HCQ may also cause photosensitivity, alopecia, and depigmentation of hair.[253]

Neuromuscular

Common neuromuscular symptoms include headache, insomnia, nightmares, and irritability, which are mild and reversible with lowering of the daily dose. Tinnitus and deafness can occur. Neuromyotoxicity has been reported and presents as proximal weakness of insidious onset with a normal creatine phosphokinase (CPK), which may be associated with peripheral neuropathy and cardiac myotoxicity. Muscle biopsy shows curvilinear bodies and muscle fiber atrophy with vacuolar changes.[274]

Cardiovascular

Rarely, conduction disturbances and cardiomyopathy have been reported.[275]

Gastrointestinal

Anorexia, nausea, vomiting, diarrhea, and abdominal cramping have been reported.[253]

Metabolic

HCQ can reduce blood glucose levels and hemoglobin A_{1c}, so diabetic patients need to be cautioned to watch their blood sugars closely with initiation of HCQ and may need adjustments in their diabetic medications.[276]

Fertility, Pregnancy, and Lactation

No reports have described adverse effects on fertility. HCQ and CQ are considered FDA Pregnancy Category C.[129] Because of the long half-life of HCQ, discontinuation of the drug at the time of pregnancy does not avoid fetal exposure. HCQ does cross the placenta, but there have been no reports of adverse outcomes or teratogenic effects in women who continue HCQ during pregnancy.[129] CQ also crosses the placenta and binds more tightly in tissue than HCQ; fetal anomalies in women who took CQ during pregnancy have been reported.[277] Quinacrine should not be used in pregnancy because it is mutagenic. Current recommendations are that HCQ may be continued throughout pregnancy, particularly in SLE, where discontinuation could precipitate a flare, which would be dangerous to both mother and baby.[175] HCQ is also found in low concentration in breast milk, but the American Academy of Pediatrics classifies it as compatible with breastfeeding[129] (see Table 64.1).

Toxicity Monitoring

The ACR recommends baseline screening with CBC, liver transaminases, and creatinine. Subsequently, no routine laboratory monitoring is recommended.[104] In 2002, the American Academy of Ophthalmology (AAO) released an information statement on screening recommendations for CQ and HCQ retinopathy.[269] Revised guidelines were published in 2011 and 2016.[272,278] With new data showing the risk of retinal toxicity increasing toward 1% after 5 to 7 years of use, a baseline retinal examination is advised to rule out underlying ocular pathology, including maculopathy, which may render subsequent toxicity screening more difficult to interpret. Annual eye examinations should commence at 5 years or sooner depending on other risk factors.[278] This should include a dilated eye examination and screening for color blindness in male patients. In addition, testing should include a subjective/functional assessment with automated threshold visual fields, appropriate to race, and an objective assessment with spectral-domain optical coherence tomography (SD OCT). Asian patients may have ocular toxicity that can manifest beyond the macula and require wider visual field test patterns. Additional screening tests may be employed and include objective testing with a multifocal electroretinogram or adaptive optics retinal imaging, and subjective testing with microperimetry. Despite these recommendations, many rheumatologists would favor annual screening or, at a minimum, screening every 2 years.

Vaccination with a yearly influenza vaccine is recommended (see Table 64.2).

Drug Interactions and Contraindications

Drug Interactions

HCQ should be used with caution in diabetic patients on hypoglycemic agents. HCQ increases digoxin levels. CQ may increase cyclosporine levels and reduce MTX levels. CQ can interfere with cytochrome P450 enzymes and should be used with caution when combined with other agents metabolized by this pathway. Concomitant use with tamoxifen produces synergism for the risk of retinal toxicity.[270]

Contraindications

Hypersensitivity to or previous retinal or visual field changes attributable to 4-aminoquinoline agents and severe liver disease caused by viral hepatitis are contraindications to further use (see Table 64.2).

Combination DMARD Therapy in Rheumatoid Arthritis

KEY POINTS

- Combinations of DMARDs can have superior efficacy without increased toxicity.
- MTX is the cornerstone of combination therapy.
- Combinations of traditional DMARDs are as effective as combinations of MTX plus biologic therapy
- Current research is focused on the best strategies for introduction, timing, and patient selection for combination therapy.

In the early 1990s, the use of combinations of DMARDs to treat RA was rare; now this strategy is used by essentially all rheumatologists to treat many of their patients.[279] Currently, the timing and make-up of combinations selected to treat RA is one of the most important decisions that clinicians face.

Monotherapy with MTX is considered by most as the initial treatment of choice for early RA. Four major studies have demonstrated the superiority of combinations of DMARDs versus monotherapy in head-to-head comparisons.[70,280–282] Trials with multiple conventional DMARDs and biologics have shown them to be more effective than placebo when added to the baseline MTX in patients who have active disease despite MTX therapy. With very few exceptions, successful combination trials have included MTX, and it remains the cornerstone of combination therapy.

History of Combination DMARD Therapy

Early combination DMARD studies were initiated in the late 1970s. The combination of cyclophosphamide, azathioprine, and HCQ produced substantial responses in a small group of patients; however, an unacceptably high number of malignancies were reported.[283] Thus, early enthusiasm for combination therapy was limited. During the 1980s, inadequate dosing, the use of DMARDs with marginal efficacy, and problematic trial design contributed to the less-than-exciting results reported with combination therapy. In 1994, the first trial to convincingly show superior efficacy without increased toxicity of combination DMARD therapy in a head-to-head comparison with mono-DMARD therapy was reported,[284] and multiple trials showing the success of combination therapy have ensued.

Early Rheumatoid Arthritis

In the late 1990s, three pivotal trials showed the success of combination DMARD therapy in early RA. Researchers in the Netherlands reported success with a step-down approach in the COBRA (Combinatietherapie Bij Reumatoide Artritis) trial.[280] In this trial, patients with early disease were randomly assigned to two groups. A combination of prednisolone, MTX, and SSZ was compared with SSZ alone. Prednisolone was started at 60 mg/day, rapidly tapered, and discontinued by week 28. MTX was given until week 40. The dose of SSZ was the same in the two groups. At 28 weeks, the combination group was significantly better than the SSZ-alone group. While prednisolone and MTX were tapered, clinical responses became similar in the two groups; however, significant benefits in certain parameters were noted in the combination group.[285] It is important to note that combination therapy was not more toxic. Subsequent data confirm that the radiographic benefits conferred by COBRA in the initial trial continued for at least 5 years.[285]

The second important early RA study is the Finland Rheumatoid Arthritis (Fin-RA) trial.[282] In this open trial, patients were randomly assigned to receive combination DMARD therapy (MTX, SSZ, HCQ, and low-dose prednisolone) or monotherapy with SSZ with optional prednisolone. The major endpoint of this trial was remission at 2 years. Significantly, patients who received combination therapy achieved more frequent remissions. A follow-up of this trial at 5 years demonstrated that patients treated initially with the combination were less likely to have evidence of C1-C2 subluxation on cervical spine radiographs.[286]

In a third trial, from Turkey, patients with early RA were randomly assigned to receive single DMARD therapy (MTX, SSZ, or HCQ), two-drug therapy (MTX and SSZ or MTX and HCQ), or three-drug therapy (MTX, SSZ, and HCQ), with remission at 2 years as the major outcome.[281] For all endpoints measured, two drugs were statistically superior to monotherapy, and three drugs were statistically superior to the two-drug regimens.

The TEAR (Treatment of Early Aggressive RA) trial (see Chapter 71) enrolled patients with early RA and compared initial combination therapy with MTX, SSZ, and HCQ (triple) or MTX and etanercept with initial MTX monotherapy with step-up to combination therapy at 6 months for patients with a Disease Activity Score (DAS) 28-ESR of 3.2 or greater. Results showed that either initial combination therapy was superior to MTX monotherapy at 6 months, with a reduction in DAS28-ESR for combined groups of 4.2 versus 3.6 ($P < 0.0001$). There were no differences in DAS28-ESR seen between either of the initial combination regimens. Between weeks 48 and 102, there were no significant differences in DAS28-ESR between combination groups, whether started as initial or step-up therapy. By week 102, there was a statistically significant change from the baseline modified Sharp/van der Heijde score between the group receiving initial MTX plus etanercept versus triple (0.64 vs. 1.69; $P = 0.047$).[287]

In sum, combination therapy, whether step-up or initial therapy, has shown in multiple trials to be superior to MTX alone in early rheumatoid arthritis. Predictors of who may respond to MTX monotherapy alone and who needs early combination therapy are still lacking.

Patients With Active Disease Despite Methotrexate

Combination DMARD therapy was first studied in groups of patients with active disease despite MTX therapy, or suboptimal MTX responders. The first study to show the advantage of combination therapy with MTX and another DMARD compared with continued therapy with MTX alone in this group of patients was the cyclosporine-MTX trial[288] (Fig. 64.8). Therapy with the

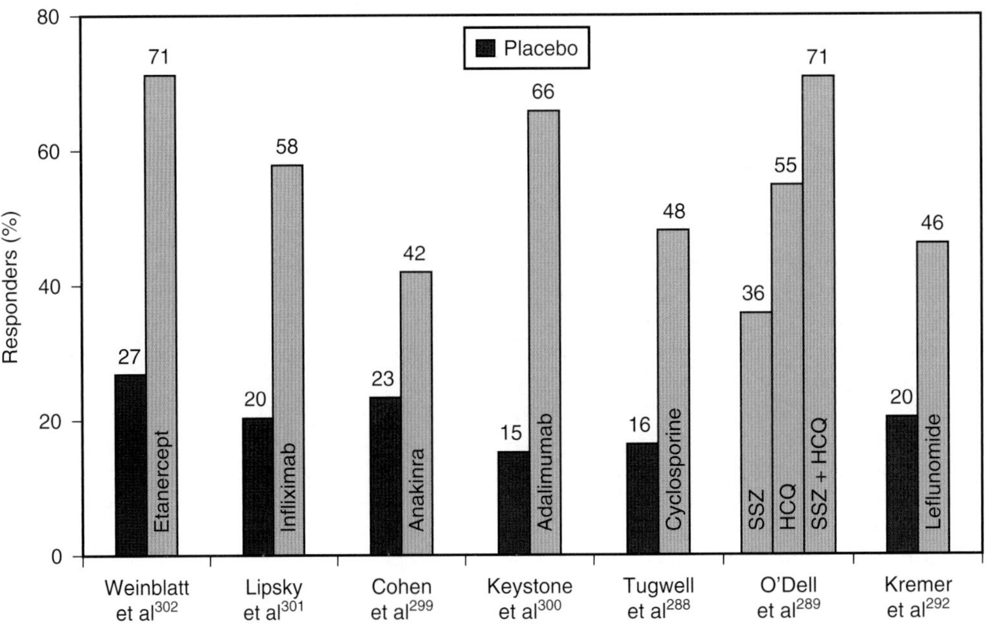

• **Fig. 64.8** Summary data taken from seven different clinical trials of therapies in patients with active disease despite methotrexate therapy. *HCQ,* Hydroxychloroquine; *MTX,* methotrexate; *SSZ,* sulfasalazine.

combination of MTX, SSZ, and HCQ, so-called *triple therapy*, is well tolerated[70,281,282,289] and more effective than MTX monotherapy[70,281,287] or SSZ monotherapy,[282] and, in an open trial of patients with early disease, more effective than the double combination of MTX and SSZ or MTX and HCQ.[281]

In 1996, a 2-year, randomized, double-blind, parallel study of 102 established patients with RA was done to compare triple-drug therapy (MTX, SSZ, and HCQ) versus double therapy (HCQ and SSZ) versus monotherapy with MTX.[70] Significantly more patients receiving triple-drug therapy achieved a modified Paulus 50% response,[290] compared with those given double therapy. Triple therapy was well tolerated, and numerically fewer withdrawals occurred in the combination group compared with the other two groups. This therapy is durable, with 62% of patients remaining on triple therapy for 5 years continuing to maintain a 50% efficacy response.[291]

In follow-up, a 2-year, double-blind trial on patients with moderately advanced disease was done in 2002, in which the triple combination group was compared with two double-combination groups (MTX plus SSZ and MTX plus HCQ) in a head-to-head comparison.[289] Patients were stratified for previous MTX use, and previous users had to have active disease despite receiving 17.5 mg/wk. The triple-therapy group and both double-therapy groups tolerated their treatments well, with only 8% withdrawing for toxicities, which were mostly minor. Triple therapy is superior to either of the double combinations.

A double-blind, placebo-controlled trial (see Fig. 64.8) compared the addition of leflunomide or placebo to baseline MTX in suboptimal MTX responders.[292] Leflunomide or placebo was added to MTX. The combination group was statistically superior to the MTX-placebo group in terms of the American College of Rheumatology 20 (ACR20) set criteria for clinical response. The combination was reasonably well tolerated, but side effects including diarrhea, nausea, and dizziness were increased in the combination arm. Elevated ALT levels (>1.2 times normal) occurred more frequently in patients on combination therapy than in those on MTX alone, with increases leading to withdrawal in 2.3% of patients who received the combination.

The Rheumatoid Arthritis: Comparison of Active Therapies (RACAT) trial was a 48-week double-blind, noninferiority trial of 353 established patients with RA with active disease despite MTX therapy (see Chapter 71). Groups were randomly assigned to receive triple DMARD therapy (MTX, SSZ, HCQ) versus MTX and etanercept.[293] Patients who did not respond by week 24 were switched in a blinded fashion to the other therapy. The primary outcome was improvement in the DAS28. Both groups had significant improvement in the first 24 weeks, with only 27% in each group requiring a switch in therapy. Improvement was seen in both of the groups who switched therapy ($P < 0.001$), and the response after switching did not differ significantly between the two groups ($P = 0.08$). The change in DAS28 (baseline to 48 weeks) was −2.1 with triple therapy and −2.3 with MTX plus etanercept. Triple therapy is noninferior to MTX plus etanercept ($P = 0.002$). Cost-effectiveness analyses have revealed that the strategy of first using triple therapy before adding etanercept is cost-effective with no differential effect on efficacy or toxicity.[294]

Corticosteroids in DMARD Combinations

Corticosteroids have not traditionally been considered DMARDs. However, they clearly fulfill all of the criteria for DMARDs, including halting radiographic progression.[295] Few clinicians who care for patients with RA dispute their efficacy. Indeed, they have been used as baseline therapy for more than half of the patients included in the combination trials discussed previously.

Prednisolone undoubtedly was a critical component for the success of the combination therapy for early rheumatoid arthritis (COBRA) protocol[280] and may have played a role in the success of the combination group in the Fin-RA trial.[282] One study's[295,296] report of the ability of prednisolone to significantly retard radiographic progression of RA compared with placebo is testament to the efficacy of steroids when used in combination with other DMARDs. Corticosteroids clearly deserve further formal investigation as a component of combination therapy. The COBRA trial and the Kirwan data have raised another interesting question: Should/could short courses of high-dose steroids be used as a form of induction therapy?[297]

Biologic Agents in DMARD Combinations

Biologic agents that block TNF (etanercept, infliximab, adalimumab, certolizumab, and golimumab) and IL-1 (anakinra) have been studied in patients with early-stage and established RA in combination with MTX[298–306] (see Fig. 64.8). These trials have shown superior improvements in clinical and radiographic endpoints in the combination groups.[303,304] Other biologic agents and small molecules—rituximab, an anti-CD20 monoclonal antibody; abatacept, a T cell co-stimulatory inhibitor; tocilizumab, an IL-6 receptor antagonist; and tofacitinib, an oral Janus kinase inhibitor—have been studied in combination with MTX and also show superior improvements in clinical and radiographic outcomes.[307–310] There are additional biologic agents being studied and approved in the treatment of RA. In almost every biologic study, combination use with MTX leads to superior outcomes when compared to therapy with the biologic agent alone.

Selecting the Right Patients for the Right Combination Therapy

Factors that predict a poor prognosis for patients with RA are well accepted and include high titer rheumatoid factor and CCP, elevated ESR and CRP, the number of joints involved, erosions, and the presence of certain genetic markers. However, unless these factors can predict response to certain therapies in a differential fashion, they are of limited therapeutic use. Patient characteristics recommending one therapeutic regimen versus another remain to be fully elucidated. Genetic differences have been suggested to influence outcomes in a differential fashion. Until this observation can be corroborated and factors that predict response to other therapies elucidated, choices will remain largely empiric.

Treatment of patients with RA by using MTX combinations should be the gold standard against which future therapies are compared. Available data demonstrate that a variety of combinations are more effective than MTX alone. Until recently, no direct head-to-head trials comparing combinations of traditional DMARDs to MTX plus biologic agents existed. The TEAR and RACAT trials have shown that the use of traditional DMARD combinations (MTX, SSZ, HCQ) is as effective as combinations that include biologic agents (MTX plus etanercept) as initial therapy and, importantly, in MTX nonresponders. Recent guidelines published by the ACR[131] and the European League against Rheumatism (EULAR)[311] recommendations for the use of DMARDs and biologic agents in RA support this premise.

Although more information is available every day, many questions remain to be answered regarding the appropriate timing of combination therapy and the optimal combinations for specific patients and for specific clinical situations. Future research is needed to clarify the role of corticosteroids and, particularly, biologic response modifiers as components of and alternatives to MTX combination regimens.

 Full references for this chapter can be found on ExpertConsult.com.

Selected References

3. Kremer J: Toward a better understanding of methotrexate, *Arthritis Rheum* 50:1370–1382, 2004.
6. Ranganathan P, McLeod H: Methotrexate pharmacogenetics: the first step toward individualized therapy in rheumatoid arthritis, *Arthritis Rheum* 54:1366–1377, 2006.
10. Morabito L, Montesinos M, Schreibman D, et al.: Methotrexate and sulfasalazine promote adenosine release by a mechanism that requires ecto-5′-nucleotidase-mediated conversion of adenine nucleotides, *J Clin Invest* 101:295–300, 1998.
11. Hasko G, Cronstein B: Adenosine: an endogenous regulator of innate immunity, *Trends Immunol* 25:33–39, 2004.
14. Cronstein B: Adenosine, an endogenous anti-inflammatory agent, *J Appl Physiol* 76:5–13, 1994.
19. Cronstein B: The mechanism of action of methotrexate, *Rheum Dis Clin North Am* 23:739–755, 1997.
23. Cronstein B: Low-dose methotrexate: a mainstay in the treatment of rheumatoid arthritis, *Pharmacol Rev* 57:163–172, 2005.
24. Cronstein B: Going with the flow: methotrexate, adenosine, and blood flow, *Ann Rheum Dis* 65:421–422, 2006.
28. Choi H, Hernan M, Seeger J: Methotrexate and mortality in patients with rheumatoid arthritis: a prospective study, *Lancet* 359:1173–1177, 2002.
34. Hornung N, Stengaard-Pedersen K, Ehrnrooth E, et al.: The effects of low-dose methotrexate on thymidylate synthase activity in human peripheral blood mononuclear cells, *Clin Exp Rheumatol* 18:691–698, 2000.
37. Seitz M, Loetscher B, Dewald B: Methotrexate action in rheumatoid arthritis: stimulation of cytokine inhibitor and inhibition of chemokine production by peripheral blood mononuclear cells, *Br J Rheumatol* 34:602–609, 1995.
39. Seitz M, Zwicker M, Loetscher B: Effects of methotrexate on differentiation of monocytes and production of cytokine inhibitors by monocytes, *Arthritis Rheum* 42:2023–2028, 1998.
42. Cronstein B, Lounet-Lescoulie P, Lambert N: Antiinflammatory and immunoregulatory action of methotrexate in the treatment of rheumatoid arthritis, *Arthritis Rheum* 41:48–57, 1998.
47. Cutolo M, Sulli A, Pizzorni C, et al.: Anti-inflammatory mechanisms of methotrexate in rheumatoid arthritis, *Ann Rheum Dis* 60:729–735, 2001.
49. Hamilton R, Kremer J: Why intramuscular methotrexate works better than oral drug in patients with rheumatoid arthritis, *Br J Rheumatol* 36:86–90, 1997.
50. Hamilton R, Kremer J: The effect of food on methotrexate absorption, *J Rheumatol* 22:2072–2077, 1995.
51. Schiff MH, Jaffe JS, Freundlich B: Head-to-head, randomized, crossover study of oral versus subcutaneous methotrexate in patients with rheumatoid arthritis: drug-exposure limitations of oral methotrexate at doses of >15 mg may be overcome with subcutaneous administration, *Ann Rheum Dis* 73:1549–1551, 2014.
52. Pichlmeier U, Heuer KU: Subcutaneous administration of methotrexate with a prefilled autoinjector pen results in a higher relative bioavailability compared with oral administration of methotrexate, *Clin Exp Rheumatol* 32:563–571, 2014.
53. Wegrzyn J, Adeleine P, Miossec P: Better efficacy of methotrexate administered by intramuscular injections versus oral route in patients with rheumatoid arthritis, *Ann Rheum Dis* 63:1232–1234, 2004.
56. Hoekstra M, Haagsma C, Neef C, et al.: Splitting high-dose oral methotrexate improves the bioavailability: a pharmacokinetic study in patients with rheumatoid arthritis, *J Rheumatol* 33:481–485, 2006.
59. Kremer J, Alarcon G, Weinblatt M, et al.: Clinical, laboratory, radiographic and histopathologic features of methotrexate-associated lung injury in patients with rheumatoid arthritis: a multi-center study with literature review, *Arthritis Rheum* 40:1829–1837, 1997.
62. Andersen P, West S, O'Dell J, et al.: Weekly pulse methotrexate in rheumatoid arthritis: clinical and immunologic effects in a randomized, double-blind study, *Ann Intern Med* 103:489–496, 1985.
65. Williams HJ, Willkens RF, Samuelson Jr CO, et al.: Comparison of low-dose oral pulse methotrexate and placebo in the treatment of rheumatoid arthritis: a controlled clinical trial, *Arthritis Rheum* 28:721–730, 1985.
68. Pincus T, Marcum S, Callahan L: Long-term drug therapy for rheumatoid arthritis in seven rheumatology private practices: second line drugs and prednisone, *J Rheumatol* 19:1885–1894, 1992.
69. Wolfe F: The epidemiology of drug treatment failure in rheumatoid arthritis, *Baillieres Clin Rheumatol* 9:619–632, 1995.
70. O'Dell J, Haire C, Erikson N, et al.: Treatment of rheumatoid arthritis with methotrexate alone, sulfasalazine and hydroxychloroquine, or a combination of all three medications, *N Engl J Med* 334:1287–1291, 1996.
71. Weinblatt M: Methotrexate (MTX) in rheumatoid arthritis (RA): a 5 year multiprospective trial, *Arthritis Rheum* 36:S3, 1993.
75. Upchurch K, Heller K, Bress N: Low-dose methotrexate therapy for cutaneous vasculitis of rheumatoid arthritis, *J Am Acad Dermatol* 17:355–359, 1987.
78. Willkens R, Williams H, Ward J, et al.: Randomized, double-blind, placebo controlled trial of low-dose pulse methotrexate in psoriatic arthritis, *Arthritis Rheum* 27:376–381, 1984.
81. De Groot K, Muhler M, Reinhold-Keller E, et al.: Induction of remission in Wegener's granulomatosis with low dose methotrexate, *J Rheumatol* 25:492–495, 1998.
96. Lower E, Baughman R: Prolonged use of methotrexate for sarcoidosis, *Arch Intern Med* 155:846–851, 1995.
101. Gourmelen O, Le Loët X, Fortier-Beaulieu M, et al.: Methotrexate treatment of multicentric reticulohistiocytosis, *J Rheumatol* 18:627–628, 1991.
102. Kremer J, Alarcon G, Lightfoot R, et al.: Methotrexate for rheumatoid arthritis: suggested guidelines for monitoring liver toxicity, *Arthritis Rheum* 37:316–328, 1994.
104. Saag K, Geng G, Patkar N: American College of Rheumatology 2008 recommendations for the use of nonbiologic and biologic disease-modifying antirheumatic drugs in rheumatoid arthritis, *Arthritis Rheum* 59:762–784, 2008.
106. Stamp L, O'Donnell J, Chapman P, et al.: Methotrexate polyglutamate concentrations are not associated with disease control in rheumatoid arthritis patients receiving long-term methotrexate therapy, *Arthritis Rheum* 62:359–368, 2010.
109. Selma T, Beizer J, Higbee M: *Geriatric dosage handbook*, ed 11, Hudson, Ohio, 2006, Lexicomp.
114. Gutierrez-Urena S, Molina J, Garcia C, et al.: Pancytopenia secondary to methotrexate therapy in rheumatoid arthritis, *Arthritis Rheum* 39:272–276, 1996.
119. Cook N, Carroll G: Successful reintroduction of methotrexate after pneumonitis in two patients with rheumatoid arthritis, *Ann Rheum Dis* 51:272–274, 1992.
120. Alarcón G, Kremer J, Macaluso M, et al.: Risk factors for methotrexate-induced lung injury in patients with rheumatoid arthritis: a multicenter, case-control study, *Ann Intern Med* 127:356–364, 1997.

126. Kerstens P, Boerbooms A, Jeurissen M, et al.: Accelerated nodulosis during low dose methotrexate therapy for rheumatoid arthritis: an analysis of ten cases, *J Rheumatol* 19:867–871, 1992.
127. Merrill J, Shen C, Schreibman D, et al.: Adenosine A1 receptor promotion of multinucleated giant cell formation by human monocytes: a mechanism for methotrexate-induced nodulosis in rheumatoid arthritis, *Arthritis Rheum* 40:1308–1315, 1997.
132. Erhardt C, Mumford PA, Venables PJ, et al.: Factors predicting a poor life prognosis in rheumatoid arthritis: an eight year prospective study, *Ann Rheum Dis* 48:7–13, 1989.
134. Chu E, Allegra C: *Cancer chemotherapy and biotherapy*, Philadelphia, 1996, Lippincott-Raven.
135. Carmichael S, Beal J, Day R, et al.: Combination therapy with methotrexate and hydroxychloroquine for rheumatoid arthritis increases exposure to methotrexate, *J Rheumatol* 29:2077–2083, 2002.
138. Fox R: Mechanism of action of leflunomide in rheumatoid arthritis, *J Rheumatol* 25(Suppl 53):20–26, 1998.
148. Manna S, Mukhopadhyay A, Aggarwal B: Leflunomide suppresses TNF-induced cellular responses: effect on NF-kappaB, activator protein-1, c-Jun N-terminal protein kinase, and apoptosis, *J Immunol* 165:5962–5969, 2000.
149. Miagkov A, Kovalenko D, Brown C, et al.: NF-kappaB activation provides the potential link between inflammation and hyperplasia in the arthritic joint, *Proc Natl Acad Sci U S A* 95:13859–13864, 1998.
150. Cao W, Kao P, Aoki Y, et al.: A novel mechanism of action of the immunoregulatory drug, leflunomide: augmentation of the immunosuppressive cytokine TGF-beta 1, and suppression of the immunostimulatory cytokine, IL-2, *Transplant Proc* 28:3079–3080, 1996.
151. Mladenovic V, Domljan Z, Rozman B, et al.: Safety and effectiveness of leflunomide in the treatment of patients with active rheumatoid arthritis: results of a randomized, placebo-controlled, phase II study, *Arthritis Rheum* 38:1595–1603, 1995.
152. Rozman B: Clinical experience with leflunomide in rheumatoid arthritis, *J Rheumatol* 25(Suppl 53):27–32, 1998.
160. Metzler C, Fink C, Lamprecht P, et al.: Maintenance of remission with leflunomide in Wegener's granulomatosis, *Rheumatology* 43:315–320, 2004.
164. Silverman E, Mouy R, Spiegel L, et al.: Leflunomide or methotrexate for juvenile rheumatoid arthritis, *N Engl J Med* 352:1655–1666, 2005.
166. Leflunomide: serious hepatic, skin and respiratory reactions. Bulletin AADR 20(2):2001.
167. U.S. Food and Drug Administration: *Leflunomide*, 2010.
170. Roubille C, Haraoui B: Interstitisal lung diseases induced or exacerbated by DMARDS and biologic agents in rheumatoid arthritis: a stystematic literature review, *Semin Arthritis Rheum* 23:613–626, 2014.
177. Yamazaki T, Miyai E, Shibata H, et al.: Pharmacological studies of salazosulfapyridine (SASP) evaluation of anti-rheumatic action, *Pharmacometrics* 41:563–574, 1991.
178. Tornhamre S, Edenius C, Smedegard G, et al.: Effects of sulfasalazine and sulfasalazine analogue on the formation of lipoxygenase and cyclo-oxygenase products, *Eur J Pharmacol* 169:225–234, 1989.
186. Gronberg A, Isaksson P, Smedegard G: Inhibitory effect of sulfasalazine on production of IL-1beta, IL-6 and TNF-alpha, *Arthritis Rheum* 37:S383, 1994.
190. Minghetti P, Blackburn W: Effects of sulfasalazine and its metabolites on steady state messenger RNA concentrations for inflammatory cytokines, matrix metalloproteinases and tissue inhibitors of metalloproteinase in rheumatoid synovial fibroblasts, *J Rheumatol* 27:653–660, 2000.
193. Sheldon P: Rheumatoid arthritis and gut-related lymphocytes: the iteropathy concept, *Ann Rheum Dis* 47:697–700, 1988.
195. Kanerud L, Scheynius A, Hafstrom I: Evidence of a local intestinal immunomodulatory effect of sulfasalazine in rheumatoid arthritis, *Arthritis Rheum* 37:1138–1145, 1994.
200. Plosker G, Croom K, Sulfasalazine: a review of its use in the management of rheumatoid arthritis, *Drugs* 65:1825–1849, 2005.
201. Farr A, Brodrick A, Bacon P: Plasma synovial fluid concentration of sulphasalazine and two of its metabolites in rheumatoid arthritis, *Rheumatol Int* 5:247–251, 1985.
202. Taggart A, McDermott B, Roberts S: The effect of age and acetylator phenotype on the pharmacokinetics of sulfasalazine in patients with rheumatoid arthritis, *Clin Pharmacokinet* 23:311–320, 1992.
203. Schroder H, Campbell D: Absorption, metabolism and excretion of salicylazo-sulfapyridine in man, *Clin Pharmacol Ther* 13:539, 1972.
206. Weinblatt M, Reda D, Henderson W, et al.: Sulfasalazine treatment for rheumatoid arthritis: a meta-analysis of 15 randomized trials, *J Rheumatol* 26:2123–2130, 1999.
208. Haagsma C, Van Riel P, De Jong A, et al.: Combination of sulphasalazine and methotrexate versus the single components in early rheumatoid arthritis: a randomized, controlled, double-blind, 52 week clinical trial, *Br J Rheumatol* 36:1082–1088, 1997.
213. Clegg D, Reda D, Weisman M, et al.: Comparison of sulfasalazine and placebo in the treatment of reactive arthritis (Reiter's syndrome), *Arthritis Rheum* 39:2021–2027, 1996.
216. Donvan S, Hawley S, MacCarthy J, et al.: Tolerability of enteric-coated sulphasalazine in rheumatoid arthritis: results of a co-operating clinics study, *Br J Rheumatol* 29:201–204, 1990.
218. Canvin J, El-Gaalawy H, Chalmers I: Fatal agranulocytosis with sulfasalazine therapy in rheumatoid arthritis, *J Rheumatol* 20:909, 1993.
219. Farr M, Scott D, Bacon P: Sulphasalazine desensitization in rheumatoid arthritis, *BMJ* 284:118, 1982.
220. Parry S, Barbatzas C, Peel E, et al.: Sulphasalazine and lung toxicity, *Eur Respir J* 19:756–764, 2002.
222. Alloway J, Mitchell S: Sufasalazine neurotoxicity: a report of aseptic meningitis and a review of the literature, *J Rheumatol* 20:409, 1993.
225. Wozniacka A, Carter A, McCauliffe D: Antimalarials in cutaneous lupus erythematosus: mechanisms of therapeutic benefit, *Lupus* 11:71–81, 2002.
236. Bondeson J, Sundler R: Antimalarial drugs inhibit phospholipase A2 activation and induction of interleukin 1β and tumor necrosis factor in macrophages: implications for their mode of action in rheumatoid arthritis, *Gen Pharmacol* 30:357–366, 1998.
237. Chen X, Gresham A, Morrison A, et al.: Oxidative stress mediates synthesis of cytosolic phospholipase A2 after UVB injury, *J Biol Chem* 111:693–695, 1996.
238. Ruzicka T, Printz M: Arachidonic acid metabolism in guinea pig skin: effects of chloroquine, *Agents Actions* 12:527–529, 1982.
239. Ramakrishnan N, Kalinich J, McClain D: Ebselen inhibition of apoptosis by reduction of peroxides, *Biochem Pharmacol* 51:1443–1451, 1996.
246. Mackenzie A: Pharmacologic actions of the 4-aminoquinoline compounds, *Am J Med* 75:11–18, 1983.
250. Felson D, Anderson J, Meenan R: The comparative efficacy and toxicity of second-line drugs in rheumatoid arthritis, *Arthritis Rheum* 33:1449–1461, 1999.
252. Edmonds J, Scott K, Furst D: Antirheumatic drugs: a proposed new classification, *Arthritis Rheum* 36:336–339, 1993.
255. Canadian Hydroxychloroquine Study Group: A randomized study of the effects of withdrawing hydroxychloroquine sulfate in systemic lupus erythematosus, *N Engl J Med* 324:150–154, 1991.
258. Edwards M, Pierangeli S, Liu X, et al.: Hydroxychloroquine reverses thrombogenic properties of antiphospholipid antibodies in mice, *Circulation* 96:4380–4384, 1997.
259. Espinola R, Pierangeli S, Harris E: Hydroxychloroquine reverses platelet activation induced by human IgG antiphospholipid antibodies, *Thromb Haemost* 87:518–522, 2002.

265. Olson N, Lindsley C: Adjunctive use of hydroxychloroquine in childhood dermatomyositis, *J Rheumatol* 16:1545–1547, 1989.
266. Lakhanpal S, Ginsburg W, Michet C, et al.: Eosinophilic fasciitis: clinical spectrum and therapeutic response in 52 cases, *Semin Arthritis Rheum* 17:221–231, 1988.
268. Rothschild B: Prospective six-month double-blind trial of plaquenil treatment of calcium pyrophosphate deposition disease (CPPD), *Arthritis Rheum* 37(Suppl 9):S414, 1994.
269. Marmor M, Carr R, Easterbrook M, et al.: Information statement: recommendations on screening for chloroquine and hydroxychloroquine retinopathy, *Ophthalmology* 109:1377–1382, 2002.
270. Melles RB, Marmor MF: The risk of toxic retinopathy inpatients on long-term hydroxychloroquine therapy, *JAMA Ophthalmol* 10:E1–E8, 2014.
271. Deleted in review.
273. Wallace D: Antimalarials—the "real" advance in lupus, *Lupus* 10:385–387, 2001.
274. Stein M, Bell M, Ang L: Hydroxychloroquine neuromyotoxicity, *J Rheumatol* 27:2927–2931, 2000.
275. Cervera A, Espinosa G, Cervera R, et al.: Cardiac toxicity secondary to long term treatment with chloroquine, *Ann Rheum Dis* 60:301–304, 2001.
276. Rekedal L, Massarotti E, Garg R, et al.: Changes in glycosylated hemoglobin after initiation of hydroxychloroquine or methotrexate in diabetic patients with rheumatologic diseases, *Arthritis Rheum* 62:3569–3573, 2010.
278. Marmor MF, Kellner U, Lai TY, et al.: Revised recommendations on screening for chloroquine and hydroxychloroquine retinopathy, *Ophthalmology* 11:415–422, 2011.
279. Mikuls T, O'Dell J: The changing face of rheumatoid arthritis, *Arthritis Rheum* 43:464–465, 2000.
280. Boers M, Verhoeven A, Marusse H, et al.: Randomized comparison of combined step-down prednisolone, methotrexate and suphasalazine with sulphasalazine alone in early rheumatoid arthritis, *Lancet* 350:309–318, 1997.
281. Calguneri M, Pay S, Caliskener Z, et al.: Combination therapy versus mono-therapy for the treatment of patients with rheumatoid arthritis, *Clin Exp Rheumatol* 17:699–704, 1999.
282. Mottonen T, Hannonsen P, Leiralalo-Repoo M, et al.: Comparison of combination therapy with single-drug therapy in early rheumatoid arthritis: a randomized trial, *Lancet* 353:1568–1573, 1999.
283. Csuka M, Carrero G, McCarty D: Treatment of intractable rheumatoid arthritis with combined cyclophosphamide, azathioprine and hydroxychloroquine: a follow-up study, *JAMA* 255:2315, 1986.
285. Landewe R, Boers M, Verhoeven A, et al.: COBRA combination therapy in patients with early rheumatoid arthritis: long-term structural benefits of a brief intervention, *Arthritis Rheum* 46:347–356, 2002.
286. Neva M, Dauppi M, Kautiainen H, et al.: Combination drug therapy retards the development of rheumatoid atlantoaxial subluxations, *Arthritis Rheum* 11:2397–2401, 2000.
288. Tugwell P, Pincus T, Yokum D, et al.: Combination therapy with cyclosporine and methotrexate in severe rheumatoid arthritis, *N Engl J Med* 333:137–142, 1995.
293. O'Dell J, Mikuls TR, Taylor TH, et al.: Therapies for active rheumatoid arthritis after methotrexate failure, *N Engl J Med* 369:307–318, 2013.

65 Immunosuppressive Drugs

JACOB M. VAN LAAR

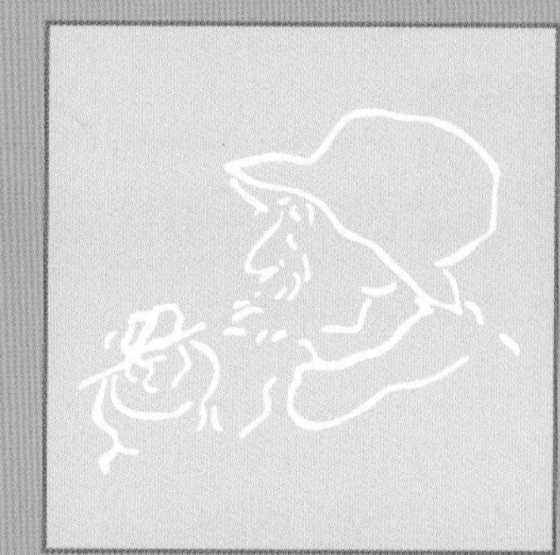

KEY POINTS

Immunosuppressive drugs are effective remission-inducing and maintenance agents in the management of inflammatory rheumatic conditions, especially systemic autoimmune diseases.

The most commonly used immunosuppressive drugs include cytostatic agents (e.g., cyclophosphamide and azathioprine), mycophenolate mofetil, and calcineurin inhibitors (e.g., cyclosporine and tacrolimus), each with a unique mode of action and toxicity profile. Due to its relatively favorable risk-benefit profile, mycophenolate mofetil has become the anchor drug in the management of systemic lupus erythematosus, systemic vasculitis, systemic sclerosis, and myositis-related interstitial lung disease.

The long-term use of immunosuppressive drugs is associated with an increased risk of bacterial, viral, and fungal infection, as well as a reduced response to vaccinations.

Cytostatic agents should be avoided in pregnancy and lactation, and referral to a fertility clinic should be considered for all fertile male and female patients. Other immunosuppressive drugs should only be used during pregnancy if the potential benefits outweigh the potential risks.

Introduction

Immunosuppressive drugs comprise different classes of drugs that dampen the immune system—notably T and B lymphocytes—functionally and/or numerically (Table 65.1) but do not permanently correct the fundamental imbalance of immune regulation in autoimmune disease. As such, they do not have curative potential, yet they can be effective in remission induction and control of specific rheumatic disease manifestations, and they remain cornerstone drugs in the management of rheumatic conditions, especially systemic autoimmune diseases. Immunosuppressive drugs such as cyclophosphamide, azathioprine, and cyclosporin have withstood the test of time, as attested by their ongoing use in transplantation medicine, nephrology, gastroenterology, ophthalmology, dermatology, and rheumatology. Consequently, their therapeutic potential and toxicity profiles hold few surprises. Newer drugs, such as mycophenolate mofetil (MMF) and, to a lesser extent, tacrolimus, have come to the fore, notably because of their favorable risk-benefit profile, affordable pricing, and ease of use for patients. Apart from drug-specific toxicities, the main risk of immunosuppressive treatment is infection. In the absence of validated biomarkers of infection, sound clinical judgment and experience remain indispensable in monitoring patients who use immunosuppressive drugs, often for long periods. The use of live vaccines is contraindicated, and although other vaccinations are generally less effective, annual influenza vaccination is recommended in patients being treated with immunosuppressive medication. Pneumococcal vaccination and herpes zoster vaccination also should be considered in select patients in accordance with (inter)national guidelines.

This chapter outlines the clinical pharmacology and therapeutic use of immunosuppressive drugs used in rheumatology. These drugs include cytostatic agents that affect bone marrow progenitor cells (cyclophosphamide and azathioprine) and drugs such as MMF, cyclosporine, and tacrolimus that target lymphocytes by inhibiting specific intra-cellular signaling pathways and/or proliferation. Their effects on the immune system overlap with those of traditional disease-modifying anti-rheumatic drugs, such as methotrexate, glucocorticoids, and biologics. The most commonly used immunosuppressive drugs—cyclophosphamide, azathioprine, and MMF—and the less commonly used calcineurin inhibitors cyclosporine and tacrolimus are discussed in more detail. Glucocorticoids, traditional disease-modifying anti-rheumatic drugs (e.g., methotrexate, leflunomide, sulfasalazine, and hydroxychloroquine), biologics, and novel intra-cellular targeting agents are discussed elsewhere. The role of other immunosuppressive drugs (e.g., thalidomide, chlorambucil, sirolimus, and everolimus) in routine rheumatologic clinical practice has not been sufficiently established to merit discussion.

Cyclophosphamide

Cyclophosphamide was introduced as a cytotoxic agent in 1958 and is still one of the most potent immunosuppressant drugs available. In combination with glucocorticoids, cyclophosphamide is particularly effective as a remission induction agent in severe systemic lupus erythematosus (SLE) and necrotizing vasculitis.

Structure

Cyclophosphamide is an oxazaphosphorine-substituted nitrogen mustard and inactive prodrug that requires enzymatic bioactivation (Fig. 65.1). Cyclophosphamide belongs to the class of alkylating agents that substitute alkyl radicals into DNA, resulting in cell death. Cyclophosphamide is the alkylating agent of choice for most rheumatic diseases requiring such therapy.

Mechanisms of Action

The DNA-alkylating effects of cyclophosphamide are mediated predominantly through phosphoramide mustard and, to a lesser extent, other active metabolites. These positively charged, reactive intermediates alkylate nucleophilic bases, resulting in the

TABLE 65.1 **Mechanisms of Action of Immunosuppressive Drugs**

Drugs	Class	Mechanism of Action
Cyclophosphamide	Alkylating cytotoxics	Active metabolites alkylate DNA
Azathioprine	Purine analogue cytotoxics	Inhibits purine synthesis
Cyclosporine, tacrolimus (FK506)	Calcineurin inhibitors	Inhibits calcium-dependent T cell activation and IL-2 production
Mycophenolate mofetil	Purine synthesis inhibitors	Mycophenolic acid inhibits inosine monophosphate dehydrogenase

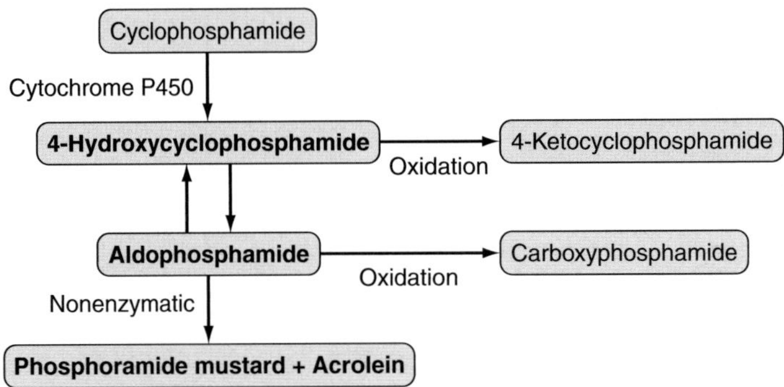

• **Fig. 65.1** The metabolism of cyclophosphamide. Cyclophosphamide is converted to 4-hydroxycyclophosphamide, in equilibrium with its tautomer aldophosphamide, by cytochrome P450 enzymes. Subsequent nonenzymatic processes lead to the formation of phosphoramide mustard and acrolein. Oxidation of 4-hydroxycyclophosphamide and aldophosphamide through enzymes, including aldehyde dehydrogenase, results in inactive metabolites. Cytotoxic metabolites are shown in bold.

cross-linking of DNA and of DNA proteins, breaks in DNA, and consequently decreased DNA synthesis and apoptosis.[1] The cytotoxicity of alkylating agents correlates with the amount of DNA cross-linking, but the relationship between cytotoxicity and immunosuppressive effects is unclear. The effects of cyclophosphamide are not exclusively limited to proliferating cells or particular cell types. Sensitivity varies among cell populations, however; for example, hematopoietic progenitor cells are relatively resistant to even high doses of cyclophosphamide. The immunosuppressive effects of cyclophosphamide include decreased numbers of T lymphocytes and B lymphocytes, decreased lymphocyte proliferation, decreased antibody production, and suppression of delayed hypersensitivity to new antigens with relative preservation of established delayed hypersensitivity.[2]

Pharmacology

Absorption and Distribution

Oral and intravenous (IV) administration of cyclophosphamide results in similar plasma concentrations.[3] Peak plasma concentrations of cyclophosphamide occur 1 hour after oral administration. Protein binding of cyclophosphamide is low (20%), and it is widely distributed.[1]

Metabolism and Elimination

Cyclophosphamide is rapidly metabolized, largely by the liver, to active and inactive metabolites. The formation of the active 4-hydroxycyclophosphamide is mediated by various cytochrome P450 (CYP) enzymes, and genetic variations in the enzymes in patients with lupus nephritis affect responses to cyclophosphamide.[4] 4-Hydroxycyclophosphamide, which is not cytotoxic at physiologic pH, readily diffuses into cells and spontaneously decomposes into the active phosphoramide mustard. The elimination half-life of cyclophosphamide is 5 to 9 hours, and alkylating activity is undetectable in the plasma of most patients 24 hours after a dose of 12 mg/kg.[1] Plasma concentrations of cyclophosphamide are not clinically useful predictors of either efficacy or toxicity. Between 30% and 60% of the total cyclophosphamide is eliminated in the urine, mostly as inactive metabolites, although some cyclophosphamide and active metabolites, such as phosphoramide mustard and acrolein, also can be detected in urine.[1]

Pharmacokinetic Considerations

Liver Disease. Although the half-life of cyclophosphamide is increased to 12 hours in patients with liver failure compared with 8 hours in control subjects, toxicity is not increased, suggesting that exposure to cytotoxic metabolites is not increased and dose modification in liver disease is generally not required.[1]

Renal Impairment. Some studies have shown little alteration in drug disposition with no increased toxicity in patients with impaired renal function.[1] In patients with autoimmune disease and a creatinine clearance of 25 to 50 mL/min and 10 to 25 mL/min, exposure to cyclophosphamide increased approximately 40% and 70%, respectively.[5] In clinical practice, initial cyclophosphamide doses are therefore decreased by approximately 30% in patients with moderate to severe renal impairment, and subsequent doses are titrated according to clinical response and effects on the leukocyte (white blood cell) count. Cyclophosphamide is removed by dialysis and is administered after dialysis, or, alternatively, dialysis can be initiated the day after cyclophosphamide administration.[5]

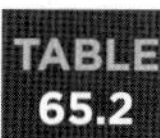

TABLE 65.2 Lupus Nephritis Treatment Protocols

National Institutes of Health Protocol

Cyclophosphamide: 6× monthly IV 500-750 mg/m^2, then maintenance doses every 3 mo until 1 y after remission, or consider alternative remission maintenance treatment with azathioprine or mycophenolate mofetil; dose adjustments on the basis of nadir leukocyte counts and glomerular filtration rate

All patients to receive prednisone, 0.5-1 mg/kg/day for 4 wk, decreasing the every-other-day dose each week, if possible, by 5 mg to achieve a prednisone dose of 0.25 mg/kg on alternate days

Euro-Lupus Protocols

Low-dose cyclophosphamide: 6× biweekly IV 500 mg

High-dose cyclophosphamide: 6× monthly IV 500 mg/m^2 of body surface area, followed by 2 quarterly pulses with higher dose (+250 mg depending on leukocyte nadir, maximum 1500 mg)

All patients to receive:

- Glucocorticoids: 3× daily IV methylprednisolone, 750 mg, followed by oral 0.5 mg/kg/day of prednisolone (or equivalent) for 4 wk; after 4 wk, tapering of glucocorticoid by 2.5 mg prednisolone every 2 wk; low-dose glucocorticoid therapy (5-7.5 mg prednisolone/day) was maintained at least until mo 30 after inclusion; dose at discretion of treating physician thereafter
- Azathioprine: oral, 2 mg/kg daily, starting 2 wk after last cyclophosphamide infusion until mo 30 after inclusion; choice of immunosuppressant at discretion of treating physician thereafter

IV, Intravenous.

Clinical Indications

Cyclophosphamide is most commonly used as a remission induction agent for patients with systemic necrotizing vasculitis or Goodpasture's syndrome, for patients with organ-threatening SLE, and for some patients with autoimmune disease–associated interstitial lung disease and inflammatory eye disease. In SLE, a remission induction course with IV cyclophosphamide followed by maintenance with azathioprine or MMF to minimize cyclophosphamide toxicity is still commonly used to treat severe organ involvement, including lupus nephritis, although remission induction regimens with MMF (discussed in subsequent text) and the B cell–depleting biologic agent rituximab have been proven as effective and safer alternatives to cyclophosphamide.[6] The original National Institutes of Health (NIH) protocol entailed six monthly IV infusions with cyclophosphamide, 1 g/m^2, and then one infusion every 3 months for at least 24 additional months,[7] whereas the Euro-Lupus protocol used in Europe entailed administration of six IV infusions of 500 mg of cyclophosphamide every 2 weeks followed by azathioprine maintenance (Table 65.2). A comparison with six monthly IV infusions of cyclophosphamide, 500 mg/m^2, followed by two further infusions of slightly higher doses 3 and 6 months later, along with azathioprine maintenance therapy, resulted in similar rates of the endpoints of end-stage renal disease or doubling of creatinine concentration with up to 10 years of follow-up.[8]

Cyclophosphamide administered as either IV pulse therapy or orally can also be effective in patients with other serious complications of SLE, including CNS involvement and thrombocytopenia and interstitial lung disease associated with systemic sclerosis and other autoimmune diseases.[9–11] A recent Cochrane analysis of four trials with 495 patients with connective tissue disease–associated interstitial lung disease, however, found only modest benefit on lung function (FVC) and clinical symptoms.[12] Several trials have investigated whether IV cyclophosphamide is as effective as oral cyclophosphamide as remission induction therapy for granulomatosis with polyangiitis (GPA). Although early trial results suggested the superiority of oral dosing, later clinical trial data pointed to equal efficacy but slightly less hematologic toxicity with IV therapy.[13–16] As in lupus nephritis, shorter induction courses of cyclophosphamide have been reported to be effective in GPA and microscopic polyangiitis.[17] Cyclophosphamide has a steep dose-response curve, making it an ideal compound for dose escalation. High doses of cyclophosphamide, with or without stem cell rescue and lymphoablative antibodies or total body irradiation, have been used for severe juvenile idiopathic arthritis (JIA), rheumatoid arthritis (RA), systemic sclerosis, and SLE.[18] With the introduction of effective biologics and new treatment paradigms for RA and JIA, the clinical need for immunoablative treatment in these diseases has waned. Although large series have shown promising results of immunoablative therapy and stem cell rescue in patients with severe SLE, a randomized trial showed that standard-dose IV cyclophosphamide was not inferior to high-dose cyclophosphamide *without* stem cell rescue or lymphoablative antibodies.[19] In systemic sclerosis, three randomized, controlled trials have demonstrated the superior efficacy of the immunoablative therapy *with* stem cell rescue compared with IV pulse cyclophosphamide on a range of outcome measures, including modified Rodnan skin score, functional ability, quality of life, and survival, albeit at the expense of greater toxicity in the first year as a result of infections and cardiopulmonary events.[20–22] The latter may, at least in part, be explained by the cardiotoxic effects of high-dose cyclophosphamide, the metabolites of which can result in death from hemorrhagic necrotic perimyocarditis and toxic endothelial damage.[23]

Dosage and Route of Administration

For typical dosage regimens, see Table 65.2. Dosages for IV pulse therapy with cyclophosphamide range from 0.5 to 1 g/m^2, and the dosage for oral therapy is 2 mg/kg. The bioavailability of oral cyclophosphamide is excellent.

Toxicity

Hematologic

Reversible myelosuppression manifesting as leukopenia and neutropenia is common and dose dependent. Generally, platelet counts are not affected with IV pulse doses of less than 50 mg/kg, but with long-term oral use a mild decrease in the platelet count is common. After a single IV dose of cyclophosphamide, the approximate times to nadir and recovery of leukocyte counts are 8 to 14 days and 21 days, respectively.[24] The white blood cell nadir is about 3000 cells/mm^3 after a dose of 1 g/m^2 (~25 mg/kg) and 1500 cells/mm^3 after a dose of 1.5 g/m^2. With long-term use, sensitivity to the myelosuppressive effects of cyclophosphamide is increased, and doses usually need to be decreased over time.

Infection

Infection with a range of common and opportunistic pathogens is a frequent complication. In 100 patients with SLE, infection occurred in 45 patients during treatment with a cyclophosphamide-based regimen and was the primary cause of death in 7 patients.[25] In this study, infection was equally common in patients receiving oral or IV cyclophosphamide and was associated with a white blood cell nadir at some point in treatment of less than 3000/mm^3 (55% infection rate vs. 36%). At the time of infection, the average white blood cell count was normal, however.[25] A higher maximal glucocorticoid dose was also associated with increased risk of infection. Half of the infections occurred at prednisone doses of less than 40 mg/day, and a quarter of the infections occurred at doses of less than 25 mg/day. Lower rates of infection (25% to 30%) have been reported in patients with SLE who received cyclophosphamide in NIH protocols.[26] Oral cyclophosphamide regimens generally pose a greater risk of infection than IV pulse regimens. Serious infections occurred in 41% and 70% of patients with GPA who were treated with pulse IV and daily oral cyclophosphamide, respectively.[13] These rates of infection are higher than rates reported in long-term NIH protocols, in which 48% of 158 patients experienced 140 infections requiring hospitalization.[27] The reported frequency of cyclophosphamide-associated infection varies, probably as a function of the stage and severity of the underlying disease, the degree of cyclophosphamide-induced immunosuppression, and variations in concomitant glucocorticoid regimens. *Pneumocystis jiroveci* pneumonia has been recognized as a preventable, serious opportunistic infection that complicates treatment of systemic vasculitis with regimens using cyclophosphamide and methotrexate. The risk is highest during the remission induction phase and is greater with oral than IV cyclophosphamide regimens.[28] Surprisingly, in two placebo-controlled, randomized clinical trials in people with scleroderma lung disease, active treatment for 1 year with either oral cyclophosphamide or sequential treatment with prednisolone plus IV cyclophosphamide followed by azathioprine was not associated with more toxicity, suggesting disease-specific differences in toxicity.[10,11]

Urologic

The bladder toxicities of cyclophosphamide, hemorrhagic cystitis, and bladder cancer are related to the route of administration, duration of therapy, and cumulative cyclophosphamide dose. Bladder toxicity, a particular problem with long-term oral cyclophosphamide, is largely due to acrolein, a metabolite of cyclophosphamide. It is commonly accepted that bladder toxicity can be minimized in patients receiving pulse doses of IV cyclophosphamide by administering mesna, a sulfhydryl compound that binds acrolein in the urine and inactivates it.[29] Direct evidence for the effectiveness of mesna in preventing cystitis, however, comes from its use with ifosfamide in patients with cancer and data from animal models. The data from rheumatology series are consistent with a protective effect but are inadequate to come to firm conclusions, which explains the differences between national guidelines.[30] The short half-life of mesna renders it suboptimal for the prevention of bladder toxicity in patients receiving daily oral cyclophosphamide, but oral mesna administered three times a day with daily oral cyclophosphamide was associated with a relatively low incidence of bladder toxicity of 12%.[31]

Nonglomerular hematuria, which may range from minor, microscopic blood loss to severe, macroscopic bleeding, is the most common manifestation of cyclophosphamide-induced cystitis.[32] Nonglomerular hematuria occurred at some time in 50% of 145 patients treated with oral cyclophosphamide and was related to the duration of therapy and cumulative cyclophosphamide dose.[32] The risk of bladder cancer was increased 31-fold (95% confidence interval [CI], 13-fold to 65-fold), and bladder cancer had developed in 7 patients (5%) any time between 7 months and 15 years after the initiation of therapy. The cancer was preceded by nonglomerular hematuria in all patients. Six of the seven patients had a cumulative dose of more than 100 g of cyclophosphamide and a duration of therapy of more than 2.7 years. Smokers were at an increased risk of hemorrhagic cystitis and bladder cancer.

Malignancy

Cyclophosphamide increases the risk of malignancies (other than bladder cancer) twofold to fourfold. In the largest study, 119 patients with RA who had been treated with oral cyclophosphamide were followed up for 20 years.[32] In the cyclophosphamide group, 50 cancers occurred in 37 patients, compared with 26 cancers that occurred in 25 of 119 control subjects with RA. Bladder, skin, myeloproliferative, and oropharyngeal malignancies occurred more commonly in the cyclophosphamide group. The risk of malignancies increased with the cumulative dose of cyclophosphamide, and a malignancy developed in 53% of patients who received more than 80 g of cyclophosphamide. Few malignancies have been reported in patients treated with pulse IV cyclophosphamide regimens. Current data do not allow quantification of the long-term risk of malignancy associated with pulse IV cyclophosphamide treatment, but it is likely to be substantially smaller than that associated with oral regimens.

Reproduction

Cyclophosphamide, when used to treat autoimmune disease, results in significant gonadal toxicity. The risk of sustained amenorrhea after cyclophosphamide therapy has ranged from 11% to 59%.[33] The risk of ovarian failure depends more on the age of the patient and the cumulative dose of cyclophosphamide than on the route of administration.[33] Patients younger than 25 years receiving six pulses of IV cyclophosphamide had a low frequency of ovarian failure (none of four patients), whereas patients older than 31 years receiving 15 to 24 pulses all had ovarian failure (four of four patients). The use of alkylating agents in male patients leads to azoospermia, and, if the clinical situation allows, referral to a fertility clinic for banking of sperm (or ova in female patients) should be considered before cyclophosphamide treatment. The offspring of adults who underwent cancer chemotherapy in childhood had no increase in genetic disease.[34]

Pulmonary

Cyclophosphamide-induced pulmonary toxicity occurs in less than 1% of patients. Early-onset pneumonitis 1 to 6 months after exposure to cyclophosphamide may respond to withdrawal of the drug and treatment with corticosteroids. A more insidious, irreversible, late-onset pneumonitis and fibrosis with radiographic findings of diffuse reticular or reticulonodular infiltrates may occur after treatment with oral cyclophosphamide for 1 to 13 years.[35]

Miscellaneous

A varying degree of reversible alopecia can occur with daily oral and monthly pulse cyclophosphamide. Cardiotoxicity, a dose-limiting adverse effect in oncology and transplant protocols, and water intoxication, as a result of inappropriate anti-diuretic hormone secretion, are rare at standard doses.[36] Unusual hypersensitivity reactions include urticaria and anaphylaxis, although the bladder protectant mesna is a more likely cause of allergic responses in patients receiving both drugs.[37,38]

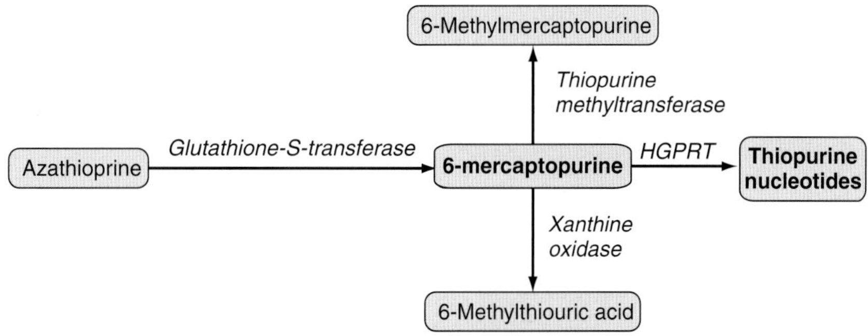

• **Fig. 65.2** Azathioprine is converted to mercaptopurine (6-MP) enzymatically by glutathione-*S*-transferase and nonenzymatic mechanisms. Xanthine oxidase and thiopurine methyltransferase metabolize 6-MP to the inactive metabolites 6-methylthiouric acid and 6-methylmercaptopurine. Hypoxanthine-guanine-phosphoribosyl-transferase (HGPRT) metabolizes 6-MP to active, cytotoxic thiopurine nucleotides.

Strategies to Minimize Toxicity

Strategies to minimize toxicity include adjusting the dose of cyclophosphamide to avoid a significant degree of leukopenia (white blood cell count <3000/mm^3 for daily oral therapy or a nadir of <2000/mm^3 for pulse IV therapy) and granulocytopenia.[39] The blood count is monitored initially at 1- to 2-week intervals and monthly thereafter in patients taking stable oral doses. To decrease the risk of infection added by concomitant high-dose glucocorticoids, the dose of glucocorticoids should be reduced after a clinical response has been obtained. Alternate-day administration of glucocorticoids can be considered in the maintenance phase. Oral cyclophosphamide is best administered as a single dose in the morning with the patient drinking plenty of fluids and emptying the bladder frequently to dilute the urinary concentration of acrolein and to minimize the amount of time the bladder is exposed to it. Prophylaxis against *P. jiroveci* pneumonia is often prescribed, particularly during the induction phase when doses of cyclophosphamide and glucocorticoids are higher. The use of mesna to prevent bladder toxicity was described earlier. Urinalysis should be performed monthly, and nonglomerular hematuria should be evaluated by a urologist. All patients who receive cyclophosphamide, particularly patients in whom hemorrhagic cystitis develops, are at increased risk of developing bladder cancer, and lifelong surveillance is required with urinalysis, urine cytology, and, if indicated, cystoscopy.[40] Lastly, drugs that are less toxic than cyclophosphamide, such as methotrexate, MMF, and rituximab, are considered effective alternative options for inducing remission or for remission maintenance in patients with GPA or lupus nephritis.[41–44]

Pregnancy and Lactation

Cyclophosphamide is a U.S. Food and Drug Administration (FDA) Pregnancy Category D drug. Cyclophosphamide is teratogenic, particularly in the first trimester, and should be avoided during pregnancy and lactation.[45,46] If a patient becomes pregnant while taking (receiving) this drug, the patient should be apprised of the potential hazard to the fetus. Women of childbearing potential should be advised to avoid becoming pregnant.

Drug Interactions

Cimetidine inhibits the activity of several hepatic enzymes. It has resulted in increased exposure to cyclophosphamide metabolites in a rabbit model.[47] Ranitidine and presumably other H2 receptor antagonists that have little effect on hepatic drug metabolism are not associated with increased cyclophosphamide toxicity.[48] Allopurinol increases the half-life of cyclophosphamide and the frequency of leukopenia.[49] Cyclophosphamide decreases plasma pseudocholinesterase activity and can potentiate the effect of succinylcholine.[50]

Azathioprine

Structure

Azathioprine is a prodrug that is converted to 6-mercaptopurine (6-MP), which involves the removal of an imidazole group.[51] 6-MP is a purine analogue that acts as a cycle-specific antimetabolite chemotherapeutic agent and interferes with the synthesis of nucleotides, thereby inhibiting proliferation of lymphocytes. Azathioprine has a better therapeutic index than 6-MP and has replaced it in the treatment of rheumatic autoimmune disease.

Mechanisms of Action

The exact mechanism of action of the active thiopurine metabolites of azathioprine in autoimmune disease is unknown. Thiopurine metabolites, such as thioguanine nucleotides, decrease the de novo synthesis of purine nucleotides by inhibiting amidotransferase enzymes and purine ribonucleotide interconversion and are incorporated into DNA and RNA.[51] The incorporation of thioguanine nucleotides into the nucleic acids of cells is thought to mediate the cytotoxicity of azathioprine, whereas inhibition of purine synthesis may be more important in decreasing cellular proliferation. Leukopenia is unnecessary for immunosuppression. Azathioprine decreases the circulating lymphocyte count, suppresses lymphocyte proliferation, inhibits antibody production, inhibits monocyte production, suppresses natural killer cell activity, and inhibits cell-mediated and humoral immunity.

Pharmacology

Absorption and Distribution

Oral azathioprine is well absorbed and rapidly converted to 6-MP, which is further metabolized to several compounds, including 6-thiourate (Fig. 65.2), that are excreted in urine. The plasma half-life of azathioprine is less than 15 minutes, but it is 1 to 3 hours for the active derivative, 6-MP.[52] The bioavailability of azathioprine, measured as the concentrations of mercaptopurine achieved after oral administration, varies. In healthy volunteers, bioavailability ranged from 27% to 83%, with an average of 47%.[52] Mercaptopurine is widely distributed with a volume of distribution of 4 to 8 L/kg.[51]

Metabolism and Elimination

The metabolism of azathioprine is complex[51,53] and has been simplified in Fig. 65.2. Two enzymes, xanthine oxidase and thiopurine S-methyltransferase (TPMT), shunt mercaptopurine metabolites to relatively inactive compounds, whereas other enzymes such as hypoxanthine-guanine-phosphoribosyl-transferase lead to the formation of cytotoxic thiopurine nucleotides. Low TPMT activity or inhibition of xanthine oxidase by drugs such as allopurinol leads to decreased detoxification and increased formation of cytotoxic metabolites after the administration of azathioprine or mercaptopurine. Maximal concentrations of mercaptopurine occur 1 to 3 hours after administration of azathioprine, and the half-life of mercaptopurine is 1 to 2 hours.[52] The half-life of the intra-cellular, active 6-thioguanine nucleotides is estimated to be 1 to 2 weeks, however, and concentrations do not change over the 24-hour dose period in patients receiving daily azathioprine.[54] At conventional rheumatologic doses, approximately 1% of mercaptopurine is excreted unchanged in the urine.[54] Increased toxicity can occur with renal impairment (creatinine clearance <25 mL/min), and a modest dose reduction is usually necessary. The substantial interindividual variability in azathioprine disposition and TPMT activity are more important determinants of sensitivity to azathioprine than renal function.[55] Azathioprine is only slightly dialyzable (10%) through conventional hemodialysis membranes.

Dosage

Azathioprine is often started at a dose of 1 mg/kg daily, and if this dose is tolerated, it is increased to 2 to 2.5 mg/kg after 2 to 4 weeks. A gradual increase in dose is often better tolerated. The onset of immunosuppressive effects is relatively slow, over several weeks, presumably because the active thioguanine metabolites slowly accumulate intra-cellularly.

Clinical Indications

In current practice, azathioprine is mainly used in the treatment of connective tissue disease rather than inflammatory joint disease. Azathioprine is less effective than methotrexate in RA and has a slow mode of onset when compared with other disease-modifying anti-rheumatic drugs and biologics. Nevertheless, it remains a treatment option for patients with RA who have refractory disease or as a glucocorticoid-sparing agent in patients with organ involvement. Azathioprine is used to treat some patients with lupus nephritis, and although it is more effective than glucocorticoids alone, it is not as effective as IV pulse cyclophosphamide to induce remission.[56] It is effective in maintenance therapy, however,[57] even after low-dose cyclophosphamide induction. For other manifestations of SLE, including cutaneous disease, azathioprine is widely used as a glucocorticoid-sparing agent.[58]

Azathioprine in combination with glucocorticoids is useful in the treatment of a range of other autoimmune diseases such as inflammatory muscle disease, inflammatory eye disease (including Behçet's disease),[59] psoriatic arthritis,[60] reactive arthritis, and various forms of vasculitis. In systemic vasculitis, azathioprine is less effective as a remission induction agent than cyclophosphamide[17] but is safer as a remission-maintenance and glucocorticoid-sparing drug.[41] Nevertheless, a small study has shown the efficacy of high-dose (1200 to 1800 mg infusions) monthly azathioprine as an initial treatment of GPA and lupus nephritis.[61] Azathioprine is frequently used in people with systemic sclerosis and overlap syndromes, especially in people with interstitial lung disease or joint involvement.[11,62]

Toxicity

Hematologic

Reversible myelosuppression is dose related but varies among individuals. Low-dose azathioprine (1 to 2 mg/kg/day) rarely results in leukopenia or thrombocytopenia. Pure red cell aplasia is also rare. Severe myelosuppression is uncommon and is caused by low or absent TPMT activity. Decreased TPMT activity leads to a decreased ability to detoxify mercaptopurine and results in the increased formation of cytotoxic thioguanine metabolites and clinical toxicity.[63] TPMT activity is polymorphic with a trimodal distribution. Approximately 90% of subjects show high activity, 10% show intermediate activity, and 0.3% (the subjects homozygous for the poorly functional polymorphisms) show very low activity.[64,65] The median TPMT activity in African Americans is approximately 17% lower than in white Americans.[65] The 1 in 300 subjects with low or absent TPMT activity are at great risk of severe azathioprine-induced myelosuppression, which has a delayed but sudden onset, most commonly 4 to 10 weeks after azathioprine has been started.[66] In more than half of all cases of leukopenia in patients receiving azathioprine, the patients have a normal TPMT genotype and phenotype, however.

Gastrointestinal

Liver test abnormalities occur in 34% of patients but are seldom serious. Serious liver toxicity, severe cholestasis, hepatic veno-occlusive disease, and nodular regenerative hyperplasia and pancreatitis are rare.

Malignancy

Data regarding the risk of malignancy in patients treated with azathioprine for rheumatologic disease are conflicting. Some studies found an increased risk, particularly of lymphoproliferative malignancies, whereas others did not find an increased risk.[67] A 24-year retrospective study of 358 patients with SLE found no difference in malignancy rates between patients who had and had not received azathioprine, and no lymphomas occurred in the azathioprine group.[63]

Hypersensitivity

Acute hypersensitivity syndromes, usually occurring within 2 weeks of starting therapy, are rare, with a range of manifestations including shock, fever, rash, pancreatitis, renal failure, and hepatitis.[68]

Other Toxicities

Infection is less common with azathioprine than with alkylating agents; however, infections with a range of bacterial and nonbacterial pathogens, including herpes zoster and cytomegalovirus, may occur. The rate of infection when azathioprine is administered alone or with low doses of glucocorticoids is approximately 2.5 per 100 person-years of exposure. Maculopapular or urticarial rashes can occur. Eosinophilia and drug fever are rare.

Strategies to Minimize Toxicity

TPMT activity testing is the most commonly used method to identify patients at risk of serious toxicity. More than 23 variants in the

TPMT gene, associated with decreased TPMT activity, have been identified, with the TPMT*2, TPMT*3A, and TPMT*3C alleles accounting for most of the intermediate- or low-activity cases. The concordance between TPMT genetics and phenotypes is slightly less than 100%. TPMT activity (phenotype) can be measured directly in red blood cell membranes. Alternatively (e.g., in patients who have undergone blood transfusions), genetic polymorphisms can be identified by polymerase chain reaction. Guidelines for TPMT activity testing vary among different specialties, but it is generally recommended that TPMT status be tested before starting azathioprine therapy. Whether testing is cost-effective and clinically useful when compared with traditional monitoring of white blood cell counts is still a matter of debate.[69–72] In the absence of TPMT testing, administration of a low initial dose and careful monitoring of the white blood cell count in patients starting azathioprine is required. Some authors suggest weekly monitoring during the first 15 weeks of azathioprine treatment.[65] When patients are taking a stable dose of azathioprine, blood counts are monitored monthly and liver function tests are monitored every 3 to 4 months.

Drug Interactions

One of the most important and potentially fatal drug interactions in rheumatology is the ability of allopurinol to dramatically increase the cytotoxic effects of azathioprine through inhibition of xanthine oxidase–mediated inactivation of mercaptopurine.[73] Various strategies have been used to treat hyperuricemia and gout in patients receiving azathioprine, which is a common clinical problem after transplantation. Reduction of the dose of azathioprine by at least two-thirds in patients who also are receiving allopurinol is advocated. Because myelosuppression can still occur after a 75% reduction in dose, however, careful monitoring is required.[73] Alternatively, uricosurics such as benzbromarone have been effective and safe,[73] and MMF has been substituted for azathioprine as an alternative immunosuppressant.[74] The combination of azathioprine with several other drugs, including sulfasalazine, ganciclovir, angiotensin-converting enzyme inhibitors, carbamazepine, co-trimoxazole, and clozapine, may also increase the risk of myelosuppression.

Pregnancy and Lactation

Azathioprine is an FDA Pregnancy Category D drug. Azathioprine crosses the placenta, but drug and metabolite concentrations are lower in the fetal circulation, suggesting placental metabolism.[46,75] Data relating to rheumatologic diseases are limited, and although azathioprine is being used during pregnancy, it is better avoided during pregnancy and lactation if possible.[76] In a prospective observational study in 189 pregnant women treated with azathioprine for various autoimmune conditions, the rate of major malformation was 3.5%, which was similar to that of the general population.[77] Its use was associated with prematurity, however. Azathioprine may be considered in cases where the benefits of disease control in the mother give the best chances of term pregnancy and fetal survival.

Mycophenolate Mofetil

Structure

MMF, a prodrug, is the inactive 2-morpholinoester of mycophenolic acid, which is hydrolyzed to the active mycophenolic acid (MPA), an antibiotic with immunosuppressive effects.[78]

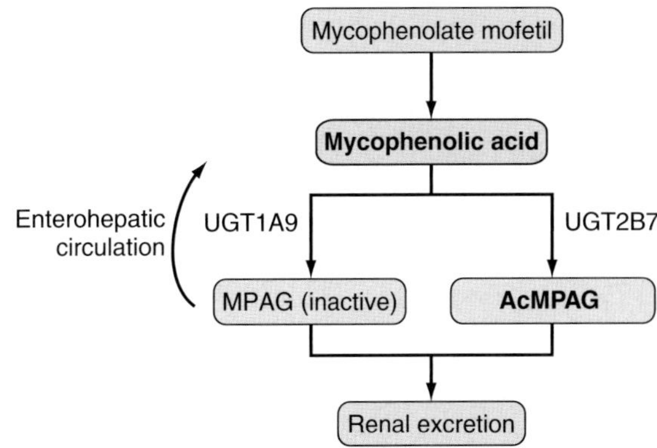

• **Fig. 65.3** Mycophenolate mofetil is converted to mycophenolic acid (MPA) and is subsequently metabolized to its glucuronide (Glu) conjugates, MPAG and AcMPAG, by different isoforms of UDP glucuronidyl transferases (UGT) in the liver. Pathways of enterohepatic circulation of MPA via the glucuronide conjugate metabolites are shown. The majority of MPAG is excreted in urine.

Mechanism of Action

Two pathways exist for the synthesis of guanine nucleotides: the de novo pathway and the salvage pathway. MPA reversibly inhibits inosine monophosphate dehydrogenase, a crucial enzyme for the de novo synthesis of guanosine purines.[78,79] Lymphocytes, in contrast to many other cells, are critically dependent on the de novo purine synthesis pathway and are a relatively selective target for MPA, accounting for the ability of the drug to inhibit reversibly B cell and T cell proliferation without myelotoxicity.[80] MPA results in decreased guanine synthesis and decreased DNA synthesis, decreased lymphocyte proliferation, altered microRNA expression, and decreased antibody production.[79–82] MPA also inhibits proliferation of fibroblasts, endothelial cells, and arterial smooth muscle cells and prevents deposition and contraction of collagen, extra-cellular matrix proteins, and smooth muscle actin.[83]

Pharmacology

MMF is rapidly and completely absorbed and de-esterified to the active MPA, which is highly (98%) protein bound. Most MPA (>99%) is found in plasma, with little in cells; most is glucuronidated to the poorly active, stable phenolic glucuronide, which is eliminated in the urine (Fig. 65.3).[84] Minor metabolites, some of which may be active, have also been described. Peak levels of MPA occur 1 to 2 hours after administration, and secondary peaks, thought to be due to enterohepatic circulation, can be seen. The half-life of MPA is 16 hours.[84] MPA concentrations may vary fivefold to tenfold in people receiving the same dose.[85] A small amount of this variability may be due to genetic variation in uridine-glucuronosyltransferase enzymes.[86] Renal disease and liver disease have relatively minor effects on the disposition of the active drug, MPA. Generally, dosage adjustments are not required,[84] but because free MPA concentrations are approximately doubled in patients with severe renal impairment (creatinine clearance <20 to 30 mL/min),[87] they may be necessary sometimes. A retrospective study in 16 patients with lupus nephritis showed that concentration-controlled dose adjustments with a target MPA area under the curve (AUC)—from intake until 12 hours after ingestion—of 60 to 90 mg*h/L were associated with optimized MPA exposure and excellent renal outcome at 12 months, although adverse effects were reported in one-third of patients, resulting in a switch to azathioprine in two patients.[88] Another observational study also pointed to the potential benefits of therapeutic monitoring in 34 patients with lupus nephritis when dosing was adjusted to achieve an AUC of 30 to 60 mg*h/L.[89] In this study, MPA exposure was not associated with adverse events, and patients with an AUC of 30 mg*h/L or greater had a greater renal response at 1 year. In a study involving 51 patients with lupus nephritis, a 4-hour AUC was found to be a better indicator of the adequacy of MMF-treatment than through levels.[90] The major glucuronide metabolite of MPA accumulates in patients with impaired renal function and may cause increased gastrointestinal adverse effects. Because MPA is highly protein bound, it is not cleared by hemodialysis.[91]

Dosage

Effective daily dosages of MMF range from 0.5 to 1.5 g twice a day. In 71 patients with lupus nephritis, the initial dose was 1 g/day with a target of 3 g/day. The mean maximal dose was 2680 mg/day, and 63% of patients tolerated 3 g/day.[42]

Clinical Indications

MMF is increasingly used as a safer alternative to cytostatic agents in the treatment of several systemic autoimmune diseases, notably SLE,[92] systemic sclerosis,[93] vasculitis,[94] and inflammatory muscle disease.[95,96] In a 24-week study in people with lupus nephritis, mycophenolate was more effective than monthly pulse cyclophosphamide, with a failure rate (without complete or partial remission at 24 weeks, plus those who stopped treatment for any reason) of 34 of 71 (47.9%) compared with 48 of 69 in the cyclophosphamide group (69.6%; P = 0.01).[42] In a systematic review of four trials involving 618 patients, MMF was not superior to cyclophosphamide for renal remission, and there was no significant difference for adverse events (infections, leukopenia, gastrointestinal symptoms, herpes zoster, end-stage renal disease, and death) except for a lower incidence of alopecia and amenorrhea with the use of MMF compared with cyclophosphamide.[97] Notwithstanding its appeal as a safer alternative to cyclophosphamide for remission induction therapy of lupus nephritis, MMF is most commonly used for maintenance therapy of lupus nephritis. Although systematic reviews comparing its efficacy and safety with azathioprine have not yielded consistent results, and a study on repeat kidney biopsies in 30 patients with lupus nephritis failed to detect differences between azathioprine and MMF as maintenance therapy after a short course of IV cyclophosphamide, a large randomized clinical trial of 240 patients with active lupus demonstrated superior efficacy of enteric-coated mycophenolate over azathioprine.[98–101] The use of enteric-coated mycophenolate in this trial was associated with a significantly greater proportion of patients achieving remission (32.5% vs. 19.2%), shorter time to remission, and lower flare rates, whereas there was no difference in adverse events, except for leucopenia, which occurred more frequently in the azathioprine group. A network meta-analysis of 53 randomized trials of cyclophosphamide, calcineurin-inhibitors, and MMF, involving 4222 patients with proliferative lupus nephritis, provided no conclusive evidence as to the best induction therapy but did confirm MMF was the most effective maintenance therapy.[102] MMF is an alternative remission induction agent for patients with anti-neutrophil cytoplasmic antibody–associated vasculitis and evidence of low disease activity and who are not at risk of experiencing organ damage.[103] MMF was slightly less effective than azathioprine in maintaining remission but was safer than cyclophosphamide.[104,105] In seven patients with myositis, six had a good clinical and biochemical response to mycophenolate,[96] an observation that was confirmed in another study in six patients who had refractory myositis.[106] In addition, in three studies in patients who had interstitial lung disease associated with dermatomyositis (n = 4) or other connective tissue diseases, including RA (n = 10) and systemic sclerosis (n = 13), MMF was effective in improving signs and symptoms of lung disease.[107–109] In a prospective, randomized clinical trial of 142 patients with scleroderma-related lung disease, a 2-year course of MMF was safer and better tolerated but not more effective than a 1-year course of oral cyclophosphamide.[110] In post-hoc analyses of the Scleroderma Lung Studies I and II, MMF was found to be associated with improvements in dyspnea, lung function, and skin thickening compared with placebo.[111,112] A modest beneficial effect of MMF on skin thickening was also found in early diffuse cutaneous systemic sclerosis patients from a large international observational study.[113] The clinical effects of MMF on skin thickening were paralleled by attenuation of inflammatory gene signatures in the skin.[114]

Toxicity

MMF is generally well tolerated. The most common adverse effects are gastrointestinal, such as diarrhea, nausea, abdominal pain, and vomiting. Occasional infections, leukopenia, lymphocytopenia, and elevated liver enzymes can occur. Of 54 patients with SLE treated with MMF over a 3-year period, 16% withdrew because of adverse events, with 73% continuing treatment at 12 months.[115] In patients with lupus nephritis, diarrhea was more common and serious infections were less common with MMF than with cyclophosphamide.[42] Enteric-coated mycophenolate sodium and MMF have similar rates of adverse effects.[116] Opportunistic infections, including one that was fatal, occurred in 3 of 10 patients with idiopathic dermatomyositis who were treated with glucocorticoids and MMF.[96]

Pregnancy and Lactation

MMF is an FDA Pregnancy Category C drug. Mycophenolic acid is associated with miscarriage and congenital malformations when used during pregnancy, and therefore it should be avoided whenever possible by women trying to conceive. Switching from MMF to azathioprine in 19 patients with SLE did not result in deterioration of global disease activity, and another study in 54 patients with SLE who had quiescent lupus nephritis showed that replacing MMF with azathioprine rarely leads to renal flares, and pregnancy outcomes were favorable.[117,118] MMF is transferred into the mother's milk, and extreme caution should be used in women with childbearing potential and lactating mothers.

Drug Interactions

Because MPA is glucuronidated and is not metabolized by CYP oxidation, there are few clinically significant drug interactions. Antacids reduce bioavailability by approximately 15%, and cholestyramine reduces bioavailability by approximately 40%.[119] Rifampin treatment reduced MPA concentrations twofold to threefold.[120] Co-administration with azathioprine is not recommended.

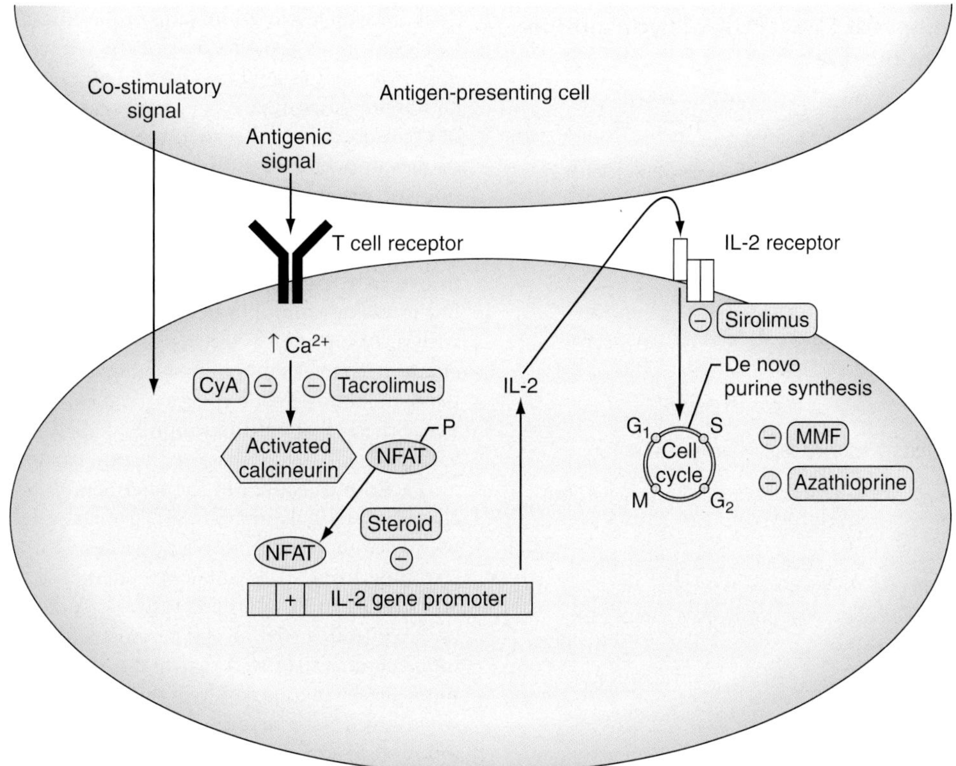

• **Fig. 65.4** Stages of T cell activation. Multiple targets for immunosuppressive agents. Stimulation of the T cell receptor results in calcineurin activation, a process inhibited by cyclosporine (CyA) and tacrolimus. Calcineurin dephosphorylates nuclear factor of activated T cells (NFAT), enabling it to enter the nucleus and bind to IL-2 promoter. Glucocorticoids inhibit cytokine gene transcription in lymphocytes and antigen-presenting cells by several mechanisms. Co-stimulatory signals are necessary to optimize T cell IL-2 gene transcription, prevent T cell anergy, and inhibit T cell apoptosis. IL-2 receptor stimulation induces the cell to enter the cell cycle and proliferate. This step may be blocked by IL-2 receptor antibodies or by sirolimus, which inhibits second messenger signals induced by IL-2 receptor ligation. After progression into the cell cycle, azathioprine and mycophenolate mofetil (MMF) interrupt DNA replication by inhibiting purine synthesis. (From Denton MD, Magee CC, Sayegh MH: Immunosuppressive strategies in transplantation. *Lancet* 353:1083–1091, 1999.)

Cyclosporine and Tacrolimus

Structure

Cyclosporine, a lipophilic endecapeptide derived from a fungus, and tacrolimus, a macrolide derived from an actinomycete, are calcineurin inhibitors used for their immunosuppressive properties in various rheumatic conditions.

Mechanism of Action

Calcineurin inhibitors impair production of IL-2 and other cytokines, reducing lymphocyte proliferation by forming complexes with cyclophilin, one of a group of cytosolic-binding proteins known as *immunophilins.* This complex binds to and inhibits calcineurin, a serine/threonine phosphatase. Inhibition of calcineurin phosphatase activity prevents the translocation of cytosolic nuclear factor of activated T cells (NFAT) to the nucleus, a translocation that is required for the transcription of genes for cytokines such as IL-2 and for T cell activation (Fig. 65.4).[121] Tacrolimus, previously known as FK506, is about 100 times more potent than cyclosporine and binds to a different immunophilin called *FK506 binding protein* (FKBP). This FK506–FKBP complex suppresses the activation of the calcineurin-dependent NFAT pathway and the activation of the calcineurin-independent pathway for c-Jun N-terminal kinase (JNK) and p38, inhibiting the early steps of T lymphocyte activation.

Pharmacology

Absorption and Distribution

Cyclosporine and tacrolimus are poorly and variably absorbed from the gut, with a bioavailability of approximately 30% and elimination half-lives ranging from 3 to 20 hours. Cyclosporine and tacrolimus are lipophilic and widely distributed in body tissues, particularly in the lean body mass.[122]

Metabolism and Elimination

The dispositions of cyclosporine and tacrolimus have two major determinants. First, P-glycoprotein (Pgp), a drug efflux pump, pumps substrates such as cyclosporine and tacrolimus out of cells. Pgp, the product of the multidrug resistance gene, is expressed on intestinal epithelial cells and in the liver. Second, cyclosporine and tacrolimus are extensively metabolized by the CYP3A enzyme system, which is active not only in the liver but also in intestinal epithelium. Pgp, by limiting drug uptake, and CYP3A4, by assisting drug metabolism in the gut and liver, act to limit the

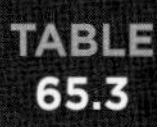

TABLE 65.3 Considerations for Clinical Use of Cyclosporine in Rheumatic Disease

Select appropriate patients
Contraindications: Current or past malignancy other than basal cell carcinoma, renal impairment, uncontrolled hypertension, or hepatic dysfunction
Cautions: Elderly age, obesity, controlled hypertension, premalignant lesions, drugs that interact with cyclosporine, pregnancy
Obtain ≥2 creatinine concentrations before starting cyclosporine, and average these to provide baseline creatinine value
Start low—cyclosporine 2.5 mg/kg/day in divided doses
Stay low—maximum 4 mg/kg/day (microemulsion formulation)
Monitor blood pressure and creatinine initially every 2 wk for 3 mo, then monthly if stable
If serum creatinine increases >30% above patient's baseline, reduce dosage of cyclosporine by 1 mg/kg/day; recheck serum creatinine in 1-2 wk, and temporarily discontinue cyclosporine if creatinine remains >30% above baseline
When creatinine level returns to within 15% of baseline, cyclosporine can be restarted at a lower dosage

bioavailability of cyclosporine and tacrolimus and determine their disposition.[123] Drugs that inhibit CYP3A4 or Pgp can increase tacrolimus concentrations (see Table 65.4).[124] Cyclosporine and tacrolimus elimination is not altered in renal failure[125]; however, because of their nephrotoxicity, cyclosporine and tacrolimus are avoided in patients with impaired renal function. Liver disease impairs the excretion of cyclosporine and tacrolimus metabolites.

Dosage

Because of their narrow therapeutic window, effective use of cyclosporine and tacrolimus requires that appropriate patients be selected for treatment and monitored carefully (Table 65.3). The starting dosage of cyclosporine is 2.5 mg/kg/day, usually administered in divided doses. In obese patients, dosage is based on the approximate ideal body weight. Clinical response is slow, occurring over 4 to 8 weeks, and may be maximal only after 12 weeks or more of treatment. To improve efficacy, the dosage can be increased by 0.5 mg/kg/day at 4- to 8-week intervals to a maximal dosage of 4 mg/kg/day of the microemulsion formulation. If no clinical response occurs in 4 to 6 months, cyclosporine should be discontinued. In patients whose disease is well controlled, the dosage of cyclosporine can be decreased by 0.5 mg/kg/day at 4- to 8-week intervals to determine the minimal effective dose for the individual patient. Tacrolimus is usually started at 2 mg/day, then increased to 4 mg/day with weekly monitoring of plasma concentrations until reaching a target concentration of 4 to 6 nm/mL.

Clinical Indications

Cyclosporine can be a useful drug in refractory RA in combination with methotrexate and hydroxychloroquine, although this combination has been superseded by combinations of methotrexate and biologics and the Janus kinase (JAK)/signal transducer and activator of transcription (STAT) inhibitors.[126] Cyclosporine can increase mean peak plasma methotrexate levels and AUC by about 20%,[127] which may contribute to the efficacy of the combination. Cyclosporine is also effective for the skin and joint manifestations of psoriasis, although biologics and other new agents are used more commonly nowadays.[128] Fewer data are available regarding the use of cyclosporine in other rheumatic diseases. In uncontrolled, small studies in people with SLE,[129] cyclosporine has been reported to improve disease activity, have a glucocorticoid-sparing effect, and improve proteinuria, thrombocytopenia, and leukopenia. The efficacy of cyclosporine as a glucocorticoid-sparing drug was confirmed in a randomized clinical trial in patients with severe SLE, but it was not found to be more effective or safer when compared with azathioprine.[130] Cyclosporine has also been reported to be effective in small series of cases in many other autoimmune conditions, including pyoderma gangrenosum, Behçet's disease, maintenance therapy of anti-neutrophil cytoplasmic antibody–associated vasculitis, and macrophage-activation syndrome in juvenile RA.[131]

Tacrolimus is used in the treatment of SLE and myositis-associated interstitial lung disease. Topical 1% tacrolimus has been used with moderate success in patients with resistant skin disease resulting from SLE, subacute cutaneous lupus erythematosus, and discoid lupus erythematosus.[132] A large open-label, randomized, controlled trial in 150 patients with biopsy-confirmed active lupus nephritis showed that remission induction with tacrolimus (0.06 to 0.1 mg/kg/day) was not inferior to MMF (2 to 3 g/day) when given with prednisolone (0.6 mg/kg/day) for 6 weeks and followed by azathioprine maintenance, with major infectious episodes occurring in 5.4% versus 9.2% of patients, respectively.[133] To avoid the toxicities of standard drug dosing, tacrolimus (4 mg/day) has been combined with low-dose MMF (1 g/day) in lupus nephritis (class III, IV, V) in a large randomized, controlled trial involving 368 Chinese patients. The combination was superior to intravenous cyclophosphamide pulses in achieving complete renal response at 6 months (46% vs. 26%; $P < 0.001$), albeit at the expense of infectious complications.[134] Tacrolimus has also been advocated in patients who had interstitial lung disease associated with polymyositis or dermatomyositis based on observational studies. Patients treated with tacrolimus in addition to conventional therapy had a significantly improved survival compared with patients who were treated with conventional therapy alone.[135]

Toxicity

Cyclosporin has a longer track record in rheumatology than tacrolimus. Thus most of the toxicity data discussed in the following sections are derived from clinical studies with cyclosporin, although cyclosporin and tacrolimus share comparable toxicity profiles.[121] Long-term safety data, particularly with regards to nephrotoxicity, on tacrolimus are lacking. In the few studies in SLE done to date, tacrolimus has reportedly been associated with a lower frequency of cosmetic, hypertensive, and dyslipidemic adverse effects, but head-to-head studies have not yet been conducted.

Hypertension

Hypertension occurs in approximately 20% of patients with autoimmune disease who receive treatment with cyclosporine. The magnitude of increase in blood pressure (BP) is usually mild but clinically significant because it increases the risk of stroke, myocardial infarction, heart failure, and other adverse cardiovascular events associated with elevated BP.[136] The hypertension should be controlled by reducing the dose of cyclosporine or by anti-hypertensive drug therapy.[137]

Nephrotoxicity

Virtually all patients who take cyclosporine have a small but measurable decrease in renal function that is reversible after cyclosporine is discontinued. Serum creatinine concentrations have increased approximately 20% in 6- to 12-month clinical trials, but few patients have had to withdraw because of this outcome.[138] Long-term data regarding renal function in patients with RA who are treated with cyclosporine are limited. In one 12-month study, an increase in serum creatinine of more than 30% occurred in 50% of patients; half of these patients responded to cyclosporine dose reduction and half did not, requiring discontinuation of the drug.[137] The small increase in serum creatinine observed in most studies occurs mainly during the first 2 to 3 months of treatment, and then creatinine remains relatively stable over 12 months.[137,138] Other data, however, suggest that over periods of treatment longer than 1 year, many patients, who over the first year had a stable, acceptable increase in creatinine concentration, subsequently have an increase in creatinine to more than 30% of baseline that is not controlled by cyclosporine dose reduction; such patients must discontinue treatment.[139] Preventable risk factors for cyclosporine-induced nephrotoxicity are a high dosage of cyclosporine (>5 mg/kg/day) and an increase in serum creatinine concentration of more than 50% of the baseline value. The risk of cyclosporine nephropathy is low in patients treated according to the clinical guidelines (see Table 65.3).

Gastrointestinal

Gastrointestinal upset is common but usually mild and transient. A few patients discontinue cyclosporine therapy for this reason, however.

Malignancy

In transplant recipients, cyclosporine use has been associated with an increased risk of skin cancer and lymphoma. In 208 patients with RA who were treated with cyclosporine for an average of 1.6 years, the incidence of malignancy and mortality was similar to that of control subjects with RA,[140] but a meta-analysis on the risk of immunomodulatory drugs in people with RA, psoriasis, and psoriatic arthritis did find an increased risk of nonmelanoma skin cancer in patients treated with cyclosporine.[141] Epstein-Barr virus–induced B cell lymphoma, which may be reversible when cyclosporine is discontinued, has been reported in a few patients receiving cyclosporine for a variety of indications.

Other Toxicities

Other adverse effects that are common but usually of minor significance include hypertrichosis, gingival hyperplasia, tremor, paresthesia, breast tenderness, hyperkalemia, hypomagnesemia, and an increase in serum uric acid.[137] Cyclosporine may result in a clinically insignificant increase in alkaline phosphatase concentrations but does not increase the frequency of abnormal transaminase concentrations in patients also receiving methotrexate.[142]

Strategies to Minimize Toxicity

Because cyclosporine may increase liver enzymes, as well as potassium, uric acid, and lipid concentrations, and decrease magnesium concentrations, it is prudent to measure these enzymes and concentrations before, and occasionally after, initiating therapy. At least two, and preferably more, recent normal BP and serum creatinine determinations should be obtained before starting treatment.

TABLE 65.4 Clinically Important Drug Interactions With Cyclosporine[a]

Increased Cyclosporine Concentrations
Erythromycin, clarithromycin
Azole antifungals: ketoconazole, fluconazole, itraconazole
Calcium channel antagonists: diltiazem, verapamil, amlodipine[b]
Grapefruit juice
Others: amiodarone, danazol, allopurinol, colchicine
Decreased Cyclosporine Concentrations
Inducers of hepatic enzymes: rifampicin, phenytoin, phenobarbitone, nafcillin, St John's wort
Increased Cyclosporine Toxicity
Increased renal toxicity with aminoglycosides, quinolone antibiotics, amphotericin B, (?) nonsteroidal anti-inflammatory drugs, (?) angiotensin-converting enzyme inhibitors
Cyclosporine Increasing Toxicity of Another Drug
Increased risk of myopathy and rhabdomyolysis with lovastatin and other statins
Increased risk of colchicine neuromyopathy and toxicity
Increased digoxin concentrations
Increased risk of hyperkalemia with K^+-sparing diuretics and K^+ supplements

[a]Most interactions with cyclosporine are also likely to apply to tacrolimus.

[b]Data are conflicting about whether amlodipine does or does not increase cyclosporine concentrations.

Cyclosporine concentrations are not useful predictors of efficacy or toxicity in rheumatic diseases and are not routinely performed. Cyclosporine trough concentrations, which are measured approximately 12 hours after the last dose, can be useful if concerns exist about compliance or unusual drug disposition in individual patients.

Pregnancy and Lactation

Cyclosporine and tacrolimus are FDA Pregnancy Category C drugs. Cyclosporine and tacrolimus use in pregnancy is not recommended unless the potential benefit exceeds the potential risk to the fetus. Breastfeeding should be avoided.

Drug Interactions

Cyclosporine and tacrolimus, because of the influence of Pgp and CYP3A4 enzyme activity on their disposition, have many clinically important drug interactions (Table 65.4).[143] Many drugs, such as erythromycin, azole antifungal drugs, and some calcium channel antagonists that inhibit CYP3A4 (inhibiting the metabolism of cyclosporine), also inhibit Pgp. Drug interactions mediated by these dual mechanisms may result in increases in cyclosporine and tacrolimus concentrations. Azithromycin, in contrast to erythromycin and clarithromycin, seems unlikely to alter cyclosporine levels. The plasma concentrations and clinical toxicity of several statin lipid-lowering agents are increased substantially by cyclosporine, but the pharmacokinetics of fluvastatin and pravastatin, because they are not metabolized primarily by CYP3A4, are altered less by cyclosporine.[144] Nevertheless, the pravastatin AUC curve, a measure of drug exposure, was five times higher in patients also receiving cyclosporine.[145] Of the calcium channel antagonists, diltiazem, nicardipine, and verapamil increase cyclosporine concentrations; nifedipine and amlodipine have variable effects; and isradipine and nitrendipine do not generally affect concentrations.[146] It is controversial whether nonsteroidal anti-inflammatory drugs (NSAIDs) increase cyclosporine nephrotoxicity. Cyclosporine and NSAIDs have been safely co-administered[147]; however, increased cyclosporine-associated nephrotoxicity with NSAIDs has been reported. If serum creatinine increases, in addition to decreasing the dose of cyclosporine, discontinuation of the NSAID may be tried. Grapefruit juice increases plasma concentrations of cyclosporine and tacrolimus, so patients should be warned to avoid consuming grapefruit.

Conclusion

Immunosuppressive drugs are key therapeutic tools in the management of many rheumatic diseases. They include alkylating agents such as cyclophosphamide and purine analogue cytotoxic drugs such as azathioprine with a long history of clinical use in rheumatology, as well as noncytotoxic immunosuppressants such as MMF, which is increasingly used in rheumatologic practice as a key anchor drug in the management of systemic autoimmune diseases, and the less commonly used calcineurin inhibitors cyclosporin and tacrolimus. In contrast to exquisitely targeted therapeutics represented by biologics and small molecules, our understanding of the in vivo mechanism of action of immunosuppressive drugs is still limited. In contrast, their potential clinical efficacy and safety profiles are generally well known, and serious toxicities can usually be prevented by careful monitoring of laboratory tests for white blood cell counts, liver and renal function, and electrolytes. Nevertheless, vigilance is required, because the risk of (opportunistic) infection is increased.[148,149] As a general rule, combination therapy of the different immunosuppressants discussed earlier should be avoided. The individual response to immunosuppressive therapy can be highly variable, and decisions to continue a chosen immunosuppressant should be revisited on a regular basis, weighing the benefits and adverse effects. Clinical decision making is an evolutionary process, and ongoing and future clinical trials will determine whether conventional immunosuppressive drugs are going to be superseded by newer drugs such as JAK/STAT inhibitors or biologics, which have acquired a firm niche in the treatment of arthritic diseases.

 Full references for this chapter can be found on ExpertConsult.com.

Selected References

1. de Jonge ME, Huitema AD, Rodenhuis S, et al.: Clinical pharmacokinetics of cyclophosphamide, *Clin Pharmacokinet* 44:1135–1164, 2005.
2. Fauci AS, Wolff SM, Johnson JS: Effect of cyclophosphamide upon the immune response in Wegener's granulomatosis, *N Engl J Med* 285:1493–1496, 1971.
3. Struck RF, Alberts DS, Horne K, et al.: Plasma pharmacokinetics of cyclophosphamide and its cytotoxic metabolites after intravenous versus oral administration in a randomized, crossover trial, *Cancer Res* 47:2723–2726, 1987.
4. Takada K, Arefayene M, Desta Z, et al.: Cytochrome P450 pharmacogenetics as a predictor of toxicity and clinical response to pulse cyclophosphamide in lupus nephritis, *Arthritis Rheum* 50:2202–2210, 2004.
5. Haubitz M, Bohnenstengel F, Brunkhorst R, et al.: Cyclophosphamide pharmacokinetics and dose requirements in patients with renal insufficiency, *Kidney Int* 61:1495–1501, 2002.
6. Moroni G, Raffiotta F, Trezzi B, et al.: Rituximab vs mycophenolate and vs cyclophosphamide pulses for induction therapy of active lupus nephritis: a clinical observational study, *Rheumatology (Oxford)* 53:1570–1577, 2014.
7. Illei GG, Austin HA, Crane M, et al.: Combination therapy with pulse cyclophosphamide plus pulse methylprednisolone improves long-term renal outcome without adding toxicity in patients with lupus nephritis, *Ann Intern Med* 135:248–257, 2001.
8. Houssiau FA, Vasconcelos C, D'Cruz D, et al.: The 10-year follow-up data of the Euro-Lupus Nephritis trial comparing low-dose and high-dose intravenous cyclophosphamide, *Ann Rheum Dis* 69:61–64, 2010.
9. Trevisani VF, Castro AA, Neves Neto JF, et al.: Cyclophosphamide versus methylprednisolone for treating neuropsychiatric involvement in systemic lupus erythematosus, *Cochrane Database Syst Rev* 2:CD002265, 2006.
10. Tashkin DP, Elashoff R, Clements PJ, et al.: Cyclophosphamide versus placebo in scleroderma lung disease, *N Engl J Med* 354:2655–2666, 2006.
11. Hoyles RK, Ellis RW, Wellsbury J, et al.: A multicenter, prospective, randomized, double-blind, placebo-controlled trial of corticosteroids and intravenous cyclophosphamide followed by oral azathioprine for the treatment of pulmonary fibrosis in scleroderma, *Arthritis Rheum* 54:3962–3970, 2006.
12. Barnes H, Holland AE, Westall GP, et al.: Cyclophosphamide for connective tissue disease-associated interstitial lung disease, *Cochrane Database Syst Rev* 1:CD010908, 2018.
13. Guillevin L, Cordier JF, Lhote F, et al.: A prospective, multicenter, randomized trial comparing steroids and pulse cyclophosphamide versus steroids and oral cyclophosphamide in the treatment of generalized Wegener's granulomatosis, *Arthritis Rheum* 40:2187–2198, 1997.
14. Haubitz M, Schellong S, Gobel U, et al.: Intravenous pulse administration of cyclophosphamide versus daily oral treatment in patients with antineutrophil cytoplasmic antibody-associated vasculitis and renal involvement: a prospective, randomized study, *Arthritis Rheum* 41:1835–1844, 1998.
15. de Groot K, Harper L, Jayne DR, et al.: Pulse versus daily oral cyclophosphamide for induction of remission in antineutrophil cytoplasmic antibody-associated vasculitis: a randomized trial, *Ann Intern Med* 150:670–680, 2009.
16. Harper L, Morgan MD, Walsh M, et al.: Pulse versus daily oral cyclophosphamide for induction of remission in ANCA-associated vasculitis: long-term follow-up, *Ann Rheum Dis* 71:95560, 2012.
17. Jayne D, Rasmussen N, Andrassy K, et al.: A randomized trial of maintenance therapy for vasculitis associated with antineutrophil cytoplasmic autoantibodies, *N Engl J Med* 349:36–44, 2003.
18. Farge D, Labopin M, Tyndall A, et al.: Autologous hematopoietic stem cell transplantation for autoimmune diseases: an observational study on 12 years' experience from the European Group for Blood and Marrow Transplantation Working Party on Autoimmune Diseases, *Haematologica* 95:284–292, 2010.
19. Petri M, Brodsky RA, Jones RJ, et al.: High-dose cyclophosphamide versus monthly intravenous cyclophosphamide for systemic lupus erythematosus: a prospective randomised trial, *Arthritis Rheum* 62:1487–1493, 2010.
20. Burt RK, Shah SJ, Dill K, et al.: Autologous non-myeloablative haemopoietic stem-cell transplantation compared with pulse cyclophosphamide once per month for systemic sclerosis (ASSIST): an open-label, randomised phase 2 trial, *Lancet* 378:498–506, 2011.
21. van Laar JM, Farge D, Sont JK, et al.: Autologous hematopoietic stem cell transplantation vs intravenous pulse cyclophosphamide in diffuse cutaneous systemic sclerosis: a randomized clinical trial, *JAMA* 311:2490–2498, 2014.

22. Sullivan KM, Goldmuntz EA, Keyes-Elstein L, et al.: Myeloablative autologous stem-cell transplantation for severe scleroderma, *N Engl J Med* 378:35–47, 2018.
23. Kurauchi K, Nishikawa T, Mijahara E, et al.: Role of metabolites of cyclophosphamide in cardiotoxicity, *BMC Res Notes* 10:406, 2017.
24. Fraiser LH, Kanekal S, Kehrer JP: Cyclophosphamide toxicity: characterising and avoiding the problem, *Drugs* 42:781–795, 1991.
25. Pryor BD, Bologna SG, Kahl LE: Risk factors for serious infection during treatment with cyclophosphamide and high-dose corticosteroids for systemic lupus erythematosus [erratum appears in *Arthritis Rheum* 40(9):1711, 1997], *Arthritis Rheum* 39:1475–1482, 1996.
26. Gourley MF, Austin HA, Scott D, et al.: Methylprednisolone and cyclophosphamide, alone or in combination, in patients with lupus nephritis: a randomized, controlled trial, *Ann Intern Med* 125:549–557, 1996.
27. Hoffman GS, Kerr GS, Leavitt RY, et al.: Wegener granulomatosis: an analysis of 158 patients, *Ann Intern Med* 116:488–498, 1992.
28. Godeau B, Mainardi JL, Roudot-Thoraval F, et al.: Factors associated with Pneumocystis carinii pneumonia in Wegener's granulomatosis, *Ann Rheum Dis* 54:991–994, 1995.
29. Goren MP: Oral mesna: a review, *Semin Oncol* 19(6 Suppl 12):65–71, 1992.
30. Monach PA, Arnold LM, Merkel PA: Incidence and prevention of bladder toxicity from cyclophosphamide in the treatment of rheumatic diseases. a data driven review, *Arthritis Rheum* 62:9–21, 2010.
31. Reinhold-Keller E, Beuge N, Latza U, et al.: An interdisciplinary approach to the care of patients with Wegener's granulomatosis: longterm outcome in 155 patients [erratum appears in *Arthritis Rheum* 43(10):2379, 2000], *Arthritis Rheum* 43:1021–1032, 2000.
32. Radis CD, Kahl LE, Baker GL, et al.: Effects of cyclophosphamide on the development of malignancy and on long-term survival of patients with rheumatoid arthritis: a 20-year followup study, *Arthritis Rheum* 38:1120–1127, 1995.
33. Mok CC, Lau CS, Wong RW: Risk factors for ovarian failure in patients with systemic lupus erythematosus receiving cyclophosphamide therapy, *Arthritis Rheum* 41:831–837, 1998.
34. Byrne J, Rasmussen SA, Steinhorn SC, et al.: Genetic disease in offspring of long-term survivors of childhood and adolescent cancer, *Am J Hum Genet* 62:45–52, 1998.
35. Malik SW, Myers JL, DeRemee RA, et al.: Lung toxicity associated with cyclophosphamide use: two distinct patterns, *Am J Respir Crit Care Med* 154(6 Pt 1):1851–1856, 1996.
36. Bressler RB, Huston DP: Water intoxication following moderate dose intravenous cyclophosphamide, *Arch Intern Med* 145:548–549, 1985.
37. Knysak DJ, McLean JA, Solomon WR, et al.: Immediate hypersensitivity reaction to cyclophosphamide, *Arthritis Rheum* 37:1101–1104, 1994.
38. Reinhold-Keller E, Mohr J, Christophers E, et al.: Mesna side effects which imitate vasculitis, *Clin Invest* 70:698–704, 1992.
39. Langford CA, Klippel JH, Balow JE, et al.: Use of cytotoxic agents and cyclosporine in the treatment of autoimmune disease, part 2: inflammatory bowel disease, systemic vasculitis, and therapeutic toxicity, *Ann Intern Med* 129:49–58, 1998.
40. Talar-Williams C, Hijazi YM, Walther MM, et al.: Cyclophosphamide induced cystitis and bladder cancer in patients with Wegener granulomatosis, *Ann Intern Med* 124:477–484, 1996.
41. Mukhtyar C, Guillevin L, Cid MC, et al.: EULAR recommendations for the management of primary small and medium vessel vasculitis, *Ann Rheum Dis* 68:310–317, 2009.
42. Ginzler EM, Dooley MA, Aranow C, et al.: Mycophenolate mofetil or intravenous cyclophosphamide for lupus nephritis, *N Engl J Med* 353:2219–2228, 2005.
43. Yates M, Watts RA, Bajema IM, et al.: EULAR/ERA-EDTA recommendations for the management of ANCA-associated vasculitis, *Ann Rheum Dis* 75:1583–1594, 2016.
44. Gordon C, Amissah-Arthur MB, Gayed M, et al.: The British Society for Rheumatology guideline for the management of systemic lupus erythematosus in adults: executive summary, *Rheumatology (Oxford)* 57:14–18, 2018.
45. Clowse ME, Magder L, Petri M: Cyclophosphamide for lupus during pregnancy, *Lupus* 14:593–597, 2005.
46. Ostensen M: Disease specific problems related to drug therapy in pregnancy, *Lupus* 13:746–750, 2004.
47. Anthony LB, Long QC, Struck RF, et al.: The effect of cimetidine on cyclophosphamide metabolism in rabbits, *Cancer Chemother Pharmacol* 27:125–130, 1990.
48. Alberts DS, Mason-Liddil N, Plezia PM, et al.: Lack of ranitidine effects on cyclophosphamide bone marrow toxicity or metabolism: a placebo-controlled clinical trial, *J Natl Cancer Inst* 83:1739–1742, 1991.
49. Allopurinol and cytotoxic drugs: interaction in relation to bone marrow depression. Boston collaborative drug surveillance program, *JAMA* 227:1036–1040, 1974.
50. Koseoglu V, Chiang J, Chan KW: Acquired pseudocholinesterase deficiency after high-dose cyclophosphamide, *Bone Marrow Transplant* 24:1367–1368, 1999.
51. van Scoik KG, Johnson CA, Porter WR: The pharmacology and metabolism of the thiopurine drugs 6-mercaptopurine and azathioprine, *Drug Metab Rev* 16:157–174, 1985.
52. van Os EC, Zins BJ, Sandborn WJ, et al.: Azathioprine pharmacokinetics after intravenous, oral, delayed release oral and rectal foam administration, *Gut* 39:63–68, 1996.
53. Stolk JN, Boerbooms AM, de Abreu RA, et al.: Reduced thiopurine methyltransferase activity and development of side effects of azathioprine treatment in patients with rheumatoid arthritis, *Arthritis Rheum* 41:1858–1866, 1998.
54. Bergan S, Rugstad HE, Bentdal O, et al.: Kinetics of mercaptopurine and thioguanine nucleotides in renal transplant recipients during azathioprine treatment, *Therap Drug Monit* 16:13–20, 1994.
55. Chocair PR, Duley JA, Simmonds HA, et al.: The importance of thiopurine methyltransferase activity for the use of azathioprine in transplant recipients, *Transplantation* 53:1051–1056, 1992.
56. Grootscholten C, Ligtenberg G, Hagen EC, et al.: Azathioprine/methylprednisolone versus cyclophosphamide in proliferative lupus nephritis: a randomized controlled trial, *Kidney Int* 70:732–742, 2006.
57. Contreras G, Pardo V, Leclercq B, et al.: Sequential therapies for proliferative lupus nephritis, *N Engl J Med* 350:971–980, 2004.
58. Rahman P, Humphrey-Murto S, Gladman DD, et al.: Cytotoxic therapy in systemic lupus erythematosus: experience from a single center, *Medicine* 76:432–437, 1997.
59. Hamuryudan V, Ozyazgan Y, Hizli N, et al.: Azathioprine in Behçet's syndrome: effects on long-term prognosis, *Arthritis Rheum* 40:769–774, 1997.
60. Jones G, Crotty M, Brooks P: Psoriatic arthritis: a quantitative overview of therapeutic options. the psoriatic arthritis meta-analysis study group, *Br J Rheumatol* 36:95–99, 1997.
61. Benenson E, Fries JW, Heilig B, et al.: High-dose azathioprine pulse therapy as a new treatment option in patients with active Wegener's granulomatosis and lupus nephritis refractory or intolerant to cyclophosphamide, *Clin Rheumatol* 24:251–257, 2005.
62. Bérezné A, Ranque B, Valeyre D, et al.: Therapeutic strategy combining intravenous cyclophosphamide followed by oral azathioprine to treat worsening interstitial lung disease associated with systemic sclerosis: a retrospective multicenter open-label study, *J Rheumatol* 35:1064–1072, 2008.
63. Nero P, Rahman A, Isenberg DA: Does long term treatment with azathioprine predispose to malignancy and death in patients with systemic lupus erythematosus? *Ann Rheum Dis* 63:325–326, 2004.
64. Szumlanski CL, Honchel R, Scott MC, et al.: Human liver thiopurine methyltransferase pharmacogenetics: biochemical properties, liver erythrocyte correlation and presence of isozymes, *Pharmacogenetics* 2:148–159, 1992.

65. McLeod HL, Lin JS, Scott EP, et al.: Thiopurine methyltransferase activity in American white subjects and black subjects, *Clin Pharmacol Ther* 55:15–20, 1994.
66. Leipold G, Schutz E, Haas JP, et al.: Azathioprine-induced severe pancytopenia due to a homozygous two-point mutation of the thiopurine methyltransferase gene in a patient with juvenile HLA-B27-associated spondylarthritis, *Arthritis Rheum* 40:1896–1898, 1997.
67. Silman AJ, Petrie J, Hazleman B, et al.: Lymphoproliferative cancer and other malignancy in patients with rheumatoid arthritis treated with azathioprine: a 20 year follow up study, *Ann Rheum Dis* 47:988–992, 1988.
68. Fields CL, Robinson JW, Roy TM, et al.: Hypersensitivity reaction to azathioprine, *South Med J* 91:471–474, 1998.
69. Schedel J, Gödde A, Schütz E, et al.: Impact of thiopurine methyltransferase activity and 6-thioguanine nucleotide concentrations in patients with chronic inflammatory diseases, *Ann N Y Acad Sci* 1069:477–491, 2006.
70. Stassen PM, Derks RPH, Kallenberg CGM, et al.: Thiopurine-methyltransferase (TPMT) genotype and TPMT activity in patients with anti-neutrophil cytoplasmic antibody-associated vasculitis: relation to azathioprine maintenance treatment and adverse effects, *Ann Rheum Dis* 68:758–759, 2009.
71. Tani C, Mosca M, Colucci R, et al.: Genetic polymorphisms of thiopurine S-methyltransferase in a cohort of patients with systemic autoimmune diseases, *Clin Exp Rheumatol* 27:321–324, 2009.
72. Payne K, Newman W, Fargher E, et al.: TPMT testing: any better than routine monitoring? *Rheumatology* 46:727–729, 2007.
73. Cummins D, Sekar M, Halil O, et al.: Myelosuppression associated with azathioprine-allopurinol interaction after heart and lung transplantation, *Transplantation* 61:1661–1662, 1996.
74. Navascues RA, Gomez E, Rodriguez M, et al.: Safety of the allopurinol-mycophenolate mofetil combination in the treatment of hyperuricemia of kidney transplant recipients, *Nephron* 91:173–174, 2002.
75. de Boer NK, Jarbandhan SV, de Graaf P, et al.: Azathioprine use during pregnancy: unexpected intrauterine exposure to metabolites, *Am J Gastroenterol* 101:1390–1392, 2006.
76. Temprano KK, Bandlamudi R, Moore TL: Antirheumatic drugs in pregnancy and lactation, *Semin Arthritis Rheum* 35:112–121, 2005.
77. Goldstein LH, Dolinsky G, Greenberg R, et al.: Pregnancy outcome of women exposed to azathioprine during pregnancy, *Birth Defects Res A Clin Mol Teratol* 79:696–701, 2007.
78. Lipsky JJ: Mycophenolate mofetil, *Lancet* 348:1357–1359, 1996.
79. Ransom JT: Mechanism of action of mycophenolate mofetil, *Ther Drug Monit* 17:681–684, 1995.
80. Suthanthiran M, Strom TB: Immunoregulatory drugs: mechanistic basis for use in organ transplantation, *Pediatr Nephrol* 11:651–657, 1997.
81. Tang Q, Yang Y, Zhao M, et al.: Mycophenolic acid upregulates miR-142-3P/5P and miR-146a in lupus CD4+T cells, *Lupus* 24:935–942, 2015.
82. Smith KG, Isbel NM, Catton MG, et al.: Suppression of the humoral immune response by mycophenolate mofetil, *Nephrol Dial Transplant* 13:160–164, 1998.
83. Roos N, Poulalhon N, Farge D, et al.: In vitro evidence for a direct antifibrotic role of the immunosuppressive drug mycophenolate mofetil, *J Pharmacol Exp Ther* 321:583–589, 2007.
84. Bullingham RE, Nicholls AJ, Kamm BR: Clinical pharmacokinetics of mycophenolate mofetil, *Clin Pharmacokinet* 34:429–455, 1998.
85. van Hest RM, Mathot RA, Vulto AG, et al.: Within-patient variability of mycophenolic acid exposure: therapeutic drug monitoring from a clinical point of view, *Ther Drug Monit* 28:31–34, 2006.
86. Kuypers DR, Naesens M, Vermeire S, et al.: The impact of uridine diphosphate-glucuronosyltransferase 1A9 (UGT1A9) gene promoter region single-nucleotide polymorphisms T-275A and C-2152T on early mycophenolic acid dose-interval exposure in de novo renal allograft recipients, *Clin Pharmacol Ther* 78:351–361, 2005.
87. Meier-Kriesche HU, Shaw LM, Korecka M, et al.: Pharmacokinetics of mycophenolic acid in renal insufficiency, *Ther Drug Monit* 22:27–30, 2000.
88. Daleboudt GM, Reinders ME, den Hartigh J, et al.: Concentration-controlled treatment of lupus nephritis with mycophenolate mofetil, *Lupus* 22:171–179, 2013.
89. Alexander S, Fleming DH, Mathew BS, et al.: Pharmacokinetics of concentration-controlled mycophenolate mofetil in proliferative lupus nephritis: an observational cohort study, *Ther Drug Monit* 36:423–432, 2014.
90. Pourafshar N, Karimi A, Wen X, et al.: The utility of trough mycophenolate acid levels for the management of lupus nephritis, *Nephrol Dial Transpl* March 13, 2018 (Epub ahead of print).
91. Johnson HJ, Swan SK, Heim-Duthoy KL, et al.: The pharmacokinetics of a single oral dose of mycophenolate mofetil in patients with varying degrees of renal function, *Clin Pharmacol Ther* 63:512–518, 1998.
92. Chan TM, Li FK, Tang CS, et al.: Efficacy of mycophenolate mofetil in patients with diffuse proliferative lupus nephritis. Hong Kong-Guangzhou Nephrology Study Group, *N Engl J Med* 343:1156–1162, 2000.
93. Derk CT, Grace E, Shenin M, et al.: A prospective open-label study of mycophenolate mofetil for the treatment of diffuse systemic sclerosis, *Rheumatology (Oxford)* 48:1595–1599, 2009.
94. Langford CA, Talar-Williams C, Sneller MC: Mycophenolate mofetil for remission maintenance in the treatment of Wegener's granulomatosis, *Arthritis Rheum* 51:278–283, 2004.
95. Majithia V, Harisdangkul V: Mycophenolate mofetil (CellCept): an alternative therapy for autoimmune inflammatory myopathy, *Rheumatology (Oxford)* 44:386–389, 2005.
96. Rowin J, Amato AA, Deisher N, et al.: Mycophenolate mofetil in dermatomyositis: is it safe? *Neurology* 66:1245–1247, 2006.
97. Touma Z, Gladman DD, Urowitz MB, et al.: Mycophenolate mofetil for induction treatment of lupus nephritis: a systematic review and meta-analysis, *J Rheumatol* 38:39–78, 2011.
98. Henderson L, Masson P, Craig JC, et al.: Treatment for lupus nephritis, *Cochrane Database Syst Rev* 12:CD0022922, 2012.
99. Maneiro JR, Lopez-Canoa N, Salgado E, et al.: Maintenance therapy of lupus nephritis with mycophenolate or azathioprine: a systematic review and meta-analysis, *Rheumatology* 53:834–838, 2014.
100. Stoenoiu MS, Aydin S, Tektonidou M, et al.: Repeat kidney biopsies fail to detect differences between azathioprine and mycophenolate mofetil maintenance therapy for lupus nephritis: data from the MAINTAIN Nephritis Trial, *Nephrol Dial Transpl* 27:1924–1930, 2012.
101. Ordi-Ros J, Sáez-Comet L, Pérez-Conessa M, et al.: Enteric-coated mycophenolate sodium versus azathioprine in patients with active systemic lupus erythematosus: a randomised clinical trial, *Ann Rheum Dis* 76:1575–1582, 2017.
102. Palmer SC, Tunnicliffe DJ, Singh-Grewal D, et al.: Induction and maintenance immunosuppression treatment of proliferative lupus nephritis: a network meta-analysis of randomized trials, *Am J Kidney Dis* 70:324–336, 2017.
103. Ntatsaki E, Carruthers D, Chakravarty K, et al.: BSR and BHPR guideline for the management of adults with ANCA-associated vasculitis, *Rheumatology* 53:2306–2309, 2014.
104. Hiemstra TF, Walsh M, Mahr A, et al.: Mycophenolate mofetil vs azathioprine for remission maintenance in antineutrophil cytoplasmic antibody-associated vasculitis: a randomized controlled trial, *JAMA* 304:2381–2388, 2010.
105. Draibe J, Poveda R, Fulladosa X, et al.: Use of mycophenolate in ANCA-associated renal vasculitis: 13 years of experience at a university hospital, *Nephrol Dial Transpl* (Suppl1)i132–i137, 2015.

106. Pisoni CN, Cuadrado MJ, Khamashta MA, et al.: Mycophenolate mofetil treatment in resistant myositis, *Rheumatology (Oxford)* 46:516–518, 2007.
107. Morganroth PA, Kreider ME, Werth VP: Mycophenolate mofetil for interstitial lung disease in dermatomyositis, *Arthritis Care Res* 62:1496–1501, 2010.
108. Saketkoo LA, Espinoza LR: Rheumatoid arthritis interstitial lung disease: mycophenolate mofetil as an antifibrotic and disease-modifying antirheumatic drug, *Arch Intern Med* 168:1718–1719, 2008.
109. Gerbino AJ, Goss CH, Molitor JA: Effect of mycophenolate mofetil on pulmonary function in scleroderma-associated interstitial lung disease, *Chest* 133:455–460, 2008.
110. Tashkin DP, Roth MD, Clements PJ, et al.: Mycophenolate mofetil versus oral cyclophosphamide in scleroderma-related interstitial lung disease (SLE II): a randomized controlled, double-blind, parallel group trial, *Lancet Respir Med* 4:708–719, 2016.
111. Volkmann ER, Tashkin DP, Li N, et al.: Mycophenolate mofetil versus placebo for systemic sclerosis-related interstitial lung disease: an analysis of scleroderma lung studies I and II, *Arthritis Rheumatol* 69:1451–1460, 2017.
112. Namas R, Tashkin DP, Furst DE, et al.: Efficacy of mycophenolate mofetil and oral cyclophosphamide on skin thickness: post-hoc analyses from two randomized placebo-controlled trials, *Arthritis Care Res* 70:439–444, 2018.
113. Herrick AL, Pan X, Peytrignet S, et al.: Treatment outcome in early diffuse cutaneous systemic sclerosis: the European Scleroderma Observational Study (ESOS), *Ann Rheum Dis* 76:1207–1218, 2017.
114. Hinchcliff M, Toledo DM, Taroni JN, et al.: Mycophenolate mofetil treatment of systemic sclerosis reduces myeloid cell numbers and attenuates the inflammatory gene signature in skin, *J Invest Dermatol* 138:1301–1310, 2018.
115. Riskalla MM, Somers EC, Fatica RA, et al.: Tolerability of mycophenolate mofetil in patients with systemic lupus erythematosus, *J Rheumatol* 30:1508–1512, 2003.
116. Behrend M, Braun F: Enteric-coated mycophenolate sodium: tolerability profile compared with mycophenolate mofetil, *Drugs* 65:1037–1050, 2005.
117. Maimouni H, Gladmann DD, Ibanez D, et al.: Switching treatment between mycophenolate mofetil and azathioprine in lupus patients: indications and outcomes, *Arthritis Care Res (Hoboken)* 66:1905–1909, 2014.
118. Fischer-Betz R, Specker C, Brinks R, et al.: Low risk of renal flares and negative outcomes in women with lupus nephritis conceiving after switching from mycophenolate mofetil to azathioprine, *Rheumatology* 52:1070–1076, 2013.
119. Bullingham R, Shah J, Goldblum R, et al.: Effects of food and antacid on the pharmacokinetics of single doses of mycophenolate mofetil in rheumatoid arthritis patients, *Br J Clin Pharmacol* 41:513–516, 1996.
120. Kuypers DR, Verleden G, Naesens M, et al.: Drug interaction between mycophenolate mofetil and rifampin: possible induction of uridine diphosphate-glucuronosyltransferase, *Clin Pharmacol Ther* 78:81–88, 2005.

66

Anti-cytokine Therapies

KATHARINE MCCARTHY, ARTHUR KAVANAUGH, AND CHRISTOPHER T. RITCHLIN

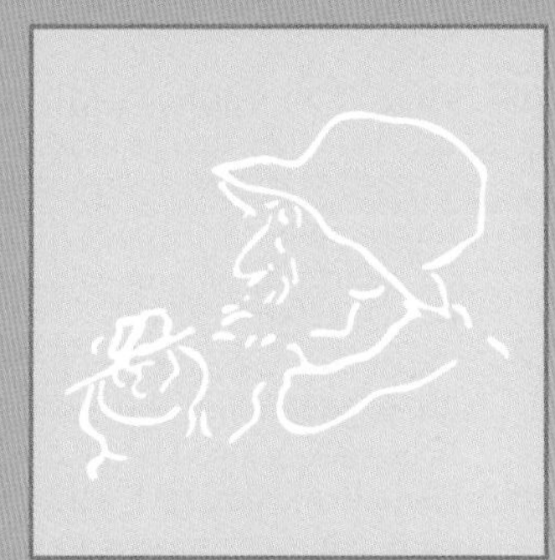

KEY POINTS

Inhibiting a single key cytokine can be an effective treatment for immune-mediated inflammatory diseases.

Treatment with TNF inhibitors in rheumatoid arthritis (RA), psoriatic arthritis (PsA), and axial spondyloarthritis (AxSpA) can significantly decrease radiographic damage, decrease symptoms, improve quality of life, and help preserve functional status. Most patients have at least a partial response. Combining a TNF inhibitor with methotrexate achieves additive benefits in RA.

Maintaining clinical efficacy with TNF inhibitors usually requires continued therapy. However, there might be a window of opportunity in early disease for patients who attain very low levels of disease activity to experience long-term remission.

TNF inhibitors are effective in Crohn's disease, ulcerative colitis, juvenile idiopathic arthritis, hidradenitis suppurative, and uveitis; however, they have been ineffective in patients with vasculitis (granulomatosis with polyangiitis and temporal arteritis).

IL-6 inhibition is an effective therapy in RA, as well as in patients with giant cell arteritis who are refractory to steroid therapy or flare when steroids are tapered.

Although IL-1 inhibition is only modestly effective in RA, it can be highly effective in certain autoinflammatory conditions (e.g., periodic fever syndromes) and crystal-induced arthritis.

IL-12/23 inhibitors are effective and approved for use in psoriatic arthritis, psoriasis, and Crohn's disease, with promising data in systemic lupus erythematosus (SLE).

IL-17 inhibition is effective in psoriatic arthritis, psoriasis, and ankylosing spondylitis. Combination therapy, such as TNF and IL-17 inhibitors, continues to be studied for additional benefit relative to risk of adverse events.

Introduction

Insights into the key effectors that initiate and sustain inflammation and tissue damage catalyzed the growth of biologic therapies that target inflammatory cytokines. Cytokines are small secreted proteins that promote communication and a wide range of interactions between cells.[1] Substantial research identified specific pro-inflammatory cytokines that are upregulated and characteristically present in the blood and/or tissues of individual inflammatory diseases, including TNF, interleukin (IL)-1, IL-6, IL-17, and IL-23.[2,3] Anti-cytokine therapies, or drugs that block the actions of cytokines, dramatically revised treatment paradigms in immune inflammatory disorders due to their ability to reduce inflammation and pain and greatly limit tissue damage and disease progression. Across the disease spectrum, anti-cytokine therapies have greatly improved quality of life and functional status. Biologic drug therapies are complex molecules that differ in size, shape, and composition, therefore impacting the binding to regulatory molecules and the overall inhibition of the inflammatory process. Understanding the pharmacology of anti-cytokines therapies is essential to predict the efficacy as well as potential side effects of drug therapy.

Following discovery of the key cytokines that orchestrate inflammation, including TNF and IL-1, 6, 17, and 23, drug development efforts have been structured to optimize selectivity, potency, and overall efficacy while minimizing unintended consequences of drug binding and adverse side effects. Initial in vitro studies optimized the pharmacodynamic binding of the drug molecule, followed by in vivo studies in animals and then humans to characterize the pharmacokinetics, including drug absorption, metabolism, and overall safety of the medication. Once the ideal biologic molecule is identified, production and manufacturing of the molecule is a complex and laborious process often leading to inherent variations in the product. Compared to traditional chemical synthesis of small molecule drugs, including conventional disease-modifying anti-rheumatic drugs (DMARDS) such as methotrexate, leflunomide, and hydroxychloroquine, biologic products are designed and manufactured with recombinant DNA technology, including replication in a vector that requires cell culture, separation, and purification. Even minor differences in production process or cell lines can generate variations in the resulting protein molecule compared to the original reference product.[4,5] Overall, the structure and function of anti-cytokine therapies is a complex relationship involving a variety of components.

Tumor Necrosis Factor

TNF and Inflammation

TNF is a multifunctional cytokine that exerts pleiotropic effects on various cell types. It is critical in maintaining host defense and has a significant role in the pathogenesis of several chronic inflammatory diseases.[6] The wide range of effects exerted arise, in part, by its ability to bind to two different receptors. Both transmembrane TNF and soluble TNF are involved in the inflammatory process; transmembrane TNF is critical for cell-to-cell signaling and local inflammation, while soluble TNF can act at sites remote from TNF-producing cells.[7] Two distinct receptors, including a 55 kilodalton protein (p55/TNFRI) and a 75 kilodalton protein (p75/TNFRII), are mediated by distinct different signaling pathways.[8,9] The two receptors differ in binding affinity, signaling properties, and primary functions.[10,11]

TNF is a pivotal cytokine in the pathogenesis of rheumatoid arthritis (RA), psoriatic arthritis, psoriasis, and inflammatory bowel disease. A number of different inflammatory cells secrete TNF; however, in the inflammatory conditions mentioned, TNF is produced largely by activated macrophages. Human TNF is synthesized and expressed as a 26-kDa transmembrane protein on the plasma membrane and is cleaved by a specific metalloproteinase (TNF-converting enzyme). After proteolytic cleavage, TNF is converted to a 17-kDa soluble protein, which oligomerizes to form the active homotrimer. The actions of TNF are mediated through two structurally distinct receptors: TNF-RI (55 kDa; CD120a), which promotes the release of many other cytokines including IL-1, IL-6, and GM-CSF; and TNF-RII (75 kDa; CD120b), which activates homeostatic and repair functions.[12] The two receptors differ in their binding affinities, signaling properties, and primary functions.[12,13] The binding of TNF to its receptor initiates several signaling pathways. Signaling cascades include the activation of transcription factors (e.g., nuclear factor κB [NF-κB]), protein kinases (intra-cellular enzymes that mediate cellular responses to inflammatory stimuli, such as c-Jun N-terminal kinase [JNK] and p38 mitogen-activated protein kinase [MAPK]), and proteases (enzymes that cleave peptide bonds, such as caspases).

TNF may contribute to the pathogenesis of inflammatory arthritis through myriad mechanisms, including induction of other pro-inflammatory cytokines (e.g., IL-1, IL-6) and chemokines (e.g., IL-8); enhancement of leukocyte migration by increasing endothelial layer permeability and adhesion molecule expression and function; activation of numerous cell types; and induction of the synthesis of acute phase reactants and other proteins, including tissue-degrading enzymes (matrix metalloproteinase enzymes) produced by synoviocytes and chondrocytes. The pivotal role of TNF in mediating such diverse inflammatory activities provided the rationale for targeting this cytokine in systemic inflammatory diseases. Initially, animal studies proved that inhibition of TNF with monoclonal antibodies or soluble TNF-R constructs ameliorated the signs of inflammation and prevented joint destruction.[7,14] Subsequently, studies in humans confirmed the substantial efficacy of these compounds.[15]

TABLE 66.1 Potential Mechanisms of Action of Tumor Necrosis Factor Inhibitors

Decrease Production of Other Inflammatory Mediators
Cytokines (e.g., IL-1, IL-6, GM-CSF)
Chemokines (e.g., IL-8)
Degradative enzymes (e.g., MMPs)
Acute phase reactants (e.g., C-reactive protein)
Alter Vascular Function, Leukocyte Traffic and Activation
Decreased adhesion molecule expression and function
Angiogenesis inhibition
Modulate the Function of Immunocompetent Cells
T Cells
Normalize activation threshold for CD3–T cell receptor signaling
Alter Th1/Th2 phenotype, cytokine secretion
Increase regulatory T cell number and function
Induce apoptosis (?)
Monocytes and Macrophages
Modulate HLA-DR expression
Possibly increase apoptosis (?)

GM-CSF, Granulocyte-macrophage colony-stimulating factor; *HLA-DR*, human leukocyte antigen DR; *MMPs*, matrix metalloproteinases; *Th*, T helper.

Mechanism of Action of TNF Inhibitors

Several potential mechanisms of action might explain the efficacy of TNF inhibitors in RA and other conditions (Table 66.1). The correlation, though, between any particular mechanism and specific aspects of clinical efficacy remains to be delineated. Downregulation of local and systemic pro-inflammatory cytokine production and reduction of lymphocyte activation and migration into the joint may be one of the most relevant mechanisms; for example, serum levels of IL-6 and IL-1 are significantly reduced after administration of anti-TNF monoclonal antibody.[16] The decline in TNF and the consequent reduction in IL-1 would likely reduce the synthesis of matrix metalloproteinase (MMP) and the production of other degradative enzymes. In support of this key interaction, serial studies reported a marked reduction in proMMP-3 and proMMP-1 following anti-TNF therapy.[17–19]

As noted, anti-TNF therapy is also associated with a reduction of lymphocyte migration into rheumatoid joints. Using radiolabeled granulocytes, anti-TNF monoclonal antibody significantly reduced cell movement into inflamed joints.[20] In addition, post-treatment synovial biopsies showed reduced cellular infiltrates, with fewer T cells and macrophages present.[21] These effects may take place in response to reduced expression of endothelial adhesion molecules in the synovial tissue.

Treatment with anti-TNF monoclonal antibody also results in a dose-dependent decrease in soluble forms of intercellular adhesion molecule-1 (ICAM-1) and E-selectin (CD62E).[20] Changes in soluble E-selectin, soluble ICAM-1, and circulating lymphocytes with anti-TNF therapy correlate with clinical outcomes. Vascular endothelial growth factor (VEGF) is a potent endothelial cell–specific angiogenic factor. VEGF produced in the synovium is an important regulator of neovascularization in the pannus tissue. After anti-TNF therapy, VEGF serum levels are reduced in patients with RA, and the decline correlates significantly with observed clinical benefit.[22] Given that angiogenesis is a prominent feature of rheumatoid synovitis, the interaction between angiogenesis joint inflammation was investigated with computerized image analysis of the endothelium. Interestingly, endothelium stained strongly for several biomarkers (e.g., von Willebrand factor, CD31) and neovasculature (αvβ3), which declined in the setting of reduced vascularity following anti-TNF therapy. A number of other potential mechanisms of action have been suggested to be operative for TNF inhibitors (see Table 66.1), although the events that underlie their regulation along with temporal and spatial interactions are not well understood.

TNF Inhibitors

All TNF inhibitor-directed biologics are recombinant proteins that can bind membrane TNF and soluble TNF; however, structure significantly impacts binding specificity and the ability to form drug-ligand complexes (Fig. 66.1). Differences in specificity impact degree of binding to membrane TNF, soluble TNF, as well as lymphotoxin, while valency defines the number of drug-ligand binding sites and the ability to cross-link and form

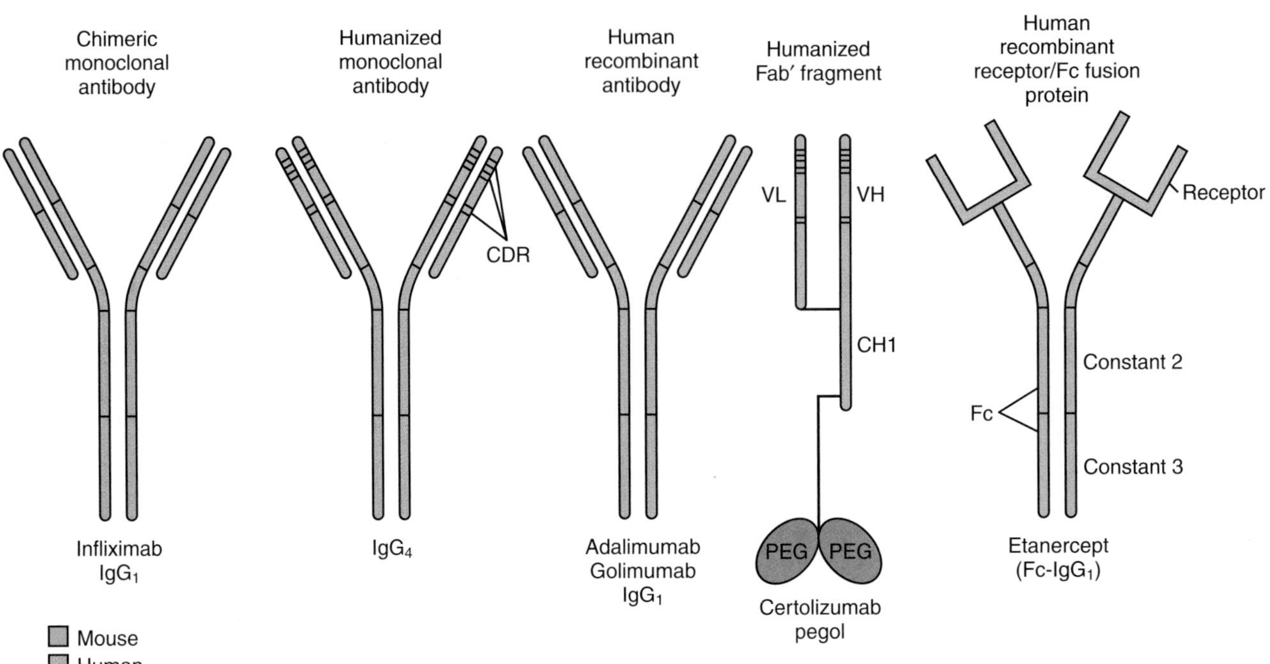

• **Fig. 66.1** Structures of infliximab, etanercept, adalimumab, golimumab, and certolizumab pegol. *CDR,* Complementarity-determining region; *CH1,* complement fixation; *FC,* fragment crystallizable; *PEG,* polyethylene glycol; *TNF,* tumor necrosis factor; *VH,* variable heavy; *VL,* variable light.

larger complexes. Additionally, differences in the Fc region affect immunogenicity and drug-ligand binding.[23] In general, due to their large size, recombinant proteins do not undergo hepatic or renal metabolism and therefore it is unlikely that hepatic or renal impairment significantly alters drug clearance or concentration. Most of the molecules that target TNF are primarily distributed within the vascular compartment considering the volume of distribution; however, each agent differs in absorption to the site of inflammation depending on local factors such as vascularity and endothelial permeability.

Although all five available agents are macromolecule TNF inhibitors, some pharmacologic and pharmacodynamic differences distinguish them and are described in Table 66.2.[10] The monoclonal antibodies infliximab, adalimumab, golimumab, and certolizumab pegol are specific for TNF, whereas etanercept binds both TNF and lymphotoxin-α (LT-α; previously referred to as lymphotoxin). With the exception of certolizumab pegol, these agents are capable of affecting Fc-mediated functions, such as complement-dependent cytolysis and antibody-dependent cell-mediated cytotoxicity, and all bind to both soluble and membrane forms of TNF, although some relative differences in affinity may be noted. Other differences, such as effects on cytokine secretion, have been observed in some in vitro studies.[11] Data on apoptosis have been somewhat discrepant. In patients with RA, both the anti-TNF monoclonal antibody infliximab and the soluble receptor construct etanercept can induce apoptosis in synovial macrophages.[24,25] However, in patients with Crohn's disease, etanercept was not clinically effective at the doses studied and did not induce apoptosis. In contrast, the anti-TNF monoclonal antibodies infliximab and adalimumab were clinically effective and induced apoptosis in highly activated lymphocytes.[26] Nevertheless certolizumab pegol is effective in Crohn's disease and is not able to induce apoptosis. The extent to which these potential differences among TNF inhibitors correlate with any specific aspects of efficacy or toxicity remains to be established.

Infliximab

Infliximab was the first monoclonal antibody targeting TNF approved by the US Food and Drug Administration (FDA). Infliximab consists of variable light and heavy chains derived from a murine monoclonal antibody linked to the constant domain of human kappa and immunoglobulin (IgG1κ), with a resulting structure ~70% human overall. Infliximab neutralizes both soluble and transmembrane forms of TNF; however, it does not bind or neutralize TNF-β. Concomitant treatment with infliximab and methotrexate results in decreased clearance of infliximab.[27]

Etanercept

Etanercept was the first subcutaneously administered TNF inhibitor FDA approved consisting of a dimeric soluble form of the p75 TNF receptor. Etanercept is unique among the TNF inhibitors for its ability to inhibit binding of both TNF and lymphotoxin to cell surface TNF receptors.

Adalimumab

Adalimumab is a recombinant human IgG1 monoclonal antibody administered subcutaneously. It binds specifically to TNF and blocks interaction with the p55/TNFRI and p75/TNFRII cell surface receptors, but, unlike etanercept, it does not bind or inactivate lymphotoxin. Methotrexate reduces overall clearance, as concentration at steady state (Css) is 5 μg/mL without methotrexate versus Css 8 to 9 μg/mL with concurrent methotrexate therapy. Additionally, presence of antiadalimumab antibodies leads to greater drug clearance.[28,29]

TABLE 66.2 Pharmacokinetic Characteristics of TNF Inhibitors

	Infliximab	Adalimumab	Golimumab	Certolizumab	Etanercept
Structure	Chimeric mAb	Human IgG1 mAb	Human IgG1K mAb	PEGylated Fab mAb fragment	TNFR2 Fc fusion protein
Ligands	sTNF tmTNF	sTNF tmTNF	sTNF tmTNF	sTNF tmTNF	sTNF, tmTNF, and TNFβ
Absorption:					
• Bioavailability	N/A	64%	53% SC admin	80%	58%
• Tmax	2.5 hours	5.5 ± 2.3 days	2-6 days	2-7 days	2.9 ± 1.4 day
Distribution:					
• Vd	4.5-6 L	4.7-6 L	58-126 mL/kg	4.7-8 L	6-11 L
Metabolism:					
• Half-life	7.7-9.5 days	14 ± 4 days	14 days	14 days	4.3 ± 1.3 days
Elimination	Degradation by proteases				
Route of administration	IV	SC	IV or SC	SC	SC
Dosing	3-5 mg/kg at 0, 2, 6 weeks then every 8 weeks (clinical dose adjustments up to every 4 weeks)	40 mg every 2 weeks (clinical dose adjustments up to every week)	2 mg/kg IV at 0 and 4 weeks, then every 8 weeks or 50 mg SC monthly	400 mg monthly, or 200 mg every 2 weeks	50 mg weekly, or 25 mg twice weekly
Complement complex formation	+++	+++	+++	–	+
Effect of methotrexate	Lower incidence of anti-infliximab antibodies	Drug clearance decreased by up to 44%	Concentration increased 21%-52% Anti-golimumab antibodies decreased from 7% to 2%	Lower incidence of anti-certolizumab antibodies	No change

Tmax, Time of maximum concentration; *Vd,* volume of distribution.

Golimumab

Golimumab, available as both a subcutaneous injection and intravenous infusion, is another human monoclonal antibody that binds to both soluble and transmembrane forms of TNF; however, it does not bind or neutralize lymphotoxin. Concurrent administration with methotrexate led to 21% to 52% higher mean steady state golimumab concentrations depending upon disease state, while also reducing anti-golimumab antibodies from 7% to 2%.[30]

Certolizumab

Certolizumab is a recombinant, humanized antibody Fab′ fragment conjugated to a 40 kDa polyethylene glycol (PEG-2MAL40K). The Fab′ fragment is composed of a light chain with 214 amino acids and a heavy chain of 229 amino acids, providing specificity to selectively neutralize both transmembrane and soluble TNF, but it does not neutralize TNFβ. Certolizumab does not contain an Fc region that is normally present in a complete antibody; therefore, it does not fix complement, induce antibody-dependent cell-mediated cytotoxicity, or provoke neutrophil degranulation. The presence of anti-certolizumab antibodies is associated with a 3.6-fold increase in clearance. The effect of methotrexate on certolizumab pharmacokinetics has not been extensively studied, however, concurrent therapy led to lower incidence of autoantibodies and therefore is more likely to sustain therapeutic plasma levels.[31]

Efficacy of the TNF Inhibitors

Rheumatoid Arthritis

Infliximab, etanercept, adalimumab, golimumab (SC and IV), and certolizumab are approved in many countries worldwide for the treatment of RA. Initial studies demonstrated the efficacy and tolerability of various doses of TNF inhibitors and also established the optimal doses.[32–39] Concurrent therapy with MTX, even at a relatively low dose of 7.5 mg/wk, enhances the clinical response to all agents; for infliximab and adalimumab, concomitant MTX decreases immunogenicity.[40] Almost all subsequent studies with TNF inhibitor drugs in RA have used such combination therapy.

The efficacy of these five agents was established in pivotal phase III clinical trials (Table 66.3). These agents have shown superior efficacy compared with MTX alone as assessed by American College of Rheumatology (ACR) criteria.[41] In addition to achieving substantial efficacy, the use of TNF inhibitors was associated with significant improvement in functional status and quality of life.[25,42,43] Perhaps most remarkably, patients receiving TNF inhibitors had a dramatic reduction in the progression of joint damage as assessed by radiographic change scores.[39,43,44]

TABLE 66.3 Efficacy of Anti-cytokine Therapies in Immune-Mediated Inflammatory Disorders

Biologic Agent	Target	RA/PsA:%ACR20(%PBO)/wks AxSpA: %ASAS or BASDAI (%PBO)/wks	Reference
Etanercept	TNF RA	N = 234:59 (11)/24	Moreland et al.[25]
	TNF PsA	N = 205:59 (15)/24	Mease et al.[139]
	rAxSpA	N = 277:57(22)/24 ASAS20	Davis et al.[140]
Infliximab (IV)	TNF RA	N = 428:52(17)/54	Lipsky et al.[141]
	TNF PsA	N = 104:65(10)/16	Antoni et al.[142]
	rAxSpA	N = 70:50(9)/12 BASDAI50	Braun et al.[143]
Adalimumab	TNF RA	N = 271:57(14)/24	Weinblatt et al.[44]
	TNF PsA	N = 313:58(14)/12	Mease et al.[144]
	rAxSpA	N = 208:58(21)/12 ASAS20	van der Heijde et al.[145]
Golimumab	TNF RA	N = 444:56(33)/24	Keystone et al.[57]
	TNF PsA	N = 403:51(9)/14	Kavanaugh et al.[107]
	rAxSpA	N = 356:60(22)/14 ASAS20	Inman et al.[146]
Certolizumab	TNF RA	N = 982:61(14)/24	Keystone et al.[147]
	TNF PsA	N = 409:58(24)/24	Mease et al.[148]
	rAxSpA	N = 325:64(38):12 ASAS20	Landewe et al.[149]
Anakinra	IL-1R RA	N = 506:38(22)/24	Cohen et al.[150]
Tocilizumab (IV)	IL-6R RA	N = 359:61(41)/16	Maini et al.[151]
Sarilumab	IL-6R RA	N = 1369:66(33)/24	Genovese et al.[152]
Ustekinumab	IL-12/23 PsA	N = 615:50(23)/24	McInnes et al.[153]
Secukinumab	IL-17 PsA	N = 394:54(7)/24	McInnes et al.[154]
	IL-17 rAxSpA	N = 371: 60(29)/16 ASAS20	Baeten et al.[155]
Ixekizumab	IL-17 PsA	N = 417:62(30)/24	Mease et al.[156]
	IL-17 rAxSpA	N = 341: 48(18)/16 ASAS40	van der Heijde et al.[157]

ACR20, American College of Rheumatology Response Criteria; *ASAS*, Assessment of Spondylitis International Society; *BASDAI*, Bath Ankylosing Spondylitis Disease Activity Index; *PsA*, psoriatic arthritis; *RA*, rheumatoid arthritis; *rAxSpA*, radiographic axial spondyloarthritis.

Psoriatic Arthritis

The impressive efficacy of TNF inhibitors in RA catalyzed studies of these agents in PsA. Similar to RA trials, multiple randomized clinical trials with five TNF inhibitors demonstrated significant improvement in disease activity, quality of life, function, and slowing of disease progress as evidenced by radiographic changes (see Table 66.3). In addition, disease-specific clinical findings such as skin and nail psoriasis, enthesitis, and dactylitis also improve significantly.[45] Whether TNF inhibitors suppress axial symptoms and signs has not been formally examined but they are effective for ankylosing spondylitis (see later), so the prevailing opinion is that they reduce spine and sacroiliac joint inflammation in PsA. In contrast to RA, addition of methotrexate to etanercept was not more effective than etanercept as a solo agent. The efficacy and safety of MTX and etanercept as monotherapies and in combination for treatment of PsA were examined in the SEAM Trial.[46] Although etanercept was significantly more effective than MTX monotherapy, patients on MTX demonstrated therapeutic responses in the joints, skin, and enthuses. The combination of MTX and etanercept, though, was not more effective then etanercept monotherapy. The addition of MTX to other TNF inhibitors has not been examined in controlled trials, but it is anticipated that the results will be similar.

Ankylosing Spondylitis

The five TNF inhibitors were widely studied in AS in phase III trials (see Table 66.3). They demonstrated remarkable similarity in their efficacy in relieving symptoms of AS. Studies have also shown that TNF inhibitors improve health-related quality of life, patient-reported outcomes, anemia, CRP levels, and sleep quality in AS patients.[47] TNF inhibitors control inflammation in the spine as measured by various MRI sequences. Initial comparisons of phase III data with subjects in the historical OASIS cohort who did receive TNF inhibitors suggested that TNF inhibitors did not inhibit radiograph progression measured by assessment of syndesmophyte formation over time. Subsequent analyses that examined longitudinal cohorts of patients matched by propensity scoring did show that early and continuous treatment of AS with TNF inhibitors inhibited radiograph progression.[48]

Following the revised classification of AS to include the term *axial nonradiographic SpA* in 2009,[49,50] all five TNF inhibitors were demonstrated to be effective in patients who did not meet radiographic criteria for AS but met the requirements for AxSpA. A recent trial demonstrated that certolizumab was effective for nonradiographic AxSpA, and it is the first TNF inhibitor approved by the FDA for this indication.[51]

Treatment of Other Immune-Mediated Inflammatory Disorders

The efficacy and safety of TNF inhibitors in the treatment of Crohn's disease, juvenile idiopathic arthritis, and psoriasis have been clearly defined.[52,53] Based on promising results in an array of immune-inflammatory disorders, these agents are prescribed in a variety of other disorders, including idiopathic juvenile arthritis, uveitis, sarcoidosis, Sjögren's syndrome, Behçet's disease, inflammatory myopathies, and various types of vasculitis. Although a number of case reports or small, uncontrolled clinical trials have reported on these conditions, there is a paucity of conclusive data from controlled trials. Perhaps the most notable clinical response has been observed in the treatment of uveitis and hidradenitis suppurativa, especially with anti-TNF monoclonal antibody constructs.[54] Of course, promising results in uncontrolled trials have been disproven in controlled trials. For example, anecdotal evidence suggested that etanercept may be an effective agent for granulomatosis with polyangiitis (GPA) (formerly Wegener's granulomatosis). When examined in a placebo-controlled trial of etanercept given in addition to standard therapy for induction and maintenance of remission in GPA, however, etanercept failed to achieve significant clinical improvement; most importantly, a greater risk of solid malignancies was observed in the subjects on etanercept beyond that observed with cyclophosphamide alone.

Despite evidence that TNF inhibitors are associated with the development of certain autoantibodies and even lupus-like syndromes, the safety and efficacy of TNF inhibitors have been assessed in a small group of patients with SLE.[55] Patients with joint involvement experienced remission of arthritis, and a significant reduction in the level of proteinuria occurred with infliximab. In this small study, TNF inhibitor therapy did not lead to adverse events suggestive of an increase in SLE activity; however, as might have been expected, autoantibodies to double-stranded DNA and cardiolipin did increase.

Toxicity

In clinical trials, etanercept, infliximab, adalimumab, golimumab, and certolizumab pegol have generally been well tolerated.[25,38,39,43,44,56–63] Longer-term follow-up of patients initially enrolled in clinical trials has provided additional safety data for these agents. However, TNF plays a key role not only in the pathogenesis of autoimmune disease but also in normal immune homeostasis. Therefore, a number of safety considerations, including the potential risk of infection and malignancy, are germane to the optimal clinical use of these agents.[64]

Additional information concerning adverse effects associated with these agents has been obtained through pharmacovigilance. Adverse events related to the use of TNF inhibitors can be grouped into those that are agent-related and those that are target-related (Table 66.4).[65] Injection site and infusion reactions and immunogenicity and their sequelae vary, depending on the particular agent. A potentially increased predisposition to infection, development of malignancy, induction of autoimmune disorders, an association with demyelinating disorders, myelosuppression, and worse outcomes with congestive heart failure might be considered target-related adverse events. Thus, any clinically effective TNF inhibitor might be expected to be associated with such adverse events, although the relative risk among different agents may vary, depending on dose and other factors.

Infusion and Injection Site Reactions

Infliximab has been associated with infusion reactions, the most common of which are headache (20%) and nausea (15%). These are rarely severe, are usually transient, and typically can be controlled by slowing the rate of infusion or by treating with acetaminophen or antihistamines.[43] With etanercept, adalimumab, golimumab, and certolizumab pegol, cutaneous reactions at injection sites represent the most frequent administration-related side effect; however, they rarely lead to discontinuation of therapy.[25,57] Injection site reactions typically consist of erythematous or urticarial lesions. Although they can arise at sites of previous injections, these reactions are mostly limited to the skin and are not associated with other or systemic features of immediate hypersensitivity. Reactions typically occur close to treatment initiation and abate over time, even with continued dosing.

Antigenicity

As is true for any therapeutic agent (especially large protein molecules, some of which contain foreign sequences), antibodies to TNF inhibitors can develop. Although the clinical relevance of these antibodies is presently unclear, they can diminish the half-life of the therapeutic agent and consequently decrease its efficacy. Approximately 3% of etanercept-treated patients develop antibodies to the drug. In an early study, it was noted that antibodies to infliximab developed in 53%, 21%, and 7% of patients who were receiving 1, 3, and 10 mg/kg infliximab, respectively.[40,65a] RA trials of infliximab with or without concomitant MTX treatment revealed that immunogenicity was decreased by concomitant MTX, perhaps owing in part to the increase in the half-life of infliximab associated with MTX use. A multicenter trial of infliximab therapy in Crohn's disease demonstrated that induction of these anti-infliximab antibodies might contribute to hypersensitivity reactions in some patients. Antibodies to adalimumab, golimumab, and certolizumab pegol developed in about 4% to 12% of patients; this rate was reduced to 1% with concurrent MTX treatment.[57,61,66–68] Although it is believed that there is a trend toward higher clearance of TNF inhibitors in the presence of antibodies to the construct, routine testing for antibodies to TNF inhibitors is not widely available, nor is it currently recommended.

Infection

Given that TNF is a key mediator of inflammation, a major concern surrounding the use of TNF inhibitors is their potential to increase the risk of infection.[69] Although inhibition of TNF in animals does not appear to increase their risk for infection with most pathogens, it does interfere with the ability to mount an inflammatory response against intra-cellular organisms. In experimental models, TNF blockade impaired resistance to infection with mycobacteria, *Pneumocystis carinii,* fungi, *Listeria monocytogenes,* and *Legionella.* In patients with RA, infection with these types of opportunistic organisms has been observed. However, confounding the attribution of infection to any therapeutic agent is the fact that infections occur more frequently and are important contributors to the accelerated morbidity of RA patients compared with the normal population. It is difficult to determine how much of this

TABLE 66.4 Potential Adverse Effects and Recommended Monitoring

	ADVERSE EFFECTS		
	Target-Related	**Agent-Related**	**Monitoring**
TNF	Infections (including serious infections) Opportunistic infections (e.g., tuberculosis) Malignancies (skin cancer, lymphoma [?]) Demyelinating conditions Hematologic abnormalities Congestive heart failure Autoantibodies (anti-nuclear antibody, anti–double-stranded DNA) Hepatotoxicity Dermatologic reactions Lupus-like syndromes	Administration reactions Immunogenicity	TB prior to start and annual screening Viral hepatitis prior to start Infections
IL-1	Infections Neutropenia	Administration reactions Hypersensitivity reactions	Infections Neutrophil count
IL-6	Increased liver enzymes Abnormalities in lipid profiles Neutropenia Low platelet count Malignancies Demyelinating conditions Gastrointestinal perforations	Administration reactions Hypersensitivity reactions	TB prior to start and annual screening Viral hepatitis prior to start Infections Liver function tests Lipids Neutrophil and platelet counts
IL-12/23	Infections	Administration reactions Hypersensitivity reactions	TB prior to start and annual screening Viral hepatitis prior to start Infections
IL-17	Infections Gastrointestinal perforations	Administration reactions Hypersensitivity reactions	TB prior to start and annual screening Viral hepatitis prior to start Infections

susceptibility relates to the disease itself and how much is caused by the effects of immunomodulatory drugs (e.g., steroids, DMARDs). The subset of RA patients with great susceptibility to infection (i.e., those with severe, active disease) is also the subset most commonly enrolled in trials of TNF inhibitors; this is the group of patients for whom these agents have the greatest clinical utility.

In RA trials with TNF inhibitors, a number of infections have occurred. In general, the most frequent infections have been those that occur most commonly among all people, such as upper and lower respiratory tract infections and urinary tract infections. In most studies, a slightly greater propensity to develop infection was seen in patients receiving TNF inhibitors; however, this trend is common in most studies of effective therapies for RA. The incidence of serious infection, defined as infection requiring hospitalization or treatment with parenteral antibiotics, among RA patients treated with TNF inhibitors was similar to that of the control groups in individual studies; it also approximated the incidence noted among RA patients before the anti-TNF era.[70] In certain subgroups, such as patients with early RA, the overall incidence of infection was less than in patients with more long-standing disease, and infections and serious infections were comparable among TNF inhibitor-treated patients and controls.

It is worth noting, however, that several characteristics of clinical trials might affect investigators' ability to extrapolate their safety data to the clinic. In general, patients enrolled in clinical trials tend to be healthier and therefore less likely to develop adverse effects such as infection, compared with the general population of RA patients in the clinic. Therefore, post-marketing data provide an important complement to safety data obtained from clinical trials. Also, clinical trials are powered to assess efficacy and therefore may not include sufficient numbers of patients to ascertain real but small differences in uncommon side effects. A systematic analysis that combined the results from nine clinical trials of TNF inhibitors has been performed.[71] This analysis found an increased risk of serious infection among patients receiving TNF inhibitors compared with controls (3.6% vs. 1.7%); however, a nonstandard definition of *serious infection* was used, and no attempt was undertaken to control for the time of exposure, which was nearly always longer for patients receiving TNF inhibitors. In this same analysis, a trend toward a greater incidence of serious infection was observed with higher doses of TNF inhibitor. In one of the only clinical trials that had a primary outcome of safety, use of a high-dose TNF inhibitor was also associated with a greater incidence of serious infection compared with a lower dose; the lower dose was no different from placebo in this regard.

In post-marketing surveillance data, also known as *pharmacovigilance,* serious infections have certainly been observed among patients receiving TNF inhibitors.[64] The relative impact of potentially confounding factors such as comorbidities and concomitant medications on the rate of serious infection remains incompletely defined. This important question has also been addressed by using registries of RA patients.[72,73] In a German registry, rates of infection and serious infection in the RABBIT Registry showed that treatment with TNF inhibitors exhibited a 1.5-times higher risk of infection compared to treatment with nonbiologic DMARDs.[74] The drop in relative risk of infection over time in the cohort was attributed to a decline in steroid dose and increased physical function. In data from a British registry, 7644 RA patients treated with TNF inhibitors were compared with 1354 RA patients on DMARDs alone.[70] In this analysis, the crude rate of serious infection was higher among TNF inhibitor–treated patients (1.28; 95% confidence interval [CI], 0.94 to 1.76), although this did not reach statistical significance. Further, when the rates were adjusted for age, sex, severity of RA, use of corticosteroids, and comorbidity, no differences between the groups were noted (relative risk [RR], 1.03; 95% CI, 0.68 to 1.57).

In summary, although treatment with TNF inhibitors can result in increased risk of infection and serious infection, other factors such as the severity of RA, the use of other medications such as corticosteroids, and the presence of comorbidities are important contributors to these outcomes. Clinicians must monitor patients closely for signs and symptoms of infection, and it is worth noting that TNF inhibitor therapy itself can mask the initial signs and symptoms of infection.

Opportunistic infections, particularly disseminated *Mycobacterium tuberculosis,* are of concern with the use of TNF inhibitors.[75] Of note, more patients treated with TNF inhibitors have extrapulmonary and disseminated tuberculosis (TB), highlighting the specific role of TNF in controlling this infection. Rates of TB associated with the use of TNF inhibitors are higher in geographic regions where TB is more prevalent in the general population. Most cases of TB observed in the early years after the introduction of TNF inhibitors arose within the first few months after initiation of therapy and were probably related to the reactivation of latent TB. Very few cases of TB were observed during clinical trials of the TNF inhibitors, highlighting the important role of pharmaco-vigilance in identifying safety signals with new therapies. For etanercept, no cases of TB occurred in clinical trials, but 38 cases of etanercept-associated TB were reported worldwide among an estimated 150,000 patients exposed through December 2002. For infliximab, 441 cases of TB were reported among approximately 500,000 initially exposed patients; only six cases of infliximab-related TB were reported from clinical trials. Ninety-seven percent of infliximab-related cases occurred within 7 months of treatment initiation, with a median time of onset of 12 weeks. The incidence of TB in clinical trials with adalimumab was greater in earlier clinical trials; this was related to lack of screening, the locations of the studies, and the higher doses used in early trials. The incidence dropped to 1% after adalimumab was reduced to its current dose, and after screening for latent TB infection was instituted before therapy (21 cases in 2400 patients).[78] The incidence of TB was even lower in golimumab and certolizumab pegol trials. The incidence of TB was 0.23 in golimumab clinical trials, and most cases occurred in countries with a high incidence rate of TB.[57,59] In studies with certolizumab pegol, 36 cases of TB occurred among 2367 exposed patients; these cases also occurred in countries with endemic rates of TB. This highlights the benefit of screening for and treating latent TB among patients being considered for TNF inhibitor therapy.[76] However, because treated patients may acquire new cases of TB, and because cases of latent TB may be missed owing to false-negative screening tests, constant vigilance for TB is required during therapy with TNF inhibitors.

The impact of screening for latent TB in patients receiving TNF inhibitors has been assessed in a Spanish registry; the rate of development of active TB among RA patients treated with TNF inhibitors dropped by 83% with use of the recommended guideline. Current U.S. guidelines recommend purified protein derivative (PPD) skin testing and/or ex vivo testing for TB, as well as a chest radiograph, before anti-TNF therapy is initiated. If the PPD test is positive without evidence of active infection, treatment for latent TB with isoniazid is recommended. The recommended duration of therapy is 3 to 9 months depending on treatment regimen.[77]

Recommendations concerning the timing of TNF inhibitor therapy and prophylaxis for latent TB vary; however, concomitant initiation appears feasible.[37] During anti-TB treatment, alanine aminotransferase (ALT) monitoring is recommended, especially for those who chronically consume alcohol and/or who take potentially hepatotoxic drugs. Treatment should be adjusted according to local guidelines.

Malignancy

TNF inhibitors can theoretically affect the host defense against malignancy. To date, the occurrence of malignancies in clinical trials and long-term follow-up of RA patients from clinical trials do not appear to significantly exceed the rate that would be expected in this population. The overall rate of most malignancies in patients with RA is the same as in the normal population. However, risks of certain cancers, such as lymphoma and lung cancer, appear to be increased in patients with RA. Although the actual reason is not known, the severity, activity, duration of the disease, and the use of immunomodulatory agents such as MTX seem to play a role in the increased risk of lymphoma in RA patients.[78] Post-marketing analysis of the association between TNF inhibitors and lymphoma is inconclusive. In one population-based analysis, standardized incidence ratios of lymphoma among patients receiving anti-TNF therapies were somewhat higher than those among RA controls; however, this analysis did not adjust for baseline differences between patients.[78] The impact of anti-TNF therapy on lymphoma is still not settled, and additional studies with large longitudinal cohorts and proper adjustment for confounders are required.[79]

In a more recent analysis in which adjustments were made for age, sex, and disease duration, no increased risk of lymphoma was identified among RA patients treated with TNF inhibitors compared with those treated with other therapies. In clinical trials of anti-TNF monoclonal antibodies, malignancies, including lymphomas and skin cancers, were noted with treatment, but the longer time of exposure to TNF inhibitors was not accounted for. Overall, TNF inhibitor therapy does not appear to be associated with a major increased risk of cancer. Still, consideration is required for each individual, especially in certain situations such as among RA patients with a history of malignancy. There are no data addressing this important question from clinical trials, as patients with cancers are excluded. Data from several registries have suggested that there may not be an increased risk of recurrent cancer among such patients treated with TNF inhibitors, but this is still an open and very important question.[80]

TNF inhibitors are prescribed more frequently in children, and the potential for increased risk of malignancies in children with autoimmune disorders, particularly in those receiving TNF inhibitors, has been pointed out by the Adverse Event Reporting System of the FDA. Forty-eight reports of malignancy were identified: 31 following infliximab use, 15 following etanercept use, and 2 following adalimumab use. Half of the malignancies were lymphomas, and most cases involved concomitant use of other immunosuppressants.[81] Given these uncertainties, caution is indicated when the use of TNF inhibitors is considered for patients with a history of malignancy or for those at high risk of malignancy for other reasons. Longer-term follow-up of larger numbers of patients will provide clinicians with a better idea of the safety of these agents in this regard.

Autoimmune Disorders

Approximately 10% to 15% of patients treated with any TNF inhibitor develop antibodies to double-stranded DNA.[64] However, few patients (0.2% to 0.4%) develop symptoms consistent with drug-induced lupus. The mechanism and the significance of the development of antibodies are uncertain, although this adverse effect seems relatively specific for TNF inhibitors and is not noted with other biologic agents. Of note, patients with TNF inhibitor–related lupus generally do not develop life-threatening lupus involvement (e.g., nephritis, CNS lupus) and rarely develop the diversity of other autoantibodies characteristic of idiopathic SLE (e.g., anti-Sm/RNP, anti-Ro/La, anti-Scl70). A few patients have reportedly developed anti-cardiolipin antibodies, but they are mostly asymptomatic. Among those few patients who developed lupus-like symptoms while on TNF inhibition therapy, improvement is generally noted upon discontinuation of therapy. Although the rare occurrence of autoimmune disorders has not dissuaded most clinicians from using TNF inhibitors in patients with RA, some remain cautious about using these drugs in patients with a history of SLE.

Demyelinating Syndromes

Several cases of multiple sclerosis (MS) or peripheral demyelinating disease have been reported with anti-TNF therapy in patients with RA, PsA, and Crohn's disease. In addition, two studies of TNF inhibitors in MS patients showed worsening of MS-related symptoms and exacerbations in the treated group.[64] Although some evidence suggests that the incidence of MS may be increased in patients with RA, the association between anti-TNF therapy and MS remains unclear. The risk of developing a demyelinating disease is very small; however, many clinicians withhold anti-TNF therapy in patients with a history of demyelinating diseases and in those showing signs and symptoms of such disease during anti-TNF therapy.

Cardiovascular Risk and Lipid Profile

Cardiovascular morbidity and mortality are increased in immune inflammatory and autoimmune disorders. Mechanistically, the association with major adverse cardiovascular events (MACE) is likely linked to the increased prevalence of traditional risk factors for cardiovascular disease and to uncontrolled systemic inflammation, which accelerates progression of atherosclerosis. Treatment of RA patients with TNF inhibitors is associated with overall improvement in cardiovascular disease risk, related to beneficial effects on lipid parameters and to control of systemic inflammation.[82] Long-term investigations are needed to define the possible beneficial effects of TNF inhibitors on overall and cardiovascular survival in patients in the wide array of chronic inflammatory diseases.

Congestive Heart Failure

Data suggest that TNF may play a role in the pathogenesis of congestive heart failure (CHF), and inhibition of TNF was highly effective in animal models of ischemic cardiomyopathy. However, in trials of TNF inhibitors in patients with stable but severe (class III or IV) CHF, no clinical benefit was observed, and in some treatment arms, higher incidences of mortality and hospitalization for worsening of CHF were reported. Thus, TNF inhibition has been largely abandoned as a therapeutic approach in patients with CHF. In patients with RA, treatment with TNF inhibitors does not appear to result in an increased incidence of CHF.[83] In fact, TNF inhibitor therapy may actually improve mortality associated with heart disease and overall mortality in RA patients.

Paradoxical Psoriasis

The development of inflammatory skin lesions with a psoriasiform appearance is reported in 2% to 5% of patients treated with TNF inhibitors.[84] The lesions may resemble psoriasis vulgaris, but a high prevalence of palmar plantar psoriasis has also been noted. Recent studies revealed that the pathologic features in the skin are characterized by overproduction of type 1 interferons and a relative paucity of infiltrating T cells in contrast to classic psoriasis. One probable mechanism to explain this finding is that TNF blockade blocks the maturation of plasmacytoid dendritic cells and prolongs and enhances type 1 interferon production.[85]

Interleukin-1

IL-1 and Inflammation

Members of the IL-1 family include IL-1α, IL-1β, and the naturally occurring IL-1 receptor antagonist (IL-1Ra).[86] Specific cellular proteases process IL-1α and IL-1β to their 17-kDa mature forms. Pro–IL-1α precursor is active intra-cellularly. However, pro–IL-1β is not active before cleavage with IL-1β –converting enzyme. After cleavage, it is secreted and is fully functional. IL-1Ra is a naturally occurring antagonist protein with amino acid sequence homologous to IL-1α and IL-1β. Multiple forms of this protein exist. One is secreted and functions as a competitive inhibitor of IL-1α and IL-1β, binding to the same counter receptor but transducing no signal. The IL-1 polypeptides bind to two cell surface receptors: type I (IL-1RI) and type II (IL-1RII). IL-1RI is found on most cell types, whereas IL-1RII occurs mainly on the surface of neutrophils, monocytes, B cells, and bone marrow progenitor cells. When IL-1 binds to IL-1RI, the signal transduction is mediated through the association of a second receptor unit, the IL-1R accessory protein. The three members of the IL-1 family bind to IL-1RI with similar affinities. Binding of IL-1 to IL-1RII does not lead to signal transduction. IL-1RII acts like a decoy receptor and a competitive inhibitor. Soluble forms of IL-1RII inhibit IL-1 activity by competing with IL-1RI for IL-1 binding. IL-18 is another member of the IL-1 family of inflammatory cytokines. It is now recognized as an important regulator of innate and acquired immune responses. IL-18 is expressed at sites of chronic inflammation, in autoimmune diseases, in a variety of cancers, and in the context of numerous infectious diseases. IL-18 likely plays a role in RA, and strategies to block IL-18 activity are underway in clinical trials.

As with TNF, IL-1 is one of the key mediators of the inflammatory response. Studies in animal models of arthritis have demonstrated the therapeutic potential of IL-1 blockade. IL-1β gene knockout mice show markedly reduced levels of inflammation following immunization with type II collagen. The use of genetically modified mice has helped to confirm the physiologic significance of IL-1Ra: Deletion of this gene in mice results in the spontaneous development of arthritis.

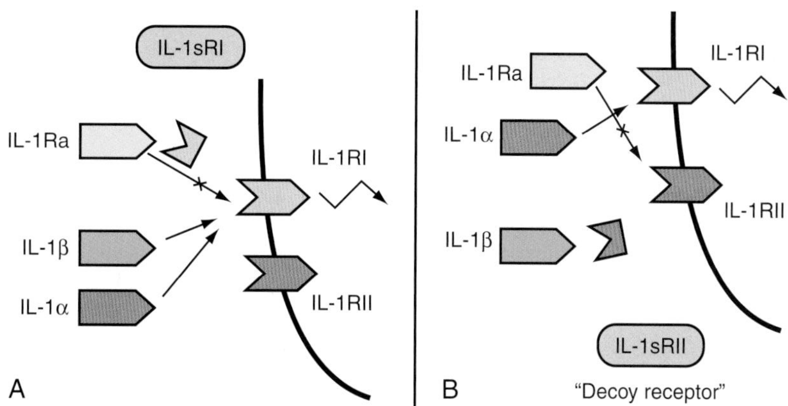

• **Fig. 66.2** (A and B) Anakinra. Structure and mechanism of action: Anakinra is a recombinant, nonglycosylated homologue of the IL-1 receptor (IL-1R). It blocks the activity of IL-1 by competitively inhibiting IL-1 binding to the IL-1RI receptor. *IL-1sRI* and *IL-1sRII,* Soluble receptor.

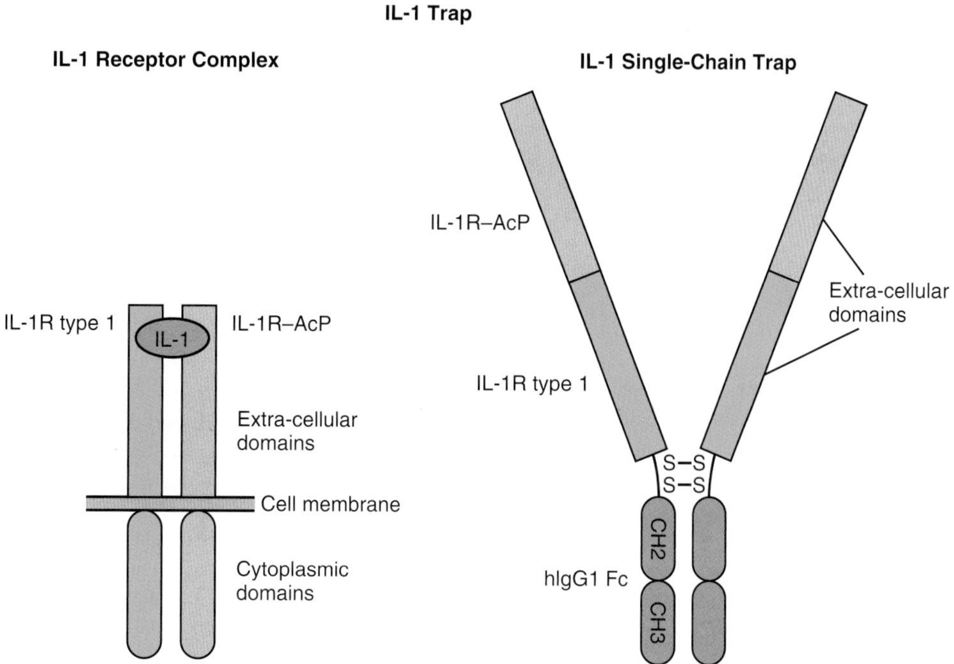

• **Fig. 66.3** Rilonacept. Structure: Rilonacept is a fusion protein consisting of the human IL-1 receptor extra-cellular domains and the Fc portion of human IgG1.

Interleukin-1 Inhibitors

Anakinra

Anakinra is a recombinant, nonglycosylated homolog of IL-1 receptor antagonist (IL-1R) that differs from native human IL-1R by the addition of a single methionine residue at its amino terminus. Anakinra blocks the activity of IL-1 alpha and beta by competitively inhibiting IL-1 binding to the IL-1 type I receptor (IL-1R1)[87] (Fig. 66.2). Levels of the naturally occurring IL-1R, which are elevated in the synovium and synovial fluid from RA and PsA patients, appear to be insufficient for the excess amount of locally produced IL-1.

Anakinra is highly (95%) bioavailable and leads to maximum plasma concentrations 3 to 7 hours after administration, while elimination half-life ranges from 4 to 6 hours. Estimated anakinra clearance increases with increasing creatinine clearance and body weight. Due to decreased clearance with worsening renal function, dose adjustments are recommended in severe renal disease.[88] The recommended dose of anakinra for the treatment of patients with moderately to severely active RA is 100 mg/day administered by subcutaneous injection. Anakinra can be used alone or in combination with MTX. Because of the potential for increased risk of infection, it is not recommended for use in conjunction with TNF inhibitors.

Rilonacept

Rilonacept, previously known as IL-1 Trap, is a fusion protein consisting of the human IL-1 receptor extra-cellular domains and the Fc portion of human IgG1. It incorporates in a single molecule the extra-cellular domains of *both* receptor components required for IL-1 signaling: IL-1RI and the IL-1R accessory protein (Fig. 66.3). Rilonacept has a very high binding affinity for IL-1 (dissociation constant ≈1 pM), and it is specific for IL-1β and IL-1α.

TABLE 66.5 **Pharmacokinetic Characteristics of IL Inhibitors**

		Structure	Bioavailability/ Tmax	Distribution (Vd)	Metabolism Half-life	Route of Admin	Dosing
IL-1	Anakinra	IL-1R receptor antagonist	95% 3-7 hours	6-10 L	4-6 hours	SC	100 mg daily
	Rilonacept	IgG1 fusion protein with IL-1R1 and IL-1RAcP	50% 48-72 hours	Not specified	8-9 days	SC	160 mg weekly
	Canakinumab	IgG1k antibody binds IL-1β	66% 8 days	6.0-6.4 L	26 days	SC	150-300 mg every 4-8 weeks
IL-6	Tocilizumab	IgG1kχ binds sIL-6R and mIL-6R	80%-95% 3-4.5 days	6.4-7.4 L	5-13 days	IV, or SC	4-8 mg/kg IV every 4 weeks, or 162 mg SC every 1-2 weeks
	Sarilumab	IgG1 binds sIL-6R and mIL-6R	80% 2-4 days	7.3 L	8-10 days	SC	200 mg every 2 weeks
IL 12/23	Ustekinumab	IgG1k antibody binds IL-12 and IL-23	57% 7-14 days	2-7 L	15-45 days	SC	45-90 mg every 12 weeks
IL-17	Ixekizumab	Human IgG4 antibody binds IL-17A	60%-81% 4 days	7.1 L	13 days	SC	80 mg every 4 weeks
	Secukinumab	Human IgG4 antibody binds IL-17A	55%-77% 6 days	7.1-8.6 L	22-31 days	SC	150 mg or 300 mg every 4 weeks

Tmax, Time of maximum concentration; *Vd*, volume of distribution.

Rilonacept blocks IL-1β signaling by acting as a soluble decoy receptor that binds IL-1β and prevents its interaction with cell surface receptors. Rilonacept also binds IL-1α and IL-1 receptor antagonist (IL-1ra) with reduced affinity.[89,90] It is administered subcutaneously with a loading dose of 320 mg followed by 160 mg once weekly.

Canakinumab

Canakinumab is a human monoclonal antibody of the IgG1κ isotype. The antibody binds to human IL-1β and neutralizes its activity by blocking the interaction with IL-1 receptors, but it does not bind IL-1α or IL-1 receptor antagonist (IL-1Ra). Bioavailability of subcutaneous administration is approximately 66% and reaches maximum concentration in 7 days. Clearance is primarily dependent upon body weight, with half-life ranging from 23 to 25 days; however, no sex- or age-related differences have been observed.[91,92] It has no cross-reactivity with other members of the IL-1 family, including IL-1α. It is given subcutaneously 150 mg every 8 weeks to subjects weighing greater than 40 kg, while the recommended dose is 2 mg/kg for patients whose body weight is between 15 and 40 kg.

Efficacy

Rheumatoid Arthritis

Anakinra is approved for the treatment of RA, and the key trial results are shown in Table 66.5. Analysis of hand radiographs by two different methods after 24 weeks of treatment showed a statistically significant decrease in the rate of progressive joint damage compared with placebo.[93] Improvements in functional status and quality of life were also observed.[94] Anakinra is a competitive inhibitor of IL-1 that must be continuously present in great excess to be effective, and it must be administered daily. It was hypothesized that the relatively modest clinical results seen with anakinra in RA patients (compared with those achieved by TNF inhibitors) might be related to the agent rather than to the target. Two lines of evidence appear to refute this hypothesis: the efficacy of anakinra in other inflammatory diseases, and the comparable clinical efficacy of other IL-1 inhibitors in RA. Due to a comparatively short duration of action, the recommended dose of anakinra for the treatment of patients with moderately to severely active RA is 100 mg/day administered by subcutaneous injection. The lower level of efficacy of anakinra compared to TNF inhibitors and the requirement for daily administration has limited widespread use for this indication.

Based on early studies, the subcutaneous administration of rilonacept in subjects with RA provided evidence of its clinical and biologic activity. However, a double-blind, placebo-controlled clinical trial in patients with moderate to severe RA who were randomized to receive weekly injections of placebo or several doses of rilonacept for 12 weeks showed only modest efficacy.[95]

Canakinumab reduced disease activity in patients with new-onset RA, including patients who fail to benefit from TNF blocking therapies. However, the long-term benefit and radiologic changes remain unstudied.

Autoinflammatory Diseases

Systemic autoinflammatory diseases are rare syndromes that have common systemic manifestations, such as fever, neutrophilia, arthralgias, myalgias, and severe fatigue, which are generally periodic rather than progressive. Familial Mediterranean fever is perhaps the most well-known autoinflammatory disease. Patients with familial cold autoinflammatory syndrome (FCAS) might present with a spectrum of disease activity: neonatal-onset multisystem inflammatory disease (NOMID; also known as chronic infantile neurologic, cutaneous, articular syndrome [CINCA]), Muckle–Wells syndrome (MWS), and familial cold urticaria. These conditions share some clinical features and are associated with various mutations in the *NALP3/CIAS1/PYPAF1* gene, which encodes the protein cryopyrin. Cryopyrin is a key component of the inflammasome; thus, the autoinflammatory syndromes may be related to abnormalities in IL-1 regulation. This was proven by the remarkable responses to anakinra reported in these syndromes. In addition, significant and rapid responses have been achieved when anakinra was used to treat patients with adult-onset Still's disease. Improvement in various hematologic, biochemical, and other markers suggests that IL-1 plays a key role in this disease as well. Often, after blocking IL-1β, patients with Cryoprin-associated periodic syndromes (CAPS) and other autoinflammatory diseases experience a rapid and sustained cessation of symptoms as well as reductions in biochemical, hematologic, and functional markers of their disease. Because treatment with rilonacept and canakinumab are equally effective in treating autoinflammatory diseases, the active mediator in these diseases is IL-1β and not IL-1α.

Rilonacept and canakinumab are approved for the CAPS disorders FCAS and MWS.[96–99] Canakinumab is also approved for hyperimmunoglobulin D syndrome/mevalonate kinase deficiency, familial Mediterranean fever, and Still's disease (orphan status). Anakinra is the first and only drug that is approved for the treatment of children and adults with NOMID, the most severe form of CAPS. IL-1 inhibitors are also effective for the treatment of systemic juvenile idiopathic arthritis.[100]

Gout

Some patients with recurrent attacks of gouty arthritis who are resistant to colchicine and nonsteroidal anti-inflammatory drugs (NSAIDs) require steroids to control the disease flares. When treated with anakinra, rilonacept, and canakinumab, a rapid, sustained, and remarkable reduction in inflammation and pain has been observed. This effect seems to be superior to steroids IL-1 blockers' effect on controlling gout attacks and is currently being investigated in clinical trials.[101]

Other Disorders

IL-1 blockers are being investigated in various disorders including indolent myeloma, type 1 and 2 diabetes, osteoarthritis, and GVHD. The role of IL-1 is also of interest in managing cardiovascular disease. The inflammatory hypothesis is based on the findings that inflammatory biomarkers are associated with increased risk of cardiovascular events; however, there are limited data to suggest that reducing vascular inflammation independent of cholesterol reduction reduces the rates of cardiovascular events. Prior phase II trials have demonstrated that IL-1 inhibition leads to decreased CRP and IL-6 biomarkers; however, the CANTOS trial evaluated if IL-1β inhibition reduced clinical outcomes of vascular events.[102] Findings identified canakinumab significantly lowered CRP without affecting cholesterol levels as anticipated; however, only the 150 mg canakinumab dosing led to significant findings of 15% lower reduction in myocardial infarction, stroke, or cardiovascular death. Overall, canakinumab supported the inflammatory hypothesis regarding biomarkers; however, clinical outcomes were limited by adverse events including risk of infections.

Toxicity

Anakinra is generally well tolerated, with injection site reactions as the most frequently reported adverse event. In a randomized clinical trial, injection site reactions were reported in 25% of patients given placebo and in 50%, 73%, and 81% of patients given anakinra in doses of 30, 75, and 150 mg/day, respectively.[103] These reactions were generally mild and transient. Infections were uncommon and occurred at a similar rate in the placebo and treatment groups. Infections that required antibiotic therapy occurred in 12% of the placebo-treated group and in 15% to 17% of the treatment group. These infections consisted primarily of bacterial events such as cellulitis and pneumonia. The incidence of pulmonary infection appeared to be higher among patients with underlying asthma. In placebo-controlled studies, up to 8% of patients receiving anakinra showed a reduction in the neutrophil count, compared with 2% of placebo patients. Other adverse events reported were headache, nausea, diarrhea, sinusitis, influenza-like syndrome, and abdominal pain. Malignancy rate and incidences were similar to those expected for the populations studied. Long-term follow-up of patients on anakinra has proven the overall tolerability of therapy over several years.

In animal studies, the combination of TNF inhibition and IL-1 inhibition achieved synergistic efficacy in arthritis models. However, when this approach was tested in RA patients, the combination did not achieve any additional clinical benefit but did result in greater toxicity—specifically, an increased incidence of infection and serious infection.[104] Therefore, the combination of biologic therapies targeting TNF and IL-1 is currently not recommended.

Interleukin-6

IL-6 and Inflammation

IL-6 and other members of the IL-6 cytokine family play a critical role in inflammatory and immune responses.[105] IL-6 is a small polypeptide characterized by a four–α-helix bundle structure that is stabilized by intramolecular disulfide bridges. IL-6 is secreted by various cell types, including monocytes, T and B lymphocytes, and fibroblasts. It is detectable at elevated levels in the serum and synovial tissue in inflammatory arthritides, including RA and PsA. IL-6 exerts its activity by binding its receptor component, IL-6R, which exists in soluble and membrane-bound forms, and the accessory protein, glycoprotein 130 (gp130). The IL-6R is constitutively expressed on several cell types, including lymphocytes and hepatocytes. However, soluble forms of IL-6R can productively interact with the 130 kDa signal transducing component gp130, which is expressed on a wide range of cell types (Fig. 66.4). IL-6 has multiple effects on various aspects of the immune system to initiate inflammation. IL-6 stimulates the production of T helper (Th)17 cells. These pathogenic cells secrete IL-17 and IL-22 and are involved in the induction of autoimmune injury. IL-6 also plays a role in B cell activation and differentiation. Effects of IL-6 on osteoclast differentiation and activation, including receptor activator of NF-κB (RANK) ligand–dependent mechanisms, have been clearly demonstrated.[24] Recruitment of neutrophils to the inflammatory sites and stimulation of VEGF synergistically with TNF and IL-1β contribute to pannus formation.[106] Levels of IL-6 are directly proportionate with levels of CRP and disease severity. IL-6 knockout mice are resistant to collagen-induced arthritis (CIA) and show reduced levels of serum TNF. Taken

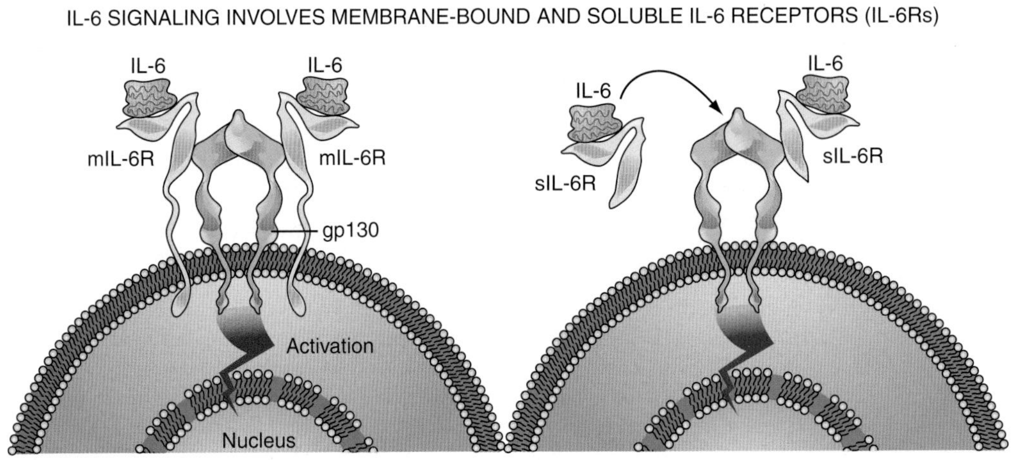

IL-6 SIGNALING INVOLVES MEMBRANE-BOUND AND SOLUBLE IL-6 RECEPTORS (IL-6Rs)

• **Fig. 66.4** IL-6. Mechanism of action: IL-6 binds first to the membrane-bound IL-6 receptor (mIL-6R). The IL-6/mIL-6R complex then associates with the signal-transducing membrane protein, gp130.

together, these functions form the basis of the rationale that IL-6 blockade is an attractive biologic target therapy for the treatment of RA and other autoimmune diseases.

IL-6 Agents

Currently two biologics targeting IL-6 are FDA approved, including tocilizumab and sarilumab. Each molecule binds to both soluble and membrane-bound IL-6 receptors (sIL-6R and mIL-6R) to therefore inhibit IL-6 mediated signaling. For signal transduction, the combination IL-6 to IL-6R must also bind a ubiquitous transmembrane protein, glycoprotein (gp) 130, leading to homodimerization of gp130 and signal transduction through JAK/STAT pathways.[107] Gp130 is expressed in a considerably wider variety of cell types; however, it can bind either membrane-bound IL-6R expressed on certain cells or pro-inflammatory soluble IL-6R through trans-signaling.[108] Therefore, therapies targeting IL-6R are more specific to the inflammatory response compared to neutralizing IL-6.

Tocilizumab may be administered either intravenously or subcutaneously with time to maximum concentration of 3 to 4 days, while sarilumab is only dosed through subcutaneous administration and similar Tmax. Both drugs are unique in comparison to other anti-cytokine therapies discussed as they demonstrate biphasic pharmacokinetics. Nonlinear concentration-dependent elimination predominates at low concentrations; however, once saturated, clearance is mainly determined by linear pharmacokinetics at higher concentrations. Therefore, elimination half-life is also concentration-dependent and ranges from 11 to 13 days for IV tocilizumab administration, 5 to 13 days for SC tocilizumab administration, and 8 to 10 days for SC sarilumab administration. Age, sex, and race do not impact the pharmacokinetics of either drug.[109–111]

Tocilizumab

Structure and Mechanism of Action. Previously referred to as *myeloma receptor antibody* (MRA), tocilizumab is a humanized IgG1 monoclonal antibody that binds with high affinity to soluble and membrane-bound forms of the 80-kDa component of the IL-6R. Tocilizumab is a recombinant humanized anti-human IL-6 receptor monoclonal antibody of the IgG1κ (gamma 1, kappa) subclass with a typical H_2L_2 polypeptide structure. Each light chain and heavy chain consists of 214 and 448 amino acids, respectively. The four polypeptide chains are linked intra- and intermolecularly by disulfide bonds. Tocilizumab has a molecular weight of approximately 148 kDa. Treatment with this monoclonal antibody effectively inhibits IL-6–mediated interactions on cells constitutively expressing the IL-6R. In addition, as noted, soluble forms of the IL-6R can productively interact with the 130-kDa signal-transducing component gp130, which is expressed on a wide range of cell types; thus, treatment with tocilizumab effectively inhibits a broad array of IL-6–driven processes.

Pharmacokinetics. Tocilizumab has a nonlinear pharmacokinetic profile.[106] The maximum concentration increases in approximate proportion to increases in dosage, whereas the area under the concentration-time curve increases disproportionately. As the dosage increases, clearance and the apparent elimination rate constant decrease, and terminal half-life and mean residence times are prolonged. Methotrexate therapy, alcohol consumption, age, and race have not been found to affect the pharmacokinetics of tocilizumab. Tocilizumab binds to soluble IL-6R in a dose-dependent manner and saturates the receptor at approximately 0.1 μg/mL. Tocilizumab also competitively inhibits IL-6 binding to soluble IL-6R; complete inhibition is seen at higher concentrations of approximately 4 μg/mL. After intravenous dosing, tocilizumab undergoes biphasic elimination from the circulation. In patients with RA, the central volume of distribution was 3.5 L, and the peripheral volume of distribution was 2.9 L, resulting in a volume distribution at steady state of 6.4 L.

Drug Dose. Indications for the use of tocilizumab vary across the globe. In the United States, initial approval for tocilizumab in late 2009 was for it to be used alone or concomitant with methotrexate or other DMARDs in treating adult patients with RA in whom one or more TNF inhibitors had failed. Recommended starting dose is 4 mg/kg followed by an increase to 8 mg/kg based on clinical response. In other countries, it is recommended to start therapy at 8 mg/kg, with the possibility of reducing to 4 mg/kg, for example, in the case of tolerability concerns. It is administered once every 4 weeks as a 60-minute single intravenous infusion. Doses exceeding 800 mg per infusion are not recommended.

Efficacy. Therapy with tocilizumab had a beneficial effect on the progression of radiographic joint damage defined by total Sharp score, in addition to improvements in clinical and functional status.

Tocilizumab has been studied in a series of multinational phase III clinical trials involving more than 4000 patients. The key phase III trial data are shown in Table 66.3.

Mean joint erosion, joint space narrowing, and total Genant-modified Sharp scores indicated that both tocilizumab doses were associated with significant inhibition of radiographic progression from baseline compared with that of placebo.[112] Clinical, functional, and structural remission in patients with advanced RA were demonstrated in a 52-week trial.

Sarilumab

Structure and Mechanism of Action. Sarilumab is a human monoclonal antibody that inhibits IL-6 mediated signaling through both the soluble and membrane-bound IL-6 receptors (sIL-6R and mIL-6R).

Pharmacokinetics. With dosing at either 150 mg or 200 mg, sarilumab reaches a maximum concentration after 2 to 4 days, with steady state reached after 14 to 16 weeks. Elimination is through both linear and nonlinear pathways, with nonlinear saturable elimination predominating at lower concentrations and linear proteolytic pathways utilized at higher concentrations. This leads to a half-life that is concentration-dependent, ranging from 8 to 10 days depending on dosing.

Drug Dose. Sarilumab was studied as both 150 mg and 200 mg subcutaneous injections every 2 weeks. Due to greater efficacy with the 200 mg dosing, the higher dosing is the recommended treatment regimen as monotherapy or in conjunction with a conventional DMARD; however, the lower 150 mg dosing may be utilized if laboratory abnormalities occur.

Efficacy. Sarilumab showed efficacy in two different doses (150 mg and 200 mg) given subcutaneously every 2 weeks in phase III randomized trials and is approved for the treatment of moderate to severe RA (see Table 66.3).

Anti-IL-6 Antibody

Sirukumab. A human monoclonal anti-IL-6 monoclonal antibody has also shown improvements in signs and symptoms of RA given 50 mg or 100 mg subcutaneously every 2 to 4 weeks.[113] Although sirukumab demonstrated significant efficacy in treating RA, the incidence of adverse events, including elevated liver enzymes (13% to 14% vs. 3% placebo) and neutropenia (2.7% to 5.3% vs. 0.4% placebo), led the US FDA advisory committee to not recommend the drug for FDA approval.

Toxicity

A number of safety concerns are associated with blocking a major regulatory cytokine such as IL-6. These can be grouped as general immunomodulatory effects (e.g., infection), IL-6–related effects (e.g., abnormalities in liver enzymes, lipid profiles), and finally agent-specific effects (e.g., infusion reactions) (see Table 66.4).

Infections are a concern, as they are with all immunomodulatory therapies for RA. In clinical trials of tocilizumab, the occurrence of infection appears compatible with that of other approved biologic agents. Although the overall infection rate with tocilizumab monotherapy was comparable with rates in methotrexate monotherapy groups, the incidence of overall infection was slightly higher with concomitant DMARD therapy. The most commonly reported infections (5% to 8%) were upper respiratory infections and nasopharyngitis. A similar incidence of serious adverse events (5%) was generally observed across study groups. Serious infections occurred more often in higher-dose groups as compared with the placebo group. Cellulitis, pneumonia, diverticulitis, gastroenteritis, and herpes zoster were the most common infections noted. Only rare cases of opportunistic infection have been reported.[101–103]

Transient elevations of ALT and aspartate aminotransferase (AST) levels were commonly observed in patients treated with IL-6 inhibitors. Elevations were more apparent immediately following tocilizumab infusions, potentially reflecting blockade of the anti-apoptotic properties of IL-6 in hepatocytes. An increase in ALT levels to three or more times the upper limit of normal was noted in 5% to 6.5% of patients who received tocilizumab and concomitant DMARD therapy. These rates were 1.5% and 2.1% in patients who received only DMARD or only tocilizumab, respectively.[114–117] Comparatively, sarilumab led to LFT elevations in 1 to 4% of patients with concurrent DMARD therapy. To date, elevated transaminases have not been associated with reduced liver function or serious adverse events.[106,116,117]

Lipid profiles were altered in the tocilizumab and sarilumab groups compared with placebo. Tocilizumab was associated with increases in all lipid levels, including total cholesterol and its fractions, low-density lipoprotein (LDL) cholesterol, and high-density lipoprotein (HDL) cholesterol. Increases in these parameters were noted by the first assessment at 6 weeks and remained elevated through the clinical trials. Sarilumab led to lipid elevations at 4 weeks after start, with no additional increases observed thereafter. Despite elevations in these parameters, clinical cardiovascular events have not increased in clinical trials. Mean increases in the 8 mg/kg tocilizumab plus DMARD group and sarilumab plus DMARD group were 21.7 mg/dL and 12 to 16 mg/dL (LDL cholesterol), 4.3 mg/dL and 3 mg/dL (HDL cholesterol), 30.1 mg/dL and 20 to 27 mg/dL (triglycerides), and 30.9 mg/dL and 0 mg/dL (total cholesterol), respectively.[103–104]

A higher proportion of patients receiving IL-6 inhibitors had a decrease in neutrophil counts (up to 29% for tocilizumab) in comparison with patients who were not receiving this drug (4%). The drop in neutrophil counts was generally mild (grade 1, according to the common toxicity criteria, i.e., 1500 to 2000 cells/mm^3 or more) to moderate (grade 2, 1000 to 1500 cells/mm^3) in severity and reversed with discontinuation of treatment. To date, no clear association between low neutrophil counts and infection-related adverse events has been noted.[115,117,118]

Treatment with tocilizumab or sarilumab was associated with a reduction in platelet counts. The decrease in platelet counts was below the lower limit of normal and was reported in 8% to 9% of patients receiving tocilizumab with or without MTX, while approximately 1% for sarilumab. However, no serious bleeding incidents occurred. Only isolated cases of epistaxis and hemoptysis were reported in patients with moderate to severe thrombocytopenia.

Rare events of gastrointestinal perforation have been reported in clinical trials, primarily as complications of diverticulitis. The overall rate of gastrointestinal perforation was 0.26 event per 100 patient-years. Most patients who developed gastrointestinal perforations were taking concomitant NSAIDs, corticosteroids, or methotrexate. Patients presenting with new-onset abdominal symptoms therefore should be evaluated promptly for early identification of gastrointestinal perforation.

Because tocilizumab is a humanized antibody, infusion-related adverse events might be expected. Adverse reactions associated with the infusion were reported to be 8% and 7% in patients receiving 4 mg/kg and 8 mg/kg tocilizumab together with MTX. The most commonly reported adverse events were hypertension during the infusion and headache and skin reactions within 24 hours after the infusion. These reactions did not result in termination of treatment. Antibodies to tocilizumab were detected in a small group of patients, and very few were associated with medically significant hypersensitivity reactions that led to withdrawal. The development of antibodies and of infusion reactions may be greater among patients receiving the lower dose of tocilizumab.

Rates of malignancy were similar in the treatment and standard of care groups. Rare cases of demyelinating disorders were reported in clinical trials. Long-term experience with tocilizumab will determine the actual risk of developing these entities; however, caution needs to be exercised in patients with any risk factors for malignancy or demyelinating disorders.

A systematic literature search on six published randomized controlled trials that assessed the risk of adverse events with tocilizumab revealed that tocilizumab in combination with MTX as a treatment for RA is associated with a small but significantly increased risk of adverse events, which is comparable with that of other biologics. The risk of infection was significantly higher in the 8 mg/kg combination group compared with controls (odds ratio [OR], 1.30; 95% CI, 1.07 to 1.58). No increased incidence of malignancy, TB reactivation, or hepatitis was observed.[119]

Drug Interactions

Inhibition of IL-6 may affect cytochrome P450 substrates. In vivo studies showed that omeprazole and simvastatin levels decreased by 28% and 57% 1 week after tocilizumab infusion. Upon initiation or discontinuation of a IL-6 inhibitor with a narrow therapeutic margin, such as warfarin, or a drug concentration, such as cyclosporine, the patient should be closely monitored.

IL-6 inhibitors have not been studied, and their use should be avoided, in combination with biologic DMARDs such as TNF inhibitors, IL-1 blockers, anti-CD20 monoclonal antibodies, and co-stimulation blockers.

Interleukin-12/23

IL-12 and IL-23 in Inflammation

IL-12 and IL-23 are released by dendritic cells and macrophages in response to innate danger signals.[120] Both of these molecules are important in host defense and wound healing. IL-12 induces the differentiation of naïve T lymphocytes to IFNγ-secreting Th1 cells whereas IL-23, in the presence of IL-6, TGFβ, and IL-1, promotes the differentiation of naïve T lymphocytes to Th17 cells that release IL-17, IL-22, and TNF. The IL-23/IL-17 pathway is pivotal in the development of psoriasis, enthesitis, dactylitis, and arthritis observed in PsA. Interestingly, blockade of IL-12/23 or IL-23 has not been effective for treatment of spinal inflammation in axial spondyloarthritis.[121] The pro-inflammatory effects of IL-23 on inflammation and bone remodeling are largely indirectly modulated by Th17 cells through the release of TNF and IL-17.

Anti-IL12/23 Antibodies

Ustekinumab

Structure and Mechanism of Action. Ustekinumab is a human IgG1k monoclonal antibody that binds to p40 on both IL-12 and IL-23 cytokines. A cumulative 1326 amino acids are combined to form the large drug molecule, with a resulting molecular mass of 148 to 149 kDa. Depending upon the drug dose and study population, the time to maximum serum concentration ranges from 7 to 13.5 days, while the half-life for elimination ranges from 15 to 45 days. Lower serum concentrations were seen in patients with higher body weight; therefore, dose adjustment is recommended with threshold of 100 kg for psoriasis and psoriatic arthritis patients. Pharmacokinetics was not impacted by patient age or concomitant methotrexate therapy.[122,123]

Drug Dose. After initial loading dose at week 0 and week 4 to hasten time to steady state, ustekinumab may be dosed either 45 mg or 90 mg subcutaneously every 12 weeks thereafter. The greater 90 mg dosing should be considered for heavier patients (>100 kg) for greater efficacy. In comparison, an intravenous weight-based loading dose followed by subcutaneous administration every 8 weeks is recommended for Crohn's disease to achieve higher therapeutic concentration for greater clinical efficacy.

Efficacy. Ustekinumab is approved for the treatment of psoriasis and PsA. The pivotal phase III trials are listed in Table 66.3. This agent is also approved for the treatment of Crohn's disease.[124] Promising phase II data have also been published in SLE.[125]

Toxicity

IL-12/23 inhibitors are generally very well tolerated. Injections site reactions are possible as with any of the above agents; however, there is a less than1% to 2% occurrence with ustekinumab. Risk of infections should be evaluated, as described in detail previously for other anti-cytokine therapies.[126]

Drug Interactions

Considering chronic inflammation and increased cytokine levels may modify CYP450 enzyme formation and activity, ustekinumab may also normalize CYP450 enzyme activity and substrate concentrations. Upon initiation or discontinuation of ustekinumab, concomitant CYP450 substrates with a narrow therapeutic index, such as warfarin or cyclosporine, should have drug concentrations and therapeutic effect closely monitored.

Anti-IL-23

Antibodies that target P19 are approved for the treatment of psoriasis and are currently under investigation in PsA.[127] Treatment responses in psoriasis have been most impressive with complete or almost complete clearance noted in a majority of patients. Phase II trials have also demonstrated efficacy in PsA.[128] Similar to ustekinumab, IL-23 blockade was not effective in ankylosing spondylitis.[129] These agents are very well tolerated with few serious adverse events noted in phase III trials.[127]

Interleukin-17

IL-17 and Inflammation

The IL-17 family of cytokines is comprised of six structurally related molecules, IL17 A-F, capable of binding to a number of distinct canonical IL-17 receptors. IL-17A and F are most strongly implicated in immune-mediated inflammation and mucosal homeostasis, and they bind to a common receptor.[130] The 17 cytokines promote the upregulation of a number of chemokines and cytokines including IL-6, G-CSF, anti-microbial peptides, and β-defensins, and they promote neutrophil migration via effects on IL-8. These cytokines also maintain host defense by protecting mucosal surfaces and inducing wound healing. Levels of IL-17 are increased in RA blood and tissues, but blockade of IL-17 is not effective in RA, in contrast to PsA and AS (described later).

IL-17 Mechanism of Action

The IL-17 cytokines promote inflammation by triggering proliferation of fibroblastoid-like synoviocytes in joints and keratinocytes in skin. They also induce neutrophil migration in these tissues. They orchestrate pathologic bone resorption by several mechanisms that involve RANKL, and in some tissue compartments they may induce bone formation.

Anti-IL-17 Antibodies

Secukinumab

Structure and Mechanism of Action. Secukinumab is a human IgG1 monoclonal antibody that selectively binds to IL-17A cytokine to inhibit binding with the IL-17 receptor.[131] Pharmacokinetics are dose proportional, with secukinumab reaching maximum concentration 6 days after each dose. After approximately 24 weeks with every 4-week dosing, steady state is reached, and the drug is eliminated with a half-life of 22 to 31 days. Although secukinumab clearance increases with increasing patient weight, no dose adjustments are indicated.

Drug Dose. Secukinumab is typically started with loading doses of either 150 mg or 300 mg administered subcutaneously once weekly at weeks 0, 1, 2, 3, 4, followed by maintenance dosing every 4 weeks thereafter. For PsA, 150 mg is the typical starting dose whereas 300 mg is prescribed for psoriasis. The dose in PsA can be increased to 300 mg for patients who experience an inadequate response to the 150 mg dose.

Efficacy. Agents that inhibit IL-17 demonstrate remarkable efficacy for patients with moderate to severe psoriasis. IL-17 inhibition was examined in RA but proven not to be effective. In contrast, both secukinumab and ixekizumab are effective for peripheral arthritis, axial inflammation, enthesitis, and dactylitis (see Table 66.3). Both agents are approved for the treatment of psoriasis, psoriatic arthritis, and axial spondyloarthritis.[127]

Ixekizumab

Structure and Mechanism of Action. Ixekizumab is a humanized IgG4 monoclonal antibody with the same binding and neutralizing activity against IL-17A.[132] As another larger molecule including two light chains of 219 amino acids each, as well as two heavy chains of 445 amino acids each, the overall molecular weight is 146 to 158 kDa. Ixekizumab also exhibits dose-proportional pharmacokinetics with time to maximum concentration of 4 days. Bioavailability of 60% to 81% is similar to secukinumab (55% to 77%); however, of interest there is notable increased bioavailability with ixekizumab subcutaneous administration into the thigh compared to abdomen or arm despite acceptable administration into either site. Steady state is reached sooner after 10 weeks, however, also with shorter half-life of 13 days. Clearance is increased in people of greater weight; however, age had no significant impact on pharmacokinetics.

Drug Dose. Dosing regimens differ by indication, but a loading dosing of 160 mg (two injections of 80 mg each) is typically included for each new start. For psoriatic arthritis, maintenance dosing is 80 mg administered subcutaneously every 4 weeks. In comparison, treatment for psoriasis typically starts with 160 mg dose, followed by 80 mg every 2 weeks for the first 3 months (until week 12), then extended to 80 mg every 4 weeks as discussed previously.

Efficacy. Ixekizumab is approved for treatment of psoriasis and psoriatic arthritis, and phase III data in axSpA show results comparable with TNF inhibitors and secukinumab. Similar to other agents that block IL-17 and IL-23, it is extremely effective for psoriasis. It is also effective for the other domains of psoriatic arthritis.

Toxicity

IL-17 inhibitors are generally well tolerated as well, with potential adverse events similar to IL 12/23 inhibitors. Candidiasis is reported in clinical trials but is generally limited in scope, although esophageal involvement has been observed. One unique concern is worsening of inflammatory bowel disease, as well as new onset of inflammatory bowel disease. Ongoing research suggests the incidence is low, but further research and post-marketing surveillance will elicit greater information.

Dual Cytokine Inhibition

Dual acting anti-cytokine therapies remain of interest to further improve clinical efficacy, however, they may be limited by binding specificity and overall rate of clearance. ABT-257 was developed to inhibit both TNF as well as IL-17A to improve the treatment response in patients with rheumatoid arthritis, however, it was limited by high clearance and short half-life, similar to its precursor ABT-122. Both molecules contained dual-variable domain immunoglobulin (DVD-Ig) to incorporate two different binding elements into a single antibody molecule, however, ABT-257 also incorporated a QL mutation in the Fc region to increase its binding affinity for the Fc receptor (FcR) to promote antibody recycling and decrease the overall rate of clearance. Unfortunately, the potential for either molecule to induce a durable response was limited by the high rate of clearance, with ABT-257 also inducing significant antibody development in 97% of subjects in single-dose study and 83% of subjects in multiple-dose study.[133] Antibody development led to even shorter half-life and lower overall serum concentration, with some subjects demonstrating no drug accumulation after repeated exposure. These bi-typical antibodies were studies in two controlled trials, one in RA and the other in PsA.[134] The efficacy in both trials was equivalent to adalimumab monotherapy, but adverse events were not higher in the patients treated with the dual variable domain antibody. It is anticipated that additional studies with dual variable domain antibodies or combinations of anti-cytokine antibodies given in lower doses or sequentially will take place in the future.

JAK-STAT Pathway

A discussion of cytokine blockade would not be complete without mentioning the Janus kinase/signal transduction and activator of transcription (JAK-STAT) signaling pathway. A range of cytokines that contribute to the development of autoimmunity and immune-mediated inflammation transduce downstream signaling through these cytoplasmic signaling pathways.[135] Following cytokine receptor engagement, receptor-associated JAKs are activated and phosphorylate STATs, which translocate to the nucleus and promote transcription of a wide range of molecules that mediate inflammation and remodeling of connective tissue. Four JAKs have been identified, JAK1, JAK2, JAK3, and TYK2, and many cytokine receptors associate with specific JAKS (Fig. 66.5). Agents that block the JAK-STAT pathway have been approved for RA, PsA, and inflammatory bowel disease and are currently in clinical trials for a wide range of inflammatory disorders. These pathways and associated therapeutic inhibitors are discussed in detail in Chapter 68.

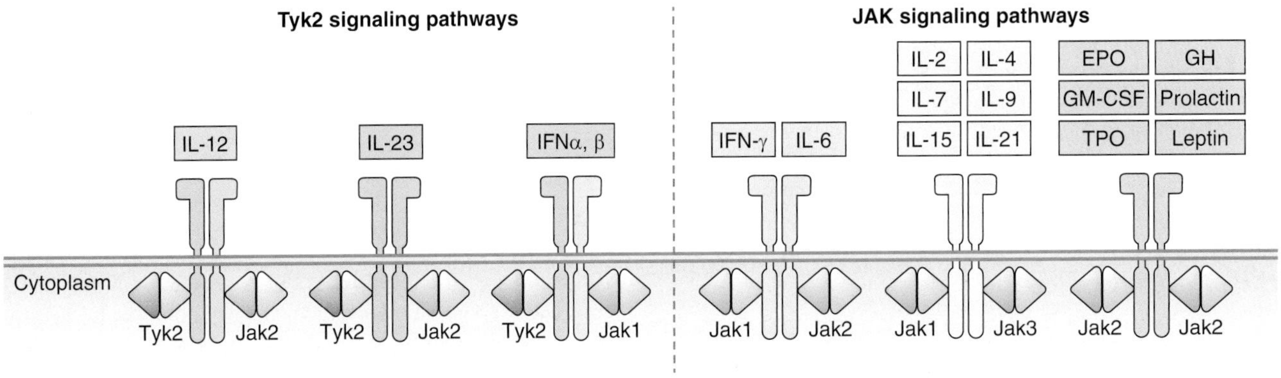

• **Fig. 66.5** Cytokine signaling through the JAK-STAT pathway. Specific cytokines signal through dimers of JAK1, -2, and -3 and Tyk 2 molecules. Thus, inhibitors of one set of homo- or hetero-dimers may demonstrate different therapeutic effects and adverse event profiles compared to agents that inhibit another set. *EPO,* Erythropoietin; *GH,* growth hormone; *GM-CSF,* granulocyte macrophage colony-stimulating factor; *JAK-STAT,* janus kinase/signal transduction and activator of transcription; *TPO,* thrombopoietin; *Tyk,* tyrosine kinase 2. (Used with permission of The Rheumatology Education Group [TREG].)

Therapies Directed at Cytokines That Regulate B Cells

Following the success with B-cell depletion with rituximab, a monoclonal antibody that binds to CD20, alternative targets were studied. BLyS and APRIL are two TNF family cytokines involved in the regulation of B-cell maturation, proliferation, function, and survival. TACI, BCMA, and BAFF are receptors with unique binding properties for BLyS and APRIL. *Belimumab, atacicept,* and *tabalumab* are BAFF/BLyS inhibitors (and APRIL in the case of atacicept) that were investigated in RA, however, due to low efficacy and considerations of toxicity, the development plans for these agents in RA were suspended. A phase III trial examining the efficacy of combining a BLyS inhibitor with rituximab is currently underway.[120] Belimumab has demonstrated modest efficacy in SLE and is approved for use in the United States (see Chapter 67).[136]

Monitoring When Treating With Cytokine Blockade

For all anti-cytokine therapies, patients should be evaluated for active and inactive (latent) TB infection before initiation of therapy. Appropriate screening tests (e.g., tuberculin skin test or ex vivo testing for TB, chest radiograph) should be performed on all patients, with anti-TB therapy initiated before patients with active TB are started on anti-cytokine therapy. Repeat testing at regular intervals (e.g., annually) for exposure to TB has been recommended by some regulatory authorities. Use of immunosuppressive therapy may increase the risk of reactivation of hepatitis B virus (HBV) among those who are chronic carriers; therefore evaluating patients for HBV before starting anti-cytokine therapy is recommended. Lastly, patients should be closely monitored for signs and symptoms of any infections, with therapy discontinued if a patient develops serious infection.

Due to rare occurrence of myelosuppression and concern about the risk of infection with TNF inhibitors, clinicians typically assess the complete blood count (CBC) intermittently during therapy. Assiduous monitoring of patients for any sign or symptom of infection, demyelinating disease, and malignancy is requisite during treatment with all TNF inhibitors.

Neutrophil counts should be assessed before anakinra treatment is initiated, as well as monthly during anakinra therapy for 3 months, and then every 4 months for up to 1 year.

For all patients starting an IL-6 inhibitor, liver function tests should be evaluated prior to start and repeated initially every 4 to 8 weeks during treatment. It is not recommended to initiate tocilizumab if ALT and AST levels are greater than 1.5 times the upper level of normal or if there is any evidence of liver disease. When the ALT or AST level is between one and three times the upper level of normal, the dose of tocilizumab, sarilumab, or concomitant DMARD should be adjusted. For persistent increases in this range, the IL-6 inhibitor dose should be modified. If the ALT or AST level is greater than three to five times the upper level of normal, IL-6 agent should be interrupted until the level falls below three times the upper level of normal. For ALT or AST elevations greater than five times the upper level of normal, the drug should be discontinued.

Patients receiving an IL-6 inhibitor should have lipid levels monitored with a goal toward maintaining levels within the target ranges of the Guideline on the Management of Blood Cholesterol or local guidelines.[137] Patients should be managed with lipid-lowering agents if appropriate.

Caution should be exercised when an IL-6 inhibitor is initiated in patients with a very low neutrophil count at baseline, and all patients should have their absolute neutrophil count (ANC) monitored 4 to 8 weeks after the first infusion. One recommendation is that tocilizumab should not be administered to patients with ANC values less than 2000 cells/mm^3. If the ANC falls to between 500 cells/mm^3 and 1000 cells/mm^3, drug therapy should be discontinued until the ANC reaches above 1000 cells/mm^3.

It is not recommended to initiate tocilizumab treatment in patients with a platelet count below 100,000/mm^3. Treatment with an IL-6 inhibitor should be interrupted if the platelet count falls to below 50,000/mm^3. Platelets should be monitored every 3 to 8 weeks.

Lastly, IL12/23 and IL 17 inhibitors do not require any additional specific monitoring except for signs and symptoms of infection, as well as potential agent-related adverse effects of injection site reactions and hypersensitivity reactions.

TABLE 66.6 Anti-cytokine Therapy in Pregnancy and Lactation

	Pregnancy Category	Transplacental Transport	Lactation	Neonatal Outcomes
Adalimumab	B	Active transport greatest in 3rd trimester	Present in breast milk 0.1%-1% of maternal serum level, and minimally absorbed by breastfed infant	No evidence of major birth defects, however detected in infant serum for at least 3 months after birth
Certolizumab	B	Minimal	Limited data; infant systemic exposure expected to be low due to degradation in infant gastrointestinal tract	No evidence of major birth defects
Etanercept	B	Fetal concentration 1/30th of maternal concentration	Present in low levels of milk, and minimally absorbed by breastfed infant	No evidence of major birth defects, and no detection 12 weeks after birth
Golimumab	B	Active transport greatest in 3rd trimester	Limited data; present in low levels of milk per animal studies, and expected minimal absorption by breastfed infant	No evidence of major birth defects, possible detection in infant serum however duration unknown
Infliximab	B	Active transport greatest in 3rd trimester	Limited data; infant systemic exposure expected to be low due to degradation in infant gastrointestinal tract	No evidence of major birth defects, however detected in infant serum up to 6 months after birth
Tocilizumab	C	Active transport greatest in 3rd trimester	Concentration excreted into breast milk and infant systemic absorption not studied	No evidence of teratogenicity in animal studies; limited human data.
Sarilumab	Not specified	Active transport greatest in 3rd trimester	Maternal immunoglobulins excreted in breast milk, however sarilumab concentration unknown	Inhibition IL-6 signaling may interfere with cervical ripening, dilatation, and myometrial activity leading to potential delays in parturition
Ixekizumab	Not specified	Active transport greatest in 3rd trimester	Limited data; present in low levels of milk per animal studies, and expected minimal absorption by breastfed infant	No evidence of teratogenicity in animal studies; limited data in humans
Secukinumab	B	Active transport greatest in 3rd trimester	Limited data; infant systemic exposure expected to be low due to degradation in infant gastrointestinal tract	No evidence of major birth defects
Ustekinumab	B	Active transport greatest in 3rd trimester	Limited data; present in low levels of milk per animal studies, and expected minimal absorption by breastfed infant	No evidence of major birth defects

Pregnancy and Breastfeeding

Developmental toxicity in animal studies has not revealed any maternal toxicity, embryo toxicity, or teratogenicity associated with TNF inhibition. Minimal controlled studies in humans have been conducted, however, information is growing from registry databases as well as retrospective studies (Table 66.6). As the number of patients treated with TNF inhibitors increases, a growing number of pregnancies will be reported among them.[75] Outcome data based on anecdotal observations of small numbers of pregnant women treated with infliximab, etanercept, and adalimumab reveal that the relative rates of live births, miscarriages, and therapeutic terminations were comparable with rates in a national cohort of age-matched healthy women. Placental transfer of monoclonal antibodies is known to increase as pregnancy progresses, with the largest amount transferred during the third trimester. Certolizumab is an exception in which the PEGylated moiety significantly reduces placental transfer. Overall, TNF inhibitors are classified as US FDA Pregnancy Category B. The use of TNF inhibitors in pregnancy is recommended only if such treatment is clearly needed. If TNF inhibitors are used during pregnancy, transfer to the fetus is possible, and monitoring might be considered on that basis.

Beyond TNF inhibitors, reproductive studies have been limited to animals and do not reveal any evidence of harm to the fetus. However, no well-controlled studies have been conducted in pregnant women; therefore, anti-cytokine therapies should be used during pregnancy only if potential benefits justify potential risk to the fetus.

There are limited data about breastfeeding, including the amount of drug that is secreted into human milk. Immunoglobulins are present in breast milk, however, they are readily degraded in the gastrointestinal tract of the nursing infant, therefore, overall infant exposure is unknown.

Vaccinations

Prior to starting therapy with an anti-cytokine therapy, it is preferred to have all recommended vaccinations brought up to date. Because data on the response to live vaccinations or the secondary transmission of infection by live vaccinations in patients receiving immunosuppressive therapy are insufficient, concurrent administration of live vaccines with anti-cytokine therapy is not recommended. Inactivated, recombinant, or conjugate vaccines, including the newer Shingrix vaccine are permissible prior to and during anti-cytokine therapy.

Conclusion

The development of potent, specific inhibitors to a spectrum of pivotal pro-inflammatory cytokines including TNF, IL-1β, IL-6, IL-12, IL-23, and IL-17 has dramatically altered the therapeutic landscape and improved outcomes for patients with immune inflammatory disorders. In particular, treatment with targeted biologics has substantially alleviated the signs and symptoms of both peripheral and axial arthritis, improved function and quality of life for inhibited radiographic progression, and averted disability for many patients. The success of targeting cytokines has "raised the bar" for the goals to treat these debilitating disorders and reinvigorated investigations into additional refinements of therapy. The experience with the current treatments also catalyzed research into the potential utility of inhibitors of additional cytokines such as IL-6, IL-15, and IL-18 and other components of the immune system relevant to autoimmune and inflammatory disease.

A number of questions remain regarding the optimal use of these drugs. Longer-term safety data will allow clinicians to more fully assess the risk-benefit ratio for individual patients. Given uncertainties regarding the long-term safety of these drugs and the heterogeneity of clinical responses, research defining the populations of patients expected to derive the greatest benefit with the least toxicity is critical. For example, ongoing research assessing genetic polymorphisms or proteomic or glycomic differences among treated patients could optimize efficacy while minimizing toxicity. This is also relevant from a cost standpoint. Although the acquisition costs of these agents are relatively high, data supporting their cost-effectiveness, including gains in employment and reduced hospitalizations, are emerging.[138]

The success observed with these biologic therapies has raised additional clinical questions. For example, can very early treatment with highly effective therapy, such as the combination of TNF inhibitor and MTX, truly alter the disease course? What are the optimal treatment paradigms for various rheumatic diseases? How can precision medicine be applied to identify the most appropriate biologic therapy for an individual patient? Is there a role for combination biologics given that up to 50% of patients do not achieve primary outcomes in phase III trials, and how should these combination regimens be developed? Certainly, advances in biopharmaceuticals could generate agents that possess desirable characteristics in terms of pharmacokinetics, immunogenicity, adverse effects, ease of administration, and cost. These developments will likely allow clinicians to maximize the use of these novel therapies and achieve clinical benefits that previously were considered unattainable.

Full references for this chapter can be found on ExpertConsult.com.

Selected References

1. Zhang JM, An J: Cytokines, inflammation, and pain, *Int Anesthesiol Clin* 45(2):27–37, 2007.
2. Feldmann M, Brennan FM, Maini RN: Role of cytokines in rheumatoid arthritis, *Annu Rev Immunol* 14:397–440, 1996.
3. Koch AE, Kunkel SL, Strieter RM: Cytokines in rheumatoid arthritis, *J Investig Med* 43(1):28–38, 1995.
5. Lybecker K: *The Biologics Revolution in the Production of Drugs*, Fraser Institute, 2016.
6. Monaco C, Nanchahal J, Taylor P, et al.: Anti-TNF therapy: past, present and future, *Int Immunol* 27(1):55–62, 2015.
8. McCann FE, Perocheau DP, Ruspi G, et al.: Selective tumor necrosis factor receptor I blockade is antiinflammatory and reveals immunoregulatory role of tumor necrosis factor receptor II in collagen-induced arthritis, *Arthritis Rheumatol* 66(10):2728–2738, 2014.
10. Kavanaugh A, Cohen S, Cush JJ: The evolving use of tumor necrosis factor inhibitors in rheumatoid arthritis, *J Rheumatol* 31(10):1881–1884, 2004.
11. Zou JX, Braun J, Sieper J: Immunological basis for the use of TNFalpha-blocking agents in ankylosing spondylitis and immunological changes during treatment, *Clin Exp Rheumatol* 20(6 Suppl 28):S34–S37, 2002.
12. Bazzoni F, Beutler B: The tumor necrosis factor ligand and receptor families, *New Eng J Med* 334(26):1717–1725, 1996.
14. Feldmann M, Elliott MJ, Woody JN, et al.: Anti-tumor necrosis factor-alpha therapy of rheumatoid arthritis, *Adv Immunol* 64:283–350, 1997.
16. Taylor PC: Pharmacology of TNF blockade in rheumatoid arthritis and other chronic inflammatory diseases, *Curr Opin Pharmacol* 10(3):308–315, 2010.
18. Charles P, Elliott MJ, Davis D, et al.: Regulation of cytokines, cytokine inhibitors, and acute-phase proteins following anti-TNF-alpha therapy in rheumatoid arthritis, *J Immunol* 163(3):1521–1528, 1999.
22. Paleolog EM, Miotla JM: Angiogenesis in arthritis: role in disease pathogenesis and as a potential therapeutic target, *Angiogenesis* 2(4):295–307, 1998.
23. Mewar D, Wilson AG: Treatment of rheumatoid arthritis with tumour necrosis factor inhibitors, *Br J Pharmacol* 162(4):785–791, 2011.
25. Moreland LW, Schiff MH, Baumgartner SW, et al.: Etanercept therapy in rheumatoid arthritis. A randomized, controlled trial, *Ann Intern Med* 130(6):478–486, 1999.
27. Klotz U, Teml A, Schwab M: Clinical pharmacokinetics and use of infliximab, *Clin Pharmacokinet* 46(8):645–660, 2007.
29. Weisman MH, Moreland LW, Furst DE, et al.: Efficacy, pharmacokinetic, and safety assessment of adalimumab, a fully human anti-tumor necrosis factor-alpha monoclonal antibody, in adults with rheumatoid arthritis receiving concomitant methotrexate: a pilot study, *Clinical Therapeutics* 25(6):1700–1721, 2003.
32. Brennan FM, Browne KA, Green PA, et al.: Reduction of serum matrix metalloproteinase 1 and matrix metalloproteinase 3 in rheumatoid arthritis patients following anti-tumour necrosis factor-alpha (cA2) therapy, *Br J Rheumatol* 36(6):643–650, 1997.
34. Genovese MC, Bathon JM, Martin RW, et al.: Etanercept versus methotrexate in patients with early rheumatoid arthritis: two-year radiographic and clinical outcomes, *Arthritis Rheum* 46(6):1443–1450, 2002.
35. Kavanaugh A, St Clair EW, McCune WJ, et al.: Chimeric anti-tumor necrosis factor-alpha monoclonal antibody treatment of patients with rheumatoid arthritis receiving methotrexate therapy, *J Rheumatol* 27(4):841–850, 2000.
37. Klareskog L, van der Heijde D, de Jager JP, et al.: Therapeutic effect of the combination of etanercept and methotrexate compared with each treatment alone in patients with rheumatoid arthritis:

double-blind randomised controlled trial, *Lancet* 363(9410):675–681, 2004.
39. Weinblatt ME, Kremer JM, Bankhurst AD, et al.: A trial of etanercept, a recombinant tumor necrosis factor receptor:Fc fusion protein, in patients with rheumatoid arthritis receiving methotrexate, *N Engl J Med* 340(4):253–259, 1999.
41. Kay J, Upchurch KS: ACR/EULAR 2010 rheumatoid arthritis classification criteria, *Rheumatology (Oxford)* 51(Suppl 6):vi5–9, 2012.
42. Korth-Bradley JM, Rubin AS, Hanna RK, et al.: The pharmacokinetics of etanercept in healthy volunteers, *Ann Pharmacotherapy* 34(2):161–164, 2000.
44. Weinblatt ME, Keystone EC, Furst DE, et al.: Adalimumab, a fully human anti-tumor necrosis factor alpha monoclonal antibody, for the treatment of rheumatoid arthritis in patients taking concomitant methotrexate: the ARMADA trial, *Arthritis Rheum* 48(1):35–45, 2003.
45. Ritchlin CT, Colbert RA, Gladman DD: Psoriatic arthritis, *N Engl J Med* 376(10):957–970, 2017.
46. Mease PJ, Gladman DD, Collier DH, et al.: Etanercept and methotrexate as monotherapy or in combination for psoriatic arthritis: primary results from a randomized, controlled phase III trial, *Arthritis Rheumatol* 71:1112–1124, 2019.
47. Rudwaleit M, Landewe R, Sieper J: Ankylosing spondylitis and axial spondyloarthritis, *N Engl J Med* 375(13):1302–1303, 2016.
48. Sari I, Haroon N: Radiographic progression in ankylosing spondylitis: from prognostication to disease modification, *Curr Rheumatol Rep* 20(12):82, 2018.
49. Rudwaleit M, Landewe R, van der Heijde D, et al.: The development of Assessment of SpondyloArthritis International Society classification criteria for axial spondyloarthritis (part I): classification of paper patients by expert opinion including uncertainty appraisal, *Ann Rheum Dis* 68(6):770–776, 2009.
50. Rudwaleit M, van der Heijde D, Landewe R, et al.: The development of Assessment of SpondyloArthritis International Society classification criteria for axial spondyloarthritis (part II): validation and final selection, *Ann Rheum Dis* 68(6):777–783, 2009.
51. Deodhar A, Gensler LS, Kay J, et al.: A fifty-two-week, randomized, placebo-controlled trial of certolizumab pegol in nonradiographic axial spondyloarthritis, *Arthritis Rheumatol*, 2019.
52. TNF inhibitors for Crohn's disease: when, which, and for how long, *Med Lett Drugs Ther* 55(1432):102–103, 2013.
53. Gimenez-Roca C, Iglesias E, Torrente-Segarra V, et al.: Efficacy and safety of TNF-alpha antagonists in children with juvenile idiopathic arthritis who started treatment under 4 years of age, *Rheumatol Int* 35(2):323–326, 2015.
55. Aringer M, Smolen JS: TNF inhibition in SLE: where do we stand? *Lupus* 18(1):5–8, 2009.
56. Breedveld FC, Weisman MH, Kavanaugh AF, et al.: The PREMIER study: a multicenter, randomized, double-blind clinical trial of combination therapy with adalimumab plus methotrexate versus methotrexate alone or adalimumab alone in patients with early, aggressive rheumatoid arthritis who had not had previous methotrexate treatment, *Arthritis Rheum* 54(1):26–37, 2006.
57. Keystone EC, Genovese MC, Klareskog L, et al.: Golimumab, a human antibody to tumour necrosis factor {alpha} given by monthly subcutaneous injections, in active rheumatoid arthritis despite methotrexate therapy: the GO-FORWARD Study, *Ann Rheum Dis* 68(6):789–796, 2009.
58. Keystone EC, Kavanaugh AF, Sharp JT, et al.: Radiographic, clinical, and functional outcomes of treatment with adalimumab (a human anti-tumor necrosis factor monoclonal antibody) in patients with active rheumatoid arthritis receiving concomitant methotrexate therapy: a randomized, placebo-controlled, 52-week trial, *Arthritis Rheum* 50(5):1400–1411, 2004.
59. Smolen J, Landewe RB, Mease P, et al.: Efficacy and safety of certolizumab pegol plus methotrexate in active rheumatoid arthritis: the RAPID 2 study. A randomised controlled trial, *Ann Rheum Dis* 68(6):797–804, 2009.
60. Smolen JS, Han C, Bala M, et al.: Evidence of radiographic benefit of treatment with infliximab plus methotrexate in rheumatoid arthritis patients who had no clinical improvement: a detailed subanalysis of data from the anti-tumor necrosis factor trial in rheumatoid arthritis with concomitant therapy study, *Arthritis Rheum* 52(4):1020–1030, 2005.
61. Smolen JS, Kay J, Doyle MK, et al.: Golimumab in patients with active rheumatoid arthritis after treatment with tumour necrosis factor alpha inhibitors (GO-AFTER study): a multicentre, randomised, double-blind, placebo-controlled, phase III trial, *Lancet* 374(9685):210–221, 2009.
62. St Clair EW, van der Heijde DM, Smolen JS, et al.: Combination of infliximab and methotrexate therapy for early rheumatoid arthritis: a randomized, controlled trial, *Arthritis Rheum* 50(11):3432–3443, 2004.
63. Weinblatt ME, Keystone EC, Furst DE, et al.: Long term efficacy and safety of adalimumab plus methotrexate in patients with rheumatoid arthritis: ARMADA 4 year extended study, *Ann Rheum Dis* 65(6):753–759, 2006.
65. Lee SJ, Kavanaugh A: Adverse reactions to biologic agents: focus on autoimmune disease therapies, *J Allergy Clin Immunol* 116(4):900–905, 2005.
66. Emery P, Fleischmann RM, Moreland LW, et al.: Golimumab, a human anti-tumor necrosis factor alpha monoclonal antibody, injected subcutaneously every four weeks in methotrexate-naive patients with active rheumatoid arthritis: twenty-four-week results of a phase III, multicenter, randomized, double-blind, placebo-controlled study of golimumab before methotrexate as first-line therapy for early-onset rheumatoid arthritis, *Arthritis Rheum* 60(8):2272–2283, 2009.
67. Kavanaugh A, McInnes I, Mease P, et al.: Golimumab, a new human tumor necrosis factor alpha antibody, administered every four weeks as a subcutaneous injection in psoriatic arthritis: twenty-four-week efficacy and safety results of a randomized, placebo-controlled study, *Arthritis Rheum* 60(4):976–986, 2009.
69. Rutherford AI, Subesinghe S, Hyrich KL, et al.: Serious infection across biologic-treated patients with rheumatoid arthritis: results from the British Society for Rheumatology Biologics Register for Rheumatoid Arthritis, *Ann Rheum Dis* 77(6):905–910, 2018.
70. Bongartz T, Sutton AJ, Sweeting MJ, et al.: Anti-TNF antibody therapy in rheumatoid arthritis and the risk of serious infections and malignancies: systematic review and meta-analysis of rare harmful effects in randomized controlled trials, *JAMA* 295(19):2275–2285, 2006.
71. Yamanaka H, Tanaka Y, Inoue E, et al.: Efficacy and tolerability of tocilizumab in rheumatoid arthritis patients seen in daily clinical practice in Japan: results from a retrospective study (REACTION study), *Mod Rheumatol* 21(2):122–133, 2011.
72. Dixon WG, Watson K, Lunt M, et al.: Rates of serious infection, including site-specific and bacterial intracellular infection, in rheumatoid arthritis patients receiving anti-tumor necrosis factor therapy: results from the British Society for Rheumatology Biologics Register, *Arthritis Rheum* 54(8):2368–2376, 2006.
73. Genovese MC, Rubbert-Roth A, Smolen JS, et al.: Longterm safety and efficacy of tocilizumab in patients with rheumatoid arthritis: a cumulative analysis of up to 4.6 years of exposure, *J Rheumatol* 40(6):768–780, 2013.
75. Rutherford AI, Patarata E, Subesinghe S, et al.: Opportunistic infections in rheumatoid arthritis patients exposed to biologic therapy: results from the British Society for Rheumatology Biologics Register for Rheumatoid Arthritis, *Rheumatology (Oxford)* 57(6):997–1001, 2018.

77. Borisov AS, Bamrah Morris S, Njie GJ, et al.: Update of recommendations for use of once-weekly isoniazid-rifapentine regimen to treat latent mycobacterium tuberculosis infection, *MMWR Morb Mortal Wkly Rep* 67(25):723–726, 2018.
79. Kavanaugh A: Rheumatoid arthritis: do TNF inhibitors influence lymphoma development? *Nat Rev Rheumatol* 13(12):697–698, 2017.
80. Collison J: Anti-TNF therapy not linked to cancer recurrence, *Nat Rev Rheumatol* 14(10):560, 2018.
81. Raaschou P, Simard JF, Neovius M, et al.: Anti-Rheumatic Therapy in Sweden Study G. Does cancer that occurs during or after anti-tumor necrosis factor therapy have a worse prognosis? A national assessment of overall and site-specific cancer survival in rheumatoid arthritis patients treated with biologic agents, *Arthritis Rheum* 63(7):1812–1822, 2011.
84. Conrad C, Di Domizio J, Mylonas A, et al.: TNF blockade induces a dysregulated type I interferon response without autoimmunity in paradoxical psoriasis, *Nat Commun* 9(1):25, 2018.
85. Nestle FO, Conrad C, Tun-Kyi A, et al.: Plasmacytoid predendritic cells initiate psoriasis through interferon-alpha production, *J Exp Med* 202(1):135–143, 2005.
86. Gunther S, Deredge D, Bowers AL, et al.: IL-1 family cytokines use distinct molecular mechanisms to signal through their shared co-receptor, *Immunity* 47(3):510–523 e4, 2017.
87. Urien S, Bardin C, Bader-Meunier B, et al.: Anakinra pharmacokinetics in children and adolescents with systemic-onset juvenile idiopathic arthritis and autoinflammatory syndromes, *BMC Pharmacol Toxicol* 14:40, 2013.
89. Autmizguine J, Cohen-Wolkowiez M, Ilowite N, et al.: Rilonacept pharmacokinetics in children with systemic juvenile idiopathic arthritis, *J Clin Pharmacol* 55(1):39–44, 2015.
91. Sun H, Van LM, Floch D, et al.: Pharmacokinetics and pharmacodynamics of canakinumab in patients with systemic juvenile idiopathic arthritis, *J Clin Pharmacol* 56(12):1516–1527, 2016.
94. Jiang Y, Genant HK, Watt I, et al.: A multicenter, double-blind, dose-ranging, randomized, placebo-controlled study of recombinant human interleukin-1 receptor antagonist in patients with rheumatoid arthritis: radiologic progression and correlation of Genant and Larsen scores, *Arthritis Rheum* 43(5):1001–1009, 2000.
95. McDermott MF: Rilonacept in the treatment of chronic inflammatory disorders, *Drugs Today (Barc)* 45(6):423–430, 2009.
96. Church LD, McDermott MF: Canakinumab: a human anti-IL-1beta monoclonal antibody for the treatment of cryopyrin-associated periodic syndromes, *Expert Rev Clin Immunol* 6(6):831–841, 2010.
97. Church LD, Savic S, McDermott MF: Long term management of patients with cryopyrin-associated periodic syndromes (CAPS): focus on rilonacept (IL-1 Trap), *Biologics* 2(4):733–742, 2008.
98. Hoffman HM: Rilonacept for the treatment of cryopyrin-associated periodic syndromes (CAPS), *Expert Opin Biol Ther* 9(4):519–531, 2009.
99. Hoffman HM, Throne ML, Amar NJ, et al.: Efficacy and safety of rilonacept (interleukin-1 Trap) in patients with cryopyrin-associated periodic syndromes: results from two sequential placebo-controlled studies, *Arthritis Rheum* 58(8):2443–2452, 2008.
100. Ilowite NT, Prather K, Lokhnygina Y, et al.: Randomized, double-blind, placebo-controlled trial of the efficacy and safety of rilonacept in the treatment of systemic juvenile idiopathic arthritis, *Arthritis Rheumatol* 66(9):2570–2579, 2014.
101. Janssen CA, Oude Voshaar MAH, Vonkeman HE, et al.: Anakinra for the treatment of acute gout flares: a randomized, double-blind, placebo-controlled, active-comparator, non-inferiority trial, *Rheumatology (Oxford)* 2019.
102. Ridker PM: Mortality differences associated with treatment Responses in CANTOS and FOURIER: insights and implications, *Circulation* 137(17):1763–1766, 2018.
103. Dinarello CA: Interleukin-1 in the pathogenesis and treatment of inflammatory diseases, *Blood* 117(14):3720–3732, 2011.
104. Genovese MC, Cohen S, Moreland L, et al.: Combination therapy with etanercept and anakinra in the treatment of patients with rheumatoid arthritis who have been treated unsuccessfully with methotrexate, *Arthritis Rheum* 50(5):1412–1419, 2004.
105. Unver N, McAllister F: IL-6 family cytokines: key inflammatory mediators as biomarkers and potential therapeutic targets, *Cytokine Growth Factor Rev* 41:10–17, 2018.
107. Hennigan S, Kavanaugh A: Interleukin-6 inhibitors in the treatment of rheumatoid arthritis, *Ther Clin Risk Manag* 4(4):767–775, 2008.
108. Rose-John S: IL-6 trans-signaling via the soluble IL-6 receptor: importance for the pro-inflammatory activities of IL-6, *Int J Biol Sci* 8(9):1237–1247, 2012.
111. Abdallah H, Hsu JC, Lu P, et al.: Pharmacokinetic and pharmacodynamic analysis of subcutaneous tocilizumab in patients with rheumatoid arthritis from 2 randomized, controlled trials: SUMMACTA and BREVACTA, *J Clini Pharmacol* 57(4):459–468, 2017.
112. Emery P, Keystone E, Tony HP, et al.: IL-6 receptor inhibition with tocilizumab improves treatment outcomes in patients with rheumatoid arthritis refractory to anti-tumour necrosis factor biologicals: results from a 24-week multicentre randomised placebo-controlled trial, *Ann Rheum Dis* 67(11):1516–1523, 2008.
113. Smolen JS, Weinblatt ME, Sheng S, et al.: Sirukumab, a human anti-interleukin-6 monoclonal antibody: a randomised, 2-part (proof-of-concept and dose-finding), phase II study in patients with active rheumatoid arthritis despite methotrexate therapy, *Ann Rheum Dis* 73(9):1616–1625, 2014.
114. Genovese MC, McKay JD, Nasonov EL, et al.: Interleukin-6 receptor inhibition with tocilizumab reduces disease activity in rheumatoid arthritis with inadequate response to disease-modifying antirheumatic drugs: the tocilizumab in combination with traditional disease-modifying antirheumatic drug therapy study, *Arthritis Rheum* 58(10):2968–2980, 2008.
115. Nishimoto N, Hashimoto J, Miyasaka N, et al.: Study of active controlled monotherapy used for rheumatoid arthritis, an IL-6 inhibitor (SAMURAI): evidence of clinical and radiographic benefit from an x ray reader-blinded randomised controlled trial of tocilizumab, *Ann Rheum Dis* 66(9):1162–1167, 2007.
116. Nishimoto N, Miyasaka N, Yamamoto K, et al.: Long-term safety and efficacy of tocilizumab, an anti-IL-6 receptor monoclonal antibody, in monotherapy, in patients with rheumatoid arthritis (the STREAM study): evidence of safety and efficacy in a 5-year extension study, *Ann Rheum Dis* 68(10):1580–1584, 2009.
117. Smolen JS, Beaulieu A, Rubbert-Roth A, et al.: Effect of interleukin-6 receptor inhibition with tocilizumab in patients with rheumatoid arthritis (OPTION study): a double-blind, placebo-controlled, randomised trial, *Lancet* 371(9617):987–997, 2008.
118. Nakahara H, Song J, Sugimoto M, et al.: Anti-interleukin-6 receptor antibody therapy reduces vascular endothelial growth factor production in rheumatoid arthritis, *Arthritis Rheum* 48(6):1521–1529, 2003.
119. Campbell L, Chen C, Bhagat SS, et al.: Risk of adverse events including serious infections in rheumatoid arthritis patients treated with tocilizumab: a systematic literature review and meta-analysis of randomized controlled trials, *Rheumatology (Oxford)* 50(3):552–562, 2011.
120. Teng MW, Bowman EP, McElwee JJ, et al.: IL-12 and IL-23 cytokines: from discovery to targeted therapies for immune-mediated inflammatory diseases, *Nat Med* 21(7):719–729, 2015.

121. Mease P: Ustekinumab fails to show efficacy in a phase III axial spondyloarthritis program: the importance of negative results, *Arthritis Rheumatol* 71(2):179–181, 2019.
123. Zhu YW, Mendelsohn A, Pendley C, et al.: Population pharmacokinetics of ustekinumab in patients with active psoriatic arthritis, *Int J Clin Pharmacol Ther* 48(12):830–846, 2010.
124. Sandborn WJ, Gasink C, Gao LL, et al.: Ustekinumab induction and maintenance therapy in refractory Crohn's disease, *N Engl J Med* 367(16):1519–1528, 2012.
125. Costedoat-Chalumeau N, Houssiau FA: Ustekinumab: a promising new drug for SLE? *Lancet* 392(10155):1284–1286, 2018.
126. Lopez-Ferrer A, Laiz A, Puig L: The safety of ustekinumab for the treatment of psoriatic arthritis, *Expert Opin Drug Saf* 16(6):733–742, 2017.
127. Frieder J, Kivelevitch D, Haugh I, et al.: Anti-IL-23 and anti-IL-17 biologic agents for the treatment of immune-mediated inflammatory conditions, *Clin Pharmacol Ther* 103(1):88–101, 2018.
128. Deodhar A, Gottlieb AB, Boehncke WH, et al.: Efficacy and safety of guselkumab in patients with active psoriatic arthritis: a randomised, double-blind, placebo-controlled, phase 2 study, *Lancet* 391(10136):2213–2224, 2018.
129. Baeten D, Ostergaard M, Wei JC, et al.: Risankizumab, an IL-23 inhibitor, for ankylosing spondylitis: results of a randomised, double-blind, placebo-controlled, proof-of-concept, dose-finding phase 2 study, *Ann Rheum Dis* 77(9):1295–1302, 2018.
130. McGeachy MJ, Cua DJ, Gaffen SL: The IL-17 family of cytokines in health and disease, *Immunity* 50(4):892–906, 2019.
133. Othman AA, Khatri A, Loebbert R, et al.: Pharmacokinetics, safety, and tolerability of the dual inhibitor of tumor necrosis factor-alpha and interleukin 17A, ABBV-257, in healthy volunteers and patients with rheumatoid arthritis, *Clin Pharmacol Drug Develop* 2018.
134. Genovese MC, Weinblatt ME, Mease PJ, et al.: Dual inhibition of tumour necrosis factor and interleukin-17A with ABT-122: open-label long-term extension studies in rheumatoid arthritis or psoriatic arthritis, *Rheumatology (Oxford)* 57(11):1972–1981, 2018.
135. O'Shea JJ, Schwartz DM, Villarino AV, et al.: The JAK-STAT pathway: impact on human disease and therapeutic intervention, *Annu Rev Med* 66:311–328, 2015.
136. Jordan N, D'Cruz DP: Belimumab for the treatment of systemic lupus erythematosus, *Expert Rev Clin Immunol* 11(2):195–204, 2015.
137. Grundy SM, Stone NJ, Bailey AL, et al.: AHA/ACC/AACVPR/AAPA/ABC/ACPM/ADA/AGS/APhA/ASPC/NLA/PCNA guideline on the management of blood cholesterol, *Circulation* CIR0000000000000625, 2018.
138. Bukstein DA, Luskin AT: Pharmacoeconomics of biologic therapy, *Immunol Allergy Clin North Am* 37(2):413–430, 2017.
139. Mease PJ, Kivitz AJ, Burch FX, et al.: Etanercept treatment of psoriatic arthritis: safety, efficacy, and effect on disease progression, *Arthritis Rheum* 50(7):2264–2272, 2004.
140. Davis Jr JC, Van Der Heijde D, Braun J, et al.: Recombinant human tumor necrosis factor receptor (etanercept) for treating ankylosing spondylitis: a randomized, controlled trial, *Arthritis Rheum* 48(11):3230–3236, 2003.
141. Lipsky PE, van der Heijde DM, St Clair EW, et al.: Infliximab and methotrexate in the treatment of rheumatoid arthritis. Anti-tumor necrosis factor trial in rheumatoid arthritis with concomitant therapy study group, *N Engl J Med* 343(22):1594–1602, 2000.
142. Antoni C, Krueger GG, de Vlam K, et al.: Infliximab improves signs and symptoms of psoriatic arthritis: results of the IMPACT 2 trial, *Ann Rheum Dis* 64(8):1150–1157, 2005.
143. Brandt J, Sieper J, Braun J: Infliximab in the treatment of active and severe ankylosing spondylitis, *Clin Exp Rheumatol* 20(6 Suppl 28):S106–S110, 2002.
144. Mease PJ, Gladman DD, Ritchlin CT, et al.: Adalimumab for the treatment of patients with moderately to severely active psoriatic arthritis: results of a double-blind, randomized, placebo-controlled trial, *Arthritis Rheum* 52(10):3279–3289, 2005.
145. van der Heijde D, Kivitz A, Schiff MH, et al.: Efficacy and safety of adalimumab in patients with ankylosing spondylitis: results of a multicenter, randomized, double-blind, placebo-controlled trial, *Arthritis Rheum* 54(7):2136–2146, 2006.
146. Inman RD, Davis Jr JC, Heijde D, et al.: Efficacy and safety of golimumab in patients with ankylosing spondylitis: results of a randomized, double-blind, placebo-controlled, phase III trial, *Arthritis Rheum* 58(11):3402–3412, 2008.
147. Keystone E, Heijde D, Mason Jr D, et al.: Certolizumab pegol plus methotrexate is significantly more effective than placebo plus methotrexate in active rheumatoid arthritis: findings of a fifty-two-week, phase III, multicenter, randomized, double-blind, placebo-controlled, parallel-group study, *Arthritis Rheum* 58(11):3319–3329, 2008.
148. Mease PJ, Fleischmann R, Deodhar AA, et al.: Effect of certolizumab pegol on signs and symptoms in patients with psoriatic arthritis: 24-week results of a Phase 3 double-blind randomised placebo-controlled study (RAPID-PsA), *Ann Rheum Dis* 73(1):48–55, 2014.
149. Landewe R, Braun J, Deodhar A, et al.: Efficacy of certolizumab pegol on signs and symptoms of axial spondyloarthritis including ankylosing spondylitis: 24-week results of a double-blind randomised placebo-controlled Phase 3 study, *Ann Rheum Dis* 73(1):39–47, 2014.
150. Cohen SB, Moreland LW, Cush JJ, et al.: A multicentre, double blind, randomised, placebo controlled trial of anakinra (Kineret), a recombinant interleukin 1 receptor antagonist, in patients with rheumatoid arthritis treated with background methotrexate, *Ann Rheum Dis* 63(9):1062–1068, 2004.
151. Maini RN, Taylor PC, Szechinski J, et al.: Double-blind randomized controlled clinical trial of the interleukin-6 receptor antagonist, tocilizumab, in European patients with rheumatoid arthritis who had an incomplete response to methotrexate, *Arthritis Rheum* 54(9):2817–2829, 2006.
152. Genovese MC, Fleischmann R, Kivitz AJ, et al.: Sarilumab plus methotrexate in patients with active rheumatoid arthritis and inadequate response to methotrexate: results of a phase III study, *Arthritis Rheumatol* 67(6):1424–1437, 2015.
153. McInnes IB, Kavanaugh A, Gottlieb AB, et al.: Efficacy and safety of ustekinumab in patients with active psoriatic arthritis: 1 year results of the phase 3, multicentre, double-blind, placebo-controlled PSUMMIT 1 trial, *Lancet* 382(9894):780–789, 2013.
154. McInnes IB, Mease PJ, Kirkham B, et al.: Secukinumab, a human anti-interleukin-17A monoclonal antibody, in patients with psoriatic arthritis (FUTURE 2): a randomised, double-blind, placebo-controlled, phase 3 trial, *Lancet* 386(9999):1137–1146, 2015.
155. Baeten D, Sieper J, Braun J, et al.: Secukinumab, an interleukin-17A inhibitor, in ankylosing spondylitis, *N Engl J Med* 373(26):2534–2548, 2015.
156. Mease PJ, van der Heijde D, Ritchlin CT, et al.: Ixekizumab, an interleukin-17A specific monoclonal antibody, for the treatment of biologic-naive patients with active psoriatic arthritis: results from the 24-week randomised, double-blind, placebo-controlled and active (adalimumab)-controlled period of the phase III trial SPIRIT-P1, *Ann Rheum Dis* 76(1):79–87, 2017.
157. van der Heijde D, Cheng-Chung Wei J, Dougados M, et al.: Ixekizumab, an interleukin-17A antagonist in the treatment of ankylosing spondylitis or radiographic axial spondyloarthritis in patients previously untreated with biological disease-modifying anti-rheumatic drugs (COAST-V): 16 week results of a phase 3 randomised, double-blind, active-controlled and placebo-controlled trial, *Lancet* 392(10163):2441–2451, 2018.

67

Cell-Targeted Biologics and Emerging Targets: Rituximab, Abatacept, and Other Biologics

PETER C. TAYLOR

KEY POINTS

Rituximab is an effective biologic therapy across the spectrum of rheumatoid arthritis (RA) patient populations but with greatest benefit in seropositive patients. Clinical trials in people with active, established RA confirm that a single cycle of rituximab given as two infusions of 1 g each, together with once-weekly oral methotrexate, produces a clinical response comparable to that observed with TNF blockade. A treatment cycle of two infusions of 500 mg is also efficacious but may result in a lower proportion of patients demonstrating more robust clinical responses and is less likely to inhibit radiographic progression.

Current data suggest that the most appropriate interval between rituximab courses is 6 to 12 months. Repeat treatment produces American College of Rheumatology (ACR) responses that equal or exceed those from the first course of treatment, with a comparable duration of effect.

Rituximab has an acceptable safety record in RA trials, but infusion reactions can occur; most are mild to moderate. Frequency and severity are reduced by the administration of intravenous methylprednisolone before rituximab infusions.

Abatacept can result in a meaningful clinical response within 16 weeks in people with RA.

Abatacept represents an effective biologic therapy with acceptable safety across the spectrum of RA patient populations. Sustained clinical responses may be incremental for up to 2 years of treatment.

The benefit-risk profile of abatacept may be most optimal when it is introduced earlier in the RA treatment paradigm. Both rituximab and abatacept slow radiographic progression in patients with RA.

Current uncertainties include the lack of reliable biomarkers to inform the rational choice of a biologic agent.

Introduction

As appreciation of the gravity of the social and economic burden imposed by rheumatoid arthritis (RA) has grown, so has the recognition that more favorable clinical outcomes are achieved when synovitis is optimally suppressed. The evidence is particularly compelling early in the course of RA, when intervention with disease-modifying combination therapy results in improved remission rates and increased clinical and radiographic benefits.[1–3] The armamentarium of potential therapeutics has also grown with the identification of relevant disease molecules. Of these, biologic therapeutics targeting TNF, particularly when used in combination with oral methotrexate, have had notable success in suppressing inflammation and markedly inhibiting the progression of structural damage previously thought to be an unavoidable characteristic of RA.[4,5] Nevertheless, despite the unprecedented clinical and commercial successes of TNF inhibitors, their availability is restricted by high costs. In addition, a substantial proportion of patients with RA do not demonstrate significant clinical responses.

An entirely different treatment approach to the blockade of proinflammatory cytokines is the targeting of cells implicated in the persistence (or even potentially initiation) of RA (see Chapters 74, 75). It is believed that immune responses drive the disease process in RA, and because chronicity is a hallmark of the RA phenotype, it presumably reflects the persistence of immunologic memory, which is induced and maintained by the adaptive immune system. In particular, T and B cells develop highly specific receptors and, after stimulation, expand enormously in number and then persist for long periods. If this is true of aberrant immune responses that lead to disease, then T and B cells represent rational targets for immune intervention. The focus of this chapter is on biologic agents with specificity for cellular targets, namely cell surface molecules associated with B cell subsets, most notably CD20, and co-stimulation molecules expressed on antigen-presenting cells that recognize cognate ligands on T cells. Two drugs that have become an accepted part of the pharmacologic armamentarium for RA treatment will be emphasized: rituximab and abatacept. Rituximab (Rituxan, Genentech, South San Francisco, CA, and Biogen Idec, Cambridge, MA; MabThera, F. Hoffman-LaRoche AG, Basel, Switzerland) is an antibody that selectively depletes a B cell subset that expresses the CD20 antigen. Other biologic agents targeting this antigen that have been in clinical trials are the humanized monoclonal antibody ocrelizumab and fully human monoclonal antibody ofatumumab. Abatacept (Orencia, Bristol-Myers Squibb, New York, NY) is a fusion protein that selectively modulates a co-stimulatory signal necessary for T cell activation.

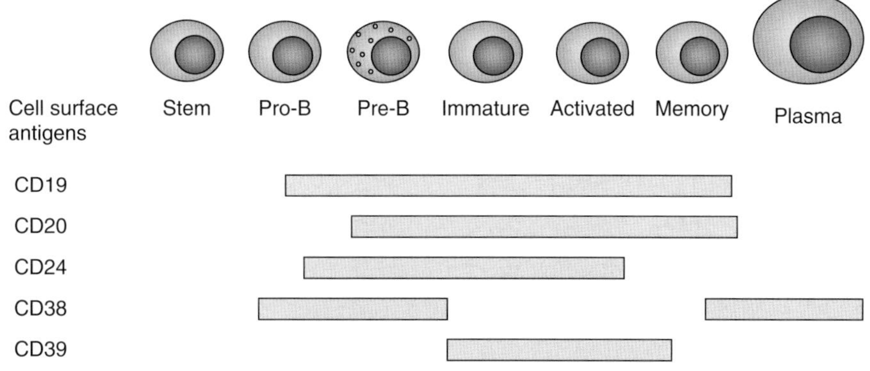

• **Fig. 67.1** Expression of the CD20 antigen on B lineage cells.

Rituximab is approved in the United States and Europe for use in combination with methotrexate to reduce the signs and symptoms of RA in adult patients who have moderately to severely active disease and have not responded to one or more anti-TNF drugs. Abatacept is the first selective co-stimulation modulator to be approved in the United States and Europe for the treatment of patients with RA who have an inadequate response to other nonbiologic or biologic disease-modifying anti-rheumatic drugs.

Targeting B Cells

KEY POINT

B cells are major contributors to RA pathogenesis, but their precise roles in the induction and maintenance of abnormal immune activation remain poorly understood.

The role of B cells in the pathogenesis of RA is not fully understood. Nonetheless, there are a number of known B cell functions of likely relevance, including their role in antigen presentation, secretion of pro-inflammatory cytokines, production of rheumatoid factor and thus immune complex formation, and co-stimulation of T cells. Of note, immune complexes are an important trigger to the production of TNF and other pro-inflammatory cytokines. B cells are also implicated in the process of ectopic lymphoid organogenesis in the rheumatoid synovium.

B cells arise from stem cells in the bone marrow, where they acquire an antibody receptor bearing a unique variable region. A number of maturation and activation steps take place as the B cells migrate from the marrow compartment, through blood, and to perifollicular germinal centers and memory compartments in lymphoid tissue before returning to the marrow as mature plasma cells.[6] Successful maturation and survival of cells are tightly regulated and dependent on a number of trophic signals delivered via cell surface ligands, such as vascular cell adhesion molecule-1 (VCAM-1), and soluble factors, such as B lymphocyte stimulator (BLyS).[7,8]

In the late 1990s, one study[9,10] suggested that the (assumed) underlying autoreactive response in RA might be driven by self-perpetuating B cells and that the initiation of inflammation results from ligation of the low-affinity immunoglobulin G (IgG) receptor FcRγIIIa by immune complexes. An attractive feature of this hypothesis, particularly in seropositive patients, is that it might account for the tissue tropisms of disease expression in the RA syndrome complex, because FcRγIIIa is expressed in high levels in synovium and other extra-articular tissues that may be involved in RA. Rheumatoid factor–producing cells can capture antibodies bound to antigen before antigen internalization by endocytosis and subsequent presentation of peptide fragments to a T cell, with provision of T cell help to the B cell. Edwards and Cambridge[11] also proposed that such rheumatoid factor–producing B cells might become self-perpetuating by an amplification signal arising from co-ligation of the B cell receptor and small immune complexes formed by IgG rheumatoid factor bound to the complement component C3d, providing a survival signal. In contrast, co-ligation of certain other B cell surface receptors with the B cell receptor may provide a negative survival signal. In the rare event that self-perpetuating, autoreactive B cells arise, having escaped normal regulatory mechanisms, this theory predicts that a B cell depletion strategy would remove the autoreactive B cell clones and their antibody products. Because CD20 is not internalized and is highly expressed on a range of B lineage cells, including pre–B cells, immature B cells, activated cells, and memory cells, but is not found on stem, dendritic, or plasma cells (Fig. 67.1), it is an ideal target for B cell depletion by monoclonal antibodies. The hypothesis that B cells represent a therapeutic target in RA has also been tested in the clinic using other strategies for B cell inhibition, as discussed in a later section.

The CD20 antigen is located in the B cell membrane, with 44 amino acids exposed to the extra-cellular space. Its function is unknown, although it may have a role in cell signaling or in calcium mobilization.[12] Interestingly, CD20 knockout mice do not have a clear-cut phenotype or obvious B cell defect.[13] $CD20^+$ B cells represent a prominent population in the RA synovial tissue in a distinct and frequent subset of patients.

Rituximab and Rheumatoid Arthritis

KEY POINT

Rituximab is a depleting chimeric monoclonal antibody lytic for a population of B cells expressing CD20.

Rituximab is a chimeric mouse-human monoclonal antibody directed against the extra-cellular domain of the CD20 antigen. It initiates complement-mediated B cell lysis and may permit antibody-dependent, cell-mediated cytotoxicity when the Fc portion of the antibody is recognized by corresponding receptors on cytotoxic cells. Rituximab may also initiate apoptosis[14] and influence the ability of B cells to respond to antigen or other stimuli.[15] Rituximab initially found a role in the clinic as a single-agent treatment for relapsed or refractory low-grade or follicular CD20+ B cell non-Hodgkin's lymphoma, for which it was approved. For this reason, there was wide experience with rituximab in hematologic oncology before initiation of clinical trials in RA and the approval of rituximab in the United States and Europe for the treatment of TNF inhibitor–refractory patients with RA who have active disease.

After rituximab administration, rapid B cell depletion takes place in peripheral blood, and conventional methods for measurement of peripheral blood B cells by means of CD19 expression detect no cells at all in most cases. Investigation of synovial tissue from patients with RA who are treated with rituximab reveal a decrease in synovial B cells and plasma cells in most, though not all, patients.[16,17] These findings raise the possibility that the inflamed synovium might contain as yet poorly understood rescue mechanisms that provide survival niches or, alternatively, that some B cells may have an inherent resistance against depletion.

Analysis of peripheral blood memory B cells before depletion, during depletion, and after reconstitution seems to be predictive of clinical outcome, with patients who show early relapses having substantially higher IgD+ and IgD-CD27+ memory B cell numbers and proportion during B cell recovery.[18] In addition to these cellular biomarkers, serologic parameters have been analyzed.

Decreases in rheumatoid factor (RF) or anti-citrullinated protein antibody (ACPA) serum levels are reported to be associated with B cell depletion,[19] but further studies are needed to determine the relationships between these serologic changes and clinical response.

Clinical Studies

KEY POINTS

Rituximab is an effective biologic therapy across the spectrum of RA patient populations.

Rituximab appears to have greatest benefit in seropositive patients.

Clinical trials in patients with active, established RA confirm that a single cycle of rituximab given as two infusions of 1 g each, together with once-weekly oral methotrexate, produces an enduring clinical response. A treatment cycle of two infusions of 500 mg is also efficacious but may result in a lower proportion of patients demonstrating more robust clinical responses.

The findings of early clinical studies of B cell depletion therapy in patients with active RA using rituximab in a number of different treatment regimens suggested an encouraging benefit with an acceptable safety profile and pointed to a possible therapeutic role for rituximab in people with RA.[20–22] Confirmation of benefit, however, required a randomized, double-blind, controlled study. In a phase IIa study, the efficacy of rituximab in people with active RA was tested in 161 patients who had failed to respond adequately to methotrexate at a dose of at least 10 mg a week for a minimum of 16 weeks.[23] Patients were assigned to one of four treatment regimens: a 1-g infusion of intravenous rituximab alone on days 1 and 15, methotrexate alone as a comparison arm, intravenous rituximab with cyclophosphamide infusions at a dose of 750 mg on days 3 and 17, or rituximab and methotrexate. All patients received 100 mg of methylprednisolone just

TABLE 67.1 Percentage of Patients Achieving Responses at 24 Weeks in the DANCER and REFLEX Studies

Study	Drug Regimen	ACR20	ACR50	ACR70
Phase IIa[19]	1 g rituximab × 2 + methotrexate	73	43	23
	Methotrexate	38	13	5
Phase IIb DANCER[20]	1 g rituximab × 2 + methotrexate	54	34	20
	Methotrexate	28	13	5
Phase III REFLEX[21]	1 g rituximab × 2 + methotrexate	51	27	12
	Methotrexate	18	5	1

ACR, American College of Rheumatology; *DANCER*, Dose-ranging Assessment: International Clinical Evaluation of Rituximab in Rheumatoid Arthritis; *REFLEX*, Randomized Evaluation of Long-term Efficacy of Rituximab in Rheumatoid Arthritis.

before each treatment, in addition to prednisolone, 60 mg daily, on days 2, 4, 5, 6, and 7, and 30 mg daily on days 8 to 14. The primary endpoint was the proportion of patients achieving an American College of Rheumatology (ACR)50 response at week 24, and exploratory analyses were undertaken at week 48. At week 24, a significantly greater proportion of patients achieved an ACR50 in the rituximab and methotrexate combination group (43%; $P = 0.005$) and in the rituximab and cyclophosphamide combination group (41%; $P = 0.005$) than in the group receiving methotrexate as monotherapy (13%) (Table 67.1). Thirty-three percent of the patients receiving rituximab alone achieved an ACR50 response, but this outcome failed to reach statistical significance compared with methotrexate alone ($P = 0.059$). In all the rituximab groups, the mean change from baseline in disease activity score was significant compared with methotrexate alone.

At 48 weeks, exploratory analyses indicated ACR50 and ACR70 responses in 35% and 15%, respectively, of patients in the rituximab and methotrexate group, which was significantly greater than the 5% and 0% responding at the corresponding levels in the methotrexate group. In the rituximab and cyclophosphamide treatment arm, 27% of patients achieved an ACR50 response.

Rituximab treatment was associated with near-complete peripheral blood B cell depletion that persisted throughout the 24-week period of the primary analysis. Patients in the rituximab groups had a substantial and rapid reduction in the concentration of rheumatoid factor in serum, but despite peripheral B cell depletion, immunoglobulin levels did not change substantially.[23] The overall incidence of infection was similar in the control and rituximab groups at 24 and 48 weeks. By week 24, four patients in the rituximab groups and one patient in the control group had acquired a serious infection. Two additional serious infections were reported during the extended 48-week period in the rituximab groups, one of which was fatal. Infusion reactions of any type were reported in 36% of patients receiving rituximab and 30% of patients receiving placebo, although most were characterized as mild or moderate. The reactions included hypotension, hypertension, flushing, pruritus, and rash. In the rare case of severe reactions, a cytokine release syndrome associated with marked cell lysis after rituximab might be a contributing factor.

In summary, the findings of the phase IIa study indicated that a single course of treatment with rituximab, particularly in combination with methotrexate, produces an enduring response in patients with severe, seropositive, active RA. Further, treatment with rituximab was well tolerated, with a favorable safety profile over 48 weeks of follow-up.

To follow up the phase IIa study, a phase IIb study was undertaken to examine the efficacy and safety of rituximab at different doses, with or without glucocorticoids, in patients with active RA who were resistant to disease-modifying anti-rheumatic drugs (DMARDs), including biologic agents. The findings of this phase IIb study, known as the DANCER (Dose-ranging Assessment: International Clinical Evaluation of Rituximab in RA) trial, have been reported.[24] A total of 465 people with active disease were recruited. To be included in the study, they had to have (1) failed to respond to at least one DMARD other than methotrexate, but no more than five, or failed to respond to biologic response modifiers, and (2) been treated with methotrexate as a single DMARD for at least 12 weeks, with 4 weeks of stable therapy at a dose of at least 10 mg a week. All other DMARDs were withdrawn at least 4 weeks before randomization—8 weeks for infliximab, adalimumab, and leflunomide. Patients were randomized to receive either placebo infusions or rituximab at a dose of 500 mg or 1 g on days 1 and 15, together with one of three glucocorticoid options: glucocorticoid placebo, 100 mg of intravenous methylprednisolone before each rituximab infusion, or 100 mg of methylprednisolone before each infusion in addition to an oral corticosteroid.

The results at 24 weeks confirmed the significant efficacy of a single course of rituximab in active RA when combined with methotrexate. This benefit was independent of glucocorticoids, although administration of methylprednisolone on day 1 reduced the incidence and severity of first rituximab infusion reactions by about one-third (Fig. 67.2). Both rituximab doses were efficacious. At the lower dose, 55% of recipients achieved ACR20 responses, as did 54% of those at the higher rituximab dose—in both cases, this was significantly greater than the 28% of the subjects who received placebo infusions. Similarly, significantly higher proportions of subjects achieved ACR50, ACR70 (see Table 67.1), and European League Against Rheumatism (EULAR) good responses at 24 weeks at both rituximab doses compared with subjects who received placebo infusions (Fig. 67.3). At the most stringent ACR70 response level, the difference in the percentage of responders in the placebo, lower-dose rituximab, and higher-dose rituximab groups was most marked at the higher rituximab dose of 1 g 2 weeks apart (5%, 13%, and 20%, respectively; $P < 0.05$). Adverse events reported up to 24 weeks were largely infusion related, particularly at the time of the first infusion.

A trial known as REFLEX (Randomized Evaluation of Long-term Efficacy of Rituximab in RA) was designed to determine the efficacy and safety of rituximab when used in combination with methotrexate in patients with active RA who had had an inadequate response to one or more anti-TNF therapies because of either lack of efficacy (90% of patients recruited) or toxicity (10% of patients recruited); in addition, all patients had radiographic evidence of at least one joint with definite erosion attributable to RA (Fig. 67.4). The recruited cohort consisted of 520 patients with a mean disease duration of 12 years with a background regimen of methotrexate, 10 to 25 mg once a week. After a washout period during which other DMARDs and anti-TNF drugs were withdrawn, patients were randomized to receive a single course of 1 g of

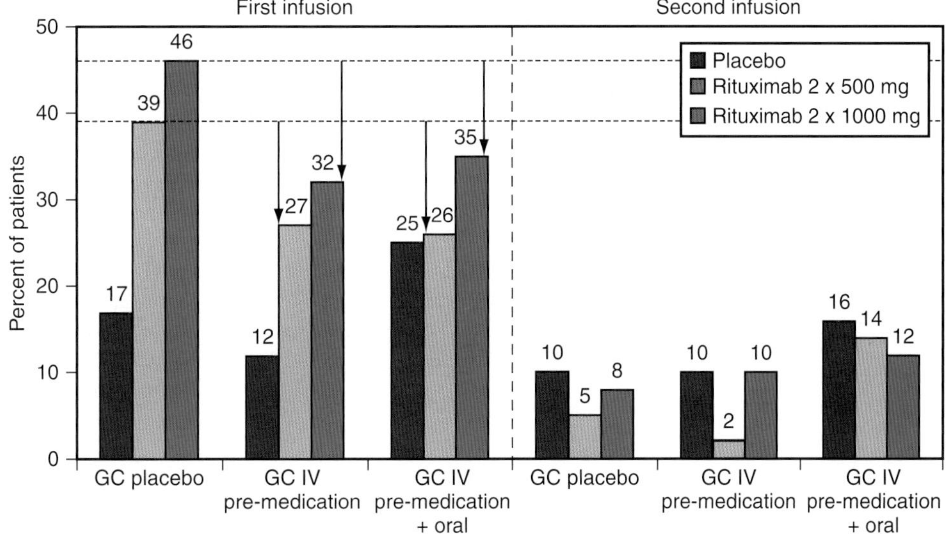

• **Fig. 67.2** The occurrence of infusion reactions in the DANCER (Dose-ranging Assessment: International Clinical Evaluation of Rituximab in RA) trial, a phase IIb study undertaken to examine the efficacy and safety of rituximab at two doses, with or without glucocorticoids (GCs), in patients with active rheumatoid arthritis (RA) resistant to disease-modifying anti-rheumatic drugs (DMARDs), including biologic agents. Patients were randomized to receive either placebo infusions or rituximab at a dose of 500 mg or 1 g on days 1 and 15, together with one of three glucocorticoid options: glucocorticoid placebo, 100 mg intravenous methylprednisolone before each rituximab infusion, or 100 mg methylprednisolone before each infusion in addition to an oral corticosteroid. Pre-treatment with methylprednisolone before rituximab infusion reduced the incidence and severity of reactions by about one-third. *IV,* Intravenous. (Data from Emery P, Fleischmann R, Filipowicz-Sosnowska A; DANCER study group, et al.: The efficacy and safety of rituximab in patients with active rheumatoid arthritis despite methotrexate treatment: results of a phase IIB randomized, double-blind, placebo-controlled, dose-ranging study. *Arthritis Rheum* 54:1390–1400, 2006.)

rituximab or placebo infusions on days 1 and 15. All patients were given 100 mg of intravenous methylprednisolone before each infusion and a brief course of oral prednisolone between the two doses: 60 mg daily from days 2 to 7, and 30 mg daily from days 8 to 14.[25]

Of the patients assigned to receive rituximab, 82% completed 6 months, compared with only 54% of the patients assigned to receive a placebo. The major reason for study withdrawal was lack of response, reported in 40% of the placebo group and 12% of the rituximab group. At 6 months, significantly more patients receiving rituximab achieved ACR20, ACR50, and ACR70 responses than did those receiving placebo: 51%, 27%, and 12%, respectively, of subjects receiving rituximab, versus 18%, 5%, and 1%, respectively, of those receiving placebo (see Table 67.1). In terms of change in Disease Activity Scale (DAS28), intention-to-treat analyses showed that in patients who received placebo infusions, the reduction from baseline was 0.34, which was less than the 0.6-point reduction considered to be clinically meaningful; in contrast, the reduction was 1.83 in the rituximab group.[25]

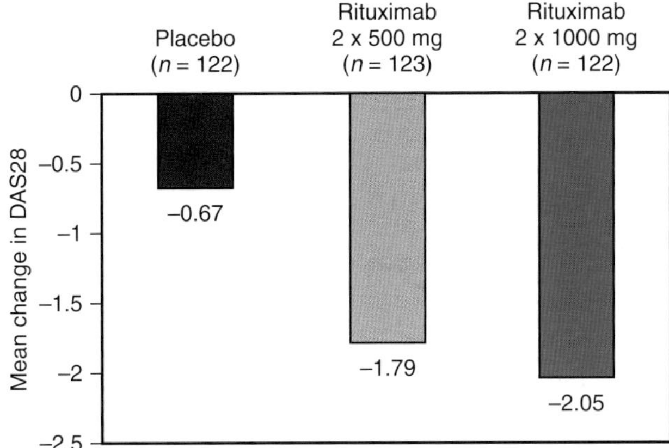

• **Fig. 67.3** DANCER (Dose-ranging Assessment: International Clinical Evaluation of Rituximab in RA trial) changes in the Disease Activity Scale (DAS)28 at 6 months. Mean changes in DAS28 from baseline in the phase IIb DANCER study were significantly greater in patients treated with two rituximab infusions 2 weeks apart at either 500 mg or 1 g each, compared with placebo infusions ($P < 0.0001$). (Data from Emery P, Fleischmann R, Filipowicz-Sosnowska A; DANCER study group, et al.: The efficacy and safety of rituximab in patients with active rheumatoid arthritis despite methotrexate treatment: results of a phase IIB randomized, double-blind, placebo-controlled, dose-ranging study. *Arthritis Rheum* 54:1390–1400, 2006.)

The ACR response evaluates RA treatment based on a 20%, 50%, or 70% improvement in five of seven core components. From the patient's perspective, however, determining the actual benefit of an ACR20 improvement is not straightforward. In the REFLEX study, the rituximab group had significantly greater improvements in all components of the ACR core measures. Rituximab demonstrated a clinically meaningful benefit for patients with RA in physical function as evaluated by a Health Assessment Questionnaire (HAQ) in all nonoverlapping ACR response categories. In the active treatment arm, both clinical and subjective parameters of the ACR core components contributed to the assignment of an ACR20 response, whereas in the placebo group, the subjective parameters dominated.[25]

In the REFLEX study, after a single treatment course, the maximal clinical response to rituximab plus methotrexate was observed at 24 weeks. After this time, patients were eligible to exit the study and receive further rituximab treatment based on clinical need. Of the patients in the rituximab plus methotrexate group, 37% (114 of 308) remained in the study over 48 weeks, indicating continued clinical benefit after the single initial treatment course. The majority of patients who withdrew did so to receive further courses of rituximab between weeks 24 and 48 of the study. In contrast, 89% of the placebo plus methotrexate group (185 of 209) withdrew before week 48.[26]

Another phase III study, known as SERENE (Study Evaluating Rituximab's Efficacy in methotrexate iNadequate rEsponders), confirmed the benefits of rituximab in patients with RA receiving concomitant methotrexate who had active disease at baseline despite methotrexate therapy and who had not received prior biologic therapy.[27] Patients were randomized to receive either placebo or rituximab at one of two doses, 2 × 500 mg or 2 × 1000. From week 24, in an open-label extension, the patients in the rituximab arms who did not achieve remission as assessed by

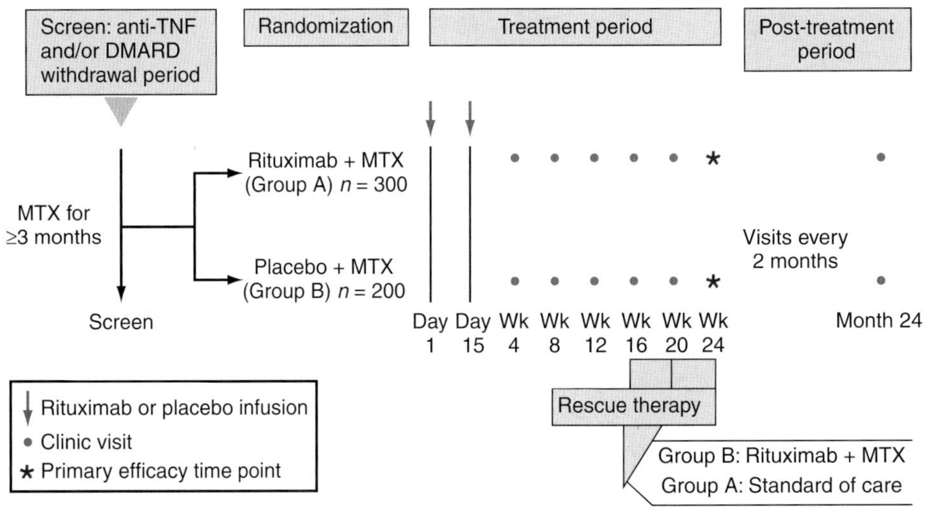

• **Fig. 67.4** The design of the phase III REFLEX (Randomized Evaluation of Long-term Efficacy of Rituximab in RA) study to determine the efficacy and safety of rituximab when used in combination with methotrexate (MTX) in patients with active rheumatoid arthritis (RA) who have an inadequate response to one or more anti–tumor necrosis factor (TNF) therapies. DMARD, Disease-modifying anti-rheumatic drug.

DAS28 received a second course of rituximab, and all patients who had received placebo were treated with the lower rituximab dose. At week 24, a significantly greater proportion of patients receiving rituximab, 2 × 500 mg or 2 × 1000 mg plus methotrexate, achieved the primary endpoint of an ACR20 response versus patients receiving placebo plus methotrexate (54.5% and 50.6% vs. 23.3%, respectively; $P < 0.0001$). By week 48, approximately 90% of patients in all treatment groups had received a second course of treatment. The majority of these repeat treatments (82% to 88%) were given by week 30.

In patients treated with rituximab, efficacy outcomes at week 48 were comparable with those at week 24; additionally, improvement was observed for several clinically important endpoints, including an approximate doubling in the proportion of patients who achieved low disease activity (DAS28 < 3.2) in the rituximab (2 × 1000 mg) plus methotrexate–dose group from week 24 to week 48. The safety profile of rituximab in the SERENE study was comparable with that observed in earlier trials, with the most common adverse event being infusion-related reactions, most of which were not serious, at the time of first infusion. Reductions in immunoglobulin levels were observed, predominantly IgM, but with mean levels remaining within normal limits. No relationships between infectious complications and reduced immunoglobulin levels were observed—in fact, the rate of infection observed in patients receiving rituximab plus methotrexate was low and comparable with that of patients receiving methotrexate alone over the placebo-controlled 24-week period. This low rate of serious infection continued throughout the full 48-week period, with no obvious difference between the rituximab doses.

Results from the IMAGE (International Study in Methotrexate-naïve Subjects Investigating Rituximab's Efficacy) study, which included 748 patients without prior use of either biologic drugs or methotrexate, have been reported. In this group, high-risk patients who had baseline high DAS28 scores or high C-reactive protein (CRP) levels were found to have greater DAS28 improvement at week 52 if they received rituximab in addition to methotrexate.[28]

Disease Modification

KEY POINT

Rituximab given as two infusions of 1 g slows radiographic progression in patients with RA.

The extraordinary success of TNF blockade in inhibiting structural damage to joints in patients with RA has set a new standard to which all new biologic agents must aspire. Inhibition of structural joint damage by rituximab in people with RA and a previous inadequate response to TNF inhibitors from the REFLEX study was first described over a 1-year period,[29] with a subsequent demonstration that the initial effects of rituximab are maintained over an extended interval of 2 years, with all measures of joint damage significantly improved compared with placebo plus methotrexate.[30] At week 56,[29] the mean change in the Genant-modified Sharp score in the placebo plus methotrexate arm was 2.31, compared with 1.0 in the rituximab plus methotrexate group ($P = 0.0043$). Significant differences were also reported for joint space narrowing and bone erosions. At week 104, significantly lower changes in the total Genant-modified Sharp score (1.14 vs. 2.81; $P < 0.0001$), erosion score (0.72 vs. 1.80; $P < 0.0001$), and joint space narrowing scores (0.42 vs. 1.00; $P < 0.0009$) were observed with rituximab plus methotrexate versus placebo plus methotrexate.[30] Importantly, within the rituximab group, 87% who had no progression of joint damage at 1 year remained nonprogressive at 2 years. Thus these data confirm that treatment with rituximab plus methotrexate has the benefit of sustained inhibition of joint damage progression in patients with RA who had a previously inadequate response to TNF inhibitors.

Radiographic outcomes were reported for a phase III study designed to determine the efficacy of rituximab in the prevention of joint damage and its safety in combination with methotrexate in the context of patients initiating treatment with methotrexate.[28] This study, known as the IMAGE trial, was a randomized, controlled, double-blind trial involving 748 methotrexate-naïve patients assigned to receive rituximab at doses of either 2 × 1000 mg or 2 × 500 mg every 24 weeks in combination with methotrexate or methotrexate alone. The primary endpoint was radiographic progression measured by modified total Sharp score (mTSS) at week 52. In subjects treated with 2 × 1000 mg rituximab and methotrexate, a significantly smaller change (0.359) in the mTSS was observed compared with subjects taking methotrexate alone (1.079; $P < 0.001$). Furthermore, a significantly higher proportion of subjects treated with MabThera and methotrexate had no progression in their joint damage over 1 year (64% vs. 53%; $P = 0.0309$). By week 52, 65% of these subjects experienced a 50% improvement in symptoms (ACR50) and 47% experienced a 70% improvement (ACR70), compared with 42% and 25%, respectively, for subjects taking methotrexate alone ($P < 0.0001$ for both ACR50 and ACR70 comparisons).

Recent evidence suggests that rituximab inhibits joint damage independently of its effects on disease activity.[31] A random 90% sample of patient data from two arms of the IMAGE trial were divided into low, moderate, or high disease activity at 1 year of treatment by simplified disease activity index, or by swollen joint count or CRP tertiles. Progression of damage by the Genant mTSS was compared between therapies (Kruskal-Wallis and Wilcoxon tests) for each of these subgroups. In subjects treated with methotrexate, 1-year radiographic progression in low, moderate, and high disease activity was 0.40 ± 0.88, 1.04 ± 1.73, and 1.31 ± 3.02, respectively. In contrast, in subjects receiving rituximab plus methotrexate, radiographic progression was 0.38 ± 1.07, 0.39 ± 1.28 ($P = 0.003$ by comparison with methotrexate), and −0.05 ± 0.44 ($P = 0.05$ by comparison with methotrexate), respectively. These data suggest that, as in the case of biologic TNF and IL-6 receptor (IL-6R) inhibition, anti-CD20 antibody conveys profound antidestructive effects and dissociates the link between disease activity and joint damage.

Safety Issues

KEY POINTS

Rituximab has an acceptable safety record in RA trials, but infusion reactions can occur; most are mild to moderate. The frequency and severity of infusion reactions are reduced by the administration of intravenous methylprednisolone before rituximab infusions.

A very rare complication in patients with RA who are treated with rituximab is progressive multifocal leukoencephalopathy. Because of the increase in relative risk, patients should be counseled appropriately.

The rapidity and magnitude of peripheral blood B cell depletion after anti-CD20 therapy raises concerns about potential adverse sequelae. The peripheral compartment recovers after many months, but repopulation occurs predominantly with an immature and naïve subset of B cells. Nevertheless, it must also be remembered that the circulation contains less than 2% of total B cells.[32] A common concern regarding all therapies directed at B cells is the potential for toxicity related to modulation of humoral immunity. Unlike other newly introduced biologic therapies for RA, rituximab has the considerable advantage of an oncology safety database based on more than 350,000 treatments of patients with non-Hodgkin's lymphoma since 1997.[33] The overall safety conclusions are that serious adverse events are infrequent and often associated with well-defined risk factors such as cardiopulmonary disease or a high number of circulating cancer cells. Of note, in the lymphoma population, prolonged peripheral B cell depletion has not been associated with cumulative toxicity or increased occurrence of opportunist infections.[34–36] Nevertheless, it cannot be assumed that the toxicity profile will be identical in distinct disease phenotypes with differing pathogenic processes.

In RA open-label,[37] phase II,[23,24] and phase III[21] studies, although decreases in total serum immunoglobulin levels were observed in patients receiving rituximab, concentrations remained within normal limits. Of note, existing antibody titers against tetanus toxoid appear to be unaffected by a single course of rituximab treatment.[38] Some anecdotal evidence, however, indicates that total serum immunoglobulin concentrations fall below the normal range in patients receiving multiple cycles of rituximab treatment over a number of years in open-label studies.[11] It is unclear whether this outcome results in an increased risk of infection. In phase II studies, the majority of adverse events, including headache, nausea, and rigors, were mild to moderate and were associated with infusions. In a meta-analysis of randomized clinical trial data from three studies that reported adverse events arising after a single cycle of rituximab treatment in a total of 938 patients with RA who were refractory to nonbiologic DMARDs or biologic anti-TNFs,[23–25] it was calculated that the incidence of patients experiencing adverse events of all systems was not higher in the patients treated with rituximab than in the placebo groups (relative risk [RR], 1.062; 95% confidence interval [CI], 0.912 to 1.236; $P = 0.438$).[39]

In the DANCER trial, adverse events associated with rituximab were largely associated with the first infusion; these adverse events occurred in 39% of subjects treated with 500 mg of rituximab (without use of a steroid) and in 46% receiving 1 g, compared with 17% in subjects who received placebo infusions.[24] The corresponding incidence with the second infusion decreased to 5%, 8%, and 10%, respectively. Two serious infusion reactions, hypersensitivity and generalized edema, occurred on day 1. Pretreatment with methylprednisolone reduced the incidence and severity of reactions by about one-third (see Fig. 67.2). Infectious adverse events (largely upper respiratory tract infections) were reported in 28% of subjects who received a placebo and in 35% of subjects who received rituximab. Six serious infections occurred: two in the placebo group, four in patients receiving 1000 mg of rituximab, and none in patients receiving 500 mg of rituximab. No opportunistic infections or tuberculosis reactivations were reported.

Although the overall safety record based on trial data has been favorable, with wider clinical use of biologic B cell depletion, rarer serious complications have come to light. A potential association has been reported between the biologic therapies efalizumab, natalizumab, and rituximab and the rare, progressive, and usually fatal condition termed *progressive multifocal leukoencephalopathy* (PML), a rare brain disease caused by reactivation of the John Cunningham (JC) virus.[40] PML has been reported in patients receiving rituximab for hematologic conditions and systemic lupus erythematosus (SLE)[41] and, more recently, in patients with RA.[40] The cumulative incidence rate of PML in the RA population has been estimated at 1/100,000 RA admissions in an analysis limited to hospitalized patients with SLE and other rheumatic diseases (including 25 patients with RA), a majority of whom had concomitant risk factors, including HIV, malignancy, or transplantation of bone marrow or another organ.[42] The cumulative reporting rate of 2.2 cases of PML per 100,000 patients with RA treated with rituximab is more than double the estimated frequency in RA (95% CI, 0.3 to 8.0).[40] Although the absolute risk is small, the RR is such that it emphasizes the importance of providing the prospective patient being considered for B cell–depleting therapy with thoughtful and balanced information about likely benefits, as well as more common through very rare complications.

The profound and enduring peripheral B cell depletion that accompanies use of rituximab raises a potential safety concern for patients in clinical practice who fail to derive adequate symptomatic benefit and may then be exposed to biologic DMARDs of an alternative mechanism of action at a time point before repopulation of circulating B cells can take place. Relatively few data regarding this circumstance are available to date, but preliminary information is available in 185 of 2578 patients with RA who went on to receive a biologic agent with an alternative mechanism of action as documented in a safety follow-up period after participation in trials in which they had previously received rituximab.[43] Of the 185 patients, 89% remained depleted of peripheral B cells at the point of beginning treatment with a biologic agent with a new mechanism of action. The rate of serious infectious events reported after treatment with rituximab but prior to the second biologic exposure was 6.99 per 100 patient-years, which is comparable with the reported rate of 5.49 per 100 patient-years after exposure to a second biologic agent, the majority of which were TNF inhibitors. No fatal or opportunistic infections were observed, with the nature and course of infectious complications being within expectations for patients with RA receiving biologic therapy. In a population of methotrexate-naïve patients entering the IMAGE study,[28] safety data were consistent with results from previous rituximab clinical trials and further enhance the robust safety profile. Rates of serious adverse events and serious infections were similar between the two MabThera groups and the methotrexate-only group.

People with RA, particularly those treated with immunosuppressants, are at an increased risk of infection, and for this reason vaccination is an important aspect of RA clinical management. The question of whether B cell–depleting therapy could adversely affect immunization responses by suppressing the antibody response from new vaccination or reducing pre-formed antibody from prior vaccination has been investigated, and the findings have been reported.[44–46] These studies indicate that vaccine responses to some, but not all, vaccinations may be diminished in patients treated with rituximab, most strikingly in the first 4 to 8 weeks after administration of rituximab.[44] Although prior vaccination and timing of vaccine administration after rituximab infusion may influence the ability to mount a response, no straightforward relationship exists between peripheral B cell reconstitution and response to immunization. Therefore, when vaccination is indicated, ideally it should be performed prior to rituximab treatment and avoided immediately after B cell depletion with a delay of several months. Of course, this guideline may not be practical for vaccines with seasonal availability (such as those for influenza variants), and it must be recognized that responses to vaccination do not necessarily correlate with the risk of infection. In general, the timing of rituximab administration must be determined according to clinical need without the requirement to delay until after supplies of a seasonally variable vaccine become available and the patient has been immunized.

In a recent meta-analysis of 6 studies enrolling 2728 patients, nonmelanotic skin carcinoma occurred more commonly than other carcinomas in the rituximab treatment groups (0.8% in the rituximab group vs. none reported in the control group). Moreover, the overall incidence of malignancies was higher in the rituximab group (2.1%) compared with the control group (0.6%).[47]

The safety and efficacy profile of rituximab in the treatment of RA discussed thus far is based on reports from randomized placebo-controlled trials of 6 to 12 months' duration. Open-label extension studies have analyzed safety and efficacy results over multiple courses of rituximab.[48] In safety analyses based on 5013 patient-years of rituximab exposure, in a total of 2578 patients with RA who received at least one course of rituximab, infusion-related reactions were the most common adverse event occurring in a quarter of patients during the first infusion of the initial treatment cycle, although only 1% of infusion reactions in total were considered to be of a serious nature. Importantly and reassuringly, the rates of both adverse events and serious adverse events were stable over infusion cycles, with the latter reported as 17.85 events/100 patient-years (95% CI, 16.72 to 19.06). Infections and serious infections over time remained stable across five treatment cycles at four to six events/100 patient-years. No cases of tuberculosis, disseminated fungal infections, or other serious opportunistic infections were identified during the analysis period.

The rate of herpes zoster infections in this large series was 0.98 events per 100 patient-years, similar to that reported for other RA populations. The much more serious and rare opportunistic infection PML occurred in a single patient who also received cancer chemotherapy and radiation, with the event occurring about 18 months after the last dose of rituximab and 9 months after receiving chemotherapy and radiation. The causal relationship to rituximab, if any, is thus not entirely clear. There was no increased risk of malignancy by comparison with reference patients with RA and with the general population in the United States. Myocardial infarction was one of the most common serious adverse events reported in the longer-term analyses at a rate of 0.56 per 100 patient-years, but this is consistent with rates reported in epidemiologic studies of patients with RA. Rituximab is reported to have the greatest risk for hepatitis B virus reactivation among RA patients who have received biologics (adjusted hazard ration greater than 16).[49]

Duration of Benefit

KEY POINT

Repeat treatment with rituximab produces clinical responses that equal or exceed those from the first course of treatment, with a comparable duration of effect.

Among patients with RA who experience clinical responses to rituximab treatment, the time to clinical relapse is heterogeneous. In some patients, relapse is closely correlated to the reappearance of peripheral blood B cells, but in other patients, it may be delayed by years.[50] Clinical relapse is more closely associated with increases in autoantibody levels, but better biomarkers are needed to reliably inform optimal management strategies on an individual basis. All B cell populations are depleted after rituximab therapy. Of residual B lineage cells, more than 80% exhibit a memory or plasma cell precursor phenotype.[51] B cell repopulation occurs at a mean of 8 months after rituximab therapy and depends on the formation of naïve B cells of an immature phenotype resembling those found in umbilical cord blood. Peripheral B cell depletion is accompanied by substantial increases in blood BLyS concentrations, which tend to fall with B cell repopulation.[52] BLyS is a naturally occurring protein required for the development of B lymphocytes into mature plasma cells. Elevated levels of BLyS in people with RA are believed to contribute to the production of autoantibodies. In cases of prolonged clinical responses to rituximab, however, more gradual reductions in BLyS concentrations have been observed, extending beyond the period of B cell depletion. Thus BLyS may contribute to the survival or regeneration of pathogenic, autoreactive B cells. This hypothesis predicts a potential therapeutic role for BLyS blockade in addition to B cell depletion.

Information concerning the efficacy and safety of repeated cycles of rituximab treatment has emerged from experience in clinical practice and from randomized trials. The recently reported phase III MIRROR (Methotrexate Inadequate Responders Randomised study Of Rituximab) trial was a randomized, double-blind, international study to evaluate the efficacy and safety of three dosing regimens of rituximab in combination with methotrexate in 375 patients with active RA and an inadequate response to methotrexate.[53] Patients were randomized to three groups with two courses of rituximab treatment at varying doses as follows: group A: 500 mg of rituximab (all courses) on days 1 and 15, with repeat treatment at 24 weeks; group B: first course 500 mg of rituximab on days 1 and 15, a second course of 1000 mg of rituximab, and repeat treatment at 24 weeks; and group C: 1000 mg of rituximab (all courses) on days 1 and 15, with repeat treatment at 24 weeks. The primary endpoint was the proportion of patients achieving ACR20 at week 48. Secondary endpoints included ACR50, ACR70, and EULAR responses. There was a trend toward better efficacy results with the regular 2 × 1000-mg dose compared with the low dose of 2 × 500 mg, and this reached statistical significance for EULAR good/moderate response (2 × 1000 mg = 88% vs. 2 × 500 mg = 72%, $P < 0.05$). Other endpoints, although numerically superior at 48 weeks, did not show any statistically significant difference between the three dosing regimens.

Current Role

KEY POINT

Rituximab is generally considered to be an effective biologic option in patients with RA, particularly seropositive patients who have inadequate responses to TNF inhibitors.

Recent advances in our understanding of the pathogenesis of RA emphasize the critical role of B cells in self-sustaining chronic inflammatory processes. Rituximab is an important addition to the therapeutic armamentarium for the treatment of RA. In current clinical practice, the major use for rituximab in the treatment of RA is confined to the TNF inhibitor–refractory population. SWITCH-RA is a global, observational study comparing the effectiveness of rituximab with an alternative TNF inhibitor in patients with RA who had an inadequate response to one previous anti-TNF agent.[54] In this large cohort, 604 patients received rituximab and 507 received an alternative anti-TNF as a second biologic therapy. Reasons for discontinuing the first anti-TNF included inefficacy and intolerance. Least squares mean (SE) change in DAS28-3-erythrocyte sedimentation rate (ESR) at 6 months was significantly greater in patients who received rituximab than in patients who received an anti-TNF agent: −1.5 versus −1.1; P = 0.007. The difference remained significant among patients who discontinued the initial anti-TNF agent because of inefficacy (−1.7 vs. −1.3; P = 0.017) but not because of intolerance (−0.7 vs. −0.7; P = 0.894). Seropositive patients showed significantly greater improvements in DAS28-3-ESR with rituximab than with an anti-TNF agent (−1.6 vs. −1.2; P = 0.011), particularly those who switched because of inefficacy (−1.9 vs. −1.5; P = 0.021). The overall incidence of adverse events was similar between the rituximab and TNF inhibitor groups. These real-life data suggest that, particularly in seropositive patients and in patients who switched because of inefficacy after discontinuation of an initial TNF inhibitor, switching to rituximab is associated with significantly improved clinical effectiveness compared with switching to a second anti-TNF agent.

Data from a number of clinical trials (IMAGE, MIRROR, SERENE, REFLEX, and DANCER)[24,27,28,52,55] suggest that seropositive patients with RA (RF and/or ACPA) show a higher likelihood of response to B cell–depleting therapy compared with seronegative patients, in particular for improving signs and symptoms and inhibition of radiographic changes. Nevertheless, it is still the case in both trials and clinical experience that a proportion of seronegative patients with RA show good clinical responses, although this proportion is less than in the case of seropositive patients.[56] In pooled analyses of data from the MIRROR and SERENE studies, at week 48, odds ratios for seropositive patients versus seronegative patients of achieving ACR20, ACR50, and ACR70 responses were 2.23 (95% CI, 1.38 to 3.58), 2.72 (95% CI, 1.58 to 4.70), and 3.29 (95% CI, 1.40 to 7.82), respectively.[57] These observations generate the hypothesis that other mechanisms may account for lower levels of response in seronegative patients, such as antigen presentation, co-stimulation, and cytokine drive, whereas high levels of response to rituximab therapy may be mediated primarily by the suppression of pathogenic antibodies.

The optimal and most cost-effective dosing regimen for rituximab remains a matter of debate. The phase III SERENE study showed equal clinical efficacy for the 500 mg × 2 and 1000 mg × 2 rituximab doses,[27] but the phase III MIRROR trial[53] had differences in some outcomes favoring the higher dosage. Methotrexate-naïve patients (not an approved patient population for rituximab) were studied in the IMAGE study with clinical results that were equivalent, but with a radiographic result that favored the higher dosage.[28] Thus a summary of the current randomized controlled trial (RCT) data on rituximab dosing is that 1000 mg × 2 works well in a clinically meaningful proportion of patients but not in all patients. The 500 mg × 2 rituximab dose achieves broadly similar results in the relevant patient populations overall and has the advantages of lower cost and possibly a lower rate of serious adverse events but perhaps with lower probability of high-impact clinical responses and inhibition of structural damage. Based on the DANCER study findings, it is recommended that each cycle of 1000 mg × 2 rituximab be given in combination with once-weekly methotrexate, usually at doses of at least 15 mg/week, to optimize efficacy. Further, administration of 100 mg intravenous methylprednisolone is recommended before each rituximab infusion to reduce the frequency and severity of infusion reactions.

Rituximab may also have a role in patients for whom TNF blockade is relatively contraindicated, such as those with connective tissue disease overlap syndromes. At present, uncertainties exist about the implications of long-term peripheral B cell depletion and the timing and need for redosing with rituximab in patients who respond. Current research suggests that restoration of peripheral B cell numbers takes about 8 months after depletion treatment, although retreatment may be needed earlier. Results have been presented for an open-label study to evaluate the response to repeated courses of rituximab in patients with active RA who are participating in one of several phase II or III studies and to determine the optimal frequency for repeated treatment.[58] In a series of 155 patients with prior exposure to TNF inhibitors, ACR20, ACR50, and ACR70 scores were 65%, 33%, and 12%, respectively, after the first course, and they were 72%, 42%, and 21%, respectively, for the second treatment course, relative to the original baseline. In 82 of these patients who received a third course of rituximab, the median interval between the first and second courses was very similar to that between the second and third courses: 30 to 31 weeks.[58] Further studies are needed to identify the optimal regimens for maintenance therapy that will provide efficacy and limit toxicity.[59] Development of biomarkers informative of management decisions that would optimize response is a highly desirable goal, but as yet no biomarkers are in routine use. The magnitude of clinical response appears to be related to the completeness of peripheral B cell depletion, and this holds true whether the lower 500 mg × 2 dose schedule or the higher 1000 mg × 2 schedule is administered. By means of sensitive measurements permitting detection of very low numbers of preplasma B cells in the circulation, a recent study reported that patients with RA whose disease did not respond to an initial cycle of rituximab have higher circulating preplasma cell numbers at baseline and incomplete depletion. Furthermore, an additional cycle of rituximab administered prior to total B cell repopulation enhances B cell depletion and clinical responses.[60]

Although the available safety data for rituximab in people with RA are reassuring, these data need to be interpreted with caution until larger numbers of patients have been treated and long-term safety and retreatment data become available. Further, a substantial body of safety data for rituximab in the treatment of non-Hodgkin's lymphoma is available, with similarly low infection rates reported. In oncology, some of the associated adverse events are related to circulating tumor loads. Overall, these data are reassuring with regard to the RA population, although close monitoring of immunocompetence and for the possibility of rare opportunistic infections is advisable.

Future Directions and Other Approaches to B Cell–Targeted Therapy

KEY POINT

Additional biologic approaches that target B cells are under investigation.

Rituximab is currently indicated for the treatment of patients with moderate to severe RA who show no response, experience a loss of response with time, or have adverse effects to anti-TNF agents.[61] The findings of recently reported studies indicate that rituximab is also efficacious in a proportion of both patients with RA who are treatment naïve and patients with RA who take methotrexate, particularly if they are seropositive.[27,28] Therefore, in the face of competitive health economic data compared with TNF inhibitors, there has been interest in the potential of rituximab as a first-line biologic agent. Nevertheless, questions remain about the safety of repeated treatment cycles, although encouraging data are emerging. Although the US Food and Drug Administration (FDA) has received reports of patients who experienced fatal PML after rituximab treatment for SLE and RA, this event appears to be rare. A key issue that determines the future place of B cell depletion therapy will be defining the most effective strategy in early stages of RA to induce a remission and potentially even biologic-free remission, whether this can be achieved safely and effectively with rituximab, and whether any biomarkers can be developed that will reliably inform biologic treatment strategy on an individual patient basis.

Clinical trials and safety data for other antibodies targeting CD20, such as ocrelizumab, a humanized version of rituximab, and ofatumumab, a fully human anti-CD20, have also been reported. In phase I/II trials in people with RA, ocrelizumab, in combination with methotrexate, was found to be safe and effective at doses consisting of two infusions of 200 mg or higher given 2 weeks apart.[62] Two ocrelizumab dose levels were studied in three phase III RA studies across various patient populations; full findings have yet to be reported. In spring 2010, however, a decision was announced to discontinue development of ocrelizumab for the RA indication after a detailed analysis of the efficacy and safety data from the RA program found that the overall benefit-risk profile of ocrelizumab was not favorable, taking into account other currently available treatment options. This decision was based on an infection-related safety signal that included serious infections, some of which were fatal, and opportunistic infections.

Ofatumumab is a human IgG1κ lytic monoclonal antibody with specificity for human CD20 antigen. It recognizes a unique membrane-proximal epitope on the human CD20 molecule that is distinct from the epitope recognized by rituximab and ocrelizumab.[63] The membrane proximity of this epitope is likely to account for the high efficiency of B cell killing observed with ofatumumab in both in vitro and in vivo pre-clinical studies. A phase I/II study of ofatumumab, administered as two intravenous infusions of 300, 700, or 1000 mg 2 weeks apart in patients with active RA who had an inadequate response to DMARDs, demonstrated significant clinical benefit and reasonable tolerability (which improved after implementation of pre-medication) at all doses investigated when compared with placebo, with the 700-mg dose considered optimal.[63] Despite these positive results in RA studies, further work on ofatumumab by intravenous delivery in autoimmune conditions was discontinued, and focus on a subcutaneous delivery program began. Plans for a study in people with multiple sclerosis are under way, but further development in RA remains under review, although this situation has not been prompted by the observation of unexpected opportunist infections as was the case for ocrelizumab.

Many other approaches to B cell–targeted therapy are in clinical testing, although it is unlikely that any of these will have a significant impact on the rituximab niche in the near future. Alternative strategies to target the B cell compartment include the use of BLyS antibodies. Belimumab is a human anti-BLyS monoclonal antibody recently investigated in clinical trials for the treatment of RA and other rheumatic indications. An alternative approach to BLyS inhibition that is still in the early stages of clinical development is to block signaling through BLyS receptors using a soluble receptor, such as transmembrane activator and calcium modulator and cyclophilin ligand interactor immunoglobulin. Preliminary results of a phase II double-blind, placebo-controlled study of belimumab in active RA have been presented.[64] Patients were randomized to receive intravenous belimumab at a dose of 1, 4, or 10 mg/kg or placebo infusions on days 0, 14, and 28, then every 28 days through 24 weeks. The ACR20 response at week 24 in the combined belimumab groups was 29%, compared with 16% in the placebo group; no dose response was observed. The antibody was well tolerated. These preliminary findings with a functional inhibitor of B cells are surprising, given the effectiveness of rituximab; however, it may simply represent a pharmacokinetic problem, indicating that the dose of belimumab was too low. The benefit-risk ratio of belimumab has come under close scrutiny by the FDA, and it seems unlikely that it will progress in clinical development with RA as an indication.

Rituximab in Other Rheumatic Conditions

KEY POINT

Rituximab is effective in RA and anti-neutrophil cytoplasmic antibody–associated vasculitis. Clinical trials in SLE have not shown clinical benefit.

Rituximab has also been used to treat a number of other rheumatic diseases.[11] Theoretical considerations and preliminary data suggested that B cell depletion using rituximab might have efficacy for immune thrombocytopenia, anti-neutrophil cytoplasmic antibody (ANCA)–associated vasculitis, and SLE. The rationale for the use of rituximab in the treatment of patients with ANCA-associated vasculitis is that elimination of CD20 B cell precursors could lead to transient removal of pathogenic antibodies and remission, assuming that ANCA are produced by short-lived B lineage cells rather than long-living plasma cells. Furthermore, in ANCA-associated vasculitis, the number of activated, circulating B lymphocytes correlates with disease activity and tissue involvement. The hypothesis that rituximab might induce disease remission in patients with severe ANCA-associated vasculitis has been tested in a phase II/III multicenter, randomized, double-blind, placebo-controlled trial known as RAVE (Rituximab for ANCA-associated Vasculitis). Findings have been reported comparing rituximab (375 mg/m^2 administered intravenously once weekly for 4 weeks) with cyclophosphamide (2 mg/kg/day administered orally).[65] Sixty-three patients in the rituximab group (64%) reached the primary endpoint, compared with 52 patients in the control group (53%), a result that met the criterion for noninferiority ($P < 0.001$). The rituximab-based regimen was more efficacious than the cyclophosphamide-based regimen for inducing remission of relapsing disease; 34 of 51 patients in the rituximab group (67%) compared with 21 of 50 patients in the control group (42%) reached the primary endpoint ($P = 0.01$). Rituximab was also as effective as cyclophosphamide in the treatment of patients with major renal disease or alveolar hemorrhage. No significant differences were found between the treatment groups with respect to rates of adverse events. Despite these encouraging data, the true positive effect of rituximab in ANCA-associated vasculitis is difficult to determine because of the simultaneous administration of high-dose glucocorticoids, which may contribute to a substantial decrease in ANCA titers and the observed remission rates.

Given the large body of evidence implicating abnormalities in the B cell compartment in SLE, a recent therapeutic focus has been to develop interventions that target the B cell compartment by multiple mechanisms, and rituximab has been studied most extensively. The best evidence in support of using rituximab for the treatment of patients with ANCA-associated vasculitis or SLE comes from clinical experience, retrospective case series, and small prospective uncontrolled studies, mainly in patients with refractory or frequently relapsing disease.[66,67] Very recently, however, two moderately sized phase III randomized placebo-controlled trials of rituximab for the treatment of moderately active nonrenal SLE (EXPLORER) or class III/IV lupus nephritis (LUNAR) have failed to demonstrate superiority of this B cell–depleting agent compared with placebo when added to standard of care (conventional immunosuppressive therapy). Both trials had a relatively short follow-up period. Preliminary data from LUNAR (a study to evaluate the efficacy and safety of rituximab in subjects with International Society of Nephrology/Renal Pathology Society [ISN/RPS] class III or IV lupus nephritis) have been reported.[68] This multicenter, randomized, double-blind, placebo-controlled trial included 144 patients with lupus nephritis (67% of patients had class IV disease) and compared the efficacy and safety of rituximab with placebo. Patients with class III and IV disease and a urine protein to creatinine ratio greater than 1 were randomly assigned to receive either 1000 mg of rituximab or placebo on days 1, 15, 168, and 182, in conjunction with mycophenolate mofetil and corticosteroids. No significant differences were observed in complete or partial renal response or clinical benefit to therapy at week 52, although rituximab administration was associated with significantly reduced titers of antibodies to double-stranded DNA and increased levels of C3 complement component. Serious adverse events, such as infection, were similar between the two patient groups.

The EXPLORER trial (a study to evaluate the efficacy and safety of rituximab in patients with severe SLE) randomly assigned patients with SLE who had moderate to severe disease activity despite treatment with immunosuppressive agents and corticosteroids to receive either placebo or rituximab infusions.[69] Patients with active glomerulonephritis were excluded. The British Isles lupus assessment group index was used to score treatment response four times per week for 52 weeks after the first infusion. Responses were recorded in 66% of patients in the placebo group and 75.1% of patients treated with rituximab. The time to the first moderate or severe flare did not differ between groups, but a trend for a prolonged time to the first "a" score flare in the rituximab group was observed. Annual rates of severe and moderate disease activity flares were similar, but the mean annual rate of "a" score flares was significantly lower in the rituximab group than in the placebo group (0.86 vs. 1.41). The number of adverse events and overall infections were comparable between groups at 78 weeks, although serious infections were more numerous in the placebo group.

It is unclear why the LUNAR and EXPLORER studies failed to prove the superiority of rituximab to placebo in patients with SLE, although design flaws seem likely. Overuse of concomitant steroids and continued immunosuppressive treatment could help mask the possible benefits of rituximab. Moreover, consensus is lacking regarding the optimal dose and administration regimen of rituximab in patients with SLE and adjustments for the organ or system involved. EXPLORER included patients with very active disease who were treated aggressively with moderate- to high-dose glucocorticoids, which made the short-term detection of treatment benefits difficult.[70] Other potential shortcomings for lupus clinical studies in general, including EXPLORER and LUNAR, is that the length of follow-up may have been too short to demonstrate separation between the different treatments. The unexpected failure to show overall clinical benefit of rituximab in SLE trials may also reflect the inadequacy of the clinical outcome instruments employed. This factor is less likely to be relevant in the LUNAR nephritis study, for which the outcome measurements were more unequivocal. It is noteworthy that in both the EXPLORER and LUNAR studies, outcomes appeared to be more favorable in African-American and Hispanic subjects.[71]

Rituximab has also been used in primary Sjögren's syndrome; granulomatosis with polyangiitis; hepatitis C–associated cryoglobulinemia; ANCA-associated vasculitides other than granulomatosis with polyangiitis, such as polyarteritis nodosa, dermatomyositis, and polymyositis[72]; antiphospholipid syndrome; and scleroderma.[73]

Targeting Co-stimulatory Molecules

KEY POINT

Activated T cells are implicated in the pathogenesis of RA, and co-stimulation is essential in induction of adaptive immune responses.

Co-stimulation is an essential step in the induction of adaptive immune responses. Although the role of T cells in the perpetuation of RA has been debated and remains poorly understood, it has long been believed that T cell activation is a key event in the pathogenesis. Successful T cell activation requires multiple signals. One signal is provided by presentation of an antigen bound to cell surface major histocompatibility complex (MHC) molecules on antigen-presenting cells to a specific T cell receptor (TCR). In the absence of further signals, T cells become unresponsive and may ultimately be eliminated through apoptosis. An important co-stimulatory signal is provided by an interaction between members of the B7 family (either CD80 or CD86) on antigen-presenting cells and CD28 on T cells (Fig. 67.5). Other key interactions between antigen-presenting cells and T cells are mediated by the binding of intercellular adhesion molecule-1 (ICAM-1) to leukocyte function-associated antigen-1 (LFA-1), CD40 to CD40 ligand, LFA-3 to CD2, and so on. After activation, T cells express cytolytic T lymphocyte–associated protein 4 (CTLA-4), which interferes with the B7-CD28 interaction and helps return the cells to the quiescent state.

Abatacept and Rheumatoid Arthritis

KEY POINT

Abatacept is a human fusion protein comprising the extra-cellular portion of CTLA-4 and the Fc fragment of IgG-1.

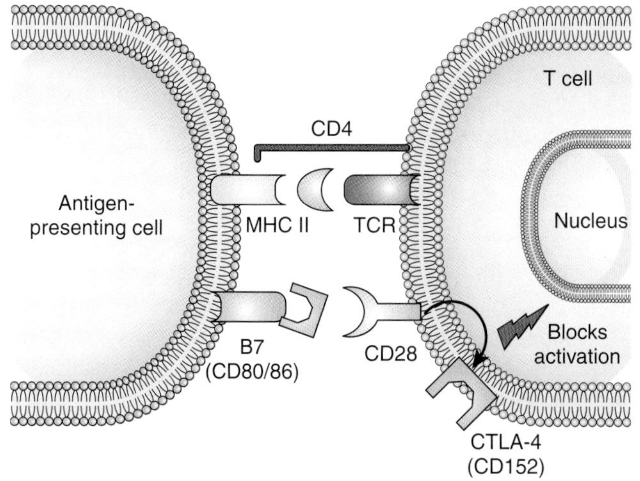

• **Fig. 67.5** Interactions between antigen-presenting cells and T cells. Successful T cell activation requires multiple signals. One signal is provided by the presentation of an antigen bound to cell surface major histocompatibility complex (MHC) molecules on antigen-presenting cells to a specific T cell receptor (TCR). In the absence of further signals, T cells become unresponsive and may ultimately be eliminated through apoptosis. An important co-stimulatory signal is provided by an interaction between members of the B7 family (either CD80 or CD86) on antigen-presenting cells and CD28 on T cells. After activation, T cells express cytolytic T lymphocyte–associated protein 4 (CTLA-4), which interferes with the B7-CD28 interaction and helps return the cells to the quiescent state.

Abatacept is a novel, fully human fusion protein consisting of the extra-cellular portion of CTLA-4 and the Fc fragment of human IgG-1 (CTLA-4Ig). In December 2005, abatacept (Orencia) became the first co-stimulatory blocker to be approved by the FDA for the treatment of patients with RA who had had an inadequate response to other drugs. Abatacept binds to CD80 and CD86 on antigen-presenting cells, thus preventing these molecules from binding their ligand, CD28, on T cells, with the consequent inhibition of optimal T cell activation. In vitro, abatacept decreases T cell proliferation and inhibits the production of TNF, IFN-γ, and IL-2. CTLA-4Ig showed promising activity in rodent collagen-induced arthritis models, prompting its evaluation in several clinical trials in people with RA.[74,75]

Clinical Studies

KEY POINT

Abatacept is an effective therapy across the spectrum of RA patient populations. For a majority of patients achieving clinical responses in the first 6 months, sustained clinical responses follow that may be incremental for up to 2 years of treatment.

Abatacept has been evaluated in several double-blind, placebo-controlled trials in a number of clinical scenarios in adults with active RA. These scenarios include an inadequate response to conventional DMARDs such as methotrexate or to TNF inhibitors and, more recently, methotrexate-naïve patients in the early phase of disease. In addition, data have been reported in the context of an exploratory phase II study designed to assess the effect of co-stimulation blockade on progression of undifferentiated, early inflammatory arthritis to fulfill classification criteria for RA.

TABLE 67.2 Percentage of Patients Achieving Responses at 24 Weeks in the AIM and ATTAIN Studies

Study	Drug Regimen	ACR20	ACR50	ACR70
Phase IIb AIM[42]	Abatacept 10 mg/kg + methotrexate	60	37	17
	Methotrexate	35	12	2
Phase III AIM[45]	Abatacept 10 mg/kg + methotrexate	68	40	20
	Methotrexate	40	17	7
Phase III ATTAIN[46]	Abatacept 10 mg/kg + methotrexate	50	20	10
	Methotrexate	20	4	1

ACR, American College of Rheumatology; *AIM*, Abatacept in Inadequate Responders to Methotrexate; *ATTAIN*, Abatacept Trial in Treatment of Anti-TNF Inadequate Responders.

An initial 3-month, phase IIa, double-blind, randomized, placebo-controlled pilot study demonstrated the efficacy of B7 blockade in treating the signs and symptoms in patients with active RA despite treatment with at least one conventional DMARD.[76] In this pilot study, the effect of one of two different biologic co-stimulatory modulators was compared with that of placebo infusions. The two biologic agents used were CTLA-4Ig, which binds approximately fourfold less avidly to CD86 than to CD80, and belatacept, a second-generation CTLA-4Ig with two mutated amino acid residues conferring an increased avidity for CD86 over that of the parent molecule. The proportion of patients achieving ACR20 responses on day 85 was dose dependent, suggesting clinical efficacy for both co-stimulatory blocking molecules.

The findings were confirmed in a multicenter phase IIb study of abatacept plus methotrexate in 339 patients who had active RA despite methotrexate treatment.[77] In this study, patients were randomized to receive either infusions of placebo; abatacept, 2 mg/kg; or abatacept, 10 mg/kg at baseline, at 2 weeks, 4 weeks, and then monthly through 6 months. ACR20 responses were achieved in 60%, 41.9%, and 35.3% of patients receiving the 10-mg/kg dose of abatacept, the 2-mg/kg dose of abatacept, and placebo, respectively. At the more stringent ACR50 response level, the figures were 36.5%, 22.9%, and 11.8% (Table 67.2). Improvements in the individual components of the ACR response criteria were generally greater in the 10-mg/kg group than in the 2-mg/kg group. No deaths, malignancies, or opportunistic infections were reported for any patient receiving abatacept during the 6 months of therapy. Patients in the phase IIb study continued to receive blinded therapy for an additional 6 months, during which time response to therapy was maintained. For patients receiving 10 mg/kg of abatacept, the ACR70, ACR50, and ASCR20 response rates were 21%, 42%, and 63%, respectively, compared with 8%, 20%, and 36% for patients receiving placebo infusions. Further, at the higher dose, statistically significant improvements in physical function and health-related quality of life were maintained over the 1-year period.[78] In the phase IIb study, from day 90 onward, statistically significant and progressively rising differences in remission rates were observed between the group receiving methotrexate plus abatacept, 10 mg/kg, and the group assigned to methotrexate and placebo infusions. By 1 year of treatment, 34.8% of patients receiving abatacept plus methotrexate achieved a DAS28 remission

(<2.6), in contrast to 10.1% of the patients receiving methotrexate plus placebo ($P < 0.001$).[78] Patients completing the double-blind phase over 12 months became eligible to enter a long-term extension phase in which all participants received methotrexate plus abatacept, 10 mg/kg. At year 3, patients treated with abatacept experienced greater than 70% improvement in swollen and tender joint counts and approximately 50% improvement in pain and physical function.[79] Patients who received placebo infusions during the double-blinded phase and then switched to abatacept during the long-term extension rapidly achieved equivalent efficacy to those treated with abatacept throughout.

The findings of two large phase III studies of abatacept in different RA populations have been reported. A population of methotrexate-refractory patients was studied in the Abatacept in Inadequate Responders to Methotrexate (AIM) trial. This study was designed to further evaluate the safety and clinical efficacy of abatacept plus methotrexate, as well as the effect on radiographic progression.[80] In the other phase III study, the Abatacept Trial in Treatment of Anti-TNF Inadequate Responders (ATTAIN),[81] the objective was to determine whether abatacept is a safe and effective treatment for patients with RA who were unresponsive to previous anti-TNF treatment.

In the AIM study, 652 patients with RA who had an inadequate response to methotrexate were randomly assigned to receive placebo or a fixed dose of abatacept approximating 10 mg/kg on days 1, 15, and 29 and every 4 weeks thereafter for a year; all patients continued to receive background methotrexate therapy.[80] Both patient groups exhibited high disease activity at baseline, with a DAS28 of 6.4. Patients receiving abatacept showed greater improvement in all ACR response criteria at 6 and 12 months than did patients treated with placebo (see Table 67.2). In findings similar to the phase IIb study, abatacept plus methotrexate-induced DAS28 remission (<2.6) in 14.8% of patients at 6 months and in 23.8% at 12 months, compared with 2.8% and 1.9% of patients receiving methotrexate plus placebo at the corresponding time points ($P < 0.001$). Physical function significantly improved in 63.7% of the abatacept plus methotrexate group, versus 39.3% of the placebo plus methotrexate group ($P < 0.001$). Further, patients taking the abatacept and methotrexate combination had a slower progression of mean structural damage (1.2 mTSS points over 1 year) compared with methotrexate alone (2.3 mTSS points).[80] Of interest, when assessed by conventional clinical outcome measures such as EULAR response, the data suggest that a plateau of clinical efficacy is achieved with abatacept between 4 and 6 months of treatment. Using more stringent measures for analyses, however, such as time to a low DAS (DAS28 < 3.2) or time to a sustained low DAS, no plateau of efficacy was observed over the first 12 months, suggesting an ongoing recruitment of clinical benefit with abatacept plus methotrexate.[82]

Patients completing the double-blind phase of the AIM study over 12 months became eligible to enter a long-term extension phase in which all participants received methotrexate plus abatacept at a fixed dose approximating 10 mg/kg every 4 weeks (Fig. 67.6). Clinically meaningful reductions in disease activity were maintained through 2 years, accompanied by an improved sense of subjective well-being assessed by patient-reported outcomes.[83] Further, inhibition of structural damage to joints was sustained, as evaluated by plain radiography; the effect after 2 years of abatacept was significantly greater than that at 1 year, with minimal radiographic progression observed over the second year of treatment.[84]

A third trial in methotrexate-inadequate responders provided the opportunity to evaluate two biologic agents in a single study. The placebo- and active comparator-controlled ATTEST (abatacept or infliximab vs. placebo, a trial for tolerability, efficacy, and safety in treating RA) study, although not powered to detect superiority, provided information on the relative efficacy

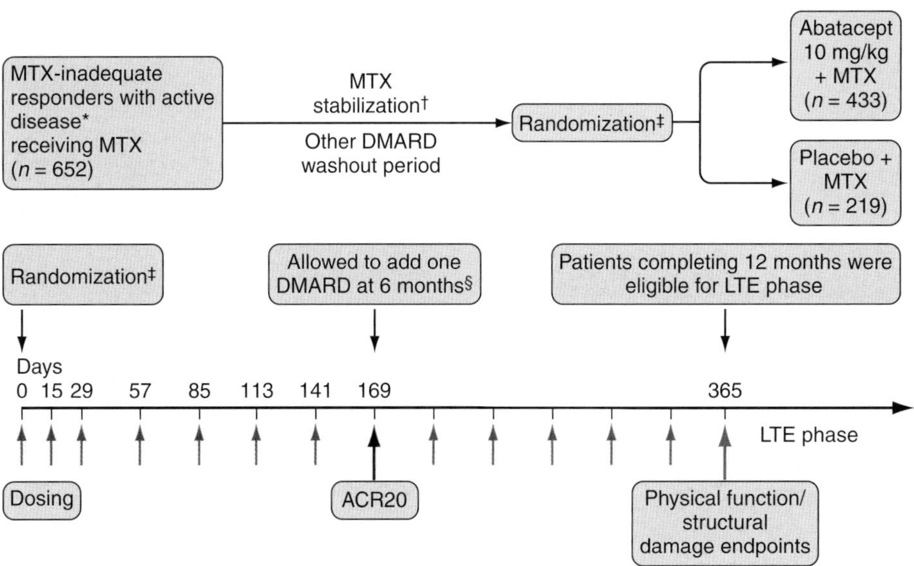

• **Fig. 67.6** Phase III AIM (Abatacept in Inadequate Responders to Methotrexate) study design. *ACR,* American College of Rheumatology; *CRP,* C-reactive protein; *DMARD,* disease-modifying anti-rheumatic drug; *LTE,* long-term extension; *MTX,* methotrexate.

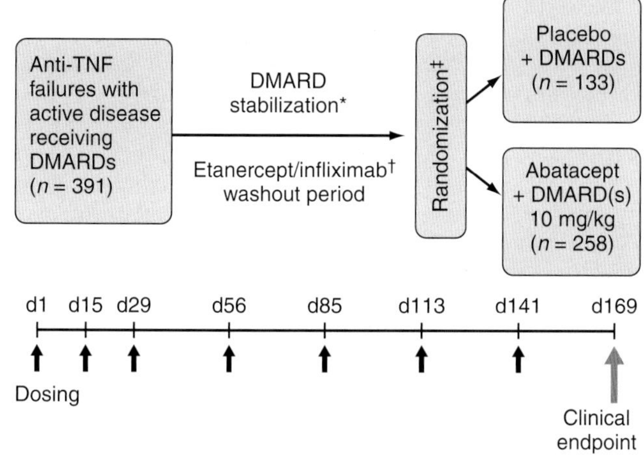

• **Fig. 67.7** Phase III ATTAIN (Abatacept Trial in Treatment of Anti-TNF Inadequate Responders) study design. *DMARD,* Disease-modifying antirheumatic drug; *TNF,* tumor necrosis factor. (From Genovese MC, Becker JC, Schiff M, et al.: Abatacept for rheumatoid arthritis refractory to tumor necrosis factor alpha inhibition. *N Engl J Med* 353:1114–1123, 2005.)

and safety profiles of abatacept and infliximab versus placebo in the same population.[85] Patients with an inadequate response to methotrexate were randomized (3:3:2) to abatacept (approved dose), infliximab (3 mg/kg), or placebo with background methotrexate. At month 6, patients in the placebo group were switched to abatacept, and infliximab and abatacept groups continued to year 1, with blinding maintained. The primary endpoint of this trial, reduction in DAS28 (ESR) at month 6 for abatacept versus placebo, was met, with mean reductions of −2.53 versus −1.48 ($P < 0.001$), respectively. The proportion of patients achieving low disease activity and DAS28 remission was also greater with abatacept. Improvements in ACR20, ACR50, and ACR70 responses at month 6 were significantly greater versus placebo for both abatacept and infliximab. The onset of ACR20 responses was generally more rapid for infliximab than for abatacept, but responses were similar by month 3. By year 1, DAS28 (ESR) reductions of −2.88 and −2.25 were seen for patients treated with abatacept and infliximab, respectively, and ACR responses were maintained from month 6 with abatacept but not with infliximab.

In the ATTAIN phase III study, abatacept therapy was evaluated in 391 patients with active disease receiving conventional DMARDs or anakinra who failed to respond adequately to at least 3 months of therapy with etanercept, infliximab, or both agents at the approved doses.[81] Anti-TNF therapy was discontinued at the time of enrollment if it had not been stopped previously. After a washout period, patients were randomly assigned in a 2:1 ratio to receive either the same fixed dose of abatacept (approximating 10 mg/kg) or placebo (Fig. 67.7). Patients receiving abatacept showed significantly greater improvement in all ACR response criteria through 6 months (see Table 67.2) than did patients treated with placebo (ACR20 response 50.4% vs. 19.5%, $P < 0.001$; ACR50 response 20.3% vs. 3.8%, $P < 0.001$; and ACR70 response 10.2% vs. 1.5%, $P = 0.003$) (Table 67.3). Further, a DAS28 remission was achieved in 10% of patients receiving abatacept versus only 1% of patients receiving placebo infusions plus DMARDs. ACR20 responses were seen regardless of whether patients had previously been exposed to etanercept, infliximab, or both anti-TNF therapies without an adequate response. Improvement in physical function was also significantly increased in the abatacept group (47% vs. 23%). The incidence of infection was slightly higher in the abatacept group than in the placebo group, although no specific infection was clearly more frequent, and the intensity of infections was similar in the two groups. There were no significant differences in the number of patients discontinuing treatment as a result of infection or in the incidence of serious infection.

All patients who completed the 6-month double-blind phase of the ATTAIN study were eligible to enter a 1-year, long-term extension phase during which all patients received a once-monthly fixed dose of abatacept in addition to at least one conventional DMARD.[86] Of 258 patients randomized to receive abatacept during the double-blind phase, 223 completed 6 months of treatment, and 218 entered the long-term extension. Of these patients, 168 completed 18 months of treatment. The ACR20 responses observed at the end of the double-blind phase were sustained throughout the 1-year extension phase, with the proportion of patients achieving the more stringent ACR50 and ACR70 responses rising to 35% and 18%, respectively, at 18 months. Further, the proportion of patients meeting DAS28 remission criteria doubled to 22.5% by the end of the extension period. Similarly, among all patients initially treated with abatacept and DMARDs who entered the long-term extension phase, the mean reduction in DAS28 from baseline to the end of the double-blind phase was −1.99; by the end of 18 months, the mean reduction from baseline was −2.81. In the double-blind phase, patients assigned to placebo infusions together with DMARDs had a mean reduction in DAS28 of −0.93; at the end of the long-term extension, after crossing over to abatacept infusions, the reduction from baseline was −2.72.[87] These data again emphasize the sustained but relatively slow and incremental clinical responses observed after abatacept therapy.

The second trial conducted in TNF-inadequate responders was a phase IIIb/IV, 6-month, open-label study. The ARRIVE (Abatacept Researched in Rheumatoid arthritis patients with an Inadequate anti-TNF response to Validate Effectiveness) trial was the first to assess the safety of abatacept in patients who switched directly from TNF inhibitor therapy without undergoing washout, an approach that may be more clinically relevant for everyday practice.[88] Patients enrolled in this study had high disease activity levels at entry and an inadequate response to up to three TNF inhibitors; the inadequate response could have occurred for efficacy, safety, or tolerability reasons. Patients were eligible even if they had a positive purified protein-derivative test result. Abatacept could be administered as monotherapy (for those recruited in the United States only), and patients were not limited to a particular background DMARD. Similar, clinically meaningful improvements were seen in disease activity, physical function, and health-related quality of life, regardless of whether there was a washout period. Post hoc analyses revealed that, numerically, more patients who had previously failed to respond to one TNF inhibitor achieved DAS28-defined remission and low disease activity than did those who had failed to respond to two or more TNF inhibitors.

Because T cell activation is believed to be an initiating event in an immunologic cascade observed in RA, co-stimulation blockade might be predicted to have benefits from an early stage of evolution of the syndrome independently of any driving antigen or antigens. The 2-year abatacept study to gauge remission and joint damage

TABLE 67.3 Comparison of TNF Inhibition Versus Other Biologics Abatacept Versus Adalimumab (AMPLE trial)

Treatment Regimen	Total Number of Patients	Number of Patients Showing MTX-Inadequate Response	Percentage of Patients Showing MTX-Inadequate Response
SC Abatacept + MTX	318	206	64.8
Adalimumab + MTX	328	208	63.4

Estimate of difference (95% CI) between groups was 1.8 (–5.6, 9.2); intent to treat, confirmed with per protocol population

MTX, Methotrexate.

Modified from Weinblatt ME, et al.: Head-to-head comparison of subcutaneous abatacept versus adalimumab for rheumatoid arthritis: findings of a phase IIIb, multinational, prospective, randomized study. *Arthritis Rheum* 65(1):28–38, 2013.

progression in methotrexate-naïve patients with early erosive RA (AGREE) consisted of a 12-month double-blind period, followed by a 12-month open-label period in methotrexate-naïve patients with early RA.[89] Eligibility included short disease duration, poor prognostic factors, including high CRP levels, radiographic evidence of erosions, and seropositivity for RF or ACPA. Patients were randomized 1 : 1 to receive abatacept plus methotrexate (n = 256) or methotrexate alone (n = 253) during the first 12-month period.[89] From year 1 onward, all patients received open-label abatacept plus methotrexate. The co-primary endpoints were 28-joint DAS (DAS28)–defined remission and radiographic joint damage progression at year 1.

Significantly more patients treated with abatacept plus methotrexate achieved DAS28 (CRP)–defined remission and ACR50 and ACR70 responses at year 1, and the difference between treatment arms was significant by month 2. Over 1 year, 27.3 versus 11.9% of patients treated with abatacept plus methotrexate versus patients treated with methotrexate alone ($P < 0.001$) experienced a major clinical response (ACR70 maintained for 56 consecutive months).[89] Significant improvements were also seen in physical function at year 1 for patients treated with abatacept plus methotrexate compared with patients treated with methotrexate alone.[89] Improvements in disease activity and ACR responses were sustained or improved over the second year for patients who continued to receive abatacept plus methotrexate therapy, with 55.2% achieving remission at year 2.[90] Changes from baseline to year 1 in Genant-mTSS and erosion score were significantly lower for methotrexate-naïve patients who were randomized to the abatacept plus methotrexate arm.[89] Furthermore, there was an increasing degree of inhibition of progression in year 2 relative to year 1 for patients originally randomized to the abatacept arm.[91] For patients originally receiving methotrexate alone, structural damage progression was reduced over year 2 relative to year 1, following the addition of abatacept.[90] Nevertheless, overall structural damage progression at year 2 remained greater for these patients compared with patients who received abatacept from baseline.[90]

The potential for early treatment with abatacept to delay the time of progression to fulfillment of classification criteria for RA in people with ACPA-positive, undifferentiated, early inflammatory arthritis with clinical synovitis of two or more joints was investigated in an exploratory, phase II, 2-year study known as ADJUST (abatacept study to determine the effectiveness in preventing the development of RA in patients with undifferentiated inflammatory arthritis).[92] After 6 months of double-blind, randomized (1 : 1) treatment with either abatacept at the approved dose of approximately 10 mg/kg (n = 28) or placebo (n = 28), abatacept treatment was terminated. At year 1, the proportion of patients who developed RA according to ACR 1987 criteria or discontinued because of lack of efficacy was assessed. When treatment with abatacept was stopped after 6 months, 22 and 17 patients treated with abatacept and placebo, respectively, remained in the study inasmuch as they had not fulfilled classification criteria for RA; by year 2, seven and four patients treated with abatacept and placebo, respectively, remained in the study. Numerically, RA developed in more patients treated with placebo than in those treated with abatacept over 1 year (66.7% vs. 46.2%), although CIs overlapped. Radiographic assessments demonstrated an inhibitory effect on structural damage progression at month 6, which was maintained for 6 months after therapy cessation, with similar trends observed for MRI-assessed osteitis, erosion, and synovitis.[92] Abatacept treatment was also associated with reductions in ACPA levels that persisted beyond cessation of the active drug. At enrollment, patients had short symptom duration, and although they did not meet ACR 1987 criteria for RA at the point of recruitment, more than half already had evidence of one or more erosions and were thus likely to have had early RA. The findings must be interpreted in light of this situation.

The popularity among patients of the subcutaneous delivery route out of available choices of parenteral delivery has prompted studies to look at the effectiveness and safety of subcutaneously delivered abatacept, which is now available in a subcutaneous formulation, consisting of a fixed dose of 125 mg of the drug, administered once weekly. Six clinical trials have been performed in patients with RA treated with the subcutaneous formulation, including ACQUIRE (a phase II dose-finding study comparing the efficacy of intravenous and subcutaneous formulations),[93] ALLOW (a withdrawal-restart study of immunogenicity with subcutaneous abatacept plus methotrexate vs. methotrexate),[94] ACCOMPANY (a study of immunogenicity in subcutaneous abatacept plus methotrexate vs. subcutaneous abatacept),[95] ATTUNE (an intravenous to subcutaneous switch study),[96] and AMPLE (a head-to-head subcutaneous abatacept plus methotrexate vs. adalimumab plus methotrexate).[97] All of these studies demonstrate an efficacy and a safety profile comparable with that obtained with the classic intravenous administration. In particular, it has been demonstrated that the fixed dose of the drug achieves a serum concentration comparable with that reached with the weight-tiered intravenous regimen, eliciting therapeutic concentrations in more than 90% of patients.

The AMPLE trial (abatacept vs. adalimumab comparison in biologic-naïve subjects with RA with background methotrexate) in particular deserves further elaboration. In a noninferiority phase III study design, AMPLE was the first head-to-head study in patients with RA that was powered to compare biologic DMARD agents on a background of methotrexate in people who were inadequate responders to methotrexate therapy and naïve to biologic DMARD therapy. Methotrexate-refractory people with active RA who were naïve to biologic therapy were recruited. A total of 318 people were randomized to weekly subcutaneous 125-mg doses of abatacept without an intravenous loading dose plus methotrexate with once-weekly placebo injections, and 328 people were randomized to biweekly adalimumab plus methotrexate with once-weekly placebo injections. Because unmarked adalimumab (Humira) syringes could not be obtained, the study was single blinded, using a rigorous protocol, including a blinded assessor at each recruiting site.

The AMPLE trial demonstrated the comparable efficacy of subcutaneous abatacept to adalimumab on background methotrexate with respect to the primary outcome measure, ACR20 at 1 year, with subcutaneous abatacept demonstrating noninferiority to adalimumab (64.8% vs. 63.4%). Furthermore, comparable response and kinetics were seen across all efficacy measures, including ACR 20/50/70 and DAS28 (CRP) responses, as well as inhibition of radiographic progression. Safety outcomes were balanced with some differences, such as fewer discontinuations due to adverse events and serious adverse events in the subcutaneous abatacept group. Local injection site reaction complaints were also significantly less frequent in people receiving subcutaneous abatacept. These findings confirm the clinical impression that among currently available biologic therapies, abatacept is at the better tolerated and safer end of the safety spectrum. Interestingly, in AMPLE, baseline anti-CCP2 positivity was associated with a better response for abatacept and adalimumab. Patients with the highest baseline anti-CCP2 antibody concentrations, however, had better clinical responses with abatacept than patients with lower concentrations, an association that was not observed with adalimumab.[98]

Safety Issues

KEY POINTS

Abatacept has acceptable safety across the spectrum of RA patient populations.

Abatacept is administered either as a 30-minute intravenous infusion that is usually without complications or as a once-weekly, fixed dose, subcutaneous injection that is tolerated with a very low rate of injection site reactions.

Safety assessments from abatacept clinical trials have in general demonstrated a comparable overall incidence of adverse events and serious adverse events for people treated with abatacept and placebo. The safety of long-term abatacept treatment is reported to be consistent, with the incidence of overall adverse events and serious adverse events remaining stable up to 7 years.[99]

A safety analysis has been undertaken on pooled data from abatacept clinical trials through December 2007 that included 4150 patients who were exposed to abatacept. This represents 10,365 patient-years of exposure, with an average exposure period of 2.5 years.[99] The incidence of serious infections was generally low, although it was higher for people treated with abatacept compared with people treated with placebo over 1 year (serious infections: 3.47 vs. 2.41 events/100 patient-years, respectively). Records of annual incidence rates for serious infections did not appear to show an increase in risk over time. Pneumonia, bronchitis, cellulitis, and urinary tract infection were the most common causes of hospital admission for infections. Opportunistic infections were rarely observed in this pooled cohort, including the following events per 100 patient-years of treatment: *Mycobacterium tuberculosis*, 0.06 events; aspergillosis, 0.02; blastomycosis, 0.01; and systemic *Candida*, 0.01.[99]

The incidence of malignancies (excluding nonmelanoma skin cancer) during the double-blind treatment periods was reported to be 0.59 events/100 patient-years for people treated with abatacept versus 0.63 events/100 patient-years for people treated with placebo. This low incidence rate did not rise with increasing exposure. In particular, for lung cancer and lymphoma, the incidence rate was 0.24 lung cancers and 0.06 lymphomas/100 patient-years during the double-blind period and 0.16 lung cancers and 0.07 lymphomas/100 patient-years during the cumulative period. To better interpret malignancy risk data, the incidence rates observed in abatacept studies were compared with those documented in five observational cohorts of patients with RA who were naïve to biologics and were taking nonbiologic DMARDs. Standardized incidence rates for the observational cohorts ranged from 0.4 to 1.06; for patients treated with abatacept, the risk of lung cancer did not appear to be increased, with standardized incidence rates ranging from 0.65 to 1.84. The lymphoma risk in patients treated with abatacept appeared to be comparable with that in biologic naïve patients with RA, with standardized incidence rates ranging from 0.60 to 1.23.[99] In the pooled trial data from double-treatment periods, autoimmune events were reported in 1.4% of patients treated with abatacept and 0.8% of patients treated with placebo. Most events were mild or moderate in intensity, and the most frequently reported event was psoriasis, with rates of 0.53 and 0.56 events/100 patient-years over the double-blind and cumulative periods, respectively.

In clinical practice it is common to use conventional DMARDs in combination regimens, based on the belief that they provide additive benefits in terms of efficacy without the downside of unacceptable toxicity. Whether these same principles apply to the use of abatacept was addressed in the ASSURE trial (Abatacept Study of Safety in Use with other RA therapies).[100] This multicenter, randomized, double-blind study investigated the safety of adding abatacept or placebo infusions to a background treatment regimen of at least one of the traditional nonbiologic or biologic DMARDs currently approved for RA treatment for at least 3 months. A total of 1456 patients were randomized 2 : 1 to receive abatacept at a fixed dose approximating 10 mg/kg by weight range or placebo.

A number of interesting observations arose from this study. In the group as a whole, the proportion of serious adverse events occurring in each treatment arm was similar: 13% for abatacept and 12% for placebo. The discontinuations rate due to adverse events was 5% in the abatacept group and 4% in the placebo group. As expected on the basis of prior studies, serious infections occurred more frequently in the abatacept group (2.9%) than in the placebo group (1.9%). Five deaths occurred in the abatacept group and four deaths occurred in the placebo group; it was thought that all but one of the deaths in each group were unlikely to be related to the study drug. All the deaths occurred in patients without concomitant biologic background therapy. Nevertheless, a subanalysis of the data, based on whether patients were receiving biologic or nonbiologic background therapy, revealed that serious adverse events occurred almost twice as frequently in the subgroup receiving abatacept plus another biologic agent (22.3%) as in the other subgroups (12.5%).

A particularly important observation in this study was the increased number of serious infections observed when abatacept was combined with other biologic therapies (5.8% vs. 1.6% for the subgroup receiving background biologic therapy plus placebo infusions). Further, the clinical benefits of abatacept tended to be less in the patients receiving background biologic therapy than in patients with a background of nonbiologic DMARDs. No cases of lymphoma, demyelinating disorders, or tuberculosis were reported.

The ASSURE trial findings mirrored those of a smaller randomized, placebo-controlled, double-blind pilot study. This phase IIb trial investigated the efficacy and safety of the addition of abatacept infusions at 2 mg/kg over 1 year in patients with at least 8 of 66 swollen joints and 10 of 68 tender joints despite at least 3 months of treatment with twice-weekly 25-mg subcutaneous etanercept.[101] The biologic combination had limited clinical benefit compared with etanercept and placebo infusions but was associated with an increase in the proportion of patients experiencing serious adverse events (16.5% vs. 2.8%) and serious infections (3.5% vs. 0%). On the basis of these observations, the use of abatacept is not advised in combination with other biologic therapies.

Data are emerging concerning the comparative efficacy, safety, and kinetics of response for the anti-TNF antibody infliximab and abatacept.[102] In a 1-year double-blind study, patients with RA who had an inadequate response to methotrexate (a mean baseline DAS28 of 6.8) and no prior anti-TNF therapy were randomized to receive abatacept at a dose approximating 10 mg/kg every 4 weeks (156 patients); infliximab, 3 mg/kg every 8 weeks (165 patients); or placebo every 4 weeks (110 patients). Patients randomized to receive a placebo were switched to abatacept after 6 months but were not included in the 1-year analyses. At the end of the first 6 months, the frequency of serious adverse events was 5.1%, 11.5%, and 11.8% for abatacept, infliximab, and placebo, respectively. In the same order, the frequency of acute infusion-related adverse events was 5.1%, 18.2%, and 10%. Over the 1-year period, infections reported as serious adverse events were more frequent with infliximab (8.5%) than with abatacept (1.9%). These infections included two cases of tuberculosis, both in patients treated with infliximab. When considered in the light of the clinical response data discussed earlier, this study and others emphasize the relatively slow time to peak clinical response with abatacept in comparison with TNF blockade, with increasing efficacy beyond 6 months. These studies also point to the possibility of a favorable benefit-risk profile over 1 year. It will be critical to see whether these encouraging early safety data are maintained over the longer term.

Of note, the incidence rate of serious infections observed with abatacept is at the lower end of the range reported in patients with RA who are treated with other biologic agents. In summary, the long-term integrated safety data from up to eight abatacept trials, representing more than 10,000 patient-years of exposure, confirm that, overall, abatacept has a favorable safety profile that is consistent with observations from the short-term experience in all RA populations studied, with no new clinically important safety issues identified with long-term exposure. This conclusion is supported by a recent Cochrane review.[103]

Current Role

KEY POINT

Abatacept is a biologic option in patients with RA who have inadequate responses to TNF inhibitors, although recent evidence suggests that the benefit-risk profile of abatacept may be most optimal when introduced earlier in the treatment paradigm.

Abatacept may be used as monotherapy or concomitantly with DMARDs other than TNF inhibitors. It is not recommended for use concomitantly with IL-1 or TNF inhibitors. The encouraging clinical trial data confirm that abatacept, like rituximab, represents a valuable agent in the therapeutic armamentarium for patients with RA who have not responded adequately to TNF blockade. Abatacept has a particular advantage among intravenously delivered biologics for RA in that it is very well tolerated and quick to administer, and infusion-related problems are rare. The more recently introduced subcutaneous formulation adds to the range of options for convenience of delivery depending on patient preference and circumstances. Nevertheless, the clinical responses and radiographic benefits observed with abatacept appear to be greater in methotrexate-naïve patients compared with patients who have failed to respond to methotrexate or other DMARDs. Patients who previously failed to respond to methotrexate treatment appear to demonstrate higher clinical responses than patients who have failed to respond to TNF inhibitors. Furthermore, the findings of the phase III AMPLE trial, which demonstrated noninferiority for efficacy with respect to symptoms and signs of abatacept plus methotrexate compared with adalimumab plus methotrexate and comparable inhibition of structural damage progression, suggest that the most favorable clinical outcomes with abatacept may be achieved if it is used earlier in the treatment paradigm than was generally the case when it first became available for use in the clinic. Indeed, since the recent availability of the subcutaneous formulation, abatacept is increasingly finding favor as a well-tolerated and first-line choice of biologic therapy with a favorable benefit-risk ratio. The merits of switching a patient from a TNF inhibitor to abatacept or rituximab on the basis of a clinical response that is incomplete are not yet clear-cut with respect to disease modification. Other factors likely to inform the future use and relative positioning of biologics in the clinic include additional long-term safety data, comparative cost-effectiveness analyses, and the perceived convenience of intravenous versus subcutaneous administration.

Implications for the Pathogenesis of Rheumatoid Arthritis

KEY POINTS

The clinical efficacy of abatacept in people with RA validates the importance of co-stimulation in pathogenesis.

Co-stimulation inhibition modulates production of a number of pro-inflammatory cytokines.

The clinical efficacy of abatacept in a proportion of patients with RA implicates co-stimulatory events in disease pathogenesis; however, abatacept might mediate immunosuppressive effects in RA by a number of different mechanisms. In the RA joint, blocking access of CD28 to CD80 or CD86 might be of little importance because memory T cells, which predominate in inflamed synovium, are much less dependent on this pathway.[104] A more important mechanism of action in the synovium might be the induction of tolerogenic antigen-presenting cells. Binding of CD80 or CD86 on antigen-presenting cells by CTLA-4Ig initiates a "reverse signal," with induction of tryptophan catabolism and inhibition of antigen presentation. Naïve T cells are located predominantly in lymphoid tissue, and blockade of the CD28-CD80/CD86 interaction in lymph nodes may reduce T cell priming and the production of autoreactive T cells. Interestingly, patients with RA are reported to have higher frequencies of CD28-null T cells.[105] Further, the level of expression of CD28 is significantly reduced on all naïve T cells and memory CD4+, CD28+ T cells, a phenomenon related to overproduction of TNF.[106] A likely consequence of low-density cell surface expression of CD28 is that, for these T cells, abatacept can more readily block the interaction with CD80 and CD86. The clinical and radiographic benefits of abatacept administration in people with RA illustrate the importance of the co-stimulation pathway in T cell activation and subsequent amplification of the inflammatory cascade, including pathways that promote tissue destruction.[107] The modulatory effect of co-stimulation blockade on the expression of a range of inflammatory genes in synovial tissue has been demonstrated by quantitative PCR studies and evaluation of synovial biopsies in patients with active RA who received abatacept treatment, having previously failed to respond to TNF inhibitors.[108] Furthermore, a small, largely nonsignificant reduction in cellular content was observed in biopsy samples after abatacept treatment, suggesting that co-stimulation inhibition reduces the inflammatory status of the synovium without disrupting cellular homoeostasis.

Abatacept in Other Rheumatic Conditions

KEY POINTS

Abatacept has clinical use for treatment of RA, polyarticular juvenile idiopathic arthritis, and psoriatic arthritis.

In addition to being approved for the treatment of active RA, abatacept is also approved in two other indications. First, abatacept in combination with methotrexate is indicated for the treatment of moderate to severe active polyarticular juvenile idiopathic arthritis in pediatric patients 6 years and older who have had an insufficient response to other DMARDs, including at least one TNF inhibitor. Second, abatacept alone or in combination with methotrexate is indicated for the treatment of active psoriatic arthritis (PsA) in adult patients with inadequate response to previous DMARD therapy and in whom additional systemic therapy for psoriatic skin lesions is not required.

Results from a 12-month multicenter clinical trial did not show therapeutic benefit of abatacept over placebo in patients with non–life-threatening SLE. In particular, abatacept failed to prevent new disease flares in patients with SLE who underwent tapering of corticosteroids in an analysis where mild, moderate, and severe disease flares were evaluated together. Serious adverse events were higher in the abatacept group (19.8% vs. 6.8%). Although the primary and secondary endpoints were not met, improvements in certain exploratory measures were found.[109] Studies are ongoing in type 1 diabetes and inflammatory bowel disease.

Abatacept was also used in a 26-week, phase I, open-label, dose-escalation study of psoriasis vulgaris.[110] Sustained improvements of at least 50% in clinical disease activity were reported after four infusions of abatacept in 20 of 43 patients with stable psoriasis vulgaris. Clinical improvement was associated with quantitative reduction in epidermal hyperplasia, which correlated with a quantitative reduction in skin-infiltrating T cells. Nevertheless, no clear-cut increase in the rate of intralesional T cell apoptosis was identified. It may be that the observed reduction in lesional T cells numbers was due to inhibition of T cell proliferation, T cell recruitment, or apoptosis of antigen-specific T cells at extralesional sites. Altered antibody responses to T cell–dependent neoantigens were observed, but immunologic tolerance to these antigens was not demonstrated. This study illustrates the importance of the CD28-CD152 pathway in the pathogenesis of psoriatic skin disease.

The safety and efficacy of subcutaneously administered abatacept was compared to placebo in the treatment of patients with active PsA in the phase III, randomized, double-blind, placebo-controlled ASTRAEA (Active PSoriaTic Arthritis RAndomizEd TriAl) study.[111] Patients (n = 424) were randomly assigned (1 : 1) to receive either weekly subcutaneous abatacept 125 mg (n = 213) or placebo subcutaneously (n = 211) for 24 weeks during the double-blind period of the study. Patients were stratified by methotrexate use, prior TNF inhibitor use, and whether plaque psoriasis involved ≥3% of body surface area. Patients not achieving ≥20% improvement in swollen and tender joint counts by week 16 were switched to open-label abatacept in an early escape. All patients subsequently received weekly subcutaneous abatacept 125 mg for 28 weeks through an open-label period. The primary endpoint was the proportion of patients achieving an ACR20 response at week 24. Secondary endpoints included the proportion of Health Assessment Questionnaire-Disability Index (HAQ-DI) responders (defined as ≥0.35 score reduction from baseline), the proportion of both TNF inhibitor naive and experienced patients achieving ACR20, and the proportion of nonprogressors in total PsA-modified Sharp/van der Heijde score (defined as a change from baseline ≤0) at week 24. By week 24, a total of 76 (35.7%) patients receiving abatacept and 89 (42.2%) patients receiving placebo underwent early escape from the study (and were thus classified as nonresponders) and hence were switched to open-label abatacept at week 16; in addition, 12 (5.6%) patients receiving abatacept and 24 (11.4%) patients receiving placebo discontinued treatment. Abatacept significantly improved the proportion of patients (39.4%) achieving an ACR20 response at week 24 versus 22.3% on placebo (P <0.001). Secondary endpoints included 31% HAQ-DI responders on abatacept versus 23.7% on placebo and 42.7% radiographic nonprogressors on abatacept versus 32.7% on placebo. Furthermore, of the 84 abatacept treated patients who were anti-TNF naïve, 44% achieved ACR20, whereas 18 out of 81 (22.2%) of anti-TNF naïve placebo-treated patients achieved ACR20 (P = 0.003). Of the anti-TNF experienced patients, 47 of 129 (36.4%) abatacept-treated patients achieved ACR20 compared with 29 of 130 (22.3%) placebo-treated patients (P = 0.012). ACR20 responses were maintained to week 44.

The proportion of patients who had dactylitis or enthesitis at baseline and achieved complete resolution at week 24 was 44.3% and 32.9%, respectively, in the group receiving abatacept, and 34.0% and 21.2%, respectively, in the group receiving placebo. By week 52, the proportion with complete resolution in dactylitis and enthesitis had increased to 68.9% and 48.6%, respectively, in the abatacept group, and 60.0% and 43.9%, respectively, in the placebo group.

Psoriasis Area and Severity Index (PASI) scores of 50 out of 75 at week 24 in patients with baseline psoriasis ≥3% body surface were achieved by 26.7% and 16.4% respectively in the abatacept-treated patients and by 19.6% and 10.1% respectively in the placebo group. For the TNF inhibitor naïve subpopulation, PASI 50 of 75 scores at week 24 were 32.7% and 18.2% respectively in abatacept-treated patients and 19.6% and 9.8% in the placebo group. For the TNF inhibitor experienced subpopulation, PASI 50 of 75 scores at week 24 were 23.1% and 16.5% respectively in abatacept-treated patients and 19.6% and 10.3% in the placebo group. The safety profile of abatacept was similar to placebo in the ASTRAEA trial.

In a small, open-label study, abatacept treatment was reported to be effective, safe, and well tolerated in patients with early and active primary Sjögren's syndrome, with treatment resulting in improved disease activity, laboratory parameters, fatigue, and health-related quality of life.[112] In another small open-label study, 31 patients with RA and secondary Sjögren's syndrome completed 6 months of abatacept therapy. Eleven patients with histologic features characteristic of Sjögren's syndrome on a minor salivary gland biopsy had statistically significant improvements in saliva volume and in Schirmer's test for tear volume.[113]

Targeting T Cells

Clinical Studies

KEY POINT

A number of approaches to targeting T cells independently from co-stimulation pathways have not shown clear-cut benefit in clinical trials.

In the early years of investigating the potential of biologic therapies in RA, T cells were among the first targets to be explored. Data from several different pre-clinical animal models of inflammatory arthritis suggested a pathogenic role for CD4⁺ T cells in response to various arthritogenic antigens presented in the context of class II MHC molecules.[104] These observations led to a number of experimental protocols designed to investigate the effect of depleting and nondepleting antibodies directed at CD4, as well as other T cell–associated molecules. Early randomized, placebo-controlled clinical studies exploring the potential of biologic therapies targeting T cells in the treatment of RA have generally had disappointing results. Some anti–T cell agents were not efficacious; other preliminary trials demonstrating some clinical efficacy were terminated as a result of adverse events, particularly prolonged and profound T cell depletion.[114] Nevertheless, the primatized monoclonal anti–CD4 antibody keliximab results in a dose-dependent clinical response when administered once weekly over 4 consecutive weeks, and the clinical response correlates with $CD4^+$ T cell coating with keliximab rather than T cell depletion. In two consecutive randomized, double-blind trials with comparable populations, keliximab treatment was associated with $CD4^+$ T cell counts below 250 cells/mm^3 in 12% of subjects in one study and in 47% of subjects in the other study.[115]

Examples of biologic therapies targeting other T cell–associated molecules include Campath-1H, a monoclonal antibody directed against CD52; a monoclonal anti–CD5 antibody linked to ricin toxin; and a fusion protein comprising an IL-2 receptor–binding domain coupled to diphtheria toxin (DAB_{486}IL-2 fusion toxin). CD52 is a polypeptide expressed on all lymphocytes. Campath-1H was tested as a treatment for refractory RA in two small trials, and although a single intravenous dose of between 1 and 100 mg resulted in significant $CD4^+$ T cell depletion and clinical improvement in more than half of patients, the correlation between biologic action and clinical response was poor.[116,117] Further, therapy was associated with significant acute toxicity, which was presumed to reflect a cytokine release syndrome, including headache, nausea, and hypotension. Arthritis activity returned over time despite prolonged suppression of peripheral blood $CD4^+$ T cell numbers.

CD5 is a transmembrane glycoprotein expressed on 70% of T cells. CD5-1C, a monoclonal antibody linked to ricin, a plant toxin that inhibits protein synthesis, was used to treat RA in a double-blind, placebo-controlled trial.[118] At the doses tested, only modest and transient T cell depletion was observed, and no clinical benefit occurred.

In a strategy designed to selectively deplete activated T cells expressing IL-2 receptor, DAB_{486}IL-2 fusion toxin was given by intravenous infusion in open-label and placebo-controlled studies.[119,120] Although a small percentage of patients (18%) exhibited clinical responses in the placebo-controlled study, the incidence of adverse events was significant, including nausea, fever, and raised plasma transaminases. Further, antibodies against diphtheria toxin developed in nearly all patients.

Other approaches to targeting T cells that have been tested include efforts to directly interfere with the trimolecular complex comprising human leukocyte antigen class II, antigenic peptide, and TCR by means of a DR4-DR1 peptide vaccine, TCR Vβ peptide vaccine, collagen, or cartilage glycoprotein 39.[121] Despite a rationale for these approaches based on promising pre-clinical animal model data, all have been abandoned because of borderline or absent clinical benefits in human disease.

Future Directions

KEY POINT

Novel approaches to targeting T cells are being tested, including T cell vaccination.

The importance of immune regulation in maintenance of the healthy state is perhaps best illustrated by the consequences of immune dysregulation, a phenomenon common to a wide range of chronic inflammatory disease phenotypes. Emerging evidence points to the importance of certain $CD4^+$ T cell subsets in the negative regulation of the adaptive immune system. The best characterized of these subsets are the so-called naturally occurring $CD4^+CD25^+$ regulatory T cells and IL-10–producing Tr1 cells. Recent advances in the understanding of the molecular basis of $CD4^+CD25^+$ regulatory T cell generation include the observation that the X-linked forkhead–winged helix transcription factor Foxp3 is required for $CD4^+CD25^+$ T cell development and function. Although further progress in understanding the pathophysiologic role of regulatory T cells will require the identification of more specific markers for distinct regulatory T cell populations, there is already evidence of the feasibility of enhancing regulatory T cell function in vivo either by TCR modulation, using antibodies to CD3, or by co-stimulatory signals, using a CD28 superagonist.[122]

When a chronic inflammatory disease reflects an antigen-driven process, an attractive goal is to modulate T cell function in such a way as to generate antigen-specific unresponsiveness in the absence of long-term generalized immunosuppression. Some but not all studies report a relative deficiency of regulatory T cells in RA.[29] Of note, antibodies to CD3 and to TNF appear to enhance regulatory T cell function or number in patients with RA.[123–126] This finding raises the possibility that combination treatment with anti-CD3 and anti-TNF might be beneficial in more completely restoring immune regulation in people with RA. In fact, chronic inflammation and overproduction of TNF perturb T cell antigen receptor–dependent signaling,[127] suggesting that active inflammation may attenuate tolerogenic signals expected to be induced by a nondepleting anti-CD3 antibody. Thus pre-treatment with TNF blockade might restore tolerogenic signals transduced by the TCR in response to drugs such as anti-CD3. Although the use of anti-CD3 in the clinic has been limited by the occurrence of drug-induced cytokine release syndrome,[128] the effects can be modulated by anti-TNF agents, as demonstrated in patients treated for acute allograft rejection.[129] Such a combination therapy approach has yet to be tested in people with RA.

A potentially beneficial immunomodulatory response has been demonstrated in a small open pilot study by vaccinating 16 patients with RA with expanded, activated, and irradiated autologous synovial fluid T cells.[130] Vaccination was associated with expansion of $CD4^+$ and $CD8^+$ T cells, many of which expressed the Vβ2 TCR chain. Some were anti-idiotypic, responding specifically to vaccine T cells with the production of IL-10 ($CD4^+$ cells) or granzyme B ($CD8^+$ cells). A broader regulatory response, however, was directed toward activated T cells in general, specifically against peptides derived from the IL-2 receptor α chain. This broader response may be important to generate in a syndrome such as RA, where the precise autoantigen and pathogenic T cell clones are not readily identifiable. This might also explain why earlier attempts at T cell vaccination using TCR-derived peptides have not been pursued.[121] Nevertheless, the efficacy of such a T cell vaccination approach needs to be validated in further trials, and the safety and durability of response must be further investigated before the potential feasibility of such an approach to therapy in routine clinical use can be properly assessed.

Anti–T cell therapies, including anti-CD4, cyclosporine, and CTLA-4Ig, synergize with TNF blockade in mice. Various agonists of immune inhibitory receptors on T cells could be potential adjuncts to anti-TNF, either without methotrexate or used together. The programmed cell death 1 (PD-1) protein, which is among the most potent inhibitory receptors on T cells, is responsible for the "exhausted" phenotype in chronic viral infection. PD-1 superagonists inhibit immune responses and upregulate regulatory T cells. Antibodies targeting PD-1 in people with cancer have shown encouraging improvements in the context of advanced cancers.[131]

It remains to be seen whether agonistic approaches will have a future place in the treatment of RA.

Conclusion

KEY POINT

Rituximab and abatacept both have an established role in the pharmacologic management of RA and rituximab has an established role in treating ANCA-associated vasculitis.

Despite recent advances in understanding the optimal use of nonbiologic DMARD therapies and the considerable success of biologic therapies targeting TNF, a substantial proportion of patients with RA remain refractory to or intolerant of these therapeutic modalities. The data discussed in this chapter illustrate that there is a role in clinical practice for newer biologic agents with specificity for cellular targets. In particular, depletion of B cells with the monoclonal antibody rituximab results in sustained improvement in the signs and symptoms of RA after just two doses (one treatment cycle), with little evidence of drug-related toxicity despite the profound and lasting depletion of B cells. Similarly, inhibition of T cell co-stimulation by abatacept demonstrates clear clinical efficacy within 16 weeks and, in some cases, additional improvement for 1 year or beyond, with acceptable safety. This observation is in marked contrast to the previously observed unfavorable benefit-risk ratio associated with a T cell–depleting strategy using Campath-1H. The response of patients with RA to this wide spectrum of therapeutic strategies attests to the complexity and heterogeneity of the syndrome and provides further impetus for studies that use these therapies to enhance our understanding of disease pathogenesis.

Although both rituximab and abatacept benefit a significant proportion of patients with RA—whether they are naïve to DMARDs or have experience with either biologic DMARDs, nonbiologic DMARDs, or both—to date very little is known about the comparative effects of these treatment approaches on symptoms and signs of disease or on inhibition of structural damage. Furthermore, despite some pointers to biomarkers that might optimize treatment outcomes with a particular therapeutic approach at the cohort level, such as seropositivity in patients with RA who are treated with rituximab, as yet no biomarkers reliably inform the best choice of therapy on an individual basis. Rituximab and abatacept are a welcome addition to the biologic armamentarium for RA, and both agents may also have a role in the pharmacologic management of rheumatic disorders beyond RA alone. It is anticipated that further clinical research and experience in the use of these biologic therapies will help better inform optimal treatment strategies.

Full references for this chapter can be found on ExpertConsult.com.

Selected References

1. Korpela M, Laasonen L, Hannonen P, et al.: Retardation of joint damage in patients with early rheumatoid arthritis by initial aggressive treatment with disease-modifying antirheumatic drugs: five-year experience from the FIN-RACo study, *Arthritis Rheum* 50(7):2072–2081, 2004.
2. Grigor C, Capell H, Stirling A, et al.: Effect of a treatment strategy of tight control for rheumatoid arthritis (the TICORA study): a single-blind randomised controlled trial, *Lancet* 364(9430):263–269, 2004.
3. Goekoop-Ruiterman YP, de Vries-Bouwstra JK, Allaart CF, et al.: Clinical and radiographic outcomes of four different treatment strategies in patients with early rheumatoid arthritis (the BeSt study): a randomized, controlled trial, *Arthritis Rheum* 52(11):3381–3390, 2005.
4. Klareskog L, van der Heijde D, de Jager JP, et al.: Therapeutic effect of the combination of etanercept and methotrexate compared with each treatment alone in patients with rheumatoid arthritis: double-blind randomised controlled trial, *Lancet* 363(9410):675–681, 2004.
5. Lipsky PE, van der Heijde DM, St Clair EW, et al.: Anti-tumor necrosis factor trial in rheumatoid arthritis with concomitant therapy study group: infliximab and methotrexate in the treatment of rheumatoid arthritis, *N Engl J Med* 343(22):1594–1602, 2000.
8. Mackay F, Sierro F, Grey S, et al.: The BAFF/APRIL system: an important player in systemic rheumatic diseases, *Curr Dir Autoimmun* 8:243–265, 2005.
9. Bhatia A, Blades S, Cambridge G, et al.: Differential distribution of FcγRIIIa in normal human tissues and co-localisation with DAF and fibrillin-1: implications for immunological microenvironments, *Immunology* 94(1):56–63, 1998.

10. Abrahams VM, Cambridge G, Lydyard PM, et al.: Induction of tumour necrosis factor α by human monocytes: a key role for FcγRIIIa in rheumatoid arthritis, *Arthritis Rheum* 43(3):608–616, 2000.
11. Edwards JCW, Cambridge G: B cell targeting in rheumatoid arthritis and other diseases, *Nat Rev Immunol* 6(5):394–405, 2006.
12. Riley JK, Sliwkoski MX: CD20: a gene in search of a function, *Semin Oncol* 27(6 Suppl 12):17–24, 2000.
13. O'Keefe TL, Williams GT, Davies SL, et al.: Mice carrying a CD20 gene disruption, *Immunogenetics* 48(2):125–132, 1998.
14. Szodoray P, Alex P, Dandapani V, et al.: Apoptotic effect of rituximab on peripheral B cells in RA, *Scand J Immunol* 60(1–2):209–218, 2004.
15. Tsokos GC: B cells, be gone: B-cell depletion in the treatment of rheumatoid arthritis, *N Engl J Med* 350(25):2546–2548, 2004.
16. Kavanaugh A, Rosengren S, Lee SJ, et al.: Assessment of rituximab's immunomodulatory synovial effects (ARISE trial). 1: clinical and synovial biomarker results, *Ann Rheum Dis* 67(3):402–408, 2008.
17. Teng YK, Levarht EW, Toes RE, et al.: Residual inflammation after rituximab treatment is associated with sustained synovial plasma cell infiltration and enhanced B cell repopulation, *Ann Rheum Dis* 68(6):1011–1016, 2009.
18. Roll P, Dorner T, Tony HP: Anti-CD20 therapy in patients with rheumatoid arthritis: predictors of response and B cell subset regeneration after repeated treatment, *Arthritis Rheum* 58(6):1566–1575, 2008.
19. Thurlings RM, Vos K, Wijbrandts CA, et al.: Synovial tissue response to rituximab: mechanism of action and identification of biomarkers of response, *Ann Rheum Dis* 67(7):917–925, 2008.
20. Edwards JC, Cambridge G: Sustained improvement in rheumatoid arthritis following a protocol designed to deplete B lymphocytes, *Rheumatology (Oxford)* 40(2):205–211, 2001.
21. De Vita S, Zaja F, Sacco S, et al.: Efficacy of selective B cell blockade in the treatment of rheumatoid arthritis: evidence for a pathogenetic role of B cells, *Arthritis Rheum* 46(8):2029–2033, 2002.
22. Leandro MJ, Edwards JC, Cambridge G: Clinical outcome in 22 patients with rheumatoid arthritis treated with B lymphocyte depletion, *Ann Rheum Dis* 61(10):883–888, 2002.
23. Edwards JC, Szczepanski L, Szechinski J, et al.: Efficacy of B-cell-targeted therapy with rituximab in patients with rheumatoid arthritis, *N Engl J Med* 350(25):2572–2581, 2004.
24. Emery P, Fleischmann R, Filipowicz-Sosnowska A, et al.: The efficacy and safety of rituximab in patients with active rheumatoid arthritis despite methotrexate treatment: results of a phase IIB randomized, double-blind, placebo-controlled, dose-ranging study, *Arthritis Rheum* 54(5):1390–1400, 2006.
25. Cohen SB, Emery P, Greenwald MW, et al.: Rituximab for rheumatoid arthritis refractory to anti-tumor necrosis factor therapy: results of a multicenter, randomized, double-blind, placebo-controlled, phase III trial evaluating primary efficacy and safety at twenty-four weeks, *Arthritis Rheum* 54(9):2793–2806, 2006.
26. Cohen S, Emery P, Greenwald M, et al.: Prolonged efficacy of rituximab in rheumatoid arthritis patients with inadequate response to one or more TNF inhibitors: 1-year follow-up of a subset of patients receiving a single course in a controlled trial (REFLEX study), *Ann Rheum Dis* 65(Suppl 2):183, 2006.
27. Emery P, Deodhar A, Rigby WF, et al.: Efficacy and safety of different doses and retreatment of rituximab: a randomised, placebo-controlled trial in patients who are biological naive with active rheumatoid arthritis and an inadequate response to methotrexate (study evaluating rituximab's efficacy in methotrexate inadequate responders [SERENE], *Ann Rheum Dis* 69(9):1629–1635, 2010.
28. Tak PP, Rigby WF, Rubbert-Roth A, et al.: Inhibition of joint damage and improved clinical outcomes with rituximab plus methotrexate in early active rheumatoid arthritis: the IMAGE trial, *Ann Rheum Dis* 70(1):39–46, 2011.
29. Keystone E, Emery P, Peterfy CG, et al.: Rituximab inhibits structural joint damage in patients with rheumatoid arthritis with an inadequate response to tumour necrosis factor inhibitor therapies, *Ann Rheum Dis* 68(2):216–221, 2009.
30. Cohen SB, Keystone E, Genovese MC, et al.: Continued inhibition of structural damage over 2 years in patients with rheumatoid arthritis treated with rituximab in combination with methotrexate, *Ann Rheum Dis* 69(6):1158–1161, 2010.
31. Aletaha D, Alasti F, Smolen JS: Rituximab dissociates the tight link between disease activity and joint damage in rheumatoid arthritis patients, *Ann Rheum Dis* 72(1):7–12, 2013.
36. Coiffier B, Lepage E, Briere J, et al.: CHOP chemotherapy plus rituximab compared with CHOP alone in elderly patients with diffuse large B cell lymphoma, *N Engl J Med* 346(4):235–242, 2002.
37. Higashida J, Wun T, Schmidt S, et al.: Safety and efficacy of rituximab in patients with rheumatoid arthritis refractory to disease modifying anti-rheumatic drugs and anti-TNFA treatment, *J Rheumatol* 32(11):2109–2115, 2005.
38. Emery P, Fleischman RM, Filipowicz-Sosnowska A, et al.: Rituximab in rheumatoid arthritis: a double-blind, placebo-controlled, dose ranging study, *Arthritis Rheum* 52(Suppl):S709, 2005.
39. Lee YH, Bae SC, Song GG: The efficacy and safety of rituximab for the treatment of active rheumatoid arthritis: a systematic review and meta-analysis of randomized controlled trials, *Rheumatol Int* 31(11):1493–1499, 2011.
41. Calabrese LH, Molloy ES, Huang D, et al.: Progressive multifocal leukoencephalopathy in rheumatic diseases: evolving clinical and pathologic patterns of disease, *Arthritis Rheum* 56(7):2116–2128, 2007.
42. Molloy ES, Calabrese LH: Progressive multifocal leukoencephalopathy: a national estimate of frequency in systemic lupus erythematosus and other rheumatic diseases, *Arthritis Rheum* 60(12):3761–3765, 2009.
43. Genovese MC, Breedveld FC, Emery P, et al.: Safety of biological therapies following rituximab treatment in rheumatoid arthritis patients, *Ann Rheum Dis* 68(12):1894–1897, 2009.
44. van Assen S, Holvast A, Benne CA, et al.: Humoral responses after influenza vaccination are severely reduced in patients with rheumatoid arthritis treated with rituximab, *Arthritis Rheum* 62(1):75–81, 2010.
45. Bingham 3rd CO, Looney RJ, Deodhar A, et al.: Immunization responses in rheumatoid arthritis patients treated with rituximab: results from a controlled clinical trial, *Arthritis Rheum* 62(1):64–74, 2010.
47. Volkmann ER, Agrawal H, Maranian P, et al.: Rituximab for rheumatoid arthritis: a meta-analysis and systematic review, *Clin Med Insights Ther* 2:749–760, 2010.
48. van Vollenhoven RF, Emery P, Bingham 3rd CO, et al.: Longterm safety of patients receiving rituximab in rheumatoid arthritis clinical trials, *J Rheumatol* 37(3):558–567, 2010.
49. Chen MH, Chen MH, Liu CY, et al.: Hepatitis B virus reactivation in rheumatoid arthritis patients undergoing biologics treatment, *J Infect Dis* 215(4):566–573, 2017.
50. Cambridge G, Leandro MJ, Edwards JC, et al.: Serologic changes following B lymphocyte depletion therapy for rheumatoid arthritis, *Arthritis Rheum* 48(8):2146–2154, 2003.
51. Leandro MJ, Cambridge G, Ehrenstein MR, et al.: Reconstitution of peripheral blood B cells following rituximab treatment in patients with rheumatoid arthritis, *Arthritis Rheum* 54(2):613–620, 2006.
52. Cambridge G, Stohl W, Leandro MJ, et al.: Circulating levels of B lymphocyte stimulator in patients with rheumatoid arthritis following rituximab treatment: relationships with B cell depletion, circulating antibodies, and clinical relapse, *Arthritis Rheum* 54(3):723–732, 2006.
53. Rubbert-Roth A, Tak PP, Zerbini C, et al.: Efficacy and safety of various repeat treatment dosing regimens of rituximab in patients with active rheumatoid arthritis: results of a Phase III randomized study (MIRROR), *Rheumatology (Oxford)* 49(9):1683–1693, 2010.
54. Emery P, Gottenberg JE, Rubbert-Roth A, et al.: Rituximab versus an alternative TNF inhibitor in patients with rheumatoid arthritis who failed to respond to a single previous TNF inhibitor: SWITCH-RA, a global, observational, comparative effectiveness study, *Ann Rheum Dis* 74:979–984, 2015.

56. Isaacs JD, Cohen SB, Emery P, et al.: Effect of baseline rheumatoid factor and anticitrullinated peptide antibody serotype on rituximab clinical response: a meta-analysis, *Ann Rheum Dis* 72(3):329–336, 2013.
57. Isaacs JD, Olech E, Tak PP, et al: Autoantibody-positive rheumatoid arthritis (RA) patients (pts) have enhanced clinical response to rituximab (RTX) when compared with seronegative patients [abstract FRI0256]. Presented at the Annual European Congress of Rheumatology, 10-13, 2009, Copenhagen, Denmark.
58. van Vollenhoven RF, Cohen S, Pavelka K, et al.: Response to rituximab in patients with rheumatoid arthritis is maintained by repeat therapy: results of an open-label trial, *Ann Rheum Dis* 65(Suppl 2):510, 2006.
59. Smolen JS, Keystone EC, Emery P, et al.: Consensus statement on the use of rituximab in patients with rheumatoid arthritis, *Ann Rheum Dis* 66(2):143–150, 2007.
60. Vital EM, Dass S, Rawstron AC, et al.: Management of nonresponse to rituximab in rheumatoid arthritis: predictors and outcome of re-treatment, *Arthritis Rheum* 62(5):1273–1279, 2010.
61. Scheinberg M, Hamerschlak N, Kutner JM, et al.: Rituximab in refractory autoimmune diseases: Brazilian experience with 29 patients (2002-2004), *Clin Exp Rheumatol* 24(1):65–69, 2006.
62. Genovese MC, Kaine JL, Lowenstein MB, et al.: Ocrelizumab, a humanized anti-CD20 monoclonal antibody, in the treatment of patients with rheumatoid arthritis: a phase I/II randomized, blinded, placebo-controlled, dose-ranging study, *Arthritis Rheum* 58(9):2652–2661, 2008.
63. Taylor PC, Quattrocchi E, Mallett S, et al.: Ofatumumab, a fully human anti-CD20 mAb, in biologic-naïve, MTX-IR rheumatoid arthritis: a randomized, double-blind, placebo-controlled trial, *Ann Rheum Dis* 70(12):2119–2125, 2011.
64. McKay J, Chwalinska-Sadowska H, Boling E, et al.: Efficacy and safety of belimumab (BMAB), a fully human monoclonal antibody to B lymphocyte stimulator (BLyS) for the treatment of rheumatoid arthritis, *Arthritis Rheum* 52(Suppl):S710, 2005.
65. Stone JH, Merkel PA, Spiera R, et al.: Rituximab versus cyclophosphamide for ANCA-associated vasculitis, *N Engl J Med* 363(3):221–232, 2010.
66. Walsh M, Jayne D: Rituximab in the treatment of anti-neutrophil cytoplasm antibody associated vasculitis and systemic lupus erythematosus: past, present and future, *Kidney Int* 72(6):676–682, 2007.
67. Ng KP, Cambridge G, Leandro MJ, et al.: B cell depletion therapy in systemic lupus erythematosus: long-term follow-up and predictors of response, *Ann Rheum Dis* 66(9):1259–1262, 2007.
68. Furie RA, Looney JR, Rovin B, et al.: Efficacy and safety of rituximab in patients with proliferative lupus nephritis: results from the randomized, double-blind phase III LUNAR study, *Ann Rheum Dis* 69(Suppl 3):549, 2010.
69. Merrill JT, Neuwelt CM, Wallace DJ, et al.: Efficacy and safety of rituximab in moderately-to-severely active systemic lupus erythematosus: the randomized, double-blind, phase II/III systemic lupus erythematosus evaluation of rituximab trial, *Arthritis Rheum* 62(1):222–233, 2010.
70. Bosch X: Inflammation: rituximab in ANCA vasculitis and lupus: bittersweet results, *Nat Rev Nephrol* 6(3):137–139, 2010.
71. Calero I, Sanz I: Targeting B cells for the treatment of SLE: the beginning of the end or the end of the beginning? *Discov Med* 10(54):416–424, 2010.
72. Furst DE, Breedveld FC, Kalden JR, et al.: Updated consensus statement on biological agents for the treatment of rheumatic diseases, 2006, *Ann Rheum Dis* 65(Suppl 3):iii2–iii15, 2006.
74. Knoerzer DB, Karr RW, Schwartz BD, et al.: Collagen-induced arthritis in the BB rat: prevention of disease by treatment with CTLA-4-Ig, *J Clin Invest* 96(2):987–993, 1995.
75. Webb LM, Walmsley MJ, Feldmann M: Prevention and amelioration of collagen-induced arthritis by blockade of the CD28 costimulatory pathway: requirement for both B7-1 and B7-2, *Eur J Immunol* 26(10):2320–2328, 1996.
76. Moreland LW, Alten R, Van den Bosch F, et al.: Co-stimulatory blockade in patients with rheumatoid arthritis: a pilot, dose-finding, double-blind, placebo-controlled clinical trial evaluating CTLA-4Ig and LEA29Y eighty-five days after the first infusion, *Arthritis Rheum* 46(6):1470–1479, 2002.
77. Kremer JM, Westhovens R, Leon M, et al.: Treatment of rheumatoid arthritis by selective inhibition of T-cell activation with fusion protein CTLA4Ig, *N Engl J Med* 349(20):1907–1915, 2003.
78. Kremer JM, Dougados M, Emery P, et al.: Treatment of rheumatoid arthritis with the selective costimulation modulator abatacept: twelve-month results of a phase IIb, double-blind, randomized, placebo-controlled trial, *Arthritis Rheum* 52(8):2263–2271, 2005.
79. Westhovens R, Emery P, Aranda R, et al.: Abatacept provides sustained clinical benefit through 3 years in rheumatoid arthritis patients with inadequate responses to methotrexate, *Ann Rheum Dis* 65(Suppl 2):512, 2006.
80. Kremer JM, Genant HK, Moreland LW, et al.: Effects of abatacept in patients with methotrexate-resistant active rheumatoid arthritis: a randomized trial, *Ann Intern Med* 144(12):865–876, 2006.
81. Dougados M, LeBars MA, Schmidely N: Low disease activity in rheumatoid arthritis treated with abatacept in the AIM (abatacept in inadequate response to methotrexate) trial, *Ann Rheum Dis* 65(Suppl 2):188, 2006.
82. Genovese MC, Becker JC, Schiff M, et al.: Abatacept for rheumatoid arthritis refractory to tumor necrosis factor alpha inhibition, *N Engl J Med* 353(11):1114–1123, 2005.
83. Kremer JM, Emery P, Becker JC, et al.: Abatacept provides significant and sustained benefits in clinical and patient-reported outcomes through 2 years in rheumatoid arthritis and an inadequate response to methotrexate: the long-term extension (LTE) of the AIM trial, *Ann Rheum Dis* 65(Suppl 2):327, 2006.
84. Genant HK, Peterfy C, Westhovens R, et al.: Abatacept inhibits progression of structural damage in rheumatoid arthritis: results from the long-term extension of the AIM trial, *Ann Rheum Dis* 67(8):1084–1089, 2008.
85. Schiff M, Keiserman M, Codding C, et al.: Efficacy and safety of abatacept or infliximab versus placebo in ATTEST: a phase III, multicenter, randomized, double-blind, placebo-controlled study in patients with rheumatoid arthritis and an inadequate response to methotrexate, *Ann Rheum Dis* 67(8):1096–1103, 2008.
86. Genovese MC, Schiff M, Luggen M, et al.: Efficacy and safety of the co-stimulation modulator abatacept following two years of treatment in patients with rheumatoid arthritis and an inadequate response to anti-TNF therapy, *Ann Rheum Dis* 67(4):547–554, 2008.
87. Siblia J, Schiff M, Genovese MC, et al.: Sustained improvement in disease activity score 28 (DAS28) and patient reported outcomes (PRO) with abatacept in rheumatoid arthritis patients with an inadequate response to anti-TNF therapy: the long-term extension of the ATTAIN trial, *Ann Rheum Dis* 65(Suppl 2):501, 2006.
88. Schiff M, Pritchard C, Huffstutter JE, et al.: The 6-month safety and efficacy of abatacept in patients with rheumatoid arthritis who underwent a washout after anti-tumour necrosis factor therapy or were directly switched to abatacept: the ARRIVE trial, *Ann Rheum Dis* 68(11):1708–1714, 2009.
89. Westhovens R, Robles M, Ximenes AC, et al.: Clinical efficacy and safety of abatacept in methotrexate-naïve patients with early rheumatoid arthritis and poor prognostic factors, *Ann Rheum Dis* 68(12):1870–1877, 2009.
90. Westhovens R, Robles M, Nayiager S, et al.: Disease remission is achieved within two years in over half of methotrexate naive patients with early erosive rheumatoid arthritis (RA) treated with abatacept plus MTX: results from the agree trial (abstract 638), *Arthritis Rheum* 60:S239, 2009.
91. Bathon J, Genant H, Nayiager S, et al.: Reduced radiographic progression in patients with early rheumatoid arthritis (RA) treated with abatacept + methotrexate compared to methotrexate alone: 24 month outcomes [abstract 639], *Arthritis Rheum* 60:S239–S240, 2009.

92. Emery P, Durez P, Dougados M, et al.: The impact of T-cell co-stimulation modulation in patients with undifferentiated inflammatory arthritis or very early rheumatoid arthritis: a clinical and imaging study of abatacept, *Ann Rheum Dis* 69(3):510–516, 2010.
93. Genovese MC, Covarrubias Á, Leon G, et al.: Subcutaneous abatacept versus intravenous abatacept: a phase IIIb non-inferiority study in patients with an inadequate response to methotrexate, *Arthritis Rheum* 63(10):2854–2864, 2011.
94. US Food and Drug Administration Arthritis Advisory Committee: *Briefing document for abatacept (BMS-188667) biologic license application 12118*, Silver Spring, MD, 2005, US Food and Drug Administration.
95. Nash P, Nayiager S, Genovese MC, et al.: Immunogenicity, safety, and efficacy of abatacept administered subcutaneously with or without background methotrexate in patients with rheumatoid arthritis: results from a phase III, international, multicenter, parallel-arm, open-label study, *Arthritis Care Res (Hoboken)* 65(5):718–728, 2013.
96. Keystone EC, Kremer JM, Russell A, et al.: Abatacept in subjects who switch from intravenous to subcutaneous therapy: results from the phase IIIb attune study, *Ann Rheum Dis* 71(6):857–861, 2012.
97. Weinblatt ME, Schiff M, Valente R, et al.: Head-to-head comparison of subcutaneous abatacept versus adalimumab for rheumatoid arthritis: findings of a phase IIIb, multinational, prospective, randomized study, *Arthritis Rheum* 65(1):28–38, 2013.
98. Sokolove J, Schiff M, Fleischmann R, et al.: Impact of baseline anti-cyclic citrullinated peptide-2 antibody concentration on efficacy outcomes following treatment with subcutaneous abatacept or adalimumab: 2-year results from the AMPLE trial, *Ann Rheum Dis* 75(4):709–714, 2016.
99. Schiff M: Abatacept treatment for rheumatoid arthritis, *Rheumatology (Oxford)* 50(3):437–449, 2010.
100. Weinblatt M, Combe B, Covucci A, et al.: Safety of the selective co-stimulation modulator abatacept in rheumatoid arthritis patients receiving background biologic and nonbiologic disease-modifying antirheumatic drugs: a one-year randomized, placebo-controlled study, *Arthritis Rheum* 54(9):2807–2816, 2006.
101. Weinblatt ME, Schiff MH, Goldman A, et al.: Selective co-stimulation modulation using abatacept in patients with active rheumatoid arthritis while receiving etanercept: a randomized clinical trial, *Ann Rheum Dis* 66(2):228–234, 2007.
102. Schiff M, Keiserman M, Codding C, et al.: Efficacy and safety of abatacept or infliximab versus placebo in attest: a phase III, multicenter, randomized, double-blind, placebo-controlled study in patients with rheumatoid arthritis and an inadequate response to methotrexate, *Ann Rheum Dis* 67(8):1096–1103, 2008.
103. Maxwell L, Singh A: Abatacept for rheumatoid arthritis, *Cochrane Database Syst Rev* 4:CD007277, 2009.
104. Weyand CM, Goronzy JJ: T-cell-targeted therapies in rheumatoid arthritis, *Nat Clin Pract Rheumatol* 2(4):201–210, 2006.
105. Warrington KJ, Takemura S, Goronzy JJ, et al.: $CD4^+$, $CD28^-$ T cells in rheumatoid arthritis patients combine features of the innate and adaptive immune systems, *Arthritis Rheum* 44(1):13–20, 2001.
106. Bryl E, Vallejo AN, Matteson EL, et al.: Modulation of CD28 expression with anti-tumor necrosis factor alpha therapy in rheumatoid arthritis, *Arthritis Rheum* 52(10):2996–3003, 2005.
107. Choy EH: Selective modulation of T-cell co-stimulation: a novel mode of action for the treatment of rheumatoid arthritis, *Clin Exp Rheumatol* 27(3):510–518, 2009.
108. Buch MH, Boyle DL, Rosengren S, et al.: Mode of action of abatacept in rheumatoid arthritis patients having failed tumour necrosis factor blockade: a histological, gene expression and dynamic magnetic resonance imaging pilot study, *Ann Rheum Dis* 68(7):1220–1227, 2009.
109. Merrill JT, Burgos-Vargas R, Westhovens R, et al.: The efficacy and safety of abatacept in patients with non-life-threatening manifestations of systemic lupus erythematosus: results of a twelve-month, multicenter, exploratory, phase IIb, randomized, double-blind, placebo-controlled trial, *Arthritis Rheum* 62(10):3077–3087, 2010.
110. Abrams JR, Lebwohl MG, Guzzo CA, et al.: CTLA4Ig-mediated blockade of T-cell costimulation in patients with psoriasis vulgaris, *J Clin Invest* 103(9):1243–1252, 1999.
111. Mease P, Gottlieb AB, van der Heijde D, et al.: Efficacy and safety of abatacept, a T-cell modulator, in a randomised, double-blind, placebo-controlled, phase III study in psoriatic arthritis, *Ann Rheum Dis* 76(9):1550–1558, 2017.
112. Meiners PM, Vissink A, Kroese FG, et al.: Abatacept treatment reduces disease activity in early primary Sjögren's syndrome (open-label proof of concept ASAP study), *Ann Rheum Dis* 73(7):1393–1396, 2014.
113. Tsuboi H1, Matsumoto I, Hagiwara S, et al.: Efficacy and safety of abatacept for patients with Sjögren's syndrome associated with rheumatoid arthritis: rheumatoid arthritis with Orencia trial toward Sjögren's syndrome endocrinopathy (ROSE) trial—an open-label, one-year, prospective study—interim analysis of 32 patients for 24 weeks, *Mod Rheumatol* 25:187–193, 2015.
114. Taylor PC: Antibody therapy for rheumatoid arthritis, *Curr Opin Pharmacol* 3(3):323–328, 2003.
115. Mason U, Aldrich J, Breedveld F, et al.: CD4 coating, but not CD4 depletion, is a predictor of efficacy with primatized monoclonal anti-CD4 treatment of active rheumatoid arthritis, *J Rheumatol* 29(2):220–229, 2002.
116. Weinblatt ME, Maddison PJ, Bulpitt KJ, et al.: CAMPATH-1H, a humanized monoclonal antibody, in refractory rheumatoid arthritis: an intravenous dose-escalation study, *Arthritis Rheum* 38(11):1589–1594, 1995.
117. Schnitzer TJ, Yocum DE, Michalska M, et al.: Subcutaneous administration of CAMPATH-1H: clinical and biological outcomes, *J Rheumatol* 24(6):1031–1036, 1997.
118. Olsen NJ, Brooks RH, Cush JJ, et al.: A double-blind, placebo-controlled study of anti-CD5 immunoconjugate in patients with rheumatoid arthritis. The Xoma RA Investigator Group, *Arthritis Rheum* 39(7):1102–1108, 1996.
119. Sewell KL, Parker KC, Woodworth TG, et al.: DAB486IL-2 fusion toxin in refractory rheumatoid arthritis, *Arthritis Rheum* 36(9):1223–1233, 1993.
120. Moreland LW, Sewell KL, Trentham DE, et al.: Interleukin-2 diphtheria fusion protein (DAB486IL-2) in refractory rheumatoid arthritis: a double-blind, placebo-controlled trial with open-label extension, *Arthritis Rheum* 38(9):1177–1186, 1995.
121. Keystone EC: Abandoned therapies and unpublished trials in rheumatoid arthritis, *Curr Opin Rheumatol* 15(3):253–258, 2003.
122. Thompson C, Powrie F: Regulatory T cells, *Curr Opin Pharmacol* 4(4):408–414, 2004.
123. Ehrenstein MR, Evans JG, Singh A, et al.: Compromised function of regulatory T cells in rheumatoid arthritis and reversal by anti-TNF alpha therapy, *J Exp Med* 200(3):277–285, 2004.
124. Valencia X, Stephens G, Goldbach-Mansky R, et al.: TNF downmodulates the function of human CD4+CD25hi T-regulatory cells, *Blood* 108(1):253–261, 2006.
125. Herold KC, Burton JB, Francois F, et al.: Activation of human T cells by FcR nonbinding anti-CD3 mAb, hOKT3gamma1(Ala-Ala), *J Clin Invest* 111(3):409–418, 2003.
126. Bisikirska B, Colgan J, Luban J, et al.: TCR stimulation with modified anti-CD3 mAb expands $CD8^+$ T cell population and induces $CD8^+CD25^+$ Tregs, *J Clin Invest* 115(10):2904–2913, 2005.
128. Chatenoud L: CD3-specific antibodies as promising tools to aim at immune tolerance in the clinic, *Int Rev Immunol* 25(3–4):215–233, 2006.
130. Chen G, Li N, Zang YC, et al.: Vaccination with selected synovial T cells in rheumatoid arthritis, *Arthritis Rheum* 56(2):453–463, 2007.
131. Yao S, Zhu Y, Chen L: Advances in targeting cell surface signalling molecules for immune modulation, *Nat Rev Drug Discov* 12(2):130–146, 2013.

68

Intra-cellular Targeting Agents in Rheumatic Disease

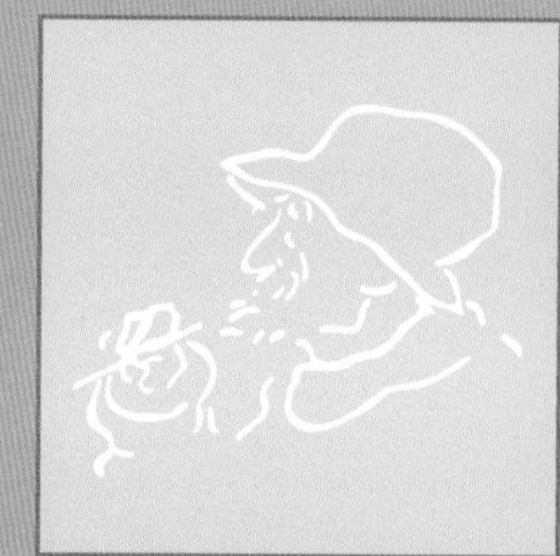

VIRGINIA REDDY AND STANLEY COHEN

KEY POINTS

During the past 30 years, key pathways responsible for signal transduction to the nucleus after ligand binding to cellular receptors on immune cells have been elucidated.

Protein kinases that phosphorylate intra-cellular proteins are major players in signal transduction.

Oral small-molecule inhibitors of downstream protein kinases, including p38 mitogen-activated protein kinases (MAPK) and mitogen-activated protein kinase kinase (MEK) inhibitors, have been investigated with limited or no success in rheumatoid arthritis (RA) clinical trials.

Spleen tyrosine kinase (SYK) inhibitors for rheumatic diseases have been associated with modest benefit and significant adverse events and are not approved for treatment in rheumatic diseases.

Multiple protein tyrosine kinase inhibitors have been approved for treatment of hematologic and oncologic conditions.

Janus kinase (JAK) inhibitors have been successfully developed as therapies for RA and psoriatic arthritis and are being evaluated in lupus and spondyloarthropathies.

The efficacy and safety of JAK inhibitors are similar to biologic disease-modifying anti-rheumatic drugs. The observed increase in herpes zoster and, possibly, opportunistic infections, may be unique to these inhibitors.

Bruton tyrosine kinase (BTK) inhibitors are approved for oncologic indications and are being evaluated in RA and lupus.

Oral small-molecule phosphodiesterase inhibitors are approved for treatment of psoriatic arthritis with modest benefit in skin and joint disease.

Introduction

Advances in treatment for rheumatoid arthritis (RA) during the past 2 decades have resulted in dramatic improvements in quality of life for these patients. The development of biologic therapies targeting molecules involved in the pathogenesis of RA has led to significant improvements in the signs and symptoms of disease in as many as 60% to 70% of patients and resulted in remission in 10% to 50% of patients; however, this depends on the definition of remission and disease duration.[1,2]

Biologic therapies, however, have limitations. More than half of patients continue to have active disease, and these medications require either subcutaneous or intravenous administration. These therapies are associated with significant expense and can induce immunogenicity. During the past 30 years, the intra-cellular signaling pathways involved in signal transduction from the cell surface to the nucleus after ligand-receptor binding to its receptor have been identified. This improved understanding of these pathways has provided opportunities for development of small molecule-therapies that target these pathways. Interruption of the signaling cascade has been demonstrated in pre-clinical models to reduce pro-inflammatory cytokine production, with improvement in animal models of inflammatory arthritis similar to improvements seen with biologics.[3–5] During the past decade, multiple clinical trials in patients with RA that evaluated small molecules targeting specific kinases have been conducted. The majority of these investigational trials failed because of limited efficacy or significant toxicity. In 2012, tofacitinib, a janus kinase (JAK) inhibitor, was approved for RA treatment in the United States and Japan, and other JAK inhibitors have been approved or are under development. This chapter will focus on the various molecules that have been evaluated as potential therapies for rheumatic diseases or are presently undergoing active investigation.

Signal Transduction Pathways

Research during the past 30 years has firmly established that reversible protein phosphorylation is a fundamental mechanism of cell signaling.[6,7] Protein kinases are the enzymes that catalyze the transfer of the γ phosphate of a purine nucleotide triphosphate (i.e., adenosine triphosphate [ATP] and guanosine triphosphate [GTP]) to the hydroxyl groups of their protein substrates. A total of 518 kinases have been identified, with the majority selectively phosphorylating serine or threonine peptides. Ninety kinases that phosphorylate tyrosine (protein tyrosine kinases [PTKs]) have been identified and play major roles in signal transduction. These PTKs can exist as receptor tyrosine kinases, such as epidermal growth factor and platelet-derived growth factor, but the majority of kinases are found intra-cellular and facilitate signal transduction by interacting with the intracytoplasmic portion of the cell membrane receptor after ligand binding. Protein phosphorylation ultimately links membrane events to calcium modulation, cytoskeletal rearrangement, gene transcription, and other canonical features of lymphocyte action.[8]

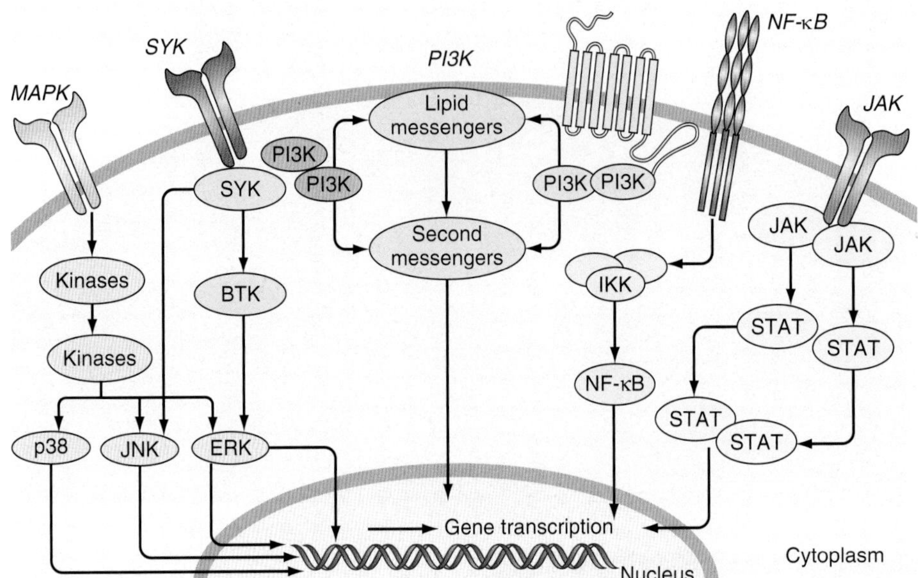

• **Fig. 68.1** Overview: signal transduction pathways. *BTK,* Bruton's tyrosine kinase; *ERK,* extra-cellular signal-regulated kinase; *IKK,* IκB kinase; *JAK,* janus kinase; *JNK,* c-JUN N-terminal kinase; *MAPK,* mitogen-activated protein kinases; *NF-κB,* nuclear factor-κB; *STAT,* signal transducer and activator of transcription; *SYK,* spleen tyrosine kinase.

Many of the major classes of receptors that trigger immune cell activation are linked to protein phosphorylation and are physically associated with protein kinases (Fig. 68.1). Multiple signaling pathways after ligand-receptor interaction have made targeting specific pathways for therapeutic benefit difficult in inflammatory arthritis because of the redundancy of these pathways. Inhibition of one signaling component may be compensated for by increased signaling through an alternative pathway, which results in incomplete inhibition.

The initial event in T cell receptor (TCR), B cell receptor (BCR), NK (natural killer), and Fc receptor (FcR) signaling is phosphorylation of receptor subunits on tyrosine residues.[9,10] Cytokine receptors, especially type I/II cytokine receptors, signal directly by activating kinases, which phosphorylate receptor subunits and, thereby, initiate signaling in T cells and NK cells. Type I and type II cytokine binding activates JAK, which then phosphorylates cytokine receptors, which allows signal transducer and activators of transcription (STAT) DNA-binding proteins to attach to receptors and become phosphorylated. STAT activation leads to their dimerization and translocation to the nucleus, where they regulate gene expression. In B cells, antigen binding leads to activation of three main PTKs: the SRC-family kinases, LYN and SYK, and the TEC-family kinase, Bruton's tyrosine kinase (BTK). SYK phosphorylates adaptor protein B cell linker protein (BLNK) and, along with BTK, activates phospholipase Cγ (PLCγ).[11] Activation of PLCγ leads to the release of intra-cellular Ca^{2+} and activation of protein kinase C (PKC), which activate mitogen-activated protein kinases (MAPKs). The MAPK cascade activates transcription factors nuclear factor-κB (NF-κB) and nuclear factor of activated T cells (NFAT), which allows gene regulation.

Upstream and downstream protein kinases in these pathways have been targeted in oncology as well as inflammatory disorders (Table 68.1). Initial concerns existed about the safety of kinase inhibitors because of the potential lack of specificity to inhibit a specific kinase.[12,13] This lack of specificity has become less of an issue in the clinic, with the successful development of multiple, less selective kinase inhibitors, which occurred initially in oncology. Imatinib was the first tyrosine kinase inhibitor approved in oncology for chronic myeloid leukemia and has been highly effective with acceptable toxicity. Subsequently, less selective tyrosine kinase inhibitors have been developed for treatment of hematologic malignancies.[14,15] Even though off-target kinases are impacted by these inhibitors, safety issues have been acceptable. Multiple kinase inhibitors have been approved in oncology, including therapeutics for treatment of renal cell carcinoma and non–small cell lung cancer. The acceptable safety profile in the oncology experience stimulated efforts to develop kinase inhibitors in inflammatory diseases, such as RA, psoriatic arthritis (PsA), psoriasis, inflammatory bowel disease, and systemic lupus erythematosus.

TABLE 68.1 Protein Tyrosine Kinases Targeted in Rheumatic Diseases

p38 mitogen-activated protein kinases
Mitogen activated protein kinase kinase
Spleen tyrosine kinases
Janus kinases
Bruton's tyrosine kinase
Phosphatidylinositol 3-kinase

p38 MAPK Inhibitors

The MAPKs were identified in the 1990s as being involved in the production of pro-inflammatory cytokines after cell stimulation by various stressors.[16,17] There are three major families of MAPKs:

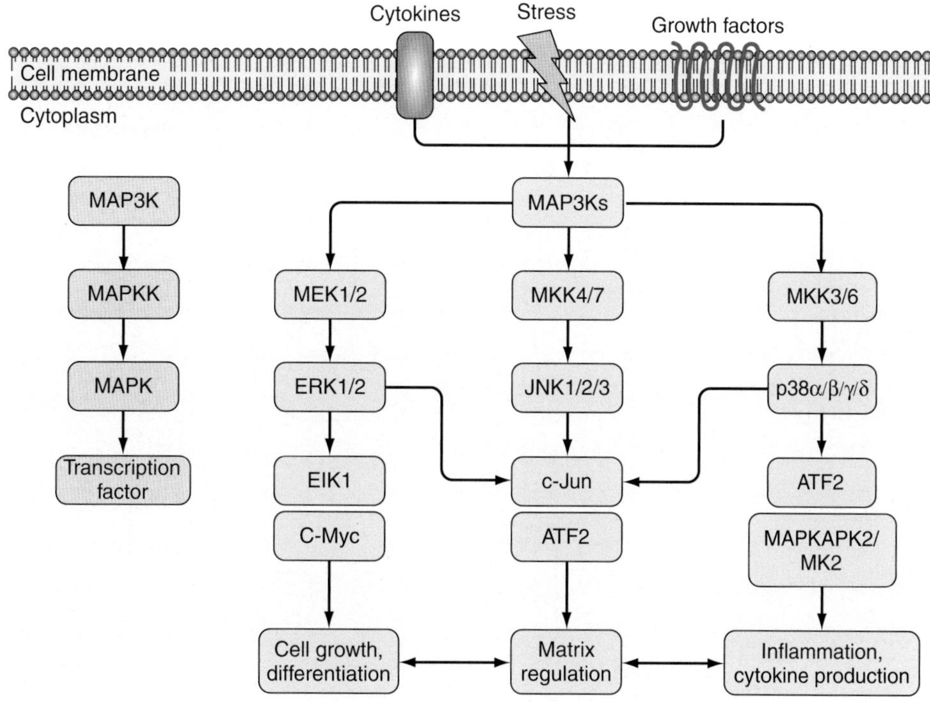

• **Fig. 68.2** Simplified mitogen-activated protein kinase (MAPK) pathway. *ATF,* Activating transcription factor; *ERK,* extra-cellular signal-regulated kinase; *JNK,* c-JUN N-terminal kinase; *MKK,* MAPK kinase.

extra-cellular signal-regulated kinase (ERK), c-JUN N-terminal kinase (JNK), and p38 (Fig. 68.2). The MAPs are intra-cellular enzymes that transmit a signal to the nucleus, which results in gene transcription.[18,19] Complex parallel and crossover signaling cascades link the three main MAPK families. MAPK activation is mediated by upstream MAPK kinases (MKKs), which are also activated by MKK kinases (MKKKs or MAP3Ks).

p38 MAPK is a key regulator of pro-inflammatory cytokine production. Varied cellular stresses, such as inflammatory cytokines, pathogens, and growth factors, activate kinases which regulate the expression of key genes, which results in transcriptional activation of TNF, IL-1 and IL-6, cyclooxygenase (COX-2), and matrix metalloproteinases (MMPs). p38 activation and phosphorylation is regulated by two upstream kinases, MKK3 and MKK6, which are phosphorylated by multiple MAP3Ks. There are four isoforms of p38—α, β, γ, and δ—and p38α is the isoform thought to be the most important regulator of cytokine expression. Phosphorylated activated p38 MAPK is also found in the synovial lining and endothelium of vessels in RA synovium.[20] The p38 MAPKs were the first kinases targeted after the observation that inhibition of this pathway could reduce lipopolysaccharide (LPS)-induced TNF and IL-1 production by monocytes.[21] Several pre-clinical studies have demonstrated that inhibition of p38 MAPK suppresses production of inflammatory cytokines, and pre-clinical animal models demonstrated reduction in paw swelling and joint damage.[22,23]

Several clinical trials have been performed with investigational p38 inhibitors. The p38α isoform has been the primary target in clinical trials. A 24-week double-blind randomized, placebo-controlled clinical trial (RCT) of SCIO-469 monotherapy, a p38α MAPK inhibitor, was performed in 302 patients with active RA; however, at week 12, no difference was seen between the SCIO-469–treated patients compared with placebo for the American College of Rheumatology (ACR)20 or ACR50 response.[24]

Pamapimod, another selective inhibitor of the α isoform of p38 MAPK, was studied in a 12-week RCT in 204 patients with active RA. No improvement was noted when compared to methotrexate (MTX) monotherapy.[25] A companion dose-ranging study that evaluated pamapimod in patients with RA, who had active disease despite MTX therapy, also proved ineffective.[26] These studies of SCIO-469 and pamapimod, as well as studies of other p38 MAPK inhibitors in RA, demonstrate early reduction in C-reactive protein (CRP) levels, but this decrease is transient.

For both the SCIO-469 and pamapimod studies, common adverse events (AEs) included adverse effects on the CNS, with symptoms including dizziness and headaches. It was hoped that a molecule with little or no CNS penetration would be associated with fewer of these side effects. VX-702, a highly selective inhibitor of the p38α isoform of MAPK,[27] minimally penetrates the CNS; two 12-week placebo-controlled RCTs studied these effects. However, no significant efficacy was demonstrated in the RCTs, and the AE profile was similar to that reported with other p38 MAPKs.

Two subsequent reviews of MAPK inhibitors proposed theories of why inhibition of p38 MAPKs in animal models was successful, whereas studies in patients with RA were not.[28,29] Issues raised include dose limitations caused by toxicity, altered biodistribution of newer molecules that prevent CNS penetration, incorrect isoform targeting, and the fact that p38α may have a regulatory role in the induction of anti-inflammatory cytokines.[30] The most plausible explanation, which is supported by the transient acute phase response, is the redundancy of signaling networks, such that blocking a downstream molecule, such as p38, would not block upstream kinases, which may redirect the signaling flow. Recognition of this concern has stimulated efforts to target more upstream protein kinases, and no further trials in RA with p38 inhibitors are ongoing.

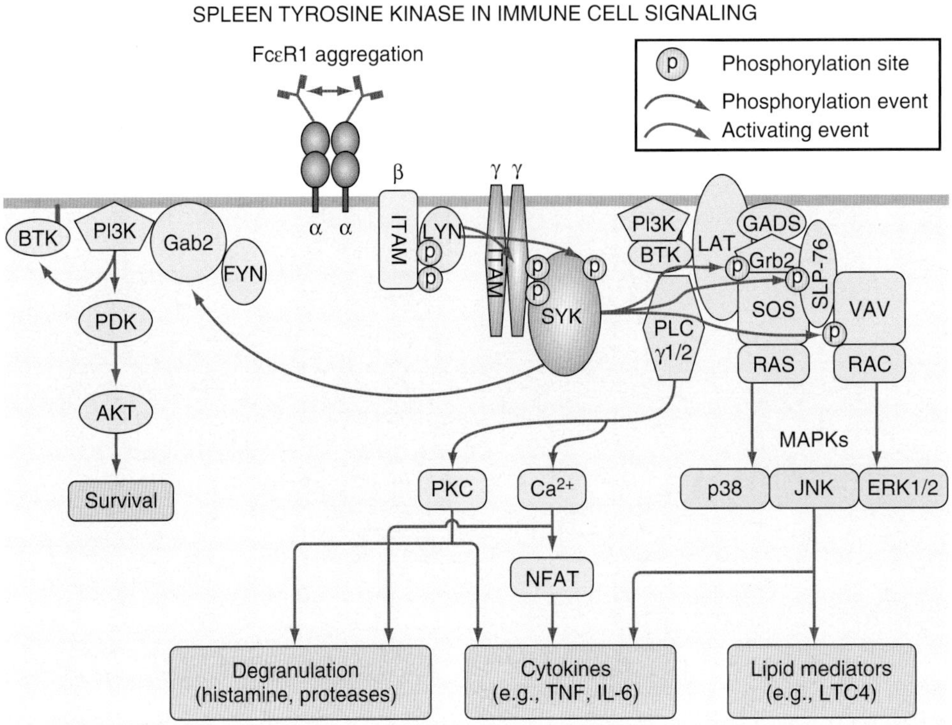

• **Fig. 68.3** Spleen tyrosine kinase (SYK) in immune cell signal transduction. *JNK,* c-JUN N-Terminal kinase; *LTC4,* leukotrience C4; *MAPK,* mitogen-activated protein kinase; *NFAT,* nuclear factor of activated T cells; *PDK,* phosphoinositide dependent kinase; *PKC,* protein kinase C.

MEK Inhibitors

MEK is a MAPKK involved in growth factor signal transduction and cytokine production. Inhibitors of MEK demonstrated efficacy in pre-clinical models of RA.[31] Based on the pre-clinical observations, ARRY-438162, an oral inhibitor of MEK1/MEK2, was evaluated in a double-blind randomized clinical trial of 201 patients with RA with active disease despite MTX treatment. No difference between the active treatment groups and placebo was demonstrated. The most common active AEs were skin rashes and diarrhea that were dose related. Serious AEs were rare. No additional trials of molecules targeting MEK in RA are ongoing at this time.

Spleen Tyrosine Kinase Inhibitors

Spleen tyrosine kinase (SYK) inhibitors have been evaluated as a potential treatment for RA. SYK is a nonreceptor PTK that is a modulator of immune signaling in cells bearing Fcγ-activating receptors, including B cells, mast cells, macrophages, neutrophils, eosinophils, basophils, and synoviocytes.[32,33] SYK binds to the cytoplasmic region of these receptors that contain the immune-receptor tyrosine-based activation motif (ITAM). Receptor binding results in ITAM phosphorylation, which activates SYK. This motif is located in the cytoplasmic portion of FcγR, FcεR, Igα (B cells), CD3ξ (T cells), and integrins.[34] SYK activation activates downstream MAPKs, PI3K, and PLCγ; this results in an increase in IL-6 and MMP production (Fig. 68.3).

These observations have led to interest in SYK as a potential target for treatment of RA.[35] SYK has been found to be activated in synoviocytes, and activation of SYK is important for cytokine and metalloproteinase production induced by TNF in fibroblast-like synoviocytes from patients with RA.[36] Pre-clinical models suggest inhibition of SYK could ameliorate inflammatory arthritis.[37–39] An oral agent that inhibits SYK is fostamatinib disodium, which is a prodrug of the active metabolite R406; it was evaluated in pre-clinical models of inflammatory arthritis and found to be effective. Based on this observation, fostamatinib was evaluated in patients with RA in four phase II clinical trials[40–43] and one phase III[44] clinical trial. Statistically superior improvements in clinical outcomes at 12 to 24 weeks, measured by ACR response and change in disease activity score (DAS28), were seen in two of the phase II randomized clinical trials evaluating fostamatinib in combination with MTX in nonbiologic disease-modifying anti-rheumatic drug (DMARD) nonresponders. Clinical response was seen as early as week 1. In a third phase IIb, 24-week trial, fostamatinib was evaluated as monotherapy compared with placebo and with an active comparator, adalimumab. Patients treated with fostamatinib showed improvement when compared to patients treated with placebo; however, the fostamatinib-treated patients had less improvement than those treated with adalimumab.[42]

A 3-month RCT of fostamatinib was conducted in 219 patients in whom biologic agents had previously failed.[43] The study failed to meet its primary endpoint, which was ACR20 response at month 3. However, in a subgroup of patients who had MRI of hands and wrists performed, there was an improvement in MRI synovitis scores in the fostamatinib group compared with placebo.

A 52-week phase III multinational RCT was conducted in 918 patients with RA with active disease despite MTX.[44] The co-primary endpoints were change from baseline in ACR20 response and change in modified Total Sharp van der Heijde score (mTSS) at week 24. The fostamatinib cohorts achieved a statistically superior ACR20 response compared with placebo-treated patients, but this was a lower response than that seen in the phase II program.

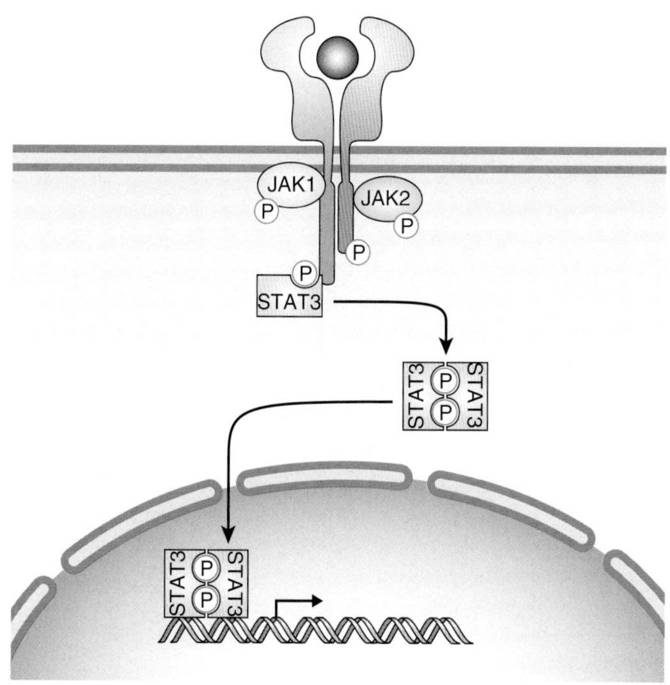

• **Fig. 68.4** Janus kinase (JAK)/signal transducer and activator of transcription (STAT) signaling pathways.

Additionally, there was no statistical difference in the co-primary endpoint change in mTSS between fostamatinib and placebo.

In all the phase II/III trials, a dose-dependent increase in AEs, including diarrhea, neutropenia, dizziness, hypertension, and elevated liver function tests (LFTs), was observed. AEs were more common in the fostamatinib cohorts, including hypertension, diarrhea, neutropenia, and LFT elevations. Serious AEs occurred in 2.9% to 4.9% of fostamatinib-treated patients and 1.6% of placebo-treated patients. A small number of malignancies were seen in the fostamatinib cohorts and none in the placebo-treated patients.[45] Based on the failure of fostamatinib to achieve the primary endpoint in the phase III clinical trial and the AE profile, development of the molecule for RA therapy was terminated.

A second SYK inhibitor has been evaluated in RA patients. MK-8457 is a novel inhibitor of SYK and zeta-chain–associated protein kinase 70 (ZAP70) and was considered to be a more specific SYK inhibitor with fewer off-target effects. Two small phase II dose-ranging trials utilizing an adaptive design were conducted.[46–48] MK8457 was found to be effective in the MTX incomplete responders, similar to fostamatinib, but not in the patients who had not responded to previous TNF inhibitors. Toxicity was significant in both studies, primarily serious infectious episodes (SIEs), which included opportunistic infections. Because of the significant toxicity noted and failure to see the benefit in TNF in incomplete responders, development of this molecule was terminated.

Janus Kinase Inhibitors

JAKs are PTKs that bind the cytoplasmic region of transmembrane cytokine receptors and mediate signaling through type I and type II cytokine receptors.[49] After receptor-ligand interaction, various JAKs are activated, which results in tyrosine phosphorylation of the receptor and subsequent activation of STATs, which act as transcription factors (Fig. 68.4). JAK/STAT signaling mediates cellular responses to multiple cytokines and growth factors. These responses include proliferation, differentiation, migration, apoptosis, and cell survival, depending on the signal and cellular context. Activated STATs enter the nucleus and bind to specific enhancer sequences in target genes, which impacts their transcription.[50]

JAKs consist of four types: JAK1, JAK2, JAK3, and TYK2. The JAKs signal as pairs (Fig. 68.5). JAK3 is primarily expressed in hematopoietic cells and is critical for signal transduction from the common γ-chain of the receptors for IL-2, IL-4, IL-7, IL-9, IL-15, and IL-21 on the plasma membrane to the nuclei of immune cells. JAK3 only signals in combination with JAK1. These cytokines are integral to lymphocyte activation, function, and proliferation. JAK3-knockout mice have defects in T and B lymphocytes and NK cells, with no other defects reported. Humans lacking JAK3 develop a severe combined immunodeficiency (SCID), with a deficiency in NK cells and T lymphocytes.[51]

JAK1 and JAK2 were initially not considered as potential therapeutic targets because knocking out these kinases results in germline lethality.[10] However, a JAK1/JAK2 inhibitor, baricitinib, has been approved for RA, and ruxolitinib, which also has selectivity for JAK1/2, has been approved for myelofibrosis and polycythemia vera.[52,53] Hormone-like cytokines erythropoietin, thrombopoietin, growth hormone, granulocyte-macrophage colony-stimulating factor (GM-CSF), IL-3, and IL-5 all signal through JAK2. IL-6, IL-10, IL-11, IL-19, IL-20, IL-22, and IFN-α, IFN-β, and IFN-γ signal through JAK1.

TYK2 facilitates signaling for IL-12, IL-23, and type 1 IFNs.[54] TYK2 pairs with either JAK1 or JAK2 to facilitate signaling. TYK2 inhibitors are under development as oral therapies for psoriasis due to inhibition of IL12/23 activity, as well as for systemic lupus erythematosus (SLE), due to inhibition of IFN-α and other inflammatory cytokines.[56,57]

JAK Selectivity

Tofacitinib has been demonstrated in in vitro assays to reversibly inhibit JAK1, JAK2, JAK3, and, to a lesser extent, TYK2, with functional selectivity for JAK1/3 and JAK1/2 signaling versus JAK2/2. Inhibition of JAK1/3 by tofacitinib will inhibit signaling for cytokines that bind receptors and utilize the common γ-chain receptor, such as IL-2, IL-4, IL-7, IL-9, IL-15, and IL-21.[55,56] Reduction in NK cells has been demonstrated with tofacitinib treatment.[57,58] It has been postulated that IL-6 inhibition, which signals through JAK1, may play a role in the efficacy of the molecule and in AEs, such as neutropenia and hyperlipidemia, which have been seen with monoclonal antibodies to the IL-6 receptor. IL-17 production by T helper 17 cells is also inhibited.[59] Tofacitinib along with all the other JAK inhibitors do not block IL-1 or TNF signaling.

Additional JAK inhibitors have been demonstrated in preclinical models as potentially more specific JAK1 inhibitors (upadacitinib/filgotinib).[60,61] Peficitinib has been demonstrated to inhibit JAK1/3 preferentially.[62] The assays evaluating specificity of the JAK inhibitors vary depending on the methodology, whether it be biochemical or cellular, which makes the comparative data difficult to interpret. Additionally, depending on the amount of ATP substrate utilized in the assay or degree of cytokine stimulation, results may vary.[63] For example, tofacitinib, at the doses used in the clinic, demonstrates substantial nanomolar inhibitory potency in enzymatic assays against all JAK family kinases except TYK2; however, in cellular assays, it exhibits functional specificity for JAK1 and JAK1/3 versus JAK2. Regulatory agencies now

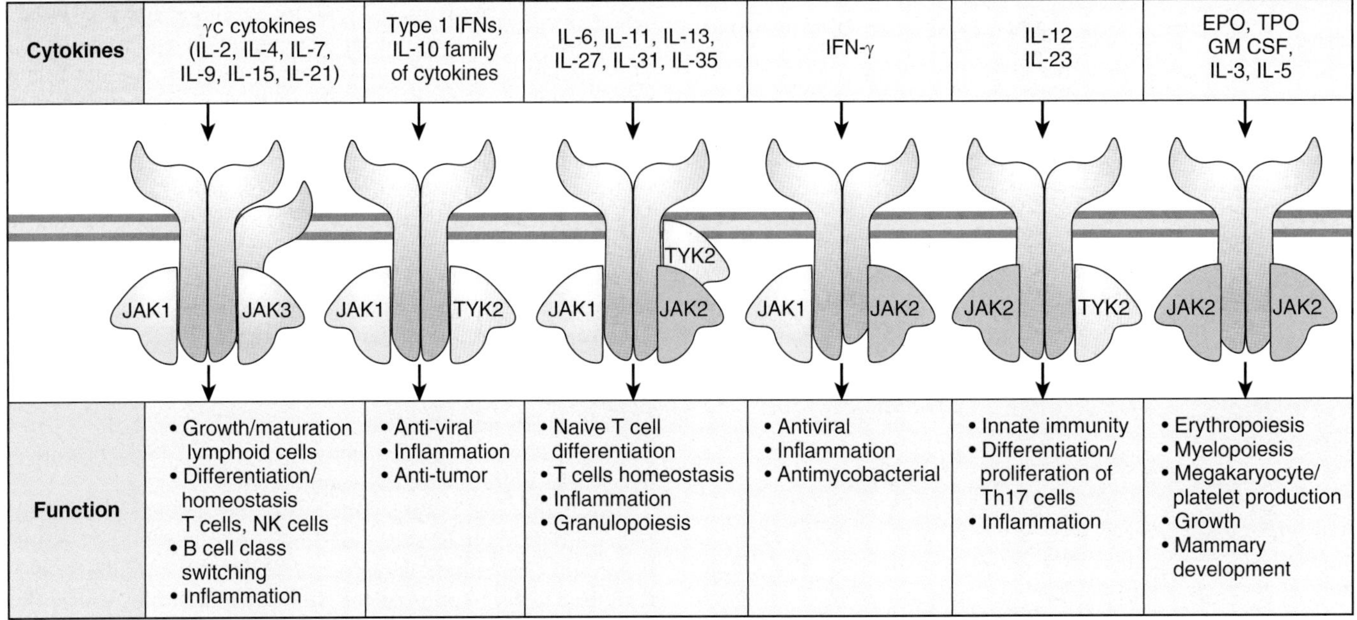

• **Fig. 68.5** Janus kinase (JAK)/signal transducer and activator of transcription (STAT) signaling pathways. *EPO,* Erythropoietin; *GM-CSF,* granulocyte-macrophage colony-stimulating factor; *IFN,* interferon; *TPO,* thrombopoietin; *TYK,* tyrosine kinase.

consider tofacitinib as well as baricitinib to be pan-JAK inhibitors. Complicating the issue of JAK selectivity is whether the maximal concentration (Cmax) or the average drug concentration results in the major impact on JAK inhibition. For example, at Cmax, JAK selectivity may not exist, whereas at lower concentrations, such as the average concentration, preferential JAK inhibition would be possible. A preliminary publication demonstrated that clinical profiles of cytokine inhibition for a number of JAK inhibitors in RA are strikingly similar when efficacious doses are considered, which suggests possible limited potential for differentiation of these therapeutics based on their JAK pharmacology.[64]

The relevance of specific JAK inhibition in these assays to their clinical effectiveness remains unknown.

TABLE 68.2 Janus Kinase (JAK) Inhibitors for Rheumatic Diseases: Pre-clinical JAK Isoform Selectivity

Tofacitinib	JAK1/3 inhibitor
Baricitinib	JAK1/2 inhibitor
Upadacitinib	JAK1 inhibitor
Peficitinib	JAK1/3 inhibitor
Filgotinib	JAK1 inhibitor

JAK Inhibitors for Treatment of Rheumatoid Arthritis

Multiple JAK inhibitors have been evaluated as treatment for RA in patients failing conventional synthetic DMARDs (csDMARDs) or biologic therapies (Table 68.2). Tofacitinib was evaluated in multiple phase III clinical trials resulting in approval in the United States in 2012 and in Europe in 2017; regulators approved the medications for treatment of patients with RA with active disease, despite MTX treatment, at a dose of 5 mg twice daily, in combination with nonbiologic DMARDs or as monotherapy[65–70] (Table 68.3). The delay in European approval concerned safety concerns, of a trend for greater risk of infection and malignancies with the 10 mg twice a day dose, but the concerns were subsequently addressed with long-term extension studies and phase IV clinical trials, which proved similar risk for these AEs. The 10 mg twice-daily dose for RA is approved in Switzerland and Russia.

Baricitinib was approved in Europe and several other countries in 2017 at 4 mg once daily for csDMARD incomplete responders; in 2018, it was approved in the United States at 2 mg daily in patients with active disease despite previous treatment with TNF inhibitors.[71–74] The US Food and Drug Administration (FDA) expressed concerns over the benefit/risk profile of the 4 mg dose due to a trend for increased rates of AEs with the 4 mg dose. With the 2 mg dose only evaluated in two of the four pivotal phase III clinical trials, the agency did not feel there was enough evidence to support approval of the 4 mg dose.

Upadacitinib at 15/30 mg once daily, filgotinib 100/200 mg daily, and peficitinib 100/150 mg daily are in phase III trials in RA.[75–84] Peficitinib is being developed outside of the United States, primarily in Asia. All should be commercially available in the next few years.

All of the JAK inhibitors had similar development programs, were evaluated in classic phase I/II dose ranging studies, thus resulting in the doses subsequently evaluated in phase III studies. In phase III, efficacy and safety was evaluated in MTX and csDMARD incomplete responder populations, TNF incomplete responders, and in early RA patients, with comparison to MTX. Impact on prevention of structural damage was assessed along with comparison to biologic therapy (adalimumab). JAK inhibitor monotherapy was also evaluated. Tofacitinib, baricitinib, and filgotinib have reported long-term safety outcomes, and one phase IV study evaluated tofacitinib monotherapy in comparison to combination tofacitinib/MTX and adalimumab/MTX.[85–88]

TABLE 68.3 **Tofacitinib: Phase 3 Study Designs-DMARD Incomplete Responders**

	DURATION ≥1 YEAR			DURATION OF 6 MONTHS	
Study *n*	Study 1044 "scan" *n* = 797	Study 1046 "sync" *n* = 792	Study 1064 "standard" *n* = 717	Study 1032 "step" *n* = 399	Study 1045 "solo" *n* = 610
Population	MTX IR	DMARD IR	MTX IR	TNF IR	DMARD IR
Background treatment	MTX	DMARDs	MTXs	MTX	None
Distinguishing feature	Radiograph	Background DMARDs	Active control (adalimumab)	TNF failures	Monotherapy

JAK Inhibitor Pharmacology

Tofacitinib was initially approved at a dose of 5 mg twice a day, but an 11 mg XR formulation which was approved in 2016 is the most commonly used dose in the clinic. This formulation was approved by the FDA based on a pharmacokinetic study, and not a clinical trial.[89] Japan regulatory authorities have not approved the 11 mg XR formulation based on a small study in RA patients failing to demonstrate noninferiority to the 5 mg twice-a-day dose in change in disease activity.[90] Real world experience has not demonstrated a significant difference in clinical response to that of the 5-mg twice-a-day dose.[91] The pharmacokinetic profile of tofacitinib XR is characterized by rapid absorption (peak plasma concentrations are reached within 4 hours), rapid elimination (half-life of approximately 6 hours), and dose-proportional increases in systemic exposure.[92] Steady-state concentrations are achieved in 24 to 48 hours with minimal accumulation after twice-daily administration. Tofacitinib is eliminated through both hepatic (70%) and renal (30%) clearance. The metabolism is primarily through CYP3A4 and less so by CYP2C19. At the approved dosage, no extrinsic factors or drugs require dose modification based on pharmacokinetic evaluation in pre-clinical studies, except for ketoconazole, which suppresses CYP3A4 activity, and for rifampin, which enhances CYP3A4 activity. The pharmacodynamic effects of tofacitinib have been demonstrated to persist for 4 to 6 weeks after dosing, including a reduction in NK cells.[58] Like all the JAK inhibitors in animal models, tofacitinib is a teratogen; pre-menopausal women should utilize contraception and avoid conception for 4 to 6 weeks after the last dose.

Baricitinib is approved at 2 and 4 mg daily outside of the United States. It is approved for RA patients with persistent disease activity despite csDMARDs or TNF inhibitors, as monotherapy, or combination with MTX or other csDMARDs outside of the United States. It is approved for TNF inhibitor failures only in the United States at 2 mg daily. Baricitinib is rapidly absorbed with a Tmax of 1 hour and a half-life of 12.5 hours. It is eliminated primarily by renal excretion and recommended to use the 2 mg dose in patients with renal insufficiency.[93] Probenecid and other strong organic anion transporter 3 inhibitors (OAT3) reduce baricitinib clearance. Baricitinib undergoes minor metabolism by CYP3A4, but no dose modification is necessary with drugs that impact the CYP450 enzymes. Baricitinib is also associated with a reduction in NK cells with a reduction of 40% to 50% over 24 weeks in phase III trials.[94]

Upadacitinib immediate release formulation was evaluated in phase I/II trials at doses of 3 mg twice a day to 18 mg twice a day and 24 mg every day.[95,96] Upadacitinib extended release formulation at a dose of 15 and 30 mg once daily was evaluated in phase III clinical trials after pharmacokinetic studies demonstrated similar bioavailability to the 12 and 24 mg twice a day doses.[97] Rapid absorption was observed with Tmax of 2 to 3 hours and half-life of 10-12.5 hours. Elimination is primarily through hepatic metabolism through the CYP3A enzyme and, to lesser degree, CYP2D6, which suggests that modification of dose will be necessary with ketoconazole and rifampin. Reduction in NK cells has been noted with upadactinib.[59]

Filgotinib has been evaluated in phase III trials at 100 mg and 200 mg once daily. Filgotinib is a prodrug rapidly metabolized to an active metabolite. Absorption is rapid; Tmax is 2 to 3 hours with a half-life of 4.9 to 5.7 hours, although the active metabolite has a half-life of 18 to 23 hours.[60] Elimination is both by hepatic clearance by carboxylesterases as well as by renal clearance. Limited impact on the CYP450 enzymes has been noted. Filgotinib monotherapy had no impact on NK cells in a 24 weeks phase II dose ranging study.[98]

Peficitinib was evaluated in phase II dose ranging trials at 25 mg, 50 mg, 100 mg, and 150 mg once daily, and based on efficacy seen with the 100 and 150 mg once daily these doses were evaluated in phase III clinical trials.[79,80]

JAK Inhibitor Clinical Development and Efficacy

The approved JAK inhibitors were evaluated in multiple clinical trials demonstrating statistically significant efficacy compared to placebo-treated patients. Phase II clinical trials evaluated tofacitinib at doses of 1 to 30 mg twice a day as monotherapy or in combination with MTX.[99,100] Consistent improvement in clinical outcomes occurred with doses of 5 mg twice daily or greater, but toxicity was greater at higher doses. Based on the efficacy and safety profile from the phase II clinical trials, tofacitinib 5 mg twice daily and 10 mg twice daily doses were progressed to phase III trials. Baricitinib was evaluated at doses of 1, 2, 4, and 8 mg once daily in phase II trials.[101,102] Efficacy was similar at 2, 4, and 8 mg daily with a trend for more safety issues at 8 mg, which resulted in the 2 and 4 mg doses progressing to phase III clinical trials. Upadacitinib was evaluated as an immediate release formulation of 6, 12, and 18 mg twice a day in phase I/II trials; based on studies demonstrating similar pharmacokinetics between the 12

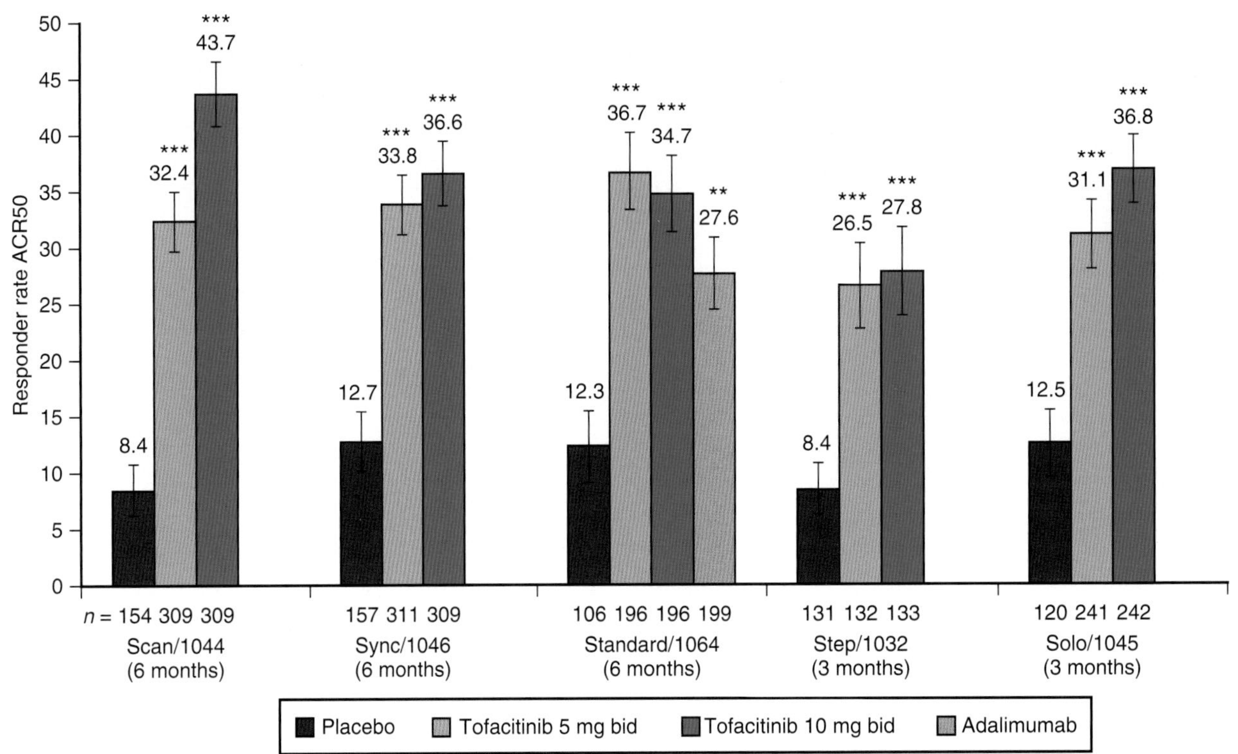

• **Fig. 68.6** American College of Rheumatology (ACR50) response across tofacitinib disease-modifying anti-rheumatic drug (DMARD)/biologic incomplete responders phase III clinical trials.

mg and 18 mg twice a day and 15 mg and 30 mg once daily, the once-daily formulation was evaluated in phase III clinical trials.[96] Filgotinib was evaluated in phase I/II clinical trials at 30, 75, 150, 200, and 300 mg daily or 100 mg twice a day.[103,104] Based on phase I/II efficacy and safety, the 100 and 200 mg daily doses were evaluated in phase III trials. Peficitinib was evaluated in phase II trials of RA patients at doses of 50, 100, and 150 mg daily. Based on results from phase II dose ranging trials, the 100 mg and 150 mg daily doses were evaluated in phase III.[78,79]

The phase III clinical trials programs were similar for the approved JAK inhibitors as well as those in development. All the trials were global programs, with the majority of patients enrolled outside of the United States. The development programs were large, with 2500 to 4000 patients enrolled.[64–79,81,82] The clinical trials evaluated RA patients with active disease despite MTX or csDMARDs, patients with active disease despite receiving TNF inhibitors, as well as patients naïve to MTX. All therapies were also evaluated as monotherapy in patients who had failed csDMARDs due to lack of efficacy or toxicity. The ability of these therapies to slow radiographic progression was evaluated over 12 months in RA patients receiving background MTX and compared to an active comparator (adalimumab). Long-term extension studies to evaluate persistence of response and to monitor long-term safety issues were part of all the development programs (see Table 68.3).

Tofacitinib (5 and 10 mg twice a day), baricitinib (4 mg daily), upadacitinib (15 and 30 mg daily), and peficitinib (100 and 150 mg) in combination with MTX or csDMARDs demonstrated statistically significant improvement (compared to placebo) in signs and symptoms as measured by ACR response, CDAI, SDAI, and change in disease activity as measured by DAS28 (Figs. 68.6 and 68.7 and Table 68.4). In RA patients on background MTX nonresponsive to TNF inhibitors/biologics, tofacitinib (5 and 10 mg twice a day), baricitinib (2 and 4 mg), upadacitinib (15 and 30 mg), and filgotinib (100 and 200 mg) demonstrated significant improvement compared to placebo over 6 months.[67,73,74,82] In RA patients naïve to MTX, tofacitinib monotherapy at 5 and 10 mg twice a day was statistically superior to MTX as determined by ACR 70 response. Baricitinib 4 mg monotherapy and baricitinib 4 mg in combination with MTX were statistically superior to MTX in a DMARD-naïve population in improvement in disease activity as determined by ACR response or change in DAS28.[69,71]

Preliminary data from two 52-week phase III trials of peficitinib 100/150 mg daily in RA patients with active disease despite MTX or csDMARDs demonstrated statistical superiority in improvement as measured by the ACR20/50/70 and change in DAS28 at week 12.[81,82] In one study, open label etanercept was included as an active comparator with numerically greater ACR responses than peficitinib as well as change in DAS28, DAS28 low disease activity state (LDAS)/remission, but no statistical comparisons were conducted.

JAK Inhibitors Versus Adalimumab

In the development program, tofacitinib was compared to adalimumab in the MTX incomplete responder populations with similar clinical benefit, but the study was not powered to evaluate statistical difference between the groups.[66] In a phase IV study, tofacitinib 5 mg twice a day plus MTX was determined to be noninferior to adalimumab plus MTX in ACR 50 response at

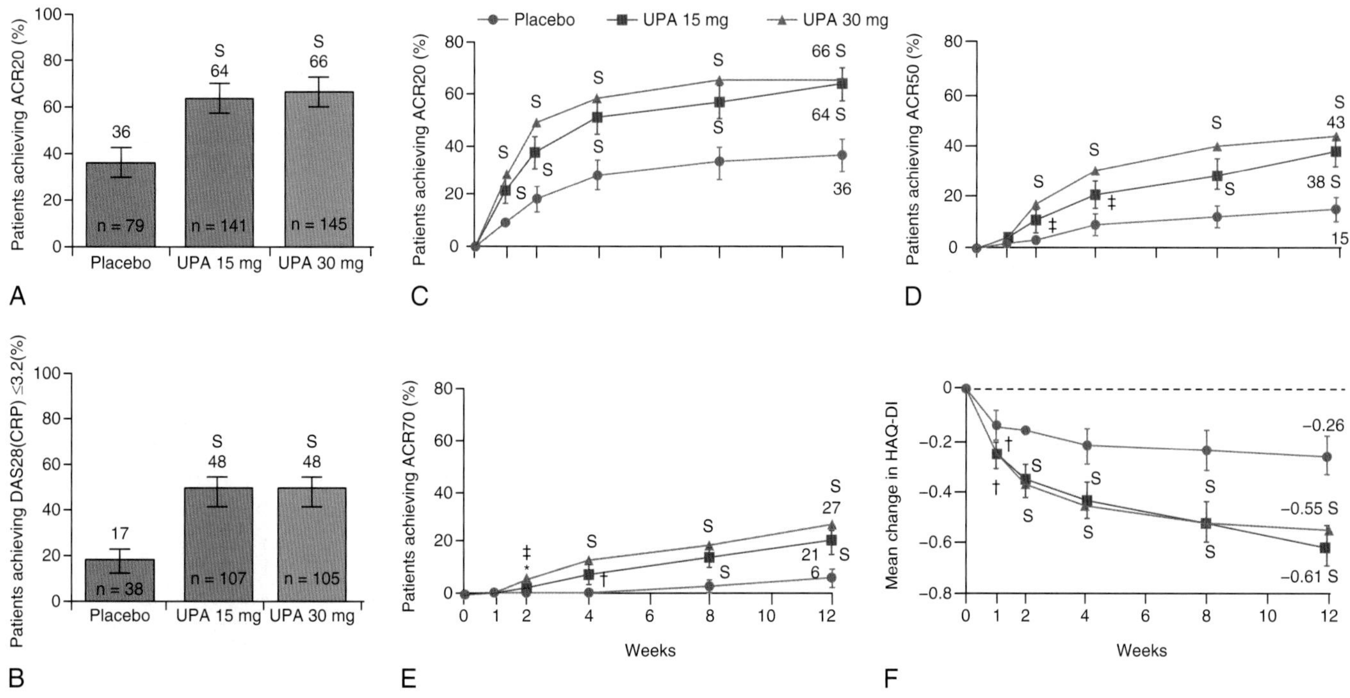

• **Fig. 68.7** American College of Rheumatology (ACR) responses/change in Health Assessment Questionnaire and Disability Index (HAQ-DI) for upadacitinib in the phase III clinical trial of rheumatoid arthritis (RA) patients with incomplete response to conventional synthetic disease-modifying anti-rheumatic drugs (csDMARDs).

TABLE 68.4 Janus Kinase (JAK) Inhibitors: Clinical Efficacy in Biologic Disease-Modifying Anti-rheumatic Drug (DMARD) Failures (Placebo Corrected)

	ACR20(%)	ACR50(%)	ACR70(%)	DAS28 ≤3.2(%0)	HAQ-DI Response
Tofacitinib 5 mg	17.3	18	12	9.3	0.25
Tofacitinib 10 mg	23.7	20	9	15.8	0.28
Baricitinib 2 mg	22	12	11	15	0.20
Baricitinib 4 mg	28	20	9	22	0.25
Upadacitinib 15 mg	37	22	8	28	0.25
Upadacitinib 30 mg	28	25	12	29	0.28
Filgotinib 100 mg	26.4	17.1	7.6	21.8	0.25
Filgotinib 200 mg	35	28	15	25.3	0.32

6 months.[86] 1146 patients were enrolled; at 6 months, ACR50 was achieved by 38% of patients with tofacitinib monotherapy, 46% of patients with tofacitinib and MTX, and 44% of patients with adalimumab and MTX. Although there was a good clinical response with tofacitinib monotherapy, noninferiority to adalimumab/MTX was not achieved in this study.

Baricitinib and upadacitinib were both compared to adalimumab in the MTX incomplete responder population.[71,77] Baricitinib was statistically superior to adalimumab at week 12 for the ACR20/50/70 response and for the ACR20 and ACR70 response at week 24. Upadacitinib was compared to adalimumab in a phase III study in MTX incomplete responders. Upadacitinib was statistically superior to adalimumab at week 12 in ACR50, DAS28CRP, and LDAS. At week 26, more patients achieved LDAS or remission on upadacitinib than adalimumab.

Radiographic Outcomes

Radiographic outcomes were evaluated in the clinical trials for all the JAK inhibitors. Improvements in structural benefit, as measured by the mTSS, were observed at the 10 mg tofacitinib twice a day dosage in the MTX incomplete responder population, but they did not achieve statistical significance at the 5 mg twice a day dosage.[68] In the MTX-naïve population, mean changes in the mTSS from baseline to month 6 were less statistically significant in the tofacitinib groups than in the MTX group (0.2 in the 5 mg tofacitinib group and <0.1 in the 10 mg tofacitinib group,

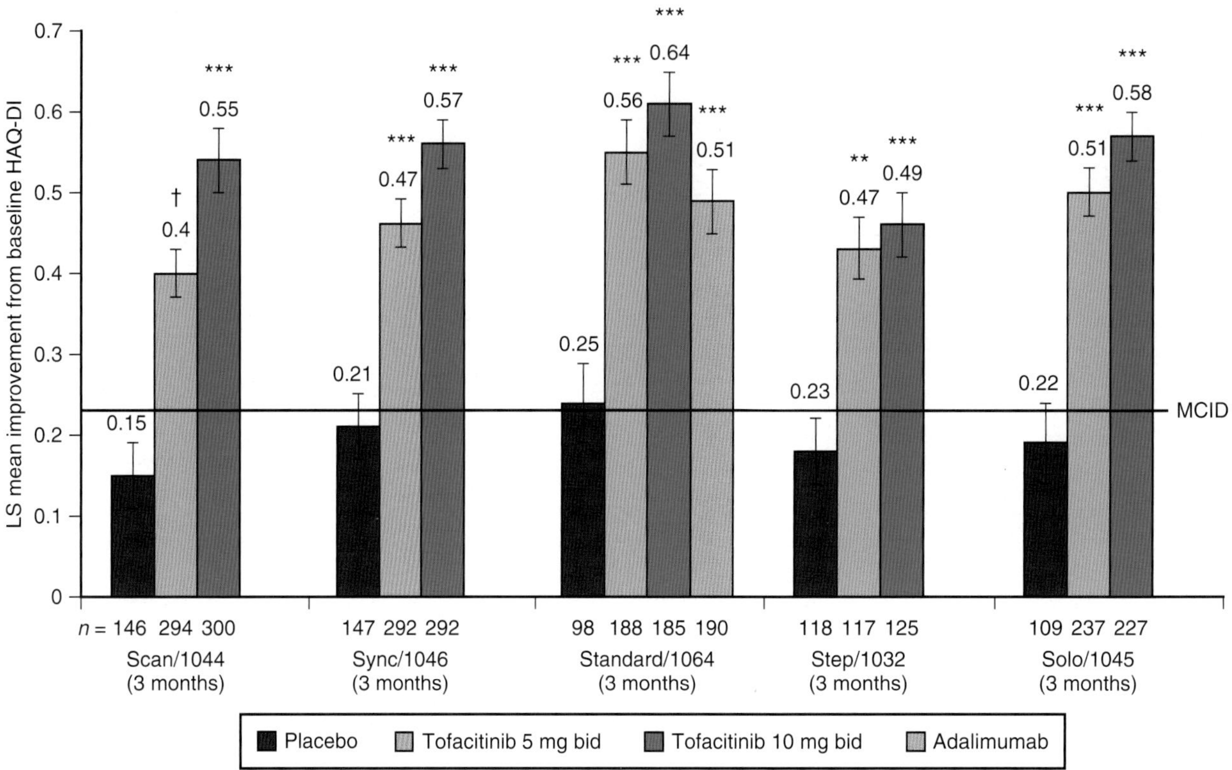

• **Fig. 68.8** Tofacitinib: Health Assessment Questionnaire and Disability Index (HAQ-DI) response across disease-modifying anti-rheumatic drug (DMARD)/biologic incomplete responders phase III clinical trials.

compared with change of 0.8 in the MTX group).[69] Based on this trial, the FDA allowed the claim for slowing of radiographic progression for tofacitinib.

Four mg baricitinib in combination with MTX reduced radiographic progression compared with placebo, as did the active comparator adalimumab in a 52-week study (mTSS-placebo 1.80; Bari 0.71; Ada 0.60).[72] In the csDMARD naïve population, baricitinib 4 mg plus MTX inhibited radiographic progression compared to MTX at 52 weeks; however, baricitinib monotherapy was not statistically different (MTX-1.02; Bari-0.80; Bari/MTX-0.40).

Preliminary data from a 26-week phase III clinical trial of 15 mg upadacitinib in combination with MTX demonstrated statistically significant inhibition of radiographic progression.[77] Similar findings were reported for peficitinib 100/150 mg daily in combination with MTX in a 28-week study.[82]

Patient-Reported Outcomes

Patient-reported outcomes were evaluated in all the development programs for the JAK (Fig. 68.8). These included the Health Assessment Questionnaire (HAQ), SF-36, and measures of patient pain and fatigue. Significant improvements compared to placebo treated patients in the HAQ were seen in all of the studies in early disease, MTX or csDMARD incomplete responders, and TNF or biologic incomplete responders, exceeding the minimally clinically important difference of 0.22. In comparison to the combination of adalimumab/MTX, baricitinib/MTX and upadacitinib/MTX were statistically superior to adalimumab in improvement in HAQ scores at several timepoints during the 52-week studies.[71,77] Improvements in the physical as well as mental component of the SF-36 were noted, and the changes were comparable for each of the JAK inhibitors. Similar improvements in pain and fatigue were also observed.

Efficacy Summary: JAK Inhibitors

Similar efficacy of the JAK inhibitors was observed in the development programs of the individual therapies. The JAK inhibitors had similar or better efficacy compared to adalimumab in MTX incomplete responders. In early RA patients naïve to MTX, tofacitinib, baricitinib, and upadacitinib were superior to MTX clinically and in preservation of structure. Tofacitinib, which was approved in 2012, has been utilized in clinic in patients with active disease, despite MTX or biologics, with efficacy results similar to those of the development program. Rarely is it used early in RA due to restriction by insurers and because of concern for toxicity. As more JAK inhibitors become available, utilization earlier in disease will most likely occur.

It is unknown, if a patient fails a JAK inhibitor, whether the patient will respond to a second JAK inhibitor; these studies have not been performed. Additionally, there have been no trials with direct comparisons of JAK inhibitors as we have had with biologic DMARDs.

JAK Inhibitor Safety

The nature of AEs associated with JAK inhibitors has been delineated in the clinical trial programs, in the long-term extension

TABLE 68.5 JAK Inhibitors: Safety Issues

- Serious infectious episodes
- Viral/opportunistic infections: herpes zoster
- Tuberculosis
- Lipids and cardiovascular risk
- Hepatic safety
- GI perforations
- Increased risk of thromboembolic disease?

protocols of the clinical trials, and, to a lesser degree, with observational registries.[84–86]

The most common AEs were upper respiratory infections, headache, nasopharyngitis, and diarrhea, which clinicians observed slightly more often in the patients on JAK inhibitors than in the placebo group.

AEs associated with JAK inhibitors include SIEs, opportunistic infections, herpes zoster, gastrointestinal (GI) perforations, and the possible increased risk of thromboembolic disease (Table 68.5). The type and frequency of AEs are similar to those of biologic DMARDs except for the increased incidence of herpes zoster.

Tofacitinib

Tofacitinib has the largest long-term safety database. Safety data has been reported on 7061 RA patients with 22,875 patient-years of exposure to tofacitinib 5 or 10 mg twice a day.[84,105] The median exposure was 3.1 years. The rate of serious adverse events (SAEs) with tofacitinib was 9.6/100 patient-years for the 5 mg dose and 8.6 per 100 patient-years for the 10 mg dose, which was similar to that for adalimumab in the active comparator trial, 9.76/100 patient-years. The most common SAE was pneumonia. The incidence rate (IR) for SIEs was 2.5/100 patient-years, similar to that seen with biologic therapies. The rate of serious infections episodes (SIEs) remained stable over time in the long-term extension protocol through 6 years of follow-up. The most common serious infections were pneumonia, urinary tract infection, herpes zoster, and cellulitis. At the time of FDA approval in the long-term extension trials, the rate of SIEs was 2.3/100 patient-years for the 5 mg dose and 4.06/100 patient-years for the 10 mg dose, which was statistically different because the confidence intervals (CIs) did not overlap (Fig. 68.9).[106] For this reason, the 10 mg dose was not approved by the FDA or the European Medicines Agency (EMA); however, in the long-term extension study, this difference no longer was observed. The 10 mg twice a day dose is now approved in the United States for ulcerative colitis.[107]

Although the clinical trials and long-term safety extension trial for tofacitinib did not show an increased risk for thromboembolic phenomenon in the overall population, an interim analysis of an ongoing phase IV clinical trial enrolling patients at risk for cardiovascular disease did demonstrate an increased risk for venous thromboembolism that was dose related.[108] Based on this data the 10 mg BID tofacitinib dose was discontinued in this trial and the 5 mg dose continues to be evaluated. In 2019 the U.S. FDA and EMA both added warnings to avoid tofacitinib in patients with high risk for clots. This observation along with the possible association of baricitinib with venous thromboembolism suggests this may be a class effect. The mechanism of action is unknown.

Nonserious and serious herpes zoster infection events were reported in 3.6/100 patient-years, which is greater than those seen with csDMARDs or other biologic DMARDs; 90.2% involved a single dermatome and were considered serious in 7.3% of herpes zoster patients.[109] The rate of herpes zoster did not increase over time. A Cox regression analysis of risk factors demonstrated that the 10 mg dose, glucocorticoid usage, age, and being Asian increased the likelihood of developing herpes zoster. Increased herpes zoster risk has been reported with all the JAK inhibitors approved or in development for RA. If possible, RA patients should be vaccinated for herpes zoster before initiating JAK inhibitors.

Tuberculosis (TB) was reported in 36 patients (0.2/100 patient-years): IRs were similar for the 5 and 10 mg doses. Most of the cases were from areas endemic for TB. Cases of both pulmonary and extrapulmonary TB were reported. The incidence of TB in the randomized clinical trials was consistent with those reported for TNF inhibitors (0.02 [global] to 2.56 [South Korea]) and nonbiologic DMARDs (0.01 [global] to 0.28 [South Korea]). Screening for latent TB is indicated before initiating JAK inhibitors.

Excluding cases of TB, 61 patients experienced an opportunistic infection (0.3 events/100 patient-years [95% CI, 0.20 to 0.4]). The cases included multi-dermatomal herpes zoster, esophageal candidiasis (several were incidental findings on endoscopies performed for other reasons), cytomegalovirus infection/viremia, cryptococcal infection (pneumonia, meningitis), *Pneumocystis jiroveci* pneumonia, nontuberculous mycobacteria in the lung, and BK virus encephalitis. Opportunistic infections were more common in Asia and Latin America, in older patients, and with the 10 mg dosage.

The overall mortality rate of tofacitinib, malignancy risk, and lymphoma incidence in the phase II, III, and LTE studies was consistent with the published rates in RA clinical trials for TNF inhibitors and other biologic DMARDs. Lymphomas reported were predominantly non-Hodgkin's B cell lymphomas.

Twenty-two GI perforations occurred in the development program on tofacitinib, though none occurred in the placebo. These events occurred in patients on background corticosteroids and nonsteroidal anti-inflammatory drugs (NSAIDs). The IR reported at the time of approval was 0.11/100 patient-years, similar to what has been reported with TNF and IL-6 inhibitors. Use of this therapy in patients with diverticulitis should probably be avoided, which is similar to the present standard of care with IL-6 inhibitors.

Baricitinib

A preliminary presentation of the baricitinib-integrated safety summary provided safety information on 3492 RA patients with 7860 patient-years of follow-up with median duration of exposure 2.6 years.[86] SIEs were reported in 3 per 100 patient-years, and the IR for herpes zoster was 3.3 per 100 patient-years, which is similar to findings with tofacitinib. The IR for these AEs was stable over the 3 years of follow-up. The most common SIEs were pneumonia, urinary tract infections, herpes zoster, cellulitis, and sepsis. Ninety-four percent of herpes zoster were nonserious and incidence rate was greater in Asia, as seen with tofacitinib.

The IR of TB was 0.14 per 100 patient-years, and the IR of GI perforations were 0.04 per 100 patient-years. Major adverse cardiac events (MACEs) were seen in 0.5 patients per 100 years and malignancy in 0.8 per 100 patient-years, with six patients developing lymphoma. Numerically for these AEs, IRs were higher for the 4 mg dose compared to the 2 mg dose, although CIs overlapped.

During the placebo-controlled portion of the clinical trial program, there was an imbalance in the IRs of venous thromboembolism and pulmonary embolism (PE): 4 mg baricitinib

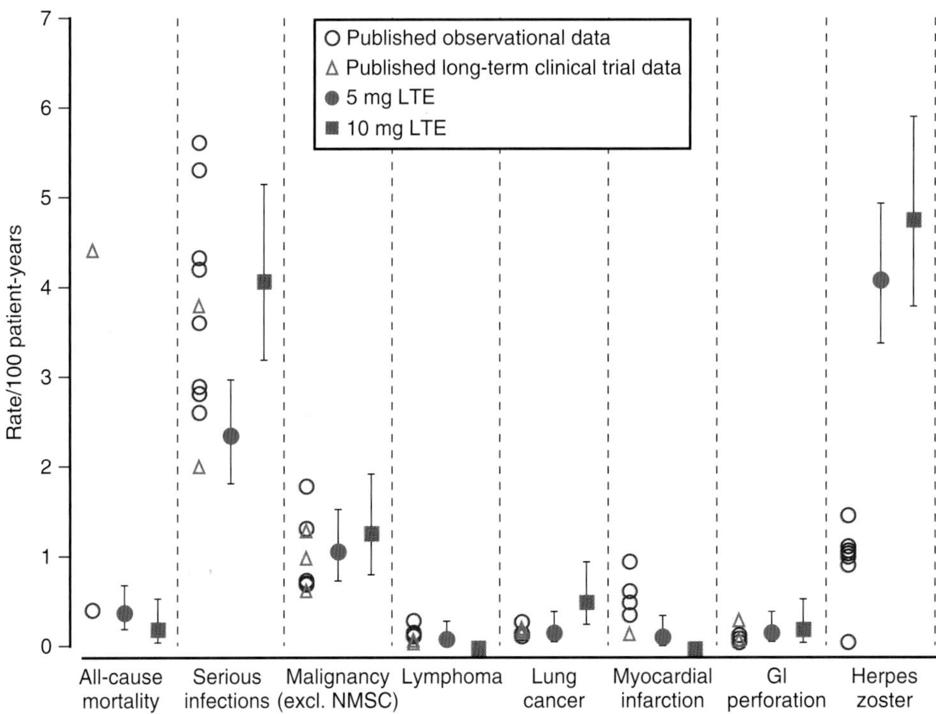

• **Fig. 68.9** Adverse events of interest for tofacitinib 5/10 mg compared to published data on adverse events of biologic disease-modifying anti-rheumatic drugs (DMARDs) from long-term extension studies/ observational registries (FDA Arthritis Advisory committee meeting 2012).

1.7% (5 events), 2 mg baricitinib 0% (0 events), and placebo 0% (0 events).[110] No difference in arterial thrombotic events was reported. Overall, in the development program, the IR for venous thromboembolism was 0.5/100 patient-years, similar to that reported in claims-based databases. Based on this observation, the FDA required a boxed warning on thrombosis to be included the package insert for baricitinib. Baricitinib is the only JAK inhibitor not associated with a reduction in platelet counts normally associated with a reduction in inflammation, and 2% of patients had had elevated platelet counts greater than 600,000.[111] However, there was no relationship between the development of DVT/PE and elevated platelet counts in the clinical trial program. Past history of DVT/PE was associated with an increased risk of development of DVT/PE on baricitinib. This observation combined with the tofacitinib dose-related increase in DVT/PE supports the possibility that this may be a class effect. These therapies should be avoided if possible in patients at higher risk for venous thromboembolic events.

Integrated safety analyses for upadacitinib, filgotinib, or peficitinib are not yet available. Data from individual clinical trials with these therapies suggest that safety issues are similar to tofacitinib, baricitinib, and biologic DMARDs, other than the observed increased incidence of herpes zoster.

Safety Summary: JAK Inhibitors

The safety profile of all the JAK inhibitors is similar. Whether one JAK inhibitor is safer than the others is not yet clear because data from the integrated safety analyses for upadacitinib, filgotinib, and peficitinib have not been reported. Is the risk of venous thromboembolism limited to baricitinib or is it related in some way to JAK inhibition? Will the fact that filgotinib is not associated with a reduction in NK cells result in fewer herpes zoster or opportunistic infections? Hopefully, with the pending trial results and increased experience in the clinic with the JAK inhibitors, these important questions will be answered.

Laboratory Evaluation With JAK Inhibitors

Based on their mechanism of action, certain laboratory abnormalities were expected (Table 68.6). JAK1 facilitates signaling for IL-6, which results in neutrophil homeostasis. IL-6 inhibitors have been associated with reduction in neutrophil counts, which is believed to be part of their mechanism of action in RA. So it is to be expected that inhibiting JAK1, which facilitates signal transduction for IL-6, is associated with a reduction in neutrophil counts. A modest reduction in neutrophil counts has been seen with all the JAK inhibitors with rare grade 3/4 neutropenia noted. The reduction in neutrophil counts were infrequently associated with AEs and not associated with increased infection risk. JAK3 plays an integral role in lymphocyte survival/maturation, and all the JAK inhibitors have been associated with lowered lymphocyte counts with rare grade 4 lymphopenia. Monitoring complete blood cell (CBC) and total lymphocyte counts on a regular basis (monthly for 3 months, then every 3 months) is recommended by regulatory agencies. A boxed warning is in the package inserts for both tofacitinib and baricitinib for lymphopenia, and discontinuation of treatment is recommended for patients with persistent lymphocyte counts less than 500/μL due to increased risk of infection noted in the tofacitinib clinical trials.

JAK2 facilitates signal transduction for erythropoietin, and significant concern over the safety of JAK2 inhibitors was suggested by pre-clinical research. Concern over significant anemia was raised based on pre-clinical investigation, but clinically this is unusual. Baricitinib inhibits JAK2 more than the other JAK inhibitors in enzymatic and biochemical assays, but significant anemia has been rare with any of the JAK inhibitors.

TABLE 68.6 JAK Inhibitors: Laboratory Changes Observed

• LFT abnormalities: More prevalent with combination Rx
• Lipid: Increased HDL/LDL; ratio generally unchanged
• Hemoglobin: Reduced if JAK2 activity impacted; rarely clinically significant
• Neutrophils: Reduced; rarely <1000/mm^3; presumed part of MOA
• Lymphocytes: Reduced; rarely <500/mm^3; dose reduction or discontinuation indicated due to increased risk of SIEs
• Nonsignificant CPK elevations
• Serum creatinine: Small nonsignificant elevations seen

IL-6 plays a homeostatic role for hepatocytes, and JAK1 inhibition reduces IL-6 signaling. Compared to placebo in the clinical trials, all the JAK inhibitors have been associated with transaminase elevations. Liver function abnormalities have been more common when the JAK inhibitors were used in combination with MTX. No cases fulfilling Hy's Law were reported in the clinical trials, and the liver function abnormalities resolved with dose reduction or discontinuation. Monitoring of LFTs monthly for the first 3 months, then every 3 months, is recommended for patients on JAK inhibitors.

Elevations in serum lipids have been seen in patients receiving all DMARDs, with most significant increases seen in IL-6 inhibitors. Elevations in total cholesterol, high-density lipoprotein (HDL) and low-density lipoprotein (LDL) have been reported with all the JAK inhibitors in ~30% of patients. Generally, the elevations were in the range of 15% to 20%. Elevations have been noted by 12 weeks and are generally stable thereafter. In general, the mean HDL/LDL ratio remains unchanged. Increases in rates of cardiovascular AEs have not been reported. A phase IV study mandated by the FDA evaluating cardiovascular risk with tofacitinib in comparison to TNF inhibitors is ongoing; it seeks to confirm the lack of cardiovascular signal seen in the development programs.[112] Atorvastatin treatment has been demonstrated to be effective in patients with elevations in cholesterol on tofacitinib.[113] Monitoring of serum lipids is recommended 8 to 12 weeks after initiating therapy.

Small, clinically insignificant increases in serum creatinine and increased creatinine kinase were noted with all the JAK inhibitors and have not been associated with significant safety risks. Creatinine increases were in the 0.02 to 0.04 mg/dL range greater than placebo in the development program. The etiology of this change is unclear.[114]

Real-World Experience With JAK inhibitors

RA patients in clinical trials may not represent the typical RA patients due to limitations on medications and comorbidities which exclude the majority of patients from clinical trial participation. Compared to patients enrolled in clinical trials, those in real-world observational studies have worse prognostic factors, including older age, longer disease duration, and greater than 1 prior DMARD exposure. These differences may lead to an overestimation of the effectiveness of therapies, or an underestimation of AE rates.[115] Therefore, an analysis of real-world observational studies is critical for understanding treatment efficacy and risk of AEs in the broader spectrum of patients encountered in the real world.

There have been a number of real-world studies of tofacitinib in RA, with the majority of published studies coming from the United States, where tofacitinib was approved by the FDA in 2012. Sources of data include administrative claim databases, clinical databases, registries, and national pharmacovigilance programs. Very limited data is available yet for baricitinib.

In the real-world setting, patients initiating tofacitinib tend to have longer disease duration, and have been exposed to more bDMARDs, in comparison with patients initiating a bDMARD. A 5-year prospective observational study using the US Corrona RA Registry compared patients initiating tofacitinib to patients initiating a bDMARD or to patients initiating a csDMARD (with no prior or current tofacitinib exposure).[116] In this study, patients initiating tofacitinib had an average duration of disease of 13.7 years versus 10.5 years for bDMARD initiators and 4.6 years for csDMARD initiators. The tofacitinib initiators also had exposure to more bDMARDs (mean 2.7) versus the bDMARD initiators (1.5) and the csDMARD initiators (0).

In keeping with data indicating the benefit of tofacitinib as monotherapy, tofacitinib in the real-world setting appears to be used more frequently as monotherapy compared with bDMARDs. In real-world patients, tofacitinib also appears to be effective as monotherapy, as measured by patient adherence to therapy (i.e., filling prescriptions regularly) and persistence with therapy. One study analyzing tofacitinib use in clinical practice in two US Health Care Claims Databases assessed a total of 455 patients and found that slightly more than 50% of patients received monotherapy, and more than 75% of patients had prior biologic use. There was no significant difference in adherence to therapy and persistence with therapy, or with all-cause or RA-related costs in monotherapy versus combination therapy.[117] Another study assessed real-world experience with tofacitinib compared with adalimumab, etanercept, and abatacept in RA patients with one previous biologic DMARD; this study used data from a US commercial database and a Medicare supplemental claims database.[118] Findings included: tofacitinib patients were older than adalimumab patients; the 12-month pre-index use of bDMARDs was greater in tofacitinib patients (77.6%) versus bDMARD cohorts (47.6% to 59.6%); and tofacitinib patients were more likely to receive monotherapy (53.1% vs. 41.4% to 48.3% of bDMARD patients). Persistence and adherence to tofacitinib was similar compared to persistence and adherence to the bDMARDs assessed in this study.

The safety profile of tofacitinib in real-world patients appears to be similar to those reported in the clinical trials, and there have been no unexpected safety events identified in the real-world setting. One study analyzed the worldwide tofacitinib post-marketing surveillance over a 3-year period from 2012 to 2015. Exposure to tofacitinib was estimated to be more than 34,000 patient-years; 25,417 AEs, 102 fatal cases, and 4352 SAEs were reported. The reporting risks (per 100 patient-years) were 2.57 for infections, 0.91 for GI disorders, 0.60 for respiratory disorders, 0.45 for neoplasms, 0.43 for cardiac disorders, and 0.12 for hepatobiliary disorders.[119,120] In the 5-year observational study of Corrona registry patients, tofacitinib initiators experienced comparable age- and sex-adjusted rates of serious infections, cardiovascular events, and malignancies, but they had a higher rate of nonserious herpes zoster than bDMARD and csDMARD initiators.[121]

JAK Inhibitors for Other Rheumatic Diseases

Psoriatic Arthritis

Tofacitinib was approved for use in the United States for treatment of PsA in 2017. This was based largely on the data from two phase III studies, the Oral Psoriatic Arthritis trial (OPAL) Broaden, which assessed tofacitinib versus adalimumab versus placebo in patients with PsA who had previously failed csDMARDs, and the OPAL Beyond trial, which was a study of tofacitinib versus placebo in patients who previously failed TNF inhibitors.[122,123]

The OPAL Broaden trial enrolled 422 patients who had an inadequate response to at least one csDMARD and who were TNF-naïve. This was a 12-month, double-blind, active-controlled and placebo-controlled trial, which compared tofacitinib at 5 mg or 10 mg twice daily doses to adalimumab 40 mg every 2 weeks, or to placebo with a blinded switch at 3 months to either tofacitinib 5 mg or 10 mg. ACR20 response rates at month 3 were 50% in the 5 mg tofacitinib group and 61% in the 10 mg group, as compared with 33% in the placebo group ($p = 0.01$ for the comparison of the 5 mg dose with placebo, and $p < 0.001$ for the 10 mg dose). ACR20 was 52% in the adalimumab group. The active treatment arms also improved significantly in physical function compared to placebo. Researchers observed greater benefit with tofacitinib versus placebo by week 2 (ACR20 of 22% for the 5 mg group and 32% for the 10 mg group, vs. 6% for patients receiving placebo). Minimal Disease Activity (MDA) at week 12 was observed in 26% of patients on tofacitinib (at 5 and 10 mg doses) and 25 % of adalimumab patients, compared to only 7% on placebo.

Seventy-four percent of the patients had psoriasis affecting at least 3% of their body surface area (BSA) and had PASI75 response assessed. Both 5 and 10 mg tofacitinib PASI75 response rates were statistically superior to placebo and similar to adalimumab at week 12. The improvement in the PASI75 persisted at 12 months. Sixty-six percent of the patients had enthesitis, and statistically significant improvement (determined by change in the Leeds Enthesitis index at week 12) was observed for the 10 mg dose but not for the 5 mg dose. Similar improvements in dactylitis were also seen, and improvements in enthesitis and dactylitis were maintained at 1 year.

Over a 12-month period, there were similar rates of SAEs with the tofacitinib 5 mg and 10 mg, and with the adalimumab groups. The SAEs were similar to SAEs reported in studies of tofacitinib in RA, including four cases of herpes zoster in patients who received tofacitinib continuously, versus none of the patients who received placebo or adalimumab. The most common AEs were nasopharyngitis, URI, and headache.

The OPAL Beyond trial was a phase III trial which enrolled 395 patients with a prior inadequate response to at least one TNF inhibitor. Patients had previously failed a mean 1.5 TNF inhibitors, and 8% had received other biologics. This was a 6-month randomized, double-blind trial in which patients were assigned to treatment with tofacitinib (5 mg or 10 mg twice daily) or placebo with a switch at 3 months to either 5 mg or 10 mg of tofacitinib. At week 12, the rates of ACR20 response were 50% with the 5 mg tofacitinib dose and 47% with the 10 mg dose, as compared with 24% with placebo ($p < 0.001$ for both). The mean changes from baseline in HAQ and Disability Index (HAQ-DI) score were −0.39 and −0.35, as compared with −0.14 ($p < 0.001$ for both comparisons). As in the OPAL Broaden trial, ACR20 response was noted to be superior, as early as week 2 of the study, in patients receiving tofacitinib 5 mg or 10 mg versus placebo. Both tofacitinib doses were superior to placebo at 12 weeks for ACR 50 but not ACR 70 response rates. Statistically superior improvement in PASI75 was observed for the 10 mg dose but not the 5 mg dose. Similar improvements in enthesitis and dactylitis for the 5 and 10 mg doses were numerically greater than placebo, but due to hierarchical statistical testing significance was not assessed.

SAEs over the 6 month trial period occurred at similar rates as in other tofacitinib trials (4% in patients who received 5 mg tofacitinib continuously and 6% in patients who received 10 mg continuously). Three cases of herpes zoster were reported in tofacitinib-treated patients. Numerically, more AEs and study discontinuations were reported for the 10 mg dose (8%) compared to the 5 mg dose (3%) and the placebo-treated patients (3%).

A third phase III trial, OPAL Balance, is anticipated to be completed in July 2019.[124] This is a long-term open-label extension study to evaluate the safety, tolerability, and efficacy of tofacitinib in subjects who have previously participated in randomized studies of tofacitinib for PsA.

Baricitinib has been studied in moderate to severe plaque psoriasis. 271 patients were randomized to a 24-week-dose ranging study evaluating 2, 4, 8, and 10 mg daily.[125] Statistically significant improvements in the PASI75 at week 12 were only seen for the 8 and 10 mg doses compared to placebo. Baricitinib has not been evaluated in PsA. Peficitinib was evaluated in a phase II trial in psoriasis but has not been evaluated in PsA.[126]

Upadacitinib is presently in phase III clinical trials for PsA. The trials are evaluating patients who have failed biologics and patients who are biologic naïve.[127] A preliminary presentation reported the results of filgotinib in PsA. 131 patients were enrolled in a 16-week trial to receive 200 mg filgotinib or placebo. Eighty-five percent of the patients were naïve to TNF inhibitors.[128] The ACR20 response was 80% for filgotinib compared to 30% for placebo ($p < 0.001$). ACR50 and ACR70 responses for filgotinib also were statistically superior to placebo.

Systemic Lupus Erythematosus

Pre-clinical Studies

Pre-clinical data suggest that tofacitinib may be of benefit in SLE. One study of experimental lupus nephritis assessed the efficacy of tofacitinib in NZB/NZWF1 mice, a murine model for lupus nephritis. Animals treated with tofacitinib showed significantly reduced proteinuria and improved renal function and histologic lesions of the kidney, including diminished C3 and IgG deposition in glomeruli.[129]

In another pre-clinical study, NZB/NZWF1 mice were treated with tofacitinib and found to have reduced levels of anti–double-stranded DNA (dsDNA) antibodies, decreased proteinuria, and amelioration of nephritis when compared with control animals.[130] A third study found that in MLR/lpr lupus-prone mice, treatment with tofacitinib led to improvement in measures of disease activity, including nephritis, skin inflammation, and autoantibody production. The researchers observed that tofacitinib modulated factors associated with premature vascular damage in SLE, including endothelium-dependent vasorelaxation and endothelial differentiation.[131]

There have been no studies published assessing the efficacy of tofacitinib in human subjects with SLE. There are several studies under way.

Baricitinib

A report of a 24-week phase II, double-blind, placebo-controlled study of baricitinib demonstrated efficacy in patients with SLE receiving standard therapy.[132] Participants were randomly assigned to receive either placebo, baricitinib 2 mg, or baricitinib 4 mg once daily along with continuation of background therapy, which is standard for lupus clinical trials. The primary end point was resolution of arthritis or rash, measured by the SLE Disease Activity Index (SLEDAI-2K) at 24 weeks. Of the 314 participants who were randomly assigned to treatment, 79%, 82%, and 83% completed 24 weeks of treatment with placebo, baricitinib 2 mg, and baricitinib 4 mg, respectively.

A significantly greater percentage of patients in the baricitinib 4 mg group compared to placebo achieved resolution of SLEDAI-2K arthritis or rash (67% vs. 53%; $P < .05$) and had a SLE Responder Index-4 response (64% vs. 48%; $P < .05$) at 24 weeks compared with placebo. In addition, the percentage of patients achieving flare reduction, lupus LDAS, and tender joint count change from baseline were also more improved in the baricitinib 4 mg group compared with placebo.

SAEs were reported in 10 (10%) patients receiving baricitinib 4 mg, 11 (10%) receiving baricitinib 2 mg, and 5 (5%) receiving placebo; no deaths were reported. Serious infections were reported in six (6%) patients with baricitinib 4 mg, two (2%) with baricitinib 2 mg, and one (1%) with placebo.

The investigators concluded that the baricitinib 4 mg dose, but not the 2 mg dose, significantly improved the signs and symptoms of SLE; that dose is presently being investigated in a phase III clinical trial.[133]

Ankylosing Spondylitis

Early clinical studies of tofacitinib in ankylosing spondylitis are promising. A phase II randomized, double-blind, placebo-controlled, dose-ranging study of tofacitinib in patients with ankylosing spondylitis enrolled 207 biologic-naïve participants.[135] Patients were randomized to placebo or tofacitinib 2, 5, or 10 mg twice daily. In this study, patients receiving tofacitinib 5 mg twice daily met criteria for ASAS20 at a rate significantly higher than placebo (80.8% vs. 41.2%; $p < 0.001$). Subjects in the 2 mg and 10 mg twice-daily arms demonstrated greater ASAS20 response than placebo, but this finding did not reach statistical significance. Secondary endpoints generally demonstrated greater improvements with tofacitinib 5 mg and 10 mg twice daily compared with placebo.

A follow-up, post hoc analysis of this study assessed improvement in MRI findings of inflammation.[136] Patients with available radiographic data for MRI of the sacroiliac (SI) joints and spine were assessed for minimally important changes (MIC) of the Spondyloarthritis Research Consortium of Canada (SPARCC) MRI scores. A greater proportion of patients achieved MIC with tofacitinib 2, 5, and 10 mg twice a day versus placebo for SI joint and spine scores. In addition, a greater proportion of patients receiving tofacitinib versus placebo, who achieved MIC for SI joint and spine scores, also achieved ASAS20, versus patients who did not achieve MIC, which indicates a correlation of radiographic response with clinical responses.

A phase III study of tofacitinib in ankylosing spondylitis is ongoing.[137]

A recent press release by Gilead reported that filgotinib 200 mg daily was superior to placebo in ankylosing spondylitis.[138] The primary objective was to evaluate the effect of filgotinib on the signs and symptoms of ankylosing spondylitis as assessed at week 12 by the Ankylosing Spondylitis Disease Activity Score (ASDAS). Patients on filgotinib had a mean change from baseline of −1.5 compared to −0.6 for placebo. 79% on filgotinib achieved ASAS20 response compared to 40% on placebo.

BTK Inhibitors

Oral BTK inhibitors (ibrutinib) have been approved for treatment of patients with mantle cell lymphoma, Waldenstrom's macroglobulinemia, and chronic lymphocytic leukemia who have received at least one previous therapy.[139] BTK inhibitors are in early development as a potential treatment for RA. BTK plays a prominent role in BCR signal transduction and also has a role in Toll-like receptor and FcR signaling in myeloid cells (Fig. 68.10).[140] BTK is a member of the TEC family of cytoplasmic PTKs. In humans, mutations in BTK can result in the development of Bruton's agammaglobulinemia (known also as X-linked agammaglobulinemia),which is an immunodeficiency characterized by a defect in B cell development that results in a significant absence of circulating B cells.[141]

Upon ligand binding to the BCR or FcR, BTK is activated by upstream SRC-family kinases LYN, FYN, and SYK. Activated BTK drives phosphorylation of PLCγ and subsequent PKC activation, which in turn results in calcium flux and the activation of transcription factors, including NF-κB and NFAT, which regulate the expression of downstream genes controlling proliferation, survival, chemokines, and cytokines. B cells play multiple roles in the pathogenesis of RA and SLE, including antigen presentation, inflammatory cytokine production, and rheumatoid factor (RF) and anti-cyclic citrullinated protein antibody (ACPA) production. Rituximab, which depletes B cells, has demonstrated efficacy as treatment for patients with RA; belimumab, for SLE, supports efforts to develop a small molecule BTK inhibitor that impacts B cell activation.[142,143]

Additionally, animal models of arthritis suggest that BTK inhibition can result in a reduction of inflammatory cytokine production from myeloid cells (including TNF, IL-1, and IL-6) by preventing signaling through the FCγRIII receptor.[144,145] Additionally, activated BTK has been demonstrated to be increased in peripheral blood B cells of patients with RA compared with controls.[10] A recent in vitro study demonstrated that BTK inhibition decreased monocyte differentiation into M1 macrophages, which are inflammatory, and skewed differentiation more to an M2 phenotype, which is anti-inflammatory.[146] BTK inhibitors are under development, and two BTK inhibitors (evobrutinib and fenebrutinib) have moved into phase II clinical trials in RA and phase II in SLE.[147–149] These BTK inhibitors bind to BTK in a covalent or noncovalent fashion, and the molecules are highly selective for BTK with limited impact on other kinases. Pre-clinical models demonstrated significant target engagement for these BTK inhibitors under development.[150–152]

PI3K Inhibitors

PI3Ks are lipid kinases that play central role in regulation of cell cycle, apoptosis, DNA repair, senescence, angiogenesis, cellular metabolism, and motility.[153,154] They are intermediate signaling molecules and are best known for their roles in the PI3K/AKT/mammalian target of rapamycin (mTOR) signaling pathway. PI3Ks transmit signals from the cell surface to the cytoplasm by generating second messengers—phosphorylated

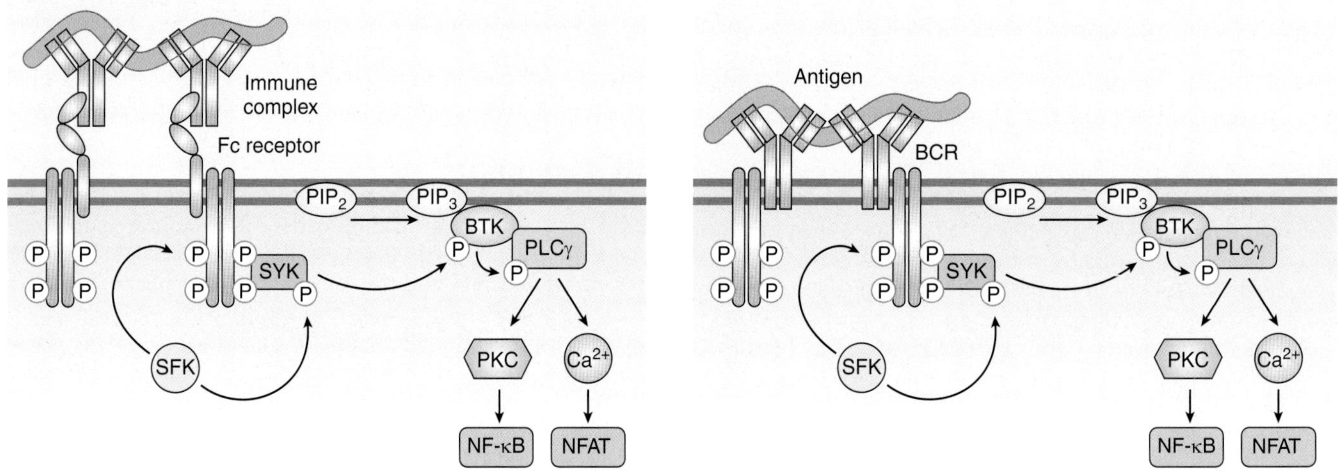

• **Fig. 68.10** Bruton's tyrosine kinase (BTK) signaling pathways after ligand binding to B cell receptor and Fcγ receptor.

phosphatidylinositols—which in turn activate multiple effector kinase pathways, including BTK, AKT, PKC, NF-κB, and JNK/stress-activated protein kinase (SAPK) pathways; this ultimately results in survival and growth of normal cells.

PI3K signaling is mediated by p110 α, β, γ, and δ isoforms. Two isoforms of the catalytic subunits, p110γ and p110δ, are enriched in leukocytes, in which they promote activation, cellular growth, proliferation, differentiation, and survival through the generation of the second messengers phosphatidylinositol biphosphate (PIP2) and phosphatidylinositol triphosphate (PIP3). The functions of PI3K-δ and PI3K-γ in the differentiation, maintenance, and activation of immune cells support an important role for these enzymes in oncology, inflammation, and autoimmunity.[155] Two PI3K-δ inhibitors, idelalisib and copanlisib, are approved for the treatment of chronic lymphocytic leukemia and relapsed follicular lymphoma; a third oral inhibitor of PI3K-γ and PI3K-δ, duvelisib, is approved for refractory chronic lymphocytic leukemia and small lymphocytic lymphoma.[156]

Nonclinical models that utilize animals that are either deficient in PI3K-δ and/or PI3K-γ, or treated with inhibitors of these isoforms of PI3K, established the potential role of PI3K in several inflammatory and autoimmune diseases.[157–159] Treatment of mice with inhibitors of PI3K-δ suggests this enzyme is important in the production of antibodies from marginal-zone B cells and peritoneal B1 cells, which are major sources of autoantibodies in disease. These inhibitors also reduce antigen-specific antibody responses.[160]

Inhibitors of PI3K-δ enzymes have been evaluated in RA; however, to date, no data has been published.

Sphingosine-1-Phosphate Modulators

Sphingosine-1-phosphate (S1P) is an abundant, biologically active lysophospholipid. In the immune system, changes in local S1P concentrations and gradients can modify lymphocyte migration patterns, alter inflammatory cell responses, and affect the barrier function of endothelial cells. Interaction of S1P with its receptor results in inhibition of lymphocyte egress from primary and secondary lymphoid tissues, which results in lymphocyte depletion in the peripheral blood. The major and irreversible route of S1P degradation is via S1P lyase (S1PL). Fingolimod, an S1P receptor modulator, was approved in 2013 for relapsing-remitting multiple sclerosis.

Pre-clinical studies demonstrated that reduced S1PL activity has a significant effect in reducing the inflammatory response in models of RA.[161,162] LX3305, a small-molecule inhibitor of S1PL, was evaluated as a DMARD. Results of a placebo-controlled, dose-ranging phase II RCT of LX3305 in patients with RA with active disease despite MTX treatment have been reported.[163] In the study, 208 patients received 70 mg, 110 mg, or 150 mg daily or placebo for 12 weeks, and the primary endpoint was ACR20 at week 12. Of the patients who received the 150 mg dose, 60% achieved an ACR20 response compared with 49% on placebo, which was not statistically different. Various sub-analyses were conducted, which suggested potential benefits; no significant safety issues were noted. Based on the results of this proof-of-concept study, development in RA was terminated.

Phosphodiesterase Inhibitors

Inhibition of type 4 phosphodiesterase (PDE) exhibits inhibition of TNF production and inhibition of other pro-inflammatory cytokines.[164,165] Cyclic adenosine monophosphate (cAMP) is the principal second messenger responsible for immune response regulation. PDE4 is the main cAMP-degrading enzyme found in cells of the immune system and in keratinocytes. It is the predominant isoenzyme expressed in macrophages, lymphocytes, and neutrophils. Elevation of intra-cellular cAMP inhibits TNF production through the protein kinase A pathway. Three PDE4 inhibitors have been approved to date for treatment of inflammatory diseases: roflumilast for the treatment of severe COPD and asthma symptoms by the EU in 2010 and the United States in 2011; crisaborole, a topical therapy, for treatment of atopic dermatitis by the United States in 2016; apremilast by the FDA for treatment of PsA in March 2014; and plaque psoriasis in September 2014.

Apremilast inhibits production of inducible nitric oxide synthase, and the pro-inflammatory cytokines, IFN-γ, TNF, IL-12, and IL-23.[166] The half-life of apremilast is 6 to 9 hours, which

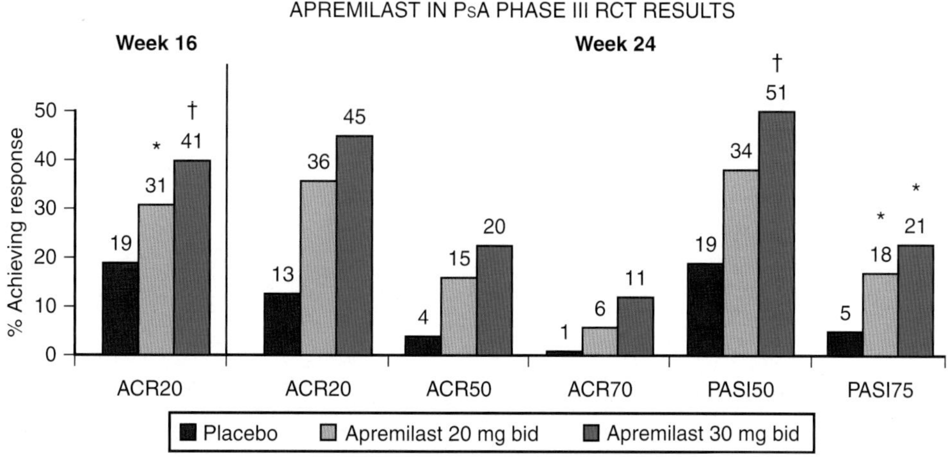

*P <0.02; †P <0.0001
Data from Kavanaugh A, et al.: *Ann Rheum Dis* 73(6):1020-1026, 2014.

• **Fig. 68.11** Apremilast in phase III clinical trials in psoriatic arthritis: clinical outcomes.

necessitates twice-daily dosing. Dosages of apremilast at 20 mg twice daily and 30 mg twice daily were evaluated in three multicenter, randomized, double-blind, placebo-controlled trials of 1493 patients with active PsA.[167,168] Patients were randomly assigned to receive either 20 mg twice daily or 30 mg twice daily. Patients with varied subtypes of PsA were enrolled across the three studies, including symmetric polyarthritis (62.0%), asymmetric oligoarthritis (27.0%), distal interphalangeal (DIP) joint arthritis (6.0%), arthritis mutilans (3.0%), and predominant spondylitis (2.1%). Patients received concomitant therapy with at least one DMARD (65.0%), MTX (55.0%), sulfasalazine (SSZ) (9.0%), leflunomide (LEF) (7.0%), low-dose oral corticosteroids (14.0%), and NSAIDs (71.0%). Prior treatment with nonbiologic DMARDs only was reported in 76.0% of patients, and prior treatment with biologic DMARDs was reported in 22.0% of patients, which includes 9.0% of patients who had not responded to prior biologic DMARD treatment.

ACR20 responses with apremilast 30 mg twice a day were statistically superior to placebo in all three studies. ACR50 and ACR70 responses were numerically greater for apremilast but did not achieve statistical significance (Fig. 68.11). The PASI75 response was 21% for apremilast and 5% for the placebo group. The responses for both skin and arthritis are less robust, in general, than responses with TNF inhibitors.

Long-term safety and efficacy data is now available for apremilast in PsA and psoriasis patients.[169,170] Diarrhea, headache, and nausea were the most commonly reported adverse reactions. The most common adverse reactions leading to discontinuation were nausea (1.8%), diarrhea (1.8%), and headache. The initial dose is titrated from 10 mg daily to 30 mg twice a day during a period of 5 days to reduce the likelihood of GI AEs. The proportion of patients with PsA who discontinued treatment in the trials because of any adverse reaction was 4.6% for patients taking apremilast 30 mg twice a day and 1.2% for patients treated with placebo.

Warnings in the package insert include the possibility of weight loss and depression. Weight loss of 5 to 10 pounds in the PsA clinical trials was reported in 10% of patients treated with apremilast and 3.3% of patients treated with placebo. Depression was seen in a small number of patients with slightly greater frequency than in patients treated with placebo.

Apremilast was evaluated in RA with little efficacy, and development in RA was terminated.[171]

Apremilast 30 mg twice a day was evaluated in a 12-week phase II placebo-controlled clinical trial for Behçet's disease treatment.[172] Patients with two or more oral ulcers were randomized to receive apremilast or placebo. The mean standard deviation (±SD) number of oral ulcers per patient at week 12 was significantly lower in the apremilast group than in the placebo group (0.5±1.0 vs. 2.1±2.6) (P < 0.001). The mean decline in pain from oral ulcers from baseline to week 12 was also greater with apremilast than with placebo. Nausea, vomiting, and diarrhea were more common in the apremilast group than in the placebo group, which is similar to what has been reported in other indications. A preliminary report of a phase III randomized clinical trial evaluating apremilast 30 mg twice a day compared to placebo for 12 weeks has been presented. All patients received apremilast for an additional 52 weeks.[173] 207 patients were enrolled, and the primary endpoint was the area under the curve (AUC) for the number of oral ulcers. AUC was statistically significant at week 12 with apremilast compared to placebo (AUC 129.5 vs 222.1, $P < 0.001$). The most common treatment emergent adverse events (TEAEs) that occurred in 5% or more of patients on apremilast were diarrhea 41%, nausea 19.2%, and headache 14.4%, compared to placebo 19.4%, 10.7%, and 9.7% respectively. Apremilast is not presently approved for Behçet's disease.

Conclusion

The unraveling of the intra-cellular pathways involved in signal transduction, which result in T/B cell activation and inflammatory cytokine production, has resulted in the development of small-molecule inhibitors to these pathways, which can abrogate inflammation in inflammatory diseases. Research demonstrates efficacy similar to biologic DMARDs; acceptable safety profiles in clinical trials, and now long-term extension data, observational registry findings, and real world experience confirms these observations. At a minimum, 4 to 5 JAK inhibitors will be available in clinics for RA treatment. These therapies will be utilized as an alternative to biologics for PsA and possibly for SLE ankylosing spondylitis, pending completion of the clinical trials. BTK inhibitors, which are based on pre-clinical research, could be effective in

RA and SLE; those studies are ongoing. Further studies evaluating comparative utility of these small molecules will enhance our knowledge on best utilization of these therapies in our treatment algorithm.

 Full references for this chapter can be found on ExpertConsult.com.

Selected References

1. Breedveld FC, Weisman MH, Kavanaugh AF, et al.: The PREMIER study: a multicenter, randomized, double-blind clinical trial of combination therapy with adalimumab plus methotrexate versus methotrexate alone or adalimumab alone in patients with early, aggressive rheumatoid arthritis who had not had previous methotrexate treatment, *Arthritis Rheum* 54:26–37, 2003.
2. Goekoop-Ruiterman YP, de Vries-Bouwstra JK, Allaart CF, et al.: Comparison of treatment strategies in early rheumatoid arthritis: a randomized trial, *Ann Intern Med* 146:406–415, 2007.
3. Badjer A, Griswold D, Kapadia R, et al.: A selective inhibitor of mitogen-activated protein kinase, in rat adjuvant arthritis, *Arthritis Rheum* 43:75–83, 2000.
4. Nishikawa M, Myoui A, Tomita T, et al.: Prevention of the onset and progression of collagen-induced arthritis in rats by the potent p38 mitogen-activated protein kinase inhibitor, *Arthritis Rheum* 48:2670–2681, 2003.
5. Chang B, Huang M, Francesco M, et al.: The Bruton tyrosine kinase inhibitor PCI-32765 ameliorates autoimmune arthritis by inhibition of multiple effector cells, *Arthritis Res Ther* 13:R115–R129, 2011.
6. O'Shea JJ, Holland SM, Staudt LM: JAKs and STATs in immunity, immunodeficiency and cancer, *N Engl J Med* 368:161–170, 2013.
7. O'Shea J, Laurence A, McInnes I: Back to the future: oral targeted therapy for RA and other autoimmune diseases, *Nat Rev Rheumatol* 9:173–182, 2013.
8. Ghoreschi K, Laurence A, O'Shea JJ: Janus kinases in immune cell signaling, *Immunol Rev* 228(1):273–287, 2009.
9. Leonard W, O'Shea J: JAKs and STATs: biological implications, *Ann Rev Immunol* 16:293–322, 1998.
10. O'Shea J, Plenge R: JAK and STAT signaling molecules in immunoregulation and immune-mediated disease, *Immunity* 36:542–550, 2012.
11. Yablonski D, Weiss A: Mechanisms of signaling by the hematopoietic-specific adaptor proteins, SLP-76 and LAT and their B cell counterpart, BLNK/SLP-65, *Adv Immunol* 79:93–128, 2001.
12. Karaman MW, et al.: A quantitative analysis of kinase inhibitor selectivity, *Nat Biotechnol* 26:127–132, 2008.
13. Ghoreschi K, Laurence A, O'Shea J: Selectivity and therapeutic inhibition of kinases: to be or not to be? *Nat Immunol* 10:356–360, 2009.
14. Druker BJ, Guilhot F, O'Brien SG: Five-year follow-up of patients receiving imatinib for chronic myeloid leukemia, *N Engl J Med* 355(23):2408–2417, 2006.
15. Kantarjian H, Shah N, Hochhaus A, et al.: Dasatinib versus imatinib in newly diagnosed chronic-phase chronic myeloid leukemia, *N Engl J Med* 362:2260–2270, 2010.
16. Lee J, Laydon J, McDonnell P, et al.: A protein kinase involved in the regulation of inflammatory cytokine biosynthesis, *Nature* 372:739–746, 1994.
17. Schett G, Tohidast-Akrad M, Smolen J, et al.: Activation, differential location and regulation of the stress-activated protein kinases, extracellular signal-regulated kinase, c-JUN N terminal kinase, and P38 mitogen activated protein kinase, in synovial tissue and cells in rheumatoid arthritis, *Arthritis Rheum* 43:2501–2512, 2000.
18. Sweeny S, Firestein G: Primer: signal transduction in rheumatic disease-a clinician's guide, *Nat Clin Pract Rheumatol* 3:651–660, 2007.
19. Remy G, Risco A, Inesta-Vaquera F, et al.: Differential activation of p38 MAPK isoforms by MKK3 and MKK6, *Cell Signal* 22(4):660–667, 2010.
20. Schett G, Zwerina J, Friestein G, et al.: The p38 mitogen-activated protein kinase (MAPK) pathway in rheumatoid arthritis, *Ann Rheum Dis* 67:909–916, 2008.
21. Pawson T: Protein modules and signaling networks, *Nature* 373:573–580, 1995.
22. Dominguez C, Powers D, Tarnayo N: p38 MAP kinase inhibitors: many are made, but few are chosen, *Curr Opinion Drug Discov Devel* 8:421–430, 2005.
23. Kumar S, Boehm J, Lee J, et al.: p38 MAP kinases: key signaling molecules as therapeutic targets for inflammatory disease, *Nat Rev Drug Discov* 2:717–726, 2003.
24. Genovese M, Cohen S, Wofsy D, et al.: A 24 week, randomized, double blind, placebo controlled trial, parallel study of the efficacy of oral SCIO-569, a p38 mitogen activated protein kinase inhibitor, in patients with active rheumatoid arthritis, *J Rheumatol* 38(50):846–854, 2011.
25. Cohen SB, Cheng TT, Chindalore V, et al.: Evaluation of the efficacy and safety of pamapimod, a p38 MAP kinase inhibitor, in a double-blind, methotrexate-controlled study of patients with active rheumatoid arthritis, *Arthritis Rheum* 60:1232–1241, 2009.
26. Alten RE, Zerbini C, Jeka S, et al.: Efficacy and safety of pamapimod in patients with active rheumatoid arthritis receiving stable methotrexate therapy, *Ann Rheum Dis* 69(2):364–367, 2010.
27. Damjanov N, Kauffman R, Spencer-Green G, et al.: Efficacy, pharmacodynamics, and safety of VX-702, a novel p38 MAPK inhibitor, in rheumatoid arthritis: results of two randomized double blind placebo-controlled studies, *Arthritis Rheum* 60(5):1232–1241, 2009.
28. Genovese M: Inhibition of p38: has the fat lady sung? *Arthr Rheum* 60:317–320, 2009.
29. Hammaker D, Firestein G: "Go upstream, young man"—lessons learned from the p38 saga, *Ann Rheum Dis* 69:i77–i82, 2009.
30. Guo X, Gerl RE, Schrader JW: Defining the involvement of p38alpha MAPK in the production of anti- and proinflammatory cytokines using an SB 203580-resistant form of the kinase, *J Biol Chem* 278:22237–22242, 2003.
31. Kay J, Morales R, Bellatin L, et al.: *Treatment of rheumatoid arthritis with a MEK kinase inhibitor: results of a 12-week randomized, placebo-controlled phase 2 study in patients with active RA on a background of methotrexate*, EULAR meeting, Abstract OP0013. 2010.
32. Sada K, Takano T, Yanagi S, et al.: Structure and function of Syk protein-tyrosine kinase, *J Biochem* 130:177–186, 2001.
33. Furumoto Y, Nunomura S, Terada T, et al.: The Fc-epsilon RIbeta immunoreceptor tyrosine-based activation motif exerts inhibitory control on MAPK and IkappaB kinase phosphorylation and mast cell cytokine production, *J Biol Chem* 279:49177–49187, 2004.
34. Mocsai A, Ruland J, Tybulewicz V: The SYK tyrosine kinase: a crucial player in diverse biological functions, *Nat Rev Immunol* 10(6):387–402, 2010.
35. Bajpai M, Chopra P, Dastidar SG, et al.: Spleen tyrosine kinase: a novel target for therapeutic intervention of rheumatoid arthritis, *Expert Opin Investig Drugs* 17:641–659, 2008.
36. Pine PR, Chang B, Schoettler N, et al.: Inflammation and bone erosion are suppressed in models of rheumatoid arthritis following treatment with a novel Syk inhibitor, *Clin Immunol* 124:244–257, 2007.
37. Cha HS, Boyle DL, Inoue T, et al.: A novel spleen tyrosine kinase inhibitor bloc ks c-Jun N-terminal kinase-mediated gene expression in synoviocytes, *J Pharmacol Exp Ther* 317:571–578, 2006.
38. Braselmann S, Taylor V, Zhao H, et al.: R406, an orally available spleen tyrosine kinase inhibitor blocks fc receptor signaling and reduces immune complex-mediated inflammation, *J Pharmacol Exp Ther* 319:998–1008, 2006.
39. Singh R, Masuda ES: Spleen tyrosine kinase (Syk) biology, inhibitors and therapeutic applications, *Annu Rep Med Chem* 42:379–391, 2007.
40. Weinblatt ME, Kavanaugh A, Burgos-Vargas R, et al.: Treatment of rheumatoid arthritis with a Syk inhibitor, *Arthritis and Rheum* 58:3309–3318, 2008.
41. Weinblatt ME, Kavanaugh A, Genovese MC, et al.: An oral spleen tyrosine kinase (Syk) inhibitor for rheumatoid arthritis, *N Engl J Med* 363:1303–1312, 2010.

42. Taylor P, Genovese M, Greenwood M, et al.: OSKIRA-4: a phase IIb randomised, placebo-controlled study of the efficacy and safety of fostamatinib monotherapy, *Ann Rheum Dis* 74(12):2123–2129, 2015.
43. Genovese MC, Kavanaugh A, Weinblatt ME, et al.: An oral Syk kinase in the treatment of rheumatoid arthritis—a three-month randomized, placebo controlled, phase II study in patients with active rheumatoid arthritis that did not respond to biologic agents, *Arthritis Rheum* 63:337–345, 2011.
44. Weinblatt M, Genovese M, Ho M, et al.: Effects of fostamatinib, an oral spleen tyrosine kinase inhibitor, in rheumatoid arthritis patients with an inadequate response to methotrexate: results from a phase III, multicenter, randomized, double-blind, placebo-controlled, parallel-group study, *Arthritis Rheum* 66(12):3255–3264, 2014.
45. Kavanaugh A, Weinblatt M, Genovese M, et al.: Longer-term safety of fostamatinib (R788) in patients with rheumatoid arthritis—analysis of clinical trial data from up to 2 years of exposure. Abstract 2594. ACR/ARHP Annual Meeting, November 4–9, 2011, Chicago.
46. Merck Sharp & Dohme Corp: Safety and efficacy of MK-8457 and methotrexate (MTX) in participants with active rheumatoid arthritis despite MTX therapy (MK-8457-008). In ClinicalTrials.gov. Available at https://clinicaltrials.gov/ct2/results?term=nct01569152.
47. Merck Sharp & Dohme Corp: A randomized, double-blind, placebo-controlled, parallel-group, multicenter trial to evaluate the safety, tolerability, and efficacy of MK-8457 in participants with rheumatoid arthritis (MK-8457-010). In ClinicalTrials.gov. Available at https://clinicaltrials.gov/ct2/results?term=NCT01651936.
48. Van Vollenhoven R, Cohen S, Mease P: Efficacy and safety of MK-8457, a novel SYK inhibitor for the treatment of rheumatoid arthritis in two randomized, controlled, phase 2 studies. Abstract 1528. ACR/ARHP Annual Meeting, November 14–19, 2014, Boston.
49. Ghoreschi K, Laurence A, O'Shea JJ: Janus kinases in immune cell signaling, *Immunol Rev* 228:273–287, 2009.
50. Darnell JE, Kerr I, Stark G: JAK-STAT pathways and transcriptional activation in response to IFNs and other extracellular signaling proteins, *Science* 264:1415–1421, 1994.
51. Pesu M, Candotti F, Husa M, et al.: Jak3, severe combined immunodeficiency, and a new class of immunosuppressive drugs, *Immunol Rev* 203:127–142, 2005.
52. Levine RL, Wadleigh M, Cools J, et al.: Activating mutation in the tyrosine kinase Jak2 in polycythemia vera, essential thrombocythemia, and myeloid metaplasia with myelofibrosis, *Cancer Cell* 7:387–397, 2005.
53. Harrison C, Kiladjian J, Al-Ali H, et al.: JAK Inhibition with ruxolitinib versus best available therapy for myelofibrosis, *N Engl J Med* 366(9):787–798, 2012.
54. Tokumasa N, Suto A, Kagami S, et al.: Expression of Tyk2 in dendritic cells is required for IL-12, Il-23 and IFN-gamma production and the induction of Th1 cell differentiation, *Blood* 110:553–560, 2007.
55. Kahn C, Cohen S, Bradley J, et al.: Tofacitinib for rheumatoid arthritis, Tofacitinib Arthritis Advisory Committee Meeting, May 9, 2012, Silver Spring, MD.
56. Changelian P, Moshinsky D, Kuhn C, et al.: The specificity of Jak3 kinase inhibitors, *Blood* 15:2155–2157, 2008.
57. Conklyn M, Andresen C, Changelian P, et al.: The Jak 3 inhibitor, CP-690,550 selectively reduces NK and CD8+ cell numbers in cynomolgus monkey blood following chronic oral dosing, *J Leukoc Biol* 6:1248–1254, 2004.
58. Genovese M, Kawabata T, Soma K, et al.: Reversibility of pharmacodynamics effects after short- and long-term treatment with tofacitinib in patients with rheumatoid arthritis, *ACR Meeting*, 2013, abstract 438.
59. Ghoreschi K, Jesson M, Li X: Modulation of innate and adaptive immune responses by tofacitinib (CP-690,550), *J Immunol* 186:4234–4243, 2011.
60. Parmentier J, Voss J, Graff C et al.: In vitro and in vivo characterization of the JAK1 selectivity of upadacitinib (ABT-494), *BMC Rheumatology* 20182:23.
61. Namour F, Diderichsen P, Cox E, et al.: Pharmacokinetics and pharmacokinetic/pharmacodynamic modeling of filgotinib (GLPG0634), a selective JAK1 inhibitor, in support of phase IIB dose selection, *Clin Pharmacokinet* 54(8):859–874, 2015.
62. Cao Y, Sawamoto T, Valluri U, et al.: Pharmacokinetics, pharmacodynamics, and safety of ASP015K, (Peficitinib), a new janus kinase inhibitor, in healthy subjects, *Clin Pharma in Drug Development* 5(6):435–449, 2016.
63. Clark JD, Flanagan ME, Telliez JB: Discovery and development of Janus kinase (JAK) inhibitors for inflammatory diseases, *J Med Chem* 57(12):5023–5038, 2014.
64. Dowty M, Lin T, Wang L, et al.: Lack of differentiation of janus kinase inhibitors in rheumatoid arthritis based on janus kinase pharmacology and clinically meaningful concentrations. Abstract OP0147. EULAR Annual Meeting, June 11–14, 2014, Paris.
65. Fleischmann R, Kremer J, Cush J, et al.: Placebo-controlled trial of tofacitinib monotherapy in rheumatoid arthritis, *N Engl J Med* 367:495–507, 2012.
66. Kremer J, Li ZG, Hall S, et al.: Tofacitinib in combination with nonbiologic disease-modifying antirheumatic drugs in patients with active rheumatoid arthritis: a randomized trial, *Ann Intern Med* 159:253–261, 2013.
67. van Vollenhoven RF, Fleischmann R, Cohen, et al.: Tofacitinib or adalimumab versus placebo in rheumatoid arthritis, *N Engl J Med* 367:508–51928, 2012.
68. Burmester GR, Blanco R, Charles-Schoeman C, et al.: Tofacitinib (CP-690,550) in combination with methotrexate in patients with active rheumatoid arthritis with an inadequate response to tumour necrosis factor inhibitors: a randomised phase 3 trial, *Lancet* 381(9865):451–460, 2013.
69. van der Heijde D, Tanaka Y, Fleischmann R, et al.: Tofacitinib (CP-690,550) in patients with rheumatoid arthritis receiving methotrexate:twelve-month data from a twenty-four-month phase III randomized radiographic study, *Arthritis Rheum* 65:559–570, 2013.
70. Lee EB, Fleischmann R, Hall, et al.: Tofacitinib versus methotrexate in rheumatoid arthritis, *N Engl J Med* 370:2377–2386, 2014.
71. Genovese M, Kremer J, Zamani O, et al.: Baricitinib in patients with refractory rheumatoid arthritis, *NEJM*, 2017.
72. Fleischmann R, Schiff M, van der Heide, et al.: Baricitinib, methotrexate, or combination in patients with rheumatoid arthritis and no or limited prior disease-modifying antirheumatic drug treatment, *Arthritis Rheumatol* 69(3):506–517, 2017.
73. Dougados M, van der Heide D, Chen YC, et al.: Baricitinib in patients with inadequate response or intolerance to conventional synthetic DMARDs: results from the RA-BUILD study, *Ann Rheum Dis* 76:88–95, 2017.
74. Smolen J, Kremer J, Gaich C, et al.: Patient-reported outcomes from a randomised phase III study of baricitinib in patients with rheumatoid arthritis and an inadequate response to biological agents (RA-BEACON), *Ann Rheum Dis* 0:1–7, 2016.
75. Genovese M, Fleischmann R, Combe B, et al.: Safety and efficacy of upadacitinib in patients with active rheumatoid arthritis refractory to biologic disease-modifying anti-rheumatic drugs (SELECT-BEYOND): a double-blind, randomised controlled phase 3 trial, *Lancet* 391:2513–2524, 2018.
76. Burmester G, Kremer J, van den Bosch, et al.: Safety and efficacy of upadacitinib in patients with rheumatoid arthritis and inadequate response to conventional synthetic disease-modifying anti-rheumatic drugs (SELECT-NEXT): a randomised, double-blind,placebo-controlled phase 3 trial, *Lancet* 391:2503–2512, 2018.
77. Smolen J, Cohen S, Emery P, et al.: *Upadacitinib as Monotherapy: a phase 3 randomized controlled Double-Blind study in patients with active rheumatoid arthritis and Inadequate Response to methotrexate*, 2018. ACR meeting abstract 889.
78. Fleischmann R, Pangan A, Mysler E, et al.: *A phase 3, randomized double-blind study Comparing upadacitinib to placebo and to adalimumab. Patients with active rheumatoid arthritis with Inadequate Response to methotrexate*, 2018. ACR meeting abstract 890.
79. Clintrials.gov-upadacitinib
80. Genovese M, Greenwald M, Codding C, et al.: Peficitinib, a JAK inhibitor, in combination with limited conventional synthetic disease-modifying antirheumatic drugs in the treatment of moderate-to-severe rheumatoid arthritis, *Arth and Rheum* 69:932–942, 2017.

81. Kivitz A, Gutierrez-Urena R, et al.: Peficitinib, a JAK inhibitor, in the treatment of moderate-to-severe rheumatoid arthritis in patients with an inadequate response to methotrexate, *Arth and Rheum* 2017(69):709–719, 2017.
82. Tanaka Y, Takeuchi T, Tanaka S, et al.: *Efficacy and Safety of the novel Oral janus kinase inhibitor, Peficitinib in a phase 3, Double-Blind, placebo Controlled, Randomized study of patients with RA who had an Inadequate Response to DMARDs*, 2018. ACR meeting, abstract 887.
83. Takeuchi T, Tanaka Y, Tanaka S, et al.: *Efficacy and Safety of the novel Oral janus kinase inhibitor, Peficitinib in a phase 3, Double-Blind, placebo Controlled, Randomized study of patients with RA who had an Inadequate Response to methotrexate*, 2018. ACR meeting, abstract 888.
84. Genovese M, Kalunian K, Walker D, et al.: *Safety and Efficacy of Filgotinib in a phase 3 Trial of patients with active rheumatoid Arthritis and Inadequate Response or Intolerance to Biologic Dmard*, 2018. ACR meeting, abstract L06.
85. Cohen S, Tanaka Y, Mariette X, et al.: *Long-term Safety of Tofacitinib up to 9.5 Years: a Comprehensive Integrated Analysis of the rheumatoid arthritis Clinical Development Program*, 2018. ACR meeting, abstract 963.
86. Kavanaugh A, Genovese M, Winthrop, et al.: *Rheumatoid arthritis Treatment with Filgotinib: week 132 Safety Data from a phase 2b Open-Label extension study*, ACR meeting, 2018. Abstract 2551.
87. Genovese M, Smolen J, Takeuchi T, et al.: *Safety Profile of Baricitinib for the Treatment of rheumatoid arthritis up to 6 Years: an Updated Integrated Safety Analysis*, ACR meeting, 2018. Abstract 962.
88. Fleischmann R, Mysler E, Hall S, et al.: Efficacy and safety of tofacitinib monotherapy, tofacitinib with methotrexate, and adalimumab with methotrexate in patients with rheumatoid arthritis (ORAL Strategy): a phase 3b/4, double-blind, head-to-head, randomised controlled trial, *Lancet* 390:457–468, 2017.
89. Lamba M, Wang R, Fletcher T et al. Evaluation of a single- dose and steady state pharmacokinetics, pharmacodynamics, bioavailibity and tolerability of the modified release formulation of tofacitinib versus the immediate release formulation of tofacitinib in healthy volunteers. EULAR meeting. Abstract THU0188.
90. Tanaka Y, Sugiyama N, Toyuizumi S: Modified- versus immediate-release tofacitinib in Japanese rheumatoid arthritis patients: a randomized, phase III, non-inferiority study, *Rheumatology* 1–10, 2017.
91. Cohen S, Litman H, Chen C, et al.: *Clinical Effectiveness of Tofacitinib 11 mg once Daily versus Tofacitinib 5 mg twice daily in the Corrona US RA Registry*, ACR Meeting 2018, abstract 580.
92. Dowty M, Jesson M, Ghosh S, et al.: Preclinical to clinical translation of tofacitinib, a Janus kinase inhibitor, in rheumatoid arthritis, *J Pharmacol Exp Ther* 348(1):165–173, 2014.
93. Shi JG, Chen X, Lee F, et al.: The pharmacokinetics, pharmacodynamics, and safety of baricitinib, an oral Jak1/2 inhibitor in healthy volunteers, *J Clin Pharmacol* 54(12):1354–1361, 2014.
94. Tanaka Y, Mcinnes I, Taylor P, et al.: Characterization and changes of lymphocyte subsets in baricitinib–treated patients with rheumatoid arthritis, *Arth and Rheum* 70(12):1923–1932, 2018.
95. Kremer JM, Emery P, Camp HS, et al.: A Phase 2b study of ABT-494, a selective JAK1 inhibitor, in patients with rheumatoid arthritis and an inadequate response to anti-TNF therapy, *Arthritis Rheumatol*, 2016. July 7 [Epub ahead of print].
96. Genovese MC, Smolen JS, Weinblatt ME, et al.: A randomized Phase 2b study of ABT-494, a selective JAK1 inhibitor in patients with rheumatoid arthritis and an inadequate response to methotrexate, *Arthritis Rheumatol*, 2016. July 7 [Epub ahead of print].
97. Mohamed M, Zeng J, Marroum P, et al.: Pharmacokinetics of upadacitinib with the clinical regimens of the extended-release formulation utilized in rheumatoid arthritis phase 3 trials, *Clin Pharmacol Drug Dev* 8:208–216, 2019.
98. Galien R, Brys R, Van der Aa A, et al.: *Absence of Effects of Filgotinib on Erythrocytes, CD8+ and NK cells in rheumatoid arthritis patients Brings Further Evidence for the JAK1 Selectivity of Filgotinib*, ACR meeting 2015, abstract 2781.
99. Kremer J, Cohen S, Wilkinson B, et al.: A phase llb dose ranging study of the oral JAK inhibitor tofacitinib (CP-669,550) versus placebo in combination with methotrexate in patients with active rheumatoid arthritis and inadequate response to methotrexate alone, *Arthritis Rheum* 64(4):970–981, 2012.
100. Kremer J, Bloom B, Breedveld F, et al.: The safety and efficacy of a JAK inhibitor in patients with active rheumatoid arthritis; results of a double-blind placebo controlled phase lla trial of three dosage levels of CP-669,550 versus placebo, *Arthritis Rheum* 60:1895–1905, 2009.
101. Keystone EC, Taylor PC, Drescher E, et al.: Safety and efficacy of baricitinib at 24 weeks in patients with rheumatoid arthritis who have had an inadequate response to methotrexate, *Ann Rheum Dis* 74:333–340, 2015.
102. Tanaka Y, Emoto K, Cai Z, et al.: Efficacy and safety of baricitinib in Japanese patients with active rheumatoid arthritis receiving background methotrexate therapy: a 12-week, double-blind, randomized placebo-controlled study, *J Rheumatol* 43:504–511, 2016.
103. Westhovens R, Taylor P, Alten R, et al.: Filgotinib (GLPG0634/GS-6034), an oral JAK1 selective inhibitor, is effective in combination with methotrexate (MTX) in patients with active rheumatoid arthritis and insufficient response to MTX: results from a randomised, dose-finding study (Darwin 1), *Ann Rheum Dis* 76:998–1008, 2017.
104. Kavanaugh A, Kremer J, Ponce L, et al.: Filgotinib (GLPG0634/GS-6034), an oral selective JAK1 inhibitor, is effective as monotherapy in patients with active rheumatoid arthritis: results from a randomised, dose-finding study (Darwin 2), *Ann Rheum Dis* 76:1009–1019, 2017.
105. Cohen S, Radoninski S, Gomez-Reino J, et al.: Analysis of infections and all-cause mortality in phase ll, lll and long-term extension studies of tofacitinib in patients with rheumatoid arthritis, *Arthritis Rheum* 66(11):2924–2937, 2014.
106. FDA Tofacitinib Advisory Board meeting, 2012.
107. Sandborn W, Su C, Sands B, et al.: Tofacitinib as induction and maintenance therapy for ulcerative colitis, *NEJM* 376:1723–1736, 2017.
108. Mease P, Kremer J, Cohen S, et al.: *Incidence of Thromboembolic Events in Tofacitinib rheumatoid arthritis*, Psoriasis, 2017, Psoriatic Arthritis and Ulcerative Colitis Development program. ACR meeting, abstract 16L.
109. Winthrop K, Yamanaka H, Valdez, et al.: *Herpes zoster and tofacitinib therapy in patients with rheumatoid arthritis*, vol. 66. 2014, pp 2675–2684.
110. Weinblatt M, Taylor P, Burmester G, et al.: *Cardiovascular Safety-Update from up to 6 Years of Treatment with Baricitinib in rheumatoid arthritis Clinical Trials*, 2018. ACR meeting, abstract 2815.
111. FDA Baricitinib Arthritis Advisory Board, 2018.
112. ClinicalTrialsgovidentifier NCT01932372
113. Mcinnes I, Kim H, Lee S, et al.: Open-label tofacitinib and double blind atorvastatinin rheumatoid arthritis patients: a randomized study, *Ann Rheum Dis* 73:124–131, 2014.
114. Isaacs J, Zuckerman A, Krishnaswami S, et al.: Changes in serum creatinine in patients with active rheumatoid arthritis treated with tofacitinib:results from clinical trials, *Arth Res Ther*, 2014.
115. Kilcher G, Hummel N, et al.: Rheumatoid arthritis patients treated in trial and real world settings: comparison of randomized trials with registries, *Rheumatology (Oxford)* 57:354–369, 2018.
116. Kremer J, Cappelli L, et al.: Real-world data from a post-approval safety surveillance study of tofacitinib vs biologic DMARDs and conventional synthetic DMARDs: five-year results from a US-based rheumatoid arthritis registry, *Arthritis Rheumatol* 70(Suppl 10), 2018.
117. Harnett J, Curtis JR, et al.: Initial experience with tofacitinib in clinical practice: treatment patterns and costs of tofacitinib administered as monotherapy or in combination with conventional synthetic DMARDs in 2 US health care claims databases, *Clin Ther* 38(6):1451–1463, 2016.
118. Harnett J, Gerber R, et al.: Evaluation of real-world experience with tofacitinib Compared with adalimumab, Etanercept, and Abatacept in RA patients with 1 previous biologic DMARD: data from a U.S. administrative claims database, *J Manag Care Spec Pharm* 22(12):1457–1471, 2016.
119. Cohen S, Curtis J, et al.: Worldwide, 3-year, post-marketing surveillance experience with tofacitinib in rheumatoid, *Arthritis Rheumatol Ther* 5(1):283–291, 2018.
120. Caporali R, Zavaglia D: Real-world experience with tofacitinib for treatment of rheumatoid arthritis, *Clin Exp Rheumatol*, 2018 Aug 29. [Epub ahead of print]).

69 Urate-Lowering Therapy

TED R. MIKULS

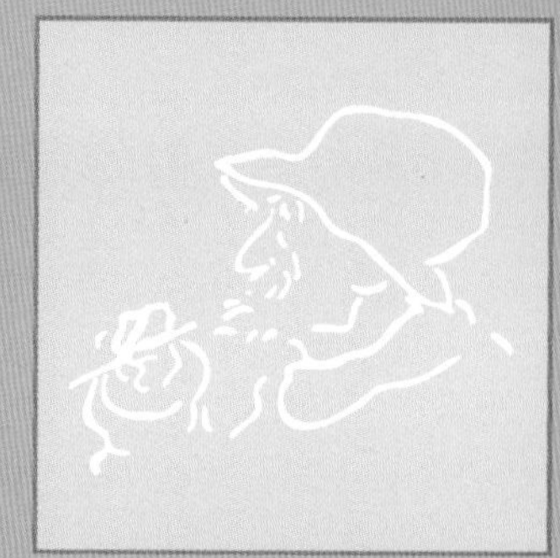

KEY POINTS

Urate-lowering therapy (ULT) is central to the management of hyperuricemia in gout.

The goal of ULT in gout is to reduce the frequency of flares and prevent progressive joint destruction and tophaceous deposition. This goal can be achieved by lowering and maintaining serum urate (sUA) concentrations to less than 5 to 6 mg/dL.

Optimal ULT requires careful patient selection with attention to comorbid illness, ongoing education, adoption of a treat-to-target approach, and effective anti-inflammatory prophylaxis with treatment initiation.

Introduction

The long-term management of gout is based primarily on the optimal use of urate-lowering therapy (ULT). Available ULT classes include (1) xanthine oxidase (XO) inhibitors (allopurinol and febuxostat); (2) uricosurics (probenecid, lesinurad, benzbromarone, and sulfinpyrazone); and (3) uricases (pegloticase) (Table 69.1). This chapter focuses primarily on the most common rheumatic indication for ULT, the treatment of hyperuricemia in gout.

Nonpharmacologic Treatment of Hyperuricemia

The importance of education and lifestyle advice, including weight loss, select dietary restrictions, and reduced alcohol intake, is consistently emphasized in gout management guidelines.[1,2] Despite a growing list of dietary factors implicated in hyperuricemia and gout, investigations of dietary interventions on health outcomes in gout are lacking. Furthermore, evidence suggests that such interventions in isolation yield modest results and suffer from a lack of widespread patient acceptance and long-term adherence.[3] In addition to dietary modifications, which include reducing the intake of dietary purines (particularly meats and seafood), fructose, beer, and liquor, weight loss represents an important goal for overweight gout patients. Although even modest amounts of weight loss can be important to overall health, resulting reductions in serum urate (sUA) are modest[4] and insufficient in many patients with gout. Among a small group of morbidly obese patients with gout, bariatric surgery resulted in an approximate 25% reduction in mean sUA accompanying an average postsurgical weight loss of 34 kg, suggesting that larger amounts of weight loss might render more meaningful sUA reductions.[5]

Patient Selection, Timing of Treatment Initiation, and Asymptomatic Hyperuricemia

Hyperuricemia should be treated in patients with gout with recurrent and frequent flares, tophi, and/or radiographic changes consistent with gout.[1,2] Although it has long been suggested that ULT should be initiated only after flare resolution (with the rationale that its earlier initiation could amplify the duration and magnitude of symptoms), this dogma has been challenged. In a randomized controlled study of 57 men with gout, allopurinol initiation during a flare resulted in no differences in pain or the occurrence of recurrent gout flares compared with placebo when administered with background anti-inflammatory agents.[6] Importantly, the development of a gout flare that complicates ongoing ULT is not an indication to discontinue ULT. Results from a cost-effectiveness analysis in nontophaceous gout, involving a hypothetical patient cohort, suggest that the institution of allopurinol is cost effective in patients seen with two or more acute gout flares within a 1-year period.[7] Traditionally reserved for those with well-established disease, at least one recent study suggests that the initiation of ULT earlier in the disease course may yield substantial benefit. In a two-year, double-blind, placebo-controlled study of 314 gout patients with a history of only 1 or 2 lifetime flares, the initiation and titration of febuxostat led to significant declines in flare incidence as well as reductions in synovitis detected by MRI.[8]

In addition to its initiation earlier in the course of gout, there has been substantial speculation regarding the potential role of ULT in individuals with asymptomatic hyperuricemia (see Chapter 100), particularly given hypotheses of a protective benefit in cardiovascular (CVD) and chronic kidney disease (CKD). Two studies examining the use of febuxostat in asymptomatic hyperuricemia have yielded conflicting results. The first, involving patients with stage 3 CKD, demonstrated no benefit of febuxostat over placebo in preserving renal function over 2 years of follow-up.[9] In contrast, a randomized open-label study of more than 1000 older individuals (>65 years) with asymptomatic hyperuricemia suggested benefit with ULT. Specifically, febuxostat therapy (vs. no therapy or allopurinol 100 mg daily) was associated with a 25% reduction (hazard ratio [HR] 0.75; 95% confidence interval [CI], 0.59 to 0.95) in the composite endpoint of death from any cause, cerebrovascular disease, nonfatal coronary artery disease, heart failure, other arteriosclerotic disease, atrial fibrillation, or renal impairment.[10] The benefit of ULT in this study appeared to be primarily driven by lower rates of renal impairment. Although provocative, additional studies will be needed to define the role of ULT in these populations, particularly in light of data suggesting that different agents render different effects in terms of cardiovascular or renal disease risk.[11,12]

TABLE 69.1 Dosing and Safety Information for Currently Available Urate-Lowering Therapies in the Management of Gout

	Dose	Route/ Schedule	Half-Life	Primary Site of Metabolism/Elimination	Adverse Effects	Contraindications (C)/Drug Interactions (DI)
Xanthine Oxidase Inhibitors						
Allopurinol	50-900 mg	PO/daily	1-2 hr (half-life of active metabolite oxypurinol 15-30 hr)	Met: Hepatic xanthine oxidase and aldehyde oxidase (into oxypurinol) Elim: Renal (renal dosing may be required)	Common: Gout flare; skin rash; nausea; diarrhea; LFT abnormalities Rare: Allopurinol hypersensitivity syndrome (AHS) (more common in HLA-B*5801+); cytopenias	C: Concomitant azathioprine, 6-MP, theophylline, prior hypersensitivity DI: Azathioprine, 6-MP, theophylline, ampicillin/amoxicillin, uricosurics, thiazides, cyclosporine, warfarin, ACE inhibitors (possible), Dilantin, cyclophosphamide, vidarabine
Febuxostat	40-120 mg	PO/daily	6-8 hr	Met: Hepatic (glucuronyl conjugation and oxidation via Cyt P450) Elim: Hepatic and renal	Common: Gout flare; skin rash; nausea; arthralgias; LFT abnormalities Rare: Cardiovascular events (unclear association); cytopenias	C: Concomitant azathioprine, 6-MP, theophylline, prior hypersensitivity; severe hepatic impairment DI: Azathioprine, 6-MP, theophylline
Uricosurics					[a]Adverse effects, contraindications, drug interactions similar for available uricosurics—grouped together below	
Probenecid	500-2000 mg	PO/bid	3-8 hr (500 mg); 6-12 hr (larger doses)	Met: Hepatic (hydroxylation) Elim: Hepatic and renal	Common: Gout flare; nephrolithiasis; rash; flushing; nausea; loss of appetite; renal dysfunction (particularly for lesinurad when dose as monotherapy) Rare: Cytopenias, nephrotic syndrome, anaphylaxis, back pain (rare reports of hepatotoxicity with benzbromarone)	C: Prior hypersensitivity; nephrolithiasis; UA overexcretion; concomitantly with other cancer therapies; known blood dyscrasias; active peptic ulcer disease; sulfinpyrazone should be avoided in patients with phenylbutazone/pyrazole allergy DI (more extensive for probenecid/sulfinpyrazone then benzbromarone or lesinurad): allopurinol, NSAIDs, salicylates, penicillins, cephalosporins, fluoroquinolones, imipenem, rifampin, nitrofurantoin, sulfonamides, heparin, dapsone, acyclovir, ganciclovir, zidovudine, alcohol, diazoxide, mecamylamine, pyrazinamide, antineoplastic agents, clofibrate; dyphylline, diuretics, benzodiazepines, methotrexate, riboflavin, thiopental, sildenafil[b], amlodipine[b], statins[b], colchicine[b]
Lesinurad (dosed with allopurinol or febuxostat)	200 mg	PO/daily	1-3 hr	Met: Hepatic (CYP2C9) and renal (30%-40% excreted unchanged)		
Sulfinpyrazone	200-800 mg	PO/bid	3-12 hr	Met: Hepatic (CYP2C9) Elim: Hepatic and renal		
Benzbromarone	50-200 mg	PO/daily	3 hr (half-life of active metabolite 6-hydroxybenzbromarone ~30 hr)	Met: Hepatic (CYP2C9) Elim: Hepatic and renal		
Uricases						
Pegloticase	8 mg[a]	IV/every 2 wk	Highly variable (days to wk)	Not well defined	Common: Gout flare; allergic reactions; anaphylaxis (~7%); infusion reactions (urticaria, dyspnea, chest discomfort, pruritis, chest discomfort) Rare: CHF exacerbation (unclear association)	C: Allergic reactions to medication or loss of effect (serum UA >6.0 mg/dL indicates development of antipegloticase antibody) DI: Other PEGylated agents (possible)

[a]Predosing with fexofenadine 60 mg, acetaminophen 1000 mg, and hydrocortisone 200 mg IV on the day of the infusion.

[b]Reported for lesinurad.

ACE, Angiotensin-converting enzyme; *bid,* twice daily; *CHF,* congestive heart failure; *Cyt,* cytochrome; *Elim,* elimination; *HLA,* human leukocyte antigen; *IV,* intravenous; *NSAIDs,* nonsteroidal anti-inflammatory drugs; *PEGylated,* polyethylene glycosylated; *PO,* by mouth; *tid,* three times daily; *UA,* uric acid.

Duration of Urate-Lowering Therapy

In asymptomatic gout patients successfully treated with ULT, withdrawal of therapy often results in an abrupt increase in sUA, with recurrent attacks occurring in approximately one-third of patients within 2 years.[13] Similarly, reductions from continuous ULT to an "intermittent" regimen in previously stable patients with gout lead to significantly higher flare rates,[14] whereas ULT discontinuation in the setting of tophaceous gout leads to recurrent gout flares in a vast majority and recurrent tophi in nearly half.[15] Taken together, these reports suggest that ULT should be "lifelong" in most patients.

Target Serum Urate Goals

Lowering and maintaining sUA at concentrations less than 6.0 mg/dL (<360 μmol/L) leads to improved long-term outcomes in gout, a treat-to-target approach advocated for in rheumatology management guidelines[1,2] with prior recommendations advocating an even lower target goal (<5.0 mg/dL or <300 μmol/L) in patients with tophi.[1] ULT reduces the long-term risk of recurrent flare by approximately 60% for each 1 mg/dL decrease in sUA.[16] Additional evidence suggests that reaching and maintaining sUA concentrations of less than 6.0 mg/dL is important for the depletion of total body urate stores.[17] It is important to recognize that these target goals often fall well below the upper-limit normal for sUA in clinical laboratories that define ranges based on population-based distributions.

Anti-inflammatory Prophylaxis With Urate-Lowering Therapy Administration

Rebound gout flare is the most common "complication" of ULT regardless of the agent used, rendering anti-inflammatory prophylaxis a key component of successful gout treatment.[1,2] Gout flares complicating ULT are thought to be caused by reduced sUA concentrations that result in the mobilization of monosodium urate crystals from articular and periarticular deposits into joints. The frequency of treatment-related gout flares appears to be higher with more rapid and potent urate-lowering interventions and can be at least partially mitigated by initiating low-dose ULT with stepwise dose increases to achieve target sUA goal even in the absence of prophylaxis.[18,19] Both colchicine and low-dose nonsteroidal anti-inflammatory drugs (NSAIDs), such as naproxen 250 mg twice per day, are effective in reducing gout flares during ULT initiation.[20–22] Although low-dose glucocorticoids (e.g., prednisone equivalent of ≤10 mg daily) are commonly used in this context, data supporting their use are limited. Results from a prior study[21] suggest that anti-inflammatory prophylaxis with low-dose oral colchicine (0.6 mg, twice/day) protects against rebound gout flares and may need to be continued for up to 6 months after ULT initiation. Agents targeting IL-1, including anakinra, canakinumab, and rilonacept, have demonstrated preliminary efficacy in the prevention of gout flare complicating ULT initiation.[23,24,24a]

Urate-Lowering Therapy Adherence

Suboptimal treatment compliance poses a major obstacle to effective ULT, with reports consistently demonstrating rates of medication adherence of 50% or less in gout.[25,26] Treatment adherence in gout is the lowest of seven different chronic conditions examined,[25] emphasizing the importance of patient education in disease management.

Xanthine Oxidase Inhibition

Allopurinol

KEY POINTS

Advantages of allopurinol over the most commonly used uricosurics include its once-daily dosing, effectiveness in both "underexcretors" and "overproducers," and its effectiveness in patients with renal insufficiency.

Allopurinol hypersensitivity syndrome (AHS) is an uncommon, albeit potentially serious, adverse event associated with its use.

Allopurinol doses higher than 300 mg/day are frequently required to achieve target sUA goals.

Evidence and consensus-based gout treatment guidelines recommend the initial use of low-dose allopurinol (≤100 mg/day) with gradual increases in dosing to achieve target sUA goals.

Available for more than 50 years, allopurinol accounts for a vast majority of all ULT prescriptions.[27] In addition to its established track record in gout, allopurinol has several advantages that render this as first-line ULT. These include: (1) low cost, (2) once-daily oral administration, (3) effectiveness in patients who underexcrete and those who overproduce UA, (4) favorable safety profile, and (5) potential effectiveness in patients with renal impairment. Allopurinol treatment results in significant declines in sUA,[20,22,29] decreased gout flare rates,[20,22,29–35] and declines in tophus area.[20]

Role in Rheumatic Disease and Indications

Approved indications for allopurinol include (1) treatment of hyperuricemia in gout, (2) the management of hyperuricemia resulting from the treatment of malignancy (most often leukemia or lymphoma), and (3) the management of nephrolithiasis in the context of increased urinary uric acid (UA) excretion. Although not approved for the treatment of asymptomatic hyperuricemia in the absence of gout, there is evidence suggesting that allopurinol use may have other health benefits. Hyperuricemia is independently associated with cardiovascular morbidity and mortality,[36–39] giving rise to speculation that ULT could be cardioprotective.[40] At least two prospective studies have shown a lower all-cause mortality risk among individuals receiving allopurinol,[40,41] although it was not clear from these investigations whether this benefit was mediated by reductions in cardiovascular risk. In a placebo-controlled study of pediatric essential hypertension, allopurinol use resulted in significant, albeit modest, declines in blood pressure.[42] Allopurinol also promotes endothelial function, improving measures of both local and systemic blood flow,[43] and has been associated with improvements in renal function in at-risk populations.[44,45] It is suggested that at least some of the benefit of allopurinol may be independent of XO inhibition. This speculation is supported by a recent large-scale randomized controlled study demonstrating a 20% to 30% lower risk of all-cause or cardiovascular death in gout patients treated with allopurinol compared with patients receiving febuoxstat over a median follow-up period of 32 months.[11]

Chemical Structure and Mechanism of Action

An antimetabolite in simple organisms, allopurinol inhibits XO (Fig. 69.1), a key enzyme in purine catabolism, but does not inhibit the biosynthesis of purines in humans.

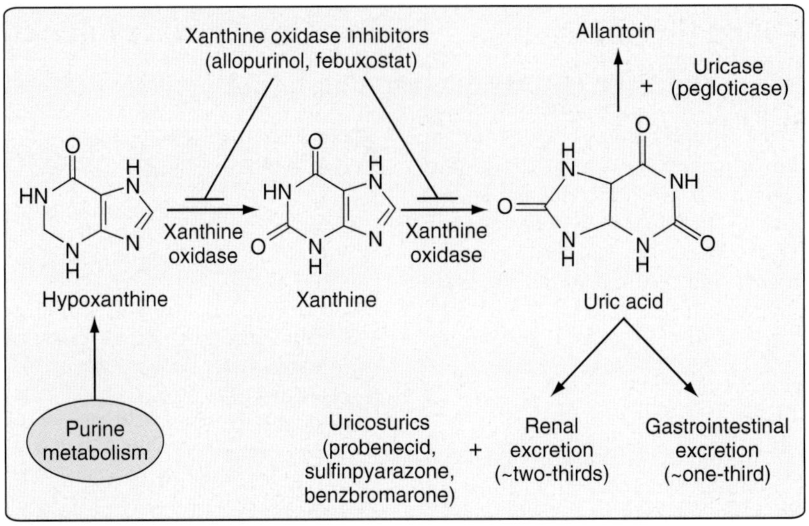

• **Fig. 69.1** Endogenous synthesis and elimination of uric acid (UA). UA is the end product of purine degradation in humans. Xanthine oxidase (XO), which converts hypoxanthine to xanthine and xanthine to UA, is a rate-limiting enzyme in this process and is targeted by select urate-lowering therapies in gout treatment, including allopurinol and febuxostat. Although humans do not express a functional form of uricase, other mammalian species are able to catalyze the conversion of UA into allantoin, which is far more soluble. Recombinant forms of uricase, including pegloticase, have been developed for use in the treatment of refractory gout. UA in humans is eliminated primarily in the kidneys. Renal excretion of UA is enhanced through uricosuric administration.

Pharmacology

Pharmacologic characteristics of the ULTs are summarized in Table 69.1. Allopurinol is approximately 90% absorbed from the gastrointestinal (GI) tract and is metabolized into oxypurinol, its active metabolite. Peak serum concentrations for allopurinol and oxypurinol are achieved within approximately 1 to 2 hours and 4 to 5 hours, respectively. The plasma half-life of allopurinol is relatively brief (1 to 2 hours), although the half-life of oxypurinol is substantially longer (~15 hours or longer), allowing for once-daily dosing. Allopurinol is eliminated primarily via glomerular filtration, whereas oxypurinol undergoes some degree of renal tubular reabsorption. With renal mechanisms primarily responsible for drug elimination, the plasma half-life of allopurinol, and to a greater degree oxypurinol, are increased with renal insufficiency.

Dose and Drug Administration

Allopurinol is available as 100 mg and 300 mg pills for once-daily oral administration (see Table 69.1), with split dosing advocated in some instances for daily doses 600 mg or higher. Used in the treatment and/or prevention of tumor lysis syndrome, allopurinol is available intravenously. Approved at daily doses as high as 800 mg in the United States and 900 mg in Europe, allopurinol is often maintained at inappropriately low doses (e.g., ≤300 mg daily) in everyday clinical practice,[46] although greater doses are often required to appropriately manage the signs and symptoms of gout. It is well established that only a modest proportion of patients achieve a target sUA of less than 6.0 mg/dL with allopurinol 300 mg/day, the most commonly used dose. With a target sUA threshold of less than 5.0 mg/dL, investigators have shown that only one-fourth of patients with gout achieve this goal with 300 mg of daily allopurinol, a proportion that increased to 78% with a daily dose of 600 mg.[47] The limitation of "standard" dose allopurinol has been proven in randomized clinical trials that have compared fixed daily doses of 300 mg with febuxostat in various doses. In those studies, approximately 40% of allopurinol-treated patients with gout achieved a final sUA of less than 6.0 mg/dL.[20,22] Gout treatment guidelines recommend that allopurinol be started in low doses (e.g., 100 mg daily) and increased by 100 mg every 2 to 5 weeks as required to achieve the target.[1,2] Data from two studies suggest that each 100 mg increase in allopurinol leads to an additional decline in sUA approaching 1.0 mg/dL.[48,49] Implementing a "start low and go slow" approach and other key elements of proposed "best practices,"[1,2] investigators reported a 92% success rate in achieving sUA treatment goals in gout.[50] Using a nurse-led intervention involving patient education and a similar treat-to-target approach, 95% of gout patients achieved target sUA concentrations after two years of treatment compared with just 30% of those receiving usual care.[51] Importantly, those receiving the intervention after 2 years experienced fewer gout flares and had a lower number of tophi compared with gout patients subject to usual care. Among the intervention patients receiving allopurinol, the most commonly used ULT in the study, the mean daily dose achieved after 2 years was 460 mg.

There is general consensus that *initial* allopurinol dosing should be adjusted for diminished renal function,[2,52,53] which prolongs the plasma half-life of oxypurinol. Commonly cited dosing algorithms suggest administering an initial daily dose of 100 mg or less for patients with a glomerular filtration rate (GFR) of less than 20 mL/min, with even lower doses for those with more severe renal impairment.[54] Whether existing dosing guidelines preclude the use of incremental dosing beyond these recommended renal thresholds has been the subject of debate. The standard recommended renal dosing guidelines[54] are not evidence based and are founded largely on a single retrospective case series showing that patients in whom allopurinol hypersensitivity syndrome (AHS) developed were more likely to have renal insufficiency. Indeed, of patients with CKD in whom AHS developed, many received "appropriately" dosed allopurinol.[55,56] In a review of 120 patients with gout receiving allopurinol, more than half (57%) required titration of daily doses higher than the "renal threshold" recommended by Hande,[54] a strategy that was well tolerated in the vast majority of patients.[57]

Toxicity

AHS is an uncommon but potentially fatal treatment complication with approximately 90% of cases occurring within 60 days of allopurinol initiation.[58] AHS is characterized by the presence of an erythematous desquamating rash (similar to Stevens-Johnson syndrome), fever, eosinophilia, and end-organ damage, including hepatitis and renal failure.[54] During more than 65,000 person-years of follow-up of allopurinol initiators, 45 patients were hospitalized for severe cutaneous adverse reactions, corresponding to a crude incidence rate of 0.69 events per 1000 person-years.[59] In addition to its association with higher initial allopurinol doses and impaired renal function,[60] AHS appears to be substantially more common in individuals positive for *HLA-B*5801*. In a small Taiwanese case-control study, all patients in whom AHS developed were positive for *HLA-B*5801,* compared with only 15% of allopurinol-treated patients without AHS.[61] In the United States, this risk allele has been estimated to be present in 0.7% of Caucasians and Hispanics, 7.4% of Asians, and 3.8% of African Americans.[62] With genetic assays commercially available, testing for *HLA-B*5801* has been proposed to be cost effective and even cost saving when implemented in intermediate or high-risk populations,[63,64] such as African Americans or Asians, respectively, particularly in the context of CKD.[63,64] It is estimated that the use of low starting doses, adjusted for renal function, may by itself reduce AHS risk by approximately 10-fold.[60] Given the potential severity of AHS, patients should be educated about the remote possibility of this adverse event and cautioned to discontinue allopurinol if a rash develops, particularly if accompanied by fever or mucocutaneous lesions.

Recognizing the rare occurrence of AHS, allopurinol is generally well tolerated. Estimates suggest that less than 5% to 10% of those exposed are intolerant to the drug.[65] Rebound flares are among the most common complication that accompanies allopurinol and other ULTs, an issue that is most prominent in the early phases of drug initiation and can be mitigated by anti-inflammatory prophylaxis. Isolated maculopapular skin rash can occur outside the context of AHS and is estimated to complicate approximately 1% to 3% of allopurinol treatment courses. Other common adverse events associated with allopurinol use are summarized in Table 69.1. Liver function abnormalities can be seen in approximately 6% to 7% of allopurinol users,[29] although rates of severe liver injury appear to be exceedingly low. The role and recommended frequency for laboratory surveillance in toxicity monitoring has not been well defined.

Fertility, Pregnancy, and Lactation

Recognizing that there have been no human studies of its use in pregnancy,[66] allopurinol should be avoided in pregnancy (animal reproduction studies have shown an adverse effect on the fetus without adequate human studies). Both allopurinol and oxypurinol are expressed in breast milk, and because drug effects in the developing infant are largely unknown, it should not be administered to nursing mothers.

Drug Interactions and Contraindications

Allopurinol drug interactions have been well characterized. Azathioprine and 6-mercaptopurine (6-MP) are metabolized by XO, hence co-administration of allopurinol leads to marked increases in circulating drug levels that can lead to bone marrow suppression.[67–69] Theophylline is also metabolized by XO, and therefore co-administration of this agent with allopurinol can lead to increased theophylline levels and potentiate toxicity. The co-administration of allopurinol with ampicillin/amoxicillin has been associated with a higher incidence of drug-related rash.[70] Thiazide diuretics may also reduce the renal excretion of allopurinol and oxypurinol with suggestions that this could potentiate drug-related toxicity, including the risk of AHS.[71] Uricosurics increase the renal excretion of oxypurinol, thus offsetting to some degree the urate-lowering effect of allopurinol.[72] Allopurinol co-administration may increase drug levels of cyclosporine and warfarin, mandating close monitoring of drug levels and bleeding parameters, respectively. Other allopurinol-associated drug interactions are summarized in Table 69.1. Although regimens for desensitization have been described, allopurinol should be avoided in patients with known allergies to allopurinol, especially AHS.

Febuxostat

KEY POINTS

Febuxostat is a potent inhibitor of xanthine oxidase (XO), with a chemical structure that is distinct from that of allopurinol.

Febuxostat represents an important alternative for patients for whom allopurinol is not effective, either because of intolerance or lack of efficacy.

Role in Rheumatic Diseases and Indications

Febuxostat is approved for the treatment of hyperuricemia in patients with gout. Similar to other ULTs, febuxostat is not currently indicated for the treatment of asymptomatic hyperuricemia. Given its unique structure, febuxostat represents an important alternative means of XO inhibition, particularly in patients with gout who are intolerant to allopurinol.[65] Because of its potent urate-lowering effect, febuxostat has been hypothesized to exert potential benefits beyond the treatment of gout, with at least one study demonstrating improvements in vascular function[73] in patients with tophaceous gout with other studies suggesting possible renal protective effects.[10] These preliminary results, however, must be interpreted with caution, particularly in light of trial data demonstrating 20% to 30% higher rates of all-cause and cardiovascular mortality with febuxostat compared with allopurinol in patients with gout.[11]

Chemical Structure and Mechanism of Action

In contrast to allopurinol, febuxostat is a nonpurine analog that reduces serum and urinary urate concentrations through selective XO inhibition (see Fig. 69.1). In contrast to allopurinol, which may inhibit other enzymes involved in purine and pyrimidine synthesis, febuxostat demonstrates significant enzymatic inhibition only for XO at therapeutic concentrations.[74]

Pharmacology

After oral administration, febuxostat is rapidly absorbed from the GI tract with approximately 50% absorption, reaching peak plasma concentrations within a few hours[75] with near-complete plasma protein binding (see Table 69.1). Febuxostat displays linear pharmacokinetics undergoing primary hepatic metabolism through conjugation via uridine diphosphate glucuronosyltransferase and oxidation via cytochrome P450 enzymes.[75] Peak urate-lowering effects with febuxostat generally occur during the first 5 to 7 days of treatment. Drug elimination occurs via both hepatic and renal pathways. Although active metabolites are produced via oxidation, these are present in much lower plasma concentrations.

Dose and Drug Administration

Febuxostat is available in 40 mg tablets in the United States, in 80 mg tablet doses in the United States and Europe, and 120 mg tablet doses in Europe. Usual dosing ranges from 40 mg to 120 mg daily (see Table 69.1). Febuxostat should be initiated at a lower dose (40 mg to 80 mg daily) and increased to higher doses (80 mg to 120 mg daily) if sUA levels remain higher than 6.0 mg/dL after 2 weeks. In a phase 2 study, sUA levels of less than 6.0 mg/dL were obtained by 56%, 76%, and 94% of patients receiving 40 mg, 80 mg, and 120 mg/day of febuxostat, respectively, compared with 0% for placebo.[18] Mean sUA reductions were greater with higher daily doses, ranging from a 37% reduction in the 40 mg/day group to 59% in the 120 mg/day group. Two subsequent trials lasting 28 weeks (n = 1067)[22] and 52 weeks (n = 762)[20] compared febuxostat (80 mg to 240 mg/day) with fixed-dose allopurinol (300 mg daily) with both trials by using the primary outcome of an sUA of less than 6.0 mg/dL at the last three consecutive monthly observations. The primary endpoint was achieved by 48% to 53%, 62% to 65%, and 69% of patients with gout receiving daily doses of 80 mg, 120 mg, and 240 mg, respectively, compared with 21% to 22% of patients receiving fixed-dose allopurinol. Secondary outcomes in one trial[20] showed declines in both gout flare rates and an approximately 70% to 80% reduction in gout tophus area during follow-up. Changes in gout flare rate and tophus area were not significantly different from those observed with allopurinol. Studies of febuxostat[20,22,29] to date have primarily used fixed-dose allopurinol (≤300 mg/day) as an active comparator. These trials have shown that the magnitude of urate lowering achieved with allopurinol 300 mg daily parallels that achieved with a daily febuxostat dose of 40 mg. As detailed previously, current gout treatment guidelines recommend initiating low-dose allopurinol (i.e., 100 mg/day) with incremental dosing as needed to achieve target urate thresholds.[1,2,52] Because optimal allopurinol dosing strategies were not used in these studies, these results almost certainly overestimate the incremental effectiveness of febuxostat relative to optimally dosed allopurinol.

Metabolized primarily in the liver, febuxostat may not require renal dosing.[76] This receives support from small short-term pharmacokinetic studies that included a limited number of patients with renal impairment.[77,78] There are insufficient data from longer-term studies of febuxostat in patients with moderate renal impairment (serum creatinine of ~1.6 to 2.0 mg/dL) and even less data from patients with more severe renal dysfunction (serum creatinine >2.0 mg/dL). Available data, albeit limited, suggest that those with mild or moderate renal impairment (estimated creatinine clearance [Cr CL] between 30 and 90 mL/min) experience similar efficacy and similar rates of toxicity compared with those with preserved renal function receiving the same doses of febuxostat.[11,20,29]

Toxicity

Similar to other ULTs, rebound gout flares are the most common complication of febuxostat administration, underscoring the importance of anti-inflammatory prophylaxis.[18] Other adverse reactions observed with febuxostat are summarized in Table 69.1, adverse effects that appear to occur at similar rates to those observed with allopurinol.[29,75] In initial studies comparing febuxostat with allopurinol, there was a slightly higher rate of cardiovascular events in patients receiving febuxostat (0.74 events per 100 patient-years; 95% CI, 0.36 to 1.37) compared with those randomly assigned to allopurinol (0.60 events per 100 patient; 95% CI, 0.16 to 1.53).[75] In the large 6-month CONFIRMS trial, investigators found no differences in the rates of cardiovascular events between patients treated with febuxostat (40 mg and 80 mg/day) and allopurinol (200 mg to 300 mg/day).[29] Although showing no difference in its primary endpoint (a composite of cardiovascular death, nonfatal myocardial infarction, nonfatal stroke, or unstable angina requiring revascularization), the large-scale randomized CARES study showed febuxostat treatment to be associated with a 20% to 30% higher risk than allopurinol for the prespecified secondary endpoints of all-cause and cardiovascular mortality in patients with gout.[11] Recognizing important limitations, including the absence of a placebo arm and a dropout rate approaching 50%,[79] the CARES trial did not show that febuxostat reduces survival but instead suggests a higher risk of this agent compared with allopurinol.

Because of its unique structure and select XO inhibition, it is suggested that febuxostat may represent a rational alternative for patients with gout with a history of allopurinol hypersensitivity. Whether febuxostat can be effectively administered in such patients is not clear, given post-marketing reports of hypersensitivity in patients given febuxostat. In a small retrospective study involving 13 patients with gout with a history of severe allopurinol-related adverse reactions, 12 were subsequently treated safely with febuxostat (10 achieved target sUA goals).[80] A hypersensitivity vasculitis of the skin developed in a single patient.

Fertility, Pregnancy, and Lactation

The effects of febuxostat on fertility are not known. Likewise, there have been no studies of febuxostat in pregnant women, although results from animal studies have not suggested a significant risk of teratogenicity.[75] In the absence of appropriate human studies, however, febuxostat should be avoided in pregnancy. It is not known whether the drug is excreted in human milk, and febuxostat should be used only with caution in nursing women.

Drug Interactions and Contraindications

Although formal drug-interaction studies have not been performed, febuxostat should be used with caution with drugs that are metabolized by XO (azathioprine, 6-MP, theophylline) (see Table 69.1). Because of its hepatic metabolism, febuxostat should not be used in patients with moderate to severe liver impairment.

Uricosurics

KEY POINTS

- Probenecid, lesinurad, sulfinpyrazone, and benzbromarone are the most common uricosuric agents used in gout treatment worldwide.
- Often requiring twice- or three-times-per day dosing, uricosurics are potentially effective in lowering sUA in patients who underexcrete UA, the most common pathologic defect leading to hyperuricemia.
- Lesinurad is a potent uricosuric approved for once-daily dosing in combination with XO inhibition, because lesinurad monotherapy is associated with a higher risk of renal toxicity.
- Probenecid and sulfinpyrazone may have limited efficacy in the context of moderate to severe renal insufficiency.

Uricosurics were the first class of ULT used in gout treatment.[81] A complex system of renal handling of urate has been proposed that sequentially includes four components[82]: (1) near-complete glomerular filtration, (2) proximal reabsorption, (3) tubular urate secretion, and (4) reabsorption for a second time more distally. Available uricosurics diminish the postsecretory reabsorption of UA, therefore promoting its elimination and reducing sUA. Uricosurics address the most common physiologic defect in gout, UA underexcretion. In addition to promoting renal UA excretion, uricosurics may inhibit the tubular secretion of a number of other compounds, including penicillins. Although many agents display uricosuric properties, the most commonly used uricosurics in gout worldwide are probenecid, lesinurad, sulfinpyrazone, and benzbromarone. Probenecid is the most widely used uricosuric in gout treatment. Lesinurad was recently approved in gout to be used in combination with either allopurinol or febuxostat. Primarily because of concerns of treatment-related toxicity, sulfinpyrazone and benzbromarone are less widely available, and neither is available in the United States.

Although the focus of this section is on "primary" uricosurics, there are several medications approved for the treatment of non-gouty conditions that exert uricosuric effects. "Secondary" uricosurics and their indications are summarized in Table 69.2.[83–88] Salicylates exert a paradoxical effect on renal urate elimination, with the inhibition of active secretion with lower doses (e.g., <1 g/day) and a "uricosuric-like" inhibition of UA reabsorption at higher doses (>4 to 5 g/day). Along with salicylates, losartan has perhaps been most closely scrutinized for its hypouricemic properties, an effect that is mediated via inhibition of URAT1 and appears to be specific to this angiotensin receptor blocker.[84] The magnitude of sUA lowering that can be achieved with these "secondary" hypouricemics is typically modest. Losartan used at an anti-hypertensive dose of 50 mg/day resulted in mean sUA declines of 9%.[84] It is important to recognize that the urate-lowering effect of losartan appears to be negated when co-administered with hydrochlorothiazide,[89] a combination used in hypertension treatment.

Role in Rheumatic Disease and Indications

Probenecid, lesinurad, sulfinpyrazone, and benzbromarone are used to treat hyperuricemia associated with gout and are indicated in patients with gout who underexcrete UA (24-hour urine UA, <700 mg). Probenecid is also approved as an adjuvant to penicillin therapy, increasing plasma concentrations and prolonging the terminal half-life of penicillin and other penicillin derivatives. Although potentially effective for a majority of patients with gout, uricosurics are much less commonly used than allopurinol and have been designated as second-line ULTs in gout management guidelines.[1] In a population-based study from the United Kingdom, uricosuric therapy accounted for less than 5% of all ULT prescriptions.[27]

TABLE 69.2 Agents Not Approved for Gout Treatment That Display Urate-Lowering Properties

Agent	Usual Indication
Losartan	Hypertension, congestive heart failure
Fenofibrate	Hyperlipidemia, hypertriglyceridemia
Atorvastatin	Hyperlipidemia
Rosuvastatin	Hyperlipidemia
Guaifenesin	Upper respiratory airway congestion
Leflunomide	Rheumatoid arthritis
Salicylates (high dose)	Analgesia, fever, anti-inflammatory

Mechanism of Action

Uricosurics work primarily through the inhibition of the renal tubular urate-transporters: uric acid transporter 1 (URAT1), glucose transporter 9 (GLUT9), and organic anion transporters 1, 3, and 4 (Fig. 69.2). Thus uricosurics reduce UA reabsorption, promote renal elimination, and decrease sUA.[90–94]

Pharmacology

Administered orally, uricosurics undergo GI absorption and are extensively protein bound in the serum. Half-lives of probenecid[95] and sulfinpyrazone[96] are relatively brief, ranging from approximately 3 to 12 hours (see Table 69.1). Although benzbromarone also has a relatively short half-life of approximately 3 hours, its active metabolite 6-hydroxybenzbromarone has a much longer half-life, allowing for effective once-daily administration.[97] With an elimination half-life of just 1.5 to 2.7 hours, lesinurad given as a single dose increases uricosuria for up to 12 hours.[98] Elimination of the uricosurics is primarily via hepatic metabolism, followed by variable excretion of metabolites in the urine, bile, and/or feces. The metabolism of probenecid is limited to side-chain hydroxylation, *N*-depropylation, and glucuronic conjugation of its carboxyl group.[99–101] Sulfinpyrazone, benzbromarone, and lesinurad are metabolized via cytochrome P450 (CYP), with CYP2C9 representing a principal mediator.[102,103] Warfarin is also metabolized primarily via CYP2C9, explaining its potential drug-drug interactions with these agents. Lesinurad also induces CYP3A and may decrease circulating concentrations of drugs metabolized by this cytochrome (e.g., sildenafil, amlodipine, or statins), in addition to mediating modest decreases in exposure to other agents used in gout such as colchicine or indomethacin.[104,105]

Dose and Drug Administration

Usual probenecid dosing is 500 to 2000 mg daily in divided doses. Probenecid (500 mg) is also formulated with colchicine (0.5 mg) as a combination tablet (col-probenecid). In a 12-week randomized study involving patients with preserved renal function, probenecid, 1500 mg/day was associated with a 32% reduction in plasma urate concentration,[106] with older studies documenting other qualitative benefits of therapy, including softening of tophi, functional improvement, and improved pain symptoms.[34,107] Sulfinpyrazone is given in divided doses at an initial daily dose of 200 to 400 mg, increasing to 800 mg daily, if necessary to achieve target sUA goals. Although there is no level of renal function below which probenecid and sulfinpyrazone are known to completely lose efficacy, these drugs may lose effectiveness in patients with moderate to severe renal insufficiency.[108] In a retrospective study of 57 patients with gout, probenecid yielded moderate efficacy as a ULT with baseline sUA, but not renal function per se, predicting treatment response.[109] In contrast to common

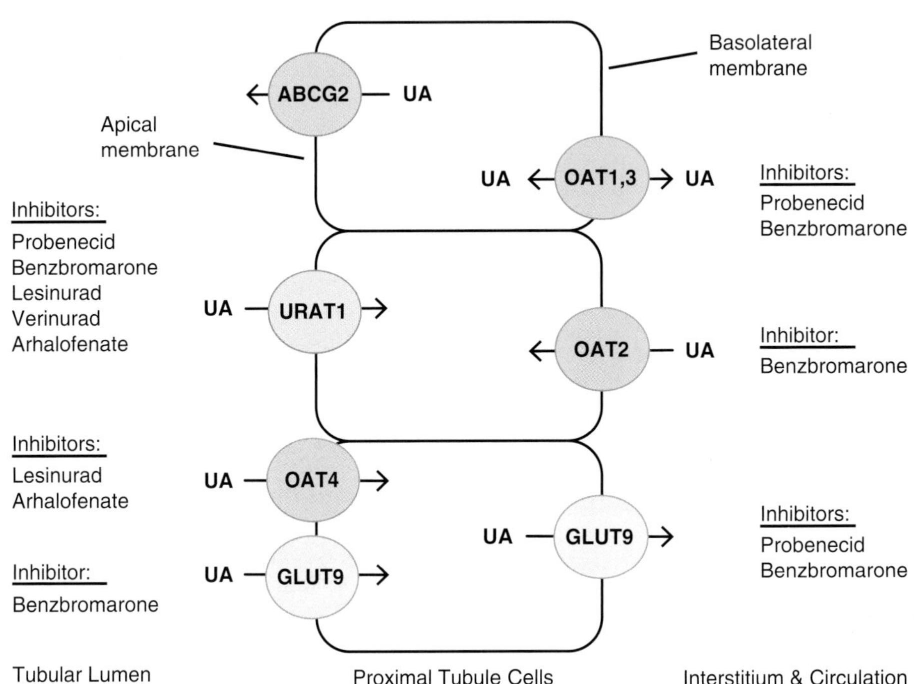

• **Fig. 69.2** Renal handling of uric acid (UA) and sites of action for available uricosurics, including probenecid, lesinurad, sulfinpyrazone, and benzbromarone in the proximal renal tubule. *ABCG2,* Adenosine triphosphate-binding cassette subfamily G member 2; *GLUT,* glucose transporter; *OAT,* organic anion transporter; *UA,* uric acid; *URAT,* uric acid transporter. (Modified from Bardin T, Richette P: Novel uricosurics. *Rheumatology* [Oxford] 57[suppl 1]:i42-i46, 2018, with permission.)

dogma, these results suggest that probenecid can be used effectively in select patients with mild to moderate CKD. Probenecid may also be used as an adjuvant to XO inhibition. Among patients failing allopurinol monotherapy (200 to 300 mg/day), 86% achieved a target sUA of less than 5 mg/dL after the addition of probenecid (1000 mg/day).[110]

Lesinurad is dosed once daily (200 mg) in combination with either allopurinol or febuxostat. When given in higher doses or as monotherapy, the risk of renal toxicity is increased. With the addition of lesinurad 200 mg daily to fixed-dose allopurinol (200 to 600 mg/day), patients experienced an additional 16% decline in sUA over 4 weeks in a phase 2 study.[111] In subsequent replicate phase 3 studies, the proportion achieving an sUA target of less than 6.0 mg/dL nearly doubled from ~25% for those receiving allopurinol alone (300 mg/day, 200 mg for those with moderate renal impairment) to 50% to 60% among those receiving the combination of lesinurad and allopurinol.[112,113]

Benzbromarone is administered once daily and may be effective in patients with moderate renal impairment. Benzbromarone treatment in usual doses (50 to 200 mg/day) leads to between 25% and 50% reductions in sUA[114–117] in addition to decreases in gout flare rates and tophi.[118–120] In a randomized controlled trial, benzbromarone maintained its hypouricemic effect even among patients with a Cr CL as low as 20 to 40 mL/min.[117] Among patients intolerant to or experiencing treatment failure with allopurinol 300 mg/day, 92% of those administered benzbromarone (200 mg/day) achieved an sUA of less than 5.0 mg/dL compared with 65% of those receiving probenecid (2000 mg/day).[121]

Toxicity

As with other ULTs, rebound gout flares represent a common complication of uricosurics. Because urinary UA acts as a potential nidus for stone formation, uricosuric therapy is associated with an increased risk of nephrolithiasis. In a longitudinal study including more than 780 patient-years of benzbromarone exposure, nephrolithiasis developed in approximately 10% (21 of 216 patients).[122] Of the 21 patients with incident nephrolithiasis, oxalate stones developed in seven patients, and stones composed of either UA or a combination of UA and calcium developed in 14 patients. In addition to limiting uricosurics to patients who underexcrete UA, the risk of treatment-related nephrolithiasis can be mitigated by optimizing fluid intake and alkalinizing the urine with a goal of maintaining a urine pH higher than 6.0.[123] When used as a monotherapy or in daily doses greater than 200 mg, lesinurad has been associated with increased renal toxicity. Other adverse effects observed with uricosurics are summarized in Table 69.1. Rare adverse effects include anaphylaxis, anemia (including aplastic and hemolytic anemia), other cytopenias, fever, nephrotic syndrome, and back pain. Rare reports of severe liver injury led to the withdrawal of benzbromarone by its primary manufacturer in 2003, a decision challenged in systematic risk-benefit analysis of the drug.[123a] Because of its NSAID-like properties, sulfinpyrazone has been associated with an increased frequency of blood dyscrasia (rare) in addition to upper GI disturbances including peptic ulcer disease.[124]

Fertility, Pregnancy, and Lactation

There are limited data regarding the impact of uricosurics on fertility, fetal development, and use with nursing infants; thus these agents should be used with caution in such patients only when the potential benefits of treatment outweigh its potential risks.

Drug Interactions and Contraindications

With the knowledge that tubular secretion plays a central role in the renal clearance of numerous drugs, drug-drug interactions with the use of uricosurics, particularly probenecid, are well known. Inhibition of tubular drug secretion appears to be greater for probenecid and sulfinpyrazone than lesinurad or benzbromarone due to the specific inhibition of URAT1 attributed to the latter two agents. Drug interactions observed with uricosurics are summarized in Table 69.1.

Because of the potential for cross-reactivity, sulfinpyrazone should be avoided in patients with allergies to phenylbutazone or other pyrazole compounds. Lesinurad is contraindicated in patients with a Cr Cl less than 45 mL/min. Except under special circumstances, these agents should be avoided in patients with nephrolithiasis, with evidence of UA overexcretion, and undergoing cancer treatment including chemotherapy and/or radiation. Caution should also be used in patients with known blood dyscrasias, active peptic ulcer disease, and/or significant hepatic or renal disease.

Uricases

Pegloticase

KEY POINTS

Pegloticase facilitates the conversion of UA into allantoin; the latter is far more soluble.

The intravenous administration of pegloticase is associated with rapid and marked declines in sUA, which may be particularly important in the rapid depletion of total-body urate levels.

Antigenicity and an immune response directed towards the drug are major limitations in the repeated dosing of pegloticase (a problem heralded by a rise in sUA to concentration above 6.0 mg/dL).

Pegloticase, a modified mammalian uricase, is a biologic parenterally administered agent. Unlike other mammalian species, humans have lost the ability to synthesize functional uricase that converts UA into allantoin, the latter being 5 to 10 times more soluble. The use of alternative uricases (e.g., rasburicase, a recombinant uricase from *Aspergillus flavus*[125]) in the treatment of tumor lysis syndrome has been substantially limited by drug-related antigenicity and prohibitively high rates of anaphylaxis with repeat drug administration. In contrast to older generation uricases, pegloticase appears to be less allergenic and has been administered successfully to many patients as repeated intravenous (IV) infusions.

Role in Rheumatic Disease and Indications

Pegloticase is approved for the treatment of hyperuricemia in patients with treatment-refractory gout. Approved with an orphan drug status in the United States, pegloticase is indicated in a small subset of patients with gout. Treatment-refractory disease is characterized by severe disabling gout, often accompanied by marked tophaceous deposition and significant comorbidity, in which conventional ULT is either contraindicated or ineffective.[126] Pegloticase administration is associated with rapid and marked declines in sUA. In clinical trials, pegloticase use resulted in plasma concentrations as low as 0.5 to 1 mg/dL within 24 hours of an initial dose.[127] As a consequence, pegloticase administration has been associated with dramatic regression of tophi[128] and depletion of urate stores, raising speculation that pegloticase or other uricase formulations could play a role as an induction therapy in select patients with severe tophaceous gout and excessive total body urate stores (Fig. 69.3).

Chemical Structure and Mechanism of Action

Pegloticase is a recombinant mammalian uricase linked to polyethylene glycol (PEG). Pegloticase facilitates the conversion of UA into allantoin. The conversion of allantoin from UA generates hydrogen peroxide (H_2O_2) that is rapidly scavenged by erythrocytes.[129]

Pharmacology

The pharmacokinetics of pegloticase follows a one-compartment linear model. Maximum serum concentrations and the magnitude of urate-lowering effect after IV pegloticase administration increase in a dose-dependent fashion.[130] Pegloticase pharmacokinetics are not affected by age, sex, weight, or underlying renal function. Variability in drug elimination and treatment durability appears to be related at least in part to the presence and concentration of circulating antipegloticase antibody (see the following section on Dose and Drug Administration).

Dose and Drug Administration

Pegloticase is approved for IV infusion administered during a 2-hour period at a dose of 8 mg every 2 weeks (see Table 69.1). Regulatory approval of pegloticase is based on results from two 6-month replicate randomized placebo-controlled studies[127] in addition to open-label follow-up extensions (n = 212). Patients in these clinical trials had pre-treatment sUA exceeding 8.0 mg/dL, had symptomatic gout, and had failed prior allopurinol therapy based on reported intolerance or ineffectiveness at a maximum medically appropriate dose. Patients received prophylaxis against infusion reactions (see Table 69.1) and against rebound gout flares (colchicine, NSAID, or glucocorticoid). The primary outcome for both randomized studies was an sUA of less than 6.0 mg/dL for 80% or more of the sampling period from month 3 to 6 of follow-up. This outcome was met by 47% and 38% of patients who received pegloticase, 8 mg by IV every 2 weeks, in the two randomized studies.[127] In pooled analyses, 40% of patients with baseline tophi who received pegloticase, 8 mg every 2 weeks (vs. 7% of patients receiving placebo) had complete resolution of tophi by the time of the final study visit.

Although nonresponders generally experienced plasma urate reductions equally as dramatic as responders after their initial pegloticase infusion, nonresponders usually lost the treatment effect within the first 3 months of therapy. Efficacy loss, defined as sUA rising higher than 6.0 mg/dL during treatment, appears to be strongly associated with the formation of antipegloticase antibodies (primarily immunoglobulin [Ig] M and IgG subtypes that bind the PEG portion of the drug). Clinically meaningful manifestations of antipegloticase antibody formation, including an increased risk of anaphylaxis and neutralization of drug effect, appear to be most striking at antibody titers exceeding 1:2430. It is recommended that sUA, rather than drug antibody titers, be monitored closely during treatment with discontinuation of pegloticase if preinfusion sUA increases higher than 6.0 mg/dL.[131]

Toxicity

The most common serious adverse event observed with pegloticase therapy is anaphylaxis, observed in approximately 7% of

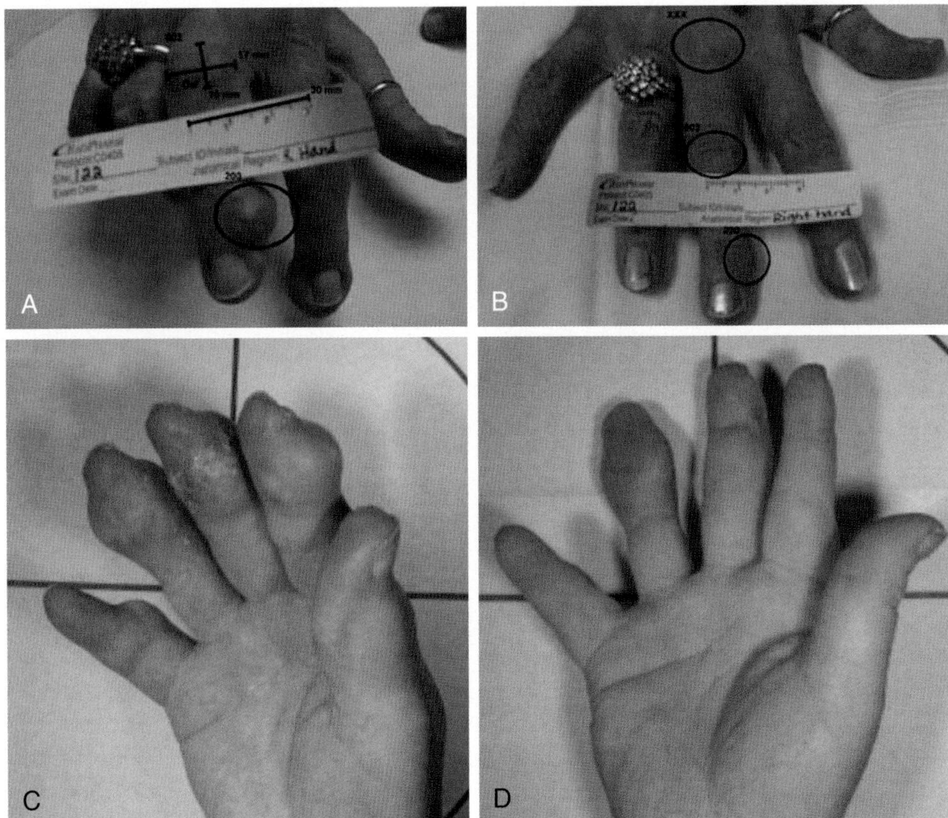

• **Fig. 69.3** (A) Baseline tophus in patient 1 involving the medial aspect of the right third distal interphalangeal (DIP) joint. (B) Same patient with resolution of tophus after 13 weeks of pegloticase therapy. (C) Baseline tophi in patient 2, and (D) same patient after 25 weeks of pegloticase treatment. (From Baraf HS, et al.: Tophus burden reduction with pegloticase: results from phase 3 randomized trials and open-label extension in patients with chronic gout refractory to conventional therapy. *Arthritis Res Ther* 15:R137, 2013, with permission.)

participants in regulatory studies (see Table 69.1). Antipegloticase antibody can be detected in a vast majority of patients (~90%) receiving treatment, although clinically meaningful antibody titers are encountered less often. In clinical studies, anaphylaxis occurred despite prophylaxis that included antihistamine and glucocorticoid therapy with an onset of symptoms typically seen within 2 hours of drug administration. Treatment-related anaphylaxis is far more common among patients with treatment failure; thus close sUA surveillance and discontinuation of pegloticase for patients with an sUA higher than 6.0 mg/dL is an essential element in risk mitigation. Post hoc analysis of the replicate studies suggests that nearly all cases of anaphylaxis would have been prevented with the use of this strategy. The concomitant use of other ULT is contraindicated, as these agents will mask antibody-mediated increases in sUA. Ongoing studies are evaluating the potential of immunosuppressive therapy (e.g., azathioprine, methotrexate, mycophenolate) in reducing drug antigenicity, thus improving treatment durability with pegloticase. This concept gained recent support from a small preliminary open label study examining methotrexate.[132] Recognizing overlap with symptoms of anaphylaxis, infusion reactions occur in as many as 25% of patients receiving pegloticase with manifestations that include urticaria, dyspnea, chest discomfort, pain, erythema, and pruritis. Infusion reactions can occur anytime in the course of therapy, with rare reports of delayed hypersensitivity reactions.

As with other ULTs, rebound gout flare is common after the administration of pegloticase. Other adverse events observed with pegloticase are summarized in Table 69.1. In the clinical studies and in open-label follow-up, exacerbations of congestive heart failure were also more common with pegloticase than placebo, although a causal association with active drug therapy has not been established.[131]

Fertility, Pregnancy, and Lactation

No studies have examined the impact of pegloticase on either fertility or pregnancy in humans, and it is unknown whether pegloticase is excreted in human milk. In the absence of appropriate human studies, pegloticase should be used only with caution in pregnancy and is not recommended for use in nursing mothers.

Drug Interactions and Contraindications

Recognizing that antipegloticase antibodies bind the PEG portion of the agent, pegloticase should be used with caution in patients receiving other PEG-containing therapies. Whether the formation of antipegloticase antibodies precludes or impacts future treatment with other PEGylated molecules is unknown. Pegloticase is contraindicated in patients with glucose-6-phosphate dehydrogenase (G6PD) deficiency because of an increased risk of hemolysis and methemoglobinemia. Patients with an increased risk should be screened for G6PD deficiency before initiation.[131]

Future Directions

The treatment armamentarium in chronic gout will likely grow in the future, with several novel ULTs under development.

A peroxisome-proliferator–activated gamma modulator, arhalofenate (MBX-102), has been highlighted in studies as an agent demonstrating dual uricosuric and anti-inflammatory effects. In addition to inhibiting renal UA transporters (URAT1, OAT4), in vitro studies have shown that the agent effectively blocks monosodium urate–induced production of IL-1. In a five-arm, 12-week randomized controlled study, investigators compared the efficacy and safety of arhalofenate (600 mg or 800 mg/day), allopurinol 300 mg/daily with or without colchicine prophylaxis (0.6 mg/daily), and placebo.[133] Arhalofenate led to 12.5% and 16.5% reductions in sUA, respectively, with the 800 mg dose yielding significantly fewer gout flares than placebo or allopurinol without colchicine. Among 16 hyperuricemic gout patients receiving the combination of arhalofenate 800 mg/daily and febuxostat 80 mg/daily, all achieved an sUA target of less than 6.0 mg/dL, and 93% achieved an sUA of less than 5 mg/dL.[134]

Verinurad (RDEA3170) is a highly selective URAT1 inhibitor currently in development. In phase 2 dose-ranging studies involving 375 total patients, verinurad administered as a monotherapy in daily doses of 2.5 mg to 15 mg led to dose-dependent reductions (17.5% to 55.8%) in sUA but was associated with more renal toxicity than either placebo or allopurinol.[135] In parallel phase 2 studies, verinurad was examined in combination with the XO inhibitors allopurinol and febuxostat.[136,137] In addition to demonstrating dose-dependent urate-lowering effects, verinurad was generally well tolerated and resulted in no meaningful changes in serum creatinine concentrations when used in combination. Of note, its co-administration with allopurinol led to decreased concentrations of oxypurinol, suggesting that the potential synergy of these two therapies may be at least partially reduced by this effect.[137]

Two other compounds in early stages of development include SEL-212 and ALLN-346. SEL-212 combines pegsiticase (a uricase enzyme also known as pegadricase) with synthetic vaccine particles containing rapamycin, which were demonstrated in pre-clinical studies to attenuate the immunogenicity of pegsiticase. Dosed monthly as an IV infusion, SEL-212 is currently in phase 2 trials.[138] ALLN-346 is a pH stable oral recombinant uricase that degrades intestinal urate into allantoin, thus decreasing total urate burden. In a proof-of-concept study, the oral administration of ALLN-346 yielded significant reductions in plasma and urine urate concentrations in an established animal model of hyperuricemia.[139]

Full references for this chapter can be found on ExpertConsult.com.

Selected References

1. Khanna D, Fitzgerald JD, Khanna PP, et al.: 2012 American College of Rheumatology guidelines for management of gout. Part 1: systematic nonpharmacologic and pharmacologic therapeutic approaches to hyperuricemia, *Arthritis Care Res (Hoboken)* 64(10):1431–1446, 2012.
2. Zhang W, Doherty M, Bardin T, et al.: EULAR evidence based recommendations for gout. Part II: Management. Report of a task force of the EULAR Standing Committee For International Clinical Studies Including Therapeutics (ESCISIT), *Ann Rheum Dis* 65:1312–1324, 2006.
3. Gonzalez AA, Puig JG, Mateos FA, et al.: Should dietary restrictions always be prescribed in the treatment of gout?, *Adv Exp Med Biol* 253A:243–246, 1989.
4. Zhu Y, Zhang Y, Choi HK: The serum urate-lowering impact of weight loss among men with a high cardiovascular risk profile: the Multiple Risk Factor Intervention Trial, *Rheumatology (Oxford)* 49:2391–2399, 2010.
5. Dalbeth N, Chen P, White M, et al.: Impact of bariatric surgery on serum urate targets in people with morbid obesity and diabetes: a prospective longitudinal study, *Ann Rheum Dis* 73(5):797–802, 2014.
6. Taylor TH, Mecchella JN, Larson RJ, et al.: Initiation of allopurinol at first medical contact for acute attacks of gout: a randomized clinical trial, *Am J Med* 125(11):1126–1134.e1127, 2012.
7. Ferraz M, O'Brien B: A cost effectiveness analysis of urate lowering drugs in nontophaceous recurrent gouty arthritis, *J Rheumatol* 22:908–914, 1995.
13. Loebl W, Scott J: Withdrawal of allopurinol in patients with gout, *Ann Rheum Dis* 33:304–307, 1974.
14. Bull P, Scott J: Intermittent control of hyperuricemia in the treatment of gout, *J Rheumatol* 16:1246–1248, 1989.
15. van Lieshout-Zuidema M, Breedveld F: Withdrawal of long-term antihyperuricemic therapy in tophaceous gout, *J Rheumatol* 20:1383–1385, 1993.
16. Shoji A, Yamanaka H, Kamatani N: A retrospective study of the relationship between serum urate level and recurrent attacks of gouty arthritis: evidence for reduction of recurrent gouty arthritis with antihyperuricemic therapy, *Arthritis Rheum* 51:321–325, 2004.
17. Li-Yu J, Clayburne G, Sieck M, et al.: Treatment of chronic gout. Can we determine when urate stores are depleted enough to prevent attacks of gout? *J Rheumatol* 28:577–580, 2001.
18. Becker MA, Schumacher Jr HR, Wortmann RL, et al.: Febuxostat, a novel nonpurine selective inhibitor of xanthine oxidase: a twenty-eight-day, multicenter, phase II, randomized, double-blind, placebo-controlled, dose-response clinical trial examining safety and efficacy in patients with gout, *Arthritis Rheum* 52(3):916–923, 2005.
20. Becker MA, Schumacher Jr HR, Wortmann RL, et al.: Febuxostat compared with allopurinol in patients with hyperuricemia and gout, *N Engl J Med* 353(23):2450–2461, 2005.
21. Borstad GC, Bryant LR, Abel MP, et al.: Colchicine for prophylaxis of acute flares when initiating allopurinol for chronic gouty arthritis, *J Rheumatol* 31(12):2429–2432, 2004.
22. Schumacher Jr HR, Becker MA, Wortmann RL, et al.: Effects of febuxostat versus allopurinol and placebo in reducing serum urate in subjects with hyperuricemia and gout: a 28-week, phase III, randomized, double-blind, parallel-group trial, *Arthritis Rheum* 59(11):1540–1548, 2008.
23. Schlesinger N, Mysler E, Lin HY, et al.: Canakinumab reduces the risk of acute gouty arthritis flares during initiation of allopurinol treatment: results of a double-blind, randomised study, *Ann Rheum Dis* 70(7):1264–1271, 2011.
24. Schumacher Jr HR, Evans RR, Saag KG, et al.: Rilonacept (interleukin-1 trap) for prevention of gout flares during initiation of uric acid-lowering therapy: results from a phase III randomized, double-blind, placebo-controlled, confirmatory efficacy study, *Arthritis Care Res (Hoboken)* 64(10):1462–1470, 2012.
25. Briesacher BA, Andrade SE, Fouayzi H, et al.: Comparison of drug adherence rates among patients with seven different medical conditions, *Pharmacotherapy* 28(4):437–443, 2008.
26. Harrold LR, Andrade SE, Briesacher BA, et al.: Adherence with urate-lowering therapies for the treatment of gout, *Arthritis Res Ther* 11(2):R46, 2009.
27. Mikuls T, Farrar J, Bilker W, et al.: Gout epidemiology: results from the U.K. General Practice Research Database, 1990-1999, *Ann Rheum Dis* 64:267–272, 2005.
28. Deleted in review.

29. Becker MA, Schumacher HR, Espinoza LR, et al.: The urate-lowering efficacy and safety of febuxostat in the treatment of the hyperuricemia of gout: the CONFIRMS trial, *Arthritis Res Ther* 12(2):R63, 2010.
30. Delbarre F, Amor B, Auscher C, de Gery A: Treatment of gout with allopurinol. A study of 106 cases, *Ann Rheum Dis* 25:627–633, 1966.
31. Kuzell W, Seebach LM, Glover RP, Jackman AE: Treatment of gout with allopurinol and sulphinpyrazone in combination and with allopurinol alone, *Ann Rheum Dis* 25:634–642, 1966.
32. Rundles R, Metz EN, Silberman HR: Allopurinol in the treatment of gout, *Ann Intern Med* 64:229–258, 1966.
33. Sarawate CA, Patel PA, Schumacher HR, et al.: Serum urate levels and gout flares: analysis from managed care data, *J Clin Rheumatol* 12(2):61–65, 2006.
34. Scott: Comparison of allopurinol and probenecid, *Ann Rheum Dis* 25:623–626, 1966.
35. Wilson J, Simmonds HA, North JD: Allopurinol in the treatment of uraemic patients with gout, *Ann Rheum Dis* 26:136–142, 1967.
36. Culleton BF, Larson MG, Kannel WB, et al.: Serum uric acid and risk for cardiovascular disease and death: the Framingham Heart Study, *Ann Intern Med* 131(1):7–13, 1999.
37. Darmawan J, Rasker JJ, Nuralim H: The effect of control and self-medication of chronic gout in a developing country. Outcome after 10 years, *J Rheumatol* 30(11):2437–2443, 2003.
38. Krishnan E: Hyperuricemia and incident heart failure, *Circ Heart Fail* 2(6):556–562, 2009.
39. Lehto S, Niskanen L, Ronnemaa T, et al.: Serum uric acid is a strong predictor of stroke in patients with non-insulin-dependent diabetes mellitus, *Stroke* 29(3):635–639, 1998.
40. Luk AJ, Levin GP, Moore EE, et al.: Allopurinol and mortality in hyperuricaemic patients, *Rheumatology (Oxford)* 48(7):804–806, 2009.
41. Dubreuil M, Zhu Y, Zhang Y, et al.: Allopurinol initiation and all-cause mortality in the general population, *Ann Rheum Dis*, 2014.
42. Feig DI, Soletsky B, Johnson RJ: Effect of allopurinol on blood pressure of adolescents with newly diagnosed essential hypertension: a randomized trial, *JAMA* 300(8):924–932, 2008.
43. Doehner W, Schoene N, Rauchhaus M, et al.: Effects of xanthine oxidase inhibition with allopurinol on endothelial function and peripheral blood flow in hyperuricemic patients with chronic heart failure: results from 2 placebo-controlled studies, *Circulation* 105(22):2619–2624, 2002.
44. Perez-Ruiz F, Calabozo M, Herrero-Beites AM, et al.: Improvement of renal function in patients with chronic gout after proper control of hyperuricemia and gouty bouts, *Nephron* 86(3):287–291, 2000.
45. Siu YP, Leung KT, Tong MK, et al.: Use of allopurinol in slowing the progression of renal disease through its ability to lower serum uric acid level, *Am J Kidney Dis* 47(1):51–59, 2006.
46. Sarawate CA, Brewer KK, Yang W, et al.: Gout medication treatment patterns and adherence to standards of care from a managed care perspective, *Mayo Clin Proc* 81(7):925–934, 2006.
47. Reinders MK, Haagsma C, Jansen TL, et al.: A randomised controlled trial on the efficacy and tolerability with dose escalation of allopurinol 300-600 mg/day versus benzbromarone 100-200 mg/day in patients with gout, *Ann Rheum Dis* 68(6):892–897, 2009.
48. Rundles RW, Metz EN, Silberman HR: Allopurinol in the treatment of gout, *Ann Intern Med* 64(2):229–258, 1966.
49. Yu TF: The effect of allopurinol in primary and secondary gout, *Arthritis Rheum* 8(5):905–906, 1965.
50. Rees F, Jenkins W, Doherty M: Patients with gout adhere to curative treatment if informed appropriately: proof-of-concept observational study, *Ann Rheum Dis* 72(6):826–830, 2013.
52. Jordan KM, Cameron JS, Snaith M, et al.: British Society for Rheumatology and British Health Professionals in Rheumatology guideline for the management of gout, *Rheumatology (Oxford)* 46(8):1372–1374, 2007.
53. Mikuls T, MacLean C, Olivieri J, et al.: Quality of care indicators for gout management, *Arthritis Rheum* 50:937–943, 2004.
54. Hande K, Noone RM, Stone WJ: Severe allopurinol toxicity. Description of guidelines for prevention in patients with renal insufficiency, *Am J Med* 76:47–56, 1984.
55. Dalbeth N, Stamp L: Allopurinol dosing in renal impairment: walking the tightrope between adequate urate lowering and adverse events, *Semin Dial* 20(5):391–395, 2007.
56. Lee HY, Ariyasinghe JT, Thirumoorthy T: Allopurinol hypersensitivity syndrome: a preventable severe cutaneous adverse reaction? *Singapore Med J* 49(5):384–387, 2008.
57. Stamp LK, O'Donnell JL, Zhang M, et al.: Using allopurinol above the dose based on creatinine clearance is effective and safe in patients with chronic gout, including those with renal impairment, *Arthritis Rheum* 63(2):412–421, 2011.
58. Ramasamy SN, Korb-Wells CS, Kannangara DR, et al.: Allopurinol hypersensitivity: a systematic review of all published cases, 1950-2012, *Drug Saf* 36(10):953–980, 2013.
59. Kim SC, Newcomb C, Margolis D, et al.: Severe cutaneous reactions requiring hospitalization in allopurinol initiators: a population-based cohort study, *Arthritis Care Res (Hoboken)* 65:578–584, 2013.
60. Stamp LK, Taylor WJ, Jones PB, et al.: Starting dose is a risk factor for allopurinol hypersensitivity syndrome: a proposed safe starting dose of allopurinol, *Arthritis Rheum* 64(8):2529–2536, 2012.
61. Hung SI, Chung WH, Liou LB, et al.: HLA-B*5801 allele as a genetic marker for severe cutaneous adverse reactions caused by allopurinol, *Proc Natl Acad Sci U S A* 102(11):4134–4139, 2005.
63. Saokaew S, Tassaneeyakul W, Maenthaisong R, et al.: Cost-effectiveness analysis of HLA-B*5801 testing in preventing allopurinol-induced SJS/TEN in Thai population, *PLoS One* 9(4):e94294, 2014.
65. Schlesinger N: Management of acute and chronic gouty arthritis: present state-of-the-art, *Drugs* 64(21):2399–2416, 2004.
66. Allopurinol [package insert], Corona, Calif, 2006, Watson Laboratories.
67. Brooks RJ, Dorr RT, Durie BG: Interaction of allopurinol with 6-mercaptopurine and azathioprine, *Biomed Pharmacother* 36(4):217–222, 1982.
68. Cummins D, Sekar M, Halil O, et al.: Myelosuppression associated with azathioprine-allopurinol interaction after heart and lung transplantation, *Transplantation* 61(11):1661–1662, 1996.
69. Kennedy DT, Hayney MS, Lake KD: Azathioprine and allopurinol: the price of an avoidable drug interaction, *Ann Pharmacother* 30(9):951–954, 1996.
70. Jick H, Porter JB: Potentiation of ampicillin skin reactions by allopurinol or hyperuricemia, *J Clin Pharmacol* 21(10):456–458, 1981.
71. Emmerson BT: The management of gout, *N Engl J Med* 334(7):445–451, 1996.
72. Stocker SL, Williams KM, McLachlan AJ, et al.: Pharmacokinetic and pharmacodynamic interaction between allopurinol and probenecid in healthy subjects, *Clin Pharmacokinet* 47(2):111–118, 2008.
73. Tausche AK, Christoph M, Forkmann M, et al.: As compared to allopurinol, urate-lowering therapy with febuxostat has superior effects on oxidative stress and pulse wave velocity in patients with severe chronic tophaceous gout, *Rheumatol Int* 34(1):101–109, 2014.
74. Takano Y, Hase-Aoki K, Horiuchi H, et al.: Selectivity of febuxostat, a novel non-purine inhibitor of xanthine oxidase/xanthine dehydrogenase, *Life Sci* 76(16):1835–1847, 2005.
75. Uloric [package insert]: Deerfield, Ill, Takeda Pharmaceuticals America, 2009.
76. Yu KH: Febuxostat: a novel non-purine selective inhibitor of xanthine oxidase for the treatment of hyperuricemia in gout, *Recent Pat Inflamm Allergy Drug Discov* 1(1):69–75, 2007.

77. Hoshide S, Takahashi Y, Ishikawa T, et al.: PK/PD and safety of a single dose of TMX-67 (febuxostat) in subjects with mild and moderate renal impairment, *Nucleosides Nucleotides Nucleic Acids* 23(8–9):1117–1118, 2004.
78. Mayer MD, Khosravan R, Vernillet L, et al.: Pharmacokinetics and pharmacodynamics of febuxostat, a new non-purine selective inhibitor of xanthine oxidase in subjects with renal impairment, *Am J Ther* 12(1):22–34, 2005.
80. Chohan S, Becker MA: Safety and efficacy of febuxostat (FEB) treatment in subjects with gout and severe allopurinol (ALLO) adverse reactions (abstract), *Arthritis Rheum* 62(Suppl):S67, 2010.
81. Ogryzlo MA, Harrison J: Evaluation of uricosuric agents in chronic gout, *Ann Rheum Dis* 16(4):425–437, 1957.
82. Levinson DJ, Sorensen LB: Renal handling of uric acid in normal and gouty subject: evidence for a 4-component system, *Ann Rheum Dis* 39(2):173–179, 1980.
83. Athyros VG, Mikhailidis DP, Liberopoulos EN, et al.: Effect of statin treatment on renal function and serum uric acid levels and their relation to vascular events in patients with coronary heart disease and metabolic syndrome: a subgroup analysis of the GREek Atorvastatin and Coronary heart disease Evaluation (GREACE) Study, *Nephrol Dial Transplant* 22(1):118–127, 2007.
84. Hamada T, Ichida K, Hosoyamada M, et al.: Uricosuric action of losartan via the inhibition of urate transporter 1 (URAT 1) in hypertensive patients, *Am J Hypertens* 21(10):1157–1162, 2008.
85. Ogata N, Fujimori S, Oka Y, et al.: Effects of three strong statins (atorvastatin, pitavastatin, and rosuvastatin) on serum uric acid levels in dyslipidemic patients, *Nucleosides Nucleotides Nucleic Acids* 29(4–6):321–324, 2010.
86. Perez-Ruiz F, Nolla JM: Influence of leflunomide on renal handling of urate and phosphate in patients with rheumatoid arthritis, *J Clin Rheumatol* 9(4):215–218, 2003.
87. Ramsdell CM, Postlethwaite AE, Kelley WN: Uricosuric effect of glyceryl guaiacolate, *J Rheumatol* 1(1):114–116, 1974.
88. Uetake D, Ohno I, Ichida K, et al.: Effect of fenofibrate on uric acid metabolism and urate transporter 1, *Intern Med* 49(2):89–94, 2010.
89. Hamada T, Mizuta E, Kondo T, et al.: Effects of a low-dose antihypertensive diuretic in combination with losartan, telmisartan, or candesartan on serum urate levels in hypertensive patients, *Arzneimittelforschung* 60(2):71–75, 2010.
90. Anzai N, Ichida K, Jutabha P, et al.: Plasma urate level is directly regulated by a voltage-driven urate efflux transporter URATv1 (SLC2A9) in humans, *J Biol Chem* 283(40):26834–26838, 2008.
91. Brandstatter A, Kiechl S, Kollerits B, et al.: Sex-specific association of the putative fructose transporter SLC2A9 variants with uric acid levels is modified by BMI, *Diabetes Care* 31(8):1662–1667, 2008.
92. Caulfield MJ, Munroe PB, O'Neill D, et al.: SLC2A9 is a high-capacity urate transporter in humans, *PLoS Med* 5(10):e197, 2008.
93. Enomoto A, Kimura H, Chairoungdua A, et al.: Molecular identification of a renal urate anion exchanger that regulates blood urate levels, *Nature* 417(6887):447–452, 2002.
94. Vitart V, Rudan I, Hayward C, et al.: SLC2A9 is a newly identified urate transporter influencing serum urate concentration, urate excretion and gout, *Nat Genet* 40(4):437–442, 2008.
95. Selen A, Amidon GL, Welling PG: Pharmacokinetics of probenecid following oral doses to human volunteers, *J Pharm Sci* 71(11):1238–1242, 1982.
96. Rosenkranz B, Fischer C, Jakobsen P, et al.: Plasma levels of sulfinpyrazone and of two of its metabolites after a single dose and during the steady state, *Eur J Clin Pharmacol* 24(2):231–235, 1983.
97. Jain AK, Ryan JR, McMahon FG, et al.: Effect of single oral doses of benzbromarone on serum and urinary uric acid, *Arthritis Rheum* 17(2):149–157, 1974.
99. Cunningham RF, Perel JM, Israili ZH, et al.: Probenecid metabolism in vitro with rat, mouse, and human liver preparations. Studies of factors affecting the site of oxidation, *Drug Metab Dispos* 5(2):205–210, 1977.
100. Dayton PG, Perel JM, Cunningham RF, et al.: Studies of the fate of metabolites and analogs of probenecid. The significance of metabolic sites, especially lack of ring hydroxylation, *Drug Metab Dispos* 1(6):742–751, 1973.
101. Israili ZH, Percel JM, Cunningham RF, et al.: Metabolites of probenecid. Chemical, physical, and pharmacological studies, *J Med Chem* 15(7):709–713, 1972.
102. He M, Rettie AE, Neal J, et al.: Metabolism of sulfinpyrazone sulfide and sulfinpyrazone by human liver microsomes and cDNA-expressed cytochrome P450s, *Drug Metab Dispos* 29(5):701–711, 2001.
103. Uchida S, Shimada K, Misaka S,I, et al.: Benzbromarone pharmacokinetics and pharmacodynamics in different cytochrome P450 2C9 genotypes, *Drug Metab Pharmacokinet*, 2010.
106. Liang L, Xu N, Zhang H, et al.: A randomized controlled study of benzbromarone and probenecid in the treatment of gout, *West China Med J* 9:405–408, 1994.
107. Gutman A, Yu TF: Protracted uricosuric therapy in tophaceous gout, *Lancet* 2:1258–1260, 1957.
108. Bartels EC, Matossian GS: Gout: six-year follow-up on probenecid (benemid) therapy, *Arthritis Rheum* 2(3):193–202, 1959.
109. Pui K, Gow PJ, Dalbeth N: Efficacy and tolerability of probenecid as urate-lowering therapy in gout; clinical experience in high-prevalence population, *J Rheumatol* 40(6):872–876, 2013.
110. Reinders MK, van Roon EN, Houtman PM, et al.: Biochemical effectiveness of allopurinol and allopurinol-probenecid in previously benzbromarone-treated gout patients, *Clin Rheumatol* 26(9):1459–1465, 2007.
114. de Gery A, Auscher C, Saporta L, et al.: Treatment of gout and hyperuricaemia by benzbromarone, ethyl 2 (dibromo-3,5 hydroxy-4 benzoyl)-3 benzofuran, *Adv Exp Med Biol* 41:683–689, 1974.
115. Ferber H, Bader U, Matzkies F: The action of benzbromarone in relation to age, sex and accompanying diseases, *Adv Exp Med Biol* 122A:287–294, 1980.
116. Perez-Ruiz F, Alonso-Ruiz A, Calabozo M, et al.: Efficacy of allopurinol and benzbromarone for the control of hyperuricaemia. A pathogenic approach to the treatment of primary chronic gout, *Ann Rheum Dis* 57(9):545–549, 1998.
117. Perez-Ruiz F, Calabozo M, Fernandez-Lopez MJ, et al.: Treatment of chronic gout in patients with renal function impairment: an open, randomized, actively controlled study, *J Clin Rheumatol* 5(2):49–55, 1999.
118. Bluestone R, Klinenberg J, Lee IK: Benzbromarone as a long-term uricosuric agent, *Adv Exp Med Biol 122A*283–286, 1980.
119. Kumar S, Ng J, Gow P: Benzbromarone therapy in management of refractory gout, *N Z Med J* 118(1217):U1528, 2005.
120. Perez-Ruiz F, Calabozo M, Pijoan JI, et al.: Effect of urate-lowering therapy on the velocity of size reduction of tophi in chronic gout, *Arthritis Rheum* 47(4):356–360, 2002.
121. Reinders MK, van Roon EN, Jansen TL, et al.: Efficacy and tolerability of urate-lowering drugs in gout: a randomised controlled trial of benzbromarone versus probenecid after failure of allopurinol, *Ann Rheum Dis* 68(1):51–56, 2009.
122. Perez-Ruiz F, Hernandez-Baldizon S, Herrero-Beites AM, et al.: Risk factors associated with renal lithiasis during uricosuric treatment of hyperuricemia in patients with gout, *Arthritis Care Res (Hoboken)* 62(9):1299–1305, 2010.
123. Masbernard A, Giudicelli CP: Ten years' experience with benzbromarone in the management of gout and hyperuricaemia, *S Afr Med J* 59(20):701–706, 1981.
124. Sulfinpyrazone [package insert]: Summit, N.J., 1996, Ciba-Geigy.
125. Cammalleri L, Malaguarnera M: Rasburicase represents a new tool for hyperuricemia in tumor lysis syndrome and in gout, *Int J Med Sci* 4(2):83–93, 2007.
126. Becker MA, Schumacher HR, Benjamin KL, et al.: Quality of life and disability in patients with treatment-failure gout, *J Rheumatol* 36(5):1041–1048, 2009.

127. Sundy JS, Baraf HS, Yood RA, et al.: Efficacy and tolerability of pegloticase for the treatment of chronic gout in patients refractory to conventional treatment: two randomized controlled trials, *JAMA* 306(7):711–720, 2011.
128. Baraf HS, Becker MA, Gutierrez-Urena SR, et al.: Tophus burden reduction with pegloticase: results from phase 3 randomized trials and open-label extension in patients with chronic gout refractory to conventional therapy, *Arthritis Res Ther* 15(5):R137, 2013.
129. Hershfield MS, Roberts 2nd LJ, Ganson NJ, et al.: Treating gout with pegloticase, a PEGylated urate oxidase, provides insight into the importance of uric acid as an antioxidant in vivo, *Proc Natl Acad Sci U S A* 107(32):14351–14356, 2010.
130. Sundy JS, Ganson NJ, Kelly SJ, et al.: Pharmacokinetics and pharmacodynamics of intravenous PEGylated recombinant mammalian urate oxidase in patients with refractory gout, *Arthritis Rheum* 56(3):1021–1028, 2007.

70

Bisphosphonates

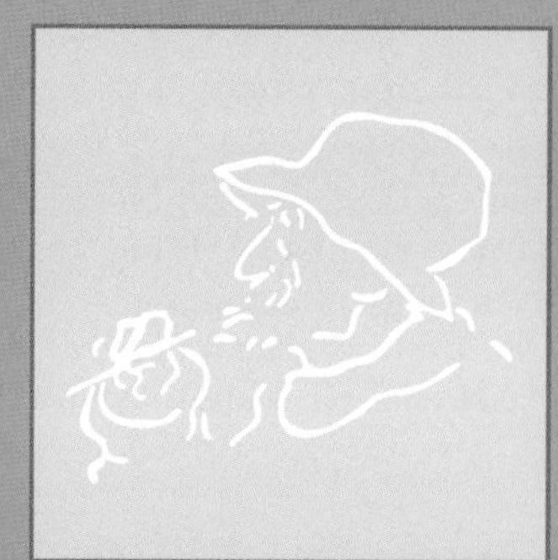

ARTHUR C. SANTORA II AND KENNETH G. SAAG

KEY POINTS

- Bisphosphonates (BPs) share a similar chemical structure that results in rapid distribution to hydroxyapatite on bone surfaces or renal excretion after either oral absorption or intravenous infusion.
- Bisphosphonates on bone surfaces are "targeted" to osteoclasts that dissolve and concentrate BPs in resorption lacunae before absorbing them.
- Inhibition of osteoclast-mediated bone resorption is useful for the efficacious treatment of osteoporosis, prevention of bone loss, and treatment of Paget's disease of bone, as well as cancer metastases in bone and hypercalcemia of malignancy.
- The nitrogen-containing bisphosphonates inhibit bone resorption at doses 100 to several 1000 times lower than those that inhibit mineralization.
- After discontinuation of BP treatment, bone resorption increases in two phases: first due to loss of BPs on bone surfaces (with a half-life of about 1 month) and the second due to loss of BPs trapped within bone formed during prior treatment (with a half-life of about 5 years). The magnitude of reduction of bone resorption more than 6 months after treatment is discontinued is a function of dose and duration of prior BP treatment.
- Bisphosphonates have common nonserious symptomatic adverse effects and rare more serious adverse effects that appear associated with prolonged skeletal retention and protracted suppression of bone resorption.

Introduction

Bisphosphonates were first synthesized over 150 years ago, as inhibitors of insoluble calcium salt formation. Their principal application was industrial, as anti-scaling agents.[1] Their initial use in humans was in toothpaste, to prevent calcified tartar accumulation.[2] Bisphosphonates were explored in nonclinical and clinical studies as inhibitors of ectopic calcification, calcium-containing kidney stone formation, and for targeting radionuclides to sites of bone mineralization. The ^{99m}Tc-methylene bisphosphonate complex (^{99m}Tc-MDP) localizes to hydroxyapatite on bone surfaces and has been the standard "bone scan" imaging agent since the 1970s. Efforts to treat and prevent heterotopic ossification with a bisphosphonate met with very limited success. No beneficial effects of bisphosphonates on either vascular calcification or kidney stone disease have been established in human studies. Nonclinical studies of bisphosphonates identified a "side effect"—inhibition of osteoclast-mediated bone resorption[3,4]—that has been exploited for the treatment of osteoporosis and Paget's disease of bone and prevention of bone loss. While etidronate inhibits both resorption and mineralization, newer bisphosphonates have been identified over the last 40 years that selectively inhibit bone resorption at much lower doses than those that inhibit bone mineralization. This chapter presents a concise review of the clinical pharmacology of bisphosphonates currently used for the treatment and prevention of osteoporosis and Paget's disease, the clinical trial data that support their use as treatments of these diseases, and a review of their potential adverse effects. While the clinical pharmacology is also relevant to the use of bisphosphonates for the treatment of cancer metastatic to bone and hypercalcemia of malignancy, clinical studies of patients with these oncologic conditions will not be reviewed.

Clinical Pharmacology

Bisphosphonates were developed to treat metabolic bone diseases characterized by abnormally high rates of bone resorption, the most common of which are osteoporosis and Paget's disease of bone. Bisphosphonates also have a role in the treatment of cancer metastatic to bone, including hypercalcemia of malignancy that may result from lysis of bone by enlarging skeletal metastases. While the clinically relevant objectives of treatment may differ by disease, the underlying clinical pharmacology resulting in inhibition of osteoclast-mediated bone resorption is common.

Chemistry of Bisphosphonates

Bisphosphonates are analogues of pyrophosphate in which the central oxygen of the P-O-P structure of pyrophosphate is a central carbon of the P-C-P structure of bisphosphonate (Fig. 70.1).

Bisphosphonates retain a relatively high affinity for hydroxyapatite found in bone but are not hydrolyzed by phosphatases in humans or other vertebrates. Table 70.1 lists the generic names and structures of marketed bisphosphonate products, including the more common brand names used in the United States.[5]

Pharmacokinetics

Absorption

The bioavailability of bisphosphonates after oral administration is generally low, less than 1%[6] when administered fasting at least 2 hours before a meal. Food and beverages (other than water) reduce bioavailability by about 90% when bisphosphonates are dosed with a meal and reduced by about 50% if taken 30 to 60 minutes before food. One exception is enteric coated risedronate 35 mg (Atelvia), which has a bioavailability when taken with food that is like that of regular risedronate 35 mg tablets taken fasting, 4 hours before a meal. Doses of bisphosphonates greater than 100 mg typically have higher bioavailability. The fractional bioavailability of ibandronate 100 mg is 30% greater and 150 mg 91% greater than the fractional bioavailability of ibandronate 50 mg than that of a 50 mg tablet.[7] The fractional bioavailability of etidronate 400 or 800 mg for Paget's disease is approximately 3%.[8]

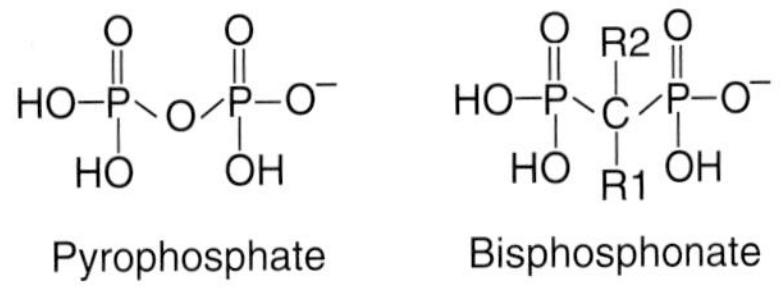

• **Fig. 70.1** Structure of pyrophosphate and a bisphosphonate. The R2 moiety of bisphosphonates used clinically in the United States is either H or OH and the R1 moiety either H, CH3, or an aliphatic or aromatic amine.

Distribution and Metabolism

After absorption or intravenous (IV) administration, bisphosphonates rapidly distribute to the extra-cellular space and are cleared from plasma with a $T_{½}$ of 1 to 2 hours.[9] In nonclinical studies, approximately 50% to 60% of the administered dose is found in bone and 40% to 50% eliminated in urine.[10] There is no known metabolism or intra-cellular soft tissue accumulation of bisphosphonates.

The kinetics of bisphosphonates in bone may be described by a three-compartment model: in bone extra-cellular fluid (ECF), on the bone surface, and within the bone matrix. The flow of bisphosphonates to bone is through afferent arteries, and from bone to systemic ECF is through the efferent veins; there is no known diffusion of bisphosphonates from bone surfaces or matrix directly to or from the systemic ECF.

Due to the high affinity of BPs for hydroxyapatite on bone surfaces and very high bone surface area, the great majority (>99%) of BPs that flow into bone are initially retained on bone surfaces.

TABLE 70.1 Bisphosphonates Used in the United States for Osteoporosis and Paget's Disease of Bone

Generic Name (Anion)[a]	Available Formulations[b]	Administration Schedule[b]	Indication[c]	Bisphosphonate Structure[d]
Imaging Agent				
Medronate	99mTc conjugate intravenous	—	Delineate areas of altered osteogenesis	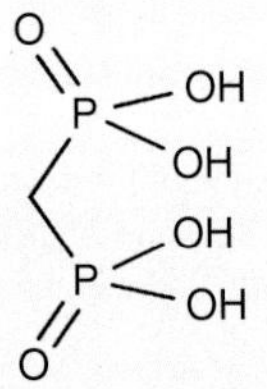
Drug				
Alendronate	5, 10 mg oral 35, 70 mg oral 70 mg effervescent	Daily Once weekly Once weekly	Osteoporosis	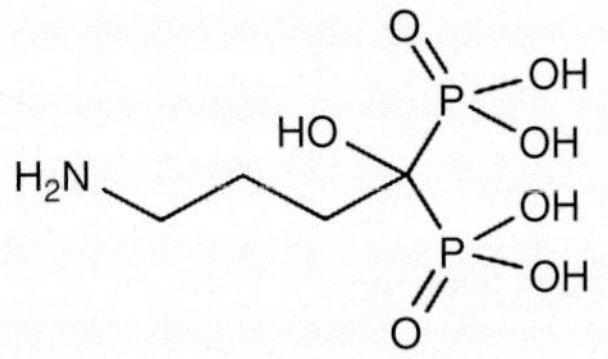
Risedronate	5 mg oral 35 mg oral 150 mg oral 30 mg oral 35 mg oral with food	Daily Once weekly Once monthly Daily for 2 months Once weekly	Osteoporosis Osteoporosis Osteoporosis Paget's disease Osteoporosis	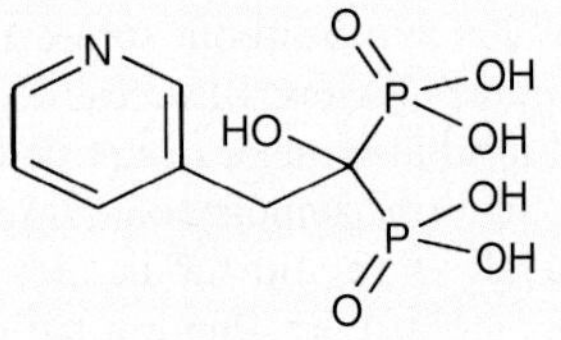
Ibandronate	150 mg oral 3 mg intravenous	Once monthly Once every 3 months	Osteoporosis	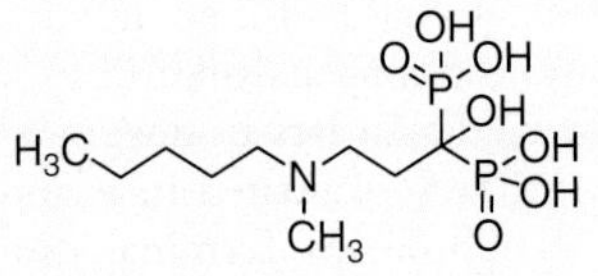

TABLE 70.1 Bisphosphonates Used in the United States for Osteoporosis and Paget's Disease of Bone—*Cont'd*

Generic Name (Anion)[a]	Available Formulations[b]	Administration Schedule[b]	Indication[c]	Bisphosphonate Structure[d]
Zoledronate	5 mg intravenous 5 mg intravenous	Once yearly or every 2 years Once	Osteoporosis Paget's disease	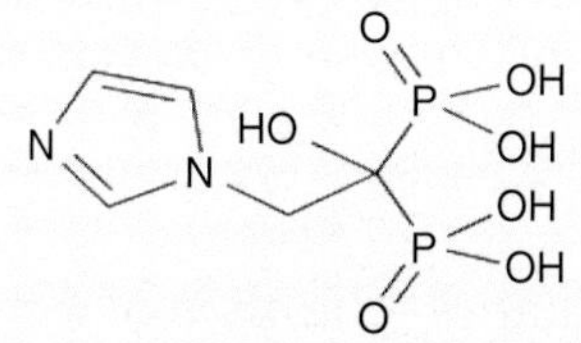
Pamidronate	30 mg intravenous	Once daily for 3 days	Paget's disease	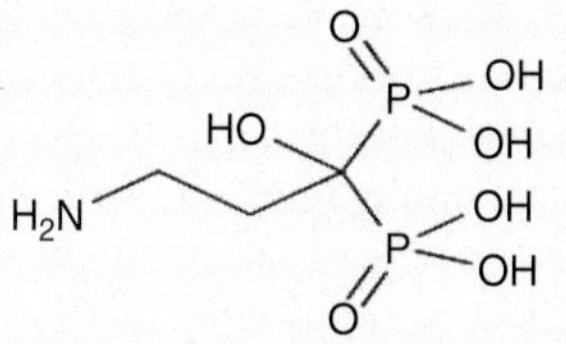
Etidronate	5 to 10 mg/kg oral 10 to 20 mg/kg oral 200 and 400 mg tablets	Daily, not to exceed 6 months Daily, not to exceed 3 months	Paget's disease	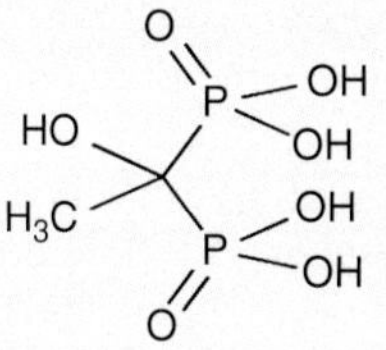

[a]Generic name of anionic active moiety. The full generic name commonly includes the salt (typically mono- or di-sodium) or uses the name of the free acid (e.g., zoledronic acid).

[b]Available formulations and administration schedules are provided to allow comparisons among bisphosphonates. Refer to the most recently approved "FULL PRESCRIBING INFORMATION" of each product before considering its use.

[c]Indications are listed in general terms as Osteoporosis and Paget's disease. Refer to the most recently approved "FULL PRESCRIBING INFORMATION" of each product for approved Indications and Usage information and Important Limitations for Use.

[d]Structures of free acid forms as presented in O'Neil MJ, Heckelman PE, Dobbelaar PH, Roman KJ, Kenny CM, Karaffa LS, and Royal Society of Chemistry (Great Britain): *The Merck index: an encyclopedia of chemicals, drugs, and biologicals,* ed 15, vol 1. Cambridge, 2013, Royal Society of Chemistry.

Nonclinical studies demonstrated that [^{3}H] alendronate was found almost exclusively on bone surfaces and was concentrated under active osteoclasts 4 hours after IV administration.[11] However, 7 weeks later, very little [^{3}H] alendronate remained on bone surfaces and most was found within recently mineralized bone matrix. Bisphosphonates trapped within mineralized bone remain there unless freed by new osteoclastic bone resorption. BPs are not metabolized and once resorbed and released into bone ECF they may: (1) bind to another bone surface or (2) leave bone and re-enter the systemic circulation. BPs recycled from bone are either terminally eliminated in urine or re-enter bone anywhere in the skeleton.

Elimination of bisphosphonates in urine occurs through both glomerular filtration and tubular secretion, the latter via a transport system shared by alendronate and etidronate.[9] While the great majority of oral bisphosphonates pass through the gastrointestinal (GI) tract without being absorbed, less than 1% of parenteral alendronate is excreted through the GI tract.[10,12]

The elimination kinetics of most bisphosphonates have been studied in animals with no notable differences observed. The terminal elimination half-life ($T_{1/2}$) of alendronate rats was 200 days in rats and 3 years in dogs.[10] Elimination of risedronate in humans has been evaluated in relatively short studies, with only 28 days of follow-up. Terminal elimination $T_{1/2}$ in humans has been reported only for alendronate. Excretion of alendronate after IV administration daily for 4 days was tracked by measuring 24-hour excretion for up to 2 years.[13] The terminal elimination $T_{1/2}$ estimated from the daily urinary excretion of alendronate measured monthly from the end of month 8 to month 18 after dosing averaged 10.5 to 10.9 years. An intermediate elimination $T_{1/2}$ of 36 days was estimated based on urinary alendronate excreted measured 1 to 6 months after dosing. In a short-term (28 day) study of risedronate excretion, the "terminal exponential half-life" was reported as 561 hours (23.4 days).[14] The intermediate elimination $T_{1/2}$—about 3 weeks for risedronate and 5 weeks for alendronate—probably represents its half-life on the surface of bone.

The half-life of alendronate in bone is shorter than the terminal elimination half-life from the body, because approximately 50% of the drug recycled from bone is returned to bone and bound to a different bone surface. Accumulation of a bisphosphonate during long-term treatment may be modeled based on the average daily dose, duration of treatment oral bioavailability, fractional uptake of the absorbed BP into bone, retention in bone after approximately 6 months, and terminal elimination $T_{1/2}$. In the case of alendronate with an oral bioavailability of 0.64%, 33% of total absorbed dose retained in the body (6 months after administration) the skeletal accumulation would be about 21 μg per day after a 10 mg average daily oral dose (same as 70 mg once weekly). The total skeletal accumulation of alendronate is estimated to be about 40 mg after 5 years and 75 mg after 10 years with either 10 mg daily or 70 mg once weekly. This model may also be used to estimate whether prior bisphosphonate treatment is likely to be sufficient to reduce bone resorption and prevent bone loss during a "drug holiday" (interruption of treatment) after multi-year use (see later in the chapter). It is estimated that if treatment is stopped after 10 years of alendronate 70 mg per week, skeletal release of alendronate into the circulation is approximately the same as that produced by an oral dose of 2.5 mg per day.[15]

Molecular Mechanism of Action

The molecular mechanisms of action of bisphosphonates were established several years after they were approved for the treatment of Paget's disease or osteoporosis. BPs may be grouped into two classes based on mechanism of action. The non-nitrogen containing BPs including etidronate may be incorporated into adenine nucleotides that are nonhydrolyzable analogues of adenosine triphosphate (ATP). They may also inhibit aminoacylation of tRNA. The result of these effects is cell death.[16–18] Nitrogen-containing bisphosphonates are not incorporated into ATP analogues. Nitrogen-containing bisphosphonates specifically inhibit farnesyl diphosphate synthase,[19,20] a key enzyme in the mevalonate pathway, leading to cholesterol synthesis. Inhibition of farnesyl diphosphate synthase reduces the isoprenoid lipids geranylgeranyl diphosphate (GGPP) and farnesyl diphosphate (FPP), leading to insufficient geranylgeranylation of regulatory proteins required for normal cytoskeletal function and osteoclast survival.[21,22] Low doses of nitrogen-containing bisphosphonates produce reversible inhibition of osteoclast function while high doses result in apoptosis. Non-nitrogen containing bisphosphonates do not inhibit farnesyl diphosphate synthase.

Mechanism of Action at the Cell and Tissue Level

Osteoclasts are uniquely sensitive to the effects of bisphosphonates because they are exposed to much higher concentrations of BPs than other cells. There are several reasons: (1) bisphosphonates are targeted to bone surfaces due to their high affinity for hydroxyapatite; (2) osteoclasts solubilize bisphosphonates on bone surfaces when they acidify resorption lacunae and trap them within the lacunae where their local concentration may reach 1 mM[23]; and (3) BPs are hydrophilic, charged anions that do enter cells by either diffusion, active or passive transport across their plasma membranes. However, BPs enter osteoclasts by endocytosis along with other contents within resorption lacunae.

Bisphosphonates on bone surfaces have no recognized direct effect on osteoblasts, quiescent lining cells, or pre-osteoblasts primarily because these cells do not solubilize alendronate on bone surfaces, do not form resorption lacunae and concentrate BPs released from the bone surface, and have much lower levels of endocytosis than do mature osteoclasts. When pre-osteoclasts on a bone surface coated with a bisphosphonate become active osteoclasts, they accumulate BPs that inhibit their general metabolic activity. In nonclinical studies, [^{3}H] alendronate is found with osteoclasts 12 to 15 hours after it is administered.[11] As osteoclasts accumulate bisphosphonates their ruffled borders adjacent to the resorption lacuna are lost, acidification is inhibited,[24] and resorption slows.[25] Alendronate in solution has little or no effect on isolated osteoclasts until the concentration reaches 0.5 mM.[25] Inhibition of bone resorption by isolated osteoclasts in vitro is reversible. While sufficiently high doses of N-BPs may cause osteoclast apoptosis, lower and moderate doses do not.[26]

Nonclinical and clinical studies of bisphosphonates included detailed histologic examination of bone after short- and long-term treatment. None of the nitrogen-containing BPs that are selective inhibitors of bone resorption have been associated with clinically meaningful inhibition of bone mineralization and/or osteomalacia. Treatment of Paget's disease with zoledronic acid may result in such rapid mineralization of pagetic bone that hypocalcemia, hypophosphatemia, secondary hyperparathyroidism, and delayed mineralization may transiently occur.[27] In contrast, the nonselective BP etidronate may directly inhibit bone mineralization at the standard doses for treatment of Paget's disease.

Bone histomorphology of osteoporotic patients treated with alendronate and other nitrogen-containing bisphosphonates shows greatly reduced rates of bone formation that reaches a stable plateau after 1 to 2 years and remains at the same low level during long-term treatment.[28] There is very little primary bone modeling in adults, and bone resorption rates cannot be accurately measured with bone histomorphometry. It is hypothesized that decreased bone remodeling during bisphosphonate treatment is associated with similar decreases in both resorption and formation. While the decrease in bone remodeling is large versus that observed in the placebo group of untreated osteoporotic women in these studies, bone remodeling in osteoporotic postmenopausal women may be three times greater than that found in young pre-menopausal women.[29] Moreover, improvement in trabecular microarchitecture has been observed during long-term treatment with alendronate.[30]

Mechanism of Action on Bone Strength

The objective of treatment of osteoporotic patients and people who are losing bone (e.g., due to menopause, hypogonadism in men, or with administration of chronic glucocorticoids) is to reduce their risk of fracture, and several bisphosphonates reduce the risk of vertebral and nonvertebral (including hip) fractures during treatment for 3 to 6 years. There are several hypothetical mechanisms that may account for these favorable effects.

Bisphosphonates are generally effective in preventing bone loss associated with menopause in women, hypogonadism in men, and people on glucocorticoids and, in doing so, prevent a decrease in bone strength resulting from a decrease in bone mass. However, if this were their only effect it would take 10 years of treatment to prevent the anticipated 10% peri-menopausal loss of bone mass[31] and result in a 50% lower hip or spine fracture risk (based on bone mineral density [BMD] vs. fracture risk in epidemiologic studies).[32] As the reduction in risk of spine and hip fractures occurs within 6 to 18 months[33] when changes in BMD are relatively small, their short-term effects on bone strength are likely mediated through the effect of decreased remodeling on bone microarchitecture. In clinical trials, this is associated with a reduction in levels of biochemical measures of bone remodeling such as N-telopeptide (a marker of bone resorption) and propeptide of type 1 pro-collagen (P1NP).

Treatment Effects and Indications

Osteoporosis

The vast majority of bisphosphonate use is for the prevention and treatment of osteoporosis, mostly in post-menopausal women, but also in men and among men and women on glucocorticoids. Indications for use of these and other osteoporosis drugs are discussed

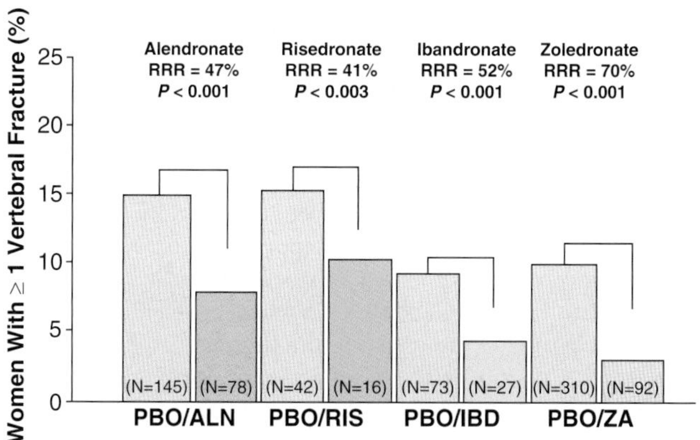

• **Fig. 70.2** Vertebral fracture risk reduction in bisphosphonate randomized controlled clinical trials among post-menopausal women with prevalent fractures. *ALN,* Alendronate; *IBD,* ibandronate; *PBO,* placebo; *RIS,* risedronate; *ZA,* zoledronic acid. (Data obtained from the following sources: Black DM, Cummings SR, Karpf DB, et al.: Randomised trial of effect of alendronate on risk of fracture in women with existing vertebral fractures. Fracture Intervention Trial Research Group. *Lancet* 348:1535-1541, 1996; Harris ST, Watts NB, Genant HK, et al.: Effects of risedronate treatment on vertebral and nonvertebral fractures in women with postmenopausal osteoporosis: a randomized controlled trial. Vertebral Efficacy With Risedronate Therapy (VERT) Study Group. *JAMA* 282:1344-1352, 1999; Chesnut CH, 3rd, Skag A, Christiansen C, et al.: Effects of oral ibandronate administered daily or intermittently on fracture risk in postmenopausal osteoporosis. *J Bone Miner Res* 19:1241-1249, 2004; and Black DM, Delmas PD, Eastell R, et al.: Once-yearly zoledronic acid for treatment of postmenopausal osteoporosis. *NEJM* 356:1809-1822, 2007.)

in Chapter 107. All bisphosphonates currently used in these disease states (see Table 70.1) have demonstrated efficacy and were approved for osteoporosis treatment and/or prevention based on their ability to promote an increase in BMD at the spine and hip, reduce bone remodeling, and decrease the risk of vertebral fractures (Fig. 70.2).[34–37]

Alendronate,[34,38] risedronate,[39] and zoledronic acid[37] significantly reduce the risk of nonvertebral fractures and hip fractures in post-menopausal osteoporosis. For example, in the large fracture intervention trial (FIT), alendronate reduced the risk of vertebral, hip, and wrist fractures by about 50%.[33] Risedronate resulted in an approximate 30% risk reduction of hip fractures overall, although fractures efficacy was less apparent among women age 80 or older, who were selected for the study on the basis of clinical risk factors.[39] Zoledronic acid is the only bisphosphonate studied among patients with recent hip fracture, in whom it was able to successfully reduce the rate of subsequent clinical fractures by 35%, and there was a nearly 30% reduced overall mortality in those patients who received zoledronic acid versus placebo.[40] While the pivotal fracture studies of alendronate and risedronate used daily dosing, weekly dosing (alendronate and risedronate) or monthly dosing (risedronate) have become much more common due to near equivalency in terms of BMD effects, easier administration, and improved adherence with less frequent dosing. With generic availability of 1 year zoledronic acid, this has proven a preferred therapeutic option for many people preferring less frequent administration and avoiding the oral side effects discussed later in the chapter.

For men, and for prevention and treatment of glucocorticoid-induced osteoporosis,[41–44] bone effects are largely limited to BMD stabilization or improvements and suppression biochemical markers of bone remodeling, because, at a minimum, primary studies for these disorders were insufficiently long or large enough to show a fracture effect. Furthermore, there are no head-to-head comparator data demonstrating differential reductions in risk of fractures when comparing one bisphosphonate with another. Limited data suggest that alendronate may be relatively more potent that risedronate at standard dose with regard to BMD density.[45,46] Beyond their use for initial prevention and treatment of osteoporosis, another key indication for bisphosphonates is after the use of an osteoanabolic drug such as teriparatide, abaloparatide, or romosozumab. Consolidating BMD gain and helping to fill in only partially calcified remodeling space is facilitated by the use of a bisphosphonate after an anabolic.[47,48] It is also important to administer a bisphosphonate after denosumab, because its effects on suppressing bone resorption are much more transient than a bisphosphonate upon its discontinuation. The timing of an oral (likely immediately when the next dose of denosumab would be due) versus an IV bisphosphonate (perhaps with a slight delay beyond the typical denosumab infusion period) is under further investigation.[49–51]

TABLE 70.2 Bisphosphonate Safety Considerations

Osteonecrosis of the jaw (ONJ)
Atypical fractures
Acute phase reactions
Upper gastrointestinal adverse effects/esophageal cancer
Atrial fibrillation
Fracture nonunion
Renal toxicity
Uveitis
Pregnancy/pediatric considerations

Paget's Disease of Bone

Bisphosphonates, particularly IV zoledronic acid, have dramatically changed the landscape of management of Paget's disease of bone. A single IV infusion is often credited with a dramatic reversal of atypical bone remodeling, and for some patients retreatment may not be necessary for years, if not indefinitely (also see Chapter 107).[52]

Adverse Effects and Tolerability

Adverse effects of bisphosphonates are generally not severe and those that can be more severe are generally not common (see Table 70.2). For most patients with a clear clinical indication for a bisphosphonate, the risk benefit ratio is highly favorable.

Gastrointestinal

Oral bisphosphonates can cause nausea, dyspepsia, esophagitis, and rarely esophageal or gastric ulcerations.[53] The mechanism is related to a direct toxic effect on the mucosa due to a direct chemical irritation of the mucosa (pill esophagitis). Exercising caution when taking an oral bisphophonate by imbibing the drug with a full glass of water and remaining upright for at least 30 minutes post-dose can partially mitigate this issue. Less than 20% of patients stop oral bisphosphonates due to GI intolerance.[53] A meta-analysis suggested an increased risk of esophageal cancer, but this concern was offset by other meta-analyses using the same or newer datasets that did not support such an association.[54,55]

Acute Phase Response Reactions

With use of IV bisphosphonates an "acute phase reaction" (APR) may occur.[37] APRs can include myalgias, arthralgias, abdominal/bone pain, malaise, and occasional pyrexia.[56] Mild and usually transient (typically lasting less than 4 days) reactions may be present as often as 30% of the time, and more significant flu-like illnesses occur in less than 10% of people. Symptoms are attenuated with acetaminophen and tend to be less severe or absent with IV bisphosphonate re-administration or among people who have previously received oral bisphosphonates. APRs are associated with circulating gamma-delta T cells and may be more common in younger individuals.[57–59] Arthralgias and bone pain are occasionally reported with oral bisphosphonates as well.

Osteonecrosis of the Jaw

Osteonecrosis of the jaw (ONJ) is defined as an area of exposed bone in the maxillofacial region that does not heal within 8 weeks and excludes osteoradionecrosis due to radiation therapy.[60] Medication-related ONJ requires a history of bisphosphonate, RANKL inhibitor, or angiogenesis inhibitor treatment.[61] The incidence, clinical presentation, and management of ONJ differ greatly in osteoporotic patients treated with bisphosphonates (or denosumab) and patients with cancer metastases in bones receiving much higher doses. ONJ was first described in cancer patients treated with IV pamidronate and zoledronic acid.[62] The incidence of ONJ in cancer patients treated with high-dose zoledronic acid or denosumab is approximately 1% to 2% per year.[60,63,64] During long-term treatment cumulative incidence approached 10% in the setting of malignancy.[65] In contrast, ONJ in patients treated with oral or IV bisphosphonates at standard osteoporosis doses is a rare event. The incidence is estimated at approximately 1/10,000 patients exposed.[61,66,67]

ONJ may occur in the absence of bisphosphonate treatment, and the background incidence of ONJ in untreated osteoporotic patients is unknown. The pathophysiology of anti-resorptive related ONJ has not been established, and a number of potential mechanisms have been hypothesized.[61] The majority of cases of ONJ follow invasive dental procedures such as tooth extraction, dental implants, or bony surgery. Periodontal or other dental disease are risk factors. When ONJ is suspected, patients should be referred to oral surgeons familiar with the differential diagnosis (e.g., vs. infectious osteitis or osteomyelitis) and treatment of ONJ. While most cases of anti-resorptive-related ONJ in patients with osteoporosis are mild and resolve with conservative measures (e.g., anti-microbial rinses),[60,63,68] long-term antibiotic treatment may be required when infection is present. Interruption of treatment with bisphosphonates is recommended until the mouth is fully healed. Restarting anti-resorptive drug therapy should be considered based on an individual patient's benefit and risk.[61,69–71] Controversy exists regarding the role of bisphosphonate discontinuation antecedent to invasive dental procedures. While there are no studies that indicate that the risk of ONJ is reduced when bisphosphonates are interrupted before invasive dental procedures, the sustained inhibition of resorption of these drugs makes a short break in therapy before dental work less meaningful in terms of a detrimental effect on osteoporosis risk in most settings.

Atypical Femoral Fracture

An atypical femoral fracture (AFF) is a fracture that occurs in the subtrochanteric region of the hip, with minimal trauma. It is further defined as a transverse fracture involving both cortices and it often results in a medial bone spike.[72] A prodromal syndrome of bone pain is often associated as a periosteal reaction or early stress fracture affecting the diaphyseal cortex of this region. AFFs are rare with bisphosphonate exposure but appear significantly associated with bisphosphonate use based on predominately large observational studies.[73,74] The incidence is estimated at 1/1000 to 6/1000[75] and is most related to prolonged bisphosphonate exposure.[76] Critical evaluation of hip or thigh pain among bisphosphonate users should include conventional radiographic imaging and, if necessary, nuclear medicine scintigraphy and/or MRI to exclude this possibility.[77] Intramedullary nail placement is necessary for completed fractures and may be recommended for certain stress fractures associated with a "dreaded black line." Bisphosphonate discontinuation is necessary if this adverse effect occurs. Anecdotal reports support use of osteoanabolic drugs to address this concern and substitute for osteoporosis management, should it occur. Mechanisms for atypical femoral fractures and ONJ may be similar.[78,79]

Other Bisphosphonate Adverse Effects

Atrial Fibrillation

In a large study of zoledronic acid use among older adults with recent hip fractures, an increased rate of serious cases of atrial fibrillation was reported.[80–82] A review of placebo-controlled clinical trials of alendronate did not find an increased risk of atrial fibrillation or flutter in patients treated with alendronate.[83] A comprehensive review of this issue by the U.S. Food and Drug Administration could not attribute atrial fibrillation to a class effect of bisphosphonates.[84]

Uveitis

Very rare reports of uveitis have been described, and it seems likely that the mechanism is similar to the acute phase response.[85,86]

Fracture Nonunion

Long bone fracture healing with bisphosphonates has been reported to be associated with a more exuberant callus.[87] In studies of fracture healing in animals, treatment with alendronate before or after the fracture did not affect callus formation or the strength of a healed bone at the fracture site.[88] Terminal remodeling of the callus was slowed during treatment post-fracture. The risk of both delayed fracture union and nonunion has been studied as a safety endpoint in almost all long-term placebo-controlled trials of bisphosphonates for the prevention or treatment of osteoporosis, and an increased risk has not been found. An increased risk of fracture nonunion was reported in a case-controlled study of patients who used bisphosphonates after a fracture of the humerus,[89] but similar results have not been consistently confirmed in other studies.[90] It is suggested by some that potent IV bisphosphonates not be administered for 2 weeks following a long-bone fracture to maximize their benefit and avoid localization of the bisphosphonate to the healing fracture callus.[91]

Renal Toxicity

Potent IV bisphosphonates must be avoided in people with impaired glomerular filtration rates (GFRs). A creatinine clearance greater than 35 mL/min and absence of acute renal impairment are necessary to administer IV zoledronic acid. Acute renal

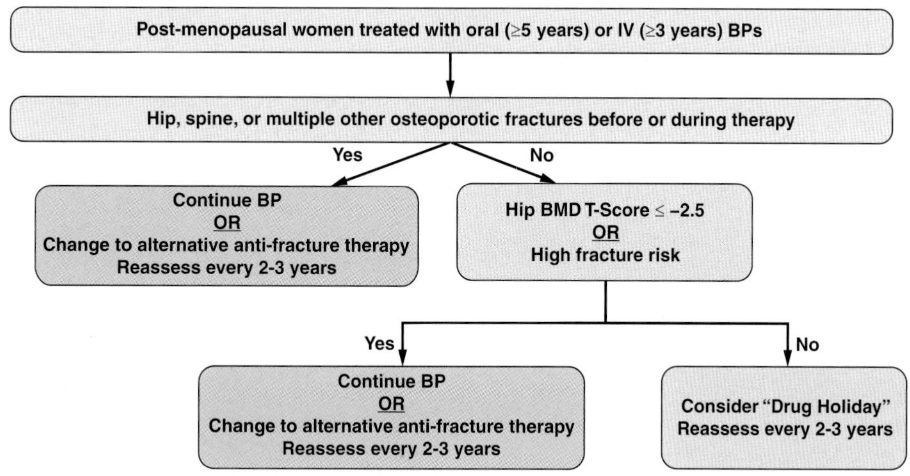

• **Fig. 70.3** American Society for Bone and Mineral Research algorithm for the management of post-menopausal women on long-term bisphosphonate therapy. *Blue shading* denotes recommendation to continue current therapy and *red shading* to stop the bisphosphonate or switch to an alternate osteoporosis therapy. *BMD,* Bone mineral density; *BP,* bisphosphonate; *IV,* intravenous. (Modified from Adler RA, El-Hajj Fuleihan G, Bauer DC, et al.: Managing osteoporosis in patients on long-term bisphosphonate treatment: report of a Task Force of the American Society for Bone and Mineral Research. *J Bone Miner Res* 31:16-35, 2016.)

toxicity may occur in patients with normal renal function when IV bisphosphonates are infused too rapidly. A single zoledronic acid dose should not exceed 5 mg, and the duration of infusion should be no less than 15 minutes. Oral agents are also relatively contraindicated in those with advanced chronic kidney disease (CKD-3 and those on dialysis), due to the risk of hypocalcemia and uncertain effect on renal osteodystrophy. Oral bisphosphonates are not recognized to cause renal injury when approved doses are administered to patients without advanced chronic kidney disease. Reports support renal safety and adequate efficacy of risedronate,[92] in particular, among people with an impaired GFR (CKD-2 and -3). In people with advanced chronic kidney disease, other forms of metabolic bone disease may be present and bisphosphonates or other osteoporosis medications may be relatively or absolutely contraindicated.

Use in Children and Pregnancy Considerations

Bisphosphonates should not be used during pregnancy. Nonclinical reproductive toxicology studies demonstrated that high doses of bisphosphonates throughout pregnancy cause maternal hypocalcemia and dystocia associated with maternal death and subsequent fetal death. Maternal hypocalcemia may be associated with delayed ossification of the fetal skeleton. Except for zoledronic acid, which may cause CNS, visceral, and external malformations, other bisphosphonates are not recognized as teratogenic. As they are contraindicated during pregnancy, there are relatively few reports of the outcome of pregnancy after bisphosphonate use during pregnancy. There are reports of planned use during pregnancy in patients with osteogenesis imperfecta and hypercalcemia of malignancy. Negative fetal outcomes were uncommon and generally attributed to concomitant use of other drugs. Several reviews of the literature indicate no clear evidence of fetal or maternal harm after generally brief exposure to these drugs.[93–96] Due to the skeletal retention and gradual skeletal release after treatment discontinuation, there are concerns about the use of these drugs in pre-menopausal women of child-bearing potential. Anecdotes exist suggesting no clear associations with fetal abnormalities among women who have been past bisphosphonate users and have had subsequent pregnancies, many of whom have also been on glucocorticoids. Women who take bisphosphonates before pregnancy or inadvertently during early pregnancy likely have slightly worse fetal outcomes overall, owing in part to the underlying disease for which glucocorticoids are required. However, very cautious use of bisphosphonate is recommended in younger women with glucocorticoid-induced osteoporosis.

There are no approved indications for use of bisphosphonates in children with glucocorticoid-induced osteoporosis, osteogenesis imperfecta, or other disorders of calcium or mineral metabolism associated with high rates of bone resorption. Bisphosphonates being investigated may be helpful among younger women and children, particularly those receiving glucocorticoids, and among those who have experienced a prior fragility fracture.

Duration of Therapy and "Drug Holidays"

Rare adverse events that appear to be associated with more protracted bisphosphonate usage, such as ONJ and AFF, coupled with the prolonged benefits even after bisphosphonates are stopped with respect to bone remodeling suppression, relative stability of BMD (particularly at the spine), and a modest protracted fracture benefit,[97] have motivated consideration of taking a break from bisphosphonate therapy, often termed a drug holiday. A task force of the American Society of Bone and Mineral Research (ASBMR)[98] (Fig. 70.3) has suggested that after 3 years of IV bisphosphonates[99] and 5 years of oral therapy, a break in therapy should be considered among patients at lower future fracture risk for up to 1 to 3 years.[98] For some patients, residual fracture risk may be significant,[100] and it is unwarranted to stop all anti-fracture medications. Instead, switching to an osteoporosis drug with an alternative mechanism of action or one that is not retained in the skeleton is a consideration.

The references for this chapter can also be found on ExpertConsult.com.

References

1. Fleisch H: *Bisphosphonates in bone disease: from the laboratory to the patient*, 4th ed, San Diego, 2000, Academic Press.
2. Francis MD, Briner WW: The effect of phosphonates on dental enamel in vitro and calculus formation in vivo, *Calcif Tissue Res* 11:1–9, 1973.
3. Fleisch H, Russell RG, Francis MD: Diphosphonates inhibit hydroxyapatite dissolution in vitro and bone resorption in tissue culture and in vivo, *Science* 165:1262–1264, 1969.
4. Fleisch H, Russell RG, Simpson B, et al.: Prevention by a diphosphonate of immobilization "osteoporosis" in rats, *Nature* 223:211–212, 1969.
5. O'Neil MJ, Heckelman PE, Dobbelaar PH, et al.: *The Merck index: an encyclopedia of chemicals, drugs, and biologicals*, 15th ed, Cambridge, UK, 2013, Royal Society of Chemistry.
6. Merck & Co. I: *FOSAMAX® (alendronte sodium) tablets and oral solution Prescribing Information. Merck & Co. I*, Merck & Co., Inc, 2016. http://www.merck.com/product/usa/pi_circulars/f/fosamax/fosamax_pi.pdf.
7. Reginster JY, Wilson KM, Dumont E, et al.: Monthly oral ibandronate is well tolerated and efficacious in postmenopausal women: results from the monthly oral pilot study, *J Clin Endocrinol Metab* 90:5018–5024, 2005.
8. Recker RR, Saville PD: Intestinal absorption of disodium ethane-1-hydroxy-1,1-diphosphonate (disodium etidronate) using a deconvolution technique, *Toxicol Appl Pharmacol* 24:580–589, 1973.
9. Lin JH: Bisphosphonates: a review of their pharmacokinetic properties, *Bone* 18:75–85, 1996.
10. Lin JH, Duggan DE, Chen IW, et al.: Physiological disposition of alendronate, a potent anti-osteolytic bisphosphonate, in laboratory animals, *Drug Metab Dispos* 19:926–932, 1991.
11. Masarachia P, Weinreb M, Balena R, et al.: Comparison of the distribution of 3H-alendronate and 3H-etidronate in rat and mouse bones, *Bone* 19:281–290, 1996.
12. Porras AG, Holland SD, Gertz BJ: Pharmacokinetics of alendronate, *Clin Pharmacokinet* 36:315–328, 1999.
13. Khan SA, Kanis JA, Vasikaran S, et al.: Elimination and biochemical responses to intravenous alendronate in postmenopausal osteoporosis, *J Bone Miner Res* 12:1700–1707, 1997.
14. Chilcott W: *ACTONEL® (risedronate sodium) tablets Prescribing Information*, Warner Chilcott (US), LLC, 2015. https://wwwallergancom/assets/pdf/actonel_pi.
15. Rodan G, Reszka A, Golub E, et al.: Bone safety of long-term bisphosphonate treatment, *Curr Med Res Opin* 20:1291–1300, 2004.
16. Frith JC, Monkkonen J, Blackburn GM, et al.: Clodronate and liposome-encapsulated clodronate are metabolized to a toxic ATP analog, adenosine 5′-(beta, gamma-dichloromethylene) triphosphate, by mammalian cells in vitro, *J Bone Miner Res* 12:1358–1367, 1997.
17. Rogers MJ, Ji X, Russell RG, et al.: Incorporation of bisphosphonates into adenine nucleotides by amoebae of the cellular slime mould Dictyostelium discoideum, *Biochem J* 303(Pt 1):303–311, 1994.
18. Rogers MJ, Russell RG, Blackburn GM, et al.: Metabolism of halogenated bisphosphonates by the cellular slime mould Dictyostelium discoideum, *Biochem Biophys Res Commun* 189:414–423, 1992.
19. Bergstrom JD, Bostedor RG, Masarachia PJ, et al.: Alendronate is a specific, nanomolar inhibitor of farnesyl diphosphate synthase, *Arch Biochem Biophys* 373:231–241, 2000.
20. Dunford JE, Thompson K, Coxon FP, et al.: Structure-activity relationships for inhibition of farnesyl diphosphate synthase in vitro and inhibition of bone resorption in vivo by nitrogen-containing bisphosphonates, *J Pharmacol Exp Ther* 296:235–242, 2001.
21. Fisher JE, Rogers MJ, Halasy JM, et al.: Alendronate mechanism of action: geranylgeraniol, an intermediate in the mevalonate pathway, prevents inhibition of osteoclast formation, bone resorption, and kinase activation in vitro, *Proc Natl Acad Sci U S A* 96:133–138, 1999.
22. Luckman SP, Hughes DE, Coxon FP, et al.: Nitrogen-containing bisphosphonates inhibit the mevalonate pathway and prevent post-translational prenylation of GTP-binding proteins, including Ras, *J Bone Miner Res* 13:581–589, 1998.
23. Russell RG: Bisphosphonates: the first 40 years, *Bone* 49:2–19, 2011.
24. Zimolo Z, Wesolowski G, Rodan GA: Acid extrusion is induced by osteoclast attachment to bone. Inhibition by alendronate and calcitonin, *J Clin Invest* 96:2277–2283, 1995.
25. Sato M, Grasser W, Endo N, et al.: Bisphosphonate action. Alendronate localization in rat bone and effects on osteoclast ultrastructure, *J Clin Invest* 88:2095–2105, 1991.
26. Fisher JE, Rosenberg E, Santora AC, et al.: In vitro and in vivo responses to high and low doses of nitrogen-containing bisphosphonates suggest engagement of different mechanisms for inhibition of osteoclastic bone resorption, *Calcif Tissue Int* 92:531–538, 2013.
27. Polyzos SA, Anastasilakis AD, Makras P, et al.: Paget's disease of bone and calcium homeostasis: focus on bisphosphonate treatment, *Exp Clin Endocrinol Diabetes* 119:519–524, 2011.
28. Chavassieux PM, Arlot ME, Reda C, et al.: Histomorphometric assessment of the long-term effects of alendronate on bone quality and remodeling in patients with osteoporosis, *J Clin Invest* 100:1475–1480, 1997.
29. Bone HG, Greenspan SL, McKeever C, et al.: Alendronate and estrogen effects in postmenopausal women with low bone mineral density. Alendronate/Estrogen Study Group, *J Clin Endocrinol Metab* 85:720–726, 2000.
30. Recker R, Masarachia P, Santora A, et al.: Trabecular bone microarchitecture after alendronate treatment of osteoporotic women, *Curr Med Res Opin* 21:185–194, 2005.
31. Greendale GA, Sowers M, Han W, et al.: Bone mineral density loss in relation to the final menstrual period in a multiethnic cohort: results from the Study of Women's Health Across the Nation (SWAN), *J Bone Miner Res* 27:111–118, 2012.
32. Stone KL, Seeley DG, Lui LY, et al.: BMD at multiple sites and risk of fracture of multiple types: long-term results from the Study of Osteoporotic Fractures, *J Bone Miner Res* 18:1947–1954, 2003.
33. Black DM, Thompson DE, Bauer DC, et al.: Fracture risk reduction with alendronate in women with osteoporosis: the Fracture Intervention Trial. FIT Research Group, *J Clin Endocrinol Metab* 85:4118–4124, 2000.
34. Black DM, Cummings SR, Karpf DB, et al.: Randomised trial of effect of alendronate on risk of fracture in women with existing vertebral fractures. Fracture Intervention Trial Research Group, *Lancet* 348:1535–1541, 1996.
35. Harris ST, Watts NB, Genant HK, et al.: Effects of risedronate treatment on vertebral and nonvertebral fractures in women with postmenopausal osteoporosis: a randomized controlled trial. Vertebral Efficacy With Risedronate Therapy (VERT) Study Group, *JAMA* 282:1344–1352, 1999.
36. Chesnut 3rd CH, Skag A, Christiansen C, et al.: Effects of oral ibandronate administered daily or intermittently on fracture risk in postmenopausal osteoporosis, *J Bone Miner Res* 19:1241–1249, 2004.
37. Black DM, Delmas PD, Eastell R, et al.: Once-yearly zoledronic acid for treatment of postmenopausal osteoporosis, *New England Journal of Medicine* 356:1809–1822, 2007.
38. Karpf DB, Shapiro DR, Seeman E, et al.: Prevention of nonvertebral fractures by alendronate. A meta-analysis. Alendronate Osteoporosis Treatment Study Groups, *JAMA* 277:1159–1164, 1997.

39. McClung MR, Geusens P, Miller PD, et al.: Effect of risedronate on the risk of hip fracture in elderly women. Hip Intervention Program Study Group, *N Engl J Med* 344:333–340, 2001.
40. Lyles KW, Colon-Emeric CS, Magaziner JS, et al.: Zoledronic acid and clinical fractures and mortality after hip fracture, *N Engl J Med* 357:1799–1809, 2007.
41. Saag KG, Emkey R, Schnitzer TJ, et al.: Alendronate for the prevention and treatment of glucocorticoid-induced osteoporosis. Glucocorticoid-Induced Osteoporosis Intervention Study Group, *N Engl J Med* 339:292–299, 1998.
42. Cohen S, Levy RM, Keller M, et al.: Risedronate therapy prevents corticosteroid-induced bone loss: a twelve-month, multicenter, randomized, double-blind, placebo-controlled, parallel-group study, *Arthritis Rheum* 42:2309–2318, 1999.
43. Reid DM, Hughes RA, Laan RF, et al.: Efficacy and safety of daily risedronate in the treatment of corticosteroid-induced osteoporosis in men and women: a randomized trial. European Corticosteroid-Induced Osteoporosis Treatment Study, *J Bone Miner Res* 15:1006–1013, 2000.
44. Reid DM, Devogelaer JP, Saag K, et al.: Zoledronic acid and risedronate in the prevention and treatment of glucocorticoid-induced osteoporosis (HORIZON): a multicentre, double-blind, double-dummy, randomised controlled trial, *Lancet* 373:1253–1263, 2009.
45. Rosen CJ, Hochberg MC, Bonnick SL, et al.: Treatment with once-weekly alendronate 70 mg compared with once-weekly risedronate 35 mg in women with postmenopausal osteoporosis: a randomized double-blind study, *J Bone Miner Res* 20:141–151, 2005.
46. Bonnick S, Saag KG, Kiel DP, et al.: Comparison of weekly treatment of postmenopausal osteoporosis with alendronate versus risedronate over two years, *J Clin Endocrinol Metab* 91:2631–2637, 2006.
47. Black DM, Bilezikian JP, Ensrud KE, et al.: One year of alendronate after one year of parathyroid hormone (1-84) for osteoporosis, *N Engl J Med* 353:555–565, 2005.
48. Saag KG, Petersen J, Brandi ML, et al.: Romosozumab or alendronate for fracture prevention in women with osteoporosis, *N Engl J Med* 377:1417–1427, 2017.
49. Reid IR, Horne AM, Mihov B, et al.: Bone loss after denosumab: only partial protection with zoledronate, *Calcif Tissue Int* 101:371–374, 2017.
50. Horne AM, Mihov B, Reid IR: Bone loss after romosozumab/denosumab: effects of bisphosphonates, *Calcif Tissue Int* 103:55–61, 2018.
51. Chapurlat R: Effects and management of denosumab discontinuation, *Joint Bone Spine* 85:515–517, 2018.
52. Reid IR, Miller P, Lyles K, et al.: Comparison of a single infusion of zoledronic acid with risedronate for Paget's disease, *N Engl J Med* 353:898–908, 2005.
53. Modi A, Sen S, Adachi JD, et al.: The impact of GI events on persistence and adherence to osteoporosis treatment: 3-, 6-, and 12-month findings in the MUSIC-OS study, *Osteoporos Int* 29:329–337, 2018.
54. Andrici J, Tio M, Eslick GD: Meta-analysis: oral bisphosphonates and the risk of oesophageal cancer, *Aliment Pharmacol Ther* 36:708–716, 2012.
55. Wright E, Schofield PT, Molokhia M: Bisphosphonates and evidence for association with esophageal and gastric cancer: a systematic review and meta-analysis, *BMJ Open* 5:e007133, 2015.
56. Bertoldo F, Pancheri S, Zenari S, et al.: Serum 25-hydroxyvitamin D levels modulate the acute-phase response associated with the first nitrogen-containing bisphosphonate infusion, *J Bone Miner Res* 25:447–454, 2010.
57. Popp AW, Senn R, Curkovic I, et al.: Factors associated with acute-phase response of bisphosphonate-naïve or pretreated women with osteoporosis receiving an intravenous first dose of zoledronate or ibandronate, *Osteoporosis International* 28:1995–2002, 2017.
58. Rossini M, Adami S, Viapiana O, et al.: Circulating gammadelta T cells and the risk of acute-phase response after zoledronic acid administration, *J Bone Miner Res* 27:227–230, 2012.
59. Reid IR, Gamble GD, Mesenbrink P, et al.: Characterization of and risk factors for the acute-phase response after zoledronic acid, *J Clin Endocrinol Metab* 95:4380–4387, 2010.
60. Khan AA, Morrison A, Hanley DA, et al.: Diagnosis and management of osteonecrosis of the jaw: a systematic review and international consensus, *J Bone Miner Res* 30:3–23, 2015.
61. Ruggiero SL, Dodson TB, Fantasia J, et al.: American Association of Oral and Maxillofacial Surgeons position paper on medication-related osteonecrosis of the jaw—2014 update, *J Oral Maxillofac Surg* 72:1938–1956, 2014.
62. Marx RE: Pamidronate (Aredia) and zoledronate (Zometa) induced avascular necrosis of the jaws: a growing epidemic, *J Oral Maxillofac Surg* 61:1115–1117, 2003.
63. Ruggiero SL, Dodson TB, Assael LA, et al.: American Association of Oral and Maxillofacial Surgeons position paper on bisphosphonate-related osteonecrosis of the jaws—2009 update, *J Oral Maxillofac Surg* 67:2–12, 2009.
64. Scagliotti GV, Hirsh V, Siena S, et al.: Overall survival improvement in patients with lung cancer and bone metastases treated with denosumab versus zoledronic acid: subgroup analysis from a randomized phase 3 study, *J Thorac Oncol* 7:1823–1829, 2012.
65. Hoff AO, Toth BB, Altundag K, et al.: Frequency and risk factors associated with osteonecrosis of the jaw in cancer patients treated with intravenous bisphosphonates, *J Bone Miner Res* 23:826–836, 2008.
66. Khan A, Morrison A, Cheung A, et al.: Osteonecrosis of the jaw (ONJ): diagnosis and management in 2015, *Osteoporos Int* 27:853–859, 2016.
67. Khan AA, Morrison A, Kendler DL, et al.: Case-based review of osteonecrosis of the jaw (ONJ) and application of the international recommendations for management from the international task force on ONJ, *J Clin Densitom* 20:8–24, 2017.
68. Ruggiero SL: Diagnosis and staging of medication-related osteonecrosis of the jaw, *Oral Maxillofac Surg Clin North Am* 27:479–487, 2015.
69. Marx RE, Sawatari Y, Fortin M, et al.: Bisphosphonate-induced exposed bone (osteonecrosis/osteopetrosis) of the jaws: risk factors, recognition, prevention, and treatment, *J Oral Maxillofac Surg* 63:1567–1575, 2005.
70. Hellstein JW, Adler RA, Edwards B, et al.: Managing the care of patients receiving antiresorptive therapy for prevention and treatment of osteoporosis: executive summary of recommendations from the American Dental Association Council on Scientific Affairs, *J Am Dent Assoc* 142:1243–1251, 2011.
71. Vandone AM, Donadio M, Mozzati M, et al.: Impact of dental care in the prevention of bisphosphonate-associated osteonecrosis of the jaw: a single-center clinical experience, *Ann Oncol* 23:193–200, 2012.
72. Shane E, Burr D, Abrahamsen B, et al.: Atypical subtrochanteric and diaphyseal femoral fractures: second report of a task force of the American Society for Bone and Mineral Research, *J Bone Miner Res* 29:1–23, 2014.
73. Gedmintas L, Solomon DH, Kim SC: Bisphosphonates and risk of subtrochanteric, femoral shaft, and atypical femur fracture: a systematic review and meta-analysis, *J Bone Miner Res* 28:1729–1737, 2013.
74. Schilcher J, Koeppen V, Ranstam J, et al.: Atypical femoral fractures are a separate entity, characterized by highly specific radiographic features. A comparison of 59 cases and 218 controls, *Bone* 52:389–392, 2013.
75. LeBlanc ES, Rosales AG, Black DM, et al.: Evaluating atypical features of femur fractures: how change in radiological criteria influenced incidence and demography of atypical femur fractures in a community setting, *J Bone Miner Res* 32:2304–2314, 2017.

76. Dell RM, Adams AL, Greene DF, et al.: Incidence of atypical nontraumatic diaphyseal fractures of the femur, *J Bone Miner Res* 27:2544–2550, 2012.
77. Dell R, Greene D: A proposal for an atypical femur fracture treatment and prevention clinical practice guideline, *Osteoporos Int* 29:1277–1283, 2018.
78. Mashiba T, Turner CH, Hirano T, et al.: Effects of suppressed bone turnover by bisphosphonates on microdamage accumulation and biomechanical properties in clinically relevant skeletal sites in beagles, *Bone* 28:524–531, 2001.
79. Tang SY, Allen MR, Phipps R, et al.: Changes in non-enzymatic glycation and its association with altered mechanical properties following 1-year treatment with risedronate or alendronate, *Osteoporos Int* 20:887–894, 2009.
80. Cummings SR, Schwartz AV, Black DM: Alendronate and atrial fibrillation, *New England Journal of Medicine* 356:1895–1896, 2007.
81. Heckbert SR, Li G, Cummings SR, et al.: Use of alendronate and risk of incident atrial fibrillation in women, *Arch Intern Med* 168:826–831, 2008.
82. Sorensen HT, Christensen S, Mehnert F, et al.: Use of bisphosphonates among women and risk of atrial fibrillation and flutter: population based case-control study, *BMJ* 336:813–816, 2008.
83. Barrett-Connor E, Swern AS, Hustad CM, et al.: Alendronate and atrial fibrillation: a meta-analysis of randomized placebo-controlled clinical trials, *Osteoporos Int* 23:233–245, 2012.
84. Kim SY, Kim MJ, Cadarette SM, et al.: Bisphosphonates and risk of atrial fibrillation: a meta-analysis, *Arthritis Res Ther* 12, R30-R2010.
85. Patel DV, Horne A, House M, et al.: The incidence of acute anterior uveitis after intravenous zoledronate, *Ophthalmology* 120:773–776, 2013.
86. Pazianas M, Clark EM, Eiken PA, et al.: Inflammatory eye reactions in patients treated with bisphosphonates and other osteoporosis medications: cohort analysis using a national prescription database, *J Bone Miner Res* 28:455–463, 2013.
87. Cao Y, Mori S, Mashiba T, et al.: Raloxifene, estrogen, and alendronate affect the processes of fracture repair differently in ovariectomized rats, *Journal of Bone and Mineral Research* 17:2237–2246, 2002.
88. Peter CP, Cook WO, Nunamaker DM, Provost MT, Seedor JG, Rodan GA: Effect of alendronate on fracture healing and bone remodeling in dogs, *J Orthop Res* 14:74–79, 1996.
89. Solomon DH, Hochberg MC, Mogun H, Schneeweiss S: The relation between bisphosphonate use and non-union of fractures of the humerus in older adults, *Osteoporos Int* 20:895–901, 2009.
90. Li YT, Cai HF, Zhang ZL: Timing of the initiation of bisphosphonates after surgery for fracture healing: a systematic review and meta-analysis of randomized controlled trials, *Osteoporos Int* 26:431–441, 2015.
91. Eriksen EF, Lyles KW, Colon-Emeric CS, et al.: Antifracture efficacy and reduction of mortality in relation to timing of the first dose of zoledronic acid after hip fracture, *J Bone Miner Res* 24:1308–1313, 2009.
92. Miller PD, Roux C, Boonen S, et al.: Safety and efficacy of risedronate in patients with age-related reduced renal function as estimated by the Cockcroft and Gault method: a pooled analysis of nine clinical trials, *J Bone Miner Res* 20:2105–2115, 2005.
93. Sokal A, Elefant E, Leturcq T, et al.: Pregnancy and newborn outcomes after exposure to bisphosphonates: a case-control study, *Osteoporos Int* 30:221–229, 2019.
94. Green SB, Pappas AL: Effects of maternal bisphosphonate use on fetal and neonatal outcomes, *Am J Health Syst Pharm* 71:2029–2036, 2014.
95. Levy S, Fayez I, Taguchi N, et al.: Pregnancy outcome following in utero exposure to bisphosphonates, *Bone* 44:428–430, 2009.
96. Ornoy A, Wajnberg R, Diav-Citrin O: The outcome of pregnancy following pre-pregnancy or early pregnancy alendronate treatment, *Reprod Toxicol* 22:578–579, 2006.
97. Black DM, Schwartz AV, Ensrud KE, et al.: Effects of continuing or stopping alendronate after 5 years of treatment: the Fracture Intervention Trial Long-term Extension (FLEX): a randomized trial, *JAMA* 296:2927–2938, 2006.
98. Adler RA, El-Hajj Fuleihan G, Bauer DC, et al.: Managing osteoporosis in patients on long-term bisphosphonate treatment: Report of a Task Force of the American Society for Bone and Mineral Research, *Journal of Bone and Mineral Research* 31:16–35, 2016.
99. Black DM, Reid IR, Cauley JA, et al.: The effect of 6 versus 9 years of zoledronic acid treatment in osteoporosis: a randomized second extension to the HORIZON-Pivotal Fracture Trial (PFT), *J Bone Miner Res* 30:934–944, 2015.
100. Schwartz AV, Bauer DC, Cummings SR, et al.: Efficacy of continued alendronate for fractures in women with and without prevalent vertebral fracture: the FLEX trial, *J Bone Miner Res* 25:976–982, 2010.

71

Analgesic Agents in Rheumatic Disease

GREGORY R. POLSTON AND MARK S. WALLACE

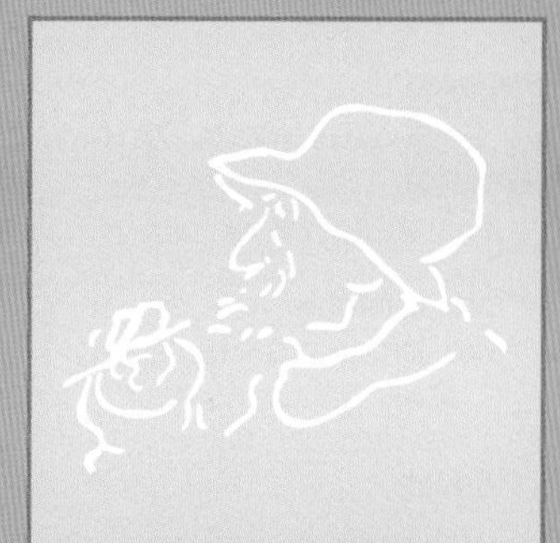

KEY POINTS

The primary analgesic agents such as acetaminophen, nonsteroidal anti-inflammatory agents, and opioids have intrinsic analgesic properties that are most efficacious for nociceptive and inflammatory pain.

Adjuvant agents such as anti-depressants, anti-convulsants, and muscle relaxants lack intrinsic analgesic properties but are effective in neuropathic and functional pain and can enhance effects of other analgesics.

The use of opioids for chronic pain should not be considered as first-line agents.

Many drugs can increase and decrease the metabolism of opioids through interaction of CYP2DG and CYP3A4 systems.

Increased reports of methadone overdose are thought to be due to co-administration of drugs that inhibit the CYP3A4 system.

Tricyclic anti-depressants are efficacious in a variety of pain syndromes; compliance is an issue because of side effects and delayed onset.

Newer serotonin and norepinephrine reuptake inhibitors (such as duloxetine) are better tolerated and have a faster onset than older tricyclic anti-depressants.

Numerous anti-convulsants have been studied with conflicting results. Only gabapentin and pregabalin consistently demonstrated efficacy.[1,2]

Muscle relaxants are intended for short-term use only and do not have long-term benefits.

Introduction

Pain is the most common reason why patients seek medical attention, yet under treatment, acute and chronic pain persists despite decades of efforts to provide clinicians with information about analgesics.[1,2] A major consequence of undertreating the patient who initially presents with pain as a result of rheumatic disease is the development of chronic pain. Chronic pain has been demonstrated to have deleterious effects on many aspects of the patient's daily life. These effects include deterioration in physical functioning, the development of psychological distress and psychiatric disorders, and impairments in interpersonal functioning.[3,4] In addition to the personal suffering it causes, chronic pain imposes a burden on society in increased health care costs, disability, and lost workdays.

Physiology of Pain Perception (the "Pain Experience")

The "pain experience" involves more than just the sensation of pain. Pain activates many areas of the brain that interact, resulting in the pain experience, which will differ among individual patients. The "Pain Experience" involves three components: biologic, psychological, and sociological. As described later, activation of various parts of the nervous system will contribute to each of these components. The three components of the pain experience include: (1) sensory/discriminative (biologic), (2) affective/emotional (psychological), and (3) evaluative/cognitive (sociological).[5]

The sensory/discriminative component of pain provides information on the intensity, location, and quality of the pain. These pathways consist of peripheral receptor activation, axon depolarization, and ascending pathways to the cortex for processing.

The ascending pathways that carry impulses from the nociceptor to the sensory cortex also give off fibers to brain stem structures and deep brain structures. Activation of these structures in the brain stem and deep brain will stimulate emotional and sympathetic responses from the individual, leading to the emotional/affective component of pain.

Finally, ascending pain pathways also send projections to the forebrain structures where the pain is processed on a cognitive and evaluative level, explaining why patients respond differently to pain based on culture, sex, and past experiences.

The main neurotransmitter in primary afferents is the excitatory amino acid glutamate. Activation of nociceptors causes the release of glutamate from pre-synaptic terminals in the spinal cord dorsal horn; this release acts on the ionotropic glutamate receptor amino-3-hydroxy-5-methylisoxazole-4-propionic acid postsynaptically to cause rapid depolarization of dorsal horn neurons and, if threshold is reached, action potential discharge.[6,7]

Pain Classification

Pain can be mechanistically divided into four classifications: nociceptive, inflammatory, functional, and neuropathic. Nociceptive pain is transient pain in response to a noxious stimulus that activates high threshold afferents. Nociceptive pain serves a protective function. Inflammatory pain is the spontaneous hypersensitivity

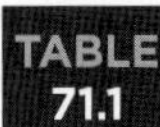

TABLE 71.1 Analgesic Options to Treat Chronic Pain

Primary Analgesics	Adjunct Analgesics
Acetaminophen	Tricyclic anti-depressants
Nonsteroidal anti-inflammatory drugs/cyclooxygenase-2 inhibitors	Serotonin-norepinephrine reuptake inhibitors
Opioids	Anti-convulsants
	Muscle relaxants
	Topical agents

to pain that occurs in response to tissue damage and inflammation (e.g., post-operative pain, trauma, arthritis). Functional pain is hypersensitivity to pain resulting from abnormal central processing of normal input (e.g., pathologic irritable bowel syndrome, fibromyalgia). Neuropathic pain is spontaneous pain and hypersensitivity to pain that occurs in association with damage to or lesions of the nervous system (e.g., peripheral neuropathy, postherpetic neuralgia). Nociceptive pain and inflammatory pain are prevalent in rheumatic disease. Functional pain and neuropathic pain are probably less prevalent in rheumatic disease; however, both should always be considered because poorly controlled pain can lead to nervous system dysfunction and functional and neuropathic pain.[8]

Pharmacologic Treatment of Chronic Pain

The efficacy of analgesics is dependent on the pain mechanism. Primary analgesics are more efficacious in nociceptive and inflammatory pain, whereas adjuvant agents are more efficacious in neuropathic and functional pain. Each pain classification involves different pain mechanisms, and within each classification are multiple different pain mechanisms.[9,10]

Pain is mediated through both peripheral and central mechanisms, and often more than one mechanism of pain is active in a given patient. Thus, the use of two or more agents with differing mechanisms increases the likelihood of interrupting pain signals and relieving pain.

Pharmacologic agents for the management of chronic pain are divided into primary analgesics, which have intrinsic analgesic properties, and adjunct analgesics, which may have primary analgesic properties in neuropathic pain but usually enhance the analgesic effects of primary analgesics when used in non-neuropathic pain syndromes. Table 71.1 summarizes these agents. Nonsteroidal anti-inflammatory drugs (NSAIDs)/cyclooxygenase (COX)-2 inhibitors will be discussed elsewhere (see Chapter 62).

Opioids

Numerous studies have demonstrated the efficacy of the opioids in a variety of chronic pain states, including neuropathic and non-neuropathic. However, studies to document long-term efficacy have not been conducted. Long-term opioid therapy to treat chronic pain remains controversial. Over the last century, the pendulum has swung back and forth with regard to the use of the opioids to treat pain. In the mid-20th century, opioids were limited because of fears of addiction and diversion. In the late 20th century, the pendulum went to the other side, with liberal use of opioids to treat chronic pain. This is thought to have resulted in an overuse of opioids to treat chronic pain as the United States became the leading consumer of the world's opioids with a dramatic rise in prescription opioid–related deaths and the declaration of an "opioid epidemic." With the turn of the 21st century, the pendulum started moving back toward the middle with recognition of the importance of opioids in chronic pain management but an understanding of the need to balance these benefits with risks. Therefore, a set of Universal Precautions has been developed as a guide to help the physician who prescribes opioids[11] (Table 71.2). In 2009, the American Pain Society and the American Academy of Pain Medicine jointly published guidelines that acknowledge that opioid analgesics have an important role in pain management, and that underuse of these agents may contribute to suboptimal pain management.[12] However, these guidelines also acknowledge that abuse of prescription opioids has become an epidemic, with dramatic increases seen in the United States that are continuing to rise. An Agency for Healthcare Research and Quality report published in 2014 suggested that the evidence for risks of long-term opioid treatment to treat chronic pain outweighed the evidence for effectiveness.[13] Due to the increasing opioid crisis and questions on risks/benefits of long-term use of opioids to treat chronic pain, the Centers for Disease Control and Prevention published a set of guidelines intended for the primary care physician to use for chronic noncancer pain.[14]

TABLE 71.2 Universal Precautions for Long-Term Opioid Use to Treat Pain

Diagnosis with appropriate differential
Psychological assessment, including risk of addictive disorders
Informed consent
Treatment agreement
Preintervention and postintervention assessment of pain level and function
Appropriate trial of opioid therapy with or without adjunctive medication
Reassessment of pain score and level of function
Regular assessment of the "4 As" (analgesia, activities of daily living, adverse effects, aberrant drug-taking behaviors)
Periodic review of pain diagnosis and comorbid conditions, including addictive disease
Consideration of prescription of naloxone if doses greater than 50 mg of morphine equivalents per day or other risk factor for overdose
Documentation

Evaluating patients with chronic noncancer pain can be problematic, as the perception of pain is not only dependent on physiologic factors but also the patient's psychological and social background. Thus, developing a pain treatment plan that includes opioids can also be challenging. Historically, the use of opioids was reserved for short-term treatment or for end of life care. In the late 1980s, however, this practice changed. Chronic pain became recognized as a disease and experts began recommending more liberal prescription practices. Unfortunately, as the use of opioid prescriptions increased, so too did opioid overdoses and prescription drug substance abuse disorders. The increase in abuse and overdoses has become so rampant that we now are in the midst of an opioid epidemic that presents dangers not only for patients but for society as a whole. In an effort to combat this problem, a number of strategies have been proposed to identify patients who are more likely to benefit from opioid therapy, thus improving patient selection and outcome. These include specific guidelines to always consider nonopioid therapies first, as well as guidelines for upper dose daily limits for opioid analgesics.[14–18]

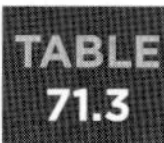

TABLE 71.3 Risk Factors for Poor Outcomes With Chronic Opioid Therapy

High
>90 mg morphine equivalent/day or methadone
High abuse risk (current abuse, young age, significant psychiatric hx, prior aberrant behaviors, initial screening score)
Lack of clear reason for pain
Comorbidity (renal, hepatic, respiratory, sleep apnea)
Use of other sedatives, stimulants, anxiolytics, or sleeping medication
Multiple medications to combat side effects
Younger age
Lack of functional improvement
Rapid dose escalation after starting medication
Poorly treated mental health issues
Others in home with high risk for diversion or unstable living conditions
Moderate
50 to 90 mg morphine equivalent/day
Prior substance abuse diagnosis in remission for greater than 6 months
Moderate risk on initial risk questionnaire
Prescriber "uneasy" about providing opioids for the patient
Low
50 mg morphine equivalent/day
Compliant with medication and attempting nonopioid therapies
Clear indication for pain
Low risk on initial risk questionnaire
Clear functional improvement

Additional recommendations include taking a full social history at the start of therapy. Included in this history are alcohol use, illegal drug use, family history of substance abuse, and identifying if others in the home are at risk for misuse. Using validated patient questionnaires to predict success with chronic opioid therapy, such as the Opioid Risk Tool[19]; Diagnosis, Intractability, Risk, Efficacy (DIRE)[20]; or Screener and Opioid Assessment for Patients with Pain[21] is also recommended. Along with a complete physical exam, the patient can be stratified into risk groups (low, medium, high) (Table 71.3), which will offer insight as to how best to monitor individual patients. Other efforts include making every patient sign an opioid agreement, consent to random drug testing, and demonstrate clear functional improvement in order to continue this therapy. State prescription drug monitoring programs have been created to help document compliance and identify "doctor shopping." State and national regulations, including Risk Evaluation and Mitigation Strategies (REMS) (fda.gov/drugs/information-drug-class/opioid-analgesic-risk-evaluation-and-mitigation-strategy-rems), for all opioids have also been implemented. The REMS program requires specific education for providers, patients, and caregivers regarding the use of these drugs, along with documentation of any benefit and review of misuse, abuse, or addiction. Many current opioid analgesics have been reformulated with abuse-deterrent and tamper-resistant properties. Unfortunately, none of these changes to opioid products prevent the most common route of abuse—simply ingesting large quantities of pills.

Along with the recommendations above, a short-acting weak opioid such as hydrocodone or tramadol should be used first. If the patient requires more than three or four short-acting weak opioids per day, consider converting to a long-acting opioid if the pain is continuous. It is generally believed that controlled-release or long-acting opioids not only provide convenience to patients by reducing the number of daily doses required, they also provide a pharmacokinetic profile that results in reduced serum level peaks and troughs, and thereby an improvement in the consistency of effective analgesia and a potential reduction in opioid-related side effects that are often correlated with high peak serum levels. Long-acting opioids should only be used for around-the-clock pain and after failure of short-acting opioids. Long-acting opioids should not be used for intermittent or breakthrough pain. There is no clinical evidence that long-acting opioids decrease the risk of misuse or addiction, and there is concern that the total daily dose of opioids increases simply due to higher dose increments. When converting to a long-acting opioid, access to a short-acting opioid for breakthrough pain can be continued but remember that both the short-acting dose and the long-acting dose should be added together to determine total daily dose of morphine equivalents. Evaluation by a pain specialist may be considered when a morphine equianalgesic dosage exceeds 50 to 90 mg/day. The benefits of levels higher than 100 mg/day have not been established, and recent evidence suggests a significant increase in morbidity and mortality.[22]

Opiate Receptor Classes

Early work by investigators led to the postulation of three opiate receptors: mu, kappa, and sigma.[23,24] Later studies by another group led to the identification of the delta opioid receptor.[25] With the exception of the sigma receptor, all of the opiate receptors are responsible for opioid-induced analgesia. Opioid receptors are mediated through a G protein, leading to a cascade of events that typically inhibit neuron activation.[26] Persistent activation of G protein–coupled receptors typically results in progressive loss of effect, known as *tolerance* (discussed later).

Opiate Receptor Distribution and Mechanisms of Opioid-Induced Analgesia

The main sites of action of the opiates are believed to be located in the brain and spinal cord; however, under some circumstances, peripheral mechanisms are involved. Responses of an individual patient may vary dramatically with different mu-opioid receptor (MOR) agonists. If problems are encountered with one drug, another should be tried. Mechanisms underlying variations in individual responses to morphine-like agonists are poorly understood; however, they are thought to be due to MOR polymorphisms.

Numerous sites in the brain have MORs. Activation of receptors located in the mesencephalic periaqueductal gray[27] appears to be the most important cause of opioid-induced analgesia. MOR agonists block release of the inhibitory transmitter γ-aminobutyric acid[28] from tonically active periaqueductal gray (PAG) systems that regulate activity in projections from the PAG to the medulla. This results in an increase in PAG outflow to the medulla, leading to activation of medulla spinal projections and release of noradrenaline or serotonin at the level of the spinal dorsal horn. This release can attenuate dorsal horn excitability and analgesia. PAG activation can also increase the excitability of the dorsal raphe and the locus coeruleus, from which ascending serotonergic and noradrenergic projections originate to project to the limbic forebrain, leading to the euphoric effects sometimes experienced with systemic MOR agonists.[29]

In the spinal cord, MOR agonists are limited for the most part to the substantia gelatinosa of the superficial dorsal horn, the region in which small, high-threshold sensory afferents terminate. Most of these opiate receptors are located pre-synaptically and postsynaptically on small peptidergic primary afferent C fibers. Pre-synaptic activation of the MOR prevents the opening of voltage-sensitive Ca^{2+} channels, thereby preventing transmitter release. Postsynaptic activation of the MOR increases potassium conductance, resulting in hyperpolarization and reduced excitation induced by the pre-synaptic release of glutamate.[30] The ability of spinal opiates to reduce the release of excitatory neurotransmitters from C fibers pre-synaptically and to decrease the excitability of dorsal horn neurons postsynaptically is believed to account for powerful and selective effects upon spinal nociceptive processing. In humans, an extensive literature indicates that a variety of opiates delivered spinally (intrathecally or epidurally) can induce a powerful analgesia.[30]

Systemic delivery of the opioids will reduce nociceptive pain through a central mechanism located in the brain and spinal cord, as described previously, whereas the peripheral application has no effect. However, under conditions of inflammation, which result in an exaggerated pain response (hyperalgesia), the peripheral application of the opioids will reduce the hyperalgesia. This action is believed to be mediated by opiate receptors on the peripheral terminals of small primary afferents that become active under inflammatory conditions. Whether the effects are uniquely on the afferent terminal or on inflammatory cells that release products that sensitize the nerve terminal is not known.[31]

Tolerance

Over time, a given dose of an opioid shows less effect and an increased dose is required to produce the same physiologic response. Tolerance to different effects of opioids occurs at different rates. For example, tolerance to sedation and nausea occurs earlier than analgesic tolerance. The difference in analgesic tolerance versus respiratory tolerance may explain why a patient can overdose unintentionally despite an unchanged daily dose of opioid. Some effects, such as constipation, never show tolerance.

The mechanism of opioid tolerance is controversial. Apparent opioid tolerance may be an indication of disease progression with a resultant increase in pain intensity; this is the first event that should be ruled out before true tolerance is assumed. Many cellular mechanisms can lead to tolerance. First, long-term opioid exposure can lead to receptor internalization, dephosphorylation, and desensitization. Second, exposure to high doses of opioids can lead to an increase in intra-cellular cyclic adenosine monophosphate (CAMP), activation of bulbospinal pathways, and glutamate receptor phosphorylation, producing an excitatory state (opioid-induced hyperalgesia).[32,33] An incomplete cross-tolerance occurs between the various opioids, and when tolerance develops to one opioid, switching to another opioid can result in an increased effect.

Physical Dependence

Physical dependence is not addiction (and the terms should not be used interchangeably). Physical dependence is a pharmacologic effect characteristic of a number of different types of medications. Physical dependence is defined as the occurrence of an abstinence syndrome (withdrawal reaction) following abrupt discontinuation of the drug, substantial dose reduction, or administration of an antagonist. Physical dependence is generally assumed to occur with regular opioid use for as brief a period as a few days.

Opioid withdrawal is manifested by significant somatomotor and autonomic outflow (reflected by agitation, hyperalgesia, hyperthermia, hypertension, diarrhea, pupillary dilation, and release of virtually all pituitary and adrenomedullary hormones) and by affective symptoms (dysphoria, anxiety, and depression).[34] Opioid withdrawal can be minimized by slowly tapering the opioid. These phenomena are considered to be highly aversive and motivate the drug recipient to make robust efforts to avoid the withdrawal state. Initially, drug addicts are driven to repeated doses of opioids owing to the euphoric effects. However, over time, the euphoric effects are lessened, and addicts are driven to continue use to avoid withdrawal.

TABLE 71.4 Opioid Risk Tool

	Male	Female
Family history (parents and siblings):		
Alcohol abuse	3	1
Illegal drug use	3	2
Prescription drug abuse	4	4
Personal history:		
Alcohol abuse	3	3
Illegal drug use	4	4
Prescription drug abuse	5	5
Mental health:		
Diagnosis of ADD, OCD, bipolar, schizophrenia	2	2
Diagnosis of depression	1	1
Other:		
Age 16 to 45 years	1	1
History of preadolescent sexual abuse	0	3

Sum of Scores
0-3 low risk: 6% chance of developing problematic behaviors
4-7 moderate risk: 28% chance of developing problematic behaviors
≥8 high risk: >90% chance of developing problematic behaviors

ADD, Attention deficit disorder; *OCD*, obsessive-compulsive disorder.

Adapted from Webster LR, Webster RM: Predicting aberrant behaviors in opioid-treated patients: preliminary validation of the Opioid Risk Tool. *Pain Med* 6:432–442, 2005.

Addiction

Identification of the disease of addiction is important for safe and effective clinical management of pain in individuals with addictive disorders. The disease of addiction affects approximately 10% of the general population, and its prevalence may be higher in subpopulations of patients with pain. Active addiction is a contraindication to the use of the opioids; a past history is a relative contraindication, but opioids can be used successfully with appropriate monitoring. A persistent misunderstanding is prevalent among health care providers, regulators, and the general population regarding the nature and manifestations of addiction, which may result in undertreatment of pain and stigmatization of patients using opioids for pain control.

Evaluating for addiction in a patient who is prescribed long-term opioids for pain control is often problematic. This risk of opioid addiction and misuse can be assessed with validated

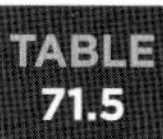

TABLE 71.5 Opioid Drug Interactions

Opioid Drug Interactions
Tramadol, oxycodone, hydrocodone, and codeine are converted to active metabolites by CYP2D6 Drugs that inhibit this enzyme will decrease opioid effects: fluoxetine, paroxetine, quinidine, duloxetine, terbinafine, amiodarone, sertraline, and others
Methadone and fentanyl are converted by CYP3A4 Drugs that inhibit this enzyme will increase opioid effects: several anti-retrovirals, clarithromycin, itraconazole, ketoconazole, nefazodone, telithromycin, aprepitant, diltiazem, erythromycin, fluconazole, grapefruit juice, verapamil, cimetidine, and others
Morphine, hydromorphone, and oxymorphone are not significantly metabolized by CYP450 isoenzymes

From Daniell H: Inhibition of opioid analgesia by selective serotonin reuptake inhibitors, *J Clin Oncol* 20:2409, 2002; U.S. Food and Drug Administration.

questionnaires (Table 71.4),[19] but if there is uncertainty of misuse or abuse, referral to addiction specialists should be considered. Although the concept of addiction may include the symptoms of physical dependence and tolerance, physical dependence or tolerance alone does not equate with addiction. In the chronic pain patient taking long-term opioids, physical dependence and tolerance should be expected, but the maladaptive behavior changes associated with addiction are not expected.[35,36]

Addiction is a behavioral pattern characterized by compulsive use of a drug and overwhelming involvement with its procurement and use in spite of potential harm.[34,37] For patients with continuous pain, inadequate pain management (e.g., "as necessary" dosing schedule, use of drugs with inadequate potency, use of dosing intervals that are too long) can lead to behavioral symptoms that mimic those seen with psychological dependence and can be mistaken for addiction termed *pseudoaddiction*. In the case of pseudoaddiction, problem behaviors resolve after sufficient pain relief is established. However, behaviors related to true addiction may also resolve after dose escalation. Thus, it can be difficult to distinguish pseudoaddiction from true addiction; careful evaluation and management may be required until the circumstances are sorted out (see Table 71.4).[38]

Opioid Pharmacology

Morphine

Morphine is the gold standard against which all other opioids are measured. Morphine can be administered by oral, rectal, subcutaneous, intravenous, intramuscular, and intraspinal routes. Oral bioavailability of morphine is about 25% (range, 10% to 40%). Peak plasma concentrations occur 0.5 to 1 hour after ingestion with a half-life of around 3 to 4 hours. To increase the dosing interval of oral morphine, several sustained- and controlled-release preparations have been developed (Table 71.5). The average protein binding of morphine is around 35%, but this decreases with renal and hepatic dysfunction. Because of the hydrophilicity of morphine, there is poor CNS penetration and little tissue accumulation with repeated dosing. Morphine is metabolized primarily in the liver to two main metabolites: morphine-3-glucuronide (M3G) and morphine-6-glucuronide (M6G). M3G is the primary metabolite with potent CNS excitatory properties. Because of its polarity, CNS penetration is poor; however, in renal failure, M3G plasma concentrations can be high enough to drive this metabolite into the CNS, leading to excitation. M6G possesses potent MOR agonism, but because of its high polarity, CNS penetration is poor. However, like M3G, M6G can accumulate in renal impairment, leading to exaggerated opioid effects. Only about 10% of unmetabolized morphine is excreted renally, whereas 90% is excreted renally as morphine glucuronide (70% to 80%) and normorphine (5% to 10%) conjugates.[39]

Methadone

Methadone is a long-acting MOR agonist with potency similar to that of morphine but with two important differences.[28] It has a long half-life and it has high oral bioavailability. Routes of administration are oral and intravenous, with oral delivery being by far the most common. Intravenous routes have been used as a single loading dose for post-operative pain control. Because of its low hepatic clearance and therefore low first-pass effect, oral bioavailability is around 80%. Methadone has higher lipid solubility than morphine, which results in faster CNS penetration and onset of action; however, its lipid solubility leads to a higher volume of distribution and a shorter duration of action with initial dosing. Low hepatic clearance leads to accumulation, a longer duration of action, and possible overdose with repeated dosing.

Because of the long half-life of methadone (average, 15 to 30 hours, with published reports ranging from 8 to 59 hours) with drug accumulation over several days, methadone needs to be administered with caution with long intervals between dose adjustments (5 to 7 days). Deaths have been reported with the use of methadone for chronic pain, and in November 2006, the U.S. Food and Drug Administration (FDA) issued a public health advisory for methadone with a black box warning. Although details are often unclear, many of these deaths may be due to conversion of patients from other opioids to methadone. Methadone has been associated with QRS prolongation, which can lead to sudden cardiac death. If unfamiliar with the use of methadone, it is advisable to seek consultation with a pain specialist, especially when considering prescribing methadone at greater than a low dose (20 to 30 mg/day).[40,41]

The L-isomer of methadone possesses opioid activity, whereas the D-isomer is weak or inactive as an opioid. Evidence suggests that D-methadone is anti-nociceptive as a result of its *N*-methyl-D-aspartate (NMDA) receptor antagonist activity, making methadone attractive in treating neuropathic pain.[42]

Methadone is metabolized primarily by CYP3A4, secondarily by CYP2D6, and to a smaller extent by CYP1A2 and additional enzymes that are under study. CYP3A4, the most abundant metabolic enzyme in the body, can vary 30-fold between individuals in terms of its presence and activity in the liver. In addition, drugs that inhibit this enzyme (several anti-retrovirals, clarithromycin, itraconazole, ketoconazole, nefazodone, telithromycin, aprepitant, diltiazem, erythromycin, fluconazole, grapefruit juice, verapamil, cimetidine, and others) will increase the effect of methadone, possibly leading to overdose. This enzyme is also found in the gastrointestinal tract, so methadone metabolism actually starts before the drug enters the circulatory system. The amount of this enzyme in the intestine can vary up to 11-fold, partially accounting for the variable breakdown of methadone.[43]

Because the half-life of methadone is so long, it has been used extensively to treat opioid dependence and withdrawal. The use of methadone to treat addiction requires a separate clinic and physician license. However, methadone can be used to treat pain under the routine medical Drug Enforcement Administration license.[44]

Fentanyl

Fentanyl is a potent opioid with very high lipid solubility. This high lipid solubility leads to fast onset, a short duration of action, high protein binding (80%), and a high volume of distribution. The high volume of distribution accounts for the short duration of action owing to the high concentration gradient from the plasma to fat and muscle. However, with repeated dosing, the duration of action increases as fat and muscle stores become saturated with fentanyl. Although the analgesic half-life is around 1 to 2 hours, the terminal half-life is about 3 to 4 hours.[45]

Routes of delivery of fentanyl include transdermal, transmucosal, intravenous, and intraspinal. Subcutaneous delivery is also used in terminal cancer patients. High potency and lipid solubility make fentanyl ideal for transdermal and transmucosal delivery. Two transdermal fentanyl patches are available on the market: reservoir and matrix. The reservoir patch can be accessed and the fentanyl extracted, whereas the matrix patch is tamper-proof. Each system delivers fentanyl over 72 hours; however, some patients will deplete the patch within 48 hours, requiring more frequent patch changes. This variability can result from skin perspiration, fat stores, skin temperature, and muscle bulk. After application, the skin serves as a depot, and systemic levels rise for the next 12 to 24 hours, then remain stable until 72 hours. Peak concentration occurs somewhere between 27 and 36 hours (25 mg 27 hours, 100 μg 36 hours). A steady state is reached after several applications. After removal of the system, plasma concentrations fall by 50% over 17 hours.[46]

Three transmucosal products are currently available. The fentanyl oralet contains fentanyl in a base of food starch, confectioners' sugar (2 g vs. 30 g in a Snickers bar), edible glue, citric acid, and artificial berry flavor. The oralet is placed between the gum and the cheek and is allowed to dissolve over 15 minutes with bioavailability of about 50%. Onset is fast, with a peak effect at about 35 minutes. The fentanyl buccal tablets use an OraVescent delivery system that generates a reaction that releases carbon dioxide when the tablet comes in contact with saliva. Transient pH changes accompanying the reaction optimize the dissolution (at a lower pH) of fentanyl through the buccal mucosa. Onset is fast with a peak effect at about 25 minutes. The Bio-Erodible Muco Adhesive (BEMA) fentanyl delivery system is composed of water-soluble polymeric films. This system consists of a bioadhesive layer bonded onto an inactive layer. The active ingredient, fentanyl citrate, is incorporated into the bioadhesive layer, which adheres to the moist buccal mucosa. The amount of fentanyl delivered transmucosally is proportional to the film surface area. It is believed that the inactive layer isolates the bioadhesive layer from the saliva, which may optimize delivery of fentanyl across the buccal mucosa, resulting in higher bioavailability (71%). Onset is fast with a slightly longer peak effect (60 minutes) as compared with the other transmucosal systems; however, there may be a longer duration. Chewing and swallowing any of the transmucosal fentanyl products results in lower bioavailability and peak effect because swallowed fentanyl is poorly absorbed from the gastrointestinal tract.[47] Current REMS recommend that ultra-rapid opioids be used for cancer-related pain or in palliative setting (fda.gov/drugs/information-drug-class/transmucosal-immediate-release-fentanyl-tirf-medicines).

Fentanyl is metabolized primarily by CYP3A4 to the inactive metabolite norfentanyl; therefore, drugs that inhibit this enzyme will increase the drug effect (see earlier under "Methadone"). Only opioid-tolerant patients (>60 mg/day of oral morphine equivalent) should be started on fentanyl products owing to risks of severe respiratory depression.

Oxycodone and Oxymorphone

Oxycodone is administered by the oral or rectal route. Oral bioavailability is 60%, and protein binding 45%. Onset and duration of action are similar to morphine. Oxycodone is metabolized by the CYP3A4 enzyme primarily to noroxycodone, which has about 25% potency of the parent compound but also has neuroexcitatory effects. Minor metabolites include oxymorphone, which is more potent than oxycodone and has a longer half-life, and noroxymorphone, which has no analgesic properties.[48]

Oxycodone is available as an immediate-release tablet or solution and as a controlled-release preparation. The controlled-release preparation has an immediate release effect of up to 40% of the contents, followed by a sustained 12-hour release component. The immediate release effect results in rapid onset followed by a sustained effect. This can be a disadvantage because the patient may perceive the duration as short when coming down from the high peak plasma concentration caused by the immediate release.

Oxymorphone is a metabolite of oxycodone and can be delivered via the oral and rectal routes. Both bioavailability and protein binding are low (10%), but terminal half-life is long (10 to 12 hours). Most of the oxymorphone is metabolized to oxymorphone-3-glucuronide, which is an inactive metabolite. Oxymorphone is available in immediate-release and sustained-release preparations.[49]

Hydromorphone

Hydromorphone is administered by the oral, intravenous, intramuscular, and subcutaneous routes. Oral bioavailability is low (ranging from 25% to 50%), and protein binding is less than 20%. The kinetics are very similar to morphine. Hydromorphone has an extensive first-pass effect, and 95% is metabolized to the inactive hydromorphone-3-glucuronide. A 24-hour-release preparation of hydromorphone has been approved by the FDA. This preparation uses an osmotic piston-driven system in pill form that slowly delivers hydromorphone over 24 hours.[50]

Meperidine

Meperidine can be delivered by the oral, rectal, intravenous, intramuscular, subcutaneous, and intraspinal routes. Meperidine use has decreased over time owing to side effects and risks associated with the parent compound and metabolites (see later). Oral bioavailability is about 50%, protein binding is about 60%, and peak concentrations in plasma usually are observed in 1 to 2 hours. Onset and duration are similar to morphine. Large doses of meperidine repeated at short intervals may produce an excitatory syndrome that includes hallucinations, tremors, muscle twitches, dilated pupils, hyperactive reflexes, and convulsions. These excitatory symptoms are caused by accumulation of the metabolite, normeperidine, which has a half-life of 15 to 20 hours compared with 3 hours for meperidine. Because normeperidine is eliminated by the kidney and the liver, decreased renal or hepatic function increases the likelihood of such toxicity. As a result of these properties, meperidine is not recommended for the treatment of chronic pain because of concerns over metabolite toxicity. It should not be used for longer than 48 hours or in doses greater than 600 mg/day.[51,52]

Severe reactions may follow the administration of meperidine to patients being treated with monoamine oxidase[53] inhibitors. Two basic types of interactions can be observed. The most prominent is an excitatory reaction ("serotonin syndrome"). This reaction may be due to the ability of meperidine to block neuronal reuptake of serotonin and resulting serotonergic overactivity. Another type of interaction, a potentiation of opioid effect due to inhibition of hepatic CYPs, also can be observed in patients taking MAO inhibitors, necessitating a reduction in the doses of opioids.

Hydrocodone

Hydrocodone is a weak MOR agonist. It is delivered only by the oral route and is mostly prescribed in acetaminophen-containing compounds. It was reclassified as a Schedule II opioid in 2014, because of high abuse rates, numerous overdoses, and unintentional acetaminophen toxicity in the United States. A long-acting hydrocodone that does not contain acetaminophen was approved by the FDA. Its approval was controversial and correct usage in clinical practice is not known. Hydrocodone has an oral bioavailability of about 25% with low protein binding in the rapid release form. It is metabolized to hydromorphone, but its analgesic activity is not dependent upon metabolism to hydromorphone. However, rapid metabolizers may experience a faster onset of action owing to the production of hydromorphone. Onset and duration of effect are similar to morphine.

Codeine

Codeine has an exceptionally low affinity for the MOR, and the analgesic effect of codeine is due to its conversion to morphine. The oral bioavailability is about 60% and is poorly protein bound. The onset and duration of effect are similar to morphine. It is administered via the oral route.

The conversion of codeine to morphine is effected by CYP2D6. Well-characterized genetic polymorphisms in CYP2D6 lead to the inability to convert codeine to morphine, thus making codeine ineffective as an analgesic for about 10% of the white population. Other polymorphisms can lead to enhanced metabolism and thus to increased sensitivity to the effects of codeine.[54] Variation in metabolic efficiency is evident among ethnic groups. For example, Chinese individuals produce less morphine from codeine than do whites and are less sensitive to the effects of morphine.[55]

Tramadol

Tramadol is a synthetic codeine analogue with a dual mechanism of action. Analgesia results through weak MOR agonism and inhibition of uptake of norepinephrine and serotonin.

Tramadol is 68% bioavailable after a single oral dose with about 20% protein binding. Its affinity for the opioid receptor is only that of morphine. However, the primary *O*-demethylated metabolite of tramadol is two to four times as potent as the parent drug and may account for part of the analgesic effect. Tramadol is supplied as a racemic mixture, which is more effective than either enantiomer alone. The (+)-enantiomer binds to the receptor and inhibits serotonin uptake. The (–)-enantiomer inhibits norepinephrine uptake and stimulates α_2-adrenergic receptors.[56] The compound undergoes hepatic metabolism and renal excretion, with an elimination half-life of 6 hours for tramadol and 7.5 hours for its active metabolite. Analgesia begins within an hour of oral dosing and peaks within 2 to 3 hours. The duration of analgesia is about 6 hours. The maximum recommended daily dose is 400 mg due to risk of seizures and serotonin syndrome. Tramadol is also available in an extended 24-hour release preparation.

Physical dependence on and abuse of tramadol have been reported. Although its abuse potential is unclear, tramadol probably should be avoided in patients with a history of addiction. Because of its inhibitory effect on serotonin uptake, tramadol should not be used in patients taking MAO inhibitors and triptans. Seizures have been reported with concomitant use of selective serotonin receptor inhibitors (SSRIs), serotonin-norepinephrine reuptake inhibitors (SNRIs), tricyclic anti-depressants (TCAs), and neuroleptics.[56]

Tapentadol

Tapentadol is a strong opioid with a dual mechanism of action, similar to tramadol. It is a strong MOR agonist and a serotonin and norepinephrine reuptake inhibitor. Because of its first-pass metabolism, its bioavailability is low (32%) and protein binding is low (20%). The metabolites of tapentadol are inactive. The half-life is approximately 4 hours.

Similar to tramadol, tapentadol is contraindicated in patients taking MAO inhibitors, triptans, SSRIs, SNRIs, TCAs, and neuroleptics owing to risk of serotonin syndrome. There does not appear to be a risk of seizures, as is seen with tramadol. Tapentadol is currently available as an oral immediate-release drug; however, an extended-release preparation is in development (Fig. 71.1).

Toxicity

Respiration

Although effects on respiration are readily demonstrated, clinically significant respiratory depression rarely occurs with standard analgesic doses in the absence of other contributing comorbidities or concomitant use of sedatives. In addition, the respiratory depressant effect of the opioid is significantly reduced with continued opioid use owing to tolerance. It should be stressed, however, that respiratory depression represents the primary cause of morbidity secondary to opiate therapy.[57] In humans, death from opiate poisoning is nearly always due to respiratory arrest or obstruction.[58] For example, in November 2006, the FDA notified health care professionals of reports of death and life-threatening adverse events, such as respiratory depression and cardiac arrhythmias, in patients receiving methadone (FDA ALERT [11/2006]: Death, narcotic overdose, and serious cardiac arrhythmias, cdc.gov/mmwr/pdf/wk/mm61e0703a1.pdf). Methadone appears to be involved in approximately one-third of all prescription opioid–related deaths, exceeding hydrocodone and oxycodone despite being prescribed one-tenth as often. This has led to revisions in methadone conversion tables.

At therapeutic doses, opiates depress all phases of respiration (rate, minute volume, and tidal exchange). High doses can produce irregular and agonal breathing.[48] A number of factors can increase the risk of opioid-induced respiratory depression, even at therapeutic doses. These include[28] concomitant use of sedatives such as alcohol, benzodiazepines, and tranquilizers, (2) obstructive and central sleep apnea, (3) extremes in age (both newborns and elderly), (4) comorbidities such as pulmonary disease and renal disease, and[28] removal of the painful stimulus. Pain serves as a respiratory stimulant, and removal of pain (e.g., neurolytic block with severe cancer pain) will reduce the ventilatory drive, leading to respiratory depression. Dose dumping is the unintentional rapid release of the opioid from controlled release medications. This can occur after ingestion of alcohol and is thought to be one of the causes of overdoses.

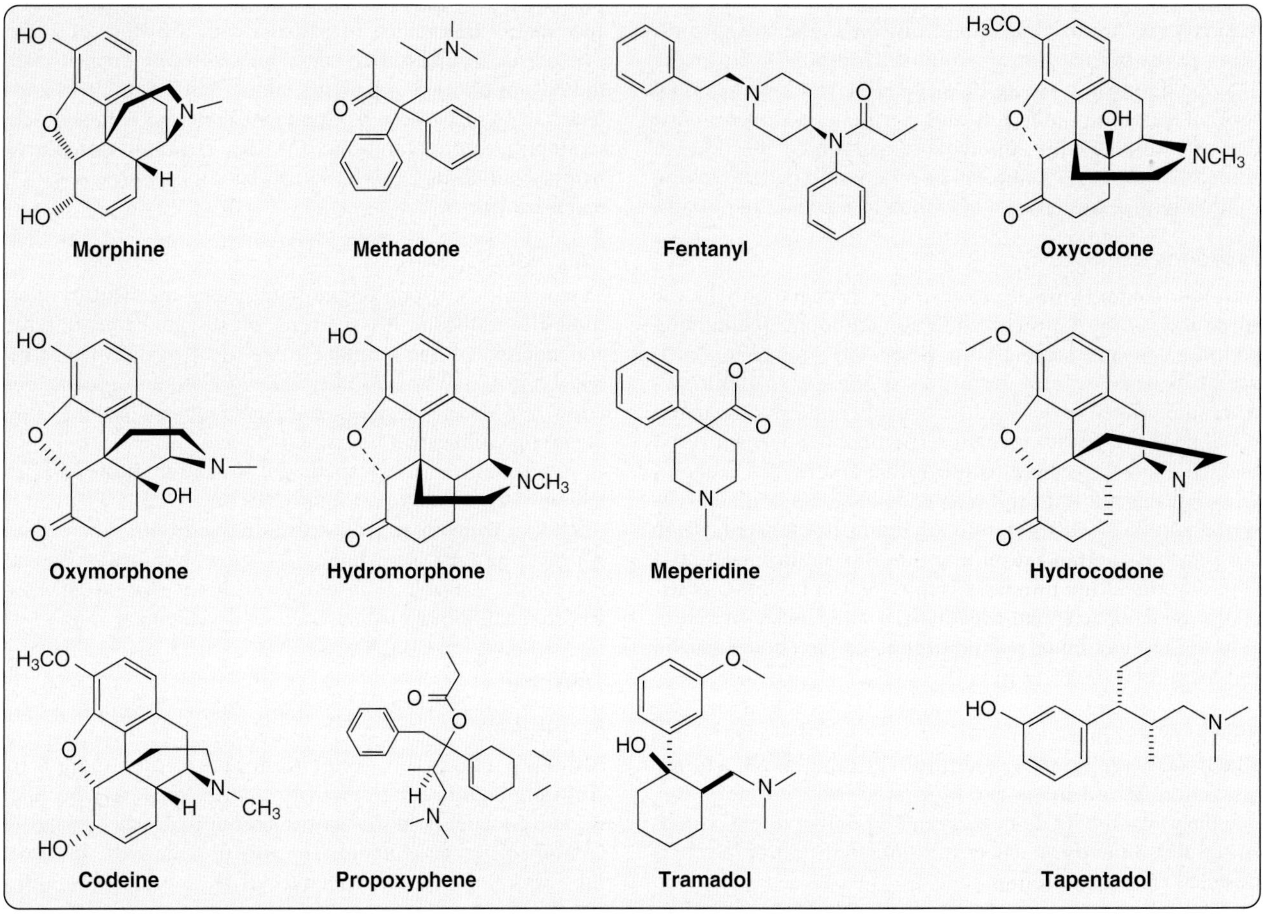

• **Fig. 71.1** Opioid structures.

Sedation

Opiates can produce drowsiness and cognitive impairment, which can increase respiratory depression. These effects most typically are noted following initiation of opiate therapy or after a dose increase but usually resolve with continued opioid use. If the sedation does not resolve, other causes of the sedation should be investigated, such as concomitant use of other sedatives or the presence of sleep apnea. In the absence of these variables, opioid rotation may result in less sedation.[59]

Neuroendocrine Effect

Regulation of the release of hormones and factors from the pituitary is under complex regulation by opiate receptors in the hypothalamic-pituitary-adrenal (HPA) axis. The opioids block the release of a large number of many HPA hormones, including sex hormones, prolactin, oxytocin, growth hormone, and anti-diuretic hormone.

In males, the opioids inhibit adrenal function, resulting in reduced cortisol production and reduced adrenal androgens. In females, the opioids lower luteinizing hormone (LH) and follicle-stimulating hormone (FSH) release. In both males and females, long-term opioid therapy can result in endocrinopathies, including hypogonadotropic hypogonadism, leading to decreased libido, and females may develop menstrual cycle irregularities. These changes are reversible with removal of the opiate. Mechanisms of neuroendocrine effects of the opioids are thought to be due to a direct effect on the pituitary and an indirect action on the hypothalamus, blocking the release of gonadotropin-releasing hormone (GnRH) and corticotropin-releasing hormone (CRH). Secretion of thyrotropin is relatively unaffected.

Opioids inhibit the release of dopamine from neurons of the tuberoinfundibular of the arcuate nucleus. Prolactin release from lactotrope cells in the anterior pituitary is under inhibitory control by dopamine; therefore the reduced dopamine caused by the opioids results in an increase in plasma prolactin. Prolactin counteracts the effects of dopamine, which is responsible for sexual arousal, and high levels of prolactin can result in impotence and loss of libido. Long-term opioid use can increase growth hormone by inhibiting somatostatin release; this regulates GH-releasing hormone secretion.[60]

Anti-diuretic hormone (ADH) and oxytocin are synthesized in the perikarya of the magnocellular neurons in the paraventricular and supraoptic nuclei of the hypothalamus and are released from the posterior pituitary. Kappa opioid receptor agonists inhibit the release of oxytocin and anti-diuretic hormone (and cause prominent diuresis). MOR agonists have minimal effect or tend to produce anti-diuretic effects in humans, and reduce oxytocin secretion.[51] Some of the opioids (i.e., morphine) stimulate histamine release, resulting in hypotension and secondary ADH release. The effects of the opioids on vasopressin and oxytocin release may reflect both a direct effect upon terminal secretion and indirect effects upon dopaminergic and noradrenergic modulatory projections into the paraventricular and supraoptic hypothalamus.[61,62]

Miosis

Lumination of the pupil activates a reflex arc, which, through local circuitry in the Edinger-Westphal nucleus, activates parasympathetic outflow through the ciliary ganglion to the pupil, producing constriction. The parasympathetic outflow is locally regulated by GABAergic interneurons, and the opiates are believed to block GABAergic interneuron–mediated inhibition, resulting in miosis.[63] At high doses of agonists, the miosis is marked, and pinpoint pupils suggest opioid intoxication. Although some tolerance to the mitotic effect develops with therapeutic doses of the opioids, high circulating concentrations of opioids continue to result in constricted pupils.

Myoclonus and Seizure

Myoclonus and seizures have been reported in patients receiving high doses of opiates.[64,65] In addition, seizure-like activity can occur with extremely high doses of the opioids. Seizures may also occur at lower doses of meperidine owing to the normeperidine metabolite, which lowers the seizure threshold. Myoclonus and seizure activity is thought to be due to inhibition of GABA from inhibitory interneurons in the hippocampal pyramidal cells and dorsal horn cells.[66] The opiates also have a direct stimulatory effect through interaction with G inhibitory and stimulatory coupled receptors.[67] It has been suggested that in addition to the normeperidine metabolite, which is seizurogenic, morphine-3-glucuronide (from morphine) may induce myoclonus and seizures at high doses.[68,69]

Nausea and Vomiting

The gastrointestinal tract is under the control of the vomiting center located in the brain stem. The vomiting center is activated by the chemoreceptor trigger zone (CRTZ), the vestibular system, and the gastrointestinal tract. The opioids activate the CRTZ, sensitize the vestibular system, and reduce gastric emptying time, all of which will lead to activation of the vomiting center.[70] Drugs that reduce CRTZ activity (antidopaminergics, 5-hydroxytryptamine$_3$ [5-HT$_3$] serotonin receptor antagonists) and vestibular sensitization (anticholinergics, antihistamines) will reduce opioid-induced nausea. Drugs that enhance gastrointestinal motility are also effective (e.g., metoclopramide).[71]

Constipation

It is estimated that 40% to 95% of patients treated with opioids show constipation and that changes in bowel function can be demonstrated even with acute dosing.[72] Opioid receptors are densely distributed in enteric neurons between the myenteric and submucosal plexuses and on a variety of secretory cells.[73,74] Stimulation of MOR in the intestines reduces propulsatile contractions and diminishes intestinal secretions.[74] The prolonged transit time of the intestinal contents, along with reduced intestinal secretion, leads to increased water absorption, increasing the viscosity of bowel contents and constipation. In addition, anal sphincter tone is increased, and reflex relaxation in response to rectal distension is reduced. All of these effects combine to contribute to morphine-induced constipation.[75] Tolerance to opioid-induced constipation does not occur.

Biliary Spasm

Relaxation of the sphincter of Oddi is suppressed by the opioids, which can result in an increase in the common bile duct pressure, leading to symptoms of biliary colic. Therefore, treatment of the pain of biliary colic with opioids can lead to an exacerbation of the pain rather than relief.

Urinary Retention

MOR agonists inhibit the urinary voiding reflex, increase the tone of the external sphincter, and induce bladder relaxation, which can result in urinary retention. This effect is mediated by MOR and delta-opioid receptor activation in the brain and spinal cord. This will result in higher bladder volumes and sometimes requires catheterization.[76]

Pruritus

Pruritus can occur with all of the MOR agonists. The mechanism is thought to be due to disinhibition of itch-specific neurons, which have been identified in the spinal dorsal horn.[77] It can occur with both systemic and spinally administered doses but is more common with spinally administered doses.[78] It tends to be focused in the trunk and face.

Immunosuppression

The effect of the opioids on immune function is controversial. The opioids suppress immune function through a direct effect on immune system cells and indirectly by activating sympathetic outflow and modulation of the hypothalamic-pituitary-adrenal axis.[79,80] A proposed mechanism for the immune suppressive effects of morphine on neutrophils is through nitric oxide-dependent inhibition of nuclear factor κB (NF-κB) activation.[81] Others have proposed that the induction and activation of mitogen-activated protein kinase (MAPK) may play a role.[82] Pain itself is immunosuppressive; therefore, a reduction in pain will counteract and probably outweigh the direct immunosuppressive effects of the opioids. In addition, it appears that acute delivery of the opioids is more immunosuppressive than long-term delivery, suggesting tolerance to this effect.

Sweating

The opioids exert a wide range of effects on thermoregulation, with high doses leading to hyperthermia and low doses leading to hypothermia.[83] Excessive sweating has been reported to occur in as many as 45% of patients taking methadone. The mechanism appears to be related to release of histamine.[84–86]

Anti-depressants

Anti-depressants have long been used for the treatment of chronic pain. In the past, they were more often chosen to improve mood rather than to treat pain because of co-existing anxiety and depression. After separate studies showed improved pain control in patients without depression, as well as in patients with depression without improvement in mood, it was realized that these medications have independent analgesic actions.[87,88] Further, improvement in pain is seen earlier and at lower doses than improvements in depression, also demonstrating this analgesic efficacy.[89] A recent meta-analysis of 18 randomized, placebo-controlled studies with multiple anti-depressants concluded that there was strong evidence for efficacy of anti-depressants for pain relief, fatigue, and sleep disturbance, and in improving health-related quality of life.[90] The FDA in the United States has now approved the selective serotonin and norepinephrine reuptake inhibitors (SNRI) duloxetine for fibromyalgia, diabetic peripheral neuropathy, and chronic musculoskeletal pain, and milnacipran for fibromyalgia.

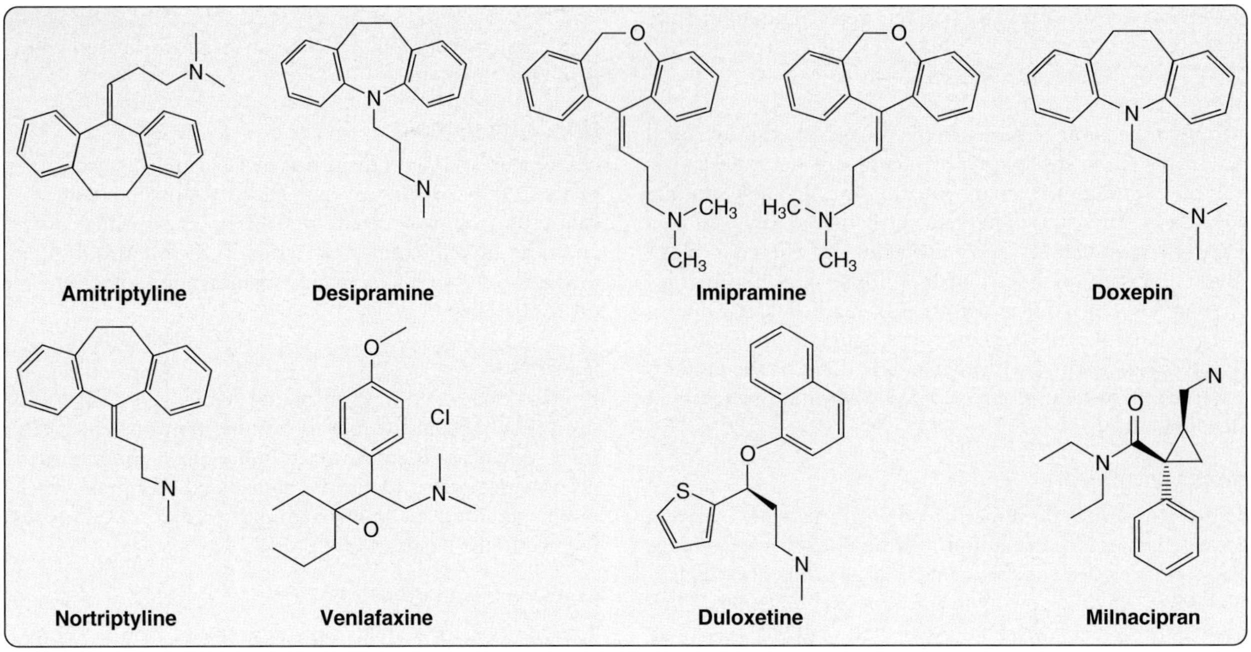

Amitriptyline Desipramine Imipramine Doxepin

Nortriptyline Venlafaxine Duloxetine Milnacipran

• **Fig. 71.2** Chemical structures of anti-depressants.

Nevertheless, not all anti-depressants are effective pain medications. For example, the selective serotonin reuptake inhibitors (SSRI) have minimal analgesic properties and therefore have a limited role in the treatment of chronic pain.[91] Trazodone, used mainly for sleep, is another anti-depressant without analgesic actions. But trazodone is frequently used as a sleep aid because of the high incidence of sleep difficulties in the chronic pain population.[92]

The main site of analgesic action for all of the anti-depressants is thought to be the reuptake inhibition of norepinephrine and serotonin at the level of the spinal cord and higher. This inhibition increases the extra-cellular concentration of these two monoamines, resulting in activation of descending inhibitory pain pathways, and ultimately decreases pain.[93,94] A peripheral action has also been proposed for the TCAs because topical application produced analgesia in animal models of pain.[93,95] Current investigation has shown that topical application can result in the inhibition of NMDA receptors and the blockade of sodium and calcium channels, which alone or in combination could explain their peripheral analgesic properties.[93,95–97] Because TCAs are effective in blocking sodium channels, and the proliferation of sodium channels plays a key role in the pathogenesis of neuropathic pain, this may be one of the main sites of action for these drugs.[98,99] Finally, TCAs potentiate endogenous opioids (Fig. 71.2).[100]

Tricyclic Anti-depressants

TCAs are considered first-line agents in the treatment of chronic neuropathic pain and fibromyalgia.[101,102] Two systematic reviews with 17 randomized controlled trials (RCTs) using 10 anti-depressants have shown numbers needed to treat (NNTs) of approximately 2.5 for neuropathic pain (Table 71.6).[103,104] All TCAs have shown fairly equal efficacy within the class.

TCAs are usually divided into tertiary amines (amitriptyline, imipramine, and doxepin) and secondary amines (nortriptyline and desipramine). Nortriptyline and desipramine are demethylated in the liver from amitriptyline and imipramine, respectively. The tertiary amines tend to block the reuptake of serotonin more than norepinephrine, and the secondary amines are more selective in their inhibition of norepinephrine uptake.

It is recommended that tricyclics should be started at the lowest dose possible and titrated slowly. It is recommended that tricyclics should be started at the lowest dose possible and titrated slowly. A typical starting dose for amitriptyline, nortriptyline, or desipramine is as low as 5 to 10 mg before bedtime. Doses can be increased by the same amount as the starting dose approximately every 7 days (Table 71.7). Studies have shown improved analgesia with amitriptyline in the range of 25 to 50 mg, but some studies have gone as high as 200 mg. Response should be seen within 3 to 4 weeks (see Table 71.7).

Side Effects

Unfortunately, side effects with all of the TCAs are common and can limit use, especially in the elderly and in patients with hepatic impairment. Side effects tend to be less with the secondary amines. Sedation is common owing to its antihistamine effects but can be beneficial if there are sleep complaints. Anticholinergic side effects, which include dry mouth, constipation, urinary retention, and blurred vision, are also prevalent. Both anticholinergic and antihistamine side effects are dose-dependent and can decrease with time; slow titration can improve compliance. Weight gain and sexual dysfunction are frequently reported. Cardiac side effects include orthostatic hypotension and dysrhythmias. Cardiac history should be reviewed and a baseline electrocardiogram (ECG) should be considered for patients over the age of 40. Seizure thresholds are lowered. Risk of suicidal thinking and behavior is increased in children, adolescents, and young adults up to the age of 24. Further, if these medications are taken intentionally or accidentally in overdose, they are dangerous and can be extremely lethal at relatively low doses. When these medications are stopped, it is recommended that they are reduced by 25% per week to decrease side effects.

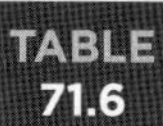

TABLE 71.6 Analgesic Efficacy of Anti-depressants

	ANIMALS[a]			HUMANS[b]	
Anti-depressant	Number of Studies	Positive Results		Number of Studies	Combined NNT[c]
TCAs	126	Acute pain tests Chronic pain models	81% 95%	23	3.1
SSRIs[d]	39	Acute pain tests Chronic pain models	44% 33%	3	6.8
SNRIs[e]	10	Acute pain tests Chronic pain models	100% 100%	3	5.5
Others[f]	7	Acute pain tests Chronic pain models	100% 100%	1	1.6 (bupropion: one study)

[a]Data adapted from Eschalier A, Ardid D, Dubray C: Tricyclic and other antidepressants as analgesics. In Sawynok J, Cowan A, editors: *Novel aspects of pain management: opioids and beyond,* New York, 1999, Wiley-Liss, pp 303–310; and Sawynok J, Cowan A: *Novel aspects of pain management: opioids and beyond,* New York, 1999, Wiley-Liss, pp 303–310. Complete up to 2005. Only approximately 10% of the animals were treated using chronic pain models.

[b]From Finnerup N, Otto M, McQuary H, et al.: Algorithm for neuropathic pain treatment: an evidence based proposal, *Pain* 118:289–305, 2005.

[c]Number of patients treated to improve the health of one patient (at least 50% decrease in pain intensity).

[d]For example, fluoxetine, fluvoxamine, sertraline, paroxetine, and citalopram.

[e]For example, venlafaxine, milnacipran, and duloxetine.

[f]For example, mirtazapine and bupropion.

NNT, Number needed to treat; *SNRIs,* serotonin-norepinephrine reuptake inhibitors; *SSRIs,* selective serotonin reuptake inhibitors; *TCAs,* tricyclic anti-depressants.

From Mico J, Ardid D, Berrocoso E, et al: Antidepressants and pain, *Trends Pharmacol Sci* 27:348–354, 2006.

TABLE 71.7 Tricyclic Anti-depressants: Pharmacodynamics

Drug	Amitriptyline	Desipramine[a]	Doxepin	Imipramine	Nortriptyline
Half-life	9-27 hours	7-60 hours	6-80 hours	6-18 hours	28-31 hours
Metabolism	Hepatic	Hepatic	Hepatic	Hepatic	Hepatic
Excretion	Urine	Urine	Urine	Urine	Urine
Protein binding	≥90%	90%-92%	80%-85%	60%-95%	93%-95%
Therapeutic dose/ day	10-150 mg	10-150 mg	10-150 mg	10-200 mg	10-150 mg
Administration	qhs or 2 times/day	qhs or 2 times/day	qhs or 2-3 times/day	qhs or 2 times/day	qhs or 2-3 times/day
Titration	≥7 days/dose change	≥3 days/dose change	≥7 days/dose change	≥7 days/dose change	≥3 days/dose change
Metabolism/Transport Effects					
Substrate CYP1A2	Minor	Minor	Minor	Minor	Minor
Substrate CYP2C9	Minor				
Substrate CYP2C19	Minor		Minor	Major	Minor
Substrate CYP2D6	Major	Major	Major	Major	Major
Substrate CYP3A4	Minor		Minor	Minor	Minor
Substrate CYP2B6	Minor			Minor	
Inhibits CYP1A2	Weak	Weak		Weak	
Inhibits CYP2A6		Moderate			
Inhibits CYP2B6		Moderate			
Inhibits CYP2C9	Weak				
Inhibits CYP2C19	Weak			Weak	
Inhibits CYP2D6	Weak	Moderate		Moderate	Weak
Inhibits CYP2E1	Weak	Weak		Weak	Weak
Inhibits CYP3A4		Moderate			

[a]Data from Wolters Kluwer Health. www.uptodate.com. Accessed June 15, 2012.

TABLE 71.8 Serotonin-Norepinephrine Reuptake Inhibitors: Pharmacodynamics

	Venlafaxine[a]	Duloxetine	Milnacipran
Half-life	5-7 hours	8-17 hours	6-87 hours
Metabolism	Hepatic	Hepatic	Hepatic
Excretion	Urine	Urine 70%, feces 20%	Urine
Protein binding	35%	≥90%	13%
Therapeutic dose/day	37.5-225 mg	20-60 mg	12.5-200 mg
Administration	2-3 times	Daily	Twice daily
Titration	≥4-7 days/dose change	≥7 days/dose change	1-2 days/dose change
Metabolism/Transport Effects			
Substrate CYP1A2		Major	
Substrate CYP2C19	Minor		
Substrate CYP2C9	Minor		
Substrate CYP2D6	Major	Major	
Substrate CYP3A4	Major		
Inhibits CYP2B6	Weak		
Inhibits CYP2D6	Weak	Moderate	
Inhibits CYP3A4	Weak		

[a]Data from Wolters Kluwer Health. www.uptodate.com. Accessed June 15, 2012.

Serotonin-Norepinephrine Reuptake Inhibitors (SNRIs)

The SNRIs, venlafaxine, duloxetine, and milnacipran, have also shown analgesic properties. Together they have shown benefit in painful diabetic peripheral neuropathy, neuropathic pain, fibromyalgia, and, most recently, chronic musculoskeletal pain. Venlafaxine, the first drug in this class, is an inhibitor of serotonin reuptake at low doses, and at higher doses it inhibits norepinephrine reuptake. This means that it acts more like an SSRI at lower doses and does not become an SNRI until higher doses, where more side effects occur. Venlafaxine has shown some effectiveness with polyneuropathy,[105] including painful diabetic neuropathy[106] and fibromyalgia, but all of these indications are off-label.[107] Doses range from 75 to 225 mg/day. Milnacipran has been approved for use in fibromyalgia in the United States but not in Europe. A recent meta-analysis using five studies (4129 patients) showed that this drug was superior to placebo except for sleep disturbance in treating fibromyalgia.[108] Doses ranged from 25 to 200 mg/day. This same paper found four duloxetine studies (1411 patients) showing superiority to placebo in fibromyalgia except for fatigue symptoms.[108] Long-term benefit of 6 months has been shown with single daily doses of 60 or 120 mg per day of duloxetine for fibromyalgia. Starting doses are 20 to 30 mg in the morning. Duloxetine has also been approved for diabetic peripheral neuropathy, fibromyalgia, and generalized musculoskeletal pain in the United States. It is superior to placebo at doses between 60 and 120 mg per day with this disorder, and patients typically respond within the first week.[109–111] Last, duloxetine has also shown efficacy in treating chronic musculoskeletal pain, including discomfort from osteoarthritis and chronic lower back pain.[112–115]

Side Effects

Side effects of all three of these SNRIs include nausea, dry mouth, and constipation. Sexual side effects tend to be less than with SSRIs. Duloxetine should not be used with co-existing hepatic insufficiency. Milnacipran is not recommended for patients with end-stage renal disease but is unique in that it is not metabolized by cytochrome P450 isoenzymes. Serotonin syndrome, caused by iatrogenic overstimulation of central and peripheral serotonin receptors, presents with neuromuscular hyperactivity, autonomic hyperactivity, and altered mental status. It may occur abruptly and progress rapidly when these drugs are used at high doses or combined with other medications that stimulate serotonin. These drugs can also impair platelet aggregation, particularly if used concomitantly with aspirin or NSAIDs. Dose-related increases in blood pressure have been reported and should be followed. SNRIs carry a black box warning in the United States for increased risk of suicidal thinking and behavior in children, adolescents, and young adults under the age of 25. When these medications are discontinued, withdrawal symptoms have been reported that can be severe and prolonged, requiring slow weaning. It is recommended that the dose is decreased by 25% per week to minimize these symptoms (see Tables 71.5 through 71.10).

Anti-convulsants

Neuropathic pain (NeP) is chronic pain initiated by nervous system lesions or dysfunction and maintained by a number of mechanisms. Excess stimulation of nociceptive pathways or

TABLE 71.9 Potential Tricyclic Anti-depressant Drug Interactions

Monoamine oxidase inhibitors
Drugs that inhibit cytochrome P450 isoenzymes
Drugs that prolong the QT interval
CNS QT interval
Antidopaminergic drugs
Alcohol
Lithium
St. John's wort
Tryptophan

TABLE 71.10 Potential Serotonin-Norepinephrine Reuptake Inhibitor Drug Interactions

Milnacipran

Monoamine oxidase inhibitors
Serotonergic drugs
Triptans
CNS-active drugs
Digoxin
Alcohol
Drugs that interfere with hemostasis
Antidopaminergic drugs
St. John's wort
Tryptophan

Duloxetine

Monoamine oxidase inhibitors
Drugs that inhibit cytochrome P450 isoenzymes
CNS-active drugs
Triptans
Serotonergic drugs
Alcohol
Drugs that interfere with hemostasis
Antidopaminergic drugs
St. John's wort
Tryptophan

Venlafaxine

Monoamine oxidase inhibitors
Drugs that inhibit cytochrome P450 isoenzymes
CNS-active drugs
Triptans
Serotonergic drugs
Drugs that interfere with hemostasis
Antidopaminergic drugs
Alcohol
Protease inhibitors
St. John's wort
Tryptophan

damage to non-nociceptive pathways alters the balance between painful and nonpainful inputs so that pain results without nociceptor stimulation. Several cellular and molecular mechanisms operating over different periods of time are thought to be involved in the abnormal peripheral and CNS activity associated with NeP.[10] Many of these mechanisms can be modulated

TABLE 71.11 Mechanism of Action of Anti-convulsants

	Sodium Channel Blockade	NMDA Antagonism	GABA Agonism
Carbamazepine	X	X	X
Clonazepam			X
Gabapentin		X	
Lamotrigine	X	X	
Levetiracetam		X	
Oxcarbazepine	X	X	
Phenytoin	X		
Pregabalin		X	
Topiramate	X	X (through AMPA/ kainate antagonism)	X
Valproic acid			X

AMPA, Amino-3-hydroxy-5-methylisoxazole propionic acid; *GABA,* γ-aminobutyric acid; *NMDA, N*-methyl-D-aspartate.

by the anti-convulsants. First, nerve injury is reported to evoke spontaneous discharges from the cell bodies of myelinated fibers at the levels of the dorsal root ganglia. The mechanism of spontaneous activity is thought to be secondary to an increase in the concentration of sodium channels in neuromas, dorsal root ganglion cells, and areas of demyelination.[116] Second, spinal inhibitory interneurons modulate the peripheral-to-central transmission of pain signals, thus "gating" ascending sensory information.[117] GABA and glycine and their receptors are abundant in the superficial dorsal horn,[118,119] but their levels are regulated by primary afferent input and change significantly after nerve injury.[119]

Finally, increased glutamatergic neurotransmission may also contribute to hyperexcitability and NeP through activation of both NMDA receptors and non-NMDA amino-3-hydroxy-5-methylisoxazole propionic acid (AMPA)/kainate-type glutamate receptors.[120] Therefore, drugs that modulate sodium channels, increase GABA, reduce glutamate release, or block glutamate effects can potentially reduce neuropathic pain.

The four main mechanisms of action of the anti-convulsants that result in pain reduction include (1) calcium channel modulation,[28] (2) sodium channel blockade, (3) NMDA antagonism, and (4) $GABA_A$ agonism. The net result of the mechanisms of action consists of reduced spontaneous pain and hypersensitivity through membrane stabilization, reduced neurotransmitter release, and reduced postsynaptic cellular activation in the dorsal horn of the spinal cord. Table 71.11 summarizes the mechanisms of action of the various anti-convulsants.

With the exception of pregabalin and gabapentin, studies on the efficacy of the various anti-convulsants to treat pain have been inconsistent. Pregabalin is FDA approved to treat postherpetic neuralgia (PHN), painful diabetic peripheral neuropathy (DPN), fibromyalgia, and pain related to spinal cord injury; gabapentin is

TABLE 71.12 Comparison of Gabapentin and Pregabalin Pharmacology

	Gabapentin	Pregabalin
FDA-approved pain indication	Postherpetic neuralgia	Postherpetic neuralgia Diabetic neuropathy Fibromyalgia
Mechanism of action	Modulates calcium channel opening by binding to the α-2-delta	Modulates calcium channel opening by binding to the P_2-odulates
Pharmacokinetic profile	Nonlinear: plasma concentration is not dose proportionate	Linear: plasma concentration is dose proportionate
Oral bioavailability	60% 900 mg 47% 1200 mg 34% 2400 mg 33% 3600 mg	90% at all doses
Effective dose	1800 mg/day No additional benefit with doses above 1800 mg/day	150 mg/day Dose range from 150-600 mg/day
Schedule	Unscheduled	Schedule V

FDA, U.S. Food and Drug Administration.

FDA approved to treat PHN; carbamazepine is FDA approved to treat trigeminal neuralgia; and valproic acid and topiramate are FDA approved to treat migraine headaches. The discussion in this chapter will focus on pregabalin and gabapentin, which have the most evidence in support of treating chronic neuropathic pain (Table 71.12).

Mechanism of Action

Pregabalin and gabapentin are synthetic molecules that are structurally related to GABA. Both structures are derived from the addition of a cyclohexyl or branched-chain aliphatic carbohydrate moiety to the GABA backbone. However, the three-dimensional shapes of pregabalin and gabapentin are significantly different from GABA. The amine (NH_2) and carboxyl groups (CO_2H) are closer to each other than in the native GABA structure. It is proposed that this difference in the three-dimensional structure of pregabalin and gabapentin versus GABA accounts for their different pharmacologic activities.[121,122]

Although the exact mechanism of action of gabapentin and pregabalin is unknown, results from animal models suggest that pregabalin modulates neuronal hyperexcitability, resulting in analgesic and anti-convulsant effects. Reduction of neurotransmitter release occurs because pregabalin selectively binds to the α_2-δ subunit of the N and P/Q subtypes of calcium channels of neurons in the brain and spinal cord, thereby modulating calcium influx into pre-synaptic cells.[123] Therefore, there is less postsynaptic activation through the AMPA/kainite, NMDA, and neurokinin receptors. Unlike the opioids, which limit calcium influx via a G protein pathway, no tolerance is associated with pregabalin and gabapentin. Gabapentin and pregabalin do not have any effect on L-type calcium channels (e.g., verapamil); therefore, there is no effect on blood pressure. New evidence in animal models suggests that the site of action of gabapentin is in the locus coeruleus.[124] This finding is supported by a recent clinical study which showed no effect of spinally delivered gabapentin on chronic pain.[27]

Pharmacology of Gabapentin and Pregabalin

Gabapentin

Gabapentin has a nonlinear bioavailability with a reduction in absorption as the dose increases. This is the result of an active and saturable transport mechanism.[125] Gabapentin 900 mg has 60% bioavailability, and a 3600-mg dose has only 33% bioavailability. More frequent delivery of smaller doses may improve bioavailability through the saturable transport mechanism. It is less than 3% protein bound, and because of its high lipid solubility, it readily penetrates the CNS. Gabapentin is not metabolized and is excreted unchanged in the urine. Therefore, renal impairment will significantly increase the drug half-life. Studies have shown efficacy at doses up to 1800 mg and 2400 mg; however, doses above 1800 mg/day do not appear to be more efficacious, and the current maximum FDA-approved dose to treat pain is 1800 mg/day. Because of its nonlinear kinetics, titration of gabapentin to an effective dose can be prolonged with an average onset of 10 to 14 days after initiation.

Pregabalin

Pregabalin is not dependent on active transport for absorption and therefore has linear kinetics with bioavailability of about 90%. Unlike gabapentin, pregabalin absorption is independent of dose. It has negligible protein binding and readily penetrates into the CNS. Pregabalin is not metabolized and is excreted unchanged in the urine; therefore, renal impairment will significantly increase the drug half-life, and dose adjustments are required.[121] The effective dose of pregabalin is between 150 and 300 mg per day. Owing to the linear kinetics and high bioavailability, the effective dose can be achieved in 2 to 3 days; therefore, onset is faster than with gabapentin.

Toxicity of Gabapentin and Pregabalin

Neither gabapentin nor pregabalin has any significant drug interactions, and protein binding is minimal. Because gabapentin and pregabalin have similar mechanisms of action, their side effect profiles are very similar. The most common side effects with at least more than twice the incidence of placebo in controlled trials were dizziness, somnolence, dry mouth, peripheral edema, blurred vision, weight gain, and thinking abnormalities. Dizziness and

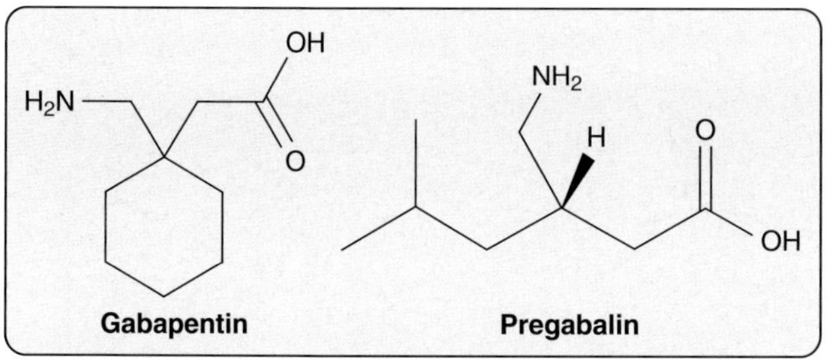

• **Fig. 71.3** Chemical structures of pregabalin and gabapentin.

somnolence usually began shortly after initiation of therapy, and most cases resolved with continued dosing. Dizziness and somnolence are dose-related and can be reduced with slow titration. This side effect can also be an advantage when administered at night in that it will improve sleep. Controlled studies with gabapentin and pregabalin have demonstrated improved sleep quality when compared with placebo.[28,126] Xerostomia (dry mouth) is dose dependent; however, it is usually mild, and few withdrawals from clinical trials have resulted from this side effect. Peripheral edema occurred in almost a third of subjects in clinical trials. It does not appear to be dose-related, nor is it associated with any cardiovascular, renal, or hepatic abnormalities. It is more common with the concomitant use of a thiazolidinedione antidiabetic agent.[127] Blurred vision is dose-related and usually resolves with continued use. It is not associated with any ocular abnormalities. Weight gain has been reported to be as high as 8% of baseline weight but is not associated with any cardiac, renal, or hepatic abnormalities. A mildly increased appetite was reported in epilepsy and fibromyalgia trials. There is no association with baseline body mass index (BMI), sex, or age. Weight gain appears to plateau and is mild. Thinking abnormalities are typical of anti-convulsants and are consistent with the calcium channel modulation mechanism of these agents. Thinking abnormalities tend to be mild but can be bothersome enough in some patients to lead to discontinuation.

Anti-convulsants, including gabapentin and pregabalin, have approximately twice the risk of suicidal ideation over placebo. This increased risk is not age-related and appears to occur at between 1 and 24 weeks of therapy. Patients should be warned of this side effect and instructed to contact their health care provider immediately if it occurs.

Studies with pregabalin have shown a mild PR interval prolongation that was not associated with increased risk of second- or third-degree atrioventricular block. Pregabalin may result in a mildly decreased platelet count, which is not associated with an increase in bleeding-related adverse events. Pregabalin may also result in mild elevations in creatinine kinase, which are asymptomatic in most patients.

In controlled clinical trials of pregabalin, more patients reported euphoria as compared with placebo. In a follow-up drug likability study in recreational drug users of sedative-hypnotics, pregabalin subjects reported a "good drug effect," "high," and "liking" to a degree that was similar to 30 mg of diazepam. In addition, clinical studies showed withdrawal symptoms of insomnia, nausea, headache, and diarrhea. Therefore, the FDA approved the drug with a category V controlled substance schedule.

There have been emerging reports of increased risk of opioid overdose in patients using both pregabalin and opioid[128] or gabapentin.[129] As with any anti-convulsant therapy, pregabalin and gabapentin should be withdrawn slowly over at least a week to avoid withdrawal symptoms (Fig. 71.3).

Muscle Relaxants

Patients frequently describe muscular pain as "spasms," and clinicians clearly know that loss of range of motion is detrimental to their patients. It makes sense that a medicine that acts as a "muscle relaxant" would be of great value in treating patients with these complaints. Unfortunately, skeletal muscle relaxants do not have a primary role in the treatment of chronic pain because of limited true effects on muscles, significant side effect profiles, drug interactions, or addiction potential.

The list of medications classified as skeletal muscle relaxants is highly diverse (Fig. 71.4). Because each of the drugs in this class has a unique mechanism of action and side effect profile, each medication from this class must be examined separately. Adding to the difficulty of understanding these medications is the lack of consensus as to how or why they provide benefit. The two approved clinical indications are for treatment in upper motor neuron diseases that result in spasticity and in peripheral musculoskeletal disorders that cause pain and spasms. Each of these medications can thus be classified as an antispastic or antispasmodic agent. These medications should not be used as first-line medications and usually should be used in conjunction with other pain medications. In addition, most antispasmodic medications come with restriction of use to 2 to 3 weeks. Despite this, many skeletal muscle relaxants are prescribed on a long-term basis for chronic conditions.[130]

Understanding the reflex arc in muscle is important in understanding where these agents act. The simplest reflex is monosynaptic. A muscle spindle transmits an efferent signal through the Ia afferent neuron; this enters the dorsal horn of the spinal cord and synapses on an alpha motoneuron. This neuron then exits the spinal cord through the ventral root and innervates the extrafusal fibers of the same muscle, causing a contraction in the muscle. The Ia afferent signal is also transmitted polysynaptically through interneurons that inhibit alpha motoneurons of antagonist muscles, causing them to relax. Gamma motoneurons located in the ventral horn adjust the sensitivity of the muscle spindles to stretch. They travel with the alpha motoneurons and receive input from cutaneous receptors and many supraspinal pathways, including the corticospinal and reticulospinal tracts. Polysynaptic spinal reflexes with supraspinal connections are much more abundant than monosynaptic reflexes. These connections are both excitatory and inhibitory, providing improved control and feedback to set and fine-tune motor tone. The main tract that inhibits spinal reflexes is the dorsal reticulospinal tract, and the main excitatory pathway is the bulbopontine tegmentum.[131]

Spasticity occurs in upper motoneuron disorders such as multiple sclerosis, spinal cord injuries, traumatic brain injuries, strokes, and cerebral palsy. These diseases cause loss of descending inhibition from the brain to the spinal cord, leading to muscular hypertonicity and increased resistance to stretch. This presentation, which is classically described as a "clasp-knife phenomenon," tends to affect the flexors of the upper extremities and the extensors of the lower extremities more than other muscle groups. Medications approved for spasticity include baclofen (Lioresal), dantrolene (Dantrium), tizanidine (Zanaflex), and diazepam (Valium).

The antispasmodic agents are used to treat muscle pain and spasms when hypertonicity, hyperreflexia, or other signs of upper motoneuron disorders are not present. This presentation is much more common than spasticity and would include syndromes such as fibromyalgia, tension headaches, myofascial

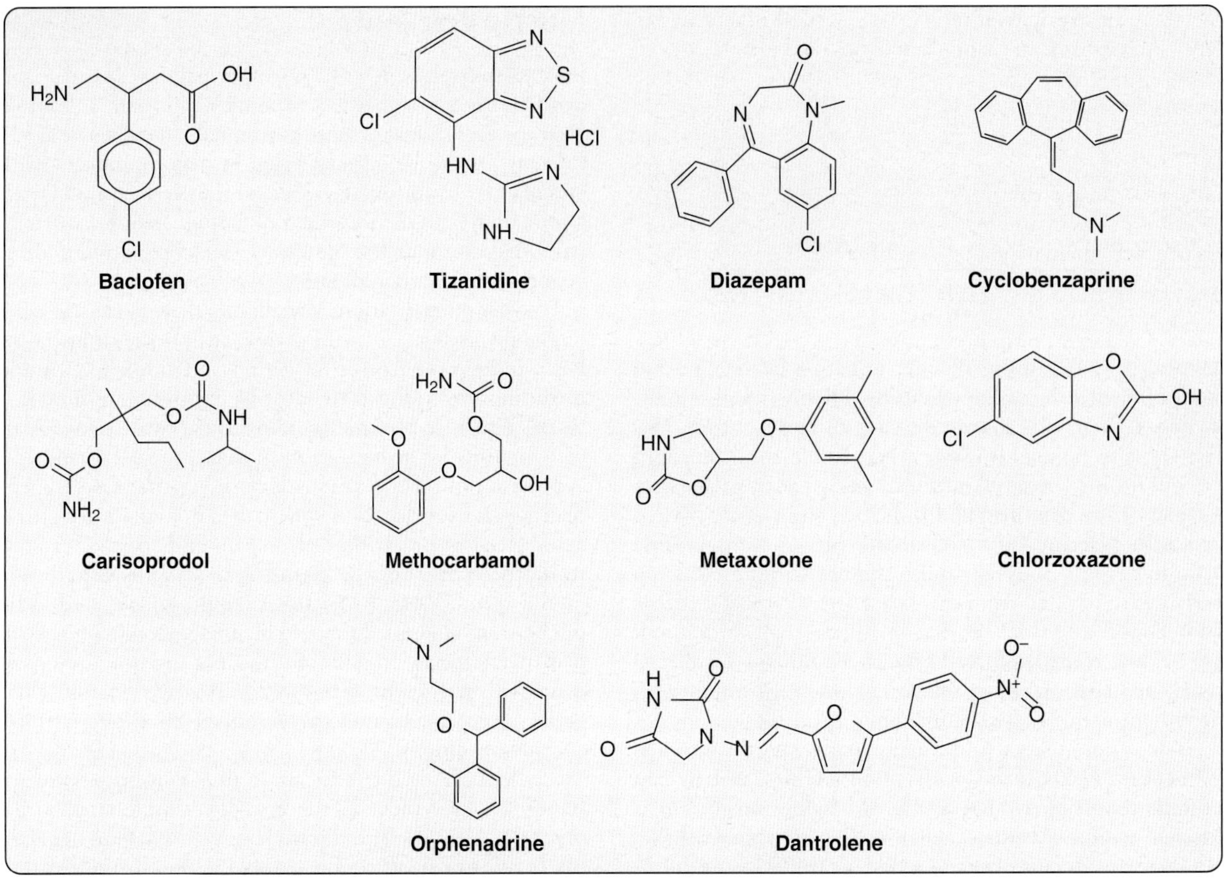

Baclofen Tizanidine Diazepam Cyclobenzaprine

Carisoprodol Methocarbamol Metaxolone Chlorzoxazone

Orphenadrine Dantrolene

• **Fig. 71.4** Chemical structures of muscle relaxants.

pain disorders, and nonspecific back pain. Medications include cyclobenzaprine (Flexeril), carisoprodol (Soma), metaxalone (Skelaxin), chlorzoxazone (Parafon Forte), methocarbamol (Robaxin), and orphenadrine (Norflex). Tizanidine and benzodiazepines are approved for both spasticity and musculoskeletal disorders. How each of these drugs improves these conditions is not completely clear, but the nonspecific sedative effects may have greater importance than the effects on muscles or spinal reflexes.

Antispasmodic Medications

Baclofen

Baclofen blocks pre- and postsynaptic $GABA_B$ receptors[132,133] and disrupts polysynaptic and monosynaptic reflexes at the spinal cord level.[134] Oral doses usually start at 5 mg three times per day with a maximum dose of 80 mg per day. This medication frequently can be used intrathecally for the same indication with a reduction in clinical side effects. Sedation, weakness, hypotension, nausea, depression, and constipation have been reported. Taper slowly and adjust for renal impairment. Withdrawal symptoms include hallucinations, seizures, and pruritus.

Dantrolene

Dantrolene acts directly on the muscle by decreasing the release of calcium from skeletal muscle sarcoplasmic reticulum.[135] It has a black box warning about hepatotoxicitiy.[136] Its risk is much greater with patients taking 800 mg per day or more compared with doses of 400 mg per day. It is recommended to stop this medication after 45 days if no benefit is derived.

Tizanidine

Tizanidine is a centrally acting agonist of the α_2 receptor[137,138] that reduces the release of excitatory amino acids from the presynaptic terminal of spinal interneurons.[139] This reduces tonic stretch reflexes and polysynaptic reflex activity.[140] Doses start at 2 to 4 mg at night and increase by 2 to 4 mg three to four times per day with a maximum dose of 36 mg per day. Side effects include hypotension, sedation, and dry mouth. Its major route of elimination is renal, and renal impairment can significantly decrease clearance. It is metabolized via CYP1A2, and concomitant use with ciprofloxacin or fluvoxamine is contraindicated.[141] Elevated liver functions—three times the upper level of normal—have occurred in 5% of patients.[141] Monitoring of liver function is recommended. Acute withdrawal can cause hypertension, tachycardia, and hypertonia. Use with alcohol should be warned against, and oral contraceptives will decrease clearance with doses as low as 4 mg per day.

Diazepam

Diazepam works by central blockade of $GABA_A$,[135,142] which is an inhibitory neurotransmitter in the CNS. It was the first drug used to treat spasticity and is often used to compare new agents in clinical trials. Efficacy for spasticity and muscle pain is believed to be similar to that of benzodiazepines as a class.[143] Clinical trials showing efficacy with benzodiazepines are based on tetrazepam, which currently is not available in the United States.[144] It is not considered a first-line agent for spasticity or muscle pain because of its sedative effects, drug interactions, and significant abuse potential.

Muscle Relaxants

Cyclobenzaprine

Cyclobenzaprine is structurally related to tricyclic antidepressants and thus causes sedation through its anticholinergic effects. It acts primarily at the brain stem to reduce tonic somatic motor activity influencing both gamma and alpha motoneurons. Dosing at 5 mg three times per day has shown similar efficacy when compared with 10 mg three times per day with reduced side effects.[145] The maximum daily dose is 30 mg. This drug should not be used during the acute recovery phase of myocardial infarction, or in patients with arrhythmias, heart block, congestive heart failure, or hyperthyroidism. The risk of seizures with tramadol is increased if this medication is added.[146] The risk of serotonin syndrome can be increased in patients taking selective serotonin reuptake inhibitors.[147]

Carisoprodol

Carisoprodol in animal studies has shown muscle relaxation through altered interneuronal activity in the spinal cord and in the descending reticular formation of the brain. It is metabolized in the liver to meprobamate, a Schedule IV medication with abuse potential.[148] Meprobamate binds to $GABA_A$ receptors, which results in further sedation. Doses start at 250 mg up to four times per day with a maximum dose of 1400 mg per day. It is contraindicated in patients with a history of acute intermittent porphyria. CYP1C19 inhibitors such as omeprazole or fluvoxamine may increase carisoprodol levels and decrease meprobamate. CYP1C19 inducers such as rifampin or St. John's wort increase exposure to meprobamate.

Methocarbamol

Methocarbamol, a carbamate derivative of guaifenesin, is a CNS depressant with no direct action on striated muscle, the motor end plate, or the nerve fiber. It comes in 500- and 750-mg tablets and can be given up to four times per day with a maximum dose of 8 g per day. It should be used with caution in patients with myasthenia gravis receiving anti-cholinesterase agents.

Metaxalone

Metaxalone also has no direct actions on muscles. Its effects occur mainly through generalized CNS depression. It tends to cause much less sedation than other drugs in this class and has limited drug interactions. It is contraindicated in drug-induced, hemolytic anemias and in significantly impaired renal or hepatic function. The dose most commonly used is 800 mg three or four times per day.

Chlorzoxazone

Chlorzoxazone is a centrally acting agent that acts primarily at the level of the spinal cord and subcortical areas of the brain, where it inhibits multisynaptic reflex arcs. Doses are 250 to 750 mg three or four times per day. Hepatocellular toxicity has been reported with this drug.

Orphenadrine

Orphenadrine is derived from diphenhydramine. It does not directly relax muscles and possesses greater anticholinergic properties than diphenhydramine. Its dosage recommendation is 100 mg twice a day. It is contraindicated in patients with glaucoma, pyloric/duodenal obstruction, peptic ulcers, prostatic hyperplasia or obstruction of the bladder neck, cardiospasm (megaesophagus), and myasthenia gravis.

Efficacy

Clinical studies using these drugs are very limited, poorly controlled, and of short duration. One meta-analysis[149] found fair evidence that tizanidine and baclofen are roughly equivalent and are similar to diazepam for the treatment of spasticity. Investigators go on to state that data on efficacy for muscle relaxants with musculoskeletal conditions are limited but for treatment compared with placebo, cyclobenzaprine, tizanidine, carisoprodol, and orphenadrine showed a consistent trend favoring active treatment. Data demonstrating effectiveness for chlorzoxazone, methocarbamol, baclofen, and dantrolene are limited. Last, data for metaxalone are mixed.

Topical Pain Medications

Topical medications have become popular and have seen increased use because of less systemic absorption, activity at site of pain, and patient preference. Currently, the literature supporting these medications is limited. Further, despite local application, there are still reports of systemic side effects. As already reported, topical TCAs produce analgesia in animal models of pain.[93,95] Lidocaine is commercially available in cream, gel, and patch form. It can be considered for treatment of neuropathic pain.[150] Capsaicin, which depletes Substance P, is available in lower concentrations over the counter and in an 8% patch. The FDA has approved the 8% patch for postherpetic neuralgia. The lower concentrations (0.25% to 0.75%) have been used for both muscular and neuropathic pain, again with limited clinical support. Topical nonsteroidal anti-inflammatory drugs have shown benefit with limited side effects in a review of 61 studies for musculoskeletal conditions.[151]

Emerging Targets

Opioids

The rise of the opioid crisis has led to the search for newer and safer opioids to treat chronic pain. Oliceridine is a μ-GPS (G protein specific) modulator improved safety and tolerability. The mu receptor acts through the GPS pathway resulting in pain and the β-arrestin pathway resulting in increased pain, respiratory depression, and gastrointestinal (GI) dysfunction. Traditional opioid agonists activate both the GPS and β-arrestin pathways. Oliceridine is a μ-G protein specific (GPS) modulator that results in improved pain and reduced side effects since it does not activate the β-arrestin pathway.[152] Phase III studies in acute pain have been completed.

NKTR-181 is a full μ-opioid receptor agonist that has a PEG polymer attached that modulates the rate of entry across the blood-brain barrier (BBB). The PEG is strongly linked, making it difficult to modify for faster BBB penetration. Studies have shown that the NKTR-181 results in a 2.8-hour delay in miosis (a measure of BBB penetration) compared with oxycodone (11 minutes).[153] Phase III trials in low back pain have been completed.

Nerve Growth Factor Inhibitors

Nerve growth factor (NGF) is a ligand to the tyrosine kinase (TrKA) receptor located on sensory neurons. Inflammation results in increased levels of NGF, which stimulate the TrKA receptor leading to an increase in inflammatory mediators and increased sensitivity to pain. Overexpression of NGF also leads to a proliferation of sympathetic fibers, which may be important in the production of inflammatory and neuropathic pain. Because NGF is essential for the survival and development of sensory neurons, NGF inhibitors may lead to peripheral nerve dysfunction and neuropathies. Tanezumab, a recombinant humanized monoclonal antibody targeting NGF, is in phase II trials and is being developed to treat pain associated with osteoarthritis, low back pain, and metastatic bone cancer.[154] In 2010, the FDA halted all clinical trials for this entire class of drug due to reports of osteonecrosis. In 2012, an advisory panel to the FDA voted unanimously to allow the trials to continue but without concomitant use of NSAIDs as patient on NSAIDs had greater joint damage. Studies using tanezumab in osteoarthritis of the knee/hip and low back pain are promising.[155–159] Tanezumab combined with NSAIDs is better than tanezumab monotherapy; however, there are more adverse events with the combination therapy.[160,161] Fasinumab is a newer NGF inhibitor with promise. An exploratory study in osteoarthritis knee pain showed it to be safe with significant improvement in pain over placebo.[162]

Cannabinoid Agonists

Cannabinoid receptors type 1 (CB1) are located at multiple locations in the peripheral and CNS, whereas CB2 receptors are located on inflammatory cells (monocytes, B/T cells, mast cells). CB2 activation results in a reduction in inflammatory mediator release, plasma extravasation, and sensory terminal sensitization. Activation of peripheral CB1 receptors results in a reduction in the release of pro-inflammatory terminal peptides and a reduction in terminal sensitivity. Activation of central CB1 receptors leads to reduced dorsal horn excitability and activates descending inhibitory pathways in the brain. The net result is a reduction in both pain and hyperalgesia. Inhaled cannabis has been extensively studied in various pain syndromes with mixed results. More recent well-controlled trials in neuropathic pain have shown promise, and systematic reviews of randomized trials suggest a significant analgesic effect compared with placebo.[163,164] All of these studies have been conducted with tetrahydrocannabidiol (THC) only with no studies evaluating cannabidiol (CBD). Studies suggest that THC has a biphasic effect with low dose, reducing pain and higher doses increasing pain stressing the need to educate patients using THC for pain. There is increasing evidence that CBD can mitigate the psychoactive effects of THC, and combination use is becoming more popular.[165] Sativex is a sublingual spray containing a mixture of tetrahydrocannabinol and cannabidiol, which failed to reach the primary efficacy endpoint in a phase III cancer pain trial. Studies with cannabis in musculoskeletal pain are limited; however, it has reduced the pain of rheumatoid arthritis and chronic pain of various other causes.[166,167] Use of these medications has seen exponential growth as laws have changed within the United States, but it is uncertain where they fit in treatment algorithms.[168,169] Just like all medications with potential for abuse or misuse, cannabinoid prescriptions need proper patient selection and oversight.

AMPA/Kainate Antagonists

Glutamate, an excitatory amino acid neurotransmitter, has been implicated in pain perception. Two types of glutamate receptors are found in the CNS: ionotropic and metabotropic. Ionotropic receptors are further functionally categorized into NMDA and non-NMDA receptor subtypes (AMPA and kainate receptors).[170] AMPA and kainate receptors are prevalent within the dorsal horn of the spinal cord, and activation is thought to mediate rapid excitatory neurotransmission, resulting in central sensitization mechanisms. Tezampanel, an intravenously administered antagonist of AMPA and kainate receptors, is effective in reducing human experimental pain.[171] NGX426, an oral prodrug of tezampanel, is effective in reducing human experimental pain.[172]

Angiotensin II Type 2 Receptor Antagonists

Angiotensin II type 2 receptors (AT2) are expressed on small fibers and the dorsal root ganglion. Angiotensin-converting enzyme inhibitors have failed to show any effects on pain, and attention has been directed at the more specific type 2 receptors. A phase II study with EMA-401 (an AT2 receptor antagonist) in postherpetic neuralgia in 183 subjects resulted in significant reductions in the primary outcome measure of pain intensity. Secondary outcome measures of pain relief onset, 30% and 50% responder rate, McGill pain questionnaire, and Patient Global Impression of change were are also positive. The drug appears to be safe and well tolerated.[173]

Mirogabalin

Mirogabalin is an N-type calcium channel modulator that is specific to the α-2-delta type II subunit. This results in fewer side effect than the nonspecific modulators such as pregabalin. A phase II study in painful diabetic peripheral neuropathy showed that mirogabalin was superior to placebo for pain relief and sleep with a low incidence of treatment-emergent adverse events.[174]

Full references for this chapter can be found on ExpertConsult.com.

Selected References

1. Coda B, Bonica J: General considerations of acute pain. In Loeser JD, editor: *The management of pain*, ed 3, Philadelphia, 2001, Lippincott Williams & Wilkins, pp 222–240.
2. Mantyselka P, Kumpusalo E, Ahonen R, et al.: Pain as a reason to visit the doctor: a study in Finnish primary health care, *Pain* 89(2–3):175–180, 2001.
3. Galer BS, Dworkin RH: *A clinical guide to neuropathic pain*, Minneapolis, 2000, McGraw-Hill Companies, Inc.
4. Eisendrath S: Psychiatric aspects of chronic pain, *Neurology* 45(12 Suppl l):S26–S34, 1995.
5. Willis WD: Physiology of pain perception. In Takala J, Oomura Y, Ito M, Otsuka M, editors: *Biowarning system in the brain*, Tokyo, 1998, University of Tokyo Press.
6. Parsons CG: NMDA receptors as targets for drug action in neuropathic pain, *Eur J Pharmacol* 429(1–3):71–78, 2001.
7. Stephenson F: Subunit characterization of NMDA receptors, *Curr Drug Targets* 2(3):233–239, 2001.
8. Woolf CJ: American College of Physicians, American Physiological Society Pain: moving from symptom control toward mechanism-specific pharmacologic management, *Ann Intern Med* 140(6):441–451, 2004.
9. Attal N, Bouhassira D: Mechanisms of pain in peripheral neuropathy, *Acta Neurol Scand* 173(Suppl l):12–24, 1999.
10. Woolf CJ, Mannion RJ: Neuropathic pain: aetiology, symptoms, mechanisms, and management, *Lancet* 353(9168):1959–1964, 1999.
11. Gourlay DL, Heit HA, Almahrezi A: Universal precautions in pain medicine: a rational approach to the treatment of chronic pain, *Pain Med* 6(2):107–112, 2005.

12. Chou R, Fanciullo GJ, Fine PG, et al.: Clinical guidelines for the use of chronic opioid therapy in chronic noncancer pain, *J Pain* 10(2):113–130, 2009.
13. Chou RD, Devine B, Hansen R, et al.: Effectiveness and risk of long term opioid treatment in chronic pain, *AHRQ Evidence Reports/Technology Assessment* 14(E005-EF), 2017.
14. Dowell D, Haegerich TM, Chou R: CDC guideline for prescribing opioids for chronic pain—United States, 2016, *J Am Med Assoc* 315(15):1624–1645, 2016.
15. Hegmann KT, Weiss MS, Bowden K, et al.: ACOEM practice guidelines: opioids for treatment of acute, subacute, chronic, and postoperative pain, *J Occup Environ Med* 56(12):e143–e159, 2014.
16. Chou R, Gordon DB, de Leon-Casasola OA, et al.: Management of postoperative pain: a clinical practice guideline from the American Pain Society, the American Society of Regional Anesthesia and Pain Medicine, and the American Society of Anesthesiologists' Committee on Regional Anesthesia, Executive Committee, and Administrative Council, *J Pain* 17(2):131–157, 2016.
17. Manchikanti L, Kaye AM, Knezevic NN, et al.: Responsible, safe, and effective prescription of opioids for chronic non-cancer pain: American Society of Interventional Pain Physicians (ASIPP) guidelines, *Pain Phy* 20(2S):S3–S92, 2017.
18. Rosenberg JM, Bilka BM, Wilson SM, et al.: Opioid therapy for chronic pain: overview of the 2017 US Department of Veterans Affairs and US Department of Defense clinical practice guideline, *Pain Med* 19(5):928–941, 2017.
19. Webster LR, Webster RM: Predicting aberrant behaviors in opioid-treated patients: preliminary validation of the Opioid Risk Tool, *Pain Med* 6(6):432–442, 2005.
20. Belgrade MJ, Schamber CD, Lindgren BR: The DIRE score: predicting outcomes of opioid prescribing for chronic pain, *J Pain* 7(9):671–681, 2006.
21. Butler SF, Fernandez K, Benoit C, et al.: Validation of the revised Screener and opioid assessment for patients with pain (SOAPP-R), *J Pain* 9(4):360–372, 2008.
22. Dunn KM, Saunders KW, Rutter CM, et al.: Opioid prescriptions for chronic pain and overdose: a cohort study, *Ann Intern Med* 152(2):85–92, 2010.
23. Martin WR, Eades CG, Thompson JA, et al.: The effects of morphine- and nalorphine-like drugs in the nondependent and morphine-dependent chronic spinal dog, *J Pharmacol Exp Ther* 197(3):517–532, 1976.
24. Martin WR: History and development of mixed opioid agonists, partial agonists and antagonists, *Br J Clin Pharmacol* 7(Suppl 3):273S–279S, 1979.
25. Lord JA, Waterfield AA, Hughes J, et al.: Endogenous opioid peptides: multiple agonists and receptors, *Nature* 267(5611):495–499, 1977.
26. Connor M, Christie MD: Opioid receptor signalling mechanisms, *Clin and Exp Pharmacol Physiol* 26(7):493–499, 1999.
27. Rauck R, Coffey RJ, Schultz DM, et al.: Intrathecal gabapentin to treat chronic intractable noncancer pain, *Anesthesiology* 119(3):675–686, 2013.
28. Crofford LJ, Rowbotham MC, Mease PJ, et al.: Pregabalin for the treatment of fibromyalgia syndrome: results of a randomized, double-blind, placebo-controlled trial, *Arthritis Rheum* 52(4):1264–1273, 2005.
29. Karavelis A, Foroglou G, Selviaridis P, et al.: Intraventricular administration of morphine for control of intractable cancer pain in 90 patients, *Neurosurgery* 39(1):57–61, 1996; discussion 61-62.
30. Yaksh T: Pharmacology and mechanisms of opioid analgesic activity, *Acta Anesthesiol Scand* 41(1):94–111, 1997.
31. Stein C, Lang LJ: Peripheral mechanisms of opioid analgesia, *Curr Opin Pharmacol* 9(1):3–8, 2009.
32. Trujillo KA, Akil H: Inhibition of morphine tolerance and dependence by the NMDA receptor antagonist MK-801, *Science* 251(4989):85–87, 1991.
33. Christie MJ: Cellular neuroadaptations to chronic opioids: tolerance, withdrawal and addiction, *Br J Pharmacol* 154(2):384–396, 2008.
34. Kreek MJ, Koob GF: Drug dependence: stress and dysregulation of brain reward pathways, *Drug Alcohol Depend* 51(1–2):23–47, 1998.
35. Savage SR: Assessment for addiction in pain-treatment settings, *Clin J Pain* 18(Suppl 4):S28–S38, 2002.
36. Sees K, Clark H: Opioid use in the treatment of chronic pain: assessment of addiction, *J Pain Sympt Manage* 8(5):257–264, 1993.
37. Wise RA: The role of reward pathways in the development of drug dependence, *Pharmacol Therap* 35(1–2):227–263, 1987.
38. Weissman DE, Haddox JD: Opioid pseudoaddiction—an iatrogenic syndrome, *Pain* 36(3):363–366, 1989.
39. Schobelock M, Shepard K, Mosdell K: Multiple-dose pharmacokinetic evaluation of two formulations of sustained-release morphine sulfate tablets, *Curr Ther Res* 56:1009–1021, 1995.
40. Hall W, Lynskey M, Degenhardt L: Trends in opiate-related deaths in the United Kingdom and Australia, 1985-1995, *Drug Alcohol Depend* 57(3):247–254, 2000.
41. Milroy CM, Forrest AR: Methadone deaths: a toxicological analysis, *J Clin Pathol* 53(4):277–281, 2000.
42. Kristensen K, Blemmer T, Angelo HR, et al.: Stereoselective pharmacokinetics of methadone in chronic pain patients, *Ther Drug Monit* 18(3):221–227, 1996.
43. Daniell HW: Inhibition of opioid analgesia by selective serotonin reuptake inhibitors, *J Clin Oncol* 20(9):2409, 2002; author reply 2409-2410.
44. Gottenberg JE, Ravaud P, Puechal X, et al.: Effects of hydroxychloroquine on symptomatic improvement in primary Sjogren syndrome: the JOQUER randomized clinical trial, *J Am Med Assoc* 312(3):249–258, 2014.
45. Mather LE: Clinical pharmacokinetics of fentanyl and its newer derivatives, *Clin Pharmacokinet* 8(5):422–446, 1983.
46. Varvel JR, Shafer SL, Hwang SS, et al.: Absorption characteristics of transdermally administered fentanyl, *Anesthesiology* 70(6):928–934, 1989.
47. Streisand JB, Varvel JR, Stanski DR, et al.: Absorption and bioavailability of oral transmucosal fentanyl citrate, *Anesthesiology* 75(2):223–229, 1991.
48. Poyhia R, Seppala T, Olkkola KT, et al.: The pharmacokinetics and metabolism of oxycodone after intramuscular and oral administration to healthy subjects, *Br J Clin Pharmacol* 33(6):617–621, 1992.
49. *Opana® (oxymorphone hydrochloride) tablets package insert*, Chadds Ford, PA, 2006, Endo Pharmaceutical, Inc.
50. *Exalgo® (hydromorphone HCL extended-release) package insert*, Conshocken, PA, 2010, Neuromed Pharmaceuticals, Inc.
51. Edwards DJ, Svensson CK, Visco JP, et al.: Clinical pharmacokinetics of pethidine: 1982, *Clin Pharmacokinet* 7(5):421–433, 1982.
52. Stone PA, Macintyre PE, Jarvis DA: Norpethidine toxicity and patient controlled analgesia, *Br J Anaesth* 71(5):738–740, 1993.
53. Lim G, Sung B, Ji RR, et al.: Upregulation of spinal cannabinoid-1-receptors following nerve injury enhances the effects of Win 55,212-2 on neuropathic pain behaviors in rats, *Pain* 105(1–2):275–283, 2003.
54. Eichelbaum M, Evert B: Influence of pharmacogenetics on drug disposition and response, *Clin Exp Pharmacol Physiol* 23(10–11):983–985, 1996.
55. Caraco Y, Sheller J, Wood AJ: Impact of ethnic origin and quinidine coadministration on codeine's disposition and pharmacodynamic effects, *J Pharmacol Exp Ther* 290(1):413–422, 1999.
56. Lewis KS, Han NH: Tramadol: a new centrally acting analgesic, *Am J Health Syst Pharm* 54(6):643–652, 1997.
57. White JM, Irvine RJ: Mechanisms of fatal opioid overdose, *Addiction* 94(7):961–972, 1999.
58. Pattinson KT: Opioids and the control of respiration, *Br J Anaesth* 100(6):747–758, 2008.

59. Cherny NI: Opioid analgesics: comparative features and prescribing guidelines, *Drugs* 51(5):713–737, 1996.
60. Bluet-Pajot MT, Tolle V, Zizzari P, et al.: Growth hormone secretagogues and hypothalamic networks, *Endocrine* 14(1):1–8, 2001.
61. Lightman SL: The neuroendocrine paraventricular hypothalamus: receptors, signal transduction, mRNA and neurosecretion, *J Exp Biol* 139:31–49, 1988.
62. Gimpl G, Fahrenholz F: The oxytocin receptor system: structure, function, and regulation, *Physiol Res* 8(2):629–683, 2001.
63. Lalley PM: Opioidergic and dopaminergic modulation of respiration, *Respir Physiol Neurobiol* 164(1–2):160–167, 2008.
64. Lyss AP, Portenoy RK: Strategies for limiting the side effects of cancer pain therapy, *Semin Oncol* 24(5 Suppl 16):S16–28–34, 1997.
65. Vella-Brincat J, Macleod A: Adverse effects of opioids on the central nervous systems of palliative care patients, *J Pain Care Pharmacother* 21(1):15–25, 2007.
66. McGinty JF: What we know and still need to learn about opioids in the hippocampus, *NIDA Res Monograph* 82:1–11, 1988.
67. King T, Ossipov MH, Vanderah TW, et al.: Is paradoxical pain induced by sustained opioid exposure an underlying mechanism of opioid antinociceptive tolerance? *Neurosignals* 14(4):194–205, 2005.
68. Smith MT: Neuroexcitatory effects of morphine and hydromorphone: evidence implicating the 3-glucuronide metabolites, *Clinical and experimental pharmacology & physiology* 27(7):524–528, 2000.
69. Seifert CF, Kennedy S: Meperidine is alive and well in the new millennium: evaluation of meperidine usage patterns and frequency of adverse drug reactions, *Pharmacotherapy* 24(6):776–783, 2004.
70. Greenwood-Van Meerveld B: Emerging drugs for postoperative ileus, *Expert Opin Emerg Drugs* 12(4):619–626, 2007.
71. Cameron D, Gan T: Management of postoperative nausea and vomiting in ambulatory surgery, *Anesthesiol Clin North Amer* 21(2):347–365, 2003.
72. Benyamin R, Trescot A, Datta S, et al.: Opioid complications and side effects, *Pain Physician* 1(2 Suppl l):105–120, 2008.
73. Kromer W: Endogenous and exogenous opioids in the control of gastrointestinal motility and secretion, *Pharmacol Rev* 40(2):121–162, 1988.
74. De Luca A, Coupar IM: Insights into opioid action in the intestinal tract, *Pharmacol Therap* 69(2):103–115, 1996.
75. Wood J, Galligan J: Function of opioids in the enteric nervous system, *Neuro Gastroenterol Motil* 16(2 Suppl l):17–28, 2004.
76. Dray A, Nunan L: Supraspinal and spinal mechanisms in morphine-induced inhibition of reflex urinary bladder contractions in the rat, *Neuroscience* 22(1):281–287, 1987.
77. Schmelz M: Itch—mediators and mechanisms, *J Dermatol Sci* 28(2):91–96, 2002.
78. Ballantyne JC, Loach AB, Carr DB: Itching after epidural and spinal opiates, *Pain* 33(2):149–160, 1988.
79. Sharp B, Yaksh T: Pain killers of the immune system, *Nat Med* 3(8):831–832, 1997.
80. Mellon RD, Bayer BM: Evidence for central opioid receptors in the immunomodulatory effects of morphine: review of potential mechanism(s) of action, *J Neuroimmunol* 83(1–2):19–28, 1998.
81. Welters ID, Menzebach A, Goumon Y, et al.: Morphine inhibits NF-kappaB nuclear binding in human neutrophils and monocytes by a nitric oxide-dependent mechanism, *Anesthesiology* 92(6):1677–1684, 2000.
82. Chuang LF, Killam Jr KF, Chuang RY: Induction and activation of mitogen-activated protein kinases of human lymphocytes as one of the signaling pathways of the immunomodulatory effects of morphine sulfate, *J Biol Chem* 272(43):26815–26817, 1997.
83. Adler MW, Geller EB, Rosow CE, et al.: The opioid system and temperature regulation, *Annu Rev Pharmacol Toxicol* 28:429–449, 1988.
84. Ikeda T, Kurz A, Sessler DI, et al.: The effect of opioids on thermoregulatory responses in humans and the special antishivering action of meperidine, *Ann N Y Acad Sci* 813:792–798, 1997.
85. Al-Adwani A, Basu N: Methadone and excessive sweating, *Addiction* 99(2):259, 2004.
86. Catterall RA: Problems of sweating and transdermal fentanyl, *Palliat Med* 11(2):169–170, 1997.
87. Fishbain DA, Cutler R, Rosomoff HL, et al.: Evidence-based data from animal and human experimental studies on pain relief with antidepressants: a structured review, *Pain Med* 1(4):310–316, 2000.
88. Saarto T, Wiffen P: Antidepressants for neuropathic pain, *Cochrane Data Base Rev* CD005454, 2005.
89. Hirschfeld RM, Mallinckrodt C, Lee TC, et al.: Time course of depression-symptom improvement during treatment with duloxetine, *Depress Anxiety* 21(4):170–177, 2005.
90. Hauser W, Bernardy K, Uceyler N, et al.: Treatment of fibromyalgia syndrome with antidepressants: a meta-analysis, *J Am Med Assoc* 301(2):198–209, 2009.
91. Sindrup SH, Jensen TS: Efficacy of pharmacological treatments of neuropathic pain: an update and effect related to mechanism of drug action, *Pain* 83(3):389–400, 1999.
92. Fagiolini A, Comandini A, Catena Dell'Osso M, et al.: Rediscovering trazodone for the treatment of major depressive disorder, *CNS Drugs* 26(12):1033–1049, 2012.
93. Mico JA, Ardid D, Berrocoso E, et al.: Antidepressants and pain, *Trends Pharmacol Sci* 27(7):348–354, 2006.
94. Aida S, Baba H, Yamakura T, et al.: The effectiveness of preemptive analgesia varies according to the type of surgery: a randomized, double-blind study, *Anesth Analg* 89(3):711–716, 1999.
95. Sawynok J, Esser MJ, Reid AR: Peripheral antinociceptive actions of desipramine and fluoxetine in an inflammatory and neuropathic pain test in the rat, *Pain* 82(2):149–158, 1999.
96. Esser MJ, Sawynok J: Caffeine blockade of the thermal antihyperalgesic effect of acute amitriptyline in a rat model of neuropathic pain, *Eur J Pharmacol* 399(2–3):131–139, 2000.
97. Eschalier A, Ardid D, Dubray C: Tricyclic and other antidepressants as analgesics. In Sawynok J, Cowan A, editors: *Novel aspects of pain management: opioids and beyond*, New York, 1999, Wiley-Liss, pp 303–310.
98. Amir R, Argoff CE, Bennett GJ, et al.: The role of sodium channels in chronic inflammatory and neuropathic pain, *J Pain* 7(5 Suppl 3):S1–S29, 2006.
99. Gerner P, Kao G, Srinivasa V, et al.: Topical amitriptyline in healthy volunteers, *Reg Anesth Pain Med* 28(4):289–293, 2003.
100. Godfrey RG: A guide to the understanding and use of tricyclic antidepressants in the overall management of fibromyalgia and other chronic pain syndromes, *Arch Intern Med* 156(10):1047–1052, 1996.
101. Moulin D, Clark AJ, Gilron I, et al.: Pharmacological management of chronic neuropathic pain—Consensus statement and guidelines from the Canadian Pain Society, *Pain Res Manag* 12(1):13–21, 2007.
102. Finnerup NB, Otto M, McQuay HJ, et al.: Algorithm for neuropathic pain treatment: an evidence based proposal, *Pain* 118(3):289–305, 2005.
103. McQuay HJ, Tramer M, Nye BA, et al.: A systematic review of antidepressants in neuropathic pain, *Pain* 68(2–3):217–227, 1996.
104. Sindrup SH, Jensen TS: Pharmacologic treatment of pain in polyneuropathy, *Neurology* 55(7):915–920, 2000.
105. Sindrup SH, Bach FW, Madsen C, et al.: Venlafaxine versus imipramine in painful polyneuropathy: a randomized, controlled trial, *Neurology* 60(8):1284–1289, 2003.
106. Rowbotham MC, Goli V, Kunz NR, et al.: Venlafaxine extended release in the treatment of painful diabetic neuropathy: a double-blind, placebo-controlled study, *Pain* 110(3):697–706, 2004.
107. Sayar K, Aksu G, Ak I, et al.: Venlafaxine treatment of fibromyalgia, *Ann Pharmacother* 37(11):1561–1565, 2003.
108. Hauser W, Petzke F, Uceyler N, et al.: Comparative efficacy and acceptability of amitriptyline, duloxetine and milnacipran in fibromyalgia syndrome: a systematic review with meta-analysis, *Rheumatology* 50(3):532–543, 2011.

109. Goldstein DJ, Lu Y, Detke MJ, et al.: Duloxetine vs. placebo in patients with painful diabetic neuropathy, *Pain* 116(1–2):109–118, 2005.
110. Raskin J, Pritchett YL, Wang F, et al.: A double-blind, randomized multicenter trial comparing duloxetine with placebo in the management of diabetic peripheral neuropathic pain, *Pain Med* 6(5):346–356, 2005.
111. Wernicke JF, Pritchett YL, D'Souza DN, et al.: A randomized controlled trial of duloxetine in diabetic peripheral neuropathic pain, *Neurology* 67(8):1411–1420, 2006.
112. Skljarevski V, Zhang S, Chappell AS, et al.: Maintenance of effect of duloxetine in patients with chronic low back pain: a 41-week uncontrolled, dose-blinded study, *Pain Med* 11(5):648–657, 2010.
113. Skljarevski V, Zhang S, Desaiah D, et al.: Duloxetine versus placebo in patients with chronic low back pain: a 12-week, fixed-dose, randomized, double-blind trial, *J Pain* 11(12):1282–1290, 2010.
114. Chappell AS, Desaiah D, Liu-Seifert H, et al.: A double-blind, randomized, placebo-controlled study of the efficacy and safety of duloxetine for the treatment of chronic pain due to osteoarthritis of the knee, *Pain Prac* 11(1):33–41, 2011.
115. Wise TN: Duloxetine in the treatment of osteoarthritis knee pain, *Curr Psychiatr Rep* 12(1):2–3, 2010.
116. Devor M, Govrin-Lippmann R, Angelides K: Na+ channel immunolocalization in peripheral mammalian axons and changes following nerve injury and neuroma formation, *J Neurosci* 13(5):1976–1992, 1993.
117. Melzack R, Wall PD: Pain mechanisms: a new theory, *Science* 150(3699):971–979, 1965.
118. Castro-Lopes JM, Tavares I, Coimbra A: GABA decreases in the spinal cord dorsal horn after peripheral neurectomy, *Brain Res* 620(2):287–291, 1993.
119. Polgar E, Hughes DI, Riddell JS, et al.: Selective loss of spinal GABAergic or glycinergic neurons is not necessary for development of thermal hyperalgesia in the chronic constriction injury model of neuropathic pain, *Pain* 104(1–2):229–239, 2003.
120. Fukuoka T, Tokunaga A, Kondo E, et al.: Change in mRNAs for neuropeptides and the GABA(A) receptor in dorsal root ganglion neurons in a rat experimental neuropathic pain model, *Pain* 78(1):13–26, 1998.

72 Nutrition and Rheumatic Diseases

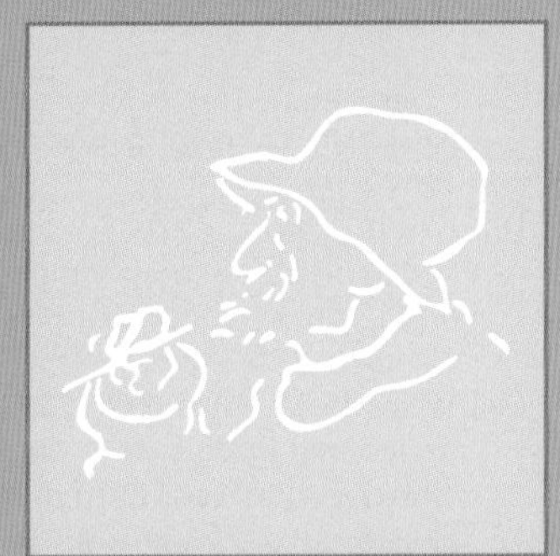

LISA K. STAMP AND LESLIE G. CLELAND

KEY POINTS

Nutritional factors and their metabolites can influence the intensity of inflammation.

Nutritional factors have been implicated in the etiology of a variety of rheumatic disorders, including gout and rheumatoid arthritis (RA).

Dietary supplementation with omega-3 fatty acids can reduce signs and symptoms of inflammation in RA, as well as reduce the need for escalation of treatment with disease-modifying anti-inflammatory drugs and the use of nonsteroidal anti-inflammatory drugs (NSAIDs).

Fish oil supplements have been associated with improved disease control in systemic lupus erythematosus.

Advice regarding nutrition and lifestyle is an expected component of medical advice for patients seeking guidance in the management of health risks and the challenges of chronic diseases.

Introduction

Nutrition plays a role in the management of most chronic diseases. Physicians provide dietary advice to patients with diabetes, heart disease, and obesity as part of standard clinical care. Although the role of diet and nutrition is entrenched in the etiology and management of gout, the influence of nutrition in other rheumatic diseases, such as rheumatoid arthritis (RA), is less widely considered, and accordingly opportunities for offering dietary advice are often overlooked. Many people with arthritis believe food plays a role in their symptom severity, and approximately 50% will have tried dietary manipulation in an attempt to improve their symptoms.[1]

It is well recognized that inflammatory disease processes can interfere with nutritional status. The impact of nutritional factors on the inflammatory response has also been recognized. Furthermore, diets and lifestyles have changed considerably through industrialization, with significant effects on rates of obesity, food choices, and consumption of different dietary components. In light of this, the role of nutrition in the etiology and management of rheumatic diseases is becoming increasingly important. It is therefore important for clinicians to be equipped to address issues of diet both proactively and as they arise.

Nutrition and Inflammation

KEY POINTS

Omega-3 fatty acids are immunoregulatory.

Vitamin D has multiple immunosuppressive effects.

Antioxidants can be acquired through the diet.

Adipose tissue is metabolically active and has effects on the inflammatory response.

Probiotics can have anti-inflammatory properties.

Omega-3 Fatty Acids

Fatty Acid Biochemistry

Fatty acids can be divided into three groups on the basis of the number of double bonds they contain. Saturated fatty acids have no double bond, monounsaturated fatty acids have one double bond, and polyunsaturated fatty acids (PUFAs) have two or more double bonds. C18 fatty acids are prominent in the diet and provide the index fatty acids for the above classification. PUFAs are further grouped according to the site of the double bond proximal to the methyl (omega) terminus as n-6 or n-3. Vertebrates do not have the enzymes required to introduce double bonds in the n-3 and n-6 positions; therefore these fatty acids must be obtained from the diet. Thus they are known as *essential fatty acids*.

In general, Western diets contain substantially more n-6 fats than n-3 fats because of their presence in processed foods and the visible fats and oils sourced from soybean, safflower, sunflower, and corn, which are rich in the n-6 fat linoleic acid (LA; 18:2n-6). The n-3 homologue of LA, α-linolenic acid (ALA; 18:3n-3), is the dominant PUFA in flaxseed oil, which is used less often as a dietary constituent. LA and ALA may be used in energy metabolism or be converted to the C20 fatty acids arachidonic acid (AA) and eicosapentaenoic acid (EPA), respectively. AA and EPA are then incorporated into cell membranes and tissues. EPA can be further metabolized to the n-3 fatty acid docosahexaenoic (DHA).

The critical process linking fatty acids and inflammation is the metabolism of AA and EPA to eicosanoids, which act as inflammatory mediators. AA is metabolized via cyclooxygenase (COX) to n-6 eicosanoids (prostaglandin [PG] E_2, thromboxane [TX] A_2, or via 5-lipoxygenase [5-LOX] to n-6 leukotrienes [LTs]). Through the same pathways, EPA is metabolized to n-3 PGs and LTs, respectively. In comparison to the n-6 eicosanoids produced from AA, EPA is a poor COX substrate such that n-3 PGs are not as readily produced (Fig. 72.1). EPA and DHA competitively inhibit production of most n-6 eicosanoids; prostacyclin (PGI_2) is a notable exception. Increased dietary consumption of n-3 fatty acids such as EPA increases the proportion of EPA incorporated in cellular membranes and tissues, partly at the expense of AA incorporation. The net result is an alteration in the balance of n-3/n-6 eicosanoid production (see Fig. 72.1). EPA and DHA can also be metabolized through lipid oxygenase pathways to novel specialized proresolving lipid mediators (SPMs) of inflammation (see later).

Pro-inflammatory Actions of Eicosanoids

In general, the n-6 eicosanoids (PGE_2 and TXA_2) are pro-inflammatory, whereas the n-3 eicosanoids are either less potent in their effects (TXA_3) or less abundant (PGE_3). TXA_2 promotes IL-1β and TNF production by mononuclear cells,[2] whereas PGE_2 results in vasodilatation, increased vascular permeability, and hyperalgesia (see Fig. 72.1). PGE_3 is edemagenic, although little is produced. LTB_5 is 10 to 30 times less potent than LTB_4 as a neutrophil chemotaxin.

Effect of n-3 Fatty Acids on Pro-inflammatory Cytokine Production

IL-1β and TNF production may be reduced as a consequence of dietary n-3 fatty acid supplementation. Although some of this cytokine inhibition is mediated through effects on eicosanoids, there also appears to be eicosanoid-independent cytokine inhibition. Fatty acids may have direct effects on intra-cellular signaling mechanisms, including nuclear factor-κB (NF-κB) and peroxisome proliferator–activated receptor (PPAR)-γ, thereby affecting cytokine production.[3] The NLRP3 inflammasome, which is involved in production of both IL-1β and IL-18 and implicated in a number of autoinflammatory diseases, is activated by a variety of stimuli, including pathogenic organisms and monosodium urate crystals.[4] n-3 Fatty acids inhibit NLRP3-dependent caspase activation and IL-1β production.[5]

Effects of n-3 Fatty Acids on Major Histocompatibility Expression

The number of major histocompatibility (MHC) molecules expressed on antigen-presenting cells (APCs) is an important determinant of T cell response to antigen. Patients with RA have high levels of class II MHC expression on T cells and synovial lining cells.[6] In vitro studies show that EPA and/or DHA reduces monocyte expression of human leukocyte antigen (HLA)-DR and HLA-DP molecules and reduces the ability of monocytes to present antigen to autologous lymphocytes.[7] Thus n-3 fatty acids may have an anti-inflammatory effect via suppression of pathogenic T cell activation through inhibition of APC function. A murine study has also shown that fish oil also has effects on MHC molecules on B cells and T cell organization at the immunologic synapse.[8]

Effect of n-3 Fatty Acids on Adhesion Molecule Expression

Adhesion molecules expressed on endothelial cells and leukocytes mediate the transit of cells from the circulation into tissues. Intercellular adhesion molecule-1 (ICAM-1) and its cognate receptor, leukocyte function-associated antigen (LFA)-1, are important in migration of leukocytes into inflamed synovium in animal models.[9] ICAM-1 blockade has also been reported to reduce disease activity in RA.[10] In vitro n-3 fatty acids decrease human monocyte ICAM-1 and LFA-1 expression.[7] In addition, dietary n-3 fatty acid supplementation reduces soluble ICAM-1 and vascular cell adhesion molecule-1 (VCAM-1) plasma concentrations.[11]

Effect of n-3 Fatty Acids on Degradative Enzymes

Proteinases have a pivotal role in cartilage degradation and bone erosion. n-3 Fatty acids added in vitro can suppress proteinases a disintegrin and metalloproteinase (ADAM family) with thrombospondin-1 domains (ADAMTS)-4, ADAMTS-5, and matrix metalloproteinase (MMP)-3 in IL-1α-stimulated bovine chondrocytes.[12] This inhibition of chondrocyte proteases is a mechanism through which n-3 fatty acids may inhibit cartilage degradation and bone erosion.

The receptor activator of NF-κB (RANK)/ligand (RANKL)/osteoprotegerin (OPG) pathway is also important in bone pathophysiology in RA. Increased RANK/RANKL and decreased OPG contribute to bone erosion. Three months of dietary fish oil supplementation decreased the RANK/OPG ratio, which may help prevent bone resorption that leads to erosions.[13]

Importance of the Balance of n-3 and n-6 Fatty Acids in Inflammation

The balance of AA and EPA can be altered through dietary fatty acid intake. In humans, the conversion of dietary ALA to tissue EPA is inefficient, and fish/fish oils are a more effective way to increase EPA and DHA in tissues. Changes in AA/EPA ratios in tissues have downstream effects on eicosanoid production and the resulting pro-inflammatory/anti-inflammatory environment. Dietary supplementation with fish oil in humans results in decreased production of PGE_2,[14] TXA_2,[14] and LTB4,[15] with increased production of TXA_3[16] and LTB_5.[17] These data provide a mechanistic basis for beneficial effects of dietary n-3 fatty acid supplementation in the control of inflammatory diseases. Dietary fish oil supplements increase vascular production of prostacyclin (PGI_2).[18] Although the role of PGI_2 in inflammation is not well defined, it is a potent vasodilator and inhibits platelet aggregation, as well as disaggregating platelets. These effects favor maintenance of vascular patency. Importantly, patients with several of the major rheumatic diseases (e.g., RA, systemic lupus erythematosus [SLE], and gout) are at increased risk for serious cardiovascular events and mortality, to which nonsteroidal anti-inflammatory drug (NSAID)–associated COX-2 inhibition may contribute.

Specialized Proresolving Mediators and N-3 Fatty Acids

Resolution of inflammation is an active rather than passive process. SPMs, which include lipoxins, resolvins, protectins, and maresins, synthesized from n-3 fatty acids EPA and DHA, have an important role in this process (Table 72.1). SPMs are formed through the actions of multiple lipid oxygenases (LO), including 5-LO and COX-2, with the yield of some SPMs increased by acetylation of COX-2 by aspirin (see Fig. 72.1). Resolvins derived from EPA are known as *E-resolvins*, with those derived from DHA known as *D-resolvins*. Production of resolvins can be increased by dietary n-3 fatty acid supplementation.[19] The resolvins have a variety of anti-inflammatory actions, including inhibition of TNF and IL-1β production and inhibition of human polymorphonuclear leukocyte transendothelial migration.[20] Resolvins reduce pain and joint stiffness but not joint/paw edema in adjuvant-induced arthritis.[21] SPMs have been detected in synovial fluid from patients with RA, suggesting that these mediators may have local anti-inflammatory effects.[22]

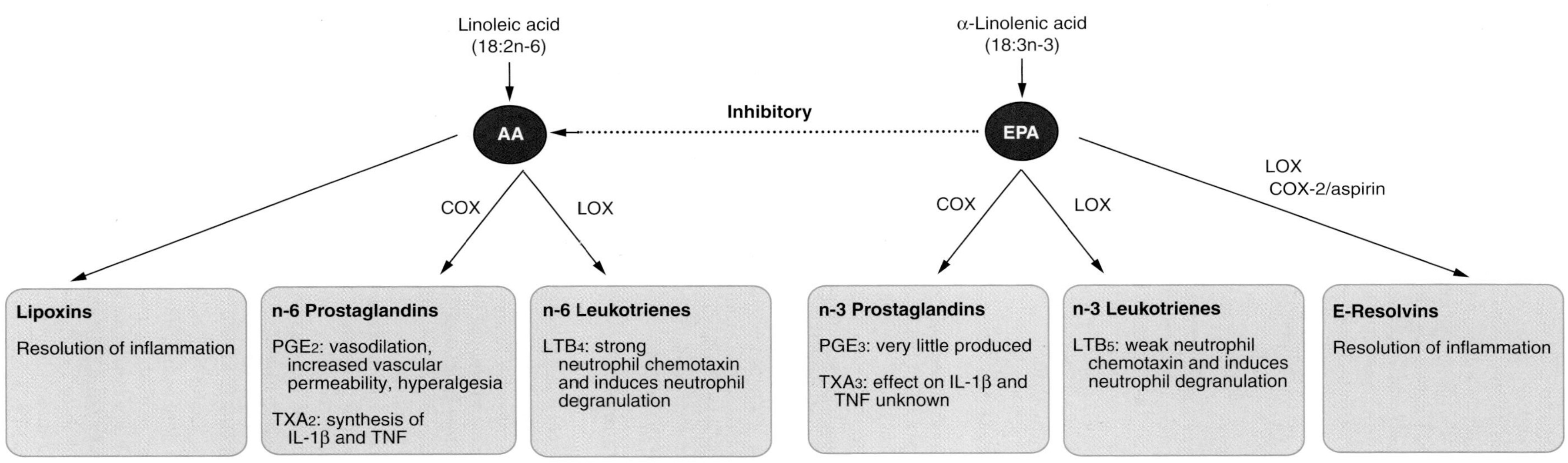

• **Fig. 72.1** Metabolism of linoleic acid and α-linolenic acid to n-6 and n-3 prostaglandins and leukotrienes. *AA,* Arachidonic acid; *COX,* cyclooxygenase; *EPA,* eicosapentaenoic acid; *LOX,* lipoxygenase; *LTB,* leukotriene B; *PGE,* prostaglandin E; *TNF,* tumor necrosis factor; *TXA,* thromboxane A.

TABLE 72.1 **Effects of Adipokines**

PRECURSOR	AA	EPA			DHA	
Family	**Lipoxins**	**E-Resolvins**	**D-Resolvins**		**Protectins**	**Maresins**
	LXA4	RvE1	RvD1	RvD2	PD1	MaR1
Actions	↓Pain signals ↓PMN adhesion ↓Angiogenesis and cell proliferation	↑Macrophage phagocytosis ↑Neutrophil apoptosis ↓Organ fibrosis inhibits NF-κB	↑IL-10, ↓LTB4 ↓Adhesion receptors ↓Pro-inflammatory cytokines TNF ↓Chemotaxis neutrophils	↑PMN adhesion to endothelial cells	↓NF-κB and COX-2 expression ↓TNF and IFN-γ ↓T cell migration	↓Pain

AA, Arachidonic acid; *COX*, cyclooxygenase; *EPA*, eicosapentaenoic acid; *DHA*, docosahexaenoic acid; *IFN*, interferon; *LT*, leukotriene; *LXA4*, lipoxin A4; *MaR1*, maresin 1; *NF-κB*, nuclear factor-κB; *PD1*, protectin D1; *PMN*, polymorphonuclear neutrophil; *RvD1*, resolvin D1; *TNF*, tumor necrosis factor; ↑, increase; ↓, decrease.

Vitamin D and the Inflammatory Process

Vitamin D has multiple immunosuppressive effects in addition to its effects on bone and calcium metabolism. The biologically active form of vitamin D (1,25-dihydroxyvitamin $[OH]_2D_3$) interacts with vitamin D receptors, which are expressed on a variety of cells, including osteoblasts, T cells, dendritic cells (DCs), macrophages, and B cells. These cells also have the capacity to convert more abundant $25(OH)D_3$ to $1,25(OH)_2D_3$ and to degrade $1,25(OH)_2D_3$. Accordingly, the molecular machinery is in place for important autocrine and paracrine effects of vitamin D at sites of inflammation.

DCs have a central role in activation of the immune system and in response to self antigens. $1,25(OH)_2D_3$ inhibits the differentiation of monocyte precursors into mature DCs, downregulates expression of class II MHC molecules on DCs, inhibits IL-12 production, and promotes DC apoptosis, thereby inhibiting DC-dependent T cell activation.[23,24] In addition, $1,25(OH)_2D_3$ can promote DC expression of tolerizing functions, which instruct T regulatory (Treg) cells, which in turn may inhibit the development of autoimmunity.[25]

Vitamin D inhibits monocyte/macrophage pro-inflammatory cytokine production, including TNF, IL-6, and IL-1α.[26,27] Vitamin D has direct effects on T cells, in particular inhibition of proliferation and cytokine production by T helper (Th)1 cells with associated promotion of Th2 differentiation.[28] $1,25(OH)_2D_3$ also reduces Th17 cell differentiation through its effects on DCs, and also has direct effects on Th17 cells that lead to inhibition of IL-17A, IL-21, IL-22, and IFN-γ production and enhancement of expression of FOXP3, cytotoxic T lymphocyte–associated antigen (CTLA)-4, and IL-10.[25,29] Importantly, the more abundant, weakly active form of vitamin D, $25(OH)D_3$, can be converted by DCs to potently active $1,25(OH)_2D_3$, with consequent alteration in T cell responses toward an anti-inflammatory phenotype, which is characterized by high CTLA-4 and reduced IL-17, IFN-γ, and IL-21 production.[30] Thus the level of free $25(OH)D_3$ available to DCs may have a pivotal role in determining the balance between T cell inflammatory and regulatory responses.[30]

$1,25(OH)_2D_3$ inhibits the proliferation of activated B cells, induces activated B cell apoptosis, and inhibits plasma cell differentiation and immunoglobulin secretion.[31] Thus vitamin D deficiency may have a role in the etiology of B cell–mediated autoimmune disorders, whereas vitamin D supplementation may have beneficial effects in B cell–mediated autoimmune diseases, such as SLE and RA.

The array of relevant effects of vitamin D on the immune system suggests that vitamin D status may be important with regard to the etiology and management of rheumatic diseases more generally.

Reactive Oxygen Species/Antioxidants

Production of reactive oxygen species (ROS), such as superoxide and hydrogen peroxide, are part of the normal immune response. Acting through transcription factors such as NF-κB, ROS increase production of pro-inflammatory eicosanoids and cytokines, including PGE_2, TNF, and IL-1β. Thus unchecked production of ROS may cause inflammation and tissue damage. Antioxidant enzymes such as superoxide dismutase and glutathione peroxidase remove superoxide, thereby providing protection from oxidative damage. Vitamin C (ascorbic acid), vitamin E (α-tocopherol), and β-carotene are acquired through the diet and can act as ROS scavengers.

Obesity

With excess energy intake and reduced energy expenditure, body weight and adiposity increase. Obesity (body mass index [BMI] >30 kg/m^2) is a significant health problem globally.

Adipose tissue was originally thought to be simply a fat store. However, it is now recognized that adipose tissue and adipocytes are metabolically active and contribute to systemic inflammatory responses (Fig. 72.2). Adipocytes release the pro-inflammatory cytokines TNF, IL-1β, and IL-6. IL-6 enters the systemic circulation and increases C-reactive protein (CRP) and serum amyloid A production by the liver.

Adipocytes produce adipokines: leptin, resistin, and visfatin (pro-inflammatory), and adiponectin (anti-inflammatory) (see Fig. 72.2). Although the primary function of leptin is appetite control, it also has a number of pro-inflammatory actions. Leptin increases the expression of adhesion molecules such as ICAM-1 and monocyte chemoattractant protein (MCP)-1, thereby favoring recruitment of monocytes/macrophages into adipose tissue. Leptin also increases IL-1β, TNF, and IL-6 production by monocytes/macrophages. Leptin increases proliferation of Th1 cells, and inhibits proliferation of Th2 cells and Treg cells. By contrast, adiponectin has anti-inflammatory effects, which include inhibition of TNF-induced adhesion molecule expression and inhibition of NF-κB, a pivotal intra-cellular factor in activation of inflammatory responses. Adiponectin also reduces production of TNF and IL-6 while promoting production of the anti-inflammatory cytokines IL-10 and IL-1RA. Adiponectin also increases the number

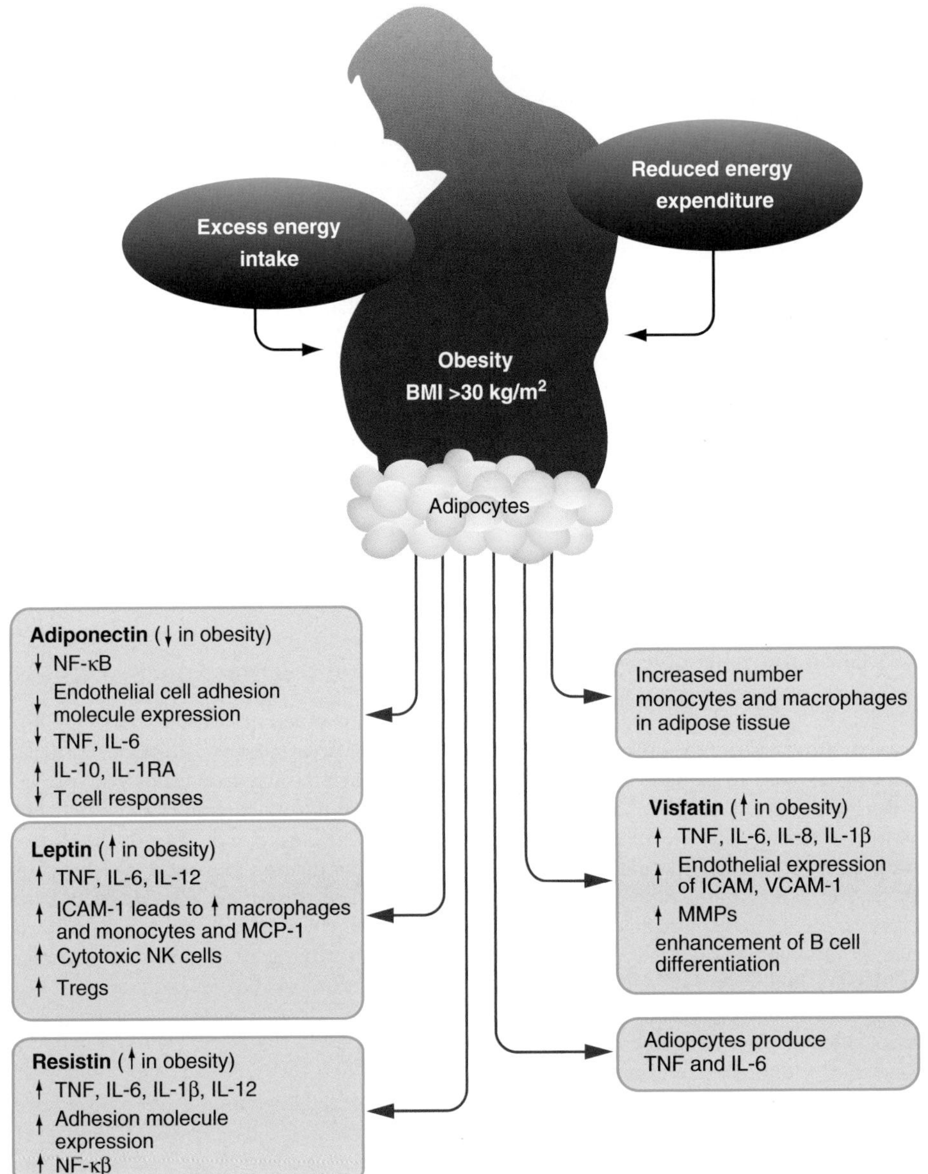

• **Fig. 72.2** Inflammatory mechanisms of obesity. *BMI,* Body mass index; *ICAM,* intercellular adhesion molecule; *MCP-1,* monocyte chemotactic protein-1; *MMPs,* matrix metalloproteinases; *NF-κB,* nuclear factor-κB; *NK,* natural killer; *Th,* T helper; *TNF,* tumor necrosis factor; *VCAM-1,* vascular cell adhesion molecule-1.

of Tregs. Production of adiponectin is inhibited by TNF, which thereby helps sustain the pro-inflammatory alteration of homeostasis found in obesity. Resistin is produced by mononuclear cells and adipocytes. Resistin increases macrophage/monocyte and adipocyte production of TNF, IL-6, and IL-1β, and also increases expression of the adhesion molecules ICAM-1, VCAM-1, and MCP-1.[32] Visfatin, which is produced by lymphocytes and adipocytes, has similar pro-inflammatory effects, including induction of IL-8, IL-6, IL-1β, and TNF; increased endothelial expression of ICAM-1, VCAM-1, and MMPs; and enhancement of B cell differentiation.[32] The net result of obesity is thus an inflammatory state associated with an increase in circulating CRP.

Gut and Oral Microbiome and Inflammation

The microbiome refers to the collective microorganisms in a particular environment. Humans along with other complex species harbor a very large number of symbiotic organisms within their microbiome. Microbiomes can be probed by genetic analysis of samples from sites of interest on or within human subjects. The gut microbiome is influenced by multiple factors including diet, oral probiotics, gut transit time, obesity, various disease states, antibiotic therapy, maturation, and aging.[33] The microbiome in turn can influence nutrition, the mucosal barrier, and immune functions and disease expression. The gut microbiome is a source of micronutrients and other metabolically active compounds, and contributes to digestion, including a pivotal role in the digestion of some complex polysaccharides. The term dysbiosis describes an unhealthy imbalance of microorganisms at mucosal surfaces or on the skin. Because of the multiplicity of specific organisms in the microbiome, findings suggesting changes in the relative abundance of specific organisms in various disease states seen in exploratory studies need to be confirmed by more focused independent investigations.

The increased abundance of *Prevotella copri* in stools of patients with recent (within 6 weeks to 6 months) onset of seropositive RA, who had not received disease-modifying anti-rheumatic drugs (DMARDs), biologics, steroids, or recent antibiotics, supports the notion that the presence of certain gut organisms or dysbiosis of gut microflora may contribute to RA pathogenesis.[34] In vitro and in vivo animal studies suggest *P. copri* may act through activation of autoreactive T cells in the intestine.[35] The antibiotic minocycline, which ameliorates early RA,[36] and the DMARD sulfasalazine, which has an antimicrobial sulfapyridine moiety, can be expected to affect gut microbiota. Alterations in gut microbiota have been reported with both methotrexate and etanercept,[37] and changes in the gut microbiota may contribute to the gastrointestinal toxicity of methotrexate.[38] Dysbiosis in the oral cavity and citrullination of peptides by gingival bacteria associated with periodontal disease is an explanation for an association between RA and periodontal disease.[39] The high success rates with gut re-colonization via fecal microbial transplantation (FMT) for persistent *Clostridium difficile* infections have led to exploration of this approach in other conditions, including inflammatory bowel disease.[33] The possible value of FMT in inflammatory rheumatic diseases is virtually unexplored beyond anecdotal experience.

Conclusion

Dietary components can have a variety of effects on the inflammatory process and on bone destructive pathways (Table 72.2). Thus alterations in diet may have effects on both the risk and management of rheumatic diseases, as is discussed later in this chapter.

TABLE 72.2 Effects of Dietary Components on Inflammatory and Bone Destructive Pathways

n-3 Fatty Acids
Decreased production of n-6–derived eicosanoids (PGE_2, TXA_2, LTB_4), which have pro-inflammatory effects
Increased production of n-3–derived eicosanoids (PGE_3, TXA_3, LTB_5), which in general are less pro-inflammatory
Decreased IL-1β and TNF production
Increased production of specialized proresolving lipid mediators (resolvins, protectins, maresins, lipoxins)
Decreased major histocompatibility complex II expression by antigen-presenting cells
Decreased adhesion molecule expression: ICAM, VCAM, LFA
Decreased expression of matrix metalloproteinases
Alteration in RANK/OPG ratio
Vitamin D
Inhibition of monocyte differentiation into DCs and promotion of DC apoptosis
Induction of tolerogenic Tregs with enhanced suppressive activity
Inhibition of monocyte/macrophage IL-1β and TNF production
Inhibition of Th1 cell proliferation and cytokine production
Enhancement of Th2 cytokine production
Reduction in Th17 cell differentiation and IL-17A production
Inhibition of proliferation of activated B cells, differentiation of activated B cells, and immunoglobulin secretion

DC, Dendritic cell; *ICAM*, intercellular adhesion molecule; *LFA*, leukocyte function-associated antigen; *LTB*, leukotriene B; *PGE*, prostaglandin E; *RANK/OPG*, receptor activator of nuclear factor-κB/osteoprotegerin; *Th*, T helper; *TNF*, tumor necrosis factor; *TXA*, thromboxane A; *VCAM*, vascular cell adhesion molecule.

Nutrition in the Etiology of Rheumatic Diseases

KEY POINTS

- Assessment of dietary intake is difficult, and identification of a single dietary factor that regulates disease might not be possible.
- Omega-3 fatty acids may protect against RA.
- The association between vitamin D and RA remains unclear.
- Obesity might affect disease activity and outcomes in RA.

Rheumatoid Arthritis

A number of epidemiologic studies have examined the role of nutrition in the etiology of RA. Assessment of dietary intake in epidemiologic studies is difficult, and to identify the effects of a single dietary variable and distinguish it from other nutritional and lifestyle factors may not be possible. However, long-term healthy eating patterns in women have been associated with a reduced risk of RA in those 55 years of age or younger, particularly for seropositive RA.[40] Notwithstanding, a number of nutritional factors are candidates for an influence on the development of RA.

Omega-3 Fatty Acid Consumption

The long-chain n-3 fats, EPA and DHA, are most abundant in fish and fish oils. Fish intake has a protective effect against RA. A population-based, case-controlled study reported a modest decrease in the risk of RA in subjects who consume oily fish one to seven times per week compared with those who seldom or never consumed fish (OR, 0.8; 95% CI, 0.6 to 1).[41] A subsequent long-term cohort study found that sustained consumption of fish was associated with reduced risk for RA (relative risk [RR], 0.48;95% CI, 0.33 to 0.71).[42] Interestingly, a recent nested case-control study reported a significant inverse association between risk for RA and erythrocyte n-6 linoleic acid levels but not other n-6 or n-3 fatty acids.[43]

Red Meat and Protein Consumption

High consumption of red meat has been associated with an increased risk of inflammatory polyarthritis (OR, 1.9; 95% CI, 0.9 to 4.0).[44] Although one study reported that meat and offal were associated with an increased risk for RA,[45] this was not confirmed in other studies.[46,47] Whether the association between red meat consumption and inflammatory arthritis is causative remains unclear, although the presence of significant amounts of AA in red meat may provide some explanation for the association.

Tea and Coffee Consumption

Tea and coffee have been identified as potential risk factors for RA. In the Finnish National Health Study, consumption of four or more cups of coffee per day was associated with an increased risk of rheumatoid factor (RF)-positive RA, but not RF-negative RA, after adjustment for potential confounders such as age, smoking, and sex (RR, 2.2; 95% CI, 1.13 to 4.27).[48] In comparison, both the Iowa Women's Health Study and the Women's Health Initiative Observational Study found no association between daily caffeine intake and risk for RA.[49,50]

Women who consumed four or more cups of decaffeinated coffee per day were at increased risk for RA compared with non–coffee drinkers (RR, 2.58; 95% CI, 1.63 to 4.06). Furthermore, women who consumed three or more cups of tea per day had a reduced risk of RA (RR, 0.39; 95% CI, 0.16 to 0.97).[49] More recent studies have not shown an association between tea/coffee and RA.[46,51] A recent meta-analysis stratified by seropositivity reported a positive association between coffee consumption and seropositive RA (RR, 1.34; 95% CI, 1.16 to 1.52) but not seronegative RA (RR, 1.09; 95% CI, 0.88 to 1.35). No association was found between tea consumption and RA.[52]

Although the epidemiologic evidence for an association between coffee/tea and RA is equivocal, interest has been sustained by the presence of metabolically active agents within these beverages. For example, the major catechin in tea inhibits induction of inducible nitric oxide synthase (iNOS) by stimulated macrophages.[53] iNOS generates highly reactive free radical products while di-imidating substrate arginine moieties to citrulline. Citrullinated peptides/proteins are recognized immunogens that provide a focus for autoimmunity in RA. Green tea extract increases chemokine receptor expression and reduces chemokine production in RA synovial fibroblasts.[54] Gallic acid, a natural polyphenolic acid found in tea, induces apoptosis of RA fibroblast-like synoviocytes (FLS) and reduces the expression of IL-1 and IL-6 genes in RA FLS.[55]

Alcohol Consumption

Alcohol consumption may reduce the risk for RA. In a case-control study of 515 patients with RA, alcohol consumption was associated with a reduced risk of anti-citrullinated protein antibody (ACPA)-positive RA.[56] A dose-dependent inverse relationship between alcohol consumption and risk of RA was also demonstrated in two independent case-control studies (the Swedish Epidemiologic Investigation of Rheumatoid Arthritis [EIRA] and the Danish case-control study of rheumatoid arthritis [CACORA] studies).[57] The reduction in risk of RA was more pronounced in patients with the shared epitope compared with those without the shared epitope and most pronounced in smokers with the shared epitope.[57] Data from the Nurses Health Studies I and II involving 1.90 million years of person-time from 1980 to 2008 reported a modest reduction in the risk of RA with long-term moderate alcohol use. The adjusted hazard ratio (HR) for alcohol use of 5 to 9.9 g/day was 0.78 (95% CI, 0.61 to 1.00), with a stronger association observed in those with seropositive disease (HR, 0.69; 95% CI, 0.50 to 0.95).[58]

With regard to candidate mechanisms for this putative reduction in risk for RA, alcohol downregulates the production of pro-inflammatory cytokines and upregulates production of the anti-inflammatory cytokine IL-10.[59,60] Furthermore, in a murine model of arthritis, ethanol almost totally prevented the development of collagen-induced arthritis, and in those mice that did develop arthritis, the disease was less severe. These anti-inflammatory effects of ethanol were associated with reduced leukocyte migration, downregulation of NF-κB, and reduced production of the pro-inflammatory cytokines IL-6 and TNF, but not the anti-inflammatory cytokine IL-10.[61]

Sugar-Sweetened Beverages

Sugar-sweetened beverage consumption has been associated with gout and other inflammatory diseases, including diabetes. In the Nurses' Health Study I and II, women who consume one or more sugar-sweetened beverage per day have an increased risk for seropositive RA (HR, 1.63; 95% CI, 1.15 to 2.30) compared with women who consume no or less than one serving per month. This effect remained significant after adjustment for BMI. No association between sugar-sweetened beverage consumption and seronegative RA was observed.[62] Sucrose consumption has been implicated in the development of periodontal infection, which has been linked to the development of RA. Soda drinks, which contain high-fructose corn syrup and sucrose, have been associated with higher CRP, IL-6, and TNF receptor-2 concentrations in patients at risk of cardiovascular disease (CVD).[63] However, the exact mechanisms linking sugar-sweetened beverages and RA remain to be determined.

Vitamin D

As noted earlier, vitamin D has anti-inflammatory actions. Although vitamin D has been implicated in reducing the risk of the autoimmune diseases, diabetes,[64] and multiple sclerosis, its association with the risk of RA is less clear.[65]

The Iowa Women's Health Study reported that a higher intake of vitamin D was associated with a reduced risk of RA (RR, 0.67; 95% CI, 0.44 to 1.00, $P = 0.05$) in women aged 55 to 69 years.[66] However, in a large study of 186,389 women followed up for 22 years, no association was found between dietary intake of vitamin D and the risk of developing RA.[67] Apart from supplements, the main source of vitamin D is de novo synthesis in the skin, thus estimated dietary intake may be a poor predictor of serum vitamin D concentrations. In a study of 79 patients with RA, no association was found between prior serum vitamin D concentrations and subsequent development of RA.[68] However, it is notable that the geometric means for both patients and controls in this study were only half the lower reference level of 60 nmol/L, which has been set subsequently to reflect a level that suppresses secondary hyperparathyroidism resulting from vitamin D insufficiency. A meta-analysis revealed a reduced risk of RA with higher vitamin D intake (RR of highest vs. lowest intake groups, 0.76; 95% CI, 0.58 to 0.94).[69] Randomized controlled trials of sufficient size and duration are required to determine whether the observed relationship between vitamin D and RA is causal and to establish the most effective dose, duration, and serum vitamin concentration to prevent RA.

Obesity and Rheumatoid Arthritis

Studies that examined the association between obesity and the risk of RA have had conflicting results, with findings of both increased risk of RA[70–72] and no association between the two.[73,74] A recent Danish cohort study reported the overall risk of RA was 10% higher for each 5% increment of total body fat (HR 1.10; 95% CI 1.02 to 1.18), 5% higher for each 5 cm increment of waist circumference (HR 1.05; 95% CI 1.01 to 1.10), and nearly 50% higher in those with an obese compared with normal BMI (HR 1.46; 95% CI 1.12 to 1.90) in women but not men.[75]

The association between obesity and a pro-inflammatory state provides a rational link between disease activity and severity in RA. Higher BMI has been associated with less radiographic damage.[76–79] Increased plasma concentrations of the adipokines, leptin, adiponectin, and visfatin have been observed in patients with RA compared with healthy controls.[80] Visfatin and leptin have been associated with increased and reduced radiographic joint damage, respectively,[79] although more recent data suggest that adipokines do not mediate the observed association between BMI and radiographic damage.[77] Although radiographic damage may be less in patients with higher BMI, other indicators of disease severity and comorbidities are adversely affected. For example, higher BMI (≥30 kg/m^2) has been associated with higher disease activity, Health Assessment Questionnaire (HAQ) scores, pain scores, and requirement for joint replacements.[81] Higher BMI is also associated with less chance of achieving disease remission or low disease activity.[81,82] Obese patients with RA are also at increased risk for important comorbidities, including hypertension, diabetes, and ischemic heart disease.[81,83] The cause of the apparent disconnect between obesity and disease severity and radiographic damage remains unclear, but one potential explanation is altered body composition in RA, which may create an inaccurate BMI measurement.

The body can be divided into fat mass and fat-free mass (consisting of body cell mass and connective tissue). Rheumatoid arthritis commonly leads to changes in body composition, with fat-free mass reported to be 13% to 14% lower in patients with RA.[84] This loss of fat-free mass is often associated with increased fat mass with unchanged body weight, a state known as *rheumatoid cachectic obesity*. Approximately one in five RA patients may have rheumatoid cachexia, as defined by fat-free mass index lower than the 25th percentile, and fat mass index higher than the 50th percentile of a reference population.[85] BMI, the commonly used measure of obesity, does not distinguish between fat mass and fat-free mass, thus individuals of similar height and weight, but different body composition, will have a similar BMI. Patients with RA have higher body fat and BMI than healthy controls. However, for a given mass of body fat, BMI was lower in patients with RA compared with healthy controls.[86] On the basis of this, the authors suggest that the categories of BMI should be adjusted downward in patients with RA.

Gout

KEY POINTS

The link between diet and gout has been recognized for centuries.
High intake of meat, seafood, and alcohol is associated with increased risk of gout.
Dietary fructose increases serum urate.
Higher intake of low-fat dairy products has been associated with a reduced risk of gout.
Increased BMI predisposes to gout.

For centuries gout has been associated with overindulgence in rich food and wine. Gout occurs when serum urate (SU) concentrations reach super saturation concentrations (~6.8 mg/dL at 37° C and physiologic pH), resulting in the formation of monosodium urate crystals, which deposit in joints and soft tissues. Urate is the end product in the breakdown of purines, which are a product of cellular turnover or are ingested in the diet. The purines adenosine and guanine are present in nucleic acids and the intra-cellular energy transporters adenosine triphosphate and guanosine triphosphate. Accordingly, foods derived from metabolically active animal tissues may increase dietary purine load.

Dietary Factors and Gout

Several large clinical studies have identified an association between high intake of meat and seafood (but not total protein intake) and both SU concentrations[87] and gout.[88] In comparison, the risk of gout is reduced with higher intake of low-fat dairy products and long-term coffee consumption.[88,89] The Dietary Approaches to Stop Hypertension (DASH) diet, which is based on high intake of fruits, vegetables, nuts, legumes, low fat dairy, and whole grains, and low intake of sodium, sweetened beverages, and red and processed meats, is associated with a lower risk of developing gout[90] and lowering serum urate in hyperuricemic individuals without gout.[91] Whether a similar urate lowering effect is seen in people with gout in response to the DASH diet remains to be determined. Fructose, which is found in corn syrup, sugar-sweetened soft drinks, and fruit juices, has also been associated with hyperuricemia and gout.[92,93] Fructose increases SU through increased purine degradation.[94] Furthermore, urate and fructose share a common transporter within the kidney *(SLC2A9)*.[95] Recent data show a gene environment interaction between fructose and the renal urate transporter SLC2A9,[96] and variations in *SLC2A9* influence the serum urate response to a fructose load.[97] In addition, allopurinol inhibits the increase in serum urate induced by a fructose load.[98] In rats, allopurinol reduces fructose-induced expression of the TXNIP inflammasome, which mediates dietary fructose–associated hepatic lipogenesis in rats.[99] Thus allopurinol appears to offset the adverse effects of fructose with regard to urate metabolism. Alcohol consumption other than moderate wine intake is associated with an increased risk of gout, with beer conferring a higher risk than liquor.[100]

Dietary vitamin C supplementation reduces the risk of gout (RR of gout with no supplementation vs. 1000 to 1499 mg vitamin C/day, 0.66 [95% CI, 0.49 to 0.88]).[101] Vitamin C (ascorbic acid) is an important vitamin that can only be obtained through dietary intake. Because ascorbic acid is water soluble, it is not stored within the body and thus must be regularly supplemented through the diet to maintain the ascorbic acid pool. Dietary sources of ascorbic acid include fresh fruits and vegetables, in particular citrus fruits and green leafy vegetables such as broccoli.

It is important to recognize that the influence of diet on serum urate is minimal compared with the influence of genes associated with serum urate transport.[102]

Fasting and Gout

Prolonged periods (2 weeks to 8 months) of fasting in obese patients result in a significant increase in SU and in some cases the development of gout.[103] In patients with previously documented gout, a 1-day fast led to an increase in SU of 0.5 to 2.1 mg/dL with a mean rise of 1.1 mg/dL, with refeeding associated with a return in SU to baseline levels after 24 hours.[104] In a smaller study of people with gout there was no increase in gout flares or serum urate during the 1-month Ramadan fast.[105] Explanations for the increase in SU during fasting include increased urate production, decreased excretion because of decreased glomerular filtration rate, altered renal tubular transport of uric acid, and competition with ketones for renal tubular excretion.[106]

Obesity and Gout

Obesity is associated with an increased risk of gout.[107] In a study comparing obese men (mean BMI, 34 ± 4 kg/m^2) with healthy controls (BMI, 21 ± 1 kg/m^2), SU concentrations were raised to a similar degree in the obese patients (~8.0 ± 1.6 mg/dL vs. controls, 5.2 ± 0.81 mg/dL), regardless of body fat distribution (predominantly visceral or predominantly subcutaneous). By contrast, 80% of patients with hyperuricemia and accumulation of fat subcutaneously had low 24-hour urinary urate excretion compared with 10% of their counterparts with fat accumulation predominantly in a visceral distribution. These data suggest that the mechanism of hyperuricemia may vary depending on body fat distribution.[108] In a separate study that used CT to determine transverse area of abdominal fat components, visceral fat correlated strongly with SU, whereas no relationship was seen between SU and BMI or cross-sectional area of subcutaneous fat.[109] However, a recent Mendelian randomization study reported that genetically higher BMI but not abdominal obesity was associated with an increased risk of gout.[110]

Osteoarthritis

KEY POINTS

Obesity is associated with knee osteoarthritis (OA).
Direct biomechanical effects of obesity contribute to OA.
Increased leptin provides another link between obesity and OA.

Associations have been established between obesity and onset and progression of knee OA. There is an almost exponential increase in the risk of knee OA while BMI increases.[111] The evidence for an association between obesity and OA of the hip or hand is less well defined, although a meta-analysis reported a twofold increase in the risk of hand OA in obese individuals compared with those of normal weight.[112] Body composition also appears to be important. In a longitudinal cohort study of 1653 people without radiographic knee OA at baseline, there was a significantly increased risk of knee OA in those who were obese, were obese and sarcopenic but not those who were sarcopenic only.[113]

In addition to direct biomechanical effects of obesity on the joint, there appears to be an important role for the adipokines, including leptin, adiponectin, resistin, visfatin, and chimerin.

Expression of leptin was increased in advanced OA cartilage compared with minimally damaged OA cartilage, with a correlation between the leptin mRNA expression in advanced OA cartilage and BMI. Furthermore, leptin reduced chondrocyte proliferation and increased IL-1β, MMP-9, and MMP-13 expression.[114]

High dietary total fat and saturated fatty acids intake has been associated with increased radiographic progression determined by joint space narrowing, while higher dietary intake of polyunsaturated fatty acids have been associated with reduced joint space narrowing in people with knee OA over a 2-year period.[115] Dietary antioxidants (vitamin E, vitamin C, and β-carotene) have been reported to reduce progression of knee OA but have no effect on the onset of OA.[116,117] The association between serum vitamin D concentrations and OA remains unclear. One study reports no association between vitamin D and risk of joint space narrowing or cartilage loss in knee OA,[118] but another study reports a positive association between knee cartilage volume and serum vitamin D concentrations.[119] A meta-analysis concluded that there was moderate evidence for an association between low levels of vitamin D and radiographic progression of knee OA and strong evidence for an inverse association between vitamin D and cartilage loss.[120]

Nutrition in the Management of Rheumatic Diseases

The role of nutrition in the management of gout is well accepted despite the lack of high quality evidence. However, its role in other rheumatic diseases such as RA is less routine. Despite a relative lack of interest or emphasis from physicians, many patients consider food may contribute to their arthritis and seek information about or try putative dietary remedies. A convincing, informed approach to nutritional advice is thus an important aspect of management, which can help patients avoid worthless interventions that are expensive, time consuming, in some cases harmful, and can divert patients from more effective measures (summarized in Fig. 72.3). Furthermore, positive advice regarding dietary choices may empower patients at a time when they often experience a sense of loss of control. Well-informed, authoritative dietary advice can also protect patients from poorly grounded advice from relatives, friends, and nonauthoritative Internet sites about dietary measures.

Rheumatoid Arthritis

KEY POINTS

Omega-3 fatty acids increase remission rates with treat-to-target DMARD therapy and reduce NSAID requirements.
There is no evidence for the benefit of antioxidants in the management of RA.
Fasting, vegetarian/vegan, and elimination diets are difficult to sustain, and it is difficult to predict which patients may respond.
The vascular benefits of omega-3 fatty acids are important in RA patients because they have an increased risk of cardiovascular disease.
Some dietary variables may interact with methotrexate.

Dietary n-3 Fatty Acids in the Management of Rheumatoid Arthritis

Fish oil is a rich source of the anti-inflammatory long-chain n-3 fatty acids EPA and DHA. The threshold dose of EPA and DHA usually required to obtain an anti-inflammatory effect is 2.7 g/day of EPA plus DHA, which is the equivalent of nine or more standard 1 g fish oil capsules or 10 mL of bottled fish oil per day. This dose is generally more than that with which patients will self-prescribe, although community awareness of required doses varies. Tissue levels of EPA and DHA from fish and fish oils are increased when dietary n-6 fatty acid intake is reduced concomitantly through substitution of n-6 rich visible fats (e.g., with a base of corn oil, soy oil, sunflower oil) with unsaturated products with less n-6 fat (with a base of olive oil, rapeseed/canola oil, or flaxseed oil).[121]

Krill oil has been promoted as an alternative source of EPA and DHA, although evidence for efficacy of krill oil in RA is lacking. While krill oil has less EPA plus DHA than standard fish oil on a weight for weight basis (approximately 25% for krill oil vs. 30% for fish oil),[122] the EPA and DHA are present within phospholipids and as free fatty acids in krill oil and within triglycerides in fish oil.[123,124] EPA and DHA are moderately better absorbed from krill oil such that equal gravimetric doses of krill oil and fish oil supplements achieve similar blood levels of omega-3 fatty acids.[122–124] Krill oil contains astaxanthin, which gives it a reddish color and has antioxidant properties. As discussed elsewhere in this chapter, there is no evidence for important anti-arthritic or anti-inflammatory effects of antioxidants. There have been no studies into the effect of astaxanthin in RA. Because krill oil is substantially more expensive than fish oil and, in contrast to fish oil, has not been subjected to systematic study of anti-inflammatory effects, krill oil is not a suitable substitute for fish oil.

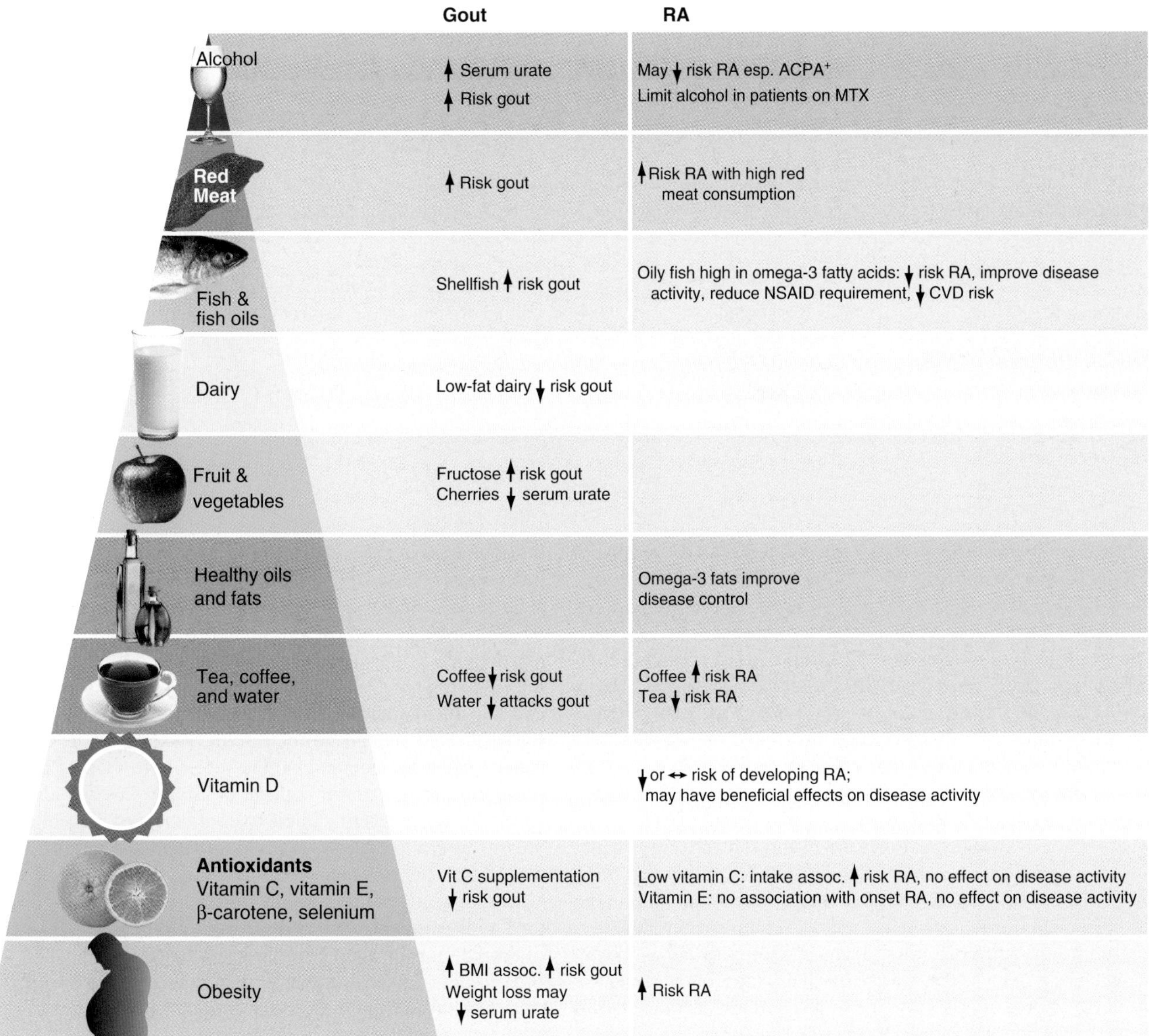

• **Fig. 72.3** Summary of nutrition in rheumatic diseases. *ACPA,* Anti-citrullinated protein antibody; *BMI,* body mass index; *CVD,* cardiovascular disease; *MTX,* methotrexate; *NSAID,* nonsteroidal anti-inflammatory drug; *RA,* rheumatoid arthritis; *Vit,* vitamin.

In general, patients with recent-onset or more established RA can be expected to achieve better disease control when anti-inflammatory doses of fish oil are co-administered with appropriately intensive combination DMARD therapy. In a longitudinal cohort study of patients with recent-onset RA (<12 months' duration), response-driven, intensive combination DMARD therapy was combined with either supplemental fish oil or placebo. At 3 years, those patients compliant with fish oil therapy had improved self-reported function in activities of daily living, lower tender joint counts, lower erythrocyte sedimentation rate (ESR), higher remission rates (72% vs. 31%), and less NSAID use than those who did not consume fish oil.[125] This study demonstrates the feasibility of long-term fish oil use, and the better outcome for patients taking fish oil is consistent with randomized controlled trial data that show reduced symptoms with fish oil compared with placebo treatment.[126] A more recent study compared high-dose fish oil with low-dose fish oil, 5.5 or 0.4 g/day, respectively, of the omega-3 fats, EPA + DHA, in DMARD naïve patients with early RA. Fish oil was used in combination with a treat-to-target predetermined intensive combination DMARD protocol. During 12 months of treatment, patients receiving high-dose fish oil were more likely to achieve American College of Rheumatology remission (HR, 2.17; 95% CI, 1.07 to 4.42; $P = 0.03$), and triple therapy with methotrexate, sulfasalazine, and hydroxychloroquine (HR, 0.28; 95% CI, 0.12 to 0.63; $P = 0.002$) was less likely to fail.[127] In this study, plasma phospholipid EPA concentrations were related to time to remission with a one-unit increase in EPA associated with a 12% increase in probability of remission during the study period even after adjustment for smoking, presence of CCP antibodies, and HLA-DR allele status (HR 1.12 (95%CI 1.02 to 1.23). Plasma phospholipid EPA levels were also negatively related to time to DMARD failure.[128] Plasma phosphatidylcholine EPA concentration and the EPA/AA ratio have been reported to be inversely correlated with change in DAS28 3 months after starting anti-TNF therapy.[129]

Dietary intake of fish has also been associated with lower disease activity in people with RA, with those participants who consumed fish 2 or more times/week having a lower DAS-28 compared with those who never or only consumed fish less than 1 time/month.[130]

TABLE 72.3 Comparison Between Nonsteroidal Anti-inflammatory Drugs and Anti-inflammatory Doses of Fish Oil

	NSAIDs	Fish Oil
COX inhibition	COX-1/COX-2 selectivity varies depending on agents	Nonselective
NSAID sparing	No	Yes (↓ prostaglandin E_2)
Serious cardiovascular events	Increased risk for MI	Could be reduced (no effect or benefit in cardiovascular studies at lower doses)
Blood pressure	Increased	Reduced
TNF and IL-1β	Increased	Reduced
Upper gastrointestinal bleeding	Increased	Not reported
Time to effect	Rapid	Delayed (≤3 months)

COX, Cyclooxygenase; *MI,* myocardial infarction; *NSAID,* nonsteroidal anti-inflammatory drug; *TNF,* tumor necrosis factor.

Anti-inflammatory doses of fish oil reduce NSAID requirements in patients with RA.[131,132] NSAIDs alter the balance of PGE_2/TXA_2 in favor of TXA_2, thereby increasing the production of IL-1β and TNF by monocytes.[133] By contrast, fish oil reduces the production of these cytokines.[14] Fish oil also lacks many of the adverse effects associated with NSAIDs (Table 72.3). The direct effects of fish oil and their influence on NSAID use may potentially reduce long-term tissue damage associated with release of these cytokines, although this remains to be established.

Important for both patients and physicians to recognize is that, as with most standard DMARDs, there is a latent period of as long as 15 weeks before the symptomatic benefits of anti-inflammatory doses of fish oil are experienced. One small pilot study has shown that this latent period can be reduced with intravenous administration of n-3 fats.[134] Although the inconvenience and cost of intravenous therapy is a barrier to this approach, the benefits of short-term intravenous therapy can be prolonged by a switch to oral n-3 supplementation.[135]

Adverse Effects of Fish Oils. The most common adverse effects associated with fish oil in anti-inflammatory doses are a fishy aftertaste, gastrointestinal upset, and nausea. These side effects are clearly neither organ nor life threatening, but they can be dose limiting. Patient preferences vary, but in general, bottled fish oil layered on juice is the most efficient way to take an anti-inflammatory dose (one quick swallow compared with 10 to 15 standard fish oil capsules). Fish oil is best tolerated with food and not on an empty stomach. In general, fish oil is best tolerated when taken just before the evening meal or other main meal of the day. The term *fish oil* defines oil prepared from fish bodies to provide a distinction from cod liver oil, which is prepared from fish livers and is rich in the fat-soluble vitamins A and D. Standard fish oil contains more EPA plus DHA (30% w/w) than cod liver oil (EPA plus DHA ~20%) and is the preferred material. Vitamin D can be given separately as needed, and vitamin A supplementation is best avoided because negative effects on bone mineral density and fracture risk have been reported.[136]

Although anti-inflammatory doses of fish oil have not been associated with serious toxicity, concerns may be raised. One consideration is a putative bleeding tendency associated with therapeutic fish oil ingestion. This notion has its origins in studies of Greenland Eskimos consuming their aboriginal diet, in whom myocardial infarction is rare and bleeding times were prolonged relative to those observed in Danes.[137] However, these concerns need to be placed within the context of the high amounts of EPA and DHA in the aboriginal Eskimo diet (more than double the threshold anti-inflammatory dose) and the lower amounts of antagonistic n-6 fatty acids compared with Western diets. Although bleeding episodes have not been a feature of long-term fish oil therapy for RA,[125] and platelet EPA is fourfold lower than found in the Eskimos, surgeons may ask that fish oil be discontinued before elective surgery. Also, pharmacists may advise patients to discontinue fish oil while taking warfarin, even though no increase in bleeding tendency has been seen in patients undergoing cardiac surgery when taking fish oil concomitantly with warfarin, aspirin, or aspirin plus clopidogrel therapy.[138,139] More recent clinical trials also suggest that higher doses of fish oil can be taken for prolonged periods without increased bleeding events or other serious adverse effects.[127,140] There is no evidence to suggest that combinations of fish oil and oral direct Factor Xa inhibitors would be problematic, although evidence that the combination is proven to be safe is also lacking.

Another concern is the possible presence of the environmental contaminants methylmercury, polychlorinated biphenyls (PCBs), and dioxins, which are concentrated in large carnivorous fish. These toxins are excluded from properly prepared fish oil for therapeutic use. The U.S. Food and Drug Administration has accorded "generally regarded as safe" status to intakes of as much as 3 g/day of long-chain n-3 fatty acids from marine sources.

Role of Omega-3 Supplementation in Rheumatic Diseases With Increased Cardiovascular Disease Risk. A number of rheumatic diseases, including RA, SLE, gout, and psoriatic arthritis, are associated with increased cardiovascular mortality. n-3 Fatty acids have the potential to alter cardiovascular risk through multiple mechanisms, including stabilization of the myocardium, leading to reduction in cardiac arrhythmias, reduced blood pressure, stabilization of atheromatous plaques, reduced triglycerides and increased high-density lipoprotein (HDL), decreased platelet thromboxane release, increased vascular prostacyclin release, and anti-inflammatory effects (Fig. 72.4). However, a recent Cochrane review that included 79 RCTs (112,059 participants) concluded there was little or no effect of increasing omega-3 fatty acids on all-cause mortality (RR 0.98, 95% CI 0.90 to 1.03), cardiovascular mortality (RR 0.95, 95% CI 0.87 to 1.03), and cardiovascular events (RR 0.99, 95% CI 0.94 to 1.04).[141]

To date there have been no specific studies of the cardiovascular benefits of n-3 fatty acid supplementation in patients with RA or other rheumatic diseases. However, patients with early RA

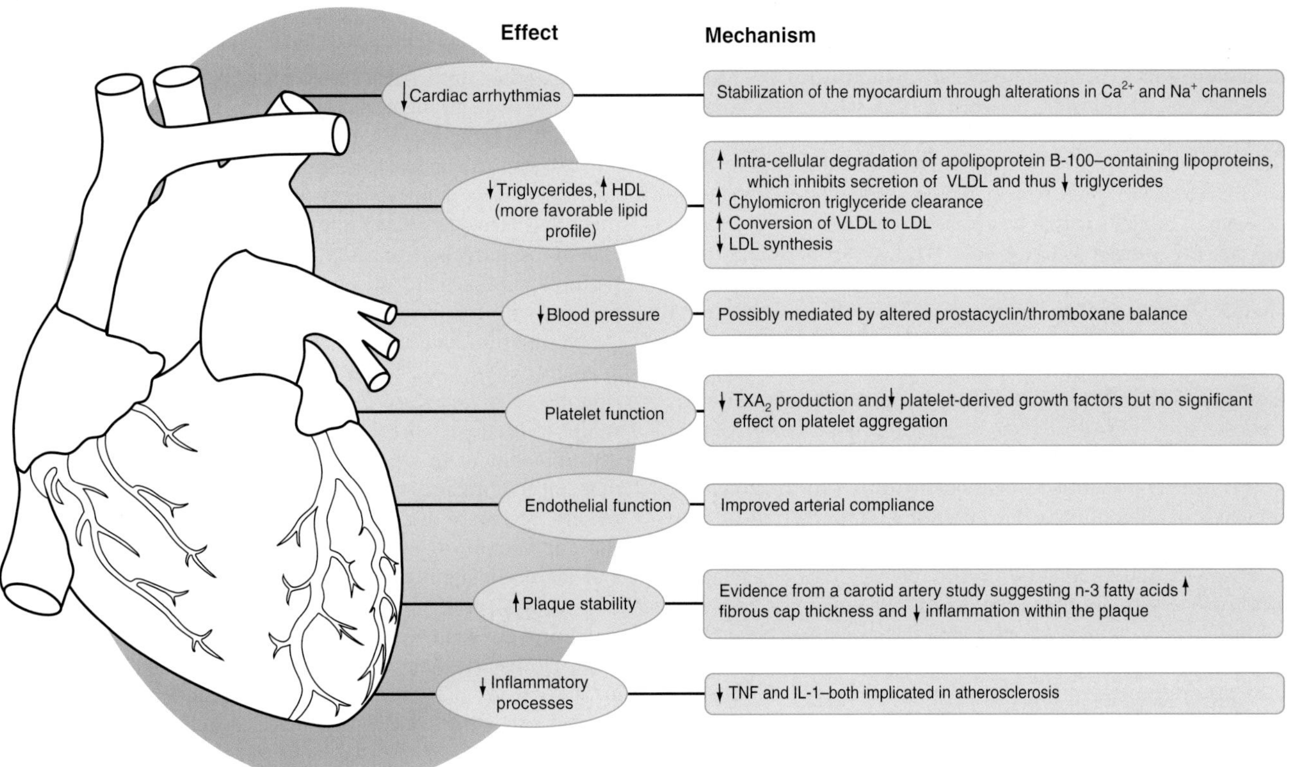

• **Fig. 72.4** Effects of omega-3 fatty acids on the cardiovascular system. *HDL,* High-density lipoprotein; *LDL,* low-density lipoprotein; *TNF,* tumor necrosis factor; *TXA_2,* thromboxane A_2; *VLDL,* very-low-density lipoprotein.

receiving fish oil have lower triglycerides, increased "good" HDL cholesterol, less NSAID use, greater disease suppression, and reduced platelet synthesis of TXA_2, all of which can be expected to reduce cardiovascular risk.[125] The blood levels of patients taking EPA plus DHA achieved with anti-inflammatory doses of fish oil[125] are above the threshold associated with reduced risk for sudden cardiac death.[142]

Antioxidants in the Management of Rheumatoid Arthritis

Despite the association between ROS and RA, a meta-analysis shows no convincing evidence that antioxidant supplementation improves disease control in patients with RA.[143]

Dietary Omega-3 Fatty Acids as a Potential Preventive for Rheumatoid Arthritis

In a nested case-control study, subjects without RA but with either the RA susceptibility defining HLA-DR shared epitope or a family history of RA or both were studied. In the subjects with the shared epitope, the presence of either anti-citrullinated protein antibodies (ACPAs) or rheumatoid factor was associated inversely with erythrocyte EPA and DHA or self-reported ingestion of a dietary n-3 fatty acid supplement. Erythrocyte EPA and DHA were higher in those taking fish oil supplements.[144,145] The presence of ACPAs or rheumatoid factor provides evidence of the pre-clinical phase of RA, which may last several years before RA manifests clinically.[146,147] In a study of volunteer subjects with no history of RA, participants testing positive for ACPAs were further evaluated. The proportion found to have prevalent inflammatory arthritis was related inversely to erythrocyte EPA, DHA, and omega-3 docosapentaenoic acid (DPA). Subsequent development of inflammatory arthritis was inversely related to DPA with similar directional trends for EPA and DHA.[148] In light of the above findings and the generally regarded as safe (GRAS) status of fish oil, fish oil supplements can be considered as a potential preventive for RA for those at risk. Thus while randomized controlled trials are needed to more firmly establish fish oil supplements as a preventive for RA, they can be recommended as a safe measure with potential benefit to patients and their relatives who are concerned regarding their risk for RA.

Vitamin E. Serum concentrations of vitamin E are similar in patients with RA and healthy controls.[149] In rats with CIA fed 200 mg/kg of vitamin E for 4 weeks, a significant reduction in leptin, TNF, and IL-6 concentrations was seen compared with control-fed mice.[150] A 12-week placebo-controlled study of vitamin E supplementation in patients with RA showed a reduction in pain scores but no effect on joint tenderness score, duration of morning stiffness, swollen joint count, or laboratory parameters.[151]

Vitamin C. Although animal models have shown benefits with vitamin C supplementation, human studies have not shown any clinical benefit in patients with RA.[152]

Selenium. Although not an antioxidant per se, selenium is found at the active site of the enzyme glutathione peroxidase, an important antioxidant enzyme. Plasma concentrations of selenium are reduced in patients with RA compared with healthy controls,[153] and an inverse association between serum selenium concentrations and active joints has been reported.[154] Notwithstanding, studies of selenium supplementation have not shown clinical benefit in patients with RA, despite increases in serum and red blood cell selenium concentrations.[155,156] However, polymorphonuclear cell selenium concentrations do not increase with dietary supplementation, which may explain the lack of clinical effect.[157]

Vitamin D and the Management of Rheumatoid Arthritis

Animal models have shown that 1,25(OH)$_2$D can prevent and have therapeutic benefits in experimental arthritis.[158] Studies examining the relationship between serum vitamin D concentrations and disease activity in RA have been conflicting: Both an inverse relationship[159,160] and no relationship[161] have been observed. However, increases in patient global visual analogue scores seen in patients with lower serum vitamin D may confound results of the disease activity scale (DAS)28.[162] Interestingly, using data from the Swedish EIRA study, higher dietary intake of vitamin D was associated with a good EULAR response after 3 months of DMARD therapy (OR 1.8; 95% CI 1.14 to 2.83).[162a]

In humans, the vitamin D receptor expresses at sites of cartilage erosion and in chondrocytes and synoviocytes in patients with RA but not healthy control subjects, suggesting that vitamin D may have local effects within the inflamed joint.[163] Supplemental vitamin D is usually prescribed to patients with RA for treatment or prophylaxis of osteoporosis. However, a 12-month trial of vitamin D (calciferol) 100,000 IU/day showed improvement in RA disease activity and a reduction in the requirement for analgesics and NSAIDs.[164] In another small study of 19 patients with RA, oral α-calcitriol 2 μg/day was observed to have a beneficial effect on disease activity compared with placebo.[165] Neither significant side effects nor increases in serum calcium were reported in either of these studies. Vitamin D induced TNF production, suggesting that it may alter responses to TNF inhibitor therapy in RA. A recent study showed that 1,25(OH)$_2$D$_3$, but not TNF blockade, suppressed IL-17A and IL-22 production in co-cultures of Th17 cells and RA synovial fibroblasts from patients with early RA. Furthermore, the combination of 1,25(OH)$_2$D$_3$ and TNF blockade resulted in a significant additive effect with reductions in IL-6, IL-8, MMP-1, and MMP-3.[166] These data suggest there may be a rationale for patients receiving TNF inhibitor therapy to receive supplemental vitamin D.

It is important to recognize that cod liver oil, a rich source of dietary n-3 fatty acids, is also rich in vitamin D. Cod liver oil has been used in the management of RA in sufficient doses to deliver anti-inflammatory doses of long-chain n-3 fatty acids.[167] Although serum vitamin D concentrations rose significantly, the study did not allow for the respective contributions of vitamin D and co-ingested n-3 fatty acids to be evaluated. The relatively high content of vitamin A in cod liver oil militates against its use for delivering anti-inflammatory doses of n-3 fatty acids.

Dietary Restriction in Rheumatoid Arthritis—Fasting, Vegetarian, and Elimination Diets

A number of studies have examined elimination of different nutrients from the diet in the management of RA. At the extreme, total fasting and subtotal fasting reduced clinical and laboratory parameters of disease activity in some patients within a few days, but deterioration occurred on reintroduction of food.[168] Thus fasting is an impractical management strategy because it should last no longer than 7 days and the positive effects are short-lived, whereas RA is a chronic disease. A number of potential mechanisms for this improvement have been postulated, including a psychological or placebo effect, weight loss, and immunosuppression as a result of reduced caloric intake, alteration in fatty acids and IL-6 concentrations, and alterations in gut flora.

Elemental diets are used with the aim of providing major food groups as simpler components (e.g., protein as free amino acids, fat as medium-chain triglycerides, carbohydrates as small sugars). Minimal general benefit was seen in only a minority of patients, with a lack of benefit observed in objective parameters such as inflammatory markers and swollen and tender joint counts.[169,170]

Vegetarian and vegan diets have also been studied in RA. Response to these diets has been variable, with poor patient compliance and high dropout rates resulting from both lack of efficacy and adverse effects (mainly nausea and vomiting).[171,172] A meta-analysis of four clinical trials of fasting, followed by vegetarian diets that lasted at least 3 months, showed that clinically significant long-term benefits in RA can occur.[173] However, the diet required is strict, and no means currently exist to predict which patients will respond.

Elimination diets involve avoidance of foods that are putatively allergenic. Foods are deemed to be "allergenic" if their elimination results in decreased disease activity and subsequent ingestion results in increased disease activity. Although such diets may result in improvement in a proportion of patients, variable responsiveness and compliance can be a significant limitation.[174,175] A systematic review of dietary studies in patients with RA highlighted the uncertainty of response, high risk of bias in existing studies, and the not insignificant risk of adverse effects.[176] Notwithstanding, from a practical perspective, if a patient believes his or her arthritis is caused by hypersensitivity to a particular food item or group, it may be worth assessing the effects of dietary avoidance in an $n = 1$ study of sequential withdrawal and challenge. Objective clinical and laboratory signs of disease activity should be documented after one or more cycles of withdrawal and reintroduction of the suspected food item. The findings can then be used as a basis to decide whether the food item should be avoided by the individual in the longer term.

Interactions Among Diet, Obesity, and Disease-Modifying Anti-rheumatic Drugs

It is well recognized that certain dietary components may interact with DMARDs. Methotrexate remains the anchor drug in the management of RA and is also used commonly in many other rheumatic diseases. Alcohol may increase the risk of hepatotoxicity in patients receiving methotrexate, and alcohol intake should be limited and quantification of a "safe" intake is debated.[177,178] Methotrexate has multiple potential actions, many of which can be traced to its action as a dihydrofolate reductase inhibitor. Routine supplementation with folic acid is recommended to reduce potential adverse effects associated with methotrexate.[179] However, higher red blood cell folate concentrations have been associated with higher disease activity in patients with RA receiving methotrexate.[180] In some countries fortification of flour, pasta, rice, and bread with folic acid is a governmental requirement. Not surprisingly, such dietary fortification may lead to increased methotrexate doses in some patients.[181] However, studies of high and low doses of folic acid supplementation have shown no significant effects on disease activity in people with RA.[182,183]

Methotrexate treatment increases extra-cellular accumulation of adenosine, which has multiple anti-inflammatory effects on neutrophils and macrophages, including inhibition of IL-1β and TNF synthesis. Caffeine is a methylxanthine and acts as an adenosine receptor antagonist. Caffeine may therefore interfere with the effects of methotrexate. In rats with adjuvant arthritis, caffeine reverses the anti-inflammatory effects of methotrexate.[184] In patients with RA, less intense caffeine intakes have no effect on methotrexate efficacy.[185] In patients treated with methotrexate 7.5 mg per week, without folate, responses were reduced in those consuming caffeine in doses greater than 180 mg/day compared with doses less than 120 mg/day.[186]

Obesity may also have an impact on response to therapy. Data from the British Biologics Register revealed an increased risk of bDMARD refractory disease in those with a BMI ≥ 30 kg/m^2 (multivariate HR 1.2 (95% CI 1.0 to 1.4).[187] In comparison, a recent meta-analysis revealed no effect of obesity on response to abatacept or tocilizumab.[188]

Gout

KEY POINTS

Dietary interventions in gout should address the association between gout and the metabolic syndrome and increased cardiovascular disease.
Dehydration is a trigger for acute gout.
Weight loss may reduce serum urate.

Sustained reduction of SU to less than 6 mg/dL, or less than 5 mg/dL if tophi are present, is critical for the effective management of gout. This is generally achieved through use of urate-lowering therapy. Dietary intervention on its own is insufficient to achieve target serum urate concentrations. Furthermore, in a small study, even when people with gout received comprehensive education about diet, which led to an increase in knowledge, there was no effect on serum urate.[189] When considering dietary interventions in the management of gout, it is important to recognize that gout is associated with the metabolic syndrome and with an increased risk of cardiovascular disease and mortality. It is important to note that there are no randomized controlled trials to support dietary and lifestyle interventions in gout.

The diet usually advocated for gout entails restricted intake of foods and drinks that contain higher amounts of purines or that are thought to precipitate acute attacks of gout. Restricted items include meat, seafood, beer/wine, and legumes. Such diets are frequently high in saturated fats and carbohydrates, which may add to the risk of metabolic syndrome. A more recent study has revealed a minor contribution of diet to serum urate levels compared with the influence of genetics.[102] Given the stigma surrounding gout, it is important for healthcare providers to educate people with gout about the role of (or lack of role) of diet in the etiology of gout. It remains sensible to advise patients to avoid foods that trigger gout flares until serum urate is at target.

Dehydration is a potential trigger for acute gout attacks, and increased water intake has been associated with a reduced risk of gouty attacks.[190]

A number of dietary supplements have been suggested for the management of gout, although a recent Cochrane review concluded that there is a lack of high quality evidence.[191]

In a small short-term study in healthy volunteers, ingestion of cherries reduced serum urate (before urate, 3.6 ± 0.2 mg/dL vs. after urate, 3.1 ± 0.25 mg/dL; $P < 0.05$) and increased urinary urate excretion.[192] A 2012 study suggested that cherries may prevent gout flares. In a study of 633 individuals, cherry intake during a 2-day period was associated with a 35% lower risk of gout attacks compared with no cherry intake (OR, 0.65; 95% CI, 0.5 to 0.85). A similar association was observed with cherry extract. Furthermore, when cherry intake was combined with allopurinol treatment, the risk of gout was 75% lower than during periods without either (OR, 0.25; 95% CI, 0.15 to 0.42).[193] In another small retrospective study of 24 patients with crystal proven gout consuming one tablespoon of tart cherry juice for greater than or equal to 4 months, there was a significant reduction in gout flares from 6.85 ± 1.34 flares/year to 2.0 ± 0.6 flares/year ($P = 0.0086$).[194] The exact mechanism of action of cherries in reducing gout flares remains unclear and is likely multifactorial. Cherry products contain high levels of anthocyanins, which have a number of anti-inflammatory and antioxidant effects, including inhibition of cyclooxygenase and scavenging of nitric oxide radicals.[195–197] Cherry juice also inhibits production of IL-1β by human monocytes ex vivo by approximately 60%.[194]

Vitamin C supplementation may reduce SU concentrations.[198,199] In a study of 184 patients without gout randomly assigned to receive placebo or vitamin C 500 mg/day for 2 months, SU was reduced significantly in the vitamin C group, with a mean reduction of −0.5 mg/dL (95% CI, −0.5 to 0.02 mg/dL) compared with the placebo group ($P < 0.0001$).[200] In the subgroup of 21 patients with baseline SU greater than 7 mg/dL, the mean reduction in serum urate was 1.3 mg/dL. However, in a small study of patients with gout, vitamin C, 500 mg/day for 8 weeks had no clinically significant urate-lowering effect alone or in combination with allopurinol.[201] Whether a larger dose of vitamin C has a more potent urate-lowering effect in patients with gout remains to be determined. In a study of 120 people with gout having recurrent flares, lactose powder control, skim milk powder (SMP) control, and SMP enriched with glycomacropeptide (GMP) and milk fat extract (G600), the frequency of gout flares was reduced in all groups over the 3-month study period compared with baseline. There was a significantly greater reduction in gout flares in the SMP/GMP/G600 group.[202]

Obesity is common in people with gout, and increased abdominal circumference is associated with failure to reach target serum urate in people receiving urate-lowering therapy.[203] Weight loss is recommended in overweight people with gout. A recent meta-analysis that included 10 studies of weight loss in people with gout reported mean weight loss of 3 to 4 kg. The effect on serum urate ranged from −168 to +30 μmol/L, with 0% to 60% of participants achieving target serum urate of less than 360 μmol/L.[204]

Given the effects of n-3 fatty acids on the inflammasome, they may be useful in the management of acute gout or, potentially, as prophylaxis against acute gout in conjunction with urate-lowering therapy. One cross-sectional study reported a nonsignificant trend for a negative association between n-3 fatty acid levels and more than two self-reported gout flares in the previous 12 months (OR 0.68; 95% CI 0.46 to 1.02), which became significant after adjustment for age, BMI, SU, presence of tophi, and use of urate-lowering therapy (OR 0.62; 95% CI 0.38 to 0.98).[205] Further clinical studies of the effects of n-3 fatty acid supplementation on serum urate and gout flares are required. Gout is often associated with hypertriglyceridemia, upon which anti-inflammatory doses of fish oil can be expected to have an ameliorating effect.[125,206]

Osteoarthritis

KEY POINTS

Weight loss is important in the management of OA.
From a mechanistic viewpoint, n-3 fatty acids may be beneficial and can be an alternative or adjunct to NSAIDs for long-term analgesia.

Weight loss is generally considered an important aspect of the management of OA of weight-bearing joints. A meta-analysis of weight loss studies in patients with knee OA reported that moderate weight loss (≥5%) is associated with statistically significant improvement in self-reported disability scores. Although knee pain was also reduced, this did not reach statistical significance.[207] Intensive weight loss has an anti-inflammatory effect, evidenced by a reduction in IL-6, as well as beneficial biomechanical effects in obese people with knee OA.[208] Furthermore, exercise in combination with diet-induced weight loss can help maintain weight loss and is associated with greater improvements in symptoms than either diet or exercise alone.[208] A dose–response relationship between weight loss and clinical outcomes including pain, function, health-related quality of life, and 6-minute walk distance has also been reported.[209]

Degradation and loss of articular cartilage and synovial inflammation are all characteristic features of OA. MMPs have an important role in cartilage degradation, and n-3 fatty acids reduce IL-1α–induced expression of MMP-3 and MMP-13 in bovine chondrocyte cultures.[12] The anti-inflammatory effects of n-3 fatty acids, as compared with n-6 fatty acids discussed previously, may reduce synovial inflammation.

A high-fat diet rich in n-3 fatty acids mitigates the effects of obesity on injury-induced OA in mice and accelerates wound repair. By contrast, a high-fat diet rich in n-6 fatty acids was found to increase the severity of the OA.[210] OA-prone guinea pigs fed on a n-3 fatty acid–rich diet had amelioration of OA of a severity similar to that observed in an OA-resistant guinea pig strain.[211] An inverse relationship between plasma total n-3 fatty acids and DHA and patellofemoral cartilage loss, but not tibiofemoral cartilage loss or synovitis, has been reported in patients with or at risk of knee OA.[212] Taken together, these studies suggest that n-3 fatty acid supplementation may be beneficial in reducing/preventing structural progression in OA.

To date there are limited human data on the role of n-3 fatty acid supplementation in OA. A 2-year study of high- versus low-dose fish oil used to treat OA revealed clinically significant improvements in pain and disability scores in both groups, with similar improvement at 12 months and greater improvement at 24 months in those receiving low-dose fish oil.[213] A systematic review and meta-analysis of five clinical trials of n-3 fatty acid supplements in OA, which did not include this trial,[213] reported no significant effect on pain.[214]

On the basis of epidemiologic studies, as well as the role of vitamin D in bone health, clinical trials examining the role of vitamin D supplementation in osteoarthritis have been undertaken. In patients with symptomatic knee OA, no difference was found between placebo and oral vitamin D treatment, at doses sufficient to elevate 25-hydroxyvitamin D plasma to higher than 36 ng/mL for 2 years, with regard to knee pain or MRI-assessed loss of cartilage volume.[215] Similarly, in another RCT with 413 people with knee OA and low baseline vitamin D (12.5 to 60 nmol/L) oral vitamin D_3 resulted in no significant change in MRI-determined tibial cartilage volume or knee pain scores.[216] A post-hoc analysis grouped participants based on 25(OH)D levels at 3 and 24 months as consistently insufficient (≤50 nmol/L at both time-points), fluctuating, and consistently sufficient (>50 nmol/L at both time-points). Those who were consistently sufficient had less tibial cartilage volume loss and less loss of physical function compared with those consistently insufficient.[217] There is currently insufficient evidence to support routine use of vitamin D in OA,[218] although ensuring vitamin D levels are greater than 50 nmol/L may be appropriate.

Conclusion

Rheumatic diseases are typically chronic, and, as with any chronic disease, nutritional issues are intrinsic to optimization of long-term health. Although patients as individuals can make their own nutritional choices, it is desirable for rheumatologists to be adequately informed regarding the plausibility and evidence for frequently considered nutritional supplements, toward which this chapter has been directed. In terms of positive advice for patients and referring physicians, the strongest case can be made for dietary supplementation with fish oil in adequate doses for inflammatory arthritis. For long-term analgesia in rheumatic diseases, fish oil can be recommended in favor of NSAIDs. To the extent that fish oil is taken instead of NSAIDs, the risks for serious upper gastrointestinal complications and increased risk for serious thrombotic cardiovascular events associated with NSAIDs can be avoided because fish oil has not been associated with these risks. Furthermore, fish oil reduces cardiovascular risk factors through mechanisms independent of and additional to its NSAID-sparing effects.

Full references for this chapter can be found on ExpertConsult.com.

Selected References

1. Salminen E, Heikkila S, Poussa T, et al.: Female patients tend to alter their diet following the diagnosis of rheumatoid arthritis and breast cancer, *Prev Med* 34:529–535, 2002.
2. Caughey GE, Pouliot M, Cleland LG, et al.: Regulation of tumor necrosis factor-α and IL-1β synthesis by thromboxane A_2 in nonadherent human monocytes, *J Immunol* 158:351–358, 1997.
4. Martinon F, Petrilli V, Mayor A, et al.: Gout-associated uric acid crystals activate the NALP3 inflammasome, *Nature* 440:237–241, 2006.
19. Mas E, Croft K, Zahra P, et al.: Resolvins D1, D2, and other mediators of self-limited resolution of inflammation in human blood following n-3 fatty acid supplementation, *Clin Chem* 58:1476–1484, 2012.
20. Buckley C, Gilroy D, Serhan C: Proresolving lipid mediators and mechanisms in the resolution of acute inflammation, *Immunity* 40(3):315–327, 2014.
27. Neve A, Corrado A, Cantatore F: Immunodmodulatory effects of vitamin D in peripheral blood monocyte-derived macrophages from patients with rheumatoid arthritis, *Clin Exp Med* 14(3):275–283, 2014.
28. van Etten E, Mathieu C: Immunoregulation by 1,25-dihydroxyvitamin D_3: basic concepts, *J Steroid Biochem Mol Biol* 97:93–101, 2005.
30. Jeffery L, Wood A, Qureshi O, et al.: Availability of 25-hydroxyvitamin D3 to APCs controls the balance between regulatory and inflammatory T cell responses, *J Immunol* 189:5155–5164, 2012.
32. Stofkova A: Resistin and visfatin: regulators of insulin sensitivity, inflammation and immunity, *Endocr Regul* 44:25–36, 2010.
33. Thomas S, Izard J, Walsh E, et al.: The host microbiome regulates and maintains human health: a primer and perspective for non-microbiologists, *Cancer Res* 77(8):1783–1812, 2017.
35. Maeda Y, Kurakawa T, Umemoto E, et al.: Dysbiosis contributes to arthritis development via activation of autoreactive T cells in the intestine, *Arthritis Rheum* 68(11):2646–2661, 2016.
37. Picchianti-Diamanti A, Panebianco C, Salemi S, et al.: Analysis of gut microbiota in rheumatoid arthritis patients: disease-related dysbiosis and modifications induced by etanercept, *Int J Mol Sci* 19(10):2938, 2018.

39. Kaur S, White S, Bartold PM: Periodontal disease and rheumatoid arthritis; a systematic review, *J Dent Res* 92(5):399–408, 2013.
40. Hu Y, Sparks J, Malspeis S, et al.: Long-term dietary quality and risk of developing rheumatoid arthritis in women, *Ann Rheum Dis* 76(8):1357–1364, 2017.
43. de Pablo P, Romaguera D, Fisk H, et al.: High erythrocyte levels of the n-6 polyunsaturated fatty acid linoleic acid are associated with lower risk of subsequent rheumatoid arthritis in a southern European nested case-control study, *Ann Rheum Dis* 77(7):981–987, 2018.
52. Lee Y, Bae S-C, Song G: Coffee or tea consumption and the risk of rheumatoid arthritis: a meta-analysis, *Clin Rheumatol* 33(11):1575–1583, 2014.
58. Lu B, Solomon D, Costenbader K, et al.: Alcohol consumption and risk of incident rheumatoid arthritis in women: a prospective study, *Arthritis Rheum* 66(8):1998–2005, 2014.
62. Hu Y, Costenbader K, Gao X, et al.: Sugar-sweetened soda consumption and risk of developing rheumatoid arthritis in women, *Am J Clin Nutr* 100(3):959–967, 2014.
63. de Koning L, Malik V, Kellogg M, et al.: Sweetened beverage consumption, incident coronary heart disease, and biomarkers of risk in men, *Circulation* 125:1735–1741, 2012.
67. Costenbader K, Feskanich D, Holmes M, et al.: Vitamin D intake and risks of systemic lupus erythematosus and rheumatoid arthritis in women, *Ann Rheum Dis* 67:530–535, 2008.
72. Lu B, Hiraki L, Sparks J, et al.: Being overweight or obese and risk of developing rheumatoid arthritis among women: a prospective cohort study, *Ann Rheum Dis* 73(11):1914–1922, 2014.
75. Linauskas A, Overvad K, Symmons D, et al.: Body fat percentage, waist circumference and obesity as risk factors for rheumatoid arthritis—A Danish cohort study, *Arthritis Care Res*, 2018. [Epub ahead of print].
76. Baker J, Ostergaard M, George M, et al.: Greater body mass index independtly predicts less radiographic progression on x-ray and MRI over 1-2 years, *Ann Rheum Dis* 73(11):1923–1928, 2014.
77. Baker J, George M, Baker D, et al.: Associations between body mass, radiographic joint damage, adipokines and risk factors for bone loss in rheumatoid arthritis, *Rheumatology* 50:2100–2107, 2011.
78. Van der Helm-van Mil A, van der Kooij S, Allaart C, et al.: A high body mass index has a protective effect on the amount of joint destruction in small joints in early rheumatoid arthritis, *Ann Rheum Dis* 67:769–774, 2008.
79. Westhoff G, Rau R, Zink A: Radiographic joint damage in early rheumatoid arthritis is highly dependent on body mass index, *Arthritis Rheum* 56:3575–3582, 2007.
80. Rho Y, Solus J, Sokka T, et al.: Adipocytokines are associated with radiographic joint damage in rheumatoid arthritis, *Arthritis Rheum* 60:1906–1914, 2009.
81. Ajeganova S, Andersson M, Hafström I, et al.: Association of obesity with worse disease severity in rheumatoid arthritis as well as with comorbidities: a long-term followup from disease onset, *Arthritis Care Res (Hoboken)* 65:78–87, 2013.
82. Sandberg M, Bengtsson C, Kallberg H, et al.: Overweight decreases the chance of achieving good response and low disease activity in early rheumatoid arthritis, *Ann Rheum Dis* 73(11):2029–2033, 2014.
83. Wolfe F, Michaud K: Effect of body mass index on mortality and clinical status in rheumatoid arthritis, *Arthritis Car Res* 64:1471–1479, 2012.
84. Roubenoff R, Roubenoff R, Cannon J, et al.: Rheumatoid cachexia: cytokine-driven hypermetabolism accompanying reduced body cell mass in chronic inflammation, *J Clin Invest* 93:2379–2386, 1994.
85. Elkan A-C, Håkansson N, Frostegård J, et al.: Rheumatoid cachexia is associated with dyslipidemia and low levels of atheroprotective natural antibodies against phosphorylcholine but not with dietary fat in patients with rheumatoid arthritis: a cross-sectional study, *Arthritis Care Res (Hoboken)* 11:R37, 2009.
90. Rai SK, Fung TT, Lu N, et al.: The Dietary Approaches to Stop Hypertension (DASH) diet, Western diet, and risk of gout in men: prospective cohort study, *BMJ (Clinical research ed)* 357:j1794, 2017. [published Online First: 2017/05/11].
91. Juraschek SP, Gelber AC, Choi HK, et al.: Effects of the Dietary Approaches to Stop Hypertension (DASH) Diet and Sodium Intake on Serum Uric Acid, *Arthritis Rheum (Hoboken, NJ)* 68(12):3002–3009, 2016.
92. Choi H, Curhan G: Soft drinks, fructose consumption, and the risk of gout in men: prospective cohort study, *Br Med J* 336:309–312, 2008.
93. Choi J, Ford E, Gao X, et al.: Sugar-sweetened soft drinks, diet soft drinks and serum uric acid level: the Third National Health and Nutrition Examination Survey, *Arthritis Care Res* 59:109–116, 2008.
95. Vitart V, Rudan I, Hayward C, et al.: SLC2A9 is a newly identified urate transporter influencing serum urate concentration, urate excretion and gout, *Nat Genet* 40:437–442, 2008.
96. Batt C, Phipps-Green A, Black M, et al.: Sugar-sweetened beverage consumption: a risk factor for prevalent gout with SLC2A9 genotypespecific effects on serum urate and risk of gout, *Ann Rheum Dis* 73(12):2101–2106, 2014.
97. Dalbeth N, House M, Gamble G, et al.: Population-specific influence of SLC2A9 genotype on the acute hyperuricaemic response to a fructose load, *Ann Rheum Dis* 72:1868–1873, 2013.
100. Choi H, Atkinson K, Karlson E, et al.: Alcohol intake and risk of incident gout in men: a prospective study, *Lancet* 363:1277–1281, 2004.
101. Choi H, Gao X, Curhan G: Vitamin C intake and the risk of gout in men. A prospective study, *Arch Intern Med* 169:502–507, 2009.
102. Major T, Topless R, Dalbeth N, et al.: Evaluation of the diet wide contribution to serum urate levels: meta-analysis of population based cohorts, *BMJ (Clinical research ed)* 363:k3951, 2018.
110. Larsson S, Burgess S, Michaëlsson K: Genetic association between adiposity and gout: a Mendelian randomization study, *Rheumatology*, 2018.
112. Yusuf E, Nelissen R, Ioan-Facsinay A, et al.: Association between weight or body mass index and hand osteoarthritis: a systematic review, *Ann Rheum Dis* 69(4):761–765, 2010.
113. Misra D, Fielding R, Felson D, et al.: Risk of knee OA with obesity, sarcopenic obesity and sarcopenia, Hoboken, NJ, 2018, *Arthritis & rheumatology*.
115. Lu B, Driban JB, Xu C, et al.: Dietary fat intake and radiographic progression of knee osteoarthritis: data from the osteoarthritis initiative, *Arthritis Care Res* 69(3):368–375, 2017. [published Online First: 2016/06/09].
117. McAlindon T, Jacques P, Zhang Y, et al.: Do antioxidant micronutrients protect against the development and progression of knee osteoarthritis? *Arthritis Rheum* 39:648–656, 1996.
122. Nichols P, Kitessa S, Abeywardena M: Commentary on a trial comparing krill oil versus in standard fish oil, *Lipids Health Dis* 13(2), 2014.
123. Ulven S, Kirkhus B, Lamglait A, et al.: Metabolic effects of krill oil are essentially similar to those of fish oil, but at lower dose of EPA and DHA, in healthy volunteers, *Lipids* 46:37–46, 2011.
124. Schuchardt J, Schneider I, Meyer H, et al.: Incorporation of EPA and DHA into plasma phospholipids in response to different omega-3 fatty acid formulations—a comparative bioavailability study of fish oil vs. krill oil, *Lipids Health Dis* 10:145, 2011.
125. Cleland L, Caughey G, James M, et al.: Reduction of cardiovascular risk factors with longterm fish oil treatment in early rheumatoid arthritis, *J Rheumatol* 33:1973–1979, 2006.
127. Proudman S, James M, Spargo L, et al.: Fish oil in recent onset rheumatoid arthritis: a randomised, double-blind controlled trial within algorithm-based drug use, *Ann Rheum Dis* 74(1):89–95, 2015.
128. Proudman SM, Cleland LG, Metcalf RG, et al.: Plasma n-3 fatty acids and clinical outcomes in recent-onset rheumatoid arthritis, *Br J Nutr* 114(6):885–890, 2015.
129. Jeffery L, Fisk H, Calder P, et al.: Plasma levels of eicosapentaenoic acid are associated with anti-TNF responsiveness in rheumatoid arthritis and inhibit the etanercept-driven rise in Th17 cell differentiation in vitro, *J Rheumatol* 44(6):748–756, 2017.

130. Tedeschi SK, Bathon JM, et al.: Relationship between fish consumption and disease activity in rheumatoid arthritis, *Arthritis Care Res.* 70(3):327–332, 2018.
134. Leeb B, Sautner J, Andel I, et al.: Intravenous application of omega-3 fatty acids in patients with active rheumatoid arthritis. The ORA-1 trial. An open pilot study, *Lipids* 41:29–34, 2006.
136. Ribaya-Mercado J, Blumberg J, Vitamin A: Is it a risk factor for osteoporosis and bone fracture? *Nutr Rev* 65:425–438, 2007.
139. Watson P, Joy P, Nkonde C, et al.: Comparison of bleeding complications with omega-3 fatty acids + aspirin + clopidogrel—versus—aspirin + clopidogrel in patients with cardiovascular disease, *Am J Cardiol* 104:1052–1054, 2009.
141. Abdelhamid A, Brown T, Brainard J, et al.: Omega-3 fatty acids for the primary and secondary prevention of cardiovascular disease, *Cochrane Database Syst Rev* 7:CD003177, 2018.
143. Canter P, Wider B, Ernst E: The antioxidant vitamins A, C, E and selenium in the treatment of arthritis: a systematic review of randomized clinical trials, *Rheumatology* 46:1223–1233, 2007.
144. Gan RW, Demoruelle MK, Deane KD, et al.: Omega-3 fatty acids are associated with a lower prevalence of autoantibodies in shared epitope positive subjects at risk for rheumatoid arthritis, *Ann Rheum Dis* 76:147–152, 2017.
146. Deane KD, Norris JM, Holers VM: Preclinical rheumatoid arthritis: identification, evaluation, and future directions for investigation, *Rheum Dis Clin N Am* 36:213–41, 2010.
147. Deane KD, El-Gabalawy H: Pathogenesis and prevention of rheumatic disease: focus on preclinical RA and SLE, *Nat Rev Rheumatol* 10:212-28, 2014.
148. Gan GW, Bemis EA, Demoruelle KM, et al.: The association between omega-3 fatty acid biomarkers and inflammatory arthritis in an anti-citrullinated protein antibody positive population, *Rheumatology* 56:2229-2236, 2017.
151. Edmonds S, Winyard P, Guo R, et al.: Putative analgesic activity of repeated oral doses of vitamin E in the treatment of rheumatoid arthritis. Results of a prospective placebo controlled double blind trial, *Ann Rheum Dis* 56:649–655, 1997.
160. Zakeri Z, Sandoughi M, Mashhadi M, et al.: Serum vitamin D level and disease activity in patients with recent onset rheumatoid arthritis, *Int J Rheum Dis Oct* 18, 2013. [Epub ahead of print].
161. Craig S, Yu J, Curtis J, et al.: Vitamin D status and its associations with disease activity and severity in African Americans with recent-onset rheumatoid arthritis, *J Rheumatol* 37:275–281, 2010.
166. van Hamburg J, Asmawidjaja P, Davelaar N, et al.: TNF blockade requires 1,25$(OH)_2D_3$ to control human Th17-mediated synovial inflammation, *Ann Rheum Dis* 70:606–612, 2012.
168. Hafstrom I, Ringertz B, Gyllenhammar H, et al.: Effects of fasting on disease activity, neutrophil function, fatty acid composition, and leukotriene biosynthesis in patients with rheumatoid arthritis, *Arthritis Rheum* 31:585–592, 1988.
171. Kjeldsen-Kragh J, Borchgrevink C, Mowinkel P, et al.: Controlled trial of fasting and one-year vegetarian diet in rheumatoid arthritis, *Lancet* 338:899–902, 1991.
173. Muller H, de Toledo W, Resch K-L: Fasting followed by vegetarian diet in patients with rheumatoid arthritis: a systematic review, *Scand J Rheumatol* 30:1–10, 2001.
177. Humphreys J, Warner A, Costello R, et al.: Quantifying the hepatotoxic risk of alcohol consumption in patients with rheumatoid arthritis taking methotrexate, *Ann Rheum Dis* 76(9):1509–1514, 2017.
178. Kremer J, Weinblatt M: Quantifying the hepatotoxic risk of alcohol consumption in patients with rheumatoid arthritis taking methotrexate, *Ann Rheum Dis* 77(1):e4, 2018.
187. Kearsley-Fleet L, Davies R, De Cock D, et al.: Biologic refractory disease in rheumatoid arthritis: results from the British Society for Rheumatology Biologics Register for Rheumatoid Arthritis, *Ann Rheum Dis*, 2018.
189. Holland R, McGill NW: Comprehensive dietary education in treated gout patients does not further improve serum urate, *Intern Med J* 45(2):189–194, 2015. [published Online First: 2014/12/17].
192. Jacob R, Spinozzi G, Simon V, et al.: Consumption of cherries lowers plasma urate in healthy women, *J Nutr* 133:1826–1829, 2003.
193. Zhang Y, Neogi T, Chen C, et al.: Cherry consumption and decreased risk of recurrent gout attacks, *Arthritis Rheum* 64:4004–4011, 2012.
201. Stamp L, O'Donnell J, Frampton C, et al.: Clinically insignificant effect of supplemental vitamin C on serum urate in patients with gout; a pilot randomised controlled trial, *Arthritis Rheum* 65:1636–1642, 2013.
204. Nielsen SM, Bartels EM, Henriksen M, et al.: Weight loss for overweight and obese individuals with gout: a systematic review of longitudinal studies, *Ann Rheum Dis* 76(11):1870–1882, 2017. [published Online First: 2017/09/04].
205. Abhishek A, Valdes A, Doherty M: Low omega-3 fatty acid levels associate with frequent gout attacks: a case controlled study, *Ann Rheum Dis* 75(4):784–785, 2016.
208. Messier SP, Mihalko SL, Legault C, et al.: Effects of intensive diet and exercise on knee joint loads, inflammation, and clinical outcomes among overweight and obese adults with knee osteoarthritis: the IDEA randomized clinical trial, *Jama* 310(12):1263–1273, 2013. [published Online First: 2013/09/26].
213. Hill C, March L, Aitken D, et al.: Fish oil in knee osteoarthritis: a randomized clinical trial of low dose versus high dose, *Ann Rheum Dis* 75:23–29, 2016.
216. Jin X, Jones G, Cicuttini F, et al.: Effect of vitamin D supplementation on tibial cartilage volume and knee pain among patients with symptomatic knee osteoarthritis: a randomized clinical trial, *JAMA* 315(10):1005–1013, 2016.
217. Zheng S, Jin X, Cicuttini F, et al.: Maintaining vitamin D sufficiency is associated with improved structural and symptomatic outcomes in knee osteoarthritis, *Am J Med* 130(10):1211–1218, 2017.

73 Evaluation and Management of Early Undifferentiated Arthritis

KARIM RAZA

KEY POINTS

- Arthritis refers to synovial swelling apparent on clinical examination; the definition of "early" in the context of inflammatory arthritis has changed over time.
- "Undifferentiated" arthritis (UA) is a diagnosis of exclusion; the features that associate with it have changed over time, as the criteria that define other arthritides (e.g., rheumatoid arthritis [RA]) have evolved.
- The accurate prediction of outcome, including the development of persistent arthritis or RA, is critical in patients with early UA, and several algorithms exist to guide management decisions.
- Studies with currently available anti-rheumatic agents suggest that transition from UA to classifiable RA might be delayed by use of methotrexate.
- Patients are increasingly being identified with synovitis on imaging but not on clinical examination. Clinical trial data are not yet available to inform the management of such patients.

Introduction

The cardinal physical finding that has historically defined inflammatory arthritis is the presence of clinically apparent synovial swelling at a peripheral joint. It is, however, increasingly recognized that a physical examination might lack sensitivity for the detection of synovial inflammation.[1,2] This can be a particular challenge in the context of certain joints, such as the metatarsophalangeal (MTP) joints, and multiple studies have shown that patients with inflammatory joint symptoms may have evidence of synovial inflammation using imaging modalities, such as ultrasound and MRI, but that a physical examination may fail to identify joint swelling. This is often true for patients with clinical synovitis in at least one joint, where the use of ultrasound[1,2] and MRI[3] identifies synovial inflammation in joints that were not clinically swollen, as well as patients with inflammatory symptoms but no clinically apparent joint swelling, where imaging can show changes consistent with synovial inflammation.[4–6]

Most research to date on approaches to prognosis and treatment of early undifferentiated arthritis has involved patients with clinically apparent synovial swelling, which will be referred to as *clinical-undifferentiated arthritis* (UA). Nevertheless, an emerging literature is developing on patients with musculoskeletal symptoms and synovitis apparent only with imaging (herein called *imaging-UA*), and the approach to such patients will also be discussed.

Changing Definitions of Classifiable and Undifferentiated Arthritis

Undifferentiated inflammatory arthritis, by definition, does not fulfill the criteria for any defined inflammatory joint disease. Thus, as criteria for other diseases evolve, the spectrum of patients included in the undifferentiated group will change. This is most evident in terms of the evolution of criteria for rheumatoid arthritis (RA). The 1987 American College of Rheumatology (ACR) classification criteria for RA[7] were developed primarily to define a relatively homogenous group of patients for inclusion in research studies. They were not intended to be used to diagnose RA in patients with new-onset joint inflammation and therefore perform relatively poorly in that context. Indeed, two of the seven domains in the usually applied list format (the presence of rheumatoid nodules and of radiographic changes at hands and wrists) are unusual in patients with early disease.

The 2010 ACR/European League Against Rheumatism (EULAR) classification criteria[8] are more sensitive and allow a larger proportion of patients presenting with early arthritis to be classifiable as RA. Consequently a lower proportion are labeled as having UA. Important elements underlying this high sensitivity include the high weight given to the involvement of large numbers of joints, especially when only one needs to be swollen and others can be scored as involved with tenderness alone, and to high levels of autoantibodies. One of the challenges associated with using the 2010 criteria is that more patients fulfilling these criteria will have symptoms that spontaneously resolve compared with patients who fulfill the 1987 ACR criteria.[9] In addition, when applied at presentation, they do not perform particularly well in terms of identifying autoantibody-negative patients who have UA according to the 1987 criteria (referred to as 1987-UA) and develop RA according to the 1987 criteria (referred to as 1987-RA) at follow-up; 49% of such patients in a Dutch cohort and 75% in a French cohort did not fulfill the 2010 criteria (referred to as 2010-UA) at baseline.[10]

TABLE 73.1 Differential Diagnosis for Patients With a New Onset of Peripheral Inflammatory Arthritis

Crystal arthritis (e.g., gout, pseudogout)
Inflammatory osteoarthritis
Rheumatoid arthritis
Psoriatic arthritis
Other spondyloarthropathy
Systemic lupus erythematosus
Other connective tissue diseases/vasculitis
Postinfective arthritis (e.g., reactive arthritis, postviral arthritis)
Sarcoidosis
Malignancy-associated arthritis
RS3PE
Septic arthritis
Other

RS3PE, Remitting seronegative symmetrical synovitis with pitting edema.

TABLE 73.2 EULAR-Defined Characteristics Describing Arthralgia at Risk of Rheumatoid Arthritis

Parameters Available Via History
Joint symptoms of recent onset (duration <1 year) Symptoms located in MCP joints Duration of morning stiffness of at least 60 minutes Most severe symptoms present in the early morning Presence of a first-degree relative with RA
Parameters Available Via Physical Examination
Difficulty making a fist Positive squeeze test of MCP joints

EULAR, European League Against Rheumatism; *MCP*, metacarpophalangeal; *RA*, rheumatoid arthritis.

Because UA is a diagnosis of exclusion, considerable attention needs to be paid to ensuring that defined causes of inflammatory arthritis have been considered (Table 73.1). In some cases, it is clear that such an alternative diagnosis is present. The pattern of joint involvement (e.g., first MTP joint involvement in gout, wrist involvement in pseudogout, and symmetrical ankle involvement in sarcoidosis) and the rapidity of joint involvement (e.g., the rapid development of septic arthritis) often give important clues to the diagnosis. Nevertheless, some diagnoses require additional clinical information (e.g., travel history in an individual with Chikungunya arthritis and diagnostic skin lesions in a patient with psoriatic arthritis), and careful clinical assessment with detailed physical examination, including assessment for hematuria and proteinuria, is important.

Definition of "Early" Arthritis

There is no consensus as to the definition of the word "early" in the context of inflammatory joint diseases. Interest in the concept of duration relates to two important principles in the management of RA. The first is that damage to cartilage and periarticular bone develops progressively over time and, at least with current therapies, is not easily reversible. The second is that of a "therapeutic window of opportunity" in early RA, during which intervention is associated with an enhanced ability to control and reverse synovial inflammation. This window may be the consequence of the "early" phase of clinically apparent synovial swelling representing a pathologically distinct phase in the natural history of RA, during which the disease might be more amenable to therapy with a greater chance of achieving remission.

The duration of this "window of opportunity" has not been fully defined. One of the particular challenges relating to this is the difficulty in designing an ethically acceptable placebo-controlled study to optimally address this issue. In particular, many studies have used observational cohorts where outcomes in patients treated "late" have been compared with those treated "early"; although we know how to control for some confounders (e.g., autoantibody status), it is quite possible that there are other relevant variables that might influence how soon patients are treated and might also influence outcomes. The fact that disease-modifying anti-rheumatic drug (DMARD) therapy is generally required for patients as soon as a diagnosis of RA is made means that it is not often possible to randomize patients with RA to early versus delayed treatment, although early "intensive" versus early "conventional" approaches can be compared. Nevertheless, with these caveats in mind, a consensus exists in the literature that in patients with RA, the therapeutic window of opportunity lasts approximately 12 weeks after the onset of inflammatory type joint symptoms.[11]

With increasing recognition that intervening early improves outcomes in RA, there has been a recent focus of attention on the phases of RA development that precede the onset of joint swelling. Key "at risk" stages that individuals can move through include: (1) individuals with genetic and/or environmental risk factors who then develop (2) systemic autoimmunity (typically associated with the development of rheumatoid factor [RF] and/or anti-citrullinated protein antibodies [ACPA] in the blood) followed (or potentially even preceded) by (3) musculoskeletal symptoms suggestive of underlying inflammation but without clinically apparent synovial swelling (also known as clinically suspect arthralgia [CSA]).[12] A definition of this term has recently been proposed (Table 73.2),[13] and studies have shown that at least a proportion of patients with CSA have imaging evidence of synovitis. Nevertheless, as with patients with clinically apparent joint swelling, there is a wide differential diagnosis for musculoskeletal symptoms with inflammatory features in the absence of clinically apparent joint swelling that must be carefully considered. These include many of the conditions listed in Table 73.1 but also others, including polymyalgia rheumatica, hypothyroidism, and fibromyalgia. Data to inform management decisions in such patients with subclinical synovitis are limited, but management strategies will be discussed.

Evaluation of Early Undifferentiated Inflammatory Arthritis

Facilitating Access to Rheumatologists

Although some new-onset inflammatory arthritides (e.g., gout) can be managed by primary care providers, all patients with a new onset of inflammatory arthritis in whom there is diagnostic uncertainty should be evaluated by a specialist for:

- Assessment of the underlying diagnosis.
- Prediction of the risk of the development of RA (or other defined arthritis) in those with genuine UA.
- Treatment using a shared decision-making approach.[14]

Ideally, such patients should be seen as soon as possible after the onset of their symptoms, with recent EULAR recommendations suggesting that patients presenting with new inflammatory arthritis should be seen by a rheumatologist within 6 weeks after the onset of symptoms.[14] This is a challenging issue, and, currently, only a minority of RA patients are actually seen within this time frame.[15]

Facilitating rapid access to specialists for patients with new-onset (undifferentiated) inflammatory arthritis requires a multifaceted approach.[16] A key aspect of overall delay is the delay on the part of the patient in seeking help in the first place.[17] Many patients do not recognize the significance of inflammatory musculoskeletal symptoms or that early treatment is critical.[18] Public health messaging to address these issues is key. Another important element of delay is the delay by the primary health care provider in recognizing patients with a new onset of (undifferentiated) inflammatory arthritis and making a timely referral. In the UK, patients with RA and UA made an average of four visits to the general clinician before being referred to a rheumatologist.[19]

One of the difficulties that primary care physicians face is that, at an early stage, clinical features might not be typical, even in patients who eventually develop RA. Indeed, a recent survey has identified how common inflammatory-type musculoskeletal symptoms are in patients presenting to their primary care doctor, even when the consultation was not primarily for a musculoskeletal problem. Education programs for clinicians in primary care and referral algorithms could address this issue. Finally, delays by the rheumatologist in assessing patients upon referrals also contribute to the overall delay. Innovative models of care such as "early arthritis recognition clinics," where patients are seen quickly for brief consultations by an experienced rheumatologist, with the specific objective of ruling inflammatory arthritis in or out, have shown that delays can be reduced using novel approaches.[20]

Predicting Outcomes in Clinical-Undifferentiated Inflammatory Arthritis

Recent EULAR guidelines on the management of early arthritis highlight that clinical examination is the method of choice for detecting arthritis, which may be confirmed by ultrasonography. These guidelines stress the importance of predicting outcomes in patients with clinical-UA.[14]

Key outcomes of interest to the patient and the clinician are the development of persistent, as opposed to resolving, disease and, in those with persistent disease, the development of defined arthritides, including RA. Work from the University of Leiden has defined a set of variables that are highly predictive of the development of persistent arthritis after 2 years in patients with early arthritis (Table 73.3).[21] Importantly the presence of persistence (i.e., a symptom duration of ≥6 months) is the variable with the highest weighting in terms of predicting the persistence of arthritis. The importance of symptom duration at presentation as a predictor of future disease persistence in patients with early arthritis has been highlighted in a number of other studies.[22,23]

In health care environments where rapid help seeking is facilitated, predicting persistence becomes more challenging as the proportion of patients with long-standing symptoms at presentation declines. Other key variables in prediction rules include clinical and laboratory features associated with RA. This is perhaps not surprising because the majority of those who ended up with a persistent disease did indeed have RA; of those with persistent disease at 2 years, 66% had RA, 15% UA, 9% psoriatic arthritis, 3% a connective tissue disease, and 3% a spondyloarthropathy.[21] In addition to predicting arthritis persistence, predicting RA development is also important. The most widely validated prediction rule to predict RA in patients with newly presenting 1987-UA is shown in Table 73.3.[24] The risk of RA on the basis of the score from the prediction rule is shown in Fig. 73.1. Importantly, this has now been validated in a range of different populations, including in India[25] and Canada.[26]

Most current algorithms to predict persistent arthritis or RA have used, as a starting point, the whole population of patients with early (often undifferentiated) arthritis recruited via secondary care rheumatology clinics—often from European academic hospitals with specialist early arthritis clinics. This raises a number of important issues in the context of the utilization of these rules in other clinical environments. First, the rules have not been developed in primary care populations and should not be used as the "referral instruments" to guide referral from primary to secondary care. Second, although the prediction rule for RA in patients with 1987-UA[24] has been validated in a number of countries, their performance has not been assessed in all populations. Data suggesting variation in clinical phenotypes of RA in different geographic areas[27] highlight the importance of validating prediction rules in relevant populations before applying them, especially when prediction rules are dominated by clinical features.

Prediction rules for persistent arthritis and for RA give prominence to variables assessed by clinical joint examination and to RF and ACPA. Approaches to optimizing these prediction rules include strategies that define joint and periarticular inflammation more accurately and may involve capitalizing on the broader range of autoantibodies associated with RA. In the context of joint assessment, gray scale and power Doppler assessment of metacarpophalangeal joints, wrists, and metatarsophalangeal joints provides additional data that improve the performance of the Leiden prediction rule.[1] In addition, tenosynovitis is a common feature of patients with early RA, and ultrasound-defined digit flexor tenosynovitis provides independent predictive data for persistent RA development in patients with early arthritis.[28]

Although RF and ACPA are important characteristics of RA and are thus included in classification criteria and prediction rules, many patients lack these autoantibodies, especially in early disease. More recently, additional autoantibodies that bind to a range of post-translational modifications have been identified, such as anti-carbamylated protein (anti-CarP) antibodies.[29,30] In 1987-UA patients, the presence of anti-CarP antibodies was associated with progression to RA, an association that remained even when corrected for the presence of ACPA and RF.[31] After stratifying for ACPA and RF, anti-CarP antibodies were associated with progression to RA only for ACPA- and RF-negative patients. In contrast, for 2010-UA patients, anti-CarP antibodies were not associated with progression to RA when a correction was made for the presence of ACPA and RF.

TABLE 73.3 Predictors of Outcome in Patients With Early Arthritis

PREDICTION RULE FOR PERSISTENCE IN PATIENTS WITH EARLY ARTHRITIS[a]		PREDICTION RULE FOR RA IN PATIENTS WITH UA[b]	
Variable	Score	Variable	Score
Symptom duration ≥6 weeks but <6 months	2	Age	Years × 0.02
Symptom duration ≥6 months	3	Female sex	1
Morning stiffness ≥1 hour	1	Distribution of Involved Joints	
Arthritis in ≥3 joint groups	1	Small joints hands, and feet	0.5
Bilateral pain on MTP joint compression	1	Symmetric	0.5
IgM RF ≥5 IU	2	Upper extremities	1
Anti-CCP ≥92 IU	3	Upper and lower extremities	1.5
Erosions on hand or foot radiographs	2	EMS VAS 26-90mm	1
		EMS VAS >90mm	2
		Tender joints 4-10	0.5
		Tender joints >10	1
		Swollen joints 4-10	0.5
		Swollen joints >10	1
		CRP 5-50 mg/L	0.5
		CRP >50 mg/L	1.5
		RF positive	1
		ACPA positive	2

[a]Predictors of persistence in patients with early arthritis.

[b]Predictors of development of RA in patients with undifferentiated arthritis according to 1987 ACR criteria. See Fig. 73.1 for predictive capacity of this system.

ACPA, Anti-citrullinated protein antibody; *CCP,* cyclic citrullinated peptide; *CRP,* C-reactive protein; *EMS VAS,* early morning stiffness visual analog scale; *IgM,* immunoglobulin M; *IU,* international units; *MTP,* metatarsophalangeal; *RA,* rheumatoid arthritis; *RF,* rheumatoid factor; *UA,* undifferentiated arthritis.

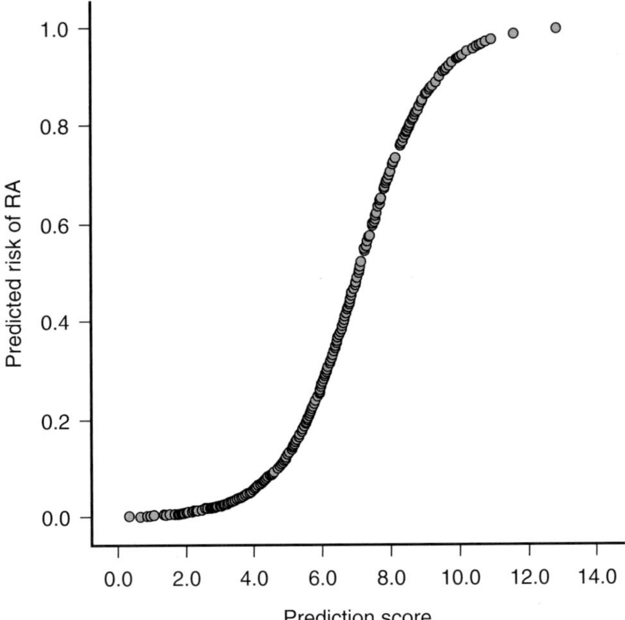

• **Fig. 73.1** Predicted risk of rheumatoid arthritis as a function of the prediction score. The performance of a scoring system for predicting development of rheumatoid arthritis (RA) from undifferentiated arthritis (see Table 73.3) is shown. The algorithm can be used to stratify patients for clinical trials to prevent RA. (From van der Helm-van Mil AHM, le Cessie S, van Dongen H, et al.: A prediction rule for disease outcome in patients with recent-onset undifferentiated arthritis. *Arthritis Rheum* 56:433-440, 2007.)

Several studies assessed whether characteristics of the synovium in patients with early arthritis distinguish those UA patients who will develop RA from those who will not. Preliminary data suggest that early arthritis patients who eventually develop RA have a pattern of synovial chemokine expression that differs from patients with other early arthritides, with high expression of CXCL4 and CXCL7 in early RA.[32] Furthermore, synovial fibroblast characteristics, including expression of fibroblast activation protein (FAP), appear to differ in early RA patients when compared with those with other forms of early arthritis.[33,34] Although approaches to accessing synovial tissue have advanced with increasing availability of minimally invasive ultrasound-guided biopsy approaches,[35] synovial tissue–based biomarkers for predicting RA development in patients with UA have not yet been widely validated and have not yet been incorporated into clinically useful predictive algorithms.

Predicting Outcomes in Imaging–Undifferentiated Inflammatory Arthritis

Patients with CSA or other types of arthralgia by definition do not have clinically apparent joint swelling. These patients are, however, at increased risk of the development of arthritis based on symptoms. In addition, many of these patients have imaging evidence of synovitis and thus have imaging-UA. Prediction rules have been developed to predict progression to arthritis or to RA in patients at risk of RA but who do not have a swollen joint. The best known of these has been developed for use in patients with musculoskeletal symptoms who are positive for either RF or ACPA.[36]

In ACPA-positive patients with musculoskeletal symptoms, ultrasound findings predict progression and rate of progression to inflammatory arthritis, with the highest risk of progression associated with power Doppler signal.[37] These studies have taken, as a starting point, cohorts of patients at risk of RA on the basis of autoantibody positivity. Other studies have taken, as a starting point, cohorts of patients with CSA and assessed the role of autoantibodies and imaging findings to predict RA development.[38] RF and ACPA and, in particular, their combination increased the risk of arthritis development, although there was no additive effect of anti-CarP antibodies. Similarly, the presence of small joint power Doppler signal in patients with inflammatory-type musculoskeletal symptoms was associated with future arthritis development.[39]

Interestingly, no studies to date have defined their population on the basis of imaging synovitis. Thus imaging synovitis clearly predicts arthritis and RA development in patients with other risk factors for RA, but outcomes of patients defined primarily on imaging synovitis (but no clinically evident swelling) are not currently known. This is an important issue as data suggest that a proportion of the otherwise entirely healthy population have imaging evidence of synovitis.

Management of Early Undifferentiated Arthritis

Assuming a clinical diagnosis cannot be reached and the patient is defined as having early UA, management decisions will be influenced by the extent of the patient's symptoms and their impact on function, as well as by the predicted future outcome of the arthritis (e.g., resolving diseases vs. persistent UA vs. persistent RA). Shared decision making between the patient and physician is critical and should include adequate education and information for the patient, for whom the concept of an "undifferentiated" arthritis may be unfamiliar and uncertainties about future disease progression may be challenging.

Traditional Disease-Modifying Anti-rheumatic Drugs

Current recommendations suggest that patients with undifferentiated arthritis at risk of persistent arthritis should be started on a DMARD as early as possible, ideally within 3 months of symptom onset, even if they do not fulfill classification criteria for a defined inflammatory rheumatologic disease.[14] Methotrexate is considered the anchor drug and, unless contraindicated, should be part of the first treatment strategy in patients at risk of persistent disease. This recommendation is largely based on data suggesting efficacy in early RA.

Most recommendations regarding the pharmacologic management of UA, particularly UA at risk of development into RA, are extrapolated from clinical trials in early RA. Nevertheless, there have been a few clinical trials specifically in UA patients. One of the first trials compared methotrexate (starting at 15 mg/week) with placebo in patients with 1987-UA and symptoms of arthritis of no more than two years' duration.[40] Treatment was escalated if the disease activity score (DAS) was greater than 2.4 and after 12 months was tapered and discontinued. In the total study group, a smaller proportion of patients on methotrexate progressed to RA compared with patients on placebo (40% vs. 53%), although this difference did not reach statistical significance. In the methotrexate group, however, patients developed 1987-RA at a later time point than in the placebo group and fewer patients developed radiographic erosions over 18 months. Interestingly, data suggested that the benefit of methotrexate was greatest in the ACPA-positive subgroup (Fig. 73.2).[40]

A study from Japan showed that, compared with placebo, methotrexate reduced the chances of RA development in patients with ACPA-positive 1987-UA and symptoms of less than one year.[41] Methotrexate efficacy was also assessed in patients with 2010-UA in the IMPROVED study.[42] That study included patients with 1987-RA, 2010-RA, and 2010-UA and assessed treatment with methotrexate (7.5 to 25 mg/week) and prednisolone (60 mg/day tapering to 7.5 mg/day over 7 weeks and then persisting for 4 months). At 4 months, similar proportions of patients were in DAS remission in the three groups (58% of 1987-RA, 61% of 201-RA, and 65% of 2010-UA); in the whole population, ACPA positivity was an independent predictor for remission. In a 5-year follow-up, patients who failed to achieve remission were randomized to either adalimumab or combination DMARD therapy (sulfasalazine 2000 mg/day and hydroxychloroquine 400 mg/day), in addition to methotrexate.[43] Overall, at 5 years, 47% of UA patients and 49% of RA patients were in remission, although more patients with UA than RA were in drug-free remission at 5 years (31% vs. 19%; $P < 0.001$). This illustrates the good outcomes that can be achieved by the early introduction of conventional synthetic DMARDs in patients with UA and by the rapid escalation of therapy in patients with ongoing disease activity.

Biologic Therapy

The effect of biologic therapy in patients with 1987-UA has been assessed. Abatacept monotherapy has been assessed in ACPA-positive 1987-UA patients who have had symptoms for less than 18 months.[44] There was a nonsignificant trend between groups in terms of progression to RA at 24 weeks (46% of abatacept-treated patients and 67% of placebo-treated patients developed RA by one year). In patients with 1987-UA of less than 12 months' duration and of "poor prognosis" as defined by recurrence of synovitis after an intramuscular injection of corticosteroid, the effects of infliximab (3 mg/kg) monotherapy versus placebo at weeks 0, 2, 6, and 14 was assessed.[45] There was no difference in the proportion of patients achieving remission by week 26 or in the proportion of patients developing RA by week 52. Infliximab also did not prevent progression to RA in a separate study of patients with ACPA-positive UA.[46] Thus there is little current evidence to support the initial use of biologic therapy in patients with UA.

Glucocorticoid Therapy

Other studies (e.g., the Steroids in Very Early Arthritis [STIVEA][47] and Stop Arthritis Very Early [SAVE] trials)[48] have assessed the benefit of intramuscular steroids in patients with very early inflammatory polyarthritis, although in both these studies symptom duration represented the key inclusion criterion and the fulfillment of classification criteria for RA was not an exclusion; therefore neither study specifically evaluated UA. In SAVE,[48] patients had a symptom duration of less than 16 weeks, and in STIVEA[47] it was of 4 to 10 weeks' duration. STIVEA showed that treatment with three intramuscular injections of 80 mg methylprednisolone acetate given at weekly intervals postponed the need for DMARDs. In contrast, in SAVE, treatment with a single intramuscular injection of 120 mg of methylprednisolone did not influence eventual DMARD treatment. Nevertheless, treatment with glucocorticoid, whether intra-articular, intramuscular, or oral, has been used as bridging therapy in UA.

Nonpharmacologic Approaches

Nonpharmacologic approaches should also be considered in the management of patients with early UA. Dynamic exercise therapy and occupation therapy input can be helpful, and advice regarding smoking cessation, dental care, weight control, and management of comorbidities, including risk factors for atherosclerotic disease, should be part of overall patient care and are particularly important in those identified as being at high risk for RA.[14] Assessment

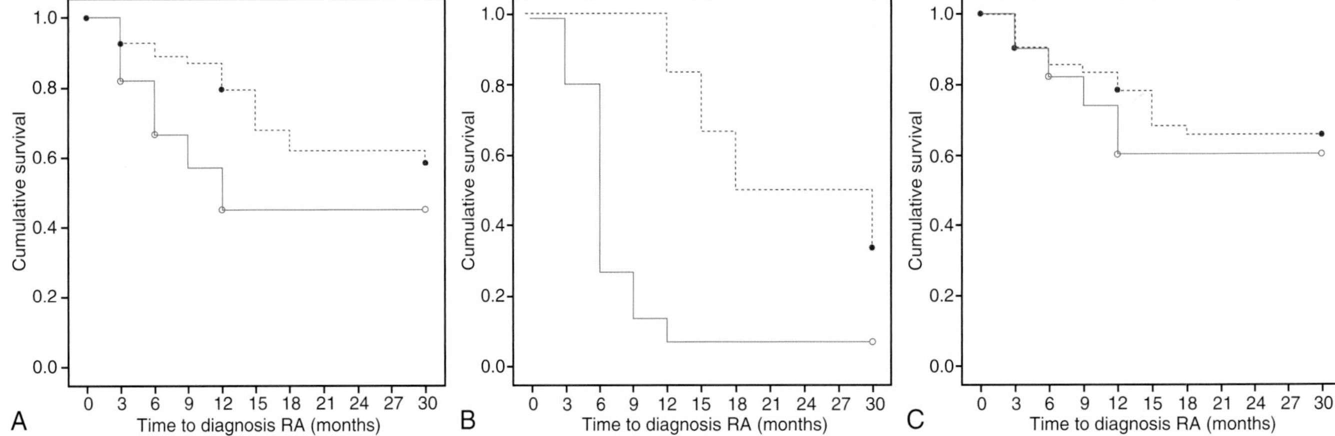

• **Fig. 73.2** Kaplan-Meir survival analysis for the diagnosis of rheumatoid arthritis (RA) after treatment with methotrexate. Undifferentiated arthritis patients were treated with methotrexate or placebo and progress to classifiable RA was assessed. The methotrexate group is indicated by the *broken line* and the placebo group by the *solid line*. Hazard ratios (HRs) and 95% confidence intervals (CIs) indicate the risk of developing RA during the study in the placebo group versus the methotrexate group. (A) Total group (n = 110); HR 1.7 (95% CI 0.99-3.01), P = 0.04. (B) Patients positive for anti-citrullinated protein antibody (ACPA) (n = 27); HR 4.9 (95% CI 1.88-12.79), $P < 0.001$. (C) Patients negative for ACPA (n = 83); HR 1.3 (95% CI 0.61-2.63), P = 0.51. (From van Dongen H, van Aken J, Lard LR, et al.: Efficacy of methotrexate treatment in patients with probable rheumatoid arthritis: a double-blind, randomized, placebo-controlled trial. *Arthritis Rheum* 56:1424-1432, 2007.)

of vaccination status and ensuring relevant vaccinations are up to date are important in those commencing DMARD therapy.[14]

Management of Imaging-Only Synovitis

The management of patients with inflammatory-type musculoskeletal symptoms and imaging-UA represents a challenging area. No clinical trials of pharmacologic intervention in such imaging-UA patients have yet been reported. The Prevention of RA by Rituximab (PRAIRI) study, however, reported the effects of a single 100 mg methylprednisolone infusion followed by either 1000 mg rituximab or placebo in patients with arthralgia and both immunoglobulin M (IgM)-RF and ACPA positivity and either a C-reactive protein (CRP) level of greater than 0.6 mg/L or subclinical synovitis as determined by ultrasound or MRI performed in the context of routine care.[49] Of the 109 patients recruited, only 48 had joint imaging before the study; although the range of joints studies is not reported, only a minority (2 of 48) had imaging evidence of synovitis at the joints studied. Although the study showed that a single infusion of rituximab modestly delayed the development of arthritis in high-risk individuals (but did not reduce the number who eventually developed arthritis), this study included only a very small number of patients with imaging-UA.

Given the evolving nature of pathologic processes operating at the earliest stages of RA as individuals transition from symptoms and autoantibodies to a disease with imaging and then clinical synovitis, care should be taken in drawing conclusions regarding the management of imaging-UA patients from studies in patients at risk of RA on the basis of symptoms and positive autoantibodies but without imaging evidence of synovitis. Ongoing trials are focusing specifically on patients with imaging evidence of articular or periarticular pathology, and results are awaited with interest. These include ARIAA (Abatacept Reversing Subclinical Inflammation as Measured by MRI in ACPA Positive Arthralgia; https://clinicaltrials.gov/ct2/show/NCT02778906), in which patients must have synovitis, tenosynovitis, or osteitis on MRI at baseline, and TREAT EARLIER (Treat Early Arthralgia to Reverse or Limit Impending Exacerbation to Rheumatoid Arthritis; https://www.trialregister.nl/trial/4599), in which patients with CSA and an extremity MRI-positive for subclinical inflammation are given a single intramuscular injection of methylprednisolone and randomized to either oral methotrexate or placebo.

In the absence of data from these studies, decisions regarding treatment require a shared decision-making approach with an explanation of the lack of trial data and careful discussion of therapeutic options, including symptomatic management. If therapy is commenced and the patient's symptoms and/or imaging evidence of synovitis resolve, strong consideration should be given to DMARD withdrawal and the subsequent assessment of disease recurrence. In the absence of clinical trial data, the long-term use of DMARDs in individuals who have never had clinically apparent synovitis but who have had imaging-UA should be approached with considerable caution.

The references for this chapter can also be found on ExpertConsult.com.

References

1. Filer A, de Pablo P, Allen G, et al.: Utility of ultrasound joint counts in the prediction of rheumatoid arthritis in patients with very early synovitis, *Ann Rheum Dis* 70:500–507, 2011.
2. Wakefield RJ, Green MJ, Marzo-Ortega H, et al.: Should oligoarthritis be reclassified? Ultrasound reveals a high prevalence of subclinical disease, *Ann Rheum Dis* 63:382–385, 2004.
3. Krabben A, Stomp W, van Nies JA, et al.: MRI-detected subclinical joint inflammation is associated with radiographic progression, *Ann Rheum Dis* 73:2034–2037, 2014.
4. Krabben A, Stomp W, van der Heijde DM, et al.: MRI of hand and foot joints of patients with anticitrullinated peptide antibody positive arthralgia without clinical arthritis, *Ann Rheum Dis* 72:1540–1544, 2013.
5. Gent YY, Ter Wee MM, Ahmadi N, et al.: Three-year clinical outcome following baseline magnetic resonance imaging in

anti-citrullinated protein antibody-positive arthralgia patients: an exploratory study, *Arthritis Rheumatol* 66:2909–2910, 2014.

6. van de Stadt LA, Bos WH, Meursinge Reynders M, et al.: The value of ultrasonography in predicting arthritis in auto-antibody positive arthralgia patients: a prospective cohort study, *Arthritis Res Ther* 12:R98, 2010.
7. Arnett FC, Edworthy SM, Bloch DA, et al.: The American Rheumatism Association 1987 revised criteria for the classification of rheumatoid arthritis, *Arthritis Rheum* 31:315–324, 1988.
8. Aletaha D, Neogi T, Silman AJ, et al.: 2010 rheumatoid arthritis classification criteria: an American College of Rheumatology/European League Against Rheumatism collaborative initiative, *Ann Rheum Dis* 69:1580–1588, 2010.
9. Cader MZ, Filer A, Hazlehurst J, et al.: Performance of the 2010 ACR/EULAR criteria for rheumatoid arthritis: comparison with 1987 ACR criteria in a very early synovitis cohort, *Ann Rheum Dis* 70:949–955, 2011.
10. Boeters DM, Gaujoux-Viala C, Constantin A, et al.: The 2010 ACR/EULAR criteria are not sufficiently accurate in the early identification of autoantibody-negative rheumatoid arthritis: Results from the Leiden-EAC and ESPOIR cohorts, *Semin Arthritis Rheum* 47:170–174, 2017.
11. van der Linden MP, le Cessie S, Raza K, et al.: Long-term impact of delay in assessment of patients with early arthritis, *Arthritis Rheum* 62:3537–3546, 2010.
12. Gerlag DM, Raza K, van Baarsen LG, et al.: EULAR recommendations for terminology and research in individuals at risk of rheumatoid arthritis: report from the Study Group for Risk Factors for Rheumatoid Arthritis, *Ann Rheum Dis* 71:638–641, 2012.
13. van Steenbergen HW, Aletaha D, Beaart-van de Voorde LJ, et al.: EULAR definition of arthralgia suspicious for progression to rheumatoid arthritis, *Ann Rheum Dis* 76:491–496, 2017.
14. Combe B, Landewe R, Daien CI, et al.: 2016 update of the EULAR recommendations for the management of early arthritis, *Ann Rheum Dis* 76:948–959, 2017.
15. Raza K, Stack R, Kumar K, et al.: Delays in assessment of patients with rheumatoid arthritis: variations across Europe, *Ann Rheum Dis* 70:1822–1825, 2011.
16. Villeneuve E, Nam JL, Bell MJ, et al.: A systematic literature review of strategies promoting early referral and reducing delays in the diagnosis and management of inflammatory arthritis, *Ann Rheum Dis* 72:13–22, 2013.
17. Kumar K, Daley E, Carruthers DM, et al.: Delay in presentation to primary care physicians is the main reason why patients with rheumatoid arthritis are seen late by rheumatologists, *Rheumatology (Oxford)* 46:1438–1440, 2007.
18. Sheppard J, Kumar K, Buckley CD, et al.: 'I just thought it was normal aches and pains': a qualitative study of decision-making processes in patients with early rheumatoid arthritis, *Rheumatology (Oxford)* 47:1577–1582, 2008.
19. Stack RJN P, Jinks C, Shaw K, et al.: Delays between the onset of symptoms and first rheumatology consultation in patients with rheumatoid arthritis in the UK: an observational stduy, *BMJ Open*, 2019; In press.
20. van Nies JA, Brouwer E, van Gaalen FA, et al.: Improved early identification of arthritis: evaluating the efficacy of Early Arthritis Recognition Clinics, *Ann Rheum Dis* 72:1295–1301, 2013.
21. Visser H, le Cessie S, Vos K, et al.: How to diagnose rheumatoid arthritis early: a prediction model for persistent (erosive) arthritis, *Arthritis Rheum* 46:357–365, 2002.
22. Green M, Marzo-Ortega H, McGonagle D, et al.: Persistence of mild, early inflammatory arthritis: the importance of disease duration, rheumatoid factor, and the shared epitope, *Arthritis Rheum* 42:2184–2188, 1999.
23. Tunn EJ, Bacon PA: Differentiating persistent from self-limiting symmetrical synovitis in an early arthritis clinic—reply, *Brit J Rheumatol* 32:764, 1993.
24. van der Helm-van Mil AH, le Cessie S, van Dongen H, et al.: A prediction rule for disease outcome in patients with recent-onset undifferentiated arthritis: how to guide individual treatment decisions, *Arthritis Rheum* 56:433–440, 2007.
25. Ghosh K, Chatterjee A, Ghosh S, et al.: Validation of Leiden Score in predicting progression of rheumatoid arthritis in undifferentiated arthritis in Indian population, *Ann Med Health Sci Res* 6:205–210, 2016.
26. Kuriya B, Cheng CK, Chen HM, et al.: Validation of a prediction rule for development of rheumatoid arthritis in patients with early undifferentiated arthritis, *Ann Rheum Dis* 68:1482–1485, 2009.
27. Malemba JJ, Mbuyi-Muamba JM, Mukaya J, et al.: The phenotype and genotype of rheumatoid arthritis in the Democratic Republic of Congo, *Arthritis Res Ther* 15:R89, 2013.
28. Sahbudin I, Pickup L, Nightingale P, et al.: The role of ultrasound-defined tenosynovitis and synovitis in the prediction of rheumatoid arthritis development, *Rheumatology (Oxford)*, 2018.
29. Shi J, Knevel R, Suwannalai P, et al.: Autoantibodies recognizing carbamylated proteins are present in sera of patients with rheumatoid arthritis and predict joint damage, *Proc Natl Acad Sci U S A* 108:17372–17377, 2011.
30. Shi J, van Steenbergen HW, van Nies JA, et al.: The specificity of anti-carbamylated protein antibodies for rheumatoid arthritis in a setting of early arthritis, *Arthritis Res Ther* 17:339, 2015.
31. Boeters DM, Trouw LA, van der Helm-van Mil AHM, et al.: Does information on novel identified autoantibodies contribute to predicting the progression from undifferentiated arthritis to rheumatoid arthritis: a study on anti-CarP antibodies as an example, *Arthritis Res Ther* 20:94, 2018.
32. Yeo L, Adlard N, Biehl M, et al.: Expression of chemokines CXCL4 and CXCL7 by synovial macrophages defines an early stage of rheumatoid arthritis, *Ann Rheum Dis* 75:763–771, 2016.
33. Filer A, Ward LSC, Kemble S, et al.: Identification of a transitional fibroblast function in very early rheumatoid arthritis, *Ann Rheum Dis* 76:2105–2112, 2017.
34. Choi IY, Karpus ON, Turner JD, et al.: Stromal cell markers are differentially expressed in the synovial tissue of patients with early arthritis, *PLoS One* 12:e0182751, 2017.
35. Kelly S, Humby F, Filer A, et al.: Ultrasound-guided synovial biopsy: a safe, well-tolerated and reliable technique for obtaining high-quality synovial tissue from both large and small joints in early arthritis patients, *Ann Rheum Dis* 74:611–617, 2015.
36. van de Stadt LA, Witte BI, Bos WH, et al.: A prediction rule for the development of arthritis in seropositive arthralgia patients, *Ann Rheum Dis* 72:1920–1926, 2013.
37. Nam JL, Hensor EM, Hunt L, et al.: Ultrasound findings predict progression to inflammatory arthritis in anti-CCP antibody-positive patients without clinical synovitis, *Ann Rheum Dis* 75:2060–2067, 2016.
38. Ten Brinck RM, van Steenbergen HW, van Delft MAM, et al.: The risk of individual autoantibodies, autoantibody combinations and levels for arthritis development in clinically suspect arthralgia, *Rheumatology (Oxford)* 56:2145–2153, 2017.
39. van der Ven M, van der Veer-Meerkerk M, Ten Cate DF, et al.: Absence of ultrasound inflammation in patients presenting with arthralgia rules out the development of arthritis, *Arthritis Res Ther* 19:202, 2017.
40. van Dongen H, van Aken J, Lard LR, et al.: Efficacy of methotrexate treatment in patients with probable rheumatoid arthritis: a double-blind, randomized, placebo-controlled trial, *Arthritis Rheum* 56:1424–1432, 2007.
41. Kudo-Tanaka E, Shimizu T, Nii T, et al.: Early therapeutic intervention with methotrexate prevents the development of rheumatoid arthritis in patients with recent-onset undifferentiated arthritis: a prospective cohort study, *Mod Rheumatol* 25:831–836, 2015.
42. Wevers-de Boer K, Visser K, Heimans L, et al.: Remission induction therapy with methotrexate and prednisone in patients with early rheumatoid and undifferentiated arthritis (the IMPROVED study), *Ann Rheum Dis* 71:1472–1477, 2012.

43. Akdemir G, Heimans L, Bergstra SA, et al.: Clinical and radiological outcomes of 5-year drug-free remission-steered treatment in patients with early arthritis: IMPROVED study, *Ann Rheum Dis* 77:111–118, 2018.
44. Emery P, Durez P, Dougados M, et al.: Impact of T-cell costimulation modulation in patients with undifferentiated inflammatory arthritis or very early rheumatoid arthritis: a clinical and imaging study of abatacept (the ADJUST trial), *Ann Rheum Dis* 69:510–516, 2010.
45. Saleem B, Mackie S, Quinn M, et al.: Does the use of tumour necrosis factor antagonist therapy in poor prognosis, undifferentiated arthritis prevent progression to rheumatoid arthritis? *Ann Rheum Dis* 67:1178–1180, 2008.
46. Durez PdB LM, Depresseux G, Toukap AN, et al.: Infliximab versus placebo in adult patients with ACPA positive undifferentiated arthritis, *Arthritis Rheum* 63, 2011. Abstract 435.
47. Verstappen SM, McCoy MJ, Roberts C, et al.: Beneficial effects of a 3-week course of intramuscular glucocorticoid injections in patients with very early inflammatory polyarthritis: results of the STIVEA trial, *Ann Rheum Dis* 69:503–509, 2010.
48. Machold KP, Landewe R, Smolen JS, et al.: The Stop Arthritis Very Early (SAVE) trial, an international multicentre, randomised, double-blind, placebo-controlled trial on glucocorticoids in very early arthritis, *Ann Rheum Dis* 69:495–502, 2010.
49. Gerlag DM, Safy M, Maijer KI, et al.: Effects of B-cell directed therapy on the preclinical stage of rheumatoid arthritis: the PRAIRI study, *Ann Rheum Dis* 78:179–185, 2019.

Index

Page numbers followed by "f" indicate figures, "t" indicate tables, "b" indicate boxes, and "e" indicate online content.

D

E

H

I

J

K

N

O

P

Q

R

S

T

U

X

Y

Z

Chapter Acknowledgments

Chapter 22: This is manuscript number 29920-IMM from Scripps Research. This work was supported by NIH grants from NIAMS, NIAID, and NIEHS.

Chapter 37: The authors thank Dr. Chin Lee for critical discussion. The authors are employees of Genentech, Inc., a member of the Roche Group.

Chapter 61: The authors thank Drs. Mette Axelsen, Anne Duer, Susanne Juhl Pedersen, Rene Poggenborg (all Copenhagen), Richard Coulden, Ryan Hung (both Edmonton), Ali Guermazi (Boston), José Raya (New York), Ida Haugen (Oslo), and Fiona McQueen (Auckland), and radiographer Jakob Møller (Copenhagen) for providing images and Henrik S. Thomsen (Copenhagen) for critical review of parts of the text.